Professional Edition

2015

ICD-9-CM

FOR HOSPITALS   Volumes 1, 2, & 3

INCLUDES NETTER'S ANATOMY ART

Carol J. Buck
MS, CPC, CPC-H, CCS-P

Former Program Director
Medical Secretary Programs
Northwest Technical College
East Grand Forks, Minnesota

ELSEVIER

3251 Riverport Lane
St. Louis, Missouri 63043

2015 ICD-9-CM FOR HOSPITALS, VOLUMES 1, 2, & 3,
PROFESSIONAL EDITION

ISBN: 978-0-323-35250-5
eISBN: 978-0-323-35280-2

Notices

Knowledge and best practice in this field are constantly changing. As new research and experience broaden our understanding, changes in research methods, professional practices, or medical treatment may become necessary.

Practitioners and researchers must always rely on their own experience and knowledge in evaluating and using any information, methods, compounds, or experiments described herein. In using such information or methods they should be mindful of their own safety and the safety of others, including parties for whom they have a professional responsibility.

With respect to any drug or pharmaceutical products identified, readers are advised to check the most current information provided (i) on procedures featured or (ii) by the manufacturer of each product to be administered, to verify the recommended dose or formula, the method and duration of administration, and contraindications. It is the responsibility of practitioners, relying on their own experience and knowledge of their patients, to make diagnoses, to determine dosages and the best treatment for each individual patient, and to take all appropriate safety precautions.

To the fullest extent of the law, neither the Publisher nor the authors, contributors, or editors, assume any liability for any injury and/or damage to persons or property as a matter of products liability, negligence or otherwise, or from any use or operation of any methods, products, instructions, or ideas contained in the material herein.

International Standard Book Number 978-0-323-35250-5

Director, Private Sector Education & Professional/Reference: Jeanne R. Olson
Senior Content Development Specialist: Jenna Price
Publishing Services Manager: Pat Joiner
Project Manager: Lisa A. P. Bushey
Design Direction: Amy Buxton

Printed in the United States of America

Last digit is the print number: 9 8 7 6 5 4 3 2 1

Query Team

Patricia Cordy Henricksen, MS, CHCA, CPC-I, CPC, CCP-P, ASC-PM
Auditing and Coding Educator
Soterion Medical Services
Lexington, Kentucky

Jacqueline Klitz Grass, MA, CPC
Coding and Reimbursement Specialist
Grand Forks, North Dakota

Kathleen Buchda, CPC, CPMA
Revenue Recognition
New Richmond, Wisconsin

Technical Collaborators

Nancy Maguire, ACS, CRT, PCS, FCS, HCS-D, APC, AFC
Physician Consultant for Auditing and Education
Winchester, Virginia

Judith Neppel, RN, MS
Executive Director
Minnesota Rural Health Association
University of Minnesota, Crookston
Crookston, Minnesota

Elsevier/MC Strategies Revenue Cycle, Coding and Compliance Staff

"Experts in providing e-learning on revenue cycle, coding and compliance."

Deborah Neville, RHIA, CCS-P
Director

Lynn-Marie D. Wozniak, MS, RHIT
Content Manager

Sandra L. Macica, MS, RHIA, CCS, ROCC
Product Specialist

Therese M. Jorwic, MPH, RHIA, CCS, CCS-P, FAHIMA
Product Specialist

CONTENTS

GUIDE TO USING THE 2015 ICD-9-CM FOR HOSPITALS, VOLUMES 1, 2, & 3, PROFESSIONAL EDITION vii

SYMBOLS AND CONVENTIONS x

Part I Introduction 1

ICD-9-CM BACKGROUND 1

COORDINATION AND MAINTENANCE COMMITTEE 1

CHARACTERISTICS OF ICD-9-CM 1
  The Disease Classification 2

ICD-9-CM OFFICIAL GUIDELINES FOR CODING AND REPORTING 2

Part II Alphabetic Index Volume 2 85

Section I   Index to Diseases and Injuries 86
Section II   Table of Drugs and Chemicals 522
Section III Index to External Causes of Injury (E Code) 645

Part III Diseases: Tabular List Volume 1 669

1. Infectious and Parasitic Diseases (001–139) 669
2. Neoplasms (140–239) 701
3. Endocrine, Nutritional and Metabolic Diseases, and Immunity Disorders (240–279) 729
4. Diseases of the Blood and Blood-Forming Organs (280–289) 742
5. Mental, Behavioral and Neurodevelopmental Disorders (290–319) 749
6. Diseases of the Nervous System and Sense Organs (320–389) 764
7. Diseases of the Circulatory System (390–459) 800
8. Diseases of the Respiratory System (460–519) 821
9. Diseases of the Digestive System (520–579) 834
10. Diseases of the Genitourinary System (580–629) 855
11. Complications of Pregnancy, Childbirth, and the Puerperium (630–679) 873
12. Diseases of the Skin and Subcutaneous Tissue (680–709) 890
13. Diseases of the Musculoskeletal System and Connective Tissue (710–739) 899
14. Congenital Anomalies (740–759) 915
15. Certain Conditions Originating in the Perinatal Period (760–779) 930
16. Symptoms, Signs, and Ill-Defined Conditions (780–799) 939
17. Injury and Poisoning (800–999) 952
Supplementary Classification of Factors Influencing Health Status and Contact with Health Services (V01–V91) 1008
Supplementary Classification of External Causes of Injury and Poisoning (E000–E999) 1036
Appendix A—Morphology of Neoplasms 1075
Appendix B—Glossary of Mental Disorders (Deleted as of October 1, 2004) 1081
Appendix C—Classification of Drugs by American Hospital Formulary Services List Number and Their ICD-9-CM Equivalents 1082
Appendix D—Classification of Industrial Accidents According to Agency 1084
Appendix E—List of Three-Digit Categories 1086
Table A—Table of Bacterial Food Poisoning 1097

Part IV Procedures Volume 3 1099

Index to Procedures   1100
Classification of Procedures   1196
  0. Procedures and Interventions, Not Elsewhere Classified (00)   1196
  1. Operations on the Nervous System (01–05)   1202
  2. Operations on the Endocrine System (06–07)   1206
  3. Operations on the Eye (08–16)   1208
  3A. Other Miscellaneous Diagnostic and Therapeutic Procedures (17)   1213
  4. Operations on the Ear (18–20)   1215
  5. Operations on the Nose, Mouth, and Pharynx (21–29)   1217
  6. Operations on the Respiratory System (30–34)   1221
  7. Operations on the Cardiovascular System (35–39)   1225
  8. Operations on the Hemic and Lymphatic System (40–41)   1242
  9. Operations on the Digestive System (42–54)   1243
  10. Operations on the Urinary System (55–59)   1258
  11. Operations on the Male Genital Organs (60–64)   1263
  12. Operations on the Female Genital Organs (65–71)   1265
  13. Obstetrical Procedures (72–75)   1271
  14. Operations on the Musculoskeletal System (76–84)   1272
  15. Operations on the Integumentary System (85–86)   1285
  16. Miscellaneous Diagnostic and Therapeutic Procedures (87–99)   1289

Part V Inpatient Procedures 1305

2014 Final Inpatient Procedures   1307

2015 Final Inpatient Procedures will be posted on the companion website www.codingupdates.com when available.

Part VI 2015 MS-DRGs (online only)

Part VI contains MS-DRGs (Version 31.0) Appendixes A, B, D, and the Procedure Code Tables from Appendix E and are posted on the companion website www.codingupdates.com.

MS-DRG, Appendix A   List of Medicare Severity Diagnosis Related Groups

MS-DRG, Appendix B   Diagnosis Code/ MDC/MS-DRG Index

MS-DRG, Appendix D   MS-DRG Surgical Hierarchy by MDC and MS-DRG

MS-DRG, Appendix E   MS-DRG, Operating Room Procedures and Procedure Code/MS-DRG Index

  Table 1 Pacemaker Lead/Device Reference Table

  Table 2 Abdominal Aorta/Thoracic Vessel Resection Reference Table

  Table 3 Cardioverter-Defibrillator Lead/ Generator Reference Table

  Table 4 Spinal Fusion Reference Table

  Table 5 Kidney/Pancreas Transplant Reference Table

  Table 6 Lead/Device Reference Table

GUIDE TO USING THE 2015 ICD-9-CM FOR HOSPITALS, VOLUMES 1, 2, & 3, PROFESSIONAL EDITION

Medical coding has long been a part of the health care profession. Through the years medical coding systems have become more complex and extensive. Today, medical coding is an intricate and immense process that is present in every health care setting. The increased use of electronic submissions for health care services only increases the need for coders who understand the coding process.

2015 ICD-9-CM for Hospitals, Volumes 1, 2, & 3, Professional Edition was developed to help meet the needs of coding professionals at all levels by offering a comprehensive coding text at a reasonable price. This text combines the official coding guidelines and all three volumes of the ICD-9-CM in one book.

All material strictly adheres to the latest government versions available at the time of printing.

Updates from the *Definitions of Medicare Code Edits* (MCE) will be posted to the companion website (www. codingupdates.com) when available.

ILLUSTRATIONS AND ITEMS

The ICD-9-CM, Volume 1, Tabular List contains illustrations, pictures, and items to assist you in understanding difficult terminology, diseases/conditions, or coding in a specific category. Items are always printed in ▆▆▆▆ ink so the added material is not mistaken for official notations or instructions. ▆▆▆▆ ink is used for other annotations in the text. Your ideas on what other descriptions or illustrations should be in future editions of this text are always appreciated.

Annotated

Throughout the volumes, revisions, additions, and deleted codes or words are indicated by the following symbols:

◀▥▥ **Revised:** Revisions within the line or code from the previous edition are indicated by the arrow.

◀ **New:** Additions to the previous edition are indicated by the triangle.

~~deleted~~ **Deleted:** Deletions from the previous edition are struck through.

▆▆ **Omit code:** No code is to be assigned. The words "omit code" are highlighted in ▆▆ for easier reference.

ICD-9-CM, Volume 1, Tabular List Symbols

● **Unacceptable Principal Diagnosis:** These codes have a blue dot before them and give additional information or describe the circumstances affecting the health care encounter but are unacceptable as principal diagnosis in the *Definitions of Medicare Code Edits** (MCE) Version 31.0 for inpatient admission.

● **Use Additional Digit(s):** The red dot cautions that the code requires additional digit(s) to ensure the greatest specificity.

OGCR **OGCR:** The *ICD-9-CM Official Guidelines for Coding and Reporting* symbol indicates the placement of a portion of a guideline as that guideline pertains to the code by which it is located. The complete OGCR are located in Part I.

Coding Clinic identifies the year, quarter, and page number that presents information about an ICD-9-CM code in the American Hospital Association's *Coding Clinic for ICD-9-CM.*

▆▆ **Excludes:** Terms following the word "Excludes" are to be coded elsewhere and are highlighted in ▆▆ for easier reference.

Includes: This note appears to further define or give examples of the content of codes and is highlighted in ▓▓▓▓ for easier reference.

Use additional: The words indicate an instructional note that another code may be needed and are highlighted in ▓▓▓▓ for easier reference.

Code first: The words indicate an instructional note that directs the coder to sequence the underlying condition before the manifestation. "Code first" is highlighted in ▓▓▓▓ for easier reference.

Omit code: No code is to be assigned. The words "omit code" are highlighted in ▓▓▓▓ for easier reference.

Indicates complications and comorbidities and major complications and comorbidities according to the Inpatient Prospective Payment System (IPPS) published in the *Medicare Severity Diagnosis Related Groups (MS-DRGs), Definitions Manual*, Version 31.0. For the latest updates, reference http://www.cms.hhs.gov/AcuteInpatientPPS/FFD/list.asp.

Indicates exclusions to complications and comorbidities and major complications and comorbidities, according to the *Medicare Severity Diagnosis Related Groups (MS-DRGs), Definitions Manual*, Version 31.0.

HAC is a Hospital-Acquired Condition that, when present as a secondary diagnosis in an inpatient setting, is a higher cost, higher volume, or both and results in a higher MS-DRG assignment according to the Inpatient Prospective Payment System (IPPS) published in the *Medicare Severity Diagnosis Related Groups (MS-DRGs), Definitions Manual*, Version 31.0.

Present on Admission: These code categories represent circumstances regarding the health care encounter or factors influencing health status that do not represent a current disease or injury or are always present on admission according to the Inpatient Prospective Payment System (IPPS) published in the *Medicare Severity Diagnosis Related Groups (MS-DRGs), Definitions Manual*, Version 31.0.

Age conflict: The *Definitions of Medicare Code Edits* (MCE), Version 31.0 detects inconsistencies between a patient's age and diagnosis. For example, a 5-year-old patient with benign prostatic hypertrophy or a 78-year-old pregnant female.

The diagnosis is clinically and virtually impossible in a patient of the stated age. Therefore, either the diagnosis or the age is presumed to be incorrect. There are four age categories for diagnoses in the *Definitions of Medicare Code Edits* (MCE), Version 31.0:

N • **Newborn.** Age of 0 years; a subset of diagnoses intended only for newborns and neonates (e.g., fetal distress, perinatal jaundice).

P • **Pediatric.** Age range is 0-17 years inclusive (e.g., Reye's syndrome, routine child health exam).

M • **Maternity.** Age range is 12-55 years inclusive (e.g., diabetes in pregnancy, antepartum pulmonary complication).

A • **Adult.** Age range is 15-124 years inclusive (e.g., senile delirium, mature cataract).

♀ ♂ **Sex conflict:** *Definitions of Medicare Code Edits* (MCE), Version 31.0 detects inconsistencies between a patient's sex and any diagnosis or procedure on the patient's record. For example, a male patient with cervical cancer (diagnosis) or a female patient with a prostatectomy (procedure). In both instances, the indicated diagnosis or the procedure conflicts with the stated sex of the patient. Therefore, either the patient's diagnosis, procedure, or sex is presumed to be incorrect.

Manifestation Code: Describes the manifestation of an underlying disease, not the disease itself, and therefore, should not be assigned as a principal diagnosis, according to the *Definitions of Medicare Code Edits* (MCE), Version 31.0.

ICD-9-CM, Volume 3, Tabular List Symbols

● **Use Additional Digit(s):** The red dot cautions that the code requires additional digit(s).

✖ **Valid O.R. Procedure:** The colored "x" is placed before a code that is a valid operating room (O.R.) procedure according to the *Medicare Severity Diagnosis Related Groups (MS-DRGs), Definitions Manual*, Version 31.0.

◆ **Non-O.R. Procedure:** Indicates updates based on the *Definitions of Medicare Code Edits** (MCE), Version 31.0 to those procedures that Medicare would not normally reimburse.

♀ ♂ **Sex conflict:** *Definitions of Medicare Code Edits** (MCE), Version 31.0 detects inconsistencies between a patient's sex and procedure. For example, a female patient with a prostatectomy (procedure). The procedure conflicts with the stated sex of the patient.

Excludes: Terms following the word "Excludes" are to be coded elsewhere and are highlighted in ▓▓▓▓▓▓ for easier reference.

Includes: This note appears immediately under a code to further define or give examples of the content of codes and is highlighted in ▓▓▓▓▓▓ for easier reference.

Use additional: The words indicate an instructional note that another code may be needed, and they are highlighted in ▓▓▓▓▓▓ for easier reference.

Code also: This identifies synchronous procedures, which require reporting of individual components of a procedure.

Omit code: No code is to be assigned. The words are highlighted in ▓▓▓▓▓▓ for easier reference.

SYMBOLS AND CONVENTIONS

ICD-9-CM, Volumes 1, 2, & 3
Symbols Used to Identify New, Revised, or Deleted Material

Volume 1, Tabular List

237.70   **Neurofibromatosis, unspecified** ◄ ◄ Indicates **new** information or a new code.

V01.1   **Cholera** ◄▥ ◄ Indicates a **revision** within the line or code.

244.3   Other iatrogenic hypothyroidism ◄ Indicates **deleted** words/codes in the current edition.
     Hypothyroidism resulting from:
      P-aminosalicylic acid [PAS]
      Phenylbutazone
      Resorcinol
      Iatrogenic hypothyroidism NOS
     Use additional E code to identify drug

Volume 2, Alphabetic Index

Tachypnea 786.06
    hysterical 300.11 ◄▥ ◄ Indicates a **revision** within the line or code.
    newborn (idiopathic) (transitory) 770.6 ◄ ◄ Indicates **new** information or a ne code.

Congestion, congestive (chronic) (passive) ◄ Indicates a **deleted** entry in the current edition.

Volume 3, Procedures, Index

Biopsy
    peritoneum ◄▥ ◄ Indicates a **revision** within the line or code.
      closed 54.24 ◄ ◄ Indicates **new** information or code.

Lung (complete) (with mediastinal dissection) 32.5 32.59 ◄ Indicates a **deleted** entry in the current edition.

Volume 3, Procedures, Tabular List

00.19   **Disruption of blood brain barrier via infusion [BBBD]** ◄▥ ◄ Indicates a **revision** within the line or code.
    Infusion of substance to disrupt blood brain barrier ◄ ◄ Indicates **new** information or a new code.

00.74   **Hip** replacement **bearing surface, metal-on-polyethylene** ◄ Indicates a **deleted** entry in the current edition.

Codes or index entries are for purposes of illustration only and may not be current.

Symbols for Volume 1, Tabular List

Use Additional Digit(s): The red dot cautions you that the code requires additional digit(s) to ensure the greatest specificity.

● **237.7** **Neurofibromatosis**
von Recklinghausen's disease

Indicates complications and comorbidities and major complications and comorbidities according to the *Medicare Severity Diagnosis Related Groups (MS-DRGs), Definitions Manual*, Version 31.0.

Unacceptable Principal Diagnosis: These codes have a blue dot before them and give additional information or describe the circumstances affecting the health care encounter but are unacceptable as principal diagnosis in the *Definitions of Medicare Code Edits* (MCE), Version 31.0.

● **284.2** **Myelophthisis**

242.1 **Toxic uninodular goiter**
Thyroid nodule, toxic or with hyperthyroidism
Uninodular goiter, toxic or with hyperthyroidism

Present on Admission: Are exempt codes that do not represent a current disease or injury or are always present on admission according to the *Medicare Severity Diagnosis Related Groups (MS-DRGs), Definitions Manual*, Version 31.0.

007.4 **Cryptosporidiosis**
Coding Clinic: 1997, Q4, P30-31

Indicates a Volume 1 reference in the American Hospital Association *Coding Clinic for ICD-9-CM*.

112.2 **Of other urogenital sites**

This symbol indicates a Hospital-Acquired Condition (HAC) in the *Medicare Severity Diagnosis Related Groups (MS-DRGs), Definitions Manual*, Version 31.0.

Definitions of Medicare Code Edits (MCE), Version 31.0 **Newborn** edit (age 0 years) indicating diagnoses intended only for newborns and neonates (e.g., fetal distress, perinatal jaundice).

747.83 **Persistent fetal circulation**   **N**

783.41 **Failure to thrive**   **P**

Definitions of Medicare Code Edits (MCE), Version 31.0 **Pediatric** edit (age 0-17 years inclusive), e.g., Reye's syndrome, routine child health exam.

Definitions of Medicare Code Edits (MCE), Version 31.0 **Maternity** edit (age 12-55 years inclusive), e.g., diabetes in pregnancy, antepartum pulmonary complication.

632 **Missed abortion**   **M**

256.31 **Premature menopause**   **A**

Definitions of Medicare Code Edits (MCE), Version 31.0 **Adult** edit (age 15-124 years inclusive), e.g., senile delirium, mature cataract.

Codes or index entries are for purposes of illustration only and may not be current.

Definitions of Medicare Code Edits (MCE), Version 31.0 **Sex Conflict** detects inconsistencies between a male patient's sex and any diagnosis on the patient's record. For example, a male patient with a diagnosis of cervical cancer.

184.0   Malignant neoplasm of the vagina   ♀

185   Malignant neoplasm of the prostate   ♂

Definitions of Medicare Code Edits (MCE), Version 31.0 **Sex Conflict** detects inconsistencies between a female patient's sex and any diagnosis on the patient's record. For example, a female patient with a diagnosis of prostate cancer.

Manifestation codes describe the symptoms of an underlying disease, not the disease itself, and therefore, should not be used as a principal diagnosis according to the *Definitions of Medicare Code Edits* (MCE), Version 31.0.

284.2   *Myelophthisis*

Conventions for Volume 1, Tabular List
2. NEOPLASMS (140–239)

Notes define terms or give coding instructions.

Notes
1. Content
   This chapter contains the following broad groups:
   140–195   Malignant neoplasms, stated or presumed to be primary, of specified sites, except of lymphatic and hematopoietic tissue

510   Empyema

Use additional code to identify infectious organism (041.0–041.9)

"Use additional" directs you to assign an additional code to give more complete picture of the diagnosis.

Code first: The words indicate an instructional note that directs the coder to sequence the underlying condition (etiology) before the manifestation.

366.4   Cataract associated with other disorders
    366.41   Diabetic cataract
    Code first diabetes (249.5, 250.5)

A code with this note may be first listed (primary) if no causal condition is applicable or known.

428   Heart failure
    Code, if applicable, heart failure due to hypertension first (402.0–402.9, with fifth-digit 1 or 404.0–404.9 with fifth-digit 1 or 3)

Terms following the word "Excludes" are to be coded elsewhere. The term "Excludes" means "Do Not Code Here."

150.2   Abdominal esophagus
    Excludes   *adenocarcinoma (151.0)*
                    cardio-esophageal junction (151.0)

The "Includes" note appears to further define, or give example of, the contents of the code.

087   Relapsing fever
    Includes   recurrent fever

Codes or index entries are for purposes of illustration only and may not be current.

474   **Chronic disease of tonsils and adenoids**

"and" indicates a code that can be assigned if either of the conditions is present or if both of the conditions are present.

366.4   **Cataract associated with other disorders**

"with" indicates a code that can be used only if both conditions are present.

"NEC" means Not Elsewhere Classifiable and is to be used only when the information at hand specifies a condition but there is no more specific code for that condition.

244.8   **Other specified acquired hypothyroidism**
     Secondary hypothyroidism NEC

Bold type is used for all codes and titles.

159.0   **Intestinal tract, part unspecified**
     Intestine NOS

"NOS" means Not Otherwise Specified and is the equivalent of "unspecified."

426.89   **Other**
     Dissociation:
       atrioventricular [AV]

Brackets are used to enclose synonyms, alternative wording, or explanatory phrases.

158.8   **Specified parts of peritoneum**
     Cul-de-sac (of Douglas)
     Mesentery

Parentheses are used to enclose supplementary words that may be present or absent in the statement of a disease without affecting the code.

628.4   **Of cervical or vaginal origin**
     Infertility associated with:
       anomaly of cervical mucus
       congenital structural anomaly

A colon is used after an incomplete term that needs one or more of the modifiers that follow in order to make it assignable to a given category.

Codes or index entries are for purposes of illustration only and may not be current.

Conventions for Volume 2, Alphabetic Index

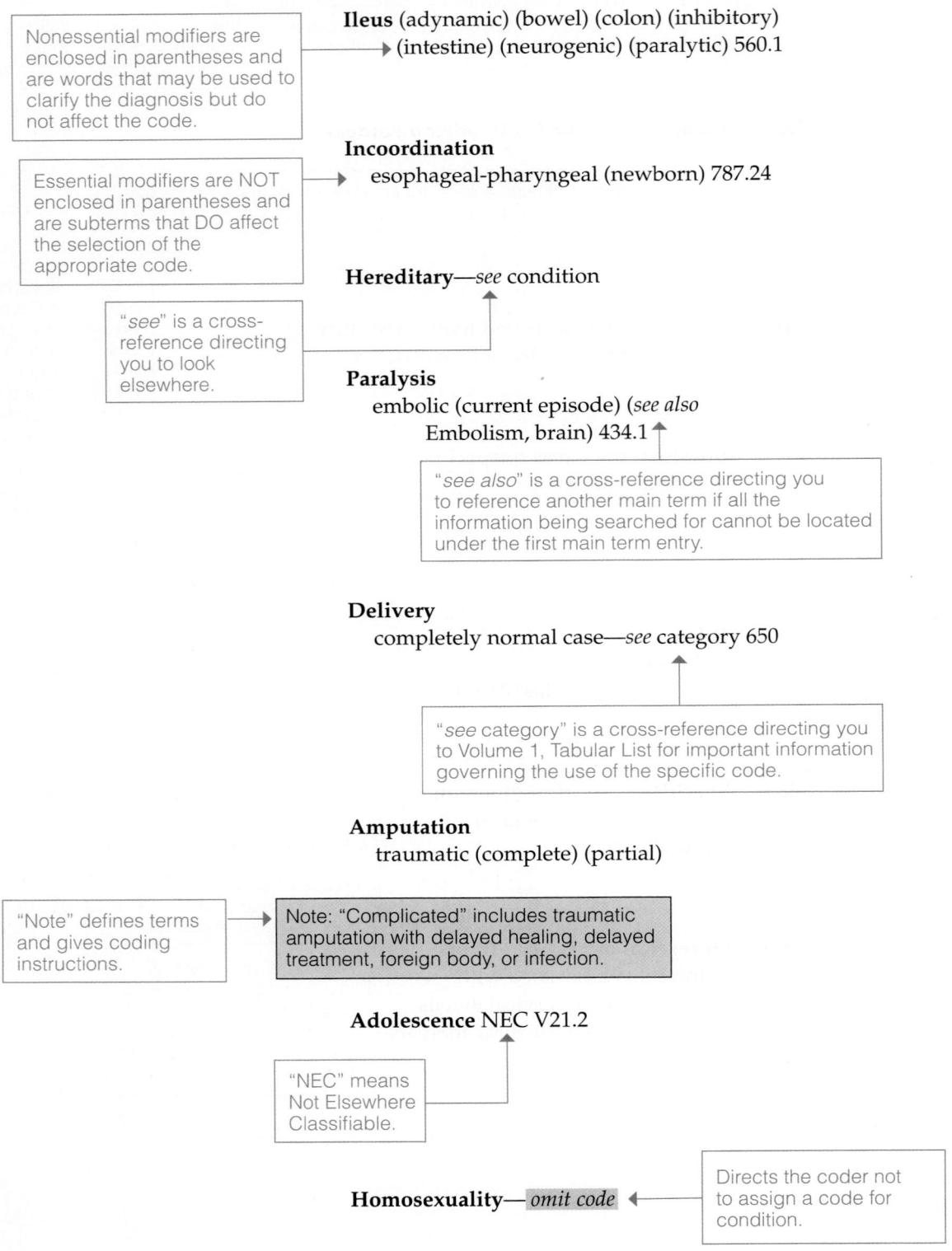

Ileus (adynamic) (bowel) (colon) (inhibitory) (intestine) (neurogenic) (paralytic) 560.1

Nonessential modifiers are enclosed in parentheses and are words that may be used to clarify the diagnosis but do not affect the code.

Incoordination
esophageal-pharyngeal (newborn) 787.24

Essential modifiers are NOT enclosed in parentheses and are subterms that DO affect the selection of the appropriate code.

Hereditary—*see* condition

"*see*" is a cross-reference directing you to look elsewhere.

Paralysis
embolic (current episode) (*see also* Embolism, brain) 434.1

"*see also*" is a cross-reference directing you to reference another main term if all the information being searched for cannot be located under the first main term entry.

Delivery
completely normal case—*see* category 650

"*see* category" is a cross-reference directing you to Volume 1, Tabular List for important information governing the use of the specific code.

Amputation
traumatic (complete) (partial)

"Note" defines terms and gives coding instructions.

Note: "Complicated" includes traumatic amputation with delayed healing, delayed treatment, foreign body, or infection.

Adolescence NEC V21.2

"NEC" means Not Elsewhere Classifiable.

Homosexuality—*omit code*

Directs the coder not to assign a code for condition.

Codes or index entries are for purposes of illustration only and may not be current.

Conventions for Volume 3, Procedures, Index

Arthrotomy 80.10

    as operative approach—*omit code*

> "*omit code*" identifies procedures or services that are included in another larger procedure or service. For example, an incision that is part of the main surgical procedure is not coded separately.

Ileal

    bladder

        closed 57.87 *[45.51]*

> For some operative procedures it is necessary to record the individual components of the procedure. These procedures are termed **"synchronous procedures"** and are listed together in the Index. The codes are sequenced in the same order as displayed in the Index.

Operation

    Thompson

        cleft lip repair 27.54

        correction of lymphedema 40.9

        quadricepsplasty 83.86

> Eponyms are operations named for people and are listed in the Index both under the eponym and under the term "Operation."

Thompson

    cleft lip repair 27.54

    correction of lymphedema 40.9

    quadricepsplasty 83.86

Volume 3, Index to Procedures, also contains "*see*," "*see also*," "*see* category," "essential modifiers," "nonessential modifiers," "notes," NEC, and NOS as in Volume 2, Alphabetic Index.

Codes or index entries are for purposes of illustration only and may not be current.

Symbols for Volume 3, Procedures, Tabular List

Use Additional Digit(s): The red dot cautions that the code requires additional digit(s) to ensure the greatest specificity.

● **31.9   Other operations on larynx and trachea**
✖ **31.91   Division of laryngeal nerve**

Valid O.R. Procedure: The "x" is placed before a code that is a valid operating room (O.R.) procedure according to the *Medicare Severity Diagnosis Related Groups (MS-DRGs), Definition Manual*, Version 31.0.

00.0   Therapeutic ultrasound
▸ Coding Clinic: 2002, Q4, P90-91

Indicates a Volume 3 reference in the American Hospital Association *Coding Clinic for ICD-9-CM*.

65.01   Laparoscopic oophorotomy   ♀

Definitions of Medicare Code Edits* (MCE), Version 31.0 **Sex Conflict** detects inconsistencies between a female patient's sex and any procedure on the patient's record. For example, a female patient assigned a procedure code for a prostatectomy.

Definitions of Medicare Code Edits* (MCE), Version 31.0 **Sex Conflict** detects inconsistencies between a male patient's sex and any procedure on the patient's record. For example, a male patient assigned a procedure code for a hysterectomy.

60.0   Incision of prostate   ♂

✖ **00.10   Implantation of chemotherapeutic agent**
Brain wafer chemotherapy
Interstitial/intracavitary

Excludes *injection or infusion of cancer chemotherapeutic substance (99.25)*

Coding Clinic: 2002, Q4, P93
◆ Non-OR Procedure with MDC 01, MS-DRG 023

Non-OR Procedure indicates updates based on the *Definitions of Medicare Code Edits** (MCE), Version 31.0 to those procedures that Medicare would not normally reimburse.

Conventions for Volume 3, Procedures, Tabular List

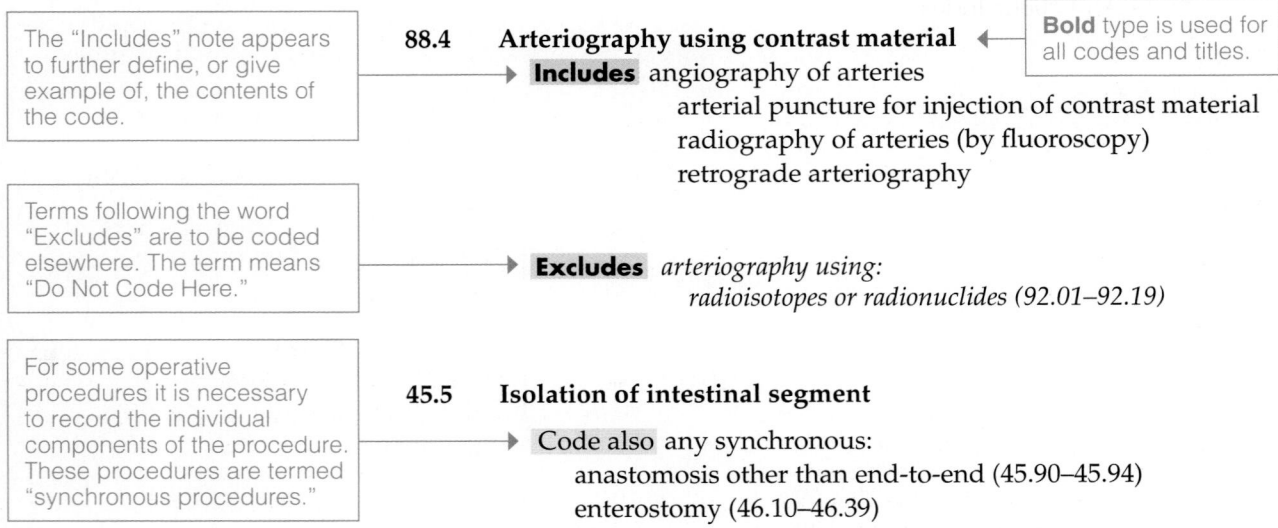

The "Includes" note appears to further define, or give example of, the contents of the code.

88.4   Arteriography using contrast material
Includes angiography of arteries
arterial puncture for injection of contrast material
radiography of arteries (by fluoroscopy)
retrograde arteriography

Bold type is used for all codes and titles.

Terms following the word "Excludes" are to be coded elsewhere. The term means "Do Not Code Here."

Excludes *arteriography using: radioisotopes or radionuclides (92.01–92.19)*

For some operative procedures it is necessary to record the individual components of the procedure. These procedures are termed "synchronous procedures."

45.5   Isolation of intestinal segment
Code also any synchronous:
anastomosis other than end-to-end (45.90–45.94)
enterostomy (46.10–46.39)

Codes or index entries are for purposes of illustration only and may not be current.

Introduction

ICD-9-CM BACKGROUND

The International Classification of Diseases, 9th Revision, Clinical Modification (ICD-9-CM) is based on the official version of the World Health Organization's 9th Revision, International Classification of Diseases (ICD-9). ICD-9 is designed for the classification of morbidity and mortality information for statistical purposes, and for the indexing of hospital records by disease and operations, for data storage and retrieval. The historical background of the International Classification of Diseases may be found in the Introduction to ICD-9 (Manual of the International Classification of Diseases, Injuries, and Causes of Death, World Health Organization, Geneva, Switzerland, 1977).

ICD-9-CM is a clinical modification of the World Health Organization's International Classification of Diseases, 9th Revision (ICD-9). The term "clinical" is used to emphasize the modification's intent: to serve as a useful tool in the area of classification of morbidity data for indexing of medical records, medical care review, and ambulatory and other medical care programs, as well as for basic health statistics. To describe the clinical picture of the patient, the codes must be more precise than those needed only for statistical groupings and trend analysis.

COORDINATION AND MAINTENANCE COMMITTEE

Annual modifications are made to the ICD-9-CM through the ICD-9-CM Coordination and Maintenance Committee (C&M). The Committee is made up of representatives from two Federal Government agencies, the National Center for Health Statistics and the Health Care Financing Administration. The Committee holds meetings twice a year which are open to the public. Modification proposals submitted to the Committee for consideration are presented at the meetings for public discussion. Those modification proposals which are approved are incorporated into the official government version of the ICD-9-CM and become effective for use October 1 of the year following their presentation. The C&M also prepares updates for use April 1 of each year. To date, no April 1 updates have been released.

CHARACTERISTICS OF ICD-9-CM

ICD-9-CM far exceeds its predecessors in the number of codes provided. The disease classification has been expanded to include health-related conditions and to provide greater specificity at the fifth-digit level of detail. These fifth digits are not optional; they are intended for use in recording the information substantiated in the clinical record.

Volume I of ICD-9-CM contains five appendices:

Appendix A	Morphology of Neoplasms
Appendix B	Glossary of Mental Disorders (Deleted in 2004)
Appendix C	Classification of Drugs by American Hospital Formulary Service List Number and Their ICD-9-CM Equivalents
Appendix D	Classification of Industrial Accidents According to Agency
Appendix E	List of Three-Digit Categories

These appendices are included as a reference to the user in order to provide further information about the patient's clinical picture, to further define a diagnostic statement, to aid in classifying new drugs, or to reference three-digit categories.

Volume 2 of ICD-9-CM contains many diagnostic terms which do not appear in Volume 1 since the index includes most diagnostic terms currently in use.

The Disease Classification

ICD-9-CM is totally compatible with its parent system, ICD-9, thus meeting the need for comparability of morbidity and mortality statistics at the international level. A few fourth-digit codes were created in existing three-digit rubrics only when the necessary detail could not be accommodated by the use of a fifth-digit subclassification. To ensure that each rubric of ICD-9-CM collapses back to its ICD-9 counterpart, the following specifications governed the ICD-9-CM disease classification:

Specifications for the Tabular List

1. Three-digit rubrics and their contents are unchanged from ICD-9.
2. The sequence of three-digit rubrics is unchanged from ICD-9.
3. Unsubdivided three-digit rubrics are subdivided where necessary to:
   a) Add clinical detail
   b) Isolate terms for clinical accuracy
4. The modification in ICD-9-CM is accomplished by the addition of a fifth digit to existing ICD-9 rubrics.
5. The optional dual classification in ICD-9 is modified.
   a) Duplicate rubrics are deleted:
      1) Four-digit manifestation categories duplicating etiology entries.
      2) Manifestation inclusion terms duplicating etiology entries.
   b) Manifestations of diseases are identified, to the extent possible, by creating five-digit codes in the etiology rubrics.
   c) When the manifestation of a disease cannot be included in the etiology rubrics, provision for its identification is made by retaining the ICD-9 rubrics used for classifying manifestations of disease.
6. The format of ICD-9-CM is revised from that used in ICD-9.
   a) American spelling of medical terms is used.
   b) Inclusion terms are indented beneath the titles of codes.
   c) Codes not to be used for principal tabulation of disease are printed with the notation, "Code first underlying disease."

Specifications for the Alphabetic Index

1. Format of the Alphabetic Index follows the format of ICD-9.
2. When two codes are required to indicate etiology and manifestation, the manifestation code appears in brackets, e.g., diabetic cataract 250.5X [366.41]. The etiology code is always sequenced first followed by the manifestation code.

The following guidelines were the most current at the time of publication. Check the website at http://codingupdates.com for the latest updates to the Guidelines.

ICD-9-CM OFFICIAL GUIDELINES FOR CODING AND REPORTING

Effective October 1, 2011
Narrative changes appear in bold text
Items underlined have been moved within the guidelines since October 1, 2010

The Centers for Medicare and Medicaid Services (CMS) and the National Center for Health Statistics (NCHS), two departments within the U.S. Federal Government's Department of Health and Human Services (DHHS) provide the following guidelines for coding and reporting using the International Classification of Diseases, 9th Revision, Clinical Modification (ICD-9-CM). These guidelines should be used as a companion document to the official version of the ICD-9-CM as published on CD-ROM by the U.S. Government Printing Office (GPO).

These guidelines have been approved by the four organizations that make up the Cooperating Parties for the ICD-9-CM: the American Hospital Association (AHA), the American Health Information Management Association (AHIMA), CMS, and NCHS. These guidelines are included on the official government version of the ICD-9-CM, and also appear in "Coding Clinic for ICD-9-CM" published by the AHA.

These guidelines are a set of rules that have been developed to accompany and complement the official conventions and instructions provided within the ICD-9-CM itself. The instructions and conventions of the classification take precedence over guidelines. These guidelines are based on the coding and sequencing instructions in Volumes I, II and III of ICD-9-CM, but provide additional instruction. Adherence to these guidelines when assigning ICD-9-CM diagnosis and procedure codes is required under the Health Insurance Portability and Accountability Act (HIPAA). The diagnosis codes (Volumes 1-2) have been adopted under HIPAA for all healthcare settings. Volume 3 procedure codes have been adopted for inpatient procedures reported by hospitals. A joint effort between the healthcare provider and the coder is essential to achieve complete and accurate documentation, code assignment, and reporting of diagnoses and procedures. These guidelines have been developed to assist both the healthcare provider and the coder in identifying those diagnoses and procedures that are to be reported. The importance of consistent, complete documentation in the medical record cannot be overemphasized. Without such documentation accurate coding cannot be achieved. The entire record should be reviewed to determine the specific reason for the encounter and the conditions treated.

The term encounter is used for all settings, including hospital admissions. In the context of these guidelines, the term provider is used throughout the guidelines to mean physician or any qualified health care practitioner who is legally accountable for establishing the patient's diagnosis. Only this set of guidelines, approved by the Cooperating Parties, is official.

The guidelines are organized into sections. Section I includes the structure and conventions of the classification and general guidelines that apply to the entire classification, and chapter-specific guidelines that correspond to the chapters as they are arranged in the classification. Section II includes guidelines for selection of principal diagnosis for non-outpatient settings. Section III includes guidelines for reporting additional diagnoses in non-outpatient settings. Section IV is for outpatient coding and reporting.

ICD-9-CM Official Guidelines for Coding and Reporting

Section I. Conventions, general coding guidelines and chapter specific guidelines

A. Conventions for the ICD-9-CM
  1. Format:
  2. Abbreviations
     a. Index abbreviations
     b. Tabular abbreviations
  3. Punctuation
  4. Includes and Excludes Notes and Inclusion terms
  5. Other and Unspecified codes
     a. "Other" codes
     b. "Unspecified" codes
  6. Etiology/manifestation convention ("code first", "use additional code" and "in diseases classified elsewhere" notes)
  7. "And"
  8. "With"
  9. "See" and "See Also"

B. General Coding Guidelines
  1. Use of Both Alphabetic Index and Tabular List
  2. Locate each term in the Alphabetic Index
  3. Level of Detail in Coding
  4. Code or codes from 001.0 through V91.99
  5. Selection of codes 001.0 through 999.9
  6. Signs and symptoms
  7. Conditions that are an integral part of a disease process
  8. Conditions that are not an integral part of a disease process
  9. Multiple coding for a single condition
  10. Acute and Chronic Conditions
  11. Combination Code
  12. Late Effects
  13. Impending or Threatened Condition
  14. Reporting Same Diagnosis Code More than Once
  15. Admissions/Encounters for Rehabilitation
  16. Documentation for BMI and Pressure Ulcer Stages
  17. Syndromes
  18. **Documentation of Complications of care**

C. Chapter-Specific Coding Guidelines
  1. Chapter 1: Infectious and Parasitic Diseases (001-139)
     a. Human Immunodeficiency Virus (HIV) Infections
     b. Septicemia, Systemic Inflammatory Response Syndrome (SIRS), Sepsis, Severe Sepsis, and Septic Shock
     c. Methicillin Resistant *Staphylococcus aureus* (MRSA) Conditions
  2. Chapter 2: Neoplasms (140-239)
     a. Treatment directed at the malignancy
     b. Treatment of secondary site
     c. Coding and sequencing of complications
     d. Primary malignancy previously excised
     e. Admissions/Encounters involving chemotherapy, immunotherapy and radiation therapy
     f. Admission/encounter to determine extent of malignancy
     g. Symptoms, signs, and ill-defined conditions listed in Chapter 16 associated with neoplasms
     h. Admission/encounter for pain control/ management
     i. Malignant neoplasm associated with transplanted organ
  3. Chapter 3: Endocrine, Nutritional, and Metabolic Diseases and Immunity Disorders (240-279)
     a. Diabetes mellitus
  4. Chapter 4: Diseases of Blood and Blood Forming Organs (280-289)
     a. Anemia of chronic disease
  5. Chapter 5: Mental Disorders (290-319)
     Reserved for future guideline expansion
  6. Chapter 6: Diseases of Nervous System and Sense Organs (320-389)
     a. Pain - Category 338
     b. **Glaucoma**
  7. Chapter 7: Diseases of Circulatory System (390-459)
     a. Hypertension
     b. Cerebral infarction/stroke/cerebrovascular accident (CVA)
     c. Postoperative cerebrovascular accident
     d. Late Effects of Cerebrovascular Disease
     e. Acute myocardial infarction (AMI)
  8. Chapter 8: Diseases of Respiratory System (460-519)
     a. Chronic Obstructive Pulmonary Disease [COPD] and Asthma
     b. Chronic Obstructive Pulmonary Disease [COPD] and Bronchitis
     c. Acute Respiratory Failure
     d. Influenza due to *certain* identified *viruses*

9. Chapter 9: Diseases of Digestive System (520-579)
Reserved for future guideline expansion

10. Chapter 10: Diseases of Genitourinary System (580-629)
    a. Chronic kidney disease

11. Chapter 11: Complications of Pregnancy, Childbirth, and the Puerperium (630-679)
    a. General Rules for Obstetric Cases
    b. Selection of OB Principal or First-listed Diagnosis
    c. Fetal Conditions Affecting the Management of the Mother
    d. HIV Infection in Pregnancy, Childbirth and the Puerperium
    e. Current Conditions Complicating Pregnancy
    f. Diabetes mellitus in pregnancy
    g. Gestational diabetes
    h. Normal Delivery, Code 650
    i. The Postpartum and Peripartum Periods
    j. Code 677, Late effect of complication of pregnancy
    k. Abortions

12. Chapter 12: Diseases Skin and Subcutaneous Tissue (680-709)
    a. Pressure ulcer stage codes

13. Chapter 13: Diseases of Musculoskeletal and Connective Tissue (710-739)
    a. Coding of Pathologic Fractures

14. Chapter 14: Congenital Anomalies (740-759)
    a. Codes in categories 740-759, Congenital Anomalies

15. Chapter 15: Newborn (Perinatal) Guidelines (760-779)
    a. General Perinatal Rules
    b. Use of codes V30-V39
    c. Newborn transfers
    d. Use of category V29
    e. Use of other V codes on perinatal records
    f. Maternal Causes of Perinatal Morbidity
    g. Congenital Anomalies in Newborns
    h. Coding Additional Perinatal Diagnoses
    i. Prematurity and Fetal Growth Retardation
    j. Newborn sepsis

16. Chapter 16: Signs, Symptoms and Ill-Defined Conditions (780-799)
Reserved for future guideline expansion

17. Chapter 17: Injury and Poisoning (800-999)
    a. Coding of Injuries
    b. Coding of Traumatic Fractures
    c. Coding of Burns
    d. Coding of Debridement of Wound, Infection, or Burn

    e. Adverse Effects, Poisoning and Toxic Effects
    f. Complications of care
    g. SIRS due to Non-infectious Process

18. Classification of Factors Influencing Health Status and Contact with Health Service (Supplemental V01-V91)
    a. Introduction
    b. V codes use in any healthcare setting
    c. V Codes indicate a reason for an encounter
    d. Categories of V Codes
    e. V Codes That May Only be Principal/ First-Listed Diagnosis

19. Supplemental Classification of External Causes of Injury and Poisoning (E-codes, E800-E999)
    a. General E Code Coding Guidelines
    b. Place of Occurrence Guideline
    c. Adverse Effects of Drugs, Medicinal and Biological Substances Guidelines
    d. Child and Adult Abuse Guideline
    e. Unknown or Suspected Intent Guideline
    f. Undetermined Cause
    g. Late Effects of External Cause Guidelines
    h. Misadventures and Complications of Care Guidelines
    i. Terrorism Guidelines
    j. Activity Code Guidelines
    k. External cause status

Section II. Selection of Principal Diagnosis

A. Codes for symptoms, signs, and ill-defined conditions
B. Two or more interrelated conditions, each potentially meeting the definition for principal diagnosis
C. Two or more diagnoses that equally meet the definition for principal diagnosis
D. Two or more comparative or contrasting conditions
E. A symptom(s) followed by contrasting/comparative diagnoses
F. Original treatment plan not carried out
G. Complications of surgery and other medical care
H. Uncertain Diagnosis
I. Admission from Observation Unit
    1. Admission Following Medical Observation
    2. Admission Following Post-Operative Observation
J. Admission from Outpatient Surgery

Section III. Reporting Additional Diagnoses

A. Previous conditions
B. Abnormal findings
C. Uncertain Diagnosis

Section IV. Diagnostic Coding and Reporting Guidelines for Outpatient Services

A. Selection of first-listed condition
   1. Outpatient Surgery
   2. Observation Stay
B. Codes from 001.0 through V91.99
C. Accurate reporting of ICD-9-CM diagnosis codes
D. Selection of codes 001.0 through 999.9
E. Codes that describe symptoms and signs
F. Encounters for circumstances other than a disease or injury
G. Level of Detail in Coding
   1. ICD-9-CM codes with 3, 4, or 5 digits
   2. Use of full number of digits required for a code
H. ICD-9-CM code for the diagnosis, condition, problem, or other reason for encounter/visit
I. Uncertain diagnosis
J. Chronic diseases
K. Code all documented conditions that coexist
L. Patients receiving diagnostic services only
M. Patients receiving therapeutic services only
N. Patients receiving preoperative evaluations only
O. Ambulatory surgery
P. Routine outpatient prenatal visits

Appendix I: Present on Admission Reporting Guidelines

Section I. Conventions, general coding guidelines and chapter specific guidelines

The conventions, general guidelines and chapter-specific guidelines are applicable to all health care settings unless otherwise indicated. The conventions and instructions of the classification take precedence over guidelines.

A. Conventions for the ICD-9-CM

The conventions for the ICD-9-CM are the general rules for use of the classification independent of the guidelines. These conventions are incorporated within the index and tabular of the ICD-9-CM as instructional notes. The conventions are as follows:

1. Format:

The ICD-9-CM uses an indented format for ease in reference

2. Abbreviations

  a. Index abbreviations

    NEC "Not elsewhere classifiable" This abbreviation in the index represents "other specified" when a specific code is not available for a condition the index directs the coder to the "other specified" code in the tabular.

  b. Tabular abbreviations

    NEC "Not elsewhere classifiable" This abbreviation in the tabular represents "other specified". When a specific code is not available for a condition the tabular includes an NEC entry under a code to identify the code as the "other specified" code. *(See Section I.A.5.a. "Other" codes)*.

    NOS "Not otherwise specified" This abbreviation is the equivalent of unspecified. *(See Section I.A.5.b., "Unspecified" codes)*

3. Punctuation

  [ ] Brackets are used in the tabular list to enclose synonyms, alternative wording or explanatory phrases. Brackets are used in the index to identify manifestation codes. *(See Section I.A.6. "Etiology/manifestations")*

  ( ) Parentheses are used in both the index and tabular to enclose supplementary words that may be present or absent in the statement of a disease or procedure without affecting the code number to which it is assigned. The terms within the parentheses are referred to as nonessential modifiers.

  : Colons are used in the Tabular list after an incomplete term which needs one or more of the modifiers following the colon to make it assignable to a given category.

4. Includes and Excludes Notes and Inclusion terms

Includes: This note appears immediately under a three-digit code title to further define, or give examples of, the content of the category.

Excludes: An excludes note under a code indicates that the terms excluded from the code are to be coded elsewhere. In some cases the codes for the excluded terms should not be used in conjunction with the code from which it is excluded. An example of this is a congenital condition excluded from an acquired form of the same condition. The congenital and acquired codes should not be used together. In other cases, the excluded terms may be used together with an excluded code. An example of this is when fractures of different bones are coded to different codes. Both codes may be used together if both types of fractures are present.

Inclusion terms: List of terms is included under certain four and five digit codes. These terms are the conditions for which that code number is to be used. The terms may be synonyms of the code title, or, in the case of "other specified" codes, the terms are a list of the various conditions assigned to that code. The inclusion terms are not necessarily exhaustive. Additional terms found only in the index may also be assigned to a code.

5. **Other and Unspecified codes**

   a. **"Other" codes**

   Codes titled "other" or "other specified" (usually a code with a 4th digit 8 or fifth-digit 9 for diagnosis codes) are for use when the information in the medical record provides detail for which a specific code does not exist. Index entries with NEC in the line designate "other" codes in the tabular. These index entries represent specific disease entities for which no specific code exists so the term is included within an "other" code.

   b. **"Unspecified" codes**

   Codes (usually a code with a 4th digit 9 or 5th digit 0 for diagnosis codes) titled "unspecified" are for use when the information in the medical record is insufficient to assign a more specific code.

6. **Etiology/manifestation convention ("code first", "use additional code" and "in diseases classified elsewhere" notes)**

   Certain conditions have both an underlying etiology and multiple body system manifestations due to the underlying etiology. For such conditions, the ICD-9-CM has a coding convention that requires the underlying condition be sequenced first followed by the manifestation. Wherever such a combination exists, there is a "use additional code" note at the etiology code, and a "code first" note at the manifestation code. These instructional notes indicate the proper sequencing order of the codes, etiology followed by manifestation.

   In most cases the manifestation codes will have in the code title, "in diseases classified elsewhere." Codes with this title are a component of the etiology/manifestation convention. The code title indicates that it is a manifestation code. "In diseases classified elsewhere" codes are never permitted to be used as first listed or principal diagnosis codes. They must be used in conjunction with an underlying condition code and they must be listed following the underlying condition.

   There are manifestation codes that do not have "in diseases classified elsewhere" in the title. For such codes a "use additional code" note will still be present and the rules for sequencing apply.

   In addition to the notes in the tabular, these conditions also have a specific index entry structure. In the index both conditions are listed together with the etiology code first followed by the manifestation codes in brackets. The code in brackets is always to be sequenced second.

   The most commonly used etiology/manifestation combinations are the codes for Diabetes mellitus,

category 250. For each code under category 250 there is a use additional code note for the manifestation that is specific for that particular diabetic manifestation. Should a patient have more than one manifestation of diabetes, more than one code from category 250 may be used with as many manifestation codes as are needed to fully describe the patient's complete diabetic condition. The category 250 diabetes codes should be sequenced first, followed by the manifestation codes.

"Code first" and "Use additional code" notes are also used as sequencing rules in the classification for certain codes that are not part of an etiology/manifestation combination.

See - Section I.B.9. "Multiple coding for a single condition".

7. **"And"**

   The word "and" should be interpreted to mean either "and" or "or" when it appears in a title.

8. **"With"**

   The word "with" should be interpreted to mean "associated with" or "due to" when it appears in a code title, the Alphabetic Index, or an instructional note in the Tabular List.

   The word "with" in the alphabetic index is sequenced immediately following the main term, not in alphabetical order.

9. **"See" and "See Also"**

   The "see" instruction following a main term in the index indicates that another term should be referenced. It is necessary to go to the main term referenced with the "see" note to locate the correct code.

   A "see also" instruction following a main term in the index instructs that there is another main term that may also be referenced that may provide additional index entries that may be useful. It is not necessary to follow the "see also" note when the original main term provides the necessary code.

B. **General Coding Guidelines**

1. **Use of Both Alphabetic Index and Tabular List**

   Use both the Alphabetic Index and the Tabular List when locating and assigning a code. Reliance on only the Alphabetic Index or the Tabular List leads to errors in code assignments and less specificity in code selection.

2. **Locate each term in the Alphabetic Index**

   Locate each term in the Alphabetic Index and verify the code selected in the Tabular List. Read and be guided by instructional notations that appear in both the Alphabetic Index and the Tabular List.

3. **Level of Detail in Coding**

   Diagnosis and procedure codes are to be used at their highest number of digits available.

   ICD-9-CM diagnosis codes are composed of codes with 3, 4, or 5 digits. Codes with three digits are included in ICD-9-CM as the heading of a category of codes that may be further subdivided by the use of fourth and/or fifth digits, which provide greater detail.

A three-digit code is to be used only if it is not further subdivided. Where fourth-digit subcategories and/or fifth-digit subclassifications are provided, they must be assigned. A code is invalid if it has not been coded to the full number of digits required for that code. For example, Acute myocardial infarction, code 410, has fourth digits that describe the location of the infarction (e.g., 410.2, Of inferolateral wall), and fifth digits that identify the episode of care. It would be incorrect to report a code in category 410 without a fourth and fifth digit.

ICD-9-CM Volume 3 procedure codes are composed of codes with either 3 or 4 digits. Codes with two digits are included in ICD-9-CM as the heading of a category of codes that may be further subdivided by the use of third and/or fourth digits, which provide greater detail.

4. Code or codes from 001.0 through V91.99

The appropriate code or codes from 001.0 through V91.99 must be used to identify diagnoses, symptoms, conditions, problems, complaints or other reason(s) for the encounter/visit.

5. Selection of codes 001.0 through 999.9

The selection of codes 001.0 through 999.9 will frequently be used to describe the reason for the admission/encounter. These codes are from the section of ICD-9-CM for the classification of diseases and injuries (e.g., infectious and parasitic diseases; neoplasms; symptoms, signs, and ill-defined conditions, etc.).

6. Signs and symptoms

Codes that describe symptoms and signs, as opposed to diagnoses, are acceptable for reporting purposes when a related definitive diagnosis has not been established (confirmed) by the provider. Chapter 16 of ICD-9-CM, Symptoms, Signs, and Ill-defined conditions (codes 780.0 - 799.9) contain many, but not all codes for symptoms.

7. Conditions that are an integral part of a disease process

Signs and symptoms that are associated routinely with a disease process should not be assigned as additional codes, unless otherwise instructed by the classification.

8. Conditions that are not an integral part of a disease process

Additional signs and symptoms that may not be associated routinely with a disease process should be coded when present.

9. Multiple coding for a single condition

In addition to the etiology/manifestation convention that requires two codes to fully describe a single condition that affects multiple body systems, there are other single conditions that also require more than one code. "Use additional code" notes are found in the tabular at codes that are not part of an etiology/manifestation pair where a secondary code is useful to fully describe a condition. The sequencing rule is the same as the etiology/manifestation pair - , "use additional code" indicates that a secondary code should be added.

For example, for infections that are not included in chapter 1, a secondary code from category 041, Bacterial infection in conditions classified elsewhere and of unspecified site, may be required to identify the bacterial organism causing the infection. A "use additional code" note will normally be found at the infectious disease code, indicating a need for the organism code to be added as a secondary code.

"Code first" notes are also under certain codes that are not specifically manifestation codes but may be due to an underlying cause. When a "code first" note is present and an underlying condition is present the underlying condition should be sequenced first.

"Code, if applicable, any causal condition first", notes indicate that this code may be assigned as a principal diagnosis when the causal condition is unknown or not applicable. If a causal condition is known, then the code for that condition should be sequenced as the principal or first-listed diagnosis.

Multiple codes may be needed for late effects, complication codes and obstetric codes to more fully describe a condition. See the specific guidelines for these conditions for further instruction.

10. Acute and Chronic Conditions

If the same condition is described as both acute (subacute) and chronic, and separate subentries exist in the Alphabetic Index at the same indentation level, code both and sequence the acute (subacute) code first.

11. Combination Code

A combination code is a single code used to classify:
Two diagnoses, or
A diagnosis with an associated secondary process (manifestation)
A diagnosis with an associated complication

Combination codes are identified by referring to subterm entries in the Alphabetic Index and by reading the inclusion and exclusion notes in the Tabular List.

Assign only the combination code when that code fully identifies the diagnostic conditions involved or when the Alphabetic Index so directs. Multiple coding should not be used when the classification provides a combination code that clearly identifies all of the elements documented in the diagnosis. When the combination code lacks necessary specificity in describing the manifestation or complication, an additional code should be used as a secondary code.

12. Late Effects

A late effect is the residual effect (condition produced) after the acute phase of an illness or injury has terminated. There is no time limit on when a late effect code can be used. The residual may be apparent early, such as in cerebrovascular accident cases, or it may occur months or years later, such as that due to a previous injury. Coding of late effects generally requires two codes sequenced in the following order: The condition or nature of the late effect is sequenced first. The late effect code is sequenced second.

Exceptions to the above guidelines are those instances where the late effect code has been expanded (at the fourth and fifth-digit levels) to include the manifestation(s) **or the classification instructs otherwise.** The code for the acute phase of an illness or injury that led to the late effect is never used with a code for the late effect.

13. Impending or Threatened Condition

Code any condition described at the time of discharge as "impending" or "threatened" as follows:

If it did occur, code as confirmed diagnosis.

If it did not occur, reference the Alphabetic Index to determine if the condition has a subentry term for "impending" or "threatened" and also reference main term entries for "Impending" and for "Threatened."

If the subterms are listed, assign the given code.

If the subterms are not listed, code the existing underlying condition(s) and not the condition described as impending or threatened.

14. Reporting Same Diagnosis Code More than Once

Each unique ICD-9-CM diagnosis code may be reported only once for an encounter. This applies to bilateral conditions or two different conditions classified to the same ICD-9-CM diagnosis code.

15. Admissions/Encounters for Rehabilitation

When the purpose for the admission/encounter is rehabilitation, sequence the appropriate V code from category V57, Care involving use of rehabilitation procedures, as the principal/first-listed diagnosis. The code for the condition for which the service is being performed should be reported as an additional diagnosis.

Only one code from category V57 is required. Code V57.89, Other specified rehabilitation procedures, should be assigned if more than one type of rehabilitation is performed during a single encounter. A procedure code should be reported to identify each type of rehabilitation therapy actually performed.

16. Documentation for BMI and Pressure Ulcer Stages

For the Body Mass Index (BMI) and pressure ulcer stage codes, code assignment may be based on medical record documentation from clinicians who are not the patient's provider (i.e., physician or other qualified healthcare practitioner legally accountable for establishing the patient's diagnosis), since this information is typically documented by other clinicians involved in the care of the patient (e.g., a dietitian often documents the BMI and nurses often documents the pressure ulcer stages). However, the associated diagnosis (such as overweight, obesity, or pressure ulcer) must be documented by the patient's provider. If there is conflicting medical record documentation, either from the same clinician or different clinicians, the patient's attending provider should be queried for clarification.

The BMI and pressure ulcer stage codes should only be reported as secondary diagnoses. As with all other secondary diagnosis codes, the BMI and pressure ulcer stage codes should only be assigned when they meet the definition of a reportable additional diagnosis (see Section III, Reporting Additional Diagnoses).

17. Syndromes

Follow the Alphabetic Index guidance when coding syndromes. In the absence of index guidance, assign codes for the documented manifestations of the syndrome.

18. Documentation of Complications of care

Code assignment is based on the provider's documentation of the relationship between the condition and the care or procedure. The guideline extends to any complications of care, regardless of the chapter the code is located in. It is important to note that not all conditions that occur during or following medical care or surgery are classified as complications. There must be a cause-and-effect relationship between the care provided and the condition, and an indication in the documentation that it is a complication. Query the provider for clarification, if the complication is not clearly documented.

C. Chapter-Specific Coding Guidelines

In addition to general coding guidelines, there are guidelines for specific diagnoses and/or conditions in the classification. Unless otherwise indicated, these guidelines apply to all health care settings. Please refer to Section II for guidelines on the selection of principal diagnosis.

1. Chapter 1: Infectious and Parasitic Diseases (001-139)

a. Human Immunodeficiency Virus (HIV) Infections

1) Code only confirmed cases

Code only confirmed cases of HIV infection/illness. This is an exception to the hospital inpatient guideline Section II, H.

In this context, "confirmation" does not require documentation of positive serology or culture for HIV; the provider's diagnostic statement that the patient is HIV positive, or has an HIV-related illness is sufficient.

2) **Selection and sequencing of HIV codes**

   (a) **Patient admitted for HIV-related condition**

   If a patient is admitted for an HIV-related condition, the principal diagnosis should be 042, followed by additional diagnosis codes for all reported HIV-related conditions.

   (b) **Patient with HIV disease admitted for unrelated condition**

   If a patient with HIV disease is admitted for an unrelated condition (such as a traumatic injury), the code for the unrelated condition (e.g., the nature of injury code) should be the principal diagnosis. Other diagnoses would be 042 followed by additional diagnosis codes for all reported HIV-related conditions.

   (c) **Whether the patient is newly diagnosed**

   Whether the patient is newly diagnosed or has had previous admissions/encounters for HIV conditions is irrelevant to the sequencing decision.

   (d) **Asymptomatic human immunodeficiency virus**

   V08 Asymptomatic human immunodeficiency virus [HIV] infection, is to be applied when the patient without any documentation of symptoms is listed as being "HIV positive," "known HIV," "HIV test positive," or similar terminology. Do not use this code if the term "AIDS" is used or if the patient is treated for any HIV-related illness or is described as having any condition(s) resulting from his/her HIV positive status; use 042 in these cases.

   (e) **Patients with inconclusive HIV serology**

   Patients with inconclusive HIV serology, but no definitive diagnosis or manifestations of the illness, may be assigned code 795.71, Inconclusive serologic test for Human Immunodeficiency Virus [HIV].

   (f) **Previously diagnosed HIV-related illness**

   Patients with any known prior diagnosis of an HIV-related illness should be coded to 042. Once a patient has developed an HIV-related illness, the patient should always be assigned code 042 on every subsequent admission/encounter. Patients previously diagnosed with any HIV illness (042) should never be assigned to 795.71 or V08.

   (g) **HIV Infection in Pregnancy, Childbirth and the Puerperium**

   During pregnancy, childbirth or the puerperium, a patient admitted (or presenting for a health care encounter) because of an HIV-related illness should receive a principal diagnosis code of 647.6X, Other specified infectious and parasitic diseases in the mother classifiable elsewhere, but complicating the pregnancy, childbirth or the puerperium, followed by 042 and the code(s) for the HIV-related illness(es). Codes from Chapter 15 always take sequencing priority.

   Patients with asymptomatic HIV infection status admitted (or presenting for a health care encounter) during pregnancy, childbirth, or the puerperium should receive codes of 647.6X and V08.

   (h) **Encounters for testing for HIV**

   If a patient is being seen to determine his/her HIV status, use code V73.89, Screening for other specified viral disease. Use code V69.8, Other problems related to lifestyle, as a secondary code if an asymptomatic patient is in a known high risk group for HIV. Should a patient with signs or symptoms or illness, or a confirmed HIV related diagnosis be tested for HIV, code the signs and symptoms or the diagnosis. An additional counseling code V65.44 may be used if counseling is provided during the encounter for the test.

   When a patient returns to be informed of his/her HIV test results use code V65.44, HIV counseling, if the results of the test are negative.

   If the results are positive but the patient is asymptomatic use code V08, Asymptomatic HIV infection. If the results are positive and the patient is symptomatic use code 042, HIV infection, with codes for the HIV related symptoms or diagnosis. The HIV counseling code may also be used if counseling is provided for patients with positive test results.

GUIDELINES - SECTION I.C.1

9

b. **Septicemia, Systemic Inflammatory Response Syndrome (SIRS), Sepsis, Severe Sepsis, and Septic Shock**

1) **SIRS, Septicemia, and Sepsis**

(a) The terms *septicemia* and *sepsis* are often used interchangeably by providers, however they are not considered synonymous terms. The following descriptions are provided for reference but do not preclude querying the provider for clarification about terms used in the documentation:

(i) Septicemia generally refers to a systemic disease associated with the presence of pathological microorganisms or toxins in the blood, which can include bacteria, viruses, fungi or other organisms.

(ii) Systemic inflammatory response syndrome (SIRS) generally refers to the systemic response to infection, trauma/burns, or other insult (such as cancer) with symptoms including fever, tachycardia, tachypnea, and leukocytosis.

(iii) Sepsis generally refers to SIRS due to infection.

(iv) Severe sepsis generally refers to sepsis with associated acute organ dysfunction.

(b) **The Coding of SIRS, sepsis and severe sepsis**

The coding of SIRS, sepsis and severe sepsis requires a minimum of 2 codes: a code for the underlying cause (such as infection or trauma) and a code from subcategory 995.9 Systemic inflammatory response syndrome (SIRS).

(i) The code for the underlying cause (such as infection or trauma) must be sequenced before the code from subcategory 995.9 Systemic inflammatory response syndrome (SIRS).

(ii) Sepsis and severe sepsis require a code for the systemic infection (038.xx, 112.5, etc.) and either code 995.91, Sepsis, or 995.92, Severe sepsis. If the causal organism is not documented, assign code 038.9, Unspecified septicemia.

(iii) Severe sepsis requires additional code(s) for the associated acute organ dysfunction(s).

(iv) If a patient has sepsis with multiple organ dysfunctions, follow the instructions for coding severe sepsis.

(v) Either the term sepsis or SIRS must be documented to assign a code from subcategory 995.9.

(vi) *See Section I.C.17.g), Injury and poisoning, for information regarding systemic inflammatory response syndrome (SIRS) due to trauma/ burns and other non-infectious processes.*

(c) Due to the complex nature of sepsis and severe sepsis, some cases may require querying the provider prior to assignment of the codes.

2) **Sequencing sepsis and severe sepsis**

(a) **Sepsis and severe sepsis as principal diagnosis**

If sepsis or severe sepsis is present on admission, and meets the definition of principal diagnosis, the systemic infection code (e.g., 038.xx, 112.5, etc) should be assigned as the principal diagnosis, followed by code 995.91, Sepsis, or 995.92, Severe sepsis, as required by the sequencing rules in the Tabular List. Codes from subcategory 995.9 can never be assigned as a principal diagnosis. A code should also be assigned for any localized infection, if present.

If the sepsis or severe sepsis is due to a postprocedural infection, see Section I.C.1.b.10 for guidelines related to sepsis due to postprocedural infection.

(b) **Sepsis and severe sepsis as secondary diagnoses**

When sepsis or severe sepsis develops during the encounter (it was not present on admission), the systemic infection code and code 995.91 or 995.92 should be assigned as secondary diagnoses.

(c) **Documentation unclear as to whether sepsis or severe sepsis is present on admission**

Sepsis or severe sepsis may be present on admission but the diagnosis may not be confirmed until sometime after admission. If the documentation is not clear whether the sepsis or severe sepsis was present on admission, the provider should be queried.

3) **Sepsis/SIRS with Localized Infection**

If the reason for admission is both sepsis, severe sepsis, or SIRS and a localized infection, such as pneumonia or cellulitis, a code for the systemic infection (038.xx,

112.5, etc) should be assigned first, then code 995.91 or 995.92, followed by the code for the localized infection. If the patient is admitted with a localized infection, such as pneumonia, and sepsis/SIRS doesn't develop until after admission, see guideline I.C.1.b.2.b).

If the localized infection is postprocedural, *see Section I.C.1.b.10 for guidelines related to sepsis due to postprocedural infection.*

<u>Note:</u> The term urosepsis is a nonspecific term. If that is the only term documented then only code 599.0 should be assigned based on the default for the term in the ICD-9-CM index, in addition to the code for the causal organism if known.

4) **Bacterial Sepsis and Septicemia**

In most cases, it will be a code from category 038, Septicemia, that will be used in conjunction with a code from subcategory 995.9 such as the following:

(a) **Streptococcal sepsis**

If the documentation in the record states streptococcal sepsis, codes 038.0, Streptococcal septicemia, and code 995.91 should be used, in that sequence.

(b) **Streptococcal septicemia**

If the documentation states streptococcal septicemia, only code 038.0 should be assigned, however, the provider should be queried whether the patient has sepsis, an infection with SIRS.

5) **Acute organ dysfunction that is not clearly associated with the sepsis**

If a patient has sepsis and an acute organ dysfunction, but the medical record documentation indicates that the acute organ dysfunction is related to a medical condition other than the sepsis, do not assign code 995.92, Severe sepsis. An acute organ dysfunction must be associated with the sepsis in order to assign the severe sepsis code. If the documentation is not clear as to whether an acute organ dysfunction is related to the sepsis or another medical condition, query the provider.

6) **Septic shock**

(a) **Sequencing of septic shock and postprocedural septic shock**

Septic shock generally refers to circulatory failure associated with severe sepsis, and, therefore, it represents a type of acute organ dysfunction.

For cases of septic shock, the code for the systemic infection should be

sequenced first, followed by codes 995.92, **Severe sepsis** and 785.52, **Septic shock or 998.02, Postoperative septic shock.** Any additional codes for other acute organ dysfunctions should also be assigned. As noted in the sequencing instructions in the Tabular List, the code for septic shock cannot be assigned as a principal diagnosis.

(b) **Septic shock and postprocedural septic shock without documentation of severe sepsis**

Since septic shock indicates the presence of severe sepsis, code 995.92, Severe sepsis, **can be** assigned with code 785.52, Septic shock, **or code 998.02 Postoperative shock, septic,** even if the term severe sepsis is not documented in the record.

7) **Sepsis and septic shock complicating abortion and pregnancy**

Sepsis and septic shock complicating abortion, ectopic pregnancy, and molar pregnancy are classified to category codes in Chapter 11 (630-639).

See section I.C.11.i.7 for information on the coding of puerperal sepsis.

8) **Negative or inconclusive blood cultures**

Negative or inconclusive blood cultures do not preclude a diagnosis of septicemia or sepsis in patients with clinical evidence of the condition, however, the provider should be queried.

9) **Newborn sepsis**

See Section I.C.15.j for information on the coding of newborn sepsis.

10) **Sepsis due to a Postprocedural Infection**

(a) **Documentation of causal relationship**

As with all postprocedural complications, code assignment is based on the provider's documentation of the relationship between the infection and the procedure.

(b) **Sepsis due to postprocedural infection**

In cases of postprocedural sepsis, the complication code, such as code 998.59, Other postoperative infection, or 674.3x, Other complications of obstetrical surgical wounds should be coded first followed by the appropriate sepsis codes (systemic infection code and either code 995.91 or 995.92). An additional code(s) for any acute organ dysfunction should also be assigned for cases of severe sepsis.

See Section I.C.1.b.6 if the sepsis or severe sepsis results in postprocedural septic shock.

(c) **Postprocedural infection and postprocedural septic shock**

In cases where a postprocedural infection has occurred and has resulted in severe sepsis and postprocedural septic shock, the code for the precipitating complication such as code 998.59, Other postoperative infection, or 674.3x, Other complications of obstetrical surgical wounds should be coded first followed by the appropriate sepsis codes (systemic infection code and code 995.92). Code 998.02, Postoperative septic shock, should be assigned as an additional code. In cases of severe sepsis, an additional code(s) for any acute organ dysfunction should also be assigned.

11) **External cause of injury codes with SIRS**

Refer to Section I.C.19.a.7 for instruction on the use of external cause of injury codes with codes for SIRS resulting from trauma.

12) **Sepsis and Severe Sepsis Associated with Non-infectious Process**

In some cases, a non-infectious process, such as trauma, may lead to an infection which can result in sepsis or severe sepsis. If sepsis or severe sepsis is documented as associated with a non-infectious condition, such as a burn or serious injury, and this condition meets the definition for principal diagnosis, the code for the non-infectious condition should be sequenced first, followed by the code for the systemic infection and either code 995.91, Sepsis, or 995.92, Severe sepsis. Additional codes for any associated acute organ dysfunction(s) should also be assigned for cases of severe sepsis. If the sepsis or severe sepsis meets the definition of principal diagnosis, the systemic infection and sepsis codes should be sequenced before the non-infectious condition. When both the associated non-infectious condition and the sepsis or severe sepsis meet the definition of principal diagnosis, either may be assigned as principal diagnosis.

See Section I.C.1.b.2.a for guidelines pertaining to sepsis or severe sepsis as the principal diagnosis.

Only one code from subcategory 995.9 should be assigned. Therefore, when a non-infectious condition leads to an infection resulting in sepsis or severe sepsis, assign either code 995.91 or 995.92. Do not additionally assign code 995.93, Systemic inflammatory response syndrome due to non-infectious process without acute organ dysfunction, or 995.94, Systemic inflammatory response syndrome with acute organ dysfunction.

See Section I.C.17.g for information on the coding of SIRS due to trauma/burns or other non-infectious disease processes.

c. **Methicillin Resistant *Staphylococcus aureus* (MRSA) Conditions**

1) **Selection and sequencing of MRSA codes**

(a) **Combination codes for MRSA infection**

When a patient is diagnosed with an infection that is due to methicillin resistant *Staphylococcus aureus* (MRSA), and that infection has a combination code that includes the causal organism (e.g., septicemia, pneumonia) assign the appropriate code for the condition (e.g., code 038.12, Methicillin resistant Staphylococcus aureus septicemia or code 482.42, Methicillin resistant pneumonia due to Staphylococcus aureus). Do not assign code 041.12, Methicillin resistant Staphylococcus aureus, as an additional code because the code includes the type of infection and the MRSA organism. Do not assign a code from subcategory V09.0, Infection with microorganisms resistant to penicillins, as an additional diagnosis.

See Section C.1.b.1 for instructions on coding and sequencing of septicemia.

(b) **Other codes for MRSA infection**

When there is documentation of a current infection (e.g., wound infection, stitch abscess, urinary tract infection) due to MRSA, and that infection does not have a combination code that includes the causal organism, select the appropriate code to identify the condition along with code 041.12, Methicillin resistant Staphylococcus aureus, for the MRSA infection. Do not assign a code from subcategory V09.0, Infection with microorganisms resistant to penicillins.

(c) **Methicillin susceptible Staphylococcus aureus (MSSA) and MRSA colonization**

The condition or state of being colonized or carrying MSSA or MRSA is called colonization or carriage, while an individual person is described as being colonized or being a carrier. Colonization means that MSSA or MSRA is present on or in the body without necessarily causing illness. A positive MRSA colonization test might be documented by the provider as "MRSA screen positive" or "MRSA nasal swab positive".

Assign code V02.54, Carrier or suspected carrier, Methicillin resistant Staphylococcus aureus, for patients documented as having MRSA colonization. Assign code V02.53, Carrier or suspected carrier, Methicillin susceptible Staphylococcus aureus, for patient documented as having MSSA colonization. Colonization is not necessarily indicative of a disease process or as the cause of a specific condition the patient may have unless documented as such by the provider.

Code V02.59, Other specified bacterial diseases, should be assigned for other types of staphylococcal colonization (e.g., *S. epidermidis, S. saprophyticus*). Code V02.59 should not be assigned for colonization with any type of *Staphylococcus aureus* (MRSA, MSSA).

(d) MRSA colonization and infection

If a patient is documented as having both MRSA colonization and infection during a hospital admission, code V02.54, Carrier or suspected carrier, Methicillin resistant *Staphylococcus aureus*, and a code for the MRSA infection may both be assigned.

2. Chapter 2: Neoplasms (140-239)

General guidelines

Chapter 2 of the ICD-9-CM contains the codes for most benign and all malignant neoplasms. Certain benign neoplasms, such as prostatic adenomas, may be found in the specific body system chapters. To properly code a neoplasm it is necessary to determine from the record if the neoplasm is benign, in-situ, malignant, or of uncertain histologic behavior. If malignant, any secondary (metastatic) sites should also be determined.

The neoplasm table in the Alphabetic Index should be referenced first. However, if the histological term is documented, that term should be referenced first, rather than going immediately to the Neoplasm Table, in order to determine which column in the Neoplasm Table is appropriate. For example, if the documentation indicates "adenoma," refer to the term in the Alphabetic Index to review the entries under this term and the instructional note to "see also neoplasm, by site, benign." The table provides the proper code based on the type of neoplasm and the site. It is important to select the proper column in the table that corresponds to the type of neoplasm. The tabular should then be referenced to verify that the correct code has been selected from the table and that a more specific site code does not exist.

See Section I.C.18.d.4. for information regarding V codes for genetic susceptibility to cancer.

a. Treatment directed at the malignancy

If the treatment is directed at the malignancy, designate the malignancy as the principal diagnosis.

The only exception to this guideline is if a patient admission/encounter is solely for the administration of chemotherapy, immunotherapy or radiation therapy, assign the appropriate V58.x code as the first-listed or principal diagnosis, and the diagnosis or problem for which the service is being performed as a secondary diagnosis.

b. Treatment of secondary site

When a patient is admitted because of a primary neoplasm with metastasis and treatment is directed toward the secondary site only, the secondary neoplasm is designated as the principal diagnosis even though the primary malignancy is still present.

c. Coding and sequencing of complications

Coding and sequencing of complications associated with the malignancies or with the therapy thereof are subject to the following guidelines:

1) Anemia associated with malignancy

When admission/encounter is for management of an anemia associated with the malignancy, and the treatment is only for anemia, the appropriate anemia code (such as code 285.22, Anemia in neoplastic disease) is designated as the principal diagnosis and is followed by the appropriate code(s) for the malignancy.

Code 285.22 may also be used as a secondary code if the patient suffers from anemia and is being treated for the malignancy.

If anemia in neoplastic disease and anemia due to antineoplastic chemotherapy are both documented, **assign codes for both conditions**.

2) Anemia associated with chemotherapy, immunotherapy and radiation therapy

When the admission/encounter is for management of an anemia associated with chemotherapy, immunotherapy or radiotherapy and the only treatment is for the anemia, the anemia is sequenced first. The appropriate neoplasm code should be assigned as an additional code.

3) Management of dehydration due to the malignancy

When the admission/encounter is for management of dehydration due to the malignancy or the therapy, or a combination of both, and only the dehydration is being treated (intravenous rehydration), the dehydration is sequenced first, followed by the code(s) for the malignancy.

4) Treatment of a complication resulting from a surgical procedure

When the admission/encounter is for treatment of a complication resulting from a surgical procedure, designate the complication as the principal or first-listed diagnosis if treatment is directed at resolving the complication.

d. Primary malignancy previously excised

When a primary malignancy has been previously excised or eradicated from its site and there is no further treatment directed to that site and there is no evidence of any existing primary malignancy, a code from category V10, Personal history of malignant neoplasm, should be used to indicate the former site of the malignancy. Any mention of extension, invasion, or metastasis to another site is coded as a secondary malignant neoplasm to that site. The secondary site may be the principal or first-listed with the V10 code used as a secondary code.

e. Admissions/Encounters involving chemotherapy, immunotherapy and radiation therapy

1) Episode of care involves surgical removal of neoplasm

When an episode of care involves the surgical removal of a neoplasm, primary or secondary site, followed by adjunct chemotherapy or radiation treatment during the same episode of care, the neoplasm code should be assigned as principal or first-listed diagnosis, using codes in the 140-198 series or where appropriate in the 200-203 series.

2) Patient admission/encounter solely for administration of chemotherapy, immunotherapy and radiation therapy

If a patient admission/encounter is solely for the administration of chemotherapy, immunotherapy or radiation therapy assign code V58.0, Encounter for radiation therapy, or V58.11, Encounter for antineoplastic chemotherapy, or V58.12, Encounter for antineoplastic immunotherapy as the first-listed or principal diagnosis. If a patient receives more than one of these therapies during the same admission more than one of these codes may be assigned, in any sequence.

The malignancy for which the therapy is being administered should be assigned as a secondary diagnosis.

3) Patient admitted for radiotherapy/ chemotherapy and immunotherapy and develops complications

When a patient is admitted for the purpose of radiotherapy, immunotherapy or chemotherapy and develops complications such as uncontrolled nausea and vomiting or dehydration, the principal or first-listed diagnosis is V58.0, Encounter for radiotherapy, or V58.11, Encounter for antineoplastic chemotherapy, or V58.12, Encounter for antineoplastic immunotherapy followed by any codes for the complications.

f. Admission/encounter to determine extent of malignancy

When the reason for admission/encounter is to determine the extent of the malignancy, or for a procedure such as paracentesis or thoracentesis, the primary malignancy or appropriate metastatic site is designated as the principal or first-listed diagnosis, even though chemotherapy or radiotherapy is administered.

g. Symptoms, signs, and ill-defined conditions listed in Chapter 16 associated with neoplasms

Symptoms, signs, and ill-defined conditions listed in Chapter 16 characteristic of, or associated with, an existing primary or secondary site malignancy cannot be used to replace the malignancy as principal or first-listed diagnosis, regardless of the number of admissions or encounters for treatment and care of the neoplasm.

h. Admission/encounter for pain control/ management

See Section I.C.6.a.5 for information on coding admission/encounter for pain control/management.

i. Malignant neoplasm associated with transplanted organ

A malignant neoplasm of a transplanted organ should be coded as a transplant complication. Assign first the appropriate code from subcategory 996.8, Complications of transplanted organ, followed by code 199.2, Malignant neoplasm associated with transplanted organ. Use an additional code for the specific malignancy.

3. Chapter 3: Endocrine, Nutritional, and Metabolic Diseases and Immunity Disorders (240-279)

a. Diabetes mellitus

Codes under category 250, Diabetes mellitus, identify complications/manifestations associated with diabetes mellitus. A fifth-digit is required for all category 250 codes to identify the type of diabetes mellitus and whether the diabetes is controlled or uncontrolled.

See I.C.3.a.7 for secondary diabetes

1) Fifth-digits for category 250:

The following are the fifth-digits for the codes under category 250:

0   type II or unspecified type, not stated as uncontrolled

1   type I, [juvenile type], not stated as uncontrolled

2   type II or unspecified type, uncontrolled

3   type I, [juvenile type], uncontrolled

The age of a patient is not the sole determining factor, though most type I diabetics develop the condition before reaching puberty. For this reason type I diabetes mellitus is also referred to as juvenile diabetes.

2) **Type of diabetes mellitus not documented**

If the type of diabetes mellitus is not documented in the medical record the default is type II.

3) **Diabetes mellitus and the use of insulin**

All type I diabetics must use insulin to replace what their bodies do not produce. However, the use of insulin does not mean that a patient is a type I diabetic. Some patients with type II diabetes mellitus are unable to control their blood sugar through diet and oral medication alone and do require insulin. If the documentation in a medical record does not indicate the type of diabetes but does indicate that the patient uses insulin, the appropriate fifth-digit for type II must be used. For type II patients who routinely use insulin, code V58.67, Long-term (current) use of insulin, should also be assigned to indicate that the patient uses insulin. Code V58.67 should not be assigned if insulin is given temporarily to bring a type II patient's blood sugar under control during an encounter.

4) **Assigning and sequencing diabetes codes and associated conditions**

When assigning codes for diabetes and its associated conditions, the code(s) from category 250 must be sequenced before the codes for the associated conditions. The diabetes codes and the secondary codes that correspond to them are paired codes that follow the etiology/manifestation convention of the classification (*See Section I.A.6., Etiology/manifestation convention*). Assign as many codes from category 250 as needed to identify all of the associated conditions that the patient has. The corresponding secondary codes are listed under each of the diabetes codes.

(a) **Diabetic retinopathy/diabetic macular edema**

Diabetic macular edema, code 362.07, is only present with diabetic retinopathy. Another code from subcategory 362.0, Diabetic retinopathy, must be used with code 362.07. Codes under subcategory 362.0 are diabetes manifestation codes, so they must be used following the appropriate diabetes code.

5) **Diabetes mellitus in pregnancy and gestational diabetes**

(a) For diabetes mellitus complicating pregnancy, see Section I.C.11.f., Diabetes mellitus in pregnancy.

(b) For gestational diabetes, see Section I.C.11, g., Gestational diabetes.

6) **Insulin pump malfunction**

(a) **Underdose of insulin due insulin pump failure**

An underdose of insulin due to an insulin pump failure should be assigned 996.57, Mechanical complication due to insulin pump, as the principal or first listed code, followed by the appropriate diabetes mellitus code based on documentation.

(b) **Overdose of insulin due to insulin pump failure**

The principal or first listed code for an encounter due to an insulin pump malfunction resulting in an overdose of insulin, should also be 996.57, Mechanical complication due to insulin pump, followed by code 962.3, Poisoning by insulins and antidiabetic agents, and the appropriate diabetes mellitus code based on documentation.

7) **Secondary Diabetes Mellitus**

Codes under category 249, Secondary diabetes mellitus, identify complications/ manifestations associated with secondary diabetes mellitus. Secondary diabetes is always caused by another condition or event (e.g., cystic fibrosis, malignant neoplasm of pancreas, pancreatectomy, adverse effect of drug, or poisoning).

(a) **Fifth-digits for category 249:**

A fifth-digit is required for all category 249 codes to identify whether the diabetes is controlled or uncontrolled.

(b) **Secondary diabetes mellitus and the use of insulin**

For patients who routinely use insulin, code V58.67, Long-term (current) use of insulin, should also be assigned. Code V58.67 should not be assigned if insulin is given temporarily to bring a patient's blood sugar under control during an encounter.

(c) Assigning and sequencing secondary diabetes codes and associated conditions

When assigning codes for secondary diabetes and its associated conditions (e.g. renal manifestations), the code(s) from category 249 must be sequenced before the codes for the associated conditions. The secondary diabetes codes and the diabetic manifestation codes that correspond to them are paired codes that follow the etiology/manifestation convention of the classification. Assign as many codes from category 249 as needed to identify all of the associated conditions that the patient has. The corresponding codes for the associated conditions are listed under each of the secondary diabetes codes. For example, secondary diabetes with diabetic nephrosis is assigned to code 249.40, followed by 581.81.

(d) Assigning and sequencing secondary diabetes codes and its causes

The sequencing of the secondary diabetes codes in relationship to codes for the cause of the diabetes is based on the reason for the encounter, applicable ICD-9-CM sequencing conventions, and chapter-specific guidelines.

If a patient is seen for treatment of the secondary diabetes or one of its associated conditions, a code from category 249 is sequenced as the principal or first-listed diagnosis, with the cause of the secondary diabetes (e.g. cystic fibrosis) sequenced as an additional diagnosis.

If, however, the patient is seen for the treatment of the condition causing the secondary diabetes (e.g., malignant neoplasm of pancreas), the code for the cause of the secondary diabetes should be sequenced as the principal or first-listed diagnosis followed by a code from category 249.

(i) Secondary diabetes mellitus due to pancreatectomy

For postpancreatectomy diabetes mellitus (lack of insulin due to the surgical removal of all or part of the pancreas), assign code 251.3, Postsurgical hypoinsulinemia. Assign a code from subcategory 249, Secondary diabetes mellitus and a code from subcategory V88.1, Acquired absence of pancreas as additional codes. Code also any diabetic manifestations (e.g. diabetic nephrosis 581.81).

(ii) Secondary diabetes due to drugs

Secondary diabetes may be caused by an adverse effect of correctly administered medications, poisoning or late effect of poisoning.

See section I.C.17.e for coding of adverse effects and poisoning, and section I.C.19 for E code reporting.

4. Chapter 4: Diseases of Blood and Blood Forming Organs (280-289)

a. Anemia of chronic disease

Subcategory 285.2, Anemia in chronic illness, has codes for anemia in chronic kidney disease, code 285.21; anemia in neoplastic disease, code 285.22; and anemia in other chronic illness, code 285.29. These codes can be used as the principal/first listed code if the reason for the encounter is to treat the anemia. They may also be used as secondary codes if treatment of the anemia is a component of an encounter, but not the primary reason for the encounter. When using a code from subcategory 285 it is also necessary to use the code for the chronic condition causing the anemia.

1) Anemia in chronic kidney disease

When assigning code 285.21, Anemia in chronic kidney disease, it is also necessary to assign a code from category 585, Chronic kidney disease, to indicate the stage of chronic kidney disease.

See I.C.10.a. Chronic kidney disease (CKD).

2) Anemia in neoplastic disease

When assigning code 285.22, Anemia in neoplastic disease, it is also necessary to assign the neoplasm code that is responsible for the anemia. Code 285.22 is for use for anemia that is due to the malignancy, not for anemia due to antineoplastic chemotherapy drugs. Assign **the appropriate code** for anemia due to antineoplastic chemotherapy.

See I.C.2.c.1 Anemia associated with malignancy.

See I.C.2.c.2 Anemia associated with chemotherapy, immunotherapy and radiation therapy.

See I.C.17.e.1. Adverse effects.

5. Chapter 5: Mental Disorders (290-319)

Reserved for future guideline expansion

6. **Chapter 6: Diseases of Nervous System and Sense Organs (320-389)**

   a. **Pain - Category 338**

      1) **General coding information**

         Codes in category 338 may be used in conjunction with codes from other categories and chapters to provide more detail about acute or chronic pain and neoplasm-related pain, unless otherwise indicated below.

         If the pain is not specified as acute or chronic, do not assign codes from category 338, except for post-thoracotomy pain, postoperative pain, neoplasm related pain, or central pain syndrome.

         A code from subcategories 338.1 and 338.2 should not be assigned if the underlying (definitive) diagnosis is known, unless the reason for the encounter is pain control/management and not management of the underlying condition.

         (a) **Category 338 Codes as Principal or First-Listed Diagnosis**

             Category 338 codes are acceptable as principal diagnosis or the first-listed code:

             • When pain control or pain management is the reason for the admission/encounter (e.g., a patient with displaced intervertebral disc, nerve impingement and severe back pain presents for injection of steroid into the spinal canal). The underlying cause of the pain should be reported as an additional diagnosis, if known.

             • When an admission or encounter is for a procedure aimed at treating the underlying condition (e.g., spinal fusion, kyphoplasty), a code for the underlying condition (e.g., vertebral fracture, spinal stenosis) should be assigned as the principal diagnosis. No code from category 338 should be assigned.

             • When a patient is admitted for the insertion of a neurostimulator for pain control, assign the appropriate pain code as the principal or first listed diagnosis. When an admission or encounter is for a procedure aimed at treating the underlying condition and a neurostimulator is inserted for pain control during the same admission/encounter, a code for the underlying condition should be assigned as the principal diagnosis and the appropriate

             pain code should be assigned as a secondary diagnosis.

         (b) **Use of Category 338 Codes in Conjunction with Site Specific Pain Codes**

             (i) **Assigning Category 338 Codes and Site-Specific Pain Codes**

                 Codes from category 338 may be used in conjunction with codes that identify the site of pain (including codes from chapter 16) if the category 338 code provides additional information. For example, if the code describes the site of the pain, but does not fully describe whether the pain is acute or chronic, then both codes should be assigned.

             (ii) **Sequencing of Category 338 Codes with Site-Specific Pain Codes**

                 The sequencing of category 338 codes with site-specific pain codes (including chapter 16 codes), is dependent on the circumstances of the encounter/admission as follows:

                 • If the encounter is for pain control or pain management, assign the code from category 338 followed by the code identifying the specific site of pain (e.g., encounter for pain management for acute neck pain from trauma is assigned code 338.11, Acute pain due to trauma, followed by code 723.1, Cervicalgia, to identify the site of pain).

                 • If the encounter is for any other reason except pain control or pain management, and a related definitive diagnosis has not been established (confirmed) by the provider, assign the code for the specific site of pain first, followed by the appropriate code from category 338.

      2) **Pain due to devices, implants and grafts**

         Pain associated with devices, implants or grafts left in a surgical site (for example painful hip prosthesis) is assigned to the appropriate code(s) found in Chapter 17, Injury and Poisoning. Use additional code(s) from category 338 to identify acute or chronic pain due to presence of the device, implant or graft (338.18-338.19 or 338.28-338.29).

3) Postoperative Pain

Post-thoracotomy pain and other postoperative pain are classified to subcategories 338.1 and 338.2, depending on whether the pain is acute or chronic. The default for post-thoracotomy and other postoperative pain not specified as acute or chronic is the code for the acute form.

Routine or expected postoperative pain immediately after surgery should not be coded.

(a) Postoperative pain not associated with specific postoperative complication

Postoperative pain not associated with a specific postoperative complication is assigned to the appropriate postoperative pain code in category 338.

(b) Postoperative pain associated with specific postoperative complication

Postoperative pain associated with a specific postoperative complication (such as painful wire sutures) is assigned to the appropriate code(s) found in Chapter 17, Injury and Poisoning. If appropriate, use additional code(s) from category 338 to identify acute or chronic pain (338.18 or 338.28). If pain control/management is the reason for the encounter, a code from category 338 should be assigned as the principal or first-listed diagnosis in accordance with *Section I.C.6.a.1.a above*.

(c) Postoperative pain as principal or first-listed diagnosis

Postoperative pain may be reported as the principal or first-listed diagnosis when the stated reason for the admission/encounter is documented as postoperative pain control/management.

(d) Postoperative pain as secondary diagnosis

Postoperative pain may be reported as a secondary diagnosis code when a patient presents for outpatient surgery and develops an unusual or inordinate amount of postoperative pain.

The provider's documentation should be used to guide the coding of postoperative pain, as well as *Section III. Reporting Additional Diagnoses* and *Section IV. Diagnostic Coding and Reporting in the Outpatient Setting*.

See Section II.I.2 for information on sequencing of diagnoses for patients admitted to hospital inpatient care following post-operative observation.

See Section II.J for information on sequencing of diagnoses for patients admitted to hospital inpatient care from outpatient surgery.

See Section IV.A.2 for information on sequencing of diagnoses for patients admitted for observation.

4) Chronic pain

Chronic pain is classified to subcategory 338.2. There is no time frame defining when pain becomes chronic pain. The provider's documentation should be used to guide use of these codes.

5) Neoplasm Related Pain

Code 338.3 is assigned to pain documented as being related, associated or due to cancer, primary or secondary malignancy, or tumor. This code is assigned regardless of whether the pain is acute or chronic.

This code may be assigned as the principal or first-listed code when the stated reason for the admission/encounter is documented as pain control/pain management. The underlying neoplasm should be reported as an additional diagnosis.

When the reason for the admission/encounter is management of the neoplasm and the pain associated with the neoplasm is also documented, code 338.3 may be assigned as an additional diagnosis.

See Section I.C.2 for instructions on the sequencing of neoplasms for all other stated reasons for the admission/encounter (except for pain control/pain management).

6) Chronic pain syndrome

This condition is different than the term "chronic pain," and therefore this code should only be used when the provider has specifically documented this condition.

b. Glaucoma

1) Glaucoma

For types of glaucoma classified to subcategories 365.1-365.6, an additional code should be assigned from subcategory 365.7, Glaucoma stage, to identify the glaucoma stage. Codes from 365.7, Glaucoma stage, may not be assigned as a principal or first-listed diagnosis.

2) Bilateral glaucoma with same stage

When a patient has bilateral glaucoma and both are documented as being the same type and stage, report only the code for the type of glaucoma and one code for the stage.

3) Bilateral glaucoma stage with different stages

When a patient has bilateral glaucoma and each eye is documented as having a different stage, assign one code for the type of glaucoma and one code for the highest glaucoma stage.

4) Bilateral glaucoma with different types and different stages

When a patient has bilateral glaucoma and each eye is documented as having a different type and a different stage, assign one code for each type of glaucoma and one code for the highest glaucoma stage.

5) Patient admitted with glaucoma and stage evolves during the admission

If a patient is admitted with glaucoma and the stage progresses during the admission, assign the code for highest stage documented.

6) Indeterminate stage glaucoma

Assignment of code 365.74, Indeterminate stage glaucoma, should be based on the clinical documentation. Code 365.74 is used for glaucomas whose stage cannot be clinically determined. This code should not be confused with code 365.70, Glaucoma stage, unspecified. Code 365.70 should be assigned when there is no documentation regarding the stage of the glaucoma.

7. Chapter 7: Diseases of Circulatory System (390-459)

a. Hypertension

Hypertension Table

The Hypertension Table, found under the main term, "Hypertension", in the Alphabetic Index, contains a complete listing of all conditions due to or associated with hypertension and classifies them according to malignant, benign, and unspecified.

1) Hypertension, Essential, or NOS

Assign hypertension (arterial) (essential) (primary) (systemic) (NOS) to category code 401 with the appropriate fourth digit to indicate malignant (.0), benign (.1), or unspecified (.9). Do not use either .0 malignant or .1 benign unless medical record documentation supports such a designation.

2) Hypertension with Heart Disease

Heart conditions (425.8, 429.0-429.3, 429.8, 429.9) are assigned to a code from category 402 when a causal relationship is stated (due to hypertension) or implied (hypertensive). Use an additional code from category 428 to identify the type of heart failure in those patients with heart failure. More than one code from category 428 may be assigned if the patient has systolic or diastolic failure and congestive heart failure.

The same heart conditions (425.8, 429.0-429.3, 429.8, 429.9) with hypertension, but without a stated causal relationship, are coded separately. Sequence according to the circumstances of the admission/encounter.

3) Hypertensive Chronic Kidney Disease

Assign codes from category 403, Hypertensive chronic kidney disease, when conditions classified to category 585 or code 587 are present with hypertension. Unlike hypertension with heart disease, ICD-9-CM presumes a cause-and-effect relationship and classifies chronic kidney disease (CKD) with hypertension as hypertensive chronic kidney disease.

Fifth digits for category 403 should be assigned as follows:

- 0 with CKD stage I through stage IV, or unspecified.
- 1 with CKD stage V or end stage renal disease.

The appropriate code from category 585, Chronic kidney disease, should be used as a secondary code with a code from category 403 to identify the stage of chronic kidney disease.

See Section I.C.10.a for information on the coding of chronic kidney disease.

4) Hypertensive Heart and Chronic Kidney Disease

Assign codes from combination category 404, Hypertensive heart and chronic kidney disease, when both hypertensive kidney disease and hypertensive heart disease are stated in the diagnosis. Assume a relationship between the hypertension and the chronic kidney disease, whether or not the condition is so designated. Assign an additional code from category 428, to identify the type of heart failure. More than one code from category 428 may be assigned if the patient has systolic or diastolic failure and congestive heart failure.

Fifth digits for category 404 should be assigned as follows:

- 0 without heart failure and with chronic kidney disease (CKD) stage I through stage IV, or unspecified
- 1 with heart failure and with CKD stage I through stage IV, or unspecified
- 2 without heart failure and with CKD stage V or end stage renal disease
- 3 with heart failure and with CKD stage V or end stage renal disease

The appropriate code from category 585, Chronic kidney disease, should be used as a secondary code with a code from category 404 to identify the stage of kidney disease.

See Section I.C.10.a for information on the coding of chronic kidney disease.

5) **Hypertensive Cerebrovascular Disease**

First assign codes from 430-438, Cerebrovascular disease, then the appropriate hypertension code from categories 401-405.

6) **Hypertensive Retinopathy**

Two codes are necessary to identify the condition. First assign the code from subcategory 362.11, Hypertensive retinopathy, then the appropriate code from categories 401-405 to indicate the type of hypertension.

7) **Hypertension, Secondary**

Two codes are required: one to identify the underlying etiology and one from category 405 to identify the hypertension. Sequencing of codes is determined by the reason for admission/encounter.

8) **Hypertension, Transient**

Assign code 796.2, Elevated blood pressure reading without diagnosis of hypertension, unless patient has an established diagnosis of hypertension. Assign code 642.3x for transient hypertension of pregnancy.

9) **Hypertension, Controlled**

Assign appropriate code from categories 401-405. This diagnostic statement usually refers to an existing state of hypertension under control by therapy.

10) **Hypertension, Uncontrolled**

Uncontrolled hypertension may refer to untreated hypertension or hypertension not responding to current therapeutic regimen. In either case, assign the appropriate code from categories 401-405 to designate the stage and type of hypertension. Code to the type of hypertension.

11) **Elevated Blood Pressure**

For a statement of elevated blood pressure without further specificity, assign code 796.2, Elevated blood pressure reading without diagnosis of hypertension, rather than a code from category 401.

b. **Cerebral infarction/stroke/cerebrovascular accident (CVA)**

The terms stroke and CVA are often used interchangeably to refer to a cerebral infarction. The terms stroke, CVA, and cerebral infarction NOS are all indexed to the default code 434.91, Cerebral artery occlusion, unspecified, with infarction.

Additional code(s) should be assigned for any neurologic deficits associated with the acute CVA, regardless of whether or not the neurologic deficit resolves prior to discharge.

See Section I.C.18.d.3 for information on coding status post administration of tPA in a different facility within the last 24 hours.

c. **Postoperative cerebrovascular accident**

A cerebrovascular hemorrhage or infarction that occurs as a result of medical intervention is coded to 997.02, Iatrogenic cerebrovascular infarction or hemorrhage. Medical record documentation should clearly specify the cause-and-effect relationship between the medical intervention and the cerebrovascular accident in order to assign this code. A secondary code from the code range 430-432 or from a code from subcategories 433 or 434 with a fifth digit of "1" should also be used to identify the type of hemorrhage or infarct.

This guideline conforms to the use additional code note instruction at category 997. Code 436, Acute, but ill-defined, cerebrovascular disease, should not be used as a secondary code with code 997.02.

d. **Late Effects of Cerebrovascular Disease**

1) **Category 438, Late Effects of Cerebrovascular disease**

Category 438 is used to indicate conditions classifiable to categories 430-437 as the causes of late effects (neurologic deficits), themselves classified elsewhere. These "late effects" include neurologic deficits that persist after initial onset of conditions classifiable to 430-437. The neurologic deficits caused by cerebrovascular disease may be present from the onset or may arise at any time after the onset of the condition classifiable to 430-437.

Codes in category 438 are only for use for late effects of cerebrovascular disease, not for neurologic deficits associated with an acute CVA.

2) **Codes from category 438 with codes from 430-437**

Codes from category 438 may be assigned on a health care record with codes from 430-437, if the patient has a current cerebrovascular accident (CVA) and deficits from an old CVA.

3) **Code V12.54**

Assign code V12.54, Transient ischemic attack (TIA), and cerebral infarction without residual deficits (and not a code from category 438) as an additional code for history of cerebrovascular disease when no neurologic deficits are present.

e. **Acute myocardial infarction (AMI)**

1) **ST elevation myocardial infarction (STEMI) and non ST elevation myocardial infarction (NSTEMI)**

   The ICD-9-CM codes for acute myocardial infarction (AMI) identify the site, such as anterolateral wall or true posterior wall. Subcategories 410.0-410.6 and 410.8 are used for ST elevation myocardial infarction (STEMI). Subcategory 410.7, Subendocardial infarction, is used for non ST elevation myocardial infarction (NSTEMI) and nontransmural MIs.

2) **Acute myocardial infarction, unspecified**

   Subcategory 410.9 is the default for the unspecified term acute myocardial infarction. If only STEMI or transmural MI without the site is documented, query the provider as to the site, or assign a code from subcategory 410.9.

3) **AMI documented as nontransmural or subendocardial but site provided**

   If an AMI is documented as nontransmural or subendocardial, but the site is provided, it is still coded as a subendocardial AMI. If NSTEMI evolves to STEMI, assign the STEMI code. If STEMI converts to NSTEMI due to thrombolytic therapy, it is still coded as STEMI.

   See Section I.C.18.d.3 for information on coding status post administration of tPA in a different facility within the last 24 hours.

8. **Chapter 8: Diseases of Respiratory System (460-519)**

   See I.C.17.f. for ventilator-associated pneumonia.

   a. **Chronic Obstructive Pulmonary Disease [COPD] and Asthma**

   1) **Conditions that comprise COPD and Asthma**

      The conditions that comprise COPD are obstructive chronic bronchitis, subcategory 491.2, and emphysema, category 492. All asthma codes are under category 493, Asthma. Code 496, Chronic airway obstruction, not elsewhere classified, is a nonspecific code that should only be used when the documentation in a medical record does not specify the type of COPD being treated.

   2) **Acute exacerbation of chronic obstructive bronchitis and asthma**

      The codes for chronic obstructive bronchitis and asthma distinguish between uncomplicated cases and those in acute exacerbation. An acute exacerbation is a worsening or a decompensation of a chronic condition. An acute exacerbation

is not equivalent to an infection superimposed on a chronic condition, though an exacerbation may be triggered by an infection.

3) **Overlapping nature of the conditions that comprise COPD and asthma**

   Due to the overlapping nature of the conditions that make up COPD and asthma, there are many variations in the way these conditions are documented. Code selection must be based on the terms as documented. When selecting the correct code for the documented type of COPD and asthma, it is essential to first review the index, and then verify the code in the tabular list. There are many instructional notes under the different COPD subcategories and codes. It is important that all such notes be reviewed to assure correct code assignment.

4) **Acute exacerbation of asthma and status asthmaticus**

   An acute exacerbation of asthma is an increased severity of the asthma symptoms, such as wheezing and shortness of breath. Status asthmaticus refers to a patient's failure to respond to therapy administered during an asthmatic episode and is a life threatening complication that requires emergency care. If status asthmaticus is documented by the provider with any type of COPD or with acute bronchitis, the status asthmaticus should be sequenced first. It supersedes any type of COPD including that with acute exacerbation or acute bronchitis. It is inappropriate to assign an asthma code with 5th digit 2, with acute exacerbation, together with an asthma code with 5th digit 1, with status asthmatics. Only the 5th digit 1 should be assigned.

b. **Chronic Obstructive Pulmonary Disease [COPD] and Bronchitis**

1) **Acute bronchitis with COPD**

   Acute bronchitis, code 466.0, is due to an infectious organism. When acute bronchitis is documented with COPD, code 491.22, Obstructive chronic bronchitis with acute bronchitis, should be assigned. It is not necessary to also assign code 466.0. If a medical record documents acute bronchitis with COPD with acute exacerbation, only code 491.22 should be assigned. The acute bronchitis included in code 491.22 supersedes the acute exacerbation. If a medical record documents COPD with acute exacerbation without mention of acute bronchitis, only code 491.21 should be assigned.

c. Acute Respiratory Failure

1) Acute respiratory failure as principal diagnosis

Acute respiratory failure, may be assigned as a principal diagnosis when it is the condition established after study to be chiefly responsible for occasioning the admission to the hospital, and the selection is supported by the Alphabetic Index and Tabular List. However, chapter-specific coding guidelines (such as obstetrics, poisoning, HIV, newborn) that provide sequencing direction take precedence.

2) Acute respiratory failure as secondary diagnosis

Respiratory failure may be listed as a secondary diagnosis if it occurs after admission, or if it is present on admission, but does not meet the definition of principal diagnosis.

3) Sequencing of acute respiratory failure and another acute condition

When a patient is admitted with respiratory failure and another acute condition, (e.g., myocardial infarction, cerebrovascular accident, aspiration pneumonia), the principal diagnosis will not be the same in every situation. This applies whether the other acute condition is a respiratory or nonrespiratory condition. Selection of the principal diagnosis will be dependent on the circumstances of admission. If both the respiratory failure and the other acute condition are equally responsible for occasioning the admission to the hospital, and there are no chapter-specific sequencing rules, the guideline regarding two or more diagnoses that equally meet the definition for principal diagnosis (Section II, C.) may be applied in these situations.

If the documentation is not clear as to whether acute respiratory failure and another condition are equally responsible for occasioning the admission, query the provider for clarification.

d. Influenza due to *certain* identified *viruses*

Code only confirmed cases of avian influenza (codes 488.01-488.02, 488.09, Influenza due to indentified avian influenza virus), **2009** H1N1 influenza virus (codes 488.11-488.12, 488.19)**, or novel influenza A (codes 488.81-488.82, 488.89, Influenza due to identified novel influenza A virus).** This is an exception to the hospital inpatient guideline Section II, H. (Uncertain Diagnosis).

In this context, "confirmation" does not require documentation of positive laboratory testing specific for avian, **2009 H1N1** or novel influenza **A virus**. However, coding should be based on the provider's diagnostic statement that the patient has avian **influenza, 2009 H1N1 influenza,** or novel influenza **A.**

If the provider records "suspected" or "possible" or "probable" avian, **2009 H1N1,** or novel influenza **A,** the appropriate influenza code from category 487, **Influenza** should be assigned. A code from category 488, Influenza due to certain identified avian influenza viruses, should not be assigned.

9. **Chapter 9: Diseases of Digestive System (520-579)**

Reserved for future guideline expansion

10. **Chapter 10: Diseases of Genitourinary System (580-629)**

a. Chronic kidney disease

1) Stages of chronic kidney disease (CKD)

The ICD-9-CM classifies CKD based on severity. The severity of CKD is designated by stages I-V. Stage II, code 585.2, equates to mild CKD; stage III, code 585.3, equates to moderate CKD; and stage IV, code 585.4, equates to severe CKD. Code 585.6, End stage renal disease (ESRD), is assigned when the provider has documented end-stage-renal disease (ESRD).

If both a stage of CKD and ESRD are documented, assign code 585.6 only.

2) Chronic kidney disease and kidney transplant status

Patients who have undergone kidney transplant may still have some form of CKD, because the kidney transplant may not fully restore kidney function. Therefore, the presence of CKD alone does not constitute a transplant complication. Assign the appropriate 585 code for the patient's stage of CKD and code V42.0. If a transplant complication such as failure or rejection is documented, see section I.C.17.f.2.b for information on coding complications of a kidney transplant. If the documentation is unclear as to whether the patient has a complication of the transplant, query the provider.

3) Chronic kidney disease with other conditions

Patients with CKD may also suffer from other serious conditions, most commonly diabetes mellitus and hypertension. The sequencing of the CKD code in relationship to codes for other contributing conditions is based on the conventions in the tabular list.

See I.C.3.a.4 for sequencing instructions for diabetes.

See I.C.4.a.1 for anemia in CKD.

See I.C.7.a.3 for hypertensive chronic kidney disease.

See I.C.17.f.2.b, Kidney transplant complications, for instructions on coding of documented rejection or failure.

11. Chapter 11: Complications of Pregnancy, Childbirth, and the Puerperium (630-679)

a. General Rules for Obstetric Cases

1) Codes from chapter 11 and sequencing priority

Obstetric cases require codes from chapter 11, codes in the range 630-679, Complications of Pregnancy, Childbirth, and the Puerperium. Chapter 11 codes have sequencing priority over codes from other chapters. Additional codes from other chapters may be used in conjunction with chapter 11 codes to further specify conditions. Should the provider document that the pregnancy is incidental to the encounter, then code V22.2 should be used in place of any chapter 11 codes. It is the provider's responsibility to state that the condition being treated is not affecting the pregnancy.

2) Chapter 11 codes used only on the maternal record

Chapter 11 codes are to be used only on the maternal record, never on the record of the newborn.

3) Chapter 11 fifth-digits

Categories 640-649, 651-676 have required fifth-digits, which indicate whether the encounter is antepartum, postpartum and whether a delivery has also occurred.

4) Fifth-digits, appropriate for each code

The fifth-digits, which are appropriate for each code number, are listed in brackets under each code. The fifth-digits on each code should all be consistent with each other. That is, should a delivery occur all of the fifth-digits should indicate the delivery.

b. Selection of OB Principal or First-listed Diagnosis

1) Routine outpatient prenatal visits

For routine outpatient prenatal visits when no complications are present codes V22.0, Supervision of normal first pregnancy, and V22.1, Supervision of other normal pregnancy, should be used as the first-listed diagnoses. These codes should not be used in conjunction with chapter 11 codes.

2) Prenatal outpatient visits for high-risk patients

For **routine** prenatal outpatient visits for patients with high-risk pregnancies, a code from category V23, Supervision of high-risk pregnancy, should be used as the first-listed diagnosis. Secondary chapter 11 codes may be used in conjunction with these codes if appropriate.

3) Episodes when no delivery occurs

In episodes when no delivery occurs, the principal diagnosis should correspond to the principal complication of the pregnancy, which necessitated the encounter. Should more than one complication exist, all of which are treated or monitored, any of the complications codes may be sequenced first.

4) When a delivery occurs

When a delivery occurs, the principal diagnosis should correspond to the main circumstances or complication of the delivery. In cases of cesarean delivery, the selection of the principal diagnosis should be the condition established after study that was responsible for the patient's admission. If the patient was admitted with a condition that resulted in the performance of a cesarean procedure, that condition should be selected as the principal diagnosis. If the reason for the admission/encounter was unrelated to the condition resulting in the cesarean delivery, the condition related to the reason for the admission/encounter should be selected as the principal diagnosis, even if a cesarean was performed.

5) Outcome of delivery

An outcome of delivery code, V27.0-V27.9, should be included on every maternal record when a delivery has occurred. These codes are not to be used on subsequent records or on the newborn record.

c. Fetal Conditions Affecting the Management of the Mother

1) Codes from categories 655 and 656

Codes from categories 655, Known or suspected fetal abnormality affecting management of the mother, and 656, Other known or suspected fetal and placental problems affecting the management of the mother, are assigned only when the fetal condition is actually responsible for modifying the management of the mother, i.e., by requiring diagnostic studies, additional observation, special care, or termination of pregnancy. The fact that the fetal condition exists does not justify assigning a code from this series to the mother's record.

See I.C.18.d. for suspected maternal and fetal conditions not found

2) In utero surgery

In cases when surgery is performed on the fetus, a diagnosis code from category 655, Known or suspected fetal abnormalities affecting management of the mother, should be assigned identifying the fetal condition. Procedure code 75.36, Correction of fetal defect, should be assigned on the hospital inpatient record.

No code from Chapter 15, the perinatal codes, should be used on the mother's record to identify fetal conditions. Surgery performed in utero on a fetus is still to be coded as an obstetric encounter.

d. HIV Infection in Pregnancy, Childbirth and the Puerperium

During pregnancy, childbirth or the puerperium, a patient admitted because of an HIV-related illness should receive a principal diagnosis of 647.6X, Other specified infectious and parasitic diseases in the mother classifiable elsewhere, but complicating the pregnancy, childbirth or the puerperium, followed by 042 and the code(s) for the HIV-related illness(es).

Patients with asymptomatic HIV infection status admitted during pregnancy, childbirth, or the puerperium should receive codes of 647.6X and V08.

e. Current Conditions Complicating Pregnancy

Assign a code from subcategory 648.x for patients that have current conditions when the condition affects the management of the pregnancy, childbirth, or the puerperium. Use additional secondary codes from other chapters to identify the conditions, as appropriate.

f. Diabetes mellitus in pregnancy

Diabetes mellitus is a significant complicating factor in pregnancy. Pregnant women who are diabetic should be assigned code 648.0x, Diabetes mellitus complicating pregnancy, and a secondary code from category 250, Diabetes mellitus, or category 249, Secondary diabetes to identify the type of diabetes.

Code V58.67, Long-term (current) use of insulin, should also be assigned if the diabetes mellitus is being treated with insulin.

g. Gestational diabetes

Gestational diabetes can occur during the second and third trimester of pregnancy in women who were not diabetic prior to pregnancy. Gestational diabetes can cause complications in the pregnancy similar to those of pre-existing diabetes mellitus. It also puts the woman at greater risk of developing diabetes after the pregnancy. Gestational diabetes is coded to 648.8x, Abnormal glucose tolerance. Codes 648.0x and 648.8x should never be used together on the same record.

Code V58.67, Long-term (current) use of insulin, should also be assigned if the gestational diabetes is being treated with insulin.

h. Normal Delivery, Code 650

1) Normal delivery

Code 650 is for use in cases when a woman is admitted for a full-term normal delivery and delivers a single, healthy infant without any complications antepartum, during the delivery, or postpartum during the delivery episode. Code 650 is always a principal diagnosis. It is not to be used if any other code from chapter 11 is needed to describe a current complication of the antenatal, delivery, or perinatal period. Additional codes from other chapters may be used with code 650 if they are not related to or are in any way complicating the pregnancy.

2) Normal delivery with resolved antepartum complication

Code 650 may be used if the patient had a complication at some point during her pregnancy, but the complication is not present at the time of the admission for delivery.

3) V27.0, Single liveborn, outcome of delivery

V27.0, Single liveborn, is the only outcome of delivery code appropriate for use with 650.

i. The Postpartum and Peripartum Periods

1) Postpartum and peripartum periods

The postpartum period begins immediately after delivery and continues for six weeks following delivery. The peripartum period is defined as the last month of pregnancy to five months postpartum.

2) Postpartum complication

A postpartum complication is any complication occurring within the six-week period.

3) Pregnancy-related complications after 6 week period

Chapter 11 codes may also be used to describe pregnancy-related complications after the six-week period should the provider document that a condition is pregnancy related.

4) Postpartum complications occurring during the same admission as delivery

Postpartum complications that occur during the same admission as the delivery are identified with a fifth digit of "2." Subsequent admissions/encounters for postpartum complications should be identified with a fifth digit of "4."

5) Admission for routine postpartum care following delivery outside hospital

When the mother delivers outside the hospital prior to admission and is admitted for routine postpartum care and no complications are noted, code V24.0, Postpartum care and examination immediately after delivery, should be assigned as the principal diagnosis.

6) Admission following delivery outside hospital with postpartum conditions

A delivery diagnosis code should not be used for a woman who has delivered prior to admission to the hospital. Any postpartum conditions and/or postpartum procedures should be coded.

7) Puerperal sepsis

Code 670.2x, Puerperal sepsis, should be assigned with a secondary code to identify the causal organism (e.g., for a bacterial infection, assign a code from category 041, Bacterial infections in conditions classified elsewhere and of unspecified site). A code from category 038, Septicemia, should not be used for puerperal sepsis. Do not assign code 995.91, Sepsis, as code 670.2x describes the sepsis. If applicable, use additional codes to identify severe sepsis (995.92) and any associated acute organ dysfunction.

j. Code 677, Late effect of complication of pregnancy

1) Code 677

Code 677, Late effect of complication of pregnancy, childbirth, and the puerperium is for use in those cases when an initial complication of a pregnancy develops a sequelae requiring care or treatment at a future date.

2) After the initial postpartum period

This code may be used at any time after the initial postpartum period.

3) Sequencing of Code 677

This code, like all late effect codes, is to be sequenced following the code describing the sequelae of the complication.

k. Abortions

1) Fifth-digits required for abortion categories

Fifth-digits are required for abortion categories 634-637. Fifth digit assignment is based on the status of the patient at the beginning (or start) of the encounter. Fifth-digit 1, incomplete, indicates that all of the products of conception have not been expelled from the uterus. Fifth-digit 2, complete, indicates that all products of conception have been expelled from the uterus.

2) Code from categories 640-649 and 651-659

A code from categories 640-649 and 651-659 may be used as additional codes with an abortion code to indicate the complication leading to the abortion.

Fifth digit 3 is assigned with codes from these categories when used with an abortion code because the other fifth digits will not apply. Codes from the 660-669 series are not to be used for complications of abortion.

3) Code 639 for complications

Code 639 is to be used for all complications following abortion. Code 639 cannot be assigned with codes from categories 634-638.

4) Abortion with Liveborn Fetus

When an attempted termination of pregnancy results in a liveborn fetus assign code 644.21, Early onset of delivery, with an appropriate code from category V27, Outcome of Delivery. The procedure code for the attempted termination of pregnancy should also be assigned.

5) Retained Products of Conception following an abortion

Subsequent admissions for retained products of conception following a spontaneous or legally induced abortion are assigned the appropriate code from category 634, Spontaneous abortion, or 635 Legally induced abortion, with a fifth digit of "1" (incomplete). This advice is appropriate even when the patient was discharged previously with a discharge diagnosis of complete abortion.

12. Chapter 12: Diseases Skin and Subcutaneous Tissue (680-709)

a. Pressure ulcer stage codes

1) Pressure ulcer stages

Two codes are needed to completely describe a pressure ulcer: A code from subcategory 707.0, Pressure ulcer, to identify the site of the pressure ulcer and a code from subcategory 707.2, Pressure ulcer stages.

The codes in subcategory 707.2, Pressure ulcer stages, are to be used as an additional diagnosis with a code(s) from subcategory 707.0, Pressure Ulcer. Codes from 707.2, Pressure ulcer stages, may not be assigned as a principal or first-listed diagnosis. The pressure ulcer stage codes should only be used with pressure ulcers and not with other types of ulcers (e.g., stasis ulcer).

The ICD-9-CM classifies pressure ulcer stages based on severity, which is designated by stages I-IV and unstageable.

2) Unstageable pressure ulcers

Assignment of code 707.25, Pressure ulcer, unstageable, should be based on the clinical documentation. Code 707.25 is used for pressure ulcers whose stage cannot be clinically determined (e.g., the ulcer is covered by eschar or has been treated with a skin or muscle graft) and pressure ulcers that are documented as deep tissue injury but not documented as due to trauma. This code should not be confused with code 707.20, Pressure ulcer, stage unspecified. Code 707.20 should be assigned when there is no documentation regarding the stage of the pressure ulcer.

3) **Documented pressure ulcer stage**

Assignment of the pressure ulcer stage code should be guided by clinical documentation of the stage or documentation of the terms found in the index. For clinical terms describing the stage that are not found in the index, and there is no documentation of the stage, the provider should be queried.

4) **Bilateral pressure ulcers with same stage**

When a patient has bilateral pressure ulcers (e.g., both buttocks) and both pressure ulcers are documented as being the same stage, only the code for the site and one code for the stage should be reported.

5) **Bilateral pressure ulcers with different stages**

When a patient has bilateral pressure ulcers at the same site (e.g., both buttocks) and each pressure ulcer is documented as being at a different stage, assign one code for the site and the appropriate codes for the pressure ulcer stage.

6) **Multiple pressure ulcers of different sites and stages**

When a patient has multiple pressure ulcers at different sites (e.g., buttock, heel, shoulder) and each pressure ulcer is documented as being at different stages (e.g., stage 3 and stage 4), assign the appropriate codes for each different site and a code for each different pressure ulcer stage.

7) **Patients admitted with pressure ulcers documented as healed**

No code is assigned if the documentation states that the pressure ulcer is completely healed.

8) **Patients admitted with pressure ulcers documented as healing**

Pressure ulcers described as healing should be assigned the appropriate pressure ulcer stage code based on the documentation in the medical record. If the documentation does not provide information about the stage of the healing pressure ulcer, assign code 707.20, Pressure ulcer stage, unspecified.

If the documentation is unclear as to whether the patient has a current (new) pressure ulcer or if the patient is being treated for a healing pressure ulcer, query the provider.

9) **Patient admitted with pressure ulcer evolving into another stage during the admission**

If a patient is admitted with a pressure ulcer at one stage and it progresses to a higher stage, assign the code for highest stage reported for that site.

13. **Chapter 13: Diseases of Musculoskeletal and Connective Tissue (710-739)**

a. **Coding of Pathologic Fractures**

1) **Acute Fractures vs. Aftercare**

Pathologic fractures are reported using subcategory 733.1, when the fracture is newly diagnosed. Subcategory 733.1 may be used while the patient is receiving active treatment for the fracture. Examples of active treatment are: surgical treatment, emergency department encounter, evaluation and treatment by a new physician.

Fractures are coded using the aftercare codes (subcategories V54.0, V54.2, V54.8 or V54.9) for encounters after the patient has completed active treatment of the fracture and is receiving routine care for the fracture during the healing or recovery phase. Examples of fracture aftercare are: cast change or removal, removal of external or internal fixation device, medication adjustment, and follow up visits following fracture treatment.

Care for complications of surgical treatment for fracture repairs during the healing or recovery phase should be coded with the appropriate complication codes.

Care of complications of fractures, such as malunion and nonunion, should be reported with the appropriate codes.

See Section I.C.17.b for information on the coding of traumatic fractures.

14. **Chapter 14: Congenital Anomalies (740-759)**

a. **Codes in categories 740-759, Congenital Anomalies**

Assign an appropriate code(s) from categories 740-759, Congenital Anomalies, when an anomaly is documented. A congenital anomaly may be the principal/first listed diagnosis on a record or a secondary diagnosis.

When a congenital anomaly does not have a unique code assignment, assign additional code(s) for any manifestations that may be present.

When the code assignment specifically identifies the congenital anomaly, manifestations that are an inherent component of the anomaly should not be coded separately. Additional codes should be assigned for manifestations that are not an inherent component.

Codes from Chapter 14 may be used throughout the life of the patient. If a congenital anomaly has been corrected, a personal history code should be used to identify the history of the anomaly. Although present at birth, a congenital anomaly may not be identified until later in life. Whenever the condition is diagnosed by the physician, it is appropriate to assign a code from codes 740-759.

For the birth admission, the appropriate code from category V30, Liveborn infants, according to type of birth should be sequenced as the principal diagnosis, followed by any congenital anomaly codes, 740-759.

15. **Chapter 15: Newborn (Perinatal) Guidelines (760-779)**

For coding and reporting purposes the perinatal period is defined as before birth through the 28th day following birth. The following guidelines are provided for reporting purposes. Hospitals may record other diagnoses as needed for internal data use.

a. **General Perinatal Rules**

1) **Chapter 15 Codes**

They are <u>never</u> for use on the maternal record. Codes from Chapter 11, the obstetric chapter, are never permitted on the newborn record. Chapter 15 code may be used throughout the life of the patient if the condition is still present.

2) **Sequencing of perinatal codes**

Generally, codes from Chapter 15 should be sequenced as the principal/first-listed diagnosis on the newborn record, with the exception of the appropriate V30 code for the birth episode, followed by codes from any other chapter that provide additional detail. The "use additional code" note at the beginning of the chapter supports this guideline. If the index does not provide a specific code for a perinatal condition, assign code 779.89, Other specified conditions originating in the perinatal period, followed by the code from another chapter that specifies the condition. Codes for signs and symptoms may be assigned when a definitive diagnosis has not been established.

3) **Birth process or community acquired conditions**

If a newborn has a condition that may be either due to the birth process or community acquired and the documentation does not indicate which it is, the default is due to the birth process and the code from Chapter 15 should be used. If the condition is community-acquired, a code from Chapter 15 should not be assigned.

4) **Code all clinically significant conditions**

All clinically significant conditions noted on routine newborn examination should be coded. A condition is clinically significant if it requires:

- clinical evaluation; or
- therapeutic treatment; or
- diagnostic procedures; or
- extended length of hospital stay; or
- increased nursing care and/or monitoring; or
- has implications for future health care needs

Note: The perinatal guidelines listed above are the same as the general coding guidelines for "additional diagnoses", except for the final point regarding implications for future health care needs. Codes should be assigned for conditions that have been specified by the provider as having implications for future health care needs. Codes from the perinatal chapter should not be assigned unless the provider has established a definitive diagnosis.

b. **Use of codes V30-V39**

When coding the birth of an infant, assign a code from categories V30-V39, according to the type of birth. A code from this series is assigned as a principal diagnosis, and assigned only once to a newborn at the time of birth.

c. **Newborn transfers**

If the newborn is transferred to another institution, the V30 series is not used at the receiving hospital.

d. **Use of category V29**

1) **Assigning a code from category V29**

Assign a code from category V29, Observation and evaluation of newborns and infants for suspected conditions not found, to identify those instances when a healthy newborn is evaluated for a suspected condition that is determined after study not to be present. Do not use a code from category V29 when the patient has identified signs or symptoms of a suspected problem; in such cases, code the sign or symptom.

A code from category V29 may also be assigned as a principal code for readmissions or encounters when the V30 code no longer applies. Codes from category V29 are for use only for healthy newborns and infants for which no condition after study is found to be present.

2) **V29 code on a birth record**

A V29 code is to be used as a secondary code after the V30, Outcome of delivery, code.

e. **Use of other V codes on perinatal records**

V codes other than V30 and V29 may be assigned on a perinatal or newborn record code. The codes may be used as a principal or first-listed diagnosis for specific types of encounters or for readmissions or encounters when the V30 code no longer applies.

See Section I.C.18 for information regarding the assignment of V codes.

f. **Maternal Causes of Perinatal Morbidity**

Codes from categories 760-763, Maternal causes of perinatal morbidity and mortality, are assigned only when the maternal condition has actually affected the fetus or newborn. The fact that the mother has an associated medical condition or experiences some complication of pregnancy, labor or delivery does not justify the routine assignment of codes from these categories to the newborn record.

g. **Congenital Anomalies in Newborns**

For the birth admission, the appropriate code from category V30, Liveborn infants according to type of birth, should be used, followed by any congenital anomaly codes, categories 740-759. Use additional secondary codes from other chapters to specify conditions associated with the anomaly, if applicable.

Also, see Section I.C.14 for information on the coding of congenital anomalies.

h. **Coding Additional Perinatal Diagnoses**

1) **Assigning codes for conditions that require treatment**

Assign codes for conditions that require treatment or further investigation, prolong the length of stay, or require resource utilization.

2) **Codes for conditions specified as having implications for future health care needs**

Assign codes for conditions that have been specified by the provider as having implications for future health care needs.

Note: This guideline should not be used for adult patients.

3) **Codes for newborn conditions originating in the perinatal period**

Assign a code for newborn conditions originating in the perinatal period (categories 760-779), as well as complications arising during the current episode of care classified in other chapters, only if the diagnoses have been documented by the responsible provider at the time of transfer or discharge as having affected the fetus or newborn.

i. **Prematurity and Fetal Growth Retardation**

Providers utilize different criteria in determining prematurity. A code for prematurity should not be assigned unless it is documented. The 5th digit assignment for codes from category 764 and subcategories 765.0 and 765.1 should be based on the recorded birth weight and estimated gestational age.

A code from subcategory 765.2, Weeks of gestation, should be assigned as an additional code with category 764 and codes from 765.0 and 765.1 to specify weeks of gestation as documented by the provider in the record.

j. **Newborn sepsis**

Code 771.81, Septicemia [sepsis] of newborn, should be assigned with a secondary code from category 041, Bacterial infections in conditions classified elsewhere and of unspecified site, to identify the organism. A code from category 038, Septicemia, should not be used on a newborn record. Do not assign code 995.91, Sepsis, as code 771.81 describes the sepsis. If applicable, use additional codes to identify severe sepsis (995.92) and any associated acute organ dysfunction.

16. **Chapter 16: Signs, Symptoms and Ill-Defined Conditions (780-799)**

Reserved for future guideline expansion

17. **Chapter 17: Injury and Poisoning (800-999)**

a. **Coding of Injuries**

When coding injuries, assign separate codes for each injury unless a combination code is provided, in which case the combination code is assigned. Multiple injury codes are provided in ICD-9-CM, but should not be assigned unless information for a more specific code is not available. These traumatic injury codes are not to be used for normal, healing surgical wounds or to identify complications of surgical wounds.

The code for the most serious injury, as determined by the provider and the focus of treatment, is sequenced first.

1) **Superficial injuries**

Superficial injuries such as abrasions or contusions are not coded when associated with more severe injuries of the same site.

2) **Primary injury with damage to nerves/blood vessels**

When a primary injury results in minor damage to peripheral nerves or blood vessels, the primary injury is sequenced first with additional code(s) from categories 950-957, Injury to nerves and spinal cord, and/or 900-904, Injury to blood vessels. When the primary injury is to the blood vessels or nerves, that injury should be sequenced first.

b. **Coding of Traumatic Fractures**

The principles of multiple coding of injuries should be followed in coding fractures. Fractures of specified sites are coded individually by site in accordance with both the provisions within categories 800-829 and the level of detail furnished by medical record content. Combination categories for multiple fractures are provided for use when there is insufficient detail in the medical record (such as trauma cases transferred to another hospital), when the reporting form limits the number of codes that can be used in reporting pertinent clinical data, or when there is insufficient specificity at the fourth-digit or fifth-digit level. More specific guidelines are as follows:

1) Acute Fractures vs. Aftercare

Traumatic fractures are coded using the acute fracture codes (800-829) while the patient is receiving active treatment for the fracture. Examples of active treatment are: surgical treatment, emergency department encounter, and evaluation and treatment by a new physician.

Fractures are coded using the aftercare codes (subcategories V54.0, V54.1, V54.8, or V54.9) for encounters after the patient has completed active treatment of the fracture and is receiving routine care for the fracture during the healing or recovery phase. Examples of fracture aftercare are: cast change or removal, removal of external or internal fixation device, medication adjustment, and follow up visits following fracture treatment.

Care for complications of surgical treatment for fracture repairs during the healing or recovery phase should be coded with the appropriate complication codes.

Care of complications of fractures, such as malunion and nonunion, should be reported with the appropriate codes.

Pathologic fractures are not coded in the 800-829 range, but instead are assigned to subcategory 733.1. *See Section I.C.13.a for additional information.*

2) Multiple fractures of same limb

Multiple fractures of same limb classifiable to the same three-digit or four-digit category are coded to that category.

3) Multiple unilateral or bilateral fractures of same bone

Multiple unilateral or bilateral fractures of same bone(s) but classified to different fourth-digit subdivisions (bone part) within the same three-digit category are coded individually by site.

4) Multiple fracture categories 819 and 828

Multiple fracture categories 819 and 828 classify bilateral fractures of both upper limbs (819) and both lower limbs (828), but without any detail at the fourth-digit level other than open and closed type of fractures.

5) Multiple fractures sequencing

Multiple fractures are sequenced in accordance with the severity of the fracture. The provider should be asked to list the fracture diagnoses in the order of severity.

c. Coding of Burns

Current burns (940-948) are classified by depth, extent and by agent (E code). Burns are classified by depth as first degree (erythema), second degree (blistering), and third degree (full-thickness involvement).

1) Sequencing of burn and related condition codes

Sequence first the code that reflects the highest degree of burn when more than one burn is present.

a. When the reason for the admission or encounter is for treatment of external multiple burns, sequence first the code that reflects the burn of the highest degree.

b. When a patient has both internal and external burns, the circumstances of admission govern the selection of the principal diagnosis or first-listed diagnosis.

c. When a patient is admitted for burn injuries and other related conditions such as smoke inhalation and/or respiratory failure, the circumstances of admission govern the selection of the principal or first-listed diagnosis.

2) Burns of the same local site

Classify burns of the same local site (three-digit category level, 940-947) but of different degrees to the subcategory identifying the highest degree recorded in the diagnosis.

3) Non-healing burns

Non-healing burns are coded as acute burns.

Necrosis of burned skin should be coded as a non-healed burn.

4) Code 958.3, Posttraumatic wound infection

Assign code 958.3, Posttraumatic wound infection, not elsewhere classified, as an additional code for any documented infected burn site.

5) Assign separate codes for each burn site

When coding burns, assign separate codes for each burn site. Category 946 Burns of Multiple specified sites, should only be used if the location of the burns are not documented. Category 949, Burn, unspecified, is extremely vague and should rarely be used.

6) Assign codes from category 948, Burns

Burns classified according to extent of body surface involved, when the site of the burn is not specified or when there is a need for additional data. It is advisable to use category 948 as additional coding when needed to provide data for evaluating burn mortality, such as that needed by burn units. It is also advisable to use category 948 as an additional code for reporting purposes when there is mention of a third-degree burn involving 20 percent or more of the body surface.

In assigning a code from category 948:

Fourth-digit codes are used to identify the percentage of total body surface involved in a burn (all degree).

Fifth-digits are assigned to identify the percentage of body surface involved in third-degree burn.

Fifth-digit zero (0) is assigned when less than 10 percent or when no body surface is involved in a third-degree burn.

Category 948 is based on the classic "rule of nines" in estimating body surface involved: head and neck are assigned nine percent, each arm nine percent, each leg 18 percent, the anterior trunk 18 percent, posterior trunk 18 percent, and genitalia one percent. Providers may change these percentage assignments where necessary to accommodate infants and children who have proportionately larger heads than adults and patients who have large buttocks, thighs, or abdomen that involve burns.

7) Encounters for treatment of late effects of burns

Encounters for the treatment of the late effects of burns (i.e., scars or joint contractures) should be coded to the residual condition (sequelae) followed by the appropriate late effect code (906.5-906.9). A late effect E code may also be used, if desired.

8) Sequelae with a late effect code and current burn

When appropriate, both a sequelae with a late effect code, and a current burn code may be assigned on the same record (when both a current burn and sequelae of an old burn exist).

d. Coding of Debridement of Wound, Infection, or Burn

Excisional debridement involves surgical removal or cutting away, as opposed to a mechanical (brushing, scrubbing, washing) debridement.

For coding purposes, excisional debridement is assigned to code 86.22.

Nonexcisional debridement is assigned to code 86.28.

e. Adverse Effects, Poisoning and Toxic Effects

The properties of certain drugs, medicinal and biological substances or combinations of such substances, may cause toxic reactions. The occurrence of drug toxicity is classified in ICD-9-CM as follows:

1) Adverse Effect

When the drug was correctly prescribed and properly administered, code the reaction plus the appropriate code from the E930-E949 series. Codes from the E930-E949 series must be used to identify the causative substance for an adverse effect of drug, medicinal and biological substances, correctly prescribed and properly administered. The effect, such as tachycardia, delirium, gastrointestinal hemorrhaging, vomiting, hypokalemia, hepatitis, renal failure, or respiratory failure, is coded and followed by the appropriate code from the E930-E949 series.

Adverse effects of therapeutic substances correctly prescribed and properly administered (toxicity, synergistic reaction, side effect, and idiosyncratic reaction) may be due to (1) differences among patients, such as age, sex, disease, and genetic factors, and (2) drug-related factors, such as type of drug, route of administration, duration of therapy, dosage, and bioavailability.

2) Poisoning

(a) Error was made in drug prescription

Errors made in drug prescription or in the administration of the drug by provider, nurse, patient, or other person, use the appropriate poisoning code from the 960-979 series.

(b) Overdose of a drug intentionally taken

If an overdose of a drug was intentionally taken or administered and resulted in drug toxicity, it would be coded as a poisoning (960-979 series).

(c) Nonprescribed drug taken with correctly prescribed and properly administered drug

If a nonprescribed drug or medicinal agent was taken in combination with a correctly prescribed and properly administered drug, any drug toxicity or other reaction resulting from the interaction of the two drugs would be classified as a poisoning.

(d) Interaction of drug(s) and alcohol

When a reaction results from the interaction of a drug(s) and alcohol, this would be classified as poisoning.

(e) Sequencing of poisoning

When coding a poisoning or reaction to the improper use of a medication (e.g., wrong dose, wrong substance, wrong route of administration) the poisoning code is sequenced first, followed by a code for the manifestation. If there is also a diagnosis of drug abuse or dependence to the substance, the abuse or dependence is coded as an additional code.

See Section I.C.3.a.6.b. if poisoning is the result of insulin pump malfunctions and Section I.C.19 for general use of E-codes.

3) Toxic Effects

(a) Toxic effect codes

When a harmful substance is ingested or comes in contact with a person, this is classified as a toxic effect. The toxic effect codes are in categories 980-989.

(b) Sequencing toxic effect codes

A toxic effect code should be sequenced first, followed by the code(s) that identify the result of the toxic effect.

(c) External cause codes for toxic effects

An external cause code from categories E860-E869 for accidental exposure, codes E950.6 or E950.7 for intentional self-harm, category E962 for assault, or categories E980-E982, for undetermined, should also be assigned to indicate intent.

f. Complications of care

1) General guidelines for complications of care

(a) Documentation of complications of care

See Section I.B.18. for information on documentation of complications of care.

(b) Use additional code to identify nature of complication

An additional code identifying the complication should be assigned with codes in categories 996-999, Complications of Surgical and Medical Care NEC, when the additional code provides greater

specificity as to the nature of the condition. If the complication code fully describes the condition, no additional code is necessary.

2) Transplant complications

(a) Transplant complications other than kidney

Codes under subcategory 996.8, Complications of transplanted organ, are for use for both complications and rejection of transplanted organs. A transplant complication code is only assigned if the complication affects the function of the transplanted organ. Two codes are required to fully describe a transplant complication, the appropriate code from subcategory 996.8 and a secondary code that identifies the complication.

Pre-existing conditions or conditions that develop after the transplant are not coded as complications unless they affect the function of the transplanted organs.

See I.C.18.d.3) for transplant organ removal status

See I.C.2.i for malignant neoplasm associated with transplanted organ.

(b) Kidney transplant complications

Patients who have undergone kidney transplant may still have some form of chronic kidney disease (CKD) because the kidney transplant may not fully restore kidney function. Code 996.81 should be assigned for documented complications of a kidney transplant, such as transplant failure or rejection or other transplant complication. Code 996.81 should not be assigned for post kidney transplant patients who have chronic kidney (CKD) unless a transplant complication such as transplant failure or rejection is documented. If the documentation is unclear as to whether the patient has a complication of the transplant, query the provider.

Conditions that affect the function of the transplanted kidney, other than CKD, should be assigned code 996.81, Complications of transplanted organ, Kidney, and a secondary code that identifies the complication.

For patients with CKD following a kidney transplant, but who do not have a complication such as failure or rejection, *see section I.C.10.a.2, Chronic kidney disease and kidney transplant status.*

3) Ventilator associated pneumonia

(a) Documentation of Ventilator associated Pneumonia

As with all procedural or postprocedural complications, code assignment is based on the provider's documentation of the relationship between the condition and the procedure.

Code 997.31, Ventilator associated pneumonia, should be assigned only when the provider has documented ventilator associated pneumonia (VAP). An additional code to identify the organism (e.g., Pseudomonas aeruginosa, code 041.7) should also be assigned. Do not assign an additional code from categories 480-484 to identify the type of pneumonia.

Code 997.31 should not be assigned for cases where the patient has pneumonia and is on a mechanical ventilator but the provider has not specifically stated that the pneumonia is ventilator-associated pneumonia.

If the documentation is unclear as to whether the patient has a pneumonia that is a complication attributable to the mechanical ventilator, query the provider.

(b) Patient admitted with pneumonia and develops VAP

A patient may be admitted with one type of pneumonia (e.g., code 481, Pneumococcal pneumonia) and subsequently develop VAP. In this instance, the principal diagnosis would be the appropriate code from categories 480-484 for the pneumonia diagnosed at the time of admission. Code 997.31, Ventilator associated pneumonia, would be assigned as an additional diagnosis when the provider has also documented the presence of ventilator associated pneumonia.

g. SIRS due to Non-infectious Process

The systemic inflammatory response syndrome (SIRS) can develop as a result of certain non-infectious disease processes, such as trauma, malignant neoplasm, or pancreatitis. When SIRS is documented with a noninfectious condition, and no subsequent infection is documented, the code for the underlying condition, such as an injury, should be assigned, followed by code 995.93, Systemic inflammatory response syndrome due to noninfectious process without acute organ dysfunction, or 995.94, Systemic inflammatory response syndrome due to non-infectious process with acute organ dysfunction. If an acute organ dysfunction is documented, the appropriate code(s) for the associated acute organ dysfunction(s) should be assigned in addition to code 995.94. If acute organ dysfunction is documented, but it cannot be determined if the acute organ dysfunction is associated with SIRS or due to another condition (e.g., directly due to the trauma), the provider should be queried.

When the non-infectious condition has led to an infection that results in SIRS, *see Section I.C.1.b.12 for the guideline for sepsis and severe sepsis associated with a non-infectious process.*

18. Classification of Factors Influencing Health Status and Contact with Health Service (Supplemental V01-*V91*)

Note: The chapter specific guidelines provide additional information about the use of V codes for specified encounters.

a. Introduction

ICD-9-CM provides codes to deal with encounters for circumstances other than a disease or injury. The Supplementary Classification of Factors Influencing Health Status and Contact with Health Services (V01.0 - V91.99) is provided to deal with occasions when circumstances other than a disease or injury (codes 001-999) are recorded as a diagnosis or problem.

There are four primary circumstances for the use of V codes:

1) A person who is not currently sick encounters the health services for some specific reason, such as to act as an organ donor, to receive prophylactic care, such as inoculations or health screenings, or to receive counseling on health related issues.

2) A person with a resolving disease or injury, or a chronic, long-term condition requiring continuous care, encounters the health care system for specific aftercare of that disease or injury (e.g., dialysis for renal disease; chemotherapy for malignancy; cast change). A diagnosis/symptom code should be used whenever a current, acute, diagnosis is being treated or a sign or symptom is being studied.

3) Circumstances or problems influence a person's health status but are not in themselves a current illness or injury.

4) Newborns, to indicate birth status

b. V codes use in any healthcare setting

V codes are for use in any healthcare setting. V codes may be used as either a first listed (principal diagnosis code in the inpatient setting) or secondary code, depending on the circumstances of the encounter. Certain V codes may only be used as first listed, others only as secondary codes.

See Section I.C.18.e, V Codes That May Only be Principal/First-Listed Diagnosis.

c. **V Codes indicate a reason for an encounter**

They are not procedure codes. A corresponding procedure code must accompany a V code to describe the procedure performed.

d. **Categories of V Codes**

1) **Contact/Exposure**

Category V01 indicates contact with or exposure to communicable diseases. These codes are for patients who do not show any sign or symptom of a disease but have been exposed to it by close personal contact with an infected individual or are in an area where a disease is epidemic. These codes may be used as a first listed code to explain an encounter for testing, or, more commonly, as a secondary code to identify a potential risk.

Codes V15.84 – V15.86 describe contact with or (suspected) exposure to asbestos, potentially hazardous body fluids, and lead.

Subcategories V87.0 – V87.3 describe contact with or (suspected) exposure to hazardous metals, aromatic compounds, other potentially hazardous chemicals, and other potentially hazardous substances.

2) **Inoculations and vaccinations**

Categories V03-V06 are for encounters for inoculations and vaccinations. They indicate that a patient is being seen to receive a prophylactic inoculation against a disease. The injection itself must be represented by the appropriate procedure code. A code from V03-V06 may be used as a secondary code if the inoculation is given as a routine part of preventive health care, such as a well-baby visit.

3) **Status**

Status codes indicate that a patient is a carrier of a disease, has the sequelae or residual of a past disease or condition, or has another factor influencing a person's health status. This includes such things as the presence of prosthetic or mechanical devices resulting from past treatment. A status code is informative, because the status may affect the course of treatment and its outcome. A status code is distinct from a history code. The history code indicates that the patient no longer has the condition.

A status code should not be used with a diagnosis code from one of the body system chapters, if the diagnosis code includes the information provided by the status code. For example, code V42.1, Heart transplant status, should not be used with code 996.83, Complications of transplanted

heart. The status code does not provide additional information. The complication code indicates that the patient is a heart transplant patient.

The status V codes/categories are:

V02	Carrier or suspected carrier of infectious diseases
	Carrier status indicates that a person harbors the specific organisms of a disease without manifest symptoms and is capable of transmitting the infection.
V07.5X	Use of agents affecting estrogen receptors and estrogen level
	This code indicates when a patient is receiving a drug that affects estrogen receptors and estrogen levels for prevention of cancer.
V08	Asymptomatic HIV infection status
	This code indicates that a patient has tested positive for HIV but has manifested no signs or symptoms of the disease.
V09	Infection with drug-resistant microorganisms
	This category indicates that a patient has an infection that is resistant to drug treatment. Sequence the infection code first.
V21	Constitutional states in development
V22.2	Pregnant state, incidental
	This code is a secondary code only for use when the pregnancy is in no way complicating the reason for visit. Otherwise, a code from the obstetric chapter is required.
V26.5x	Sterilization status
V42	Organ or tissue replaced by transplant
V43	Organ or tissue replaced by other means
V44	Artificial opening status
V45	Other postsurgical states
	Assign code V45.87, Transplant organ removal status, to indicate that a transplanted organ has been previously removed. This code should not be assigned for the encounter in which the transplanted organ is removed. The complication necessitating removal of the transplant organ

should be assigned for that encounter.

See section I.C17.f.2. for information on the coding of organ transplant complications.

Assign code V45.88, Status post administration of tPA (rtPA) in a different facility within the last 24 hours prior to admission to the current facility, as a secondary diagnosis when a patient is received by transfer into a facility and documentation indicates they were administered tissue plasminogen activator (tPA) within the last 24 hours prior to admission to the current facility.

This guideline applies even if the patient is still receiving the tPA at the time they are received into the current facility.

The appropriate code for the condition for which the tPA was administered (such as cerebrovascular disease or myocardial infarction) should be assigned first.

Code V45.88 is only applicable to the receiving facility record and not to the transferring facility record.

V46   Other dependence on machines

V49.6   Upper limb amputation status

V49.7   Lower limb amputation status

Note: Categories V42-V46, and subcategories V49.6, V49.7 are for use only if there are no complications or malfunctions of the organ or tissue replaced, the amputation site or the equipment on which the patient is dependent.

V49.81   Asymptomatic postmenopausal status (age-related) (natural)

V49.82   Dental sealant status

V49.83   Awaiting organ transplant status

V49.86   Do not resuscitate status

This code may be used when it is documented by the provider that a patient is on do not resuscitate status at any time during the stay.

V49.87   Physical restraint status

This code may be used when it is documented by the provider that a patient has been put in restraints during the current

encounter. Please note that this code should not be reported when it is documented by the provider that a patient is temporarily restrained during a procedure.

V58.6x   Long-term (current) drug use

Codes from this subcategory indicate a patient's continuous use of a prescribed drug (including such things as aspirin therapy) for the long-term treatment of a condition or for prophylactic use. It is not for use for patients who have addictions to drugs. This subcategory is not for use of medications for detoxification or maintenance programs to prevent withdrawal symptoms in patients with drug dependence (e.g., methadone maintenance for opiate dependence). Assign the appropriate code for the drug dependence instead.

Assign a code from subcategory V58.6, Long-term (current) drug use, if the patient is receiving a medication for an extended period as a prophylactic measure (such as for the prevention of deep vein thrombosis) or as treatment of a chronic condition (such as arthritis) or a disease requiring a lengthy course of treatment (such as cancer). Do not assign a code from subcategory V58.6 for medication being administered for a brief period of time to treat an acute illness or injury (such as a course of antibiotics to treat acute bronchitis).

V83   Genetic carrier status

Genetic carrier status indicates that a person carries a gene, associated with a particular disease, which may be passed to offspring who may develop that disease. The person does not have the disease and is not at risk of developing the disease.

V84   Genetic susceptibility status

Genetic susceptibility indicates that a person has a gene that increases the risk of that person developing the disease.

Codes from category V84, Genetic susceptibility to disease, should not be used as principal or first-listed codes. If the patient has the condition to which he/she is susceptible, and that condition is the reason for the encounter, the code for the current condition should be sequenced first. If the patient is being seen for follow-up after completed treatment for this condition, and the condition no longer exists, a follow-up code should be sequenced first, followed by the appropriate personal history and genetic susceptibility codes. If the purpose of the encounter is genetic counseling associated with procreative management, a code from subcategory V26.3, Genetic counseling and testing, should be assigned as the first-listed code, followed by a code from category V84. Additional codes should be assigned for any applicable family or personal history.

See Section I.C. 18.d.14 for information on prophylactic organ removal due to a genetic susceptibility.

V85	Body Mass Index (BMI)
V86	Estrogen receptor status
V88	Acquired absence of other organs and tissue
V90	Retained foreign body

4) History (of)

There are two types of history V codes, personal and family. Personal history codes explain a patient's past medical condition that no longer exists and is not receiving any treatment, but that has the potential for recurrence, and therefore may require continued monitoring. The exceptions to this general rule are category V14, Personal history of allergy to medicinal agents, and subcategory V15.0, Allergy, other than to medicinal agents. A person who has had an allergic episode to a substance or food in the past should always be considered allergic to the substance.

Family history codes are for use when a patient has a family member(s) who has had a particular disease that causes the patient to be at higher risk of also contracting the disease.

Personal history codes may be used in conjunction with follow-up codes and family history codes may be used in conjunction with screening codes to explain the need for a test or procedure. History

codes are also acceptable on any medical record regardless of the reason for visit. A history of an illness, even if no longer present, is important information that may alter the type of treatment ordered.

The history V code categories are:

V10	Personal history of malignant neoplasm
V12	Personal history of certain other diseases
V13	Personal history of other diseases
	Except: V13.4, Personal history of arthritis, and subcategory V13.6, Personal history of congenital (corrected) malformations. These conditions are life-long so are not true history codes.
V14	Personal history of allergy to medicinal agents
V15	Other personal history presenting hazards to health
	Except: **Codes V15.7, Personal history of contraception; V15.84, Contact with and (suspected) exposure to asbestos; V15.85, Contact with and (suspected) exposure to potentially hazardous body fluids; V15.86, Contact with and (suspected) exposure to lead.**
V16	Family history of malignant neoplasm
V17	Family history of certain chronic disabling diseases
V18	Family history of certain other specific diseases
V19	Family history of other conditions
V87	Other specified personal exposures and history presenting hazards to health
	Except: Subcategories V87.0, Contact with and (suspected) exposure to hazardous metals; V87.1, Contact with and (suspected) exposure to hazardous aromatic compounds; V87.2, Contact with and (suspected) exposure to other potentially hazardous chemicals; and V87.3, Contact with and (suspected) exposure to other potentially hazardous substances

5) Screening

Screening is the testing for disease or disease precursors in seemingly well individuals so that early detection and treatment can be provided for those who test positive for the disease. Screenings that are recommended for many subgroups in a population include: routine mammograms for women over 40, a fecal occult blood test for everyone over 50, an amniocentesis to rule out a fetal anomaly for pregnant women over 35, because the incidence of breast cancer and colon cancer in these subgroups is higher than in the general population, as is the incidence of Down's syndrome in older mothers.

The testing of a person to rule out or confirm a suspected diagnosis because the patient has some sign or symptom is a diagnostic examination, not a screening. In these cases, the sign or symptom is used to explain the reason for the test.

A screening code may be a first listed code if the reason for the visit is specifically the screening exam. It may also be used as an additional code if the screening is done during an office visit for other health problems. A screening code is not necessary if the screening is inherent to a routine examination, such as a pap smear done during a routine pelvic examination.

Should a condition be discovered during the screening then the code for the condition may be assigned as an additional diagnosis.

The V code indicates that a screening exam is planned. A procedure code is required to confirm that the screening was performed.

The screening V code categories:

V28   Antenatal screening

V73-V82   Special screening examinations

6) Observation

There are three observation V code categories. They are for use in very limited circumstances when a person is being observed for a suspected condition that is ruled out. The observation codes are not for use if an injury or illness or any signs or symptoms related to the suspected condition are present. In such cases the diagnosis/symptom code is used with the corresponding E code to identify any external cause.

The observation codes are to be used as principal diagnosis only. The only exception to this is when the principal diagnosis is required to be a code from the V30, Live born infant, category. Then the V29 observation code is sequenced after the V30 code. Additional codes may be used in addition to the observation code but only if they are unrelated to the suspected condition being observed.

Codes from subcategory V89.0, Suspected maternal and fetal conditions not found, may either be used as a first listed or as an additional code assignment depending on the case. They are for use in very limited circumstances on a maternal record when an encounter is for a suspected maternal or fetal condition that is ruled out during that encounter (for example, a maternal or fetal condition may be suspected due to an abnormal test result). These codes should not be used when the condition is confirmed. In those cases, the confirmed condition should be coded. In addition, these codes are not for use if an illness or any signs or symptoms related to the suspected condition or problem are present. In such cases the diagnosis/symptom code is used.

Additional codes may be used in addition to the code from subcategory V89.0, but only if they are unrelated to the suspected condition being evaluated.

Codes from subcategory V89.0 may not be used for encounters for antenatal screening of mother. *See Section I.C.18.d., Screening).*

For encounters for suspected fetal condition that are inconclusive following testing and evaluation, assign the appropriate code from category 655, 656, 657 or 658.

The observation V code categories:

V29   Observation and evaluation of newborns for suspected condition not found

      For the birth encounter, a code from category V30 should be sequenced before the V29 code.

V71   Observation and evaluation for suspected condition not found

V89   Suspected maternal and fetal conditions not found

7) Aftercare

Aftercare visit codes cover situations when the initial treatment of a disease or injury has been performed and the patient requires continued care during the healing or recovery phase, or for the long-term consequences of the disease. The aftercare V code should not be used if treatment is directed at a current, acute disease or injury. The diagnosis code is to be used in these cases. Exceptions to this rule are codes V58.0, Radiotherapy, and codes from subcategory V58.1, Encounter for chemotherapy and immunotherapy for neoplastic conditions. These codes are to be first listed, followed by the diagnosis code when a patient's encounter is solely to receive radiation therapy or chemotherapy for the treatment of a neoplasm. Should a patient receive both chemotherapy and radiation therapy during the same encounter code V58.0 and V58.1 may be used together on a record with either one being sequenced first.

The aftercare codes are generally first listed to explain the specific reason for the encounter. An aftercare code may be used as an additional code when some type of aftercare is provided in addition to the reason for admission and no diagnosis code is applicable. An example of this would be the closure of a colostomy during an encounter for treatment of another condition.

Aftercare codes should be used in conjunction with any other aftercare codes or other diagnosis codes to provide better detail on the specifics of an aftercare encounter visit, unless otherwise directed by the classification. The sequencing of multiple aftercare codes is discretionary.

Certain aftercare V code categories need a secondary diagnosis code to describe the resolving condition or sequelae, for others, the condition is inherent in the code title.

Additional V code aftercare category terms include fitting and adjustment, and attention to artificial openings.

Status V codes may be used with aftercare V codes to indicate the nature of the aftercare. For example code V45.81, Aortocoronary bypass status, may be used with code V58.73, Aftercare following surgery of the circulatory system, NEC, to indicate the surgery for which the aftercare is being performed. Also, a transplant status code may be used following code V58.44, Aftercare following organ transplant, to identify the organ transplanted. A status code should not be used when the aftercare code indicates the type of status, such as using V55.0, Attention to tracheostomy with V44.0, Tracheostomy status.

See Section I.B.16 Admissions/Encounter for Rehabilitation

The aftercare V category/codes:

V51.0	Encounter for breast reconstruction following mastectomy
V52	Fitting and adjustment of prosthetic device and implant
V53	Fitting and adjustment of other device
V54	Other orthopedic aftercare
V55	Attention to artificial openings
V56	Encounter for dialysis and dialysis catheter care
V57	Care involving the use of rehabilitation procedures
V58.0	Radiotherapy
V58.11	Encounter for antineoplastic chemotherapy
V58.12	Encounter for antineoplastic immunotherapy
V58.3x	Attention to dressings and sutures
V58.41	Encounter for planned post-operative wound closure
V58.42	Aftercare, surgery, neoplasm
V58.43	Aftercare, surgery, trauma
V58.44	Aftercare involving organ transplant
V58.49	Other specified aftercare following surgery
V58.7x	Aftercare following surgery
V58.81	Fitting and adjustment of vascular catheter
V58.82	Fitting and adjustment of non-vascular catheter
V58.83	Monitoring therapeutic drug
V58.89	Other specified aftercare

8) Follow-up

The follow-up codes are used to explain continuing surveillance following completed treatment of a disease, condition, or injury. They imply that the condition has been fully treated and no longer exists. They should not be confused with aftercare codes that explain current treatment for a healing condition or its sequelae. Follow-up codes may be used in conjunction with history codes to provide the full picture of the healed condition and its treatment. The follow-up code is sequenced first, followed by the history code.

A follow-up code may be used to explain repeated visits. Should a condition be found to have recurred on the follow-up visit, then the diagnosis code should be used in place of the follow-up code.

The follow-up V code categories:

V24	Postpartum care and evaluation
V67	Follow-up examination

9) Donor

Category V59 is the donor codes. They are used for living individuals who are donating blood or other body tissue. These codes are only for individuals donating for others, not for self donations. They are not for use to identify cadaveric donations.

10) Counseling

Counseling V codes are used when a patient or family member receives assistance in the aftermath of an illness or injury, or when support is required in coping with family or social problems. They are not necessary for use in conjunction with a diagnosis code when the counseling component of care is considered integral to standard treatment.

The counseling V categories/codes:

V25.0	General counseling and advice for contraceptive management
V26.3	Genetic counseling
V26.4	General counseling and advice for procreative management
V61.X	Other family circumstances
V65.1	Person consulted on behalf of another person
V65.3	Dietary surveillance and counseling
V65.4	Other counseling, not elsewhere classified

11) Obstetrics and related conditions

See Section I.C.11., the Obstetrics guidelines for further instruction on the use of these codes.

V codes for pregnancy are for use in those circumstances when none of the problems or complications included in the codes from the Obstetrics chapter exist (a routine prenatal visit or postpartum care). Codes V22.0, Supervision of normal first pregnancy, and V22.1, Supervision of other normal pregnancy, are always first listed and are not to be used with any other code from the OB chapter.

The outcome of delivery, category V27, should be included on all maternal delivery records. It is always a secondary code.

V codes for family planning (contraceptive) or procreative management and counseling should be included on an obstetric record either during the pregnancy or the postpartum stage, if applicable.

Obstetrics and related conditions V code categories:

V22	Normal pregnancy
V23	Supervision of high-risk pregnancy
	Except: V23.2, Pregnancy with history of abortion. Code 646.3, Recurrent pregnancy loss, from the OB chapter is required to indicate a history of abortion during a pregnancy.
V24	Postpartum care and evaluation

V25	Encounter for contraceptive management
	Except V25.0x
	(See Section I.C.18.d.11, Counseling)
V26	Procreative management
	Except V26.5x, Sterilization status, V26.3 and V26.4
	(See Section I.C.18.d.11., Counseling)
V27	Outcome of delivery
V28	Antenatal screening
	(See Section I.C.18.d.6., Screening)
V91	Multiple gestation placenta status

12) Newborn, infant and child

See Section I.C.15, the Newborn guidelines for further instruction on the use of these codes.

Newborn V code categories:

V20	Health supervision of infant or child
V29	Observation and evaluation of newborns for suspected condition not found
	(See Section I.C.18.d.7, Observation)
V30-V39	Liveborn infant according to type of birth

13) Routine and administrative examinations

The V codes allow for the description of encounters for routine examinations, such as, a general check-up, or examinations for administrative purposes, such as a pre-employment physical. The codes are not to be used if the examination is for diagnosis of a suspected condition or for treatment purposes. In such cases the diagnosis code is used. During a routine exam, should a diagnosis or condition be discovered, it should be coded as an additional code. Pre-existing and chronic conditions and history codes may also be included as additional codes as long as the examination is for administrative purposes and not focused on any particular condition.

Pre-operative examination and pre-procedural laboratory examination V codes are for use only in those situations when a patient is being cleared for a procedure or surgery and no treatment is given.

The V codes categories/code for routine and administrative examinations:

V20.2	Routine infant or child health check
	Any injections given should have a corresponding procedure code.

V70	General medical examination
V72	Special investigations and examinations

Codes V72.5 and V72.62 may be used if the reason for the patient encounter is for routine laboratory/radiology testing in the absence of any signs, symptoms, or associated diagnosis. If routine testing is performed during the same encounter as a test to evaluate a sign, symptom, or diagnosis, it is appropriate to assign both the V code and the code describing the reason for the non-routine test.

14) **Miscellaneous V codes**

The miscellaneous V codes capture a number of other health care encounters that do not fall into one of the other categories. Certain of these codes identify the reason for the encounter, others are for use as additional codes that provide useful information on circumstances that may affect a patient's care and treatment.

Prophylactic Organ Removal

For encounters specifically for prophylactic removal of breasts, ovaries, or another organ due to a genetic susceptibility to cancer or a family history of cancer, the principal or first listed code should be a code from subcategory V50.4, Prophylactic organ removal, followed by the appropriate genetic susceptibility code and the appropriate family history code.

If the patient has a malignancy of one site and is having prophylactic removal at another site to prevent either a new primary malignancy or metastatic disease, a code for the malignancy should also be assigned in addition to a code from subcategory V50.4. A V50.4 code should not be assigned if the patient is having organ removal for treatment of a malignancy, such as the removal of the testes for the treatment of prostate cancer.

Miscellaneous V code categories/codes:

V07	Need for isolation and other prophylactic or treatment measures

Except V07.5X, Use of agents affecting estrogen receptors and estrogen levels

V40.31	**Wandering in diseases classified elsewhere**
V50	Elective surgery for purposes other than remedying health states

V58.5	Orthodontics
V60	Housing, household, and economic circumstances
V62	Other psychosocial circumstances
V63	Unavailability of other medical facilities for care
V64	Persons encountering health services for specific procedures, not carried out
V66	Convalescence and Palliative Care
V68	Encounters for administrative purposes
V69	Problems related to lifestyle
V85	Body Mass Index

15) **Nonspecific V codes**

Certain V codes are so non-specific, or potentially redundant with other codes in the classification, that there can be little justification for their use in the inpatient setting. Their use in the outpatient setting should be limited to those instances when there is no further documentation to permit more precise coding. Otherwise, any sign or symptom or any other reason for visit that is captured in another code should be used.

Nonspecific V code categories/codes:

V11	Personal history of mental disorder

A code from the mental disorders chapter, with an in remission fifth-digit, should be used.

V13.4	Personal history of arthritis
V13.6	Personal history of congenital malformations
V15.7	Personal history of contraception
V23.2	Pregnancy with history of abortion
V40	Mental and behavioral problems

Exception:

V40.31   Wandering in diseases classified elsewhere

V41	Problems with special senses and other special functions
V47	Other problems with internal organs
V48	Problems with head, neck, and trunk
V49	Problems with limbs and other problems

Exceptions:

V49.6	Upper limb amputation status

V49.7   Lower limb amputation status

V49.81   Asymptomatic postmenopausal status (age-related) (natural)

V49.82   Dental sealant status

V49.83   Awaiting organ transplant status

V49.86   Do not resuscitate status

V49.87   Physical restraints status

V51.8   Other aftercare involving the use of plastic surgery

V58.2   Blood transfusion, without reported diagnosis

V58.9   Unspecified aftercare

See Section IV.K. and Section IV.L. of the Outpatient guidelines.

e. V Codes That May Only be Principal/First-Listed Diagnosis

The list of V codes/categories below may only be reported as the principal/first-listed diagnosis, except when there are multiple encounters on the same day and the medical records for the encounters are combined or when there is more than one V code that meets the definition of principal diagnosis (e.g., a patient is admitted to home healthcare for both aftercare and rehabilitation and they equally meet the definition of principal diagnosis). These codes should not be reported if they do not meet the definition of principal or first-listed diagnosis.

See Section II and Section IV.A for information on selection of principal and first-listed diagnosis.

See Section II.C for information on two or more diagnoses that equally meet the definition for principal diagnosis.

V20.X   Health supervision of infant or child

V22.0   Supervision of normal first pregnancy

V22.1   Supervision of other normal pregnancy

V24.X   Postpartum care and examination

V26.81   Encounter for assisted reproductive fertility procedure cycle

V26.82   Encounter for fertility preservation procedure

V30.X   Single liveborn

V31.X   Twin, mate liveborn

V32.X   Twin, mate stillborn

V33.X   Twin, unspecified

V34.X   Other multiple, mates all liveborn

V35.X   Other multiple, mates all stillborn

V36.X   Other multiple, mates live- and stillborn

V37.X   Other multiple, unspecified

V39.X   Unspecified

V46.12   Encounter for respirator dependence during power failure

V46.13   Encounter for weaning from respirator [ventilator]

V51.0   Encounter for breast reconstruction following mastectomy

V56.0   Extracorporeal dialysis

V57.X   Care involving use of rehabilitation procedures

V58.0   Radiotherapy

V58.11   Encounter for antineoplastic chemotherapy

V58.12   Encounter for antineoplastic immunotherapy

V59.X   Donors

V66.0   Convalescence and palliative care following surgery

V66.1   Convalescence and palliative care following radiotherapy

V66.2   Convalescence and palliative care following chemotherapy

V66.3   Convalescence and palliative care following psychotherapy and other treatment for mental disorder

V66.4   Convalescence and palliative care following treatment of fracture

V66.5   Convalescence and palliative care following other treatment

V66.6   Convalescence and palliative care following combined treatment

V66.9   Unspecified convalescence

V68.X   Encounters for administrative purposes

V70.0   Routine general medical examination at a health care facility

V70.1   General psychiatric examination, requested by the authority

V70.2   General psychiatric examination, other and unspecified

V70.3   Other medical examination for administrative purposes

V70.4   Examination for medicolegal reasons

V70.5   Health examination of defined subpopulations

V70.6   Health examination in population surveys

V70.8   Other specified general medical examinations

V70.9   Unspecified general medical examination

V71.X   Observation and evaluation for suspected conditions not found

19. Supplemental Classification of External Causes of Injury and Poisoning (E-codes, E800-E999)

Introduction: These guidelines are provided for those who are currently collecting E codes in order that there will be standardization in the process. If your institution plans to begin collecting E codes, these guidelines are to be applied. The use of E codes is supplemental to the application of ICD-9-CM diagnosis codes.

External causes of injury and poisoning codes (categories E000 and E800-E999) are intended to provide data for injury research and evaluation of injury prevention strategies. Activity codes (categories E001-E030) are intended to be used to describe the activity of a person seeking care for injuries as well as other health conditions, when the injury or other health condition resulted from an activity or the activity contributed to a condition. E codes capture how the injury, poisoning, or adverse effect happened (cause), the intent (unintentional or accidental; or intentional, such as suicide or assault), the person's status (e.g. civilian, military), the associated activity and the place where the event occurred.

Some major categories of E codes include:

transport accidents

poisoning and adverse effects of drugs, medicinal substances and biologicals

accidental falls

accidents caused by fire and flames

accidents due to natural and environmental factors

late effects of accidents, assaults or self injury

assaults or purposely inflicted injury

suicide or self inflicted injury

These guidelines apply for the coding and collection of E codes from records in hospitals, outpatient clinics, emergency departments, other ambulatory care settings and provider offices, and nonacute care settings, except when other specific guidelines apply.

a. General E Code Coding Guidelines

1) Used with any code in the range of 001-V91

An E code from categories E800-E999 may be used with any code in the range of 001-V91, which indicates an injury, poisoning, or adverse effect due to an external cause.

An activity E code (categories E001-E030) may be used with any code in the range of 001-V91 that indicates an injury, or other health condition that resulted from an activity, or the activity contributed to a condition.

2) Assign the appropriate E code for all initial treatments

Assign the appropriate E code for the initial encounter of an injury, poisoning, or adverse effect of drugs, not for subsequent treatment.

External cause of injury codes (E-codes) may be assigned while the acute fracture codes are still applicable.

See Section I.C.17.b.1 for coding of acute fractures.

3) Use the full range of E codes

Use the full range of E codes (E800–E999) to completely describe the cause, the intent and the place of occurrence, if applicable, for all injuries, poisonings, and adverse effects of drugs.

See a.1.), j.), and k.) in this section for information on the use of status and activity E codes.

4) Assign as many E codes as necessary

Assign as many E codes as necessary to fully explain each cause.

5) The selection of the appropriate E code

The selection of the appropriate E code is guided by the Index to External Causes, which is located after the alphabetical index to diseases and by Inclusion and Exclusion notes in the Tabular List.

6) E code can never be a principal diagnosis

An E code can never be a principal (first listed) diagnosis.

7) External cause code(s) with systemic inflammatory response syndrome (SIRS)

An external cause code is not appropriate with a code from subcategory 995.9, unless the patient also has another condition for which an E code would be appropriate (such as an injury, poisoning, or adverse effect of drugs.

8) Multiple Cause E Code Coding Guidelines

More than one E-code is required to fully describe the external cause of an illness, injury or poisoning. The assignment of E-codes should be sequenced in the following priority:

If two or more events cause separate injuries, an E code should be assigned for each cause. The first listed E code will be selected in the following order:

E codes for child and adult abuse take priority over all other E codes.

See Section I.C.19.e., Child and Adult abuse guidelines.

E codes for terrorism events take priority over all other E codes except child and adult abuse.

E codes for cataclysmic events take priority over all other E codes except child and adult abuse and terrorism.

E codes for transport accidents take priority over all other E codes except cataclysmic events, child and adult abuse and terrorism.

Activity and external cause status codes are assigned following all causal (intent) E codes.

The first-listed E code should correspond to the cause of the most serious diagnosis due to an assault, accident, or self-harm, following the order of hierarchy listed above.

9) If the reporting format limits the number of E codes

If the reporting format limits the number of E codes that can be used in reporting clinical data, report the code for the cause/intent most related to the principal diagnosis. If the format permits capture of additional E codes, the cause/intent, including medical misadventures, of the additional events should be reported rather than the codes for place, activity or external status.

b. Place of Occurrence Guideline

Use an additional code from category E849 to indicate the Place of Occurrence for injuries and poisonings. The Place of Occurrence describes the place where the event occurred and not the patient's activity at the time of the event.

Do not use E849.9 if the place of occurrence is not stated.

c. Adverse Effects of Drugs, Medicinal and Biological Substances Guidelines

1) Do not code directly from the Table of Drugs

Do not code directly from the Table of Drugs and Chemicals. Always refer back to the Tabular List.

2) Use as many codes as necessary to describe

Use as many codes as necessary to describe completely all drugs, medicinal or biological substances.

If the reporting format limits the number of E codes, and there are different fourth digit codes in the same three digit category, use the code for "Other specified" of that category of drugs, medicinal or biological substances. If there is no "Other specified" code in that category, use the appropriate "Unspecified" code in that category.

If the reporting format limits the number of E codes, and the codes are in different three digit categories, assign the appropriate E code for other multiple drugs and medicinal substances.

3) If the same E code would describe the causative agent

If the same E code would describe the causative agent for more than one adverse reaction, assign the code only once.

4) If two or more drugs, medicinal or biological substances

If two or more drugs, medicinal or biological substances are reported, code each individually unless the combination code is listed in the Table of Drugs and Chemicals. In that case, assign the E code for the combination.

5) When a reaction results from the interaction of a drug(s)

When a reaction results from the interaction of a drug(s) and alcohol, use poisoning codes and E codes for both.

6) Codes from the E930-E949 series

Codes from the E930-E949 series must be used to identify the causative substance for an adverse effect of drug, medicinal and biological substances, correctly prescribed and properly administered. The effect, such as tachycardia, delirium, gastrointestinal hemorrhaging, vomiting, hypokalemia, hepatitis, renal failure, or respiratory failure, is coded and followed by the appropriate code from the E930-E949 series.

d. Child and Adult Abuse Guideline

1) Intentional injury

When the cause of an injury or neglect is intentional child or adult abuse, the first listed E code should be assigned from categories E960-E968, Homicide and injury purposely inflicted by other persons, (except category E967). An E code from category E967, Child and adult battering and other maltreatment, should be added as an additional code to identify the perpetrator, if known.

2) Accidental intent

In cases of neglect when the intent is determined to be accidental E code E904.0, Abandonment or neglect of infant and helpless person, should be the first listed E code.

e. Unknown or Suspected Intent Guideline

1) If the intent (accident, self-harm, assault) of the cause of an injury or poisoning is unknown

If the intent (accident, self-harm, assault) of the cause of an injury or poisoning is unknown or unspecified, code the intent as undetermined E980-E989.

  2) If the intent (accident, self-harm, assault) of the cause of an injury or poisoning is questionable

If the intent (accident, self-harm, assault) of the cause of an injury or poisoning is questionable, probable or suspected, code the intent as undetermined E980-E989.

f. Undetermined Cause

When the intent of an injury or poisoning is known, but the cause is unknown, use codes: E928.9, Unspecified accident, E958.9, Suicide and self-inflicted injury by unspecified means, and E968.9, Assault by unspecified means.

These E codes should rarely be used, as the documentation in the medical record, in both the inpatient outpatient and other settings, should normally provide sufficient detail to determine the cause of the injury.

g. Late Effects of External Cause Guidelines

  1) Late effect E codes

Late effect E codes exist for injuries and poisonings but not for adverse effects of drugs, misadventures and surgical complications.

  2) Late effect E codes (E929, E959, E969, E977, E989, or E999.1)

A late effect E code (E929, E959, E969, E977, E989, or E999.1) should be used with any report of a late effect or sequela resulting from a previous injury or poisoning (905-909).

  3) Late effect E code with a related current injury

A late effect E code should never be used with a related current nature of injury code.

  4) Use of late effect E codes for subsequent visits

Use a late effect E code for subsequent visits when a late effect of the initial injury or poisoning is being treated. There is no late effect E code for adverse effects of drugs.

Do not use a late effect E code for subsequent visits for follow-up care (e.g., to assess healing, to receive rehabilitative therapy) of the injury or poisoning when no late effect of the injury has been documented.

h. Misadventures and Complications of Care Guidelines

  1) Code range E870-E876

Assign a code in the range of E870-E876 if misadventures are stated by the provider. When applying the E code guidelines pertaining to sequencing, these E codes are considered causal codes.

  2) Code range E878-E879

Assign a code in the range of E878-E879 if the provider attributes an abnormal reaction or later complication to a surgical or medical procedure, but does not mention misadventure at the time of the procedure as the cause of the reaction.

i. Terrorism Guidelines

  1) Cause of injury identified by the Federal Government (FBI) as terrorism

When the cause of an injury is identified by the Federal Government (FBI) as terrorism, the first-listed E-code should be a code from category E979, Terrorism. The definition of terrorism employed by the FBI is found at the inclusion note at E979. The terrorism E-code is the only E-code that should be assigned. Additional E codes from the assault categories should not be assigned.

  2) Cause of an injury is suspected to be the result of terrorism

When the cause of an injury is suspected to be the result of terrorism a code from category E979 should not be assigned. Assign a code in the range of E codes based circumstances on the documentation of intent and mechanism.

  3) Code E979.9, Terrorism, secondary effects

Assign code E979.9, Terrorism, secondary effects, for conditions occurring subsequent to the terrorist event. This code should not be assigned for conditions that are due to the initial terrorist act.

  4) Statistical tabulation of terrorism codes

For statistical purposes these codes will be tabulated within the category for assault, expanding the current category from E960-E969 to include E979 and E999.1.

j. Activity Code Guidelines

Assign a code from category E001-E030 to describe the activity that caused or contributed to the injury or other health condition.

Unlike other E codes, activity E codes may be assigned to indicate a health condition (not just injuries) resulted from an activity, or the activity contributed to the condition.

The activity codes are not applicable to poisonings, adverse effects, misadventures or late effects.

Do not assign E030, Unspecified activity, if the activity is not stated.

k. External cause status

A code from category E000, External cause status, should be assigned whenever any other E code is assigned for an encounter, including an Activity

E code, except for the events noted below. Assign a code from category E000, External cause status, to indicate the work status of the person at the time the event occurred. The status code indicates whether the event occurred during military activity, whether a non-military person was at work, whether an individual including a student or volunteer was involved in a non-work activity at the time of the causal event.

A code from E000, External cause status, should be assigned, when applicable, with other external cause codes, such as transport accidents and falls. The external cause status codes are not applicable to poisonings, adverse effects, misadventures or late effects.

Do not assign a code from category E000 if no other E codes (cause, activity) are applicable for the encounter.

Do not assign code E000.9, Unspecified external cause status, if the status is not stated.

Section II. Selection of Principal Diagnosis

The circumstances of inpatient admission always govern the selection of principal diagnosis. The principal diagnosis is defined in the Uniform Hospital Discharge Data Set (UHDDS) as "that condition established after study to be chiefly responsible for occasioning the admission of the patient to the hospital for care."

The UHDDS definitions are used by hospitals to report inpatient data elements in a standardized manner. These data elements and their definitions can be found in the July 31, 1985, Federal Register (Vol. 50, No, 147), pp. 31038-40.

Since that time the application of the UHDDS definitions has been expanded to include all non-outpatient settings (acute care, short term, long term care and psychiatric hospitals; home health agencies; rehab facilities; nursing homes, etc).

In determining principal diagnosis the coding conventions in the ICD-9-CM, Volumes I and II take precedence over these official coding guidelines.

(See Section I.A., Conventions for the ICD-9-CM)

The importance of consistent, complete documentation in the medical record cannot be overemphasized. Without such documentation the application of all coding guidelines is a difficult, if not impossible, task.

A. **Codes for symptoms, signs, and ill-defined conditions**

Codes for symptoms, signs, and ill-defined conditions from Chapter 16 are not to be used as principal diagnosis when a related definitive diagnosis has been established.

B. **Two or more interrelated conditions, each potentially meeting the definition for principal diagnosis.**

When there are two or more interrelated conditions (such as diseases in the same ICD-9-CM chapter or manifestations characteristically associated with a certain disease) potentially meeting the definition of principal diagnosis, either condition may be sequenced first, unless the circumstances of the admission, the therapy provided, the Tabular List, or the Alphabetic Index indicate otherwise.

C. **Two or more diagnoses that equally meet the definition for principal diagnosis**

In the unusual instance when two or more diagnoses equally meet the criteria for principal diagnosis as determined by the circumstances of admission, diagnostic workup and/or therapy provided, and the Alphabetic Index, Tabular List, or another coding guidelines does not provide sequencing direction, any one of the diagnoses may be sequenced first.

D. **Two or more comparative or contrasting conditions.**

In those rare instances when two or more contrasting or comparative diagnoses are documented as "either/or" (or similar terminology), they are coded as if the diagnoses were confirmed and the diagnoses are sequenced according to the circumstances of the admission. If no further determination can be made as to which diagnosis should be principal, either diagnosis may be sequenced first.

E. **A symptom(s) followed by contrasting/comparative diagnoses**

When a symptom(s) is followed by contrasting/comparative diagnoses, the symptom code is sequenced first. All the contrasting/comparative diagnoses should be coded as additional diagnoses.

F. **Original treatment plan not carried out**

Sequence as the principal diagnosis the condition, which after study occasioned the admission to the hospital, even though treatment may not have been carried out due to unforeseen circumstances.

G. **Complications of surgery and other medical care**

When the admission is for treatment of a complication resulting from surgery or other medical care, the complication code is sequenced as the principal diagnosis. If the complication is classified to the 996-999 series and the code lacks the necessary specificity in describing the complication, an additional code for the specific complication should be assigned.

H. **Uncertain Diagnosis**

If the diagnosis documented at the time of discharge is qualified as "probable", "suspected", "likely", "questionable", "possible", or "still to be ruled out", or other similar terms indicating uncertainty, code the condition as if it existed or was established. The bases for these guidelines are the diagnostic workup, arrangements for further workup or observation, and initial therapeutic approach that correspond most closely with the established diagnosis.

Note: This guideline is applicable only to inpatient admissions to short-term, acute, long-term care and psychiatric hospitals.

I. Admission from Observation Unit

1. Admission Following Medical Observation

When a patient is admitted to an observation unit for a medical condition, which either worsens or does not improve, and is subsequently admitted as an inpatient of the same hospital for this same medical condition, the principal diagnosis would be the medical condition which led to the hospital admission.

2. Admission Following Post-Operative Observation

When a patient is admitted to an observation unit to monitor a condition (or complication) that develops following outpatient surgery, and then is subsequently admitted as an inpatient of the same hospital, hospitals should apply the Uniform Hospital Discharge Data Set (UHDDS) definition of principal diagnosis as "that condition established after study to be chiefly responsible for occasioning the admission of the patient to the hospital for care."

J. Admission from Outpatient Surgery

When a patient receives surgery in the hospital's outpatient surgery department and is subsequently admitted for continuing inpatient care at the same hospital, the following guidelines should be followed in selecting the principal diagnosis for the inpatient admission:

- If the reason for the inpatient admission is a complication, assign the complication as the principal diagnosis.

- If no complication, or other condition, is documented as the reason for the inpatient admission, assign the reason for the outpatient surgery as the principal diagnosis.

- If the reason for the inpatient admission is another condition unrelated to the surgery, assign the unrelated condition as the principal diagnosis.

Section III. Reporting Additional Diagnoses

GENERAL RULES FOR OTHER (ADDITIONAL) DIAGNOSES

For reporting purposes the definition for "other diagnoses" is interpreted as additional conditions that affect patient care in terms of requiring:

clinical evaluation; or
therapeutic treatment; or
diagnostic procedures; or
extended length of hospital stay; or
increased nursing care and/or monitoring.

The UHDDS item #11-b defines Other Diagnoses as "all conditions that coexist at the time of admission, that develop subsequently, or that affect the treatment received and/or the length of stay. Diagnoses that relate to an earlier episode which have no bearing on the current hospital stay are to be excluded." UHDDS definitions apply to inpatients in acute care, short-term, long term care and psychiatric hospital setting. The UHDDS definitions are used by acute care short-term hospitals to report inpatient data elements in a standardized manner. These data elements and their definitions can be found in the July 31, 1985, Federal Register (Vol. 50, No, 147), pp. 31038-40.

Since that time the application of the UHDDS definitions has been expanded to include all non-outpatient settings (acute care, short term, long term care and psychiatric hospitals; home health agencies; rehab facilities; nursing homes, etc).

The following guidelines are to be applied in designating "other diagnoses" when neither the Alphabetic Index nor the Tabular List in ICD-9-CM provide direction. The listing of the diagnoses in the patient record is the responsibility of the attending provider.

A. Previous conditions

If the provider has included a diagnosis in the final diagnostic statement, such as the discharge summary or the face sheet, it should ordinarily be coded. Some providers include in the diagnostic statement resolved conditions or diagnoses and status-post procedures from previous admission that have no bearing on the current stay. Such conditions are not to be reported and are coded only if required by hospital policy.

However, history codes (V10-V19) may be used as secondary codes if the historical condition or family history has an impact on current care or influences treatment.

B. Abnormal findings

Abnormal findings (laboratory, x-ray, pathologic, and other diagnostic results) are not coded and reported unless the provider indicates their clinical significance. If the findings are outside the normal range and the attending provider has ordered other tests to evaluate the condition or prescribed treatment, it is appropriate to ask the provider whether the abnormal finding should be added.

Please note: This differs from the coding practices in the outpatient setting for coding encounters for diagnostic tests that have been interpreted by a provider.

C. Uncertain Diagnosis

If the diagnosis documented at the time of discharge is qualified as "probable", "suspected", "likely", "questionable", "possible", or "still to be ruled out" or other similar terms indicating uncertainty, code the condition as if it existed or was established. The bases for these guidelines are the diagnostic workup, arrangements for further workup or observation, and initial therapeutic approach that correspond most closely with the established diagnosis.

Note: This guideline is applicable only to inpatient admissions to short-term, acute, long-term care and psychiatric hospitals.

Section IV. Diagnostic Coding and Reporting Guidelines for Outpatient Services

These coding guidelines for outpatient diagnoses have been approved for use by hospitals/providers in coding and reporting hospital-based outpatient services and provider-based office visits.

Information about the use of certain abbreviations, punctuation, symbols, and other conventions used in the ICD-9-CM Tabular List (code numbers and titles), can be found in Section IA of these guidelines, under "Conventions Used in the Tabular List." Information about the correct sequence to use in finding a code is also described in Section I.

The terms encounter and visit are often used interchangeably in describing outpatient service contacts and, therefore, appear together in these guidelines without distinguishing one from the other.

Though the conventions and general guidelines apply to all settings, coding guidelines for outpatient and provider reporting of diagnoses will vary in a number of instances from those for inpatient diagnoses, recognizing that:

The Uniform Hospital Discharge Data Set (UHDDS) definition of principal diagnosis applies only to inpatients in acute, short-term, long-term care and psychiatric hospitals.

Coding guidelines for inconclusive diagnoses (probable, suspected, rule out, etc.) were developed for inpatient reporting and do not apply to outpatients.

A. Selection of first-listed condition

In the outpatient setting, the term first-listed diagnosis is used in lieu of principal diagnosis.

In determining the first-listed diagnosis the coding conventions of ICD-9-CM, as well as the general and disease specific guidelines take precedence over the outpatient guidelines.

Diagnoses often are not established at the time of the initial encounter/visit. It may take two or more visits before the diagnosis is confirmed.

The most critical rule involves beginning the search for the correct code assignment through the Alphabetic Index. Never begin searching initially in the Tabular List as this will lead to coding errors.

1. Outpatient Surgery

When a patient presents for outpatient surgery, code the reason for the surgery as the first-listed diagnosis (reason for the encounter), even if the surgery is not performed due to a contraindication.

2. Observation Stay

When a patient is admitted for observation for a medical condition, assign a code for the medical condition as the first-listed diagnosis.

When a patient presents for outpatient surgery and develops complications requiring admission to observation, code the reason for the surgery as the first reported diagnosis (reason for the encounter), followed by codes for the complications as secondary diagnoses.

B. Codes from 001.0 through *V91.99*

The appropriate code or codes from 001.0 through V91.99 must be used to identify diagnoses, symptoms, conditions, problems, complaints, or other reason(s) for the encounter/visit.

C. Accurate reporting of ICD-9-CM diagnosis codes

For accurate reporting of ICD-9-CM diagnosis codes, the documentation should describe the patient's condition, using terminology which includes specific diagnoses as well as symptoms, problems, or reasons for the encounter. There are ICD-9-CM codes to describe all of these.

D. Selection of codes 001.0 through 999.9

The selection of codes 001.0 through 999.9 will frequently be used to describe the reason for the encounter. These codes are from the section of ICD-9-CM for the classification of diseases and injuries (e.g. infectious and parasitic diseases; neoplasms; symptoms, signs, and ill-defined conditions, etc.).

E. Codes that describe symptoms and signs

Codes that describe symptoms and signs, as opposed to diagnoses, are acceptable for reporting purposes when a diagnosis has not been established (confirmed) by the provider. Chapter 16 of ICD-9-CM, Symptoms, Signs, and Ill-defined conditions (codes 780.0 - 799.9) contain many, but not all codes for symptoms.

F. Encounters for circumstances other than a disease or injury

ICD-9-CM provides codes to deal with encounters for circumstances other than a disease or injury. The Supplementary Classification of factors Influencing Health Status and Contact with Health Services (V01.0- V91.99) is provided to deal with occasions when circumstances other than a disease or injury are recorded as diagnosis or problems. *See Section I.C.18 for information on V-codes.*

G. Level of Detail in Coding

1. ICD-9-CM codes with 3, 4, or 5 digits

ICD-9-CM is composed of codes with either 3, 4, or 5 digits. Codes with three digits are included in ICD-9-CM as the heading of a category of codes that may be further subdivided by the use of fourth and/or fifth digits, which provide greater specificity.

2. Use of full number of digits required for a code

A three-digit code is to be used only if it is not further subdivided. Where fourth-digit subcategories and/or fifth-digit subclassifications are provided, they must be assigned. A code is invalid if it has not been coded to the full number of digits required for that code.

See also discussion under Section I.b.3., General Coding Guidelines, Level of Detail in Coding.

H. ICD-9-CM code for the diagnosis, condition, problem, or other reason for encounter/visit

List first the ICD-9-CM code for the diagnosis, condition, problem, or other reason for encounter/visit shown in the medical record to be chiefly responsible for the services provided. List additional codes that describe any coexisting conditions. In some cases the first-listed diagnosis may be a symptom when a diagnosis has not been established (confirmed) by the physician.

I. Uncertain diagnosis

Do not code diagnoses documented as "probable", "suspected," "questionable," "rule out," or "working diagnosis" or other similar terms indicating uncertainty. Rather, code the condition(s) to the highest degree of certainty for that encounter/visit, such as symptoms, signs, abnormal test results, or other reason for the visit.

Please note: This differs from the coding practices used by short-term, acute care, long-term care and psychiatric hospitals.

J. Chronic diseases

Chronic diseases treated on an ongoing basis may be coded and reported as many times as the patient receives treatment and care for the condition(s)

K. Code all documented conditions that coexist

Code all documented conditions that coexist at the time of the encounter/visit, and require or affect patient care treatment or management. Do not code conditions that were previously treated and no longer exist. However, history codes (V10-V19) may be used as secondary codes if the historical condition or family history has an impact on current care or influences treatment.

L. Patients receiving diagnostic services only

For patients receiving diagnostic services only during an encounter/visit, sequence first the diagnosis, condition, problem, or other reason for encounter/visit shown in the medical record to be chiefly responsible for the outpatient services provided during the encounter/visit. Codes for other diagnoses (e.g., chronic conditions) may be sequenced as additional diagnoses.

For encounters for routine laboratory/radiology testing in the absence of any signs, symptoms, or associated diagnosis, assign V72.5 and/**or** a code from subcategory V72.6. If routine testing is performed during the same encounter as a test to evaluate a sign, symptom, or diagnosis, it is appropriate to assign both the V code and the code describing the reason for the non-routine test.

For outpatient encounters for diagnostic tests that have been interpreted by a physician, and the final report is available at the time of coding, code any confirmed or definitive diagnosis(es) documented in the interpretation. Do not code related signs and symptoms as additional diagnoses.

Please note: This differs from the coding practice in the hospital inpatient setting regarding abnormal findings on test results.

M. Patients receiving therapeutic services only

For patients receiving therapeutic services only during an encounter/visit, sequence first the diagnosis, condition, problem, or other reason for encounter/visit shown in the medical record to be chiefly responsible for the outpatient services provided during the encounter/visit. Codes for other diagnoses (e.g., chronic conditions) may be sequenced as additional diagnoses.

The only exception to this rule is that when the primary reason for the admission/encounter is chemotherapy, radiation therapy, or rehabilitation, the appropriate V code for the service is listed first, and the diagnosis or problem for which the service is being performed listed second.

N. Patients receiving preoperative evaluations only

For patients receiving preoperative evaluations only, sequence first a code from category V72.8, Other specified examinations, to describe the pre-op consultations. Assign a code for the condition to describe the reason for the surgery as an additional diagnosis. Code also any findings related to the pre-op evaluation.

O. Ambulatory surgery

For ambulatory surgery, code the diagnosis for which the surgery was performed. If the postoperative diagnosis is known to be different from the preoperative diagnosis at the time the diagnosis is confirmed, select the postoperative diagnosis for coding, since it is the most definitive.

P. Routine outpatient prenatal visits

For routine outpatient prenatal visits when no complications are present, codes V22.0, Supervision of normal first pregnancy, or V22.1, Supervision of other normal pregnancy, should be used as the principal diagnosis. These codes should not be used in conjunction with chapter 11 codes.

Appendix I Present on Admission Reporting Guidelines

Introduction

These guidelines are to be used as a supplement to the *ICD-9-CM Official Guidelines for Coding and Reporting* to facilitate the assignment of the Present on Admission (POA) indicator for each diagnosis and external cause of injury code reported on claim forms (UB-04 and 837 Institutional).

These guidelines are not intended to replace any guidelines in the main body of the *ICD-9-CM Official Guidelines for Coding and Reporting*. The POA guidelines are not intended to provide guidance on when a condition should be coded, but rather, how to apply the POA indicator to the final set of diagnosis codes that have been assigned in accordance with Sections I, II, and III of the official coding guidelines. Subsequent to the assignment of the ICD-9-CM codes, the POA indicator should then be assigned to those conditions that have been coded.

As stated in the Introduction to the ICD-9-CM Official Guidelines for Coding and Reporting, a joint effort between the healthcare provider and the coder is essential to achieve complete and accurate documentation, code assignment, and reporting of diagnoses and procedures. The importance of consistent, complete documentation in the medical record cannot be overemphasized. Medical record documentation from any provider involved in the care and treatment of the patient may be used to support the determination of whether a condition was present on admission or not. In the context of the official coding guidelines, the term "provider" means a physician or any qualified healthcare practitioner who is legally accountable for establishing the patient's diagnosis.

These guidelines are not a substitute for the provider's clinical judgment as to the determination of whether a condition was/was not present on admission. The provider should be queried regarding issues related to the linking of signs/symptoms, timing of test results, and the timing of findings.

General Reporting Requirements

All claims involving inpatient admissions to general acute care hospitals or other facilities that are subject to a law or regulation mandating collection of present on admission information.

Present on admission is defined as present at the time the order for inpatient admission occurs — conditions that develop during an outpatient encounter, including emergency department, observation, or outpatient surgery, are considered as present on admission.

POA indicator is assigned to principal and secondary diagnoses (as defined in Section II of the Official Guidelines for Coding and Reporting) and the external cause of injury codes.

Issues related to inconsistent, missing, conflicting or unclear documentation must still be resolved by the provider.

If a condition would not be coded and reported based on UHDDS definitions and current official coding guidelines, then the POA indicator would not be reported.

Reporting Options

Y - Yes

N - No

U - Unknown

W – Clinically undetermined

Unreported/Not used (or "1" for Medicare usage) – (Exempt from POA reporting)

Reporting Definitions

Y = present at the time of inpatient admission

N = not present at the time of inpatient admission

U = documentation is insufficient to determine if condition is present on admission

W = provider is unable to clinically determine whether condition was present on admission or not

Timeframe for POA Identification and Documentation

There is no required timeframe as to when a provider (per the definition of "provider" used in these guidelines) must identify or document a condition to be present on admission. In some clinical situations, it may not be possible for a provider to make a definitive diagnosis (or a condition may not be recognized or reported by the patient) for a period of time after admission. In some cases it may be several days before the provider arrives at a definitive diagnosis. This does not mean that the condition was not present on admission. Determination of whether the condition was present on admission or not will be based on the applicable POA guideline as identified in this document, or on the provider's best clinical judgment.

If at the time of code assignment the documentation is unclear as to whether a condition was present on admission or not, it is appropriate to query the provider for clarification.

Assigning the POA Indicator

Condition is on the "Exempt from Reporting" list

Leave the "present on admission" field blank if the condition is on the list of ICD-9-CM codes for which this field is not applicable. This is the only circumstance in which the field may be left blank.

POA Explicitly Documented

Assign Y for any condition the provider explicitly documents as being present on admission.

Assign N for any condition the provider explicitly documents as not present at the time of admission.

Conditions diagnosed prior to inpatient admission

Assign "Y" for conditions that were diagnosed prior to admission (example: hypertension, diabetes mellitus, asthma)

Conditions diagnosed during the admission but clearly present before admission

Assign "Y" for conditions diagnosed during the admission that were clearly present but not diagnosed until after admission occurred.

Diagnoses subsequently confirmed after admission are considered present on admission if at the time of admission they are documented as suspected, possible, rule out, differential diagnosis, or constitute an underlying cause of a symptom that is present at the time of admission.

Condition develops during outpatient encounter prior to inpatient admission

Assign Y for any condition that develops during an outpatient encounter prior to a written order for inpatient admission.

Documentation does not indicate whether condition was present on admission

Assign "U" when the medical record documentation is unclear as to whether the condition was present on admission. "U" should not be routinely assigned and used only in very limited circumstances. Coders are encouraged to query the providers when the documentation is unclear.

Documentation states that it cannot be determined whether the condition was or was not present on admission

Assign "W" when the medical record documentation indicates that it cannot be clinically determined whether or not the condition was present on admission.

Chronic condition with acute exacerbation during the admission

If the code is a combination code that identifies both the chronic condition and the acute exacerbation, see POA guidelines pertaining to combination codes.

If the combination code only identifies the chronic condition and not the acute exacerbation (e.g., acute exacerbation of chronic leukemia), assign "Y."

Conditions documented as possible, probable, suspected, or rule out at the time of discharge

If the final diagnosis contains a possible, probable, suspected, or rule out diagnosis, and this diagnosis was based on signs, symptoms, or clinical findings suspected at the time of inpatient admission, assign "Y."

If the final diagnosis contains a possible, probable, suspected, or rule out diagnosis, and this diagnosis was based on signs, symptoms or clinical findings that were not present on admission, assign "N".

Conditions documented as impending or threatened at the time of discharge

If the final diagnosis contains an impending or threatened diagnosis, and this diagnosis is based on symptoms or clinical findings that were present on admission, assign "Y".

If the final diagnosis contains an impending or threatened diagnosis, and this diagnosis is based on symptoms or clinical findings that were not present on admission, assign "N".

Acute and Chronic Conditions

Assign "Y" for acute conditions that are present at time of admission and N for acute conditions that are not present at time of admission.

Assign "Y" for chronic conditions, even though the condition may not be diagnosed until after admission.

If a single code identifies both an acute and chronic condition, see the POA guidelines for combination codes.

Combination Codes

Assign "N" if any part of the combination code was not present on admission (e.g., obstructive chronic bronchitis with acute exacerbation and the exacerbation was not present on admission; gastric ulcer that does not start bleeding until after admission; asthma patient develops status asthmaticus after admission)

Assign "Y" if all parts of the combination code were present on admission (e.g., patient with diabetic nephropathy is admitted with uncontrolled diabetes)

If the final diagnosis includes comparative or contrasting diagnoses, and both were present, or suspected, at the time of admission, assign "Y".

For infection codes that include the causal organism, assign "Y" if the infection (or signs of the infection) was present on admission, even though the culture results may not be known until after admission (e.g., patient is admitted with pneumonia and the provider documents pseudomonas as the causal organism a few days later).

Same Diagnosis Code for Two or More Conditions

When the same ICD-9-CM diagnosis code applies to two or more conditions during the same encounter (e.g. bilateral condition, or two separate conditions classified to the same ICD-9-CM diagnosis code):

Assign "Y" if all conditions represented by the single ICD-9-CM code were present on admission (e.g. bilateral fracture of the same bone, same site, and both fractures were present on admission)

Assign "N" if any of the conditions represented by the single ICD-9-CM code was not present on admission (e.g. dehydration with hyponatremia is assigned to code 276.1, but only one of these conditions was present on admission).

Obstetrical conditions

Whether or not the patient delivers during the current hospitalization does not affect assignment of the POA indicator. The determining factor for POA assignment is whether the pregnancy complication or obstetrical condition described by the code was present at the time of admission or not.

If the pregnancy complication or obstetrical condition was present on admission (e.g., patient admitted in preterm labor), assign "Y".

If the pregnancy complication or obstetrical condition was not present on admission (e.g., 2nd degree laceration during delivery, postpartum hemorrhage that occurred during current hospitalization, fetal distress develops after admission), assign "N".

If the obstetrical code includes more than one diagnosis and any of the diagnoses identified by the code were not present on admission assign "N".

(e.g., Code 642.7, Pre-eclampsia or eclampsia superimposed on pre-existing hypertension).

GUIDELINES - APPENDIX I

49

If the obstetrical code includes information that is not a diagnosis, do not consider that information in the POA determination.

(e.g. Code 652.1x, Breech or other malpresentation successfully converted to cephalic presentation should be reported as present on admission if the fetus was breech on admission but was converted to cephalic presentation after admission (since the conversion to cephalic presentation does not represent a diagnosis, the fact that the conversion occurred after admission has no bearing on the POA determination).

Perinatal conditions

Newborns are not considered to be admitted until after birth. Therefore, any condition present at birth or that developed in utero is considered present at admission and should be assigned "Y". This includes conditions that occur during delivery (e.g., injury during delivery, meconium aspiration, exposure to streptococcus B in the vaginal canal).

Congenital conditions and anomalies

Assign "Y" for congenital conditions and anomalies, **except for categories 740-759, Congenital anomalies, which are on the exempt list.** Congenital conditions are always considered present on admission.

External cause of injury codes

Assign "Y" for any E code representing an external cause of injury or poisoning that occurred prior to inpatient admission (e.g., patient fell out of bed at home, patient fell out of bed in emergency room prior to admission)

Assign "N" for any E code representing an external cause of injury or poisoning that occurred during inpatient hospitalization (e.g., patient fell out of hospital bed during hospital stay, patient experienced an adverse reaction to a medication administered after inpatient admission)

Categories and Codes Exempt from Diagnosis Present on Admission Requirement

Effective Date: October 1, 2008

Note: "Diagnosis present on admission" for these code categories are exempt because they represent circumstances regarding the healthcare encounter or factors influencing health status that do not represent a current disease or injury or are always present on admission.

Categories or subcategories listed are inclusive of all codes within those categories or subcategories, unless otherwise indicated. In order to streamline the POA exempt list and make it easier to read, where all of the codes in a code range are POA exempt, only the code range is shown, rather than listing each of the individual codes in the range.

137-139, Late effects of infectious and parasitic diseases

268.1, Rickets, late effect

326, Late effects of intracranial abscess or pyogenic infection

412, Old myocardial infarction

438, Late effects of cerebrovascular disease

650, Normal delivery

660.7, Failed forceps or vacuum extractor, unspecified

677, Late effect of complication of pregnancy, childbirth, and the puerperium

740-759, Congenital anomalies

905-909, Late effects of injuries, poisonings, toxic effects, and other external causes

V02, Carrier or suspected carrier of infectious diseases

V03, Need for prophylactic vaccination and inoculation against bacterial diseases

V04, Need for prophylactic vaccination and inoculation against certain viral diseases

V05, Need for other prophylactic vaccination and inoculation against single diseases

V06, Need for prophylactic vaccination and inoculation against combinations of diseases

V07, Need for isolation and other prophylactic or treatment measures

V10, Personal history of malignant neoplasm

V11, Personal history of mental disorder

V12, Personal history of certain other diseases

V13, Personal history of other diseases

V14, Personal history of allergy to medicinal agents

V15, Other personal history presenting hazards to health

V16, Family history of malignant neoplasm

V17, Family history of certain chronic disabling diseases

V18, Family history of certain other specific conditions

V19, Family history of other conditions

V20, Health supervision of infant or child

V21, Constitutional states in development

V22, Normal pregnancy

V23, Supervision of high-risk pregnancy

V24, Postpartum care and examination

V25, Encounter for contraceptive management

V26, Procreative management

V27, Outcome of delivery

V28, Antenatal screening

V29, Observation and evaluation of newborns for suspected condition not found

V30-V39, Liveborn infants according to type of birth

V42, Organ or tissue replaced by transplant

V43, Organ or tissue replaced by other means

V44, Artificial opening status

V45, Other postprocedural states

V46, Other dependence on machines and devices

V49.60-V49.77, Upper and lower limb amputation status

V49.81-V49.85, Other specified conditions influencing health status

V50, Elective surgery for purposes other than remedying health states

V51, Aftercare involving the use of plastic surgery

V52, Fitting and adjustment of prosthetic device and implant

V53, Fitting and adjustment of other device

V54, Other orthopedic aftercare

V55, Attention to artificial openings

V56, Encounter for dialysis and dialysis catheter care

V57, Care involving use of rehabilitation procedures

V58, Encounter for other and unspecified procedures and aftercare

V59, Donors

V60, Housing, household, and economic circumstances

V61, Other family circumstances

V62, Other psychosocial circumstances

V64, Persons encountering health services for specific procedures, not carried out

V65, Other persons seeking consultation

V66, Convalescence and palliative care

V67, Follow-up examination

V68, Encounters for administrative purposes

V69, Problems related to lifestyle

V70, General medical examination

V71, Observation and evaluation for suspected condition not found

V72, Special investigations and examinations

V73, Special screening examination for viral and chlamydial diseases

V74, Special screening examination for bacterial and spirochetal diseases

V75, Special screening examination for other infectious diseases

V76, Special screening for malignant neoplasms

V77, Special screening for endocrine, nutritional, metabolic, and immunity disorders

V78, Special screening for disorders of blood and blood-forming organs

V79, Special screening for mental disorders and developmental handicaps

V80, Special screening for neurological, eye, and ear diseases

V81, Special screening for cardiovascular, respiratory, and genitourinary diseases

V82, Special screening for other conditions

V83, Genetic carrier status

V84, Genetic susceptibility to disease

V85, Body Mass Index

V86, Estrogen receptor status

V87.32, Contact with and (suspected) exposure to algae bloom

V87.4, Personal history of drug therapy

V88, Acquired absence of other organs and tissue

V89, Suspected maternal and fetal conditions not found

V90, Retained foreign body

V91, Multiple gestation placenta status

E000, External cause status

E001-E030, Activity

E800-E807, Railway accidents

E810-E819, Motor vehicle traffic accidents

E820-E825, Motor vehicle nontraffic accidents

E826-E829, Other road vehicle accidents

E830-E838, Water transport accidents

E840-E845, Air and space transport accidents

E846-E848, Vehicle accidents not elsewhere classifiable

E849, Place of occurrence (Except E849.7)

E883.1, Accidental fall into well

E883.2, Accidental fall into storm drain or manhole

E884.0, Fall from playground equipment

E884.1, Fall from cliff

E885.0, Fall from (nonmotorized) scooter

E885.1, Fall from roller skates

E885.2, Fall from skateboard

E885.3, Fall from skis

E885.4, Fall from snowboard

E886.0, Fall on same level from collision, pushing, or shoving, by or with other person, In sports

E890.0-E890.9, Conflagration in private dwelling

E893.0, Accident caused by ignition of clothing, from controlled fire in private dwelling

E893.2, Accident caused by ignition of clothing, from controlled fire not in building or structure

E894, Ignition of highly inflammable material

E895, Accident caused by controlled fire in private dwelling

E897, Accident caused by controlled fire not in building or structure

E917.0, Striking against or struck accidentally by objects or persons, in sports without subsequent fall

E917.1, Striking against or struck accidentally by objects or persons, caused by a crowd, by collective fear or panic without subsequent fall

E917.2, Striking against or struck accidentally by objects or persons, in running water without subsequent fall

E917.5, Striking against or struck accidentally by objects or persons, object in sports with subsequent fall

E917.6, Striking against or struck accidentally by objects or persons, caused by a crowd, by collective fear or panic with subsequent fall

E919, Accident caused by machinery (Except E919.2)

E921, Accident caused by explosion of pressure vessel

E922, Accident caused by firearm and air gun missile

E926.2, Visible and ultraviolet light sources

E928.0-E928.8, Other and unspecified environmental and accidental causes

E929.0-E929.9, Late effects of accidental injury

E959, Late effects of self-inflicted injury

GUIDELINES · APPENDIX I

51

E970-E978, Legal intervention

E979, Terrorism

E981, Poisoning by gases in domestic use, undetermined whether accidentally or purposely inflicted

E982, Poisoning by other gases, undetermined whether accidentally or purposely inflicted

E985, Injury by firearms, air guns and explosives, undetermined whether accidentally or purposely inflicted

E987.0, Falling from high place, undetermined whether accidentally or purposely inflicted, residential premises

E987.2, Falling from high place, undetermined whether accidentally or purposely inflicted, natural sites

E989, Late effects of injury, undetermined whether accidentally or purposely inflicted

E990-E999, Injury resulting from operations of war

POA Examples

The POA examples have been removed from the guidelines.

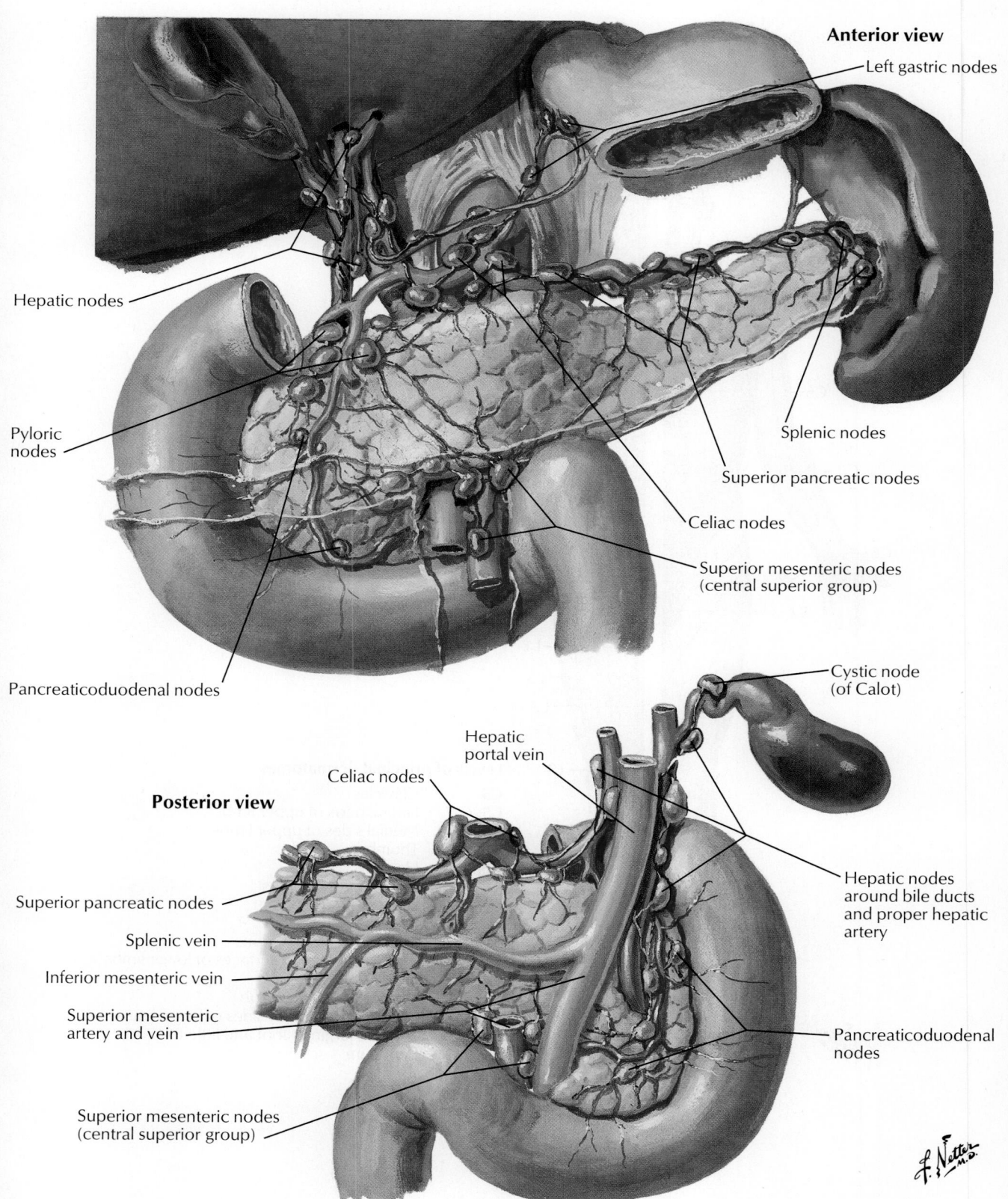

Anterior view

Left gastric nodes

Hepatic nodes

Pyloric nodes

Pancreaticoduodenal nodes

Splenic nodes

Superior pancreatic nodes

Celiac nodes

Superior mesenteric nodes (central superior group)

Cystic node (of Calot)

Hepatic portal vein

Celiac nodes

Posterior view

Superior pancreatic nodes

Splenic vein

Inferior mesenteric vein

Superior mesenteric artery and vein

Superior mesenteric nodes (central superior group)

Hepatic nodes around bile ducts and proper hepatic artery

Pancreaticoduodenal nodes

Plate 315 Lymph Vessels and Nodes of Pancreas. (Netter: Atlas of Human Anatomy, 4 ed, 2006, Saunders.)

Dermatome pattern

Levels of principal dermatomes

C5	Clavicles
C5, 6, 7	Lateral parts of upper limbs
C8; T1	Medial sides of upper limbs
C6	Thumb
C6, 7, 8	Hand
C8	Ring and little fingers
T4	Level of nipples
T10	Level of umbilicus
T12	Inguinal or groin regions
L1, 2, 3, 4	Anterior and inner surfaces of lower limbs
L4, 5; S1	Foot
L4	Medial side of great toe
L5; S1, 2	Outer and posterior sides of lower limbs
S1	Lateral margin of foot and little toe
S2, 3, 4	Perineum

Plate 164   Dermatomes. (Netter: Atlas of Human Anatomy, 4 ed, 2006, Saunders.)

Female: frontal section

- Peritoneum
- Body of bladder
- Fundus of bladder
- Interureteric crest
- Left ureteric orifice
- Trigone of bladder
- Neck of bladder
- Paravesical endopelvic fascia and vesical venous plexus
- Vesical fascia
- Tendinous arch of levator ani muscle
- Obturator internus muscle
- Levator ani muscle
- Tendinous arch of pelvic fascia
- Urethra
- Sphincter urethrae muscle
- Perineal membrane
- Inferior pubic ramus
- Crus of clitoris and ischiocavernosus muscle
- Bulb of vestibule and bulbospongiosus muscle
- Deep perineal (investing or Gallaudet's) fascia
- Superficial perineal (Colles') fascia

Round ligament of uterus

Vagina

Male: frontal section

- Peritoneum
- Body of bladder
- Fundus of bladder
- Ductus (vas) deferens
- Interureteric crest
- Right ureteric orifice
- Trigone of bladder
- Neck of bladder
- Paravesical endopelvic fascia and vesical venous plexus
- Tendinous arch of levator ani muscle
- Uvula of bladder
- Obturator internus muscle
- Levator ani muscle
- Capsule of prostate
- Prostate and prostatic urethra
- Seminal colliculus
- Bulbourethral (Cowper's) gland
- Perineal membrane and sphincter urethrae muscle
- Bulbous portion of spongy urethra
- Corpus spongiosum and bulbospongiosus muscle
- Deep perineal (investing or Gallaudet's) fascia

- Internal urethral sphincter
- Tendinous arch of pelvic fascia
- Anterior recess of ischio-anal fossa
- Inferior pubic ramus
- Crus of penis and ischiocavernosus muscle
- Superficial perineal (Colles') fascia

Plate 366 Urinary Bladder: Female and Male. (Netter: Atlas of Human Anatomy, 4 ed, 2006, Saunders.)

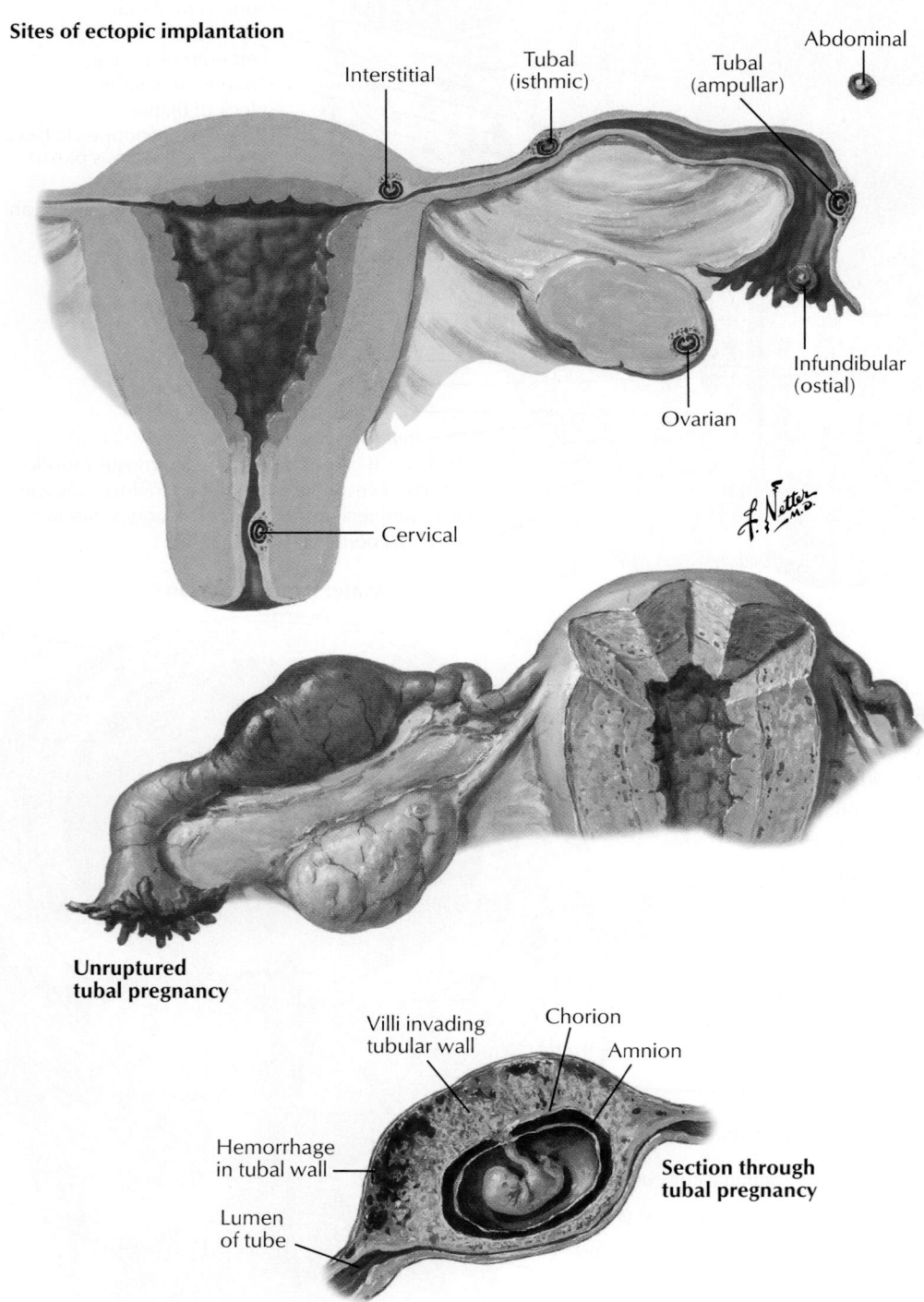

Sites of ectopic implantation

Interstitial

Tubal (isthmic)

Tubal (ampullar)

Abdominal

Infundibular (ostial)

Ovarian

Cervical

Unruptured tubal pregnancy

Villi invading tubular wall

Chorion

Amnion

Hemorrhage in tubal wall

Section through tubal pregnancy

Lumen of tube

Plate 375   Ectopic Pregnancy. (Netter: Atlas of Human Anatomy, 4 ed, 2006, Saunders.)

Skin of penis

Superficial fascia of penis (Colles' fascia)

Deep (Buck's) fascia of penis

Testicular artery

Ductus deferens

Artery to ductus deferens

Genital branch of genitofemoral nerve

Pampiniform (venous) plexus

Epididymis

Appendix of epididymis

Appendix of testis

Testis (covered by visceral layer of tunica vaginalis)

Parietal layer of tunica vaginalis

Superficial inguinal ring

External spermatic fascia

Cremaster muscle and fascia

Septum of scrotum (formed by dartos fascia)

Superficial (dartos) fascia of scrotum

Skin of scrotum

Superficial (dartos) fascia of scrotum

External spermatic fascia

Cremaster muscle and fascia

Internal spermatic fascia

Parietal layer of tunica vaginalis

Epididymis

Testis (covered by visceral layer of tunica vaginalis)

Skin of scrotum

Plate 387   Scrotum and Contents. (Netter: Atlas of Human Anatomy, 4 ed, 2006, Saunders.)

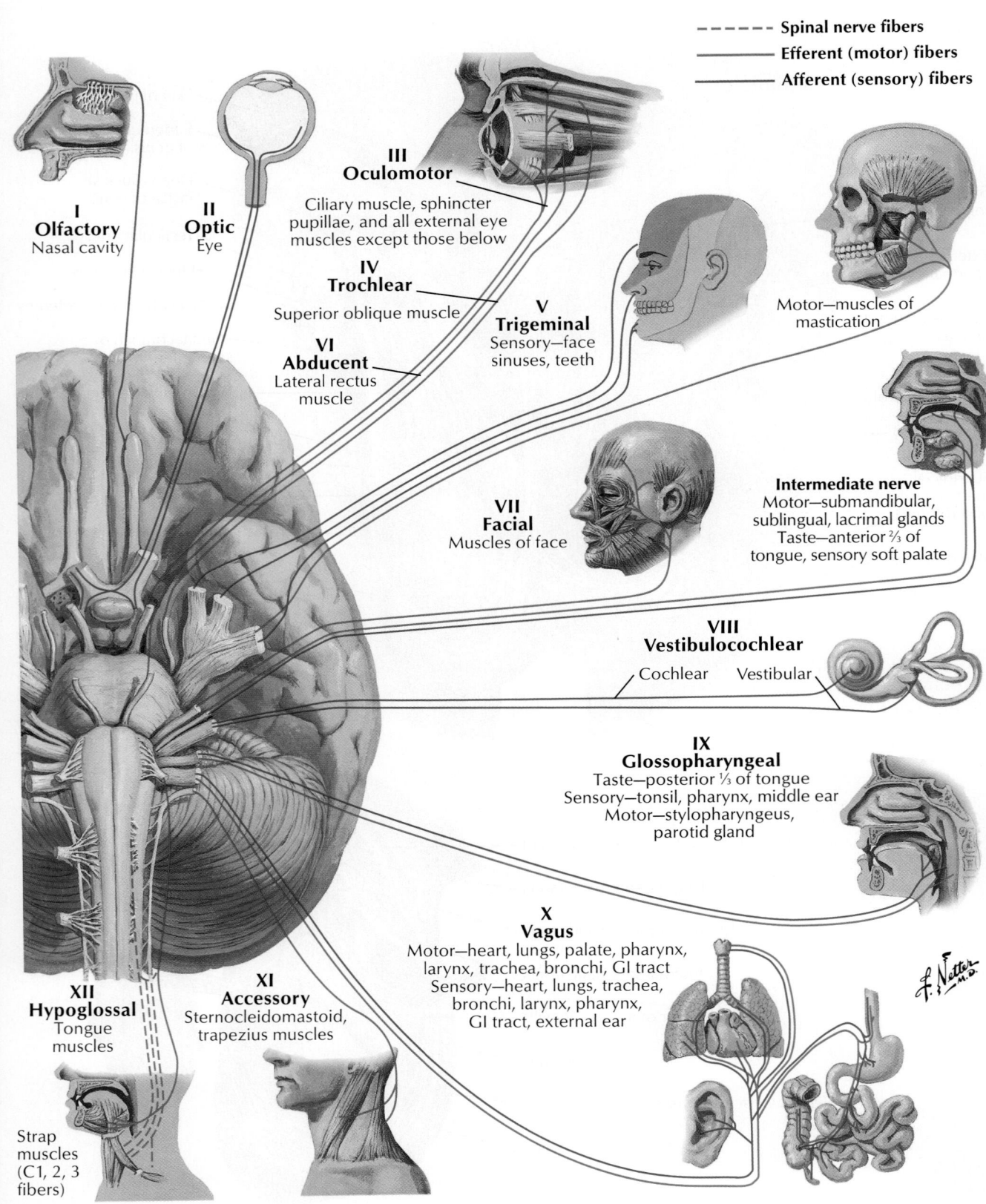

----- Spinal nerve fibers
——— Efferent (motor) fibers
——— Afferent (sensory) fibers

I
Olfactory
Nasal cavity

II
Optic
Eye

III
Oculomotor
Ciliary muscle, sphincter pupillae, and all external eye muscles except those below

IV
Trochlear
Superior oblique muscle

V
Trigeminal
Sensory—face sinuses, teeth

VI
Abducent
Lateral rectus muscle

Motor—muscles of mastication

VII
Facial
Muscles of face

Intermediate nerve
Motor—submandibular, sublingual, lacrimal glands
Taste—anterior ⅔ of tongue, sensory soft palate

VIII
Vestibulocochlear
Cochlear   Vestibular

IX
Glossopharyngeal
Taste—posterior ⅓ of tongue
Sensory—tonsil, pharynx, middle ear
Motor—stylopharyngeus, parotid gland

X
Vagus
Motor—heart, lungs, palate, pharynx, larynx, trachea, bronchi, GI tract
Sensory—heart, lungs, trachea, bronchi, larynx, pharynx, GI tract, external ear

XII
Hypoglossal
Tongue muscles

XI
Accessory
Sternocleidomastoid, trapezius muscles

Strap muscles (C1, 2, 3 fibers)

Plate 118   Cranial Nerves (Motor and Sensory Distribution): Schema. (Netter: Atlas of Human Anatomy, 4 ed, 2006, Saunders.)

Superior view

- Supratrochlear nerve
- Medial rectus muscle
- Superior oblique muscle
- Infratrochlear nerve
- Nasociliary nerve
- Trochlear nerve (IV)
- Common tendinous ring
- Ophthalmic nerve (V₁)
- Optic nerve (II)
- Internal carotid artery and nerve plexus
- Oculomotor nerve (III)
- Trochlear nerve (IV)
- Abducent nerve (VI)
- Tentorium cerebelli

- Medial branch } Supraorbital nerve
- Lateral branch
- Levator palpebrae superioris muscle
- Superior rectus muscle
- Lacrimal gland
- Lacrimal nerve
- Lateral rectus muscle
- Frontal nerve
- Maxillary nerve (V₂)
- Meningeal branch of maxillary nerve
- Mandibular nerve (V₃)
- Lesser petrosal nerve
- Meningeal branch of mandibular nerve
- Greater petrosal nerve
- Trigeminal (semilunar) ganglion
- Tentorial (meningeal) branch of ophthalmic nerve

Superior view:
levator palpebrae superioris, superior rectus, and superior oblique muscles partially cut away

- Supratrochlear nerve (cut)
- Supraorbital nerve branches (cut)
- Infratrochlear nerve
- Anterior ethmoidal nerve
- Optic nerve (II)
- Posterior ethmoidal nerve
- Superior branch of oculomotor nerve (III) (cut)
- Nasociliary nerve
- Internal carotid plexus
- Trochlear nerve (IV) (cut)
- Oculomotor nerve (III)
- Abducent nerve (VI)

- Long ciliary nerves
- Short ciliary nerves
- Lacrimal nerve
- Ciliary ganglion
- Parasympathetic root of ciliary ganglion (from inferior branch of oculomotor nerve)
- Sympathetic root of ciliary ganglion (from internal carotid plexus)
- Sensory root of ciliary ganglion (from nasociliary nerve)
- Branches to inferior and medial rectus muscles
- Abducent nerve (VI)
- Inferior branch of oculomotor nerve (III)
- Lacrimal nerve
- Frontal nerve (cut)
- Ophthalmic nerve (V₁)

Plate 86 Nerves of Orbit. (Netter: Atlas of Human Anatomy, 4 ed, 2006, Saunders.)

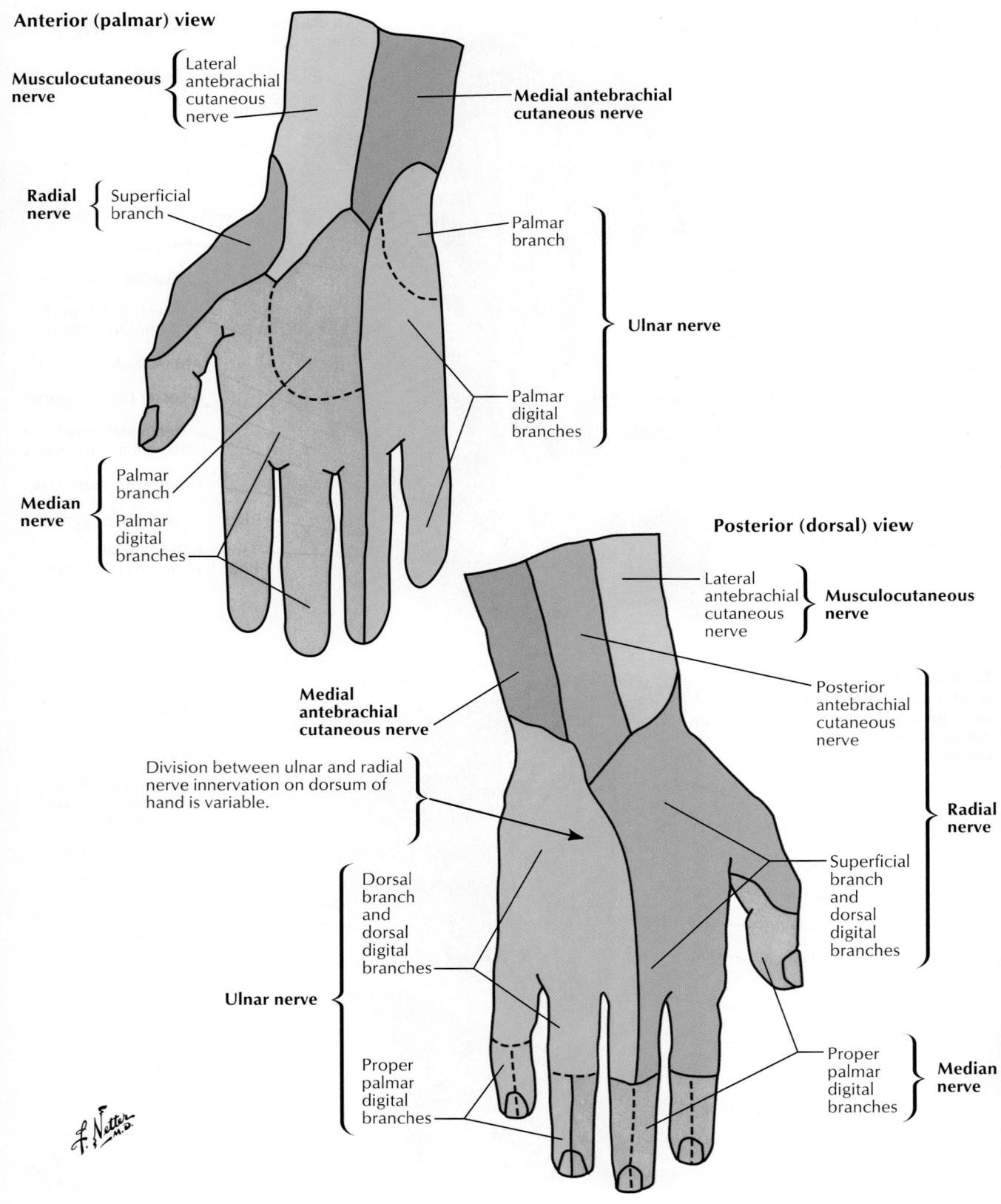

Anterior (palmar) view

Musculocutaneous nerve { Lateral antebrachial cutaneous nerve

Medial antebrachial cutaneous nerve

Radial nerve { Superficial branch

Palmar branch

Ulnar nerve

Palmar digital branches

Median nerve { Palmar branch
Palmar digital branches

Posterior (dorsal) view

Lateral antebrachial cutaneous nerve — **Musculocutaneous nerve**

Posterior antebrachial cutaneous nerve

Medial antebrachial cutaneous nerve

Radial nerve

Division between ulnar and radial nerve innervation on dorsum of hand is variable.

Superficial branch and dorsal digital branches

Ulnar nerve { Dorsal branch and dorsal digital branches

Proper palmar digital branches

Proper palmar digital branches — Median nerve

Plate 472   Cutaneous Innervation of Wrist and Hand. (Netter: Atlas of Human Anatomy, 4 ed, 2006, Saunders.)

Anterior view

Deltoid muscle

Coracobrachialis muscle

Biceps brachii muscle { Short head (*cut*)
Long head (*cut*)

Musculocutaneous nerve

Brachialis muscle

Biceps brachii muscle (*cut*) and tendon

Lateral antebrachial cutaneous nerve
(from musculocutaneous nerve)

Radial nerve { Deep branch
Superficial branch

Supinator muscle

Brachioradialis muscle

Radial artery

Pronator teres muscle (*partially cut*)

Median nerve

Flexor pollicis longus muscle

Flexor carpi radialis
tendon (*cut*)

Flexor retinaculum
(transverse carpal
ligament)

Superficial branch
of radial nerve

Recurrent (motor)
branch of
median nerve to
thenar muscles

Common palmar
digital branches
of median nerve

Proper palmar
digital branches
of median nerve

Intercostobrachial nerve

Medial brachial
cutaneous nerve

Radial nerve

Ulnar nerve

Medial antebrachial
cutaneous nerve

Median nerve

Brachial artery

Bicipital aponeurosis

Humeral head (*cut*) }
Ulnar head } Pronator teres muscle

Flexor carpi radialis muscle (*cut*)

Humeroulnar head }
Radial head } Flexor digitorum
superficialis muscle (*cut*)

Flexor digitorum profundus muscle

Flexor carpi ulnaris muscle

Ulnar artery and nerve

Dorsal branch of ulnar nerve

Flexor digitorum superficialis tendons (*cut*)

Deep palmar branch of ulnar artery and deep branch of ulnar nerve

Superficial branch of ulnar nerve

Superficial palmar arch (*cut*)

Common palmar digital branch of ulnar nerve

Communicating branch of median nerve with ulnar nerve

Proper palmar digital branches of ulnar nerve

Plate 473   Arteries and Nerves of Upper Limb. (Netter: Atlas of Human Anatomy, 4 ed, 2006, Saunders.)

Lateral cutaneous branch of subcostal nerve

Inguinal ligament (Poupart's)

Superficial circumflex iliac vein

Femoral branches of genitofemoral nerve

Lateral femoral cutaneous nerve

Saphenous opening (fossa ovalis)

Fascia lata

Anterior cutaneous branches of femoral nerve

Patellar nerve plexus

Branches of lateral sural cutaneous nerve (from common fibular [peroneal] nerve)

Deep fascia of leg (crural fascia)

Superficial fibular (peroneal) nerve
Medial dorsal cutaneous branch

Intermediate dorsal cutaneous branch

Small saphenous vein and lateral dorsal cutaneous nerve (from sural nerve)

Lateral dorsal digital nerve and vein of 5th toe

Dorsal metatarsal veins

Dorsal digital nerves and veins

Superficial epigastric vein

Ilioinguinal nerve (scrotal branch) (usually passes through superficial inguinal ring)

Genital branch of genitofemoral nerve

Femoral vein

Superficial external pudendal vein

Accessory saphenous vein

Great saphenous vein

Cutaneous branches of obturator nerve

Infrapatellar branch of saphenous nerve

Saphenous nerve (terminal branch of femoral nerve)

Great saphenous vein

Dorsal digital nerves

Dorsal venous arch

Dorsal digital nerve and vein of medial side of great toe

Dorsal digital branch of deep fibular (peroneal) nerve

Plate 544   Superficial Nerves and Veins of Lower Limb: Anterior View. (Netter: Atlas of Human Anatomy, 4 ed, 2006, Saunders.)

Lateral cutaneous branch of iliohypogastric nerve

Iliac crest

Medial clunial nerves (from dorsal rami of S1, 2, 3)

Superior clunial nerves (from dorsal rami of L1, 2, 3)

Inferior clunial nerves (from posterior femoral cutaneous nerve)

Perforating cutaneous nerve (from dorsal rami of S1, 2, 3)

Branches of posterior femoral cutaneous nerve

Branches of lateral femoral cutaneous nerve

Accessory saphenous vein

Branch of femoral cutaneous nerve

Branch of cutaneous branch of femoral nerve

Terminal branches of posterior femoral cutaneous nerve

Great saphenous vein

Lateral sural cutaneous nerve (from common fibular [peroneal] nerve)

Small saphenous vein

Sural communicating nerve

Branches of saphenous nerve

Medial sural cutaneous nerve (from tibial nerve)

Sural nerve

Lateral calcaneal branches of sural nerve

Medial calcaneal branches of tibial nerve

Lateral dorsal cutaneous nerve (continuation of sural nerve)

Plantar cutaneous branches of medial plantar nerve

Plantar cutaneous branches of lateral plantar nerve

Plate 545   Superficial Nerves and Veins of Lower Limb: Posterior View. (Netter: Atlas of Human Anatomy, 4 ed, 2006, Saunders.)

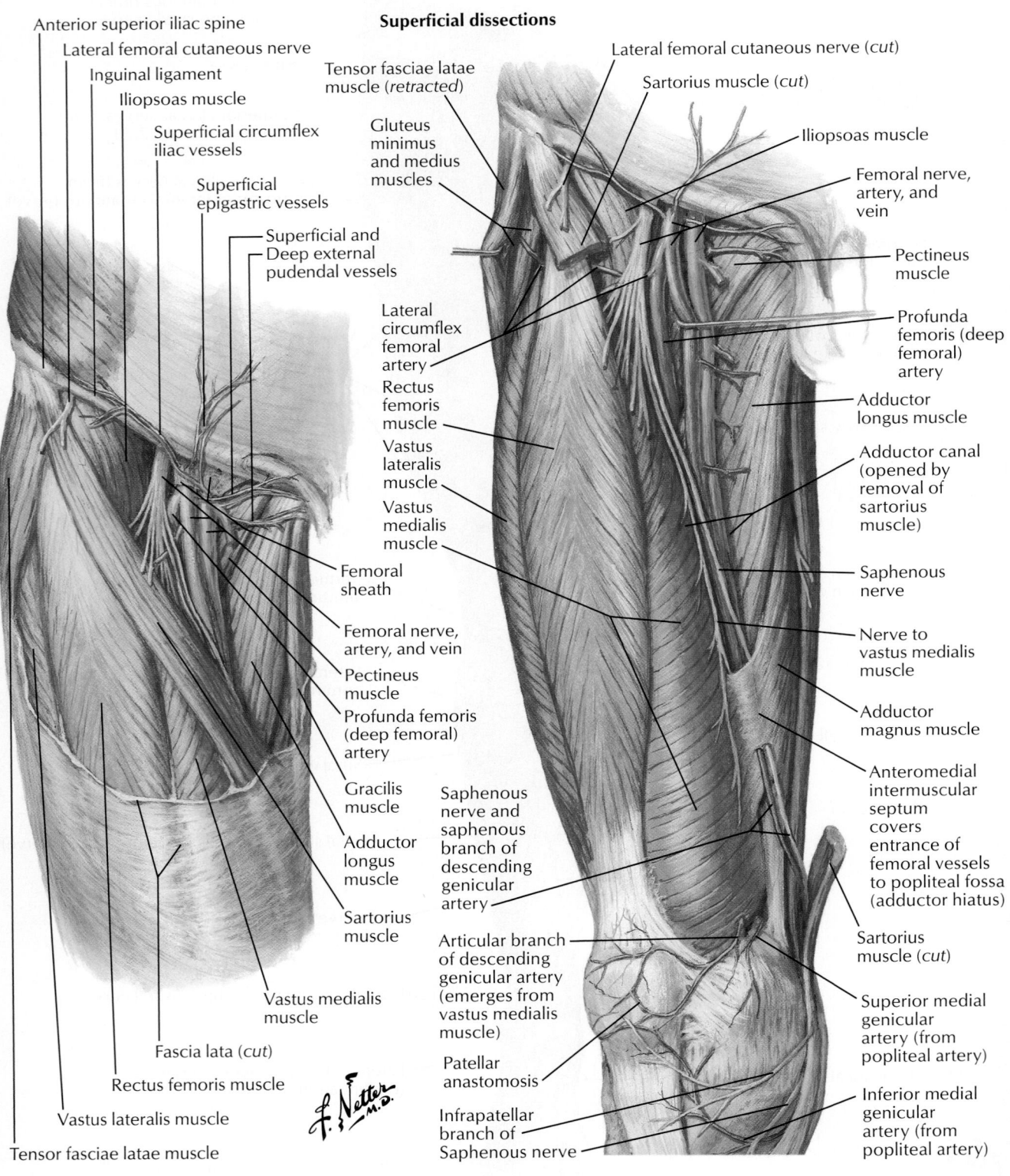

Superficial dissections

Anterior superior iliac spine

Lateral femoral cutaneous nerve

Inguinal ligament

Iliopsoas muscle

Superficial circumflex iliac vessels

Superficial epigastric vessels

Superficial and Deep external pudendal vessels

Tensor fasciae latae muscle (*retracted*)

Gluteus minimus and medius muscles

Lateral circumflex femoral artery

Rectus femoris muscle

Vastus lateralis muscle

Vastus medialis muscle

Femoral sheath

Femoral nerve, artery, and vein

Pectineus muscle

Profunda femoris (deep femoral) artery

Gracilis muscle

Adductor longus muscle

Sartorius muscle

Vastus medialis muscle

Fascia lata (*cut*)

Rectus femoris muscle

Vastus lateralis muscle

Tensor fasciae latae muscle

Lateral femoral cutaneous nerve (*cut*)

Sartorius muscle (*cut*)

Iliopsoas muscle

Femoral nerve, artery, and vein

Pectineus muscle

Profunda femoris (deep femoral) artery

Adductor longus muscle

Adductor canal (opened by removal of sartorius muscle)

Saphenous nerve

Nerve to vastus medialis muscle

Adductor magnus muscle

Anteromedial intermuscular septum covers entrance of femoral vessels to popliteal fossa (adductor hiatus)

Sartorius muscle (*cut*)

Superior medial genicular artery (from popliteal artery)

Inferior medial genicular artery (from popliteal artery)

Saphenous nerve and saphenous branch of descending genicular artery

Articular branch of descending genicular artery (emerges from vastus medialis muscle)

Patellar anastomosis

Infrapatellar branch of Saphenous nerve

Plate 500 Arteries and Nerves of Thigh: Anterior View. (Netter: Atlas of Human Anatomy, 4 ed, 2006, Saunders.)

Deep dissection

Deep circumflex iliac artery

Lateral femoral cutaneous nerve

Sartorius muscle (cut)

Iliopsoas muscle

Tensor fasciae latae muscle (retracted)

Gluteus medius and minimus muscles

Femoral nerve

Rectus femoris muscle (cut)

Ascending, transverse and descending branches of Lateral circumflex femoral artery

Medial circumflex femoral artery

Pectineus muscle (cut)

Profunda femoris (deep femoral) artery

Perforating branches

Adductor longus muscle (cut)

Vastus lateralis muscle

Vastus intermedius muscle

Rectus femoris muscle (cut)

Saphenous nerve

Anteromedial intermuscular septum (opened)

Vastus medialis muscle

Quadriceps femoris tendon

Patella and patellar anastomosis

Medial patellar retinaculum

Patellar ligament

External iliac artery and vein

Inguinal ligament (Poupart's)

Femoral artery and vein (cut)

Pectineus muscle (cut)

Obturator canal

Obturator externus muscle

Adductor longus muscle (cut)

Anterior branch and Posterior branch of obturator nerve

Quadratus femoris muscle

Adductor brevis muscle

Branches of posterior branch of obturator nerve

Adductor magnus muscle

Gracilis muscle

Cutaneous branch of obturator nerve

Femoral artery and vein (cut)

Descending genicular artery
Articular branch
Saphenous branch

Adductor hiatus

Sartorius muscle (cut)

Adductor magnus tendon

Adductor tubercle on medial epicondyle of femur

Superior medial genicular artery (from popliteal artery)

Infrapatellar branch of Saphenous nerve

Inferior medial genicular artery (from popliteal artery)

Plate 501 Arteries and Nerves of Thigh: Anterior View. (Netter: Atlas of Human Anatomy, 4 ed, 2006, Saunders.)

Deep dissection

Iliac crest

Superior clunial nerves

Gluteus maximus muscle (*cut*)

Medial clunial nerves

Inferior gluteal artery and nerve

Pudendal nerve

Nerve to obturator internus (and superior gemellus)

Posterior femoral cutaneous nerve

Sacrotuberous ligament

Ischial tuberosity

Inferior clunial nerves (*cut*)

Adductor magnus muscle

Gracilis muscle

Sciatic nerve

Muscular branches of sciatic nerve

Semitendinosus muscle (*retracted*)

Semimembranosus muscle

Sciatic nerve

Articular branch

Adductor hiatus

Popliteal vein and artery

Superior medial genicular artery

Medial epicondyle of femur

Tibial nerve

Gastrocnemius muscle (medial head)

Medial sural cutaneous nerve

Small saphenous vein

Gluteal aponeurosis and gluteus medius muscle (*cut*)

Superior gluteal artery and nerve

Gluteus minimus muscle

Tensor fasciae latae muscle

Piriformis muscle

Gluteus medius muscle (*cut*)

Superior gemellus muscle

Greater trochanter of femur

Obturator internus muscle

Inferior gemellus muscle

Gluteus maximus muscle (*cut*)

Quadratus femoris muscle

Medial circumflex femoral artery

Vastus lateralis muscle and iliotibial tract

Adductor minimus part of adductor magnus muscle

1st perforating artery (from profunda femoris artery)

Adductor magnus muscle

2nd and 3rd perforating arteries (from profunda femoris artery)

4th perforating artery (from profunda femoris artery)

Long head (*retracted*) ⎫ Biceps femoris
Short head   ⎬ muscle

Superior lateral genicular artery

Common fibular (peroneal) nerve

Plantaris muscle

Gastrocnemius muscle (lateral head)

Lateral sural cutaneous nerve

Plate 502   Arteries and Nerves of Thigh: Posterior View. (Netter: Atlas of Human Anatomy, 4 ed, 2006, Saunders.)

66

Horizontal section

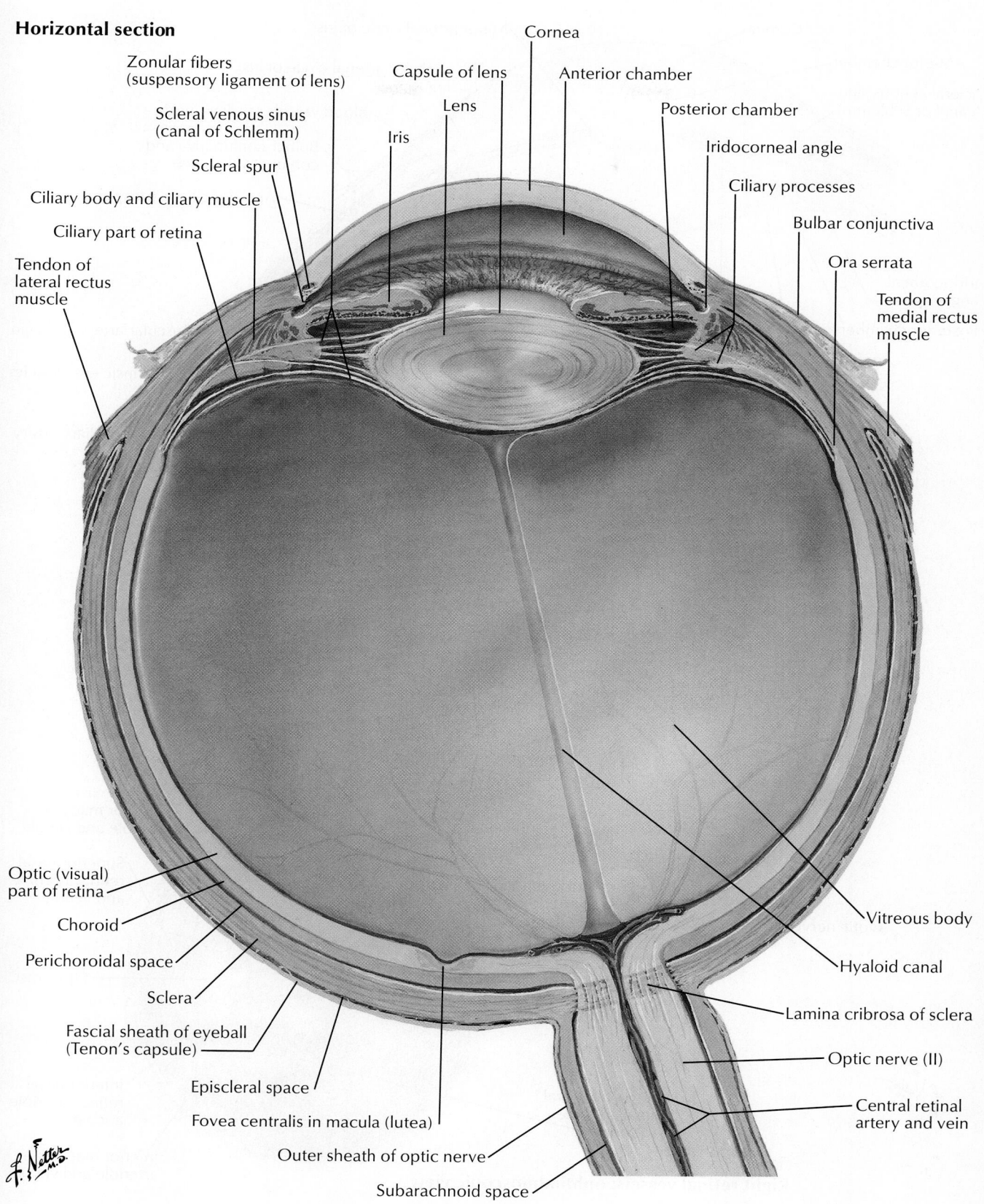

Zonular fibers
(suspensory ligament of lens)

Scleral venous sinus
(canal of Schlemm)

Scleral spur

Ciliary body and ciliary muscle

Ciliary part of retina

Tendon of
lateral rectus
muscle

Capsule of lens

Lens

Iris

Cornea

Anterior chamber

Posterior chamber

Iridocorneal angle

Ciliary processes

Bulbar conjunctiva

Ora serrata

Tendon of
medial rectus
muscle

Optic (visual)
part of retina

Choroid

Perichoroidal space

Sclera

Fascial sheath of eyeball
(Tenon's capsule)

Episcleral space

Fovea centralis in macula (lutea)

Outer sheath of optic nerve

Subarachnoid space

Vitreous body

Hyaloid canal

Lamina cribrosa of sclera

Optic nerve (II)

Central retinal
artery and vein

Plate 87   Eyeball. (Netter: Atlas of Human Anatomy, 4 ed, 2006, Saunders.)

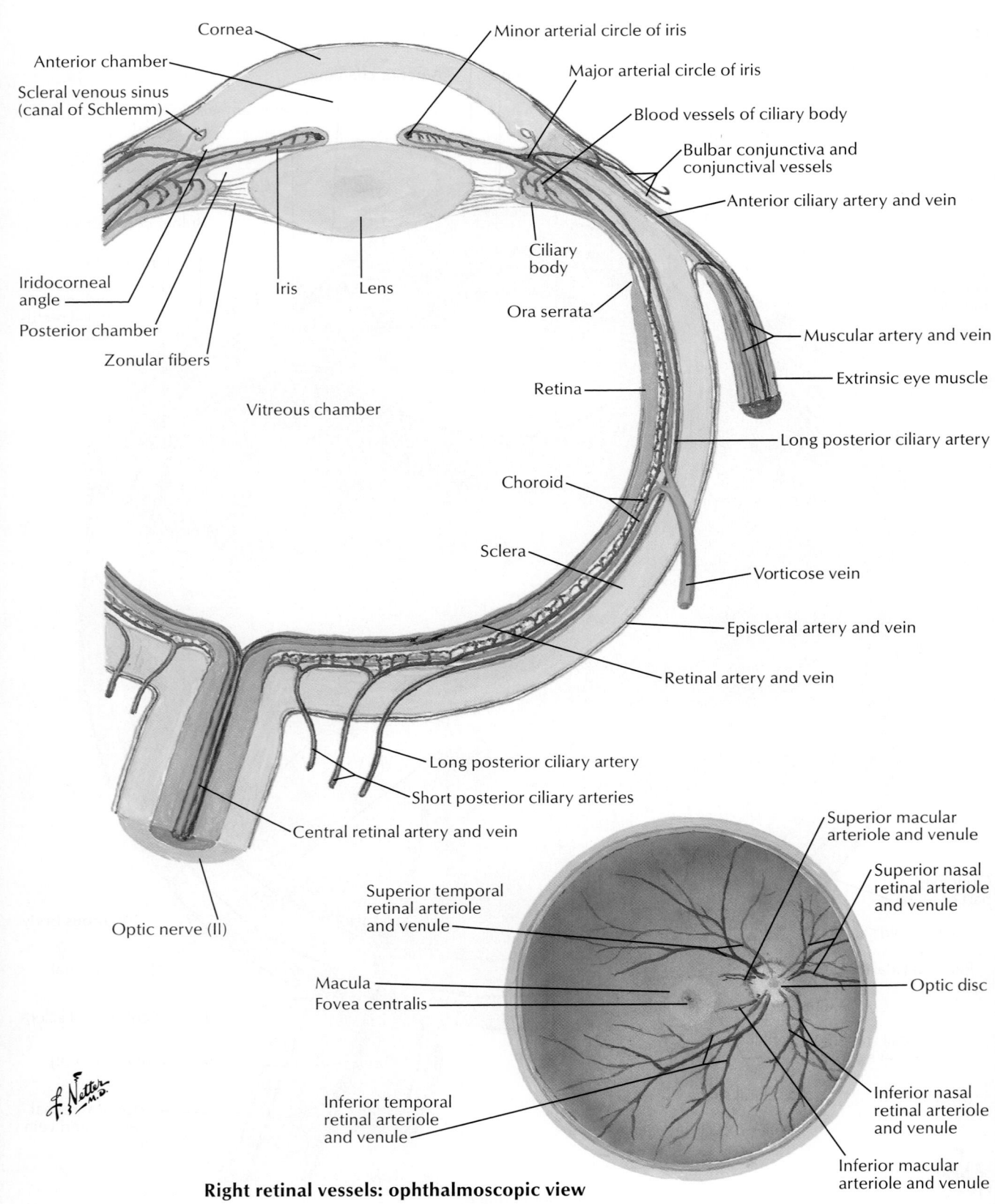

Cornea

Anterior chamber

Scleral venous sinus
(canal of Schlemm)

Minor arterial circle of iris

Major arterial circle of iris

Blood vessels of ciliary body

Bulbar conjunctiva and
conjunctival vessels

Anterior ciliary artery and vein

Iridocorneal
angle

Iris

Lens

Posterior chamber

Zonular fibers

Ciliary
body

Ora serrata

Vitreous chamber

Muscular artery and vein

Extrinsic eye muscle

Retina

Long posterior ciliary artery

Choroid

Sclera

Vorticose vein

Episcleral artery and vein

Retinal artery and vein

Long posterior ciliary artery

Short posterior ciliary arteries

Central retinal artery and vein

Optic nerve (II)

Superior macular
arteriole and venule

Superior nasal
retinal arteriole
and venule

Superior temporal
retinal arteriole
and venule

Macula

Fovea centralis

Optic disc

Inferior nasal
retinal arteriole
and venule

Inferior temporal
retinal arteriole
and venule

Inferior macular
arteriole and venule

Right retinal vessels: ophthalmoscopic view

Plate 90 Intrinsic Arteries and Veins of Eye. (Netter: Atlas of Human Anatomy, 4 ed, 2006, Saunders.)

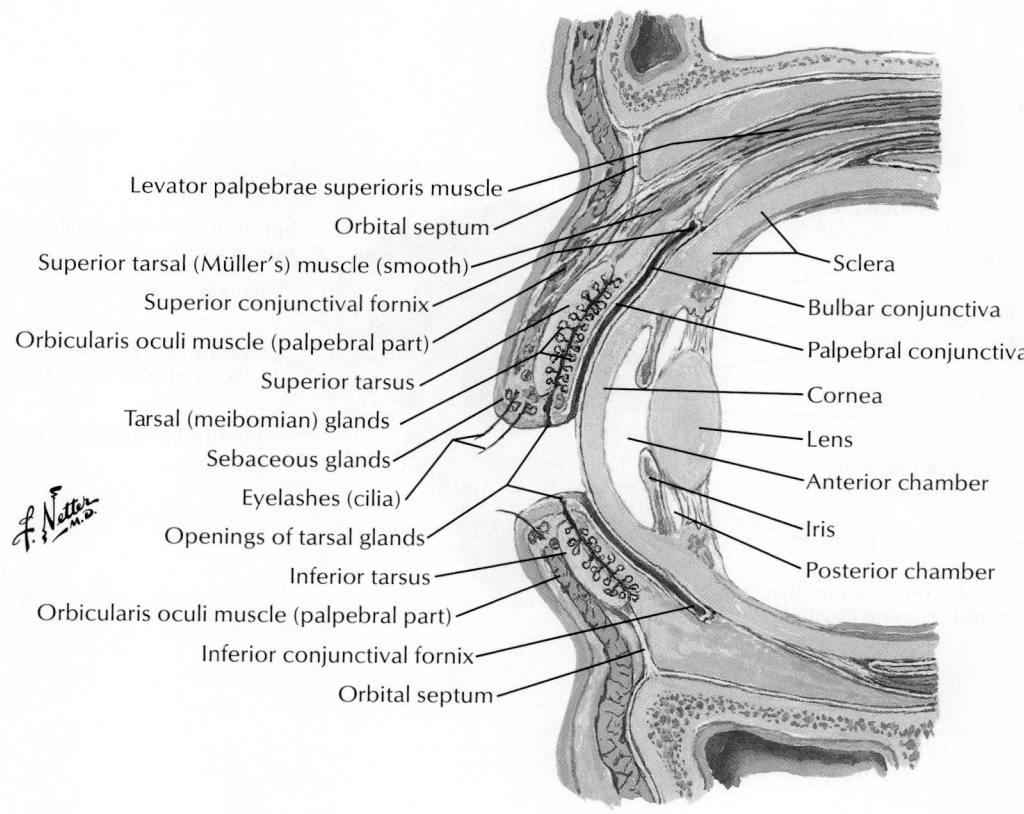

Levator palpebrae superioris muscle

Orbital septum

Superior tarsal (Müller's) muscle (smooth)

Superior conjunctival fornix

Orbicularis oculi muscle (palpebral part)

Superior tarsus

Tarsal (meibomian) glands

Sebaceous glands

Eyelashes (cilia)

Openings of tarsal glands

Inferior tarsus

Orbicularis oculi muscle (palpebral part)

Inferior conjunctival fornix

Orbital septum

Sclera

Bulbar conjunctiva

Palpebral conjunctiva

Cornea

Lens

Anterior chamber

Iris

Posterior chamber

Plate 81, Middle   Eyelid. (Netter: Atlas of Human Anatomy, 4 ed, 2006, Saunders.)

Superior palpebral conjunctiva:
tarsal (meibomian) glands
shining through

Seen through { Pupil
cornea { Iris

Corneoscleral junction
(corneal limbus)

Bulbar conjunctiva
over sclera

Inferior conjunctival fornix

Inferior palpebral conjunctiva:
tarsal glands shining through

Superior lacrimal papilla and
punctum

Plica semilunaris

Lacrimal caruncle in
lacrimal lake (lacus lacrimalis)

Inferior lacrimal papilla and
punctum

Plate 81, Upper   Eyelid. (Netter: Atlas of Human Anatomy, 4 ed, 2006, Saunders.)

Orbital part of lacrimal gland

Palpebral part of lacrimal gland

Excretory ducts of lacrimal gland

Plica semilunaris

Lacrimal caruncle

Inferior lacrimal papilla and punctum

Superior lacrimal papilla and punctum

Lacrimal canaliculi

Lacrimal sac

Nasolacrimal duct

Opening of nasolacrimal duct

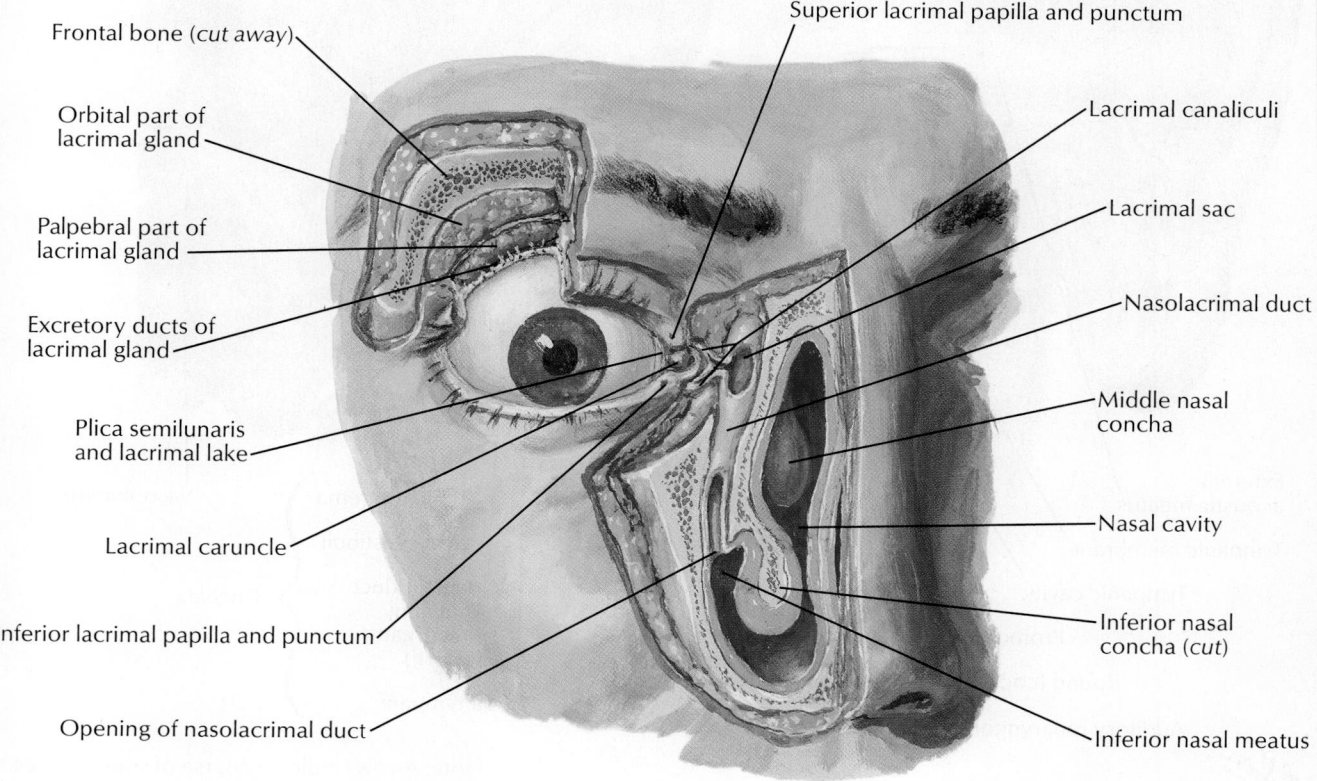

Frontal bone (*cut away*)

Orbital part of lacrimal gland

Palpebral part of lacrimal gland

Excretory ducts of lacrimal gland

Plica semilunaris and lacrimal lake

Lacrimal caruncle

Inferior lacrimal papilla and punctum

Opening of nasolacrimal duct

Superior lacrimal papilla and punctum

Lacrimal canaliculi

Lacrimal sac

Nasolacrimal duct

Middle nasal concha

Nasal cavity

Inferior nasal concha (*cut*)

Inferior nasal meatus

Plate 82   Lacrimal Apparatus. (Netter: Atlas of Human Anatomy, 4 ed, 2006, Saunders.)

Frontal section

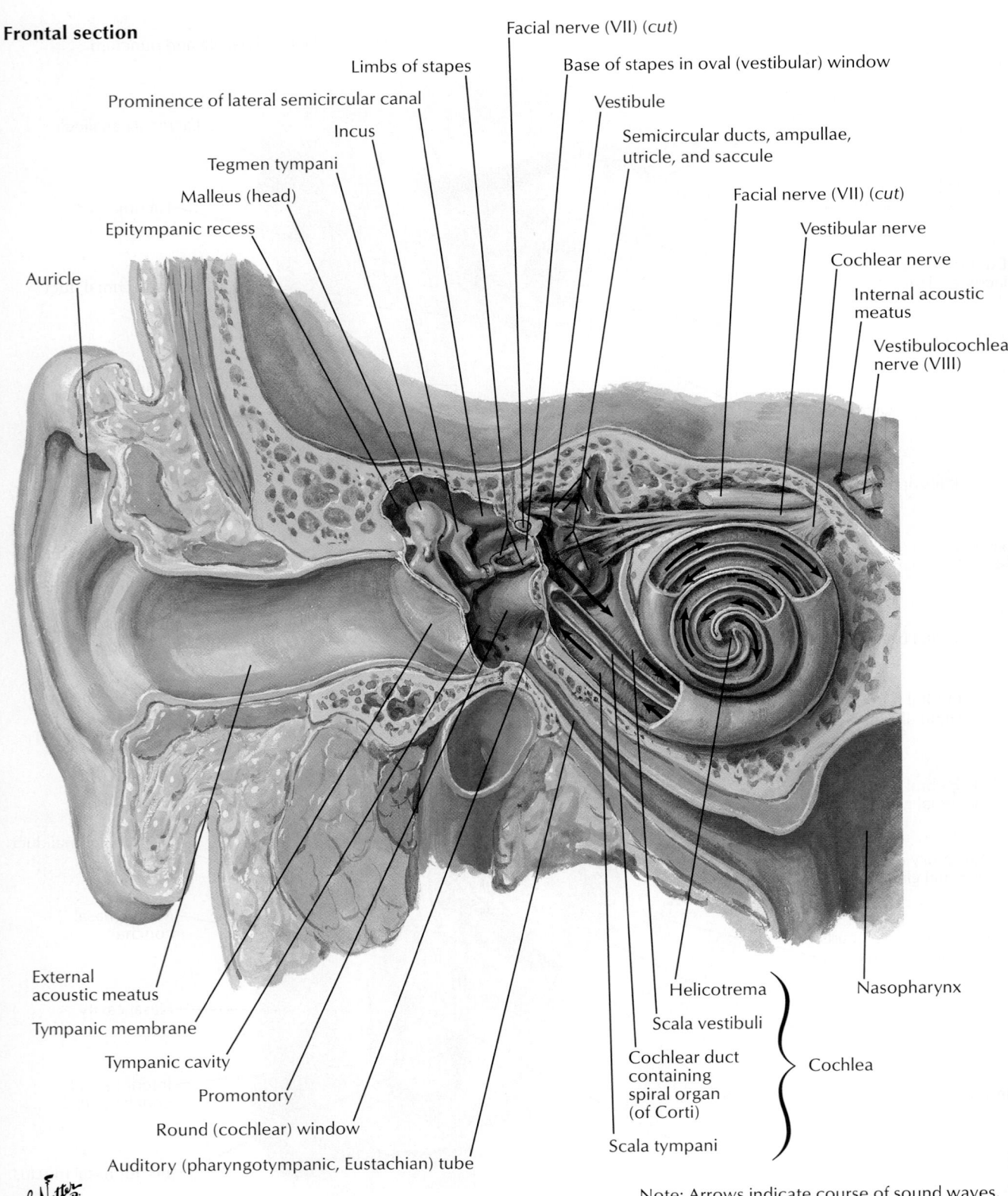

Facial nerve (VII) (*cut*)

Limbs of stapes

Base of stapes in oval (vestibular) window

Prominence of lateral semicircular canal

Vestibule

Incus

Semicircular ducts, ampullae, utricle, and saccule

Tegmen tympani

Malleus (head)

Facial nerve (VII) (*cut*)

Epitympanic recess

Vestibular nerve

Cochlear nerve

Auricle

Internal acoustic meatus

Vestibulocochlear nerve (VIII)

External acoustic meatus

Tympanic membrane

Tympanic cavity

Promontory

Round (cochlear) window

Auditory (pharyngotympanic, Eustachian) tube

Helicotrema

Scala vestibuli

Cochlear duct containing spiral organ (of Corti)

Scala tympani

Cochlea

Nasopharynx

Note: Arrows indicate course of sound waves.

Plate 92   Pathway of Sound Reception. (Netter: Atlas of Human Anatomy, 4 ed, 2006, Saunders.)

Medial wall of tympanic cavity: lateral view

Prominence of lateral semicircular canal

Prominence of facial canal

Geniculum (geniculate ganglion) of facial nerve

Greater petrosal nerve

Mastoid antrum

Base of stapes in fossa of oval (vestibular) window

Limbs of stapes

Pyramidal eminence

Chorda tympani nerve (*cut*)

Mastoid cells

Tendon of stapedius muscle

Fossa of round (cochlear) window

Facial nerve (VII) in stylomastoid foramen

Jugular fossa

Tympanic cells

Tensor tympani muscle (*tendon cut*)

Auditory (pharyngotympanic, Eustachian) tube

Levator veli palatini muscle

Promontory with tympanic nerve (of Jacobson) and plexus under mucosa

Internal carotid artery

Plate 94   Tympanic Cavity. (Netter: Atlas of Human Anatomy, 4 ed, 2006, Saunders.)

Otoscopic view of right tympanic membrane

Pars flaccida

Posterior mallear fold

Lateral process of malleus

Anterior mallear fold

Long limb of incus

Handle of malleus

Umbo

Cone of light

Tympanic

Pars tensa

Plate 93   Tympanic Cavity. (Netter: Atlas of Human Anatomy, 4 ed, 2006, Saunders.)

Dissected right bony labyrinth (otic capsule): membranous labyrinth removed

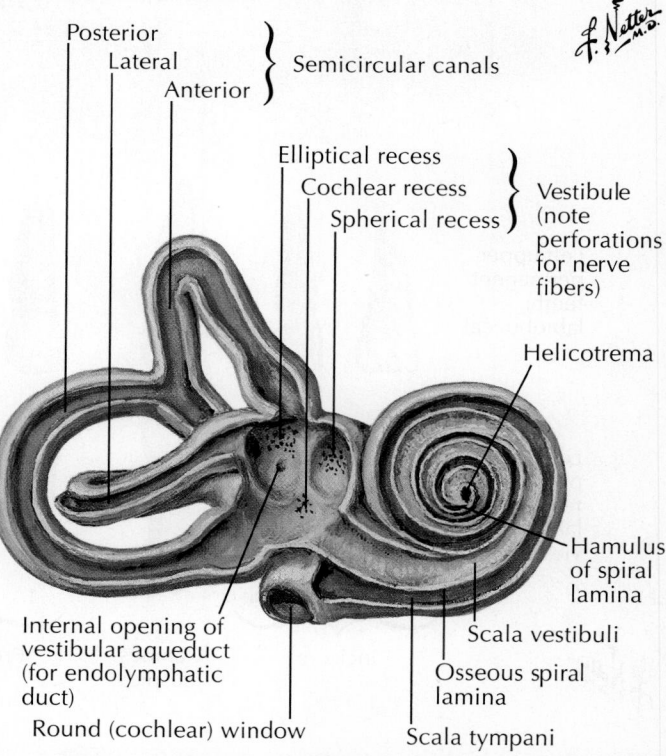

Posterior

Lateral

Anterior

Semicircular canals

Elliptical recess

Cochlear recess

Spherical recess

Vestibule (note perforations for nerve fibers)

Helicotrema

Hamulus of spiral lamina

Scala vestibuli

Osseous spiral lamina

Scala tympani

Internal opening of vestibular aqueduct (for endolymphatic duct)

Round (cochlear) window

Plate 95   Bony Membranous Labyrinth. (Netter: Atlas of Human Anatomy, 4 ed, 2006, Saunders.)

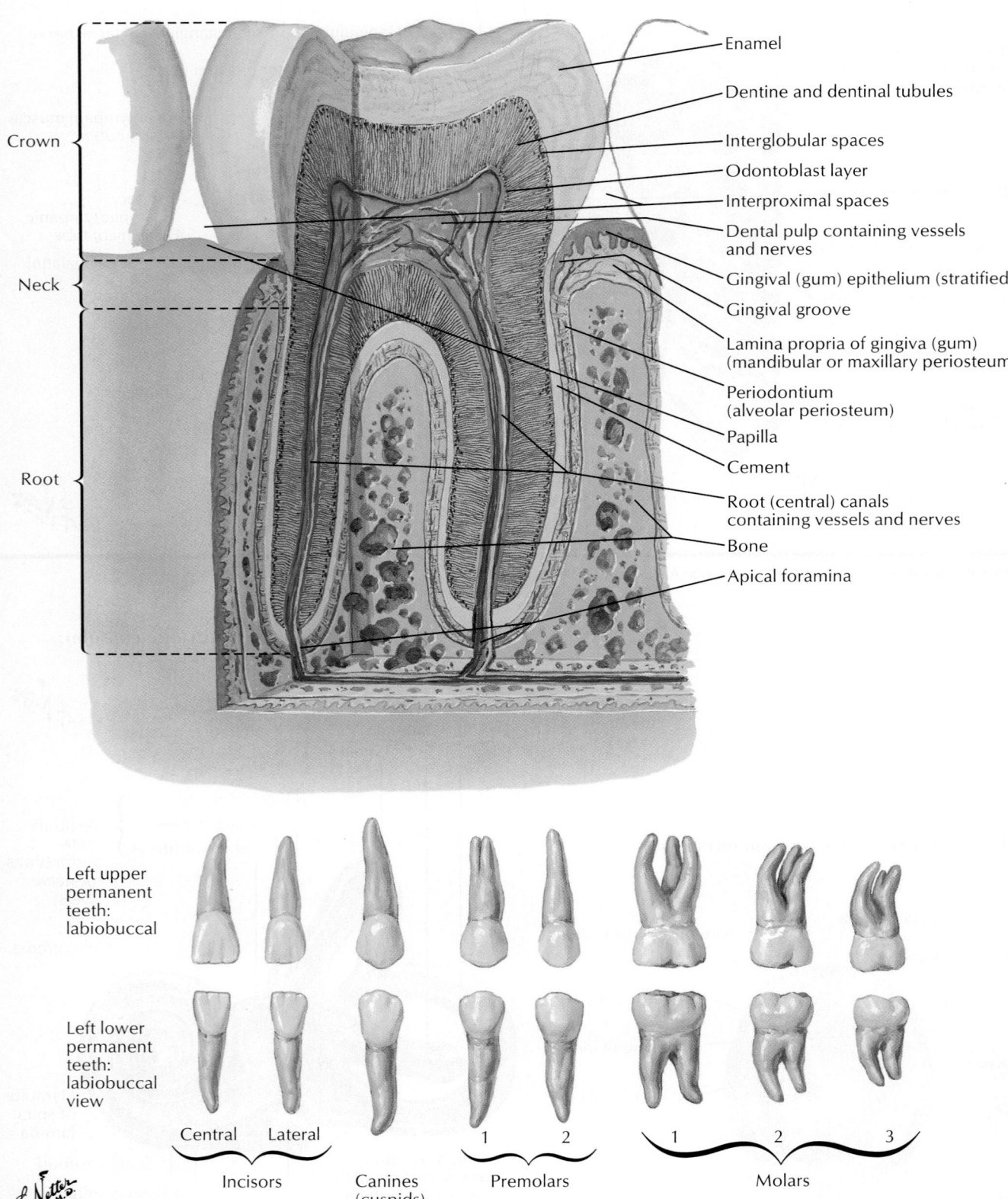

Crown

Neck

Root

Enamel

Dentine and dentinal tubules

Interglobular spaces

Odontoblast layer

Interproximal spaces

Dental pulp containing vessels and nerves

Gingival (gum) epithelium (stratified)

Gingival groove

Lamina propria of gingiva (gum) (mandibular or maxillary periosteum)

Periodontium (alveolar periosteum)

Papilla

Cement

Root (central) canals containing vessels and nerves

Bone

Apical foramina

Left upper permanent teeth: labiobuccal

Left lower permanent teeth: labiobuccal view

Central   Lateral

Incisors

Canines (cuspids)

1   2

Premolars

1   2   3

Molars

Plate 57   Teeth. (Netter: Atlas of Human Anatomy, 4 ed, 2006, Saunders.)

Tongue

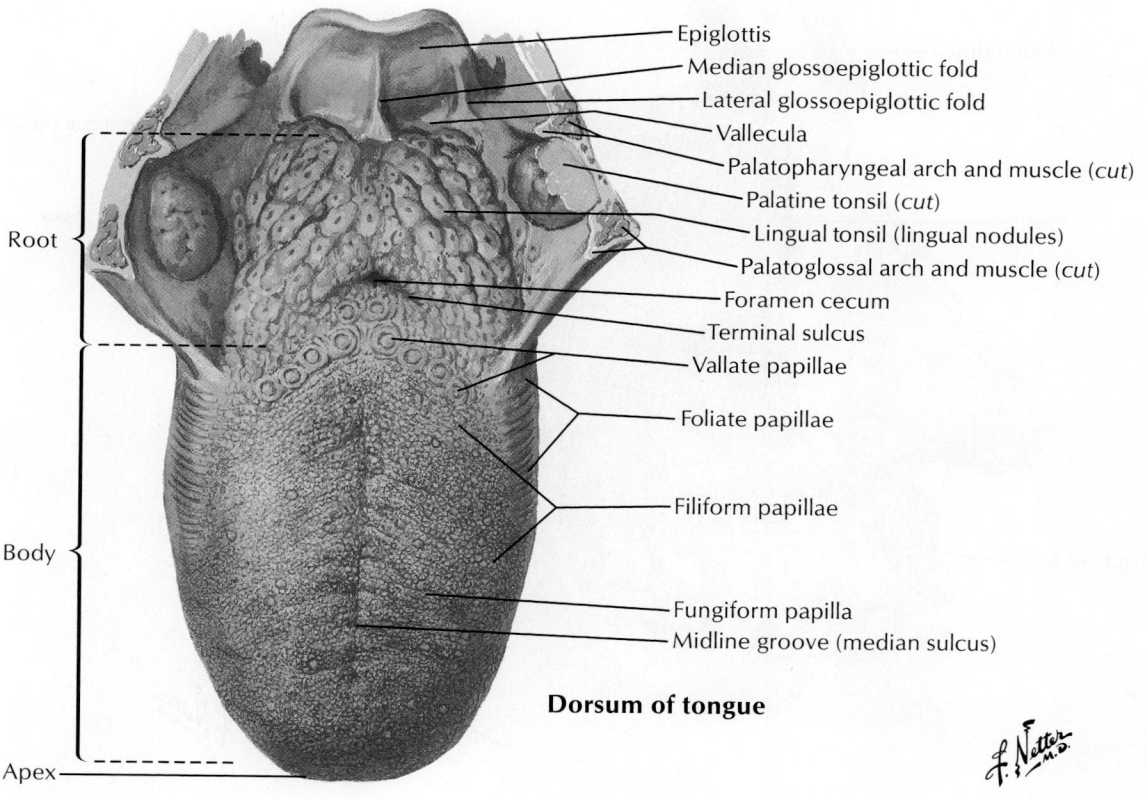

Epiglottis

Median glossoepiglottic fold

Lateral glossoepiglottic fold

Vallecula

Palatopharyngeal arch and muscle (*cut*)

Palatine tonsil (*cut*)

Lingual tonsil (lingual nodules)

Palatoglossal arch and muscle (*cut*)

Foramen cecum

Terminal sulcus

Vallate papillae

Foliate papillae

Filiform papillae

Fungiform papilla

Midline groove (median sulcus)

Root

Body

Apex

Dorsum of tongue

Plate 58   Tongue. (Netter: Atlas of Human Anatomy, 4 ed, 2006, Saunders.)

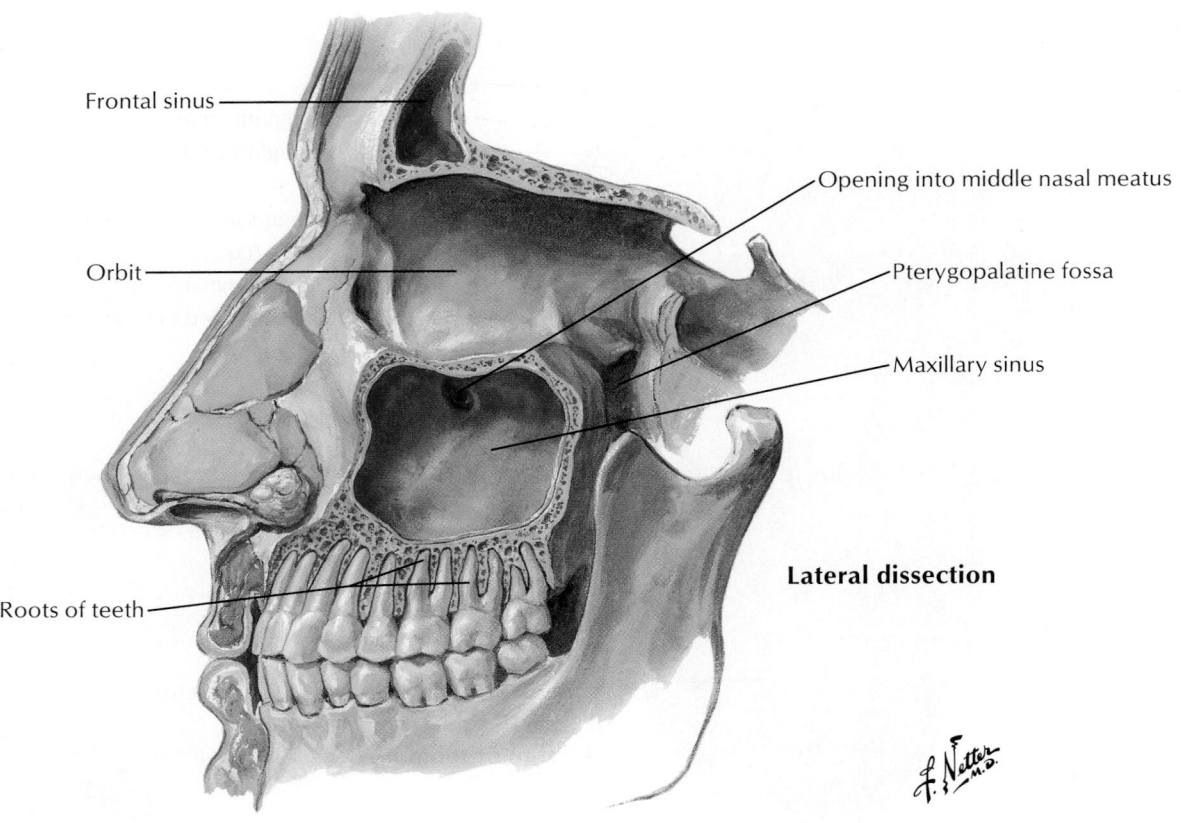

Frontal sinus

Opening into middle nasal meatus

Orbit

Pterygopalatine fossa

Maxillary sinus

Lateral dissection

Roots of teeth

Plate 49 Paranasal Sinuses. (Netter: Atlas of Human Anatomy, 4 ed, 2006, Saunders.)

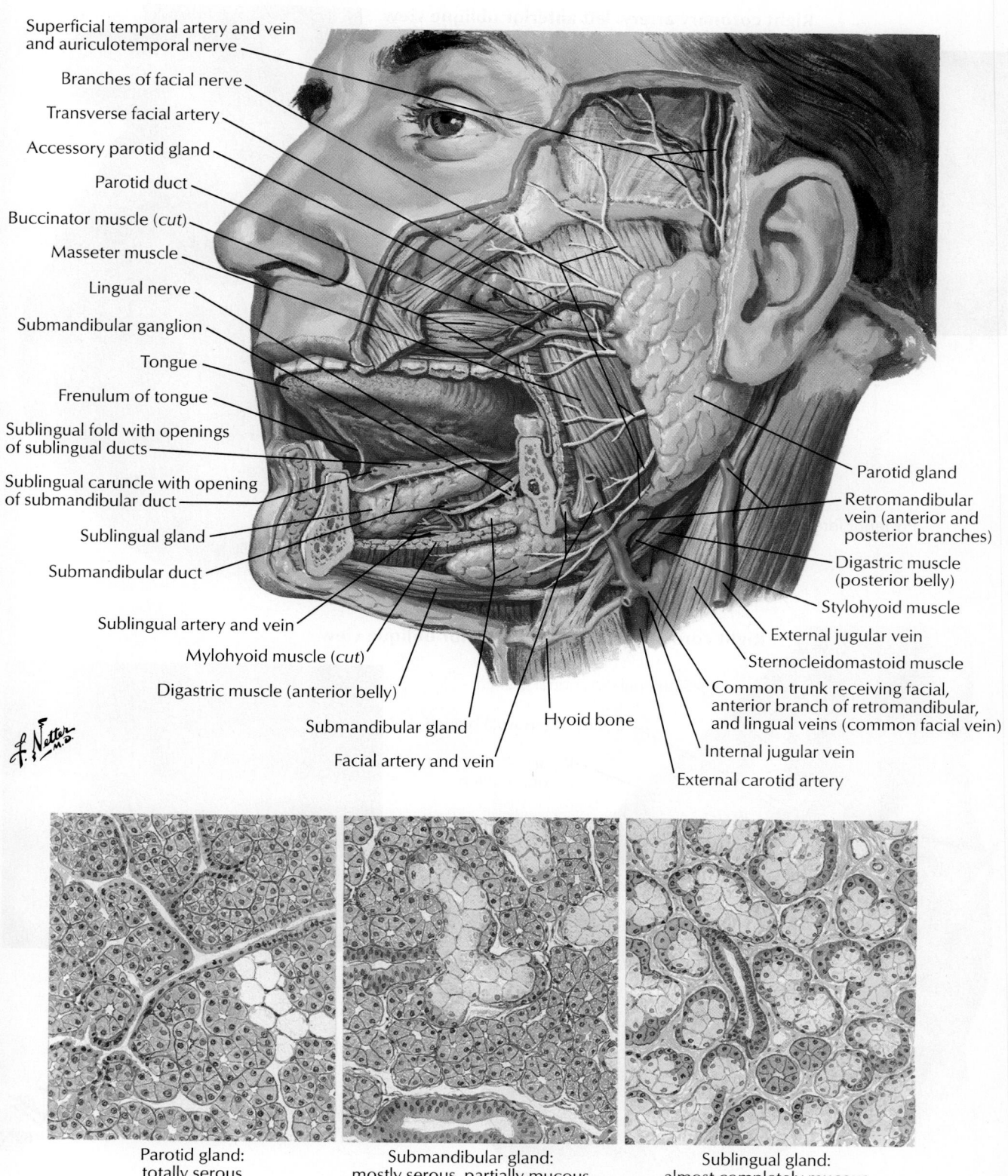

Superficial temporal artery and vein and auriculotemporal nerve

Branches of facial nerve

Transverse facial artery

Accessory parotid gland

Parotid duct

Buccinator muscle (*cut*)

Masseter muscle

Lingual nerve

Submandibular ganglion

Tongue

Frenulum of tongue

Sublingual fold with openings of sublingual ducts

Sublingual caruncle with opening of submandibular duct

Sublingual gland

Submandibular duct

Sublingual artery and vein

Mylohyoid muscle (*cut*)

Digastric muscle (anterior belly)

Submandibular gland

Facial artery and vein

Hyoid bone

Parotid gland

Retromandibular vein (anterior and posterior branches)

Digastric muscle (posterior belly)

Stylohyoid muscle

External jugular vein

Sternocleidomastoid muscle

Common trunk receiving facial, anterior branch of retromandibular, and lingual veins (common facial vein)

Internal jugular vein

External carotid artery

Parotid gland: totally serous

Submandibular gland: mostly serous, partially mucous

Sublingual gland: almost completely mucous

Plate 61   Salivary Glands. (Netter: Atlas of Human Anatomy, 4 ed, 2006, Saunders.)

Right coronary artery: left anterior oblique view

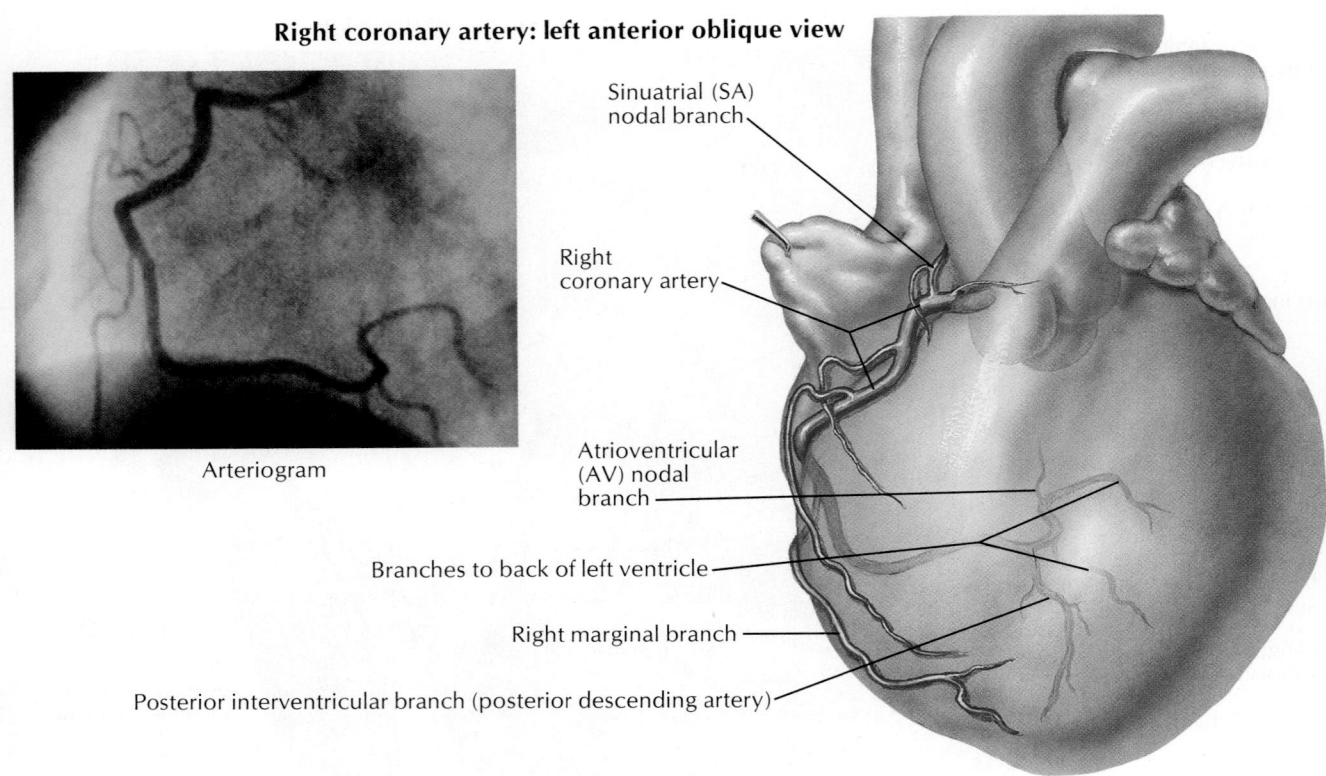

Arteriogram

Sinuatrial (SA) nodal branch

Right coronary artery

Atrioventricular (AV) nodal branch

Branches to back of left ventricle

Right marginal branch

Posterior interventricular branch (posterior descending artery)

Right coronary artery: right anterior oblique view

Sinuatrial (SA) nodal branch

Conus (arteriosus) branch

Right coronary artery

Right marginal branch

Arteriogram

Atrioventricular (AV) nodal branch

Right posterolateral branches (to back of left ventricle)

Posterior interventricular branch (posterior descending artery)

Plate 218   Coronary Arteries: Arteriographic Views. (Netter: Atlas of Human Anatomy, 4 ed, 2006, Saunders.)

Left coronary artery: left anterior oblique view

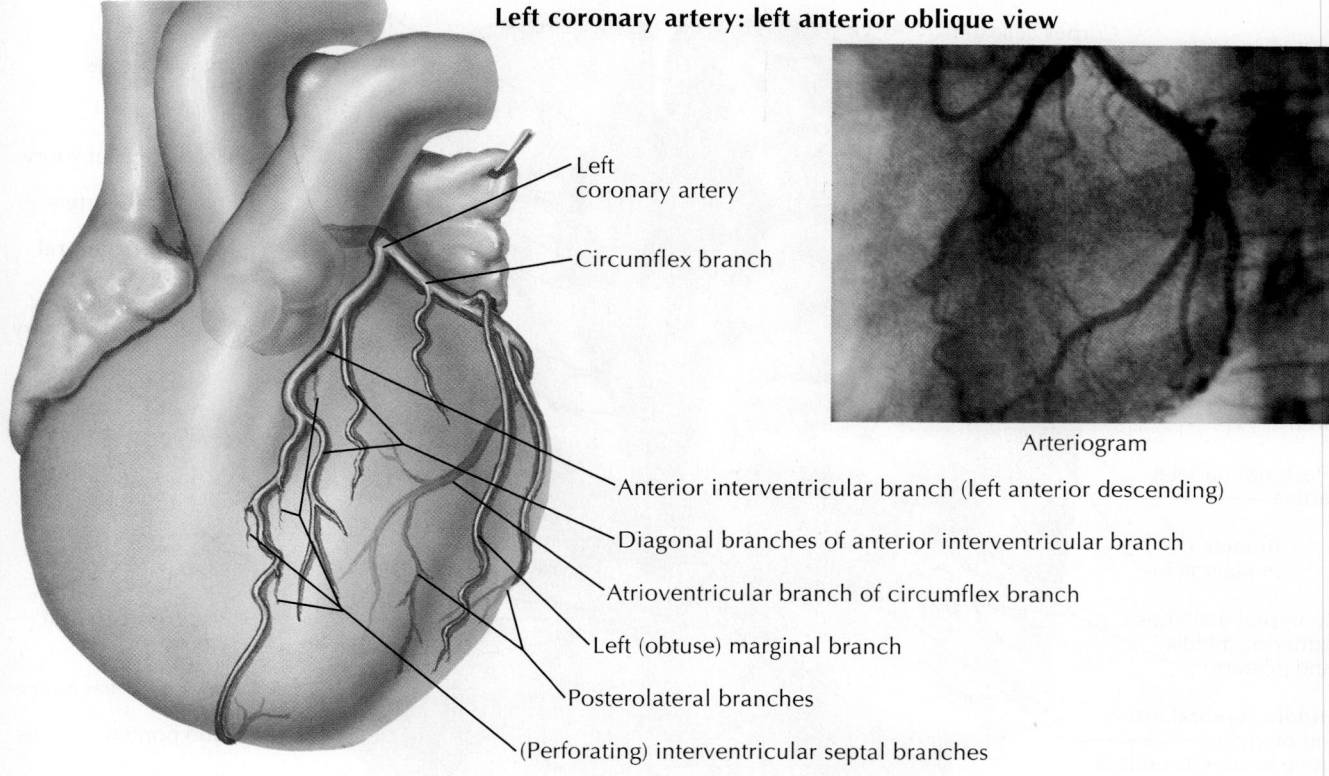

Left coronary artery

Circumflex branch

Arteriogram

Anterior interventricular branch (left anterior descending)

Diagonal branches of anterior interventricular branch

Atrioventricular branch of circumflex branch

Left (obtuse) marginal branch

Posterolateral branches

(Perforating) interventricular septal branches

Left coronary artery: right anterior oblique view

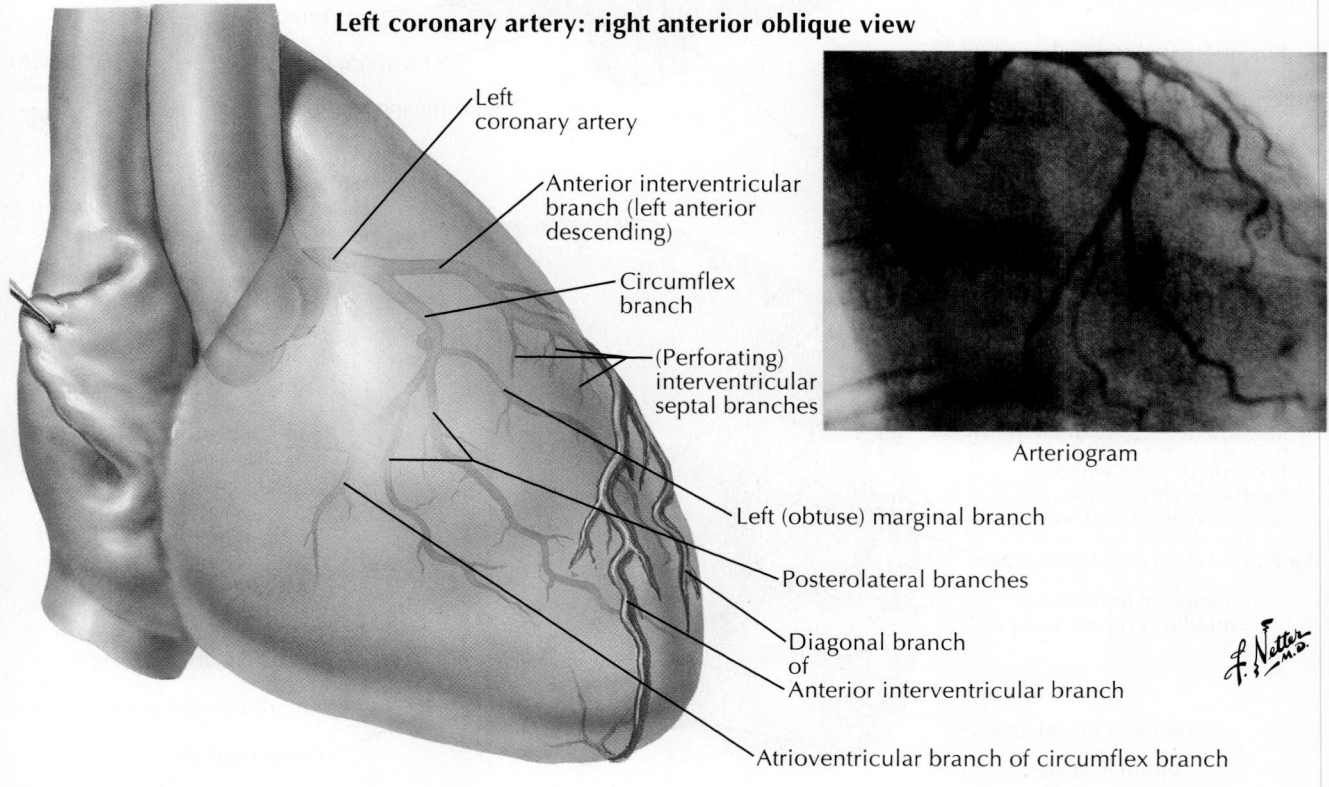

Left coronary artery

Anterior interventricular branch (left anterior descending)

Circumflex branch

(Perforating) interventricular septal branches

Arteriogram

Left (obtuse) marginal branch

Posterolateral branches

Diagonal branch of Anterior interventricular branch

Atrioventricular branch of circumflex branch

Plate 219 Coronary Arteries: Arteriographic Views. (Netter: Atlas of Human Anatomy, 4 ed, 2006, Saunders.)

Corpus callosum

Anterolateral central (lenticulostriate) arteries

Lateral frontobasal (orbitofrontal) artery

Prefrontal artery

Precentral (pre-Rolandic) and central (Rolandic) sulcal arteries

Anterior parietal (postcentral sulcal) artery

Posterior parietal artery

Branch to angular gyrus

Temporal branches (anterior, middle, and posterior)

Middle cerebral artery and branches (deep in lateral cerebral [Sylvian] sulcus)

Anterior communicating artery

Posterior communicating artery

Anterior inferior cerebellar artery (AICA)

Posterior spinal artery

Paracentral artery

Medial frontal branches

Pericallosal artery

Callosomarginal artery

Polar frontal artery

Anterior cerebral arteries

Medial frontobasal (orbitofrontal) artery

Distal medial striate artery (recurrent artery of Heubner)

Internal carotid artery

Anterior choroidal artery

Posterior cerebral artery

Superior cerebellar artery

Basilar and pontine arteries

Labyrinthine (internal acoustic) artery

Vertebral artery

Posterior inferior cerebellar artery (PICA)

Anterior spinal artery

Corpus striatum (caudate and lentiform nuclei)

Anterolateral central (lenticulostriate) arteries

Insula (island of Reil)

Limen of insula

Precentral (pre-Rolandic), central (Rolandic) sulcal, and parietal arteries

Lateral cerebral (Sylvian) sulcus

Temporal branches of middle cerebral artery

Temporal lobe

Middle cerebral artery

Internal carotid artery

Falx cerebri

Callosomarginal arteries and Pericallosal arteries (branches of anterior cerebral arteries)

Trunk of corpus callosum

Internal capsule

Septum pellucidum

Rostrum of corpus callosum

Anterior cerebral arteries

Distal medial striate artery (recurrent artery of Heubner)

Anterior communicating artery

Optic chiasm

Plate 141 Arteries of Brain: Frontal View and Section. (Netter: Atlas of Human Anatomy, 4 ed, 2006, Saunders.)

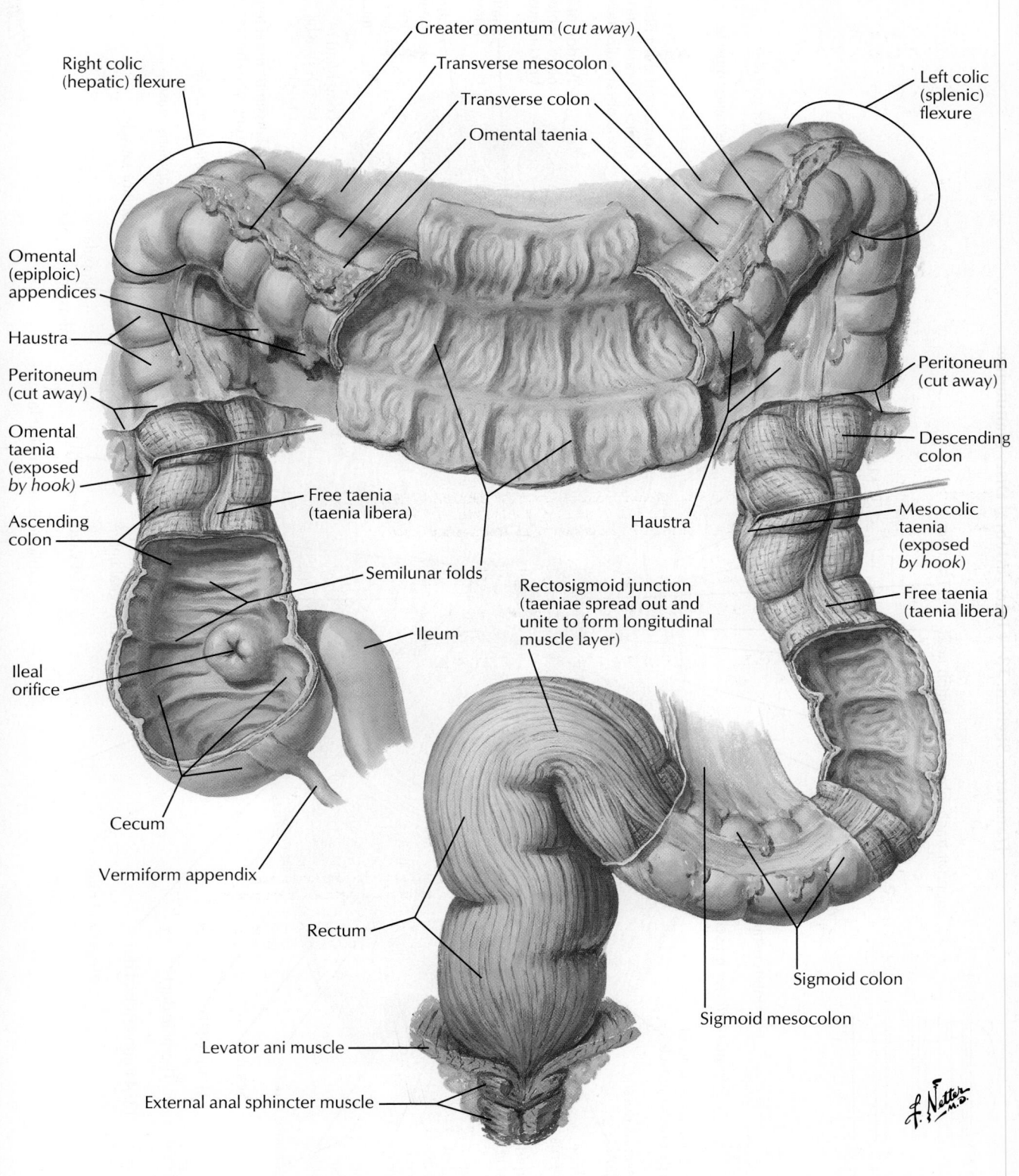

Right colic (hepatic) flexure

Greater omentum (*cut away*)

Transverse mesocolon

Transverse colon

Omental taenia

Left colic (splenic) flexure

Omental (epiploic) appendices

Haustra

Peritoneum (cut away)

Omental taenia (exposed *by hook*)

Ascending colon

Peritoneum (cut away)

Descending colon

Free taenia (taenia libera)

Haustra

Mesocolic taenia (exposed *by hook*)

Free taenia (taenia libera)

Semilunar folds

Ileum

Rectosigmoid junction (taeniae spread out and unite to form longitudinal muscle layer)

Ileal orifice

Cecum

Vermiform appendix

Rectum

Sigmoid colon

Sigmoid mesocolon

Levator ani muscle

External anal sphincter muscle

Plate 284 Mucosa and Musculature of Large Intestine. (Netter: Atlas of Human Anatomy, 4 ed, 2006, Saunders.)

Transverse Section: T3-4 Intervertebral Disc, Manubrium

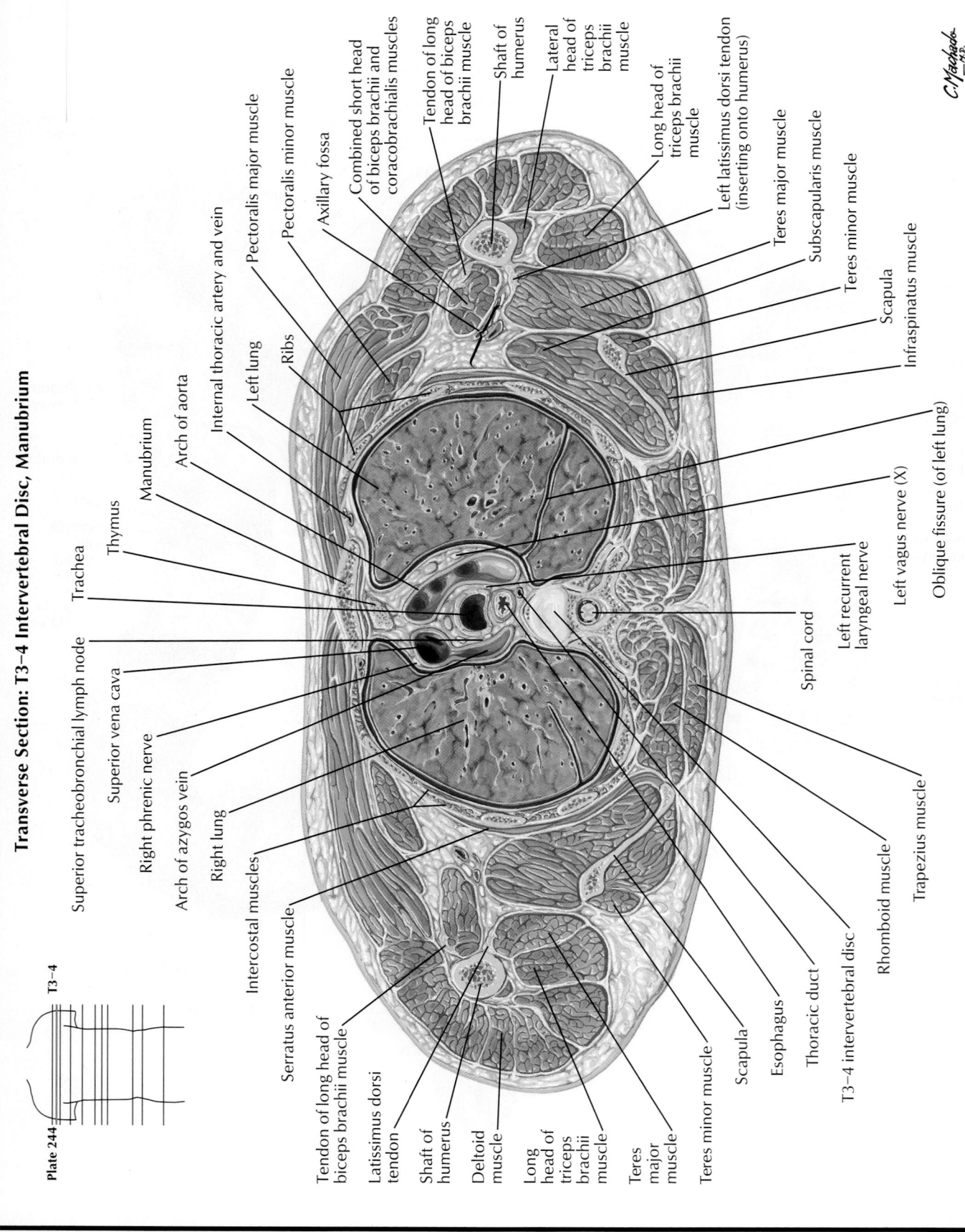

T3-4

Plate 244

Superior tracheobronchial lymph node
Trachea
Thymus
Manubrium
Arch of aorta
Internal thoracic artery and vein
Left lung
Ribs
Pectoralis major muscle
Axillary fossa
Combined short head of biceps brachii and coracobrachialis muscles
Tendon of long head of biceps brachii muscle
Shaft of humerus
Lateral head of triceps brachii muscle
Long head of triceps brachii muscle
Left latissimus dorsi tendon (inserting onto humerus)
Teres major muscle
Subscapularis muscle
Teres minor muscle
Scapula
Infraspinatus muscle

Pectoralis minor muscle

Superior vena cava
Right phrenic nerve
Arch of azygos vein
Right lung
Intercostal muscles
Serratus anterior muscle
Tendon of long head of biceps brachii muscle
Latissimus dorsi tendon
Shaft of humerus
Deltoid muscle
Long head of triceps brachii muscle
Teres major muscle
Teres minor muscle
Scapula
Esophagus
Thoracic duct
T3-4 intervertebral disc
Rhomboid muscle
Trapezius muscle

Spinal cord
Left recurrent laryngeal nerve
Left vagus nerve (X)
Oblique fissure (of left lung)

Plate 244 Cross Section of Thorax at T3-4 Disc Level. (Netter: Atlas of Human Anatomy, 4 ed, 2006, Saunders.)

82

Right knee in extension: posterior view

Posterior cruciate ligament

Anterior cruciate ligament

Posterior meniscofemoral ligament

Adductor tubercle on medial epicondyle of femur

Lateral condyle of femur (articular surface)

Medial condyle of femur (articular surface)

Popliteus tendon

Medial meniscus

Fibular collateral ligament

Tibial collateral ligament

Lateral meniscus

Medial condyle of tibia

Head of fibula

Plate 509   Knee: Cruciate and Collateral Ligaments. (Netter: Atlas of Human Anatomy, 4 ed, 2006, Saunders.)

Paramedian (sagittal) dissection

Ureter

Uterine (fallopian) tube

Ovary

Ligament of ovary

Round ligament of uterus

Broad ligament (*cut*)

Superior pubic ramus (*cut*)

Inferior pubic ramus (*cut*)

Ischiocavernosus muscle

Body of clitoris

Labia minora

Labium majus

Rectouterine pouch (of Douglas)

Peritoneum (*cut edge*)

Vesicouterine pouch

Rectum

Ureter

Urinary bladder

Vagina

Pelvic diaphragm (levator ani muscle)

Deep transverse perineal muscle (*cut*)

External anal sphincter muscle

Median (sagittal) section

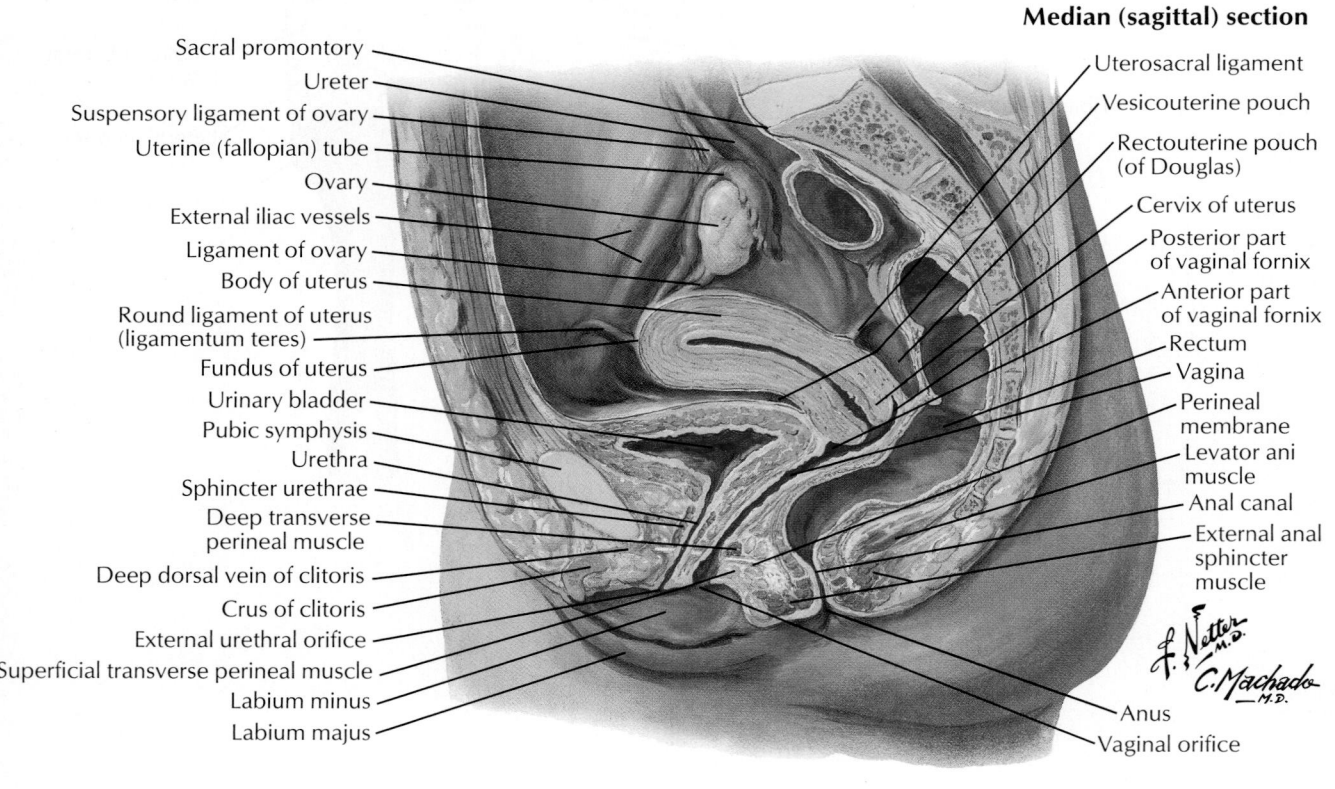

Sacral promontory

Ureter

Suspensory ligament of ovary

Uterine (fallopian) tube

Ovary

External iliac vessels

Ligament of ovary

Body of uterus

Round ligament of uterus (ligamentum teres)

Fundus of uterus

Urinary bladder

Pubic symphysis

Urethra

Sphincter urethrae

Deep transverse perineal muscle

Deep dorsal vein of clitoris

Crus of clitoris

External urethral orifice

Superficial transverse perineal muscle

Labium minus

Labium majus

Uterosacral ligament

Vesicouterine pouch

Rectouterine pouch (of Douglas)

Cervix of uterus

Posterior part of vaginal fornix

Anterior part of vaginal fornix

Rectum

Vagina

Perineal membrane

Levator ani muscle

Anal canal

External anal sphincter muscle

Anus

Vaginal orifice

Plate 360 Pelvic Viscera and Perineum: Female. (Netter: Atlas of Human Anatomy, 4 ed, 2006, Saunders.)

Alphabetic Index Volume 2

A

AAT (alpha-1 antitrypsin) deficiency 273.4
AAV (disease) (illness) (infection) - *see* Human immunodeficiency virus (disease) (illness) (infection)
Abactio - *see* Abortion, induced
Abactus venter - *see* Abortion, induced
Abarognosis 781.99
Abasia (-astasia) 307.9
   atactica 781.3
   choreic 781.3
   hysterical 300.11
   paroxysmal trepidant 781.3
   spastic 781.3
   trembling 781.3
   trepidans 781.3
Abderhalden-Kaufmann-Lignac syndrome (cystinosis) 270.0
Abdomen, abdominal - *see also* condition
   accordion 306.4
   acute 789.0●
   angina 557.1
   burst 868.00
   convulsive equivalent (*see also* Epilepsy) 345.5●
   heart 746.87
   muscle deficiency syndrome 756.79
   obstipum 756.79
Abdominalgia 789.0●
   periodic 277.31
Abduction contracture, hip or other joint - *see* Contraction, joint
Abercrombie's syndrome (amyloid degeneration) 277.39
Aberrant (congenital) - *see also* Malposition, congenital
   adrenal gland 759.1
   blood vessel NEC 747.60
      arteriovenous NEC 747.60
      cerebrovascular 747.81
      gastrointestinal 747.61
      lower limb 747.64
      renal 747.62
      spinal 747.82
      upper limb 747.63
   breast 757.6
   endocrine gland NEC 759.2
   gastrointestinal vessel (peripheral) 747.61
   hepatic duct 751.69
   lower limb vessel (peripheral) 747.64
   pancreas 751.7
   parathyroid gland 759.2
   peripheral vascular vessel NEC 747.60
   pituitary gland (pharyngeal) 759.2
   renal blood vessel 747.62
   sebaceous glands, mucous membrane, mouth 750.26
   spinal vessel 747.82
   spleen 759.0
   testis (descent) 752.51
   thymus gland 759.2
   thyroid gland 759.2
   upper limb vessel (peripheral) 747.63
Aberratio
   lactis 757.6
   testis 752.51
Aberration - *see also* Anomaly
   chromosome - *see* Anomaly, chromosome(s)
   distantial 368.9
   mental (*see also* Disorder, mental, nonpsychotic) 300.9
Abetalipoproteinemia 272.5
Abionarce 780.79
Abiotrophy 799.89
Ablatio
   placentae - *see* Placenta, ablatio
   retinae (*see also* Detachment, retina) 361.9

Ablation
   pituitary (gland) (with hypofunction) 253.7
   placenta - *see* Placenta, ablatio
   uterus 621.8
Ablepharia, ablepharon, ablephary 743.62
Ablepsia - *see* Blindness
Ablepsy - *see* Blindness
Ablutomania 300.3
Abnormal, abnormality, abnormalities - *see also* Anomaly
   acid-base balance 276.4
      fetus or newborn - *see* Distress, fetal
   adaptation curve, dark 368.63
   alveolar ridge 525.9
   amnion 658.9●
      affecting fetus or newborn 762.9
   anatomical relationship NEC 759.9
   apertures, congenital, diaphragm 756.6
   auditory perception NEC 388.40
   autosomes NEC 758.5
      13 758.1
      18 758.2
      21 or 22 758.0
      D_1 758.1
      E_3 758.2
      G 758.0
   ballistocardiogram 794.39
   basal metabolic rate (BMR) 794.7
   biosynthesis, testicular androgen 257.2
   blood level (of)
      cobalt 790.6
      copper 790.6
      iron 790.6
      lead 790.6
      lithium 790.6
      magnesium 790.6
      mineral 790.6
      zinc 790.6
   blood pressure
      elevated (without diagnosis of hypertension) 796.2
      low (*see also* Hypotension) 458.9
      reading (incidental) (isolated) (nonspecific) 796.3
   blood sugar 790.29
   bowel sounds 787.5
   breathing behavior - *see* Respiration
   caloric test 794.19
   cervix (acquired) NEC 622.9
      congenital 752.40
      in pregnancy or childbirth 654.6●
         causing obstructed labor 660.2●
            affecting fetus or newborn 763.1
   chemistry, blood NEC 790.6
   chest sounds 786.7
   chorion 658.9●
      affecting fetus or newborn 762.9
   chromosomal NEC 758.89
      analysis, nonspecific result 795.2
      autosomes (*see also* Abnormal, autosomes NEC) 758.5
      fetal, (suspected) affecting management of pregnancy 655.1●
      sex 758.81
   clinical findings NEC 796.4
   communication - *see* Fistula
   configuration of pupils 379.49
   coronary
      artery 746.85
      vein 746.9
   cortisol-binding globulin 255.8
   course, Eustachian tube 744.24
   creatinine clearance 794.4
   dentofacial NEC 524.9
      functional 524.50
      specified type NEC 524.89
   development, developmental NEC 759.9
      bone 756.9
      central nervous system 742.9
   direction, teeth 524.30

Abnormal, abnormality, abnormalities (Continued)
   dynia (*see also* Defect, coagulation) 286.9
   Ebstein 746.2
   echocardiogram 793.2
   echoencephalogram 794.01
   echogram NEC - *see* Findings, abnormal, structure
   electrocardiogram (ECG) (EKG) 794.31
   electroencephalogram (EEG) 794.02
   electromyogram (EMG) 794.17
      ocular 794.14
   electro-oculogram (EOG) 794.12
   electroretinogram (ERG) 794.11
   erythrocytes 289.9
      congenital, with perinatal jaundice 282.9 [774.0]
   eustachian valve 746.9
   excitability under minor stress 301.9
   fat distribution 782.9
   feces 787.7
   fetal heart rate - *see* Distress, fetal
   fetus NEC
      affecting management of pregnancy - *see* Pregnancy, management affected by, fetal
      causing disproportion 653.7●
         affecting fetus or newborn 763.1
         causing obstructed labor 660.1●
            affecting fetus or newborn 763.1
   findings without manifest disease - *see* Findings, abnormal
   fluid
      amniotic 792.3
      cerebrospinal 792.0
      peritoneal 792.9
      pleural 792.9
      synovial 792.9
      vaginal 792.9
   forces of labor NEC 661.9●
      affecting fetus or newborn 763.7
   form, teeth 520.2
   function studies
      auditory 794.15
      bladder 794.9
      brain 794.00
      cardiovascular 794.30
      endocrine NEC 794.6
      kidney 794.4
      liver 794.8
      nervous system
         central 794.00
         peripheral 794.19
      oculomotor 794.14
      pancreas 794.9
      placenta 794.9
      pulmonary 794.2
      retina 794.11
      special senses 794.19
      spleen 794.9
      thyroid 794.5
      vestibular 794.16
   gait 781.2
      hysterical 300.11
   gastrin secretion 251.5
   globulin
      cortisol-binding 255.8
      thyroid-binding 246.8
   glucagon secretion 251.4
   glucose 790.29
      in pregnancy, childbirth, or puerperium 648.8●
         fetus or newborn 775.0
      non-fasting 790.29
   gravitational (G) forces or states 994.9
   hair NEC 704.2
   hard tissue formation in pulp 522.3
   head movement 781.0

◀ New   ◀═ Revised   ~~deleted~~ Deleted   ● Use Additional Digit(s)   ▓ Omit code

Abnormal, abnormality, abnormalities
  (Continued)
  heart
    rate
      fetus, affecting liveborn infant
        before the onset of labor 763.81
        during labor 763.82
        unspecified as to time of onset
          763.83
      intrauterine
        before the onset of labor 763.81
        during labor 763.82
        unspecified as to time of onset
          763.83
      newborn
        before the onset of labor 763.81
        during labor 763.82
        unspecified as to time of onset
          763.83
    shadow 793.2
    sounds NEC 785.3
  hemoglobin (see also Disease, hemoglobin)
    282.7
    trait - see Trait, hemoglobin, abnormal
  hemorrhage, uterus - see Hemorrhage, uterus
  histology NEC 795.4
  increase in
    appetite 783.6
    development 783.9
  involuntary movement 781.0
  jaw closure 524.51
  karyotype 795.2
  knee jerk 796.1
  labor NEC 661.9●
    affecting fetus or newborn 763.7
  laboratory findings - see Findings, abnormal
  length, organ or site, congenital - see
    Distortion
  liver function test 790.6
  loss of height 781.91
  loss of weight 783.21
  lung shadow 793.19
  mammogram 793.80
    calcification 793.89
    calculus 793.89
    microcalcification 793.81
  Mantoux test 795.51
  membranes (fetal)
    affecting fetus or newborn 762.9
    complicating pregnancy 658.8●
  menstruation - see Menstruation
  metabolism (see also condition) 783.9
  movement 781.0
    disorder NEC 333.90
      sleep related, unspecified 780.58
      specified NEC 333.99
    head 781.0
    involuntary 781.0
    specified type NEC 333.99
  muscle contraction, localized 728.85
  myoglobin (Aberdeen) (Annapolis) 289.9
  narrowness, eyelid 743.62
  optokinetic response 379.57
  organs or tissues of pelvis NEC
    in pregnancy or childbirth 654.9●
      affecting fetus or newborn 763.89
      causing obstructed labor 660.2●
        affecting fetus or newborn 763.1
  origin - see Malposition, congenital
  palmar creases 757.2
  Papanicolaou (smear)
    anus 796.70
      with
        atypical squamous cells
          cannot exclude high grade
            squamous intraepithelial
            lesion (ASC-H) 796.72
          of undetermined significance
            (ASC-US) 796.71
        cytologic evidence of malignancy
          796.76

Abnormal, abnormality, abnormalities
  (Continued)
  Papanicolaou (Continued)
    anus (Continued)
      with (Continued)
        high grade squamous
          intraepithelial lesion (HGSIL)
          796.74
        low grade squamous intraepithelial
          lesion (LGSIL) 796.73
        glandular 796.70
        specified finding NEC 796.79
    cervix 795.00
      with
        atypical squamous cells
          cannot exclude high grade
            squamous intraepithelial
            lesion (ASC-H) 795.02
          of undetermined significance
            (ASC-US) 795.01
        cytologic evidence of malignancy
          795.06
        high grade squamous
          intraepithelial lesion (HGSIL)
          795.04
        low grade squamous intraepithelial
          lesion (LGSIL) 795.03
        nonspecific finding NEC 795.09
    other site 796.9
    vagina 795.10
      with
        atypical squamous cells
          cannot exclude high grade
            squamous intraepithelial
            lesion (ASC-H) 795.12
          of undetermined significance
            (ASC-US) 795.11
        cytologic evidence of malignancy
          795.16
        high grade squamous
          intraepithelial lesion
          (HGSIL)795.14
        low grade squamous intraepithelial
          lesion (LGSIL) 795.13
        glandular 795.10
        specified finding NEC 795.19
    parturition
      affecting fetus or newborn 763.9
      mother - see Delivery, complicated
    pelvis (bony) - see Deformity, pelvis
    percussion, chest 786.7
    periods (grossly) (see also Menstruation)
      626.9
    phonocardiogram 794.39
    placenta - see Placenta, abnormal
    plantar reflex 796.1
    plasma protein - see Deficiency, plasma,
      protein
    pleural folds 748.8
    position - see also Malposition
      gravid uterus 654.4●
        causing obstructed labor 660.2●
          affecting fetus or newborn
            763.1
    posture NEC 781.92
    presentation (fetus) - see Presentation, fetus,
      abnormal
    product of conception NEC 631.8
    puberty - see Puberty
    pulmonary
      artery 747.39
      function, newborn 770.89
      test results 794.2
      ventilation, newborn 770.89
        hyperventilation 786.01
    pulsations in neck 785.1
    pupil reflexes 379.40
    quality of milk 676.8●
    radiological examination 793.99
      abdomen NEC 793.6
      biliary tract 793.3

Abnormal, abnormality, abnormalities
  (Continued)
  radiological examination (Continued)
    breast 793.89
      mammogram NOS 793.80
      mammographic
        calcification 793.89
        calculus 793.89
        microcalcification 793.81
    gastrointestinal tract 793.4
    genitourinary organs 793.5
    head 793.0
    image test inconclusive due to excess
      body fat 793.91
    intrathoracic organ NEC 793.2
    lung (field) 793.19
    musculoskeletal system 793.7
    retroperitoneum 793.6
    skin and subcutaneous tissue 793.99
    skull 793.0
  red blood cells 790.09
    morphology 790.09
    volume 790.09
  reflex NEC 796.1
  renal function test 794.4
  respiration signs - see Respiration
  response to nerve stimulation 794.10
  retinal correspondence 368.34
  rhythm, heart - see also Arrhythmia
    fetus - see Distress, fetal
  saliva 792.4
  scan
    brain 794.09
    kidney 794.4
    liver 794.8
    lung 794.2
    thyroid 794.5
  secretion
    gastrin 251.5
    glucagon 251.4
  semen 792.2
  serum level (of)
    acid phosphatase 790.5
    alkaline phosphatase 790.5
    amylase 790.5
    enzymes NEC 790.5
    lipase 790.5
  shape
    cornea 743.41
    gallbladder 751.69
    gravid uterus 654.4●
      affecting fetus or newborn 763.89
      causing obstructed labor 660.2●
        affecting fetus or newborn 763.1
    head (see also Anomaly, skull) 756.0
    organ or site, congenital NEC - see
      Distortion
  sinus venosus 747.40
  size
    fetus, complicating delivery 653.5●
      causing obstructed labor 660.1●
    gallbladder 751.69
    head (see also Anomaly, skull) 756.0
    organ or site, congenital NEC - see
      Distortion
    teeth 520.2
  skin and appendages, congenital NEC
    757.9
  soft parts of pelvis - see Abnormal, organs or
    tissues of pelvis
  spermatozoa 792.2
  sputum (amount) (color) (excessive) (odor)
    (purulent) 786.4
  stool NEC 787.7
    bloody 578.1
      occult 792.1
    bulky 787.7
    color (dark) (light) 792.1
    content (fat) (mucus) (pus) 792.1
    occult blood 792.1
  synchondrosis 756.9

Abnormal, abnormality, abnormalities *(Continued)*
  test results without manifest disease - *see* Findings, abnormal
  thebesian valve 746.9
  thermography - *see* Findings, abnormal, structure
  threshold, cones or rods (eye) 368.63
  thyroid-binding globulin 246.8
  thyroid product 246.8
  toxicology (findings) NEC 796.0
  tracheal cartilage (congenital) 748.3
  transport protein 273.8
  ultrasound results - *see* Findings, abnormal, structure
  umbilical cord
    affecting fetus or newborn 762.6
    complicating delivery 663.9●
    specified NEC 663.8●
  union
    cricoid cartilage and thyroid cartilage 748.3
    larynx and trachea 748.3
    thyroid cartilage and hyoid bone 748.3
  urination NEC 788.69
    psychogenic 306.53
    stream
      intermittent 788.61
      slowing 788.62
      splitting 788.61
      weak 788.62
    urgency 788.63
  urine (constituents) NEC 791.9
  uterine hemorrhage (*see also* Hemorrhage, uterus) 626.9
    climacteric 627.0
    postmenopausal 627.1
  vagina (acquired) (congenital)
    in pregnancy or childbirth 654.7●
      affecting fetus or newborn 763.89
      causing obstructed labor 660.2●
        affecting fetus or newborn 763.1
  vascular sounds 785.9
  vectorcardiogram 794.39
  visually evoked potential (VEP) 794.13
  vulva (acquired) (congenital)
    in pregnancy or childbirth 654.8●
      affecting fetus or newborn 763.89
      causing obstructed labor 660.2●
        affecting fetus or newborn 763.1
  weight
    gain 783.1
      of pregnancy 646.1●
        with hypertension - *see* Toxemia, of pregnancy
    loss 783.21
  x-ray examination - *see* Abnormal, radiological examination
Abnormally formed uterus - *see* Anomaly, uterus
Abnormity (any organ or part) - *see* Anomaly
ABO
  hemolytic disease 773.1
  incompatibility (due to transfusion of blood or blood products)
    with hemolytic transfusion reaction (HTR) (not specified as acute or delayed) 999.61
      24 hours or more after transfusion 999.63
      acute 999.62
      delayed 999.63
      less than 24 hours after transfusion 999.62
      unspecified time after transfusion 999.61
    reaction 999.60
      specified NEC 999.69
Abocclusion 524.20
Abolition, language 784.69

Aborter, habitual or recurrent NEC
  without current pregnancy 629.81
  current abortion (*see also* Abortion, spontaneous) 634.9●
    affecting fetus or newborn 761.8
  observation in current pregnancy 646.3●
Abortion (complete) (incomplete) (inevitable) (with retained products of conception) 637.9●

> Note: Use the following fifth-digit subclassification with categories 634-637:
>
> 0   unspecified
> 1   incomplete
> 2   complete

  with
    complication(s) (any) following previous abortion - *see* category 639
    damage to pelvic organ (laceration) (rupture) (tear) 637.2●
    embolism (air) (amniotic fluid) (blood clot) (pulmonary) (pyemic) (septic) (soap) 637.6●
    genital tract and pelvic infection 637.0●
    hemorrhage, delayed or excessive 637.1●
    metabolic disorder 637.4●
    renal failure (acute) 637.3●
    sepsis (genital tract) (pelvic organ) 637.0●
      urinary tract 637.7●
    shock (postoperative) (septic) 637.5●
    specified complication NEC 637.7●
    toxemia 637.3●
    unspecified complication(s) 637.8●
    urinary tract infection 637.7●
  accidental - *see* Abortion, spontaneous
  artificial - *see* Abortion, induced
  attempted (failed) - *see* Abortion, failed
  criminal - *see* Abortion, illegal
  early - *see* Abortion, spontaneous
  elective - *see* Abortion, legal
  failed (legal) 638.9
    with
      damage to pelvic organ (laceration) (rupture) (tear) 638.2
      embolism (air) (amniotic fluid) (blood clot) (pulmonary) (pyemic) (septic) (soap) 638.6
      genital tract and pelvic infection 638.0
      hemorrhage, delayed or excessive 638.1
      metabolic disorder 638.4
      renal failure (acute) 638.3
      sepsis (genital tract) (pelvic organ) 638.0
        urinary tract 638.7
      shock (postoperative) (septic) 638.5
      specified complication NEC 638.7
      toxemia 638.3
      unspecified complication(s) 638.8
      urinary tract infection 638.7
  fetal indication - *see* Abortion, legal
  fetus 779.6
  following threatened abortion - *see* Abortion, by type
  habitual or recurrent (care during pregnancy) 646.3●
    with current abortion (*see also* Abortion, spontaneous) 634.9●
    affecting fetus or newborn 761.8
    without current pregnancy 629.81
  homicidal - *see* Abortion, illegal
  illegal 636.9●
    with
      damage to pelvic organ (laceration) (rupture) (tear) 636.2●
      embolism (air) (amniotic fluid) (blood clot) (pulmonary) (pyemic) (septic) (soap) 636.6●
      genital tract and pelvic infection 636.0●

Abortion *(Continued)*
  illegal *(Continued)*
    with *(Continued)*
      hemorrhage, delayed or excessive 636.1●
      metabolic disorder 636.4●
      renal failure 636.3●
      sepsis (genital tract) (pelvic organ) 636.0●
        urinary tract 636.7●
      shock (postoperative) (septic) 636.5●
      specified complication NEC 636.7●
      toxemia 636.3●
      unspecified complication(s) 636.8●
      urinary tract infection 636.7●
    fetus 779.6
  induced 637.9●
    illegal - *see* Abortion, illegal
    legal indications - *see* Abortion, legal
    medical indications - *see* Abortion, legal
    therapeutic - *see* Abortion, legal
  late - *see* Abortion, spontaneous
  legal (legal indication) (medical indication) (under medical supervision) 635.9●
    with
      damage to pelvic organ (laceration) (rupture) (tear) 635.2●
      embolism (air) (amniotic fluid) (blood clot) (pulmonary) (pyemic) (septic) (soap) 635.6●
      genital tract and pelvic infection 635.0●
      hemorrhage, delayed or excessive 635.1●
      metabolic disorder 635.4●
      renal failure (acute) 635.3●
      sepsis (genital tract) (pelvic organ) 635.0●
        urinary tract 635.7●
      shock (postoperative) (septic) 635.5●
      specified complication NEC 635.7●
      toxemia 635.3●
      unspecified complication(s) 635.8●
      urinary tract infection 635.7●
    fetus 779.6
  medical indication - *see* Abortion, legal
  mental hygiene problem - *see* Abortion, legal
  missed 632
  operative - *see* Abortion, legal
  psychiatric indication - *see* Abortion, legal
  recurrent - *see* Abortion, spontaneous
  self-induced - *see* Abortion, illegal
  septic - *see* Abortion, by type, with sepsis
  spontaneous 634.9●
    with
      damage to pelvic organ (laceration) (rupture) (tear) 634.2●
      embolism (air) (amniotic fluid) (blood clot) (pulmonary) (pyemic) (septic) (soap) 634.6●
      genital tract and pelvic infection 634.0●
      hemorrhage, delayed or excessive 634.1●
      metabolic disorder 634.4●
      renal failure 634.3●
      sepsis (genital tract) (pelvic organ) 634.0●
        urinary tract 634.7●
      shock (postoperative) (septic) 634.5●
      specified complication NEC 634.7●
      toxemia 634.3●
      unspecified complication(s) 634.8●
      urinary tract infection 634.7●
    fetus 761.8
    threatened 640.0●
      affecting fetus or newborn 762.1
  surgical - *see* Abortion, legal
  therapeutic - *see* Abortion, legal
  threatened 640.0●
    affecting fetus or newborn 762.1

◀ New   ◀ Revised   deleted Deleted   ● Use Additional Digit(s)   Omit code

Abortion *(Continued)*
 tubal - *see* Pregnancy, tubal
 voluntary - *see* Abortion, legal
Abortus fever 023.9
Aboulomania 301.6
Abrachia 755.20
Abrachiatism 755.20
Abrachiocephalia 759.89
Abrachiocephalus 759.89
Abrami's disease (acquired hemolytic jaundice)
 283.9
Abramov-Fiedler myocarditis (acute isolated
 myocarditis) 422.91
Abrasion - *see also* Injury, superficial, by site
 cornea 918.1
 dental 521.20
  extending into
   dentine 521.22
   pulp 521.23
  generalized 521.25
  limited to enamel 521.21
  localized 521.24
 teeth, tooth (dentifrice) (habitual) (hard
  tissues) (occupational) (ritual)
  (traditional) (wedge defect) (*see also*
  Abrasion, dental) 521.20
Abrikossov's tumor (M9580/0) - *see also*
 Neoplasm, connective tissue, benign
 malignant (M9580/3) - *see* Neoplasm,
  connective tissue, malignant
Abrism 988.8
Abruption, placenta - *see* Placenta, abruptio
Abruptio placentae - *see* Placenta, abruptio
Abscess (acute) (chronic) (infectional)
 (lymphangitic) (metastatic) (multiple)
 (pyogenic) (septic) (with lymphangitis)
 (*see also* Cellulitis) 682.9
 abdomen, abdominal
  cavity 567.22
  wall 682.2
 abdominopelvic 567.22
 accessory sinus (chronic) (*see also* Sinusitis)
  473.9
 adrenal (capsule) (gland) 255.8
 alveolar 522.5
  with sinus 522.7
 amebic 006.3
  bladder 006.8
  brain (with liver or lung abscess) 006.5
  liver (without mention of brain or lung
   abscess) 006.3
   with
    brain abscess (and lung abscess)
     006.5
    lung abscess 006.4
  lung (with liver abscess) 006.4
   with brain abscess 006.5
  seminal vesicle 006.8
  specified site NEC 006.8
  spleen 006.8
 anaerobic 040.0
 ankle 682.6
 anorectal 566
 antecubital space 682.3
 antrum (chronic) (Highmore) (*see also*
  Sinusitis, maxillary) 473.0
 anus 566
 apical (tooth) 522.5
  with sinus (alveolar) 522.7
 appendix 540.1
 areola (acute) (chronic) (nonpuerperal) 611.0
  puerperal, postpartum 675.1●
 arm (any part, above wrist) 682.3
 artery (wall) 447.2
 atheromatous 447.2
 auditory canal (external) 380.10
 auricle (ear) (staphylococcal) (streptococcal)
  380.10
 axilla, axillary (region) 682.3
  lymph gland or node 683
 back (any part) 682.2

Abscess *(Continued)*
 Bartholin's gland 616.3
  with
   abortion - *see* Abortion, by type, with
    sepsis
   ectopic pregnancy (*see also* categories
    633.0-633.9) 639.0
   molar pregnancy (*see also* categories
    630-632) 639.0
  complicating pregnancy or puerperium
   646.6●
  following
   abortion 639.0
   ectopic or molar pregnancy 639.0
 bartholinian 616.3
 Bezold's 383.01
 bile, biliary, duct or tract (*see also*
  Cholecystitis) 576.8
 bilharziasis 120.1
 bladder (wall) 595.89
  amebic 006.8
 bone (subperiosteal) (*see also* Osteomyelitis)
  730.0●
  accessory sinus (chronic) (*see also*
   Sinusitis) 473.9
  acute 730.0●
  chronic or old 730.1●
  jaw (lower) (upper) 526.4
  mastoid - *see* Mastoiditis, acute
  petrous (*see also* Petrositis) 383.20
  spinal (tuberculous) (*see also* Tuberculosis)
   015.0● [730.88]
   nontuberculous 730.08
 bowel 569.5
 brain (any part) 324.0
  amebic (with liver or lung abscess) 006.5
  cystic 324.0
  late effect - *see* category 326
  otogenic 324.0
  tuberculous (*see also* Tuberculosis) 013.3●
 breast (acute) (chronic) (nonpuerperal) 611.0
  newborn 771.5
  puerperal, postpartum 675.1●
  tuberculous (*see also* Tuberculosis) 017.9●
 broad ligament (chronic) (*see also* Disease,
  pelvis, inflammatory) 614.4
  acute 614.3
 Brodie's (chronic) (localized) (*see also*
  Osteomyelitis) 730.1●
 bronchus 519.19
 buccal cavity 528.3
 bulbourethral gland 597.0
 bursa 727.89
  pharyngeal 478.29
 buttock 682.5
 canaliculus, breast 611.0
 canthus 372.20
 cartilage 733.99
 cecum 569.5
  with appendicitis 540.1
 cerebellum, cerebellar 324.0
  late effect - *see* category 326
 cerebral (embolic) 324.0
  late effect - *see* category 326
 cervical (neck region) 682.1
  lymph gland or node 683
  stump (*see also* Cervicitis) 616.0
 cervix (stump) (uteri) (*see also* Cervicitis)
  616.0
 cheek, external 682.0
  inner 528.3
 chest 510.9
  with fistula 510.0
  wall 682.2
 chin 682.0
 choroid 363.00
 ciliary body 364.3
 circumtonsillar 475
 cold (tuberculous) - *see also* Tuberculosis,
  abscess
  articular - *see* Tuberculosis, joint

Abscess *(Continued)*
 colon (wall) 569.5
 colostomy or enterostomy 569.61
 conjunctiva 372.00
 connective tissue NEC 682.9
 cornea 370.55
  with ulcer 370.00
 corpus
  cavernosum 607.2
  luteum (*see also* Salpingo-oophoritis)
   614.2
 Cowper's gland 597.0
 cranium 324.0
 cul-de-sac (Douglas') (posterior) (*see also*
  Disease, pelvis, inflammatory)
  614.4
  acute 614.3
 dental 522.5
  with sinus (alveolar) 522.7
 dentoalveolar 522.5
  with sinus (alveolar) 522.7
 diaphragm, diaphragmatic 567.22
 digit NEC 681.9
 Douglas' cul-de-sac or pouch (*see also*
  Disease, pelvis, inflammatory)
  614.4
  acute 614.3
 Dubois' 090.5
 ductless gland 259.8
 ear
  acute 382.00
  external 380.10
  inner 386.30
  middle - *see* Otitis media
 elbow 682.3
 endamebic - *see* Abscess, amebic
 entamebic - *see* Abscess, amebic
 enterostomy 569.61
 epididymis 604.0
 epidural 324.9
  brain 324.0
  late effect - *see* category 326
  spinal cord 324.1
 epiglottis 478.79
 epiploon, epiploic 567.22
 erysipelatous (*see also* Erysipelas) 035
 esophagostomy 530.86
 esophagus 530.19
 ethmoid (bone) (chronic) (sinus)
   (*see also* Sinusitis, ethmoidal)
   473.2
 external auditory canal 380.10
 extradural 324.9
  brain 324.0
  late effect - *see* category 326
  spinal cord 324.1
 extraperitoneal - *see* Abscess, peritoneum
 eye 360.00
 eyelid 373.13
 face (any part, except eye) 682.0
 fallopian tube (*see also* Salpingo-oophoritis)
  614.2
 fascia 728.89
 fauces 478.29
 fecal 569.5
 femoral (region) 682.6
 filaria, filarial (*see also* Infestation, filarial)
  125.9
 finger (any) (intrathecal) (periosteal)
   (subcutaneous) (subcuticular)
   681.00
 fistulous NEC 682.9
 flank 682.2
 foot (except toe) 682.7
 forearm 682.3
 forehead 682.0
 frontal (sinus) (chronic) (*see also* Sinusitis,
  frontal) 473.1
 gallbladder (*see also* Cholecystitis, acute)
  575.0
 gastric 535.0●

A

Abscess *(Continued)*
  genital organ or tract NEC
    female 616.9
      with
        abortion - *see* Abortion, by type,
          with sepsis
        ectopic pregnancy *(see also*
          categories 633.0-633.9) 639.0
        molar pregnancy *(see also* categories
          630-632) 639.0
      following
        abortion 639.0
        ectopic or molar pregnancy 639.0
      puerperal, postpartum,
        childbirth 670.8●
    male 608.4
  genitourinary system, tuberculous *(see also*
    Tuberculosis) 016.9●
  gingival 523.30
  gland, glandular (lymph) (acute) NEC 683
  glottis 478.79
  gluteal (region) 682.5
  gonorrheal NEC *(see also* Gonococcus) 098.0
  groin 682.2
  gum 523.30
  hand (except finger or thumb) 682.4
  head (except face) 682.8
  heart 429.89
  heel 682.7
  helminthic *(see also* Infestation, by specific
    parasite) 128.9
  hepatic 572.0
    amebic *(see also* Abscess, liver, amebic)
      006.3
    duct 576.8
  hip 682.6
    tuberculous (active) *(see also* Tuberculosis)
      015.1●
  ileocecal 540.1
  ileostomy (bud) 569.61
  iliac (region) 682.2
    fossa 540.1
  iliopsoas 567.31
    tuberculous *(see also* Tuberculosis) 015.0●
      [730.88]
  infraclavicular (fossa) 682.3
  inguinal (region) 682.2
    lymph gland or node 683
  intersphincteric (anus) 566
  intestine, intestinal 569.5
    rectal 566
  intra-abdominal *(see also* Abscess,
    peritoneum) 567.22
    postoperative 998.59
  intracranial 324.0
    late effect - *see* category 326
  intramammary - *see* Abscess, breast
  intramastoid *(see also* Mastoiditis, acute)
    383.00
  intraorbital 376.01
  intraperitoneal 567.22
  intraspinal 324.1
    late effect - *see* category 326
  intratonsillar 475
  iris 364.3
  ischiorectal 566
  jaw (bone) (lower) (upper) 526.4
    skin 682.0
  joint *(see also* Arthritis, pyogenic) 711.0●
    vertebral (tuberculous) *(see also*
      Tuberculosis) 015.0● *[730.88]*
      nontuberculous 724.8
  kidney 590.2
    with
      abortion - *see* Abortion, by type, with
        urinary tract infection
      calculus 592.0
      ectopic pregnancy *(see also* categories
        633.0-633.9) 639.8
      molar pregnancy *(see also* categories
        630-632) 639.8

Abscess *(Continued)*
  kidney *(Continued)*
    with *(Continued)*
      complicating pregnancy or
        puerperium 646.6●
        affecting fetus or newborn 760.1
    following
      abortion 639.8
      ectopic or molar pregnancy 639.8
  knee 682.6
    joint 711.06
    tuberculous (active) *(see also* Tuberculosis)
      015.2●
  labium (majus) (minus) 616.4
    complicating pregnancy, childbirth, or
      puerperium 646.6●
  lacrimal (passages) (sac) *(see also*
    Dacryocystitis) 375.30
    caruncle 375.30
    gland *(see also* Dacryoadenitis) 375.00
  lacunar 597.0
  larynx 478.79
  lateral (alveolar) 522.5
    with sinus 522.7
  leg, except foot 682.6
  lens 360.00
  lid 373.13
  lingual 529.0
    tonsil 475
  lip 528.5
  Littre's gland 597.0
  liver 572.0
    amebic 006.3
      with
        brain abscess (and lung abscess)
          006.5
        lung abscess 006.4
    due to Entamoeba histolytica 006.3
    dysenteric *(see also* Abscess, liver, amebic)
      006.3
    pyogenic 572.0
    tropical *(see also* Abscess, liver, amebic)
      006.3
  loin (region) 682.2
  lumbar (tuberculous) *(see also* Tuberculosis)
    015.0● *[730.88]*
    nontuberculous 682.2
  lung (miliary) (putrid) 513.0
    amebic (with liver abscess) 006.4
      with brain abscess 006.5
  lymph, lymphatic, gland or node (acute) 683
    any site, except mesenteric 683
    mesentery 289.2
  lymphangitic, acute - *see* Cellulitis
  malar 526.4
  mammary gland - *see* Abscess, breast
  marginal (anus) 566
  mastoid (process) *(see also* Mastoiditis, acute)
    383.00
    subperiosteal 383.01
  maxilla, maxillary 526.4
    molar (tooth) 522.5
      with sinus 522.7
    premolar 522.5
    sinus (chronic) *(see also* Sinusitis,
      maxillary) 473.0
  mediastinum 513.1
  meibomian gland 373.12
  meninges *(see also* Meningitis) 320.9
  mesentery, mesenteric 567.22
  mesosalpinx *(see also* Salpingo-oophoritis)
    614.2
  milk 675.1●
  Monro's (psoriasis) 696.1
  mons pubis 682.2
  mouth (floor) 528.3
  multiple sites NEC 682.9
  mural 682.2
  muscle 728.89
    psoas 567.31
  myocardium 422.92

Abscess *(Continued)*
  nabothian (follicle) *(see also* Cervicitis) 616.0
  nail (chronic) (with lymphangitis) 681.9
    finger 681.02
    toe 681.11
  nasal (fossa) (septum) 478.19
    sinus (chronic) *(see also* Sinusitis) 473.9
  nasopharyngeal 478.29
  nates 682.5
  navel 682.2
    newborn NEC 771.4
  neck (region) 682.1
    lymph gland or node 683
  nephritic *(see also* Abscess, kidney) 590.2
  nipple 611.0
    puerperal, postpartum 675.0●
  nose (septum) 478.19
    external 682.0
  omentum 567.22
  operative wound 998.59
  orbit, orbital 376.01
  ossifluent - *see* Abscess, bone
  ovary, ovarian (corpus luteum) *(see also*
    Salpingo-oophoritis) 614.2
  oviduct *(see also* Salpingo-oophoritis)
    614.2
  palate (soft) 528.3
    hard 526.4
  palmar (space) 682.4
  pancreas (duct) 577.0
  paradontal 523.30
  parafrenal 607.2
  parametric, parametrium (chronic) *(see also*
    Disease, pelvis, inflammatory) 614.4
    acute 614.3
  paranephric 590.2
  parapancreatic 577.0
  parapharyngeal 478.22
  pararectal 566
  parasinus *(see also* Sinusitis) 473.9
  parauterine *(see also* Disease, pelvis,
    inflammatory) 614.4
    acute 614.3
  paravaginal *(see also* Vaginitis) 616.10
  parietal region 682.8
  parodontal 523.30
  parotid (duct) (gland) 527.3
    region 528.3
  parumbilical 682.2
    newborn 771.4
  pectoral (region) 682.2
  pelvirectal 567.22
  pelvis, pelvic
    female (chronic) *(see also* Disease, pelvis,
      inflammatory) 614.4
      acute 614.3
    male, peritoneal (cellular tissue) - *see*
      Abscess, peritoneum
    tuberculous *(see also* Tuberculosis)
      016.9●
  penis 607.2
    gonococcal (acute) 098.0
      chronic or duration of 2 months or
        over 098.2
  perianal 566
  periapical 522.5
    with sinus (alveolar) 522.7
  periappendiceal 540.1
  pericardial 420.99
  pericecal 540.1
  pericemental 523.30
  pericholecystic *(see also* Cholecystitis, acute)
    575.0
  pericoronal 523.30
  peridental 523.30
  perigastric 535.0●
  perimetric *(see also* Disease, pelvis,
    inflammatory) 614.4
    acute 614.3
  perinephric, perinephritic *(see also* Abscess,
    kidney) 590.2

◄ New   ◄▮▮▮ Revised   ~~deleted~~ Deleted   ● Use Additional Digit(s)   Omit code

Abscess *(Continued)*
 perineum, perineal (superficial) 682.2
  deep (with urethral involvement) 597.0
  urethra 597.0
 periodontal (parietal) 523.31
  apical 522.5
 periosteum, periosteal *(see also* Periostitis)
   730.3●
  with osteomyelitis *(see also* Osteomyelitis)
    730.2●
   acute or subacute 730.0●
   chronic or old 730.1●
 peripleuritic 510.9
  with fistula 510.0
 periproctic 566
 periprostatic 601.2
 perirectal (staphylococcal) 566
 perirenal (tissue) *(see also* Abscess, kidney)
   590.2
 perisinuous (nose) *(see also* Sinusitis) 473.9
 peritoneum, peritoneal (perforated)
   (ruptured) 567.22
  with
   abortion - *see* Abortion, by type, with
     sepsis
   appendicitis 540.1
   ectopic pregnancy *(see also* categories
     633.0-633.9) 639.0
   molar pregnancy *(see also* categories
     630-632) 639.0
  following
   abortion 639.0
   ectopic or molar pregnancy 639.0
  pelvic, female *(see also* Disease, pelvis,
    inflammatory) 614.4
   acute 614.3
  postoperative 998.59
  puerperal, postpartum, childbirth 670.8●
  tuberculous *(see also* Tuberculosis) 014.0●
 peritonsillar 475
 perityphlic 540.1
 periureteral 593.89
 periurethral 597.0
  gonococcal (acute) 098.0
   chronic or duration of 2 months or
     over 098.2
 periuterine *(see also* Disease, pelvis,
   inflammatory) 614.4
  acute 614.3
 perivesical 595.89
 pernicious NEC 682.9
 petrous bone - *see* Petrositis
 phagedenic NEC 682.9
  chancroid 099.0
 pharynx, pharyngeal (lateral) 478.29
 phlegmonous NEC 682.9
 pilonidal 685.0
 pituitary (gland) 253.8
 pleura 510.9
  with fistula 510.0
 popliteal 682.6
 postanal 566
 postcecal 540.1
 postlaryngeal 478.79
 postnasal 478.19
 postpharyngeal 478.24
 posttonsillar 475
 posttyphoid 002.0
 Pott's *(see also* Tuberculosis) 015.0● *[730.88]*
 pouch of Douglas (chronic) *(see also* Disease,
   pelvis, inflammatory) 614.4
 premammary - *see* Abscess, breast
 prepatellar 682.6
 prostate *(see also* Prostatitis) 601.2
  gonococcal (acute) 098.12
   chronic or duration of 2 months or
     over 098.32
 psoas 567.31
  tuberculous *(see also* Tuberculosis) 015.0●
    [730.88]
 pterygopalatine fossa 682.8

Abscess *(Continued)*
 pubis 682.2
 puerperal - *see* Puerperal, abscess, by site
 pulmonary - *see* Abscess, lung
 pulp, pulpal (dental) 522.0
   finger 681.01
   toe 681.10
 pyemic - *see* Septicemia
 pyloric valve 535.0●
 rectovaginal septum 569.5
 rectovesical 595.89
 rectum 566
 regional NEC 682.9
 renal *(see also* Abscess, kidney) 590.2
 retina 363.00
 retrobulbar 376.01
 retrocecal 567.22
 retrolaryngeal 478.79
 retromammary - *see* Abscess, breast
 retroperineal 682.2
 retroperitoneal 567.38
   postprocedural 998.59
 retropharyngeal 478.24
   tuberculous *(see also* Tuberculosis)
     012.8●
 retrorectal 566
 retrouterine *(see also* Disease, pelvis,
    inflammatory) 614.4
   acute 614.3
 retrovesical 595.89
 root, tooth 522.5
   with sinus (alveolar) 522.7
 round ligament *(see also* Disease, pelvis,
    inflammatory) 614.4
   acute 614.3
 rupture (spontaneous) NEC 682.9
 sacrum (tuberculous) *(see also* Tuberculosis)
    015.0● *[730.88]*
   nontuberculous 730.08
 salivary duct or gland 527.3
 scalp (any part) 682.8
 scapular 730.01
 sclera 379.09
 scrofulous *(see also* Tuberculosis) 017.2●
 scrotum 608.4
 seminal vesicle 608.0
   amebic 006.8
 septal, dental 522.5
   with sinus (alveolar) 522.7
 septum (nasal) 478.19
 serous *(see also* Periostitis) 730.3●
 shoulder 682.3
 side 682.2
 sigmoid 569.5
 sinus (accessory) (chronic) (nasal) *(see also*
    Sinusitis) 473.9
   intracranial venous (any) 324.0
    late effect - *see* category 326
 Skene's duct or gland 597.0
 skin NEC 682.9
   tuberculous (primary) *(see also*
     Tuberculosis) 017.0●
 sloughing NEC 682.9
 specified site NEC 682.8
   amebic 006.8
 spermatic cord 608.4
 sphenoidal (sinus) *(see also* Sinusitis,
    sphenoidal) 473.3
 spinal
   cord (any part) (staphylococcal) 324.1
    tuberculous *(see also* Tuberculosis)
      013.5●
   epidural 324.1
 spine (column) (tuberculous) *(see also*
    Tuberculosis) 015.0● *[730.88]*
   nontuberculous 730.08
 spleen 289.59
   amebic 006.8
 staphylococcal NEC 682.9
 stitch 998.59
 stomach (wall) 535.0●

Abscess *(Continued)*
 strumous (tuberculous) *(see also* Tuberculosis)
    017.2●
 subarachnoid 324.9
   brain 324.0
   cerebral 324.0
   late effect - *see* category 326
   spinal cord 324.1
 subareolar - *see also* Abscess, breast
   puerperal, postpartum 675.1●
 subcecal 540.1
 subcutaneous NEC 682.9
 subdiaphragmatic 567.22
 subdorsal 682.2
 subdural 324.9
   brain 324.0
   late effect - *see* category 326
   spinal cord 324.1
 subgaleal 682.8
 subhepatic 567.22
 sublingual 528.3
   gland 527.3
 submammary - *see* Abscess, breast
 submandibular (region) (space) (triangle)
    682.0
   gland 527.3
 submaxillary (region) 682.0
   gland 527.3
 submental (pyogenic) 682.0
   gland 527.3
 subpectoral 682.2
 subperiosteal - *see* Abscess, bone
 subperitoneal 567.22
 subphrenic - *see also* Abscess, peritoneum
    567.22
   postoperative 998.59
 subscapular 682.2
 subungual 681.9
 suburethral 597.0
 sudoriparous 705.89
 suppurative NEC 682.9
 supraclavicular (fossa) 682.3
 suprahepatic 567.22
 suprapelvic *(see also* Disease, pelvis,
    inflammatory) 614.4
   acute 614.3
 suprapubic 682.2
 suprarenal (capsule) (gland) 255.8
 sweat gland 705.89
 syphilitic 095.8
 teeth, tooth (root) 522.5
   with sinus (alveolar) 522.7
   supporting structures NEC 523.30
 temple 682.0
 temporal region 682.0
 temporosphenoidal 324.0
   late effect - *see* category 326
 tendon (sheath) 727.89
 testicle - *see* Orchitis
 thecal 728.89
 thigh (acquired) 682.6
 thorax 510.9
   with fistula 510.0
 throat 478.29
 thumb (intrathecal) (periosteal)
    (subcutaneous) (subcuticular)
    681.00
 thymus (gland) 254.1
 thyroid (gland) 245.0
 toe (any) (intrathecal) (periosteal)
    (subcutaneous) (subcuticular) 681.10
 tongue (staphylococcal) 529.0
 tonsil(s) (lingual) 475
 tonsillopharyngeal 475
 tooth, teeth (root) 522.5
   with sinus (alveolar) 522.7
   supporting structure NEC 523.30
 trachea 478.9
 trunk 682.2
 tubal *(see also* Salpingo-oophoritis) 614.2
 tuberculous - *see* Tuberculosis, abscess

◀ New   ◀▏▏ Revised   deleted Deleted   ● Use Additional Digit(s)   ▒ Omit code

Abscess (Continued)
  tubo-ovarian (see also Salpingo-oophoritis) 614.2
  tunica vaginalis 608.4
  umbilicus NEC 682.2
    newborn 771.4
  upper arm 682.3
  upper respiratory 478.9
  urachus 682.2
  urethra (gland) 597.0
  urinary 597.0
  uterus, uterine (wall) (see also Endometritis) 615.9
    ligament (see also Disease, pelvis, inflammatory) 614.4
      acute 614.3
    neck (see also Cervicitis) 616.0
  uvula 528.3
  vagina (wall) (see also Vaginitis) 616.10
  vaginorectal (see also Vaginitis) 616.10
  vas deferens 608.4
  vermiform appendix 540.1
  vertebra (column) (tuberculous) (see also Tuberculosis) 015.0● [730.88]
    nontuberculous 730.0●
  vesical 595.89
  vesicouterine pouch (see also Disease, pelvis, inflammatory) 614.4
  vitreous (humor) (pneumococcal) 360.04
  vocal cord 478.5
  von Bezold's 383.01
  vulva 616.4
    complicating pregnancy, childbirth, or puerperium 646.6●
  vulvovaginal gland (see also Vaginitis) 616.3
  web-space 682.4
  wrist 682.4
Absence (organ or part) (complete or partial)
  acoustic nerve 742.8
  adrenal (gland) (congenital) 759.1
    acquired V45.79
  albumin (blood) 273.8
  alimentary tract (complete) (congenital) (partial) 751.8
    lower 751.5
    upper 750.8
  alpha-fucosidase 271.8
  alveolar process (acquired) 525.8
    congenital 750.26
  anus, anal (canal) (congenital) 751.2
  aorta (congenital) 747.22
  aortic valve (congenital) 746.89
  appendix, congenital 751.2
  arm (acquired) V49.60
    above elbow V49.66
    below elbow V49.65
    congenital (see also Deformity, reduction, upper limb) 755.20
      lower - see Absence, forearm, congenital
      upper (complete) (partial) (with absence of distal elements, incomplete) 755.24
        with
          complete absence of distal elements 755.21
          forearm (incomplete) 755.23
  artery (congenital) (peripheral) NEC (see also Anomaly, peripheral vascular system) 747.60
    brain 747.81
    cerebral 747.81
    coronary 746.85
    pulmonary 747.31
    umbilical 747.5
  atrial septum 745.69
  auditory canal (congenital) (external) 744.01
  auricle (ear) (with stenosis or atresia of auditory canal), congenital 744.01
  bile, biliary duct (common) or passage (congenital) 751.61

Absence (Continued)
  bladder (acquired) V45.74
    congenital 753.8
  bone (congenital) NEC 756.9
    marrow 284.9
      acquired (secondary) 284.89
      congenital 284.09
      hereditary 284.09
      idiopathic 284.9
    skull 756.0
  bowel sounds 787.5
  brain 740.0
    specified part 742.2
  breast(s) (acquired) V45.71
    congenital 757.6
  broad ligament (congenital) 752.19
  bronchus (congenital) 748.3
  calvarium, calvaria (skull) 756.0
  canaliculus lacrimalis, congenital 743.65
  carpal(s) (congenital) (complete) (partial) (with absence of distal elements, incomplete) (see also Deformity, reduction, upper limb) 755.28
    with complete absence of distal elements 755.21
  cartilage 756.9
  caudal spine 756.13
  cecum (acquired) (postoperative) (posttraumatic) V45.72
    congenital 751.2
  cementum 520.4
  cerebellum (congenital) (vermis) 742.2
  cervix (acquired) (uteri) V88.01
    with remaining uterus V88.03
    and uterus V88.01
    congenital 752.43
  chin, congenital 744.89
  cilia (congenital) 743.63
    acquired 374.89
  circulatory system, part NEC 747.89
  clavicle 755.51
  clitoris (congenital) 752.49
  coccyx, congenital 756.13
  cold sense (see also Disturbance, sensation) 782.0
  colon (acquired) (postoperative) V45.72
    congenital 751.2
  congenital
    lumen - see Atresia
    organ or site NEC - see Agenesis
    septum - see Imperfect, closure
  corpus callosum (congenital) 742.2
  cricoid cartilage 748.3
  diaphragm (congenital) (with hernia) 756.6
    with obstruction 756.6
  digestive organ(s) or tract, congenital (complete) (partial) 751.8
    acquired V45.79
    lower 751.5
    upper 750.8
  ductus arteriosus 747.89
  duodenum (acquired) (postoperative) V45.72
    congenital 751.1
  ear, congenital 744.09
    acquired V45.79
    auricle 744.01
    external 744.01
    inner 744.05
    lobe, lobule 744.21
    middle, except ossicles 744.03
      ossicles 744.04
    ossicles 744.04
  ejaculatory duct (congenital) 752.89
  endocrine gland NEC (congenital) 759.2
  epididymis (congenital) 752.89
    acquired V45.77
  epiglottis, congenital 748.3
  epileptic (atonic) (typical) (see also Epilepsy) 345.0●
  erythrocyte 284.9

Absence (Continued)
  erythropoiesis 284.9
    congenital 284.01
  esophagus (congenital) 750.3
  eustachian tube (congenital) 744.24
  extremity (acquired)
    congenital (see also Deformity, reduction) 755.4
    lower V49.70
    upper V49.60
  extrinsic muscle, eye 743.69
  eye (acquired) V45.78
    adnexa (congenital) 743.69
    congenital 743.00
    muscle (congenital) 743.69
  eyelid (fold), congenital 743.62
    acquired 374.89
  face
    bones NEC 756.0
    specified part NEC 744.89
  fallopian tube(s) (acquired) V45.77
    congenital 752.19
  femur, congenital (complete) (partial) (with absence of distal elements, incomplete) (see also Deformity, reduction, lower limb) 755.34
    with
      complete absence of distal elements 755.31
      tibia and fibula (incomplete) 755.33
  fibrin 790.92
  fibrinogen (congenital) 286.3
    acquired 286.6
  fibula, congenital (complete) (partial) (with absence of distal elements, incomplete) (see also Deformity, reduction, lower limb) 755.37
    with
      complete absence of distal elements 755.31
      tibia 755.35
        with
          complete absence of distal elements 755.31
          femur (incomplete) 755.33
            with complete absence of distal elements 755.31
  finger (acquired) V49.62
    congenital (complete) (partial) (see also Deformity, reduction, upper limb) 755.29
    meaning all fingers (complete) (partial) 755.21
    transverse 755.21
  fissures of lungs (congenital) 748.5
  foot (acquired) V49.73
    congenital (complete) 755.31
  forearm (acquired) V49.65
    congenital (complete) (partial) (with absence of distal elements, incomplete) (see also Deformity, reduction, upper limb) 755.25
    with
      complete absence of distal elements (hand and fingers) 755.21
      humerus (incomplete) 755.23
  fovea centralis 743.55
  fucosidase 271.8
  gallbladder (acquired) V45.79
    congenital 751.69
  gamma globulin (blood) 279.00
  genital organs
    acquired V45.77
    congenital
      female 752.89
        external 752.49
        internal NEC 752.89
      male 752.89
        penis 752.69
  genitourinary organs, congenital NEC 752.89
  glottis 748.3

◀ New   ◀▥ Revised   ~~deleted~~ Deleted   ● Use Additional Digit(s)   ▨ Omit code

Absence *(Continued)*
  gonadal, congenital NEC 758.6
  hair (congenital) 757.4
    acquired - *see* Alopecia
  hand (acquired) V49.63
    congenital (complete) *(see also* Deformity,
      reduction, upper limb) 755.21
  heart (congenital) 759.89
    acquired - *see* Status, organ replacement
  heat sense *(see also* Disturbance, sensation)
    782.0
  humerus, congenital (complete) (partial)
    (with absence of distal elements,
    incomplete) *(see also* Deformity,
    reduction, upper limb) 755.24
    with
      complete absence of distal elements
        755.21
      radius and ulna (incomplete) 755.23
  hymen (congenital) 752.49
  ileum (acquired) (postoperative)
    (posttraumatic) V45.72
    congenital 751.1
  immunoglobulin, isolated NEC 279.03
    IgA 279.01
    IgG 279.03
    IgM 279.02
  incus (acquired) 385.24
    congenital 744.04
  internal ear (congenital) 744.05
  intestine (acquired) (small) V45.72
    congenital 751.1
      large 751.2
    large V45.72
      congenital 751.2
  iris (congenital) 743.45
  jaw - *see* Absence, mandible
  jejunum (acquired) V45.72
    congenital 751.1
  joint (acquired) (following prior explantation
    of joint prosthesis) (with or without
    presence of antibiotic-impregnated
    cement spacer) NEC V88.29
    congenital NEC 755.8
    hip V88.21
    knee V88.22
  kidney(s) (acquired) V45.73
    congenital 753.0
  labium (congenital) (majus) (minus) 752.49
  labyrinth, membranous 744.05
  lacrimal apparatus (congenital) 743.65
  larynx (congenital) 748.3
  leg (acquired) V49.70
    above knee V49.76
    below knee V49.75
    congenital (partial) (unilateral) *(see also*
      Deformity, reduction, lower limb)
      755.31
      lower (complete) (partial) (with
        absence of distal elements,
        incomplete) 755.35
        with
          complete absence of distal
            elements (foot and toes)
            755.31
          thigh (incomplete) 755.33
            with complete absence of
              distal elements 755.31
      upper - *see* Absence, femur
  lens (congenital) 743.35
    acquired 379.31
  ligament, broad (congenital) 752.19
  limb (acquired)
    congenital (complete) (partial) *(see also*
      Deformity, reduction) 755.4
      lower 755.30
        complete 755.31
        incomplete 755.32
        longitudinal - *see* Deficiency, lower
          limb, longitudinal
        transverse 755.31

Absence *(Continued)*
  limb *(Continued)*
    congenital *(Continued)*
      upper 755.20
        complete 755.21
        incomplete 755.22
        longitudinal - *see* Deficiency, upper
          limb, longitudinal
        transverse 755.21
      lower NEC V49.70
      upper NEC V49.60
  lip 750.26
  liver (congenital) (lobe) 751.69
  lumbar (congenital) (vertebra)
    756.13
    isthmus 756.11
    pars articularis 756.11
  lumen - *see* Atresia
  lung (bilateral) (congenital) (fissure) (lobe)
    (unilateral) 748.5
    acquired (any part) V45.76
  mandible (congenital) 524.09
  maxilla (congenital) 524.09
  menstruation 626.0
  metacarpal(s), congenital (complete) (partial)
    (with absence of distal elements,
    incomplete) *(see also* Deformity,
    reduction, upper limb) 755.28
    with all fingers, complete 755.21
  metatarsal(s), congenital (complete) (partial)
    (with absence of distal elements,
    incomplete) *(see also* Deformity,
    reduction, lower limb) 755.38
    with complete absence of distal elements
      755.31
  muscle (congenital) (pectoral) 756.81
    ocular 743.69
  musculoskeletal system (congenital) NEC
    756.9
  nail(s) (congenital) 757.5
  neck, part 744.89
  nerve 742.8
  nervous system, part NEC 742.8
  neutrophil 288.00
  nipple (congenital) 757.6
    acquired V45.71
  nose (congenital) 748.1
    acquired 738.0
  nuclear 742.8
  ocular muscle (congenital) 743.69
  organ
    of Corti (congenital) 744.05
    or site
      acquired V45.79
      congenital NEC 759.89
  osseous meatus (ear) 744.03
  ovary (acquired) V45.77
    congenital 752.0
  oviduct (acquired) V45.77
    congenital 752.19
  pancreas (congenital) 751.7
    acquired (postoperative) (posttraumatic)
      V88.11
    partial V88.12
    total V88.11
  parathyroid gland (congenital) 759.2
  parotid gland(s) (congenital) 750.21
  patella, congenital 755.64
  pelvic girdle (congenital) 755.69
  penis (congenital) 752.69
    acquired V45.77
  pericardium (congenital) 746.89
  perineal body (congenital) 756.81
  phalange(s), congenital 755.4
    lower limb (complete) (intercalary)
      (partial) (terminal) *(see also*
      Deformity, reduction, lower limb)
      755.39
      meaning all toes (complete) (partial)
        755.31
      transverse 755.31

Absence *(Continued)*
  phalange(s) *(Continued)*
    upper limb (complete) (intercalary)
      (partial) (terminal) *(see also*
      Deformity, reduction, upper limb)
      755.29
      meaning all digits (complete) (partial)
        755.21
      transverse 755.21
  pituitary gland (congenital) 759.2
  postoperative - *see* Absence, by site, acquired
  prostate (congenital) 752.89
    acquired V45.77
  pulmonary
    artery 747.31
    trunk 747.31
    valve (congenital) 746.01
    vein 747.49
  punctum lacrimale (congenital) 743.65
  radius, congenital (complete) (partial) (with
    absence of distal elements, incomplete)
    755.26
    with
      complete absence of distal elements
        755.21
      ulna 755.25
        with
          complete absence of distal
            elements 755.21
          humerus (incomplete) 755.23
  ray, congenital 755.4
    lower limb (complete) (partial) *(see also*
      Deformity, reduction, lower limb)
      755.38
      meaning all rays 755.31
      transverse 755.31
    upper limb (complete) (partial) *(see also*
      Deformity, reduction, upper limb)
      755.28
      meaning all rays 755.21
      transverse 755.21
  rectum (congenital) 751.2
    acquired V45.79
  red cell 284.9
    acquired (secondary) 284.81
    congenital 284.01
    hereditary 284.01
    idiopathic 284.9
  respiratory organ (congenital) NEC 748.9
  rib (acquired) 738.3
    congenital 756.3
  roof of orbit (congenital) 742.0
  round ligament (congenital) 752.89
  sacrum, congenital 756.13
  salivary gland(s) (congenital) 750.21
  scapula 755.59
  scrotum, congenital 752.89
  seminal tract or duct (congenital) 752.89
    acquired V45.77
  septum (congenital) - *see also* Imperfect,
    closure, septum
    atrial 745.69
      and ventricular 745.7
    between aorta and pulmonary artery
      745.0
    ventricular 745.3
      and atrial 745.7
  sex chromosomes 758.81
  shoulder girdle, congenital (complete)
    (partial) 755.59
  skin (congenital) 757.39
  skull bone 756.0
    with
      anencephalus 740.0
      encephalocele 742.0
      hydrocephalus 742.3
        with spina bifida *(see also* Spina
          bifida) 741.0●
      microcephalus 742.1
  spermatic cord (congenital) 752.89
  spinal cord 742.59

Absence *(Continued)*
  spine, congenital 756.13
  spleen (congenital) 759.0
    acquired V45.79
  sternum, congenital 756.3
  stomach (acquired) (partial) (postoperative) V45.75
    with postgastric surgery syndrome 564.2
    congenital 750.7
  submaxillary gland(s) (congenital) 750.21
  superior vena cava (congenital) 747.49
  tarsal(s), congenital (complete) (partial) (with absence of distal elements, incomplete) *(see also* Deformity, reduction, lower limb) 755.38
  teeth, tooth (congenital) 520.0
    with abnormal spacing 524.30
    acquired 525.10
      with malocclusion 524.30
      due to
        caries 525.13
        extraction 525.10
        periodontal disease 525.12
        trauma 525.11
  tendon (congenital) 756.81
  testis (congenital) 752.89
    acquired V45.77
  thigh (acquired) 736.89
  thumb (acquired) V49.61
    congenital 755.29
  thymus gland (congenital) 759.2
  thyroid (gland) (surgical) 246.8
    with hypothyroidism 244.0
    cartilage, congenital 748.3
    congenital 243
  tibia, congenital (complete) (partial) (with absence of distal elements, incomplete) *(see also* Deformity, reduction, lower limb) 755.36
    with
      complete absence of distal elements 755.31
      fibula 755.35
        with
          complete absence of distal elements 755.31
          femur (incomplete) 755.33
            with complete absence of distal elements 755.31
  toe (acquired) V49.72
    congenital (complete) (partial) 755.39
      meaning all toes 755.31
      transverse 755.31
    great V49.71
  tongue (congenital) 750.11
  tooth, teeth (congenital) 520.0
    with abnormal spacing 524.30
    acquired 525.10
      with malocclusion 524.30
      due to
        caries 525.13
        extraction 525.10
        periodontal disease 525.12
        trauma 525.11
  trachea (cartilage) (congenital) (rings) 748.3
  transverse aortic arch (congenital) 747.21
  tricuspid valve 746.1
  ulna, congenital (complete) (partial) (with absence of distal elements, incomplete) *(see also* Deformity, reduction, upper limb) 755.27
    with
      complete absence of distal elements 755.21
      radius 755.25
        with
          complete absence of distal elements 755.21
          humerus (incomplete) 755.23
  umbilical artery (congenital) 747.5

Absence *(Continued)*
  ureter (congenital) 753.4
    acquired V45.74
  urethra, congenital 753.8
    acquired V45.74
  urinary system, part NEC, congenital 753.8
    acquired V45.74
  uterus (acquired) V88.01
    with remaining cervical stump V88.02
    and cervix V88.01
    congenital 752.31
  uvula (congenital) 750.26
  vagina, congenital 752.45
    acquired V45.77
  vas deferens (congenital) 752.89
    acquired V45.77
  vein (congenital) (peripheral) NEC *(see also* Anomaly, peripheral vascular system) 747.60
    brain 747.81
    great 747.49
    portal 747.49
    pulmonary 747.49
  vena cava (congenital) (inferior) (superior) 747.49
  ventral horn cell 742.59
  ventricular septum 745.3
  vermis of cerebellum 742.2
  vertebra, congenital 756.13
  vulva, congenital 752.49
Absentia epileptica *(see also* Epilepsy) 345.0●
Absinthemia *(see also* Dependence) 304.6●
Absinthism *(see also* Dependence) 304.6●
Absorbent system disease 459.89
Absorption
  alcohol, through placenta or breast milk 760.71
  antibiotics, through placenta or breast milk 760.74
  anticonvulsants, through placenta or breast milk 760.77
  antifungals, through placenta or breast milk 760.74
  anti-infective, through placenta or breast milk 760.74
  antimetabolics, through placenta or breast milk 760.78
  chemical NEC 989.9
    specified chemical or substance - *see* Table of Drugs and Chemicals
    through placenta or breast milk (fetus or newborn) 760.70
      alcohol 760.71
      anticonvulsants 760.77
      antifungals 760.74
      anti-infective agents 760.74
      antimetabolics 760.78
      cocaine 760.75
      "crack" 760.75
      diethylstilbestrol [DES] 760.76
      hallucinogenic agents 760.73
      medicinal agents NEC 760.79
      narcotics 760.72
      obstetric anesthetic or analgesic drug 763.5
      specified agent NEC 760.79
      suspected, affecting management of pregnancy 655.5●
  cocaine, through placenta or breast milk 760.75
  drug NEC *(see also* Reaction, drug)
    through placenta or breast milk (fetus or newborn) 760.70
      alcohol 760.71
      anticonvulsants 760.77
      antifungals 760.74
      anti-infective agents 760.74
      antimetabolics 760.78
      cocaine 760.75
      "crack" 760.75
      diethylstilbestrol (DES) 760.76

Absorption *(Continued)*
  drug NEC *(Continued)*
    through placenta or breast milk *(Continued)*
      hallucinogenic agents 760.73
      medicinal agents NEC 760.79
      narcotics 760.72
      obstetric anesthetic or analgesic drug 763.5
      specified agent NEC 760.79
      suspected, affecting management of pregnancy 655.5●
  fat, disturbance 579.8
  hallucinogenic agents, through placenta or breast milk 760.73
  immune sera, through placenta or breast milk 760.79
  lactose defect 271.3
  medicinal agents NEC, through placenta or breast milk 760.79
  narcotics, through placenta or breast milk 760.72
  noxious substance - *see* Absorption, chemical
  protein, disturbance 579.8
  pus or septic, general - *see* Septicemia
  quinine, through placenta or breast milk 760.74
  toxic substance - *see* Absorption, chemical
  uremic - *see* Uremia
Abstinence symptoms or syndrome
  alcohol 291.81
  drug 292.0
  neonatal 779.5
Abt-Letterer-Siwe syndrome (acute histiocytosis X) (M9722/3) 202.5●
Abulia 799.89
Abulomania 301.6
Abuse
  adult 995.80
    emotional 995.82
    multiple forms 995.85
    neglect (nutritional) 995.84
    physical 995.81
    psychological 995.82
    sexual 995.83
  alcohol *(see also* Alcoholism) 305.0●
    dependent 303.9●
    nondependent 305.0●
  child 995.50
    counseling
      perpetrator
        non-parent V62.83
        parent V61.22
      victim V61.21
    emotional 995.51
    multiple forms 995.59
    neglect (nutritional) 995.52
    physical 995.54
      shaken infant syndrome 995.55
    psychological 995.51
    sexual 995.53
  drugs, nondependent 305.9●

Note: Use the following fifth-digit subclassification with the following codes: 305.0, 305.2-305.9:

  0   unspecified
  1   continuous
  2   episodic
  3   in remission

    amphetamine type 305.7●
    antidepressants 305.8●
    anxiolytic 305.4●
    barbiturates 305.4●
    caffeine 305.9●
    cannabis 305.2●
    cocaine type 305.6●
    hallucinogens 305.3●
    hashish 305.2●
    hypnotic 305.4●

◀ New   ◀▥ Revised   ~~deleted~~ Deleted   ● Use Additional Digit(s)   ▨ Omit code

Abuse (Continued)
  drugs, nondependent (Continued)
    inhalant 305.9●
    LSD 305.3●
    marijuana 305.2●
    mixed 305.9●
    morphine type 305.5●
    opioid type 305.5●
    phencyclidine (PCP) 305.9●
    sedative 305.4●
    specified NEC 305.9●
    tranquilizers 305.4●
  spouse 995.80
  tobacco 305.1
Acalcerosis 275.40
Acalcicosis 275.40
Acalculia 784.69
  developmental 315.1
Acanthocheilonemiasis 125.4
Acanthocytosis 272.5
Acanthokeratodermia 701.1
Acantholysis 701.8
  bullosa 757.39
Acanthoma (benign) (M8070/0) - see also
    Neoplasm, by site, benign
  malignant (M8070/3) - see Neoplasm, by site,
    malignant
Acanthosis (acquired) (nigricans) 701.2
  adult 701.2
  benign (congenital) 757.39
  congenital 757.39
  glycogenic
    esophagus 530.89
  juvenile 701.2
  tongue 529.8
Acanthrocytosis 272.5
Acapnia 276.3
Acarbia 276.2
Acardia 759.89
Acardiacus amorphus 759.89
Acardiotrophia 429.1
Acardius 759.89
Acariasis 133.9
  sarcoptic 133.0
Acaridiasis 133.9
Acarinosis 133.9
Acariosis 133.9
Acarodermatitis 133.9
  urticarioides 133.9
Acarophobia 300.29
Acatalasemia 277.89
Acatalasia 277.89
Acatamathesia 784.69
Acataphasia 784.59
Acathisia 781.0
  due to drugs 333.99
Acceleration, accelerated
  atrioventricular conduction 426.7
  idioventricular rhythm 427.89
Accessory (congenital)
  adrenal gland 759.1
  anus 751.5
  appendix 751.5
  atrioventricular conduction 426.7
  auditory ossicles 744.04
  auricle (ear) 744.1
  autosome(s) NEC 758.5
    21 or 22 758.0
  biliary duct or passage 751.69
  bladder 753.8
  blood vessels (peripheral) (congenital) NEC
    (see also Anomaly, peripheral vascular
    system) 747.60
    cerebral 747.81
    coronary 746.85
  bone NEC 756.9
    foot 755.67
  breast tissue, axilla 757.6
  carpal bones 755.56
  cecum 751.5
  cervix 752.44

Accessory (Continued)
  chromosome(s) NEC 758.5
    13-15 758.1
    16-18 758.2
    21 or 22 758.0
    autosome(s) NEC 758.5
    D₁ 758.1
    E₃ 758.2
    G 758.0
    sex 758.81
  coronary artery 746.85
  cusp(s), heart valve NEC 746.89
    pulmonary 746.09
  cystic duct 751.69
  digits 755.00
  ear (auricle) (lobe) 744.1
  endocrine gland NEC 759.2
  external os 752.44
  eyelid 743.62
  eye muscle 743.69
  face bone(s) 756.0
  fallopian tube (fimbria) (ostium) 752.19
  fingers 755.01
  foreskin 605
  frontonasal process 756.0
  gallbladder 751.69
  genital organ(s)
    female 752.89
      external 752.49
      internal NEC 752.89
    male NEC 752.89
      penis 752.69
  genitourinary organs NEC 752.89
  heart 746.89
    valve NEC 746.89
      pulmonary 746.09
  hepatic ducts 751.69
  hymen 752.49
  intestine (large) (small) 751.5
  kidney 753.3
  lacrimal canal 743.65
  leaflet, heart valve NEC 746.89
    pulmonary 746.09
  ligament, broad 752.19
  liver (duct) 751.69
  lobule (ear) 744.1
  lung (lobe) 748.69
  muscle 756.82
  navicular of carpus 755.56
  nervous system, part NEC 742.8
  nipple 757.6
  nose 748.1
  organ or site NEC - see Anomaly, specified
    type NEC
  ovary 752.0
  oviduct 752.19
  pancreas 751.7
  parathyroid gland 759.2
  parotid gland (and duct) 750.22
  pituitary gland 759.2
  placental lobe - see Placenta, abnormal
  preauricular appendage 744.1
  prepuce 605
  renal arteries (multiple) 747.62
  rib 756.3
    cervical 756.2
  roots (teeth) 520.2
  salivary gland 750.22
  sesamoids 755.8
  sinus - see Condition
  skin tags 757.39
  spleen 759.0
  sternum 756.3
  submaxillary gland 750.22
  tarsal bones 755.67
  teeth, tooth 520.1
    causing crowding 524.31
  tendon 756.89
  thumb 755.01
  thymus gland 759.2
  thyroid gland 759.2

Accessory (Continued)
  toes 755.02
  tongue 750.13
  tragus 744.1
  ureter 753.4
  urethra 753.8
  urinary organ or tract NEC 753.8
  uterus 752.2
  vagina 752.49
  valve, heart NEC 746.89
    pulmonary 746.09
  vertebra 756.19
  vocal cords 748.3
  vulva 752.49
Accident, accidental - see also condition
  birth NEC 767.9
  cardiovascular (see also Disease,
    cardiovascular) 429.2
  cerebral (see also Disease, cerebrovascular,
    acute) 434.91
  cerebrovascular (current) (CVA) (see also
    Disease, cerebrovascular, acute)
    434.91
    aborted 434.91
    embolic 434.11
    healed or old V12.54
    hemorrhagic - see Hemorrhage, brain
    impending 435.9
    ischemic 434.91
    late effect - see Late effect(s) (of)
      cerebrovascular disease
    postoperative 997.02
    thrombotic 434.01
  coronary (see also Infarct, myocardium)
    410.9●
  craniovascular (see also Disease,
    cerebrovascular, acute) 436
  during pregnancy, to mother, affecting fetus
    or newborn 760.5
  heart, cardiac (see also Infarct, myocardium)
    410.9●
  intrauterine 779.89
  vascular - see Disease, cerebrovascular, acute
Accommodation
  disorder of 367.51
    drug-induced 367.89
    toxic 367.89
  insufficiency of 367.4
  paralysis of 367.51
    hysterical 300.11
  spasm of 367.53
Accouchement - see Delivery
Accreta placenta (without hemorrhage) 667.0●
  with hemorrhage 666.0●
Accretio cordis (nonrheumatic) 423.1
Accretions on teeth 523.6
Accumulation secretion, prostate 602.8
Acephalia, acephalism, acephaly 740.0
Acephalic 740.0
Acephalobrachia 759.89
Acephalocardia 759.89
Acephalocardius 759.89
Acephalochiria 759.89
Acephalochirus 759.89
Acephalogaster 759.89
Acephalostomus 759.89
Acephalothorax 759.89
Acephalus 740.0
Acetonemia 790.6
  diabetic 250.1●
    due to secondary diabetes 249.1●
Acetonglycosuria 982.8
Acetonuria 791.6
Achalasia 530.0
  cardia 530.0
  digestive organs congenital NEC 751.8
  esophagus 530.0
  pelvirectal 751.3
  psychogenic 306.4
  pylorus 750.5
  sphincteral NEC 564.89

Achard-Thiers syndrome (adrenogenital) 255.2
Ache(s) - *see* Pain
Acheilia 750.26
Acheiria 755.21
Achillobursitis 726.71
Achillodynia 726.71
Achlorhydria, achlorhydric 536.0
　anemia 280.9
　diarrhea 536.0
　neurogenic 536.0
　postvagotomy 564.2
　psychogenic 306.4
　secondary to vagotomy 564.2
Achloroblepsia 368.52
Achloropsia 368.52
Acholia 575.8
Acholuric jaundice (familial) (splenomegalic)
　(*see also* Spherocytosis) 282.0
　acquired 283.9
Achondroplasia 756.4
Achrestic anemia 281.8
Achroacytosis, lacrimal gland 375.00
　tuberculous (*see also* Tuberculosis)
　　017.3●
Achroma, cutis 709.00
Achromate (congenital) 368.54
Achromatopia 368.54
Achromatopsia (congenital) 368.54
Achromia
　congenital 270.2
　parasitica 111.0
　unguium 703.8
Achylia
　gastrica 536.8
　　neurogenic 536.3
　　psychogenic 306.4
　pancreatica 577.1
Achylosis 536.8
Acid
　burn - *see also* Burn, by site
　　from swallowing acid - *see* Burn, internal
　　　organs
　deficiency
　　amide nicotinic 265.2
　　amino 270.9
　　ascorbic 267
　　folic 266.2
　　nicotinic (amide) 265.2
　　pantothenic 266.2
　intoxication 276.2
　peptic disease 536.8
　stomach 536.8
　　psychogenic 306.4
Acidemia 276.2
　arginosuccinic 270.6
　fetal
　　affecting management of pregnancy
　　　656.3●
　　before onset of labor, in liveborn infant
　　　768.2
　　during labor and delivery, in liveborn
　　　infant 768.3
　　intrauterine 656.3●
　　unspecified as to time of onset, in liveborn
　　　infant 768.4
　newborn 775.81
　pipecolic 270.7
Acidity, gastric (high) (low) 536.8
　psychogenic 306.4
Acidocytopenia 288.59
Acidocytosis 288.3
Acidopenia 288.59
Acidosis 276.2
　diabetic 250.1●
　　due to secondary diabetes 249.1●
　fetal, affecting management of pregnancy
　　656.8●
　fetal, affecting newborn 775.81
　kidney tubular 588.89
　lactic 276.2

Acidosis (*Continued*)
　metabolic NEC 276.2
　　with respiratory acidosis 276.4
　　　of newborn 775.81
　　late, of newborn 775.7
　newborn 775.81
　renal
　　hyperchloremic 588.89
　　tubular (distal) (proximal) 588.89
　respiratory 276.2
　　complicated by
　　　metabolic acidosis 276.4
　　　　of newborn 775.81
　　　metabolic alkalosis 276.4
Aciduria 791.9
　arginosuccinic 270.6
　beta-aminoisobutyric (BAIB) 277.2
　glutaric
　　type I 270.7
　　type II (type IIA, IIB, IIC) 277.85
　　type III 277.86
　glycolic 271.8
　methylmalonic 270.3
　　with glycinemia 270.7
　organic 270.9
　orotic (congenital) (hereditary) (pyrimidine
　　deficiency) 281.4
Acladiosis 111.8
　skin 111.8
Aclasis
　diaphyseal 756.4
　tarsoepiphyseal 756.59
Acleistocardia 745.5
Aclusion 524.4
Acmesthesia 782.0
Acne (pustular) (vulgaris) 706.1
　agminata (*see also* Tuberculosis) 017.0●
　artificialis 706.1
　atrophica 706.0
　cachecticorum (Hebra) 706.1
　conglobata 706.1
　conjunctiva 706.1
　cystic 706.1
　decalvans 704.09
　erythematosa 695.3
　eyelid 706.1
　frontalis 706.0
　indurata 706.1
　keloid 706.1
　lupoid 706.0
　necrotic, necrotica 706.0
　　miliaris 704.8
　neonatal 706.1
　nodular 706.1
　occupational 706.1
　papulosa 706.1
　rodens 706.0
　rosacea 695.3
　scorbutica 267
　scrofulosorum (Bazin) (*see also* Tuberculosis)
　　017.0●
　summer 692.72
　tropical 706.1
　varioliformis 706.0
Acneiform drug eruptions 692.3
Acnitis (primary) (*see also* Tuberculosis) 017.0●
Acomia 704.00
Acontractile bladder 344.61
Aconuresis (*see also* Incontinence) 788.30
Acosta's disease 993.2
Acousma 780.1
Acoustic - *see* condition
Acousticophobia 300.29
Acquired - *see* condition
Acquired immune deficiency syndrome - *see*
　Human immunodeficiency virus
　(disease) (illness) (infection)
Acquired immunodeficiency syndrome - *see*
　Human immunodeficiency virus
　(disease) (illness) (infection)
Acragnosis 781.99

Acrania 740.0
Acroagnosis 781.99
Acroangiodermatitis 448.9
Acroasphyxia, chronic 443.89
Acrobrachycephaly 756.0
Acrobystiolith 608.89
Acrobystitis 607.2
Acrocephalopolysyndactyly 755.55
Acrocephalosyndactyly 755.55
Acrocephaly 756.0
Acrochondrohyperplasia 759.82
Acrocyanosis 443.89
　newborn 770.83
　　meaning transient blue hands and
　　　feet - *omit code*
Acrodermatitis 686.8
　atrophicans (chronica) 701.8
　continua (Hallopeau) 696.1
　enteropathica 686.8
　Hallopeau's 696.1
　perstans 696.1
　pustulosa continua 696.1
　recalcitrant pustular 696.1
Acrodynia 985.0
Acrodysplasia 755.55
Acrohyperhidrosis (*see also* Hyperhidrosis)
　780.8
Acrokeratosis verruciformis 757.39
Acromastitis 611.0
Acromegaly, acromegalia (skin) 253.0
Acromelalgia 443.82
Acromicria, acromikria 756.59
Acronyx 703.0
Acropachy, thyroid (*see also* Thyrotoxicosis)
　242.9●
Acropachyderma 757.39
Acroparesthesia 443.89
　simple (Schultz's type) 443.89
　vasomotor (Nothnagel's type) 443.89
Acropathy thyroid (*see also* Thyrotoxicosis)
　242.9●
Acrophobia 300.29
Acroposthitis 607.2
Acroscleriasis (*see also* Scleroderma) 710.1
Acroscleroderma (*see also* Scleroderma) 710.1
Acrosclerosis (*see also* Scleroderma) 710.1
Acrosphacelus 785.4
Acrosphenosyndactylia 755.55
Acrospiroma, eccrine (M8402/0) - *see*
　Neoplasm, skin, benign
Acrostealgia 732.9
Acrosyndactyly (*see also* Syndactylism)
　755.10
Acrotrophodynia 991.4
Actinic - *see also* condition
　cheilitis (due to sun) 692.72
　　chronic NEC 692.74
　　due to radiation, except from sun 692.82
　conjunctivitis 370.24
　dermatitis (due to sun) (*see also* Dermatitis,
　　actinic) 692.70
　　due to
　　　roentgen rays or radioactive substance
　　　　692.82
　　　ultraviolet radiation, except from sun
　　　　692.82
　　　sun NEC 692.70
　elastosis solare 692.74
　granuloma 692.73
　keratitis 370.24
　ophthalmia 370.24
　reticuloid 692.73
Actinobacillosis, general 027.8
Actinobacillus
　lignieresii 027.8
　mallei 024
　muris 026.1
Actinocutitis NEC (*see also* Dermatitis, actinic)
　692.70
Actinodermatitis NEC (*see also* Dermatitis,
　actinic) 692.70

◀ New　◀▦ Revised　~~deleted~~ Deleted　● Use Additional Digit(s)　▨ Omit code

Actinomyces
    israelii (infection) - *see* Actinomycosis
    muris-ratti (infection) 026.1
Actinomycosis, actinomycotic 039.9
    with
        pneumonia 039.1
    abdominal 039.2
    cervicofacial 039.3
    cutaneous 039.0
    pulmonary 039.1
    specified site NEC 039.8
    thoracic 039.1
Actinoneuritis 357.89
Action, heart
    disorder 427.9
        postoperative 997.1
    irregular 427.9
        postoperative 997.1
        psychogenic 306.2
Active - *see* condition
Activity decrease, functional 780.99
Acute - *see also* condition
    abdomen NEC 789.0●
    gallbladder (*see also* Cholecystitis, acute)
        575.0
Acyanoblepsia 368.53
Acyanopsia 368.53
Acystia 753.8
Acystinervia - *see* Neurogenic, bladder
Acystineuria - *see* Neurogenic, bladder
Adactylia, adactyly (congenital) 755.4
    lower limb (complete) (intercalary) (partial)
        (terminal) (*see also* Deformity,
        reduction, lower limb) 755.39
        meaning all digits (complete) (partial)
            755.31
        transverse (complete) (partial) 755.31
    upper limb (complete) (intercalary) (partial)
        (terminal) (*see also* Deformity,
        reduction, upper limb) 755.29
        meaning all digits (complete) (partial)
            755.21
        transverse (complete) (partial) 755.21
Adair-Dighton syndrome (brittle bones and
    blue sclera, deafness) 756.51
Adamantinoblastoma (M9310/0) - *see*
    Ameloblastoma
Adamantinoma (M9310/0) - *see* Ameloblastoma
Adamantoblastoma (M9310/0) - *see*
    Ameloblastoma
Adams-Stokes (-Morgagni) disease or
    syndrome (syncope with heart block)
    426.9
Adaptation reaction (*see also* Reaction,
    adjustment) 309.9
Addiction - *see also* Dependence
    absinthe 304.6●
    alcoholic (ethyl) (methyl) (wood) 303.9●
        complicating pregnancy, childbirth, or
            puerperium 648.4●
            affecting fetus or newborn 760.71
            suspected damage to fetus affecting
                management of pregnancy 655.4●
    drug (*see also* Dependence) 304.9●
    ethyl alcohol 303.9●
    heroin 304.0●
    hospital 301.51
    methyl alcohol 303.9●
    methylated spirit 303.9●
    morphine (-like substances) 304.0●
    nicotine 305.1
    opium 304.0●
    tobacco 305.1
    wine 303.9●
Addison's
    anemia (pernicious) 281.0
    disease (bronze) (primary adrenal
        insufficiency) 255.41
        tuberculous (*see also* Tuberculosis)
            017.6●
    keloid (morphea) 701.0

Addison's (Continued)
    melanoderma (adrenal cortical
        hypofunction) 255.41
Addison-Biermer anemia (pernicious)
    281.0
Addison-Gull disease - *see* Xanthoma
Addisonian crisis or melanosis (acute
    adrenocortical insufficiency) 255.41
Additional - *see also* Accessory
    chromosome(s) 758.5
        13-15 758.1
        16-18 758.2
        21 758.0
        autosome(s) NEC 758.5
        sex 758.81
Adduction contracture, hip or other joint - *see*
    Contraction, joint
ADEM (acute disseminated encephalomy-elitis)
    (postinfectious) 136.9 [323.61]
    infectious 136.9 [323.61]
    noninfectious 323.81
Adenasthenia gastrica 536.0
Aden fever 061
Adenitis (*see also* Lymphadenitis) 289.3
    acute, unspecified site 683
        epidemic infectious 075
    axillary 289.3
        acute 683
        chronic or subacute 289.1
    Bartholin's gland 616.89
    bulbourethral gland (*see also* Urethritis)
        597.89
    cervical 289.3
        acute 683
        chronic or subacute 289.1
    chancroid (Ducrey's bacillus) 099.0
    chronic (any lymph node, except mesenteric)
        289.1
        mesenteric 289.2
    Cowper's gland (*see also* Urethritis) 597.89
    epidemic, acute 075
    gangrenous 683
    gonorrheal NEC 098.89
    groin 289.3
        acute 683
        chronic or subacute 289.1
    infectious 075
    inguinal (region) 289.3
        acute 683
        chronic or subacute 289.1
    lymph gland or node, except mesenteric
        289.3
        acute 683
        chronic or subacute 289.1
        mesenteric (acute) (chronic) (nonspecific)
            (subacute) 289.2
    mesenteric (acute) (chronic) (nonspecific)
        (subacute) 289.2
        due to Pasteurella multocida (P. septica)
            027.2
    parotid gland (suppurative) 527.2
    phlegmonous 683
    salivary duct or gland (any) (recurring)
        (suppurative) 527.2
    scrofulous (*see also* Tuberculosis) 017.2●
    septic 289.3
    Skene's duct or gland (*see also* Urethritis)
        597.89
    strumous, tuberculous (*see also* Tuberculosis)
        017.2●
    subacute, unspecified site 289.1
    sublingual gland (suppurative) 527.2
    submandibular gland (suppurative)
        527.2
    submaxillary gland (suppurative)
        527.2
    suppurative 683
    tuberculous - *see* Tuberculosis, lymph gland
    urethral gland (*see also* Urethritis) 597.89
    venereal NEC 099.8
    Wharton's duct (suppurative) 527.2

Adenoacanthoma (M8570/3) - *see* Neoplasm,
    by site, malignant
Adenoameloblastoma (M9300/0) 213.1
    upper jaw (bone) 213.0
Adenocarcinoma (M8140/3) - *see also*
    Neoplasm, by site, malignant

Note: The list of adjectival modifiers
below is not exhaustive. A description
of adenocarcinoma that does not appear
in this list should be coded in the same
manner as carcinoma with that description.
Thus, "mixed acidophil-basophil
adenocarcinoma," should be coded in the
same manner as "mixed acidophil-basophil
carcinoma," which appears in the list under
"Carcinoma."

Except where otherwise indicated, the
morphological varieties of adenocarcinoma
in the list below should be coded by site as
for "Neoplasm, malignant."

---

    with
        apocrine metaplasia (M8573/3)
        cartilaginous (and osseous) metaplasia
            (M8571/3)
        osseous (and cartilaginous) metaplasia
            (M8571/3)
        spindle cell metaplasia (M8572/3)
        squamous metaplasia (M8570/3)
    acidophil (M8280/3)
        specified site - *see* Neoplasm, by site,
            malignant
        unspecified site 194.3
    acinar (M8550/3)
    acinic cell (M8550/3)
    adrenal cortical (M8370/3) 194.0
    alveolar (M8251/3)
        and
            epidermoid carcinoma, mixed
                (M8560/3)
            squamous cell carcinoma, mixed
                (M8560/3)
    apocrine (M8401/3)
        breast - *see* Neoplasm, breast, malignant
        specified site NEC - *see* Neoplasm, skin,
            malignant
        unspecified site 173.99
    basophil (M8300/3)
        specified site - *see* Neoplasm, by site,
            malignant
        unspecified site 194.3
    bile duct type (M8160/3)
        liver 155.1
        specified site NEC - *see* Neoplasm, by site,
            malignant
        unspecified site 155.1
    bronchiolar (M8250/3) - *see* Neoplasm, lung,
        malignant
    ceruminous (M8420/3) 173.29
    chromophobe (M8270/3)
        specified site - *see* Neoplasm, by site,
            malignant
        unspecified site 194.3
    clear cell (mesonephroid type) (M8310/3)
    colloid (M8480/3)
    cylindroid type (M8200/3)
    diffuse type (M8145/3)
        specified site - *see* Neoplasm, by site,
            malignant
        unspecified site 151.9
    duct (infiltrating) (M8500/3)
        with Paget's disease (M8541/3) -
            see Neoplasm, breast,
            malignant
        specified site - *see* Neoplasm,
            by site, malignant
        unspecified site 174.9
    embryonal (M9070/3)
    endometrioid (M8380/3) - *see* Neoplasm, by
        site, malignant

Adenocarcinoma *(Continued)*
eosinophil (M8280/3)
    specified site - *see* Neoplasm, by site,
        malignant
    unspecified site 194.3
follicular (M8330/3)
    and papillary (M8340/3) 193
    moderately differentiated type (M8332/3)
        193
    pure follicle type (M8331/3) 193
    specified site - *see* Neoplasm, by site,
        malignant
    trabecular type (M8332/3) 193
    unspecified type 193
    well differentiated type (M8331/3) 193
gelatinous (M8480/3)
granular cell (M8320/3)
Hürthle cell (M8290/3) 193
in
    adenomatous
        polyp (M8210/3)
            polyposis coli (M8220/3) 153.9
        polypoid adenoma (M8210/3)
        tubular adenoma (M8210/3)
        villous adenoma (M8261/3)
infiltrating duct (M8500/3)
    with Paget's disease (M8541/3) - *see*
        Neoplasm, breast, malignant
    specified site - *see* Neoplasm, by site,
        malignant
    unspecified site 174.9
inflammatory (M8530/3)
    specified site - *see* Neoplasm, by site,
        malignant
    unspecified site 174.9
in situ (M8140/2) - *see* Neoplasm, by site, in
        situ
intestinal type (M8144/3)
    specified site - *see* Neoplasm, by site,
        malignant
    unspecified site 151.9
intraductal (noninfiltrating) (M8500/2)
    papillary (M8503/2)
        specified site - *see* Neoplasm, by site, in
            situ
        unspecified site 233.0
    specified site - *see* Neoplasm, by site, in situ
    unspecified site 233.0
islet cell (M8150/3)
    and exocrine, mixed (M8154/3)
        specified site - *see* Neoplasm, by site,
            malignant
        unspecified site 157.9
    pancreas 157.4
    specified site NEC - *see* Neoplasm, by site,
        malignant
    unspecified site 157.4
lobular (M8520/3)
    specified site - *see* Neoplasm, by site,
        malignant
    unspecified site 174.9
medullary (M8510/3)
mesonephric (M9110/3)
mixed cell (M8323/3)
mucinous (M8480/3)
mucin-producing (M8481/3)
mucoid (M8480/3) - *see also* Neoplasm, by
        site, malignant
    cell (M8300/3)
        specified site - *see* Neoplasm, by site,
            malignant
        unspecified site 194.3
nonencapsulated sclerosing (M8350/3) 193
oncocytic (M8290/3)
oxyphilic (M8290/3)
papillary (M8260/3)
    and follicular (M8340/3) 193
    intraductal (noninfiltrating) (M8503/2)
        specified site - *see* Neoplasm, by site,
            in situ
        unspecified site 233.0

Adenocarcinoma *(Continued)*
papillary *(Continued)*
    serous (M8460/3)
        specified site - *see* Neoplasm, by site,
            malignant
        unspecified site 183.0
papillocystic (M8450/3)
    specified site - *see* Neoplasm, by site,
        malignant
    unspecified site 183.0
pseudomucinous (M8470/3)
    specified site - *see* Neoplasm, by site,
        malignant
    unspecified site 183.0
renal cell (M8312/3) 189.0
sebaceous (M8410/3)
serous (M8441/3) - *see also* Neoplasm, by
        site, malignant
    papillary
        specified site - *see* Neoplasm, by site,
            malignant
        unspecified site 183.0
signet ring cell (M8490/3)
superficial spreading (M8143/3)
sweat gland (M8400/3) - *see* Neoplasm, skin,
        malignant
trabecular (M8190/3)
tubular (M8211/3)
villous (M8262/3)
water-clear cell (M8322/3) 194.1
Adenofibroma (M9013/0)
clear cell (M8313/0) - *see* Neoplasm, by site,
        benign
endometrioid (M8381/0) 220
    borderline malignancy (M8381/1) 236.2
    malignant (M8381/3) 183.0
mucinous (M9015/0)
    specified site - *see* Neoplasm, by site,
        benign
    unspecified site 220
prostate 600.20
    with
        other lower urinary tract symptoms
            (LUTS) 600.21
        urinary
            obstruction 600.21
            retention 600.21
serous (M9014/0)
    specified site - *see* Neoplasm, by site,
        benign
    unspecified site 220
specified site - *see* Neoplasm, by site, benign
unspecified site 220
Adenofibrosis
breast 610.2
endometrioid 617.0
Adenoiditis 474.01
acute 463
chronic 474.01
    with chronic tonsillitis 474.02
Adenoids (congenital) (of nasal fossa) 474.9
hypertrophy 474.12
vegetations 474.2
Adenolipomatosis (symmetrical) 272.8
Adenolymphoma (M8561/0)
specified site - *see* Neoplasm, by site, benign
unspecified 210.2
Adenoma (sessile) (M8140/0) - *see also*
        Neoplasm, by site, benign

> Note: Except where otherwise indicated,
> the morphological varieties of adenoma in
> the list below should be coded by site as for
> "Neoplasm, benign."

acidophil (M8280/0)
    specified site - *see* Neoplasm, by site,
        benign
    unspecified site 227.3
acinar (cell) (M8550/0)
acinic cell (M8550/0)

Adenoma *(Continued)*
adrenal (cortex) (cortical) (functioning)
        (M8370/0) 227.0
    clear cell type (M8373/0) 227.0
    compact cell type (M8371/0) 227.0
    glomerulosa cell type (M8374/0) 227.0
    heavily pigmented variant (M8372/0) 227.0
    mixed cell type (M8375/0) 227.0
alpha cell (M8152/0)
    pancreas 211.7
    specified site NEC - *see* Neoplasm, by site,
        benign
    unspecified site 211.7
alveolar (M8251/0)
apocrine (M8401/0)
    breast 217
    specified site NEC - *see* Neoplasm, skin,
        benign
    unspecified site 216.9
basal cell (M8147/0)
basophil (M8300/0)
    specified site - *see* Neoplasm, by site,
        benign
    unspecified site 227.3
beta cell (M8151/0)
    pancreas 211.7
    specified site NEC - *see* Neoplasm, by site,
        benign
    unspecified site 211.7
bile duct (M8160/0) 211.5
black (M8372/0) 227.0
bronchial (M8140/1) 235.7
    carcinoid type (M8240/3) - *see* Neoplasm,
        lung, malignant
    cylindroid type (M8200/3) - *see*
        Neoplasm, lung, malignant
ceruminous (M8420/0) 216.2
chief cell (M8321/0) 227.1
chromophobe (M8270/0)
    specified site - *see* Neoplasm, by site,
        benign
    unspecified site 227.3
clear cell (M8310/0)
colloid (M8334/0)
    specified site - *see* Neoplasm, by site,
        benign
    unspecified site 226
cylindroid type, bronchus (M8200/3) - *see*
        Neoplasm, lung, malignant
duct (M8503/0)
embryonal (M8191/0)
endocrine, multiple (M8360/1)
    single specified site - *see* Neoplasm, by
        site, uncertain behavior
    two or more specified sites 237.4
    unspecified site 237.4
endometrioid (M8380/0) - *see also* Neoplasm,
        by site, benign
    borderline malignancy (M8380/1) - *see*
        Neoplasm, by site, uncertain
        behavior
eosinophil (M8280/0)
    specified site - *see* Neoplasm, by site,
        benign
    unspecified site 227.3
fetal (M8333/0)
    specified site - *see* Neoplasm, by site,
        benign
    unspecified site 226
follicular (M8330/0)
    specified site - *see* Neoplasm, by site,
        benign
    unspecified site 226
hepatocellular (M8170/0) 211.5
Hürthle cell (M8290/0) 226
intracystic papillary (M8504/0)
islet cell (functioning) (M8150/0)
    pancreas 211.7
    specified site NEC - *see* Neoplasm, by site,
        benign
    unspecified site 211.7

Adenoma *(Continued)*
　liver cell (M8170/0) 211.5
　macrofollicular (M8334/0)
　　specified site NEC - *see* Neoplasm, by site,
　　　benign
　　unspecified site 226
　malignant, malignum (M8140/3) - *see*
　　Neoplasm, by site, malignant
　mesonephric (M9110/0)
　microfollicular (M8333/0)
　　specified site - *see* Neoplasm, by site,
　　　benign
　　unspecified site 226
　mixed cell (M8323/0)
　monomorphic (M8146/0)
　mucinous (M8480/0)
　mucoid cell (M8300/0)
　　specified site - *see* Neoplasm, by site,
　　　benign
　　unspecified site 227.3
　multiple endocrine (M8360/1)
　　single specified site - *see* Neoplasm, by
　　　site, uncertain behavior
　　two or more specified sites 237.4
　　unspecified site 237.4
　nipple (M8506/0) 217
　oncocytic (M8290/0)
　oxyphilic (M8290/0)
　papillary (M8260/0) - *see also* Neoplasm, by
　　site, benign
　　intracystic (M8504/0)
　papillotubular (M8263/0)
　Pick's tubular (M8640/0)
　　specified site - *see* Neoplasm, by site,
　　　benign
　　unspecified site
　　　female 220
　　　male 222.0
　pleomorphic (M8940/0)
　polypoid (M8210/0)
　prostate (benign) 600.20
　　with
　　　other lower urinary tract symptoms
　　　　(LUTS) 600.21
　　　urinary
　　　　obstruction 600.21
　　　　retention 600.21
　rete cell 222.0
　sebaceous, sebaceum (gland) (senile)
　　(M8410/0) - *see also* Neoplasm, skin,
　　benign
　　disseminata 759.5
　Sertoli cell (M8640/0)
　　specified site - *see* Neoplasm, by site,
　　　benign
　　unspecified site
　　　female 220
　　　male 222.0
　skin appendage (M8390/0) - *see* Neoplasm,
　　skin, benign
　sudoriferous gland (M8400/0) - *see*
　　Neoplasm, skin, benign
　sweat gland or duct (M8400/0) - *see*
　　Neoplasm, skin, benign
　testicular (M8640/0)
　　specified site - *see* Neoplasm, by site,
　　　benign
　　unspecified site
　　　female 220
　　　male 222.0
　thyroid 226
　trabecular (M8190/0)
　tubular (M8211/0) - *see also* Neoplasm, by
　　site, benign
　　papillary (M8460/3)
　　Pick's (M8640/0)
　　　specified site - *see* Neoplasm, by site,
　　　　benign
　　　unspecified site
　　　　female 220
　　　　male 222.0

Adenoma *(Continued)*
　tubulovillous (M8263/0)
　villoglandular (M8263/0)
　villous (M8261/1) - *see* Neoplasm, by site,
　　uncertain behavior
　water-clear cell (M8322/0) 227.1
　wolffian duct (M9110/0)
Adenomatosis (M8220/0)
　endocrine (multiple) (M8360/1)
　　single specified site - *see* Neoplasm, by
　　　site, uncertain behavior
　　two or more specified sites 237.4
　　unspecified site 237.4
　erosive of nipple (M8506/0) 217
　pluriendocrine - *see* Adenomatosis,
　　endocrine
　pulmonary (M8250/1) 235.7
　　malignant (M8250/3) - *see* Neoplasm,
　　　lung, malignant
　specified site - *see* Neoplasm, by site, benign
　unspecified site 211.3
Adenomatous
　cyst, thyroid (gland) - *see* Goiter, nodular
　goiter (nontoxic) (*see also* Goiter, nodular)
　　241.9
　　toxic or with hyperthyroidism 242.3●
Adenomyoma (M8932/0) - *see also* Neoplasm,
　by site, benign
　prostate 600.20
　　with
　　　other lower urinary tract symptoms
　　　　(LUTS) 600.21
　　　urinary
　　　　obstruction 600.21
　　　　retention 600.21
Adenomyometritis 617.0
Adenomyosis (uterus) (internal) 617.0
Adenopathy (lymph gland) 785.6
　inguinal 785.6
　mediastinal 785.6
　mesentery 785.6
　syphilitic (secondary) 091.4
　tracheobronchial 785.6
　　tuberculous (*see also* Tuberculosis) 012.1●
　　　primary, progressive 010.8●
　tuberculous (*see also* Tuberculosis, lymph
　　gland) 017.2●
　　tracheobronchial 012.1●
　　　primary, progressive 010.8●
Adenopharyngitis 462
Adenophlegmon 683
Adenosalpingitis 614.1
Adenosarcoma (M8960/3) 189.0
Adenosclerosis 289.3
Adenosis
　breast (sclerosing) 610.2
　vagina, congenital 752.49
Adentia (complete) (partial) (*see also* Absence,
　teeth) 520.0
Adherent
　labium (minus) 624.4
　pericardium (nonrheumatic) 423.1
　　rheumatic 393
　placenta 667.0●
　　with hemorrhage 666.0●
　prepuce 605
　scar (skin) NEC 709.2
　tendon in scar 709.2
Adhesion(s), adhesive (postinfectional)
　　(postoperative)
　abdominal (wall) (*see also* Adhesions,
　　peritoneum) 568.0
　amnion to fetus 658.8●
　　affecting fetus or newborn 762.8
　appendix 543.9
　arachnoiditis - *see* Meningitis
　auditory tube (Eustachian) 381.89
　bands - *see also* Adhesions, peritoneum
　　cervix 622.3
　　uterus 621.5
　bile duct (any) 576.8

Adhesion(s) *(Continued)*
　bladder (sphincter) 596.89
　bowel (*see also* Adhesions, peritoneum)
　　568.0
　cardiac 423.1
　　rheumatic 398.99
　cecum (*see also* Adhesions, peritoneum)
　　568.0
　cervicovaginal 622.3
　　congenital 752.49
　　postpartal 674.8●
　　　old 622.3
　cervix 622.3
　clitoris 624.4
　colon (*see also* Adhesions, peritoneum) 568.0
　common duct 576.8
　congenital - *see also* Anomaly, specified type
　　NEC
　　fingers (*see also* Syndactylism, fingers)
　　　755.11
　　labium (majus) (minus) 752.49
　　omental, anomalous 751.4
　　ovary 752.0
　　peritoneal 751.4
　　toes (*see also* Syndactylism, toes) 755.13
　　tongue (to gum or roof of mouth) 750.12
　conjunctiva (acquired) (localized) 372.62
　　congenital 743.63
　　extensive 372.63
　cornea - *see* Opacity, cornea
　cystic duct 575.8
　diaphragm (*see also* Adhesions, peritoneum)
　　568.0
　due to foreign body - *see* Foreign body
　duodenum (*see also* Adhesions, peritoneum)
　　568.0
　　with obstruction 537.3
　ear, middle - *see* Adhesions, middle ear
　epididymis 608.89
　epidural - *see* Adhesions, meninges
　epiglottis 478.79
　Eustachian tube 381.89
　eyelid 374.46
　　postoperative 997.99
　　　surgically created V45.69
　gallbladder (*see also* Disease, gallbladder)
　　575.8
　globe 360.89
　heart 423.1
　　rheumatic 398.99
　ileocecal (coil) (*see also* Adhesions,
　　peritoneum) 568.0
　ileum (*see also* Adhesions, peritoneum)
　　568.0
　intestine (postoperative) (*see also* Adhesions,
　　peritoneum) 568.0
　　with obstruction 560.81
　　　with hernia - *see* Hernia, by site,
　　　　with obstruction
　　　　gangrenous - *see* Hernia, by site,
　　　　　with gangrene
　intra-abdominal (*see also* Adhesions,
　　peritoneum) 568.0
　iris 364.70
　　to corneal graft 996.79
　joint (*see also* Ankylosis) 718.5●
　kidney 593.89
　labium (majus) (minus), congenital 752.49
　liver 572.8
　lung 511.0
　mediastinum 519.3
　meninges 349.2
　　cerebral (any) 349.2
　　　congenital 742.4
　　congenital 742.8
　　spinal (any) 349.2
　　　congenital 742.59
　　tuberculous (cerebral) (spinal) (*see also*
　　　Tuberculosis, meninges) 013.0●
　mesenteric (*see also* Adhesions, peritoneum)
　　568.0

Adhesion(s) *(Continued)*
- middle ear (fibrous) 385.10
  - drum head 385.19
    - to
      - incus 385.11
      - promontorium 385.13
      - stapes 385.12
    - specified NEC 385.19
- nasal (septum) (to turbinates) 478.19
- nerve NEC 355.9
  - spinal 355.9
    - root 724.9
      - cervical NEC 723.4
      - lumbar NEC 724.4
      - lumbosacral 724.4
      - thoracic 724.4
- ocular muscle 378.60
- omentum (*see also* Adhesions, peritoneum) 568.0
- organ or site, congenital NEC - *see* Anomaly, specified type NEC
- ovary 614.6
  - congenital (to cecum, kidney, or omentum) 752.0
- parauterine 614.6
- parovarian 614.6
- pelvic (peritoneal)
  - female (postoperative) (postinfection) 614.6
  - male (postoperative) (postinfection) (*see also* Adhesions, peritoneum) 568.0
  - postpartal (old) 614.6
  - tuberculous (*see also* Tuberculosis) 016.9●
- penis to scrotum (congenital) 752.69
- periappendiceal (*see also* Adhesions, peritoneum) 568.0
- pericardium (nonrheumatic) 423.1
  - rheumatic 393
  - tuberculous (*see also* Tuberculosis) 017.9● [420.0]
- pericholecystic 575.8
- perigastric (*see also* Adhesions, peritoneum) 568.0
- periovarian 614.6
- periprostatic 602.8
- perirectal (*see also* Adhesions, peritoneum) 568.0
- perirenal 593.89
- peritoneum, peritoneal (fibrous) (postoperative) 568.0
  - with obstruction (intestinal) 560.81
    - with hernia - *see also* Hernia, by site, with obstruction
      - gangrenous - *see* Hernia, by site, with gangrene
  - duodenum 537.3
  - congenital 751.4
  - female (postoperative) (postinfective) 614.6
  - pelvic, female 614.6
  - pelvic, male 568.0
  - postpartal, pelvic 614.6
  - to uterus 614.6
- peritubal 614.6
- periureteral 593.89
- periuterine 621.5
- perivesical 596.89
- perivesicular (seminal vesicle) 608.89
- pleura, pleuritic 511.0
  - tuberculous (*see also* Tuberculosis, pleura) 012.0●
- pleuropericardial 511.0
- postoperative (gastrointestinal tract) (*see also* Adhesions, peritoneum)
  - eyelid 997.99
    - surgically created V45.69
  - pelvic, female 614.9
  - pelvic, male 568.0
  - urethra 598.2

Adhesion(s) *(Continued)*
- postpartal, old 624.4
- preputial, prepuce 605
- pulmonary 511.0
- pylorus (*see also* Adhesions, peritoneum) 568.0
- Rosenmüller's fossa 478.29
- sciatic nerve 355.0
- seminal vesicle 608.89
- shoulder (joint) 726.0
- sigmoid flexure (*see also* Adhesions, peritoneum) 568.0
- spermatic cord (acquired) 608.89
  - congenital 752.89
- spinal canal 349.2
  - nerve 355.9
    - root 724.9
      - cervical NEC 723.4
      - lumbar NEC 724.4
      - lumbosacral 724.4
      - thoracic 724.4
- stomach (*see also* Adhesions, peritoneum) 568.0
- subscapular 726.2
- tendonitis 726.90
  - shoulder 726.0
- testicle 608.89
- tongue (congenital) (to gum or roof of mouth) 750.12
  - acquired 529.8
- trachea 519.19
- tubo-ovarian 614.6
- tunica vaginalis 608.89
- ureter 593.89
- uterus 621.5
  - to abdominal wall 614.6
    - in pregnancy or childbirth 654.4●
      - affecting fetus or newborn 763.89
- vagina (chronic) (postoperative) (postradiation) 623.2
- vaginitis (congenital) 752.49
- vesical 596.89
- vitreomacular adhesion 379.27
- vitreous 379.29

Adie (-Holmes) syndrome (tonic pupillary reaction) 379.46
Adiponecrosis neonatorum 778.1
Adiposa dolorosa 272.8
Adiposalgia 272.8
Adiposis
- cerebralis 253.8
- dolorosa 272.8
- tuberosa simplex 272.8

Adiposity 278.02
- heart (*see also* Degeneration, myocardial) 429.1
- localized 278.1

Adiposogenital dystrophy 253.8
Adjustment
- prosthesis or other device - *see* Fitting of
- reaction - *see* Reaction, adjustment

Administration, prophylactic
- antibiotics, long-term V58.62
  - short-term use - *omit code*
- antitoxin, any V07.2
- antivenin V07.2
- chemotherapeutic agent NEC V07.39
- chemotherapy NEC V07.39
- diphtheria antitoxin V07.2
- fluoride V07.31
- gamma globulin V07.2
- immune sera (gamma globulin) V07.2
- passive immunization agent V07.2
- RhoGAM V07.2

Admission (encounter)
- as organ donor - *see* Donor
- by mistake V68.9
- for
  - adequacy testing (for)
    - hemodialysis V56.31
    - peritoneal dialysis V56.32

Admission *(Continued)*
- for *(Continued)*
  - adjustment (of)
    - artificial
      - arm (complete) (partial) V52.0
      - eye V52.2
      - leg (complete) (partial) V52.1
    - brain neuropacemaker V53.02
    - breast
      - implant V52.4
        - exchange (different material) (different size) V52.4
      - prosthesis V52.4
    - cardiac device V53.39
      - defibrillator, automatic implantable (with synchronous cardiac pacemaker) V53.32
      - pacemaker V53.31
        - carotid sinus V53.39
    - catheter
      - non-vascular V58.82
      - vascular V58.81
    - cerebral ventricle (communicating) shunt V53.01
    - colostomy belt V55.3
    - contact lenses V53.1
    - cystostomy device V53.6
    - dental prosthesis V52.3
    - device, unspecified type V53.90
      - abdominal V53.59
      - cardiac V53.39
        - defibrillator, automatic implantable (with synchronous cardiac pacemaker) V53.32
        - pacemaker V53.31
      - carotid sinus V53.39
      - cerebral ventricle (communicating) shunt V53.01
      - gastrointestinal NEC V53.59
      - insulin pump V53.91
      - intestinal V53.50
      - nervous system V53.09
      - orthodontic V53.4
      - other device V53.99
      - prosthetic V52.9
        - breast V52.4
        - dental V52.3
        - eye V52.2
        - specified type NEC V52.8
      - special senses V53.09
      - substitution
        - auditory V53.09
        - nervous system V53.09
        - visual V53.09
      - urinary V53.6
    - dialysis catheter
      - extracorporeal V56.1
      - peritoneal V56.2
    - diaphragm (contraceptive) V25.02
    - gastric lap band V53.51
    - gastrointestinal appliance and device NEC V53.59
    - growth rod V54.02
    - hearing aid V53.2
    - ileostomy device V55.2
    - intestinal appliance and device V53.50
    - neuropacemaker (brain) (peripheral nerve) (spinal cord) V53.02
    - orthodontic device V53.4
    - orthopedic (device) V53.7
      - brace V53.7
      - cast V53.7
      - shoes V53.7
    - pacemaker
      - brain V53.02
      - cardiac V53.31
      - carotid sinus V53.39
      - peripheral nerve V53.02
      - spinal cord V53.02

◀ New   ◀|||| Revised   ~~deleted~~ Deleted   ● Use Additional Digit(s)   ▨ Omit code

Admission *(Continued)*
  for *(Continued)*
    adjustment (of) *(Continued)*
      prosthesis V52.9
        arm (complete) (partial) V52.0
        breast V52.4
        dental V52.3
        eye V52.2
        leg (complete) (partial) V52.1
        specified type NEC V52.8
      spectacles V53.1
      wheelchair V53.8
    adoption referral or proceedings
      V68.89
    aftercare (*see also* Aftercare) V58.9
      cardiac pacemaker V53.31
      chemotherapy (oral) (intravenous)
        V58.11
      dialysis
        extracorporeal (renal) V56.0
        peritoneal V56.8
        renal V56.0
      fracture (*see also* Aftercare, fracture)
        V54.9
      medical NEC V58.89
      organ transplant V58.44
      orthopedic V54.9
        following explantation of joint
          prosthesis (for joint prosthesis
          insertion) (staged procedure)
          V54.82
        specified care NEC V54.89
      pacemaker device
        brain V53.02
        cardiac V53.31
        carotid sinus V53.39
        nervous system V53.02
        spinal cord V53.02
      postoperative NEC V58.49
        wound closure, planned
          V58.41
      postpartum
        immediately after delivery
          V24.0
        routine follow-up V24.2
      postradiation V58.0
      radiation therapy V58.0
      removal of
        non-vascular catheter V58.82
        vascular catheter V58.81
      specified NEC V58.89
      surgical NEC V58.49
        wound closure, planned V58.41
    antineoplastic
      chemotherapy (oral) (intravenous)
        V58.11
      immunotherapy V58.12
    artificial insemination V26.1
    assisted reproductive fertility procedure
      cycle V26.81
    attention to artificial opening (of)
      V55.9
      artificial vagina V55.7
      colostomy V55.3
      cystostomy V55.5
      enterostomy V55.4
      gastrostomy V55.1
      ileostomy V55.2
      jejunostomy V55.4
      nephrostomy V55.6
      specified site NEC V55.8
        intestinal tract V55.4
        urinary tract V55.6
      tracheostomy V55.0
      ureterostomy V55.6
      urethrostomy V55.6
    battery replacement
      cardiac pacemaker V53.31
    blood typing V72.86
      Rh typing V72.86
    boarding V65.0

Admission *(Continued)*
  for *(Continued)*
    breast
      augmentation or reduction V50.1
      implant exchange (different material)
        (different size) V52.4
      reconstruction following mastectomy
        V51.0
      removal
        prophylactic V50.41
        tissue expander without
          synchronous insertion of
          permanent implant V52.4
    change of
      cardiac pacemaker (battery) 53.31
      carotid sinus pacemaker V53.39
      catheter in artificial opening - *see*
        Attention to, artificial, opening
      drains V58.49
      dressing
        wound V58.30
          nonsurgical V58.30
          surgical V58.31
      fixation device
        external V54.89
        internal V54.01
      Kirschner wire V54.89
      neuropacemaker device (brain)
        (peripheral nerve) (spinal cord)
        V53.02
      nonsurgical wound dressing V58.30
      pacemaker device
        brain V53.02
        cardiac V53.31
        carotid sinus V53.39
        nervous system V53.02
      plaster cast V54.89
      splint, external V54.89
      Steinmann pin V54.89
      surgical wound dressing V58.31
      traction device V54.89
      wound packing V58.30
        nonsurgical V58.30
        surgical V58.31
    checkup only V70.0
    chemotherapy, (oral) (intravenous)
      antineoplastic V58.11
    circumcision, ritual or routine (in absence
      of medical indication) V50.2
    clinical research investigation (control)
      (normal comparison) (participant)
      V70.7
    closure of artificial opening - *see* Attention
      to, artificial, opening
    contraceptive
      counseling V25.09
        emergency V25.03
        postcoital V25.03
      management V25.9
        specified type NEC V25.8
    convalescence following V66.9
      chemotherapy V66.2
      psychotherapy V66.3
      radiotherapy V66.1
      surgery V66.0
      treatment (for) V66.5
        combined V66.6
        fracture V66.4
        mental disorder NEC V66.3
        specified condition NEC V66.5
    cosmetic surgery NEC V50.1
      breast reconstruction following
        mastectomy V51.0
      following healed injury or operation
        V51.8
    counseling (*see also* Counseling) V65.40
      without complaint or sickness V65.49
      contraceptive management V25.09
        emergency V25.03
        postcoital V25.03
      dietary V65.3

Admission *(Continued)*
  for *(Continued)*
    counseling *(Continued)*
      exercise V65.41
      fertility preservation (prior to cancer
        therapy) (prior to surgical
        removal of gonads) V26.42
      for
        nonattending third party V65.19
        pediatric
          pre-adoption visit for adoptive
            parent(s) V65.11
          pre-birth visit for expectant
            parent(s) V65.11
        victim of abuse
          child V61.21
          partner or spouse V61.11
      genetic V26.33
      gonorrhea V65.45
      HIV V65.44
      human immunodeficiency virus V65.44
      injury prevention V65.43
      insulin pump training V65.46
      natural family planning
        procreative V26.41
        to avoid pregnancy V25.04
      procreative management V26.49
        using natural family planning V26.41
      sexually transmitted disease NEC
        V65.45
        HIV V65.44
      specified reason NEC V65.49
      substance use and abuse V65.42
      syphilis V65.45
      victim of abuse
        child V61.21
        partner or spouse V61.11
    desensitization to allergens V07.1
    dialysis V56.0
      catheter
        fitting and adjustment
          extracorporeal V56.1
          peritoneal V56.2
        removal or replacement
          extracorporeal V56.1
          peritoneal V56.2
      extracorporeal (renal) V56.0
      peritoneal V56.8
      renal V56.0
    dietary surveillance and counseling V65.3
    drug monitoring, therapeutic V58.83
    ear piercing V50.3
    elective surgery
      breast
        augmentation or reduction V50.1
        reconstruction following
          mastectomy V51.0
        removal, prophylactic V50.41
      circumcision, ritual or routine (in
        absence of medical indication)
        V50.2
      cosmetic NEC V50.1
        breast reconstruction following
          mastectomy V51.0
        following healed injury or
          operation V51.8
      ear piercing V50.3
      face-lift V50.1
      hair transplant V50.0
      plastic
        breast reconstruction following
          mastectomy V51.0
        cosmetic NEC V50.1
        following healed injury or
          operation V51.8
      prophylactic organ removal V50.49
        breast V50.41
        ovary V50.42
      repair of scarred tissue (following
        healed injury or operation) V51.8
      specified type NEC V50.8

Admission (Continued)
  for (Continued)
    end-of-life care V66.7
    examination (see also Examination)
      V70.9
      administrative purpose NEC V70.3
      adoption V70.3
      allergy V72.7
      antibody response V72.61
      at health care facility V70.0
      athletic team V70.3
      camp V70.3
      cardiovascular, preoperative V72.81
      clinical research investigation (control)
        (participant) V70.7
      dental V72.2
      developmental testing (child) (infant)
        V20.2
      donor (potential) V70.8
      driver's license V70.3
      ear V72.19
      employment V70.5
      eye V72.0
      follow-up (routine) - see Examination,
        follow-up
      for admission to
        old age home V70.3
        school V70.3
      general V70.9
        specified reason NEC V70.8
      gynecological V72.31
      health supervision
        child (over 28 days old) V20.2
        infant (over 28 days old) V20.2
        newborn
          8 to 28 days old V20.32
          under 8 days old V20.31
      hearing V72.19
        following failed hearing screening
          V72.11
      immigration V70.3
      infant
        8 to 28 days old V20.32
        over 28 days old, routine V20.2
        under 8 days old V20.31
      insurance certification V70.3
      laboratory V72.60
        ordered as part of a routine
          general medical examination
          V72.62
        pre-operative V72.63
        pre-procedural V72.63
        specified NEC V72.69
      marriage license V70.3
      medical (general) (see also Examination,
        medical) V70.9
      medicolegal reasons V70.4
      naturalization V70.3
      pelvic (annual) (periodic) V72.31
      postpartum checkup V24.2
      pregnancy (possible) (unconfirmed)
        V72.40
        negative result V72.41
        positive result V72.42
      preoperative V72.84
        cardiovascular V72.81
        respiratory V72.82
        specified NEC V72.83
      preprocedural V72.84
        cardiovascular V72.81
        general physical V72.83
        respiratory V72.82
        specified NEC V72.83
      prior to chemotherapy V72.83
      prison V70.3
      psychiatric (general) V70.2
        requested by authority V70.1
      radiological NEC V72.5
      respiratory, preoperative V72.82
      school V70.3
      screening - see Screening

Admission (Continued)
  for (Continued)
    examination (Continued)
      skin hypersensitivity V72.7
      specified type NEC V72.85
      sport competition V70.3
      vision V72.0
      well baby and child care V20.2
    exercise therapy V57.1
    face-lift, cosmetic reason V50.1
    fertility preservation (prior to cancer
      therapy) (prior to surgical removal
      of gonads) V26.82
    fitting (of)
      artificial
        arm (complete) (partial) V52.0
        eye V52.2
        leg (complete) (partial) V52.1
      biliary drainage tube V58.82
      brain neuropacemaker V53.02
      breast V52.4
        implant V52.4
        prosthesis V52.4
      cardiac pacemaker V53.31
      catheter
        non-vascular V58.82
        vascular V58.81
      cerebral ventricle (communicating)
        shunt V53.01
      chest tube V58.82
      colostomy belt V55.2
      contact lenses V53.1
      cystostomy device V53.6
      dental prosthesis V52.3
      device, unspecified type V53.90
        abdominal V53.59
        cerebral ventricle (communicating)
          shunt V53.01
        gastrointestinal NEC V53.59
        insulin pump V53.91
        intestinal V53.50
        intrauterine contraceptive
          insertion V25.11
          removal V25.12
            and reinsertion V25.13
          replacement V25.13
        nervous system V53.09
        orthodontic V53.4
        other device V53.99
        prosthetic V52.9
          breast V52.4
          dental V52.3
          eye V52.2
        special senses V53.09
        substitution
          auditory V53.09
          nervous system V53.09
          visual V53.09
      diaphragm (contraceptive) V25.02
      fistula (sinus tract) drainage tube
        V58.82
      gastric lap band V53.51
      gastrointestinal appliance and device
        NEC V53.59
      growth rod V54.02
      hearing aid V53.2
      ileostomy device V55.2
      intestinal appliance and device
        V53.50
      intrauterine contraceptive device
        insertion V25.11
        removal V25.12
          and reinsertion V25.13
        replacement V25.13
      neuropacemaker (brain) (peripheral
        nerve) (spinal cord) V53.02
      orthodontic device V53.4
      orthopedic (device) V53.7
        brace V53.7
        cast V53.7
        shoes V53.7

Admission (Continued)
  for (Continued)
    fitting (of) (Continued)
      pacemaker
        brain V53.02
        cardiac V53.31
        carotid sinus V53.39
        spinal cord V53.02
      pleural drainage tube V58.82
      portacath V58.81
      prosthesis V52.9
        arm (complete) (partial) V52.0
        breast V52.4
        dental V52.3
        eye V52.2
        leg (complete) (partial) V52.1
        specified type NEC V52.8
      spectacles V53.1
      wheelchair V53.8
    follow-up examination (routine)
      (following) V67.9
      cancer chemotherapy V67.2
      chemotherapy V67.2
      high-risk medication NEC V67.51
      injury NEC V67.59
      psychiatric V67.3
      psychotherapy V67.3
      radiotherapy V67.1
      specified surgery NEC V67.09
      surgery V67.00
        vaginal pap smear V67.01
      treatment (for) V67.9
        combined V67.6
        fracture V67.4
        involving high-risk medication
          NEC V67.51
        mental disorder V67.3
        specified NEC V67.59
    hair transplant, for cosmetic reason
      V50.0
    health advice, education, or instruction
      V65.4
    hearing conservation and treatment
      V72.12
    hormone replacement therapy
      (postmenopausal) V07.4
    hospice care V66.7
    immunizations (childhood) appropriate
      for age V20.2
    immunotherapy, antineoplastic V58.12
    insertion (of)
      intrauterine contraceptive device
        V25.11
      subdermal implantable contraceptive
        V25.5
    insulin pump titration V53.91
    insulin pump training V65.46
    intrauterine device
      insertion V25.11
      management V25.42
      removal V25.12
        and reinsertion V25.13
      replacement V25.13
    investigation to determine further
      disposition V63.8
    in vitro fertilization cycle V26.81
    isolation V07.0
    issue of
      disability examination certificate
        V68.01
      medical certificate NEC V68.09
      repeat prescription NEC V68.1
        contraceptive device NEC V25.49
    kidney dialysis V56.0
    lengthening of growth rod V54.02
    mental health evaluation V70.2
      requested by authority V70.1
    natural family planning counseling and
      advice
      procreative V26.41
      to avoid pregnancy V25.04

◀ New   ◀══ Revised   deleted Deleted   ● Use Additional Digit(s)   Omit code

Admission *(Continued)*
  for *(Continued)*
    nonmedical reason NEC V68.89
    nursing care evaluation V63.8
    observation (without need for further medical care) *(see also* Observation) V71.9
      accident V71.4
      alleged rape or seduction V71.5
      criminal assault V71.6
      following accident V71.4
        at work V71.3
      foreign body ingestion V71.89
      growth and development variations, childhood V21.0
      inflicted injury NEC V71.6
      ingestion of deleterious agent or foreign body V71.89
      injury V71.6
      malignant neoplasm V71.1
      mental disorder V71.09
      newborn - *see* Observation, suspected, condition, newborn
      rape V71.5
      specified NEC V71.89
        disorder V71.9
          abuse V71.81
          accident V71.4
            at work V71.3
          benign neoplasm V71.89
          cardiovascular V71.7
          exposure
            anthrax V71.82
            biological agent NEC V71.83
            SARS V71.83
          heart V71.7
          inflicted injury NEC V71.6
          malignant neoplasm V71.1
          mental NEC V71.09
          neglect V71.81
          specified condition NEC V71.89
          tuberculosis V71.2
      maternal and fetal problem not found
        amniotic cavity and membrane V89.01
        cervical shortening V89.05
        fetal anomaly V89.03
        fetal growth V89.04
        oligohydramnios V89.01
        other specified NEC V89.09
        placenta V89.02
        polyhydramnios V89.01
      tuberculosis V71.2
    occupational therapy V57.21
    organ transplant, donor - *see* Donor
    ovary, ovarian removal, prophylactic V50.42
    palliative care V66.7
    Papanicolaou smear
      cervix V76.2
        for suspected malignant neoplasm V76.2
        no disease found V71.1
        routine, as part of gynecological examination V72.31
        to confirm findings of recent normal smear following initial abnormal smear V72.32
      vaginal V76.47
        following hysterectomy for malignant condition V67.01
    passage of sounds or bougie in artificial opening - *see* Attention to, artificial, opening
    paternity testing V70.4
    peritoneal dialysis V56.32
    physical therapy NEC V57.1

Admission *(Continued)*
  for *(Continued)*
    plastic surgery
      breast reconstruction following mastectomy V51.0
      cosmetic NEC V50.1
      following healed injury or operation V51.8
    postmenopausal hormone replacement therapy V07.4
    postpartum observation
      immediately after delivery V24.0
      routine follow-up V24.2
    poststerilization (for restoration) V26.0
    procreative management V26.9
      assisted reproductive fertility procedure cycle V26.81
      in vitro fertilization cycle V26.81
      specified type NEC V26.89
    prophylactic
      administration of
        antibiotics, long-term V58.62
          short-term use - omit code
        antitoxin, any V07.2
        antivenin V07.2
        chemotherapeutic agent NEC V07.39
        chemotherapy NEC V07.39
        diphtheria antitoxin V07.2
        fluoride V07.31
        gamma globulin V07.2
        immune sera (gamma globulin) V07.2
        RhoGAM V07.2
        tetanus antitoxin V07.2
      breathing exercises V57.0
      chemotherapy NEC V07.39
        fluoride V07.31
      measure V07.9
        specified type NEC V07.8
      organ removal V50.49
        breast V50.41
        ovary V50.42
    psychiatric examination (general) V70.2
      requested by authority V70.1
    radiation management V58.0
    radiotherapy V58.0
    reconstruction following mastectomy V51.0
    reforming of artificial opening - *see* Attention to, artificial, opening
    rehabilitation V57.9
      multiple types V57.89
      occupational V57.21
      orthoptic V57.4
      orthotic V57.81
      physical NEC V57.1
      specified type NEC V57.89
      speech (-language) V57.3
      vocational V57.22
    removal of
      breast tissue expander without synchronous insertion of permanent implant V52.4
      cardiac pacemaker V53.31
      cast (plaster) V54.89
      catheter from artificial opening - *see* Attention to, artificial, opening
      cerebral ventricle (communicating) shunt V53.01
      cystostomy catheter V55.5
      device
        cerebral ventricle (communicating) shunt V53.01
        fixation
          external V54.89
          internal V54.01
        intrauterine contraceptive V25.12
        traction, external V54.89
      drains V58.49

Admission *(Continued)*
  for *(Continued)*
    removal of *(Continued)*
      dressing
        wound V58.30
          nonsurgical V58.30
          surgical V58.31
      fixation device
        external V54.89
        internal V54.01
      intrauterine contraceptive device V25.12
      Kirschner wire V54.89
      neuropacemaker (brain) (peripheral nerve) (spinal cord) V53.02
      nonsurgical wound dressing V58.30
      orthopedic fixation device
        external V54.89
        internal V54.01
      pacemaker device
        brain V53.02
        cardiac V53.31
        carotid sinus V53.39
        nervous system V53.02
      plaster cast V54.89
      plate (fracture) V54.01
      rod V54.01
      screw (fracture) V54.01
      splint, traction V54.89
      staples V58.32
      Steinmann pin V54.89
      subdermal implantable contraceptive V25.43
      surgical wound dressing V58.31
      sutures V58.32
      traction device, external V54.89
      ureteral stent V53.6
      wound packing V58.30
        nonsurgical V58.30
        surgical V58.31
    repair of scarred tissue (following healed injury or operation) V51.8
    replacement of intrauterine contraceptive device V25.13
    reprogramming of cardiac pacemaker V53.31
    respirator [ventilator] dependence during
      mechanical failure V46.14
      power failure V46.12
      for weaning V46.13
    restoration of organ continuity (poststerilization) (tuboplasty) (vasoplasty) V26.0
    Rh typing V72.86
    routine infant and child vision and hearing testing V20.2
    sensitivity test - *see also* Test, skin
      allergy NEC V72.7
      bacterial disease NEC V74.9
      Dick V74.8
      Kveim V82.89
      Mantoux V74.1
      mycotic infection NEC V75.4
      parasitic disease NEC V75.8
      Schick V74.3
      Schultz-Charlton V74.8
    social service (agency) referral or evaluation V63.8
    speech (-language) therapy V57.3
    sterilization V25.2
    suspected disorder (ruled out) (without need for further care) - *see* Observation
    terminal care V66.7
    tests only - *see* Test
    therapeutic drug monitoring V58.83
    therapy
      blood transfusion, without reported diagnosis V58.2
      breathing exercises V57.0

Admission (Continued)
  for (Continued)
    therapy (Continued)
      chemotherapy, antineoplastic V58.11
        prophylactic NEC V07.39
          fluoride V07.31
      dialysis (intermittent) (treatment)
        extracorporeal V56.0
        peritoneal V56.8
        renal V56.0
        specified type NEC V56.8
      exercise (remedial) NEC V57.1
        breathing V57.0
      immunotherapy, antineoplastic V58.12
      long-term (current) (prophylactic)
        drug use NEC V58.69
        antibiotics V58.62
          short-term use - *omit code*
        anticoagulants V58.61
        anti-inflammatories, non-steroidal
          (NSAID) V58.64
        antiplatelets V58.63
        antithrombotics V58.63
        aspirin V58.66
        bisphosphonates V58.68
        high-risk medications NEC V58.69
        insulin V58.67
        methadone for pain control V58.69
        opiate analgesic V58.69
        steroids V58.65
      occupational V57.21
      orthoptic V57.4
      physical NEC V57.1
      radiation V58.0
      speech (-language) V57.3
      vocational V57.22
    toilet or cleaning
      of artificial opening - *see* Attention to,
        artificial, opening
      of non-vascular catheter V58.82
      of vascular catheter V58.81
    treatment
      measure V07.9
        specified type NEC V07.8
    tubal ligation V25.2
    tuboplasty for previous sterilization V26.0
    ultrasound, routine fetal V28.3
    vaccination, prophylactic (against)
      arthropod-borne virus, viral NEC
        V05.1
        disease NEC V05.1
        encephalitis V05.0
      Bacille Calmette Guérin (BCG) V03.2
      BCG V03.2
      chickenpox V05.4
      cholera alone V03.0
        with typhoid-paratyphoid (cholera
          + TAB) V06.0
      common cold V04.7
      dengue V05.1
      diphtheria alone V03.5
      diphtheria-tetanus-pertussis (DTP)
        (DTaP) V06.1
        with
          poliomyelitis (DTP polio) V06.3
          typhoid-paratyphoid (DTP +
            TAB) V06.2
      diphtheria-tetanus [Td] [DT] without
        pertussis V06.5
      disease (single) NEC V05.9
        bacterial NEC V03.9
          specified type NEC V03.89
        combinations NEC V06.9
          specified type NEC V06.8
        specified type NEC V05.8
        viral NEC V04.89
      encephalitis, viral, arthropod-borne
        V05.0
      Hemophilus influenzae, type B [Hib]
        V03.81
      hepatitis, viral V05.3

Admission (Continued)
  for (Continued)
    vaccination, prophylactic (Continued)
      human papillomavirus (HPV) V04.89
      immune sera (gamma globulin) V07.2
      influenza V04.81
        with
          Streptococcus pneumoniae
            [pneumococcus] V06.6
      Leishmaniasis V05.2
      measles alone V04.2
      measles-mumps-rubella (MMR) V06.4
      mumps alone V04.6
        with measles and rubella (MMR)
          V06.4
      not done because of contraindication
        V64.09
      pertussis alone V03.6
      plague V03.3
      pneumonia V03.82
      poliomyelitis V04.0
        with diphtheria-tetanus-pertussis
          (DTP polio) V06.3
      rabies V04.5
      respiratory syncytial virus (RSV)
        V04.82
      rubella alone V04.3
        with measles and mumps (MMR)
          V06.4
      smallpox V04.1
      specified type NEC V05.8
      Streptococcus pneumoniae
        [pneumococcus] V03.82
        with
          influenza V06.6
      tetanus toxoid alone V03.7
        with diphtheria [Td] [DT] V06.5
          and pertussis (DTP) (DTaP)
            V06.1
      tuberculosis (BCG) V03.2
      tularemia V03.4
      typhoid alone V03.1
        with diphtheria-tetanus-pertussis
          (TAB + DTP) V06.2
      typhoid-paratyphoid alone (TAB)
        V03.1
      typhus V05.8
      varicella (chicken pox) V05.4
      viral encephalitis, arthropod-borne
        V05.0
      viral hepatitis V05.3
      yellow fever V04.4
    vasectomy V25.2
    vasoplasty for previous sterilization V26.0
    vision examination V72.0
    vocational therapy V57.22
    waiting period for admission to other
      facility V63.2
      undergoing social agency investigation
        V63.8
    well baby and child care V20.2
    x-ray of chest
      for suspected tuberculosis V71.2
      routine V72.5
Adnexitis (suppurative) (*see also* Salpingo-
  oophoritis) 614.2
Adolescence NEC V21.2
Adoption
  agency referral V68.89
  examination V70.3
  held for V68.89
Adrenal gland - *see* condition
Adrenalism 255.9
  tuberculous (*see also* Tuberculosis) 017.6●
Adrenalitis, adrenitis 255.8
  meningococcal hemorrhagic 036.3
Adrenarche, precocious 259.1
Adrenocortical syndrome 255.2
Adrenogenital syndrome (acquired)
  (congenital) 255.2
  iatrogenic, fetus or newborn 760.79

Adrenoleukodystrophy 277.86
  neonatal 277.86
  x-linked 277.86
Adrenomyeloneuropathy 277.86
Adventitious bursa - *see* Bursitis
Adynamia (episodica) (hereditary) (periodic)
  359.3
Adynamic
  ileus or intestine (*see also* Ileus) 560.1
  ureter 753.22
Aeration lung, imperfect, newborn 770.5
Aerobullosis 993.3
Aerocele - *see* Embolism, air
Aerodermectasia
  subcutaneous (traumatic) 958.7
    surgical 998.81
  surgical 998.81
Aerodontalgia 993.2
Aeroembolism 993.3
Aerogenes capsulatus infection (*see also*
  Gangrene, gas) 040.0
Aero-otitis media 993.0
Aerophagy, aerophagia 306.4
  psychogenic 306.4
Aerosinusitis 993.1
Aerotitis 993.0
Affection, affections - *see also* Disease
  sacroiliac (joint), old 724.6
  shoulder region NEC 726.2
Afibrinogenemia 286.3
  acquired 286.6
  congenital 286.3
  postpartum 666.3●
African
  sleeping sickness 086.5
  tick fever 087.1
  trypanosomiasis 086.5
    Gambian 086.3
    Rhodesian 086.4
Aftercare V58.9
  amputation stump V54.89
  artificial openings - *see* Attention to, artificial,
    opening
  blood transfusion without reported
    diagnosis V58.2
  breathing exercise V57.0
  cardiac device V53.39
    defibrillator, automatic implantable (with
      synchronous cardiac pacemaker)
      V53.32
    pacemaker V53.31
      carotid sinus V53.39
  carotid sinus pacemaker V53.39
  cerebral ventricle (communicating) shunt
    V53.01
  chemotherapy (oral) (intravenous) session
    (adjunctive) (maintenance) V58.11
  defibrillator, automatic implantable cardiac
    (with synchronous cardiac pacemaker)
    V53.32
  exercise (remedial) (therapeutic) V57.1
    breathing V57.0
  extracorporeal dialysis (intermittent)
    (treatment) V56.0
  following surgery NEC V58.49
    for
      injury V58.43
      neoplasm V58.42
      organ transplant V58.44
      trauma V58.43
    joint
      explantation of prosthesis (staged
        procedure) V54.82
      replacement V54.81
    of
      circulatory system V58.73
      digestive system V58.75
      genital organs V58.76
      genitourinary system V58.76
      musculoskeletal system V58.78
      nervous system V58.72

◀ New   ◀▥ Revised   ~~deleted~~ Deleted   ● Use Additional Digit(s)   ▨ Omit code

Aftercare *(Continued)*
  following surgery NEC *(Continued)*
    of *(Continued)*
      oral cavity V58.75
      respiratory system V58.74
      sense organs V58.71
      skin V58.77
      subcutaneous tissue V58.77
      teeth V58.75
      urinary system V58.76
    spinal - *see* Aftercare, following surgery, of, specified body system
    wound closure, planned V58.41
  fracture V54.9
    healing V54.89
      pathologic
        ankle V54.29
        arm V54.20
          lower V54.22
          upper V54.21
        finger V54.29
        foot V54.29
        hand V54.29
        hip V54.23
        leg V54.24
          lower V54.26
          upper V54.25
        pelvis V54.29
        specified site NEC V54.29
        toe(s) V54.29
        vertebrae V54.27
        wrist V54.29
      traumatic
        ankle V54.19
        arm V54.10
          lower V54.12
          upper V54.11
        finger V54.19
        foot V54.19
        hand V54.19
        hip V54.13
        leg V54.14
          lower V54.16
          upper V54.15
        pelvis V54.19
        specified site NEC V54.19
        toe(s) V54.19
        vertebrae V54.17
        wrist V54.19
    removal of
      external fixation device V54.89
      internal fixation device V54.01
    specified care NEC V54.89
  gait training V57.1
    for use of artificial limb(s) V57.81
  internal fixation device V54.09
  involving
    dialysis (intermittent) (treatment)
      extracorporeal V56.0
      peritoneal V56.8
      renal V56.0
    gait training V57.1
      for use of artificial limb(s) V57.81
    growth rod
      adjustment V54.02
      lengthening V54.02
    internal fixation device V54.09
    orthoptic training V57.4
    orthotic training V57.81
    radiotherapy session V58.0
    removal of
      drains V58.49
      dressings
        wound V58.30
          nonsurgical V58.30
          surgical V58.31
      fixation device
        external V54.89
        internal V54.01
      fracture plate V54.01
      nonsurgical wound dressing V58.30

Aftercare *(Continued)*
  involving *(Continued)*
    removal of *(Continued)*
      pins V54.01
      plaster cast V54.89
      rods V54.01
      screws V54.01
      staples V58.32
      surgical wound dressings V58.31
      sutures V58.32
      traction device, external V54.89
      wound packing V58.30
        nonsurgical V58.30
        surgical V58.31
  neuropacemaker (brain) (peripheral nerve) (spinal cord) V53.02
  occupational therapy V57.21
  orthodontic V58.5
  orthopedic V54.9
    change of external fixation or traction device V54.89
    following joint
      explantation of prosthesis (staged procedure) V54.82
      replacement V54.81
    internal fixation device V54.09
    removal of fixation device
      external V54.89
      internal V54.01
    specified care NEC V54.89
  orthoptic training V57.4
  orthotic training V57.81
  pacemaker
    brain V53.02
    cardiac V53.31
    carotid sinus V53.39
    peripheral nerve V53.02
    spinal cord V53.02
  peritoneal dialysis (intermittent) (treatment) V56.8
  physical therapy NEC V57.1
    breathing exercises V57.0
  radiotherapy session V58.0
  rehabilitation procedure V57.9
    breathing exercises V57.0
    multiple types V57.89
    occupational V57.21
    orthoptic V57.4
    orthotic V57.81
    physical therapy NEC V57.1
    remedial exercises V57.1
    specified type NEC V57.89
    speech (-language) V57.3
    therapeutic exercises V57.1
    vocational V57.22
  renal dialysis (intermittent) (treatment) V56.0
  specified type NEC V58.89
    removal of non-vascular catheter V58.82
    removal of vascular catheter V58.81
  speech (-language) therapy V57.3
  stump, amputation V54.89
  vocational rehabilitation V57.22
After-cataract 366.50
  obscuring vision 366.53
  specified type, not obscuring vision 366.52
Agalactia 676.4●
Agammaglobulinemia 279.00
  with lymphopenia 279.2
  acquired (primary) (secondary) 279.06
  Bruton's X-linked 279.04
  infantile sex-linked (Bruton's) (congenital) 279.04
  Swiss-type 279.2
Aganglionosis (bowel) (colon) 751.3
Age (old) *(see also* Senile) 797
Agenesis - *see also* Absence, by site, congenital
  acoustic nerve 742.8
  adrenal (gland) 759.1

Agenesis *(Continued)*
  alimentary tract (complete) (partial) NEC 751.8
    lower 751.2
    upper 750.8
  anus, anal (canal) 751.2
  aorta 747.22
  appendix 751.2
  arm (complete) (partial) *(see also* Deformity, reduction, upper limb) 755.20
  artery (peripheral) NEC *(see also* Anomaly, peripheral vascular system) 747.60
    brain 747.81
    coronary 746.85
    pulmonary 747.31
    umbilical 747.5
  auditory (canal) (external) 744.01
  auricle (ear) 744.01
  bile, biliary duct or passage 751.61
  bone NEC 756.9
  brain 740.0
    specified part 742.2
  breast 757.6
  bronchus 748.3
  canaliculus lacrimalis 743.65
  carpus NEC *(see also* Deformity, reduction, upper limb) 755.28
  cartilage 756.9
  cecum 751.2
  cerebellum 742.2
  cervix 752.43
  chin 744.89
  cilia 743.63
  circulatory system, part NEC 747.89
  clavicle 755.51
  clitoris 752.49
  coccyx 756.13
  colon 751.2
  corpus callosum 742.2
  cricoid cartilage 748.3
  diaphragm (with hernia) 756.6
  digestive organ(s) or tract (complete) (partial) NEC 751.8
    lower 751.2
    upper 750.8
  ductus arteriosus 747.89
  duodenum 751.1
  ear NEC 744.09
    auricle 744.01
    lobe 744.21
  ejaculatory duct 752.89
  endocrine (gland) NEC 759.2
  epiglottis 748.3
  esophagus 750.3
  Eustachian tube 744.24
  extrinsic muscle, eye 743.69
  eye 743.00
    adnexa 743.69
  eyelid (fold) 743.62
  face
    bones NEC 756.0
    specified part NEC 744.89
  fallopian tube 752.19
  femur NEC *(see also* Absence, femur, congenital) 755.34
  fibula NEC *(see also* Absence, fibula, congenital) 755.37
  finger NEC *(see also* Absence, finger, congenital) 755.29
  foot (complete) *(see also* Deformity, reduction, lower limb) 755.31
  gallbladder 751.69
  gastric 750.8
  genitalia, genital (organ)
    female 752.89
      external 752.49
      internal NEC 752.89
    male 752.89
      penis 752.69
  glottis 748.3
  gonadal 758.6

A

Agenesis *(Continued)*
 hair 757.4
 hand (complete) *(see also* Deformity,
   reduction, upper limb) 755.21
 heart 746.89
   valve NEC 746.89
     aortic 746.89
     mitral 746.89
     pulmonary 746.01
 hepatic 751.69
 humerus NEC *(see also* Absence, humerus,
   congenital) 755.24
 hymen 752.49
 ileum 751.1
 incus 744.04
 intestine (small) 751.1
   large 751.2
 iris (dilator fibers) 743.45
 jaw 524.09
 jejunum 751.1
 kidney(s) (partial) (unilateral) 753.0
 labium (majus) (minus) 752.49
 labyrinth, membranous 744.05
 lacrimal apparatus (congenital) 743.65
 larynx 748.3
 leg NEC *(see also* Deformity, reduction, lower
   limb) 755.30
 lens 743.35
 limb (complete) (partial) *(see also* Deformity,
   reduction) 755.4
   lower NEC 755.30
   upper 755.20
 lip 750.26
 liver 751.69
 lung (bilateral) (fissures) (lobe) (unilateral)
   748.5
 mandible 524.09
 maxilla 524.09
 metacarpus NEC 755.28
 metatarsus NEC 755.38
 muscle (any) 756.81
 musculoskeletal system NEC 756.9
 nail(s) 757.5
 neck, part 744.89
 nerve 742.8
 nervous system, part NEC 742.8
 nipple 757.6
 nose 748.1
 nuclear 742.8
 organ
   of Corti 744.05
   or site not listed - *see* Anomaly, specified
     type NEC
 osseous meatus (ear) 744.03
 ovary 752.0
 oviduct 752.19
 pancreas 751.7
 parathyroid (gland) 759.2
 patella 755.64
 pelvic girdle (complete) (partial) 755.69
 penis 752.69
 pericardium 746.89
 perineal body 756.81
 pituitary (gland) 759.2
 prostate 752.89
 pulmonary
   artery 747.31
   trunk 747.31
   vein 747.49
 punctum lacrimale 743.65
 radioulnar NEC *(see also* Absence, forearm,
   congenital) 755.25
 radius NEC *(see also* Absence, radius,
   congenital) 755.26
 rectum 751.2
 renal 753.0
 respiratory organ NEC 748.9
 rib 756.3
 roof of orbit 742.0
 round ligament 752.89
 sacrum 756.13

Agenesis *(Continued)*
 salivary gland 750.21
 scapula 755.59
 scrotum 752.89
 seminal duct or tract 752.89
 septum
   atrial 745.69
   between aorta and pulmonary artery 745.0
   ventricular 745.3
 shoulder girdle (complete) (partial) 755.59
 skull (bone) 756.0
   with
     anencephalus 740.0
     encephalocele 742.0
     hydrocephalus 742.3
       with spina bifida *(see also* Spina
         bifida) 741.0●
     microcephalus 742.1
 spermatic cord 752.89
 spinal cord 742.59
 spine 756.13
   lumbar 756.13
     isthmus 756.11
     pars articularis 756.11
 spleen 759.0
 sternum 756.3
 stomach 750.7
 tarsus NEC 755.38
 tendon 756.81
 testicular 752.89
 testis 752.89
 thymus (gland) 759.2
 thyroid (gland) 243
   cartilage 748.3
 tibia NEC *(see also* Absence, tibia, congenital)
   755.36
 tibiofibular NEC 755.35
 toe (complete) (partial) *(see also* Absence, toe,
   congenital) 755.39
 tongue 750.11
 trachea (cartilage) 748.3
 ulna NEC *(see also* Absence, ulna, congenital)
   755.27
 ureter 753.4
 urethra 753.8
 urinary tract NEC 753.8
 uterus 752.31
 uvula 750.26
 vagina (total) (partial) 752.45
 vas deferens 752.89
 vein(s) (peripheral) NEC *(see also* Anomaly,
   peripheral vascular system) 747.60
   brain 747.81
   great 747.49
   portal 747.49
   pulmonary 747.49
 vena cava (inferior) (superior) 747.49
 vermis of cerebellum 742.2
 vertebra 756.13
   lumbar 756.13
     isthmus 756.11
     pars articularis 756.11
 vulva 752.49
Ageusia *(see also* Disturbance, sensation) 781.1
Aggressiveness 301.3
Aggressive outburst *(see also* Disturbance,
   conduct) 312.0●
 in children or adolescents 313.9
Aging skin 701.8
Agitated - *see* condition
Agitation 307.9
 catatonic *(see also* Schizophrenia) 295.2●
Aglossia (congenital) 750.11
Aglycogenosis 271.0
Agnail (finger) (with lymphangitis) 681.02
Agnosia (body image) (tactile) 784.69
 verbal 784.69
   auditory 784.69
     secondary to organic lesion 784.69
   developmental 315.8
 secondary to organic lesion 784.69

Agnosia *(Continued)*
 visual 368.16
   object 368.16
Agoraphobia 300.22
 with panic disorder 300.21
Agrammatism 784.69
Agranulocytopenia *(see also* Agranulocytosis)
   288.09
Agranulocytosis *(see also* Neutropenia) 288.09
 chronic 288.09
 cyclical 288.02
 due to infection 288.04
 genetic 288.01
 infantile 288.01
 periodic 288.02
 pernicious 288.09
Agraphia (absolute) 784.69
 with alexia 784.61
 developmental 315.39
Agrypnia *(see also* Insomnia) 780.52
Ague *(see also* Malaria) 084.6
 brass-founders' 985.8
 dumb 084.6
 tertian 084.1
Agyria 742.2
AHTR (acute hemolytic transfusion reaction) -
   see Complications, transfusion
Ahumada-del Castillo syndrome
   (nonpuerperal galactorrhea and
   amenorrhea) 253.1
AIDS 042
AIDS-associated retrovirus (disease) (illness)
   042
 infection - *see* Human immunodeficiency
   virus, infection
AIDS-associated virus (disease) (illness) 042
 infection - *see* Human immunodeficiency
   virus, infection
AIDS-like disease (illness) (syndrome) 042
AIDS-related complex 042
AIDS-related conditions 042
AIDS-related virus (disease) (illness) 042
 infection - *see* Human immunodeficiency
   virus, infection
AIDS virus (disease) (illness) 042
 infection - *see* Human immunodeficiency
   virus, infection
Ailment, heart - *see* Disease, heart
Ailurophobia 300.29
AIN I (anal intraepithelial neoplasia I)
   (histologically confirmed) 569.44
AIN II (anal intraepithelial neoplasia II)
   (histologically confirmed) 569.44
AIN III (anal intraepithelial neoplasia III) 230.6
 anal canal 230.5
Ainhum (disease) 136.0
AIPHI (acute idiopathic pulmonary hemorrhage
   in infants (over 28 days old)) 786.31
Air
 anterior mediastinum 518.1
 compressed, disease 993.3
 embolism (any site) (artery) (cerebral) 958.0
   with
     abortion - *see* Abortion, by type, with
       embolism
     ectopic pregnancy *(see also* categories
       633.0-633.9) 639.6
     molar pregnancy *(see also* categories
       630-632) 639.6
   due to implanted device - *see*
     Complications, due to (presence of)
     any device, implant, or graft
     classified to 996.0-996.5 NEC
   following
     abortion 639.6
     ectopic or molar pregnancy 639.6
     infusion, perfusion, or transfusion
       999.1
   in pregnancy, childbirth, or puerperium
     673.0●
   traumatic 958.0

◄ New ◄▥ Revised ~~deleted~~ Deleted ● Use Additional Digit(s) ▨ Omit code

Air *(Continued)*
  hunger 786.09
    psychogenic 306.1
  leak (lung) (pulmonary) (thorax) 512.84
    iatrogenic 512.1
    persistent 512.84
    postoperative 512.2
  rarefied, effects of - *see* Effect, adverse, high altitude
  sickness 994.6
Airplane sickness 994.6
Akathisia, acathisia 781.0
  due to drugs 333.99
  neuroleptic-induced acute 333.99
Akinesia algeria 352.6
Akiyami 100.89
Akureyri disease (epidemic neuromyasthenia) 049.8
Alacrima (congenital) 743.65
Alactasia (hereditary) 271.3
Alagille syndrome 759.89
Alalia 784.3
  developmental 315.31
    receptive-expressive 315.32
  secondary to organic lesion 784.3
Alaninemia 270.8
Alastrim 050.1
Albarrán's disease (colibacilluria) 791.9
Albers-Schönberg's disease (marble bones) 756.52
Albert's disease 726.71
Albinism, albino (choroid) (cutaneous) (eye) (generalized) (isolated) (ocular) (oculocutaneous) (partial) 270.2
Albinismus 270.2
Albright (-Martin) (-Bantam) disease (pseudohypoparathyroidism) 275.49
Albright (-McCune) (-Sternberg) syndrome (osteitis fibrosa disseminata) 756.59
Albuminous - *see* Condition
Albuminuria, albuminuric (acute) (chronic) (subacute) 791.0
  Bence-Jones 791.0
  cardiac 785.9
  complicating pregnancy, childbirth, or puerperium 646.2●
    with hypertension - *see* Toxemia, of pregnancy
    affecting fetus or newborn 760.1
  cyclic 593.6
  gestational 646.2●
  gravidarum 646.2●
    with hypertension - *see* Toxemia, of pregnancy
    affecting fetus or newborn 760.1
  heart 785.9
  idiopathic 593.6
  orthostatic 593.6
  postural 593.6
  pre-eclamptic (mild) 642.4●
    affecting fetus or newborn 760.0
    severe 642.5●
      affecting fetus or newborn 760.0
  recurrent physiologic 593.6
  scarlatinal 034.1
Albumosuria 791.0
  Bence-Jones 791.0
  myelopathic (M9730/3) 203.0●
Alcaptonuria 270.2
Alcohol, alcoholic
  abstinence 291.81
  acute intoxication 305.0●
    with dependence 303.0●
  addiction (*see also* Alcoholism) 303.9●
    maternal
      with suspected fetal damage affecting management of pregnancy 655.4●
      affecting fetus or newborn 760.71
  amnestic disorder, persisting 291.1
  anxiety 291.89

Alcohol, alcoholic *(Continued)*
  brain syndrome, chronic 291.2
  cardiopathy 425.5
  chronic (*see also* Alcoholism) 303.9●
  cirrhosis (liver) 571.2
  delirium 291.0
    acute 291.0
    chronic 291.1
    tremens 291.0
    withdrawal 291.0
  dementia NEC 291.2
  deterioration 291.2
  drunkenness (simple) 305.0●
  hallucinosis (acute) 291.3
  induced
    circadian rhythm sleep disorder 291.82
    hypersomnia 291.82
    insomnia 291.82
    mental disorder 291.9
      anxiety 291.89
      mood 291.89
      sexual 291.89
      sleep 291.82
      specified type 291.89
    parasomnia 291.82
    persisting
      amnestic disorder 291.1
      dementia 291.2
    psychotic disorder
      with
        delusions 291.5
        hallucinations 291.3
    sleep disorder 291.82
  insanity 291.9
  intoxication (acute) 305.0●
    with dependence 303.0●
    pathological 291.4
  jealousy 291.5
  Korsakoff's, Korsakov's, Korsakow's 291.1
  liver NEC 571.3
    acute 571.1
    chronic 571.2
  mania (acute) (chronic) 291.9
  mood 291.89
  paranoia 291.5
  paranoid (type) psychosis 291.5
  pellagra 265.2
  poisoning, accidental (acute) NEC 980.9
    specified type of alcohol - *see* Table of Drugs and Chemicals
  psychosis (*see also* Psychosis, alcoholic) 291.9
    Korsakoff's, Korsakov's, Korsakow's 291.1
    polyneuritic 291.1
      with
        delusions 291.5
        hallucinations 291.3
  related disorder 291.9
  withdrawal symptoms, syndrome NEC 291.81
    delirium 291.0
    hallucinosis 291.3
Alcoholism 303.9●

Note: Use the following fifth-digit subclassification with category 303:

  0   unspecified
  1   continuous
  2   episodic
  3   in remission

  with psychosis (*see also* Psychosis, alcoholic) 291.9
  acute 303.0●
  chronic 303.9●
    with psychosis 291.9
  complicating pregnancy, childbirth, or puerperium 648.4●
  affecting fetus or newborn 760.71
  history V11.3
  Korsakoff's, Korsakov's, Korsakow's 291.1

Alcoholism *(Continued)*
  suspected damage to fetus affecting management of pregnancy 655.4●
Alder's anomaly or syndrome (leukocyte granulation anomaly) 288.2
Alder-Reilly anomaly (leukocyte granulation) 288.2
Aldosteronism (primary) 255.10
  congenital 255.10
  familial type I 255.11
  glucocorticoid-remediable 255.11
  secondary 255.14
Aldosteronoma (M8370/1) 237.2
Aldrich (-Wiskott) syndrome (eczema-thrombocytopenia) 279.12
Aleppo boil 085.1
Aleukemic - *see* condition
Aleukia
  congenital 288.09
  hemorrhagica 284.9
    acquired (secondary) 284.89
    congenital 284.09
    idiopathic 284.9
  splenica 289.4
Alexia (congenital) (developmental) 315.01
  secondary to organic lesion 784.61
Algoneurodystrophy 733.7
Algophobia 300.29
Alibert's disease (mycosis fungoides) (M9700/3) 202.1●
Alibert-Bazin disease (M9700/3) 202.1●
Alice in Wonderland syndrome 293.89
Alienation, mental (*see also* Psychosis) 298.9
Alkalemia 276.3
Alkalosis 276.3
  metabolic 276.3
    with respiratory acidosis 276.4
  respiratory 276.3
Alkaptonuria 270.2
Allen-Masters syndrome 620.6
Allergic bronchopulmonary aspergillosis 518.6
Allergy, allergic (reaction) 995.3
  air-borne substance (*see also* Fever, hay) 477.9
    specified allergen NEC 477.8
  alveolitis (extrinsic) 495.9
    due to
      Aspergillus clavatus 495.4
      cryptostroma corticale 495.6
      organisms (fungal, thermophilic actinomycete, other) growing in ventilation (air conditioning systems) 495.7
    specified type NEC 495.8
  anaphylactic reaction or shock 995.0
    due to food - *see* Anaphylactic reaction or shock, due to, food
  angioedema 995.1
  angioneurotic edema 995.1
  animal (cat) (dog) (epidermal) 477.8
    dander 477.2
    hair 477.2
  arthritis (*see also* Arthritis, allergic) 716.2●
  asthma - *see* Asthma
  bee sting (anaphylactic shock) 989.5
  biological - *see* Allergy, drug
  bronchial asthma - *see* Asthma
  conjunctivitis (eczematous) 372.14
  dander, animal (cat) (dog) 477.2
  dandruff 477.8
  dermatitis (venenata) - *see* Dermatitis
  diathesis V15.09
  drug, medicinal substance, and biological (any) (correct medicinal substance properly administered) (external) (internal) 995.27
    wrong substance given or taken NEC 977.9
      specified drug or substance - *see* Table of Drugs and Chemicals
  dust (house) (stock) 477.8
  eczema - *see* Eczema

Allergy, allergic *(Continued)*
  endophthalmitis 360.19
  epidermal (animal) 477.8
  existing dental restorative material 525.66
  feathers 477.8
  food (any) (ingested) 693.1
    atopic 691.8
    in contact with skin 692.5
  gastritis 535.4 ●
  gastroenteritis 558.3
  gastrointestinal 558.3
  grain 477.0
  grass (pollen) 477.0
    asthma *(see also* Asthma) 493.0 ●
    hay fever 477.0
  hair, animal (cat) (dog) 477.2
  hay fever (grass) (pollen) (ragweed) (tree)
    (see also Fever, hay) 477.9
  history (of) V15.09
    to
      arachnid bite V15.06
      eggs V15.03
      food additives V15.05
      insect bite V15.06
      latex V15.07
      milk products V15.02
      nuts V15.05
        peanuts V15.01
      radiographic dye V15.08
      seafood V15.04
      specified food NEC V15.05
      spider bite V15.06
  horse serum - *see* Allergy, serum
  inhalant 477.9
    dust 477.8
    pollen 477.0
    specified allergen other than pollen 477.8
  kapok 477.8
  medicine - *see* Allergy, drug
  migraine 339.00
  milk protein 558.3
  pannus 370.62
  pneumonia 518.3
  pollen (any) (hay fever) 477.0
    asthma *(see also* Asthma) 493.0 ●
  primrose 477.0
  primula 477.0
  purpura 287.0
  ragweed (pollen) (Senecio jacobae) 477.0
    asthma *(see also* Asthma) 493.0 ●
    hay fever 477.0
  respiratory *(see also* Allergy, inhalant) 477.9
    due to
      drug - *see* Allergy, drug
      food - *see* Allergy, food
    rhinitis *(see also* Fever, hay) 477.9
      due to food 477.1
  rose 477.0
  Senecio jacobae 477.0
  serum (prophylactic) (therapeutic) 999.59
    anaphylactic reaction or shock 999.49
  shock (anaphylactic) (due to adverse effect of
    correct medicinal substance properly
    administered) 995.0
    food - *see* Anaphylactic reaction or shock,
      due to, food
    from
      administration of blood and blood
        products 999.41
      immunization 999.42
      serum NEC 999.49
  sinusitis *(see also* Fever, hay) 477.9
  skin reaction 692.9
    specified substance - *see* Dermatitis, due
      to
  tree (any) (hay fever) (pollen) 477.0
    asthma *(see also* Asthma) 493.0 ●
  upper respiratory *(see also* Fever, hay) 477.9
  urethritis 597.89
  urticaria 708.0
  vaccine - *see* Allergy, serum

Allescheriosis 117.6
Alligator skin disease (ichthyosis congenita)
  757.1
  acquired 701.1
Allocheiria, allochiria *(see also* Disturbance,
  sensation) 782.0
Almeida's disease (Brazilian blastomycosis)
  116.1
Alopecia (atrophicans) (pregnancy) (premature)
  (senile) 704.00
  adnata 757.4
  areata 704.01
  celsi 704.01
  cicatrisata 704.09
  circumscripta 704.01
  congenital, congenitalis 757.4
  disseminata 704.01
  effluvium (telogen) 704.02
  febrile 704.09
  generalisata 704.09
  hereditaria 704.09
  marginalis 704.01
  mucinosa 704.09
  postinfectional 704.09
  seborrheica 704.09
  specific 091.82
  syphilitic (secondary) 091.82
  telogen effluvium 704.02
  totalis 704.09
  toxica 704.09
  universalis 704.09
  x-ray 704.09
Alpers' disease 330.8
Alpha-lipoproteinemia 272.4
Alpha thalassemia 282.43
Alphos 696.1
Alpine sickness 993.2
Alport's syndrome (hereditary hematuria-
  nephropathy-deafness) 759.89
ALPS (autoimmune lymphoproliferative
  syndrome) 279.41
ALTE (apparent life threatening event) in
  newborn and infant 799.82
Alteration (of), altered
  awareness 780.09
    transient 780.02
  consciousness 780.09
    persistent vegetative state
      780.03
    transient 780.02
  mental status 780.97
    amnesia (retrograde) 780.93
    memory loss 780.93
Alternaria (infection) 118
Alternating - *see* condition
Altitude, high (effects) - *see* Effect, adverse,
  high altitude
Aluminosis (of lung) 503
Alvarez syndrome (transient cerebral
  ischemia) 435.9
Alveolar capillary block syndrome
  516.64
Alveolitis
  allergic (extrinsic) 495.9
    due to organisms (fungal, thermophilic
      actinomycete, other) growing in
      ventilation (air conditioning
      systems) 495.7
    specified type NEC 495.8
  due to
    Aspergillus clavatus 495.4
    Cryptostroma corticale 495.6
  fibrosing (chronic) (cryptogenic) (lung)
    516.31
    idiopathic 516.30
    rheumatoid 714.81
  jaw 526.5
  sicca dolorosa 526.5
Alveolus, alveolar - *see* condition
Alymphocytosis (pure) 279.2
Alymphoplasia, thymic 279.2

Alzheimer's
  dementia (senile)
    with behavioral disturbance 331.0
      [294.11]
    without behavioral disturbance 331.0
      [294.10]
  disease or sclerosis 331.0
    with dementia - *see* Alzheimer's,
      dementia
Amastia *(see also* Absence, breast) 611.89
Amaurosis (acquired) (congenital) *(see also*
  Blindness) 369.00
  fugax 362.34
  hysterical 300.11
  Leber's (congenital) 362.76
  tobacco 377.34
  uremic - *see* Uremia
Amaurotic familial idiocy (infantile) (juvenile)
  (late) 330.1
Ambisexual 752.7
Amblyopia (acquired) (congenital) (partial)
  368.00
  color 368.59
    acquired 368.55
  deprivation 368.02
  ex anopsia 368.00
  hysterical 300.11
  nocturnal 368.60
    vitamin A deficiency 264.5
  refractive 368.03
  strabismic 368.01
  suppression 368.01
  tobacco 377.34
  toxic NEC 377.34
  uremic - *see* Uremia
Ameba, amebic (histolytica) - *see also*
  Amebiasis
  abscess 006.3
    bladder 006.8
    brain (with liver and lung abscess)
      006.5
    liver 006.3
      with
        brain abscess (and lung abscess)
          006.5
        lung abscess 006.4
    lung (with liver abscess) 006.4
      with brain abscess 006.5
    seminal vesicle 006.8
    spleen 006.8
  carrier (suspected of) V02.2
  meningoencephalitis
    due to Naegleria (gruberi) 136.29
    primary 136.29
Amebiasis NEC 006.9
  with
    brain abscess (with liver or lung abscess)
      006.5
    liver abscess (without mention of brain or
      lung abscess) 006.3
    lung abscess (with liver abscess)
      006.4
      with brain abscess 006.5
  acute 006.0
  bladder 006.8
  chronic 006.1
  cutaneous 006.6
  cutis 006.6
  due to organism other than Entamoeba
    histolytica 007.8
  hepatic *(see also* Abscess, liver, amebic)
    006.3
  nondysenteric 006.2
  seminal vesicle 006.8
  specified
    organism NEC 007.8
    site NEC 006.8
Ameboma 006.8
Amelia 755.4
  lower limb 755.31
  upper limb 755.21

◀ New　◀ Revised　~~deleted~~ Deleted　● Use Additional Digit(s)　▨ Omit code

Ameloblastoma (M9310/0) 213.1
  jaw (bone) (lower) 213.1
    upper 213.0
  long bones (M9261/3) - see Neoplasm, bone,
    malignant
  malignant (M9310/3) 170.1
    jaw (bone) (lower) 170.1
      upper 170.0
  mandible 213.1
  tibial (M9261/3) 170.7
Amelogenesis imperfecta 520.5
  nonhereditaria (segmentalis) 520.4
Amenorrhea (primary) (secondary) 626.0
  due to ovarian dysfunction 256.8
  hyperhormonal 256.8
Amentia (see also Disability, intellectual) 319
  Meynert's (nonalcoholic) 294.0
    alcoholic 291.1
  nevoid 759.6
American
  leishmaniasis 085.5
  mountain tick fever 066.1
  trypanosomiasis - see Trypanosomiasis,
    American
Ametropia (see also Disorder, accommodation)
  367.9
Amianthosis 501
Amimia 784.69
Amino acid
  deficiency 270.9
    anemia 281.4
  metabolic disorder (see also Disorder, amino
    acid) 270.9
Aminoaciduria 270.9
  imidazole 270.5
Amnesia (retrograde) 780.93
  auditory 784.69
    developmental 315.31
    secondary to organic lesion 784.69
  dissociative 300.12
  hysterical or dissociative type 300.12
  psychogenic 300.12
  transient global 437.7
Amnestic (confabulatory) syndrome 294.0
  alcohol-induced persisting 291.1
  drug-induced persisting 292.83
  posttraumatic 294.0
Amniocentesis screening (for) V28.2
  alphafetoprotein level, raised V28.1
  chromosomal anomalies V28.0
Amnion, amniotic - see also condition
  nodosum 658.8●
Amnionitis (complicating pregnancy) 658.4●
  affecting fetus or newborn 762.7
Amoral trends 301.7
Amotio retinae (see also Detachment, retina) 361.9
Ampulla
  lower esophagus 530.89
  phrenic 530.89
Amputation
  any part of fetus, to facilitate delivery 763.89
  cervix (supravaginal) (uteri) 622.8
    in pregnancy or childbirth 654.6●
      affecting fetus or newborn 763.89
  clitoris - see Wound, open, clitoris
  congenital
    lower limb 755.31
    upper limb 755.21
  neuroma (traumatic) - see also Injury, nerve,
    by site
    surgical complication (late) 997.61
  penis - see Amputation, traumatic, penis
  status (without complication) - see Absence,
    by site, acquired
  stump (surgical) (posttraumatic)
    abnormal, painful, or with complication
      (late) 997.60
    healed or old NEC - see also Absence, by
      site, acquired
      lower V49.70
      upper V49.60

Amputation (Continued)
  traumatic (complete) (partial)

> Note: "Complicated" includes traumatic
> amputation with delayed healing, delayed
> treatment, foreign body, or infection.

    arm 887.4
      at or above elbow 887.2
        complicated 887.3
      below elbow 887.0
        complicated 887.1
      both (bilateral) (any level(s)) 887.6
        complicated 887.7
      complicated 887.5
    finger(s) (one or both hands) 886.0
      with thumb(s) 885.0
        complicated 885.1
      complicated 886.1
    foot (except toe(s) only) 896.0
      and other leg 897.6
        complicated 897.7
      both (bilateral) 896.2
        complicated 896.3
      complicated 896.1
    toe(s) only (one or both feet) 895.0
      complicated 895.1
    genital organ(s) (external) NEC 878.8
      complicated 878.9
    hand (except finger(s) only) 887.0
      and other arm 887.6
        complicated 887.7
      both (bilateral) 887.6
        complicated 887.7
      complicated 887.1
    finger(s) (one or both hands)
      886.0
      with thumb(s) 885.0
        complicated 885.1
      complicated 886.1
    thumb(s) (with fingers of either hand)
      885.0
      complicated 885.1
    head 874.9
    late effect - see Late, effects (of),
      amputation
    leg 897.4
      and other foot 897.6
        complicated 897.7
      at or above knee 897.2
        complicated 897.3
      below knee 897.0
        complicated 897.1
      both (bilateral) 897.6
        complicated 897.7
      complicated 897.5
    lower limb(s) except toe(s) - see
      Amputation, traumatic, leg
    nose - see Wound, open, nose
    penis 878.0
      complicated 878.1
    sites other than limbs - see Wound, open,
      by site
    thumb(s) (with finger(s) of either hand)
      885.0
      complicated 885.1
    toe(s) (one or both feet) 895.0
      complicated 895.1
    upper limb(s) - see Amputation, traumatic,
      arm
Amputee (bilateral) (old) - see also Absence, by
  site, acquired V49.70
Amusia 784.69
  developmental 315.39
  secondary to organic lesion 784.69
Amyelencephalus 740.0
Amyelia 742.59
Amygdalitis - see Tonsillitis
Amygdalolith 474.8
Amyloid disease or degeneration 277.30
  heart 277.39 [425.7]

Amyloidosis (familial) (general) (generalized)
  (genetic) (primary) 277.30
  with lung involvement 277.39 [517.8]
  cardiac, hereditary 277.39
  heart 277.39 [425.7]
  nephropathic 277.39 [583.81]
  neuropathic (Portuguese) (Swiss) 277.39
    [357.4]
  pulmonary 277.39 [517.8]
  secondary 277.39
  systemic, inherited 277.39
Amylopectinosis (brancher enzyme deficiency)
  271.0
Amylophagia 307.52
Amyoplasia, congenita 756.89
Amyotonia 728.2
  congenita 358.8
Amyotrophia, amyotrophy, amyotrophic
  728.2
  congenita 756.89
  diabetic 250.6● [353.5]
    due to secondary diabetes 249.6●
      [353.5]
  lateral sclerosis (syndrome) 335.20
  neuralgic 353.5
  sclerosis (lateral) 335.20
  spinal progressive 335.21
Anacidity, gastric 536.0
  psychogenic 306.4
Anaerosis of newborn 770.88
Analbuminemia 273.8
Analgesia (see also Anesthesia) 782.0
Analphalipoproteinemia 272.5
Anaphylactic reaction or shock (correct
  substance properly administered)
  995.0
  due to
    administration of blood and blood
      products 999.41
    chemical - see Table of Drugs and
      Chemicals
    correct medicinal substance properly
      administered 995.0
    drug or medicinal substance
      correct substance properly
        administered 995.0
      overdose or wrong substance given or
        taken 977.9
      specified drug - see Table of Drugs
        and Chemicals
    following sting(s) 989.5
    food 995.60
      additives 995.66
      crustaceans 995.62
      eggs 995.68
      fish 995.65
      fruits 995.63
      milk products 995.67
      nuts (tree) 995.64
      peanuts 995.61
      seeds 995.64
      specified NEC 995.69
      tree nuts 995.64
      vegetables 995.63
    immunization 999.42
    overdose or wrong substance given or
      taken 977.9
      specified drug - see Table of Drugs and
        Chemicals
    serum NEC 999.49
  following sting(s) 989.5
  purpura 287.0
  serum NEC 999.49
Anaphylactoid reaction or shock - see
  Anaphylactic reaction or shock
Anaphylaxis - see Anaphylactic reaction or
  shock
Anaplasia, cervix 622.10
Anaplasmosis, human 082.49
Anarthria 784.51
Anarthritic rheumatoid disease 446.5

Anasarca 782.3
  cardiac (*see also* Failure, heart) 428.0
  fetus or newborn 778.0
  lung 514
  nutritional 262
  pulmonary 514
  renal (*see also* Nephrosis) 581.9
Anaspadias 752.62
Anastomosis
  aneurysmal - *see* Aneurysm
  arteriovenous, congenital NEC (*see also*
     Anomaly, arteriovenous) 747.60
    ruptured, of brain (*see also* Hemorrhage,
      subarachnoid) 430
  intestinal 569.89
    complicated NEC 997.49
      involving urinary tract 997.5
  retinal and choroidal vessels 743.58
    acquired 362.17
Anatomical narrow angle (glaucoma)
  365.02
Ancylostoma (infection) (infestation)
  126.9
  americanus 126.1
  braziliense 126.2
  caninum 126.8
  ceylanicum 126.3
  duodenale 126.0
  Necator americanus 126.1
Ancylostomiasis (intestinal) 126.9
  ancylostoma
    americanus 126.1
    caninum 126.8
    ceylanicum 126.3
    duodenale 126.0
  braziliense 126.2
  Necator americanus 126.1
Anders' disease or syndrome (adiposis
  tuberosa simplex) 272.8
Andersen's glycogen storage disease
  271.0
Anderson's disease 272.7
Andes disease 993.2
Andrews' disease (bacterid) 686.8
Androblastoma (M8630/1)
  benign (M8630/0)
    specified site - *see* Neoplasm, by site,
      benign
    unspecified site
      female 220
      male 222.0
  malignant (M8630/3)
    specified site - *see* Neoplasm, by site,
      malignant
    unspecified site
      female 183.0
      male 186.9
  specified site - *see* Neoplasm, by site,
    uncertain behavior
  tubular (M8640/0)
    with lipid storage (M8641/0)
      specified site - *see* Neoplasm, by site,
        benign
      unspecified site
        female 220
        male 222.0
    specified site - *see* Neoplasm, by site,
      benign
    unspecified site
      female 220
      male 222.0
  unspecified site
    female 236.2
    male 236.4
Android pelvis 755.69
  with disproportion (fetopelvic) 653.3●
    affecting fetus or newborn 763.1
    causing obstructed labor 660.1●
      affecting fetus or newborn 763.1
Anectasis, pulmonary (newborn or fetus)
  770.5

Anemia 285.9
  with
    disorder of
      anaerobic glycolysis 282.3
      pentose phosphate pathway 282.2
    koilonychia 280.9
  6-phosphogluconic dehydrogenase
    deficiency 282.2
  achlorhydric 280.9
  achrestic 281.8
  Addison's (pernicious) 281.0
  Addison-Biermer (pernicious) 281.0
  agranulocytic 288.09
  amino acid deficiency 281.4
  antineoplastic chemotherapy induced 285.3
  aplastic 284.9
    acquired (secondary) 284.89
    congenital 284.01
    constitutional 284.01
    due to
      antineoplastic chemotherapy 284.89
      chronic systemic disease 284.89
      drugs 284.89
      infection 284.89
      radiation 284.89
    idiopathic 284.9
    myxedema 244.9
    of or complicating pregnancy 648.2●
    red cell (acquired) (adult) (with
      thymoma) 284.81
      congenital 284.01
      pure 284.01
    specified type NEC 284.89
    toxic (paralytic) 284.89
  aregenerative 284.9
    congenital 284.01
  asiderotic 280.9
  atypical (primary) 285.9
  autohemolysis of Selwyn and Dacie (type I)
    282.2
  autoimmune hemolytic 283.0
  Baghdad Spring 282.2
  Balantidium coli 007.0
  Biermer's (pernicious) 281.0
  blood loss (chronic) 280.0
    acute 285.1
  bothriocephalus 123.4
  brickmakers' (*see also* Ancylostomiasis) 126.9
  cerebral 437.8
  childhood 282.9
  chlorotic 280.9
  chronic 285.9
    blood loss 280.0
    hemolytic 282.9
      idiopathic 283.9
    simple 281.9
  chronica congenita aregenerativa 284.01
  combined system disease NEC 281.0 [336.2]
    due to dietary deficiency 281.1 [336.2]
  complicating pregnancy or childbirth 648.2●
  congenital (following fetal blood loss) 776.5
    aplastic 284.01
    due to isoimmunization NEC 773.2
    Heinz-body 282.7
    hereditary hemolytic NEC 282.9
    nonspherocytic
      type I 282.2
      type II 282.3
    pernicious 281.0
    spherocytic (*see also* Spherocytosis) 282.0
  Cooley's (erythroblastic) 282.44
  crescent - *see* Disease, sickle-cell
  cytogenic 281.0
  Dacie's (nonspherocytic)
    type I 282.2
    type II 282.3
  Davidson's (refractory) 284.9
  deficiency 281.9
    2, 3 diphosphoglycurate mutase 282.3
    2, 3 PG 282.3
    6-PGD 282.2

Anemia (*Continued*)
  deficiency (*Continued*)
    6-phosphogluronic dehydrogenase 282.2
    amino acid 281.4
    combined B_{12} and folate 281.3
    enzyme, drug-induced (hemolytic) 282.2
    erythrocytic glutathione 282.2
    folate 281.2
      dietary 281.2
      drug-induced 281.2
    folic acid 281.2
      dietary 281.2
      drug-induced 281.2
    G-6-PD 282.2
    GGS-R 282.2
    glucose-6-phosphate dehydrogenase
      (G-6-PD) 282.2
    glucose-phosphate isomerase 282.3
    glutathione peroxidase 282.2
    glutathione reductase 282.2
    glyceraldehyde phosphate
      dehydrogenase 282.3
    GPI 282.3
    G SH 282.2
    hexokinase 282.3
    iron (Fe) 280.9
      specified NEC 280.8
    nutritional 281.9
      with
        poor iron absorption 280.9
        specified deficiency NEC 281.8
      due to inadequate dietary iron intake
        280.1
      specified type NEC 281.8
    of or complicating pregnancy 648.2●
    pentose phosphate pathway 282.2
    PFK 282.3
    phosphofructo-aldolase 282.3
    phosphofructokinase 282.3
    phosphoglycerate kinase 282.3
    PK 282.3
    protein 281.4
    pyruvate kinase (PK) 282.3
    TPI 282.3
    triosephosphate isomerase 282.3
    vitamin B_{12} NEC 281.1
      dietary 281.1
      pernicious 281.0
  Diamond-Blackfan (congenital hypoplastic)
    284.01
  dibothriocephalus 123.4
  dimorphic 281.9
  diphasic 281.8
  diphtheritic 032.89
  Diphyllobothrium 123.4
  drepanocytic (*see also* Disease, sickle-cell)
    282.60
  due to
    antineoplastic chemotherapy 285.3
    blood loss (chronic) 280.0
      acute 285.1
    chemotherapy, antineoplastic 285.3
    defect of Embden-Meyerhof pathway
      glycolysis 282.3
    disorder of glutathione metabolism 282.2
    drug - *see* Anemia, by type (*see also* Table
      of Drugs and Chemicals)
      chemotherapy, antineoplastic 285.3
    fetal blood loss 776.5
    fish tapeworm (D. latum) infestation
      123.4
    glutathione metabolism disorder 282.2
    hemorrhage (chronic) 280.0
      acute 285.1
    hexose monophosphate (HMP) shunt
      deficiency 282.2
    impaired absorption 280.9
    loss of blood (chronic) 280.0
      acute 285.1
    myxedema 244.9
    Necator americanus 126.1

◀ New   ◀▦ Revised   ~~deleted~~ Deleted   ● Use Additional Digit(s)   ▦ Omit code

Anemia *(Continued)*
  due to *(Continued)*
    prematurity 776.6
    selective vitamin B_{12} malabsorption with
      proteinuria 281.1
  Dyke-Young type (secondary)
    (symptomatic) 283.9
  dyserythropoietic (congenital) (types I, II, III)
    285.8
  dyshemopoietic (congenital) 285.8
  Egypt *(see also* Ancylostomiasis) 126.9
  elliptocytosis *(see also* Elliptocytosis) 282.1
  enzyme deficiency, drug-induced 282.2
  epidemic *(see also* Ancylostomiasis) 126.9
  EPO resistant 285.21
  erythroblastic
    familial 282.44
    fetus or newborn *(see also* Disease,
      hemolytic) 773.2
      late 773.5
  erythrocytic glutathione deficiency 282.2
  erythropoietin-resistant (EPO resistant
    anemia) 285.21
  essential 285.9
  Faber's (achlorhydric anemia) 280.9
  factitious (self-induced bloodletting) 280.0
  familial erythroblastic (microcytic) 282.44
  Fanconi's (congenital pancytopenia)
    284.09
  favism 282.2
  fetal 678.0●
    following blood loss, affecting newborn
      776.5
  fetus or newborn
    due to
      ABO
        antibodies 773.1
        incompatibility, maternal/fetal
          773.1
        isoimmunization 773.1
      Rh
        antibodies 773.0
        incompatibility, maternal/fetal
          773.0
        isoimmunization 773.0
      following fetal blood loss 776.5
  fish tapeworm (D. latum) infestation 123.4
  folate (folic acid) deficiency 281.2
    dietary 281.2
    drug-induced 281.2
  folate malabsorption, congenital 281.2
  folic acid deficiency 281.2
    dietary 281.2
    drug-induced 281.2
  G-6-PD 282.2
  general 285.9
  glucose-6-phosphate dehydrogenase
    deficiency 282.2
  glutathione-reductase deficiency 282.2
  goat's milk 281.2
  granulocytic 288.09
  Heinz-body, congenital 282.7
  hemoglobin deficiency 285.9
  hemolytic 283.9
    acquired 283.9
      with hemoglobinuria NEC 283.2
      autoimmune (cold type) (idiopathic)
        (primary) (secondary)
        (symptomatic) (warm type)
        283.0
      due to
        cold reactive antibodies 283.0
        drug exposure 283.0
        warm reactive antibodies 283.0
      fragmentation 283.19
      idiopathic (chronic) 283.9
      infectious 283.19
        autoimmune 283.0
      non-autoimmune 283.10
      toxic 283.19
    traumatic cardiac 283.19

Anemia *(Continued)*
  hemolytic *(Continued)*
    acute 283.9
      due to enzyme deficiency NEC 282.3
      fetus or newborn *(see also* Disease,
        hemolytic) 773.2
        late 773.5
      Lederer's (acquired infectious
        hemolytic anemia) 283.19
    autoimmune (acquired) 283.0
    chronic 282.9
      idiopathic 283.9
    cold type (secondary) (symptomatic)
      283.0
    congenital (spherocytic) *(see also*
      Spherocytosis) 282.0
      nonspherocytic - *see* Anemia,
        hemolytic, nonspherocytic,
        congenital
    drug-induced 283.0
      enzyme deficiency 282.2
    due to
      cardiac conditions 283.19
      drugs 283.0
      enzyme deficiency NEC 282.3
        drug-induced 282.2
      presence of shunt or other internal
        prosthetic device 283.19
      thrombotic thrombocytopenic purpura
        446.6
    elliptocytotic *(see also* Elliptocytosis) 282.1
    familial 282.9
    hereditary 282.9
      due to enzyme deficiency NEC 282.3
      specified NEC 282.8
    idiopathic (chronic) 283.9
    infectious (acquired) 283.19
    mechanical 283.19
    microangiopathic 283.19
    nonautoimmune 283.10
    nonspherocytic
      congenital or hereditary NEC 282.3
        glucose-6-phosphate
          dehydrogenase deficiency
          282.2
        pyruvate kinase (PK) deficiency
          282.3
        type I 282.2
        type II 282.3
      type I 282.2
      type II 282.3
    of or complicating pregnancy 648.2●
    resulting from presence of shunt or other
      internal prosthetic device 283.19
    secondary 283.19
      autoimmune 283.0
    sickle-cell - *see* Disease, sickle-cell
    Stransky-Regala type (Hb-E) *(see also*
      Disease, hemoglobin) 282.7
    symptomatic 283.19
      autoimmune 283.0
    toxic (acquired) 283.19
    uremic (adult) (child) 283.11
    warm type (secondary) (symptomatic)
      283.0
  hemorrhagic (chronic) 280.0
    acute 285.1
  HEMPAS 285.8
  hereditary erythroblast multinuclearity-
    positive acidified serum test 285.8
  Herrick's (hemoglobin S disease) 282.61
  hexokinase deficiency 282.3
  high A_2 282.46
  hookworm *(see also* Ancylostomiasis) 126.9
  hypochromic (idiopathic) (microcytic)
    (normoblastic) 280.9
    with iron loading 285.0
    due to blood loss (chronic) 280.0
      acute 285.1
    familial sex linked 285.0
    pyridoxine-responsive 285.0

Anemia *(Continued)*
  hypoplasia, red blood cells 284.81
    congenital or familial 284.01
  hypoplastic (idiopathic) 284.9
    congenital 284.01
    familial 284.01
    of childhood 284.09
  idiopathic 285.9
    hemolytic, chronic 283.9
  in (due to) (with)
    chronic illness NEC 285.29
    chronic kidney disease 285.21
    end-stage renal disease 285.21
    neoplastic disease 285.22
  infantile 285.9
  infective, infectional 285.9
  intertropical *(see also* Ancylostomiasis) 126.9
  iron (Fe) deficiency 280.9
    due to blood loss (chronic) 280.0
      acute 285.1
    of or complicating pregnancy 648.2●
    specified NEC 280.8
  Jaksch's (pseudoleukemia infantum) 285.8
  Joseph-Diamond-Blackfan (congenital
    hypoplastic) 284.01
  labyrinth 386.50
  Lederer's (acquired infectious hemolytic
    anemia) 283.19
  leptocytosis (hereditary) 282.40
  leukoerythroblastic 284.2
  macrocytic 281.9
    nutritional 281.2
    of or complicating pregnancy 648.2●
    tropical 281.2
  malabsorption (familial), selective B_{12} with
    proteinuria 281.1
  malarial *(see also* Malaria) 084.6
  malignant (progressive) 281.0
  malnutrition 281.9
  marsh *(see also* Malaria) 084.6
  Mediterranean 282.40
    with hemoglobinopathy 282.49
  megaloblastic 281.9
    combined B_{12} and folate deficiency 281.3
    nutritional (of infancy) 281.2
    of infancy 281.2
    of or complicating pregnancy 648.2●
    refractory 281.3
    specified NEC 281.3
  megalocytic 281.9
  microangiopathic hemolytic 283.19
  microcytic (hypochromic) 280.9
    due to blood loss (chronic) 280.0
      acute 285.1
    familial 282.49
    hypochromic 280.9
  microdrepanocytosis 282.41
  miners' *(see also* Ancylostomiasis) 126.9
  myelopathic 285.8
  myelophthisic (normocytic) 284.2
  newborn *(see also* Disease, hemolytic) 773.2
    due to isoimmunization *(see also* Disease,
      hemolytic) 773.2
    late, due to isoimmunization 773.5
    posthemorrhagic 776.5
  nonregenerative 284.9
  nonspherocytic hemolytic - *see* Anemia,
    hemolytic, nonspherocytic
  normocytic (infectional) (not due to blood
    loss) 285.9
    due to blood loss (chronic) 280.0
      acute 285.1
    myelophthisic 284.2
  nutritional (deficiency) 281.9
    with
      poor iron absorption 280.9
      specified deficiency NEC 281.8
    due to inadequate dietary iron intake
      280.1
    megaloblastic (of infancy) 281.2
  of childhood 282.9

Anemia (*Continued*)
of chronic
disease NEC 285.29
illness NEC 285.29
of or complicating pregnancy 648.2 ●
affecting fetus or newborn 760.8
of prematurity 776.6
orotic aciduric (congenital) (hereditary) 281.4
osteosclerotic 289.89
ovalocytosis (hereditary) (*see also*
Elliptocytosis) 282.1
paludal (*see also* Malaria) 084.6
pentose phosphate pathway deficiency 282.2
pernicious (combined system disease)
(congenital) (dorsolateral spinal
degeneration) (juvenile) (myelopathy)
(neuropathy) (posterior sclerosis)
(primary) (progressive) (spleen) 281.0
of or complicating pregnancy 648.2 ●
pleochromic 285.9
of sprue 281.8
portal 285.8
posthemorrhagic (chronic) 280.0
acute 285.1
newborn 776.5
postoperative
due to (acute) blood loss 285.1
chronic blood loss 280.0
other 285.9
postpartum 648.2 ●
pressure 285.9
primary 285.9
profound 285.9
progressive 285.9
malignant 281.0
pernicious 281.0
protein-deficiency 281.4
pseudoleukemica infantum 285.8
puerperal 648.2 ●
pure red cell 284.81
congenital 284.01
pyridoxine-responsive (hypochromic)
285.0
pyruvate kinase (PK) deficiency 282.3
refractoria sideroblastica 238.72
refractory (primary) 238.72
with
excess
blasts-1 (RAEB-1) 238.72
blasts-2 (RAEB-2) 238.73
hemochromatosis 238.72
ringed sideroblasts (RARS) 238.72
due to
drug 285.0
myelodysplastic syndrome 238.72
toxin 285.0
hereditary 285.0
idiopathic 238.72
megaloblastic 281.3
sideroblastic 238.72
hereditary 285.0
sideropenic 280.9
Rietti-Greppi-Micheli (thalassemia minor)
282.46
scorbutic 281.8
secondary (to) 285.9
blood loss (chronic) 280.0
acute 285.1
hemorrhage 280.0
acute 285.1
inadequate dietary iron intake 280.1
semiplastic 284.9
septic 285.9
sickle-cell (*see also* Disease, sickle-cell)
282.60
sideroachrestic 285.0
sideroblastic (acquired) (any type)
(congenital) (drug-induced) (due to
disease) (hereditary) (primary)
(secondary) (sex-linked hypochromic)
(vitamin B₆ responsive) 285.0

Anemia (*Continued*)
sideroblastic (*Continued*)
refractory 238.72
congenital 285.0
drug-induced 285.0
hereditary 285.0
sex-linked hypochromic 285.0
vitamin B₆-responsive 285.0
sideropenic 280.9
due to blood loss (chronic) 280.0
acute 285.1
simple chronic 281.9
specified type NEC 285.8
spherocytic (hereditary) (*see also*
Spherocytosis) 282.0
splenic 285.8
familial (Gaucher's) 272.7
splenomegalic 285.8
stomatocytosis 282.8
syphilitic 095.8
target cell (oval) 285.8
with thalassemia - *see* Thalassemia
thalassemia 282.40
thrombocytopenic (*see also*
Thrombocytopenia) 287.5
toxic 284.89
triosephosphate isomerase deficiency 282.3
tropical, macrocytic 281.2
tuberculous (*see also* Tuberculosis) 017.9 ●
Vegan's 281.1
vitamin
B₆-responsive 285.0
B₁₂ deficiency (dietary) 281.1
pernicious 281.0
von Jaksch's (pseudoleukemia infantum) 285.8
Witts' (achlorhydric anemia) 280.9
Zuelzer (-Ogden) (nutritional megaloblastic
anemia) 281.2
Anencephalus, anencephaly 740.0
fetal, affecting management of pregnancy
655.0 ●
Anergasia (*see also* Psychosis, organic) 294.9
senile 290.0
Anesthesia, anesthetic 782.0
complication or reaction NEC 995.22
due to
correct substance properly
administered 995.22
overdose or wrong substance given
968.4
specified anesthetic - *see* Table of
Drugs and Chemicals
cornea 371.81
death from
correct substance properly administered
995.4
during delivery 668.9 ●
overdose or wrong substance given 968.4
specified anesthetic - *see* Table of Drugs
and Chemicals
eye 371.81
functional 300.11
hyperesthetic, thalamic 338.0
hysterical 300.11
local skin lesion 782.0
olfactory 781.1
sexual (psychogenic) 302.72
shock
due to
correct substance properly
administered 995.4
overdose or wrong substance given
968.4
specified anesthetic - *see* Table of
Drugs and Chemicals
skin 782.0
tactile 782.0
testicular 608.9
thermal 782.0
Anetoderma (maculosum) 701.3
Aneuploidy NEC 758.5

Aneurin deficiency 265.1
Aneurysm (anastomotic) (artery) (cirsoid)
(diffuse) (false) (fusiform) (multiple)
(ruptured) (saccular) (varicose) 442.9
abdominal (aorta) 441.4
ruptured 441.3
syphilitic 093.0
aorta, aortic (nonsyphilitic) 441.9
abdominal 441.4
dissecting 441.02
ruptured 441.3
syphilitic 093.0
arch 441.2
ruptured 441.1
arteriosclerotic NEC 441.9
ruptured 441.5
ascending 441.2
ruptured 441.1
congenital 747.29
descending 441.9
abdominal 441.4
ruptured 441.3
ruptured 441.5
thoracic 441.2
ruptured 441.1
dissecting 441.00
abdominal 441.02
thoracic 441.01
thoracoabdominal 441.03
due to coarctation (aorta) 747.10
ruptured 441.5
sinus, right 747.29
syphilitic 093.0
thoracoabdominal 441.7
ruptured 441.6
thorax, thoracic (arch) (nonsyphilitic)
441.2
dissecting 441.01
ruptured 441.1
syphilitic 093.0
transverse 441.2
ruptured 441.1
valve (heart) (*see also* Endocarditis, aortic)
424.1
arteriosclerotic NEC 442.9
cerebral 437.3
ruptured (*see also* Hemorrhage,
subarachnoid) 430
arteriovenous (congenital) (peripheral) NEC
(*see also* Anomaly, arteriovenous)
747.60
acquired NEC 447.0
brain 437.3
ruptured (*see also* Hemorrhage,
subarachnoid) 430
coronary 414.11
pulmonary 417.0
brain (cerebral) 747.81
ruptured (*see also* Hemorrhage,
subarachnoid) 430
coronary 746.85
pulmonary 747.32
retina 743.58
specified site NEC 747.89
acquired 447.0
traumatic (*see also* Injury, blood vessel, by
site) 904.9
basal - *see* Aneurysm, brain
berry (congenital) (ruptured) (*see also*
Hemorrhage, subarachnoid) 430
nonruptured 437.3
brain 437.3
arteriosclerotic 437.3
ruptured (*see also* Hemorrhage,
subarachnoid) 430
arteriovenous 747.81
acquired 437.3
ruptured (*see also* Hemorrhage,
subarachnoid) 430
ruptured (*see also* Hemorrhage,
subarachnoid) 430

A

◀ New   ◀▮ Revised   ~~deleted~~ Deleted   ● Use Additional Digit(s)   ▨ Omit code

Aneurysm (Continued)
  brain (Continued)
    berry (congenital) (ruptured) (see also
        Hemorrhage, subarachnoid) 430
      nonruptured 437.3
    congenital 747.81
      ruptured (see also Hemorrhage,
        subarachnoid) 430
    meninges 437.3
      ruptured (see also Hemorrhage,
        subarachnoid) 430
    miliary (congenital) (ruptured) (see also
        Hemorrhage, subarachnoid) 430
    mycotic 421.0
      ruptured (see also Hemorrhage,
        subarachnoid) 430
    nonruptured 437.3
    ruptured (see also Hemorrhage,
        subarachnoid) 430
    syphilitic 094.87
    syphilitic (hemorrhage) 094.87
    traumatic - see Injury, intracranial
  cardiac (false) (see also Aneurysm, heart)
      414.10
  carotid artery (common) (external) 442.81
    internal (intracranial portion) 437.3
      extracranial portion 442.81
      ruptured into brain (see also
          Hemorrhage, subarachnoid) 430
    syphilitic 093.89
      intracranial 094.87
  cavernous sinus (see also Aneurysm, brain)
      437.3
    arteriovenous 747.81
      ruptured (see also Hemorrhage,
        subarachnoid) 430
    congenital 747.81
      ruptured (see also Hemorrhage,
        subarachnoid) 430
  celiac 442.84
  central nervous system, syphilitic 094.89
  cerebral - see Aneurysm, brain
  chest - see Aneurysm, thorax
  circle of Willis (see also Aneurysm, brain) 437.3
    congenital 747.81
      ruptured (see also Hemorrhage,
        subarachnoid) 430
    ruptured (see also Hemorrhage,
        subarachnoid) 430
  common iliac artery 442.2
  congenital (peripheral) NEC 747.60
    brain 747.81
      ruptured (see also Hemorrhage,
        subarachnoid) 430
    cerebral - see Aneurysm, brain, congenital
    coronary 746.85
    gastrointestinal 747.61
    lower limb 747.64
    pulmonary 747.32
    renal 747.62
    retina 743.58
    specified site NEC 747.89
    spinal 747.82
    upper limb 747.63
  conjunctiva 372.74
  conus arteriosus (see also Aneurysm, heart)
      414.10
  coronary (arteriosclerotic) (artery) (vein) (see
      also Aneurysm, heart) 414.11
    arteriovenous 746.85
    congenital 746.85
    syphilitic 093.89
  cylindrical 441.9
    ruptured 441.5
    syphilitic 093.9
  dissecting 442.9
    aorta 441.00
      abdominal 441.02
      thoracic 441.01
      thoracoabdominal 441.03
    syphilitic 093.9

Aneurysm (Continued)
  ductus arteriosus 747.0
  embolic - see Embolism, artery
  endocardial, infective (any valve) 421.0
  femoral 442.3
  gastroduodenal 442.84
  gastroepiploic 442.84
  heart (chronic or with a stated duration of
      over 8 weeks) (infectional) (wall)
      414.10
    acute or with a stated duration of 8 weeks
        or less (see also Infarct, myocardium)
        410.9●
    congenital 746.89
    valve - see Endocarditis
  hepatic 442.84
  iliac (common) 442.2
  infective (any valve) 421.0
  innominate (nonsyphilitic) 442.89
    syphilitic 093.89
  interauricular septum (see also Aneurysm,
      heart) 414.10
  interventricular septum (see also Aneurysm,
      heart) 414.10
  intracranial - see Aneurysm, brain
  intrathoracic (nonsyphilitic) 441.2
    ruptured 441.1
    syphilitic 093.0
  jugular vein (acute) 453.89
    chronic 453.76
  lower extremity 442.3
  lung (pulmonary artery) 417.1
  malignant 093.9
  mediastinal (nonsyphilitic) 442.89
    syphilitic 093.89
  miliary (congenital) (ruptured) (see also
      Hemorrhage, subarachnoid) 430
  mitral (heart) (valve) 424.0
  mural (arteriovenous) (heart) (see also
      Aneurysm, heart) 414.10
  mycotic, any site 421.0
    without endocarditis - see Aneurysm, by
        site
    ruptured, brain (see also Hemorrhage,
        subarachnoid) 430
  myocardium (see also Aneurysm, heart)
      414.10
  neck 442.81
  pancreaticoduodenal 442.84
  patent ductus arteriosus 747.0
  peripheral NEC 442.89
    congenital NEC (see also Aneurysm,
        congenital) 747.60
  popliteal 442.3
  pulmonary 417.1
    arteriovenous 747.32
      acquired 417.0
    syphilitic 093.89
    valve (heart) (see also Endocarditis,
        pulmonary) 424.3
  racemose 442.9
    congenital (peripheral) NEC
        747.60
  radial 442.0
  Rasmussen's (see also Tuberculosis)
      011.2●
  renal 442.1
  retinal (acquired) 362.17
    congenital 743.58
    diabetic 250.5● [362.01]
      due to secondary diabetes 249.5●
          [362.01]
  sinus, aortic (of Valsalva) 747.29
  specified site NEC 442.89
  spinal (cord) 442.89
    congenital 747.82
    syphilitic (hemorrhage) 094.89
  spleen, splenic 442.83
  subclavian 442.82
    syphilitic 093.89
  superior mesenteric 442.84

Aneurysm (Continued)
  syphilitic 093.9
    aorta 093.0
    central nervous system 094.89
    congenital 090.5
    spine, spinal 094.89
  thoracoabdominal 441.7
    ruptured 441.6
  thorax, thoracic (arch) (nonsyphilitic) 441.2
    dissecting 441.01
    ruptured 441.1
    syphilitic 093.0
  traumatic (complication) (early) - see Injury,
      blood vessel, by site
  tricuspid (heart) (valve) - see Endocarditis,
      tricuspid
  ulnar 442.0
  upper extremity 442.0
  valve, valvular - see Endocarditis
  venous 456.8
    congenital NEC (see also Aneurysm,
        congenital) 747.60
  ventricle (arteriovenous) (see also Aneurysm,
      heart) 414.10
  visceral artery NEC 442.84
Angiectasis 459.89
Angiectopia 459.9
Angiitis 447.6
  allergic granulomatous 446.4
  hypersensitivity 446.20
    Goodpasture's syndrome 446.21
    specified NEC 446.29
  necrotizing 446.0
  Wegener's (necrotizing respiratory
      granulomatosis) 446.4
Angina (attack) (cardiac) (chest) (effort) (heart)
    (pectoris) (syndrome) (vasomotor) 413.9
  abdominal 557.1
  accelerated 411.1
  agranulocytic 288.03
  aphthous 074.0
  catarrhal 462
  crescendo 411.1
  croupous 464.4
  cruris 443.9
    due to atherosclerosis NEC (see also
        Arteriosclerosis, extremities) 440.20
  decubitus 413.0
  diphtheritic (membranous) 032.0
  equivalent 413.9
  erysipelatous 034.0
  erythematous 462
  exudative, chronic 476.0
  faucium 478.29
  gangrenous 462
    diphtheritic 032.0
  infectious 462
  initial 411.1
  intestinal 557.1
  ludovici 528.3
  Ludwig's 528.3
  malignant 462
    diphtheritic 032.0
  membranous 464.4
    diphtheritic 032.0
  mesenteric 557.1
  monocytic 075
  nocturnal 413.0
  phlegmonous 475
    diphtheritic 032.0
  preinfarctional 411.1
  Prinzmetal's 413.1
  progressive 411.1
  pseudomembranous 101
  psychogenic 306.2
  pultaceous, diphtheritic 032.0
  scarlatinal 034.1
  septic 034.0
  simple 462
  stable NEC 413.9
  staphylococcal 462

Angina *(Continued)*
   streptococcal 034.0
   stridulous, diphtheritic 032.3
   syphilitic 093.9
     congenital 090.5
   tonsil 475
   trachealis 464.4
   unstable 411.1
   variant 413.1
   Vincent's 101
Angioblastoma (M9161/1) - *see* Neoplasm,
   connective tissue, uncertain behavior
Angiocholecystitis *(see also* Cholecystitis, acute)
   575.0
Angiocholitis *(see also* Cholecystitis, acute)
   576.1
Angiodysgensis spinalis 336.1
Angiodysplasia (intestinalis) (intestine) 569.84
   with hemorrhage 569.85
   duodenum 537.82
     with hemorrhage 537.83
   stomach 537.82
     with hemorrhage 537.83
Angioedema (allergic) (any site) (with urticaria)
   995.1
   hereditary 277.6
Angioendothelioma (M9130/1) - *see also*
   Neoplasm, by site, uncertain behavior
   benign (M9130/0) *(see also* Hemangioma, by
     site) 228.00
   bone (M9260/3) - *see* Neoplasm, bone,
     malignant
   Ewing's (M9260/3) - *see* Neoplasm, bone,
     malignant
   nervous system (M9130/0) 228.09
Angiofibroma (M9160/0) - *see also* Neoplasm,
   by site, benign
   juvenile (M9160/0) 210.7
     specified site - *see* Neoplasm, by site,
       benign
     unspecified site 210.7
Angiohemophilia (A) (B) 286.4
Angioid streaks (choroid) (retina) 363.43
Angiokeratoma (M9141/0) - *see also* Neoplasm,
   skin, benign
   corporis diffusum 272.7
Angiokeratosis
   diffuse 272.7
Angioleiomyoma (M8894/0) - *see* Neoplasm,
   connective tissue, benign
Angioleucitis 683
Angiolipoma (M8861/0) *(see also* Lipoma, by
   site) 214.9
   infiltrating (M8861/1) - *see* Neoplasm,
     connective tissue, uncertain behavior
Angioma (M9120/0) *(see also* Hemangioma, by
   site) 228.00
   capillary 448.1
   hemorrhagicum hereditaria 448.0
   malignant (M9120/3) - *see* Neoplasm,
     connective tissue, malignant
   pigmentosum et atrophicum 757.33
   placenta - *see* Placenta, abnormal
   plexiform (M9131/0) - *see* Hemangioma, by
     site
   senile 448.1
   serpiginosum 709.1
   spider 448.1
   stellate 448.1
Angiomatosis 757.32
   bacillary 083.8
   corporis diffusum universale 272.7
   cutaneocerebral 759.6
   encephalocutaneous 759.6
   encephalofacial 759.6
   encephalotrigeminal 759.6
   hemorrhagic familial 448.0
   hereditary familial 448.0
   heredofamilial 448.0
   meningo-oculofacial 759.6
   multiple sites 228.09

Angiomatosis *(Continued)*
   neuro-oculocutaneous 759.6
   retina (Hippel's disease) 759.6
   retinocerebellosa 759.6
   retinocerebral 759.6
   systemic 228.09
Angiomyolipoma (M8860/0)
   specified site - *see* Neoplasm, connective
     tissue, benign
   unspecified site 223.0
Angiomyoliposarcoma (M8860/3) - *see*
   Neoplasm, connective tissue, malignant
Angiomyoma (M8894/0) - *see* Neoplasm,
   connective tissue, benign
Angiomyosarcoma (M8894/3) - *see* Neoplasm,
   connective tissue, malignant
Angioneurosis 306.2
Angioneurotic edema (allergic) (any site) (with
   urticaria) 995.1
   hereditary 277.6
Angiopathia, angiopathy 459.9
   diabetic (peripheral) 250.7● *[443.81]*
     due to secondary diabetes 249.7●
       [443.81]
   peripheral 443.9
     diabetic 250.7● *[443.81]*
       due to secondary diabetes 249.7●
         [443.81]
     specified type NEC 443.89
   retinae syphilitica 093.89
   retinalis (juvenilis) 362.18
     background 362.10
     diabetic 250.5● *[362.01]*
       due to secondary diabetes 249.5●
         [362.01]
     proliferative 362.29
     tuberculous *(see also* Tuberculosis) 017.3●
       [362.18]
Angiosarcoma (M9120/3) - *see* Neoplasm,
   connective tissue, malignant
Angiosclerosis - *see* Arteriosclerosis
Angioscotoma, enlarged 368.42
Angiospasm 443.9
   brachial plexus 353.0
   cerebral 435.9
   cervical plexus 353.2
   nerve
     arm 354.9
       axillary 353.0
       median 354.1
       ulnar 354.2
     autonomic *(see also* Neuropathy,
       peripheral, autonomic) 337.9
     axillary 353.0
     leg 355.8
       plantar 355.6
     lower extremity - *see* Angiospasm, nerve,
       leg
     median 354.1
     peripheral NEC 355.9
     spinal NEC 355.9
     sympathetic *(see also* Neuropathy,
       peripheral, autonomic) 337.9
     ulnar 354.2
     upper extremity - *see* Angiospasm, nerve,
       arm
   peripheral NEC 443.9
   traumatic 443.9
     foot 443.9
     leg 443.9
   vessel 443.9
Angiospastic disease or edema 443.9
Angle's
     class I 524.21
     class II 524.22
     class III 524.23
Anguillulosis 127.2
Angulation
   cecum *(see also* Obstruction, intestine) 560.9
   coccyx (acquired) 738.6
     congenital 756.19

Angulation *(Continued)*
   femur (acquired) 736.39
     congenital 755.69
   intestine (large) (small) *(see also* Obstruction,
     intestine) 560.9
   sacrum (acquired) 738.5
     congenital 756.19
   sigmoid (flexure) *(see also* Obstruction,
     intestine) 560.9
   spine *(see also* Curvature, spine) 737.9
   tibia (acquired) 736.89
     congenital 755.69
   ureter 593.3
   wrist (acquired) 736.09
     congenital 755.59
Angulus infectiosus 686.8
Anhedonia 780.99
Anhidrosis (lid) (neurogenic) (thermogenic)
   705.0
Anhydration 276.51
   with
     hypernatremia 276.0
     hyponatremia 276.1
Anhydremia 276.52
   with
     hypernatremia 276.0
     hyponatremia 276.1
Anidrosis 705.0
Aniridia (congenital) 743.45
Anisakiasis (infection) (infestation) 127.1
Anisakis larva infestation 127.1
Aniseikonia 367.32
Anisocoria (pupil) 379.41
   congenital 743.46
Anisocytosis 790.09
Anisometropia (congenital) 367.31
Ankle - *see* condition
Ankyloblepharon (acquired) (eyelid)
   374.46
   filiforme (adnatum) (congenital)
     743.62
   total 743.62
Ankylodactly *(see also* Syndactylism)
   755.10
Ankyloglossia 750.0
Ankylosis (fibrous) (osseous) 718.50
   ankle 718.57
   any joint, produced by surgical fusion
     V45.4
   cricoarytenoid (cartilage) (joint) (larynx)
     478.79
   dental 521.6
   ear ossicle NEC 385.22
     malleus 385.21
   elbow 718.52
   finger 718.54
   hip 718.55
   incostapedial joint (infectional) 385.22
   joint, produced by surgical fusion NEC
     V45.4
   knee 718.56
   lumbosacral (joint) 724.6
   malleus 385.21
   multiple sites 718.59
   postoperative (status) V45.4
   sacroiliac (joint) 724.6
   shoulder 718.51
   specified site NEC 718.58
   spine NEC 724.9
   surgical V45.4
   teeth, tooth (hard tissues) 521.6
   temporomandibular joint 524.61
   wrist 718.53
Ankylostoma - *see* Ancylostoma
Ankylostomiasis (intestinal) - *see*
   Ancylostomiasis
Ankylurethria *(see also* Stricture, urethra) 598.9
Annular - *see also* condition
   detachment, cervix 622.8
   organ or site, congenital NEC - *see* Distortion
   pancreas (congenital) 751.7

◀ New   ⬅ Revised   ~~deleted~~ Deleted   ● Use Additional Digit(s)   ▓ Omit code

Anodontia (complete) (partial) (vera) 520.0
  with abnormal spacing 524.30
  acquired 525.10
    causing malocclusion 524.30
    due to
      caries 525.13
      extraction 525.10
      periodontal disease 525.12
      trauma 525.11
Anomaly, anomalous (congenital) (unspecified type) 759.9
  abdomen 759.9
  abdominal wall 756.70
  acoustic nerve 742.9
  adrenal (gland) 759.1
  Alder (-Reilly) (leukocyte granulation) 288.2
  alimentary tract 751.9
    lower 751.5
    specified type NEC 751.8
    upper (any part, except tongue) 750.9
      tongue 750.10
        specified type NEC 750.19
  alveolar 524.70
    ridge (process) 525.8
    specified NEC 524.79
  ankle (joint) 755.69
  anus, anal (canal) 751.5
  aorta, aortic 747.20
    arch 747.21
    coarctation (postductal) (preductal) 747.10
    cusp or valve NEC 746.9
    septum 745.0
    specified type NEC 747.29
  aorticopulmonary septum 745.0
  apertures, diaphragm 756.6
  appendix 751.5
  aqueduct of Sylvius 742.3
    with spina bifida (see also Spina bifida) 741.0●
  arm 755.50
    reduction (see also Deformity, reduction, upper limb) 755.20
  arteriovenous (congenital) (peripheral) NEC 747.60
    brain 747.81
    cerebral 747.81
    coronary 746.85
    gastrointestinal 747.61
      acquired - see Angiodysplasia
    lower limb 747.64
    renal 747.62
    specified site NEC 747.69
    spinal 747.82
    upper limb 747.63
  artery (see also Anomaly, peripheral vascular system) NEC 747.60
    brain 747.81
    cerebral 747.81
    coronary 746.85
    eye 743.9
    pulmonary 747.39
    renal 747.62
    retina 743.9
    umbilical 747.5
  arytenoepiglottic folds 748.3
  atrial
    bands 746.9
    folds 746.9
    septa 745.5
  atrioventricular
    canal 745.69
    common 745.69
    conduction 426.7
    excitation 426.7
    septum 745.4
  atrium - see Anomaly, atrial
  auditory canal 744.3
    specified type NEC 744.29
      with hearing impairment 744.02

Anomaly, anomalous (Continued)
  auricle
    ear 744.3
      causing impairment of hearing 744.02
    heart 746.9
      septum 745.5
  autosomes, autosomal NEC 758.5
  Axenfeld's 743.44
  back 759.9
  band
    atrial 746.9
    heart 746.9
    ventricular 746.9
  Bartholin's duct 750.9
  biliary duct or passage 751.60
    atresia 751.61
  bladder (neck) (sphincter) (trigone) 753.9
    specified type NEC 753.8
  blood vessel 747.9
    artery - see Anomaly, artery
    peripheral vascular - see Anomaly, peripheral vascular system
    vein - see Anomaly, vein
  bone NEC 756.9
    ankle 755.69
    arm 755.50
    chest 756.3
    cranium 756.0
    face 756.0
    finger 755.50
    foot 755.67
    forearm 755.50
    frontal 756.0
    head 756.0
    hip 755.63
    leg 755.60
    lumbosacral 756.10
    nose 748.1
    pelvic girdle 755.60
    rachitic 756.4
    rib 756.3
    shoulder girdle 755.50
    skull 756.0
      with
        anencephalus 740.0
        encephalocele 742.0
        hydrocephalus 742.3
          with spina bifida (see also Spina bifida) 741.0●
        microcephalus 742.1
    toe 755.66
  brain 742.9
    multiple 742.4
    reduction 742.2
    specified type NEC 742.4
    vessel 747.81
  branchial cleft NEC 744.49
    cyst 744.42
    fistula 744.41
    persistent 744.41
    sinus (external) (internal) 744.41
  breast 757.6
  broad ligament 752.10
    specified type NEC 752.19
  bronchus 748.3
  bulbar septum 745.0
  bulbus cordis 745.9
    persistent (in left ventricle) 745.8
  bursa 756.9
  canal of Nuck 752.9
  canthus 743.9
  capillary NEC (see also Anomaly, peripheral vascular system) 747.60
  cardiac 746.9
    septal closure 745.9
      acquired 429.71
    valve NEC 746.9
      pulmonary 746.00
      specified type NEC 746.89

Anomaly, anomalous (Continued)
  cardiovascular system 746.9
    complicating pregnancy, childbirth, or puerperium 648.5●
  carpus 755.50
  cartilage, trachea 748.3
  cartilaginous 756.9
  caruncle, lacrimal, lachrymal 743.9
  cascade stomach 750.7
  cauda equina 742.59
  cecum 751.5
  cerebral - see also Anomaly, brain vessels 747.81
  cerebrovascular system 747.81
  cervix (uterus) 752.40
    with doubling of vagina and uterus 752.2
    in pregnancy or childbirth 654.6●
      affecting fetus or newborn 763.89
      causing obstructed labor 660.2●
        affecting fetus or newborn 763.1
  Chédiak-Higashi (-Steinbrinck) (congenital gigantism of peroxidase granules) 288.2
  cheek 744.9
  chest (wall) 756.3
  chin 744.9
    specified type NEC 744.89
  chordae tendineae 746.9
  choroid 743.9
    plexus 742.9
  chromosomes, chromosomal 758.9
    13 (13-15) 758.1
    18 (16-18) 758.2
    21 or 22 758.0
    autosomes NEC (see also Abnormal, autosomes) 758.5
      deletion 758.39
    Christchurch 758.39
    D_1 758.1
    E_3 758.2
    G 758.0
    mitochondrial 758.9
    mosaics 758.89
    sex 758.81
      complement, XO 758.6
      complement, XXX 758.81
      complement, XXY 758.7
      complement, XYY 758.81
      gonadal dysgenesis 758.6
      Klinefelter's 758.7
      Turner's 758.6
    trisomy 21 758.0
  cilia 743.9
  circulatory system 747.9
    specified type NEC 747.89
  clavicle 755.51
  clitoris 752.40
  coccyx 756.10
  colon 751.5
  common duct 751.60
  communication
    coronary artery 746.85
    left ventricle with right atrium 745.4
  concha (ear) 744.3
  connection
    renal vessels with kidney 747.62
    total pulmonary venous 747.41
  connective tissue 756.9
    specified type NEC 756.89
  cornea 743.9
    shape 743.41
    size 743.41
    specified type NEC 743.49
  coronary
    artery 746.85
    vein 746.89
  cranium - see Anomaly, skull
  cricoid cartilage 748.3
  cushion, endocardial 745.60
    specified type NEC 745.69
  cystic duct 751.60

Anomaly, anomalous (Continued)
dental arch 524.20
    specified NEC 524.29
dental arch relationship 524.20
    angle's class I 524.21
    angle's class II 524.22
    angle's class III 524.23
    articulation
        anterior 524.27
        posterior 524.27
        reverse 524.27
    disto-occlusion 524.22
        division I 524.22
        division II 524.22
    excessive horizontal overlap 524.26
    interarch distance (excessive)
        (inadequate) 524.28
    mesio-occlusion 524.23
    neutro-occlusion 524.21
    open
        anterior occlusal relationship 524.24
        posterior occlusal relationship 524.25
    specified NEC 524.29
dentition 520.6
dentofacial NEC 524.9
    functional 524.50
    specified type NEC 524.89
dermatoglyphic 757.2
Descemet's membrane 743.9
    specified type NEC 743.49
development
    cervix 752.40
    vagina 752.40
    vulva 752.40
diaphragm, diaphragmatic (apertures) NEC
    756.6
digestive organ(s) or system 751.9
    lower 751.5
        specified type NEC 751.8
    upper 750.9
distribution, coronary artery 746.85
ductus
    arteriosus 747.0
    Botalli 747.0
duodenum 751.5
dura 742.9
    brain 742.4
    spinal cord 742.59
ear 744.3
    causing impairment of hearing 744.00
        specified type NEC 744.09
    external 744.3
        causing impairment of hearing
            744.02
        specified type NEC 744.29
    inner (causing impairment of hearing)
        744.05
    middle, except ossicles (causing
        impairment of hearing) 744.03
        ossicles 744.04
    ossicles 744.04
    prominent auricle 744.29
    specified type NEC 744.29
        with hearing impairment 744.09
Ebstein's (heart) 746.2
    tricuspid valve 746.2
ectodermal 757.9
Eisenmenger's (ventricular septal defect)
    745.4
ejaculatory duct 752.9
    specified type NEC 752.89
elbow (joint) 755.50
endocardial cushion 745.60
    specified type NEC 745.69
endocrine gland NEC 759.2
epididymis 752.9
epiglottis 748.3
esophagus 750.9
    specified type NEC 750.4
Eustachian tube 744.3
    specified type NEC 744.24

Anomaly, anomalous (Continued)
eye (any part) 743.9
    adnexa 743.9
        specified type NEC 743.69
    anophthalmos 743.00
    anterior
        chamber and related structures 743.9
            angle 743.9
                specified type NEC 743.44
            specified type NEC 743.44
        segment 743.9
            combined 743.48
            multiple 743.48
            specified type NEC 743.49
    cataract (see also Cataract) 743.30
    glaucoma (see also Buphthalmia) 743.20
    lid 743.9
        specified type NEC 743.63
    microphthalmos (see also
        Microphthalmos) 743.10
    posterior segment 743.9
        specified type NEC 743.59
        vascular 743.58
        vitreous 743.9
            specified type NEC 743.51
    ptosis (eyelid) 743.61
    retina 743.9
        specified type NEC 743.59
    sclera 743.9
        specified type NEC 743.47
    specified type NEC 743.8
eyebrow 744.89
eyelid 743.9
    specified type NEC 743.63
face (any part) 744.9
    bone(s) 756.0
    specified type NEC 744.89
fallopian tube 752.10
    specified type NEC 752.19
fascia 756.9
    specified type NEC 756.89
femur 755.60
fibula 755.60
finger 755.50
    supernumerary 755.01
    webbed (see also Syndactylism, fingers)
        755.11
fixation, intestine 751.4
flexion (joint) 755.9
    hip or thigh (see also Dislocation, hip,
        congenital) 754.30
folds, heart 746.9
foot 755.67
foramen
    Botalli 745.5
    ovale 745.5
forearm 755.50
forehead (see also Anomaly, skull) 756.0
form, teeth 520.2
fovea centralis 743.9
frontal bone (see also Anomaly, skull) 756.0
gallbladder 751.60
Gartner's duct 752.41
gastrointestinal tract 751.9
    specified type NEC 751.8
    vessel 747.61
genitalia, genital organ(s) or system
    female 752.9
        external 752.40
            specified type NEC 752.49
        internal NEC 752.9
    male (external and internal) 752.9
        epispadias 752.62
        hidden penis 752.65
        hydrocele, congenital 778.6
        hypospadias 752.61
        micropenis 752.64
        testis, undescended 752.51
            retractile 752.52
    specified type NEC 752.89
genitourinary NEC 752.9

Anomaly, anomalous (Continued)
Gerbode 745.4
globe (eye) 743.9
glottis 748.3
granulation or granulocyte, genetic
    288.2
    constitutional 288.2
    leukocyte 288.2
gum 750.9
gyri 742.9
hair 757.9
    specified type NEC 757.4
hand 755.50
hard tissue formation in pulp 522.3
head (see also Anomaly, skull) 756.0
heart 746.9
    auricle 746.9
    bands 746.9
    fibroelastosis cordis 425.3
    folds 746.9
    malposition 746.87
    maternal, affecting fetus or newborn
        760.3
    obstructive NEC 746.84
    patent ductus arteriosus (Botalli)
        747.0
    septum 745.9
        acquired 429.71
        aortic 745.0
        aorticopulmonary 745.0
        atrial 745.5
        auricular 745.5
        between aorta and pulmonary artery
            745.0
        endocardial cushion type 745.60
            specified type NEC 745.69
        interatrial 745.5
        interventricular 745.4
            with pulmonary stenosis or atresia,
                dextraposition of aorta, and
                hypertrophy of right ventricle
                745.2
            acquired 429.71
        specified type NEC 745.8
        ventricular 745.4
            with pulmonary stenosis or atresia,
                dextraposition of aorta, and
                hypertrophy of right ventricle
                745.2
            acquired 429.71
    specified type NEC 746.89
    tetralogy of Fallot 745.2
    valve NEC 746.9
        aortic 746.9
            atresia 746.89
            bicuspid valve 746.4
            insufficiency 746.4
            specified type NEC 746.89
            stenosis 746.3
                subaortic 746.81
                supravalvular 747.22
        mitral 746.9
            atresia 746.89
            insufficiency 746.6
            specified type NEC 746.89
            stenosis 746.5
        pulmonary 746.00
            atresia 746.01
            insufficiency 746.09
            stenosis 746.02
                infundibular 746.83
                subvalvular 746.83
        tricuspid 746.9
            atresia 746.1
            stenosis 746.1
    ventricle 746.9
heel 755.67
Hegglin's 288.2
hemianencephaly 740.0
hemicephaly 740.0
hemicrania 740.0

◀ New   ◀≡ Revised   ~~deleted~~ Deleted   ● Use Additional Digit(s)   ▨ Omit code

Anomaly, anomalous *(Continued)*
  hepatic duct 751.60
  hip (joint) 755.63
  hourglass
    bladder 753.8
    gallbladder 751.69
    stomach 750.7
  humerus 755.50
  hymen 752.40
  hypersegmentation of neutrophils, hereditary 288.2
  hypophyseal 759.2
  ileocecal (coil) (valve) 751.5
  ileum (intestine) 751.5
  ilium 755.60
  integument 757.9
    specified type NEC 757.8
  interarch distance (excessive) (inadequate) 524.28
  intervertebral cartilage or disc 756.10
  intestine (large) (small) 751.5
    fixational type 751.4
  iris 743.9
    specified type NEC 743.46
  ischium 755.60
  jaw NEC 524.9
    closure 524.51
    size (major) NEC 524.00
    specified type NEC 524.89
  jaw-cranial base relationship 524.10
    specified NEC 524.19
  jejunum 751.5
  joint 755.9
    hip
      dislocation *(see also* Dislocation, hip, congenital) 754.30
      predislocation *(see also* Subluxation, congenital, hip) 754.32
      preluxation *(see also* Subluxation, congenital, hip) 754.32
      subluxation *(see also* Subluxation, congenital, hip) 754.32
    lumbosacral 756.10
      spondylolisthesis 756.12
      spondylosis 756.11
    multiple arthrogryposis 754.89
    sacroiliac 755.69
  Jordan's 288.2
  kidney(s) (calyx) (pelvis) 753.9
    vessel 747.62
  Klippel-Feil (brevicollis) 756.16
  knee (joint) 755.64
  labium (majus) (minus) 752.40
  labyrinth, membranous (causing impairment of hearing) 744.05
  lacrimal
    apparatus, duct or passage 743.9
      specified type NEC 743.65
    gland 743.9
      specified type NEC 743.64
  Langdon Down (mongolism) 758.0
  larynx, laryngeal (muscle) 748.3
    web, webbed 748.2
  leg (lower) (upper) 755.60
    reduction NEC *(see also* Deformity, reduction, lower limb) 755.30
  lens 743.9
    shape 743.36
    specified type NEC 743.39
  leukocytes, genetic 288.2
    granulation (constitutional) 288.2
  lid (fold) 743.9
  ligament 756.9
    broad 752.10
    round 752.9
  limb, except reduction deformity 755.8
    lower 755.60
      reduction deformity *(see also* Deformity, reduction, lower limb) 755.30
      specified type NEC 755.69

Anomaly, anomalous *(Continued)*
  limb *(Continued)*
    upper 755.50
      reduction deformity *(see also* Deformity, reduction, upper limb) 755.20
      specified type NEC 755.59
  lip 750.9
    harelip *(see also* Cleft, lip) 749.10
    specified type NEC 750.26
  liver (duct) 751.60
    atresia 751.69
  lower extremity 755.60
    vessel 747.64
  lumbosacral (joint) (region) 756.10
  lung (fissure) (lobe) NEC 748.60
    agenesis 748.5
    specified type NEC 748.69
  lymphatic system 759.9
  Madelung's (radius) 755.54
  mandible 524.9
    size NEC 524.00
  maxilla 524.90
    size NEC 524.00
  May (-Hegglin) 288.2
  meatus urinarius 753.9
    specified type NEC 753.8
  meningeal bands or folds, constriction of 742.8
  meninges 742.9
    brain 742.4
    spinal 742.59
  meningocele *(see also* Spina bifida) 741.9●
    acquired 349.2
  mesentery 751.9
  metacarpus 755.50
  metatarsus 755.67
  middle ear, except ossicles (causing impairment of hearing) 744.03
    ossicles 744.04
  mitral (leaflets) (valve) 746.9
    atresia 746.89
    insufficiency 746.6
    specified type NEC 746.89
    stenosis 746.5
  mouth 750.9
    specified type NEC 750.26
  multiple NEC 759.7
    specified type NEC 759.89
  muscle 756.9
    eye 743.9
      specified type NEC 743.69
    specified type NEC 756.89
  musculoskeletal system, except limbs 756.9
    specified type NEC 756.9
  nail 757.9
    specified type NEC 757.5
  narrowness, eyelid 743.62
  nasal sinus or septum 748.1
  neck (any part) 744.9
    specified type NEC 744.89
  nerve 742.9
    acoustic 742.9
      specified type NEC 742.8
    optic 742.9
      specified type NEC 742.8
    specified type NEC 742.8
  nervous system NEC 742.9
    brain 742.9
      specified type NEC 742.4
    specified type NEC 742.8
  neurological 742.9
  nipple 757.6
  nonteratogenic NEC 754.89
  nose, nasal (bone) (cartilage) (septum) (sinus) 748.1
  ocular muscle 743.9
  omphalomesenteric duct 751.0
  opening, pulmonary veins 747.49

Anomaly, anomalous *(Continued)*
  optic
    disc 743.9
      specified type NEC 743.57
    nerve 742.9
  opticociliary vessels 743.9
  orbit (eye) 743.9
    specified type NEC 743.66
  organ
    of Corti (causing impairment of hearing) 744.05
    or site 759.9
      specified type NEC 759.89
  origin
    both great arteries from same ventricle 745.11
    coronary artery 746.85
    innominate artery 747.69
    left coronary artery from pulmonary artery 746.85
    pulmonary artery 747.39
    renal vessels 747.62
    subclavian artery (left) (right) 747.21
  osseous meatus (ear) 744.03
  ovary 752.0
  oviduct 752.10
  palate (hard) (soft) 750.9
    cleft *(see also* Cleft, palate) 749.00
  pancreas (duct) 751.7
  papillary muscles 746.9
  parathyroid gland 759.2
  paraurethral ducts 753.9
  parotid (gland) 750.9
  patella 755.64
  Pelger-Huët (hereditary hyposegmentation) 288.2
  pelvic girdle 755.60
    specified type NEC 755.69
  pelvis (bony) 755.60
    complicating delivery 653.0●
    rachitic 268.1
      fetal 756.4
  penis (glans) 752.69
  pericardium 746.89
  peripheral vascular system NEC 747.60
    gastrointestinal 747.61
    lower limb 747.64
    renal 747.62
    specified site NEC 747.69
    spinal 747.82
    upper limb 747.63
  Peter's 743.44
  pharynx 750.9
    branchial cleft 744.41
    specified type NEC 750.29
  Pierre Robin 756.0
  pigmentation 709.00
    congenital 757.33
    specified NEC 709.09
  pituitary (gland) 759.2
  pleural folds 748.8
  portal vein 747.40
  position tooth, teeth 524.30
    crowding 524.31
    displacement 524.30
      horizontal 524.33
      vertical 524.34
    distance
      interocclusal
        excessive 524.37
        insufficient 524.36
    excessive spacing 524.32
    rotation 524.35
    specified NEC 524.39
  preauricular sinus 744.46
  prepuce 752.9
  prostate 752.9
  pulmonary 748.60
    artery 747.39
    circulation 747.39

Anomaly, anomalous (*Continued*)
  pulmonary (*Continued*)
    specified type NEC 748.69
    valve 746.00
      atresia 746.01
      insufficiency 746.09
      specified type NEC 746.09
      stenosis 746.02
        infundibular 746.83
        subvalvular 746.83
    vein 747.40
    venous
      connection 747.49
        partial 747.42
        total 747.41
      return 747.49
        partial 747.42
        total (TAPVR) (complete)
          (subdiaphragmatic)
          (supradiaphragmatic)
          747.41
  pupil 743.9
  pylorus 750.9
    hypertrophy 750.5
    stenosis 750.5
  rachitic, fetal 756.4
  radius 755.50
  rectovaginal (septum) 752.40
  rectum 751.5
  refraction 367.9
  renal 753.9
    vessel 747.62
  respiratory system 748.9
    specified type NEC 748.8
  rib 756.3
    cervical 756.2
  Rieger's 743.44
  rings, trachea 748.3
  rotation - *see also* Malrotation
    hip or thigh (*see also* Subluxation,
      congenital, hip) 754.32
  round ligament 752.9
  sacroiliac (joint) 755.69
  sacrum 756.10
  saddle
    back 754.2
    nose 754.0
      syphilitic 090.5
  salivary gland or duct 750.9
    specified type NEC 750.26
  scapula 755.50
  sclera 743.9
    specified type NEC 743.47
  scrotum 752.9
  sebaceous gland 757.9
  seminal duct or tract 752.9
  sense organs 742.9
    specified type NEC 742.8
  septum
    heart - *see* Anomaly, heart,
      septum
    nasal 748.1
  sex chromosomes NEC (*see also*
    Anomaly, chromosomes)
    758.81
  shoulder (girdle) (joint) 755.50
    specified type NEC 755.59
  sigmoid (flexure) 751.5
  sinus of Valsalva 747.29
  site NEC 759.9
  skeleton generalized NEC 756.50
  skin (appendage) 757.9
    specified type NEC 757.39
  skull (bone) 756.0
    with
      anencephalus 740.0
      encephalocele 742.0
      hydrocephalus 742.3
        with spina bifida (*see also* Spina
          bifida) 741.0●
      microcephalus 742.1

Anomaly, anomalous (*Continued*)
  specified type NEC
    adrenal (gland) 759.1
    alimentary tract (complete) (partial) 751.8
      lower 751.5
      upper 750.8
    ankle 755.69
    anus, anal (canal) 751.5
    aorta, aortic 747.29
      arch 747.21
    appendix 751.5
    arm 755.59
    artery (peripheral) NEC (*see also* Anomaly,
      peripheral vascular system) 747.60
      brain 747.81
      coronary 746.85
      eye 743.58
      pulmonary 747.39
      retinal 743.58
      umbilical 747.5
    auditory canal 744.29
      causing impairment of hearing 744.02
    bile duct or passage 751.69
    bladder 753.8
      neck 753.8
    bone(s) 756.9
      arm 755.59
      face 756.0
      leg 755.69
      pelvic girdle 755.69
      shoulder girdle 755.59
      skull 756.0
        with
          anencephalus 740.0
          encephalocele 742.0
          hydrocephalus 742.3
            with spina bifida (*see also*
              Spina bifida) 741.0●
          microcephalus 742.1
    brain 742.4
    breast 757.6
    broad ligament 752.19
    bronchus 748.3
    canal of Nuck 752.89
    cardiac septal closure 745.8
    carpus 755.59
    cartilaginous 756.9
    cecum 751.5
    cervix 752.49
    chest (wall) 756.3
    chin 744.89
    ciliary body 743.46
    circulatory system 747.89
    clavicle 755.51
    clitoris 752.49
    coccyx 756.19
    colon 751.5
    common duct 751.69
    connective tissue 756.89
    cricoid cartilage 748.3
    cystic duct 751.69
    diaphragm 756.6
    digestive organ(s) or tract 751.8
      lower 751.5
      upper 750.8
    duodenum 751.5
    ear 744.29
      auricle 744.29
        causing impairment of hearing
          744.02
      causing impairment of hearing
        744.09
      inner (causing impairment of hearing)
        744.05
      middle, except ossicles 744.03
        ossicles 744.04
    ejaculatory duct 752.89
    endocrine 759.2
    epiglottis 748.3
    esophagus 750.4
    eustachian tube 744.24

Anomaly, anomalous (*Continued*)
  specified type NEC (*Continued*)
    eye 743.8
      lid 743.63
      muscle 743.69
    face 744.89
      bone(s) 756.0
    fallopian tube 752.19
    fascia 756.89
    femur 755.69
    fibula 755.69
    finger 755.59
    foot 755.67
    fovea centralis 743.55
    gallbladder 751.69
    Gartner's duct 752.89
    gastrointestinal tract 751.8
    genitalia, genital organ(s)
      female 752.89
        external 752.49
        internal NEC 752.89
      male 752.89
        penis 752.69
        scrotal transposition 752.81
    genitourinary tract NEC 752.89
    glottis 748.3
    hair 757.4
    hand 755.59
    heart 746.89
      valve NEC 746.89
        pulmonary 746.09
    hepatic duct 751.69
    hydatid of Morgagni 752.89
    hymen 752.49
    integument 757.8
    intestine (large) (small) 751.5
      fixational type 751.4
    iris 743.46
    jejunum 751.5
    joint 755.8
    kidney 753.3
    knee 755.64
    labium (majus) (minus) 752.49
    labyrinth, membranous 744.05
    larynx 748.3
    leg 755.69
    lens 743.39
    limb, except reduction deformity 755.8
      lower 755.69
        reduction deformity (*see also*
          Deformity, reduction, lower
          limb) 755.30
      upper 755.59
        reduction deformity (*see also*
          Deformity, reduction, upper
          limb) 755.20
    lip 750.26
    liver 751.69
    lung (fissure) (lobe) 748.69
    meatus urinarius 753.8
    metacarpus 755.59
    mouth 750.26
    Müllerian
      cervix 752.49
      uterus 752.39
      vagina 752.49
    muscle 756.89
      eye 743.69
    musculoskeletal system, except limbs
      756.9
    nail 757.5
    neck 744.89
    nerve 742.8
      acoustic 742.8
      optic 742.8
    nervous system 742.8
    nipple 757.6
    nose 748.1
    organ NEC 759.89
      of Corti 744.05
    osseous meatus (ear) 744.03

◀ New ◀▥ Revised ~~deleted~~ Deleted ● Use Additional Digit(s) ▨ Omit code

Anomaly, anomalous *(Continued)*
  specified type NEC *(Continued)*
    ovary 752.0
    oviduct 752.19
    pancreas 751.7
    parathyroid 759.2
    patella 755.64
    pelvic girdle 755.69
    penis 752.69
    pericardium 746.89
    peripheral vascular system NEC *(see also* Anomaly, peripheral vascular system)* 747.60
    pharynx 750.29
    pituitary 759.2
    prostate 752.89
    radius 755.59
    rectum 751.5
    respiratory system 748.8
    rib 756.3
    round ligament 752.89
    sacrum 756.19
    salivary duct or gland 750.26
    scapula 755.59
    sclera 743.47
    scrotum 752.89
      transposition 752.81
    seminal duct or tract 752.89
    shoulder girdle 755.59
    site NEC 759.89
    skin 757.39
    skull (bone(s)) 756.0
      with
        anencephalus 740.0
        encephalocele 742.0
        hydrocephalus 742.3
          with spina bifida *(see also* Spina bifida)* 741.0●
        microcephalus 742.1
  specified organ or site NEC 759.89
  spermatic cord 752.89
  spinal cord 742.59
  spine 756.19
  spleen 759.0
  sternum 756.3
  stomach 750.7
  tarsus 755.67
  tendon 756.89
  testis 752.89
  thorax (wall) 756.3
  thymus 759.2
  thyroid (gland) 759.2
    cartilage 748.3
  tibia 755.69
  toe 755.66
  tongue 750.19
  trachea (cartilage) 748.3
  ulna 755.59
  urachus 753.7
  ureter 753.4
    obstructive 753.29
  urethra 753.8
    obstructive 753.6
  urinary tract 753.8
  uterus (Müllerian) 752.39
  uvula 750.26
  vagina 752.49
  vascular NEC *(see also* Anomaly, peripheral vascular system)* 747.60
    brain 747.81
  vas deferens 752.89
  vein(s) (peripheral) NEC *(see also* Anomaly, peripheral vascular system)* 747.60
    brain 747.81
    great 747.49
    portal 747.49
    pulmonary 747.49
  vena cava (inferior) (superior) 747.49
  vertebra 756.19
  vulva 752.49

Anomaly, anomalous *(Continued)*
  spermatic cord 752.9
  spine, spinal 756.10
    column 756.10
    cord 742.9
      meningocele *(see also* Spina bifida)* 741.9●
      specified type NEC 742.59
      spina bifida *(see also* Spina bifida)* 741.9●
      vessel 747.82
    meninges 742.59
    nerve root 742.9
  spleen 759.0
  Sprengel's 755.52
  sternum 756.3
  stomach 750.9
    specified type NEC 750.7
  submaxillary gland 750.9
  superior vena cava 747.40
  talipes - *see* Talipes
  tarsus 755.67
    with complete absence of distal elements 755.31
  teeth, tooth NEC 520.9
    position 524.30
      crowding 524.31
      displacement 524.30
        horizontal 524.33
        vertical 524.34
      distance
        interocclusal
          excessive 524.37
          insufficient 524.36
      excessive spacing 524.32
      rotation 524.35
      specified NEC 524.39
    spacing 524.30
  tendon 756.9
    specified type NEC 756.89
  termination
    coronary artery 746.85
  testis 752.9
  thebesian valve 746.9
  thigh 755.9
    flexion *(see also* Subluxation, congenital, hip)* 754.32
  thorax (wall) 756.3
  throat 750.9
  thumb 755.50
    supernumerary 755.01
  thymus gland 759.2
  thyroid (gland) 759.2
    cartilage 748.3
  tibia 755.60
    saber 090.5
  toe 755.66
    supernumerary 755.02
    webbed *(see also* Syndactylism, toes)* 755.13
  tongue 750.10
    specified type NEC 750.19
  trachea, tracheal 748.3
    cartilage 748.3
    rings 748.3
  tragus 744.3
  transverse aortic arch 747.21
  trichromata 368.59
  trichromatopsia 368.59
  tricuspid (leaflet) (valve) 746.9
    atresia 746.1
    Ebstein's 746.2
    specified type NEC 746.89
    stenosis 746.1
  trunk 759.9
  Uhl's (hypoplasia of myocardium, right ventricle) 746.84
  ulna 755.50
  umbilicus 759.9
    artery 747.5
  union, trachea with larynx 748.3

Anomaly, anomalous *(Continued)*
  unspecified site 759.9
  upper extremity 755.50
    vessel 747.63
  urachus 753.7
    specified type NEC 753.7
  ureter 753.9
    obstructive 753.20
    specified type NEC 753.4
      obstructive 753.29
  urethra (valve) 753.9
    obstructive 753.6
    specified type NEC 753.8
  urinary tract or system (any part, except urachus) 753.9
    specified type NEC 753.8
    urachus 753.7
  uterus 752.39
    with only one functioning horn 752.33
    in pregnancy or childbirth 654.0●
      affecting fetus or newborn 763.89
      causing obstructed labor 660.2●
        affecting fetus or newborn 763.1
  uvula 750.9
  vagina 752.40
  valleculae 748.3
  valve (heart) NEC 746.9
    formation, ureter 753.29
    pulmonary 746.00
    specified type NEC 746.89
  vascular NEC *(see also* Anomaly, peripheral vascular system)* 747.60
    ring 747.21
  vas deferens 752.9
  vein(s) (peripheral) NEC *(see also* Anomaly, peripheral vascular system)* 747.60
    brain 747.81
    cerebral 747.81
    coronary 746.89
    great 747.40
      specified type NEC 747.49
    portal 747.40
    pulmonary 747.40
    retina 743.9
  vena cava (inferior) (superior) 747.40
  venous - *see* Anomaly, vein
  venous return (pulmonary) 747.49
    partial 747.42
    total 747.41
  ventricle, ventricular (heart) 746.9
    bands 746.9
    folds 746.9
    septa 745.4
  vertebra 756.10
  vesicourethral orifice 753.9
  vessels NEC *(see also* Anomaly, peripheral vascular system)* 747.60
    optic papilla 743.9
  vitelline duct 751.0
  vitreous humor 743.9
    specified type NEC 743.51
  vulva 752.40
  wrist (joint) 755.50
Anomia 784.69
Anonychia 757.5
  acquired 703.8
Anophthalmos, anophthalmus (clinical) (congenital) (globe) 743.00
  acquired V45.78
Anopsia (altitudinal) (quadrant) 368.46
Anorchia 752.89
Anorchism, anorchidism 752.89
Anorexia 783.0
  hysterical 300.11
  nervosa 307.1
Anosmia *(see also* Disturbance, sensation)* 781.1
  hysterical 300.11
  postinfectional 478.9
  psychogenic 306.7
  traumatic 951.8
Anosognosia 780.99

Anosphrasia 781.1
Anosteoplasia 756.50
Anotia 744.09
Anovulatory cycle 628.0
Anoxemia 799.02
   newborn 770.88
Anoxia 799.02
   altitude 993.2
   cerebral 348.1
      with
         abortion - *see* Abortion, by type,
               with specified complication
               NEC
         ectopic pregnancy (*see also* categories
               633.0-633.9) 639.8
         molar pregnancy (*see also* categories
               630-632) 639.8
      complicating
         delivery (cesarean) (instrumental)
               669.4●
         ectopic or molar pregnancy 639.8
         obstetric anesthesia or sedation
               668.2●
      during or resulting from a procedure
            997.01
      following
         abortion 639.8
         ectopic or molar pregnancy 639.8
      newborn (*see also* Distress, fetal, liveborn
            infant) 770.88
   due to drowning 994.1
   fetal, affecting newborn 770.88
   heart - *see* Insufficiency, coronary
   high altitude 993.2
   intrauterine
      fetal death (before onset of labor)
            768.0
         during labor 768.1
      liveborn infant - *see* Distress, fetal,
            liveborn infant
   myocardial - *see* Insufficiency, coronary
   newborn 768.9
      mild or moderate 768.6
      severe 768.5
   pathological 799.02
Anteflexion - *see* Anteversion
Antenatal
   care, normal pregnancy V22.1
      first V22.0
   sampling
      chorionic villus V28.89
   screening of mother (for) V28.9
      based on amniocentesis NEC V28.2
         chromosomal anomalies V28.0
         raised alphafetoprotein levels
               V28.1
      chromosomal anomalies V28.0
      fetal growth retardation using ultrasonics
            V28.4
      genomic V28.89
      isoimmunization V28.5
      malformations using ultrasonics V28.3
      proteomic V28.89
      raised alphafetoprotein levels in amniotic
            fluid V28.1
      risk
         pre-term labor V28.82
      specified condition NEC V28.89
      Streptococcus B V28.6
   survey
      fetal anatomic V28.81
   testing
      nuchal translucency V28.89
Antepartum - *see* condition
Anterior - *see also* condition
   spinal artery compression syndrome
         721.1
Antero-occlusion 524.24
Anteversion
   cervix - *see* Anteversion, uterus
   femur (neck), congenital 755.63

Anteversion (*Continued*)
   uterus, uterine (cervix) (postinfectional)
         (postpartal, old) 621.6
      congenital 752.39
      in pregnancy or childbirth 654.4●
         affecting fetus or newborn 763.89
         causing obstructed labor 660.2●
            affecting fetus or newborn
                  763.1
Anthracosilicosis (occupational) 500
Anthracosis (lung) (occupational) 500
   lingua 529.3
Anthrax 022.9
   with pneumonia 022.1 [484.5]
   colitis 022.2
   cutaneous 022.0
   gastrointestinal 022.2
   intestinal 022.2
   pulmonary 022.1
   respiratory 022.1
   septicemia 022.3
   specified manifestation NEC 022.8
Anthropoid pelvis 755.69
   with disproportion (fetopelvic) 653.2●
      affecting fetus or newborn 763.1
      causing obstructed labor 660.1●
         affecting fetus or newborn
               763.1
Anthropophobia 300.29
Antibioma, breast 611.0
Antibodies
   maternal (blood group) (*see also*
         Incompatibility) 656.2●
   anti-D, cord blood 656.1●
      fetus or newborn 773.0
Antibody
   anticardiolipin 795.79
      with
         hemorrhagic disorder 286.53
         hypercoagulable state 289.81
   antiphosphatidylglycerol 795.79
      with
         hemorrhagic disorder 286.53
         hypercoagulable state 289.81
   antiphosphatidylinositol 795.79
      with
         hemorrhagic disorder 286.53
         hypercoagulable state 289.81
   antiphosphatidylserine 795.79
      with
         hemorrhagic disorder 286.53
         hypercoagulable state 289.81
   antiphospholipid 795.79
      with
         hemorrhagic disorder 286.53
         hypercoagulable state 289.81
   deficiency syndrome
      agammaglobulinemic 279.00
      congenital 279.04
      hypogammaglobulinemic 279.00
Anticoagulant
   intrinsic, circulating, causing hemorrhagic
         disorder (*see also* Circulating,
         anticoagulants) 286.59
   lupus (LAC) 795.79
      with
         hemorrhagic disorder 286.53
         hypercoagulable state 289.81
Antimongolism syndrome 758.39
Antimonial cholera 985.4
Antisocial personality 301.7
Antithrombinemia (*see also* Circulating
      anticoagulants) 286.59
Antithromboplastinemia (*see also* Circulating
      anticoagulants) 286.59
Antithromboplastinogenemia (*see also*
      Circulating anticoagulants) 286.59
Antitoxin complication or reaction - *see*
      Complications, vaccination
Anton (-Babinski) syndrome
   (hemiasomatognosia) 307.9

Antritis (chronic) 473.0
   maxilla 473.0
      acute 461.0
   stomach 535.4●
Antrum, antral - *see* condition
Anuria 788.5
   with
      abortion - *see* Abortion, by type, with
            renal failure
      ectopic pregnancy (*see also* categories
            633.0-633.9) 639.3
      molar pregnancy (*see also* categories
            630-632) 639.3
   calculus (impacted) (recurrent) 592.9
      kidney 592.0
      ureter 592.1
   congenital 753.3
   due to a procedure 997.5
   following
      abortion 639.3
      ectopic or molar pregnancy 639.3
   newborn 753.3
   postrenal 593.4
   puerperal, postpartum, childbirth 669.3●
   specified as due to a procedure 997.5
   sulfonamide
      correct substance properly administered
            788.5
      overdose or wrong substance given or
            taken 961.0
   traumatic (following crushing) 958.5
Anus, anal - *see also* condition
   high risk human papillomavirus (HPV) DNA
         test positive 796.75
   low risk human papillomavirus (HPV) DNA
         test positive 796.79
Anusitis 569.49
Anxiety (neurosis) (reaction) (state) 300.00
   alcohol-induced 291.89
   depression 300.4
   drug-induced 292.89
   due to or associated with physical condition
         293.84
   generalized 300.02
   hysteria 300.20
   in
      acute stress reaction 308.0
      transient adjustment reaction 309.24
   panic type 300.01
   separation, abnormal 309.21
   syndrome (organic) (transient) 293.84
Aorta, aortic - *see* condition
Aortectasia (*see also* Ectasia, aortic) 447.70
   with aneurysm 441.9
Aortitis (nonsyphilitic) 447.6
   arteriosclerotic 440.0
   calcific 447.6
   Döhle-Heller 093.1
   luetic 093.1
   rheumatic (*see also* Endocarditis, acute,
         rheumatic) 391.1
   rheumatoid - *see* Arthritis, rheumatoid
   specific 093.1
   syphilitic 093.1
      congenital 090.5
Apathetic 799.25
   thyroid storm (*see also* Thyrotoxicosis) 242.9●
Apathy 799.25
Apepsia 536.8
   achlorhydric 536.0
   psychogenic 306.4
Aperistalsis, esophagus 530.0
Apert's syndrome (acrocephalosyndactyly)
      755.55
Apert-Gallais syndrome (adrenogenital) 255.2
Apertognathia 524.20
Aphagia 787.20
   psychogenic 307.1
Aphakia (acquired) (bilateral) (postoperative)
      (unilateral) 379.31
   congenital 743.35

◀ New   ◀▥ Revised   ~~deleted~~ Deleted   ● Use Additional Digit(s)   ▨ Omit code

Aphalangia (congenital) 755.4
  lower limb (complete) (intercalary) (partial)
      (terminal) 755.39
    meaning all digits (complete) (partial)
        755.31
    transverse 755.31
  upper limb (complete) (intercalary) (partial)
      (terminal) 755.29
    meaning all digits (complete) (partial)
        755.21
    transverse 755.21
Aphasia (amnestic) (ataxic) (auditory) (Broca's)
    (choreatic) (classic) (expressive) (global)
    (ideational) (ideokinetic) (ideomotor)
    (jargon) (motor) (nominal) (receptive)
    (semantic) (sensory) (syntactic) (verbal)
    (visual) (Wernicke's) 784.3
  developmental 315.31
  syphilis, tertiary 094.89
  uremic - see Uremia
Aphemia 784.3
  uremic - see Uremia
Aphonia 784.41
  clericorum 784.49
  hysterical 300.11
  organic 784.41
  psychogenic 306.1
Aphthae, aphthous - see also condition
  Bednar's 528.2
  cachectic 529.0
  epizootic 078.4
  fever 078.4
  oral 528.2
  stomatitis 528.2
  thrush 112.0
  ulcer (oral) (recurrent) 528.2
    genital organ(s) NEC
      female 616.50
      male 608.89
    larynx 478.79
Apical - see condition
Apical ballooning syndrome 429.83
Aplasia - see also Agenesis
  alveolar process (acquired) 525.8
    congenital 750.26
  aorta (congenital) 747.22
  aortic valve (congenital) 746.89
  axialis extracorticalis (congenital) 330.0
  bone marrow (myeloid) 284.9
    acquired (secondary) 284.89
    congenital 284.01
    idiopathic 284.9
  brain 740.0
    specified part 742.2
  breast 757.6
  bronchus 748.3
  cementum 520.4
  cerebellar 742.2
  congenital (pure) red cell 284.01
  corpus callosum 742.2
  erythrocyte 284.81
    congenital 284.01
  extracortical axial 330.0
  eye (congenital) 743.00
  fovea centralis (congenital) 743.55
  germinal (cell) 606.0
  iris 743.45
  labyrinth, membranous 744.05
  limb (congenital) 755.4
    lower NEC 755.30
    upper NEC 755.20
  lung (bilateral) (congenital) (unilateral) 748.5
  nervous system NEC 742.8
  nuclear 742.8
  ovary 752.0
  Pelizaeus-Merzbacher 330.0
  prostate (congenital) 752.89
  red cell (with thymoma) 284.81
    acquired (secondary) 284.81
      due to drugs 284.81
    adult 284.81

Aplasia (Continued)
  red cell (Continued)
    congenital 284.01
    hereditary 284.01
    of infants 284.01
    primary 284.01
    pure 284.01
      due to drugs 284.81
  round ligament (congenital) 752.89
  salivary gland 750.21
  skin (congenital) 757.39
  spinal cord 742.59
  spleen 759.0
  testis (congenital) 752.89
  thymic, with immunodeficiency 279.2
  thyroid 243
  uterus 752.39
  ventral horn cell 742.59
Apleuria 756.3
Apnea, apneic (spells) 786.03
  newborn, neonatorum 770.81
    essential 770.81
    obstructive 770.82
    primary 770.81
    sleep 770.81
    specified NEC 770.82
  psychogenic 306.1
  sleep 780.57
    with
      hypersomnia, unspecified 780.53
      hyposomnia, unspecified 780.51
      insomnia, unspecified 780.51
      sleep disturbance 780.57
    central, in conditions classified elsewhere
        327.27
    obstructive (adult) (pediatric) 327.23
    organic 327.20
      other 327.29
    primary central 327.21
Apneumatosis newborn 770.4
Apodia 755.31
Apophysitis (bone) (see also Osteochondrosis)
    732.9
  calcaneus 732.5
  juvenile 732.6
Apoplectiform convulsions (see also Disease,
    cerebrovascular, acute) 436
Apoplexia, apoplexy, apoplectic (see also
    Disease, cerebrovascular, acute)
    436
  abdominal 569.89
  adrenal 036.3
  attack 436
  basilar (see also Disease, cerebrovascular,
      acute) 436
  brain (see also Disease, cerebrovascular,
      acute) 436
  bulbar (see also Disease, cerebrovascular,
      acute) 436
  capillary (see also Disease, cerebrovascular,
      acute) 436
  cardiac (see also Infarct, myocardium)
      410.9●
  cerebral (see also Disease, cerebrovascular,
      acute) 436
  chorea (see also Disease, cerebrovascular,
      acute) 436
  congestive (see also Disease, cerebrovascular,
      acute) 436
    newborn 767.4
  embolic (see also Embolism, brain)
      434.1●
  fetus 767.0
  fit (see also Disease, cerebrovascular, acute)
      436
  healed or old V12.54
  heart (auricle) (ventricle) (see also Infarct,
      myocardium) 410.9●
  heat 992.0
  hemiplegia (see also Disease, cerebrovascular,
      acute) 436

Apoplexia, apoplexy, apoplectic (Continued)
  hemorrhagic (stroke) (see also Hemorrhage,
      brain) 432.9
  ingravescent (see also Disease,
      cerebrovascular, acute) 436
  late effect - see Late effect(s) (of)
      cerebrovascular disease
  lung - see Embolism, pulmonary
  meninges, hemorrhagic (see also
      Hemorrhage, subarachnoid) 430
  neonatorum 767.0
  newborn 767.0
  pancreatitis 577.0
  placenta 641.2●
  progressive (see also Disease, cerebrovascular,
      acute) 436
  pulmonary (artery) (vein) - see Embolism,
      pulmonary
  sanguineous (see also Disease,
      cerebrovascular, acute) 436
  seizure (see also Disease, cerebrovascular,
      acute) 436
  serous (see also Disease, cerebrovascular,
      acute) 436
  spleen 289.59
  stroke (see also Disease, cerebrovascular,
      acute) 436
  thrombotic (see also Thrombosis, brain)
      434.0●
  uremic - see Uremia
  uteroplacental 641.2●
Appendage
  fallopian tube (cyst of Morgagni) 752.11
  intestine (epiploic) 751.5
  preauricular 744.1
  testicular (organ of Morgagni) 752.89
Appendicitis 541
  with
    perforation, peritonitis (generalized), or
        rupture 540.0
      with peritoneal abscess 540.1
    peritoneal abscess 540.1
  acute (catarrhal) (fulminating) (gangrenous)
      (inflammatory) (obstructive)
      (retrocecal) (suppurative) 540.9
    with
      perforation, peritonitis, or rupture
          540.0
        with peritoneal abscess 540.1
      peritoneal abscess 540.1
  amebic 006.8
  chronic (recurrent) 542
  exacerbation - see Appendicitis, acute
  fulminating - see Appendicitis, acute
  gangrenous - see Appendicitis, acute
  healed (obliterative) 542
  interval 542
  neurogenic 542
  obstructive 542
  pneumococcal 541
  recurrent 542
  relapsing 542
  retrocecal 541
  subacute (adhesive) 542
  subsiding 542
  suppurative - see Appendicitis, acute
  tuberculous (see also Tuberculosis) 014.8●
Appendiclausis 543.9
Appendicolithiasis 543.9
Appendicopathia oxyurica 127.4
Appendix, appendicular - see also condition
  Morgagni (male) 752.89
    fallopian tube 752.11
Appetite
  depraved 307.52
  excessive 783.6
    psychogenic 307.51
  lack or loss (see also Anorexia) 783.0
    nonorganic origin 307.59
  perverted 307.52
    hysterical 300.11

Apprehension, apprehensiveness (abnormal) (state) 300.00
  specified type NEC 300.09
Approximal wear 521.10
Apraxia (classic) (ideational) (ideokinetic) (ideomotor) (motor) 784.69
  oculomotor, congenital 379.51
  verbal 784.69
Aptyalism 527.7
Aqueous misdirection 365.83
Arabicum elephantiasis (see also Infestation, filarial) 125.9
Arachnidism 989.5
Arachnitis - see Meningitis
Arachnodactyly 759.82
Arachnoidism 989.5
Arachnoiditis (acute) (adhesive) (basic) (brain) (cerebrospinal) (chiasmal) (chronic) (spinal) (see also Meningitis) 322.9
  meningococcal (chronic) 036.0
  syphilitic 094.2
  tuberculous (see also Tuberculosis, meninges) 013.0●
Araneism 989.5
Arboencephalitis, Australian 062.4
Arborization block (heart) 426.6
Arbor virus, arbovirus (infection) NEC 066.9
ARC 042
Arches - see condition
Arcuate uterus 752.36
Arcuatus uterus 752.36
Arcus (cornea)
  juvenilis 743.43
    interfering with vision 743.42
  senilis 371.41
Arc-welders' lung 503
Arc-welders' syndrome (photokeratitis) 370.24
Areflexia 796.1
Areola - see condition
Argentaffinoma (M8241/1) - see also Neoplasm, by site, uncertain behavior
  benign (M8241/0) - see Neoplasm, by site, benign
  malignant (M8241/3) - see Neoplasm, by site, malignant
  syndrome 259.2
Argentinian hemorrhagic fever 078.7
Arginosuccinicaciduria 270.6
Argonz-Del Castillo syndrome (nonpuerperal galactorrhea and amenorrhea) 253.1
Argyll-Robertson phenomenon, pupil, or syndrome (syphilitic) 094.89
  atypical 379.45
  nonluetic 379.45
  nonsyphilitic 379.45
  reversed 379.45
Argyria, argyriasis NEC 985.8
  conjunctiva 372.55
  cornea 371.16
  from drug or medicinal agent
    correct substance properly administered 709.09
    overdose or wrong substance given or taken 961.2
Arhinencephaly 742.2
Arias-Stella phenomenon 621.30
Ariboflavinosis 266.0
Arizona enteritis 008.1
Arm - see condition
Armenian disease 277.31
Arnold-Chiari obstruction or syndrome (see also Spina bifida) 741.0●
  type I 348.4
  type II (see also Spina bifida) 741.0●
  type III 742.0
  type IV 742.2
Arousals
  confusional 327.41

Arrest, arrested
  active phase of labor 661.1●
    affecting fetus or newborn 763.7
  any plane in pelvis
    complicating delivery 660.1●
      affecting fetus or newborn 763.1
  bone marrow (see also Anemia, aplastic) 284.9
  cardiac 427.5
    with
      abortion - see Abortion, by type, with specified complication NEC
      ectopic pregnancy (see also categories 633.0-633.9) 639.8
      molar pregnancy (see also categories 630-632) 639.8
    complicating
      anesthesia
        correct substance properly administered 427.5
        obstetric 668.1●
        overdose or wrong substance given 968.4
          specified anesthetic - see Table of Drugs and Chemicals
      delivery (cesarean) (instrumental) 669.4●
      ectopic or molar pregnancy 639.8
      surgery (nontherapeutic) (therapeutic) 997.1
    fetus or newborn 779.85
    following
      abortion 639.8
      ectopic or molar pregnancy 639.8
    personal history, successfully rescuscitated V12.53
    postoperative (immediate) 997.1
      long-term effect of cardiac surgery 429.4
  cardiorespiratory (see also Arrest, cardiac) 427.5
  deep transverse 660.3●
    affecting fetus or newborn 763.1
  development or growth
    bone 733.91
    child 783.40
    fetus 764.9●
      affecting management of pregnancy 656.5●
    tracheal rings 748.3
  epiphyseal 733.91
  granulopoiesis 288.09
  heart - see Arrest, cardiac
  respiratory 799.1
    newborn 770.87
  sinus 426.6
  transverse (deep) 660.3●
    affecting fetus or newborn 763.1
Arrhenoblastoma (M8630/1)
  benign (M8630/0)
    specified site - see Neoplasm, by site, benign
    unspecified site
      female 220
      male 222.0
  malignant (M8630/3)
    specified site - see Neoplasm, by site, malignant
    unspecified site
      female 183.0
      male 186.9
  specified site - see Neoplasm, by site, uncertain behavior
  unspecified site
    female 236.2
    male 236.4
Arrhinencephaly 742.2
  due to
    trisomy 13 (13-15) 758.1
    trisomy 18 (16-18) 758.2

Arrhythmia (auricle) (cardiac) (cordis) (gallop rhythm) (juvenile) (nodal) (reflex) (sinus) (supraventricular) (transitory) (ventricle) 427.9
  bigeminal rhythm 427.89
  block 426.9
  bradycardia 427.89
  contractions, premature 427.60
  coronary sinus 427.89
  ectopic 427.89
  extrasystolic 427.60
  postoperative 997.1
  psychogenic 306.2
  vagal 780.2
Arrillaga-Ayerza syndrome (pulmonary artery sclerosis with pulmonary hypertension) 416.0
Arsenical
  dermatitis 692.4
  keratosis 692.4
  pigmentation 985.1
    from drug or medicinal agent
      correct substance properly administered 709.09
      overdose or wrong substance given or taken 961.1
Arsenism 985.1
  from drug or medicinal agent
    correct substance properly administered 692.4
    overdose or wrong substance given or taken 961.1
Arterial - see condition
Arteriectasis 447.8
Arteriofibrosis - see Arteriosclerosis
Arteriolar sclerosis - see Arteriosclerosis
Arteriolith - see Arteriosclerosis
Arteriolitis 447.6
  necrotizing, kidney 447.5
  renal - see Hypertension, kidney
Arteriolosclerosis - see Arteriosclerosis
Arterionephrosclerosis (see also Hypertension, kidney) 403.90
Arteriopathy 447.9
Arteriosclerosis, arteriosclerotic (artery) (deformans) (diffuse) (disease) (endarteritis) (general) (obliterans) (obliterative) (occlusive) (senile) (with calcification) 440.9
  with
    gangrene 440.24
    psychosis (see also Psychosis, arteriosclerotic) 290.40
    ulceration 440.23
  aorta 440.0
  arteries of extremities - see Arteriosclerosis, extremities
  basilar (artery) (see also Occlusion, artery, basilar) 433.0●
  brain 437.0
  bypass graft
    coronary artery 414.05
      autologous artery (gastroepiploic) (internal mammary) 414.04
      autologous vein 414.02
      nonautologous biological 414.03
      of transplanted heart 414.07
    extremity 440.30
      autologous vein 440.31
      nonautologous biological 440.32
  cardiac - see Arteriosclerosis, coronary
  cardiopathy - see Arteriosclerosis, coronary
  cardiorenal (see also Hypertension, cardiorenal) 404.90
  cardiovascular (see also Disease, cardiovascular) 429.2
  carotid (artery) (common) (internal) (see also Occlusion, artery, carotid) 433.1●
  central nervous system 437.0

◄ New   ◄▥ Revised   ~~deleted~~ Deleted   ● Use Additional Digit(s)   ▨ Omit code

Arteriosclerosis, arteriosclerotic (Continued)
cerebral 437.0
late effect - see Late effect(s) (of)
cerebrovascular disease
cerebrospinal 437.0
cerebrovascular 437.0
coronary (artery) 414.00
due to
calcified coronary lesion (severely)
414.4
graft - see Arteriosclerosis, bypass graft
native artery 414.01
of transplanted heart 414.06
lipid rich plaque 414.3
extremities (native artery) NEC 440.20
bypass graft 440.30
autologous vein 440.31
nonautologous biological 440.32
claudication (intermittent) 440.21
and
gangrene 440.24
rest pain 440.22
and
gangrene 440.24
ulceration 440.23
and gangrene 440.24
ulceration 440.23
and gangrene 440.24
gangrene 440.24
rest pain 440.22
and
gangrene 440.24
ulceration 440.23
and gangrene 440.24
specified site NEC 440.29
ulceration 440.23
and gangrene 440.24
heart (disease) - see also Arteriosclerosis,
coronary
valve 424.99
aortic 424.1
mitral 424.0
pulmonary 424.3
tricuspid 424.2
iliac 440.8
kidney (see also Hypertension, kidney) 403.90
labyrinth, labyrinthine 388.00
medial NEC (see also Arteriosclerosis,
extremities) 440.20
mesentery (artery) 557.1
Mönckeberg's (see also Arteriosclerosis,
extremities) 440.20
myocarditis 429.0
nephrosclerosis (see also Hypertension,
kidney) 403.90
peripheral (of extremities) - see
Arteriosclerosis, extremities
precerebral 433.9●
specified artery NEC 433.8●
pulmonary (idiopathic) 416.0
renal (see also Hypertension, kidney) 403.90
arterioles (see also Hypertension, kidney)
403.90
artery 440.1
retinal (vascular) 440.8 [362.13]
specified artery NEC 440.8
with gangrene 440.8 [785.4]
spinal (cord) 437.0
vertebral (artery) (see also Occlusion, artery,
vertebral) 433.2●
Arteriospasm 443.9
Arteriovenous - see condition
Arteritis 447.6
allergic (see also Angiitis, hypersensitivity)
446.20
aorta (nonsyphilitic) 447.6
syphilitic 093.1
aortic arch 446.7
brachiocephalica 446.7
brain 437.4
syphilitic 094.89

Arteritis (Continued)
branchial 446.7
cerebral 437.4
late effect - see Late effect(s) (of)
cerebrovascular disease
syphilitic 094.89
coronary (artery) - see also Arteriosclerosis,
coronary
rheumatic 391.9
chronic 398.99
syphilitic 093.89
cranial (left) (right) 446.5
deformans - see Arteriosclerosis
giant cell 446.5
necrosing or necrotizing 446.0
nodosa 446.0
obliterans - see also Arteriosclerosis
subclaviocarotica 446.7
pulmonary 417.8
retina 362.18
rheumatic - see Fever, rheumatic
senile - see Arteriosclerosis
suppurative 447.2
syphilitic (general) 093.89
brain 094.89
coronary 093.89
spinal 094.89
temporal 446.5
young female, syndrome 446.7
Artery, arterial - see condition
Arthralgia (see also Pain, joint) 719.4●
allergic (see also Pain, joint) 719.4●
in caisson disease 993.3
psychogenic 307.89
rubella 056.71
Salmonella 003.23
temporomandibular joint 524.62
Arthritis, arthritic (acute) (chronic) (subacute)
716.9●
meaning Osteoarthritis - see Osteoarthrosis

> Note: Use the following fifth-digit
> subclassification with categories 711-712,
> 715-716:
>
> 0   site unspecified
> 1   shoulder region
> 2   upper arm
> 3   forearm
> 4   hand
> 5   pelvic region and thigh
> 6   lower leg
> 7   ankle and foot
> 8   other specified sites
> 9   multiple sites

allergic 716.2●
ankylosing (crippling) (spine) 720.0 [713.2]
sites other than spine 716.9●
atrophic 714.0
spine 720.9
back (see also Arthritis, spine) 721.90
Bechterew's (ankylosing spondylitis) 720.0
blennorrhagic 098.50 [711.6]●
cervical, cervicodorsal (see also Spondylosis,
cervical) 721.0
Charcôt's 094.0 [713.5]
diabetic 250.6● [713.5]
due to secondary diabetes 249.6●
[713.5]
syringomyelic 336.0 [713.5]
tabetic 094.0 [713.5]
chylous (see also Filariasis) 125.9 [711.7]●
climacteric NEC 716.3●
coccyx 721.8
cricoarytenoid 478.79
crystal (-induced) - see Arthritis, due to
crystals
deformans (see also Osteoarthrosis)
715.9●
spine 721.90
with myelopathy 721.91

Arthritis, arthritic (Continued)
degenerative (see also Osteoarthrosis) 715.9●
idiopathic 715.09
polyarticular 715.09
spine 721.90
with myelopathy 721.91
dermatoarthritis, lipoid 272.8 [713.0]
due to or associated with
acromegaly 253.0 [713.0]
actinomycosis 039.8 [711.4]●
amyloidosis 277.39 [713.7]
bacterial disease NEC 040.89 [711.4]●
Behçet's syndrome 136.1 [711.2]●
blastomycosis 116.0 [711.4]●
brucellosis (see also Brucellosis) 023.9
[711.4]●
caisson disease 993.3
coccidioidomycosis 114.3 [711.6]●
coliform (Escherichia coli) 711.0●
colitis, ulcerative (see also Colitis,
ulcerative) 556.9 [713.1]
cowpox 051.01 [711.5]●
crystals (see also Gout)
dicalcium phosphate 275.49 [712.1]●
pyrophosphate 275.49 [712.2]●
specified NEC 275.49 [712.8]●
dermatoarthritis, lipoid 272.8 [713.0]
dermatological disorder NEC 709.9
[713.3]
diabetes 250.6● [713.5]
due to secondary diabetes 249.6●
[713.5]
diphtheria 032.89 [711.4]●
dracontiasis 125.7 [711.7]●
dysentery 009.0 [711.3]●
endocrine disorder NEC 259.9 [713.0]
enteritis NEC 009.1 [711.3]●
infectious (see also Enteritis, infectious)
009.0 [711.3]●
specified organism NEC 008.8
[711.3]●
regional (see also Enteritis, regional)
555.9 [713.1]
specified organism NEC 008.8 [711.3]●
epiphyseal slip, nontraumatic (old)
716.8●
erysipelas 035 [711.4]●
erythema
epidemic 026.1
multiforme 695.10 [713.3]
nodosum 695.2 [713.3]
Escherichia coli 711.0●
filariasis NEC 125.9 [711.7]●
gastrointestinal condition NEC 569.9
[713.1]
glanders 024 [711.4]●
Gonococcus 098.50
gout 274.00
H. influenzae 711.0●
helminthiasis NEC 128.9 [711.7]●
hematological disorder NEC 289.9 [713.2]
hemochromatosis 275.03 [713.0]
hemoglobinopathy NEC (see also Disease,
hemoglobin) 282.7 [713.2]
hemophilia (see also Hemophilia) 286.0
[713.2]
Hemophilus influenzae (H. influenzae)
711.0●
Henoch (-Schönlein) purpura 287.0 [713.6]
histoplasmosis NEC (see also
Histoplasmosis) 115.99 [711.6]●
human parvovirus 079.83 [711.5]●
hyperparathyroidism 252.00 [713.0]
hypersensitivity reaction NEC 995.3
[713.6]
hypogammaglobulinemia (see also
Hypogammaglobulinemia) 279.00
[713.0]
hypothyroidism NEC 244.9 [713.0]
infection (see also Arthritis, infectious)
711.9●

Arthritis, arthritic *(Continued)*
  due to or associated with *(Continued)*
    infectious disease NEC 136.9 *[711.8]●*
    leprosy *(see also Leprosy)* 030.9 *[711.4]●*
    leukemia NEC (M9800/3) 208.9● *[713.2]*
    lipoid dermatoarthritis 272.8 *[713.0]*
    Lyme disease 088.81 *[711.8]●*
    Mediterranean fever, familial 277.31
        [713.7]
    meningococcal infection 036.82
    metabolic disorder NEC 277.9 *[713.0]*
    multiple myelomatosis (M9730/3) 203.0●
        [713.2]
    mumps 072.79 *[711.5]●*
    mycobacteria 031.8 *[711.4]●*
    mycosis NEC 117.9 *[711.6]●*
    neurological disorder NEC 349.9 *[713.5]*
    ochronosis 270.2 *[713.0]*
    O'Nyong Nyong 066.3 *[711.5]●*
    parasitic disease NEC 136.9 *[711.8]●*
    paratyphoid fever *(see also Fever,*
        paratyphoid) 002.9 *[711.3]●*
    parvovirus B19 079.83 *[711.5]●*
    Pneumococcus 711.0●
    poliomyelitis *(see also Poliomyelitis)*
        045.9● *[711.5]●*
    Pseudomonas 711.0●
    psoriasis 696.0
    pyogenic organism (E. coli) (H.
        influenzae) (Pseudomonas)
        (Streptococcus) 711.0●
    rat-bite fever 026.1 *[711.4]●*
    regional enteritis *(see also Enteritis,*
        regional) 555.9 *[713.1]*
    Reiter's disease 099.3 *[711.1]●*
    respiratory disorder NEC 519.9 *[713.4]*
    reticulosis, malignant (M9720/3) 202.3●
        [713.2]
    rubella 056.71
    salmonellosis 003.23
    sarcoidosis 135 *[713.7]*
    serum sickness 999.59 *[713.6]*
    Staphylococcus 711.0●
    Streptococcus 711.0●
    syphilis *(see also Syphilis)* 094.0 *[711.4]●*
    syringomyelia 336.0 *[713.5]*
    thalassemia *(see also Thalassemia)* 282.40
        [713.2]
    tuberculosis *(see also Tuberculosis,*
        arthritis) 015.9● *[711.4]●*
    typhoid fever 002.0 *[711.3]●*
    ulcerative colitis *(see also Colitis,*
        ulcerative) 556.9 *[713.1]*
    urethritis
        nongonococcal *(see also Urethritis,*
            nongonococcal) 099.40 *[711.1]●*
        nonspecific *(see also Urethritis,*
            nongonococcal) 099.40 *[711.1]●*
        Reiter's 099.3 *[711.1]●*
    viral disease NEC 079.99 *[711.5]●*
  erythema epidemic 026.1
  gonococcal 098.50
  gouty 274.00
    acute 274.01
  hypertrophic *(see also Osteoarthrosis)* 715.9●
    spine 721.90
      with myelopathy 721.91
  idiopathic, blennorrheal 099.3
  in caisson disease 993.3 *[713.8]*
  infectious or infective (acute) (chronic)
      (subacute) NEC 711.9●
    nonpyogenic 711.9●
    spine 720.9
  inflammatory NEC 714.9
  juvenile rheumatoid (chronic) (polyarticular)
      714.30
    acute 714.31
    monoarticular 714.33
    pauciarticular 714.32
  lumbar *(see also Spondylosis, lumbar)* 721.3
  meningococcal 036.82

Arthritis, arthritic *(Continued)*
  menopausal NEC 716.3●
  migratory - *see* Fever, rheumatic
  neuropathic (Charcôt's) 094.0 *[713.5]*
    diabetic 250.6● *[713.5]*
      due to secondary diabetes 249.6●
          [713.5]
    nonsyphilitic NEC 349.9 *[713.5]*
    syringomyelic 336.0 *[713.5]*
    tabetic 094.0 *[713.5]*
  nodosa *(see also Osteoarthrosis)* 715.9●
    spine 721.90
      with myelopathy 721.91
  nonpyogenic NEC 716.9●
    spine 721.90
      with myelopathy 721.91
  ochronotic 270.2 *[713.0]*
  palindromic *(see also Rheumatism,*
      palindromic) 719.3●
  pneumococcal 711.0●
  postdysenteric 009.0 *[711.3]●*
  postrheumatic, chronic (Jaccoud's) 714.4
  primary progressive 714.0
    spine 720.9
  proliferative 714.0
    spine 720.0
  psoriatic 696.0
  purulent 711.0●
  pyogenic or pyemic 711.0●
  reactive 099.3
  rheumatic 714.0
    acute or subacute - *see* Fever, rheumatic
    chronic 714.0
    spine 720.9
  rheumatoid (nodular) 714.0
    with
      splenoadenomegaly and leukopenia
          714.1
      visceral or systemic involvement 714.2
    aortitis 714.89
    carditis 714.2
    heart disease 714.2
    juvenile (chronic) (polyarticular) 714.30
      acute 714.31
      monoarticular 714.33
      pauciarticular 714.32
    spine 720.0
  rubella 056.71
  sacral, sacroiliac, sacrococcygeal *(see also*
      Spondylosis, sacral) 721.3
  scorbutic 267
  senile or senescent *(see also Osteoarthrosis)*
      715.9●
    spine 721.90
      with myelopathy 721.91
  septic 711.0●
  serum (nontherapeutic) (therapeutic) 999.59
      [713.6]
  specified form NEC 716.8●
  spine 721.90
    with myelopathy 721.91
    atrophic 720.9
    degenerative 721.90
      with myelopathy 721.91
    hypertrophic (with deformity) 721.90
      with myelopathy 721.91
    infectious or infective NEC 720.9
    Marie-Strümpell 720.0
    nonpyogenic 721.90
      with myelopathy 721.91
    pyogenic 720.9
    rheumatoid 720.0
    traumatic (old) 721.7
    tuberculous *(see also Tuberculosis)* 015.0●
        [720.81]
  staphylococcal 711.0●
  streptococcal 711.0●
  suppurative 711.0●
  syphilitic 094.0 *[713.5]*
    congenital 090.49 *[713.5]*
  syphilitica deformans (Charcôt) 094.0 *[713.5]*

Arthritis, arthritic *(Continued)*
  temporomandibular joint 524.69
  thoracic *(see also Spondylosis, thoracic)* 721.2
  toxic of menopause 716.3●
  transient 716.4●
  traumatic (chronic) (old) (post) 716.1●
    current injury - *see* nature of injury
  tuberculous *(see also Tuberculosis, arthritis)*
      015.9● *[711.4]●*
  urethritica 099.3 *[711.1]●*
  urica, uratic 274.00
  venereal 099.3 *[711.1]●*
  vertebral *(see also Arthritis, spine)* 721.90
  villous 716.8●
  von Bechterew's 720.0
Arthrocele *(see also Effusion, joint)* 719.0●
Arthrochondritis - *see* Arthritis
Arthrodesis status V45.4
Arthrodynia *(see also Pain, joint)* 719.4●
  psychogenic 307.89
Arthrodysplasia 755.9
Arthrofibrosis, joint *(see also Ankylosis)* 718.5●
Arthrogryposis 728.3
  multiplex, congenita 754.89
Arthrokatadysis 715.35
Arthrolithiasis 274.00
Arthro-onychodysplasia 756.89
Arthro-osteo-onychodysplasia 756.89
Arthropathy *(see also Arthritis)* 716.9●

Note: Use the following fifth-digit
subclassification with categories 711-712, 716:

    0   site unspecified
    1   shoulder region
    2   upper arm
    3   forearm
    4   hand
    5   pelvic region and thigh
    6   lower leg
    7   ankle and foot
    8   other specified sites
    9   multiple sites

  Behçet's 136.1 *[711.2]●*
  Charcôt's 094.0 *[713.5]*
    diabetic 250.6● *[713.5]*
      due to secondary diabetes 249.6●
          [713.5]
    syringomyelic 336.0 *[713.5]*
    tabetic 094.0 *[713.5]*
  crystal (-induced) - *see* Arthritis, due to
      crystals
  gouty 274.00
    acute 274.01
    chronic (without mention of tophus
        (tophi)) 274.02
      with tophus (tophi) 274.03
  neurogenic, neuropathic (Charcôt's) (tabetic)
      094.0 *[713.5]*
    diabetic 250.6● *[713.5]*
      due to secondary diabetes 249.6●
          [713.5]
    nonsyphilitic NEC 349.9 *[713.5]*
    syringomyelic 336.0 *[713.5]*
  postdysenteric NEC 009.0 *[711.3]●*
  postrheumatic, chronic (Jaccoud's) 714.4
  psoriatic 696.0
  pulmonary 731.2
  specified NEC 716.8●
  syringomyelia 336.0 *[713.5]*
  tabes dorsalis 094.0 *[713.5]*
  tabetic 094.0 *[713.5]*
  transient 716.4●
  traumatic 716.1●
  uric acid 274.00
Arthrophyte *(see also Loose, body, joint)* 718.1●
Arthrophytis 719.80
  ankle 719.87
  elbow 719.82
  foot 719.87
  hand 719.84

◀ New   ◀▥ Revised   ~~deleted~~ Deleted   ● Use Additional Digit(s)   ▨ Omit code

Arthrophytis *(Continued)*
 hip 719.85
 knee 719.86
 multiple sites 719.89
 pelvic region 719.85
 shoulder (region) 719.81
 specified site NEC 719.88
 wrist 719.83
Arthropyosis *(see also* Arthritis, pyogenic) 711.0●
Arthroscopic surgical procedure converted to open procedure V64.43
Arthrosis (deformans) (degenerative) *(see also* Osteoarthrosis) 715.9●
 Charcôt's 094.0 *[713.5]*
 polyarticular 715.09
 spine *(see also* Spondylosis) 721.90
Arthus phenomenon 995.21
 due to
  correct substance properly administered 995.21
  overdose or wrong substance given or taken 977.9
   specified drug - *see* Table of Drugs and Chemicals
  serum 999.59
Articular - *see also* condition
 disc disorder (reducing or non-reducing) 524.63
 spondylolisthesis 756.12
Articulation
 anterior 524.27
 posterior 524.27
 reverse 524.27
Artificial
 device (prosthetic) - *see* Fitting, device
 insemination V26.1
 menopause (states) (symptoms) (syndrome) 627.4
 opening status (functioning) (without complication) V44.9
  anus (colostomy) V44.3
  colostomy V44.3
  cystostomy V44.50
   appendico-vesicostomy V44.52
   cutaneous-vesicostomy V44.51
   specified type NEC V44.59
  enterostomy V44.4
  gastrostomy V44.1
  ileostomy V44.2
  intestinal tract NEC V44.4
  jejunostomy V44.4
  nephrostomy V44.6
  specified site NEC V44.8
  tracheostomy V44.0
  ureterostomy V44.6
  urethrostomy V44.6
  urinary tract NEC V44.6
  vagina V44.7
  vagina status V44.7
ARV (disease) (illness) (infection) - *see* Human immunodeficiency virus (disease) (illness) (infection)
Arytenoid - *see* condition
Asbestosis (occupational) 501
Asboe-Hansen's disease (incontinentia pigmenti) 757.33
Ascariasis (intestinal) (lung) 127.0
Ascaridiasis 127.0
Ascaridosis 127.0
Ascaris 127.0
 lumbricoides (infestation) 127.0
 pneumonia 127.0
Ascending - *see* condition
Aschoff's bodies *(see also* Myocarditis, rheumatic) 398.0
Ascites 789.59
 abdominal NEC 789.59
 cancerous (M8000/6) 789.51
 cardiac 428.0
 chylous (nonfilarial) 457.8
  filarial *(see also* Infestation, filarial) 125.9

Ascites *(Continued)*
 congenital 778.0
 due to S. japonicum 120.2
 fetal, causing fetopelvic disproportion 653.7●
 heart 428.0
 joint *(see also* Effusion, joint) 719.0●
 malignant (M8000/6) 789.51
 pseudochylous 789.59
 syphilitic 095.2
 tuberculous *(see also* Tuberculosis) 014.0●
Ascorbic acid (vitamin C) deficiency (scurvy) 267
ASC-H (atypical squamous cells cannot exclude high grade squamous intraepithelial lesion)
 anus 796.72
 cervix 795.02
 vagina 795.12
ASC-US (atypical squamous cells of undetermined significance)
 anus 796.71
 cervix 795.01
 vagina 795.11
ASCVD (arteriosclerotic cardiovascular disease) 429.2
Aseptic - *see* condition
Asherman's syndrome 621.5
Asialia 527.7
Asiatic cholera *(see also* Cholera) 001.9
Asocial personality or trends 301.7
Asomatognosia 781.8
Aspergillosis 117.3
 with pneumonia 117.3 *[484.6]*
 allergic bronchopulmonary 518.6
 nonsyphilitic NEC 117.3
Aspergillus (flavus) (fumigatus) (infection) (terreus) 117.3
Aspermatogenesis 606.0
Aspermia (testis) 606.0
Asphyxia, asphyxiation (by) 799.01
 antenatal - *see* Distress, fetal
 bedclothes 994.7
 birth *(see also* Asphyxia, newborn) 768.9
 bunny bag 994.7
 carbon monoxide 986
 caul *(see also* Asphyxia, newborn) 768.9
 cave-in 994.7
  crushing - *see* Injury, internal, intrathoracic organs
 constriction 994.7
 crushing - *see* Injury, internal, intrathoracic organs
 drowning 994.1
 fetal, affecting newborn 768.9
 food or foreign body (in larynx) 933.1
  bronchioles 934.8
  bronchus (main) 934.1
  lung 934.8
  nasopharynx 933.0
  nose, nasal passages 932
  pharynx 933.0
  respiratory tract 934.9
   specified part NEC 934.8
  throat 933.0
  trachea 934.0
 gas, fumes, or vapor NEC 987.9
  specified - *see* Table of Drugs and Chemicals
 gravitational changes 994.7
 hanging 994.7
 inhalation - *see* Inhalation
 intrauterine
  fetal death (before onset of labor) 768.0
   during labor 768.1
  liveborn infant - *see* Distress, fetal, liveborn infant
 local 443.0
 mechanical 994.7
  during birth *(see also* Distress, fetal) 768.9

Asphyxia, asphyxiation *(Continued)*
 mucus 933.1
  bronchus (main) 934.1
  larynx 933.1
  lung 934.8
  nasal passages 932
  newborn 770.18
  pharynx 933.0
  respiratory tract 934.9
   specified part NEC 934.8
  throat 933.0
  trachea 934.0
  vaginal (fetus or newborn) 770.18
 newborn 768.9
  with neurologic involvement 768.5
  blue 768.6
  livida 768.6
  mild or moderate 768.6
  pallida 768.5
  severe 768.5
  white 768.5
 pathological 799.01
 plastic bag 994.7
 postnatal *(see also* Asphyxia, newborn) 768.9
  mechanical 994.7
 pressure 994.7
 reticularis 782.61
 strangulation 994.7
 submersion 994.1
 traumatic NEC - *see* Injury, internal, intrathoracic organs
 vomiting, vomitus - *see* Asphyxia, food or foreign body
Aspiration
 acid pulmonary (syndrome) 997.39
  obstetric 668.0●
 amniotic fluid 770.13
  with respiratory symptoms 770.14
 bronchitis 507.0
 clear amniotic fluid 770.13
  with
   pneumonia 770.14
   pneumonitis 770.14
   respiratory symptoms 770.14
 contents of birth canal 770.17
  with respiratory symptoms 770.18
 fetal 770.10
  blood 770.15
   with
    pneumonia 770.16
    pneumonitis 770.16
  pneumonitis 770.18
 food, foreign body, or gasoline (with asphyxiation) - *see* Asphyxia, food or foreign body
 meconium 770.11
  with
   pneumonia 770.12
   pneumonitis 770.12
   respiratory symptoms 770.12
  below vocal cords 770.11
   with respiratory symptoms 770.12
 mucus 933.1
  into
   bronchus (main) 934.1
   lung 934.8
   respiratory tract 934.9
    specified part NEC 934.8
   trachea 934.0
  newborn 770.17
  vaginal (fetus or newborn) 770.17
 newborn 770.10
  with respiratory symptoms 770.18
  blood 770.15
   with
    pneumonia 770.16
    pneumonitis 770.16
    respiratory symptoms 770.16
 pneumonia 507.0
  fetus or newborn 770.18
   meconium 770.12

Aspiration *(Continued)*
  pneumonitis 507.0
    fetus or newborn 770.18
      meconium 770.12
    obstetric 668.0●
  postnatal stomach contents 770.85
    with
      pneumonia 770.86
      pneumonitis 770.86
      respiratory symptoms 770.86
  syndrome of newborn (massive) 770.18
    meconium 770.12
  vernix caseosa 770.17
Asplenia 759.0
  with mesocardia 746.87
Assam fever 085.0
Assimilation, pelvis
  with disproportion 653.2●
    affecting fetus or newborn 763.1
    causing obstructed labor 660.1●
      affecting fetus or newborn 763.1
Assmann's focus *(see also* Tuberculosis) 011.0●
Astasia (-abasia) 307.9
  hysterical 300.11
Asteatosis 706.8
  cutis 706.8
Astereognosis 780.99
Asterixis 781.3
  in liver disease 572.8
Asteroid hyalitis 379.22
Asthenia, asthenic 780.79
  cardiac *(see also* Failure, heart) 428.9
    psychogenic 306.2
  cardiovascular *(see also* Failure, heart) 428.9
    psychogenic 306.2
  heart *(see also* Failure, heart) 428.9
    psychogenic 306.2
  hysterical 300.11
  myocardial *(see also* Failure, heart) 428.9
    psychogenic 306.2
  nervous 300.5
  neurocirculatory 306.2
  neurotic 300.5
  psychogenic 300.5
  psychoneurotic 300.5
  psychophysiologic 300.5
  reaction, psychoneurotic 300.5
  senile 797
  Stiller's 780.79
  tropical anhidrotic 705.1
Asthenopia 368.13
  accommodative 367.4
  hysterical (muscular) 300.11
  psychogenic 306.7
Asthenospermia 792.2
Asthma, asthmatic (bronchial) (catarrh)
  (spasmodic) 493.9●

> Note: The following fifth digit
> subclassification is for use with codes 493.0-
> 493.2, 493.9:
>
>   0   unspecified
>   1   with status asthmaticus
>   2   with (acute) exacerbation

  with
    chronic obstructive pulmonary disease
      (COPD) 493.2●
    hay fever 493.0●
    rhinitis, allergic 493.0●
  allergic 493.9●
    stated cause (external allergen) 493.0●
  atopic 493.0●
  cardiac *(see also* Failure, ventricular, left)
    428.1
  cardiobronchial *(see also* Failure, ventricular,
    left) 428.1
  cardiorenal *(see also* Hypertension,
    cardiorenal) 404.90
  childhood 493.0●
  Colliers' 500

Asthma, asthmatic *(Continued)*
  cough variant 493.82
  croup 493.9●
  detergent 507.8
  due to
    detergent 507.8
    inhalation of fumes 506.3
    internal immunological process 493.0●
  endogenous (intrinsic) 493.1●
  eosinophilic 518.3
  exercise induced bronchospasm 493.81
  exogenous (cosmetics) (dander or dust)
    (drugs) (dust) (feathers) (food) (hay)
    (platinum) (pollen) 493.0●
  extrinsic 493.0●
  grinders' 502
  hay 493.0●
  heart *(see also* Failure, ventricular, left) 428.1
  IgE 493.0●
  infective 493.1●
  intrinsic 493.1●
  Kopp's 254.8
  late-onset 493.1●
  meat-wrappers' 506.9
  Millar's (laryngismus stridulus) 478.75
  millstone makers' 502
  miners' 500
  Monday morning 504
  New Orleans (epidemic) 493.0●
  platinum 493.0●
  pneumoconiotic (occupational) NEC 505
  potters' 502
  psychogenic 316 *[493.9]*●
  pulmonary eosinophilic 518.3
  red cedar 495.8
  Rostan's *(see also* Failure, ventricular, left)
    428.1
  sandblasters' 502
  sequoiosis 495.8
  stonemasons' 502
  thymic 254.8
  tuberculous *(see also* Tuberculosis,
    pulmonary) 011.9●
  Wichmann's (laryngismus stridulus)
    478.75
  wood 495.8
Astigmatism (compound) (congenital)
  367.20
  irregular 367.22
  regular 367.21
Astroblastoma (M9430/3)
  nose 748.1
  specified site - *see* Neoplasm, by site,
    malignant
  unspecified site 191.9
Astrocytoma (cystic) (M9400/3)
  anaplastic type (M9401/3)
    specified site - *see* Neoplasm, by site,
      malignant
    unspecified site 191.9
  fibrillary (M9420/3)
    specified site - *see* Neoplasm, by site,
      malignant
    unspecified site 191.9
  fibrous (M9420/3)
    specified site - *see* Neoplasm, by site,
      malignant
    unspecified site 191.9
  gemistocytic (M9411/3)
    specified site - *see* Neoplasm, by site,
      malignant
    unspecified site 191.9
  juvenile (M9421/3)
    specified site - *see* Neoplasm, by site,
      malignant
    unspecified site 191.9
  nose 748.1
  pilocytic (M9421/3)
    specified site - *see* Neoplasm, by site,
      malignant
    unspecified site 191.9

Astrocytoma *(Continued)*
  piloid (M9421/3)
    specified site - *see* Neoplasm, by site,
      malignant
    unspecified site 191.9
  protoplasmic (M9410/3)
    specified site - *see* Neoplasm, by site,
      malignant
    unspecified site 191.9
  specified site - *see* Neoplasm, by site,
    malignant
  subependymal (M9383/1) 237.5
    giant cell (M9384/1) 237.5
  unspecified site 191.9
Astroglioma (M9400/3)
  nose 748.1
  specified site - *see* Neoplasm, by site,
    malignant
  unspecified site 191.9
Asymbolia 784.60
Asymmetrical breathing 786.09
Asymmetry - *see also* Distortion
  breast, between native and reconstructed
    612.1
  chest 786.9
  face 754.0
  jaw NEC 524.12
    maxillary 524.11
  pelvis with disproportion 653.0●
    affecting fetus or newborn 763.1
    causing obstructed labor 660.1●
      affecting fetus or newborn 763.1
Asynergia 781.3
Asynergy 781.3
  ventricular 429.89
Asystole (heart) *(see also* Arrest, cardiac) 427.5
At risk for falling V15.88
Ataxia, ataxy, ataxic 781.3
  acute 781.3
  brain 331.89
  cerebellar 334.3
    hereditary (Marie's) 334.2
    in
      alcoholism 303.9● *[334.4]*
      myxedema *(see also* Myxedema) 244.9
        [334.4]
      neoplastic disease NEC 239.9 *[334.4]*
  cerebral 331.89
  family, familial 334.2
    cerebral (Marie's) 334.2
    spinal (Friedreich's) 334.0
  Friedreich's (heredofamilial) (spinal) 334.0
  frontal lobe 781.3
  gait 781.2
    hysterical 300.11
  general 781.3
  hereditary NEC 334.2
    cerebellar 334.2
    spastic 334.1
    spinal 334.0
  heredofamilial (Marie's) 334.2
  hysterical 300.11
  locomotor (progressive) 094.0
    diabetic 250.6● *[337.1]*
      due to secondary diabetes 249.6●
        [337.1]
  Marie's (cerebellar) (heredofamilial)
    334.2
  nonorganic origin 307.9
  partial 094.0
  postchickenpox 052.7
  progressive locomotor 094.0
  psychogenic 307.9
  Sanger-Brown's 334.2
  spastic 094.0
    hereditary 334.1
    syphilitic 094.0
  spinal
    hereditary 334.0
    progressive locomotor 094.0
  telangiectasia 334.8

◄ New   ◄▮ Revised   ~~deleted~~ Deleted   ● Use Additional Digit(s)   ▨ Omit code

Ataxia-telangiectasia 334.8
Atelectasis (absorption collapse) (complete)
  (compression) (massive) (partial)
  (postinfective) (pressure collapse)
  (pulmonary) (relaxation) 518.0
  newborn (congenital) (partial) 770.5
    primary 770.4
  primary 770.4
  tuberculous (see also Tuberculosis,
    pulmonary) 011.9●
Ateleiosis, ateliosis 253.3
Atelia - see Distortion
Ateliosis 253.3
Atelocardia 746.9
Atelomyelia 742.59
Athelia 757.6
Atheroembolism
  extremity
    lower 445.02
    upper 445.01
  kidney 445.81
  specified site NEC 445.89
Atheroma, atheromatous (see also
    Arteriosclerosis) 440.9
  aorta, aortic 440.0
    valve (see also Endocarditis, aortic) 424.1
  artery - see Arteriosclerosis
  basilar (artery) (see also Occlusion, artery,
    basilar) 433.0●
  carotid (artery) (common) (internal) (see also
    Occlusion, artery, carotid) 433.1●
  cerebral (arteries) 437.0
  coronary (artery) - see Arteriosclerosis,
    coronary
  degeneration - see Arteriosclerosis
  heart, cardiac - see Arteriosclerosis, coronary
  mitral (valve) 424.0
  myocardium, myocardial - see
    Arteriosclerosis, coronary
  pulmonary valve (heart) (see also
    Endocarditis, pulmonary) 424.3
  skin 706.2
  tricuspid (heart) (valve) 424.2
  valve, valvular - see Endocarditis
  vertebral (artery) (see also Occlusion, artery,
    vertebral) 433.2●
Atheromatosis - see also Arteriosclerosis
  arterial, congenital 272.8
Atherosclerosis - see Arteriosclerosis
Athetosis (acquired) 781.0
  bilateral 333.79
  congenital (bilateral) 333.6
  double 333.71
  unilateral 781.0
Athlete's
  foot 110.4
  heart 429.3
Athletic team examination V70.3
Athrepsia 261
Athyrea (acquired) (see also Hypothyroidism)
    244.9
  congenital 243
Athyreosis (congenital) 243
  acquired - see Hypothyroidism
Athyroidism (acquired) (see also
    Hypothyroidism) 244.9
  congenital 243
Atmospheric pyrexia 992.0
Atonia, atony, atonic
  abdominal wall 728.2
  bladder (sphincter) 596.4
    neurogenic NEC 596.54
      with cauda equina syndrome 344.61
  capillary 448.9
  cecum 564.89
    psychogenic 306.4
  colon 564.89
    psychogenic 306.4
  congenital 779.89
  dyspepsia 536.3
    psychogenic 306.4

Atonia, atony, atonic (Continued)
  intestine 564.89
    psychogenic 306.4
  stomach 536.3
    neurotic or psychogenic 306.4
    psychogenic 306.4
  uterus 661.2●
    with hemorrhage (postpartum) 666.1●
      affecting fetus or newborn 763.7
    without hemorrhage
      intrapartum 661.2●
      postpartum 669.8●
  vesical 596.4
Atopy NEC V15.09
Atransferrinemia, congenital 273.8
Atresia, atretic (congenital) 759.89
  alimentary organ or tract NEC 751.8
    lower 751.2
    upper 750.8
  ani, anus, anal (canal) 751.2
  aorta 747.22
    with hypoplasia of ascending aorta and
      defective development of left
      ventricle (with mitral valve atresia)
      746.7
    arch 747.11
    ring 747.21
  aortic (orifice) (valve) 746.89
    arch 747.11
  aqueduct of Sylvius 742.3
    with spina bifida (see also Spina bifida)
      741.0●
  artery NEC (see also Atresia, blood vessel)
      747.60
    cerebral 747.81
    coronary 746.85
    eye 743.58
    pulmonary 747.31
    umbilical 747.5
  auditory canal (external) 744.02
  bile, biliary duct (common) or passage
      751.61
    acquired (see also Obstruction, biliary)
      576.2
  bladder (neck) 753.6
  blood vessel (peripheral) NEC 747.60
    cerebral 747.81
    gastrointestinal 747.61
    lower limb 747.64
    pulmonary artery 747.31
    renal 747.62
    spinal 747.82
    upper limb 747.63
  bronchus 748.3
  canal, ear 744.02
  cardiac
    valve 746.89
      aortic 746.89
      mitral 746.89
      pulmonary 746.01
      tricuspid 746.1
  cecum 751.2
  cervix (acquired) 622.4
    congenital 752.43
    in pregnancy or childbirth 654.6●
      affecting fetus or newborn 763.89
      causing obstructed labor 660.2●
        affecting fetus or newborn 763.1
  choana 748.0
  colon 751.2
  cystic duct 751.61
    acquired 575.8
      with obstruction (see also Obstruction,
        gallbladder) 575.2
  digestive organs NEC 751.8
  duodenum 751.1
  ear canal 744.02
  ejaculatory duct 752.89
  epiglottis 748.3
  esophagus 750.3
  Eustachian tube 744.24

Atresia, atretic (Continued)
  fallopian tube (acquired) 628.2
    congenital 752.19
  follicular cyst 620.0
  foramen of
    Luschka 742.3
      with spina bifida (see also Spina bifida)
        741.0●
    Magendie 742.3
      with spina bifida (see also Spina bifida)
        741.0●
  gallbladder 751.69
  genital organ
    external
      female 752.49
      male NEC 752.89
        penis 752.69
    internal
      female 752.89
      male 752.89
  glottis 748.3
  gullet 750.3
  heart
    valve NEC 746.89
      aortic 746.89
      mitral 746.89
      pulmonary 746.01
      tricuspid 746.1
  hymen 752.42
    acquired 623.3
    postinfective 623.3
  ileum 751.1
  intestine (small) 751.1
    large 751.2
  iris, filtration angle (see also Buphthalmia)
      743.20
  jejunum 751.1
  kidney 753.3
  lacrimal, apparatus 743.65
    acquired - see Stenosis, lacrimal
  larynx 748.3
  ligament, broad 752.19
  lung 748.5
  meatus urinarius 753.6
  mitral valve 746.89
    with atresia or hypoplasia of aortic orifice
      or valve, with hypoplasia of
      ascending aorta and defective
      development of left ventricle
      746.7
  nares (anterior) (posterior) 748.0
  nasolacrimal duct 743.65
  nasopharynx 748.8
  nose, nostril 748.0
    acquired 738.0
  organ or site NEC - see Anomaly, specified
      type NEC
  osseous meatus (ear) 744.03
  oviduct (acquired) 628.2
    congenital 752.19
  parotid duct 750.23
    acquired 527.8
  pulmonary (artery) 747.31
    valve 746.01
    vein 747.49
  pulmonic 746.01
  pupil 743.46
  rectum 751.2
  salivary duct or gland 750.23
    acquired 527.8
  sublingual duct 750.23
    acquired 527.8
  submaxillary duct or gland 750.23
    acquired 527.8
  trachea 748.3
  tricuspid valve 746.1
  ureter 753.29
  ureteropelvic junction 753.21
  ureterovesical orifice 753.22
  urethra (valvular) 753.6
  urinary tract NEC 753.29

◄ New   ◄▥ Revised   ~~deleted~~ Deleted   ● Use Additional Digit(s)   ▨ Omit code

Atresia, atretic (Continued)
uterus 752.31
acquired 621.8
vagina (acquired) 623.2
congenital (total) (partial) 752.45
postgonococcal (old) 098.2
postinfectional 623.2
senile 623.2
vascular NEC (see also Atresia, blood vessel)
747.60
cerebral 747.81
vas deferens 752.89
vein NEC (see also Atresia, blood vessel)
747.60
cardiac 746.89
great 747.49
portal 747.49
pulmonary 747.49
vena cava (inferior) (superior) 747.49
vesicourethral orifice 753.6
vulva 752.49
acquired 624.8
Atrichia, atrichosis 704.00
congenital (universal) 757.4
Atrioventricularis commune 745.69
Atrophia - see also Atrophy
alba 709.09
cutis 701.8
idiopathica progressiva 701.8
senilis 701.8
dermatological, diffuse (idiopathic) 701.8
flava hepatis (acuta) (subacuta) (see also
Necrosis, liver) 570
gyrata of choroid and retina (central)
363.54
generalized 363.57
senilis 797
dermatological 701.8
unguium 703.8
congenita 757.5
Atrophoderma, atrophodermia 701.9
diffusum (idiopathic) 701.8
maculatum 701.3
et striatum 701.3
due to syphilis 095.8
syphilitic 091.3
neuriticum 701.8
pigmentosum 757.33
reticulatum symmetricum faciei 701.8
senile 701.8
symmetrical 701.8
vermiculata 701.8
Atrophy, atrophic
adrenal (autoimmune) (capsule) (cortex)
(gland) 255.41
with hypofunction 255.41
alveolar process or ridge (edentulous)
525.20
mandible 525.20
minimal 525.21
moderate 525.22
severe 525.23
maxilla 525.20
minimal 525.24
moderate 525.25
severe 525.26
appendix 543.9
Aran-Duchenne muscular 335.21
arm 728.2
arteriosclerotic - see Arteriosclerosis
arthritis 714.0
spine 720.9
bile duct (any) 576.8
bladder 596.89
blanche (of Milian) 701.3
bone (senile) 733.99
due to
disuse 733.7
infection 733.99
tabes dorsalis (neurogenic) 094.0
posttraumatic 733.99

Atrophy, atrophic (Continued)
brain (cortex) (progressive) 331.9
with dementia 290.10
Alzheimer's 331.0
with dementia - see Alzheimer's,
dementia
circumscribed (Pick's) 331.11
with dementia
with behavioral disturbance 331.11
[294.11]
without behavioral disturbance
331.11 [294.10]
congenital 742.4
hereditary 331.9
senile 331.2
breast 611.4
puerperal, postpartum 676.3●
buccal cavity 528.9
cardiac (brown) (senile) (see also
Degeneration, myocardial) 429.1
cartilage (infectional) (joint) 733.99
cast, plaster of Paris 728.2
cerebellar - see Atrophy, brain
cerebral - see Atrophy, brain
cervix (endometrium) (mucosa)
(myometrium) (senile) (uteri) 622.8
menopausal 627.8
Charcôt-Marie-Tooth 356.1
choroid 363.40
diffuse secondary 363.42
hereditary (see also Dystrophy, choroid)
363.50
gyrate
central 363.54
diffuse 363.57
generalized 363.57
senile 363.41
ciliary body 364.57
colloid, degenerative 701.3
conjunctiva (senile) 372.89
corpus cavernosum 607.89
cortical (see also Atrophy, brain) 331.9
Cruveilhier's 335.21
cystic duct 576.8
dacryosialadenopathy 710.2
degenerative
colloid 701.3
senile 701.3
Déjérine-Thomas 333.0
diffuse idiopathic, dermatological 701.8
disuse
bone 733.7
muscle 728.2
pelvic muscles and anal sphincter 618.83
Duchenne-Aran 335.21
ear 388.9
edentulous alveolar ridge 525.20
mandible 525.20
minimal 525.21
moderate 525.22
severe 525.23
maxilla 525.20
minimal 525.24
moderate 525.25
severe 525.26
emphysema, lung 492.8
endometrium (senile) 621.8
cervix 622.8
enteric 569.89
epididymis 608.3
eyeball, cause unknown 360.41
eyelid (senile) 374.50
facial (skin) 701.9
facioscapulohumeral (Landouzy-Déjérine)
359.1
fallopian tube (senile), acquired 620.3
fatty, thymus (gland) 254.8
gallbladder 575.8
gastric 537.89
gastritis (chronic) 535.1●
gastrointestinal 569.89

Atrophy, atrophic (Continued)
genital organ, male 608.89
glandular 289.3
globe (phthisis bulbi) 360.41
gum (see also Recession, gingival) 523.20
hair 704.2
heart (brown) (senile) (see also Degeneration,
myocardial) 429.1
hemifacial 754.0
Romberg 349.89
hydronephrosis 591
infantile 261
paralysis, acute (see also Poliomyelitis,
with paralysis) 045.1●
intestine 569.89
iris (generalized) (postinfectional) (sector
shaped) 364.59
essential 364.51
progressive 364.51
sphincter 364.54
kidney (senile) (see also Sclerosis, renal)
587
with hypertension (see also Hypertension,
kidney) 403.90
congenital 753.0
hydronephrotic 591
infantile 753.0
lacrimal apparatus (primary) 375.13
secondary 375.14
Landouzy-Déjérine 359.1
laryngitis, infection 476.0
larynx 478.79
Leber's optic 377.16
lip 528.5
liver (acute) (subacute) (see also Necrosis,
liver) 570
chronic (yellow) 571.8
yellow (congenital) 570
with
abortion - see Abortion, by type,
with specified complication
NEC
ectopic pregnancy (see also
categories 633.0-633.9) 639.8
molar pregnancy (see also categories
630-632) 639.8
chronic 571.8
complicating pregnancy 646.7●
following
abortion 639.8
ectopic or molar pregnancy 639.8
from injection, inoculation or
transfusion (onset within 8
months after administration) -
see Hepatitis, viral
healed 571.5
obstetric 646.7●
postabortal 639.8
postimmunization - see Hepatitis,
viral
posttransfusion - see Hepatitis, viral
puerperal, postpartum 674.8●
lung (senile) 518.89
congenital 748.69
macular (dermatological) 701.3
syphilitic, skin 091.3
striated 095.8
muscle, muscular 728.2
disuse 728.2
Duchenne-Aran 335.21
extremity (lower) (upper) 728.2
familial spinal 335.11
general 728.2
idiopathic 728.2
infantile spinal 335.0
myelopathic (progressive) 335.10
myotonic 359.21
neuritic 356.1
neuropathic (peroneal) (progressive) 356.1
peroneal 356.1
primary (idiopathic) 728.2

◀ New   ◀▥ Revised   ~~deleted~~ Deleted   ● Use Additional Digit(s)   ▨ Omit code

Atrophy, atrophic *(Continued)*
  muscle, muscular *(Continued)*
    progressive (familial) (hereditary) (pure)
        335.21
      adult (spinal) 335.19
      infantile (spinal) 335.0
      juvenile (spinal) 335.11
      spinal 335.10
        adult 335.19
        hereditary or familial 335.11
        infantile 335.0
    pseudohypertrophic 359.1
    spinal (progressive) 335.10
      adult 335.19
      Aran-Duchenne 335.21
      familial 335.11
      hereditary 335.11
      infantile 335.0
      juvenile 335.11
    syphilitic 095.6
  myocardium *(see also* Degeneration,
      myocardial) 429.1
  myometrium (senile) 621.8
    cervix 622.8
  myotatic 728.2
  myotonia 359.21
  nail 703.8
    congenital 757.5
  nasopharynx 472.2
  nerve - *see also* Disorder, nerve
    abducens 378.54
    accessory 352.4
    acoustic or auditory 388.5
    cranial 352.9
      first (olfactory) 352.0
      second (optic) *(see also* Atrophy, optic
          nerve) 377.10
      third (oculomotor) (partial) 378.51
        total 378.52
      fourth (trochlear) 378.53
      fifth (trigeminal) 350.8
      sixth (abducens) 378.54
      seventh (facial) 351.8
      eighth (auditory) 388.5
      ninth (glossopharyngeal) 352.2
      tenth (pneumogastric) (vagus)
          352.3
      eleventh (accessory) 352.4
      twelfth (hypoglossal) 352.5
    facial 351.8
    glossopharyngeal 352.2
    hypoglossal 352.5
    oculomotor (partial) 378.51
      total 378.52
    olfactory 352.0
    peripheral 355.9
    pneumogastric 352.3
    trigeminal 350.8
    trochlear 378.53
    vagus (pneumogastric) 352.3
  nervous system, congenital 742.8
  neuritic *(see also* Disorder, nerve) 355.9
  neurogenic NEC 355.9
    bone
      tabetic 094.0
  nutritional 261
  old age 797
  olivopontocerebellar 333.0
  optic nerve (ascending) (descending)
      (infectional) (nonfamilial)
      (papillomacular bundle) (postretinal)
      (secondary NEC) (simple) 377.10
    associated with retinal dystrophy
        377.13
    dominant hereditary 377.16
    glaucomatous 377.14
    hereditary (dominant) (Leber's) 377.16
    Leber's (hereditary) 377.16
    partial 377.15
    postinflammatory 377.12
    primary 377.11

Atrophy, atrophic *(Continued)*
  optic nerve *(Continued)*
    syphilitic 094.84
      congenital 090.49
      tabes dorsalis 094.0
  orbit 376.45
  ovary (senile), acquired 620.3
  oviduct (senile), acquired 620.3
  palsy, diffuse 335.20
  pancreas (duct) (senile) 577.8
  papillary muscle 429.81
  paralysis 355.9
  parotid gland 527.0
  patches skin 701.3
    senile 701.8
  penis 607.89
  pharyngitis 472.1
  pharynx 478.29
  pluriglandular 258.8
  polyarthritis 714.0
  prostate 602.2
  pseudohypertrophic 359.1
  renal *(see also* Sclerosis, renal) 587
  reticulata 701.8
  retina *(see also* Degeneration, retina) 362.60
    hereditary *(see also* Dystrophy, retina)
        362.70
  rhinitis 472.0
  salivary duct or gland 527.0
  scar NEC 709.2
  sclerosis, lobar (of brain) 331.0
    with dementia
      with behavioral disturbance 331.0
          [294.11]
      without behavioral disturbance 331.0
          [294.10]
  scrotum 608.89
  seminal vesicle 608.89
  senile 797
    degenerative, of skin 701.3
  skin (patches) (senile) 701.8
  spermatic cord 608.89
  spinal (cord) 336.8
    acute 336.8
    muscular (chronic) 335.10
      adult 335.19
      familial 335.11
      juvenile 335.10
    paralysis 335.10
      acute *(see also* Poliomyelitis, with
          paralysis) 045.1●
  spine (column) 733.99
  spleen (senile) 289.59
  spots (skin) 701.3
    senile 701.8
  stomach 537.89
  striate and macular 701.3
    syphilitic 095.8
  subcutaneous 701.9
    due to injection 999.9
  sublingual gland 527.0
  submaxillary gland 527.0
  Sudeck's 733.7
  suprarenal (autoimmune) (capsule) (gland)
      255.41
    with hypofunction 255.41
  tarso-orbital fascia, congenital 743.66
  testis 608.3
  thenar, partial 354.0
  throat 478.29
  thymus (fat) 254.8
  thyroid (gland) 246.8
    with
      cretinism 243
      myxedema 244.9
    congenital 243
  tongue (senile) 529.8
    papillae 529.4
    smooth 529.4
  trachea 519.19
  tunica vaginalis 608.89

Atrophy, atrophic *(Continued)*
  turbinate 733.99
  tympanic membrane (nonflaccid) 384.82
    flaccid 384.81
  ulcer *(see also* Ulcer, skin) 707.9
  upper respiratory tract 478.9
  uterus, uterine (acquired) (senile) 621.8
    cervix 622.8
    due to radiation (intended effect) 621.8
  vagina (senile) 627.3
  vascular 459.89
  vas deferens 608.89
  vertebra (senile) 733.99
  vulva (primary) (senile) 624.1
  Werdnig-Hoffmann 335.0
  yellow (acute) (congenital) (liver) (subacute)
      (see also Necrosis, liver) 570
    chronic 571.8
    resulting from administration of blood,
        plasma, serum, or other biological
        substance (within 8 months of
        administration) - *see* Hepatitis, viral

Attack
  akinetic *(see also* Epilepsy) 345.0●
  angina - *see* Angina
  apoplectic *(see also* Disease, cerebrovascular,
      acute) 436
  benign shuddering 333.93
  bilious - *see* Vomiting
  cataleptic 300.11
  cerebral *(see also* Disease, cerebrovascular,
      acute) 436
  coronary *(see also* Infarct, myocardium)
      410.9●
  cyanotic, newborn 770.83
  epileptic *(see also* Epilepsy) 345.9●
  epileptiform 780.39
  heart *(see also* Infarct, myocardium) 410.9●
  hemiplegia *(see also* Disease, cerebrovascular,
      acute) 436
  hysterical 300.11
  jacksonian *(see also* Epilepsy) 345.5●
  myocardium, myocardial *(see also* Infarct,
      myocardium) 410.9●
  myoclonic *(see also* Epilepsy) 345.1●
  panic 300.01
  paralysis *(see also* Disease, cerebrovascular,
      acute) 436
  paroxysmal 780.39
  psychomotor *(see also* Epilepsy) 345.4●
  salaam *(see also* Epilepsy) 345.6●
  schizophreniform *(see also* Schizophrenia)
      295.4●
  sensory and motor 780.39
  syncope 780.2
  toxic, cerebral 780.39
  transient ischemic (TIA) 435.9
  unconsciousness 780.2
    hysterical 300.11
  vasomotor 780.2
  vasovagal (idiopathic) (paroxysmal) 780.2

Attention to
  artificial
    opening (of) V55.9
      digestive tract NEC V55.4
      specified site NEC V55.8
      urinary tract NEC V55.6
    vagina V55.7
  colostomy V55.3
  cystostomy V55.5
  dressing
    wound V58.30
      nonsurgical V58.30
      surgical V58.31
  gastrostomy V55.1
  ileostomy V55.2
  jejunostomy V55.4
  nephrostomy V55.6
  surgical dressings V58.31
  sutures V58.32
  tracheostomy V55.0

Attention to (Continued)
   ureterostomy V55.6
   urethrostomy V55.6
Attrition
   gum (see also Recession, gingival) 523.20
   teeth (hard tissues) 521.10
      excessive 521.10
         extending into
            dentine 521.12
            pulp 521.13
         generalized 521.15
         limited to enamel 521.11
         localized 521.14
Atypical - see also condition
   cells
      endocervical 795.00
      endometrial 795.00
      glandular
         anus 796.70
         cervical 795.00
         vaginal 795.10
   distribution, vessel (congenital) (peripheral)
      NEC 747.60
   endometrium 621.9
   kidney 593.89
Atypism, cervix 622.10
Audible tinnitus (see also Tinnitus) 388.30
Auditory - see condition
Audry's syndrome (acropachyderma) 757.39
Aujeszky's disease 078.89
Aura
   jacksonian (see also Epilepsy) 345.5●
   persistent migraine 346.5●
      with cerebral infarction 346.6●
      without cerebral infarction 346.5●
Aurantiasis, cutis 278.3
Auricle, auricular - see condition
Auriculotemporal syndrome 350.8
Australian
   Q fever 083.0
   X disease 062.4
Autism, autistic (child) (infantile) 299.0●
Autodigestion 799.89
Autoerythrocyte sensitization 287.2
Autographism 708.3
Autoimmune
   cold sensitivity 283.0
   disease NEC 279.49
   hemolytic anemia 283.0
   inhibitors to clotting factors 286.52
   lymphoproliferative syndrome (ALPS)
      279.41
   thyroiditis 245.2
Autoinfection, septic - see Septicemia
Autointoxication 799.89
Automatism 348.89
   with temporal sclerosis 348.81
   epileptic (see also Epilepsy) 345.4●

Automatism (Continued)
   paroxysmal, idiopathic (see also Epilepsy)
      345.4●
Autonomic, autonomous
   bladder 596.54
      neurogenic 596.54
         with cauda equina 344.61
   dysreflexia 337.3
   faciocephalalgia (see also Neuropathy,
      peripheral, autonomic) 337.9
   hysterical seizure 300.11
   imbalance (see also Neuropathy, peripheral,
      autonomic) 337.9
Autophony 388.40
Autosensitivity, erythrocyte 287.2
Autotopagnosia 780.99
Autotoxemia 799.89
Autumn - see condition
Avellis' syndrome 344.89
Aversion
   oral 783.3
      newborn 779.31
      nonorganic origin 307.59
Aviators
   disease or sickness (see also Effect, adverse,
      high altitude) 993.2
   ear 993.0
   effort syndrome 306.2
Avitaminosis (multiple NEC) (see also
      Deficiency, vitamin) 269.2
   A 264.9
   B 266.9
      with
         beriberi 265.0
         pellagra 265.2
   B_1 265.1
   B_2 266.0
   B_6 266.1
   B_{12} 266.2
   C (with scurvy) 267
   D 268.9
      with
         osteomalacia 268.2
         rickets 268.0
   E 269.1
   G 266.0
   H 269.1
   K 269.0
   multiple 269.2
   nicotinic acid 265.2
   P 269.1
Avulsion (traumatic) 879.8
   blood vessel - see Injury, blood vessel, by site
   cartilage - see also Dislocation, by site
      knee, current (see also Tear, meniscus)
         836.2
      symphyseal (inner), complicating
         delivery 665.6●

Avulsion (Continued)
   complicated 879.9
   diaphragm - see Injury, internal, diaphragm
   ear - see Wound, open, ear
   epiphysis of bone - see Fracture, by site
   external site other than limb - see Wound,
      open, by site
   eye 871.3
   fingernail - see Wound, open, finger
   fracture - see Fracture, by site
   genital organs, external - see Wound, open,
      genital organs
   head (intracranial) NEC - see also Injury,
      intracranial, with open intracranial
      wound
      complete 874.9
      external site NEC 873.8
         complicated 873.9
   internal organ or site - see Injury, internal, by
      site
   joint - see also Dislocation, by site
      capsule - see Sprain, by site
   ligament - see Sprain, by site
   limb - see also Amputation, traumatic,
      by site
      skin and subcutaneous tissue - see Wound,
         open, by site
   muscle - see Sprain, by site
   nerve (root) - see Injury, nerve, by site
   scalp - see Wound, open, scalp
   skin and subcutaneous tissue - see Wound,
      open, by site
   symphyseal cartilage (inner), complicating
      delivery 665.6●
   tendon - see also Sprain, by site
      with open wound - see Wound, open, by
         site
   toenail - see Wound, open, toe(s)
   tooth 873.63
      complicated 873.73
Awaiting organ transplant status V49.83
Awareness of heart beat 785.1
Axe grinders' disease 502
Axenfeld's anomaly or syndrome 743.44
Axilla, axillary - see also condition
   breast 757.6
Axonotmesis - see Injury, nerve, by site
Ayala's disease 756.89
Ayerza's disease or syndrome (pulmonary
      artery sclerosis with pulmonary
      hypertension) 416.0
Azoospermia 606.0
Azorean disease (of the nervous system)
      334.8
Azotemia 790.6
   meaning uremia (see also Uremia) 586
Aztec ear 744.29
Azygos lobe, lung (fissure) 748.69

◀ New   ◀▥ Revised   ~~deleted~~ Deleted   ● Use Additional Digit(s)   ▨ Omit code

B

Baader's syndrome (erythema multiforme exudativum) 695.19
Baastrup's syndrome 721.5
Babesiasis 088.82
Babesiosis 088.82
Babington's disease (familial hemorrhagic telangiectasia) 448.0
Babinski's syndrome (cardiovascular syphilis) 093.89
Babinski-Fröhlich syndrome (adiposogenital dystrophy) 253.8
Babinski-Nageotte syndrome 344.89
Bacillary - see condition
Bacilluria 791.9
    asymptomatic, in pregnancy or puerperium 646.5●
    tuberculous (see also Tuberculosis) 016.9●
Bacillus - see also Infection, bacillus
    abortus infection 023.1
    anthracis infection 022.9
    coli
        infection 041.49
            generalized 038.42
            intestinal 008.00
            pyemia 038.42
            septicemia 038.42
    Flexner's 004.1
    fusiformis infestation 101
    mallei infection 024
    Shiga's 004.0
    suipestifer infection (see also Infection, Salmonella) 003.9
Back - see condition
Backache (postural) 724.5
    psychogenic 307.89
    sacroiliac 724.6
Backflow (pyelovenous) (see also Disease, renal) 593.9
Backknee (see also Genu, recurvatum) 736.5
Bacteremia 790.7
    newborn 771.83
Bacteria
    in blood (see also Bacteremia) 790.7
    in urine (see also Bacteriuria) 791.9
Bacterial - see condition
Bactericholia (see also Cholecystitis, acute) 575.0
Bacterid, bacteride (Andrews' pustular) 686.8
Bacteriuria, bacteruria 791.9
    with
        urinary tract infection 599.0
    asymptomatic 791.9
        in pregnancy or puerperium 646.5●
            affecting fetus or newborn 760.1
Bad
    breath 784.99
    heart - see Disease, heart
    trip (see also Abuse, drugs, nondependent) 305.3●
Baehr-Schiffrin disease (thrombotic thrombocytopenic purpura) 446.6
Baelz's disease (cheilitis glandularis apostematosa) 528.5
Baerensprung's disease (eczema marginatum) 110.3
Bagassosis (occupational) 495.1
Baghdad boil 085.1
Bagratuni's syndrome (temporal arteritis) 446.5
Baker's
    cyst (knee) 727.51
        tuberculous (see also Tuberculosis) 015.2●
    itch 692.89
Bakwin-Krida syndrome (craniometa-physeal dysplasia) 756.89
Balanitis (circinata) (gangraenosa) (infectious) (vulgaris) 607.1
    amebic 006.8
    candidal 112.2
    chlamydial 099.53
    due to Ducrey's bacillus 099.0

Balanitis (Continued)
    erosiva circinata et gangraenosa 607.1
    gangrenous 607.1
    gonococcal (acute) 098.0
        chronic or duration of 2 months or over 098.2
    nongonococcal 607.1
    phagedenic 607.1
    venereal NEC 099.8
    xerotica obliterans 607.81
Balanoposthitis 607.1
    chlamydial 099.53
    gonococcal (acute) 098.0
        chronic or duration of 2 months or over 098.2
    ulcerative NEC 099.8
Balanorrhagia - see Balanitis
Balantidiasis 007.0
Balantidiosis 007.0
Balbuties, balbutio (see also Disorder, fluency) 315.35
Bald
    patches on scalp 704.00
    tongue 529.4
Baldness (see also Alopecia) 704.00
Balfour's disease (chloroma) 205.3●
Balint's syndrome (psychic paralysis of visual fixation) 368.16
Balkan grippe 083.0
Ball
    food 938
    hair 938
Ballantyne (-Runge) syndrome (postmaturity) 766.22
Balloon disease (see also Effect, adverse, high altitude) 993.2
Ballooning posterior leaflet syndrome 424.0
Baló's disease or concentric sclerosis 341.1
Bamberger's disease (hypertrophic pulmonary osteoarthropathy) 731.2
Bamberger-Marie disease (hypertrophic pulmonary osteoarthropathy) 731.2
Bamboo spine 720.0
Bancroft's filariasis 125.0
Band(s)
    adhesive (see also Adhesions, peritoneum) 568.0
    amniotic 658.8●
        affecting fetus or newborn 762.8
    anomalous or congenital - see also Anomaly, specified type NEC
        atrial 746.9
        heart 746.9
        intestine 751.4
        omentum 751.4
        ventricular 746.9
    cervix 622.3
    gallbladder (congenital) 751.69
    intestinal (adhesive) (see also Adhesions, peritoneum) 568.0
        congenital 751.4
    obstructive (see also Obstruction, intestine) 560.81
    periappendiceal (congenital) 751.4
    peritoneal (adhesive) (see also Adhesions, peritoneum) 568.0
        with intestinal obstruction 560.81
        congenital 751.4
    uterus 621.5
    vagina 623.2
Bandemia (without diagnosis of specific infection) 288.66
Bandl's ring (contraction)
    complicating delivery 661.4●
        affecting fetus or newborn 763.7
Bang's disease (Brucella abortus) 023.1
Bangkok hemorrhagic fever 065.4
Bannister's disease 995.1
Bantam-Albright-Martin disease (pseudohypoparathyroidism) 275.49

Banti's disease or syndrome (with cirrhosis) (with portal hypertension) - see Cirrhosis, liver
Bar
    calcaneocuboid 755.67
    calcaneonavicular 755.67
    cubonavicular 755.67
    prostate 600.90
        with
            other lower urinary tract symptoms (LUTS) 600.91
            urinary
                obstruction 600.91
                retention 600.91
    talocalcaneal 755.67
Baragnosis 780.99
Barasheh, barashek 266.2
Barcoo disease or rot (see also Ulcer, skin) 707.9
Bard-Pic syndrome (carcinoma, head of pancreas) 157.0
Bärensprung's disease (eczema marginatum) 110.3
Baritosis 503
Barium lung disease 503
Barlow's syndrome (meaning mitral valve prolapse) 424.0
Barlow (-Möller) disease or syndrome (meaning infantile scurvy) 267
Barodontalgia 993.2
Baron Münchausen syndrome 301.51
Barosinusitis 993.1
Barotitis 993.0
Barotrauma 993.2
    odontalgia 993.2
    otitic 993.0
    sinus 993.1
Barraquer's disease or syndrome (progressive lipodystrophy) 272.6
Barré-Guillain syndrome 357.0
Barré-Liéou syndrome (posterior cervical sympathetic) 723.2
Barrel chest 738.3
Barrett's esophagus 530.85
Barrett's syndrome or ulcer (chronic peptic ulcer of esophagus) 530.85
Bársony-Polgár syndrome (corkscrew esophagus) 530.5
Bársony-Teschendorf syndrome (corkscrew esophagus) 530.5
Barth syndrome 759.89
Bartholin's
    adenitis (see also Bartholinitis) 616.89
    gland - see condition
Bartholinitis (suppurating) 616.89
    gonococcal (acute) 098.0
        chronic or duration of 2 months or over 098.2
Bartonellosis 088.0
Bartter's syndrome (secondary hyperaldosteronism with juxtaglomerular hyperplasia) 255.13
Basal - see condition
Basan's (hidrotic) ectodermal dysplasia 757.31
Baseball finger 842.13
Basedow's disease or syndrome (exophthalmic goiter) 242.0●
Basic - see condition
Basilar - see condition
Bason's (hidrotic) ectodermal dysplasia 757.31
Basopenia 288.59
Basophilia 288.65
Basophilism (corticoadrenal) (Cushing's) (pituitary) (thymic) 255.0
Bassen-Kornzweig syndrome (abetalipoproteinemia) 272.5
Bat ear 744.29
Bateman's
    disease 078.0
    purpura (senile) 287.2
Bathing cramp 994.1
Bathophobia 300.23

Batten's disease, retina 330.1 *[362.71]*
Batten-Mayou disease 330.1 *[362.71]*
Batten-Steinert syndrome 359.21
Battered
    adult (syndrome) 995.81
    baby or child (syndrome) 995.54
    spouse (syndrome) 995.81
Battey mycobacterium infection 031.0
Battledore placenta - *see* Placenta, abnormal
Battle exhaustion (*see also* Reaction, stress,
    acute) 308.9
Baumgarten-Cruveilhier (cirrhosis) disease, or
    syndrome 571.5
Bauxite
    fibrosis (of lung) 503
    workers' disease 503
Bayle's disease (dementia paralytica) 094.1
Bazin's disease (primary) (*see also* Tuberculosis)
    017.1●
Beach ear 380.12
Beaded hair (congenital) 757.4
Beals syndrome 759.82
Beard's disease (neurasthenia) 300.5
Bearn-Kunkel (-Slater) syndrome (lupoid
    hepatitis) 571.49
Beat
    elbow 727.2
    hand 727.2
    knee 727.2
Beats
    ectopic 427.60
    escaped, heart 427.60
        postoperative 997.1
    premature (nodal) 427.60
        atrial 427.61
        auricular 427.61
        postoperative 997.1
        specified type NEC 427.69
        supraventricular 427.61
        ventricular 427.69
Beau's
    disease or syndrome (*see also* Degeneration,
        myocardial) 429.1
    lines (transverse furrows on fingernails) 703.8
Bechterew's disease (ankylosing spondylitis)
    720.0
Bechterew-Strümpell-Marie syndrome
    (ankylosing spondylitis) 720.0
Beck's syndrome (anterior spinal artery
    occlusion) 433.8●
Becker's
    disease
        idiopathic mural endomyocardial disease
            425.2
        myotonia congenita, recessive form 359.22
    dystrophy 359.22
Beckwith (-Wiedemann) syndrome 759.89
Bedbugs bite(s) - *see* Injury, superficial, by site
Bedclothes, asphyxiation or suffocation by 994.7
Bed confinement status V49.84
Bednar's aphthae 528.2
Bedsore (*see also* Ulcer, pressure) 707.00
    with gangrene 707.00 *[785.4]*
Bedwetting (*see also* Enuresis) 788.36
Beer-drinkers' heart (disease) 425.5
Bee sting (with allergic or anaphylactic shock)
    989.5
Begbie's disease (exophthalmic goiter) 242.0●
Behavior disorder, disturbance - *see also*
    Disturbance, conduct
    antisocial, without manifest psychiatric
        disorder
        adolescent V71.02
        adult V71.01
        child V71.02
    dyssocial, without manifest psychiatric
        disorder
        adolescent V71.02
        adult V71.01
        child V71.02
    high-risk- *see* problem

Behçet's syndrome 136.1
Behr's disease 362.50
Beigel's disease or morbus (white piedra) 111.2
Bejel 104.0
Bekhterev's disease (ankylosing spondylitis)
    720.0
Bekhterev-Strümpell-Marie syndrome
    (ankylosing spondylitis) 720.0
Belching (*see also* Eructation) 787.3
Bell's
    disease (*see also* Psychosis, affective) 296.0●
    mania (*see also* Psychosis, affective) 296.0●
    palsy, paralysis 351.0
        infant 767.5
        newborn 767.5
        syphilitic 094.89
    spasm 351.0
Bence-Jones albuminuria, albuminosuria, or
    proteinuria 791.0
Bends 993.3
Benedikt's syndrome (paralysis) 344.89
Benign - *see also* condition
    cellular changes, cervix 795.09
    prostate
        hyperplasia 600.20
            with
                other lower urinary tract symptoms
                    (LUTS) 600.21
                urinary
                    obstruction 600.21
                    retention 600.21
        neoplasm 222.2
Bennett's
    disease (leukemia) 208.9●
    fracture (closed) 815.01
        open 815.11
Benson's disease 379.22
Bent
    back (hysterical) 300.11
    nose 738.0
        congenital 754.0
Bereavement V62.82
    as adjustment reaction 309.0
Berger's paresthesia (lower limb) 782.0
Bergeron's disease (hysteroepilepsy) 300.11
Beriberi (acute) (atrophic) (chronic) (dry)
    (subacute) (wet) 265.0
    with polyneuropathy 265.0 *[357.4]*
    heart (disease) 265.0 *[425.7]*
    leprosy 030.1
    neuritis 265.0 *[357.4]*
Berlin's disease or edema (traumatic) 921.3
Berloque dermatitis 692.72
Bernard-Horner syndrome (*see also*
    Neuropathy, peripheral, autonomic) 337.9
Bernard-Sergent syndrome (acute
    adrenocortical insufficiency) 255.41
Bernard-Soulier disease or thrombopathy
    287.1
Bernhardt's disease or paresthesia 355.1
Bernhardt-Roth disease or syndrome
    (parasthesia) 355.1
Bernheim's syndrome (*see also* Failure, heart)
    428.0
Bertielliasis 123.8
Bertolotti's syndrome (sacralization of fifth
    lumbar vertebra) 756.15
Berylliosis (acute) (chronic) (lung)
    (occupational) 503
Besnier's
    lupus pernio 135
    prurigo (atopic dermatitis) (infantile eczema)
        691.8
Besnier-Boeck disease or sarcoid 135
Besnier-Boeck-Schaumann disease
    (sarcoidosis) 135
Best's disease 362.76
Bestiality 302.1
Beta-adrenergic hyperdynamic circulatory
    state 429.82
Beta-aminoisobutyric aciduria 277.2

Beta-mercaptolactate-cysteine disulfiduria
    270.0
Beta thalassemia (mixed) 282.44
    major 282.44
    minor 282.46
Beurmann's disease (sporotrichosis) 117.1
Bezoar 938
    intestine 936
    stomach 935.2
Bezold's abscess (*see also* Mastoiditis) 383.01
Bianchi's syndrome (aphasia-apraxia-alexia)
    784.69
Bicornuate or bicornis uterus (complete)
    (partial) 752.34
    in pregnancy or childbirth 654.0●
        with obstructed labor 660.2●
            affecting fetus or newborn 763.1
        affecting fetus or newborn 763.89
Bicuspid aortic valve 746.4
Biedl-Bardet syndrome 759.89
Bielschowsky's disease 330.1
Bielschowsky-Jansky
    amaurotic familial idiocy 330.1
    disease 330.1
Biemond's syndrome (obesity, polydactyly, and
    intellectual disabilities) 759.89
Biermer's anemia or disease (pernicious
    anemia) 281.0
Biett's disease 695.4
Bifid (congenital) - *see also* Imperfect, closure
    apex, heart 746.89
    clitoris 752.49
    epiglottis 748.3
    kidney 753.3
    nose 748.1
    patella 755.64
    scrotum 752.89
    toe 755.66
    tongue 750.13
    ureter 753.4
    uterus 752.34
    uvula 749.02
        with cleft lip (*see also* Cleft, palate, with
            cleft lip) 749.20
Biforis uterus (suprasimplex) 752.34
Bifurcation (congenital) - *see also* Imperfect,
    closure
    gallbladder 751.69
    kidney pelvis 753.3
    renal pelvis 753.3
    rib 756.3
    tongue 750.13
    trachea 748.3
    ureter 753.4
    urethra 753.8
    uvula 749.02
        with cleft lip (*see also* Cleft, palate, with
            cleft lip) 749.20
    vertebra 756.19
Bigeminal pulse 427.89
Bigeminy 427.89
Big spleen syndrome 289.4
Bilateral - *see* condition
Bile duct - *see* condition
Bile pigments in urine 791.4
Bilharziasis (*see also* Schistosomiasis) 120.9
    chyluria 120.0
    cutaneous 120.3
    galacturia 120.0
    hematochyluria 120.0
    intestinal 120.1
    lipemia 120.9
    lipuria 120.0
    Oriental 120.2
    piarhemia 120.9
    pulmonary 120.2
    tropical hematuria 120.0
    vesical 120.0
Biliary - *see* condition
Bilious (attack) - *see also* Vomiting
    fever, hemoglobinuric 084.8

◄ New   ◄|||| Revised   ~~deleted~~ Deleted   ● Use Additional Digit(s)   ▨ Omit code

Bilirubinuria 791.4
Biliuria 791.4
Billroth's disease
  meningocele (*see also* Spina bifida) 741.9●
Bilobate placenta - *see* Placenta, abnormal
Bilocular
  heart 745.7
  stomach 536.8
Bing-Horton syndrome (histamine cephalgia) 339.00
Binswanger's disease or dementia 290.12
Biörck (-Thorson) syndrome (malignant carcinoid) 259.2
Biparta, bipartite - *see also* Imperfect, closure
  carpal scaphoid 755.59
  patella 755.64
  placenta - *see* Placenta, abnormal
  vagina 752.49
Bird
  face 756.0
  fanciers' lung or disease 495.2
  flu (*see also* Influenza, avian) 488.02
Bird's disease (oxaluria) 271.8
Birth
  abnormal fetus or newborn 763.9
  accident, fetus or newborn - *see* Birth, injury
  complications in mother - *see* Delivery, complicated
  compression during NEC 767.9
  defect - *see* Anomaly
  delayed, fetus 763.9
  difficult NEC, affecting fetus or newborn 763.9
  dry, affecting fetus or newborn 761.1
  forced, NEC, affecting fetus or newborn 763.89
  forceps, affecting fetus or newborn 763.2
  hematoma of sternomastoid 767.8
  immature 765.1●
    extremely 765.0●
  inattention, after or at 995.52
  induced, affecting fetus or newborn 763.89
  infant - *see* Newborn
  injury NEC 767.9
    adrenal gland 767.8
    basal ganglia 767.0
    brachial plexus (paralysis) 767.6
    brain (compression) (pressure) 767.0
    cerebellum 767.0
    cerebral hemorrhage 767.0
    conjunctiva 767.8
    eye 767.8
    fracture
      bone, any except clavicle or spine 767.3
      clavicle 767.2
      femur 767.3
      humerus 767.3
      long bone 767.3
      radius and ulna 767.3
      skeleton NEC 767.3
      skull 767.3
      spine 767.4
      tibia and fibula 767.3
    hematoma 767.8
      liver (subcapsular) 767.8
      mastoid 767.8
      skull 767.19
      sternomastoid 767.8
      testes 767.8
      vulva 767.8
    intracranial (edema) 767.0
    laceration
      brain 767.0
      by scalpel 767.8
      peripheral nerve 767.7
    liver 767.8
    meninges
      brain 767.0
      spinal cord 767.4
    nerves (cranial, peripheral) 767.7
      brachial plexus 767.6
      facial 767.5

Birth (*Continued*)
  injury NEC (*Continued*)
    paralysis 767.7
      brachial plexus 767.6
      Erb (-Duchenne) 767.6
      facial nerve 767.5
      Klumpke (-Déjérine) 767.6
      radial nerve 767.6
      spinal (cord) (hemorrhage) (laceration) (rupture) 767.4
    rupture
      intracranial 767.0
      liver 767.8
      spinal cord 767.4
      spleen 767.8
      viscera 767.8
    scalp 767.19
    scalpel wound 767.8
    skeleton NEC 767.3
    specified NEC 767.8
    spinal cord 767.4
    spleen 767.8
    subdural hemorrhage 767.0
    tentorial, tear 767.0
    testes 767.8
    vulva 767.8
  instrumental, NEC, affecting fetus or newborn 763.2
  lack of care, after or at 995.52
  multiple
    affected by maternal complications of pregnancy 761.5
    healthy liveborn - *see* Newborn, multiple
  neglect, after or at 995.52
  newborn - *see* Newborn
  palsy or paralysis NEC 767.7
  precipitate, fetus or newborn 763.6
  premature (infant) 765.1●
  prolonged, affecting fetus or newborn 763.9
  retarded, fetus or newborn 763.9
  shock, newborn 779.89
  strangulation or suffocation
    due to aspiration of clear amniotic fluid 770.13
      with respiratory symptoms 770.14
    mechanical 767.8
  trauma NEC 767.9
  triplet
    affected by maternal complications of pregnancy 761.5
    healthy liveborn - *see* Newborn, multiple
  twin
    affected by maternal complications of pregnancy 761.5
    healthy liveborn - *see* Newborn, twin
  ventouse, affecting fetus or newborn 763.3
Birthmark 757.32
Birt-Hogg-Dube syndrome 759.89
Bisalbuminemia 273.8
Biskra button 085.1
Bite(s)
  with intact skin surface - *see* Contusion
  animal - *see* Wound, open, by site
    intact skin surface - *see* Contusion
  bedbug - *see* Injury, superficial, by site
  centipede 989.5
  chigger 133.8
  fire ant 989.5
  flea - *see* Injury, superficial, by site
  human (open wound) - *see also* Wound, open, by site
    intact skin surface - *see* Contusion
  insect
    nonvenomous - *see* Injury, superficial, by site
    venomous 989.5
  mad dog (death from) 071
  open
    anterior 524.24
    posterior 524.25
  poisonous 989.5

Bite(s) (*Continued*)
  red bug 133.8
  reptile 989.5
    nonvenomous - *see* Wound, open, by site
  snake 989.5
    nonvenomous - *see* Wound, open, by site
  spider (venomous) 989.5
    nonvenomous - *see* Injury, superficial, by site
  venomous 989.5
Biting
  cheek or lip 528.9
  nail 307.9
Black
  death 020.9
  eye NEC 921.0
  hairy tongue 529.3
  heel 924.20
  lung disease 500
  palm 923.20
Blackfan-Diamond anemia or syndrome (congenital hypoplastic anemia) 284.01
Blackhead 706.1
Blackout 780.2
Blackwater fever 084.8
Bladder - *see* condition
Blast
  blindness 921.3
  concussion - *see* Blast, injury
  injury 869.0
    with open wound into cavity 869.1
    abdomen or thorax - *see* Injury, internal, by site
    brain (*see also* Concussion, brain) 850.9
      with skull fracture - *see* Fracture, skull
    ear (acoustic nerve trauma) 951.5
      with perforation, tympanic membrane - *see* Wound, open, ear, drum
    lung (*see also* Injury, internal, lung) 861.20
    otitic (explosive) 388.11
Blastomycosis, blastomycotic (chronic) (cutaneous) (disseminated) (lung) (pulmonary) (systemic) 116.0
  Brazilian 116.1
  European 117.5
  keloidal 116.2
  North American 116.0
  primary pulmonary 116.0
  South American 116.1
Bleb(s) 709.8
  emphysematous (bullous) (diffuse) (lung) (ruptured) (solitary) 492.0
  filtering, eye (postglaucoma) (status) V45.69
    with complication 997.99
    postcataract extraction (complication) 997.99
  lung (ruptured) 492.0
    congenital 770.5
  subpleural (emphysematous) 492.0
Bleeder (familial) (hereditary) (*see also* Defect, coagulation) 286.9
  nonfamilial 286.9
Bleeding (*see also* Hemorrhage) 459.0
  anal 569.3
  anovulatory 628.0
  atonic, following delivery 666.1●
  capillary 448.9
  due to subinvolution 621.1
    puerperal 666.2●
  ear 388.69
  excessive, associated with menopausal onset 627.0
  familial (*see also* Defect, coagulation) 286.9
  following intercourse 626.7
  gastrointestinal 578.9
  gums 523.8
  hemorrhoids - *see* Hemorrhoids, bleeding
  intermenstrual
    irregular 626.6
    regular 626.5

Bleeding (Continued)
  intraoperative 998.11
  irregular NEC 626.4
  menopausal 627.0
  mouth 528.9
  nipple 611.79
  nose 784.7
  ovulation 626.5
  postclimacteric 627.1
  postcoital 626.7
  postmenopausal 627.1
    following induced menopause 627.4
  postoperative 998.11
  preclimacteric 627.0
  puberty 626.3
    excessive, with onset of menstrual periods 626.3
  rectum, rectal 569.3
  tendencies (see also Defect, coagulation) 286.9
  throat 784.8
  umbilical stump 772.3
  umbilicus 789.9
  unrelated to menstrual cycle 626.6
  uterus, uterine 626.9
    climacteric 627.0
    dysfunctional 626.8
    functional 626.8
    unrelated to menstrual cycle 626.6
  vagina, vaginal 623.8
    functional 626.8
  vicarious 625.8
Blennorrhagia, blennorrhagic - see Blennorrhea
Blennorrhea (acute) 098.0
  adultorum 098.40
  alveolaris 523.40
  chronic or duration of 2 months or over 098.2
  gonococcal (neonatorum) 098.40
  inclusion (neonatal) (newborn) 771.6
  neonatorum 098.40
Blepharelosis (see also Entropion) 374.00
Blepharitis (eyelid) 373.00
  angularis 373.01
  ciliaris 373.00
    with ulcer 373.01
  marginal 373.00
    with ulcer 373.01
  scrofulous (see also Tuberculosis) 017.3 ●
    [373.00]
  squamous 373.02
  ulcerative 373.01
Blepharochalasis 374.34
  congenital 743.62
Blepharoclonus 333.81
Blepharoconjunctivitis (see also Conjunctivitis) 372.20
  angular 372.21
  contact 372.22
Blepharophimosis (eyelid) 374.46
  congenital 743.62
Blepharoplegia 374.89
Blepharoptosis 374.30
  congenital 743.61
Blepharopyorrhea 098.49
Blepharospasm 333.81
  due to drugs 333.85
Blessig's cyst 362.62
Blighted ovum 631.8
Blind
  bronchus (congenital) 748.3
  eye - see also Blindness
    hypertensive 360.42
    hypotensive 360.41
  loop syndrome (postoperative) 579.2
  sac, fallopian tube (congenital) 752.19
  spot, enlarged 368.42
  tract or tube (congenital) NEC - see Atresia
Blindness (acquired) (congenital) (both eyes) 369.00
  with deafness V49.85
  blast 921.3
    with nerve injury - see Injury, nerve, optic

Blindness (Continued)
  Bright's - see Uremia
  color (congenital) 368.59
    acquired 368.55
    blue 368.53
    green 368.52
    red 368.51
    total 368.54
  concussion 950.9
  cortical 377.75
  day 368.10
    acquired 368.10
    congenital 368.10
    hereditary 368.10
    specified type NEC 368.10
  due to
    injury NEC 950.9
    refractive error - see Error, refractive
  eclipse (total) 363.31
  emotional 300.11
  face 368.16
  hysterical 300.11
  legal (both eyes) (USA definition) 369.4
    with impairment of better (less impaired) eye
      near-total 369.02
        with
          lesser eye impairment 369.02
            near-total 369.04
            total 369.03
      profound 369.05
        with
          lesser eye impairment 369.05
            near-total 369.07
            profound 369.08
            total 369.06
      severe 369.21
        with
          lesser eye impairment 369.21
            blind 369.11
            near-total 369.13
            profound 369.14
            severe 369.22
            total 369.12
      total
        with lesser eye impairment
          total 369.01
  mind 784.69
  moderate
    both eyes 369.25
      with impairment of lesser eye (specified as)
        blind, not further specified 369.15
        low vision, not further specified 369.23
        near-total 369.17
        profound 369.18
        severe 369.24
        total 369.16
    one eye 369.74
      with vision of other eye (specified as)
        near-normal 369.75
        normal 369.76
  near-total
    both eyes 369.04
      with impairment of lesser eye (specified as)
        blind, not further specified 369.02
        total 369.03
    one eye 369.64
      with vision of other eye (specified as)
        near-normal 369.65
        normal 369.66
  night 368.60
    acquired 368.62
    congenital (Japanese) 368.61
    hereditary 368.61
    specified type NEC 368.69
    vitamin A deficiency 264.5
  nocturnal - see Blindness, night

Blindness (Continued)
  one eye 369.60
    with low vision of other eye 369.10
  profound
    both eyes 369.08
      with impairment of lesser eye (specified as)
        blind, not further specified 369.05
        near-total 369.07
        total 369.06
    one eye 369.67
      with vision of other eye (specified as)
        near-normal 369.68
        normal 369.69
  psychic 784.69
  severe
    both eyes 369.22
      with impairment of lesser eye (specified as)
        blind, not further specified 369.11
        low vision, not further specified 369.21
        near-total 369.13
        profound 369.14
        total 369.12
    one eye 369.71
      with vision of other eye (specified as)
        near-normal 369.72
        normal 369.73
  snow 370.24
  sun 363.31
  temporary 368.12
  total
    both eyes 369.01
    one eye 369.61
      with vision of other eye (specified as)
        near-normal 369.62
        normal 369.63
  transient 368.12
  traumatic NEC 950.9
  word (developmental) 315.01
    acquired 784.61
    secondary to organic lesion 784.61
Blister - see also Injury, superficial, by site
  beetle dermatitis 692.89
  due to burn - see Burn, by site, second degree
  fever 054.9
  fracture - *omit code*
  multiple, skin, nontraumatic 709.8
Bloating 787.3
Bloch-Siemens syndrome (incontinentia pigmenti) 757.33
Bloch-Stauffer dyshormonal dermatosis 757.33
Bloch-Sulzberger disease or syndrome (incontinentia pigmenti) (melanoblastosis) 757.33
Block
  alveolar capillary 516.8
  arborization (heart) 426.6
  arrhythmic 426.9
  atrioventricular (AV) (incomplete) (partial) 426.10
    with
      2:1 atrioventricular response block 426.13
      atrioventricular dissociation 426.0
    first degree (incomplete) 426.11
    second degree (Mobitz type I) 426.13
      Mobitz (type II) 426.12
    third degree 426.0
    complete 426.0
      congenital 746.86
    congenital 746.86
    Mobitz (incomplete)
      type I (Wenckebach's) 426.13
      type II 426.12
    partial 426.13

◄ New   ◄ Revised   ~~deleted~~ Deleted   ● Use Additional Digit(s)   Omit code

Block *(Continued)*
auriculoventricular *(see also* Block, atrioventricular) 426.10
   complete 426.0
      congenital 746.86
   congenital 746.86
bifascicular (cardiac) 426.53
bundle branch (complete) (false) (incomplete) 426.50
   bilateral 426.53
   left (complete) (main stem) 426.3
      with right bundle branch block 426.53
      anterior fascicular 426.2
         with
            posterior fascicular block 426.3
            right bundle branch block 426.52
      hemiblock 426.2
      incomplete 426.2
         with right bundle branch block 426.53
      posterior fascicular 426.2
         with
            anterior fascicular block 426.3
            right bundle branch block 426.51
   right 426.4
      with
         left bundle branch block (incomplete) (main stem) 426.53
         left fascicular block 426.53
            anterior 426.52
            posterior 426.51
   Wilson's type 426.4
cardiac 426.9
conduction 426.9
   complete 426.0
Eustachian tube *(see also* Obstruction, Eustachian tube) 381.60
fascicular (left anterior) (left posterior) 426.2
foramen Magendie (acquired) 331.3
   congenital 742.3
      with spina bifida *(see also* Spina bifida) 741.0●
heart 426.9
   first degree (atrioventricular) 426.11
   second degree (atrioventricular) 426.13
   third degree (atrioventricular) 426.0
   bundle branch (complete) (false) (incomplete) 426.50
      bilateral 426.53
      left *(see also* Block, bundle branch, left) 426.3
      right *(see also* Block, bundle branch, right) 426.4
   complete (atrioventricular) 426.0
      congenital 746.86
   incomplete 426.13
   intra-atrial 426.6
   intraventricular NEC 426.6
   sinoatrial 426.6
   specified type NEC 426.6
hepatic vein 453.0
intraventricular (diffuse) (myofibrillar) 426.6
   bundle branch (complete) (false) (incomplete) 426.50
      bilateral 426.53
      left *(see also* Block, bundle branch, left) 426.3
      right *(see also* Block, bundle branch, right) 426.4
kidney *(see also* Disease, renal) 593.9
   postcystoscopic 997.5
myocardial *(see also* Block, heart) 426.9
nodal 426.10
optic nerve 377.49
organ or site (congenital) NEC - *see* Atresia
parietal 426.6
peri-infarction 426.6
portal (vein) 452
sinoatrial 426.6
sinoauricular 426.6
spinal cord 336.9

Block *(Continued)*
trifascicular 426.54
tubal 628.2
vein NEC 453.9
Blocq's disease or syndrome (astasia-abasia) 307.9
Blood
   constituents, abnormal NEC 790.6
   disease 289.9
      specified NEC 289.89
   donor V59.01
      other blood components V59.09
      stem cells V59.02
      whole blood V59.01
   dyscrasia 289.9
      with
         abortion - *see* Abortion, by type, with hemorrhage, delayed or excessive
         ectopic pregnancy *(see also* categories 633.0–633.9) 639.1
         molar pregnancy *(see also* categories 630–632) 639.1
      following
         abortion 639.1
         ectopic or molar pregnancy 639.1
      newborn NEC 776.9
      puerperal, postpartum 666.3●
   flukes NEC *(see also* Infestation, Schistosoma) 120.9
   in
      feces *(see also* Melena) 578.1
         occult 792.1
      urine *(see also* Hematuria) 599.70
   mole 631.8
   occult 792.1
   poisoning *(see also* Septicemia) 038.9
   pressure
      decreased, due to shock following injury 958.4
      fluctuating 796.4
      high *(see also* Hypertension) 401.9
         borderline 796.2
         incidental reading (isolated) (nonspecific), without diagnosis of hypertension 796.2
      low *(see also* Hypotension) 458.9
         incidental reading (isolated) (nonspecific), without diagnosis of hypotension 796.3
   spitting *(see also* Hemoptysis) 786.30
   staining cornea 371.12
   transfusion
      without reported diagnosis V58.2
      donor V59.01
         stem cells V59.02
      reaction or complication - *see* Complications, transfusion
   tumor - *see* Hematoma
   vessel rupture - *see* Hemorrhage
   vomiting *(see also* Hematemesis) 578.0
Blood-forming organ disease 289.9
Bloodgood's disease 610.1
Bloodshot eye 379.93
Bloom (-Machacek) (-Torre) syndrome 757.39
Blotch, palpebral 372.55
Blount's disease (tibia vara) 732.4
Blount-Barber syndrome (tibia vara) 732.4
Blue
   baby 746.9
   bloater 491.20
      with
         acute bronchitis 491.22
         exacerbation (acute) 491.21
   diaper syndrome 270.0
   disease 746.9
   dome cyst 610.0
   drum syndrome 381.02
   sclera 743.47
      with fragility of bone and deafness 756.51
   toe syndrome 445.02

Blueness *(see also* Cyanosis) 782.5
Blurring, visual 368.8
Blushing (abnormal) (excessive) 782.62
BMI (body mass index)
   adult
      25.0–25.9 V85.21
      26.0–26.9 V85.22
      27.0–27.9 V85.23
      28.0–28.9 V85.24
      29.0–29.9 V85.25
      30.0–30.9 V85.30
      31.0–31.9 V85.31
      32.0–32.9 V85.32
      33.0–33.9 V85.33
      34.0–34.9 V85.34
      35.0–35.9 V85.35
      36.0–36.9 V85.36
      37.0–37.9 V85.37
      38.0–38.9 V85.38
      39.0–39.9 V85.39
      40.0–44.9 V85.41
      45.0–49.9 V85.42
      50.0–59.9 V85.43
      60.0–69.9 V85.44
      70 and over V85.45
      between 19–24 V85.1
      less than 19 V85.0
   pediatric
      5th percentile to less than 85th percentile for age V85.52
      85th percentile to less than 95th percentile for age V85.53
      greater than or equal to 95th percentile for age V85.54
      less than 5th percentile for age V85.51
Boarder, hospital V65.0
   infant V65.0
Bockhart's impetigo (superficial folliculitis) 704.8
Bodechtel-Guttmann disease (subacute sclerosing panencephalitis) 046.2
Boder-Sedgwick syndrome (ataxia-telangiectasia) 334.8
Body, bodies
   Aschoff *(see also* Myocarditis, rheumatic) 398.0
   asteroid, vitreous 379.22
   choroid, colloid (degenerative) 362.57
      hereditary 362.77
   cytoid (retina) 362.82
   drusen (retina) *(see also* Drusen) 362.57
      optic disc 377.21
   fibrin, pleura 511.0
   foreign - *see* Foreign body
   Hassall-Henle 371.41
   loose
      joint *(see also* Loose, body, joint) 718.1●
         knee 717.6
      knee 717.6
      sheath, tendon 727.82
   Mallory's 034.1
   mass index (BMI)
      adult
         25.0–25.9 V85.21
         26.0–26.9 V85.22
         27.0–27.9 V85.23
         28.0–28.9 V85.24
         29.0–29.9 V85.25
         30.0–30.9 V85.30
         31.0–31.9 V85.31
         32.0–32.9 V85.32
         33.0–33.9 V85.33
         34.0–34.9 V85.34
         35.0–35.9 V85.35
         36.0–36.9 V85.36
         37.0–37.9 V85.37
         38.0–38.9 V85.38
         39.0–39.9 V85.39
         40.0–44.9 V85.41
         45.0–49.9 V85.42
         50.0-59.9 V85.43

Body, bodies (Continued)
  mass index (BMI) (Continued)
    adult (Continued)
      60.0-69.9 V85.44
      70 and over V85.45
      between 19–24 V85.1
      less than 19 V85.0
    pediatric
      5th percentile to less than 85th
        percentile for age V85.52
      85th percentile to less than 95th
        percentile for age V85.53
      greater than or equal to 95th percentile
        for age V85.54
      less than 5th percentile for age V85.51
  Mooser 081.0
  Negri 071
  rice (joint) (see also Loose, body, joint) 718.1●
    knee 717.6
  rocking 307.3
Boeck's
  disease (sarcoidosis) 135
  lupoid (miliary) 135
  sarcoid 135
Boerhaave's syndrome (spontaneous
  esophageal rupture) 530.4
Boggy
  cervix 622.8
  uterus 621.8
Boil (see also Carbuncle) 680.9
  abdominal wall 680.2
  Aleppo 085.1
  ankle 680.6
  anus 680.5
  arm (any part, above wrist) 680.3
  auditory canal, external 680.0
  axilla 680.3
  back (any part) 680.2
  Baghdad 085.1
  breast 680.2
  buttock 680.5
  chest wall 680.2
  corpus cavernosum 607.2
  Delhi 085.1
  ear (any part) 680.0
  eyelid 373.13
  face (any part, except eye) 680.0
  finger (any) 680.4
  flank 680.2
  foot (any part) 680.7
  forearm 680.3
  Gafsa 085.1
  genital organ, male 608.4
  gluteal (region) 680.5
  groin 680.2
  hand (any part) 680.4
  head (any part, except face) 680.8
  heel 680.7
  hip 680.6
  knee 680.6
  labia 616.4
  lacrimal (see also Dacryocystitis) 375.30
    gland (see also Dacryoadenitis) 375.00
    passages (duct) (sac) (see also
      Dacryocystitis) 375.30
  leg, any part, except foot 680.6
  multiple sites 680.9
  natal 085.1
  neck 680.1
  nose (external) (septum) 680.0
  orbit, orbital 376.01
  partes posteriores 680.5
  pectoral region 680.2
  penis 607.2
  perineum 680.2
  pinna 680.0
  scalp (any part) 680.8
  scrotum 608.4
  seminal vesicle 608.0
  shoulder 680.3
  skin NEC 680.9

Boil (Continued)
  specified site NEC 680.8
  spermatic cord 608.4
  temple (region) 680.0
  testis 608.4
  thigh 680.6
  thumb 680.4
  toe (any) 680.7
  tropical 085.1
  trunk 680.2
  tunica vaginalis 608.4
  umbilicus 680.2
  upper arm 680.3
  vas deferens 608.4
  vulva 616.4
  wrist 680.4
Bold hives (see also Urticaria) 708.9
Bolivian hemorrhagic fever 078.7
Bombé, iris 364.74
Bomford-Rhoads anemia (refractory) 238.72
Bone - see condition
Bonnevie-Ullrich syndrome 758.6
Bonnier's syndrome 386.19
Bonvale Dam fever 780.79
Bony block of joint 718.80
  ankle 718.87
  elbow 718.82
  foot 718.87
  hand 718.84
  hip 718.85
  knee 718.86
  multiple sites 718.89
  pelvic region 718.85
  shoulder (region) 718.81
  specified site NEC 718.88
  wrist 718.83
BOOP (bronchiolitis obliterans organized
  pneumonia) 516.8
Borderline
  diabetes mellitus 790.29
  hypertension 796.2
  intellectual functioning V62.89
  osteopenia 733.90
  pelvis 653.1●
    with obstruction during labor 660.1●
      affecting fetus or newborn 763.1
  psychosis (see also Schizophrenia) 295.5●
    of childhood (see also Psychosis,
      childhood) 299.8●
  schizophrenia (see also Schizophrenia) 295.5●
Borna disease 062.9
Bornholm disease (epidemic pleurodynia) 074.1
Borrelia vincentii (mouth) (pharynx) (tonsils)
  101
Bostock's catarrh (see also Fever, hay) 477.9
Boston exanthem 048
Botalli, ductus (patent) (persistent) 747.0
Bothriocephalus latus infestation 123.4
Botulism 005.1
  food poisoning 005.1
  infant 040.41
  non-foodborne 040.42
  wound 040.42
Bouba (see also Yaws) 102.9
Bouffée délirante 298.3
Bouillaud's disease or syndrome (rheumatic
  heart disease) 391.9
Bourneville's disease (tuberous sclerosis) 759.5
Boutonneuse fever 082.1
Boutonniere
  deformity (finger) 736.21
  hand (intrinsic) 736.21
Bouveret (-Hoffmann) disease or syndrome
  (paroxysmal tachycardia) 427.2
Bovine heart - see Hypertrophy, cardiac
Bowel - see condition
Bowen's
  dermatosis (precancerous) (M8081/2) - see
    Neoplasm, skin, in situ
  disease (M8081/2) - see Neoplasm, skin, in
    situ

Bowen's (Continued)
  epithelioma (M8081/2) - see Neoplasm, skin,
    in situ
  type
    epidermoid carcinoma in situ (M8081/2) -
      see Neoplasm, skin, in situ
    intraepidermal squamous cell carcinoma
      (M8081/2) - see Neoplasm, skin, in
      situ
Bowing
  femur 736.89
    congenital 754.42
  fibula 736.89
    congenital 754.43
  forearm 736.09
    away from midline (cubitus valgus)
      736.01
    toward midline (cubitus varus) 736.02
  leg(s), long bones, congenital 754.44
  radius 736.09
    away from midline (cubitus valgus)
      736.01
    toward midline (cubitus varus) 736.02
  tibia 736.89
    congenital 754.43
Bowleg(s) 736.42
  congenital 754.44
  rachitic 268.1
Boyd's dysentery 004.2
Brachial - see condition
Brachman-de Lange syndrome (Amsterdam
  dwarf, intellectual disabilities, and
  brachycephaly) 759.89
Brachycardia 427.89
Brachycephaly 756.0
Brachymorphism and ectopia lentis 759.89
Bradley's disease (epidemic vomiting)
  078.82
Bradycardia 427.89
  chronic (sinus) 427.81
  newborn 779.81
  nodal 427.89
  postoperative 997.1
  reflex 337.09
  sinoatrial 427.89
    with paroxysmal tachyarrhythmia or
      tachycardia 427.81
    chronic 427.81
  sinus 427.89
    with paroxysmal tachyarrhythmia or
      tachycardia 427.81
    chronic 427.81
    persistent 427.81
    severe 427.81
  tachycardia syndrome 427.81
  vagal 427.89
Bradykinesia 781.0
Bradypnea 786.09
Brailsford's disease 732.3
  radial head 732.3
  tarsal scaphoid 732.5
Brailsford-Morquio disease or syndrome
  (mucopolysaccharidosis IV) 277.5
Brain - see also condition
  death 348.82
  syndrome (acute) (chronic) (nonpsychotic)
    (organic) (with neurotic reaction) (with
    behavioral reaction) (see also
    Syndrome, brain) 310.9
    with
      presenile brain disease 290.10
      psychosis, psychotic reaction (see also
        Psychosis, organic) 294.9
    congenital (see also Disability, intellectual)
      319
Branched-chain amino-acid disease 270.3
Branchial - see condition
Brandt's syndrome (acrodermatitis
  enteropathica) 686.8
Brash (water) 787.1
Brass-founders' ague 985.8

◄ New   ⇐ Revised   deleted Deleted   ● Use Additional Digit(s)   ▬ Omit code

Bravais-Jacksonian epilepsy (*see also* Epilepsy) 345.5●
Braxton Hicks contractions 644.1●
Braziers' disease 985.8
Brazilian
    blastomycosis 116.1
    leishmaniasis 085.5
BRBPR (bright red blood per rectum) 569.3
Break
    cardiorenal - *see* Hypertension, cardiorenal
    retina (*see also* Defect, retina) 361.30
Breakbone fever 061
Breakdown
    device, implant, or graft - *see* Complications, mechanical
    nervous (*see also* Disorder, mental, nonpsychotic) 300.9
    perineum 674.2●
Breast - *see also* condition
    buds 259.1
        in newborn 779.89
    dense 793.82
    nodule 793.89
Breast feeding difficulties 676.8●
Breath
    foul 784.99
    holder, child 312.81
    holding spells 786.9
    shortness 786.05
Breathing
    asymmetrical 786.09
    bronchial 786.09
    exercises V57.0
    labored 786.09
    mouth 784.99
        causing malocclusion 524.59
    periodic 786.09
        high altitude 327.22
    tic 307.20
Breathlessness 786.09
Breda's disease (*see also* Yaws) 102.9
Breech
    delivery, affecting fetus or newborn 763.0
    extraction, affecting fetus or newborn 763.0
    presentation (buttocks) (complete) (frank) 652.2●
        with successful version 652.1●
        before labor, affecting fetus or newborn 761.7
        during labor, affecting fetus or newborn 763.0
Breisky's disease (kraurosis vulvae) 624.09
Brennemann's syndrome (acute mesenteric lymphadenitis) 289.2
Brenner's
    tumor (benign) (M9000/0) 220
        borderline malignancy (M9000/1) 236.2
        malignant (M9000/3) 183.0
        proliferating (M9000/1) 236.2
Bretonneau's disease (diphtheritic malignant angina) 032.0
Breus' mole 631.8
Brevicollis 756.16
Bricklayers' itch 692.89
Brickmakers' anemia 126.9
Bridge
    myocardial 746.85
Bright red blood per rectum (BRBPR) 569.3
Bright's
    blindness - *see* Uremia
    disease (*see also* Nephritis) 583.9
        arteriosclerotic (*see also* Hypertension, kidney) 403.90
Brill's disease (recrudescent typhus) 081.1
    flea-borne 081.0
    louse-borne 081.1
Brill-Symmers disease (follicular lymphoma) (M9690/3) 202.0●
Brill-Zinsser disease (recrudescent typhus) 081.1

Brinton's disease (linitis plastica) (M8142/3) 151.9
Brion-Kayser disease (*see also* Fever, paratyphoid) 002.9
Briquet's disorder or syndrome 300.81
Brissaud's
    infantilism (infantile myxedema) 244.9
    motor-verbal tic 307.23
Brissaud-Meige syndrome (infantile myxedema) 244.9
Brittle
    bones (congenital) 756.51
    nails 703.8
        congenital 757.5
Broad - *see also* condition
    beta disease 272.2
    ligament laceration syndrome 620.6
Brock's syndrome (atelectasis due to enlarged lymph nodes) 518.0
Brocq's disease 691.8
    atopic (diffuse) neurodermatitis 691.8
    lichen simplex chronicus 698.3
    parakeratosis psoriasiformis 696.2
    parapsoriasis 696.2
Brocq-Duhring disease (dermatitis herpetiformis) 694.0
Brodie's
    abscess (localized) (chronic) (*see also* Osteomyelitis) 730.1●
    disease (joint) (*see also* Osteomyelitis) 730.1●
Broken
    arches 734
        congenital 755.67
    back - *see* Fracture, vertebra, by site
    bone - *see* Fracture, by site
    compensation - *see* Disease, heart
    heart syndrome 429.83
    implant or internal device - *see* listing under Complications, mechanical
    neck - *see* Fracture, vertebra, cervical
    nose 802.0
        open 802.1
    tooth, teeth 873.63
        complicated 873.73
Bromhidrosis 705.89
Bromidism, bromism
    acute 967.3
        correct substance properly administered 349.82
        overdose or wrong substance given or taken 967.3
    chronic (*see also* Dependence) 304.1●
Bromidrosiphobia 300.23
Bromidrosis 705.89
Bronchi, bronchial - *see* condition
Bronchiectasis (cylindrical) (diffuse) (fusiform) (localized) (moniliform) (postinfectious) (recurrent) (saccular) 494.0
    with acute exacerbation 494.1
    congenital 748.61
    tuberculosis (*see also* Tuberculosis) 011.5●
Bronchiolectasis - *see* Bronchiectasis
Bronchiolitis (acute) (infectious) (subacute) 466.19
    with
        bronchospasm or obstruction 466.19
        influenza, flu, or grippe (*see also* Influenza) 487.1
    catarrhal (acute) (subacute) 466.19
    chemical 506.0
        chronic 506.4
    chronic (obliterative) 491.8
    due to external agent - *see* Bronchitis, acute, due to
    fibrosa obliterans 491.8
    influenzal (*see also* Influenza) 487.1
    obliterans 491.8
        with organizing pneumonia (BOOP) 516.8
        status post lung transplant 996.84

Bronchiolitis (*Continued*)
    obliterative (chronic) (diffuse) (subacute) 491.8
        due to fumes or vapors 506.4
    respiratory syncytial virus 466.11
    vesicular - *see* Pneumonia, broncho-
Bronchitis (diffuse) (hypostatic) (infectious) (inflammatory) (simple) 490
    with
        emphysema - *see* Emphysema
        influenza, flu, or grippe (*see also* Influenza) 487.1
        obstruction airway, chronic 491.20
            with
                acute bronchitis 491.22
                exacerbation (acute) 491.21
        tracheitis 490
            acute or subacute 466.0
                with bronchospasm or obstruction 466.0
            chronic 491.8
    acute or subacute 466.0
        with
            bronchiectasis 494.1
            bronchospasm 466.0
            obstruction 466.0
            tracheitis 466.0
        chemical (due to fumes or vapors) 506.0
        due to
            fumes or vapors 506.0
            radiation 508.8
    allergic (acute) (*see also* Asthma) 493.9●
    arachidic 934.1
    aspiration 507.0
        due to fumes or vapors 506.0
    asthmatic (acute) 493.90
        with
            acute exacerbation 493.92
            status asthmaticus 493.91
        chronic 493.2●
    capillary 466.19
        with bronchospasm or obstruction 466.19
        chronic 491.8
    caseous (*see also* Tuberculosis) 011.3●
    Castellani's 104.8
    catarrhal 490
        acute - *see* Bronchitis, acute
        chronic 491.0
    chemical (acute) (subacute) 506.0
        chronic 506.4
        due to fumes or vapors (acute) (subacute) 506.0
            chronic 506.4
    chronic 491.9
        with
            tracheitis (chronic) 491.8
        asthmatic 493.2●
        catarrhal 491.0
        chemical (due to fumes and vapors) 506.4
        due to
            fumes or vapors (chemical) (inhalation) 506.4
            radiation 508.8
            tobacco smoking 491.0
        mucopurulent 491.1
        obstructive 491.20
            with
                acute bronchitis 491.22
                exacerbation (acute) 491.21
        purulent 491.1
        simple 491.0
        specified type NEC 491.8
    croupous 466.0
        with bronchospasm or obstruction 466.0
        due to fumes or vapors 506.0
    emphysematous 491.20
        with
            acute bronchitis 491.22
            exacerbation (acute) 491.21
    exudative 466.0
    fetid (chronic) (recurrent) 491.1

B

Bronchitis (Continued)
fibrinous, acute or subacute 466.0
  with bronchospasm or obstruction 466.0
grippal (see also Influenza) 487.1
influenzal (see also Influenza) 487.1
membranous, acute or subacute 466.0
  with bronchospasm or obstruction 466.0
moulders' 502
mucopurulent (chronic) (recurrent) 491.1
  acute or subacute 466.0
obliterans 491.8
obstructive (chronic) 491.20
  with
    acute bronchitis 491.22
    exacerbation (acute) 491.21
pituitous 491.1
plastic (inflammatory) 466.0
pneumococcal, acute or subacute 466.0
  with bronchospasm or obstruction 466.0
pseudomembranous 466.0
purulent (chronic) (recurrent) 491.1
  acute or subacute 466.0
    with bronchospasm or obstruction
      466.0
putrid 491.1
scrofulous (see also Tuberculosis) 011.3●
senile 491.9
septic, acute or subacute 466.0
  with bronchospasm or obstruction 466.0
smokers' 491.0
spirochetal 104.8
suffocative, acute or subacute 466.0
summer (see also Asthma) 493.9●
suppurative (chronic) 491.1
  acute or subacute 466.0
tuberculous (see also Tuberculosis) 011.3●
ulcerative 491.8
  Vincent's 101
Vincent's 101
viral, acute or subacute 466.0
Bronchoalveolitis 485
Bronchoaspergillosis 117.3
Bronchocele
meaning
  dilatation of bronchus 519.19
  goiter 240.9
Bronchogenic carcinoma 162.9
Bronchohemisporosis 117.9
Broncholithiasis 518.89
  tuberculous (see also Tuberculosis) 011.3●
Bronchomalacia 748.3
Bronchomoniliasis 112.89
Bronchomycosis 112.89
Bronchonocardiosis 039.1
Bronchopleuropneumonia - see Pneumonia,
  broncho-
Bronchopneumonia - see Pneumonia, broncho-
Bronchopneumonitis - see Pneumonia,
  broncho-
Bronchopulmonary - see condition
Bronchopulmonitis - see Pneumonia, broncho-
Bronchorrhagia 786.30
  newborn 770.3
  tuberculous (see also Tuberculosis) 011.3●
Bronchorrhea (chronic) (purulent) 491.0
  acute 466.0
Bronchospasm 519.11
  with
    asthma - see Asthma
    bronchiolitis, acute 466.19
      due to respiratory syncytial virus
        466.11
    bronchitis - see Bronchitis
    chronic obstructive pulmonary disease
      (COPD) 496
    emphysema - see Emphysema
    due to external agent - see
      Condition, respiratory, acute,
      due to
  acute 519.11
  exercise induced 493.81

Bronchospirochetosis 104.8
Bronchostenosis 519.19
Bronchus - see condition
Bronze, bronzed
diabetes 275.01
disease (Addison's) (skin) 255.41
  tuberculous (see also Tuberculosis) 017.6●
Brooke's disease or tumor (M8100/0) - see
  Neoplasm, skin, benign
Brown's tendon sheath syndrome 378.61
Brown enamel of teeth (hereditary) 520.5
Brown-Séquard's paralysis (syndrome) 344.89
Brow presentation complicating delivery
  652.4●
Brucella, brucellosis (infection) 023.9
  abortus 023.1
  canis 023.3
  dermatitis, skin 023.9
  melitensis 023.0
  mixed 023.8
  suis 023.2
Bruck's disease 733.99
Bruck-de Lange disease or syndrome
  (Amsterdam dwarf, intellectual
  disabilities, and brachycephaly) 759.89
Brugada syndrome 746.89
Brug's filariasis 125.1
Brugsch's syndrome (acropachyderma) 757.39
Bruhl's disease (splenic anemia with fever)
  285.8
Bruise (skin surface intact) - see also Contusion
  with
    fracture - see Fracture, by site
    open wound - see Wound, open, by site
    internal organ (abdomen, chest, or pelvis) -
      see Injury, internal, by site
    umbilical cord 663.6●
      affecting fetus or newborn 762.6
Bruit 785.9
  arterial (abdominal) (carotid) 785.9
  supraclavicular 785.9
Brushburn - see Injury, superficial, by site
Bruton's X-linked agammaglobulinemia
  279.04
Bruxism 306.8
  sleep related 327.53
Bubbly lung syndrome 770.7
Bubo 289.3
  blennorrhagic 098.89
  chancroidal 099.0
  climatic 099.1
  due to Hemophilus ducreyi 099.0
  gonococcal 098.89
  indolent NEC 099.8
  inguinal NEC 099.8
    chancroidal 099.0
    climatic 099.1
    due to H. ducreyi 099.0
  scrofulous (see also Tuberculosis) 017.2●
  soft chancre 099.0
  suppurating 683
  syphilitic 091.0
    congenital 090.0
  tropical 099.1
  venereal NEC 099.8
  virulent 099.0
Bubonic plague 020.0
Bubonocele - see Hernia, inguinal
Buccal - see condition
Buchanan's disease (juvenile osteochondrosis
  of iliac crest) 732.1
Buchem's syndrome (hyperostosis corticalis)
  733.3
Buchman's disease (osteochondrosis, juvenile)
  732.1
Bucket handle fracture (semilunar cartilage)
  (see also Tear, meniscus) 836.2
Budd-Chiari syndrome (hepatic vein
  thrombosis) 453.0
Budgerigar-fanciers' disease or lung 495.2
Büdinger-Ludloff-Läwen disease 717.89

Buds
breast 259.1
in newborn 779.89
Buerger's disease (thromboangiitis obliterans)
  443.1
Bulbar - see condition
Bulbus cordis 745.9
persistent (in left ventricle) 745.8
Bulging fontanels (congenital) 756.0
Bulimia 783.6
nervosa 307.51
nonorganic origin 307.51
Bulky uterus 621.2
Bulla(e) 709.8
lung (emphysematous) (solitary) 492.0
Bullet wound - see also Wound, open, by site
fracture - see Fracture, by site, open
internal organ (abdomen, chest, or pelvis) -
  see Injury, internal, by site, with open
  wound
intracranial - see Laceration, brain, with open
  wound
Bullis fever 082.8
Bullying (see also Disturbance, conduct)
  312.0●
Bundle
branch block (complete) (false) (incomplete)
  426.50
    bilateral 426.53
    left (see also Block, bundle branch, left)
      426.3
      hemiblock 426.2
    right (see also Block, bundle branch, right)
      426.4
of His - see condition
of Kent syndrome (anomalous
  atrioventricular excitation) 426.7
Bungpagga 040.81
Bunion 727.1
Bunionette 727.1
Bunyamwera fever 066.3
Buphthalmia, buphthalmos (congenital)
  743.20
associated with
  keratoglobus, congenital 743.22
  megalocornea 743.22
  ocular anomalies NEC 743.22
isolated 743.21
simple 743.21
Bürger-Grütz disease or syndrome (essential
  familial hyperlipemia) 272.3
Buried roots 525.3
Burke's syndrome 577.8
Burkitt's
tumor (M9750/3) 200.2●
type malignant, lymphoma, lymphoblastic,
  or undifferentiated (M9750/3) 200.2●
Burn (acid) (cathode ray) (caustic) (chemical)
  (electric heating appliance) (electricity)
  (fire) (flame) (hot liquid or object)
  (irradiation) (lime) (radiation) (steam)
  (thermal) (x-ray) 949.0

Note: Use the following fifth-digit
subclassification with category 948 to
indicate the percent of body surface with
third degree burn:

0	less than 10 percent or unspecified
1	10–19 percent
2	20–29 percent
3	30–39 percent
4	40–49 percent
5	50–59 percent
6	60–69 percent
7	70–79 percent
8	80–89 percent
9	90 percent or more of body surface

with
  blisters - see Burn, by site, second degree
  erythema - see Burn, by site, first degree

◀ New   ◀◀ Revised   ~~deleted~~ Deleted   ● Use Additional Digit(s)   ▨ Omit code

Burn *(Continued)*
  with *(Continued)*
    skin loss (epidermal) - *see also* Burn, by site, second degree
    full thickness - *see also* Burn, by site, third degree
      with necrosis of underlying tissues - *see* Burn, by site, third degree, deep
    first degree - *see* Burn, by site, first degree
    second degree - *see* Burn, by site, second degree
    third degree - *see also* Burn, by site, third degree
      deep - *see* Burn, by site, third degree, deep
  abdomen, abdominal (muscle) (wall) 942.03
    with
      trunk - *see* Burn, trunk, multiple sites
    first degree 942.13
    second degree 942.23
    third degree 942.33
      deep 942.43
        with loss of body part 942.53
  ankle 945.03
    with
      lower limb(s) - *see* Burn, leg, multiple sites
    first degree 945.13
    second degree 945.23
    third degree 945.33
      deep 945.43
        with loss of body part 945.53
  anus - *see* Burn, trunk, specified site NEC
  arm(s) 943.00
    first degree 943.10
    second degree 943.20
    third degree 943.30
      deep 943.40
        with loss of body part 943.50
    lower - *see* Burn, forearm(s)
    multiple sites, except hand(s) or wrist(s) 943.09
      first degree 943.19
      second degree 943.29
      third degree 943.39
        deep 943.49
          with loss of body part 943.59
    upper 943.03
      first degree 943.13
      second degree 943.23
      third degree 943.33
        deep 943.43
          with loss of body part 943.53
  auditory canal (external) - *see* Burn, ear
  auricle (ear) - *see* Burn, ear
  axilla 943.04
    with
      upper limb(s), except hand(s) or wrist(s) - *see* Burn, arm(s), multiple sites
    first degree 943.14
    second degree 943.24
    third degree 943.34
      deep 943.44
        with loss of body part 943.54
  back 942.04
    with
      trunk - *see* Burn, trunk, multiple sites
    first degree 942.14
    second degree 942.24
    third degree 942.34
      deep 942.44
        with loss of body part 942.54
  biceps
    brachii - *see* Burn, arm(s), upper
    femoris - *see* Burn, thigh
  breast(s) 942.01
    with
      trunk - *see* Burn, trunk, multiple sites
    first degree 942.11
    second degree 942.21

Burn *(Continued)*
  breast(s) *(Continued)*
    third degree 942.31
      deep 942.41
        with loss of body part 942.51
  brow - *see* Burn, forehead
  buttock(s) - *see* Burn, back
  canthus (eye) 940.1
    chemical 940.0
  cervix (uteri) 947.4
  cheek (cutaneous) 941.07
    with
      face or head - *see* Burn, head, multiple sites
    first degree 941.17
    second degree 941.27
    third degree 941.37
      deep 941.47
        with loss of body part 941.57
  chest wall (anterior) 942.02
    with
      trunk - *see* Burn, trunk, multiple sites
    first degree 942.12
    second degree 942.22
    third degree 942.32
      deep 942.42
        with loss of body part 942.52
  chin 941.04
    with
      face or head - *see* Burn, head, multiple sites
    first degree 941.14
    second degree 941.24
    third degree 941.34
      deep 941.44
        with loss of body part 941.54
  clitoris - *see* Burn, genitourinary organs, external
  colon 947.3
  conjunctiva (and cornea) 940.4
    chemical
      acid 940.3
      alkaline 940.2
  cornea (and conjunctiva) 940.4
    chemical
      acid 940.3
      alkaline 940.2
  costal region - *see* Burn, chest wall
  due to ingested chemical agent - *see* Burn, internal organs
  ear (auricle) (canal) (drum) (external) 941.01
    with
      face or head - *see* Burn, head, multiple sites
    first degree 941.11
    second degree 941.21
    third degree 941.31
      deep 941.41
        with loss of a body part 941.51
  elbow 943.02
    with
      hand(s) and wrist(s) - *see* Burn, multiple specified sites
      upper limb(s), except hand(s) or wrist(s) - *see also* Burn, arm(s), multiple sites
    first degree 943.12
    second degree 943.22
    third degree 943.32
      deep 943.42
        with loss of body part 943.52
  electricity, electric current - *see* Burn, by site
  entire body - *see* Burn, multiple, specified sites
  epididymis - *see* Burn, genitourinary organs, external
  epigastric region - *see* Burn, abdomen
  epiglottis 947.1
  esophagus 947.2

Burn *(Continued)*
  extent (percent of body surface)
    less than 10 percent 948.0 ●
    10–19 percent 948.1 ●
    20–29 percent 948.2 ●
    30–39 percent 948.3 ●
    40–49 percent 948.4 ●
    50–59 percent 948.5 ●
    60–69 percent 948.6 ●
    70–79 percent 948.7 ●
    80–89 percent 948.8 ●
    90 percent or more 948.9 ●
  extremity
    lower - *see* Burn, leg
    upper - *see* Burn, arm(s)
  eye(s) (and adnexa) (only) 940.9
    with
      face, head, or neck 941.02
        first degree 941.12
        second degree 941.22
        third degree 941.32
          deep 941.42
            with loss of body part 941.52
      other sites (classifiable to more than one category in 940–945) - *see* Burn, multiple, specified sites
      resulting rupture and destruction of eyeball 940.5
    specified part - *see* Burn, by site
  eyeball - *see also* Burn, eye
    with resulting rupture and destruction of eyeball 940.5
  eyelid(s) 940.1
    chemical 940.0
  face - *see* Burn, head
  finger (nail) (subungual) 944.01
    with
      hand(s) - *see* Burn, hand(s), multiple sites
      other sites - *see* Burn, multiple, specified sites
      thumb 944.04
        first degree 944.14
        second degree 944.24
        third degree 944.34
          deep 944.44
            with loss of body part 944.54
    first degree 944.11
    second degree 944.21
    third degree 944.31
      deep 944.41
        with loss of body part 944.51
    multiple (digits) 944.03
      with thumb - *see* Burn, finger, with thumb
      first degree 944.13
      second degree 944.23
      third degree 944.33
        deep 944.43
          with loss of body part 944.53
  flank - *see* Burn, abdomen
  foot 945.02
    with
      lower limb(s) - *see* Burn, leg, multiple sites
    first degree 945.12
    second degree 945.22
    third degree 945.32
      deep 945.42
        with loss of body part 945.52
  forearm(s) 943.01
    with
      upper limb(s), except hand(s) or wrist(s) - *see* Burn, arm(s), multiple sites
    first degree 943.11
    second degree 943.21
    third degree 943.31
      deep 943.41
        with loss of body part 943.51

Burn *(Continued)*
forehead 941.07
with
face or head - *see* Burn, head, multiple
sites
first degree 941.17
second degree 941.27
third degree 941.37
deep 941.47
with loss of body part 941.57
fourth degree - *see* Burn, by site, third
degree, deep
friction - *see* Injury, superficial, by site
from swallowing caustic or corrosive
substance NEC - *see* Burn, internal
organs
full thickness - *see* Burn, by site, third
degree
gastrointestinal tract 947.3
genitourinary organs
external 942.05
with
trunk - *see* Burn, trunk, multiple
sites
first degree 942.15
second degree 942.25
third degree 942.35
deep 942.45
with loss of body part 942.55
internal 947.8
globe (eye) - *see* Burn, eyeball
groin - *see* Burn, abdomen
gum 947.0
hand(s) (phalanges) (and wrist) 944.00
first degree 944.10
second degree 944.20
third degree 944.30
deep 944.40
with loss of body part 944.50
back (dorsal surface) 944.06
first degree 944.16
second degree 944.26
third degree 944.36
deep 944.46
with loss of body part 944.56
multiple sites 944.08
first degree 944.18
second degree 944.28
third degree 944.38
deep 944.48
with loss of body part 944.58
head (and face) 941.00
eye(s) only 940.9
specified part - *see* Burn, by site
first degree 941.10
second degree 941.20
third degree 941.30
deep 941.40
with loss of body part 941.50
multiple sites 941.09
with eyes - *see* Burn, eyes, with face,
head, or neck
first degree 941.19
second degree 941.29
third degree 941.39
deep 941.49
with loss of body part
941.59
heel - *see* Burn, foot
hip - *see* Burn, trunk, specified site NEC
iliac region - *see* Burn, trunk, specified site
NEC
infected 958.3
inhalation *(see also* Burn, internal organs)
947.9
internal organs 947.9
from caustic or corrosive substance
(swallowing) NEC 947.9
specified NEC *(see also* Burn, by site)
947.8
interscapular region - *see* Burn, back

Burn *(Continued)*
intestine (large) (small) 947.3
iris - *see* Burn, eyeball
knee 945.05
with
lower limb(s) - *see* Burn, leg, multiple
sites
first degree 945.15
second degree 945.25
third degree 945.35
deep 945.45
with loss of body part 945.55
labium (majus) (minus) - *see* Burn,
genitourinary organs, external
lacrimal apparatus, duct, gland, or sac
940.1
chemical 940.0
larynx 947.1
late effect - *see* Late, effects (of), burn
leg 945.00
first degree 945.10
second degree 945.20
third degree 945.30
deep 945.40
with loss of body part 945.50
lower 945.04
with other part(s) of lower limb(s) - *see*
Burn, leg, multiple sites
first degree 945.14
second degree 945.24
third degree 945.34
deep 945.44
with loss of body part 945.54
multiple sites 945.09
first degree 945.19
second degree 945.29
third degree 945.39
deep 945.49
with loss of body part 945.59
upper - *see* Burn, thigh
lightning - *see* Burn, by site
limb(s)
lower (including foot or toe(s)) - *see* Burn,
leg
upper (except wrist and hand) - *see* Burn,
arm(s)
lip(s) 941.03
with
face or head - *see* Burn, head, multiple
sites
first degree 941.13
second degree 941.23
third degree 941.33
deep 941.43
with loss of body part 941.53
lumbar region - *see* Burn, back
lung 947.1
malar region - *see* Burn, cheek
mastoid region - *see* Burn, scalp
membrane, tympanic - *see* Burn, ear
midthoracic region - *see* Burn, chest wall
mouth 947.0
multiple *(see also* Burn, unspecified) 949.0
specified sites classifiable to more than
one category in 940–945 946.0
first degree 946.1
second degree 946.2
third degree 946.3
deep 946.4
with loss of body part 946.5
muscle, abdominal - *see* Burn, abdomen
nasal (septum) - *see* Burn, nose
neck 941.08
with
face or head - *see* Burn, head, multiple
sites
first degree 941.18
second degree 941.28
third degree 941.38
deep 941.48
with loss of body part 941.58

Burn *(Continued)*
nose (septum) 941.05
with
face or head - *see* Burn, head, multiple
sites
first degree 941.15
second degree 941.25
third degree 941.35
deep 941.45
with loss of body part 941.55
occipital region - *see* Burn, scalp
orbit region 940.1
chemical 940.0
oronasopharynx 947.0
palate 947.0
palm(s) 944.05
with
hand(s) and wrist(s) - *see* Burn,
hand(s), multiple sites
first degree 944.15
second degree 944.25
third degree 944.35
deep 944.45
with loss of a body part 944.55
parietal region - *see* Burn, scalp
penis - *see* Burn, genitourinary organs,
external
perineum - *see* Burn, genitourinary organs,
external
periocular area 940.1
chemical 940.0
pharynx 947.0
pleura 947.1
popliteal space - *see* Burn, knee
prepuce - *see* Burn, genitourinary organs,
external
pubic region - *see* Burn, genitourinary
organs, external
pudenda - *see* Burn, genitourinary organs,
external
rectum 947.3
sac, lacrimal 940.1
chemical 940.0
sacral region - *see* Burn, back
salivary (ducts) (glands) 947.0
scalp 941.06
with
face or neck - *see* Burn, head, multiple
sites
first degree 941.16
second degree 941.26
third degree 941.36
deep 941.46
with loss of body part 941.56
scapular region 943.06
with
upper limb(s), except hand(s) or
wrist(s) - *see* Burn, arm(s),
multiple sites
first degree 943.16
second degree 943.26
third degree 943.36
deep 943.46
with loss of body part 943.56
sclera - *see* Burn, eyeball
scrotum - *see* Burn, genitourinary organs,
external
septum, nasal - *see* Burn, nose
shoulder(s) 943.05
with
hand(s) and wrist(s) - *see* Burn,
multiple, specified sites
upper limb(s), except hand(s) or
wrist(s) - *see* Burn, arm(s),
multiple sites
first degree 943.15
second degree 943.25
third degree 943.35
deep 943.45
with loss of body part 943.55
skin NEC *(see also* Burn, unspecified) 949.0

◀ New   ◀▬ Revised   ~~deleted~~ Deleted   ● Use Additional Digit(s)   ▨ Omit code

Burn *(Continued)*
skull - *see* Burn, head
small intestine 947.3
sternal region - *see* Burn, chest wall
stomach 947.3
subconjunctival - *see* Burn, conjunctiva
subcutaneous - *see* Burn, by site, third degree
submaxillary region - *see* Burn, head
submental region - *see* Burn, chin
sun - *see* Sunburn
supraclavicular fossa - *see* Burn, neck
supraorbital - *see* Burn, forehead
temple - *see* Burn, scalp
temporal region - *see* Burn, scalp
testicle - *see* Burn, genitourinary organs,
    external
testis - *see* Burn, genitourinary organs,
    external
thigh 945.06
    with
        lower limb(s) - *see* Burn, leg, multiple
            sites
        first degree 945.16
        second degree 945.26
        third degree 945.36
            deep 945.46
                with loss of body part 945.56
thorax (external) - *see* Burn, chest wall
throat 947.0
thumb(s) (nail) (subungual) 944.02
    with
        finger(s) - *see* Burn, finger, with other
            sites, thumb
        hand(s) and wrist(s) - *see* Burn,
            hand(s), multiple sites
        first degree 944.12
        second degree 944.22
        third degree 944.32
            deep 944.42
                with loss of body part 944.52
toe (nail) (subungual) 945.01
    with
        lower limb(s) - *see* Burn, leg, multiple
            sites
        first degree 945.11
        second degree 945.21
        third degree 945.31
            deep 945.41
                with loss of body part 945.51
tongue 947.0
tonsil 947.0
trachea 947.1
trunk 942.00
    first degree 942.10
    second degree 942.20
    third degree 942.30
        deep 942.40
            with loss of body part 942.50
    multiple sites 942.09
        first degree 942.19
        second degree 942.29
        third degree 942.39
            deep 942.49
                with loss of body part 942.59

Burn *(Continued)*
trunk *(Continued)*
    specified site NEC 942.09
        first degree 942.19
        second degree 942.29
        third degree 942.39
            deep 942.49
                with loss of body part
                    942.59
tunica vaginalis - *see* Burn, genitourinary
    organs, external
tympanic membrane - *see* Burn, ear
tympanum - *see* Burn, ear
ultraviolet 692.82
unspecified site (multiple) 949.0
    with extent of body surface involved
        specified
        less than 10 percent 948.0 ●
        10–19 percent 948.1 ●
        20–29 percent 948.2 ●
        30–39 percent 948.3 ●
        40–49 percent 948.4 ●
        50–59 percent 948.5 ●
        60–69 percent 948.6 ●
        70–79 percent 948.7 ●
        80–89 percent 948.8 ●
        90 percent or more 948.9 ●
    first degree 949.1
    second degree 949.2
    third degree 949.3
        deep 949.4
            with loss of body part 949.5
uterus 947.4
uvula 947.0
vagina 947.4
vulva - *see* Burn, genitourinary organs,
    external
wrist(s) 944.07
    with
        hand(s) - *see* Burn, hand(s), multiple
            sites
        first degree 944.17
        second degree 944.27
        third degree 944.37
            deep 944.47
                with loss of body part
                    944.57
Burnett's syndrome (milk-alkali)
    275.42
Burnier's syndrome (hypophyseal
    dwarfism) 253.3
Burning
    feet syndrome 266.2
    sensation (*see also* Disturbance, sensation)
        782.0
    tongue 529.6
Burns' disease (osteochondrosis, lower ulna)
    732.3
Bursa - *see also* condition
    pharynx 478.29
Bursitis NEC 727.3
    Achilles tendon 726.71
    adhesive 726.90
        shoulder 726.0

Bursitis NEC *(Continued)*
    ankle 726.79
    buttock 726.5
    calcaneal 726.79
    collateral ligament
        fibular 726.63
        tibial 726.62
    Duplay's 726.2
    elbow 726.33
    finger 726.8
    foot 726.79
    gonococcal 098.52
    hand 726.4
    hip 726.5
    infrapatellar 726.69
    ischiogluteal 726.5
    knee 726.60
    occupational NEC 727.2
    olecranon 726.33
    pes anserinus 726.61
    pharyngeal 478.29
    popliteal 727.51
    prepatellar 726.65
    radiohumeral 727.3
    scapulohumeral 726.19
        adhesive 726.0
    shoulder 726.10
        adhesive 726.0
    subacromial 726.19
        adhesive 726.0
    subcoracoid 726.19
    subdeltoid 726.19
        adhesive 726.0
    subpatellar 726.69
    syphilitic 095.7
    Thornwaldt's, Tornwaldt's (pharyngeal)
        478.29
    toe 726.79
    trochanteric area 726.5
    wrist 726.4
Burst stitches or sutures (complication of
    surgery) (external) (*see also* Dehiscence)
    998.32
    internal 998.31
Buruli ulcer 031.1
Bury's disease (erythema elevatum diutinum)
    695.89
Buschke's disease or scleredema (adultorum)
    710.1
Busquet's disease (osteoperiostitis) (*see also*
    Osteomyelitis) 730.1 ●
Busse-Buschke disease (cryptococcosis)
    117.5
Buttock - *see* condition
Button
    Biskra 085.1
    Delhi 085.1
    oriental 085.1
Buttonhole hand (intrinsic) 736.21
Bwamba fever (encephalitis) 066.3
Byssinosis (occupational) 504
Bywaters' syndrome 958.5

C

Cacergasia 300.9
Cachexia 799.4
    cancerous - *see also* Neoplasm, by site,
        malignant 799.4
    cardiac - *see* Disease, heart
    dehydration 276.51
        with
            hypernatremia 276.0
            hyponatremia 276.1
    due to malnutrition 799.4
    exophthalmic 242.0●
    heart - *see* Disease, heart
    hypophyseal 253.2
    hypopituitary 253.2
    lead 984.9
        specified type of lead - *see* Table of Drugs
            and Chemicals
    malaria 084.9
    malignant *see also* Neoplasm, by site,
        malignant 799.4
    marsh 084.9
    nervous 300.5
    old age 797
    pachydermic - *see* Hypothyroidism
    paludal 084.9
    pituitary (postpartum) 253.2
    renal (*see also* Disease, renal) 593.9
    saturnine 984.9
        specified type of lead - *see* Table of Drugs
            and Chemicals
    senile 797
    Simmonds' (pituitary cachexia) 253.2
    splenica 289.59
    strumipriva (*see also* Hypothyroidism) 244.9
    tuberculous NEC (*see also* Tuberculosis)
        011.9●
Café au lait spots 709.09
Caffey's disease or syndrome (infantile cortical
    hyperostosis) 756.59
Caisson disease 993.3
Caked breast (puerperal, postpartum) 676.2●
Cake kidney 753.3
Calabar swelling 125.2
Calcaneal spur 726.73
Calcaneoapophysitis 732.5
Calcaneonavicular bar 755.67
Calcareous - *see* condition
Calcicosis (occupational) 502
Calciferol (vitamin D) deficiency 268.9
    with
        osteomalacia 268.2
        rickets (*see also* Rickets) 268.0
Calcification
    adrenal (capsule) (gland) 255.41
        tuberculous (*see also* Tuberculosis) 017.6●
    aorta 440.0
    artery (annular) - *see* Arteriosclerosis
    auricle (ear) 380.89
    bladder 596.89
        due to S. hematobium 120.0
    brain (cortex) - *see* Calcification, cerebral
    bronchus 519.19
    bursa 727.82
    cardiac (*see also* Degeneration, myocardial)
        429.1
    cartilage (postinfectional) 733.99
    cerebral (cortex) 348.89
        artery 437.0
    cervix (uteri) 622.8
    choroid plexus 349.2
    conjunctiva 372.54
    corpora cavernosa (penis) 607.89
    cortex (brain) - *see* Calcification, cerebral
    dental pulp (nodular) 522.2
    dentinal papilla 520.4
    disc, intervertebral 722.90
        cervical, cervicothoracic 722.91
        lumbar, lumbosacral 722.93
        thoracic, thoracolumbar 722.92

Calcification (*Continued*)
    fallopian tube 620.8
    falx cerebri - *see* Calcification, cerebral
    fascia 728.89
    gallbladder 575.8
    general 275.40
    heart (*see also* Degeneration, myocardial)
        429.1
        valve - *see* Endocarditis
    intervertebral cartilage or disc
        (postinfectional) 722.90
        cervical, cervicothoracic 722.91
        lumbar, lumbosacral 722.93
        thoracic, thoracolumbar 722.92
    intracranial - *see* Calcification, cerebral
    intraspinal ligament 728.89
    joint 719.80
        ankle 719.87
        elbow 719.82
        foot 719.87
        hand 719.84
        hip 719.85
        knee 719.86
        multiple sites 719.89
        pelvic region 719.85
        shoulder (region) 719.81
        specified site NEC 719.88
        wrist 719.83
    kidney 593.89
        tuberculous (*see also* Tuberculosis)
            016.0●
    larynx (senile) 478.79
    lens 366.8
    ligament 728.89
        intraspinal 728.89
        knee (medial collateral) 717.89
    lung 518.89
        active 518.89
        postinfectional 518.89
        tuberculous (*see also* Tuberculosis,
            pulmonary) 011.9●
    lymph gland or node (postinfectional)
        289.3
        tuberculous (*see also* Tuberculosis, lymph
            gland) 017.2●
    mammographic 793.89
    massive (paraplegic) 728.10
    medial (*see also* Arteriosclerosis, extremities)
        440.20
    meninges (cerebral) 349.2
    metastatic 275.40
    Mönckeberg's - *see* Arteriosclerosis
    muscle 728.10
        heterotopic, postoperative 728.13
    myocardium, myocardial (*see also*
        Degeneration, myocardial) 429.1
    ovary 620.8
    pancreas 577.8
    penis 607.89
    periarticular 728.89
    pericardium (*see also* Pericarditis) 423.8
    pineal gland 259.8
    pleura 511.0
        postinfectional 518.89
        tuberculous (*see also* Tuberculosis, pleura)
            012.0●
    pulp (dental) (nodular) 522.2
    renal 593.89
    Rider's bone 733.99
    sclera 379.16
    semilunar cartilage 717.89
    spleen 289.59
    subcutaneous 709.3
    suprarenal (capsule) (gland) 255.41
    tendon (sheath) 727.82
        with bursitis, synovitis or tenosynovitis
            727.82
    trachea 519.19
    ureter 593.89
    uterus 621.8
    vitreous 379.29

Calcified - *see also* Calcification
    hematoma NEC 959.9
Calcinosis (generalized) (interstitial) (tumoral)
    (universalis) 275.49
    circumscripta 709.3
    cutis 709.3
    intervertebralis 275.49 [722.90]
    Raynaud's phenomenon
        sclerodactylytelangiectasis (CRST)
        710.1
Calciphylaxis (*see also* Calcification, by site)
    275.49
Calcium
    blood
        high (*see also* Hypercalcemia) 275.42
        low (*see also* Hypocalcemia) 275.41
    deposits - *see also* Calcification, by site
        in bursa 727.82
        in tendon (sheath) 727.82
            with bursitis, synovitis or
                tenosynovitis 727.82
    salts or soaps in vitreous 379.22
Calciuria 791.9
Calculi - *see* Calculus
Calculosis, intrahepatic - *see*
    Choledocholithiasis
Calculus, calculi, calculous 592.9
    ampulla of Vater - *see* Choledocholithiasis
    anuria (impacted) (recurrent) 592.0
    appendix 543.9
    bile duct (any) - *see* Choledocholithiasis
    biliary - *see* Cholelithiasis
    bilirubin, multiple - *see* Cholelithiasis
    bladder (encysted) (impacted) (urinary)
        594.1
        diverticulum 594.0
    bronchus 518.89
    calyx (kidney) (renal) 592.0
        congenital 753.3
    cholesterol (pure) (solitary) - *see*
        Cholelithiasis
    common duct (bile) - *see* Choledocholithiasis
    conjunctiva 372.54
    cystic 594.1
        duct - *see* Cholelithiasis
    dental 523.6
        subgingival 523.6
        supragingival 523.6
    epididymis 608.89
    gallbladder - *see also* Cholelithiasis
        congenital 751.69
    hepatic (duct) - *see* Choledocholithiasis
    intestine (impaction) (obstruction) 560.39
    kidney (impacted) (multiple) (pelvis)
        (recurrent) (staghorn) 592.0
        congenital 753.3
    lacrimal (passages) 375.57
    liver (impacted) - *see* Choledocholithiasis
    lung 518.89
    mammographic 793.89
    nephritic (impacted) (recurrent) 592.0
    nose 478.19
    pancreas (duct) 577.8
    parotid gland 527.5
    pelvis, encysted 592.0
    prostate 602.0
    pulmonary 518.89
    renal (impacted) (recurrent) 592.0
        congenital 753.3
    salivary (duct) (gland) 527.5
    seminal vesicle 608.89
    staghorn 592.0
    Stensen's duct 527.5
    sublingual duct or gland 527.5
        congenital 750.26
    submaxillary duct, gland, or region 527.5
    suburethral 594.8
    tonsil 474.8
    tooth, teeth 523.6
    tunica vaginalis 608.89
    ureter (impacted) (recurrent) 592.1

◀ New   ◀· Revised   ~~deleted~~ Deleted   ● Use Additional Digit(s)   ▨ Omit code

Calculus, calculi, calculous *(Continued)*
  urethra (impacted) 594.2
  urinary (duct) (impacted) (passage) (tract) 592.9
    lower tract NEC 594.9
      specified site 594.8
    vagina 623.8
    vesical (impacted) 594.1
    Wharton's duct 527.5
Caliectasis 593.89
California
  disease 114.0
  encephalitis 062.5
Caligo cornea 371.03
Callositas, callosity (infected) 700
Callus (infected) 700
  bone 726.91
  excessive, following fracture - *see also* Late, effect (of), fracture
Calvé (-Perthes) disease (osteochondrosis, femoral capital) 732.1
Calvities *(see also* Alopecia) 704.00
Cameroon fever *(see also* Malaria) 084.6
Camptocormia 300.11
Camptodactyly (congenital) 755.59
Camurati-Engelmann disease (diaphyseal sclerosis) 756.59
Canal - *see* condition
Canaliculitis (lacrimal) (acute) 375.31
  Actinomyces 039.8
  chronic 375.41
Canavan's disease 330.0
Cancer (M8000/3) - *see also* Neoplasm, by site, malignant

Note: The term "cancer" when modified by an adjective or adjectival phrase indicating a morphological type should be coded in the same manner as "carcinoma" with that adjective or phrase. Thus, "squamous-cell cancer" should be coded in the same manner as "squamous-cell carcinoma," which appears in the list under "Carcinoma."

  bile duct type (M8160/3), liver 155.1
  hepatocellular (M8170/3) 155.0
Cancerous (M8000/3) - *see* Neoplasm, by site, malignant
Cancerphobia 300.29
Cancrum oris 528.1
Candidiasis, candidal 112.9
  with pneumonia 112.4
  balanitis 112.2
  congenital 771.7
  disseminated 112.5
  endocarditis 112.81
  esophagus 112.84
  intertrigo 112.3
  intestine 112.85
  lung 112.4
  meningitis 112.83
  mouth 112.0
  nails 112.3
  neonatal 771.7
  onychia 112.3
  otitis externa 112.82
  otomycosis 112.82
  paronychia 112.3
  perionyxis 112.3
  pneumonia 112.4
  pneumonitis 112.4
  skin 112.3
  specified site NEC 112.89
  systemic 112.5
  urogenital site NEC 112.2
  vagina 112.1
  vulva 112.1
  vulvovaginitis 112.1
Candidiosis - *see* Candidiasis
Candiru infection or infestation 136.8

Canities (premature) 704.3
  congenital 757.4
Canker (mouth) (sore) 528.2
  rash 034.1
Cannabinosis 504
Canton fever 081.9
Cap
  cradle 690.11
Capillariasis 127.5
Capillary - *see* condition
Caplan's syndrome 714.81
Caplan-Colinet syndrome 714.81
Capsule - *see* condition
Capsulitis (joint) 726.90
  adhesive (shoulder) 726.0
  hip 726.5
  knee 726.60
  labyrinthine 387.8
  thyroid 245.9
  wrist 726.4
Caput
  crepitus 756.0
  medusae 456.8
  succedaneum 767.19
Carapata disease 087.1
Carate - *see* Pinta
Carbohydrate-deficient glycoprotein syndrome (CDGS) 271.8
Carboxyhemoglobinemia 986
Carbuncle 680.9
  abdominal wall 680.2
  ankle 680.6
  anus 680.5
  arm (any part, above wrist) 680.3
  auditory canal, external 680.0
  axilla 680.3
  back (any part) 680.2
  breast 680.2
  buttock 680.5
  chest wall 680.2
  corpus cavernosum 607.2
  ear (any part) (external) 680.0
  eyelid 373.13
  face (any part, except eye) 680.0
  finger (any) 680.4
  flank 680.2
  foot (any part) 680.7
  forearm 680.3
  genital organ (male) 608.4
  gluteal (region) 680.5
  groin 680.2
  hand (any part) 680.4
  head (any part, except face) 680.8
  heel 680.7
  hip 680.6
  kidney *(see also* Abscess, kidney) 590.2
  knee 680.6
  labia 616.4
  lacrimal
    gland *(see also* Dacryoadenitis) 375.00
    passages (duct) (sac) *(see also* Dacryocystitis) 375.30
  leg, any part except foot 680.6
  lower extremity, any part except foot 680.6
  malignant 022.0
  multiple sites 680.9
  neck 680.1
  nose (external) (septum) 680.0
  orbit, orbital 376.01
  partes posteriores 680.5
  pectoral region 680.2
  penis 607.2
  perineum 680.2
  pinna 680.0
  scalp (any part) 680.8
  scrotum 608.4
  seminal vesicle 608.0
  shoulder 680.3
  skin NEC 680.9
  specified site NEC 680.8
  spermatic cord 608.4

Carbuncle *(Continued)*
  temple (region) 680.0
  testis 608.4
  thigh 680.6
  thumb 680.4
  toe (any) 680.7
  trunk 680.2
  tunica vaginalis 608.4
  umbilicus 680.2
  upper arm 680.3
  urethra 597.0
  vas deferens 608.4
  vulva 616.4
  wrist 680.4
Carbunculus *(see also* Carbuncle) 680.9
Carcinoid (tumor) (M8240/1) - *see* Tumor, carcinoid
Carcinoidosis 259.2
Carcinoma (M8010/3) - *see also* Neoplasm, by site, malignant

Note: Except where otherwise indicated, the morphological varieties of carcinoma in the list below should be coded by site as for "Neoplasm, malignant."

  with
    apocrine metaplasia (M8573/3)
    cartilaginous (and osseous) metaplasia (M8571/3)
    osseous (and cartilaginous) metaplasia (M8571/3)
    productive fibrosis (M8141/3)
    spindle cell metaplasia (M8572/3)
    squamous metaplasia (M8570/3)
  acidophil (M8280/3)
    specified site - *see* Neoplasm, by site, malignant
    unspecified site 194.3
  acidophil-basophil, mixed (M8281/3)
    specified site - *see* Neoplasm, by site, malignant
    unspecified site 194.3
  acinar (cell) (M8550/3)
  acinic cell (M8550/3)
  adenocystic (M8200/3)
  adenoid
    cystic (M8200/3)
    squamous cell (M8075/3)
  adenosquamous (M8560/3)
  adnexal (skin) (M8390/3) - *see* Neoplasm, skin, malignant
  adrenal cortical (M8370/3) 194.0
  alveolar (M8251/3)
    cell (M8250/3) - *see* Neoplasm, lung, malignant
  anaplastic type (M8021/3)
  apocrine (M8401/3)
    breast - *see* Neoplasm, breast, malignant
    specified site NEC - *see* Neoplasm, skin, malignant
    unspecified site 173.99
  basal cell (pigmented) (M8090/3) - *see also* Neoplasm, skin, malignant 173.91
    fibro-epithelial type (M8093/3) - *see* Neoplasm, skin, malignant
    morphea type (M8092/3) - *see* Neoplasm, skin, malignant
    multicentric (M8091/3) - *see* Neoplasm, skin, malignant
  basaloid (M8123/3)
  basal-squamous cell, mixed (M8094/3) - *see* Neoplasm, skin, malignant
  basophil (M8300/3)
    specified site - *see* Neoplasm, by site, malignant
    unspecified site 194.3
  basophil-acidophil, mixed (M8281/3)
    specified site - *see* Neoplasm, by site, malignant
    unspecified site 194.3

Carcinoma (Continued)
  basosquamous (M8094/3) - see Neoplasm,
    skin, malignant
  bile duct type (M8160/3)
    and hepatocellular, mixed (M8180/3)
      155.0
    liver 155.1
    specified site NEC - see Neoplasm, by site,
      malignant
    unspecified site 155.1
  branchial or branchiogenic 146.8
  bronchial or bronchogenic - see Neoplasm,
    lung, malignant
  bronchiolar (terminal) (M8250/3) - see
    Neoplasm, lung, malignant
  bronchiolo-alveolar (M8250/3) - see
    Neoplasm, lung, malignant
  bronchogenic (epidermoid) 162.9
  C cell (M8510/3)
    specified site - see Neoplasm, by site,
      malignant
    unspecified site 193
  ceruminous (M8420/3) 173.29
  chorionic (M9100/3)
    specified site - see Neoplasm, by site,
      malignant
    unspecified site
      female 181
      male 186.9
  chromophobe (M8270/3)
    specified site - see Neoplasm, by site,
      malignant
    unspecified site 194.3
  clear cell (mesonephroid type) (M8310/3)
  cloacogenic (M8124/3)
    specified site - see Neoplasm, by site,
      malignant
    unspecified site 154.8
  colloid (M8480/3)
  cribriform (M8201/3)
  cylindroid type (M8200/3)
  diffuse type (M8145/3)
    specified site - see Neoplasm, by site,
      malignant
    unspecified site 151.9
  duct (cell) (M8500/3)
    with Paget's disease (M8541/3) - see
      Neoplasm, breast, malignant
    infiltrating (M8500/3)
      specified site - see Neoplasm, by site,
        malignant
      unspecified site 174.9
  ductal (M8500/3)
  ductular, infiltrating (M8521/3)
  embryonal (M9070/3)
    and teratoma, mixed (M9081/3)
    combined with choriocarcinoma
      (M9101/3) - see Neoplasm, by site,
      malignant
    infantile type (M9071/3)
    liver 155.0
    polyembryonal type (M9072/3)
  endometrioid (M8380/3)
  eosinophil (M8280/3)
    specified site - see Neoplasm, by site,
      malignant
    unspecified site 194.3
  epidermoid (M8070/3) - see also Carcinoma,
    squamous cell
    and adenocarcinoma, mixed (M8560/3)
    in situ, Bowen's type (M8081/2) - see
      Neoplasm, skin, in situ
    intradermal - see Neoplasm, skin,
      in situ
  fibroepithelial type basal cell (M8093/3) - see
    Neoplasm, skin, malignant
  follicular (M8330/3)
    and papillary (mixed) (M8340/3) 193
    moderately differentiated type (M8332/3)
      193
    pure follicle type (M8331/3) 193

Carcinoma (Continued)
  follicular (Continued)
    specified site - see Neoplasm, by site,
      malignant
    trabecular type (M8332/3) 193
    unspecified site 193
    well differentiated type (M8331/3)
      193
  gelatinous (M8480/3)
  giant cell (M8031/3)
    and spindle cell (M8030/3)
  granular cell (M8320/3)
  granulosa cell (M8620/3) 183.0
  hepatic cell (M8170/3) 155.0
  hepatocellular (M8170/3) 155.0
    and bile duct, mixed (M8180/3)
      155.0
  hepatocholangiolitic (M8180/3) 155.0
  Hürthle cell (thyroid) 193
  hypernephroid (M8311/3)
  in
    adenomatous
      polyp (M8210/3)
      polyposis coli (M8220/3) 153.9
    pleomorphic adenoma (M8940/3)
    polypoid adenoma (M8210/3)
    situ (M8010/3) - see Carcinoma, in situ
    tubular adenoma (M8210/3)
    villous adenoma (M8261/3)
  infiltrating duct (M8500/3)
    with Paget's disease (M8541/3) - see
      Neoplasm, breast, malignant
    specified site - see Neoplasm, by site,
      malignant
    unspecified site 174.9
  inflammatory (M8530/3)
    specified site - see Neoplasm, by site,
      malignant
    unspecified site 174.9
  in situ (M8010/2) - see also Neoplasm, by site,
    in situ
    epidermoid (M8070/2) - see also
      Neoplasm, by site, in situ
      with questionable stromal invasion
        (M8076/2)
        specified site - see Neoplasm, by
          site, in situ
        unspecified site 233.1
      Bowen's type (M8081/2) - see
        Neoplasm, skin, in situ
    intraductal (M8500/2)
      specified site - see Neoplasm, by site, in
        situ
      unspecified site 233.0
    lobular (M8520/2)
      specified site - see Neoplasm, by site, in
        situ
      unspecified site 233.0
    papillary (M8050/2) - see Neoplasm, by
      site, in situ
    squamous cell (M8070/2) - see also
      Neoplasm, by site, in situ
      with questionable stromal invasion
        (M8076/2)
        specified site - see Neoplasm, by
          site, in situ
        unspecified site 233.1
    transitional cell (M8120/2) - see
      Neoplasm, by site, in situ
  intestinal type (M8144/3)
    specified site - see Neoplasm, by site,
      malignant
    unspecified site 151.9
  intraductal (noninfiltrating) (M8500/2)
    papillary (M8503/2)
      specified site - see Neoplasm, by site, in
        situ
      unspecified site 233.0
    specified site - see Neoplasm, by site, in
      situ
    unspecified site 233.0

Carcinoma (Continued)
  intraepidermal (M8070/2) - see also
    Neoplasm, skin, in situ
    squamous cell, Bowen's type (M8081/2) -
      see Neoplasm, skin, in situ
  intraepithelial (M8010/2) - see also
    Neoplasm, by site, in situ
    squamous cell (M8072/2) - see Neoplasm,
      by site, in situ
  intraosseous (M9270/3) 170.1
    upper jaw (bone) 170.0
  islet cell (M8150/3)
    and exocrine, mixed (M8154/3)
      specified site - see Neoplasm, by site,
        malignant
      unspecified site 157.9
    pancreas 157.4
    specified site NEC - see Neoplasm, by site,
      malignant
    unspecified site 157.4
  juvenile, breast (M8502/3) - see Neoplasm,
    breast, malignant
  Kulchitsky's cell (carcinoid tumor of
    intestine) 259.2
  large cell (M8012/3)
    squamous cell, non-keratinizing type
      (M8072/3)
  Leydig cell (testis) (M8650/3)
    specified site - see Neoplasm, by site,
      malignant
    unspecified site 186.9
      female 183.0
      male 186.9
  liver cell (M8170/3) 155.0
  lobular (infiltrating) (M8520/3)
    noninfiltrating (M8520/2)
      specified site - see Neoplasm, by site, in
        situ
      unspecified site 233.0
    specified site - see Neoplasm, by site,
      malignant
    unspecified site 174.9
  lymphoepithelial (M8082/3)
  medullary (M8510/3)
    with
      amyloid stroma (M8511/3)
        specified site - see Neoplasm, by
          site, malignant
        unspecified site 193
      lymphoid stroma (M8512/3)
        specified site - see Neoplasm, by
          site, malignant
        unspecified site 174.9
  Merkel cell 209.36
    buttock 209.36
    ear 209.31
    eyelid, including canthus 209.31
    face 209.31
    genitals 209.36
    lip 209.31
    lower limb 209.34
    neck 209.32
    nodal presentation 209.75
    scalp 209.32
    secondary (any site) 209.75
    specified site NEC 209.36
    trunk 209.35
    unknown primary site 209.75
    upper limb 209.33
    visceral metastatic presentation 209.75
  mesometanephric (M9110/3)
  mesonephric (M9110/3)
  metastatic (M8010/6) - see Metastasis, cancer
  metatypical (M8095/3) - see Neoplasm, skin,
    malignant
  morphea type basal cell (M8092/3) - see
    Neoplasm, skin, malignant
  mucinous (M8480/3)
  mucin-producing (M8481/3)
  mucin-secreting (M8481/3)
  mucoepidermoid (M8430/3)

◀ New   ◀◀ Revised   ~~deleted~~ Deleted   ● Use Additional Digit(s)   ▓ Omit code

Carcinoma *(Continued)*
  mucoid (M8480/3)
    cell (M8300/3)
      specified site - *see* Neoplasm, by site,
        malignant
      unspecified site 194.3
  mucous (M8480/3)
  neuroendocrine
    high grade (M8240/3) 209.30
    malignant poorly differentiated
      (M8240/3) 209.30
  nonencapsulated sclerosing (M8350/3)
    193
  noninfiltrating
    intracystic (M8504/2) - *see* Neoplasm, by
      site, in situ
    intraductal (M8500/2)
      papillary (M8503/2)
        specified site - *see* Neoplasm, by
          site, in situ
        unspecified site 233.0
      specified site - *see* Neoplasm, by site, in
        situ
      unspecified site 233.0
    lobular (M8520/2)
      specified site - *see* Neoplasm, by site, in
        situ
      unspecified site 233.0
  oat cell (M8042/3)
    specified site - *see* Neoplasm, by site,
      malignant
    unspecified site 162.9
  odontogenic (M9270/3) 170.1
    upper jaw (bone) 170.0
  onocytic (M8290/3)
  oxyphilic (M8290/3)
  papillary (M8050/3)
    and follicular (mixed) (M8340/3) 193
    epidermoid (M8052/3)
    intraductal (noninfiltrating) (M8503/2)
      specified site - *see* Neoplasm, by site, in
        situ
      unspecified site 233.0
    serous (M8460/3)
      specified site - *see* Neoplasm, by site,
        malignant
      surface (M8461/3)
        specified site - *see* Neoplasm, by
          site, malignant
        unspecified site 183.0
      unspecified site 183.0
    squamous cell (M8052/3)
    transitional cell (M8130/3)
  papillocystic (M8450/3)
    specified site - *see* Neoplasm, by site,
      malignant
    unspecified site 183.0
  parafollicular cell (M8510/3)
    specified site - *see* Neoplasm, by site,
      malignant
    unspecified site 193
  pleomorphic (M8022/3)
  polygonal cell (M8034/3)
  prickle cell (M8070/3)
  pseudoglandular, squamous cell (M8075/3)
  pseudomucinous (M8470/3)
    specified site - *see* Neoplasm, by site,
      malignant
    unspecified site 183.0
  pseudosarcomatous (M8033/3)
  regaud type (M8082/3) - *see* Neoplasm,
    nasopharynx, malignant
  renal cell (M8312/3) 189.0
  reserve cell (M8041/3)
  round cell (M8041/3)
  Schmincke (M8082/3) - *see* Neoplasm,
    nasopharynx, malignant
  Schneiderian (M8121/3)
    specified site - *see* Neoplasm, by site,
      malignant
    unspecified site 160.0

Carcinoma *(Continued)*
  scirrhous (M8141/3)
  sebaceous (M8410/3) - *see* Neoplasm, skin,
    malignant
  secondary (M8010/6) - *see* Neoplasm, by site,
    malignant, secondary
  secretory, breast (M8502/3) - *see* Neoplasm,
    breast, malignant
  serous (M8441/3)
    papillary (M8460/3)
      specified site - *see* Neoplasm, by site,
        malignant
      unspecified site 183.0
    surface, papillary (M8461/3)
      specified site - *see* Neoplasm, by site,
        malignant
      unspecified site 183.0
  Sertoli cell (M8640/3)
    specified site - *see* Neoplasm, by site,
      malignant
    unspecified site 186.9
  signet ring cell (M8490/3)
    metastatic (M8490/6) - *see* Neoplasm, by
      site, secondary
  simplex (M8231/3)
  skin appendage (M8390/3) - *see* Neoplasm,
    skin, malignant
  small cell (M8041/3)
    fusiform cell type (M8043/3)
    squamous cell, nonkeratinizing type
      (M8073/3)
  solid (M8230/3)
    with amyloid stroma (M8511/3)
      specified site - *see* Neoplasm, by site,
        malignant
      unspecified site 193
  spheroidal cell (M8035/3)
  spindle cell (M8032/3)
    and giant cell (M8030/3)
  spinous cell (M8070/3)
  squamous (cell) (M8070/3)
    adenoid type (M8075/3)
    and adenocarcinoma, mixed
      (M8560/3)
    intraepidermal, Bowen's type - *see*
      Neoplasm, skin, in situ
    keratinizing type (large cell)
      (M8071/3)
    large cell, nonkeratinizing type
      (M8072/3)
    microinvasive (M8076/3)
      specified site - *see* Neoplasm, by site,
        malignant
      unspecified site 180.9
    nonkeratinizing type (M8072/3)
    papillary (M8052/3)
    pseudoglandular (M8075/3)
    skin (*see also* Neoplasm, skin, malignant)
      173.92
    small cell, nonkeratinizing type
      (M8073/3)
    spindle cell type (M8074/3)
    verrucous (M8051/3)
  superficial spreading (M8143/3)
  sweat gland (M8400/3) - *see* Neoplasm, skin,
    malignant
  theca cell (M8600/3) 183.0
  thymic (M8580/3) 164.0
  trabecular (M8190/3)
  transitional (cell) (M8120/3)
    papillary (M8130/3)
    spindle cell type (M8122/3)
  tubular (M8211/3)
  undifferentiated type (M8020/3)
  urothelial (M8120/3)
  ventriculi 151.9
  verrucous (epidermoid) (squamous cell)
    (M8051/3)
  villous (M8262/3)
  water-clear cell (M8322/3) 194.1
  wolffian duct (M9110/3)

Carcinomaphobia 300.29
Carcinomatosis
  peritonei (M8010/6) 197.6
  specified site NEC (M8010/3) - *see*
    Neoplasm, by site, malignant
  unspecified site (M8010/6) 199.0
Carcinosarcoma (M8980/3) - *see also* Neoplasm,
  by site, malignant
  embryonal type (M8981/3) - *see* Neoplasm,
    by site, malignant
Cardia, cardial - *see* condition
Cardiac - *see also* condition
  death - *see* Disease, heart
  device
    defibrillator, automatic implantable (with
      synchronous cardiac pacemaker)
      V45.02
    in situ NEC V45.00
    pacemaker
      cardiac
        fitting or adjustment V53.31
        in situ V45.01
      carotid sinus
        fitting or adjustment V53.39
        in situ V45.09
  pacemaker - *see* Cardiac, device, pacemaker
  tamponade 423.3
Cardialgia (*see also* Pain, precordial) 786.51
Cardiectasis - *see* Hypertrophy, cardiac
Cardiochalasia 530.81
Cardiomalacia (*see also* Degeneration,
  myocardial) 429.1
Cardiomegalia glycogenica diffusa 271.0
Cardiomegaly (*see also* Hypertrophy, cardiac)
  429.3
  congenital 746.89
  glycogen 271.0
  hypertensive (*see also* Hypertension, heart)
    402.90
  idiopathic 425.4
Cardiomyoliposis (*see also* Degeneration,
  myocardial) 429.1
Cardiomyopathy (congestive) (constrictive)
  (familial) (infiltrative) (obstructive)
  (restrictive) (sporadic) 425.4
  alcoholic 425.5
  amyloid 277.39 [425.7]
  beriberi 265.0 [425.7]
  cobalt-beer 425.5
  congenital 425.3
  due to
    amyloidosis 277.39 [425.7]
    beriberi 265.0 [425.7]
    cardiac glycogenosis 271.0 [425.7]
    Chagas' disease 086.0
    Friedreich's ataxia 334.0 [425.8]
    hypertension - *see* Hypertension, with,
      heart involvement
    mucopolysaccharidosis 277.5 [425.7]
    myotonia atrophica 359.21 [425.8]
    progressive muscular dystrophy 359.1
      [425.8]
    sarcoidosis 135 [425.8]
  glycogen storage 271.0 [425.7]
  hypertensive - *see* Hypertension, with, heart
    involvement
  hypertrophic 425.18
    nonobstructive 425.18
    obstructive 425.11
      congenital 746.84
  idiopathic (concentric) 425.4
  in
    Chagas' disease 086.0
    sarcoidosis 135 [425.8]
  ischemic 414.8
  metabolic NEC 277.9 [425.7]
    amyloid 277.39 [425.7]
    thyrotoxic (*see also* Thyrotoxicosis) 242.9●
      [425.7]
    thyrotoxicosis (*see also* Thyrotoxicosis)
      242.9● [425.7]

Cardiomyopathy (Continued)
  newborn 425.4
    congenital 425.3
  nutritional 269.9 [425.7]
    beriberi 265.0 [425.7]
  obscure of Africa 425.2
  peripartum 674.5●
  postpartum 674.5●
  primary 425.4
  secondary 425.9
  stress induced 429.83
  takotsubo 429.83
  thyrotoxic (see also Thyrotoxicosis) 242.9●
    [425.7]
  toxic NEC 425.9
  tuberculous (see also Tuberculosis) 017.9●
    [425.8]
Cardionephritis - see Hypertension, cardiorenal
Cardionephropathy - see Hypertension, cardiorenal
Cardionephrosis - see Hypertension, cardiorenal
Cardioneurosis 306.2
Cardiopathia nigra 416.0
Cardiopathy (see also Disease, heart) 429.9
  hypertensive (see also Hypertension, heart) 402.90
  idiopathic 425.4
  mucopolysaccharidosis 277.5 [425.7]
Cardiopericarditis (see also Pericarditis) 423.9
Cardiophobia 300.29
Cardioptosis 746.87
Cardiorenal - see condition
Cardiorrhexis (see also Infarct, myocardium) 410.9●
Cardiosclerosis - see Arteriosclerosis, coronary
Cardiosis - see Disease, heart
Cardiospasm (esophagus) (reflex) (stomach) 530.0
  congenital 750.7
Cardiostenosis - see Disease, heart
Cardiosymphysis 423.1
Cardiothyrotoxicosis - see Hyperthyroidism
Cardiovascular - see condition
Carditis (acute) (bacterial) (chronic) (subacute) 429.89
  Coxsackie 074.20
  hypertensive (see also Hypertension, heart) 402.90
  meningococcal 036.40
  rheumatic - see Disease, heart, rheumatic
  rheumatoid 714.2
Care (of)
  child (routine) V20.1
  convalescent following V66.9
    chemotherapy V66.2
    medical NEC V66.5
    psychotherapy V66.3
    radiotherapy V66.1
    surgery V66.0
    surgical NEC V66.0
    treatment (for) V66.5
      combined V66.6
      fracture V66.4
      mental disorder NEC V66.3
      specified type NEC V66.5
  end-of-life V66.7
  family member (handicapped) (sick)
    creating problem for family V61.49
    provided away from home for holiday relief V60.5
    unavailable, due to
      absence (person rendering care) (sufferer) V60.4
      inability (any reason) of person rendering care V60.4
  holiday relief V60.5
  hospice V66.7
  lack of (at or after birth) (infant) (child) 995.52
    adult 995.84

Care (Continued)
  lactation of mother V24.1
  palliative V66.7
  postpartum
    immediately after delivery V24.0
    routine follow-up V24.2
  prenatal V22.1
    first pregnancy V22.0
    high-risk pregnancy V23.9
      inconclusive fetal viability V23.87
      specified problem NEC V23.89
  terminal V66.7
  unavailable, due to
    absence of person rendering care V60.4
    inability (any reason) of person rendering care V60.4
  well baby V20.1
Caries (bone) (see also Tuberculosis, bone) 015.9● [730.8]●
  arrested 521.04
  cementum 521.03
  cerebrospinal (tuberculous) 015.0● [730.88]
  dental (acute) (chronic) (incipient) (infected) 521.00
    with pulp exposure 521.03
    extending to
      dentine 521.02
      pulp 521.03
    other specified NEC 521.09
    pit and fissure 521.06
    primary
      pit and fissure origin 521.06
      root surface 521.08
      smooth surface origin 521.07
    root surface 521.08
    smooth surface 521.07
  dentin (acute) (chronic) 521.02
  enamel (acute) (chronic) (incipient) 521.01
  external meatus 380.89
  hip (see also Tuberculosis) 015.1● [730.85]
  initial 521.01
  knee 015.2● [730.86]
  labyrinth 386.8
  limb NEC 015.7● [730.88]
  mastoid (chronic) (process) 383.1
  middle ear 385.89
  nose 015.7● [730.88]
  orbit 015.7● [730.88]
  ossicle 385.24
  petrous bone 383.20
  sacrum (tuberculous) 015.0● [730.88]
  spine, spinal (column) (tuberculous) 015.0● [730.88]
  syphilitic 095.5
    congenital 090.0 [730.8]●
  teeth (internal) 521.00
    initial 521.01
  vertebra (column) (tuberculous) 015.0● [730.88]
Carini's syndrome (ichthyosis congenita) 757.1
Carious teeth 521.00
Carneous mole 631.8
Carnosinemia 270.5
Carotid body or sinus syndrome 337.01
Carotidynia 337.01
Carotinemia (dietary) 278.3
Carotinosis (cutis) (skin) 278.3
Carpal tunnel syndrome 354.0
Carpenter's syndrome 759.89
Carpopedal spasm (see also Tetany) 781.7
Carpoptosis 736.05
Carrier (suspected) of
  amebiasis V02.2
  bacterial disease (meningococcal, staphylococcal) NEC V02.59
  cholera V02.0
  cystic fibrosis gene V83.81
  defective gene V83.89
  diphtheria V02.4
  dysentery (bacillary) V02.3
    amebic V02.2

Carrier (Continued)
  Endamoeba histolytica V02.2
  gastrointestinal pathogens NEC V02.3
  genetic defect V83.89
  gonorrhea V02.7
  group B streptococcus V02.51
  HAA (hepatitis Australian-antigen) V02.61
  hemophilia A (asymptomatic) V83.01
    symptomatic V83.02
  hepatitis V02.60
    Australian-antigen (HAA) V02.61
    B V02.61
    C V02.62
    specified type NEC V02.69
    serum V02.61
    viral V02.60
  infective organism NEC V02.9
  malaria V02.9
  paratyphoid V02.3
  Salmonella V02.3
    typhosa V02.1
  serum hepatitis V02.61
  Shigella V02.3
  Staphylococcus NEC V02.59
    methicillin
      resistant Staphylococcus aureus V02.54
      susceptible Staphylococcus aureus V02.53
  Streptococcus NEC V02.52
    group B V02.51
  typhoid V02.1
  venereal disease NEC V02.8
Carrión's disease (Bartonellosis) 088.0
Car sickness 994.6
Carter's
  relapsing fever (Asiatic) 087.0
Cartilage - see condition
Caruncle (inflamed)
  abscess, lacrimal (see also Dacryocystitis) 375.30
  conjunctiva 372.00
    acute 372.00
  eyelid 373.00
  labium (majus) (minus) 616.89
  lacrimal 375.30
  urethra (benign) 599.3
  vagina (wall) 616.89
Cascade stomach 537.6
Caseation lymphatic gland (see also Tuberculosis) 017.2●
Caseous
  bronchitis - see Tuberculosis, pulmonary
  meningitis 013.0●
  pneumonia - see Tuberculosis, pulmonary
Cassidy (-Scholte) syndrome (malignant carcinoid) 259.2
Castellani's bronchitis 104.8
Castleman's tumor or lymphoma (mediastinal lymph node hyperplasia) 785.6
Castration, traumatic 878.2
  complicated 878.3
Casts in urine 791.7
Cat's ear 744.29
Catalepsy 300.11
  catatonic (acute) (see also Schizophrenia) 295.2●
  hysterical 300.11
  schizophrenic (see also Schizophrenia) 295.2●
Cataphasia (see also Disorder, fluency) 315.35
Cataplexy (idiopathic) see also Narcolepsy
Cataract (anterior cortical) (anterior polar) (black) (capsular) (central) (cortical) (hypermature) (immature) (incipient) (mature) 366.9
  anterior
    and posterior axial embryonal 743.33
    pyramidal 743.31
    subcapsular polar
      infantile, juvenile, or presenile 366.01
      senile 366.13

◀ New   ◀▥ Revised   ~~deleted~~ Deleted   ● Use Additional Digit(s)   ▨ Omit code

Cataract *(Continued)*
  associated with
    calcinosis 275.40 *[366.42]*
    craniofacial dysostosis 756.0 *[366.44]*
    galactosemia 271.1 *[366.44]*
    hypoparathyroidism 252.1 *[366.42]*
    myotonic disorders 359.21 *[366.43]*
    neovascularization 366.33
  blue dot 743.39
  cerulean 743.39
  complicated NEC 366.30
  congenital 743.30
    capsular or subcapsular 743.31
    cortical 743.32
    nuclear 743.33
    specified type NEC 743.39
    total or subtotal 743.34
    zonular 743.32
  coronary (congenital) 743.39
    acquired 366.12
  cupuliform 366.14
  diabetic 250.5● *[366.41]*
    due to secondary diabetes 249.5● *[366.41]*
  drug-induced 366.45
  due to
    chalcosis 360.24 *[366.34]*
    chronic choroiditis *(see also* Choroiditis)
        363.20 *[366.32]*
    degenerative myopia 360.21 *[366.34]*
    glaucoma *(see also* Glaucoma) 365.9 *[366.31]*
    infection, intraocular NEC 366.32
    inflammatory ocular disorder NEC 366.32
    iridocyclitis, chronic 364.10 *[366.33]*
    pigmentary retinal dystrophy 362.74
        [366.34]
    radiation 366.46
  electric 366.46
  glassblowers' 366.46
  heat ray 366.46
  heterochromic 366.33
  in eye disease NEC 366.30
  infantile *(see also* Cataract, juvenile) 366.00
  intumescent 366.12
  irradiational 366.46
  juvenile 366.00
    anterior subcapsular polar 366.01
    combined forms 366.09
    cortical 366.03
    lamellar 366.03
    nuclear 366.04
    posterior subcapsular polar 366.02
    specified NEC 366.09
    zonular 366.03
  lamellar 743.32
    infantile juvenile, or presenile 366.03
  morgagnian 366.18
  myotonic 359.21 *[366.43]*
  myxedema 244.9 *[366.44]*
        nuclear 366.16
  posterior, polar (capsular) 743.31
    infantile, juvenile, or presenile 366.02
    senile 366.14
  presenile *(see also* Cataract, juvenile) 366.00
  punctate
    acquired 366.12
    congenital 743.39
  secondary (membrane) 366.50
    obscuring vision 366.53
    specified type, not obscuring vision 366.52
  senile 366.10
    anterior subcapsular polar 366.13
    combined forms 366.19
    cortical 366.15
    hypermature 366.18
    immature 366.12
    incipient 366.12
    mature 366.17
    nuclear 366.16
    posterior subcapsular polar 366.14
    specified NEC 366.19
    total or subtotal 366.17

Cataract *(Continued)*
  snowflake 250.5● *[366.41]*
    due to secondary diabetes 249.5● *[366.41]*
  specified NEC 366.8
  subtotal (senile) 366.17
    congenital 743.34
  sunflower 360.24 *[366.34]*
  tetanic NEC 252.1 *[366.42]*
  total (mature) (senile) 366.17
    congenital 743.34
    localized 366.21
    traumatic 366.22
  toxic 366.45
  traumatic 366.20
    partially resolved 366.23
    total 366.22
  zonular (perinuclear) 743.32
    infantile, juvenile, or presenile 366.03
Cataracta 366.10
  brunescens 366.16
  cerulea 743.39
  complicata 366.30
  congenita 743.30
  coralliformis 743.39
  coronaria (congenital) 743.39
    acquired 366.12
  diabetic 250.5● *[366.41]*
    due to secondary diabetes 249.5●
        [366.41]
  floriformis 360.24 *[366.34]*
  membranacea
    accreta 366.50
    congenita 743.39
  nigra 366.16
Catarrh, catarrhal (inflammation) *(see also*
        condition) 460
  acute 460
  asthma, asthmatic *(see also* Asthma) 493.9●
  Bostock's *(see also* Fever, hay) 477.9
  bowel - *see* Enteritis
  bronchial 490
    acute 466.0
    chronic 491.0
    subacute 466.0
  cervix, cervical (canal) (uteri) - *see* Cervicitis
  chest *(see also* Bronchitis) 490
  chronic 472.0
  congestion 472.0
  conjunctivitis 372.03
  due to syphilis 095.9
    congenital 090.0
  enteric - *see* Enteritis
  epidemic *(see also* Influenza) 487.1
  Eustachian 381.50
  eye (acute) (vernal) 372.03
  fauces *(see also* Pharyngitis) 462
  febrile 460
  fibrinous acute 466.0
  gastroenteric - *see* Enteritis
  gastrointestinal - *see* Enteritis
  gingivitis 523.00
  hay *(see also* Fever, hay) 477.9
  infectious 460
  intestinal - *see* Enteritis
  larynx *(see also* Laryngitis, chronic) 476.0
  liver 070.1
    with hepatic coma 070.0
  lung *(see also* Bronchitis) 490
    acute 466.0
    chronic 491.0
  middle ear (chronic) - *see* Otitis media,
        chronic
  mouth 528.00
  nasal (chronic) *(see also* Rhinitis) 472.0
    acute 460
  nasobronchial 472.2
  nasopharyngeal (chronic) 472.2
    acute 460
  nose - *see* Catarrh, nasal
  ophthalmia 372.03
  pneumococcal, acute 466.0

Catarrh, catarrhal *(Continued)*
  pulmonary *(see also* Bronchitis) 490
    acute 466.0
    chronic 491.0
  spring (eye) 372.13
  suffocating *(see also* Asthma) 493.9●
  summer (hay) *(see also* Fever, hay) 477.9
  throat 472.1
  tracheitis 464.10
    with obstruction 464.11
  tubotympanal 381.4
    acute *(see also* Otitis media, acute,
        nonsuppurative) 381.00
    chronic 381.10
  vasomotor *(see also* Fever, hay) 477.9
  vesical (bladder) - *see* Cystitis
Catarrhus aestivus *(see also* Fever, hay) 477.9
Catastrophe, cerebral *(see also* Disease,
        cerebrovascular, acute) 436
Catatonia, catatonic (acute) 781.99
  with
    affective psychosis - *see* Psychosis, affective
  agitation 295.2●
  dementia (praecox) 295.2●
  due to or associated with physical condition
        293.89
  excitation 295.2●
  excited type 295.2●
  in conditions classified elsewhere 293.89
  schizophrenia 295.2●
  stupor 295.2●
Cat-scratch - *see also* Injury, superficial
  disease or fever 078.3
Cauda equina - *see also* condition
  syndrome 344.60
Cauliflower ear 738.7
Caul over face 768.9
Causalgia 355.9
  lower limb 355.71
  upper limb 354.4
Cause
  external, general effects NEC 994.9
  not stated 799.9
  unknown 799.9
Caustic burn - *see also* Burn, by site
  from swallowing caustic or corrosive
        substance - *see* Burn, internal organs
Cavare's disease (familial periodic paralysis)
        359.3
Cave-in, injury
  crushing (severe) *(see also* Crush, by site)
        869.1
  suffocation 994.7
Cavernitis (penis) 607.2
  lymph vessel - *see* Lymphangioma
Cavernositis 607.2
Cavernous - *see* condition
Cavitation of lung *(see also* Tuberculosis) 011.2●
  nontuberculous 518.89
  primary, progressive 010.8●
Cavity
  lung - *see* Cavitation of lung
  optic papilla 743.57
  pulmonary - *see* Cavitation of lung
  teeth 521.00
  vitreous (humor) 379.21
Cavovarus foot, congenital 754.59
Cavus foot (congenital) 754.71
  acquired 736.73
Cazenave's
  disease (pemphigus) NEC 694.4
  lupus (erythematosus) 695.4
CDGS (carbohydrate-deficient glycoprotein
        syndrome) 271.8
Cecitis - *see* Appendicitis
Cecocele - *see* Hernia
Cecum - *see* condition
Celiac
  artery compression syndrome 447.4
  disease 579.0
  infantilism 579.0

Cell, cellular - *see also* condition
  anterior chamber (eye) (positive aqueous ray) 364.04
Cellulitis (diffuse) (with lymphangitis) (*see also* Abscess) 682.9
  abdominal wall 682.2
  anaerobic (*see also* Gas gangrene) 040.0
  ankle 682.6
  anus 566
  areola 611.0
  arm (any part, above wrist) 682.3
  auditory canal (external) 380.10
  axilla 682.3
  back (any part) 682.2
  breast 611.0
    postpartum 675.1●
  broad ligament (*see also* Disease, pelvis, inflammatory) 614.4
    acute 614.3
  buttock 682.5
  cervical (neck region) 682.1
  cervix (uteri) (*see also* Cervicitis) 616.0
  cheek, external 682.0
    internal 528.3
  chest wall 682.2
  chronic NEC 682.9
  colostomy 569.61
  corpus cavernosum 607.2
  digit 681.9
  Douglas' cul-de-sac or pouch (chronic) (*see also* Disease, pelvis, inflammatory) 614.4
    acute 614.3
  drainage site (following operation) 998.59
  ear, external 380.10
  enterostomy 569.61
  erysipelar (*see also* Erysipelas) 035
  esophagostomy 530.86
  eyelid 373.13
  face (any part, except eye) 682.0
  finger (intrathecal) (periosteal) (subcutaneous) (subcuticular) 681.00
  flank 682.2
  foot (except toe) 682.7
  forearm 682.3
  gangrenous (*see also* Gangrene) 785.4
  genital organ NEC
    female - *see* Abscess, genital organ, female
    male 608.4
  glottis 478.71
  gluteal (region) 682.5
  gonococcal NEC 098.0
  groin 682.2
  hand (except finger or thumb) 682.4
  head (except face) NEC 682.8
  heel 682.7
  hip 682.6
  jaw (region) 682.0
  knee 682.6
  labium (majus) (minus) (*see also* Vulvitis) 616.10
  larynx 478.71
  leg, except foot 682.6
  lip 528.5
  mammary gland 611.0
  mouth (floor) 528.3
  multiple sites NEC 682.9
  nasopharynx 478.21
  navel 682.2
    newborn NEC 771.4
  neck (region) 682.1
  nipple 611.0
  nose 478.19
    external 682.0
  orbit, orbital 376.01
  palate (soft) 528.3
  pectoral (region) 682.2
  pelvis, pelvic
    with
      abortion - *see* Abortion, by type, with sepsis

Cellulitis (Continued)
  pelvis, pelvic (Continued)
    with (Continued)
      ectopic pregnancy (*see also* categories 633.0–633.9) 639.0
      molar pregnancy (*see also* categories 630–632) 639.0
    female (*see also* Disease, pelvis, inflammatory) 614.4
      acute 614.3
    following
      abortion 639.0
      ectopic or molar pregnancy 639.0
    male 567.21
    puerperal, postpartum, childbirth 670.8●
  penis 607.2
  perineal, perineum 682.2
  perirectal 566
  peritonsillar 475
  periurethral 597.0
  periuterine (*see also* Disease, pelvis, inflammatory) 614.4
    acute 614.3
  pharynx 478.21
  phlegmonous NEC 682.9
  rectum 566
  retromammary 611.0
  retroperitoneal (*see also* Peritonitis) 567.38
  round ligament (*see also* Disease, pelvis, inflammatory) 614.4
    acute 614.3
  scalp (any part) 682.8
    dissecting 704.8
  scrotum 608.4
  seminal vesicle 608.0
  septic NEC 682.9
  shoulder 682.3
  specified sites NEC 682.8
  spermatic cord 608.4
  submandibular (region) (space) (triangle) 682.0
    gland 527.3
  submaxillary 528.3
    gland 527.3
  submental (pyogenic) 682.0
    gland 527.3
  suppurative NEC 682.9
  testis 608.4
  thigh 682.6
  thumb (intrathecal) (periosteal) (subcutaneous) (subcuticular) 681.00
  toe (intrathecal) (periosteal) (subcutaneous) (subcuticular) 681.10
  tonsil 475
  trunk 682.2
  tuberculous (primary) (*see also* Tuberculosis) 017.0●
  tunica vaginalis 608.4
  umbilical 682.2
    newborn NEC 771.4
  vaccinal 999.39
  vagina - *see* Vaginitis
  vas deferens 608.4
  vocal cords 478.5
  vulva (*see also* Vulvitis) 616.10
  wrist 682.4
Cementoblastoma, benign (M9273/0) 213.1
  upper jaw (bone) 213.0
Cementoma (M9273/0) 213.1
  gigantiform (M9275/0) 213.1
    upper jaw (bone) 213.0
  upper jaw (bone) 213.0
Cementoperiostitis 523.40
  acute 523.33
  apical 523.40
Cephalgia, cephalagia (*see also* Headache) 784.0
  histamine 339.00
  nonorganic origin 307.81
  other trigeminal autonomic (TACS) 339.09
  psychogenic 307.81
  tension 307.81

Cephalhematocele, cephalematocele
  due to birth injury 767.19
  fetus or newborn 767.19
  traumatic (*see also* Contusion, head) 920
Cephalhematoma, cephalematoma (calcified)
  due to birth injury 767.19
  fetus or newborn 767.19
  traumatic (*see also* Contusion, head) 920
Cephalic - *see* condition
Cephalitis - *see* Encephalitis
Cephalocele 742.0
Cephaloma - *see* Neoplasm, by site, malignant
Cephalomenia 625.8
Cephalopelvic - *see* condition
Cercomoniasis 007.3
Cerebellitis - *see* Encephalitis
Cerebellum (cerebellar) - *see* condition
Cerebral - *see* condition
Cerebritis - *see* Encephalitis
Cerebrohepatorenal syndrome 759.89
Cerebromacular degeneration 330.1
Cerebromalacia (*see also* Softening, brain) 348.89
  due to cerebrovascular accident 438.89
Cerebrosidosis 272.7
Cerebrospasticity - *see* Palsy, cerebral
Cerebrospinal - *see* condition
Cerebrum - *see* condition
Ceroid storage disease 272.7
Cerumen (accumulation) (impacted) 380.4
Cervical - *see also* condition
  auricle 744.43
  high risk human papillomavirus (HPV) DNA test positive 795.05
  intraepithelial glandular neoplasia 233.1
  low risk human papillomavirus (HPV) DNA test positive 795.09
  rib 756.2
  shortening - *see* Short, cervical
Cervicalgia 723.1
Cervicitis (acute) (chronic) (nonvenereal) (subacute) (with erosion or ectropion) 616.0
  with
    abortion - *see* Abortion, by type, with sepsis
    ectopic pregnancy (*see also* categories 633.0-633.9) 639.0
    molar pregnancy (*see also* categories 630-632) 639.0
    ulceration 616.0
  chlamydial 099.53
  complicating pregnancy or puerperium 646.6●
    affecting fetus or newborn 760.8
  following
    abortion 639.0
    ectopic or molar pregnancy 639.0
  gonococcal (acute) 098.15
    chronic or duration of 2 months or more 098.35
  senile (atrophic) 616.0
  syphilitic 095.8
  trichomonal 131.09
  tuberculous (*see also* Tuberculosis) 016.7●
Cervicoaural fistula 744.49
Cervicocolpitis (emphysematosa) (*see also* Cervicitis) 616.0
Cervix - *see* condition
Cesarean delivery, operation or section NEC 669.7●
  affecting fetus or newborn 763.4
  (planned) occurring after 37 completed weeks of gestation but before 39 completed weeks gestation due to (spontaneous) onset of labor 649.8●
  post mortem, affecting fetus or newborn 761.6
  previous, affecting management of pregnancy 654.2●
Céstan's syndrome 344.89
Céstan-Chenais paralysis 344.89

Céstan-Raymond syndrome 433.8●
Cestode infestation NEC 123.9
   specified type NEC 123.8
Cestodiasis 123.9
CGF (congenital generalized fibromatosis) 759.89
Chabert's disease 022.9
Chacaleh 266.2
Chafing 709.8
Chagas' disease (see also Trypanosomiasis, American) 086.2
   with heart involvement 086.0
Chagres fever 084.0
Chalasia (cardiac sphincter) 530.81
Chalazion 373.2
Chalazoderma 757.39
Chalcosis 360.24
   cornea 371.15
   crystalline lens 360.24 [366.34]
   retina 360.24
Chalicosis (occupational) (pulmonum) 502
Chancre (any genital site) (hard) (indurated) (infecting) (primary) (recurrent) 091.0
   congenital 090.0
   conjunctiva 091.2
   Ducrey's 099.0
   extragenital 091.2
   eyelid 091.2
   Hunterian 091.0
   lip (syphilis) 091.2
   mixed 099.8
   nipple 091.2
   Nisbet's 099.0
   of
      carate 103.0
      pinta 103.0
      yaws 102.0
   palate, soft 091.2
   phagedenic 099.0
   Ricord's 091.0
   Rollet's (syphilitic) 091.0
   seronegative 091.0
   seropositive 091.0
   simple 099.0
   soft 099.0
      bubo 099.0
   urethra 091.0
   yaws 102.0
Chancriform syndrome 114.1
Chancroid 099.0
   anus 099.0
   penis (Ducrey's bacillus) 099.0
   perineum 099.0
   rectum 099.0
   scrotum 099.0
   urethra 099.0
   vulva 099.0
Chandipura fever 066.8
Chandler's disease (osteochondritis dissecans, hip) 732.7
Change(s) (of) - see also Removal of
   arteriosclerotic - see Arteriosclerosis
   battery
      cardiac pacemaker V53.31
   bone 733.90
      diabetic 250.8● [731.8]
         due to secondary diabetes 249.8● [731.8]
      in disease, unknown cause 733.90
   bowel habits 787.99
   cardiorenal (vascular) (see also Hypertension, cardiorenal) 404.90
   cardiovascular - see Disease, cardiovascular
   circulatory 459.9
   cognitive or personality change of other type, nonpsychotic 310.1
   color, teeth, tooth
      during formation 520.8
      extrinsic 523.6
      intrinsic posteruptive 521.7
   contraceptive device V25.42

Change(s) (Continued)
   cornea, corneal
      degenerative NEC 371.40
      membrane NEC 371.30
      senile 371.41
   coronary (see also Ischemia, heart) 414.9
   degenerative
      chamber angle (anterior) (iris) 364.56
      ciliary body 364.57
      spine or vertebra (see also Spondylosis) 721.90
   dental pulp, regressive 522.2
   drains V58.49
   dressing
      wound V58.30
         nonsurgical V58.30
         surgical V58.31
   fixation device V54.89
      external V54.89
      internal V54.01
   heart - see also Disease, heart
   hip joint 718.95
   hyperplastic larynx 478.79
   hypertrophic
      nasal sinus (see also Sinusitis) 473.9
      turbinate, nasal 478.0
      upper respiratory tract 478.9
   inflammatory - see Inflammation
   joint (see also Derangement, joint) 718.90
      sacroiliac 724.6
   Kirschner wire V54.89
   knee 717.9
   macular, congenital 743.55
   malignant (M----/3) - see also Neoplasm, by site, malignant

> Note: For malignant change occurring in a neoplasm, use the appropriate M code with behavior digit/3 e.g., malignant change in uterine fibroid-M8890/3. For malignant change occurring in a nonneoplastic condition (e.g., gastric ulcer) use the M code M8000/3.

   mental (status) NEC 780.97
      due to or associated with physical condition - see Syndrome, brain
   myocardium, myocardial - see Degeneration, myocardial
   of life (see also Menopause) 627.2
   pacemaker battery (cardiac) V53.31
   peripheral nerve 355.9
   personality (nonpsychotic) NEC 310.1
   plaster cast V54.89
   refractive, transient 367.81
   regressive, dental pulp 522.2
   retina 362.9
      myopic (degenerative) (malignant) 360.21
      vascular appearance 362.13
   sacroiliac joint 724.6
   scleral 379.19
      degenerative 379.16
   senile (see also Senility) 797
   sensory (see also Disturbance, sensation) 782.0
   skin texture 782.8
   spinal cord 336.9
   splint, external V54.89
   subdermal implantable contraceptive V25.5
   suture V58.32
   traction device V54.89
   trophic 355.9
      arm NEC 354.9
      leg NEC 355.8
      lower extremity NEC 355.8
      upper extremity NEC 354.9
   vascular 459.9
   vasomotor 443.9
   voice 784.49
      psychogenic 306.1

Change(s) (Continued)
   wound packing V58.30
      nonsurgical V58.30
      surgical V58.31
Changing sleep-work schedule, affecting sleep 327.36
Changuinola fever 066.0
Chapping skin 709.8
Character
   depressive 301.12
Charcôt's
   arthropathy 094.0 [713.5]
   cirrhosis - see Cirrhosis, biliary
   disease 094.0
      spinal cord 094.0
   fever (biliary) (hepatic) (intermittent) - see Choledocholithiasis
   joint (disease) 094.0 [713.5]
      diabetic 250.6● [713.5]
         due to secondary diabetes 249.6● [713.5]
      syringomyelic 336.0 [713.5]
   syndrome (intermittent claudication) 443.9
      due to atherosclerosis 440.21
Charcôt-Marie-Tooth disease, paralysis, or syndrome 356.1
CHARGE association (syndrome) 759.89
Charleyhorse (quadriceps) 843.8
   muscle, except quadriceps - see Sprain, by site
Charlouis' disease (see also Yaws) 102.9
Chauffeur's fracture - see Fracture, ulna, lower end
Cheadle (-Möller) (-Barlow) disease or syndrome (infantile scurvy) 267
Checking (of)
   contraceptive device (intrauterine) V25.42
   device
      fixation V54.89
         external V54.89
         internal V54.09
      traction V54.89
   Kirschner wire V54.89
   plaster cast V54.89
   splint, external V54.89
Checkup
   following treatment - see Examination
   health V70.0
   infant (over 28 days old) (not sick) V20.2
   newborn, routine
      8 to 28 days old V20.32
      over 28 days old, routine V20.2
      under 8 days old V20.31
      weight V20.32
   pregnancy (normal) V22.1
      first V22.0
      high-risk pregnancy V23.9
         inconclusive fetal viability V23.87
         specified problem NEC V23.89
Chédiak-Higashi (-Steinbrinck) anomaly, disease, or syndrome (congenital gigantism of peroxidase granules) 288.2
Cheek - see also condition
   biting 528.9
Cheese itch 133.8
Cheese washers' lung 495.8
Cheilitis 528.5
   actinic (due to sun) 692.72
      chronic NEC 692.74
         due to radiation, except from sun 692.82
      due to radiation, except from sun 692.82
   acute 528.5
   angular 528.5
   catarrhal 528.5
   chronic 528.5
   exfoliative 528.5
   gangrenous 528.5
   glandularis apostematosa 528.5
   granulomatosa 351.8
   infectional 528.5

Cheilitis (Continued)
    membranous 528.5
    Miescher's 351.8
    suppurative 528.5
    ulcerative 528.5
    vesicular 528.5
Cheilodynia 528.5
Cheilopalatoschisis (see also Cleft, palate, with
        cleft lip) 749.20
Cheilophagia 528.9
Cheiloschisis (see also Cleft, lip) 749.10
Cheilosis 528.5
    with pellagra 265.2
    angular 528.5
    due to
        dietary deficiency 266.0
        vitamin deficiency 266.0
Cheiromegaly 729.89
Cheiropompholyx 705.81
Cheloid (see also Keloid) 701.4
Chemical burn - see also Burn, by site
    from swallowing chemical - see Burn,
        internal organs
Chemodectoma (M8693/1) - see Paraganglioma,
    nonchromaffin
Chemoprophylaxis NEC V07.39
Chemosis, conjunctiva 372.73
Chemotherapy
    convalescence V66.2
    encounter (for) (oral) (intravenous)
        V58.11
    maintenance (oral) (intravenous)
        V58.11
    prophylactic NEC V07.39
        fluoride V07.31
Cherubism 526.89
Chest - see condition
Cheyne-Stokes respiration (periodic) 786.04
Chiari's
    disease or syndrome (hepatic vein
            thrombosis) 453.0
    malformation
        type I 348.4
        type II (see also Spina bifida) 741.0●
        type III 742.0
        type IV 742.2
        network 746.89
Chiari-Frommel syndrome 676.6●
Chicago disease (North American
        blastomycosis) 116.0
Chickenpox (see also Varicella) 052.9
    exposure to V01.71
    vaccination and inoculation (prophylactic)
        V05.4
Chiclero ulcer 085.4
Chiggers 133.8
Chignon 111.2
    fetus or newborn (from vacuum extraction)
        767.19
Chigoe disease 134.1
Chikungunya fever 066.3
Chilaiditi's syndrome (subphrenic
        displacement, colon) 751.4
Chilblains 991.5
    lupus 991.5
Child
    behavior causing concern V61.20
        adopted child V61.24
        biological child V61.23
        foster child V61.25
Childbed fever 670.8●
Childbirth - see also Delivery
    puerperal complications - see Puerperal
Childhood, period of rapid growth V21.0
Chill(s) 780.64
    with fever 780.60
    without fever 780.64
    congestive 780.99
        in malarial regions 084.6
    septic - see Septicemia
    urethral 599.84

Chilomastigiasis 007.8
Chin - see condition
Chinese dysentery 004.9
Chiropractic dislocation (see also Lesion,
        nonallopathic, by site) 739.9
Chitral fever 066.0
Chlamydia, chlamydial - see condition
Chloasma 709.09
    cachecticorum 709.09
    eyelid 374.52
        congenital 757.33
        hyperthyroid 242.0●
    gravidarum 646.8●
    idiopathic 709.09
    skin 709.09
    symptomatic 709.09
Chloroma (M9930/3) 205.3●
Chlorosis 280.9
    Egyptian (see also Ancylostomiasis) 126.9
    miners' (see also Ancylostomiasis) 126.9
Chlorotic anemia 280.9
Chocolate cyst (ovary) 617.1
Choked
    disk or disc - see Papilledema
    on food, phlegm, or vomitus NEC (see also
        Asphyxia, food) 933.1
    phlegm 933.1
    while vomiting NEC (see also Asphyxia,
        food) 933.1
Chokes (resulting from bends) 993.3
Choking sensation 784.99
Cholangiectasis (see also Disease, gallbladder)
        575.8
Cholangiocarcinoma (M8160/3)
    and hepatocellular carcinoma, combined
        (M8180/3) 155.0
    liver 155.1
    specified site NEC - see Neoplasm, by site,
        malignant
    unspecified site 155.1
Cholangiohepatitis 575.8
    due to fluke infestation 121.1
Cholangiohepatoma (M8180/3) 155.0
Cholangiolitis (acute) (chronic) (extrahepatic)
        (gangrenous) 576.1
    intrahepatic 575.8
    paratyphoidal (see also Fever, paratyphoid)
        002.9
    typhoidal 002.0
Cholangioma (M8160/0) 211.5
    malignant - see Cholangiocarcinoma
Cholangitis (acute) (ascending) (catarrhal)
        (chronic) (infective) (malignant) (primary)
        (recurrent) (sclerosing) (secondary)
        (stenosing) (suppurative) 576.1
    chronic nonsuppurative destructive
        571.6
    nonsuppurative destructive (chronic)
        571.6
Cholecystdocholithiasis - see
        Choledocholithiasis
Cholecystitis 575.10
    with
        calculus, stones in
            bile duct (common) (hepatic) - see
                Choledocholithiasis
            gallbladder - see Cholelithiasis
        acute 575.0
        acute and chronic 575.12
        chronic 575.11
        emphysematous (acute) (see also
            Cholecystitis, acute) 575.0
        gangrenous (see also Cholecystitis, acute)
            575.0
        paratyphoidal, current (see also Fever,
            paratyphoid) 002.9
        suppurative (see also Cholecystitis, acute)
            575.0
        typhoidal 002.0
Choledochitis (suppurative) 576.1
Choledocholith - see Choledocholithiasis

Choledocholithiasis 574.5●

> Note: Use the following fifth-digit
> subclassification with category 574:
>
> 0   without mention of obstruction
> 1   with obstruction

    with
        cholecystitis 574.4●
            acute 574.3●
            chronic 574.4●
        cholelithiasis 574.9●
            with
                cholecystitis 574.7●
                    acute 574.6●
                        and chronic 574.8●
                    chronic 574.7●
Cholelithiasis (impacted) (multiple) 574.2●

> Note: Use the following fifth-digit
> subclassification with category 574:
>
> 0   without mention of obstruction
> 1   with obstruction

    with
        cholecystitis 574.1●
            acute 574.0●
            chronic 574.1●
        choledocholithiasis 574.9●
            with
                cholecystitis 574.7●
                    acute 574.6●
                        and chronic 574.8●
                    chronic cholecystitis 574.7●
Cholemia (see also Jaundice) 782.4
    familial 277.4
    Gilbert's (familial nonhemolytic) 277.4
Cholemic gallstone - see Cholelithiasis
Choleperitoneum, choleperitonitis (see also
        Disease, gallbladder) 567.81
Cholera (algid) (Asiatic) (asphyctic) (epidemic)
        (gravis) (Indian) (malignant) (morbus)
        (pestilential) (spasmodic) 001.9
    antimonial 985.4
    carrier (suspected) of V02.0
    classical 001.0
    contact V01.0
    due to
        Vibrio
            cholerae (Inaba, Ogawa, Hikojima
                serotypes) 001.0
            el Tor 001.1
    el Tor 001.1
    exposure to V01.0
    vaccination, prophylactic (against) V03.0
Cholerine (see also Cholera) 001.9
Cholestasis 576.8
    due to total parenteral nutrition (TPN) 573.8
Cholesteatoma (ear) 385.30
    attic (primary) 385.31
    diffuse 385.35
    external ear (canal) 380.21
    marginal (middle ear) 385.32
        with involvement of mastoid cavity
            385.33
        secondary (with middle ear involvement)
            385.33
    mastoid cavity 385.30
    middle ear (secondary) 385.32
        with involvement of mastoid cavity
            385.33
    postmastoidectomy cavity (recurrent) 383.32
    primary 385.31
    recurrent, postmastoidectomy cavity 383.32
    secondary (middle ear) 385.32
        with involvement of mastoid cavity
            385.33
Cholesteatosis (middle ear) (see also
        Cholesteatoma) 385.30
    diffuse 385.35
Cholesteremia 272.0

◀ New   ◀▦ Revised   ~~deleted~~ Deleted   ● Use Additional Digit(s)   ▨ Omit code

Cholesterin
  granuloma, middle ear 385.82
  in vitreous 379.22
Cholesterol
  deposit
    retina 362.82
    vitreous 379.22
  elevated (high) 272.0
    with elevated (high) triglycerides 272.2
  imbibition of gallbladder (see also Disease,
    gallbladder) 575.6
Cholesterolemia 272.0
  essential 272.0
  familial 272.0
  hereditary 272.0
Cholesterosis, cholesterolosis (gallbladder)
    575.6
  with
    cholecystitis - see Cholecystitis
    cholelithiasis - see Cholelithiasis
  middle ear (see also Cholesteatoma) 385.30
Cholocolic fistula (see also Fistula, gallbladder)
    575.5
Choluria 791.4
Chondritis (purulent) 733.99
  auricle 380.03
  costal 733.6
    Tietze's 733.6
  patella, posttraumatic 717.7
  pinna 380.03
  posttraumatica patellae 717.7
  tuberculous (active) (see also Tuberculosis)
    015.9●
    intervertebral 015.0● [730.88]
Chondroangiopathia calcarea seu punctate
    756.59
Chondroblastoma (M9230/0) - see also
    Neoplasm, bone, benign
  malignant (M9230/3) - see Neoplasm, bone,
    malignant
Chondrocalcinosis (articular) (crystal
    deposition) (dihydrate) (see also Arthritis,
    due to, crystals) 275.49 [712.3]●
  due to
    calcium pyrophosphate 275.49 [712.2]●
    dicalcium phosphate crystals 275.49
      [712.1]●
    pyrophosphate crystals 275.49 [712.2]●
Chondrodermatitis nodularis helicis 380.00
Chondrodysplasia 756.4
  angiomatose 756.4
  calcificans congenita 756.59
  epiphysialis punctata 756.59
  hereditary deforming 756.4
  rhizomelic punctata 277.86
Chondrodystrophia (fetalis) 756.4
  calcarea 756.4
  calcificans congenita 756.59
  fetalis hypoplastica 756.59
  hypoplastica calcinosa 756.59
  punctata 756.59
  tarda 277.5
Chondrodystrophy (familial) (hypoplastic)
    756.4
  myotonic (congenital) 359.23
Chondroectodermal dysplasia 756.55
Chondrolysis 733.99
Chondroma (M9220/0) - see also Neoplasm,
    cartilage, benign
  juxtacortical (M9221/0) - see Neoplasm,
    bone, benign
  periosteal (M9221/0) - see Neoplasm, bone,
    benign
Chondromalacia 733.92
  epiglottis (congenital) 748.3
  generalized 733.92
  knee 717.7
  larynx (congenital) 748.3
  localized, except patella 733.92
  patella, patellae 717.7
  systemic 733.92

Chondromalacia (Continued)
  tibial plateau 733.92
  trachea (congenital) 748.3
Chondromatosis (M9220/1) - see Neoplasm,
    cartilage, uncertain behavior
Chondromyxosarcoma (M9220/3) - see
    Neoplasm, cartilage, malignant
Chondro-osteodysplasia (Morquio-Brailsford
    type) 277.5
Chondro-osteodystrophy 277.5
Chondro-osteoma (M9210/0) - see Neoplasm,
    bone, benign
Chondropathia tuberosa 733.6
Chondrosarcoma (M9220/3) - see also
    Neoplasm, cartilage, malignant
  juxtacortical (M9221/3) - see Neoplasm,
    bone, malignant
  mesenchymal (M9240/3) - see Neoplasm,
    connective tissue, malignant
Chordae tendineae rupture (chronic) 429.5
Chordee (nonvenereal) 607.89
  congenital 752.63
  gonococcal 098.2
Chorditis (fibrinous) (nodosa) (tuberosa)
    478.5
Chordoma (M9370/3) - see Neoplasm, by site,
    malignant
Chorea (gravis) (minor) (spasmodic) 333.5
  with
    heart involvement - see Chorea with
      rheumatic heart disease
    rheumatic heart disease (chronic, inactive,
      or quiescent) (conditions classifiable
      to 393–398) - see- rheumatic heart
      condition involved,
      active or acute (conditions classifiable
        to 391) 392.0
  acute - see Chorea, Sydenham's
  apoplectic (see also Disease, cerebrovascular,
    acute) 436
  chronic 333.4
  electric 049.8
  gravidarum - see Eclampsia, pregnancy
  habit 307.22
  hereditary 333.4
  Huntington's 333.4
  posthemiplegic 344.89
  pregnancy - see Eclampsia, pregnancy
  progressive 333.4
    chronic 333.4
    hereditary 333.4
  rheumatic (chronic) 392.9
    with heart disease or involvement - see
      Chorea, with rheumatic heart
      disease
  senile 333.5
  Sydenham's 392.9
    with heart involvement - see Chorea, with
      rheumatic heart disease
    nonrheumatic 333.5
  variabilis 307.23
Choreoathetosis (paroxysmal) 333.5
Chorioadenoma (destruens) (M9100/1) 236.1
Chorioamnionitis 658.4●
  affecting fetus or newborn 762.7
Chorioangioma (M9120/0) 219.8
Choriocarcinoma (M9100/3)
  combined with
    embryonal carcinoma (M9101/3) - see
      Neoplasm, by site, malignant
    teratoma (M9101/3) - see Neoplasm, by
      site, malignant
  specified site - see Neoplasm, by site,
    malignant
  unspecified site
    female 181
    male 186.9
Chorioencephalitis, lymphocytic (acute)
    (serous) 049.0
Chorioepithelioma (M9100/3) - see
    Choriocarcinoma

Choriomeningitis (acute) (benign)
    (lymphocytic) (serous) 049.0
Chorionepithelioma (M9100/3) - see
    Choriocarcinoma
Chorionitis (see also Scleroderma) 710.1
Chorioretinitis 363.20
  disseminated 363.10
    generalized 363.13
    in
      neurosyphilis 094.83
      secondary syphilis 091.51
    peripheral 363.12
    posterior pole 363.11
    tuberculous (see also Tuberculosis) 017.3●
      [363.13]
  due to
    histoplasmosis (see also Histoplasmosis)
      115.92
    toxoplasmosis (acquired) 130.2
      congenital (active) 771.2
  focal 363.00
    juxtapapillary 363.01
    peripheral 363.04
    posterior pole NEC 363.03
  juxtapapillaris, juxtapapillary 363.01
  progressive myopia (degeneration) 360.21
  syphilitic (secondary) 091.51
    congenital (early) 090.0 [363.13]
      late 090.5 [363.13]
    late 095.8 [363.13]
  tuberculous (see also Tuberculosis) 017.3●
    [363.13]
Choristoma - see Neoplasm, by site, benign
Choroid - see condition
Choroideremia, choroidermia (initial stage)
    (late stage) (partial or total atrophy)
    363.55
Choroiditis (see also Chorioretinitis) 363.20
  leprous 030.9 [363.13]
  senile guttate 363.41
  sympathetic 360.11
  syphilitic (secondary) 091.51
    congenital (early) 090.0 [363.13]
      late 090.5 [363.13]
    late 095.8 [363.13]
  Tay's 363.41
  tuberculous (see also Tuberculosis) 017.3●
    [363.13]
Choroidopathy NEC 363.9
  degenerative (see also Degeneration, choroid)
    363.40
  hereditary (see also Dystrophy, choroid)
    363.50
  specified type NEC 363.8
Choroidoretinitis - see Chorioretinitis
Choroidosis, central serous 362.41
Choroidretinopathy, serous 362.41
Christian's syndrome (chronic histiocytosis X)
    277.89
Christian-Weber disease (nodular
    nonsuppurative panniculitis) 729.30
Christmas disease 286.1
Chromaffinoma (M8700/0) - see also Neoplasm,
    by site, benign
  malignant (M8700/3) - see Neoplasm, by site,
    malignant
Chromatopsia 368.59
Chromhidrosis, chromidrosis 705.89
Chromoblastomycosis 117.2
Chromomycosis 117.2
Chromophytosis 111.0
Chromotrichomycosis 111.8
Chronic - see condition
Churg-Strauss syndrome 446.4
Chyle cyst, mesentery 457.8
Chylocele (nonfilarial) 457.8
  filarial (see also Infestation, filarial) 125.9
  tunica vaginalis (nonfilarial) 608.84
    filarial (see also Infestation, filarial) 125.9
Chylomicronemia (fasting) (with
    hyperprebetalipoproteinemia) 272.3

Chylopericardium (acute) 420.90
Chylothorax (nonfilarial) 457.8
  filarial (*see also* Infestation, filarial) 125.9
Chylous
  ascites 457.8
  cyst of peritoneum 457.8
  hydrocele 603.9
  hydrothorax (nonfilarial) 457.8
    filarial (*see also* Infestation, filarial) 125.9
Chyluria 791.1
  bilharziasis 120.0
  due to
    Brugia (malayi) 125.1
    Wuchereria (bancrofti) 125.0
      malayi 125.1
  filarial (*see also* Infestation, filarial) 125.9
  filariasis (*see also* Infestation, filarial) 125.9
  nonfilarial 791.1
Cicatricial (deformity) - *see* Cicatrix
Cicatrix (adherent) (contracted) (painful)
    (vicious) 709.2
  adenoid 474.8
  alveolar process 525.8
  anus 569.49
  auricle 380.89
  bile duct (*see also* Disease, biliary) 576.8
  bladder 596.89
  bone 733.99
  brain 348.89
  cervix (postoperative) (postpartal) 622.3
    in pregnancy or childbirth 654.6●
      causing obstructed labor 660.2●
  chorioretinal 363.30
    disseminated 363.35
    macular 363.32
    peripheral 363.34
    posterior pole NEC 363.33
  choroid - *see* Cicatrix, chorioretinal
  common duct (*see also* Disease, biliary) 576.8
  congenital 757.39
  conjunctiva 372.64
  cornea 371.00
    tuberculous (*see also* Tuberculosis) 017.3●
      [371.05]
  duodenum (bulb) 537.3
  esophagus 530.3
  eyelid 374.46
    with
      ectropion - *see* Ectropion
      entropion - *see* Entropion
  hypopharynx 478.29
  knee, semilunar cartilage 717.5
  lacrimal
    canaliculi 375.53
    duct
      acquired 375.56
      neonatal 375.55
    punctum 375.52
    sac 375.54
  larynx 478.79
  limbus (cystoid) 372.64
  lung 518.89
  macular 363.32
    disseminated 363.35
    peripheral 363.34
  middle ear 385.89
  mouth 528.9
  muscle 728.89
  nasolacrimal duct
    acquired 375.56
    neonatal 375.55
  nasopharynx 478.29
  palate (soft) 528.9
  penis 607.89
  prostate 602.8
  rectum 569.49
  retina 363.30
    disseminated 363.35
    macular 363.32
    peripheral 363.34
    posterior pole NEC 363.33

Cicatrix (*Continued*)
  semilunar cartilage - *see* Derangement,
    meniscus
  seminal vesicle 608.89
  skin 709.2
    infected 686.8
    postinfectional 709.2
    tuberculous (*see also* Tuberculosis)
      017.0●
  specified site NEC 709.2
  throat 478.29
  tongue 529.8
  tonsil (and adenoid) 474.8
  trachea 478.9
  tuberculous NEC (*see also* Tuberculosis)
    011.9●
  ureter 593.89
  urethra 599.84
  uterus 621.8
  vagina 623.4
    in pregnancy or childbirth
      654.7●
      causing obstructed labor
        660.2●
  vocal cord 478.5
  wrist, constricting (annular) 709.2
CIDP (chronic inflammatory demyelinating
    polyneuropathy) 357.81
CIN I (cervical intraepithelial neoplasia I)
    622.11
CIN II (cervical intraepithelial neoplasia II)
    622.12
CIN III (cervical intraepithelial neoplasia III)
    233.1
Cinchonism
  correct substance properly administered
    386.9
  overdose or wrong substance given or taken
    961.4
Circine herpes 110.5
Circle of Willis - *see* condition
Circular - *see also* condition
  hymen 752.49
Circulating anticoagulants, antibodies, or
    inhibitors (*see also* Anticoagulants)
    286.59
  extrinsic 287.8
  following childbirth 666.3●
  intrinsic, causing hemorrhagic disorder
    286.59
    with
      acquired hemophilia 286.52
      antiphospholipid antibody
        286.53
  postpartum 666.3●
Circulation
  collateral (venous), any site 459.89
  defective 459.9
    congenital 747.9
    lower extremity 459.89
  embryonic 747.9
  failure 799.89
    fetus or newborn 779.89
    peripheral 785.59
  fetal, persistent 747.83
  heart, incomplete 747.9
Circulatory system - *see* condition
Circulus senilis 371.41
Circumcision
  in absence of medical indication
    V50.2
  ritual V50.2
  routine V50.2
Circumscribed - *see* condition
Circumvallata placenta - *see* Placenta,
    abnormal
Cirrhosis, cirrhotic 571.5
  with alcoholism 571.2
  alcoholic (liver) 571.2
  atrophic (of liver) - *see* Cirrhosis, portal
  Baumgarten-Cruveilhier 571.5

Cirrhosis, cirrhotic (*Continued*)
  biliary (cholangiolitic) (cholangitic)
      (cholestatic) (extrahepatic)
      (hypertrophic) (intrahepatic)
      (nonobstructive) (obstructive)
      (pericholangiolitic) (posthepatic)
      (primary) (secondary) (xanthomatous)
      571.6
    due to
      clonorchiasis 121.1
      flukes 121.3
  brain 331.9
  capsular - *see* Cirrhosis, portal
  cardiac 571.5
    alcoholic 571.2
  central (liver) - *see* Cirrhosis, liver
  Charcôt's 571.6
  cholangiolitic - *see* Cirrhosis, biliary
  cholangitic - *see* Cirrhosis, biliary
  cholestatic - *see* Cirrhosis, biliary
  clitoris (hypertrophic) 624.2
  coarsely nodular 571.5
  congestive (liver) - *see* Cirrhosis, cardiac
  Cruveilhier-Baumgarten 571.5
  cryptogenic (of liver) 571.5
    alcoholic 571.2
  dietary (*see also* Cirrhosis, portal) 571.5
  due to
    bronzed diabetes 275.01
    congestive hepatomegaly - *see* Cirrhosis,
      cardiac
    cystic fibrosis 277.00
    hemochromatosis (*see also*
      Hemochromatosis) 275.03
    hepatolenticular degeneration 275.1
    passive congestion (chronic) - *see*
      Cirrhosis, cardiac
    Wilson's disease 275.1
    xanthomatosis 272.2
  extrahepatic (obstructive) - *see* Cirrhosis,
    biliary
  fatty 571.8
    alcoholic 571.0
  florid 571.2
  Glisson's - *see* Cirrhosis, portal
  Hanot's (hypertrophic) - *see* Cirrhosis,
    biliary
  hepatic - *see* Cirrhosis, liver
  hepatolienal - *see* Cirrhosis, liver
  hobnail - *see* Cirrhosis, portal
  hypertrophic - *see also* Cirrhosis, liver
    biliary - *see* Cirrhosis, biliary
    Hanot's - *see* Cirrhosis, biliary
  infectious NEC - *see* Cirrhosis, portal
  insular - *see* Cirrhosis, portal
  intrahepatic (obstructive) (primary)
      (secondary) - *see* Cirrhosis, biliary
  juvenile (*see also* Cirrhosis, portal) 571.5
  kidney (*see also* Sclerosis, renal) 587
  Laennec's (of liver) 571.2
    nonalcoholic 571.5
  liver (chronic) (hepatolienal) (hypertrophic)
      (nodular) (splenomegalic) (unilobar)
      571.5
    with alcoholism 571.2
    alcoholic 571.2
    congenital (due to failure of obliteration
      of umbilical vein) 777.8
    cryptogenic 571.5
      alcoholic 571.2
    fatty 571.8
      alcoholic 571.0
    macronodular 571.5
      alcoholic 571.2
    micronodular 571.5
      alcoholic 571.2
    nodular, diffuse 571.5
      alcoholic 571.2
    pigmentary 275.01
    portal 571.5
      alcoholic 571.2

◄ New ◄▪ Revised ~~deleted~~ Deleted ● Use Additional Digit(s) ▨ Omit code

Cirrhosis, cirrhotic (Continued)
  liver (Continued)
    postnecrotic 571.5
      alcoholic 571.2
      syphilitic 095.3
    lung (chronic) (see also Fibrosis, lung) 515
    macronodular (of liver) 571.5
      alcoholic 571.2
    malarial 084.9
    metabolic NEC 571.5
    micronodular (of liver) 571.5
      alcoholic 571.2
    monolobular - see Cirrhosis, portal
    multilobular - see Cirrhosis, portal
    nephritis (see also Sclerosis, renal) 587
    nodular - see Cirrhosis, liver
    nutritional (fatty) 571.5
    obstructive (biliary) (extrahepatic)
      (intrahepatic) - see Cirrhosis, biliary
    ovarian 620.8
    paludal 084.9
    pancreas (duct) 577.8
    pericholangiolitic - see Cirrhosis, biliary
    periportal - see Cirrhosis, portal
    pigment, pigmentary (of liver) 275.01
    portal (of liver) 571.5
      alcoholic 571.2
    posthepatitic (see also Cirrhosis, postnecrotic) 571.5
    postnecrotic (of liver) 571.5
      alcoholic 571.2
    primary (intrahepatic) - see Cirrhosis, biliary
    pulmonary (see also Fibrosis, lung) 515
    renal (see also Sclerosis, renal) 587
    septal (see also Cirrhosis, postnecrotic) 571.5
    spleen 289.51
    splenomegalic (of liver) - see Cirrhosis, liver
    stasis (liver) - see Cirrhosis, liver
    stomach 535.4●
    Todd's (see also Cirrhosis, biliary) 571.6
    toxic (nodular) - see Cirrhosis, postnecrotic
    trabecular - see Cirrhosis, postnecrotic
    unilobar - see Cirrhosis, liver
    vascular (of liver) - see Cirrhosis, liver
    xanthomatous (biliary) (see also Cirrhosis, biliary) 571.6
      due to xanthomatosis (familial) (metabolic) (primary) 272.2
Cistern, subarachnoid 793.0
Citrullinemia 270.6
Citrullinuria 270.6
Ciuffini-Pancoast tumor (M8010/3) (carcinoma, pulmonary apex) 162.3
Civatte's disease or poikiloderma 709.09
CJD (Creutzfeldt-Jakob disease) 046.19
  variant (vCJD) 046.11
CLABSI (central line-associated bloodstream infection) 999.32
Clam diggers' itch 120.3
Clap - see Gonorrhea
Clark's paralysis 343.9
Clarke-Hadfield syndrome (pancreatic infantilism) 577.8
Clastothrix 704.2
Claude's syndrome 352.6
Claude Bernard-Horner syndrome (see also Neuropathy, peripheral, autonomic) 337.9
Claudication, intermittent 443.9
  cerebral (artery) (see also Ischemia, cerebral, transient) 435.9
  due to atherosclerosis 440.21
  spinal cord (arteriosclerotic) 435.1
    syphilitic 094.89
  spinalis 435.1
  venous (axillary) 453.89
Claudicatio venosa intermittens 453.89
Claustrophobia 300.29
Clavus (infected) 700
Clawfoot (congenital) 754.71
  acquired 736.74

Clawhand (acquired) 736.06
  congenital 755.59
Clawtoe (congenital) 754.71
  acquired 735.5
Clay eating 307.52
Clay shovelers' fracture - see Fracture, vertebra, cervical
Cleansing of artificial opening (see also Attention to artificial opening) V55.9
Cleft (congenital) - see also Imperfect, closure
  alveolar process 525.8
  branchial (persistent) 744.41
    cyst 744.42
  clitoris 752.49
  cricoid cartilage, posterior 748.3
  facial (see also Cleft, lip) 749.10
  lip 749.10
    with cleft palate 749.20
      bilateral (lip and palate) 749.24
        with unilateral lip or palate 749.25
        complete 749.23
        incomplete 749.24
      unilateral (lip and palate) 749.22
        with bilateral lip or palate 749.25
        complete 749.21
        incomplete 749.22
    bilateral 749.14
      with cleft palate, unilateral 749.25
      complete 749.13
      incomplete 749.14
    unilateral 749.12
      with cleft palate, bilateral 749.25
      complete 749.11
      incomplete 749.12
  nose 748.1
  palate 749.00
    with cleft lip 749.20
      bilateral (lip and palate) 749.24
        with unilateral lip or palate 749.25
        complete 749.23
        incomplete 749.24
      unilateral (lip and palate) 749.22
        with bilateral lip or palate 749.25
        complete 749.21
        incomplete 749.22
    bilateral 749.04
      with cleft lip, unilateral 749.25
      complete 749.03
      incomplete 749.04
    unilateral 749.02
      with cleft lip, bilateral 749.25
      complete 749.01
      incomplete 749.02
  penis 752.69
  posterior, cricoid cartilage 748.3
  scrotum 752.89
  sternum (congenital) 756.3
  thyroid cartilage (congenital) 748.3
  tongue 750.13
  uvula 749.02
    with cleft lip (see also Cleft, lip, with cleft palate) 749.20
  water 366.12
Cleft hand (congenital) 755.58
Cleidocranial dysostosis 755.59
Cleidotomy, fetal 763.89
Cleptomania 312.32
Clérambault's syndrome 297.8
  erotomania 302.89
Clergyman's sore throat 784.49
Click, clicking
  systolic syndrome 785.2
Clifford's syndrome (postmaturity) 766.22
Climacteric (see also Menopause) 627.2
  arthritis NEC (see also Arthritis, climacteric) 716.3●
  depression (see also Psychosis, affective) 296.2●
  disease 627.2
    recurrent episode 296.3●
    single episode 296.2●

Climacteric (Continued)
  female (symptoms) 627.2
  male (symptoms) (syndrome) 608.89
  melancholia (see also Psychosis, affective) 296.2●
    recurrent episode 296.3●
    single episode 296.2●
  paranoid state 297.2
  paraphrenia 297.2
  polyarthritis NEC 716.39
    male 608.89
  symptoms (female) 627.2
Clinical research investigation (control) (participant) V70.7
Clinodactyly 755.59
Clitoris - see condition
Cloaca, persistent 751.5
Clonorchiasis 121.1
Clonorchiosis 121.1
Clonorchis infection, liver 121.1
Clonus 781.0
Closed bite 524.20
Closed surgical procedure converted to open procedure
  arthroscopic V64.43
  laparoscopic V64.41
  thoracoscopic V64.42
Closure
  artificial opening (see also Attention to artificial opening) V55.9
  congenital, nose 748.0
  cranial sutures, premature 756.0
  defective or imperfect NEC - see Imperfect, closure
  fistula, delayed - see Fistula
  fontanelle, delayed 756.0
  foramen ovale, imperfect 745.5
  hymen 623.3
  interauricular septum, defective 745.5
  interventricular septum, defective 745.4
  lacrimal duct 375.56
    congenital 743.65
    neonatal 375.55
  nose (congenital) 748.0
    acquired 738.0
  primary angle without glaucoma damage 365.06
  vagina 623.2
  valve - see Endocarditis
  vulva 624.8
Clot (blood)
  artery (obstruction) (occlusion) (see also Embolism) 444.9
  atrial appendage 429.89
  bladder 596.7
  brain (extradural or intradural) (see also Thrombosis, brain) 434.0●
    late effect - see Late effect(s) (of) cerebrovascular disease
  circulation 444.9
  heart (see also Infarct, myocardium) 410.9●
    without myocardial infarction 429.89
  vein (see also Thrombosis) 453.9
Clotting defect NEC (see also Defect, coagulation) 286.9
Clouded state 780.09
  epileptic (see also Epilepsy) 345.9●
  paroxysmal (idiopathic) (see also Epilepsy) 345.9●
Clouding
  corneal graft 996.51
Cloudy
  antrum, antra 473.0
  dialysis effluent 792.5
Clouston's (hidrotic) ectodermal dysplasia 757.31
Clubbing of fingers 781.5
Clubfinger 736.29
  acquired 736.29
  congenital 754.89

Clubfoot (congenital) 754.70
  acquired 736.71
  equinovarus 754.51
  paralytic 736.71
Club hand (congenital) 754.89
  acquired 736.07
Clubnail (acquired) 703.8
  congenital 757.5
Clump kidney 753.3
Clumsiness 781.3
  syndrome 315.4
Cluttering (see also Disorder, fluency) 315.35
Clutton's joints 090.5
Coagulation, intravascular (diffuse)
    (disseminated) (see also Fibrinolysis) 286.6
  newborn 776.2
Coagulopathy (see also Defect, coagulation)
    286.9
  consumption 286.6
  intravascular (disseminated) NEC 286.6
    newborn 776.2
Coalition
  calcaneoscaphoid 755.67
  calcaneus 755.67
  tarsal 755.67
Coal miners'
  elbow 727.2
  lung 500
Coal workers' lung or pneumoconiosis 500
Coarctation
  aorta (postductal) (preductal) 747.10
  pulmonary artery 747.31
Coated tongue 529.3
Coats' disease 362.12
Cocainism (see also Dependence) 304.2●
Coccidioidal granuloma 114.3
Coccidioidomycosis 114.9
  with pneumonia 114.0
  cutaneous (primary) 114.1
  disseminated 114.3
  extrapulmonary (primary) 114.1
  lung 114.5
    acute 114.0
    chronic 114.4
    primary 114.0
  meninges 114.2
  primary (pulmonary) 114.0
    acute 114.0
  prostate 114.3
  pulmonary 114.5
    acute 114.0
    chronic 114.4
    primary 114.0
  specified site NEC 114.3
Coccidioidosis 114.9
  lung 114.5
    acute 114.0
    chronic 114.4
    primary 114.0
  meninges 114.2
Coccidiosis (colitis) (diarrhea) (dysentery)
    007.2
Cocciuria 791.9
Coccus in urine 791.9
Coccydynia 724.79
Coccygodynia 724.79
Coccyx - see condition
Cochin-China
  diarrhea 579.1
    anguilluliasis 127.2
  ulcer 085.1
Cock's peculiar tumor 706.2
Cockayne's disease or syndrome (microcephaly
    and dwarfism) 759.89
Cockayne-Weber syndrome (epidermolysis
    bullosa) 757.39
Cocked-up toe 735.2
Codman's tumor (benign chondroblastoma)
    (M9230/0) - see Neoplasm, bone, benign
Coenurosis 123.8
Coffee workers' lung 495.8

Cogan's syndrome 370.52
  congenital oculomotor apraxia 379.51
  nonsyphilitic interstitial keratitis 370.52
Coiling, umbilical cord - see Complications,
    umbilical cord
Coitus, painful (female) 625.0
  male 608.89
  psychogenic 302.76
Cold 460
  with influenza, flu, or grippe (see also
    Influenza) 487.1
  abscess - see Tuberculosis, abscess
    articular - see Tuberculosis, joint
  agglutinin
    disease (chronic) or syndrome 283.0
    hemoglobinuria 283.0
      paroxysmal (cold) (nocturnal) 283.2
  allergic (see also Fever, hay) 477.9
  bronchus or chest - see Bronchitis
    with grippe or influenza (see also
      Influenza) 487.1
  common (head) 460
    vaccination, prophylactic (against) V04.7
  deep 464.10
  effects of 991.9
    specified effect NEC 991.8
  excessive 991.9
    specified effect NEC 991.8
  exhaustion from 991.8
  exposure to 991.9
    specified effect NEC 991.8
  grippy (see also Influenza) 487.1
  head 460
  injury syndrome (newborn) 778.2
  intolerance 780.99
  on lung - see Bronchitis
  rose 477.0
  sensitivity, autoimmune 283.0
  virus 460
Coldsore (see also Herpes, simplex) 054.9
Colibacillosis 041.49
  generalized 038.42
Colibacilluria 791.9
Colic (recurrent) 789.7
  abdomen 789.7
    psychogenic 307.89
  appendicular 543.9
  appendix 543.9
  bile duct - see Choledocholithiasis
  biliary - see Cholelithiasis
  bilious - see Cholelithiasis
  common duct - see Choledocholithiasis
  Devonshire NEC 984.9
    specified type of lead - see Table of Drugs
      and Chemicals
  flatulent 787.3
  gallbladder or gallstone - see Cholelithiasis
  gastric 536.8
  hepatic (duct) - see Choledocholithiasis
  hysterical 300.11
  in
    adult 789.0
    child over 12 months old 789.0
    infant 789.7
  infantile 789.7
  intestinal 789.7
  kidney 788.0
  lead NEC 984.9
    specified type of lead - see Table of Drugs
      and Chemicals
  liver (duct) - see Choledocholithiasis
  mucous 564.9
    psychogenic 316 [564.9]
  nephritic 788.0
  Painter's NEC 984.9
  pancreas 577.8
  psychogenic 306.4
  renal 788.0
  saturnine NEC 984.9
    specified type of lead - see Table of Drugs
      and Chemicals

Colic (Continued)
  spasmodic 789.7
  ureter 788.0
  urethral 599.84
    due to calculus 594.2
  uterus 625.8
    menstrual 625.3
  vermicular 543.9
  virus 460
  worm NEC 128.9
Colicystitis (see also Cystitis) 595.9
Colitis (acute) (catarrhal) (croupous) (cystica
    superficialis) (exudative) (hemorrhagic)
    (noninfectious) (phlegmonous)
    (presumed noninfectious) 558.9
  adaptive 564.9
  allergic 558.3
  amebic (see also Amebiasis) 006.9
    nondysenteric 006.2
  anthrax 022.2
  bacillary (see also Infection, Shigella) 004.9
  balantidial 007.0
  chronic 558.9
    ulcerative (see also Colitis, ulcerative)
      556.9
  coccidial 007.2
  dietetic 558.9
  due to radiation 558.1
  eosinophilic 558.42
  functional 558.9
  gangrenous 009.0
  giardial 007.1
  granulomatous 555.1
  gravis (see also Colitis, ulcerative) 556.9
  infectious (see also Enteritis, due to, specific
    organism) 009.0
    presumed 009.1
  ischemic 557.9
    acute 557.0
    chronic 557.1
    due to mesenteric artery insufficiency 557.1
  membranous 564.9
    psychogenic 316 [564.9]
  mucous 564.9
    psychogenic 316 [564.9]
  necrotic 009.0
  polyposa (see also Colitis, ulcerative) 556.9
  protozoal NEC 007.9
  pseudomembranous 008.45
  pseudomucinous 564.9
  regional 555.1
  segmental 555.1
  septic (see also Enteritis, due to, specific
    organism) 009.0
  spastic 564.9
    psychogenic 316 [564.9]
  Staphylococcus 008.41
    food 005.0
  thromboulcerative 557.0
  toxic 558.2
  transmural 555.1
  trichomonal 007.3
  tuberculous (ulcerative) 014.8●
  ulcerative (chronic) (idiopathic) (nonspecific)
    556.9
    entero- 556.0
    fulminant 557.0
    ileo- 556.1
    left-sided 556.5
    procto- 556.2
    proctosigmoid 556.3
    psychogenic 316 [556]
    specified NEC 556.8
    universal 556.6
Collagen disease NEC 710.9
  nonvascular 710.9
  vascular (allergic) (see also Angiitis,
    hypersensitivity) 446.20
Collagenosis (see also Collagen disease) 710.9
  cardiovascular 425.4
  mediastinal 519.3

◀ New   ◀◀ Revised   ~~deleted~~ Deleted   ● Use Additional Digit(s)   Omit code

Collapse 780.2
  adrenal 255.8
  cardiorenal (see also Hypertension, cardiorenal) 404.90
  cardiorespiratory 785.51
    fetus or newborn 779.85
  cardiovascular (see also Disease, heart) 785.51
    fetus or newborn 779.85
  circulatory (peripheral) 785.59
    with
      abortion - see Abortion, by type, with shock
      ectopic pregnancy (see also categories 633.0–633.9) 639.5
      molar pregnancy (see also categories 630–632) 639.5
    during or after labor and delivery 669.1●
    fetus or newborn 779.85
    following
      abortion 639.5
      ectopic or molar pregnancy 639.5
    during or after labor and delivery 669.1●
      fetus or newborn 779.89
    during or resulting from a surgical procedure 998.00
  external ear canal 380.50
    secondary to
      inflammation 380.53
      surgery 380.52
      trauma 380.51
  general 780.2
  heart - see Disease, heart
  heat 992.1
  hysterical 300.11
  labyrinth, membranous (congenital) 744.05
  lung (massive) (see also Atelectasis) 518.0
    pressure, during labor 668.0●
  myocardial - see Disease, heart
  nervous (see also Disorder, mental, nonpsychotic) 300.9
  neurocirculatory 306.2
  nose 738.0
  postoperative (cardiovascular) 998.09
  pulmonary (see also Atelectasis) 518.0
    fetus or newborn 770.5
      partial 770.5
      primary 770.4
  thorax 512.89
    iatrogenic 512.1
    postoperative 512.1
  trachea 519.19
  valvular - see Endocarditis
  vascular (peripheral) 785.59
    with
      abortion - see Abortion, by type, with shock
      ectopic pregnancy (see also categories 633.0–633.9) 639.5
      molar pregnancy (see also categories 630–632) 639.5
    cerebral (see also Disease, cerebrovascular, acute) 436
    during or after labor and delivery 669.1●
    fetus or newborn 779.89
    following
      abortion 639.5
      ectopic or molar pregnancy 639.5
  vasomotor 785.59
  vertebra 733.13
Collateral - see also condition
  circulation (venous) 459.89
  dilation, veins 459.89
Colles' fracture (closed) (reversed) (separation) 813.41
  open 813.51
Collet's syndrome 352.6
Collet-Sicard syndrome 352.6
Colliculitis urethralis (see also Urethritis) 597.89

Colliers'
  asthma 500
  lung 500
  phthisis (see also Tuberculosis) 011.4●
Collodion baby (ichthyosis congenita) 757.1
Colloid milium 709.3
Coloboma NEC 743.49
  choroid 743.59
  fundus 743.52
  iris 743.46
  lens 743.36
  lids 743.62
  optic disc (congenital) 743.57
    acquired 377.23
  retina 743.56
  sclera 743.47
Coloenteritis - see Enteritis
Colon - see condition
Colonization
  MRSA (methicillin resistant Staphylococcus aureus) V02.54
  MSSA (methicillin susceptible Staphylococcus aureus) V02.53
Coloptosis 569.89
Color
  amblyopia NEC 368.59
    acquired 368.55
  blindness NEC (congenital) 368.59
    acquired 368.55
Colostomy
  attention to V55.3
  fitting or adjustment V55.3
  malfunctioning 569.62
  status V44.3
Colpitis (see also Vaginitis) 616.10
Colpocele 618.6
Colpocystitis (see also Vaginitis) 616.10
Colporrhexis 665.4●
Colpospasm 625.1
Column, spinal, vertebral - see condition
Coma 780.01
  apoplectic (see also Disease, cerebrovascular, acute) 436
  diabetic (with ketoacidosis) 250.3●
    due to secondary diabetes 249.3●
    hyperosmolar 250.2●
      due to secondary diabetes 249.2●
  eclamptic (see also Eclampsia) 780.39
  epileptic 345.3
  hepatic 572.2
  hyperglycemic 250.2●
    due to secondary diabetes 249.2●
  hyperosmolar (diabetic) (nonketotic) 250.2●
    due to secondary diabetes 249.2●
  hypoglycemic 251.0
    diabetic 250.3●
      due to secondary diabetes 249.3●
  insulin 250.3●
    due to secondary diabetes 249.3●
    hyperosmolar 250.2●
      due to secondary diabetes 249.2●
    nondiabetic 251.0
    organic hyperinsulinism 251.0
  Kussmaul's (diabetic) 250.3●
    due to secondary diabetes 249.3●
  liver 572.2
  newborn 779.2
  prediabetic 250.2●
    due to secondary diabetes 249.2●
  uremic - see Uremia
Combat fatigue (see also Reaction, stress, acute) 308.9
Combined - see condition
Comedo 706.1
Comedocarcinoma (M8501/3) - see also Neoplasm, breast, malignant
  noninfiltrating (M8501/2)
    specified site - see Neoplasm, by site, in situ
    unspecified site 233.0
Comedomastitis 610.4

Comedones 706.1
  lanugo 757.4
Comma bacillus, carrier (suspected) of V02.3
Comminuted fracture - see Fracture, by site
Common
  aortopulmonary trunk 745.0
  atrioventricular canal (defect) 745.69
  atrium 745.69
  cold (head) 460
    vaccination, prophylactic (against) V04.7
  truncus (arteriosus) 745.0
  ventricle 745.3
Commotio (current)
  cerebri (see also Concussion, brain) 850.9
    with skull fracture - see Fracture, skull, by site
  retinae 921.3
  spinalis - see Injury, spinal, by site
Commotion (current)
  brain (without skull fracture) (see also Concussion, brain) 850.9
    with skull fracture - see Fracture, skull, by site
  spinal cord - see Injury, spinal, by site
Communication
  abnormal - see also Fistula
    between
      base of aorta and pulmonary artery 745.0
      left ventricle and right atrium 745.4
      pericardial sac and pleural sac 748.8
      pulmonary artery and pulmonary vein 747.39
    congenital, between uterus and
      anterior abdominal wall 752.39
      bladder 752.39
      intestine 752.39
      rectum 752.39
    left ventricular-right atrial 745.4
    pulmonary artery-pulmonary vein 747.39
Compartment syndrome - see Syndrome, compartment
Compensation
  broken - see Failure, heart
  failure - see Failure, heart
  neurosis, psychoneurosis 300.11
Complaint - see also Disease
  bowel, functional 564.9
    psychogenic 306.4
  intestine, functional 564.9
    psychogenic 306.4
  kidney (see also Disease, renal) 593.9
  liver 573.9
  miners' 500
Complete - see condition
Complex
  cardiorenal (see also Hypertension, cardiorenal) 404.90
  castration 300.9
  Costen's 524.60
  ego-dystonic homosexuality 302.0
  Eisenmenger's (ventricular septal defect) 745.4
  homosexual, ego-dystonic 302.0
  hypersexual 302.89
  inferiority 301.9
  jumped process
    spine - see Dislocation, vertebra
  primary, tuberculosis (see also Tuberculosis) 010.0●
  regional pain syndrome 355.9
    type I 337.20
      lower limb 337.22
      specified site NEC 337.29
      upper limb 337.21
    type II
      lower limb 355.71
      upper limb 354.4
  Taussig-Bing (transposition, aorta and overriding pulmonary artery) 745.11

Complications
- abortion NEC - *see* categories 634–639
- accidental puncture or laceration during a procedure 998.2
- amniocentesis, fetal 679.1●
- amputation stump (late) (surgical) 997.60
  - traumatic - *see* Amputation, traumatic
- anastomosis (and bypass) - *see also* Complications, due to (presence of) any device, implant, or graft classified to 996.0–996.5 NEC
  - hemorrhage NEC 998.11
  - intestinal (internal) NEC 997.49
    - involving urinary tract 997.5
  - mechanical - *see* Complications, mechanical, graft
  - urinary tract (involving intestinal tract) 997.5
- anesthesia, anesthetic NEC (*see also* Anesthesia, complication) 995.22
  - in labor and delivery 668.9●
    - affecting fetus or newborn 763.5
    - cardiac 668.1●
    - central nervous system 668.2●
    - pulmonary 668.0●
    - specified type NEC 668.8●
- aortocoronary (bypass) graft 996.03
  - atherosclerosis - *see* Arteriosclerosis, coronary
  - embolism 996.72
  - occlusion NEC 996.72
  - thrombus 996.72
- arthroplasty (*see also* Complications, prosthetic joint) 996.49
- artificial opening
  - cecostomy 569.60
  - colostomy 569.60
  - cystostomy 596.83
    - infection 596.81
    - mechanical 596.82
    - specified complication NEC 596.83
  - enterostomy 569.60
  - esophagostomy 530.87
    - infection 530.86
    - mechanical 530.87
  - gastrostomy 536.40
  - ileostomy 569.60
  - jejunostomy 569.60
  - nephrostomy 997.5
  - tracheostomy 519.00
  - ureterostomy 997.5
  - urethrostomy 997.5
- bariatric surgery
  - gastric band procedure 539.09
    - infection 539.01
  - specified procedure NEC 539.89
    - infection 539.81
- bile duct implant (prosthetic) NEC 996.79
  - infection or inflammation 996.69
  - mechanical 996.59
- bleeding (intraoperative) (postoperative) 998.11
- blood vessel graft 996.1
  - aortocoronary 996.03
    - atherosclerosis - *see* Arteriosclerosis, coronary
    - embolism 996.72
    - occlusion NEC 996.72
    - thrombus 996.72
  - atherosclerosis - *see* Arteriosclerosis, extremities
  - embolism 996.74
  - occlusion NEC 996.74
  - thrombus 996.74
- bone growth stimulator NEC 996.78
  - infection or inflammation 996.67
- bone marrow transplant 996.85
- breast implant (prosthetic) NEC 996.79
  - infection or inflammation 996.69
  - mechanical 996.54

Complications (*Continued*)
- bypass - *see also* Complications, anastomosis
  - aortocoronary 996.03
    - atherosclerosis - *see* Arteriosclerosis, coronary
    - embolism 996.72
    - occlusion NEC 996.72
    - thrombus 996.72
  - carotid artery 996.1
    - atherosclerosis - *see* Arteriosclerosis, coronary
    - embolism 996.74
    - occlusion NEC 996.74
    - thrombus 996.74
- cardiac (*see also* Disease, heart) 429.9
  - device, implant, or graft NEC 996.72
    - infection or inflammation 996.61
    - long-term effect 429.4
    - mechanical (*see also* Complications, mechanical, by type) 996.00
    - valve prosthesis 996.71
      - infection or inflammation 996.61
  - postoperative NEC 997.1
    - long-term effect 429.4
- cardiorenal (*see also* Hypertension, cardiorenal) 404.90
- carotid artery bypass graft 996.1
  - atherosclerosis - *see* Arteriosclerosis, coronary
  - embolism 996.74
  - occlusion NEC 996.74
  - thrombus 996.74
- cataract fragments in eye 998.82
- catheter device NEC - *see also* Complications, due to (presence of) any device, implant, or graft classified to 996.0-996.5 NEC
  - mechanical - *see* Complications, mechanical, catheter
- cecostomy 569.60
- cesarean section wound 674.3●
- chemotherapy (antineoplastic) 995.29
- chin implant (prosthetic) NEC 996.79
  - infection or inflammation 996.69
  - mechanical 996.59
- colostomy (enterostomy) 569.60
  - specified type NEC 569.69
- contraceptive device, intrauterine NEC 996.76
  - infection 996.65
  - inflammation 996.65
  - mechanical 996.32
- cord (umbilical) - *see* Complications, umbilical cord
- cornea
  - due to
    - contact lens 371.82
- coronary (artery) bypass (graft) NEC 996.03
  - atherosclerosis - *see* Arteriosclerosis, coronary
  - embolism 996.72
  - infection or inflammation 996.61
  - mechanical 996.03
  - occlusion NEC 996.72
  - specified type NEC 996.72
  - thrombus 996.72
- cystostomy 596.83
  - infection 596.81
  - mechanical 596.82
  - specified complication NEC 596.83
- delivery 669.9●
  - procedure (instrumental) (manual) (surgical) 669.4●
  - specified type NEC 669.8●

Complications (*Continued*)
- dialysis (hemodialysis) (peritoneal) (renal) NEC 999.9
  - catheter NEC - *see also* Complications, due to (presence of) any device, implant, or graft classified to 996.0–996.5 NEC
    - infection or inflammation 996.62
      - peritoneal 996.68
    - mechanical 996.1
      - peritoneal 996.56
- drug NEC 995.29
- due to (presence of) any device, implant, or graft classified to 996.0–996.5 NEC
  - with infection or inflammation - *see* Complications, infection or inflammation, due to (presence of) any device, implant, or graft classified to 996.0–996.5 NEC
  - arterial NEC 996.74
    - coronary NEC 996.03
      - atherosclerosis - *see* Arteriosclerosis, coronary
      - embolism 996.72
      - occlusion NEC 996.72
      - specified type NEC 996.72
      - thrombus 996.72
    - renal dialysis 996.73
  - arteriovenous fistula or shunt NEC 996.74
  - bone growth stimulator 996.78
  - breast NEC 996.79
  - cardiac NEC 996.72
    - defibrillator 996.72
    - pacemaker 996.72
    - valve prosthesis 996.71
  - catheter NEC 996.79
    - spinal 996.75
    - urinary, indwelling 996.76
    - vascular NEC 996.74
      - renal dialysis 996.73
    - ventricular shunt 996.75
  - coronary (artery) bypass (graft) NEC 996.03
    - atherosclerosis - *see* Arteriosclerosis, coronary
    - embolism 996.72
    - occlusion NEC 996.72
    - thrombus 996.72
  - electrodes
    - brain 996.75
    - heart 996.72
  - esophagostomy 530.87
  - gastrointestinal NEC 996.79
  - genitourinary NEC 996.76
  - heart valve prosthesis NEC 996.71
  - infusion pump 996.74
  - insulin pump 996.57
  - internal
    - joint prosthesis 996.77
    - orthopedic NEC 996.78
    - specified type NEC 996.79
  - intrauterine contraceptive device NEC 996.76
  - joint prosthesis, internal NEC 996.77
  - mechanical - *see* Complications, mechanical
  - nervous system NEC 996.75
  - ocular lens NEC 996.79
  - orbital NEC 996.79
  - orthopedic NEC 996.78
    - joint, internal 996.77
  - renal dialysis 996.73
  - specified type NEC 996.79
  - urinary catheter, indwelling 996.76
  - vascular NEC 996.74
  - ventricular shunt 996.75
- during dialysis NEC 999.9
- ectopic or molar pregnancy NEC 639.9
- electroshock therapy NEC 999.9
- enterostomy 569.60
  - specified type NEC 569.69

◀ New ◀ Revised ~~deleted~~ Deleted ● Use Additional Digit(s) ▨ Omit code

Complications (*Continued*)
esophagostomy 530.87
    infection 530.86
    mechanical 530.87
external (fixation) device with internal
        component(s) NEC 996.78
    infection or inflammation 996.67
    mechanical 996.49
extracorporeal circulation NEC 999.9
eye implant (prosthetic) NEC 996.79
    infection or inflammation 996.69
    mechanical
        ocular lens 996.53
        orbital globe 996.59
fetal, from amniocentesis 679.1●
gastrointestinal, postoperative NEC (*see also*
        Complications, surgical procedures)
        997.49
gastrostomy 536.40
    specified type NEC 536.49
genitourinary device, implant or graft NEC
        996.76
    erosion of implanted vaginal mesh 629.31
    exposure of implanted vaginal mesh
        629.32
    infection or inflammation 996.65
        urinary catheter, indwelling 996.64
    mechanical (*see also* Complications,
        mechanical, by type) 996.30
        specified NEC 996.39
graft (bypass) (patch) - *see also*
        Complications, due to (presence of)
        any device, implant, or graft classified
        to 996.0–996.5 NEC
    bone marrow 996.85
    corneal NEC 996.79
        infection or inflammation 996.69
        rejection or reaction 996.51
        retroprosthetic membrane 996.51
    mechanical - *see* Complications,
        mechanical, graft
    organ (immune or nonimmune cause)
        (partial) (total) 996.80
        bone marrow 996.85
        heart 996.83
        intestines 996.87
        kidney 996.81
        liver 996.82
        lung 996.84
        pancreas 996.86
        specified NEC 996.89
    skin NEC 996.79
        infection or inflammation 996.69
        rejection 996.52
            artificial 996.55
            decellularized allodermis 996.55
heart - *see also* Disease, heart transplant
        (immune or nonimmune cause) 996.83
hematoma (intraoperative) (postoperative)
        998.12
hemorrhage (intraoperative) (postoperative)
        998.11
hyperalimentation therapy NEC 999.9
immunization (procedure) - *see*
        Complications, vaccination
implant - *see also* Complications, due to
        (presence of) any device, implant, or
        graft classified to 996.0–996.5 NEC
    dental placement, hemorrhagic 525.71
    mechanical, - *see* Complications,
        mechanical, implant
infection and inflammation
    due to (presence of) any device, implant
        or graft classified to 996.0–996.5
        NEC 996.60
        arterial NEC 996.62
            coronary 996.61
            renal dialysis 996.62
        arteriovenous fistula or shunt 996.62
        artificial heart 996.61
        bone growth stimulator 996.67

Complications (*Continued*)
infection and inflammation (*Continued*)
    due to (*Continued*)
        breast 996.69
        cardiac 996.61
        catheter NEC 996.69
            central venous 999.31
                bloodstream 999.32
                localized 999.33
            Hickman 999.31
                bloodstream 999.32
                localized 999.33
            peripherally inserted central (PICC)
                999.31
                bloodstream 999.32
                localized 999.33
            peritoneal 996.68
            portacath (port-a-cath) 999.31
                bloodstream 999.32
                localized 999.33
            spinal 996.63
            triple lumen 999.31
                bloodstream 999.32
                localized 999.33
            umbilical venous 999.31
                bloodstream 999.32
                localized 999.33
            urinary, indwelling 996.64
            vascular (arterial) (dialysis)
                (peripheral venous) NEC
                996.62
            ventricular shunt 996.63
        central venous catheter 999.31
            bloodstream 999.32
            localized 999.33
        coronary artery bypass 996.61
        electrodes
            brain 996.63
            heart 996.61
        gastrointestinal NEC 996.69
        genitourinary NEC 996.65
            indwelling urinary catheter 996.64
        heart assist device 996.61
        heart valve 996.61
        Hickman catheter 999.31
            bloodstream 999.32
            localized 999.33
        infusion pump 996.62
        insulin pump 996.69
        intrauterine contraceptive device
            996.65
        joint prosthesis, internal 996.66
        ocular lens 996.69
        orbital (implant) 996.69
        orthopedic NEC 996.67
            joint, internal 996.66
        peripherally inserted central catheter
            (PICC) 999.31
            bloodstream 999.32
            localized 999.33
        portacath (port-a-cath) 999.31
            bloodstream 999.32
            localized 999.33
        specified type NEC 996.69
        triple lumen catheter 999.31
            bloodstream 999.32
            localized 999.33
        umbilical venous catheter 999.31
            bloodstream 999.32
            localized 999.33
        urinary catheter, indwelling 996.64
        ventricular shunt 996.63
    infusion (procedure) 999.88
        blood - *see* Complications, transfusion
        infection NEC 999.39
        sepsis NEC 999.39
    inhalation therapy NEC 999.9
    injection (procedure) 999.9
        drug reaction (*see also* Reaction, drug)
            995.27
        infection NEC 999.39

Complications (*Continued*)
injection (*Continued*)
    sepsis NEC 999.39
    serum (prophylactic) (therapeutic) - *see*
        Complications, vaccination
    vaccine (any) - *see* Complications,
        vaccination
inoculation (any) - *see* Complications,
        vaccination
insulin pump 996.57
internal device (catheter) (electronic)
        (fixation) (prosthetic) - *see also*
        Complications, due to (presence of)
        any device, implant, or graft classified
        to 996.0–996.5 NEC
    mechanical - *see* Complications,
        mechanical
intestinal pouch, specified NEC 569.79
intestinal transplant (immune or nonimmune
        cause) 996.87
intraoperative bleeding or hemorrhage
        998.11
intrauterine contraceptive device (*see also*
        Complications, contraceptive device)
        996.76
    with fetal damage affecting management
        of pregnancy 655.8●
    infection or inflammation 996.65
in utero procedure
    fetal 679.1●
    maternal 679.0●
jejunostomy 569.60
kidney transplant (immune or nonimmune
        cause) 996.81
labor 669.9●
    specified condition NEC 669.8●
liver transplant (immune or nonimmune
        cause) 996.82
lumbar puncture 349.0
mechanical
    anastomosis - *see* Complications,
        mechanical, graft
    artificial heart 996.09
    bypass - *see* Complications, mechanical,
        graft
    catheter NEC 996.59
        cardiac 996.09
        cystostomy 596.82
        dialysis (hemodialysis) 996.1
            peritoneal 996.56
        during a procedure 998.2
        urethral, indwelling 996.31
    colostomy 569.62
    device NEC 996.59
        balloon (counterpulsation), intra-aortic
            996.1
        cardiac 996.00
            automatic implantable defibrillator
                996.04
            long-term effect 429.4
            specified NEC 996.09
        contraceptive, intrauterine 996.32
        counterpulsation, intra-aortic 996.1
        fixation, external, with internal
            components 996.49
        fixation, internal (nail, rod, plate)
            996.40
        genitourinary 996.30
            specified NEC 996.39
        insulin pump 996.57
        nervous system 996.2
        orthopedic, internal 996.40
            prosthetic joint (*see also*
                Complications, mechanical,
                device, orthopedic, prosthetic,
                joint) 996.47
        prosthetic NEC 996.59
            joint 996.47
                articular bearing surface wear
                    996.46
                aseptic loosening 996.41

Complications (Continued)
  mechanical (Continued)
    device NEC (Continued)
      prosthetic NEC (Continued)
        joint (Continued)
          breakage 996.43
          dislocation 996.42
          failure 996.47
          fracture 996.43
            around prosthetic 996.44
            peri-prosthetic 996.44
          instability 996.42
          loosening 996.41
          peri-prosthetic osteolysis 996.45
          subluxation 996.42
          wear 996.46
      umbrella, vena cava 996.1
      vascular 996.1
    dorsal column stimulator 996.2
    electrode NEC 996.59
      brain 996.2
      cardiac 996.01
      spinal column 996.2
    enterostomy 569.62
    esophagostomy 530.87
    fistula, arteriovenous, surgically created 996.1
    gastrostomy 536.42
    graft NEC 996.52
      aortic (bifurcation) 996.1
      aortocoronary bypass 996.03
      blood vessel NEC 996.1
      bone 996.49
      cardiac 996.00
      carotid artery bypass 996.1
      cartilage 996.49
      corneal 996.51
      coronary bypass 996.03
      decellularized allodermis 996.55
      genitourinary 996.30
        specified NEC 996.39
      muscle 996.49
      nervous system 996.2
      organ (immune or nonimmune cause) 996.80
        heart 996.83
        intestines 996.87
        kidney 996.81
        liver 996.82
        lung 996.84
        pancreas 996.86
        specified NEC 996.89
      orthopedic, internal 996.49
      peripheral nerve 996.2
      prosthetic NEC 996.59
      skin 996.52
        artificial 996.55
      specified NEC 996.59
      tendon 996.49
      tissue NEC 996.52
      tooth 996.59
      ureter, without mention of resection 996.39
      vascular 996.1
    heart valve prosthesis 996.02
      long-term effect 429.4
    implant NEC 996.59
      cardiac 996.00
        automatic implantable defibrillator 996.04
        long-term effect 429.4
        specified NEC 996.09
      electrode NEC 996.59
        brain 996.2
        cardiac 996.01
        spinal column 996.2
      genitourinary 996.30
      nervous system 996.2
      orthopedic, internal 996.49

Complications (Continued)
  mechanical (Continued)
    implant NEC (Continued)
      prosthetic NEC 996.59
        in
          bile duct 996.59
          breast 996.54
          chin 996.59
          eye
            ocular lens 996.53
            orbital globe 996.59
        vascular 996.1
    insulin pump 996.57
    nonabsorbable surgical material 996.59
    pacemaker NEC 996.59
      brain 996.2
      cardiac 996.01
      nerve (phrenic) 996.2
    patch - see Complications, mechanical, graft
    prosthesis NEC 996.59
      bile duct 996.59
      breast 996.54
      chin 996.59
      ocular lens 996.53
      reconstruction, vas deferens 996.39
    reimplant NEC 996.59
      extremity (see also Complications, reattached, extremity) 996.90
      organ (see also Complications, transplant, organ, by site) 996.80
    repair - see Complications, mechanical, graft
    respirator [ventilator] V46.14
    shunt NEC 996.59
      arteriovenous, surgically created 996.1
      ventricular (communicating) 996.2
    stent NEC 996.59
    tracheostomy 519.02
    vas deferens reconstruction 996.39
    ventilator [respirator] V46.14
  medical care NEC 999.9
    cardiac NEC 997.1
    gastrointestinal NEC 997.49
    nervous system NEC 997.00
    peripheral vascular NEC 997.2
    respiratory NEC 997.39
    urinary NEC 997.5
    vascular
      mesenteric artery 997.71
      other vessels 997.79
      peripheral vessels 997.2
      renal artery 997.72
  nephrostomy 997.5
  nervous system
    device, implant, or graft NEC 349.1
      mechanical 996.2
    postoperative NEC 997.00
  obstetric 669.9●
    procedure (instrumental) (manual) (surgical) 669.4●
    specified NEC 669.8●
    surgical wound 674.3●
  ocular lens implant NEC 996.79
    infection or inflammation 996.69
    mechanical 996.53
  organ transplant - see Complications, transplant, organ, by site
  orthopedic device, implant, or graft
    internal (fixation) (nail) (plate) (rod) NEC 996.78
      infection or inflammation 996.67
      joint prosthesis 996.77
        infection or inflammation 996.66
      mechanical 996.40
    pacemaker (cardiac) 996.72
      infection or inflammation 996.61
      mechanical 996.01
  pancreas transplant (immune or nonimmune cause) 996.86
  perfusion NEC 999.9

Complications (Continued)
  perineal repair (obstetrical) 674.3●
    disruption 674.2●
  pessary (uterus) (vagina) - see Complications, contraceptive device
  phototherapy 990
  postcystoscopic 997.5
  postmastoidectomy NEC 383.30
  postoperative - see Complications, surgical procedures
  pregnancy NEC 646.9●
    affecting fetus or newborn 761.9
  prosthetic device, internal - see also Complications, due to (presence of) any device, implant or graft classified to 996.0–996.5 NEC
    mechanical NEC (see also Complications, mechanical) 996.59
  puerperium NEC (see also Puerperal) 674.9●
  puncture, spinal 349.0
  pyelogram 997.5
  radiation 990
  radiotherapy 990
  reattached
    body part, except extremity 996.99
    extremity (infection) (rejection) 996.90
      arm(s) 996.94
      digit(s) (hand) 996.93
        foot 996.95
      finger(s) 996.93
      foot 996.95
      forearm 996.91
      hand 996.92
      leg 996.96
      lower NEC 996.96
      toe(s) 996.95
      upper NEC 996.94
  reimplant NEC - see also Complications, due to (presence of) any device, implant, or graft classified to 996.0–996.5 NEC
    bone marrow 996.85
    extremity (see also Complications, reattached, extremity) 996.90
      due to infection 996.90
    mechanical - see Complications, mechanical, reimplant
    organ (immune or nonimmune cause) (partial) (total) (see also Complications, transplant, organ, by site) 996.80
  renal allograft 996.81
  renal dialysis - see Complications, dialysis
  respirator [ventilator], mechanical V46.14
  respiratory 519.9
    device, implant or graft NEC 996.79
      infection or inflammation 996.69
      mechanical 996.59
    distress syndrome, adult, following trauma and surgery 518.52
    insufficiency, acute, postoperative 518.52
    postoperative NEC 997.39
    therapy NEC 999.9
  sedation during labor and delivery 668.9●
    affecting fetus or newborn 763.5
    cardiac 668.1●
    central nervous system 668.2●
    pulmonary 668.0●
    specified type NEC 668.8●
  seroma (intraoperative) (postoperative) (noninfected) 998.13
    infected 998.51
  shunt - see also Complications, due to (presence of) any device, implant, or graft classified to 996.0–996.5 NEC
    mechanical - see Complications, mechanical, shunt

◄ New　◄▥ Revised　~~deleted~~ Deleted　● Use Additional Digit(s)　▨ Omit code

Complications (Continued)
  specified body system NEC
    device, implant, or graft - see
        Complications, due to (presence of)
        any device, implant, or graft
        classified to 996.0–996.5 NEC
    postoperative NEC 997.99
  spinal puncture or tap 349.0
  stoma, external
    gastrointestinal tract
      colostomy 569.60
      enterostomy 569.60
      esophagostomy 530.87
        infection 530.86
        mechanical 530.87
      gastrostomy 536.40
    urinary tract 596.83
  stomach banding 539.09
  stomach stapling 539.89
  surgical procedures 998.9
    accidental puncture or laceration
        998.2
    amputation stump (late) 997.60
    anastomosis - see Complications,
        anastomosis
    burst stitches or sutures (external) (see also
        Dehiscence) 998.32
      internal 998.31
    cardiac 997.1
      long-term effect following cardiac
          surgery 429.4
    catheter device - see Complications,
        catheter device
    cataract fragments in eye 998.82
    cecostomy malfunction 569.62
    colostomy malfunction 569.62
    cystostomy malfunction 596.82
      infection 596.81
      mechanical 596.82
      specified complication NEC 596.83
    dehiscence (of incision) (external) (see also
        Dehiscence) 998.32
      internal 998.31
    dialysis NEC (see also Complications,
        dialysis) 999.9
    disruption (see also Dehiscence)
      anastomosis (internal) - see
          Complications, mechanical,
          graft
      internal suture (line) 998.31
      wound (external) 998.32
        internal 998.31
    dumping syndrome (postgastrectomy)
        564.2
    elephantiasis or lymphedema 997.99
      postmastectomy 457.0
    emphysema (surgical) 998.81
    enterostomy malfunction 569.62
    esophagostomy malfunction 530.87
    evisceration 998.32
    fistula (persistent postoperative) 998.6
    foreign body inadvertently left in wound
        (sponge) (suture) (swab) 998.4
    from nonabsorbable surgical material
        (Dacron) (mesh) (permanent suture)
        (reinforcing) (Teflon) - see
        Complications due to (presence of)
        any device, implant, or graft
        classified to 996.0–996.5 NEC
    gastrointestinal NEC 997.49
    gastrostomy malfunction 536.42
    hematoma 998.12
    hemorrhage 998.11
    ileostomy malfunction 569.62
    internal prosthetic device NEC (see also
        Complications, internal device)
        996.70
      hemolytic anemia 283.19
      infection or inflammation 996.60
      malfunction - see Complications,
          mechanical

Complications (Continued)
  surgical procedures (Continued)
    internal prosthetic device NEC (Continued)
      mechanical complication - see
          Complications, mechanical
      thrombus 996.70
    jejunostomy malfunction 569.62
    nervous system NEC 997.00
    obstruction, internal anastomosis - see
        Complications, mechanical, graft
    other body system NEC 997.99
    peripheral vascular NEC 997.2
    postcardiotomy syndrome 429.4
    postcholecystectomy syndrome 576.0
    postcommissurotomy syndrome 429.4
    postgastrectomy dumping syndrome 564.2
    postmastectomy lymphedema syndrome
        457.0
    postmastoidectomy 383.30
      cholesteatoma, recurrent 383.32
      cyst, mucosal 383.31
      granulation 383.33
      inflammation, chronic 383.33
    postvagotomy syndrome 564.2
    postvalvulotomy syndrome 429.4
    reattached extremity (infection) (rejection)
        (see also Complications, reattached,
        extremity) 996.90
    respiratory NEC 997.39
    seroma 998.13
    shock (endotoxic) (septic) 998.02
      hypovolemic 998.09
    shunt, prosthetic (thrombus) - see also
        Complications, due to (presence of)
        any device, implant, or graft
        classified to 996.0–996.5 NEC
      hemolytic anemia 283.19
    specified complication NEC 998.89
    stitch abscess 998.59
    transplant - see Complications, graft
    ureterostomy malfunction 997.5
    urethrostomy malfunction 997.5
    urinary NEC 997.5
    vascular
      mesenteric artery 997.71
      other vessels 997.79
      peripheral vessels 997.2
      renal artery 997.72
    wound infection 998.59
  therapeutic misadventure NEC 999.9
    surgical treatment 998.9
  tracheostomy 519.00
  transfusion (blood) (lymphocytes) (plasma)
      999.80
    acute lung injury (TRALI) 518.7
    atrophy, liver, yellow, subacute (within 8
        months of administration) - see
        Hepatitis, viral
    bone marrow 996.85
    embolism
      air 999.1
      thrombus 999.2
    febrile nonhemolytic reaction (FNHTR)
        780.66
    hemolysis NEC 999.89
      bone marrow 996.85
    hemolytic reaction, incompatibility
        unspecified 999.83
      acute 999.84
      delayed 999.85
    hepatitis (serum) (type B) (within 8
        months after administration) - see
        Hepatitis, viral
    incompatibility reaction
      ABO 999.60
        with hemolytic transfusion reaction
            (HTR) (not specified as acute
            or delayed) 999.61
        acute 999.62
        delayed 999.63
        specified type NEC 999.69

Complications (Continued)
  transfusion (Continued)
    incompatibility reaction (Continued)
      minor blood group 999.89
      non-ABO (minor antigens) (Duffy)
          (Kell) (Kidd) (Lewis) (M) (N) (P)
          (S) 999.75
        with hemolytic transfusion reaction
            (HTR) (not specified as acute
            or delayed) 999.76
        acute 999.77
        delayed 999.78
        specified type NEC 999.79
      Rh antigen (C) (c) (D) (E) (e) (factor)
          999.70
        with hemolytic transfusion reaction
            (HTR) (not specified as acute
            or delayed) 999.71
        acute 999.72
        delayed 999.73
        specified type NEC 999.74
    infection 999.39
      acute 999.34
    jaundice (serum) (within 8 months after
        administration) - see Hepatitis, viral
    sepsis 999.39
    shock or reaction NEC 999.89
      bone marrow 996.85
    specified reaction NEC 999.89
    subacute yellow atrophy of liver (within 8
        months after administration) - see
        Hepatitis, viral
    thromboembolism 999.2
  transplant NEC - see also Complications, due
      to (presence of) any device, implant, or
      graft classified to 996.0–996.5 NEC
    bone marrow 996.85
    organ (immune or nonimmune cause)
        (partial) (total) 996.80
      bone marrow 996.85
      heart 996.83
      intestines 996.87
      kidney 996.81
      liver 996.82
      lung 996.84
      pancreas 996.86
      specified NEC 996.89
    stem cell(s) 996.88
      from
          peripheral blood 996.88
          umbilical cord 996.88
  trauma NEC (early) 958.8
  ultrasound therapy NEC 999.9
  umbilical cord
    affecting fetus or newborn 762.6
    complicating delivery 663.9●
      affecting fetus or newborn 762.6
      specified type NEC 663.8●
  urethral catheter NEC 996.76
    infection or inflammation 996.64
    mechanical 996.31
  urinary, postoperative NEC 997.5
  vaccination 999.9
    anaphylaxis NEC 999.42
    cellulitis 999.39
    encephalitis or encephalomyelitis 323.51
    hepatitis (serum) (type B) (within 8
        months after administration) - see
        Hepatitis, viral
    infection (general) (local) NEC 999.39
    jaundice (serum) (within 8 months after
        administration) - see Hepatitis, viral
    meningitis 997.09 [321.8]
    myelitis 323.52
    protein sickness 999.52
    reaction (allergic) 999.52
      serum 999.52
    sepsis 999.39
    serum intoxication, sickness, rash, or other
        serum reaction NEC 999.52
    shock (allergic) (anaphylactic) 999.49

◄ New   ◄ Revised   deleted Deleted   ● Use Additional Digit(s)   Omit code

Complications (Continued)
  vaccination (Continued)
    subacute yellow atrophy of liver (within 8
      months after administration) - see
      Hepatitis, viral
    vaccinia (generalized) 999.0
      localized 999.39
  vascular
    device, implant, or graft NEC 996.74
      infection or inflammation 996.62
      mechanical NEC 996.1
        cardiac (see also Complications,
          mechanical, by type) 996.00
    following infusion, perfusion, or
      transfusion 999.2
    postoperative NEC 997.2
      mesenteric artery 997.71
      other vessels 997.79
      peripheral vessels 997.2
      renal artery 997.72
  ventilation therapy NEC 999.9
  ventilator [respirator], mechanical V46.14
Compound presentation, complicating
  delivery 652.8●
    causing obstructed labor 660.0●
Compressed air disease 993.3
Compression
  with injury - see specific injury
  arm NEC 354.9
  artery 447.1
    celiac, syndrome 447.4
  brachial plexus 353.0
  brain (stem) 348.4
    due to
      contusion, brain - see Contusion,
        brain
      injury NEC - see also Hemorrhage,
        brain, traumatic
        birth - see Birth, injury, brain
      laceration, brain - see Laceration,
        brain
    osteopathic 739.0
  bronchus 519.19
  by cicatrix - see Cicatrix
  cardiac 423.9
  cauda equina 344.60
    with neurogenic bladder 344.61
  celiac (artery) (axis) 447.4
  cerebral - see Compression, brain
  cervical plexus 353.2
  cord (umbilical) - see Compression, umbilical
    cord
  cranial nerve 352.9
    second 377.49
    third (partial) 378.51
      total 378.52
    fourth 378.53
    fifth 350.8
    sixth 378.54
    seventh 351.8
  divers' squeeze 993.3
  duodenum (external) (see also Obstruction,
    duodenum) 537.3
  during birth 767.9
  esophagus 530.3
    congenital, external 750.3
  Eustachian tube 381.63
  facies (congenital) 754.0
  fracture - see Fracture, by site
  heart - see Disease, heart
  intestine (see also Obstruction, intestine)
    560.9
    with hernia - see Hernia, by site, with
      obstruction
  laryngeal nerve, recurrent 478.79
  leg NEC 355.8
  lower extremity NEC 355.8
  lumbosacral plexus 353.1
  lung 518.89
  lymphatic vessel 457.1
  medulla - see Compression, brain

Compression (Continued)
  nerve NEC - see also Disorder, nerve
    arm NEC 354.9
    autonomic nervous system (see also
      Neuropathy, peripheral, autonomic)
      337.9
    axillary 353.0
    cranial NEC 352.9
    due to displacement of intervertebral disc
      722.2
      with myelopathy 722.70
      cervical 722.0
        with myelopathy 722.71
      lumbar, lumbosacral 722.10
        with myelopathy 722.73
      thoracic, thoracolumbar 722.11
        with myelopathy 722.72
    iliohypogastric 355.79
    ilioinguinal 355.79
    leg NEC 355.8
    lower extremity NEC 355.8
    median (in carpal tunnel) 354.0
    obturator 355.79
    optic 377.49
    plantar 355.6
    posterior tibial (in tarsal tunnel) 355.5
    root (by scar tissue) NEC 724.9
      cervical NEC 723.4
      lumbar NEC 724.4
      lumbosacral 724.4
      thoracic 724.4
    saphenous 355.79
    sciatic (acute) 355.0
    sympathetic 337.9
    traumatic - see Injury, nerve
    ulnar 354.2
    upper extremity NEC 354.9
  peripheral - see Compression, nerve
  spinal (cord) (old or nontraumatic) 336.9
    by displacement of intervertebral
      disc - see Displacement,
      intervertebral disc
    nerve
      root NEC 724.9
        postoperative 722.80
          cervical region 722.81
          lumbar region 722.83
          thoracic region 722.82
        traumatic - see Injury, nerve, spinal
      traumatic - see Injury, nerve, spinal
    spondylogenic 721.91
      cervical 721.1
      lumbar, lumbosacral 721.42
      thoracic 721.41
    traumatic - see also Injury, spinal, by site
      with fracture, vertebra - see Fracture,
        vertebra, by site, with spinal
        cord injury
  spondylogenic - see Compression, spinal
    cord, spondylogenic
  subcostal nerve (syndrome) 354.8
  sympathetic nerve NEC 337.9
  syndrome 958.5
  thorax 512.89
    iatrogenic 512.1
    postoperative 512.1
  trachea 519.19
    congenital 748.3
  ulnar nerve (by scar tissue) 354.2
  umbilical cord
    affecting fetus or newborn 762.5
      cord prolapsed 762.4
    complicating delivery 663.2●
      cord around neck 663.1●
      cord prolapsed 663.0●
  upper extremity NEC 354.9
  ureter 593.3
  urethra - see Stricture, urethra
  vein 459.2
  vena cava (inferior) (superior) 459.2
  vertebral NEC - see Compression, spinal (cord)

Compulsion, compulsive
  eating 307.51
  neurosis (obsessive) 300.3
  personality 301.4
  states (mixed) 300.3
  swearing 300.3
    in Gilles de la Tourette's syndrome
      307.23
  tics and spasms 307.22
  water drinking NEC (syndrome) 307.9
Concato's disease (pericardial polyserositis)
  423.2
  peritoneal 568.82
  pleural - see Pleurisy
Concavity, chest wall 738.3
Concealed
  hemorrhage NEC 459.0
  penis 752.65
Concentric fading 368.12
Concern (normal) about sick person in family
  V61.49
Concrescence (teeth) 520.2
Concretio cordis 423.1
  rheumatic 393
Concretion - see also Calculus
  appendicular 543.9
  canaliculus 375.57
  clitoris 624.8
  conjunctiva 372.54
  eyelid 374.56
  intestine (impaction) (obstruction)
    560.39
  lacrimal (passages) 375.57
  prepuce (male) 605
    female (clitoris) 624.8
  salivary gland (any) 527.5
  seminal vesicle 608.89
  stomach 537.89
  tonsil 474.8
Concussion (current) 850.9
  with
    loss of consciousness 850.5
      brief (less than one hour)
        30 minutes or less 850.11
        31–59 minutes 850.12
      moderate (1–24 hours) 850.2
      prolonged (more than 24 hours) (with
        complete recovery) (with return
        to pre-existing conscious level)
        850.3
        without return to pre-existing
          conscious level 850.4
    mental confusion or disorientation
      (without loss of consciousness)
      850.0
      with loss of consciousness - see
        Concussion, with, loss of
        consciousness
    without loss of consciousness
      850.0
  blast (air) (hydraulic) (immersion)
    (underwater) 869.0
    with open wound into cavity
      869.1
    abdomen or thorax - see Injury, internal,
      by site
    brain - see Concussion, brain
    ear (acoustic nerve trauma) 951.5
      with perforation, tympanic
        membrane - see Wound, open,
        ear drum
    thorax - see Injury, internal, intrathoracic
      organs NEC
  brain or cerebral (without skull fracture)
    850.9
    with
      loss of consciousness 850.5
        brief (less than one hour)
          30 minutes or less 850.11
          31–59 minutes 850.12
        moderate (1–24 hours) 850.2

◀ New   ◀▥ Revised   ~~deleted~~ Deleted   ● Use Additional Digit(s)   ▨ Omit code

Compression *(Continued)*
 brain or cerebral *(Continued)*
  with *(Continued)*
   loss of consciousness *(Continued)*
    prolonged (more than 24 hours)
     (with complete recovery)
     (with return to pre-existing
     conscious level) 850.3
    without return to pre-existing
     conscious level 850.4
    mental confusion or disorientation
     (without loss of consciousness)
     850.0
    with loss of consciousness - *see*
     Concussion, brain, with, loss
     of consciousness
   skull fracture - *see* Fracture, skull, by site
   without loss of consciousness 850.0
  cauda equina 952.4
  cerebral - *see* Concussion, brain
  conus medullaris (spine) 952.4
  hydraulic - *see* Concussion, blast
  internal organs - *see* Injury, internal, by site
  labyrinth - *see* Injury, intracranial
  ocular 921.3
  osseous labyrinth - *see* Injury, intracranial
  spinal (cord) - *see also* Injury, spinal, by site
   due to
    broken
     back - *see* Fracture, vertebra, by site,
      with spinal cord injury
     neck - *see* Fracture, vertebra,
      cervical, with spinal cord
      injury
    fracture, fracture dislocation, or
     compression fracture of spine or
     vertebra - *see* Fracture, vertebra,
     by site, with spinal cord injury
  syndrome 310.2
  underwater blast - *see* Concussion, blast
Condition - *see also* Disease
 fetal hematologic 678.0●
 psychiatric 298.9
 respiratory NEC 519.9
  acute or subacute NEC 519.9
   due to
    external agent 508.9
     specified type NEC 508.8
    fumes or vapors (chemical)
     (inhalation) 506.3
    radiation 508.0
  chronic NEC 519.9
   due to
    external agent 508.9
     specified type NEC 508.8
    fumes or vapors (chemical)
     (inhalation) 506.4
    radiation 508.1
  due to
   external agent 508.9
    specified type NEC 508.8
   fumes or vapors (chemical) inhalation
    506.9
   smoke inhalation 508.2
Conduct disturbance *(see also* Disturbance,
  conduct) 312.9
 adjustment reaction 309.3
 hyperkinetic 314.2
Condyloma NEC 078.11
 acuminatum 078.11
 gonorrheal 098.0
 latum 091.3
 syphilitic 091.3
  congenital 090.0
 venereal, syphilitic 091.3
Confinement - *see* Delivery
Conflagration - *see also* Burn, by site
 asphyxia (by inhalation of gases, fumes, or
  vapors) 987.9
  specified agent - *see* Table of Drugs and
   Chemicals

Conflict
 family V61.9
  specified circumstance NEC V61.8
 interpersonal NEC V62.81
 marital V61.10
  involving
   divorce V61.03
   estrangement V61.09
 parent (guardian)-child V61.20
  adopted child V61.24
  biological child V61.23
  foster child V61.25
 partner V61.10
Confluent - *see* condition
Confusion, confused (mental) (state) *(see also*
  State, confusional) 298.9
 acute 293.0
 epileptic 293.0
 postoperative 293.9
 psychogenic 298.2
 reactive (from emotional stress,
  psychological trauma) 298.2
 subacute 293.1
Confusional arousals 327.41
Congelation 991.9
Congenital - *see also* condition
 aortic septum 747.29
 generalized fibromatosis (CGF) 759.89
 intrinsic factor deficiency 281.0
 malformation - *see* Anomaly
Congestion, congestive
 asphyxia, newborn 768.9
 bladder 596.89
 bowel 569.89
 brain *(see also* Disease, cerebrovascular NEC)
  437.8
  malarial 084.9
 breast 611.79
 bronchi 519.19
 bronchial tube 519.19
 catarrhal 472.0
 cerebral - *see* Congestion, brain
 cerebrospinal - *see* Congestion, brain
 chest 786.9
 chill 780.99
  malarial *(see also* Malaria) 084.6
 circulatory NEC 459.9
 conjunctiva 372.71
 due to disturbance of circulation 459.9
 duodenum 537.3
 enteritis - *see* Enteritis
 eye 372.71
 fibrosis syndrome (pelvic) 625.5
 gastroenteritis - *see* Enteritis
 general 799.89
 glottis 476.0
 heart *(see also* Failure, heart) 428.0
 hepatic 573.0
 hypostatic (lung) 514
 intestine 569.89
 intracranial - *see* Congestion, brain
 kidney 593.89
 labyrinth 386.50
 larynx 476.0
 liver 573.0
 lung 786.9
  active or acute *(see also* Pneumonia) 486
   congenital 770.0
  chronic 514
  hypostatic 514
  idiopathic, acute 518.52
  passive 514
 malaria, malarial (brain) (fever) *(see also*
  Malaria) 084.6
 medulla - *see* Congestion, brain
 nasal 478.19
 nose 478.19
 orbit, orbital 376.33
  inflammatory (chronic) 376.10
   acute 376.00
 ovary 620.8

Congestion, congestive *(Continued)*
 pancreas 577.8
 pelvic, female 625.5
 pleural 511.0
 prostate (active) 602.1
 pulmonary - *see* Congestion, lung
 renal 593.89
 retina 362.89
 seminal vesicle 608.89
 spinal cord 336.1
 spleen 289.51
  chronic 289.51
 stomach 537.89
 trachea 464.11
 urethra 599.84
 uterus 625.5
  with subinvolution 621.1
 viscera 799.89
Congestive - *see* Congestion
Conical
 cervix 622.6
 cornea 371.60
 teeth 520.2
Conjoined twins 759.4
 causing disproportion (fetopelvic) 678.1●
 fetal 678.1●
Conjugal maladjustment V61.10
 involving
  divorce V61.03
  estrangement V61.09
Conjunctiva - *see* condition
Conjunctivitis (exposure) (infectious)
  (nondiphtheritic) (pneumococcal)
  (pustular) (staphylococcal) (streptococcal)
  NEC 372.30
 actinic 370.24
 acute 372.00
  atopic 372.05
  chemical 372.06
  contagious 372.03
  follicular 372.02
  hemorrhagic (viral) 077.4
  toxic 372.06
 adenoviral (acute) 077.3
 allergic (chronic) 372.14
  with hay fever 372.05
 anaphylactic 372.05
 angular 372.03
 Apollo (viral) 077.4
 atopic 372.05
 blennorrhagic (neonatorum) 098.40
 catarrhal 372.03
 chemical 372.06
  allergic 372.05
  meaning corrosion - *see* Burn, conjunctiva
 chlamydial 077.98
  due to
   Chlamydia trachomatis - *see* Trachoma
   paratrachoma 077.0
 chronic 372.10
  allergic 372.14
  follicular 372.12
  simple 372.11
  specified type NEC 372.14
  vernal 372.13
 diphtheritic 032.81
 due to
  dust 372.05
  enterovirus type 70 077.4
  erythema multiforme 695.10 [372.33]
  filariasis *(see also* Filariasis) 125.9 [372.15]
  mucocutaneous
   disease NEC 372.33
   leishmaniasis 085.5 [372.15]
  Reiter's disease 099.3 [372.33]
  syphilis 095.8 [372.10]
  toxoplasmosis (acquired) 130.1
   congenital (active) 771.2
  trachoma - *see* Trachoma
 dust 372.05
 eczematous 370.31

Conjunctivitis (Continued)
  epidemic 077.1
    hemorrhagic 077.4
  follicular (acute) 372.02
    adenoviral (acute) 077.3
    chronic 372.12
  glare 370.24
  gonococcal (neonatorum) 098.40
  granular (trachomatous) 076.1
    late effect 139.1
  hemorrhagic (acute) (epidemic) 077.4
  herpetic (simplex) 054.43
    zoster 053.21
  inclusion 077.0
  infantile 771.6
  influenzal 372.03
  Koch-Weeks 372.03
  light 372.05
  medicamentosa 372.05
  membranous 372.04
  meningococcic 036.89
  Morax-Axenfeld 372.02
  mucopurulent NEC 372.03
  neonatal 771.6
    gonococcal 098.40
  Newcastle's 077.8
  nodosa 360.14
  of Beal 077.3
  parasitic 372.15
    filariasis (see also Filariasis) 125.9 [372.15]
    mucocutaneous leishmaniasis 085.5
      [372.15]
  Parinaud's 372.02
  petrificans 372.39
  phlyctenular 370.31
  pseudomembranous 372.04
    diphtheritic 032.81
  purulent 372.03
  Reiter's 099.3 [372.33]
  rosacea 695.3 [372.31]
  serous 372.01
    viral 077.99
  simple chronic 372.11
  specified NEC 372.39
  sunlamp 372.04
  swimming pool 077.0
  toxic 372.06
  trachomatous (follicular) 076.1
    acute 076.0
    late effect 139.1
  traumatic NEC 372.39
  tuberculous (see also Tuberculosis) 017.3●
    [370.31]
  tularemic 021.3
  tularensis 021.3
  vernal 372.13
    limbar 372.13 [370.32]
  viral 077.99
    acute hemorrhagic 077.4
    specified NEC 077.8
Conjunctivochalasis 372.81
Conjunctoblepharitis - see Conjunctivitis
Conn (-Louis) syndrome (primary
    aldosteronism) 255.12
Connective tissue - see condition
Conradi (-Hünermann) syndrome or disease
    (chondrodysplasia calcificans congenita)
    756.59
Consanguinity V19.7
Consecutive - see condition
Consolidated lung (base) - see Pneumonia,
    lobar
Constipation 564.00
  atonic 564.09
  drug induced
    correct substance properly administered
      564.09
    overdose or wrong substance given or
      taken 977.9
      specified drug - see Table of Drugs and
        Chemicals

Constipation (Continued)
  neurogenic 564.09
  other specified NEC 564.09
  outlet dysfunction 564.02
  psychogenic 306.4
  simple 564.00
  slow transit 564.01
  spastic 564.09
Constitutional - see also condition
  arterial hypotension (see also Hypotension)
    458.9
  obesity 278.00
    morbid 278.01
  psychopathic state 301.9
  short stature in childhood 783.43
  state, developmental V21.9
    specified development NEC V21.8
  substandard 301.6
Constitutionally substandard 301.6
Constriction
  anomalous, meningeal bands or folds 742.8
  aortic arch (congenital) 747.10
  asphyxiation or suffocation by 994.7
  bronchus 519.19
  canal, ear (see also Stricture, ear canal,
    acquired) 380.50
  duodenum 537.3
  gallbladder (see also Obstruction,
    gallbladder) 575.2
    congenital 751.69
  intestine (see also Obstruction, intestine) 560.9
  larynx 478.74
    congenital 748.3
  meningeal bands or folds, anomalous 742.8
  organ or site, congenital NEC - see Atresia
  prepuce (congenital) 605
  pylorus 537.0
    adult hypertrophic 537.0
    congenital or infantile 750.5
    newborn 750.5
  ring (uterus) 661.4●
    affecting fetus or newborn 763.7
  spastic - see also Spasm
    ureter 593.3
    urethra - see Stricture, urethra
  stomach 537.89
  ureter 593.3
  urethra - see Stricture, urethra
  visual field (functional) (peripheral) 368.45
Constrictive - see condition
Consultation V65.9
  medical - see also Counseling, medical
  specified reason NEC V65.8
  without complaint or sickness V65.9
    feared complaint unfounded V65.5
    specified reason NEC V65.8
Consumption - see Tuberculosis
Contact - see also Exposure (suspected)
  with
    AIDS virus V01.79
    anthrax V01.81
    asbestos V15.84
    cholera V01.0
    communicable disease V01.9
      specified type NEC V01.89
      viral NEC V01.79
    Escherichia coli (E. coli) V01.83
    German measles V01.4
    gonorrhea V01.6
    HIV V01.79
    human immunodeficiency virus V01.79
    lead V15.86
    meningococcus V01.84
    parasitic disease NEC V01.89
    poliomyelitis V01.2
    potentially hazardous body fluids V15.85
    rabies V01.5
    rubella V01.4
    SARS-associated coronavirus V01.82
    smallpox V01.3
    syphilis V01.6

Contact (Continued)
  with (Continued)
    tuberculosis V01.1
    varicella V01.71
    venereal disease V01.6
    viral disease NEC V01.79
  dermatitis - see Dermatitis
Contamination, food (see also Poisoning, food)
    005.9
Contraception, contraceptive
  advice NEC V25.09
    family planning V25.09
    fitting of diaphragm V25.02
    prescribing or use of
      oral contraceptive agent V25.01
      specified agent NEC V25.02
  counseling NEC V25.09
    emergency V25.03
    family planning V25.09
    fitting of diaphragm V25.02
    prescribing or use of
      oral contraceptive agent V25.01
        emergency V25.03
        postcoital V25.03
      specified agent NEC V25.02
  device (in situ) V45.59
    causing menorrhagia 996.76
    checking V25.42
    complications 996.32
    insertion V25.11
    intrauterine V45.51
    reinsertion V25.13
    removal V25.12
      and reinsertion V25.13
    replacement V25.13
    subdermal V45.52
  fitting of diaphragm V25.02
  insertion
    intrauterine contraceptive device V25.11
    subdermal implantable V25.5
  maintenance V25.40
    examination V25.40
      intrauterine device V25.42
      oral contraceptive V25.41
      specified method NEC V25.49
      subdermal implantable V25.43
    intrauterine device V25.42
    oral contraceptive V25.41
    specified method NEC V25.49
    subdermal implantable V25.43
  management NEC V25.49
  prescription
    oral contraceptive agent V25.01
      emergency V25.03
      postcoital V25.03
      repeat V25.41
    specified agent NEC V25.02
      repeat V25.49
  sterilization V25.2
  surveillance V25.40
    intrauterine device V25.42
    oral contraceptive agent V25.41
    specified method NEC V25.49
    subdermal implantable V25.43
Contraction, contracture, contracted
  Achilles tendon (see also Short, tendon,
    Achilles) 727.81
  anus 564.89
  axilla 729.90
  bile duct (see also Disease, biliary) 576.8
  bladder 596.89
    neck or sphincter 596.0
  bowel (see also Obstruction, intestine) 560.9
  Braxton Hicks 644.1●
  breast implant, capsular 611.83
  bronchus 519.19
  burn (old) - see Cicatrix
  capsular, of breast implant 611.83
  cecum (see also Obstruction, intestine) 560.9
  cervix (see also Stricture, cervix) 622.4
    congenital 752.49

◀ New   ◀◀ Revised   ~~deleted~~ Deleted   ● Use Additional Digit(s)   ▨ Omit code

Contraction, contracture, contracted
(Continued)
cicatricial - see Cicatrix
colon (see also Obstruction, intestine) 560.9
conjunctiva, trachomatous, active 076.1
late effect 139.1
Dupuytren's 728.6
eyelid 374.41
eye socket (after enucleation) 372.64
face 729.90
fascia (lata) (postural) 728.89
Dupuytren's 728.6
palmar 728.6
plantar 728.71
finger NEC 736.29
congenital 755.59
joint (see also Contraction, joint) 718.44
flaccid, paralytic
joint (see also Contraction, joint) 718.4●
muscle 728.85
ocular 378.50
gallbladder (see also Obstruction,
gallbladder) 575.2
hamstring 728.89
tendon 727.81
heart valve - see Endocarditis
Hicks' 644.1●
hip (see also Contraction, joint) 718.4●
hourglass
bladder 596.89
congenital 753.8
gallbladder (see also Obstruction,
gallbladder) 575.2
congenital 751.69
stomach 536.8
congenital 750.7
psychogenic 306.4
uterus 661.4●
affecting fetus or newborn 763.7
hysterical 300.11
infantile (see also Epilepsy) 345.6●
internal os (see also Stricture, cervix) 622.4
intestine (see also Obstruction, intestine) 560.9
joint (abduction) (acquired) (adduction)
(flexion) (rotation) 718.40
ankle 718.47
congenital NEC 755.8
generalized or multiple 754.89
lower limb joints 754.89
hip (see also Subluxation, congenital,
hip) 754.32
lower limb (including pelvic girdle)
not involving hip 754.89
upper limb (including shoulder girdle)
755.59
elbow 718.42
foot 718.47
hand 718.44
hip 718.45
hysterical 300.11
knee 718.46
multiple sites 718.49
pelvic region 718.45
shoulder (region) 718.41
specified site NEC 718.48
wrist 718.43
kidney (granular) (secondary) (see also
Sclerosis, renal) 587
congenital 753.3
hydronephritic 591
pyelonephritic (see also Pyelitis, chronic)
590.00
tuberculous (see also Tuberculosis) 016.0●
ligament 728.89
congenital 756.89
liver - see Cirrhosis, liver
muscle (postinfectional) (postural) NEC
728.85
congenital 756.89
sternocleidomastoid 754.1
extraocular 378.60

Contraction, contracture, contracted
(Continued)
muscle NEC (Continued)
eye (extrinsic) (see also Strabismus) 378.9
paralytic (see also Strabismus, paralytic)
378.50
flaccid 728.85
hysterical 300.11
ischemic (Volkmann's) 958.6
paralytic 728.85
posttraumatic 958.6
psychogenic 306.0
specified as conversion reaction 300.11
myotonic 728.85
neck (see also Torticollis) 723.5
congenital 754.1
psychogenic 306.0
ocular muscle (see also Strabismus) 378.9
paralytic (see also Strabismus, paralytic)
378.50
organ or site, congenital NEC - see Atresia
outlet (pelvis) - see Contraction, pelvis
palmar fascia 728.6
paralytic
joint (see also Contraction, joint) 718.4●
muscle 728.85
ocular (see also Strabismus, paralytic)
378.50
pelvis (acquired) (general) 738.6
affecting fetus or newborn 763.1
complicating delivery 653.1●
causing obstructed labor 660.1●
generally contracted 653.1●
causing obstructed labor 660.1●
inlet 653.2●
causing obstructed labor 660.1●
midpelvic 653.8●
causing obstructed labor 660.1●
midplane 653.8●
causing obstructed labor 660.1●
outlet 653.3●
causing obstructed labor 660.1●
plantar fascia 728.71
premature
atrial 427.61
auricular 427.61
auriculoventricular 427.61
heart (junctional) (nodal) 427.60
supraventricular 427.61
ventricular 427.69
prostate 602.8
pylorus (see also Pylorospasm) 537.81
rectosigmoid (see also Obstruction, intestine)
560.9
rectum, rectal (sphincter) 564.89
psychogenic 306.4
ring (Bandl's) 661.4●
affecting fetus or newborn 763.7
scar - see Cicatrix
sigmoid (see also Obstruction, intestine) 560.9
socket, eye 372.64
spine (see also Curvature, spine) 737.9
stomach 536.8
hourglass 536.8
congenital 750.7
psychogenic 306.4
psychogenic 306.4
tendon (sheath) (see also Short, tendon)
727.81
toe 735.8
ureterovesical orifice (postinfectional) 593.3
urethra 599.84
uterus 621.8
abnormal 661.9●
affecting fetus or newborn 763.7
clonic, hourglass or tetanic 661.4●
affecting fetus or newborn 763.7
dyscoordinate 661.4●
affecting fetus or newborn 763.7
hourglass 661.4●
affecting fetus or newborn 763.7

Contraction, contracture, contracted
(Continued)
uterus (Continued)
hypotonic NEC 661.2●
affecting fetus or newborn 763.7
incoordinate 661.4●
affecting fetus or newborn 763.7
inefficient or poor 661.2●
affecting fetus or newborn 763.7
irregular 661.2●
affecting fetus or newborn 763.7
tetanic 661.4●
affecting fetus or newborn 763.7
vagina (outlet) 623.2
vesical 596.89
neck or urethral orifice 596.0
visual field, generalized 368.45
Volkmann's (ischemic) 958.6
Contusion (skin surface intact) 924.9
with
crush injury - see Crush
dislocation - see Dislocation, by site
fracture - see Fracture, by site
internal injury - see also Injury, internal, by
site
heart - see Contusion, cardiac
kidney - see Contusion, kidney
liver - see Contusion, liver
lung - see Contusion, lung
spleen - see Contusion, spleen
intracranial injury - see Injury, intracranial
nerve injury - see Injury, nerve
open wound - see Wound, open, by site
abdomen, abdominal (muscle) (wall) 922.2
organ(s) NEC 868.00
adnexa, eye NEC 921.9
ankle 924.21
with other parts of foot 924.20
arm 923.9
lower (with elbow) 923.10
upper 923.03
with shoulder or axillary region 923.09
auditory canal (external) (meatus) (and other
part(s) of neck, scalp, or face, except
eye) 920
auricle, ear (and other part(s) of neck, scalp,
or face except eye) 920
axilla 923.02
with shoulder or upper arm 923.09
back 922.31
bone NEC 924.9
brain (cerebral) (membrane) (with
hemorrhage) 851.8●

Note: Use the following fifth-digit
subclassification with categories 851–854:

0	unspecified state of consciousness
1	with no loss of consciousness
2	with brief [less than one hour] loss of consciousness
3	with moderate [1-24 hours] loss of consciousness
4	with prolonged [more than 24 hours] loss of consciousness and return to pre-existing conscious level
5	with prolonged [more than 24 hours] loss of consciousness, without return to pre-existing conscious level

Use fifth-digit 5 to designate when a patient
is unconscious and dies before regaining
consciousness, regardless of the duration of
the loss of consciousness

6	with loss of consciousness of unspecified duration
9	with concussion, unspecified

with
open intracranial wound 851.9●
skull fracture - see Fracture, skull, by
site

Contusion *(Continued)*
  brain *(Continued)*
    cerebellum 851.4●
      with open intracranial wound 851.5●
    cortex 851.0●
      with open intracranial wound 851.1●
    occipital lobe 851.4●
      with open intracranial wound 851.5●
    stem 851.4●
      with open intracranial wound 851.5●
  breast 922.0
  brow (and other part(s) of neck, scalp, or face, except eye) 920
  buttock 922.32
  canthus 921.1
  cardiac 861.01
    with open wound into thorax 861.11
  cauda equina (spine) 952.4
  cerebellum - *see* Contusion, brain, cerebellum
  cerebral - *see* Contusion, brain
  cheek(s) (and other part(s) of neck, scalp, or face, except eye) 920
  chest (wall) 922.1
  chin (and other part(s) of neck, scalp, or face, except eye) 920
  clitoris 922.4
  conjunctiva 921.1
  conus medullaris (spine) 952.4
  cornea 921.3
  corpus cavernosum 922.4
  cortex (brain) (cerebral) - *see* Contusion, brain, cortex
  costal region 922.1
  ear (and other part(s) of neck, scalp, or face except eye) 920
  elbow 923.11
    with forearm 923.10
  epididymis 922.4
  epigastric region 922.2
  eye NEC 921.9
  eyeball 921.3
  eyelid(s) (and periocular area) 921.1
  face (and neck, or scalp, any part, except eye) 920
  femoral triangle 922.2
  fetus or newborn 772.6
  finger(s) (nail) (subungual) 923.3
  flank 922.2
  foot (with ankle) (excluding toe(s)) 924.20
  forearm (and elbow) 923.10
  forehead (and other part(s) of neck, scalp, or face, except eye) 920
  genital organs, external 922.4
  globe (eye) 921.3
  groin 922.2
  gum(s) (and other part(s) of neck, scalp, or face, except eye) 920
  hand(s) (except fingers alone) 923.20
  head (any part, except eye) (and face) (and neck) 920
  heart - *see* Contusion, cardiac
  heel 924.20
  hip 924.01
    with thigh 924.00
  iliac region 922.2
  inguinal region 922.2
  internal organs (abdomen, chest, or pelvis) NEC - *see* Injury, internal, by site
  interscapular region 922.33
  iris (eye) 921.3
  kidney 866.01
    with open wound into cavity 866.11
  knee 924.11
    with lower leg 924.10
  labium (majus) (minus) 922.4
  lacrimal apparatus, gland, or sac 921.1
  larynx (and other part(s) of neck, scalp, or face, except eye) 920
  late effect - *see* Late, effects (of), contusion
  leg 924.5
    lower (with knee) 924.10

Contusion *(Continued)*
  lens 921.3
  lingual (and other part(s) of neck, scalp, or face, except eye) 920
  lip(s) (and other part(s) of neck, scalp, or face, except eye) 920
  liver 864.01
    with
      laceration - *see* Laceration, liver
      open wound into cavity 864.11
  lower extremity 924.5
    multiple sites 924.4
  lumbar region 922.31
  lung 861.21
    with open wound into thorax 861.31
  malar region (and other part(s) of neck, scalp, or face, except eye) 920
  mandibular joint (and other part(s) of neck, scalp, or face, except eye) 920
  mastoid region (and other part(s) of neck, scalp, or face, except eye) 920
  membrane, brain - *see* Contusion, brain
  midthoracic region 922.1
  mouth (and other part(s) of neck, scalp, or face, except eye) 920
  multiple sites (not classifiable to same three-digit category) 924.8
    lower limb 924.4
    trunk 922.8
    upper limb 923.8
  muscle NEC 924.9
  myocardium - *see* Contusion, cardiac
  nasal (septum) (and other part(s) of neck, scalp, or face, except eye) 920
  neck (and scalp, or face, any part, except eye) 920
  nerve - *see* Injury, nerve, by site
  nose (and other part(s) of neck, scalp, or face, except eye) 920
  occipital region (scalp) (and neck or face, except eye) 920
    lobe - *see* Contusion, brain, occipital lobe
  orbit (region) (tissues) 921.2
  palate (soft) (and other part(s) of neck, scalp, or face, except eye) 920
  parietal region (scalp) (and neck, or face, except eye) 920
    lobe - *see* Contusion, brain
  penis 922.4
  pericardium - *see* Contusion, cardiac
  perineum 922.4
  periocular area 921.1
  pharynx (and other part(s) of neck, scalp, or face, except eye) 920
  popliteal space (*see also* Contusion, knee) 924.11
  prepuce 922.4
  pubic region 922.4
  pudenda 922.4
  pulmonary - *see* Contusion, lung
  quadriceps femoralis 924.00
  rib cage 922.1
  sacral region 922.32
  salivary ducts or glands (and other part(s) of neck, scalp, or face, except eye) 920
  scalp (and neck, or face, any part, except eye) 920
  scapular region 923.01
    with shoulder or upper arm 923.09
  sclera (eye) 921.3
  scrotum 922.4
  shoulder 923.00
    with upper arm or axillar regions 923.09
  skin NEC 924.9
  skull 920
  spermatic cord 922.4
  spinal cord - *see also* Injury, spinal, by site
    cauda equina 952.4
    conus medullaris 952.4
  spleen 865.01
    with open wound into cavity 865.11

Contusion *(Continued)*
  sternal region 922.1
  stomach - *see* Injury, internal, stomach
  subconjunctival 921.1
  subcutaneous NEC 924.9
  submaxillary region (and other part(s) of neck, scalp, or face, except eye) 920
  submental region (and other part(s) of neck, scalp, or face, except eye) 920
  subperiosteal NEC 924.9
  supraclavicular fossa (and other part(s) of neck, scalp, or face, except eye) 920
  supraorbital (and other part(s) of neck, scalp, or face, except eye) 920
  temple (region) (and other part(s) of neck, scalp, or face, except eye) 920
  testis 922.4
  thigh (and hip) 924.00
  thorax 922.1
    organ - *see* Injury, internal, intrathoracic
  throat (and other part(s) of neck, scalp, or face, except eye) 920
  thumb(s) (nail) (subungual) 923.3
  toe(s) (nail) (subungual) 924.3
  tongue (and other part(s) of neck, scalp, or face, except eye) 920
  trunk 922.9
    multiple sites 922.8
    specified site - *see* Contusion, by site
  tunica vaginalis 922.4
  tympanum (membrane) (and other part(s) of neck, scalp, or face, except eye) 920
  upper extremity 923.9
    multiple sites 923.8
  uvula (and other part(s) of neck, scalp, or face, except eye) 920
  vagina 922.4
  vocal cord(s) (and other part(s) of neck, scalp, or face, except eye) 920
  vulva 922.4
  wrist 923.21
    with hand(s), except finger(s) alone 923.20
Conus (any type) (congenital) 743.57
  acquired 371.60
  medullaris syndrome 336.8
Convalescence (following) V66.9
  chemotherapy V66.2
  medical NEC V66.5
  psychotherapy V66.3
  radiotherapy V66.1
  surgery NEC V66.0
  treatment (for) NEC V66.5
    combined V66.6
    fracture V66.4
    mental disorder NEC V66.3
    specified disorder NEC V66.5
Conversion
  closed surgical procedure to open procedure
    arthroscopic V64.43
    laparoscopic V64.41
    thoracoscopic V64.42
  hysteria, hysterical, any type 300.11
  neurosis, any 300.11
  reaction, any 300.11
Converter, tuberculosis (test reaction) 795.51
Convulsions (idiopathic) 780.39
  apoplectiform (*see also* Disease, cerebrovascular, acute) 436
  brain 780.39
  cerebral 780.39
  cerebrospinal 780.39
  due to trauma NEC - *see* Injury, intracranial
  eclamptic (*see also* Eclampsia) 780.39
  epileptic (*see also* Epilepsy) 345.9●
  epileptiform (*see also* Seizure, epileptiform) 780.39
  epileptoid (*see also* Seizure, epileptiform) 780.39

◀ New   ⬅ Revised   ~~deleted~~ Deleted   ● Use Additional Digit(s)   ▨ Omit code

Convulsions (Continued)
  ether
    anesthetic
      correct substance properly
          administered 780.39
      overdose or wrong substance given
          968.2
      other specified type - see Table of Drugs
          and Chemicals
  febrile (simple) 780.31
    complex 780.32
  generalized 780.39
  hysterical 300.11
  infantile 780.39
    epilepsy - see Epilepsy
  internal 780.39
  jacksonian (see also Epilepsy) 345.5●
  myoclonic 333.2
  newborn 779.0
  paretic 094.1
  pregnancy (nephritic) (uremic) - see
      Eclampsia, pregnancy
  psychomotor (see also Epilepsy) 345.4●
  puerperal, postpartum - see Eclampsia,
      pregnancy
  recurrent 780.39
    epileptic - see Epilepsy
  reflex 781.0
  repetitive 780.39
    epileptic - see Epilepsy
  salaam (see also Epilepsy) 345.6●
  scarlatinal 034.1
  spasmodic 780.39
  tetanus, tetanic (see also Tetanus) 037
  thymic 254.8
  uncinate 780.39
  uremic 586
Convulsive - see also Convulsions
  disorder or state 780.39
    epileptic - see Epilepsy
  equivalent, abdominal (see also Epilepsy)
      345.5●
Cooke-Apert-Gallais syndrome
    (adrenogenital) 255.2
Cooley's anemia (erythroblastic)
    282.44
Coolie itch 126.9
Cooper's
  disease 610.1
  hernia - see Hernia, Cooper's
Coordination disturbance 781.3
Copper wire arteries, retina 362.13
Copra itch 133.8
Coprolith 560.39
Coprophilia 302.89
Coproporphyria, hereditary 277.1
Coprostasis 560.32
  with hernia - see also Hernia, by site, with
      obstruction
    gangrenous - see Hernia, by site, with
        gangrene
Cor
  biloculare 745.7
  bovinum - see Hypertrophy, cardiac
  bovis - see also Hypertrophy, cardiac
  pulmonale (chronic) 416.9
    acute 415.0
  triatriatum, triatrium 746.82
  triloculare 745.8
    biatriatum 745.3
    biventriculare 745.69
Corbus' disease 607.1
Cord - see also condition
  around neck (tightly) (with compression)
    affecting fetus or newborn 762.5
    complicating delivery 663.1●
      without compression 663.3●
        affecting fetus or newborn
            762.6
  bladder NEC 344.61
    tabetic 094.0

Cord (Continued)
  prolapse
    affecting fetus or newborn 762.4
    complicating delivery 663.0●
Cord's angiopathy (see also Tuberculosis) 017.3●
    [362.18]
Cordis ectopia 746.87
Corditis (spermatic) 608.4
Corectopia 743.46
Cori type glycogen storage disease - see
    Disease, glycogen storage
Cork-handlers' disease or lung 495.3
Corkscrew esophagus 530.5
Corlett's pyosis (impetigo) 684
Corn (infected) 700
Cornea - see also condition
  donor V59.5
  guttata (dystrophy) 371.57
  plana 743.41
Cornelia de Lange's syndrome
    (Amsterdam dwarf, intellectual
    disabilities, and brachycephaly)
    759.89
Cornual gestation or pregnancy - see
    Pregnancy, cornual
Cornu cutaneum 702.8
Coronary (artery) - see also condition
  arising from aorta or pulmonary trunk
      746.85
Corpora - see also condition
  amylacea (prostate) 602.8
  cavernosa - see condition
Corpulence (see also Obesity)
Corpus - see condition
Corrigan's disease - see Insufficiency,
    aortic
Corrosive burn - see Burn, by site
Corsican fever (see also Malaria) 084.6
Cortical - see also condition
  blindness 377.75
  necrosis, kidney (bilateral) 583.6
Corticoadrenal - see condition
Corticosexual syndrome 255.2
Coryza (acute) 460
  with grippe or influenza (see also Influenza)
      487.1
  syphilitic 095.8
    congenital (chronic) 090.0
Costen's syndrome or complex 524.60
Costiveness (see also Constipation) 564.00
Costochondritis 733.6
Cotard's syndrome (paranoia) 297.1
Cot death 798.0
Cotia virus 059.8
Cotungo's disease 724.3
Cough 786.2
  with hemorrhage (see also Hemoptysis)
      786.39
  affected 786.2
  bronchial 786.2
    with grippe or influenza (see also
        Influenza) 487.1
  chronic 786.2
  epidemic 786.2
  functional 306.1
  hemorrhagic 786.39
  hysterical 300.11
  laryngeal, spasmodic 786.2
  nervous 786.2
  psychogenic 306.1
  smokers' 491.0
  tea tasters' 112.89
Counseling NEC V65.40
  without complaint or sickness
      V65.49
  abuse victim NEC V62.89
    child V61.21
    partner V61.11
    spouse V61.11
  child abuse, maltreatment, or neglect
      V61.21

Counseling NEC (Continued)
  contraceptive NEC V25.09
    device (intrauterine) V25.02
    maintenance V25.40
      intrauterine contraceptive device V25.42
      oral contraceptive (pill) V25.41
      specified type NEC V25.49
      subdermal implantable V25.43
    management NEC V25.9
    oral contraceptive (pill) V25.01
      emergency V25.03
      postcoital V25.03
    prescription NEC V25.02
      oral contraceptive (pill) V25.01
        emergency V25.03
        postcoital V25.03
        repeat prescription V25.41
      repeat prescription V25.40
    subdermal implantable V25.43
    surveillance NEC V25.40
  dietary V65.3
  exercise V65.41
  expectant parent(s)
    pediatric pre-adoption visit V65.11
    pediatric pre-birth visit V65.11
  explanation of
    investigation finding NEC V65.49
    medication NEC V65.49
  family planning V25.09
    natural
      procreative V26.41
      to avoid pregnancy V25.04
  for nonattending third party V65.19
  genetic V26.33
  gonorrhea V65.45
  health (advice) (education) (instruction) NEC
      V65.49
  HIV V65.44
  human immunodeficiency virus V65.44
  injury prevention V65.43
  insulin pump training V65.46
  marital V61.10
  medical (for) V65.9
    boarding school resident V60.6
    condition not demonstrated V65.5
    feared complaint and no disease found
        V65.5
    institutional resident V60.6
    on behalf of another V65.19
    person living alone V60.3
  natural family planning
    procreative V26.41
    to avoid pregnancy V25.04
  parent (guardian)-child conflict V61.20
    adopted child V61.24
    biological child V61.23
    foster child V61.25
    specified problem NEC V61.29
  partner abuse
    perpetrator V61.12
    victim V61.11
  pediatric
    pre-adoption visit for adoptive parent(s)
        V65.11
    pre-birth visit for expectant parents
        V65.11
  perpetrator of
    child abuse V62.83
      parental V61.22
    partner abuse V61.12
    spouse abuse V61.12
  procreative V65.49
  sex NEC V65.49
    transmitted disease NEC V65.45
      HIV V65.44
  specified reason NEC V65.49
  spousal abuse
    perpetrator V61.12
    victim V61.11
  substance use and abuse V65.42
  syphilis V65.45

Counseling NEC *(Continued)*
  victim (of)
    abuse NEC V62.89
    child abuse V61.21
    partner abuse V61.11
    spousal abuse V61.11
Coupled rhythm 427.89
Couvelaire uterus (complicating delivery) - *see*
  Placenta, separation
Cowper's gland - *see* condition
Cowperitis (*see also* Urethritis) 597.89
  gonorrheal (acute) 098.0
    chronic or duration of 2 months or over
    098.2
Cowpox (abortive) 051.01
  due to vaccination 999.0
  eyelid 051.01 *[373.5]*
    postvaccination 999.0 *[373.5]*
Coxa
  plana 732.1
  valga (acquired) 736.31
    congenital 755.61
    late effect of rickets 268.1
  vara (acquired) 736.32
    congenital 755.62
    late effect of rickets 268.1
Coxae malum senilis 715.25
Coxalgia (nontuberculous) 719.45
  tuberculous (*see also* Tuberculosis) 015.1 ●
    [730.85]
Coxalgic pelvis 736.30
Coxitis 716.65
Coxsackie (infection) (virus) 079.2
  central nervous system NEC 048
  endocarditis 074.22
  enteritis 008.67
  meningitis (aseptic) 047.0
  myocarditis 074.23
  pericarditis 074.21
  pharyngitis 074.0
  pleurodynia 074.1
  specific disease NEC 074.8
Crabs, meaning pubic lice 132.2
Crack baby 760.75
Cracked
  nipple 611.2
    puerperal, postpartum 676.1 ●
  tooth 521.81
Cradle cap 690.11
Craft neurosis 300.89
Craigiasis 007.8
Cramp(s) 729.82
  abdominal 789.0 ●
  bathing 994.1
  colic 789.7
    infantile 789.7
    psychogenic 306.4
  due to immersion 994.1
  extremity (lower) (upper) NEC 729.82
  fireman 992.2
  heat 992.2
  hysterical 300.11
  immersion 994.1
  intestinal 789.0 ●
    psychogenic 306.4
  linotypist's 300.89
    organic 333.84
  muscle (extremity) (general) 729.82
    due to immersion 994.1
    hysterical 300.11
  occupational (hand) 300.89
    organic 333.84
  psychogenic 307.89
  salt depletion 276.1
  sleep related leg 327.52
  stoker 992.2
  stomach 789.0 ●
  telegraphers' 300.89
    organic 333.84
  typists' 300.89
    organic 333.84

Cramp(s) *(Continued)*
  uterus 625.8
    menstrual 625.3
  writers' 333.84
    organic 333.84
    psychogenic 300.89
Cranial - *see* condition
Cranioclasis, fetal 763.89
Craniocleidodysostosis 755.59
Craniofenestria (skull) 756.0
Craniolacunia (skull) 756.0
Craniopagus 759.4
Craniopathy, metabolic 733.3
Craniopharyngeal - *see* condition
Craniopharyngioma (M9350/1) 237.0
Craniorachischisis (totalis) 740.1
Cranioschisis 756.0
Craniostenosis 756.0
Craniosynostosis 756.0
Craniotabes (cause unknown) 733.3
  rachitic 268.1
  syphilitic 090.5
Craniotomy, fetal 763.89
Cranium - *see* condition
Craw-craw 125.3
CRBSI (catheter-related bloodstream infection)
  999.31
Creaking joint 719.60
  ankle 719.67
  elbow 719.62
  foot 719.67
  hand 719.64
  hip 719.65
  knee 719.66
  multiple sites 719.69
  pelvic region 719.65
  shoulder (region) 719.61
  specified site NEC 719.68
  wrist 719.63
Creeping
  eruption 126.9
  palsy 335.21
  paralysis 335.21
Crenated tongue 529.8
Creotoxism 005.9
Crepitus
  caput 756.0
  joint 719.60
    ankle 719.67
    elbow 719.62
    foot 719.67
    hand 719.64
    hip 719.65
    knee 719.66
    multiple sites 719.69
    pelvic region 719.65
    shoulder (region) 719.61
    specified site NEC 719.68
    wrist 719.63
Crescent or conus choroid, congenital 743.57
Cretin, cretinism (athyrotic) (congenital)
  (endemic) (metabolic) (nongoitrous)
  (sporadic) 243
  goitrous (sporadic) 246.1
  pelvis (dwarf type) (male type) 243
    with disproportion (fetopelvic) 653.1 ●
      affecting fetus or newborn 763.1
      causing obstructed labor 660.1 ●
        affecting fetus or newborn 763.1
  pituitary 253.3
Cretinoid degeneration 243
Creutzfeldt-Jakob disease (CJD) (syndrome)
  046.19
  with dementia
    with behavioral disturbance 046.19
      [294.11]
    without behavioral disturbance 046.19
      [294.10]
  familial 046.19
  iatrogenic 046.19
  specified NEC 046.19

Creutzfeldt-Jakob disease *(Continued)*
  sporadic 046.19
  variant (vCJD) 046.11
    with dementia
      with behavioral disturbance 046.11
        [294.11]
      without behavioral disturbance 046.11
        [294.10]
Crib death 798.0
Cribriform hymen 752.49
Cri-du-chat syndrome 758.31
Crigler-Najjar disease or syndrome (congenital
  hyperbilirubinemia) 277.4
Crimean hemorrhagic fever 065.0
Criminalism 301.7
Crisis
  abdomen 789.0 ●
  addisonian (acute adrenocortical
    insufficiency) 255.41
  adrenal (cortical) 255.41
  asthmatic - *see* Asthma
  brain, cerebral (*see also* Disease,
    cerebrovascular, acute) 436
  celiac 579.0
  Dietl's 593.4
  emotional NEC 309.29
    acute reaction to stress 308.0
    adjustment reaction 309.9
    specific to childhood or adolescence 313.9
  gastric (tabetic) 094.0
  glaucomatocyclitic 364.22
  heart (*see also* Failure, heart) 428.9
  hypertensive - *see* Hypertension
  nitritoid
    correct substance properly administered
      458.29
    overdose or wrong substance given or
      taken 961.1
  oculogyric 378.87
    psychogenic 306.7
  Pel's 094.0
  psychosexual identity 302.6
  rectum 094.0
  renal 593.81
  sickle cell 282.62
  stomach (tabetic) 094.0
  tabetic 094.0
  thyroid (*see also* Thyrotoxicosis) 242.9 ●
  thyrotoxic (*see also* Thyrotoxicosis) 242.9 ●
  vascular - *see* Disease, cerebrovascular, acute
Crocq's disease (acrocyanosis) 443.89
Crohn's disease (*see also* Enteritis, regional)
  555.9
Cronkhite-Canada syndrome 211.3
Crooked septum, nasal 470
Cross
  birth (of fetus) complicating delivery 652.3 ●
    with successful version 652.1 ●
      causing obstructed labor 660.0 ●
  bite, anterior or posterior 524.27
  eye (*see also* Esotropia) 378.00
Crossed ectopia of kidney 753.3
Crossfoot 754.50
Croup, croupous (acute) (angina) (catarrhal)
  (infective) (inflammatory) (laryngeal)
  (membranous) (nondiphtheritic)
  (pseudomembranous) 464.4
  asthmatic (*see also* Asthma) 493.9 ●
  bronchial 466.0
  diphtheritic (membranous) 032.3
  false 478.75
  spasmodic 478.75
    diphtheritic 032.3
  stridulous 478.75
    diphtheritic 032.3
Crouzon's disease (craniofacial dysostosis)
  756.0
Crowding, teeth 524.31
CRST syndrome (cutaneous systemic sclerosis)
  710.1
Cruchet's disease (encephalitis lethargica) 049.8

◀ New   ◀▥ Revised   ~~deleted~~ Deleted   ● Use Additional Digit(s)   ▨ Omit code

Cruelty in children (see also Disturbance, conduct) 312.9
Crural ulcer (see also Ulcer, lower extremity) 707.10
Crush, crushed, crushing (injury) 929.9
　abdomen 926.19
　　internal - see Injury, internal, abdomen
　ankle 928.21
　　with other parts of foot 928.20
　arm 927.9
　　lower (and elbow) 927.10
　　upper 927.03
　　　with shoulder or axillary region 927.09
　axilla 927.02
　　with shoulder or upper arm 927.09
　back 926.11
　breast 926.19
　buttock 926.12
　cheek 925.1
　chest - see Injury, internal, chest
　ear 925.1
　elbow 927.11
　　with forearm 927.10
　face 925.1
　finger(s) 927.3
　　with hand(s) 927.20
　　　and wrist(s) 927.21
　flank 926.19
　foot, excluding toe(s) alone (with ankle) 928.20
　forearm (and elbow) 927.10
　genitalia, external (female) (male) 926.0
　　internal - see Injury, internal, genital organ NEC
　hand, except finger(s) alone (and wrist) 927.20
　head - see Fracture, skull, by site
　heel 928.20
　hip 928.01
　　with thigh 928.00
　internal organ (abdomen, chest, or pelvis) - see Injury, internal, by site
　knee 928.11
　　with leg, lower 928.10
　labium (majus) (minus) 926.0
　larynx 925.2
　late effect - see Late, effects (of), crushing
　leg 928.9
　　lower 928.10
　　　and knee 928.11
　　upper 928.00
　limb
　　lower 928.9
　　　multiple sites 928.8
　　upper 927.9
　　　multiple sites 927.8
　multiple sites NEC 929.0
　neck 925.2
　nerve - see Injury, nerve, by site
　nose 802.0
　　open 802.1
　penis 926.0
　pharynx 925.2
　scalp 925.1
　scapular region 927.01
　　with shoulder or upper arm 927.09
　scrotum 926.0
　shoulder 927.00
　　with upper arm or axillary region 927.09
　skull or cranium - see Fracture, skull, by site
　spinal cord - see Injury, spinal, by site
　syndrome (complication of trauma) 958.5
　testis 926.0
　thigh (with hip) 928.00
　throat 925.2
　thumb(s) (and fingers) 927.3
　toe(s) 928.3
　　with foot 928.20
　　　and ankle 928.21
　tonsil 925.2

Crush, crushed, crushing (Continued)
　trunk 926.9
　　chest - see Injury, internal, intrathoracic organs NEC
　　internal organ - see Injury, internal, by site
　　multiple sites 926.8
　　specified site NEC 926.19
　vulva 926.0
　wrist 927.21
　　with hand(s), except fingers alone 927.20
Crusta lactea 690.11
Crusts 782.8
Crutch paralysis 953.4
Cruveilhier's disease 335.21
Cruveilhier-Baumgarten cirrhosis, disease, or syndrome 571.5
Cruz-Chagas disease (see also Trypanosomiasis) 086.2
Crying
　constant, continuous
　　adolescent 780.95
　　adult 780.95
　　baby 780.92
　　child 780.95
　　infant 780.92
　　newborn 780.92
　excessive
　　adolescent 780.95
　　adult 780.95
　　baby 780.92
　　child 780.95
　　infant 780.92
　　newborn 780.92
Cryofibrinogenemia 273.2
Cryoglobulinemia (mixed) 273.2
Crypt (anal) (rectal) 569.49
Cryptitis (anal) (rectal) 569.49
Cryptococcosis (European) (pulmonary) (systemic) 117.5
Cryptococcus 117.5
　epidermicus 117.5
　neoformans, infection by 117.5
Cryptopapillitis (anus) 569.49
Cryptophthalmos (eyelid) 743.06
Cryptorchid, cryptorchism, cryptorchidism 752.51
Cryptosporidiosis 007.4
　hepatobiliary 136.8
　respiratory 136.8
Cryptotia 744.29
Crystallopathy
　calcium pyrophosphate (see also Arthritis) 275.49 [712.2]●
　dicalcium phosphate (see also Arthritis) 275.49 [712.1]●
　gouty 274.00
　pyrophosphate NEC (see also Arthritis) 275.49 [712.2]●
　uric acid 274.00
Crystalluria 791.9
Csillag's disease (lichen sclerosus et atrophicus) 701.0
Cuban itch 050.1
Cubitus
　valgus (acquired) 736.01
　　congenital 755.59
　　late effect of rickets 268.1
　varus (acquired) 736.02
　　congenital 755.59
　　late effect of rickets 268.1
Cultural deprivation V62.4
Cupping of optic disc 377.14
Curling's ulcer - see Ulcer, duodenum
Curling esophagus 530.5
Curschmann (-Batten) (-Steinert) disease or syndrome 359.21
Curvature
　organ or site, congenital NEC - see Distortion
　penis (lateral) 752.69
　Pott's (spinal) (see also Tuberculosis) 015.0● [737.43]

Curvature (Continued)
　radius, idiopathic, progressive (congenital) 755.54
　spine (acquired) (angular) (idiopathic) (incorrect) (postural) 737.9
　　congenital 754.2
　　due to or associated with
　　　Charcôt-Marie-Tooth disease 356.1 [737.40]
　　　mucopolysaccharidosis 277.5 [737.40]
　　　neurofibromatosis 237.71 [737.40]
　　　osteitis
　　　　deformans 731.0 [737.40]
　　　　fibrosa cystica 252.01 [737.40]
　　　osteoporosis (see also Osteoporosis) 733.00 [737.40]
　　　poliomyelitis (see also Poliomyelitis) 138 [737.40]
　　　tuberculosis (Pott's curvature) (see also Tuberculosis) 015.0● [737.43]
　　kyphoscoliotic (see also Kyphoscoliosis) 737.30
　　kyphotic (see also Kyphosis) 737.10
　　late effect of rickets 268.1 [737.40]
　　Pott's 015.0● [737.40]
　　scoliotic (see also Scoliosis) 737.30
　　specified NEC 737.8
　　tuberculous 015.0● [737.40]
Cushing's
　basophilism, disease, or syndrome (iatrogenic) (idiopathic) (pituitary basophilism) (pituitary dependent) 255.0
　ulcer - see Ulcer, peptic
Cushingoid due to steroid therapy
　correct substance properly administered 255.0
　overdose or wrong substance given or taken 962.0
Cut (external) - see Wound, open, by site
Cutaneous - see also condition
　hemorrhage 782.7
　horn (cheek) (eyelid) (mouth) 702.8
　larva migrans 126.9
Cutis - see also condition
　hyperelastic 756.83
　　acquired 701.8
　laxa 756.83
　　senilis 701.8
　marmorata 782.61
　osteosis 709.3
　pendula 756.83
　　acquired 701.8
　rhomboidalis nuchae 701.8
　verticis gyrata 757.39
　　acquired 701.8
Cyanopathy, newborn 770.83
Cyanosis 782.5
　autotoxic 289.7
　common atrioventricular canal 745.69
　congenital 770.83
　conjunctiva 372.71
　due to
　　endocardial cushion defect 745.60
　　nonclosure, foramen botalli 745.5
　　patent foramen botalli 745.5
　　persistent foramen ovale 745.5
　enterogenous 289.7
　fetus or newborn 770.83
　ostium primum defect 745.61
　paroxysmal digital 443.0
　retina, retinal 362.10
Cycle
　anovulatory 628.0
　menstrual, irregular 626.4
Cyclencephaly 759.89
Cyclical vomiting 536.2
　associated with migraine 346.2●
　psychogenic 306.4
Cyclitic membrane 364.74

Cyclitis (see also Iridocyclitis) 364.3
　acute 364.00
　　primary 364.01
　　recurrent 364.02
　chronic 364.10
　　in
　　　sarcoidosis 135 [364.11]
　　　tuberculosis (see also Tuberculosis)
　　　　017.3● [364.11]
　Fuchs' heterochromic 364.21
　granulomatous 364.10
　lens induced 364.23
　nongranulomatous 364.00
　posterior 363.21
　primary 364.01
　recurrent 364.02
　secondary (noninfectious) 364.04
　　infectious 364.03
　subacute 364.00
　　primary 364.01
　　recurrent 364.02
Cyclokeratitis - see Keratitis
Cyclophoria 378.44
Cyclopia, cyclops 759.89
Cycloplegia 367.51
Cyclospasm 367.53
Cyclosporiasis 007.5
Cyclothymia 301.13
Cyclothymic personality 301.13
Cyclotropia 378.33
Cyesis - see Pregnancy
Cylindroma (M8200/3) - see also Neoplasm, by
　　site, malignant
　eccrine dermal (M8200/0) - see Neoplasm,
　　skin, benign
　skin (M8200/0) - see Neoplasm, skin, benign
Cylindruria 791.7
Cyllosoma 759.89
Cynanche
　diphtheritic 032.3
　tonsillaris 475
Cynorexia 783.6
Cyphosis - see Kyphosis
Cyprus fever (see also Brucellosis) 023.9
Cyriax's syndrome (slipping rib) 733.99
Cyst (mucus) (retention) (serous) (simple)

> Note: In general, cysts are not neoplastic
> and are classified to the appropriate category
> for disease of the specified anatomical site.
> This generalization does not apply to certain
> types of cysts which are neoplastic in nature,
> for example, dermoid, nor does it apply
> to cysts of certain structures, for example,
> branchial cleft, which are classified as
> developmental anomalies.
>
> The following listing includes some of the
> most frequently reported sites of cysts as
> well as qualifiers which indicate the type
> of cyst. The latter qualifiers usually are not
> repeated under the anatomical sites. Since
> the code assignment for a given site may
> vary depending upon the type of cyst, the
> coder should refer to the listings under the
> specified type of cyst before consideration is
> given to the site.

　accessory, fallopian tube 752.11
　adenoid (infected) 474.8
　adrenal gland 255.8
　　congenital 759.1
　air, lung 518.89
　allantoic 753.7
　alveolar process (jaw bone) 526.2
　amnion, amniotic 658.8●
　anterior chamber (eye) 364.60
　　exudative 364.62
　　implantation (surgical) (traumatic) 364.61
　　parasitic 360.13
　anterior nasopalatine 526.1
　antrum 478.19

Cyst (Continued)
　anus 569.49
　apical (periodontal) (tooth) 522.8
　appendix 543.9
　arachnoid, brain 348.0
　arytenoid 478.79
　auricle 706.2
　Baker's (knee) 727.51
　　tuberculous (see also Tuberculosis) 015.2●
　Bartholin's gland or duct 616.2
　bile duct (see also Disease, biliary) 576.8
　bladder (multiple) (trigone) 596.89
　Blessig's 362.62
　blood, endocardial (see also Endocarditis)
　　424.90
　blue dome 610.0
　bone (local) 733.20
　　aneurysmal 733.22
　　jaw 526.2
　　　developmental (odontogenic) 526.0
　　　fissural 526.1
　　　latent 526.89
　　solitary 733.21
　　unicameral 733.21
　brain 348.0
　　congenital 742.4
　　hydatid (see also Echinococcus) 122.9
　　third ventricle (colloid) 742.4
　branchial (cleft) 744.42
　branchiogenic 744.42
　breast (benign) (blue dome) (pedunculated)
　　(solitary) (traumatic) 610.0
　　involution 610.4
　　sebaceous 610.8
　broad ligament (benign) 620.8
　　embryonic 752.11
　bronchogenic (mediastinal) (sequestration)
　　518.89
　　congenital 748.4
　buccal 528.4
　bulbourethral gland (Cowper's) 599.89
　bursa, bursal 727.49
　　pharyngeal 478.26
　calcifying odontogenic (M9301/0) 213.1
　　upper jaw (bone) 213.0
　canal of Nuck (acquired) (serous) 629.1
　　congenital 752.41
　canthus 372.75
　carcinomatous (M8010/3) - see Neoplasm, by
　　site, malignant
　cartilage (joint) - see Derangement, joint
　cauda equina 336.8
　cavum septi pellucidi NEC 348.0
　celomic (pericardium) 746.89
　cerebellopontine (angle) - see Cyst, brain
　cerebellum - see Cyst, brain
　cerebral - see Cyst, brain
　cervical lateral 744.42
　cervix 622.8
　　embryonal 752.41
　　nabothian (gland) 616.0
　chamber, anterior (eye) 364.60
　　exudative 364.62
　　implantation (surgical) (traumatic)
　　　364.61
　　parasitic 360.13
　chiasmal, optic NEC (see also Lesion,
　　chiasmal) 377.54
　chocolate (ovary) 617.1
　choledochal (congenital) 751.69
　　acquired 576.8
　choledochus 751.69
　chorion 658.8●
　choroid plexus 348.0
　chyle, mesentery 457.8
　ciliary body 364.60
　　exudative 364.64
　　implantation 364.61
　　primary 364.63
　clitoris 624.8
　coccyx (see also Cyst, bone) 733.20

Cyst (Continued)
　colloid
　　third ventricle (brain) 742.4
　　thyroid gland - see Goiter
　colon 569.89
　common (bile) duct (see also Disease, biliary)
　　576.8
　congenital NEC 759.89
　　adrenal glands 759.1
　　epiglottis 748.3
　　esophagus 750.4
　　fallopian tube 752.11
　　kidney 753.10
　　　multiple 753.19
　　　single 753.11
　　larynx 748.3
　　liver 751.62
　　lung 748.4
　　mediastinum 748.8
　　ovary 752.0
　　oviduct 752.11
　　pancreas 751.7
　　periurethral (tissue) 753.8
　　prepuce NEC 752.69
　　　penis 752.69
　　sublingual 750.26
　　submaxillary gland 750.26
　　thymus (gland) 759.2
　　tongue 750.19
　　ureterovesical orifice 753.4
　　vulva 752.41
　conjunctiva 372.75
　cornea 371.23
　corpora quadrigemina 348.0
　corpus
　　albicans (ovary) 620.2
　　luteum (ruptured) 620.1
　Cowper's gland (benign) (infected)
　　599.89
　cranial meninges 348.0
　craniobuccal pouch 253.8
　craniopharyngeal pouch 253.8
　cystic duct (see also Disease, gallbladder)
　　575.8
　Cysticercus (any site) 123.1
　Dandy-Walker 742.3
　　with spina bifida (see also Spina bifida)
　　　741.0●
　dental 522.8
　　developmental 526.0
　　eruption 526.0
　　lateral periodontal 526.0
　　primordial (keratocyst) 526.0
　　root 522.8
　dentigerous 526.0
　　mandible 526.0
　　maxilla 526.0
　dermoid (M9084/0) - see also Neoplasm, by
　　site, benign
　　with malignant transformation (M9084/3)
　　　183.0
　　implantation
　　　external area or site (skin) NEC 709.8
　　　iris 364.61
　　　skin 709.8
　　　vagina 623.8
　　　vulva 624.8
　　mouth 528.4
　　oral soft tissue 528.4
　　sacrococcygeal 685.1
　　　with abscess 685.0
　developmental of ovary, ovarian 752.0
　dura (cerebral) 348.0
　　spinal 349.2
　ear (external) 706.2
　echinococcal (see also Echinococcus) 122.9
　embryonal
　　cervix uteri 752.41
　　genitalia, female external 752.41
　　uterus 752.39
　　vagina 752.41

◀ New　　◀▪ Revised　　~~deleted~~ Deleted　　● Use Additional Digit(s)　　▨ Omit code

Cyst *(Continued)*
endometrial 621.8
  ectopic 617.9
endometrium (uterus) 621.8
  ectopic - *see* Endometriosis
enteric 751.5
enterogenous 751.5
epidermal (inclusion) (*see also* Cyst, skin)
  706.2
epidermoid (inclusion) (*see also* Cyst, skin)
  706.2
  mouth 528.4
  not of skin - *see* Cyst, by site
  oral soft tissue 528.4
epididymis 608.89
epiglottis 478.79
epiphysis cerebri 259.8
epithelial (inclusion) (*see also* Cyst, skin)
  706.2
epoophoron 752.11
eruption 526.0
esophagus 530.89
ethmoid sinus 478.19
eye (retention) 379.8
  congenital 743.03
  posterior segment, congenital 743.54
eyebrow 706.2
eyelid (sebaceous) 374.84
  infected 373.13
  sweat glands or ducts 374.84
falciform ligament (inflammatory) 573.8
fallopian tube 620.8
  congenital 752.11
female genital organs NEC 629.89
fimbrial (congenital) 752.11
fissural (oral region) 526.1
follicle (atretic) (graafian) (ovarian) 620.0
  nabothian (gland) 616.0
follicular (atretic) (ovarian) 620.0
  dentigerous 526.0
frontal sinus 478.19
gallbladder or duct 575.8
ganglion 727.43
Gartner's duct 752.41
gas, of mesentery 568.89
gingiva 523.8
gland of moll 374.84
globulomaxillary 526.1
graafian follicle 620.0
granulosal lutein 620.2
hemangiomatous (M9121/0) (*see also*
  Hemangioma) 228.00
hydatid (*see also* Echinococcus) 122.9
  fallopian tube (Morgagni) 752.11
  liver NEC 122.8
  lung NEC 122.9
  Morgagni 752.89
   fallopian tube 752.11
  specified site NEC 122.9
hymen 623.8
  embryonal 752.41
hypopharynx 478.26
hypophysis, hypophyseal (duct) (recurrent)
  253.8
  cerebri 253.8
implantation (dermoid)
  anterior chamber (eye) 364.61
  external area or site (skin) NEC 709.8
  iris 364.61
  vagina 623.8
  vulva 624.8
incisor, incisive canal 526.1
inclusion (epidermal) (epithelial)
  (epidermoid) (mucous) (squamous)
  (*see also* Cyst, skin) 706.2
  not of skin - *see* Neoplasm, by site, benign
intestine (large) (small) 569.89
intracranial - *see* Cyst, brain
intraligamentous 728.89
  knee 717.89
intrasellar 253.8

Cyst *(Continued)*
iris (idiopathic) 364.60
  exudative 364.62
  implantation (surgical) (traumatic) 364.61
  miotic pupillary 364.55
  parasitic 360.13
Iwanoff's 362.62
jaw (bone) (aneurysmal) (extravasation)
  (hemorrhagic) (traumatic) 526.2
  developmental (odontogenic) 526.0
  fissural 526.1
keratin 706.2
kidney (congenital) 753.10
  acquired 593.2
  calyceal (*see also* Hydronephrosis) 591
  multiple 753.19
  pyelogenic (*see also* Hydronephrosis) 591
  simple 593.2
  single 753.11
  solitary (not congenital) 593.2
labium (majus) (minus) 624.8
  sebaceous 624.8
lacrimal
  apparatus 375.43
  gland or sac 375.12
larynx 478.79
lens 379.39
  congenital 743.39
lip (gland) 528.5
liver 573.8
  congenital 751.62
  hydatid (*see also* Echinococcus) 122.8
   granulosis 122.0
   multilocularis 122.5
lung 518.89
  congenital 748.4
  giant bullous 492.0
lutein 620.1
lymphangiomatous (M9173/0) 228.1
lymphoepithelial
  mouth 528.4
  oral soft tissue 528.4
macula 362.54
malignant (M8000/3) - *see* Neoplasm, by site,
  malignant
mammary gland (sweat gland) (*see also* Cyst,
  breast) 610.0
mandible 526.2
  dentigerous 526.0
  radicular 522.8
maxilla 526.2
  dentigerous 526.0
  radicular 522.8
median
  anterior maxillary 526.1
  palatal 526.1
mediastinum (congenital) 748.8
meibomian (gland) (retention) 373.2
  infected 373.12
membrane, brain 348.0
meninges (cerebral) 348.0
  spinal 349.2
meniscus knee 717.5
mesentery, mesenteric (gas) 568.89
  chyle 457.8
  gas 568.89
mesonephric duct 752.89
mesothelial
  peritoneum 568.89
  pleura (peritoneal) 568.89
milk 611.5
miotic pupillary (iris) 364.55
Morgagni (hydatid) 752.89
  fallopian tube 752.11
mouth 528.4
Müllerian duct 752.89
  appendix testis 608.89
  cervix (embryonal) 752.41
  fallopian tube 752.11
  prostatic utricle 599.89
  vagina (embryonal) 752.41

Cyst *(Continued)*
multilocular (ovary) (M8000/1) 239.5
myometrium 621.8
nabothian (follicle) (ruptured) 616.0
nasal sinus 478.19
nasoalveolar 528.4
nasolabial 528.4
nasopalatine (duct) 526.1
  anterior 526.1
nasopharynx 478.26
neoplastic (M8000/1) - *see also* Neoplasm, by
  site, unspecified nature
  benign (M8000/0) - *see* Neoplasm, by site,
   benign
  uterus 621.8
nervous system - *see* Cyst, brain
neuroenteric 742.59
neuroepithelial ventricle 348.0
nipple 610.0
nose 478.19
  skin of 706.2
odontogenic, developmental 526.0
omentum (lesser) 568.89
  congenital 751.8
oral soft tissue (dermoid) (epidermoid)
  (lymphoepithelial) 528.4
ora serrata 361.19
orbit 376.81
ovary, ovarian (twisted) 620.2
  adherent 620.2
  chocolate 617.1
  corpus
   albicans 620.2
   luteum 620.1
  dermoid (M9084/0) 220
  developmental 752.0
  due to failure of involution NEC
   620.2
  endometrial 617.1
  follicular (atretic) (graafian)
   (hemorrhagic) 620.0
  hemorrhagic 620.2
  in pregnancy or childbirth 654.4●
   affecting fetus or newborn 763.89
   causing obstructed labor 660.2●
    affecting fetus or newborn 763.1
  multilocular (M8000/1) 239.5
  pseudomucinous (M8470/0) 220
  retention 620.2
  serous 620.2
  theca lutein 620.2
  tuberculous (*see also* Tuberculosis)
   016.6●
  unspecified 620.2
oviduct 620.8
palatal papilla (jaw) 526.1
palate 526.1
  fissural 526.1
  median (fissural) 526.1
palatine, of papilla 526.1
pancreas, pancreatic 577.2
  congenital 751.7
  false 577.2
  hemorrhagic 577.2
  true 577.2
paralabral
  hip 718.85
  shoulder 840.7
paramesonephric duct - *see* Cyst, Müllerian
  duct
paranephric 593.2
paraovarian 752.11
paraphysis, cerebri 742.4
parasitic NEC 136.9
parathyroid (gland) 252.8
paratubal (fallopian) 620.8
paraurethral duct 599.89
paroophoron 752.11
parotid gland 527.6
  mucous extravasation or retention 527.6
parovarian 752.11

Cyst *(Continued)*
  pars planus 364.60
    exudative 364.64
    primary 364.63
  pelvis, female
    in pregnancy or childbirth 654.4●
      affecting fetus or newborn 763.89
      causing obstructed labor 660.2●
        affecting fetus or newborn 763.1
  penis (sebaceous) 607.89
  periapical 522.8
  pericardial (congenital) 746.89
    acquired (secondary) 423.8
  pericoronal 526.0
  perineural (Tarlov's) 355.9
  periodontal 522.8
    lateral 526.0
  peripancreatic 577.2
  peripelvic (lymphatic) 593.2
  peritoneum 568.89
    chylous 457.8
  pharynx (wall) 478.26
  pilar 704.41
  pilonidal (infected) (rectum) 685.1
    with abscess 685.0
    malignant (M9084/3) 173.59
  pituitary (duct) (gland) 253.8
  placenta (amniotic) - *see* Placenta, abnormal
  pleura 519.8
  popliteal 727.51
  porencephalic 742.4
    acquired 348.0
  postanal (infected) 685.1
    with abscess 685.0
  posterior segment of eye, congenital 743.54
  postmastoidectomy cavity 383.31
  preauricular 744.47
  prepuce 607.89
    congenital 752.69
  primordial (jaw) 526.0
  prostate 600.3
  pseudomucinous (ovary) (M8470/0) 220
  pudenda (sweat glands) 624.8
  pupillary, miotic 364.55
    sebaceous 624.8
  radicular (residual) 522.8
  radiculodental 522.8
  ranular 527.6
  Rathke's pouch 253.8
  rectum (epithelium) (mucous) 569.49
  renal - *see* Cyst, kidney
  residual (radicular) 522.8
  retention (ovary) 620.2
  retina 361.19
    macular 362.54
    parasitic 360.13
    primary 361.13
    secondary 361.14
  retroperitoneal 568.89
  sacrococcygeal (dermoid) 685.1
    with abscess 685.0
  salivary gland or duct 527.6
    mucous extravasation or retention 527.6
  Sampson's 617.1
  sclera 379.19
  scrotum (sebaceous) 706.2
    sweat glands 706.2
  sebaceous (duct) (gland) 706.2
    breast 610.8
    eyelid 374.84
    genital organ NEC
      female 629.89
      male 608.89
    scrotum 706.2
  semilunar cartilage (knee) (multiple) 717.5
  seminal vesicle 608.89
  serous (ovary) 620.2
  sinus (antral) (ethmoidal) (frontal)
    (maxillary) (nasal) (sphenoidal)
    478.19
  Skene's gland 599.89

Cyst *(Continued)*
  skin (epidermal) (epidermoid, inclusion)
    (epithelial) (inclusion) (retention)
    (sebaceous) 706.2
    breast 610.8
    eyelid 374.84
    genital organ NEC
      female 629.89
      male 608.89
    neoplastic 216.3
    scrotum 706.2
    sweat gland or duct 705.89
  solitary
    bone 733.21
    kidney 593.2
  spermatic cord 608.89
  sphenoid sinus 478.19
  spinal meninges 349.2
  spine (*see also* Cyst, bone) 733.20
  spleen NEC 289.59
    congenital 759.0
    hydatid (*see also* Echinococcus) 122.9
  spring water (pericardium) 746.89
  subarachnoid 348.0
    intrasellar 793.0
  subdural (cerebral) 348.0
    spinal cord 349.2
  sublingual gland 527.6
    mucous extravasation or retention 527.6
  submaxillary gland 527.6
    mucous extravasation or retention 527.6
  suburethral 599.89
  suprarenal gland 255.8
  suprasellar - *see* Cyst, brain
  sweat gland or duct 705.89
  sympathetic nervous system 337.9
  synovial 727.40
    popliteal space 727.51
  Tarlov's 355.9
  tarsal 373.2
  tendon (sheath) 727.42
  testis 608.89
  theca-lutein (ovary) 620.2
  Thornwaldt's, Tornwaldt's 478.26
  thymus (gland) 254.8
  thyroglossal (duct) (infected) (persistent)
    759.2
  thyroid (gland) 246.2
    adenomatous - *see* Goiter, nodular
    colloid (*see also* Goiter) 240.9
  thyrolingual duct (infected) (persistent) 759.2
  tongue (mucous) 529.8
  tonsil 474.8
  tooth (dental root) 522.8
  trichilemmal (proliferating) 704.42
  tubo-ovarian 620.8
    inflammatory 614.1
  tunica vaginalis 608.89
  turbinate (nose) (*see also* Cyst, bone) 733.20
  Tyson's gland (benign) (infected) 607.89
  umbilicus 759.89
  urachus 753.7
  ureter 593.89
  ureterovesical orifice 593.89
    congenital 753.4
  urethra 599.84
  urethral gland (Cowper's) 599.89
  uterine
    ligament 620.8
      embryonic 752.11
    tube 620.8
  uterus (body) (corpus) (recurrent) 621.8
    embryonal 752.39
  utricle (ear) 386.8
    prostatic 599.89
  utriculus masculinus 599.89
  vagina, vaginal (squamous cell) (wall) 623.8
    embryonal 752.41
    implantation 623.8
    inclusion 623.8
  vallecula, vallecular 478.79

Cyst *(Continued)*
  ventricle, neuroepithelial 348.0
  verumontanum 599.89
  vesical (orifice) 596.89
  vitreous humor 379.29
  vulva (sweat glands) 624.8
    congenital 752.41
    implantation 624.8
    inclusion 624.8
    sebaceous gland 624.8
  vulvovaginal gland 624.8
  wolffian 752.89
Cystadenocarcinoma (M8440/3) - *see also*
  Neoplasm, by site, malignant
  bile duct type (M8161/3) 155.1
  endometrioid (M8380/3) - *see* Neoplasm, by
    site, malignant
  mucinous (M8470/3)
    papillary (M8471/3)
      specified site - *see* Neoplasm, by site,
        malignant
      unspecified site 183.0
    specified site - *see* Neoplasm, by site,
      malignant
    unspecified site 183.0
  papillary (M8450/3)
    mucinous (M8471/3)
      specified site - *see* Neoplasm, by site,
        malignant
      unspecified site 183.0
    pseudomucinous (M8471/3)
      specified site - *see* Neoplasm, by site,
        malignant
      unspecified site 183.0
    serous (M8460/3)
      specified site - *see* Neoplasm, by site,
        malignant
      unspecified site 183.0
    specified site - *see* Neoplasm, by site,
      malignant
    unspecified site 183.0
  pseudomucinous (M8470/3)
    papillary (M8471/3)
      specified site - *see* Neoplasm, by site,
        malignant
      unspecified site 183.0
    specified site - *see* Neoplasm, by site,
      malignant
    unspecified site 183.0
  serous (M8441/3)
    papillary (M8460/3)
      specified site - *see* Neoplasm, by site,
        malignant
      unspecified site 183.0
    specified site - *see* Neoplasm, by site,
      malignant
    unspecified site 183.0
Cystadenofibroma (M9013/0)
  clear cell (M8313/0) - *see* Neoplasm, by site,
    benign
  endometrioid (M8381/0) 220
    borderline malignancy (M8381/1) 236.2
    malignant (M8381/3) 183.0
  mucinous (M9015/0)
    specified site - *see* Neoplasm, by site,
      benign
    unspecified site 220
  serous (M9014/0)
    specified site - *see* Neoplasm, by site,
      benign
    unspecified site 220
  specified site - *see* Neoplasm, by site, benign
  unspecified site 220
Cystadenoma (M8440/0) - *see also* Neoplasm,
  by site, benign
  bile duct (M8161/0) 211.5
  endometrioid (M8380/0) - *see also* Neoplasm,
    by site, benign
    borderline malignancy (M8380/1) - *see*
      Neoplasm, by site, uncertain
      behavior

Cystadenoma *(Continued)*
  malignant (M8440/3) - *see* Neoplasm, by site,
    malignant
  mucinous (M8470/0)
    borderline malignancy (M8470/1)
      specified site - *see* Neoplasm, uncertain
        behavior
      unspecified site 236.2
    papillary (M8471/0)
      borderline malignancy (M8471/1)
        specified site - *see* Neoplasm, by
          site, uncertain behavior
        unspecified site 236.2
      specified site - *see* Neoplasm, by site,
        benign
      unspecified site 220
    specified site - *see* Neoplasm, by site,
      benign
    unspecified site 220
  papillary (M8450/0)
    borderline malignancy (M8450/1)
      specified site - *see* Neoplasm, by site,
        uncertain behavior
      unspecified site 236.2
    lymphomatosum (M8561/0) 210.2
    mucinous (M8471/0)
      borderline malignancy (M8471/1)
        specified site - *see* Neoplasm, by site,
          uncertain behavior
        unspecified site 236.2
      specified site - *see* Neoplasm, by site,
        benign
      unspecified site 220
    pseudomucinous (M8471/0)
      borderline malignancy (M8471/1)
        specified site - *see* Neoplasm, by site
          uncertain behavior
        unspecified site 236.2
      specified site - *see* Neoplasm, by site,
        benign
      unspecified site 220
    serous (M8460/0)
      borderline malignancy (M8460/1)
        specified site - *see* Neoplasm, by
          site, uncertain behavior
        unspecified site 236.2
      specified site - *see* Neoplasm, by site,
        benign
      unspecified site 220
    specified site - *see* Neoplasm, by site,
      benign
    unspecified site 220
  pseudomucinous (M8470/0)
    borderline malignancy (M8470/1)
      specified site - *see* Neoplasm, by site
        uncertain behavior
      unspecified site 236.2
    papillary (M8471/0)
      borderline malignancy (M8471/1)
        specified site - *see* Neoplasm, by site
          uncertain behavior
        unspecified site 236.2
      specified site - *see* Neoplasm, by site,
        benign
      unspecified site 220
    specified site - *see* Neoplasm, by site,
      benign
    unspecified site 220
  serous (M8441/0)
    borderline malignancy (M8441/1)
      specified site - *see* Neoplasm, by site,
        uncertain behavior
      unspecified site 236.2
    papillary (M8460/0)
      borderline malignancy (M8460/1)
        specified site - *see* Neoplasm, by
          site, uncertain behavior
        unspecified site 236.2
      specified site - *see* Neoplasm, by site,
        benign
      unspecified site 220

Cystadenoma *(Continued)*
  serous *(Continued)*
    specified site - *see* Neoplasm, by site,
      benign
    unspecified site 220
  thyroid 226
Cystathioninemia 270.4
Cystathioninuria 270.4
Cystic - *see also* condition
  breast, chronic 610.1
  corpora lutea 620.1
  degeneration, congenital
    brain 742.4
    kidney (*see also* Cystic, disease, kidney)
      753.10
  disease
    breast, chronic 610.1
    kidney, congenital 753.10
      medullary 753.16
      multiple 753.19
      polycystic - *see* Polycystic, kidney
      single 753.11
      specified NEC 753.19
    liver, congenital 751.62
    lung 518.89
      congenital 748.4
    pancreas, congenital 751.7
    semilunar cartilage 717.5
  duct - *see* condition
  eyeball, congenital 743.03
  fibrosis (pancreas) 277.00
    with
      manifestations
        gastrointestinal 277.03
        pulmonary 277.02
        specified NEC 277.09
      meconium ileus 277.01
      pulmonary exacerbation 277.02
  hygroma (M9173/0) 228.1
  kidney, congenital 753.10
    medullary 753.16
    multiple 753.19
    polycystic - *see* Polycystic, kidney
    single 753.11
    specified NEC 753.19
  liver, congenital 751.62
  lung 518.89
    congenital 748.4
  mass - *see* Cyst
  mastitis, chronic 610.1
  ovary 620.2
  pancreas, congenital 751.7
Cysticerciasis 123.1
Cysticercosis (mammary) (subretinal) 123.1
Cysticercus 123.1
  cellulosae infestation 123.1
Cystinosis (malignant) 270.0
Cystinuria 270.0
Cystitis (bacillary) (colli) (diffuse) (exudative)
  (hemorrhagic) (purulent) (recurrent)
  (septic) (suppurative) (ulcerative) 595.9
  with
    abortion - *see* Abortion, by type, with
      urinary tract infection
    ectopic pregnancy (*see also* categories
      633.0–633.9) 639.8
    fibrosis 595.1
    leukoplakia 595.1
    malakoplakia 595.1
    metaplasia 595.1
    molar pregnancy (*see also* categories
      630–632) 639.8
  actinomycotic 039.8 *[595.4]*
  acute 595.0
    of trigone 595.3
  allergic 595.89
  amebic 006.8 *[595.4]*
  bilharzial 120.9 *[595.4]*
  blennorrhagic (acute) 098.11
    chronic or duration of 2 months or more
      098.31

Cystitis *(Continued)*
  bullous 595.89
  calculous 594.1
  chlamydial 099.53
  chronic 595.2
    interstitial 595.1
    of trigone 595.3
  complicating pregnancy, childbirth, or
    puerperium 646.6●
    affecting fetus or newborn 760.1
  cystic(a) 595.81
  diphtheritic 032.84
  echinococcal
    glanulosus 122.3 *[595.4]*
    multilocularis 122.6 *[595.4]*
  emphysematous 595.89
  encysted 595.81
  follicular 595.3
  following
    abortion 639.8
    ectopic or molar pregnancy 639.8
  gangrenous 595.89
  glandularis 595.89
  gonococcal (acute) 098.11
    chronic or duration of 2 months or more
      098.31
  incrusted 595.89
  interstitial 595.1
  irradiation 595.82
  irritation 595.89
  malignant 595.89
  monilial 112.2
  of trigone 595.3
  panmural 595.1
  polyposa 595.89
  prostatic 601.3
  radiation 595.82
  Reiter's (abacterial) 099.3
  specified NEC 595.89
  subacute 595.2
  submucous 595.1
  syphilitic 095.8
  trichomoniasis 131.09
  tuberculous (*see also* Tuberculosis)
    016.1●
  ulcerative 595.1
Cystocele
  female (without uterine prolapse)
    618.01
    with uterine prolapse 618.4
      complete 618.3
      incomplete 618.2
    lateral 618.02
    midline 618.01
    paravaginal 618.02
  in pregnancy or childbirth 654.4●
    affecting fetus or newborn 763.89
    causing obstructed labor 660.2●
      affecting fetus or newborn
        763.1
  male 596.89
Cystoid
  cicatrix limbus 372.64
  degeneration macula 362.53
Cystolithiasis 594.1
Cystoma (M8440/0) - *see also* Neoplasm, by site,
  benign
  endometrial, ovary 617.1
  mucinous (M8470/0)
    specified site - *see* Neoplasm, by site,
      benign
    unspecified site 220
  serous (M8441/0)
    specified site - *see* Neoplasm, by site,
      benign
    unspecified site 220
  simple (ovary) 620.2
Cystoplegia 596.53
Cystoptosis 596.89
Cystopyelitis (*see also* Pyelitis) 590.80
Cystorrhagia 596.89

Cystosarcoma phyllodes (M9020/1) 238.3
  benign (M9020/0) 217
  malignant (M9020/3) - *see* Neoplasm, breast, malignant
Cystostomy status V44.50
  with complication 596.83
    infection 596.81
    mechanical 596.82
    specified complication NEC 596.83
  appendico-vesicostomy V44.52

Cystostomy status *(Continued)*
  cutaneous-vesicostomy V44.51
  specified type NEC V44.59
Cystourethritis *(see also* Urethritis) 597.89
Cystourethrocele *(see also* Cystocele)
  female (without uterine prolapse) 618.09
    with uterine prolapse 618.4
      complete 618.3
      incomplete 618.2
  male 596.89

Cytomegalic inclusion disease 078.5
  congenital 771.1
Cytomycosis, reticuloendothelial *(see also* Histoplasmosis, American) 115.00
Cytopenia 289.9
  refractory
    with
      multilineage dysplasia (RCMD) 238.72
        and ringed sideroblasts (RCMD-RS) 238.72

◀ New ◀▦ Revised deleted Deleted ● Use Additional Digit(s) Omit code

D

Daae (-Finsen) disease (epidemic pleurodynia) 074.1
Dabney's grip 074.1
Da Costa's syndrome (neurocirculatory asthenia) 306.2
Dacryoadenitis, dacryadenitis 375.00
  acute 375.01
  chronic 375.02
Dacryocystitis 375.30
  acute 375.32
  chronic 375.42
  neonatal 771.6
  phlegmonous 375.33
  syphilitic 095.8
    congenital 090.0
  trachomatous, active 076.1
    late effect 139.1
  tuberculous (see also Tuberculosis) 017.3●
Dacryocystoblenorrhea 375.42
Dacryocystocele 375.43
Dacryolith, dacryolithiasis 375.57
Dacryoma 375.43
Dacryopericystitis (acute) (subacute) 375.32
  chronic 375.42
Dacryops 375.11
Dacryosialadenopathy, atrophic 710.2
Dacryostenosis 375.56
  congenital 743.65
Dactylitis
  bone (see also Osteomyelitis) 730.2●
  sickle-cell 282.62
    Hb-C 282.64
    Hb-SS 282.62
    specified NEC 282.69
  syphilitic 095.5
  tuberculous (see also Tuberculosis) 015.5●
Dactylolysis spontanea 136.0
Dactylosymphysis (see also Syndactylism) 755.10
Damage
  arteriosclerotic - see Arteriosclerosis
  brain 348.9
    anoxic, hypoxic 348.1
      during or resulting from a procedure 997.01
      ischemic, in newborn 768.70
        mild 768.71
        moderate 768.72
        severe 768.73
    child NEC 343.9
    due to birth injury 767.0
    minimal (child) (see also Hyperkinesia) 314.9
    newborn 767.0
  cardiac - see also Disease, heart
  cardiorenal (vascular) (see also Hypertension, cardiorenal) 404.90
  central nervous system - see Damage, brain
  cerebral NEC - see Damage, brain
  coccyx, complicating delivery 665.6●
  coronary (see also Ischemia, heart) 414.9
  eye, birth injury 767.8
  heart - see also Disease, heart
    valve - see Endocarditis
  hypothalamus NEC 348.9
  liver 571.9
    alcoholic 571.3
  medication 995.20
  myocardium (see also Degeneration, myocardial) 429.1
  pelvic
    joint or ligament, during delivery 665.6●
    organ NEC
      with
        abortion - see Abortion, by type, with damage to pelvic organs
        ectopic pregnancy (see also categories 633.0–633.9) 639.2
        molar pregnancy (see also categories 630–632) 639.2

Damage (Continued)
  pelvic (Continued)
    organ NEC (Continued)
      during delivery 665.5●
      following
        abortion 639.2
        ectopic or molar pregnancy 639.2
  renal (see also Disease, renal) 593.9
  skin, solar 692.79
    acute 692.72
    chronic 692.74
  subendocardium, subendocardial (see also Degeneration, myocardial) 429.1
  vascular 459.9
Dameshek's syndrome (erythroblastic anemia) 282.49
Dana-Putnam syndrome (subacute combined sclerosis with pernicious anemia) 281.0 [336.2]
Danbolt (-Closs) syndrome (acrodermatitis enteropathica) 686.8
Dandruff 690.18
Dandy fever 061
Dandy-Walker deformity or syndrome (atresia, foramen of Magendie) 742.3
  with spina bifida (see also Spina bifida) 741.0●
Dangle foot 736.79
Danielssen's disease (anesthetic leprosy) 030.1
Danlos' syndrome 756.83
Darier's disease (congenital) (keratosis follicularis) 757.39
  due to vitamin A deficiency 264.8
  meaning erythema annulare centrifugum 695.0
Darier-Roussy sarcoid 135
Dark area on retina 239.81
Darling's
  disease (see also Histoplasmosis, American) 115.00
  histoplasmosis (see also Histoplasmosis, American) 115.00
Dartre 054.9
Darwin's tubercle 744.29
Davidson's anemia (refractory) 284.9
Davies' disease 425.0
Davies-Colley syndrome (slipping rib) 733.99
Dawson's encephalitis 046.2
Day blindness (see also Blindness, day) 368.60
Dead
  fetus
    retained (in utero) 656.4●
      early pregnancy (death before 22 completed weeks' gestation) 632
      late (death after 22 completed weeks' gestation) 656.4●
    syndrome 641.3●
  labyrinth 386.50
  ovum, retained 631.8
Deaf and dumb NEC 389.7
Deaf mutism (acquired) (congenital) NEC 389.7
  endemic 243
  hysterical 300.11
  syphilitic, congenital 090.0
Deafness (acquired) (complete) (congenital) (hereditary) (middle ear) (partial) 389.9
  with
    blindness V49.85
    blue sclera and fragility of bone 756.51
  auditory fatigue 389.9
  aviation 993.0
    nerve injury 951.5
  boilermakers' 951.5
  central 389.14
    with conductive hearing loss 389.20
      bilateral 389.22
      unilateral 389.21
  conductive (air) 389.00
    with sensorineural hearing loss 389.20
      bilateral 389.22
      unilateral 389.21
    bilateral 389.06

Deafness (Continued)
  conductive (Continued)
    combined types 389.08
    external ear 389.01
    inner ear 389.04
    middle ear 389.03
    multiple types 389.08
    tympanic membrane 389.02
    unilateral 389.05
  emotional (complete) 300.11
  functional (complete) 300.11
  high frequency 389.8
  hysterical (complete) 300.11
  injury 951.5
  low frequency 389.8
  mental 784.69
  mixed conductive and sensorineural 389.20
    bilateral 389.22
    unilateral 389.21
  nerve
    with conductive hearing loss 389.20
      bilateral 389.22
      unilateral 389.21
    bilateral 389.12
    unilateral 389.13
  neural
    with conductive hearing loss 389.20
      bilateral 389.22
      unilateral 389.21
    bilateral 389.12
    unilateral 389.13
  noise-induced 388.12
    nerve injury 951.5
  nonspeaking 389.7
  perceptive 389.10
    with conductive hearing loss 389.20
      bilateral 389.22
      unilateral 389.21
    central 389.14
    neural
      bilateral 389.12
      unilateral 389.13
    sensorineural 389.10
      asymmetrical 389.16
      bilateral 389.18
      unilateral 389.15
    sensory
      bilateral 389.11
      unilateral 389.17
  psychogenic (complete) 306.7
  sensorineural (see also Deafness, perceptive) 389.10
    asymmetrical 389.16
    bilateral 389.18
    unilateral 389.15
  sensory
    with conductive hearing loss 389.20
      bilateral 389.22
      unilateral 389.21
    bilateral 389.11
    unilateral 389.17
  specified type NEC 389.8
  sudden NEC 388.2
  syphilitic 094.89
  transient ischemic 388.02
  transmission - see Deafness, conductive
  traumatic 951.5
  word (secondary to organic lesion) 784.69
    developmental 315.31
Death
  after delivery (cause not stated) (sudden) 674.9●
  anesthetic
    due to
      correct substance properly administered 995.4
      overdose or wrong substance given 968.4
        specified anesthetic - see Table of Drugs and Chemicals
  during delivery 668.9●

Death (Continued)
brain 348.82
cardiac (sudden) (SCD) - code to underlying
condition
family history of V17.41
personal history of, successfully
resuscitated V12.53
cause unknown 798.2
cot (infant) 798.0
crib (infant) 798.0
fetus, fetal (cause not stated) (intrauterine)
779.9
early, with retention (before 22 completed
weeks' gestation) 632
from asphyxia or anoxia (before labor)
768.0
during labor 768.1
late, affecting management of pregnancy
(after 22 completed weeks'
gestation) 656.4●
from pregnancy NEC 646.9●
instantaneous 798.1
intrauterine (see also Death, fetus) 779.9
complicating pregnancy 656.4●
maternal, affecting fetus or newborn 761.6
neonatal NEC 779.9
sudden (cause unknown) 798.1
cardiac (SCD)
family history of V17.41
personal history of, successfully
resuscitated V12.53
during delivery 669.9●
under anesthesia NEC 668.9●
infant, syndrome (SIDS) 798.0
puerperal, during puerperium 674.9●
unattended (cause unknown) 798.9
under anesthesia NEC
due to
correct substance properly
administered 995.4
overdose or wrong substance given
968.4
specified anesthetic - see Table of
Drugs and Chemicals
during delivery 668.9●
violent 798.1
de Beurmann-Gougerot disease
(sporotrichosis) 117.1
Debility (general) (infantile) (postinfectional)
799.3
with nutritional difficulty 269.9
congenital or neonatal NEC 779.9
nervous 300.5
old age 797
senile 797
Débove's disease (splenomegaly) 789.2
Decalcification
bone (see also Osteoporosis) 733.00
teeth 521.89
Decapitation 874.9
fetal (to facilitate delivery) 763.89
Decapsulation, kidney 593.89
Decay
dental 521.00
senile 797
tooth, teeth 521.00
Decensus, uterus - see Prolapse, uterus
Deciduitis (acute)
with
abortion - see Abortion, by type, with
sepsis
ectopic pregnancy (see also categories
633.0–633.9) 639.0
molar pregnancy (see also categories
630–632) 639.0
affecting fetus or newborn 760.8
following
abortion 639.0
ectopic or molar pregnancy 639.0
in pregnancy 646.6●
puerperal, postpartum 670.1●

Deciduoma malignum (M9100/3) 181
Deciduous tooth (retained) 520.6
Decline (general) (see also Debility) 799.3
Decompensation
cardiac (acute) (chronic) (see also Disease,
heart) 429.9
failure - see Failure, heart
cardiorenal (see also Hypertension,
cardiorenal) 404.90
cardiovascular (see also Disease,
cardiovascular) 429.2
heart (see also Disease, heart) 429.9
failure - see Failure, heart
hepatic 572.2
myocardial (acute) (chronic) (see also Disease,
heart) 429.9
failure - see Failure, heart
respiratory 519.9
Decompression sickness 993.3
Decrease, decreased
blood
platelets (see also Thrombocytopenia)
287.5
pressure 796.3
due to shock following
injury 958.4
operation 998.00
white cell count 288.50
specified NEC 288.59
cardiac reserve - see Disease, heart
estrogen 256.39
postablative 256.2
fetal movements 655.7●
fragility of erythrocytes 289.89
function
adrenal (cortex) 255.41
medulla 255.5
ovary in hypopituitarism 253.4
parenchyma of pancreas 577.8
pituitary (gland) (lobe) (anterior) 253.2
posterior (lobe) 253.8
functional activity 780.99
glucose 790.29
haptoglobin (serum) NEC 273.8
leukocytes 288.50
libido 799.81
lymphocytes 288.51
platelets (see also Thrombocytopenia) 287.5
pulse pressure 785.9
respiration due to shock following injury
958.4
sexual desire 799.81
tear secretion NEC 375.15
tolerance
fat 579.8
salt and water 276.9
vision NEC 369.9
white blood cell count 288.50
Decubital gangrene (see also Ulcer, pressure)
707.00 [785.4]
Decubiti (see also Ulcer, pressure) 707.00
Decubitus (ulcer) (see also Ulcer, pressure)
707.00
with gangrene 707.00 [785.4]
ankle 707.06
back
lower 707.03
upper 707.02
buttock 707.05
coccyx 707.03
elbow 707.01
head 707.09
heel 707.07
hip 707.04
other site 707.09
sacrum 707.03
shoulder blades 707.02
Deepening acetabulum 718.85
Defect, defective 759.9
3-beta-hydroxysteroid dehydrogenase 255.2
11-hydroxylase 255.2

Defect, defective (Continued)
21-hydroxylase 255.2
abdominal wall, congenital 756.70
aorticopulmonary septum 745.0
aortic septal 745.0
atrial septal (ostium secundum type) 745.5
acquired 429.71
ostium primum type 745.61
sinus venosus 745.8
atrioventricular
canal 745.69
septum 745.4
acquired 429.71
atrium secundum 745.5
acquired 429.71
auricular septal 745.5
acquired 429.71
bilirubin excretion 277.4
biosynthesis, testicular androgen 257.2
bridge 525.60
bulbar septum 745.0
butanol-insoluble iodide 246.1
chromosome - see Anomaly, chromosome
circulation (acquired) 459.9
congenital 747.9
newborn 747.9
clotting NEC (see also Defect, coagulation)
286.9
coagulation (factor) (see also Deficiency,
coagulation factor) 286.9
with
abortion - see Abortion, by type, with
hemorrhage
ectopic pregnancy (see also categories
634–638) 639.1
molar pregnancy (see also categories
630–632) 639.1
acquired (any) 286.7
antepartum or intrapartum 641.3●
affecting fetus or newborn 762.1
causing hemorrhage of pregnancy or
delivery 641.3●
complicating pregnancy, childbirth, or
puerperium 649.3●
due to
liver disease 286.7
vitamin K deficiency 286.7
newborn, transient 776.3
postpartum 666.3●
specified type NEC 286.9
conduction (heart) 426.9
bone (see also Deafness, conductive) 389.00
congenital, organ or site NEC - see also
Anomaly
circulation 747.9
Descemet's membrane 743.9
specified type NEC 743.49
diaphragm 756.6
ectodermal 757.9
esophagus 750.9
pulmonic cusps - see Anomaly, heart valve
respiratory system 748.9
specified type NEC 748.8
crown 525.60
cushion endocardial 745.60
dental restoration 525.60
dentin (hereditary) 520.5
Descemet's membrane (congenital) 743.9
acquired 371.30
specific type NEC 743.49
deutan 368.52
developmental - see also Anomaly, by site
cauda equina 742.59
left ventricle 746.9
with atresia or hypoplasia of aortic
orifice or valve, with hypoplasia
of ascending aorta 746.7
in hypoplastic left heart syndrome
746.7
testis 752.9
vessel 747.9

◀ New   ◀▥ Revised   ~~deleted~~ Deleted   ● Use Additional Digit(s)   ▥ Omit code

Defect, defective *(Continued)*
diaphragm
with elevation, eventration, or hernia - *see*
Hernia, diaphragm
congenital 756.6
with elevation, eventration, or hernia
756.6
gross (with elevation, eventration, or
hernia) 756.6
ectodermal, congenital 757.9
Eisenmenger's (ventricular septal defect)
745.4
endocardial cushion 745.60
specified type NEC 745.69
esophagus, congenital 750.9
extensor retinaculum 728.9
fibrin polymerization *(see also* Defect,
coagulation) 286.3
filling
biliary tract 793.3
bladder 793.5
dental 525.60
gallbladder 793.3
kidney 793.5
stomach 793.4
ureter 793.5
fossa ovalis 745.5
gene, carrier (suspected) of V83.89
Gerbode 745.4
glaucomatous, without elevated tension
365.89
Hageman (factor) *(see also* Defect,
coagulation) 286.3
hearing *(see also* Deafness) 389.9
high grade 317
homogentisic acid 270.2
interatrial septal 745.5
acquired 429.71
interauricular septal 745.5
acquired 429.71
interventricular septal 745.4
with pulmonary stenosis or atresia,
dextraposition of aorta, and
hypertrophy of right ventricle
745.2
acquired 429.71
in tetralogy of Fallot 745.2
iodide trapping 246.1
iodotyrosine dehalogenase 246.1
kynureninase 270.2
learning, specific 315.2
major osseous 731.3
mental *(see also* Disability, intellectual)
319
osseous, major 731.3
osteochondral NEC 738.8
ostium
primum 745.61
secundum 745.5
pericardium 746.89
peroxidase-binding 246.1
placental blood supply - *see* Placenta,
insufficiency
platelet (qualitative) 287.1
constitutional 286.4
postural, spine 737.9
protan 368.51
pulmonic cusps, congenital 746.00
renal pelvis 753.9
obstructive 753.29
specified type NEC 753.3
respiratory system, congenital 748.9
specified type NEC 748.8
retina, retinal 361.30
with detachment *(see also* Detachment,
retina, with retinal defect) 361.00
multiple 361.33
with detachment 361.02
nerve fiber bundle 362.85
single 361.30
with detachment 361.01

Defect, defective *(Continued)*
septal (closure) (heart) NEC 745.9
acquired 429.71
atrial 745.5
specified type NEC 745.8
speech NEC 784.59
developmental 315.39
late effect of cerebrovascular disease - *see*
Late effect(s) (of) cerebrovascular
disease, speech and language deficit
secondary to organic lesion 784.59
Taussig-Bing (transposition, aorta and
overriding pulmonary artery)
745.11
teeth, wedge 521.20
thyroid hormone synthesis 246.1
tritan 368.53
ureter 753.9
obstructive 753.29
vascular (acquired) (local) 459.9
congenital (peripheral) NEC 747.60
gastrointestinal 747.61
lower limb 747.64
renal 747.62
specified NEC 747.69
spinal 747.82
upper limb 747.63
ventricular septal 745.4
with pulmonary stenosis or atresia,
dextraposition of aorta, and
hypertrophy of right ventricle 745.2
acquired 429.71
atrioventricular canal type 745.69
between infundibulum and anterior
portion 745.4
in tetralogy of Fallot 745.2
isolated anterior 745.4
vision NEC 369.9
visual field 368.40
arcuate 368.43
heteronymous, bilateral 368.47
homonymous, bilateral 368.46
localized NEC 368.44
nasal step 368.44
peripheral 368.44
sector 368.43
voice and resonance 784.40
wedge, teeth (abrasion) 521.20
Defeminization syndrome 255.2
Deferentitis 608.4
gonorrheal (acute) 098.14
chronic or duration of 2 months or over
098.34
Defibrination syndrome *(see also* Fibrinolysis)
286.6
Deficiency, deficient
3-beta-hydroxysteroid dehydrogenase 255.2
6-phosphogluconic dehydrogenase (anemia)
282.2
11-beta-hydroxylase 255.2
17-alpha-hydroxylase 255.2
18-hydroxysteroid dehydrogenase 255.2
20-alpha-hydroxylase 255.2
21-hydroxylase 255.2
AAT (alpha-1 antitrypsin) 273.4
abdominal muscle syndrome 756.79
accelerator globulin (Ac G) (blood) *(see also*
Defect, coagulation) 286.3
AC globulin (congenital) *(see also* Defect,
coagulation) 286.3
acquired 286.7
activating factor (blood) *(see also* Defect,
coagulation) 286.3
adenohypophyseal 253.2
adenosine deaminase 277.2
aldolase (hereditary) 271.2
alpha-1-antitrypsin 273.4
alpha-1-trypsin inhibitor 273.4
alpha-fucosidase 271.8
alpha-lipoprotein 272.5
alpha-mannosidase 271.8

Deficiency, deficient *(Continued)*
amino acid 270.9
anemia - *see* Anemia, deficiency
aneurin 265.1
with beriberi 265.0
antibody NEC 279.00
antidiuretic hormone 253.5
antihemophilic
factor (A) 286.0
B 286.1
C 286.2
globulin (AHG) NEC 286.0
antithrombin III 289.81
antitrypsin 273.4
argininosuccinate synthetase or lyase 270.6
ascorbic acid (with scurvy) 267
autoprothrombin
I *(see also* Defect, coagulation) 286.3
II 286.1
C *(see also* Defect, coagulation) 286.3
bile salt 579.8
biotin 266.2
biotinidase 277.6
bradykinase-1 277.6
brancher enzyme (amylopectinosis) 271.0
calciferol 268.9
with
osteomalacia 268.2
rickets *(see also* Rickets) 268.0
calcium 275.40
dietary 269.3
calorie, severe 261
carbamyl phosphate synthetase 270.6
cardiac *(see also* Insufficiency, myocardial)
428.0
carnitine 277.81
due to
hemodialysis 277.83
inborn errors of metabolism 277.82
valproic acid therapy 277.83
iatrogenic 277.83
palmitoyltransferase (CPT1, CPT2) 277.85
palmityl transferase (CPT1, CPT2) 277.85
primary 277.81
secondary 277.84
carotene 264.9
Carr factor *(see also* Defect, coagulation) 286.9
central nervous system 349.9
ceruloplasmin 275.1
cevitamic acid (with scurvy) 267
choline 266.2
Christmas factor 286.1
chromium 269.3
citrin 269.1
clotting (blood) *(see also* Defect, coagulation)
286.9
coagulation factor NEC 286.9
with
abortion - *see* Abortion, by type, with
hemorrhage
ectopic pregnancy *(see also* categories
634–638) 639.1
molar pregnancy *(see also* categories
630–632) 639.1
acquired (any) 286.7
antepartum or intrapartum 641.3●
affecting fetus or newborn 762.1
complicating pregnancy, childbirth, or
puerperium 649.3●
due to
liver disease 286.7
vitamin K deficiency 286.7
newborn, transient 776.3
postpartum 666.3●
specified type NEC 286.3
color vision (congenital) 368.59
acquired 368.55
combined glucocorticoid and
mineralocorticoid 255.41
combined, two or more coagulation factors
(see also Defect, coagulation) 286.9

Deficiency, deficient *(Continued)*
  complement factor NEC 279.8
  contact factor *(see also* Defect, coagulation) 286.3
  copper NEC 275.1
  corticoadrenal 255.41
  craniofacial axis 756.0
  cyanocobalamin (vitamin B_{12}) 266.2
  debrancher enzyme (limit dextrinosis) 271.0
  desmolase 255.2
  diet 269.9
  dihydrofolate reductase 281.2
  dihydropteridine reductase 270.1
  dihydropyrimidine dehydrogenase (DPD) 277.6
  disaccharidase (intestinal) 271.3
  disease NEC 269.9
  ear(s) V48.8
  edema 262
  endocrine 259.9
  enzymes, circulating NEC *(see also* Deficiency, by specific enzyme)* 277.6
  ergosterol 268.9
    with
      osteomalacia 268.2
      rickets *(see also* Rickets) 268.0
  erythrocytic glutathione (anemia) 282.2
  eyelid(s) V48.8
  factor *(see also* Defect, coagulation) 286.9
    I (congenital) (fibrinogen) 286.3
      antepartum or intrapartum 641.3●
        affecting fetus or newborn 762.1
      newborn, transient 776.3
      postpartum 666.3●
    II (congenital) (prothrombin) 286.3
    V (congenital) (labile) 286.3
    VII (congenital) (stable) 286.3
    VIII (congenital) (functional) 286.0
      with
        functional defect 286.0
        vascular defect 286.4
    IX (Christmas) (congenital) (functional) 286.1
    X (congenital) (Stuart-Prower) 286.3
    XI (congenital) (plasma thromboplastin antecedent) 286.2
    XII (congenital) (Hageman) 286.3
    XIII (congenital) (fibrin stabilizing) 286.3
    Hageman 286.3
    multiple (congenital) 286.9
      acquired 286.7
  fibrinase *(see also* Defect, coagulation) 286.3
  fibrinogen (congenital) *(see also* Defect, coagulation) 286.3
    acquired 286.6
  fibrin-stabilizing factor (congenital) *(see also* Defect, coagulation) 286.3
    acquired 286.7
  finger - *see* Absence, finger
  fletcher factor *(see also* Defect, coagulation) 286.9
  fluorine 269.3
  folate, anemia 281.2
  folic acid (vitamin B_C) 266.2
    anemia 281.2
  follicle-stimulating hormone (FSH) 253.4
  fructokinase 271.2
  fructose-1, 6-diphosphate 271.2
  fructose-1-phosphate aldolase 271.2
  FSH (follicle-stimulating hormone) 253.4
  fucosidase 271.8
  galactokinase 271.1
  galactose-1-phosphate uridyl transferase 271.1
  gamma globulin in blood 279.00
  glass factor *(see also* Defect, coagulation) 286.3
  glucocorticoid 255.41
  glucose-6-phosphatase 271.0
  glucose-6-phosphate dehydrogenase anemia 282.2

Deficiency, deficient *(Continued)*
  glucuronyl transferase 277.4
  glutathione-reductase (anemia) 282.2
  glycogen synthetase 271.0
  growth hormone 253.3
  Hageman factor (congenital) *(see also* Defect, coagulation) 286.3
  head V48.0
  hemoglobin *(see also* Anemia) 285.9
  hepatophosphorylase 271.0
  hexose monophosphate (HMP) shunt 282.2
  HGH (human growth hormone) 253.3
  HG-PRT 277.2
  homogentisic acid oxidase 270.2
  hormone - *see also* Deficiency, by specific hormone
    anterior pituitary (isolated) (partial) NEC 253.4
      growth (human) 253.3
    follicle-stimulating 253.4
    growth (human) (isolated) 253.3
    human growth 253.3
    interstitial cell-stimulating 253.4
    luteinizing 253.4
    melanocyte-stimulating 253.4
    testicular 257.2
  human growth hormone 253.3
  humoral 279.00
    with
      hyper-IgM 279.05
        autosomal recessive 279.05
        X-linked 279.05
      increased IgM 279.05
    congenital hypogammaglobulinemia 279.04
    non-sex-linked 279.06
    selective immunoglobulin NEC 279.03
      IgA 279.01
      IgG 279.03
      IgM 279.02
        increased 279.05
    specified NEC 279.09
  hydroxylase 255.2
  hypoxanthine-guanine phosphoribosyltransferase (HG-PRT) 277.2
  ICSH (interstitial cell-stimulating hormone) 253.4
  immunity NEC 279.3
    cell-mediated 279.10
      with
        hyperimmunoglobulinemia 279.2
        thrombocytopenia and eczema 279.12
      specified NEC 279.19
    combined (severe) 279.2
      syndrome 279.2
    common variable 279.06
    humoral NEC 279.00
    IgA (secretory) 279.01
    IgG 279.03
    IgM 279.02
  immunoglobulin, selective NEC 279.03
    IgA 279.01
    IgG 279.03
    IgM 279.02
  inositol (B complex) 266.2
  interferon 279.49
  internal organ V47.0
  interstitial cell-stimulating hormone (ICSH) 253.4
  intrinsic factor (Castle's) (congenital) 281.0
  intrinsic (urethral) sphincter (ISD) 599.82
  invertase 271.3
  iodine 269.3
  iron, anemia 280.9
  labile factor (congenital) *(see also* Defect, coagulation) 286.3
    acquired 286.7
  lacrimal fluid (acquired) 375.15
    congenital 743.64

Deficiency, deficient *(Continued)*
  lactase 271.3
  Laki-Lorand factor *(see also* Defect, coagulation) 286.3
  lecithin-cholesterol acyltranferase 272.5
  LH (luteinizing hormone) 253.4
  limb V49.0
    lower V49.0
      congenital *(see also* Deficiency, lower limb, congenital) 755.30
    upper V49.0
      congenital *(see also* Deficiency, upper limb, congenital) 755.20
  lipocaic 577.8
  lipoid (high-density) 272.5
  lipoprotein (familial) (high-density) 272.5
  liver phosphorylase 271.0
  long chain 3-hydroxyacyl CoA dehydrogenase (LCHAD) 277.85
  long chain/very long chain acyl CoA dehydrogenase (LCAD, VLCAD) 277.85
  lower limb V49.0
    congenital 755.30
      with complete absence of distal elements 755.31
      longitudinal (complete) (partial) (with distal deficiencies, incomplete) 755.32
        with complete absence of distal elements 755.31
        combined femoral, tibial, fibular (incomplete) 755.33
        femoral 755.34
        fibular 755.37
        metatarsal(s) 755.38
        phalange(s) 755.39
          meaning all digits 755.31
        tarsal(s) 755.38
        tibia 755.36
        tibiofibular 755.35
      transverse 755.31
  luteinizing hormone (LH) 253.4
  lysosomal alpha-1, 4 glucosidase 271.0
  magnesium 275.2
  mannosidase 271.8
  medium chain acyl CoA dehydrogenase (MCAD) 277.85
  melanocyte-stimulating hormone (MSH) 253.4
  menadione (vitamin K) 269.0
    newborn 776.0
  mental (familial) (hereditary) *(see also* Disability, intellectual) 319
  methylenetetrahydrofolate reductase (MTHFR) 270.4
  mineral NEC 269.3
  mineralocorticoid 255.42
  molybdenum 269.3
  moral 301.7
  multiple, syndrome 260
  myocardial *(see also* Insufficiency, myocardial) 428.0
  myophosphorylase 271.0
  NADH (DPNH)-methemoglobin-reductase (congenital) 289.7
  NADH diaphorase or reductase (congenital) 289.7
  neck V48.1
  niacin (amide) (-tryptophan) 265.2
  nicotinamide 265.2
  nicotinic acid (amide) 265.2
  nose V48.8
  number of teeth *(see also* Anodontia) 520.0
  nutrition, nutritional 269.9
    specified NEC 269.8
  ornithine transcarbamylase 270.6
  ovarian 256.39
  oxygen *(see also* Anoxia) 799.02
  pantothenic acid 266.2
  parathyroid (gland) 252.1

◀ New   ◀▥ Revised   ~~deleted~~ Deleted   ● Use Additional Digit(s)   ▦ Omit code

Deficiency, deficient *(Continued)*
  phenylalanine hydroxylase 270.1
  phosphoenolpyruvate carboxykinase 271.8
  phosphofructokinase 271.2
  phosphoglucomutase 271.0
  phosphohexosisomerase 271.0
  phosphomannomutase 271.8
  phosphomannose isomerase 271.8
  phosphomannosyl mutase 271.8
  phosphorylase kinase, liver 271.0
  pituitary (anterior) 253.2
    posterior 253.5
  placenta - *see* Placenta, insufficiency
  plasma
    cell 279.00
      protein (paraproteinemia)
          (pyroglobulinemia) 273.8
        gamma globulin 279.00
      thromboplastin
        antecedent (PTA) 286.2
        component (PTC) 286.1
  platelet NEC 287.1
    constitutional 286.4
  polyglandular 258.9
  potassium (K) 276.8
  proaccelerin (congenital) (*see also* Defect,
      congenital) 286.3
    acquired 286.7
  proconvertin factor (congenital) (*see also*
      Defect, coagulation) 286.3
    acquired 286.7
  prolactin 253.4
  protein 260
    anemia 281.4
    C 289.81
    plasma - *see* Deficiency, plasma, protein
    S 289.81
  prothrombin (congenital) (*see also* Defect,
      coagulation) 286.3
    acquired 286.7
  Prower factor (*see also* Defect, coagulation)
      286.3
  PRT 277.2
  pseudocholinesterase 289.89
  psychobiological 301.6
  PTA 286.2
  PTC 286.1
  purine nucleoside phosphorylase 277.2
  pyracin (alpha) (beta) 266.1
  pyridoxal 266.1
  pyridoxamine 266.1
  pyridoxine (derivatives) 266.1
  pyruvate carboxylase 271.8
  pyruvate dehydrogenase 271.8
  pyruvate kinase (PK) 282.3
  riboflavin (vitamin B$_2$) 266.0
  saccadic eye movements 379.57
  salivation 527.7
  salt 276.1
  secretion
    ovary 256.39
    salivary gland (any) 527.7
    urine 788.5
  selenium 269.3
  serum
    antitrypsin, familial 273.4
    protein (congenital) 273.8
  short chain acyl CoA dehydrogenase (SCAD)
      277.85
  short stature homeobox gene (SHOX)
    with
      dyschondrosteosis 756.89
      short stature (idiopathic) 783.43
      Turner's syndrome 758.6
  smooth pursuit movements (eye) 379.58
  sodium (Na) 276.1
  SPCA (*see also* Defect, coagulation) 286.3
  specified NEC 269.8
  stable factor (congenital) (*see also* Defect,
      coagulation) 286.3
    acquired 286.7

Deficiency, deficient *(Continued)*
  Stuart (-Prower) factor (*see also* Defect,
      coagulation) 286.3
  sucrase 271.3
  sucrase-isomaltase 271.3
  sulfite oxidase 270.0
  syndrome, multiple 260
  thiamine, thiaminic (chloride) 265.1
  thrombokinase (*see also* Defect, coagulation)
      286.3
    newborn 776.0
  thrombopoieten 287.39
  thymolymphatic 279.2
  thyroid (gland) 244.9
  tocopherol 269.1
  toe - *see* Absence, toe
  tooth bud (*see also* Anodontia) 520.0
  trunk V48.1
  UDPG-glycogen transferase 271.0
  upper limb V49.0
    congenital 755.20
      with complete absence of distal
          elements 755.21
      longitudinal (complete) (partial) (with
          distal deficiencies, incomplete)
          755.22
        carpal(s) 755.28
        combined humeral, radial, ulnar
            (incomplete) 755.23
        humeral 755.24
        metacarpal(s) 755.28
        phalange(s) 755.29
          meaning all digits 755.21
        radial 755.26
        radioulnar 755.25
        ulnar 755.27
      transverse (complete) (partial) 755.21
  vascular 459.9
  vasopressin 253.5
  viosterol (*see also* Deficiency, calciferol) 268.9
  vitamin (multiple) NEC 269.2
    A 264.9
      with
        Bitôt's spot 264.1
          corneal 264.2
            with corneal ulceration 264.3
          keratomalacia 264.4
          keratosis, follicular 264.8
          night blindness 264.5
          scar of cornea, xerophthalmic 264.6
          specified manifestation NEC 264.8
            ocular 264.7
      xeroderma 264.8
      xerophthalmia 264.7
      xerosis
          conjunctival 264.0
            with Bitôt's spot 264.1
          corneal 264.2
            with corneal ulceration 264.3
    B (complex) NEC 266.9
      with
        beriberi 265.0
        pellagra 265.2
      specified type NEC 266.2
    B$_1$ NEC 265.1
      beriberi 265.0
    B$_2$ 266.0
    B$_6$ 266.1
    B$_{12}$ 266.2
    B$_C$ (folic acid) 266.2
    C (ascorbic acid) (with scurvy) 267
    D (calciferol) (ergosterol) 268.9
      with
        osteomalacia 268.2
        rickets (*see also* Rickets) 268.0
    E 269.1
    folic acid 266.2
    G 266.0
    H 266.2
    K 269.0
      of newborn 776.0

Deficiency, deficient *(Continued)*
  vitamin NEC *(Continued)*
    nicotinic acid 265.2
    P 269.1
    PP 265.2
    specified NEC 269.1
    zinc 269.3
Deficient - *see also* Deficiency
  blink reflex 374.45
  craniofacial axis 756.0
  number of teeth (*see also* Anodontia) 520.0
  secretion of urine 788.5
Deficit
  attention 799.51
  cognitive communication 799.52
  concentration 799.51
  executive function 799.55
  frontal lobe 799.55
  neurologic NEC 781.99
    due to
      cerebrovascular lesion (*see also*
          Disease, cerebrovascular, acute)
          436
        late effect - *see* Late effect(s) (of)
            cerebrovascular disease
      transient ischemic attack 435.9
    ischemic
      reversible (RIND) 434.91
        history of (personal) V12.54
        prolonged (PRIND) 434.91
          history of (personal) V12.54
  oxygen 799.02
  psychomotor 799.54
  visuospatial 799.53
Deflection
  radius 736.09
  septum (acquired) (nasal) (nose) 470
  spine - *see* Curvature, spine
  turbinate (nose) 470
Defluvium
  capillorum (*see also* Alopecia) 704.00
  ciliorum 374.55
  unguium 703.8
Deformity 738.9
  abdomen, congenital 759.9
  abdominal wall
    acquired 738.8
    congenital 756.70
    muscle deficiency syndrome 756.79
  acquired (unspecified site) 738.9
    specified site NEC 738.8
  adrenal gland (congenital) 759.1
  alimentary tract, congenital 751.9
    lower 751.5
    specified type NEC 751.8
    upper (any part, except tongue) 750.9
      specified type NEC 750.8
      tongue 750.10
        specified type NEC 750.19
  ankle (joint) (acquired) 736.70
    abduction 718.47
    congenital 755.69
    contraction 718.47
    specified NEC 736.79
  anus (congenital) 751.5
    acquired 569.49
  aorta (congenital) 747.20
    acquired 447.8
    arch 747.21
      acquired 447.8
    coarctation 747.10
  aortic
    arch 747.21
      acquired 447.8
    cusp or valve (congenital) 746.9
      acquired (*see also* Endocarditis, aortic)
          424.1
    ring 747.21
  appendix 751.5
  arm (acquired) 736.89
    congenital 755.50

Deformity (Continued)
  arteriovenous (congenital) (peripheral) NEC
      747.60
    gastrointestinal 747.61
    lower limb 747.64
    renal 747.62
    specified NEC 747.69
    spinal 747.82
    upper limb 747.63
  artery (congenital) (peripheral) NEC
      (see also Deformity, vascular)
      747.60
    acquired 447.8
    cerebral 747.81
    coronary (congenital) 746.85
      acquired (see also Ischemia, heart)
        414.9
    retinal 743.9
    umbilical 747.5
  atrial septal (congenital) (heart) 745.5
  auditory canal (congenital) (external) (see also
      Deformity, ear) 744.3
    acquired 380.50
  auricle
    ear (congenital) (see also Deformity, ear)
        744.3
      acquired 380.32
    heart (congenital) 746.9
  back (acquired) - see Deformity, spine
  Bartholin's duct (congenital) 750.9
  bile duct (congenital) 751.60
    acquired 576.8
      with calculus, choledocholithiasis, or
        stones - see Choledocholithiasis
  biliary duct or passage (congenital) 751.60
    acquired 576.8
      with calculus, choledocholithiasis, or
        stones - see Choledocholithiasis
  bladder (neck) (sphincter) (trigone)
      (acquired) 596.89
    congenital 753.9
  bone (acquired) NEC 738.9
    congenital 756.9
    turbinate 738.0
  boutonniere (finger) 736.21
  brain (congenital) 742.9
    acquired 348.89
    multiple 742.4
    reduction 742.2
    vessel (congenital) 747.81
  breast (acquired) 611.89
    congenital 757.6
    reconstructed 612.0
  bronchus (congenital) 748.3
    acquired 519.19
  bursa, congenital 756.9
  canal of Nuck 752.9
  canthus (congenital) 743.9
    acquired 374.89
  capillary (acquired) 448.9
    congenital NEC (see also Deformity,
        vascular) 747.60
  cardiac - see Deformity, heart
  cardiovascular system (congenital)
      746.9
  caruncle, lacrimal (congenital) 743.9
    acquired 375.69
  cascade, stomach 537.6
  cecum (congenital) 751.5
    acquired 569.89
  cerebral (congenital) 742.9
    acquired 348.89
  cervix (acquired) (uterus) 622.8
    congenital 752.40
  cheek (acquired) 738.19
    congenital 744.9
  chest (wall) (acquired) 738.3
    congenital 754.89
    late effect of rickets 268.1
  chin (acquired) 738.19
    congenital 744.9

Deformity (Continued)
  choroid (congenital) 743.9
    acquired 363.8
    plexus (congenital) 742.9
      acquired 349.2
  cicatricial - see Cicatrix
  cilia (congenital) 743.9
    acquired 374.89
  circulatory system (congenital) 747.9
  clavicle (acquired) 738.8
    congenital 755.51
  clitoris (congenital) 752.40
    acquired 624.8
  clubfoot - see Clubfoot
  coccyx (acquired) 738.6
    congenital 756.10
  colon (congenital) 751.5
    acquired 569.89
  concha (ear) (congenital) (see also Deformity,
      ear) 744.3
    acquired 380.32
  congenital, organ or site not listed (see also
      Anomaly) 759.9
  cornea (congenital) 743.9
    acquired 371.70
  coronary artery (congenital) 746.85
    acquired (see also Ischemia, heart) 414.9
  cranium (acquired) 738.19
    congenital (see also Deformity, skull,
        congenital) 756.0
  cricoid cartilage (congenital) 748.3
    acquired 478.79
  cystic duct (congenital) 751.60
    acquired 575.8
  Dandy-Walker 742.3
    with spina bifida (see also Spina bifida)
        741.0●
  diaphragm (congenital) 756.6
    acquired 738.8
  digestive organ(s) or system (congenital)
      NEC 751.9
    specified type NEC 751.8
  ductus arteriosus 747.0
  duodenal bulb 537.89
  duodenum (congenital) 751.5
    acquired 537.89
  dura (congenital) 742.9
    brain 742.4
      acquired 349.2
    spinal 742.59
      acquired 349.2
  ear (congenital) 744.3
    acquired 380.32
    auricle 744.3
      causing impairment of hearing 744.02
    causing impairment of hearing 744.00
    external 744.3
      causing impairment of hearing
          744.02
    internal 744.05
    lobule 744.3
    middle 744.03
      ossicles 744.04
    ossicles 744.04
  ectodermal (congenital) NEC 757.9
    specified type NEC 757.8
  ejaculatory duct (congenital) 752.9
    acquired 608.89
  elbow (joint) (acquired) 736.00
    congenital 755.50
    contraction 718.42
  endocrine gland NEC 759.2
  epididymis (congenital) 752.9
    acquired 608.89
    torsion 608.24
  epiglottis (congenital) 748.3
    acquired 478.79
  esophagus (congenital) 750.9
    acquired 530.89
  Eustachian tube (congenital) NEC 744.3
    specified type NEC 744.24

Deformity (Continued)
  extremity (acquired) 736.9
    congenital, except reduction deformity
        755.9
      lower 755.60
      upper 755.50
    reduction - see Deformity, reduction
  eye (congenital) 743.9
    acquired 379.8
    muscle 743.9
  eyebrow (congenital) 744.89
  eyelid (congenital) 743.9
    acquired 374.89
    specified type NEC 743.62
  face (acquired) 738.19
    congenital (any part) 744.9
      due to intrauterine malposition and
          pressure 754.0
  fallopian tube (congenital) 752.10
    acquired 620.8
  femur (acquired) 736.89
    congenital 755.60
  fetal
    with fetopelvic disproportion 653.7●
      affecting fetus or newborn 763.1
    causing obstructed labor 660.1●
      affecting fetus or newborn 763.1
    known or suspected, affecting
        management of pregnancy 655.9●
  finger (acquired) 736.20
    boutonniere type 736.21
    congenital 755.50
    flexion contracture 718.44
    swan neck 736.22
  flexion (joint) (acquired) 736.9
    congenital NEC 755.9
    hip or thigh (acquired) 736.39
      congenital (see also Subluxation,
          congenital, hip) 754.32
  foot (acquired) 736.70
    cavovarus 736.75
      congenital 754.59
    congenital NEC 754.70
      specified type NEC 754.79
    valgus (acquired) 736.79
      congenital 754.60
        specified type NEC 754.69
    varus (acquired) 736.79
      congenital 754.50
        specified type NEC 754.59
  forearm (acquired) 736.00
    congenital 755.50
  forehead (acquired) 738.19
    congenital (see also Deformity, skull,
        congenital) 756.0
  frontal bone (acquired) 738.19
    congenital (see also Deformity, skull,
        congenital) 756.0
  gallbladder (congenital) 751.60
    acquired 575.8
  gastrointestinal tract (congenital) NEC 751.9
    acquired 569.89
    specified type NEC 751.8
  genitalia, genital organ(s) or system NEC
    congenital 752.9
    female (congenital) 752.9
      acquired 629.89
      external 752.40
      internal 752.9
    male (congenital) 752.9
      acquired 608.89
  globe (eye) (congenital) 743.9
    acquired 360.89
  gum (congenital) 750.9
    acquired 523.9
  gunstock 736.02
  hand (acquired) 736.00
    claw 736.06
    congenital 755.50
    minus (and plus) (intrinsic) 736.09
    pill roller (intrinsic) 736.09

◄ New   ◄▐ Revised   ~~deleted~~ Deleted   ● Use Additional Digit(s)   ▨ Omit code

Deformity *(Continued)*
  hand *(Continued)*
    plus (and minus) (intrinsic) 736.09
    swan neck (intrinsic) 736.09
  head (acquired) 738.10
    congenital *(see also* Deformity, skull,
      congenital) 756.0
    specified NEC 738.19
  heart (congenital) 746.9
    auricle (congenital) 746.9
    septum 745.9
      auricular 745.5
      specified type NEC 745.8
      ventricular 745.4
    valve (congenital) NEC 746.9
      acquired - *see* Endocarditis
      pulmonary (congenital) 746.00
      specified type NEC 746.89
    ventricle (congenital) 746.9
  heel (acquired) 736.76
    congenital 755.67
  hepatic duct (congenital) 751.60
    acquired 576.8
      with calculus, choledocholithiasis, or
        stones - *see* Choledocholithiasis
  hip (joint) (acquired) 736.30
    congenital NEC 755.63
    flexion 718.45
      congenital *(see also* Subluxation,
        congenital, hip) 754.32
  hourglass - *see* Contraction, hourglass
  humerus (acquired) 736.89
    congenital 755.50
  hymen (congenital) 752.40
  hypophyseal (congenital) 759.2
  ileocecal (coil) (valve) (congenital) 751.5
    acquired 569.89
  ileum (intestine) (congenital) 751.5
    acquired 569.89
  ilium (acquired) 738.6
    congenital 755.60
  integument (congenital) 757.9
  intervertebral cartilage or disc (acquired) -
    see also Displacement, intervertebral
    disc
    congenital 756.10
  intestine (large) (small) (congenital) 751.5
    acquired 569.89
  iris (acquired) 364.75
    congenital 743.9
    prolapse 364.89
  ischium (acquired) 738.6
    congenital 755.60
  jaw (acquired) (congenital) NEC 524.9
    due to intrauterine malposition and
      pressure 754.0
  joint (acquired) NEC 738.8
    congenital 755.9
    contraction (abduction) (adduction)
      (extension) (flexion) - *see*
      Contraction, joint
  kidney(s) (calyx) (pelvis) (congenital) 753.9
    acquired 593.89
    vessel 747.62
      acquired 459.9
  Klippel-Feil (brevicollis) 756.16
  knee (acquired) NEC 736.6
    congenital 755.64
  labium (majus) (minus) (congenital) 752.40
    acquired 624.8
  lacrimal apparatus or duct (congenital) 743.9
    acquired 375.69
  larynx (muscle) (congenital) 748.3
    acquired 478.79
    web (glottic) (subglottic) 748.2
  leg (lower) (upper) (acquired) NEC 736.89
    congenital 755.60
      reduction - *see* Deformity, reduction,
        lower limb
  lens (congenital) 743.9
    acquired 379.39

Deformity *(Continued)*
  lid (fold) (congenital) 743.9
    acquired 374.89
  ligament (acquired) 728.9
    congenital 756.9
  limb (acquired) 736.9
    congenital, except reduction deformity
      755.9
      lower 755.60
        reduction *(see also* Deformity,
          reduction, lower limb)
          755.30
      upper 755.50
        reduction *(see also* Deformity,
          reduction, lower limb)
          755.20
    specified NEC 736.89
  lip (congenital) NEC 750.9
    acquired 528.5
    specified type NEC 750.26
  liver (congenital) 751.60
    acquired 573.8
    duct (congenital) 751.60
      acquired 576.8
        with calculus, choledocholithiasis,
          or stones - *see*
          Choledocholithiasis
  lower extremity - *see* Deformity, leg
  lumbosacral (joint) (region) (congenital)
    756.10
    acquired 738.5
  lung (congenital) 748.60
    acquired 518.89
    specified type NEC 748.69
  lymphatic system, congenital 759.9
  Madelung's (radius) 755.54
  maxilla (acquired) (congenital) 524.9
  meninges or membrane (congenital) 742.9
    brain 742.4
      acquired 349.2
    spinal (cord) 742.59
      acquired 349.2
  mesentery (congenital) 751.9
    acquired 568.89
  metacarpus (acquired) 736.00
    congenital 755.50
  metatarsus (acquired) 736.70
    congenital 754.70
  middle ear, except ossicles (congenital)
    744.03
    ossicles 744.04
  mitral (leaflets) (valve) (congenital)
    746.9
    acquired - *see* Endocarditis, mitral
    Ebstein's 746.89
    parachute 746.5
    specified type NEC 746.89
    stenosis, congenital 746.5
  mouth (acquired) 528.9
    congenital NEC 750.9
      specified type NEC 750.26
  multiple, congenital NEC 759.7
    specified type NEC 759.89
  muscle (acquired) 728.9
    congenital 756.9
      specified type NEC 756.89
      sternocleidomastoid (due to
        intrauterine malposition and
        pressure) 754.1
  musculoskeletal system, congenital NEC
    756.9
    specified type NEC 756.9
  nail (acquired) 703.9
    congenital 757.9
  nasal - *see* Deformity, nose
  neck (acquired) NEC 738.2
    congenital (any part) 744.9
      sternocleidomastoid 754.1
  nervous system (congenital) 742.9
  nipple (congenital) 757.6
    acquired 611.89

Deformity *(Continued)*
  nose, nasal (cartilage) (acquired) 738.0
    bone (turbinate) 738.0
    congenital 748.1
      bent 754.0
      squashed 754.0
    saddle 738.0
      syphilitic 090.5
    septum 470
      congenital 748.1
    sinus (wall) (congenital) 748.1
      acquired 738.0
    syphilitic (congenital) 090.5
      late 095.8
  ocular muscle (congenital) 743.9
    acquired 378.60
  opticociliary vessels (congenital) 743.9
  orbit (congenital) (eye) 743.9
    acquired NEC 376.40
      associated with craniofacial
        deformities 376.44
      due to
        bone disease 376.43
        surgery 376.47
        trauma 376.47
  organ of Corti (congenital) 744.05
  ovary (congenital) 752.0
    acquired 620.8
  oviduct (congenital) 752.10
    acquired 620.8
  palate (congenital) 750.9
    acquired 526.89
    cleft (congenital) *(see also* Cleft, palate)
      749.00
    hard, acquired 526.89
    soft, acquired 528.9
  pancreas (congenital) 751.7
    acquired 577.8
  parachute, mitral valve 746.5
  parathyroid (gland) 759.2
  parotid (gland) (congenital) 750.9
    acquired 527.8
  patella (acquired) 736.6
    congenital 755.64
  pelvis, pelvic (acquired) (bony) 738.6
    with disproportion (fetopelvic) 653.0●
      affecting fetus or newborn 763.1
      causing obstructed labor 660.1●
        affecting fetus or newborn 763.1
    congenital 755.60
    rachitic (late effect) 268.1
  penis (glans) (congenital) 752.9
    acquired 607.89
  pericardium (congenital) 746.9
    acquired - *see* Pericarditis
  pharynx (congenital) 750.9
    acquired 478.29
  Pierre Robin (congenital) 756.0
  pinna (acquired) 380.32
    congenital 744.3
  pituitary (congenital) 759.2
  pleural folds (congenital) 748.8
  portal vein (congenital) 747.40
  posture - *see* Curvature, spine
  prepuce (congenital) 752.9
    acquired 607.89
  prostate (congenital) 752.9
    acquired 602.8
  pulmonary valve - *see* Endocarditis,
    pulmonary
  pupil (congenital) 743.9
    acquired 364.75
  pylorus (congenital) 750.9
    acquired 537.89
  rachitic (acquired), healed or old 268.1
  radius (acquired) 736.00
    congenital 755.50
      reduction - *see* Deformity, reduction,
        upper limb
  rectovaginal septum (congenital) 752.40
    acquired 623.8

Deformity *(Continued)*
rectum (congenital) 751.5
    acquired 569.49
reduction (extremity) (limb) 755.4
    brain 742.2
    lower limb 755.30
        with complete absence of distal
            elements 755.31
        longitudinal (complete) (partial) (with
            distal deficiencies, incomplete)
            755.32
            with complete absence of distal
                elements 755.31
            combined femoral, tibial, fibular
                (incomplete) 755.33
            femoral 755.34
            fibular 755.37
            metatarsal(s) 755.38
            phalange(s) 755.39
                meaning all digits 755.31
            tarsal(s) 755.38
            tibia 755.36
            tibiofibular 755.35
        transverse 755.31
    upper limb 755.20
        with complete absence of distal
            elements 755.21
        longitudinal (complete) (partial) (with
            distal deficiencies, incomplete)
            755.22
            with complete absence of distal
                elements 755.21
            carpal(s) 755.28
            combined humeral, radial, ulnar
                (incomplete) 755.23
            humeral 755.24
            metacarpal(s) 755.28
            phalange(s) 755.29
                meaning all digits 755.21
            radial 755.26
            radioulnar 755.25
            ulnar 755.27
        transverse (complete) (partial)
            755.21
renal - *see* Deformity, kidney
respiratory system (congenital) 748.9
    specified type NEC 748.8
rib (acquired) 738.3
    congenital 756.3
        cervical 756.2
rotation (joint) (acquired) 736.9
    congenital 755.9
    hip or thigh 736.39
        congenital (*see also* Subluxation,
            congenital, hip) 754.32
sacroiliac joint (congenital) 755.69
    acquired 738.5
sacrum (acquired) 738.5
    congenital 756.10
saddle
    back 737.8
    nose 738.0
        syphilitic 090.5
salivary gland or duct (congenital) 750.9
    acquired 527.8
scapula (acquired) 736.89
    congenital 755.50
scrotum (congenital) 752.9
    acquired 608.89
sebaceous gland, acquired 706.8
seminal tract or duct (congenital) 752.9
    acquired 608.89
septum (nasal) (acquired) 470
    congenital 748.1
shoulder (joint) (acquired) 736.89
    congenital 755.50
        specified type NEC 755.59
    contraction 718.41
sigmoid (flexure) (congenital) 751.5
    acquired 569.89
sinus of Valsalva 747.29

Deformity *(Continued)*
skin (congenital) 757.9
    acquired NEC 709.8
skull (acquired) 738.19
    congenital 756.0
        with
            anencephalus 740.0
            encephalocele 742.0
            hydrocephalus 742.3
                with spina bifida (*see also* Spina
                    bifida) 741.0●
            microcephalus 742.1
        due to intrauterine malposition and
            pressure 754.0
soft parts, organs or tissues (of pelvis)
    in pregnancy or childbirth NEC 654.9●
        affecting fetus or newborn 763.89
        causing obstructed labor 660.2●
            affecting fetus or newborn 763.1
spermatic cord (congenital) 752.9
    acquired 608.89
        torsion 608.22
            extravaginal 608.21
            intravaginal 608.22
spinal
    column - *see* Deformity, spine
    cord (congenital) 742.9
        acquired 336.8
        vessel (congenital) 747.82
    nerve root (congenital) 742.9
        acquired 724.9
spine (acquired) NEC 738.5
    congenital 756.10
        due to intrauterine malposition and
            pressure 754.2
    kyphoscoliotic (*see also* Kyphoscoliosis)
        737.30
    kyphotic (*see also* Kyphosis) 737.10
    lordotic (*see also* Lordosis) 737.20
    rachitic 268.1
    scoliotic (*see also* Scoliosis) 737.30
spleen
    acquired 289.59
    congenital 759.0
Sprengel's (congenital) 755.52
sternum (acquired) 738.3
    congenital 756.3
stomach (congenital) 750.9
    acquired 537.89
submaxillary gland (congenital) 750.9
    acquired 527.8
swan neck (acquired)
    finger 736.22
    hand 736.09
talipes - *see* Talipes
teeth, tooth NEC 520.9
testis (congenital) 752.9
    acquired 608.89
        torsion 608.20
thigh (acquired) 736.89
    congenital 755.60
thorax (acquired) (wall) 738.3
    congenital 754.89
    late effect of rickets 268.1
thumb (acquired) 736.20
    congenital 755.50
thymus (tissue) (congenital) 759.2
thyroid (gland) (congenital) 759.2
    cartilage 748.3
        acquired 478.79
tibia (acquired) 736.89
    congenital 755.60
    saber 090.5
toe (acquired) 735.9
    congenital 755.66
    specified NEC 735.8
tongue (congenital) 750.10
    acquired 529.8
tooth, teeth NEC 520.9
trachea (rings) (congenital) 748.3
    acquired 519.19

Deformity *(Continued)*
transverse aortic arch (congenital) 747.21
tricuspid (leaflets) (valve) (congenital) 746.9
    acquired - *see* Endocarditis, tricuspid
    atresia or stenosis 746.1
    specified type NEC 746.89
trunk (acquired) 738.3
    congenital 759.9
ulna (acquired) 736.00
    congenital 755.50
upper extremity - *see* Deformity, arm
urachus (congenital) 753.7
ureter (opening) (congenital) 753.9
    acquired 593.89
urethra (valve) (congenital) 753.9
    acquired 599.84
urinary tract or system (congenital)
    753.9
    urachus 753.7
uterus (congenital) 752.39
    acquired 621.8
uvula (congenital) 750.9
    acquired 528.9
vagina (congenital) 752.40
    acquired 623.8
valve, valvular (heart) (congenital)
    746.9
    acquired - *see* Endocarditis
    pulmonary 746.00
    specified type NEC 746.89
vascular (congenital) (peripheral) NEC
    747.60
    acquired 459.9
    gastrointestinal 747.61
    lower limb 747.64
    renal 747.62
    specified site NEC 747.69
    spinal 747.82
    upper limb 747.63
vas deferens (congenital) 752.9
    acquired 608.89
vein (congenital) NEC (*see also* Deformity,
    vascular) 747.60
    brain 747.81
    coronary 746.9
    great 747.40
vena cava (inferior) (superior) (congenital)
    747.40
vertebra - *see* Deformity, spine
vesicourethral orifice (acquired) 596.89
    congenital NEC 753.9
        specified type NEC 753.8
vessels of optic papilla (congenital)
    743.9
visual field (contraction) 368.45
vitreous humor (congenital) 743.9
    acquired 379.29
vulva (congenital) 752.40
    acquired 624.8
wrist (joint) (acquired) 736.00
    congenital 755.50
    contraction 718.43
    valgus 736.03
        congenital 755.59
    varus 736.04
        congenital 755.59
Degeneration, degenerative
adrenal (capsule) (gland) 255.8
    with hypofunction 255.41
    fatty 255.8
    hyaline 255.8
    infectional 255.8
    lardaceous 277.39
amyloid (any site) (general) 277.39
anterior cornua, spinal cord 336.8
anterior labral 840.8
aorta, aortic 440.0
    fatty 447.8
    valve (heart) (*see also* Endocarditis, aortic)
        424.1
arteriovascular - *see* Arteriosclerosis

Degeneration, degenerative *(Continued)*
  artery, arterial (atheromatous) (calcareous) -
    see also Arteriosclerosis
    amyloid 277.39
    lardaceous 277.39
    medial NEC (*see also* Arteriosclerosis,
      extremities) 440.20
  articular cartilage NEC (*see also* Disorder,
    cartilage, articular) 718.0 ●
    elbow 718.02
    knee 717.5
    patella 717.7
    shoulder 718.01
    spine (*see also* Spondylosis) 721.90
  atheromatous - *see* Arteriosclerosis
  bacony (any site) 277.39
  basal nuclei or ganglia NEC 333.0
  bone 733.90
  brachial plexus 353.0
  brain (cortical) (progressive) 331.9
    arteriosclerotic 437.0
    childhood 330.9
      specified type NEC 330.8
    congenital 742.4
    cystic 348.0
      congenital 742.4
    familial NEC 331.89
    grey matter 330.8
    heredofamilial NEC 331.89
    in
      alcoholism 303.9 ● [331.7]
      beriberi 265.0 [331.7]
      cerebrovascular disease 437.9 [331.7]
      congenital hydrocephalus 742.3 [331.7]
        with spina bifida (*see also* Spina
          bifida) 741.0 ● [331.7]
      Babry's disease 272.7 [330.2]
      Gaucher's disease 272.7 [330.2]
      Hunter's disease or syndrome 277.5
        [330.3]
      lipidosis
        cerebral 330.1
        generalized 272.7 [330.2]
      mucopolysaccharidosis 277.5 [330.3]
      myxedema (*see also* Myxedema) 244.9
        [331.7]
      neoplastic disease NEC (M8000/1)
        239.9 [331.7]
      Niemann-Pick disease 272.7 [330.2]
      sphingolipidosis 272.7 [330.2]
      vitamin B$_{12}$ deficiency 266.2 [331.7]
    motor centers 331.89
    senile 331.2
    specified type NEC 331.89
  breast - *see* Disease, breast
  Bruch's membrane 363.40
  bundle of His 426.50
    left 426.3
    right 426.4
  calcareous NEC 275.49
  capillaries 448.9
    amyloid 277.39
    fatty 448.9
    lardaceous 277.39
  cardiac (brown) (calcareous) (fatty) (fibrous)
    (hyaline) (mural) (muscular)
    (pigmentary) (senile) (with
    arteriosclerosis) (*see also* Degeneration,
    myocardial) 429.1
    valve, valvular - *see* Endocarditis
  cardiorenal (*see also* Hypertension,
    cardiorenal) 404.90
  cardiovascular (*see also* Disease,
    cardiovascular) 429.2
    renal (*see also* Hypertension, cardiorenal)
      404.90
  cartilage (joint) - *see* Derangement, joint
  cerebellar NEC 334.9
    primary (hereditary) (sporadic) 334.2
  cerebral - *see* Degeneration, brain
  cerebromacular 330.1

Degeneration, degenerative *(Continued)*
  cerebrovascular 437.1
    due to hypertension 437.2
    late effect - *see* Late effect(s) (of)
      cerebrovascular disease
  cervical plexus 353.2
  cervix 622.8
    due to radiation (intended effect) 622.8
      adverse effect or misadventure 622.8
  changes, spine or vertebra (*see also*
    Spondylosis) 721.90
  chitinous 277.39
  chorioretinal 363.40
    congenital 743.53
    hereditary 363.50
  choroid (colloid) (drusen) 363.40
    hereditary 363.50
    senile 363.41
      diffuse secondary 363.42
  cochlear 386.8
  collateral ligament (knee) (medial) 717.82
    lateral 717.81
  combined (spinal cord) (subacute) 266.2
    [336.2]
    with anemia (pernicious) 281.0 [336.2]
      due to dietary deficiency 281.1 [336.2]
    due to vitamin B$_{12}$ deficiency anemia
      (dietary) 281.1 [336.2]
  conjunctiva 372.50
    amyloid 277.39 [372.50]
  cornea 371.40
    calcerous 371.44
    familial (hereditary) (*see also* Dystrophy,
      cornea) 371.50
      macular 371.55
      reticular 371.54
    hyaline (of old scars) 371.41
    marginal (Terrien's) 371.48
    mosaic (shagreen) 371.41
    nodular 371.46
    peripheral 371.48
    senile 371.41
  cortical (cerebellar) (parenchymatous) 334.2
    alcoholic 303.9 ● [334.4]
    diffuse, due to arteriopathy 437.0
  corticobasal 331.6
  corticostriatal-spinal 334.8
  cretinoid 243
  cruciate ligament (knee) (posterior) 717.84
    anterior 717.83
  cutis 709.3
    amyloid 277.39
  dental pulp 522.2
  disc disease - *see* Degeneration, intervertebral
    disc
  dorsolateral (spinal cord) - *see* Degeneration,
    combined
  endocardial 424.90
  extrapyramidal NEC 333.90
  eye NEC 360.40
    macular (*see also* Degeneration, macula)
      362.50
      congenital 362.75
      hereditary 362.76
  fatty (diffuse) (general) 272.8
    liver 571.8
      alcoholic 571.0
    localized site - *see* Degeneration, by site,
      fatty
    placenta - *see* Placenta, abnormal
  globe (eye) NEC 360.40
    macular - *see* Degeneration, macula
  grey matter 330.8
  heart (brown) (calcareous) (fatty) (fibrous)
    (hyaline) (mural) (muscular)
    (pigmentary) (senile) (with
    arteriosclerosis) (*see also* Degeneration,
    myocardial) 429.1
    amyloid 277.39 [425.7]
    atheromatous - *see* Arteriosclerosis,
      coronary

Degeneration, degenerative *(Continued)*
  heart *(Continued)*
    gouty 274.82
    hypertensive (*see also* Hypertension,
      heart) 402.90
    ischemic 414.9
    valve, valvular - *see* Endocarditis
  hepatolenticular (Wilson's) 275.1
  hepatorenal 572.4
  heredofamilial
    brain NEC 331.89
    spinal cord NEC 336.8
  hyaline (diffuse) (generalized) 728.9
    localized - *see also* Degeneration, by site
      cornea 371.41
      keratitis 371.41
  hypertensive vascular - *see* Hypertension
  infrapatellar fat pad 729.31
  internal semilunar cartilage 717.3
  intervertebral disc 722.6
    with myelopathy 722.70
    cervical, cervicothoracic 722.4
      with myelopathy 722.71
    lumbar, lumbosacral 722.52
      with myelopathy 722.73
    thoracic, thoracolumbar 722.51
      with myelopathy 722.72
  intestine 569.89
    amyloid 277.39
    lardaceous 277.39
  iris (generalized) (*see also* Atrophy, iris)
    364.59
    pigmentary 364.53
    pupillary margin 364.54
  ischemic - *see* Ischemia
  joint disease (*see also* Osteoarthrosis) 715.9 ●
    multiple sites 715.09
    spine (*see also* Spondylosis) 721.90
  kidney (*see also* Sclerosis, renal) 587
    amyloid 277.39 [583.81]
    cyst, cystic (multiple) (solitary) 593.2
      congenital (*see also* Cystic, disease,
        kidney) 753.10
    fatty 593.89
    fibrocystic (congenital) 753.19
    lardaceous 277.39 [583.81]
    polycystic (congenital) 753.12
      adult type (APKD) 753.13
      autosomal dominant 753.13
      autosomal recessive 753.14
      childhood type (CPKD) 753.14
      infantile type 753.14
    waxy 277.39 [583.81]
  Kuhnt-Junius (retina) 362.52
  labyrinth, osseous 386.8
  lacrimal passages, cystic 375.12
  lardaceous (any site) 277.39
  lateral column (posterior), spinal cord (*see
    also* Degeneration, combined) 266.2
    [336.2]
  lattice 362.63
  lens 366.9
    infantile, juvenile, or presenile 366.00
    senile 366.10
  lenticular (familial) (progressive) (Wilson's)
    (with cirrhosis of liver) 275.1
    striate artery 437.0
  lethal ball, prosthetic heart valve 996.02
  ligament
    collateral (knee) (medial) 717.82
      lateral 717.81
    cruciate (knee) (posterior) 717.84
      anterior 717.83
  liver (diffuse) 572.8
    amyloid 277.39
    congenital (cystic) 751.62
    cystic 572.8
      congenital 751.62
    fatty 571.8
      alcoholic 571.0
    hypertrophic 572.8

Degeneration, degenerative *(Continued)*
  liver *(Continued)*
    lardaceous 277.39
    parenchymatous, acute or subacute *(see also* Necrosis, liver) 570
    pigmentary 572.8
    toxic (acute) 573.8
    waxy 277.39
  lung 518.89
  lymph gland 289.3
    hyaline 289.3
    lardaceous 277.39
  macula (acquired) (senile) 362.50
    atrophic 362.51
    Best's 362.76
    congenital 362.75
    cystic 362.54
    cystoid 362.53
    disciform 362.52
    dry 362.51
    exudative 362.52
    familial pseudoinflammatory 362.77
    hereditary 362.76
    hole 362.54
    juvenile (Stargardt's) 362.75
    nonexudative 362.51
    pseudohole 362.54
    wet 362.52
  medullary - *see* Degeneration, brain
  membranous labyrinth, congenital (causing impairment of hearing) 744.05
  meniscus - *see* Derangement, joint
  microcystoid 362.62
  mitral - *see* Insufficiency, mitral
  Mönckeberg's *(see also* Arteriosclerosis, extremities) 440.20
  moral 301.7
  motor centers, senile 331.2
  mural *(see also* Degeneration, myocardial) 429.1
    heart, cardiac *(see also* Degeneration, myocardial) 429.1
    myocardium, myocardial *(see also* Degeneration, myocardial) 429.1
  muscle 728.9
    fatty 728.9
    fibrous 728.9
    heart *(see also* Degeneration, myocardial) 429.1
    hyaline 728.9
  muscular progressive 728.2
  myelin, central nervous system NEC 341.9
  myocardium, myocardial (brown) (calcareous) (fatty) (fibrous) (hyaline) (mural) (muscular) (pigmentary) (senile) (with arteriosclerosis) 429.1
    with rheumatic fever (conditions classifiable to 390) 398.0
      active, acute, or subacute 391.2
        with chorea 392.0
      inactive or quiescent (with chorea) 398.0
    amyloid 277.39 [425.7]
    congenital 746.89
    fetus or newborn 779.89
    gouty 274.82
    hypertensive *(see also* Hypertension, heart) 402.90
    ischemic 414.8
    rheumatic *(see also* Degeneration, myocardium, with rheumatic fever) 398.0
    syphilitic 093.82
  nasal sinus (mucosa) *(see also* Sinusitis) 473.9
    frontal 473.1
    maxillary 473.0
  nerve - *see* Disorder, nerve

Degeneration, degenerative *(Continued)*
  nervous system 349.89
    amyloid 277.39 [357.4]
    autonomic *(see also* Neuropathy, peripheral, autonomic) 337.9
    fatty 349.89
    peripheral autonomic NEC *(see also* Neuropathy, peripheral, autonomic) 337.9
  nipple 611.9
  nose 478.19
  oculoacousticocerebral, congenital (progressive) 743.8
  olivopontocerebellar (familial) (hereditary) 333.0
  osseous labyrinth 386.8
  ovary 620.8
    cystic 620.2
    microcystic 620.2
  pallidal, pigmentary (progressive) 333.0
  pancreas 577.8
    tuberculous *(see also* Tuberculosis) 017.9●
  papillary muscle 429.81
  paving stone 362.61
  penis 607.89
  peritoneum 568.89
  pigmentary (diffuse) (general)
    localized - *see* Degeneration, by site
    pallidal (progressive) 333.0
    secondary 362.65
  pineal gland 259.8
  pituitary (gland) 253.8
  placenta (fatty) (fibrinoid) (fibroid) - *see* Placenta, abnormal
  popliteal fat pad 729.31
  posterolateral (spinal cord) *(see also* Degeneration, combined) 266.2 [336.2]
  pulmonary valve (heart) *(see also* Endocarditis, pulmonary) 424.3
  pulp (tooth) 522.2
  pupillary margin 364.54
  renal *(see also* Sclerosis, renal) 587
    fibrocystic 753.19
    polycystic 753.12
      adult type (APKD) 753.13
      autosomal dominant 753.13
      autosomal recessive 753.14
      childhood type (CPKD) 753.14
      infantile type 753.14
  reticuloendothelial system 289.89
  retina (peripheral) 362.60
    with retinal defect *(see also* Detachment, retina, with retinal defect) 361.00
    cystic (senile) 362.50
    cystoid 362.53
    hereditary *(see also* Dystrophy, retina) 362.70
      cerebroretinal 362.71
      congenital 362.75
      juvenile (Stargardt's) 362.75
      macula 362.76
    Kuhnt-Junius 362.52
    lattice 362.63
    macular *(see also* Degeneration, macula) 362.50
    microcystoid 362.62
    palisade 362.63
    paving stone 362.61
    pigmentary (primary) 362.74
      secondary 362.65
    posterior pole *(see also* Degeneration, macula) 362.50
    secondary 362.66
    senile 362.60
      cystic 362.53
      reticular 362.64
  saccule, congenital (causing impairment of hearing) 744.05
  sacculocochlear 386.8

Degeneration, degenerative *(Continued)*
  senile 797
    brain 331.2
    cardiac, heart, or myocardium *(see also* Degeneration, myocardial) 429.1
    motor centers 331.2
    reticule 362.64
    retina, cystic 362.50
    vascular - *see* Arteriosclerosis
  silicone rubber poppet (prosthetic valve) 996.02
  sinus (cystic) *(see also* Sinusitis) 473.9
    polypoid 471.1
  skin 709.3
    amyloid 277.39
    colloid 709.3
  spinal (cord) 336.8
    amyloid 277.39
    column 733.90
    combined (subacute) *(see also* Degeneration, combined) 266.2 [336.2]
      with anemia (pernicious) 281.0 [336.2]
    dorsolateral *(see also* Degeneration, combined) 266.2 [336.2]
    familial NEC 336.8
    fatty 336.8
    funicular *(see also* Degeneration, combined) 266.2 [336.2]
    heredofamilial NEC 336.8
    posterolateral *(see also* Degeneration, combined) 266.2 [336.2]
    subacute combined - *see* Degeneration, combined
    tuberculous *(see also* Tuberculosis) 013.8●
  spine 733.90
  spleen 289.59
    amyloid 277.39
    lardaceous 277.39
  stomach 537.89
    lardaceous 277.39
  strionigral 333.0
  sudoriparous (cystic) 705.89
  suprarenal (capsule) (gland) 255.8
    with hypofunction 255.41
  sweat gland 705.89
  synovial membrane (pulpy) 727.9
  tapetoretinal 362.74
    adult or presenile form 362.50
  testis (postinfectional) 608.89
  thymus (gland) 254.8
    fatty 254.8
    lardaceous 277.39
  thyroid (gland) 246.8
  tricuspid (heart) (valve) - *see* Endocarditis, tricuspid
  tuberculous NEC *(see also* Tuberculosis) 011.9●
  turbinate 733.90
  uterus 621.8
    cystic 621.8
  vascular (senile) - *see also* Arteriosclerosis
    hypertensive - *see* Hypertension
  vitreoretinal (primary) 362.73
    secondary 362.66
  vitreous humor (with infiltration) 379.21
  wallerian NEC - *see* Disorder, nerve
  waxy (any site) 277.39
  Wilson's hepatolenticular 275.1
Deglutition
  paralysis 784.99
    hysterical 300.11
  pneumonia 507.0
Degos' disease or syndrome 447.8
Degradation disorder, branched-chain amino-acid 270.3
Dehiscence
  anastomosis - *see* Complications, anastomosis
  cesarean wound 674.1●

◀ New   ◀◀ Revised   ~~deleted~~ Deleted   ● Use Additional Digit(s)   ▨ Omit code

Dehiscence *(Continued)*
 closure of
  cornea 998.32
  fascia, superficial or muscular 998.31
  internal organ 998.31
  mucosa 998.32
  muscle or muscle flap 998.31
  ribs or rib cage 998.31
  skin 998.32
  skull or craniotomy 998.31
  sternum or sternotomy 998.31
  subcutaneous tissue 998.32
  tendon or ligament 998.31
  traumatic laceration (external) (internal)
    998.33
 episiotomy 674.2●
 operation wound 998.32
  deep 998.31
  external 998.32
  internal 998.31
  superficial 998.32
 perineal wound (postpartum) 674.2●
 postoperative 998.32
  abdomen 998.32
   internal 998.31
  internal 998.31
 traumatic injury wound repair 998.33
 uterine wound 674.1●
Dehydration (cachexia) 276.51
 with
  hypernatremia 276.0
  hyponatremia 276.1
 newborn 775.5
Deiters' nucleus syndrome 386.19
Déjérine's disease 356.0
Déjérine-Klumpke paralysis 767.6
Déjérine-Roussy syndrome 338.0
Déjérine-Sottas disease or neuropathy
  (hypertrophic) 356.0
Déjérine-Thomas atrophy or syndrome 333.0
de Lange's syndrome (Amsterdam dwarf,
  intellectual disabilities, and
  brachycephaly) 759.89
Delay, delayed
 adaptation, cones or rods 368.63
 any plane in pelvis
  affecting fetus or newborn 763.1
  complicating delivery 660.1●
 birth or delivery NEC 662.1●
  affecting fetus or newborn 763.9
  second twin, triplet, or multiple mate
    662.3●
 closure - *see also* Fistula
  cranial suture 756.0
  fontanel 756.0
 coagulation NEC 790.92
 conduction (cardiac) (ventricular) 426.9
 delivery NEC 662.1●
  second twin, triplet, etc. 662.3●
   affecting fetus or newborn 763.89
 development
  in childhood 783.40
   physiological 783.40
  intellectual NEC 315.9
  learning NEC 315.2
  reading 315.00
  sexual 259.0
  speech 315.39
   and language due to hearing loss
     315.34
   associated with hyperkinesis 314.1
  spelling 315.09
 gastric emptying 536.8
 menarche 256.39
  due to pituitary hypofunction 253.4
 menstruation (cause unknown) 626.8
 milestone in childhood 783.42
 motility - *see* Hypomotility
 passage of meconium (newborn) 777.1
 primary respiration 768.9
 puberty 259.0

Delay, delayed *(Continued)*
 separation of umbilical cord 779.83
 sexual maturation, female 259.0
 vaccination V64.00
Del Castillo's syndrome (germinal aplasia)
  606.0
Deleage's disease 359.89
Deletion syndrome
 5p 758.31
 22q11.2 758.32
 autosomal NEC 758.39
 constitutional 5q deletion 758.39
Delhi (boil) (button) (sore) 085.1
Delinquency (juvenile) 312.9
 group (*see also* Disturbance, conduct) 312.2●
 neurotic 312.4
Delirium, delirious 780.09
 acute 780.09
  due to conditions classified elsewhere
    293.0
 alcoholic 291.0
  acute 291.0
  chronic 291.1
 alcoholicum 291.0
 chronic (*see also* Psychosis) 293.89
  due to or associated with physical
    condition - *see* Psychosis, organic
 drug-induced 292.81
 due to conditions classified elsewhere
   293.0
 eclamptic (*see also* Eclampsia) 780.39
 exhaustion (*see also* Reaction, stress, acute)
   308.9
 hysterical 300.11
 in
  presenile dementia 290.11
  senile dementia 290.3
 induced by drug 292.81
 manic, maniacal (acute) (*see also* Psychosis,
   affective) 296.0●
  recurrent episode 296.1●
  single episode 296.0●
 puerperal 293.9
 senile 290.3
 subacute (psychotic) 293.1
 thyroid (*see also* Thyrotoxicosis) 242.9●
 traumatic - *see also* Injury, intracranial
  with
   lesion, spinal cord - *see* Injury, spinal,
     by site
   shock, spinal - *see* Injury, spinal,
     by site
 tremens (impending) 291.0
 uremic - *see* Uremia
 withdrawal
  alcoholic (acute) 291.0
   chronic 291.1
  drug 292.0
Delivery

Note: Use the following fifth-digit subclassification with categories 640–649, 651–676:
0 unspecified as to episode of care
1 delivered, with or without mention of antepartum condition
2 delivered, with mention of postpartum complication
3 antepartum condition or complication
4 postpartum condition or complication

 breech (assisted) (buttocks) (complete)
   (frank) (spontaneous) 652.2●
  affecting fetus or newborn 763.0
  extraction NEC 669.6●
 cesarean (for) 669.7●
  abnormal
   cervix 654.6●
   pelvic organs of tissues 654.9●
   pelvis (bony) (major) NEC 653.0●

Delivery *(Continued)*
 cesarean *(Continued)*
  abnormal *(Continued)*
   (planned) occurring after 37 completed
     weeks of gestation but before 39
     completed weeks gestation due
     to (spontaneous) onset of labor
     649.8●
   presentation or position 652.9●
    in multiple gestation 652.6●
   size, fetus 653.5●
   soft parts (of pelvis) 654.9●
   uterus, congenital 654.0●
   vagina 654.7●
   vulva 654.8●
  abruptio placentae 641.2●
  acromion presentation 652.8●
  affecting fetus or newborn 763.4
  anteversion, cervix or uterus 654.4●
  atony, uterus 661.2●
   with hemorrhage 666.1●
  bicornis or bicornuate uterus 654.0●
  breech presentation (buttocks) (complete)
    (frank) 652.2●
  brow presentation 652.4●
  cephalopelvic disproportion (normally
    formed fetus) 653.4●
  chin presentation 652.4●
  cicatrix of cervix 654.6●
  contracted pelvis (general) 653.1●
   inlet 653.2●
   outlet 653.3●
  cord presentation or prolapse 663.0●
  cystocele 654.4●
  deformity (acquired) (congenital)
   pelvic organs or tissues NEC 654.9●
   pelvis (bony) NEC 653.0●
  displacement, uterus NEC 654.4●
  disproportion NEC 653.9●
  distress
   fetal 656.8●
   maternal 669.0●
  eclampsia 642.6●
  face presentation 652.4●
  failed
   forceps 660.7●
   trial of labor NEC 660.6●
   vacuum extraction 660.7●
   ventouse 660.7●
  fetal deformity 653.7●
  fetal-maternal hemorrhage 656.0●
  fetus, fetal
   distress 656.8●
   prematurity 656.8●
  fibroid (tumor) (uterus) 654.1●
  footling 652.8●
   with successful version 652.1●
  hemorrhage (antepartum) (intrapartum)
    NEC 641.9●
  hydrocephalic fetus 653.6●
  incarceration of uterus 654.3●
  incoordinate uterine action 661.4●
  inertia, uterus 661.2●
   primary 661.0●
   secondary 661.1●
  lateroversion, uterus or cervix 654.4●
  mal lie 652.9●
  malposition
   fetus 652.9●
    in multiple gestation 652.6●
   pelvic organs or tissues NEC 654.9●
   uterus NEC or cervix 654.4●
  malpresentation NEC 652.9●
   in multiple gestation 652.6●
  maternal
   diabetes mellitus (conditions
     classifiable to 249 and 250)
     648.0●
   heart disease NEC 648.6●
  meconium in liquor 656.8●
   staining only 792.3

Delivery (*Continued*)
cesarean (*Continued*)
    oblique presentation 652.3●
    oversize fetus 653.5●
    pelvic tumor NEC 654.9●
    placental insufficiency 656.5●
    placenta previa 641.0●
        with hemorrhage 641.1●
    poor dilation, cervix 661.0●
    pre-eclampsia 642.4●
        severe 642.5●
    previous
        cesarean delivery, section 654.2●
        surgery (to)
            cervix 654.6●
            gynecological NEC 654.9●
            rectum 654.8●
            uterus NEC 654.9●
                previous cesarean delivery,
                    section 654.2●
            vagina 654.7●
    prolapse
        arm or hand 652.7●
        uterus 654.4●
    prolonged labor 662.1●
    rectocele 654.4●
    retroversion, uterus or cervix 654.3●
    rigid
        cervix 654.6●
        pelvic floor 654.4●
        perineum 654.8●
        vagina 654.7●
        vulva 654.8●
    sacculation, pregnant uterus 654.4●
    scar(s)
        cervix 654.6●
        cesarean delivery, section 654.2●
        uterus NEC 654.9●
            due to previous cesarean delivery,
                section 654.2●
    Shirodkar suture in situ 654.5●
    shoulder presentation 652.8●
    stenosis or stricture, cervix 654.6●
    transverse presentation or lie 652.3●
    tumor, pelvic organs or tissues NEC
        654.4●
    umbilical cord presentation or prolapse
        663.0●
  completely normal case - *see* category 650
  complicated (by) NEC 669.9●
    abdominal tumor, fetal 653.7●
        causing obstructed labor 660.1●
    abnormal, abnormality of
        cervix 654.6●
            causing obstructed labor 660.2●
        forces of labor 661.9●
        formation of uterus 654.0●
        pelvic organs or tissues 654.9●
            causing obstructed labor 660.2●
        pelvis (bony) (major) NEC 653.0●
            causing obstructed labor 660.1●
        presentation or position NEC 652.9●
            causing obstructed labor 660.0●
        size, fetus 653.5●
            causing obstructed labor 660.1●
        soft parts (of pelvis) 654.9●
            causing obstructed labor 660.2●
        uterine contractions NEC 661.9●
        uterus (formation) 654.0●
            causing obstructed labor 660.2●
        vagina 654.7●
            causing obstructed labor 660.2●
    abnormally formed uterus (any type)
        (congenital) 654.0●
        causing obstructed labor 660.2●
    acromion presentation 652.8●
        causing obstructed labor 660.0●
    adherent placenta 667.0●
        with hemorrhage 666.0●
    adhesions, uterus (to abdominal wall)
        654.4●

Delivery (*Continued*)
complicated NEC (*Continued*)
    advanced maternal age NEC 659.6●
        multigravida 659.6●
        primigravida 659.5●
    air embolism 673.0●
    amnionitis 658.4●
    amniotic fluid embolism 673.1●
    anesthetic death 668.9●
    annular detachment, cervix 665.3●
    antepartum hemorrhage - *see* Delivery,
        complicated, hemorrhage
    anteversion, cervix or uterus 654.4●
        causing obstructed labor 660.2●
    apoplexy 674.0●
        placenta 641.2●
    arrested active phase 661.1●
    asymmetrical pelvis bone 653.0●
        causing obstructed labor 660.1●
    atony, uterus with hemorrhage
        (hypotonic) (inertia) 666.1●
        hypertonic 661.4●
    Bandl's ring 661.4●
    Battledore placenta - *see* Placenta,
        abnormal
    bicornis or bicornuate uterus 654.0●
        causing obstructed labor 660.2●
    birth injury to mother NEC 665.9●
    bleeding (*see also* Delivery, complicated,
        hemorrhage) 641.9●
    breech presentation (assisted) (buttocks)
        (complete) (frank) (spontaneous)
        652.2●
        with successful version 652.1●
    brow presentation 652.4●
    cephalopelvic disproportion (normally
        formed fetus) 653.4●
        causing obstructed labor 660.1●
    cerebral hemorrhage 674.0●
    cervical dystocia 661.2●
    chin presentation 652.4●
        causing obstructed labor 660.0●
    cicatrix
        cervix 654.6●
            causing obstructed labor 660.2●
        vagina 654.7●
            causing obstructed labor 660.2●
    coagulation defect 649.3●
    colporrhexis 665.4●
        with perineal laceration 664.0●
    compound presentation 652.8●
        causing obstructed labor 660.0●
    compression of cord (umbilical) 663.2●
        around neck 663.1●
        cord prolapsed 663.0●
    contraction, contracted pelvis 653.1●
        causing obstructed labor 660.1●
        general 653.1●
            causing obstructed labor 660.1●
        inlet 653.2●
            causing obstructed labor 660.1●
        midpelvic 653.8●
            causing obstructed labor 660.1●
        midplane 653.8●
            causing obstructed labor 660.1●
        outlet 653.3●
            causing obstructed labor 660.1●
    contraction ring 661.4●
    cord (umbilical) 663.9●
        around neck, tightly or with
            compression 663.1●
            without compression 663.3●
        bruising 663.6●
        complication NEC 663.9●
            specified type NEC 663.8●
        compression NEC 663.2●
        entanglement NEC 663.3●
            with compression 663.2●
        forelying 663.0●
        hematoma 663.6●
        marginal attachment 663.8●

Delivery (*Continued*)
complicated NEC (*Continued*)
    cord (*Continued*)
        presentation 663.0●
        prolapse (complete) (occult) (partial)
            663.0●
        short 663.4●
        specified complication NEC 663.8●
        thrombosis (vessels) 663.6●
        vascular lesion 663.6●
        velamentous insertion 663.8●
    Couvelaire uterus 641.2●
    cretin pelvis (dwarf type) (male type)
        653.1●
        causing obstructed labor 660.1●
    crossbirth 652.3●
        with successful version 652.1●
        causing obstructed labor 660.0●
    cyst (Gartner's duct) 654.7●
    cystocele 654.4●
        causing obstructed labor 660.2●
    death of fetus (near term) 656.4●
        early (before 22 completed weeks'
            gestation) 632
    deformity (acquired) (congenital)
        fetus 653.7●
            causing obstructed labor 660.1●
        pelvic organs or tissues NEC 654.9●
            causing obstructed labor 660.2●
        pelvis (bony) NEC 653.0●
            causing obstructed labor 660.1●
    delay, delayed
        delivery in multiple pregnancy 662.3●
            due to locked mates 660.5●
        following rupture of membranes
            (spontaneous) 658.2●
            artificial 658.3●
    depressed fetal heart tones 659.7●
    diastasis recti 665.8●
    dilatation
        bladder 654.4●
            causing obstructed labor 660.2●
        cervix, incomplete, poor or slow
            661.0●
    diseased placenta 656.7●
    displacement uterus NEC 654.4●
        causing obstructed labor 660.2●
    disproportion NEC 653.9●
        causing obstructed labor 660.1●
    disruptio uteri - *see* Delivery, complicated,
        rupture, uterus
    distress
        fetal 656.8●
        maternal 669.0●
    double uterus (congenital) 654.0●
        causing obstructed labor 660.2●
    dropsy amnion 657●
    dysfunction, uterus 661.9●
        hypertonic 661.4●
        hypotonic 661.2●
            primary 661.0●
            secondary 661.1●
        incoordinate 661.4●
    dystocia
        cervical 661.2●
        fetal - *see* Delivery, complicated,
            abnormal, presentation
        maternal - *see* Delivery, complicated,
            prolonged labor
        pelvic - *see* Delivery, complicated,
            contraction pelvis
        positional 652.8●
        shoulder girdle 660.4●
    eclampsia 642.6●
    ectopic kidney 654.4●
        causing obstructed labor 660.2●
    edema, cervix 654.6●
        causing obstructed labor 660.2●
    effusion, amniotic fluid 658.1●
    elderly multigravida 659.6●
    elderly primigravida 659.5●

Delivery *(Continued)*
  complicated NEC *(Continued)*
    embolism (pulmonary) 673.2●
      air 673.0●
      amniotic fluid 673.1●
      blood-clot 673.2●
      cerebral 674.0●
      fat 673.8●
      pyemic 673.3●
      septic 673.3●
    entanglement, umbilical cord 663.3●
      with compression 663.2●
      around neck (with compression) 663.1●
    eversion, cervix or uterus 665.2●
    excessive
      fetal growth 653.5●
        causing obstructed labor 660.1●
      size of fetus 653.5●
        causing obstructed labor 660.1●
    face presentation 652.4●
      causing obstructed labor 660.0●
      to pubes 660.3●
    failure, fetal head to enter pelvic brim 652.5●
      causing obstructed labor 660.0●
    female genital mutilation 660.8●
    fetal
      acid-base balance 656.8●
      death (near term) NEC 656.4●
        early (before 22 completed weeks' gestation) 632
      deformity 653.7●
        causing obstructed labor 660.1●
      distress 656.8●
      heart rate or rhythm 659.7●
      reduction of multiple fetuses reduced to single fetus 651.7●
    fetopelvic disproportion 653.4●
      causing obstructed labor 660.1●
    fever during labor 659.2●
    fibroid (tumor) (uterus) 654.1●
      causing obstructed labor 660.2●
    fibromyomata 654.1●
      causing obstructed labor 660.2●
    forelying umbilical cord 663.0●
    fracture of coccyx 665.6●
    hematoma 664.5●
      broad ligament 665.7●
      ischial spine 665.7●
      pelvic 665.7●
      perineum 664.5●
      soft tissues 665.7●
      subdural 674.0●
      umbilical cord 663.6●
      vagina 665.7●
      vulva or perineum 664.5●
    hemorrhage (uterine) (antepartum) (intrapartum) (pregnancy) 641.9●
      accidental 641.2●
      associated with
        afibrinogenemia 641.3●
        coagulation defect 641.3●
          hyperfibrinolysis 641.3●
          hypofibrinogenemia 641.3●
      cerebral 674.0●
      due to
        low-lying placenta 641.1●
        placenta previa 641.1●
        premature separation of placenta (normally implanted) 641.2●
        retained placenta 666.0●
        trauma 641.8●
        uterine leiomyoma 641.8●
      marginal sinus rupture 641.2●
      placenta NEC 641.9●
      postpartum (atonic) (immediate) (within 24 hours) 666.1●
        with retained or trapped placenta 666.0●
        delayed 666.2●

Delivery *(Continued)*
  complicated NEC *(Continued)*
    hemorrhage *(Continued)*
      postpartum *(Continued)*
        secondary 666.2●
        third stage 666.0●
    hourglass contraction, uterus 661.4●
    hydramnios 657
    hydrocephalic fetus 653.6●
      causing obstructed labor 660.1●
    hydrops fetalis 653.7●
      causing obstructed labor 660.1●
    hypertension - *see* Hypertension, complicating pregnancy
    hypertonic uterine dysfunction 661.4●
    hypotonic uterine dysfunction 661.2●
    impacted shoulders 660.4●
    incarceration, uterus 654.3●
      causing obstructed labor 660.2●
    incomplete dilation (cervix) 661.0●
    incoordinate uterus 661.4●
    indication NEC 659.9●
      specified type NEC 659.8●
    inertia, uterus 661.2●
      hypertonic 661.4●
      hypotonic 661.2●
      primary 661.0●
      secondary 661.1●
    infantile
      genitalia 654.4●
        causing obstructed labor 660.2●
      uterus (os) 654.4●
        causing obstructed labor 660.2●
    injury (to mother) NEC 665.9●
    intrauterine fetal death (near term) NEC 656.4●
      early (before 22 completed weeks' gestation) 632
    inversion, uterus 665.2●
    kidney, ectopic 654.4●
      causing obstructed labor 660.2●
    knot (true), umbilical cord 663.2●
    labor
      onset (spontaneous) after 37 completed weeks of gestation but before 39 completed weeks gestation with delivery by (planned) cesarean section 649.8●
      premature (before 37 completed weeks gestation) 644.2●
    laceration 664.9●
      anus (sphincter) (healed) (old) 654.8●
        with mucosa 664.3●
        not associated with third-degree perineal laceration 664.6●
      bladder (urinary) 665.5●
      bowel 665.5●
      central 664.4●
      cervix (uteri) 665.3●
      fourchette 664.0●
      hymen 664.0●
      labia (majora) (minora) 664.0●
      pelvic
        floor 664.1●
        organ NEC 665.5●
      perineum, perineal 664.4●
        first degree 664.0●
        second degree 664.1●
        third degree 664.2●
        fourth degree 664.3●
        central 664.4●
        extensive NEC 664.4●
        muscles 664.1●
        skin 664.0●
        slight 664.0●
      peritoneum (pelvic) 665.5●
      periurethral tissue 664.8●

Delivery *(Continued)*
  complicated NEC *(Continued)*
    laceration *(Continued)*
      rectovaginal (septum) (without perineal laceration) 665.4●
        with perineum 664.2●
          with anal or rectal mucosa 664.3●
      skin (perineum) 664.0●
      specified site or type NEC 664.8●
      sphincter ani (healed) (old) 654.8●
        with mucosa 664.3●
        not associated with third-degree perineal laceration 664.6●
      urethra 665.5●
      uterus 665.1●
        before labor 665.0●
      vagina, vaginal (deep) (high) (sulcus) (wall) (without perineal laceration) 665.4●
        with perineum 664.0●
          muscles, with perineum 664.1●
      vulva 664.0●
    lateroversion, uterus or cervix 654.4●
      causing obstructed labor 660.2●
    locked mates 660.5●
    low implantation of placenta - *see* Delivery, complicated, placenta, previa
    mal lie 652.9●
    malposition
      fetus NEC 652.9●
        causing obstructed labor 660.0●
      pelvic organs or tissues NEC 654.9●
        causing obstructed labor 660.2●
      placenta 641.1●
        without hemorrhage 641.0●
      uterus NEC or cervix 654.4●
        causing obstructed labor 660.2●
    malpresentation 652.9●
      causing obstructed labor 660.0●
    marginal sinus (bleeding) (rupture) 641.2●
    maternal hypotension syndrome 669.2●
    meconium in liquor 656.8●
    membranes, retained - *see* Delivery, complicated, placenta, retained
    mentum presentation 652.4●
      causing obstructed labor 660.0●
    metrorrhagia (myopathia) - *see* Delivery, complicated, hemorrhage
    metrorrhexis - *see* Delivery, complicated, rupture, uterus
    multiparity (grand) 659.4●
    myelomeningocele, fetus 653.7●
      causing obstructed labor 660.1●
    Nägele's pelvis 653.0●
      causing obstructed labor 660.1●
    nonengagement, fetal head 652.5●
      causing obstructed labor 660.0●
    oblique presentation 652.3●
      causing obstructed labor 660.0●
    obstetric
      shock 669.1●
      trauma NEC 665.9●
    obstructed labor 660.9●
      due to
        abnormality of pelvic organs or tissues (conditions classifiable to 654.0–654.9) 660.2●
        deep transverse arrest 660.3●
        impacted shoulders 660.4●
        locked twins 660.5●
        malposition and malpresentation of fetus (conditions classifiable to 652.0–652.9) 660.0●
        persistent occipitoposterior 660.3●
        shoulder dystocia 660.4●
    occult prolapse of umbilical cord 663.0●
    oversize fetus 653.5●
      causing obstructed labor 660.1●

Delivery (Continued)
  complicated NEC (Continued)
    pathological retraction ring, uterus 661.4●
    pelvic
      arrest (deep) (high) (of fetal head)
        (transverse) 660.3●
      deformity (bone) - see also Deformity,
        pelvis, with disproportion
        soft tissue 654.9●
          causing obstructed labor 660.2●
      tumor NEC 654.9●
        causing obstructed labor 660.2●
    penetration, pregnant uterus by
      instrument 665.1●
    perforation - see Delivery, complicated,
      laceration
    persistent
      hymen 654.8●
        causing obstructed labor 660.2●
      occipitoposterior 660.3●
    placenta, placental
      ablatio 641.2●
      abnormality 656.7●
        with hemorrhage 641.2●
      abruptio 641.2●
      accreta 667.0●
        with hemorrhage 666.0●
      adherent (without hemorrhage) 667.0●
        with hemorrhage 666.0●
      apoplexy 641.2●
      Battledore - see Placenta, abnormal
      detachment (premature) 641.2●
      disease 656.7●
      hemorrhage NEC 641.9●
      increta (without hemorrhage) 667.0●
        with hemorrhage 666.0●
      low (implantation) 641.1●
        without hemorrhage 641.0●
      malformation 656.7●
        with hemorrhage 641.2●
      malposition 641.1●
        without hemorrhage 641.0●
      marginal sinus rupture 641.2●
      percreta 667.0●
        with hemorrhage 666.0●
      premature separation 641.2●
      previa (central) (lateral) (marginal)
        (partial) 641.1●
        without hemorrhage 641.0●
      retained (with hemorrhage) 666.0●
        without hemorrhage 667.0●
      rupture of marginal sinus 641.2●
      separation (premature) 641.2●
      trapped 666.0●
        without hemorrhage 667.0●
      vicious insertion 641.1●
    polyhydramnios 657●
    polyp, cervix 654.6●
      causing obstructed labor 660.2●
    precipitate labor 661.3●
    premature
      labor (before 37 completed weeks'
        gestation) 644.2●
      rupture, membranes 658.1●
        delayed delivery following 658.2●
    presenting umbilical cord 663.0●
    previous
      cesarean delivery, section 654.2●
      surgery
        cervix 654.6●
          causing obstructed labor 660.2●
        gynecological NEC 654.9●
          causing obstructed labor 660.2●
        perineum 654.8●
        rectum 654.8●
        uterus NEC 654.9●
          due to previous cesarean
            delivery, section 654.2●
        vagina 654.7●
          causing obstructed labor 660.2●
        vulva 654.8●

Delivery (Continued)
  complicated NEC (Continued)
    primary uterine inertia 661.0●
    primipara, elderly or old 659.5●
    prolapse
      arm or hand 652.7●
        causing obstructed labor 660.0●
      cord (umbilical) 663.0●
      fetal extremity 652.8●
      foot or leg 652.8●
        causing obstructed labor 660.0●
      umbilical cord (complete) (occult)
        (partial) 663.0●
      uterus 654.4●
        causing obstructed labor 660.2●
    prolonged labor 662.1●
      first stage 662.0●
      second stage 662.2●
      active phase 661.2●
      due to
        cervical dystocia 661.2●
        contraction ring 661.4●
        tetanic uterus 661.4●
        uterine inertia 661.2●
          primary 661.0●
          secondary 661.1●
      latent phase 661.0●
    pyrexia during labor 659.2●
    rachitic pelvis 653.2●
      causing obstructed labor 660.1●
    rectocele 654.4●
      causing obstructed labor 660.2●
    retained membranes or portions of
      placenta 666.2●
      without hemorrhage 667.1●
    retarded (prolonged) birth 662.1●
    retention secundines (with hemorrhage)
      666.2●
      without hemorrhage 667.1●
    retroversion, uterus or cervix 654.3●
      causing obstructed labor 660.2●
    rigid
      cervix 654.6●
        causing obstructed labor 660.2●
      pelvic floor 654.4●
        causing obstructed labor 660.2●
      perineum or vulva 654.8●
        causing obstructed labor 660.2●
      vagina 654.7●
        causing obstructed labor 660.2●
    Robert's pelvis 653.0●
      causing obstructed labor 660.1●
    rupture - see also Delivery, complicated,
      laceration
      bladder (urinary) 665.5●
      cervix 665.3●
      marginal sinus 641.2●
      membranes, premature 658.1●
      pelvic organ NEC 665.5●
      perineum (without mention of other
        laceration) - see Delivery,
        complicated, laceration,
        perineum
      peritoneum (pelvic) 665.5●
      urethra 665.5●
      uterus (during labor) 665.1●
        before labor 665.0●
    sacculation, pregnant uterus 654.4●
    sacral teratomas, fetal 653.7●
      causing obstructed labor 660.1●
    scar(s)
      cervix 654.6●
        causing obstructed labor 660.2●
      cesarean delivery, section 654.2●
        causing obstructed labor 660.2●
      perineum 654.8●
        causing obstructed labor 660.2●
      uterus NEC 654.9●
        causing obstructed labor 660.2●
        due to previous cesarean delivery,
          section 654.2●

Delivery (Continued)
  complicated NEC (Continued)
    scar(s) (Continued)
      vagina 654.7●
        causing obstructed labor 660.2●
      vulva 654.8●
        causing obstructed labor 660.2●
    scoliotic pelvis 653.0●
      causing obstructed labor 660.1●
    secondary uterine inertia 661.1●
    secundines, retained - see Delivery,
      complicated, placenta, retained
    separation
      placenta (premature) 641.2●
      pubic bone 665.6●
      symphysis pubis 665.6●
    septate vagina 654.7●
      causing obstructed labor 660.2●
    shock (birth) (obstetric) (puerperal)
      669.1●
    short cord syndrome 663.4●
    shoulder
      girdle dystocia 660.4●
      presentation 652.8●
        causing obstructed labor 660.0●
    Siamese twins 678.1●
    slow slope active phase 661.2●
    spasm
      cervix 661.4●
      uterus 661.4●
    spondylolisthesis, pelvis 653.3●
      causing obstructed labor 660.1●
    spondylolysis (lumbosacral) 653.3●
      causing obstructed labor 660.1●
    spondylosis 653.0●
      causing obstructed labor 660.1●
    stenosis or stricture
      cervix 654.6●
        causing obstructed labor 660.2●
      vagina 654.7●
        causing obstructed labor 660.2●
    sudden death, unknown cause 669.9●
    tear (pelvic organ) (see also Delivery,
      complicated, laceration) 664.9●
      anal sphincter (healed) (old) 654.8●
        not associated with third-degree
          perineal laceration 664.6●
    teratomas, sacral, fetal 653.7●
      causing obstructed labor 660.1●
    tetanic uterus 661.4●
    tipping pelvis 653.0●
      causing obstructed labor 660.1●
    transverse
      arrest (deep) 660.3●
      presentation or lie 652.3●
        with successful version 652.1●
        causing obstructed labor 660.0●
    trauma (obstetrical) NEC 665.9●
      periurethral 664.8
    tumor
      abdominal, fetal 653.7●
        causing obstructed labor 660.1●
      pelvic organs or tissues NEC 654.9●
        causing obstructed labor 660.2●
    umbilical cord (see also Delivery,
      complicated, cord) 663.9●
      around neck tightly, or with
        compression 663.1●
      entanglement NEC 663.3●
        with compression 663.2●
      prolapse (complete) (occult) (partial)
        663.0●
    unstable lie 652.0●
      causing obstructed labor 660.0●
    uterine
      inertia (see also Delivery, complicated,
        inertia, uterus) 661.2●
      spasm 661.4●
    vasa previa 663.5●
    velamentous insertion of cord 663.8●
    young maternal age 659.8●

◀ New   ◀≡ Revised   ~~deleted~~ Deleted   ● Use Additional Digit(s)   ▨ Omit code

Delivery *(Continued)*
delayed NEC 662.1●
following rupture of membranes
(spontaneous) 658.2●
artificial 658.3●
second twin, triplet, etc. 662.3●
difficult NEC 669.9●
previous, affecting management of
pregnancy or childbirth V23.49
specified type NEC 669.8●
early onset (spontaneous) 644.2●
footling 652.8●
with successful version 652.1●
forceps NEC 669.5●
affecting fetus or newborn 763.2
missed (at or near term) 656.4●
multiple gestation NEC 651.9●
with fetal loss and retention of one or
more fetus(es) 651.6●
following (elective) fetal reduction 651.7●
specified type NEC 651.8●
with fetal loss and retention of one or
more fetus(es) 651.6●
following (elective) fetal reduction
651.7●
nonviable infant 656.4●
normal - *see* category 650
precipitate 661.3●
affecting fetus or newborn 763.6
premature NEC (before 37 completed weeks'
gestation) 644.2●
previous, affecting management of
pregnancy V23.41
quadruplet NEC 651.2●
with fetal loss and retention of one or
more fetus(es) 651.5●
following (elective) fetal reduction
651.7●
quintuplet NEC 651.8●
with fetal loss and retention of one or
more fetus(es) 651.6●
following (elective) fetal reduction
651.7●
sextuplet NEC 651.8●
with fetal loss and retention of one or
more fetus(es) 651.6●
following (elective) fetal reduction
651.7●
specified complication NEC 669.8●
stillbirth (near term) NEC 656.4●
early (before 22 completed weeks'
gestation) 632
term pregnancy (live birth) NEC - *see*
category 650
stillbirth NEC 656.4●
threatened premature 644.2●
triplets NEC 651.1●
with fetal loss and retention of one or
more fetus(es) 651.4●
delayed delivery (one or more mates)
662.3●
following (elective) fetal reduction
651.7●
locked mates 660.5●
twins NEC 651.0●
with fetal loss and retention of one fetus
651.3●
delayed delivery (one or more mates)
662.3●
following (elective) fetal reduction 651.7●
locked mates 660.5●
uncomplicated - *see* category 650
vacuum extractor NEC 669.5●
affecting fetus or newborn 763.3
ventouse NEC 669.5●
affecting fetus or newborn 763.3
Dellen, cornea 371.41
Delusions (paranoid) 297.9
grandiose 297.1
parasitosis 300.29
systematized 297.1

Dementia 294.20
with behavioral disturbance (aggressive)
(combative) (violent) 294.21
alcohol-induced persisting (*see also*
Psychosis, alcoholic) 291.2
Alzheimer's - *see* Alzheimer's, dementia
arteriosclerotic (simple type)
(uncomplicated) 290.40
with
acute confusional state 290.41
delirium 290.41
delusions 290.42
depressed mood 290.43
depressed type 290.43
paranoid type 290.42
Binswanger's 290.12
catatonic (acute) (*see also* Schizophrenia)
295.2●
congenital (*see also* Disability, intellectual)
319
degenerative 290.9
presenile-onset - *see* Dementia, presenile
senile-onset - *see* Dementia, senile
developmental (*see also* Schizophrenia) 295.9●
dialysis 294.8
transient 293.9
drug-induced persisting (*see also* Psychosis,
drug) 292.82
due to or associated with condition(s)
classified elsewhere
Alzheimer's
with behavioral disturbance 331.0
[294.11]
without behavioral disturbance 331.0
[294.10]
cerebral lipidoses
with behavioral disturbance 330.1
[294.11]
without behavioral disturbance 330.1
[294.10]
epilepsy
with behavioral disturbance 345.9●
[294.11]
without behavioral disturbance 345.9●
[294.10]
hepatolenticular degeneration
with behavioral disturbance 275.1
[294.11]
without behavioral disturbance 275.1
[294.10]
HIV
with behavioral disturbance 042
[294.11]
without behavioral disturbance 042
[294.10]
Huntington's chorea
with behavioral disturbance 333.4
[294.11]
without behavioral disturbance 333.4
[294.10]
Jakob-Creutzfeldt disease (CJD)
with behavioral disturbance 046.19
[294.11]
without behavioral disturbance 046.19
[294.10]
variant (vCJD) 046.11
with dementia
with behavioral disturbance
046.11 [294.11]
without behavioral disturbance
046.11 [294.10]
Lewy bodies
with behavioral disturbance 331.82
[294.11]
without behavioral disturbance 331.82
[294.10]
multiple sclerosis
with behavioral disturbance 340
[294.11]
without behavioral disturbance 340
[294.10]

Dementia *(Continued)*
due to or associated with condition(s)
classified elsewhere *(Continued)*
neurosyphilis
with behavioral disturbance 094.9
[294.11]
without behavioral disturbance 094.9
[294.10]
Parkinsonism
with behavioral disturbance 331.82
[294.11]
without behavioral disturbance 331.82
[294.10]
Parkinson's disease
with behavioral disturbance 332.0
[294.11]
without behavioral disturbance 332.0
[294.10]
Pelizaeus-Merzbacher disease
with behavioral disturbance 333.0
[294.11]
without behavioral disturbance 333.0
[294.10]
Pick's disease
with behavioral disturbance 331.11
[294.11]
without behavioral disturbance 331.11
[294.10]
polyarteritis nodosa
with behavioral disturbance 446.0
[294.11]
without behavioral disturbance 446.0
[294.10]
syphilis
with behavioral disturbance 094.1
[294.11]
without behavioral disturbance 094.1
[294.10]
Wilson's disease
with behavioral disturbance 275.1
[294.11]
without behavioral disturbance 275.1
[294.10]
frontal 331.19
with behavioral disturbance 331.19
[294.11]
without behavioral disturbance 331.19
[294.10]
frontotemporal 331.19
with behavioral disturbance 331.19
[294.11]
without behavioral disturbance 331.19
[294.10]
hebephrenic (acute) 295.1●
Heller's (infantile psychosis) (*see also*
Psychosis, childhood) 299.1●
idiopathic 290.9
presenile-onset - *see* Dementia, presenile
senile-onset - *see* Dementia, senile
in
arteriosclerotic brain disease 290.40
senility 290.0
induced by drug 292.82
infantile, infantilia (*see also* Psychosis,
childhood) 299.0●
Lewy body 331.82
with behavioral disturbance 331.82
[294.11]
without behavioral disturbance 331.82
[294.10]
multi-infarct (cerebrovascular) (*see also*
Dementia, arteriosclerotic) 290.40
old age 290.0
paralytica, paralytic 094.1
juvenilis 090.40
syphilitic 094.1
congenital 090.40
tabetic form 094.1
paranoid (*see also* Schizophrenia) 295.3●
paraphrenic (*see also* Schizophrenia) 295.3●
paretic 094.1

Dementia *(Continued)*
  praecox *(see also* Schizophrenia) 295.9●
  presenile 290.10
    with
      acute confusional state 290.11
      delirium 290.11
      delusional features 290.12
      depressive features 290.13
    depressed type 290.13
    paranoid type 290.12
    simple type 290.10
    uncomplicated 290.10
  primary (acute) *(see also* Schizophrenia)
    295.0●
  progressive, syphilitic 094.1
  puerperal - *see* Psychosis, puerperal
  schizophrenic *(see also* Schizophrenia) 295.9●
  senile 290.0
    with
      acute confusional state 290.3
      delirium 290.3
      delusional features 290.20
      depressive features 290.21
    depressed type 290.21
    exhaustion 290.0
    paranoid type 290.20
  simple type (acute) *(see also* Schizophrenia)
    295.0●
  simplex (acute) *(see also* Schizophrenia)
    295.0●
  syphilitic 094.1
  uremic - *see* Uremia
  vascular 290.40
    with
      delirium 290.41
      delusions 290.42
      depressed mood 290.43
Demerol dependence *(see also* Dependence)
  304.0●
Demineralization, ankle *(see also* Osteoporosis)
  733.00
Demodex folliculorum (infestation) 133.8
Demoralization 799.25
de Morgan's spots (senile angiomas) 448.1
Demyelinating
  polyneuritis, chronic inflammatory 357.81
Demyelination, demyelinization
  central nervous system 341.9
    specified NEC 341.8
  corpus callosum (central) 341.8
  global 340
Dengue (fever) 061
  sandfly 061
  vaccination, prophylactic (against) V05.1
  virus hemorrhagic fever 065.4
Dens
  evaginatus 520.2
  in dente 520.2
  invaginatus 520.2
Dense
  breast(s) 793.82
Density
  increased, bone (disseminated) (generalized)
    (spotted) 733.99
  lung (nodular) 518.89
Dental - *see also* condition
  examination only V72.2
Dentia praecox 520.6
Denticles (in pulp) 522.2
Dentigerous cyst 526.0
Dentin
  irregular (in pulp) 522.3
  opalescent 520.5
  secondary (in pulp) 522.3
  sensitive 521.89
Dentinogenesis imperfecta 520.5
Dentinoma (M9271/0) 213.1
  upper jaw (bone) 213.0
Dentition 520.7
  abnormal 520.6
  anomaly 520.6

Dentition *(Continued)*
  delayed 520.6
  difficult 520.7
  disorder of 520.6
  precocious 520.6
  retarded 520.6
Denture sore (mouth) 528.9
Dependence

> Note: Use the following fifth-digit
> subclassification with category 304:
>
> 0   unspecified
> 1   continuous
> 2   episodic
> 3   in remission

  with
    withdrawal symptoms
      alcohol 291.81
      drug 292.0
  14-hydroxy-dihydromorphinone 304.0●
  absinthe 304.6●
  acemorphan 304.0●
  acetanilid(e) 304.6●
  acetophenetidin 304.6●
  acetorphine 304.0●
  acetyldihydrocodeine 304.0●
  acetyldihydrocodeinone 304.0●
  Adalin 304.1●
  Afghanistan black 304.3●
  agrypnal 304.1●
  alcohol, alcoholic (ethyl) (methyl) (wood)
    303.9●
    maternal, with suspected fetal damage
      affecting management of pregnancy
      655.4●
  allobarbitone 304.1●
  allonal 304.1●
  allylisopropylacetylurea 304.1●
  alphaprodine (hydrochloride) 304.0●
  Alurate 304.1●
  Alvodine 304.0●
  amethocaine 304.6●
  amidone 304.0●
  amidopyrine 304.6●
  aminopyrine 304.6●
  amobarbital 304.1●
  amphetamine(s) (type) (drugs classifiable to
    969.72) 304.4●
  amylene hydrate 304.6●
  amylobarbitone 304.1●
  amylocaine 304.6●
  Amytal (sodium) 304.1●
  analgesic (drug) NEC 304.6●
    synthetic with morphine-like effect
      304.0●
  anesthetic (agent) (drug) (gas) (general)
    (local) NEC 304.6●
  Angel dust 304.6●
  anileridine 304.0●
  antipyrine 304.6●
  anxiolytic 304.1●
  aprobarbital 304.1●
  aprobarbitone 304.1●
  atropine 304.6●
  Avertin (bromide) 304.6●
  barbenyl 304.1●
  barbital(s) 304.1●
  barbitone 304.1●
  barbiturate(s) (compounds) (drugs
    classifiable to 967.0) 304.1●
  barbituric acid (and compounds) 304.1●
  benzedrine 304.4●
  benzylmorphine 304.0●
  Beta-chlor 304.1●
  bhang 304.3●
  blue velvet 304.0●
  Brevital 304.1●
  bromal (hydrate) 304.1●
  bromide(s) NEC 304.1●
  bromine compounds NEC 304.1●

Dependence *(Continued)*
  bromisovalum 304.1●
  bromoform 304.1●
  Bromo-seltzer 304.1●
  bromural 304.1●
  butabarbital (sodium) 304.1●
  butabarpal 304.1●
  butallylonal 304.1●
  butethal 304.1●
  buthalitone (sodium) 304.1●
  Butisol 304.1●
  butobarbitone 304.1●
  butyl chloral (hydrate) 304.1●
  caffeine 304.4●
  cannabis (indica) (sativa) (resin) (derivatives)
    (type) 304.3●
  carbamazepine 304.6●
  Carbrital 304.1●
  carbromal 304.1●
  carisoprodol 304.6●
  Catha (edulis) 304.4●
  chloral (betaine) (hydrate) 304.1●
  chloralamide 304.1●
  chloralformamide 304.1●
  chloralose 304.1●
  chlordiazepoxide 304.1●
  Chloretone 304.1●
  chlorobutanol 304.1●
  chlorodyne 304.1●
  chloroform 304.6●
  Cliradon 304.0●
  coca (leaf) and derivatives 304.2●
  cocaine 304.2●
    hydrochloride 304.2●
    salt (any) 304.2●
  codeine 304.0●
  combination of drugs (excluding morphine
    or opioid type drug) NEC 304.8●
    morphine or opioid type drug with any
      other drug 304.7●
  croton-chloral 304.1●
  cyclobarbital 304.1●
  cyclobarbitone 304.1●
  dagga 304.3●
  Delvinal 304.1●
  Demerol 304.0●
  desocodeine 304.0●
  desomorphine 304.0●
  desoxyephedrine 304.4●
  DET 304.5●
  dexamphetamine 304.4●
  dexedrine 304.4●
  dextromethorphan 304.0●
  dextromoramide 304.0●
  dextronorpseudoephedrine 304.4●
  dextrorphan 304.0●
  diacetylmorphine 304.0●
  Dial 304.1●
  diallylbarbituric acid 304.1●
  diamorphine 304.0●
  diazepam 304.1●
  dibucaine 304.6●
  dichloroethane 304.6●
  diethyl barbituric acid 304.1●
  diethylsulfone-diethylmethane 304.1●
  difencloxazine 304.0●
  dihydrocodeine 304.0●
  dihydrocodeinone 304.0●
  dihydrohydroxycodeinone 304.0●
  dihydroisocodeine 304.0●
  dihydromorphine 304.0●
  dihydromorphinone 304.0●
  dihydroxcodeinone 304.0●
  Dilaudid 304.0●
  dimenhydrinate 304.6●
  dimethylmeperidine 304.0●
  dimethyltriptamine 304.5●
  Dionin 304.0●
  diphenoxylate 304.6●
  dipipanone 304.0●
  d-lysergic acid diethylamide 304.5●

◀ New   ◀▥ Revised   ~~deleted~~ Deleted   ● Use Additional Digit(s)   ▨ Omit code

Dependence *(Continued)*
DMT 304.5●
Dolophine 304.0●
DOM 304.2●
doriden 304.1●
dormiral 304.1●
Dormison 304.1●
Dromoran 304.0●
drug NEC 304.9●
    analgesic NEC 304.6●
    combination (excluding morphine or
        opioid type drug) NEC 304.8●
    morphine or opioid type drug with
        any other drug 304.7●
    complicating pregnancy, childbirth, or
        puerperium 648.3●
        affecting fetus or newborn 779.5
    hallucinogenic 304.5●
    hypnotic NEC 304.1●
    narcotic NEC 304.9●
    psychostimulant NEC 304.4●
    sedative 304.1●
    soporific NEC 304.1●
    specified type NEC 304.6●
    suspected damage to fetus affecting
        management of pregnancy 655.5●
    synthetic, with morphine-like effect
        304.0●
    tranquilizing 304.1●
duboisine 304.6●
ectylurea 304.1●
Endocaine 304.6●
Equanil 304.1●
Eskabarb 304.1●
ethchlorvynol 304.1●
ether (ethyl) (liquid) (vapor) (vinyl) 304.6●
ethidene 304.6●
ethinamate 304.1●
ethoheptazine 304.6●
ethyl
    alcohol 303.9●
    bromide 304.6●
    carbamate 304.6●
    chloride 304.6●
    morphine 304.0●
ethylene (gas) 304.6●
    dichloride 304.6●
ethylidene chloride 304.6●
etilfen 304.1●
etorphine 304.0●
etoval 304.1●
eucodal 304.0●
euneryl 304.1●
Evipal 304.1●
Evipan 304.1●
fentanyl 304.0●
ganja 304.3●
gardenal 304.1●
gardenpanyl 304.1●
gelsemine 304.6●
Gelsemium 304.6●
Gemonil 304.1●
glucochloral 304.1●
glue (airplane) (sniffing) 304.6●
glutethimide 304.1●
hallucinogenics 304.5●
hashish 304.3●
headache powder NEC 304.6●
Heavenly Blue 304.5●
hedonal 304.1●
hemp 304.3●
heptabarbital 304.1●
Heptalgin 304.0●
heptobarbitone 304.1●
heroin 304.0●
    salt (any) 304.0●
hexethal (sodium) 304.1●
hexobarbital 304.1●
Hycodan 304.0●
hydrocodone 304.0●
hydromorphinol 304.0●

Dependence *(Continued)*
hydromorphinone 304.0●
hydromorphone 304.0●
hydroxycodeine 304.0●
hypnotic NEC 304.1●
Indian hemp 304.3●
inhalant 304.6●
intranarcon 304.1●
Kemithal 304.1●
ketobemidone 304.0●
khat 304.4●
kif 304.3●
Lactuca (virosa) extract 304.1●
lactucarium 304.1●
laudanum 304.0●
Lebanese red 304.3●
Leritine 304.0●
lettuce opium 304.1●
Levanil 304.1●
Levo-Dromoran 304.0●
levo-iso-methadone 304.0●
levorphanol 304.0●
Librium 304.1●
Lomotil 304.6●
Lotusate 304.1●
LSD (-25) (and derivatives) 304.5●
Luminal 304.1●
lysergic acid 304.5●
    amide 304.5●
maconha 304.3●
magic mushroom 304.5●
marihuana 304.3●
MDA (methylene dioxyamphetamine)
    304.4●
Mebaral 304.1●
Medinal 304.1●
Medomin 304.1●
megahallucinogenics 304.5●
meperidine 304.0●
mephobarbital 304.1●
meprobamate 304.1●
mescaline 304.5●
methadone 304.0●
methamphetamine(s) 304.4●
methaqualone 304.1●
metharbital 304.1●
methitural 304.1●
methobarbitone 304.1●
methohexital 304.1●
methopholine 304.6●
methyl●
    alcohol 303.9●
    bromide 304.6●
    morphine 304.0●
    sulfonal 304.1●
methylated spirit 303.9●
methylbutinol 304.6●
methyldihydromorphinone 304.0●
methylene
    chloride 304.6●
    dichloride 304.6●
    dioxyamphetamine (MDA) 304.4●
methylparafynol 304.1●
methylphenidate 304.4●
methyprylone 304.1●
metopon 304.0●
Miltown 304.1●
morning glory seeds 304.5●
morphinan(s) 304.0●
morphine (sulfate) (sulfite) (type) (drugs
    classifiable to 965.00–965.09) 304.0●
morphine or opioid type drug (drugs
    classifiable to 965.00–965.09) with any
    other drug 304.7●
morphinol(s) 304.0●
morphinon 304.0●
morpholinylethylmorphine 304.0●
mylomide 304.1●
myristicin 304.5●
narcotic (drug) NEC 304.9●
nealbarbital 304.1●

Dependence *(Continued)*
nealbarbitone 304.1●
Nembutal 304.1●
Neonal 304.1●
Neraval 304.1●
Neravan 304.1●
neurobarb 304.1●
nicotine 305.1
Nisentil 304.0●
nitrous oxide 304.6●
Noctec 304.1●
Noludar 304.1●
nonbarbiturate sedatives and tranquilizers
    with similar effect 304.1●
noptil 304.1●
normorphine 304.0●
noscapine 304.0●
Novocaine 304.6●
Numorphan 304.0●
nunol 304.1●
Nupercaine 304.6●
Oblivon 304.1●
on
    aspirator V46.0
    hemodialysis V45.11
    hyperbaric chamber V46.8
    iron lung V46.11
    machine (enabling) V46.9
        specified type NEC V46.8
    peritoneal dialysis V45.11
    Possum (patient-operated-selector-
        mechanism) V46.8
    renal dialysis machine V45.11
    respirator [ventilator] V46.11
        encounter
            during
                power failure V46.12
                mechanical failure V46.14
            for weaning V46.13
    supplemental oxygen V46.2
    wheelchair V46.3
opiate 304.0●
opioids 304.0●
opioid type drug 304.0●
    with any other drug 304.7●
opium (alkaloids) (derivatives) (tincture)
    304.0●
ortal 304.1●
oxazepam 304.1●
oxycodone 304.0●
oxymorphone 304.0●
Palfium 304.0●
Panadol 304.6●
pantopium 304.0●
pantopon 304.0●
papaverine 304.0●
paracetamol 304.6●
paracodin 304.0●
paraldehyde 304.1●
paregoric 304.0●
Parzone 304.0●
PCP (phencyclidine) 304.6●
Pearly Gates 304.5●
pentazocine 304.0●
pentobarbital 304.1●
pentobarbitone (sodium) 304.1●
Pentothal 304.1●
Percaine 304.6●
Percodan 304.0●
Perichlor 304.1●
Pernocton 304.1●
Pernoston 304.1●
peronine 304.0●
pethidine (hydrochloride) 304.0●
petrichloral 304.1●
peyote 304.5●
Phanodorn 304.1●
phenacetin 304.6●
phenadoxone 304.0●
phenaglycodol 304.1●
phenazocine 304.0●

Dependence (Continued)
  phencyclidine 304.6●
  phenmetrazine 304.4●
  phenobal 304.1●
  phenobarbital 304.1●
  phenobarbitone 304.1●
  phenomorphan 304.0●
  phenonyl 304.1●
  phenoperidine 304.0●
  pholcodine 304.0●
  piminodine 304.0●
  Pipadone 304.0●
  Pitkin's solution 304.6●
  Placidyl 304.1●
  polysubstance 304.8●
  Pontocaine 304.6●
  pot 304.3●
  potassium bromide 304.1●
  Preludin 304.4●
  Prinadol 304.0●
  probarbital 304.1●
  procaine 304.6●
  propanal 304.1●
  propoxyphene 304.6●
  psilocibin 304.5●
  psilocin 304.5●
  psilocybin 304.5●
  psilocyline 304.5●
  psilocyn 304.5●
  psychedelic agents 304.5●
  psychostimulant NEC 304.4●
  psychotomimetic agents 304.5●
  pyrahexyl 304.3●
  Pyramidon 304.6●
  quinalbarbitone 304.1●
  racemoramide 304.0●
  racemorphan 304.0●
  Rela 304.6●
  scopolamine 304.6●
  secobarbital 304.1●
  seconal 304.1●
  sedative NEC 304.1●
    nonbarbiturate with barbiturate effect
        304.1●
  Sedormid 304.1●
  sernyl 304.1●
  sodium bromide 304.1●
  Soma 304.6●
  Somnal 304.1●
  Somnos 304.1●
  Soneryl 304.1●
  soporific (drug) NEC 304.1●
  specified drug NEC 304.6●
  speed 304.4●
  spinocaine 304.6●
  stovaine 304.6●
  STP 304.5●
  stramonium 304.6●
  Sulfonal 304.1●
  sulfonethylmethane 304.1●
  sulfonmethane 304.1●
  Surital 304.1●
  synthetic drug with morphine-like effect
        304.0●
  talbutal 304.1●
  tetracaine 304.6●
  tetrahydrocannabinol 304.3●
  tetronal 304.1●
  THC 304.3●
  thebacon 304.0●
  thebaine 304.0●
  thiamil 304.1●
  thiamylal 304.1●
  thiopental 304.1●
  tobacco 305.1
  toluene, toluol 304.6●
  tranquilizer NEC 304.1●
    nonbarbiturate with barbiturate effect
        304.1●
  tribromacetaldehyde 304.6●
  tribromethanol 304.6●

Dependence (Continued)
  tribromomethane 304.6●
  trichloroethanol 304.6●
  trichoroethyl phosphate 304.1●
  triclofos 304.1●
  Trional 304.1●
  Tuinal 304.1●
  Turkish green 304.3●
  urethan(e) 304.6●
  Valium 304.1●
  Valmid 304.1●
  veganin 304.0●
  veramon 304.1●
  Veronal 304.1●
  versidyne 304.6●
  vinbarbital 304.1●
  vinbarbitone 304.1●
  vinyl bitone 304.1●
  vitamin B₆ 266.1
  wine 303.9●
  Zactane 304.6●
Dependency
  passive 301.6
  reactions 301.6
Depersonalization (episode, in neurotic state)
    (neurotic) (syndrome) 300.6
Depletion
  carbohydrates 271.9
  complement factor 279.8
  extracellular fluid 276.52
    plasma 276.52
  potassium 276.8
    nephropathy 588.89
  salt or sodium 276.1
    causing heat exhaustion or prostration
        992.0
    nephropathy 593.9
  volume 276.50
    extracellular fluid 276.52
    plasma 276.52
Deployment (military)
  personal history of V62.22
  returned from V62.22
  status V62.21
Deposit
  argentous, cornea 371.16
  bone, in Boeck's sarcoid 135
  calcareous, calcium - see Calcification
  cholesterol
    retina 362.82
    skin 709.3
    vitreous (humor) 379.22
  conjunctival 372.56
  cornea, corneal NEC 371.10
    argentous 371.16
    in
        cystinosis 270.0 [371.15]
        mucopolysaccharidosis 277.5 [371.15]
  crystalline, vitreous (humor) 379.22
  hemosiderin, in old scars of cornea 371.11
  metallic, in lens 366.45
  skin 709.3
  teeth, tooth (betel) (black) (green) (materia
        alba) (orange) (soft) (tobacco) 523.6
  urate, in kidney (see also Disease, renal) 593.9
Depraved appetite 307.52
Depression 311
  acute (see also Psychosis, affective) 296.2●
    recurrent episode 296.3●
    single episode 296.2●
  agitated (see also Psychosis, affective) 296.2●
    recurrent episode 296.3●
    single episode 296.2●
  anaclitic 309.21
  anxiety 300.4
  arches 734
    congenital 754.61
  autogenous (see also Psychosis, affective)
        296.2●
    recurrent episode 296.3●
    single episode 296.2●

Depression (Continued)
  basal metabolic rate (BMR) 794.7
  bone marrow 289.9
  central nervous system 799.1
    newborn 779.2
  cerebral 331.9
    newborn 779.2
  cerebrovascular 437.8
    newborn 779.2
  chest wall 738.3
  endogenous (see also Psychosis, affective)
        296.2●
    recurrent episode 296.3●
    single episode 296.2●
  functional activity 780.99
  hysterical 300.11
  involutional, climacteric, or menopausal (see
        also Psychosis, affective) 296.2●
    recurrent episode 296.3●
    single episode 296.2●
  major 296.2●
    recurrent episode 296.3●
    single episode 296.2●
  manic (see also Psychosis, affective) 296.80
  medullary 348.89
    newborn 779.2
  mental 300.4
  metatarsal heads - see Depression, arches
  metatarsus - see Depression, arches
  monopolar (see also Psychosis, affective)
        296.2●
    recurrent episode 296.3●
    single episode 296.2●
  nervous 300.4
  neurotic 300.4
  nose 738.0
  postpartum 648.4●
  psychogenic 300.4
    reactive 298.0
  psychoneurotic 300.4
  psychotic (see also Psychosis, affective)
        296.2●
    reactive 298.0
    recurrent episode 296.3●
    single episode 296.2●
  reactive 300.4
    neurotic 300.4
    psychogenic 298.0
    psychoneurotic 300.4
    psychotic 298.0
  recurrent 296.3●
  respiratory center 348.89
    newborn 770.89
  scapula 736.89
  senile 290.21
  situational (acute) (brief) 309.0
    prolonged 309.1
  skull 754.0
  sternum 738.3
  visual field 368.40
Depressive reaction - see also Reaction,
    depressive
  acute (transient) 309.0
    with anxiety 309.28
  prolonged 309.1
  situational (acute) 309.0
    prolonged 309.1
Deprivation
  cultural V62.4
  emotional V62.89
    affecting
        adult 995.82
        infant or child 995.51
  food 994.2
    specific substance NEC 269.8
  protein (familial) (kwashiorkor) 260
  sleep V69.4
  social V62.4
    affecting
        adult 995.82
        infant or child 995.51

◀ New   ◀▦ Revised   ~~deleted~~ Deleted   ● Use Additional Digit(s)   ▦ Omit code

Deprivation (Continued)
symptoms, syndrome
alcohol 291.81
drug 292.0
vitamins (see also Deficiency, vitamin) 269.2
water 994.3
de Quervain's
disease (tendon sheath) 727.04
syndrome 259.51
thyroiditis (subacute granulomatous
thyroiditis) 245.1
Derangement
ankle (internal) 718.97
current injury (see also Dislocation, ankle)
837.0
recurrent 718.37
cartilage (articular) NEC (see also Disorder,
cartilage, articular) 718.0●
knee 717.9
recurrent 718.36
recurrent 718.3●
collateral ligament (knee) (medial) (tibial)
717.82
current injury 844.1
lateral (fibular) 844.0
lateral (fibular) 717.81
current injury 844.0
cruciate ligament (knee) (posterior) 717.84
anterior 717.83
current injury 844.2
current injury 844.2
elbow (internal) 718.92
current injury (see also Dislocation, elbow)
832.00
recurrent 718.32
gastrointestinal 536.9
heart - see Disease, heart
hip (joint) (internal) (old) 718.95
current injury (see also Dislocation, hip)
835.00
recurrent 718.35
intervertebral disc - see Displacement,
intervertebral disc
joint (internal) 718.90
ankle 718.97
current injury - see also Dislocation,
by site
knee, meniscus or cartilage (see also
Tear, meniscus) 836.2
elbow 718.92
foot 718.97
hand 718.94
hip 718.95
knee 717.9
multiple sites 718.99
pelvic region 718.95
recurrent 718.30
ankle 718.37
elbow 718.32
foot 718.37
hand 718.34
hip 718.35
knee 718.36
multiple sites 718.39
pelvic region 718.35
shoulder (region) 718.31
specified site NEC 718.38
temporomandibular (old) 524.69
wrist 718.33
shoulder (region) 718.91
specified site NEC 718.98
spine NEC 724.9
temporomandibular 524.69
wrist 718.93
knee (cartilage) (internal) 717.9
current injury (see also Tear, meniscus)
836.2
ligament 717.89
capsular 717.85
collateral - see Derangement, collateral
ligament

Derangement (Continued)
knee (Continued)
ligament (Continued)
cruciate - see Derangement, cruciate
ligament
specified NEC 717.85
recurrent 718.36
low back NEC 724.9
meniscus NEC (knee) 717.5
current injury (see also Tear, meniscus)
836.2
lateral 717.40
anterior horn 717.42
posterior horn 717.43
specified NEC 717.49
medial 717.3
anterior horn 717.1
posterior horn 717.2
recurrent 718.3●
site other than knee - see Disorder,
cartilage, articular
mental (see also Psychosis) 298.9
rotator cuff (recurrent) (tear) 726.10
current 840.4
sacroiliac (old) 724.6
current - see Dislocation, sacroiliac
semilunar cartilage (knee) 717.5
current injury 836.2
lateral 836.1
medial 836.0
recurrent 718.3●
shoulder (internal) 718.91
current injury (see also Dislocation,
shoulder) 831.00
recurrent 718.31
spine (recurrent) NEC 724.9
current - see Dislocation, spine
temporomandibular (internal) (joint) (old)
524.69
current - see Dislocation, jaw
Dercum's disease or syndrome (adiposis
dolorosa) 272.8
Derealization (neurotic) 300.6
Dermal - see condition
Dermaphytid - see Dermatophytosis
Dermatergosis - see Dermatitis
Dermatitis (allergic) (contact) (occupational)
(venenata) 692.9
ab igne 692.82
acneiform 692.9
actinic (due to sun) 692.70
acute 692.72
chronic NEC 692.74
other than from sun NEC 692.82
ambustionis
due to
burn or scald - see Burn, by site
sunburn (see also Sunburn) 692.71
amebic 006.6
ammonia 691.0
anaphylactoid NEC 692.9
arsenical 692.4
artefacta 698.4
psychogenic 316 [698.4]
asthmatic 691.8
atopic (allergic) (intrinsic) 691.8
psychogenic 316 [691.8]
atrophicans 701.8
diffusa 701.8
maculosa 701.3
autoimmune progesterone 279.49
berlock, berloque 692.72
blastomycetic 116.0
blister beetle 692.89
Brucella NEC 023.9
bullosa 694.9
striata pratensis 692.6
bullous 694.9
mucosynechial, atrophic 694.60
with ocular involvement 694.61
seasonal 694.8

Dermatitis (Continued)
calorica
due to
burn or scald - see Burn, by site
cold 692.89
sunburn (see also Sunburn) 692.71
caterpillar 692.89
cercarial 120.3
combustionis
due to
burn or scald - see Burn, by site
sunburn (see also Sunburn) 692.71
congelationis 991.5
contusiformis 695.2
diabetic 250.8●
diaper 691.0
diphtheritica 032.85
due to
acetone 692.2
acids 692.4
adhesive plaster 692.4
alcohol (skin contact) (substances
classifiable to 980.0–980.9) 692.4
taken internally 693.8
alkalis 692.4
allergy NEC 692.9
ammonia (household) (liquid) 692.4
animal
dander (cat) (dog) 692.84
hair (cat) (dog) 692.84
arnica 692.3
arsenic 692.4
taken internally 693.8
blister beetle 692.89
cantharides 692.3
carbon disulphide 692.2
caterpillar 692.89
caustics 692.4
cereal (ingested) 693.1
contact with skin 692.5
chemical(s) NEC 692.4
internal 693.8
irritant NEC 692.4
taken internally 693.8
chlorocompounds 692.2
coffee (ingested) 693.1
contact with skin 692.5
cold weather 692.89
cosmetics 692.81
cyclohexanes 692.2
dander, animal (cat) (dog) 692.84
deodorant 692.81
detergents 692.0
dichromate 692.4
drugs and medicinals (correct substance
properly administered) (internal
use) 693.0
external (in contact with skin) 692.3
wrong substance given or taken
976.9
specified substance - see Table of
Drugs and Chemicals
wrong substance given or taken 977.9
specified substance - see Table of
Drugs and Chemicals
dyes 692.89
hair 692.89
epidermophytosis - see Dermatophytosis
esters 692.2
external irritant NEC 692.9
specified agent NEC 692.89
eye shadow 692.81
fish (ingested) 693.1
contact with skin 692.5
flour (ingested) 693.1
contact with skin 692.5
food (ingested) 693.1
in contact with skin 692.5
fruit (ingested) 693.1
contact with skin 692.5
fungicides 692.3

Dermatitis (Continued)
  due to (Continued)
    furs 692.84
    glycols 692.2
    greases NEC 692.1
    hair, animal (cat) (dog) 692.84
    hair dyes 692.89
    hot
      objects and materials - see Burn, by site
      weather or places 692.89
    hydrocarbons 692.2
    infrared rays, except from sun 692.82
      solar NEC (see also Dermatitis, due to,
        sun) 692.70
    ingested substance 693.9
      drugs and medicinals (see also
        Dermatitis, due to, drugs and
        medicinals) 693.0
      food 693.1
      specified substance NEC 693.8
    ingestion or injection of
      chemical 693.8
      drug (correct substance properly
        administered) 693.0
        wrong substance given or taken
          977.9
          specified substance - see Table of
            Drugs and Chemicals
    insecticides 692.4
    internal agent 693.9
      drugs and medicinals (see also
        Dermatitis, due to, drugs and
        medicinals) 693.0
      food (ingested) 693.1
        in contact with skin 692.5
      specified agent NEC 693.8
    iodine 692.3
    iodoform 692.3
    irradiation 692.82
    jewelry 692.83
    keratolytics 692.3
    ketones 692.2
    lacquer tree (Rhus verniciflua) 692.6
    light (sun) NEC (see also Dermatitis, due
      to, sun) 692.70
      other 692.82
    low temperature 692.89
    mascara 692.81
    meat (ingested) 693.1
      contact with skin 692.5
    mercury, mercurials 692.3
    metals 692.83
    milk (ingested) 693.1
      contact with skin 692.5
    Neomycin 692.3
    nylon 692.4
    oils NEC 692.1
    paint solvent 692.2
    pediculocides 692.3
    petroleum products (substances
      classifiable to 981) 692.4
    phenol 692.3
    photosensitiveness, photosensitivity (sun)
      692.72
      other light 692.82
    plants NEC 692.6
    plasters, medicated (any) 692.3
    plastic 692.4
    poison
      ivy (Rhus toxicodendron) 692.6
      oak (Rhus diversiloba) 692.6
      plant or vine 692.6
      sumac (Rhus venenata) 692.6
      vine (Rhus radicans) 692.6
    preservatives 692.89
    primrose (primula) 692.6
    primula 692.6
    radiation 692.82
      sun NEC (see also Dermatitis, due to,
        sun) 692.70
      tanning bed 692.82

Dermatitis (Continued)
  due to (Continued)
    radioactive substance 692.82
    radium 692.82
    ragweed (Senecio jacobae) 692.6
    Rhus (diversiloba) (radicans)
      (toxicodendron) (venenata)
      (verniciflua) 692.6
    rubber 692.4
    scabicides 692.3
    Senecio jacobae 692.6
    solar radiation - see Dermatitis, due to,
      sun
    solvents (any) (substances classifiable to
      982.0–982.8) 692.2
      chlorocompound group 692.2
      cyclohexane group 692.2
      ester group 692.2
      glycol group 692.2
      hydrocarbon group 692.2
      ketone group 692.2
      paint 692.2
    specified agent NEC 692.89
    sun 692.70
      acute 692.72
      chronic NEC 692.74
      specified NEC 692.79
    sunburn (see also Sunburn) 692.71
    sunshine NEC (see also Dermatitis, due to,
      sun) 692.70
    tanning bed 692.82
    tetrachlorethylene 692.2
    toluene 692.2
    topical medications 692.3
    turpentine 692.2
    ultraviolet rays, except from sun
      692.82
      sun NEC (see also Dermatitis, due to,
        sun) 692.70
    vaccine or vaccination (correct substance
      properly administered) 693.0
      wrong substance given or taken
        bacterial vaccine 978.8
          specified - see Table of Drugs and
            Chemicals
        other vaccines NEC 979.9
          specified - see Table of Drugs and
            Chemicals
    varicose veins (see also Varicose, vein,
      inflamed or infected) 454.1
    x-rays 692.82
  dyshydrotic 705.81
  dysmenorrheica 625.8
  eczematoid NEC 692.9
    infectious 690.8
  eczematous NEC 692.9
  epidemica 695.89
  erysipelatosa 695.81
  escharotica - see Burn, by site
  exfoliativa, exfoliative 695.89
    generalized 695.89
    infantum 695.81
    neonatorum 695.81
  eyelid 373.31
    allergic 373.32
    contact 373.32
    eczematous 373.31
    herpes (zoster) 053.20
      simplex 054.41
    infective 373.5
      due to
        actinomycosis 039.3 [373.5]
        herpes
          simplex 054.41
          zoster 053.20
        impetigo 684 [373.5]
        leprosy (see also Leprosy) 030.0
          [373.4]
        lupus vulgaris (tuberculous)
          (see also Tuberculosis)
          017.0● [373.4]

Dermatitis (Continued)
  eyelid (Continued)
    infective (Continued)
      due to (Continued)
        mycotic dermatitis (see also
          Dermatomycosis) 111.9 [373.5]
        vaccinia 051.02 [373.5]
          postvaccination 999.0 [373.5]
        yaws (see also Yaws) 102.9 [373.4]
    facta, factitia 698.4
      psychogenic 316 [698.4]
    ficta 698.4
      psychogenic 316 [698.4]
    flexural 691.8
    follicularis 704.8
    friction 709.8
    fungus 111.9
      specified type NEC 111.8
    gangrenosa, gangrenous (infantum) (see also
      Gangrene) 785.4
    gestationis 646.8●
    gonococcal 098.89
    gouty 274.89
    harvest mite 133.8
    heat 692.89
    herpetiformis (bullous) (erythematous)
      (pustular) (vesicular) 694.0
      juvenile 694.2
      senile 694.5
    hiemalis 692.89
    hypostatic, hypostatica 454.1
      with ulcer 454.2
    impetiginous 684
    infantile (acute) (chronic) (intertriginous)
      (intrinsic) (seborrheic) 690.12
    infectiosa eczematoides 690.8
    infectious (staphylococcal) (streptococcal)
      686.9
      eczematoid 690.8
    infective eczematoid 690.8
    Jacquet's (diaper dermatitis) 691.0
    leptus 133.8
    lichenified NEC 692.9
    lichenoid, chronic 701.0
    lichenoides purpurica pigmentosa 709.1
    meadow 692.6
    medicamentosa (correct substance properly
      administered) (internal use) (see also
      Dermatitis, due to, drugs or
      medicinals) 693.0
      due to contact with skin 692.3
    mite 133.8
    multiformis 694.0
      juvenile 694.2
      senile 694.5
    napkin 691.0
    neuro 698.3
    neurotica 694.0
    nummular NEC 692.9
    osteatosis, osteatotic 706.8
    papillaris capillitii 706.1
    pellagrous 265.2
    perioral 695.3
    perstans 696.1
    photosensitivity (sun) 692.72
      other light 692.82
    pigmented purpuric lichenoid 709.1
    polymorpha dolorosa 694.0
    primary irritant 692.9
    pruriginosa 694.0
    pruritic NEC 692.9
    psoriasiform nodularis 696.2
    psychogenic 316
    purulent 686.00
    pustular contagious 051.2
    pyococcal 686.00
    pyocyaneus 686.09
    pyogenica 686.00
    radiation 692.82
    repens 696.1
    Ritter's (exfoliativa) 695.81

◀ New   ◀▥ Revised   ~~deleted~~ Deleted   ● Use Additional Digit(s)   ▦ Omit code

Dermatitis *(Continued)*
Schamberg's (progressive pigmentary dermatosis) 709.09
schistosome 120.3
seasonal bullous 694.8
seborrheic 690.10
infantile 690.12
sensitization NEC 692.9
septic *(see also* Septicemia) 686.00
gonococcal 098.89
solar, solare NEC *(see also* Dermatitis, due to, sun) 692.70
stasis 454.1
due to
postphlebitic syndrome 459.12
with ulcer 459.13
varicose veins - *see* Varicose
ulcerated or with ulcer (varicose) 454.2
sunburn *(see also* Sunburn) 692.71
suppurative 686.00
traumatic NEC 709.8
trophoneurotica 694.0
ultraviolet, except from sun 692.82
due to sun NEC *(see also* Dermatitis, due to, sun) 692.70
varicose 454.1
with ulcer 454.2
vegetans 686.8
verrucosa 117.2
xerotic 706.8
Dermatoarthritis, lipoid 272.8 [713.0]
Dermatochalasia, dermatochalasis 374.87
Dermatofibroma (lenticulare) (M8832/0) - *see also* Neoplasm, skin, benign
protuberans (M8832/1) - *see* Neoplasm, skin, uncertain behavior
Dermatofibrosarcoma (protuberans) (M8832/3) - *see* Neoplasm, skin, malignant
Dermatographia 708.3
Dermatolysis (congenital) (exfoliativa) 757.39
acquired 701.8
eyelids 374.34
palpebrarum 374.34
senile 701.8
Dermatomegaly NEC 701.8
Dermatomucomyositis 710.3
Dermatomycosis 111.9
furfuracea 111.0
specified type NEC 111.8
Dermatomyositis (acute) (chronic) 710.3
Dermatoneuritis of children 985.0
Dermatophiliasis 134.1
Dermatophytide - *see* Dermatophytosis
Dermatophytosis (Epidermophyton) (infection) (microsporum) (tinea) (Trichophyton) 110.9
beard 110.0
body 110.5
deep seated 110.6
fingernails 110.1
foot 110.4
groin 110.3
hand 110.2
nail 110.1
perianal (area) 110.3
scalp 110.0
scrotal 110.8
specified site NEC 110.8
toenails 110.1
vulva 110.8
Dermatopolyneuritis 985.0
Dermatorrhexis 756.83
acquired 701.8
Dermatosclerosis *(see also* Scleroderma) 710.1
localized 701.0
Dermatosis 709.9
Andrews' 686.8
atopic 691.8
Bowen's (M8081/2) - *see* Neoplasm, skin, in situ

Dermatosis *(Continued)*
bullous 694.9
specified type NEC 694.8
erythematosquamous 690.8
exfoliativa 695.89
factitial 698.4
gonococcal 098.89
herpetiformis 694.0
juvenile 694.2
senile 694.5
hysterical 300.11
linear IgA 694.8
menstrual NEC 709.8
neutrophilic, acute febrile 695.89
occupational *(see also* Dermatitis) 692.9
papulosa nigra 709.8
pigmentary NEC 709.00
progressive 709.09
Schamberg's 709.09
Siemens-Bloch 757.33
progressive pigmentary 709.09
psychogenic 316
pustular subcorneal 694.1
Schamberg's (progressive pigmentary) 709.09
senile NEC 709.3
specified NEC 702.8
Unna's (seborrheic dermatitis) 690.10
Dermographia 708.3
Dermographism 708.3
Dermoid (cyst) (M9084/0) - *see also* Neoplasm, by site, benign
with malignant transformation (M9084/3) 183.0
Dermopathy
infiltrative, with thyrotoxicosis 242.0●
nephrogenic fibrosing 701.8
senile NEC 709.3
Dermophytosis - *see* Dermatophytosis
Descemet's membrane - *see* condition
Descemetocele 371.72
Descending - *see* condition
Descensus uteri (complete) (incomplete) (partial) (without vaginal wall prolapse) 618.1
with mention of vaginal wall prolapse - *see* Prolapse, uterovaginal
Desensitization to allergens V07.1
Desert
rheumatism 114.0
sore *(see also* Ulcer, skin) 707.9
Desertion (child) (newborn) 995.52
adult 995.84
Desmoid (extra-abdominal) (tumor) (M8821/1) - *see also* Neoplasm, connective tissue, uncertain behavior
abdominal (M8822/1) - *see* Neoplasm, connective tissue, uncertain behavior
Despondency 300.4
Desquamative dermatitis NEC 695.89
Destruction
articular facet *(see also* Derangement, joint) 718.9●
vertebra 724.9
bone 733.90
syphilitic 095.5
joint *(see also* Derangement, joint) 718.9●
sacroiliac 724.6
kidney 593.89
live fetus to facilitate birth NEC 763.89
ossicles (ear) 385.24
rectal sphincter 569.49
septum (nasal) 478.19
tuberculous NEC *(see also* Tuberculosis) 011.9●
tympanic membrane 384.82
tympanum 385.89
vertebral disc - *see* Degeneration, intervertebral disc
Destructiveness *(see also* Disturbance, conduct) 312.9
adjustment reaction 309.3

Detachment
cartilage - *see also* Sprain, by site
knee - *see* Tear, meniscus
cervix, annular 622.8
complicating delivery 665.3●
choroid (old) (postinfectional) (simple) (spontaneous) 363.70
hemorrhagic 363.72
serous 363.71
knee, medial meniscus (old) 717.3
current injury 836.0
ligament - *see* Sprain, by site
placenta (premature) - *see* Placenta, separation
retina (recent) 361.9
with retinal defect (rhegmatogenous) 361.00
giant tear 361.03
multiple 361.02
partial
with
giant tear 361.03
multiple defects 361.02
retinal dialysis (juvenile) 361.04
single defect 361.01
retinal dialysis (juvenile) 361.04
single 361.01
subtotal 361.05
total 361.05
delimited (old) (partial) 361.06
old
delimited 361.06
partial 361.06
total or subtotal 361.07
pigment epithelium (RPE) (serous) 362.42
exudative 362.42
hemorrhagic 362.43
rhegmatogenous *(see also* Detachment, retina, with retinal defect) 361.00
serous (without retinal defect) 361.2
specified type NEC 361.89
traction (with vitreoretinal organization) 361.81
vitreous humor 379.21
Detergent asthma 507.8
Deterioration
epileptic
with behavioral disturbance 345.9● [294.11]
without behavioral disturbance 345.9● [294.10]
heart, cardiac *(see also* Degeneration, myocardial) 429.1
mental *(see also* Psychosis) 298.9
myocardium, myocardial *(see also* Degeneration, myocardial) 429.1
senile (simple) 797
transplanted organ - *see* Complications, transplant, organ, by site
de Toni-Fanconi syndrome (cystinosis) 270.0
Deuteranomaly 368.52
Deuteranopia (anomalous trichromat) (complete) (incomplete) 368.52
Deutschländer's disease - *see* Fracture, foot
Development
abnormal, bone 756.9
arrested 783.40
bone 733.91
child 783.40
due to malnutrition (protein-calorie) 263.2
fetus or newborn 764.9●
tracheal rings (congenital) 748.3
defective, congenital - *see also* Anomaly
cauda equina 742.59
left ventricle 746.9
with atresia or hypoplasia of aortic orifice or valve with hypoplasia of ascending aorta 746.7
in hypoplastic left heart syndrome 746.7

Development (*Continued*)
delayed (*see also* Delay, development)
783.40
arithmetical skills 315.1
language (skills) 315.31
and speech due to hearing loss 315.34
expressive 315.31
mixed receptive-expressive 315.32
learning skill, specified NEC 315.2
mixed skills 315.5
motor coordination 315.4
reading 315.00
specified
learning skill NEC 315.2
type NEC, except learning 315.8
speech 315.39
and language due to hearing loss 315.34
associated with hyperkinesia 314.1
phonological 315.39
spelling 315.09
written expression 315.2
imperfect, congenital - *see also* Anomaly
heart 746.9
lungs 748.60
improper (fetus or newborn) 764.9●
incomplete (fetus or newborn) 764.9●
affecting management of pregnancy 656.5●
bronchial tree 748.3
organ or site not listed - *see* Hypoplasia
respiratory system 748.9
sexual, precocious NEC 259.1
tardy, mental (*see also* Disability, intellectual) 319
Developmental - *see* condition
Devergie's disease (pityriasis rubra pilaris) 696.4
Deviation
conjugate (eye) 378.87
palsy 378.81
spasm, spastic 378.82
esophagus 530.89
eye, skew 378.87
mandible, opening and closing 524.53
midline (jaw) (teeth) 524.29
specified site NEC - *see* Malposition
occlusal plane 524.76
organ or site, congenital NEC - *see* Malposition, congenital
septum (acquired) (nasal) 470
congenital 754.0
sexual 302.9
bestiality 302.1
coprophilia 302.89
ego-dystonic
homosexuality 302.0
lesbianism 302.0
erotomania 302.89
Clérambault's 297.8
exhibitionism (sexual) 302.4
fetishism 302.81
transvestic 302.3
frotteurism 302.89
homosexuality, ego-dystonic 302.0
pedophilic 302.2
lesbianism, ego-dystonic 302.0
masochism 302.83
narcissism 302.89
necrophilia 302.89
nymphomania 302.89
pederosis 302.2
pedophilia 302.2
sadism 302.84
sadomasochism 302.84
satyriasis 302.89
specified type NEC 302.89
transvestic fetishism 302.3
transvestism 302.3
voyeurism 302.82
zoophilia (erotica) 302.1

Deviation (*Continued*)
teeth, midline 524.29
trachea 519.19
ureter (congenital) 753.4
Devic's disease 341.0
Device
cerebral ventricle (communicating) in situ V45.2
contraceptive - *see* Contraceptive, device
drainage, cerebrospinal fluid V45.2
Devil's
grip 074.1
pinches (purpura simplex) 287.2
Devitalized tooth 522.9
Devonshire colic 984.9
specified type of lead - *see* Table of Drugs and Chemicals
Dextraposition, aorta 747.21
with ventricular septal defect, pulmonary stenosis or atresia, and hypertrophy of right ventricle 745.2
in tetralogy of Fallot 745.2
Dextratransposition, aorta 745.11
Dextrinosis, limit (debrancher enzyme deficiency) 271.0
Dextrocardia (corrected) (false) (isolated) (secondary) (true) 746.87
with
complete transposition of viscera 759.3
situs inversus 759.3
Dextroversion, kidney (left) 753.3
Dhobie itch 110.3
DHTR (delayed hemolytic transfusion reaction) - *see* Complications, transfusion
Diabetes, diabetic (brittle) (congenital) (familial) (mellitus) (severe) (slight) (without complication) 250.0●

> Note: Use the following fifth-digit subclassification with category 250:
>
> 0 type II or unspecified type, not stated as uncontrolled
>
> Fifth-digit 0 is for use for type II patients, even if the patient requires insulin
>
> 1 type I [juvenile type], not stated as uncontrolled
> 2 type II or unspecified type, uncontrolled
> Fifth-digit 2 is for use for type II patients, even if the patient requires insulin
> 3 type I [juvenile type], uncontrolled

with
coma (with ketoacidosis) 250.3●
due to secondary diabetes 249.3●
hyperosmolar (nonketotic) 250.2●
due to secondary diabetes 249.2●
complication NEC 250.9●
due to secondary diabetes 249.9●
specified NEC 250.8●
due to secondary diabetes 249.8●
gangrene 250.7● [785.4]
due to secondary diabetes 249.7● [785.4]
hyperglycemia - *code to* Diabetes, by type, with 5th digit for not stated as uncontrolled
hyperosmolarity 250.2●
due to secondary diabetes 249.2●
ketosis, ketoacidosis 250.1●
due to secondary diabetes 249.1●
loss of protective sensation (LOPS) - *see* Diabetes, neuropathy
osteomyelitis 250.8● [731.8]
due to secondary diabetes 249.8● [731.8]
specified manifestations NEC 250.8●
due to secondary diabetes 249.8●

Diabetes, diabetic (*Continued*)
acetonemia 250.1●
due to secondary diabetes 249.1●
acidosis 250.1●
due to secondary diabetes 249.1●
amyotrophy 250.6● [353.5]
due to secondary diabetes 249.6● [353.5]
angiopathy, peripheral 250.7● [443.81]
due to secondary diabetes 249.7● [443.81]
asymptomatic 790.29
autonomic neuropathy (peripheral) 250.6● [337.1]
due to secondary diabetes 249.6● [337.1]
bone change 250.8● [731.8]
due to secondary diabetes 249.8● [731.8]
borderline 790.29
bronze, bronzed 275.01
cataract 250.5● [366.41]
due to secondary diabetes 249.5● [366.41]
chemical induced - *see* Diabetes, secondary
complicating pregnancy, childbirth, or puerperium 648.0●
coma (with ketoacidosis) 250.3●
due to secondary diabetes 249.3●
hyperglycemic 250.3●
due to secondary diabetes 249.3●
hyperosmolar (nonketotic) 250.2●
due to secondary diabetes 249.2●
hypoglycemic 250.3●
due to secondary diabetes 249.3●
insulin 250.3●
due to secondary diabetes 249.3●
complicating pregnancy, childbirth, or puerperium (maternal) (conditions classifiable to 249 and 250) 648.0●
affecting fetus or newborn 775.0
complication NEC 250.9●
due to secondary diabetes 249.9●
specified NEC 250.8●
due to secondary diabetes 249.8●
dorsal sclerosis 250.6● [340]
due to secondary diabetes 249.6● [340]
drug-induced - *see also* Diabetes, secondary
overdose or wrong substance given or taken - *see* Table of Drugs and Chemicals
due to
cystic fibrosis - *see* Diabetes, secondary
infection - *see* Diabetes, secondary
dwarfism-obesity syndrome 258.1
gangrene 250.7● [785.4]
due to secondary diabetes 249.7● [785.4]
gastroparesis 250.6● [536.3]
due to secondary diabetes 249.6● [536.3]
gestational 648.8●
complicating pregnancy, childbirth, or puerperium 648.8●
glaucoma 250.5● [365.44]
due to secondary diabetes 249.5● [365.44]
glomerulosclerosis (intercapillary) 250.4● [581.81]
due to secondary diabetes 249.4● [581.81]
glycogenosis, secondary 250.8● [259.8]
due to secondary diabetes 249.8● [259.8]
hemochromatosis (*see also* Hemochromatosis) 275.03
hyperosmolar coma 250.2●
due to secondary diabetes 249.2●
hyperosmolarity 250.2●
due to secondary diabetes 249.2●
hypertension-nephrosis syndrome 250.4● [581.81]
due to secondary diabetes 249.4● [581.81]
hypoglycemia 250.8●
due to secondary diabetes 249.8●
hypoglycemic shock 250.8●
due to secondary diabetes 249.8●
inadequately controlled - *code to* Diabetes, by type, with 5th digit for not stated as uncontrolled

◀ New ◀ Revised ~~deleted~~ Deleted ● Use Additional Digit(s) ▨ Omit code

Diabetes, diabetic *(Continued)*
  insipidus 253.5
    nephrogenic 588.1
    pituitary 253.5
    vasopression-resistant 588.1
  intercapillary glomerulosclerosis 250.4● [581.81]
    due to secondary diabetes 249.4● [581.81]
  iritis 250.5● [364.42]
    due to secondary diabetes 249.5● [364.42]
  ketosis, ketoacidosis 250.1●
    due to secondary diabetes 249.1●
  Kimmelstiel (-Wilson) disease or syndrome (intercapillary glomerulosclerosis) 250.4● [581.81]
    due to secondary diabetes 249.4● [581.81]
  Lancereaux's (diabetes mellitus with marked emaciation) 250.8● [261]
    due to secondary diabetes 249.8● [261]
  latent (chemical) - *see* Diabetes, secondary
    complicating pregnancy, childbirth, or puerperium 648.0●
  lipoidosis 250.8● [272.7]
    due to secondary diabetes 249.8● [272.7]
  macular edema 250.5● [362.07]
    due to secondary diabetes 249.5● [362.07]
  maternal
    with manifest disease in the infant 775.1
    affecting fetus or newborn 775.0
  microaneurysms, retinal 250.5● [362.01]
    due to secondary diabetes 249.5● [362.01]
  mononeuropathy 250.6● [355.9]
    due to secondary diabetes 249.6● [355.9]
  neonatal, transient 775.1
  nephropathy 250.4● [583.81]
    due to secondary diabetes 249.4● [583.81]
  nephrosis (syndrome) 250.4● [581.81]
    due to secondary diabetes 249.4● [583.81]
  neuralgia 250.6● [357.2]
    due to secondary diabetes 249.6● [357.2]
  neuritis 250.6● [357.2]
    due to secondary diabetes 249.6● [357.2]
  neurogenic arthropathy 250.6● [713.5]
    due to secondary diabetes 249.6● [713.5]
  neuropathy 250.6● [357.2]
    autonomic (peripheral) 250.6 [337.1]
      due to secondary diabetes 249.6 [337.1]
    due to secondary diabetes 249.6● [357.2]
  nonclinical 790.29
  osteomyelitis 250.8● [731.8]
    due to secondary diabetes 249.8● [731.8]
  out of control - *code to* Diabetes, by type, with 5th digit for uncontrolled
  peripheral autonomic neuropathy 250.6● [337.1]
    due to secondary diabetes 249.6● [337.1]
  phosphate 275.3
  polyneuropathy 250.6● [357.2]
    due to secondary diabetes 249.6● [357.2]
  poorly controlled - *code to* Diabetes, by type, with 5th digit for not stated as uncontrolled
  renal (true) 271.4
  retinal
    edema 250.5● [362.07]
      due to secondary diabetes 249.5● [362.07]
    hemorrhage 250.5● [362.01]
      due to secondary diabetes 249.5● [362.01]
    microaneurysms 250.5● [362.01]
      due to secondary diabetes 249.5● [362.01]
    retinitis 250.5● [362.01]
      due to secondary diabetes 249.5● [362.01]
    retinopathy 250.5● [362.01]
      due to secondary diabetes 249.5● [362.01]
      background 250.5● [362.01]
        due to secondary diabetes 249.5● [362.01]

Diabetes, diabetic *(Continued)*
  retinopathy *(Continued)*
    nonproliferative 250.5● [362.03]
      due to secondary diabetes 249.5● [362.03]
      mild 250.5● [362.04]
        due to secondary diabetes 249.5● [362.04]
      moderate 250.5● [362.05]
        due to secondary diabetes 249.5● [362.05]
      severe 250.5● [362.06]
        due to secondary diabetes 249.5● [362.06]
    proliferative 250.5● [362.02]
      due to secondary diabetes 249.5● [362.02]
  secondary (chemical-induced) (due to chronic condition) (due to infection) (drug-induced) 249.0●
    with
      coma (with ketoacidosis) 249.3●
        hyperosmolar (nonketotic) 249.2●
      complication NEC 249.9●
        specified NEC 249.8●
      gangrene 249.7● [785.4]
      hyperosmolarity 249.2●
      ketosis, ketoacidosis 249.1●
      osteomyelitis 249.8● [731.8]
      specified manifestations NEC 249.8●
    acetonemia 249.1●
    acidosis 249.1●
    amyotrophy 249.6● [353.5]
    angiopathy, peripheral 249.7● [443.81]
    autonomic neuropathy (peripheral) 249.6● [337.1]
    bone change 249.8● [731.8]
    cataract 249.5● [366.41]
    coma (with ketoacidosis) 249.3●
      hyperglycemic 249.3●
      hyperosmolar (nonketotic) 249.2●
      hypoglycemic 249.3●
      insulin 249.3●
    complicating pregnancy, childbirth, or puerperium (maternal) 648.0●
      affecting fetus or newborn 775.0
    complication NEC 249.9●
      specified NEC 249.8●
    dorsal sclerosis 249.6● [340]
    due to overdose or wrong substance given or taken - *see* Table of Drugs and Chemicals
    gangrene 249.7● [785.4]
    gastroparesis 249.6● [536.3]
    glaucoma 249.5● [365.44]
    glomerulosclerosis (intercapillary) 249.4● [581.81]
    glycogenosis, secondary 249.8● [259.8]
    hyperosmolar coma 249.2●
    hyperosmolarity 249.2●
    hypertension-nephrosis syndrome 249.4● [581.81]
    hypoglycemia 249.8●
    hypoglycemic shock 249.8●
    intercapillary glomerulosclerosis 249.4● [581.81]
    iritis 249.5● [364.42]
    ketosis, ketoacidosis 249.1●
    Kimmelstiel (-Wilson) disease or syndrome (intercapillary glomerulosclerosis) 249.4● [581.81]
    Lancereaux's (diabetes mellitus with marked emaciation) 249.8● [261]
    lipoidosis 249.8● [272.7]
    macular edema 249.5● [362.07]
    maternal
      with manifest disease in the infant 775.1
      affecting fetus or newborn 775.0
    microaneurysms, retinal 249.5● [362.01]
    mononeuropathy 249.6● [355.9]

Diabetes, diabetic *(Continued)*
  secondary *(Continued)*
    nephropathy 249.4● [583.81]
    nephrosis (syndrome) 249.4● [581.81]
    neuralgia 249.6● [357.2]
    neuritis 249.6● [357.2]
    neurogenic arthropathy 249.6● [713.5]
    neuropathy 249.6● [357.2]
      autonomic (peripheral) 249.6 [337.1]
    osteomyelitis 249.8● [731.8]
    peripheral autonomic neuropathy 249.6● [337.1]
    polyneuropathy 249.6● [357.2]
    retinal
      edema 249.5● [362.07]
      hemorrhage 249.5● [362.01]
      microaneurysms 249.5● [362.01]
    retinitis 249.5● [362.01]
    retinopathy 249.5● [362.01]
      background 249.5● [362.01]
      nonproliferative 249.5● [362.03]
        mild 249.5● [362.04]
        moderate 249.5● [362.05]
        severe 249.5● [362.06]
      proliferative 249.5● [362.02]
    ulcer (skin) 249.8● [707.9]
      lower extremity 249.8● [707.10]
        ankle 249.8● [707.13]
        calf 249.8● [707.12]
        foot 249.8● [707.15]
        heel 249.8● [707.14]
        knee 249.8● [707.19]
        specified site NEC 249.8● [707.19]
        thigh 249.8● [707.11]
        toes 249.8● [707.15]
      specified site NEC 249.8● [707.8]
    xanthoma 249.8● [272.2]
  steroid induced - *see also* Diabetes, secondary
    overdose or wrong substance given or taken 962.0
  stress 790.29
  subclinical 790.29
  subliminal 790.29
  sugar 250.0●
  ulcer (skin) 250.8● [707.9]
    due to secondary diabetes 249.8● [707.9]
    lower extremity 250.8● [707.10]
      due to secondary diabetes 249.8● [707.10]
      ankle 250.8● [707.13]
        due to secondary diabetes 249.8● [707.13]
      calf 250.8● [707.12]
        due to secondary diabetes 249.8● [707.12]
      foot 250.8● [707.15]
        due to secondary diabetes 249.8● [707.15]
      heel 250.8● [707.14]
        due to secondary diabetes 249.8● [707.14]
      knee 250.8● [707.19]
        due to secondary diabetes 249.8● [707.19]
      specified site NEC 250.8● [707.19]
        due to secondary diabetes 249.8● [707.19]
      thigh 250.8● [707.11]
        due to secondary diabetes 249.8● [707.11]
      toes 250.8● [707.15]
        due to secondary diabetes 249.8● [707.15]
    specified site NEC 250.8● [707.8]
      due to secondary diabetes 249.8● [707.8]
  xanthoma 250.8● [272.2]
    due to secondary diabetes 249.8● [272.2]
Diacyclothrombopathia 287.1
Diagnosis deferred 799.9

Dialysis (intermittent) (treatment)
　anterior retinal (juvenile) (with detachment)
　　361.04
　extracorporeal V56.0
　hemodialysis V56.0
　　status only V45.11
　peritoneal V56.8
　　status only V45.11
　renal V56.0
　　status only V45.11
　specified type NEC V56.8
Diamond-Blackfan anemia or syndrome
　　(congenital hypoplastic anemia) 284.01
Diamond-Gardener syndrome
　　(autoerythrocyte sensitization) 287.2
Diaper rash 691.0
Diaphoresis (excessive) NEC (see also
　　Hyperhidrosis) 780.8
Diaphragm - see condition
Diaphragmalgia 786.52
Diaphragmitis 519.4
Diaphyseal aclasis 756.4
Diaphysitis 733.99
Diarrhea, diarrheal (acute) (autumn) (bilious)
　　(bloody) (catarrhal) (choleraic) (chronic)
　　(gravis) (green) (infantile) (lienteric)
　　(noninfectious) (presumed noninfectious)
　　(putrefactive) (secondary) (sporadic)
　　(summer) (symptomatic) (thermic) 787.91
　achlorhydric 536.0
　allergic 558.3
　amebic (see also Amebiasis) 006.9
　　with abscess - see Abscess, amebic
　　acute 006.0
　　chronic 006.1
　　nondysenteric 006.2
　bacillary - see Dysentery, bacillary
　bacterial NEC 008.5
　balantidial 007.0
　bile salt-induced 579.8
　cachectic NEC 787.91
　chilomastix 007.8
　choleriformis 001.1
　coccidial 007.2
　Cochin-China 579.1
　　anguilluliasis 127.2
　　psilosis 579.1
　Dientamoeba 007.8
　dietetic 787.91
　due to
　　achylia gastrica 536.8
　　Aerobacter aerogenes 008.2
　　Bacillus coli - see Enteritis, E. coli
　　bacteria NEC 008.5
　　bile salts 579.8
　　Capillaria
　　　hepatica 128.8
　　　philippinensis 127.5
　　Clostridium perfringens (C) (F) 008.46
　　Enterobacter aerogenes 008.2
　　enterococci 008.49
　　Escherichia coli - see Enteritis, E. coli
　　Giardia lamblia 007.1
　　Heterophyes heterophyes 121.6
　　irritating foods 787.91
　　Metagonimus yokogawai 121.5
　　Necator americanus 126.1
　　Paracolobactrum arizonae 008.1
　　Paracolon bacillus NEC 008.47
　　　Arizona 008.1
　　Proteus (bacillus) (mirabilis) (Morganii)
　　　008.3
　　Pseudomonas aeruginosa 008.42
　　S. japonicum 120.2
　　specified organism NEC 008.8
　　　bacterial 008.49
　　　viral NEC 008.69
　　Staphylococcus 008.41
　　Streptococcus 008.49
　　　anaerobic 008.46
　　Strongyloides stercoralis 127.2

Diarrhea, diarrheal (Continued)
　due to (Continued)
　　Trichuris trichiuria 127.3
　　virus NEC (see also Enteritis, viral)
　　　008.69
　dysenteric 009.2
　　due to specified organism NEC 008.8
　dyspeptic 787.91
　endemic 009.3
　　due to specified organism NEC 008.8
　epidemic 009.2
　　due to specified organism NEC 008.8
　fermentative 787.91
　flagellate 007.9
　Flexner's (ulcerative) 004.1
　functional 564.5
　　following gastrointestinal surgery 564.4
　　psychogenic 306.4
　giardial 007.1
　Giardia lamblia 007.1
　hill 579.1
　hyperperistalsis (nervous) 306.4
　infectious 009.2
　　due to specified organism NEC 008.8
　　presumed 009.3
　inflammatory 787.91
　　due to specified organism NEC 008.8
　malarial (see also Malaria) 084.6
　mite 133.8
　mycotic 117.9
　nervous 306.4
　neurogenic 564.5
　parenteral NEC 009.2
　postgastrectomy 564.4
　postvagotomy 564.4
　prostaglandin induced 579.8
　protozoal NEC 007.9
　psychogenic 306.4
　septic 009.2
　　due to specified organism NEC 008.8
　specified organism NEC 008.8
　　bacterial 008.49
　　viral NEC 008.69
　Staphylococcus 008.41
　Streptococcus 008.49
　　anaerobic 008.46
　toxic 558.2
　travelers' 009.2
　　due to specified organism NEC 008.8
　trichomonal 007.3
　tropical 579.1
　tuberculous 014.8●
　ulcerative (chronic) (see also Colitis,
　　ulcerative) 556.9
　viral (see also Enteritis, viral) 008.8
　zymotic NEC 009.2
Diastasis
　cranial bones 733.99
　　congenital 756.0
　joint (traumatic) - see Dislocation, by site
　muscle 728.84
　　congenital 756.89
　recti (abdomen) 728.84
　　complicating delivery 665.8●
　　congenital 756.79
Diastema, teeth, tooth 524.30
Diastematomyelia 742.51
Diataxia, cerebral, infantile 343.0
Diathesis
　allergic V15.09
　bleeding (familial) 287.9
　cystine (familial) 270.0
　gouty 274.9
　hemorrhagic (familial) 287.9
　　newborn NEC 776.0
　oxalic 271.8
　scrofulous (see also Tuberculosis) 017.2●
　spasmophilic (see also Tetany) 781.7
　ulcer 536.9
　uric acid 274.9
Diaz's disease or osteochondrosis 732.5

Dibothriocephaliasis 123.4
　larval 123.5
Dibothriocephalus (infection) (infestation)
　　(latus) 123.4
　larval 123.5
Dicephalus 759.4
Dichotomy, teeth 520.2
Dichromat, dichromata (congenital) 368.59
Dichromatopsia (congenital) 368.59
Dichuchwa 104.0
Dicroceliasis 121.8
Didelphys, didelphic (see also Double uterus)
　　752.2
Didymitis (see also Epididymitis) 604.90
Died - see also Death
　without
　　medical attention (cause unknown) 798.9
　　sign of disease 798.2
Dientamoeba diarrhea 007.8
Dietary
　inadequacy or deficiency 269.9
　surveillance and counseling V65.3
Dietl's crisis 593.4
Dieulafoy lesion (hemorrhagic)
　of
　　duodenum 537.84
　　esophagus 530.82
　　intestine 569.86
　　stomach 537.84
Difficult
　birth, affecting fetus or newborn 763.9
　delivery NEC 669.9●
Difficulty
　feeding 783.3
　　adult 783.3
　　breast 676.8●
　　child 783.3
　　elderly 783.3
　　infant 783.3
　　newborn 779.31
　　nonorganic (infant) NEC 307.59
　mechanical, gastroduodenal stoma 537.89
　reading 315.00
　　specific, spelling 315.09
　swallowing (see also Dysphagia) 787.20
　walking 719.7
Diffuse - see condition
Diffused ganglion 727.42
Di George's syndrome (thymic hypoplasia)
　　279.11
Digestive - see condition
Di Guglielmo's disease or syndrome
　　(M9841/3) 207.0●
Dihydropyrimidine dehydrogenase disease
　　(DPD) 277.6
Diktyoma (M9051/3) - see Neoplasm, by site,
　　malignant
Dilaceration, tooth 520.4
Dilatation
　anus 564.89
　　venule - see Hemorrhoids
　aorta (focal) (general) (see also Ectasia, aortic)
　　447.70
　　with aneurysm 441.9
　　congenital 747.29
　　infectional 093.0
　　ruptured 441.5
　　syphilitic 093.0
　appendix (cystic) 543.9
　artery 447.8
　bile duct (common) (congenital) 751.69
　　acquired 576.8
　bladder (sphincter) 596.89
　　congenital 753.8
　　in pregnancy or childbirth 654.4●
　　　causing obstructed labor 660.2●
　　　　affecting fetus or newborn 763.1
　blood vessel 459.89
　bronchus, bronchi 494.0
　　with acute exacerbation 494.1
　calyx (due to obstruction) 593.89

◀ New　◀▏▏ Revised　deleted Deleted　● Use Additional Digit(s)　░ Omit code

Dilatation (*Continued*)
  capillaries 448.9
  cardiac (acute) (chronic) (*see also*
      Hypertrophy, cardiac) 429.3
    congenital 746.89
      valve NEC 746.89
        pulmonary 746.09
    hypertensive (*see also* Hypertension,
        heart) 402.90
  cavum septi pellucidi 742.4
  cecum 564.89
    psychogenic 306.4
  cervix (uteri) - *see also* Incompetency, cervix
    incomplete, poor, slow
      affecting fetus or newborn 763.7
      complicating delivery 661.0●
        affecting fetus or newborn 763.7
  colon 564.7
    congenital 751.3
    due to mechanical obstruction 560.89
    psychogenic 306.4
  common bile duct (congenital) 751.69
    acquired 576.8
      with calculus, choledocholithiasis, or
          stones - *see* Choledocholithiasis
  cystic duct 751.69
    acquired (any bile duct) 575.8
  duct, mammary 610.4
  duodenum 564.89
  esophagus 530.89
    congenital 750.4
    due to
      achalasia 530.0
      cardiospasm 530.0
  Eustachian tube, congenital 744.24
  fontanel 756.0
  gallbladder 575.8
    congenital 751.69
  gastric 536.8
    acute 536.1
    psychogenic 306.4
  heart (acute) (chronic) (*see also* Hypertrophy,
      cardiac) 429.3
    congenital 746.89
    hypertensive (*see also* Hypertension,
        heart) 402.90
    valve - *see also* Endocarditis
      congenital 746.89
  ileum 564.89
    psychogenic 306.4
  inguinal rings - *see* Hernia, inguinal
  jejunum 564.89
    psychogenic 306.4
  kidney (calyx) (collecting structures) (cystic)
      (parenchyma) (pelvis) 593.89
  lacrimal passages 375.69
  lymphatic vessel 457.1
  mammary duct 610.4
  Meckel's diverticulum (congenital) 751.0
  meningeal vessels, congenital 742.8
  myocardium (acute) (chronic) (*see also*
      Hypertrophy, cardiac) 429.3
  organ or site, congenital NEC - *see* Distortion
  pancreatic duct 577.8
  pelvis, kidney 593.89
  pericardium - *see* Pericarditis
  pharynx 478.29
  prostate 602.8
  pulmonary
    artery (idiopathic) 417.8
      congenital 747.39
    valve, congenital 746.09
  pupil 379.43
  rectum 564.89
  renal 593.89
  saccule vestibularis, congenital 744.05
  salivary gland (duct) 527.8
  sphincter ani 564.89
  stomach 536.8
    acute 536.1
    psychogenic 306.4

Dilatation (*Continued*)
  submaxillary duct 527.8
  trachea, congenital 748.3
  ureter (idiopathic) 593.89
    congenital 753.20
    due to obstruction 593.5
  urethra (acquired) 599.84
  vasomotor 443.9
  vein 459.89
  ventricular, ventricle (acute) (chronic)
      (*see also* Hypertrophy, cardiac)
      429.3
    cerebral, congenital 742.4
    hypertensive (*see also* Hypertension,
        heart) 402.90
  venule 459.89
    anus - *see* Hemorrhoids
  vesical orifice 596.89
Dilated, dilation - *see* Dilatation
Diminished
  hearing (acuity) (*see also* Deafness)
      389.9
  pulse pressure 785.9
  vision NEC 369.9
  vital capacity 794.2
Diminuta taenia 123.6
Diminution, sense or sensation (cold) (heat)
    (tactile) (vibratory) (*see also* Disturbance,
    sensation) 782.0
Dimitri-Sturge-Weber disease
    (encephalocutaneous angiomatosis)
    759.6
Dimple
  parasacral 685.1
    with abscess 685.0
  pilonidal 685.1
    with abscess 685.0
  postanal 685.1
    with abscess 685.0
Dioctophyma renale (infection) (infestation)
    128.8
Dipetalonemiasis 125.4
Diphallus 752.69
Diphtheria, diphtheritic (gangrenous)
    (hemorrhagic) 032.9
  carrier (suspected) of V02.4
  cutaneous 032.85
  cystitis 032.84
  faucial 032.0
  infection of wound 032.85
  inoculation (anti) (not sick) V03.5
  laryngeal 032.3
  myocarditis 032.82
  nasal anterior 032.2
  nasopharyngeal 032.1
  neurological complication 032.89
  peritonitis 032.83
  specified site NEC 032.89
Diphyllobothriasis (intestine) 123.4
  larval 123.5
Diplacusis 388.41
Diplegia (upper limbs) 344.2
  brain or cerebral 437.8
  congenital 343.0
  facial 351.0
    congenital 352.6
  infantile or congenital (cerebral) (spastic)
      (spinal) 343.0
  lower limbs 344.1
  syphilitic, congenital 090.49
Diplococcus, diplococcal - *see* condition
Diplomyelia 742.59
Diplopia 368.2
  refractive 368.15
Dipsomania (*see also* Alcoholism) 303.9●
  with psychosis (*see also* Psychosis, alcoholic)
      291.9
Dipylidiasis 123.8
  intestine 123.8
Direction, teeth, abnormal 524.30
Dirt-eating child 307.52

Disability, disabilities
  heart - *see* Disease, heart
  intellectual 319
    borderline V62.89
    mild, IQ 50-70 317
    moderate, IQ 35-49 318.0
    profound, IQ under 20 318.2
    severe, IQ 20-34 318.1
  learning NEC 315.2
  special spelling 315.09
Disarticulation (*see also* Derangement, joint)
    718.9●
  meaning
    amputation
      status - *see* Absence, by site
      traumatic - *see* Amputation, traumatic
    dislocation, traumatic or congenital - *see*
        Dislocation
Disaster, cerebrovascular (*see also* Disease,
    cerebrovascular, acute) 436
Discharge
  anal NEC 787.99
  breast (female) (male) 611.79
  conjunctiva 372.89
  continued locomotor idiopathic (*see also*
      Epilepsy) 345.5●
  diencephalic autonomic idiopathic (*see also*
      Epilepsy) 345.5●
  ear 388.60
    blood 388.69
    cerebrospinal fluid 388.61
  excessive urine 788.42
  eye 379.93
  nasal 478.19
  nipple 611.79
  patterned motor idiopathic (*see also* Epilepsy)
      345.5●
  penile 788.7
  postnasal - *see* Sinusitis
  sinus, from mediastinum 510.0
  umbilicus 789.9
  urethral 788.7
    bloody 599.84
  vaginal 623.5
Discitis 722.90
  cervical, cervicothoracic 722.91
  lumbar, lumbosacral 722.93
  thoracic, thoracolumbar 722.92
Discogenic syndrome - *see* Displacement,
    intervertebral disc
Discoid
  kidney 753.3
  meniscus, congenital 717.5
  semilunar cartilage 717.5
Discoloration
  mouth 528.9
  nails 703.8
  teeth 521.7
    due to
      drugs 521.7
      metals (copper) (silver) 521.7
      pulpal bleeding 521.7
    during formation 520.8
      extrinsic 523.6
      intrinsic posteruptive 521.7
Discomfort
  chest 786.59
  visual 368.13
Discomycosis - *see* Actinomycosis
Discontinuity, ossicles, ossicular chain
    385.23
Discrepancy
  centric occlusion
    maximum intercuspation 524.55
    of teeth 524.55
  leg length (acquired) 736.81
    congenital 755.30
  uterine size-date 649.6●
Discrimination
  political V62.4
  racial V62.4

Discrimination *(Continued)*
 religious V62.4
 sex V62.4
Disease, diseased - *see also* Syndrome
 Abrami's (acquired hemolytic jaundice)
  283.9
 absorbent system 459.89
 accumulation - *see* Thesaurismosis
 acid-peptic 536.8
 Acosta's 993.2
 Adams-Stokes (-Morgagni) (syncope with
  heart block) 426.9
 Addison's (bronze) (primary adrenal
  insufficiency) 255.41
  anemia (pernicious) 281.0
  tuberculous (*see also* Tuberculosis) 017.6●
 Addison-Gull - *see* Xanthoma
 adenoids (and tonsils) (chronic) 474.9
 adrenal (gland) (capsule) (cortex) 255.9
  hyperfunction 255.3
  hypofunction 255.41
  specified type NEC 255.8
 ainhum (dactylolysis spontanea) 136.0
 akamushi (scrub typhus) 081.2
 Akureyri (epidemic neuromyasthenia) 049.8
 Albarrán's (colibacilluria) 791.9
 Albers-Schönberg's (marble bones) 756.52
 Albert's 726.71
 Albright (-Martin) (-Bantam) 275.49
 Alibert's (mycosis fungoides) (M9700/3)
  202.1●
 Alibert-Bazin (M9700/3) 202.1●
 alimentary canal 569.9
 alligator skin (ichthyosis congenita) 757.1
  acquired 701.1
 Almeida's (Brazilian blastomycosis) 116.1
 Alpers' 330.8
 alpine 993.2
 altitude 993.2
 alveoli, teeth 525.9
 Alzheimer's - *see* Alzheimer's
 amyloid (any site) 277.30
 anarthritic rheumatoid 446.5
 Anders' (adiposis tuberosa simplex) 272.8
 Andersen's (glycogenosis IV) 271.0
 Anderson's (angiokeratoma corporis
  diffusum) 272.7
 Andes 993.2
 Andrews' (bacterid) 686.8
 angiopastic, angiospasmodic 443.9
  cerebral 435.9
   with transient neurologic deficit
    435.9
  vein 459.89
 anterior
  chamber 364.9
  horn cell 335.9
   specified type NEC 335.8
 antral (chronic) 473.0
  acute 461.0
 anus NEC 569.49
 aorta (nonsyphilitic) 447.9
  syphilitic NEC 093.89
 aortic (heart) (valve) (*see also* Endocarditis,
  aortic) 424.1
 apollo 077.4
 aponeurosis 726.90
 appendix 543.9
 aqueous (chamber) 364.9
 arc-welders' lung 503
 Armenian 277.31
 Arnold-Chiari (*see also* Spina bifida) 741.0●
 arterial 447.9
  occlusive (*see also* Occlusion, by site)
   444.22
   with embolus or thrombus - *see*
    Occlusion, by site
   due to stricture or stenosis 447.1
  specified type NEC 447.8
 arteriocardiorenal (*see also* Hypertension,
  cardiorenal) 404.90

Disease, diseased *(Continued)*
 arteriolar (generalized) (obliterative) 447.90
  specified type NEC 447.8
 arteriorenal - *see* Hypertension, kidney
 arteriosclerotic - *see also* Arteriosclerosis
  cardiovascular 429.2
  coronary - *see* Arteriosclerosis, coronary
  heart - *see* Arteriosclerosis, coronary
  vascular - *see* Arteriosclerosis
 artery 447.9
  cerebral 437.9
  coronary - *see* Arteriosclerosis, coronary
  specified type NEC 447.8
 arthropod-borne NEC 088.9
  specified type NEC 088.89
 Asboe-Hansen's (incontinentia pigmenti)
  757.33
 atticoantral, chronic (with posterior or
  superior marginal perforation of ear
  drum) 382.2
 auditory canal, ear 380.9
 Aujeszky's 078.89
 auricle, ear NEC 380.30
 Australian X 062.4
 autoimmune NEC 279.49
  hemolytic (cold type) (warm type) 283.0
  parathyroid 252.1
  thyroid 245.2
 aviators' (*see also* Effect, adverse, high
  altitude) 993.2
 ax(e)-grinders' 502
 Ayala's 756.89
 Ayerza's (pulmonary artery sclerosis with
  pulmonary hypertension) 416.0
 Azorean (of the nervous system) 334.8
 Babington's (familial hemorrhagic
  telangiectasia) 448.0
 back bone NEC 733.90
 bacterial NEC 040.89
  zoonotic NEC 027.9
   specified type NEC 027.8
 Baehr-Schiffrin (thrombotic
  thrombocytopenic purpura) 446.6
 Baelz's (cheilitis glandularis apostematosa)
  528.5
 Baerensprung's (eczema marginatum) 110.3
 Balfour's (chloroma) 205.3●
 balloon (*see also* Effect, adverse, high
  altitude) 993.2
 Baló's 341.1
 Bamberger (-Marie) (hypertrophic
  pulmonary osteoarthropathy) 731.2
 Bang's (Brucella abortus) 023.1
 Bannister's 995.1
 Banti's (with cirrhosis) (with portal
  hypertension) - *see* Cirrhosis, liver
 Barcoo (*see also* Ulcer, skin) 707.9
 barium lung 503
 Barlow (-Möller) (infantile scurvy) 267
 barometer makers' 985.0
 Barraquer (-Simons) (progressive
  lipodystrophy) 272.6
 basal ganglia 333.90
  degenerative NEC 333.0
  specified NEC 333.89
 Basedow's (exophthalmic goiter) 242.0●
 basement membrane NEC 583.89
  with
   pulmonary hemorrhage
    (Goodpasture's syndrome)
    446.21 *[583.81]*
 Bateman's 078.0
  purpura (senile) 287.2
 Batten's 330.1 *[362.71]*
 Batten-Mayou (retina) 330.1 *[362.71]*
 Batten-Steinert 359.21
 Battey 031.0
 Baumgarten-Cruveilhier (cirrhosis of liver)
  571.5
 bauxite-workers' 503
 Bayle's (dementia paralytica) 094.1

Disease, diseased *(Continued)*
 Bazin's (primary) (*see also* Tuberculosis)
  017.1●
 Beard's (neurasthenia) 300.5
 Beau's (*see also* Degeneration, myocardial)
  429.1
 Bechterew's (ankylosing spondylitis) 720.0
 Becker's
  idiopathic mural endomyocardial disease
   425.2
  myotonia congenita, recessive form 359.22
 Begbie's (exophthalmic goiter) 242.0●
 Behr's 362.50
 Beigel's (white piedra) 111.2
 Bekhterev's (ankylosing spondylitis) 720.0
 Bell's (*see also* Psychosis, affective) 296.0●
 Bennett's (leukemia) 208.9●
 Benson's 379.22
 Bergeron's (hysteroepilepsy) 300.11
 Berlin's 921.3
 Bernard-Soulier (thrombopathy) 287.1
 Bernhardt (-Roth) 355.1
 beryllium 503
 Besnier-Boeck (-Schaumann) (sarcoidosis)
  135
 Best's 362.76
 Beurmann's (sporotrichosis) 117.1
 Bielschowsky (-Jansky) 330.1
 Biermer's (pernicious anemia) 281.0
 Biett's (discoid lupus erythematosus) 695.4
 bile duct (*see also* Disease, biliary) 576.9
 biliary (duct) (tract) 576.9
  with calculus, choledocholithiasis, or
   stones - *see* Choledocholithiasis
 Billroth's (meningocele) (*see also* Spina bifida)
  741.9●
 Binswanger's 290.12
 Bird's (oxaluria) 271.8
 bird fanciers' 495.2
 black lung 500
 bladder 596.9
  specified NEC 596.89
 bleeder's 286.0
 Bloch-Sulzberger (incontinentia pigmenti)
  757.33
 Blocq's (astasia-abasia) 307.9
 blood (-forming organs) 289.9
  specified NEC 289.89
  vessel 459.9
 Bloodgood's 610.1
 Blount's (tibia vara) 732.4
 blue 746.9
 Bodechtel-Guttmann (subacute sclerosing
  panencephalitis) 046.2
 Boeck's (sarcoidosis) 135
 bone 733.90
  fibrocystic NEC 733.29
   jaw 526.2
  marrow 289.9
  Paget's (osteitis deformans) 731.0
  specified type NEC 733.99
  von Recklinghausen's (osteitis fibrosa
   cystica) 252.01
 Bonfils' - *see* Disease, Hodgkin's
 Borna 062.9
 Bornholm (epidemic pleurodynia) 074.1
 Bostock's (*see also* Fever, hay) 477.9
 Bouchard's (myopathic dilatation of the
  stomach) 536.1
 Bouillaud's (rheumatic heart disease) 391.9
 Bourneville (-Brissaud) (tuberous sclerosis)
  759.5
 Bouveret (-Hoffmann) (paroxysmal
  tachycardia) 427.2
 bowel 569.9
  functional 564.9
   psychogenic 306.4
 Bowen's (M8081/2) - *see* Neoplasm, skin, in
  situ
 Bozzolo's (multiple myeloma) (M9730/3)
  203.0●

Disease, diseased *(Continued)*
  Bradley's (epidemic vomiting) 078.82
  Brailsford's 732.3
    radius, head 732.3
    tarsal, scaphoid 732.5
  Brailsford-Morquio (mucopolysaccharidosis IV) 277.5
  brain 348.9
    Alzheimer's 331.0
      with dementia - *see* Alzheimer's, dementia
    arterial, artery 437.9
    arteriosclerotic 437.0
    congenital 742.9
    degenerative - *see* Degeneration, brain
    inflammatory - *see also* Encephalitis
      late effect - *see* category 326
    organic 348.9
      arteriosclerotic 437.0
    parasitic NEC 123.9
    Pick's 331.11
      with dementia
        with behavioral disturbance 331.11 [294.11]
        without behavioral disturbance 331.11 [294.10]
    senile 331.2
  braziers' 985.8
  breast 611.9
    cystic (chronic) 610.1
    fibrocystic 610.1
    inflammatory 611.0
    Paget's (M8540/3) 174.0
    puerperal, postpartum NEC 676.3●
    specified NEC 611.89
  Breda's (*see also* Yaws) 102.9
  Breisky's (kraurosis vulvae) 624.09
  Bretonneau's (diphtheritic malignant angina) 032.0
  Bright's (*see also* Nephritis) 583.9
    arteriosclerotic (*see also* Hypertension, kidney) 403.90
  Brill's (recrudescent typhus) 081.1
    flea-borne 081.0
    louse-borne 081.1
  Brill-Symmers (follicular lymphoma) (M9690/3) 202.0●
  Brill-Zinsser (recrudescent typhus) 081.1
  Brinton's (leather bottle stomach) (M8142/3) 151.9
  Brion-Kayser (*see also* Fever, paratyphoid) 002.9
  broad
    beta 272.2
    ligament, noninflammatory 620.9
      specified NEC 620.8
  Brocq's 691.8
    meaning
      atopic (diffuse) neurodermatitis 691.8
      dermatitis herpetiformis 694.0
      lichen simplex chronicus 698.3
      parapsoriasis 696.2
      prurigo 698.2
  Brocq-Duhring (dermatitis herpetiformis) 694.0
  Brodie's (joint) (*see also* Osteomyelitis) 730.1●
  bronchi 519.19
  bronchopulmonary 519.19
  bronze (Addison's) 255.41
    tuberculous (*see also* Tuberculosis) 017.6●
  Brown-Séquard 344.89
  Bruck's 733.99
  Bruck-de Lange (Amsterdam dwarf, intellectual disabilities, and brachycephaly) 759.89
  Bruhl's (splenic anemia with fever) 285.8
  Bruton's (X-linked agammaglobulinemia) 279.04
  buccal cavity 528.9
  Buchanan's (juvenile osteochondrosis, iliac crest) 732.1

Disease, diseased *(Continued)*
  Buchman's (osteochondrosis juvenile) 732.1
  Budgerigar-Fanciers' 495.2
  Budinger-Ludloff-Läwen 717.89
  Büerger's (thromboangiitis obliterans) 443.1
  Burger-Grütz (essential familial hyperlipemia) 272.3
  Burns' (lower ulna) 732.3
  bursa 727.9
  Bury's (erythema elevatum diutinum) 695.89
  Buschke's 710.1
  Busquet's (*see also* Osteomyelitis) 730.1●
  Busse-Buschke (cryptococcosis) 117.5
  C₂ (*see also* Alcoholism) 303.9●
  Caffey's (infantile cortical hyperostosis) 756.59
  caisson 993.3
  calculous 592.9
  California 114.0
  Calvé (-Perthes) (osteochondrosis, femoral capital) 732.1
  Camurati-Engelmann (diaphyseal sclerosis) 756.59
  Canavan's 330.0
  capillaries 448.9
  Carapata 087.1
  cardiac - *see* Disease, heart
  cardiopulmonary, chronic 416.9
  cardiorenal (arteriosclerotic) (hepatic) (hypertensive) (vascular) (*see also* Hypertension, cardiorenal) 404.90
  cardiovascular (arteriosclerotic) 429.2
    congenital 746.9
    hypertensive (*see also* Hypertension, heart) 402.90
      benign 402.10
      malignant 402.00
    renal (*see also* Hypertension, cardiorenal) 404.90
    syphilitic (asymptomatic) 093.9
  carotid gland 259.8
  Carrión's (Bartonellosis) 088.0
  cartilage NEC 733.90
    specified NEC 733.99
  Castellani's 104.8
  cat-scratch 078.3
  Cavare's (familial periodic paralysis) 359.3
  Cazenave's (pemphigus) 694.4
  cecum 569.9
  celiac (adult) 579.0
    infantile 579.0
  cellular tissue NEC 709.9
  central core 359.0
  cerebellar, cerebellum - *see* Disease, brain
  cerebral (*see also* Disease, brain) 348.9
    arterial, artery 437.9
    degenerative - *see* Degeneration, brain
  cerebrospinal 349.9
  cerebrovascular NEC 437.9
    acute 436
      embolic - *see* Embolism, brain
      late effect - *see* Late effect(s) (of) cerebrovascular disease
      puerperal, postpartum, childbirth 674.0●
      thrombotic - *see* Thrombosis, brain
    arteriosclerotic 437.0
    embolic - *see* Embolism, brain
    ischemic, generalized NEC 437.1
    late effect - *see* Late effect(s) (of) cerebrovascular disease
    occlusive 437.1
    puerperal, postpartum, childbirth 674.0●
    specified type NEC 437.8
    thrombotic - *see* Thrombosis, brain
  ceroid storage 272.7
  cervix (uteri)
    inflammatory 616.0
    noninflammatory 622.9
      specified NEC 622.8
  Chabert's 022.9

Disease, diseased *(Continued)*
  Chagas' (*see also* Trypanosomiasis, American) 086.2
  Chandler's (osteochondritis dissecans, hip) 732.7
  Charcôt's (joint) 094.0 [713.5]
    spinal cord 094.0
  Charcôt-Marie-Tooth 356.1
  Charlouis' (*see also* Yaws) 102.9
  Cheadle (-Möller) (-Barlow) (infantile scurvy) 267
  Chédiak-Steinbrinck (-Higashi) (congenital gigantism of peroxidase granules) 288.2
  cheek, inner 528.9
  chest 519.9
  Chiari's (hepatic vein thrombosis) 453.0
  Chicago (North American blastomycosis) 116.0
  chignon (white piedra) 111.2
  chigoe, chigo (jigger) 134.1
  childhood granulomatous 288.1
  Chinese liver fluke 121.1
  chlamydial NEC 078.88
  cholecystic (*see also* Disease, gallbladder) 575.9
  choroid 363.9
    degenerative (*see also* Degeneration, choroid) 363.40
    hereditary (*see also* Dystrophy, choroid) 363.50
    specified type NEC 363.8
  Christian's (chronic histiocytosis X) 277.89
  Christian-Weber (nodular nonsuppurative panniculitis) 729.30
  Christmas 286.1
  ciliary body 364.9
    specified NEC 364.89
  circulatory (system) NEC 459.9
    chronic, maternal, affecting fetus or newborn 760.3
    specified NEC 459.89
    syphilitic 093.9
      congenital 090.5
  Civatte's (poikiloderma) 709.09
  climacteric 627.2
    male 608.89
  coagulation factor deficiency (congenital) (*see also* Defect, coagulation) 286.9
  Coats' 362.12
  coccidioidal pulmonary 114.5
    acute 114.0
    chronic 114.4
    primary 114.0
    residual 114.4
  Cockayne's (microcephaly and dwarfism) 759.89
  Cogan's 370.52
  cold
    agglutinin 283.0
      or hemoglobinuria 283.0
        paroxysmal (cold) (nocturnal) 283.2
    hemagglutinin (chronic) 283.0
  collagen NEC 710.9
    nonvascular 710.9
    specified NEC 710.8
    vascular (allergic) (*see also* Angiitis, hypersensitivity) 446.20
  colon 569.9
    functional 564.9
      congenital 751.3
    ischemic 557.0
  combined system (of spinal cord) 266.2 [336.2]
    with anemia (pernicious) 281.0 [336.2]
  compressed air 993.3
  Concato's (pericardial polyserositis) 423.2
    peritoneal 568.82
    pleural - *see* Pleurisy
  congenital NEC 799.89

Disease, diseased *(Continued)*
conjunctiva 372.9
  chlamydial 077.98
    specified NEC 077.8
  specified type NEC 372.89
  viral 077.99
    specified NEC 077.8
connective tissue, diffuse *(see also* Disease,
  collagen) 710.9
Conor and Bruch's (boutonneuse fever)
  082.1
Conradi (-Hünermann) 756.59
Cooley's (erythroblastic anemia) 282.44
Cooper's 610.1
Corbus' 607.1
cork-handlers' 495.3
cornea *(see also* Keratopathy) 371.9
coronary *(see also* Ischemia, heart) 414.9
  congenital 746.85
  ostial, syphilitic 093.20
    aortic 093.22
    mitral 093.21
    pulmonary 093.24
    tricuspid 093.23
Corrigan's - *see* Insufficiency, aortic
Cotugno's 724.3
Coxsackie (virus) NEC 074.8
cranial nerve NEC 352.9
Creutzfeldt-Jakob (CJD) 046.19
  with dementia
    with behavioral disturbance 046.19
      [294.11]
    without behavioral disturbance 046.19
      [294.10]
  familial 046.19
  iatrogenic 046.19
  specified NEC 046.19
  sporadic 046.19
  variant (vCJD) 046.11
    with dementia
      with behavioral disturbance 046.11
        [294.11]
      without behavioral disturbance
        046.11 *[294.10]*
Crigler-Najjar (congenital
  hyperbilirubinemia) 277.4
Crocq's (acrocyanosis) 443.89
Crohn's (intestine) *(see also* Enteritis,
  regional) 555.9
Crouzon's (craniofacial dysostosis) 756.0
Cruchet's (encephalitis lethargica) 049.8
Cruveilhier's 335.21
Cruz-Chagas *(see also* Trypanosomiasis,
  American) 086.2
crystal deposition *(see also* Arthritis, due to,
  crystals) 712.9●
Csillag's (lichen sclerosus et atrophicus)
  701.0
Curschmann's 359.21
Cushing's (pituitary basophilism) 255.0
cystic
  breast (chronic) 610.1
  kidney, congenital *(see also* Cystic, disease,
    kidney) 753.10
  liver, congenital 751.62
  lung 518.89
    congenital 748.4
  pancreas 577.2
    congenital 751.7
  renal, congenital *(see also* Cystic, disease,
    kidney) 753.10
  semilunar cartilage 717.5
cysticercus 123.1
cystine storage (with renal sclerosis) 270.0
cytomegalic inclusion (generalized) 078.5
  with
    pneumonia 078.5 *[484.1]*
  congenital 771.1
Daae (-Finsen) (epidemic pleurodynia) 074.1
dancing 297.8
Danielssen's (anesthetic leprosy) 030.1

Disease, diseased *(Continued)*
Darier's (congenital) (keratosis follicularis)
  757.39
  erythema annulare centrifugum 695.0
  vitamin A deficiency 264.8
Darling's (histoplasmosis) *(see also*
  Histoplasmosis, American) 115.00
Davies' 425.0
de Beurmann-Gougerot (sporotrichosis)
  117.1
Débove's (splenomegaly) 789.2
deer fly *(see also* Tularemia) 021.9
deficiency 269.9
degenerative - *see also* Degeneration
  disc - *see* Degeneration, intervertebral disc
Degos' 447.8
Déjérine (-Sottas) 356.0
Déléage's 359.89
demyelinating, demyelinizating (brain stem)
  (central nervous system) 341.9
  multiple sclerosis 340
  specified NEC 341.8
de Quervain's (tendon sheath) 727.04
  thyroid (subacute granulomatous
    thyroiditis) 245.1
Dercum's (adiposis dolorosa) 272.8
Deutschländer's - *see* Fracture, foot
Devergie's (pityriasis rubra pilaris) 696.4
Devic's 341.0
diaphorase deficiency 289.7
diaphragm 519.4
diarrheal, infectious 009.2
diatomaceous earth 502
Diaz's (osteochondrosis astragalus) 732.5
digestive system 569.9
Di Guglielmo's (erythemic myelosis)
  (M9841/3) 207.0●
Dimitri-Sturge-Weber (encephalocutaneous
  angiomatosis) 759.6
disc, degenerative - *see* Degeneration,
  intervertebral disc
discogenic *(see also* Disease, intervertebral
  disc) 722.90
diverticular - *see* Diverticula
Down's (mongolism) 758.0
Dubini's (electric chorea) 049.8
Dubois' (thymus gland) 090.5
Duchenne's 094.0
  locomotor ataxia 094.0
  muscular dystrophy 359.1
  paralysis 335.22
  pseudohypertrophy, muscles 359.1
Duchenne-Griesinger 359.1
ductless glands 259.9
Duhring's (dermatitis herpetiformis) 694.0
Dukes (-Filatov) 057.8
duodenum NEC 537.9
  specified NEC 537.89
Duplay's 726.2
Dupré's (meningism) 781.6
Dupuytren's (muscle contracture) 728.6
Durand-Nicolas-Favre (climatic bubo) 099.1
Duroziez's (congenital mitral stenosis) 746.5
Dutton's (trypanosomiasis) 086.9
Eales' 362.18
ear (chronic) (inner) NEC 388.9
  middle 385.9
    adhesive *(see also* Adhesions, middle
      ear) 385.10
    specified NEC 385.89
Eberth's (typhoid fever) 002.0
Ebstein's
  heart 746.2
  meaning diabetes 250.4● *[581.81]*
    due to secondary diabetes 249.4●
      [581.81]
Echinococcus *(see also* Echinococcus) 122.9
ECHO virus NEC 078.89
Economo's (encephalitis lethargica) 049.8
Eddowes' (brittle bones and blue sclera)
  756.51

Disease, diseased *(Continued)*
Edsall's 992.2
Eichstedt's (pityriasis versicolor) 111.0
Ellis-van Creveld (chondroectodermal
  dysplasia) 756.55
endocardium - *see* Endocarditis
endocrine glands or system NEC 259.9
  specified NEC 259.8
endomyocardial, idiopathic mural 425.2
Engel-von Recklinghausen (osteitis fibrosa
  cystica) 252.01
Engelmann's (diaphyseal sclerosis) 756.59
English (rickets) 268.0
Engman's (infectious eczematoid dermatitis)
  690.8
enteroviral, enterovirus NEC 078.89
  central nervous system NEC 048
epidemic NEC 136.9
epididymis 608.9
epigastric, functional 536.9
  psychogenic 306.4
Erb (-Landouzy) 359.1
Erb-Goldflam 358.00
Erdheim-Chester (ECD) 277.89
Erichsen's (railway spine) 300.16
esophagus 530.9
  functional 530.5
  psychogenic 306.4
Eulenburg's (congenital paramyotonia)
  359.29
Eustachian tube 381.9
Evans' (thrombocytopenic purpura) 287.32
external auditory canal 380.9
extrapyramidal NEC 333.90
eye 379.90
  anterior chamber 364.9
  inflammatory NEC 364.3
  muscle 378.9
eyeball 360.9
eyelid 374.9
eyeworm of Africa 125.2
Fabry's (angiokeratoma corporis diffusum)
  272.7
facial nerve (seventh) 351.9
  newborn 767.5
Fahr-Volhard (malignant nephrosclerosis)
  403.00
fallopian tube, noninflammatory 620.9
  specified NEC 620.8
familial periodic 277.31
  paralysis 359.3
Fanconi's (congenital pancytopenia) 284.09
Farber's (disseminated lipogranulomatosis)
  272.8
fascia 728.9
  inflammatory 728.9
Fauchard's (periodontitis) 523.40
Favre-Durand-Nicolas (climatic bubo) 099.1
Favre-Racouchot (elastoidosis cutanea
  nodularis) 701.8
Fede's 529.0
Feer's 985.0
Felix's (juvenile osteochondrosis, hip) 732.1
Fenwick's (gastric atrophy) 537.89
Fernels' (aortic aneurysm) 441.9
fibrocaseous, of lung *(see also* Tuberculosis,
  pulmonary) 011.9●
fibrocystic - *see also* Fibrocystic, disease
  newborn 277.01
Fiedler's (leptospiral jaundice) 100.0
fifth 057.0
Filatoff's (infectious mononucleosis) 075
Filatov's (infectious mononucleosis) 075
file-cutters' 984.9
  specified type of lead - *see* Table of Drugs
    and Chemicals
filterable virus NEC 078.89
fish skin 757.1
  acquired 701.1
Flajani (-Basedow) (exophthalmic goiter)
  242.0●

Disease, diseased *(Continued)*
  Flatau-Schilder 341.1
  flax-dressers' 504
  Fleischner's 732.3
  flint 502
  fluke - *see* Infestation, fluke
  Følling's (phenylketonuria) 270.1
  foot and mouth 078.4
  foot process 581.3
  Forbes' (glycogenosis III) 271.0
  Fordyce's (ectopic sebaceous glands)
      (mouth) 750.26
  Fordyce-Fox (apocrine miliaria) 705.82
  Fothergill's
      meaning scarlatina anginosa 034.1
      neuralgia (*see also* Neuralgia, trigeminal)
          350.1
  Fournier's 608.83
      female 616.89
  fourth 057.8
  Fox (-Fordyce) (apocrine miliaria) 705.82
  Francis' (*see also* Tularemia) 021.9
  Franklin's (heavy chain) 273.2
  Frei's (climatic bubo) 099.1
  Freiberg's (flattening metatarsal) 732.5
  Friedländer's (endarteritis obliterans) - *see*
      Arteriosclerosis
  Friedreich's
      combined systemic or ataxia 334.0
      facial hemihypertrophy 756.0
      myoclonia 333.2
  Fröhlich's (adiposogenital dystrophy) 253.8
  Frommel's 676.6●
  frontal sinus (chronic) 473.1
      acute 461.1
  Fuller's earth 502
  fungus, fungous NEC 117.9
  Gaisböck's (polycythemia hypertonica) 289.0
  gallbladder 575.9
      congenital 751.60
  Gamna's (siderotic splenomegaly) 289.51
  Gamstorp's (adynamia episodica hereditaria)
      359.3
  Gandy-Nanta (siderotic splenomegaly)
      289.51
  Gannister (occupational) 502
  Garré's (*see also* Osteomyelitis) 730.1●
  gastric (*see also* Disease, stomach) 537.9
  gastroesophageal reflux (GERD) 530.81
  gastrointestinal (tract) 569.9
      amyloid 277.39
      functional 536.9
          psychogenic 306.4
  Gaucher's (adult) (cerebroside lipidosis)
      (infantile) 272.7
  Gayet's (superior hemorrhagic
      polioencephalitis) 265.1
  Gee (-Herter) (-Heubner) (-Thaysen)
      (nontropical sprue) 579.0
  generalized neoplastic (M8000/6) 199.0
  genital organs NEC
      female 629.9
          specified NEC 629.89
      male 608.9
  Gerhardt's (erythromelalgia) 443.82
  Gerlier's (epidemic vertigo) 078.81
  Gibert's (pityriasis rosea) 696.3
  Gibney's (perispondylitis) 720.9
  Gierke's (glycogenosis I) 271.0
  Gilbert's (familial nonhemolytic jaundice)
      277.4
  Gilchrist's (North American blastomycosis)
      116.0
  Gilford (-Hutchinson) (progeria) 259.8
  Gilles de la Tourette's (motor-verbal tic)
      307.23
  Giovannini's 117.9
  gland (lymph) 289.9
  Glanzmann's (hereditary hemorrhagic
      thrombasthenia) 287.1
  glassblowers' 527.1

Disease, diseased *(Continued)*
  Glénard's (enteroptosis) 569.89
  Glisson's (*see also* Rickets) 268.0
  glomerular
      membranous, idiopathic 581.1
      minimal change 581.3
  glycogen storage (Andersen's) (Cori types
      1-7) (Forbes') (McArdle-Schmid-
      Pearson) (Pompe's) (types I-VII) 271.0
      cardiac 271.0 [425.7]
      generalized 271.0
      glucose-6-phosphatase deficiency 271.0
      heart 271.0 [425.7]
      hepatorenal 271.0
      liver and kidneys 271.0
      myocardium 271.0 [425.7]
      von Gierke's (glycogenosis I) 271.0
  Goldflam-Erb 358.00
  Goldscheider's (epidermolysis bullosa)
      757.39
  Goldstein's (familial hemorrhagic
      telangiectasia) 448.0
  gonococcal NEC 098.0
  Goodall's (epidemic vomiting) 078.82
  Gordon's (exudative enteropathy) 579.8
  Gougerot's (trisymptomatic) 709.1
  Gougerot-Carteaud (confluent reticulate
      papillomatosis) 701.8
  Gougerot-Hailey-Hailey (benign familial
      chronic pemphigus) 757.39
  graft-versus-host 279.50
      acute 279.51
          on chronic 279.53
      chronic 279.52
  grain-handlers' 495.8
  Grancher's (splenopneumonia) - *see*
      Pneumonia
  granulomatous (childhood) (chronic) 288.1
  graphite lung 503
  Graves' (exophthalmic goiter) 242.0●
  Greenfield's 330.0
  green monkey 078.89
  Griesinger's (*see also* Ancylostomiasis) 126.9
  grinders' 502
  Grisel's 723.5
  Gruby's (tinea tonsurans) 110.0
  Guertin's (electric chorea) 049.8
  Guillain-Barré 357.0
  Guinon's (motor-verbal tic) 307.23
  Gull's (thyroid atrophy with myxedema)
      244.8
  Gull and Sutton's - *see* Hypertension, kidney
  gum NEC 523.9
  Günther's (congenital erythropoietic
      porphyria) 277.1
  gynecological 629.9
      specified NEC 629.89
  H 270.0
  Haas' 732.3
  Habermann's (acute parapsoriasis
      varioliformis) 696.2
  Haff 985.1
  Hageman (congenital factor XII deficiency)
      (*see also* Defect, congenital) 286.3
  Haglund's (osteochondrosis os tibiale
      externum) 732.5
  Hagner's (hypertrophic pulmonary
      osteoarthropathy) 731.2
  Hailey-Hailey (benign familial chronic
      pemphigus) 757.39
  hair (follicles) NEC 704.9
      specified type NEC 704.8
  Hallervorden-Spatz 333.0
  Hallopeau's (lichen sclerosus et atrophicus)
      701.0
  Hamman's (spontaneous mediastinal
      emphysema) 518.1
  hand, foot, and mouth 074.3
  Hand-Schüller-Christian (chronic
      histiocytosis X) 277.89
  Hanot's - *see* Cirrhosis, biliary

Disease, diseased *(Continued)*
  Hansen's (leprosy) 030.9
      benign form 030.1
      malignant form 030.0
  Harada's 363.22
  Harley's (intermittent hemoglobinuria)
      283.2
  Hart's (pellagra-cerebellar ataxia-renal
      aminoaciduria) 270.0
  Hartnup (pellagra-cerebellar ataxia-renal
      aminoaciduria) 270.0
  Hashimoto's (struma lymphomatosa)
      245.2
  Hb - *see* Disease, hemoglobin
  heart (organic) 429.9
      with
          acute pulmonary edema (*see also*
              Failure, ventricular, left) 428.1
          hypertensive 402.91
              with renal failure 404.92
              benign 402.11
                  with renal failure 404.12
              malignant 402.01
                  with renal failure 404.02
          kidney disease - *see* Hypertension,
              cardiorenal
          rheumatic fever (conditions
              classifiable to 390)
              active 391.9
                  with chorea 392.0
              inactive or quiescent (with
                  chorea) 398.90
      amyloid 277.39 [425.7]
      aortic (valve) (*see also* Endocarditis, aortic)
          424.1
      arteriosclerotic or sclerotic (minimal)
          (senile) - *see* Arteriosclerosis,
          coronary
      artery, arterial - *see* Arteriosclerosis,
          coronary
      atherosclerotic - *see* Arteriosclerosis,
          coronary
      beer drinkers' 425.5
      beriberi 265.0 [425.7]
      black 416.0
      congenital NEC 746.9
          cyanotic 746.9
          maternal, affecting fetus or newborn
              760.3
          specified type NEC 746.89
      congestive (*see also* Failure, heart) 428.0
      coronary 414.9
      cryptogenic 429.9
      due to
          amyloidosis 277.39 [425.7]
          beriberi 265.0 [425.7]
          cardiac glycogenosis 271.0 [425.7]
          Friedreich's ataxia 334.0 [425.8]
          gout 274.82
          mucopolysaccharidosis 277.5 [425.7]
          myotonia atrophica 359.21 [425.8]
          progressive muscular dystrophy 359.1
              [425.8]
          sarcoidosis 135 [425.8]
      fetal 746.9
          inflammatory 746.89
      fibroid (*see also* Myocarditis) 429.0
      functional 427.9
          postoperative 997.1
          psychogenic 306.2
      glycogen storage 271.0 [425.7]
      gonococcal NEC 098.85
      gouty 274.82
      hypertensive (*see also* Hypertension,
          heart) 402.90
          benign 402.10
          malignant 402.00
      hyperthyroid (*see also* Hyperthyroidism)
          242.9● [425.7]
      incompletely diagnosed - *see* Disease,
          heart

Disease, diseased *(Continued)*
  heart *(Continued)*
    ischemic (chronic) *(see also* Ischemia,
      heart) 414.9
      acute *(see also* Infarct, myocardium)
        410.9●
        without myocardial infarction
          411.89
          with coronary (artery) occlusion
            411.81
      asymptomatic 412
      diagnosed on ECG or other special
        investigation but currently
        presenting no symptoms
        412
    kyphoscoliotic 416.1
    mitral *(see also* Endocarditis, mitral)
      394.9
    muscular *(see also* Degeneration,
      myocardial) 429.1
    postpartum 674.8●
    psychogenic (functional) 306.2
    pulmonary (chronic) 416.9
      acute 415.0
      specified NEC 416.8
    rheumatic (chronic) (inactive) (old)
      (quiescent) (with chorea) 398.90
      active or acute 391.9
        with chorea (active) (rheumatic)
          (Sydenham's) 392.0
        specified type NEC 391.8
      maternal, affecting fetus or newborn
        760.3
    rheumatoid - *see* Arthritis, rheumatoid
    sclerotic - *see* Arteriosclerosis, coronary
    senile *(see also* Myocarditis) 429.0
    specified type NEC 429.89
    syphilitic 093.89
      aortic 093.1
        aneurysm 093.0
      asymptomatic 093.89
      congenital 090.5
    thyroid (gland) *(see also* Hyperthyroidism)
      242.9● *[425.7]*
    thyrotoxic *(see also* Thyrotoxicosis) 242.9●
      [425.7]
    tuberculous *(see also* Tuberculosis) 017.9●
      [425.8]
    valve, valvular (obstructive)
      (regurgitant) - *see also* Endocarditis
      congenital NEC *(see also* Anomaly,
        heart, valve) 746.9
        pulmonary 746.00
        specified type NEC 746.89
    vascular - *see* Disease, cardiovascular
  heavy-chain (gamma G) 273.2
  Heberden's 715.04
  Hebra's
    dermatitis exfoliativa 695.89
    erythema multiforme exudativum 695.19
    pityriasis
      maculata et circinata 696.3
      rubra 695.89
        pilaris 696.4
    prurigo 698.2
  Heerfordt's (uveoparotitis) 135
  Heidenhain's 290.10
    with dementia 290.10
  Heilmeyer-Schöner (M9842/3) 207.1●
  Heine-Medin *(see also* Poliomyelitis)
    045.9●
  Heller's *(see also* Psychosis, childhood)
    299.1●
  Heller-Döhle (syphilitic aortitis) 093.1
  hematopoietic organs 289.9
  hemoglobin (Hb) 282.7
    with thalassemia 282.49
    abnormal (mixed) NEC 282.7
      with thalassemia 282.49
    AS genotype 282.5
    Bart's 282.43

Disease, diseased *(Continued)*
  hemoglobin (Hb) *(Continued)*
    C (Hb-C) 282.7
      with other abnormal hemoglobin NEC
        282.7
      elliptocytosis 282.7
      Hb-S (without crisis) 282.63
        with
          crisis 282.64
          vaso-occlusive pain 282.64
      sickle-cell (without crisis) 282.63
        with
          crisis 282.64
          vaso-occlusive pain 282.64
      thalassemia 282.49
    constant spring 282.7
    D (Hb-D) 282.7
      with other abnormal hemoglobin NEC
        282.7
      Hb-S (without crisis) 282.68
        with crisis 282.69
      sickle-cell (without crisis) 282.68
        with crisis 282.69
      thalassemia 282.49
    E (Hb-E) 282.7
      with other abnormal hemoglobin NEC
        282.7
      Hb-S (without crisis) 282.68
        with crisis 282.69
      sickle-cell (without crisis) 282.68
        with crisis 282.69
      thalassemia 282.47
    elliptocytosis 282.7
    F (Hb-F) 282.7
    G (Hb-G) 282.7
    H (Hb-H) 282.43
    hereditary persistence, fetal (HPFH)
      ("Swiss variety") 282.7
    high fetal gene 282.7
    I thalassemia 282.49
    M 289.7
    S - *see also* Disease, sickle-cell, Hb-S
      thalassemia (without crisis)
        282.41
        with
          crisis 282.42
          vaso-occlusive pain 282.42
    spherocytosis 282.7
    unstable, hemolytic 282.7
    Zurich (Hb-Zurich) 282.7
  hemolytic (fetus) (newborn) 773.2
    autoimmune (cold type) (warm type)
      283.0
    due to or with
      incompatibility
        ABO (blood group) 773.1
        blood (group) (Duffy) (Kell)
          (Kidd) (Lewis) (M) (S)
          NEC 773.2
        Rh (blood group) (factor) 773.0
      Rh negative mother 773.0
    unstable hemoglobin 282.7
  hemorrhagic 287.9
    newborn 776.0
  Henoch (-Schönlein) (purpura nervosa)
    287.0
  hepatic - *see* Disease, liver
  hepatolenticular 275.1
  heredodegenerative NEC
    brain 331.89
    spinal cord 336.8
  Hers' (glycogenosis VI) 271.0
  Herter (-Gee) (-Heubner) (nontropical sprue)
    579.0
  Herxheimer's (diffuse idiopathic cutaneous
    atrophy) 701.8
  Heubner's 094.89
  Heubner-Herter (nontropical sprue) 579.0
  high fetal gene or hemoglobin thalassemia
    (see also Thalassemia) 282.40
  Hildenbrand's (typhus) 081.9

Disease, diseased *(Continued)*
  hip (joint) NEC 719.95
    congenital 755.63
    suppurative 711.05
    tuberculous *(see also* Tuberculosis) 015.1●
      [730.85]
  Hippel's (retinocerebral angiomatosis) 759.6
  Hirschfeld's (acute diabetes mellitus) *(see also*
    Diabetes) 250.0●
    due to secondary diabetes 249.0●
  Hirschsprung's (congenital megacolon) 751.3
  His (-Werner) (trench fever) 083.1
  HIV 042
  Hodgkin's (M9650/3) 201.9●

> Note: Use the following fifth-digit
> subclassification with category 201:
>
> 0   unspecified site
> 1   lymph nodes of head, face, and neck
> 2   intrathoracic lymph nodes
> 3   intra-abdominal lymph nodes
> 4   lymph nodes of axilla and upper limb
> 5   lymph nodes of inguinal region and
>   lower limb
> 6   intrapelvic lymph nodes
> 7   spleen
> 8   lymph nodes of multiple sites

    lymphocytic
      depletion (M9653/3) 201.7●
        diffuse fibrosis (M9654/3) 201.7●
        reticular type (M9655/3) 201.7●
      predominance (M9651/3) 201.4●
    lymphocytic-histiocytic predominance
      (M9651/3) 201.4●
    mixed cellularity (M9652/3) 201.6●
    nodular sclerosis (M9656/3) 201.5●
      cellular phase (M9657/3) 201.5●
  Hodgson's 441.9
    ruptured 441.5
  Hoffa (-Kastert) (liposynovitis prepatellaris)
    272.8
  Holla *(see also* Spherocytosis) 282.0
  homozygous-Hb-S 282.61
  hoof and mouth 078.4
  hookworm *(see also* Ancylostomiasis) 126.9
  Horton's (temporal arteritis) 446.5
  host-versus-graft (immune or nonimmune
    cause) 279.50
  HPFH (hereditary persistence of fetal
    hemoglobin) ("Swiss variety") 282.7
  Huchard's (continued arterial hypertension)
    401.9
  Huguier's (uterine fibroma) 218.9
  human immunodeficiency (virus) 042
  hunger 251.1
  Hunt's
    dyssynergia cerebellaris myoclonica 334.2
    herpetic geniculate ganglionitis 053.11
  Huntington's 333.4
  Huppert's (multiple myeloma) (M9730/3)
    203.0●
  Hurler's (mucopolysaccharidosis I) 277.5
  Hutchinson's, meaning
    angioma serpiginosum 709.1
    cheiropompholyx 705.81
    prurigo estivalis 692.72
  Hutchinson-Boeck (sarcoidosis) 135
  Hutchinson-Gilford (progeria) 259.8
  hyaline (diffuse) (generalized) 728.9
    membrane (lung) (newborn) 769
  hydatid *(see also* Echinococcus) 122.9
  Hyde's (prurigo nodularis) 698.3
  hyperkinetic *(see also* Hyperkinesia) 314.9
    heart 429.82
  hypertensive *(see also* Hypertension) 401.9
  hypophysis 253.9
    hyperfunction 253.1
    hypofunction 253.2
  Iceland (epidemic neuromyasthenia) 049.8
  I cell 272.7

◀ New   ◀ Revised   ~~deleted~~ Deleted   ● Use Additional Digit(s)   ▨ Omit code

Disease, diseased *(Continued)*
  ill-defined 799.89
  immunologic NEC 279.9
  immunoproliferative 203.8●
  inclusion 078.5
    salivary gland 078.5
  infancy, early NEC 779.9
  infective NEC 136.9
  inguinal gland 289.9
  internal semilunar cartilage, cystic 717.5
  intervertebral disc 722.90
    with myelopathy 722.70
    cervical, cervicothoracic 722.91
      with myelopathy 722.71
    lumbar, lumbosacral 722.93
      with myelopathy 722.73
    thoracic, thoracolumbar 722.92
      with myelopathy 722.72
  intestine 569.9
    functional 564.9
      congenital 751.3
      psychogenic 306.4
    lardaceous 277.39
    organic 569.9
    protozoal NEC 007.9
  iris 364.9
    specified NEC 364.89
  iron
    metabolism *(see also* Hemochromatosis) 275.09
    storage *(see also* Hemochromatosis) 275.03
  Isambert's *(see also* Tuberculosis, larynx) 012.3●
  Iselin's (osteochondrosis, fifth metatarsal) 732.5
  island (scrub typhus) 081.2
  itai-itai 985.5
  Jadassohn's (maculopapular erythroderma) 696.2
  Jadassohn-Pellizari's (anetoderma) 701.3
  Jakob-Creutzfeldt (CJD) 046.19
    with dementia
      with behavioral disturbance 046.19 *[294.11]*
      without behavioral disturbance 046.19 *[294.10]*
    familial 046.19
    iatrogenic 046.19
    specified NEC 046.19
    sporadic 046.19
    variant (vCJD) 046.11
      with dementia
        with behavioral disturbance 046.11 *[294.11]*
        without behavioral disturbance 046.11 *[294.10]*
  Jaksch (-Luzet) (pseudoleukemia infantum) 285.8
  Janet's 300.89
  Jansky-Bielschowsky 330.1
  jaw NEC 526.9
    fibrocystic 526.2
  Jensen's 363.05
  Jeune's (asphyxiating thoracic dystrophy) 756.4
  Jigger 134.1
  Johnson-Stevens (erythema multiforme exudativum) 695.13
  joint NEC 719.9●
    ankle 719.97
    Charcôt 094.0 *[713.5]*
    degenerative *(see also* Osteoarthrosis) 715.9●
      multiple 715.09
      spine *(see also* Spondylosis) 721.90
    elbow 719.92
    foot 719.97
    hand 719.94
    hip 719.95

Disease, diseased *(Continued)*
  joint NEC *(Continued)*
    hypertrophic (chronic) (degenerative) *(see also* Osteoarthrosis) 715.9●
      spine *(see also* Spondylosis) 721.90
    knee 719.96
    Luschka 721.90
    multiple sites 719.99
    pelvic region 719.95
    sacroiliac 724.6
    shoulder (region) 719.91
    specified site NEC 719.98
    spine NEC 724.9
      pseudarthrosis following fusion 733.82
      sacroiliac 724.6
    wrist 719.93
  Jourdain's (acute gingivitis) 523.00
  Jüngling's (sarcoidosis) 135
  Kahler (-Bozzolo) (multiple myeloma) (M9730/3) 203.0●
  Kalischer's 759.6
  Kaposi's 757.33
    lichen ruber 697.8
      acuminatus 696.4
      moniliformis 697.8
    xeroderma pigmentosum 757.33
  Kaschin-Beck (endemic polyarthritis) 716.00
    ankle 716.07
    arm 716.02
      lower (and wrist) 716.03
      upper (and elbow) 716.02
    foot (and ankle) 716.07
    forearm (and wrist) 716.03
    hand 716.04
    leg 716.06
      lower 716.06
      upper 716.05
    multiple sites 716.09
    pelvic region (hip) (thigh) 716.05
    shoulder region 716.01
    specified site NEC 716.08
  Katayama 120.2
  Kawasaki 446.1
  Kedani (scrub typhus) 081.2
  kidney (functional) (pelvis) *(see also* Disease, renal) 593.9
    chronic 585.9
      requiring chronic dialysis 585.6
      stage
        I 585.1
        II (mild) 585.2
        III (moderate) 585.3
        IV (severe) 585.4
        V 585.5
    cystic (congenital) 753.10
      multiple 753.19
      single 753.11
      specified NEC 753.19
    fibrocystic (congenital) 753.19
    in gout 274.10
    polycystic (congenital) 753.12
      adult type (APKD) 753.13
      autosomal dominant 753.13
      autosomal recessive 753.14
      childhood type (CPKD) 753.14
      infantile type 753.14
  Kienböck's (carpal lunate) (wrist) 732.3
  Kimmelstiel (-Wilson) (intercapillary glomerulosclerosis) 250.4● *[581.81]*
    due to secondary diabetes 249.4● *[581.81]*
  Kinnier Wilson's (hepatolenticular degeneration) 275.1
  kissing 075
  Kleb's *(see also* Nephritis) 583.9
  Klinger's 446.4
  Klippel's 723.8
  Klippel-Feil (brevicollis) 756.16
  Knight's 911.1
  Köbner's (epidermolysis bullosa) 757.39
  Koenig-Wichmann (pemphigus) 694.4

Disease, diseased *(Continued)*
  Köhler's
    first (osteoarthrosis juvenilis) 732.5
    second (Freiberg's infraction, metatarsal head) 732.5
    patellar 732.4
    tarsal navicular (bone) (osteoarthrosis juvenilis) 732.5
  Köhler-Freiberg (infraction, metatarsal head) 732.5
  Köhler-Mouchet (osteoarthrosis juvenilis) 732.5
  Köhler-Pellegrini-Stieda (calcification, knee joint) 726.62
  Kok 759.89
  König's (osteochondritis dissecans) 732.7
  Korsakoff's (nonalcoholic) 294.0
    alcoholic 291.1
  Kostmann's (infantile genetic agranulocytosis) 288.01
  Krabbe's 330.0
  Kraepelin-Morel *(see also* Schizophrenia) 295.9●
  Kraft-Weber-Dimitri 759.6
  Kufs' 330.1
  Kugelberg-Welander 335.11
  Kuhnt-Junius 362.52
  Kümmell's (-Verneuil) (spondylitis) 721.7
  Kundrat's (lymphosarcoma) 200.1●
  kuru 046.0
  Kussmaul (-Meier) (polyarteritis nodosa) 446.0
  Kyasanur Forest 065.2
  Kyrle's (hyperkeratosis follicularis in cutem penetrans) 701.1
  labia
    inflammatory 616.10
    noninflammatory 624.9
      specified NEC 624.8
  labyrinth, ear 386.8
  lacrimal system (apparatus) (passages) 375.9
    gland 375.00
    specified NEC 375.89
  Lafora's 333.2
  Lagleyze-von Hippel (retinocerebral angiomatosis) 759.6
  Lancereaux-Mathieu (leptospiral jaundice) 100.0
  Landry's 357.0
  Lane's 569.89
  lardaceous (any site) 277.39
  Larrey-Weil (leptospiral jaundice) 100.0
  Larsen (-Johansson) (juvenile osteopathia patellae) 732.4
  larynx 478.70
  Lasègue's (persecution mania) 297.9
  Leber's 377.16
  Lederer's (acquired infectious hemolytic anemia) 283.19
  Legg's (capital femoral osteochondrosis) 732.1
  Legg-Calvé-Perthes (capital femoral osteochondrosis) 732.1
  Legg-Calvé-Waldenström (femoral capital osteochondrosis) 732.1
  Legg-Perthes (femoral capital osteochondrosis) 732.1
  Legionnaires' 482.84
  Leigh's 330.8
  Leiner's (exfoliative dermatitis) 695.89
  Leloir's (lupus erythematosus) 695.4
  Lenegre's 426.0
  lens (eye) 379.39
  Leriche's (osteoporosis, posttraumatic) 733.7
  Letterer-Siwe (acute histiocytosis X) (M9722/3) 202.5●
  Lev's (acquired complete heart block) 426.0
  Lewandowski's *(see also* Tuberculosis) 017.0●
  Lewandowski-Lutz (epidermodysplasia verruciformis) 078.19

Disease, diseased (*Continued*)
Lewy body 331.82
    with dementia
        with behavioral disturbance 331.82
            [294.11]
        without behavioral disturbance 331.82
            [294.10]
    Leyden's (periodic vomiting) 536.2
    Libman-Sacks (verrucous endocarditis) 710.0
        [424.91]
    Lichtheim's (subacute combined sclerosis
        with pernicious anemia) 281.0
            [336.2]
    ligament 728.9
    light chain 203.0●
    Lightwood's (renal tubular acidosis)
        588.89
    Lignac's (cystinosis) 270.0
    Lindau's (retinocerebral angiomatosis)
        759.6
    Lindau-von Hippel (angiomatosis
        retinocerebellosa) 759.6
    lip NEC 528.5
    lipidosis 272.7
    lipoid storage NEC 272.7
    Lipschütz's 616.50
    Little's - *see* Palsy, cerebral
    liver 573.9
        alcoholic 571.3
            acute 571.1
            chronic 571.3
        chronic 571.9
            alcoholic 571.3
        cystic, congenital 751.62
        drug-induced 573.3
        due to
            chemicals 573.3
            fluorinated agents 573.3
            hypersensitivity drugs 573.3
            isoniazids 573.3
        end stage NEC 572.8
            due to hepatitis - *see* Hepatitis
        fibrocystic (congenital) 751.62
        glycogen storage 271.0
        organic 573.9
        polycystic (congenital) 751.62
    Lobo's (keloid blastomycosis) 116.2
    Lobstein's (brittle bones and blue sclera)
        756.51
    locomotor system 334.9
    Lorain's (pituitary dwarfism) 253.3
    Lou Gehrig's 335.20
    Lucas-Championnière (fibrinous bronchitis)
        466.0
    Ludwig's (submaxillary cellulitis)
        528.3
    luetic - *see* Syphilis
    lumbosacral region 724.6
    lung NEC 518.89
        black 500
        congenital 748.60
        cystic 518.89
            congenital 748.4
        fibroid (chronic) (*see also* Fibrosis, lung)
            515
        fluke 121.2
            oriental 121.2
        in
            amyloidosis 277.39 [517.8]
            polymyositis 710.4 [517.8]
            sarcoidosis 135 [517.8]
            Sjögren's syndrome 710.2 [517.8]
            syphilis 095.1
            systemic lupus erythematosus 710.0
                [517.8]
            systemic sclerosis 710.1 [517.2]
        interstitial (chronic) 515
            acute 136.3
            respiratory bronchiolitis
                516.34
        nonspecific, chronic 496

Disease, diseased (*Continued*)
lung NEC (*Continued*)
    obstructive (chronic) (COPD) 496
        with
            acute
                bronchitis 491.22
                exacerbation NEC 491.21
            alveolitis, allergic (*see also* Alveolitis,
                allergic) 495.9
            asthma (chronic) (obstructive)
                493.2●
            bronchiectasis 494.0
                with acute exacerbation 494.1
            bronchitis (chronic) 491.20
                with
                    acute bronchitis 491.22
                    exacerbation (acute) 491.21
            decompensated 491.21
                with exacerbation 491.21
            emphysema NEC 492.8
        diffuse (with fibrosis) 496
    of childhood, specified NEC 516.69
    polycystic 518.89
        asthma (chronic) (obstructive) 493.2●
        congenital 748.4
    purulent (cavitary) 513.0
    restrictive 518.89
    rheumatoid 714.81
        diffuse interstitial 714.81
    specified NEC 518.89
    Lutembacher's (atrial septal defect with
        mitral stenosis) 745.5
    Lutz-Miescher (elastosis perforans
        serpiginosa) 701.1
    Lutz-Splendore-de Almeida (Brazilian
        blastomycosis) 116.1
    Lyell's (toxic epidermal necrolysis) 695.15
        due to drug
            correct substance properly
                administered 695.15
            overdose or wrong substance given or
                taken 977.9
            specific drug - *see* Table of Drugs
                and Chemicals
    Lyme 088.81
    lymphatic (gland) (system) 289.9
        channel (noninfective) 457.9
        vessel (noninfective) 457.9
            specified NEC 457.8
    lymphoproliferative (chronic) (M9970/1)
        238.79
        X linked 759.89
    Machado-Joseph 334.8
    Madelung's (lipomatosis) 272.8
    Madura (actinomycotic) 039.9
        mycotic 117.4
    Magitot's 526.4
    Majocchi's (purpura annularis
        telangiectodes) 709.1
    malarial (*see also* Malaria) 084.6
    Malassez's (cystic) 608.89
    Malibu 919.8
        infected 919.9
    malignant (M8000/3) - *see also* Neoplasm, by
        site, malignant
        previous, affecting management of
            pregnancy V23.89
    Manson's 120.1
    maple bark 495.6
    maple syrup (urine) 270.3
    Marburg (virus) 078.89
    Marchiafava (-Bignami) 341.8
    Marfan's 090.49
        congenital syphilis 090.49
        meaning Marfan's syndrome 759.82
    Marie-Bamberger (hypertrophic pulmonary
        osteoarthropathy) (secondary) 731.2
        primary or idiopathic (acropachyderma)
            757.39
        pulmonary (hypertrophic
            osteoarthropathy) 731.2

Disease, diseased (*Continued*)
Marie-Strümpell (ankylosing spondylitis)
    720.0
Marion's (bladder neck obstruction) 596.0
Marsh's (exophthalmic goiter) 242.0●
Martin's 715.27
mast cell 757.33
    systemic (M9741/3) 202.6●
mastoid (*see also* Mastoiditis) 383.9
    process 385.9
maternal, unrelated to pregnancy NEC,
    affecting fetus or newborn 760.9
Mathieu's (leptospiral jaundice) 100.0
Mauclaire's 732.3
Mauriac's (erythema nodosum syphiliticum)
    091.3
Maxcy's 081.0
McArdle (-Schmid-Pearson) (glycogenosis V)
    271.0
mediastinum NEC 519.3
Medin's (*see also* Poliomyelitis) 045.9●
Mediterranean 282.40
    with hemoglobinopathy 282.49
medullary center (idiopathic) (respiratory)
    348.89
Meige's (chronic hereditary edema) 757.0
Meleda 757.39
Ménétrier's (hypertrophic gastritis) 535.2●
Ménière's (active) 386.00
    cochlear 386.02
    cochleovestibular 386.01
    inactive 386.04
    in remission 386.04
    vestibular 386.03
meningeal - *see* Meningitis
mental (*see also* Psychosis) 298.9
Merzbacher-Pelizaeus 330.0
mesenchymal 710.9
mesenteric embolic 557.0
metabolic NEC 277.9
metal polishers' 502
metastatic - *see* Metastasis
Mibelli's 757.39
microdrepanocytic 282.41
microvascular - *code to* condition
microvillus
    atrophy 751.5
    inclusion (MVD) 751.5
Miescher's 709.3
Mikulicz's (dryness of mouth, absent or
    decreased lacrimation) 527.1
Milkman (-Looser) (osteomalacia with
    pseudofractures) 268.2
Miller's (osteomalacia) 268.2
Mills' 335.29
Milroy's (chronic hereditary edema) 757.0
Minamata 985.0
Minor's 336.1
Minot's (hemorrhagic disease, newborn)
    776.0
Minot-von Willebrand-Jürgens
    (angiohemophilia) 286.4
Mitchell's (erythromelalgia) 443.82
mitral - *see* Endocarditis, mitral
Mljet (mal de Meleda) 757.39
Möbius', Moebius' 346.2●
Möeller's 267
Möller (-Barlow) (infantile scurvy) 267
Mönckeberg's (*see also* Arteriosclerosis,
    extremities) 440.20
Mondor's (thrombophlebitis of breast) 451.89
Monge's 993.2
Morel-Kraepelin (*see also* Schizophrenia)
    295.9●
Morgagni's (syndrome) (hyperostosis
    frontalis interna) 733.3
Morgagni-Adams-Stokes (syncope with
    heart block) 426.9
Morquio (-Brailsford) (-Ullrich)
    (mucopolysaccharidosis IV) 277.5
Morton's (with metatarsalgia) 355.6

◀ New   ◀▥ Revised   ~~deleted~~ Deleted   ● Use Additional Digit(s)   ▨ Omit code

Disease, diseased *(Continued)*
Morvan's 336.0
motor neuron (bulbar) (mixed type) 335.20
Mouchet's (juvenile osteochondrosis, foot) 732.5
mouth 528.9
Moyamoya 437.5
Mucha's (acute parapsoriasis varioliformis) 696.2
mu-chain 273.2
mucolipidosis (I) (II) (III) 272.7
Münchmeyer's (exostosis luxurians) 728.11
Murri's (intermittent hemoglobinuria) 283.2
muscle 359.9
    inflammatory 728.9
    ocular 378.9
musculoskeletal system 729.90
mushroom workers' 495.5
Myà's (congenital dilation, colon) 751.3
mycotic 117.9
myeloproliferative (chronic) (M9960/1) 238.79
myocardium, myocardial *(see also Degeneration, myocardial)* 429.1
    hypertensive *(see also Hypertension, heart)* 402.90
    primary (idiopathic) 425.4
myoneural 358.9
Naegeli's 287.1
nail 703.9
    specified type NEC 703.8
Nairobi sheep 066.1
nasal 478.19
    cavity NEC 478.19
    sinus (chronic) - *see* Sinusitis
navel (newborn) NEC 779.89
    delayed separation of umbilical cord 779.83
nemaline body 359.0
neoplastic, generalized (M8000/6) 199.0
nerve - *see* Disorder, nerve
nervous system (central) 349.9
    autonomic, peripheral *(see also Neuropathy, peripheral, autonomic)* 337.9
    congenital 742.9
    inflammatory - *see* Encephalitis
    parasympathetic *(see also Neuropathy, peripheral, autonomic)* 337.9
    peripheral NEC 355.9
    prion NEC 046.79
    specified NEC 349.89
    sympathetic *(see also Neuropathy, peripheral, autonomic)* 337.9
    vegetative *(see also Neuropathy, peripheral, autonomic)* 337.9
Nettleship's (urticaria pigmentosa) 757.33
Neumann's (pemphigus vegetans) 694.4
neurologic (central) NEC *(see also Disease, nervous system)* 349.9
    peripheral NEC 355.9
neuromuscular system NEC 358.9
Newcastle 077.8
Nicolas (-Durand) -Favre (climatic bubo) 099.1
Niemann-Pick (lipid histiocytosis) 272.7
nipple 611.9
    Paget's (M8540/3) 174.0
Nishimoto (-Takeuchi) 437.5
nonarthropod-borne NEC 078.89
    central nervous system NEC 049.9
    enterovirus NEC 078.89
nonautoimmune hemolytic NEC 283.10
Nonne-Milroy-Meige (chronic hereditary edema) 757.0
Norrie's (congenital progressive oculoacousticocerebral degeneration) 743.8
nose 478.19
nucleus pulposus - *see* Disease, intervertebral disc

Disease, diseased *(Continued)*
nutritional 269.9
    maternal, affecting fetus or newborn 760.4
oasthouse, urine 270.2
obliterative vascular 447.1
Odelberg's (juvenile osteochondrosis) 732.1
Oguchi's (retina) 368.61
Ohara's *(see also Tularemia)* 021.9
Ollier's (chondrodysplasia) 756.4
Opitz's (congestive splenomegaly) 289.51
Oppenheim's 358.8
Oppenheim-Urbach (necrobiosis lipoidica diabeticorum) 250.8● *[709.3]*
    due to secondary diabetes 249.8● *[709.3]*
optic nerve NEC 377.49
orbit 376.9
    specified NEC 376.89
Oriental liver fluke 121.1
Oriental lung fluke 121.2
Ormond's 593.4
Osgood's tibia (tubercle) 732.4
Osgood-Schlatter 732.4
Osler (-Vaquez) (polycythemia vera) (M9950/1) 238.4
Osler-Rendu (familial hemorrhagic telangiectasia) 448.0
osteofibrocystic 252.01
Otto's 715.35
outer ear 380.9
ovary (noninflammatory) NEC 620.9
    cystic 620.2
    polycystic 256.4
    specified NEC 620.8
Owren's (congenital) *(see also Defect, coagulation)* 286.3
Paas' 756.59
Paget's (osteitis deformans) 731.0
    with infiltrating duct carcinoma of the breast (M8541/3) - *see* Neoplasm, breast, malignant
    bone 731.0
        osteosarcoma in (M9184/3) - *see* Neoplasm, bone, malignant
    breast (M8540/3) 174.0
    extramammary (M8542/3) - *see also* Neoplasm, skin, malignant
        anus 154.3
            skin 173.59
    malignant (M8540/3)
        breast 174.0
        specified site NEC (M8542/3) - *see* Neoplasm, skin, malignant
        unspecified site 174.0
    mammary (M8540/3) 174.0
    nipple (M8540/3) 174.0
palate (soft) 528.9
Paltauf-Sternberg 201.9●
pancreas 577.9
    cystic 577.2
        congenital 751.7
    fibrocystic 277.00
Panner's 732.3
    capitellum humeri 732.3
    head of humerus 732.3
    tarsal navicular (bone) (osteochondrosis) 732.5
panvalvular - *see* Endocarditis, mitral
parametrium 629.9
parasitic NEC 136.9
    cerebral NEC 123.9
    intestinal NEC 129
    mouth 112.0
    skin NEC 134.9
    specified type - *see* Infestation
    tongue 112.0
parathyroid (gland) 252.9
    specified NEC 252.8
Parkinson's 332.0
parodontal 523.9
Parrot's (syphilitic osteochondritis) 090.0
Parry's (exophthalmic goiter) 242.0●

Disease, diseased *(Continued)*
Parson's (exophthalmic goiter) 242.0●
Pavy's 593.6
Paxton's (white piedra) 111.2
Payr's (splenic flexure syndrome) 569.89
pearl-workers' (chronic osteomyelitis) *(see also Osteomyelitis)* 730.1●
Pel-Ebstein - *see* Disease, Hodgkin's
Pelizaeus-Merzbacher 330.0
    with dementia
        with behavioral disturbance 330.0 *[294.11]*
        without behavioral disturbance 330.0 *[294.10]*
Pellegrini-Stieda (calcification, knee joint) 726.62
pelvis, pelvic
    female NEC 629.9
        specified NEC 629.89
    gonococcal (acute) 098.19
        chronic or duration of 2 months or over 098.39
    infection *(see also Disease, pelvis, inflammatory)* 614.9
    inflammatory (female) (PID) 614.9
        with
            abortion - *see* Abortion, by type, with sepsis
            ectopic pregnancy *(see also categories 633.0–633.9)* 639.0
            molar pregnancy *(see also categories 630–632)* 639.0
        acute 614.3
        chronic 614.4
        complicating pregnancy 646.6●
            affecting fetus or newborn 760.8
        following
            abortion 639.0
            ectopic or molar pregnancy 639.0
        peritonitis (acute) 614.5
            chronic NEC 614.7
        puerperal, postpartum, childbirth 670.8●
        specified NEC 614.8
    organ, female NEC 629.9
        specified NEC 629.89
    peritoneum, female NEC 629.9
        specified NEC 629.89
penis 607.9
    inflammatory 607.2
peptic NEC 536.9
    acid 536.8
periapical tissues NEC 522.9
pericardium 423.9
    specified type NEC 423.8
perineum
    female
        inflammatory 616.9
            specified NEC 616.89
        noninflammatory 624.9
            specified NEC 624.8
    male (inflammatory) 682.2
periodic (familial) (Reimann's) NEC 277.31
    paralysis 359.3
periodontal NEC 523.9
    specified NEC 523.8
periosteum 733.90
peripheral
    arterial 443.9
    autonomic nervous system *(see also Neuropathy, autonomic)* 337.9
    nerve NEC *(see also Neuropathy)* 356.9
        multiple - *see* Polyneuropathy
    vascular 443.9
        specified type NEC 443.89
peritoneum 568.9
    pelvic, female 629.9
        specified NEC 629.89
Perrin-Ferraton (snapping hip) 719.65

Disease, diseased (*Continued*)

persistent mucosal (middle ear) (with posterior or superior marginal perforation of ear drum) 382.2

Perthes' (capital femoral osteochondrosis) 732.1

Petit's (*see also* Hernia, lumbar) 553.8

Peutz-Jeghers 759.6

Peyronie's 607.85

Pfeiffer's (infectious mononucleosis) 075

pharynx 478.20

Phocas' 610.1

photochromogenic (acid-fast bacilli) (pulmonary) 031.0
    nonpulmonary 031.9

Pick's
    brain 331.11
        with dementia
            with behavioral disturbance 331.11 [294.11]
            without behavioral disturbance 331.11 [294.10]
        cerebral atrophy 331.11
            with dementia
                with behavioral disturbance 331.11 [294.11]
                without behavioral disturbance 331.11 [294.10]
    lipid histiocytosis 272.7
    liver (pericardial pseudocirrhosis of liver) 423.2
    pericardium (pericardial pseudocirrhosis of liver) 423.2
    polyserositis (pericardial pseudocirrhosis of liver) 423.2

Pierson's (osteochondrosis) 732.1

pigeon fanciers' or breeders' 495.2

pineal gland 259.8

pink 985.0

Pinkus' (lichen nitidus) 697.1

pinworm 127.4

pituitary (gland) 253.9
    hyperfunction 253.1
    hypofunction 253.2

pituitary snuff-takers' 495.8

placenta
    affecting fetus or newborn 762.2
    complicating pregnancy or childbirth 656.7 ●

pleura (cavity) (*see also* Pleurisy) 511.0

Plummer's (toxic nodular goiter) 242.3 ●

pneumatic
    drill 994.9
    hammer 994.9

policeman's 729.2

Pollitzer's (hidradenitis suppurativa) 705.83

polycystic (congenital) 759.89
    kidney or renal 753.12
        adult type (APKD) 753.13
        autosomal dominant 753.13
        autosomal recessive 753.14
        childhood type (CPKD) 753.14
        infantile type 753.14
    liver or hepatic 751.62
    lung or pulmonary 518.89
        congenital 748.4
    ovary, ovaries 256.4
    spleen 759.0

polyethylene 996.45

Pompe's (glycogenosis II) 271.0

Poncet's (tuberculous rheumatism) (*see also* Tuberculosis) 015.9 ●

Posada-Wernicke 114.9

Potain's (pulmonary edema) 514

Pott's (*see also* Tuberculosis) 015.0 ● [730.88]
    osteomyelitis 015.0 ● [730.88]
    paraplegia 015.0 ● [730.88]
    spinal curvature 015.0 ● [737.43]
    spondylitis 015.0 ● [720.81]

Potter's 753.0

Poulet's 714.2

Disease, diseased (*Continued*)

pregnancy NEC (*see also* Pregnancy) 646.9 ●

Preiser's (osteoporosis) 733.09

Pringle's (tuberous sclerosis) 759.5

Profichet's 729.90

prostate 602.9
    specified type NEC 602.8

protozoal NEC 136.8
    intestine, intestinal NEC 007.9

pseudo-Hurler's (mucolipidosis III) 272.7

psychiatric (*see also* Psychosis) 298.9

psychotic (*see also* Psychosis) 298.9

Puente's (simple glandular cheilitis) 528.5

puerperal NEC (*see also* Puerperal) 674.9 ●

pulmonary - *see also* Disease, lung
    amyloid 277.39 [517.8]
    artery 417.9
    circulation, circulatory 417.9
        specified NEC 417.8
    diffuse obstructive (chronic) 496
        with
            acute bronchitis 491.22
            asthma (chronic) (obstructive) 493.2 ●
            exacerbation NEC (acute) 491.21
    heart (chronic) 416.9
        specified NEC 416.8
    hypertensive (vascular) 416.0
        cardiovascular 416.0
    obstructive diffuse (chronic) 496
        with
            acute bronchitis 491.22
            asthma (chronic) (obstructive) 493.2 ●
            bronchitis (chronic) 491.20
                with
                    exacerbation (acute) 491.21
                acute 491.22
            exacerbation NEC (acute) 491.21
            decompensated 491.21
                with exacerbation 491.21
    valve (*see also* Endocarditis, pulmonary) 424.3

pulp (dental) NEC 522.9

pulseless 446.7

Putnam's (subacute combined sclerosis with pernicious anemia) 281.0 [336.2]

Pyle (-Cohn) (craniometaphyseal dysplasia) 756.89

pyramidal tract 333.90

Quervain's
    tendon sheath 727.04
    thyroid (subacute granulomatous thyroiditis) 245.1

Quincke's - *see* Edema, angioneurotic

Quinquaud (acne decalvans) 704.09

rag sorters' 022.1

Raynaud's (paroxysmal digital cyanosis) 443.0

reactive airway - *see* Asthma

Recklinghausen's (M9540/1) 237.71
    bone (osteitis fibrosa cystica) 252.01

Recklinghausen-Applebaum (hemochromatosis) (*see also* Hemochromatosis) 275.03

Reclus' (cystic) 610.1

rectum NEC 569.49

Refsum's (heredopathia atactica polyneuritiformis) 356.3

Reichmann's (gastrosuccorrhea) 536.8

Reimann's (periodic) 277.31

Reiter's 099.3

renal (functional) (pelvis) (*see also* Disease, kidney) 593.9
    with
        edema (*see also* Nephrosis) 581.9
        exudative nephritis 583.89
        lesion of interstitial nephritis 583.89
        stated generalized cause - *see* Nephritis
    acute 593.9

Disease, diseased (*Continued*)

renal (*Continued*)
    basement membrane NEC 583.89
        with
            pulmonary hemorrhage (Goodpasture's syndrome) 446.21 [583.81]
    chronic (*see also* Disease, kidney, chronic) 585.9
    complicating pregnancy or puerperium NEC 646.2 ●
        with hypertension - *see* Toxemia, of pregnancy
        affecting fetus or newborn 760.1
    cystic, congenital (*see also* Cystic, disease, kidney) 753.10
    diabetic 250.4 ● [583.81]
        due to secondary diabetes 249.4 ● [581.81]
    due to
        amyloidosis 277.39 [583.81]
        diabetes mellitus 250.4 ● [583.81]
            due to secondary diabetes 249.4 ● [581.81]
        systemic lupus erythematosis 710.0 [583.81]
    end-stage 585.6
    exudative 583.89
    fibrocystic (congenital) 753.19
    gonococcal 098.19 [583.81]
    gouty 274.10
    hypertensive (*see also* Hypertension, kidney) 403.90
    immune complex NEC 583.89
    interstitial (diffuse) (focal) 583.89
    lupus 710.0 [583.81]
    maternal, affecting fetus or newborn 760.1
        hypertensive 760.0
    phosphate-losing (tubular) 588.0
    polycystic (congenital) 753.12
        adult type (APKD) 753.13
        autosomal dominant 753.13
        autosomal recessive 753.14
        childhood type (CPKD) 753.14
        infantile type 753.14
    specified lesion or cause NEC (*see also* Glomerulonephritis) 583.89
    subacute 581.9
    syphilitic 095.4
    tuberculous (*see also* Tuberculosis) 016.0 ● [583.81]
    tubular (*see also* Nephrosis, tubular) 584.5

Rendu-Osler-Weber (familial hemorrhagic telangiectasia) 448.0

renovascular (arteriosclerotic) (*see also* Hypertension, kidney) 403.90

respiratory (tract) 519.9
    acute or subacute (upper) NEC 465.9
        due to fumes or vapors 506.3
        multiple sites NEC 465.8
        noninfectious 478.9
        streptococcal 034.0
    chronic 519.9
        arising in the perinatal period 770.7
        due to fumes or vapors 506.4
    due to
        aspiration of liquids or solids 508.9
        external agents NEC 508.9
            specified NEC 508.8
        fumes or vapors 506.9
            acute or subacute NEC 506.3
            chronic 506.4
    fetus or newborn NEC 770.9
    obstructive 496
    smoke inhalation 508.2
    specified type NEC 519.8
    upper (acute) (infectious) NEC 465.9
        multiple sites NEC 465.8
        noninfectious NEC 478.9
        streptococcal 034.0

◄ New   ◄▦ Revised   ~~deleted~~ Deleted   ● Use Additional Digit(s)   ▨ Omit code

Disease, diseased (Continued)
   retina, retinal NEC 362.9
      Batten's or Batten-Mayou 330.1 [362.71]
      degeneration 362.89
      vascular lesion 362.17
   rheumatic (see also Arthritis) 716.8●
      heart - see Disease, heart, rheumatic
   rheumatoid (heart) - see Arthritis, rheumatoid
   rickettsial NEC 083.9
      specified type NEC 083.8
   Riedel's (ligneous thyroiditis) 245.3
   Riga (-Fede) (cachectic aphthae) 529.0
   Riggs' (compound periodontitis) 523.40
   Ritter's 695.81
   Rivalta's (cervicofacial actinomycosis) 039.3
   Robles' (onchocerciasis) 125.3 [360.13]
   Roger's (congenital interventricular septal
      defect) 745.4
   Rokitansky's (see also Necrosis, liver) 570
   Romberg's 349.89
   Rosenthal's (factor XI deficiency) 286.2
   Rossbach's (hyperchlorhydria) 536.8
      psychogenic 306.4
   Roth (-Bernhardt) 355.1
   Runeberg's (progressive pernicious anemia)
      281.0
   Rust's (tuberculous spondylitis) (see also
      Tuberculosis) 015.0● [720.81]
   Rustitskii's (multiple myeloma) (M9730/3)
      203.0●
   Ruysch's (Hirschsprung's disease) 751.3
   Sachs (-Tay) 330.1
   sacroiliac NEC 724.6
   salivary gland or duct NEC 527.9
      inclusion 078.5
         streptococcal 034.0
      virus 078.5
   Sander's (paranoia) 297.1
   Sandhoff's 330.1
   sandworm 126.9
   Savill's (epidemic exfoliative dermatitis)
      695.89
   Schamberg's (progressive pigmentary
      dermatosis) 709.09
   Schaumann's (sarcoidosis) 135
   Schenck's (sporotrichosis) 117.1
   Scheuermann's (osteochondrosis) 732.0
   Schilder (-Flatau) 341.1
   Schimmelbusch's 610.1
   Schlatter's tibia (tubercle) 732.4
   Schlatter-Osgood 732.4
   Schmorl's 722.30
      cervical 722.39
      lumbar, lumbosacral 722.32
      specified region NEC 722.39
      thoracic, thoracolumbar 722.31
   Scholz's 330.0
   Schönlein (-Henoch) (purpura rheumatica)
      287.0
   Schottmüller's (see also Fever, paratyphoid)
      002.9
   Schüller-Christian (chronic histiocytosis X)
      277.89
   Schultz's (agranulocytosis) 288.09
   Schwalbe-Ziehen-Oppenheimer 333.6
   Schwartz-Jampel 359.23
   Schweninger-Buzzi (macular atrophy) 701.3
   sclera 379.19
   scrofulous (see also Tuberculosis) 017.2●
   scrotum 608.9
   sebaceous glands NEC 706.9
   Secretan's (posttraumatic edema) 782.3
   semilunar cartilage, cystic 717.5
   seminal vesicle 608.9
   Senear-Usher (pemphigus erythematosus)
      694.4
   serum NEC 999.59
   Sever's (osteochondrosis calcaneum) 732.5
   sexually transmitted - see Disease, venereal
   Sézary's (reticulosis) (M9701/3) 202.2●
   Shaver's (bauxite pneumoconiosis) 503

Disease, diseased (Continued)
   Sheehan's (postpartum pituitary necrosis)
      253.2
   shimamushi (scrub typhus) 081.2
   shipyard 077.1
   sickle-cell 282.60
      with
         crisis 282.62
         Hb-S disease 282.61
         other abnormal hemoglobin (Hb-D)
            (Hb-E) (Hb-G) (Hb-J) (Hb-K)
            (Hb-O) (Hb-P) (high fetal gene)
            (without crisis) 282.68
            with crisis 282.69
      elliptocytosis 282.60
      Hb-C (without crisis) 282.63
         with
            crisis 282.64
            vaso-occlusive pain 282.64
      Hb-S 282.61
         with
            crisis 282.62
            Hb-C (without crisis) 282.63
               with
                  crisis 282.64
                  vaso-occlusive pain 282.64
            other abnormal hemoglobin (Hb-D)
               (Hb-E) (Hb-G) (Hb-J) (Hb-K)
               (Hb-O) (Hb-P) (high fetal
               gene) (without crisis) 282.68
               with crisis 282.69
      spherocytosis 282.60
      thalassemia (without crisis) 282.41
         with
            crisis 282.42
            vaso-occlusive pain 282.42
   Siegal-Cattan-Mamou (periodic) 277.31
   silo fillers' 506.9
   Simian B 054.3
   Simmonds' (pituitary cachexia) 253.2
   Simons' (progressive lipodystrophy) 272.6
   Sinding-Larsen (juvenile osteopathia
      patellae) 732.4
   sinus - see also Sinusitis
      brain 437.9
      specified NEC 478.19
   Sirkari's 085.0
   sixth (see also Exanthem subitum) 058.10
   Sjögren (-Gougerot) 710.2
      with lung involvement 710.2 [517.8]
   Skevas-Zerfus 989.5
   skin NEC 709.9
      due to metabolic disorder 277.9
      specified type NEC 709.8
   sleeping (see also Narcolepsy) 347.00
      meaning sleeping sickness (see also
         Trypanosomiasis) 086.5
   small vessel 443.9
   Smith-Strang (oasthouse urine) 270.2
   Sneddon-Wilkinson (subcorneal pustular
      dermatosis) 694.1
   South African creeping 133.8
   Spencer's (epidemic vomiting) 078.82
   Spielmeyer-Stock 330.1
   Spielmeyer-Vogt 330.1
   spine, spinal 733.90
      combined system (see also Degeneration,
         combined) 266.2 [336.2]
         with pernicious anemia 281.0 [336.2]
      cord NEC 336.9
         congenital 742.9
      demyelinating NEC 341.8
      joint (see also Disease, joint, spine) 724.9
         tuberculous 015.0● [730.8]●
      spinocerebellar 334.9
         specified NEC 334.8
   spleen (organic) (postinfectional) 289.50
      amyloid 277.39
      lardaceous 277.39
      polycystic 759.0
      specified NEC 289.59

Disease, diseased (Continued)
   sponge divers' 989.5
   Stanton's (melioidosis) 025
   Stargardt's 362.75
   Startle 759.89
   Steinert's 359.21
   Sternberg's - see Disease, Hodgkin's
   Stevens-Johnson (erythema multiforme
      exudativum) 695.13
   Sticker's (erythema infectiosum) 057.0
   Stieda's (calcification, knee joint) 726.62
   Still's (juvenile rheumatoid arthritis) 714.30
      adult onset 714.2
   Stiller's (asthenia) 780.79
   Stokes' (exophthalmic goiter) 242.0●
   Stokes-Adams (syncope with heart block)
      426.9
   Stokvis (-Talma) (enterogenous cyanosis)
      289.7
   stomach NEC (organic) 537.9
      functional 536.9
         psychogenic 306.4
      lardaceous 277.39
   stonemasons' 502
   storage
      glycogen (see also Disease, glycogen
         storage) 271.0
      lipid 272.7
      mucopolysaccharide 277.5
   striatopallidal system 333.90
      specified NEC 333.89
   Strümpell-Marie (ankylosing spondylitis)
      720.0
   Stuart's (congenital factor X deficiency) (see
      also Defect, coagulation) 286.3
   Stuart-Prower (congenital factor X
      deficiency) (see also Defect,
      coagulation) 286.3
   Sturge (-Weber) (-Dimitri)
      (encephalocutaneous angiomatosis)
      759.6
   Stuttgart 100.89
   Sudeck's 733.7
   supporting structures of teeth NEC 525.9
   suprarenal (gland) (capsule) 255.9
      hyperfunction 255.3
      hypofunction 255.41
   Sutton's 709.09
   Sutton and Gull's - see Hypertension, kidney
   sweat glands NEC 705.9
      specified type NEC 705.89
   sweating 078.2
   Sweeley-Klionsky 272.7
   Swift (-Feer) 985.0
   swimming pool (bacillus) 031.1
   swineherd's 100.89
   Sylvest's (epidemic pleurodynia) 074.1
   Symmers (follicular lymphoma) (M9690/3)
      202.0●
   sympathetic nervous system (see also
      Neuropathy, peripheral, autonomic)
      337.9
   synovium 727.9
   syphilitic - see Syphilis
   systemic tissue mast cell (M9741/3) 202.6●
   Taenzer's 757.4
   Takayasu's (pulseless) 446.7
   Talma's 728.85
   Tangier (familial high-density lipoprotein
      deficiency) 272.5
   Tarral-Besnier (pityriasis rubra pilaris) 696.4
   Tay-Sachs 330.1
   Taylor's 701.8
   tear duct 375.69
   teeth, tooth 525.9
      hard tissues 521.9
         specified NEC 521.89
      pulp NEC 522.9
   tendon 727.9
      inflammatory NEC 727.9
   terminal vessel 443.9

Disease, diseased *(Continued)*
testis 608.9
Thaysen-Gee (nontropical sprue) 579.0
Thomsen's 359.22
Thomson's (congenital poikiloderma) 757.33
Thornwaldt's, Tornwaldt's (pharyngeal
bursitis) 478.29
throat 478.20
septic 034.0
thromboembolic *(see also* Embolism) 444.9
thymus (gland) 254.9
specified NEC 254.8
thyroid (gland) NEC 246.9
heart *(see also* Hyperthyroidism) 242.9●
[425.7]
lardaceous 277.39
specified NEC 246.8
Tietze's 733.6
Tommaselli's
correct substance properly administered
599.70
overdose or wrong substance given or
taken 961.4
tongue 529.9
tonsils, tonsillar (and adenoids) (chronic)
474.9
specified NEC 474.8
tooth, teeth 525.9
hard tissues 521.9
specified NEC 521.89
pulp NEC 522.9
Tornwaldt's (pharyngeal bursitis) 478.29
Tourette's 307.23
trachea 519.19
tricuspid - *see* Endocarditis, tricuspid
triglyceride-storage, type I, II, III 272.7
triple vessel - *see* Arteriosclerosis, coronary
trisymptomatic, Gougerot's 709.1
trophoblastic *(see also* Hydatidiform mole)
630
previous, affecting management of
pregnancy V23.1
tsutsugamushi (scrub typhus) 081.2
tube (fallopian), noninflammatory 620.9
specified NEC 620.8
tuberculous NEC *(see also* Tuberculosis)
011.9●
tubo-ovarian
inflammatory *(see also* Salpingo-
oophoritis) 614.2
noninflammatory 620.9
specified NEC 620.8
tubotympanic, chronic (with anterior
perforation of ear drum) 382.1
tympanum 385.9
Uhl's 746.84
umbilicus (newborn) NEC 779.89
delayed separation 779.83
Underwood's (sclerema neonatorum) 778.1
undiagnosed 799.9
Unna's (seborrheic dermatitis) 690.18
unstable hemoglobin hemolytic 282.7
Unverricht (-Lundborg) 345.1●
Urbach-Oppenheim (necrobiosis lipoidica
diabeticorum) 250.8● *[709.3]*
due to secondary diabetes 249.8● *[709.3]*
Urbach-Wiethe (lipoid proteinosis) 272.8
ureter 593.9
urethra 599.9
specified type NEC 599.84
urinary (tract) 599.9
bladder 596.9
specified NEC 596.89
maternal, affecting fetus or newborn 760.1
Usher-Senear (pemphigus erythematosus)
694.4
uterus (organic) 621.9
infective *(see also* Endometritis) 615.9
inflammatory *(see also* Endometritis) 615.9
noninflammatory 621.9
specified type NEC 621.8

Disease, diseased *(Continued)*
uveal tract
anterior 364.9
posterior 363.9
vagabonds' 132.1
vagina, vaginal
inflammatory 616.10
noninflammatory 623.9
specified NEC 623.8
Valsuani's (progressive pernicious anemia,
puerperal) 648.2●
complicating pregnancy or puerperium
648.2●
valve, valvular - *see also* Endocarditis
congenital NEC *(see also* Anomaly, heart,
valve) 746.9
pulmonary 746.00
specified type NEC 746.89
van Bogaert-Nijssen (-Peiffer) 330.0
van Creveld-von Gierke (glycogenosis I)
271.0
van den Bergh's (enterogenous cyanosis)
289.7
van Neck's (juvenile osteochondrosis) 732.1
Vaquez (-Osler) (polycythemia vera)
(M9950/1) 238.4
vascular 459.9
arteriosclerotic - *see* Arteriosclerosis
hypertensive - *see* Hypertension
obliterative 447.1
peripheral 443.9
occlusive 459.9
peripheral (occlusive) 443.9
in (due to) (with) diabetes mellitus
250.7● *[443.81]*
in (due to) (with) secondary
diabetes 249.7● *[443.81]*
specified type NEC 443.89
vas deferens 608.9
vasomotor 443.9
vasospastic 443.9
vein 459.9
venereal 099.9
chlamydial NEC 099.50
anus 099.52
bladder 099.53
cervix 099.53
epididymis 099.54
genitourinary NEC 099.55
lower 099.53
specified NEC 099.54
pelvic inflammatory disease 099.54
perihepatic 099.56
peritoneum 099.56
pharynx 099.51
rectum 099.52
specified site NEC 099.59
testis 099.54
vagina 099.53
vulva 099.53
fifth 099.1
sixth 099.1
complicating pregnancy, childbirth, or
puerperium 647.2●
specified nature or type NEC 099.8
chlamydial - *see* Disease, venereal,
chlamydial
Verneuil's (syphilitic bursitis) 095.7
Verse's (calcinosis intervertebralis) 275.49
[722.90]
vertebra, vertebral NEC 733.90
disc - *see* Disease, Intervertebral disc
vibration NEC 994.9
Vidal's (lichen simplex chronicus) 698.3
Vincent's (trench mouth) 101
Virchow's 733.99
virus (filterable) NEC 078.89
arbovirus NEC 066.9
arthropod-borne NEC 066.9
central nervous system NEC 049.9
specified type NEC 049.8

Disease, diseased *(Continued)*
virus NEC *(Continued)*
complicating pregnancy, childbirth, or
puerperium 647.6●
contact (with) V01.79
varicella V01.71
exposure to V01.79
varicella V01.71
Marburg 078.89
maternal
with fetal damage affecting
management of pregnancy
655.3●
nonarthropod-borne NEC 078.89
central nervous system NEC 049.9
specified NEC 049.8
vaccination, prophylactic (against) V04.89
vitreous 379.29
vocal cords NEC 478.5
Vogt's (Cecile) 333.71
Vogt-Spielmeyer 330.1
Volhard-Fahr (malignant nephrosclerosis)
403.00
Volkmann's
acquired 958.6
von Bechterew's (ankylosing spondylitis)
720.0
von Economo's (encephalitis lethargica)
049.8
von Eulenburg's (congenital paramyotonia)
359.29
von Gierke's (glycogenosis I) 271.0
von Graefe's 378.72
von Hippel's (retinocerebral angiomatosis)
759.6
von Hippel-Lindau (angiomatosis
retinocerebellosa) 759.6
von Jaksch's (pseudoleukemia infantum)
285.8
von Recklinghausen's (M9540/1) 237.71
bone (osteitis fibrosa cystica) 252.01
von Recklinghausen-Applebaum
(hemochromatosis) *(see also*
Hemochromatosis) 275.03
von Willebrand (-Jürgens) (angiohemophilia)
286.4
von Zambusch's (lichen sclerosus et
atrophicus) 701.0
Voorhoeve's (dyschondroplasia) 756.4
Vrolik's (osteogenesis imperfecta) 756.51
vulva
inflammatory 616.10
noninflammatory 624.9
specified NEC 624.8
Wagner's (colloid milium) 709.3
Waldenström's (osteochondrosis capital
femoral) 732.1
Wallgren's (obstruction of splenic vein with
collateral circulation) 459.89
Wardrop's (with lymphangitis) 681.9
finger 681.02
toe 681.11
Wassilieff's (leptospiral jaundice) 100.0
wasting NEC 799.4
due to malnutrition 261
paralysis 335.21
Waterhouse-Friderichsen 036.3
waxy (any site) 277.39
Weber-Christian (nodular nonsuppurative
panniculitis) 729.30
Wegner's (syphilitic osteochondritis) 090.0
Weil's (leptospiral jaundice) 100.0
of lung 100.0
Weir Mitchell's (erythromelalgia) 443.82
Werdnig-Hoffmann 335.0
Werlhof's *(see also* Purpura,
thrombocytopenic) 287.39
Werner's 258.01
Werner's (progeria adultorum) 259.8
Werner-His (trench fever) 083.1
Werner-Schultz (agranulocytosis) 288.09

◀ New   ◀▥ Revised   ~~deleted~~ Deleted   ● Use Additional Digit(s)   ▨ Omit code

Disease, diseased *(Continued)*
Wernicke's (superior hemorrhagic polioencephalitis) 265.1
Wernicke-Posadas 114.9
Whipple's (intestinal lipodystrophy) 040.2
whipworm 127.3
white
blood cell 288.9
specified NEC 288.8
spot 701.0
White's (congenital) (keratosis follicularis) 757.39
Whitmore's (melioidosis) 025
Widal-Abrami (acquired hemolytic jaundice) 283.9
Wilkie's 557.1
Wilkinson-Sneddon (subcorneal pustular dermatosis) 694.1
Willis' (diabetes mellitus) *(see also* Diabetes) 250.0●
due to secondary diabetes 249.0●
Wilson's (hepatolenticular degeneration) 275.1
Wilson-Brocq (dermatitis exfoliativa) 695.89
winter vomiting 078.82
Wise's 696.2
Wohlfart-Kugelberg-Welander 335.11
Woillez's (acute idiopathic pulmonary congestion) 518.52
Wolman's (primary familial xanthomatosis) 272.7
wool-sorters' 022.1
Zagari's (xerostomia) 527.7
Zahorsky's (exanthem subitum) 058.10
Ziehen-Oppenheim 333.6
zoonotic, bacterial NEC 027.9
specified type NEC 027.8
Disfigurement (due to scar) 709.2
head V48.6
limb V49.4
neck V48.7
trunk V48.7
Disgerminoma - *see* Dysgerminoma
Disinsertion, retina 361.04
Disintegration, complete, of the body 799.89
traumatic 869.1
Disk kidney 753.3
Dislocatable hip, congenital *(see also* Dislocation, hip, congenital) 754.30
Dislocation (articulation) (closed) (displacement) (simple) (subluxation) 839.8

> **Note:**
>
> "Closed" includes simple, complete, partial, uncomplicated, and unspecified dislocation.
>
> "Open" includes dislocation specified as infected or compound and dislocation with foreign body.
>
> "Chronic," "habitual," "old," or "recurrent" dislocations should be coded as indicated under the entry "Dislocation, recurrent"; and "pathological" as indicated under the entry "Dislocation, pathological."
>
> For late effect of dislocation *see* Late, effect, dislocation.

with fracture - *see* Fracture, by site
acromioclavicular (joint) (closed) 831.04
open 831.14
anatomical site (closed)
specified NEC 839.69
open 839.79
unspecified or ill-defined 839.8
open 839.9
ankle (scaphoid bone) (closed) 837.0
open 837.1

Dislocation *(Continued)*
arm (closed) 839.8
open 839.9
astragalus (closed) 837.0
open 837.1
atlanto-axial (closed) 839.01
open 839.11
atlas (closed) 839.01
open 839.11
axis (closed) 839.02
open 839.12
back (closed) 839.8
open 839.9
Bell-Daly 723.8
breast bone (closed) 839.61
open 839.71
capsule, joint - *see* Dislocation, by site
carpal (bone) - *see* Dislocation, wrist
carpometacarpal (joint) (closed) 833.04
open 833.14
cartilage (joint) - *see also* Dislocation, by site
knee - *see* Tear, meniscus
cervical, cervicodorsal, or cervicothoracic (spine) (vertebra) - *see* Dislocation, vertebra, cervical
chiropractic *(see also* Lesion, nonallopathic) 739.9
chondrocostal - *see* Dislocation, costochondral
chronic - *see* Dislocation, recurrent
clavicle (closed) 831.04
open 831.14
coccyx (closed) 839.41
open 839.51
collar bone (closed) 831.04
open 831.14
compound (open) NEC 839.9
congenital NEC 755.8
hip *(see also* Dislocation, hip, congenital) 754.30
lens 743.37
rib 756.3
sacroiliac 755.69
spine NEC 756.19
vertebra 756.19
coracoid (closed) 831.09
open 831.19
costal cartilage (closed) 839.69
open 839.79
costochondral (closed) 839.69
open 839.79
cricoarytenoid articulation (closed) 839.69
open 839.79
cricothyroid (cartilage) articulation (closed) 839.69
open 839.79
dorsal vertebrae (closed) 839.21
open 839.31
ear ossicle 385.23
elbow (closed) 832.00
anterior (closed) 832.01
open 832.11
congenital 754.89
divergent (closed) 832.09
open 832.19
lateral (closed) 832.04
open 832.14
medial (closed) 832.03
open 832.13
open 832.10
posterior (closed) 832.02
open 832.12
recurrent 718.32
specified type NEC 832.09
open 832.19
eye 360.81
lateral 376.36
eyeball 360.81
lateral 376.36

Dislocation *(Continued)*
femur
distal end (closed) 836.50
anterior 836.52
open 836.62
lateral 836.54
open 836.64
medial 836.53
open 836.63
open 836.60
posterior 836.51
open 836.61
proximal end (closed) 835.00
anterior (pubic) 835.03
open 835.13
obturator 835.02
open 835.12
open 835.10
posterior 835.01
open 835.11
fibula
distal end (closed) 837.0
open 837.1
proximal end (closed) 836.59
open 836.69
finger(s) (phalanx) (thumb) (closed) 834.00
interphalangeal (joint) 834.02
open 834.12
metacarpal (bone), distal end 834.01
open 834.11
metacarpophalangeal (joint) 834.01
open 834.11
open 834.10
recurrent 718.34
foot (closed) 838.00
open 838.10
recurrent 718.37
forearm (closed) 839.8
open 839.9
fracture - *see* Fracture, by site
glenoid (closed) 831.09
open 831.19
habitual - *see* Dislocation, recurrent
hand (closed) 839.8
open 839.9
hip (closed) 835.00
anterior 835.03
obturator 835.02
open 835.12
open 835.13
congenital (unilateral) 754.30
with subluxation of other hip 754.35
bilateral 754.31
developmental 718.75
open 835.10
posterior 835.01
open 835.11
recurrent 718.35
humerus (closed) 831.00
distal end *(see also* Dislocation, elbow) 832.00
open 831.10
proximal end (closed) 831.00
anterior (subclavicular) (subcoracoid) (subglenoid) (closed) 831.01
open 831.11
inferior (closed) 831.03
open 831.13
open 831.10
posterior (closed) 831.02
open 831.12
implant - *see* Complications, mechanical
incus 385.23
infracoracoid (closed) 831.01
open 831.11
innominate (pubic junction) (sacral junction) (closed) 839.69
acetabulum *(see also* Dislocation, hip) 835.00
open 839.79

Dislocation *(Continued)*
  interphalangeal (joint)
    finger or hand (closed) 834.02
      open 834.12
    foot or toe (closed) 838.06
      open 838.16
  jaw (cartilage) (meniscus) (closed) 830.0
    open 830.1
    recurrent 524.69
  joint NEC (closed) 839.8
    developmental 718.7●
    open 839.9
    pathological - *see* Dislocation, pathological
    recurrent - *see* Dislocation, recurrent
  knee (closed) 836.50
    anterior 836.51
      open 836.61
    congenital (with genu recurvatum) 754.41
    habitual 718.36
    lateral 836.54
      open 836.64
    medial 836.53
      open 836.63
    old 718.36
    open 836.60
    posterior 836.52
      open 836.62
    recurrent 718.36
    rotatory 836.59
      open 836.69
  lacrimal gland 375.16
  leg (closed) 839.8
    open 839.9
  lens (crystalline) (complete) (partial) 379.32
    anterior 379.33
    congenital 743.37
    ocular implant 996.53
    posterior 379.34
    traumatic 921.3
  ligament - *see* Dislocation, by site
  lumbar (vertebrae) (closed) 839.20
    open 839.30
  lumbosacral (vertebrae) (closed) 839.20
    congenital 756.19
    open 839.30
  mandible (closed) 830.0
    open 830.1
  maxilla (inferior) (closed) 830.0
    open 830.1
  meniscus (knee) - *see also* Tear, meniscus
    other sites - *see* Dislocation, by site
  metacarpal (bone)
    distal end (closed) 834.01
      open 834.11
    proximal end (closed) 833.05
      open 833.15
  metacarpophalangeal (joint) (closed) 834.01
    open 834.11
  metatarsal (bone) (closed) 838.04
    open 838.14
  metatarsophalangeal (joint) (closed) 838.05
    open 838.15
  midcarpal (joint) (closed) 833.03
    open 833.13
  midtarsal (joint) (closed) 838.02
    open 838.12
  Monteggia's - *see* Dislocation, hip
  multiple locations (except fingers only or toes only) (closed) 839.8
    open 839.9
  navicular (bone) foot (closed) 837.0
    open 837.1
  neck (*see also* Dislocation, vertebra, cervical) 839.00
  Nélaton's - *see* Dislocation, ankle
  nontraumatic (joint) - *see* Dislocation, pathological
  nose (closed) 839.69
    open 839.79
  not recurrent, not current injury - *see* Dislocation, pathological

Dislocation *(Continued)*
  occiput from atlas (closed) 839.01
    open 839.11
  old - *see* Dislocation, recurrent
  open (compound) NEC 839.9
  ossicle, ear 385.23
  paralytic (flaccid) (spastic) - *see* Dislocation, pathological
  patella (closed) 836.3
    congenital 755.64
    open 836.4
  pathological NEC 718.20
    ankle 718.27
    elbow 718.22
    foot 718.27
    hand 718.24
    hip 718.25
    knee 718.26
    lumbosacral joint 724.6
    multiple sites 718.29
    pelvic region 718.25
    sacroiliac 724.6
    shoulder (region) 718.21
    specified site NEC 718.28
    spine 724.8
      sacroiliac 724.6
    wrist 718.23
  pelvis (closed) 839.69
    acetabulum (*see also* Dislocation, hip) 835.00
    open 839.79
  phalanx
    foot or toe (closed) 838.09
      open 838.19
    hand or finger (*see also* Dislocation, finger) 834.00
  postpoliomyelitic - *see* Dislocation, pathological
  prosthesis, internal - *see* Complications, mechanical
  radiocarpal (joint) (closed) 833.02
    open 833.12
  radioulnar (joint)
    distal end (closed) 833.01
      open 833.11
    proximal end (*see also* Dislocation, elbow) 832.00
  radius
    distal end (closed) 833.00
      open 833.10
    proximal end (closed) 832.01
      open 832.11
  recurrent (*see also* Derangement, joint, recurrent) 718.3●
    elbow 718.32
    hip 718.35
    joint NEC 718.38
    knee 718.36
    lumbosacral (joint) 724.6
    patella 718.36
    sacroiliac 724.6
    shoulder 718.31
    temporomandibular 524.69
  rib (cartilage) (closed) 839.69
    congenital 756.3
    open 839.79
  sacrococcygeal (closed) 839.42
    open 839.52
  sacroiliac (joint) (ligament) (closed) 839.42
    congenital 755.69
    open 839.52
    recurrent 724.6
  sacrum (closed) 839.42
    open 839.52
  scaphoid (bone)
    ankle or foot (closed) 837.0
      open 837.1
    wrist (closed) (*see also* Dislocation, wrist) 833.00
      open 833.10

Dislocation *(Continued)*
  scapula (closed) 831.09
    open 831.19
  semilunar cartilage, knee - *see* Tear, meniscus
  septal cartilage (nose) (closed) 839.69
    open 839.79
  septum (nasal) (old) 470
  sesamoid bone - *see* Dislocation, by site
  shoulder (blade) (ligament) (closed) 831.00
    anterior (subclavicular) (subcoracoid) (subglenoid) (closed) 831.01
      open 831.11
    chronic 718.31
    inferior 831.03
      open 831.13
    open 831.10
    posterior (closed) 831.02
      open 831.12
    recurrent 718.31
  skull - *see* Injury, intracranial
  Smith's - *see* Dislocation, foot
  spine (articular process) (*see also* Dislocation, vertebra) (closed) 839.40
    atlanto-axial (closed) 839.01
      open 839.11
      recurrent 723.8
    cervical, cervicodorsal, cervicothoracic (closed) (*see also* Dislocation, vertebrae, cervical) 839.00
      open 839.10
      recurrent 723.8
    coccyx 839.41
      open 839.51
    congenital 756.19
    due to birth trauma 767.4
    open 839.50
    recurrent 724.9
    sacroiliac 839.42
      recurrent 724.6
    sacrum (sacrococcygeal) (sacroiliac) 839.42
      open 839.52
  spontaneous - *see* Dislocation, pathological
  sternoclavicular (joint) (closed) 839.61
    open 839.71
  sternum (closed) 839.61
    open 839.71
  subastragalar - *see* Dislocation, foot
  subglenoid (closed) 831.01
    open 831.11
  symphysis
    jaw (closed) 830.0
      open 830.1
    mandibular (closed) 830.0
      open 830.1
    pubis (closed) 839.69
      open 839.79
  tarsal (bone) (joint) 838.01
    open 838.11
  tarsometatarsal (joint) 838.03
    open 838.13
  temporomandibular (joint) (closed) 830.0
    open 830.1
    recurrent 524.69
  thigh
    distal end (*see also* Dislocation, femur, distal end) 836.50
    proximal end (*see also* Dislocation, hip) 835.00
  thoracic (vertebrae) (closed) 839.21
    open 839.31
  thumb(s) (*see also* Dislocation, finger) 834.00
  thyroid cartilage (closed) 839.69
    open 839.79
  tibia
    distal end (closed) 837.0
      open 837.1

◀ New   ◀◀ Revised   ~~deleted~~ Deleted   ● Use Additional Digit(s)   Omit code

Dislocation (Continued)

tibia (Continued)

proximal end (closed) 836.50

anterior 836.51

open 836.61

lateral 836.54

open 836.64

medial 836.53

open 836.63

open 836.60

posterior 836.52

open 836.62

rotatory 836.59

open 836.69

tibiofibular

distal (closed) 837.0

open 837.1

superior (closed) 836.59

open 836.69

toe(s) (closed) 838.09

open 838.19

trachea (closed) 839.69

open 839.79

ulna

distal end (closed) 833.09

open 833.19

proximal end - see Dislocation, elbow

vertebra (articular process) (body) (closed)

(traumatic) 839.40

cervical, cervicodorsal or cervicothoracic

(closed) 839.00

first (atlas) 839.01

open 839.11

second (axis) 839.02

open 839.12

third 839.03

open 839.13

fourth 839.04

open 839.14

fifth 839.05

open 839.15

sixth 839.06

open 839.16

seventh 839.07

open 839.17

congenital 756.19

multiple sites 839.08

open 839.18

open 839.10

congenital 756.19

dorsal 839.21

open 839.31

recurrent 724.9

lumbar, lumbosacral 839.20

open 839.30

non-traumatic - see Displacement,

intervertebral disc

open NEC 839.50

recurrent 724.9

specified region NEC 839.49

open 839.59

thoracic 839.21

open 839.31

wrist (carpal bone) (scaphoid) (semilunar)

(closed) 833.00

carpometacarpal (joint) 833.04

open 833.14

metacarpal bone, proximal end 833.05

open 833.15

midcarpal (joint) 833.03

open 833.13

open 833.10

radiocarpal (joint) 833.02

open 833.12

radioulnar (joint) 833.01

open 833.11

recurrent 718.33

specified site NEC 833.09

open 833.19

xiphoid cartilage (closed) 839.61

open 839.71

Dislodgement

artificial skin graft 996.55

decellularized allodermis graft 996.55

Disobedience, hostile (covert) (overt) (see also

Disturbance, conduct) 312.0 ●

Disorder - see also Disease

academic underachievement, childhood and

adolescence 313.83

accommodation 367.51

drug-induced 367.89

toxic 367.89

adjustment (see also Reaction, adjustment)

309.9

with

anxiety 309.24

anxiety and depressed mood 309.28

depressed mood 309.0

disturbance of conduct 309.3

disturbance of emotions and conduct

309.4

adrenal (capsule) (cortex) (gland) 255.9

specified type NEC 255.8

adrenogenital 255.2

affective (see also Psychosis, affective) 296.90

atypical 296.81

aggressive, unsocialized (see also

Disturbance, conduct) 312.0 ●

alcohol, alcoholic (see also Alcohol) 291.9

induced mood 291.89

allergic - see Allergy

amino acid (metabolic) (see also Disturbance,

metabolism, amino acid) 270.9

albinism 270.2

alkaptonuria 270.2

argininosuccinicaciduria 270.6

beta-amino-isobutyricaciduria 277.2

cystathioninuria 270.4

cystinosis 270.0

cystinuria 270.0

glycinuria 270.0

homocystinuria 270.4

imidazole 270.5

maple syrup (urine) disease 270.3

neonatal, transitory 775.89

oasthouse urine disease 270.2

ochronosis 270.2

phenylketonuria 270.1

phenylpyruvic oligophrenia 270.1

purine NEC 277.2

pyrimidine NEC 277.2

renal transport NEC 270.0

specified type NEC 270.8

transport NEC 270.0

renal 270.0

xanthinuria 277.2

amnestic (see also Amnestic syndrome) 294.8

alcohol-induced persisting 291.1

drug-induced persisting 292.83

in conditions classified elsewhere 294.0

anaerobic glycolysis with anemia 282.3

anxiety (see also Anxiety) 300.00

due to or associated with physical

condition 293.84

arteriole 447.9

specified type NEC 447.8

artery 447.9

specified type NEC 447.8

articulation - see Disorder, joint

Asperger's 299.8 ●

attachment of infancy or early childhood

313.89

attention deficit 314.00

with hyperactivity 314.01

predominantly

combined hyperactive/inattentive 314.01

hyperactive/impulsive 314.01

inattentive 314.00

residual type 314.8

auditory processing disorder 388.45

acquired 388.45

developmental 315.32

Disorder (Continued)

autistic 299.0 ●

autoimmune NEC 279.49

hemolytic (cold type) (warm type) 283.0

parathyroid 252.1

thyroid 245.2

avoidant, childhood or adolescence 313.21

balance

acid-base 276.9

mixed (with hypercapnia) 276.4

electrolyte 276.9

fluid 276.9

behavior NEC (see also Disturbance, conduct)

312.9

disruptive 312.9

bilirubin excretion 277.4

bipolar (affective) (alternating) 296.80

Note: Use the following fifth-digit
subclassification with categories 296.0–296.6:

0   unspecified
1   mild
2   moderate
3   severe, without mention of psychotic
    behavior
4   severe, specified as with psychotic
    behavior
5   in partial or unspecified remission
6   in full remission

atypical 296.7

specified type NEC 296.89

type I 296.7

most recent episode (or current)

depressed 296.5 ●

hypomanic 296.4 ●

manic 296.4 ●

mixed 296.6 ●

unspecified 296.7

single manic episode 296.0 ●

type II (recurrent major depressive

episodes with hypomania) 296.89

bladder 596.9

functional NEC 596.59

specified NEC 596.89

bleeding 286.9

bone NEC 733.90

specified NEC 733.99

brachial plexus 353.0

branched-chain amino-acid degradation

270.3

breast 611.9

puerperal, postpartum 676.3 ●

specified NEC 611.89

Briquet's 300.81

bursa 727.9

shoulder region 726.10

carbohydrate metabolism, congenital 271.9

cardiac, functional 427.9

postoperative 997.1

psychogenic 306.2

cardiovascular, psychogenic 306.2

cartilage NEC 733.90

articular 718.00

ankle 718.07

elbow 718.02

foot 718.07

hand 718.04

hip 718.05

knee 717.9

multiple sites 718.09

pelvic region 718.05

shoulder region 718.01

specified

site NEC 718.08

type NEC 733.99

wrist 718.03

catatonic - see Catatonia

central auditory processing 315.32

acquired 388.45

developmental 315.32

Disorder (Continued)
  cervical region NEC 723.9
  cervical root (nerve) NEC 353.2
  character NEC (see also Disorder, personality)
      301.9
  ciliary body 364.9
    specified NEC 364.89
  coagulation (factor) (see also Defect,
      coagulation) 286.9
    factor VIII (congenital) (functional) 286.0
    factor IX (congenital) (functional) 286.1
    neonatal, transitory 776.3
  coccyx 724.70
    specified NEC 724.79
  cognitive 294.9
  colon 569.9
    functional 564.9
      congenital 751.3
  communication 307.9
  conduct (see also Disturbance, conduct) 312.9
    adjustment reaction 309.3
    adolescent onset type 312.82
    childhood onset type 312.81
    compulsive 312.30
      specified type NEC 312.39
    hyperkinetic 314.2
    onset unspecified 312.89
    socialized (type) 312.20
      aggressive 312.23
      unaggressive 312.21
    specified NEC 312.89
  conduction, heart 426.9
    specified NEC 426.89
  conflict
    sexual orientation 302.0
  congenital
    glycosylation (CDG) 271.8
  convulsive (secondary) (see also Convulsions)
      780.39
    due to injury at birth 767.0
    idiopathic 780.39
  coordination 781.3
  cornea NEC 371.89
    due to contact lens 371.82
  corticosteroid metabolism NEC 255.2
  cranial nerve - see Disorder, nerve, cranial
  cyclothymic 301.13
  degradation, branched-chain amino acid
      270.3
  delusional 297.1
  dentition 520.6
  depersonalization 300.6
  depressive NEC 311
    atypical 296.82
    major (see also Psychosis, affective) 296.2●
      recurrent episode 296.3●
      single episode 296.2●
  development, specific 315.9
    associated with hyperkinesia 314.1
    coordination 315.4
    language 315.31
      and speech due to hearing loss 315.34
    learning 315.2
      arithmetical 315.1
      reading 315.00
    mixed 315.5
    motor coordination 315.4
    specified type NEC 315.8
    speech 315.39
      and language due to hearing loss
          315.34
  diaphragm 519.4
  digestive 536.9
    fetus or newborn 777.9
      specified NEC 777.8
    psychogenic 306.4
  disintegrative childhood 299.1●
  dissociative 300.15
    identity 300.14
    nocturnal 307.47
  drug-related 292.9

Disorder (Continued)
  dysmorphic body 300.7
  dysthymic 300.4
  ear 388.9
    degenerative NEC 388.00
    external 380.9
      specified 380.89
    pinna 380.30
    specified type NEC 388.8
    vascular NEC 388.00
  eating NEC 307.50
  electrolyte NEC 276.9
    with
      abortion - see Abortion, by type, with
          metabolic disorder
      ectopic pregnancy (see also categories
          633.0–633.9) 639.4
      molar pregnancy (see also categories
          630–632) 639.4
    acidosis 276.2
      metabolic 276.2
      respiratory 276.2
    alkalosis 276.3
      metabolic 276.3
      respiratory 276.3
    following
      abortion 639.4
      ectopic or molar pregnancy 639.4
    neonatal, transitory NEC 775.5
  emancipation as adjustment reaction 309.22
  emotional (see also Disorder, mental,
      nonpsychotic) V40.9
  endocrine 259.9
    specified type NEC 259.8
  esophagus 530.9
    functional 530.5
    psychogenic 306.4
  explosive
    intermittent 312.34
    isolated 312.35
  expressive language 315.31
  eye 379.90
    globe - see Disorder, globe
    ill-defined NEC 379.99
    limited duction NEC 378.63
    specified NEC 379.8
  eyelid 374.9
    degenerative 374.50
    sensory 374.44
    specified type NEC 374.89
    vascular 374.85
  factitious (with combined psychological and
      physical signs and symptoms) (with
      predominantly physical signs and
      symptoms) 300.19
    with predominantly psychological signs
        and symptoms 300.16
  factor, coagulation (see also Defect,
      coagulation) 286.9
    VIII (congenital) (functional) 286.0
    IX (congenital) (functional) 286.1
  fascia 728.9
  fatty acid oxidation 277.85
  feeding - see Feeding
  female sexual arousal 302.72
  fluency 315.35
    adult onset 307.0
    childhood onset 315.35
    due to late effect of cerebrovascular
        accident 438.14
    in conditions classified elsewhere
        784.52
  fluid NEC 276.9
  gastric (functional) 536.9
    motility 536.8
    psychogenic 306.4
    secretion 536.8
  gastrointestinal (functional) NEC 536.9
    newborn (neonatal) 777.9
      specified NEC 777.8
    psychogenic 306.4

Disorder (Continued)
  gender (child) 302.6
    adult 302.85
  gender identity (childhood) 302.6
    adolescents 302.85
    adults (-life) 302.85
  genitourinary system, psychogenic 306.50
  globe 360.9
    degenerative 360.20
      specified NEC 360.29
    specified type NEC 360.89
  hearing - see also Deafness
    conductive type (air) (see also Deafness,
        conductive) 389.00
    mixed conductive and sensorineural
        389.20
      bilateral 389.22
      unilateral 389.21
    nerve
      bilateral 389.12
      unilateral 389.13
    perceptive (see also Deafness, perceptive)
        389.10
    sensorineural type NEC (see also Deafness,
        sensorineural) 389.10
  heart action 427.9
    postoperative 997.1
  hematological, transient neonatal 776.9
    specified type NEC 776.8
  hematopoietic organs 289.9
  hemorrhagic NEC 287.9
    due to intrinsic circulating anticoagulants,
        antibodies, or inhibitors 286.59
      with
        acquired hemophilia 286.52
        antiphospholipid antibody 286.53
    specified type NEC 287.8
  hemostasis (see also Defect, coagulation)
      286.9
  homosexual conflict 302.0
  hypomanic (chronic) 301.11
  identity
    childhood and adolescence 313.82
      gender 302.6
  immune mechanism (immunity) 279.9
    single complement (C_1–C_9) 279.8
    specified type NEC 279.8
  impulse control (see also Disturbance,
      conduct, compulsive) 312.30
  infant sialic acid storage 271.8
  integument, fetus or newborn 778.9
    specified type NEC 778.8
  interactional psychotic (childhood) (see also
      Psychosis, childhood) 299.1●
  intermittent explosive 312.34
  intervertebral disc 722.90
    cervical, cervicothoracic 722.91
    lumbar, lumbosacral 722.93
    thoracic, thoracolumbar 722.92
  intestinal 569.9
    functional NEC 564.9
      congenital 751.3
      postoperative 564.4
    psychogenic 306.4
  introverted, of childhood and adolescence
      313.22
  involuntary emotional expression (IEED)
      310.81
  iris 364.9
    specified NEC 364.89
  iron, metabolism 275.09
    specified type NEC 275.09
  isolated explosive 312.35
  joint NEC 719.90
    ankle 719.97
    elbow 719.92
    foot 719.97
    hand 719.94
    hip 719.95
    knee 719.96
    multiple sites 719.99

◀ New   ◀▦ Revised   ~~deleted~~ Deleted   ● Use Additional Digit(s)   ▦ Omit code

Disorder *(Continued)*
    joint NEC *(Continued)*
        pelvic region 719.95
        psychogenic 306.0
        shoulder (region) 719.91
        specified site NEC 719.98
        temporomandibular 524.60
            sounds on opening or closing 524.64
            specified NEC 524.69
        wrist 719.93
    kidney 593.9
        functional 588.9
            specified NEC 588.89
    labyrinth, labyrinthine 386.9
        specified type NEC 386.8
    lactation 676.9●
    language (developmental) (expressive) 315.31
        mixed receptive-expressive 315.32
    learning 315.9
    ligament 728.9
    ligamentous attachments, peripheral - *see
        also* Enthesopathy
        spine 720.1
    limb NEC 729.90
        psychogenic 306.0
    lipid
        metabolism, congenital 272.9
        storage 272.7
    lipoprotein deficiency (familial) 272.5
    low back NEC 724.9
        psychogenic 306.0
    lumbosacral
        plexus 353.1
        root (nerve) NEC 353.4
    lymphoproliferative (chronic) NEC
        (M9970/1) 238.79
        post-transplant (PTLD) 238.77
    major depressive (*see also* Psychosis,
        affective) 296.2●
        recurrent episode 296.3●
        single episode 296.2●
    male erectile 607.84
        nonorganic origin 302.72
    manic (*see also* Psychosis, affective) 296.0●
        atypical 296.81
    mathematics 315.1
    meniscus NEC (*see also* Disorder, cartilage,
        articular) 718.0●
    menopausal 627.9
        specified NEC 627.8
    menstrual 626.9
        psychogenic 306.52
        specified NEC 626.8
    mental (nonpsychotic) 300.9
        affecting management of pregnancy,
            childbirth, or puerperium 648.4●
        drug-induced 292.9
            hallucinogen persisting perception
                292.89
            specified type NEC 292.89
        due to or associated with
            alcoholism 291.9
            drug consumption NEC 292.9
                specified type NEC 292.89
            physical condition NEC 293.9
        induced by drug 292.9
            specified type NEC 292.89
        neurotic (*see also* Neurosis) 300.9
        of infancy, childhood or adolescence 313.9
        persistent
            other
                due to conditions classified
                    elsewhere 294.8
            unspecified
                due to conditions classified
                    elsewhere 294.9
        presenile 310.1
            psychotic NEC 290.10
        previous, affecting management of
            pregnancy V23.89
        psychoneurotic (*see also* Neurosis) 300.9

Disorder *(Continued)*
    mental *(Continued)*
        psychotic (*see also* Psychosis) 298.9
            brief 298.8
            senile 290.20
        specific, following organic brain damage
            310.9
            cognitive or personality change of
                other type 310.1
            frontal lobe syndrome 310.0
            postconcussional syndrome 310.2
            specified type NEC 310.89
        transient
            in conditions classified elsewhere 293.9
    metabolism NEC 277.9
        with
            abortion - *see* Abortion, by type, with
                metabolic disorder
            ectopic pregnancy (*see also* categories
                633.0–633.9) 639.4
            molar pregnancy (*see also* categories
                630–632) 639.4
        alkaptonuria 270.2
        amino acid (*see also* Disorder, amino acid)
            270.9
            specified type NEC 270.8
        ammonia 270.6
        arginine 270.6
        argininosuccinic acid 270.6
        basal 794.7
        bilirubin 277.4
        calcium 275.40
        carbohydrate 271.9
            specified type NEC 271.8
        cholesterol 272.9
        citrulline 270.6
        copper 275.1
        corticosteroid 255.2
        cystine storage 270.0
        cystinuria 270.0
        fat 272.9
            fatty acid oxidation 277.85
        following
            abortion 639.4
            ectopic or molar pregnancy 639.4
        fructosemia 271.2
        fructosuria 271.2
        fucosidosis 271.8
        galactose-1-phosphate uridyl transferase
            271.1
        glutamine 270.7
        glycine 270.7
        glycogen storage NEC 271.0
            hepatorenal 271.0
        hemochromatosis (*see also*
            Hemochromatosis) 275.03
        in labor and delivery 669.0●
        iron 275.09
        lactose 271.3
        lipid 272.9
            specified type NEC 272.8
            storage 272.7
        lipoprotein - *see also* Hyperlipemia
            deficiency (familial) 272.5
        lysine 270.7
        magnesium 275.2
        mannosidosis 271.8
        mineral 275.9
            specified type NEC 275.8
            mitochondrial 277.87
        mucopolysaccharide 277.5
        nitrogen 270.9
        ornithine 270.6
        oxalosis 271.8
        pentosuria 271.8
        phenylketonuria 270.1
        phosphate 275.3
        phosphorus 275.3
        plasma protein 273.9
            specified type NEC 273.8
        porphyrin 277.1

Disorder *(Continued)*
    metabolism NEC *(Continued)*
        purine 277.2
        pyrimidine 277.2
        serine 270.7
        sodium 276.9
        specified type NEC 277.89
        steroid 255.2
        threonine 270.7
        urea cycle 270.6
        xylose 271.8
    micturition NEC 788.69
        psychogenic 306.53
    misery and unhappiness, of childhood and
        adolescence 313.1
    mitochondrial metabolism 277.87
    mitral valve 424.0
    mood (*see also* Disorder, bipolar) 296.90
        alcohol-induced 291.89
        episodic 296.90
            specified NEC 296.99
        in conditions classified elsewhere 293.83
    motor tic 307.20
        chronic 307.22
        transient (childhood) 307.21
    movement NEC 333.90
        hysterical 300.11
        medication-induced 333.90
        periodic limb 327.51
        sleep related unspecified 780.58
            other organic 327.59
        specified type NEC 333.99
        stereotypic 307.3
    mucopolysaccharide 277.5
    muscle 728.9
        psychogenic 306.0
        specified type NEC 728.3
    muscular attachments, peripheral - *see also*
        Enthesopathy
        spine 720.1
    musculoskeletal system NEC 729.90
        psychogenic 306.0
    myeloproliferative (chronic) NEC (M9960/1)
        238.79
    myoneural 358.9
        due to lead 358.2
        specified type NEC 358.8
        toxic 358.2
    myotonic 359.29
    neck region NEC 723.9
    nerve 349.9
        abducens NEC 378.54
        accessory 352.4
        acoustic 388.5
        auditory 388.5
        auriculotemporal 350.8
        axillary 353.0
        cerebral - *see* Disorder, nerve, cranial
        cranial 352.9
            first 352.0
            second 377.49
            third
                partial 378.51
                total 378.52
            fourth 378.53
            fifth 350.9
            sixth 378.54
            seventh NEC 351.9
            eighth 388.5
            ninth 352.2
            tenth 352.3
            eleventh 352.4
            twelfth 352.5
            multiple 352.6
        entrapment - *see* Neuropathy, entrapment
        facial 351.9
            specified NEC 351.8
        femoral 355.2
        glossopharyngeal NEC 352.2
        hypoglossal 352.5
        iliohypogastric 355.79

Disorder *(Continued)*
  nerve *(Continued)*
    ilioinguinal 355.79
    intercostal 353.8
    lateral
      cutaneous of thigh 355.1
      popliteal 355.3
    lower limb NEC 355.8
    medial, popliteal 355.4
    median NEC 354.1
    obturator 355.79
    oculomotor
      partial 378.51
      total 378.52
    olfactory 352.0
    optic 377.49
      hypoplasia 377.43
      ischemic 377.41
      nutritional 377.33
      toxic 377.34
    peroneal 355.3
    phrenic 354.8
    plantar 355.6
    pneumogastric 352.3
    posterior tibial 355.5
    radial 354.3
    recurrent laryngeal 352.3
    root 353.9
      specified NEC 353.8
    saphenous 355.79
    sciatic NEC 355.0
    specified NEC 355.9
      lower limb 355.79
      upper limb 354.8
    spinal 355.9
    sympathetic NEC 337.9
    trigeminal 350.9
      specified NEC 350.8
    trochlear 378.53
    ulnar 354.2
    upper limb NEC 354.9
    vagus 352.3
  nervous system NEC 349.9
    autonomic (peripheral) *(see also*
      Neuropathy, peripheral,
      autonomic) 337.9
    cranial 352.9
    parasympathetic *(see also* Neuropathy,
      peripheral, autonomic) 337.9
    specified type NEC 349.89
    sympathetic *(see also* Neuropathy,
      peripheral, autonomic) 337.9
    vegetative *(see also* Neuropathy,
      peripheral, autonomic) 337.9
  neurohypophysis NEC 253.6
  neurological NEC 781.99
    peripheral NEC 355.9
  neuromuscular NEC 358.9
    hereditary NEC 359.1
    specified NEC 358.8
    toxic 358.2
  neurotic 300.9
    specified type NEC 300.89
  neutrophil, polymorphonuclear (functional)
    288.1
  nightmare 307.47
  night terror 307.46
  obsessive-compulsive 300.3
  oppositional defiant, childhood and
    adolescence 313.81
  optic
    chiasm 377.54
      associated with
        inflammatory disorders 377.54
        neoplasm NEC 377.52
          pituitary 377.51
        pituitary disorders 377.51
        vascular disorders 377.53
    nerve 377.49
    radiations 377.63
    tracts 377.63

Disorder *(Continued)*
  orbit 376.9
    specified NEC 376.89
  orgasmic
    female 302.73
    male 302.74
  overanxious, of childhood and adolescence
    313.0
  oxidation, fatty acid 277.85
  pancreas, internal secretion (other than
    diabetes mellitus) 251.9
    specified type NEC 251.8
  panic 300.01
    with agoraphobia 300.21
  papillary muscle NEC 429.81
  paranoid 297.9
    induced 297.3
    shared 297.3
  parathyroid 252.9
    specified type NEC 252.8
  paroxysmal, mixed 780.39
  pentose phosphate pathway with anemia
    282.2
  periodic limb movement 327.51
  peroxisomal 277.86
  personality 301.9
    affective 301.10
    aggressive 301.3
    amoral 301.7
    anancastic, anankastic 301.4
    antisocial 301.7
    asocial 301.7
    asthenic 301.6
    avoidant 301.82
    borderline 301.83
    compulsive 301.4
    cyclothymic 301.13
    dependent-passive 301.6
    dyssocial 301.7
    emotional instability 301.59
    epileptoid 301.3
    explosive 301.3
    following organic brain damage 310.1
    histrionic 301.50
    hyperthymic 301.11
    hypomanic (chronic) 301.11
    hypothymic 301.12
    hysterical 301.50
    immature 301.89
    inadequate 301.6
    introverted 301.21
    labile 301.59
    moral deficiency 301.7
    narcissistic 301.81
    obsessional 301.4
    obsessive-compulsive 301.4
    overconscientious 301.4
    paranoid 301.0
    passive (-dependent) 301.6
    passive-aggressive 301.84
    pathological NEC 301.9
    pseudosocial 301.7
    psychopathic 301.9
    schizoid 301.20
      introverted 301.21
      schizotypal 301.22
    schizotypal 301.22
    seductive 301.59
    type A 301.4
    unstable 301.59
  pervasive developmental 299.9 ●
    childhood-onset 299.8 ●
    specified NEC 299.8 ●
  phonological 315.39
  pigmentation, choroid (congenital)
    743.53
  pinna 380.30
    specified type NEC 380.39
  pituitary, thalamic 253.9
    anterior NEC 253.4
    iatrogenic 253.7

Disorder *(Continued)*
  pituitary, thalamic *(Continued)*
    postablative 253.7
    specified NEC 253.8
  pityriasis-like NEC 696.8
  platelets (blood) 287.1
  polymorphonuclear neutrophils (functional)
    288.1
  porphyrin metabolism 277.1
  postmenopausal 627.9
    specified type NEC 627.8
  post-transplant lymphoproliferative (PTLD)
    238.77
  post-traumatic stress (PTSD) 309.81
  posttraumatic stress 309.81
    acute 309.81
    brief 309.81
    chronic 309.81
  premenstrual dysphoric (PMDD) 625.4
  psoriatic-like NEC 696.8
  psychic, with diseases classified elsewhere
    316
  psychogenic NEC *(see also* condition)
    300.9
    allergic NEC
      respiratory 306.1
    anxiety 300.00
      atypical 300.00
      generalized 300.02
    appetite 307.59
    articulation, joint 306.0
    asthenic 300.5
    blood 306.8
    cardiovascular (system) 306.2
    compulsive 300.3
    cutaneous 306.3
    depressive 300.4
    digestive (system) 306.4
    dysmenorrheic 306.52
    dyspneic 306.1
    eczematous 306.3
    endocrine (system) 306.6
    eye 306.7
    feeding 307.59
    functional NEC 306.9
    gastric 306.4
    gastrointestinal (system) 306.4
    genitourinary (system) 306.50
    heart (function) (rhythm) 306.2
    hemic 306.8
    hyperventilatory 306.1
    hypochondriacal 300.7
    hysterical 300.10
    intestinal 306.4
    joint 306.0
    learning 315.2
    limb 306.0
    lymphatic (system) 306.8
    menstrual 306.52
    micturition 306.53
    monoplegic NEC 306.0
    motor 307.9
    muscle 306.0
    musculoskeletal 306.0
    neurocirculatory 306.2
    obsessive 300.3
    occupational 300.89
    organ or part of body NEC 306.9
    organs of special sense 306.7
    paralytic NEC 306.0
    phobic 300.20
    physical NEC 306.9
    pruritic 306.3
    rectal 306.4
    respiratory (system) 306.1
    rheumatic 306.0
    sexual (function) 302.70
      specified type NEC 302.79
    sexual orientation conflict 302.0
    skin (allergic) (eczematous) (pruritic)
      306.3

◀ New   ◀ Revised   ~~deleted~~ Deleted   ● Use Additional Digit(s)   ▓ Omit code

Disorder *(Continued)*
  psychogenic NEC *(Continued)*
    sleep 307.40
      initiation or maintenance 307.41
        persistent 307.42
        transient 307.41
      movement 780.58
      sleep terror 307.46
      specified type NEC 307.49
    specified part of body NEC 306.8
    stomach 306.4
  psychomotor NEC 307.9
    hysterical 300.11
  psychoneurotic *(see also* Neurosis) 300.9
    mixed NEC 300.89
  psychophysiologic *(see also* Disorder,
      psychosomatic) 306.9
  psychosexual identity (childhood) 302.6
    adult-life 302.85
  psychosomatic NEC 306.9
    allergic NEC
      respiratory 306.1
    articulation, joint 306.0
    cardiovascular (system) 306.2
    cutaneous 306.3
    digestive (system) 306.4
    dysmenorrheic 306.52
    dyspneic 306.1
    endocrine (system) 306.6
    eye 306.7
    gastric 306.4
    gastrointestinal (system) 306.4
    genitourinary (system) 306.50
    heart (functional) (rhythm) 306.2
    hyperventilatory 306.1
    intestinal 306.4
    joint 306.0
    limb 306.0
    lymphatic (system) 306.8
    menstrual 306.52
    micturition 306.53
    monoplegic NEC 306.0
    muscle 306.0
    musculoskeletal 306.0
    neurocirculatory 306.2
    organs of special sense 306.7
    paralytic NEC 306.0
    pruritic 306.3
    rectal 306.4
    respiratory (system) 306.1
    rheumatic 306.0
    sexual (function) 302.70
      specified type NEC 302.79
    skin 306.3
    specified part of body NEC 306.8
    stomach 306.4
  psychotic *(see also* Psychosis) 298.9
    brief 298.8
  purine metabolism NEC 277.2
  pyrimidine metabolism NEC 277.2
  reactive attachment of infancy or early
      childhood 313.89
  reading, developmental 315.00
  reflex 796.1
  REM sleep behavior 327.42
  renal function, impaired 588.9
    specified type NEC 588.89
  renal transport NEC 588.89
  respiration, respiratory NEC 519.9
    due to
      aspiration of liquids or solids 508.9
      inhalation of fumes or vapors 506.9
      smoke inhalation 508.2
    psychogenic 306.1
  retina 362.9
    specified type NEC 362.89
  rumination 307.53
  sacroiliac joint NEC 724.6
  sacrum 724.6
  schizo-affective *(see also* Schizophrenia)
      295.7●

Disorder *(Continued)*
  schizoid, childhood or adolescence 313.22
  schizophreniform 295.4●
  schizotypal personality 301.22
  secretion, thyrocalcitonin 246.0
  seizure 345.9●
    recurrent 345.9●
      epileptic - *see* Epilepsy
  semantic pragmatic 315.39
    with autism 299.0●
  sense of smell 781.1
    psychogenic 306.7
  separation anxiety 309.21
  sexual *(see also* Deviation, sexual) 302.9
    aversion 302.79
    desire, hypoactive 302.71
    function, psychogenic 302.70
  shyness, of childhood and adolescence 313.21
  single complement (C₁–C₉) 279.8
  skin NEC 709.9
    fetus or newborn 778.9
      specified type 778.8
    psychogenic (allergic) (eczematous)
        (pruritic) 306.3
    specified type NEC 709.8
    vascular 709.1
  sleep 780.50
    with apnea - *see* Apnea, sleep
    alcohol induced 291.82
    arousal 307.46
      confusional 327.41
    circadian rhythm 327.30
      advanced sleep phase type 327.32
      alcohol induced 291.82
      delayed sleep phase type 327.31
      drug induced 292.85
      free running type 327.34
      in conditions classified elsewhere
          327.37
      irregular sleep-wake type 327.33
      jet lag type 327.35
      other 327.39
      shift work type 327.36
    drug induced 292.85
    initiation or maintenance *(see also*
        Insomnia) 780.52
      nonorganic origin (transient) 307.41
        persistent 307.42
    nonorganic origin 307.40
      specified type NEC 307.49
    organic specified type NEC 327.8
    periodic limb movement 327.51
    specified NEC 780.59
    wake
      cycle - *see* Disorder, sleep, circadian
          rhythm
      schedule - *see* Disorder, sleep, circadian
          rhythm
  social, of childhood and adolescence 313.22
  soft tissue 729.90
    specified type NEC 729.99
  somatization 300.81
  somatoform (atypical) (undifferentiated)
      300.82
    severe 300.81
    specified type NEC 300.89
  speech 784.59
    nonorganic origin 307.9
  spine NEC 724.9
    ligamentous or muscular attachments,
        peripheral 720.1
  steroid metabolism NEC 255.2
  stomach (functional) *(see also* Disorder,
      gastric) 536.9
    psychogenic 306.4
  storage, iron 275.09
  stress *(see also* Reaction, stress, acute) 308.3
    posttraumatic
      acute 309.81
      brief 309.81
      chronic (motor or vocal) 309.81

Disorder *(Continued)*
  substitution 300.11
  suspected - *see* Observation
  synovium 727.9
  temperature regulation, fetus or newborn
      778.4
  temporomandibular joint NEC 524.60
    sounds on opening or closing 524.64
    specified NEC 524.69
  tendon 727.9
    shoulder region 726.10
  thoracic root (nerve) NEC 353.3
  thyrocalcitonin secretion 246.0
  thyroid (gland) NEC 246.9
    specified type NEC 246.8
  tic 307.20
    chronic (motor or vocal) 307.22
    motor-verbal 307.23
    organic origin 333.1
    transient (of childhood) 307.21
  tooth NEC 525.9
    development NEC 520.9
      specified type NEC 520.8
    eruption 520.6
    specified type NEC 525.8
  Tourette's 307.23
  transport, carbohydrate 271.9
    specified type NEC 271.8
  tubular, phosphate-losing 588.0
  tympanic membrane 384.9
  unaggressive, unsocialized *(see also*
      Disturbance, conduct) 312.1●
  undersocialized, unsocialized *(see also*
      Disturbance, conduct)
    aggressive (type) 312.0●
    unaggressive (type) 312.1●
  vision, visual NEC 368.9
    binocular NEC 368.30
    cortex 377.73
      associated with
        inflammatory disorders 377.73
        neoplasms 377.71
        vascular disorders 377.72
    pathway NEC 377.63
      associated with
        inflammatory disorders 377.63
        neoplasms 377.61
        vascular disorders 377.62
  vocal tic
    chronic 307.22
  wakefulness *(see also* Hypersomnia) 780.54
    nonorganic origin (transient) 307.43
      persistent 307.44
  written expression 315.2
Disorganized globe 360.29
Displacement, displaced

> Note: For acquired displacement of bones,
> cartilage, joints, tendons, due to injury, *see*
> *also* Dislocation.
>
> Displacements at ages under one year
> should be considered congenital, provided
> there is no indication the condition was
> acquired after birth.

  acquired traumatic of bone, cartilage, joint,
      tendon NEC (without fracture) *(see also*
      Dislocation) 839.8
    with fracture - *see* Fracture, by site
  adrenal gland (congenital) 759.1
  alveolus and teeth, vertical 524.75
  appendix, retrocecal (congenital) 751.5
  auricle (congenital) 744.29
  bladder (acquired) 596.89
    congenital 753.8
  brachial plexus (congenital) 742.8
  brain stem, caudal 742.4
  canaliculus lacrimalis 743.65
  cardia, through esophageal hiatus 750.6
  cerebellum, caudal 742.4
  cervix - *see* Displacement, uterus

Displacement, displaced *(Continued)*
  colon (congenital) 751.4
  device, implant, or graft - *see* Complications, mechanical
  epithelium
    columnar of cervix 622.10
    cuboidal, beyond limits of external os (uterus) 752.49
  esophageal mucosa into cardia of stomach, congenital 750.4
  esophagus (acquired) 530.89
    congenital 750.4
  eyeball (acquired) (old) 376.36
    congenital 743.8
    current injury 871.3
    lateral 376.36
  fallopian tube (acquired) 620.4
    congenital 752.19
    opening (congenital) 752.19
  gallbladder (congenital) 751.69
  gastric mucosa 750.7
    into
      duodenum 750.7
      esophagus 750.7
      Meckel's diverticulum, congenital 750.7
  globe (acquired) (lateral) (old) 376.36
    current injury 871.3
  graft
    artificial skin graft 996.55
    decellularized allodermis graft 996.55
  heart (congenital) 746.87
    acquired 429.89
  hymen (congenital) (upward) 752.49
  internal prosthesis NEC - *see* Complications, mechanical
  intervertebral disc (with neuritis, radiculitis, sciatica, or other pain) 722.2
    with myelopathy 722.70
    cervical, cervicodorsal, cervicothoracic 722.0
      with myelopathy 722.71
      due to major trauma - *see* Dislocation, vertebra, cervical
    due to trauma - *see* Dislocation, vertebra
    lumbar, lumbosacral 722.10
      with myelopathy 722.73
      due to major trauma - *see* Dislocation, vertebra, lumbar
    thoracic, thoracolumbar 722.11
      with myelopathy 722.72
      due to major trauma - *see* Dislocation, vertebra, thoracic
  intrauterine device 996.32
  kidney (acquired) 593.0
    congenital 753.3
  lacrimal apparatus or duct (congenital) 743.65
  macula (congenital) 743.55
  Meckel's diverticulum (congenital) 751.0
  nail (congenital) 757.5
    acquired 703.8
  opening of Wharton's duct in mouth 750.26
  organ or site, congenital NEC - *see* Malposition, congenital
  ovary (acquired) 620.4
    congenital 752.0
    free in peritoneal cavity (congenital) 752.0
    into hernial sac 620.4
  oviduct (acquired) 620.4
    congenital 752.19
  parathyroid (gland) 252.8
  parotid gland (congenital) 750.26
  punctum lacrimale (congenital) 743.65
  sacroiliac (congenital) (joint) 755.69
    current injury - *see* Dislocation, sacroiliac
    old 724.6
  spine (congenital) 756.19
  spleen, congenital 759.0
  stomach (congenital) 750.7
    acquired 537.89
  subglenoid (closed) 831.01
  sublingual duct (congenital) 750.26

Displacement, displaced *(Continued)*
  teeth, tooth 524.30
    horizontal 524.33
    vertical 524.34
  tongue (congenital) (downward) 750.19
  trachea (congenital) 748.3
  ureter or ureteric opening or orifice (congenital) 753.4
  uterine opening of oviducts or fallopian tubes 752.19
  uterus, uterine (*see also* Malposition, uterus) 621.6
    congenital 752.39
  ventricular septum 746.89
    with rudimentary ventricle 746.89
  xyphoid bone (process) 738.3
Disproportion 653.9●
  affecting fetus or newborn 763.1
  breast, reconstructed 612.1
    between native and reconstructed 612.1
  caused by
    conjoined twins 678.1●
    contraction, pelvis (general) 653.1●
      inlet 653.2●
      midpelvic 653.8●
      midplane 653.8●
      outlet 653.3●
    fetal
      ascites 653.7●
      hydrocephalus 653.6●
      hydrops 653.7●
      meningomyelocele 653.7●
      sacral teratoma 653.7●
      tumor 653.7●
    hydrocephalic fetus 653.6●
    pelvis, pelvic, abnormality (bony) NEC 653.0●
    unusually large fetus 653.5●
  causing obstructed labor 660.1●
  cephalopelvic, normally formed fetus 653.4●
    causing obstructed labor 660.1●
  fetal NEC 653.5●
    causing obstructed labor 660.1●
  fetopelvic, normally formed fetus 653.4●
    causing obstructed labor 660.1●
  mixed maternal and fetal origin, normally, formed fetus 653.4●
  pelvis, pelvic (bony) NEC 653.1●
    causing obstructed labor 660.1●
  specified type NEC 653.8●
Disruption
  cesarean wound 674.1●
  family V61.09
    due to
      child in
        care of non-parental family member V61.06
        foster care V61.06
        welfare custody V61.05
      death of family member V61.07
      divorce V61.03
      estrangement V61.09
        parent-child V61.04
      extended absence of family member NEC V61.08
      family member
        on military deployment V61.01
        return from military deployment V61.02
      legal separation V61.03
  gastrointestinal anastomosis 997.49
  ligament(s) - *see also* Sprain
    knee
      current injury - *see* Dislocation, knee
      old 717.89
        capsular 717.85
        collateral (medial) 717.82
          lateral 717.81
        cruciate (posterior) 717.84
          anterior 717.83
        specified site NEC 717.85

Disruption *(Continued)*
  marital V61.10
    involving
      divorce V61.03
      estrangement V61.09
  operation wound (external) (*see also* Dehiscence) 998.32
    internal 998.31
  organ transplant, anastomosis site - *see* Complications, transplant, organ, by site
  ossicles, ossicular chain 385.23
    traumatic - *see* Fracture, skull, base
  parenchyma
    liver (hepatic) - *see* Laceration, liver, major
    spleen - *see* Laceration, spleen, parenchyma, massive
  phase-shift, of 24 hour sleep-wake cycle, unspecified 780.55
    nonorganic origin 307.45
  sleep-wake cycle (24 hour), unspecified 780.55
    circadian rhythm 327.33
    nonorganic origin 307.45
  suture line (external) (*see also* Dehiscence) 998.32
    internal 998.31
  wound 998.30
    cesarean operation 674.1●
    episiotomy 674.2●
    operation (surgical) 998.32
      cesarean 674.1●
      internal 998.31
    perineal (obstetric) 674.2●
    uterine 674.1●
Disruptio uteri - *see also* Rupture, uterus
  complicating delivery - *see* Delivery, complicated, rupture, uterus
Dissatisfaction with
  employment V62.29
  school environment V62.3
Dissecting - *see* condition
Dissection
  aorta 441.00
    abdominal 441.02
    thoracic 441.01
    thoracoabdominal 441.03
  artery, arterial
    carotid 443.21
    coronary 414.12
    iliac 443.22
    renal 443.23
    specified NEC 443.29
    vertebral 443.24
  vascular 459.9
  wound - *see* Wound, open, by site
Disseminated - *see* condition
Dissociated personality NEC 300.15
Dissociation
  auriculoventricular or atrioventricular (any degree) (AV) 426.89
    with heart block 426.0
  interference 426.89
  isorhythmic 426.89
  rhythm
    atrioventricular (AV) 426.89
    interference 426.89
Dissociative
  identity disorder 300.14
  reaction NEC 300.15
Dissolution, vertebra (*see also* Osteoporosis) 733.00
Distention
  abdomen (gaseous) 787.3
  bladder 596.89
  cecum 569.89
  colon 569.89
  gallbladder 575.8
  gaseous (abdomen) 787.3
  intestine 569.89
  kidney 593.89

◀ New   ◀▮▮ Revised   ~~deleted~~ Deleted   ● Use Additional Digit(s)   ▮▮▮ Omit code

Distention (*Continued*)
  liver 573.9
  seminal vesicle 608.89
  stomach 536.8
    acute 536.1
    psychogenic 306.4
  ureter 593.5
  uterus 621.8
Distichia, distichiasis (eyelid) 743.63
Distoma hepaticum infestation 121.3
Distomiasis 121.9
  bile passages 121.3
    due to Clonorchis sinensis 121.1
  hemic 120.9
  hepatic (liver) 121.3
    due to Clonorchis sinensis (clonorchiasis)
      121.1
  intestinal 121.4
  liver 121.3
    due to Clonorchis sinensis 121.1
  lung 121.2
  pulmonary 121.2
Distomolar (fourth molar) 520.1
  causing crowding 524.31
Disto-occlusion (division I) (division II) 524.22
Distortion (congenital)
  adrenal (gland) 759.1
  ankle (joint) 755.69
  anus 751.5
  aorta 747.29
  appendix 751.5
  arm 755.59
  artery (peripheral) NEC (*see also* Distortion,
    peripheral vascular system) 747.60
    cerebral 747.81
    coronary 746.85
    pulmonary 747.39
    retinal 743.58
    umbilical 747.5
  auditory canal 744.29
    causing impairment of hearing 744.02
  bile duct or passage 751.69
  bladder 753.8
  brain 742.4
  bronchus 748.3
  cecum 751.5
  cervix (uteri) 752.49
  chest (wall) 756.3
  clavicle 755.51
  clitoris 752.49
  coccyx 756.19
  colon 751.5
  common duct 751.69
  cornea 743.41
  cricoid cartilage 748.3
  cystic duct 751.69
  duodenum 751.5
  ear 744.29
    auricle 744.29
      causing impairment of hearing
        744.02
    causing impairment of hearing 744.09
    external 744.29
      causing impairment of hearing
        744.02
    inner 744.05
    middle, except ossicles 744.03
      ossicles 744.04
    ossicles 744.04
  endocrine (gland) NEC 759.2
  epiglottis 748.3
  Eustachian tube 744.24
  eye 743.8
    adnexa 743.69
  face bone(s) 756.0
  fallopian tube 752.19
  femur 755.69
  fibula 755.69
  finger(s) 755.59
  foot 755.67
  gallbladder 751.69

Distortion (*Continued*)
  genitalia, genital organ(s)
    female 752.89
      external 752.49
      internal NEC 752.89
    male 752.89
      penis 752.69
  glottis 748.3
  gyri 742.4
  hand bone(s) 755.59
  heart (auricle) (ventricle) 746.89
    valve (cusp) 746.89
  hepatic duct 751.69
  humerus 755.59
  hymen 752.49
  ileum 751.5
  intestine (large) (small) 751.5
    with anomalous adhesions, fixation or
      malrotation 751.4
  jaw NEC 524.89
  jejunum 751.5
  kidney 753.3
  knee (joint) 755.64
  labium (majus) (minus) 752.49
  larynx 748.3
  leg 755.69
  lens 743.36
  liver 751.69
  lumbar spine 756.19
    with disproportion (fetopelvic) 653.0●
      affecting fetus or newborn 763.1
      causing obstructed labor 660.1●
  lumbosacral (joint) (region) 756.19
  lung (fissures) (lobe) 748.69
  nerve 742.8
  nose 748.1
  organ
    of Corti 744.05
    of site not listed - *see* Anomaly, specified
      type NEC
  ossicles, ear 744.04
  ovary 752.0
  oviduct 752.19
  pancreas 751.7
  parathyroid (gland) 759.2
  patella 755.64
  peripheral vascular system NEC 747.60
    gastrointestinal 747.61
    lower limb 747.64
    renal 747.62
    spinal 747.82
    upper limb 747.63
  pituitary (gland) 759.2
  radius 755.59
  rectum 751.5
  rib 756.3
  sacroiliac joint 755.69
  sacrum 756.19
  scapula 755.59
  shoulder girdle 755.59
  site not listed - *see* Anomaly, specified type
    NEC
  skull bone(s) 756.0
    with
      anencephalus 740.0
      encephalocele 742.0
      hydrocephalus 742.3
        with spina bifida (*see also* Spina
          bifida) 741.0●
      microcephalus 742.1
  spinal cord 742.59
  spine 756.19
  spleen 759.0
  sternum 756.3
  thorax (wall) 756.3
  thymus 759.2
  thyroid (gland) 759.2
    cartilage 748.3
  tibia 755.69
  toe(s) 755.66
  tongue 750.19

Distortion (*Continued*)
  trachea (cartilage) 748.3
  ulna 755.59
  ureter 753.4
    causing obstruction 753.20
  urethra 753.8
    causing obstruction 753.6
  uterus 752.39
  vagina 752.49
  vein (peripheral) NEC (*see also* Distortion,
    peripheral vascular system) 747.60
    great 747.49
    portal 747.49
    pulmonary 747.49
  vena cava (inferior) (superior) 747.49
  vertebra 756.19
  visual NEC 368.15
    shape or size 368.14
  vulva 752.49
  wrist (bones) (joint) 755.59
Distress
  abdomen 789.0●
  colon 564.9
  emotional V40.9
  epigastric 789.0●
  fetal (syndrome) 768.4
    affecting management of pregnancy or
      childbirth 656.8●
    liveborn infant 768.4
      first noted
        before onset of labor 768.2
        during labor and delivery 768.3
    stillborn infant (death before onset of
      labor) 768.0
      death during labor 768.1
  gastrointestinal (functional) 536.9
    psychogenic 306.4
  intestinal (functional) NEC 564.9
    psychogenic 306.4
  intrauterine - *see* Distress, fetal
  leg 729.5
  maternal 669.0●
  mental V40.9
  respiratory 786.09
    acute (adult) 518.82
    adult syndrome (following trauma and
      surgery) 518.52
      specified NEC 518.82
    fetus or newborn 770.89
    syndrome (idiopathic) (newborn) 769
  stomach 536.9
    psychogenic 306.4
Distribution vessel, atypical NEC 747.60
  coronary artery 746.85
  spinal 747.82
Districhiasis 704.2
Disturbance - *see also* Disease
  absorption NEC 579.9
    calcium 269.3
    carbohydrate 579.8
    fat 579.8
    protein 579.8
    specified type NEC 579.8
    vitamin (*see also* Deficiency, vitamin) 269.2
  acid-base equilibrium 276.9
  activity and attention, simple, with
    hyperkinesis 314.01
  amino acid (metabolic) (*see also* Disorder,
    amino acid) 270.9
    imidazole 270.5
    maple syrup (urine) disease 270.3
    transport 270.0
  assimilation, food 579.9
  attention, simple 314.00
    with hyperactivity 314.01
  auditory, nerve, except deafness 388.5
  behavior (*see also* Disturbance, conduct) 312.9
  blood clotting (hypoproteinemia)
    (mechanism) (*see also* Defect,
    coagulation) 286.9
  central nervous system NEC 349.9

Disturbance *(Continued)*
   cerebral nerve NEC 352.9
   circulatory 459.9
   conduct 312.9
      adjustment reaction 309.3
      adolescent onset type 312.82
      childhood onset type 312.81

> Note: Use the following fifth-digit
> subclassification with categories 312.0–312.2:
>
> 0   unspecified
> 1   mild
> 2   moderate
> 3   severe

      compulsive 312.30
         intermittent explosive disorder
            312.34
         isolated explosive disorder
            312.35
         kleptomania 312.32
         pathological gambling 312.31
         pyromania 312.33
      hyperkinetic 314.2
      intermittent explosive 312.34
      isolated explosive 312.35
      mixed with emotions 312.4
      socialized (type) 312.20
         aggressive 312.23
         unaggressive 312.21
      specified type NEC 312.89
      undersocialized, unsocialized
         aggressive (type) 312.0●
         unaggressive (type) 312.1●
   coordination 781.3
   cranial nerve NEC 352.9
   deep sensibility - *see* Disturbance, sensation
   digestive 536.9
      psychogenic 306.4
   electrolyte - *see* Imbalance, electrolyte
   emotions specific to childhood or
      adolescence 313.9
      with
         academic underachievement 313.83
         anxiety and fearfulness 313.0
         elective mutism 313.23
         identity disorder 313.82
         jealousy 313.3
         misery and unhappiness 313.1
         oppositional defiant disorder 313.81
         overanxiousness 313.0
         sensitivity 313.21
         shyness 313.21
         social withdrawal 313.22
         withdrawal reaction 313.22
      involving relationship problems 313.3
      mixed 313.89
      specified type NEC 313.89
   endocrine (gland) 259.9
      neonatal, transitory 775.9
         specified NEC 775.89
   equilibrium 780.4
   feeding (elderly) (infant) 783.3
      newborn 779.31
      nonorganic origin NEC 307.59
      psychogenic NEC 307.59
   fructose metabolism 271.2
   gait 781.2
      hysterical 300.11
   gastric (functional) 536.9
      motility 536.8
      psychogenic 306.4
      secretion 536.8
   gastrointestinal (functional) 536.9
      psychogenic 306.4
   habit, child 307.9
   hearing, except deafness 388.40
   heart, functional (conditions classifiable to
      426, 427, 428)
      due to presence of (cardiac) prosthesis
         429.4

Disturbance *(Continued)*
   heart, functional *(Continued)*
      postoperative (immediate) 997.1
         long-term effect of cardiac surgery
            429.4
      psychogenic 306.2
   hormone 259.9
   innervation uterus, sympathetic,
      parasympathetic 621.8
   keratinization NEC
      gingiva 523.10
      lip 528.5
      oral (mucosa) (soft tissue) 528.79
         residual ridge mucosa
            excessive 528.72
            minimal 528.71
      tongue 528.79
   labyrinth, labyrinthine (vestibule) 386.9
   learning, specific NEC 315.2
   memory (*see also* Amnesia) 780.93
      mild, following organic brain damage
         310.89
   mental (*see also* Disorder, mental) 300.9
      associated with diseases classified
         elsewhere 316
   metabolism (acquired) (congenital) (*see also*
      Disorder, metabolism) 277.9
      with
         abortion - *see* Abortion, by type, with
            metabolic disorder
         ectopic pregnancy (*see also* categories
            633.0–633.9) 639.4
         molar pregnancy (*see also* categories
            630–632) 639.4
      amino acid (*see also* Disorder, amino acid)
         270.9
         aromatic NEC 270.2
         branched-chain 270.3
         specified type NEC 270.8
         straight-chain NEC 270.7
         sulfur-bearing 270.4
         transport 270.0
      ammonia 270.6
      arginine 270.6
      argininosuccinic acid 270.6
      carbohydrate NEC 271.9
      cholesterol 272.9
      citrulline 270.6
      cystathionine 270.4
      fat 272.9
      following
         abortion 639.4
         ectopic or molar pregnancy 639.4
      general 277.9
         carbohydrate 271.9
         iron 275.09
         phosphate 275.3
         sodium 276.9
      glutamine 270.7
      glycine 270.7
      histidine 270.5
      homocystine 270.4
      in labor or delivery 669.0●
      iron 275.09
      isoleucine 270.3
      leucine 270.3
      lipoid 272.9
         specified type NEC 272.8
      lysine 270.7
      methionine 270.4
      neonatal, transitory 775.9
         specified type NEC 775.89
      nitrogen 788.99
      ornithine 270.6
      phosphate 275.3
      phosphatides 272.7
      serine 270.7
      sodium NEC 276.9
      threonine 270.7
      tryptophan 270.2
      tyrosine 270.2

Disturbance *(Continued)*
   metabolism *(Continued)*
      urea cycle 270.6
      valine 270.3
   motor 796.1
   nervous functional 799.21
   neuromuscular mechanism (eye) due to
      syphilis 094.84
   nutritional 269.9
      nail 703.8
   ocular motion 378.87
      psychogenic 306.7
   oculogyric 378.87
      psychogenic 306.7
   oculomotor NEC 378.87
      psychogenic 306.7
   olfactory nerve 781.1
   optic nerve NEC 377.49
   oral epithelium, including tongue
      528.79
      residual ridge mucosa
         excessive 528.72
         minimal 528.71
   personality (pattern) (trait) (*see also* Disorder,
      personality) 301.9
      following organic brain damage 310.1
   polyglandular 258.9
   psychomotor 307.9
   pupillary 379.49
   reflex 796.1
   rhythm, heart 427.9
      postoperative (immediate) 997.1
         long-term effect of cardiac surgery
            429.4
      psychogenic 306.2
   salivary secretion 527.7
   sensation (cold) (heat) (localization) (tactile
      discrimination localization) (texture)
      (vibratory) NEC 782.0
      hysterical 300.11
      skin 782.0
      smell 781.1
      taste 781.1
   sensory (*see also* Disturbance, sensation)
      782.0
      innervation 782.0
   situational (transient) (*see also* Reaction,
      adjustment) 309.9
      acute 308.3
   sleep 780.50
      with apnea - *see* Apnea, sleep
      initiation or maintenance (*see also*
         Insomnia) 780.52
         nonorganic origin 307.41
      nonorganic origin 307.40
         specified type NEC 307.49
      specified NEC 780.59
         nonorganic origin 307.49
      wakefulness (*see also* Hypersomnia)
         780.54
         nonorganic origin 307.43
   sociopathic 301.7
   speech NEC 784.59
      developmental 315.39
         associated with hyperkinesis
           314.1
      secondary to organic lesion 784.59
   stomach (functional) (*see also* Disturbance,
      gastric) 536.9
   sympathetic (nerve) (*see also* Neuropathy,
      peripheral, autonomic) 337.9
   temperature sense 782.0
      hysterical 300.11
   tooth
      eruption 520.6
      formation 520.4
      structure, hereditary NEC 520.5
   touch (*see also* Disturbance, sensation)
      782.0
   vascular 459.9
      arteriosclerotic - *see* Arteriosclerosis

Disturbance *(Continued)*
vasomotor 443.9
vasospastic 443.9
vestibular labyrinth 386.9
vision, visual NEC 368.9
psychophysical 368.16
specified NEC 368.8
subjective 368.10
voice and resonance 784.40
wakefulness (initiation or maintenance) *(see also* Hypersomnia) 780.54
nonorganic origin 307.43
Disulfiduria, beta-mercaptolactate-cysteine 270.0
Disuse atrophy, bone 733.7
Ditthomska syndrome 307.81
Diuresis 788.42
Divers'
palsy or paralysis 993.3
squeeze 993.3
Diverticula, diverticulosis, diverticulum
(acute) (multiple) (perforated) (ruptured) 562.10
with diverticulitis 562.11
aorta (Kommerell's) 747.21
appendix (noninflammatory) 543.9
bladder (acquired) (sphincter) 596.3
congenital 753.8
broad ligament 620.8
bronchus (congenital) 748.3
acquired 494.0
with acute exacerbation 494.1
calyx, calyceal (kidney) 593.89
cardia (stomach) 537.1
cecum 562.10
with
diverticulitis 562.11
with hemorrhage 562.13
hemorrhage 562.12
congenital 751.5
colon (acquired) 562.10
with
diverticulitis 562.11
with hemorrhage 562.13
hemorrhage 562.12
congenital 751.5
duodenum 562.00
with
diverticulitis 562.01
with hemorrhage 562.03
hemorrhage 562.02
congenital 751.5
epiphrenic (esophagus) 530.6
esophagus (congenital) 750.4
acquired 530.6
epiphrenic 530.6
pulsion 530.6
traction 530.6
Zenker's 530.6
Eustachian tube 381.89
fallopian tube 620.8
gallbladder (congenital) 751.69
gastric 537.1
heart (congenital) 746.89
ileum 562.00
with
diverticulitis 562.01
with hemorrhage 562.03
hemorrhage 562.03
intestine (large) 562.10
with
diverticulitis 562.11
with hemorrhage 562.13
hemorrhage 562.12
congenital 751.5
small 562.00
with
diverticulitis 562.01
with hemorrhage 562.03
hemorrhage 562.02
congenital 751.5

Diverticula, diverticulosis *(Continued)*
jejunum 562.00
with
diverticulitis 562.01
with hemorrhage 562.03
hemorrhage 562.02
kidney (calyx) (pelvis) 593.89
with calculus 592.0
Kommerell's 747.21
laryngeal ventricle (congenital) 748.3
Meckel's (displaced) (hypertrophic) 751.0
midthoracic 530.6
organ or site, congenital NEC - *see* Distortion
pericardium (congenital) (cyst) 746.89
acquired (true) 423.8
pharyngoesophageal (pulsion) 530.6
pharynx (congenital) 750.27
pulsion (esophagus) 530.6
rectosigmoid 562.10
with
diverticulitis 562.11
with hemorrhage 562.13
hemorrhage 562.12
congenital 751.5
rectum 562.10
with
diverticulitis 562.11
with hemorrhage 562.13
hemorrhage 562.12
renal (calyces) (pelvis) 593.89
with calculus 592.0
Rokitansky's 530.6
seminal vesicle 608.0
sigmoid 562.10
with
diverticulitis 562.11
with hemorrhage 562.13
hemorrhage 562.12
congenital 751.5
small intestine 562.00
with
diverticulitis 562.01
with hemorrhage 562.03
hemorrhage 562.02
stomach (cardia) (juxtacardia) (juxtapyloric) (acquired) 537.1
congenital 750.7
subdiaphragmatic 530.6
trachea (congenital) 748.3
acquired 519.19
traction (esophagus) 530.6
ureter (acquired) 593.89
congenital 753.4
ureterovesical orifice 593.89
urethra (acquired) 599.2
congenital 753.8
ventricle, left (congenital) 746.89
vesical (urinary) 596.3
congenital 753.8
Zenker's (esophagus) 530.6
Diverticulitis (acute) *(see also* Diverticula) 562.11
with hemorrhage 562.13
bladder (urinary) 596.3
cecum (perforated) 562.11
with hemorrhage 562.13
colon (perforated) 562.11
with hemorrhage 562.13
duodenum 562.01
with hemorrhage 562.03
esophagus 530.6
ileum (perforated) 562.01
with hemorrhage 562.03
intestine (large) (perforated) 562.11
with hemorrhage 562.13
small 562.01
with hemorrhage 562.03
jejunum (perforated) 562.01
with hemorrhage 562.03
Meckel's (perforated) 751.0
pharyngoesophageal 530.6

Diverticulitis *(Continued)*
rectosigmoid (perforated) 562.11
with hemorrhage 562.13
rectum 562.11
with hemorrhage 562.13
sigmoid (old) (perforated) 562.11
with hemorrhage 562.13
small intestine (perforated) 562.01
with hemorrhage 562.03
vesical (urinary) 596.3
Diverticulosis - *see* Diverticula
Division
cervix uteri 622.8
external os into two openings by frenum 752.44
external (cervical) into two openings by frenum 752.44
glans penis 752.69
hymen 752.49
labia minora (congenital) 752.49
ligament (partial or complete) (current) - *see also* Sprain, by site
with open wound - *see* Wound, open, by site
muscle (partial or complete) (current) - *see also* Sprain, by site
with open wound - *see* Wound, open, by site
nerve - *see* Injury, nerve, by site
penis glans 752.69
spinal cord - *see* Injury, spinal, by site
vein 459.9
traumatic - *see* Injury, vascular, by site
Divorce V61.03
Dix-Hallpike neurolabyrinthitis 386.12
Dizziness 780.4
hysterical 300.11
psychogenic 306.9
Doan-Wiseman syndrome (primary splenic neutropenia) 289.53
Dog bite - *see* Wound, open, by site
Döhle-Heller aortitis 093.1
Döhle body-panmyelopathic syndrome 288.2
Dolichocephaly, dolichocephalus 754.0
Dolichocolon 751.5
Dolichostenomelia 759.82
Donohue's syndrome (leprechaunism) 259.8
Donor
blood V59.01
other blood components V59.09
stem cells V59.02
whole blood V59.01
bone V59.2
marrow V59.3
cornea V59.5
egg (oocyte) (ovum) V59.70
over age 35 V59.73
anonymous recipient V59.73
designated recipient V59.74
under age 35 V59.71
anonymous recipient V59.71
designated recipient V59.72
heart V59.8
kidney V59.4
liver V59.6
lung V59.8
lymphocyte V59.8
organ V59.9
specified NEC V59.8
potential, examination of V70.8
skin V59.1
specified organ or tissue NEC V59.8
sperm V59.8
stem cells V59.02
tissue V59.9
specified type NEC V59.8
Donovanosis (granuloma venereum) 099.2
DOPS (diffuse obstructive pulmonary syndrome) 496

Double
albumin 273.8
aortic arch 747.21
auditory canal 744.29
auricle (heart) 746.82
bladder 753.8
external (cervical) os 752.44
kidney with double pelvis (renal) 753.3
larynx 748.3
meatus urinarius 753.8
organ or site NEC - see Accessory
orifice
heart valve NEC 746.89
pulmonary 746.09
outlet, right ventricle 745.11
pelvis (renal) with double ureter 753.4
penis 752.69
tongue 750.13
ureter (one or both sides) 753.4
with double pelvis (renal) 753.4
urethra 753.8
urinary meatus 753.8
uterus (any degree) 752.2
with doubling of cervix and vagina
752.2
in pregnancy or childbirth 654.0●
affecting fetus or newborn 763.89
vagina 752.47
with doubling of cervix and uterus
752.2
vision 368.2
vocal cords 748.3
vulva 752.49
whammy (syndrome) 360.81
Douglas' pouch, cul-de-sac - see condition
Down's disease or syndrome (mongolism)
758.0
Down-growth, epithelial (anterior chamber)
364.61
DPD (dihydropyrimidine dehydrogenase
deficiency) 277.6
Dracontiasis 125.7
Dracunculiasis 125.7
Dracunculosis 125.7
Drainage
abscess (spontaneous) - see Abscess
anomalous pulmonary veins to hepatic veins
or right atrium 747.41
stump (amputation) (surgical) 997.62
suprapubic, bladder 596.89
Dream state, hysterical 300.13
Drepanocytic anemia (see also Disease, sickle
cell) 282.60
Dresbach's syndrome (elliptocytosis) 282.1
Dreschlera (infection) 118
hawaiiensis 117.8
Dressler's syndrome (postmyocardial
infarction) 411.0
Dribbling (post-void) 788.35
Drift, ulnar 736.09
Drinking (alcohol) - see also Alcoholism
excessive, to excess NEC (see also Abuse,
drugs, nondependent) 305.0●
bouts, periodic 305.0●
continual 303.9●
episodic 305.0●
habitual 303.9●
periodic 305.0●
Drip, postnasal (chronic) 784.91
due to:
allergic rhinitis - see Rhinitis, allergic
common cold 460
gastroesophageal reflux - see Reflux,
gastroesophageal
nasopharyngitis - see Nasopharyngitis
other known condition - code to condition
sinusitis - see Sinusitis
Drivers' license examination V70.3
Droop
Cooper's 611.81
facial 781.94

Drop
finger 736.29
foot 736.79
hematocrit (precipitous) 790.01
hemoglobin 790.01
toe 735.8
wrist 736.05
Dropped
dead 798.1
heart beats 426.6
Dropsy, dropsical (see also Edema) 782.3
abdomen 789.59
amnion (see also Hydramnios) 657●
brain - see Hydrocephalus
cardiac (see also Failure, heart) 428.0
cardiorenal (see also Hypertension,
cardiorenal) 404.90
chest 511.9
fetus or newborn 778.0
due to isoimmunization 773.3
gangrenous (see also Gangrene) 785.4
heart (see also Failure, heart) 428.0
hepatic - see Cirrhosis, liver
infantile - see Hydrops, fetalis
kidney (see also Nephrosis) 581.9
liver - see Cirrhosis, liver
lung 514
malarial (see also Malaria) 084.9
neonatorum - see Hydrops, fetalis
nephritic 581.9
newborn - see Hydrops, fetalis
nutritional 269.9
ovary 620.8
pericardium (see also Pericarditis) 423.9
renal (see also Nephrosis) 581.9
uremic - see Uremia
Drowned, drowning (near) 994.1
lung 518.52
Drowsiness 780.09
Drug - see also condition
addiction (see also Dependence) 304.9●
adverse effect, correct substance properly
administered 995.20
allergy 995.27
dependence (see also Dependence) 304.9●
habit (see also Dependence) 304.9●
hypersensitivity 995.27
induced
circadian rhythm sleep disorder 292.85
hypersomnia 292.85
insomnia 292.85
mental disorder 292.9
anxiety 292.89
mood 292.84
sexual 292.89
sleep 292.85
specified type 292.89
parasomnia 292.85
persisting
amnestic disorder 292.83
dementia 292.82
psychotic disorder
with
delusions 292.11
hallucinations 292.12
sleep disorder 292.85
intoxication 292.89
overdose - see Table of Drugs and Chemicals
poisoning - see Table of Drugs and Chemicals
therapy (maintenance) status NEC
chemotherapy, antineoplastic V58.11
immunotherapy, antineoplastic V58.12
long-term (current) (prophylactic) use
V58.69
antibiotics V58.62
anticoagulants V58.61
anti-inflammatories, non-steroidal
(NSAID) V58.64
antiplatelets V58.63
antithrombotics V58.63
aspirin V58.66

Drug (Continued)
therapy status NEC (Continued)
long-term use (Continued)
bisphosphonates V58.68
high-risk medications NEC V58.69
insulin V58.67
methadone for pain control V58.69
opiate analgesic V58.69
steroids V58.65
methadone 304.00
wrong substance given or taken in error - see
Table of Drugs and Chemicals
Drunkenness (see also Abuse, drugs,
nondependent) 305.0●
acute in alcoholism (see also Alcoholism)
303.0●
chronic (see also Alcoholism) 303.9●
pathologic 291.4
simple (acute) 305.0●
in alcoholism 303.0●
sleep 307.47
Drusen
optic disc or papilla 377.21
retina (colloid) (hyaloid degeneration) 362.57
hereditary 362.77
Drusenfieber 075
Dry, dryness - see also condition
eye 375.15
syndrome 375.15
larynx 478.79
mouth 527.7
nose 478.19
skin syndrome 701.1
socket (teeth) 526.5
throat 478.29
DSAP (disseminated superficial actinic
porokeratosis) 692.75
DSTR (delayed serologic transfusion reaction)
due to or resulting from
incompatibility
ABO 999.69
non-ABO antigen (minor) (Duffy)
(Kell) (Kidd) (Lewis) (M) (N) (P)
(S) 999.79
Rh antigen (C) (c) (D) (E) (e) 999.74
Duane's retraction syndrome 378.71
Duane-Stilling-Türk syndrome (ocular
retraction syndrome) 378.71
Dubin-Johnson disease or syndrome 277.4
Dubini's disease (electric chorea) 049.8
Dubois' abscess or disease 090.5
Duchenne's
disease 094.0
locomotor ataxia 094.0
muscular dystrophy 359.1
pseudohypertrophy, muscles 359.1
paralysis 335.22
syndrome 335.22
Duchenne-Aran myelopathic, muscular atrophy
(nonprogressive) (progressive) 335.21
Duchenne-Griesinger disease 359.1
Ducrey's
bacillus 099.0
chancre 099.0
disease (chancroid) 099.0
Duct, ductus - see condition
Duengero 061
Duhring's disease (dermatitis herpetiformis)
694.0
Dukes (-Filatov) disease 057.8
Dullness
cardiac (decreased) (increased) 785.3
Dumb ague (see also Malaria) 084.6
Dumbness (see also Aphasia) 784.3
Dumdum fever 085.0
Dumping syndrome (postgastrectomy) 564.2
nonsurgical 536.8
Duodenitis (nonspecific) (peptic) 535.60
with hemorrhage 535.61
due to
strongyloides stercoralis 127.2

◀ New ◀◀◀ Revised ~~deleted~~ Deleted ● Use Additional Digit(s) ▨ Omit code

Duodenocholangitis 575.8
Duodenum, duodenal - *see* condition
Duplay's disease, periarthritis, or syndrome
  726.2
Duplex - *see also* Accessory
  kidney 753.3
  placenta - *see* Placenta, abnormal
  uterus 752.2
Duplication - *see also* Accessory
  anus 751.5
  aortic arch 747.21
  appendix 751.5
  biliary duct (any) 751.69
  bladder 753.8
  cecum 751.5
    and appendix 751.5
  cervical, cervix 752.44
  clitoris 752.49
  cystic duct 751.69
  digestive organs 751.8
  duodenum 751.5
  esophagus 750.4
  fallopian tube 752.19
  frontonasal process 756.0
  gallbladder 751.69
  ileum 751.5
  intestine (large) (small) 751.5
  jejunum 751.5
  kidney 753.3
  liver 751.69
  nose 748.1
  pancreas 751.7
  penis 752.69
  respiratory organs NEC 748.9
  salivary duct 750.22
  spinal cord (incomplete) 742.51
  stomach 750.7
  ureter 753.4
  vagina 752.47
  vas deferens 752.89
  vocal cords 748.3
Dupré's disease or syndrome (meningism)
  781.6
Dupuytren's
  contraction 728.6
  disease (muscle contracture) 728.6
  fracture (closed) 824.4
    ankle (closed) 824.4
      open 824.5
    fibula (closed) 824.4
      open 824.5
    open 824.5
    radius (closed) 813.42
      open 813.52
  muscle contracture 728.6
Durand-Nicolas-Favre disease (climatic bubo)
  099.1
Durotomy, incidental (inadvertent) (*see also*
  Tear, dural) 349.31
Duroziez's disease (congenital mitral stenosis)
  746.5
Dust
  conjunctivitis 372.05
  reticulation (occupational) 504
Dutton's
  disease (trypanosomiasis) 086.9
  relapsing fever (West African) 087.1
Dwarf, dwarfism 259.4
  with infantilism (hypophyseal)
    253.3
  achondroplastic 756.4
  Amsterdam 759.89
  bird-headed 759.89
  congenital 259.4
  constitutional 259.4
  hypophyseal 253.3
  infantile 259.4
  Levi type 253.3
  Lorain-Levi (pituitary) 253.3
  Lorain type (pituitary) 253.3
  metatropic 756.4

Dwarf, dwarfism (Continued)
  nephrotic-glycosuric, with
    hypophosphatemic rickets 270.0
  nutritional 263.2
  ovarian 758.6
  pancreatic 577.8
  pituitary 253.3
  polydystrophic 277.5
  primordial 253.3
  psychosocial 259.4
  renal 588.0
    with hypertension - *see* Hypertension,
      kidney
  Russell's (uterine dwarfism and craniofacial
    dysostosis) 759.89
Dyke-Young anemia or syndrome (acquired
  macrocytic hemolytic anemia)
  (secondary) (symptomatic) 283.9
Dynia abnormality (*see also* Defect, coagulation)
  286.9
Dysacousis 388.40
Dysadrenocortism 255.9
  hyperfunction 255.3
  hypofunction 255.41
Dysarthria 784.51
  due to late effect of cerebrovascular disease
    (*see also* Late effect(s) (of)
    cerebrovascular disease) 438.13
Dysautonomia (*see also* Neuropathy, peripheral,
  autonomic) 337.9
  familial 742.8
Dysbarism 993.3
Dysbasia 719.7
  angiosclerotica intermittens 443.9
    due to atherosclerosis 440.21
  hysterical 300.11
  lordotica (progressiva) 333.6
  nonorganic origin 307.9
  psychogenic 307.9
Dysbetalipoproteinemia (familial) 272.2
Dyscalculia 315.1
Dyschezia (*see also* Constipation) 564.00
Dyschondroplasia (with hemangiomata) 756.4
  Voorhoeve's 756.4
Dyschondrosteosis 756.59
Dyschromia 709.00
Dyscollagenosis 710.9
Dyscoria 743.41
Dyscraniopyophalangy 759.89
Dyscrasia
  blood 289.9
    with antepartum hemorrhage 641.3●
    hemorrhage, subungual 287.8
    newborn NEC 776.9
    puerperal, postpartum 666.3●
  ovary 256.8
  plasma cell 273.9
  pluriglandular 258.9
  polyglandular 258.9
Dysdiadochokinesia 781.3
Dysectasia, vesical neck 596.89
Dysendocrinism 259.9
Dysentery, dysenteric (bilious) (catarrhal)
  (diarrhea) (epidemic) (gangrenous)
  (hemorrhagic) (infectious) (sporadic)
  (tropical) (ulcerative) 009.0
  abscess, liver (*see also* Abscess, amebic) 006.3
  amebic (*see also* Amebiasis) 006.9
    with abscess - *see* Abscess, amebic
    acute 006.0
    carrier (suspected) of V02.2
    chronic 006.1
  arthritis (*see also* Arthritis, due to, dysentery)
    009.0 [711.3]●
    bacillary 004.9 [711.3]●
  asylum 004.9
  bacillary 004.9
    arthritis 004.9 [711.3]●
    Boyd 004.2
    Flexner 004.1
    Schmitz (-Stutzer) 004.0

Dysentery, dysenteric (Continued)
  bacillary (Continued)
    Shiga 004.0
    Shigella 004.9
      group A 004.0
      group B 004.1
      group C 004.2
      group D 004.3
      specified type NEC 004.8
    Sonne 004.3
    specified type NEC 004.8
  bacterium 004.9
  balantidial 007.0
  Balantidium coli 007.0
  Boyd's 004.2
  Chilomastix 007.8
  Chinese 004.9
  choleriform 001.1
  coccidial 007.2
  Dientamoeba fragilis 007.8
  due to specified organism NEC - *see* Enteritis,
    due to, by organism
  Embadomonas 007.8
  Endolimax nana - *see* Dysentery, amebic
  Entamoba, entamebic - *see* Dysentery, amebic
  Flexner's 004.1
  Flexner-Boyd 004.2
  giardial 007.1
  Giardia lamblia 007.1
  Hiss-Russell 004.1
  lamblia 007.1
  leishmanial 085.0
  malarial (*see also* Malaria) 084.6
  metazoal 127.9
  Monilia 112.89
  protozoal NEC 007.9
  Russell's 004.8
  salmonella 003.0
  schistosomal 120.1
  Schmitz (-Stutzer) 004.0
  Shiga 004.0
  Shigella NEC (*see also* Dysentery, bacillary)
    004.9
    boydii 004.2
    dysenteriae 004.0
      Schmitz 004.0
      Shiga 004.0
    flexneri 004.1
    group A 004.0
    group B 004.1
    group C 004.2
    group D 004.3
    Schmitz 004.0
    Shiga 004.0
    Sonnei 004.3
  Sonne 004.3
  strongyloidiasis 127.2
  trichomonal 007.3
  tuberculous (*see also* Tuberculosis) 014.8●
  viral (*see also* Enteritis, viral) 008.8
Dysequilibrium 780.4
Dysesthesia 782.0
  hysterical 300.11
Dysfibrinogenemia (congenital) (*see also* Defect,
  coagulation) 286.3
Dysfunction
  adrenal (cortical) 255.9
    hyperfunction 255.3
    hypofunction 255.41
  associated with sleep stages or arousal from
    sleep 780.56
    nonorganic origin 307.47
  bladder NEC 596.59
  bleeding, uterus 626.8
  brain, minimal (*see also* Hyperkinesia)
    314.9
  cerebral 348.30
  colon 564.9
    psychogenic 306.4
  colostomy or enterostomy 569.62
  cystic duct 575.8

Dysfunction (Continued)
　diastolic 429.9
　　with heart failure - see Failure, heart
　　due to
　　　cardiomyopathy - see Cardiomyopathy
　　　hypertension - see Hypertension, heart
　endocrine NEC 259.9
　endometrium 621.8
　enteric stoma 569.62
　enterostomy 569.62
　erectile 607.84
　　nonorganic origin 302.72
　esophagostomy 530.87
　Eustachian tube 381.81
　gallbladder 575.8
　gastrointestinal 536.9
　gland, glandular NEC 259.9
　heart 427.9
　　postoperative (immediate) 997.1
　　　long-term effect of cardiac surgery
　　　　429.4
　hemoglobin 289.89
　hepatic 573.9
　hepatocellular NEC 573.9
　hypophysis 253.9
　　hyperfunction 253.1
　　hypofunction 253.2
　　posterior lobe 253.6
　　　hypofunction 253.5
　kidney (see also Disease, renal) 593.9
　labyrinthine 386.50
　　specified NEC 386.58
　liver 573.9
　　constitutional 277.4
　minimal brain (child) (see also Hyperkinesia)
　　314.9
　ovary, ovarian 256.9
　　hyperfunction 256.1
　　　estrogen 256.0
　　hypofunction 256.39
　　　postablative 256.2
　　postablative 256.2
　　specified NEC 256.8
　papillary muscle 429.81
　　with myocardial infarction 410.8●
　parathyroid 252.8
　　hyperfunction 252.00
　　hypofunction 252.1
　pineal gland 259.8
　pituitary (gland) 253.9
　　hyperfunction 253.1
　　hypofunction 253.2
　　posterior 253.6
　　　hypofunction 253.5
　placental - see Placenta, insufficiency
　platelets (blood) 287.1
　polyglandular 258.9
　　specified NEC 258.8
　psychosexual 302.70
　　with
　　　dyspareunia (functional) (psychogenic)
　　　　302.76
　　　frigidity 302.72
　　　impotence 302.72
　　　inhibition
　　　　orgasm
　　　　　female 302.73
　　　　　male 302.74
　　　　sexual
　　　　　desire 302.71
　　　　　excitement 302.72
　　　premature ejaculation 302.75
　　　sexual aversion 302.79
　　　specified disorder NEC 302.79
　　　vaginismus 306.51
　pylorus 537.9
　rectum 564.9
　　psychogenic 306.4
　segmental (see also Dysfunction, somatic)
　　739.9
　senile 797

Dysfunction (Continued)
　sexual 302.70
　sinoatrial node 427.81
　somatic 739.9
　　abdomen 739.9
　　acromioclavicular 739.7
　　cervical 739.1
　　cervicothoracic 739.1
　　costochondral 739.8
　　costovertebral 739.8
　　extremities
　　　lower 739.6
　　　upper 739.7
　　head 739.0
　　hip 739.5
　　lumbar, lumbosacral 739.3
　　occipitocervical 739.0
　　pelvic 739.5
　　pubic 739.5
　　rib cage 739.8
　　sacral 739.4
　　sacrococcygeal 739.4
　　sacroiliac 739.4
　　specified site NEC 739.9
　　sternochondral 739.8
　　sternoclavicular 739.7
　　temporomandibular 739.0
　　thoracic, thoracolumbar 739.2
　stomach 536.9
　　psychogenic 306.4
　suprarenal 255.9
　　hyperfunction 255.3
　　hypofunction 255.41
　symbolic NEC 784.60
　　specified type NEC 784.69
　systolic 429.9
　　with heart failure - see Failure, heart
　temporomandibular (joint) (joint-pain-
　　syndrome) NEC 524.60
　　sounds on opening or closing 524.64
　　specified NEC 524.69
　testicular 257.9
　　hyperfunction 257.0
　　hypofunction 257.2
　　specified type NEC 257.8
　thymus 254.9
　thyroid 246.9
　　complicating pregnancy, childbirth, or
　　　puerperium 648.1●
　　hyperfunction - see Hyperthyroidism
　　hypofunction - see Hypothyroidism
　uterus, complicating delivery 661.9●
　　affecting fetus or newborn 763.7
　　hypertonic 661.4●
　　hypotonic 661.2●
　　　primary 661.0●
　　　secondary 661.1●
　velopharyngeal (acquired) 528.9
　　congenital 750.29
　ventricular 429.9
　　with congestive heart failure (see also
　　　Failure, heart) 428.0
　　due to
　　　cardiomyopathy - see Cardiomyopathy
　　　hypertension - see Hypertension, heart
　　left, reversible following sudden
　　　emotional stress 429.83
　vesicourethral NEC 596.59
　vestibular 386.50
　　specified type NEC 386.58
Dysgammaglobulinemia 279.06
Dysgenesis
　gonadal (due to chromosomal anomaly)
　　758.6
　　pure 752.7
　kidney(s) 753.0
　ovarian 758.6
　renal 753.0
　reticular 279.2
　seminiferous tubules 758.6
　tidal platelet 287.31

Dysgerminoma (M9060/3)
　specified site - see Neoplasm, by site,
　　malignant
　unspecified site
　　female 183.0
　　male 186.9
Dysgeusia 781.1
Dysgraphia 781.3
Dyshidrosis 705.81
Dysidrosis 705.81
Dysinsulinism 251.8
Dyskaryotic cervical smear 795.09
Dyskeratosis (see also Keratosis) 701.1
　bullosa hereditaria 757.39
　cervix 622.10
　congenital 757.39
　follicularis 757.39
　　vitamin A deficiency 264.8
　gingiva 523.8
　oral soft tissue NEC 528.79
　tongue 528.79
　uterus NEC 621.8
Dyskinesia 781.3
　biliary 575.8
　esophagus 530.5
　hysterical 300.11
　intestinal 564.89
　neuroleptic-induced tardive 333.85
　nonorganic origin 307.9
　orofacial 333.82
　　due to drugs 333.85
　psychogenic 307.9
　subacute, due to drugs 333.85
　tardive (oral) 333.85
Dyslalia 784.59
　developmental 315.39
Dyslexia 784.61
　developmental 315.02
　secondary to organic lesion 784.61
Dyslipidemia 272.4
Dysmaturity (see also Immaturity) 765.1●
　lung 770.4
　pulmonary 770.4
Dysmenorrhea (essential) (exfoliative)
　　(functional) (intrinsic) (membranous)
　　(primary) (secondary) 625.3
　psychogenic 306.52
Dysmetabolic syndrome X 277.7
Dysmetria 781.3
Dysmorodystrophia mesodermalis congenita
　759.82
Dysnomia 784.3
Dysorexia 783.0
　hysterical 300.11
Dysostosis
　cleidocranial, cleidocranialis 755.59
　craniofacial 756.0
　Fairbank's (idiopathic familial generalized
　　osteophytosis) 756.50
　mandibularis 756.0
　mandibulofacial, incomplete 756.0
　multiplex 277.5
　orodigitofacial 759.89
Dyspareunia (female) 625.0
　male 608.89
　psychogenic 302.76
Dyspepsia (allergic) (congenital)
　　(fermentative) (flatulent) (functional)
　　(gastric) (gastrointestinal)
　　(neurogenic) (occupational) (reflex)
　　536.8
　acid 536.8
　atonic 536.3
　　psychogenic 306.4
　diarrhea 787.91
　　psychogenic 306.4
　intestinal 564.89
　　psychogenic 306.4
　nervous 306.4
　neurotic 306.4
　psychogenic 306.4

◀ New　◀▥▥ Revised　d̶e̶l̶e̶t̶e̶d̶ Deleted　● Use Additional Digit(s)　▨ Omit code

Dysphagia 787.20
cervical 787.29
functional 300.11
hysterical 300.11
nervous 300.11
neurogenic 787.29
oral phase 787.21
oropharyngeal phase 787.22
pharyngeal phase 787.23
pharyngoesophageal phase 787.24
psychogenic 306.4
sideropenic 280.8
spastica 530.5
specified NEC 787.29
Dysphagocytosis, congenital 288.1
Dysphasia 784.59
Dysphonia 784.42
clericorum 784.49
functional 300.11
hysterical 300.11
psychogenic 306.1
spastica 478.79
Dyspigmentation - *see also* Pigmentation
eyelid (acquired) 374.52
Dyspituitarism 253.9
hyperfunction 253.1
hypofunction 253.2
posterior lobe 253.6
Dysplasia - *see also* Anomaly
alveolar capillary, with vein misalignment 516.64
anus 569.44
intraepithelial neoplasia I (AIN I) (histologically confirmed) 569.44
intraepithelial neoplasia II (AIN II) (histologically confirmed) 569.44
intraepithelial neoplasia III (AIN III) 230.6
anal canal 230.5
mild (histologically confirmed) 569.44
moderate (histologically confirmed) 569.44
severe 230.6
anal canal 230.5
artery
fibromuscular NEC 447.8
carotid 447.8
renal 447.3
bladder 596.89
bone (fibrous) NEC 733.29
diaphyseal, progressive 756.59
jaw 526.89
monostotic 733.29
polyostotic 756.54
solitary 733.29
brain 742.9
bronchopulmonary, fetus or newborn 770.7
cervix (uteri) 622.10
cervical intraepithelial neoplasia I (CIN I) 622.11
cervical intraepithelial neoplasia II (CIN II) 622.12
cervical intraepithelial neoplasia III (CIN III) 233.1
CIN I 622.11
CIN II 622.12
CIN III 233.1
mild 622.11
moderate 622.12
severe 233.1
chondroectodermal 756.55
chondromatose 756.4
colon 211.3
craniocarpotarsal 759.89
craniometaphyseal 756.89
dentinal 520.5
diaphyseal, progressive 756.59
ectodermal (anhidrotic) (Bason) (Clouston's) (congenital) (Feinmesser) (hereditary) (hidrotic) (Marshall) (Robinson's) 757.31

Dysplasia (*Continued*)
epiphysealis 756.9
multiplex 756.56
punctata 756.59
epiphysis 756.9
multiple 756.56
epithelial
epiglottis 478.79
uterine cervix 622.10
erythroid NEC 289.89
eye (*see also* Microphthalmos) 743.10
familial metaphyseal 756.89
fibromuscular, artery NEC 447.8
carotid 447.8
renal 447.3
fibrous
bone NEC 733.29
diaphyseal, progressive 756.59
jaw 526.89
monostotic 733.29
polyostotic 756.54
solitary 733.29
high grade, focal - *see* Neoplasm, by site, benign
hip (congenital) 755.63
with dislocation (*see also* Dislocation, hip, congenital) 754.30
hypohidrotic ectodermal 757.31
joint 755.8
kidney 753.15
leg 755.69
linguofacialis 759.89
lung 748.5
macular 743.55
mammary (benign) (gland) 610.9
cystic 610.1
specified type NEC 610.8
metaphyseal 756.9
familial 756.89
monostotic fibrous 733.29
muscle 756.89
myeloid NEC 289.89
nervous system (general) 742.9
neuroectodermal 759.6
oculoauriculovertebral 756.0
oculodentodigital 759.89
olfactogenital 253.4
osteo-onycho-arthro (hereditary) 756.89
periosteum 733.99
polyostotic fibrous 756.54
progressive diaphyseal 756.59
prostate 602.3
intraepithelial neoplasia I [PIN I] 602.3
intraepithelial neoplasia II [PIN II] 602.3
intraepithelial neoplasia III [PIN III] 233.4
renal 753.15
renofacialis 753.0
retinal NEC 743.56
retrolental (*see also* Retinopathy of prematurity) 362.21
skin 709.8
spinal cord 742.9
thymic, with immunodeficiency 279.2
vagina 623.0
mild 623.0
moderate 623.0
severe 233.31
vocal cord 478.5
vulva 624.8
intraepithelial neoplasia I (VIN I) 624.01
intraepithelial neoplasia II (VIN II) 624.02
intraepithelial neoplasia III (VIN III) 233.32
mild 624.01
moderate 624.02
severe 233.32
VIN I 624.01
VIN II 624.02
VIN III 233.32

Dyspnea (nocturnal) (paroxysmal) 786.09
asthmatic (bronchial) (*see also* Asthma) 493.9●
with bronchitis (*see also* Asthma) 493.9●
chronic 493.2●
cardiac (*see also* Failure, ventricular, left) 428.1
cardiac (*see also* Failure, ventricular, left) 428.1
functional 300.11
hyperventilation 786.01
hysterical 300.11
Monday morning 504
newborn 770.89
psychogenic 306.1
uremic - *see* Uremia
Dyspraxia 781.3
syndrome 315.4
Dysproteinemia 273.8
transient with copper deficiency 281.4
Dysprothrombinemia (constitutional) (*see also* Defect, coagulation) 286.3
Dysreflexia, autonomic 337.3
Dysrhythmia
cardiac 427.9
postoperative (immediate) 997.1
long-term effect of cardiac surgery 429.4
specified type NEC 427.89
cerebral or cortical 348.30
Dyssecretosis, mucoserous 710.2
Dyssocial reaction, without manifest psychiatric disorder
adolescent V71.02
adult V71.01
child V71.02
Dyssomnia NEC 780.56
nonorganic origin 307.47
Dyssplenism 289.4
Dyssynergia
biliary (*see also* Disease, biliary) 576.8
cerebellaris myoclonica 334.2
detrusor sphincter (bladder) 596.55
ventricular 429.89
Dystasia, hereditary areflexic 334.3
Dysthymia 300.4
Dysthymic disorder 300.4
Dysthyroidism 246.9
Dystocia 660.9●
affecting fetus or newborn 763.1
cervical 661.2●
affecting fetus or newborn 763.7
contraction ring 661.4●
affecting fetus or newborn 763.7
fetal 660.9●
abnormal size 653.5●
affecting fetus or newborn 763.1
deformity 653.7●
maternal 660.9●
affecting fetus or newborn 763.1
positional 660.0●
affecting fetus or newborn 763.1
shoulder (girdle) 660.4●
affecting fetus or newborn 763.1
uterine NEC 661.4●
affecting fetus or newborn 763.7
Dystonia
acute
due to drugs 333.72
neuroleptic-induced acute 333.72
deformans progressiva 333.6
lenticularis 333.6
musculorum deformans 333.6
torsion (idiopathic) 333.6
acquired 333.79
fragments (of) 333.89
genetic 333.6
symptomatic 333.79
Dystonic
movements 781.0
Dystopia kidney 753.3

Dystrophy, dystrophia 783.9
  adiposogenital 253.8
  asphyxiating thoracic 756.4
  Becker's type 359.22
  brevicollis 756.16
  Bruch's membrane 362.77
  cervical (sympathetic) NEC 337.09
  chondro-osseus with punctate epiphyseal
      dysplasia 756.59
  choroid (hereditary) 363.50
    central (areolar) (partial) 363.53
      total (gyrate) 363.54
    circinate 363.53
    circumpapillary (partial) 363.51
      total 363.52
    diffuse
      partial 363.56
      total 363.57
    generalized
      partial 363.56
      total 363.57
    gyrate
      central 363.54
      generalized 363.57
    helicoid 363.52
    peripapillary - see Dystrophy, choroid,
        circumpapillary
    serpiginous 363.54
  cornea (hereditary) 371.50
    anterior NEC 371.52
    Cogan's 371.52
    combined 371.57
    crystalline 371.56
    endothelial (Fuchs') 371.57
    epithelial 371.50
      juvenile 371.51
      microscopic cystic 371.52
    granular 371.53
    lattice 371.54
    macular 371.55
    marginal (Terrien's) 371.48
    Meesman's 371.51
    microscopic cystic (epithelial)
        371.52
    nodular, Salzmann's 371.46
    polymorphous 371.58
    posterior NEC 371.58
    ring-like 371.52

Dystrophy, dystrophia (Continued)
  cornea (Continued)
    Salzmann's nodular 371.46
    stromal NEC 371.56
  dermatochondrocorneal 371.50
  Duchenne's 359.1
  due to malnutrition 263.9
  Erb's 359.1
  familial
    hyperplastic periosteal 756.59
    osseous 277.5
  foveal 362.77
  Fuchs', cornea 371.57
  Gowers' muscular 359.1
  hair 704.2
  hereditary, progressive muscular 359.1
  hypogenital, with diabetic tendency 759.81
  Landouzy-Déjérine 359.1
  Leyden-Möbius 359.1
  mesodermalis congenita 759.82
  muscular 359.1
    congenital (hereditary) 359.0
      myotonic 359.22
    distal 359.1
    Duchenne's 359.1
    Erb's 359.1
    fascioscapulohumeral 359.1
    Gowers' 359.1
    hereditary (progressive) 359.1
    Landouzy-Déjérine 359.1
    limb-girdle 359.1
    myotonic 359.21
    progressive (hereditary) 359.1
      Charcôt-Marie-Tooth 356.1
    pseudohypertrophic (infantile) 359.1
  myocardium, myocardial (see also
      Degeneration, myocardial) 429.1
  myotonic 359.21
  myotonica 359.21
  nail 703.8
    congenital 757.5
  neurovascular (traumatic) (see also
      Neuropathy, peripheral, autonomic)
      337.9
  nutritional 263.9
  ocular 359.1
  oculocerebrorenal 270.8
  oculopharyngeal 359.1

Dystrophy, dystrophia (Continued)
  ovarian 620.8
  papillary (and pigmentary) 701.1
  pelvicrural atrophic 359.1
  pigmentary (see also Acanthosis) 701.2
  pituitary (gland) 253.8
  polyglandular 258.8
  posttraumatic sympathetic - see Dystrophy,
      symphatic
  progressive ophthalmoplegic 359.1
  reflex neuromuscular - see Dystrophy,
      sympathetic
  retina, retinal (hereditary) 362.70
    albipunctate 362.74
    Bruch's membrane 362.77
    cone, progressive 362.75
    hyaline 362.77
    in
      Bassen-Kornzweig syndrome 272.5
          [362.72]
      cerebroretinal lipidosis 330.1 [362.71]
      Refsum's disease 356.3 [362.72]
      systemic lipidosis 272.7 [362.71]
    juvenile (Stargardt's) 362.75
    pigmentary 362.74
    pigment epithelium 362.76
    progressive cone (-rod) 362.75
    pseudoinflammatory foveal 362.77
    rod, progressive 362.75
    sensory 362.75
    vitelliform 362.76
  Salzmann's nodular 371.46
  scapuloperoneal 359.1
  skin NEC 709.9
  sympathetic (posttraumatic) (reflex)
      337.20
    lower limb 337.22
    specified site NEC 337.29
    upper limb 337.21
  tapetoretinal NEC 362.74
  thoracic asphyxiating 756.4
  unguium 703.8
    congenital 757.5
  vitreoretinal (primary) 362.73
    secondary 362.66
  vulva 624.09
Dysuria 788.1
  psychogenic 306.53

E

Eagle-Barrett syndrome 756.71
Eales' disease (syndrome) 362.18
Ear - *see also* condition
   ache 388.70
     otogenic 388.71
      referred 388.72
   lop 744.29
   piercing V50.3
   swimmers' acute 380.12
   tank 380.12
   tropical 111.8 [380.15]
   wax 380.4
Earache 388.70
   otogenic 388.71
   referred 388.72
Early satiety 780.94
Eaton-Lambert syndrome (*see also* Syndrome, Lambert-Eaton) 358.30
Eberth's disease (typhoid fever) 002.0
Ebstein's
   anomaly or syndrome (downward displacement, tricuspid valve into right ventricle) 746.2
   disease (diabetes) 250.4● [581.81]
     due to secondary diabetes 249.4● [581.81]
Eccentro-osteochondrodysplasia 277.5
Ecchondroma (M9210/0) - *see* Neoplasm, bone, benign
Ecchondrosis (M9210/1) 238.0
Ecchordosis physaliphora 756.0
Ecchymosis (multiple) 459.89
   conjunctiva 372.72
   eye (traumatic) 921.0
   eyelids (traumatic) 921.1
   newborn 772.6
   spontaneous 782.7
   traumatic - *see* Contusion
ECD (Erdheim-Chester disease) 277.89
Echinococciasis - *see* Echinococcus
Echinococcosis - *see* Echinococcus
Echinococcus (infection) 122.9
   granulosus 122.4
     liver 122.0
     lung 122.1
     orbit 122.3 [376.13]
     specified site NEC 122.3
     thyroid 122.2
   liver NEC 122.8
     granulosus 122.0
     multilocularis 122.5
   lung NEC 122.9
     granulosus 122.1
     multilocularis 122.6
   multilocularis 122.7
     liver 122.5
     specified site NEC 122.6
   orbit 122.9 [376.13]
     granulosus 122.3 [376.13]
     multilocularis 122.6 [376.13]
   specified site NEC 122.9
     granulosus 122.3
     multilocularis 122.6 [376.13]
   thyroid NEC 122.9
     granulosus 122.2
     multilocularis 122.6
Echinorhynchiasis 127.7
Echinostomiasis 121.8
Echolalia 784.69
ECHO virus infection NEC 079.1
Eclampsia, eclamptic (coma) (convulsions) (delirium) 780.39
   female, child-bearing age NEC - *see* Eclampsia, pregnancy
   gravidarum - *see* Eclampsia, pregnancy
   male 780.39
   not associated with pregnancy or childbirth 780.39

Eclampsia, eclamptic (*Continued*)
   pregnancy, childbirth, or puerperium 642.6●
     with pre-existing hypertension 642.7●
     affecting fetus or newborn 760.0
   uremic 586
Eclipse blindness (total) 363.31
Economic circumstance affecting care V60.9
   specified type NEC V60.89
Economo's disease (encephalitis lethargica) 049.8
Ectasia, ectasis
   annuloaortic 424.1
   aorta (*see also* Ectasia, aortic) 447.70
     with aneurysm 441.9
      ruptured 441.5
   aortic 447.70
     with aneurysm 441.9
     abdominal 447.72
     thoracic 447.71
     thoracoabdominal 447.73
   breast 610.4
   capillary 448.9
   cornea (marginal) (postinfectional) 371.71
   duct (mammary) 610.4
   gastric antral vascular (GAVE) 537.82
     with hemorrhage 537.83
     without hemorrhage 537.82
   kidney 593.89
   mammary duct (gland) 610.4
   papillary 448.9
   renal 593.89
   salivary gland (duct) 527.8
   scar, cornea 371.71
   sclera 379.11
Ecthyma 686.8
   contagiosum 051.2
   gangrenosum 686.09
   infectiosum 051.2
Ectocardia 746.87
Ectodermal dysplasia, congenital 757.31
Ectodermosis erosiva pluriorificialis 695.19
Ectopic, ectopia (congenital) 759.89
   abdominal viscera 751.8
     due to defect in anterior abdominal wall 756.79
   ACTH syndrome 255.0
   adrenal gland 759.1
   anus 751.5
   auricular beats 427.61
   beats 427.60
   bladder 753.5
   bone and cartilage in lung 748.69
   brain 742.4
   breast tissue 757.6
   cardiac 746.87
   cerebral 742.4
   cordis 746.87
   endometrium 617.9
   gallbladder 751.69
   gastric mucosa 750.7
   gestation - *see* Pregnancy, ectopic
   heart 746.87
   hormone secretion NEC 259.3
   hyperparathyroidism 259.3
   kidney (crossed) (intrathoracic) (pelvis) 753.3
     in pregnancy or childbirth 654.4●
      causing obstructed labor 660.2●
   lens 743.37
   lentis 743.37
   mole - *see* Pregnancy, ectopic
   organ or site NEC - *see* Malposition, congenital
   ovary 752.0
   pancreas, pancreatic tissue 751.7
   pregnancy - *see* Pregnancy, ectopic
   pupil 364.75
   renal 753.3
   sebaceous glands of mouth 750.26

Ectopic, ectopia (*Continued*)
   secretion
     ACTH 255.0
     adrenal hormone 259.3
     adrenalin 259.3
     adrenocorticotropin 255.0
     antidiuretic hormone (ADH) 259.3
     epinephrine 259.3
     hormone NEC 259.3
     norepinephrine 259.3
     pituitary (posterior) 259.3
   spleen 759.0
   testis 752.51
   thyroid 759.2
   ureter 753.4
   ventricular beats 427.69
   vesicae 753.5
Ectrodactyly 755.4
   finger (*see also* Absence, finger, congenital) 755.29
   toe (*see also* Absence, toe, congenital) 755.39
Ectromelia 755.4
   lower limb 755.30
   upper limb 755.20
Ectropion 374.10
   anus 569.49
   cervix 622.0
     with mention of cervicitis 616.0
   cicatricial 374.14
   congenital 743.62
   eyelid 374.10
     cicatricial 374.14
     congenital 743.62
     mechanical 374.12
     paralytic 374.12
     senile 374.11
     spastic 374.13
   iris (pigment epithelium) 364.54
   lip (congenital) 750.26
     acquired 528.5
   mechanical 374.12
   paralytic 374.12
   rectum 569.49
   senile 374.11
   spastic 374.13
   urethra 599.84
   uvea 364.54
Eczema (acute) (allergic) (chronic) (erythematous) (fissum) (occupational) (rubrum) (squamous) 692.9
   asteatotic 706.8
   atopic 691.8
   contact NEC 692.9
   dermatitis NEC 692.9
   due to specified cause - *see* Dermatitis, due to
   dyshidrotic 705.81
   external ear 380.22
   flexural 691.8
   gouty 274.89
   herpeticum 054.0
   hypertrophicum 701.8
   hypostatic - *see* Varicose, vein
   impetiginous 684
   infantile (acute) (chronic) (due to any substance) (intertriginous) (seborrheic) 690.12
   intertriginous NEC 692.9
     infantile 690.12
   intrinsic 691.8
   lichenified NEC 692.9
   marginatum 110.3
   nummular 692.9
   pustular 686.8
   seborrheic 690.18
     infantile 690.12
   solare 692.72
   stasis (lower extremity) 454.1
     ulcerated 454.2
   vaccination, vaccinatum 999.0
   varicose (lower extremity) - *see* Varicose, vein
   verrucosum callosum 698.3

Eczematoid, exudative 691.8
Eddowes' syndrome (brittle bones and blue
  sclera) 756.51
Edema, edematous 782.3
  with nephritis (see also Nephrosis) 581.9
  allergic 995.1
  angioneurotic (allergic) (any site) (with
      urticaria) 995.1
    hereditary 277.6
  angiospastic 443.9
  Berlin's (traumatic) 921.3
  brain (cytotoxic) (vasogenic) 348.5
    due to birth injury 767.8
    fetus or newborn 767.8
  cardiac (see also Failure, heart) 428.0
  cardiovascular (see also Failure, heart) 428.0
  cerebral - see Edema, brain
  cerebrospinal vessel - see Edema, brain
  cervix (acute) (uteri) 622.8
    puerperal, postpartum 674.8●
  chronic hereditary 757.0
  circumscribed, acute 995.1
    hereditary 277.6
  complicating pregnancy (gestational) 646.1●
    with hypertension - see Toxemia, of
        pregnancy
  conjunctiva 372.73
  connective tissue 782.3
  cornea 371.20
    due to contact lenses 371.24
    idiopathic 371.21
    secondary 371.22
  cystoid macular 362.53
  due to
    lymphatic obstruction - see Edema,
        lymphatic
    salt retention 276.0
  epiglottis - see Edema, glottis
  essential, acute 995.1
    hereditary 277.6
  extremities, lower - see Edema, legs
  eyelid NEC 374.82
  familial, hereditary (legs) 757.0
  famine 262
  fetus or newborn 778.5
  genital organs
    female 629.89
    male 608.86
  gestational 646.1●
    with hypertension - see Toxemia, of
        pregnancy
  glottis, glottic, glottides (obstructive)
      (passive) 478.6
    allergic 995.1
      hereditary 277.6
    due to external agent - see Condition,
        respiratory, acute, due to specified
        agent
  heart (see also Failure, heart) 428.0
    newborn 779.89
  heat 992.7
  hereditary (legs) 757.0
  inanition 262
  infectious 782.3
  intracranial 348.5
    due to injury at birth 767.8
  iris 364.89
  joint (see also Effusion, joint) 719.0●
  larynx (see also Edema, glottis) 478.6
  legs 782.3
    due to venous obstruction 459.2
    hereditary 757.0
  localized 782.3
    due to venous obstruction 459.2
      lower extremity 459.2
  lower extremities - see Edema, legs
  lung 514
    acute 518.4
      with heart disease or failure (see also
          Failure, ventricular, left) 428.1
        congestive 428.0

Edema, edematous (Continued)
  lung (Continued)
    acute (Continued)
      chemical (due to fumes or vapors)
          506.1
        due to
          external agent(s) NEC 508.9
            specified NEC 508.8
          fumes and vapors (chemical)
              (inhalation) 506.1
          radiation 508.0
      chemical (acute) 506.1
        chronic 506.4
    chronic 514
      chemical (due to fumes or vapors)
          506.4
        due to
          external agent(s) NEC 508.9
            specified NEC 508.8
          fumes or vapors (chemical)
              (inhalation) 506.4
          radiation 508.1
    due to
      external agent 508.9
        specified NEC 508.8
      high altitude 993.2
      near drowning 994.1
    postoperative 518.4
    terminal 514
  lymphatic 457.1
    due to mastectomy operation 457.0
  macula 362.83
    cystoid 362.53
    diabetic 250.5● [362.07]
      due to secondary diabetes 249.5●
          [362.07]
  malignant (see also Gangrene, gas) 040.0
  Milroy's 757.0
  nasopharynx 478.25
  neonatorum 778.5
  nutritional (newborn) 262
    with dyspigmentation, skin and hair
        260
  optic disc or nerve - see Papilledema
  orbit 376.33
    circulatory 459.89
  palate (soft) (hard) 528.9
  pancreas 577.8
  penis 607.83
  periodic 995.1
    hereditary 277.6
  pharynx 478.25
  pitting 782.3
  pulmonary - see Edema, lung
  Quincke's 995.1
    hereditary 277.6
  renal (see also Nephrosis) 581.9
  retina (localized) (macular) (peripheral)
      362.83
    cystoid 362.53
    diabetic 250.5● [362.07]
      due to secondary diabetes 249.5●
          [362.07]
  salt 276.0
  scrotum 608.86
  seminal vesicle 608.86
  spermatic cord 608.86
  spinal cord 336.1
  starvation 262
  stasis - see also Hypertension, venous
      459.30
  subconjunctival 372.73
  subglottic (see also Edema, glottis) 478.6
  supraglottic (see also Edema, glottis) 478.6
  testis 608.86
  toxic NEC 782.3
  traumatic NEC 782.3
  tunica vaginalis 608.86
  vas deferens 608.86
  vocal cord - see Edema, glottis
  vulva (acute) 624.8

Edentia (complete) (partial) (see also Absence,
    tooth) 520.0
  acquired (see also Edentulism) 525.40
    due to
      caries 525.13
      extraction 525.10
      periodontal disease 525.12
      specified NEC 525.19
      trauma 525.11
    causing malocclusion 524.30
  congenital (deficiency of tooth buds)
      520.0
Edentulism 525.40
  complete 525.40
    class I 525.41
    class II 525.42
    class III 525.43
    class IV 525.44
  partial 525.50
    class I 525.51
    class II 525.52
    class III 525.53
    class IV 525.54
Edsall's disease 992.2
Educational handicap V62.3
Edwards' syndrome 758.2
Effect, adverse NEC
  abnormal gravitational (G) forces or states
      994.9
  air pressure - see Effect, adverse, atmospheric
      pressure
  altitude (high) - see Effect, adverse, high
      altitude
  anesthetic
    in labor and delivery NEC 668.9●
      affecting fetus or newborn 763.5
  antitoxin - see Complications, vaccination
  atmospheric pressure 993.9
    due to explosion 993.4
    high 993.3
    low - see Effect, adverse, high altitude
    specified effect NEC 993.8
  biological, correct substance properly
      administered (see also Effect, adverse,
      drug) 995.20
  blood (derivatives) (serum) (transfusion) - see
      Complications, transfusion
  chemical substance NEC 989.9
    specified - see Table of Drugs and
        Chemicals
  cobalt, radioactive (see also Effect,
      adverse, radioactive substance)
      990
  cold (temperature) (weather) 991.9
    chilblains 991.5
    frostbite - see Frostbite
    specified effect NEC 991.8
  drugs and medicinals 995.20
    correct substance properly administered
        995.20
    overdose or wrong substance given or
        taken 977.9
      specified drug - see Table of Drugs and
          Chemicals
  electric current (shock) 994.8
    burn - see Burn, by site
  electricity (electrocution) (shock)
      994.8
    burn - see Burn, by site
  exertion (excessive) 994.5
  exposure 994.9
    exhaustion 994.4
  external cause NEC 994.9
  fallout (radioactive) NEC 990
  fluoroscopy NEC 990
  foodstuffs
    allergic reaction (see also Allergy, food)
        693.1
    anaphylactic reaction or shock due to
        food NEC - see Anaphylactic
        reaction or shock, due to food

◀ New   ◀▥ Revised   ~~deleted~~ Deleted   ● Use Additional Digit(s)   ▨ Omit code

Effect, adverse NEC *(Continued)*
  foodstuffs *(Continued)*
    noxious 988.9
      specified type NEC *(see also* Poisoning,
        by name of noxious foodstuff)
        988.8
  gases, fumes, or vapors - *see* Table of Drugs
    and Chemicals
  glue (airplane) sniffing 304.6●
  heat - *see* Heat
  high altitude NEC 993.2
    anoxia 993.2
    on
      ears 993.0
      sinuses 993.1
    polycythemia 289.0
  hot weather - *see* Heat
  hunger 994.2
  immersion, foot 991.4
  immunization - *see* Complications,
    vaccination
  immunological agents - *see* Complications,
    vaccination
  implantation (removable) of isotope or
    radium NEC 990
  infrared (radiation) (rays) NEC 990
    burn - *see* Burn, by site
    dermatitis or eczema 692.82
  infusion - *see* Complications, infusion
  ingestion or injection of isotope (therapeutic)
    NEC 990
  irradiation NEC *(see also* Effect, adverse,
    radiation) 990
  isotope (radioactive) NEC 990
  lack of care (child) (infant) (newborn) 995.52
    adult 995.84
  lightning 994.0
    burn - *see* Burn, by site
  Lirugin - *see* Complications, vaccination
  medicinal substance, correct, properly
    administered *(see also* Effect, adverse,
    drugs) 995.20
  mesothorium NEC 990
  motion 994.6
  noise, inner ear 388.10
  other drug, medicinal and biological
    substance 995.29
  overheated places - *see* Heat
  polonium NEC 990
  psychosocial, of work environment V62.1
  radiation (diagnostic) (fallout) (infrared)
    (natural source) (therapeutic) (tracer)
    (ultraviolet) (x-ray) NEC 990
    with pulmonary manifestations
      acute 508.0
      chronic 508.1
    dermatitis or eczema 692.82
      due to sun NEC *(see also* Dermatitis,
        due to, sun) 692.70
    fibrosis of lungs 508.1
    maternal with suspected damage to fetus
      affecting management of pregnancy
      655.6●
    pneumonitis 508.0
  radioactive substance NEC 990
    dermatitis or eczema 692.82
  radioactivity NEC 990
  radiotherapy NEC 990
    dermatitis or eczema 692.82
  radium NEC 990
  reduced temperature 991.9
    frostbite - *see* Frostbite
    immersion, foot (hand) 991.4
    specified effect NEC 991.8
  roentgenography NEC 990
  roentgenoscopy NEC 990
  roentgen rays NEC 990
  serum (prophylactic) (therapeutic) NEC
    999.59
  specified NEC 995.89
    external cause NEC 994.9

Effect, adverse NEC *(Continued)*
  strangulation 994.7
  submersion 994.1
  teletherapy NEC 990
  thirst 994.3
  transfusion - *see* Complications, transfusion
  ultraviolet (radiation) (rays) NEC 990
    burn - *see also* Burn, by site
      from sun *(see also* Sunburn) 692.71
    dermatitis or eczema 692.82
      due to sun NEC *(see also* Dermatitis,
        due to, sun) 692.70
  uranium NEC 990
  vaccine (any) - *see* Complications,
    vaccination
  weightlessness 994.9
  whole blood - *see also* Complications,
    transfusion
    overdose or wrong substance given *(see
      also* Table of Drugs and Chemicals)
      964.7
  working environment V62.1
  x-rays NEC 990
    dermatitis or eczema 692.82
Effect, remote
  of cancer - *see* condition
Effects, late - *see* Late, effect (of)
Effluvium, telogen 704.02
Effort
  intolerance 306.2
  syndrome (aviators) (psychogenic) 306.2
Effusion
  amniotic fluid *(see also* Rupture, membranes,
    premature) 658.1●
  brain (serous) 348.5
  bronchial *(see also* Bronchitis) 490
  cerebral 348.5
  cerebrospinal *(see also* Meningitis) 322.9
    vessel 348.5
  chest - *see* Effusion, pleura
  intracranial 348.5
  joint 719.00
    ankle 719.07
    elbow 719.02
    foot 719.07
    hand 719.04
    hip 719.05
    knee 719.06
    multiple sites 719.09
    pelvic region 719.05
    shoulder (region) 719.01
    specified site NEC 719.08
    wrist 719.03
  meninges *(see also* Meningitis) 322.9
  pericardium, pericardial *(see also* Pericarditis)
    423.9
    acute 420.90
  peritoneal (chronic) 568.82
  pleura, pleurisy, pleuritic, pleuropericardial
    511.9
    bacterial, nontuberculous 511.1
    fetus or newborn 511.9
    malignant 511.81
    nontuberculous 511.9
      bacterial 511.1
    pneumococcal 511.1
    staphylococcal 511.1
    streptococcal 511.1
    traumatic 862.29
      with open wound 862.39
    tuberculous *(see also* Tuberculosis, pleura)
      012.0●
      primary progressive 010.1●
  pulmonary - *see* Effusion, pleura
  spinal *(see also* Meningitis) 322.9
  thorax, thoracic - *see* Effusion, pleura
Egg (oocyte) (ovum)
  donor V59.70
    over age 35 V59.73
      anonymous recipient V59.73
      designated recipient V59.74

Egg *(Continued)*
  donor *(Continued)*
    under age 35 V59.71
      anonymous recipient V59.71
      designated recipient V59.72
Eggshell nails 703.8
  congenital 757.5
Ego-dystonic
  homosexuality 302.0
  lesbianism 302.0
  sexual orientation 302.0
Egyptian splenomegaly 120.1
Ehlers-Danlos syndrome 756.83
Ehrlichiosis 082.40
  chaffeensis 082.41
  specified type NEC 082.49
Eichstedt's disease (pityriasis versicolor) 111.0
EIN (endometrial intraepithelial neoplasia)
  621.35
Eisenmenger's complex or syndrome
  (ventricular septal defect) 745.4
Ejaculation, semen
  painful 608.89
    psychogenic 306.59
  premature 302.75
  retrograde 608.87
Ekbom syndrome (restless legs) 333.94
Ekman's syndrome (brittle bones and blue
  sclera) 756.51
Elastic skin 756.83
  acquired 701.8
Elastofibroma (M8820/0) - *see* Neoplasm,
  connective tissue, benign
Elastoidosis
  cutanea nodularis 701.8
  cutis cystica et comedonica 701.8
Elastoma 757.39
  juvenile 757.39
  Miescher's (elastosis perforans serpiginosa)
    701.1
Elastomyofibrosis 425.3
Elastosis 701.8
  atrophicans 701.8
  perforans serpiginosa 701.1
  reactive perforating 701.1
  senilis 701.8
  solar (actinic) 692.74
Elbow - *see* condition
Electric
  current, electricity, effects (concussion) (fatal)
    (nonfatal) (shock) 994.8
    burn - *see* Burn, by site
  feet (foot) syndrome 266.2
  shock from electroshock gun (taser) 994.8
Electrocution 994.8
Electrolyte imbalance 276.9
  with
    abortion - *see* Abortion, by type, with
      metabolic disorder
    ectopic pregnancy *(see also* categories
      633.0–633.9) 639.4
    hyperemesis gravidarum (before 22
      completed weeks' gestation) 643.1●
    molar pregnancy *(see also* categories
      630–632) 639.4
  following
    abortion 639.4
    ectopic or molar pregnancy 639.4
Elephant man syndrome 237.71
Elephantiasis (nonfilarial) 457.1
  arabicum *(see also* Infestation, filarial) 125.9
  congenita hereditaria 757.0
  congenital (any site) 757.0
  due to
    Brugia (malayi) 125.1
    mastectomy operation 457.0
    Wuchereria (bancrofti) 125.0
      malayi 125.1
  eyelid 374.83
  filarial *(see also* Infestation, filarial) 125.9
  filariensis *(see also* Infestation, filarial) 125.9

Elephantiasis (Continued)
  gingival 523.8
  glandular 457.1
  graecorum 030.9
  lymphangiectatic 457.1
  lymphatic vessel 457.1
    due to mastectomy operation 457.0
  neuromatosa 237.71
  postmastectomy 457.0
  scrotum 457.1
  streptococcal 457.1
  surgical 997.99
    postmastectomy 457.0
  telangiectodes 457.1
  vulva (nonfilarial) 624.8
Elevated - see Elevation
  findings on laboratory examination - see
      Findings, abnormal, without diagnosis
      (examination) (laboratory test)
  GFR (glomerular filtration rate) - see
      Findings, abnormal, without diagnosis
      (examination) (laboratory test)
Elevation
  17-ketosteroids 791.9
  acid phosphatase 790.5
  alkaline phosphatase 790.5
  amylase 790.5
  antibody titers 795.79
  basal metabolic rate (BMR) 794.7
  blood pressure (see also Hypertension) 401.9
    reading (incidental) (isolated)
        (nonspecific), no diagnosis of
        hypertension 796.2
  blood sugar 790.29
  body temperature (of unknown origin) (see
      also Pyrexia) 780.60
  C-reactive protein (CRP) 790.95
  cancer antigen 125 [CA 125] 795.82
  carcinoembryonic antigen [CEA] 795.81
  cholesterol 272.0
    with high triglycerides 272.2
  conjugate, eye 378.81
  CRP (C-reactive protein) 790.95
  diaphragm, congenital 756.6
  GFR (glomerular filtration rate) - see
      Findings, abnormal, without diagnosis
      (examination) (laboratory test)
  glucose
    fasting 790.21
    tolerance test 790.22
  immunoglobulin level 795.79
  indolacetic acid 791.9
  lactic acid dehydrogenase (LDH) level 790.4
  leukocytes 288.60
  lipase 790.5
  lipoprotein a level 272.8
  liver function test (LFT) 790.6
    alkaline phosphatase 790.5
    aminotransferase 790.4
    bilirubin 782.4
    hepatic enzyme NEC 790.5
    lactate dehydrogenase 790.4
  lymphocytes 288.61
  prostate specific antigen (PSA) 790.93
  renin 790.99
    in hypertension (see also Hypertension,
        renovascular) 405.91
  Rh titer (see also Complications, transfusion)
      999.70
  scapula, congenital 755.52
  sedimentation rate 790.1
  SGOT 790.4
  SGPT 790.4
  transaminase 790.4
  triglycerides 272.1
    with high cholesterol 272.2
  vanillylmandelic acid 791.9
  venous pressure 459.89
  VMA 791.9
  white blood cell count 288.60
    specified NEC 288.69

Elliptocytosis (congenital) (hereditary) 282.1
  Hb-C (disease) 282.7
  hemoglobin disease 282.7
  sickle-cell (disease) 282.60
  trait 282.5
Ellis-van Creveld disease or syndrome
    (chondroectodermal dysplasia) 756.55
Ellison-Zollinger syndrome
    (gastric hypersecretion with pancreatic islet
    cell tumor) 251.5
Elongation, elongated (congenital) - see also
    Distortion
  bone 756.9
  cervix (uteri) 752.49
    acquired 622.6
    hypertrophic 622.6
  colon 751.5
  common bile duct 751.69
  cystic duct 751.69
  frenulum, penis 752.69
  labia minora, acquired 624.8
  ligamentum patellae 756.89
  petiolus (epiglottidis) 748.3
  styloid bone (process) 733.99
  tooth, teeth 520.2
  uvula 750.26
    acquired 528.9
Elschnig bodies or pearls 366.51
El Tor cholera 001.1
Emaciation (due to malnutrition) 261
Emancipation disorder 309.22
Embadomoniasis 007.8
Embarrassment heart, cardiac - see Disease,
    heart
Embedded
  fragment (status) - see Foreign body,
      retained
  root only 525.3
  splinter (status) - see Foreign body,
      retained
  tooth, teeth 520.6
Embolic - see condition
Embolism 444.9
  with
    abortion - see Abortion, by type, with
        embolism
    ectopic pregnancy (see also categories
        633.0–633.9) 639.6
    molar pregnancy (see also categories
        630–632) 639.6
  air (any site) 958.0
    with
      abortion - see Abortion, by type, with
          embolism
      ectopic pregnancy (see also categories
          633.0–633.9) 639.6
      molar pregnancy (see also categories
          630–632) 639.6
    due to implanted device - see
        Complications, due to (presence of)
        any device, implant, or graft
        classified to 996.0–996.5 NEC
    following
      abortion 639.6
      ectopic or molar pregnancy 639.6
      infusion, perfusion, or transfusion
          999.1
    in pregnancy, childbirth, or puerperium
        673.0●
    traumatic 958.0
  amniotic fluid (pulmonary) 673.1●
    with
      abortion - see Abortion, by type, with
          embolism
      ectopic pregnancy (see also categories
          633.0–633.9) 639.6
      molar pregnancy (see also categories
          630–632) 639.6
    following
      abortion 639.6
      ectopic or molar pregnancy 639.6

Embolism (Continued)
  aorta, aortic 444.1
    abdominal 444.09
      saddle 444.01
    bifurcation 444.09
    saddle 444.01
    thoracic 444.1
  artery 444.9
    auditory, internal 433.8●
    basilar (see also Occlusion, artery, basilar)
        433.0●
    bladder 444.89
    carotid (common) (internal) (see also
        Occlusion, artery, carotid) 433.1●
    cerebellar (anterior inferior) (posterior
        inferior) (superior) 433.8●
    cerebral (see also Embolism, brain) 434.1●
    choroidal (anterior) 433.8●
    communicating posterior 433.8●
    coronary (see also Infarct, myocardium)
        410.9●
      without myocardial infarction 411.81
    extremity 444.22
      lower 444.22
      upper 444.21
    hypophyseal 433.8●
    mesenteric (with gangrene) 557.0
    ophthalmic (see also Occlusion, retina)
        362.30
    peripheral 444.22
    pontine 433.8●
    precerebral NEC - see Occlusion, artery,
        precerebral
    pulmonary - see Embolism, pulmonary
    pyemic 449
      pulmonary 415.12
    renal 593.81
    retinal (see also Occlusion, retina) 362.30
    septic 449
      pulmonary 415.12
    specified site NEC 444.89
    vertebral (see also Occlusion, artery,
        vertebral) 433.2●
  auditory, internal 433.8●
  basilar (artery) (see also Occlusion, artery,
      basilar) 433.0●
  birth, mother - see Embolism, obstetrical
  blood-clot
    with
      abortion - see Abortion, by type, with
          embolism
      ectopic pregnancy (see also categories
          633.0–633.9) 639.6
      molar pregnancy (see also categories
          630–632) 639.6
    following
      abortion 639.6
      ectopic or molar pregnancy 639.6
    in pregnancy, childbirth, or puerperium
        673.2●
  brain 434.1●
    with
      abortion - see Abortion, by type, with
          embolism
      ectopic pregnancy (see also categories
          633.0–633.9) 639.6
      molar pregnancy (see also categories
          630–632) 639.6
    following
      abortion 639.6
      ectopic or molar pregnancy 639.6
    late effect - see Late effect(s) (of)
        cerebrovascular disease
    puerperal, postpartum, childbirth 674.0●
  capillary 448.9
  cardiac (see also Infarct, myocardium) 410.9●
  carotid (artery) (common) (internal) (see also
      Occlusion, artery, carotid) 433.1●
  cavernous sinus (venous) - see Embolism,
      intracranial venous sinus
  cerebral (see also Embolism, brain) 434.1●

◄ New   ◄▥ Revised   d̶e̶l̶e̶t̶e̶d̶ Deleted   ● Use Additional Digit(s)   ▨ Omit code

Embolism *(Continued)*
  cholesterol - *see* Atheroembolism
  choroidal (anterior) (artery) 433.8●
  coronary (artery or vein) (systemic) *(see also*
      Infarct, myocardium) 410.9●
    without myocardial infarction 411.81
    due to (presence of) any device, implant, or
      graft classifiable to 996.0–996.5 - *see*
      Complications, due to (presence of)
      any device, implant, or graft classified
      to 996.0–996.5 NEC
  encephalomalacia *(see also* Embolism, brain)
      434.1●
  extremities 444.22
    lower 444.22
    upper 444.21
  eye 362.30
  fat (cerebral) (pulmonary) (systemic) 958.1
    with
      abortion - *see* Abortion, by type, with
        embolism
      ectopic pregnancy *(see also* categories
        633.0–633.9) 639.6
      molar pregnancy *(see also* categories
        630–632) 639.6
    complicating delivery or puerperium
      673.8●
    following
      abortion 639.6
      ectopic or molar pregnancy 639.6
    in pregnancy, childbirth, or the
      puerperium 673.8●
  femoral (artery) 444.22
    vein 453.6
      deep 453.41
  following
    abortion 639.6
    ectopic or molar pregnancy 639.6
    infusion, perfusion, or transfusion
      air 999.1
      thrombus 999.2
  heart (fatty) *(see also* Infarct, myocardium)
      410.9●
  hepatic (vein) 453.0
  iliac (artery) 444.81
  iliofemoral 444.81
  in pregnancy, childbirth, or puerperium
      (pulmonary) - *see* Embolism,
      obstetrical
  intestine (artery) (vein) (with gangrene) 557.0
  intracranial *(see also* Embolism, brain) 434.1●
    venous sinus (any) 325
      late effect - *see* category 326
      nonpyogenic 437.6
        in pregnancy or puerperium 671.5●
  kidney (artery) 593.81
  lateral sinus (venous) - *see* Embolism,
      intracranial venous sinus
  longitudinal sinus (venous) - *see* Embolism,
      intracranial venous sinus
  lower extremity 444.22
  lung (massive) - *see* Embolism, pulmonary
  meninges *(see also* Embolism, brain) 434.1●
  mesenteric (artery) (with gangrene) 557.0
  multiple NEC 444.9
  obstetrical (pulmonary) 673.2●
    air 673.0●
    amniotic fluid (pulmonary) 673.1●
    blood-clot 673.2●
    cardiac 674.8●
    fat 673.8●
    heart 674.8●
    pyemic 673.3●
    septic 673.3●
    specified NEC 674.8●
  ophthalmic *(see also* Occlusion, retina) 362.30
  paradoxical NEC 444.9
  penis 607.82
  peripheral arteries NEC 444.22
    lower 444.22
    upper 444.21

Embolism *(Continued)*
  pituitary 253.8
  popliteal (artery) 444.22
  portal (vein) 452
  postoperative NEC 997.2
    cerebral 997.02
    mesenteric artery 997.71
    other vessels 997.79
    peripheral vascular 997.2
    pulmonary 415.11
      septic 415.11
    renal artery 997.72
  precerebral artery *(see also* Occlusion, artery,
      precerebral) 433.9●
  puerperal - *see* Embolism, obstetrical
  pulmonary (acute) (artery) (vein) 415.19
    with
      abortion - *see* Abortion, by type, with
        embolism
      ectopic pregnancy *(see also* categories
        633.0–633.9) 639.6
      molar pregnancy *(see also* categories
        630–632) 639.6
    chronic 416.2
    following
      abortion 639.6
      ectopic or molar pregnancy 639.6
    healed or old V12.55
    iatrogenic 415.11
    in pregnancy, childbirth, or puerperium -
      see Embolism, obstetrical
    personal history of V12.55
    postoperative 415.11
    septic 415.12
  pyemic (multiple) *(see also* Septicemia) 415.12
    with
      abortion - *see* Abortion, by type, with
        embolism
      ectopic pregnancy *(see also* categories
        633.0–633.9) 639.6
      molar pregnancy *(see also* categories
        630–632) 639.6
    Aerobacter aerogenes 415.12
    enteric gram-negative bacilli 415.12
    Enterobacter aerogenes 415.12
    Escherichia coli 415.12
    following
      abortion 639.6
      ectopic or molar pregnancy 639.6
    Hemophilus influenzae 415.12
    pneumococcal 415.12
    Proteus vulgaris 415.12
    Pseudomonas (aeruginosa) 415.12
    puerperal, postpartum, childbirth (any
      organism) 673.3●
    Serratia 415.12
    specified organism NEC 415.12
    staphylococcal 415.12
      aureus 415.12
      specified organism NEC 415.12
    streptococcal 415.12
  renal (artery) 593.81
    vein 453.3
  retina, retinal *(see also* Occlusion, retina)
      362.30
  saddle
    abdominal aorta 444.01
    pulmonary artery 415.13
  septic 415.12
    arterial 449
  septicemic - *see* Embolism, pyemic
  sinus - *see* Embolism, intracranial venous
      sinus
  soap
    with
      abortion - *see* Abortion, by type, with
        embolism
      ectopic pregnancy *(see also* categories
        633.0–633.9) 639.6
      molar pregnancy *(see also* categories
        630–632) 639.6

Embolism *(Continued)*
  soap *(Continued)*
    following
      abortion 639.6
      ectopic or molar pregnancy 639.6
  spinal cord (nonpyogenic) 336.1
    in pregnancy or puerperium 671.5●
    pyogenic origin 324.1
    late effect - *see* category 326
  spleen, splenic (artery) 444.89
  thrombus (thromboembolism) following
      infusion, perfusion, or transfusion
      999.2
  upper extremity 444.21
  vein 453.9
    with inflammation or phlebitis - *see*
      Thrombophlebitis
    antecubital (acute) 453.81
      chronic 453.71
    axillary (acute) 453.84
      chronic 453.74
    basilic (acute) 453.81
      chronic 453.71
    brachial (acute) 453.82
      chronic 453.72
    brachiocephalic (acute) (innominate) 453.87
      chronic 453.77
    cephalic (acute) 453.81
      chronic 453.71
    cerebral *(see also* Embolism, brain) 434.1●
    coronary *(see also* Infarct, myocardium)
      410.9●
      without myocardial infarction 411.81
    hepatic 453.0
    internal jugular (acute) 453.86
      chronic 453.76
    lower extremity (superficial) 453.6
      deep 453.40
        acute 453.40
          calf 453.42
          distal (lower leg) 453.42
          femoral 453.41
          iliac 453.41
          lower leg 453.42
          peroneal 453.42
          popliteal 453.41
          proximal (upper leg) 453.41
          thigh 453.41
          tibial 453.42
        chronic 453.50
          calf 453.52
          distal (lower leg) 453.52
          femoral 453.51
          iliac 453.51
          lower leg 453.52
          peroneal 453.52
          popliteal 453.51
          proximal (upper leg) 453.51
          thigh 453.51
          tibial 453.52
        saphenous (greater) (lesser) 453.6
        superficial 453.6
    mesenteric (with gangrene) 557.0
    portal 452
    pulmonary - *see* Embolism, pulmonary
    radial (acute) 453.82
      chronic 453.72
    renal 453.3
    saphenous (greater) (lesser) 453.6
    specified NEC (acute) 453.89
      with inflammation or phlebitis - *see*
        Thrombophlebitis
      chronic 453.79
    subclavian (acute) 453.85
      chronic 453.75
    superior vena cava (acute) 453.87
      chronic 453.77
    thoracic (acute) 453.87
      chronic 453.77
    ulnar (acute) 453.82
      chronic 453.72

E

Embolism *(Continued)*
  vein *(Continued)*
    upper extremity (acute) 453.83
      chronic 453.73
        deep 453.72
          superficial 453.71
      deep 453.82
      superficial 453.81
    vena cava
      inferior 453.2
      superior (acute) 453.87
        chronic 453.77
    vessels of brain *(see also* Embolism, brain)
      434.1 ●
Embolization - *see* Embolism
Embolus - *see* Embolism
Embryoma (M9080/1) - *see also* Neoplasm, by
    site, uncertain behavior
  benign (M9080/0) - *see* Neoplasm, by site,
    benign
  kidney (M8960/3) 189.0
  liver (M8970/3) 155.0
  malignant (M9080/3) - *see also* Neoplasm, by
    site, malignant
    kidney (M8960/3) 189.0
    liver (M8970/3) 155.0
    testis (M9070/3) 186.9
      undescended 186.0
  testis (M9070/3) 186.9
    undescended 186.0
Embryonic
  circulation 747.9
  heart 747.9
  vas deferens 752.89
Embryopathia NEC 759.9
Embryotomy, fetal 763.89
Embryotoxon 743.43
  interfering with vision 743.42
Emesis - *see also* Vomiting
  bilious 787.04
  gravidarum - *see* Hyperemesis, gravidarum
Emissions, nocturnal (semen) 608.89
Emotional
  crisis - *see* Crisis, emotional
  disorder *(see also* Disorder, mental) 300.9
  instability (excessive) 301.3
  lability 799.24
  overlay - *see* Reaction, adjustment
  upset 300.9
Emotionality, pathological 301.3
Emotogenic disease *(see also* Disorder,
    psychogenic) 306.9
Emphysema (atrophic) (centriacinar)
    (centrilobular) (chronic) (diffuse)
    (essential) (hypertrophic) (interlobular)
    (lung) (obstructive) (panlobular)
    (paracicatricial) (paracinar) (postural)
    (pulmonary) (senile) (subpleural)
    (traction) (unilateral) (unilobular)
    (vesicular) 492.8
  with bronchitis
    chronic 491.20
      with
        acute bronchitis 491.22
        exacerbation (acute) 491.21
  bullous (giant) 492.0
  cellular tissue 958.7
    surgical 998.81
  compensatory 518.2
  congenital 770.2
  conjunctiva 372.89
  connective tissue 958.7
    surgical 998.81
  due to fumes or vapors 506.4
  eye 376.89
  eyelid 374.85
    surgical 998.81
    traumatic 958.7
  fetus or newborn (interstitial) (mediastinal)
    (unilobular) 770.2
  heart 416.9

Emphysema *(Continued)*
  interstitial 518.1
    congenital 770.2
    fetus or newborn 770.2
  laminated tissue 958.7
    surgical 998.81
  mediastinal 518.1
    fetus or newborn 770.2
  newborn (interstitial) (mediastinal)
    (unilobular) 770.2
  obstructive diffuse with fibrosis 492.8
  orbit 376.89
  subcutaneous 958.7
    due to trauma 958.7
    nontraumatic 518.1
    surgical 998.81
  surgical 998.81
  thymus (gland) (congenital)254.8
  traumatic 958.7
  tuberculous *(see also* Tuberculosis,
    pulmonary) 011.9 ●
Employment examination (certification) V70.5
Empty sella (turcica) syndrome 253.8
Empyema (chest) (diaphragmatic) (double)
    (encapsulated) (general) (interlobar)
    (lung) (medial) (necessitatis) (perforating
    chest wall) (pleura) (pneumococcal)
    (residual) (sacculated) (streptococcal)
    (supradiaphragmatic) 510.9
  with fistula 510.0
  accessory sinus (chronic) *(see also* Sinusitis)
    473.9
  acute 510.9
    with fistula 510.0
  antrum (chronic) *(see also* Sinusitis,
    maxillary) 473.0
  brain (any part) *(see also* Abscess, brain) 324.0
  ethmoidal (sinus) (chronic) *(see also* Sinusitis,
    ethmoidal) 473.2
  extradural *(see also* Abscess, extradural) 324.9
  frontal (sinus) (chronic) *(see also* Sinusitis,
    frontal) 473.1
  gallbladder *(see also* Cholecystitis, acute)
    575.0
  mastoid (process) (acute) *(see also*
    Mastoiditis, acute) 383.00
  maxilla, maxillary 526.4
    sinus (chronic) *(see also* Sinusitis,
      maxillary) 473.0
  nasal sinus (chronic) *(see also* Sinusitis) 473.9
  sinus (accessory) (nasal) *(see also* Sinusitis)
    473.9
  sphenoidal (chronic) (sinus) *(see also*
    Sinusitis, sphenoidal) 473.3
  subarachnoid *(see also* Abscess, extradural)
    324.9
  subdural *(see also* Abscess, extradural) 324.9
  tuberculous *(see also* Tuberculosis, pleura)
    012.0 ●
  ureter *(see also* Ureteritis) 593.89
  ventricular *(see also* Abscess, brain) 324.0
Enameloma 520.2
Encephalitis (bacterial) (chronic) (hemorrhagic)
    (idiopathic) (nonepidemic) (spurious)
    (subacute) 323.9
  acute - *see also* Encephalitis, viral
    disseminated (postinfectious) NEC 136.9
      [323.61]
      postimmunization or postvaccination
        323.51
    inclusional 049.8
    inclusion body 049.8
    necrotizing 049.8
  arboviral, arbovirus NEC 064
  arthropod-borne *(see also* Encephalitis, viral,
    arthropod-borne) 064
  Australian X 062.4
  Bwamba fever 066.3
  California (virus) 062.5
  Central European 063.2
  Czechoslovakian 063.2

Encephalitis *(Continued)*
  Dawson's (inclusion body) 046.2
  diffuse sclerosing 046.2
  due to
    actinomycosis 039.8 *[323.41]*
    cat-scratch disease 078.3 *[323.01]*
    human herpesvirus 6 058.21
    human herpesvirus 7 058.29
    human herpesvirus NEC 058.29
    human immunodeficiency virus [HIV]
      disease 042 *[323.01]*
    infectious mononucleosis 075 *[323.01]*
    malaria *(see also* Malaria) 084.6 *[323.2]*
    Negishi virus 064
    ornithosis 073.7 *[323.01]*
    other infection classified elsewhere 136.9
      [323.41]
    prophylactic inoculation against smallpox
      323.51
    rickettsiosis *(see also* Rickettsiosis) 083.9
      [323.1]
    rubella 056.01
    toxoplasmosis (acquired) 130.0
      congenital (active) 771.2 *[323.41]*
    typhus (fever) *(see also* Typhus) 081.9
      [323.1]
    vaccination (smallpox) 323.51
  Eastern equine 062.2
  endemic 049.8
  epidemic 049.8
  equine (acute) (infectious) (viral) 062.9
    eastern 062.2
    Venezuelan 066.2
    western 062.1
  Far Eastern 063.0
  following vaccination or other immunization
    procedure 323.51
  herpes 054.3
  human herpesvirus 6 058.21
  human herpesvirus 7 058.29
  human herpesvirus NEC 058.29
  Ilheus (virus) 062.8
  inclusion body 046.2
  infectious (acute) (virus) NEC 049.8
  influenzal *(see also* Influenza) 487.8 *[323.41]*
    lethargic 049.8
  Japanese (B type) 062.0
  La Crosse 062.5
  Langat 063.8
  late effect - *see* Late, effect, encephalitis
  lead 984.9 *[323.71]*
  lethargic (acute) (infectious) (influenzal)
    049.8
  lethargica 049.8
  louping ill 063.1
  lupus 710.0 *[323.81]*
  lymphatica 049.0
  Mengo 049.8
  meningococcal 036.1
  mumps 072.2
  Murray Valley 062.4
  myoclonic 049.8
  Negishi virus 064
  otitic NEC 382.4 *[323.41]*
  parasitic NEC 123.9 *[323.41]*
  periaxialis (concentrica) (diffusa) 341.1
  postchickenpox 052.0
  postexanthematous NEC 057.9 *[323.62]*
  postimmunization 323.51
  postinfectious NEC 136.9 *[323.62]*
  postmeasles 055.0
  posttraumatic 323.81
  postvaccinal (smallpox) 323.51
  postvaricella 052.0
  postviral NEC 079.99 *[323.62]*
    postexanthematous 057.9 *[323.62]*
    specified NEC 057.8 *[323.62]*
  Powassan 063.8
  progressive subcortical (Binswanger's)
    290.12
  Rasmussen 323.81

◄ New   ◄▥ Revised   ~~deleted~~ Deleted   ● Use Additional Digit(s)   ▨ Omit code

Encephalitis *(Continued)*
 Rio Bravo 049.8
 rubella 056.01
 Russian
  autumnal 062.0
  spring-summer type (taiga) 063.0
 saturnine 984.9 *[323.71]*
 Semliki Forest 062.8
 serous 048
 slow-acting virus NEC 046.8
 specified cause NEC 323.81
 St. Louis type 062.3
 subacute sclerosing 046.2
 subcorticalis chronica 290.12
 summer 062.0
 suppurative 324.0
 syphilitic 094.81
  congenital 090.41
 tick-borne 063.9
 torula, torular 117.5 *[323.41]*
 toxic NEC 989.9 *[323.71]*
 toxoplasmic (acquired) 130.0
  congenital (active) 771.2 *[323.41]*
 trichinosis 124 *[323.41]*
 Trypanosomiasis *(see also* Trypanosomiasis)
  086.9 *[323.2]*
 tuberculous *(see also* Tuberculosis) 013.6●
 type B (Japanese) 062.0
 type C 062.3
 van Bogaert's 046.2
 Venezuelan 066.2
 Vienna type 049.8
 viral, virus 049.9
  arthropod-borne NEC 064
   mosquito-borne 062.9
    Australian X disease 062.4
    California virus 062.5
    Eastern equine 062.2
    Ilheus virus 062.8
    Japanese (B type) 062.0
    Murray Valley 062.4
    specified type NEC 062.8
    St. Louis 062.3
    type B 062.0
    type C 062.3
    Western equine 062.1
   tick-borne 063.9
    biundulant 063.2
    Central European 063.2
    Czechoslovakian 063.2
    diphasic meningoencephalitis 063.2
    Far Eastern 063.0
    Langat 063.8
    louping ill 063.1
    Powassan 063.8
    Russian spring-summer (taiga) 063.0
    specified type NEC 063.8
   vector unknown 064
  slow acting NEC 046.8
  specified type NEC 049.8
  vaccination, prophylactic (against) V05.0
 von Economo's 049.8
 Western equine 062.1
 West Nile type 066.41
Encephalocele 742.0
 orbit 376.81
Encephalocystocele 742.0
Encephaloduroarteriomyosynangiosis
  (EDAMS) 437.5
Encephalomalacia (brain) (cerebellar) (cerebral)
  (cerebrospinal) *(see also* Softening, brain)
  348.89
 due to
  hemorrhage *(see also* Hemorrhage, brain)
   431
  recurrent spasm of artery 435.9
 embolic (cerebral) *(see also* Embolism, brain)
  434.1●
 subcorticalis chronicus arteriosclerotica 290.12
 thrombotic *(see also* Thrombosis, brain)
  434.0●

Encephalomeningitis - *see* Meningoencephalitis
Encephalomeningocele 742.0
Encephalomeningomyelitis - *see*
  Meningoencephalitis
Encephalomeningopathy *(see also*
  Meningoencephalitis) 349.9
Encephalomyelitis (chronic) (granulomatous)
  (myalgic, benign) *(see also* Encephalitis)
  323.9
 abortive disseminated 049.8
 acute disseminated (ADEM) (postinfectious)
  136.9 *[323.61]*
  infectious 136.9 *[323.61]*
  noninfectious 323.81
  postimmunization 323.51
 due to
  cat-scratch disease 078.3 *[323.01]*
  infectious mononucleosis 075 *[323.01]*
  ornithosis 073.7 *[323.01]*
  vaccination (any) 323.51
 equine (acute) (infectious) 062.9
  eastern 062.2
  Venezuelan 066.2
  western 062.1
 funicularis infectiosa 049.8
 late effect - *see* Late, effect, encephalitis
 Munch-Peterson's 049.8
 postchickenpox 052.0
 postimmunization 323.51
 postmeasles 055.0
 postvaccinal (smallpox) 323.51
 rubella 056.01
 specified cause NEC 323.81
 syphilitic 094.81
 West Nile 066.41
Encephalomyelocele 742.0
Encephalomyelomeningitis - *see*
  Meningoencephalitis
Encephalomyeloneuropathy 349.9
Encephalomyelopathy 349.9
 subacute necrotizing (infantile) 330.8
Encephalomyeloradiculitis (acute) 357.0
Encephalomyeloradiculoneuritis (acute) 357.0
Encephalomyeloradiculopathy 349.9
Encephalomyocarditis 074.23
Encephalopathia hyperbilirubinemica,
  newborn 774.7
 due to isoimmunization (conditions
  classifiable to 773.0–773.2) 773.4
Encephalopathy (acute) 348.30
 alcoholic 291.2
 anoxic - *see* Damage, brain, anoxic
 arteriosclerotic 437.0
  late effect - *see* Late effect(s) (of)
   cerebrovascular disease
 bilirubin, newborn 774.7
  due to isoimmunization 773.4
 congenital 742.9
 demyelinating (callosal) 341.8
 due to
  birth injury (intracranial) 767.8
  dialysis 294.8
   transient 293.9
  drugs - *(see also* Table of Drugs and
   Chemicals) 349.82
  hyperinsulinism - *see* Hyperinsulinism
  influenza (virus) *(see also* Influenza) 487.8
   identified
    avian 488.09
    (novel) 2009 H1N1 488.19
  lack of vitamin *(see also* Deficiency,
   vitamin) 269.2
  nicotinic acid deficiency 291.2
  serum (nontherapeutic) (therapeutic) 999.59
  syphilis 094.81
  trauma (postconcussional) 310.2
   current *(see also* Concussion, brain) 850.9
    with skull fracture - *see* Fracture,
     skull, by site, with
     intracranial injury
  vaccination 323.51

Encephalopathy *(Continued)*
 hepatic 572.2
 hyperbilirubinemic, newborn 774.7
  due to isoimmunization (conditions
   classifiable to 773.0–773.2) 773.4
 hypertensive 437.2
 hypoglycemic 251.2
 hypoxic - *see also* Damage, brain, anoxic
  ischemic (HIE) 768.70
   mild 768.71
   moderate 768.72
   severe 768.73
 infantile cystic necrotizing (congenital) 341.8
 lead 984.9 *[323.71]*
 leukopolio 330.0
 metabolic *(see also* Delirium) 348.31
  drug induced 349.82
  toxic 349.82
 necrotizing
  hemorrhagic (acute) 323.61
  subacute 330.8
 other specified type NEC 348.39
 pellagrous 265.2
 portal-systemic 572.2
 postcontusional 310.2
 posttraumatic 310.2
 saturnine 984.9 *[323.71]*
 septic 348.31
 spongiform, subacute (viral) 046.19
 subacute
  necrotizing 330.8
  spongiform 046.19
  viral, spongiform 046.19
 subcortical progressive (Schilder) 341.1
  chronic (Binswanger's) 290.12
 toxic 349.82
  metabolic 349.82
 traumatic (postconcussional) 310.2
  current *(see also* Concussion, brain) 850.9
   with skull fracture - *see* Fracture, skull,
    by site, with intracranial injury
 vitamin B deficiency NEC 266.9
 Wernicke's (superior hemorrhagic
  polioencephalitis) 265.1
Encephalorrhagia *(see also* Hemorrhage, brain)
  432.9
 healed or old V12.54
 late effect - *see* Late effect(s) (of)
  cerebrovascular disease
Encephalosis, posttraumatic 310.2
Enchondroma (M9220/0) - *see also* Neoplasm,
  bone, benign
 multiple, congenital 756.4
Enchondromatosis (cartilaginous) (congenital)
  (multiple) 756.4
Enchondroses, multiple (cartilaginous)
  (congenital) 756.4
Encopresis *(see also* Incontinence, feces) 787.60
 nonorganic origin 307.7
Encounter for - *see also* Admission for
 administrative purpose only V68.9
  referral of patient without examination or
   treatment V68.81
  specified purpose NEC V68.89
 chemotherapy, (oral) (intravenous),
  antineoplastic V58.11
 determination of fetal viability of pregnancy
  V23.87
 dialysis
  extracorporeal (renal) V56.0
  peritoneal V56.8
 disability examination V68.01
 end-of-life care V66.7
 hospice care V66.7
 immunizations (childhood) appropriate for
  age V20.2
 immunotherapy, antineoplastic V58.12
 joint prosthesis insertion following prior
  explantation of joint prosthesis V54.82
 palliative care V66.7
 paternity testing V70.4

m

Encounter for (Continued)
　radiotherapy V58.0
　respirator [ventilator] dependence
　　during
　　　mechanical failure V46.14
　　　power failure V46.12
　　for weaning V46.13
　routine infant and child vision and hearing
　　testing V20.2
　school examination V70.3
　　following surgery V67.09
　screening mammogram NEC V76.12
　　for high-risk patient V76.11
　terminal care V66.7
　weaning from respirator [ventilator] V46.13
Encystment - see Cyst
End-of-life care V66.7
Endamebiasis - see Amebiasis
Endamoeba - see Amebiasis
Endarteritis (bacterial, subacute) (infective)
　　(septic) 447.6
　brain, cerebral or cerebrospinal 437.4
　　late effect - see Late effect(s) (of)
　　　cerebrovascular disease
　coronary (artery) - see Arteriosclerosis,
　　coronary
　deformans - see Arteriosclerosis
　embolic (see also Embolism) 444.9
　obliterans - see also Arteriosclerosis
　　pulmonary 417.8
　pulmonary 417.8
　retina 362.18
　senile - see Arteriosclerosis
　syphilitic 093.89
　　brain or cerebral 094.89
　　congenital 090.5
　　spinal 094.89
　tuberculous (see also Tuberculosis) 017.9 ●
Endemic - see condition
Endocarditis (chronic) (indeterminate)
　　(interstitial) (marantic) (nonbacterial
　　thrombotic) (residual) (sclerotic)
　　(sclerous) (senile) (valvular) 424.90
　with
　　rheumatic fever (conditions classifiable to
　　　390)
　　　active - see Endocarditis, acute,
　　　　rheumatic
　　　inactive or quiescent (with chorea)
　　　　397.9
　acute or subacute 421.9
　　rheumatic (aortic) (mitral) (pulmonary)
　　　(tricuspid) 391.1
　　　with chorea (acute) (rheumatic)
　　　　(Sydenham's) 392.0
　aortic (heart) (nonrheumatic) (valve) 424.1
　　with
　　　mitral (valve) disease 396.9
　　　　active or acute 391.1
　　　　　with chorea (acute) (rheumatic)
　　　　　　(Sydenham's) 392.0
　　　　bacterial 421.0
　　　rheumatic fever (conditions classifiable
　　　　to 390)
　　　　active - see Endocarditis, acute,
　　　　　rheumatic
　　　　inactive or quiescent (with chorea)
　　　　　395.9
　　　　　with mitral disease 396.9
　　acute or subacute 421.9
　　arteriosclerotic 424.1
　　congenital 746.89
　　hypertensive 424.1
　　rheumatic (chronic) (inactive) 395.9
　　　with mitral (valve) disease 396.9
　　　　active or acute 391.1
　　　　　with chorea (acute) (rheumatic)
　　　　　　(Sydenham's) 392.0
　　　　active or acute 391.1
　　　　　with chorea (acute) (rheumatic)
　　　　　　(Sydenham's) 392.0

Endocarditis (Continued)
　aortic (Continued)
　　specified cause, except rheumatic 424.1
　　syphilitic 093.22
　arteriosclerotic or due to arteriosclerosis
　　424.99
　atypical verrucous (Libman-Sacks) 710.0
　　[424.91]
　bacterial (acute) (any valve) (chronic)
　　(subacute) 421.0
　blastomycotic 116.0 [421.1]
　candidal 112.81
　congenital 425.3
　constrictive 421.0
　Coxsackie 074.22
　due to
　　blastomycosis 116.0 [421.1]
　　candidiasis 112.81
　　Coxsackie (virus) 074.22
　　disseminated lupus erythematosus 710.0
　　　[424.91]
　　histoplasmosis (see also Histoplasmosis)
　　　115.94
　　hypertension (benign) 424.99
　　moniliasis 112.81
　　prosthetic cardiac valve 996.61
　　Q fever 083.0 [421.1]
　　serratia marcescens 421.0
　　typhoid (fever) 002.0 [421.1]
　fetal 425.3
　gonococcal 098.84
　hypertensive 424.99
　infectious or infective (acute) (any valve)
　　(chronic) (subacute) 421.0
　lenta (acute) (any valve) (chronic) (subacute)
　　421.0
　Libman-Sacks 710.0 [424.91]
　Loeffler's (parietal fibroplastic) 421.0
　malignant (acute) (any valve) (chronic)
　　(subacute) 421.0
　meningococcal 036.42
　mitral (chronic) (double) (fibroid) (heart)
　　(inactive) (valve) (with chorea)
　　394.9
　　with
　　　aortic (valve) disease 396.9
　　　　active or acute 391.1
　　　　　with chorea (acute) (rheumatic)
　　　　　　(Sydenham's) 392.0
　　　rheumatic fever (conditions classifiable
　　　　to 390)
　　　　active - see Endocarditis, acute,
　　　　　rheumatic
　　　　inactive or quiescent (with chorea)
　　　　　394.9
　　　　　with aortic valve disease
　　　　　　396.9
　　active or acute 391.1
　　　with chorea (acute) (rheumatic)
　　　　(Sydenham's) 392.0
　　bacterial 421.0
　　arteriosclerotic 424.0
　　congenital 746.89
　　hypertensive 424.0
　　nonrheumatic 424.0
　　　acute or subacute 421.9
　　syphilitic 093.21
　monilial 112.81
　mycotic (acute) (any valve) (chronic)
　　(subacute) 421.0
　pneumococcic (acute) (any valve) (chronic)
　　(subacute) 421.0
　pulmonary (chronic) (heart) (valve)
　　424.3
　　with
　　　rheumatic fever (conditions classifiable
　　　　to 390)
　　　　active - see Endocarditis, acute,
　　　　　rheumatic
　　　　inactive or quiescent (with chorea)
　　　　　397.1

Endocarditis (Continued)
　pulmonary (Continued)
　　acute or subacute 421.9
　　　rheumatic 391.1
　　　　with chorea (acute) (rheumatic)
　　　　　(Sydenham's) 392.0
　　arteriosclerotic or due to arteriosclerosis
　　　424.3
　　congenital 746.09
　　hypertensive or due to hypertension
　　　(benign) 424.3
　　rheumatic (chronic) (inactive) (with
　　　chorea) 397.1
　　　active or acute 391.1
　　　　with chorea (acute) (rheumatic)
　　　　　(Sydenham's) 392.0
　　syphilitic 093.24
　purulent (acute) (any valve) (chronic)
　　(subacute) 421.0
　rheumatic (chronic) (inactive) (with chorea)
　　397.9
　　active or acute (aortic) (mitral)
　　　(pulmonary) (tricuspid) 391.1
　　　with chorea (acute) (rheumatic)
　　　　(Sydenham's) 392.0
　septic (acute) (any valve) (chronic)
　　(subacute) 421.0
　specified cause, except rheumatic 424.99
　streptococcal (acute) (any valve) (chronic)
　　(subacute) 421.0
　subacute - see Endocarditis, acute
　suppurative (any valve) (acute) (chronic)
　　(subacute) 421.0
　syphilitic NEC 093.20
　toxic (see also Endocarditis, acute) 421.9
　tricuspid (chronic) (heart) (inactive)
　　(rheumatic) (valve) (with chorea) 397.0
　　with
　　　rheumatic fever (conditions classifiable
　　　　to 390)
　　　　active - see Endocarditis, acute,
　　　　　rheumatic
　　　　inactive or quiescent (with chorea)
　　　　　397.0
　　active or acute 391.1
　　　with chorea (acute) (rheumatic)
　　　　(Sydenham's) 392.0
　　arteriosclerotic 424.2
　　congenital 746.89
　　hypertensive 424.2
　　nonrheumatic 424.2
　　　acute or subacute 421.9
　　specified cause, except rheumatic 424.2
　　syphilitic 093.23
　tuberculous (see also Tuberculosis) 017.9 ●
　　[424.91]
　typhoid 002.0 [421.1]
　ulcerative (acute) (any valve) (chronic)
　　(subacute) 421.0
　vegetative (acute) (any valve) (chronic)
　　(subacute) 421.0
　verrucous (acute) (any valve) (chronic)
　　(subacute) NEC 710.0 [424.91]
　　nonbacterial 710.0 [424.91]
　　nonrheumatic 710.0 [424.91]
Endocardium, endocardial - see also condition
　cushion defect 745.60
　specified type NEC 745.69
Endocervicitis (see also Cervicitis) 616.0
　due to
　　intrauterine (contraceptive) device 996.65
　gonorrheal (acute) 098.15
　　chronic or duration of 2 months or over
　　　098.35
　hyperplastic 616.0
　syphilitic 095.8
　trichomonal 131.09
　tuberculous (see also Tuberculosis) 016.7 ●
Endocrine - see condition
Endocrinopathy, pluriglandular 258.9
Endodontitis 522.0

◀ New　◀◀ Revised　deleted Deleted　● Use Additional Digit(s)　▨ Omit code

Endomastoiditis (*see also* Mastoiditis) 383.9
Endometrioma 617.9
Endometriosis 617.9
   appendix 617.5
   bladder 617.8
   bowel 617.5
   broad ligament 617.3
   cervix 617.0
   colon 617.5
   cul-de-sac (Douglas') 617.3
   exocervix 617.0
   fallopian tube 617.2
   female genital organ NEC 617.8
   gallbladder 617.8
   in scar of skin 617.6
   internal 617.0
   intestine 617.5
   lung 617.8
   myometrium 617.0
   ovary 617.1
   parametrium 617.3
   pelvic peritoneum 617.3
   peritoneal (pelvic) 617.3
   rectovaginal septum 617.4
   rectum 617.5
   round ligament 617.3
   skin 617.6
   specified site NEC 617.8
   stromal (M8931/1) 236.0
   umbilicus 617.8
   uterus 617.0
      internal 617.0
   vagina 617.4
   vulva 617.8
Endometritis (nonspecific) (purulent) (septic) (suppurative) 615.9
   with
      abortion - *see* Abortion, by type, with sepsis
      ectopic pregnancy (*see also* categories 633.0-633.9) 639.0
      molar pregnancy (*see also* categories 630-632) 639.0
   acute 615.0
   blennorrhagic 098.16
      acute 098.16
      chronic or duration of 2 months or over 098.36
   cervix, cervical (*see also* Cervicitis) 616.0
      hyperplastic 616.0
   chronic 615.1
   complicating pregnancy 670.1●
      affecting fetus or newborn 760.8
      septic 670.2●
   decidual 615.9
   following
      abortion 639.0
      ectopic or molar pregnancy 639.0
   gonorrheal (acute) 098.16
      chronic or duration of 2 months or over 098.36
   hyperplastic (*see also* Hyperplasia, endometrium) 621.30
      cervix 616.0
   polypoid - *see* Endometritis, hyperplastic
   puerperal, postpartum, childbirth 670.1●
      septic 670.2●
   senile (atrophic) 615.9
   subacute 615.0
   tuberculous (*see also* Tuberculosis) 016.7●
Endometrium - *see* condition
Endomyocardiopathy, South African 425.2
Endomyocarditis - *see* Endocarditis
Endomyofibrosis 425.0
Endomyometritis (*see also* Endometritis) 615.9
Endopericarditis - *see* Endocarditis
Endoperineuritis - *see* Disorder, nerve
Endophlebitis (*see also* Phlebitis) 451.9
   leg 451.2
      deep (vessels) 451.19
      superficial (vessels) 451.0

Endophlebitis (*Continued*)
   portal (vein) 572.1
   retina 362.18
   specified site NEC 451.89
   syphilitic 093.89
Endophthalmia (*see also* Endophthalmitis) 360.00
   gonorrheal 098.42
Endophthalmitis (globe) (infective) (metastatic) (purulent) (subacute) 360.00
   acute 360.01
   bleb associated 379.63
   chronic 360.03
   parasitic 360.13
   phacoanaphylactic 360.19
   specified type NEC 360.19
   sympathetic 360.11
Endosalpingioma (M9111/1) 236.2
Endosalpingiosis 629.89
Endosteitis - *see* Osteomyelitis
Endothelioma, bone (M9260/3) - *see* Neoplasm, bone, malignant
Endotheliosis 287.8
   hemorrhagic infectional 287.8
Endotoxemia - *code to* condition
Endotoxic shock 785.52
   postoperative 998.02
Endotrachelitis (*see also* Cervicitis) 616.0
Enema rash 692.89
Engel-von Recklinghausen disease or syndrome (osteitis fibrosa cystica) 252.01
Engelmann's disease (diaphyseal sclerosis) 756.59
English disease (*see also* Rickets) 268.0
Engman's disease (infectious eczematoid dermatitis) 690.8
Engorgement
   breast 611.79
      newborn 778.7
      puerperal, postpartum 676.2●
   liver 573.9
   lung 514
   pulmonary 514
   retina, venous 362.37
   stomach 536.8
   venous, retina 362.37
Enlargement, enlarged - *see also* Hypertrophy
   abdomen 789.3●
   adenoids 474.12
      and tonsils 474.10
   alveolar process or ridge 525.8
   apertures of diaphragm (congenital) 756.6
   blind spot, visual field 368.42
   gingival 523.8
   heart, cardiac (*see also* Hypertrophy, cardiac) 429.3
   lacrimal gland, chronic 375.03
   liver (*see also* Hypertrophy, liver) 789.1
   lymph gland or node 785.6
   orbit 376.46
   organ or site, congenital NEC - *see* Anomaly, specified type NEC
   parathyroid (gland) 252.01
   pituitary fossa 793.0
   prostate (simple) (soft) 600.00
      with
         other lower urinary tract symptoms (LUTS) 600.01
         urinary
            obstruction 600.01
            retention 600.01
   sella turcica 793.0
   spleen (*see also* Splenomegaly) 789.2
      congenital 759.0
   thymus (congenital) (gland) 254.0
   thyroid (gland) (*see also* Goiter) 240.9
   tongue 529.8
   tonsils 474.11
      and adenoids 474.10
   uterus 621.2

Enophthalmos 376.50
   due to
      atrophy of orbital tissue 376.51
      surgery 376.52
      trauma 376.52
Enostosis 526.89
Entamebiasis - *see* Amebiasis
Entamebic - *see* Amebiasis
Entanglement, umbilical cord(s) 663.3●
   with compression 663.2●
   affecting fetus or newborn 762.5
   around neck with compression 663.1●
   twins in monoamniotic sac 663.2●
Enteralgia 789.0●
Enteric - *see* condition
Enteritis (acute) (catarrhal) (choleraic) (chronic) (congestive) (diarrheal) (exudative) (follicular) (hemorrhagic) (infantile) (lienteric) (noninfectious) (perforative) (phlegmonous) (presumed noninfectious) (pseudomembranous) 558.9
   adaptive 564.9
   aertrycke infection 003.0
   allergic 558.3
   amebic (*see also* Amebiasis) 006.9
      with abscess - *see* Abscess, amebic
      acute 006.0
         with abscess - *see* Abscess, amebic
         nondysenteric 006.2
      chronic 006.1
         with abscess - *see* Abscess, amebic
         nondysenteric 006.2
      nondysenteric 006.2
   anaerobic (cocci) (gram-negative) (gram-positive) (mixed) NEC 008.46
   bacillary NEC 004.9
   bacterial NEC 008.5
      specified NEC 008.49
   Bacteroides (fragilis) (melaninogeniscus) (oralis) 008.46
   Butyrivibrio (fibriosolvens) 008.46
   Campylobacter 008.43
   Candida 112.85
   Chilomastix 007.8
   choleriformis 001.1
   chronic 558.9
      ulcerative (*see also* Colitis, ulcerative) 556.9
   cicatrizing (chronic) 555.0
   Clostridium
      botulinum 005.1
      difficile 008.45
      haemolyticum 008.46
      novyi 008.46
      perfringens (C) (F) 008.46
      specified type NEC 008.46
   coccidial 007.2
   dietetic 558.9
   due to
      achylia gastrica 536.8
      adenovirus 008.62
      Aerobacter aerogenes 008.2
      anaerobes (*see also* Enteritis, anaerobic) 008.46
      Arizona (bacillus) 008.1
      astrovirus 008.66
      Bacillus coli - *see* Enteritis, E. coli
      bacteria NEC 008.5
         specified NEC 008.49
      Bacteroides (*see also* Enteritis, Bacteroides) 008.46
      Butyrivibrio (fibriosolvens) 008.46
      calicivirus 008.65
      Campylobacter 008.43
      Clostridium - *see* Enteritis, Clostridium
      Cockle agent 008.64
      Coxsackie (virus) 008.67
      Ditchling agent 008.64
      ECHO virus 008.67
      Enterobacter aerogenes 008.2
      enterococci 008.49

Enteritis (Continued)
  due to (Continued)
    enterovirus NEC 008.67
    Escherichia coli - see Enteritis, E. coli
    Eubacterium 008.46
    Fusobacterium (nucleatum) 008.46
    gram-negative bacteria NEC 008.47
      anaerobic NEC 008.46
    Hawaii agent 008.63
    irritating foods 558.9
    Klebsiella aerogenes 008.47
    Marin County agent 008.66
    Montgomery County agent 008.63
    noroviris 008.63
    Norwalk-like agent 008.63
    Norwalk virus 008.63
    Otofuke agent 008.63
    Paracolobactrum arizonae 008.1
    paracolon bacillus NEC 008.47
      Arizona 008.1
    Paramatta agent 008.64
    Peptococcus 008.46
    Peptostreptococcus 008.46
    Proprionibacterium 008.46
    Proteus (bacillus) (mirabilis) (morganii)
      008.3
    Pseudomonas aeruginosa 008.42
    Rotavirus 008.61
    Sapporo agent 008.63
    small round virus (SRV) NEC 008.64
      featureless NEC 008.63
      structured NEC 008.63
    Snow Mountain (SM) agent 008.63
    specified
      bacteria NEC 008.49
      organism, nonbacterial NEC
        008.8
      virus NEC 008.69
    Staphylococcus 008.41
    Streptococcus 008.49
      anaerobic 008.46
    Taunton agent 008.63
    Torovirus 008.69
    Treponema 008.46
    Veillonella 008.46
    virus 008.8
      specified type NEC 008.69
    Wollan (W) agent 008.64
    Yersinia enterocolitica 008.44
  dysentery - see Dysentery
  E. coli 008.00
    enterohemorrhagic 008.04
    enteroinvasive 008.03
    enteropathogenic 008.01
    enterotoxigenic 008.02
    specified type NEC 008.09
  El Tor 001.1
  embadomonial 007.8
  eosinophilic 558.41
  epidemic 009.0
  Eubacterium 008.46
  fermentative 558.9
  fulminant 557.0
  Fusobacterium (nucleatum) 008.46
  gangrenous (see also Enteritis, due to, by
    organism) 009.0
  giardial 007.1
  gram-negative bacteria NEC 008.47
    anaerobic NEC 008.46
  infectious NEC (see also Enteritis, due to,
    organism) 009.0
    presumed 009.1
  influenzal (see also Influenza) 487.8
  ischemic 557.9
    acute 557.0
    chronic 557.1
    due to mesenteric artery insufficiency
      557.1
  membranous 564.9
  mucous 564.9
  myxomembranous 564.9

Enteritis (Continued)
  necrotic (see also Enteritis, due to, by
    organism) 009.0
  necroticans 005.2
  necrotizing of fetus or newborn (see also
    Enterocolitis, necrotizing, newborn)
    777.50
  neurogenic 564.9
  newborn 777.8
    necrotizing (see also Enterocolitis,
      necrotizing, newborn) 777.50
  parasitic NEC 129
  paratyphoid (fever) (see also Fever,
    paratyphoid) 002.9
  Peptococcus 008.46
  Peptostreptococcus 008.46
  Proprionibacterium 008.46
  protozoal NEC 007.9
  radiation 558.1
  regional (of) 555.9
    intestine
      large (bowel, colon, or rectum) 555.1
        with small intestine 555.2
      small (duodenum, ileum, or jejunum)
        555.0
        with large intestine 555.2
  Salmonella infection 003.0
  salmonellosis 003.0
  segmental (see also Enteritis, regional) 555.9
  septic (see also Enteritis, due to, by organism)
    009.0
  Shigella 004.9
  simple 558.9
  spasmodic 564.9
  spastic 564.9
  staphylococcal 008.41
    due to food 005.0
  streptococcal 008.49
    anaerobic 008.46
  toxic 558.2
  Treponema (denticola) (macrodentium)
    008.46
  trichomonal 007.3
  tuberculous (see also Tuberculosis) 014.8●
  typhosa 002.0
  ulcerative (chronic) (see also Colitis,
    ulcerative) 556.9
  Veillonella 008.46
  viral 008.8
    adenovirus 008.62
    enterovirus 008.67
    specified virus NEC 008.69
  Yersinia enterocolitica 008.44
  zymotic 009.0
Enteroarticular syndrome 099.3
Enterobiasis 127.4
Enterobius vermicularis 127.4
Enterocele (see also Hernia) 553.9
  pelvis, pelvic (acquired) (congenital) 618.6
  vagina, vaginal (acquired) (congenital)
    618.6
Enterocolitis - see also Enteritis
  fetus or newborn (see also Enterocolitis,
    necrotizing, newborn) 777.8
    necrotizing 777.50
  fulminant 557.0
  granulomatous 555.2
  hemorrhagic (acute) 557.0
    chronic 557.1
  necrotizing (acute) (membranous) 557.0
    newborn 777.50
      with
        perforation 777.53
        pneumatosis without perforation
          777.52
        pneumatosis and perforation 777.53
      without pneumatosis, without
        perforation 777.51
    stage I 777.51
    stage II 777.52
    stage III 777.53

Enterocolitis (Continued)
  primary necrotizing (see also Enterocolitis,
    necrotizing, newborn) 777.50
  pseudomembranous 008.45
    newborn 008.45
  radiation 558.1
    newborn (see also Enterocolitis,
      necrotizing, newborn) 777.50
  ulcerative 556.0
Enterocystoma 751.5
Enterogastritis - see Enteritis
Enterogenous cyanosis 289.7
Enterolith, enterolithiasis (impaction) 560.39
  with hernia - see also Hernia, by site, with
    obstruction
    gangrenous - see Hernia, by site, with
      gangrene
Enteropathy 569.9
  exudative (of Gordon) 579.8
  gluten 579.0
  hemorrhagic, terminal 557.0
  protein-losing 579.8
Enteroperitonitis (see also Peritonitis) 567.9
Enteroptosis 569.89
Enterorrhagia 578.9
Enterospasm 564.9
  psychogenic 306.4
Enterostenosis (see also Obstruction, intestine)
  560.9
Enterostomy status V44.4
  with complication 569.60
Enthesopathy 726.90
  ankle and tarsus 726.70
  elbow region 726.30
    specified NEC 726.39
  hip 726.5
  knee 726.60
  peripheral NEC 726.8
  shoulder region 726.10
    adhesive 726.0
  spinal 720.1
  wrist and carpus 726.4
Entrance, air into vein - see Embolism, air
Entrapment, nerve - see Neuropathy,
  entrapment
Entropion (eyelid) 374.00
  cicatricial 374.04
  congenital 743.62
  late effect of trachoma (healed) 139.1
  mechanical 374.02
  paralytic 374.02
  senile 374.01
  spastic 374.03
Enucleation of eye (current) (traumatic) 871.3
Enuresis 788.30
  habit disturbance 307.6
  nocturnal 788.36
    psychogenic 307.6
  nonorganic origin 307.6
  psychogenic 307.6
Enzymopathy 277.9
Eosinopenia 288.59
Eosinophilia 288.3
  with
    angiolymphoid hyperplasia (ALHE)
      228.01
  allergic 288.3
  hereditary 288.3
  idiopathic 288.3
  infiltrative 518.3
  Loeffler's 518.3
  myalgia syndrome 710.5
  pulmonary (tropical) 518.3
  secondary 288.3
  tropical 518.3
Eosinophilic - see also condition
  fasciitis 728.89
  granuloma (bone) 277.89
  infiltration lung 518.3
Ependymitis (acute) (cerebral) (chronic)
  (granular) (see also Meningitis) 322.9

◀ New   ◀▪ Revised   ~~deleted~~ Deleted   ● Use Additional Digit(s)   ▨ Omit code

Ependymoblastoma (M9392/3)
    specified site - *see* Neoplasm, by site,
        malignant
    unspecified site 191.9
Ependymoma (epithelial) (malignant)
        (M9391/3)
    anaplastic type (M9392/3)
        specified site - *see* Neoplasm, by site,
            malignant
        unspecified site 191.9
    benign (M9391/0)
        specified site - *see* Neoplasm, by site,
            benign
        unspecified site 225.0
    myxopapillary (M9394/1) 237.5
    papillary (M9393/1) 237.5
        specified site - *see* Neoplasm, by site,
            malignant
        unspecified site 191.9
Ependymopathy 349.2
    spinal cord 349.2
Ephelides, ephelis 709.09
Ephemeral fever (*see also* Pyrexia) 780.60
Epiblepharon (congenital) 743.62
Epicanthus, epicanthic fold (congenital)
        (eyelid) 743.63
Epicondylitis (elbow) (lateral) 726.32
    medial 726.31
Epicystitis (*see also* Cystitis) 595.9
Epidemic - *see* condition
Epidermidalization, cervix - *see* condition
Epidermidization, cervix - *see* condition
Epidermis, epidermal - *see* condition
Epidermization, cervix - *see* condition
Epidermodysplasia verruciformis 078.19
Epidermoid
    cholesteatoma - *see* Cholesteatoma
    inclusion (*see also* Cyst, skin) 706.2
Epidermolysis
    acuta (combustiformis) (toxica) 695.15
    bullosa 757.39
    necroticans combustiformis 695.15
        due to drug
            correct substance properly
                administered 695.15
            overdose or wrong substance given or
                taken 977.9
                specified drug - *see* Table of Drugs
                    and Chemicals
Epidermophytid - *see* Dermatophytosis
Epidermophytosis (infected) - *see*
        Dermatophytosis
Epidermosis, ear (middle) (*see also*
        Cholesteatoma) 385.30
Epididymis - *see* condition
Epididymitis (nonvenereal) 604.90
    with abscess 604.0
    acute 604.99
    blennorrhagic (acute) 098.0
        chronic or duration of 2 months or over
            098.2
    caseous (*see also* Tuberculosis) 016.4●
    chlamydial 099.54
    diphtheritic 032.89 [604.91]
    filarial 125.9 [604.91]
    gonococcal (acute) 098.0
        chronic or duration of 2 months or over
            098.2
    recurrent 604.99
    residual 604.99
    syphilitic 095.8 [604.91]
    tuberculous (*see also* Tuberculosis) 016.4●
Epididymo-orchitis (*see also* Epididymitis)
        604.90
    with abscess 604.0
    chlamydial 099.54
    gonococcal (acute) 098.13
        chronic or duration of 2 months or over
            098.33
Epidural - *see* condition
Epigastritis (*see also* Gastritis) 535.5●

Epigastrium, epigastric - *see* condition
Epigastrocele (*see also* Hernia, epigastric) 553.29
Epiglottiditis (acute) 464.30
    with obstruction 464.31
    chronic 476.1
    viral 464.30
        with obstruction 464.31
Epiglottis - *see* condition
Epiglottitis (acute) 464.30
    with obstruction 464.31
    chronic 476.1
    viral 464.30
        with obstruction 464.31
Epignathus 759.4
Epilepsia
    partialis continua (*see also* Epilepsy) 345.7●
    procursiva (*see also* Epilepsy) 345.8●
Epilepsy, epileptic (idiopathic) 345.9●

Note: Use the following fifth-digit
subclassifications with categories 345.0,
345.1, 345.4–345.9

0   without mention of intractable
        epilepsy
1   with intractable epilepsy
        pharmacoresistant
            (pharmacologically resistant)
        poorly controlled
        refractory (medically)
        treatment resistant

---

abdominal 345.5●
absence (attack) 345.0●
akinetic 345.0●
    psychomotor 345.4●
automatism 345.4●
autonomic diencephalic 345.5●
brain 345.9●
Bravais-Jacksonian 345.5●
cerebral 345.9●
climacteric 345.9●
clonic 345.1●
clouded state 345.9●
coma 345.3●
communicating 345.4●
complicating pregnancy, childbirth, or the
    puerperium 649.4●
congenital 345.9●
convulsions 345.9●
cortical (focal) (motor) 345.5●
cursive (running) 345.8●
cysticercosis 123.1
deterioration
    with behavioral disturbance 345.9●
        [294.11]
    without behavioral disturbance 345.9●
        [294.10]
due to syphilis 094.89
equivalent 345.5●
fit 345.9●
focal (motor) 345.5●
gelastic 345.8●
generalized 345.9●
    convulsive 345.1●
    flexion 345.1●
    nonconvulsive 345.0●
grand mal (idiopathic) 345.1●
Jacksonian (motor) (sensory) 345.5●
Kojevnikoff's, Kojevnikov's, Kojewnikoff's
    345.7●
laryngeal 786.2
limbic system 345.4●
localization related (focal) (partial) and
        epileptic syndromes
    with
        complex partial seizures 345.4●
        simple partial seizures 345.5●
major (motor) 345.1●
minor 345.0●
mixed (type) 345.9●
motor partial 345.5●

Epilepsy, epileptic (*Continued*)
    musicogenic 345.1●
    myoclonus, myoclonic 345.1●
        progressive (familial) 345.1●
    nonconvulsive, generalized 345.0●
    parasitic NEC 123.9
    partial (focalized) 345.5●
        with
            impairment of consciousness 345.4●
            memory and ideational disturbances
                345.4●
        without impairment of consciousness
            345.5●
        abdominal type 345.5●
        motor type 345.5●
        psychomotor type 345.4●
        psychosensory type 345.4●
        secondarily generalized 345.4●
        sensory type 345.5●
        somatomotor type 345.5●
        somatosensory type 345.5●
        temporal lobe type 345.4●
        visceral type 345.5●
        visual type 345.5●
    peripheral 345.9●
    petit mal 345.0●
    photokinetic 345.8●
    progressive myoclonic (familial) 345.1●
    psychic equivalent 345.5●
    psychomotor 345.4●
    psychosensory 345.4●
    reflex 345.1●
    seizure 345.9●
    senile 345.9●
    sensory-induced 345.5●
    sleep (*see also* Narcolepsy) 347.00
    somatomotor type 345.5●
    somatosensory 345.5●
    specified type NEC 345.8●
    status (grand mal) 345.3
        focal motor 345.7●
        petit mal 345.2
        psychomotor 345.7●
        temporal lobe 345.7●
    symptomatic 345.9●
    temporal lobe 345.4●
    tonic (-clonic) 345.1●
    traumatic (injury unspecified) 907.0
        injury specified - *see* Late, effect (of)
            specified injury
    twilight 293.0
    uncinate (gyrus) 345.4●
    Unverricht (-Lundborg) (familial myoclonic)
        345.1●
    visceral 345.5●
    visual 345.5●
Epileptiform
    convulsions 780.39
    seizure 780.39
Epiloia 759.5
Epimenorrhea 626.2
Epipharyngitis (*see also* Nasopharyngitis)
    460
Epiphora 375.20
    due to
        excess lacrimation 375.21
        insufficient drainage 375.22
Epiphyseal arrest 733.91
    femoral head 732.2
Epiphyseolysis, epiphysiolysis (*see also*
        Osteochondrosis) 732.9
Epiphysitis (*see also* Osteochondrosis) 732.9
    juvenile 732.6
    marginal (Scheuermann's) 732.0
    os calcis 732.5
    syphilitic (congenital) 090.0
    vertebral (Scheuermann's) 732.0
Epiplocele (*see also* Hernia) 553.9
Epiploitis (*see also* Peritonitis) 567.9
Epiplosarcomphalocele (*see also* Hernia,
    umbilicus) 553.1

Episcleritis 379.00
  gouty 274.89 [379.09]
  nodular 379.02
  periodica fugax 379.01
    angioneurotic - see Edema, angioneurotic
  specified NEC 379.09
  staphylococcal 379.00
  suppurative 379.00
  syphilitic 095.0
  tuberculous (see also Tuberculosis) 017.3●
    [379.09]
Episode
  brain (see also Disease, cerebrovascular,
    acute) 436
  cerebral (see also Disease, cerebrovascular,
    acute) 436
  depersonalization (in neurotic state) 300.6
  hyporesponsive 780.09
  psychotic (see also Psychosis) 298.9
    organic, transient 293.9
  schizophrenic (acute) NEC (see also
    Schizophrenia) 295.4●
Epispadias
  female 753.8
  male 752.62
Episplenitis 289.59
Epistaxis (multiple) 784.7
  hereditary 448.0
  vicarious menstruation 625.8
Epithelioma (malignant) (M8011/3) - see also
    Neoplasm, by site, malignant
  adenoides cysticum (M8100/0) - see
    Neoplasm, skin, benign
  basal cell (M8090/3) - see Neoplasm, skin,
    malignant
  benign (M8011/0) - see Neoplasm, by site,
    benign
  Bowen's (M8081/2) - see Neoplasm, skin, in
    situ
  calcifying (benign) (Malherbe's) (M8110/0) -
    see Neoplasm, skin, benign
  external site - see Neoplasm, skin, malignant
  intraepidermal, Jadassohn (M8096/0) - see
    Neoplasm, skin, benign
  squamous cell (M8070/3) - see Neoplasm, by
    site, malignant
Epitheliopathy
  pigment, retina 363.15
  posterior multifocal placoid (acute) 363.15
Epithelium, epithelial - see condition
Epituberculosis (allergic) (with atelectasis) (see
    also Tuberculosis) 010.8●
Eponychia 757.5
Epstein's
  nephrosis or syndrome (see also Nephrosis)
    581.9
  pearl (mouth) 528.4
Epstein-Barr infection (viral) 075
  chronic 780.79 [139.8]
Epulis (giant cell) (gingiva) 523.8
Equinia 024
Equinovarus (congenital) 754.51
  acquired 736.71
Equivalent
  angina 413.9
  convulsive (abdominal) (see also Epilepsy)
    345.5●
  epileptic (psychic) (see also Epilepsy) 345.5●
Erb's
  disease 359.1
  palsy, paralysis (birth) (brachial) (newborn)
    767.6
    spinal (spastic) syphilitic 094.89
  pseudohypertrophic muscular dystrophy
    359.1
Erb (-Duchenne) paralysis (birth injury)
    (newborn) 767.6
Erb-Goldflam disease or syndrome 358.00
Erdheim-Chester disease (ECD) 277.89
Erdheim's syndrome (acromegalic
    macrospondylitis) 253.0

Erection, painful (persistent) 607.3
Ergosterol deficiency (vitamin D) 268.9
  with
    osteomalacia 268.2
    rickets (see also Rickets) 268.0
Ergotism (ergotized grain) 988.2
  from ergot used as drug (migraine therapy)
    correct substance properly administered
      349.82
    overdose or wrong substance given or
      taken 975.0
Erichsen's disease (railway spine) 300.16
Erlacher-Blount syndrome (tibia vara) 732.4
Erosio interdigitalis blastomycetica 112.3
Erosion
  arteriosclerotic plaque - see Arteriosclerosis,
    by site
  artery NEC 447.2
    without rupture 447.8
  bone 733.99
  bronchus 519.19
  cartilage (joint) 733.99
  cervix (uteri) (acquired) (chronic)
    (congenital) 622.0
    with mention of cervicitis 616.0
  cornea (recurrent) (see also Keratitis) 371.42
    traumatic 918.1
  dental (idiopathic) (occupational) 521.30
    extending into
      dentine 521.32
      pulp 521.33
    generalized 521.35
    limited to enamel 521.31
    localized 521.34
  duodenum, postpyloric - see Ulcer,
    duodenum
  esophagus 530.89
  gastric 535.4●
  implanted vaginal mesh
    in, into
      pelvic floor muscles 629.31
      surrounding organ(s) or tissue 629.31
  intestine 569.89
  lymphatic vessel 457.8
  pylorus, pyloric (ulcer) 535.4●
  sclera 379.16
  spine, aneurysmal 094.89
  spleen 289.59
  stomach 535.4●
  teeth (idiopathic) (occupational) (see also
    Erosion, dental) 521.30
    due to
      medicine 521.30
      persistent vomiting 521.30
  urethra 599.84
  uterus 621.8
  vaginal prosthetic materials NEC
    in, into
      pelvic floor muscles 629.31
      surrounding organ(s) or tissue 629.31
  vertebra 733.99
Erotomania 302.89
  Clerambault's 297.8
Error
  in diet 269.9
  refractive 367.9
    astigmatism (see also Astigmatism) 367.20
    drug-induced 367.89
    hypermetropia 367.0
    hyperopia 367.0
    myopia 367.1
    presbyopia 367.4
    toxic 367.89
Eructation 787.3
  nervous 306.4
  psychogenic 306.4
Eruption
  creeping 126.9
  drug - see Dermatitis, due to, drug
  Hutchinson, summer 692.72
  Kaposi's varicelliform 054.0

Eruption (Continued)
  napkin (psoriasiform) 691.0
  polymorphous
    light (sun) 692.72
      other source 692.82
  psoriasiform, napkin 691.0
  recalcitrant pustular 694.8
  ringed 695.89
  skin (see also Dermatitis) 782.1
    creeping (meaning hookworm) 126.9
    due to
      chemical(s) NEC 692.4
        internal use 693.8
      drug - see Dermatitis, due to, drug
      prophylactic inoculation or vaccination
        against disease - see Dermatitis,
        due to, vaccine
      smallpox vaccination NEC - see
        Dermatitis, due to, vaccine
    erysipeloid 027.1
    feigned 698.4
    Hutchinson, summer 692.72
    Kaposi's, varicelliform 054.0
      vaccinia 999.0
    lichenoid, axilla 698.3
    polymorphous, due to light 692.72
    toxic NEC 695.0
    vesicular 709.8
  teeth, tooth
    accelerated 520.6
    delayed 520.6
    difficult 520.6
    disturbance of 520.6
    in abnormal sequence 520.6
    incomplete 520.6
    late 520.6
    natal 520.6
    neonatal 520.6
    obstructed 520.6
    partial 520.6
    persistent primary 520.6
    premature 520.6
    prenatal 520.6
  vesicular 709.8
Erysipelas (gangrenous) (infantile) (newborn)
    (phlegmonous) (suppurative) 035
  external ear 035 [380.13]
  puerperal, postpartum, childbirth 670.8●
Erysipelatoid (Rosenbach's) 027.1
Erysipeloid (Rosenbach's) 027.1
Erythema, erythematous (generalized) 695.9
  ab igne - see Burn, by site, first degree
  annulare (centrifugum) (rheumaticum) 695.0
  arthriticum epidemicum 026.1
  brucellum (see also Brucellosis) 023.9
  bullosum 695.19
  caloricum - see Burn, by site, first degree
  chronicum migrans 088.81
  circinatum 695.19
  diaper 691.0
  due to
    chemical (contact) NEC 692.4
      internal 693.8
    drug (internal use) 693.0
      contact 692.3
  elevatum diutinum 695.89
  endemic 265.2
  epidemic, arthritic 026.1
  figuratum perstans 695.0
  gluteal 691.0
  gyratum (perstans) (repens) 695.19
  heat - see Burn, by site, first degree
  ichthyosiforme congenitum 757.1
  induratum (primary) (scrofulosorum) (see
    also Tuberculosis) 017.1●
    nontuberculous 695.2
  infantum febrile 057.8
  infectional NEC 695.9
  infectiosum 057.0
  inflammation NEC 695.9
  intertrigo 695.89

◀ New   ◀◧ Revised   ~~deleted~~ Deleted   ● Use Additional Digit(s)   ▨ Omit code

Erythema, erythematous (Continued)
iris 695.10
lupus (discoid) (localized) (see also Lupus,
erythematosus) 695.4
marginatum 695.0
rheumaticum - see Fever, rheumatic
medicamentosum - see Dermatitis, due to,
drug
migrans 529.1
chronicum 088.81
multiforme 695.10
bullosum 695.19
conjunctiva 695.19
exudativum (Hebra) 695.19
major 695.12
minor 695.11
pemphigoides 694.5
napkin 691.0
neonatorum 778.8
nodosum 695.2
tuberculous (see also Tuberculosis) 017.1●
nummular, nummulare 695.19
palmar 695.0
palmaris hereditarium 695.0
pernio 991.5
perstans solare 692.72
rash, newborn 778.8
scarlatiniform (exfoliative) (recurrent) 695.0
simplex marginatum 057.8
solare (see also Sunburn) 692.71
streptogenes 696.5
toxic, toxicum NEC 695.0
newborn 778.8
tuberculous (primary) (see also Tuberculosis)
017.0●
venenatum 695.0
Erythematosus - see condition
Erythematous - see condition
Erythermalgia (primary) 443.82
Erythralgia 443.82
Erythrasma 039.0
Erythredema 985.0
polyneuritica 985.0
polyneuropathy 985.0
Erythremia (acute) (M9841/3) 207.0●
chronic (M9842/3) 207.1●
secondary 289.0
Erythroblastopenia (acquired) 284.89
congenital 284.01
Erythroblastophthisis 284.01
Erythroblastosis (fetalis) (newborn) 773.2
due to
ABO
antibodies 773.1
incompatibility, maternal/fetal 773.1
isoimmunization 773.1
Rh
antibodies 773.0
incompatibility, maternal/fetal 773.0
isoimmunization 773.0
Erythrocyanosis (crurum) 443.89
Erythrocythemia - see Erythremia
Erythrocytopenia 285.9
Erythrocytosis (megalosplenic)
familial 289.6
oval, hereditary (see also Elliptocytosis) 282.1
secondary 289.0
stress 289.0
Erythroderma (see also Erythema) 695.9
desquamativa (in infants) 695.89
exfoliative 695.89
ichthyosiform, congenital 757.1
infantum 695.89
maculopapular 696.2
neonatorum 778.8
psoriaticum 696.1
secondary 695.9
Erythrodysesthesia, palmar plantar (PPE) 693.0
Erythrogenesis imperfecta 284.09
Erythroleukemia (M9840/3) 207.0●
Erythromelalgia 443.82

Erythromelia 701.8
Erythropenia 285.9
Erythrophagocytosis 289.9
Erythrophobia 300.23
Erythroplakia
oral mucosa 528.79
tongue 528.79
Erythroplasia (Queyrat) (M8080/2)
specified site - see Neoplasm, skin, in situ
unspecified site 233.5
Erythropoiesis, idiopathic ineffective 285.0
Escaped beats, heart 427.60
postoperative 997.1
Escherichia coli (E. coli) - see Infection,
Escherichia coli
Esoenteritis - see Enteritis
Esophagalgia 530.89
Esophagectasis 530.89
due to cardiospasm 530.0
Esophagismus 530.5
Esophagitis (alkaline) (chemical) (chronic)
(infectional) (necrotic) (peptic)
(postoperative) (regurgitant) 530.10
acute 530.12
candidal 112.84
eosinophilic 530.13
reflux 530.11
specified NEC 530.19
tuberculous (see also Tuberculosis)
017.8●
ulcerative 530.19
Esophagocele 530.6
Esophagodynia 530.89
Esophagomalacia 530.89
Esophagoptosis 530.89
Esophagospasm 530.5
Esophagostenosis 530.3
Esophagostomiasis 127.7
Esophagostomy
complication 530.87
infection 530.86
malfunctioning 530.87
mechanical 530.87
Esophagotracheal - see condition
Esophagus - see condition
Esophoria 378.41
convergence, excess 378.84
divergence, insufficiency 378.85
Esotropia (nonaccommodative) 378.00
accommodative 378.35
alternating 378.05
with
A pattern 378.06
specified noncomitancy NEC 378.08
V pattern 378.07
X pattern 378.08
Y pattern 378.08
intermittent 378.22
intermittent 378.20
alternating 378.22
monocular 378.21
monocular 378.01
with
A pattern 378.02
specified noncomitancy NEC 378.04
V pattern 378.03
X pattern 378.04
Y pattern 378.04
intermittent 378.21
Espundia 085.5
Essential - see condition
Esterapenia 289.89
Esthesioneuroblastoma (M9522/3) 160.0
Esthesioneurocytoma (M9521/3) 160.0
Esthesioneuroepithelioma (M9523/3) 160.0
Esthiomene 099.1
Estivo-autumnal
fever 084.0
malaria 084.0
Estrangement V61.09
Estriasis 134.0

Ethanolaminuria 270.8
Ethanolism (see also Alcoholism) 303.9●
Ether dependence, dependency (see also
Dependence) 304.6●
Etherism (see also Dependence) 304.6●
Ethmoid, ethmoidal - see condition
Ethmoiditis (chronic) (nonpurulent) (purulent)
(see also Sinusitis, ethmoidal) 473.2
influenzal (see also Influenza) 487.1
Woakes' 471.1
Ethylism (see also Alcoholism) 303.9●
Eulenburg's disease (congenital paramyotonia)
359.29
Eunuchism 257.2
Eunuchoidism 257.2
hypogonadotropic 257.2
European blastomycosis 117.5
Eustachian - see condition
Euthyroid sick syndrome 790.94
Euthyroidism 244.9
Evaluation
fetal lung maturity 659.8●
for suspected condition (see also Observation)
V71.9
abuse V71.81
exposure
anthrax V71.82
biologic agent NEC V71.83
SARS V71.83
neglect V71.81
newborn - see Observation, suspected,
condition, newborn
specified condition NEC V71.89
mental health V70.2
requested by authority V70.1
nursing care V63.8
social service V63.8
Evans' syndrome (thrombocytopenic purpura)
287.32
Event, apparent life threatening in newborn and
infant (ALTE) 799.82
Eventration
colon into chest - see Hernia, diaphragm
diaphragm (congenital) 756.6
Eversion
bladder 596.89
cervix (uteri) 622.0
with mention of cervicitis 616.0
foot NEC 736.79
congenital 755.67
lacrimal punctum 375.51
punctum lacrimale (postinfectional) (senile)
375.51
ureter (meatus) 593.89
urethra (meatus) 599.84
uterus 618.1
complicating delivery 665.2●
affecting fetus or newborn 763.89
puerperal, postpartum 674.8●
Evidence
of malignancy
cytologic
without histologic confirmation
anus 796.76
cervix 795.06
vagina 795.16
Evisceration
birth injury 767.8
bowel (congenital) - see Hernia, ventral
congenital (see also Hernia, ventral) 553.29
operative wound 998.32
traumatic NEC 869.1
eye 871.3
Evulsion - see Avulsion
Ewing's
angioendothelioma (M9260/3) - see
Neoplasm, bone, malignant
sarcoma (M9260/3) - see Neoplasm, bone,
malignant
tumor (M9260/3) - see Neoplasm, bone,
malignant

◄ New ◄▥ Revised ~~deleted~~ Deleted ● Use Additional Digit(s) ▨ Omit code

Exaggerated lumbosacral angle (with impinging spine) 756.12
Examination (general) (routine) (of) (for) V70.9
  allergy V72.7
  annual V70.0
  cardiovascular preoperative V72.81
  cervical Papanicolaou smear V76.2
    as a part of routine gynecological examination V72.31
    to confirm findings of recent normal smear following initial abnormal smear V72.32
  child care (routine) V20.2
  clinical research investigation (normal control patient) (participant) V70.7
  dental V72.2
  developmental testing (child) (infant) V20.2
  donor (potential) V70.8
  ear V72.19
  eye V72.0
  following
    accident (motor vehicle) V71.4
    alleged rape or seduction (victim or culprit) V71.5
    inflicted injury (victim or culprit) NEC V71.6
    rape or seduction, alleged (victim or culprit) V71.5
    treatment (for) V67.9
      combined V67.6
      fracture V67.4
      involving high-risk medication NEC V67.51
      mental disorder V67.3
      specified condition NEC V67.59
  follow-up (routine) (following) V67.9
    cancer chemotherapy V67.2
    chemotherapy V67.2
    disease NEC V67.59
    high-risk medication NEC V67.51
    injury NEC V67.59
    population survey V70.6
    postpartum V24.2
    psychiatric V67.3
    psychotherapy V67.3
    radiotherapy V67.1
    specified surgery NEC V67.09
    surgery V67.00
    vaginal pap smear V67.01
  gynecological V72.31
    for contraceptive maintenance V25.40
      intrauterine device V25.42
      pill V25.41
      specified method NEC V25.49
  health (of)
    armed forces personnel V70.5
    checkup V70.0
    child, routine V20.2
    defined subpopulation NEC V70.5
    inhabitants of institutions V70.5
    occupational V70.5
    pre-employment screening V70.5
    preschool children V70.5
      for admission to school V70.3
    prisoners V70.5
      for entrance into prison V70.3
    prostitutes V70.5
    refugees V70.5
    school children V70.5
    students V70.5
  hearing V72.19
    following failed hearing screening V72.11
  infant
    8 to 28 days old V20.32
    over 28 days old, routine V20.2
    under 8 days old V20.31
  laboratory V72.60
    ordered as part of a routine general medical examination V72.62
    pre-operative V72.63

Examination (Continued)
  laboratory (Continued)
    pre-procedural V72.63
    specified NEC V72.69
  lactating mother V24.1
  medical (for) (of) V70.9
    administrative purpose NEC V70.3
    admission to
      old age home V70.3
      prison V70.3
      school V70.3
    adoption V70.3
    armed forces personnel V70.5
    at health care facility V70.0
    camp V70.3
    child, routine V20.2
    clinical research (control) (normal comparison) (participant) V70.7
    defined subpopulation NEC V70.5
    donor (potential) V70.8
    driving license V70.3
    general V70.9
      routine V70.0
      specified reason NEC V70.8
    immigration V70.3
    inhabitants of institutions V70.5
    insurance certification V70.3
    marriage V70.3
    medicolegal reasons V70.4
    naturalization V70.3
    occupational V70.5
    population survey V70.6
    pre-employment V70.5
    preschool children V70.5
      for admission to school V70.3
    prison V70.3
    prisoners V70.5
      for entrance into prison V70.3
    prostitutes V70.5
    refugees V70.5
    school children V70.5
    specified reason NEC V70.8
    sport competition V70.3
    students V70.5
  medicolegal reason V70.4
  pelvic (annual) (periodic) V72.31
  periodic (annual) (routine) V70.0
  postpartum
    immediately after delivery V24.0
    routine follow-up V24.2
  pregnancy (unconfirmed) (possible) V72.40
    negative result V72.41
    positive result V72.42
  prenatal V22.1
    first pregnancy V22.0
    high-risk pregnancy V23.9
      specified problem NEC V23.89
      to determine fetal viability V23.87
  preoperative V72.84
    cardiovascular V72.81
    respiratory V72.82
    specified NEC V72.83
  preprocedural V72.84
    cardiovascular V72.81
    general physical V72.83
    respiratory V72.82
    specified NEC V72.83
  prior to chemotherapy V72.83
  psychiatric V70.2
    follow-up not needing further care V67.3
    requested by authority V70.1
  radiological NEC V72.5
  respiratory preoperative V72.82
  screening - see Screening
  sensitization V72.7
  skin V72.7
    hypersensitivity V72.7
  special V72.9
  specified type or reason NEC V72.85
    preoperative V72.83
      specified NEC V72.83

Examination (Continued)
  teeth V72.2
  vaginal Papanicolaou smear V76.47
    following hysterectomy for malignant condition V67.01
  victim or culprit following
    alleged rape or seduction V71.5
    inflicted injury NEC V71.6
  vision V72.0
  well baby V20.2
Exanthem, exanthema (see also Rash) 782.1
  Boston 048
  epidemic, with meningitis 048
  lichenoid psoriasiform 696.2
  subitum 058.10
    due to
      human herpesvirus 6 058.11
      human herpesvirus 7 058.12
  viral, virus NEC 057.9
    specified type NEC 057.8
Excess, excessive, excessively
  alcohol level in blood 790.3
  carbohydrate tissue, localized 278.1
  carotene (dietary) 278.3
  cold 991.9
    specified effect NEC 991.8
  convergence 378.84
  crying 780.95
    of
      adolescent 780.95
      adult 780.95
      baby 780.92
      child 780.95
      infant (baby) 780.92
      newborn 780.92
  development, breast 611.1
  diaphoresis (see also Hyperhidrosis) 780.8
  distance, interarch 524.28
  divergence 378.85
  drinking (alcohol) NEC (see also Abuse, drugs, nondependent) 305.0●
    continual (see also Alcoholism) 303.9●
    habitual (see also Alcoholism) 303.9●
  eating 783.6
  eyelid fold (congenital) 743.62
  fat 278.02
    in heart (see also Degeneration, myocardial) 429.1
    tissue, localized 278.1
  foreskin 605
  gas 787.3
  gastrin 251.5
  glucagon 251.4
  heat (see also Heat) 992.9
  horizontal
    overjet 524.26
    overlap 524.26
  interarch distance 524.28
  intermaxillary vertical dimension 524.37
  interocclusal distance of teeth 524.37
  large
    colon 564.7
      congenital 751.3
    fetus or infant 766.0
      with obstructed labor 660.1●
      affecting management of pregnancy 656.6●
      causing disproportion 653.5●
    newborn (weight of 4500 grams or more) 766.0
    organ or site, congenital NEC - see Anomaly, specified type NEC
  lid fold (congenital) 743.62
  long
    colon 751.5
    organ or site, congenital NEC - see Anomaly, specified type NEC
  umbilical cord (entangled)
    affecting fetus or newborn 762.5
    in pregnancy or childbirth 663.3●
      with compression 663.2●

◄ New   ◄▒ Revised   ~~deleted~~ Deleted   ● Use Additional Digit(s)   ▒ Omit code

Excess, excessive, excessively (Continued)
menstruation 626.2
number of teeth 520.1
causing crowding 524.31
nutrients (dietary) NEC 783.6
potassium (K) 276.7
salivation (see also Ptyalism) 527.7
secretion - see also Hypersecretion
milk 676.6●
sputum 786.4
sweat (see also Hyperhidrosis) 780.8
short
organ or site, congenital NEC - see
Anomaly, specified type NEC
umbilical cord
affecting fetus or newborn 762.6
in pregnancy or childbirth 663.4●
skin NEC 701.9
eyelid 743.62
acquired 374.30
sodium (Na) 276.0
spacing of teeth 524.32
sputum 786.4
sweating (see also Hyperhidrosis) 780.8
tearing (ducts) (eye) (see also Epiphora)
375.20
thirst 783.5
due to deprivation of water 994.3
tissue in reconstructed breast 612.0
tuberosity 524.07
vitamin
A (dietary) 278.2
administered as drug (chronic)
(prolonged excessive intake)
278.2
reaction to sudden overdose
963.5
D (dietary) 278.4
administered as drug (chronic)
(prolonged excessive intake)
278.4
reaction to sudden overdose
963.5
weight 278.02
gain 783.1
of pregnancy 646.1●
loss 783.21
Excitability, abnormal, under minor stress
309.29
Excitation
catatonic (see also Schizophrenia) 295.2●
psychogenic 298.1
reactive (from emotional stress,
psychological trauma) 298.1
Excitement
manic (see also Psychosis, affective) 296.0●
recurrent episode 296.1●
single episode 296.0●
mental, reactive (from emotional stress,
psychological trauma) 298.1
state, reactive (from emotional stress,
psychological trauma) 298.1
Excluded pupils 364.76
Excoriation (traumatic) (see also Injury,
superficial, by site) 919.8
neurotic 698.4
Excyclophoria 378.44
Excyclotropia 378.33
Exencephalus, exencephaly 742.0
Exercise
breathing V57.0
remedial NEC V57.1
therapeutic NEC V57.1
Exfoliation
skin
due to erythematous condition 695.50
involving (percent of body surface)
less than 10 percent 695.50
10-19 percent 695.51
20-29 percent 695.52
30-39 percent 695.53

Exfoliation (Continued)
skin (Continued)
due to erythematous condition
(Continued)
involving (Continued)
40-49 percent 695.54
50-59 percent 695.55
60-69 percent 695.56
70-79 percent 695.57
80-89 percent 695.58
90 percent or more 695.59
teeth
due to systemic causes 525.0
Exfoliative - see also condition
dermatitis 695.89
Exhaustion, exhaustive (physical NEC)
780.79
battle (see also Reaction, stress, acute)
308.9
cardiac (see also Failure, heart) 428.9
delirium (see also Reaction, stress, acute)
308.9
due to
cold 991.8
excessive exertion 994.5
exposure 994.4
overexertion 994.5
fetus or newborn 779.89
heart (see also Failure, heart) 428.9
heat 992.5
due to
salt depletion 992.4
water depletion 992.3
manic (see also Psychosis, affective)
296.0●
recurrent episode 296.1●
single episode 296.0●
maternal, complicating delivery 669.8●
affecting fetus or newborn 763.89
mental 300.5
myocardium, myocardial (see also Failure,
heart) 428.9
nervous 300.5
old age 797
postinfectional NEC 780.79
psychogenic 300.5
psychosis (see also Reaction, stress, acute)
308.9
senile 797
dementia 290.0
Exhibitionism (sexual) 302.4
Exomphalos 756.72
Exophoria 378.42
convergence, insufficiency 378.83
divergence, excess 378.85
Exophthalmic
cachexia 242.0●
goiter 242.0●
ophthalmoplegia 242.0● [376.22]
Exophthalmos 376.30
congenital 743.66
constant 376.31
endocrine NEC 259.9 [376.22]
hyperthyroidism 242.0● [376.21]
intermittent NEC 376.34
malignant 242.0● [376.21]
pulsating 376.35
endocrine NEC 259.9 [376.22]
thyrotoxic 242.0● [376.21]
Exostosis 726.91
cartilaginous (M9210/0) - see Neoplasm,
bone, benign
congenital 756.4
ear canal, external 380.81
gonococcal 098.89
hip 726.5
intracranial 733.3
jaw (bone) 526.81
luxurians 728.11
multiple (cancellous) (congenital)
(hereditary) 756.4

Exostosis (Continued)
nasal bones 726.91
orbit, orbital 376.42
osteocartilaginous (M9210/0) - see
Neoplasm, bone, benign
spine 721.8
with spondylosis - see Spondylosis
syphilitic 095.5
wrist 726.4
Exotropia 378.10
alternating 378.15
with
A pattern 378.16
specified noncomitancy NEC
378.18
V pattern 378.17
X pattern 378.18
Y pattern 378.18
intermittent 378.24
intermittent 378.20
alternating 378.24
monocular 378.23
monocular 378.11
with
A pattern 378.12
specified noncomitancy NEC
378.14
V pattern 378.13
X pattern 378.14
Y pattern 378.14
intermittent 378.23
Explanation of
investigation finding V65.4
medication V65.4
Exposure (suspected) 994.9
algae bloom V87.32
cold 991.9
specified effect NEC 991.8
effects of 994.9
exhaustion due to 994.4
implanted vaginal mesh
into vagina 629.32
through vaginal wall 629.32
to
AIDS virus V01.79
anthrax V01.81
aromatic
amines V87.11
dyes V87.19
arsenic V87.01
asbestos V15.84
benzene V87.12
body fluids (hazardous) V15.85
cholera V01.0
chromium compounds V87.09
communicable disease V01.9
specified type NEC V01.89
dyes V87.2
aromatic V87.19
Escherichia coli (E. coli) V01.83
German measles V01.4
gonorrhea V01.6
hazardous
aromatic compounds NEC V87.19
body fluids V15.85
chemicals NEC V87.2
metals V87.09
substances V87.39
HIV V01.79
human immunodeficiency virus
V01.79
lead V15.86
meningococcus V01.84
mold V87.31
nickel dust V87.09
parasitic disease V01.89
poliomyelitis V01.2
polycyclic aromatic hydrocarbons V87.19
potentially hazardous body fluids
V15.85
rabies V01.5

Exposure *(Continued)*
  to *(Continued)*
    rubella V01.4
    SARS-associated coronavirus V01.82
    smallpox V01.3
    syphilis V01.6
    tuberculosis V01.1
    uranium V87.02
    varicella V01.71
    venereal disease V01.6
    viral disease NEC V01.79
      varicella V01.71
  vaginal prosthetic materials NEC
    into vagina 629.32
    through vaginal wall 629.32
Exsanguination, fetal 772.0
Exstrophy
  abdominal content 751.8
  bladder (urinary) 753.5
Extensive - *see* condition
Extra - *see also* Accessory
  rib 756.3
    cervical 756.2
Extraction
  with hook 763.89
  breech NEC 669.6●
    affecting fetus or newborn 763.0

Extraction *(Continued)*
  cataract postsurgical
    V45.61
  manual NEC 669.8●
    affecting fetus or newborn
      763.89
Extrasystole 427.60
  atrial 427.61
  postoperative 997.1
  ventricular 427.69
Extrauterine gestation or pregnancy -
  see Pregnancy, ectopic
Extravasation
  blood 459.0
    lower extremity 459.0
  chemotherapy, vesicant
    999.81
  chyle into mesentery 457.8
  pelvicalyceal 593.4
  pyelosinus 593.4
  urine 788.8
    from ureter 788.8
  vesicant
    agent NEC 999.82
    chemotherapy 999.81
Extremity - *see* condition
Extrophy - *see* Exstrophy

Extroversion
  bladder 753.5
  uterus 618.1
    complicating delivery 665.2●
      affecting fetus or newborn 763.89
    postpartal (old) 618.1
Extruded tooth 524.34
Extrusion
  alveolus and teeth 524.75
  breast implant (prosthetic) 996.54
  device, implant, or graft - *see* Complications,
    mechanical
  eye implant (ball) (globe) 996.59
  intervertebral disc - *see* Displacement,
    intervertebral disc
  lacrimal gland 375.43
  mesh (reinforcing) 996.59
  ocular lens implant 996.53
  prosthetic device NEC - *see* Complications,
    mechanical
  vitreous 379.26
Exudate, pleura - *see* Effusion, pleura
Exudates, retina 362.82
Exudative - *see* condition
Eye, eyeball, eyelid - *see* condition
Eyestrain 368.13
Eyeworm disease of Africa 125.2

F

Faber's anemia or syndrome (achlorhydric anemia) 280.9
Fabry's disease (angiokeratoma corporis diffusum) 272.7
Face, facial - see condition
Facet of cornea 371.44
Faciocephalalgia, autonomic (see also Neuropathy, peripheral, autonomic) 337.9
Facioscapulohumeral myopathy 359.1
Factitious disorder, illness - see Illness, factitious
Factor
  deficiency - see Deficiency, factor
  psychic, associated with diseases classified elsewhere 316
  risk-see problem
  V Leiden mutation 289.81
Fahr-Volhard disease (malignant nephrosclerosis) 403.00
Failure, failed
  adenohypophyseal 253.2
  attempted abortion (legal) (see also Abortion, failed) 638.9
  bone marrow (anemia) 284.9
    acquired (secondary) 284.89
    congenital 284.09
    idiopathic 284.9
  cardiac (see also Failure, heart) 428.9
    newborn 779.89
  cardiorenal (chronic) 428.9
    hypertensive (see also Hypertension, cardiorenal) 404.93
  cardiorespiratory 799.1
    specified during or due to a procedure 997.1
      long-term effect of cardiac surgery 429.4
  cardiovascular (chronic) 428.9
  cerebrovascular 437.8
  cervical dilatation in labor 661.0●
    affecting fetus or newborn 763.7
  circulation, circulatory 799.89
    fetus or newborn 779.89
    peripheral 785.50
      postoperative 998.00
  compensation - see Disease, heart
  congestive (see also Failure, heart) 428.0
  conscious sedation, during procedure 995.24
  coronary (see also Insufficiency, coronary) 411.89
  dental implant 525.79
    due to
      infection 525.71
      lack of attached gingiva 525.72
      occlusal trauma (caused by poor prosthetic design) 525.72
      parafunctional habits 525.72
      periodontal infection (periimplantitis) 525.72
      poor oral hygiene 525.72
      unintentional loading 525.71
    endosseous NEC 525.79
    mechanical 525.73
    osseointegration 525.71
      due to
        complications of systemic disease 525.71
        poor bone quality 525.71
        premature loading 525.71
      iatrogenic 525.71
      prior to intentional prosthetic loading 525.71
    post-osseointegration
      biological 525.72
        iatrogenic 525.72
        due to complications of systemic disease 525.72
      mechanical 525.73

Failure, failed (Continued)
  dental implant (Continued)
    pre-integration 525.71
    pre-osseointegration 525.71
  dental prosthesis causing loss of dental implant 525.73
  dental restoration
    marginal integrity 525.61
    periodontal anatomical integrity 525.65
  descent of head (at term) 652.5●
    affecting fetus or newborn 763.1
    in labor 660.0●
      affecting fetus or newborn 763.1
  device, implant, or graft - see Complications, mechanical
  engagement of head NEC 652.5●
    in labor 660.0●
  extrarenal 788.99
  fetal head to enter pelvic brim 652.5●
    affecting fetus or newborn 763.1
    in labor 660.0●
      affecting fetus or newborn 763.1
  forceps NEC 660.7●
    affecting fetus or newborn 763.1
  fusion (joint) (spinal) 996.49
  growth in childhood 783.43
  heart (acute) (sudden) 428.9
    with
      abortion - see Abortion, by type, with specified complication NEC
      acute pulmonary edema (see also Failure, ventricular, left) 428.1
        with congestion (see also Failure, heart) 428.0
      decompensation (see also Failure, heart) 428.0
      dilation - see Disease, heart
      ectopic pregnancy (see also categories 633.0–633.9) 639.8
      molar pregnancy (see also categories 630–632) 639.8
    arteriosclerotic 440.9
    combined left-right sided 428.0
    combined systolic and diastolic 428.40
      acute 428.41
      acute on chronic 428.43
      chronic 428.42
    compensated (see also Failure, heart) 428.0
    complicating
      abortion - see Abortion, by type, with specified complication NEC
      delivery (cesarean) (instrumental) 669.4●
      ectopic pregnancy (see also categories 633.0–633.9) 639.8
      molar pregnancy (see also categories 630–632) 639.8
      obstetric anesthesia or sedation 668.1●
      surgery 997.1
    congestive (compensated) (decompensated) (see also Failure, heart) 428.0
      with rheumatic fever (conditions classifiable to 390)
        active 391.8
        inactive or quiescent (with chorea) 398.91
      fetus or newborn 779.89
      hypertensive (see also Hypertension, heart) 402.91
        with renal disease (see also Hypertension, cardiorenal) 404.91
          with renal failure 404.93
        benign 402.11
        malignant 402.01
      rheumatic (chronic) (inactive) (with chorea) 398.91
        active or acute 391.8
          with chorea (Sydenham's) 392.0

Failure, failed (Continued)
  heart (Continued)
    decompensated (see also Failure, heart) 428.0
    degenerative (see also Degeneration, myocardial) 429.1
    diastolic 428.30
      acute 428.31
      acute on chronic 428.33
      chronic 428.32
    due to presence of (cardiac) prosthesis 429.4
    fetus or newborn 779.89
    following
      abortion 639.8
      cardiac surgery 429.4
      ectopic or molar pregnancy 639.8
    high output NEC 428.9
    hypertensive (see also Hypertension, heart) 402.91
      with renal disease (see also Hypertension, cardiorenal) 404.91
        with renal failure 404.93
      benign 402.11
      malignant 402.01
    left (ventricular) (see also Failure, ventricular, left) 428.1
      with right-sided failure (see also Failure, heart) 428.0
    low output (syndrome) NEC 428.9
    organic - see Disease, heart
    postoperative (immediate) 997.1
      long term effect of cardiac surgery 429.4
    rheumatic (chronic) (congestive) (inactive) 398.91
    right (secondary to left heart failure, conditions classifiable to 428.1) (ventricular) (see also Failure, heart) 428.0
    senile 797
    specified during or due to a procedure 997.1
      long-term effect of cardiac surgery 429.4
    systolic 428.20
      acute 428.21
      acute on chronic 428.23
      chronic 428.22
    thyrotoxic (see also Thyrotoxicosis) 242.9●
      [425.7]
    valvular - see Endocarditis
  hepatic 572.8
    acute 570
    due to a procedure 997.49
  hepatorenal 572.4
  hypertensive heart (see also Hypertension, heart) 402.91
    benign 402.11
    malignant 402.01
  induction (of labor) 659.1●
    abortion (legal) (see also Abortion, failed) 638.9
    affecting fetus or newborn 763.89
    by oxytocic drugs 659.1●
    instrumental 659.0●
    mechanical 659.0●
    medical 659.1●
    surgical 659.0●
  initial alveolar expansion, newborn 770.4
  involution, thymus (gland) 254.8
  kidney - see Failure, renal
  lactation 676.4●
  Leydig's cell, adult 257.2
  liver 572.8
    acute 570
  medullary 799.89
  mitral - see Endocarditis, mitral
  moderate sedation, during procedure 995.24

Failure, failed (Continued)
  myocardium, myocardial (see also Failure, heart) 428.9
    chronic (see also Failure, heart) 428.0
    congestive (see also Failure, heart) 428.0
  ovarian (primary) 256.39
    iatrogenic 256.2
    postablative 256.2
    postirradiation 256.2
    postsurgical 256.2
  ovulation 628.0
  prerenal 788.99
  renal (kidney) 586
    with
      abortion - see Abortion, by type, with renal failure
      ectopic pregnancy (see also categories 633.0–633.9) 639.3
      edema (see also Nephrosis) 581.9
      hypertension (see also Hypertension, kidney) 403.91
      hypertensive heart disease (conditions classifiable to 402) 404.92
        with heart failure 404.93
        benign 404.12
          with heart failure 404.13
        malignant 404.02
          with heart failure 404.03
      molar pregnancy (see also categories 630–632) 639.3
      tubular necrosis (acute) 584.5
    acute 584.9
      with lesion of
        necrosis
          cortical (renal) 584.6
          medullary (renal) (papillary) 584.7
          tubular 584.5
        specified pathology NEC 584.8
    chronic 585.9
      hypertensive or with hypertension (see also Hypertension, kidney) 403.91
    due to a procedure 997.5
    following
      abortion 639.3
      crushing 958.5
      ectopic or molar pregnancy 639.3
      labor and delivery (acute) 669.3●
    hypertensive (see also Hypertension, kidney) 403.91
    puerperal, postpartum 669.3●
  respiration, respiratory 518.81
    acute 518.81
      following trauma and surgery 518.51
    acute and chronic 518.84
      following trauma and surgery 518.53
    center 348.89
      newborn 770.84
    chronic 518.83
      following trauma and surgery or shock 518.51
    newborn 770.84
  rotation
    cecum 751.4
    colon 751.4
    intestine 751.4
    kidney 753.3
  sedation, during procedure
    conscious 995.24
    moderate 995.24
  segmentation - see also Fusion
    fingers (see also Syndactylism, fingers) 755.11
    toes (see also Syndactylism, toes) 755.13
  seminiferous tubule, adult 257.2
  senile (general) 797
    with psychosis 290.20
  testis, primary (seminal) 257.2
  to progress 661.2●

Failure, failed (Continued)
  to thrive
    adult 783.7
    child 783.41
    newborn 779.34
  transplant 996.80
    bone marrow 996.85
    organ (immune or nonimmune cause) 996.80
      bone marrow 996.85
      heart 996.83
      intestines 996.87
      kidney 996.81
      liver 996.82
      lung 996.84
      pancreas 996.86
      specified NEC 996.89
    skin 996.52
      artificial 996.55
      decellularized allodermis 996.55
      temporary allograft or pigskin graft - omit code
    stem cell(s) 996.88
      from
        peripheral blood 996.88
        umbilical cord 996.88
  trial of labor NEC 660.6●
    affecting fetus or newborn 763.1
  tubal ligation 998.89
  urinary 586
  vacuum extraction
    abortion - see Abortion, failed
    delivery NEC 660.7●
      affecting fetus or newborn 763.1
  vasectomy 998.89
  ventouse NEC 660.7●
    affecting fetus or newborn 763.1
  ventricular (see also Failure, heart) 428.9
    left 428.1
      with rheumatic fever (conditions classifiable to 390)
        active 391.8
          with chorea 392.0
        inactive or quiescent (with chorea) 398.91
      hypertensive (see also Hypertension, heart) 402.91
        benign 402.11
        malignant 402.01
      rheumatic (chronic) (inactive) (with chorea) 398.91
        active or acute 391.8
          with chorea 392.0
    right (see also Failure, heart) 428.0
  vital centers, fetus or newborn 779.89
  weight gain in childhood 783.41
Fainting (fit) (spell) 780.2
Falciform hymen 752.49
Fall, maternal, affecting fetus or newborn 760.5
Fallen arches 734
Falling, any organ or part - see Prolapse
Fallopian
  insufflation
    fertility testing V26.21
    following sterilization reversal V26.22
  tube - see condition
Fallot's
  pentalogy 745.2
  tetrad or tetralogy 745.2
  triad or trilogy 746.09
Fallout, radioactive (adverse effect) NEC 990
False - see also condition
  bundle branch block 426.50
  bursa 727.89
  croup 478.75
  joint 733.82
  labor (pains) 644.1●
  opening, urinary, male 752.69
  passage, urethra (prostatic) 599.4

False (Continued)
  positive
    serological test for syphilis 795.6
    Wassermann reaction 795.6
  pregnancy 300.11
Family, familial - see also condition
  affected by
    family member
      currently on deployment (military) V61.01
      returned from deployment (military) (current or past conflict) V61.02
  disruption (see also Disruption, family) V61.09
  estrangement V61.09
  hemophagocytic
    lymphohistiocytosis 288.4
    reticulosis 288.4
  Li-Fraumeni (syndrome) V84.01
  planning advice V25.09
    natural
      procreative V26.41
      to avoid pregnancy V25.04
  problem V61.9
    specified circumstance NEC V61.8
  retinoblastoma (syndrome) 190.5
Famine 994.2
  edema 262
Fanconi's anemia (congenital pancytopenia) 284.09
Fanconi (-de Toni) (-Debré) syndrome (cystinosis) 270.0
Farber (-Uzman) syndrome or disease (disseminated lipogranulomatosis) 272.8
Farcin 024
Farcy 024
Farmers'
  lung 495.0
  skin 692.74
Farsightedness 367.0
Fascia - see condition
Fasciculation 781.0
Fasciculitis optica 377.32
Fasciitis 729.4
  eosinophilic 728.89
  necrotizing 728.86
  nodular 728.79
  perirenal 593.4
  plantar 728.71
  pseudosarcomatous 728.79
  traumatic (old) NEC 728.79
    current - see Sprain, by site
Fasciola hepatica infestation 121.3
Fascioliasis 121.3
Fasciolopsiasis (small intestine) 121.4
Fasciolopsis (small intestine) 121.4
Fast pulse 785.0
Fat
  embolism (cerebral) (pulmonary) (systemic) 958.1
    with
      abortion - see Abortion, by type, with embolism
      ectopic pregnancy (see also categories 633.0–633.9) 639.6
      molar pregnancy (see also categories 630–632) 639.6
    complicating delivery or puerperium 673.8●
    following
      abortion 639.6
      ectopic or molar pregnancy 639.6
    in pregnancy, childbirth, or the puerperium 673.8●
  excessive 278.02
    in heart (see also Degeneration, myocardial) 429.1
  general 278.02
  hernia, herniation 729.30
    eyelid 374.34
    knee 729.31

◀ New   ⬤ Revised   deleted Deleted   ● Use Additional Digit(s)   Omit code

Fat *(Continued)*
  hernia, herniation *(Continued)*
    orbit 374.34
    retro-orbital 374.34
    retropatellar 729.31
    specified site NEC 729.39
  indigestion 579.8
  in stool 792.1
  localized (pad) 278.1
    heart *(see also* Degeneration, myocardial)
      429.1
    knee 729.31
    retropatellar 729.31
  necrosis - *see also* Fatty, degeneration
    breast (aseptic) (segmental) 611.3
    mesentery 567.82
    omentum 567.82
    peritoneum 567.82
  pad 278.1
Fatal familial insomnia (FFI) 046.72
Fatal syncope 798.1
Fatigue 780.79
  auditory deafness *(see also* Deafness) 389.9
  chronic, syndrome 780.71
  combat *(see also* Reaction, stress, acute) 308.9
  during pregnancy 646.8●
  general 780.79
    psychogenic 300.5
  heat (transient) 992.6
  muscle 729.89
  myocardium *(see also* Failure, heart) 428.9
  nervous 300.5
  neurosis 300.5
  operational 300.89
  postural 729.89
  posture 729.89
  psychogenic (general) 300.5
  senile 797
  syndrome NEC 300.5
    chronic 780.71
  undue 780.79
  voice 784.49
Fatness 278.02
Fatty - *see also* condition
  apron 278.1
  degeneration (diffuse) (general) NEC 272.8
    localized - *see* Degeneration, by site, fatty
    placenta - *see* Placenta, abnormal
  heart (enlarged) *(see also* Degeneration,
    myocardial) 429.1
  infiltration (diffuse) (general) *(see also*
    Degeneration, by site, fatty) 272.8
    heart (enlarged) *(see also* Degeneration,
      myocardial) 429.1
  liver 571.8
    alcoholic 571.0
  necrosis - *see* Degeneration, fatty
  phanerosis 272.8
Fauces - *see* condition
Fauchard's disease (periodontitis) 523.40
Faucitis 478.29
Faulty - *see also* condition
  position of teeth 524.30
Favism (anemia) 282.2
Favre-Racouchot disease (elastoidosis cutanea
  nodularis) 701.8
Favus 110.9
  beard 110.0
  capitis 110.0
  corporis 110.5
  eyelid 110.8
  foot 110.4
  hand 110.2
  scalp 110.0
  specified site NEC 110.8
Fear, fearfulness (complex) (reaction) 300.20
  child 313.0
  of
    animals 300.29
    closed spaces 300.29
    crowds 300.29

Fear, fearfulness *(Continued)*
  of *(Continued)*
    eating in public 300.23
    heights 300.29
    open spaces 300.22
      with panic attacks 300.21
    public speaking 300.23
    streets 300.22
      with panic attacks 300.21
    travel 300.22
      with panic attacks 300.21
    washing in public 300.23
  transient 308.0
Feared complaint unfounded V65.5
Febricula (continued) (simple) *(see also* Pyrexia)
  780.60
Febrile *(see also* Pyrexia) 780.60
  convulsion (simple) 780.31
    complex 780.32
  nonhemolytic transfusion reaction (FNHTR)
    780.66
  seizure (simple) 780.31
    atypical 780.32
    complex 780.32
    complicated 780.32
Febris *(see also* Fever) 780.60
  aestiva *(see also* Fever, hay) 477.9
  flava *(see also* Fever, yellow) 060.9
  melitensis 023.0
  pestis *(see also* Plague) 020.9
  puerperalis 672●
  recurrens *(see also* Fever, relapsing) 087.9
    pediculo vestimenti 087.0
  rubra 034.1
  typhoidea 002.0
  typhosa 002.0
Fecal - *see* condition
Fecalith (impaction) 560.32
  with hernia - *see also* Hernia, by site, with
    obstruction
    gangrenous - *see* Hernia, by site, with
      gangrene
  appendix 543.9
  congenital 777.1
Fede's disease 529.0
Feeble-minded 317
Feeble rapid pulse due to shock following
  injury 958.4
Feeding
  faulty (elderly) (infant) 783.3
    newborn 779.31
  formula check V20.2
  improper (elderly) (infant) 783.3
    newborn 779.31
  problem (elderly) (infant) 783.3
    newborn 779.31
    nonorganic origin 307.59
Feeling of foreign body in throat 784.99
Feer's disease 985.0
Feet - *see* condition
Feigned illness V65.2
Feil-Klippel syndrome (brevicollis) 756.16
Feinmesser's (hidrotic) ectodermal dysplasia
  757.31
Felix's disease (juvenile osteochondrosis, hip)
  732.1
Felon (any digit) (with lymphangitis) 681.01
  herpetic 054.6
Felty's syndrome (rheumatoid arthritis with
  splenomegaly and leukopenia) 714.1
Feminism in boys 302.6
Feminization, testicular 259.51
  with pseudohermaphroditism, male 259.51
Femoral hernia - *see* Hernia, femoral
Femora vara 736.32
Femur, femoral - *see* condition
Fenestrata placenta - *see* Placenta, abnormal
Fenestration, fenestrated - *see also* Imperfect,
  closure
  aorta-pulmonary 745.0
  aorticopulmonary 745.0

Fenestration, fenestrated *(Continued)*
  aortopulmonary 745.0
  cusps, heart valve NEC 746.89
    pulmonary 746.09
  hymen 752.49
  pulmonic cusps 746.09
Fenwick's disease 537.89
Fermentation (gastric) (gastrointestinal)
  (stomach) 536.8
  intestine 564.89
    psychogenic 306.4
  psychogenic 306.4
Fernell's disease (aortic aneurysm) 441.9
Fertile eunuch syndrome 257.2
Fertility, meaning multiparity - *see* Multiparity
Fetal
  alcohol syndrome 760.71
  anemia 678.0●
  thrombocytopenia 678.0●
  twin to twin transfusion 678.0●
Fetalis uterus 752.39
Fetid
  breath 784.99
  sweat 705.89
Fetishism 302.81
  transvestic 302.3
Fetomaternal hemorrhage
  affecting management of pregnancy 656.0●
  fetus or newborn 772.0
Fetus, fetal - *see also* condition
  papyraceous 779.89
  type lung tissue 770.4
Fever 780.60
  with chills 780.60
    in malarial regions *(see also* Malaria) 084.6
  abortus NEC 023.9
  aden 061
  African tick-borne 087.1
  American
    mountain tick 066.1
    spotted 082.0
  and ague *(see also* Malaria) 084.6
  aphthous 078.4
  arbovirus hemorrhagic 065.9
  Assam 085.0
  Australian A or Q 083.0
  Bangkok hemorrhagic 065.4
  biliary, Charcôt's intermittent - *see*
    Choledocholithiasis
  bilious, hemoglobinuric 084.8
  blackwater 084.8
  blister 054.9
  Bonvale Dam 780.79
  boutonneuse 082.1
  brain 323.9
    late effect - *see* category 326
  breakbone 061
  Bullis 082.8
  Bunyamwera 066.3
  Burdwan 085.0
  Bwamba (encephalitis) 066.3
  Cameroon *(see also* Malaria) 084.6
  Canton 081.9
  catarrhal (acute) 460
    chronic 472.0
  cat-scratch 078.3
  cerebral 323.9
    late effect - *see* category 326
  cerebrospinal (meningococcal) *(see also*
    Meningitis, cerebrospinal) 036.0
  Chagres 084.0
  Chandipura 066.8
  changuinola 066.0
  Charcôt's (biliary) (hepatic) (intermittent) *see*
    Choledocholithiasis
  Chikungunya (viral) 066.3
    hemorrhagic 065.4
  childbed 670.8●
  Chitral 066.0
  Colombo *(see also* Fever, paratyphoid) 002.9
  Colorado tick (virus) 066.1

Fever *(Continued)*
  congestive
    malarial *(see also* Malaria) 084.6
    remittent *(see also* Malaria) 084.6
  Congo virus 065.0
  continued 780.60
    malarial 084.0
  Corsican *(see also* Malaria) 084.6
  Crimean hemorrhagic 065.0
  Cyprus *(see also* Brucellosis) 023.9
  dandy 061
  deer fly *(see also* Tularemia) 021.9
  dehydration, newborn 778.4
  dengue (virus) 061
    hemorrhagic 065.4
  desert 114.0
  due to heat 992.0
  Dumdum 085.0
  enteric 002.0
  ephemeral (of unknown origin) *(see also* Pyrexia) 780.60
  epidemic, hemorrhagic of the Far East 065.0
  erysipelatous *(see also* Erysipelas) 035
  estivo-autumnal (malarial) 084.0
  etiocholanolone 277.31
  famine - *see also* Fever, relapsing
    meaning typhus - *see* Typhus
  Far Eastern hemorrhagic 065.0
  five day 083.1
  Fort Bragg 100.89
  gastroenteric 002.0
  gastromalarial *(see also* Malaria) 084.6
  Gibraltar *(see also* Brucellosis) 023.9
  glandular 075
  Guama (viral) 066.3
  Haverhill 026.1
  hay (allergic) (with rhinitis) 477.9
    with
      asthma (bronchial) *(see also* Asthma) 493.0●
    due to
      dander, animal (cat) (dog) 477.2
      dust 477.8
      fowl 477.8
      hair, animal (cat) (dog) 477.2
      pollen, any plant or tree 477.0
      specified allergen other than pollen 477.8
  heat (effects) 992.0
  hematuric, bilious 084.8
  hemoglobinuric (malarial) 084.8
    bilious 084.8
  hemorrhagic (arthropod-borne) NEC 065.9
    with renal syndrome 078.6
    arenaviral 078.7
    Argentine 078.7
    Bangkok 065.4
    Bolivian 078.7
    Central Asian 065.0
    chikungunya 065.4
    Crimean 065.0
    dengue (virus) 065.4
    Ebola 065.8
    epidemic 078.6
      of Far East 065.0
    Far Eastern 065.0
    Junin virus 078.7
    Korean 078.6
    Kyasanur forest 065.2
    Machupo virus 078.7
    mite-borne NEC 065.8
    mosquito-borne 065.4
    Omsk 065.1
    Philippine 065.4
    Russian (Yaroslav) 078.6
    Singapore 065.4
    Southeast Asia 065.4
    Thailand 065.4
    tick-borne NEC 065.3

Fever *(Continued)*
  hepatic *(see also* Cholecystitis) 575.8
    intermittent (Charcôt's) - *see* Choledocholithiasis
  herpetic *(see also* Herpes) 054.9
  hyalomma tick 065.0
  icterohemorrhagic 100.0
  inanition 780.60
    newborn 778.4
  in conditions classified elsewhere 780.61
  infective NEC 136.9
  intermittent (bilious) *(see also* Malaria) 084.6
    hepatic (Charcôt) - *see* Choledocholithiasis
    of unknown origin *(see also* Pyrexia) 780.60
    pernicious 084.0
  iodide
    correct substance properly administered 780.60
    overdose or wrong substance given or taken 975.5
  Japanese river 081.2
  jungle yellow 060.0
  Junin virus, hemorrhagic 078.7
  Katayama 120.2
  Kedani 081.2
  Kenya 082.1
  Korean hemorrhagic 078.6
  Lassa 078.89
  Lone Star 082.8
  lung - *see* Pneumonia
  Machupo virus, hemorrhagic 078.7
  malaria, malarial *(see also* Malaria) 084.6
  Malta *(see also* Brucellosis) 023.9
  Marseilles 082.1
  marsh *(see also* Malaria) 084.6
  Mayaro (viral) 066.3
  Mediterranean *(see also* Brucellosis) 023.9
    familial 277.31
    tick 082.1
  meningeal - *see* Meningitis
  metal fumes NEC 985.8
  Meuse 083.1
  Mexican - *see* Typhus, Mexican
  Mianeh 087.1
  miasmatic *(see also* Malaria) 084.6
  miliary 078.2
  milk, female 672●
  mill 504
  mite-borne hemorrhagic 065.8
  Monday 504
  mosquito-borne NEC 066.3
    hemorrhagic NEC 065.4
  mountain 066.1
    meaning
      Rocky Mountain spotted 082.0
      undulant fever *(see also* Brucellosis) 023.9
    tick (American) 066.1
  Mucambo (viral) 066.3
  mud 100.89
  Neapolitan *(see also* Brucellosis) 023.9
  neutropenic 288.00
  newborn (environmentally-induced) 778.4
  nine-mile 083.0
  nonexanthematous tick 066.1
  North Asian tick-borne typhus 082.2
  Omsk hemorrhagic 065.1
  O'nyong nyong (viral) 066.3
  Oropouche (viral) 066.3
  Oroya 088.0
  paludal *(see also* Malaria) 084.6
  Panama 084.0
  pappataci 066.0
  paratyphoid 002.9
    A 002.1
    B (Schottmüller's) 002.2
    C (Hirschfeld) 002.3
  parrot 073.9
  periodic 277.31
  pernicious, acute 084.0

Fever *(Continued)*
  persistent (of unknown origin) *(see also* Pyrexia) 780.60
  petechial 036.0
  pharyngoconjunctival 077.2
    adenoviral type 3 077.2
  Philippine hemorrhagic 065.4
  phlebotomus 066.0
  Piry 066.8
  Pixuna (viral) 066.3
  Plasmodium ovale 084.3
  pleural *(see also* Pleurisy) 511.0
  pneumonic - *see* Pneumonia
  polymer fume 987.8
  postimmunization 780.63
  postoperative 780.62
    due to infection 998.59
  posttransfusion 780.66
  postvaccination 780.63
  pretibial 100.89
  puerperal, postpartum 672●
  putrid - *see* Septicemia
  pyemic - *see* Septicemia
  Q 083.0
    with pneumonia 083.0 [484.8]
  quadrilateral 083.0
  quartan (malaria) 084.2
  Queensland (coastal) 083.0
    seven-day 100.89
  Quintan (A) 083.1
  quotidian 084.0
  rabbit *(see also* Tularemia) 021.9
  rat-bite 026.9
    due to
      Spirillum minor or minus 026.0
      Spirochaeta morsus muris 026.0
      Streptobacillus moniliformis 026.1
  recurrent - *see* Fever, relapsing
  relapsing 087.9
    Carter's (Asiatic) 087.0
    Dutton's (West African) 087.1
    Koch's 087.9
    louse-borne (epidemic) 087.0
    Novy's (American) 087.1
    Obermeyer's (European) 087.0
    spirillum NEC 087.9
    tick-borne (endemic) 087.1
  remittent (bilious) (congestive) (gastric) *(see also* Malaria) 084.6
  rheumatic (active) (acute) (chronic) (subacute) 390
    with heart involvement 391.9
      carditis 391.9
      endocarditis (aortic) (mitral) (pulmonary) (tricuspid) 391.1
      multiple sites 391.8
      myocarditis 391.2
      pancarditis, acute 391.8
      pericarditis 391.0
      specified type NEC 391.8
      valvulitis 391.1
    inactive or quiescent with
      cardiac hypertrophy 398.99
      carditis 398.90
      endocarditis 397.9
        aortic (valve) 395.9
          with mitral (valve) disease 396.9
        mitral (valve) 394.9
          with aortic (valve) disease 396.9
        pulmonary (valve) 397.1
        tricuspid (valve) 397.0
      heart conditions (classifiable to 429.3, 429.6, 429.9) 398.99
      failure (congestive) (conditions classifiable to 428.0, 428.9) 398.91
      left ventricular failure (conditions classifiable to 428.1) 398.91
      myocardial degeneration (conditions classifiable to 429.1) 398.0

◄ New   ◄■ Revised   ~~deleted~~ Deleted   ● Use Additional Digit(s)   Omit code

Fever *(Continued)*
  rheumatic *(Continued)*
    inactive or quiescent with *(Continued)*
      myocarditis (conditions classifiable to 429.0) 398.0
      pancarditis 398.99
      pericarditis 393
  Rift Valley (viral) 066.3
  Rocky Mountain spotted 082.0
  rose 477.0
  Ross river (viral) 066.3
  Russian hemorrhagic 078.6
  sandfly 066.0
  San Joaquin (valley) 114.0
  Sao Paulo 082.0
  scarlet 034.1
  septic - *see* Septicemia
  seven-day 061
    Japan 100.89
    Queensland 100.89
  shin bone 083.1
  Singapore hemorrhagic 065.4
  solar 061
  sore 054.9
  South African tick-bite 087.1
  Southeast Asia hemorrhagic 065.4
  spinal - *see* Meningitis
  spirillary 026.0
  splenic (*see also* Anthrax) 022.9
  spotted (Rocky Mountain) 082.0
    American 082.0
    Brazilian 082.0
    Colombian 082.0
    meaning
      cerebrospinal meningitis 036.0
      typhus 082.9
  spring 309.23
  steroid
    correct substance properly administered 780.60
    overdose or wrong substance given or taken 962.0
  streptobacillary 026.1
  subtertian 084.0
  Sumatran mite 081.2
  sun 061
  swamp 100.89
  sweating 078.2
  swine 003.8
  sylvatic yellow 060.0
  Tahyna 062.5
  tertian - *see* Malaria, tertian
  Thailand hemorrhagic 065.4
  thermic 992.0
  three day 066.0
    with Coxsackie exanthem 074.8
  tick
    American mountain 066.1
    Colorado 066.1
    Kemerovo 066.1
    Mediterranean 082.1
    mountain 066.1
    nonexanthematous 066.1
    Quaranfil 066.1
  tick-bite NEC 066.1
  tick-borne NEC 066.1
    hemorrhagic NEC 065.3
  transitory of newborn 778.4
  trench 083.1
  tsutsugamushi 081.2
  typhogastric 002.0
  typhoid (abortive) (ambulant) (any site) (hemorrhagic) (infection) (intermittent) (malignant) (rheumatic) 002.0
  typhomalarial (*see also* Malaria) 084.6
  typhus - *see* Typhus
  undulant (*see also* Brucellosis) 023.9
  unknown origin (*see also* Pyrexia) 780.60
  uremic - *see* Uremia
  uveoparotid 135
  valley (Coccidioidomycosis) 114.0

Fever *(Continued)*
  Venezuelan equine 066.2
  Volhynian 083.1
  Wesselsbron (viral) 066.3
  West
    African 084.8
    Nile (viral) 066.40
      with
        cranial nerve disorders 066.42
        encephalitis 066.41
        optic neuritis 066.42
        other complications 066.49
        other neurologic manifestations 066.42
        polyradiculitis 066.42
  Whitmore's 025
  Wolhynian 083.1
  worm 128.9
  Yaroslav hemorrhagic 078.6
  yellow 060.9
    jungle 060.0
    sylvatic 060.0
    urban 060.1
    vaccination, prophylactic (against) V04.4
  Zika (viral) 066.3
Fibrillation
  atrial (established) (paroxysmal) 427.31
  auricular (atrial) (established) 427.31
  cardiac (ventricular) 427.41
  coronary (*see also* Infarct, myocardium) 410.9●
  heart (ventricular) 427.41
  muscular 728.9
  postoperative 997.1
  ventricular 427.41
Fibrin
  ball or bodies, pleural (sac) 511.0
  chamber, anterior (eye) (gelatinous exudate) 364.04
Fibrinogenolysis (hemorrhagic) - *see* Fibrinolysis
Fibrinogenopenia (congenital) (hereditary) (*see also* Defect, coagulation) 286.3
  acquired 286.6
Fibrinolysis (acquired) (hemorrhagic) (pathologic) 286.6
  with
    abortion - *see* Abortion, by type, with hemorrhage, delayed or excessive
    ectopic pregnancy (*see also* categories 633.0–633.9) 639.1
    molar pregnancy (*see also* categories 630–632) 639.1
  antepartum or intrapartum 641.3●
    affecting fetus or newborn 762.1
  following
    abortion 639.1
    ectopic or molar pregnancy 639.1
  newborn, transient 776.2
  postpartum 666.3●
Fibrinopenia (hereditary) (*see also* Defect, coagulation) 286.3
  acquired 286.6
Fibrinopurulent - *see* condition
Fibrinous - *see* condition
Fibroadenoma (M9010/0)
  cellular intracanalicular (M9020/0) 217
  giant (intracanalicular) (M9020/0) 217
  intracanalicular (M9011/0)
    cellular (M9020/0) 217
    giant (M9020/0) 217
    specified site - *see* Neoplasm, by site, benign
    unspecified site 217
  juvenile (M9030/0) 217
  pericanicular (M9012/0)
    specified site - *see* Neoplasm, by site, benign
    unspecified site 217
  phyllodes (M9020/0) 217

Fibroadenoma *(Continued)*
  prostate 600.20
    with
      other lower urinary tract symptoms (LUTS) 600.21
      urinary
        obstruction 600.21
        retention 600.21
  specified site - *see* Neoplasm, by site, benign
  unspecified site 217
Fibroadenosis, breast (chronic) (cystic) (diffuse) (periodic) (segmental) 610.2
Fibroangioma (M9160/0) - *see also* Neoplasm, by site, benign
  juvenile (M9160/0)
    specified site - *see* Neoplasm, by site, benign
    unspecified site 210.7
Fibrocellulitis progressiva ossificans 728.11
Fibrochondrosarcoma (M9220/3) - *see* Neoplasm, cartilage, malignant
Fibrocystic
  disease 277.00
    bone NEC 733.29
    breast 610.1
    jaw 526.2
    kidney (congenital) 753.19
    liver 751.62
    lung 518.89
      congenital 748.4
    pancreas 277.00
  kidney (congenital) 753.19
Fibrodysplasia ossificans multiplex (progressiva) 728.11
Fibroelastosis (cordis) (endocardial) (endomyocardial) 425.3
Fibroid (tumor) (M8890/0) - *see also* Neoplasm, connective tissue, benign
  disease, lung (chronic) (*see also* Fibrosis, lung) 515
  heart (disease) (*see also* Myocarditis) 429.0
  induration, lung (chronic) (*see also* Fibrosis, lung) 515
  in pregnancy or childbirth 654.1●
    affecting fetus or newborn 763.89
    causing obstructed labor 660.2●
      affecting fetus or newborn 763.1
  liver - *see* Cirrhosis, liver
  lung (*see also* Fibrosis, lung) 515
  pneumonia (chronic) (*see also* Fibrosis, lung) 515
  uterus (M8890/0) (*see also* Leiomyoma, uterus) 218.9
Fibrolipoma (M8851/0) (*see also* Lipoma, by site) 214.9
Fibroliposarcoma (M8850/3) - *see* Neoplasm, connective tissue, malignant
Fibroma (M8810/0) - *see also* Neoplasm, connective tissue, benign
  ameloblastic (M9330/0) 213.1
    upper jaw (bone) 213.0
  bone (nonossifying) 733.99
    ossifying (M9262/0) - *see* Neoplasm, bone, benign
  cementifying (M9274/0) - *see* Neoplasm, bone, benign
  chondromyxoid (M9241/0) - *see* Neoplasm, bone, benign
  desmoplastic (M8823/1) - *see* Neoplasm, connective tissue, uncertain behavior
  facial (M8813/0) - *see* Neoplasm, connective tissue, benign
  invasive (M8821/1) - *see* Neoplasm, connective tissue, uncertain behavior
  molle (M8851/0) (*see also* Lipoma, by site) 214.9
  myxoid (M8811/0) - *see* Neoplasm, connective tissue, benign
  nasopharynx, nasopharyngeal (juvenile) (M9160/0) 210.7

Fibroma (Continued)
nonosteogenic (nonossifying) - see Dysplasia, fibrous
odontogenic (M9321/0) 213.1
upper jaw (bone) 213.0
ossifying (M9262/0) - see Neoplasm, bone, benign
periosteal (M8812/0) - see Neoplasm, bone, benign
prostate 600.20
with
other lower urinary tract symptoms (LUTS) 600.21
urinary
obstruction 600.21
retention 600.21
soft (M8851/0) (see also Lipoma, by site) 214.9
Fibromatosis 728.79
abdominal (M8822/1) - see Neoplasm, connective tissue, uncertain behavior
aggressive (M8821/1) - see Neoplasm, connective tissue, uncertain behavior
congenital generalized (CGF) 759.89
Dupuytren's 728.6
gingival 523.8
plantar fascia 728.71
proliferative 728.79
pseudosarcomatous (proliferative) (subcutaneous) 728.79
subcutaneous pseudosarcomatous (proliferative) 728.79
Fibromyalgia 729.1
Fibromyoma (M8890/0) - see also Neoplasm, connective tissue, benign
uterus (corpus) (see also Leiomyoma, uterus) 218.9
in pregnancy or childbirth 654.1●
affecting fetus or newborn 763.89
causing obstructed labor 660.2●
affecting fetus or newborn 763.1
Fibromyositis (see also Myositis) 729.1
scapulohumeral 726.2
Fibromyxolipoma (M8852/0) (see also Lipoma, by site) 214.9
Fibromyxoma (M8811/0) - see Neoplasm, connective tissue, benign
Fibromyxosarcoma (M8811/3) - see Neoplasm, connective tissue, malignant
Fibro-odontoma, ameloblastic (M9290/0) 213.1
upper jaw (bone) 213.0
Fibro-osteoma (M9262/0) - see Neoplasm, bone, benign
Fibroplasia, retrolental (see also Retinopathy of prematurity) 362.21
Fibropurulent - see condition
Fibrosarcoma (M8810/3) - see also Neoplasm, connective tissue, malignant
ameloblastic (M9330/3) 170.1
upper jaw (bone) 170.0
congenital (M8814/3) - see Neoplasm, connective tissue, malignant
fascial (M8813/3) - see Neoplasm, connective tissue, malignant
infantile (M8814/3) - see Neoplasm, connective tissue, malignant
odontogenic (M9330/3) 170.1
upper jaw (bone) 170.0
periosteal (M8812/3) - see Neoplasm, bone, malignant
Fibrosclerosis
breast 610.3
corpora cavernosa (penis) 607.89
familial multifocal NEC 710.8
multifocal (idiopathic) NEC 710.8
penis (corpora cavernosa) 607.89
Fibrosis, fibrotic
adrenal (gland) 255.8
alveolar (diffuse) 516.31
amnion 658.8●
anal papillae 569.49

Fibrosis, fibrotic (Continued)
anus 569.49
appendix, appendiceal, noninflammatory 543.9
arteriocapillary - see Arteriosclerosis
bauxite (of lung) 503
biliary 576.8
due to Clonorchis sinensis 121.1
bladder 596.89
interstitial 595.1
localized submucosal 595.1
panmural 595.1
bone, diffuse 756.59
breast 610.3
capillary - see also Arteriosclerosis
lung (chronic) (see also Fibrosis, lung) 515
cardiac (see also Myocarditis) 429.0
cervix 622.8
chorion 658.8●
corpus cavernosum 607.89
cystic (of pancreas) 277.00
with
manifestations
gastrointestinal 277.03
pulmonary 277.02
specified NEC 277.09
meconium ileus 277.01
pulmonary exacerbation 277.02
due to (presence of) any device, implant, or graft - see Complications, due to (presence of) any device, implant, or graft classified to 996.0–996.5 NEC
ejaculatory duct 608.89
endocardium (see also Endocarditis) 424.90
endomyocardial (African) 425.0
epididymis 608.89
eye muscle 378.62
graphite (of lung) 503
heart (see also Myocarditis) 429.0
hepatic - see also Cirrhosis, liver
due to Clonorchis sinensis 121.1
hepatolienal - see Cirrhosis, liver
hepatosplenic - see Cirrhosis, liver
infrapatellar fat pad 729.31
interstitial pulmonary, newborn 770.7
intrascrotal 608.89
kidney (see also Sclerosis, renal) 587
liver - see Cirrhosis, liver
lung (atrophic) (capillary) (chronic) (confluent) (massive) (perialveolar) (peribronchial) 515
with
anthracosilicosis (occupational) 500
anthracosis (occupational) 500
asbestosis (occupational) 501
bagassosis (occupational) 495.1
bauxite 503
berylliosis (occupational) 503
byssinosis (occupational) 504
calcicosis (occupational) 502
chalicosis (occupational) 502
dust reticulation (occupational) 504
farmers' lung 495.0
gannister disease (occupational) 502
graphite 503
pneumonoconiosis (occupational) 505
pneumosiderosis (occupational) 503
siderosis (occupational) 503
silicosis (occupational) 502
tuberculosis (see also Tuberculosis) 011.4●
diffuse (idiopathic) (interstitial) 516.31
due to
bauxite 503
fumes or vapors (chemical) (inhalation) 506.4
graphite 503
following radiation 508.1
postinflammatory 515
silicotic (massive) (occupational) 502
tuberculous (see also Tuberculosis) 011.4●

Fibrosis, fibrotic (Continued)
lymphatic gland 289.3
median bar 600.90
with
other lower urinary tract symptoms (LUTS) 600.91
urinary
obstruction 600.91
retention 600.91
mediastinum (idiopathic) 519.3
meninges 349.2
muscle NEC 728.2
iatrogenic (from injection) 999.9
myocardium, myocardial (see also Myocarditis) 429.0
oral submucous 528.8
ovary 620.8
oviduct 620.8
pancreas 577.8
cystic 277.00
with
manifestations
gastrointestinal 277.03
pulmonary 277.02
specified NEC 277.09
meconium ileus 277.01
pulmonary exacerbation 277.02
penis 607.89
periappendiceal 543.9
periarticular (see also Ankylosis) 718.5●
pericardium 423.1
perineum, in pregnancy or childbirth 654.8●
affecting fetus or newborn 763.89
causing obstructed labor 660.2●
affecting fetus or newborn 763.1
perineural NEC 355.9
foot 355.6
periureteral 593.89
placenta - see Placenta, abnormal
pleura 511.0
popliteal fat pad 729.31
preretinal 362.56
prostate (chronic) 600.90
with
other lower urinary tract symptoms (LUTS) 600.91
urinary
obstruction 600.91
retention 600.91
pulmonary (chronic) (see also Fibrosis, lung) 515
alveolar capillary block 516.8
idiopathic 516.31
interstitial
diffuse (idiopathic) 516.31
newborn 770.7
radiation - see Effect, adverse, radiation
rectal sphincter 569.49
retroperitoneal, idiopathic 593.4
sclerosing mesenteric (idiopathic) 567.82
scrotum 608.89
seminal vesicle 608.89
senile 797
skin NEC 709.2
spermatic cord 608.89
spleen 289.59
bilharzial (see also Schistosomiasis) 120.9
subepidermal nodular (M8832/0) - see Neoplasm, skin, benign
submucous NEC 709.2
oral 528.8
tongue 528.8
syncytium - see Placenta, abnormal
testis 608.89
chronic, due to syphilis 095.8
thymus (gland) 254.8
tunica vaginalis 608.89
ureter 593.89
urethra 599.84

◀ New   ◀▥ Revised   ~~deleted~~ Deleted   ● Use Additional Digit(s)   ▨ Omit code

Fibrosis, fibrotic *(Continued)*
uterus (nonneoplastic) 621.8
bilharzial *(see also* Schistosomiasis) 120.9
neoplastic *(see also* Leiomyoma, uterus) 218.9
vagina 623.8
valve, heart *(see also* Endocarditis) 424.90
vas deferens 608.89
vein 459.89
lower extremities 459.89
vesical 595.1
Fibrositis (periarticular) (rheumatoid) 729.0
humeroscapular region 726.2
nodular, chronic
Jaccoud's 714.4
rheumatoid 714.4
ossificans 728.11
scapulohumeral 726.2
Fibrothorax 511.0
Fibrotic - *see* Fibrosis
Fibrous - *see* condition
Fibroxanthoma (M8831/0) - *see also* Neoplasm, connective tissue, benign
atypical (M8831/1) - *see* Neoplasm, connective tissue, uncertain behavior
malignant (M8831/3) - *see* Neoplasm, connective tissue, malignant
Fibroxanthosarcoma (M8831/3) - *see* Neoplasm, connective tissue, malignant
Fiedler's
disease (leptospiral jaundice) 100.0
myocarditis or syndrome (acute isolated myocarditis) 422.91
Fiessinger-Leroy (-Reiter) syndrome 099.3
Fiessinger-Rendu syndrome (erythema muliforme exudativum) 695.19
Fifth disease (eruptive) 057.0
venereal 099.1
Filaria, filarial - *see* Infestation, filarial
Filariasis *(see also* Infestation, filarial) 125.9
bancroftian 125.0
Brug's 125.1
due to
bancrofti 125.0
Brugia (Wuchereria) (malayi) 125.1
Loa loa 125.2
malayi 125.1
organism NEC 125.6
Wuchereria (bancrofti) 125.0
malayi 125.1
Malayan 125.1
ozzardi 125.5
specified type NEC 125.6
Filatoff's, Filatov's, Filatow's disease (infectious mononucleosis) 075
File-cutters' disease 984.9
specified type of lead - *see* Table of Drugs and Chemicals
Filling defect
biliary tract 793.3
bladder 793.5
duodenum 793.4
gallbladder 793.3
gastrointestinal tract 793.4
intestine 793.4
kidney 793.5
stomach 793.4
ureter 793.5
Filtering bleb, eye (postglaucoma) (status) V45.69
with complication or rupture 997.99
postcataract extraction (complication) 997.99
Fimbrial cyst (congenital) 752.11
Fimbriated hymen 752.49
Financial problem affecting care V60.2
Findings, (abnormal), without diagnosis (examination) (laboratory test) 796.4
17-ketosteroids, elevated 791.9
acetonuria 791.6
acid phosphatase 790.5
albumin-globulin ratio 790.99

Findings *(Continued)*
albuminuria 791.0
alcohol in blood 790.3
alkaline phosphatase 790.5
amniotic fluid 792.3
amylase 790.5
antenatal screening 796.5
antiphosphatidylglycerol antibody 795.79
antiphosphatidylinositol antibody 795.79
antiphosphatidylserine antibody 795.79
anisocytosis 790.09
anthrax, positive 795.31
antibody titers, elevated 795.79
anticardiolipin antibody 795.79
antigen-antibody reaction 795.79
antiphospholipid antibody 795.79
bacteriuria 791.9
ballistocardiogram 794.39
bicarbonate 276.9
bile in urine 791.4
bilirubin 277.4
bleeding time (prolonged) 790.92
blood culture, positive 790.7
blood gas level (arterial) 790.91
blood sugar level 790.29
high 790.29
fasting glucose 790.21
glucose tolerance test 790.22
low 251.2
C-reactive protein (CRP) 790.95
calcium 275.40
cancer antigen 125 [CA 125] 795.82
carbonate 276.9
carcinoembryonic antigen [CEA] 795.81
casts, urine 791.7
catecholamines 791.9
cells, urine 791.7
cerebrospinal fluid (color) (content) (pressure) 792.0
cervical
high risk human papillomavirus (HPV) DNA test positive 795.05
low risk human papillomavirus (HPV) DNA test positive 795.09
non-atypical endometrial cells 795.09
chloride 276.9
cholesterol 272.9
high 272.0
with high triglycerides 272.2
chromosome analysis 795.2
chyluria 791.1
circulation time 794.39
cloudy dialysis effluent 792.5
cloudy urine 791.9
coagulation study 790.92
cobalt, blood 790.6
color of urine (unusual) NEC 791.9
copper, blood 790.6
creatinine clearance 794.4
crystals, urine 791.9
culture, positive NEC 795.39
blood 790.7
HIV V08
human immunodeficiency virus V08
nose 795.39
Staphylococcus - *see* Carrier (suspected) of, Staphylococcus
skin lesion NEC 795.39
spinal fluid 792.0
sputum 795.39
stool 792.1
throat 795.39
urine 791.9
viral
human immunodeficiency V08
wound 795.39
cytology specified site NEC 796.9
echocardiogram 793.2
echoencephalogram 794.01
echogram NEC - *see* Findings, abnormal, structure

Findings *(Continued)*
electrocardiogram (ECG) (EKG) 794.31
electroencephalogram (EEG) 794.02
electrolyte level, urinary 791.9
electromyogram (EMG) 794.17
ocular 794.14
electro-oculogram (EOG) 794.12
electroretinogram (ERG) 794.11
enzymes, serum NEC 790.5
fibrinogen titer coagulation study 790.92
filling defect - *see* Filling defect
function study NEC 794.9
auditory 794.15
bladder 794.9
brain 794.00
cardiac 794.30
endocrine NEC 794.6
thyroid 794.5
kidney 794.4
liver 794.8
nervous system
central 794.00
peripheral 794.19
oculomotor 794.14
pancreas 794.9
placenta 794.9
pulmonary 794.2
retina 794.11
special senses 794.19
spleen 794.9
vestibular 794.16
gallbladder, nonvisualization 793.3
glucose 790.29
elevated
fasting 790.21
tolerance test 790.22
glycosuria 791.5
heart
shadow 793.2
sounds 785.3
hematinuria 791.2
hematocrit
drop (precipitous) 790.01
elevated 282.7
low 285.9
hematologic NEC 790.99
hematuria 599.70
hemoglobin
drop 790.01
elevated 282.7
low 285.9
hemoglobinuria 791.2
histological NEC 795.4
hormones 259.9
immunoglobulins, elevated 795.79
indolacetic acid, elevated 791.9
iron 790.6
karyotype 795.2
ketonuria 791.6
lactic acid dehydrogenase (LDH) 790.4
lead 790.6
lipase 790.5
lipids NEC 272.9
lithium, blood 790.6
liver function test 790.6
lung field (shadow) 793.19
coin lesion 793.11
magnesium, blood 790.6
mammogram 793.80
calcification 793.89
calculus 793.89
dense breasts 793.82
inconclusive 793.82
due to dense breasts 793.82
microcalcification 793.81
mediastinal shift 793.2
melanin, urine 791.9
microbiologic NEC 795.39
mineral, blood NEC 790.6
myoglobinuria 791.3
nasal swab, anthrax 795.31

Findings *(Continued)*
  neonatal screening 796.6
  nitrogen derivatives, blood 790.6
  nonvisualization of gallbladder 793.3
  nose culture, positive 795.39
  odor of urine (unusual) NEC 791.9
  oxygen saturation 790.91
  Papanicolaou (smear) 796.9
    anus 796.70
      with
        atypical squamous cells
          cannot exclude high grade
              squamous intraepithelial
              lesion (ASC-H) 796.72
          of undetermined significance
              (ASC-US) 796.71
        cytologic evidence of malignancy
            796.76
        high grade squamous
            intraepithelial lesion (HGSIL)
            796.74
        low grade squamous intraepithelial
            lesion (LGSIL) 796.73
      glandular 796.70
      specified finding NEC 796.79
    cervix 795.00
      with
        atypical squamous cells
          cannot exclude high grade
              squamous intraepithelial
              lesion (ASC-H) 795.02
          of undetermined significance
              (ASC-US) 795.01
        cytologic evidence of malignancy
            795.06
        high grade squamous
            intraepithelial lesion (HGSIL)
            795.04
        low grade squamous intraepithelial
            lesion (LGSIL) 795.03
        non-atypical endometrial cells
            795.09
      dyskaryotic 795.09
      non-atypical endometrial cells 795.09
      nonspecific finding NEC 795.09
    other site 796.9
    vagina 795.10
      with
        atypical squamous cells
          cannot exclude high grade
              squamous intraepithelial
              lesion (ASC-H) 795.12
          of undetermined significance
              (ASC-US) 795.11
        cytologic evidence of
            malignancy 795.16
        high grade squamous
            intraepithelial lesion
            (HGSIL) 795.14
        low grade squamous
            intraepithelial lesion
            (LGSIL) 795.13
      glandular 795.10
      specified NEC 795.19
  peritoneal fluid 792.9
  phonocardiogram 794.39
  phosphorus 275.3
  pleural fluid 792.9
  pneumoencephalogram 793.0
  PO₂-oxygen ratio 790.91
  poikilocytosis 790.09
  potassium
    deficiency 276.8
    excess 276.7
  PPD 795.51
  prostate specific antigen (PSA) 790.93
  protein, serum NEC 790.99
  proteinuria 791.0
  prothrombin time (prolonged) (partial) (PT)
      (PTT) 790.92
  pyuria 791.9

Findings *(Continued)*
  radiologic (x-ray) 793.99
    abdomen 793.6
    biliary tract 793.3
    breast 793.89
      abnormal mammogram NOS 793.80
      mammographic
        calcification 793.89
        calculus 793.89
        microcalcification 793.81
    gastrointestinal tract 793.4
    genitourinary organs 793.5
    head 793.0
    image test inconclusive due to excess
        body fat 793.91
    intrathoracic organs NEC 793.2
    lung 793.19
    musculoskeletal 793.7
    placenta 793.99
    retroperitoneum 793.6
    skin 793.99
    skull 793.0
    subcutaneous tissue 793.99
  red blood cell 790.09
    count 790.09
    morphology 790.09
    sickling 790.09
    volume 790.09
  saliva 792.4
  scan NEC 794.9
    bladder 794.9
    bone 794.9
    brain 794.09
    kidney 794.4
    liver 794.8
    lung 794.2
    pancreas 794.9
    placental 794.9
    spleen 794.9
    thyroid 794.5
  sedimentation rate, elevated 790.1
  semen 792.2
  serological (for)
    human immunodeficiency virus (HIV)
      inconclusive 795.71
      positive V08
    syphilis - *see* Findings, serology for
        syphilis
  serology for syphilis
    false positive 795.6
    positive 097.1
      false 795.6
      follow-up of latent syphilis - *see*
          Syphilis, latent
      only finding - *see* Syphilis, latent
  serum 790.99
    blood NEC 790.99
    enzymes NEC 790.5
    proteins 790.99
  SGOT 790.4
  SGPT 790.4
  sickling of red blood cells 790.09
  skin test, positive 795.79
    tuberculin (without active tuberculosis)
        795.51
  sodium 790.6
    deficiency 276.1
    excess 276.0
  specified NEC 796.9
  spermatozoa 792.2
  spinal fluid 792.0
    culture, positive 792.0
  sputum culture, positive 795.39
    for acid-fast bacilli 795.39
  stool NEC 792.1
    bloody 578.1
      occult 792.1
    color 792.1
    culture, positive 792.1
    occult blood 792.1
  stress test 794.39

Findings *(Continued)*
  structure, body (echogram) (thermogram)
      (ultrasound) (x-ray) NEC 793.99
    abdomen 793.6
    breast 793.89
      abnormal mammogram 793.80
      mammographic
        calcification 793.89
        calculus 793.89
        microcalcification 793.81
    gastrointestinal tract 793.4
    genitourinary organs 793.5
    head 793.0
      echogram (ultrasound) 794.01
    intrathoracic organs NEC 793.2
    lung 793.19
    musculoskeletal 793.7
    placenta 793.99
    retroperitoneum 793.6
    skin 793.99
    subcutaneous tissue NEC 793.99
  synovial fluid 792.9
  thermogram - *see* Findings, abnormal,
      structure
  throat culture, positive 795.39
  thyroid (function) 794.5
    metabolism (rate) 794.5
    scan 794.5
    uptake 794.5
  total proteins 790.99
  toxicology (drugs) (heavy metals)
      796.0
  transaminase (level) 790.4
  triglycerides 272.9
    high 272.1
      with high cholesterol 272.2
  tuberculin skin test (without active
      tuberculosis) 795.51
  tumor markers NEC 795.89
  ultrasound - *see also* Findings, abnormal,
      structure
    cardiogram 793.2
  uric acid, blood 790.6
  urine, urinary constituents 791.9
    acetone 791.6
    albumin 791.0
    bacteria 791.9
    bile 791.4
    blood 599.70
    casts or cells 791.7
    chyle 791.1
    culture, positive 791.9
    glucose 791.5
    hemoglobin 791.2
    ketone 791.6
    protein 791.0
    pus 791.9
    sugar 791.5
  vaginal
    fluid 792.9
    high risk human papillomavirus (HPV)
        DNA test positive 795.15
    low risk human papillomavirus (HPV)
        DNA test positive 795.19
  vanillylmandelic acid, elevated 791.9
  vectorcardiogram (VCG) 794.39
  ventriculogram (cerebral) 793.0
  VMA, elevated 791.9
  Wassermann reaction
    false positive 795.6
    positive 097.1
      follow-up of latent syphilis - *see*
          Syphilis, latent
      only finding - *see* Syphilis, latent
  white blood cell 288.9
    count 288.9
      elevated 288.60
      low 288.50
    differential 288.9
    morphology 288.9
  wound culture 795.39

◄ New ◄ Revised ~~deleted~~ Deleted ● Use Additional Digit(s) ▨ Omit code

Findings (Continued)
   xerography 793.89
   zinc, blood 790.6
Finger - see condition
Finnish type nephrosis (congenital) 759.89
Fire, St. Anthony's (see also Erysipelas) 035
Fish
   hook stomach 537.89
   meal workers' lung 495.8
Fisher's syndrome 357.0
Fissure, fissured
   abdominal wall (congenital) 756.79
   anus, anal 565.0
      congenital 751.5
   buccal cavity 528.9
   clitoris (congenital) 752.49
   ear, lobule (congenital) 744.29
   epiglottis (congenital) 748.3
   larynx 478.79
      congenital 748.3
   lip 528.5
      congenital (see also Cleft, lip) 749.10
   nipple 611.2
      puerperal, postpartum 676.1●
   palate (congenital) (see also Cleft, palate) 749.00
   postanal 565.0
   rectum 565.0
   skin 709.8
      streptococcal 686.9
   spine (congenital) (see also Spina bifida) 741.9●
   sternum (congenital) 756.3
   tongue (acquired) 529.5
      congenital 750.13
Fistula (sinus) 686.9
   abdomen (wall) 569.81
      bladder 596.2
      intestine 569.81
      ureter 593.82
      uterus 619.2
   abdominorectal 569.81
   abdominosigmoidal 569.81
   abdominothoracic 510.0
   abdominouterine 619.2
      congenital 752.39
   abdominovesical 596.2
   accessory sinuses (see also Sinusitis) 473.9
   actinomycotic - see Actinomycosis
   alveolar
      antrum (see also Sinusitis, maxillary) 473.0
      process 522.7
   anorectal 565.1
   antrobuccal (see also Sinusitis, maxillary) 473.0
   antrum (see also Sinusitis, maxillary) 473.0
   anus, anal (infectional) (recurrent) 565.1
      congenital 751.5
      tuberculous (see also Tuberculosis) 014.8●
   aortic sinus 747.29
   aortoduodenal 447.2
   appendix, appendicular 543.9
   arteriovenous (acquired) 447.0
      brain 437.3
         congenital 747.81
            ruptured (see also Hemorrhage, subarachnoid) 430
         ruptured (see also Hemorrhage, subarachnoid) 430
      cerebral 437.3
         congenital 747.81
      congenital (peripheral) 747.60
         brain - see Fistula, arteriovenous, brain, congenital
         coronary 746.85
         gastrointestinal 747.61
         lower limb 747.64
         pulmonary 747.39
         renal 747.62
         specified site NEC 747.69
         upper limb 747.63

Fistula (Continued)
   arteriovenous (Continued)
      coronary 414.19
         congenital 746.85
      heart 414.19
      pulmonary (vessels) 417.0
         congenital 747.39
      surgically created (for dialysis) V45.11
         complication NEC 996.73
            atherosclerosis - see Arteriosclerosis, extremities
            embolism 996.74
            infection or inflammation 996.62
            mechanical 996.1
            occlusion NEC 996.74
            thrombus 996.74
      traumatic - see Injury, blood vessel, by site
   artery 447.2
   aural 383.81
      congenital 744.49
   auricle 383.81
      congenital 744.49
   Bartholin's gland 619.8
   bile duct (see also Fistula, biliary) 576.4
   biliary (duct) (tract) 576.4
      congenital 751.69
   bladder (neck) (sphincter) 596.2
      into seminal vesicle 596.2
   bone 733.99
   brain 348.89
      arteriovenous - see Fistula, arteriovenous, brain
   branchial (cleft) 744.41
   branchiogenous 744.41
   breast 611.0
      puerperal, postpartum 675.1●
   bronchial 510.0
   bronchocutaneous, bronchomediastinal, bronchopleural, bronchopleuromediastinal (infective) 510.0
      tuberculous (see also Tuberculosis) 011.3●
   bronchoesophageal 530.84
      congenital 750.3
   buccal cavity (infective) 528.3
   canal, ear 380.89
   carotid-cavernous
      congenital 747.81
         with hemorrhage 430
      traumatic 900.82
         with hemorrhage (see also Hemorrhage, brain, traumatic) 853.0●
         late effect 908.3
   cecosigmoidal 569.81
   cecum 569.81
   cerebrospinal (fluid) 349.81
   cervical, lateral (congenital) 744.41
   cervicoaural (congenital) 744.49
   cervicosigmoidal 619.1
   cervicovesical 619.0
   cervix 619.8
   chest (wall) 510.0
   cholecystocolic (see also Fistula, gallbladder) 575.5
   cholecystocolonic (see also Fistula, gallbladder) 575.5
   cholecystoduodenal (see also Fistula, gallbladder) 575.5
   cholecystoenteric (see also Fistula, gallbladder) 575.5
   cholecystogastric (see also Fistula, gallbladder) 575.5
   cholecystointestinal (see also Fistula, gallbladder) 575.5
   choledochoduodenal 576.4
   cholocolic (see also Fistula, gallbladder) 575.5
   coccyx 685.1
      with abscess 685.0
   colon 569.81
   colostomy 569.69
   colovaginal (acquired) 619.1

Fistula (Continued)
   common duct (bile duct) 576.4
   congenital, NEC - see Anomaly, specified type NEC
   cornea, causing hypotony 360.32
   coronary, arteriovenous 414.19
      congenital 746.85
   costal region 510.0
   cul-de-sac, Douglas' 619.8
   cutaneous 686.9
   cystic duct (see also Fistula, gallbladder) 575.5
      congenital 751.69
   cystostomy 596.83
   dental 522.7
   diaphragm 510.0
      bronchovisceral 510.0
      pleuroperitoneal 510.0
      pulmonoperitoneal 510.0
   duodenum 537.4
   ear (canal) (external) 380.89
   enterocolic 569.81
   enterocutaneous 569.81
   enteroenteric 569.81
   entero-uterine 619.1
      congenital 752.39
   enterovaginal 619.1
      congenital 752.49
   enterovesical 596.1
   epididymis 608.89
      tuberculous (see also Tuberculosis) 016.4●
   esophagobronchial 530.89
      congenital 750.3
   esophagocutaneous 530.89
   esophagopleurocutaneous 530.89
   esophagotracheal 530.84
      congenital 750.3
   esophagus 530.89
      congenital 750.4
   ethmoid (see also Sinusitis, ethmoidal) 473.2
   eyeball (cornea) (sclera) 360.32
   eyelid 373.11
   fallopian tube (external) 619.2
   fecal 569.81
      congenital 751.5
   from periapical lesion 522.7
   frontal sinus (see also Sinusitis, frontal) 473.1
   gallbladder 575.5
      with calculus, cholelithiasis, stones (see also Cholelithiasis) 574.2●
      congenital 751.69
   gastric 537.4
   gastrocolic 537.4
      congenital 750.7
      tuberculous (see also Tuberculosis) 014.8●
   gastroenterocolic 537.4
   gastroesophageal 537.4
   gastrojejunal 537.4
   gastrojejunocolic 537.4
   genital
      organs
         female 619.9
            specified site NEC 619.8
         male 608.89
      tract-skin (female) 619.2
   hepatopleural 510.0
   hepatopulmonary 510.0
   horseshoe 565.1
   ileorectal 569.81
   ileosigmoidal 569.81
   ileostomy 569.69
   ileovesical 596.1
   ileum 569.81
   in ano 565.1
      tuberculous (see also Tuberculosis) 014.8●
   inner ear (see also Fistula, labyrinth) 386.40
   intestine 569.81
   intestinocolonic (abdominal) 569.81
   intestinoureteral 593.82
   intestinouterine 619.1
   intestinovaginal 619.1
      congenital 752.49

Fistula (Continued)
  intestinovesical 596.1
  involving female genital tract 619.9
    digestive-genital 619.1
    genital tract-skin 619.2
    specified site NEC 619.8
    urinary-genital 619.0
  ischiorectal (fossa) 566
  jejunostomy 569.69
  jejunum 569.81
  joint 719.80
    ankle 719.87
    elbow 719.82
    foot 719.87
    hand 719.84
    hip 719.85
    knee 719.86
    multiple sites 719.89
    pelvic region 719.85
    shoulder (region) 719.81
    specified site NEC 719.88
    tuberculous - see Tuberculosis, joint
    wrist 719.83
  kidney 593.89
  labium (majus) (minus) 619.8
  labyrinth, labyrinthine NEC 386.40
    combined sites 386.48
    multiple sites 386.48
    oval window 386.42
    round window 386.41
    semicircular canal 386.43
  lacrimal, lachrymal (duct) (gland) (sac)
      375.61
  lacrimonasal duct 375.61
  laryngotracheal 748.3
  larynx 478.79
  lip 528.5
    congenital 750.25
  lumbar, tuberculous (see also Tuberculosis)
      015.0● [730.8]●
  lung 510.0
  lymphatic (node) (vessel) 457.8
  mamillary 611.0
  mammary (gland) 611.0
    puerperal, postpartum 675.1●
  mastoid (process) (region) 383.1
  maxillary (see also Sinusitis, maxillary) 473.0
  mediastinal 510.0
  mediastinobronchial 510.0
  mediastinocutaneous 510.0
  middle ear 385.89
  mouth 528.3
  nasal 478.19
    sinus (see also Sinusitis) 473.9
  nasopharynx 478.29
  nipple - see Fistula, breast
  nose 478.19
  oral (cutaneous) 528.3
    maxillary (see also Sinusitis, maxillary)
        473.0
    nasal (with cleft palate) (see also Cleft,
        palate) 749.00
  orbit, orbital 376.10
  oro-antral (see also Sinusitis, maxillary) 473.0
  oval window (internal ear) 386.42
  oviduct (external) 619.2
  palate (hard) 526.89
    soft 528.9
  pancreatic 577.8
  pancreaticoduodenal 577.8
  parotid (gland) 527.4
    region 528.3
  pelvoabdominointestinal 569.81
  penis 607.89
  perianal 565.1
  pericardium (pleura) (sac) (see also
      Pericarditis) 423.8
  pericecal 569.81
  perineal - see Fistula, perineum
  perineorectal 569.81
  perineosigmoidal 569.81

Fistula (Continued)
  perineo-urethroscrotal 608.89
  perineum, perineal (with urethral
      involvement) NEC 599.1
    tuberculous (see also Tuberculosis) 017.9●
    ureter 593.82
  perirectal 565.1
    tuberculous (see also Tuberculosis) 014.8●
  peritoneum (see also Peritonitis) 567.22
  periurethral 599.1
  pharyngo-esophageal 478.29
  pharynx 478.29
    branchial cleft (congenital) 744.41
  pilonidal (infected) (rectum) 685.1
    with abscess 685.0
  pleura, pleural, pleurocutaneous,
      pleuroperitoneal 510.0
    stomach 510.0
    tuberculous (see also Tuberculosis) 012.0●
  pleuropericardial 423.8
  postauricular 383.81
  postoperative, persistent 998.6
  preauricular (congenital) 744.46
  prostate 602.8
  pulmonary 510.0
    arteriovenous 417.0
      congenital 747.39
    tuberculous (see also Tuberculosis,
        pulmonary) 011.9●
  pulmonoperitoneal 510.0
  rectolabial 619.1
  rectosigmoid (intercommunicating) 569.81
  rectoureteral 593.82
  rectourethral 599.1
    congenital 753.8
  rectouterine 619.1
    congenital 752.39
  rectovaginal 619.1
    congenital 752.49
    old, postpartal 619.1
    tuberculous (see also Tuberculosis)
        014.8●
  rectovesical 596.1
    congenital 753.8
  rectovesicovaginal 619.1
  rectovulvar 619.1
    congenital 752.49
  rectum (to skin) 565.1
    tuberculous (see also Tuberculosis)
        014.8●
  renal 593.89
  retroauricular 383.81
  round window (internal ear) 386.41
  salivary duct or gland 527.4
    congenital 750.24
  sclera 360.32
  scrotum (urinary) 608.89
    tuberculous (see also Tuberculosis)
        016.5●
  semicircular canals (internal ear) 386.43
  sigmoid 569.81
    vesicoabdominal 596.1
  sigmoidovaginal 619.1
    congenital 752.49
  skin 686.9
    ureter 593.82
    vagina 619.2
  sphenoidal sinus (see also Sinusitis,
      sphenoidal) 473.3
  splenocolic 289.59
  stercoral 569.81
  stomach 537.4
  sublingual gland 527.4
    congenital 750.24
  submaxillary
    gland 527.4
      congenital 750.24
    region 528.3
  thoracic 510.0
    duct 457.8
  thoracicoabdominal 510.0

Fistula (Continued)
  thoracicogastric 510.0
  thoracicointestinal 510.0
  thoracoabdominal 510.0
  thoracogastric 510.0
  thorax 510.0
  thyroglossal duct 759.2
  thyroid 246.8
  trachea (congenital) (external) (internal)
      748.3
  tracheoesophageal 530.84
    congenital 750.3
    following tracheostomy 519.09
  traumatic
    arteriovenous (see also Injury, blood
        vessel, by site) 904.9
    brain - see Injury, intracranial
  tuberculous - see Tuberculosis, by site
  typhoid 002.0
  umbilical 759.89
  umbilico-urinary 753.8
  urachal, urachus 753.7
  ureter (persistent) 593.82
  ureteroabdominal 593.82
  ureterocervical 593.82
  ureterorectal 593.82
  ureterosigmoido-abdominal 593.82
  ureterovaginal 619.0
  ureterovesical 596.2
  urethra 599.1
    congenital 753.8
    tuberculous (see also Tuberculosis) 016.3●
  urethroperineal 599.1
  urethroperineovesical 596.2
  urethrorectal 599.1
    congenital 753.8
  urethroscrotal 608.89
  urethrovaginal 619.0
  urethrovesical 596.2
  urethrovesicovaginal 619.0
  urinary (persistent) (recurrent) 599.1
  uteroabdominal (anterior wall) 619.2
    congenital 752.39
  uteroenteric 619.1
  uterofecal 619.1
  uterointestinal 619.1
    congenital 752.39
  uterorectal 619.1
    congenital 752.39
  uteroureteric 619.0
  uterovaginal 619.8
  uterovesical 619.0
    congenital 752.39
  uterus 619.8
  vagina (wall) 619.8
    postpartal, old 619.8
  vaginocutaneous (postpartal) 619.2
  vaginoileal (acquired) 619.1
  vaginoperineal 619.2
  vesical NEC 596.2
  vesicoabdominal 596.2
  vesicocervicovaginal 619.0
  vesicocolic 596.1
  vesicocutaneous 596.2
  vesicoenteric 596.1
  vesicointestinal 596.1
  vesicometrorectal 619.1
  vesicoperineal 596.2
  vesicorectal 596.1
    congenital 753.8
  vesicosigmoidal 596.1
  vesicosigmoidovaginal 619.1
  vesicoureteral 596.2
  vesicoureterovaginal 619.0
  vesicourethral 596.2
  vesicourethrorectal 596.1
  vesicouterine 619.0
    congenital 752.39
  vesicovaginal 619.0
  vulvorectal 619.1
    congenital 752.49

◀ New　◀▥ Revised　~~deleted~~ Deleted　● Use Additional Digit(s)　▨ Omit code

Fit 780.39
apoplectic (*see also* Disease, cerebrovascular, acute) 436
late effect - *see* Late effect(s) (of) cerebrovascular disease
epileptic (*see also* Epilepsy) 345.9●
fainting 780.2
hysterical 300.11
newborn 779.0
Fitting (of)
artificial
arm (complete) (partial) V52.0
breast V52.4
implant exchange (different material) (different size) V52.4
eye(s) V52.2
leg(s) (complete) (partial) V52.1
brain neuropacemaker V53.02
cardiac pacemaker V53.31
carotid sinus pacemaker V53.39
cerebral ventricle (communicating) shunt V53.01
colostomy belt V55.3
contact lenses V53.1
cystostomy device V53.6
defibrillator, automatic implantable cardiac (with synchronous cardiac pacemaker) V53.32
dentures V52.3
device, unspecified type V53.90
abdominal V53.59
cardiac
defibrillator, automatic implantable (with synchronous cardiac pacemaker) V53.32
pacemaker V53.31
specified NEC V53.39
cerebral ventricle (communicating) shunt V53.01
gastrointestinal NEC V53.59
insulin pump V53.91
intestinal V53.50
intrauterine contraceptive
insertion V25.11
removal V25.12
and reinsertion V25.13
replacement V25.13
nervous system V53.09
orthodontic V53.4
orthoptic V53.1
other device V53.99
prosthetic V52.9
breast V52.4
dental V52.3
eye V52.2
specified type NEC V52.8
special senses V53.09
substitution
auditory V53.09
nervous system V53.09
visual V53.09
urinary V53.6
diaphragm (contraceptive) V25.02
gastric lap band V53.51
gastrointestinal appliance and device NEC V53.59
glasses (reading) V53.1
growth rod V54.02
hearing aid V53.2
ileostomy device V55.2
intestinal appliance and device V53.50
intrauterine contraceptive device
insertion V25.11
removal V25.12
and reinsertion V25.13
replacement V25.13
neuropacemaker (brain) (peripheral nerve) (spinal cord) V53.02
orthodontic device V53.4

Fitting (Continued)
orthopedic (device) V53.7
brace V53.7
cast V53.7
corset V53.7
shoes V53.7
pacemaker (cardiac) V53.31
brain V53.02
carotid sinus V53.39
peripheral nerve V53.02
spinal cord V53.02
prosthesis V52.9
arm (complete) (partial) V52.0
breast V52.4
implant exchange (different material) (different size) V52.4
dental V52.3
eye V52.2
leg (complete) (partial) V52.1
specified type NEC V52.8
spectacles V53.1
wheelchair V53.8
Fitz's syndrome (acute hemorrhagic pancreatitis) 577.0
Fitz-Hugh and Curtis syndrome 098.86
due to
Chlamydia trachomatis 099.56
Neisseria gonorrhoeae (gonococcal peritonitis) 098.86
Fixation
joint - *see* Ankylosis
larynx 478.79
pupil 364.76
stapes 385.22
deafness (*see also* Deafness, conductive) 389.04
uterus (acquired) - *see* Malposition, uterus
vocal cord 478.5
Flaccid - *see also* condition
foot 736.79
forearm 736.09
palate, congenital 750.26
Flail
chest 807.4
newborn 767.3
joint (paralytic) 718.80
ankle 718.87
elbow 718.82
foot 718.87
hand 718.84
hip 718.85
knee 718.86
multiple sites 718.89
pelvic region 718.85
shoulder (region) 718.81
specified site NEC 718.88
wrist 718.83
Flajani (-Basedow) syndrome or disease (exophthalmic goiter) 242.0●
Flap, liver 572.8
Flare, anterior chamber (aqueous) (eye) 364.04
Flashback phenomena (drug) (hallucinogenic) 292.89
Flat
chamber (anterior) (eye) 360.34
chest, congenital 754.89
electroencephalogram (EEG) 348.89
foot (acquired) (fixed type) (painful) (postural) (spastic) 734
congenital 754.61
rocker bottom 754.61
vertical talus 754.61
rachitic 268.1
rocker bottom (congenital) 754.61
vertical talus, congenital 754.61
organ or site, congenital NEC - *see* Anomaly, specified type NEC

Flat (Continued)
pelvis 738.6
with disproportion (fetopelvic) 653.2●
affecting fetus or newborn 763.1
causing obstructed labor 660.1●
affecting fetus or newborn 763.1
congenital 755.69
Flatau-Schilder disease 341.1
Flattening
head, femur 736.39
hip 736.39
lip (congenital) 744.89
nose (congenital) 754.0
acquired 738.0
Flatulence 787.3
Flatus 787.3
vaginalis 629.89
Flax dressers' disease 504
Flea bite - *see* Injury, superficial, by site
Fleischer (-Kayser) ring (corneal pigmentation) 275.1 [371.14]
Fleischner's disease 732.3
Fleshy mole 631.8
Flexibilitas cerea (*see also* Catalepsy) 300.11
Flexion
cervix - *see* Flexion, uterus
contracture, joint (*see also* Contraction, joint) 718.4●
deformity, joint (*see also* Contraction, joint) 736.9
hip, congenital (*see also* Subluxation, congenital, hip) 754.32
uterus (*see also* Malposition, uterus) 621.6
Flexner's
bacillus 004.1
diarrhea (ulcerative) 004.1
dysentery 004.1
Flexner-Boyd dysentery 004.2
Flexure - *see* condition
Floater, vitreous 379.24
Floating
cartilage (joint) (*see also* Disorder, cartilage, articular) 718.0●
knee 717.6
gallbladder (congenital) 751.69
kidney 593.0
congenital 753.3
liver (congenital) 751.69
rib 756.3
spleen 289.59
Flooding 626.2
Floor - *see* condition
Floppy
infant NEC 781.99
iris syndrome 364.81
valve syndrome (mitral) 424.0
Flu - *see also* Influenza
bird (*see also* Influenza, avian) 488.02
gastric NEC 008.8
swine - *see* Influenza, (novel) 2009 H1N1
Fluctuating blood pressure 796.4
Fluid
abdomen 789.59
chest (*see also* Pleurisy, with effusion) 511.9
heart (*see also* Failure, heart) 428.0
joint (*see also* Effusion, joint) 719.0●
loss (acute) 276.50
with
hypernatremia 276.0
hyponatremia 276.1
lung - *see also* Edema, lung
encysted 511.89
peritoneal cavity 789.59
malignant 789.51
pleural cavity (*see also* Pleurisy, with effusion) 511.9
retention 276.69
Flukes NEC (*see also* Infestation, fluke) 121.9
blood NEC (*see also* Infestation, Schistosoma) 120.9
liver 121.3

Fluor (albus) (vaginalis) 623.5
  trichomonal (Trichomonas vaginalis) 131.00
Fluorosis (dental) (chronic) 520.3
Flushing 782.62
  menopausal 627.2
Flush syndrome 259.2
Flutter
  atrial or auricular 427.32
  heart (ventricular) 427.42
    atrial 427.32
  impure 427.32
  postoperative 997.1
  ventricular 427.42
Flux (bloody) (serosanguineous) 009.0
FNHTR (febrile nonhemolytic transfusion
    reaction) 780.66
Focal - see condition
Fochier's abscess - see Abscess, by site
Focus, Assmann's (see also Tuberculosis)
    011.0●
Fogo selvagem 694.4
Foix-Alajouanine syndrome 336.1
Folds, anomalous - see also Anomaly, specified
    type NEC
  Bowman's membrane 371.31
  Descemet's membrane 371.32
  epicanthic 743.63
  heart 746.89
  posterior segment of eye, congenital
    743.54
Folie a deux 297.3
Follicle
  cervix (nabothian) (ruptured) 616.0
  graafian, ruptured, with hemorrhage
    620.0
  nabothian 616.0
Folliclis (primary) (see also Tuberculosis)
    017.0●
Follicular - see also condition
  cyst (atretic) 620.0
Folliculitis 704.8
  abscedens et suffodiens 704.8
  decalvans 704.09
  gonorrheal (acute) 098.0
    chronic or duration of 2 months or more
      098.2
  keloid, keloidalis 706.1
  pustular 704.8
  ulerythematosa reticulata 701.8
Folliculosis, conjunctival 372.02
Følling's disease (phenylketonuria) 270.1
Follow-up (examination) (routine) (following)
    V67.9
  cancer chemotherapy V67.2
  chemotherapy V67.2
  fracture V67.4
  high-risk medication V67.51
  injury NEC V67.59
  postpartum
    immediately after delivery V24.0
    routine V24.2
  psychiatric V67.3
  psychotherapy V67.3
  radiotherapy V67.1
  specified condition NEC V67.59
  specified surgery NEC V67.09
  surgery V67.00
    vaginal pap smear V67.01
  treatment V67.9
    combined NEC V67.6
    fracture V67.4
    involving high-risk medication NEC
      V67.51
    mental disorder V67.3
    specified NEC V67.59
Fong's syndrome (hereditary
    osteoonychodysplasia) 756.89
Food
  allergy 693.1
  anaphylactic shock - see Anaphylactic
    reaction or shock, due to food

Food (Continued)
  asphyxia (from aspiration or inhalation) (see
      also Asphyxia, food) 933.1
  choked on (see also Asphyxia, food)
      933.1
  deprivation 994.2
    specified kind of food NEC 269.8
  intoxication (see also Poisoning, food)
      005.9
  lack of 994.2
  poisoning (see also Poisoning, food)
      005.9
  refusal or rejection NEC 307.59
  strangulation or suffocation (see also
      Asphyxia, food) 933.1
  toxemia (see also Poisoning, food)
      005.9
Foot - see also condition
  and mouth disease 078.4
  process disease 581.3
Foramen ovale (nonclosure) (patent)
    (persistent) 745.5
Forbes' (glycogen storage) disease 271.0
Forbes-Albright syndrome (nonpuerperal
    amenorrhea and lactation associated with
    pituitary tumor) 253.1
Forced birth or delivery NEC 669.8●
  affecting fetus or newborn NEC 763.89
Forceps
  delivery NEC 669.5●
    affecting fetus or newborn 763.2
Fordyce's disease (ectopic sebaceous glands)
    (mouth) 750.26
Fordyce-Fox disease (apocrine miliaria)
    705.82
Forearm - see condition
Foreign body

Note: For foreign body with open wound
or other injury, see Wound, open, or the type
of injury specified.

---

  accidentally left during a procedure
    998.4
  anterior chamber (eye) 871.6
    magnetic 871.5
      retained or old 360.51
    retained or old 360.61
  ciliary body (eye) 871.6
    magnetic 871.5
      retained or old 360.52
    retained or old 360.62
  entering through orifice (current) (old)
    accessory sinus 932
    air passage (upper) 933.0
      lower 934.8
    alimentary canal 938
    alveolar process 935.0
    antrum (Highmore) 932
    anus 937
    appendix 936
    asphyxia due to (see also Asphyxia, food)
      933.1
    auditory canal 931
    auricle 931
    bladder 939.0
    bronchioles 934.8
    bronchus (main) 934.1
    buccal cavity 935.0
    cecum 936
    cervix (canal) uterine 939.1
    coil, ileocecal 936
    colon 936
    conjunctiva 930.1
    conjunctival sac 930.1
    cornea 930.0
    digestive organ or tract NEC 938
    duodenum 936
    ear (external) 931
    esophagus 935.1

Foreign body (Continued)
  entering through orifice (Continued)
    eye (external) 930.9
      combined sites 930.8
      intraocular - see Foreign body, by site
      specified site NEC 930.8
    eyeball 930.8
      intraocular - see Foreign body,
        intraocular
    eyelid 930.1
      retained or old 374.86
    frontal sinus 932
    gastrointestinal tract 938
    genitourinary tract 939.9
    globe 930.8
      penetrating 871.6
        magnetic 871.5
          retained or old 360.50
        retained or old 360.60
    gum 935.0
    Highmore's antrum 932
    hypopharynx 933.0
    ileocecal coil 936
    ileum 936
    inspiration (of) 933.1
    intestine (large) (small) 936
    lacrimal apparatus, duct, gland, or sac 930.2
    larynx 933.1
    lung 934.8
    maxillary sinus 932
    mouth 935.0
    nasal sinus 932
    nasopharynx 933.0
    nose (passage) 932
    nostril 932
    oral cavity 935.0
    palate 935.0
    penis 939.3
    pharynx 933.0
    pyriform sinus 933.0
    rectosigmoid 937
      junction 937
    rectum 937
    respiratory tract 934.9
      specified part NEC 934.8
    sclera 930.1
    sinus 932
      accessory 932
      frontal 932
      maxillary 932
      nasal 932
      pyriform 933.0
    small intestine 936
    stomach (hairball) 935.2
    suffocation by (see also Asphyxia, food)
      933.1
    swallowed 938
      tongue 935.0
    tear ducts or glands 930.2
    throat 933.0
    tongue 935.0
      swallowed 933.0
    tonsil, tonsillar 933.0
      fossa 933.0
    trachea 934.0
    ureter 939.0
    urethra 939.0
    uterus (any part) 939.1
    vagina 939.2
    vulva 939.2
    wind pipe 934.0
  feeling of, in throat 784.99
  granuloma (old) 728.82
    bone 733.99
    in operative wound (inadvertently left)
      998.4
      due to surgical material intentionally
        left - see Complications, due to
        (presence of) any device,
        implant, or graft classified to
        996.0–996.5 NEC

◀ New   ◀= Revised   d̶e̶l̶e̶t̶e̶d̶ Deleted   ● Use Additional Digit(s)   ▦ Omit code

Foreign body *(Continued)*
  granuloma *(Continued)*
    muscle 728.82
    skin 709.4
    soft tissue NEC 709.4
    subcutaneous tissue 709.4
  in
    bone (residual) 733.99
    open wound - *see* Wound, open, by site complicated
    soft tissue (residual) 729.6
  inadvertently left in operation wound (causing adhesions, obstruction, or perforation) 998.4
  ingestion, ingested NEC 938
  inhalation or inspiration *(see also* Asphyxia, food) 933.1
  internal organ, not entering through an orifice - *see* Injury, internal, by site, with open wound
  intraocular (nonmagnetic) 871.6
    combined sites 871.6
      magnetic 871.5
        retained or old 360.59
      retained or old 360.69
    magnetic 871.5
      retained or old 360.50
    retained or old 360.60
    specified site NEC 871.6
      magnetic 871.5
        retained or old 360.59
      retained or old 360.69
  iris (nonmagnetic) 871.6
    magnetic 871.5
      retained or old 360.52
    retained or old 360.62
  lens (nonmagnetic) 871.6
    magnetic 871.5
      retained or old 360.53
    retained or old 360.63
  lid, eye 930.1
  ocular muscle 870.4
    retained or old 376.6
  old or residual
    bone 733.99
    eyelid 374.86
    middle ear 385.83
    muscle 729.6
      ocular 376.6
    retrobulbar 376.6
    skin 729.6
      with granuloma 709.4
    soft tissue 729.6
      with granuloma 709.4
    subcutaneous tissue 729.6
      with granuloma 709.4
  operation wound, left accidentally 998.4
  orbit 870.4
    retained or old 376.6
  posterior wall, eye 871.6
    magnetic 871.5
      retained or old 360.55
    retained or old 360.65
  respiratory tree 934.9
    specified site NEC 934.8
  retained (old) (nonmagnetic) (in) V90.9
    anterior chamber (eye) 360.61
      magnetic 360.51
    ciliary body 360.62
      magnetic 360.52
    eyelid 374.86
    fragment(s)
      acrylics V90.2
      animal quills V90.31
      animal spines V90.31
      cement V90.83
      concrete V90.83
      crystalline V90.83
      depleted
        isotope V90.09
        uranium V90.01

Foreign body *(Continued)*
  retained *(Continued)*
    fragment(s) *(Continued)*
      diethylhexylphthalates V90.2
      glass V90.81
      isocyanate V90.2
      metal V90.10
        magnetic V90.11
        nonmagnetic V90.12
      organic NEC V90.39
      plastic V90.2
      radioactive
        nontherapeutic V90.09
        specified NEC V90.09
      stone V90.83
      tooth V90.32
      wood V90.33
    globe 360.60
      magnetic 360.50
    intraocular 360.60
      magnetic 360.50
      specified site NEC 360.69
        magnetic 360.59
    iris 360.62
      magnetic 360.52
    lens 360.63
      magnetic 360.53
    muscle 729.6
    orbit 376.6
    posterior wall of globe 360.65
      magnetic 360.55
    retina 360.65
      magnetic 360.55
    retrobulbar 376.6
    skin 729.6
      with granuloma 709.4
    soft tissue 729.6
      with granuloma 709.4
    specified NEC V90.89
    subcutaneous tissue 729.6
      with granuloma 709.4
    vitreous 360.64
      magnetic 360.54
  retina 871.6
    magnetic 871.5
      retained or old 360.55
    retained or old 360.65
  superficial, without major open wound *(see also* Injury, superficial, by site) 919.6
  swallowed NEC 938
  throat, feeling of 784.99
  vitreous (humor) 871.6
    magnetic 871.5
      retained or old 360.54
    retained or old 360.64
Forking, aqueduct of Sylvius 742.3
  with spina bifida *(see also* Spina bifida) 741.0 ●
Formation
  bone in scar tissue (skin) 709.3
  connective tissue in vitreous 379.25
  Elschnig pearls (postcataract extraction) 366.51
  hyaline in cornea 371.49
  sequestrum in bone (due to infection) *(see also* Osteomyelitis) 730.1 ●
  valve
    colon, congenital 751.5
    ureter (congenital) 753.29
Formication 782.0
Fort Bragg fever 100.89
Fossa - *see also* condition
  pyriform - *see* condition
Foster care (status) V60.81
Foster-Kennedy syndrome 377.04
Fothergill's
  disease, meaning scarlatina anginosa 034.1
  neuralgia *(see also* Neuralgia, trigeminal) 350.1
Foul breath 784.99

Found dead (cause unknown) 798.9
Foundling V20.0
Fournier's disease (idiopathic gangrene) 608.83
  female 616.89
Fourth
  cranial nerve - *see* condition
  disease 057.8
  molar 520.1
Foville's syndrome 344.89
Fox's
  disease (apocrine miliaria) 705.82
  impetigo (contagiosa) 684
Fox-Fordyce disease (apocrine miliaria) 705.82
Fracture (abduction) (adduction) (avulsion) (compression) (crush) (dislocation) (oblique) (separation) (closed) 829.0

Note: For fracture of any of the following sites with fracture of other bones - *see* Fracture, multiple.

"Closed" includes the following descriptions of fractures, with or without delayed healing, unless they are specified as open or compound:

    comminuted
    depressed
    elevated
    fissured
    greenstick
    impacted
    linear
    simple
    slipped epiphysis
    spiral
    unspecified

"Open" includes the following descriptions of fractures, with or without delayed healing:

    compound
    infected
    missile
    puncture
    with foreign body

For late effect of fracture, *see* Late, effect, fracture, by site.

---

  with
    internal injuries in same region (conditions classifiable to 860–869) - *see also* Injury, internal, by site
    pelvic region - *see* Fracture, pelvis
  acetabulum (with visceral injury) (closed) 808.0
    open 808.1
  acromion (process) (closed) 811.01
    open 811.11
  alveolus (closed) 802.8
    open 802.9
  ankle (malleolus) (closed) 824.8
    bimalleolar (Dupuytren's) (Pott's) 824.4
      open 824.5
    bone 825.21
      open 825.31
    lateral malleolus only (fibular) 824.2
      open 824.3
    medial malleolus only (tibial) 824.0
      open 824.1
    open 824.9
    pathologic 733.16
    talus 825.21
      open 825.31
    trimalleolar 824.6
      open 824.7
  antrum - *see* Fracture, skull, base
  arm (closed) 818.0
    and leg(s) (any bones) 828.0
      open 828.1

Fracture (*Continued*)
  arm (*Continued*)
    both (any bones) (with rib(s)) (with
      sternum) 819.0
      open 819.1
    lower 813.80
      open 813.90
    open 818.1
    upper - *see* Fracture, humerus
  astragalus (closed) 825.21
    open 825.31
  atlas - *see* Fracture, vertebra, cervical, first
  axis - *see* Fracture, vertebra, cervical, second
  back - *see* Fracture, vertebra, by site
  Barton's - *see* Fracture, radius, lower end
  basal (skull) - *see* Fracture, skull, base
  Bennett's (closed) 815.01
    open 815.11
  bimalleolar (closed) 824.4
    open 824.5
  bone (closed) NEC 829.0
    birth injury NEC 767.3
    open 829.1
    pathological NEC (*see also* Fracture,
      pathologic) 733.10
    stress NEC (*see also* Fracture, stress) 733.95
  boot top - *see* Fracture, fibula
  boxers' - *see* Fracture, metacarpal bone(s)
  breast bone - *see* Fracture, sternum
  buckle - *see* Fracture, torus
  bucket handle (semilunar cartilage) - *see* Tear,
    meniscus
  burst - *see* Fracture, traumatic, by site
  bursting - *see* Fracture, phalanx, hand, distal
  calcaneus (closed) 825.0
    open 825.1
  capitate (bone) (closed) 814.07
    open 814.17
  capitellum (humerus) (closed) 812.49
    open 812.59
  carpal bone(s) (wrist NEC) (closed) 814.00
    open 814.10
    specified site NEC 814.09
      open 814.19
  cartilage, knee (semilunar) - *see* Tear,
    meniscus
  cervical - *see* Fracture, vertebra, cervical
  chauffeur's - *see* Fracture, ulna, lower end
  chisel - *see* Fracture, radius, upper end
  chronic - *see* Fracture, pathologic
  clavicle (interligamentous part) (closed)
    810.00
    acromial end 810.03
      open 810.13
    due to birth trauma 767.2
    open 810.10
    shaft (middle third) 810.02
      open 810.12
    sternal end 810.01
      open 810.11
  clayshovelers' - *see* Fracture, vertebra,
    cervical
  coccyx - *see also* Fracture, vertebra, coccyx
    complicating delivery 665.6●
  collar bone - *see* Fracture, clavicle
  Colles' (reversed) (closed) 813.41
    open 813.51
  comminuted - *see* Fracture, by site
  compression - *see also* Fracture, by site
    nontraumatic - *see* Fracture, pathologic
  congenital 756.9
  coracoid process (closed) 811.02
    open 811.12
  coronoid process (ulna) (closed) 813.02
    mandible (closed) 802.23
      open 802.33
    open 813.12
  corpus cavernosum penis 959.13
  costochondral junction - *see* Fracture, rib
  costosternal junction - *see* Fracture, rib
  cranium - *see* Fracture, skull, by site

Fracture (*Continued*)
  cricoid cartilage (closed) 807.5
    open 807.6
  cuboid (ankle) (closed) 825.23
    open 825.33
  cuneiform
    foot (closed) 825.24
      open 825.34
    wrist (closed) 814.03
      open 814.13
  dental implant 525.73
  dental restorative material
    with loss of material 525.64
    without loss of material 525.63
  due to
    birth injury - *see* Birth injury, fracture
    gunshot - *see* Fracture, by site, open
    neoplasm - *see* Fracture, pathologic
    osteoporosis - *see* Fracture, pathologic
  Dupuytren's (ankle) (fibula) (closed) 824.4
    open 824.5
    radius 813.42
      open 813.52
  Duverney's - *see* Fracture, ilium
  elbow - *see also* Fracture, humerus, lower end
    olecranon (process) (closed) 813.01
      open 813.11
    supracondylar (closed) 812.41
      open 812.51
  ethmoid (bone) (sinus) - *see* Fracture, skull,
    base
  face bone(s) (closed) NEC 802.8
    with
      other bone(s) - *see* Fracture, multiple,
        skull
      skull - *see also* Fracture, skull
        involving other bones - *see* Fracture,
          multiple, skull
    open 802.9
  fatigue - *see* Fracture, march
  femur, femoral (closed) 821.00
    cervicotrochanteric 820.03
      open 820.13
    condyles, epicondyles 821.21
      open 821.31
    distal end - *see* Fracture, femur, lower end
    epiphysis (separation)
      capital 820.01
        open 820.11
      head 820.01
        open 820.11
      lower 821.22
        open 821.32
      trochanteric 820.01
        open 820.11
      upper 820.01
        open 820.11
    head 820.09
      open 820.19
    lower end or extremity (distal end)
      (closed) 821.20
      condyles, epicondyles 821.21
        open 821.31
      epiphysis (separation) 821.22
        open 821.32
      multiple sites 821.29
        open 821.39
      open 821.30
      specified site NEC 821.29
        open 821.39
      supracondylar 821.23
        open 821.33
      T-shaped 821.21
        open 821.31
    neck (closed) 820.8
      base (cervicotrochanteric) 820.03
        open 820.13
      extracapsular 820.20
        open 820.30
      intertrochanteric (section) 820.21
        open 820.31

Fracture (*Continued*)
  femur, femoral (*Continued*)
    neck (*Continued*)
      intracapsular 820.00
        open 820.10
      intratrochanteric 820.21
        open 820.31
      midcervical 820.02
        open 820.12
      open 820.9
      pathologic 733.14
        specified part NEC 733.15
      specified site NEC 820.09
        open 820.19
      stress 733.96
      transcervical 820.02
        open 820.12
      transtrochanteric 820.20
        open 820.30
    open 821.10
    pathologic 733.14
      specified part NEC 733.15
    peritrochanteric (section) 820.20
      open 820.30
    shaft (lower third) (middle third) (upper
      third) 821.01
      open 821.11
      stress 733.97
    subcapital 820.09
      open 820.19
    subtrochanteric (region) (section) 820.22
      open 820.32
    supracondylar 821.23
      open 821.33
    transepiphyseal 820.01
      open 820.11
    trochanter (greater) (lesser) (*see also*
      Fracture, femur, neck, by site)
      820.20
      open 820.30
    T-shaped, into knee joint 821.21
      open 821.31
    upper end 820.8
      open 820.9
  fibula (closed) 823.81
    with tibia 823.82
      open 823.92
    distal end 824.8
      open 824.9
    epiphysis
      lower 824.8
        open 824.9
      upper - *see* Fracture, fibula, upper end
    head - *see* Fracture, fibula, upper end
    involving ankle 824.2
      open 824.3
    lower end or extremity 824.8
      open 824.9
    malleolus (external) (lateral) 824.2
      open 824.3
    open NEC 823.91
    pathologic 733.16
    proximal end - *see* Fracture, fibula, upper
      end
    shaft 823.21
      with tibia 823.22
        open 823.32
      open 823.31
    stress 733.93
    torus 823.41
      with tibia 823.42
    upper end or extremity (epiphysis) (head)
      (proximal end) (styloid) 823.01
      with tibia 823.02
        open 823.12
      open 823.11
  finger(s), of one hand (closed) (*see also*
    Fracture, phalanx, hand) 816.00
    with
      metacarpal bone(s), of same hand 817.0
        open 817.1

◀ New   ◀▪ Revised   ~~deleted~~ Deleted   ● Use Additional Digit(s)   ▨ Omit code

Fracture *(Continued)*
 finger(s), of one hand *(Continued)*
  with *(Continued)*
   thumb of same hand 816.03
    open 816.13
  open 816.10
 foot, except toe(s) alone (closed) 825.20
  open 825.30
 forearm (closed) NEC 813.80
  lower end (distal end) (lower epiphysis) 813.40
   open 813.50
  open 813.90
  shaft 813.20
   open 813.30
  upper end (proximal end) (upper epiphysis) 813.00
   open 813.10
 fossa, anterior, middle, or posterior - *see* Fracture, skull, base
 frontal (bone) - *see also* Fracture, skull, vault
  sinus - *see* Fracture, skull, base
 Galeazzi's - *see* Fracture, radius, lower end
 glenoid (cavity) (fossa) (scapula) (closed) 811.03
  open 811.13
 Gosselin's - *see* Fracture, ankle
 greenstick - *see* Fracture, by site
 grenade-throwers' - *see* Fracture, humerus, shaft
 gutter - *see* Fracture, skull, vault
 hamate (closed) 814.08
  open 814.18
 hand, one (closed) 815.00
  carpals 814.00
   open 814.10
   specified site NEC 814.09
    open 814.19
  metacarpals 815.00
   open 815.10
  multiple, bones of one hand 817.0
   open 817.1
  open 815.10
  phalanges *(see also* Fracture, phalanx, hand) 816.00
   open 816.10
 healing
  aftercare *(see also* Aftercare, fracture) V54.89
  change of cast V54.89
  complications - *see* condition
  convalescence V66.4
  removal of
   cast V54.89
   fixation device
    external V54.89
    internal V54.01
 heel bone (closed) 825.0
  open 825.1
 Hill-Sachs 812.09
 hip (closed) *(see also* Fracture, femur, neck) 820.8
  open 820.9
  pathologic 733.14
 humerus (closed) 812.20
  anatomical neck 812.02
   open 812.12
  articular process *(see also* Fracture humerus, condyle(s)) 812.44
   open 812.54
  capitellum 812.49
   open 812.59
  condyle(s) 812.44
   lateral (external) 812.42
    open 812.52
   medial (internal epicondyle) 812.43
    open 812.53
    open 812.54
  distal end - *see* Fracture, humerus, lower end

Fracture *(Continued)*
 humerus *(Continued)*
  epiphysis
   lower *(see also* Fracture, humerus, condyle(s)) 812.44
    open 812.54
   upper 812.09
    open 812.19
  external condyle 812.42
   open 812.52
  great tuberosity 812.03
   open 812.13
  head 812.09
   open 812.19
  internal epicondyle 812.43
   open 812.53
  lesser tuberosity 812.09
   open 812.19
  lower end or extremity (distal end) *(see also* Fracture, humerus, by site) 812.40
   multiple sites NEC 812.49
    open 812.59
   open 812.50
   specified site NEC 812.49
    open 812.59
  neck 812.01
   open 812.11
  open 812.30
  pathologic 733.11
  proximal end - *see* Fracture, humerus, upper end
  shaft 812.21
   open 812.31
  supracondylar 812.41
   open 812.51
  surgical neck 812.01
   open 812.11
  trochlea 812.49
   open 812.59
  T-shaped 812.44
   open 812.54
  tuberosity - *see* Fracture, humerus, upper end
  upper end or extremity (proximal end) *(see also* Fracture, humerus, by site) 812.00
   open 812.10
   specified site NEC 812.09
    open 812.19
 hyoid bone (closed) 807.5
  open 807.6
 hyperextension - *see* Fracture, radius, lower end
 ilium (with visceral injury) (closed) 808.41
  open 808.51
 impaction, impacted - *see* Fracture, by site
 incus - *see* Fracture, skull, base
 innominate bone (with visceral injury) (closed) 808.49
  open 808.59
 instep, of one foot (closed) 825.20
  with toe(s) of same foot 827.0
   open 827.1
  open 825.30
 insufficiency - *see* Fracture, pathologic, by site
 internal
  ear - *see* Fracture, skull, base
  semilunar cartilage, knee - *see* Tear, meniscus, medial
 intertrochanteric - *see* Fracture, femur, neck, intertrochanteric
 ischium (with visceral injury) (closed) 808.42
  open 808.52
 jaw (bone) (lower) (closed) *(see also* Fracture, mandible) 802.20
  angle 802.25
   open 802.35
  open 802.30
  upper - *see* Fracture, maxilla

Fracture *(Continued)*
 knee
  cap (closed) 822.0
   open 822.1
  cartilage (semilunar) - *see* Tear, meniscus
 labyrinth (osseous) - *see* Fracture, skull, base
 larynx (closed) 807.5
  open 807.6
 late effect - *see* Late, effects (of), fracture
 Le Fort's - *see* Fracture, maxilla
 leg (closed) 827.0
  with rib(s) or sternum 828.0
   open 828.1
  both (any bones) 828.0
   open 828.1
  lower - *see* Fracture, tibia
   open 827.1
  upper - *see* Fracture, femur
 limb
  lower (multiple) (closed) NEC 827.0
   open 827.1
  upper (multiple) (closed) NEC 818.0
   open 818.1
 long bones, due to birth trauma - *see* Birth injury, fracture
 lumbar - *see* Fracture, vertebra, lumbar
 lunate bone (closed) 814.02
  open 814.12
 malar bone (closed) 802.4
  open 802.5
 Malgaigne's (closed) 808.43
  open 808.53
 malleolus (closed) 824.8
  bimalleolar 824.4
   open 824.5
  lateral 824.2
   and medial - *see also* Fracture, malleolus, bimalleolar
    with lip of tibia - *see* Fracture, malleolus, trimalleolar
   open 824.3
  medial (closed) 824.0
   and lateral - *see also* Fracture, malleolus, bimalleolar
    with lip of tibia - *see* Fracture, malleolus, trimalleolar
   open 824.1
  open 824.9
  trimalleolar (closed) 824.6
   open 824.7
 malleus - *see* Fracture, skull, base
 malunion 733.81
 mandible (closed) 802.20
  angle 802.25
   open 802.35
  body 802.28
   alveolar border 802.27
    open 802.37
   open 802.38
   symphysis 802.26
    open 802.36
  condylar process 802.21
   open 802.31
  coronoid process 802.23
   open 802.33
  multiple sites 802.29
   open 802.39
  open 802.30
  ramus NEC 802.24
   open 802.34
  subcondylar 802.22
   open 802.32
 manubrium - *see* Fracture, sternum
 march 733.95
  femoral neck 733.96
  fibula 733.93
  metatarsals 733.94
  pelvis 733.98
  shaft of femur 733.97
  tibia 733.93

Fracture (*Continued*)
- maxilla, maxillary (superior) (upper jaw) (closed) 802.4
  - inferior - *see* Fracture, mandible
  - open 802.5
- meniscus, knee - *see* Tear, meniscus
- metacarpus, metacarpal (bone(s)), of one hand (closed) 815.00
  - with phalanx, phalanges, hand (finger(s)) (thumb) of same hand 817.0
    - open 817.1
  - base 815.02
    - first metacarpal 815.01
      - open 815.11
    - open 815.12
    - thumb 815.01
      - open 815.11
  - multiple sites 815.09
    - open 815.19
  - neck 815.04
    - open 815.14
  - open 815.10
  - shaft 815.03
    - open 815.13
- metatarsus, metatarsal (bone(s)), of one foot (closed) 825.25
  - with tarsal bone(s) 825.29
    - open 825.39
  - open 825.35
- Monteggia's (closed) 813.03
  - open 813.13
- Moore's - *see* Fracture, radius, lower end
- multangular bone (closed)
  - larger 814.05
    - open 814.15
  - smaller 814.06
    - open 814.16
- multiple (closed) 829.0

> Note: Multiple fractures of sites classifiable to the same three- or four-digit category are coded to that category, except for sites classifiable to 810–818 or 820–827 in different limbs.
>
> Multiple fractures of sites classifiable to different fourth-digit subdivisions within the same three-digit category should be dealt with according to coding rules.
>
> Multiple fractures of sites classifiable to different three-digit categories (identifiable from the listing under "Fracture"), and of sites classifiable to 810–818 or 820–827 in different limbs should be coded according to the following list, which should be referred to in the following priority order: skull or face bones, pelvis or vertebral column, legs, arms.

- arm (multiple bones in same arm except in hand alone) (sites classifiable to 810–817 with sites classifiable to a different three-digit category in 810–817 in same arm) (closed) 818.0
  - open 818.1
- arms, both or arm(s) with rib(s) or sternum (sites classifiable to 810–818 with sites classifiable to same range of categories in other limb or to 807) (closed) 819.0
  - open 819.1
- bones of trunk NEC (closed) 809.0
  - open 809.1
- hand, metacarpal bone(s) with phalanx or phalanges of same hand (sites classifiable to 815 with sites classifiable to 816 in same hand) (closed) 817.0
  - open 817.1

Fracture (*Continued*)
- multiple (*Continued*)
  - leg (multiple bones in same leg) (sites classifiable to 820–826 with sites classifiable to a different three-digit category in that range in same leg) (closed) 827.0
    - open 827.1
  - legs, both or leg(s) with arm(s), rib(s), or sternum (sites classifiable to 820–827 with sites classifiable to same range of categories in other leg or to 807 or 810–819) (closed) 828.0
    - open 828.1
  - open 829.1
  - pelvis with other bones except skull or face bones (sites classifiable to 808 with sites classifiable to 805–807 or 810–829) (closed) 809.0
    - open 809.1
  - skull, specified or unspecified bones, or face bone(s) with any other bone(s) (sites classifiable to 800–803 with sites classifiable to 805–829) (closed) 804.0●

> Note: Use the following fifth-digit subclassification with categories 800, 801, 803, and 804:
>
> 0   unspecified state of consciousness
> 1   with no loss of consciousness
> 2   with brief [less than one hour] loss of consciousness
> 3   with moderate [1–24 hours] loss of consciousness
> 4   with prolonged [more than 24 hours] loss of consciousness and return to pre-existing conscious level
> 5   with prolonged [more than 24 hours] loss of consciousness, without return to pre-existing conscious level
>
> Use fifth-digit 5 to designate when a patient is unconscious and dies before regaining consciousness, regardless of the duration of the loss of consciousness
>
> 6   with loss of consciousness of unspecified duration
> 9   with concussion, unspecified

  - with
    - contusion, cerebral 804.1●
    - epidural hemorrhage 804.2●
    - extradural hemorrhage 804.2●
    - hemorrhage (intracranial) NEC 804.3●
    - intracranial injury NEC 804.4●
    - laceration, cerebral 804.1●
    - subarachnoid hemorrhage 804.2●
    - subdural hemorrhage 804.2●
  - open 804.5●
    - with
      - contusion, cerebral 804.6●
      - epidural hemorrhage 804.7●
      - extradural hemorrhage 804.7●
      - hemorrhage (intracranial) NEC 804.8●
      - intracranial injury NEC 804.9●
      - laceration, cerebral 804.6●
      - subarachnoid hemorrhage 804.7●
      - subdural hemorrhage 804.7●
  - vertebral column with other bones, except skull or face bones (sites classifiable to 805 or 806 with sites classifiable to 807–808 or 810–829) (closed) 809.0
    - open 809.1

Fracture (*Continued*)
- nasal (bone(s)) (closed) 802.0
  - open 802.1
  - sinus - *see* Fracture, skull, base
- navicular
  - carpal (wrist) (closed) 814.01
    - open 814.11
  - tarsal (ankle) (closed) 825.22
    - open 825.32
- neck - *see* Fracture, vertebra, cervical
- neural arch - *see* Fracture, vertebra, by site
- nonunion 733.82
- nose, nasal, (bone) (septum) (closed) 802.0
  - open 802.1
- occiput - *see* Fracture, skull, base
- odontoid process - *see* Fracture, vertebra, cervical
- olecranon (process) (ulna) (closed) 813.01
  - open 813.11
- open 829.1
- orbit, orbital (bone) (region) (closed) 802.8
  - floor (blow-out) 802.6
    - open 802.7
  - open 802.9
  - roof - *see* Fracture, skull, base
  - specified part NEC 802.8
    - open 802.9
- os
  - calcis (closed) 825.0
    - open 825.1
  - magnum (closed) 814.07
    - open 814.17
  - pubis (with visceral injury) (closed) 808.2
    - open 808.3
  - triquetrum (closed) 814.03
    - open 814.13
- osseous
  - auditory meatus - *see* Fracture, skull, base
  - labyrinth - *see* Fracture, skull, base
- ossicles, auditory (incus) (malleus) (stapes) - *see* Fracture, skull, base
- osteoporotic - *see* Fracture, pathologic
- palate (closed) 802.8
  - open 802.9
- paratrooper - *see* Fracture, tibia, lower end
- parietal bone - *see* Fracture, skull, vault
- parry - *see* Fracture, Monteggia's
- patella (closed) 822.0
  - open 822.1
- pathologic (cause unknown) 733.10
  - ankle 733.16
  - femur (neck) 733.14
    - specified NEC 733.15
  - fibula 733.16
  - hip 733.14
  - humerus 733.11
  - radius (distal) 733.12
  - specified site NEC 733.19
  - tibia 733.16
  - ulna 733.12
  - vertebrae (collapse) 733.13
  - wrist 733.12
- pedicle (of vertebral arch) - *see* Fracture, vertebra, by site
- pelvis, pelvic (bone(s)) (with visceral injury) (closed) 808.8
  - multiple
    - with
      - disruption of pelvic circle 808.43
        - open 808.53
      - disruption of pelvic ring 808.43
        - open 808.53
    - without
      - disruption of pelvic circle 808.44
        - open 808.54
      - disruption of pelvic ring 808.44
        - open 808.54
  - open 808.9
  - rim (closed) 808.49
    - open 808.59
  - stress 733.98

◀ New   ◀▥ Revised   ~~deleted~~ Deleted   ● Use Additional Digit(s)   ▒ Omit code

Fracture *(Continued)*
  peritrochanteric (closed) 820.20
    open 820.30
  phalanx, phalanges, of one
    foot (closed) 826.0
      with bone(s) of same lower limb
        827.0
        open 827.1
      open 826.1
    hand (closed) 816.00
      with metacarpal bone(s) of same hand
        817.0
        open 817.1
      distal 816.02
        open 816.12
      middle 816.01
        open 816.11
      multiple sites NEC 816.03
        open 816.13
      open 816.10
      proximal 816.01
        open 816.11
  pisiform (closed) 814.04
    open 814.14
  pond - *see* Fracture, skull, vault
  Pott's (closed) 824.4
    open 824.5
  prosthetic device, internal - *see*
    Complications, mechanical
  pubis (with visceral injury) (closed) 808.2
    open 808.3
  Quervain's (closed) 814.01
    open 814.11
  radius (alone) (closed) 813.81
    with ulna NEC 813.83
      open 813.93
    distal end - *see* Fracture, radius,
      lower end
    epiphysis
      lower - *see* Fracture, radius,
        lower end
      upper - *see* Fracture, radius,
        upper end
    head - *see* Fracture, radius, upper end
    lower end or extremity (distal end)
      (lower epiphysis) 813.42
      with ulna (lower end) 813.44
        open 813.54
      open 813.52
      torus 813.45
        with ulna 813.47
    neck - *see* Fracture, radius, upper end
    open NEC 813.91
    pathologic 733.12
    proximal end - *see* Fracture, radius, upper
      end
    shaft (closed) 813.21
      with ulna (shaft) 813.23
        open 813.33
      open 813.31
    upper end 813.07
      with ulna (upper end) 813.08
        open 813.18
      epiphysis 813.05
        open 813.15
      head 813.05
        open 813.15
      multiple sites 813.07
        open 813.17
      neck 813.06
        open 813.16
      open 813.17
      specified site NEC 813.07
        open 813.17
  ramus
    inferior or superior (with visceral injury)
      (closed) 808.2
      open 808.3
    ischium - *see* Fracture, ischium
    mandible 802.24
      open 802.34

Fracture *(Continued)*
  rib(s) (closed) 807.0●

> Note: Use the following fifth-digit
> subclassification with categories 807.0–807.1:
>
>   0   rib(s), unspecified
>   1   one rib
>   2   two ribs
>   3   three ribs
>   4   four ribs
>   5   five ribs
>   6   six ribs
>   7   seven ribs
>   8   eight or more ribs
>   9   multiple ribs, unspecified

    with flail chest (open) 807.4
      open 807.1●
  root, tooth 873.63
    complicated 873.73
  sacrum - *see* Fracture, vertebra, sacrum
  scaphoid
    ankle (closed) 825.22
      open 825.32
    wrist (closed) 814.01
      open 814.11
  scapula (closed) 811.00
    acromial, acromion (process) 811.01
      open 811.11
    body 811.09
      open 811.19
    coracoid process 811.02
      open 811.12
    glenoid (cavity) (fossa) 811.03
      open 811.13
    neck 811.03
      open 811.13
    open 811.10
  semilunar
    bone, wrist (closed) 814.02
      open 814.12
    cartilage (interior) (knee) - *see* Tear,
      meniscus
  sesamoid bone - *see* Fracture, by site
  Shepherd's (closed) 825.21
    open 825.31
  shoulder - *see also* Fracture, humerus, upper
    end
    blade - *see* Fracture, scapula
  silverfork - *see* Fracture, radius, lower end
  sinus (ethmoid) (frontal) (maxillary) (nasal)
    (sphenoidal) - *see* Fracture, skull, base
  Skillern's - *see* Fracture, radius, shaft
  skull (multiple NEC) (with face bones)
    (closed) 803.0●

> Note: Use the following fifth-digit
> subclassification with categories 800, 801,
> 803, and 804:
>
>   0   unspecified state of consciousness
>   1   with no loss of consciousness
>   2   with brief [less than one hour] loss of
>   consciousness
>   3   with moderate [1-24 hours] loss of
>   consciousness
>   4   with prolonged [more than 24 hours]
>   loss of consciousness and return
>   to pre-existing conscious level
>   5   with prolonged [more than 24 hours]
>   loss of consciousness, without
>   return to pre-existing conscious
>   level
>
> Use fifth-digit 5 to designate when a patient
> is unconscious and dies before regaining
> consciousness, regardless of the duration of
> the loss of consciousness
>
>   6   with loss of consciousness of
>   unspecified duration
>   9   with concussion, unspecified

Fracture *(Continued)*
  skull *(Continued)*
    with
      contusion, cerebral 803.1●
      epidural hemorrhage 803.2●
      extradural hemorrhage 803.2●
      hemorrhage (intracranial) NEC
        803.3●
      intracranial injury NEC 803.4●
      laceration, cerebral 803.1●
      other bones - *see* Fracture, multiple,
        skull
      subarachnoid hemorrhage 803.2●
      subdural hemorrhage 803.2●
    base (antrum) (ethmoid bone) (fossa)
      (internal ear) (nasal sinus) (occiput)
      (sphenoid) (temporal bone) (closed)
      801.0●
      with
        contusion, cerebral 801.1●
        epidural hemorrhage 801.2●
        extradural hemorrhage 801.2●
        hemorrhage (intracranial) NEC
          801.3●
        intracranial injury NEC 801.4●
        laceration, cerebral 801.1●
        subarachnoid hemorrhage 801.2●
        subdural hemorrhage 801.2●
      open 801.5●
        with
          contusion, cerebral 801.6●
          epidural hemorrhage 801.7●
          extradural hemorrhage 801.7●
          hemorrhage (intracranial) NEC
            801.8●
          intracranial injury NEC 801.9●
          laceration, cerebral 801.6●
          subarachnoid hemorrhage
            801.7●
          subdural hemorrhage 801.7●
    birth injury 767.3
    face bones - *see* Fracture, face bones
    open 803.5●
      with
        contusion, cerebral 803.6●
        epidural hemorrhage 803.7●
        extradural hemorrhage 803.7●
        hemorrhage (intracranial) NEC
          803.8●
        intracranial injury NEC 803.9●
        laceration, cerebral 803.6●
        subarachnoid hemorrhage 803.7●
        subdural hemorrhage 803.7●
    vault (frontal bone) (parietal bone)
      (vertex) (closed) 800.0●
      with
        contusion, cerebral 800.1●
        epidural hemorrhage 800.2●
        extradural hemorrhage 800.2●
        hemorrhage (intracranial) NEC
          800.3●
        intracranial injury NEC 800.4●
        laceration, cerebral 800.1●
        subarachnoid hemorrhage 800.2●
        subdural hemorrhage 800.2●
      open 800.5●
        with
          contusion, cerebral 800.6●
          epidural hemorrhage 800.7●
          extradural hemorrhage 800.7●
          hemorrhage (intracranial) NEC
            800.8●
          intracranial injury NEC 800.9●
          laceration, cerebral 800.6●
          subarachnoid hemorrhage
            800.7●
          subdural hemorrhage 800.7●
  Smith's 813.41
    open 813.51
  sphenoid (bone) (sinus) - *see* Fracture, skull,
    base

Fracture (Continued)
  spine - see also Fracture, vertebra, by site due to birth trauma 767.4
  spinous process - see Fracture, vertebra, by site
  spontaneous - see Fracture, pathologic
  sprinters' - see Fracture, ilium
  stapes - see Fracture, skull, base
  stave - see also Fracture, metacarpus, metacarpal bone(s)
    spine - see Fracture, tibia, upper end
  sternum (closed) 807.2
    with flail chest (open) 807.4
    open 807.3
  Stieda's - see Fracture, femur, lower end
  stress 733.95
    femoral neck 733.96
    fibula 733.93
    metatarsals 733.94
    pelvis 733.98
    shaft of femur 733.97
    specified site NEC 733.95
    tibia 733.93
  styloid process
    metacarpal (closed) 815.02
      open 815.12
    radius - see Fracture, radius, lower end
    temporal bone - see Fracture, skull, base
    ulna - see Fracture, ulna, lower end
  supracondylar, elbow 812.41
    open 812.51
  symphysis pubis (with visceral injury) (closed) 808.2
    open 808.3
  talus (ankle bone) (closed) 825.21
    open 825.31
  tarsus, tarsal bone(s) (with metatarsus) of one foot (closed) NEC 825.29
    open 825.39
  temporal bone (styloid) - see Fracture, skull, base
  tendon - see Sprain, by site
  thigh - see Fracture, femur, shaft
  thumb (and finger(s)) of one hand (closed) (see also Fracture, phalanx, hand) 816.00
    with metacarpal bone(s) of same hand 817.0
      open 817.1
    metacarpal(s) - see Fracture, metacarpus
    open 816.10
  thyroid cartilage (closed) 807.5
    open 807.6
  tibia (closed) 823.80
    with fibula 823.82
      open 823.92
    condyles - see Fracture, tibia, upper end
    distal end 824.8
      open 824.9
    epiphysis
      lower 824.8
        open 824.9
      upper - see Fracture, tibia, upper end
    head (involving knee joint) - see Fracture, tibia, upper end
    intercondyloid eminence - see Fracture, tibia, upper end
    involving ankle 824.0
      open 824.1
    lower end or extremity (anterior lip) (posterior lip) 824.8
      open 824.9
    malleolus (internal) (medial) 824.0
      open 824.1
    open NEC 823.90
    pathologic 733.16
    proximal end - see Fracture, tibia, upper end
    shaft 823.20
      with fibula 823.22
        open 823.32
      open 823.30

Fracture (Continued)
  tibia (Continued)
    spine - see Fracture, tibia, upper end
    stress 733.93
    torus 823.40
      with fibula 823.42
    tuberosity - see Fracture, tibia, upper end
    upper end or extremity (condyle) (epiphysis) (head) (spine) (proximal end) (tuberosity) 823.00
      with fibula 823.02
        open 823.12
      open 823.10
  toe(s), of one foot (closed) 826.0
    with bone(s) of same lower limb 827.0
      open 827.1
    open 826.1
  tooth (root) 873.63
    complicated 873.73
  torus
    fibula 823.41
      with tibia 823.42
    humerus 812.49
    radius (alone) 813.45
      with ulna 813.47
    tibia 823.40
      with fibula 823.42
    ulna (alone) 813.46
      with radius 813.47
  trachea (closed) 807.5
    open 807.6
  transverse process - see Fracture, vertebra, by site
  trapezium (closed) 814.05
    open 814.15
  trapezoid bone (closed) 814.06
    open 814.16
  trimalleolar (closed) 824.6
    open 824.7
  triquetral (bone) (closed) 814.03
    open 814.13
  trochanter (greater) (lesser) (closed) (see also Fracture, femur, neck, by site) 820.20
    open 820.30
  trunk (bones) (closed) 809.0
    open 809.1
  tuberosity (external) - see Fracture, by site
  ulna (alone) (closed) 813.82
    with radius NEC 813.83
      open 813.93
    coronoid process (closed) 813.02
      open 813.12
    distal end - see Fracture, ulna, lower end
    epiphysis
      lower - see Fracture, ulna, lower end
      upper - see Fracture, ulna, upper, end
    head - see Fracture, ulna, lower end
    lower end (distal end) (head) (lower epiphysis) (styloid process) 813.43
      with radius (lower end) 813.44
        open 813.54
      open 813.53
    olecranon process (closed) 813.01
      open 813.11
    open NEC 813.92
    pathologic 733.12
    proximal end - see Fracture, ulna, upper end
    shaft 813.22
      with radius (shaft) 813.23
        open 813.33
      open 813.32
    styloid process - see Fracture, ulna, lower end
    torus 813.46
      with radius 813.47
    transverse - see Fracture, ulna, by site

Fracture (Continued)
  ulna (Continued)
    upper end (epiphysis) 813.04
      with radius (upper end) 813.08
        open 813.18
      multiple sites 813.04
        open 813.14
      open 813.14
      specified site NEC 813.04
        open 813.14
  unciform (closed) 814.08
    open 814.18
  vertebra, vertebral (back) (body) (column) (neural arch) (pedicle) (spine) (spinous process) (transverse process) (closed) 805.8
    with
      hematomyelia - see Fracture, vertebra, by site, with spinal cord injury
      injury to
        cauda equina - see Fracture, vertebra, sacrum, with spinal cord injury
        nerve - see Fracture, vertebra, by site, with spinal cord injury
      paralysis - see Fracture, vertebra, by site, with spinal cord injury
      paraplegia - see Fracture, vertebra, by site, with spinal cord injury
      quadriplegia - see Fracture, vertebra, by site, with spinal cord injury
      spinal concussion - see Fracture, vertebra, by site, with spinal cord injury
      spinal cord injury (closed) NEC 806.8

> Note: Use the following fifth-digit subclassification with categories 806.0–806.3:
>
> C_1–C_4 or unspecified level and D_1–D_6 (T_1–T_6) or unspecified level with:
>
> 0   unspecified spinal cord injury
> 1   complete lesion of cord
> 2   anterior cord syndrome
> 3   central cord syndrome
> 4   specified injury NEC
>
> level and D_1–D_{12} level with:
>
> 5   unspecified spinal cord injury
> 6   complete lesion of cord
> 7   anterior cord syndrome
> 8   central cord syndrome
> 9   specified injury NEC

        cervical 806.0●
          open 806.1●
        chronic 733.13
        dorsal, dorsolumbar 806.2●
          open 806.3●
        open 806.9
        thoracic, thoracolumbar 806.2●
          open 806.3●
    atlanto-axial - see Fracture, vertebra, cervical
    cervical (hangman) (teardrop) (closed) 805.00
      with spinal cord injury - see Fracture, vertebra, with spinal cord injury, cervical
      first (atlas) 805.01
        open 805.11
      second (axis) 805.02
        open 805.12
      third 805.03
        open 805.13
      fourth 805.04
        open 805.14
      fifth 805.05
        open 805.15
      sixth 805.06
        open 805.16

◀ New   ◀▬ Revised   ~~deleted~~ Deleted   ● Use Additional Digit(s)   ▨ Omit code

Fracture *(Continued)*
  vertebra, vertebral *(Continued)*
    cervical *(Continued)*
      seventh 805.07
        open 805.17
      multiple sites 805.08
        open 805.18
      open 805.10
    coccyx (closed) 805.6
      with spinal cord injury (closed) 806.60
        cauda equina injury 806.62
          complete lesion 806.61
            open 806.71
          open 806.72
        open 806.70
          specified type NEC 806.69
      open 806.79
      open 805.7
    collapsed 733.13
    compression, not due to trauma 733.13
    dorsal (closed) 805.2
      with spinal cord injury - *see* Fracture,
        vertebra, with spinal cord injury,
        dorsal
      open 805.3
    dorsolumbar (closed) 805.2
      with spinal cord injury - *see* Fracture,
        vertebra, with spinal cord injury,
        dorsal
      open 805.3
    due to osteoporosis 733.13
    fetus or newborn 767.4
    lumbar (closed) 805.4
      with spinal cord injury (closed) 806.4
        open 806.5
      open 805.5
    nontraumatic 733.13
    open NEC 805.9
    pathologic (any site) 733.13
    sacrum (closed) 805.6
      with spinal cord injury 806.60
        cauda equina injury 806.62
          complete lesion 806.61
            open 806.71
          open 806.72
        open 806.70
          specified type NEC 806.69
            open 806.79
      open 805.7
    site unspecified (closed) 805.8
      with spinal cord injury (closed) 806.8
        open 806.9
      open 805.9
    stress (any site) 733.95
    thoracic (closed) 805.2
      with spinal cord injury - *see* Fracture,
        vertebra, with spinal cord injury,
        thoracic
      open 805.3
  vertex - *see* Fracture, skull, vault
  vomer (bone) 802.0
    open 802.1
  Wagstaffe's - *see* Fracture, ankle
  wrist (closed) 814.00
    open 814.10
    pathologic 733.12
  xiphoid (process) - *see* Fracture, sternum
  zygoma (zygomatic arch) (closed) 802.4
    open 802.5
Fragile X syndrome 759.83
Fragilitas
  crinium 704.2
  hair 704.2
  ossium 756.51
    with blue sclera 756.51
  unguium 703.8
    congenital 757.5
Fragility
  bone 756.51
    with deafness and blue sclera 756.51
  capillary (hereditary) 287.8

Fragility *(Continued)*
  hair 704.2
  nails 703.8
Fragmentation - *see* Fracture, by site
Frailty 797
Frambesia, frambesial (tropica) (*see also* Yaws)
    102.9
  initial lesion or ulcer 102.0
  primary 102.0
Frambeside
  gummatous 102.4
  of early yaws 102.2
Frambesioma 102.1
Franceschetti's syndrome (mandibulofacial
    dysostosis) 756.0
Francis' disease (*see also* Tularemia) 021.9
Frank's essential thrombocytopenia (*see also*
    Purpura, thrombocytopenic) 287.39
Franklin's disease (heavy chain) 273.2
Fraser's syndrome 759.89
Freckle 709.09
  malignant melanoma in (M8742/3) - *see*
    Melanoma
  melanotic (of Hutchinson) (M8742/2) - *see*
    Neoplasm, skin, in situ
  retinal 239.81
Freeman-Sheldon syndrome 759.89
Freezing 991.9
  specified effect NEC 991.8
Frei's disease (climatic bubo) 099.1
Freiberg's
  disease (osteochondrosis, second metatarsal)
    732.5
  infraction of metatarsal head 732.5
  osteochondrosis 732.5
Fremitus, friction, cardiac 785.3
Frenulum linguae 750.0
Frenum
  external os 752.44
  tongue 750.0
Frequency (urinary) NEC 788.41
  micturition 788.41
  nocturnal 788.43
  polyuria 788.42
  psychogenic 306.53
Frey's syndrome (auriculotemporal syndrome)
    705.22
Friction
  burn (*see also* Injury, superficial, by site)
    919.0
  fremitus, cardiac 785.3
  precordial 785.3
  sounds, chest 786.7
Friderichsen-Waterhouse syndrome or disease
    036.3
Friedländer's
  B (bacillus) NEC (*see also* condition) 041.3
    sepsis or septicemia 038.49
  disease (endarteritis obliterans) - *see*
    Arteriosclerosis
Friedreich's
  ataxia 334.0
  combined systemic disease 334.0
  disease 333.2
    combined systemic 334.0
  myoclonia 333.2
  sclerosis (spinal cord) 334.0
Friedrich-Erb-Arnold syndrome
    (acropachyderma) 757.39
Frigidity 302.72
  psychic or psychogenic 302.72
Fröhlich's disease or syndrome (adiposogenital
    dystrophy) 253.8
Froin's syndrome 336.8
Frommel's disease 676.6●
Frommel-Chiari syndrome 676.6●
Frontal - *see also* condition
  lobe syndrome 310.0
Frostbite 991.3
  face 991.0
  foot 991.2

Frostbite *(Continued)*
  hand 991.1
  specified site NEC 991.3
Frotteurism 302.89
Frozen 991.9
  pelvis 620.8
  shoulder 726.0
Fructosemia 271.2
Fructosuria (benign) (essential) 271.2
Fuchs'
  black spot (myopic) 360.21
  corneal dystrophy (endothelial) 371.57
  heterochromic cyclitis 364.21
Fucosidosis 271.8
Fugue 780.99
  dissociative 300.13
  hysterical (dissociative) 300.13
  reaction to exceptional stress (transient) 308.1
Fukuhara syndrome 277.87
Fuller Albright's syndrome (osteitis fibrosa
    disseminata) 756.59
Fuller's earth disease 502
Fulminant, fulminating - *see* condition
Functional - *see* condition
Functioning
  borderline intellectual V62.89
Fundus - *see also* condition
  flavimaculatus 362.76
Fungemia 117.9
Fungus, fungous
  cerebral 348.89
  disease NEC 117.9
  infection - *see* Infection, fungus
  testis (*see also* Tuberculosis) 016.5● [608.81]
Funiculitis (acute) 608.4
  chronic 608.4
  endemic 608.4
  gonococcal (acute) 098.14
    chronic or duration of 2 months or over
      098.34
  tuberculous (*see also* Tuberculosis) 016.5●
FUO (*see also* Pyrexia) 780.60
Funnel
  breast (acquired) 738.3
    congenital 754.81
    late effect of rickets 268.1
  chest (acquired) 738.3
    congenital 754.81
    late effect of rickets 268.1
  pelvis (acquired) 738.6
    with disproportion (fetopelvic) 653.3●
      affecting fetus or newborn 763.1
      causing obstructed labor 660.1●
        affecting fetus or newborn 763.1
    congenital 755.69
    tuberculous (*see also* Tuberculosis) 016.9●
Furfur 690.18
  microsporon 111.0
Furor, paroxysmal (idiopathic) (*see also*
    Epilepsy) 345.8●
Furriers' lung 495.8
Furrowed tongue 529.5
  congenital 750.13
Furrowing nail(s) (transverse) 703.8
  congenital 757.5
Furuncle 680.9
  abdominal wall 680.2
  ankle 680.6
  anus 680.5
  arm (any part, above wrist) 680.3
  auditory canal, external 680.0
  axilla 680.3
  back (any part) 680.2
  breast 680.2
  buttock 680.5
  chest wall 680.2
  corpus cavernosum 607.2
  ear (any part) 680.0
  eyelid 373.13
  face (any part, except eye) 680.0
  finger (any) 680.4

Furuncle (Continued)
  flank 680.2
  foot (any part) 680.7
  forearm 680.3
  gluteal (region) 680.5
  groin 680.2
  hand (any part) 680.4
  head (any part, except face) 680.8
  heel 680.7
  hip 680.6
  kidney (see also Abscess, kidney) 590.2
  knee 680.6
  labium (majus) (minus) 616.4
  lacrimal
    gland (see also Dacryoadenitis) 375.00
    passages (duct) (sac) (see also
      Dacryocystitis) 375.30
  leg, any part except foot 680.6
  malignant 022.0
  multiple sites 680.9
  neck 680.1
  nose (external) (septum) 680.0
  orbit 376.01
  partes posteriores 680.5
  pectoral region 680.2
  penis 607.2
  perineum 680.2
  pinna 680.0
  scalp (any part) 680.8
  scrotum 608.4
  seminal vesicle 608.0
  shoulder 680.3
  skin NEC 680.9
  specified site NEC 680.8
  spermatic cord 608.4
  temple (region) 680.0
  testis 604.90
  thigh 680.6
  thumb 680.4
  toe (any) 680.7
  trunk 680.2

Furuncle (Continued)
  tunica vaginalis 608.4
  umbilicus 680.2
  upper arm 680.3
  vas deferens 608.4
  vulva 616.4
  wrist 680.4
Furunculosis (see also Furuncle) 680.9
  external auditory meatus 680.0 [380.13]
Fusarium (infection) 118
Fusion, fused (congenital)
  anal (with urogenital canal) 751.5
  aorta and pulmonary artery 745.0
  astragaloscaphoid 755.67
  atria 745.5
  atrium and ventricle 745.69
  auditory canal 744.02
  auricles, heart 745.5
  binocular, with defective stereopsis 368.33
  bone 756.9
  cervical spine - see Fusion, spine
  choanal 748.0
  commissure, mitral valve 746.5
  cranial sutures, premature 756.0
  cusps, heart valve NEC 746.89
    mitral 746.5
    tricuspid 746.89
  ear ossicles 744.04
  fingers (see also Syndactylism, fingers) 755.11
  hymen 752.42
  hymeno-urethral 599.89
    causing obstructed labor 660.1●
      affecting fetus or newborn 763.1
  joint (acquired) - see also Ankylosis
    congenital 755.8
  kidneys (incomplete) 753.3
  labium (majus) (minus) 752.49
  larynx and trachea 748.3
  limb 755.8
    lower 755.69
    upper 755.59

Fusion, fused (Continued)
  lobe, lung 748.5
  lumbosacral (acquired) 724.6
    congenital 756.15
    surgical V45.4
  nares (anterior) (posterior) 748.0
  nose, nasal 748.0
  nostril(s) 748.0
  organ or site NEC - see Anomaly, specified
    type NEC
  ossicles 756.9
    auditory 744.04
  pulmonary valve segment 746.02
  pulmonic cusps 746.02
  ribs 756.3
  sacroiliac (acquired) (joint) 724.6
    congenital 755.69
    surgical V45.4
  skull, imperfect 756.0
  spine (acquired) 724.9
    arthrodesis status V45.4
    congenital (vertebra) 756.15
    postoperative status V45.4
  sublingual duct with submaxillary duct at
    opening in mouth 750.26
  talonavicular (bar) 755.67
  teeth, tooth 520.2
  testes 752.89
  toes (see also Syndactylism, toes) 755.13
  trachea and esophagus 750.3
  twins 759.4
  urethral-hymenal 599.89
  vagina 752.49
  valve cusps - see Fusion, cusps,
    heart valve
  ventricles, heart 745.4
  vertebra (arch) - see Fusion, spine
  vulva 752.49
Fusospirillosis (mouth) (tongue) (tonsil)
  101
Fussy infant (baby) 780.91

◀ New   ◀▥ Revised   ~~deleted~~ Deleted   ● Use Additional Digit(s)   Omit code

G

Gafsa boil 085.1
Gain, weight (abnormal) (excessive) (see also
  Weight, gain) 783.1
Gaisböck's disease or syndrome (polycythemia
  hypertonica) 289.0
Gait
  abnormality 781.2
    hysterical 300.11
  ataxic 781.2
    hysterical 300.11
  disturbance 781.2
    hysterical 300.11
  paralytic 781.2
  scissor 781.2
  spastic 781.2
  staggering 781.2
    hysterical 300.11
Galactocele (breast) (infected) 611.5
  puerperal, postpartum 676.8●
Galactophoritis 611.0
  puerperal, postpartum 675.2●
Galactorrhea 676.6●
  not associated with childbirth 611.6
Galactosemia (classic) (congenital) 271.1
Galactosuria 271.1
Galacturia 791.1
  bilharziasis 120.0
Galen's vein - see condition
Gallbladder - see also condition
  acute (see also Disease, gallbladder) 575.0
Gall duct - see condition
Gallop rhythm 427.89
Gallstone (cholemic) (colic) (impacted) - see also
  Cholelithiasis
  causing intestinal obstruction 560.31
Gambling, pathological 312.31
Gammaloidosis 277.39
Gammopathy 273.9
  macroglobulinemia 273.3
  monoclonal (benign) (essential) (idiopathic)
    (with lymphoplasmacytic dyscrasia)
    273.1
Gamna's disease (siderotic splenomegaly)
  289.51
Gampsodactylia (congenital) 754.71
Gamstorp's disease (adynamia episodica
  hereditaria) 359.3
Gandy-Nanta disease (siderotic splenomegaly)
  289.51
Gang activity, without manifest psychiatric
  disorder V71.09
  adolescent V71.02
  adult V71.01
  child V71.02
Gangliocytoma (M9490/0) - see Neoplasm,
  connective tissue, benign
Ganglioglioma (M9505/1) - see Neoplasm, by
  site, uncertain behavior
Ganglion 727.43
  joint 727.41
  of yaws (early) (late) 102.6
  periosteal (see also Periostitis) 730.3●
  tendon sheath (compound) (diffuse) 727.42
  tuberculous (see also Tuberculosis) 015.9●
Ganglioneuroblastoma (M9490/3) - see
  Neoplasm, connective tissue, malignant
Ganglioneuroma (M9490/0) - see also
  Neoplasm, connective tissue, benign
  malignant (M9490/3) - see Neoplasm,
    connective tissue, malignant
Ganglioneuromatosis (M9491/0) - see
  Neoplasm, connective tissue, benign
Ganglionitis
  fifth nerve (see also Neuralgia, trigeminal)
    350.1
  gasserian 350.1
  geniculate 351.1
    herpetic 053.11
    newborn 767.5

Ganglionitis (Continued)
  herpes zoster 053.11
  herpetic geniculate (Hunt's syndrome) 053.11
Gangliosidosis 330.1
Gangosa 102.5
Gangrene, gangrenous (anemia) (artery)
  (cellulitis) (dermatitis) (dry) (infective)
  (moist) (pemphigus) (septic) (skin) (stasis)
  (ulcer) 785.4
  with
    arteriosclerosis (native artery) 440.24
      bypass graft 440.30
        autologous vein 440.31
        nonautologous biological 440.32
    diabetes (mellitus) 250.7● [785.4]
      due to secondary diabetes 249.7●
        [785.4]
  abdomen (wall) 785.4
  adenitis 683
  alveolar 526.5
  angina 462
    diphtheritic 032.0
  anus 569.49
  appendices epiploicae - see Gangrene,
    mesentery
  appendix - see Appendicitis, acute
  arteriosclerotic - see Arteriosclerosis, with,
    gangrene
  auricle 785.4
  Bacillus welchii (see also Gangrene, gas) 040.0
  bile duct (see also Cholangitis) 576.8
  bladder 595.89
  bowel - see Gangrene, intestine
  cecum - see Gangrene, intestine
  Clostridium perfringens or welchii (see also
    Gangrene, gas) 040.0
  colon - see Gangrene, intestine
  connective tissue 785.4
  cornea 371.40
  corpora cavernosa (infective) 607.2
    noninfective 607.89
  cutaneous, spreading 785.4
  decubital (see also Ulcer, pressure) 707.00
    [785.4]
  diabetic (any site) 250.7● [785.4]
    due to secondary diabetes 249.7● [785.4]
  dropsical 785.4
  emphysematous (see also Gangrene, gas)
    040.0
  epidemic (ergotized grain) 988.2
  epididymis (infectional) (see also
    Epididymitis) 604.99
  erysipelas (see also Erysipelas) 035
  extremity (lower) (upper) 785.4
  gallbladder or duct (see also Cholecystitis,
    acute) 575.0
  gas (bacillus) 040.0
    with
      abortion - see Abortion, by type, with
        sepsis
      ectopic pregnancy (see also categories
        633.0–633.9) 639.0
      molar pregnancy (see also categories
        630–632) 639.0
    following
      abortion 639.0
      ectopic or molar pregnancy 639.0
    puerperal, postpartum, childbirth 670.8●
  glossitis 529.0
  gum 523.8
  hernia - see Hernia, by site, with gangrene
  hospital noma 528.1
  intestine, intestinal (acute) (hemorrhagic)
    (massive) 557.0
    with
      hernia - see Hernia, by site, with
        gangrene
      mesenteric embolism or infarction
        557.0
      obstruction (see also Obstruction,
        intestine) 560.9

Gangrene, gangrenous (Continued)
  laryngitis 464.00
    with obstruction 464.01
  liver 573.8
  lung 513.0
    spirochetal 104.8
  lymphangitis 457.2
  Meleney's (cutaneous) 686.09
  mesentery 557.0
    with
      embolism or infarction 557.0
      intestinal obstruction (see also
        Obstruction, intestine) 560.9
  mouth 528.1
  noma 528.1
  orchitis 604.90
  ovary (see also Salpingo-oophoritis) 614.2
  pancreas 577.0
  penis (infectional) 607.2
    noninfective 607.89
  perineum 785.4
  pharynx 462
    septic 034.0
  pneumonia 513.0
  Pott's 440.24
  presenile 443.1
  pulmonary 513.0
  pulp, tooth 522.1
  quinsy 475
  Raynaud's (symmetric gangrene) 443.0
    [785.4]
  rectum 569.49
  retropharyngeal 478.24
  rupture - see Hernia, by site, with gangrene
  scrotum 608.4
    noninfective 608.83
  senile 440.24
  sore throat 462
  spermatic cord 608.4
    noninfective 608.89
  spine 785.4
  spirochetal NEC 104.8
  spreading cutaneous 785.4
  stomach 537.89
  stomatitis 528.1
  symmetrical 443.0 [785.4]
  testis (infectional) (see also Orchitis)
    604.99
    noninfective 608.89
  throat 462
    diphtheritic 032.0
  thyroid (gland) 246.8
  tonsillitis (acute) 463
  tooth (pulp) 522.1
  tuberculous NEC (see also Tuberculosis)
    011.9●
  tunica vaginalis 608.4
    noninfective 608.89
  umbilicus 785.4
  uterus (see also Endometritis) 615.9
  uvulitis 528.3
  vas deferens 608.4
    noninfective 608.89
  vulva (see also Vulvitis) 616.10
Gannister disease (occupational) 502
  with tuberculosis - see Tuberculosis,
    pulmonary
Ganser's syndrome, hysterical 300.16
Gardner-Diamond syndrome (autoerythrocyte
  sensitization) 287.2
Gargoylism 277.5
Garré's
  disease (see also Osteomyelitis) 730.1●
  osteitis (sclerosing) (see also Osteomyelitis)
    730.1●
  osteomyelitis (see also Osteomyelitis)
    730.1●
Garrod's pads, knuckle 728.79
Gartner's duct
  cyst 752.41
  persistent 752.41

Gas 787.3
  asphyxia, asphyxiation, inhalation,
     poisoning, suffocation NEC 987.9
    specified gas - *see* Table of Drugs and
      Chemicals
  bacillus gangrene or infection - *see* Gas,
    gangrene
  cyst, mesentery 568.89
  excessive 787.3
  gangrene 040.0
    with
      abortion - *see* Abortion, by type, with
        sepsis
      ectopic pregnancy (*see also* categories
        633.0–633.9) 639.0
      molar pregnancy (*see also* categories
        630–632) 639.0
    following
      abortion 639.0
      ectopic or molar pregnancy 639.0
    puerperal, postpartum, childbirth
      670.8●
  on stomach 787.3
  pains 787.3
Gastradenitis 535.0●
Gastralgia 536.8
  psychogenic 307.89
Gastrectasis, gastrectasia 536.1
  psychogenic 306.4
Gastric - *see* condition
Gastrinoma (M8153/1)
  malignant (M8153/3)
    pancreas 157.4
    specified site NEC - *see* Neoplasm, by site,
      malignant
    unspecified site 157.4
  specified site - *see* Neoplasm, by site,
    uncertain behavior
  unspecified site 235.5
Gastritis 535.5●

> Note: Use the following fifth-digit
> subclassification for category 535:
>
>   0   without mention of hemorrhage
>   1   with hemorrhage

  acute 535.0●
  alcoholic 535.3●
  allergic 535.4●
  antral 535.4●
  atrophic 535.1●
  atrophic-hyperplastic 535.1●
  bile-induced 535.4●
  catarrhal 535.0●
  chronic (atrophic) 535.1●
  cirrhotic 535.4●
  corrosive (acute) 535.4●
  dietetic 535.4●
  due to diet deficiency 269.9 [535.4]●
  eosinophilic 535.7●
  erosive 535.4●
  follicular 535.4●
    chronic 535.1●
  giant hypertrophic 535.2●
  glandular 535.4●
    chronic 535.1●
  hypertrophic (mucosa) 535.2●
    chronic giant 211.1
  irritant 535.4●
  nervous 306.4
  phlegmonous 535.0●
  psychogenic 306.4
  sclerotic 535.4●
  spastic 536.8
  subacute 535.0●
  superficial 535.4●
  suppurative 535.0●
  toxic 535.4●
  tuberculous (*see also* Tuberculosis) 017.9●
Gastrocarcinoma (M8010/3) 151.9
Gastrocolic - *see* condition

Gastrocolitis - *see* Enteritis
Gastrodisciasis 121.8
Gastroduodenitis (*see also* Gastritis) 535.5●
  catarrhal 535.0●
  infectional 535.0●
  virus, viral 008.8
    specified type NEC 008.69
Gastrodynia 536.8
Gastroenteritis (acute) (catarrhal) (congestive)
  (hemorrhagic) (noninfectious) (*see also*
  Enteritis) 558.9
  aertrycke infection 003.0
  allergic 558.3
  chronic 558.9
    ulcerative (*see also* Colitis, ulcerative)
      556.9
  dietetic 558.9
  due to
    antineoplastic chemotherapy 558.9
    food poisoning (*see also* Poisoning, food)
      005.9
    radiation 558.1
  eosinophilic 558.41
  epidemic 009.0
  functional 558.9
  infectious (*see also* Enteritis, due to, by
    organism) 009.0
    presumed 009.1
  salmonella 003.0
  septic (*see also* Enteritis, due to, by organism)
    009.0
  toxic 558.2
  tuberculous (*see also* Tuberculosis) 014.8●
  ulcerative (*see also* Colitis, ulcerative) 556.9
  viral NEC 008.8
    specified type NEC 008.69
  zymotic 009.0
Gastroenterocolitis - *see* Enteritis
Gastroenteropathy, protein-losing 579.8
Gastroenteroptosis 569.89
Gastroesophageal laceration-hemorrhage
  syndrome 530.7
Gastroesophagitis 530.19
Gastrohepatitis (*see also* Gastritis) 535.5●
Gastrointestinal - *see* condition
Gastrojejunal - *see* condition
Gastrojejunitis (*see also* Gastritis) 535.5●
Gastrojejunocolic - *see* condition
Gastroliths 537.89
Gastromalacia 537.89
Gastroparalysis 536.3
  diabetic 250.6● [536.3]
    due to secondary diabetes 249.6●
      [536.3]
Gastroparesis 536.3
  diabetic 250.6● [536.3]
    due to secondary diabetes 249.6●
      [536.3]
Gastropathy 537.9
  congestive portal 537.89
  erythematous 535.5●
  exudative 579.8
  portal hypertensive 537.89
Gastroptosis 537.5
Gastrorrhagia 578.0
Gastrorrhea 536.8
  psychogenic 306.4
Gastroschisis (congenital) 756.73
  acquired 569.89
Gastrospasm (neurogenic) (reflex) 536.8
  neurotic 306.4
  psychogenic 306.4
Gastrostaxis 578.0
Gastrostenosis 537.89
Gastrostomy
  attention to V55.1
  complication 536.40
    specified type 536.49
  infection 536.41
  malfunctioning 536.42
  status V44.1

Gastrosuccorrhea (continuous) (intermittent)
  536.8
  neurotic 306.4
  psychogenic 306.4
Gaucher's
  disease (adult) (cerebroside lipidosis)
    (infantile) 272.7
  hepatomegaly 272.7
  splenomegaly (cerebroside lipidosis) 272.7
GAVE (gastric antral vascular ectasia) 537.82
  with hemorrhage 537.83
  without hemorrhage 537.82
Gayet's disease (superior hemorrhagic
  polioencephalitis) 265.1
Gayet-Wernicke's syndrome (superior
  hemorrhagic polioencephalitis) 265.1
Gee (-Herter) (-Heubner) (-Thaysen) disease or
  syndrome (nontropical sprue) 579.0
Gélineau's syndrome (*see also* Narcolepsy)
  347.00
Gemination, teeth 520.2
Gemistocytoma (M9411/3)
  specified site - *see* Neoplasm, by site,
    malignant
  unspecified site 191.9
General, generalized - *see* condition
Genetic
  susceptibility to
    MEN (multiple endocrine neoplasia)
      V84.81
    neoplasia
      multiple endocrine (MEN) V84.81
    neoplasm
      malignant, of
        breast V84.01
        endometrium V84.04
        other V84.09
        ovary V84.02
        prostate V84.03
    specified disease NEC V84.89
Genital - *see* condition
  warts 078.11
Genito-anorectal syndrome 099.1
Genitourinary system - *see* condition
Genu
  congenital 755.64
  extrorsum (acquired) 736.42
    congenital 755.64
    late effects of rickets 268.1
  introrsum (acquired) 736.41
    congenital 755.64
    late effects of rickets 268.1
  rachitic (old) 268.1
  recurvatum (acquired) 736.5
    congenital 754.40
      with dislocation of knee 754.41
    late effects of rickets 268.1
  valgum (acquired) (knock-knee) 736.41
    congenital 755.64
    late effects of rickets 268.1
  varum (acquired) (bowleg) 736.42
    congenital 755.64
    late effect of rickets 268.1
Geographic tongue 529.1
Geophagia 307.52
Geotrichosis 117.9
  intestine 117.9
  lung 117.9
  mouth 117.9
Gephyrophobia 300.29
Gerbode defect 745.4
GERD (gastroesophageal reflux disease)
  530.81
Gerhardt's
  disease (erythromelalgia) 443.82
  syndrome (vocal cord paralysis) 478.30
Gerlier's disease (epidemic vertigo) 078.81
German measles 056.9
  exposure to V01.4
Germinoblastoma (diffuse) (M9614/3) 202.8●
  follicular (M9692/3) 202.0●

◀ New   ◀▥ Revised   ~~deleted~~ Deleted   ● Use Additional Digit(s)   ▨ Omit code

Germinoma (M9064/3) - *see* Neoplasm, by site, malignant
Gerontoxon 371.41
Gerstmann-Sträussler-Scheinker syndrome (GSS) 046.71
Gerstmann's syndrome (finger agnosia) 784.69
Gestation (period) - *see also* Pregnancy
  ectopic NEC (*see also* Pregnancy, ectopic) 633.90
    with intrauterine pregnancy 633.91
  multiple
    placenta status
      quadruplet
        two or more monoamniotic fetuses V91.22
        two or more monochorionic fetuses V91.21
        unable to determine number of placenta and number of amniotic sacs V91.29
        unspecified number of placenta and unspecified number of amniotic sacs V91.20
      specified (greater than quadruplets) NEC
        two or more monoamniotic fetuses V91.92
        two or more monochorionic fetuses V91.91
        unable to determine number of placenta and number of amniotic sacs V91.99
        unspecified number of placenta and unspecified number of amniotic sacs V91.90
      triplet
        two or more monoamniotic fetuses V91.12
        two or more monochorionic fetuses V91.11
        unable to determine number of placenta and number of amniotic sacs V91.19
        unspecified number of placenta, unspecified number of amniotic sacs V91.10
      twin
        dichorionic/diamniotic (two placentae, two amniotic sacs) V91.03
        monochorionic/diamniotic (one placenta, two amniotic sacs) V91.02
        monochorionic/monoamniotic (one placenta, one amniotic sac) V91.01
        unable to determine number of placenta and number of amniotic sacs V91.09
        unspecified number of placenta, unspecified number of amniotic sacs V91.00
Gestational proteinuria 646.2●
  with hypertension - *see* Toxemia, of pregnancy
Ghon tubercle primary infection (*see also* Tuberculosis) 010.0●
Ghost
  teeth 520.4
  vessels, cornea 370.64
Ghoul hand 102.3
Gianotti Crosti syndrome 057.8
  due to known virus - *see* Infection, virus
  due to unknown virus 057.8
Giant
  cell
    epulis 523.8
    peripheral (gingiva) 523.8
    tumor, tendon sheath 727.02
  colon (congenital) 751.3
  esophagus (congenital) 750.4

Giant (*Continued*)
  kidney 753.3
  urticaria 995.1
    hereditary 277.6
Giardia lamblia infestation 007.1
Giardiasis 007.1
Gibert's disease (pityriasis rosea) 696.3
Gibraltar fever - *see* Brucellosis
Giddiness 780.4
  hysterical 300.11
  psychogenic 306.9
Gierke's disease (glycogenosis I) 271.0
Gigantism (cerebral) (hypophyseal) (pituitary) 253.0
Gilbert's disease or cholemia (familial nonhemolytic jaundice) 277.4
Gilchrist's disease (North American blastomycosis) 116.0
Gilford (-Hutchinson) disease or syndrome (progeria) 259.8
Gilles de la Tourette's disease (motor-verbal tic) 307.23
Gillespie's syndrome (dysplasia oculodentodigitalis) 759.89
Gingivitis 523.10
  acute 523.00
    necrotizing 101
    non-plaque induced 523.01
    plaque induced 523.00
  catarrhal 523.00
  chronic 523.10
    non-plaque induced 523.11
  desquamative 523.10
  expulsiva 523.40
  hyperplastic 523.10
  marginal, simple 523.10
  necrotizing, acute 101
  non-plaque induced 523.11
  pellagrous 265.2
  plaque induced 523.10
  ulcerative 523.10
    acute necrotizing 101
  Vincent's 101
Gingivoglossitis 529.0
Gingivopericementitis 523.40
Gingivosis 523.10
Gingivostomatitis 523.10
  herpetic 054.2
Giovannini's disease 117.9
GISA (glycopeptide intermediate staphylococcus aureus) V09.8
Gland, glandular - *see* condition
Glanders 024
Glanzmann (-Naegeli) disease or thrombasthenia 287.1
Glassblowers' disease 527.1
Glaucoma (capsular) (inflammatory) (noninflammatory) (primary) 365.9
  with increased episcleral venous pressure 365.82
  absolute 360.42
  acute 365.22
    narrow angle 365.22
    secondary 365.60
  angle closure 365.20
    acute 365.22
    attack 365.22
    chronic 365.23
    crisis 365.22
    intermittent 365.21
    interval 365.21
    primary 365.20
      chronic 365.23
    residual stage 365.24
    subacute 365.21
  angle recession 365.65
  borderline 365.00
  chronic 365.11
    noncongestive 365.11
    open angle 365.11
    simple 365.11

Glaucoma (*Continued*)
  closed angle - *see* Glaucoma, angle closure
  congenital 743.20
    associated with other eye anomalies 743.22
    simple 743.21
  congestive - *see* Glaucoma, narrow angle
  corticosteroid-induced (glaucomatous stage) 365.31
    residual stage 365.32
  exfoliation 365.52
  hemorrhagic 365.60
  hypersecretion 365.81
  in or with
    aniridia 365.42
    Axenfeld's anomaly 365.41
    congenital syndromes NEC 759.89 [365.44]
    disorder of lens NEC 365.59
    inflammation, ocular 365.62
    iris
      anomalies NEC 365.42
      atrophy, essential 365.42
      bombé 365.61
    microcornea 365.43
    neurofibromatosis 237.71 [365.44]
    ocular
      cysts NEC 365.64
      disorders NEC 365.60
      trauma 365.65
      tumors NEC 365.64
    pupillary block or seclusion 365.61
    Rieger's anomaly or syndrome 365.41
    seclusion of pupil 365.61
    Sturge-Weber (-Dimitri) syndrome 759.6 [365.44]
    systemic syndrome NEC 365.44
    tumor of globe 365.64
    vascular disorders NEC 365.63
  infantile 365.14
    congenital 743.20
      associated with other eye anomalies 743.22
      simple 743.21
  inflammatory 365.62
  juvenile 365.14
  low tension 365.12
  malignant 365.83
  narrow angle (primary) 365.20
    acute 365.22
    chronic 365.23
    intermittent 365.21
    interval 365.21
    residual stage 365.24
    subacute 365.21
  neovascular 365.63
  newborn 743.20
    associated with other eye anomalies 743.22
    simple 743.21
  noncongestive (chronic) 365.11
  nonobstructive (chronic) 365.11
  normal tension 365.12
  obstructive 365.60
    due to lens changes 365.59
  open angle 365.10
    with
      abnormal optic disc appearance or asymmetry 365.01
      borderline findings
        high risk 365.05
        intraocular pressure 365.01
        low risk 365.01
      cupping of optic discs 365.01
      thin central corneal thickness (pachymetry) 365.01
    primary 365.11
    residual stage 365.15
    high risk 365.05
    low risk 365.01
  phacoanaphylactic 365.59

Glaucoma (Continued)
  phacolytic 365.51
  phacomorphic
    acute 365.22
    borderline 365.06
  pigment dispersion 365.13
  pigmentary 365.13
  postinfectious 365.60
  pseudoexfoliation 365.52
  secondary NEC 365.60
    due to
        steroids 365.31
        surgery 365.60
  simple (chronic) 365.11
  simplex 365.11
  stage
    advanced 365.73
    early 365.71
    end-stage 365.73
    indeterminate 365.74
    mild 365.71
    moderate 365.72
    severe 365.73
    unspecified 365.70
  steroid
    induced 365.31
    responders 365.03
  suspect 365.00
    primary angle closure 365.02
  syphilitic 095.8
  traumatic NEC 365.65
    newborn 767.8
  uveitic 365.62
  wide angle (see also Glaucoma, open angle)
      365.10
Glaucomatous flecks (subcapsular) 366.31
Glazed tongue 529.4
Gleet 098.2
Glénard's disease or syndrome (enteroptosis)
    569.89
Glinski-Simmonds syndrome (pituitary
    cachexia) 253.2
Glioblastoma (multiforme) (M9440/3)
  with sarcomatous component (M9442/3)
    specified site - see Neoplasm, by site,
        malignant
    unspecified site 191.9
  giant cell (M9441/3)
    specified site - see Neoplasm, by site,
        malignant
    unspecified site 191.9
  specified site - see Neoplasm, by site,
      malignant
  unspecified site 191.9
Glioma (malignant) (M9380/3)
  astrocytic (M9400/3)
    specified site - see Neoplasm, by site,
        malignant
    unspecified site 191.9
  mixed (M9382/3)
    specified site - see Neoplasm, by site,
        malignant
    unspecified site 191.9
  nose 748.1
  specified site NEC - see Neoplasm, by site,
      malignant
  subependymal (M9383/1) 237.5
  unspecified site 191.9
Gliomatosis cerebri (M9381/3) 191.0
Glioneuroma (M9505/1) - see Neoplasm, by
    site, uncertain behavior
Gliosarcoma (M9380/3)
  specified site - see Neoplasm, by site,
      malignant
  unspecified site 191.9
Gliosis (cerebral) 349.89
  spinal 336.0
Glisson's
  cirrhosis - see Cirrhosis, portal
  disease (see also Rickets) 268.0
Glissonitis 573.3

Globinuria 791.2
Globus 306.4
  hystericus 300.11
Glomangioma (M8712/0) (see also
    Hemangioma) 228.00
Glomangiosarcoma (M8710/3) - see Neoplasm,
    connective tissue, malignant
Glomerular nephritis (see also Nephritis) 583.9
Glomerulitis (see also Nephritis) 583.9
Glomerulonephritis (see also Nephritis) 583.9
  with
    edema (see also Nephrosis) 581.9
    lesion of
      exudative nephritis 583.89
      interstitial nephritis (diffuse) (focal)
          583.89
      necrotizing glomerulitis 583.4
        acute 580.4
        chronic 582.4
      renal necrosis 583.9
        cortical 583.6
        medullary 583.7
      specified pathology NEC 583.89
        acute 580.89
        chronic 582.89
    necrosis, renal 583.9
      cortical 583.6
      medullary (papillary) 583.7
    specified pathology or lesion NEC 583.89
  acute 580.9
    with
      exudative nephritis 580.89
      interstitial nephritis (diffuse) (focal)
          580.89
      necrotizing glomerulitis 580.4
      extracapillary with epithelial crescents
          580.4
    poststreptococcal 580.0
    proliferative (diffuse) 580.0
    rapidly progressive 580.4
    specified pathology NEC 580.89
  arteriolar (see also Hypertension, kidney)
      403.90
  arteriosclerotic (see also Hypertension,
      kidney) 403.90
  ascending (see also Pyelitis) 590.80
  basement membrane NEC 583.89
    with
      pulmonary hemorrhage
          (Goodpasture's syndrome)
          446.21 [583.81]
  chronic 582.9
    with
      exudative nephritis 582.89
      interstitial nephritis (diffuse) (focal)
          582.89
      necrotizing glomerulitis 582.4
      specified pathology or lesion NEC
          582.89
    endothelial 582.2
    extracapillary with epithelial crescents
        582.4
    hypocomplementemic persistent 582.2
    lobular 582.2
    membranoproliferative 582.2
    membranous 582.1
      and proliferative (mixed) 582.2
      sclerosing 582.1
    mesangiocapillary 582.2
    mixed membranous and proliferative
        582.2
    proliferative (diffuse) 582.0
    rapidly progressive 582.4
    sclerosing 582.1
  cirrhotic - see Sclerosis, renal
  desquamative - see Nephrosis
  due to or associated with
    amyloidosis 277.39 [583.81]
      with nephrotic syndrome 277.39
          [581.81]
      chronic 277.39 [582.81]

Glomerulonephritis (Continued)
  due to or associated with (Continued)
    diabetes mellitus 250.4● [583.81]
      due to secondary diabetes 249.4●
          [581.81]
      with nephrotic syndrome 250.4●
          [581.81]
        due to secondary diabetes 249.4●
            [581.81]
    diphtheria 032.89 [580.81]
    gonococcal infection (acute) 098.19
        [583.81]
      chronic or duration of 2 months or
          over 098.39 [583.81]
    infectious hepatitis 070.9 [580.81]
    malaria (with nephrotic syndrome) 084.9
        [581.81]
    mumps 072.79 [580.81]
    polyarteritis (nodosa) (with nephrotic
        syndrome) 446.0 [581.81]
    specified pathology NEC 583.89
      acute 580.89
      chronic 582.89
    streptotrichosis 039.8 [583.81]
    subacute bacterial endocarditis 421.0
        [580.81]
    syphilis (late) 095.4
      congenital 090.5 [583.81]
      early 091.69 [583.81]
    systemic lupus erythematosus 710.0
        [583.81]
      with nephrotic syndrome 710.0
          [581.81]
      chronic 710.0 [582.81]
    tuberculosis (see also Tuberculosis) 016.0●
        [583.81]
    typhoid fever 002.0 [580.81]
  extracapillary with epithelial crescents
      583.4
    acute 580.4
    chronic 582.4
  exudative 583.89
    acute 580.89
    chronic 582.89
  focal (see also Nephritis) 583.9
    embolic 580.4
  granular 582.89
  granulomatous 582.89
  hydremic (see also Nephrosis) 581.9
  hypocomplementemic persistent 583.2
    with nephrotic syndrome 581.2
    chronic 582.2
  immune complex NEC 583.89
  infective (see also Pyelitis) 590.80
  interstitial (diffuse) (focal) 583.89
    with nephrotic syndrome 581.89
    acute 580.89
    chronic 582.89
  latent or quiescent 582.9
  lobular 583.2
    with nephrotic syndrome 581.2
    chronic 582.2
  membranoproliferative 583.2
    with nephrotic syndrome 581.2
    chronic 582.2
  membranous 583.1
    with nephrotic syndrome 581.1
    and proliferative (mixed) 583.2
      with nephrotic syndrome 581.2
      chronic 582.2
    chronic 582.1
    sclerosing 582.1
      with nephrotic syndrome 581.1
  mesangiocapillary 583.2
    with nephrotic syndrome 581.2
    chronic 582.2
  minimal change 581.3
  mixed membranous and proliferative
      583.2
    with nephrotic syndrome 581.2
    chronic 582.2

◀ New   ◀▥ Revised   ~~deleted~~ Deleted   ● Use Additional Digit(s)   Omit code

Glomerulonephritis *(Continued)*
  necrotizing 583.4
    acute 580.4
    chronic 582.4
  nephrotic *(see also* Nephrosis) 581.9
  old - *see* Glomerulonephritis, chronic
  parenchymatous 581.89
  poststreptococcal 580.0
  proliferative (diffuse) 583.0
    with nephrotic syndrome 581.0
    acute 580.0
    chronic 582.0
  purulent *(see also* Pyelitis) 590.80
  quiescent - *see* Nephritis, chronic
  rapidly progressive 583.4
    acute 580.4
    chronic 582.4
  sclerosing membranous (chronic) 582.1
    with nephrotic syndrome 581.1
  septic *(see also* Pyelitis) 590.80
  specified pathology or lesion NEC 583.89
    with nephrotic syndrome 581.89
    acute 580.89
    chronic 582.89
  suppurative (acute) (disseminated) *(see also*
      Pyelitis) 590.80
  toxic - *see* Nephritis, acute
  tubal, tubular - *see* Nephrosis, tubular
  type II (Ellis) - *see* Nephrosis
  vascular - *see* Hypertension, kidney
Glomerulosclerosis *(see also* Sclerosis, renal) 587
  focal 582.1
    with nephrotic syndrome 581.1
  intercapillary (nodular) (with diabetes)
      250.4 ● *[581.81]*
    due to secondary diabetes 249.4 ● *[581.81]*
Glossagra 529.6
Glossalgia 529.6
Glossitis 529.0
  areata exfoliativa 529.1
  atrophic 529.4
  benign migratory 529.1
  gangrenous 529.0
  Hunter's 529.4
  median rhomboid 529.2
  Moeller's 529.4
  pellagrous 265.2
Glossocele 529.8
Glossodynia 529.6
  exfoliativa 529.4
Glossoncus 529.8
Glossophytia 529.3
Glossoplegia 529.8
Glossoptosis 529.8
Glossopyrosis 529.6
Glossotrichia 529.3
Glossy skin 701.9
Glottis - *see* condition
Glottitis - *see* Glossitis
Glucagonoma (M8152/0)
  malignant (M8152/3)
    pancreas 157.4
    specified site NEC - *see* Neoplasm, by site,
        malignant
    unspecified site 157.4
  pancreas 211.7
  specified site NEC - *see* Neoplasm, by site,
      benign
  unspecified site 211.7
Glucoglycinuria 270.7
Glue ear syndrome 381.20
Glue sniffing (airplane glue) *(see also*
    Dependence) 304.6 ●
Glycinemia (with methylmalonic acidemia)
    270.7
Glycinuria (renal) (with ketosis) 270.0
Glycogen
  infiltration *(see also* Disease, glycogen
      storage) 271.0
  storage disease *(see also* Disease, glycogen
      storage) 271.0

Glycogenosis *(see also* Disease, glycogen
    storage) 271.0
  cardiac 271.0 *[425.7]*
  Cori, types I-VII 271.0
  diabetic, secondary 250.8● *[259.8]*
    due to secondary diabetes 249.8● *[259.8]*
  diffuse (with hepatic cirrhosis) 271.0
  generalized 271.0
  glucose-6-phosphatase deficiency 271.0
  hepatophosphorylase deficiency 271.0
  hepatorenal 271.0
  myophosphorylase deficiency 271.0
  pulmonary interstitial 516.62
Glycopenia 251.2
Glycopeptide
  intermediate staphylococcus aureus (GISA)
      V09.8
  resistant
    enterococcus V09.8
    staphylococcus aureus (GRSA) V09.8
Glycoprolinuria 270.8
Glycosuria 791.5
  renal 271.4
Gnathostoma (spinigerum) (infection)
    (infestation) 128.1
  wandering swellings from 128.1
Gnathostomiasis 128.1
Goiter (adolescent) (colloid) (diffuse) (dipping)
    (due to iodine deficiency) (endemic)
    (euthyroid) (heart) (hyperplastic)
    (internal) (intrathoracic) (juvenile) (mixed
    type) (nonendemic) (parenchymatous)
    (plunging) (sporadic) (subclavicular)
    (substernal) 240.9
  with
    hyperthyroidism (recurrent) *(see also*
        Goiter, toxic) 242.0●
    thyrotoxicosis *(see also* Goiter, toxic)
        242.0●
  adenomatous *(see also* Goiter, nodular)
      241.9
  cancerous (M8000/3) 193
  complicating pregnancy, childbirth, or
      puerperium 648.1●
  congenital 246.1
  cystic *(see also* Goiter, nodular) 241.9
  due to enzyme defect in synthesis of thyroid
      hormone (butane-insoluble iodine)
      (coupling) (deiodinase) (iodide
      trapping or organification)
      (iodotyrosine dehalogenase)
      (peroxidase) 246.1
  dyshormonogenic 246.1
  exophthalmic *(see also* Goiter, toxic)
      242.0●
  familial (with deaf-mutism) 243
  fibrous 245.3
  lingual 759.2
  lymphadenoid 245.2
  malignant (M8000/3) 193
  multinodular (nontoxic) 241.1
    toxic or with hyperthyroidism *(see also*
        Goiter, toxic) 242.2●
  nodular (nontoxic) 241.9
    with
      hyperthyroidism *(see also* Goiter, toxic)
          242.3●
      thyrotoxicosis *(see also* Goiter, toxic)
          242.3●
    endemic 241.9
    exophthalmic (diffuse) *(see also* Goiter,
        toxic) 242.0●
    multinodular (nontoxic) 241.1
    sporadic 241.9
    toxic *(see also* Goiter, toxic) 242.3●
    uninodular (nontoxic) 241.0
  nontoxic (nodular) 241.9
    multinodular 241.1
    uninodular 241.0
  pulsating *(see also* Goiter, toxic) 242.0●
  simple 240.0

Goiter *(Continued)*
  toxic 242.0●

> Note: Use the following fifth-digit
> subclassification with category 242:
>
> 0   without mention of thyrotoxic crisis
>   or storm
> 1   with mention of thyrotoxic crisis or
>   storm

    adenomatous 242.3●
      multinodular 242.2●
      uninodular 242.1●
    multinodular 242.2●
    nodular 242.3●
      multinodular 242.2●
      uninodular 242.1●
    uninodular 242.1●
  uninodular (nontoxic) 241.0
    toxic or with hyperthyroidism *(see also*
        Goiter, toxic) 242.1●
Goldberg (-Maxwell) (-Morris) syndrome
    (testicular feminization) 259.51
Goldblatt's
  hypertension 440.1
  kidney 440.1
Goldenhar's syndrome (oculoauriculovertebral
    dysplasia) 756.0
Goldflam-Erb disease or syndrome
    358.00
Goldscheider's disease (epidermolysis bullosa)
    757.39
Goldstein's disease (familial hemorrhagic
    telangiectasia) 448.0
Golfer's elbow 726.32
Goltz-Gorlin syndrome (dermal hypoplasia)
    757.39
Gonadoblastoma (M9073/1)
  specified site - *see* Neoplasm, by site
    uncertain behavior
  unspecified site
    female 236.2
    male 236.4
Gonecystitis *(see also* Vesiculitis) 608.0
Gongylonemiasis 125.6
  mouth 125.6
Goniosynechiae 364.73
Gonococcemia 098.89
Gonococcus, gonococcal (disease) (infection)
    (see also condition) 098.0
  anus 098.7
  bursa 098.52
  chronic NEC 098.2
  complicating pregnancy, childbirth, or
      puerperium 647.1●
    affecting fetus or newborn 760.2
  conjunctiva, conjunctivitis (neonatorum)
      098.40
  dermatosis 098.89
  endocardium 098.84
  epididymo-orchitis 098.13
    chronic or duration of 2 months or over
        098.33
  eye (newborn) 098.40
  fallopian tube (chronic) 098.37
    acute 098.17
  genitourinary (acute) (organ) (system) (tract)
      (see also Gonorrhea) 098.0
    lower 098.0
      chronic 098.2
    upper 098.10
      chronic 098.30
  heart NEC 098.85
  joint 098.50
  keratoderma 098.81
  keratosis (blennorrhagica) 098.81
  lymphatic (gland) (node) 098.89
  meninges 098.82
  orchitis (acute) 098.13
    chronic or duration of 2 months or over
        098.33

Gonococcus, gonococcal *(Continued)*
  pelvis (acute) 098.19
    chronic or duration of 2 months or over 098.39
  pericarditis 098.83
  peritonitis 098.86
  pharyngitis 098.6
  pharynx 098.6
  proctitis 098.7
  pyosalpinx (chronic) 098.37
    acute 098.17
  rectum 098.7
  septicemia 098.89
  skin 098.89
  specified site NEC 098.89
  synovitis 098.51
  tendon sheath 098.51
  throat 098.6
  urethra (acute) 098.0
    chronic or duration of 2 months or over 098.2
  vulva (acute) 098.0
    chronic or duration of 2 months or over 098.2
Gonocytoma (M9073/1)
  specified site - *see* Neoplasm, by site, uncertain behavior
  unspecified site
    female 236.2
    male 236.4
Gonorrhea 098.0
  acute 098.0
  Bartholin's gland (acute) 098.0
    chronic or duration of 2 months or over 098.2
  bladder (acute) 098.11
    chronic or duration of 2 months or over 098.31
  carrier (suspected of) V02.7
  cervix (acute) 098.15
    chronic or duration of 2 months or over 098.35
  chronic 098.2
  complicating pregnancy, childbirth, or puerperium 647.1 ●
    affecting fetus or newborn 760.2
  conjunctiva, conjunctivitis (neonatorum) 098.40
  contact V01.6
  Cowper's gland (acute) 098.0
    chronic or duration of 2 months or over 098.2
  duration of 2 months or over 098.2
  exposure to V01.6
  fallopian tube (chronic) 098.37
    acute 098.17
  genitourinary (acute) (organ) (system) (tract) 098.0
    chronic 098.2
    duration of 2 months or over 098.2
  kidney (acute) 098.19
    chronic or duration of 2 months or over 098.39
  ovary (acute) 098.19
    chronic or duration of 2 months or over 098.39
  pelvis (acute) 098.19
    chronic or duration of 2 months or over 098.39
  penis (acute) 098.0
    chronic or duration of 2 months or over 098.2
  prostate (acute) 098.12
    chronic or duration of 2 months or over 098.32
  seminal vesicle (acute) 098.14
    chronic or duration of 2 months or over 098.34
  specified site NEC - *see* Gonococcus

Gonorrhea *(Continued)*
  spermatic cord (acute) 098.14
    chronic or duration of 2 months or over 098.34
  urethra (acute) 098.0
    chronic or duration of 2 months or over 098.2
  vagina (acute) 098.0
    chronic or duration of 2 months or over 098.2
  vas deferens (acute) 098.14
    chronic or duration of 2 months or over 098.34
  vulva (acute) 098.0
    chronic or duration of 2 months or over 098.2
Goodpasture's syndrome (pneumorenal) 446.21
Good's syndrome 279.06
Gopalan's syndrome (burning feet) 266.2
Gordon's disease (exudative enteropathy) 579.8
Gorlin-Chaudhry-Moss syndrome 759.89
Gougerot's syndrome (trisymptomatic) 709.1
Gougerot-Blum syndrome (pigmented purpuric lichenoid dermatitis) 709.1
Gougerot-Carteaud disease or syndrome (confluent reticulate papillomatosis) 701.8
Gougerot-Hailey-Hailey disease (benign familial chronic pemphigus) 757.39
Gougerot (-Houwer)-Sjögren syndrome (keratoconjunctivitis sicca) 710.2
Gouley's syndrome (constrictive pericarditis) 423.2
Goundou 102.6
Gout, gouty 274.9
  with
    specified manifestations NEC 274.89
    tophi (tophus) 274.03
  acute 274.01
  arthritis 274.00
    acute 274.01
  arthropathy 274.00
    acute 274.01
    chronic (without mention of tophus (tophi)) 274.02
      with tophus (tophi) 274.03
  attack 274.01
  chronic 274.02
    tophaceous 274.03
  degeneration, heart 274.82
  diathesis 274.9
  eczema 274.89
  episcleritis 274.89 *[379.09]*
  external ear (tophus) 274.81
  flare 274.01
  glomerulonephritis 274.10
  iritis 274.89 *[364.11]*
  joint 274.00
  kidney 274.10
  lead 984.9
    specified type of lead - *see* Table of Drugs and Chemicals
  nephritis 274.10
  neuritis 274.89 *[357.4]*
  phlebitis 274.89 *[451.9]*
  rheumatic 714.0
  saturnine 984.9
    specified type of lead - *see* Table of Drugs and Chemicals
  spondylitis 274.00
  synovitis 274.00
  syphilitic 095.8
  tophi 274.03
    ear 274.81
    heart 274.82
    specified site NEC 274.82
Gowers'
  muscular dystrophy 359.1
  syndrome (vasovagal attack) 780.2
Gowers-Paton-Kennedy syndrome 377.04
Gradenigo's syndrome 383.02

Graft-versus-host disease 279.50
  due to organ transplant NEC - *see* Complications, transplant, organ
Graham Steell's murmur (pulmonic regurgitation) *(see also* Endocarditis, pulmonary) 424.3
Grain-handlers' disease or lung 495.8
Grain mite (itch) 133.8
Grand
  mal (idiopathic) *(see also* Epilepsy) 345.1 ●
    hysteria of Charcôt 300.11
    nonrecurrent or isolated 780.39
  multipara
    affecting management of labor and delivery 659.4 ●
    status only (not pregnant) V61.5
Granite workers' lung 502
Granular - *see also* condition
  inflammation, pharynx 472.1
  kidney (contracting) *(see also* Sclerosis, renal) 587
  liver - *see* Cirrhosis, liver
  nephritis - *see* Nephritis
Granulation tissue, abnormal - *see also* Granuloma
  abnormal or excessive 701.5
  postmastoidectomy cavity 383.33
  postoperative 701.5
  skin 701.5
Granulocytopenia, granulocytopenic (primary) 288.00
  malignant 288.09
Granuloma NEC 686.1
  abdomen (wall) 568.89
    skin (pyogenicum) 686.1
      from residual foreign body 709.4
  annulare 695.89
  anus 569.49
  apical 522.6
  appendix 543.9
  aural 380.23
  beryllium (skin) 709.4
    lung 503
  bone *(see also* Osteomyelitis) 730.1 ●
    eosinophilic 277.89
    from residual foreign body 733.99
  canaliculus lacrimalis 375.81
  cerebral 348.89
  cholesterin, middle ear 385.82
  coccidioidal (progressive) 114.3
    lung 114.4
    meninges 114.2
    primary (lung) 114.0
  colon 569.89
  conjunctiva 372.61
  dental 522.6
  ear, middle (cholesterin) 385.82
    with otitis media - *see* Otitis media
  eosinophilic 277.89
    bone 277.89
    lung 277.89
    oral mucosa 528.9
  exuberant 701.5
  eyelid 374.89
  facial
    lethal midline 446.3
    malignant 446.3
  faciale 701.8
  fissuratum (gum) 523.8
  foot NEC 686.1
  foreign body (in soft tissue) NEC 728.82
    bone 733.99
    in operative wound 998.4
    muscle 728.82
    skin 709.4
    subcutaneous tissue 709.4
  fungoides 202.1 ●
  gangraenescens 446.3
  giant cell (central) (jaw) (reparative) 526.3
    gingiva 523.8
    peripheral (gingiva) 523.8
  gland (lymph) 289.3

◀ New   ◀┅ Revised   ~~deleted~~ Deleted   ● Use Additional Digit(s)   ▨ Omit code

Granuloma NEC *(Continued)*
 Hodgkin's (M9661/3) 201.1●
 ileum 569.89
 infectious NEC 136.9
 inguinale (Donovan) 099.2
  venereal 099.2
 intestine 569.89
 iridocyclitis 364.10
 jaw (bone) 526.3
  reparative giant cell 526.3
 kidney *(see also* Infection, kidney) 590.9
 lacrimal sac 375.81
 larynx 478.79
 lethal midline 446.3
 lipid 277.89
 lipoid 277.89
 liver 572.8
 lung (infectious) *(see also* Fibrosis, lung) 515
  coccidioidal 114.4
  eosinophilic 277.89
 lymph gland 289.3
 Majocchi's 110.6
 malignant, face 446.3
 mandible 526.3
 mediastinum 519.3
 midline 446.3
 monilial 112.3
 muscle 728.82
  from residual foreign body 728.82
 nasal sinus *(see also* Sinusitis) 473.9
 operation wound 998.59
  foreign body 998.4
  stitch (external) 998.89
   internal wound 998.89
  talc 998.7
 oral mucosa, eosinophilic or pyogenic 528.9
 orbit, orbital 376.11
 paracoccidioidal 116.1
 penis, venereal 099.2
 periapical 522.6
 peritoneum 568.89
  due to ova of helminths NEC *(see also*
   Helminthiasis) 128.9
 postmastoidectomy cavity 383.33
 postoperative - *see* Granuloma, operation
   wound
 prostate 601.8
 pudendi (ulcerating) 099.2
 pudendorum (ulcerative) 099.2
 pulp, internal (tooth) 521.49
 pyogenic, pyogenicum (skin) 686.1
  maxillary alveolar ridge 522.6
  oral mucosa 528.9
 rectum 569.49
 reticulohistiocytic 277.89
 rubrum nasi 705.89
 sarcoid 135
 Schistosoma 120.9
 septic (skin) 686.1
 silica (skin) 709.4
 sinus (accessory) (infectional) (nasal) *(see also*
   Sinusitis) 473.9
 skin (pyogenicum) 686.1
  from foreign body or material 709.4
 sperm 608.89
 spine
  syphilitic (epidural) 094.89
  tuberculous *(see also* Tuberculosis) 015.0●
   [730.88]
 stitch (postoperative) 998.89
  internal wound 998.89
 suppurative (skin) 686.1
 suture (postoperative) 998.89
  internal wound 998.89
 swimming pool 031.1
 talc 728.82
  in operation wound 998.7
 telangiectaticum (skin) 686.1
 tracheostomy 519.09
 trichophyticum 110.6
 tropicum 102.4
 umbilicus 686.1
  newborn 771.4

Granuloma NEC *(Continued)*
 urethra 599.84
 uveitis 364.10
 vagina 099.2
 venereum 099.2
 vocal cords 478.5
 Wegener's (necrotizing respiratory
   granulomatosis) 446.4
Granulomatosis NEC 686.1
 disciformis chronica et progressiva 709.3
 infantiseptica 771.2
 lipoid 277.89
 lipophagic, intestinal 040.2
 miliary 027.0
 necrotizing, respiratory 446.4
 progressive, septic 288.1
 Wegener's (necrotizing respiratory) 446.4
Granulomatous tissue - *see* Granuloma
Granulosis rubra nasi 705.89
Graphite fibrosis (of lung) 503
Graphospasm 300.89
 organic 333.84
Grating scapula 733.99
Gravel (urinary) *(see also* Calculus) 592.9
Graves' disease (exophthalmic goiter) *(see also*
   Goiter, toxic) 242.0●
Gravis - *see* condition
Grawitz's tumor (hypernephroma) (M8312/3)
   189.0
Grayness, hair (premature) 704.3
 congenital 757.4
Gray or grey syndrome (chloramphenicol)
   (newborn) 779.4
Greenfield's disease 330.0
Green sickness 280.9
Greenstick fracture - *see* Fracture, by site
Greig's syndrome (hypertelorism) 756.0
Grief 309.0
Griesinger's disease *(see also* Ancylostomiasis)
   126.9
Grinders'
 asthma 502
 lung 502
 phthisis *(see also* Tuberculosis) 011.4●
Grinding, teeth 306.8
Grip
 Dabney's 074.1
 devil's 074.1
Grippe, grippal - *see also* Influenza
 Balkan 083.0
 intestinal *(see also* Influenza) 487.8
 summer 074.8
Grippy cold *(see also* Influenza) 487.1
Grisel's disease 723.5
Groin - *see* condition
Grooved
 nails (transverse) 703.8
 tongue 529.5
  congenital 750.13
Ground itch 126.9
Growing pains, children 781.99
Growth (fungoid) (neoplastic) (new)
   (M8000/1) - *see also* Neoplasm, by site,
   unspecified nature
 adenoid (vegetative) 474.12
 benign (M8000/0) - *see* Neoplasm, by site,
   benign
 fetal, poor 764.9●
  affecting management of pregnancy 656.5●
 malignant (M8000/3) - *see* Neoplasm, by site,
   malignant
 rapid, childhood V21.0
 secondary (M8000/6) - *see* Neoplasm, by site,
   malignant, secondary
GRSA (glycopeptide resistant staphylococcus
   aureus) V09.8
Gruber's hernia - *see* Hernia, Gruber's
Gruby's disease (tinea tonsurans) 110.0
GSS (Gerstmann-Sträussler-Scheinker
   syndrome) 046.71
G-trisomy 758.0
Guama fever 066.3

Gubler (-Millard) paralysis or syndrome 344.89
Guérin-Stern syndrome (arthrogryposis
   multiplex congenita) 754.89
Guertin's disease (electric chorea) 049.8
Guillain-Barré disease or syndrome 357.0
Guinea worms (infection) (infestation) 125.7
Guinon's disease (motor-verbal tic) 307.23
Gull's disease (thyroid atrophy with
   myxedema) 244.8
Gull and Sutton's disease - *see* Hypertension,
   kidney
Gum - *see* condition
Gumboil 522.7
Gumma (syphilitic) 095.9
 artery 093.89
  cerebral or spinal 094.89
 bone 095.5
  of yaws (late) 102.6
 brain 094.89
 cauda equina 094.89
 central nervous system NEC 094.9
 ciliary body 095.8 *[364.11]*
 congenital 090.5
  testis 090.5
 eyelid 095.8 *[373.5]*
 heart 093.89
 intracranial 094.89
 iris 095.8 *[364.11]*
 kidney 095.4
 larynx 095.8
 leptomeninges 094.2
 liver 095.3
 meninges 094.2
 myocardium 093.82
 nasopharynx 095.8
 neurosyphilitic 094.9
 nose 095.8
 orbit 095.8
 palate (soft) 095.8
 penis 095.8
 pericardium 093.81
 pharynx 095.8
 pituitary 095.8
 scrofulous *(see also* Tuberculosis) 017.0●
 skin 095.8
 specified site NEC 095.8
 spinal cord 094.89
 tongue 095.8
 tonsil 095.8
 trachea 095.8
 tuberculous *(see also* Tuberculosis) 017.0●
 ulcerative due to yaws 102.4
 ureter 095.8
 yaws 102.4
  bone 102.6
Gunn's syndrome (jaw-winking syndrome) 742.8
Gunshot wound - *see also* Wound, open, by site
 fracture - *see* Fracture, by site, open
 internal organs (abdomen, chest, or
   pelvis) - *see* Injury, internal, by site,
   with open wound
 intracranial - *see* Laceration, brain, with open
   intracranial wound
Günther's disease or syndrome (congenital
   erythropoietic porphyria) 277.1
Gustatory hallucination 780.1
Gynandrism 752.7
Gynandroblastoma (M8632/1)
 specified site - *see* Neoplasm, by site,
   uncertain behavior
 unspecified site
  female 236.2
  male 236.4
Gynandromorphism 752.7
Gynatresia (congenital) 752.49
Gynecoid pelvis, male 738.6
Gynecological examination V72.31
 for contraceptive maintenance V25.40
Gynecomastia 611.1
Gynephobia 300.29
Gyrate scalp 757.39

H

Haas' disease (osteochondrosis head of humerus) 732.3
Habermann's disease (acute parapsoriasis varioliformis) 696.2
Habit, habituation
chorea 307.22
disturbance, child 307.9
drug (see also Dependence) 304.9 ●
laxative (see also Abuse, drugs, nondependent) 305.9 ●
spasm 307.20
chronic 307.22
transient (of childhood) 307.21
tic 307.20
chronic 307.22
transient (of childhood) 307.21
use of
nonprescribed drugs (see also Abuse, drugs, nondependent) 305.9 ●
patent medicines (see also Abuse, drugs, nondependent) 305.9 ●
vomiting 536.2
Hadfield-Clarke syndrome (pancreatic infantilism) 577.8
Haff disease 985.1
Hag teeth, tooth 524.39
Hageman factor defect, deficiency, or disease (see also Defect, coagulation) 286.3
Haglund's disease (osteochondrosis os tibiale externum) 732.5
Haglund-Läwen-Fründ syndrome 717.89
Hagner's disease (hypertrophic pulmonary osteoarthropathy) 731.2
Hailey-Hailey disease (benign familial chronic pemphigus) 757.39
Hair - see also condition
plucking 307.9
Hairball in stomach 935.2
Hairy black tongue 529.3
Half vertebra 756.14
Halitosis 784.99
Hallermann-Streiff syndrome 756.0
Hallervorden-Spatz disease or syndrome 333.0
Hallopeau's
acrodermatitis (continua) 696.1
disease (lichen sclerosis et atrophicus) 701.0
Hallucination (auditory) (gustatory) (olfactory) (tactile) 780.1
alcohol-induced 291.3
drug-induced 292.12
visual 368.16
Hallucinosis 298.9
alcohol-induced (acute) 291.3
drug-induced 292.12
Hallus - see Hallux
Hallux 735.9
limitus 735.8
malleus (acquired) 735.3
rigidus (acquired) 735.2
congenital 755.66
late effects of rickets 268.1
valgus (acquired) 735.0
congenital 755.66
varus (acquired) 735.1
congenital 755.66
Halo, visual 368.15
Hamartoblastoma 759.6
Hamartoma 759.6
epithelial (gingival), odontogenic, central, or peripheral (M9321/0) 213.1
upper jaw (bone) 213.0
vascular 757.32
Hamartosis, hamartoses NEC 759.6
Hamman's disease or syndrome (spontaneous mediastinal emphysema) 518.1
Hamman-Rich syndrome (diffuse interstitial pulmonary fibrosis) 516.33

Hammer toe (acquired) 735.4
congenital 755.66
late effects of rickets 268.1
Hand - see condition
Hand-Schüller-Christian disease or syndrome (chronic histiocytosis x) 277.89
Hand-foot syndrome 693.0
Hanging (asphyxia) (strangulation) (suffocation) 994.7
Hangnail (finger) (with lymphangitis) 681.02
Hangover (alcohol) (see also Abuse, drugs, nondependent) 305.0 ●
Hanot's cirrhosis or disease - see Cirrhosis, biliary
Hanot-Chauffard (-Troisier) syndrome (bronze diabetes) 275.01
Hansen's disease (leprosy) 030.9
benign form 030.1
malignant form 030.0
Harada's disease or syndrome 363.22
Hard chancre 091.0
Hard firm prostate 600.10
with
urinary
obstruction 600.11
retention 600.11
Hardening
artery - see Arteriosclerosis
brain 348.89
liver 571.8
Hare's syndrome (M8010/3) (carcinoma, pulmonary apex) 162.3
Harelip (see also Cleft, lip) 749.10
Harkavy's syndrome 446.0
Harlequin (fetus) 757.1
color change syndrome 779.89
Harley's disease (intermittent hemoglobinuria) 283.2
Harris'
lines 733.91
syndrome (organic hyperinsulinism) 251.1
Hart's disease or syndrome (pellagra-cerebellar ataxia-renal aminoaciduria) 270.0
Hartmann's pouch (abnormal sacculation of gallbladder neck) 575.8
of intestine V44.3
attention to V55.3
Hartnup disease (pellagra-cerebellar ataxia-renal aminoaciduria) 270.0
Harvester lung 495.0
Hashimoto's disease or struma (struma lymphomatosa) 245.2
Hassall-Henle bodies (corneal warts) 371.41
Haut mal (see also Epilepsy) 345.1 ●
Haverhill fever 026.1
Hawaiian wood rose dependence 304.5 ●
Hawkins' keloid 701.4
Hay
asthma (see also Asthma) 493.0 ●
fever (allergic) (with rhinitis) 477.9
with asthma (bronchial) (see also Asthma) 493.0 ●
allergic, due to grass, pollen, ragweed, or tree 477.0
conjunctivitis 372.05
due to
dander, animal (cat) (dog) 477.2
dust 477.8
fowl 477.8
hair, animal (cat) (dog) 477.2
pollen 477.0
specified allergen other than pollen 477.8
Hayem-Faber syndrome (achlorhydric anemia) 280.9
Hayem-Widal syndrome (acquired hemolytic jaundice) 283.9
Haygarth's nodosities 715.04
Hazard-Crile tumor (M8350/3) 193

Hb (abnormal)
disease - see Disease, hemoglobin
trait - see Trait
H disease 270.0
Head - see also condition
banging 307.3
Headache 784.0
allergic 339.00
associated with sexual activity 339.82
cluster 339.00
chronic 339.02
episodic 339.01
daily
chronic 784.0
new persistent (NPDH) 339.42
drug induced 339.3
due to
loss, spinal fluid 349.0
lumbar puncture 349.0
saddle block 349.0
emotional 307.81
histamine 339.00
hypnic 339.81
lumbar puncture 349.0
medication overuse 339.3
menopausal 627.2
menstrual 346.4 ●
migraine 346.9 ●
nasal septum 784.0
nonorganic origin 307.81
orgasmic 339.82
postspinal 349.0
post-traumatic 339.20
acute 339.21
chronic 339.22
premenstrual 346.4 ●
preorgasmic 339.82
primary
cough 339.83
exertional 339.84
stabbing 339.85
thunderclap 339.43
psychogenic 307.81
psychophysiologic 307.81
rebound 339.3
short lasting unilateral neuralgiform with conjunctival injection and tearing (SUNCT) 339.05
sick 346.9 ●
spinal 349.0
complicating labor and delivery 668.8 ●
postpartum 668.8 ●
spinal fluid loss 349.0
syndrome
cluster 339.00
complicated NEC 339.44
periodic in child or adolescent 346.2 ●
specified NEC 339.89
tension 307.81
type 339.10
chronic 339.12
episodic 339.11
vascular 784.0
migraine type 346.9 ●
vasomotor 346.9 ●
Health
advice V65.4
audit V70.0
checkup V70.0
education V65.4
hazard (see also History of) V15.9
falling V15.88
specified cause NEC V15.89
instruction V65.4
services provided because (of)
boarding school residence V60.6
holiday relief for person providing home care V60.5
inadequate
housing V60.1
resources V60.2

◀ New   ◀◀ Revised   ~~deleted~~ Deleted   ● Use Additional Digit(s)   ▨ Omit code

Health *(Continued)*
  services provided because *(Continued)*
    lack of housing V60.0
    no care available in home V60.4
    person living alone V60.3
    poverty V60.3
    residence in institution V60.6
    specified cause NEC V60.89
    vacation relief for person providing home care V60.5
Healthy
  donor *(see also* Donor) V59.9
  infant or child
    accompanying sick mother V65.0
    receiving care V20.1
  person
    accompanying sick relative V65.0
    admitted for sterilization V25.2
    receiving prophylactic inoculation or vaccination *(see also* Vaccination, prophylactic) V05.9
Hearing
  conservation and treatment V72.12
  examination V72.19
    following failed hearing screening V72.11
Heart - *see* condition
Heartburn 787.1
  psychogenic 306.4
Heat (effects) 992.9
  apoplexy 992.0
  burn - *see also* Burn, by site
    from sun *(see also* Sunburn) 692.71
  collapse 992.1
  cramps 992.2
  dermatitis or eczema 692.89
  edema 992.7
  erythema - *see* Burn, by site
  excessive 992.9
    specified effect NEC 992.8
  exhaustion 992.5
    anhydrotic 992.3
    due to
      salt (and water) depletion 992.4
      water depletion 992.3
  fatigue (transient) 992.6
  fever 992.0
  hyperpyrexia 992.0
  prickly 705.1
  prostration - *see* Heat, exhaustion
  pyrexia 992.0
  rash 705.1
  specified effect NEC 992.8
  stroke 992.0
  sunburn *(see also* Sunburn) 692.71
  syncope 992.1
Heavy-chain disease 273.2
Heavy-for-dates (fetus or infant) 766.1
  4500 grams or more 766.0
  exceptionally 766.0
Hebephrenia, hebephrenic (acute) *(see also* Schizophrenia) 295.1●
  dementia (praecox) *(see also* Schizophrenia) 295.1●
  schizophrenia *(see also* Schizophrenia) 295.1●
Heberden's
  disease or nodes 715.04
  syndrome (angina pectoris) 413.9
Hebra's disease
  dermatitis exfoliativa 695.89
  erythema multiforme exudativum 695.19
  pityriasis 695.89
    maculata et circinata 696.3
    rubra 695.89
      pilaris 696.4
  prurigo 698.2
Hebra, nose 040.1
Hedinger's syndrome (malignant carcinoid) 259.2
Heel - *see* condition
Heerfordt's disease or syndrome (uveoparotitis) 135

Hegglin's anomaly or syndrome 288.2
Heidenhain's disease 290.10
  with dementia 290.10
Heilmeyer-Schoner disease (M9842/3) 207.1●
Heine-Medin disease *(see also* Poliomyelitis) 045.9●
Heinz-body anemia, congenital 282.7
Heller's disease or syndrome (infantile psychosis) *(see also* Psychosis, childhood) 299.1●
H.E.L.L.P. 642.5●
Helminthiasis *(see also* Infestation, by specific parasite) 128.9
  Ancylostoma *(see also* Ancylostoma) 126.9
  intestinal 127.9
    mixed types (types classifiable to more than one of the categories 120.0–127.7) 127.8
    specified type 127.7
  mixed types (intestinal) (types classifiable to more than one of the categories 120.0–127.7) 127.8
  Necator americanus 126.1
  specified type NEC 128.8
  Trichinella 124
Heloma 700
Hemangioblastoma (M9161/1) - *see also* Neoplasm, connective tissue, uncertain behavior
  malignant (M9161/3) - *see* Neoplasm, connective tissue, malignant
Hemangioblastomatosis, cerebelloretinal 759.6
Hemangioendothelioma (M9130/1) - *see also* Neoplasm, by site, uncertain behavior
  benign (M9130/0) 228.00
  bone (diffuse) (M9130/3) - *see* Neoplasm, bone, malignant
  malignant (M9130/3) - *see* Neoplasm, connective tissue, malignant
  nervous system (M9130/0) 228.09
Hemangioendotheliosarcoma (M9130/3) - *see* Neoplasm, connective tissue, malignant
Hemangiofibroma (M9160/0) - *see* Neoplasm, by site, benign
Hemangiolipoma (M8861/0) - *see* Lipoma
Hemangioma (M9120/0) 228.00
  arteriovenous (M9123/0) - *see* Hemangioma, by site
  brain 228.02
  capillary (M9131/0) - *see* Hemangioma, by site
  cavernous (M9121/0) - *see* Hemangioma, by site
  central nervous system NEC 228.09
  choroid 228.09
  heart 228.09
  infantile (M9131/0) - *see* Hemangioma, by site
  intra-abdominal structures 228.04
  intracranial structures 228.02
  intramuscular (M9132/0) - *see* Hemangioma, by site
  iris 228.09
  juvenile (M9131/0) - *see* Hemangioma, by site
  malignant (M9120/3) - *see* Neoplasm, connective tissue, malignant
  meninges 228.09
    brain 228.02
    spinal cord 228.09
  peritoneum 228.04
  placenta - *see* Placenta, abnormal
  plexiform (M9131/0) - *see* Hemangioma, by site
  racemose (M9123/0) - *see* Hemangioma, by site
  retina 228.03
  retroperitoneal tissue 228.04
  sclerosing (M8832/0) - *see* Neoplasm, skin, benign

Hemangioma *(Continued)*
  simplex (M9131/0) - *see* Hemangioma, by site
  skin and subcutaneous tissue 228.01
  specified site NEC 228.09
  spinal cord 228.09
  venous (M9122/0) - *see* Hemangioma, by site
  verrucous keratotic (M9142/0) - *see* Hemangioma, by site
Hemangiomatosis (systemic) 757.32
  involving single site - *see* Hemangioma
Hemangiopericytoma (M9150/1) - *see also* Neoplasm, connective tissue, uncertain behavior
  benign (M9150/0) - *see* Neoplasm, connective tissue, benign
  malignant (M9150/3) - *see* Neoplasm, connective tissue, malignant
Hemangiosarcoma (M9120/3) - *see* Neoplasm, connective tissue, malignant
Hemarthrosis (nontraumatic) 719.10
  ankle 719.17
  elbow 719.12
  foot 719.17
  hand 719.14
  hip 719.15
  knee 719.16
  multiple sites 719.19
  pelvic region 719.15
  shoulder (region) 719.11
  specified site NEC 719.18
  traumatic - *see* Sprain, by site
  wrist 719.13
Hematemesis 578.0
  with ulcer - *see* Ulcer, by site, with hemorrhage
  due to S. japonicum 120.2
  Goldstein's (familial hemorrhagic telangiectasia) 448.0
  newborn 772.4
    due to swallowed maternal blood 777.3
Hematidrosis 705.89
Hematinuria *(see also* Hemoglobinuria) 791.2
  malarial 084.8
  paroxysmal 283.2
Hematite miners' lung 503
Hematobilia 576.8
Hematocele (congenital) (diffuse) (idiopathic) 608.83
  broad ligament 620.7
  canal of Nuck 629.0
  cord, male 608.83
  fallopian tube 620.8
  female NEC 629.0
  ischiorectal 569.89
  male NEC 608.83
  ovary 629.0
  pelvis, pelvic
    female 629.0
      with ectopic pregnancy *(see also* Pregnancy, ectopic) 633.90
        with intrauterine pregnancy 633.91
    male 608.83
  periuterine 629.0
  retrouterine 629.0
  scrotum 608.83
  spermatic cord (diffuse) 608.83
  testis 608.84
  traumatic - *see* Injury, internal, pelvis
  tunica vaginalis 608.83
  uterine ligament 629.0
  uterus 621.4
  vagina 623.6
  vulva 624.5
Hematocephalus 742.4
Hematochezia *(see also* Melena) 578.1
Hematochyluria *(see also* Infestation, filarial) 125.9
Hematocolpos 626.8
Hematocornea 371.12
Hematogenous - *see* condition

Hematoma (skin surface intact) (traumatic) - *see also* Contusion

Note: Hematomas are coded according to origin and the nature and site of the hematoma or the accompanying injury. Hematomas of unspecified origin are coded as injuries of the sites involved, except:

(a) hematomas of genital organs which are coded as diseases of the organ involved unless they complicate pregnancy or delivery
(b) hematomas of the eye which are coded as diseases of the eye.

For late effect of hematoma classifiable to 920–924 *see* Late, effect, contusion.

with
   crush injury - *see* Crush
   fracture - *see* Fracture, by site
   injury of internal organs - *see also* Injury, internal, by site
      kidney - *see* Hematoma, kidney, traumatic
      liver - *see* Hematoma, liver, traumatic
      spleen - *see* Hematoma, spleen
   nerve injury - *see* Injury, nerve
   open wound - *see* Wound, open, by site
   skin surface intact - *see* Contusion
abdomen (wall) - *see* Contusion, abdomen
amnion 658.8●
aorta, dissecting 441.00
   abdominal 441.02
   thoracic 441.01
   thoracoabdominal 441.03
aortic intramural - *see* Dissection, aorta
arterial (complicating trauma) 904.9
   specified site - *see* Injury, blood vessel, by site
auricle (ear) 380.31
birth injury 767.8
   skull 767.19
brain (traumatic) 853.0●

Note: Use the following fifth-digit subclassification with categories 851–854:

0 unspecified state of consciousness
1 with no loss of consciousness
2 with brief [less than one hour] loss of consciousness
3 with moderate [1–24 hours] loss of consciousness
4 with prolonged [more than 24 hours] loss of consciousness and return to pre-existing conscious level
5 with prolonged [more than 24 hours] loss of consciousness, without return to pre-existing conscious level

Use fifth-digit 5 to designate when a patient is unconscious and dies before regaining consciousness, regardless of the duration of the loss of consciousness

6 with loss of consciousness of unspecified duration
9 with concussion, unspecified

with
   cerebral
      contusion - *see* Contusion, brain
      laceration - *see* Laceration, brain
      open intracranial wound 853.1●
      skull fracture - *see* Fracture, skull, by site
   extradural or epidural 852.4●
      with open intracranial wound 852.5●
      fetus or newborn 767.0
      nontraumatic 432.0

Hematoma *(Continued)*
brain *(Continued)*
   fetus or newborn NEC 767.0
   nontraumatic (*see also* Hemorrhage, brain) 431
      epidural or extradural 432.0
      newborn NEC 772.8
      subarachnoid, arachnoid, or meningeal (*see also* Hemorrhage, subarachnoid) 430
      subdural (*see also* Hemorrhage, subdural) 432.1
   subarachnoid, arachnoid, or meningeal 852.0●
      with open intracranial wound 852.1●
      fetus or newborn 772.2
      nontraumatic (*see also* Hemorrhage, subarachnoid) 430
   subdural 852.2●
      with open intracranial wound 852.3●
      fetus or newborn (localized) 767.0
      nontraumatic (*see also* Hemorrhage, subdural) 432.1
breast (nontraumatic) 611.89
broad ligament (nontraumatic) 620.7
   complicating delivery 665.7●
   traumatic - *see* Injury, internal, broad ligament
calcified NEC 959.9
capitis 920
   due to birth injury 767.19
   newborn 767.19
cerebral - *see* Hematoma, brain
cesarean section wound 674.3●
chorion - *see* Placenta, abnormal
complicating delivery (perineum) (vulva) 664.5●
   pelvic 665.7●
   vagina 665.7●
corpus
   cavernosum (nontraumatic) 607.82
   luteum (nontraumatic) (ruptured) 620.1
dura (mater) - *see* Hematoma, brain, subdural
epididymis (nontraumatic) 608.83
epidural (traumatic) - *see also* Hematoma, brain, extradural
   spinal - *see* Injury, spinal, by site
episiotomy 674.3●
external ear 380.31
extradural - *see also* Hematoma, brain, extradural
   fetus or newborn 767.0
   nontraumatic 432.0
      fetus or newborn 767.0
fallopian tube 620.8
genital organ (nontraumatic)
   female NEC 629.89
   male NEC 608.83
   traumatic (external site) 922.4
      internal - *see* Injury, internal, genital organ
graafian follicle (ruptured) 620.0
internal organs (abdomen, chest, or pelvis) - *see also* Injury, internal, by site
   kidney - *see* Hematoma, kidney, traumatic
   liver - *see* Hematoma, liver, traumatic
   spleen - *see* Hematoma, spleen
intracranial - *see* Hematoma, brain
kidney, cystic 593.81
   traumatic 866.01
      with open wound into cavity 866.11
labia (nontraumatic) 624.5
lingual (and other parts of neck, scalp, or face, except eye) 920
liver (subcapsular) 573.8
   birth injury 767.8
   fetus or newborn 767.8

Hematoma *(Continued)*
liver *(Continued)*
   traumatic NEC 864.01
      with
         laceration - *see* Laceration, liver
         open wound into cavity 864.11
mediastinum - *see* Injury, internal, mediastinum
meninges, meningeal (brain) - *see also* Hematoma, brain, subarachnoid
   spinal - *see* Injury, spinal, by site
mesosalpinx (nontraumatic) 620.8
   traumatic - *see* Injury, internal, pelvis
muscle (traumatic) - *see* Contusion, by site
   nontraumatic 729.92
nasal (septum) (and other part(s) of neck, scalp, or face, except eye) 920
obstetrical surgical wound 674.3●
orbit, orbital (nontraumatic) 376.32
   traumatic 921.2
ovary (corpus luteum) (nontraumatic) 620.1
   traumatic - *see* Injury, internal, ovary
pelvis (female) (nontraumatic) 629.89
   complicating delivery 665.7●
   male 608.83
   traumatic - *see also* Injury, internal, pelvis
      specified organ NEC (*see also* Injury, internal, pelvis) 867.6
penis (nontraumatic) 607.82
pericranial (and neck, or face any part, except eye) 920
   due to injury at birth 767.19
perineal wound (obstetrical) 674.3●
   complicating delivery 664.5●
perirenal, cystic 593.81
pinna 380.31
placenta - *see* Placenta, abnormal
postoperative 998.12
retroperitoneal (nontraumatic) 568.81
   traumatic - *see* Injury, internal, retroperitoneum
retropubic, male 568.81
scalp (and neck, or face any part, except eye) 920
   fetus or newborn 767.19
scrotum (nontraumatic) 608.83
   traumatic 922.4
seminal vesicle (nontraumatic) 608.83
   traumatic - *see* Injury, internal, seminal, vesicle
soft tissue, nontraumatic 729.92
spermatic cord - *see also* Injury, internal, spermatic cord
   nontraumatic 608.83
spinal (cord) (meninges) - *see also* Injury, spinal, by site
   fetus or newborn 767.4
   nontraumatic 336.1
spleen 865.01
   with
      laceration - *see* Laceration, spleen
      open wound into cavity 865.11
sternocleidomastoid, birth injury 767.8
sternomastoid, birth injury 767.8
subarachnoid - *see also* Hematoma, brain, subarachnoid
   fetus or newborn 772.2
   nontraumatic (*see also* Hemorrhage, subarachnoid) 430
   newborn 772.2
subdural - *see also* Hematoma, brain, subdural
   fetus or newborn (localized) 767.0
   nontraumatic (*see also* Hemorrhage, subdural) 432.1
subperiosteal (syndrome) 267
   traumatic - *see* Hematoma, by site
superficial, fetus or newborn 772.6
syncytium - *see* Placenta, abnormal

◀ New   ◀ Revised   ~~deleted~~ Deleted   ● Use Additional Digit(s)   Omit code

Hematoma *(Continued)*
  testis (nontraumatic) 608.83
    birth injury 767.8
    traumatic 922.4
  tunica vaginalis (nontraumatic) 608.83
  umbilical cord 663.6●
    affecting fetus or newborn 762.6
  uterine ligament (nontraumatic) 620.7
    traumatic - *see* Injury, internal, pelvis
  uterus 621.4
    traumatic - *see* Injury, internal, pelvis
  vagina (nontraumatic) (ruptured)
    623.6
    complicating delivery 665.7●
    traumatic 922.4
  vas deferens (nontraumatic) 608.83
    traumatic - *see* Injury, internal, vas
      deferens
  vitreous 379.23
  vocal cord 920
  vulva (nontraumatic) 624.5
    complicating delivery 664.5●
    fetus or newborn 767.8
    traumatic 922.4
Hematometra 621.4
Hematomyelia 336.1
  with fracture of vertebra (*see also* Fracture,
    vertebra, by site, with spinal cord
    injury) 806.8
  fetus or newborn 767.4
Hematomyelitis 323.9
  late effect - *see* category 326
Hematoperitoneum (*see also* Hemoperitoneum)
  568.81
Hematopneumothorax (*see also* Hemothorax)
  511.89
Hematopoiesis, cyclic 288.02
Hematoporphyria (acquired) (congenital)
  277.1
Hematoporphyrinuria (acquired) (congenital)
  277.1
Hematorachis, hematorrhachis 336.1
  fetus or newborn 767.4
Hematosalpinx 620.8
  with
    ectopic pregnancy (*see also* categories
      633.0–633.9) 639.2
    molar pregnancy (*see also* categories
      630–632) 639.2
  infectional (*see also* Salpingo-oophoritis)
    614.2
Hematospermia 608.82
Hematothorax (*see also* Hemothorax)
  511.89
Hematotympanum 381.03
Hematuria (benign) (essential) (idiopathic)
  599.70
  due to S. hematobium 120.0
  endemic 120.0
  gross 599.71
  intermittent 599.70
  malarial 084.8
  microscopic 599.72
  paroxysmal 599.70
  sulfonamide
    correct substance properly administered
      599.70
    overdose or wrong substance given or
      taken 961.0
  tropical (bilharziasis) 120.0
  tuberculous (*see also* Tuberculosis)
    016.9●
Hematuric bilious fever 084.8
Hemeralopia 368.10
Hemiabiotrophy 799.89
Hemi-akinesia 781.8
Hemianalgesia (*see also* Disturbance, sensation)
  782.0
Hemianencephaly 740.0
Hemianesthesia (*see also* Disturbance,
  sensation) 782.0

Hemianopia, hemianopsia (altitudinal)
  (homonymous) 368.46
  binasal 368.47
  bitemporal 368.47
  heteronymous 368.47
  syphilitic 095.8
Hemiasomatognosia 307.9
Hemiathetosis 781.0
Hemiatrophy 799.89
  cerebellar 334.8
  face 349.89
    progressive 349.89
  fascia 728.9
  leg 728.2
  tongue 529.8
Hemiballism (us) 333.5
Hemiblock (cardiac) (heart) (left) 426.2
Hemicardia 746.89
Hemicephalus, hemicephaly 740.0
Hemichorea 333.5
Hemicrania 346.9●
  congenital malformation 740.0
  continua 339.41
  paroxysmal 339.03
    chronic 339.04
    episodic 339.03
Hemidystrophy - *see* Hemiatrophy
Hemiectromelia 755.4
Hemihypalgesia (*see also* Disturbance,
  sensation) 782.0
Hemihypertrophy (congenital) 759.89
  cranial 756.0
Hemihypesthesia (*see also* Disturbance,
  sensation) 782.0
Hemi-inattention 781.8
Hemimelia 755.4
  lower limb 755.30
    paraxial (complete) (incomplete)
      (intercalary) (terminal) 755.32
      fibula 755.37
      tibia 755.36
    transverse (complete) (partial) 755.31
  upper limb 755.20
    paraxial (complete) (incomplete)
      (intercalary) (terminal) 755.22
      radial 755.26
      ulnar 755.27
    transverse (complete) (partial) 755.21
Hemiparalysis (*see also* Hemiplegia)
  342.9●
Hemiparesis (*see also* Hemiplegia) 342.9●
Hemiparesthesia (*see also* Disturbance,
  sensation) 782.0
Hemiplegia 342.9●
  acute (*see also* Disease, cerebrovascular,
    acute) 436
  alternans facialis 344.89
  apoplectic (*see also* Disease, cerebrovascular,
    acute) 436
    late effect or residual
      affecting
        dominant side 438.21
        nondominant side 438.22
        unspecified side 438.20
  arteriosclerotic 437.0
    late effect or residual
      affecting
        dominant side 438.21
        nondominant side 438.22
        unspecified side 438.20
  ascending (spinal) NEC 344.89
  attack (*see also* Disease, cerebrovascular,
    acute) 436
  brain, cerebral (current episode)
    437.8
    congenital 343.1
  cerebral - *see* Hemiplegia, brain
  congenital (cerebral) (spastic) (spinal)
    343.1
  conversion neurosis (hysterical) 300.11
  cortical - *see* Hemiplegia, brain

Hemiplegia *(Continued)*
  due to
    arteriosclerosis 437.0
      late effect or residual
        affecting
          dominant side 438.21
          nondominant side 438.22
          unspecified side 438.20
    cerebrovascular lesion (*see also* Disease,
      cerebrovascular, acute) 436
      late effect
        affecting
          dominant side 438.21
          nondominant side 438.22
          unspecified side 438.20
    embolic (current) (*see also* Embolism, brain)
      434.1●
      late effect
        affecting
          dominant side 438.21
          nondominant side 438.22
          unspecified side 438.20
  flaccid 342.0●
  hypertensive (current episode) 437.8
  infantile (postnatal) 343.4
  late effect
    birth injury, intracranial or spinal
      343.4
    cerebrovascular lesion - *see* Late
      effect(s) (of) cerebrovascular
      disease
    viral encephalitis 139.0
  middle alternating NEC 344.89
  newborn NEC 767.0
  seizure (current episode) (*see also* Disease,
    cerebrovascular, acute) 436
  spastic 342.1●
    congenital or infantile 343.1
    specified NEC 342.8●
  thrombotic (current) (*see also* Thrombosis,
    brain) 434.0●
    late effect - *see* Late effect(s) (of)
      cerebrovascular disease
Hemisection, spinal cord - *see* Fracture,
  vertebra, by site, with spinal cord
  injury
Hemispasm 781.0
  facial 781.0
Hemispatial neglect 781.8
Hemisporosis 117.9
Hemitremor 781.0
Hemivertebra 756.14
Hemobilia 576.8
Hemocholecyst 575.8
Hemochromatosis (acquired) (liver)
  (myocardium) (secondary) 275.03
  with refractory anemia 238.72
  diabetic 275.03
  due to repeated red blood cell transfusions
    275.02
  hereditary 275.01
  primary idiopathic 275.01
  specified NEC 275.03
  transfusion associated (red blood cell)
    275.02
Hemodialysis V56.0
Hemoglobin - *see also* condition
  abnormal (disease) - *see* Disease,
    hemoglobin
  AS genotype 282.5
  fetal, hereditary persistence 282.7
  H Constant Spring 282.43
  H disease 282.43
  high-oxygen-affinity 289.0
  low NEC 285.9
  S (Hb-S), heterozygous 282.5
Hemoglobinemia 283.2
  due to blood transfusion NEC
    999.89
    bone marrow 996.85
  paroxysmal 283.2

Hemoglobinopathy (mixed) (*see also* Disease, hemoglobin) 282.7
  with thalassemia 282.49
  sickle-cell 282.60
    with thalassemia (without crisis) 282.41
      with
        crisis 282.42
        vaso-occlusive pain 282.42
Hemoglobinuria, hemoglobinuric 791.2
  with anemia, hemolytic, acquired (chronic) NEC 283.2
  cold (agglutinin) (paroxysmal) (with Raynaud's syndrome) 283.2
  due to
    exertion 283.2
    hemolysis (from external causes) NEC 283.2
  exercise 283.2
  fever (malaria) 084.8
  infantile 791.2
  intermittent 283.2
  malarial 084.8
  march 283.2
  nocturnal (paroxysmal) 283.2
  paroxysmal (cold) (nocturnal) 283.2
Hemolymphangioma (M9175/0) 228.1
Hemolysis
  fetal - *see* Jaundice, fetus or newborn
  intravascular (disseminated) NEC 286.6
    with
      abortion - *see* Abortion, by type, with hemorrhage, delayed or excessive
      ectopic pregnancy (*see also* categories 633.0–633.9) 639.1
      hemorrhage of pregnancy 641.3 ●
        affecting fetus or newborn 762.1
      molar pregnancy (*see also* categories 630–632) 639.1
  acute 283.2
  following
    abortion 639.1
    ectopic or molar pregnancy 639.1
  neonatal - *see* Jaundice, fetus or newborn
  transfusion NEC 999.89
    bone marrow 996.85
Hemolytic - *see also* condition
  anemia - *see* Anemia, hemolytic
  uremic syndrome 283.11
Hemometra 621.4
Hemopericardium (with effusion) 423.0
  newborn 772.8
  traumatic (*see also* Hemothorax, traumatic) 860.2
    with open wound into thorax 860.3
Hemoperitoneum 568.81
  infectional (*see also* Peritonitis) 567.29
  traumatic - *see* Injury, internal, peritoneum
Hemophagocytic syndrome 288.4
  infection-associated 288.4
Hemophilia (familial) (hereditary) 286.0
  A 286.0
    carrier (asymptomatic) V83.01
      symptomatic V83.02
    acquired 286.52
    autoimmune 286.52
  B (Leyden) 286.1
  C 286.2
  calcipriva (*see also* Fibrinolysis) 286.7
  classical 286.0
  nonfamilial 286.7
  secondary 286.52
  vascular 286.4
Hemophilus influenzae NEC 041.5
  arachnoiditis (basic) (brain) (spinal) 320.0
    late effect - *see* category 326
  bronchopneumonia 482.2
  cerebral ventriculitis 320.0
    late effect - *see* category 326
  cerebrospinal inflammation 320.0
    late effect - *see* category 326

Hemophilus influenzae NEC (*Continued*)
  infection NEC 041.5
  leptomeningitis 320.0
    late effect - *see* category 326
  meningitis (cerebral) (cerebrospinal) (spinal) 320.0
    late effect - *see* category 326
  meningomyelitis 320.0
    late effect - *see* category 326
  pachymeningitis (adhesive) (fibrous) (hemorrhagic) (hypertrophic) (spinal) 320.0
    late effect - *see* category 326
  pneumonia (broncho-) 482.2
Hemophthalmos 360.43
Hemopneumothorax (*see also* Hemothorax) 511.89
  traumatic 860.4
    with open wound into thorax 860.5
Hemoptysis 786.30
  due to Paragonimus (westermani) 121.2
  newborn 770.3
  specified NEC 786.39
  tuberculous (*see also* Tuberculosis, pulmonary) 011.9 ●
Hemorrhage, hemorrhagic (nontraumatic) 459.0
  abdomen 459.0
  accidental (antepartum) 641.2 ●
    affecting fetus or newborn 762.1
  adenoid 474.8
  adrenal (capsule) (gland) (medulla) 255.41
    newborn 772.5
  after labor - *see* Hemorrhage, postpartum
  alveolar
    lung, newborn 770.3
    process 525.8
  alveolus 525.8
  amputation stump (surgical) 998.11
    secondary, delayed 997.69
  anemia (chronic) 280.0
    acute 285.1
  antepartum - *see* Hemorrhage, pregnancy
  anus (sphincter) 569.3
  apoplexy (stroke) 432.9
  arachnoid - *see* Hemorrhage, subarachnoid
  artery NEC 459.0
    brain (*see also* Hemorrhage, brain) 431
    middle meningeal - *see* Hemorrhage, subarachnoid
  basilar (ganglion) (*see also* Hemorrhage, brain) 431
  bladder 596.89
  blood dyscrasia 289.9
  bowel 578.9
    newborn 772.4
  brain (miliary) (nontraumatic) 431
    with
      birth injury 767.0
      arachnoid - *see* Hemorrhage, subarachnoid
    due to
      birth injury 767.0
      rupture of aneurysm (congenital) (*see also* Hemorrhage, subarachnoid) 430
      mycotic 431
      syphilis 094.89
    epidural or extradural - *see* Hemorrhage, extradural
    fetus or newborn (anoxic) (hypoxic) (due to birth trauma) (nontraumatic) 767.0
      intraventricular 772.10
        grade I 772.11
        grade II 772.12
        grade III 772.13
        grade IV 772.14
    iatrogenic 997.02
    postoperative 997.02
    puerperal, postpartum, childbirth 674.0 ●

Hemorrhage, hemorrhagic (*Continued*)
  brain (*Continued*)
    stem 431
    subarachnoid, arachnoid, or meningeal - *see* Hemorrhage, subarachnoid
    subdural - *see* Hemorrhage, subdural
    traumatic NEC 853.0 ●

Note: Use the following fifth-digit subclassification with categories 851–854:

0 unspecified state of consciousness
1 with no loss of consciousness
2 with brief [less than one hour] loss of consciousness
3 with moderate [1–24 hours] loss of consciousness
4 with prolonged [more than 24 hours] loss of consciousness and return to pre-existing conscious level
5 with prolonged [more than 24 hours] loss of consciousness, without return to pre-existing conscious level

Use fifth-digit 5 to designate when a patient is unconscious and dies before regaining consciousness, regardless of the duration of the loss of consciousness

6 with loss of consciousness of unspecified duration
9 with concussion, unspecified

    with
      cerebral
        contusion - *see* Contusion, brain
        laceration - *see* Laceration, brain
        open intracranial wound 853.1 ●
        skull fracture - *see* Fracture, skull, by site
      extradural or epidural 852.4 ●
        with open intracranial wound 852.5 ●
      subarachnoid 852.0 ●
        with open intracranial wound 852.1 ●
      subdural 852.2 ●
        with open intracranial wound 852.3 ●
    breast 611.79
    bronchial tube - *see* Hemorrhage, lung
    bronchopulmonary - *see* Hemorrhage, lung
    bronchus (cause unknown) (*see also* Hemorrhage, lung) 786.30
    bulbar (*see also* Hemorrhage, brain) 431
    bursa 727.89
    capillary 448.9
      primary 287.8
    capsular - *see* Hemorrhage, brain
    cardiovascular 429.89
    cecum 578.9
    cephalic (*see also* Hemorrhage, brain) 431
    cerebellar (*see also* Hemorrhage, brain) 431
    cerebellum (*see also* Hemorrhage, brain) 431
    cerebral (*see also* Hemorrhage, brain) 431
      fetus or newborn (anoxic) (traumatic) 767.0
    cerebromeningeal (*see also* Hemorrhage, brain) 431
    cerebrospinal (*see also* Hemorrhage, brain) 431
    cerebrovascular accident - *see* Hemorrhage, brain
    cerebrum (*see also* Hemorrhage, brain) 431
    cervix (stump) (uteri) 622.8
    cesarean section wound 674.3 ●
    chamber, anterior (eye) 364.41
    childbirth - *see* Hemorrhage, complicating, delivery

◄ New   ◄▯▯ Revised   ~~deleted~~ Deleted   ● Use Additional Digit(s)   ▨ Omit code

Hemorrhage, hemorrhagic *(Continued)*
choroid 363.61
  expulsive 363.62
ciliary body 364.41
cochlea 386.8
colon - *see* Hemorrhage, intestine
complicating
  delivery 641.9●
    affecting fetus or newborn 762.1
    associated with
      afibrinogenemia 641.3●
        affecting fetus or newborn 763.89
      coagulation defect 641.3●
        affecting fetus or newborn 763.89
      hyperfibrinolysis 641.3●
        affecting fetus or newborn 763.89
      hypofibrinogenemia 641.3●
        affecting fetus or newborn 763.89
      due to
        low-lying placenta 641.1●
          affecting fetus or newborn 762.0
        placenta previa 641.1●
          affecting fetus or newborn 762.0
        premature separation of placenta 641.2●
          affecting fetus or newborn 762.1
      retained
        placenta 666.0●
        secundines 666.2●
      trauma 641.8●
        affecting fetus or newborn 763.89
      uterine leiomyoma 641.8●
        affecting fetus or newborn 763.89
complication(s)
  of dental implant placement 525.71
  surgical procedure 998.11
concealed NEC 459.0
congenital 772.9
conjunctiva 372.72
  newborn 772.8
cord, newborn 772.0
  slipped ligature 772.3
  stump 772.3
corpus luteum (ruptured) 620.1
cortical (*see also* Hemorrhage, brain) 431
cranial 432.9
cutaneous 782.7
  newborn 772.6
cyst, pancreas 577.2
cystitis - *see* Cystitis
delayed
  with
    abortion - *see* Abortion, by type, with hemorrhage, delayed or excessive
    ectopic pregnancy (*see also* categories 633.0–633.9) 639.1
    molar pregnancy (*see also* categories 630–632) 639.1
  following
    abortion 639.1
    ectopic or molar pregnancy 639.1
  postpartum 666.2●
diathesis (familial) 287.9
  newborn 776.0
disease 287.9
  newborn 776.0
  specified type NEC 287.8
disorder 287.9
  due to intrinsic circulating anticoagulants, antibodies, or inhibitors 286.59
    with
      acquired hemophilia 286.52
      antiphospholipid antibody 286.53
  specified type NEC 287.8
due to
  any device, implant, or graft (presence of) classifiable to 996.0–996.5 - *see* Complications, due to (presence of) any device, implant, or graft classified to 996.0–996.5 NEC

Hemorrhage, hemorrhagic *(Continued)*
due to *(Continued)*
  intrinsic circulating anticoagulant, antibodies, or inhibitors 286.59
    with
      acquired hemophilia 286.52
      antiphospholipid antibody 286.53
duodenum, duodenal 537.89
  ulcer - *see* Ulcer, duodenum, with hemorrhage
dura mater - *see* Hemorrhage, subdural
endotracheal - *see* Hemorrhage, lung
epicranial subaponeurotic (massive) 767.11
epidural - *see* Hemorrhage, extradural
episiotomy 674.3●
esophagus 530.82
  varix (*see also* Varix, esophagus, bleeding) 456.0
excessive
  with
    abortion - *see* Abortion, by type, with hemorrhage, delayed or excessive
    ectopic pregnancy (*see also* categories 633.0–633.9) 639.1
    molar pregnancy (*see also* categories 630–632) 639.1
  following
    abortion 639.1
    ectopic or molar pregnancy 639.1
external 459.0
extradural (traumatic) - *see also* Hemorrhage, brain, traumatic, extradural
  birth injury 767.0
  fetus or newborn (anoxic) (traumatic) 767.0
  nontraumatic 432.0
eye 360.43
  chamber (anterior) (aqueous) 364.41
  fundus 362.81
eyelid 374.81
fallopian tube 620.8
fetomaternal 772.0
  affecting management of pregnancy or puerperium 656.0●
fetus, fetal, affecting newborn 772.0
  from
    cut end of co-twin's cord 772.0
    placenta 772.0
    ruptured cord 772.0
    vasa previa 772.0
  into
    co-twin 772.0
    mother's circulation 772.0
      affecting management of pregnancy or puerperium 656.0●
fever (*see also* Fever, hemorrhagic) 065.9
  with renal syndrome 078.6
  arthropod-borne NEC 065.9
  Bangkok 065.4
  Crimean 065.0
  dengue virus 065.4
  epidemic 078.6
  Junin virus 078.7
  Korean 078.6
  Machupo virus 078.7
  mite-borne 065.8
  mosquito-borne 065.4
  Philippine 065.4
  Russian (Yaroslav) 078.6
  Singapore 065.4
  Southeast Asia 065.4
  Thailand 065.4
  tick-borne NEC 065.3
fibrinogenolysis (*see also* Fibrinolysis) 286.6
fibrinolytic (acquired) (*see also* Fibrinolysis) 286.6
fontanel 767.19
from tracheostomy stoma 519.09
fundus, eye 362.81

Hemorrhage, hemorrhagic *(Continued)*
funis
  affecting fetus or newborn 772.0
  complicating delivery 663.8●
gastric (*see also* Hemorrhage, stomach) 578.9
gastroenteric 578.9
  newborn 772.4
gastrointestinal (tract) 578.9
  newborn 772.4
genitourinary (tract) NEC 599.89
gingiva 523.8
globe 360.43
gravidarum - *see* Hemorrhage, pregnancy
gum 523.8
heart 429.89
hypopharyngeal (throat) 784.8
intermenstrual 626.6
  irregular 626.6
  regular 626.5
internal (organs) 459.0
  capsule (*see also* Hemorrhage brain) 431
  ear 386.8
  newborn 772.8
intestine 578.9
  congenital 772.4
  newborn 772.4
into
  bladder wall 596.7
  bursa 727.89
  corpus luysii (*see also* Hemorrhage, brain) 431
intra-abdominal 459.0
  during or following surgery 998.11
intra-alveolar, newborn (lung) 770.3
intracerebral (*see also* Hemorrhage, brain) 431
intracranial NEC 432.9
  puerperal, postpartum, childbirth 674.0●
  traumatic - *see* Hemorrhage, brain, traumatic
intramedullary NEC 336.1
intraocular 360.43
intraoperative 998.11
intrapartum - *see* Hemorrhage, complicating, delivery
intrapelvic
  female 629.89
  male 459.0
intraperitoneal 459.0
intrapontine (*see also* Hemorrhage, brain) 431
intrauterine 621.4
  complicating delivery - *see* Hemorrhage, complicating, delivery
  in pregnancy or childbirth - *see* Hemorrhage, pregnancy
  postpartum (*see also* Hemorrhage, postpartum) 666.1●
intraventricular (*see also* Hemorrhage, brain) 431
  fetus or newborn (anoxic) (traumatic) 772.10
    grade I 772.11
    grade II 772.12
    grade III 772.13
    grade IV 772.14
intravesical 596.7
iris (postinfectional) (postinflammatory) (toxic) 364.41
joint (nontraumatic) 719.10
  ankle 719.17
  elbow 719.12
  foot 719.17
  forearm 719.13
  hand 719.14
  hip 719.15
  knee 719.16
  lower leg 719.16
  multiple sites 719.19
  pelvic region 719.15
  shoulder (region) 719.11
  specified site NEC 719.18
  thigh 719.15

Hemorrhage, hemorrhagic (Continued)
  joint (Continued)
    upper arm 719.12
    wrist 719.13
  kidney 593.81
  knee (joint) 719.16
  labyrinth 386.8
  leg NEC 459.0
  lenticular striate artery (see also Hemorrhage,
      brain) 431
  ligature, vessel 998.11
  liver 573.8
  lower extremity NEC 459.0
  lung 786.30
    newborn 770.3
    tuberculous (see also Tuberculosis,
        pulmonary) 011.9●
  malaria 084.8
  marginal sinus 641.2●
  massive subaponeurotic, birth injury 767.11
  maternal, affecting fetus or newborn 762.1
  mediastinum 786.30
  medulla (see also Hemorrhage, brain) 431
  membrane (brain) (see also Hemorrhage,
      subarachnoid) 430
    spinal cord - see Hemorrhage, spinal cord
  meninges, meningeal (brain) (middle) (see
      also Hemorrhage, subarachnoid) 430
    spinal cord - see Hemorrhage, spinal cord
  mesentery 568.81
  metritis 626.8
  midbrain (see also Hemorrhage, brain)
      431
  mole 631.8
  mouth 528.9
  mucous membrane NEC 459.0
    newborn 772.8
  muscle 728.89
  nail (subungual) 703.8
  nasal turbinate 784.7
    newborn 772.8
  nasopharynx 478.29
  navel, newborn 772.3
  newborn 772.9
    adrenal 772.5
    alveolar (lung) 770.3
    brain (anoxic) (hypoxic) (due to birth
        trauma) 767.0
    cerebral (anoxic) (hypoxic) (due to birth
        trauma) 767.0
    conjunctiva 772.8
    cutaneous 772.6
    diathesis 776.0
    due to vitamin K deficiency 776.0
    epicranial subaponeurotic (massive)
        767.11
    gastrointestinal 772.4
    internal (organs) 772.8
    intestines 772.4
    intra-alveolar (lung) 770.3
    intracranial (from any perinatal cause)
        767.0
    intraventricular (from any perinatal
        cause) 772.10
      grade I 772.11
      grade II 772.12
      grade III 772.13
      grade IV 772.14
    lung 770.3
    pulmonary (massive) 770.3
    spinal cord, traumatic 767.4
    stomach 772.4
    subaponeurotic (massive) 767.11
    subarachnoid (from any perinatal cause)
        772.2
    subconjunctival 772.8
    subgaleal 767.11
    umbilicus 772.0
      slipped ligature 772.3
      vasa previa 772.0
  nipple 611.79

Hemorrhage, hemorrhagic (Continued)
  nose 784.7
    newborn 772.8
  obstetrical surgical wound 674.3●
  omentum 568.89
    newborn 772.4
  optic nerve (sheath) 377.42
  orbit 376.32
  ovary 620.1
  oviduct 620.8
  pancreas 577.8
  parathyroid (gland) (spontaneous)
      252.8
  parturition - see Hemorrhage, complicating,
      delivery
  penis 607.82
  pericardium, pericarditis 423.0
  perineal wound (obstetrical) 674.3●
  peritoneum, peritoneal 459.0
  peritonsillar tissue 474.8
    after operation on tonsils 998.11
    due to infection 475
  petechial 782.7
  pituitary (gland) 253.8
  placenta NEC 641.9●
    affecting fetus or newborn 762.1
    from surgical or instrumental damage
        641.8●
      affecting fetus or newborn 762.1
    previa 641.1●
      affecting fetus or newborn 762.0
  pleura - see Hemorrhage, lung
  polioencephalitis, superior 265.1
  polymyositis - see Polymyositis
  pons (see also Hemorrhage, brain) 431
  pontine (see also Hemorrhage, brain) 431
  popliteal 459.0
  postcoital 626.7
  postextraction (dental) 998.11
  postmenopausal 627.1
  postnasal 784.7
  postoperative 998.11
  postpartum (atonic) (following delivery of
      placenta) 666.1●
    delayed or secondary (after 24 hours)
        666.2●
    retained placenta 666.0●
    third stage 666.0●
  pregnancy (concealed) 641.9●
    accidental 641.2●
      affecting fetus or newborn 762.1
    affecting fetus or newborn 762.1
    before 22 completed weeks' gestation
        640.9●
      affecting fetus or newborn 762.1
    due to
      abruptio placenta 641.2●
        affecting fetus or newborn 762.1
      afibrinogenemia or other coagulation
          defect (conditions classifiable to
          286.0–286.9) 641.3●
        affecting fetus or newborn 762.1
      coagulation defect 641.3●
        affecting fetus or newborn 762.1
      hyperfibrinolysis 641.3●
        affecting fetus or newborn 762.1
      hypofibrinogenemia 641.3●
        affecting fetus or newborn 762.1
      leiomyoma, uterus 641.8●
        affecting fetus or newborn 762.1
      low-lying placenta 641.1●
        affecting fetus or newborn 762.1
      marginal sinus (rupture) 641.2●
        affecting fetus or newborn 762.1
      placenta previa 641.1●
        affecting fetus or newborn 762.0
      premature separation of placenta
          (normally implanted) 641.2●
        affecting fetus or newborn 762.1
      threatened abortion 640.0●
        affecting fetus or newborn 762.1

Hemorrhage, hemorrhagic (Continued)
  pregnancy (Continued)
    due to (Continued)
      trauma 641.8●
        affecting fetus or newborn 762.1
      early (before 22 completed weeks'
          gestation) 640.9●
        affecting fetus or newborn 762.1
      previous, affecting management of
          pregnancy or childbirth V23.49
      unavoidable - see Hemorrhage, pregnancy,
          due to placenta previa
  prepartum (mother) - see Hemorrhage,
      pregnancy
  preretinal, cause unspecified 362.81
  prostate 602.1
  puerperal (see also Hemorrhage, postpartum)
      666.1●
  pulmonary (see also Hemorrhage, lung)
      786.30
    acute idiopathic in infants (AIPHI) (over
        28 days old) 786.31
    newborn (massive) 770.3
    renal syndrome 446.21
  purpura (primary) (see also Purpura,
      thrombocytopenic) 287.39
  rectum (sphincter) 569.3
  recurring, following initial hemorrhage at
      time of injury 958.2
  renal 593.81
    pulmonary syndrome 446.21
  respiratory tract (see also Hemorrhage, lung)
      786.30
  retina, retinal (deep) (superficial) (vessels)
      362.81
    diabetic 250.5● [362.01]
      due to secondary diabetes 249.5●
          [362.01]
    due to birth injury 772.8
  retrobulbar 376.89
  retroperitoneal 459.0
  retroplacental (see also Placenta, separation)
      641.2●
  scalp 459.0
    due to injury at birth 767.19
  scrotum 608.83
  secondary (nontraumatic) 459.0
    following initial hemorrhage at time of
        injury 958.2
  seminal vesicle 608.83
  skin 782.7
    newborn 772.6
  spermatic cord 608.83
  spinal (cord) 336.1
    aneurysm (ruptured) 336.1
      syphilitic 094.89
    due to birth injury 767.4
    fetus or newborn 767.4
  spleen 289.59
  spontaneous NEC 459.0
    petechial 782.7
  stomach 578.9
    newborn 772.4
    ulcer - see Ulcer, stomach, with
        hemorrhage
  subaponeurotic, newborn 767.11
    massive (birth injury) 767.11
  subarachnoid (nontraumatic) 430
    fetus or newborn (anoxic) (traumatic)
        772.2
    puerperal, postpartum, childbirth
        674.0●
    traumatic - see Hemorrhage, brain,
        traumatic, subarachnoid
  subconjunctival 372.72
    due to birth injury 772.8
    newborn 772.8
  subcortical (see also Hemorrhage, brain)
      431
  subcutaneous 782.7
  subdiaphragmatic 459.0

◀ New   ◀||| Revised   ~~deleted~~ Deleted   ● Use Additional Digit(s)   ▨ Omit code

Hemorrhage, hemorrhagic (Continued)
  subdural (nontraumatic) 432.1
    due to birth injury 767.0
    fetus or newborn (anoxic) (hypoxic) (due to birth trauma) 767.0
    puerperal, postpartum, childbirth 674.0●
    spinal 336.1
    traumatic - see Hemorrhage, brain, traumatic, subdural
  subgaleal 767.11
  subhyaloid 362.81
  subperiosteal 733.99
  subretinal 362.81
  subtentorial (see also Hemorrhage, subdural) 432.1
  subungual 703.8
    due to blood dyscrasia 287.8
  suprarenal (capsule) (gland) 255.41
    fetus or newborn 772.5
  tentorium (traumatic) - see also Hemorrhage, brain, traumatic
    fetus or newborn 767.0
    nontraumatic - see Hemorrhage, subdural
  testis 608.83
  thigh 459.0
  third stage 666.0●
  thorax - see Hemorrhage, lung
  throat 784.8
  thrombocythemia 238.71
  thymus (gland) 254.8
  thyroid (gland) 246.3
    cyst 246.3
  tongue 529.8
  tonsil 474.8
    postoperative 998.11
  tooth socket (postextraction) 998.11
  trachea - see Hemorrhage, lung
  traumatic - see also nature of injury
    brain - see Hemorrhage, brain, traumatic
    recurring or secondary (following initial hemorrhage at time of injury) 958.2
  tuberculous NEC (see also Tuberculosis, pulmonary) 011.9●
  tunica vaginalis 608.83
  ulcer - see Ulcer, by site, with hemorrhage
  umbilicus, umbilical cord 772.0
    after birth, newborn 772.3
    complicating delivery 663.8●
      affecting fetus or newborn 772.0
    slipped ligature 772.3
    stump 772.3
  unavoidable (due to placenta previa) 641.1●
    affecting fetus or newborn 762.0
  upper extremity 459.0
  urethra (idiopathic) 599.84
  uterus, uterine (abnormal) 626.9
    climacteric 627.0
    complicating delivery - see Hemorrhage, complicating, delivery
    due to
      intrauterine contraceptive device 996.76
        perforating uterus 996.32
    functional or dysfunctional 626.8
    in pregnancy - see Hemorrhage, pregnancy
    intermenstrual 626.6
      irregular 626.6
      regular 626.5
    postmenopausal 627.1
    postpartum (see also Hemorrhage, postpartum) 666.1●
    prepubertal 626.8
    pubertal 626.3
    puerperal (immediate) 666.1●
  vagina 623.8
  vasa previa 663.5●
    affecting fetus or newborn 772.0
  vas deferens 608.83
  ventricular (see also Hemorrhage, brain) 431
  vesical 596.89

Hemorrhage, hemorrhagic (Continued)
  viscera 459.0
    newborn 772.8
  vitreous (humor) (intraocular) 379.23
  vocal cord 478.5
  vulva 624.8
Hemorrhoids (anus) (rectum) (without complication) 455.6
  bleeding, prolapsed, strangulated, or ulcerated NEC 455.8
    external 455.5
    internal 455.2
  complicated NEC 455.8
  complicating pregnancy and puerperium 671.8●
  external 455.3
    with complication NEC 455.5
    bleeding, prolapsed, strangulated, or ulcerated 455.5
    thrombosed 455.4
  internal 455.0
    with complication NEC 455.2
    bleeding, prolapsed, strangulated, or ulcerated 455.2
    thrombosed 455.1
  residual skin tag 455.9
  sentinel pile 455.9
  thrombosed NEC 455.7
    external 455.4
    internal 455.1
Hemosalpinx 620.8
Hemosiderosis 275.09
  dietary 275.09
  pulmonary (idiopathic) 275.09 [516.1]
  transfusion NEC 275.02
    bone marrow 996.85
Hemospermia 608.82
Hemothorax 511.89
  bacterial, nontuberculous 511.1
  newborn 772.8
  nontuberculous 511.89
    bacterial 511.1
  pneumococcal 511.1
  postoperative 998.11
  staphylococcal 511.1
  streptococcal 511.1
  traumatic 860.2
    with
      open wound into thorax 860.3
      pneumothorax 860.4
        with open wound into thorax 860.5
  tuberculous (see also Tuberculosis, pleura) 012.0●
Hemotympanum 385.89
Hench-Rosenberg syndrome (palindromic arthritis) (see also Rheumatism, palindromic) 719.3●
Henle's warts 371.41
Henoch (-Schönlein)
  disease or syndrome (allergic purpura) 287.0
  purpura (allergic) 287.0
Henpue, henpuye 102.6
Heparin-induced thrombocytopenia (HIT) 289.84
Heparitinuria 277.5
Hepar lobatum 095.3
Hepatalgia 573.8
Hepatic - see also condition
  flexure syndrome 569.89
Hepatitis 573.3
  acute (see also Necrosis, liver) 570
    alcoholic 571.1
    infective 070.1
      with hepatic coma 070.0
  alcoholic 571.1
  amebic - see Abscess, liver, amebic
  anicteric (acute) - see Hepatitis, viral
  antigen-associated (HAA) - see Hepatitis, viral, type B
  Australian antigen (positive) - see Hepatitis, viral, type B

Hepatitis (Continued)
  autoimmune 571.42
  catarrhal (acute) 070.1
    with hepatic coma 070.0
    chronic 571.40
    newborn 070.1
      with hepatic coma 070.0
  chemical 573.3
  cholangiolitic 573.8
  cholestatic 573.8
  chronic 571.40
    active 571.49
      viral - see Hepatitis, viral
    aggressive 571.49
    persistent 571.41
    viral - see Hepatitis, viral
  cytomegalic inclusion virus 078.5 [573.1]
  diffuse 573.3
  "dirty needle" - see Hepatitis, viral
  drug-induced 573.3
  due to
    Coxsackie 074.8 [573.1]
    cytomegalic inclusion virus 078.5 [573.1]
    infectious mononucleosis 075 [573.1]
    malaria 084.9 [573.2]
    mumps 072.71
    secondary syphilis 091.62
    toxoplasmosis (acquired) 130.5
      congenital (active) 771.2
  epidemic - see Hepatitis, viral, type A
  fetus or newborn 774.4
  fibrous (chronic) 571.49
    acute 570
  from injection, inoculation, or transfusion (blood) (other substance) (plasma) (serum) (onset within 8 months after administration) - see Hepatitis, viral
  fulminant (viral) (see also Hepatitis, viral) 070.9
    with hepatic coma 070.6
    type A 070.1
      with hepatic coma 070.0
    type B - see Hepatitis, viral, type B
  giant cell (neonatal) 774.4
  hemorrhagic 573.8
  history of
    B V12.09
    C V12.09
  homologous serum - see Hepatitis, viral
  hypertrophic (chronic) 571.49
    acute 570
  infectious, infective (acute) (chronic) (subacute) 070.1
    with hepatic coma 070.0
  inoculation - see Hepatitis, viral
  interstitial (chronic) 571.49
    acute 570
  lupoid 571.49
  malarial 084.9 [573.2]
  malignant (see also Necrosis, liver) 570
  neonatal (toxic) 774.4
  newborn 774.4
  parenchymatous (acute) (see also Necrosis, liver) 570
  peliosis 573.3
  persistent, chronic 571.41
  plasma cell 571.49
  postimmunization - see Hepatitis, viral
  postnecrotic 571.49
  posttransfusion - see Hepatitis, viral
  recurrent 571.49
  septic 573.3
  serum - see Hepatitis, viral
    carrier (suspected of) V02.61
  subacute (see also Necrosis, liver) 570
  suppurative (diffuse) 572.0
  syphilitic (late) 095.3
    congenital (early) 090.0 [573.2]
    late 090.5 [573.2]
    secondary 091.62

Hepatitis (Continued)
  toxic (noninfectious) 573.3
    fetus or newborn 774.4
  tuberculous (see also Tuberculosis) 017.9●
  viral (acute) (anicteric) (cholangiolitic)
      (cholestatic) (chronic) (subacute) 070.9
    with hepatic coma 070.6
    AU-SH type virus - see Hepatitis, viral,
        type B
    Australian antigen - see Hepatitis, viral,
        type B
    B-antigen - see Hepatitis, viral, type B
    Coxsackie 074.8 [573.1]
    cytomegalic inclusion 078.5 [573.1]
    IH (virus) - see Hepatitis, viral, type A
    infectious hepatitis virus - see Hepatitis,
        viral, type A
    serum hepatitis virus - see Hepatitis, viral,
        type B
    SH - see Hepatitis, viral, type B
    specified type NEC 070.59
      with hepatic coma 070.49
    type A 070.1
      with hepatic coma 070.0
    type B (acute) 070.30
      with
        hepatic coma 070.20
        carrier status V02.61
        chronic 070.32
          with
            hepatic coma 070.22
              with hepatitis delta 070.23
            hepatitis delta 070.33
              with hepatic coma 070.23
            with hepatitis delta 070.21
          hepatitis delta 070.31
            with hepatic coma 070.21
    type C
      acute 070.51
        with hepatic coma 070.41
      carrier status V02.62
      chronic 070.54
        with hepatic coma 070.44
      in remission 070.54
      unspecified 070.70
        with hepatic coma 070.71
    type delta (with hepatitis B carrier state)
        070.52
      with
        active hepatitis B disease - see
            Hepatitis, viral, type B
        hepatic coma 070.42
    type E 070.53
      with hepatic coma 070.43
    vaccination and inoculation
        (prophylactic) V05.3
  Waldenström's (lupoid hepatitis) 571.49●
Hepatization, lung (acute) - see also Pneumonia,
    lobar
  chronic (see also Fibrosis, lung) 515
Hepatoblastoma (M8970/3) 155.0
Hepatocarcinoma (M8170/3) 155.0
Hepatocholangiocarcinoma (M8180/3) 155.0
Hepatocholangioma, benign (M8180/0) 211.5
Hepatocholangitis 573.8
Hepatocystitis (see also Cholecystitis) 575.10
Hepatodystrophy 570
Hepatolenticular degeneration 275.1
Hepatolithiasis - see Choledocholithiasis
Hepatoma (malignant) (M8170/3) 155.0
  benign (M8170/0) 211.5
  congenital (M8970/3) 155.0
  embryonal (M8970/3) 155.0
Hepatomegalia glycogenica diffusa 271.0
Hepatomegaly (see also Hypertrophy, liver)
    789.1
  congenital 751.69
    syphilitic 090.0
  due to Clonorchis sinensis 121.1
  Gaucher's 272.7
  syphilitic (congenital) 090.0

Hepatoptosis 573.8
Hepatorrhexis 573.8
Hepatosis, toxic 573.8
Hepatosplenomegaly 571.8
  due to S. japonicum 120.2
  hyperlipemic (Bürger-Grutz type) 272.3
Herald patch 696.3
Hereditary - see condition
Heredodegeneration 330.9
  macular 362.70
Heredopathia atactica polyneuritiformis
    356.3
Heredosyphilis (see also Syphilis, congenital)
    090.9
Hermaphroditism (true) 752.7
  with specified chromosomal anomaly - see
      Anomaly, chromosomes, sex
Hernia, hernial (acquired) (recurrent)
    553.9
  with
    gangrene (obstructed) NEC 551.9
    obstruction NEC 552.9
      and gangrene 551.9
  abdomen (wall) - see Hernia, ventral
  abdominal, specified site NEC 553.8
    with
      gangrene (obstructed) 551.8
      obstruction 552.8
        and gangrene 551.8
  appendix 553.8
    with
      gangrene (obstructed) 551.8
      obstruction 552.8
        and gangrene 551.8
  bilateral (inguinal) - see Hernia, inguinal
  bladder (sphincter)
    congenital (female) (male) 756.71
    female (see also Cystocele, female)
        618.01
    male 596.89
  brain 348.4
    congenital 742.0
  broad ligament 553.8
  cartilage, vertebral - see Displacement,
      intervertebral disc
  cerebral 348.4
    congenital 742.0
    endaural 742.0
  ciliary body 364.89
    traumatic 871.1
  colic 553.9
    with
      gangrene (obstructed) 551.9
      obstruction 552.9
        and gangrene 551.9
  colon 553.9
    with
      gangrene (obstructed) 551.9
      obstruction 552.9
        and gangrene 551.9
  colostomy (stoma) 569.69
  Cooper's (retroperitoneal) 553.8
    with
      gangrene (obstructed) 551.8
      obstruction 552.8
        and gangrene 551.8
  crural - see Hernia, femoral
  cystostomy 596.83
  diaphragm, diaphragmatic 553.3
    with
      gangrene (obstructed) 551.3
      obstruction 552.3
        and gangrene 551.3
    congenital 756.6
    due to gross defect of diaphragm
        756.6
    traumatic 862.0
      with open wound into cavity 862.1
  direct (inguinal) - see Hernia, inguinal
  disc, intervertebral - see Displacement,
      intervertebral disc

Hernia, hernial (Continued)
  diverticulum, intestine 553.9
    with
      gangrene (obstructed) 551.9
      obstruction 552.9
        and gangrene 551.9
  double (inguinal) - see Hernia, inguinal
  due to adhesion with obstruction 552.9
  duodenojejunal 553.8
    with
      gangrene (obstructed) 551.8
      obstruction 552.8
        and gangrene 551.8
  en glissade - see Hernia, inguinal
  enterostomy (stoma) 569.69
  epigastric 553.29
    with
      gangrene (obstruction) 551.29
      obstruction 552.29
        and gangrene 551.29
    recurrent 553.21
      with
        gangrene (obstructed)
            551.21
        obstruction 552.21
          and gangrene 551.21
  esophageal hiatus (sliding) 553.3
    with
      gangrene (obstructed) 551.3
      obstruction 552.3
        and gangrene 551.3
    congenital 750.6
  external (inguinal) - see Hernia, inguinal
  fallopian tube 620.4
  fascia 728.89
  fat 729.30
    eyelid 374.34
    orbital 374.34
    pad 729.30
      eye, eyelid 374.34
      knee 729.31
      orbit 374.34
      popliteal (space) 729.31
      specified site NEC 729.39
  femoral (unilateral) 553.00
    with
      gangrene (obstructed) 551.00
      obstruction 552.00
        with gangrene 551.00
    bilateral 553.02
      gangrenous (obstructed) 551.02
      obstructed 552.02
        with gangrene 551.02
      recurrent 553.03
        gangrenous (obstructed)
            551.03
        obstructed 552.03
          with gangrene 551.03
    recurrent (unilateral) 553.01
      bilateral 553.03
        gangrenous (obstructed)
            551.03
        obstructed 552.03
          with gangrene 551.03
      gangrenous (obstructed) 551.01
      obstructed 552.01
        with gangrene 551.01
  foramen
    Bochdalek 553.3
      with
        gangrene (obstructed) 551.3
        obstruction 552.3
          and gangrene 551.3
      congenital 756.6
    magnum 348.4
    Morgagni, Morgagnian 553.3
      with
        gangrene 551.3
        obstruction 552.3
          and gangrene 551.3
      congenital 756.6

◀ New   ◀ Revised   deleted Deleted   ● Use Additional Digit(s)   Omit code

Hernia, hernial *(Continued)*
  funicular (umbilical) 553.1
    with
      gangrene (obstructed) 551.1
      obstruction 552.1
        and gangrene 551.1
    spermatic cord - *see* Hernia, inguinal
  gangrenous - *see* Hernia, by site, with
    gangrene
  gastrointestinal tract 553.9
    with
      gangrene (obstructed) 551.9
      obstruction 552.9
        and gangrene 551.9
  gluteal - *see* Hernia, femoral
  Gruber's (internal mesogastric) 553.8
    with
      gangrene (obstructed) 551.8
      obstruction 552.8
        and gangrene 551.8
  Hesselbach's 553.8
    with
      gangrene (obstructed) 551.8
      obstruction 552.8
        and gangrene 551.8
  hiatal (esophageal) (sliding) 553.3
    with
      gangrene (obstructed) 551.3
      obstruction 552.3
        and gangrene 551.3
    congenital 750.6
  incarcerated (*see also* Hernia, by site, with
    obstruction) 552.9
    gangrenous (*see also* Hernia, by site, with
      gangrene) 551.9
  incisional 553.21
    with
      gangrene (obstructed) 551.21
      obstruction 552.21
        and gangrene 551.21
    lumbar - *see* Hernia, lumbar
    recurrent 553.21
      with
        gangrene (obstructed) 551.21
        obstruction 552.21
          and gangrene 551.21
  indirect (inguinal) - *see* Hernia, inguinal
  infantile - *see* Hernia, inguinal
  infrapatellar fat pad 729.31
  inguinal (direct) (double) (encysted)
    (external) (funicular) (indirect)
    (infantile) (internal) (interstitial)
    (oblique) (scrotal) (sliding)
    550.9●

> Note: Use the following fifth-digit
> subclassification with category 550:
>
> 0   unilateral or unspecified (not
>   specified as recurrent)
> 1   unilateral or unspecified, recurrent
> 2   bilateral (not specified as recurrent)
> 3   bilateral, recurrent

    with
      gangrene (obstructed) 550.0●
      obstruction 550.1●
        and gangrene 550.0●
  internal 553.8
    with
      gangrene (obstructed) 551.8
      obstruction 552.8
        and gangrene 551.8
    inguinal - *see* Hernia, inguinal
  interstitial 553.9
    with
      gangrene (obstructed) 551.9
      obstruction 552.9
        and gangrene 551.9
    inguinal - *see* Hernia, inguinal
  intervertebral cartilage or disc - *see*
    Displacement, intervertebral disc

Hernia, hernial *(Continued)*
  intestine, intestinal 553.9
    with
      gangrene (obstructed) 551.9
      obstruction 552.9
        and gangrene 551.9
  intra-abdominal 553.9
    with
      gangrene (obstructed) 551.9
      obstruction 552.9
        and gangrene 551.9
  intraparietal 553.9
    with
      gangrene (obstructed) 551.9
      obstruction 552.9
        and gangrene 551.9
  iris 364.89
    traumatic 871.1
  irreducible (*see also* Hernia, by site, with
    obstruction) 552.9
    gangrenous (with obstruction) (*see also*
      Hernia, by site, with gangrene)
      551.9
  ischiatic 553.8
    with
      gangrene (obstructed) 551.8
      obstruction 552.8
        and gangrene 551.8
  ischiorectal 553.8
    with
      gangrene (obstructed) 551.8
      obstruction 552.8
        and gangrene 551.8
  lens 379.32
    traumatic 871.1
  linea
    alba - *see* Hernia, epigastric
    semilunaris - *see* Hernia, spigelian
  Littre's (diverticular) 553.9
    with
      gangrene (obstructed) 551.9
      obstruction 552.9
        and gangrene 551.9
  lumbar 553.8
    with
      gangrene (obstructed) 551.8
      obstruction 552.8
        and gangrene 551.8
    intervertebral disc 722.10
  lung (subcutaneous) 518.89
    congenital 748.69
  mediastinum 519.3
  mesenteric (internal) 553.8
    with
      gangrene (obstructed) 551.8
      obstruction 552.8
        and gangrene 551.8
  mesocolon 553.8
    with
      gangrene (obstructed) 551.8
      obstruction 552.8
        and gangrene 551.8
  muscle (sheath) 728.89
  nucleus pulposus - *see* Displacement,
    intervertebral disc
  oblique (inguinal) - *see* Hernia, inguinal
  obstructive (*see also* Hernia, by site, with
    obstruction) 552.9
    gangrenous (with obstruction) (*see also*
      Hernia, by site, with gangrene)
      551.9
  obturator 553.8
    with
      gangrene (obstructed) 551.8
      obstruction 552.8
        and gangrene 551.8
  omental 553.8
    with
      gangrene (obstructed) 551.8
      obstruction 552.8
        and gangrene 551.8

Hernia, hernial *(Continued)*
  orbital fat (pad) 374.34
  ovary 620.4
  oviduct 620.4
  paracolostomy (stoma) 569.69
  paraduodenal 553.8
    with
      gangrene (obstructed) 551.8
      obstruction 552.8
        and gangrene 551.8
  paraesophageal 553.3
    with
      gangrene (obstructed) 551.3
      obstruction 552.3
        and gangrene 551.3
    congenital 750.6
  parahiatal 553.3
    with
      gangrene (obstructed) 551.3
      obstruction 552.3
        and gangrene 551.3
  paraumbilical 553.1
    with
      gangrene (obstructed) 551.1
      obstruction 552.1
        and gangrene 551.1
  parietal 553.9
    with
      gangrene (obstructed) 551.9
      obstruction 552.9
        and gangrene 551.9
  perineal 553.8
    with
      gangrene (obstructed) 551.8
      obstruction 552.8
        and gangrene 551.8
  peritoneal sac, lesser 553.8
    with
      gangrene (obstructed) 551.8
      obstruction 552.8
        and gangrene 551.8
  popliteal fat pad 729.31
  postoperative 553.21
    with
      gangrene (obstructed) 551.21
      obstruction 552.21
        and gangrene 551.21
  pregnant uterus 654.4●
  prevesical 596.89
  properitoneal 553.8
    with
      gangrene (obstructed) 551.8
      obstruction 552.8
        and gangrene 551.8
  pudendal 553.8
    with
      gangrene (obstructed) 551.8
      obstruction 552.8
        and gangrene 551.8
  rectovaginal 618.6
  retroperitoneal 553.8
    with
      gangrene (obstructed) 551.8
      obstruction 552.8
        and gangrene 551.8
  Richter's (parietal) 553.9
    with
      gangrene (obstructed) 551.9
      obstruction 552.9
        and gangrene 551.9
  Rieux's, Riex's (retrocecal) 553.8
    with
      gangrene (obstructed) 551.8
      obstruction 552.8
        and gangrene 551.8
  sciatic 553.8
    with
      gangrene (obstructed) 551.8
      obstruction 552.8
        and gangrene 551.8
  scrotum, scrotal - *see* Hernia, inguinal

Hernia, hernial (Continued)
  sliding (inguinal) - see also Hernia, inguinal
    hiatus - see Hernia, hiatal
  spigelian 553.29
    with
      gangrene (obstructed) 551.29
      obstruction 552.29
        and gangrene 551.29
  spinal (see also Spina bifida) 741.9●
    with hydrocephalus 741.0●
  strangulated (see also Hernia, by site, with
      obstruction) 552.9
    gangrenous (with obstruction) (see also
        Hernia, by site, with gangrene)
        551.9
  supraumbilicus (linea alba) - see Hernia,
      epigastric
  tendon 727.9
  testis (nontraumatic) 550.9●
    meaning
      scrotal hernia 550.9●
      symptomatic late syphilis 095.8
  Treitz's (fossa) 553.8
    with
      gangrene (obstructed) 551.8
      obstruction 552.8
        and gangrene 551.8
  tunica
    albuginea 608.89
    vaginalis 752.89
  umbilicus, umbilical 553.1
    with
      gangrene (obstructed) 551.1
      obstruction 552.1
        and gangrene 551.1
  ureter 593.89
    with obstruction 593.4
  uterus 621.8
    pregnant 654.4●
  vaginal (posterior) 618.6
  Velpeau's (femoral) (see also Hernia, femoral)
      553.00
  ventral 553.20
    with
      gangrene (obstructed) 551.20
      obstruction 552.20
        and gangrene 551.20
    incisional 553.21
    recurrent 553.21
      with
        gangrene (obstructed) 551.21
        obstruction 552.21
          and gangrene 551.21
  vesical
    congenital (female) (male) 756.71
    female (see also Cystocele, female) 618.01
    male 596.89
  vitreous (into anterior chamber) 379.21
    traumatic 871.1
Herniation - see also Hernia
  brain (stem) 348.4
  cerebral 348.4
  gastric mucosa (into duodenal bulb) 537.89
  mediastinum 519.3
  nucleus pulposus - see Displacement,
      intervertebral disc
Herpangina 074.0
Herpes, herpetic 054.9
  auricularis (zoster) 053.71
    simplex 054.73
  blepharitis (zoster) 053.20
    simplex 054.41
  circinate 110.5
  circinatus 110.5
    bullous 694.5
  conjunctiva (simplex) 054.43
    zoster 053.21
  cornea (simplex) 054.43
    disciform (simplex) 054.43
    zoster 053.21
  encephalitis 054.3

Herpes, herpetic (Continued)
  eye (zoster) 053.29
    simplex 054.40
  eyelid (zoster) 053.20
    simplex 054.41
  febrilis 054.9
  fever 054.9
  geniculate ganglionitis 053.11
  genital, genitalis 054.10
    specified site NEC 054.19
  gestationis 646.8●
  gingivostomatitis 054.2
  iridocyclitis (simplex) 054.44
    zoster 053.22
  iris (any site) 695.10
  iritis (simplex) 054.44
  keratitis (simplex) 054.43
    dendritic 054.42
    disciform 054.43
    interstitial 054.43
    zoster 053.21
  keratoconjunctivitis (simplex)
      054.43
    zoster 053.21
  labialis 054.9
    meningococcal 036.89
  lip 054.9
  meningitis (simplex) 054.72
    zoster 053.0
  ophthalmicus (zoster) 053.20
    simplex 054.40
  otitis externa (zoster) 053.71
    simplex 054.73
  penis 054.13
  perianal 054.10
  pharyngitis 054.79
  progenitalis 054.10
  scrotum 054.19
  septicemia 054.5
  simplex 054.9
    complicated 054.8
      ophthalmic 054.40
        specified NEC 054.49
      specified NEC 054.79
    congenital 771.2
    external ear 054.73
    keratitis 054.43
      dendritic 054.42
    meningitis 054.72
    myelitis 054.74
    neuritis 054.79
    specified complication NEC
        054.79
      ophthalmic 054.49
    visceral 054.71
  stomatitis 054.2
  tonsurans 110.0
    maculosus (of Hebra) 696.3
  visceral 054.71
  vulva 054.12
  vulvovaginitis 054.11
  whitlow 054.6
  zoster 053.9
    auricularis 053.71
    complicated 053.8
      specified NEC 053.79
    conjunctiva 053.21
    cornea 053.21
    ear 053.71
    eye 053.29
    geniculate 053.11
    keratitis 053.21
      interstitial 053.21
    myelitis 053.14
    neuritis 053.10
    ophthalmicus(a) 053.20
    oticus 053.71
    otitis externa 053.71
    specified complication NEC 053.79
    specified site NEC 053.9
  zosteriform, intermediate type 053.9

Herrick's
  anemia (hemoglobin S disease) 282.61
  syndrome (hemoglobin S disease) 282.61
Hers' disease (glycogenosis VI) 271.0
Herter's infantilism (nontropical sprue) 579.0
Herter (-Gee) disease or syndrome (nontropical
    sprue) 579.0
Herxheimer's disease (diffuse idiopathic
    cutaneous atrophy) 701.8
Herxheimer's reaction 995.91
Hesitancy, urinary 788.64
Hesselbach's hernia - see Hernia, Hesselbach's
Heterochromia (congenital) 743.46
  acquired 364.53
  cataract 366.33
  cyclitis 364.21
  hair 704.3
  iritis 364.21
  retained metallic foreign body 360.62
    magnetic 360.52
  uveitis 364.21
Heterophoria 378.40
  alternating 378.45
  vertical 378.43
Heterophyes, small intestine 121.6
Heterophyiasis 121.6
Heteropsia 368.8
Heterotopia, heterotopic - see also Malposition,
    congenital
  cerebralis 742.4
  pancreas, pancreatic 751.7
  spinalis 742.59
Heterotropia 378.30
  intermittent 378.20
    vertical 378.31
  vertical (constant) (intermittent) 378.31
Heubner's disease 094.89
Heubner-Herter disease or syndrome
    (nontropical sprue) 579.0
Hexadactylism 755.00
Heyd's syndrome (hepatorenal) 572.4
HGSIL (high grade squamous intraepithelial
    lesion) (cytologic finding) (Pap smear
    finding)
  anus 796.74
  cervix 795.04
    biopsy finding - code to CIN II or
        CIN III
  vagina 795.14
Hibernoma (M8880/0) - see Lipoma
Hiccough 786.8
  epidemic 078.89
  psychogenic 306.1
Hiccup (see also Hiccough) 786.8
Hicks (-Braxton) contractures 644.1●
Hidden penis 752.65
Hidradenitis (axillaris) (suppurative) 705.83
Hidradenoma (nodular) (M8400/0) - see also
    Neoplasm, skin, benign
  clear cell (M8402/0) - see Neoplasm, skin,
      benign
  papillary (M8405/0) - see Neoplasm, skin,
      benign
Hidrocystoma (M8404/0) - see Neoplasm, skin,
    benign
HIE (hypoxic-ischemic encephalopathy)
    768.70
  mild 768.71
  moderate 768.72
  severe 768.73
High
  A₂ anemia 282.46
  altitude effects 993.2
    anoxia 993.2
    on
      ears 993.0
      sinuses 993.1
    polycythemia 289.0
  arch
    foot 755.67
    palate 750.26

◀ New   ◀▪▪ Revised   ~~deleted~~ Deleted   ● Use Additional Digit(s)   ▨ Omit code

High *(Continued)*
  artery (arterial) tension *(see also* Hypertension) 401.9
    without diagnosis of hypertension 796.2
  basal metabolic rate (BMR) 794.7
  blood pressure *(see also* Hypertension) 401.9
    borderline 796.2
    incidental reading (isolated) (nonspecific), no diagnosis of hypertension 796.2
  cholesterol 272.0
    with high triglycerides 272.2
  compliance bladder 596.4
  diaphragm (congenital) 756.6
  frequency deafness (congenital) (regional) 389.8
  head at term 652.5 ●
    affecting fetus or newborn 763.1
  output failure (cardiac) *(see also* Failure, heart) 428.9
  oxygen-affinity hemoglobin 289.0
  palate 750.26
  risk
    behavior *-see* problem
    family situation V61.9
      specified circumstance NEC V61.8
    human papillomavirus (HPV) DNA test positive
      anal 796.75
      cervical 795.05
      vaginal 795.15
    individual NEC V62.89
    infant NEC V20.1
    patient taking drugs (prescribed) V67.51
      nonprescribed *(see also* Abuse, drugs, nondependent) 305.9 ●
    pregnancy V23.9
      inadequate prenatal care V23.7
      inconclusive fetal viability V23.87
      specified problem NEC V23.89
  temperature (of unknown origin) *(see also* Pyrexia) 780.60
  thoracic rib 756.3
  triglycerides 272.1
    with high cholesterol 272.2
Hildenbrand's disease (typhus) 081.9
Hilger's syndrome 337.09
Hill diarrhea 579.1
Hilliard's lupus *(see also* Tuberculosis) 017.0 ●
Hilum - *see* condition
Hip - *see* condition
Hippel's disease (retinocerebral angiomatosis) 759.6
Hippus 379.49
Hirschfeld's disease (acute diabetes mellitus) *(see also* Diabetes) 250.0 ●
  due to secondary diabetes 249.0 ●
Hirschsprung's disease or megacolon (congenital) 751.3
Hirsuties *(see also* Hypertrichosis) 704.1
Hirsutism *(see also* Hypertrichosis) 704.1
Hirudiniasis (external) (internal) 134.2
His-Werner disease (trench fever) 083.1
Hiss-Russell dysentery 004.1
Histamine cephalgia 339.00
Histidinemia 270.5
Histidinuria 270.5
Histiocytic syndromes 288.4
Histiocytoma (M8832/0) - *see also* Neoplasm, skin, benign
  fibrous (M8830/0) - *see also* Neoplasm, skin, benign
    atypical (M8830/1) - *see* Neoplasm, connective tissue, uncertain behavior
    malignant (M8830/3) - *see* Neoplasm, connective tissue, malignant
Histiocytosis (acute) (chronic) (subacute) 277.89
  acute differentiated progressive (M9722/3) 202.5 ●
  adult pulmonary Langerhans cell (PLCH) 516.5

Histiocytosis *(Continued)*
  cholesterol 277.89
  essential 277.89
  lipid, lipoid (essential) 272.7
  lipochrome (familial) 288.1
  malignant (M9720/3) 202.3 ●
  non-Langerhans cell 277.89
  polyostotic sclerosing 277.89
  X (chronic) 277.89
    acute (progressive) (M9722/3) 202.5 ●
Histoplasmosis 115.90
  with
    endocarditis 115.94
    meningitis 115.91
    pericarditis 115.93
    pneumonia 115.95
    retinitis 115.92
    specified manifestation NEC 115.99
  African (due to Histoplasma duboisii) 115.10
    with
      endocarditis 115.14
      meningitis 115.11
      pericarditis 115.13
      pneumonia 115.15
      retinitis 115.12
      specified manifestation NEC 115.19
  American (due to Histoplasma capsulatum) 115.00
    with
      endocarditis 115.04
      meningitis 115.01
      pericarditis 115.03
      pneumonia 115.05
      retinitis 115.02
      specified manifestation NEC 115.09
  Darling's - *see* Histoplasmosis, American
  large form *(see also* Histoplasmosis, African) 115.10
  lung 115.05
  small form *(see also* Histoplasmosis, American) 115.00
History (personal) of
  abuse
    emotional V15.42
    neglect V15.42
    physical V15.41
    sexual V15.41
  affective psychosis V11.1
  alcoholism V11.3
    specified as drinking problem *(see also* Abuse, drugs, nondependent) 305.0 ●
  allergy (to) V15.09
    analgesic agent NEC V14.6
    anesthetic NEC V14.4
    antibiotic agent NEC V14.1
      penicillin V14.0
    anti-infective agent NEC V14.3
    arachnid bite V15.06
    diathesis V15.09
    drug V14.9
      specified type NEC V14.8
    eggs V15.03
    food additives V15.05
    insect bite V15.06
    latex V15.07
    medicinal agents V14.9
      specified type NEC V14.8
    milk products V15.02
    narcotic agent NEC V14.5
    nuts V15.05
      peanuts V15.01
    penicillin V14.0
    radiographic dye V15.08
    seafood V15.04
    serum V14.7
    specified food NEC V15.05
    specified nonmedicinal agents NEC V15.09
    spider bite V15.06
    sulfa V14.2

History *(Continued)*
  allergy *(Continued)*
    sulfonamides V14.2
    therapeutic agent NEC V15.09
    vaccine V14.7
  anaphylactic reaction or shock V13.81
  anaphylaxis V13.81
  anemia V12.3
  arrest, sudden cardiac V12.53
  arthritis V13.4
  attack, transient ischemic (TIA) V12.54
  benign neoplasm of brain V12.41
  blood disease V12.3
  calculi, urinary V13.01
  cardiovascular disease V12.50
    myocardial infarction 412
  chemotherapy, antineoplastic V87.41
  child abuse V15.41
  cigarette smoking V15.82
  circulatory system disease V12.50
    myocardial infarction 412
  cleft lip and palate, corrected V13.64
  combat and operational stress reaction V11.4
  congenital malformation (corrected)
    circulatory system V13.65
    digestive system V13.67
    ear V13.64
    eye V13.64
    face V13.64
    genitourinary system V13.62
    heart V13.65
    integument V13.68
    limbs V13.68
    musculoskeletal V13.68
    neck V13.64
    nervous system V13.63
    respiratory system V13.66
    specified type NEC V13.69
  contraception V15.7
  death, sudden, successfully resuscitated V12.53
  deficit
    prolonged reversible ischemic neurologic (PRIND) V12.54
    reversible ischemic neurologic (RIND) V12.54
  diathesis, allergic V15.09
  digestive system disease V12.70
    peptic ulcer V12.71
    polyps, colonic V12.72
    specified NEC V12.79
  disease (of) V13.9
    blood V12.3
    blood-forming organs V12.3
    cardiovascular system V12.50
    circulatory system V12.50
      specified NEC V12.59
    digestive system V12.70
      peptic ulcer V12.71
      polyps, colonic V12.72
      specified NEC V12.79
    infectious V12.00
      malaria V12.03
      methicillin resistant Staphylococcus aureus (MRSA) V12.04
      MRSA (methicillin resistant Staphylococcus aureus) V12.04
      poliomyelitis V12.02
      specified NEC V12.09
      tuberculosis V12.01
    parasitic V12.00
      specified NEC V12.09
    respiratory system V12.60
      pneumonia V12.61
      specified NEC V12.69
    skin V13.3
    specified site NEC V13.89
    subcutaneous tissue V13.3

◀ New   ◀▥ Revised   ~~deleted~~ Deleted   ● Use Additional Digit(s)   ▨ Omit code   **279**

History *(Continued)*
disease *(Continued)*
trophoblastic V13.1
affecting management of pregnancy V23.1
disorder (of) V13.9
endocrine V12.29
gestational diabetes V12.21
genital system V13.29
hematological V12.3
immunity V12.29
mental V11.9
affective type V11.1
manic-depressive V11.1
neurosis V11.2
schizophrenia V11.0
specified type NEC V11.8
metabolic V12.29
musculoskeletal NEC V13.59
nervous system V12.40
specified type NEC V12.49
obstetric V13.29
affecting management of current pregnancy V23.49
ectopic pregnancy V23.42
pre-term labor V23.41
pre-term labor V13.21
sense organs V12.40
specified type NEC V12.49
specified site NEC V13.89
urinary system V13.00
calculi V13.01
infection V13.02
nephrotic syndrome V13.03
specified NEC V13.09
drug use
nonprescribed *(see also* Abuse, drugs, nondependent) 305.9●
patent *(see also* Abuse, drugs, nondependent) 305.9●
dysplasia
cervical (conditions classifiable to 622.10–622.12) V13.22
vaginal (conditions classifiable to 623.0) V13.23
vulvar (conditions classifiable to 624.01-624.02) V13.24
effect NEC of external cause V15.89
embolism V12.51
pulmonary V12.55
emotional abuse V15.42
encephalitis V12.42
endocrine disorder V12.29
gestational diabetes V12.21
estrogen therapy V87.43
extracorporeal membrane oxygenation (ECMO) V15.87
failed
conscious sedation V15.80
moderate sedation V15.80
falling V15.88
family
allergy V19.6
anemia V18.2
arteriosclerosis V17.49
arthritis V17.7
asthma V17.5
blindness V19.0
blood disorder NEC V18.3
cardiovascular disease V17.49
carrier, genetic disease V18.9
cerebrovascular disease V17.1
chronic respiratory condition NEC V17.6
colonic polyps V18.51
congenital anomalies V19.5
consanguinity V19.7
coronary artery disease V17.3
cystic fibrosis V18.19
deafness V19.2
diabetes mellitus V18.0
digestive disorders V18.59

History *(Continued)*
family *(Continued)*
disabilities, intellectual V18.4
disease or disorder (of)
allergic V19.6
blood NEC V18.3
cardiovascular NEC V17.49
cerebrovascular V17.1
colonic polyps V18.51
coronary artery V17.3
death, sudden cardiac (SCD) V17.41
digestive V18.59
ear NEC V19.3
endocrine V18.19
multiple neoplasia (MEN) syndrome V18.11
eye NEC V19.19
glaucoma V19.11
genitourinary NEC V18.7
glaucoma V19.11
hypertensive V17.49
infectious V18.8
ischemic heart V17.3
kidney V18.69
polycystic V18.61
mental V17.0
metabolic V18.19
musculoskeletal NEC V17.89
osteoporosis V17.81
neurological NEC V17.2
parasitic V18.8
psychiatric condition V17.0
skin condition V19.4
ear disorder NEC V19.3
endocrine disease V18.19
multiple neoplasia (MEN) syndrome V18.11
epilepsy V17.2
eye disorder NEC V19.19
glaucoma V19.11
genetic disease carrier V18.9
genitourinary disease NEC V18.7
glaucoma V19.11
glomerulonephritis V18.69
gout V18.19
hay fever V17.6
hearing loss V19.2
hematopoietic neoplasia V16.7
Hodgkin's disease V16.7
Huntington's chorea V17.2
hydrocephalus V19.5
hypertension V17.49
infarction, myocardial V17.3
infectious disease V18.8
intellectual disabilities V18.4
ischemic heart disease V17.3
kidney disease V18.69
polycystic V18.61
leukemia V16.6
lymphatic malignant neoplasia NEC V16.7
malignant neoplasm (of) NEC V16.9
anorectal V16.0
anus V16.0
appendix V16.0
bladder V16.52
bone V16.8
brain V16.8
breast V16.3
male V16.8
bronchus V16.1
cecum V16.0
cervix V16.49
colon V16.0
duodenum V16.0
esophagus V16.0
eye V16.8
gallbladder V16.0
gastrointestinal tract V16.0
genital organs V16.40
hemopoietic NEC V16.7

History *(Continued)*
family *(Continued)*
malignant neoplasm NEC *(Continued)*
ileum V16.0
ilium V16.8
intestine V16.0
intrathoracic organs NEC V16.2
kidney V16.51
larynx V16.2
liver V16.0
lung V16.1
lymphatic NEC V16.7
ovary V16.41
oviduct V16.41
pancreas V16.0
penis V16.49
prostate V16.42
rectum V16.0
respiratory organs NEC V16.2
skin V16.8
specified site NEC V16.8
stomach V16.0
testis V16.43
trachea V16.1
ureter V16.59
urethra V16.59
urinary organs V16.59
uterus V16.49
vagina V16.49
vulva V16.49
MEN (multiple endocrine neoplasia syndrome) V18.11
mental retardation - *see* History, family, intellectual disabilities
metabolic disease NEC V18.19
mongolism V19.5
multiple
endocrine neoplasia (MEN) syndrome V18.11
myeloma V16.7
musculoskeletal disease NEC V17.89
osteoporosis V17.81
myocardial infarction V17.3
nephritis V18.69
nephrosis V18.69
osteoporosis V17.81
parasitic disease V18.8
polycystic kidney disease V18.61
psychiatric disorder V17.0
psychosis V17.0
retinitis pigmentosa V19.19
schizophrenia V17.0
skin conditions V19.4
specified condition NEC V19.8
stroke (cerebrovascular) V17.1
sudden cardiac death (SCD) V17.41
visual loss V19.0
foreign body fully removed V15.53
fracture, healed
pathologic V13.51
stress V13.52
traumatic V15.51
genital system disorder V13.29
pre-term labor V13.21
gestational diabetes V12.21
health hazard V15.9
falling V15.88
specified cause NEC V15.89
hepatitis
B V12.09
C V12.09
Hodgkin's disease V10.72
hypospadias (corrected) V13.61
immunity disorder V12.29
immunosuppression therapy V87.46
infarction, cerebral, without residual deficits V12.54
infection
central nervous system V12.42
urinary (tract) V13.02

◀ New   ◀═ Revised   ~~deleted~~ Deleted   ● Use Additional Digit(s)   ▓ Omit code

History *(Continued)*
  infectious disease V12.00
    malaria V12.03
    methicillin resistant Staphylococcus
        aureus (MRSA) V12.04
    MRSA (methicillin resistant
        Staphylococcus aureus) V12.04
    poliomyelitis V12.02
    specified NEC V12.09
    tuberculosis V12.01
  injury NEC V15.59
    traumatic brain V15.52
  insufficient prenatal care V23.7
  in utero procedure
    during pregnancy V15.21
    while a fetus V15.22
  irradiation V15.3
  leukemia V10.60
    lymphoid V10.61
    monocytic V10.63
    myeloid V10.62
    specified type NEC V10.69
  little or no prenatal care V23.7
  low birth weight *(see also* Status, low birth
        weight) V21.30
  lymphosarcoma V10.71
  malaria V12.03
  malignant carcinoid tumor V10.91
  malignant neoplasm (of) V10.90
    accessory sinus V10.22
    adrenal V10.88
    anus V10.06
    bile duct V10.09
    bladder V10.51
    bone V10.81
    brain V10.85
    breast V10.3
    bronchus V10.11
    cervix uteri V10.41
    colon V10.05
    connective tissue NEC V10.89
    corpus uteri V10.42
    digestive system V10.00
        specified part NEC V10.09
    duodenum V10.09
    endocrine gland NEC V10.88
    epididymis V10.48
    esophagus V10.03
    eye V10.84
    fallopian tube V10.44
    female genital organ V10.40
        specified site NEC V10.44
    gallbladder V10.09
    gastrointestinal tract V10.00
    gum V10.02
    hematopoietic NEC V10.79
    hypopharynx V10.02
    ileum V10.09
    intrathoracic organs NEC V10.20
    jejunum V10.09
    kidney V10.52
    large intestine V10.05
    larynx V10.21
    lip V10.02
    liver V10.07
    lung V10.11
    lymphatic NEC V10.79
    lymph glands or nodes NEC V10.79
    male genital organ V10.45
        specified site NEC V10.49
    mediastinum V10.29
    melanoma (of skin) V10.82
    middle ear V10.22
    mouth V10.02
        specified part NEC V10.02
    nasal cavities V10.22
    nasopharynx V10.02
    nervous system NEC V10.86
    nose V10.22
    oropharynx V10.02
    ovary V10.43

History *(Continued)*
  malignant neoplasm *(Continued)*
    pancreas V10.09
    parathyroid V10.88
    penis V10.49
    pharynx V10.02
    pineal V10.88
    pituitary V10.88
    placenta V10.44
    pleura V10.29
    prostate V10.46
    rectosigmoid junction V10.06
    rectum V10.06
    renal pelvis V10.53
    respiratory organs NEC V10.20
    salivary gland V10.02
    skin V10.83
        melanoma V10.82
    small intestine NEC V10.09
    soft tissue NEC V10.89
    specified site NEC V10.89
    stomach V10.04
    testis V10.47
    thymus V10.29
    thyroid V10.87
    tongue V10.01
    trachea V10.12
    ureter V10.59
    urethra V10.59
    urinary organ V10.50
    uterine adnexa V10.44
    uterus V10.42
    vagina V10.44
    vulva V10.44
  malignant neuroendocrine tumor
        V10.91
  manic-depressive psychosis V11.1
  meningitis V12.42
  mental disorder V11.9
    affective type V11.1
    manic-depressive V11.1
    neurosis V11.2
    schizophrenia V11.0
    specified type NEC V11.8
  Merkel cell carcinoma V10.91
  metabolic disorder V12.29
  methicillin resistant Staphylococcus aureus
        (MRSA) V12.04
  MRSA (methicillin resistant Staphylococcus
        aureus) V12.04
  musculoskeletal disorder NEC V13.59
  myocardial infarction 412
  neglect (emotional) V15.42
  nephrotic syndrome V13.03
  nervous system disorder V12.40
    specified type NEC V12.49
  neurosis V11.2
  noncompliance with medical treatment
        V15.81
  nutritional deficiency V12.1
  obstetric disorder V13.29
    affecting management of current
        pregnancy V23.49
        ectopic pregnancy V23.42
        pre-term labor V23.41
    pre-term labor V13.21
  parasitic disease V12.00
    specified NEC V12.09
  perinatal problems V13.7
    low birth weight *(see also* Status, low birth
        weight) V21.30
  physical abuse V15.41
  poisoning V15.6
  poliomyelitis V12.02
  polyps, colonic V12.72
  poor obstetric V13.29
    affecting management of current
        pregnancy V23.49
        ectopic pregnancy V23.42
        pre-term labor V23.41
    pre-term labor V13.21

History *(Continued)*
  prolonged reversible ischemic neurologic
        deficit (PRIND) V12.54
  psychiatric disorder V11.9
    affective type V11.1
    manic-depressive V11.1
    neurosis V11.2
    schizophrenia V11.0
    specified type NEC V11.8
  psychological trauma V15.49
    emotional abuse V15.42
    neglect V15.42
    physical abuse V15.41
    rape V15.41
  psychoneurosis V11.2
  radiation therapy V15.3
  rape V15.41
  respiratory system disease
        V12.60
    pneumonia V12.61
    specified NEC V12.69
  reticulosarcoma V10.71
  return from military deployment
        V62.22
  reversible ischemic neurologic deficit
        (RIND) V12.54
  schizophrenia V11.0
  skin disease V13.3
  smoking (tobacco) V15.82
  steroid therapy V87.45
    inhaled V87.44
    systemic V87.45
  stroke without residual deficits
        V12.54
  subcutaneous tissue disease V13.3
  sudden
    cardiac
        arrest V12.53
        death (successfully resuscitated)
            V12.53
  surgery to
    great vessels V15.1
    heart V15.1
    in utero
        during pregnancy V15.21
        while a fetus V15.22
    organs NEC V15.29
  syndrome, nephrotic V13.03
  therapy
    antineoplastic drug V87.41
    drug NEC V87.49
    estrogen V87.43
    immunosuppression V87.46
    monoclonal drug V87.42
    steroid V87.45
        inhaled V87.44
        systemic V87.45
  thrombophlebitis V12.52
  thrombosis V12.51
    pulmonary V12.55
  tobacco use V15.82
  trophoblastic disease V13.1
    affecting management of pregnancy
        V23.1
  tuberculosis V12.01
  ulcer, peptic V12.71
  urinary system disorder V13.00
    calculi V13.01
    infection V13.02
    nephrotic syndrome V13.03
    specified NEC V13.09
HIT (heparin-induced thrombocytopenia)
        289.84
HIV infection (disease) (illness) - *see*
        Human immunodeficiency virus
        (disease) (illness) (infection)
Hives (bold) *(see also* Urticaria)
        708.9
Hoarseness 784.42
Hobnail liver - *see* Cirrhosis, portal
Hobo, hoboism V60.0

◀ New   ◀║ Revised   ~~deleted~~ Deleted   ● Use Additional Digit(s)   ▨ Omit code   **281**

Hodgkin's
    disease (M9650/3) 201.9●
        lymphocytic
            depletion (M9653/3) 201.7●
                diffuse fibrosis (M9654/3)
                    201.7●
                reticular type (M9655/3)
                    201.7●
            predominance (M9651/3) 201.4●
        lymphocytic-histiocytic predominance
            (M9651/3) 201.4●
        mixed cellularity (M9652/3) 201.6●
        nodular sclerosis (M9656/3) 201.5●
            cellular phase (M9657/3) 201.5●
    granuloma (M9661/3) 201.1●
    lymphogranulomatosis (M9650/3)
        201.9●
    lymphoma (M9650/3) 201.9●
    lymphosarcoma (M9650/3) 201.9●
    paragranuloma (M9660/3) 201.0●
    sarcoma (M9662/3) 201.2●
Hodgson's disease (aneurysmal dilatation of
    aorta) 441.9
    ruptured 441.5
Hodi-potsy 111.0
Hoffa (-Kastert) disease or syndrome
    (liposynovitis prepatellaris) 272.8
Hoffmann's syndrome 244.9 [359.5]
Hoffmann-Bouveret syndrome (paroxysmal
    tachycardia) 427.2
Hole
    macula 362.54
    optic disc, crater-like 377.22
    retina (macula) 362.54
        round 361.31
            with detachment 361.01
Holla disease (see also Spherocytosis) 282.0
Holländer-Simons syndrome (progressive
    lipodystrophy) 272.6
Hollow foot (congenital) 754.71
    acquired 736.73
Holmes' syndrome (visual disorientation)
    368.16
Holoprosencephaly 742.2
    due to
        trisomy 13 758.1
        trisomy 18 758.2
Holthouse's hernia - see Hernia, inguinal
Homesickness 309.89
Homicidal ideation V62.85
Homocystinemia 270.4
Homocystinuria 270.4
Homologous serum jaundice (prophylactic)
    (therapeutic) - see Hepatitis, viral
Homosexuality - omit code
    ego-dystonic 302.0
    pedophilic 302.2
    problems with 302.0
Homozygous Hb-S disease 282.61
Honeycomb lung 518.89
    congenital 748.4
Hong Kong ear 117.3
HOOD (hereditary osteo-onychodysplasia)
    756.89
Hooded
    clitoris 752.49
    penis 752.69
Hookworm (anemia) (disease) (infestation) - see
    Ancylostomiasis
Hoppe-Goldflam syndrome 358.00
Hordeolum (external) (eyelid) 373.11
    internal 373.12
Horn
    cutaneous 702.8
        cheek 702.8
        eyelid 702.8
        penis 702.8
    iliac 756.89
    nail 703.8
        congenital 757.5
    papillary 700

Horner's
    syndrome (see also Neuropathy, peripheral,
        autonomic) 337.9
        traumatic 954.0
    teeth 520.4
Horseshoe kidney (congenital) 753.3
Horton's
    disease (temporal arteritis) 446.5
    headache or neuralgia 339.00
Hospice care V66.7
Hospitalism (in children) NEC 309.83
Hourglass contraction, contracture
    bladder 596.89
    gallbladder 575.2
        congenital 751.69
    stomach 536.8
        congenital 750.7
        psychogenic 306.4
    uterus 661.4●
        affecting fetus or newborn 763.7
Household circumstance affecting care
    V60.9
    specified type NEC V60.89
Housemaid's knee 727.2
Housing circumstance affecting care
    V60.9
    specified type NEC V60.89
HTR (hemolytic transfusion reaction)
    due to or resulting from
        incompatibility
            ABO 999.61
                acute 999.62
                delayed 999.63
            non-ABO antigen (minor) (Duffy)
                (Kell) (Kidd) (Lewis) (M) (N) (P)
                (S) 999.76
                acute 999.77
                delayed 999.78
            Rh antigen (C) (c) (D) (E) (e) 999.71
                acute 999.72
                delayed 999.73
Huchard's disease (continued arterial
    hypertension) 401.9
Hudson-Ståhli lines 371.11
Huguier's disease (uterine fibroma) 218.9
Hum, venous - omit code
Human bite (open wound) - (see also Wound,
    open, by site)
    intact skin surface - see Contusion
Human immunodeficiency virus (disease)
    (illness) 042
    infection V08
        with symptoms, symptomatic 042
Human immunodeficiency virus-2 infection
    079.53
Human immunovirus (disease) (illness)
    (infection) - see Human immunodeficiency
    virus (disease) (illness) (infection)
Human papillomavirus 079.4
    high risk, DNA test positive
        anal 796.75
        cervical 795.05
        vaginal 795.15
    low risk, DNA test positive
        anal 796.79
        cervical 795.09
        vaginal 795.19
Human parvovirus 079.83
Human T-cell lymphotrophic virus I infection
    079.51
Human T-cell lymphotrophic virus II infection
    079.52
Human T-cell lymphotropic virus-III (disease)
    (illness) (infection) - see Human
    immunodeficiency virus (disease) (illness)
    (infection)
HTLV-I infection 079.51
HTLV-II infection 079.52
HTLV-III (disease) (illness) (infection) - see
    Human immunodeficiency virus (disease)
    (illness) (infection)

HTLV-III/LAV (disease) (illness) (infection) - see
    Human immunodeficiency virus (disease)
    (illness) (infection)
Humpback (acquired) 737.9
    congenital 756.19
Hunchback (acquired) 737.9
    congenital 756.19
Hunger 994.2
    air, psychogenic 306.1
    disease 251.1
Hungry bone syndrome 275.5
Hunner's ulcer (see also Cystitis) 595.1
Hunt's
    neuralgia 053.11
    syndrome (herpetic geniculate ganglionitis)
        053.11
    dyssynergia cerebellaris myoclonica 334.2
Hunter's glossitis 529.4
Hunter (-Hurler) syndrome
    (mucopolysaccharidosis II) 277.5
Hunterian chancre 091.0
Huntington's
    chorea 333.4
    disease 333.4
Huppert's disease (multiple myeloma)
    (M9730/3) 203.0●
Hurler (-Hunter) disease or syndrome
    (mucopolysaccharidosis II) 277.5
Hürthle cell
    adenocarcinoma (M8290/3) 193
    adenoma (M8290/0) 226
    carcinoma (M8290/3) 193
    tumor (M8290/0) 226
Hutchinson's
    disease meaning
        angioma serpiginosum 709.1
        cheiropompholyx 705.81
        prurigo estivalis 692.72
        summer eruption, or summer prurigo
            692.72
    incisors 090.5
    melanotic freckle (M8742/2) - see also
        Neoplasm, skin, in situ
        malignant melanoma in (M8742/3) - see
            Melanoma
    teeth or incisors (congenital syphilis) 090.5
Hutchinson-Boeck disease or syndrome
    (sarcoidosis) 135
Hutchinson-Gilford disease or syndrome
    (progeria) 259.8
Hyaline
    degeneration (diffuse) (generalized) 728.9
        localized - see Degeneration, by site
    membrane (disease) (lung) (newborn) 769
Hyalinosis cutis et mucosae 272.8
Hyalin plaque, sclera, senile 379.16
Hyalitis (asteroid) 379.22
    syphilitic 095.8
Hydatid
    cyst or tumor - see also Echinococcus
        fallopian tube 752.11
    mole - see Hydatidiform mole
    Morgagni (congenital) 752.89
        fallopian tube 752.11
Hydatidiform mole (benign) (complicating
    pregnancy) (delivered) (undelivered) 630
    invasive (M9100/1) 236.1
    malignant (M9100/1) 236.1
    previous, affecting management of
        pregnancy V23.1
Hydatidosis - see Echinococcus
Hyde's disease (prurigo nodularis) 698.3
Hydradenitis 705.83
Hydradenoma (M8400/0) - see Hidradenoma
Hydralazine lupus or syndrome
    correct substance properly administered
        695.4
    overdose or wrong substance given or taken
        972.6
Hydramnios 657●
    affecting fetus or newborn 761.3

◀ New   ◀▥ Revised   ~~deleted~~ Deleted   ● Use Additional Digit(s)   ▨ Omit code

Hydrancephaly 742.3
  with spina bifida (*see also* Spina bifida)
    741.0●
Hydranencephaly 742.3
  with spina bifida (*see also* Spina bifida)
    741.0●
Hydrargyrism NEC 985.0
Hydrarthrosis (*see also* Effusion, joint) 719.0●
  gonococcal 098.50
  intermittent (*see also* Rheumatism,
    palindromic) 719.3●
  of yaws (early) (late) 102.6
  syphilitic 095.8
    congenital 090.5
Hydremia 285.9
Hydrencephalocele (congenital) 742.0
Hydrencephalomeningocele (congenital) 742.0
Hydroa 694.0
  aestivale 692.72
  gestationis 646.8●
  herpetiformis 694.0
  pruriginosa 694.0
  vacciniforme 692.72
Hydroadenitis 705.83
Hydrocalycosis (*see also* Hydronephrosis) 591
  congenital 753.29
Hydrocalyx (*see also* Hydronephrosis) 591
Hydrocele (calcified) (chylous) (idiopathic)
  (infantile) (inguinal canal) (recurrent)
  (senile) (spermatic cord) (testis) (tunica
  vaginalis) 603.9
  canal of Nuck (female) 629.1
    male 603.9
  congenital 778.6
  encysted 603.0
    congenital 778.6
  female NEC 629.89
  infected 603.1
  round ligament 629.89
  specified type NEC 603.8
    congenital 778.6
  spinalis (*see also* Spina bifida) 741.9●
  vulva 624.8
Hydrocephalic fetus
  affecting management or pregnancy 655.0●
  causing disproportion 653.6●
    with obstructed labor 660.1●
      affecting fetus or newborn 763.1
Hydrocephalus (acquired) (external) (internal)
  (malignant) (noncommunicating)
  (obstructive) (recurrent) 331.4
  aqueduct of Sylvius stricture 742.3
    with spina bifida (*see also* Spina bifida)
      741.0●
  chronic 742.3
    with spina bifida (*see also* Spina bifida)
      741.0●
  communicating 331.3
  congenital (external) (internal) 742.3
    with spina bifida (*see also* Spina bifida)
      741.0●
  due to
    stricture of aqueduct of Sylvius 742.3
      with spina bifida (*see also* Spina bifida)
        741.0●
    toxoplasmosis (congenital) 771.2
  fetal affecting management of pregnancy
    655.0●
  foramen Magendie block (acquired) 331.3
    congenital 742.3
      with spina bifida (*see also* Spina bifida)
        741.0●
  newborn 742.3
    with spina bifida (*see also* Spina bifida)
      741.0●
  normal pressure 331.5
    idiopathic (INPH) 331.5
    secondary 331.3
  otitic 348.2
  syphilitic, congenital 090.49
  tuberculous (*see also* Tuberculosis) 013.8●

Hydrocolpos (congenital) 623.8
Hydrocystoma (M8404/0) - *see* Neoplasm, skin,
  benign
Hydroencephalocele (congenital) 742.0
Hydroencephalomeningocele (congenital)
  742.0
Hydrohematopneumothorax (*see also*
  Hemothorax) 511.89
Hydromeningitis - *see* Meningitis
Hydromeningocele (spinal) (*see also* Spina
  bifida) 741.9●
  cranial 742.0
Hydrometra 621.8
Hydrometrocolpos 623.8
Hydromicrocephaly 742.1
Hydromphalus (congenital) (since birth) 757.39
Hydromyelia 742.53
Hydromyelocele (*see also* Spina bifida) 741.9●
Hydronephrosis 591
  atrophic 591
  congenital 753.29
  due to S. hematobium 120.0
  early 591
  functionless (infected) 591
  infected 591
  intermittent 591
  primary 591
  secondary 591
  tuberculous (*see also* Tuberculosis) 016.0●
Hydropericarditis (*see also* Pericarditis) 423.9
Hydropericardium (*see also* Pericarditis) 423.9
Hydroperitoneum 789.59
Hydrophobia 071
Hydrophthalmos (*see also* Buphthalmia) 743.20
Hydropneumohemothorax (*see also*
  Hemothorax) 511.89
Hydropneumopericarditis (*see also* Pericarditis)
  423.9
Hydropneumopericardium (*see also*
  Pericarditis) 423.9
Hydropneumothorax 511.89
  nontuberculous 511.89
    bacterial 511.1
  pneumococcal 511.1
  staphylococcal 511.1
  streptococcal 511.1
  traumatic 860.0
    with open wound into thorax 860.1
  tuberculous (*see also* Tuberculosis, pleura)
    012.0●
Hydrops 782.3
  abdominis 789.59
  amnii (complicating pregnancy) (*see also*
    Hydramnios) 657●
  articulorum intermittens (*see also*
    Rheumatism, palindromic) 719.3●
  cardiac (*see also* Failure, heart) 428.0
  congenital - *see* Hydrops, fetalis
  endolymphatic (*see also* Disease, Ménière's)
    386.00
  fetal, fetalis or newborn 778.0
    due to
      alpha thalassemia 282.43
      isoimmunization 773.3
    not due to isoimmunization 778.0
  gallbladder 575.3
  idiopathic (fetus or newborn) 778.0
  joint (*see also* Effusion, joint) 719.0●
  labyrinth (*see also* Disease, Ménière's) 386.00
  meningeal NEC 331.4
  nutritional 262
  pericardium - *see* Pericarditis
  pleura (*see also* Hydrothorax) 511.89
  renal (*see also* Nephrosis) 581.9
  spermatic cord (*see also* Hydrocele) 603.9
Hydropyonephrosis (*see also* Pyelitis) 590.80
  chronic 590.00
Hydrorachis 742.53
Hydrorrhea (nasal) 478.19
  gravidarum 658.1●
  pregnancy 658.1●

Hydrosadenitis 705.83
Hydrosalpinx (fallopian tube) (follicularis)
  614.1
Hydrothorax (double) (pleural) 511.89
  chylous (nonfilarial) 457.8
    filaria (*see also* Infestation, filarial) 125.9
  nontuberculous 511.89
    bacterial 511.1
  pneumococcal 511.1
  staphylococcal 511.1
  streptococcal 511.1
  traumatic 862.29
    with open wound into thorax 862.39
  tuberculous (*see also* Tuberculosis, pleura)
    012.0●
Hydroureter 593.5
  congenital 753.22
Hydroureteronephrosis (*see also*
  Hydronephrosis) 591
Hydrourethra 599.84
Hydroxykynureninuria 270.2
Hydroxyprolinemia 270.8
Hydroxyprolinuria 270.8
Hygroma (congenital) (cystic) (M9173/0) 228.1
  prepatellar 727.3
  subdural - *see* Hematoma, subdural
Hymen - *see* condition
Hymenolepiasis (diminuta) (infection)
  (infestation) (nana) 123.6
Hymenolepsis (diminuta) (infection)
  (infestation) (nana) 123.6
Hypalgesia (*see also* Disturbance, sensation)
  782.0
Hyperabduction syndrome 447.8
Hyperacidity, gastric 536.8
  psychogenic 306.4
Hyperactive, hyperactivity 314.01
  basal cell, uterine cervix 622.10
  bladder 596.51
  bowel (syndrome) 564.9
    sounds 787.5
  cervix epithelial (basal) 622.10
  child 314.01
  colon 564.9
  gastrointestinal 536.8
    psychogenic 306.4
  intestine 564.9
  labyrinth (unilateral) 386.51
    with loss of labyrinthine reactivity 386.58
    bilateral 386.52
  nasal mucous membrane 478.19
  stomach 536.8
  thyroid (gland) (*see also* Thyrotoxicosis)
    242.9●
Hyperacusis 388.42
Hyperadrenalism (cortical) 255.3
  medullary 255.6
Hyperadrenocorticism 255.3
  congenital 255.2
  iatrogenic
    correct substance properly administered
      255.3
    overdose or wrong substance given or
      taken 962.0
Hyperaffectivity 301.11
Hyperaldosteronism (atypical) (hyperplastic)
  (normoaldosteronal) (nor-motensive)
  (primary) 255.10
  secondary 255.14
Hyperalgesia (*see also* Disturbance, sensation)
  782.0
Hyperalimentation 783.6
  carotene 278.3
  specified NEC 278.8
  vitamin A 278.2
  vitamin D 278.4
Hyperaminoaciduria 270.9
  arginine 270.6
  citrulline 270.6
  cystine 270.0
  glycine 270.0

Hyperaminoaciduria *(Continued)*
lysine 270.7
ornithine 270.6
renal (types I, II, III) 270.0
Hyperammonemia (congenital) 270.6
Hyperamnesia 780.99
Hyperamylasemia 790.5
Hyperaphia 782.0
Hyperazotemia 791.9
Hyperbetalipoproteinemia (acquired)
(essential) (familial) (hereditary)
(primary) (secondary) 272.0
with prebetalipoproteinemia 272.2
Hyperbilirubinemia 782.4
congenital 277.4
constitutional 277.4
neonatal (transient) *(see also* Jaundice, fetus
or newborn) 774.6
of prematurity 774.2
Hyperbilirubinemica encephalopathia,
newborn 774.7
due to isoimmunization 773.4
Hypercalcemia, hypercalcemic (idiopathic)
275.42
nephropathy 588.89
Hypercalcinuria 275.40
Hypercapnia 786.09
with mixed acid-based disorder 276.4
fetal, affecting newborn 770.89
Hypercarotinemia 278.3
Hypercementosis 521.5
Hyperchloremia 276.9
Hyperchlorhydria 536.8
neurotic 306.4
psychogenic 306.4
Hypercholesterinemia - *see*
Hypercholesterolemia
Hypercholesterolemia 272.0
with hyperglyceridemia, endogenous
272.2
essential 272.0
familial 272.0
hereditary 272.0
primary 272.0
pure 272.0
Hypercholesterolosis 272.0
Hyperchylia gastrica 536.8
psychogenic 306.4
Hyperchylomicronemia (familial) (with
hyperbetalipoproteinemia) 272.3
Hypercoagulation syndrome (primary)
289.81
secondary 289.82
Hypercorticosteronism
correct substance properly administered
255.3
overdose or wrong substance given or taken
962.0
Hypercortisonism
correct substance properly administered
255.3
overdose or wrong substance given or taken
962.0
Hyperdynamic beta-adrenergic state or
syndrome (circulatory) 429.82
Hyperekplexia 759.89
Hyperelectrolytemia 276.9
Hyperemesis 536.2
arising during pregnancy - *see* Hyperemesis,
gravidarum
gravidarum (mild) (before 22 completed
weeks' gestation) 643.0●
with
carbohydrate depletion 643.1●
dehydration 643.1●
electrolyte imbalance 643.1●
metabolic disturbance 643.1●
affecting fetus or newborn 761.8
severe (with metabolic disturbance)
643.1●
psychogenic 306.4

Hyperemia (acute) 780.99
anal mucosa 569.49
bladder 596.7
cerebral 437.8
conjunctiva 372.71
ear, internal, acute 386.30
enteric 564.89
eye 372.71
eyelid (active) (passive) 374.82
intestine 564.89
iris 364.41
kidney 593.81
labyrinth 386.30
liver (active) (passive) 573.8
lung 514
ovary 620.8
passive 780.99
pulmonary 514
renal 593.81
retina 362.89
spleen 289.59
stomach 537.89
Hyperesthesia (body surface) *(see also*
Disturbance, sensation) 782.0
larynx (reflex) 478.79
hysterical 300.11
pharynx (reflex) 478.29
Hyperestrinism 256.0
Hyperestrogenism 256.0
Hyperestrogenosis 256.0
Hyperexplexia 759.89
Hyperextension, joint 718.80
ankle 718.87
elbow 718.82
foot 718.87
hand 718.84
hip 718.85
knee 718.86
multiple sites 718.89
pelvic region 718.85
shoulder (region) 718.81
specified site NEC 718.88
wrist 718.83
Hyperfibrinolysis - *see* Fibrinolysis
Hyperfolliculinism 256.0
Hyperfructosemia 271.2
Hyperfunction
adrenal (cortex) 255.3
androgenic, acquired benign
255.3
medulla 255.6
virilism 255.2
corticoadrenal NEC 255.3
labyrinth - *see* Hyperactive, labyrinth
medulloadrenal 255.6
ovary 256.1
estrogen 256.0
pancreas 577.8
parathyroid (gland) 252.00
pituitary (anterior) (gland) (lobe)
253.1
testicular 257.0
Hypergammaglobulinemia 289.89
monoclonal, benign (BMH) 273.1
polyclonal 273.0
Waldenström's 273.0
Hyperglobulinemia 273.8
Hyperglycemia 790.29
maternal
affecting fetus or newborn 775.0
manifest diabetes in infant 775.1
postpancreatectomy (complete) (partial)
251.3
Hyperglyceridemia 272.1
endogenous 272.1
essential 272.1
familial 272.1
hereditary 272.1
mixed 272.3
pure 272.1
Hyperglycinemia 270.7

Hypergonadism
ovarian 256.1
testicular (infantile) (primary) 257.0
Hyperheparinemia *(see also* Circulating,
intrinsic anticoagulants) 287.5
Hyperhidrosis, hyperidrosis 705.21
axilla 705.21
face 705.21
focal (localized) 705.21
primary 705.21
axilla 705.21
face 705.21
palms 705.21
soles 705.21
secondary 705.22
axilla 705.22
face 705.22
palms 705.22
soles 705.22
generalized 780.8
palms 705.21
psychogenic 306.3
secondary 780.8
soles 705.21
Hyperhistidinemia 270.5
Hyperinsulinism (ectopic) (functional)
(organic) NEC 251.1
iatrogenic 251.0
reactive 251.2
spontaneous 251.2
therapeutic misadventure (from
administration of insulin) 962.3
Hyperiodemia 276.9
Hyperirritability (cerebral), in newborn 779.1
Hyperkalemia 276.7
Hyperkeratosis *(see also* Keratosis) 701.1
cervix 622.2
congenital 757.39
cornea 371.89
due to yaws (early) (late) (palmar or plantar)
102.3
eccentrica 757.39
figurata centrifuga atrophica 757.39
follicularis 757.39
in cutem penetrans 701.1
limbic (cornea) 371.89
palmoplantaris climacterica 701.1
pinta (carate) 103.1
senile (with pruritus) 702.0
tongue 528.79
universalis congenita 757.1
vagina 623.1
vocal cord 478.5
vulva 624.09
Hyperkinesia, hyperkinetic (disease) (reaction)
(syndrome) 314.9
with
attention deficit - *see* Disorder, attention
deficit
conduct disorder 314.2
developmental delay 314.1
simple disturbance of activity and
attention 314.01
specified manifestation NEC 314.8
heart (disease) 429.82
of childhood or adolescence NEC 314.9
Hyperlacrimation *(see also* Epiphora) 375.20
Hyperlipemia *(see also* Hyperlipidemia) 272.4
Hyperlipidemia 272.4
carbohydrate-induced 272.1
combined 272.2
endogenous 272.1
exogenous 272.3
fat-induced 272.3
group
A 272.0
B 272.1
C 272.2
D 272.3
mixed 272.2
specified type NEC 272.4

◀ New   ◀━ Revised   ~~deleted~~ Deleted   ● Use Additional Digit(s)   ▨ Omit code

Hyperlipidosis 272.7
  hereditary 272.7
Hyperlipoproteinemia (acquired) (essential)
    (familial) (hereditary) (primary)
    (secondary) 272.4
  Fredrickson type
    I 272.3
    IIA 272.0
    IIB 272.2
    III 272.2
    IV 272.1
    V 272.3
  low-density-lipoid-type (LDL) 272.0
  very-low-density-lipoid-type [VLDL]
    272.1
Hyperlucent lung, unilateral 492.8
Hyperluteinization 256.1
Hyperlysinemia 270.7
Hypermagnesemia 275.2
  neonatal 775.5
Hypermaturity (fetus or newborn)
  post-term infant 766.21
  prolonged gestation infant 766.22
Hypermenorrhea 626.2
Hypermetabolism 794.7
Hypermethioninemia 270.4
Hypermetropia (congenital) 367.0
Hypermobility
  cecum 564.9
  coccyx 724.71
  colon 564.9
    psychogenic 306.4
  ileum 564.89
  joint (acquired) 718.80
    ankle 718.87
    elbow 718.82
    foot 718.87
    hand 718.84
    hip 718.85
    knee 718.86
    multiple sites 718.89
    pelvic region 718.85
    shoulder (region) 718.81
    specified site NEC 718.88
    wrist 718.83
  kidney, congenital 753.3
  meniscus (knee) 717.5
  scapula 718.81
  stomach 536.8
    psychogenic 306.4
  syndrome 728.5
  testis, congenital 752.52
  urethral 599.81
Hypermotility
  gastrointestinal 536.8
  intestine 564.9
    psychogenic 306.4
  stomach 536.8
Hypernasality 784.43
Hypernatremia 276.0
  with water depletion 276.0
Hypernephroma (M8312/3) 189.0
Hyperopia 367.0
Hyperorexia 783.6
Hyperornithinemia 270.6
Hyperosmia (see also Disturbance, sensation)
    781.1
Hyperosmolality 276.0
Hyperosteogenesis 733.99
Hyperostosis 733.99
  calvarial 733.3
  cortical 733.3
    infantile 756.59
  frontal, internal of skull 733.3
  interna frontalis 733.3
  monomelic 733.99
  skull 733.3
    congenital 756.0
  vertebral 721.8
    with spondylosis - see Spondylosis
    ankylosing 721.6

Hyperovarianism 256.1
Hyperovarism, hyperovaria 256.1
Hyperoxaluria (primary) 271.8
Hyperoxia 987.8
Hyperparathyroidism 252.00
  ectopic 259.3
  other 252.08
  primary 252.01
  secondary (of renal origin) 588.81
    non-renal 252.02
  tertiary 252.08
Hyperpathia (see also Disturbance, sensation)
    782.0
  psychogenic 307.80
Hyperperistalsis 787.4
  psychogenic 306.4
Hyperpermeability, capillary 448.9
Hyperphagia 783.6
Hyperphenylalaninemia 270.1
Hyperphoria 378.40
  alternating 378.45
Hyperphosphatemia 275.3
Hyperpiesia (see also Hypertension) 401.9
Hyperpiesis (see also Hypertension) 401.9
Hyperpigmentation - see Pigmentation
Hyperpinealism 259.8
Hyperpipecolatemia 270.7
Hyperpituitarism 253.1
Hyperplasia, hyperplastic
  adenoids (lymphoid tissue) 474.12
    and tonsils 474.10
  adrenal (capsule) (cortex) (gland) 255.8
    with
      sexual precocity (male) 255.2
      virilism, adrenal 255.2
      virilization (female) 255.2
    congenital 255.2
    due to excess ACTH (ectopic) (pituitary)
      255.0
    medulla 255.8
  alpha cells (pancreatic)
    with
      gastrin excess 251.5
      glucagon excess 251.4
  angiolymphoid, with eosinophilia (ALHE)
    228.01
  appendix (lymphoid) 543.0
  artery, fibromuscular NEC 447.8
    carotid 447.8
    renal 447.3
  bone 733.99
    marrow 289.9
  breast (see also Hypertrophy, breast) 611.1
    ductal 610.8
      atypical 610.8
  carotid artery 447.8
  cementation, cementum (teeth) (tooth) 521.5
  cervical gland 785.6
  cervix (uteri) 622.10
    basal cell 622.10
    congenital 752.49
    endometrium 622.10
    polypoid 622.10
  chin 524.05
  clitoris, congenital 752.49
  dentin 521.5
  endocervicitis 616.0
  endometrium, endometrial (adenomatous)
      (atypical) (cystic) (glandular)
      (polypoid) (uterus) 621.30
    with atypia 621.33
    without atypia
      complex 621.32
      simple 621.31
    benign 621.34
    cervix 622.10
  epithelial 709.8
    focal, oral, including tongue 528.79
    mouth (focal) 528.79
    nipple 611.89
    skin 709.8

Hyperplasia, hyperplastic (Continued)
  epithelial (Continued)
    tongue (focal) 528.79
    vaginal wall 623.0
  erythroid 289.9
  fascialis ossificans (progressiva) 728.11
  fibromuscular, artery NEC 447.8
    carotid 447.8
    renal 447.3
  genital
    female 629.89
    male 608.89
  gingiva 523.8
  glandularis
    cystica uteri 621.30
    endometrium (uterus) 621.30
    interstitialis uteri 621.30
  granulocytic 288.69
  gum 523.8
  hymen, congenital 752.49
  islands of Langerhans 251.1
  islet cell (pancreatic) 251.9
    alpha cells
      with excess
        gastrin 251.5
        glucagon 251.4
    beta cells 251.1
  juxtaglomerular (complex) (kidney) 593.89
  kidney (congenital) 753.3
  liver (congenital) 751.69
  lymph node (gland) 785.6
  lymphoid (diffuse) (nodular) 785.6
    appendix 543.0
    intestine 569.89
  mandibular 524.02
    alveolar 524.72
    unilateral condylar 526.89
  Marchand multiple nodular (liver) - see
    Cirrhosis, postnecrotic
  maxillary 524.01
    alveolar 524.71
  medulla, adrenal 255.8
  myometrium, myometrial 621.2
  neuroendocrine cell, of infancy 516.61
  nose (lymphoid) (polypoid) 478.19
  oral soft tissue (inflammatory) (irritative)
      (mucosa) NEC 528.9
    gingiva 523.8
    tongue 529.8
  organ or site, congenital NEC - see Anomaly,
    specified type NEC
  ovary 620.8
  palate, papillary 528.9
  pancreatic islet cells 251.9
    alpha
      with excess
        gastrin 251.5
        glucagon 251.4
    beta 251.1
  parathyroid (gland) 252.01
  persistent, vitreous (primary) 743.51
  pharynx (lymphoid) 478.29
  prostate 600.90
    with
      other lower urinary tract symptoms
        (LUTS) 600.91
      urinary
        obstruction 600.91
        retention 600.91
    adenofibromatous 600.20
      with
        other lower urinary tract
          symptoms (LUTS) 600.21
        urinary
          obstruction 600.21
          retention 600.21
    nodular 600.10
      with
        urinary
          obstruction 600.11
          retention 600.11

Hyperplasia, hyperplastic *(Continued)*
  renal artery (fibromuscular) 447.3
  reticuloendothelial (cell) 289.9
  salivary gland (any) 527.1
  Schimmelbusch's 610.1
  suprarenal (capsule) (gland) 255.8
  thymus (gland) (persistent) 254.0
  thyroid *(see also* Goiter) 240.9
    primary 242.0●
    secondary 242.2●
  tonsil (lymphoid tissue) 474.11
    and adenoids 474.10
  urethrovaginal 599.89
  uterus, uterine (myometrium) 621.2
    endometrium *(see also* Hyperplasia, endometrium) 621.30
  vitreous (humor), primary persistent 743.51
  vulva 624.3
  zygoma 738.11
Hyperpnea *(see also* Hyperventilation) 786.01
Hyperpotassemia 276.7
Hyperprebetalipoproteinemia 272.1
  with chylomicronemia 272.3
  familial 272.1
Hyperprolactinemia 253.1
Hyperprolinemia 270.8
Hyperproteinemia 273.8
Hyperprothrombinemia 289.89
Hyperpselaphesia 782.0
Hyperpyrexia 780.60
  heat (effects of) 992.0
  malarial *(see also* Malaria) 084.6
  malignant, due to anesthetic 995.86
  rheumatic - *see* Fever, rheumatic
  unknown origin *(see also* Pyrexia) 780.60
Hyperreactor, vascular 780.2
Hyperreflexia 796.1
  bladder, autonomic 596.54
    with cauda equina 344.61
  detrusor 344.61
Hypersalivation *(see also* Ptyalism) 527.7
Hypersarcosinemia 270.8

Hypersecretion
  ACTH 255.3
  androgens (ovarian) 256.1
  calcitonin 246.0
  corticoadrenal 255.3
  cortisol 255.0
  estrogen 256.0
  gastric 536.8
    psychogenic 306.4
  gastrin 251.5
  glucagon 251.4
  hormone
    ACTH 255.3
    anterior pituitary 253.1
    growth NEC 253.0
    ovarian androgen 256.1
    testicular 257.0
    thyroid stimulating 242.8●
  insulin - *see* Hyperinsulinism
  lacrimal glands *(see also* Epiphora) 375.20
  medulloadrenal 255.6
  milk 676.6●
  ovarian androgens 256.1
  pituitary (anterior) 253.1
  salivary gland (any) 527.7
  testicular hormones 257.0
  thyrocalcitonin 246.0
  upper respiratory 478.9
Hypersegmentation, hereditary 288.2
  eosinophils 288.2
  neutrophil nuclei 288.2
Hypersensitive, hypersensitiveness, hypersensitivity - *see also* Allergy
  angiitis 446.20
    specified NEC 446.29
  carotid sinus 337.01
  colon 564.9
    psychogenic 306.4
  DNA (deoxyribonucleic acid) NEC 287.2
  drug *(see also* Allergy, drug) 995.27
  due to correct medical substance properly administered 995.27

Hypersensitive, hypersensitiveness, hypersensitivity *(Continued)*
  esophagus 530.89
  insect bites - *see* Injury, superficial, by site
  labyrinth 386.58
  pain *(see also* Disturbance, sensation) 782.0
  pneumonitis NEC 495.9
  reaction *(see also* Allergy) 995.3
    upper respiratory tract NEC 478.8
  stomach (allergic) (nonallergic) 536.8
    psychogenic 306.4
Hypersomatotropism (classic) 253.0
Hypersomnia, unspecified 780.54
  with sleep apnea, unspecified 780.53
  alcohol induced 291.82
  drug induced 292.85
  due to
    medical condition classified elsewhere 327.14
    mental disorder 327.15
  idiopathic
    with long sleep time 327.11
    without long sleep time 327.12
  menstrual related 327.13
  nonorganic origin 307.43
    persistent (primary) 307.44
    transient 307.43
  organic 327.10
    other 327.19
  primary 307.44
  recurrent 327.13
Hypersplenia 289.4
Hypersplenism 289.4
Hypersteatosis 706.3
Hyperstimulation, ovarian 256.1
Hypersuprarenalism 255.3
Hypersusceptibility - *see* Allergy
Hyper-TBG-nemia 246.8
Hypertelorism 756.0
  orbit, orbital 376.41
Hypertension, hypertensive - *see* table on pages 287–290

◀ New   ◀▥ Revised   ~~deleted~~ Deleted   ● Use Additional Digit(s)   ▨ Omit code

OGCR Section I.C.7.a.1
Assign hypertension (arterial) (essential) (systemic) (NOS) to category code 401 with appropriate fourth digit to indicate malignant (.0), benign (.1), or unspecified (.9). Do not use either .0 malignant or .1 benign unless medical record documentation supports such a designation.

	Malignant	Benign	Unspecified
Hypertension, hypertensive (arterial) (arteriolar) (crisis) (degeneration) (disease) (essential) (fluctuating) (idiopathic) (intermittent) (labile) (low renin) (orthostatic) (paroxysmal) (primary) (systemic) (uncontrolled) (vascular)	401.0	401.1	401.9
with			
chronic kidney disease	—	—	—
stage I through stage IV, or unspecified	403.00	403.10	403.90
stage V or end stage renal disease	403.01	403.11	403.91
heart involvement (conditions classifiable to 429.0–429.3, 429.8, 429.9 due to hypertension) (*see also* Hypertension, heart)	402.00	402.10	402.90
with kidney involvement - *see* Hypertension, cardiorenal			
renal (kidney) involvement (only conditions classifiable to 585, 587) (excludes conditions classifiable to 584) (*see also* Hypertension, kidney)	403.00	403.10	403.90
with heart involvement - *see* Hypertension, cardiorenal failure (and sclerosis) (*see also* Hypertension, kidney)	403.01	403.11	403.91
sclerosis without failure (*see also* Hypertension, kidney)	403.00	403.10	403.90
accelerated (*see also* Hypertension, by type, malignant)	401.0	—	—
antepartum - *see* Hypertension, complicating pregnancy, childbirth, or the puerperium			
borderline	—	—	796.2
cardiorenal (disease)	404.00	404.10	404.90
with			
chronic kidney disease	—	—	—
stage I through stage IV, or unspecified	404.00	404.10	404.90
and heart failure	404.01	404.11	404.91
stage V or end stage renal disease	404.02	404.12	404.92
and heart failure	404.03	404.13	404.93
heart failure	404.01	404.11	404.91
and chronic kidney disease	404.01	404.11	404.91
stage I through stage IV or unspecified	404.01	404.11	404.91
stage V or end stage renal disease	404.03	404.13	404.93
cardiovascular disease (arteriosclerotic) (sclerotic)	402.00	402.10	402.90
with			
heart failure	402.01	402.11	402.91
renal involvement (conditions classifiable to 403) (*see also* Hypertension, cardiorenal)	404.00	404.10	404.90
cardiovascular renal (disease) (sclerosis) (*see also* Hypertension, cardiorenal)	404.00	404.10	404.90
cerebrovascular disease NEC	437.2	437.2	437.2
complicating pregnancy, childbirth, or the puerperium	642.2●	642.0●	642.9●
with			
albuminuria (and edema) (mild)	—	—	642.4●
severe	—	—	642.5●
chronic kidney disease	642.2●	642.2●	642.2●
and heart disease	642.2●	642.2●	642.2●
edema (mild)	—	—	642.4●
severe	—	—	642.5●
heart disease	642.2●	642.2●	642.2●
and chronic kidney disease	642.2●	642.2●	642.2●

	Malignant	Benign	Unspecified
Hypertension, hypertensive *(Continued)*			
complicating pregnancy, childbirth, or the puerperium *(Continued)*			
with *(Continued)*			
renal disease	642.2●	642.2●	642.2●
and heart disease	642.2●	642.2●	642.2●
chronic	642.2●	642.0●	642.0●
with pre-eclampsia or eclampsia	642.7●	642.7●	642.7●
fetus or newborn	760.0	760.0	760.0
essential	—	642.0●	642.0●
with pre-eclampsia or eclampsia	—	642.7●	642.7●
fetus or newborn	760.0	760.0	760.0
fetus or newborn	760.0	760.0	760.0
gestational	—	—	642.3●
pre-existing	642.2●	642.0●	642.0●
with pre-eclampsia or eclampsia	642.7●	642.7●	642.7●
fetus or newborn	760.0	760.0	760.0
secondary to renal disease	642.1●	642.1●	642.1●
with pre-eclampsia or eclampsia	642.7●	642.7●	642.7●
fetus or newborn	760.0	760.0	760.0
transient	—	—	642.3●
due to			
aldosteronism, primary	405.09	405.19	405.99
brain tumor	405.09	405.19	405.99
bulbar poliomyelitis	405.09	405.19	405.99
calculus			
kidney	405.09	405.19	405.99
ureter	405.09	405.19	405.99
coarctation, aorta	405.09	405.19	405.99
Cushing's disease	405.09	405.19	405.99
glomerulosclerosis (*see also* Hypertension, kidney)	403.00	403.10	403.90
periarteritis nodosa	405.09	405.19	405.99
pheochromocytoma	405.09	405.19	405.99
polycystic kidney(s)	405.09	405.19	405.99
polycythemia	405.09	405.19	405.99
porphyria	405.09	405.19	405.99
pyelonephritis	405.09	405.19	405.99
renal (artery)			
aneurysm	405.01	405.11	405.91
anomaly	405.01	405.11	405.91
embolism	405.01	405.11	405.91
fibromuscular hyperplasia	405.01	405.11	405.91
occlusion	405.01	405.11	405.91
stenosis	405.01	405.11	405.91
thrombosis	405.01	405.11	405.91

◀ New ◀⁣⁣⁣ Revised ~~deleted~~ Deleted ● Use Additional Digit(s) Omit code

	Malignant	Benign	Unspecified
Hypertension, hypertensive *(Continued)*			
encephalopathy	437.2	437.2	437.2
gestational (transient) NEC	—	—	642.3●
Goldblatt's	440.1	440.1	440.1
heart (disease) (conditions classifiable to 429.0–429.3, 429.8, 429.9 due to hypertension)	402.00	402.10	402.90
with			
heart failure	402.01	402.11	402.91
hypertensive kidney disease (conditions classifiable to 403) (*see also* Hypertension, cardiorenal)	404.00	404.10	404.90
renal sclerosis (*see also* Hypertension, cardiorenal)	404.00	404.10	404.90
intracranial, benign	—	348.2	—
intraocular	—	—	365.04
kidney	403.00	403.10	403.90
with			
chronic kidney disease	—	—	—
stage I through stage IV, or unspecified	403.00	403.10	403.90
stage V or end stage renal disease	403.01	403.11	403.91
heart involvement (conditions classifiable to 429.0–429.3, 429.8, 429.9 due to hypertension) (*see also* Hypertension, cardiorenal)	404.00	404.10	404.90
hypertensive heart (disease) (conditions classifiable to 402) (*see also* Hypertension, cardiorenal)	404.00	404.10	404.90
lesser circulation	—	—	416.0
necrotizing	401.0	—	—
pancreatic duct - *code to* underlying condition			
with			
chronic pancreatitis	—	—	577.11
ocular			365.04
portal (due to chronic liver disease)	—	—	572.3
postoperative			997.91
psychogenic	—	—	306.2
puerperal, postpartum - *see* Hypertension, complicating pregnancy, childbirth, or the puerperium			
pulmonary (artery) (secondary)	—	—	416.8
with			
cor pulmonale (chronic)	—	—	416.8
acute	—	—	415.0
right heart ventricular strain/failure	—	—	416.8
acute	—	—	415.0
idiopathic	—	—	416.0
primary	—	—	416.0
of newborn	—	—	747.83
secondary	—	—	416.8

	Malignant	Benign	Unspecified
Hypertension, hypertensive *(Continued)*			
renal (disease) (*see also* Hypertension, kidney)	403.00	403.10	403.90
renovascular NEC	405.01	405.11	405.91
secondary NEC	405.09	405.19	405.99
due to			
aldosteronism, primary	405.09	405.19	405.99
brain tumor	405.09	405.19	405.99
bulbar poliomyelitis	405.09	405.19	405.99
calculus			
kidney	405.09	405.19	405.99
ureter	405.09	405.19	405.99
coarctation, aorta	405.09	405.19	405.99
Cushing's disease	405.09	405.19	405.99
glomerulosclerosis (*see also* Hypertension, kidney)	403.00	403.10	403.90
periarteritis nodosa	405.09	405.19	405.99
pheochromocytoma	405.09	405.19	405.99
polycystic kidney(s)	405.09	405.19	405.99
polycythemia	405.09	405.19	405.99
porphyria	405.09	405.19	405.99
pyelonephritis	405.09	405.19	405.99
renal (artery)			
aneurysm	405.01	405.11	405.91
anomaly	405.01	405.11	405.91
embolism	405.01	405.11	405.91
fibromuscular hyperplasia	405.01	405.11	405.91
occlusion	405.01	405.11	405.91
stenosis	405.01	405.11	405.91
thrombosis	405.01	405.11	405.91
transient	—	—	796.2
of pregnancy	—	—	642.3●
venous, chronic (asymptomatic) (idiopathic)	—	—	459.30
with			
complication, NEC	—	—	459.39
inflammation	—	—	459.32
with ulcer	—	—	459.33
ulcer	—	—	459.31
with inflammation	—	—	459.33
due to			
deep vein thrombosis (*see also* Syndrome, postphlebitic)	—	—	459.10

◀ New   ◀▥ Revised   ~~deleted~~ Deleted   ● Use Additional Digit(s)   Omit code

Hypertensive urgency - *see* Hypertension
Hyperthecosis, ovary 256.8
Hyperthermia (of unknown origin) (*see also* Pyrexia) 780.60
  malignant (due to anesthesia) 995.86
  newborn 778.4
Hyperthymergasia (*see also* Psychosis, affective) 296.0●
  reactive (from emotional stress, psychological trauma) 298.1
  recurrent episode 296.1●
  single episode 296.0●
Hyperthymism 254.8
Hyperthyroid (recurrent) - *see* Hyperthyroidism
Hyperthyroidism (latent) (preadult) (recurrent) (without goiter) 242.9●

Note: Use the following fifth-digit subclassification with category 242:

0 without mention of thyrotoxic crisis or storm
1 with mention of thyrotoxic crisis or storm

---

  with
    goiter (diffuse) 242.0●
      adenomatous 242.3●
        multinodular 242.2●
        uninodular 242.1●
      nodular 242.3●
        multinodular 242.2●
        uninodular 242.1●
      thyroid nodule 242.1●
  complicating pregnancy, childbirth, or puerperium 648.1●
  neonatal (transient) 775.3
Hypertonia - *see* Hypertonicity
Hypertonicity
  bladder 596.51
  fetus or newborn 779.89
  gastrointestinal (tract) 536.8
  infancy 779.89
    due to electrolyte imbalance 779.89
  muscle 728.85
  stomach 536.8
    psychogenic 306.4
  uterus, uterine (contractions) 661.4●
    affecting fetus or newborn 763.7
Hypertony - *see* Hypertonicity
Hypertransaminemia 790.4
Hypertrichosis 704.1
  congenital 757.4
  eyelid 374.54
  lanuginosa 757.4
    acquired 704.1
Hypertriglyceridemia, essential 272.1
Hypertrophy, hypertrophic
  adenoids (infectional) 474.12
    and tonsils (faucial) (infective) (lingual) (lymphoid) 474.10
  adrenal 255.8
  alveolar process or ridge 525.8
  anal papillae 569.49
  apocrine gland 705.82
  artery NEC 447.8
    carotid 447.8
    congenital (peripheral) NEC 747.60
      gastrointestinal 747.61
      lower limb 747.64
      renal 747.62
      specified NEC 747.69
      spinal 747.82
      upper limb 747.63
    renal 447.3
  arthritis (chronic) (*see also* Osteoarthrosis) 715.9●
    spine (*see also* Spondylosis) 721.90
  arytenoid 478.79
  asymmetrical (heart) 429.9
  auricular - *see* Hypertrophy, cardiac
  Bartholin's gland 624.8
  bile duct 576.8

Hypertrophy, hypertrophic (*Continued*)
  bladder (sphincter) (trigone) 596.89
  blind spot, visual field 368.42
  bone 733.99
  brain 348.89
  breast 611.1
    cystic 610.1
    fetus or newborn 778.7
    fibrocystic 610.1
    massive pubertal 611.1
    puerperal, postpartum 676.3●
    senile (parenchymatous) 611.1
  cardiac (chronic) (idiopathic) 429.3
    with
      rheumatic fever (conditions classifiable to 390)
        active 391.8
          with chorea 392.0
        inactive or quiescent (with chorea) 398.99
    congenital NEC 746.89
    fatty (*see also* Degeneration, myocardial) 429.1
    hypertensive (*see also* Hypertension, heart) 402.90
    rheumatic (with chorea) 398.99
      active or acute 391.8
        with chorea 392.0
    valve (*see also* Endocarditis) 424.90
      congenital NEC 746.89
  cartilage 733.99
  cecum 569.89
  cervix (uteri) 622.6
    congenital 752.49
    elongation 622.6
  clitoris (cirrhotic) 624.2
    congenital 752.49
  colon 569.89
    congenital 751.3
  conjunctiva, lymphoid 372.73
  cornea 371.89
  corpora cavernosa 607.89
  duodenum 537.89
  endometrium (uterus) (*see also* Hyperplasia, endometrium) 621.30
    cervix 622.6
  epididymis 608.89
  esophageal hiatus (congenital) 756.6
    with hernia - *see* Hernia, diaphragm
  eyelid 374.30
  falx, skull 733.99
  fat pad 729.30
    infrapatellar 729.31
    knee 729.31
    orbital 374.34
    popliteal 729.31
    prepatellar 729.31
    retropatellar 729.31
    specified site NEC 729.39
  foot (congenital) 755.67
  frenum, frenulum (tongue) 529.8
    linguae 529.8
    lip 528.5
  gallbladder or cystic duct 575.8
  gastric mucosa 535.2●
  gingiva 523.8
  gland, glandular (general) NEC 785.6
  gum (mucous membrane) 523.8
  heart (idiopathic) - *see also* Hypertrophy, cardiac
    valve - *see also* Endocarditis
      congenital NEC 746.89
  hemifacial 754.0
  hepatic - *see* Hypertrophy, liver
  hiatus (esophageal) 756.6
  hilus gland 785.6
  hymen, congenital 752.49
  ileum 569.89
  infrapatellar fat pad 729.31
  intestine 569.89
  jejunum 569.89

Hypertrophy, hypertrophic (*Continued*)
  kidney (compensatory) 593.1
    congenital 753.3
  labial frenulum 528.5
  labium (majus) (minus) 624.3
  lacrimal gland, chronic 375.03
  ligament 728.9
    spinal 724.8
  linguae frenulum 529.8
  lingual tonsil (infectional) 474.11
  lip (frenum) 528.5
    congenital 744.81
  liver 789.1
    acute 573.8
    cirrhotic - *see* Cirrhosis, liver
    congenital 751.69
    fatty - *see* Fatty, liver
  lymph gland 785.6
    tuberculous - *see* Tuberculosis, lymph gland
  mammary gland - *see* Hypertrophy, breast
  maxillary frenulum 528.5
  Meckel's diverticulum (congenital) 751.0
  medial meniscus, acquired 717.3
  median bar 600.90
    with
      other lower urinary tract symptoms (LUTS) 600.91
      urinary
        obstruction 600.91
        retention 600.91
  mediastinum 519.3
  meibomian gland 373.2
  meniscus, knee, congenital 755.64
  metatarsal head 733.99
  metatarsus 733.99
  mouth 528.9
  mucous membrane
    alveolar process 523.8
    nose 478.19
    turbinate (nasal) 478.0
  muscle 728.9
  muscular coat, artery NEC 447.8
    carotid 447.8
    renal 447.3
  myocardium (*see also* Hypertrophy, cardiac) 429.3
    idiopathic 425.18
  myometrium 621.2
  nail 703.8
    congenital 757.5
  nasal 478.19
    alae 478.19
    bone 738.0
    cartilage 478.19
    mucous membrane (septum) 478.19
    sinus (*see also* Sinusitis) 473.9
    turbinate 478.0
  nasopharynx, lymphoid (infectional) (tissue) (wall) 478.29
  neck, uterus 622.6
  nipple 611.1
  normal aperture diaphragm (congenital) 756.6
  nose (*see also* Hypertrophy, nasal) 478.19
  orbit 376.46
  organ or site, congenital NEC - *see* Anomaly, specified type NEC
  osteoarthropathy (pulmonary) 731.2
  ovary 620.8
  palate (hard) 526.89
    soft 528.9
  pancreas (congenital) 751.7
  papillae
    anal 569.49
    tongue 529.3
  parathyroid (gland) 252.01
  parotid gland 527.1
  penis 607.89
  phallus 607.89
    female (clitoris) 624.2
  pharyngeal tonsil 474.12
  pharyngitis 472.1

◀ New   ⬅ Revised   ~~deleted~~ Deleted   ● Use Additional Digit(s)   ▨ Omit code

Hypertrophy, hypertrophic (Continued)
    pharynx 478.29
        lymphoid (infectional) (tissue) (wall) 478.29
    pituitary (fossa) (gland) 253.8
    popliteal fat pad 729.31
    preauricular (lymph) gland (Hampstead) 785.6
    prepuce (congenital) 605
        female 624.2
    prostate (asymptomatic) (early) (recurrent) 600.90
        with
            other lower urinary tract symptoms (LUTS) 600.91
                urinary
                    obstruction 600.91
                    retention 600.91
        adenofibromatous 600.20
            with
                other lower urinary tract symptoms (LUTS) 600.21
                    urinary
                        obstruction 600.21
                        retention 600.21
        benign 600.00
            with
                other lower urinary tract symptoms (LUTS) 600.01
                    urinary
                        obstruction 600.01
                        retention 600.01
        congenital 752.89
    pseudoedematous hypodermal 757.0
    pseudomuscular 359.1
    pylorus (muscle) (sphincter) 537.0
        congenital 750.5
        infantile 750.5
    rectal sphincter 569.49
    rectum 569.49
    renal 593.1
    rhinitis (turbinate) 472.0
    salivary duct or gland 527.1
        congenital 750.26
    scaphoid (tarsal) 733.99
    scar 701.4
    scrotum 608.89
    sella turcica 253.8
    seminal vesicle 608.89
    sigmoid 569.89
    skin condition NEC 701.9
    spermatic cord 608.89
    spinal ligament 724.8
    spleen - see Splenomegaly
    spondylitis (spine) (see also Spondylosis) 721.90
    stomach 537.89
    subaortic stenosis (idiopathic) 425.11
    sublingual gland 527.1
        congenital 750.26
    submaxillary gland 527.1
    suprarenal (gland) 255.8
    tendon 727.9
    testis 608.89
        congenital 752.89
    thymic, thymus (congenital) (gland) 254.0
    thyroid (gland) (see also Goiter) 240.9
        primary 242.0●
        secondary 242.2●
    toe (congenital) 755.65
        acquired 735.8
    tongue 529.8
        congenital 750.15
        frenum 529.8
        papillae (foliate) 529.3
    tonsil (faucial) (infective) (lingual) (lymphoid) 474.11
        with
            adenoiditis 474.01
            tonsillitis 474.00
                and adenoiditis 474.02
        and adenoids 474.10
    tunica vaginalis 608.89

Hypertrophy, hypertrophic (Continued)
    turbinate (mucous membrane) 478.0
    ureter 593.89
    urethra 599.84
    uterus 621.2
        puerperal, postpartum 674.8●
    uvula 528.9
    vagina 623.8
    vas deferens 608.89
    vein 459.89
    ventricle, ventricular (heart) (left) (right) - see also Hypertrophy, cardiac
        congenital 746.89
        due to hypertension (left) (right) (see also Hypertension, heart) 402.90
            benign 402.10
            malignant 402.00
        right with ventricular septal defect, pulmonary stenosis or atresia, and dextraposition of aorta 745.2
    verumontanum 599.89
    vesical 596.89
    vocal cord 478.5
    vulva 624.3
        stasis (nonfilarial) 624.3
Hypertropia (intermittent) (periodic) 378.31
Hypertyrosinemia 270.2
Hyperuricemia 790.6
Hypervalinemia 270.3
Hyperventilation (tetany) 786.01
    hysterical 300.11
    psychogenic 306.1
    syndrome 306.1
Hyperviscidosis 277.00
Hyperviscosity (of serum) (syndrome) NEC 273.3
    polycythemic 289.0
    sclerocythemic 282.8
Hypervitaminosis (dietary) NEC 278.8
    A (dietary) 278.2
    D (dietary) 278.4
    from excessive administration or use of vitamin preparations (chronic) 278.8
        reaction to sudden overdose 963.5
        vitamin A 278.2
            reaction to sudden overdose 963.5
        vitamin D 278.4
            reaction to sudden overdose 963.5
        vitamin K
            correct substance properly administered 278.8
            overdose or wrong substance given or taken 964.3
Hypervolemia 276.69
Hypesthesia (see also Disturbance, sensation) 782.0
    cornea 371.81
Hyphema (anterior chamber) (ciliary body) (iris) 364.41
    traumatic 921.3
Hyphemia - see Hyphema
Hypoacidity, gastric 536.8
    psychogenic 306.4
Hypoactive labyrinth (function) - see Hypofunction, labyrinth
Hypoadrenalism 255.41
    tuberculous (see also Tuberculosis) 017.6●
Hypoadrenocorticism 255.41
    pituitary 253.4
Hypoalbuminemia 273.8
Hypoaldosteronism 255.42
Hypoalphalipoproteinemia 272.5
Hypobarism 993.2
Hypobaropathy 993.2
Hypobetalipoproteinemia (familial) 272.5
Hypocalcemia 275.41
    cow's milk 775.4
    dietary 269.3
    neonatal 775.4
    phosphate-loading 775.4
Hypocalcification, teeth 520.4
Hypochloremia 276.9

Hypochlorhydria 536.8
    neurotic 306.4
    psychogenic 306.4
Hypocholesteremia 272.5
Hypochondria (reaction) 300.7
Hypochondriac 300.7
Hypochondriasis 300.7
Hypochromasia blood cells 280.9
Hypochromic anemia 280.9
    due to blood loss (chronic) 280.0
        acute 285.1
    microcytic 280.9
Hypocoagulability (see also Defect, coagulation) 286.9
Hypocomplementemia 279.8
Hypocythemia (progressive) 284.9
Hypodontia (see also Anodontia) 520.0
Hypoeosinophilia 288.59
Hypoesthesia (see also Disturbance, sensation) 782.0
    cornea 371.81
    tactile 782.0
Hypoestrinism 256.39
Hypoestrogenism 256.39
Hypoferremia 280.9
    due to blood loss (chronic) 280.0
Hypofertility
    female 628.9
    male 606.1
Hypofibrinogenemia 286.3
    acquired 286.6
    congenital 286.3
Hypofunction
    adrenal (gland) 255.41
        cortex 255.41
        medulla 255.5
        specified NEC 255.5
    cerebral 331.9
    corticoadrenal NEC 255.41
    intestinal 564.89
    labyrinth (unilateral) 386.53
        with loss of labyrinthine reactivity 386.55
        bilateral 386.54
            with loss of labyrinthine reactivity 386.56
    Leydig cell 257.2
    ovary 256.39
        postablative 256.2
    pituitary (anterior) (gland) (lobe) 253.2
        posterior 253.5
    testicular 257.2
        iatrogenic 257.1
        postablative 257.1
        postirradiation 257.1
        postsurgical 257.1
Hypogammaglobulinemia 279.00
    acquired primary 279.06
    non-sex-linked, congenital 279.06
    sporadic 279.06
    transient of infancy 279.09
Hypogenitalism (congenital) (female) (male) 752.89
    penis 752.69
Hypoglycemia (spontaneous) 251.2
    coma 251.0
        diabetic 250.3●
            due to secondary diabetes 249.3●
        diabetic 250.8●
            due to secondary diabetes 249.8●
    due to insulin 251.0
        therapeutic misadventure 962.3
    familial (idiopathic) 251.2
    following gastrointestinal surgery 579.3
    infantile (idiopathic) 251.2
    in infant of diabetic mother 775.0
    leucine-induced 270.3
    neonatal 775.6
    reactive 251.2
    specified NEC 251.1
Hypoglycemic shock 251.0
    diabetic 250.8●
        due to secondary diabetes 249.8●

◄ New   ◄▦ Revised   deleted Deleted   ● Use Additional Digit(s)   ▨ Omit code

Hypoglycemic shock (Continued)
due to insulin 251.0
functional (syndrome) 251.1
Hypogonadism
female 256.39
gonadotrophic (isolated) 253.4
hypogonadotropic (isolated) (with anosmia) 253.4
isolated 253.4
male 257.2
hereditary familial (Reifenstein's syndrome) 259.52
ovarian (primary) 256.39
pituitary (secondary) 253.4
testicular (primary) (secondary) 257.2
Hypohidrosis 705.0
Hypohidrotic ectodermal dysplasia 757.31
Hypoidrosis 705.0
Hypoinsulinemia, postsurgical 251.3
postpancreatectomy (complete) (partial) 251.3
Hypokalemia 276.8
Hypokinesia 780.99
Hypoleukia splenica 289.4
Hypoleukocytosis 288.50
Hypolipidemia 272.5
Hypolipoproteinemia 272.5
Hypomagnesemia 275.2
neonatal 775.4
Hypomania, hypomanic reaction (see also Psychosis, affective) 296.0●
recurrent episode 296.1●
single episode 296.0●
Hypomastia (congenital) 611.82
Hypomenorrhea 626.1
Hypometabolism 783.9
Hypomotility
gastrointestinal tract 536.8
psychogenic 306.4
intestine 564.89
psychogenic 306.4
stomach 536.8
psychogenic 306.4
Hyponasality 784.44
Hyponatremia 276.1
Hypo-ovarianism 256.39
Hypo-ovarism 256.39
Hypoparathyroidism (idiopathic) (surgically induced) 252.1
neonatal 775.4
Hypoperfusion (in)
newborn 779.89
Hypopharyngitis 462
Hypophoria 378.40
Hypophosphatasia 275.3
Hypophosphatemia (acquired) (congenital) (familial) 275.3
renal 275.3
Hypophyseal, hypophysis - see also condition
dwarfism 253.3
gigantism 253.0
syndrome 253.8
Hypophyseothalamic syndrome 253.8
Hypopiesis - see Hypotension
Hypopigmentation 709.00
eyelid 374.53
Hypopinealism 259.8
Hypopituitarism (juvenile) (syndrome) 253.2
due to
hormone therapy 253.7
hypophysectomy 253.7
radiotherapy 253.7
postablative 253.7
postpartum hemorrhage 253.2
Hypoplasia, hypoplasis 759.89
adrenal (gland) 759.1
alimentary tract 751.8
lower 751.2
upper 750.8
angiolymphoid, with eosinophilia (ALHE) 228.01
anus, anal (canal) 751.2

Hypoplasia, hypoplasis (Continued)
aorta 747.22
aortic
arch (tubular) 747.10
orifice or valve with hypoplasia of ascending aorta and defective development of left ventricle (with mitral valve atresia) 746.7
appendix 751.2
areola 757.6
arm (see also Absence, arm, congenital) 755.20
artery (congenital) (peripheral) 747.60
brain 747.81
cerebral 747.81
coronary 746.85
gastrointestinal 747.61
lower limb 747.64
pulmonary 747.31
renal 747.62
retinal 743.58
specified NEC 747.69
spinal 747.82
umbilical 747.5
upper limb 747.63
auditory canal 744.29
causing impairment of hearing 744.02
biliary duct (common) or passage 751.61
bladder 753.8
bone NEC 756.9
face 756.0
malar 756.0
mandible 524.04
alveolar 524.74
marrow 284.9
acquired (secondary) 284.89
congenital 284.09
idiopathic 284.9
maxilla 524.03
alveolar 524.73
skull (see also Hypoplasia, skull) 756.0
brain 742.1
gyri 742.2
specified part 742.2
breast (areola) 611.82
bronchus (tree) 748.3
cardiac 746.89
valve - see Hypoplasia, heart, valve
vein 746.89
carpus (see also Absence, carpal, congenital) 755.28
cartilaginous 756.9
cecum 751.2
cementum 520.4
hereditary 520.5
cephalic 742.1
cerebellum 742.2
cervix (uteri) 752.43
chin 524.06
clavicle 755.51
coccyx 756.19
colon 751.2
corpus callosum 742.2
cricoid cartilage 748.3
dermal, focal (Goltz) 757.39
digestive organ(s) or tract NEC 751.8
lower 751.2
upper 750.8
ear 744.29
auricle 744.23
lobe 744.29
middle, except ossicles 744.03
ossicles 744.04
ossicles 744.04
enamel of teeth (neonatal) (postnatal) (prenatal) 520.4
hereditary 520.5
endocrine (gland) NEC 759.2
endometrium 621.8
epididymis 752.89
epiglottis 748.3
erythroid, congenital 284.01
erythropoietic, chronic acquired 284.81

Hypoplasia, hypoplasis (Continued)
esophagus 750.3
Eustachian tube 744.24
eye (see also Microphthalmos) 743.10
lid 743.62
face 744.89
bone(s) 756.0
fallopian tube 752.19
femur (see also Absence, femur, congenital) 755.34
fibula (see also Absence, fibula, congenital) 755.37
finger (see also Absence, finger, congenital) 755.29
focal dermal 757.39
foot 755.31
gallbladder 751.69
genitalia, genital organ(s)
female 752.89
external 752.49
internal NEC 752.89
in adiposogenital dystrophy 253.8
male 752.89
penis 752.69
glottis 748.3
hair 757.4
hand 755.21
heart 746.89
left (complex) (syndrome) 746.7
valve NEC 746.89
pulmonary 746.01
humerus (see also Absence, humerus, congenital) 755.24
hymen 752.49
intestine (small) 751.1
large 751.2
iris 743.46
jaw 524.09
kidney(s) 753.0
labium (majus) (minus) 752.49
labyrinth, membranous 744.05
lacrimal duct (apparatus) 743.65
larynx 748.3
leg (see also Absence, limb, congenital, lower) 755.30
limb 755.4
lower (see also Absence, limb, congenital, lower) 755.30
upper (see also Absence, limb, congenital, upper) 755.20
liver 751.69
lung (lobe) 748.5
mammary (areolar) 611.82
mandibular 524.04
alveolar 524.74
unilateral condylar 526.89
maxillary 524.03
alveolar 524.73
medullary 284.9
megakaryocytic 287.30
metacarpus (see also Absence, metacarpal, congenital) 755.28
metatarsus (see also Absence, metatarsal, congenital) 755.38
muscle 756.89
eye 743.69
myocardium (congenital) (Uhl's anomaly) 746.84
nail(s) 757.5
nasolacrimal duct 743.65
nervous system NEC 742.8
neural 742.8
nose, nasal 748.1
ophthalmic (see also Microphthalmos) 743.10
optic nerve 377.43
organ
of Corti 744.05
or site NEC - see Anomaly, by site
osseous meatus (ear) 744.03
ovary 752.0
oviduct 752.19
pancreas 751.7

Hypoplasia, hypoplasis (*Continued*)
parathyroid (gland) 759.2
parotid gland 750.26
patella 755.64
pelvis, pelvic girdle 755.69
penis 752.69
peripheral vascular system (congenital) NEC 747.60
    gastrointestinal 747.61
    lower limb 747.64
    renal 747.62
    specified NEC 747.69
    spinal 747.82
    upper limb 747.63
pituitary (gland) 759.2
pulmonary 748.5
    arteriovenous 747.32
    artery 747.31
    valve 746.01
punctum lacrimale 743.65
radioulnar (*see also* Absence, radius, congenital, with ulna) 755.25
radius (*see also* Absence, radius, congenital) 755.26
rectum 751.2
respiratory system NEC 748.9
rib 756.3
sacrum 756.19
scapula 755.59
shoulder girdle 755.59
skin 757.39
skull (bone) 756.0
    with
        anencephalus 740.0
        encephalocele 742.0
        hydrocephalus 742.3
            with spina bifida (*see also* Spina bifida) 741.0●
        microcephalus 742.1
spinal (cord) (ventral horn cell) 742.59
    vessel 747.82
spine 756.19
spleen 759.0
sternum 756.3
tarsus (*see also* Absence, tarsal, congenital) 755.38
testis, testicle 752.89
thymus (gland) 279.11
thyroid (gland) 243
    cartilage 748.3
tibiofibular (*see also* Absence, tibia, congenital, with fibula) 755.35
toe (*see also* Absence, toe, congenital) 755.39
tongue 750.16
trachea (cartilage) (rings) 748.3
Turner's (tooth) 520.4
ulna (*see also* Absence, ulna, congenital) 755.27
umbilical artery 747.5
ureter 753.29
uterus 752.32
vagina 752.45
vascular (peripheral) NEC (*see also* Hypoplasia, peripheral vascular system) 747.60
    brain 747.81
vein(s) (peripheral) NEC (*see also* Hypoplasia, peripheral vascular system) 747.60
    brain 747.81
    cardiac 746.89
    great 747.49
    portal 747.49
    pulmonary 747.49
vena cava (inferior) (superior) 747.49
vertebra 756.19
vulva 752.49
zonule (ciliary) 743.39
zygoma 738.12
Hypopotassemia 276.8
Hypoproaccelerinemia (*see also* Defect, coagulation) 286.3

Hypoproconvertinemia (congenital) (*see also* Defect, coagulation) 286.3
Hypoproteinemia (essential) (hypermetabolic) (idiopathic) 273.8
Hypoproteinosis 260
Hypoprothrombinemia (congenital) (hereditary) (idiopathic) (*see also* Defect, coagulation) 286.3
acquired 286.7
newborn 776.3
Hypopselaphesia 782.0
Hypopyon (anterior chamber) (eye) 364.05
iritis 364.05
ulcer (cornea) 370.04
Hypopyrexia 780.99
Hyporeflex 796.1
Hyporeninemia, extreme 790.99
in primary aldosteronism 255.10
Hyporesponsive episode 780.09
Hyposecretion
ACTH 253.4
ovary 256.39
    postablative 256.2
salivary gland (any) 527.7
Hyposegmentation of neutrophils, hereditary 288.2
Hyposiderinemia 280.9
Hyposmolality 276.1
syndrome 276.1
Hyposomatotropism 253.3
Hyposomnia, unspecified (*see also* Insomnia) 780.52
with sleep apnea, unspecified 780.51
Hypospadias (male) 752.61
female 753.8
Hypospermatogenesis 606.1
Hyposphagma 372.72
Hyposplenism 289.59
Hypostasis, pulmonary 514
Hypostatic - *see* condition
Hyposthenuria 593.89
Hyposuprarenalism 255.41
Hypo-TBG-nemia 246.8
Hypotension (arterial) (constitutional) 458.9
chronic 458.1
iatrogenic 458.29
maternal, syndrome (following labor and delivery) 669.2●
of hemodialysis 458.21
orthostatic (chronic) 458.0
    dysautonomic-dyskinetic syndrome 333.0
permanent idiopathic 458.1
postoperative 458.29
postural 458.0
specified type NEC 458.8
transient 796.3
Hypothermia (accidental) 991.6
anesthetic 995.89
associated with low environmental temperature 991.6
newborn NEC 778.3
not associated with low environmental temperature 780.65
Hypothymergasia (*see also* Psychosis, affective) 296.2●
recurrent episode 296.3●
single episode 296.2●
Hypothyroidism (acquired) 244.9
complicating pregnancy, childbirth, or puerperium 648.1●
congenital 243
due to
    ablation 244.1
        radioactive iodine 244.1
        surgical 244.0
    iodine (administration) (ingestion) 244.2
        radioactive 244.1
    irradiation therapy 244.1
    p-aminosalicylic acid (PAS) 244.3
    phenylbutazone 244.3
    resorcinol 244.3

Hypothyroidism (*Continued*)
due to (*Continued*)
    specified cause NEC 244.8
    surgery 244.0
goitrous (sporadic) 246.1
iatrogenic NEC 244.3
iodine 244.2
pituitary 244.8
postablative NEC 244.1
postsurgical 244.0
primary 244.9
secondary NEC 244.8
specified cause NEC 244.8
sporadic goitrous 246.1
Hypotonia, hypotonicity, hypotony 781.3
benign congenital 358.8
bladder 596.4
congenital 779.89
    benign 358.8
eye 360.30
    due to
        fistula 360.32
        ocular disorder NEC 360.33
    following loss of aqueous or vitreous 360.33
    primary 360.31
infantile muscular (benign) 359.0
muscle 728.9
uterus, uterine (contractions) - *see* Inertia, uterus
Hypotrichosis 704.09
congenital 757.4
lid (congenital) 757.4
    acquired 374.55
postinfectional NEC 704.09
Hypotropia 378.32
Hypoventilation 786.09
congenital central alveolar syndrome 327.25
idiopathic sleep related nonobstructive alveolar 327.24
obesity 278.03
sleep related, in conditions classifiable elsewhere 327.26
Hypovitaminosis (*see also* Deficiency, vitamin) 269.2
Hypovolemia 276.52
surgical shock 998.09
traumatic (shock) 958.4
Hypoxemia (*see also* Anoxia) 799.02
sleep related, in conditions classifiable elsewhere 327.26
Hypoxia (*see also* Anoxia) 799.02
cerebral 348.1
    during or resulting from a procedure 997.01
    newborn 770.88
        mild or moderate 768.6
        severe 768.5
fetal, affecting newborn 770.88
intrauterine - *see* Distress, fetal
myocardial (*see also* Insufficiency, coronary) 411.89
    arteriosclerotic - *see* Arteriosclerosis, coronary
newborn 770.88
sleep related 327.24
Hypoxic-ischemic encephalopathy (HIE) 768.70
mild 768.71
moderate 768.72
severe 768.73
Hypsarrhythmia (*see also* Epilepsy) 345.6●
Hysteralgia, pregnant uterus 646.8●
Hysteria, hysterical 300.10
anxiety 300.20
Charcôt's gland 300.11
conversion (any manifestation) 300.11
dissociative type NEC 300.15
psychosis, acute 298.1
Hysteroepilepsy 300.11
Hysterotomy, affecting fetus or newborn 763.89

◀ New   ◀◀ Revised   ~~deleted~~ Deleted   ● Use Additional Digit(s)   ▨ Omit code

I

Iatrogenic syndrome of excess cortisol 255.0
IBM (inclusion body myositis) 359.71
Iceland disease (epidemic neuromyasthenia) 049.8
Ichthyosis (congenita) 757.1
  acquired 701.1
  fetalis gravior 757.1
  follicularis 757.1
  hystrix 757.39
  lamellar 757.1
  lingual 528.6
  palmaris and plantaris 757.39
  simplex 757.1
  vera 757.1
  vulgaris 757.1
Ichthyotoxism 988.0
  bacterial (see also Poisoning, food) 005.9
Icteroanemia, hemolytic (acquired) 283.9
  congenital (see also Spherocytosis) 282.0
Icterus (see also Jaundice) 782.4
  catarrhal - see Icterus, infectious
  conjunctiva 782.4
   newborn 774.6
  epidemic - see Icterus, infectious
  febrilis - see Icterus, infectious
  fetus or newborn - see Jaundice, fetus or newborn
  gravis (see also Necrosis, liver) 570
   complicating pregnancy 646.7●
    affecting fetus or newborn 760.8
   fetus or newborn NEC 773.0
   obstetrical 646.7●
    affecting fetus or newborn 760.8
  hematogenous (acquired) 283.9
  hemolytic (acquired) 283.9
   congenital (see also Spherocytosis) 282.0
  hemorrhagic (acute) 100.0
   leptospiral 100.0
   newborn 776.0
   spirochetal 100.0
  infectious 070.1
   with hepatic coma 070.0
   leptospiral 100.0
   spirochetal 100.0
  intermittens juvenilis 277.4
  malignant (see also Necrosis, liver) 570
  neonatorum (see also Jaundice, fetus or newborn) 774.6
  pernicious (see also Necrosis, liver) 570
  spirochetal 100.0
Ictus solaris, solis 992.0
Id reaction (due to bacteria) 692.89
Ideation
  homicidal V62.85
  suicidal V62.84
Identity disorder 313.82
  dissociative 300.14
  gender role (child) 302.6
   adult 302.85
  psychosexual (child) 302.6
   adult 302.85
Idioglossia 307.9
Idiopathic - see condition
Idiosyncrasy (see also Allergy) 995.3
  drug, medicinal substance, and biological - see Allergy, drug
Idiot, idiocy (congenital) 318.2
  amaurotic (Bielschowsky) (-Jansky) (family) (infantile (late)) (juvenile (late)) (Vogt-Spielmeyer) 330.1
  microcephalic 742.1
  Mongolian 758.0
  oxycephalic 756.0
IEED (involuntary emotional expression disorder) 310.81
IFIS (intraoperative floppy iris syndrome) 364.81
IgE asthma 493.0●

Ileitis (chronic) (see also Enteritis) 558.9
  infectious 009.0
  noninfectious 558.9
  regional (ulcerative) 555.0
   with large intestine 555.2
  segmental 555.0
   with large intestine 555.2
  terminal (ulcerative) 555.0
   with large intestine 555.2
Ileocolitis (see also Enteritis) 558.9
  infectious 009.0
  regional 555.2
  ulcerative 556.1
Ileostomy status V44.2
  with complication 569.60
Ileotyphus 002.0
Ileum - see condition
Ileus (adynamic) (bowel) (colon) (inhibitory) (intestine) (neurogenic) (paralytic) 560.1
  arteriomesenteric duodenal 537.2
  due to gallstone (in intestine) 560.31
  duodenal, chronic 537.2
  following gastrointestinal surgery 997.49
  gallstone 560.31
  mechanical (see also Obstruction, intestine) 560.9
  meconium 777.1
   due to cystic fibrosis 277.01
  myxedema 564.89
  postoperative 997.49
  transitory, newborn 777.4
Iliac - see condition
Iliotibial band friction syndrome 728.89
Ill, louping 063.1
Illegitimacy V61.6
Illness - see also Disease
  factitious 300.19
   with
    combined psychological and physical signs and symptoms 300.19
    physical symptoms 300.19
    predominantly
     physical signs and symptoms 300.19
     psychological symptoms 300.16
   chronic (with physical symptoms) 301.51
  heart - see Disease, heart
  manic-depressive (see also Psychosis, affective) 296.80
  mental (see also Disorder, mental) 300.9
Imbalance 781.2
  autonomic (see also Neuropathy, peripheral, autonomic) 337.9
  electrolyte 276.9
   with
    abortion - see Abortion, by type, with metabolic disorder
    ectopic pregnancy (see also categories 633.0–633.9) 639.4
    hyperemesis gravidarum (before 22 completed weeks' gestation) 643.1●
    molar pregnancy (see also categories 630–632) 639.4
   following
    abortion 639.4
    ectopic or molar pregnancy 639.4
   neonatal, transitory NEC 775.5
  endocrine 259.9
  eye muscle NEC 378.9
   heterophoria - see Heterophoria
  glomerulotubular NEC 593.89
  hormone 259.9
  hysterical (see also Hysteria) 300.10
  labyrinth NEC 386.50
  posture 729.90
  sympathetic (see also Neuropathy, peripheral, autonomic) 337.9
Imbecile, imbecility 318.0
  moral 301.7
  old age 290.9

Imbecile, imbecility (Continued)
  senile 290.9
  specified IQ - see IQ
  unspecified IQ 318.0
Imbedding, intrauterine device 996.32
Imbibition, cholesterol (gallbladder) 575.6
Imerslund (-Gräsbeck) syndrome (anemia due to familial selective vitamin B₁₂ malabsorption) 281.1
Iminoacidopathy 270.8
Iminoglycinuria, familial 270.8
Immature - see also Immaturity
  personality 301.89
Immaturity 765.1●
  extreme 765.0●
  fetus or infant light-for-dates - see Light-for-dates
  lung, fetus or newborn 770.4
  organ or site NEC - see Hypoplasia
  pulmonary, fetus or newborn 770.4
  reaction 301.89
  sexual (female) (male) 259.0
Immersion 994.1
  foot 991.4
  hand 991.4
Immobile, immobility
  complete
   due to severe physical disability or frality 780.72
  intestine 564.89
  joint - see Ankylosis
  syndrome (paraplegic) 728.3
Immunization
  ABO
   affecting management of pregnancy 656.2●
    fetus or newborn 773.1
  complication - see Complications, vaccination
  Rh factor
   affecting management of pregnancy 656.1●
    fetus or newborn 773.0
   from transfusion (see also Complications, transfusion) 999.70
Immunodeficiency 279.3
  with
   adenosine-deaminase deficiency 279.2
   defect, predominant
    B-cell 279.00
    T-cell 279.10
   hyperimmunoglobulinemia 279.2
   lymphopenia, hereditary 279.2
   thrombocytopenia and eczema 279.12
   thymic
    aplasia 279.2
    dysplasia 279.2
  autosomal recessive, Swiss-type 279.2
  common variable 279.06
  severe combined (SCID) 279.2
  to Rh factor
   affecting management of pregnancy 656.1●
    fetus or newborn 773.0
  X-linked, with increased IgM 279.05
Immunotherapy, prophylactic V07.2
  antineoplastic V58.12
Impaction, impacted
  bowel, colon, rectum 560.30
   with hernia - see also Hernia, by site, with, obstruction
    gangrenous - see Hernia, by site, with gangrene
   by
    calculus 560.32
    gallstone 560.31
   fecal 560.32
   specified type NEC 560.32
  calculus - see Calculus
  cerumen (ear) (external) 380.4
  cuspid 520.6
  dental 520.6

Impaction, impacted (Continued)
    fecal, feces 560.32
        with hernia - *see also* Hernia, by site, with
            obstruction
            gangrenous - *see* Hernia, by site, with
                gangrene
    fracture - *see* Fracture, by site
    gallbladder - *see* Cholelithiasis
    gallstone(s) - *see* Cholelithiasis
        in intestine (any part) 560.31
    intestine(s) 560.30
        with hernia - *see also* Hernia, by site, with
            obstruction
            gangrenous - *see* Hernia, by site, with
                gangrene
        by
            calculus 560.32
            gallstone 560.31
            fecal 560.32
            specified type NEC 560.32
    intrauterine device (IUD) 996.32
    molar 520.6
    shoulder 660.4●
        affecting fetus or newborn 763.1
    tooth, teeth 520.6
    turbinate 733.99
Impaired, impairment (function)
    arm V49.1
        movement, involving
            musculoskeletal system V49.1
            nervous system V49.2
    auditory discrimination 388.43
    back V48.3
    body (entire) V49.89
    cognitive, mild, so stated 331.83
    combined visual hearing V49.85
    dual sensory V49.85
    glucose
        fasting 790.21
        tolerance test (oral) 790.22
    hearing (*see also* Deafness) 389.9
        combined with visual impairment
            V49.85
    heart - *see* Disease, heart
    kidney (*see also* Disease, renal) 593.9
        disorder resulting from 588.9
            specified NEC 588.89
    leg V49.1
        movement, involving
            musculoskeletal system V49.1
            nervous system V49.2
    limb V49.1
        movement, involving
            musculoskeletal system V49.1
            nervous system V49.2
    liver 573.8
    mastication 524.9
    mild cognitive, so stated 331.83
    mobility
        ear ossicles NEC 385.22
        incostapedial joint 385.22
        malleus 385.21
    myocardium, myocardial (*see also*
        Insufficiency, myocardial)
        428.0
    neuromusculoskeletal NEC V49.89
        back V48.3
        head V48.2
        limb V49.2
        neck V48.3
        spine V48.3
        trunk V48.3
    rectal sphincter 787.99
    renal (*see also* Disease, renal) 593.9
        disorder resulting from 588.9
            specified NEC 588.89
    spine V48.3
    vision NEC 369.9
        both eyes NEC 369.3
            combined with hearing impairment
                V49.85

Impaired, impairment (Continued)
    vision NEC (Continued)
        moderate 369.74
            both eyes 369.25
                with impairment of lesser eye
                    (specified as)
                    blind, not further specified
                        369.15
                    low vision, not further specified
                        369.23
                    near-total 369.17
                    profound 369.18
                    severe 369.24
                    total 369.16
            one eye 369.74
                with vision of other eye (specified
                    as)
                    near-normal 369.75
                    normal 369.76
        near-total 369.64
            both eyes 369.04
                with impairment of lesser eye
                    (specified as)
                    blind, not further specified
                        369.02
                    total 369.03
            one eye 369.64
                with vision of other eye (specified
                    as)
                    near-normal 369.65
                    normal 369.66
        one eye 369.60
            with low vision of other eye 369.10
        profound 369.67
            both eyes 369.08
                with impairment of lesser eye
                    (specified as)
                    blind, not further specified
                        369.05
                    near-total 369.07
                    total 369.06
            one eye 369.67
                with vision of other eye (specified
                    as)
                    near-normal 369.68
                    normal 369.69
        severe 369.71
            both eyes 369.22
                with impairment of lesser eye
                    (specified as)
                    blind, not further specified
                        369.11
                    low vision, not further specified
                        369.21
                    near-total 369.13
                    profound 369.14
                    total 369.12
            one eye 369.71
                with vision of other eye (specified
                    as)
                    near-normal 369.72
                    normal 369.73
        total
            both eyes 369.01
            one eye 369.61
                with vision of other eye (specified
                    as)
                    near-normal 369.62
                    normal 369.63
Impaludism - *see* Malaria
Impediment, speech NEC 784.59
    psychogenic 307.9
    secondary to organic lesion 784.59
Impending
    cerebrovascular accident or attack
        435.9
    coronary syndrome 411.1
    delirium tremens 291.0
    myocardial infarction 411.1
Imperception, auditory (acquired) (congenital)
    389.9

Imperfect
    aeration, lung (newborn) 770.5
    closure (congenital)
        alimentary tract NEC 751.8
            lower 751.5
            upper 750.8
        atrioventricular ostium 745.69
        atrium (secundum) 745.5
            primum 745.61
        branchial cleft or sinus 744.41
        choroid 743.59
        cricoid cartilage 748.3
        cusps, heart valve NEC 746.89
            pulmonary 746.09
        ductus
            arteriosus 747.0
            Botalli 747.0
        ear drum 744.29
            causing impairment of hearing
                744.03
        endocardial cushion 745.60
        epiglottis 748.3
        esophagus with communication to
            bronchus or trachea 750.3
        Eustachian valve 746.89
        eyelid 743.62
        face, facial (*see also* Cleft, lip) 749.10
        foramen
            Botalli 745.5
            ovale 745.5
        genitalia, genital organ(s) or system
            female 752.89
                external 752.49
                internal NEC 752.89
                uterus 752.39
            male 752.89
                penis 752.69
        glottis 748.3
        heart valve (cusps) NEC 746.89
        interatrial ostium or septum 745.5
        interauricular ostium or septum 745.5
        interventricular ostium or septum 745.4
        iris 743.46
        kidney 753.3
        larynx 748.3
        lens 743.36
        lip (*see also* Cleft, lip) 749.10
        nasal septum or sinus 748.1
        nose 748.1
        omphalomesenteric duct 751.0
        optic nerve entry 743.57
        organ or site NEC - *see* Anomaly, specified
            type, by site
        ostium
            interatrial 745.5
            interauricular 745.5
            interventricular 745.4
        palate (*see also* Cleft, palate) 749.00
        preauricular sinus 744.46
        retina 743.56
        roof of orbit 742.0
        sclera 743.47
        septum
            aortic 745.0
            aorticopulmonary 745.0
            atrial (secundum) 745.5
                primum 745.61
            between aorta and pulmonary artery
                745.0
            heart 745.9
            interatrial (secundum) 745.5
                primum 745.61
            interauricular (secundum) 745.5
                primum 745.61
            interventricular 745.4
                with pulmonary stenosis or atresia,
                    dextraposition of aorta, and
                    hypertrophy of right ventricle
                    745.2
                in tetralogy of Fallot 745.2
            nasal 748.1

◀ New   ◀═ Revised   ~~deleted~~ Deleted   ● Use Additional Digit(s)   ▨ Omit code

Imperfect *(Continued)*
closure *(Continued)*
septum *(Continued)*
ventricular 745.4
with pulmonary stenosis or atresia, dextraposition of aorta, and hypertrophy of right ventricle 745.2
in tetralogy of Fallot 745.2
skull 756.0
with
anencephalus 740.0
encephalocele 742.0
hydrocephalus 742.3
with spina bifida (*see also* Spina bifida) 741.0●
microcephalus 742.1
spine (with meningocele) (*see also* Spina bifida) 741.90
thyroid cartilage 748.3
trachea 748.3
tympanic membrane 744.29
causing impairment of hearing 744.03
uterus (with communication to bladder, intestine, or rectum) 752.39
uvula 749.02
with cleft lip (*see also* Cleft, palate, with cleft lip) 749.20
vitelline duct 751.0
development - *see* Anomaly, by site
erection 607.84
fusion - *see* Imperfect, closure
inflation lung (newborn) 770.5
intestinal canal 751.5
poise 729.90
rotation - *see* Malrotation
septum, ventricular 745.4
Imperfectly descended testis 752.51
Imperforate (congenital) - *see also* Atresia
anus 751.2
bile duct 751.61
cervix (uteri) 752.49
esophagus 750.3
hymen 752.42
intestine (small) 751.1
large 751.2
jejunum 751.1
pharynx 750.29
rectum 751.2
salivary duct 750.23
urethra 753.6
urinary meatus 753.6
vagina 752.49
Impervious (congenital) - *see also* Atresia
anus 751.2
bile duct 751.61
esophagus 750.3
intestine (small) 751.1
large 751.5
rectum 751.2
urethra 753.6
Impetiginization of other dermatoses 684
Impetigo (any organism) (any site) (bullous) (circinate) (contagiosa) (neonatorum) (simplex) 684
Bockhart's (superficial folliculitis) 704.8
external ear 684 *[380.13]*
eyelid 684 *[373.5]*
Fox's (contagiosa) 684
furfuracea 696.5
herpetiformis 694.3
nonobstetrical 694.3
staphylococcal infection 684
ulcerative 686.8
vulgaris 684
Impingement, soft tissue between teeth 524.89
anterior 524.81
posterior 524.82
Implant, endometrial 617.9

Implantation
anomalous - *see also* Anomaly, specified type, by site
ureter 753.4
cyst
external area or site (skin) NEC 709.8
iris 364.61
vagina 623.8
vulva 624.8
dermoid (cyst)
external area or site (skin) NEC 709.8
iris 364.61
vagina 623.8
vulva 624.8
placenta, low or marginal - *see* Placenta previa
Impotence (sexual) 607.84
organic origin NEC 607.84
psychogenic 302.72
Impoverished blood 285.9
Impression, basilar 756.0
Imprisonment V62.5
Improper
development, infant 764.9●
Improperly tied umbilical cord (causing hemorrhage) 772.3
Impulses, obsessional 300.3
Impulsive 799.23
neurosis 300.3
Impulsiveness 799.23
Inaction, kidney (*see also* Disease, renal) 593.9
Inactive - *see* condition
Inadequate, inadequacy
aesthetics of dental restoration 525.67
biologic 301.6
cardiac and renal - *see* Hypertension, cardiorenal
constitutional 301.6
development
child 783.40
fetus 764.9●
affecting management of pregnancy 656.5●
genitalia
after puberty NEC 259.0
congenital - *see* Hypoplasia, genitalia
lungs 748.5
organ or site NEC - *see* Hypoplasia, by site
dietary 269.9
distance, interarch 524.28
education V62.3
environment
economic problem V60.2
household condition NEC V60.1
poverty V60.2
unemployment V62.0
functional 301.6
household care, due to
family member
handicapped or ill V60.4
temporarily away from home V60.4
on vacation V60.5
technical defects in home V60.1
temporary absence from home of person rendering care V60.4
housing (heating) (space) V60.1
interarch distance 524.28
material resources V60.2
mental (*see also* Disability, intellectual) 319
nervous system 799.29
personality 301.6
prenatal care in current pregnancy V23.7
pulmonary
function 786.09
newborn 770.89
ventilation, newborn 770.89

Inadequate, inadequacy *(Continued)*
respiration 786.09
newborn 770.89
sample
cytology
anal 796.78
cervical 795.08
vaginal 795.18
social 301.6
Inanition 263.9
with edema 262
due to
deprivation of food 994.2
malnutrition 263.9
fever 780.60
Inappropriate
change in quantitative human chorionic gonadotropin (hCG) in early pregnancy 631.0
level of quantitative human chorionic gonadotropin (hCG) for gestational age in early pregnancy 631.0
secretion
ACTH 255.0
antidiuretic hormone (ADH) (excessive) 253.6
deficiency 253.5
ectopic hormone NEC 259.3
pituitary (posterior) 253.6
Inattention after or at birth 995.52
Inborn errors of metabolism - *see* Disorder, metabolism
Incarceration, incarcerated
bubonocele - *see also* Hernia, inguinal, with obstruction
gangrenous - *see* Hernia, inguinal, with gangrene
colon (by hernia) - *see also* Hernia, by site with obstruction
gangrenous - *see* Hernia, by site, with gangrene
enterocele 552.9
gangrenous 551.9
epigastrocele 552.29
gangrenous 551.29
epiplocele 552.9
gangrenous 551.9
exomphalos 552.1
gangrenous 551.1
fallopian tube 620.8
hernia - *see also* Hernia, by site, with obstruction
gangrenous - *see* Hernia, by site, with gangrene
iris, in wound 871.1
lens, in wound 871.1
merocele (*see also* Hernia, femoral, with obstruction) 552.00
omentum (by hernia) - *see also* Hernia, by site, with obstruction
gangrenous - *see* Hernia, by site, with gangrene
omphalocele 756.72
rupture (meaning hernia) (*see also* Hernia, by site, with obstruction) 552.9
gangrenous (*see also* Hernia, by site, with gangrene) 551.9
sarcoepiplocele 552.9
gangrenous 551.9
sarcoepiplomphalocele 552.1
with gangrene 551.1
uterus 621.8
gravid 654.3●
causing obstructed labor 660.2●
affecting fetus or newborn 763.1
Incident, cerebrovascular (*see also* Disease, cerebrovascular, acute) 436
Incineration (entire body) (from fire, conflagration, electricity, or lightning) - *see* Burn, multiple, specified sites

Incised wound
external - *see* Wound, open, by site
internal organs (abdomen, chest, or pelvis) - *see* Injury, internal, by site, with open wound

Incision, incisional
hernia - *see* Hernia, incisional
surgical, complication - *see* Complications, surgical procedures
traumatic
external - *see* Wound, open, by site
internal organs (abdomen, chest, or pelvis) - *see* Injury, internal, by site, with open wound

Inclusion
azurophilic leukocytic 288.2
blennorrhea (neonatal) (newborn) 771.6
cyst - *see* Cyst, skin
gallbladder in liver (congenital) 751.69

Incompatibility
ABO
affecting management of pregnancy 656.2●
fetus or newborn 773.1
infusion or transfusion reaction (*see also* Complications, transfusion) 999.60
blood (group) (Duffy) (E) (K(ell)) (Kidd) (Lewis) (M) (N) (P) (S) NEC
affecting management of pregnancy 656.2●
fetus or newborn 773.2
infusion or transfusion reaction (*see also* Complications, transfusion) 999.75
contour of existing restoration of tooth with oral health 525.65
marital V61.10
involving
divorce V61.03
estrangement V61.09
non-ABO (*see also* Complications, transfusion) 999.75
Rh (antigen) (C) (c) (D) (E) (e) (blood group) (factor)
affecting management of pregnancy 656.1●
fetus or newborn 773.0
infusion or transfusion reaction (*see also* Complications, transfusion) 999.70
Rhesus - *see* Incompatibility, Rh

Incompetency, incompetence, incompetent
annular
aortic (valve) (*see also* Insufficiency, aortic) 424.1
mitral (valve) - (*see also* Insufficiency, mitral) 424.0
pulmonary valve (heart) (*see also* Endocarditis, pulmonary) 424.3
aortic (valve) (*see also* Insufficiency, aortic) 424.1
syphilitic 093.22
cardiac (orifice) 530.0
valve - *see* Endocarditis
cervix, cervical (os) 622.5
in pregnancy 654.5●
affecting fetus or newborn 761.0
chronotropic 426.89
with
autonomic dysfunction 337.9
ischemic heart disease 414.9
left ventricular dysfunction 429.89
sinus node dysfunction 427.81
esophagogastric (junction) (sphincter) 530.0
heart valve, congenital 746.89
mitral (valve) - *see* Insufficiency, mitral
papillary muscle (heart) 429.81
pelvic fundus
pubocervical tissue 618.81
rectovaginal tissue 618.82

Incompetency, incompetence, incompetent (*Continued*)
pulmonary valve (heart) (*see also* Endocarditis, pulmonary) 424.3
congenital 746.09
tricuspid (annular) (rheumatic) (valve) (*see also* Endocarditis, tricuspid) 397.0
valvular - *see* Endocarditis
vein, venous (saphenous) (varicose) (*see also* Varicose, vein) 454.9
velopharyngeal (closure)
acquired 528.9
congenital 750.29

Incomplete - *see also* condition
bladder emptying 788.21
defecation 787.61
expansion lungs (newborn) 770.5
gestation (liveborn) - *see* Immaturity
rotation - *see* Malrotation

Inconclusive
image test due to excess body fat 793.91
mammogram, mammography 793.82
due to dense breasts 793.82

Incontinence 788.30
without sensory awareness 788.34
anal sphincter 787.60
continuous leakage 788.37
feces, fecal 787.60
due to hysteria 300.11
nonorganic origin 307.7
hysterical 300.11
mixed (male) (female) (urge and stress) 788.33
overflow 788.38
paradoxical 788.39
rectal 787.60
specified NEC 788.39
stress (female) 625.6
male NEC 788.32
urethral sphincter 599.84
urge 788.31
and stress (male) (female) 788.33
urine 788.30
active 788.30
due to
cognitive impairment 788.91
severe physical disability 788.91
immobility 788.91
functional 788.91
male 788.30
stress 788.32
and urge 788.33
neurogenic 788.39
nonorganic origin 307.6
stress (female) 625.6
male NEC 788.32
urge 788.31
and stress 788.33

Incontinentia pigmenti 757.33

Incoordinate
uterus (action) (contractions) 661.4●
affecting fetus or newborn 763.7

Incoordination
esophageal-pharyngeal (newborn) 787.24
muscular 781.3
papillary muscle 429.81

Increase, increased
abnormal, in development 783.9
androgens (ovarian) 256.1
anticoagulants (antithrombin) (anti-II) (anti-VIIIa) (anti-IXa) (anti-XIa) (prothrombin) (*see also* Anticoagulants) 286.59
anti-IIa 287.8
anti-Xa 287.8
extrinsic 287.8
postpartum 666.3●
cold sense (*see also* Disturbance, sensation) 782.0
estrogen 256.0

Increase, increased (*Continued*)
function
adrenal (cortex) 255.3
medulla 255.6
pituitary (anterior) (gland) (lobe) 253.1
posterior 253.6
heat sense (*see also* Disturbance, sensation) 782.0
intracranial pressure 781.99
injury at birth 767.8
light reflex of retina 362.13
permeability, capillary 448.9
pressure
intracranial 781.99
injury at birth 767.8
intraocular 365.00
pulsations 785.9
pulse pressure 785.9
sphericity, lens 743.36
splenic activity 289.4
venous pressure 459.89
portal 572.3

Incrustation, cornea, lead, or zinc 930.0
Incyclophoria 378.44
Incyclotropia 378.33
Indeterminate sex 752.7
India rubber skin 756.83
Indicanuria 270.2
Indigestion (bilious) (functional) 536.8
acid 536.8
catarrhal 536.8
due to decomposed food NEC 005.9
fat 579.8
nervous 306.4
psychogenic 306.4
Indirect - *see* condition
Indolent bubo NEC 099.8
Induced
abortion - *see* Abortion, induced
birth, affecting fetus or newborn 763.89
delivery - *see* Delivery
labor - *see* Delivery
Induration, indurated
brain 348.89
breast (fibrous) 611.79
puerperal, postpartum 676.3●
broad ligament 620.8
chancre 091.0
anus 091.1
congenital 090.0
extragenital NEC 091.2
corpora cavernosa (penis) (plastic) 607.89
liver (chronic) 573.8
acute 573.8
lung (black) (brown) (chronic) (fibroid) (*see also* Fibrosis, lung) 515
essential brown 275.09 [516.1]
penile 607.89
phlebitic - *see* Phlebitis
skin 782.8
stomach 537.89
Induratio penis plastica 607.89
Industrial - *see* condition
Inebriety (*see also* Abuse, drugs, nondependent) 305.0●
Inefficiency
kidney (*see also* Disease, renal) 593.9
thyroid (acquired) (gland) 244.9
Inelasticity, skin 782.8
Inequality, leg (acquired) (length) 736.81
congenital 755.30
Inertia
bladder 596.4
neurogenic 596.54
with cauda equina syndrome 344.61
stomach 536.8
psychogenic 306.4
uterus, uterine 661.2●
affecting fetus or newborn 763.7
primary 661.0●
secondary 661.1●

Inertia (*Continued*)
vesical 596.4
neurogenic 596.54
with cauda equina 344.61
Infant - *see also* condition
excessive crying of 780.92
fussy (baby) 780.91
held for adoption V68.89
newborn - *see* Newborn
post-term (gestation period over 40
completed weeks to 42 completed
weeks) 766.21
prolonged gestation of (period over 42
completed weeks) 766.22
syndrome of diabetic mother 775.0
"Infant Hercules" syndrome 255.2
Infantile - *see also* condition
genitalia, genitals 259.0
in pregnancy or childbirth NEC 654.4●
affecting fetus or newborn 763.89
causing obstructed labor 660.2●
affecting fetus or newborn 763.1
heart 746.9
kidney 753.3
lack of care 995.52
macula degeneration 362.75
melanodontia 521.05
os, uterus (*see also* Infantile, genitalia) 259.0
pelvis 738.6
with disproportion (fetopelvic) 653.1●
affecting fetus or newborn 763.1
causing obstructed labor 660.1●
affecting fetus or newborn 763.1
penis 259.0
testis 257.2
uterus (*see also* Infantile, genitalia)259.0
vulva 752.49
Infantilism 259.9
with dwarfism (hypophyseal) 253.3
Brissaud's (infantile myxedema) 244.9
celiac 579.0
Herter's (nontropical sprue) 579.0
hypophyseal 253.3
hypothalamic (with obesity) 253.8
idiopathic 259.9
intestinal 579.0
pancreatic 577.8
pituitary 253.3
renal 588.0
sexual (with obesity) 259.0
Infants, healthy liveborn - *see* Newborn
Infarct, infarction
adrenal (capsule) (gland) 255.41
amnion 658.8●
anterior (with contiguous portion of
intraventricular septum) NEC (*see also*
Infarct, myocardium) 410.1●
appendices epiploicae 557.0
bowel 557.0
brain (stem) 434.91
embolic (*see also* Embolism, brain)
434.11
healed or old without residuals V12.54
iatrogenic 997.02
lacunar 434.91
late effect - *see* Late effect(s) (of)
cerebrovascular disease
postoperative 997.02
puerperal, postpartum, childbirth 674.0●
thrombotic (*see also* Thrombosis, brain)
434.01
breast 611.89
Brewer's (kidney) 593.81
cardiac (*see also* Infarct, myocardium) 410.9●
cerebellar (*see also* Infarct, brain) 434.91
embolic (*see also* Embolism, brain) 434.11
cerebral (*see also* Infarct, brain) 434.91
aborted 434.91
embolic (*see also* Embolism, brain) 434.11
thrombotic (*see also* Infarct, brain) 434.01
chorion 658.8●

Infarct, infarction (*Continued*)
colon (acute) (agnogenic) (embolic)
(hemorrhagic) (nonocclusive)
(nonthrombotic) (occlusive)
(segmental) (thrombotic) (with
gangrene) 557.0
coronary artery (*see also* Infarct,
myocardium) 410.9●
cortical 434.91
embolic (*see also* Embolism) 444.9
fallopian tube 620.8
gallbladder 575.8
heart (*see also* Infarct, myocardium)
410.9●
hepatic 573.4
hypophysis (anterior lobe) 253.8
impending (myocardium) 411.1
intestine (acute) (agnogenic) (embolic)
(hemorrhagic) (nonocclusive)
(nonthrombotic) (occlusive)
(thrombotic) (with gangrene) 557.0
kidney 593.81
lacunar 434.91
liver 573.4
lung (embolic) (thrombotic) 415.19
with
abortion - *see* Abortion, by type, with,
embolism
ectopic pregnancy (*see also* categories
633.0–633.9) 639.6
molar pregnancy (*see also* categories
630–632) 639.6
following
abortion 639.6
ectopic or molar pregnancy 639.6
iatrogenic 415.11
in pregnancy, childbirth, or puerperium -
see Embolism, obstetrical
postoperative 415.11
septic 415.12
lymph node or vessel 457.8
medullary (brain) - *see* Infarct, brain
meibomian gland (eyelid) 374.85
mesentery, mesenteric (embolic) (thrombotic)
(with gangrene) 557.0
midbrain - *see* Infarct, brain
myocardium, myocardial (acute or with a
stated duration of 8 weeks or less)
(with hypertension) 410.9●

Note: Use the following fifth-digit
subclassification with category 410:

0   episode unspecified
1   initial episode
2   subsequent episode without
recurrence

with symptoms after 8 weeks from date of
infarction 414.8
anterior (wall) (with contiguous portion
of intraventricular septum) NEC
410.1●
anteroapical (with contiguous portion of
intraventricular septum) 410.1●
anterolateral (wall) 410.0●
anteroseptal (with contiguous portion of
intraventricular septum) 410.1●
apical-lateral 410.5●
atrial 410.8●
basal-lateral 410.5●
chronic (with symptoms after 8 weeks
from date of infarction) 414.8
diagnosed on ECG, but presenting no
symptoms 412
diaphragmatic wall (with contiguous
portion of intraventricular septum)
410.4●
healed or old, currently presenting no
symptoms 412
high lateral 410.5●
impending 411.1

Infarct, infarction (*Continued*)
myocardium, myocardial (*Continued*)
inferior (wall) (with contiguous portion of
intraventricular septum) 410.4●
inferolateral (wall) 410.2●
inferoposterior wall 410.3●
intraoperative 997.1
lateral wall 410.5●
non-Q wave 410.7●
non-ST elevation (NSTEMI) 410.7●
nontransmural 410.7●
papillary muscle 410.8●
past (diagnosed on ECG or other special
investigation, but currently
presenting no symptoms) 412
with symptoms NEC 414.8
posterior (strictly) (true) (wall) 410.6●
posterobasal 410.6●
posteroinferior 410.3●
posterolateral 410.5●
postprocedural 997.1
previous, currently presenting no
symptoms 412
Q wave (*see also* Infarct, myocardium, by
site) 410.9●
septal 410.8●
specified site NEC 410.8●
ST elevation (STEMI) 410.9●
anterior (wall) 410.1●
anterolateral (wall) 410.0●
inferior (wall) 410.4●
inferolateral (wall) 410.2●
inferoposterior wall 410.3●
lateral wall 410.5●
posterior (strictly) (true) (wall)
410.6●
specified site NEC 410.8●
subendocardial 410.7●
syphilitic 093.82
non-ST elevation myocardial infarction
(NSTEMI) 410.7●
nontransmural 410.7●
omentum 557.0
ovary 620.8
pancreas 577.8
papillary muscle (*see also* Infarct,
myocardium) 410.8●
parathyroid gland 252.8
pituitary (gland) 253.8
placenta (complicating pregnancy) 656.7●
affecting fetus or newborn 762.2
pontine - *see* Infarct, brain
posterior NEC (*see also* Infarct, myocardium)
410.6●
prostate 602.8
pulmonary (artery) (hemorrhagic) (vein)
415.19
with
abortion - *see* Abortion, by type, with,
embolism
ectopic pregnancy (*see also* categories
633.0–633.9) 639.6
molar pregnancy (*see also* categories
630–632) 639.6
following
abortion 639.6
ectopic or molar pregnancy 639.6
iatrogenic 415.11
in pregnancy, childbirth, or puerperium -
see Embolism, obstetrical
postoperative 415.11
septic 415.12
renal 593.81
embolic or thrombotic 593.81
retina, retinal 362.84
with occlusion - *see* Occlusion, retina
spinal (acute) (cord) (embolic) (nonembolic)
336.1
spleen 289.59
embolic or thrombotic 444.89
subchorionic - *see* Infarct, placenta

Infarct, infarction *(Continued)*
  subendocardial *(see also* Infarct, myocardium)
      410.7●
  suprarenal (capsule) (gland) 255.41
  syncytium - *see* Infarct, placenta
  testis 608.83
  thrombotic *(see also* Thrombosis) 453.9
      artery, arterial - *see* Embolism
  thyroid (gland) 246.3
  ventricle (heart) *(see also* Infarct,
      myocardium) 410.9●
Infecting - *see* condition
Infection, infected, infective (opportunistic)
      136.9
  with
      influenza viruses occurring in pigs or
          other animals - *see* Influenza,
          due to identified, novel influenza A
          virus
      lymphangitis - *see* Lymphangitis
  abortion - *see* Abortion, by type, with,
      sepsis
  abscess (skin) - *see* Abscess, by site
  Absidia 117.7
  acanthamoeba 136.21
  Acanthocheilonema (perstans) 125.4
      streptocerca 125.6
  accessory sinus (chronic) *(see also* Sinusitis)
      473.9
  Achorion - *see* Dermatophytosis
  Acremonium falciforme 117.4
  acromioclavicular (joint) 711.91
  Actinobacillus
      lignieresii 027.8
      mallei 024
      muris 026.1
  Actinomadura - *see* Actinomycosis
  Actinomyces (israelii) - *see also*
          Actinomycosis
      muris-ratti 026.1
  Actinomycetales (Actinomadura)
      (Actinomyces) (Nocardia)
      (Streptomyces) - *see* Actinomycosis
  actinomycotic NEC *(see also* Actinomycosis)
      039.9
  adenoid (chronic) 474.01
      acute 463
      and tonsil (chronic) 474.02
          acute or subacute 463
  adenovirus NEC 079.0
      in diseases classified elsewhere - *see*
          category 079
      unspecified nature or site 079.0
  Aerobacter aerogenes NEC 041.85
      enteritis 008.2
  Aerogenes capsulatus *(see also* Gangrene,
      gas) 040.0
  aertrycke *(see also* Infection, Salmonella)
      003.9
  Ajellomyces dermatitidis 116.0
  alimentary canal NEC *(see also* Enteritis, due
      to, by organism) 009.0
  Allescheria boydii 117.6
  Alternaria 118
  alveolus, alveolar (process) (pulpal origin)
      522.4
  ameba, amebic (histolytica) *(see also*
          Amebiasis) 006.9
      acute 006.0
      chronic 006.1
      free-living 136.29
      hartmanni 007.8
      specified
          site NEC 006.8
          type NEC 007.8
  amniotic fluid or cavity 658.4●
      affecting fetus or newborn 762.7
  anaerobes (cocci) (gram-negative) (gram-
      positive) (mixed) NEC 041.84
  anal canal 569.49
  Ancylostoma braziliense 126.2

Infection, infected, infective *(Continued)*
  Angiostrongylus cantonensis 128.8
  anisakiasis 127.1
  Anisakis larva 127.1
  anthrax *(see also* Anthrax) 022.9
  antrum (chronic) *(see also* Sinusitis,
      maxillary) 473.0
  anus (papillae) (sphincter) 569.49
  arbor virus NEC 066.9
  arbovirus NEC 066.9
  argentophil-rod 027.0
  Ascaris lumbricoides 127.0
  ascomycetes 117.4
  Aspergillus (flavus) (fumigatus) (terreus)
      117.3
  atypical
      acid-fast (bacilli) *(see also* Mycobacterium,
          atypical) 031.9
      mycobacteria *(see also* Mycobacterium,
          atypical) 031.9
  auditory meatus (circumscribed) (diffuse)
      (external) *(see also* Otitis, externa)
      380.10
  auricle (ear) *(see also* Otitis, externa)
      380.10
  axillary gland 683
  Babesiasis 088.82
  Babesiosis 088.82
  Bacillus NEC 041.89
      abortus 023.1
      anthracis *(see also* Anthrax) 022.9
      cereus (food poisoning) 005.89
      coli - *see* Infection, Escherichia coli
      coliform NEC 041.85
      Ducrey's (any location) 099.0
      Flexner's 004.1
      Friedländer's NEC 041.3
      fusiformis 101
      gas (gangrene) *(see also* Gangrene, gas)
          040.0
      mallei 024
      melitensis 023.0
      paratyphoid, paratyphosus 002.9
          A 002.1
          B 002.2
          C 002.3
      Schmorl's 040.3
      Shiga 004.0
      suipestifer *(see also* Infection, Salmonella)
          003.9
      swimming pool 031.1
      typhosa 002.0
      welchii *(see also* Gangrene, gas) 040.0
      Whitmore's 025
  bacterial NEC 041.9
      specified NEC 041.89
          anaerobic NEC 041.84
          gram-negative NEC 041.85
              anaerobic NEC 041.84
  Bacterium
      paratyphosum 002.9
          A 002.1
          B 002.2
          C 002.3
      typhosum 002.9
  Bacteroides (fragilis) (melaninogenicus)
      (oralis) NEC 041.82
  Balantidium coli 007.0
  Bartholin's gland 616.89
  Basidiobolus 117.7
  Bedsonia 079.98
      specified NEC 079.88
  bile duct 576.1
  bladder *(see also* Cystitis) 595.9
  Blastomyces, blastomycotic 116.0
      brasiliensis 116.1
      dermatitidis 116.0
      European 117.5
      loboi 116.2
      North American 116.0
      South American 116.1

Infection, infected, infective *(Continued)*
  bleb
      postprocedural 379.60
          stage 1 379.61
          stage 2 379.62
          stage 3 379.63
  blood stream - *see also* Septicemia
      catheter-related (CRBSI) 999.31
      central line-associated (CLABSI) 999.32
      due to central venous catheter 999.32
  bone 730.9●
      specified - *see* Osteomyelitis
  Bordetella 033.9
      bronchiseptica 033.8
      parapertussis 033.1
      pertussis 033.0
  Borrelia
      bergdorfi 088.81
      vincentii (mouth) (pharynx) (tonsil) 101
  bovine stomatitis 059.11
  brain *(see also* Encephalitis) 323.9
      late effect - *see* category 326
      membranes - *(see also* Meningitis) 322.9
      septic 324.0
          late effect - *see* category 326
      meninges *(see also* Meningitis) 320.9
  branchial cyst 744.42
  breast 611.0
      puerperal, postpartum 675.2●
          with nipple 675.9●
              specified type NEC 675.8●
          nonpurulent 675.2●
          purulent 675.1●
  bronchus *(see also* Bronchitis) 490
      fungus NEC 117.9
  Brucella 023.9
      abortus 023.1
      canis 023.3
      melitensis 023.0
      mixed 023.8
      suis 023.2
  Brugia (Wuchereria) malayi 125.1
  bursa - *see* Bursitis
  buttocks (skin) 686.9
  Candida (albicans) (tropicalis) *(see also*
          Candidiasis) 112.9
      congenital 771.7
  Candiru 136.8
  Capillaria
      hepatica 128.8
      philippinensis 127.5
  cartilage 733.99
  cat liver fluke 121.0
  catheter-related bloodstream (CRBSI) 999.31
  cellulitis - *see* Cellulitis, by site
  central line-associated 999.31
      bloodstream 999.32
  Cephalosporum falciforme 117.4
  Cercomonas hominis (intestinal) 007.3
  cerebrospinal *(see also* Meningitis) 322.9
      late effect - *see* category 326
  cervical gland 683
  cervix *(see also* Cervicitis) 616.0
  cesarean section wound 674.3●
  Chilomastix (intestinal) 007.8
  Chlamydia 079.98
      specified NEC 079.88
  Cholera *(see also* Cholera) 001.9
  chorionic plate 658.8●
  Cladosporium
      bantianum 117.8
      carrionii 117.2
      mansoni 111.1
      trichoides 117.8
      wernecki 111.1
  Clonorchis (sinensis) (liver) 121.1
  Clostridium (haemolyticum) (novyi) NEC
      041.84
      botulinum 005.1
      histolyticum *(see also* Gangrene, gas) 040.0
      oedematiens *(see also* Gangrene, gas) 040.0

◀ New ◀▥ Revised ~~deleted~~ Deleted ● Use Additional Digit(s) ▨ Omit code

Infection, infected, infective *(Continued)*
  Clostridium NEC *(Continued)*
    perfringens 041.83
      due to food 005.2
    septicum *(see also* Gangrene, gas)
        040.0
    sordellii *(see also* Gangrene, gas)
        040.0
    welchii *(see also* Gangrene, gas)
        040.0
      due to food 005.2
  Coccidioides (immitis) *(see also*
      Coccidioidomycosis) 114.9
  coccus NEC 041.89
  colon *(see also* Enteritis, due to, by organism)
      009.0
    bacillus - *see* Infection, Escherichia
        coli
  colostomy or enterostomy 569.61
  common duct 576.1
  complicating pregnancy, childbirth, or
      puerperium NEC 647.9●
    affecting fetus or newborn 760.2
  Condiobolus 117.7
  congenital NEC 771.89
    Candida albicans 771.7
    chronic 771.2
    Cytomegalovirus 771.1
    hepatitis, viral 771.2
    herpes simplex 771.2
    listeriosis 771.2
    malaria 771.2
    poliomyelitis 771.2
    rubella 771.0
    toxoplasmosis 771.2
    tuberculosis 771.2
    urinary (tract) 771.82
    vaccinia 771.2
  coronavirus 079.89
    SARS-associated 079.82
  corpus luteum *(see also* Salpingo-oophoritis)
      614.2
  Corynebacterium diphtheriae - *see*
      Diphtheria
  cotia virus 059.8
  Coxsackie *(see also* Coxsackie) 079.2
    endocardium 074.22
    heart NEC 074.20
    in diseases classified elsewhere - *see*
        category 079
    meninges 047.0
    myocardium 074.23
    pericardium 074.21
    pharynx 074.0
    specified disease NEC 074.8
    unspecified nature or site 079.2
  Cryptococcus neoformans 117.5
  Cryptosporidia 007.4
  Cunninghamella 117.7
  cyst - *see* Cyst
  Cysticercus cellulosae 123.1
  cystostomy 596.83
  cytomegalovirus 078.5
    congenital 771.1
  dental (pulpal origin) 522.4
  deuteromycetes 117.4
  Dicrocoelium dendriticum 121.8
  Dipetalonema (perstans) 125.4
    streptocerca 125.6
  diphtherial - *see* Diphtheria
  Diphyllobothrium (adult) (latum)
      (pacificum) 123.4
    larval 123.5
  Diplogonoporus (grandis) 123.8
  Dipylidium (caninum) 123.8
  Dirofilaria 125.6
  dog tapeworm 123.8
  Dracunculus medinensis 125.7
  Dreschlera 118
    hawaiiensis 117.8
  Ducrey's bacillus (any site) 099.0

Infection, infected, infective *(Continued)*
  due to or resulting from
    central venous catheter *(see also*
        Complications, due to, catheter,
        central venous) 999.31
      bloodstream 999.32
      localized 999.33
    device, implant, or graft (any) (presence
        of) - *see* Complications, infection
        and inflammation, due to (presence
        of) any device, implant, or graft
        classified to 996.0–996.5 NEC
    injection, inoculation, infusion,
        transfusion, or vaccination
        (prophylactic) (therapeutic) 999.39
      blood and blood products
        acute 999.34
    injury NEC - *see* Wound, open, by site,
        complicated
    surgery 998.59
  duodenum 535.6●
  ear - *see also* Otitis
    external *(see also* Otitis, externa) 380.10
    inner *(see also* Labyrinthitis) 386.30
    middle - *see* Otitis, media
  Eaton's agent NEC 041.81
  Eberthella typhosa 002.0
  Ebola 078.89
  echinococcosis 122.9
  Echinococcus *(see also* Echinococcus) 122.9
  Echinostoma 121.8
  ECHO virus 079.1
    in diseases classified elsewhere - *see*
        category 079
    unspecified nature or site 079.1
  Ehrlichiosis 082.40
    chaffeensis 082.41
    specified type NEC 082.49
  Endamoeba - *see* Infection, ameba
  endocardium *(see also* Endocarditis) 421.0
  endocervix *(see also* Cervicitis) 616.0
  Entamoeba - *see* Infection, ameba
  enteric *(see also* Enteritis, due to, by
      organism) 009.0
  Enterobacter aerogenes NEC 041.85
  Enterobacter sakazakii 041.85
  Enterobius vermicularis 127.4
  enterococcus NEC 041.04
  enterovirus NEC 079.89
    central nervous system NEC 048
    enteritis 008.67
    meningitis 047.9
  Entomophthora 117.7
  Epidermophyton - *see* Dermatophytosis
  epidermophytosis - *see* Dermatophytosis
  episiotomy 674.3●
  Epstein-Barr virus 075
    chronic 780.79 *[139.8]*
  erysipeloid 027.1
  Erysipelothrix (insidiosa) (rhusiopathiae)
      027.1
  erythema infectiosum 057.0
  Escherichia coli (E. coli) 041.49
    enteritis - *see* Enteritis, E. coli
    generalized 038.42
    intestinal - *see* Enteritis, E. coli
    non-Shiga toxin-producing 041.49
    Shiga toxin-producing (STEC) 041.43
      with
        unspecified O group 041.43
      non-O157 (with known O group)
          041.42
      O157 (with confirmation of Shiga toxin
          when H antigen is unknown, or
          is not H7) 041.41
      O157:H- (nonmotile) with confirmation
          of Shiga toxin 041.41
      O157:H7 with or without confirmation
          of Shiga toxin-production 041.41
      specified NEC 041.42
  esophagostomy 530.86

Infection, infected, infective *(Continued)*
  ethmoidal (chronic) (sinus) *(see also* Sinusitis,
      ethmoidal) 473.2
  Eubacterium 041.84
  Eustachian tube (ear) 381.50
    acute 381.51
    chronic 381.52
  exanthema subitum *(see also* Exanthem
      subitum) 058.10
  exit site 999.33
  external auditory canal (meatus) *(see also*
      Otitis, externa) 380.10
  eye NEC 360.00
  eyelid 373.9
    specified NEC 373.8
  fallopian tube *(see also* Salpingo-oophoritis)
      614.2
  fascia 728.89
  Fasciola
    gigantica 121.3
    hepatica 121.3
  Fasciolopsis (buski) 121.4
  fetus (intra-amniotic) - *see* Infection,
      congenital
  filarial - *see* Infestation, filarial
  finger (skin) 686.9
    abscess (with lymphangitis) 681.00
      pulp 681.01
    cellulitis (with lymphangitis) 681.00
    distal closed space (with lymphangitis)
        681.00
    nail 681.02
      fungus 110.1
  fish tapeworm 123.4
    larval 123.5
  flagellate, intestinal 007.9
  fluke - *see* Infestation, fluke
  focal
    teeth (pulpal origin) 522.4
    tonsils 474.00
      and adenoids 474.02
  Fonsecaea
    compactum 117.2
    pedrosoi 117.2
  food *(see also* Poisoning, food) 005.9
  foot (skin) 686.9
    fungus 110.4
  Francisella tularensis *(see also* Tularemia)
      021.9
  frontal sinus (chronic) *(see also* Sinusitis,
      frontal) 473.1
  fungus NEC 117.9
    beard 110.0
    body 110.5
    dermatiacious NEC 117.8
    foot 110.4
    groin 110.3
    hand 110.2
    nail 110.1
    pathogenic to compromised host only 118
    perianal (area) 110.3
    scalp 110.0
    scrotum 110.8
    skin 111.9
      foot 110.4
      hand 110.2
    toenails 110.1
    trachea 117.9
  Fusarium 118
  Fusobacterium 041.84
  gallbladder *(see also* Cholecystitis, acute)
      575.0
  Gardnerella vaginalis 041.89
  gas bacillus *(see also* Gas, gangrene) 040.0
  gastric *(see also* Gastritis) 535.5●
  Gastrodiscoides hominis 121.8
  gastroenteric *(see also* Enteritis, due to, by
      organism) 009.0
  gastrointestinal *(see also* Enteritis, due to, by
      organism) 009.0
  gastrostomy 536.41

Infection, infected, infective *(Continued)*
  generalized NEC *(see also* Septicemia) 038.9
  genital organ or tract NEC
    female 614.9
      with
        abortion - *see* Abortion, by type,
          with sepsis
        ectopic pregnancy *(see also*
          categories 633.0–633.9) 639.0
        molar pregnancy *(see also* categories
          630–632) 639.0
      complicating pregnancy 646.6●
        affecting fetus or newborn 760.8
      following
        abortion 639.0
        ectopic or molar pregnancy 639.0
      puerperal, postpartum, childbirth
        670.8●
        minor or localized 646.6●
          affecting fetus or newborn 760.8
    male 608.4
  genitourinary tract NEC 599.0
  Ghon tubercle, primary *(see also*
    Tuberculosis) 010.0●
  Giardia lamblia 007.1
  gingival (chronic) 523.10
    acute 523.00
    Vincent's 101
  glanders 024
  Glenosporopsis amazonica 116.2
  Gnathostoma spinigerum 128.1
  Gongylonema 125.6
  gonococcal NEC *(see also* Gonococcus) 098.0
  gram-negative bacilli NEC 041.85
    anaerobic 041.84
  guinea worm 125.7
  gum *(see also* Infection, gingival) 523.10
  Hantavirus 079.81
  heart 429.89
  Helicobactor pylori [H. pylori] 041.86
  helminths NEC 128.9
    intestinal 127.9
      mixed (types classifiable to more than
        one category in 120.0–127.7)
        127.8
      specified type NEC 127.7
    specified type NEC 128.8
  Hemophilus influenzae NEC 041.5
    generalized 038.41
  Herpes (simplex) *(see also* Herpes, simplex)
    054.9
    congenital 771.2
    zoster *(see also* Herpes, zoster) 053.9
      eye NEC 053.29
  Heterophyes heterophyes 121.6
  Histoplasma *(see also* Histoplasmosis) 115.90
    capsulatum *(see also* Histoplasmosis,
      American) 115.00
    duboisii *(see also* Histoplasmosis, African)
      115.10
  HIV V08
    with symptoms, symptomatic 042
  hookworm *(see also* Ancylostomiasis) 126.9
  human herpesvirus 6 058.81
  human herpesvirus 7 058.82
  human herpesvirus 8 058.89
  human herpesvirus NEC 058.89
  human immunodeficiency virus V08
    with symptoms, symptomatic 042
  human papillomavirus 079.4
  hydrocele 603.1
  hydronephrosis 591
  Hymenolepis 123.6
  hypopharynx 478.29
  inguinal glands 683
    due to soft chancre 099.0
  insertion site 999.33
  intestine, intestinal *(see also* Enteritis, due to,
    by organism) 009.0
  intrauterine *(see also* Endometritis) 615.9
    complicating delivery 646.6●

Infection, infected, infective *(Continued)*
  isospora belli or hominis 007.2
  Japanese B encephalitis 062.0
  jaw (bone) (acute) (chronic) (lower)
    (subacute) (upper) 526.4
  joint - *see* Arthritis, infectious or infective
  Kaposi's sarcoma-associated herpesvirus
    058.89
  kidney (cortex) (hematogenous) 590.9
    with
      abortion - *see* Abortion, by type, with
        urinary tract infection
      calculus 592.0
      ectopic pregnancy *(see also* categories
        633.0–633.9) 639.8
      molar pregnancy *(see also* categories
        630–632) 639.8
    complicating pregnancy or puerperium
      646.6●
      affecting fetus or newborn 760.1
    following
      abortion 639.8
      ectopic or molar pregnancy 639.8
    pelvis and ureter 590.3
  Klebsiella pneumoniae NEC 041.3
  knee (skin) NEC 686.9
    joint - *see* Arthritis, infectious
  Koch's *(see also* Tuberculosis, pulmonary)
    011.9●
  labia (majora) (minora) *(see also* Vulvitis)
    616.10
  lacrimal
    gland *(see also* Dacryoadenitis) 375.00
    passages (duct) (sac) *(see also*
      Dacryocystitis) 375.30
  larynx NEC 478.79
  leg (skin) NEC 686.9
  Leishmania *(see also* Leishmaniasis) 085.9
    braziliensis 085.5
    donovani 085.0
    Ethiopica 085.3
    furunculosa 085.1
    infantum 085.0
    Mexicana 085.4
    tropica (minor) 085.1
      major 085.2
  Leptosphaeria senegalensis 117.4
  Leptospira *(see also* Leptospirosis) 100.9
    australis 100.89
    bataviae 100.89
    pyrogenes 100.89
    specified type NEC 100.89
  leptospirochetal NEC *(see also* Leptospirosis)
    100.9
  Leptothrix - *see* Actinomycosis
  Listeria monocytogenes (listeriosis) 027.0
    congenital 771.2
  liver fluke - *see* Infestation, fluke, liver
  Loa loa 125.2
    eyelid 125.2 [373.6]
  Loboa loboi 116.2
  local, skin (staphylococcal) (streptococcal)
    NEC 686.9
    abscess - *see* Abscess, by site
    cellulitis - *see* Cellulitis, by site
    ulcer *(see also* Ulcer, skin) 707.9
  Loefflerella
    mallei 024
    whitmori 025
  lung 518.89
    atypical Mycobacterium 031.0
      tuberculous *(see also* Tuberculosis,
        pulmonary) 011.9●
    basilar 518.89
    chronic 518.89
    fungus NEC 117.9
    spirochetal 104.8
    virus - *see* Pneumonia, virus
  lymph gland (axillary) (cervical) (inguinal)
    683
    mesenteric 289.2

Infection, infected, infective *(Continued)*
  lymphoid tissue, base of tongue or posterior
    pharynx, NEC 474.00
  Madurella
    grisea 117.4
    mycetomii 117.4
  major
    with
      abortion - *see* Abortion, by type, with
        sepsis
      ectopic pregnancy *(see also* categories
        633.0–633.9) 639.0
      molar pregnancy *(see also* categories
        630–632) 639.0
    following
      abortion 639.0
      ectopic or molar pregnancy 639.0
    puerperal, postpartum, childbirth 670.0●
  malarial - *see* Malaria
  Malassezia furfur 111.0
  Malleomyces
    mallei 024
    pseudomallei 025
  mammary gland 611.0
    puerperal, postpartum 675.2●
  Mansonella (ozzardi) 125.5
  mastoid (suppurative) - *see* Mastoiditis
  maxilla, maxillary 526.4
    sinus (chronic) *(see also* Sinusitis,
      maxillary) 473.0
  mediastinum 519.2
  medina 125.7
  meibomian
    cyst 373.12
    gland 373.12
  melioidosis 025
  meninges *(see also* Meningitis) 320.9
  meningococcal *(see also* condition) 036.9
    brain 036.1
    cerebrospinal 036.0
    endocardium 036.42
    generalized 036.2
    meninges 036.0
    meningococcemia 036.2
    specified site NEC 036.89
  mesenteric lymph nodes or glands NEC
    289.2
  Metagonimus 121.5
  metatarsophalangeal 711.97
  methicillin
    resistant Staphylococcus aureus (MRSA)
      041.12
    susceptible Staphylococcus aureus
      (MSSA) 041.11
  microorganism resistant to drugs - *see*
    Resistance (to), drugs by
    microorganisms
  Microsporidia 136.8
  microsporum, microsporic - *see*
    Dermatophytosis
  mima polymorpha NEC 041.85
  mixed flora NEC 041.89
  Monilia *(see also* Candidiasis) 112.9
    neonatal 771.7
  monkeypox 059.01
  Monosporium apiospermum 117.6
  mouth (focus) NEC 528.9
    parasitic 136.9
  MRSA (methicillin resistant Staphylococcus
    aureus) 041.12
  MSSA (methicillin susceptible
    Staphylococcus aureus) 041.11
  Mucor 117.7
  muscle NEC 728.89
  mycelium NEC 117.9
  mycetoma
    actinomycotic NEC *(see also*
      Actinomycosis) 039.9
    mycotic NEC 117.4
  Mycobacterium, mycobacterial *(see also*
    Mycobacterium) 031.9

◀ New　◀▥ Revised　~~deleted~~ Deleted　● Use Additional Digit(s)　▨ Omit code

Infection, infected, infective *(Continued)*
Mycoplasma NEC 041.81
mycotic NEC 117.9
  pathogenic to compromised host only 118
  skin NEC 111.9
  systemic 117.9
myocardium NEC 422.90
nail (chronic) (with lymphangitis) 681.9
  finger 681.02
    fungus 110.1
  ingrowing 703.0
  toe 681.11
    fungus 110.1
nasal sinus (chronic (*see also* Sinusitis) 473.9
nasopharynx (chronic) 478.29
  acute 460
navel 686.9
  newborn 771.4
Neisserian - *see* Gonococcus
Neotestudina rosatii 117.4
newborn, generalized 771.89
nipple 611.0
  puerperal, postpartum 675.0●
    with breast 675.9●
      specified type NEC 675.8●
Nocardia - *see* Actinomycosis
nose 478.19
nostril 478.19
obstetrical surgical wound 674.3●
Oesophagostomum (apiostomum) 127.7
Oestrus ovis 134.0
Oidium albicans (*see also* Candidiasis) 112.9
Onchocerca (volvulus) 125.3
  eye 125.3 [360.13]
  eyelid 125.3 [373.6]
operation wound 998.59
Opisthorchis (felineus) (tenuicollis)
  (viverrini) 121.0
orbit 376.00
  chronic 376.10
orthopoxvirus 059.00
  specified NEC 059.09
ovary (*see also* Salpingo-oophoritis) 614.2
Oxyuris vermicularis 127.4
pancreas 577.0
Paracoccidioides brasiliensis 116.1
Paragonimus (westermani) 121.2
parainfluenza virus 079.89
parameningococcus NEC 036.9
  with meningitis 036.0
parapoxvirus 059.10
  specified NEC 059.19
parasitic NEC 136.9
paratyphoid 002.9
  type A 002.1
  type B 002.2
  type C 002.3
paraurethral ducts 597.89
parotid gland 527.2
Pasteurella NEC 027.2
  multocida (cat-bite) (dog-bite) 027.2
  pestis (*see also* Plague) 020.9
  pseudotuberculosis 027.2
  septica (cat-bite) (dog-bite) 027.2
  tularensis (*see also* Tularemia) 021.9
pelvic, female (*see also* Disease, pelvis,
  inflammatory) 614.9
penis (glans) (retention) NEC 607.2
  herpetic 054.13
Peptococcus 041.84
Peptostreptococcus 041.84
periapical (pulpal origin) 522.4
peridental 523.30
perineal wound (obstetrical) 674.3●
periodontal 523.31
periorbital 376.00
  chronic 376.10
perirectal 569.49
perirenal (*see also* Infection, kidney) 590.9
peritoneal (*see also* Peritonitis) 567.9
periureteral 593.89

Infection, infected, infective *(Continued)*
periurethral 597.89
Petriellidium boydii 117.6
pharynx 478.29
  Coxsackie virus 074.0
  phlegmonous 462
  posterior, lymphoid 474.00
Phialophora
  gougerotii 117.8
  jeanselmei 117.8
  verrucosa 117.2
Piedraia hortai 111.3
pinna, acute 380.11
pinta 103.9
  intermediate 103.1
  late 103.2
  mixed 103.3
  primary 103.0
pinworm 127.4
pityrosporum furfur 111.0
pleuropneumonia-like organisms NEC
  (PPLO) 041.81
pneumococcal NEC 041.2
  generalized (purulent) 038.2
Pneumococcus NEC 041.2
port 999.33
postoperative wound 998.59
posttraumatic NEC 958.3
postvaccinal 999.39
poxvirus 059.9
  specified NEC 059.8
prepuce NEC 607.1
Proprionibacterium 041.84
prostate (capsule) (*see also* Prostatitis) 601.9
Proteus (mirabilis) (morganii) (vulgaris)
  NEC 041.6
  enteritis 008.3
protozoal NEC 136.8
  intestinal NEC 007.9
Pseudomonas NEC 041.7
  mallei 024
  pneumonia 482.1
  pseudomallei 025
psittacosis 073.9
puerperal, postpartum (major) 670.0●
  minor 646.6●
pulmonary - *see* Infection, lung
purulent - *see* Abscess
putrid, generalized - *see* Septicemia
pyemic - *see* Septicemia
Pyrenochaeta romeroi 117.4
Q fever 083.0
rabies 071
rectum (sphincter) 569.49
renal (*see also* Infection, kidney) 590.9
  pelvis and ureter 590.3
reservoir 999.33
resistant to drugs - *see* Resistance (to), drugs
  by microorganisms
respiratory 519.8
  chronic 519.8
  influenzal (acute) (upper) (*see also*
    Influenza) 487.1
  lung 518.89
  rhinovirus 460
  syncytial virus 079.6
  upper (acute) (infectious) NEC 465.9
    with flu, grippe, or influenza (*see also*
      Influenza) 487.1
    influenzal (*see also* Influenza) 487.1
    multiple sites NEC 465.8
    streptococcal 034.0
    viral NEC 465.9
respiratory syncytial virus (RSV) 079.6
resulting from presence of shunt or other
  internal prosthetic device - *see*
  Complications, infection and
  inflammation, due to (presence of) any
  device, implant, or graft classified to
  996.0–996.5 NEC
retroperitoneal 567.39

Infection, infected, infective *(Continued)*
retrovirus 079.50
  human immunodeficiency virus type 2
    (HIV 2) 079.53
  human T-cell lymphotrophic virus type I
    (HTLV-I) 079.51
  human T-cell lymphotrophic virus type II
    (HTLV-II) 079.52
  specified NEC 079.59
Rhinocladium 117.1
Rhinosporidium (seeberi) 117.0
rhinovirus
  in diseases classified elsewhere - *see*
    category 079
  unspecified nature or site 079.3
Rhizopus 117.7
rickettsial 083.9
rickettsialpox 083.2
rubella (*see also* Rubella) 056.9
  congenital 771.0
Saccharomyces (*see also* Candidiasis)
  112.9
Saksenaea 117.7
salivary duct or gland (any) 527.2
Salmonella (aertrycke) (callinarum)
  (choleraesuis) (enteritidis) (suipestifer)
  (typhimurium) 003.9
  with
    arthritis 003.23
    gastroenteritis 003.0
    localized infection 003.20
      specified type NEC 003.29
    meningitis 003.21
    osteomyelitis 003.24
    pneumonia 003.22
    septicemia 003.1
    specified manifestation NEC 003.8
  due to food (poisoning) (any serotype)
    (*see also* Poisoning, food, due to,
    Salmonella)
  hirschfeldii 002.3
  localized 003.20
    specified type NEC 003.29
  paratyphi 002.9
    A 002.1
    B 002.2
    C 002.3
  schottmuelleri 002.2
  specified type NEC 003.8
  typhi 002.0
  typhosa 002.0
saprophytic 136.8
Sarcocystis, lindemanni 136.5
SARS-associated coronavirus 079.82
scabies 133.0
Schistosoma - *see* Infestation, Schistosoma
Schmorl's bacillus 040.3
scratch or other superficial injury - *see* Injury,
  superficial, by site
scrotum (acute) NEC 608.4
sealpox 059.12
secondary, burn or open wound (dislocation)
  (fracture) 958.3
seminal vesicle (*see also* Vesiculitis) 608.0
septic
  generalized - *see* Septicemia
  localized, skin (*see also* Abscess) 682.9
septicemic - *see* Septicemia
seroma 998.51
Serratia (marcescens) 041.85
  generalized 038.44
sheep liver fluke 121.3
Shigella 004.9
  boydii 004.2
  dysenteriae 004.0
  Flexneri 004.1
  group
    A 004.0
    B 004.1
    C 004.2
    D 004.3

Infection, infected, infective *(Continued)*
  Shigella *(Continued)*
    Schmitz (-Stutzer) 004.0
    Schmitzii 004.0
    Shiga 004.0
    Sonnei 004.3
    specified type NEC 004.8
  Sin Nombre virus 079.81
  sinus *(see also* Sinusitis) 473.9
    pilonidal 685.1
      with abscess 685.0
    skin NEC 686.9
  Skene's duct or gland *(see also* Urethritis)
    597.89
  skin (local) (staphylococcal) (streptococcal)
    NEC 686.9
    abscess - *see* Abscess, by site
    cellulitis - *see* Cellulitis, by site
    due to fungus 111.9
      specified type NEC 111.8
    mycotic 111.9
      specified type NEC 111.8
    ulcer *(see also* Ulcer, skin) 707.9
  slow virus 046.9
    specified condition NEC 046.8
  Sparganum (mansoni) (proliferum) 123.5
  spermatic cord NEC 608.4
  sphenoidal (chronic) (sinus) *(see also*
    Sinusitis, sphenoidal) 473.3
  Spherophorus necrophorus 040.3
  spinal cord NEC *(see also* Encephalitis)
    323.9
    abscess 324.1
      late effect - *see* category 326
    late effect - *see* category 326
    meninges - *see* Meningitis
    streptococcal 320.2
  Spirillum
    minus or minor 026.0
    morsus muris 026.0
    obermeieri 087.0
  spirochetal NEC 104.9
    lung 104.8
    specified nature or site NEC 104.8
  spleen 289.59
  Sporothrix schenckii 117.1
  Sporotrichum (schenckii) 117.1
  Sporozoa 136.8
  staphylococcal NEC 041.10
    aureus 041.11
      methicillin
        resistant (MRSA) 041.12
        susceptible MSSA) 041.11
    food poisoning 005.0
    generalized (purulent) 038.10
      aureus 038.11
        methicillin
          resistant 038.12
          susceptible 038.11
      specified organism NEC 038.19
    pneumonia 482.40
      aureus 482.41
        methicillin
          resistant (MRSA) 482.42
          susceptible (MSSA) 482.41
      MRSA (methicillin resistant
        staphylococcus aureus) 482.42
      MSSA (methicillin susceptible
        staphylococcus aureus) 482.41
      specified type NEC 482.49
    septicemia 038.10
      aureus 038.11
        methicillin
          resistant (MRSA) 038.12
          susceptible (MSSA) 038.11
      MRSA (methicillin resistant
        staphylococcus aureus) 038.12
      MSSA (methicillin susceptible
        staphylococcus aureus) 038.11
      specified organism NEC 038.19
    specified NEC 041.19

Infection, infected, infective *(Continued)*
  steatoma 706.2
  Stellantchasmus falcatus 121.6
  Streptobacillus moniliformis 026.1
  streptococcal NEC 041.00
    generalized (purulent) 038.0
    group
      A 041.01
      B 041.02
      C 041.03
      D [enterococcus] 041.04
      G 041.05
    pneumonia - *see* Pneumonia, streptococcal
    septicemia 038.0
    sore throat 034.0
    specified NEC 041.09
  Streptomyces - *see* Actinomycosis
  streptotrichosis - *see* Actinomycosis
  Strongyloides (stercoralis) 127.2
  stump (amputation) (posttraumatic)
    (surgical) 997.62
    traumatic - *see* Amputation, traumatic, by
      site, complicated
  subcutaneous tissue, local NEC 686.9
  submaxillary region 528.9
  suipestifer *(see also* Infection, Salmonella) 003.9
  swimming pool bacillus 031.1
  syphilitic - *see* Syphilis
  systemic - *see* Septicemia
  Taenia - *see* Infestation, Taenia
  Taeniarhynchus saginatus 123.2
  tanapox 059.21
  tapeworm - *see* Infestation, tapeworm
  tendon (sheath) 727.89
  Ternidens diminutus 127.7
  testis *(see also* Orchitis) 604.90
  thigh (skin) 686.9
  threadworm 127.4
  throat 478.29
    pneumococcal 462
    staphylococcal 462
    streptococcal 034.0
    viral NEC *(see also* Pharyngitis) 462
  thumb (skin) 686.9
    abscess (with lymphangitis) 681.00
      pulp 681.01
    cellulitis (with lymphangitis) 681.00
    nail 681.02
  thyroglossal duct 529.8
  toe (skin) 686.9
    abscess (with lymphangitis) 681.10
    cellulitis (with lymphangitis) 681.10
    nail 681.11
      fungus 110.1
  tongue NEC 529.0
    parasitic 112.0
  tonsil (faucial) (lingual) (pharyngeal) 474.00
    acute or subacute 463
    and adenoid 474.02
    tag 474.00
  tooth, teeth 522.4
    periapical (pulpal origin) 522.4
    peridental 523.30
    periodontal 523.31
    pulp 522.0
    socket 526.5
  TORCH - *see* Infection, congenital NEC
    without active infection 760.2
  Torula histolytica 117.5
  Toxocara (cani) (cati) (felis) 128.0
  Toxoplasma gondii *(see also* Toxoplasmosis)
    130.9
  trachea, chronic 491.8
    fungus 117.9
  traumatic NEC 958.3
  trematode NEC 121.9
  trench fever 083.1
  Treponema
    denticola 041.84
    macrodenticum 041.84
    pallidum *(see also* Syphilis) 097.9

Infection, infected, infective *(Continued)*
  Trichinella (spiralis) 124
  Trichomonas 131.9
    bladder 131.09
    cervix 131.09
    hominis 007.3
    intestine 007.3
    prostate 131.03
    specified site NEC 131.8
    urethra 131.02
    urogenitalis 131.00
    vagina 131.01
    vulva 131.01
  Trichophyton, trichophytid - *see*
    Dermatophytosis
  Trichosporon (beigelii) cutaneum 111.2
  Trichostrongylus 127.6
  Trichuris (trichiuria) 127.3
  Trombicula (irritans) 133.8
  Trypanosoma *(see also* Trypanosomiasis)
    086.9
    cruzi 086.2
  tubal *(see also* Salpingo-oophoritis) 614.2
  tuberculous NEC *(see also* Tuberculosis)
    011.9●
  tubo-ovarian *(see also* Salpingo-oophoritis)
    614.2
  tunica vaginalis 608.4
  tunnel 999.33
  tympanic membrane - *see* Myringitis
  typhoid (abortive) (ambulant) (bacillus)
    002.0
  typhus 081.9
    flea-borne (endemic) 081.0
    louse-borne (epidemic) 080
    mite-borne 081.2
    recrudescent 081.1
    tick-borne 082.9
      African 082.1
      North Asian 082.2
  umbilicus (septic) 686.9
    newborn NEC 771.4
  ureter 593.89
  urethra *(see also* Urethritis) 597.80
  urinary (tract) NEC 599.0
    with
      abortion - *see* Abortion, by type, with
        urinary tract infection
      ectopic pregnancy *(see also* categories
        633.0–633.9) 639.8
      molar pregnancy *(see also* categories
        630–632) 639.8
    candidal 112.2
    complicating pregnancy, childbirth, or
      puerperium 646.6●
      affecting fetus or newborn 760.1
      asymptomatic 646.5●
        affecting fetus or newborn 760.1
    diplococcal (acute) 098.0
      chronic 098.2
    due to Trichomonas (vaginalis) 131.00
    following
      abortion 639.8
      ectopic or molar pregnancy 639.8
    gonococcal (acute) 098.0
      chronic or duration of 2 months or
        over 098.2
    newborn 771.82
    trichomonal 131.00
    tuberculous *(see also* Tuberculosis) 016.3●
  uterus, uterine *(see also* Endometritis) 615.9
  utriculus masculinus NEC 597.89
  vaccination 999.39
  vagina (granulation tissue) (wall) *(see also*
    Vaginitis) 616.10
  varicella 052.9
  varicose veins - *see* Varicose, veins
  variola 050.9
    major 050.0
    minor 050.1
  vas deferens NEC 608.4

Infection, infected, infective (Continued)
Veillonella 041.84
verumontanum 597.89
vesical (see also Cystitis) 595.9
Vibrio
cholerae 001.0
El Tor 001.1
parahaemolyticus (food poisoning) 005.4
vulnificus 041.85
Vincent's (gums) (mouth) (tonsil) 101
virus, viral 079.99
adenovirus
in diseases classified elsewhere - see
category 079
unspecified nature or site 079.0
central nervous system NEC 049.9
enterovirus 048
meningitis 047.9
specified type NEC 047.8
slow virus 046.9
specified condition NEC 046.8
chest 519.8
conjunctivitis 077.99
specified type NEC 077.89
coronavirus 079.89
SARS-associated 079.82
Coxsackie (see also Infection, Coxsackie)
079.2
Ebola 065.8
ECHO
in diseases classified elsewhere - see
category 079
unspecified nature or site 079.1
encephalitis 049.9
arthropod-borne NEC 064
tick-borne 063.9
specified type NEC 063.8
enteritis NEC (see also Enteritis, viral)
008.8
exanthem NEC 057.9
Hantavirus 079.81
human papilloma 079.4
in diseases classified elsewhere - see
category 079
intestine (see also Enteritis, viral) 008.8
lung - see Pneumonia, viral
respiratory syncytial (RSV) 079.6
Retrovirus 079.50
rhinovirus
in diseases classified elsewhere - see
category 079
unspecified nature or site 079.3
salivary gland disease 078.5
slow 046.9
specified condition NEC 046.8
specified type NEC 079.89
in diseases classified elsewhere - see
category 079
unspecified nature or site 079.99
warts 078.10
specified NEC 078.19
yaba monkey tumor 059.22
vulva (see also Vulvitis) 616.10
whipworm 127.3
Whitmore's bacillus 025
wound (local) (posttraumatic) NEC 958.3
with
dislocation - see Dislocation, by site,
open
fracture - see Fracture, by site, open
open wound - see Wound, open, by
site, complicated
postoperative 998.59
surgical 998.59
Wuchereria 125.0
bancrofti 125.0
malayi 125.1
yaba monkey tumor virus 059.22
yatapoxvirus 059.20
yaws - see Yaws
yeast (see also Candidiasis) 112.9

Infection, infected, infective (Continued)
yellow fever (see also Fever, yellow)
060.9
Yersinia pestis (see also Plague) 020.9
Zeis' gland 373.12
zoonotic bacterial NEC 027.9
Zopfia senegalensis 117.4
Infective, infectious - see condition
Inferiority complex 301.9
constitutional psychopathic 301.9
Infertility
female 628.9
age related 628.8
associated with
adhesions, peritubal 614.6 [628.2]
anomaly
cervical mucus 628.4
congenital
cervix 628.4
fallopian tube 628.2
uterus 628.3
vagina 628.4
anovulation 628.0
dysmucorrhea 628.4
endometritis, tuberculous (see also
Tuberculosis) 016.7 ● [628.3]
Stein-Leventhal syndrome 256.4 [628.0]
due to
adiposogenital dystrophy 253.8 [628.1]
anterior pituitary disorder NEC 253.4
[628.1]
hyperfunction 253.1 [628.1]
cervical anomaly 628.4
fallopian tube anomaly 628.2
ovarian failure 256.39 [628.0]
Stein-Leventhal syndrome 256.4 [628.0]
uterine anomaly 628.3
vaginal anomaly 628.4
nonimplantation 628.3
origin
cervical 628.4
pituitary-hypothalamus NEC 253.8
[628.1]
anterior pituitary NEC 253.4 [628.1]
hyperfunction NEC 253.1 [628.1]
dwarfism 253.3 [628.1]
panhypopituitarism 253.2 [628.1]
specified NEC 628.8
tubal (block) (occlusion) (stenosis)
628.2
adhesions 614.6 [628.2]
uterine 628.3
vaginal 628.4
previous, requiring supervision of
pregnancy V23.0
male 606.9
absolute 606.0
due to
azoospermia 606.0
drug therapy 606.8
extratesticular cause NEC 606.8
germinal cell
aplasia 606.0
desquamation 606.1
hypospermatogenesis 606.1
infection 606.8
obstruction, afferent ducts 606.8
oligospermia 606.1
radiation 606.8
spermatogenic arrest (complete)
606.0
incomplete 606.1
systemic disease 606.8
Infestation 134.9
Acanthocheilonema (perstans) 125.4
streptocerca 125.6
Acariasis 133.9
demodex folliculorum 133.8
sarcoptes scabiei 133.0
trombiculae 133.8
Agamofilaria streptocerca 125.6

Infestation (Continued)
Ancylostoma, Ankylostoma 126.9
americanum 126.1
braziliense 126.2
canium 126.8
ceylanicum 126.3
duodenale 126.0
new world 126.1
old world 126.0
Angiostrongylus cantonensis 128.8
anisakiasis 127.1
Anisakis larva 127.1
arthropod NEC 134.1
Ascaris lumbricoides 127.0
Bacillus fusiformis 101
Balantidium coli 007.0
beef tapeworm 123.2
Bothriocephalus (latus) 123.4
larval 123.5
broad tapeworm 123.4
larval 123.5
Brugia malayi 125.1
Candiru 136.8
Capillaria
hepatica 128.8
philippinensis 127.5
cat liver fluke 121.0
Cercomonas hominis (intestinal) 007.3
cestodes 123.9
specified type NEC 123.8
chigger 133.8
chigoe 134.1
Chilomastix 007.8
Clonorchis (sinensis) (liver) 121.1
coccidia 007.2
complicating pregnancy, childbirth, or
puerperium 647.9 ●
affecting fetus or newborn 760.8
Cysticercus cellulosae 123.1
Demodex folliculorum 133.8
Dermatobia (hominis) 134.0
Dibothriocephalus (latus) 123.4
larval 123.5
Dicrocoelium dendriticum 121.8
Diphyllobothrium (adult) (intestinal) (latum)
(pacificum) 123.4
larval 123.5
Diplogonoporus (grandis) 123.8
Dipylidium (caninum) 123.8
Distoma hepaticum 121.3
dog tapeworm 123.8
Dracunculus medinensis 125.7
dragon worm 125.7
dwarf tapeworm 123.6
Echinococcus (see also Echinococcus) 122.9
Echinostoma ilocanum 121.8
Embadomonas 007.8
Endamoeba (histolytica) - see Infection,
ameba
Entamoeba (histolytica) - see Infection, ameba
Enterobius vermicularis 127.4
Epidermophyton - see Dermatophytosis
eyeworm 125.2
Fasciola
gigantica 121.3
hepatica 121.3
Fasciolopsis (buski) (small intestine) 121.4
filarial 125.9
due to
acanthocheilonema (perstans) 125.4
streptocerca 125.6
Brugia (Wuchereria) malayi 125.1
Dracunculus medinensis 125.7
guinea worms 125.7
Mansonella (ozzardi) 125.5
Onchocerca volvulus 125.3
eye 125.3 [360.13]
eyelid 125.3 [373.6]
Wuchereria (bancrofti) 125.0
malayi 125.1
specified type NEC 125.6

Infestation (Continued)
  fish tapeworm 123.4
    larval 123.5
  fluke 121.9
    blood NEC (see also Schistosomiasis) 120.9
    cat liver 121.0
    intestinal (giant) 121.4
    liver (sheep) 121.3
      cat 121.0
      Chinese 121.1
      clonorchiasis 121.1
      fascioliasis 121.3
      Oriental 121.1
    lung (oriental) 121.2
    sheep liver 121.3
  fly larva 134.0
  Gasterophilus (intestinalis) 134.0
  Gastrodiscoides hominis 121.8
  Giardia lamblia 007.1
  Gnathostoma (spinigerum) 128.1
  Gongylonema 125.6
  guinea worm 125.7
  helminth NEC 128.9
    intestinal 127.9
      mixed (types classifiable to more than
        one category in 120.0–127.7)
        127.8
      specified type NEC 127.7
    specified type NEC 128.8
  Heterophyes heterophyes (small intestine)
    121.6
  hookworm (see also Infestation, ancylostoma)
    126.9
  Hymenolepis (diminuta) (nana) 123.6
  intestinal NEC 129
  leeches (aquatic) (land) 134.2
  Leishmania - see Leishmaniasis
  lice (see also Infestation, pediculus) 132.9
  Linguatulidae, linguatula (pentastoma)
    (serrata) 134.1
  Loa loa 125.2
    eyelid 125.2 [373.6]
  louse (see also Infestation, pediculus) 132.9
    body 132.1
    head 132.0
    pubic 132.2
  maggots 134.0
  Mansonella (ozzardi) 125.5
  medina 125.7
  Metagonimus yokogawai (small intestine)
    121.5
  Microfilaria streptocerca 125.3
    eye 125.3 [360.13]
    eyelid 125.3 [373.6]
  Microsporon furfur 111.0
  microsporum - see Dermatophytosis
  mites 133.9
    scabic 133.0
    specified type NEC 133.8
  Monilia (albicans) (see also Candidiasis) 112.9
    vagina 112.1
    vulva 112.1
  mouth 112.0
  Necator americanus 126.1
  nematode (intestinal) 127.9
    Ancylostoma (see also Ancylostoma) 126.9
    Ascaris lumbricoides 127.0
    conjunctiva NEC 128.9
    Dioctophyma 128.8
    Enterobius vermicularis 127.4
    Gnathostoma spinigerum 128.1
    Oesophagostomum (apiostomum) 127.7
    Physaloptera 127.4
    specified type NEC 127.7
    Strongyloides stercoralis 127.2
    Ternidens diminutus 127.7
    Trichinella spiralis 124
    Trichostrongylus 127.6
    Trichuris (trichiuria) 127.3
  Oesophagostomum (apiostomum) 127.7
  Oestrus ovis 134.0

Infestation (Continued)
  Onchocerca (volvulus) 125.3
    eye 125.3 [360.13]
    eyelid 125.3 [373.6]
  Opisthorchis (felineus) (tenuicollis)
    (viverrini) 121.0
  Oxyuris vermicularis 127.4
  Paragonimus (westermani) 121.2
  parasite, parasitic NEC 136.9
    eyelid 134.9 [373.6]
    intestinal 129
    mouth 112.0
    orbit 376.13
    skin 134.9
    tongue 112.0
  pediculus 132.9
    capitis (humanus) (any site) 132.0
    corporis (humanus) (any site) 132.1
    eyelid 132.0 [373.6]
    mixed (classifiable to more than one
      category in 132.0–132.2) 132.3
    pubis (any site) 132.2
  phthirus (pubis) (any site) 132.2
    with any infestation classifiable to 132.0
      and 132.1 132.3
  pinworm 127.4
  pork tapeworm (adult) 123.0
  protozoal NEC 136.8
  pubic louse 132.2
  rat tapeworm 123.6
  red bug 133.8
  roundworm (large) NEC 127.0
  sand flea 134.1
  saprophytic NEC 136.8
  Sarcoptes scabiei 133.0
  scabies 133.0
  Schistosoma 120.9
    bovis 120.8
    cercariae 120.3
    hematobium 120.0
    intercalatum 120.8
    japonicum 120.2
    mansoni 120.1
    mattheii 120.8
    specified
      site - see Schistosomiasis
      type NEC 120.8
    spindale 120.8
  screw worms 134.0
  skin NEC 134.9
  Sparganum (mansoni) (proliferum) 123.5
    larval 123.5
  specified type NEC 134.8
  Spirometra larvae 123.5
  Sporozoa NEC 136.8
  Stellantchasmus falcatus 121.6
  Strongyloides 127.2
  Strongylus (gibsoni) 127.7
  Taenia 123.3
    diminuta 123.6
    Echinococcus (see also Echinococcus) 122.9
    mediocanellata 123.2
    nana 123.6
    saginata (mediocanellata) 123.2
    solium (intestinal form) 123.0
      larval form 123.1
  Taeniarhynchus saginatus 123.2
  tapeworm 123.9
    beef 123.2
    broad 123.4
      larval 123.5
    dog 123.8
    dwarf 123.6
    fish 123.4
      larval 123.5
    pork 123.0
    rat 123.6
  Ternidens diminutus 127.7
  Tetranychus molestissimus 133.8
  threadworm 127.4
  tongue 112.0

Infestation (Continued)
  Toxocara (cani) (cati) (felis) 128.0
  trematode(s) NEC 121.9
  Trichina spiralis 124
  Trichinella spiralis 124
  Trichocephalus 127.3
  Trichomonas 131.9
    bladder 131.09
    cervix 131.09
    intestine 007.3
    prostate 131.03
    specified site NEC 131.8
    urethra (female) (male) 131.02
    urogenital 131.00
    vagina 131.01
    vulva 131.01
  Trichophyton - see Dermatophytosis
  Trichostrongylus instabilis 127.6
  Trichuris (trichiuria) 127.3
  Trombicula (irritans) 133.8
  Trypanosoma - see Trypanosomiasis
  Tunga penetrans 134.1
  Uncinaria americana 126.1
  whipworm 127.3
  worms NEC 128.9
    intestinal 127.9
  Wuchereria 125.0
    bancrofti 125.0
    malayi 125.1
Infiltrate, infiltration
  with an iron compound 275.09
  amyloid (any site) (generalized) 277.39
  calcareous (muscle) NEC 275.49
    localized - see Degeneration, by site
  calcium salt (muscle) 275.49
  chemotherapy, vesicant 999.81
  corneal (see also Edema, cornea) 371.20
  eyelid 373.9
  fatty (diffuse) (generalized) 272.8
    localized - see Degeneration, by site,
      fatty
  glycogen, glycogenic (see also Disease,
    glycogen storage) 271.0
  heart, cardiac
    fatty (see also Degeneration, myocardial)
      429.1
    glycogenic 271.0 [425.7]
  inflammatory in vitreous 379.29
  kidney (see also Disease, renal) 593.9
  leukemic (M9800/3) - see Leukemia
  liver 573.8
    fatty - see Fatty, liver
    glycogen (see also Disease, glycogen
      storage) 271.0
  lung (see also Infiltrate, pulmonary) 793.19
    eosinophilic 518.3
    x-ray finding only 793.19
  lymphatic (see also Leukemia, lymphatic)
    204.9●
    gland, pigmentary 289.3
  muscle, fatty 728.9
  myelogenous (see also Leukemia, myeloid)
    205.9●
  myocardium, myocardial
    fatty (see also Degeneration, myocardial)
      429.1
    glycogenic 271.0 [425.7]
  pulmonary 793.19
    with
      eosinophilia 518.3
      pneumonia - see Pneumonia, by type
    x-ray finding only 793.19
  Ranke's primary (see also Tuberculosis)
    010.0●
  skin, lymphocytic (benign) 709.8
  thymus (gland) (fatty) 254.8
  urine 788.8
  vesicant
    agent NEC 999.82
    chemotherapy 999.81
  vitreous humor 379.29

◀ New   ◀▪▪ Revised   ~~deleted~~ Deleted   ● Use Additional Digit(s)   ▨ Omit code

Infirmity 799.89
  senile 797
Inflammation, inflamed, inflammatory (with exudation)
  abducens (nerve) 378.54
  accessory sinus (chronic) (*see also* Sinusitis) 473.9
  adrenal (gland) 255.8
  alimentary canal - *see* Enteritis
  alveoli (teeth) 526.5
    scorbutic 267
  amnion - *see* Amnionitis
  anal canal 569.49
  antrum (chronic) (*see also* Sinusitis, maxillary) 473.0
  anus 569.49
  appendix (*see also* Appendicitis) 541
  arachnoid - *see* Meningitis
  areola 611.0
    puerperal, postpartum 675.0●
  areolar tissue NEC 686.9
  artery - *see* Arteritis
  auditory meatus (external) (*see also* Otitis, externa) 380.10
  Bartholin's gland 616.89
  bile duct or passage 576.1
  bladder (*see also* Cystitis) 595.9
  bleb
    postprocedural 379.60
      stage 1 379.61
      stage 2 379.62
      stage 3 379.63
  bone - *see* Osteomyelitis
  bowel (*see also* Enteritis) 558.9
  brain (*see also* Encephalitis) 323.9
    late effect - *see* category 326
    membrane - *see* Meningitis
  breast 611.0
    puerperal, postpartum 675.2●
  broad ligament (*see also* Disease, pelvis, inflammatory) 614.4
    acute 614.3
  bronchus - *see* Bronchitis
  bursa - *see* Bursitis
  capsule
    liver 573.3
    spleen 289.59
  catarrhal (*see also* Catarrh) 460
    vagina 616.10
  cecum (*see also* Appendicitis) 541
  cerebral (*see also* Encephalitis) 323.9
    late effect - *see* category 326
    membrane - *see* Meningitis
  cerebrospinal (*see also* Meningitis) 322.9
    late effect - *see* category 326
    meningococcal 036.0
    tuberculous (*see also* Tuberculosis) 013.6●
  cervix (uteri) (*see also* Cervicitis) 616.0
  chest 519.9
  choroid NEC (*see also* Choroiditis) 363.20
  cicatrix (tissue) - *see* Cicatrix
  colon (*see also* Enteritis) 558.9
    granulomatous 555.1
    newborn 558.9
  connective tissue (diffuse) NEC 728.9
  cornea (*see also* Keratitis) 370.9
    with ulcer (*see also* Ulcer, cornea) 370.00
  corpora cavernosa (penis) 607.2
  cranial nerve - *see* Disorder, nerve, cranial
  diarrhea - *see* Diarrhea
  disc (intervertebral) (space) 722.90
    cervical, cervicothoracic 722.91
    lumbar, lumbosacral 722.93
    thoracic, thoracolumbar 722.92
  Douglas' cul-de-sac or pouch (chronic) (*see also* Disease, pelvis, inflammatory) 614.4
    acute 614.3

Inflammation, inflamed, inflammatory
  (*Continued*)
  due to (presence of) any device, implant, or graft classifiable to 996.0–996.5 - *see* Complications, infection and inflammation, due to (presence of) any device, implant, or graft classified to 996.0–996.5 NEC
  duodenum 535.6●
  dura mater - *see* Meningitis
  ear - *see also* Otitis
    external (*see also* Otitis, externa) 380.10
    inner (*see also* Labyrinthitis) 386.30
    middle - *see* Otitis media
  esophagus 530.10
  ethmoidal (chronic) (sinus) (*see also* Sinusitis, ethmoidal) 473.2
  Eustachian tube (catarrhal) 381.50
    acute 381.51
    chronic 381.52
  extrarectal 569.49
  eye 379.99
  eyelid 373.9
    specified NEC 373.8
  fallopian tube (*see also* Salpingo-oophoritis) 614.2
  fascia 728.9
  fetal membranes (acute) 658.4●
    affecting fetus or newborn 762.7
  follicular, pharynx 472.1
  frontal (chronic) (sinus) (*see also* Sinusitis, frontal) 473.1
  gallbladder (*see also* Cholecystitis, acute) 575.0
  gall duct (*see also* Cholecystitis) 575.10
  gastrointestinal (*see also* Enteritis) 558.9
  genital organ (diffuse) (internal)
    female 614.9
      with
        abortion - *see* Abortion, by type, with sepsis
        ectopic pregnancy (*see also* categories 633.0–633.9) 639.0
        molar pregnancy (*see also* categories 630–632) 639.0
      complicating pregnancy, childbirth, or puerperium 646.6●
        affecting fetus or newborn 760.8
      following
        abortion 639.0
        ectopic or molar pregnancy 639.0
    male 608.4
  gland (lymph) (*see also* Lymphadenitis) 289.3
  glottis (*see also* Laryngitis) 464.00
    with obstruction 464.01
  granular, pharynx 472.1
  gum 523.10
  heart (*see also* Carditis) 429.89
  hepatic duct 576.8
  hernial sac - *see* Hernia, by site
  ileum (*see also* Enteritis) 558.9
    terminal or regional 555.0
      with large intestine 555.2
  intervertebral disc 722.90
    cervical, cervicothoracic 722.91
    lumbar, lumbosacral 722.93
    thoracic, thoracolumbar 722.92
  intestine (*see also* Enteritis) 558.9
  jaw (acute) (bone) (chronic) (lower) (suppurative) (upper) 526.4
  jejunum - *see* Enteritis
  joint NEC (*see also* Arthritis) 716.9●
    sacroiliac 720.2
  kidney (*see also* Nephritis) 583.9
  knee (joint) 716.66
    tuberculous (active) (*see also* Tuberculosis) 015.2●
  labium (majus) (minus) (*see also* Vulvitis) 616.10

Inflammation, inflamed, inflammatory
  (*Continued*)
  lacrimal
    gland (*see also* Dacryoadenitis) 375.00
    passages (duct) (sac) (*see also* Dacryocystitis) 375.30
  larynx (*see also* Laryngitis) 464.00
    with obstruction 464.01
    diphtheritic 032.3
  leg NEC 686.9
  lip 528.5
  liver (capsule) (*see also* Hepatitis) 573.3
    acute 570
    chronic 571.40
    suppurative 572.0
  lung (acute) (*see also* Pneumonia) 486
    chronic (interstitial) 518.89
  lymphatic vessel (*see also* Lymphangitis) 457.2
  lymph node or gland (*see also* Lymphadenitis) 289.3
  mammary gland 611.0
    puerperal, postpartum 675.2●
  maxilla, maxillary 526.4
    sinus (chronic) (*see also* Sinusitis, maxillary) 473.0
  membranes of brain or spinal cord - *see* Meningitis
  meninges - *see* Meningitis
  mouth 528.00
  muscle 728.9
  myocardium (*see also* Myocarditis) 429.0
  nasal sinus (chronic) (*see also* Sinusitis) 473.9
  nasopharynx - *see* Nasopharyngitis
  navel 686.9
    newborn NEC 771.4
  nerve NEC 729.2
  nipple 611.0
    puerperal, postpartum 675.0●
  nose 478.19
    suppurative 472.0
  oculomotor nerve 378.51
  optic nerve 377.30
  orbit (chronic) 376.10
    acute 376.00
    chronic 376.10
  ovary (*see also* Salpingo-oophoritis) 614.2
  oviduct (*see also* Salpingo-oophoritis) 614.2
  pancreas - *see* Pancreatitis
  parametrium (chronic) (*see also* Disease, pelvis, inflammatory) 614.4
    acute 614.3
  parotid region 686.9
    gland 527.2
  pelvis, female (*see also* Disease, pelvis, inflammatory) 614.9
  penis (corpora cavernosa) 607.2
  perianal 569.49
  pericardium (*see also* Pericarditis) 423.9
  perineum (female) (male) 686.9
  perirectal 569.49
  peritoneum (*see also* Peritonitis) 567.9
  periuterine (*see also* Disease, pelvis, inflammatory) 614.9
  perivesical (*see also* Cystitis) 595.9
  petrous bone (*see also* Petrositis) 383.20
  pharynx (*see also* Pharyngitis) 462
    follicular 472.1
    granular 472.1
  pia mater - *see* Meningitis
  pleura - *see* Pleurisy
  postmastoidectomy cavity 383.30
    chronic 383.33
  pouch, internal ileoanal 569.71
  prostate (*see also* Prostatitis) 601.9
  rectosigmoid - *see* Rectosigmoiditis
  rectum (*see also* Proctitis) 569.49

Inflammation, inflamed, inflammatory
  (Continued)
  respiratory, upper (see also Infection,
      respiratory, upper) 465.9
    chronic, due to external agent - see
        Condition, respiratory, chronic, due
        to, external agent
    due to
      fumes or vapors (chemical)
          (inhalation) 506.2
      radiation 508.1
  retina (see also Retinitis) 363.20
  retrocecal (see also Appendicitis) 541
  retroperitoneal (see also Peritonitis) 567.9
  salivary duct or gland (any) (suppurative)
      527.2
  scorbutic, alveoli, teeth 267
  scrotum 608.4
  sigmoid - see Enteritis
  sinus (see also Sinusitis) 473.9
  Skene's duct or gland (see also Urethritis)
      597.89
  skin 686.9
  spermatic cord 608.4
  sphenoidal (sinus) (see also Sinusitis,
      sphenoidal) 473.3
  spinal
    cord (see also Encephalitis) 323.9
      late effect - see category 326
    membrane - see Meningitis
    nerve - see Disorder, nerve
  spine (see also Spondylitis) 720.9
  spleen (capsule) 289.59
  stomach - see Gastritis
  stricture, rectum 569.49
  subcutaneous tissue NEC 686.9
  suprarenal (gland) 255.8
  synovial (fringe) (membrane) - see Bursitis
  tendon (sheath) NEC 726.90
  testis (see also Orchitis) 604.90
  thigh 686.9
  throat (see also Sore throat) 462
  thymus (gland) 254.8
  thyroid (gland) (see also Thyroiditis) 245.9
  tongue 529.0
  tonsil - see Tonsillitis
  trachea - see Tracheitis
  trochlear nerve 378.53
  tubal (see also Salpingo-oophoritis) 614.2
  tuberculous NEC (see also Tuberculosis)
      011.9●
  tubo-ovarian (see also Salpingo-oophoritis)
      614.2
  tunica vaginalis 608.4
  tympanic membrane - see Myringitis
  umbilicus, umbilical 686.9
    newborn NEC 771.4
  uterine ligament (see also Disease, pelvis,
      inflammatory) 614.4
    acute 614.3
  uterus (catarrhal) (see also Endometritis)
      615.9
  uveal tract (anterior) (see also Iridocyclitis)
      364.3
    posterior - see Chorioretinitis
    sympathetic 360.11
  vagina (see also Vaginitis) 616.10
  vas deferens 608.4
  vein (see also Phlebitis) 451.9
    thrombotic 451.9
      cerebral (see also Thrombosis, brain)
          434.0●
      leg 451.2
        deep (vessels) NEC 451.19
        superficial (vessels) 451.0
      lower extremity 451.2
        deep (vessels) NEC 451.19
        superficial (vessels) 451.0
  vocal cord 478.5
  vulva (see also Vulvitis) 616.10
Inflation, lung imperfect (newborn) 770.5

Influenza, influenzal 487.1
  with
    bronchitis 487.1
    bronchopneumonia 487.0
    cold (any type) 487.1
    digestive manifestations 487.8
    hemoptysis 487.1
    involvement of
      gastrointestinal tract 487.8
      nervous system 487.8
    laryngitis 487.1
    manifestations NEC 487.8
      respiratory 487.1
        pneumonia 487.0
    pharyngitis 487.1
    pneumonia (any form classifiable to
        480–483, 485–486) 487.0
    respiratory manifestations NEC 487.1
    sinusitis 487.1
    sore throat 487.1
    tonsillitis 487.1
    tracheitis 487.1
    upper respiratory infection (acute) 487.1
  A/H5N1 (see also Influenza, avian) 488.02
  abdominal 487.8
  Asian 487.1
  avian 488.02
    with involvement of gastrointestinal tract
        488.09
    bronchopneumonia 488.01
    laryngitis 488.02
    manifestations NEC 488.09
      respiratory 488.02
    pharyngitis 488.02
    pneumonia (any form classifiable to
        480-483, 485-486) 488.01
    respiratory infection (acute) (upper)
        488.02
  bronchial 487.1
  bronchopneumonia 487.0
  catarrhal 487.1
  due to identified
    animal origin influenza virus - see
        Influenza, due to identified, novel
        influenza A virus
    avian influenza virus 488.02
      with
        manifestations NEC 488.09
          respiratory 488.02
        pneumonia (any form classifiable to
            480-483, 485-486) 488.01
    (novel) 2009 H1N1 influenza virus 488.12
      with
        manifestations NEC 488.19
          respiratory 488.12
        pneumonia 488.11
    novel influenza A virus 488.82
      with
        encephalopathy 488.89
        involvement of gastrointestinal
            tract 488.89
        laryngitis 488.82
        manifestations NEC 488.89
          respiratory (acute) (upper)
              488.82
        pharyngitis 488.82
        pneumonia 488.81
  epidemic 487.1
  gastric 487.8
  intestinal 487.8
  laryngitis 487.1
  maternal affecting fetus or newborn 760.2
    manifest influenza in infant 771.2
  (novel) 2009 H1N1 488.12
    with involvement of gastrointestinal tract
        488.19
    bronchopneumonia 488.11
    laryngitis 488.12
    manifestations NEC 488.19
      respiratory 488.12
    pharyngitis 488.12

Influenza, influenzal (Continued)
  (novel) 2009 H1N1 (Continued)
    pneumonia (any form classifiable to
        480-483, 485-486) 488.11
    respiratory infection (acute) (upper)
        488.12
  novel A/H1N1 (see also Influenza, (novel)
      2009 H1N1) 488.12
  novel influenza A viruses not previously
      found in humans - see Influenza, due
      to identified, novel influenza A virus
  pharyngitis 487.1
  pneumonia (any form) 487.0
  respiratory (upper) 487.1
  specified NEC 487.1
  stomach 487.8
  vaccination, prophylactic (against)
      V04.81
Influenza-like disease (see also Influenza)
    487.1
Infraction, Freiberg's (metatarsal head)
    732.5
Infraeruption, teeth 524.34
Infusion complication, misadventure, or
    reaction - see Complication, infusion
Ingestion
  chemical - see Table of Drugs and Chemicals
  drug or medicinal substance
    overdose or wrong substance given or
        taken 977.9
      specified drug - see Table of Drugs and
          Chemicals
  foreign body NEC (see also Foreign body) 938
Ingrowing
  hair 704.8
  nail (finger) (toe) (infected) 703.0
Inguinal - see also condition
  testis 752.51
Inhalation
  carbon monoxide 986
  flame
    mouth 947.0
    lung 947.1
  food or foreign body (see also Asphyxia, food
      or foreign body) 933.1
  gas, fumes, or vapor (noxious) 987.9
    specified agent - see Table of Drugs and
        Chemicals
  liquid or vomitus (see also Asphyxia, food or
      foreign body) 933.1
    lower respiratory tract NEC 934.9
  meconium (fetus or newborn) 770.11
    with respiratory symptoms 770.12
  mucus (see also Asphyxia, mucus) 933.1
  oil (causing suffocation) (see also Asphyxia,
      food or foreign body) 933.1
  pneumonia - see Pneumonia, aspiration
  smoke 508.2
  steam 987.9
  stomach contents or secretions (see also
      Asphyxia, food or foreign body)
      933.1
    in labor and delivery 668.0●
Inhibition, inhibited
  academic as adjustment reaction 309.23
  orgasm
    female 302.73
    male 302.74
  sexual
    desire 302.71
    excitement 302.72
  work as adjustment reaction 309.23
Inhibitor
  autoimmune, to clotting factors 286.52
  systemic lupus erythematosus (presence of)
      795.79
    with
      hemorrhagic disorder 286.53
      hypercoagulable state 289.81
Iniencephalus, iniencephaly 740.2
Injected eye 372.74

◀ New   ◀= Revised   ~~deleted~~ Deleted   ● Use Additional Digit(s)   ▨ Omit code

Injury 959.9

Note: For abrasion, insect bite (nonvenomous), blister, or scratch, *see* Injury, superficial.

For laceration, traumatic rupture, tear, or penetrating wound of internal organs, such as heart, lung, liver, kidney, pelvic organs, whether or not accompanied by open wound in the same region, *see* Injury, internal.

For nerve injury, *see* Injury, nerve.

For late effect of injuries classifiable to 850–854, 860–869, 900–919, 950–959, *see* Late, effect, injury, by type.

abdomen, abdominal (viscera) - *see also* Injury, internal, abdomen
   muscle or wall 959.12
acoustic, resulting in deafness 951.5
adenoid 959.09
adrenal (gland) - *see* Injury, internal, adrenal
alveolar (process) 959.09
ankle (and foot) (and knee) (and leg, except thigh) 959.7
anterior chamber, eye 921.3
anus 959.19
aorta (thoracic) 901.0
   abdominal 902.0
appendix - *see* Injury, internal, appendix
arm, upper (and shoulder) 959.2
artery (complicating trauma) (*see also* Injury, blood vessel, by site) 904.9
   cerebral or meningeal (*see also* Hemorrhage, brain, traumatic, subarachnoid) 852.0●
auditory canal (external) (meatus) 959.09
auricle, auris, ear 959.09
axilla 959.2
back 959.19
bile duct - *see* Injury, internal, bile duct
birth - *see also* Birth, injury
   canal NEC, complicating delivery 665.9●
bladder (sphincter) - *see* Injury, internal, bladder
blast (air) (hydraulic) (immersion) (underwater) NEC 869.0
   with open wound into cavity NEC 869.1
   abdomen or thorax - *see* Injury, internal, by site
   brain - *see* Concussion, brain
   ear (acoustic nerve trauma) 951.5
     with perforation of tympanic membrane - *see* Wound, open, ear, drum
blood vessel NEC 904.9
   abdomen 902.9
     multiple 902.87
     specified NEC 902.89
   aorta (thoracic) 901.0
     abdominal 902.0
   arm NEC 903.9
   axillary 903.00
     artery 903.1
     vein 903.02
   azygos vein 901.89
   basilic vein 903.1
   brachial (artery) (vein) 903.1
   bronchial 901.89
   carotid artery 900.00
     common 900.01
     external 900.02
     internal 900.03
   celiac artery 902.20
     specified branch NEC 902.24
   cephalic vein (arm) 903.1
   colica dextra 902.26
   cystic
     artery 902.24
     vein 902.39

Injury (*Continued*)
  blood vessel NEC (*Continued*)
   deep plantar 904.6
   digital (artery) (vein) 903.5
   due to accidental puncture or laceration during procedure 998.2
   extremity
     lower 904.8
       multiple 904.7
       specified NEC 904.7
     upper 903.9
       multiple 903.8
       specified NEC 903.8
   femoral
     artery (superficial) 904.1
       above profunda origin904.0
       common 904.0
     vein 904.2
   gastric
     artery 902.21
     vein 902.39
   head 900.9
     intracranial - *see* Injury, intracranial
     multiple 900.82
     specified NEC 900.89
   hemiazygos vein 901.89
   hepatic
     artery 902.22
     vein 902.11
   hypogastric 902.59
     artery 902.51
     vein 902.52
   ileocolic
     artery 902.26
     vein 902.31
   iliac 902.50
     artery 902.53
     specified branch NEC 902.59
     vein 902.54
   innominate
     artery 901.1
     vein 901.3
   intercostal (artery) (vein) 901.81
   jugular vein (external) 900.81
     internal 900.1
   leg NEC 904.8
   mammary (artery) (vein) 901.82
   mesenteric
     artery 902.20
       inferior 902.27
       specified branch NEC 902.29
       superior (trunk) 902.25
         branches, primary 902.26
     vein 902.39
       inferior 902.32
       superior (and primary subdivisions) 902.31
   neck 900.9
     multiple 900.82
     specified NEC 900.89
   ovarian 902.89
     artery 902.81
     vein 902.82
   palmar artery 903.4
   pelvis 902.9
     multiple 902.87
     specified NEC 902.89
   plantar (deep) (artery) (vein) 904.6
   popliteal 904.40
     artery 904.41
     vein 904.42
   portal 902.33
   pulmonary 901.40
     artery 901.41
     vein 901.42
   radial (artery) (vein) 903.2
   renal 902.40
     artery 902.41
     specified NEC 902.49
     vein 902.42

Injury (*Continued*)
  blood vessel NEC (*Continued*)
   saphenous
     artery 904.7
     vein (greater) (lesser) 904.3
   splenic
     artery 902.23
     vein 902.34
   subclavian
     artery 901.1
     vein 901.3
   suprarenal 902.49
   thoracic 901.9
     multiple 901.83
     specified NEC 901.89
   tibial 904.50
     artery 904.50
       anterior 904.51
       posterior 904.53
     vein 904.50
       anterior 904.52
       posterior 904.54
   ulnar (artery) (vein) 903.3
   uterine 902.59
     artery 902.55
     vein 902.56
   vena cava
     inferior 902.10
       specified branches NEC 902.19
     superior 901.2
  brachial plexus 953.4
   newborn 767.6
  brain (traumatic) NEC (*see also* Injury, intracranial) 854.0●
   due to fracture of skull - *see* Fracture, skull, by site
  breast 959.19
  broad ligament - *see* Injury, internal, broad ligament
  bronchus, bronchi - *see* Injury, internal, bronchus
  brow 959.09
  buttock 959.19
  canthus, eye 921.1
  cathode ray 990
  cauda equina 952.4
   with fracture, vertebra - *see* Fracture, vertebra, sacrum
  cavernous sinus (*see also* Injury, intracranial) 854.0●
  cecum - *see* Injury, internal, cecum
  celiac ganglion or plexus 954.1
  cerebellum (*see also* Injury, intracranial) 854.0●
  cervix (uteri) - *see* Injury, internal, cervix
  cheek 959.09
  chest - *see* Injury, internal, chest
   wall 959.11
  childbirth - *see also* Birth, injury
   maternal NEC 665.9●
  chin 959.09
  choroid (eye) 921.3
  clitoris 959.14
  coccyx 959.19
   complicating delivery 665.6●
  colon - *see* Injury, internal, colon
  common duct - *see* Injury, internal, common duct
  conjunctiva 921.1
   superficial 918.2
  cord
   spermatic - *see* Injury, internal, spermatic cord
   spinal - *see* Injury, spinal, by site
  cornea 921.3
   abrasion 918.1
   due to contact lens 371.82
   penetrating - *see* Injury, eyeball, penetrating
   superficial 918.1
     due to contact lens 371.82

Injury (Continued)
  cortex (cerebral) (see also Injury, intracranial)
        854.0●
    visual 950.3
  costal region 959.11
  costochondral 959.11
  cranial
    bones - see Fracture, skull, by site
    cavity (see also Injury, intracranial) 854.0●
    nerve - see Injury, nerve, cranial
  crushing - see Crush
  cutaneous sensory nerve
    lower limb 956.4
    upper limb 955.5
  deep tissue - see Contusion, by site
    meaning pressure ulcer 707.25
  delivery - see also Birth, injury
    maternal NEC 665.9●
  Descemet's membrane - see Injury, eyeball,
        penetrating
  diaphragm - see Injury, internal, diaphragm
  diffuse axonal - see Injury, intracranial
  duodenum - see Injury, internal, duodenum
  ear (auricle) (canal) (drum) (external)
        959.09
  elbow (and forearm) (and wrist) 959.3
  epididymis 959.14
  epigastric region 959.12
  epiglottis 959.09
  epiphyseal, current - see Fracture, by site
  esophagus - see Injury, internal, esophagus
  Eustachian tube 959.09
  extremity (lower) (upper) NEC 959.8
  eye 921.9
    penetrating eyeball - see Injury, eyeball,
        penetrating
    superficial 918.9
  eyeball 921.3
    penetrating 871.7
      with
          partial loss (of intraocular tissue)
              871.2
          prolapse or exposure (of intraocular
              tissue) 871.1
      without prolapse 871.0
      foreign body (nonmagnetic) 871.6
          magnetic 871.5
    superficial 918.9
  eyebrow 959.09
  eyelid(s) 921.1
    laceration - see Laceration, eyelid
    superficial 918.0
  face (and neck) 959.09
  fallopian tube - see Injury, internal, fallopian
        tube
  fingers(s) (nail) 959.5
  flank 959.19
  foot (and ankle) (and knee) (and leg, except
        thigh) 959.7
  forceps NEC 767.9
    scalp 767.19
  forearm (and elbow) (and wrist) 959.3
  forehead 959.09
  gallbladder - see Injury, internal, gallbladder
  gasserian ganglion 951.2
  gastrointestinal tract - see Injury, internal,
        gastrointestinal tract
  genital organ(s)
    with
        abortion - see Abortion, by type, with,
            damage to pelvic organs
        ectopic pregnancy (see also categories
            633.0–633.9) 639.2
        molar pregnancy (see also categories
            630–632) 639.2
    external 959.14
    fracture of corpus cavernosum penis
        959.13
    following
        abortion 639.2
        ectopic or molar pregnancy 639.2

Injury (Continued)
  genital organ(s) (Continued)
    internal - see Injury, internal, genital
        organs
    obstetrical trauma NEC 665.9●
        affecting fetus or newborn 763.89
  gland
    lacrimal 921.1
        laceration 870.8
    parathyroid 959.09
    salivary 959.09
    thyroid 959.09
  globe (eye) (see also Injury, eyeball) 921.3
  grease gun - see Wound, open, by site,
        complicated
  groin 959.19
  gum 959.09
  hand(s) (except fingers) 959.4
  head NEC 959.01
    with
        loss of consciousness 850.5
        skull fracture - see Fracture, skull, by
            site
  heart - see Injury, internal, heart
  heel 959.7
  hip (and thigh) 959.6
  hymen 959.14
  hyperextension (cervical) (vertebra) 847.0
  ileum - see Injury, internal, ileum
  iliac region 959.19
  infrared rays NEC 990
  instrumental (during surgery) 998.2
    birth injury - see Birth, injury
    nonsurgical (see also Injury, by site) 959.9
    obstetrical 665.9●
        affecting fetus or newborn 763.89
        bladder 665.5●
        cervix 665.3●
        high vaginal 665.4●
        perineal NEC 664.9●
        urethra 665.5●
        uterus 665.5●
  internal 869.0

Note: For injury of internal organ(s)
by foreign body entering through a
natural orifice (e.g., inhaled, ingested, or
swallowed)-see Foreign body, entering
through orifice.

For internal injury of any of the following
sites with internal injury of any other of the
sites-see Injury, internal, multiple.

    with
        fracture
            pelvis - see Fracture, pelvis
            specified site, except pelvis - see
                Injury, internal, by site
        open wound into cavity 869.1
    abdomen, abdominal (viscera) NEC
        868.00
        with
            fracture, pelvis - see Fracture, pelvis
            open wound into cavity 868.10
        specified site NEC 868.09
            with open wound into cavity
                868.19
    adrenal (gland) 868.01
        with open wound into cavity 868.11
    aorta (thoracic) 901.0
        abdominal 902.0
    appendix 863.85
        with open wound into cavity 863.95
    bile duct 868.02
        with open wound into cavity 868.12
    bladder (sphincter) 867.0
        with
            abortion - see Abortion, by type,
                with, damage to pelvic organs
            ectopic pregnancy (see also
                categories 633.0–633.9) 639.2

Injury (Continued)
  internal (Continued)
    bladder (Continued)
      with (Continued)
          molar pregnancy (see also categories
              630–632) 639.2
          open wound into cavity 867.1
      following
          abortion 639.2
          ectopic or molar pregnancy
              639.2
      obstetrical trauma 665.5●
          affecting fetus or newborn 763.89
    blood vessel - see Injury, blood vessel, by
        site
    broad ligament 867.6
        with open wound into cavity 867.7
    bronchus, bronchi 862.21
        with open wound into cavity 862.31
    cecum 863.89
        with open wound into cavity 863.99
    cervix (uteri) 867.4
        with
            abortion - see Abortion, by type,
                with damage to pelvic organs
            ectopic pregnancy (see also
                categories 633.0–633.9)
                639.2
            molar pregnancy (see also categories
                630–632) 639.2
            open wound into cavity 867.5
        following
            abortion 639.2
            ectopic or molar pregnancy 639.2
        obstetrical trauma 665.3●
            affecting fetus or newborn 763.89
    chest (see also Injury, internal, intrathoracic
        organs) 862.8
        with open wound into cavity 862.9
    colon 863.40
        with
            open wound into cavity 863.50
            rectum 863.46
                with open wound into cavity
                    863.56
        ascending (right) 863.41
            with open wound into cavity 863.51
        descending (left) 863.43
            with open wound into cavity 863.53
        multiple sites 863.46
            with open wound into cavity 863.56
        sigmoid 863.44
            with open wound into cavity 863.54
        specified site NEC 863.49
            with open wound into cavity 863.59
        transverse 863.42
            with open wound into cavity 863.52
    common duct 868.02
        with open wound into cavity 868.12
    complicating delivery 665.9●
        affecting fetus or newborn 763.89
    diaphragm 862.0
        with open wound into cavity 862.1
    duodenum 863.21
        with open wound into cavity 863.31
    esophagus (intrathoracic) 862.22
        with open wound into cavity 862.32
        cervical region 874.4
            complicated 874.5
    fallopian tube 867.6
        with open wound into cavity 867.7
    gallbladder 868.02
        with open wound into cavity 868.12
    gastrointestinal tract NEC 863.80
        with open wound into cavity 863.90
    genital organ NEC 867.6
        with open wound into cavity 867.7
    heart 861.00
        with open wound into thorax 861.10
    ileum 863.29
        with open wound into cavity 863.39

◀ New   ◀▪ Revised   ~~deleted~~ Deleted   ● Use Additional Digit(s)   ▨ Omit code

Injury *(Continued)*
  internal *(Continued)*
    intestine NEC 863.89
      with open wound into cavity 863.99
      large NEC 863.40
        with open wound into cavity 863.50
      small NEC 863.20
        with open wound into cavity 863.30
    intra-abdominal (organ) 868.00
      with open wound into cavity 868.10
      multiple sites 868.09
        with open wound into cavity 868.19
      specified site NEC 868.09
        with open wound into cavity 868.19
    intrathoracic organs (multiple) 862.8
      with open wound into cavity 862.9
      diaphragm (only) - *see* Injury, internal, diaphragm
      heart (only) - *see* Injury, internal, heart
      lung (only) - *see* Injury, internal, lung
      specified site NEC 862.29
        with open wound into cavity 862.39
    intrauterine *(see also* Injury, internal, uterus) 867.4
      with open wound into cavity 867.5
    jejunum 863.29
      with open wound into cavity 863.39
    kidney (subcapsular) 866.00
      with
        disruption of parenchyma (complete) 866.03
          with open wound into cavity 866.13
        hematoma (without rupture of capsule) 866.01
          with open wound into cavity 866.11
        laceration 866.02
          with open wound into cavity 866.12
        open wound into cavity 866.10
    liver 864.00
      with
        contusion 864.01
          with open wound into cavity 864.11
        hematoma 864.01
          with open wound into cavity 864.11
        laceration 864.05
          with open wound into cavity 864.15
          major (disruption of hepatic parenchyma) 864.04
            with open wound into cavity 864.14
          minor (capsule only) 864.02
            with open wound into cavity 864.12
          moderate (involving parenchyma) 864.03
            with open wound into cavity 864.13
          multiple 864.04
        stellate 864.04
          with open wound into cavity 864.14
        open wound into cavity 864.10
    lung 861.20
      with open wound into thorax 861.30
      aspiration 507.0
      hemopneumothorax - *see* Hemopneumothorax, traumatic
      hemothorax - *see* Hemothorax, traumatic
      pneumohemothorax - *see* Pneumohemothorax, traumatic
      pneumothorax - *see* Pneumothorax, traumatic
      transfusion related, acute (TRALI) 518.7

Injury *(Continued)*
  internal *(Continued)*
    mediastinum 862.29
      with open wound into cavity 862.39
    mesentery 863.89
      with open wound into cavity 863.99
    mesosalpinx 867.6
      with open wound into cavity 867.7
    multiple 869.0

> Note: Multiple internal injuries of sites classifiable to the same three- or four-digit category should be classified to that category.
>
> Multiple injuries classifiable to different fourth-digit subdivisions of 861.-(heart and lung injuries) should be dealt with according to coding rules.

    internal 869.0
      with open wound into cavity 869.1
    intra-abdominal organ (sites classifiable to 863–868)
      with
        intrathoracic organ(s) (sites classifiable to 861–862) 869.0
          with open wound into cavity 869.1
        other intra-abdominal organ(s) (sites classifiable to 863–868, except where classifiable to the same three-digit category) 868.09
          with open wound into cavity 868.19
    intrathoracic organ (sites classifiable to 861–862)
      with
        intra-abdominal organ(s) (sites classifiable to 863–868) 869.0
          with open wound into cavity 869.1
        other intrathoracic organs(s) (sites classifiable to 861–862, except where classifiable to the same three-digit category) 862.8
      with open wound into cavity 862.9
    myocardium - *see* Injury, internal, heart
    ovary 867.6
      with open wound into cavity 867.7
    pancreas (multiple sites) 863.84
      with open wound into cavity 863.94
      body 863.82
        with open wound into cavity 863.92
      head 863.81
        with open wound into cavity 863.91
      tail 863.83
        with open wound into cavity 863.93
    pelvis, pelvic (organs) (viscera) 867.8
      with
        fracture, pelvis - *see* Fracture, pelvis
        open wound into cavity 867.9
      specified site NEC 867.6
        with open wound into cavity 867.7
    peritoneum 868.03
      with open wound into cavity 868.13
    pleura 862.29
      with open wound into cavity 862.39
    prostate 867.6
      with open wound into cavity 867.7
    rectum 863.45
      with
        colon 863.46
          with open wound into cavity 863.56
        open wound into cavity 863.55
    retroperitoneum 868.04
      with open wound into cavity 868.14

Injury *(Continued)*
  internal *(Continued)*
    round ligament 867.6
      with open wound into cavity 867.7
    seminal vesicle 867.6
      with open wound into cavity 867.7
    spermatic cord 867.6
      with open wound into cavity 867.7
    scrotal - *see* Wound, open, spermatic cord
    spleen 865.00
      with
        disruption of parenchyma (massive) 865.04
          with open wound into cavity 865.14
        hematoma (without rupture of capsule) 865.01
          with open wound into cavity 865.11
        open wound into cavity 865.10
        tear, capsular 865.02
          with open wound into cavity 865.12
          extending into parenchyma 865.03
            with open wound into cavity 865.13
    stomach 863.0
      with open wound into cavity 863.1
    suprarenal gland (multiple) 868.01
      with open wound into cavity 868.11
    thorax, thoracic (cavity) (organs) (multiple) *(see also* Injury, internal, intrathoracic organs) 862.8
      with open wound into cavity 862.9
    thymus (gland) 862.29
      with open wound into cavity 862.39
    trachea (intrathoracic) 862.29
      with open wound into cavity 862.39
      cervical region *(see also* Wound, open, trachea) 874.02
    ureter 867.2
      with open wound into cavity 867.3
    urethra (sphincter) 867.0
      with
        abortion - *see* Abortion, by type, with, damage to pelvic organs
        ectopic pregnancy *(see also* categories 633.0–633.9) 639.2
        molar pregnancy *(see also* categories 630–632) 639.2
        open wound into cavity 867.1
      following
        abortion 639.2
        ectopic or molar pregnancy 639.2
      obstetrical trauma 665.5●
        affecting fetus or newborn 763.89
    uterus 867.4
      with
        abortion - *see* Abortion, by type, with, damage to pelvic organs
        ectopic pregnancy *(see also* categories 633.0–633.9) 639.2
        molar pregnancy *(see also* categories 630–632) 639.2
        open wound into cavity 867.5
      following
        abortion 639.2
        ectopic or molar pregnancy 639.2
      obstetrical trauma NEC 665.5●
        affecting fetus or newborn 763.89
    vas deferens 867.6
      with open wound into cavity 867.7
    vesical (sphincter) 867.0
      with open wound into cavity 867.1

Injury *(Continued)*
  internal *(Continued)*
    viscera (abdominal) (*see also* Injury, internal, multiple) 868.00
      with
        fracture, pelvis - *see* Fracture, pelvis
        open wound into cavity 868.10
      thoracic NEC (*see also* Injury, internal, intrathoracic organs) 862.8
        with open wound into cavity 862.9
  interscapular region 959.19
  intervertebral disc 959.19
  intestine - *see* Injury, internal, intestine
  intra-abdominal (organs) NEC - *see* Injury, internal, intra-abdominal
  intracranial (traumatic) 854.0●

Note: Use the following fifth-digit subclassification with categories 851–854:

0   unspecified state of consciousness
1   with no loss of consciousness
2   with brief [less than one hour] loss of consciousness
3   with moderate [1–24 hours] loss of consciousness
4   with prolonged [more than 24 hours] loss of consciousness and return to pre-existing conscious level
5   with prolonged [more than 24 hours] loss of consciousness, without return to pre-existing conscious level

Use fifth-digit 5 to designate when a patient is unconscious and dies before regaining consciousness, regardless of the duration of the loss of consciousness

6   with loss of consciousness of unspecified duration
9   with concussion, unspecified

---

      with
        open intracranial wound 854.1●
        skull fracture - *see* Fracture, skull, by site
      contusion 851.8●
        with open intracranial wound 851.9●
        brain stem 851.4●
          with open intracranial wound 851.5●
        cerebellum 851.4●
          with open intracranial wound 851.5●
        cortex (cerebral) 851.0●
          with open intracranial wound 851.2●
      hematoma - *see* Injury, intracranial, hemorrhage
      hemorrhage 853.0●
        with
          laceration - *see* Injury, intracranial, laceration
          open intracranial wound 853.1●
        extradural 852.4●
          with open intracranial wound 852.5●
        subarachnoid 852.0●
          with open intracranial wound 852.1●
        subdural 852.2●
          with open intracranial wound 852.3●
      laceration 851.8●
        with open intracranial wound 851.9●
        brain stem 851.6●
          with open intracranial wound 851.7●

Injury *(Continued)*
  intracranial *(Continued)*
    contusion *(Continued)*
      laceration *(Continued)*
        cerebellum 851.6●
          with open intracranial wound 851.7●
        cortex (cerebral) 851.2●
          with open intracranial wound 851.3●
  intraocular - *see* Injury, eyeball, penetrating
  intrathoracic organs (multiple) - *see* Injury, internal, intrathoracic organs
  intrauterine - *see* Injury, internal, intrauterine
  iris 921.3
    penetrating - *see* Injury, eyeball, penetrating
  jaw 959.09
  jejunum - *see* Injury, internal, jejunum
  joint NEC 959.9
    old or residual 718.80
      ankle 718.87
      elbow 718.82
      foot 718.87
      hand 718.84
      hip 718.85
      knee 718.86
      multiple sites 718.89
      pelvic region 718.85
      shoulder (region) 718.81
      specified site NEC 718.88
      wrist 718.83
  kidney - *see* Injury, internal, kidney
    acute (nontraumatic) 584.9
  knee (and ankle) (and foot) (and leg, except thigh) 959.7
  labium (majus) (minus) 959.14
  labyrinth, ear 959.09
  lacrimal apparatus, gland, or sac 921.1
    laceration 870.8
  larynx 959.09
  late effect - *see* Late, effects (of), injury
  leg, except thigh (and ankle) (and foot) (and knee) 959.7
    upper or thigh 959.6
  lens, eye 921.3
    penetrating - *see* Injury, eyeball, penetrating
  lid, eye - *see* Injury, eyelid
  lip 959.09
  liver - *see* Injury, internal, liver
  lobe, parietal - *see* Injury, intracranial
  lumbar (region) 959.19
    plexus 953.5
  lumbosacral (region) 959.19
    plexus 953.5
  lung - *see* Injury, internal, lung
  malar region 959.09
  mastoid region 959.09
  maternal, during pregnancy, affecting fetus or newborn 760.5
  maxilla 959.09
  mediastinum - *see* Injury, internal, mediastinum
  membrane
    brain (*see also* Injury, intracranial) 854.0●
    tympanic 959.09
  meningeal artery - *see* Hemorrhage, brain, traumatic, subarachnoid
  meninges (cerebral) - *see* Injury, intracranial
  mesenteric
    artery - *see* Injury, blood vessel, mesenteric, artery
    plexus, inferior 954.1
    vein - *see* Injury, blood vessel, mesenteric, vein
  mesentery - *see* Injury, internal, mesentery
  mesosalpinx - *see* Injury, internal, mesosalpinx
  middle ear 959.09
  midthoracic region 959.11

Injury *(Continued)*
  mouth 959.09
  multiple (sites not classifiable to the same four-digit category in 959.0–959.7) 959.8
    internal 869.0
      with open wound into cavity 869.1
  musculocutaneous nerve 955.4
  nail
    finger 959.5
    toe 959.7
  nasal (septum) (sinus) 959.09
  nasopharynx 959.09
  neck (and face) 959.09
  nerve 957.9
    abducens 951.3
    abducent 951.3
    accessory 951.6
    acoustic 951.5
    ankle and foot 956.9
    anterior crural, femoral 956.1
    arm (*see also* Injury, nerve, upper limb) 955.9
    auditory 951.5
    axillary 955.0
    brachial plexus 953.4
    cervical sympathetic 954.0
    cranial 951.9
      first or olfactory 951.8
      second or optic 950.0
      third or oculomotor 951.0
      fourth or trochlear 951.1
      fifth or trigeminal 951.2
      sixth or abducens 951.3
      seventh or facial 951.4
      eighth, acoustic, or auditory 951.5
      ninth or glossopharyngeal 951.8
      tenth, pneumogastric, or vagus 951.8
      eleventh or accessory 951.6
      twelfth or hypoglossal 951.7
      newborn 767.7
    cutaneous sensory
      lower limb 956.4
      upper limb 955.5
    digital (finger) 955.6
      toe 956.5
    facial 951.4
      newborn 767.5
    femoral 956.1
    finger 955.9
    foot and ankle 956.9
    forearm 955.9
    glossopharyngeal 951.8
    hand and wrist 955.9
    head and neck, superficial 957.0
    hypoglossal 951.7
    involving several parts of body 957.8
    leg (*see also* Injury, nerve, lower limb) 956.9
    lower limb 956.9
      multiple 956.8
      specified site NEC 956.5
    lumbar plexus 953.5
    lumbosacral plexus 953.5
    median 955.1
      forearm 955.1
      wrist and hand 955.1
    multiple (in several parts of body) (sites not classifiable to the same three-digit category) 957.8
    musculocutaneous 955.4
    musculospiral 955.3
      upper arm 955.3
    oculomotor 951.0
    olfactory 951.8
    optic 950.0
    pelvic girdle 956.9
      multiple sites 956.8
      specified site NEC 956.5

Injury *(Continued)*
nerve *(Continued)*
peripheral 957.9
multiple (in several regions) (sites not
classifiable to the same
three-digit category) 957.8
specified site NEC 957.1
peroneal 956.3
ankle and foot 956.3
lower leg 956.3
plantar 956.5
plexus 957.9
celiac 954.1
mesenteric, inferior 954.1
spinal 953.9
brachial 953.4
lumbosacral 953.5
multiple sites 953.8
sympathetic NEC 954.1
pneumogastric 951.8
radial 955.3
wrist and hand 955.3
sacral plexus 953.5
sciatic 956.0
thigh 956.0
shoulder girdle 955.9
multiple 955.8
specified site NEC 955.7
specified site NEC 957.1
spinal 953.9
plexus - *see* Injury, nerve, plexus,
spinal
root 953.9
cervical 953.0
dorsal 953.1
lumbar 953.2
multiple sites 953.8
sacral 953.3
splanchnic 954.1
sympathetic NEC 954.1
cervical 954.0
thigh 956.9
tibial 956.5
ankle and foot 956.2
lower leg 956.5
posterior 956.2
toe 956.9
trigeminal 951.2
trochlear 951.1
trunk, excluding shoulder and pelvic
girdles 954.9
specified site NEC 954.8
sympathetic NEC 954.1
ulnar 955.2
forearm 955.2
wrist (and hand) 955.2
upper limb 955.9
multiple 955.8
specified site NEC 955.7
vagus 951.8
wrist and hand 955.9
nervous system, diffuse 957.8
nose (septum) 959.09
obstetrical NEC 665.9●
affecting fetus or newborn 763.89
occipital (region) (scalp) 959.09
lobe (*see also* Injury, intracranial) 854.0●
optic 950.9
chiasm 950.1
cortex 950.3
nerve 950.0
pathways 950.2
orbit, orbital (region) 921.2
penetrating 870.3
with foreign body 870.4
ovary - *see* Injury, internal, ovary
paint-gun - *see* Wound, open, by site,
complicated
palate (soft) 959.09
pancreas - *see* Injury, internal, pancreas
parathyroid (gland) 959.09

Injury *(Continued)*
parietal (region) (scalp) 959.09
lobe - *see* Injury, intracranial
pelvic
floor 959.19
complicating delivery 664.1●
affecting fetus or newborn 763.89
joint or ligament, complicating delivery
665.6●
affecting fetus or newborn 763.89
organs - *see also* Injury, internal, pelvis
with
abortion - *see* Abortion, by type,
with damage to pelvic organs
ectopic pregnancy (*see also*
categories 633.0–633.9) 639.2
molar pregnancy (*see also* categories
633.0–633.9) 639.2
following
abortion 639.2
ectopic or molar pregnancy 639.2
obstetrical trauma 665.5●
affecting fetus or newborn 763.89
pelvis 959.19
penis 959.14
fracture of corpus cavernosum 959.13
perineum 959.14
peritoneum - *see* Injury, internal, peritoneum
periurethral tissue
with
abortion - *see* Abortion, by type, with
damage to pelvic organs
ectopic pregnancy (*see also* categories
633.0–633.9) 639.2
molar pregnancy (*see also* categories
630–632) 639.2
complicating delivery 664.8●
affecting fetus or newborn 763.89
following
abortion 639.2
ectopic or molar pregnancy 639.2
phalanges
foot 959.7
hand 959.5
pharynx 959.09
pleura - *see* Injury, internal, pleura
popliteal space 959.7
post-cardiac surgery (syndrome) 429.4
prepuce 959.14
prostate - *see* Injury, internal, prostate
pubic region 959.19
pudenda 959.14
radiation NEC 990
radioactive substance or radium NEC 990
rectovaginal septum 959.14
rectum - *see* Injury, internal, rectum
retina 921.3
penetrating - *see* Injury, eyeball,
penetrating
retroperitoneal - *see* Injury, internal,
retroperitoneum
roentgen rays NEC 990
round ligament - *see* Injury, internal, round
ligament
sacral (region) 959.19
plexus 953.5
sacroiliac ligament NEC 959.19
sacrum 959.19
salivary ducts or glands 959.09
scalp 959.09
due to birth trauma 767.19
fetus or newborn 767.19
scapular region 959.2
sclera 921.3
penetrating - *see* Injury, eyeball,
penetrating
superficial 918.2
scrotum 959.14
seminal vesicle - *see* Injury, internal, seminal
vesicle
shoulder (and upper arm) 959.2

Injury *(Continued)*
sinus
cavernous (*see also* Injury, intracranial)
854.0●
nasal 959.09
skeleton NEC, birth injury 767.3
skin NEC 959.9
skull - *see* Fracture, skull, by site
soft tissue (of external sites) (severe) - *see*
Wound, open, by site
specified site NEC 959.8
spermatic cord - *see* Injury, internal,
spermatic cord
spinal (cord) 952.9
with fracture, vertebra - *see* Fracture,
vertebra, by site, with spinal cord
injury
cervical (C_1–C_4) 952.00
with
anterior cord syndrome 952.02
central cord syndrome 952.03
complete lesion of cord 952.01
incomplete lesion NEC 952.04
posterior cord syndrome 952.04
C_5–C_7 level 952.05
with
anterior cord syndrome
952.07
central cord syndrome 952.08
complete lesion of cord
952.06
incomplete lesion NEC
952.09
posterior cord syndrome
952.09
specified type NEC 952.09
specified type NEC 952.04
dorsal (D_1–D_6) (T_1–T_6) (thoracic)
952.10
with
anterior cord syndrome 952.12
central cord syndrome 952.13
complete lesion of cord 952.11
incomplete lesion NEC 952.14
posterior cord syndrome 952.14
D_7–D_{12} level (T_7–T_{12}) 952.15
with
anterior cord syndrome
952.17
central cord syndrome 952.18
complete lesion of cord
952.16
incomplete lesion NEC
952.19
posterior cord syndrome
952.19
specified type NEC 952.19
specified type NEC 952.14
lumbar 952.2
multiple sites 952.8
nerve (root) NEC - *see* Injury, nerve,
spinal, root
plexus 953.9
brachial 953.4
lumbosacral 953.5
multiple sites 953.8
sacral 952.3
thoracic (*see also* Injury, spinal, dorsal)
952.10
spleen - *see* Injury, internal, spleen
stellate ganglion 954.1
sternal region 959.11
stomach - *see* Injury, internal, stomach
subconjunctival 921.1
subcutaneous 959.9
subdural - *see* Injury, intracranial
submaxillary region 959.09
submental region 959.09
subungual
fingers 959.5
toes 959.7

Injury *(Continued)*
  superficial 919

Note: Use the following fourth-digit subdivisions with categories 910–919:

.0   abrasion or friction burn without mention of infection
.1   abrasion or friction burn, infected
.2   blister without mention of infection
.3   blister, infected
.4   insect bite, nonvenomous, without mention of infection
.5   insect bite, nonvenomous, infected
.6   superficial foreign body (splinter) without major open wound and without mention of infection
.7   superficial foreign body (splinter) without major open wound, infected
.8   other and unspecified superficial injury without mention of infection
.9   other and unspecified superficial injury, infected

For late effects of superficial injury, *see* category 906.2.

---

  abdomen, abdominal (muscle) (wall) (and other part(s) of trunk) 911
  ankle (and hip, knee, leg, or thigh) 916
  anus (and other part(s) of trunk) 911
  arm 913
    upper (and shoulder) 912
  auditory canal (external) (meatus) (and other part(s) of face, neck, or scalp, except eye) 910
  axilla (and upper arm) 912
  back (and other part(s) of trunk) 911
  breast (and other part(s) of trunk) 911
  brow (and other part(s) of face, neck, or scalp, except eye) 910
  buttock (and other part(s) of trunk) 911
  canthus, eye 918.0
  cheek(s) (and other part(s) of face, neck, or scalp, except eye) 910
  chest wall (and other part(s) of trunk) 911
  chin (and other part(s) of face, neck, or scalp, except eye) 910
  clitoris (and other part(s) of trunk) 911
  conjunctiva 918.2
  cornea 918.1
    due to contact lens 371.82
  costal region (and other part(s) of trunk) 911
  ear(s) (auricle) (canal) (drum) (external) (and other part(s) of face, neck, or scalp, except eye) 910
  elbow (and forearm) (and wrist) 913
  epididymis (and other part(s) of trunk) 911
  epigastric region (and other part(s) of trunk) 911
  epiglottis (and other part(s) of face, neck, or scalp, except eye) 910
  eye(s) (and adnexa) NEC 918.9
  eyelid(s) (and periocular area) 918.0
  face (any part(s), except eye) (and neck or scalp) 910
  finger(s) (nail) (any) 915
  flank (and other part(s) of trunk) 911
  foot (phalanges) (and toe(s)) 917
  forearm (and elbow) (and wrist) 913
  forehead (and other part(s) of face, neck, or scalp, except eye) 910
  globe (eye) 918.9
  groin (and other part(s) of trunk) 911
  gum(s) (and other part(s) of face, neck, or scalp, except eye) 910
  hand(s) (except fingers alone) 914

Injury *(Continued)*
  superficial *(Continued)*
    head (and other part(s) of face, neck, or scalp, except eye) 910
    heel (and foot or toe) 917
    hip (and ankle, knee, leg, or thigh) 916
    iliac region (and other part(s) of trunk) 911
    interscapular region (and other part(s) of trunk) 911
    iris 918.9
    knee (and ankle, hip, leg, or thigh) 916
    labium (majus) (minus) (and other part(s) of trunk) 911
    lacrimal (apparatus) (gland) (sac) 918.0
    leg (lower) (upper) (and ankle, hip, knee, or thigh) 916
    lip(s) (and other part(s) of face, neck, or scalp, except eye) 910
    lower extremity (except foot) 916
    lumbar region (and other part(s) of trunk) 911
    malar region (and other part(s) of face, neck, or scalp, except eye) 910
    mastoid region (and other part(s) of face, neck, or scalp, except eye) 910
    midthoracic region (and other part(s) of trunk) 911
    mouth (and other part(s) of face, neck, or scalp, except eye) 910
    multiple sites (not classifiable to the same three-digit category) 919
    nasal (septum) (and other part(s) of face, neck, or scalp, except eye) 910
    neck (and face or scalp, any part(s), except eye) 910
    nose (septum) (and other part(s) of face, neck, or scalp, except eye) 910
    occipital region (and other part(s) of face, neck, or scalp, except eye) 910
    orbital region 918.0
    palate (soft) (and other part(s) of face, neck, or scalp, except eye) 910
    parietal region (and other part(s) of face, neck, or scalp, except eye) 910
    penis (and other part(s) of trunk) 911
    perineum (and other part(s) of trunk) 911
    periocular area 918.0
    pharynx (and other part(s) of face, neck, or scalp, except eye) 910
    popliteal space (and ankle, hip, leg, or thigh) 916
    prepuce (and other part(s) of trunk) 911
    pubic region (and other part(s) of trunk) 911
    pudenda (and other part(s) of trunk) 911
    sacral region (and other part(s) of trunk) 911
    salivary (ducts) (glands) (and other part(s) of face, neck, or scalp, except eye) 910
    scalp (and other part(s) of face or neck, except eye) 910
    scapular region (and upper arm) 912
    sclera 918.2
    scrotum (and other part(s) of trunk) 911
    shoulder (and upper arm) 912
    skin NEC 919
    specified site(s) NEC 919
    sternal region (and other part(s) of trunk) 911
    subconjunctival 918.2
    subcutaneous NEC 919
    submaxillary region (and other part(s) of face, neck, or scalp, except eye) 910
    submental region (and other part(s) of face, neck, or scalp, except eye) 910
    supraclavicular fossa (and other part(s) of face, neck, or scalp, except eye) 910
    supraorbital 918.0

Injury *(Continued)*
  superficial *(Continued)*
    temple (and other part(s) of face, neck, or scalp, except eye) 910
    temporal region (and other part(s) of face, neck, or scalp, except eye) 910
    testis (and other part(s) of trunk) 911
    thigh (and ankle, hip, knee, or leg) 916
    thorax, thoracic (external) (and other part(s) of trunk) 911
    throat (and other part(s) of face, neck, or scalp, except eye) 910
    thumb(s) (nail) 915
    toe(s) (nail) (subungual) (and foot) 917
    tongue (and other part(s) of face, neck, or scalp, except eye) 910
    tooth, teeth (*see also* Abrasion, dental) 521.20
    trunk (any part(s)) 911
    tunica vaginalis (and other part(s) of trunk) 911
    tympanum, tympanic membrane (and other part(s) of face, neck, or scalp, except eye) 910
    upper extremity NEC 913
    uvula (and other part(s) of face, neck, or scalp, except eye) 910
    vagina (and other part(s) of trunk) 911
    vulva (and other part(s) of trunk) 911
    wrist (and elbow) (and forearm) 913
  supraclavicular fossa 959.19
  supraorbital 959.09
  surgical complication (external or internal site) 998.2
  symphysis pubis 959.19
    complicating delivery 665.6●
      affecting fetus or newborn 763.89
  temple 959.09
  temporal region 959.09
  testis 959.14
  thigh (and hip) 959.6
  thorax, thoracic (external) 959.11
    cavity - *see* Injury, internal, thorax
    internal - *see* Injury, internal, intrathoracic organs
  throat 959.09
  thumb(s) (nail) 959.5
  thymus - *see* Injury, internal, thymus
  thyroid (gland) 959.09
  toe (nail) (any) 959.7
  tongue 959.09
  tonsil 959.09
  tooth NEC 873.63
    complicated 873.73
  trachea - *see* Injury, internal, trachea
  trunk 959.19
  tunica vaginalis 959.14
  tympanum, tympanic membrane 959.09
  ultraviolet rays NEC 990
  ureter - *see* Injury, internal, ureter
  urethra (sphincter) - *see* Injury, internal, urethra
  uterus - *see* Injury, internal, uterus
  uvula 959.09
  vagina 959.14
  vascular - *see* Injury, blood vessel
  vas deferens - *see* Injury, internal, vas deferens
  vein (*see also* Injury, blood vessel, by site) 904.9
  vena cava
    inferior 902.10
    superior 901.2
  vesical (sphincter) - *see* Injury, internal, vesical
  viscera (abdominal) - *see* Injury, internal, viscera
    with fracture, pelvis - *see* Fracture, pelvis
  visual 950.9
    cortex 950.3
  vitreous (humor) 871.2

◄ New   ◄ Revised   ~~deleted~~ Deleted   ● Use Additional Digit(s)   Omit code

Injury *(Continued)*
vulva 959.14
whiplash (cervical spine) 847.0
wringer - *see* Crush, by site
wrist (and elbow) (and forearm) 959.3
x-ray NEC 990
Inoculation - *see also* Vaccination
complication or reaction - *see* Complication, vaccination
INPH (idiopathic normal pressure hydrocephalus) 331.5
Insanity, insane *(see also* Psychosis) 298.9
adolescent *(see also* Schizophrenia) 295.9●
alternating *(see also* Psychosis, affective, circular) 296.7
confusional 298.9
acute 293.0
subacute 293.1
delusional 298.9
paralysis, general 094.1
progressive 094.1
paresis, general 094.1
senile 290.20
Insect
bite - *see* Injury, superficial, by site
venomous, poisoning by 989.5
Insemination, artificial V26.1
Insensitivity
adrenocorticotropin hormone (ACTH) 255.41
androgen 259.50
complete 259.51
partial 259.52
Insertion
cord (umbilical) lateral or velamentous 663.8●
affecting fetus or newborn 762.6
intrauterine contraceptive device V25.11
placenta, vicious - *see* Placenta, previa
subdermal implantable contraceptive V25.5
velamentous, umbilical cord 663.8●
affecting fetus or newborn 762.6
Insolation 992.0
meaning sunstroke 992.0
Insomnia, unspecified 780.52
with sleep apnea, unspecified 780.51
adjustment 307.41
alcohol induced 291.82
behavioral, of childhood V69.5
drug induced 292.85
due to
medical condition classified elsewhere 327.01
mental disorder 327.02
fatal familial (FFI) 046.72
idiopathic 307.42
nonorganic origin 307.41
persistent (primary) 307.42
transient 307.41
organic 327.00
other 327.09
paradoxical 307.42
primary 307.42
psychophysiological 307.42
subjective complaint 307.49
Inspiration
food or foreign body *(see also* Asphyxia, food or foreign body) 933.1
mucus *(see also* Asphyxia, mucus) 933.1
Inspissated bile syndrome, newborn 774.4
Instability
detrusor 596.59
emotional (excessive) 301.3
joint (posttraumatic) 718.80
ankle 718.87
elbow 718.82
foot 718.87
hand 718.84
hip 718.85
knee 718.86
lumbosacral 724.6
multiple sites 718.89

Instability *(Continued)*
joint *(Continued)*
pelvic region 718.85
sacroiliac 724.6
shoulder (region) 718.81
specified site NEC 718.88
wrist 718.83
lumbosacral 724.6
nervous 301.89
personality (emotional) 301.59
thyroid, paroxysmal 242.9●
urethral 599.83
vasomotor 780.2
Insufficiency, insufficient
accommodation 367.4
adrenal (gland) (acute) (chronic) 255.41
medulla 255.5
primary 255.41
specified site NEC 255.5
adrenocortical 255.41
anterior (occlusal) guidance 524.54
anus 569.49
aortic (valve) 424.1
with
mitral (valve) disease 396.1
insufficiency, incompetence, or regurgitation 396.3
stenosis or obstruction 396.1
stenosis or obstruction 424.1
with mitral (valve) disease 396.8
congenital 746.4
rheumatic 395.1
with
mitral (valve) disease 396.1
insufficiency, incompetence, or regurgitation 396.3
stenosis or obstruction 396.1
stenosis or obstruction 395.2
with mitral (valve) disease 396.8
specified cause NEC 424.1
syphilitic 093.22
arterial 447.1
basilar artery 435.0
carotid artery 435.8
cerebral 437.1
coronary (acute or subacute) 411.89
mesenteric 557.1
peripheral 443.9
precerebral 435.9
vertebral artery 435.1
vertebrobasilar 435.3
arteriovenous 459.9
basilar artery 435.0
biliary 575.8
cardiac *(see also* Insufficiency, myocardial) 428.0
complicating surgery 997.1
due to presence of (cardiac) prosthesis 429.4
postoperative 997.1
long-term effect of cardiac surgery 429.4
specified during or due to a procedure 997.1
long-term effect of cardiac surgery 429.4
cardiorenal *(see also* Hypertension, cardiorenal) 404.90
cardiovascular *(see also* Disease, cardiovascular) 429.2
renal *(see also* Hypertension, cardiorenal) 404.90
carotid artery 435.8
cerebral (vascular) 437.9
cerebrovascular 437.9
with transient focal neurological signs and symptoms 435.9
acute 437.1
with transient focal neurological signs and symptoms 435.9

Insufficiency, insufficient *(Continued)*
circulatory NEC 459.9
fetus or newborn 779.89
convergence 378.83
coronary (acute or subacute) 411.89
chronic or with a stated duration of over 8 weeks 414.8
corticoadrenal 255.41
dietary 269.9
divergence 378.85
food 994.2
gastroesophageal 530.89
gonadal
ovary 256.39
testis 257.2
gonadotropic hormone secretion 253.4
heart - *see also* Insufficiency, myocardial
fetus or newborn 779.89
valve *(see also* Endocarditis) 424.90
congenital NEC 746.89
hepatic 573.8
idiopathic autonomic 333.0
interocclusal distance of teeth (ridge) 524.36
kidney
acute 593.9
chronic 585.9
labyrinth, labyrinthine (function) 386.53
bilateral 386.54
unilateral 386.53
lacrimal 375.15
liver 573.8
lung (acute) *(see also* Insufficiency, pulmonary) 518.82
following trauma and surgery 518.52
newborn 770.89
mental (congenital) *(see also* Disability, intellectual) 319
mesenteric 557.1
mitral (valve) 424.0
with
aortic (valve) disease 396.3
insufficiency, incompetence, or regurgitation 396.3
stenosis or obstruction 396.2
obstruction or stenosis 394.2
with aortic valve disease 396.8
congenital 746.6
rheumatic 394.1
with
aortic (valve) disease 396.3
insufficiency, incompetence, or regurgitation 396.3
stenosis or obstruction 396.2
obstruction or stenosis 394.2
with aortic valve disease 396.8
active or acute 391.1
with chorea, rheumatic (Sydenham's) 392.0
specified cause, except rheumatic 424.0
muscle
heart - *see* Insufficiency, myocardial
ocular *(see also* Strabismus) 378.9
myocardial, myocardium (with arteriosclerosis) 428.0
with rheumatic fever (conditions classifiable to 390)
active, acute, or subacute 391.2
with chorea 392.0
inactive or quiescent (with chorea) 398.0
congenital 746.89
due to presence of (cardiac) prosthesis 429.4
fetus or newborn 779.89
following cardiac surgery 429.4
hypertensive *(see also* Hypertension, heart) 402.91
benign 402.11
malignant 402.01

Insufficiency, insufficient (Continued)
  myocardial, myocardium (Continued)
    postoperative 997.1
      long-term effect of cardiac surgery
        429.4
    rheumatic 398.0
      active, acute, or subacute 391.2
        with chorea (Sydenham's) 392.0
    syphilitic 093.82
  nourishment 994.2
  organic 799.89
  ovary 256.39
    postablative 256.2
  pancreatic 577.8
  parathyroid (gland) 252.1
  peripheral vascular (arterial) 443.9
  pituitary (anterior) 253.2
    posterior 253.5
  placental - see Placenta, insufficiency
  platelets 287.5
  prenatal care in current pregnancy V23.7
  progressive pluriglandular 258.9
  pseudocholinesterase 289.89
  pulmonary (acute) 518.82
    following
      shock 518.52
      surgery 518.52
      trauma 518.52
    newborn 770.89
    valve (see also Endocarditis, pulmonary)
      424.3
      congenital 746.09
  pyloric 537.0
  renal 593.9
    acute 593.9
    chronic 585.9
    due to a procedure 997.5
  respiratory 786.09
    acute 518.82
      following trauma and surgery
        518.52
    newborn 770.89
  rotation - see Malrotation
  suprarenal 255.41
    medulla 255.5
  tarso-orbital fascia, congenital 743.66
  tear film 375.15
  testis 257.2
  thyroid (gland) (acquired) - see also
    Hypothyroidism
    congenital 243
  tricuspid (see also Endocarditis, tricuspid)
    397.0
    congenital 746.89
    syphilitic 093.23
  urethral sphincter 599.84
  valve, valvular (heart) (see also Endocarditis)
    424.90
  vascular 459.9
    intestine NEC 557.9
    mesenteric 557.1
    peripheral 443.9
    renal (see also Hypertension, kidney)
      403.90
  velopharyngeal
    acquired 528.9
    congenital 750.29
  venous (peripheral) 459.81
  ventricular - see Insufficiency, myocardial
  vertebral artery 435.1
  vertebrobasilar artery 435.3
  weight gain during pregnancy 646.8●
  zinc 269.3
Insufflation
  fallopian
    fertility testing V26.21
    following sterilization reversal
      V26.22
  meconium 770.11
    with respiratory symptoms 770.12
Insular - see condition

Insulinoma (M8151/0)
  malignant (M8151/3)
    pancreas 157.4
    specified site - see Neoplasm, by site,
      malignant
    unspecified site 157.4
  pancreas 211.7
  specified site - see Neoplasm, by site, benign
  unspecified site 211.7
Insuloma - see Insulinoma
Insult
  brain 437.9
    acute 436
  cerebral 437.9
    acute 436
  cerebrovascular 437.9
    acute 436
  vascular NEC 437.9
    acute 436
Insurance examination (certification) V70.3
Intemperance (see also Alcoholism) 303.9●
Interception of pregnancy (menstrual
  extraction) V25.3
Interference
  balancing side 524.56
  non-working side 524.56
Intermenstrual
  bleeding 626.6
    irregular 626.6
    regular 626.5
  hemorrhage 626.6
    irregular 626.6
    regular 626.5
  pain(s) 625.2
Intermittent - see condition
Internal - see condition
Interproximal wear 521.10
Interrogation
  cardiac defibrillator (automatic)
    (implantable) V53.32
  cardiac pacemaker V53.31
  cardiac (event) (loop) recorder V53.39
  infusion pump (implanted) (intrathecal)
    V53.09
  neurostimulator V53.02
Interruption
  aortic arch 747.11
  bundle of His 426.50
  fallopian tube (for sterilization) V25.2
  phase-shift, sleep cycle 307.45
  repeated REM-sleep 307.48
  sleep
    due to perceived environmental
      disturbances 307.48
    phase-shift, of 24-hour sleep-wake cycle
      307.45
    repeated REM-sleep type 307.48
  vas deferens (for sterilization) V25.2
Intersexuality 752.7
Interstitial - see condition
Intertrigo 695.89
  labialis 528.5
Intervertebral disc - see condition
Intestine, intestinal - see also condition
  flu 487.8
Intolerance
  carbohydrate NEC 579.8
  cardiovascular exercise, with pain (at rest)
    (with less than ordinary activity) (with
    ordinary activity) V47.2
  cold 780.99
  dissacharide (hereditary) 271.3
  drug
    correct substance properly administered
      995.27
    wrong substance given or taken in error
      977.9
    specified drug - see Table of Drugs and
      Chemicals
  effort 306.2
  fat NEC 579.8

Intolerance (Continued)
  foods NEC 579.8
  fructose (hereditary) 271.2
  glucose (-galactose) (congenital) 271.3
  gluten 579.0
  lactose (hereditary) (infantile) 271.3
  lysine (congenital) 270.7
  milk NEC 579.8
  protein (familial) 270.7
  starch NEC 579.8
  sucrose (-isomaltose) (congenital) 271.3
Intoxicated NEC (see also Alcoholism)
  305.0●
Intoxication
  acid 276.2
  acute
    alcoholic 305.0●
      with alcoholism 303.0●
      hangover effects 305.0●
    caffeine 305.9●
    hallucinogenic (see also Abuse, drugs,
      nondependent) 305.3●
  alcohol (acute) 305.0●
    with alcoholism 303.0●
    hangover effects 305.0●
    idiosyncratic 291.4
    pathological 291.4
  alimentary canal 558.2
  ammonia (hepatic) 572.2
  caffeine 305.9●
  chemical - see also Table of Drugs and
    Chemicals
    via placenta or breast milk 760.70
      alcohol 760.71
      anticonvulsants 760.77
      antifungals 760.74
      anti-infective agents 760.74
      antimetabolics 760.78
      cocaine 760.75
      "crack" 760.75
      hallucinogenic agents NEC 760.73
      medicinal agents NEC 760.79
      narcotics 760.72
      obstetric anesthetic or analgesic drug
        763.5
      specified agent NEC 760.79
      suspected, affecting management of
        pregnancy 655.5●
  cocaine, through placenta or breast milk
    760.75
  delirium
    alcohol 291.0
    drug 292.81
  drug 292.89
    with delirium 292.81
    correct substance properly administered
      (see also Allergy, drug) 995.27
    newborn 779.4
    obstetric anesthetic or sedation 668.9●
      affecting fetus or newborn 763.5
    overdose or wrong substance given or
      taken - see Table of Drugs and
      Chemicals
    pathologic 292.2
    specific to newborn 779.4
    via placenta or breast milk 760.70
      alcohol 760.71
      anticonvulsants 760.77
      antifungals 760.74
      anti-infective agents 760.74
      antimetabolics 760.78
      cocaine 760.75
      "crack" 760.75
      hallucinogenic agents 760.73
      medicinal agents NEC 760.79
      narcotics 760.72
      obstetric anesthetic or analgesic drug
        763.5
      specified agent NEC 760.79
      suspected, affecting management of
        pregnancy 655.5●

◀ New   ◀▥ Revised   ~~deleted~~ Deleted   ● Use Additional Digit(s)   ▨ Omit code

Intoxication *(Continued)*
  enteric - *see* Intoxication, intestinal
  fetus or newborn, via placenta or breast milk
      760.70
    alcohol 760.71
    anticonvulsants 760.77
    antifungals 760.74
    anti-infective agents 760.74
    antimetabolics 760.78
    cocaine 760.75
    "crack" 760.75
    hallucinogenic agents 760.73
    medicinal agents NEC 760.79
    narcotics 760.72
    obstetric anesthetic or analgesic drug
        763.5
    specified agent NEC 760.79
    suspected, affecting management of
        pregnancy 655.5 ●
  food - *see* Poisoning, food
  gastrointestinal 558.2
  hallucinogenic (acute) 305.3 ●
  hepatocerebral 572.2
  idiosyncratic alcohol 291.4
  intestinal 569.89
    due to putrefaction of food 005.9
  methyl alcohol *(see also* Alcoholism) 305.0 ●
    with alcoholism 303.0 ●
  non-foodborne due to toxins of Clostridium
      botulinum [C. botulinum] - *see*
      Botulism
  pathologic 291.4
    drug 292.2
  potassium (K) 276.7
  septic
    with
      abortion - *see* Abortion, by type, with
          sepsis
      ectopic pregnancy *(see also* categories
          633.0–633.9) 639.0
      molar pregnancy *(see also* categories
          630–632) 639.0
    during labor 659.3 ●
    following
      abortion 639.0
      ectopic or molar pregnancy 639.0
    generalized - *see* Septicemia
    puerperal, postpartum, childbirth
        670.2 ●
  serum (prophylactic) (therapeutic) 999.59
  uremic - *see* Uremia
  water 276.69
Intracranial - *see* condition
Intrahepatic gallbladder 751.69
Intraligamentous - *see also* condition
  pregnancy - *see* Pregnancy, cornual
Intraocular - *see also* condition
  sepsis 360.00
Intrathoracic - *see also* condition
  kidney 753.3
  stomach - *see* Hernia, diaphragm
Intrauterine contraceptive device
  checking V25.42
  insertion V25.11
  in situ V45.51
  management V25.42
  prescription V25.02
    repeat V25.42
  reinsertion V25.13
  removal V25.12
    and reinsertion V25.13
  replacement V25.13
Intraventricular - *see* condition
Intrinsic deformity - *see* Deformity
Intruded tooth 524.34
Intrusion, repetitive, of sleep (due to
    environmental disturbances) (with
    atypical polysomnographic features)
    307.48
Intumescent, lens (eye) NEC 366.9
  senile 366.12

Intussusception (colon) (enteric) (intestine)
    (rectum) 560.0
  appendix 543.9
  congenital 751.5
  fallopian tube 620.8
  ileocecal 560.0
  ileocolic 560.0
  ureter (obstruction) 593.4
Invagination
  basilar 756.0
  colon or intestine 560.0
Invalid (since birth) 799.89
Invalidism (chronic) 799.89
Inversion
  albumin-globulin (A-G) ratio 273.8
  bladder 596.89
  cecum *(see also* Intussusception) 560.0
  cervix 622.8
  nipple 611.79
    congenital 757.6
    puerperal, postpartum 676.3 ●
  optic papilla 743.57
  organ or site, congenital NEC - *see* Anomaly,
      specified type NEC
  sleep rhythm 327.39
    nonorganic origin 307.45
  testis (congenital) 752.51
  uterus (postinfectional) (postpartal, old) 621.7
    chronic 621.7
    complicating delivery 665.2 ●
      affecting fetus or newborn 763.89
  vagina - *see* Prolapse, vagina
Investigation
  allergens V72.7
  clinical research (control) (normal
      comparison) (participant) V70.7
Inviability - *see* Immaturity
Involuntary movement, abnormal 781.0
Involution, involutional - *see also* condition
  breast, cystic or fibrocystic 610.1
  depression *(see also* Psychosis, affective) 296.2 ●
    recurrent episode 296.3 ●
    single episode 296.2 ●
  melancholia *(see also* Psychosis, affective)
      296.2 ●
    recurrent episode 296.3 ●
    single episode 296.2 ●
  ovary, senile 620.3
  paranoid state (reaction) 297.2
  paraphrenia (climacteric) (menopause) 297.2
  psychosis 298.8
  thymus failure 254.8
IQ
  under 20 318.2
  20–34 318.1
  35–49 318.0
  50–70 317
IRDS 769
Irideremia 743.45
Iridis rubeosis 364.42
  diabetic 250.5 ● *[364.42]*
    due to secondary diabetes 249.5 ● *[364.42]*
Iridochoroiditis (panuveitis) 360.12
Iridocyclitis NEC 364.3
  acute 364.00
    primary 364.01
    recurrent 364.02
  chronic 364.10
    in
      lepromatous leprosy 030.0 *[364.11]*
      sarcoidosis 135 *[364.11]*
      tuberculosis *(see also* Tuberculosis)
          017.3 ● *[364.11]*
  due to allergy 364.04
  endogenous 364.01
  gonococcal 098.41
  granulomatous 364.10
  herpetic (simplex) 054.44
    zoster 053.22
  hypopyon 364.05
  lens induced 364.23

Iridocyclitis NEC *(Continued)*
  nongranulomatous 364.00
  primary 364.01
  recurrent 364.02
  rheumatic 364.10
  secondary 364.04
    infectious 364.03
    noninfectious 364.04
  subacute 364.00
    primary 364.01
    recurrent 364.02
  sympathetic 360.11
  syphilitic (secondary) 091.52
  tuberculous (chronic) *(see also* Tuberculosis)
      017.3 ● *[364.11]*
Iridocyclochoroiditis (panuveitis) 360.12
Iridodialysis 364.76
Iridodonesis 364.89
Iridoplegia (complete) (partial) (reflex) 379.49
Iridoschisis 364.52
IRIS (Immune Reconstitution Inflammatory
    Syndrome) 995.90
Iris - *see* condition
Iritis 364.3
  acute 364.00
    primary 364.01
    recurrent 364.02
  chronic 364.10
    in
      sarcoidosis 135 *[364.11]*
      tuberculosis *(see also* Tuberculosis)
          017.3 ● *[364.11]*
  diabetic 250.5 ● *[364.42]*
    due to secondary diabetes 249.5 ● *[364.42]*
  due to
    allergy 364.04
    herpes simplex 054.44
    leprosy 030.0 *[364.11]*
  endogenous 364.01
  gonococcal 098.41
  gouty 274.89 *[364.11]*
  granulomatous 364.10
  hypopyon 364.05
  lens induced 364.23
  nongranulomatous 364.00
  papulosa 095.8 *[364.11]*
  primary 364.01
  recurrent 364.02
  rheumatic 364.10
  secondary 364.04
    infectious 364.03
    noninfectious 364.04
  subacute 364.00
    primary 364.01
    recurrent 364.02
  sympathetic 360.11
  syphilitic (secondary) 091.52
    congenital 090.0 *[364.11]*
    late 095.8 *[364.11]*
  tuberculous *(see also* Tuberculosis) 017.3 ●
      [364.11]
  uratic 274.89 *[364.11]*
Iron
  deficiency anemia 280.9
  metabolism disease 275.09
  storage disease 275.09
Iron-miners' lung 503
Irradiated enamel (tooth, teeth) 521.89
Irradiation
  burn - *see* Burn, by site
  effects, adverse 990
Irreducible, irreducibility - *see* condition
Irregular, irregularity
  action, heart 427.9
  alveolar process 525.8
  bleeding NEC 626.4
  breathing 786.09
  colon 569.89
  contour
    of cornea 743.41
      acquired 371.70
    reconstructed breast 612.0

Irregular, irregularity (Continued)
  dentin in pulp 522.3
  eye movements NEC 379.59
  menstruation (cause unknown) 626.4
  periods 626.4
  prostate 602.9
  pupil 364.75
  respiratory 786.09
  septum (nasal) 470
  shape, organ or site, congenital NEC - see
    Distortion
  sleep-wake rhythm (non-24-hour) 327.39
    nonorganic origin 307.45
  vertebra 733.99
Irritability 799.22
  bladder 596.89
    neurogenic 596.54
      with cauda equina syndrome 344.61
  bowel (syndrome) 564.1
  bronchial (see also Bronchitis) 490
  cerebral, newborn 779.1
  colon 564.1
    psychogenic 306.4
  duodenum 564.89
  heart (psychogenic) 306.2
  ileum 564.89
  jejunum 564.89
  myocardium 306.2
  nervousness 799.21
  rectum 564.89
  stomach 536.9
    psychogenic 306.4
  sympathetic (nervous system) (see also
    Neuropathy, peripheral, autonomic)
    337.9
  urethra 599.84
  ventricular (heart) (psychogenic) 306.2
Irritable (see also Irritability) 799.22
Irritation
  anus 569.49
  axillary nerve 353.0
  bladder 596.89
  brachial plexus 353.0
  brain (traumatic) (see also Injury, intracranial)
    854.0●
    nontraumatic - see Encephalitis
  bronchial (see also Bronchitis) 490
  cerebral (traumatic) (see also Injury,
    intracranial) 854.0●
    nontraumatic - see Encephalitis
  cervical plexus 353.2
  cervix (see also Cervicitis) 616.0
  choroid, sympathetic 360.11
  cranial nerve - see Disorder, nerve, cranial
  digestive tract 536.9
    psychogenic 306.4
  gastric 536.9
    psychogenic 306.4
  gastrointestinal (tract) 536.9
    functional 536.9
    psychogenic 306.4
  globe, sympathetic 360.11
  intestinal (bowel) 564.9
  labyrinth 386.50
  lumbosacral plexus 353.1
  meninges (traumatic) (see also Injury,
    intracranial) 854.0●
    nontraumatic - see Meningitis
  myocardium 306.2
  nerve - see Disorder, nerve
  nervous 799.21
  nose 478.19
  penis 607.89
  perineum 709.9
  peripheral
    autonomic nervous system (see also
      Neuropathy, peripheral, autonomic)
      337.9
    nerve - see Disorder, nerve
  peritoneum (see also Peritonitis) 567.9
  pharynx 478.29

Irritation (Continued)
  plantar nerve 355.6
  spinal (cord) (traumatic) - see also Injury,
    spinal, by site
    nerve - see also Disorder, nerve
      root NEC 724.9
      traumatic - see Injury, nerve, spinal
    nontraumatic - see Myelitis
  stomach 536.9
    psychogenic 306.4
  sympathetic nerve NEC (see also Neuropathy,
    peripheral, autonomic) 337.9
  ulnar nerve 354.2
  vagina 623.9
Isambert's disease 012.3●
Ischemia, ischemic 459.9
  basilar artery (with transient neurologic
    deficit) 435.0
  bone NEC 733.40
  bowel (transient) 557.9
    acute 557.0
    chronic 557.1
    due to mesenteric artery insufficiency 557.1
  brain - see also Ischemia, cerebral
    recurrent focal 435.9
  cardiac (see also Ischemia, heart) 414.9
  cardiomyopathy 414.8
  carotid artery (with transient neurologic
    deficit) 435.8
  cerebral (chronic) (generalized) 437.1
    arteriosclerotic 437.0
    intermittent (with transient neurologic
      deficit) 435.9
    newborn 779.2
    puerperal, postpartum, childbirth 674.0●
    recurrent focal (with transient neurologic
      deficit) 435.9
    transient (with transient neurologic
      deficit) 435.9
  colon 557.9
    acute 557.0
    chronic 557.1
    due to mesenteric artery insufficiency 557.1
  coronary (chronic) (see also Ischemia, heart)
    414.9
  demand 411.89
  heart (chronic or with a stated duration of
    over 8 weeks) 414.9
    acute or with a stated duration of 8 weeks
      or less (see also Infarct, myocardium)
      410.9●
      without myocardial infarction 411.89
        with coronary (artery) occlusion
        411.81
    subacute 411.89
  intestine (transient) 557.9
    acute 557.0
    chronic 557.1
    due to mesenteric artery insufficiency 557.1
  kidney 593.81
  labyrinth 386.50
  muscles, leg 728.89
  myocardium, myocardial (chronic or with a
    stated duration of over 8 weeks) 414.8
    acute (see also Infarct, myocardium)
      410.9●
      without myocardial infarction 411.89
        with coronary (artery) occlusion
        411.81
  renal 593.81
  retina, retinal 362.84
  small bowel 557.9
    acute 557.0
    chronic 557.1
    due to mesenteric artery insufficiency 557.1
  spinal cord 336.1
  subendocardial (see also Insufficiency,
    coronary) 411.89
  supply (see also Angina) 414.9
  vertebral artery (with transient neurologic
    deficit) 435.1

Ischialgia (see also Sciatica) 724.3
Ischiopagus 759.4
Ischium, ischial - see condition
Ischomenia 626.8
Ischuria 788.5
Iselin's disease or osteochondrosis 732.5
Islands of
  parotid tissue in
    lymph nodes 750.26
    neck structures 750.26
  submaxillary glands in
    fascia 750.26
    lymph nodes 750.26
    neck muscles 750.26
Islet cell tumor, pancreas (M8150/0) 211.7
Isoimmunization NEC (see also Incompatibility)
  656.2●
  anti-E 656.2●
  fetus or newborn 773.2
    ABO blood groups 773.1
    Rhesus (Rh) factor 773.0
Isolation V07.0
  social V62.4
Isosporosis 007.2
Issue
  medical certificate NEC V68.09
    cause of death V68.09
    disability examination V68.01
    fitness V68.09
    incapacity V68.09
  repeat prescription NEC V68.1
    appliance V68.1
    contraceptive V25.40
      device NEC V25.49
        intrauterine V25.42
        specified type NEC V25.49
      pill V25.41
    glasses V68.1
    medicinal substance V68.1
Itch (see also Pruritus) 698.9
  bakers' 692.89
  barbers' 110.0
  bricklayers' 692.89
  cheese 133.8
  clam diggers' 120.3
  coolie 126.9
  copra 133.8
  Cuban 050.1
  dew 126.9
  dhobie 110.3
  eye 379.99
  filarial (see also Infestation, filarial) 125.9
  grain 133.8
  grocers' 133.8
  ground 126.9
  harvest 133.8
  jock 110.3
  Malabar 110.9
    beard 110.0
    foot 110.4
    scalp 110.0
  meaning scabies 133.0
  Norwegian 133.0
  perianal 698.0
  poultrymen's 133.8
  sarcoptic 133.0
  scrub 134.1
  seven year V61.10
    meaning scabies 133.0
  straw 133.8
  swimmers' 120.3
  washerwoman's 692.4
  water 120.3
  winter 698.8
Itsenko-Cushing syndrome (pituitary
  basophilism) 255.0
Ivemark's syndrome (asplenia with congenital
  heart disease) 759.0
Ivory bones 756.52
Ixodes 134.8
Ixodiasis 134.8

◀ New   ◀ Revised   ~~deleted~~ Deleted   ● Use Additional Digit(s)   Omit code

J

Jaccoud's nodular fibrositis, chronic (Jaccoud's syndrome) 714.4
Jackson's
  membrane 751.4
  paralysis or syndrome 344.89
  veil 751.4
Jacksonian
  epilepsy (*see also* Epilepsy) 345.5●
  seizures (focal) (*see also* Epilepsy) 345.5●
Jacob's ulcer (M8090/3) - *see* Neoplasm, skin, malignant, by site
Jacquet's dermatitis (diaper dermatitis) 691.0
Jadassohn's
  blue nevus (M8780/0) - *see* Neoplasm, skin, benign
  disease (maculopapular erythroderma) 696.2
  intraepidermal epithelioma (M8096/0) - *see* Neoplasm, skin, benign
Jadassohn-Lewandowski syndrome (pachyonychia congenita) 757.5
Jadassohn-Pellizari's disease (anetoderma) 701.3
Jadassohn-Tièche nevus (M8780/0) - *see* Neoplasm, skin, benign
Jaffe-Lichtenstein (-Uehlinger) syndrome 252.01
Jahnke's syndrome (encephalocutaneous angiomatosis) 759.6
Jakob-Creutzfeldt disease (CJD) (syndrome) 046.19
  with dementia
    with behavioral disturba nce 046.19 [294.11]
    without behavioral disturbance 046.19 [294.10]
  familial 046.19
  iatrogenic 046.19
  specified NEC 046.19
  sporadic 046.19
  variant (vCJD) 046.11
    with dementia
      with behavioral disturbance 046.11 [294.11]
      without behavioral disturbance 046.11 [294.10]
Jaksch (-Luzet) disease or syndrome (pseudoleukemia infantum) 285.8
Jamaican
  neuropathy 349.82
  paraplegic tropical ataxic-spastic syndrome 349.82
Janet's disease (psychasthenia) 300.89
Janiceps 759.4
Jansky-Bielschowsky amaurotic familial idiocy 330.1
Japanese
  B-type encephalitis 062.0
  river fever 081.2
  seven-day fever 100.89
Jaundice (yellow) 782.4
  acholuric (familial) (splenomegalic) (*see also* Spherocytosis) 282.0
    acquired 283.9
  breast milk 774.39
  catarrhal (acute) 070.1
    with hepatic coma 070.0
    chronic 571.9
    epidemic - *see* Jaundice, epidemic
  cholestatic (benign) 782.4
  chronic idiopathic 277.4

Jaundice (*Continued*)
  epidemic (catarrhal) 070.1
    with hepatic coma 070.0
    leptospiral 100.0
    spirochetal 100.0
  febrile (acute) 070.1
    with hepatic coma 070.0
    leptospiral 100.0
    spirochetal 100.0
  fetus or newborn 774.6
    due to or associated with
      ABO
        antibodies 773.1
        incompatibility, maternal/fetal 773.1
        isoimmunization 773.1
      absence or deficiency of enzyme system for bilirubin conjugation (congenital) 774.39
      blood group incompatibility NEC 773.2
      breast milk inhibitors to conjugation 774.39
        associated with preterm delivery 774.2
      bruising 774.1
      Crigler-Najjar syndrome 277.4 [774.31]
      delayed conjugation 774.30
        associated with preterm delivery 774.2
        development 774.39
      drugs or toxins transmitted from mother 774.1
      G-6-PD deficiency 282.2 [774.0]
      galactosemia 271.1 [774.5]
      Gilbert's syndrome 277.4 [774.31]
      hepatocellular damage 774.4
      hereditary hemolytic anemia (*see also* Anemia, hemolytic) 282.9 [774.0]
      hypothyroidism, congenital 243 [774.31]
      incompatibility, maternal/fetal NEC 773.2
      infection 774.1
      inspissated bile syndrome 774.4
      isoimmunization NEC 773.2
      mucoviscidosis 277.01 [774.5]
      obliteration of bile duct, congenital 751.61 [774.5]
      polycythemia 774.1
      preterm delivery 774.2
      red cell defect 282.9 [774.0]
      Rh
        antibodies 773.0
        incompatibility, maternal/fetal 773.0
        isoimmunization 773.0
      spherocytosis (congenital) 282.0 [774.0]
      swallowed maternal blood 774.1
    physiological NEC 774.6
  from injection, inoculation, infusion, or transfusion (blood) (plasma) (serum) (other substance) (onset within 8 months after administration) - *see* Hepatitis, viral
  Gilbert's (familial nonhemolytic) 277.4
  hematogenous 283.9
  hemolytic (acquired) 283.9
    congenital (*see also* Spherocytosis) 282.0
  hemorrhagic (acute) 100.0
    leptospiral 100.0
    newborn 776.0
    spirochetal 100.0

Jaundice (*Continued*)
  hepatocellular 573.8
  homologous (serum) - *see* Hepatitis, viral
  idiopathic, chronic 277.4
  infectious (acute) (subacute) 070.1
    with hepatic coma 070.0
    leptospiral 100.0
    spirochetal 100.0
  leptospiral 100.0
  malignant (*see also* Necrosis, liver) 570
  newborn (physiological) (*see also* Jaundice, fetus or newborn) 774.6
  nonhemolytic, congenital familial (Gilbert's) 277.4
  nuclear, newborn (*see also* Kernicterus of newborn) 774.7
  obstructive NEC (*see also* Obstruction, biliary) 576.8
  postimmunization - *see* Hepatitis, viral
  posttransfusion - *see* Hepatitis, viral
  regurgitation (*see also* Obstruction, biliary) 576.8
  serum (homologous) (prophylactic) (therapeutic) - *see* Hepatitis, viral
  spirochetal (hemorrhagic) 100.0
  symptomatic 782.4
    newborn 774.6
Jaw - *see* condition
Jaw-blinking 374.43
  congenital 742.8
Jaw-winking phenomenon or syndrome 742.8
Jealousy
  alcoholic 291.5
  childhood 313.3
  sibling 313.3
Jejunitis (*see also* Enteritis) 558.9
Jejunostomy status V44.4
Jejunum, jejunal - *see* condition
Jensen's disease 363.05
Jericho boil 085.1
Jerks, myoclonic 333.2
Jervell-Lange-Nielsen syndrome 426.82
Jeune's disease or syndrome (asphyxiating thoracic dystrophy) 756.4
Jigger disease 134.1
Job's syndrome (chronic granulomatous disease) 288.1
Jod-Basedow phenomenon 242.8●
Johnson-Stevens disease (erythema multiforme exudativum) 695.13
Joint - *see also* condition
  Charcôt's 094.0 [713.5]
  false 733.82
  flail - *see* Flail, joint
  mice - *see* Loose, body, joint, by site
  sinus to bone 730.9●
  von Gies' 095.8
Jordan's anomaly or syndrome 288.2
Josephs-Diamond-Blackfan anemia (congenital hypoplastic) 284.01
Joubert syndrome 759.89
Jumpers' knee 727.2
Jungle yellow fever 060.0
Jungling's disease (sarcoidosis) 135
Junin virus hemorrhagic fever 078.7
Juvenile - *see also* condition
  delinquent 312.9
    group (*see also* Disturbance, conduct) 312.2●
  neurotic 312.4

K

Kabuki syndrome 759.89
Kahler (-Bozzolo) disease (multiple myeloma) (M9730/3) 203.0●
Kakergasia 300.9
Kakke 265.0
Kala-azar (Indian) (infantile) (Mediterranean) (Sudanese) 085.0
Kalischer's syndrome (encephalocutaneous angiomatosis) 759.6
Kallmann's syndrome (hypogonadotropic hypogonadism with anosmia) 253.4
Kanner's syndrome (autism) (see also Psychosis, childhood) 299.0●
Kaolinosis 502
Kaposi's
  disease 757.33
    lichen ruber 696.4
      acuminatus 696.4
      moniliformis 697.8
    xeroderma pigmentosum 757.33
  sarcoma (M9140/3) 176.9
    adipose tissue 176.1
    aponeurosis 176.1
    artery 176.1
    associated herpesvirus infection 058.89
    blood vessel 176.1
    bursa 176.1
    connective tissue 176.1
    external genitalia 176.8
    fascia 176.1
    fatty tissue 176.1
    fibrous tissue 176.1
    gastrointestinal tract NEC 176.3
    ligament 176.1
    lung 176.4
    lymph
      gland(s) 176.5
      node(s) 176.5
    lymphatic(s) NEC 176.1
    muscle (skeletal) 176.1
    oral cavity NEC 176.8
    palate 176.2
    scrotum 176.8
    skin 176.0
    soft tissue 176.1
    specified site NEC 176.8
    subcutaneous tissue 176.1
    synovia 176.1
    tendon (sheath) 176.1
    vein 176.1
    vessel 176.1
    viscera NEC 176.9
    vulva 176.8
  varicelliform eruption 054.0
    vaccinia 999.0
Kartagener's syndrome or triad (sinusitis, bronchiectasis, situs inversus) 759.3
Kasabach-Merritt syndrome (capillary hemangioma associated with thrombocytopenic purpura) 287.39
Kaschin-Beck disease (endemic polyarthritis) - see Disease, Kaschin-Beck
Kast's syndrome (dyschondroplasia with hemangiomas) 756.4
Katatonia- see Catatonia
Katayama disease or fever 120.2
Kathisophobia 781.0
Kawasaki disease 446.1
Kayser-Fleischer ring (cornea) (pseudosclerosis) 275.1 [371.14]
Kaznelson's syndrome (congenital hypoplastic anemia) 284.01
Kearns-Sayre syndrome 277.87
Kedani fever 081.2
Kelis 701.4
Kelly (-Patterson) syndrome (sideropenic dysphagia) 280.8

Keloid, cheloid 701.4
  Addison's (morphea) 701.0
  cornea 371.00
  Hawkins' 701.4
  scar 701.4
Keloma 701.4
Kenya fever 082.1
Keratectasia 371.71
  congenital 743.41
Keratinization NEC
  alveolar ridge mucosa
    excessive 528.72
    minimal 528.71
Keratitis (nodular) (nonulcerative) (simple) (zonular) NEC 370.9
  with ulceration (see also Ulcer, cornea) 370.00
  actinic 370.24
  arborescens 054.42
  areolar 370.22
  bullosa 370.8
  deep - see Keratitis, interstitial
  dendritic(a) 054.42
  desiccation 370.34
  diffuse interstitial 370.52
  disciform(is) 054.43
    varicella 052.7 [370.44]
  epithelialis vernalis 372.13 [370.32]
  exposure 370.34
  filamentary 370.23
  gonococcal (congenital) (prenatal) 098.43
  herpes, herpetic (simplex) NEC 054.43
    zoster 053.21
  hypopyon 370.04
  in
    chickenpox 052.7 [370.44]
    exanthema (see also Exanthem) 057.9 [370.44]
    paravaccinia (see also Paravaccinia) 051.9 [370.44]
    smallpox (see also Smallpox) 050.9 [370.44]
    vernal conjunctivitis 372.13 [370.32]
  interstitial (nonsyphilitic) 370.50
    with ulcer (see also Ulcer, cornea) 370.00
    diffuse 370.52
    herpes, herpetic (simplex) 054.43
      zoster 053.21
    syphilitic (congenital) (hereditary) 090.3
    tuberculous (see also Tuberculosis) 017.3● [370.59]
  lagophthalmic 370.34
  macular 370.22
  neuroparalytic 370.35
  neurotrophic 370.35
  nummular 370.22
  oyster-shuckers' 370.8
  parenchymatous - see Keratitis, interstitial
  petrificans 370.8
  phlyctenular 370.31
  postmeasles 055.71
  punctata, punctate 370.21
    leprosa 030.0 [370.21]
    profunda 090.3
    superficial (Thygeson's) 370.21
  purulent 370.8
  pustuliformis profunda 090.3
  rosacea 695.3 [370.49]
  sclerosing 370.54
  specified type NEC 370.8
  stellate 370.22
  striate 370.22
  superficial 370.20
    with conjunctivitis (see also Keratoconjunctivitis) 370.40
    punctate (Thygeson's) 370.21
  suppurative 370.8
  syphilitic (congenital) (prenatal) 090.3
  trachomatous 076.1
    late effect 139.1
  tuberculous (phlyctenular) (see also Tuberculosis) 017.3● [370.31]
  ulcerated (see also Ulcer, cornea) 370.00

Keratitis (Continued)
  vesicular 370.8
  welders' 370.24
  xerotic (see also Keratomalacia) 371.45
    vitamin A deficiency 264.4
Keratoacanthoma 238.2
Keratocele 371.72
Keratoconjunctivitis (see also Keratitis) 370.40
  adenovirus type 8 077.1
  epidemic 077.1
  exposure 370.34
  gonococcal 098.43
  herpetic (simplex) 054.43
    zoster 053.21
  in
    chickenpox 052.7 [370.44]
    exanthema (see also Exanthem) 057.9 [370.44]
    paravaccinia (see also Paravaccinia) 051.9 [370.44]
    smallpox (see also Smallpox) 050.9 [370.44]
  infectious 077.1
  neurotrophic 370.35
  phlyctenular 370.31
  postmeasles 055.71
  shipyard 077.1
  sicca (Sjögren's syndrome) 710.2
    not in Sjögren's syndrome 370.33
  specified type NEC 370.49
  tuberculous (phlyctenular) (see also Tuberculosis) 017.3● [370.31]
Keratoconus 371.60
  acute hydrops 371.62
  congenital 743.41
  stable 371.61
Keratocyst (dental) 526.0
Keratoderma, keratodermia (congenital) (palmaris et plantaris) (symmetrical) 757.39
  acquired 701.1
  blennorrhagica 701.1
    gonococcal 098.81
  climacterium 701.1
  eccentrica 757.39
  gonorrheal 098.81
  punctata 701.1
  tylodes, progressive 701.1
Keratodermatocele 371.72
Keratoglobus 371.70
  congenital 743.41
    associated with buphthalmos 743.22
Keratohemia 371.12
Keratoiritis (see also Iridocyclitis) 364.3
  syphilitic 090.3
  tuberculous (see also Tuberculosis) 017.3● [364.11]
Keratolysis exfoliativa (congenital) 757.39
  acquired 695.89
  neonatorum 757.39
Keratoma 701.1
  congenital 757.39
  malignum congenitale 757.1
  palmaris et plantaris hereditarium 757.39
  senile 702.0
Keratomalacia 371.45
  vitamin A deficiency 264.4
Keratomegaly 743.41
Keratomycosis 111.1
  nigricans (palmaris) 111.1
Keratopathy 371.40
  band (see also Keratitis) 371.43
  bullous (see also Keratitis) 371.23
  degenerative (see also Degeneration, cornea) 371.40
    hereditary (see also Dystrophy, cornea) 371.50
  discrete colliquative 371.49
Keratoscleritis, tuberculous (see also Tuberculosis) 017.3● [370.31]

◀ New   ◀ Revised   ~~deleted~~ Deleted   ● Use Additional Digit(s)   Omit code

Keratosis 701.1
　actinic 702.0
　arsenical 692.4
　blennorrhagica 701.1
　　gonococcal 098.81
　congenital (any type) 757.39
　ear (middle) (*see also* Cholesteatoma) 385.30
　female genital (external) 629.89
　follicular, vitamin A deficiency 264.8
　follicularis 757.39
　　acquired 701.1
　　congenital (acneiformis) (Siemens') 757.39
　　spinulosa (decalvans) 757.39
　　vitamin A deficiency 264.8
　gonococcal 098.81
　larynx, laryngeal 478.79
　male genital (external) 608.89
　middle ear (*see also* Cholesteatoma) 385.30
　nigricans 701.2
　　congenital 757.39
　obturans 380.21
　oral epithelium
　　residual ridge mucosa
　　　excessive 528.72
　　　minimal 528.71
　palmaris et plantaris (symmetrical) 757.39
　penile 607.89
　pharyngeus 478.29
　pilaris 757.39
　　acquired 701.1
　punctata (palmaris et plantaris) 701.1
　scrotal 608.89
　seborrheic 702.19
　　inflamed 702.11
　senilis 702.0
　solar 702.0
　suprafollicularis 757.39
　tonsillaris 478.29
　vagina 623.1
　vegetans 757.39
　vitamin A deficiency 264.8
Kerato-uveitis (*see also* Iridocyclitis) 364.3
Keraunoparalysis 994.0
Kerion (celsi) 110.0
Kernicterus of newborn (not due to
　isoimmunization) 774.7
　due to isoimmunization (conditions
　　classifiable to 773.0–773.2) 773.4
Ketoacidosis 276.2
　diabetic 250.1●
　　due to secondary diabetes 249.1●
Ketonuria 791.6
　branched-chain, intermittent 270.3
Ketosis 276.2
　diabetic 250.1●
　　due to secondary diabetes 249.1●
Kidney - *see* condition
Kienböck's
　disease 732.3
　　adult 732.8
　osteochondrosis 732.3
Kimmelstiel (-Wilson) disease or syndrome
　(intercapillary glomerulosclerosis) 250.4●
　[581.81]
　due to secondary diabetes 249.4● [581.81]
Kink, kinking
　appendix 543.9
　artery 447.1
　cystic duct, congenital 751.61
　hair (acquired) 704.2
　ileum or intestine (*see also* Obstruction,
　　intestine) 560.9
　Lane's (*see also* Obstruction, intestine) 560.9
　organ or site, congenital NEC - *see* Anomaly,
　　specified type NEC, by site
　ureter (pelvic junction) 593.3
　　congenital 753.20
　vein(s) 459.2
　　caval 459.2
　　peripheral 459.2

Kinnier Wilson's disease (hepatolenticular
　degeneration) 275.1
Kissing
　osteophytes 721.5
　spine 721.5
　vertebra 721.5
Klauder's syndrome (erythema multiforme
　exudativum) 695.19
Klebs' disease (*see also* Nephritis) 583.9
Klein-Waardenburg syndrome (ptosis-
　epicanthus) 270.2
Kleine-Levin syndrome 327.13
Kleptomania 312.32
Klinefelter's syndrome 758.7
Klinger's disease 446.4
Klippel's disease 723.8
Klippel-Feil disease or syndrome (brevicollis)
　756.16
Klippel-Trenaunay syndrome 759.89
Klumpke (-Déjérine) palsy, paralysis (birth)
　(newborn) 767.6
Klüver-Bucy (-Terzian) syndrome 310.0
Knee - *see* condition
Knifegrinders' rot (*see also* Tuberculosis)
　011.4●
Knock-knee (acquired) 736.41
　congenital 755.64
Knot
　intestinal, syndrome (volvulus) 560.2
　umbilical cord (true) 663.2●
　　affecting fetus or newborn 762.5
Knots, surfer 919.8
　infected 919.9
Knotting (of)
　hair 704.2
　intestine 560.2
Knuckle pads (Garrod's) 728.79
Köbner's disease (epidermolysis bullosa)
　757.39
Koch's
　infection (*see also* Tuberculosis, pulmonary)
　　011.9●
　relapsing fever 087.9
Koch-Weeks conjunctivitis 372.03
Koenig-Wichman disease (pemphigus)
　694.4
Köhler's disease (osteochondrosis) 732.5
　first (osteochondrosis juvenilis) 732.5
　second (Freiburg's infarction, metatarsal
　　head) 732.5
　patellar 732.4
　tarsal navicular (bone) (osteoarthrosis
　　juvenilis) 732.5
Köhler-Mouchet disease (osteoarthrosis
　juvenilis) 732.5
Köhler-Pellegrini-Stieda disease or syndrome
　(calcification, knee joint) 726.62
Koilonychia 703.8
　congenital 757.5
Kojevnikov's, Kojewnikoff's epilepsy (*see also*
　Epilepsy) 345.7●
König's
　disease (osteochondritis dissecans) 732.7
　syndrome 564.89
Koniophthisis (*see also* Tuberculosis) 011.4●
Koplik's spots 055.9
Kopp's asthma 254.8
Korean hemorrhagic fever 078.6
Korsakoff (-Wernicke) disease, psychosis, or
　syndrome (nonalcoholic) 294.0
　alcoholic 291.1
Korsakov's disease - *see* Korsakoff's disease
Korsakow's disease - *see* Korsakoff's disease
Kostmann's disease or syndrome (infantile
　genetic agranulocytosis) 288.01
Krabbe's
　disease (leukodystrophy) 330.0
　syndrome
　　congenital muscle hypoplasia 756.89
　　cutaneocerebral angioma 759.6

Kraepelin-Morel disease (*see also*
　Schizophrenia) 295.9●
Kraft-Weber-Dimitri disease 759.6
Kraurosis
　ani 569.49
　penis 607.0
　vagina 623.8
　vulva 624.09
Kreotoxism 005.9
Krukenberg's
　spindle 371.13
　tumor (M8490/6) 198.6
Kufs' disease 330.1
Kugelberg-Welander disease 335.11
Kuhnt-Junius degeneration or disease
　362.52
Kulchitsky's cell carcinoma (carcinoid tumor of
　intestine) 259.2
Kümmell's disease or spondylitis 721.7
Kundrat's disease (lymphosarcoma) 200.1●
Kunekune - *see* Dermatophytosis
Kunkel syndrome (lupoid hepatitis)
　571.49
Kupffer cell sarcoma (M9124/3) 155.0
Kuru 046.0
Kussmaul's
　coma (diabetic) 250.3●
　　due to secondary diabetes 249.3●
　disease (polyarteritis nodosa) 446.0
　respiration (air hunger) 786.09
Kwashiorkor (marasmus type) 260
Kyasanur Forest disease 065.2
Kyphoscoliosis, kyphoscoliotic (acquired)
　(*see also* Scoliosis) 737.30
　congenital 756.19
　due to radiation 737.33
　heart (disease) 416.1
　idiopathic 737.30
　infantile
　　progressive 737.32
　　resolving 737.31
　late effect of rickets 268.1 [737.43]
　specified NEC 737.39
　thoracogenic 737.34
　tuberculous (*see also* Tuberculosis) 015.0●
　　[737.43]
Kyphosis, kyphotic (acquired) (postural)
　737.10
　adolescent postural 737.0
　congenital 756.19
　dorsalis juvenilis 732.0
　due to or associated with
　　Charcôt-Marie-Tooth disease 356.1
　　　[737.41]
　　mucopolysaccharidosis 277.5 [737.41]
　　neurofibromatosis 237.71 [737.41]
　　osteitis
　　　deformans 731.0 [737.41]
　　　fibrosa cystica 252.01 [737.41]
　　osteoporosis (*see also* Osteoporosis) 733.0
　　　[737.41]
　　poliomyelitis (*see also* Poliomyelitis) 138
　　　[737.41]
　　radiation 737.11
　　tuberculosis (*see also* Tuberculosis) 015.0●
　　　[737.41]
　Kümmell's 721.7
　late effect of rickets 268.1 [737.41]
　Morquio-Brailsford type (spinal) 277.5
　　[737.41]
　pelvis 738.6
　postlaminectomy 737.12
　specified cause NEC 737.19
　syphilitic, congenital 090.5 [737.41]
　tuberculous (*see also* Tuberculosis) 015.0●
　　[737.41]
Kyrle's disease (hyperkeratosis follicularis in
　cutem penetrans) 701.1

L

Labia, labium - *see* condition
Labiated hymen 752.49
Labile
  blood pressure 796.2
  emotions, emotionality 301.3
  vasomotor system 443.9
Lability, emotional 799.24
Labioglossal paralysis 335.22
Labium leporinum (*see also* Cleft, lip) 749.10
Labor (*see also* Delivery)
  with complications - *see* Delivery,
    complicated
  abnormal NEC 661.9●
    affecting fetus or newborn 763.7
  arrested active phase 661.1●
    affecting fetus or newborn 763.7
  desultory 661.2●
    affecting fetus or newborn 763.7
  dyscoordinate 661.4●
    affecting fetus or newborn 763.7
  early onset (22–36 weeks gestation) 644.2●
  failed
    induction 659.1●
      mechanical 659.0●
      medical 659.1●
      surgical 659.0●
    trial (vaginal delivery) 660.6●
  false 644.1●
  forced or induced, affecting fetus or newborn
    763.89
  hypertonic 661.4●
    affecting fetus or newborn 763.7
  hypotonic 661.2●
    affecting fetus or newborn 763.7
    primary 661.0●
      affecting fetus or newborn 763.7
    secondary 661.1●
      affecting fetus or newborn 763.7
  incoordinate 661.4●
    affecting fetus or newborn 763.7
  irregular 661.2●
    affecting fetus or newborn 763.7
  long - *see* Labor, prolonged
  missed (at or near term) 656.4●
  obstructed NEC 660.9●
    affecting fetus or newborn 763.1
    due to female genital mutilation 660.8●
    specified cause NEC 660.8●
      affecting fetus or newborn 763.1
  pains, spurious 644.1●
  precipitate 661.3●
    affecting fetus or newborn 763.6
  premature 644.2●
    threatened 644.0●
  prolonged or protracted 662.1●
    affecting fetus or newborn 763.89
    first stage 662.0●
      affecting fetus or newborn 763.89
    second stage 662.2●
      affecting fetus or newborn 763.89
  threatened NEC 644.1●
  undelivered 644.1●
Labored breathing (*see also* Hyperventilation)
  786.09
Labyrinthitis (inner ear) (destructive) (latent)
  386.30
  circumscribed 386.32
  diffuse 386.31
  focal 386.32
  purulent 386.33
  serous 386.31
  suppurative 386.33
  syphilitic 095.8
  toxic 386.34
  viral 386.35
Laceration - *see also* Wound, open, by site
  accidental, complicating surgery 998.2
  Achilles tendon 845.09
    with open wound 892.2

Laceration (*Continued*)
  anus (sphincter) 879.6
    with
      abortion - *see* Abortion, by type, with
        damage to pelvic organs
      ectopic pregnancy (*see also* categories
        633.0–633.9) 639.2
      molar pregnancy (*see also* categories
        630–632) 639.2
    complicated 879.7
    complicating delivery (healed) (old)
      654.8●
      with laceration of anal or rectal
        mucosa 664.3●
      not associated with third-degree
        perineal laceration 664.6●
    following
      abortion 639.2
      ectopic or molar pregnancy 639.2
    nontraumatic, nonpuerperal (healed)
      (old) 569.43
  bladder (urinary)
    with
      abortion - *see* Abortion, by type, with
        damage to pelvic organs
      ectopic pregnancy (*see also* categories
        633.0–633.9) 639.2
      molar pregnancy (*see also* categories
        630–632) 639.2
    following
      abortion 639.2
      ectopic or molar pregnancy 639.2
    obstetrical trauma 665.5●
  blood vessel - *see* Injury, blood vessel, by site
  bowel
    with
      abortion - *see* Abortion, by type, with
        damage to pelvic organs
      ectopic pregnancy (*see also* categories
        633.0–633.9) 639.2
      molar pregnancy (*see also* categories
        630–632) 639.2
    following
      abortion 639.2
      ectopic or molar pregnancy 639.2
    obstetrical trauma 665.5●
  brain (cerebral) (membrane) (with
    hemorrhage) 851.8●

> Note: Use the following fifth-digit
> subclassification with categories 851–854:
>
> 0   unspecified state of consciousness
> 1   with no loss of consciousness
> 2   with brief [less than one hour] loss of
>   consciousness
> 3   with moderate [1–24 hours] loss of
>   consciousness
> 4   with prolonged [more than 24 hours]
>   loss of consciousness and
>   return to pre-existing conscious
>   level
> 5   with prolonged [more than 24 hours]
>   loss of consciousness, without
>   return to pre-existing conscious
>   level
>
> Use fifth-digit 5 to designate when a patient
> is unconscious and dies before regaining
> consciousness, regardless of the duration of
> the loss of consciousness
>
> 6   with loss of consciousness of
>   unspecified duration
> 9   with concussion, unspecified

    with
      open intracranial wound 851.9●
      skull fracture - *see* Fracture, skull, by
        site
    cerebellum 851.6●
      with open intracranial wound 851.7●

Laceration (*Continued*)
  brain (*Continued*)
    cortex 851.2●
      with open intracranial wound 851.3●
    during birth 767.0
    stem 851.6●
      with open intracranial wound 851.7●
  broad ligament
    with
      abortion - *see* Abortion, by type, with
        damage to pelvic organs
      ectopic pregnancy (*see also* categories
        633.0–633.9) 639.2
      molar pregnancy (*see also* categories
        630–632) 639.2
    following
      abortion 639.2
      ectopic or molar pregnancy 639.2
    nontraumatic 620.6
    obstetrical trauma 665.6●
    syndrome (nontraumatic) 620.6
  capsule, joint - *see* Sprain, by site
  cardiac - *see* Laceration, heart
  causing eversion of cervix uteri (old) 622.0
  central, complicating delivery 664.4●
  cerebellum - *see* Laceration, brain, cerebellum
  cerebral - *see also* Laceration, brain
    during birth 767.0
  cervix (uteri)
    with
      abortion - *see* Abortion, by type, with
        damage to pelvic organs
      ectopic pregnancy (*see also* categories
        633.0–633.9) 639.2
      molar pregnancy (*see also* categories
        630–632) 639.2
    following
      abortion 639.2
      ectopic or molar pregnancy 639.2
    nonpuerperal, nontraumatic 622.3
    obstetrical trauma (current) 665.3●
    old (postpartal) 622.3
    traumatic - *see* Injury, internal, cervix
  chordae heart 429.5
  complicated 879.9
  cornea - *see* Laceration, eyeball
    superficial 918.1
  cortex (cerebral) - *see* Laceration, brain, cortex
  esophagus 530.89
  eye(s) - *see* Laceration, ocular
  eyeball NEC 871.4
    with prolapse or exposure of intraocular
      tissue 871.1
    penetrating - *see* Penetrating wound,
      eyeball
    specified as without prolapse of
      intraocular tissue 871.0
  eyelid NEC 870.8
    full thickness 870.1
      involving lacrimal passages 870.2
    skin (and periocular area) 870.0
      penetrating - *see* Penetrating wound,
        orbit
  fourchette
    with
      abortion - *see* Abortion, by type, with
        damage to pelvic organs
      ectopic pregnancy (*see also* categories
        633.0–633.9) 639.2
      molar pregnancy (*see also* categories
        630–632) 639.2
    complicating delivery 664.0●
    following
      abortion 639.2
      ectopic or molar pregnancy 639.2
  heart (without penetration of heart
    chambers) 861.02
    with
      open wound into thorax 861.12
      penetration of heart chambers 861.03
        with open wound into thorax 861.13

◀ New   ◀▬ Revised   ~~deleted~~ Deleted   ● Use Additional Digit(s)   ▓ Omit code

Laceration *(Continued)*
  hernial sac - *see* Hernia, by site
  internal organ (abdomen) (chest) (pelvis)
    NEC - *see* Injury, internal, by site
  kidney (parenchyma) 866.02
    with
      complete disruption of parenchyma
        (rupture) 866.03
        with open wound into cavity 866.13
      open wound into cavity 866.12
  labia
    complicating delivery 664.0 ●
  ligament - *see also* Sprain, by site
    with open wound - *see* Wound, open, by
      site
  liver 864.05
    with open wound into cavity 864.15
    major (disruption of hepatic parenchyma)
      864.04
      with open wound into cavity 864.14
    minor (capsule only) 864.02
      with open wound into cavity 864.12
    moderate (involving parenchyma without
      major disruption) 864.03
      with open wound into cavity 864.13
    multiple 864.04
      with open wound into cavity 864.14
    stellate 864.04
      with open wound into cavity 864.14
  lung 861.22
    with open wound into thorax 861.32
  meninges - *see* Laceration, brain
  meniscus (knee) (*see also* Tear, meniscus)
    836.2
    old 717.5
    site other than knee - *see also* Sprain, by
      site
      old NEC (*see also* Disorder, cartilage,
        articular) 718.0 ●
  muscle - *see also* Sprain, by site
    with open wound - *see* Wound, open, by
      site
  myocardium - *see* Laceration, heart
  nerve - *see* Injury, nerve, by site
  ocular NEC (*see also* Laceration, eyeball)
    871.4
    adnexa NEC 870.8
      penetrating 870.3
        with foreign body 870.4
  orbit (eye) 870.8
    penetrating 870.3
      with foreign body 870.4
  pelvic
    floor (muscles)
      with
        abortion - *see* Abortion, by type,
          with damage to pelvic organs
        ectopic pregnancy (*see also*
          categories 633.0–633.9) 639.2
        molar pregnancy (*see also* categories
          630–632) 639.2
      complicating delivery 664.1 ●
      following
        abortion 639.2
        ectopic or molar pregnancy 639.2
      nonpuerperal 618.7
      old (postpartal) 618.7
    organ NEC
      with
        abortion - *see* Abortion, by type,
          with damage to pelvic organs
        ectopic pregnancy (*see also*
          categories 633.0–633.9) 639.2
        molar pregnancy (*see also* categories
          630–632) 639.2
      complicating delivery 665.5 ●
        affecting fetus or newborn 763.89
      following
        abortion 639.2
        ectopic or molar pregnancy 639.2
      obstetrical trauma 665.5 ●

Laceration *(Continued)*
  perineum, perineal (old) (postpartal) 618.7
    with
      abortion - *see* Abortion, by type, with
        damage to pelvic floor
      ectopic pregnancy (*see also* categories
        633.0–633.9) 639.2
      molar pregnancy (*see also* categories
        630–632) 639.2
    complicating delivery 664.4 ●
      first degree 664.0 ●
      second degree 664.1 ●
      third degree 664.2 ●
      fourth degree 664.3 ●
      central 664.4 ●
      involving
        anal sphincter (healed) (old) 654.8 ●
        fourchette 664.0 ●
        hymen 664.0 ●
        labia 664.0 ●
        not associated with third-degree
          perineal laceration 664.6 ●
        pelvic floor 664.1 ●
        perineal muscles 664.1 ●
        rectovaginal with septum 664.2 ●
          with anal mucosa 664.3 ●
        skin 664.0 ●
        sphincter (anal) (healed) (old)
          654.8 ●
          with anal mucosa 664.3 ●
          not associated with third-degree
            perineal laceration 664.6 ●
        vagina 664.0 ●
        vaginal muscles 664.1 ●
        vulva 664.0 ●
      secondary 674.2 ●
    following
      abortion 639.2
      ectopic or molar pregnancy 639.2
    male 879.6
      complicated 879.7
    muscles, complicating delivery 664.1 ●
    nonpuerperal, current injury 879.6
      complicated 879.7
    secondary (postpartal) 674.2 ●
  peritoneum
    with
      abortion - *see* Abortion, by type, with
        damage to pelvic organs
      ectopic pregnancy (*see also* categories
        633.0–633.9) 639.2
      molar pregnancy (*see also* categories
        630–632) 639.2
    following
      abortion 639.2
      ectopic or molar pregnancy 639.2
    obstetrical trauma 665.5 ●
  periurethral tissue
    with
      abortion - *see* Abortion, by type, with
        damage to pelvic organs
      ectopic pregnancy (*see also* categories
        633.0–633.9) 639.2
      molar pregnancy (*see also* categories
        630–632) 639.2
    following
      abortion 639.2
      ectopic or molar pregnancy 639.2
    obstetrical trauma 664.8 ●
  rectovaginal (septum)
    with
      abortion - *see* Abortion, by type, with
        damage to pelvic organs
      ectopic pregnancy (*see also* categories
        633.0–633.9) 639.2
      molar pregnancy (*see also* categories
        630–632) 639.2
    complicating delivery 665.4 ●
      with perineum 664.2 ●
        involving anal or rectal mucosa
          664.3 ●

Laceration *(Continued)*
  rectovaginal *(Continued)*
    following
      abortion 639.2
      ectopic or molar pregnancy 639.2
    nonpuerperal 623.4
    old (postpartal) 623.4
  spinal cord (meninges) - *see also* Injury,
    spinal, by site
    due to injury at birth 767.4
    fetus or newborn 767.4
  spleen 865.09
    with
      disruption of parenchyma (massive)
        865.04
        with open wound into cavity 865.14
        open wound into cavity 865.19
      capsule (without disruption of
        parenchyma) 865.02
        with open wound into cavity 865.12
      parenchyma 865.03
        with open wound into cavity 865.13
        massive disruption (rupture) 865.04
          with open wound into cavity 865.14
  tendon 848.9
    with open wound - *see* Wound, open, by
      site
    Achilles 845.09
      with open wound 892.2
    lower limb NEC 844.9
      with open wound NEC 894.2
    upper limb NEC 840.9
      with open wound NEC 884.2
  tentorium cerebelli - *see* Laceration, brain,
    cerebellum
  tongue 873.64
    complicated 873.74
  urethra
    with
      abortion - *see* Abortion, by type, with
        damage to pelvic organs
      ectopic pregnancy (*see also* categories
        633.0–633.9) 639.2
      molar pregnancy (*see also* categories
        630–632) 639.2
    following
      abortion 639.2
      ectopic or molar pregnancy 639.2
    nonpuerperal, nontraumatic 599.84
    obstetrical trauma 665.5 ●
  uterus
    with
      abortion - *see* Abortion, by type, with
        damage to pelvic organs
      ectopic pregnancy (*see also* categories
        633.0–633.9) 639.2
      molar pregnancy (*see also* categories
        630–632) 639.2
    following
      abortion 639.2
      ectopic or molar pregnancy 639.2
    nonpuerperal, nontraumatic 621.8
    obstetrical trauma NEC 665.5 ●
    old (postpartal) 621.8
  vagina
    with
      abortion - *see* Abortion, by type, with
        damage to pelvic organs
      ectopic pregnancy (*see also* categories
        633.0–633.9) 639.2
      molar pregnancy (*see also* categories
        630–632) 639.2
      perineal involvement, complicating
        delivery 664.0 ●
    complicating delivery 665.4 ●
      first degree 664.0 ●
      second degree 664.1 ●
      third degree 664.2 ●
      fourth degree 664.3 ●
      high 665.4 ●
      muscles 664.1 ●

Laceration *(Continued)*
  vagina *(Continued)*
    complicating delivery *(Continued)*
      sulcus 665.4 ●
      wall 665.4 ●
    following
      abortion 639.2
      ectopic or molar pregnancy 639.2
    nonpuerperal, nontraumatic 623.4
    old (postpartal) 623.4
  valve, heart - *see* Endocarditis
  vulva
    with
      abortion - *see* Abortion, by type, with
        damage to pelvic organs
      ectopic pregnancy *(see also* categories
        633.0–633.9) 639.2
      molar pregnancy *(see also* categories
        630–632) 639.2
    complicating delivery 664.0 ●
    following
      abortion 639.2
      ectopic or molar pregnancy 639.2
    nonpuerperal, nontraumatic 624.4
    old (postpartal) 624.4
Lachrymal - *see* condition
Lachrymonasal duct - *see* condition
Lack of
  adequate intermaxillary vertical dimension
    524.36
  appetite *(see also* Anorexia) 783.0
  care
    in home V60.4
    of adult 995.84
    of infant (at or after birth) 995.52
  coordination 781.3
  development - *see also* Hypoplasia
    physiological in childhood 783.40
  education V62.3
  energy 780.79
  financial resources V60.2
  food 994.2
    in environment V60.89
  growth in childhood 783.43
  heating V60.1
  housing (permanent) (temporary)
    V60.0
    adequate V60.1
  material resources V60.2
  medical attention 799.89
  memory *(see also* Amnesia) 780.93
    mild, following organic brain damage
      310.89
  ovulation 628.0
  person able to render necessary care
    V60.4
  physical exercise V69.0
  physiologic development in childhood
    783.40
  posterior occlusal support 524.57
  prenatal care in current pregnancy
    V23.7
  shelter V60.0
  sleep V69.4
  water 994.3
Lacrimal - *see* condition
Lacrimation, abnormal *(see also* Epiphora)
  375.20
Lacrimonasal duct - *see* condition
Lactation, lactating (breast) (puerperal)
  (postpartum)
  defective 676.4 ●
  disorder 676.9 ●
    specified type NEC 676.8 ●
  excessive 676.6 ●
  failed 676.4 ●
  mastitis NEC 675.2 ●
  mother (care and/or examination)
    V24.1
  nonpuerperal 611.6
  suppressed 676.5 ●

Lacticemia 271.3
  excessive 276.2
Lactosuria 271.3
Lacunar skull 756.0
Laennec's cirrhosis (alcoholic) 571.2
  nonalcoholic 571.5
Lafora's disease 333.2
Lag, lid (nervous) 374.41
Lagleyze-von Hippel disease (retinocerebral
  angiomatosis) 759.6
Lagophthalmos (eyelid) (nervous) 374.20
  cicatricial 374.23
    keratitis *(see also* Keratitis) 370.34
  mechanical 374.22
  paralytic 374.21
La grippe - *see* Influenza
Lahore sore 085.1
Lakes, venous (cerebral) 437.8
Laki-Lorand factor deficiency *(see also* Defect,
  coagulation) 286.3
Lalling 307.9
Lambliasis 007.1
Lame back 724.5
Lancereaux's diabetes (diabetes mellitus with
  marked emaciation) 250.8 ● [261]
  due to secondary diabetes 249.8 ● [261]
Landau-Kleffner syndrome 345.8 ●
Landouzy-Déjérine dystrophy
  (fascioscapulohumeral atrophy) 359.1
Landry's disease or paralysis 357.0
Landry-Guillain-Barré syndrome 357.0
Lane's
  band 751.4
  disease 569.89
  kink *(see also* Obstruction, intestine) 560.9
Langdon Down's syndrome (mongolism)
  758.0
Language abolition 784.69
Lanugo (persistent) 757.4
Laparoscopic surgical procedure converted to
  open procedure V64.41
Lardaceous
  degeneration (any site) 277.39
  disease 277.39
  kidney 277.39 [583.81]
  liver 277.39
Large
  baby (regardless of gestational age) 766.1
    exceptionally (weight of 4500 grams or
      more) 766.0
    of diabetic mother 775.0
  ear 744.22
  fetus - *see also* Oversize, fetus
    causing disproportion 653.5 ●
      with obstructed labor 660.1 ●
  for dates
    fetus or newborn (regardless of
      gestational age) 766.1
      affecting management of pregnancy
        656.6 ●
    exceptionally (weight of 4500 grams or
      more) 766.0
  physiological cup 743.57
  stature 783.9
  waxy liver 277.39
  white kidney - *see* Nephrosis
Larsen's syndrome (flattened facies and
  multiple congenital dislocations) 755.8
Larsen-Johansson disease (juvenile osteopathia
  patellae) 732.4
Larva migrans
  cutaneous NEC 126.9
    ancylostoma 126.9
  of Diptera in vitreous 128.0
  visceral NEC 128.0
Laryngeal - *see also* condition
  syncope 786.2
Laryngismus (acute) (infectious) (stridulous)
  478.75
  congenital 748.3
  diphtheritic 032.3

Laryngitis (acute) (edematous) (fibrinous)
  (gangrenous) (infective) (infiltrative)
  (malignant) (membranous)
  (phlegmonous) (pneumococcal)
  (pseudomembranous) (septic) (subglottic)
  (suppurative) (ulcerative) (viral) 464.00
  with
    influenza, flu, or grippe *(see also*
      Influenza) 487.1
    obstruction 464.01
    tracheitis *(see also* Laryngotracheitis)
      464.20
      with obstruction 464.21
      acute 464.20
        with obstruction 464.21
      chronic 476.1
  atrophic 476.0
  Borrelia vincentii 101
  catarrhal 476.0
  chronic 476.0
    with tracheitis (chronic) 476.1
    due to external agent - *see* Condition,
      respiratory, chronic, due to
  diphtheritic (membranous) 032.3
  due to external agent - *see* Inflammation,
    respiratory, upper, due to
  H. influenzae 464.00
    with obstruction 464.01
  Hemophilus influenzae 464.00
    with obstruction 464.01
  hypertrophic 476.0
  influenzal *(see also* Influenza) 487.1
  pachydermic 478.79
  sicca 476.0
  spasmodic 478.75
    acute 464.00
      with obstruction 464.01
  streptococcal 034.0
  stridulous 478.75
  syphilitic 095.8
    congenital 090.5
  tuberculous *(see also* Tuberculosis, larynx)
    012.3 ●
  Vincent's 101
Laryngocele (congenital) (ventricular) 748.3
Laryngofissure 478.79
  congenital 748.3
Laryngomalacia (congenital) 748.3
Laryngopharyngitis (acute) 465.0
  chronic 478.9
    due to external agent - *see* Condition,
      respiratory, chronic, due to
  due to external agent - *see* Inflammation,
    respiratory, upper, due to
  septic 034.0
Laryngoplegia *(see also* Paralysis, vocal cord)
  478.30
Laryngoptosis 478.79
Laryngospasm 478.75
  due to external agent - *see* Condition,
    respiratory, acute, due to
Laryngostenosis 478.74
  congenital 748.3
Laryngotracheitis (acute) (infectional) (viral)
  (see also Laryngitis) 464.20
  with obstruction 464.21
  atrophic 476.1
  Borrelia vincentii 101
  catarrhal 476.1
  chronic 476.1
    due to external agent - *see* Condition,
      respiratory, chronic, due to
  diphtheritic (membranous) 032.3
  due to external agent - *see* Inflammation,
    respiratory, upper, due to
  H. influenzae 464.20
    with obstruction 464.21
  hypertrophic 476.1
  influenzal *(see also* Influenza) 487.1
  pachydermic 478.75
  sicca 476.1

◄ New   ◄▥ Revised   ~~deleted~~ Deleted   ● Use Additional Digit(s)   ▨ Omit code

Laryngotracheitis *(Continued)*
  spasmodic 478.75
    acute 464.20
      with obstruction 464.21
  streptococcal 034.0
  stridulous 478.75
  syphilitic 095.8
    congenital 090.5
  tuberculous *(see also* Tuberculosis, larynx)
    012.3●
  Vincent's 101
Laryngotracheobronchitis *(see also* Bronchitis)
    490
  acute 466.0
  chronic 491.8
  viral 466.0
Laryngotracheobronchopneumonitis - *see*
    Pneumonia, broncho-
Larynx, laryngeal - *see* condition
Lasègue's disease (persecution mania) 297.9
Lassa fever 078.89
Lassitude *(see also* Weakness) 780.79
Late - *see also* condition
  effect(s) (of) - *see also* condition
    abscess
      intracranial or intraspinal (conditions
        classifiable to 324) - *see* category
        326
    adverse effect of drug, medicinal or
      biological substance 909.5
    allergic reaction 909.9
    amputation
      postoperative (late) 997.60
      traumatic (injury classifiable to
        885–887 and 895–897) 905.9
    burn (injury classifiable to 948–949) 906.9
      extremities NEC (injury classifiable to
        943 or 945) 906.7
        hand or wrist (injury classifiable to
          944) 906.6
      eye (injury classifiable to 940) 906.5
      face, head, and neck (injury classifiable
        to 941) 906.5
      specified site NEC (injury classifiable
        to 942 and 946–947) 906.8
    cerebrovascular disease (conditions
      classifiable to 430–437) 438.9
      with
        alterations of sensations 438.6
        aphasia 438.11
        apraxia 438.81
        ataxia 438.84
        cognitive deficits 438.0
        disturbances of vision 438.7
        dysarthria 438.13
        dysphagia 438.82
        dysphasia 438.12
        facial droop 438.83
        facial weakness 438.83
        fluency disorder 438.14
        hemiplegia/hemiparesis
          affecting
            dominant side 438.21
            nondominant side 438.22
            unspecified side 438.20
        monoplegia of lower limb
          affecting
            dominant side 438.41
            nondominant side 438.42
            unspecified side 438.40
        monoplegia of upper limb
          affecting
            dominant side 438.31
            nondominant side 438.32
            unspecified side 438.30
        paralytic syndrome NEC
          affecting
            bilateral 438.53
            dominant side 438.51
            nondominant side 438.52
            unspecified side 438.50

Late *(Continued)*
  effect(s) *(Continued)*
    cerebrovascular disease *(Continued)*
      with *(Continued)*
        speech and language deficit
          438.10
          specified type NEC 438.19
        stuttering 438.14
        vertigo 438.85
        specified type NEC 438.89
    childbirth complication(s) 677
    complication(s) of
      childbirth 677
      delivery 677
      pregnancy 677
      puerperium 677
      surgical and medical care (conditions
        classifiable to 996–999) 909.3
      trauma (conditions classifiable to 958)
        908.6
    contusion (injury classifiable to 920–924)
      906.3
    crushing (injury classifiable to 925–929)
      906.4
    delivery complication(s) 677
    dislocation (injury classifiable to 830–839)
      905.6
    encephalitis or encephalomyelitis
      (conditions classifiable to 323) - *see*
      category 326
      in infectious diseases 139.8
        viral (conditions classifiable to
          049.8, 049.9, 062–064) 139.0
    external cause NEC (conditions
      classifiable to 995) 909.9
      certain conditions classifiable to
        categories 991–994 909.4
    foreign body in orifice (injury classifiable
      to 930–939) 908.5
    fracture (multiple) (injury classifiable to
      828–829) 905.5
      extremity
        lower (injury classifiable to
          821–827) 905.4
          neck of femur (injury classifiable
            to 820) 905.3
        upper (injury classifiable to
          810–819) 905.2
      face and skull (injury classifiable to
        800–804) 905.0
      skull and face (injury classifiable to
        800–804) 905.0
      spine and trunk (injury classifiable to
        805 and 807–809) 905.1
        with spinal cord lesion (injury
          classifiable to 806) 907.2
    infection
      pyogenic, intracranial - *see* category
        326
    infectious diseases (conditions classifiable
      to 001–136) NEC 139.8
    injury (injury classifiable to 959)
      908.9
      blood vessel 908.3
        abdomen and pelvis (injury
          classifiable to 902) 908.4
        extremity (injury classifiable to
          903–904) 908.3
        head and neck (injury classifiable to
          900) 908.3
        intracranial (injury classifiable to
          850–854) 907.0
          with skull fracture 905.0
        thorax (injury classifiable to 901)
          908.4
      internal organ NEC (injury classifiable
        to 867 and 869) 908.2
        abdomen (injury classifiable to
          863–866 and 868) 908.1
        thorax (injury classifiable to
          860–862) 908.0

Late *(Continued)*
  effect(s) *(Continued)*
    injury *(Continued)*
      intracranial (injury classifiable to
        850–854) 907.0
        with skull fracture (injury
          classifiable to 800–801 and
          803–804) 905.0
      nerve NEC (injury classifiable to 957)
        907.9
        cranial (injury classifiable to
          950–951) 907.1
        peripheral NEC (injury classifiable
          to 957) 907.9
          lower limb and pelvic girdle
            (injury classifiable to 956)
            907.5
          upper limb and shoulder girdle
            (injury classifiable to 955)
            907.4
        roots and plexus(es), spinal (injury
          classifiable to 953) 907.3
        trunk (injury classifiable to 954)
          907.3
      spinal
        cord (injury classifiable to 806 and
          952) 907.2
        nerve root(s) and plexus(es) (injury
          classifiable to 953) 907.3
      superficial (injury classifiable to
        910–919) 906.2
      tendon (tendon injury classifiable to
        840–848, 880–884 with .2, and
        890–894 with .2) 905.8
    meningitis
      bacterial (conditions classifiable to
        320) - *see* category 326
      unspecified cause (conditions
        classifiable to 322) - *see* category
        326
    myelitis *(see also* Late, effect(s) (of),
      encephalitis) - *see* category 326
    parasitic diseases (conditions classifiable
      to 001–136 NEC) 139.8
    phlebitis or thrombophlebitis of
      intracranial venous sinuses
      (conditions classifiable to 325) - *see*
      category 326
    poisoning due to drug, medicinal or
      biological substance (conditions
      classifiable to 960–979) 909.0
    poliomyelitis, acute (conditions
      classifiable to 045) 138
    pregnancy complication(s) 677
    puerperal complication(s) 677
    radiation (conditions classifiable to 990)
      909.2
    rickets 268.1
    sprain and strain without mention of
      tendon injury (injury classifiable to
      840–848, except tendon injury) 905.7
      tendon involvement 905.8
    toxic effect of
      drug, medicinal or biological substance
        (conditions classifiable to
        960–979) 909.0
      nonmedical substance (conditions
        classifiable to 980–989) 909.1
    trachoma (conditions classifiable to 076)
      139.1
    tuberculosis 137.0
      bones and joints (conditions
        classifiable to 015) 137.3
      central nervous system (conditions
        classifiable to 013) 137.1
      genitourinary (conditions classifiable
        to 016) 137.2
      pulmonary (conditions classifiable to
        010–012) 137.0
      specified organs NEC (conditions
        classifiable to 014, 017–018) 137.4

Late (Continued)
  effect(s) (Continued)
    viral encephalitis (conditions classifiable to 049.8, 049.9, 062–064) 139.0
    wound, open
      extremity (injury classifiable to 880–884 and 890–894, except .2) 906.1
        tendon (injury classifiable to 880–884 with .2 and 890–894 with .2) 905.8
      head, neck, and trunk (injury classifiable to 870–879) 906.0
  infant
    post-term (gestation period over 40 completed weeks to 42 completed weeks) 766.21
    prolonged gestation (period over 42 completed weeks) 766.22
Latent - see condition
Lateral - see condition
Laterocession - see Lateroversion
Lateroflexion - see Lateroversion
Lateroversion
  cervix - see Lateroversion, uterus
  uterus, uterine (cervix) (postinfectional) (postpartal, old) 621.6
    congenital 752.39
    in pregnancy or childbirth 654.4 ●
      affecting fetus or newborn 763.89
Lathyrism 988.2
Launois' syndrome (pituitary gigantism) 253.0
Launois-Bensaude's lipomatosis 272.8
Launois-Cleret syndrome (adiposogenital dystrophy) 253.8
Laurence-Moon-Biedl syndrome (obesity, polydactyly, and intellectual disabilities) 759.89
LAV (disease) (illness) (infection) - see Human immunodeficiency virus (disease) (illness) (infection)
LAV/HTLV-III (disease) (illness) (infection) - see Human immunodeficiency virus (disease) (illness) (infection)
Lawford's syndrome (encephalocutaneous angiomatosis) 759.6
Lax, laxity - see also Relaxation
  ligament 728.4
  skin (acquired) 701.8
    congenital 756.83
Laxative habit (see also Abuse, drugs, nondependent) 305.9 ●
Lazy leukocyte syndrome 288.09
LCAD (long chain/very long chain acyl CoA dehydrogenase deficiency, VLCAD) 277.85
LCHAD (long chain 3-hydroxyacyl CoA dehydrogenase deficiency) 277.85
Lead - see also condition
  exposure (suspected) to V15.86
  incrustation of cornea 371.15
  poisoning 984.9
    specified type of lead - see Table of Drugs and Chemicals
Lead miners' lung 503
Leakage
  amniotic fluid 658.1 ●
    with delayed delivery 658.2 ●
    affecting fetus or newborn 761.1
  bile from drainage tube (T tube) 997.49
  blood (microscopic), fetal, into maternal circulation 656.0 ●
    affecting management of pregnancy or puerperium 656.0 ●
  device, implant, or graft - see Complications, mechanical
  spinal fluid at lumbar puncture site 997.09
  urine, continuous 788.37
Leaky heart - see Endocarditis
Learning defect, specific NEC (strephosymbolia) 315.2

Leather bottle stomach (M8142/3) 151.9
Leber's
  congenital amaurosis 362.76
  optic atrophy (hereditary) 377.16
Lederer's anemia or disease (acquired infectious hemolytic anemia) 283.19
Lederer-Brill syndrome (acquired infectious hemolytic anemia) 283.19
Leeches (aquatic) (land) 134.2
Left-sided neglect 781.8
Leg - see condition
Legal investigation V62.5
Legg (-Calvé)-Perthes disease or syndrome (osteochondrosis, femoral capital) 732.1
Legionnaires' disease 482.84
Leigh's disease 330.8
Leiner's disease (exfoliative dermatitis) 695.89
Leiofibromyoma (M8890/0) - see also Leiomyoma
  uterus (cervix) (corpus) (see also Leiomyoma, uterus) 218.9
Leiomyoblastoma (M8891/1) - see Neoplasm, connective tissue, uncertain behavior
Leiomyofibroma (M8890/0) - see also Neoplasm, connective tissue, benign
  uterus (cervix) (corpus) (see also Leiomyoma, uterus) 218.9
Leiomyoma (M8890/0) - see also Neoplasm, connective tissue, benign
  bizarre (M8893/0) - see Neoplasm, connective tissue, benign
  cellular (M8892/1) - see Neoplasm, connective tissue, uncertain behavior
  epithelioid (M8891/1) - see Neoplasm, connective tissue, uncertain behavior
  prostate (polypoid) 600.20
    with
      other lower urinary tract symptoms (LUTS) 600.21
      urinary
        obstruction 600.21
        retention 600.21
  uterus (cervix) (corpus) 218.9
    interstitial 218.1
    intramural 218.1
    submucous 218.0
    subperitoneal 218.2
    subserous 218.2
  vascular (M8894/0) - see Neoplasm, connective tissue, benign
Leiomyomatosis (intravascular) (M8890/1) - see Neoplasm, connective tissue, uncertain behavior
Leiomyosarcoma (M8890/3) - see also Neoplasm, connective tissue, malignant
  epithelioid (M8891/3) - see Neoplasm, connective tissue, malignant
Leishmaniasis 085.9
  American 085.5
    cutaneous 085.4
    mucocutaneous 085.5
  Asian desert 085.2
  Brazilian 085.5
  cutaneous 085.9
    acute necrotizing 085.2
    American 085.4
    Asian desert 085.2
    diffuse 085.3
    dry form 085.1
    Ethiopian 085.3
    eyelid 085.5 [373.6]
    late 085.1
    lepromatous 085.3
    recurrent 085.1
    rural 085.2
    ulcerating 085.1
    urban 085.1
    wet form 085.2
    zoonotic form 085.2
  dermal - see also Leishmaniasis, cutaneous
    post kala-azar 085.0

Leishmaniasis (Continued)
  eyelid 085.5 [373.6]
  infantile 085.0
  Mediterranean 085.0
  mucocutaneous (American) 085.5
  naso-oral 085.5
  nasopharyngeal 085.5
  Old World 085.1
  tegumentaria diffusa 085.4
  vaccination, prophylactic (against) V05.2
  visceral (Indian) 085.0
Leishmanoid, dermal - see also Leishmaniasis, cutaneous
  post kala-azar 085.0
Leloir's disease 695.4
Lemiere syndrome 451.89
Lenegre's disease 426.0
Lengthening, leg 736.81
Lennox-Gastaut syndrome 345.0 ●
  with tonic seizures 345.1 ●
Lennox's syndrome (see also Epilepsy) 345.0 ●
Lens - see condition
Lenticonus (anterior) (posterior) (congenital) 743.36
Lenticular degeneration, progressive 275.1
Lentiglobus (posterior) (congenital) 743.36
Lentigo (congenital) 709.09
  juvenile 709.09
  Maligna (M8742/2) - see also Neoplasm, skin, in situ
    melanoma (M8742/3) - see Melanoma
  senile 709.09
Leonine leprosy 030.0
Leontiasis
  ossium 733.3
  syphilitic 095.8
    congenital 090.5
Léopold-Lévi's syndrome (paroxysmal thyroid instability) 242.9 ●
Lepore hemoglobin syndrome 282.45
Lepothrix 039.0
Lepra 030.9
  Willan's 696.1
Leprechaunism 259.8
Lepromatous leprosy 030.0
Leprosy 030.9
  anesthetic 030.1
  beriberi 030.1
  borderline (group B) (infiltrated) (neuritic) 030.3
  cornea (see also Leprosy, by type) 030.9 [371.89]
  dimorphous (group B) (infiltrated) (lepromatous) (neuritic) (tuberculoid) 030.3
  eyelid 030.0 [373.4]
  indeterminate (group I) (macular) (neuritic) (uncharacteristic) 030.2
  leonine 030.0
  lepromatous (diffuse) (infiltrated) (macular) (neuritic) (nodular) (type L) 030.0
  macular (early) (neuritic) (simple) 030.2
  maculoanesthetic 030.1
  mixed 030.0
  neuro 030.1
  nodular 030.0
  primary neuritic 030.3
  specified type or group NEC 030.8
  tubercular 030.1
  tuberculoid (macular) (maculoanesthetic) (major) (minor) (neuritic) (type T) 030.1
Leptocytosis, hereditary 282.40
Leptomeningitis (chronic) (circumscribed) (hemorrhagic) (nonsuppurative) (see also Meningitis) 322.9
  aseptic 047.9
    adenovirus 049.1
    Coxsackie virus 047.0
    ECHO virus 047.1
    enterovirus 047.9
    lymphocytic choriomeningitis 049.0

◀ New   ◀╌ Revised   ~~deleted~~ Deleted   ● Use Additional Digit(s)   ▨ Omit code

Leptomeningitis *(Continued)*
  epidemic 036.0
  late effect - *see* category 326
  meningococcal 036.0
  pneumococcal 320.1
  syphilitic 094.2
  tuberculous *(see also* Tuberculosis, meninges)
    013.0●
Leptomeningopathy *(see also* Meningitis)
  322.9
Leptospiral - *see* condition
Leptospirochetal - *see* condition
Leptospirosis 100.9
  autumnalis 100.89
  canicula 100.89
  grippotyphosa 100.89
  hebdomadis 100.89
  icterohemorrhagica 100.0
  nanukayami 100.89
  pomona 100.89
  Weil's disease 100.0
Leptothricosis - *see* Actinomycosis
Leptothrix infestation - *see* Actinomycosis
Leptotricosis - *see* Actinomycosis
Leptus dermatitis 133.8
Léris pleonosteosis 756.89
Léri-Weill syndrome 756.59
Leriche's syndrome (aortic bifurcation
  occlusion) 444.09
Lermoyez's syndrome *(see also* Disease,
  Ménière's) 386.00
Lesbianism - omit code
  ego-dystonic 302.0
  problems with 302.0
Lesch-Nyhan syndrome (hypoxanthine-
  guanine-phosphoribosyltransferase
  deficiency) 277.2
Lesion(s)
  abducens nerve 378.54
  alveolar process 525.8
  anorectal 569.49
  aortic (valve) - *see* Endocarditis, aortic
  auditory nerve 388.5
  basal ganglion 333.90
  bile duct *(see also* Disease, biliary) 576.8
  bladder 596.9
  bone 733.90
  brachial plexus 353.0
  brain 348.89
    congenital 742.9
    vascular *(see also* Lesion, cerebrovascular)
      437.9
      degenerative 437.1
      healed or old without residuals V12.54
      hypertensive 437.2
      late effect - *see* Late effect(s) (of)
        cerebrovascular disease
  buccal 528.9
  calcified - *see* Calcification
  canthus 373.9
  carate - *see* Pinta, lesions
  cardia 537.89
  cardiac - *see also* Disease, heart
    congenital 746.9
    valvular - *see* Endocarditis
  cauda equina 344.60
    with neurogenic bladder 344.61
  cecum 569.89
  cerebral - *see* Lesion, brain
  cerebrovascular *(see also* Disease,
    cerebrovascular NEC) 437.9
    degenerative 437.1
    healed or old without residuals V12.54
    hypertensive 437.2
    specified type NEC 437.8
  cervical root (nerve) NEC 353.2
  chiasmal 377.54
    associated with
      inflammatory disorders 377.54
      neoplasm NEC 377.52
        pituitary 377.51

Lesion(s) *(Continued)*
  chiasmal *(Continued)*
    associated with *(Continued)*
      pituitary disorders 377.51
      vascular disorders 377.53
  chorda tympani 351.8
  coin, lung 793.11
  colon 569.89
  congenital - *see* Anomaly
  conjunctiva 372.9
  coronary artery *(see also* Ischemia, heart)
    414.9
  cranial nerve 352.9
    first 352.0
    second 377.49
    third
      partial 378.51
      total 378.52
    fourth 378.53
    fifth 350.9
    sixth 378.54
    seventh 351.9
    eighth 388.5
    ninth 352.2
    tenth 352.3
    eleventh 352.4
    twelfth 352.5
  cystic - *see* Cyst
  degenerative - *see* Degeneration
  dermal (skin) 709.9
  Dieulafoy (hemorrhagic)
    of
      duodenum 537.84
      intestine 569.86
      stomach 537.84
  duodenum 537.89
    with obstruction 537.3
  eyelid 373.9
  gasserian ganglion 350.8
  gastric 537.89
  gastroduodenal 537.89
  gastrointestinal 569.89
  glossopharyngeal nerve 352.2
  heart (organic) - *see also* Disease, heart
    vascular - *see* Disease, cardiovascular
  helix (ear) 709.9
  high grade myelodysplastic syndrome 238.73
  hyperchromic, due to pinta (carate) 103.1
  hyperkeratotic *(see also* Hyperkeratosis) 701.1
  hypoglossal nerve 352.5
  hypopharynx 478.29
  hypothalamic 253.9
  ileocecal coil 569.89
  ileum 569.89
  iliohypogastric nerve 355.79
  ilioinguinal nerve 355.79
  in continuity - *see* Injury, nerve, by site
  inflammatory - *see* Inflammation
  intestine 569.89
  intracerebral - *see* Lesion, brain
  intrachiasmal (optic) *(see also* Lesion,
    chiasmal) 377.54
  intracranial, space-occupying NEC 784.2
  joint 719.90
    ankle 719.97
    elbow 719.92
    foot 719.97
    hand 719.94
    hip 719.95
    knee 719.96
    multiple sites 719.99
    pelvic region 719.95
    sacroiliac (old) 724.6
    shoulder (region) 719.91
    specified site NEC 719.98
    wrist 719.93
  keratotic *(see also* Keratosis) 701.1
  kidney *(see also* Disease, renal) 593.9
  laryngeal nerve (recurrent) 352.3
  leonine 030.0
  lip 528.5

Lesion(s) *(Continued)*
  liver 573.8
  low grade myelodysplastic syndrome 238.72
  lumbosacral
    plexus 353.1
    root (nerve) NEC 353.4
  lung 518.89
    coin 793.11
  maxillary sinus 473.0
  mitral - *see* Endocarditis, mitral
  Morel Lavallée - *see* Hematoma, by site
  motor cortex 348.89
  nerve *(see also* Disorder, nerve) 355.9
  nervous system 349.9
    congenital 742.9
  nonallopathic NEC 739.9
    in region (of)
      abdomen 739.9
      acromioclavicular 739.7
      cervical, cervicothoracic 739.1
      costochondral 739.8
      costovertebral 739.8
      extremity
        lower 739.6
        upper 739.7
      head 739.0
      hip 739.5
      lower extremity 739.6
      lumbar, lumbosacral 739.3
      occipitocervical 739.0
      pelvic 739.5
      pubic 739.5
      rib cage 739.8
      sacral, sacrococcygeal, sacroiliac 739.4
      sternochondral 739.8
      sternoclavicular 739.7
      thoracic, thoracolumbar 739.2
      upper extremity 739.7
  nose (internal) 478.19
  obstructive - *see* Obstruction
  obturator nerve 355.79
  occlusive
    artery - *see* Embolism, artery
  organ or site NEC - *see* Disease, by site
  osteolytic 733.90
  paramacular, of retina 363.32
  peptic 537.89
  periodontal, due to traumatic occlusion 523.8
  perirectal 569.49
  peritoneum (granulomatous) 568.89
  pigmented (skin) 709.00
  pinta - *see* Pinta, lesions
  polypoid - *see* Polyp
  prechiasmal (optic) *(see also* Lesion, chiasmal)
    377.54
  primary - *see also* Syphilis, primary
    carate 103.0
    pinta 103.0
    yaws 102.0
  pulmonary 518.89
    valve *(see also* Endocarditis, pulmonary)
      424.3
  pylorus 537.89
  radiation NEC 990
  radium NEC 990
  rectosigmoid 569.89
  retina, retinal - *see also* Retinopathy
    vascular 362.17
  retroperitoneal 568.89
  romanus 720.1
  sacroiliac (joint) 724.6
  salivary gland 527.8
    benign lymphoepithelial 527.8
  saphenous nerve 355.79
  secondary - *see* Syphilis, secondary
  sigmoid 569.89
  sinus (accessory) (nasal) *(see also* Sinusitis)
    473.9
  skin 709.9
    suppurative 686.00
  SLAP (superior glenoid labrum) 840.7

Lesion(s) (Continued)
  space-occupying, intracranial NEC 784.2
  spinal cord 336.9
    congenital 742.9
    traumatic (complete) (incomplete)
        (transverse) - see also Injury, spinal,
        by site
      with
        broken
          back - see Fracture, vertebra, by
            site, with spinal cord
            injury
          neck - see Fracture, vertebra,
            cervical, with spinal cord
            injury
        fracture, vertebra - see Fracture,
          vertebra, by site, with spinal
          cord injury
  spleen 289.50
  stomach 537.89
  superior glenoid labrum (SLAP) 840.7
  syphilitic - see Syphilis
  tertiary - see Syphilis, tertiary
  thoracic root (nerve) 353.3
  tonsillar fossa 474.9
  tooth, teeth 525.8
    white spot 521.01
  traumatic NEC (see also nature and site of
    injury) 959.9
  tricuspid (valve) - see Endocarditis, tricuspid
  trigeminal nerve 350.9
  ulcerated or ulcerative - see Ulcer
  uterus NEC 621.9
  vagina 623.8
  vagus nerve 352.3
  valvular - see Endocarditis
  vascular 459.9
    affecting central nervous system (see also
      Lesion, cerebrovascular) 437.9
    following trauma (see also Injury, blood
      vessel, by site) 904.9
    retina 362.17
    traumatic - see Injury, blood vessel, by site
    umbilical cord 663.6 ●
      affecting fetus or newborn 762.6
  visual
    cortex NEC (see also Disorder, visual,
      cortex) 377.73
    pathway NEC (see also Disorder, visual,
      pathway) 377.63
  warty - see Verruca
  white spot, on teeth 521.01
  x-ray NEC 990
Lethargic - see condition
Lethargy 780.79
Letterer-Siwe disease (acute histiocytosis X)
  (M9722/3) 202.5 ●
Leucinosis 270.3
Leucocoria 360.44
Leucosarcoma (M9850/3) 207.8 ●
Leukasmus 270.2
Leukemia, leukemic (congenital) (M9800/3)
  208.9 ●

Note: Use the following fifth-digit
subclassification for categories 203–208:

  0 without mention of having
     achieved remission
       failed remission
  1 with remission
  2 in relapse

---

  acute NEC (M9801/3) 208.0 ●
  aleukemic NEC (M9804/3) 208.8 ●
    granulocytic (M9864/3) 205.8 ●
  basophilic (M9870/3) 205.1 ●
  blast (cell) (M9801/3) 208.0 ●
  blastic (M9801/3) 208.0 ●
    granulocytic (M9861/3) 205.0 ●
  chronic NEC (M9803/3) 208.1 ●
  compound (M9810/3) 207.8 ●

Leukemia, leukemic (Continued)
  eosinophilic (M9880/3) 205.1 ●
  giant cell (M9910/3) 207.2 ●
  granulocytic (M9860/3) 205.9 ●
    acute (M9861/3) 205.0 ●
    aleukemic (M9864/3) 205.8 ●
    blastic (M9861/3) 205.0 ●
    chronic (M9863/3) 205.1 ●
    subacute (M9862/3) 205.2 ●
    subleukemic (M9864/3) 205.8 ●
  hairy cell (M9940/3) 202.4 ●
  hemoblastic (M9801/3) 208.0 ●
  histiocytic (M9890/3) 206.9 ●
  lymphatic (M9820/3) 204.9 ●
    acute (M9821/3) 204.0 ●
    aleukemic (M9824/3) 204.8 ●
    chronic (M9823/3) 204.1 ●
    subacute (M9822/3) 204.2 ●
    subleukemic (M9824/3) 204.8 ●
  lymphoblastic (M9821/3) 204.0 ●
  lymphocytic (M9820/3) 204.9 ●
    acute (M9821/3) 204.0 ●
    aleukemic (M9824/3) 204.8 ●
    chronic (M9823/3) 204.1 ●
    granular
      large T-cell 204.8 ●
    subacute (M9822/3) 204.2 ●
    subleukemic (M9824/3) 204.8 ●
  lymphogenous (M9820/3) - see Leukemia,
    lymphoid
  lymphoid (M9820/3) 204.9 ●
    acute (M9821/3) 204.0 ●
    aleukemic (M9824/3) 204.8 ●
    blastic (M9821/3) 204.0 ●
    chronic (M9823/3) 204.1 ●
    subacute (M9822/3) 204.2 ●
    subleukemic (M9824/3) 204.8 ●
  lymphosarcoma cell (M9850/3) 207.8 ●
  mast cell (M9900/3) 207.8 ●
  megakaryocytic (M9910/3) 207.2 ●
  megakaryocytoid (M9910/3) 207.2 ●
  mixed (cell) (M9810/3) 207.8 ●
  monoblastic (M9891/3) 206.0 ●
  monocytic (Schilling-type) (M9890/3) 206.9 ●
    acute (M9891/3) 206.0 ●
    aleukemic (M9894/3) 206.8 ●
    chronic (M9893/3) 206.1 ●
    Naegeli-type (M9863/3) 205.1 ●
    subacute (M9892/3) 206.2 ●
    subleukemic (M9894/3) 206.8 ●
  monocytoid (M9890/3) 206.9 ●
    acute (M9891/3) 206.0 ●
    aleukemic (M9894/3) 206.8 ●
    chronic (M9893/3) 206.1 ●
    myelogenous (M9863/3) 205.1 ●
    subacute (M9892/3) 206.2 ●
    subleukemic (M9894/3) 206.8 ●
  monomyelocytic (M9860/3) - see Leukemia,
    myelomonocytic
  myeloblastic (M9861/3) 205.0 ●
  myelocytic (M9863/3) 205.1 ●
    acute (M9861/3) 205.0 ●
  myelogenous (M9860/3) 205.9 ●
    acute (M9861/3) 205.0 ●
    aleukemic (M9864/3) 205.8 ●
    chronic (M9863/3) 205.1 ●
    monocytoid (M9863/3) 205.1 ●
    subacute (M9862/3) 205.2 ●
    subleukemic (M9864) 205.8 ●
  myeloid (M9860/3) 205.9 ●
    acute (M9861/3) 205.0 ●
    aleukemic (M9864/3) 205.8 ●
    chronic (M9863/3) 205.1 ●
    subacute (M9862/3) 205.2 ●
    subleukemic (M9864/3) 205.8 ●
  myelomonocytic (M9860/3) 205.9 ●
    acute (M9861/3) 205.0 ●
    chronic (M9863/3) 205.1 ●
  Naegeli-type monocytic (M9863/3) 205.1 ●
  neutrophilic (M9865/3) 205.1 ●
  plasma cell (M9830/3) 203.1 ●

Leukemia, leukemic (Continued)
  plasmacytic (M9830/3) 203.1 ●
  prolymphocytic (M9825/3) - see Leukemia,
    lymphoid
  promyelocytic, acute (M9866/3) 205.0 ●
  Schilling-type monocytic (M9890/3) - see
    Leukemia, monocytic
  stem cell (M9801/3) 208.0 ●
  subacute NEC (M9802/3) 208.2 ●
  subleukemic NEC (M9804/3) 208.8 ●
  thrombocytic (M9910/3) 207.2 ●
  undifferentiated (M9801/3) 208.0 ●
Leukemoid reaction (basophilic) (lymphocytic)
  (monocytic) (myelocytic) (neutrophilic)
  288.62
Leukoaraiosis (hypertensive) 437.1
Leukoariosis - see Leukoaraiosis
Leukoclastic vasculitis 446.29
Leukocoria 360.44
Leukocythemia - see Leukemia
Leukocytopenia 288.50
Leukocytosis 288.60
  basophilic 288.8
  eosinophilic 288.3
  lymphocytic 288.8
  monocytic 288.8
  neutrophilic 288.8
Leukoderma 709.09
  syphilitic 091.3
    late 095.8
Leukodermia (see also Leukoderma) 709.09
Leukodystrophy (cerebral) (globoid cell)
  (metachromatic) (progressive)
  (sudanophilic) 330.0
Leukoedema, mouth or tongue 528.79
Leukoencephalitis
  acute hemorrhagic (postinfectious) NEC
    136.9 [323.61]
    postimmunization or postvaccinal 323.51
  subacute sclerosing 046.2
    van Bogaert's 046.2
  van Bogaert's (sclerosing) 046.2
Leukoencephalopathy (see also Encephalitis)
  323.9
  acute necrotizing hemorrhagic
    (postinfectious) 136.9 [323.61]
    postimmunization or postvaccinal 323.51
  arteriosclerotic 437.0
  Binswanger's 290.12
  metachromatic 330.0
  multifocal (progressive) 046.3
  progressive multifocal 046.3
  reversible, posterior 348.5
Leukoerythroblastosis 289.9
Leukoerythrosis 289.0
Leukokeratosis (see also Leukoplakia) 702.8
  mouth 528.6
  nicotina palati 528.79
  tongue 528.6
Leukokoria 360.44
Leukokraurosis vulva, vulvae 624.09
Leukolymphosarcoma (M9850/3) 207.8 ●
Leukoma (cornea) (interfering with central
  vision) 371.03
  adherent 371.04
Leukomalacia, periventricular 779.7
Leukomelanopathy, hereditary 288.2
Leukonychia (punctata) (striata) 703.8
  congenital 757.5
Leukopathia
  unguium 703.8
    congenital 757.5
Leukopenia 288.50
  basophilic 288.59
  cyclic 288.02
  eosinophilic 288.59
  familial 288.59
  malignant (see also Agranulocytosis)
    288.09
  periodic 288.02
  transitory neonatal 776.7

◀ New   ◀┅ Revised   deleted Deleted   ● Use Additional Digit(s)   ▨ Omit code

Leukopenic - *see* condition
Leukoplakia 702.8
  anus 569.49
  bladder (postinfectional) 596.89
  buccal 528.6
  cervix (uteri) 622.2
  esophagus 530.83
  gingiva 528.6
  kidney (pelvis) 593.89
  larynx 478.79
  lip 528.6
  mouth 528.6
  oral soft tissue (including tongue) (mucosa)
    528.6
  palate 528.6
  pelvis (kidney) 593.89
  penis (infectional) 607.0
  rectum 569.49
  syphilitic 095.8
  tongue 528.6
  tonsil 478.29
  ureter (postinfectional) 593.89
  urethra (postinfectional) 599.84
  uterus 621.8
  vagina 623.1
  vesical 596.89
  vocal cords 478.5
  vulva 624.09
Leukopolioencephalopathy 330.0
Leukorrhea (vagina) 623.5
  due to Trichomonas (vaginalis) 131.00
  trichomonal (Trichomonas vaginalis)
    131.00
Leukosarcoma (M9850/3) 207.8●
Leukosis (M9800/3) - *see* Leukemia
Lev's disease or syndrome (acquired complete
  heart block) 426.0
Levi's syndrome (pituitary dwarfism) 253.3
Levocardia (isolated) 746.87
  with situs inversus 759.3
Levulosuria 271.2
Lewandowski's disease (primary) (*see also*
  Tuberculosis) 017.0●
Lewandowski-Lutz disease
  (epidermodysplasia verruciformis)
  078.19
Lewy body dementia 331.82
Lewy body disease 331.82
Leyden's disease (periodic vomiting) 536.2
Leyden-Möbius dystrophy 359.1
Leydig cell
  carcinoma (M8650/3)
    specified site - *see* Neoplasm, by site,
      malignant
    unspecified site
      female 183.0
      male 186.9
  tumor (M8650/1)
    benign (M8650/0)
      specified site - *see* Neoplasm, by site,
        benign
      unspecified site
        female 220
        male 222.0
    malignant (M8650/3)
      specified site - *see* Neoplasm, by site,
        malignant
      unspecified site
        female 183.0
        male 186.9
    specified site - *see* Neoplasm, by site,
      uncertain behavior
    unspecified site
      female 236.2
      male 236.4
Leydig-Sertoli cell tumor (M8631/0)
  specified site - *see* Neoplasm, by site,
    benign
  unspecified site
    female 220
    male 222.0

LGSIL (low grade squamous intraepithelial
  lesion)
  anus 796.73
  cervix 795.03
  vagina 795.13
Liar, pathologic 301.7
Libman-Sacks disease or syndrome 710.0
  [424.91]
Lice (infestation) 132.9
  body (pediculus corporis) 132.1
  crab 132.2
  head (pediculus capitis) 132.0
  mixed (classifiable to more than one of the
    categories 132.0–132.2) 132.3
  pubic (pediculus pubis) 132.2
Lichen 697.9
  albus 701.0
  annularis 695.89
  atrophicus 701.0
  corneus obtusus 698.3
  myxedematous 701.8
  nitidus 697.1
  pilaris 757.39
    acquired 701.1
  planopilaris 697.0
  planus (acute) (chronicus) (hypertrophic)
    (verrucous) 697.0
    morphoeicus 701.0
    sclerosus (et atrophicus) 701.0
  ruber 696.4
    acuminatus 696.4
    moniliformis 697.8
    obtusus corneus 698.3
    of Wilson 697.0
    planus 697.0
  sclerosus (et atrophicus) 701.0
  scrofulosus (primary) (*see also* Tuberculosis)
    017.0●
  simplex (Vidal's) 698.3
    chronicus 698.3
    circumscriptus 698.3
  spinulosus 757.39
    mycotic 117.9
  striata 697.8
  urticatus 698.2
Lichenification 698.3
  nodular 698.3
Lichenoides tuberculosis (primary) (*see also*
  Tuberculosis) 017.0
Lichtheim's disease or syndrome (subacute
  combined sclerosis with pernicious
  anemia) 281.0 [336.2]
Lien migrans 289.59
Lientery (*see also* Diarrhea) 787.91
  infectious 009.2
Life circumstance problem NEC V62.89
Li-Fraumeni cancer syndrome V84.01
Ligament - *see* condition
Light-for-dates (infant) 764.0●
  with signs of fetal malnutrition 764.1●
  affecting management of pregnancy 656.5●
Light-headedness 780.4
Lightning (effects) (shock) (stroke) (struck by)
  994.0
  burn - *see* Burn, by site
  foot 266.2
Lightwood's disease or syndrome (renal
  tubular acidosis) 588.89
Lignac's disease (cystinosis) 270.0
Lignac (-de Toni) (-Fanconi) (-Debré) syndrome
  (cystinosis) 270.0
Lignac (-Fanconi) syndrome (cystinosis)
  270.0
Ligneous thyroiditis 245.3
Likoff's syndrome (angina in menopausal
  women) 413.9
Limb - *see* condition
Limitation of joint motion (*see also* Stiffness,
  joint) 719.5●
  sacroiliac 724.6
Limit dextrinosis 271.0

Limited
  cardiac reserve - *see* Disease, heart
  duction, eye NEC 378.63
  mandibular range of motion 524.52
Lindau's disease (retinocerebral angiomatosis)
  759.6
Lindau (-von Hippel) disease (angiomatosis
  retinocerebellosa) 759.6
Linea corneae senilis 371.41
Lines
  Beau's (transverse furrows on fingernails)
    703.8
  Harris' 733.91
  Hudson-Stähli 371.11
  Stähli's 371.11
Lingua
  geographical 529.1
  nigra (villosa) 529.3
  plicata 529.5
    congenital 750.13
  tylosis 528.6
Lingual (tongue) - *see also* condition
  thyroid 759.2
Linitis (gastric) 535.4●
  plastica (M8142/3) 151.9
Lioderma essentialis (cum melanosis et
  telangiectasia) 757.33
Lip - *see also* condition
  biting 528.9
Lipalgia 272.8
Lipedema - *see* Edema
Lipemia (*see also* Hyperlipidemia) 272.4
  retina, retinalis 272.3
Lipidosis 272.7
  cephalin 272.7
  cerebral (infantile) (juvenile) (late) 330.1
  cerebroretinal 330.1 [362.71]
  cerebroside 272.7
  cerebrospinal 272.7
  chemically-induced 272.7
  cholesterol 272.7
  diabetic 250.8● [272.7]
    due to secondary diabetes 249.8●
      [272.7]
  dystopic (hereditary) 272.7
  glycolipid 272.7
  hepatosplenomegalic 272.3
  hereditary, dystopic 272.7
  sulfatide 330.0
Lipoadenoma (M8324/0 - *see* Neoplasm, by site,
  benign
Lipoblastoma (M8881/0) - *see* Lipoma, by site
Lipoblastomatosis (M8881/0) - *see* Lipoma, by
  site
Lipochondrodystrophy 277.5
Lipochrome histiocytosis (familial) 288.1
Lipodermatosclerosis 729.39
Lipodystrophia progressiva 272.6
Lipodystrophy (progressive) 272.6
  insulin 272.6
  intestinal 040.2
  mesenteric 567.82
Lipofibroma (M8851/0) - *see* Lipoma, by site
Lipoglycoproteinosis 272.8
Lipogranuloma, sclerosing 709.8
Lipogranulomatosis (disseminated) 272.8
  kidney 272.8
Lipoid - *see also* condition
  histiocytosis 272.7
    essential 272.7
  nephrosis (*see also* Nephrosis) 581.3
  proteinosis of Urbach 272.8
Lipoidemia (*see also* Hyperlipidemia) 272.4
Lipoidosis (*see also* Lipidosis) 272.7
Lipoma (M8850/0) 214.9
  breast (skin) 214.1
  face 214.0
  fetal (M8881/0) - *see also* Lipoma, by site
    fat cell (M8880/0) - *see* Lipoma, by site
  infiltrating (M8856/0) - *see* Lipoma, by site
  intra-abdominal 214.3

Lipoma *(Continued)*
  intramuscular (M8856/0) - *see* Lipoma, by
      site
  intrathoracic 214.2
  kidney 214.3
  mediastinum 214.2
  muscle 214.8
  peritoneum 214.3
  retroperitoneum 214.3
  skin 214.1
      face 214.0
  spermatic cord 214.4
  spindle cell (M8857/0) - *see* Lipoma, by site
  stomach 214.3
  subcutaneous tissue 214.1
      face 214.0
  thymus 214.2
  thyroid gland 214.2
Lipomatosis (dolorosa) 272.8
  epidural 214.8
  fetal (M8881/0) - *see* Lipoma, by site
  Launois-Bensaude's 272.8
Lipomyohemangioma (M8860/0)
  specified site - *see* Neoplasm, connective
      tissue, benign
  unspecified site 223.0
Lipomyoma (M8860/0)
  specified site - *see* Neoplasm, connective
      tissue, benign
  unspecified site 223.0
Lipomyxoma (M8852/0) - *see* Lipoma,
      by site
Lipomyxosarcoma (M8852/3) - *see* Neoplasm,
      connective tissue, malignant
Lipophagocytosis 289.89
Lipoproteinemia (alpha) 272.4
  broad-beta 272.2
  floating-beta 272.2
  hyper-pre-beta 272.1
Lipoproteinosis (Rossle-Urbach-Wiethe)
      272.8
Liposarcoma (M8850/3) - *see also* Neoplasm,
      connective tissue, malignant
  differentiated type (M8851/3) - *see*
      Neoplasm, connective tissue,
      malignant
  embryonal (M8852/3) - *see* Neoplasm,
      connective tissue, malignant
  mixed type (M8855/3) - *see* Neoplasm,
      connective tissue, malignant
  myxoid (M8852/3) - *see* Neoplasm,
      connective tissue, malignant
  pleomorphic (M8854/3) - *see* Neoplasm,
      connective tissue, malignant
  round cell (M8853/3) - *see* Neoplasm,
      connective tissue, malignant
  well differentiated type (M8851/3) - *see*
      Neoplasm, connective tissue,
      malignant
Liposynovitis prepatellaris 272.8
Lipping
  cervix 622.0
  spine *(see also* Spondylosis) 721.90
  vertebra *(see also* Spondylosis) 721.90
Lip pits (mucus), congenital 750.25
Lipschütz disease or ulcer 616.50
Lipuria 791.1
  bilharziasis 120.0
Liquefaction, vitreous humor 379.21
Lisping 307.9
Lissauer's paralysis 094.1
Lissencephalia, lissencephaly 742.2
Listerellose 027.0
Listeriose 027.0
Listeriosis 027.0
  congenital 771.2
  fetal 771.2
  suspected fetal damage affecting
      management of pregnancy 655.4 ●
Listlessness 780.79
Lithemia 790.6

Lithiasis - *see also* Calculus
  hepatic (duct) - *see* Choledocholithiasis
  urinary 592.9
Lithopedion 779.9
  affecting management of pregnancy 656.8 ●
Lithosis (occupational) 502
  with tuberculosis - *see* Tuberculosis,
      pulmonary
Lithuria 791.9
Litigation V62.5
Little
  league elbow 718.82
  stroke syndrome 435.9
Little's disease - *see* Palsy, cerebral
Littre's
  gland - *see* condition
  hernia - *see* Hernia, Littre's
Littritis *(see also* Urethritis) 597.89
Livedo 782.61
  annularis 782.61
  racemose 782.61
  reticularis 782.61
Live flesh 781.0
Liver - *see also* condition
  donor V59.6
Livida, asphyxia
  newborn 768.6
Living
  alone V60.3
      with handicapped person V60.4
Lloyd's syndrome 258.1
Loa loa 125.2
Loasis 125.2
Lobe, lobar - *see* condition
Lobo's disease or blastomycosis 116.2
Lobomycosis 116.2
Lobotomy syndrome 310.0
Lobstein's disease (brittle bones and blue
      sclera) 756.51
Lobster-claw hand 755.58
Lobulation (congenital) - *see also* Anomaly,
      specified type NEC, by site
  kidney, fetal 753.3
  liver, abnormal 751.69
  spleen 759.0
Lobule, lobular - *see* condition
Local, localized - *see* condition
Locked bowel or intestine *(see also* Obstruction,
      intestine) 560.9
Locked-in state 344.81
Locked twins 660.5 ●
  affecting fetus or newborn 763.1
Locking
  joint *(see also* Derangement, joint) 718.90
  knee 717.9
Lockjaw *(see also* Tetanus) 037
Locomotor ataxia (progressive) 094.0
Löffler's
  endocarditis 421.0
  eosinophilia or syndrome 518.3
  pneumonia 518.3
  syndrome (eosinophilic pneumonitis) 518.3
Löfgren's syndrome (sarcoidosis) 135
Loiasis 125.2
  eyelid 125.2 *[373.6]*
Loneliness V62.89
Lone Star fever 082.8
Long labor 662.1 ●
  affecting fetus or newborn 763.89
  first stage 662.0 ●
  second stage 662.2 ●
Longitudinal stripes or grooves, nails 703.8
  congenital 757.5
Long-term (current) (prophylactic) drug use
      V58.69
  antibiotics V58.62
  anticoagulants V58.61
  anti-inflammatories, non-steroidal (NSAID)
      V58.64
  antiplatelets/antithrombotics V58.63
  aspirin V58.66

Long-term drug use *(Continued)*
  bisphosphonates V58.68
  high-risk medications NEC V58.69
  insulin V58.67
  methadone for pain control V58.69
  opiate analgesic V58.69
  pain killers V58.69
      anti-inflammatories, non-steroidal
          (NSAID) V58.64
      aspirin V58.66
  steroids V58.65
  tamoxifen V07.51
Loop
  intestine *(see also* Volvulus) 560.2
  intrascleral nerve 379.29
  vascular on papilla (optic) 743.57
Loose - *see also* condition
  body
      in tendon sheath 727.82
      joint 718.10
          ankle 718.17
          elbow 718.12
          foot 718.17
          hand 718.14
          hip 718.15
          knee 717.6
          multiple sites 718.19
          pelvic region 718.15
          prosthetic implant - *see* Complications,
              mechanical
          shoulder (region) 718.11
          specified site NEC 718.18
          wrist 718.13
  cartilage (joint) *(see also* Loose, body, joint)
      718.1 ●
      knee 717.6
  facet (vertebral) 724.9
  prosthetic implant - *see* Complications,
      mechanical
  sesamoid, joint *(see also* Loose, body, joint)
      718.1 ●
  tooth, teeth 525.8
Loosening epiphysis 732.9
Looser (-Debray)-Milkman syndrome
      (osteomalacia with pseudofractures)
      268.2
Lop ear (deformity) 744.29
Lorain's disease or syndrome (pituitary
      dwarfism) 253.3
Lorain-Levi syndrome (pituitary dwarfism)
      253.3
Lordosis (acquired) (postural) 737.20
  congenital 754.2
  due to or associated with
      Charcôt-Marie-Tooth disease 356.1
          [737.42]
      mucopolysaccharidosis 277.5 *[737.42]*
      neurofibromatosis 237.71 *[737.42]*
      osteitis
          deformans 731.0 *[737.42]*
          fibrosa cystica 252.01 *[737.42]*
      osteoporosis *(see also* Osteoporosis) 733.00
          [737.42]
      poliomyelitis *(see also* Poliomyelitis) 138
          [737.42]
      tuberculosis *(see also* Tuberculosis)
          015.0 ● *[737.42]*
  late effect of rickets 268.1 *[737.42]*
  postlaminectomy 737.21
  postsurgical NEC 737.22
  rachitic 268.1 *[737.42]*
  specified NEC 737.29
  tuberculous *(see also* Tuberculosis) 015.0 ●
      [737.42]
Loss
  appetite 783.0
      hysterical 300.11
      nonorganic origin 307.59
      psychogenic 307.59
  blood - *see* Hemorrhage
  central vision 368.41

◀ New   ◀▥ Revised   ~~deleted~~ Deleted   ● Use Additional Digit(s)   ▨ Omit code

Loss (Continued)
consciousness 780.09
    transient 780.2
control, sphincter, rectum 787.60
    nonorganic origin 307.7
ear ossicle, partial 385.24
elasticity, skin 782.8
extremity or member, traumatic, current - see
    Amputation, traumatic
fluid (acute) 276.50
    with
        hypernatremia 276.0
        hyponatremia 276.1
    fetus or newborn 775.5
hair 704.00
hearing - see also Deafness
    central 389.14
    conductive (air) 389.00
        with sensorineural hearing loss
            389.20
            bilateral 389.22
            unilateral 389.21
        bilateral 389.06
        combined types 389.08
        external ear 389.01
        inner ear 389.04
        middle ear 389.03
        multiple types 389.08
        tympanic membrane 389.02
        unilateral 389.05
    mixed conductive and sensorineural
        389.20
        bilateral 389.22
        unilateral 389.21
    mixed type 389.20
        bilateral 389.22
        unilateral 389.21
    nerve
        bilateral 389.12
        unilateral 389.13
    neural
        bilateral 389.12
        unilateral 389.13
    noise-induced 388.12
    perceptive NEC (see also Loss, hearing,
        sensorineural) 389.10
    sensorineural 389.10
        with conductive hearing loss
            389.20
            bilateral 389.22
            unilateral 389.21
        asymmetrical 389.16
        bilateral 389.18
        central 389.14
        neural
            bilateral 389.12
            unilateral 389.13
        sensory
            bilateral 389.11
            unilateral 389.17
        unilateral 389.15
    sensory
        bilateral 389.11
        unilateral 389.17
    specified type NEC 389.8
    sudden NEC 388.2
height 781.91
labyrinthine reactivity (unilateral)
    386.55
    bilateral 386.56
memory (see also Amnesia) 780.93
    mild, following organic brain damage
        310.89
mind (see also Psychosis) 298.9
occusal vertical dimension 524.37
organ or part - see Absence, by site,
    acquired
recurrent pregnancy - see Pregnancy,
    management affected by, abortion,
    habitual
sensation 782.0

Loss (Continued)
sense of
    smell (see also Disturbance, sensation)
        781.1
    taste (see also Disturbance, sensation)
        781.1
    touch (see also Disturbance, sensation)
        781.1
sight (acquired) (complete) (congenital) - see
    Blindness
spinal fluid
    headache 349.0
substance of
    bone (see also Osteoporosis) 733.00
    cartilage 733.99
        ear 380.32
    vitreous (humor) 379.26
tooth, teeth
    acquired 525.10
        due to
            caries 525.13
            extraction 525.10
            periodontal disease 525.12
            specified NEC 525.19
            trauma 525.11
vision, visual (see also Blindness) 369.9
    both eyes (see also Blindness, both eyes)
        369.3
    complete (see also Blindness, both eyes)
        369.00
    one eye 369.8
    sudden 368.11
    transient 368.12
vitreous 379.26
voice (see also Aphonia) 784.41
weight (cause unknown) 783.21
Lou Gehrig's disease 335.20
Louis-Bar syndrome (ataxia-telangiectasia)
    334.8
Louping ill 063.1
Lousiness - see Lice
Low
    back syndrome 724.2
    basal metabolic rate (BMR) 794.7
    birthweight 765.1●
        extreme (less than 1000 grams) 765.0●
        for gestational age 764.0●
        status (see also Status, low birth weight)
            V21.30
    bladder compliance 596.52
    blood pressure (see also Hypotension)
        458.9
        reading (incidental) (isolated)
            (nonspecific) 796.3
    cardiac reserve - see Disease, heart
    compliance bladder 596.52
    frequency deafness - see Disorder, hearing
    function - see also Hypofunction
        kidney (see also Disease, renal) 593.9
        liver 573.9
    hemoglobin 285.9
    implantation, placenta - see Placenta, previa
    insertion, placenta - see Placenta, previa
    lying
        kidney 593.0
        organ or site, congenital - see Malposition,
            congenital
        placenta - see Placenta, previa
    output syndrome (cardiac) (see also Failure,
        heart) 428.9
    platelets (blood) (see also Thrombocytopenia)
        287.5
    reserve, kidney (see also Disease, renal) 593.9
    risk
        human papillomavirus (HPV) DNA test
            positive
        anal 796.79
        cervical 795.09
        vaginal 795.19
    salt syndrome 593.9
    tension glaucoma 365.12

Low (Continued)
    vision 369.9
        both eyes 369.20
        one eye 369.70
Lowe (-Terrey-MacLachlan) syndrome
    (oculocerebrorenal dystrophy)
    270.8
Lower extremity - see condition
Lown (-Ganong)-Levine syndrome (short P-R
    interval, normal QRS complex, and
    paroxysmal supraventricular tachycardia)
    426.81
LSD reaction (see also Abuse, drugs,
    nondependent) 305.3●
L-shaped kidney 753.3
Lucas-Championnière disease (fibrinous
    bronchitis) 466.0
Lucey-Driscoll syndrome (jaundice due to
    delayed conjugation) 774.30
Ludwig's
    angina 528.3
    disease (submaxillary cellulitis) 528.3
Lues (venerea), luetic - see Syphilis
Luetscher's syndrome (dehydration)
    276.51
Lumbago 724.2
    due to displacement, intervertebral disc
        722.10
Lumbalgia 724.2
    due to displacement, intervertebral disc
        722.10
Lumbar - see condition
Lumbarization, vertebra 756.15
Lumbermen's itch 133.8
Lump - see also Mass
    abdominal 789.3●
    breast 611.72
    chest 786.6
    epigastric 789.3●
    head 784.2
    kidney 753.3
    liver 789.1
    lung 786.6
    mediastinal 786.6
    neck 784.2
    nose or sinus 784.2
    pelvic 789.3●
    skin 782.2
    substernal 786.6
    throat 784.2
    umbilicus 789.3●
Lunacy (see also Psychosis) 298.9
Lunatomalacia 732.3
Lung - see also condition
    donor V59.8
    drug addict's 417.8
    mainliners' 417.8
    vanishing 492.0
Lupoid (miliary) of Boeck 135
Lupus 710.0
    anticoagulant 795.79
        with
            hemorrhagic disorder 286.53
            hypercoagulable state 289.81
    Cazenave's (erythematosus) 695.4
    discoid (local) 695.4
    disseminated 710.0
    erythematodes (discoid) (local) 695.4
    erythematosus (discoid) (local) 695.4
        disseminated 710.0
        eyelid 373.34
        systemic 710.0
            with
                encephalitis 710.0 [323.81]
                lung involvement 710.0 [517.8]
            inhibitor (presence of) 795.79
                with hypercoagulable state
                    289.81
    exedens 017.0●
    eyelid (see also Tuberculosis) 017.0● [373.4]
    Hilliard's 017.0●

Lupus *(Continued)*
  hydralazine
    correct substance properly administered 695.4
    overdose or wrong substance given or taken 972.6
  miliaris disseminatus faciei 017.0●
  nephritis 710.0 *[583.81]*
    acute 710.0 *[580.81]*
    chronic 710.0 *[582.81]*
  nontuberculous, not disseminated 695.4
  pernio (Besnier) 135
  tuberculous *(see also* Tuberculosis) 017.0●
    eyelid *(see also* Tuberculosis) 017.0● *[373.4]*
  vulgaris 017.0●
Luschka's joint disease 721.90
Luteinoma (M8610/0) 220
Lutembacher's disease or syndrome (atrial septal defect with mitral stenosis) 745.5
Luteoma (M8610/0) 220
Lutz-Miescher disease (elastosis perforans serpiginosa) 701.1
Lutz-Splendore-de Almeida disease (Brazilian blastomycosis) 116.1
Luxatio
  bulbi due to birth injury 767.8
  coxae congenita *(see also* Dislocation, hip, congenital) 754.30
  erecta - *see* Dislocation, shoulder
  imperfecta - *see* Sprain, by site
  perinealis - *see* Dislocation, hip
Luxation - *see also* Dislocation, by site
  eyeball 360.81
    due to birth injury 767.8
    lateral 376.36
  genital organs (external) NEC - *see* Wound, open, genital organs
  globe (eye) 360.81
    lateral 376.36
  lacrimal gland (postinfectional) 375.16
  lens (old) (partial) 379.32
    congenital 743.37
      syphilitic 090.49 *[379.32]*
    Marfan's disease 090.49
    spontaneous 379.32
  penis - *see* Wound, open, penis
  scrotum - *see* Wound, open, scrotum
  testis - *see* Wound, open, testis
L-xyloketosuria 271.8
Lycanthropy *(see also* Psychosis) 298.9
Lyell's disease or syndrome (toxic epidermal necrolysis) 695.15
  due to drug
    correct substance properly administered 695.15
    overdose or wrong substance given or taken 977.9
    specified drug - *see* Table of Drugs and Chemicals
Lyme disease 088.81
Lymph
  gland or node - *see* condition
  scrotum *(see also* Infestation, filarial) 125.9
Lymphadenitis 289.3
  with
    abortion - *see* Abortion, by type, with sepsis
    ectopic pregnancy *(see also* categories 633.0–633.9) 639.0
    molar pregnancy *(see also* categories 630–632) 639.0
  acute 683
    mesenteric 289.2
  any site, except mesenteric 289.3
    acute 683
    chronic 289.1
    mesenteric (acute) (chronic) (nonspecific) (subacute) 289.2
    subacute 289.1
      mesenteric 289.2
  breast, puerperal, postpartum 675.2●

Lymphadenitis *(Continued)*
  chancroidal (congenital) 099.0
  chronic 289.1
    mesenteric 289.2
  dermatopathic 695.89
  due to
    anthracosis (occupational) 500
    Brugia (Wuchereria) malayi 125.1
    diphtheria (toxin) 032.89
    lymphogranuloma venereum 099.1
    Wuchereria bancrofti 125.0
  following
    abortion 639.0
    ectopic or molar pregnancy 639.0
  generalized 289.3
  gonorrheal 098.89
  granulomatous 289.1
  infectional 683
  mesenteric (acute) (chronic) (nonspecific) (subacute) 289.2
    due to Bacillus typhi 002.0
    tuberculous *(see also* Tuberculosis) 014.8●
  mycobacterial 031.8
  purulent 683
  pyogenic 683
  regional 078.3
  septic 683
  streptococcal 683
  subacute, unspecified site 289.1
  suppurative 683
  syphilitic (early) (secondary) 091.4
    late 095.8
  tuberculous - *see* Tuberculosis, lymph gland
  venereal 099.1
Lymphadenoid goiter 245.2
Lymphadenopathy (general) 785.6
  due to toxoplasmosis (acquired) 130.7
    congenital (active) 771.2
Lymphadenopathy-associated virus (disease) (illness) (infection) - *see* Human immunodeficiency virus (disease) (illness) (infection)
Lymphadenosis 785.6
  acute 075
Lymphangiectasis 457.1
  conjunctiva 372.89
  postinfectional 457.1
  scrotum 457.1
Lymphangiectatic elephantiasis, nonfilarial 457.1
Lymphangioendothelioma (M9170/0) 228.1
  malignant (M9170/3) - *see* Neoplasm, connective tissue, malignant
Lymphangioleiomyomatosis 516.4
Lymphangioma (M9170/0) 228.1
  capillary (M9171/0) 228.1
  cavernous (M9172/0) 228.1
  cystic (M9173/0) 228.1
  malignant (M9170/3) - *see* Neoplasm, connective tissue, malignant
Lymphangiomyoma (M9174/0) 228.1
Lymphangiomyomatosis 516.4
Lymphangiosarcoma (M9170/3) - *see* Neoplasm, connective tissue, malignant
Lymphangitis 457.2
  with
    abortion - *see* Abortion, by type, with sepsis
    abscess - *see* Abscess, by site
    cellulitis - *see* Abscess, by site
    ectopic pregnancy *(see also* categories 633.0–633.9) 639.0
    molar pregnancy *(see also* categories 630–632) 639.0
  acute (with abscess or cellulitis) 682.9
    specified site - *see* Abscess, by site
  breast, puerperal, postpartum 675.2●
  chancroidal 099.0
  chronic (any site) 457.2
  due to
    Brugia (Wuchereria) malayi 125.1
    Wuchereria bancrofti 125.0

Lymphangitis *(Continued)*
  following
    abortion 639.0
    ectopic or molar pregnancy 639.0
  gangrenous 457.2
  penis
    acute 607.2
    gonococcal (acute) 098.0
      chronic or duration of 2 months or more 098.2
  puerperal, postpartum, childbirth 670.8●
  strumous, tuberculous *(see also* Tuberculosis) 017.2●
  subacute (any site) 457.2
  tuberculous - *see* Tuberculosis, lymph gland
Lymphatic (vessel) - *see* condition
Lymphatism 254.8
  scrofulous *(see also* Tuberculosis) 017.2●
Lymphectasia 457.1
Lymphedema *(see also* Elephantiasis) 457.1
  acquired (chronic) 457.1
  chronic hereditary 757.0
  congenital 757.0
  idiopathic hereditary 757.0
  praecox 457.1
  secondary 457.1
  surgical NEC 997.99
    postmastectomy (syndrome) 457.0
Lymph-hemangioma (M9120/0) - *see* Hemangioma, by site
Lymphoblastic - *see* condition
Lymphoblastoma (diffuse) (M9630/3) 200.1●
  giant follicular (M9690/3) 202.0●
  macrofollicular (M9690/3) 202.0●
Lymphoblastosis, acute benign 075
Lymphocele 457.8
Lymphocythemia 288.51
Lymphocytic - *see also* condition
  chorioencephalitis (acute) (serous) 049.0
  choriomeningitis (acute) (serous) 049.0
Lymphocytoma (diffuse) (malignant) (M9620/3) 200.1●
Lymphocytomatosis (M9620/3) 200.1●
Lymphocytopenia 288.51
Lymphocytosis (symptomatic) 288.61
  infectious (acute) 078.89
Lymphoepithelioma (M8082/3) - *see* Neoplasm, by site, malignant
Lymphogranuloma (malignant) (M9650/3) 201.9●
  inguinale 099.1
  venereal (any site) 099.1
    with stricture of rectum 099.1
  venereum 099.1
Lymphogranulomatosis (malignant) (M9650/3) 201.9●
  benign (Boeck's sarcoid) (Schaumann's) 135
  Hodgkin's (M9650/3) 201.9●
Lymphohistiocytosis, familial hemophagocytic 288.4
Lymphoid - *see* condition
Lympholeukoblastoma (M9850/3) 207.8●
Lympholeukosarcoma (M9850/3) 207.8●
Lymphoma (malignant) (M9590/3) 202.8●

> Note: Use the following fifth-digit subclassification with categories 200–202:
>
> 0   unspecified site, extranodal and solid organ sites
> 1   lymph nodes of head, face, and neck
> 2   intrathoracic lymph nodes
> 3   intra-abdominal lymph nodes
> 4   lymph nodes of axilla and upper limb
> 5   lymph nodes of inguinal region and lower limb
> 6   intrapelvic lymph nodes
> 7   spleen
> 8   lymph nodes of multiple sites

◀ New   ◀▪ Revised   ~~deleted~~ Deleted   ● Use Additional Digit(s)   ▒ Omit code

Lymphoma *(Continued)*
  benign (M9590/0) - *see* Neoplasm, by site, benign
  Burkitt's type (lymphoblastic) (undifferentiated) (M9750/3) 200.2●
  Castleman's (mediastinal lymph node hyperplasia) 785.6
  centroblastic-centrocytic
    diffuse (M9614/3) 202.8●
    follicular (M9692/3) 202.0●
  centroblastic type (diffuse) (M9632/3) 202.8●
    follicular (M9697/3) 202.0●
  centrocytic (M9622/3) 202.8●
  compound (M9613/3) 200.8●
  convoluted cell type (lymphoblastic) (M9602/3) 202.8●
  diffuse NEC (M9590/3) 202.8●
    large B cell 202.8●
  follicular (giant) (M9690/3) 202.0●
    center cell (diffuse) (M9615/3) 202.8●
      cleaved (diffuse) (M9623/3) 202.8●
        follicular (M9695/3) 202.0●
      non-cleaved (diffuse) (M9633/3) 202.8●
        follicular (M9698/3) 202.0●
    centroblastic-centrocytic (M9692/3) 202.0●
    centroblastic type (M9697/3) 202.0●
    large cell 202.0●
    lymphocytic
      intermediate differentiation (M9694/3) 202.0●
      poorly differentiated (M9696/3) 202.0●
    mixed (cell type) (lymphocytic-histiocytic) (small cell and large cell) (M9691/3) 202.0●
  germinocytic (M9622/3) 202.8●
  giant, follicular or follicle (M9690/3) 202.0●
  histiocytic (diffuse) (M9640/3) 200.0●
    nodular (M9642/3) 200.0●
    pleomorphic cell type (M9641/3) 200.0●
  Hodgkin's (M9650/3) *(see also* Disease, Hodgkin's) 201.9●
  immunoblastic (type) (M9612/3) 200.8●
  large cell (M9640/3) 200.7●
    anaplastic 200.6●
    nodular (M9642/3) 202.0●
    pleomorphic cell type (M9641/3) 200.0●
  lymphoblastic (diffuse) (M9630/3) 200.1●
    Burkitt's type (M9750/3) 200.2●
    convoluted cell type (M9602/3) 202.8●

Lymphoma *(Continued)*
  lymphocytic (cell type) (diffuse) (M9620/3) 200.1●
    with plasmacytoid differentiation, diffuse (M9611/3) 200.8●
    intermediate differentiation (diffuse) (M9621/3) 200.1●
      follicular (M9694/3) 202.0●
      nodular (M9694/3) 202.0●
    nodular (M9690/3) 202.0●
    poorly differentiated (diffuse) (M9630/3) 200.1●
      follicular (M9696/3) 202.0●
      nodular (M9696/3) 202.0●
    well differentiated (diffuse) (M9620/3) 200.1●
      follicular (M9693/3) 202.0●
      nodular (M9693/3) 202.0●
  lymphocytic-histiocytic, mixed (diffuse) (M9613/3) 200.8●
    follicular (M9691/3) 202.0●
    nodular (M9691/3) 202.0●
  lymphoplasmacytoid type (M9611/3) 200.8●
  lymphosarcoma type (M9610/3) 200.1●
  macrofollicular (M9690/3) 202.0●
  mantle cell 200.4●
  marginal zone 200.3●
    extranodal B-cell 200.3●
    nodal B-cell 200.3●
    splenic B-cell 200.3●
  mixed cell type (diffuse) (M9613/3) 200.8●
    follicular (M9691/3) 202.0●
    nodular (M9691/3) 202.0●
  nodular (M9690/3) 202.0●
    histiocytic (M9642/3) 200.0●
    lymphocytic (M9690/3) 202.0●
      intermediate differentiation (M9694/3) 202.0●
      poorly differentiated (M9696/3) 202.0●
    mixed (cell type) (lymphocytic-histiocytic) (small cell and large cell) (M9691/3) 202.0●
  non-Hodgkin's type NEC (M9591/3) 202.8●
  peripheral T-cell 202.7●
  primary central nervous system 200.5●
  reticulum cell (type) (M9640/3) 200.0●
  small cell and large cell, mixed (diffuse) (M9613/3) 200.8●
    follicular (M9691/3) 202.0●
    nodular (M9691/3) 202.0●
  stem cell (type) (M9601/3) 202.8●

Lymphoma *(Continued)*
  T-cell 202.1●
    peripheral 202.7●
  undifferentiated (cell type) (non-Burkitt's) (M9600/3) 202.8●
    Burkitt's type (M9750/3) 200.2●
Lymphomatosis (M9590/3) - *see also* Lymphoma
  granulomatous 099.1
Lymphopathia
  venereum 099.1
  veneris 099.1
Lymphopenia 288.51
  familial 279.2
Lymphoreticulosis, benign (of inoculation) 078.3
Lymphorrhea 457.8
Lymphosarcoma (M9610/3) 200.1●
  diffuse (M9610/3) 200.1●
    with plasmacytoid differentiation (M9611/3) 200.8●
    lymphoplasmacytic (M9611/3) 200.8●
  follicular (giant) (M9690/3) 202.0●
    lymphoblastic (M9696/3) 202.0●
    lymphocytic, intermediate differentiation (M9694/3) 202.0●
    mixed cell type (M9691/3) 202.0●
  giant follicular (M9690/3) 202.0●
  Hodgkin's (M9650/3) 201.9●
  immunoblastic (M9612/3) 200.8●
  lymphoblastic (diffuse) (M9630/3) 200.1●
    follicular (M9696/3) 202.0●
    nodular (M9696/3) 202.0●
  lymphocytic (diffuse) (M9620/3) 200.1●
    intermediate differentiation (diffuse) (M9621/3) 200.1●
      follicular (M9694/3) 202.0●
      nodular (M9694/3) 202.0●
  mixed cell type (diffuse) (M9613/3) 200.8●
    follicular (M9691/3) 202.0●
    nodular (M9691/3) 202.0●
  nodular (M9690/3) 202.0●
    lymphoblastic (M9696/3) 202.0●
    lymphocytic, intermediate differentiation (M9694/3) 202.0●
    mixed cell type (M9691/3) 202.0●
  prolymphocytic (M9631/3) 200.1●
  reticulum cell (M9640/3) 200.0●
Lymphostasis 457.8
Lypemania (*see also* Melancholia) 296.2●
Lyssa 071

M

Macacus ear 744.29
Maceration
  fetus (cause not stated) 779.9
  wet feet, tropical (syndrome) 991.4
Machado-Joseph disease 334.8
Machupo virus hemorrhagic fever 078.7
Macleod's syndrome (abnormal transradiancy,
  one lung) 492.8
Macrocephalia, macrocephaly 756.0
Macrocheilia (congenital) 744.81
Macrochilia (congenital) 744.81
Macrocolon (congenital) 751.3
Macrocornea 743.41
  associated with buphthalmos 743.22
Macrocytic - see condition
Macrocytosis 289.89
Macrodactylia, macrodactylism (fingers)
  (thumbs) 755.57
  toes 755.65
Macrodontia 520.2
Macroencephaly 742.4
Macrogenia 524.05
Macrogenitosomia (female) (male) (praecox)
  255.2
Macrogingivae 523.8
Macroglobulinemia (essential) (idiopathic)
  (monoclonal) (primary) (syndrome)
  (Waldenström's) 273.3
Macroglossia (congenital) 750.15
  acquired 529.8
Macrognathia, macrognathism (congenital)
  524.00
  mandibular 524.02
    alveolar 524.72
  maxillary 524.01
    alveolar 524.71
Macrogyria (congenital) 742.4
Macrohydrocephalus (see also Hydrocephalus)
  331.4
Macromastia (see also Hypertrophy, breast)
  611.1
Macrophage activation syndrome 288.4
Macropsia 368.14
Macrosigmoid 564.7
  congenital 751.3
Macrospondylitis, acromegalic 253.0
Macrostomia (congenital) 744.83
Macrotia (external ear) (congenital) 744.22
Macula
  cornea, corneal
    congenital 743.43
      interfering with vision 743.42
    interfering with central vision 371.03
    not interfering with central vision 371.02
  degeneration (see also Degeneration, macula)
    362.50
    hereditary (see also Dystrophy, retina)
      362.70
  edema, cystoid 362.53
Maculae ceruleae 132.1
Macules and papules 709.8
Maculopathy, toxic 362.55
Madarosis 374.55
Madelung's
  deformity (radius) 755.54
  disease (lipomatosis) 272.8
  lipomatosis 272.8
Madness (see also Psychosis) 298.9
  myxedema (acute) 293.0
    subacute 293.1
Madura
  disease (actinomycotic) 039.9
    mycotic 117.4
  foot (actinomycotic) 039.4
    mycotic 117.4
Maduromycosis (actinomycotic) 039.9
  mycotic 117.4
Maffucci's syndrome (dyschondroplasia with
  hemangiomas) 756.4

Magenblase syndrome 306.4
Main en griffe (acquired) 736.06
  congenital 755.59
Maintenance
  chemotherapy regimen or treatment
    V58.11
  dialysis regimen or treatment
    extracorporeal (renal) V56.0
    peritoneal V56.8
    renal V56.0
  drug therapy or regimen
    chemotherapy, antineoplastic V58.11
    immunotherapy, antineoplastic V58.12
  external fixation NEC V54.89
  methadone 304.00
  radiotherapy V58.0
  traction NEC V54.89
Majocchi's
  disease (purpura annularis telangiectodes)
    709.1
  granuloma 110.6
Major - see condition
Mal
  cerebral (idiopathic) (see also Epilepsy)
    345.9●
  comital (see also Epilepsy) 345.9●
  de los pintos (see also Pinta) 103.9
  de Meleda 757.39
  de mer 994.6
  lie - see Presentation, fetal
  perforant (see also Ulcer, lower extremity)
    707.15
Malabar itch 110.9
  beard 110.0
  foot 110.4
  scalp 110.0
Malabsorption 579.9
  calcium 579.8
  carbohydrate 579.8
  disaccharide 271.3
  drug-induced 579.8
  due to bacterial overgrowth 579.8
  fat 579.8
  folate, congenital 281.2
  galactose 271.1
  glucose-galactose (congenital) 271.3
  intestinal 579.9
  isomaltose 271.3
  lactose (hereditary) 271.3
  methionine 270.4
  monosaccharide 271.8
  postgastrectomy 579.3
  postsurgical 579.3
  protein 579.8
  sucrose (-isomaltose) (congenital) 271.3
  syndrome 579.9
    postgastrectomy 579.3
    postsurgical 579.3
Malacia, bone 268.2
  juvenile (see also Rickets) 268.0
  Kienböck's (juvenile) (lunate) (wrist)
    732.3
    adult 732.8
Malacoplakia
  bladder 596.89
  colon 569.89
  pelvis (kidney) 593.89
  ureter 593.89
  urethra 599.84
Malacosteon 268.2
  juvenile (see also Rickets) 268.0
Maladaptation - see Maladjustment
Maladie de Roger 745.4
Maladjustment
  conjugal V61.10
    involving
      divorce V61.03
      estrangement V61.09
  educational V62.3
  family V61.9
    specified circumstance NEC V61.8

Maladjustment (Continued)
  marital V61.10
    involving
      divorce V61.03
      estrangement V61.09
  occupational V62.29
    current military deployment status V62.21
  simple, adult (see also Reaction, adjustment)
    309.9
  situational acute (see also Reaction,
    adjustment) 309.9
  social V62.4
Malaise 780.79
Malakoplakia - see Malacoplakia
Malaria, malarial (fever) 084.6
  algid 084.9
  any type, with
    algid malaria 084.9
    blackwater fever 084.8
    fever
      blackwater 084.8
      hemoglobinuric (bilious) 084.8
    hemoglobinuria, malarial 084.8
    hepatitis 084.9 [573.2]
    nephrosis 084.9 [581.81]
    pernicious complication NEC 084.9
      cardiac 084.9
      cerebral 084.9
  cardiac 084.9
  carrier (suspected) of V02.9
  cerebral 084.9
  complicating pregnancy, childbirth, or
    puerperium 647.4●
  congenital 771.2
  congestion, congestive 084.6
    brain 084.9
  continued 084.0
  estivo-autumnal 084.0
  falciparum (malignant tertian) 084.0
  hematinuria 084.8
  hematuria 084.8
  hemoglobinuria 084.8
  hemorrhagic 084.6
  induced (therapeutically) 084.7
    accidental - see Malaria, by type
  liver 084.9 [573.2]
  malariae (quartan) 084.2
  malignant (tertian) 084.0
  mixed infections 084.5
  monkey 084.4
  ovale 084.3
  pernicious, acute 084.0
  Plasmodium, P.
    falciparum 084.0
    malariae 084.2
    ovale 084.3
    vivax 084.1
  quartan 084.2
  quotidian 084.0
  recurrent 084.6
    induced (therapeutically) 084.7
      accidental - see Malaria, by type
  remittent 084.6
  specified types NEC 084.4
  spleen 084.6
  subtertian 084.0
  tertian (benign) 084.1
    malignant 084.0
  tropical 084.0
  typhoid 084.6
  vivax (benign tertian) 084.1
Malassez's disease (testicular cyst) 608.89
Malassimilation 579.9
Maldescent, testis 752.51
Maldevelopment - see also Anomaly, by site
  brain 742.9
  colon 751.5
  hip (joint) 755.63
    congenital dislocation (see also
      Dislocation, hip, congenital) 754.30
  mastoid process 756.0

◀ New   ◀■ Revised   ~~deleted~~ Deleted   ● Use Additional Digit(s)   ▨ Omit code

Maldevelopment *(Continued)*
  middle ear, except ossicles 744.03
    ossicles 744.04
  newborn (not malformation) 764.9●
  ossicles, ear 744.04
  spine 756.10
  toe 755.66
Male type pelvis 755.69
  with disproportion (fetopelvic) 653.2●
    affecting fetus or newborn 763.1
    causing obstructed labor 660.1●
      affecting fetus or newborn 763.1
Malformation (congenital) - *see also* Anomaly
  arteriovenous
    pulmonary 747.32
  bone 756.9
  bursa 756.9
  Chiari
    type I 348.4
    type II (*see also* Spina bifida) 741.0●
    type III 742.0
    type IV 742.2
  circulatory system NEC 747.9
    specified type NEC 747.89
  cochlea 744.05
  digestive system NEC 751.9
    lower 751.5
    specified type NEC 751.8
    upper 750.9
  eye 743.9
  gum 750.9
  heart NEC 746.9
    specified type NEC 746.89
    valve 746.9
  internal ear 744.05
  joint NEC 755.9
    specified type NEC 755.8
  Mondini's (congenital) (malformation, cochlea) 744.05
  muscle 756.9
  nervous system (central) 742.9
  pelvic organs or tissues
    in pregnancy or childbirth 654.9●
      affecting fetus or newborn 763.89
      causing obstructed labor 660.2●
        affecting fetus or newborn 763.1
  placenta (*see also* Placenta, abnormal) 656.7●
  respiratory organs 748.9
    specified type NEC 748.8
  Rieger's 743.44
  sense organs NEC 742.9
    specified type NEC 742.8
  skin 757.9
    specified type NEC 757.8
  spinal cord 742.9
  teeth, tooth NEC 520.9
  tendon 756.9
  throat 750.9
  umbilical cord (complicating delivery) 663.9●
    affecting fetus or newborn 762.6
  umbilicus 759.9
  urinary system NEC 753.9
    specified type NEC 753.8
  venous - *see* Anomaly, vein
Malfunction - *see also* Dysfunction
  arterial graft 996.1
  cardiac pacemaker 996.01
  catheter device - *see* Complications, mechanical, catheter
  colostomy 569.62
    valve 569.62
  cystostomy 596.82
    infection 596.81
    mechanical 596.82
    specified complication NEC 596.83
  device, implant, or graft NEC - *see* Complications, mechanical
  enteric stoma 569.62
  enterostomy 569.62
  esophagostomy 530.87

Malfunction *(Continued)*
  gastroenteric 536.8
  gastrostomy 536.42
  ileostomy
    valve 569.62
  nephrostomy 997.5
  pacemaker - *see* Complications, mechanical, pacemaker
  prosthetic device, internal - *see* Complications, mechanical
  tracheostomy 519.02
  valve
    colostomy 569.62
    ileostomy 569.62
  vascular graft or shunt 996.1
Malgaigne's fracture (closed) 808.43
  open 808.53
Malherbe's
  calcifying epithelioma (M8110/0) - *see* Neoplasm, skin, benign
  tumor (M8110/0) - *see* Neoplasm, skin, benign
Malibu disease 919.8
  infected 919.9
Malignancy (M8000/3) - *see* Neoplasm, by site, malignant
Malignant - *see* condition
Malingerer, malingering V65.2
Mallet, finger (acquired) 736.1
  congenital 755.59
  late effect of rickets 268.1
Malleus 024
Mallory's bodies 034.1
Mallory-Weiss syndrome 530.7
Malnutrition (calorie) 263.9
  complicating pregnancy 648.9●
  degree
    first 263.1
    second 263.0
    third 262
    mild (protein) 263.1
    moderate (protein) 263.0
    severe 261
      protein-calorie 262
  fetus 764.2●
    "light-for-dates" 764.1●
  following gastrointestinal surgery 579.3
  intrauterine or fetal 764.2●
    fetus or infant "light-for-dates" 764.1●
  lack of care, or neglect (child) (infant) 995.52
    adult 995.84
  malignant 260
  mild (protein) 263.1
  moderate (protein) 263.0
  protein 260
  protein-calorie 263.9
    mild 263.1
    moderate 263.0
    severe 262
    specified type NEC 263.8
  severe 261
    protein-calorie NEC 262
Malocclusion (teeth) 524.4
  angle's class I 524.21
  angle's class II 524.22
  angle's class III 524.23
  due to
    abnormal swallowing 524.59
    accessory teeth (causing crowding) 524.31
    dentofacial abnormality NEC 524.89
    impacted teeth (causing crowding) 520.6
    missing teeth 524.30
    mouth breathing 524.59
    sleep postures 524.59
    supernumerary teeth (causing crowding) 524.31
    thumb sucking 524.59
    tongue, lip, or finger habits 524.59
  temporomandibular (joint) 524.69

Malposition
  cardiac apex (congenital) 746.87
  cervix - *see* Malposition, uterus
  congenital
    adrenal (gland) 759.1
    alimentary tract 751.8
      lower 751.5
      upper 750.8
    aorta 747.21
    appendix 751.5
    arterial trunk 747.29
    artery (peripheral) NEC (*see also* Malposition, congenital, peripheral vascular system) 747.60
      coronary 746.85
      pulmonary 747.39
    auditory canal 744.29
      causing impairment of hearing 744.02
    auricle (ear) 744.29
      causing impairment of hearing 744.02
      cervical 744.43
    biliary duct or passage 751.69
    bladder (mucosa) 753.8
      exteriorized or extroverted 753.5
    brachial plexus 742.8
    brain tissue 742.4
    breast 757.6
    bronchus 748.3
    cardiac apex 746.87
    cecum 751.5
    clavicle 755.51
    colon 751.5
    digestive organ or tract NEC 751.8
      lower 751.5
      upper 750.8
    ear (auricle) (external) 744.29
      ossicles 744.04
    endocrine (gland) NEC 759.2
    epiglottis 748.3
    Eustachian tube 744.24
    eye 743.8
    facial features 744.89
    fallopian tube 752.19
    finger(s) 755.59
      supernumerary 755.01
    foot 755.67
    gallbladder 751.69
    gastrointestinal tract 751.8
    genitalia, genital organ(s) or tract
      female 752.89
        external 752.49
        internal NEC 752.89
      male 752.89
        penis 752.69
        scrotal transposition 752.81
    glottis 748.3
    hand 755.59
    heart 746.87
      dextrocardia 746.87
        with complete transposition of viscera 759.3
    hepatic duct 751.69
    hip (joint) (*see also* Dislocation, hip, congenital) 754.30
    intestine (large) (small) 751.5
      with anomalous adhesions, fixation, or malrotation 751.4
    joint NEC 755.8
    kidney 753.3
    larynx 748.3
    limb 755.8
      lower 755.69
      upper 755.59
    liver 751.69
    lung (lobe) 748.69
    nail(s) 757.5
    nerve 742.8
    nervous system NEC 742.8
    nose, nasal (septum) 748.1
    organ or site NEC - *see* Anomaly, specified type NEC, by site

M

Malposition (Continued)
  congenital (Continued)
    ovary 752.0
    pancreas 751.7
    parathyroid (gland) 759.2
    patella 755.64
    peripheral vascular system 747.60
      gastrointestinal 747.61
      lower limb 747.64
      renal 747.62
      specified NEC 747.69
      spinal 747.82
      upper limb 747.63
    pituitary (gland) 759.2
    respiratory organ or system NEC 748.9
    rib (cage) 756.3
      supernumerary in cervical region 756.2
    scapula 755.59
    shoulder 755.59
    spinal cord 742.59
    spine 756.19
    spleen 759.0
    sternum 756.3
    stomach 750.7
    symphysis pubis 755.69
    testis (undescended) 752.51
    thymus (gland) 759.2
    thyroid (gland) (tissue) 759.2
      cartilage 748.3
    toe(s) 755.66
      supernumerary 755.02
    tongue 750.19
    trachea 748.3
    uterus 752.39
    vein(s) (peripheral) NEC (see also
        Malposition, congenital, peripheral
        vascular system) 747.60
      great 747.49
      portal 747.49
      pulmonary 747.49
      vena cava (inferior) (superior) 747.49
  device, implant, or graft - see Complications,
      mechanical
  fetus NEC (see also Presentation, fetal)
      652.9 ●
    with successful version 652.1 ●
    affecting fetus or newborn 763.1
    before labor, affecting fetus or newborn
        761.7
    causing obstructed labor 660.0 ●
    in multiple gestation (one fetus or more)
        652.6 ●
      with locking 660.5 ●
      causing obstructed labor 660.0 ●
  gallbladder (see also Disease, gallbladder)
      575.8
  gastrointestinal tract 569.89
    congenital 751.8
  heart (see also Malposition, congenital, heart)
      746.87
  intestine 569.89
    congenital 751.5
  pelvic organs or tissues
    in pregnancy or childbirth 654.4 ●
      affecting fetus or newborn 763.89
      causing obstructed labor 660.2 ●
        affecting fetus or newborn 763.1
  placenta - see Placenta, previa
  stomach 537.89
    congenital 750.7
  tooth, teeth 524.30
    with impaction 520.6
  uterus (acquired) (acute) (adherent) (any
      degree) (asymptomatic)
      (postinfectional) (postpartal, old) 621.6
    anteflexion or anteversion (see also
        Anteversion, uterus) 621.6
    congenital 752.39
    flexion 621.6
      lateral (see also Lateroversion, uterus)
          621.6

Malposition (Continued)
  uterus (Continued)
    in pregnancy or childbirth 654.4 ●
      affecting fetus or newborn 763.89
      causing obstructed labor 660.2 ●
        affecting fetus or newborn 763.1
    inversion 621.6
    lateral (flexion) (version) (see also
        Lateroversion, uterus) 621.6
    lateroflexion (see also Lateroversion,
        uterus) 621.6
    lateroversion (see also Lateroversion,
        uterus) 621.6
    retroflexion or retroversion (see also
        Retroversion, uterus) 621.6
Malposture 729.90
Malpresentation, fetus (see also Presentation,
    fetal) 652.9 ●
Malrotation
  cecum 751.4
  colon 751.4
  intestine 751.4
  kidney 753.3
MALT (mucosa associated lymphoid tissue)
    200.3 ●
Malt workers' lung 495.4
Malta fever (see also Brucellosis) 023.9
Maltosuria 271.3
Maltreatment (of)
  adult 995.80
    emotional 995.82
    multiple forms 995.85
    neglect (nutritional) 995.84
    physical 995.81
    psychological 995.82
    sexual 995.83
  child 995.50
    emotional 995.51
    multiple forms 995.59
    neglect (nutritional) 995.52
    physical 995.54
    shaken infant syndrome 995.55
    psychological 995.51
    sexual 995.53
  spouse (see also Maltreatment, adult) 995.80
Malum coxae senilis 715.25
Malunion, fracture 733.81
Mammillitis (see also Mastitis) 611.0
  puerperal, postpartum 675.2 ●
Mammitis (see also Mastitis) 611.0
  puerperal, postpartum 675.2 ●
Mammographic
  calcification 793.89
  calculus 793.89
  microcalcification 793.81
Mammoplasia 611.1
Management
  contraceptive V25.9
    specified type NEC V25.8
  procreative V26.9
    specified type NEC V26.89
Mangled NEC (see also nature and site of injury)
    959.9
Mania (monopolar) (see also Psychosis,
    affective) 296.0 ●
  alcoholic (acute) (chronic) 291.9
  Bell's - see Mania, chronic
  chronic 296.0 ●
    recurrent episode 296.1 ●
    single episode 296.0 ●
  compulsive 300.3
  delirious (acute) 296.0 ●
    recurrent episode 296.1 ●
    single episode 296.0 ●
  epileptic (see also Epilepsy) 345.4 ●
  hysterical 300.10
  inhibited 296.89
  puerperal (after delivery) 296.0 ●
    recurrent episode 296.1 ●
    single episode 296.0 ●
  recurrent episode 296.1 ●

Mania (Continued)
  senile 290.8
  single episode 296.0 ●
  stupor 296.89
  stuporous 296.89
  unproductive 296.89
Manic-depressive insanity, psychosis, reaction,
    or syndrome (see also Psychosis, affective)
    296.80
  circular (alternating) 296.7
    currently
      depressed 296.5 ●
      episode unspecified 296.7
      hypomanic, previously depressed
          296.4 ●
      manic 296.4 ●
    mixed 296.6 ●
  depressed (type), depressive 296.2 ●
    atypical 296.82
    recurrent episode 296.3 ●
    single episode 296.2 ●
  hypomanic 296.0 ●
    recurrent episode 296.1 ●
    single episode 296.0 ●
  manic 296.0 ●
    atypical 296.81
    recurrent episode 296.1 ●
    single episode 296.0 ●
  mixed NEC 296.89
  perplexed 296.89
  stuporous 296.89
Manifestations, rheumatoid
  lungs 714.81
  pannus - see Arthritis, rheumatoid
  subcutaneous nodules - see Arthritis,
      rheumatoid
Mankowsky's syndrome (familial dysplastic
    osteopathy) 731.2
Mannoheptulosuria 271.8
Mannosidosis 271.8
Manson's
  disease (schistosomiasis) 120.1
  pyosis (pemphigus contagiosus) 684
  schistosomiasis 120.1
Mansonellosis 125.5
Manual - see condition
Maple bark disease 495.6
Maple bark-strippers' lung 495.6
Maple syrup (urine) disease or syndrome
    270.3
Marable's syndrome (celiac artery
    compression) 447.4
Marasmus 261
  brain 331.9
  due to malnutrition 261
  intestinal 569.89
  nutritional 261
  senile 797
  tuberculous NEC (see also Tuberculosis)
      011.9 ●
Marble
  bones 756.52
  skin 782.61
Marburg disease (virus) 078.89
March
  foot 733.94
  hemoglobinuria 283.2
Marchand multiple nodular hyperplasia (liver)
    571.5
Marchesani (-Weill) syndrome
    (brachymorphism and ectopia lentis)
    759.89
Marchiafava (-Bignami) disease or syndrome
    341.8
Marchiafava-Micheli syndrome (paroxysmal
    nocturnal hemoglobinuria) 283.2
Marcus Gunn's syndrome (jaw-winking
    syndrome) 742.8
Marfan's
  congenital syphilis 090.49
  disease 090.49

◀ New ⬅ Revised d̶e̶l̶e̶t̶e̶d̶ Deleted ● Use Additional Digit(s) ▨ Omit code

Marfan's (Continued)
  syndrome (arachnodactyly) 759.82
    meaning congenital syphilis 090.49
      with luxation of lens 090.49 [379.32]
Marginal
  implantation, placenta - see Placenta, previa
  placenta - see Placenta, previa
  sinus (hemorrhage) (rupture) 641.2●
    affecting fetus or newborn 762.1
Marie's
  cerebellar ataxia 334.2
  syndrome (acromegaly) 253.0
Marie-Bamberger disease or syndrome
    (hypertrophic) (pulmonary) (secondary)
    731.2
  idiopathic (acropachyderma) 757.39
  primary (acropachyderma) 757.39
Marie-Charcôt-Tooth neuropathic atrophy,
    muscle 356.1
Marie-Strümpell arthritis or disease
    (ankylosing spondylitis) 720.0
Marihuana, marijuana
  abuse (see also Abuse, drugs, nondependent)
    305.2●
  dependence (see also Dependence) 304.3●
Marion's disease (bladder neck obstruction)
    596.0
Marital conflict V61.10
Mark
  port wine 757.32
  raspberry 757.32
  strawberry 757.32
  stretch 701.3
  tattoo 709.09
Maroteaux-Lamy syndrome
    (mucopolysaccharidosis VI) 277.5
Marriage license examination V70.3
Marrow (bone)
  arrest 284.9
  megakaryocytic 287.30
  poor function 289.9
Marseilles fever 082.1
Marsh's disease (exophthalmic goiter) 242.0●
Marshall's (hidrotic) ectodermal dysplasia
    757.31
Marsh fever (see also Malaria) 084.6
Martin's disease 715.27
Martin-Albright syndrome
    (pseudohypoparathyroidism) 275.49
Martorell-Fabre syndrome (pulseless disease)
    446.7
Masculinization, female, with adrenal
    hyperplasia 255.2
Masculinovoblastoma (M8670/0) 220
Masochism 302.83
Masons' lung 502
Mass
  abdominal 789.3●
  anus 787.99
  bone 733.90
  breast 611.72
  cheek 784.2
  chest 786.6
  cystic - see Cyst
  ear 388.8
  epigastric 789.3●
  eye 379.92
  female genital organ 625.8
  gum 784.2
  head 784.2
  intracranial 784.2
  joint 719.60
    ankle 719.67
    elbow 719.62
    foot 719.67
    hand 719.64
    hip 719.65
    knee 719.66
    multiple sites 719.69
    pelvic region 719.65
    shoulder (region) 719.61

Mass (Continued)
  joint (Continued)
    specified site NEC 719.68
    wrist 719.63
  kidney (see also Disease, kidney) 593.9
  lung 786.6
  lymph node 785.6
  malignant (M8000/3) - see Neoplasm, by site,
    malignant
  mediastinal 786.6
  mouth 784.2
  muscle (limb) 729.89
  neck 784.2
  nose or sinus 784.2
  palate 784.2
  pelvis, pelvic 789.3●
  penis 607.89
  perineum 625.8
  rectum 787.99
  scrotum 608.89
  skin 782.2
  specified organ NEC - see Disease of
    specified organ or site
  splenic 789.2
  substernal 786.6
    thyroid (see also Goiter) 240.9
  superficial (localized) 782.2
  testes 608.89
  throat 784.2
  tongue 784.2
  umbilicus 789.3●
  uterus 625.8
  vagina 625.8
  vulva 625.8
Massive - see condition
Mastalgia 611.71
  psychogenic 307.89
Mast cell
  disease 757.33
    systemic (M9741/3) 202.6●
  leukemia (M9900/3) 207.8●
  sarcoma (M9740/3) 202.6●
  tumor (M9740/1) 238.5
    malignant (M9740/3) 202.6●
Masters-Allen syndrome 620.6
Mastitis (acute) (adolescent) (diffuse)
    (interstitial) (lobular) (nonpuerperal)
    (nonsuppurative) (parenchymatous)
    (phlegmonous) (simple) (subacute)
    (suppurative) 611.0
  chronic (cystic) (fibrocystic) 610.1
  cystic 610.1
    Schimmelbusch's type 610.1
  fibrocystic 610.1
  infective 611.0
  lactational 675.2●
  lymphangitis 611.0
  neonatal (noninfective) 778.7
    infective 771.5
  periductal 610.4
  plasma cell 610.4
  puerperal, postpartum, (interstitial)
    (nonpurulent) (parenchymatous)
    675.2●
    purulent 675.1●
    stagnation 676.2●
  puerperalis 675.2●
  retromammary 611.0
    puerperal, postpartum 675.1●
  submammary 611.0
    puerperal, postpartum 675.1●
Mastocytoma (M9740/1) 238.5
  malignant (M9740/3) 202.6●
Mastocytosis 757.33
  malignant (M9741/3) 202.6●
  systemic (M9741/3) 202.6●
Mastodynia 611.71
  psychogenic 307.89
Mastoid - see condition
Mastoidalgia (see also Otalgia)
  388.70

Mastoiditis (coalescent) (hemorrhagic)
    (pneumococcal) (streptococcal)
    (suppurative) 383.9
  acute or subacute 383.00
    with
      Gradenigo's syndrome 383.02
      petrositis 383.02
      specified complication NEC 383.02
      subperiosteal abscess 383.01
  chronic (necrotic) (recurrent) 383.1
  tuberculous (see also Tuberculosis) 015.6●
Mastopathy, mastopathia 611.9
  chronica cystica 610.1
  diffuse cystic 610.1
  estrogenic 611.89
  ovarian origin 611.89
Mastoplasia 611.1
Masturbation 307.9
Maternal condition, affecting fetus or
    newborn
  acute yellow atrophy of liver 760.8
  albuminuria 760.1
  anesthesia or analgesia 763.5
  blood loss 762.1
  chorioamnionitis 762.7
  circulatory disease, chronic (conditions
    classifiable to 390–459, 745–747) 760.3
  congenital heart disease (conditions
    classifiable to 745–746) 760.3
  cortical necrosis of kidney 760.1
  death 761.6
  diabetes mellitus 775.0
    manifest diabetes in the infant 775.1
  disease NEC 760.9
    circulatory system, chronic (conditions
      classifiable to 390–459, 745–747)
      760.3
    genitourinary system (conditions
      classifiable to 580–599) 760.1
    respiratory (conditions classifiable to
      490–519, 748) 760.3
  eclampsia 760.0
  hemorrhage NEC 762.1
  hepatitis acute, malignant, or subacute 760.8
  hyperemesis (gravidarum) 761.8
  hypertension (arising during pregnancy)
    (conditions classifiable to 642) 760.0
  infection
    disease classifiable to 001–136 760.2
    genital tract NEC 760.8
    urinary tract 760.1
  influenza 760.2
    manifest influenza in the infant 771.2
  injury (conditions classifiable to 800–996)
    760.5
  malaria 760.2
    manifest malaria in infant or fetus 771.2
  malnutrition 760.4
  necrosis of liver 760.8
  nephritis (conditions classifiable to 580–583)
    760.1
  nephrosis (conditions classifiable to 581)
    760.1
  noxious substance transmitted via breast
    milk or placenta 760.70
    alcohol 760.71
    anticonvulsants 760.77
    antifungals 760.74
    anti-infective agents 760.74
    antimetabolics 760.78
    cocaine 760.75
    "crack" 760.75
    diethylstilbestrol [DES] 760.76
    hallucinogenic agents 760.73
    medicinal agents NEC 760.79
    narcotics 760.72
    obstetric anesthetic or analgesic drug
      760.72
    specified agent NEC 760.79
  nutritional disorder (conditions classifiable
    to 260–269) 760.4

Maternal condition, affecting fetus or
newborn (Continued)
operation unrelated to current delivery (see
also Newborn, affected by) 760.64
pre-eclampsia 760.0
pyelitis or pyelonephritis, arising during
pregnancy (conditions classifiable to
590) 760.1
renal disease or failure 760.1
respiratory disease, chronic (conditions
classifiable to 490–519, 748) 760.3
rheumatic heart disease (chronic) (conditions
classifiable to 393–398) 760.3
rubella (conditions classifiable to 056) 760.2
manifest rubella in the infant or fetus
771.0
surgery unrelated to current delivery (see also
Newborn, affected by) 760.64
to uterus or pelvic organs 760.64
syphilis (conditions classifiable to 090–097)
760.2
manifest syphilis in the infant or fetus
090.0
thrombophlebitis 760.3
toxemia (of pregnancy) 760.0
pre-eclamptic 760.0
toxoplasmosis (conditions classifiable to 130)
760.2
manifest toxoplasmosis in the infant or
fetus 771.2
transmission of chemical substance through
the placenta 760.70
alcohol 760.71
anticonvulsants 760.77
antifungals 760.74
anti-infective 760.74
antimetabolics 760.78
cocaine 760.75
"crack" 760.75
diethylstilbestrol [DES] 760.76
hallucinogenic agents 760.73
narcotics 760.72
specified substance NEC 760.79
uremia 760.1
urinary tract conditions (conditions
classifiable to 580–599) 760.1
vomiting (pernicious) (persistent) (vicious)
761.8
Maternity - see Delivery
Matheiu's disease (leptospiral jaundice) 100.0
Mauclaire's disease or osteochondrosis 732.3
Maxcy's disease 081.0
Maxilla, maxillary - see condition
May (-Hegglin) anomaly or syndrome 288.2
Mayaro fever 066.3
Mazoplasia 610.8
MBD (minimal brain dysfunction), child (see
also Hyperkinesia) 314.9
MCAD (medium chain acyl CoA
dehydrogenase deficiency) 277.85
McArdle (-Schmid-Pearson) disease or
syndrome (glycogenosis V) 271.0
McCune-Albright syndrome (osteitis fibrosa
disseminata) 756.59
MCLS (mucocutaneous lymph node syndrome)
446.1
McQuarrie's syndrome (idiopathic familial
hypoglycemia) 251.2
Measles (black) (hemorrhagic) (suppressed)
055.9
with
encephalitis 055.0
keratitis 055.71
keratoconjunctivitis 055.71
otitis media 055.2
pneumonia 055.1
complication 055.8
specified type NEC 055.79
encephalitis 055.0
French 056.9
German 056.9

Measles (Continued)
keratitis 055.71
keratoconjunctivitis 055.71
liberty 056.9
otitis media 055.2
pneumonia 055.1
specified complications NEC 055.79
vaccination, prophylactic (against) V04.2
Meatitis, urethral (see also Urethritis) 597.89
Meat poisoning - see Poisoning, food
Meatus, meatal - see condition
Meat-wrappers' asthma 506.9
Meckel's
diverticulitis 751.0
diverticulum (displaced) (hypertrophic)
751.0
Meconium
aspiration 770.11
with
pneumonia 770.12
pneumonitis 770.12
respiratory symptoms 770.12
below vocal cords 770.11
with respiratory symptoms 770.12
syndrome 770.12
delayed passage in newborn 777.1
ileus 777.1
due to cystic fibrosis 277.01
in liquor 792.3
noted during delivery - 656.8●
insufflation 770.11
with respiratory symptoms 770.12
obstruction
fetus or newborn 777.1
in mucoviscidosis 277.01
passage of 792.3
noted during delivery 763.84
peritonitis 777.6
plug syndrome (newborn) NEC 777.1
staining 779.84
Median - see also condition
arcuate ligament syndrome 447.4
bar (prostate) 600.90
with
other lower urinary tract symptoms
(LUTS) 600.91
urinary
obstruction 600.91
retention 600.91
rhomboid glossitis 529.2
vesical orifice 600.90
with
other lower urinary tract symptoms
(LUTS) 600.91
urinary
obstruction 600.91
retention 600.91
Mediastinal shift 793.2
Mediastinitis (acute) (chronic) 519.2
actinomycotic 039.8
syphilitic 095.8
tuberculous (see also Tuberculosis) 012.8●
Mediastinopericarditis (see also Pericarditis)
423.9
acute 420.90
chronic 423.8
rheumatic 393
rheumatic, chronic 393
Mediastinum, mediastinal - see condition
Medical services provided for - see Health,
services provided because (of)
Medicine poisoning (by overdose) (wrong
substance given or taken in error) 977.9
specified drug or substance - see Table of
Drugs and Chemicals
Medin's disease (poliomyelitis) 045.9●
Mediterranean
anemia 282.40
with other hemoglobinopathy 282.49
disease or syndrome (hemopathic) 282.40
with other hemoglobinopathy 282.49

Mediterranean (Continued)
fever (see also Brucellosis) 023.9
familial 277.31
kala-azar 085.0
leishmaniasis 085.0
tick fever 082.1
Medulla - see condition
Medullary
cystic kidney 753.16
sponge kidney 753.17
Medullated fibers
optic (nerve) 743.57
retina 362.85
Medulloblastoma (M9470/3) 191.6
desmoplastic (M9471/3) 191.6
specified site - see Neoplasm, by site,
malignant
unspecified site 191.6
Medulloepithelioma (M9501/3) - see also
Neoplasm, by site, malignant
teratoid (M9502/3) - see Neoplasm, by site,
malignant
Medullomyoblastoma (M9472/3)
specified site - see Neoplasm, by site,
malignant
unspecified site 191.6
Meekeren-Ehlers-Danlos syndrome 756.83
Megacaryocytic - see condition
Megacolon (acquired) (functional) (not
Hirschsprung's disease) 564.7
aganglionic 751.3
congenital, congenitum 751.3
Hirschsprung's (disease) 751.3
psychogenic 306.4
toxic (see also Colitis, ulcerative) 556.9
Megaduodenum 537.3
Megaesophagus (functional) 530.0
congenital 750.4
Megakaryocytic - see condition
Megalencephaly 742.4
Megalerythema (epidermicum) (infectiosum)
057.0
Megalia, cutis et ossium 757.39
Megaloappendix 751.5
Megalocephalus, megalocephaly NEC
756.0
Megalocornea 743.41
associated with buphthalmos 743.22
Megalocytic anemia 281.9
Megalodactylia (fingers) (thumbs) 755.57
toes 755.65
Megaloduodenum 751.5
Megaloesophagus (functional) 530.0
congenital 750.4
Megalogastria (congenital) 750.7
Megalomania 307.9
Megalophthalmos 743.8
Megalopsia 368.14
Megalosplenia (see also Splenomegaly)
789.2
Megaloureter 593.89
congenital 753.22
Megarectum 569.49
Megasigmoid 564.7
congenital 751.3
Megaureter 593.89
congenital 753.22
Megrim 346.9●
Meibomian
cyst 373.2
infected 373.12
gland - see condition
infarct (eyelid) 374.85
stye 373.11
Meibomitis 373.12
Meige
-Milroy disease (chronic hereditary edema)
757.0
syndrome (blepharospasm-oromandibular
dystonia) 333.82
Melalgia, nutritional 266.2

◀ New ◀▥ Revised ~~deleted~~ Deleted ● Use Additional Digit(s) ▨ Omit code

Melancholia (see also Psychosis, affective) 296.90
  climacteric 296.2●
    recurrent episode 296.3●
    single episode 296.2●
  hypochondriac 300.7
  intermittent 296.2●
    recurrent episode 296.3●
    single episode 296.2●
  involutional 296.2●
    recurrent episode 296.3●
    single episode 296.2●
  menopausal 296.2●
    recurrent episode 296.3●
    single episode 296.2●
  puerperal 296.2●
  reactive (from emotional stress, psychological trauma) 298.0
  recurrent 296.3●
  senile 290.21
  stuporous 296.2●
    recurrent episode 296.3●
    single episode 296.2●
Melanemia 275.09
Melanoameloblastoma (M9363/0) - see Neoplasm, bone, benign
Melanoblastoma (M8720/3) - see Melanoma
Melanoblastosis
  Block-Sulzberger 757.33
  cutis linearis sive systematisata 757.33
Melanocarcinoma (M8720/3) - see Melanoma
Melanocytoma, eyeball (M8726/0) 224.0
Melanocytosis, neurocutaneous 757.33
Melanoderma, melanodermia 709.09
  Addison's (primary adrenal insufficiency) 255.41
Melanodontia, infantile 521.05
Melanodontoclasia 521.05
Melanoepithelioma (M8720/3) - see Melanoma
Melanoma (malignant) (M8720/3) 172.9

Note: Except where otherwise indicated, the morphological varieties of melanoma in the list below should be coded by site as for "Melanoma (malignant)." Internal sites should be coded to malignant neoplasm of those sites.

  abdominal wall 172.5
  ala nasi 172.3
  amelanotic (M8730/3) - see Melanoma, by site
  ankle 172.7
  anus, anal 154.3
    canal 154.2
  arm 172.6
  auditory canal (external) 172.2
  auricle (ear) 172.2
  auricular canal (external) 172.2
  axilla 172.5
  axillary fold 172.5
  back 172.5
  balloon cell (M8722/3) - see Melanoma, by site
  benign (M8720/0) - see Neoplasm, skin, benign
  breast (female) (male) 172.5
  brow 172.3
  buttock 172.5
  canthus (eye) 172.1
  cheek (external) 172.3
  chest wall 172.5
  chin 172.3
  choroid 190.6
  conjunctiva 190.3
  ear (external) 172.2
  epithelioid cell (M8771/3) - see also Melanoma, by site
    and spindle cell, mixed (M8775/3) - see Melanoma, by site
  external meatus (ear) 172.2

Melanoma (Continued)
  eye 190.9
  eyebrow 172.3
  eyelid (lower) (upper) 172.1
  face NEC 172.3
  female genital organ (external) NEC 184.4
  finger 172.6
  flank 172.5
  foot 172.7
  forearm 172.6
  forehead 172.3
  foreskin 187.1
  gluteal region 172.5
  groin 172.5
  hand 172.6
  heel 172.7
  helix 172.2
  hip 172.7
  in
    giant pigmented nevus (M8761/3) - see Melanoma, by site
    Hutchinson's melanotic freckle (M8742/3) - see Melanoma, by site
    junctional nevus (M8740/3) - see Melanoma, by site
    precancerous melanosis (M8741/3) - see Melanoma, by site
  in situ - see Melanoma, by site
    skin 172.9
  interscapular region 172.5
  iris 190.0
  jaw 172.3
  juvenile (M8770/0) - see Neoplasm, skin, benign
  knee 172.7
  labium
    majus 184.1
    minus 184.2
  lacrimal gland 190.2
  leg 172.7
  lip (lower) (upper) 172.0
  liver 197.7
  lower limb NEC 172.7
  male genital organ (external) NEC 187.9
  meatus, acoustic (external) 172.2
  meibomian gland 172.1
  metastatic
    of or from specified site - see Melanoma, by site
    site not of skin - see Neoplasm, by site, malignant, secondary
    to specified site - see Neoplasm, by site, malignant, secondary
    unspecified site 172.9
  nail 172.9
    finger 172.6
    toe 172.7
  neck 172.4
  nodular (M8721/3) - see Melanoma, by site
  nose, external 172.3
  orbit 190.1
  penis 187.4
  perianal skin 172.5
  perineum 172.5
  pinna 172.2
  popliteal (fossa) (space) 172.7
  prepuce 187.1
  pubes 172.5
  pudendum 184.4
  retina 190.5
  scalp 172.4
  scrotum 187.7
  septum nasal (skin) 172.3
  shoulder 172.6
  skin NEC 172.8
    in situ 172.9
  spindle cell (M8772/3) - see also Melanoma, by site
    type A (M8773/3) 190.0
    type B (M8774/3) 190.0
  submammary fold 172.5

Melanoma (Continued)
  superficial spreading (M8743/3) - see Melanoma, by site
  temple 172.3
  thigh 172.7
  toe 172.7
  trunk NEC 172.5
  umbilicus 172.5
  upper limb NEC 172.6
  vagina vault 184.0
  vulva 184.4
Melanoplakia 528.9
Melanosarcoma (M8720/3) - see also Melanoma
  epithelioid cell (M8771/3) - see Melanoma
Melanosis 709.09
  addisonian (primary adrenal insufficiency) 255.41
    tuberculous (see also Tuberculosis) 017.6●
  adrenal 255.41
  colon 569.89
  conjunctiva 372.55
    congenital 743.49
  corii degenerativa 757.33
  cornea (presenile) (senile) 371.12
    congenital 743.43
      interfering with vision 743.42
    prenatal 743.43
      interfering with vision 743.42
  eye 372.55
    congenital 743.49
  jute spinners' 709.09
  lenticularis progressiva 757.33
  liver 573.8
  precancerous (M8741/2) - see also Neoplasm, skin, in situ
    malignant melanoma in (M8741/3) - see Melanoma
  Riehl's 709.09
  sclera 379.19
    congenital 743.47
  suprarenal 255.41
  tar 709.09
  toxic 709.09
Melanuria 791.9
MELAS syndrome (mitochondrial encephalopathy, lactic acidosis and stroke-like episodes) 277.87
Melasma 709.09
  adrenal (gland) 255.41
  suprarenal (gland) 255.41
Melena 578.1
  due to
    swallowed maternal blood 777.3
    ulcer - see Ulcer, by site, with hemorrhage
  newborn 772.4
    due to swallowed maternal blood 777.3
Meleney's
  gangrene (cutaneous) 686.09
  ulcer (chronic undermining) 686.09
Melioidosis 025
Melitensis, febris 023.0
Melitococcosis 023.0
Melkersson (-Rosenthal) syndrome 351.8
Mellitus, diabetes - see Diabetes
Melorheostosis (bone) (leri) 733.99
Meloschisis 744.83
Melotia 744.29
Membrana
  capsularis lentis posterior 743.39
  epipapillaris 743.57
Membranacea placenta - see Placenta, abnormal
Membranaceous uterus 621.8
Membrane, membranous - see also condition
  folds, congenital - see Web
  Jackson's 751.4
  over face (causing asphyxia), fetus or newborn 768.9
  premature rupture - see Rupture, membranes, premature
  pupillary 364.74
    persistent 743.46

Membrane, membranous (*Continued*)
retained (complicating delivery) (with hemorrhage) 666.2●
without hemorrhage 667.1●
secondary (eye) 366.50
unruptured (causing asphyxia) 768.9
vitreous humor 379.25
Membranitis, fetal 658.4●
affecting fetus or newborn 762.7
Memory disturbance, loss or lack (*see also* Amnesia) 780.93
mild, following organic brain damage 310.89
MEN (multiple endocrine neoplasia) syndromes
type I 258.01
type IIA 258.02
type IIB 258.03
Menadione (vitamin K) deficiency 269.0
Menarche, precocious 259.1
Mendacity, pathologic 301.7
Mende's syndrome (ptosis-epicanthus) 270.2
Mendelson's syndrome (resulting from a procedure) 997.32
obstetric 668.0●
Ménétrier's disease or syndrome (hypertrophic gastritis) 535.2●
Ménière's disease, syndrome, or vertigo 386.00
cochlear 386.02
cochleovestibular 386.01
inactive 386.04
in remission 386.04
vestibular 386.03
Meninges, meningeal - *see* condition
Meningioma (M9530/0) - *see also* Neoplasm, meninges, benign
angioblastic (M9535/0) - *see* Neoplasm, meninges, benign
angiomatous (M9534/0) - *see* Neoplasm, meninges, benign
endotheliomatous (M9531/0) - *see* Neoplasm, meninges, benign
fibroblastic (M9532/0) - *see* Neoplasm, meninges, benign
fibrous (M9532/0) - *see* Neoplasm, meninges, benign
hemangioblastic (M9535/0) - *see* Neoplasm, meninges, benign
hemangiopericytic (M9536/0) - *see* Neoplasm, meninges, benign
malignant (M9530/3) - *see* Neoplasm, meninges, malignant
meningiothelial (M9531/0) - *see* Neoplasm, meninges, benign
meningotheliomatous (M9531/0) - *see* Neoplasm, meninges, benign
mixed (M9537/0) - *see* Neoplasm, meninges, benign
multiple (M9530/1) 237.6
papillary (M9538/1) 237.6
psammomatous (M9533/0) - *see* Neoplasm, meninges, benign
syncytial (M9531/0) - *see* Neoplasm, meninges, benign
transitional (M9537/0) - *see* Neoplasm, meninges, benign
Meningiomatosis (diffuse) (M9530/1) 237.6
Meningism (*see also* Meningismus) 781.6
Meningismus (infectional) (pneumococcal) 781.6
due to serum or vaccine 997.09 [321.8]
influenzal NEC (*see also* Influenza) 487.8
Meningitis (basal) (basic) (basilar) (brain) (cerebral) (cervical) (congestive) (diffuse) (hemorrhagic) (infantile) (membranous) (metastatic) (nonspecific) (pontine) (progressive) (simple) (spinal) (subacute) (sympathetica) (toxic) 322.9
abacterial NEC (*see also* Meningitis, aseptic) 047.9
actinomycotic 039.8 [320.7]
adenoviral 049.1
aerobacter aerogenes 320.82

Meningitis (*Continued*)
anaerobes (cocci) (gram-negative) (gram-positive) (mixed) (NEC) 320.81
arbovirus NEC 066.9 [321.2]
specified type NEC 066.8 [321.2]
aseptic (acute) NEC 047.9
adenovirus 049.1
Coxsackie virus 047.0
due to
adenovirus 049.1
Coxsackie virus 047.0
ECHO virus 047.1
enterovirus 047.9
mumps 072.1
poliovirus (*see also* Poliomyelitis) 045.2● [321.2]
ECHO virus 047.1
herpes (simplex) virus 054.72
zoster 053.0
leptospiral 100.81
lymphocytic choriomeningitis 049.0
noninfective 322.0
Bacillus pyocyaneus 320.89
bacterial NEC 320.9
anaerobic 320.81
gram-negative 320.82
anaerobic 320.81
Bacteroides (fragilis) (oralis) (melaninogenicus) 320.81
cancerous (M8000/6) 198.4
candidal 112.83
carcinomatous (M8010/6) 198.4
caseous (*see also* Tuberculosis, meninges) 013.0●
cerebrospinal (acute) (chronic) (diplococcal) (endemic) (epidemic) (fulminant) (infectious) (malignant) (meningococcal) (sporadic) 036.0
carrier (suspected) of V02.59
chronic NEC 322.2
clear cerebrospinal fluid NEC 322.0
Clostridium (haemolyticum) (novyi) NEC 320.81
coccidioidomycosis 114.2
Coxsackie virus 047.0
cryptococcal 117.5 [321.0]
diplococcal 036.0
gram-negative 036.0
gram-positive 320.1
Diplococcus pneumoniae 320.1
due to
actinomycosis 039.8 [320.7]
adenovirus 049.1
coccidiomycosis 114.2
enterovirus 047.9
specified NEC 047.8
histoplasmosis (*see also* Histoplasmosis) 115.91
Listerosis 027.0 [320.7]
Lyme disease 088.81 [320.7]
moniliasis 112.83
mumps 072.1
neurosyphilis 094.2
nonbacterial organisms NEC 321.8
oidiomycosis 112.83
poliovirus (*see also* Poliomyelitis) 045.2● [321.2]
preventive immunization, inoculation, or vaccination 997.09 [321.8]
sarcoidosis 135 [321.4]
sporotrichosis 117.1 [321.1]
syphilis 094.2
acute 091.81
congenital 090.42
secondary 091.81
trypanosomiasis (*see also* Trypanosomiasis) 086.9 [321.3]
whooping cough 033.9 [320.7]
E. coli 320.82
ECHO virus 047.1

Meningitis (*Continued*)
endothelial-leukocytic, benign, recurrent 047.9
Enterobacter aerogenes 320.82
enteroviral 047.9
specified type NEC 047.8
enterovirus 047.9
specified NEC 047.8
eosinophilic 322.1
epidemic NEC 036.0
Escherichia coli (E. coli) 320.82
Eubacterium 320.81
fibrinopurulent NEC 320.9
specified type NEC 320.89
Friedländer (bacillus) 320.82
fungal NEC 117.9 [321.1]
Fusobacterium 320.81
gonococcal 098.82
gram-negative bacteria NEC 320.82
anaerobic 320.81
cocci 036.0
specified NEC 320.82
gram-negative cocci NEC 036.0
specified NEC 320.82
gram-positive cocci NEC 320.9
H. influenzae 320.0
herpes (simplex) virus 054.72
zoster 053.0
infectious NEC 320.9
influenzal 320.0
Klebsiella pneumoniae 320.82
late effect - *see* Late, effect, meningitis
leptospiral (aseptic) 100.81
Listerella (monocytogenes) 027.0 [320.7]
Listeria monocytogenes 027.0 [320.7]
lymphocytic (acute) (benign) (serous) 049.0
choriomeningitis virus 049.0
meningococcal (chronic) 036.0
Mima polymorpha 320.82
Mollaret's 047.9
monilial 112.83
mumps (virus) 072.1
mycotic NEC 117.9 [321.1]
Neisseria 036.0
neurosyphilis 094.2
nonbacterial NEC (*see also* Meningitis, aseptic) 047.9
nonpyogenic NEC 322.0
oidiomycosis 112.83
ossificans 349.2
Peptococcus 320.81
PeptoStreptococcus 320.81
pneumococcal 320.1
poliovirus (*see also* Poliomyelitis) 045.2● [321.2]
Proprionibacterium 320.81
Proteus morganii 320.82
Pseudomonas (aeruginosa) (pyocyaneus) 320.82
purulent NEC 320.9
specified organism NEC 320.89
pyogenic NEC 320.9
specified organism NEC 320.89
Salmonella 003.21
septic NEC 320.9
specified organism NEC 320.89
serosa circumscripta NEC 322.0
serous NEC (*see also* Meningitis, aseptic) 047.9
lymphocytic 049.0
syndrome 348.2
Serratia (marcescens) 320.82
specified organism NEC 320.89
sporadic cerebrospinal 036.0
sporotrichosis 117.1 [321.1]
staphylococcal 320.3
sterile 997.09
streptococcal (acute) 320.2
suppurative 320.9
specified organism NEC 320.89

◀ New ◀◀ Revised deleted Deleted ● Use Additional Digit(s) Omit code

Meningitis (Continued)
  syphilitic 094.2
    acute 091.81
    congenital 090.42
    secondary 091.81
  torula 117.5 [321.0]
  traumatic (complication of injury) 958.8
  Treponema (denticola) (macrodenticum)
    320.81
  trypanosomiasis 086.1 [321.3]
  tuberculous (see also Tuberculosis, meninges)
    013.0●
  typhoid 002.0 [320.7]
  Veillonella 320.81
  Vibrio vulnificus 320.82
  viral, virus NEC (see also Meningitis, aseptic)
    047.9
  Wallgren's (see also Meningitis, aseptic) 047.9
Meningocele (congenital) (spinal) (see also
    Spina bifida) 741.9●
  acquired (traumatic) 349.2
  cerebral 742.0
  cranial 742.0
Meningocerebritis - see Meningoencephalitis
Meningococcemia (acute) (chronic) 036.2
Meningococcus, meningococcal (see also
    condition) 036.9
  adrenalitis, hemorrhagic 036.3
  carditis 036.40
  carrier (suspected) of V02.59
  cerebrospinal fever 036.0
  encephalitis 036.1
  endocarditis 036.42
  exposure to V01.84
  infection NEC 036.9
  meningitis (cerebrospinal) 036.0
  myocarditis 036.43
  optic neuritis 036.81
  pericarditis 036.41
  septicemia (chronic) 036.2
Meningoencephalitis (see also Encephalitis)
    323.9
  acute NEC 048
  bacterial, purulent, pyogenic, or septic - see
    Meningitis
  chronic NEC 094.1
  diffuse NEC 094.1
  diphasic 063.2
  due to
    actinomycosis 039.8 [320.7]
    blastomycosis NEC (see also
      Blastomycosis) 116.0 [323.41]
    free-living amebae 136.29
    Listeria monocytogenes 027.0 [320.7]
    Lyme disease 088.81 [320.7]
    mumps 072.2
    Naegleria (amebae) (gruberi) (organisms)
      136.29
    rubella 056.01
    sporotrichosis 117.1 [321.1]
    toxoplasmosis (acquired) 130.0
      congenital (active) 771.2 [323.41]
    Trypanosoma 086.1 [323.2]
  epidemic 036.0
  herpes 054.3
  herpetic 054.3
  H. influenzae 320.0
  infectious (acute) 048
  influenzal 320.0
  late effect - see category 326
  Listeria monocytogenes 027.0 [320.7]
  lymphocytic (serous) 049.0
  mumps 072.2
  parasitic NEC 123.9 [323.41]
  pneumococcal 320.1
  primary amebic 136.29
  rubella 056.01
  serous 048
    lymphocytic 049.0
  specific 094.2
  staphylococcal 320.3

Meningoencephalitis (Continued)
  streptococcal 320.2
  syphilitic 094.2
  toxic NEC 989.9 [323.71]
    due to
      carbon tetrachloride (vapor) 987.8
        [323.71]
      hydroxyquinoline derivatives
        poisoning 961.3 [323.71]
      lead 984.9 [323.71]
      mercury 985.0 [323.71]
      thallium 985.8 [323.71]
  toxoplasmosis (acquired) 130.0
  trypanosomic 086.1 [323.2]
  tuberculous (see also Tuberculosis, meninges)
    013.0●
  virus NEC 048
Meningoencephalocele 742.0
  syphilitic 094.89
    congenital 090.49
Meningoencephalomyelitis (see also
    Meningoencephalitis) 323.9
  acute NEC 048
    disseminated (postinfectious) 136.9
      [323.61]
      postimmunization or postvaccination
        323.51
  due to
    actinomycosis 039.8 [320.7]
    torula 117.5 [323.41]
    toxoplasma or toxoplasmosis (acquired)
      130.0
      congenital (active) 771.2 [323.41]
  late effect - see category 326
Meningoencephalomyelopathy (see also
    Meningoencephalomyelitis) 349.9
Meningoencephalopathy (see also
    Meningoencephalitis) 348.39
Meningoencephalopoliomyelitis (see also
    Poliomyelitis, bulbar) 045.0●
  late effect 138
Meningomyelitis (see also Meningoencephalitis)
    323.9
  blastomycotic NEC (see also Blastomycosis)
    116.0 [323.41]
  due to
    actinomycosis 039.8 [320.7]
    blastomycosis (see also Blastomycosis)
      116.0 [323.41]
    Meningococcus 036.0
    sporotrichosis 117.1 [323.41]
    torula 117.5 [323.41]
  late effect - see category 326
  lethargic 049.8
  meningococcal 036.0
  syphilitic 094.2
  tuberculous (see also Tuberculosis, meninges)
    013.0●
Meningomyelocele (see also Spina bifida)
    741.9●
  syphilitic 094.89
Meningomyeloneuritis - see
    Meningoencephalitis
Meningoradiculitis - see Meningitis
Meningovascular - see condition
Meniscocytosis 282.60
Menkes' syndrome - see Syndrome,
    Menkes'
Menolipsis 626.0
Menometrorrhagia 626.2
Menopause, menopausal (symptoms)
    (syndrome) 627.2
  arthritis (any site) NEC 716.3●
  artificial 627.4
  bleeding 627.0
  crisis 627.2
  depression (see also Psychosis, affective)
    296.2●
    agitated 296.2●
      recurrent episode 296.3●
      single episode 296.2●

Menopause, menopausal (Continued)
  depression (Continued)
    psychotic 296.2●
      recurrent episode 296.3●
      single episode 296.2●
    recurrent episode 296.3●
    single episode 296.2●
    melancholia (see also Psychosis, affective)
      296.2●
      recurrent episode 296.3●
      single episode 296.2●
  paranoid state 297.2
  paraphrenia 297.2
  postsurgical 627.4
  premature 256.31
    postirradiation 256.2
    postsurgical 256.2
  psychoneurosis 627.2
  psychosis NEC 298.8
  surgical 627.4
  toxic polyarthritis NEC 716.39
Menorrhagia (primary) 626.2
  climacteric 627.0
  menopausal 627.0
  postclimacteric 627.1
  postmenopausal 627.1
  preclimacteric 627.0
  premenopausal 627.0
  puberty (menses retained) 626.3
Menorrhalgia 625.3
Menoschesis 626.8
Menostaxis 626.2
Menstrual - see also Menstruation
  cycle, irregular 626.4
  disorders NEC 626.9
  extraction V25.3
  fluid, retained 626.8
  molimen 625.4
  period, normal V65.5
  regulation V25.3
Menstruation
  absent 626.0
  anovulatory 628.0
  delayed 626.8
  difficult 625.3
  disorder 626.9
    psychogenic 306.52
    specified NEC 626.8
  during pregnancy 640.8●
  excessive 626.2
  frequent 626.2
  infrequent 626.1
  irregular 626.4
  latent 626.8
  membranous 626.8
  painful (primary) (secondary) 625.3
    psychogenic 306.52
  passage of clots 626.2
  precocious 259.1
  protracted 626.8
  retained 626.8
  retrograde 626.8
  scanty 626.1
  suppression 626.8
  vicarious (nasal) 625.8
Mentagra (see also Sycosis) 704.8
Mental - see also condition
  deficiency (see also Disability, intellectual) 319
  deterioration (see also Psychosis) 298.9
  disorder (see also Disorder, mental) 300.9
  exhaustion 300.5
  insufficiency (congenital) (see also Disability,
    intellectual) 319
  observation without need for further medical
    care NEC V71.09
  retardation - see Disability, intellectual
  subnormality (see also Disability, intellectual)
    319
    mild 317
    moderate 318.0

M

Mental (*Continued*)
  subnormality (*Continued*)
    profound 318.2
    severe 318.1
  upset (*see also* Disorder, mental) 300.9
Meralgia paresthetica 355.1
Mercurial - *see* condition
Mercurialism NEC 985.0
Merergasia 300.9
Merkel cell tumor - *see* Carcinoma,
  Merkel cell
Merocele (*see also* Hernia, femoral) 553.00
Meromelia 755.4
  lower limb 755.30
    intercalary 755.32
      femur 755.34
        tibiofibular (complete) (incomplete)
          755.33
      fibula 755.37
      metatarsal(s) 755.38
      tarsal(s) 755.38
      tibia 755.36
      tibiofibular 755.35
    terminal (complete) (partial) (transverse)
      755.31
    longitudinal 755.32
      metatarsal(s) 755.38
      phalange(s) 755.39
      tarsal(s) 755.38
    transverse 755.31
  upper limb 755.20
    intercalary 755.22
      carpal(s) 755.28
      humeral 755.24
        radioulnar (complete) (incomplete)
          755.23
      metacarpal(s) 755.28
      phalange(s) 755.29
      radial 755.26
      radioulnar 755.25
      ulnar 755.27
    terminal (complete) (partial) (transverse)
      755.21
    longitudinal 755.22
      carpal(s) 755.28
      metacarpal(s) 755.28
      phalange(s) 755.29
    transverse 755.21
Merosmia 781.1
MERRF syndrome (myoclonus with epilepsy
  and with ragged red fibers) 277.87
Merycism - *see also* Vomiting
  psychogenic 307.53
Merzbacher-Pelizaeus disease 330.0
Mesaortitis - *see* Aortitis
Mesarteritis - *see* Arteritis
Mesencephalitis (*see also* Encephalitis)
  323.9
  late effect - *see* category 326
Mesenchymoma (M8990/1) - *see also*
  Neoplasm, connective tissue,
  uncertain behavior
  benign (M8990/0) - *see* Neoplasm,
    connective tissue, benign
  malignant (M8990/3) - *see* Neoplasm,
    connective tissue, malignant
Mesenteritis
  retractile 567.82
  sclerosing 567.82
Mesentery, mesenteric - *see* condition
Mesiodens, mesiodentes 520.1
  causing crowding 524.31
Mesio-occlusion 524.23
Mesocardia (with asplenia) 746.87
Mesocolon - *see* condition
Mesonephroma (malignant) (M9110/3) - *see also*
  Neoplasm, by site, malignant
  benign (M9110/0) - *see* Neoplasm, by site,
    benign
Mesophlebitis - *see* Phlebitis
Mesostromal dysgenesis 743.51

Mesothelioma (malignant) (M9050/3) - *see also*
  Neoplasm, by site, malignant
  benign (M9050/0) - *see* Neoplasm, by site,
    benign
  biphasic type (M9053/3) - *see also* Neoplasm,
    by site, malignant
    benign (M9053/0) - *see* Neoplasm, by site,
      benign
  epithelioid (M9052/3) - *see also* Neoplasm, by
    site, malignant
    benign (M9052/0) - *see* Neoplasm, by site,
      benign
  fibrous (M9051/3) - *see also* Neoplasm, by
    site, malignant
    benign (M9051/0) - *see* Neoplasm, by site,
      benign
Metabolic syndrome 277.7
Metabolism disorder 277.9
  specified type NEC 277.89
Metagonimiasis 121.5
Metagonimus infestation (small intestine) 121.5
Metal
  pigmentation (skin) 709.00
    polishers' disease 502
Metalliferous miners' lung 503
Metamorphopsia 368.14
Metaplasia
  bone, in skin 709.3
  breast 611.89
  cervix - *omit code*
  endometrium (squamous) 621.8
  esophagus 530.85
  intestinal, of gastric mucosa 537.89
  kidney (pelvis) (squamous) (*see also* Disease,
    renal) 593.89
  myelogenous 289.89
  myeloid 289.89
    agnogenic 238.76
    megakaryocytic 238.76
  spleen 289.59
  squamous cell
    amnion 658.8●
    bladder 596.89
    cervix - *see* condition
    trachea 519.19
    tracheobronchial tree 519.19
    uterus 621.8
      cervix - *see* condition
Metastasis, metastatic
  abscess - *see* Abscess
  calcification 275.40
  cancer, neoplasm, or disease
    from specified site (M8000/3) - *see*
      Neoplasm, by site, malignant
    to specified site (M8000/6) - *see*
      Neoplasm, by site, secondary
  deposits (in) (M8000/6) - *see* Neoplasm, by
    site, secondary
  mesentery, of neuroendocrine tumor 209.74
  pneumonia 038.8 *[484.8]*
  spread (to) (M8000/6) - *see* Neoplasm, by
    site, secondary
Metatarsalgia 726.70
  anterior 355.6
  due to Freiberg's disease 732.5
  Morton's 355.6
Metatarsus, metatarsal - *see also* condition
  abductus valgus (congenital) 754.60
  adductus varus (congenital) 754.53
  primus varus 754.52
  valgus (adductus) (congenital) 754.60
  varus (abductus) (congenital) 754.53
    primus 754.52
Methadone use 304.00
Methemoglobinemia 289.7
  acquired (with sulfhemoglobinemia) 289.7
  congenital 289.7
  enzymatic 289.7
  Hb-M disease 289.7
  hereditary 289.7
  toxic 289.7

Methemoglobinuria (*see also* Hemoglobinuria)
  791.2
Methicillin
  resistant staphylococcus aureus (MRSA)
    041.12
    colonization V02.54
    personal history of V12.04
  susceptible staphylococcus aureus (MSSA)
    041.11
    colonization V02.53
Methioninemia 270.4
Metritis (catarrhal) (septic) (suppurative) (*see
  also* Endometritis) 615.9
  blennorrhagic 098.16
    chronic or duration of 2 months or over
      098.36
  cervical (*see also* Cervicitis) 616.0
  gonococcal 098.16
    chronic or duration of 2 months or over
      098.36
  hemorrhagic 626.8
  puerperal, postpartum, childbirth 670.1●
  septic 670.2●
  tuberculous (*see also* Tuberculosis) 016.7●
Metropathia hemorrhagica 626.8
Metroperitonitis (*see also* Peritonitis, pelvic,
  female) 614.5
Metrorrhagia 626.6
  arising during pregnancy - *see* Hemorrhage,
    pregnancy
  postpartum NEC 666.2●
  primary 626.6
  psychogenic 306.59
  puerperal 666.2●
Metrorrhexis - *see* Rupture, uterus
Metrosalpingitis (*see also* Salpingo-oophoritis)
  614.2
Metrostaxis 626.6
Metrovaginitis (*see also* Endometritis) 615.9
  gonococcal (acute) 098.16
    chronic or duration of 2 months or over
      098.36
Mexican fever - *see* Typhus, Mexican
Meyenburg-Altherr-Uehlinger syndrome
  733.99
Meyer-Schwickerath and Weyers syndrome
  (dysplasia oculodentodigitalis) 759.89
Meynert's amentia (nonalcoholic) 294.0
  alcoholic 291.1
Mibelli's disease 757.39
Mice, joint (*see also* Loose, body, joint)
  718.1●
  knee 717.6
Micheli-Rietti syndrome (thalassemia minor)
  282.46
Michotte's syndrome 721.5
Micrencephalon, micrencephaly 742.1
Microalbuminuria 791.0
Microaneurysm, retina 362.14
  diabetic 250.5● *[362.01]*
    due to secondary diabetes 249.5●
      [362.01]
Microangiopathy 443.9
  diabetic (peripheral) 250.7● *[443.81]*
    due to secondary diabetes 249.7●
      [443.81]
    retinal 250.5● *[362.01]*
      due to secondary diabetes 249.5●
        [362.01]
  peripheral 443.9
    diabetic 250.7● *[443.81]*
      due to secondary diabetes 249.7●
        [443.81]
  retinal 362.18
    diabetic 250.5● *[362.01]*
      due to secondary diabetes 249.5●
        [362.01]
  thrombotic 446.6
    Moschcowitz's (thrombotic
      thrombocytopenic purpura)
      446.6

◄ New   ◄▥ Revised   ~~deleted~~ Deleted   ● Use Additional Digit(s)   ▨ Omit code

Microcalcification, mammographic 793.81
Microcephalus, microcephalic, microcephaly 742.1
  due to toxoplasmosis (congenital) 771.2
Microcheilia 744.82
Microcolon (congenital) 751.5
Microcornea (congenital) 743.41
Microcytic - see condition
Microdeletions NEC 758.33
Microdontia 520.2
Microdrepanocytosis (thalassemia-Hb-S disease) 282.41
  with sickle cell crisis 282.42
Microembolism
  atherothrombotic - see Atheroembolism
  retina 362.33
Microencephalon 742.1
Microfilaria streptocerca infestation 125.3
Microgastria (congenital) 750.7
Microgenia 524.06
Microgenitalia (congenital) 752.89
  penis 752.64
Microglioma (M9710/3)
  specified site - see Neoplasm, by site, malignant
  unspecified site 191.9
Microglossia (congenital) 750.16
Micrognathia, micrognathism (congenital) 524.00
  mandibular 524.04
    alveolar 524.74
  maxillary 524.03
    alveolar 524.73
Microgyria (congenital) 742.2
Microinfarct, heart (see also Insufficiency, coronary) 411.89
Microlithiasis, alveolar, pulmonary 516.2
Micromastia 611.82
Micromyelia (congenital) 742.59
Micropenis 752.64
Microphakia (congenital) 743.36
Microphthalmia (congenital) (see also Microphthalmos) 743.10
Microphthalmos (congenital) 743.10
  associated with eye and adnexal anomalies NEC 743.12
  due to toxoplasmosis (congenital) 771.2
  isolated 743.11
  simple 743.11
  syndrome 759.89
Micropsia 368.14
Microsporidiosis 136.8
Microsporosis (see also Dermatophytosis) 110.9
  nigra 111.1
Microsporum furfur infestation 111.0
Microstomia (congenital) 744.84
Microthelia 757.6
Microthromboembolism - see Embolism
Microtia (congenital) (external ear) 744.23
Microtropia 378.34
Microvillus inclusion disease (MVD) 751.5
Micturition
  disorder NEC 788.69
    psychogenic 306.53
  frequency 788.41
    psychogenic 306.53
  nocturnal 788.43
  painful 788.1
    psychogenic 306.53
Middle
  ear - see condition
  lobe (right) syndrome 518.0
Midplane - see condition
Miescher's disease 709.3
  cheilitis 351.8
  granulomatosis disciformi0s 709.3
Miescher-Leder syndrome or granulomatosis 709.3
Mieten's syndrome 759.89

Migraine (idiopathic) 346.9●

Note: The following fifth digit subclassification is for use with category 346:

0   without mention of intractable migraine without mention of status migrainosus
      without mention of refractory migraine without mention of status migrainosus
1   with intractable migraine, so stated, without mention of status migrainosus
      with refractory migraine, so stated, without mention of status migrainosus
2   without mention of intractable migraine with status migrainosus
      without mention of refractory migraine with status migrainosus
3   with intractable migraine, so stated, with status migrainosus
      with refractory migraine, so stated, with status migrainosus

  with aura (acute-onset) (without headache) (prolonged) (typical) 346.0●
  without aura 346.1●
    chronic 346.7●
    transformed 346.7●
  abdominal (syndrome) 346.2●
  allergic (histamine) 346.2●
  atypical 346.8●
  basilar 346.0●
  chronic without aura 346.7●
  classic(al) 346.0●
  common 346.1●
  complicated 346.0●
  hemiplegic 346.3●
    familial 346.3●
    sporadic 346.3●
  lower-half 339.00
  menstrual 346.4●
  menstrually related 346.4●
  ophthalmic 346.8●
  ophthalmoplegic 346.2●
  premenstrual 346.4●
  pure menstrual 346.4●
  retinal 346.0●
  specified form NEC 346.8●
  transformed without aura 346.7●
  variant 346.2●
Migrant, social V60.0
Migratory, migrating - see also condition
  person V60.0
  testis, congenital 752.52
Mikulicz's disease or syndrome (dryness of mouth, absent or decreased lacrimation) 527.1
Milian atrophia blanche 701.3
Miliaria (crystallina) (rubra) (tropicalis) 705.1
  apocrine 705.82
Miliary - see condition
Milium (see also Cyst, sebaceous) 706.2
  colloid 709.3
  eyelid 374.84
Milk
  crust 690.11
  excess secretion 676.6●
  fever, female 672●
  poisoning 988.8
  retention 676.2●
  sickness 988.8
  spots 423.1
Milkers' nodes 051.1
Milk-leg (deep vessels) 671.4●
  complicating pregnancy 671.3●
  nonpuerperal 451.19
  puerperal, postpartum, childbirth 671.4●

Milkman (-Looser) disease or syndrome (osteomalacia with pseudofractures) 268.2
Milky urine (see also Chyluria) 791.1
Millar's asthma (laryngismus stridulus) 478.75
Millard-Gubler paralysis or syndrome 344.89
Millard-Gubler-Foville paralysis 344.89
Miller-Dieker syndrome 758.33
Miller's disease (osteomalacia) 268.2
Miller Fisher's syndrome 357.0
Milles' syndrome (encephalocutaneous angiomatosis) 759.6
Mills' disease 335.29
Millstone makers' asthma or lung 502
Milroy's disease (chronic hereditary edema) 757.0
Miners' - see also condition
  asthma 500
  elbow 727.2
  knee 727.2
  lung 500
  nystagmus 300.89
  phthisis (see also Tuberculosis) 011.4●
  tuberculosis (see also Tuberculosis) 011.4●
Minkowski-Chauffard syndrome (see also Spherocytosis) 282.0
Minor - see condition
Minor's disease 336.1
Minot's disease (hemorrhagic disease, newborn) 776.0
Minot-von Willebrand (-Jürgens) disease or syndrome (angiohemophilia) 286.4
Minus (and plus) hand (intrinsic) 736.09
Miosis (persistent) (pupil) 379.42
Mirizzi's syndrome (hepatic duct stenosis) (see also Obstruction, biliary) 576.2
  with calculus, cholelithiasis, or stones - see Choledocholithiasis
Mirror writing 315.09
  secondary to organic lesion 784.69
Misadventure (prophylactic) (therapeutic) (see also Complications) 999.9
  administration of insulin 962.3
  infusion - see Complications, infusion
  local applications (of fomentations, plasters, etc.) 999.9
    burn or scald - see Burn, by site
  medical care (early) (late) NEC 999.9
    adverse effect of drugs or chemicals - see Table of Drugs and Chemicals
    burn or scald - see Burn, by site
  radiation NEC 990
  radiotherapy NEC 990
  surgical procedure (early) (late) - see Complications, surgical procedure
  transfusion - see Complications, transfusion
  vaccination or other immunological procedure - see Complications, vaccination
Misanthropy 301.7
Miscarriage - see Abortion, spontaneous
Mischief, malicious, child (see also Disturbance, conduct) 312.0●
Misdirection
  aqueous 365.83
Mismanagement, feeding 783.3
Misplaced, misplacement
  kidney (see also Disease, renal) 593.0
    congenital 753.3
  organ or site, congenital NEC - see Malposition, congenital
Missed
  abortion 632
  delivery (at or near term) 656.4●
  labor (at or near term) 656.4●
Misshapen reconstructed breast 612.0
Missing - see also Absence
  teeth (acquired) 525.10
    congenital (see also Anodontia) 520.0
    due to
      caries 525.13
      extraction 525.10

M

Missing *(Continued)*
  teeth *(Continued)*
    due to *(Continued)*
      periodontal disease 525.12
      specified NEC 525.19
      trauma 525.11
    vertebrae (congenital) 756.13
Misuse of drugs NEC *(see also* Abuse, drug, nondependent) 305.9●
Mitchell's disease (erythromelalgia) 443.82
Mite(s)
  diarrhea 133.8
  grain (itch) 133.8
  hair follicle (itch) 133.8
  in sputum 133.8
Mitochondrial encephalopathy, lactic acidosis and stroke-like episodes (MELAS syndrome) 277.87
Mitochondrial neurogastrointestinal encephalopathy syndrome (MNGIE) 277.87
Mitral - *see* condition
Mittelschmerz 625.2
Mixed - *see* condition
Mljet disease (mal de Meleda) 757.39
Mobile, mobility
  cecum 751.4
  coccyx 733.99
  excessive - *see* Hypermobility
  gallbladder 751.69
  kidney 593.0
    congenital 753.3
  organ or site, congenital NEC - *see* Malposition, congenital
  spleen 289.59
Mobitz heart block (atrioventricular) 426.10
  type I (Wenckebach's) 426.13
  type II 426.12
Möbius'
  disease 346.2●
  syndrome
    congenital oculofacial paralysis 352.6
    ophthalmoplegic migraine 346.2●
Moeller (-Barlow) disease (infantile scurvy) 267
  glossitis 529.4
Mohr's syndrome (types I and II) 759.89
Mola destruens (M9100/1) 236.1
Molarization, premolars 520.2
Molar pregnancy 631.8
  hydatidiform (delivered) (undelivered) 630
Mold(s) in vitreous 117.9
Molding, head (during birth) - *omit code*
Mole (pigmented) (M8720/0) - *see also* Neoplasm, skin, benign
  blood 631.8
  Breus' 631.8
  cancerous (M8720/3) - *see* Melanoma
  carneous 631.8
  destructive (M9100/1) 236.1
  ectopic - *see* Pregnancy, ectopic
  fleshy 631.8
  hemorrhagic 631.8
  hydatid, hydatidiform (benign) (complicating pregnancy) (delivered) (undelivered) *(see also* Hydatidiform mole) 630
    invasive (M9100/1) 236.1
    malignant (M9100/1) 236.1
    previous, affecting management of pregnancy V23.1
  invasive (hydatidiform) (M9100/1) 236.1
  malignant
    meaning
      malignant hydatidiform mole (M9100/1) 236.1
      melanoma (M8720/3) - *see* Melanoma
  nonpigmented (M8730/0) - *see* Neoplasm, skin, benign
  pregnancy NEC 631.8
  skin (M8720/0) - *see* Neoplasm, skin, benign
  stone 631.8

Mole *(Continued)*
  tubal - *see* Pregnancy, tubal
  vesicular *(see also* Hydatidiform mole) 630
Molimen, molimina (menstrual) 625.4
Mollaret's meningitis 047.9
Mollities (cerebellar) (cerebral) 437.8
  ossium 268.2
Molluscum
  contagiosum 078.0
  epitheliale 078.0
  fibrosum (M8851/0) - *see* Lipoma, by site
  pendulum (M8851/0) - *see* Lipoma, by site
Mönckeberg's arteriosclerosis, degeneration, disease, or sclerosis *(see also* Arteriosclerosis, extremities) 440.20
Monday fever 504
Monday morning dyspnea or asthma 504
Mondini's malformation (cochlea) 744.05
Mondor's disease (thrombophlebitis of breast) 451.89
Mongolian, mongolianism, mongolism, mongoloid 758.0
  spot 757.33
Monilethrix (congenital) 757.4
Monilia infestation - *see* Candidiasis
Moniliasis - *see also* Candidiasis
  neonatal 771.7
  vulvovaginitis 112.1
Monkeypox 059.01
Monoarthritis 716.60
  ankle 716.67
  arm 716.62
    lower (and wrist) 716.63
    upper (and elbow) 716.62
  foot (and ankle) 716.67
  forearm (and wrist) 716.63
  hand 716.64
  leg 716.66
    lower 716.66
    upper 716.65
  pelvic region (hip) (thigh) 716.65
  shoulder (region) 716.61
  specified site NEC 716.68
Monoblastic - *see* condition
Monochromatism (cone) (rod) 368.54
Monocytic - *see* condition
Monocytopenia 288.59
Monocytosis (symptomatic) 288.63
Monofixation syndrome 378.34
Monomania *(see also* Psychosis) 298.9
Mononeuritis 355.9
  cranial nerve - *see* Disorder, nerve, cranial
  femoral nerve 355.2
  lateral
    cutaneous nerve of thigh 355.1
    popliteal nerve 355.3
  lower limb 355.8
    specified nerve NEC 355.79
  medial popliteal nerve 355.4
  median nerve 354.1
  multiplex 354.5
  plantar nerve 355.6
  posterior tibial nerve 355.5
  radial nerve 354.3
  sciatic nerve 355.0
  ulnar nerve 354.2
  upper limb 354.9
    specified nerve NEC 354.8
  vestibular 388.5
Mononeuropathy *(see also* Mononeuritis) 355.9
  diabetic NEC 250.6● *[355.9]*
    due to secondary diabetes 249.6● *[355.9]*
    lower limb 250.6● *[355.8]*
      due to secondary diabetes 249.6● *[355.8]*
    upper limb 250.6● *[354.9]*
      due to secondary diabetes 249.6● *[354.9]*
  iliohypogastric nerve 355.79
  ilioinguinal nerve 355.79

Mononeuropathy *(Continued)*
  obturator nerve 355.79
  saphenous nerve 355.79
Mononucleosis, infectious 075
  with hepatitis 075 *[573.1]*
Monoplegia 344.5
  brain (current episode) *(see also* Paralysis, brain) 437.8
    fetus or newborn 767.8
  cerebral (current episode) *(see also* Paralysis, brain) 437.8
  congenital or infantile (cerebral) (spastic) (spinal) 343.3
  embolic (current) *(see also* Embolism, brain) 434.1●
    late effect - *see* Late effect(s) (of) cerebrovascular disease
  infantile (cerebral) (spastic) (spinal) 343.3
  lower limb 344.30
    affecting
      dominant side 344.31
      nondominant side 344.32
    due to late effect of cerebrovascular accident - *see* Late effect(s) (of) cerebrovascular accident
  newborn 767.8
  psychogenic 306.0
    specified as conversion reaction 300.11
  thrombotic (current) *(see also* Thrombosis, brain) 434.0●
    late effect - *see* Late effect(s) (of) cerebrovascular disease
  transient 781.4
  upper limb 344.40
    affecting
      dominant side 344.41
      nondominant side 344.42
    due to late effect of cerebrovascular accident - *see* Late effect(s) (of) cerebrovascular accident
Monorchism, monorchidism 752.89
Monteggia's fracture (closed) 813.03
  open 813.13
Mood swings
  brief compensatory 296.99
  rebound 296.99
Moore's syndrome *(see also* Epilepsy) 345.5●
Mooren's ulcer (cornea) 370.07
Mooser-Neill reaction 081.0
Mooser bodies 081.0
Moral
  deficiency 301.7
  imbecility 301.7
Morax-Axenfeld conjunctivitis 372.03
Morbilli *(see also* Measles) 055.9
Morbus
  anglicus, anglorum 268.0
  Beigel 111.2
  caducus *(see also* Epilepsy) 345.9●
  caeruleus 746.89
  celiacus 579.0
  comitialis *(see also* Epilepsy) 345.9●
  cordis - *see also* Disease, heart
    valvulorum - *see* Endocarditis
  coxae 719.95
    tuberculous *(see also* Tuberculosis) 015.1●
  hemorrhagicus neonatorum 776.0
  maculosus neonatorum 772.6
  renum 593.0
  senilis *(see also* Osteoarthrosis) 715.9●
Morel-Kraepelin disease *(see also* Schizophrenia) 295.9●
Morel-Moore syndrome (hyperostosis frontalis interna) 733.3
Morel-Morgagni syndrome (hyperostosis frontalis interna) 733.3
Morgagni
  cyst, organ, hydatid, or appendage 752.89
    fallopian tube 752.11
  disease or syndrome (hyperostosis frontalis interna) 733.3

◀ New   ◀|||| Revised   ~~deleted~~ Deleted   ● Use Additional Digit(s)   ▨ Omit code

Morgagni-Adams-Stokes syndrome (syncope with heart block) 426.9
Morgagni-Stewart-Morel syndrome (hyperostosis frontalis interna) 733.3
Moria (*see also* Psychosis) 298.9
Morning sickness 643.0●
Moron 317
Morphea (guttate) (linear) 701.0
Morphine dependence (*see also* Dependence) 304.0●
Morphinism (*see also* Dependence) 304.0●
Morphinomania (*see also* Dependence) 304.0●
Morphoea 701.0
Morquio (-Brailsford) (-Ullrich) disease or syndrome (mucopolysaccharidosis IV) 277.5
  kyphosis 277.5
Morris syndrome (testicular feminization) 259.51
Morsus humanus (open wound) - *see also* Wound, open, by site
  skin surface intact - *see* Contusion
Mortification (dry) (moist) (*see also* Gangrene) 785.4
Morton's
  disease 355.6
  foot 355.6
  metatarsalgia (syndrome) 355.6
  neuralgia 355.6
  neuroma 355.6
  syndrome (metatarsalgia) (neuralgia) 355.6
  toe 355.6
Morvan's disease 336.0
Mosaicism, mosaic (chromosomal) 758.9
  autosomal 758.5
  sex 758.81
Moschcowitz's syndrome (thrombotic thrombocytopenic purpura) 446.6
Mother yaw 102.0
Motion sickness (from travel, any vehicle) (from roundabouts or swings) 994.6
Mottled teeth (enamel) (endemic) (nonendemic) 520.3
Mottling enamel (endemic) (nonendemic) (teeth) 520.3
Mouchet's disease 732.5
Mould(s) (in vitreous) 117.9
Moulders'
  bronchitis 502
  tuberculosis (*see also* Tuberculosis) 011.4●
Mounier-Kuhn syndrome 748.3
  with
    acute exacerbation 494.1
    bronchiectasis 494.0
      with (acute) exacerbation 494.1
  acquired 519.19
    with bronchiectasis 494.0
      with (acute) exacerbation 494.1
Mountain
  fever - *see* Fever, mountain
  sickness 993.2
    with polycythemia, acquired 289.0
      acute 289.0
  tick fever 066.1
Mouse, joint (*see also* Loose, body, joint) 718.1●
  knee 717.6
Mouth - *see* condition
Movable
  coccyx 724.71
  kidney (*see also* Disease, renal) 593.0
    congenital 753.3
  organ or site, congenital NEC - *see* Malposition, congenital
  spleen 289.59
Movement
  abnormal (dystonic) (involuntary) 781.0
  decreased fetal 655.7●
  paradoxical facial 374.43
Moya Moya disease 437.5
Mozart's ear 744.29

MRSA (methicillin resistant staphylococcus aureus) 041.12
  colonization V02.54
  personal history of V12.04
MSSA (methicillin susceptible staphylococcus aureus) 041.11
  colonization V02.53
Mucha's disease (acute parapsoriasis varioliformis) 696.2
Mucha-Haberman syndrome (acute parapsoriasis varioliformis) 696.2
Mu-chain disease 273.2
Mucinosis (cutaneous) (papular) 701.8
Mucocele
  appendix 543.9
  buccal cavity 528.9
  gallbladder (*see also* Disease, gallbladder) 575.3
  lacrimal sac 375.43
  orbit (eye) 376.81
  salivary gland (any) 527.6
  sinus (accessory) (nasal) 478.19
  turbinate (bone) (middle) (nasal) 478.19
  uterus 621.8
Mucocutaneous lymph node syndrome (acute) (febrile) (infantile) 446.1
Mucoenteritis 564.9
Mucolipidosis I, II, III 272.7
Mucopolysaccharidosis (types 1–6) 277.5
  cardiopathy 277.5 [425.7]
Mucormycosis (lung) 117.7
Mucosa associated lymphoid tissue (MALT) 200.3●
Mucositis - *see also* Inflammation, by site 528.00
  cervix (ulcerative) 616.81
  due to
    antineoplastic therapy (ulcerative) 528.01
    other drugs (ulcerative) 528.02
    specified NEC 528.09
  gastrointestinal (ulcerative) 538
  nasal (ulcerative) 478.11
  necroticans agranulocytica (*see also* Agranulocytosis) 288.09
  ulcerative 528.00
  vagina (ulcerative) 616.81
  vulva (ulcerative) 616.81
Mucous - *see also* condition
  patches (syphilitic) 091.3
    congenital 090.0
Mucoviscidosis 277.00
  with meconium obstruction 277.01
Mucus
  asphyxia or suffocation (*see also* Asphyxia, mucus) 933.1
    newborn 770.18
  in stool 792.1
  plug (*see also* Asphyxia, mucus) 933.1
    aspiration, of newborn 770.17
    tracheobronchial 519.19
      newborn 770.18
Muguet 112.0
Mulberry molars 090.5
Müllerian mixed tumor (M8950/3) - *see* Neoplasm, by site, malignant
Multicystic kidney 753.19
Multilobed placenta - *see* Placenta, abnormal
Multinodular prostate 600.10
  with
    urinary
      obstruction 600.11
      retention 600.11
Multiparity V61.5
  affecting
    fetus or newborn 763.89
    management of
      labor and delivery 659.4●
      pregnancy V23.3
  requiring contraceptive management (*see also* Contraception) V25.9
Multipartita placenta - *see* Placenta, abnormal

Multiple, multiplex - *see also* condition
  birth
    affecting fetus or newborn 761.5
    healthy liveborn - *see* Newborn, multiple
  digits (congenital) 755.00
    fingers 755.01
    toes 755.02
  organ or site NEC - *see* Accessory
  personality 300.14
  renal arteries 747.62
Mumps 072.9
  with complication 072.8
    specified type NEC 072.79
  encephalitis 072.2
  hepatitis 072.71
  meningitis (aseptic) 072.1
  meningoencephalitis 072.2
  oophoritis 072.79
  orchitis 072.0
  pancreatitis 072.3
  polyneuropathy 072.72
  vaccination, prophylactic (against) V04.6
Mumu (*see also* Infestation, filarial) 125.9
Münchausen syndrome 301.51
Münchmeyer's disease or syndrome (exostosis luxurians) 728.11
Mural - *see* condition
Murmur (cardiac) (heart) (nonorganic) (organic) 785.2
  abdominal 787.5
  aortic (valve) (*see also* Endocarditis, aortic) 424.1
  benign - *omit code*
  cardiorespiratory 785.2
  diastolic - *see* condition
  Flint (*see also* Endocarditis, aortic) 424.1
  functional - *omit code*
  Graham Steell (pulmonic regurgitation) (*see also* Endocarditis, pulmonary) 424.3
  innocent - *omit code*
  insignificant - *omit code*
  midsystolic 785.2
  mitral (valve) - *see* Stenosis
  physiologic - *see* condition
  presystolic, mitral - *see* Insufficiency, mitral
  pulmonic (valve) (*see also* Endocarditis, pulmonary) 424.3
  Still's (vibratory) - *omit code*
  systolic (valvular) - *see* condition
  tricuspid (valve) - *see* Endocarditis, tricuspid
  undiagnosed 785.2
  valvular - *see* condition
  vibratory - *omit code*
Murri's disease (intermittent hemoglobinuria) 283.2
Muscae volitantes 379.24
Muscle, muscular - *see* condition
Musculoneuralgia 729.1
Mushrooming hip 718.95
Mushroom workers' (pickers') lung 495.5
Mutation(s)
  factor V Leiden 289.81
  prothrombin gene 289.81
  surfactant, of lung 516.63
Mutism (*see also* Aphasia) 784.3
  akinetic 784.3
  deaf (acquired) (congenital) 389.7
  hysterical 300.11
  selective (elective) 313.23
    adjustment reaction 309.83
MVD (microvillus inclusion disease) 751.5
MVID (microvillus inclusion disease) 751.5
Myà's disease (congenital dilation, colon) 751.3
Myalgia (intercostal) 729.1
  eosinophilia syndrome 710.5
  epidemic 074.1
    cervical 078.89
  psychogenic 307.89
  traumatic NEC 959.9

M

Myasthenia 358.00
　cordis - *see* Failure, heart
　gravis 358.00
　　with exacerbation (acute) 358.01
　　in crisis 358.01
　　neonatal 775.2
　　pseudoparalytica 358.00
　stomach 536.8
　　psychogenic 306.4
　syndrome
　　in
　　　botulism 005.1 *[358.1]*
　　　diabetes mellitus 250.6● *[358.1]*
　　　　due to secondary diabetes 249.6●
　　　　　[358.1]
　　　hypothyroidism (*see also*
　　　　Hypothyroidism) 244.9 *[358.1]*
　　　malignant neoplasm NEC 199.1
　　　　[358.1]
　　　pernicious anemia 281.0 *[358.1]*
　　　thyrotoxicosis (*see also* Thyrotoxicosis)
　　　　242.9● *[358.1]*
Myasthenic 728.87
Mycelium infection NEC 117.9
Mycetismus 988.1
Mycetoma (actinomycotic) 039.9
　bone 039.8
　　mycotic 117.4
　foot 039.4
　　mycotic 117.4
　madurae 039.9
　　mycotic 117.4
　maduromycotic 039.9
　　mycotic 117.4
　mycotic 117.4
　nocardial 039.9
Mycobacteriosis - *see* Mycobacterium
Mycobacterium, mycobacterial (infection) 031.9
　acid-fast (bacilli) 031.9
　anonymous (*see also* Mycobacterium,
　　atypical) 031.9
　atypical (acid-fast bacilli) 031.9
　　cutaneous 031.1
　　pulmonary 031.0
　　　tuberculous (*see also* Tuberculosis,
　　　　pulmonary) 011.9●
　　specified site NEC 031.8
　avium 031.0
　　intracellulare complex bacteremia (MAC)
　　　031.2
　balnei 031.1
　Battey 031.0
　cutaneous 031.1
　disseminated 031.2
　　avium-intracellulare complex (DMAC)
　　　031.2
　fortuitum 031.0
　intracellulare (battey bacillus) 031.0
　kakerifu 031.8
　kansasii 031.0
　kasongo 031.8
　leprae - *see* Leprosy
　luciflavum 031.0
　marinum 031.1
　pulmonary 031.0
　　tuberculous (*see also* Tuberculosis,
　　　pulmonary) 011.9●
　scrofulaceum 031.1
　tuberculosis (human, bovine) - *see also*
　　Tuberculosis
　　avian type 031.0
　ulcerans 031.1
　xenopi 031.0
Mycosis, mycotic 117.9
　cutaneous NEC 111.9
　ear 111.8 *[380.15]*
　fungoides (M9700/3) 202.1●
　mouth 112.0
　pharynx 117.9
　skin NEC 111.9
　stomatitis 112.0

Mycosis, mycotic *(Continued)*
　systemic NEC 117.9
　tonsil 117.9
　vagina, vaginitis 112.1
Mydriasis (persistent) (pupil) 379.43
Myelatelia 742.59
Myelinoclasis, perivascular, acute
　　(postinfectious) NEC 136.9 *[323.61]*
　postimmunization or postvaccinal 323.51
Myelinosis, central pontine 341.8
Myelitis (ascending) (cerebellar) (childhood)
　　(chronic) (descending) (diffuse)
　　(disseminated) (pressure) (progressive)
　　(spinal cord) (subacute) (*see also*
　　Encephalitis) 323.9
　acute (transverse) 341.20
　　idiopathic 341.22
　　in conditions classified elsewhere 341.21
　due to
　　other infection classified elsewhere 136.9
　　　[323.42]
　　specified cause NEC 323.82
　　vaccination (any) 323.52
　　viral diseases classified elsewhere
　　　323.02
　herpes simplex 054.74
　herpes zoster 053.14
　late effect - *see* category 326
　optic neuritis in 341.0
　postchickenpox 052.2
　postimmunization 323.52
　postinfectious 136.9 *[323.63]*
　postvaccinal 323.52
　postvaricella 052.2
　syphilitic (transverse) 094.89
　toxic 989.9 *[323.72]*
　transverse 323.82
　　acute 341.20
　　　idiopathic 341.22
　　　in conditions classified elsewhere
　　　　341.21
　　idiopathic 341.22
　tuberculous (*see also* Tuberculosis) 013.6●
　virus 049.9
Myeloblastic - *see* condition
Myelocele (*see also* Spina bifida) 741.9●
　with hydrocephalus 741.0●
Myelocystocele (*see also* Spina bifida) 741.9●
Myelocytic - *see* condition
Myelocytoma 205.1●
Myelodysplasia (spinal cord) 742.59
　meaning myelodysplastic syndrome - *see*
　　Syndrome, myelodysplastic
Myeloencephalitis - *see* Encephalitis
Myelofibrosis 289.83
　with myeloid metaplasia 238.76
　idiopathic (chronic) 238.76
　megakaryocytic 238.79
　primary 238.76
　secondary 289.83
Myelogenous - *see* condition
Myeloid - *see* condition
Myelokathexis 288.09
Myeloleukodystrophy 330.0
Myelolipoma (M8870/0) - *see* Neoplasm, by
　site, benign
Myeloma (multiple) (plasma cell) (plasmacytic)
　　(M9730/3) 203.0●
　monostotic (M9731/1) 238.6
　solitary (M9731/1) 238.6
Myelomalacia 336.8
Myelomata, multiple (M9730/3) 203.0●
Myelomatosis (M9730/3) 203.0●
Myelomeningitis - *see* Meningoencephalitis
Myelomeningocele (spinal cord) (*see also* Spina
　　bifida) 741.9●
　fetal, causing fetopelvic disproportion
　　653.7●
Myelo-osteo-musculodysplasia hereditaria
　756.89
Myelopathic - *see* condition

Myelopathy (spinal cord) 336.9
　cervical 721.1
　diabetic 250.6● *[336.3]*
　　due to secondary diabetes 249.6●
　　　[336.3]
　drug-induced 336.8
　due to or with
　　carbon tetrachloride 987.8 *[323.72]*
　　degeneration or displacement,
　　　intervertebral disc 722.70
　　　cervical, cervicothoracic 722.71
　　　lumbar, lumbosacral 722.73
　　　thoracic, thoracolumbar 722.72
　　hydroxyquinoline derivatives 961.3
　　　[323.72]
　　infection - *see* Encephalitis
　　intervertebral disc disorder 722.70
　　　cervical, cervicothoracic 722.71
　　　lumbar, lumbosacral 722.73
　　　thoracic, thoracolumbar 722.72
　　lead 984.9 *[323.72]*
　　mercury 985.0 *[323.72]*
　　neoplastic disease (*see also* Neoplasm, by
　　　site) 239.9 *[336.3]*
　　pernicious anemia 281.0 *[336.3]*
　　spondylosis 721.91
　　　cervical 721.1
　　　lumbar, lumbosacral 721.42
　　　thoracic 721.41
　　thallium 985.8 *[323.72]*
　lumbar, lumbosacral 721.42
　necrotic (subacute) 336.1
　radiation-induced 336.8
　spondylogenic NEC 721.91
　　cervical 721.1
　　lumbar, lumbosacral 721.42
　　thoracic 721.41
　thoracic 721.41
　toxic NEC 989.9 *[323.72]*
　transverse (*see also* Myelitis) 323.82
　vascular 336.1
Myelophthisis 284.2
Myeloproliferative disease (M9960/1)
　238.79
Myeloradiculitis (*see also* Polyneuropathy)
　357.0
Myeloradiculodysplasia (spinal) 742.59
Myelosarcoma (M9930/3) 205.3●
Myelosclerosis 289.89
　with myeloid metaplasia (M9961/1)
　　238.76
　disseminated, of nervous system 340
　megakaryocytic (M9961/1) 238.79
Myelosis (M9860/3) (*see also* Leukemia,
　　myeloid) 205.9●
　acute (M9861/3) 205.0●
　aleukemic (M9864/3) 205.8●
　chronic (M9863/3) 205.1●
　erythremic (M9840/3) 207.0●
　　acute (M9841/3) 207.0●
　megakaryocytic (M9920/3) 207.2●
　nonleukemic (chronic) 288.8
　subacute (M9862/3) 205.2●
Myesthenia - *see* Myasthenia
Myiasis (cavernous) 134.0
　orbit 134.0 *[376.13]*
Myoadenoma, prostate 600.20
　with
　　other lower urinary tract symptoms
　　　(LUTS) 600.21
　　urinary
　　　obstruction 600.21
　　　retention 600.21
Myoblastoma
　granular cell (M9580/0) - *see also*
　　Neoplasm, connective tissue,
　　benign
　malignant (M9580/3) - *see* Neoplasm,
　　connective tissue, malignant
　tongue (M9580/0) 210.1
Myocardial - *see* condition

Myocardiopathy (congestive) (constrictive)
(familial) (idiopathic) (infiltrative)
(obstructive) (primary) (restrictive)
(sporadic) 425.4
alcoholic 425.5
amyloid 277.39 [425.7]
beriberi 265.0 [425.7]
cobalt-beer 425.5
due to
amyloidosis 277.39 [425.7]
beriberi 265.0 [425.7]
cardiac glycogenosis 271.0 [425.7]
Chagas' disease 086.0
Friedreich's ataxia 334.0 [425.8]
influenza (see also Influenza) 487.8
[425.8]
mucopolysaccharidosis 277.5 [425.7]
myotonia atrophica 359.21 [425.8]
progressive muscular dystrophy 359.1
[425.8]
sarcoidosis 135 [425.8]
glycogen storage 271.0 [425.7]
hypertrophic 425.18
nonobstructive 425.18
obstructive 425.11
metabolic NEC 277.9 [425.7]
nutritional 269.9 [425.7]
obscure (African) 425.2
peripartum 674.5●
postpartum 674.5●
secondary 425.9
thyrotoxic (see also Thyrotoxicosis)
242.9 ● [425.7]
toxic NEC 425.9
Myocarditis (fibroid) (interstitial) (old)
(progressive) (senile) (with
arteriosclerosis) 429.0
with
rheumatic fever (conditions classifiable to
390) 398.0
active (see also Myocarditis, acute,
rheumatic) 391.2
inactive or quiescent (with chorea)
398.0
active (nonrheumatic) 422.90
rheumatic 391.2
with chorea (acute) (rheumatic)
(Sydenham's) 392.0
acute or subacute (interstitial) 422.90
due to Streptococcus (beta-hemolytic)
391.2
idiopathic 422.91
rheumatic 391.2
with chorea (acute) (rheumatic)
(Sydenham's) 392.0
specified type NEC 422.99
aseptic of newborn 074.23
bacterial (acute) 422.92
chagasic 086.0
chronic (interstitial) 429.0
congenital 746.89
constrictive 425.4
Coxsackie (virus) 074.23
diphtheritic 032.82
due to or in
Coxsackie (virus) 074.23
diphtheria 032.82
epidemic louse-borne typhus 080 [422.0]
influenza (see also Influenza) 487.8 [422.0]
Lyme disease 088.81 [422.0]
scarlet fever 034.1 [422.0]
toxoplasmosis (acquired) 130.3
tuberculosis (see also Tuberculosis) 017.9●
[422.0]
typhoid 002.0 [422.0]
typhus NEC 081.9 [422.0]
eosinophilic 422.91
epidemic of newborn 074.23
Fiedler's (acute) (isolated) (subacute) 422.91
giant cell (acute) (subacute) 422.91
gonococcal 098.85

Myocarditis (Continued)
granulomatous (idiopathic) (isolated)
(nonspecific) 422.91
hypertensive (see also Hypertension, heart)
402.90
idiopathic 422.91
granulomatous 422.91
infective 422.92
influenzal (see also Influenza) 487.8 [422.0]
isolated (diffuse) (granulomatous) 422.91
malignant 422.99
meningococcal 036.43
nonrheumatic, active 422.90
parenchymatous 422.90
pneumococcal (acute) (subacute) 422.92
rheumatic (chronic) (inactive) (with chorea)
398.0
active or acute 391.2
with chorea (acute) (rheumatic)
(Sydenham's) 392.0
septic 422.92
specific (giant cell) (productive) 422.91
staphylococcal (acute) (subacute) 422.92
suppurative 422.92
syphilitic (chronic) 093.82
toxic 422.93
rheumatic (see also Myocarditis, acute
rheumatic) 391.2
tuberculous (see also Tuberculosis) 017.9●
[422.0]
typhoid 002.0 [422.0]
valvular - see Endocarditis
viral, except Coxsackie 422.91
Coxsackie 074.23
of newborn (Coxsackie) 074.23
Myocardium, myocardial - see condition
Myocardosis (see also Cardiomyopathy) 425.4
Myoclonia (essential) 333.2
epileptica 345.1●
Friedrich's 333.2
massive 333.2
Myoclonic
epilepsy, familial (progressive) 345.1●
jerks 333.2
Myoclonus (familial essential) (multifocal)
(simplex) 333.2
with epilepsy and with ragged red fibers
(MERRF syndrome) 277.87
facial 351.8
massive (infantile) 333.2
palatal 333.2
pharyngeal 333.2
Myocytolysis 429.1
Myodiastasis 728.84
Myoendocarditis - see also Endocarditis
acute or subacute 421.9
Myoepithelioma (M8982/0) - see Neoplasm, by
site, benign
Myofascitis (acute) 729.1
low back 724.2
Myofibroma (M8890/0) - see also Neoplasm,
connective tissue, benign
uterus (cervix) (corpus) (see also Leiomyoma)
218.9
Myofibromatosis
infantile 759.89
Myofibrosis 728.2
heart (see also Myocarditis) 429.0
humeroscapular region 726.2
scapulohumeral 726.2
Myofibrositis (see also Myositis) 729.1
scapulohumeral 726.2
Myogelosis (occupational) 728.89
Myoglobinuria 791.3
Myoglobulinuria, primary 791.3
Myokymia - see also Myoclonus
facial 351.8
Myolipoma (M8860/0)
specified site - see Neoplasm, connective
tissue, benign
unspecified site 223.0

Myoma (M8895/0) - see also Neoplasm,
connective tissue, benign
cervix (stump) (uterus) (see also Leiomyoma)
218.9
malignant (M8895/3) - see Neoplasm,
connective tissue, malignant
prostate 600.20
with
other lower urinary tract symptoms
(LUTS) 600.21
urinary
obstruction 600.21
retention 600.21
uterus (cervix) (corpus) (see also Leiomyoma)
218.9
in pregnancy or childbirth 654.1●
affecting fetus or newborn 763.89
causing obstructed labor 660.2●
affecting fetus or newborn
763.1
Myomalacia 728.9
cordis, heart (see also Degeneration,
myocardial) 429.1
Myometritis (see also Endometritis) 615.9
Myometrium - see condition
Myonecrosis, clostridial 040.0
Myopathy 359.9
alcoholic 359.4
amyloid 277.39 [359.6]
benign, congenital 359.0
central core 359.0
centronuclear 359.0
congenital (benign) 359.0
critical illness 359.81
distal 359.1
due to drugs 359.4
endocrine 259.9 [359.5]
specified type NEC 259.8 [359.5]
extraocular muscles 376.82
facioscapulohumeral 359.1
in
Addison's disease 255.41 [359.5]
amyloidosis 277.39 [359.6]
cretinism 243 [359.5]
Cushing's syndrome 255.0 [359.5]
disseminated lupus erythematosus 710.0
[359.6]
giant cell arteritis 446.5 [359.6]
hyperadrenocorticism NEC 255.3 [359.5]
hyperparathyroidism 252.01 [359.5]
hypopituitarism 253.2 [359.5]
hypothyroidism (see also Hypothyroidism)
244.9 [359.5]
malignant neoplasm NEC (M8000/3)
199.1 [359.6]
myxedema (see also Myxedema) 244.9
[359.5]
polyarteritis nodosa 446.0 [359.6]
rheumatoid arthritis 714.0 [359.6]
sarcoidosis 135 [359.6]
scleroderma 710.1 [359.6]
Sjögren's disease 710.2 [359.6]
thyrotoxicosis (see also Thyrotoxicosis)
242.9● [359.5]
inflammatory 359.79
immune NEC 359.79
specified NEC 359.79
intensive care (ICU) 359.81
limb-girdle 359.1
myotubular 359.0
necrotizing, acute 359.81
nemaline 359.0
ocular 359.1
oculopharyngeal 359.1
of critical illness 359.81
primary 359.89
progressive NEC 359.89
proximal myotonic (PROMM) 359.21
quadriplegic, acute 359.81
rod body 359.0
scapulohumeral 359.1

Myopathy *(Continued)*
    specified type NEC 359.89
    toxic 359.4
Myopericarditis *(see also* Pericarditis) 423.9
Myopia (axial) (congenital) (increased
        curvature or refraction, nucleus of lens)
        367.1
    degenerative, malignant 360.21
    malignant 360.21
    progressive high (degenerative) 360.21
Myosarcoma (M8895/3) - *see* Neoplasm,
    connective tissue, malignant
Myosis (persistent) 379.42
    stromal (endolymphatic) (M8931/1)
        236.0
Myositis 729.1
    clostridial 040.0
    due to posture 729.1
    epidemic 074.1
    fibrosa or fibrous (chronic) 728.2
        Volkmann's (complicating trauma)
            958.6
    inclusion body (IBM) 359.71
    infective 728.0
    interstitial 728.81
    multiple - *see* Polymyositis
    occupational 729.1
    orbital, chronic 376.12
    ossificans 728.12
        circumscribed 728.12
        progressive 728.11
        traumatic 728.12

Myositis *(Continued)*
    progressive fibrosing 728.11
    purulent 728.0
    rheumatic 729.1
    rheumatoid 729.1
    suppurative 728.0
    syphilitic 095.6
    traumatic (old) 729.1
Myospasia impulsiva 307.23
Myotonia (acquisita) (intermittens) 728.85
    atrophica 359.21
    congenita 359.22
        acetazolamide responsive 359.22
        dominant form 359.22
        recessive form 359.22
    drug-induced 359.24
    dystrophica 359.21
    fluctuans 359.29
    levior 359.22
    permanens 359.29
Myotonic pupil 379.46
Myriapodiasis 134.1
Myringitis
    with otitis media - *see* Otitis media
    acute 384.00
        specified type NEC 384.09
    bullosa hemorrhagica 384.01
    bullous 384.01
    chronic 384.1
Mysophobia 300.29
Mytilotoxism 988.0
Myxadenitis labialis 528.5

Myxedema (adult) (idiocy) (infantile) (juvenile)
        (thyroid gland) *(see also* Hypothyroidism)
        244.9
    circumscribed 242.9●
    congenital 243
    cutis 701.8
    localized (pretibial) 242.9●
    madness (acute) 293.0
        subacute 293.1
    papular 701.8
    pituitary 244.8
    postpartum 674.8●
    pretibial 242.9●
    primary 244.9
Myxochondrosarcoma (M9220/3) - *see*
    Neoplasm, cartilage, malignant
Myxofibroma (M8811/0) - *see also* Neoplasm,
    connective tissue, benign
    odontogenic (M9320/0) 213.1
        upper jaw (bone) 213.0
Myxofibrosarcoma (M8811/3) - *see* Neoplasm,
    connective tissue, malignant
Myxolipoma (M8852/0) *(see also* Lipoma, by
    site) 214.9
Myxoliposarcoma (M8852/3) - *see* Neoplasm,
    connective tissue, malignant
Myxoma (M8840/0) - *see also* Neoplasm,
    connective tissue, benign
    odontogenic (M9320/0) 213.1
        upper jaw (bone) 213.0
Myxosarcoma (M8840/3) - *see* Neoplasm,
    connective tissue, malignant

N

Naegeli's
disease (hereditary hemorrhagic thrombasthenia) 287.1
leukemia, monocytic (M9863/3) 205.1●
syndrome (incontinentia pigmenti) 757.33
Naffziger's syndrome 353.0
Naga sore (*see also* Ulcer, skin) 707.9
Nägele's pelvis 738.6
with disproportion (fetopelvic) 653.0●
affecting fetus or newborn 763.1
causing obstructed labor 660.1●
affecting fetus or newborn 763.1
Nager-de Reynier syndrome (dysostosis mandibularis) 756.0
Nail - *see also* condition
biting 307.9
patella syndrome (hereditary osteoonychodysplasia) 756.89
Nanism, nanosomia (*see also* Dwarfism) 259.4
hypophyseal 253.3
pituitary 253.3
renis, renalis 588.0
Nanukayami 100.89
Napkin rash 691.0
Narcissism 301.81
Narcolepsy 347.00
with cataplexy 347.01
in conditions classified elsewhere 347.10
with cataplexy 347.11
Narcosis
carbon dioxide (respiratory) 786.09
due to drug
correct substance properly administered 780.09
overdose or wrong substance given or taken 977.9
specified drug - *see* Table of Drugs and Chemicals
Narcotism (chronic) (*see also* Dependence) 304.9●
acute
correct substance properly administered 349.82
overdose or wrong substance given or taken 967.8
specified drug - *see* Table of Drugs and Chemicals
NARP (ataxia and retinitis pigmentosa syndrome) 277.87
Narrow
anterior chamber angle 365.02
pelvis (inlet) (outlet) - *see* Contraction, pelvis
Narrowing
artery NEC 447.1
auditory, internal 433.8●
basilar 433.0●
with other precerebral artery 433.3●
bilateral 433.3●
carotid 433.1●
with other precerebral artery 433.3●
bilateral 433.3●
cerebellar 433.8●
choroidal 433.8●
communicating posterior 433.8●
coronary - *see also* Arteriosclerosis, coronary
congenital 746.85
due to syphilis 090.5
hypophyseal 433.8●
pontine 433.8●
precerebral NEC 433.9●
multiple or bilateral 433.3●
specified NEC 433.8●
vertebral 433.2●
with other precerebral artery 433.3●
bilateral 433.3●
auditory canal (external) (*see also* Stricture, ear canal, acquired) 380.50
cerebral arteries 437.0

Narrowing (*Continued*)
cicatricial - *see* Cicatrix
congenital - *see* Anomaly, congenital
coronary artery - *see* Narrowing, artery, coronary
ear, middle 385.22
Eustachian tube (*see also* Obstruction, Eustachian tube) 381.60
eyelid 374.46
congenital 743.62
intervertebral disc or space NEC - *see* Degeneration, intervertebral disc
joint space, hip 719.85
larynx 478.74
lids 374.46
congenital 743.62
mesenteric artery (with gangrene) 557.0
palate 524.89
palpebral fissure 374.46
retinal artery 362.13
ureter 593.3
urethra (*see also* Stricture, urethra) 598.9
Narrowness, abnormal, eyelid 743.62
Nasal - *see* condition
Nasolacrimal - *see* condition
Nasopharyngeal - *see also* condition
bursa 478.29
pituitary gland 759.2
torticollis 723.5
Nasopharyngitis (acute) (infective) (subacute) 460
chronic 472.2
due to external agent - *see* Condition, respiratory, chronic, due to
due to external agent - *see* Condition, respiratory, due to
septic 034.0
streptococcal 034.0
suppurative (chronic) 472.2
ulcerative (chronic) 472.2
Nasopharynx, nasopharyngeal - *see* condition
Natal tooth, teeth 520.6
Nausea (*see also* Vomiting) 787.02
with vomiting 787.01
epidemic 078.82
gravidarum - *see* Hyperemesis, gravidarum
marina 994.6
Naval - *see* condition
Neapolitan fever (*see also* Brucellosis) 023.9
Near drowning 994.1
Nearsightedness 367.1
Near-syncope 780.2
Nebécourt's syndrome 253.3
Nebula, cornea (eye) 371.01
congenital 743.43
interfering with vision 743.42
Necator americanus infestation 126.1
Necatoriasis 126.1
Neck - *see* condition
Necrencephalus (*see also* Softening, brain) 437.8
Necrobacillosis 040.3
Necrobiosis 799.89
brain or cerebral (*see also* Softening, brain) 437.8
lipoidica 709.3
diabeticorum 250.8● [709.3]
due to secondary diabetes 249.8● [709.3]
Necrodermolysis 695.15
Necrolysis, toxic epidermal 695.15
due to drug
correct substance properly administered 695.15
overdose or wrong substance given or taken 977.9
specified drug - *see* Table of Drugs and Chemicals
Stevens-Johnson syndrome overlap (SJS-TEN overlap syndrome) 695.14

Necrophilia 302.89
Necrosis, necrotic
adrenal (capsule) (gland) 255.8
antrum, nasal sinus 478.19
aorta (hyaline) (*see also* Aneurysm, aorta) 441.9
cystic medial 441.00
abdominal 441.02
thoracic 441.01
thoracoabdominal 441.03
ruptured 441.5
arteritis 446.0
artery 447.5
aseptic, bone 733.40
femur (head) (neck) 733.42
medial condyle 733.43
humoral head 733.41
jaw 733.45
medial femoral condyle 733.43
specific site NEC 733.49
talus 733.44
avascular, bone NEC (*see also* Necrosis, aseptic, bone) 733.40
bladder (aseptic) (sphincter) 596.89
bone (*see also* Osteomyelitis) 730.1●
acute 730.0●
aseptic or avascular 733.40
femur (head) (neck) 733.42
medial condyle 733.43
humoral head 733.41
jaw 733.45
medial femoral condyle 733.43
specified site NEC 733.49
talus 733.44
ethmoid 478.19
ischemic 733.40
jaw 526.4
aseptic 733.45
marrow 289.89
Paget's (osteitis deformans) 731.0
tuberculous - *see* Tuberculosis, bone
brain (softening) (*see also* Softening, brain) 437.8
breast (aseptic) (fat) (segmental) 611.3
bronchus, bronchi 519.19
central nervous system NEC (*see also* Softening, brain) 437.8
cerebellar (*see also* Softening, brain) 437.8
cerebral (softening) (*see also* Softening, brain) 437.8
cerebrospinal (softening) (*see also* Softening, brain) 437.8
colon 557.0
cornea (*see also* Keratitis) 371.40
cortical, kidney 583.6
cystic medial (aorta) 441.00
abdominal 441.02
thoracic 441.01
thoracoabdominal 441.03
dental 521.09
pulp 522.1
due to swallowing corrosive substance - *see* Burn, by site
ear (ossicle) 385.24
esophagus 530.89
ethmoid (bone) 478.19
eyelid 374.50
fat, fatty (generalized) (*see also* Degeneration, fatty) 272.8
abdominal wall 567.82
breast (aseptic) (segmental) 611.3
intestine 569.89
localized - *see* Degeneration, by site, fatty
mesentery 567.82
omentum 567.82
pancreas 577.8
peritoneum 567.82
skin (subcutaneous) 709.3
newborn 778.1

Necrosis, necrotic (Continued)
femur (aseptic) (avascular) 733.42
head 733.42
medial condyle 733.43
neck 733.42
gallbladder (see also Cholecystitis, acute)
575.0
gangrenous 785.4
gastric 537.89
glottis 478.79
heart (myocardium) - see Infarct,
myocardium
hepatic (see also Necrosis, liver) 570
hip (aseptic) (avascular) 733.42
intestine (acute) (hemorrhagic) (massive)
557.0
ischemic 785.4
jaw 526.4
aseptic 733.45
kidney (bilateral) 583.9
acute 584.9
cortical 583.6
acute 584.6
with
abortion - see Abortion, by type,
with renal failure
ectopic pregnancy (see also
categories 633.0–633.9)
639.3
molar pregnancy (see also
categories 630–632) 639.3
complicating pregnancy 646.2●
affecting fetus or newborn 760.1
following labor and delivery 669.3●
medullary (papillary) (see also Pyelitis)
590.80
in
acute renal failure 584.7
nephritis, nephropathy 583.7
papillary (see also Pyelitis) 590.80
in
acute renal failure 584.7
nephritis, nephropathy 583.7
tubular 584.5
with
abortion - see Abortion, by type,
with renal failure
ectopic pregnancy (see also
categories 633.0–633.9) 639.3
molar pregnancy (see also categories
630–632) 639.3
complicating
abortion 639.3
ectopic or molar pregnancy 639.3
pregnancy 646.2●
affecting fetus or newborn 760.1
following labor and delivery 669.3●
traumatic 958.5
larynx 478.79
liver (acute) (congenital) (diffuse) (massive)
(subacute) 570
with
abortion - see Abortion, by type, with
specified complication NEC
ectopic pregnancy (see also categories
633.0–633.9) 639.8

Necrosis, necrotic (Continued)
liver (Continued)
with (Continued)
molar pregnancy (see also categories
630–632) 639.8
complicating pregnancy 646.7●
affecting fetus or newborn 760.8
following
abortion 639.8
ectopic or molar pregnancy
639.8
obstetrical 646.7●
postabortal 639.8
puerperal, postpartum 674.8●
toxic 573.3
lung 513.0
lymphatic gland 683
mammary gland 611.3
mastoid (chronic) 383.1
mesentery 557.0
fat 567.82
mitral valve - see Insufficiency, mitral
myocardium, myocardial - see Infarct,
myocardium
nose (septum) 478.19
omentum 557.0
with mesenteric infarction 557.0
fat 567.82
orbit, orbital 376.10
ossicles, ear (aseptic) 385.24
ovary (see also Salpingo-oophoritis)
614.2
pancreas (aseptic) (duct) (fat) 577.8
acute 577.0
infective 577.0
papillary, kidney (see also Pyelitis)
590.80
perineum 624.8
peritoneum 557.0
with mesenteric infarction 557.0
fat 567.82
pharynx 462
in granulocytopenia 288.09
phosphorus 983.9
pituitary (gland) (postpartum) (Sheehan)
253.2
placenta (see also Placenta, abnormal)
656.7●
pneumonia 513.0
pulmonary 513.0
pulp (dental) 522.1
pylorus 537.89
radiation - see Necrosis, by site
radium - see Necrosis, by site
renal - see Necrosis, kidney
sclera 379.19
scrotum 608.89
skin or subcutaneous tissue 709.8
due to burn - see Burn, by site
gangrenous 785.4
spine, spinal (column) 730.18
acute 730.18
cord 336.1
spleen 289.59
stomach 537.89
stomatitis 528.1

Necrosis, necrotic (Continued)
subcutaneous fat 709.3
fetus or newborn 778.1
subendocardial - see Infarct, myocardium
suprarenal (capsule) (gland) 255.8
teeth, tooth 521.09
testis 608.89
thymus (gland) 254.8
tonsil 474.8
trachea 519.19
tuberculous NEC - see Tuberculosis
tubular (acute) (anoxic) (toxic) 584.5
due to a procedure 997.5
umbilical cord, affecting fetus or newborn
762.6
vagina 623.8
vertebra (lumbar) 730.18
acute 730.18
tuberculous (see also Tuberculosis) 015.0●
[730.8]
vesical (aseptic) (bladder) 596.89
vulva 624.8
x-ray - see Necrosis, by site
Necrospermia 606.0
Necrotizing angiitis 446.0
Negativism 301.7
Neglect (child) (newborn) NEC 995.52
adult 995.84
after or at birth 995.52
hemispatial 781.8
left-sided 781.8
sensory 781.8
visuospatial 781.8
Negri bodies 071
Neill-Dingwall syndrome (microcephaly and
dwarfism) 759.89
Neisserian infection NEC - see Gonococcus
Nematodiasis NEC (see also Infestation,
Nematode) 127.9
ancylostoma (see also Ancylostomiasis)
126.9
Neoformans cryptococcus infection 117.5
Neonatal - see also condition
abstinence syndrome 779.5
adrenoleukodystrophy 277.86
teeth, tooth 520.6
Neonatorum - see condition
Neoplasia
anal intraepithelial I (AIN I) (histologically
confirmed) 569.44
anal intraepithelial II (AIN II) (histologically
confirmed) 569.44
anal intraepithelial III (AIN III) 230.6
anal canal 230.5
endometrial intraepithelial [EIN] 621.35
multiple endocrine (MEN)
type I 258.01
type IIA 258.02
type IIB 258.03
vaginal intraepithelial I (VAIN I) 623.0
vaginal intraepithelial II (VAIN II) 623.0
vaginal intraepithelial III (VAIN III) 233.31
vulvar intraepithelial I (VIN I) 624.01
vulvar intraepithelial II (VIN II) 624.02
vulvar intraepithelial III (VIN III) 233.32
Neoplasm, neoplastic - see pages 351–397

◀ New   ◀▦ Revised   ~~deleted~~ Deleted   ● Use Additional Digit(s)   ▨ Omit code

	Malignant					
	Primary	Secondary	Ca in situ	Benign	Uncertain Behavior	Unspecified
Neoplasm, neoplastic	**199.1**	**199.1**	**234.9**	**229.9**	**238.9**	**239.9**

Notes — 1. The list below gives the code numbers for neoplasms by anatomical site. For each site there are six possible code numbers according to whether the neoplasm in question is malignant, benign, in situ, of uncertain behavior, or of unspecified nature. The description of the neoplasm will often indicate which of the six columns is appropriate; e.g., malignant melanoma of skin, benign fibroadenoma of breast, carcinoma in situ of cervix uteri.

Where such descriptors are not present, the remainder of the Index should be consulted where guidance is given to the appropriate column for each morphological (histological) variety listed; e.g., Mesonephroma — see Neoplasm, malignant; Embryoma — see also Neoplasm, uncertain behavior; Disease, Bowen's — see Neoplasm, skin, in situ. However, the guidance in the Index can be overridden if one of the descriptors mentioned above is present; e.g., malignant adenoma of colon is coded to 153.9 and not to 211.3 as the adjective "malignant" overrides the Index entry "Adenoma - see also Neoplasm, benign."

2. Sites marked with the sign * (e.g., face NEC*) should be classified to malignant neoplasm of skin of these sites if the variety of neoplasm is a squamous cell carcinoma or an epidermoid carcinoma and to benign neoplasm of skin of these sites if the variety of neoplasm is a papilloma (any type).

	Primary	Secondary	Ca in situ	Benign	Uncertain Behavior	Unspecified
abdomen, abdominal	195.2	198.89	234.8	229.8	238.8	239.89
cavity	195.2	198.89	234.8	229.8	238.8	239.89
organ	195.2	198.89	234.8	229.8	238.8	239.89
viscera	195.2	198.89	234.8	229.8	238.8	239.89
wall	173.50	198.2	232.5	216.5	238.2	239.2
basal cell carcinoma	173.51	—	—	—	—	—
specified type NEC	173.59	—	—	—	—	—
squamous cell carcinoma	173.52	—	—	—	—	—
connective tissue	171.5	198.89	—	215.5	238.1	239.2
abdominopelvic	195.8	198.89	234.8	229.8	238.8	239.89
accessory sinus - *see* Neoplasm, sinus						
acoustic nerve	192.0	198.4	—	225.1	237.9	239.7
acromion (process)	170.4	198.5	—	213.4	238.0	239.2
adenoid (pharynx) (tissue)	147.1	198.89	230.0	210.7	235.1	239.0
adipose tissue (*see also* Neoplasm, connective tissue)	171.9	198.89	—	215.9	238.1	239.2
adnexa (uterine)	183.9	198.82	233.39	221.8	236.3	239.5
adrenal (cortex) (gland) (medulla)	194.0	198.7	234.8	227.0	237.2	239.7
ala nasi (external)	173.30	198.2	232.3	216.3	238.2	239.2
alimentary canal or tract NEC	159.9	197.8	230.9	211.9	235.5	239.0
alveolar	143.9	198.89	230.0	210.4	235.1	239.0
mucosa	143.9	198.89	230.0	210.4	235.1	239.0
lower	143.1	198.89	230.0	210.4	235.1	239.0
upper	143.0	198.89	230.0	210.4	235.1	239.0
ridge or process	170.1	198.5	—	213.1	238.0	239.2
carcinoma	143.9	—	—	—	—	—
lower	143.1	—	—	—	—	—
upper	143.0	—	—	—	—	—
lower	170.1	198.5	—	213.1	238.0	239.2
mucosa	143.9	198.89	230.0	210.4	235.1	239.0
lower	143.1	198.89	230.0	210.4	235.1	239.0
upper	143.0	198.89	230.0	210.4	235.1	239.0
upper	170.0	198.5	—	213.0	238.0	239.2

	Malignant					
	Primary	Secondary	Ca in situ	Benign	Uncertain Behavior	Unspecified
Neoplasm *(Continued)*						
alveolar *(Continued)*						
sulcus	145.1	198.89	230.0	210.4	235.1	239.0
alveolus	143.9	198.89	230.0	210.4	235.1	239.0
lower	143.1	198.89	230.0	210.4	235.1	239.0
upper	143.0	198.89	230.0	210.4	235.1	239.0
ampulla of Vater	156.2	197.8	230.8	211.5	235.3	239.0
ankle NEC*	195.5	198.89	232.7	229.8	238.8	239.89
anorectum, anorectal (junction)	154.8	197.5	230.7	211.4	235.2	239.0
antecubital fossa or space*	195.4	198.89	232.6	229.8	238.8	239.89
antrum (Highmore) (maxillary)	160.2	197.3	231.8	212.0	235.9	239.1
pyloric	151.2	197.8	230.2	211.1	235.2	239.0
tympanicum	160.1	197.3	231.8	212.0	235.9	239.1
anus, anal	154.3	197.5	230.6	211.4	235.5	239.0
canal	154.2	197.5	230.5	211.4	235.5	239.0
contiguous sites with rectosigmoid junction or rectum	154.8	—	—	—	—	—
margin (*see also* Neoplasm, anus, skin)	173.50	198.2	232.5	216.5	238.2	239.2
skin	173.50	198.2	232.5	216.5	238.2	239.2
basal cell carcinoma	173.51	—	—	—	—	—
specified type NEC	173.59	—	—	—	—	—
squamous cell carcinoma	173.52	—	—	—	—	—
sphincter	154.2	197.5	230.5	211.4	235.5	239.0
aorta (thoracic)	171.4	198.89	—	215.4	238.1	239.2
abdominal	171.5	198.89	—	215.5	238.1	239.2
aortic body	194.6	198.89	—	227.6	237.3	239.7
aponeurosis	171.9	198.89	—	215.9	238.1	239.2
palmar	171.2	198.89	—	215.2	238.1	239.2
plantar	171.3	198.89	—	215.3	238.1	239.2
appendix	153.5	197.5	230.3	211.3	235.2	239.0
arachnoid (cerebral)	192.1	198.4	—	225.2	237.6	239.7
spinal	192.3	198.4	—	225.4	237.6	239.7
areola (female)	174.0	198.81	233.0	217	238.3	239.3
male	175.0	198.81	233.0	217	238.3	239.3
arm NEC*	195.4	198.89	232.6	229.8	238.8	239.89
artery - *see* Neoplasm, connective tissue						
aryepiglottic fold	148.2	198.89	230.0	210.8	235.1	239.0
hypopharyngeal aspect	148.2	198.89	230.0	210.8	235.1	239.0
laryngeal aspect	161.1	197.3	231.0	212.1	235.6	239.1
marginal zone	148.2	198.89	230.0	210.8	235.1	239.0
arytenoid (cartilage)	161.3	197.3	231.0	212.1	235.6	239.1
fold - *see* Neoplasm, aryepiglottic						

	Malignant					
	Primary	Secondary	Ca in situ	Benign	Uncertain Behavior	Unspecified
Neoplasm *(Continued)*						
associated with transplated organ	199.2	—	—	—	—	—
atlas	170.2	198.5	—	213.2	238.0	239.2
atrium, cardiac	164.1	198.89	—	212.7	238.8	239.89
auditory						
canal (external) (skin) (*see also* Neoplasm, skin, ear)	173.20	198.2	232.2	216.2	238.2	239.2
internal	160.1	197.3	231.8	212.0	235.9	239.1
nerve	192.0	198.4	—	225.1	237.9	239.7
tube	160.1	197.3	231.8	212.0	235.9	239.1
opening	147.2	198.89	230.0	210.7	235.1	239.0
auricle, ear (*see also* Neoplasm, skin, ear)	173.20	198.2	232.2	216.2	238.2	239.2
cartilage	171.0	198.89	—	215.0	238.1	239.2
auricular canal (external) (*see also* Neoplasm, skin, ear)	173.20	198.2	232.2	216.2	238.2	239.2
internal	160.1	197.3	231.8	212.0	235.9	239.1
autonomic nerve or nervous system NEC	171.9	198.89	—	215.9	238.1	239.2
axilla, axillary	195.1	198.89	234.8	229.8	238.8	239.89
fold (*see also* Neoplasm, skin, trunk)	173.50	198.2	232.5	216.5	238.2	239.2
back NEC*	195.8	198.89	232.5	229.8	238.8	239.89
Bartholin's gland	184.1	198.82	233.39	221.2	236.3	239.5
basal ganglia	191.0	198.3	—	225.0	237.5	239.6
basis pedunculi	191.7	198.3	—	225.0	237.5	239.6
bile or biliary (tract)	156.9	197.8	230.8	211.5	235.3	239.0
canaliculi (biliferi) (intrahepatic)	155.1	197.8	230.8	211.5	235.3	239.0
canals, interlobular	155.1	197.8	230.8	211.5	235.3	239.0
contiguous sites	156.8	—	—	—	—	—
duct or passage (common) (cystic) (extrahepatic)	156.1	197.8	230.8	211.5	235.3	239.0
contiguous sites						
with gallbladder	156.8	—	—	—	—	—
interlobular	155.1	197.8	230.8	211.5	235.3	239.0
intrahepatic	155.1	197.8	230.8	211.5	235.3	239.0
and extrahepatic	156.9	197.8	230.8	211.5	235.3	239.0
bladder (urinary)	188.9	198.1	233.7	223.3	236.7	239.4
contiguous sites	188.8	—	—	—	—	—
dome	188.1	198.1	233.7	223.3	236.7	239.4
neck	188.5	198.1	233.7	223.3	236.7	239.4
orifice	188.9	198.1	233.7	223.3	236.7	239.4
ureteric	188.6	198.1	233.7	223.3	236.7	239.4
urethral	188.5	198.1	233.7	223.3	236.7	239.4
sphincter	188.8	198.1	233.7	223.3	236.7	239.4
trigone	188.0	198.1	233.7	223.3	236.7	239.4
urachus	188.7	—	233.7	223.3	236.7	239.4

N

	Malignant					
	Primary	Secondary	Ca in situ	Benign	Uncertain Behavior	Unspecified
Neoplasm *(Continued)*						
bladder (urinary) *(Continued)*						
wall	188.9	198.1	233.7	223.3	236.7	239.4
anterior	188.3	198.1	233.7	223.3	236.7	239.4
lateral	188.2	198.1	233.7	223.3	236.7	239.4
posterior	188.4	198.1	233.7	223.3	236.7	239.4
blood vessel - *see* Neoplasm, connective tissue						
bone (periosteum)	170.9	198.5	—	213.9	238.0	239.2
Note — Carcinomas and adenocarcinomas, of any type other than intraosseous or odontogenic, of the sites listed under "Neoplasm, bone" should be considered as constituting metastatic spread from an unspecified primary site and coded to 198.5 for morbidity coding.						
acetabulum	170.6	198.5	—	213.6	238.0	239.2
acromion (process)	170.4	198.5	—	213.4	238.0	239.2
ankle	170.8	198.5	—	213.8	238.0	239.2
arm NEC	170.4	198.5	—	213.4	238.0	239.2
astragalus	170.8	198.5	—	213.8	238.0	239.2
atlas	170.2	198.5	—	213.2	238.0	239.2
axis	170.2	198.5	—	213.2	238.0	239.2
back NEC	170.2	198.5	—	213.2	238.0	239.2
calcaneus	170.8	198.5	—	213.8	238.0	239.2
calvarium	170.0	198.5	—	213.0	238.0	239.2
carpus (any)	170.5	198.5	—	213.5	238.0	239.2
cartilage NEC	170.9	198.5	—	213.9	238.0	239.2
clavicle	170.3	198.5	—	213.3	238.0	239.2
clivus	170.0	198.5	—	213.0	238.0	239.2
coccygeal vertebra	170.6	198.5	—	213.6	238.0	239.2
coccyx	170.6	198.5	—	213.6	238.0	239.2
costal cartilage	170.3	198.5	—	213.3	238.0	239.2
costovertebral joint	170.3	198.5	—	213.3	238.0	239.2
cranial	170.0	198.5	—	213.0	238.0	239.2
cuboid	170.8	198.5	—	213.8	238.0	239.2
cuneiform	170.9	198.5	—	213.9	238.0	239.2
ankle	170.8	198.5	—	213.8	238.0	239.2
wrist	170.5	198.5	—	213.5	238.0	239.2
digital	170.9	198.5	—	213.9	238.0	239.2
finger	170.5	198.5	—	213.5	238.0	239.2
toe	170.8	198.5	—	213.8	238.0	239.2
elbow	170.4	198.5	—	213.4	238.0	239.2
ethmoid (labyrinth)	170.0	198.5	—	213.0	238.0	239.2
face	170.0	198.5	—	213.0	238.0	239.2
lower jaw	170.1	198.5	—	213.1	238.0	239.2
femur (any part)	170.7	198.5	—	213.7	238.0	239.2

◀ New ◀▥ Revised ~~deleted~~ Deleted ● Use Additional Digit(s) ▨ Omit code

	Malignant					
	Primary	Secondary	Ca in situ	Benign	Uncertain Behavior	Unspecified
Neoplasm *(Continued)*						
bone *(Continued)*						
fibula (any part)	170.7	198.5	—	213.7	238.0	239.2
finger (any)	170.5	198.5	—	213.5	238.0	239.2
foot	170.8	198.5	—	213.8	238.0	239.2
forearm	170.4	198.5	—	213.4	238.0	239.2
frontal	170.0	198.5	—	213.0	238.0	239.2
hand	170.5	198.5	—	213.5	238.0	239.2
heel	170.8	198.5	—	213.8	238.0	239.2
hip	170.6	198.5	—	213.6	238.0	239.2
humerus (any part)	170.4	198.5	—	213.4	238.0	239.2
hyoid	170.0	198.5	—	213.0	238.0	239.2
ilium	170.6	198.5	—	213.6	238.0	239.2
innominate	170.6	198.5	—	213.6	238.0	239.2
intervertebral cartilage or disc	170.2	198.5	—	213.2	238.0	239.2
ischium	170.6	198.5	—	213.6	238.0	239.2
jaw (lower)	170.1	198.5	—	213.1	238.0	239.2
upper	170.0	198.5	—	213.0	238.0	239.2
knee	170.7	198.5	—	213.7	238.0	239.2
leg NEC	170.7	198.5	—	213.7	238.0	239.2
limb NEC	170.9	198.5	—	213.9	238.0	239.2
lower (long bones)	170.7	198.5	—	213.7	238.0	239.2
short bones	170.8	198.5	—	213.8	238.0	239.2
upper (long bones)	170.4	198.5	—	213.4	238.0	239.2
short bones	170.5	198.5	—	213.5	238.0	239.2
long	170.9	198.5	—	213.9	238.0	239.2
lower limbs NEC	170.7	198.5	—	213.7	238.0	239.2
upper limbs NEC	170.4	198.5	—	213.4	238.0	239.2
malar	170.0	198.5	—	213.0	238.0	239.2
mandible	170.1	198.5	—	213.1	238.0	239.2
marrow NEC	202.9●	198.5	—	—	—	238.79
mastoid	170.0	198.5	—	213.0	238.0	239.2
maxilla, maxillary (superior)	170.0	198.5	—	213.0	238.0	239.2
inferior	170.1	198.5	—	213.1	238.0	239.2
metacarpus (any)	170.5	198.5	—	213.5	238.0	239.2
metatarsus (any)	170.8	198.5	—	213.8	238.0	239.2
navicular (ankle)	170.8	198.5	—	213.8	238.0	239.2
hand	170.5	198.5	—	213.5	238.0	239.2
nose, nasal	170.0	198.5	—	213.0	238.0	239.2
occipital	170.0	198.5	—	213.0	238.0	239.2
orbit	170.0	198.5	—	213.0	238.0	239.2

	Malignant					
	Primary	Secondary	Ca in situ	Benign	Uncertain Behavior	Unspecified
Neoplasm *(Continued)*						
bone *(Continued)*						
parietal	170.0	198.5	—	213.0	238.0	239.2
patella	170.8	198.5	—	213.8	238.0	239.2
pelvic	170.6	198.5	—	213.6	238.0	239.2
phalanges	170.9	198.5	—	213.9	238.0	239.2
foot	170.8	198.5	—	213.8	238.0	239.2
hand	170.5	198.5	—	213.5	238.0	239.2
pubic	170.6	198.5	—	213.6	238.0	239.2
radius (any part)	170.4	198.5	—	213.4	238.0	239.2
rib	170.3	198.5	—	213.3	238.0	239.2
sacral vertebra	170.6	198.5	—	213.6	238.0	239.2
sacrum	170.6	198.5	—	213.6	238.0	239.2
scaphoid (of hand)	170.5	198.5	—	213.5	238.0	239.2
of ankle	170.8	198.5	—	213.8	238.0	239.2
scapula (any part)	170.4	198.5	—	213.4	238.0	239.2
sella turcica	170.0	198.5	—	213.0	238.0	239.2
short	170.9	198.5	—	213.9	238.0	239.2
lower limb	170.8	198.5	—	213.8	238.0	239.2
upper limb	170.5	198.5	—	213.5	238.0	239.2
shoulder	170.4	198.5	—	213.4	238.0	239.2
skeleton, skeletal NEC	170.9	198.5	—	213.9	238.0	239.2
skull	170.0	198.5	—	213.0	238.0	239.2
sphenoid	170.0	198.5	—	213.0	238.0	239.2
spine, spinal (column)	170.2	198.5	—	213.2	238.0	239.2
coccyx	170.6	198.5	—	213.6	238.0	239.2
sacrum	170.6	198.5	—	213.6	238.0	239.2
sternum	170.3	198.5	—	213.3	238.0	239.2
tarsus (any)	170.8	198.5	—	213.8	238.0	239.2
temporal	170.0	198.5	—	213.0	238.0	239.2
thumb	170.5	198.5	—	213.5	238.0	239.2
tibia (any part)	170.7	198.5	—	213.7	238.0	239.2
toe (any)	170.8	198.5	—	213.8	238.0	239.2
trapezium	170.5	198.5	—	213.5	238.0	239.2
trapezoid	170.5	198.5	—	213.5	238.0	239.2
turbinate	170.0	198.5	—	213.0	238.0	239.2
ulna (any part)	170.4	198.5	—	213.4	238.0	239.2
unciform	170.5	198.5	—	213.5	238.0	239.2
vertebra (column)	170.2	198.5	—	213.2	238.0	239.2
coccyx	170.6	198.5	—	213.6	238.0	239.2
sacrum	170.6	198.5	—	213.6	238.0	239.2
vomer	170.0	198.5	—	213.0	238.0	239.2

◀ New ◀ Revised deleted Deleted ● Use Additional Digit(s) ▨ Omit code

	Malignant					
	Primary	Secondary	Ca in situ	Benign	Uncertain Behavior	Unspecified
Neoplasm *(Continued)*						
bone *(Continued)*						
wrist	170.5	198.5	—	213.5	238.0	239.2
xiphoid process	170.3	198.5	—	213.3	238.0	239.2
zygomatic	170.0	198.5	—	213.0	238.0	239.2
book-leaf (mouth)	145.8	198.89	230.0	210.4	235.1	239.0
bowel - *see* Neoplasm, intestine						
brachial plexus	171.2	198.89	—	215.2	238.1	239.2
brain NEC	191.9	198.3	—	225.0	237.5	239.6
basal ganglia	191.0	198.3	—	225.0	237.5	239.6
cerebellopontine angle	191.6	198.3	—	225.0	237.5	239.6
cerebellum NOS	191.6	198.3	—	225.0	237.5	239.6
cerebrum	191.0	198.3	—	225.0	237.5	239.6
choroid plexus	191.5	198.3	—	225.0	237.5	239.6
contiguous sites	191.8	—	—	—	—	—
corpus callosum	191.8	198.3	—	225.0	237.5	239.6
corpus striatum	191.0	198.3	—	225.0	237.5	239.6
cortex (cerebral)	191.0	198.3	—	225.0	237.5	239.6
frontal lobe	191.1	198.3	—	225.0	237.5	239.6
globus pallidus	191.0	198.3	—	225.0	237.5	239.6
hippocampus	191.2	198.3	—	225.0	237.5	239.6
hypothalamus	191.0	198.3	—	225.0	237.5	239.6
internal capsule	191.0	198.3	—	225.0	237.5	239.6
medulla oblongata	191.7	198.3	—	225.0	237.5	239.6
meninges	192.1	198.4	—	225.2	237.6	239.7
midbrain	191.7	198.3	—	225.0	237.5	239.6
occipital lobe	191.4	198.3	—	225.0	237.5	239.6
parietal lobe	191.3	198.3	—	225.0	237.5	239.6
peduncle	191.7	198.3	—	225.0	237.5	239.6
pons	191.7	198.3	—	225.0	237.5	239.6
stem	191.7	198.3	—	225.0	237.5	239.6
tapetum	191.8	198.3	—	225.0	237.5	239.6
temporal lobe	191.2	198.3	—	225.0	237.5	239.6
thalamus	191.0	198.3	—	225.0	237.5	239.6
uncus	191.2	198.3	—	225.0	237.5	239.6
ventricle (floor)	191.5	198.3	—	225.0	237.5	239.6
branchial (cleft) (vestiges)	146.8	198.89	230.0	210.6	235.1	239.0
breast (connective tissue) (female) (glandular tissue) (soft parts)	174.9	198.81	233.0	217	238.3	239.3
areola	174.0	198.81	233.0	217	238.3	239.3
male	175.0	198.81	233.0	217	238.3	239.3
axillary tail	174.6	198.81	233.0	217	238.3	239.3
central portion	174.1	198.81	233.0	217	238.3	239.3

◀ New   ◀▥ Revised   ~~deleted~~ Deleted   ● Use Additional Digit(s)   ▨ Omit code

	Malignant					
	Primary	Secondary	Ca in situ	Benign	Uncertain Behavior	Unspecified
Neoplasm *(Continued)*						
breast *(Continued)*						
contiguous sites	174.8	—	—	—	—	—
ectopic sites	174.8	198.81	233.0	217	238.3	239.3
inner	174.8	198.81	233.0	217	238.3	239.3
lower	174.8	198.81	233.0	217	238.3	239.3
lower-inner quadrant	174.3	198.81	233.0	217	238.3	239.3
lower-outer quadrant	174.5	198.81	233.0	217	238.3	239.3
male	175.9	198.81	233.0	217	238.3	239.3
areola	175.0	198.81	233.0	217	238.3	239.3
ectopic tissue	175.9	198.81	233.0	217	238.3	239.3
nipple	175.0	198.81	233.0	217	238.3	239.3
mastectomy site (skin) (*see also* Neoplasm, mastectomy site)	173.50	198.2	—	—	—	—
specified as breast tissue	174.8	198.81	—	—	—	—
midline	174.8	198.81	233.0	217	238.3	239.3
nipple	174.0	198.81	233.0	217	238.3	239.3
male	175.0	198.81	233.0	217	238.3	239.3
outer	174.8	198.81	233.0	217	238.3	239.3
skin (*see also* Neoplasm, mastectomy site)	173.50	198.2	232.5	216.5	238.2	239.2
tail (axillary)	174.6	198.81	233.0	217	238.3	239.3
upper	174.8	198.81	233.0	217	238.3	239.3
upper-inner quadrant	174.2	198.81	233.0	217	238.3	239.3
upper-outer quadrant	174.4	198.81	233.0	217	238.3	239.3
broad ligament	183.3	198.82	233.39	221.0	236.3	239.5
bronchiogenic, bronchogenic (lung)	162.9	197.0	231.2	212.3	235.7	239.1
bronchiole	162.9	197.0	231.2	212.3	235.7	239.1
bronchus	162.9	197.0	231.2	212.3	235.7	239.1
carina	162.2	197.0	231.2	212.3	235.7	239.1
contiguous sites with lung or trachea	162.8	—	—	—	—	—
lower lobe of lung	162.5	197.0	231.2	212.3	235.7	239.1
main	162.2	197.0	231.2	212.3	235.7	239.1
middle lobe of lung	162.4	197.0	231.2	212.3	235.7	239.1
upper lobe of lung	162.3	197.0	231.2	212.3	235.7	239.1
brow	173.30	198.2	232.3	216.3	238.2	239.2
basal cell carcinoma	173.31	—	—	—	—	—
specified type NEC	173.39	—	—	—	—	—
squamous cell carcinoma	173.32	—	—	—	—	—
buccal (cavity)	145.9	198.89	230.0	210.4	235.1	239.0
commissure	145.0	198.89	230.0	210.4	235.1	239.0
groove (lower) (upper)	145.1	198.89	230.0	210.4	235.1	239.0
mucosa	145.0	198.89	230.0	210.4	235.1	239.0
sulcus (lower) (upper)	145.1	198.89	230.0	210.4	235.1	239.0

◄ New　◄‖‖ Revised　deleted Deleted　● Use Additional Digit(s)　▨ Omit code

	Malignant					
	Primary	Secondary	Ca in situ	Benign	Uncertain Behavior	Unspecified
Neoplasm *(Continued)*						
bulbourethral gland	189.3	198.1	233.9	223.81	236.99	239.5
bursa - *see* Neoplasm, connective tissue						
buttock NEC*	195.3	198.89	232.5	229.8	238.8	239.89
calf*	195.5	198.89	232.7	229.8	238.8	239.89
calvarium	170.0	198.5	—	213.0	238.0	239.2
calyx, renal	189.1	198.0	233.9	223.1	236.91	239.5
canal						
anal	154.2	197.5	230.5	211.4	235.5	239.0
auditory (external) (*see also* Neoplasm, skin, ear)	173.20	198.2	232.2	216.2	238.2	239.2
auricular (external) (*see also* Neoplasm, skin, ear)	173.20	198.2	232.2	216.2	238.2	239.2
canaliculi, biliary (biliferi) (intrahepatic)	155.1	197.8	230.8	211.5	235.3	239.0
canthus (eye) (inner) (outer)	173.10	198.2	232.1	216.1	238.2	239.2
basal cell carcinoma	173.11	—	—	—	—	—
specified type NEC	173.19	—	—	—	—	—
squamous cell carcinoma	173.12	—	—	—	—	—
capillary - *see* Neoplasm, connective tissue						
caput coli	153.4	197.5	230.3	211.3	235.2	239.0
cardia (gastric)	151.0	197.8	230.2	211.1	235.2	239.0
cardiac orifice (stomach)	151.0	197.8	230.2	211.1	235.2	239.0
cardio-esophageal junction	151.0	197.8	230.2	211.1	235.2	239.0
cardio-esophagus	151.0	197.8	230.2	211.1	235.2	239.0
carina (bronchus) (trachea)	162.2	197.0	231.2	212.3	235.7	239.1
carotid (artery)	171.0	198.89	—	215.0	238.1	239.2
body	194.5	198.89	—	227.5	237.3	239.7
carpus (any bone)	170.5	198.5	—	213.5	238.0	239.2
cartilage (articular) (joint) NEC - *see also* Neoplasm, bone	170.9	198.5	—	213.9	238.0	239.2
arytenoid	161.3	197.3	231.0	212.1	235.6	239.1
auricular	171.0	198.89	—	215.0	238.1	239.2
bronchi	162.2	197.3	—	212.3	235.7	239.1
connective tissue - *see* Neoplasm, connective tissue						
costal	170.3	198.5	—	213.3	238.0	239.2
cricoid	161.3	197.3	231.0	212.1	235.6	239.1
cuneiform	161.3	197.3	231.0	212.1	235.6	239.1
ear (external)	171.0	198.89	—	215.0	238.1	239.2
ensiform	170.3	198.5	—	213.3	238.0	239.2
epiglottis	161.1	197.3	231.0	212.1	235.6	239.1
anterior surface	146.4	198.89	230.0	210.6	235.1	239.0
eyelid	171.0	198.89	—	215.0	238.1	239.2
intervertebral	170.2	198.5	—	213.2	238.0	239.2
larynx, laryngeal	161.3	197.3	231.0	212.1	235.6	239.1
nose, nasal	160.0	197.3	231.8	212.0	235.9	239.1

	Malignant			Benign	Uncertain Behavior	Unspecified
	Primary	Secondary	Ca in situ			
Neoplasm (Continued)						
cartilage NEC (Continued)						
pinna	171.0	198.89	—	215.0	238.1	239.2
rib	170.3	198.5	—	213.3	238.0	239.2
semilunar (knee)	170.7	198.5	—	213.7	238.0	239.2
thyroid	161.3	197.3	231.0	212.1	235.6	239.1
trachea	162.0	197.3	231.1	212.2	235.7	239.1
cauda equina	192.2	198.3	—	225.3	237.5	239.7
cavity						
buccal	145.9	198.89	230.0	210.4	235.1	239.0
nasal	160.0	197.3	231.8	212.0	235.9	239.1
oral	145.9	198.89	230.0	210.4	235.1	239.0
peritoneal	158.9	197.6	—	211.8	235.4	239.0
tympanic	160.1	197.3	231.8	212.0	235.9	239.1
cecum	153.4	197.5	230.3	211.3	235.2	239.0
central						
nervous system - see Neoplasm, nervous system						
white matter	191.0	198.3	—	225.0	237.5	239.6
cerebellopontine (angle)	191.6	198.3	—	225.0	237.5	239.6
cerebellum, cerebellar	191.6	198.3	—	225.0	237.5	239.6
cerebrum, cerebral (cortex) (hemisphere) (white matter)	191.0	198.3	—	225.0	237.5	239.6
meninges	192.1	198.4	—	225.2	237.6	239.7
peduncle	191.7	198.3	—	225.0	237.5	239.6
ventricle (any)	191.5	198.3	—	225.0	237.5	239.6
cervical region	195.0	198.89	234.8	229.8	238.8	239.89
cervix (cervical) (uteri) (uterus)	180.9	198.82	233.1	219.0	236.0	239.5
canal	180.0	198.82	233.1	219.0	236.0	239.5
contiguous sites	180.8	—	—	—	—	—
endocervix (canal) (gland)	180.0	198.82	233.1	219.0	236.0	239.5
exocervix	180.1	198.82	233.1	219.0	236.0	239.5
external os	180.1	198.82	233.1	219.0	236.0	239.5
nabothian gland	180.0	198.82	233.1	219.0	236.0	239.5
squamocolumnar junction	180.8	198.82	233.1	219.0	236.0	239.5
stump	180.8	198.82	233.1	219.0	236.0	239.5
cheek	195.0	198.89	234.8	229.8	238.8	239.89
external	173.30	198.2	232.3	216.3	238.2	239.2
basal cell carcinoma	173.31	—	—	—	—	—
specified type NEC	173.39	—	—	—	—	—
squamous cell carcinoma	173.32	—	—	—	—	—
inner aspect	145.0	198.89	230.0	210.4	235.1	239.0
internal	145.0	198.89	230.0	210.4	235.1	239.0
mucosa	145.0	198.89	230.0	210.4	235.1	239.0

◄ New   ◄ Revised   ~~deleted~~ Deleted   ● Use Additional Digit(s)   Omit code

	Malignant			Benign	Uncertain Behavior	Unspecified
	Primary	Secondary	Ca in situ			
Neoplasm *(Continued)*						
chest (wall) NEC	195.1	198.89	234.8	229.8	238.8	239.89
chiasma opticum	192.0	198.4	—	225.1	237.9	239.7
chin	173.30	198.2	232.3	216.3	238.2	239.2
basal cell carcinoma	173.31	—	—	—	—	—
specified type NEC	173.39	—	—	—	—	—
squamous cell carcinoma	173.32	—	—	—	—	—
choana	147.3	198.89	230.0	210.7	235.1	239.0
cholangiole	155.1	197.8	230.8	211.5	235.3	239.0
choledochal duct	156.1	197.8	230.8	211.5	235.3	239.0
choroid	190.6	198.4	234.0	224.6	238.8	239.81
plexus	191.5	198.3	—	225.0	237.5	239.6
ciliary body	190.0	198.4	234.0	224.0	238.8	239.89
clavicle	170.3	198.5	—	213.3	238.0	239.2
clitoris	184.3	198.82	233.32	221.2	236.3	239.5
clivus	170.0	198.5	—	213.0	238.0	239.2
cloacogenic zone	154.8	197.5	230.7	211.4	235.5	239.0
coccygeal						
body or glomus	194.6	198.89	—	227.6	237.3	239.7
vertebra	170.6	198.5	—	213.6	238.0	239.2
coccyx	170.6	198.5	—	213.6	238.0	239.2
colon - *see also* Neoplasm, intestine, large	153.9	197.5	230.3	211.3	235.2	239.0
with rectum	154.0	197.5	230.4	211.4	235.2	239.0
column, spinal - *see* Neoplasm, spine						
columnella (*see also* Neoplasm, skin, face)	173.30	198.2	232.3	216.3	238.2	239.2
commissure						
labial, lip	140.6	198.89	230.0	210.4	235.1	239.0
laryngeal	161.0	197.3	231.0	212.1	235.6	239.1
common (bile) duct	156.1	197.8	230.8	211.5	235.3	239.0
concha (*see also* Neoplasm, skin, ear)	173.20	198.2	232.2	216.2	238.2	239.2
nose	160.0	197.3	231.8	212.0	235.9	239.1
conjunctiva	190.3	198.4	234.0	224.3	238.8	239.89
connective tissue NEC	171.9	198.89	—	215.9	238.1	239.2

Note — For neoplasms of connective tissue (blood vessel, bursa, fascia, ligament, muscle, peripheral nerves, sympathetic and parasympathetic nerves and ganglia, synovia, tendon, etc.) or of morphological types that indicate connective tissue, code according to the list under "Neoplasm, connective tissue;" for sites that do not appear in this list, code to neoplasm of that site; e.g.,

       liposarcoma, shoulder 171.2

       leiomyosarcoma, stomach 151.9

       neurofibroma, chest wall 215.4

Morphological types that indicate connective tissue appear in their proper place in the alphabetic index with the instruction "see Neoplasm, connective tissue ...."

abdomen	171.5	198.89	—	215.5	238.1	239.2
abdominal wall	171.5	198.89	—	215.5	238.1	239.2

| | Malignant | | | | | |
	Primary	Secondary	Ca in situ	Benign	Uncertain Behavior	Unspecified
Neoplasm *(Continued)*						
connective tissue NEC *(Continued)*						
ankle	171.3	198.89	—	215.3	238.1	239.2
antecubital fossa or space	171.2	198.89	—	215.2	238.1	239.2
arm	171.2	198.89	—	215.2	238.1	239.2
auricle (ear)	171.0	198.89	—	215.0	238.1	239.2
axilla	171.4	198.89	—	215.4	238.1	239.2
back	171.7	198.89	—	215.7	238.1	239.2
breast (female) (*see also* Neoplasm, breast)	174.9	198.81	233.0	217	238.3	239.3
male	175.9	198.81	233.0	217	238.3	239.3
buttock	171.6	198.89	—	215.6	238.1	239.2
calf	171.3	198.89	—	215.3	238.1	239.2
cervical region	171.0	198.89	—	215.0	238.1	239.2
cheek	171.0	198.89	—	215.0	238.1	239.2
chest (wall)	171.4	198.89	—	215.4	238.1	239.2
chin	171.0	198.89	—	215.0	238.1	239.2
contiguous sites	171.8	—	—	—	—	—
diaphragm	171.4	198.89	—	215.4	238.1	239.2
ear (external)	171.0	198.89	—	215.0	238.1	239.2
elbow	171.2	198.89	—	215.2	238.1	239.2
extrarectal	171.6	198.89	—	215.6	238.1	239.2
extremity	171.8	198.89	—	215.8	238.1	239.2
lower	171.3	198.89	—	215.3	238.1	239.2
upper	171.2	198.89	—	215.2	238.1	239.2
eyelid	171.0	198.89	—	215.0	238.1	239.2
face	171.0	198.89	—	215.0	238.1	239.2
finger	171.2	198.89	—	215.2	238.1	239.2
flank	171.7	198.89	—	215.7	238.1	239.2
foot	171.3	198.89	—	215.3	238.1	239.2
forearm	171.2	198.89	—	215.2	238.1	239.2
forehead	171.0	198.89	—	215.0	238.1	239.2
gastric	171.5	198.89	—	215.5	238.1	—
gastrointestinal	171.5	198.89	—	215.5	238.1	—
gluteal region	171.6	198.89	—	215.6	238.1	239.2
great vessels NEC	171.4	198.89	—	215.4	238.1	239.2
groin	171.6	198.89	—	215.6	238.1	239.2
hand	171.2	198.89	—	215.2	238.1	239.2
head	171.0	198.89	—	215.0	238.1	239.2
heel	171.3	198.89	—	215.3	238.1	239.2
hip	171.3	198.89	—	215.3	238.1	239.2
hypochondrium	171.5	198.89	—	215.5	238.1	239.2
iliopsoas muscle	171.6	198.89	—	215.5	238.1	239.2

◄ New　◄▥ Revised　d̶e̶l̶e̶t̶e̶d̶ Deleted　● Use Additional Digit(s)　▨ Omit code

	Malignant					
	Primary	Secondary	Ca in situ	Benign	Uncertain Behavior	Unspecified
Neoplasm *(Continued)*						
connective tissue NEC *(Continued)*						
infraclavicular region	171.4	198.89	—	215.4	238.1	239.2
inguinal (canal) (region)	171.6	198.89	—	215.6	238.1	239.2
intestine	171.5	198.89	—	215.5	238.1	—
intrathoracic	171.4	198.89	—	215.4	238.1	239.2
ischiorectal fossa	171.6	198.89	—	215.6	238.1	239.2
jaw	143.9	198.89	230.0	210.4	235.1	239.0
knee	171.3	198.89	—	215.3	238.1	239.2
leg	171.3	198.89	—	215.3	238.1	239.2
limb NEC	171.9	198.89	—	215.8	238.1	239.2
lower	171.3	198.89	—	215.3	238.1	239.2
upper	171.2	198.89	—	215.2	238.1	239.2
nates	171.6	198.89	—	215.6	238.1	239.2
neck	171.0	198.89	—	215.0	238.1	239.2
orbit	190.1	198.4	234.0	224.1	238.8	239.89
pararectal	171.6	198.89	—	215.6	238.1	239.2
para-urethral	171.6	198.89	—	215.6	238.1	239.2
paravaginal	171.6	198.89	—	215.6	238.1	239.2
pelvis (floor)	171.6	198.89	—	215.6	238.1	239.2
pelvo-abdominal	171.8	198.89	—	215.8	238.1	239.2
perineum	171.6	198.89	—	215.6	238.1	239.2
perirectal (tissue)	171.6	198.89	—	215.6	238.1	239.2
periurethral (tissue)	171.6	198.89	—	215.6	238.1	239.2
popliteal fossa or space	171.3	198.89	—	215.3	238.1	239.2
presacral	171.6	198.89	—	215.6	238.1	239.2
psoas muscle	171.5	198.89	—	215.5	238.1	239.2
pterygoid fossa	171.0	198.89	—	215.0	238.1	239.2
rectovaginal septum or wall	171.6	198.89	—	215.6	238.1	239.2
rectovesical	171.6	198.89	—	215.6	238.1	239.2
retroperitoneum	158.0	197.6	—	211.8	235.4	239.0
sacrococcygeal region	171.6	198.89	—	215.6	238.1	239.2
scalp	171.0	198.89	—	215.0	238.1	239.2
scapular region	171.4	198.89	—	215.4	238.1	239.2
shoulder	171.2	198.89	—	215.2	238.1	239.2
skin (dermis) NEC	173.90	198.2	232.9	216.9	238.2	239.2
stomach	171.5	198.89	—	215.5	238.1	—
submental	171.0	198.89	—	215.0	238.1	239.2
supraclavicular region	171.0	198.89	—	215.0	238.1	239.2
temple	171.0	198.89	—	215.0	238.1	239.2
temporal region	171.0	198.89	—	215.0	238.1	239.2
thigh	171.3	198.89	—	215.3	238.1	239.2

◀ New   ◀ Revised   ~~deleted~~ Deleted   ● Use Additional Digit(s)   ▨ Omit code

	Malignant			Benign	Uncertain Behavior	Unspecified
	Primary	Secondary	Ca in situ			
Neoplasm *(Continued)*						
connective tissue NEC *(Continued)*						
thoracic (duct) (wall)	171.4	198.89	—	215.4	238.1	239.2
thorax	171.4	198.89	—	215.4	238.1	239.2
thumb	171.2	198.89	—	215.2	238.1	239.2
toe	171.3	198.89	—	215.3	238.1	239.2
trunk	171.7	198.89	—	215.7	238.1	239.2
umbilicus	171.5	198.89	—	215.5	238.1	239.2
vesicorectal	171.6	198.89	—	215.6	238.1	239.2
wrist	171.2	198.89	—	215.2	238.1	239.2
conus medullaris	192.2	198.3	—	225.3	237.5	239.7
cord (true) (vocal)	161.0	197.3	231.0	212.1	235.6	239.1
false	161.1	197.3	231.0	212.1	235.6	239.1
spermatic	187.6	198.82	233.6	222.8	236.6	239.5
spinal (cervical) (lumbar) (thoracic)	192.2	198.3	—	225.3	237.5	239.7
cornea (limbus)	190.4	198.4	234.0	224.4	238.8	239.89
corpus						
albicans	183.0	198.6	233.39	220	236.2	239.5
callosum, brain	191.8	198.3	—	225.0	237.5	239.6
cavernosum	187.3	198.82	233.5	222.1	236.6	239.5
gastric	151.4	197.8	230.2	211.1	235.2	239.0
penis	187.3	198.82	233.5	222.1	236.6	239.5
striatum, cerebrum	191.0	198.3	—	225.0	237.5	239.6
uteri	182.0	198.82	233.2	219.1	236.0	239.5
isthmus	182.1	198.82	233.2	219.1	236.0	239.5
cortex						
adrenal	194.0	198.7	234.8	227.0	237.2	239.7
cerebral	191.0	198.3	—	225.0	237.5	239.6
costal cartilage	170.3	198.5	—	213.3	238.0	239.2
costovertebral joint	170.3	198.5	—	213.3	238.0	239.2
Cowper's gland	189.3	198.1	233.9	223.81	236.99	239.5
cranial (fossa, any)	191.9	198.3	—	225.0	237.5	239.6
meninges	192.1	198.4	—	225.2	237.6	239.7
nerve (any)	192.0	198.4	—	225.1	237.9	239.7
craniobuccal pouch	194.3	198.89	234.8	227.3	237.0	239.7
craniopharyngeal (duct) (pouch)	194.3	198.89	234.8	227.3	237.0	239.7
cricoid	148.0	198.89	230.0	210.8	235.1	239.0
cartilage	161.3	197.3	231.0	212.1	235.6	239.1
cricopharynx	148.0	198.89	230.0	210.8	235.1	239.0
crypt of Morgagni	154.8	197.5	230.7	211.4	235.2	239.0
crystalline lens	190.0	198.4	234.0	224.0	238.8	239.89
cul-de-sac (Douglas')	158.8	197.6	—	211.8	235.4	239.0

◀ New   ◀ Revised   deleted Deleted   ● Use Additional Digit(s)   Omit code

	Malignant					
	Primary	Secondary	Ca in situ	Benign	Uncertain Behavior	Unspecified
Neoplasm *(Continued)*						
cuneiform cartilage	161.3	197.3	231.0	212.1	235.6	239.1
cutaneous - *see* Neoplasm, skin						
cutis - *see* Neoplasm, skin						
cystic (bile) duct (common)	156.1	197.8	230.8	211.5	235.3	239.0
dermis - *see* Neoplasm, skin						
diaphragm	171.4	198.89	—	215.4	238.1	239.2
digestive organs, system, tube, or tract NEC	159.9	197.8	230.9	211.9	235.5	239.0
contiguous sites with peritoneum	159.8	—	—	—	—	—
disc, intervertebral	170.2	198.5	—	213.2	238.0	239.2
disease, generalized	199.0	199.0	234.9	229.9	238.9	199.0
disseminated	199.0	199.0	234.9	229.9	238.9	199.0
Douglas' cul-de-sac or pouch	158.8	197.6	—	211.8	235.4	239.0
duodenojejunal junction	152.8	197.4	230.7	211.2	235.2	239.0
duodenum	152.0	197.4	230.7	211.2	235.2	239.0
dura (cranial) (mater)	192.1	198.4	—	225.2	237.6	239.7
cerebral	192.1	198.4	—	225.2	237.6	239.7
spinal	192.3	198.4	—	225.4	237.6	239.7
ear (external) (*see also* Neoplasm, ear, skin)	173.20	198.2	232.2	216.2	238.2	239.2
auricle or auris (*see also* Neoplasm, ear, skin)	173.20	198.2	232.2	216.2	238.2	239.2
canal, external (*see also* Neoplasm, ear, skin)	173.20	198.2	232.2	216.2	238.2	239.2
cartilage	171.0	198.89	—	215.0	238.1	239.2
external meatus (*see also* Neoplasm, ear, skin)	173.20	198.2	232.2	216.2	238.2	239.2
inner	160.1	197.3	231.8	212.0	235.9	239.89
lobule (*see also* Neoplasm, ear, skin)	173.20	198.2	232.2	216.2	238.2	239.2
middle	160.1	197.3	231.8	212.0	235.9	239.89
contiguous sites with accessory sinuses or nasal cavities	160.8	—	—	—	—	—
skin	173.20	198.2	232.2	216.2	238.2	239.2
basal cell carcinoma	173.21	—	—	—	—	—
specified type NEC	173.29	—	—	—	—	—
squamous cell carcinoma	173.22	—	—	—	—	—
earlobe	173.20	198.2	232.2	216.2	238.2	239.2
basal cell carcinoma	173.21	—	—	—	—	—
specified type NEC	173.29	—	—	—	—	—
squamous cell carcinoma	173.22	—	—	—	—	—
ejaculatory duct	187.8	198.82	233.6	222.8	236.6	239.5
elbow NEC*	195.4	198.89	232.6	229.8	238.8	239.89
endocardium	164.1	198.89	—	212.7	238.8	239.89
endocervix (canal) (gland)	180.0	198.82	233.1	219.0	236.0	239.5
endocrine gland NEC	194.9	198.89	—	227.9	237.4	239.7
pluriglandular NEC	194.8	198.89	234.8	227.8	237.4	239.7
endometrium (gland) (stroma)	182.0	198.82	233.2	219.1	236.0	239.5

◀ New   ◀▦ Revised   ~~deleted~~ Deleted   ⬤ Use Additional Digit(s)   ▨ Omit code

	Malignant					
	Primary	Secondary	Ca in situ	Benign	Uncertain Behavior	Unspecified
Neoplasm *(Continued)*						
ensiform cartilage	170.3	198.5	—	213.3	238.0	239.2
enteric - *see* Neoplasm, intestine						
ependyma (brain)	191.5	198.3	—	225.0	237.5	239.6
epicardium	164.1	198.89	—	212.7	238.8	239.89
epididymis	187.5	198.82	233.6	222.3	236.6	239.5
epidural	192.9	198.4	—	225.9	237.9	239.7
epiglottis	161.1	197.3	231.0	212.1	235.6	239.1
anterior aspect or surface	146.4	198.89	230.0	210.6	235.1	239.0
cartilage	161.3	197.3	231.0	212.1	235.6	239.1
free border (margin)	146.4	198.89	230.0	210.6	235.1	239.0
junctional region	146.5	198.89	230.0	210.6	235.1	239.0
posterior (laryngeal) surface	161.1	197.3	231.0	212.1	235.6	239.1
suprahyoid portion	161.1	197.3	231.0	212.1	235.6	239.1
esophagogastric junction	151.0	197.8	230.2	211.1	235.2	239.0
esophagus	150.9	197.8	230.1	211.0	235.5	239.0
abdominal	150.2	197.8	230.1	211.0	235.5	239.0
cervical	150.0	197.8	230.1	211.0	235.5	239.0
contiguous sites	150.8	—	—	—	—	—
distal (third)	150.5	197.8	230.1	211.0	235.5	239.0
lower (third)	150.5	197.8	230.1	211.0	235.5	239.0
middle (third)	150.4	197.8	230.1	211.0	235.5	239.0
proximal (third)	150.3	197.8	230.1	211.0	235.5	239.0
specified part NEC	150.8	197.8	230.1	211.0	235.5	239.0
thoracic	150.1	197.8	230.1	211.0	235.5	239.0
upper (third)	150.3	197.8	230.1	211.0	235.5	239.0
ethmoid (sinus)	160.3	197.3	231.8	212.0	235.9	239.1
bone or labyrinth	170.0	198.5	—	213.0	238.0	239.2
Eustachian tube	160.1	197.3	231.8	212.0	235.9	239.1
exocervix	180.1	198.82	233.1	219.0	236.0	239.5
external						
meatus (ear) (*see also* Neoplasm, skin, ear)	173.20	198.2	232.2	216.2	238.2	239.2
os, cervix uteri	180.1	198.82	233.1	219.0	236.0	239.5
extradural	192.9	198.4	—	225.9	237.9	239.7
extrahepatic (bile) duct	156.1	197.8	230.8	211.5	235.3	239.0
contiguous sites with gallbladder	156.8	—	—	—	—	—
extraocular muscle	190.1	198.4	234.0	224.1	238.8	239.89
extrarectal	195.3	198.89	234.8	229.8	238.8	239.89
extremity*	195.8	198.89	232.8	229.8	238.8	239.89
lower*	195.5	198.89	232.7	229.8	238.8	239.89
upper*	195.4	198.89	232.6	229.8	238.8	239.89

◀ New   ◀ Revised   ~~deleted~~ Deleted   ● Use Additional Digit(s)   Omit code

Neoplasm (Continued)	Malignant			Benign	Uncertain Behavior	Unspecified
	Primary	Secondary	Ca in situ	Benign	Uncertain Behavior	Unspecified
eye NEC	190.9	198.4	234.0	224.9	238.8	239.89
contiguous sites	190.8	—	—	—	—	—
specified sites NEC	190.8	198.4	234.0	224.8	238.8	239.89
eyeball	190.0	198.4	234.0	224.0	238.8	239.89
eyebrow	173.30	198.2	232.3	216.3	238.2	239.2
basal cell carcinoma	173.31	—	—	—	—	—
specified type NEC	173.39	—	—	—	—	—
squamous cell carcinoma	173.32	—	—	—	—	—
eyelid (lower) (skin) (upper)	173.10	198.2	232.1	216.1	238.2	239.2
basal cell carcinoma	173.11	—	—	—	—	—
cartilage	171.0	198.89	—	215.0	238.1	239.2
specified type NEC	173.19	—	—	—	—	—
squamous cell carcinoma	173.12	—	—	—	—	—
face NEC*	195.0	198.89	232.3	229.8	238.8	239.89
Fallopian tube (accessory)	183.2	198.82	233.39	221.0	236.3	239.5
falx (cerebella) (cerebri)	192.1	198.4	—	225.2	237.6	239.7
fascia - see also Neoplasm, connective tissue						
palmar	171.2	198.89	—	215.2	238.1	239.2
plantar	171.3	198.89	—	215.3	238.1	239.2
fatty tissue - see Neoplasm, connective tissue						
fauces, faucial NEC	146.9	198.89	230.0	210.6	235.1	239.0
pillars	146.2	198.89	230.0	210.6	235.1	239.0
tonsil	146.0	198.89	230.0	210.5	235.1	239.0
femur (any part)	170.7	198.5	—	213.7	238.0	239.2
fetal membrane	181	198.82	233.2	219.8	236.1	239.5
fibrous tissue - see Neoplasm, connective tissue						
fibula (any part)	170.7	198.5	—	213.7	238.0	239.2
filum terminale	192.2	198.3	—	225.3	237.5	239.7
finger NEC*	195.4	198.89	232.6	229.8	238.8	239.89
flank NEC*	195.8	198.89	232.5	229.8	238.8	239.89
follicle, nabothian	180.0	198.82	233.1	219.0	236.0	239.5
foot NEC*	195.5	198.89	232.7	229.8	238.8	239.89
forearm NEC*	195.4	198.89	232.6	229.8	238.8	239.89
forehead (skin)	173.30	198.2	232.3	216.3	238.2	239.2
basal cell carcinoma	173.31	—	—	—	—	—
specified type NEC	173.39	—	—	—	—	—
squamous cell carcinoma	173.32	—	—	—	—	—
foreskin	187.1	198.82	233.5	222.1	236.6	239.5
fornix						
pharyngeal	147.3	198.89	230.0	210.7	235.1	239.0
vagina	184.0	198.82	233.31	221.1	236.3	239.5

◀ New   ◀◀ Revised   ~~deleted~~ Deleted   ● Use Additional Digit(s)   ▓ Omit code

	Malignant					
	Primary	Secondary	Ca in situ	Benign	Uncertain Behavior	Unspecified
Neoplasm *(Continued)*						
fossa (of)						
anterior (cranial)	191.9	198.3	—	225.0	237.5	239.6
cranial	191.9	198.3	—	225.0	237.5	239.6
ischiorectal	195.3	198.89	234.8	229.8	238.8	239.89
middle (cranial)	191.9	198.3	—	225.0	237.5	239.6
pituitary	194.3	198.89	234.8	227.3	237.0	239.7
posterior (cranial)	191.9	198.3	—	225.0	237.5	239.6
pterygoid	171.0	198.89	—	215.0	238.1	239.2
pyriform	148.1	198.89	230.0	210.8	235.1	239.0
Rosenmüller	147.2	198.89	230.0	210.7	235.1	239.0
tonsillar	146.1	198.89	230.0	210.6	235.1	239.0
fourchette	184.4	198.82	233.32	221.2	236.3	239.5
frenulum						
labii - *see* Neoplasm, lip, internal						
linguae	141.3	198.89	230.0	210.1	235.1	239.0
frontal						
bone	170.0	198.5	—	213.0	238.0	239.2
lobe, brain	191.1	198.3	—	225.0	237.5	239.6
meninges	192.1	198.4	—	225.2	237.6	239.7
pole	191.1	198.3	—	225.0	237.5	239.6
sinus	160.4	197.3	231.8	212.0	235.9	239.1
fundus						
stomach	151.3	197.8	230.2	211.1	235.2	239.0
uterus	182.0	198.82	233.2	219.1	236.0	239.5
gall duct (extrahepatic)	156.1	197.8	230.8	211.5	235.3	239.0
intrahepatic	155.1	197.8	230.8	211.5	235.3	239.0
gallbladder	156.0	197.8	230.8	211.5	235.3	239.0
contiguous sites with extrahepatic bile ducts	156.8	—	—	—	—	—
ganglia (*see also* Neoplasm, connective tissue)	171.9	198.89	—	215.9	238.1	239.2
basal	191.0	198.3	—	225.0	237.5	239.6
ganglion (*see also* Neoplasm, connective tissue)	171.9	198.89	—	215.9	238.1	239.2
cranial nerve	192.0	198.4	—	225.1	237.9	239.7
Gartner's duct	184.0	198.82	233.31	221.1	236.3	239.5
gastric - *see* Neoplasm, stomach						
gastrocolic	159.8	197.8	230.9	211.9	235.5	239.0
gastroesophageal junction	151.0	197.8	230.2	211.1	235.2	239.0
gastrointestinal (tract) NEC	159.9	197.8	230.9	211.9	235.5	239.0
generalized	199.0	199.0	234.9	229.9	238.9	199.0

◀ New   ◀ Revised   ~~deleted~~ Deleted   ● Use Additional Digit(s)   Omit code

	Malignant					
	Primary	Secondary	Ca in situ	Benign	Uncertain Behavior	Unspecified
Neoplasm *(Continued)*						
genital organ or tract						
female NEC	184.9	198.82	233.39	221.9	236.3	239.5
contiguous sites	184.8					
specified site NEC	184.8	198.82	233.39	221.8	236.3	239.5
male NEC	187.9	198.82	233.6	222.9	236.6	239.5
contiguous sites	187.8	—	—	—	—	—
specified site NEC	187.8	198.82	233.6	222.8	236.6	239.5
genitourinary tract						
female	184.9	198.82	233.39	221.9	236.3	239.5
male	187.9	198.82	233.6	222.9	236.6	239.5
gingiva (alveolar) (marginal)	143.9	198.89	230.0	210.4	235.1	239.0
lower	143.1	198.89	230.0	210.4	235.1	239.0
mandibular	143.1	198.89	230.0	210.4	235.1	239.0
maxillary	143.0	198.89	230.0	210.4	235.1	239.0
upper	143.0	198.89	230.0	210.4	235.1	239.0
gland, glandular (lymphatic) (system) - *see also* Neoplasm, lymph gland						
endocrine NEC	194.9	198.89	—	227.9	237.4	239.7
salivary - *see* Neoplasm, salivary, gland						
glans penis	187.2	198.82	233.5	222.1	236.6	239.5
globus pallidus	191.0	198.3	—	225.0	237.5	239.6
glomus						
coccygeal	194.6	198.89	—	227.6	237.3	239.7
jugularis	194.6	198.89	—	227.6	237.3	239.7
glosso-epiglottic fold(s)	146.4	198.89	230.0	210.6	235.1	239.0
glossopalatine fold	146.2	198.89	230.0	210.6	235.1	239.0
glossopharyngeal sulcus	146.1	198.89	230.0	210.6	235.1	239.0
glottis	161.0	197.3	231.0	212.1	235.6	239.1
gluteal region*	195.3	198.89	232.5	229.8	238.8	239.89
great vessels NEC	171.4	198.89	—	215.4	238.1	239.2
groin NEC	195.3	198.89	232.5	229.8	238.8	239.89
gum	143.9	198.89	230.0	210.4	235.1	239.0
contiguous sites	143.8	—	—	—	—	—
lower	143.1	198.89	230.0	210.4	235.1	239.0
upper	143.0	198.89	230.0	210.4	235.1	239.0
hand NEC*	195.4	198.89	232.6	229.8	238.8	239.89
head NEC*	195.0	198.89	232.4	229.8	238.8	239.89
heart	164.1	198.89	—	212.7	238.8	239.89
contiguous sites with mediastinum or thymus	164.8	—	—	—	—	—

	Malignant					
	Primary	Secondary	Ca in situ	Benign	Uncertain Behavior	Unspecified
Neoplasm *(Continued)*						
heel NEC*	195.5	198.89	232.7	229.8	238.8	239.89
helix (*see also* Neoplasm, skin, ear)	173.20	198.2	232.2	216.2	238.2	239.2
hematopoietic, hemopoietic tissue NEC	202.8●	198.89	—	—	—	238.79
hemisphere, cerebral	191.0	198.3	—	225.0	237.5	239.6
hemorrhoidal zone	154.2	197.5	230.5	211.4	235.5	239.0
hepatic	155.2	197.7	230.8	211.5	235.3	239.0
duct (bile)	156.1	197.8	230.8	211.5	235.3	239.0
flexure (colon)	153.0	197.5	230.3	211.3	235.2	239.0
primary	155.0	—	—	—	—	—
hilus of lung	162.2	197.0	231.2	212.3	235.7	239.1
hip NEC*	195.5	198.89	232.7	229.8	238.8	239.89
hippocampus, brain	191.2	198.3	—	225.0	237.5	239.6
humerus (any part)	170.4	198.5	—	213.4	238.0	239.2
hymen	184.0	198.82	233.31	221.1	236.3	239.5
hypopharynx, hypopharyngeal NEC	148.9	198.89	230.0	210.8	235.1	239.0
contiguous sites	148.8	—	—	—	—	—
postcricoid region	148.0	198.89	230.0	210.8	235.1	239.0
posterior wall	148.3	198.89	230.0	210.8	235.1	239.0
pyriform fossa (sinus)	148.1	198.89	230.0	210.8	235.1	239.0
specified site NEC	148.8	198.89	230.0	210.8	235.1	239.0
wall	148.9	198.89	230.0	210.8	235.1	239.0
posterior	148.3	198.89	230.0	210.8	235.1	239.0
hypophysis	194.3	198.89	234.8	227.3	237.0	239.7
hypothalamus	191.0	198.3	—	225.0	237.5	239.6
ileocecum, ileocecal (coil) (junction) (valve)	153.4	197.5	230.3	211.3	235.2	239.0
ileum	152.2	197.4	230.7	211.2	235.2	239.0
ilium	170.6	198.5	—	213.6	238.0	239.2
immunoproliferative NEC	203.8●	—	—	—	—	—
infraclavicular (region)*	195.1	198.89	232.5	229.8	238.8	239.89
inguinal (region)*	195.3	198.89	232.5	229.8	238.8	239.89
insula	191.0	198.3	—	225.0	237.5	239.6
insular tissue (pancreas)	157.4	197.8	230.9	211.7	235.5	239.0
brain	191.0	198.3	—	225.0	237.5	239.6
interarytenoid fold	148.2	198.89	230.0	210.8	235.1	239.0
hypopharyngeal aspect	148.2	198.89	230.0	210.8	235.1	239.0
laryngeal aspect	161.1	197.3	231.0	212.1	235.6	239.1
marginal zone	148.2	198.89	230.0	210.8	235.1	239.0
interdental papillae	143.9	198.89	230.0	210.4	235.1	239.0
lower	143.1	198.89	230.0	210.4	235.1	239.0
upper	143.0	198.89	230.0	210.4	235.1	239.0

◀ New   ◀ Revised   ~~deleted~~ Deleted   ● Use Additional Digit(s)   Omit code

	Malignant					
	Primary	Secondary	Ca in situ	Benign	Uncertain Behavior	Unspecified
Neoplasm *(Continued)*						
internal						
capsule	191.0	198.3	—	225.0	237.5	239.6
os (cervix)	180.0	198.82	233.1	219.0	236.0	239.5
intervertebral cartilage or disc	170.2	198.5	—	213.2	238.0	239.2
intestine, intestinal	159.0	197.8	230.7	211.9	235.2	239.0
large	153.9	197.5	230.3	211.3	235.2	239.0
appendix	153.5	197.5	230.3	211.3	235.2	239.0
caput coli	153.4	197.5	230.3	211.3	235.2	239.0
cecum	153.4	197.5	230.3	211.3	235.2	239.0
colon	153.9	197.5	230.3	211.3	235.2	239.0
and rectum	154.0	197.5	230.4	211.4	235.2	239.0
ascending	153.6	197.5	230.3	211.3	235.2	239.0
caput	153.4	197.5	230.3	211.3	235.2	239.0
contiguous sites	153.8	—	—	—	—	—
descending	153.2	197.5	230.3	211.3	235.2	239.0
distal	153.2	197.5	230.3	211.3	235.2	239.0
left	153.2	197.5	230.3	211.3	235.2	239.0
pelvic	153.3	197.5	230.3	211.3	235.2	239.0
right	153.6	197.5	230.3	211.3	235.2	239.0
sigmoid (flexure)	153.3	197.5	230.3	211.3	235.2	239.0
transverse	153.1	197.5	230.3	211.3	235.2	239.0
contiguous sites	153.8	—	—	—	—	—
hepatic flexure	153.0	197.5	230.3	211.3	235.2	239.0
ileocecum, ileocecal (coil) (valve)	153.4	197.5	230.3	211.3	235.2	239.0
sigmoid flexure (lower) (upper)	153.3	197.5	230.3	211.3	235.2	239.0
splenic flexure	153.7	197.5	230.3	211.3	235.2	239.0
small	152.9	197.4	230.7	211.2	235.2	239.0
contiguous sites	152.8	—	—	—	—	—
duodenum	152.0	197.4	230.7	211.2	235.2	239.0
ileum	152.2	197.4	230.7	211.2	235.2	239.0
jejunum	152.1	197.4	230.7	211.2	235.2	239.0
tract NEC	159.0	197.8	230.7	211.9	235.2	239.0
intra-abdominal	195.2	198.89	234.8	229.8	238.8	239.89
intracranial NEC	191.9	198.3	—	225.0	237.5	239.6
intrahepatic (bile) duct	155.1	197.8	230.8	211.5	235.3	239.0
intraocular	190.0	198.4	234.0	224.0	238.8	239.89
intraorbital	190.1	198.4	234.0	224.1	238.8	239.89
intrasellar	194.3	198.89	234.8	227.3	237.0	239.7
intrathoracic (cavity) (organs NEC)	195.1	198.89	234.8	229.8	238.8	239.89
contiguous sites with respiratory organs	165.8	—	—	—	—	—

	Malignant			Benign	Uncertain Behavior	Unspecified
	Primary	Secondary	Ca in situ			
Neoplasm *(Continued)*						
iris	190.0	198.4	234.0	224.0	238.8	239.89
ischiorectal (fossa)	195.3	198.89	234.8	229.8	238.8	239.89
ischium	170.6	198.5	—	213.6	238.0	239.2
island of Reil	191.0	198.3	—	225.0	237.5	239.6
islands or islets of Langerhans	157.4	197.8	230.9	211.7	235.5	239.0
isthmus uteri	182.1	198.82	233.2	219.1	236.0	239.5
jaw	195.0	198.89	234.8	229.8	238.8	239.89
bone	170.1	198.5	—	213.1	238.0	239.2
carcinoma	143.9	—	—	—	—	—
lower	143.1	—	—	—	—	—
upper	143.0	—	—	—	—	—
lower	170.1	198.5	—	213.1	238.0	239.2
upper	170.0	198.5	—	213.0	238.0	239.2
carcinoma (any type) (lower) (upper)	195.0	—	—	—	—	—
skin (*see also* Neoplasm, skin, face)	173.30	198.2	232.3	216.3	238.2	239.2
soft tissues	143.9	198.89	230.0	210.4	235.1	239.0
lower	143.1	198.89	230.0	210.4	235.1	239.0
upper	143.0	198.89	230.0	210.4	235.1	239.0
jejunum	152.1	197.4	230.7	211.2	235.2	239.0
joint NEC (*see also* Neoplasm, bone)	170.9	198.5	—	213.9	238.0	239.2
acromioclavicular	170.4	198.5	—	213.4	238.0	239.2
bursa or synovial membrane - *see* Neoplasm, connective tissue						
costovertebral	170.3	198.5	—	213.3	238.0	239.2
sternocostal	170.3	198.5	—	213.3	238.0	239.2
temporomandibular	170.1	198.5	—	213.1	238.0	239.2
junction						
anorectal	154.8	197.5	230.7	211.4	235.5	239.0
cardioesophageal	151.0	197.8	230.2	211.1	235.2	239.0
esophagogastric	151.0	197.8	230.2	211.1	235.2	239.0
gastroesophageal	151.0	197.8	230.2	211.1	235.2	239.0
hard and soft palate	145.5	198.89	230.0	210.4	235.1	239.0
ileocecal	153.4	197.5	230.3	211.3	235.2	239.0
pelvirectal	154.0	197.5	230.4	211.4	235.2	239.0
pelviureteric	189.1	198.0	233.9	223.1	236.91	239.5
rectosigmoid	154.0	197.5	230.4	211.4	235.2	239.0
squamocolumnar, of cervix	180.8	198.82	233.1	219.0	236.0	239.5
kidney (parenchymal)	189.0	198.0	233.9	223.0	236.91	239.5
calyx	189.1	198.0	233.9	223.1	236.91	239.5
hilus	189.1	198.0	233.9	223.1	236.91	239.5
pelvis	189.1	198.0	233.9	223.1	236.91	239.5
knee NEC*	195.5	198.89	232.7	229.8	238.8	239.89

◀ New   ◀ Revised   ~~deleted~~ Deleted   ● Use Additional Digit(s)   ▨ Omit code

	Malignant			Benign	Uncertain Behavior	Unspecified
	Primary	Secondary	Ca in situ			
Neoplasm *(Continued)*						
labia (skin)	184.4	198.82	233.32	221.2	236.3	239.5
majora	184.1	198.82	233.32	221.2	236.3	239.5
minora	184.2	198.82	233.32	221.2	236.3	239.5
labial - *see also* Neoplasm, lip sulcus (lower) (upper)	145.1	198.89	230.0	210.4	235.1	239.0
labium (skin)	184.4	198.82	233.32	221.2	236.3	239.5
majus	184.1	198.82	233.32	221.2	236.3	239.5
minus	184.2	198.82	233.32	221.2	236.3	239.5
lacrimal						
canaliculi	190.7	198.4	234.0	224.7	238.8	239.89
duct (nasal)	190.7	198.4	234.0	224.7	238.8	239.89
gland	190.2	198.4	234.0	224.2	238.8	239.89
punctum	190.7	198.4	234.0	224.7	238.8	239.89
sac	190.7	198.4	234.0	224.7	238.8	239.89
Langerhans, islands or islets	157.4	197.8	230.9	211.7	235.5	239.0
laryngopharynx	148.9	198.89	230.0	210.8	235.1	239.0
larynx, laryngeal NEC	161.9	197.3	231.0	212.1	235.6	239.1
aryepiglottic fold	161.1	197.3	231.0	212.1	235.6	239.1
cartilage (arytenoid) (cricoid) (cuneiform) (thyroid)	161.3	197.3	231.0	212.1	235.6	239.1
commissure (anterior) (posterior)	161.0	197.3	231.0	212.1	235.6	239.1
contiguous sites	161.8	—	—	—	—	—
extrinsic NEC	161.1	197.3	231.0	212.1	235.6	239.1
meaning hypopharynx	148.9	198.89	230.0	210.8	235.1	239.0
interarytenoid fold	161.1	197.3	231.0	212.1	235.6	239.1
intrinsic	161.0	197.3	231.0	212.1	235.6	239.1
ventricular band	161.1	197.3	231.0	212.1	235.6	239.1
leg NEC*	195.5	198.89	232.7	229.8	238.8	239.89
lens, crystalline	190.0	198.4	234.0	224.0	238.8	239.89
lid (lower) (upper)	173.10	198.2	232.1	216.1	238.2	239.2
basal cell carcinoma	173.11	—	—	—	—	—
specified type NEC	173.19	—	—	—	—	—
squamous cell carcinoma	173.12	—	—	—	—	—
ligament - *see also* Neoplasm, connective tissue						
broad	183.3	198.82	233.39	221.0	236.3	239.5
Mackenrodt's	183.8	198.82	233.39	221.8	236.3	239.5
non-uterine - *see* Neoplasm, connective tissue						
round	183.5	198.82	—	221.0	236.3	239.5
sacro-uterine	183.4	198.82	—	221.0	236.3	239.5
uterine	183.4	198.82	—	221.0	236.3	239.5
utero-ovarian	183.8	198.82	233.39	221.8	236.3	239.5
uterosacral	183.4	198.82	—	221.0	236.3	239.5

◄ New   ◀||| Revised   ~~deleted~~ Deleted   ● Use Additional Digit(s)   ▨ Omit code

	Malignant					
	Primary	Secondary	Ca in situ	Benign	Uncertain Behavior	Unspecified
Neoplasm *(Continued)*						
limb*	195.8	198.89	232.8	229.8	238.8	239.89
lower*	195.5	198.89	232.7	229.8	238.8	239.89
upper*	195.4	198.89	232.6	229.8	238.8	239.89
limbus of cornea	190.4	198.4	234.0	224.4	238.8	239.89
lingual NEC (*see also* Neoplasm, tongue)	141.9	198.89	230.0	210.1	235.1	239.0
lingula, lung	162.3	197.0	231.2	212.3	235.7	239.1
lip (external) (lipstick area) (vermillion border)	140.9	198.89	230.0	210.0	235.1	239.0
buccal aspect - *see* Neoplasm, lip, internal						
commissure	140.6	198.89	230.0	210.4	235.1	239.0
contiguous sites	140.8	—	—	—	—	—
with oral cavity or pharynx	149.8	—	—	—	—	—
frenulum - *see* Neoplasm, lip, internal						
inner aspect - *see* Neoplasm, lip, internal						
internal (buccal) (frenulum) (mucosa) (oral)	140.5	198.89	230.0	210.0	235.1	239.0
lower	140.4	198.89	230.0	210.0	235.1	239.0
upper	140.3	198.89	230.0	210.0	235.1	239.0
lower	140.1	198.89	230.0	210.0	235.1	239.0
internal (buccal) (frenulum) (mucosa) (oral)	140.4	198.89	230.0	210.0	235.1	239.0
mucosa - *see* Neoplasm, lip, internal						
oral aspect - *see* Neoplasm, lip, internal						
skin (commissure) (lower) (upper)	173.00	198.2	232.0	216.0	238.2	239.2
basal cell carcinoma	173.01	—	—	—	—	—
specified type NEC	173.09	—	—	—	—	—
squamous cell carcinoma	173.02	—	—	—	—	—
upper	140.0	198.89	230.0	210.0	235.1	239.0
internal (buccal) (frenulum) (mucosa) (oral)	140.3	198.89	230.0	210.0	235.1	239.0
liver	155.2	197.7	230.8	211.5	235.3	239.0
primary	155.0	—	—	—	—	—
lobe						
azygos	162.3	197.0	231.2	212.3	235.7	239.1
frontal	191.1	198.3	—	225.0	237.5	239.6
lower	162.5	197.0	231.2	212.3	235.7	239.1
middle	162.4	197.0	231.2	212.3	235.7	239.1
occipital	191.4	198.3	—	225.0	237.5	239.6
parietal	191.3	198.3	—	225.0	237.5	239.6
temporal	191.2	198.3	—	225.0	237.5	239.6
upper	162.3	197.0	231.2	212.3	235.7	239.1
lumbosacral plexus	171.6	198.4	—	215.6	238.1	239.2

◀ New   ◀ Revised   ~~deleted~~ Deleted   ● Use Additional Digit(s)   Omit code

	Malignant					
	Primary	Secondary	Ca in situ	Benign	Uncertain Behavior	Unspecified
Neoplasm *(Continued)*						
lung	162.9	197.0	231.2	212.3	235.7	239.1
azygos lobe	162.3	197.0	231.2	212.3	235.7	239.1
carina	162.2	197.0	231.2	212.3	235.7	239.1
contiguous sites with bronchus or trachea	162.8	—	—	—	—	—
hilus	162.2	197.0	231.2	212.3	235.7	239.1
lingula	162.3	197.0	231.2	212.3	235.7	239.1
lobe NEC	162.9	197.0	231.2	212.3	235.7	239.1
lower lobe	162.5	197.0	231.2	212.3	235.7	239.1
main bronchus	162.2	197.0	231.2	212.3	235.7	239.1
middle lobe	162.4	197.0	231.2	212.3	235.7	239.1
upper lobe	162.3	197.0	231.2	212.3	235.7	239.1
lymph, lymphatic						
channel NEC *(see also* Neoplasm, connective tissue)	171.9	198.89	—	215.9	238.1	239.2
gland (secondary)	—	196.9	—	229.0	238.8	239.89
abdominal	—	196.2	—	229.0	238.8	239.89
aortic	—	196.2	—	229.0	238.8	239.89
arm	—	196.3	—	229.0	238.8	239.89
auricular (anterior) (posterior)	—	196.0	—	229.0	238.8	239.89
axilla, axillary	—	196.3	—	229.0	238.8	239.89
brachial	—	196.3	—	229.0	238.8	239.89
bronchial	—	196.1	—	229.0	238.8	239.89
bronchopulmonary	—	196.1	—	229.0	238.8	239.89
celiac	—	196.2	—	229.0	238.8	239.89
cervical	—	196.0	—	229.0	238.8	239.89
cervicofacial	—	196.0	—	229.0	238.8	239.89
Cloquet	—	196.5	—	229.0	238.8	239.89
colic	—	196.2	—	229.0	238.8	239.89
common duct	—	196.2	—	229.0	238.8	239.89
cubital	—	196.3	—	229.0	238.8	239.89
diaphragmatic	—	196.1	—	229.0	238.8	239.89
epigastric, inferior	—	196.6	—	229.0	238.8	239.89
epitrochlear	—	196.3	—	229.0	238.8	239.89
esophageal	—	196.1	—	229.0	238.8	239.89
face	—	196.0	—	229.0	238.8	239.89
femoral	—	196.5	—	229.0	238.8	239.89
gastric	—	196.2	—	229.0	238.8	239.89
groin	—	196.5	—	229.0	238.8	239.89
head	—	196.0	—	229.0	238.8	239.89
hepatic	—	196.2	—	229.0	238.8	239.89
hilar (pulmonary)	—	196.1	—	229.0	238.8	239.89
splenic	—	196.2	—	229.0	238.8	239.89

N

◀ New ◀▥ Revised ~~deleted~~ Deleted ● Use Additional Digit(s) ▨ Omit code

	Malignant					
	Primary	Secondary	Ca in situ	Benign	Uncertain Behavior	Unspecified
Neoplasm *(Continued)*						
lymph, lymphatic *(Continued)*						
gland *(Continued)*						
hypogastric	—	196.6	—	229.0	238.8	239.89
ileocolic	—	196.2	—	229.0	238.8	239.89
iliac	—	196.6	—	229.0	238.8	239.89
infraclavicular	—	196.3	—	229.0	238.8	239.89
inguina, inguinal	—	196.5	—	229.0	238.8	239.89
innominate	—	196.1	—	229.0	238.8	239.89
intercostal	—	196.1	—	229.0	238.8	239.89
intestinal	—	196.2	—	229.0	238.8	239.89
intrabdominal	—	196.2	—	229.0	238.8	239.89
intrapelvic	—	196.6	—	229.0	238.8	239.89
intrathoracic	—	196.1	—	229.0	238.8	239.9
jugular	—	196.0	—	229.0	238.8	239.89
leg	—	196.5	—	229.0	238.8	239.89
limb						
lower	—	196.5	—	229.0	238.8	239.89
upper	—	196.3	—	229.0	238.8	239.89
lower limb	—	196.5	—	229.0	238.8	239.9
lumbar	—	196.2	—	229.0	238.8	239.89
mandibular	—	196.0	—	229.0	238.8	239.89
mediastinal	—	196.1	—	229.0	238.8	239.89
mesenteric (inferior) (superior)	—	196.2	—	229.0	238.8	239.89
midcolic	—	196.2	—	229.0	238.8	239.89
multiple sites in categories 196.0–196.6	—	196.8	—	229.0	238.8	239.89
neck	—	196.0	—	229.0	238.8	239.89
obturator	—	196.6	—	229.0	238.8	239.89
occipital	—	196.0	—	229.0	238.8	239.89
pancreatic	—	196.2	—	229.0	238.8	239.89
para-aortic	—	196.2	—	229.0	238.8	239.89
paracervical	—	196.6	—	229.0	238.8	239.89
parametrial	—	196.6	—	229.0	238.8	239.89
parasternal	—	196.1	—	229.0	238.8	239.89
parotid	—	196.0	—	229.0	238.8	239.89
pectoral	—	196.3	—	229.0	238.8	239.89
pelvic	—	196.6	—	229.0	238.8	239.89
peri-aortic	—	196.2	—	229.0	238.8	239.89
peripancreatic	—	196.2	—	229.0	238.8	239.89
popliteal	—	196.5	—	229.0	238.8	239.89
porta hepatis	—	196.2	—	229.0	238.8	239.89
portal	—	196.2	—	229.0	238.8	239.89

◀ New   ◀▥ Revised   ~~deleted~~ Deleted   ● Use Additional Digit(s)   ▨ Omit code

	Malignant					
	Primary	Secondary	Ca in situ	Benign	Uncertain Behavior	Unspecified
Neoplasm *(Continued)*						
lymph, lymphatic *(Continued)*						
gland *(Continued)*						
preauricular	—	196.0	—	229.0	238.8	239.89
prelaryngeal	—	196.0	—	229.0	238.8	239.89
presymphysial	—	196.6	—	229.0	238.8	239.89
pretracheal	—	196.0	—	229.0	238.8	239.89
primary (any site) NEC	202.9●	—	—	—	—	—
pulmonary (hiler)	—	196.1	—	229.0	238.8	239.89
pyloric	—	196.2	—	229.0	238.8	239.89
retroperitoneal	—	196.2	—	229.0	238.8	239.89
retropharyngeal	—	196.0	—	229.0	238.8	239.89
Rosenmüller's	—	196.5	—	229.0	238.8	239.89
sacral	—	196.6	—	229.0	238.8	239.89
scalene	—	196.0	—	229.0	238.8	239.89
site NEC	—	196.9	—	229.0	238.8	239.89
splenic (hilar)	—	196.2	—	229.0	238.8	239.89
subclavicular	—	196.3	—	229.0	238.8	239.89
subinguinal	—	196.5	—	229.0	238.8	239.89
sublingual	—	196.0	—	229.0	238.8	239.89
submandibular	—	196.0	—	229.0	238.8	239.89
submaxillary	—	196.0	—	229.0	238.8	239.89
submental	—	196.0	—	229.0	238.8	239.89
subscapular	—	196.3	—	229.0	238.8	239.89
supraclavicular	—	196.0	—	229.0	238.8	239.89
thoracic	—	196.1	—	229.0	238.8	239.89
tibial	—	196.5	—	229.0	238.8	239.89
tracheal		196.1	—	229.0	238.8	239.89
tracheobronchial	—	196.1	—	229.0	238.8	239.89
upper limb	—	196.3	—	229.0	238.8	239.89
Virchow's	—	196.0	—	229.0	238.8	239.89
node - *see also* Neoplasm, lymph gland	202.9●	—	—	—	—	—
primary NEC						
vessel (*see also* Neoplasm, connective tissue)	171.9	198.89	—	215.9	238.1	239.2
Mackenrodt's ligament	183.8	198.82	233.39	221.8	236.3	239.5
malar region - *see* Neoplasm, cheek	170.0	198.5	—	213.0	238.0	239.2
mammary gland - *see* Neoplasm, breast						
mandible	170.1	198.5	—	213.1	238.0	239.2
alveolar						
mucosa	143.1	198.89	230.0	210.4	235.1	239.0
ridge or process	170.1	198.5	—	213.1	238.0	239.2
carcinoma	143.1	—	—	—	—	—

	Malignant					
	Primary	Secondary	Ca in situ	Benign	Uncertain Behavior	Unspecified
Neoplasm *(Continued)*						
mandible *(Continued)*						
carcinoma	143.1	—	—	—	—	—
marrow (bone) NEC	202.9●	198.5	—	—	—	238.79
mastectomy site (skin)	173.50	198.2	—	—	—	—
basal cell carcinoma	173.51	—	—	—	—	—
specified as breast tissue	174.8	198.81	—	—	—	—
specified type NEC	173.59	—	—	—	—	—
squamous cell carcinoma	173.52	—	—	—	—	—
mastoid (air cells) (antrum) (cavity)	160.1	197.3	231.8	212.0	235.9	239.1
bone or process	170.0	198.5	—	213.0	238.0	239.2
maxilla, maxillary (superior)	170.0	198.5	—	213.0	238.0	239.2
alveolar						
mucosa	143.0	198.89	230.0	210.4	235.1	239.0
ridge or process	170.0	198.5	—	213.0	238.0	239.2
carcinoma	143.0	—	—	—	—	—
antrum	160.2	197.3	231.8	212.0	235.9	239.1
carcinoma	143.0	—	—	—	—	—
inferior - *see* Neoplasm, mandible						
sinus	160.2	197.3	231.8	212.0	235.9	239.1
meatus						
external (ear) (*see also* Neoplasm, skin, ear)	173.20	198.2	232.2	216.2	238.2	239.2
Meckel's diverticulum	152.3	197.4	230.7	211.2	235.2	239.0
mediastinum, mediastinal	164.9	197.1	—	212.5	235.8	239.89
anterior	164.2	197.1	—	212.5	235.8	239.89
contiguous sites with heart and thymus	164.8	—	—	—	—	—
posterior	164.3	197.1	—	212.5	235.8	239.89
medulla						
adrenal	194.0	198.7	234.8	227.0	237.2	239.7
oblongata	191.7	198.3	—	225.0	237.5	239.6
meibomian gland	173.10	198.2	232.1	216.1	238.2	239.2
basal cell carcinoma	173.11	—	—	—	—	—
specified type NEC	173.19	—	—	—	—	—
squamous cell carcinoma	173.12	—	—	—	—	—
melanoma - *see* Melanoma						
meninges (brain) (cerebral) (cranial) (intracranial)	192.1	198.4	—	225.2	237.6	239.7
spinal (cord)	192.3	198.4	—	225.4	237.6	239.7
meniscus, knee joint (lateral) (medial)	170.7	198.5	—	213.7	238.0	239.2
mesentery, mesenteric	158.8	197.6	—	211.8	235.4	239.0
mesoappendix	158.8	197.6	—	211.8	235.4	239.0
mesocolon	158.8	197.6	—	211.8	235.4	239.0
mesopharynx - *see* Neoplasm, oropharynx						

◀ New   ◀▐ Revised   ~~deleted~~ Deleted   ● Use Additional Digit(s)   Omit code

	Malignant					
	Primary	Secondary	Ca in situ	Benign	Uncertain Behavior	Unspecified
Neoplasm *(Continued)*						
mesosalpinx	183.3	198.82	233.39	221.0	236.3	239.5
mesovarium	183.3	198.82	233.39	221.0	236.3	239.5
metacarpus (any bone)	170.5	198.5	—	213.5	238.0	239.2
metastatic NEC - *see also* Neoplasm, by site, secondary	—	199.1	—	—	—	—
metatarsus (any bone)	170.8	198.5	—	213.8	238.0	239.2
midbrain	191.7	198.3	—	225.0	237.5	239.6
milk duct - *see* Neoplasm, breast						
mons						
pubis	184.4	198.82	233.32	221.2	236.3	239.5
veneris	184.4	198.82	233.32	221.2	236.3	239.5
motor tract	192.9	198.4	—	225.9	237.9	239.7
brain	191.9	198.3	—	225.0	237.5	239.6
spinal	192.2	198.3	—	225.3	237.5	239.7
mouth	145.9	198.89	230.0	210.4	235.1	239.0
contiguous sites	145.8	—	—	—	—	—
floor	144.9	198.89	230.0	210.3	235.1	239.0
anterior portion	144.0	198.89	230.0	210.3	235.1	239.0
contiguous sites	144.8	—	—	—	—	—
lateral portion	144.1	198.89	230.0	210.3	235.1	239.0
roof	145.5	198.89	230.0	210.4	235.1	239.0
specified part NEC	145.8	198.89	230.0	210.4	235.1	239.0
vestibule	145.1	198.89	230.0	210.4	235.1	239.0
mucosa						
alveolar (ridge or process)	143.9	198.89	230.0	210.4	235.1	239.0
lower	143.1	198.89	230.0	210.4	235.1	239.0
upper	143.0	198.89	230.0	210.4	235.1	239.0
buccal	145.0	198.89	230.0	210.4	235.1	239.0
cheek	145.0	198.89	230.0	210.4	235.1	239.0
lip - *see* Neoplasm, lip, internal						
nasal	160.0	197.3	231.8	212.0	235.9	239.1
oral	145.0	198.89	230.0	210.4	235.1	239.0
Müllerian duct						
female	184.8	198.82	233.39	221.8	236.3	239.5
male	187.8	198.82	233.6	222.8	236.6	239.5
multiple sites NEC	199.0	199.0	234.9	229.9	238.9	199.0
muscle - *see also* Neoplasm, connective tissue extraocular	190.1	198.4	234.0	224.1	238.8	239.89
myocardium	164.1	198.89	—	212.7	238.8	239.89
myometrium	182.0	198.82	233.2	219.1	236.0	239.5
myopericardium	164.1	198.89	—	212.7	238.8	239.89
nabothian gland (follicle)	180.0	198.82	233.1	219.0	236.0	239.5

◄ New   ◄⊪ Revised   ~~deleted~~ Deleted   ● Use Additional Digit(s)   ▨ Omit code

	Malignant					
	Primary	Secondary	Ca in situ	Benign	Uncertain Behavior	Unspecified
Neoplasm *(Continued)*						
nail	173.90	198.2	232.9	216.9	238.2	239.2
finger (*see also* Neoplasm, skin, limb, upper)	173.60	198.2	232.6	216.6	238.2	239.2
toe (*see also* Neoplasm, skin, limb, lower)	173.70	198.2	232.7	216.7	238.2	239.2
nares, naris (anterior) (posterior)	160.0	197.3	231.8	212.0	235.9	239.1
nasal - *see* Neoplasm, nose						
nasolabial groove (*see also* Neoplasm, skin, face)	173.30	198.2	232.3	216.3	238.2	239.2
nasolacrimal duct	190.7	198.4	234.0	224.7	238.8	239.89
nasopharynx, nasopharyngeal	147.9	198.89	230.0	210.7	235.1	239.0
contiguous sites	147.8	—	—	—	—	—
floor	147.3	198.89	230.0	210.7	235.1	239.0
roof	147.0	198.89	230.0	210.7	235.1	239.0
specified site NEC	147.8	198.89	230.0	210.7	235.1	239.0
wall	147.9	198.89	230.0	210.7	235.1	239.0
anterior	147.3	198.89	230.0	210.7	235.1	239.0
lateral	147.2	198.89	230.0	210.7	235.1	239.0
posterior	147.1	198.89	230.0	210.7	235.1	239.0
superior	147.0	198.89	230.0	210.7	235.1	239.0
nates (*see also* Neoplasm, skin, trunk)	173.50	198.2	232.5	216.5	238.2	239.2
neck NEC*	195.0	198.89	234.8	229.8	238.8	239.89
skin	173.40	198.2	232.4	216.4	238.2	239.2
basal cell carcinoma	173.41	—	—	—	—	—
specified type NEC	173.49	—	—	—	—	—
squamous cell carcinoma	173.42	—	—	—	—	—
nerve (autonomic) (ganglion) (parasympathetic) (peripheral) (sympathetic) - *see also* Neoplasm, connective tissue						
abducens	192.0	198.4	—	225.1	237.9	239.7
accessory (spinal)	192.0	198.4	—	225.1	237.9	239.7
acoustic	192.0	198.4	—	225.1	237.9	239.7
auditory	192.0	198.4	—	225.1	237.9	239.7
brachial	171.2	198.89	—	215.2	238.1	239.2
cranial (any)	192.0	198.4	—	225.1	237.9	239.7
facial	192.0	198.4	—	225.1	237.9	239.7
femoral	171.3	198.89	—	215.3	238.1	239.2
glossopharyngeal	192.0	198.4	—	225.1	237.9	239.7
hypoglossal	192.0	198.4	—	225.1	237.9	239.7
intercostal	171.4	198.89	—	215.4	238.1	239.2
lumbar	171.7	198.89	—	215.7	238.1	239.2
median	171.2	198.89	—	215.2	238.1	239.2
obturator	171.3	198.89	—	215.3	238.1	239.2
oculomotor	192.0	198.4	—	225.1	237.9	239.7
olfactory	192.0	198.4	—	225.1	237.9	239.7

◀ New ◀≡ Revised ~~deleted~~ Deleted ● Use Additional Digit(s) ▨ Omit code

| | Malignant | | | | | |
	Primary	Secondary	Ca in situ	Benign	Uncertain Behavior	Unspecified
Neoplasm *(Continued)*						
nerve *(Continued)*						
optic	192.0	198.4	—	225.1	237.9	239.7
peripheral NEC	171.9	198.89	—	215.9	238.1	239.2
radial	171.2	198.89	—	215.2	238.1	239.2
sacral	171.6	198.89	—	215.6	238.1	239.2
sciatic	171.3	198.89	—	215.3	238.1	239.2
spinal NEC	171.9	198.89	—	215.9	238.1	239.2
trigeminal	192.0	198.4	—	225.1	237.9	239.7
trochlear	192.0	198.4	—	225.1	237.9	239.7
ulnar	171.2	198.89	—	215.2	238.1	239.2
vagus	192.0	198.4	—	225.1	237.9	239.7
nervous system (central) NEC	192.9	198.4	—	225.9	237.9	239.7
autonomic NEC	171.9	198.89	—	215.9	238.1	239.2
brain - *see also* Neoplasm, brain membrane or meninges	192.1	198.4	—	225.2	237.6	239.7
contiguous sites	192.8	—	—	—	—	—
parasympathetic NEC	171.9	198.89	—	215.9	238.1	239.2
sympathetic NEC	171.9	198.89	—	215.9	238.1	239.2
nipple (female)	174.0	198.81	233.0	217	238.3	239.3
male	175.0	198.81	233.0	217	238.3	239.3
nose, nasal	195.0	198.89	234.8	229.8	238.8	239.89
ala (external) *(see also* Neoplasm, nose, skin)	173.30	198.2	232.3	216.3	238.2	239.2
bone	170.0	198.5	—	213.0	238.0	239.2
cartilage	160.0	197.3	231.8	212.0	235.9	239.1
cavity	160.0	197.3	231.8	212.0	235.9	239.1
contiguous sites with accessory sinuses or middle ear	160.8	—	—	—	—	—
choana	147.3	198.89	230.0	210.7	235.1	239.0
external (skin) *(see also* Neoplasm, nose, skin)	173.30	198.2	232.3	216.3	238.2	239.2
fossa	160.0	197.3	231.8	212.0	235.9	239.1
internal	160.0	197.3	231.8	212.0	235.9	239.1
mucosa	160.0	197.3	231.8	212.0	235.9	239.1
septum	160.0	197.3	231.8	212.0	235.9	239.1
posterior margin	147.3	198.89	230.0	210.7	235.1	239.0
sinus - *see* Neoplasm, sinus						
skin	173.30	198.2	232.3	216.3	238.2	239.2
basal cell carcinoma	173.31	—	—	—	—	—
specified type NEC	173.39	—	—	—	—	—
squamous cell carcinoma	173.32	—	—	—	—	—
turbinate (mucosa)	160.0	197.3	231.8	212.0	235.9	239.1
bone	170.0	198.5	—	213.0	238.0	239.2
vestibule	160.0	197.3	231.8	212.0	235.9	239.1
nostril	160.0	197.3	231.8	212.0	235.9	239.1

◀ New   ◀▥ Revised   ~~deleted~~ Deleted   ● Use Additional Digit(s)   ▨ Omit code

	Malignant					
	Primary	Secondary	Ca in situ	Benign	Uncertain Behavior	Unspecified
Neoplasm *(Continued)*						
nucleus pulposus	170.2	198.5	—	213.2	238.0	230.2
occipital						
bone	170.0	198.5	—	213.0	238.0	239.2
lobe or pole, brain	191.4	198.3	—	225.0	237.5	239.6
odontogenic - *see* Neoplasm, jaw bone						
oesophagus - *see* Neoplasm, esophagus						
olfactory nerve or bulb	192.0	198.4	—	225.1	237.9	239.7
olive (brain)	191.7	198.3	—	225.0	237.5	239.6
omentum	158.8	197.6	—	211.8	235.4	239.0
operculum (brain)	191.0	198.3	—	225.0	237.5	239.6
optic nerve, chiasm, or tract	192.0	198.4	—	225.1	237.9	239.7
oral (cavity)	145.9	198.89	230.0	210.4	235.1	239.0
contiguous sites with lip or pharynx	149.8	—	—	—	—	—
ill-defined	149.9	198.89	230.0	210.4	235.1	239.0
mucosa	145.9	198.89	230.0	210.4	235.1	239.0
orbit	190.1	198.4	234.0	224.1	238.8	239.89
bone	170.0	198.5	—	213.0	238.0	239.2
eye	190.1	198.4	234.0	224.1	238.8	239.89
soft parts	190.1	198.4	234.0	224.1	238.8	239.89
organ of Zuckerkandl	194.6	198.89	—	227.6	237.3	239.7
oropharynx	146.9	198.89	230.0	210.6	235.1	239.0
branchial cleft (vestige)	146.8	198.89	230.0	210.6	235.1	239.0
contiguous sites	146.8	—	—	—	—	—
junctional region	146.5	198.89	230.0	210.6	235.1	239.0
lateral wall	146.6	198.89	230.0	210.6	235.1	239.0
pillars of fauces	146.2	198.89	230.0	210.6	235.1	239.0
posterior wall	146.7	198.89	230.0	210.6	235.1	239.0
specified part NEC	146.8	198.89	230.0	210.6	235.1	239.0
vallecula	146.3	198.89	230.0	210.6	235.1	239.0
os						
external	180.1	198.82	233.1	219.0	236.0	239.5
internal	180.0	198.82	233.1	219.0	236.0	239.5
ovary	183.0	198.6	233.39	220	236.2	239.5
oviduct	183.2	198.82	233.39	221.0	236.3	239.5
palate	145.5	198.89	230.0	210.4	235.1	239.0
hard	145.2	198.89	230.0	210.4	235.1	239.0
junction of hard and soft palate	145.5	198.89	230.0	210.4	235.1	239.0
soft	145.3	198.89	230.0	210.4	235.1	239.0
nasopharyngeal surface	147.3	198.89	230.0	210.7	235.1	239.0
posterior surface	147.3	198.89	230.0	210.7	235.1	239.0
superior surface	147.3	198.89	230.0	210.7	235.1	239.0

◀ New   ◀ Revised   ~~deleted~~ Deleted   ● Use Additional Digit(s)   Omit code

	Malignant					
	Primary	Secondary	Ca in situ	Benign	Uncertain Behavior	Unspecified
Neoplasm *(Continued)*						
palatoglossal arch	146.2	198.89	230.0	210.6	235.1	239.0
palatopharyngeal arch	146.2	198.89	230.0	210.6	235.1	239.0
pallium	191.0	198.3	—	225.0	237.5	239.6
palpebra	173.10	198.2	232.1	216.1	238.2	239.2
basal cell carcinoma	173.11	—	—	—	—	—
specified type NEC	173.19	—	—	—	—	—
squamous cell carcinoma	173.12	—	—	—	—	—
pancreas	157.9	197.8	230.9	211.6	235.5	239.0
body	157.1	197.8	230.9	211.6	235.5	239.0
contiguous sites	157.8	—	—	—	—	—
duct (of Santorini) (of Wirsung)	157.3	197.8	230.9	211.6	235.5	239.0
ectopic tissue	157.8	197.8				
head	157.0	197.8	230.9	211.6	235.5	239.0
islet cells	157.4	197.8	230.9	211.7	235.5	239.0
neck	157.8	197.8	230.9	211.6	235.5	239.0
tail	157.2	197.8	230.9	211.6	235.5	239.0
para-aortic body	194.6	198.89	—	227.6	237.3	239.7
paraganglion NEC	194.6	198.89	—	227.6	237.3	239.7
parametrium	183.4	198.82	—	221.0	236.3	239.5
paranephric	158.0	197.6	—	211.8	235.4	239.0
pararectal	195.3	198.89	—	229.8	238.8	239.89
parasagittal (region)	195.0	198.89	234.8	229.8	238.8	239.89
parasellar	192.9	198.4	—	225.9	237.9	239.7
parathyroid (gland)	194.1	198.89	234.8	227.1	237.4	239.7
paraurethral	195.3	198.89	—	229.8	238.8	239.89
gland	189.4	198.1	233.9	223.89	236.99	239.5
paravaginal	195.3	198.89	—	229.8	238.8	239.89
parenchyma, kidney	189.0	198.0	233.9	223.0	236.91	239.5
parietal						
bone	170.0	198.5	—	213.0	238.0	239.2
lobe, brain	191.3	198.3	—	225.0	237.5	239.6
paroophoron	183.3	198.82	233.39	221.0	236.3	239.5
parotid (duct) (gland)	142.0	198.89	230.0	210.2	235.0	239.0
parovarium	183.3	198.82	233.39	221.0	236.3	239.5
patella	170.8	198.5	—	213.8	238.0	239.2
peduncle, cerebral	191.7	198.3	—	225.0	237.5	239.6
pelvirectal junction	154.0	197.5	230.4	211.4	235.2	239.0
pelvis, pelvic	195.3	198.89	234.8	229.8	238.8	239.89
bone	170.6	198.5	—	213.6	238.0	239.2
floor	195.3	198.89	234.8	229.8	238.8	239.89
renal	189.1	198.0	233.9	223.1	236.91	239.5

	Malignant					
	Primary	Secondary	Ca in situ	Benign	Uncertain Behavior	Unspecified
Neoplasm *(Continued)*						
pelvis, pelvic *(Continued)*						
viscera	195.3	198.89	234.8	229.8	238.8	239.89
wall	195.3	198.89	234.8	229.8	238.8	239.89
pelvo-abdominal	195.8	198.89	234.8	229.8	238.8	239.89
penis	187.4	198.82	233.5	222.1	236.6	239.5
body	187.3	198.82	233.5	222.1	236.6	239.5
corpus (cavernosum)	187.3	198.82	233.5	222.1	236.6	239.5
glans	187.2	198.82	233.5	222.1	236.6	239.5
skin NEC	187.4	198.82	233.5	222.1	236.6	239.5
periadrenal (tissue)	158.0	197.6	—	211.8	235.4	239.0
perianal (skin) *(see also* Neoplasm, skin, anus)	173.50	198.2	232.5	216.5	238.2	239.2
pericardium	164.1	198.89	—	212.7	238.8	239.89
perinephric	158.0	197.6	—	211.8	235.4	239.0
perineum	195.3	198.89	234.8	229.8	238.8	239.89
periodontal tissue NEC	143.9	198.89	230.0	210.4	235.1	239.0
periosteum - *see* Neoplasm, bone						
peripancreatic	158.0	197.6	—	211.8	235.4	239.0
peripheral nerve NEC	171.9	198.89	—	215.9	238.1	239.2
perirectal (tissue)	195.3	198.89	—	229.8	238.8	239.89
perirenal (tissue)	158.0	197.6	—	211.8	235.4	239.0
peritoneum, peritoneal (cavity)	158.9	197.6	—	211.8	235.4	239.0
contiguous sites	158.8	—	—	—	—	—
with digestive organs	159.8	—	—	—	—	—
parietal	158.8	197.6	—	211.8	235.4	239.0
pelvic	158.8	197.6	—	211.8	235.4	239.0
specified part NEC	158.8	197.6	—	211.8	235.4	239.0
peritonsillar (tissue)	195.0	198.89	234.8	229.8	238.8	239.89
periurethral tissue	195.3	198.89	—	229.8	238.8	239.89
phalanges	170.9	198.5	—	213.9	238.0	239.2
foot	170.8	198.5	—	213.8	238.0	239.2
hand	170.5	198.5	—	213.5	238.0	239.2
pharynx, pharyngeal	149.0	198.89	230.0	210.9	235.1	239.0
bursa	147.1	198.89	230.0	210.7	235.1	239.0
fornix	147.3	198.89	230.0	210.7	235.1	239.0
recess	147.2	198.89	230.0	210.7	235.1	239.0
region	149.0	198.89	230.0	210.9	235.1	239.0
tonsil	147.1	198.89	230.0	210.7	235.1	239.0
wall (lateral) (posterior)	149.0	198.89	230.0	210.9	235.1	239.0
pia mater (cerebral) (cranial)	192.1	198.4	—	225.2	237.6	239.7
spinal	192.3	198.4	—	225.4	237.6	239.7

◀ New ◀ Revised ~~deleted~~ Deleted ● Use Additional Digit(s) ▨ Omit code

Neoplasm (Continued)	Malignant Primary	Malignant Secondary	Malignant Ca in situ	Benign	Uncertain Behavior	Unspecified
pillars of fauces	146.2	198.89	230.0	210.6	235.1	239.0
pineal (body) (gland)	194.4	198.89	234.8	227.4	237.1	239.7
pinna (ear) NEC (see also Neoplasm, skin, ear)	173.20	198.2	232.2	216.2	238.2	239.2
cartilage	171.0	198.89	—	215.0	238.1	239.2
piriform fossa or sinus	148.1	198.89	230.0	210.8	235.1	239.0
pituitary (body) (fossa) (gland) (lobe)	194.3	198.89	234.8	227.3	237.0	239.7
placenta	181	198.82	233.2	219.8	236.1	239.5
pleura, pleural (cavity)	163.9	197.2	—	212.4	235.8	239.1
contiguous sites	163.8	—	—	—	—	—
parietal	163.0	197.2	—	212.4	235.8	239.1
visceral	163.1	197.2	—	212.4	235.8	239.1
plexus						
brachial	171.2	198.89	—	215.2	238.1	239.2
cervical	171.0	198.89	—	215.0	238.1	239.2
choroid	191.5	198.3	—	225.0	237.5	239.6
lumbosacral	171.6	198.89	—	215.6	238.1	239.2
sacral	171.6	198.89	—	215.6	238.1	239.2
pluri-endocrine	194.8	198.89	234.8	227.8	237.4	239.7
pole						
frontal	191.1	198.3	—	225.0	237.5	239.6
occipital	191.4	198.3	—	225.0	237.5	239.6
pons (varolii)	191.7	198.3	—	225.0	237.5	239.6
popliteal fossa or space*	195.5	198.89	234.8	229.8	238.8	239.89
postcricoid (region)	148.0	198.89	230.0	210.8	235.1	239.0
posterior fossa (cranial)	191.9	198.3	—	225.0	237.5	239.6
postnasal space	147.9	198.89	230.0	210.7	235.1	239.0
prepuce	187.1	198.82	233.5	222.1	236.6	239.5
prepylorus	151.1	197.8	230.2	211.1	235.2	239.0
presacral (region)	195.3	198.89	—	229.8	238.8	239.89
prostate (gland)	185	198.82	233.4	222.2	236.5	239.5
utricle	189.3	198.1	233.9	223.81	236.99	239.5
pterygoid fossa	171.0	198.89	—	215.0	238.1	239.2
pubic bone	170.6	198.5	—	213.6	238.0	239.2
pudenda, pudendum (female)	184.4	198.82	233.32	221.2	236.3	239.5
pulmonary	162.9	197.0	231.2	212.3	235.7	239.1
putamen	191.0	198.3	—	225.0	237.5	239.6
pyloric						
antrum	151.2	197.8	230.2	211.1	235.2	239.0
canal	151.1	197.8	230.2	211.1	235.2	239.0
pylorus	151.1	197.8	230.2	211.1	235.2	239.0

Neoplasm (Continued)	Malignant					
	Primary	Secondary	Ca in situ	Benign	Uncertain Behavior	Unspecified
pyramid (brain)	191.7	198.3	—	225.0	237.5	239.6
pyriform fossa or sinus	148.1	198.89	230.0	210.8	235.1	239.0
radius (any part)	170.4	198.5	—	213.4	238.0	239.2
Rathke's pouch	194.3	198.89	234.8	227.3	237.0	239.7
rectosigmoid (colon) (junction)	154.0	197.5	230.4	211.4	235.2	239.0
contiguous sites with anus or rectum	154.8	—	—	—	—	—
rectouterine pouch	158.8	197.6	—	211.8	235.4	239.0
rectovaginal septum or wall	195.3	198.89	234.8	229.8	238.8	239.89
rectovesical septum	195.3	198.89	234.8	229.8	238.8	239.89
rectum (ampulla)	154.1	197.5	230.4	211.4	235.2	239.0
and colon	154.0	197.5	230.4	211.4	235.2	239.0
contiguous sites with anus or rectosigmoid junction	154.8	—	—	—	—	—
renal	189.0	198.0	233.9	223.0	236.91	239.5
calyx	189.1	198.0	233.9	223.1	236.91	239.5
hilus	189.1	198.0	233.9	223.1	236.91	239.5
parenchyma	189.0	198.0	233.9	223.0	236.91	239.5
pelvis	189.1	198.0	233.9	223.1	236.91	239.5
respiratory						
organs or system NEC	165.9	197.3	231.9	212.9	235.9	239.1
contiguous sites with intrathoracic organs	165.8	—	—	—	—	—
specified sites NEC	165.8	197.3	231.8	212.8	235.9	239.1
tract NEC	165.9	197.3	231.9	212.9	235.9	239.1
upper	165.0	197.3	231.9	212.9	235.9	239.1
retina	190.5	198.4	234.0	224.5	238.8	239.81
retrobulbar	190.1	198.4	—	224.1	238.8	239.89
retrocecal	158.0	197.6	—	211.8	235.4	239.0
retromolar (area) (triangle) (trigone)	145.6	198.89	230.0	210.4	235.1	239.0
retro-orbital	195.0	198.89	234.8	229.8	238.8	239.89
retroperitoneal (space) (tissue)	158.0	197.6	—	211.8	235.4	239.0
contiguous sites	158.8	—	—	—	—	—
retroperitoneum	158.0	197.6	—	211.8	235.4	239.0
contiguous sites	158.8	—	—	—	—	—
retropharyngeal	149.0	198.89	230.0	210.9	235.1	239.0
retrovesical (septum)	195.3	198.89	234.8	229.8	238.8	239.89
rhinencephalon	191.0	198.3	—	225.0	237.5	239.6
rib	170.3	198.5	—	213.3	238.0	239.2
Rosenmüller's fossa	147.2	198.89	230.0	210.7	235.1	239.0
round ligament	183.5	198.82	—	221.0	236.3	239.5
sacrococcyx, sacrococcygeal	170.6	198.5	—	213.6	238.0	239.2
region	195.3	198.89	234.8	229.8	238.8	239.89

◀ New   ◀ Revised   ~~deleted~~ Deleted   ● Use Additional Digit(s)   Omit code

	Malignant					
	Primary	Secondary	Ca in situ	Benign	Uncertain Behavior	Unspecified
Neoplasm *(Continued)*						
sacrouterine ligament	183.4	198.82	—	221.0	236.3	239.5
sacrum, sacral (vertebra)	170.6	198.5	—	213.6	238.0	239.2
salivary gland or duct (major)	142.9	198.89	230.0	210.2	235.0	239.0
contiguous sites	142.8	—	—	—	—	—
minor NEC	145.9	198.89	230.0	210.4	235.1	239.0
parotid	142.0	198.89	230.0	210.2	235.0	239.0
pluriglandular	142.8	198.89	230.0	210.2	235.0	239.0
sublingual	142.2	198.89	230.0	210.2	235.0	239.0
submandibular	142.1	198.89	230.0	210.2	235.0	239.0
submaxillary	142.1	198.89	230.0	210.2	235.0	239.0
salpinx (uterine)	183.2	198.82	233.39	221.0	236.3	239.5
Santorini's duct	157.3	197.8	230.9	211.6	235.5	239.0
scalp	173.40	198.2	232.4	216.4	238.2	239.2
basal cell carcinoma	173.41	—	—	—	—	—
specified type NEC	173.49	—	—	—	—	—
squamous cell carcinoma	173.42	—	—	—	—	—
scapula (any part)	170.4	198.5	—	213.4	238.0	239.2
scapular region	195.1	198.89	234.8	229.8	238.8	239.89
scar NEC (*see also* Neoplasm, skin)	173.90	198.2	232.9	216.9	238.2	239.2
sciatic nerve	171.3	198.89	—	215.3	238.1	239.2
sclera	190.0	198.4	234.0	224.0	238.8	239.89
scrotum (skin)	187.7	198.82	233.6	222.4	236.6	239.5
sebaceous gland - *see* Neoplasm, skin						
sella turcica	194.3	198.89	234.8	227.3	237.0	239.7
bone	170.0	198.5	—	213.0	238.0	239.2
semilunar cartilage (knee)	170.7	198.5	—	213.7	238.0	239.2
seminal vesicle	187.8	198.82	233.6	222.8	236.6	239.5
septum						
nasal	160.0	197.3	231.8	212.0	235.9	239.1
posterior margin	147.3	198.89	230.0	210.7	235.1	239.0
rectovaginal	195.3	198.89	234.8	229.8	238.8	239.89
rectovesical	195.3	198.89	234.8	229.8	238.8	239.89
urethrovaginal	184.9	198.82	233.39	221.9	236.3	239.5
vesicovaginal	184.9	198.82	233.39	221.9	236.3	239.5
shoulder NEC*	195.4	198.89	232.6	229.8	238.8	239.89
sigmoid flexure (lower) (upper)	153.3	197.5	230.3	211.3	235.2	239.0
sinus (accessory)	160.9	197.3	231.8	212.0	235.9	239.1
bone (any)	170.0	198.5	—	213.0	238.0	239.2
contiguous sites with middle ear or nasal cavities	160.8	—	—	—	—	—
ethmoidal	160.3	197.3	231.8	212.0	235.9	239.1

◀ New ◀ Revised ~~deleted~~ Deleted ● Use Additional Digit(s) ▨ Omit code

	Malignant					
	Primary	Secondary	Ca in situ	Benign	Uncertain Behavior	Unspecified
Neoplasm *(Continued)*						
sinus *(Continued)*						
frontal	160.4	197.3	231.8	212.0	235.9	239.1
maxillary	160.2	197.3	231.8	212.0	235.9	239.1
nasal, paranasal NEC	160.9	197.3	231.8	212.0	235.9	239.1
pyriform	148.1	198.89	230.0	210.8	235.1	239.0
sphenoidal	160.5	197.3	231.8	212.0	235.9	239.1
skeleton, skeletal NEC	170.9	198.5	—	213.9	238.0	239.2
Skene's gland	189.4	198.1	233.9	223.89	236.99	239.5
skin NOS	173.90	198.2	232.9	216.9	238.2	239.2
abdominal wall	173.50	198.2	232.5	216.5	238.2	239.2
basal cell carcinoma	173.51	—	—	—	—	—
specified type NEC	173.59	—	—	—	—	—
squamous cell carcinoma	173.52	—	—	—	—	—
ala nasi *(see also* Neoplasm, skin, face)	173.30	198.2	232.3	216.3	238.2	239.2
ankle *(see also* Neoplasm, skin, limb, lower)	173.70	198.2	232.7	216.7	238.2	239.2
antecubital space *(see also* Neoplasm, skin, limb, upper)	173.60	198.2	232.6	216.6	238.2	239.2
anus	173.50	198.2	232.5	216.5	238.2	239.2
basal cell carcinoma	173.51	—	—	—	—	—
specified type NEC	173.59	—	—	—	—	—
squamous cell carcinoma	173.52	—	—	—	—	—
arm *(see also* Neoplasm, skin, limb, upper)	173.60	198.2	232.6	216.6	238.2	239.2
auditory canal (external) *(see also* Neoplasm, skin, ear)	173.20	198.2	232.2	216.2	238.2	239.2
auricle (ear) *(see also* Neoplasm, skin, ear)	173.20	198.2	232.2	216.2	238.2	239.2
auricular canal (external) *(see also* Neoplasm, skin, ear)	173.20	198.2	232.2	216.2	238.2	239.2
axilla, axillary fold *(see also* Neoplasm, skin, trunk)	173.50	198.2	232.5	216.5	238.2	239.2
back	173.50	198.2	232.5	216.5	238.2	239.2
basal cell carcinoma	173.51	—	—	—	—	—
specified type NEC	173.59	—	—	—	—	—
squamous cell carcinoma	173.52	—	—	—	—	—
basal cell carcinoma, unspecified site	173.91	—	—	—	—	—
breast *(see also* Neoplasm, skin, trunk)	173.50	198.2	232.5	216.5	238.2	239.2
brow *(see also* Neoplasm, skin, face)	173.30	198.2	232.3	216.3	238.2	239.2
buttock *(see also* Neoplasm, skin, trunk)	173.50	198.2	232.5	216.5	238.2	239.2
calf *(see also* Neoplasm, skin, limb, lower)	173.70	198.2	232.7	216.7	238.2	239.2
canthus (eye) (inner) (outer)	173.10	198.2	232.1	216.1	238.2	239.2
basal cell carcinoma	173.11	—	—	—	—	—
specified type NEC	173.19	—	—	—	—	—
squamous cell carcinoma	173.12	—	—	—	—	—
cervical region *(see also* Neoplasm, skin, neck)	173.40	198.2	232.4	216.4	238.2	239.2
cheek (external) *(see also* Neoplasm, skin, face)	173.30	198.2	232.3	216.3	238.2	239.2
chest (wall) *(see also* Neoplasm, skin, trunk)	173.50	198.2	232.5	216.5	238.2	239.2

◀ New ◀⃫ Revised ~~deleted~~ Deleted ● Use Additional Digit(s) Omit code

	Malignant					
	Primary	Secondary	Ca in situ	Benign	Uncertain Behavior	Unspecified
Neoplasm *(Continued)*						
skin NOS *(Continued)*						
chin (*see also* Neoplasm, skin, face)	173.30	198.2	232.3	216.3	238.2	239.2
clavicular area (*see also* Neoplasm, skin, trunk)	173.50	198.2	232.5	216.5	238.2	239.2
clitoris	184.3	198.82	233.32	221.2	236.3	239.5
columnella (*see also* Neoplasm, skin, face)	173.30	198.2	232.3	216.3	238.2	239.2
concha (*see also* Neoplasm, skin, ear)	173.20	198.2	232.2	216.2	238.2	239.2
contiguous sites	173.80	—	—	—	—	—
basal cell carcinoma	173.81	—	—	—	—	—
specified type NEC	173.89	—	—	—	—	—
squamous cell carcinoma	173.82	—	—	—	—	—
ear (external)	173.20	198.2	232.2	216.2	238.2	239.2
basal cell carcinoma	173.21	—	—	—	—	—
specified type NEC	173.29	—	—	—	—	—
squamous cell carcinoma	173.22	—	—	—	—	—
elbow (*see also* Neoplasm, skin, limb, upper)	173.60	198.2	232.6	216.6	238.2	239.2
eyebrow (*see also* Neoplasm, skin, face)	173.30	198.2	232.3	216.3	238.2	239.2
eyelid	173.10	198.2	232.1	216.1	238.2	239.2
basal cell carcinoma	173.11	—	—	—	—	—
specified type NEC	173.19	—	—	—	—	—
squamous cell carcinoma	173.12	—	—	—	—	—
face NEC	173.30	198.2	232.3	216.3	238.2	239.2
basal cell carcinoma	173.31	—	—	—	—	—
specified type NEC	173.39	—	—	—	—	—
squamous cell carcinoma	173.32	—	—	—	—	—
female genital organs (external)	184.4	198.82	233.30	221.2	236.3	239.5
clitoris	184.3	198.82	233.32	221.2	236.3	239.5
labium NEC	184.4	198.82	233.32	221.2	236.3	239.5
majus	184.1	198.82	233.32	221.2	236.3	239.5
minus	184.2	198.82	233.32	221.2	236.3	239.5
pudendum	184.4	198.82	233.32	221.2	236.3	239.5
vulva	184.4	198.82	233.32	221.2	236.3	239.5
finger (*see also* Neoplasm, skin, limb, upper)	173.60	198.2	232.6	216.6	238.2	239.2
flank (*see also* Neoplasm, skin, trunk)	173.50	198.2	232.5	216.5	238.2	239.2
foot (*see also* Neoplasm, skin, limb, lower)	173.70	198.2	232.7	216.7	238.2	239.2
forearm (*see also* Neoplasm, skin, limb, upper)	173.60	198.2	232.6	216.6	238.2	239.2
forehead (*see also* Neoplasm, skin, face)	173.30	198.2	232.3	216.3	238.2	239.2
glabella (*see also* Neoplasm, skin, face)	173.30	198.2	232.3	216.3	238.2	239.2
gluteal region (*see also* Neoplasm, skin, trunk)	173.50	198.2	232.5	216.5	238.2	239.2
groin (*see also* Neoplasm, skin, trunk)	173.50	198.2	232.5	216.5	238.2	239.2
hand (*see also* Neoplasm, skin, limb, upper)	173.60	198.2	232.6	216.6	238.2	239.2
head NEC (*see also* Neoplasm, skin, scalp)	173.40	198.2	232.4	216.4	238.2	239.2

◀ New   ◀▦ Revised   ~~deleted~~ Deleted   ● Use Additional Digit(s)   ▦ Omit code

| | Malignant | | | | | |
	Primary	Secondary	Ca in situ	Benign	Uncertain Behavior	Unspecified
Neoplasm *(Continued)*						
skin NOS *(Continued)*						
heel (*see also* Neoplasm, skin, limb, lower)	173.70	198.2	232.7	216.7	238.2	239.2
helix (*see also* Neoplasm, skin, ear)	173.20	198.2	232.2	216.2	238.2	239.2
hip	173.70	198.2	232.7	216.7	238.2	239.2
basal cell carcinoma	173.71	—	—	—	—	—
specified type NEC	173.79	—	—	—	—	—
squamous cell carcinoma	173.72	—	—	—	—	—
infraclavicular region (*see also* Neoplasm, skin, trunk)	173.50	198.2	232.5	216.5	238.2	239.2
inguinal region (*see also* Neoplasm, skin, trunk)	173.50	198.2	232.5	216.5	238.2	239.2
jaw (*see also* Neoplasm, skin, face)	173.30	198.2	232.3	216.3	238.2	239.2
knee (*see also* Neoplasm, skin, limb, lower)	173.70	198.2	232.7	216.7	238.2	239.2
labia						
majora	184.1	198.82	233.32	221.2	236.3	239.5
minora	184.2	198.82	233.32	221.2	236.3	239.5
leg (*see also* Neoplasm, skin, limb, lower)	173.70	198.2	232.7	216.7	238.2	239.2
lid (lower) (upper)	173.10	198.2	232.1	216.1	238.2	239.2
basal cell carcinoma	173.11	—	—	—	—	—
specified type NEC	173.19	—	—	—	—	—
squamous cell carcinoma	173.12	—	—	—	—	—
limb NEC	173.90	198.2	232.9	216.9	238.2	239.5
lower	173.70	198.2	232.7	216.7	238.2	239.2
basal cell carcinoma	173.71	—	—	—	—	—
specified type NEC	173.79	—	—	—	—	—
squamous cell carcinoma	173.72	—	—	—	—	—
upper	173.60	198.2	232.6	216.6	238.2	239.2
basal cell carcinoma	173.61	—	—	—	—	—
specified type NEC	173.69	—	—	—	—	—
squamous cell carcinoma	173.62	—	—	—	—	—
lip (lower) (upper)	173.00	198.2	232.0	216.0	238.2	239.2
basal cell carcinoma	173.01	—	—	—	—	—
specified type NEC	173.09	—	—	—	—	—
squamous cell carcinoma	173.02	—	—	—	—	—
male genital organs	187.9	198.82	233.6	222.9	236.6	239.5
penis	187.4	198.82	233.5	222.1	236.6	239.5
prepuce	187.1	198.82	233.5	222.1	236.6	239.5
scrotum	187.7	198.82	233.6	222.4	236.6	239.5
mastectomy site (*see also* Neoplasm, skin, trunk)	173.50	198.2	—	—	—	—
specified as breast tissue	174.8	198.81	—	—	—	—
meatus, acoustic (external) (*see also* Neoplasm, skin, ear)	173.20	198.2	232.2	216.2	238.2	239.2
nates (*see also* Neoplasm, skin, trunk)	173.50	198.2	232.5	216.5	238.2	239.2

◀ New ◀ Revised ~~deleted~~ Deleted ● Use Additional Digit(s) ▨ Omit code

	Malignant					
	Primary	Secondary	Ca in situ	Benign	Uncertain Behavior	Unspecified
Neoplasm *(Continued)*						
skin NOS *(Continued)*						
neck	173.40	198.2	232.4	216.4	238.2	239.2
basal cell carcinoma	173.41	—	—	—	—	—
specified type NEC	173.49	—	—	—	—	—
squamous cell carcinoma	173.42	—	—	—	—	—
nose (external) (*see also* Neoplasm, skin, face)	173.30	198.2	232.3	216.3	238.2	239.2
palm (*see also* Neoplasm, skin, limb, upper)	173.60	198.2	232.6	216.6	238.2	239.2
palpebra	173.10	198.2	232.1	216.1	238.2	239.2
basal cell carcinoma	173.11	—	—	—	—	—
specified type NEC	173.19	—	—	—	—	—
squamous cell carcinoma	173.12	—	—	—	—	—
penis NEC	187.4	198.82	233.5	222.1	236.6	239.5
perianal (*see also* Neoplasm, skin, anus)	173.50	198.2	232.5	216.5	238.2	239.2
perineum (*see also* Neoplasm, skin, anus)	173.50	198.2	232.5	216.5	238.2	239.2
pinna (*see also* Neoplasm, skin, ear)	173.20	198.2	232.2	216.2	238.2	239.2
plantar (*see also* Neoplasm, skin, limb, lower)	173.70	198.2	232.7	216.7	238.2	239.2
popliteal fossa or space (*see also* Neoplasm, skin, limb, lower)	173.70	198.2	232.7	216.7	238.2	239.2
prepuce	187.1	198.82	233.5	222.1	236.6	239.5
pubes (*see also* Neoplasm, skin, trunk)	173.50	198.2	232.5	216.5	238.2	239.2
sacrococcygeal region (*see also* Neoplasm, skin, trunk)	173.50	198.2	232.5	216.5	238.2	239.2
scalp	173.40	198.2	232.4	216.4	238.2	239.2
basal cell carcinoma	173.41	—	—	—	—	—
specified type NEC	173.49	—	—	—	—	—
squamous cell carcinoma	173.42	—	—	—	—	—
scapular region (*see also* Neoplasm, skin, trunk)	173.50	198.2	232.5	216.5	238.2	239.2
scrotum	187.7	198.82	233.6	222.4	236.6	239.5
shoulder	173.60	198.2	232.6	216.6	238.2	239.2
basal cell carcinoma	173.61	—	—	—	—	—
specified type NEC	173.69	—	—	—	—	—
squamous cell carcinoma	173.62	—	—	—	—	—
sole (foot) (*see also* Neoplasm, skin, limb, lower)	173.70	198.2	232.7	216.7	238.2	239.2
specified sites NEC	173.80	198.2	232.8	216.8	232.8	239.2
basal cell carcinoma	173.81	—	—	—	—	—
specified type NEC	173.89	—	—	—	—	—
squamous cell carcinoma	173.82	—	—	—	—	—
specified type NEC, unspecified site	173.99	—	—	—	—	—
squamous cell carcinoma, unspecified site	173.92	—	—	—	—	—
submammary fold (*see also* Neoplasm, skin, trunk)	173.50	198.2	232.5	216.5	238.2	239.2
supraclavicular region (*see also* Neoplasm, skin, neck)	173.40	198.2	232.4	216.4	238.2	239.2
temple (*see also* Neoplasm, skin, face)	173.30	198.2	232.3	216.3	238.2	239.2
thigh (*see also* Neoplasm, skin, limb, lower)	173.70	198.2	232.7	216.7	238.2	239.2

◀ New   ◀ Revised   ~~deleted~~ Deleted   ● Use Additional Digit(s)   ▨ Omit code

	Malignant					
	Primary	Secondary	Ca in situ	Benign	Uncertain Behavior	Unspecified
Neoplasm *(Continued)*						
skin NOS *(Continued)*						
thoracic wall (*see also* Neoplasm, skin, trunk)	173.50	198.2	232.5	216.5	238.2	239.2
thumb (*see also* Neoplasm, skin, limb, upper)	173.60	198.2	232.6	216.6	238.2	239.2
toe (*see also* Neoplasm, skin, limb, lower)	173.70	198.2	232.7	216.7	238.2	239.2
tragus (*see also* Neoplasm, skin, ear)	173.20	198.2	232.2	216.2	238.2	239.2
trunk	173.50	198.2	232.5	216.5	238.2	239.2
basal cell carcinoma	173.51	—	—	—	—	—
specified type NEC	173.59	—	—	—	—	—
squamous cell carcinoma	173.52	—	—	—	—	—
umbilicus (*see also* Neoplasm, skin, trunk)	173.50	198.2	232.5	216.5	238.2	239.2
vulva	184.4	198.82	233.32	221.2	236.3	239.5
wrist (*see also* Neoplasm, skin, limb, upper)	173.60	198.2	232.6	216.6	238.2	239.2
skull	170.0	198.5	—	213.0	238.0	239.2
soft parts or tissues - *see* Neoplasm, connective tissue						
specified site NEC	195.8	198.89	234.8	229.8	238.8	239.89
spermatic cord	187.6	198.82	233.6	222.8	236.6	239.5
sphenoid	160.5	197.3	231.8	212.0	235.9	239.1
bone	170.0	198.5	—	213.0	238.0	239.2
sinus	160.5	197.3	231.8	212.0	235.9	239.1
sphincter						
anal	154.2	197.5	230.5	211.4	235.5	239.0
of Oddi	156.1	197.8	230.8	211.5	235.3	239.0
spine, spinal (column)	170.2	198.5	—	213.2	238.0	239.2
bulb	191.7	198.3	—	225.0	237.5	239.6
coccyx	170.6	198.5	—	213.6	238.0	239.2
cord (cervical) (lumbar) (sacral) (thoracic)	192.2	198.3	—	225.3	237.5	239.7
dura mater	192.3	198.4	—	225.4	237.6	239.7
lumbosacral	170.2	198.5	—	213.2	238.0	239.2
membrane	192.3	198.4	—	225.4	237.6	239.7
meninges	192.3	198.4	—	225.4	237.6	239.7
nerve (root)	171.9	198.89	—	215.9	238.1	239.2
pia mater	192.3	198.4	—	225.4	237.6	239.7
root	171.9	198.89	—	215.9	238.1	239.2
sacrum	170.6	198.5	—	213.6	238.0	239.2
spleen, splenic NEC	159.1	197.8	230.9	211.9	235.5	239.0
flexure (colon)	153.7	197.5	230.3	211.3	235.2	239.0
stem, brain	191.7	198.3	—	225.0	237.5	239.6
Stensen's duct	142.0	198.89	230.0	210.2	235.0	239.0
sternum	170.3	198.5	—	213.3	238.0	239.2

◀ New ◀▥ Revised ~~deleted~~ Deleted ● Use Additional Digit(s) ▨ Omit code

	Malignant					
	Primary	Secondary	Ca in situ	Benign	Uncertain Behavior	Unspecified
Neoplasm *(Continued)*						
stomach	151.9	197.8	230.2	211.1	235.2	239.0
antrum (pyloric)	151.2	197.8	230.2	211.1	235.2	239.0
body	151.4	197.8	230.2	211.1	235.2	239.0
cardia	151.0	197.8	230.2	211.1	235.2	239.0
cardiac orifice	151.0	197.8	230.2	211.1	235.2	239.0
contiguous sites	151.8	—	—	—	—	—
corpus	151.4	197.8	230.2	211.1	235.2	239.0
fundus	151.3	197.8	230.2	211.1	235.2	239.0
greater curvature NEC	151.6	197.8	230.2	211.1	235.2	239.0
lesser curvature NEC	151.5	197.8	230.2	211.1	235.2	239.0
prepylorus	151.1	197.8	230.2	211.1	235.2	239.0
pylorus	151.1	197.8	230.2	211.1	235.2	239.0
wall NEC	151.9	197.8	230.2	211.1	235.2	239.0
anterior NEC	151.8	197.8	230.2	211.1	235.2	239.0
posterior NEC	151.8	197.8	230.2	211.1	235.2	239.0
stroma, endometrial	182.0	198.82	233.2	219.1	236.0	239.5
stump, cervical	180.8	198.82	233.1	219.0	236.0	239.5
subcutaneous (nodule) (tissue) NEC - *see* Neoplasm, connective tissue						
subdural	192.1	198.4	—	225.2	237.6	239.7
subglottis, subglottic	161.2	197.3	231.0	212.1	235.6	239.1
sublingual	144.9	198.89	230.0	210.3	235.1	239.0
gland or duct	142.2	198.89	230.0	210.2	235.0	239.0
submandibular gland	142.1	198.89	230.0	210.2	235.0	239.0
submaxillary gland or duct	142.1	198.89	230.0	210.2	235.0	239.0
submental	195.0	198.89	234.8	229.8	238.8	239.89
subpleural	162.9	197.0	—	212.3	235.7	239.1
substernal	164.2	197.1	—	212.5	235.8	239.89
sudoriferous, sudoriparous gland, site unspecified	173.90	198.2	232.9	216.9	238.2	239.2
specified site - *see* Neoplasm, skin						
supraclavicular region	195.0	198.89	234.8	229.8	238.8	239.89
supraglottis	161.1	197.3	231.0	212.1	235.6	239.1
suprarenal (capsule) (cortex) (gland) (medulla)	194.0	198.7	234.8	227.0	237.2	239.7
suprasellar (region)	191.9	198.3	—	225.0	237.5	239.6
sweat gland (apocrine) (eccrine), site unspecified	173.90	198.2	232.9	216.9	238.2	239.2
specified site - *see* Neoplasm, skin						
sympathetic nerve or nervous system NEC	171.9	198.89	—	215.9	238.1	239.2
symphysis pubis	170.6	198.5	—	213.6	238.0	239.2
synovial membrane - *see* Neoplasm, connective tissue						
tapetum, brain	191.8	198.3	—	225.0	237.5	239.6
tarsus (any bone)	170.8	198.5	—	213.8	238.0	239.2
temple (skin) (*see also* Neoplasm, skin, face)	173.30	198.2	232.3	216.3	238.2	239.2

◄ New   ⬚ Revised   ~~deleted~~ Deleted   ● Use Additional Digit(s)   ▨ Omit code

	Malignant					
	Primary	Secondary	Ca in situ	Benign	Uncertain Behavior	Unspecified
Neoplasm *(Continued)*						
temporal						
bone	170.0	198.5	—	213.0	238.0	239.2
lobe or pole	191.2	198.3	—	225.0	237.5	239.6
region	195.0	198.89	234.8	229.8	238.8	239.89
skin (*see also* Neoplasm, skin, face)	173.30	198.2	232.3	216.3	238.2	239.2
tendon (sheath) - *see* Neoplasm, connective tissue						
tentorium (cerebelli)	192.1	198.4	—	225.2	237.6	239.7
testis, testes (descended) (scrotal)	186.9	198.82	233.6	222.0	236.4	239.5
ectopic	186.0	198.82	233.6	222.0	236.4	239.5
retained	186.0	198.82	233.6	222.0	236.4	239.5
undescended	186.0	198.82	233.6	222.0	236.4	239.5
thalamus	191.0	198.3	—	225.0	237.5	239.6
thigh NEC*	195.5	198.89	234.8	229.8	238.8	239.89
thorax, thoracic (cavity) (organs NEC)	195.1	198.89	234.8	229.8	238.8	239.89
duct	171.4	198.89	—	215.4	238.1	239.2
wall NEC	195.1	198.89	234.8	229.8	238.8	239.89
throat	149.0	198.89	230.0	210.9	235.1	239.0
thumb NEC*	195.4	198.89	232.6	229.8	238.8	239.89
thymus (gland)	164.0	198.89	—	212.6	235.8	239.89
contiguous sites with heart and mediastinum	164.8	—	—	—	—	—
thyroglossal duct	193	198.89	234.8	226	237.4	239.7
thyroid (gland)	193	198.89	234.8	226	237.4	239.7
cartilage	161.3	197.3	231.0	212.1	235.6	239.1
tibia (any part)	170.7	198.5	—	213.7	238.0	239.2
toe NEC*	195.5	198.89	232.7	229.8	238.8	239.89
tongue	141.9	198.89	230.0	210.1	235.1	239.0
anterior (two-thirds) NEC	141.4	198.89	230.0	210.1	235.1	239.0
dorsal surface	141.1	198.89	230.0	210.1	235.1	239.0
ventral surface	141.3	198.89	230.0	210.1	235.1	239.0
base (dorsal surface)	141.0	198.89	230.0	210.1	235.1	239.0
border (lateral)	141.2	198.89	230.0	210.1	235.1	239.0
contiguous sites	141.8	—	—	—	—	—
dorsal surface NEC	141.1	198.89	230.0	210.1	235.1	239.0
fixed part NEC	141.0	198.89	230.0	210.1	235.1	239.0
foramen cecum	141.1	198.89	230.0	210.1	235.1	239.0
frenulum linguae	141.3	198.89	230.0	210.1	235.1	239.0
junctional zone	141.5	198.89	230.0	210.1	235.1	239.0
margin (lateral)	141.2	198.89	230.0	210.1	235.1	239.0
midline NEC	141.1	198.89	230.0	210.1	235.1	239.0
mobile part NEC	141.4	198.89	230.0	210.1	235.1	239.0
posterior (third)	141.0	198.89	230.0	210.1	235.1	239.0

◀ New   ◀▬ Revised   ~~deleted~~ Deleted   ● Use Additional Digit(s)   ▨ Omit code

	Malignant			Benign	Uncertain Behavior	Unspecified
	Primary	Secondary	Ca in situ	Benign	Uncertain Behavior	Unspecified
Neoplasm *(Continued)*						
tongue *(Continued)*						
root	141.0	198.89	230.0	210.1	235.1	239.0
surface (dorsal)	141.1	198.89	230.0	210.1	235.1	239.0
base	141.0	198.89	230.0	210.1	235.1	239.0
ventral	141.3	198.89	230.0	210.1	235.1	239.0
tip	141.2	198.89	230.0	210.1	235.1	239.0
tonsil	141.6	198.89	230.0	210.1	235.1	239.0
tonsil	146.0	198.89	230.0	210.5	235.1	239.0
fauces, faucial	146.0	198.89	230.0	210.5	235.1	239.0
lingual	141.6	198.89	230.0	210.1	235.1	239.0
palatine	146.0	198.89	230.0	210.5	235.1	239.0
pharyngeal	147.1	198.89	230.0	210.7	235.1	239.0
pillar (anterior) (posterior)	146.2	198.89	230.0	210.6	235.1	239.0
tonsillar fossa	146.1	198.89	230.0	210.6	235.1	239.0
tooth socket NEC	143.9	198.89	230.0	210.4	235.1	239.0
trachea (cartilage) (mucosa)	162.0	197.3	231.1	212.2	235.7	239.1
contiguous sites with bronchus or lung	162.8	—	—	—	—	—
tracheobronchial	162.8	197.3	231.1	212.2	235.7	239.1
contiguous sites with lung	162.8	—	—	—	—	—
tragus (*see also* Neoplasm, skin, ear)	173.20	198.2	232.2	216.2	238.2	239.2
trunk NEC*	195.8	198.89	232.5	229.8	238.8	239.89
tubo-ovarian	183.8	198.82	233.39	221.8	236.3	239.5
tunica vaginalis	187.8	198.82	233.6	222.8	236.6	239.5
turbinate (bone)	170.0	198.5	—	213.0	238.0	239.2
nasal	160.0	197.3	231.8	212.0	235.9	239.1
tympanic cavity	160.1	197.3	231.8	212.0	235.9	239.1
ulna (any part)	170.4	198.5	—	213.4	238.0	239.2
umbilicus, umbilical (*see also* Neoplasm, skin, trunk)	173.50	198.2	232.5	216.5	238.2	239.2
uncus, brain	191.2	198.3	—	225.0	237.5	239.6
unknown site or unspecified	199.1	199.1	234.9	229.9	238.9	239.9
urachus	188.7	198.1	233.7	223.3	236.7	239.4
ureter, ureteral	189.2	198.1	233.9	223.2	236.91	239.5
orifice (bladder)	188.6	198.1	233.7	223.3	236.7	239.4
ureter-bladder (junction)	188.6	198.1	233.7	223.3	236.7	239.4
urethra, urethral (gland)	189.3	198.1	233.9	223.81	236.99	239.5
orifice, internal	188.5	198.1	233.7	223.3	236.7	239.4
urethrovaginal (septum)	184.9	198.82	233.39	221.9	236.3	239.5
urinary organ or system NEC	189.9	198.1	233.9	223.9	236.99	239.5
bladder - *see* Neoplasm, bladder						
contiguous sites	189.8	—	—	—	—	—
specified sites NEC	189.8	198.1	233.9	223.89	236.99	239.5

	Malignant					
	Primary	Secondary	Ca in situ	Benign	Uncertain Behavior	Unspecified
Neoplasm *(Continued)*						
utero-ovarian	183.8	198.82	233.39	221.8	236.3	239.5
ligament	183.3	198.82	—	221.0	236.3	239.5
uterosacral ligament	183.4	198.82	—	221.0	236.3	239.5
uterus, uteri, uterine	179	198.82	233.2	219.9	236.0	239.5
adnexa NEC	183.9	198.82	233.39	221.8	236.3	239.5
contiguous sites	183.8	—	—	—	—	—
body	182.0	198.82	233.2	219.1	236.0	239.5
contiguous sites	182.8	—	—	—	—	—
cervix	180.9	198.82	233.1	219.0	236.0	239.5
cornu	182.0	198.82	233.2	219.1	236.0	239.5
corpus	182.0	198.82	233.2	219.1	236.0	239.5
endocervix (canal) (gland)	180.0	198.82	233.1	219.0	236.0	239.5
endometrium	182.0	198.82	233.2	219.1	236.0	239.5
exocervix	180.1	198.82	233.1	219.0	236.0	239.5
external os	180.1	198.82	233.1	219.0	236.0	239.5
fundus	182.0	198.82	233.2	219.1	236.0	239.5
internal os	180.0	198.82	233.1	219.0	236.0	239.5
isthmus	182.1	198.82	233.2	219.1	236.0	239.5
ligament	183.4	198.82	—	221.0	236.3	239.5
broad	183.3	198.82	233.39	221.0	236.3	239.5
round	183.5	198.82	—	221.0	236.3	239.5
lower segment	182.1	198.82	233.2	219.1	236.0	239.5
myometrium	182.0	198.82	233.2	219.1	236.0	239.5
squamocolumnar junction	180.8	198.82	233.1	219.0	236.0	239.5
tube	183.2	198.82	233.39	221.0	236.3	239.5
utricle, prostatic	189.3	198.1	233.9	223.81	236.99	239.5
uveal tract	190.0	198.4	234.0	224.0	238.8	239.89
uvula	145.4	198.89	230.0	210.4	235.1	239.0
vagina, vaginal (fornix) (vault) (wall)	184.0	198.82	233.31	221.1	236.3	239.5
vaginovesical	184.9	198.82	233.39	221.9	236.3	239.5
septum	184.9	198.82	233.39	221.9	236.3	239.5
vallecula (epiglottis)	146.3	198.89	230.0	210.6	235.1	239.0
vascular - *see* Neoplasm, connective tissue						
vas deferens	187.6	198.82	233.6	222.8	236.6	239.5
Vater's ampulla	156.2	197.8	230.8	211.5	235.3	239.0
vein, venous - *see* Neoplasm, connective tissue						
vena cava (abdominal) (inferior)	171.5	198.89	—	215.5	238.1	239.2
superior	171.4	198.89	—	215.4	238.1	239.2
ventricle (cerebral) (floor) (fourth) (lateral) (third)	191.5	198.3	—	225.0	237.5	239.6
cardiac (left) (right)	164.1	198.89	—	212.7	238.8	239.89

◀ New   ◀▥ Revised   ~~deleted~~ Deleted   ● Use Additional Digit(s)   ▨ Omit code

	Malignant					
	Primary	Secondary	Ca in situ	Benign	Uncertain Behavior	Unspecified
Neoplasm *(Continued)*						
ventricular band of larynx	161.1	197.3	231.0	212.1	235.6	239.1
ventriculus - *see* Neoplasm, stomach						
vermillion border - *see* Neoplasm, lip						
vermis, cerebellum	191.6	198.3	—	225.0	237.5	239.6
vertebra (column)	170.2	198.5	—	213.2	238.0	239.2
coccyx	170.6	198.5	—	213.6	238.0	239.2
sacrum	170.6	198.5	—	213.6	238.0	239.2
vesical - *see* Neoplasm, bladder						
vesicle, seminal	187.8	198.82	233.6	222.8	236.6	239.5
vesicocervical tissue	184.9	198.82	233.39	221.9	236.3	239.5
vesicorectal	195.3	198.89	234.8	229.8	238.8	239.89
vesicovaginal	184.9	198.82	233.39	221.9	236.3	239.5
septum	184.9	198.82	233.39	221.9	236.3	239.5
vessel (blood) - *see* Neoplasm, connective tissue						
vestibular gland, greater	184.1	198.82	233.32	221.2	236.3	239.5
vestibule						
mouth	145.1	198.89	230.0	210.4	235.1	239.0
nose	160.0	197.3	231.8	212.0	235.9	239.1
Virchow's gland	—	196.0	—	229.0	238.8	239.89
viscera NEC	195.8	198.89	234.8	229.8	238.8	239.89
vocal cords (true)	161.0	197.3	231.0	212.1	235.6	239.1
false	161.1	197.3	231.0	212.1	235.6	239.1
vomer	170.0	198.5	—	213.0	238.0	239.2
vulva	184.4	198.82	233.32	221.2	236.3	239.5
vulvovaginal gland	184.4	198.82	233.32	221.2	236.3	239.5
Waldeyer's ring	149.1	198.89	230.0	210.9	235.1	239.0
Wharton's duct	142.1	198.89	230.0	210.2	235.0	239.0
white matter (central) (cerebral)	191.0	198.3	—	225.0	237.5	239.6
windpipe	162.0	197.3	231.1	212.2	235.7	239.1
Wirsung's duct	157.3	197.8	230.9	211.6	235.5	239.0
wolffian (body) (duct)						
female	184.8	198.82	233.39	221.8	236.3	239.5
male	187.8	198.82	233.6	222.8	236.6	239.5
womb - *see* Neoplasm, uterus						
wrist NEC*	195.4	198.89	232.6	229.8	238.8	239.89
xiphoid process	170.3	198.5	—	213.3	238.0	239.2
Zuckerkandl's organ	194.6	198.89	—	227.6	237.3	239.7

N

◀ New　◀▦ Revised　~~deleted~~ Deleted　● Use Additional Digit(s)　▨ Omit code

Neovascularization
  choroid 362.16
  ciliary body 364.42
  cornea 370.60
    deep 370.63
    localized 370.61
  iris 364.42
  retina 362.16
  subretinal 362.16
Nephralgia 788.0
Nephritis, nephritic (albuminuric) (azotemic)
    (congenital) (degenerative) (diffuse)
    (disseminated) (epithelial) (familial)
    (focal) (granulomatous) (hemorrhagic)
    (infantile) (nonsuppurative, excretory)
    (uremic) 583.9
  with
    edema - see Nephrosis
    lesion of
      glomerulonephritis
        hypocomplementemic persistent
          583.2
            with nephrotic syndrome 581.2
            chronic 582.2
        lobular 583.2
          with nephrotic syndrome 581.2
          chronic 582.2
        membranoproliferative 583.2
          with nephrotic syndrome 581.2
          chronic 582.2
        membranous 583.1
          with nephrotic syndrome 581.1
          chronic 582.1
        mesangiocapillary 583.2
          with nephrotic syndrome 581.2
          chronic 582.2
        mixed membranous and
          proliferative 583.2
            with nephrotic syndrome 581.2
            chronic 582.2
        proliferative (diffuse) 583.0
          with nephrotic syndrome 581.0
          acute 580.0
          chronic 582.0
        rapidly progressive 583.4
          acute 580.4
          chronic 582.4
      interstitial nephritis (diffuse) (focal)
        583.89
          with nephrotic syndrome 581.89
          acute 580.89
          chronic 582.89
      necrotizing glomerulitis 583.4
        acute 580.4
        chronic 582.4
      renal necrosis 583.9
        cortical 583.6
        medullary 583.7
      specified pathology NEC 583.89
        with nephrotic syndrome 581.89
        acute 580.89
        chronic 582.89
    necrosis, renal 583.9
      cortical 583.6
      medullary (papillary) 583.7
    nephrotic syndrome (see also Nephrosis)
      581.9
    papillary necrosis 583.7
    specified pathology NEC 583.89
  acute 580.9
    extracapillary with epithelial crescents
      580.4
    hypertensive (see also Hypertension,
      kidney) 403.90
    necrotizing 580.4
    poststreptococcal 580.0
    proliferative (diffuse) 580.0
    rapidly progressive 580.4
    specified pathology NEC 580.89
  amyloid 277.39 [583.81]
    chronic 277.39 [582.81]

Nephritis, nephritic (Continued)
  arteriolar (see also Hypertension, kidney)
    403.90
  arteriosclerotic (see also Hypertension,
    kidney) 403.90
  ascending (see also Pyelitis) 590.80
  atrophic 582.9
  basement membrane NEC 583.89
    with pulmonary hemorrhage
      (Goodpasture's syndrome)
      446.21 [583.81]
  calculous, calculus 592.0
  cardiac (see also Hypertension, kidney)
    403.90
  cardiovascular (see also Hypertension,
    kidney) 403.90
  chronic 582.9
    arteriosclerotic (see also Hypertension,
      kidney) 403.90
    hypertensive (see also Hypertension,
      kidney) 403.90
  cirrhotic (see also Sclerosis, renal) 587
  complicating pregnancy, childbirth, or
    puerperium 646.2●
    with hypertension 642.1●
      affecting fetus or newborn 760.0
    affecting fetus or newborn 760.1
  croupous 580.9
  desquamative - see Nephrosis
  due to
    amyloidosis 277.39 [583.81]
      chronic 277.39 [582.81]
    arteriosclerosis (see also Hypertension,
      kidney) 403.90
    diabetes mellitus 250.4● [583.81]
      due to secondary diabetes 249.4●
        [583.81]
      with nephrotic syndrome 250.4●
        [581.81]
        due to secondary diabetes 249.4●
          [581.81]
    diphtheria 032.89 [580.81]
    gonococcal infection (acute) 098.19
      [583.81]
      chronic or duration of 2 months or
        over 098.39 [583.81]
    gout 274.10
    infectious hepatitis 070.9 [580.81]
    mumps 072.79 [580.81]
    specified kidney pathology NEC
      583.89
      acute 580.89
      chronic 582.89
    streptotrichosis 039.8 [583.81]
    subacute bacterial endocarditis 421.0
      [580.81]
    systemic lupus erythematosus 710.0
      [583.81]
      chronic 710.0 [582.81]
    typhoid fever 002.0 [580.81]
  endothelial 582.2
  end state (chronic) (terminal) NEC
    585.6
  epimembranous 581.1
  exudative 583.89
    with nephrotic syndrome 581.89
    acute 580.89
    chronic 582.89
  gonococcal (acute) 098.19 [583.81]
    chronic or duration of 2 months or over
      098.39 [583.81]
  gouty 274.10
  hereditary (Alport's syndrome) 759.89
  hydremic - see Nephrosis
  hypertensive (see also Hypertension, kidney)
    403.90
  hypocomplementemic persistent 583.2
    with nephrotic syndrome 581.2
    chronic 582.2
  immune complex NEC 583.89
  infective (see also Pyelitis) 590.80

Nephritis, nephritic (Continued)
  interstitial (diffuse) (focal) 583.89
    with nephrotic syndrome 581.89
    acute 580.89
    chronic 582.89
  latent or quiescent - see Nephritis, chronic
  lead 984.9
    specified type of lead - see Table of Drugs
      and Chemicals
  lobular 583.2
    with nephrotic syndrome 581.2
    chronic 582.2
  lupus 710.0 [583.81]
    acute 710.0 [580.81]
    chronic 710.0 [582.81]
  membranoproliferative 583.2
    with nephrotic syndrome 581.2
    chronic 582.2
  membranous 583.1
    with nephrotic syndrome 581.1
    chronic 582.1
  mesangiocapillary 583.2
    with nephrotic syndrome 581.2
    chronic 582.2
  minimal change 581.3
  mixed membranous and proliferative 583.2
    with nephrotic syndrome 581.2
    chronic 582.2
  necrotic, necrotizing 583.4
    acute 580.4
    chronic 582.4
  nephrotic - see Nephrosis
  old - see Nephritis, chronic
  parenchymatous 581.89
  polycystic 753.12
    adult type (APKD) 753.13
    autosomal dominant 753.13
    autosomal recessive 753.14
    childhood type (CPKD) 753.14
    infantile type 753.14
  poststreptococcal 580.0
  pregnancy - see Nephritis, complicating
    pregnancy
  proliferative 583.0
    with nephrotic syndrome 581.0
    acute 580.0
    chronic 582.0
  purulent (see also Pyelitis) 590.80
  rapidly progressive 583.4
    acute 580.4
    chronic 582.4
  salt-losing or salt-wasting (see also Disease,
    renal) 593.9
  saturnine 584.9
    specified type of lead - see Table of Drugs
      and Chemicals
  septic (see also Pyelitis) 590.80
  specified pathology NEC 583.89
    acute 580.89
    chronic 582.89
  staphylococcal (see also Pyelitis) 590.80
  streptotrichosis 039.8 [583.81]
  subacute (see also Nephrosis) 581.9
  suppurative (see also Pyelitis) 590.80
  syphilitic (late) 095.4
    congenital 090.5 [583.81]
    early 091.69 [583.81]
  terminal (chronic) (end-stage) NEC 585.6
  toxic - see Nephritis, acute
  tubal, tubular - see Nephrosis, tubular
  tuberculous (see also Tuberculosis) 016.0●
    [583.81]
  type II (Ellis) - see Nephrosis
  vascular - see also Hypertension, kidney
  war 580.9
Nephroblastoma (M8960/3) 189.0
  epithelial (M8961/3) 189.0
  mesenchymal (M8962/3) 189.0
Nephrocalcinosis 275.49
Nephrocystitis, pustular (see also Pyelitis)
  590.80

◄ New   ◄▥ Revised   ~~deleted~~ Deleted   ● Use Additional Digit(s)   ▨ Omit code

Nephrolithiasis (congenital) (pelvis) (recurrent) 592.0
 uric acid 274.11
Nephroma (M8960/3) 189.0
 mesoblastic (M8960/1) 236.9
Nephronephritis (see also Nephrosis) 581.9
Nephronopthisis 753.16
Nephropathy (see also Nephritis) 583.9
 with
  exudative nephritis 583.89
  interstitial nephritis (diffuse) (focal) 583.89
  medullary necrosis 583.7
  necrosis 583.9
   cortical 583.6
   medullary or papillary 583.7
  papillary necrosis 583.7
  specified lesion or cause NEC 583.89
 analgesic 583.89
  with medullary necrosis, acute 584.7
 arteriolar (see also Hypertension, kidney) 403.90
 arteriosclerotic (see also Hypertension, kidney) 403.90
 complicating pregnancy 646.2●
 diabetic 250.4● [583.81]
  due to secondary diabetes 249.4● [583.81]
 gouty 274.10
  specified type NEC 274.19
 hereditary amyloid 277.31
 hypercalcemic 588.89
 hypertensive (see also Hypertension, kidney) 403.90
 hypokalemic (vacuolar) 588.89
 IgA 583.9
 obstructive 593.89
  congenital 753.20
 phenacetin 584.7
 phosphate-losing 588.0
 potassium depletion 588.89
 proliferative (see also Nephritis, proliferative) 583.0
 protein-losing 588.89
 salt-losing or salt-wasting (see also Disease, renal) 593.9
 sickle-cell (see also Disease, sickle-cell) 282.60 [583.81]
 toxic 584.5
 vasomotor 584.5
 water-losing 588.89
Nephroptosis (see also Disease, renal) 593.0
 congenital (displaced) 753.3
Nephropyosis (see also Abscess, kidney) 590.2
Nephrorrhagia 593.81
Nephrosclerosis (arteriolar) (arteriosclerotic) (chronic) (hyaline) (see also Hypertension, kidney) 403.90
 gouty 274.10
 hyperplastic (arteriolar) (see also Hypertension, kidney) 403.90
 senile (see also Sclerosis, renal) 587
Nephrosis, nephrotic (Epstein's) (syndrome) 581.9
 with
  lesion of
   focal glomerulosclerosis 581.1
   glomerulonephritis
    endothelial 581.2
    hypocomplementemic persistent 581.2
    lobular 581.2
    membranoproliferative 581.2
    membranous 581.1
    mesangiocapillary 581.2
    minimal change 581.3
    mixed membranous and proliferative 581.2
    proliferative 581.0
   segmental hyalinosis 581.1
   specified pathology NEC 581.89
 acute - see Nephrosis, tubular

Nephrosis, nephrotic (Continued)
 anoxic - see Nephrosis, tubular
 arteriosclerotic (see also Hypertension, kidney) 403.90
 chemical - see Nephrosis, tubular
 cholemic 572.4
 complicating pregnancy, childbirth, or puerperium - see Nephritis, complicating pregnancy
 diabetic 250.4● [581.81]
  due to secondary diabetes 249.4● [581.81]
 Finnish type (congenital) 759.89
 hemoglobinuric - see Nephrosis, tubular
 in
  amyloidosis 277.39 [581.81]
  diabetes mellitus 250.4● [581.81]
   due to secondary diabetes 249.4● [581.81]
  epidemic hemorrhagic fever 078.6
  malaria 084.9 [581.81]
  polyarteritis 446.0 [581.81]
  systemic lupus erythematosus 710.0 [581.81]
 ischemic - see Nephrosis, tubular
 lipoid 581.3
 lower nephron - see Nephrosis, tubular
 lupoid 710.0 [581.81]
 lupus 710.0 [581.81]
 malarial 084.9 [581.81]
 minimal change 581.3
 necrotizing - see Nephrosis, tubular
 osmotic (sucrose) 588.89
 polyarteritic 446.0 [581.81]
 radiation 581.9
 specified lesion or cause NEC 581.89
 syphilitic 095.4
 toxic - see Nephrosis, tubular
 tubular (acute) 584.5
  due to a procedure 997.5
  radiation 581.9
Nephrosonephritis hemorrhagic (endemic) 078.6
Nephrostomy status V44.6
 with complication 997.5
Nerve - see condition
Nerves 799.21
Nervous (see also condition) 799.21
 breakdown 300.9
 heart 306.2
 stomach 306.4
 tension 799.21
Nervousness 799.21
Nesidioblastoma (M8150/0)
 pancreas 211.7
 specified site NEC - see Neoplasm, by site, benign
 unspecified site 211.7
Netherton's syndrome (ichthyosiform erythroderma) 757.1
Nettle rash 708.8
Nettleship's disease (urticaria pigmentosa) 757.33
Neumann's disease (pemphigus vegetans) 694.4
Neuralgia, neuralgic (acute) (see also Neuritis) 729.2
 accessory (nerve) 352.4
 acoustic (nerve) 388.5
 ankle 355.8
 anterior crural 355.8
 anus 787.99
 arm 723.4
 auditory (nerve) 388.5
 axilla 353.0
 bladder 788.1
 brachial 723.4
 brain - see Disorder, nerve, cranial
 broad ligament 625.9
 cerebral - see Disorder, nerve, cranial
 ciliary 339.00

Neuralgia, neuralgic (Continued)
 cranial nerve - see also Disorder, nerve, cranial
  fifth or trigeminal (see also Neuralgia, trigeminal) 350.1
 ear 388.71
  middle 352.1
 facial 351.8
 finger 354.9
 flank 355.8
 foot 355.8
 forearm 354.9
 Fothergill's (see also Neuralgia, trigeminal) 350.1
  postherpetic 053.12
 glossopharyngeal (nerve) 352.1
 groin 355.8
 hand 354.9
 heel 355.8
 Horton's 339.00
 Hunt's 053.11
 hypoglossal (nerve) 352.5
 iliac region 355.8
 infraorbital (see also Neuralgia, trigeminal) 350.1
 inguinal 355.8
 intercostal (nerve) 353.8
  postherpetic 053.19
 jaw 352.1
 kidney 788.0
 knee 355.8
 loin 355.8
 malarial (see also Malaria) 084.6
 mastoid 385.89
 maxilla 352.1
 median thenar 354.1
 metatarsal 355.6
 middle ear 352.1
 migrainous 339.00
 Morton's 355.6
 nerve, cranial - see Disorder, nerve, cranial
 nose 352.0
 occipital 723.8
 olfactory (nerve) 352.0
 ophthalmic 377.30
  postherpetic 053.19
 optic (nerve) 377.30
 penis 607.9
 perineum 355.8
 pleura 511.0
 postherpetic NEC 053.19
  geniculate ganglion 053.11
  ophthalmic 053.19
  trifacial 053.12
  trigeminal 053.12
 pubic region 355.8
 radial (nerve) 723.4
 rectum 787.99
 sacroiliac joint 724.3
 sciatic (nerve) 724.3
 scrotum 608.9
 seminal vesicle 608.9
 shoulder 354.9
 sluder's 337.09
 specified nerve NEC - see Disorder, nerve
 spermatic cord 608.9
 sphenopalatine (ganglion) 337.09
 subscapular (nerve) 723.4
 suprascapular (nerve) 723.4
 testis 608.89
 thenar (median) 354.1
 thigh 355.8
 tongue 352.5
 trifacial (nerve) (see also Neuralgia, trigeminal) 350.1
 trigeminal (nerve) 350.1
  postherpetic 053.12
 tympanic plexus 388.71
 ulnar (nerve) 723.4
 vagus (nerve) 352.3

Neuralgia, neuralgic (Continued)
  wrist 354.9
  writers' 300.89
    organic 333.84
Neurapraxia - see Injury, nerve, by site
Neurasthenia 300.5
  cardiac 306.2
  gastric 306.4
  heart 306.2
  postfebrile 780.79
  postviral 780.79
Neurilemmoma (M9560/0) - see also Neoplasm,
    connective tissue, benign
  acoustic (nerve) 225.1
  malignant (M9560/3) - see also Neoplasm,
    connective tissue, malignant
    acoustic (nerve) 192.0
Neurilemmosarcoma (M9560/3) - see
  Neoplasm, connective tissue, malignant
Neurilemoma - see Neurilemmoma
Neurinoma (M9560/0) - see Neurilemmoma
Neurinomatosis (M9560/1) - see also Neoplasm,
    connective tissue, uncertain behavior
  centralis 759.5
Neuritis (see also Neuralgia) 729.2
  abducens (nerve) 378.54
  accessory (nerve) 352.4
  acoustic (nerve) 388.5
    syphilitic 094.86
  alcoholic 357.5
    with psychosis 291.1
  amyloid, any site 277.39 [357.4]
  anterior crural 355.8
  arising during pregnancy 646.4●
  arm 723.4
  ascending 355.2
  auditory (nerve) 388.5
  brachial (nerve) NEC 723.4
    due to displacement, intervertebral disc
      722.0
  cervical 723.4
  chest (wall) 353.8
  costal region 353.8
  cranial nerve - see also Disorder, nerve,
    cranial
    first or olfactory 352.0
    second or optic 377.30
    third or oculomotor 378.52
    fourth or trochlear 378.53
    fifth or trigeminal (see also Neuralgia,
      trigeminal) 350.1
    sixth or abducens 378.54
    seventh or facial 351.8
      newborn 767.5
    eighth or acoustic 388.5
    ninth or glossopharyngeal 352.1
    tenth or vagus 352.3
    eleventh or accessory 352.4
    twelfth or hypoglossal 352.5
  Déjérine-Sottas 356.0
  diabetic 250.6● [357.2]
    due to secondary diabetes 249.6● [357.2]
  diphtheritic 032.89 [357.4]
  due to
    beriberi 265.0 [357.4]
    displacement, prolapse, protrusion, or
      rupture of intervertebral disc 722.2
      cervical 722.0
      lumbar, lumbosacral 722.10
      thoracic, thoracolumbar 722.11
    herniation, nucleus pulposus 722.2
      cervical 722.0
      lumbar, lumbosacral 722.10
      thoracic, thoracolumbar 722.11
  endemic 265.0 [357.4]
  facial (nerve) 351.8
    newborn 767.5
  general - see Polyneuropathy
  geniculate ganglion 351.1
    due to herpes 053.11
  glossopharyngeal (nerve) 352.1

Neuritis (Continued)
  gouty 274.89 [357.4]
  hypoglossal (nerve) 352.5
  ilioinguinal (nerve) 355.8
  in diseases classified elsewhere - see
    Polyneuropathy, in
  infectious (multiple) 357.0
  intercostal (nerve) 353.8
  interstitial hypertrophic progressive NEC
    356.9
  leg 355.8
  lumbosacral NEC 724.4
  median (nerve) 354.1
    thenar 354.1
  multiple (acute) (infective) 356.9
    endemic 265.0 [357.4]
  multiplex endemica 265.0 [357.4]
  nerve root (see also Radiculitis) 729.2
  oculomotor (nerve) 378.52
  olfactory (nerve) 352.0
  optic 377.30
    in myelitis 341.0
    meningococcal 036.81
  pelvic 355.8
  peripheral (nerve) - see also Neuropathy,
    peripheral
    complicating pregnancy or puerperium
      646.4●
    specified nerve NEC - see Mononeuritis
  pneumogastric (nerve) 352.3
  postchickenpox 052.7
  postherpetic 053.19
  progressive hypertrophic interstitial NEC
    356.9
  puerperal, postpartum 646.4●
  radial (nerve) 723.4
  retrobulbar 377.32
    syphilitic 094.85
  rheumatic (chronic) 729.2
  sacral region 355.8
  sciatic (nerve) 724.3
    due to displacement of intervertebral disc
      722.10
  serum 999.59
  specified nerve NEC - see Disorder, nerve
  spinal (nerve) 355.9
    root (see also Radiculitis) 729.2
  subscapular (nerve) 723.4
  suprascapular (nerve) 723.4
  syphilitic 095.8
  thenar (median) 354.1
  thoracic NEC 724.4
  toxic NEC 357.7
  trochlear (nerve) 378.53
  ulnar (nerve) 723.4
  vagus (nerve) 352.3
Neuroangiomatosis, encephalofacial
  759.6
Neuroastrocytoma (M9505/1) - see Neoplasm,
  by site, uncertain behavior
Neuro-avitaminosis 269.2
Neuroblastoma (M9500/3)
  olfactory (M9522/3) 160.0
  specified site - see Neoplasm, by site,
    malignant
  unspecified site 194.0
Neurochorioretinitis (see also Chorioretinitis)
  363.20
Neurocirculatory asthenia 306.2
Neurocytoma (M9506/0) - see Neoplasm, by
  site, benign
Neurodermatitis (circumscribed)
    (circumscripta) (local) 698.3
  atopic 691.8
  diffuse (Brocq) 691.8
  disseminated 691.8
  nodulosa 698.3
Neuroencephalomyelopathy, optic
  341.0
Neuroendocrine tumor - see Tumor,
  neuroendocrine

Neuroepithelioma (M9503/3) - see also
  Neoplasm, by site, malignant
  olfactory (M9521/3) 160.0
Neurofibroma (M9540/0) - see also Neoplasm,
  connective tissue, benign
  melanotic (M9541/0) - see Neoplasm,
    connective tissue, benign
  multiple (M9540/1) 237.70
    type 1 237.71
    type 2 237.72
  plexiform (M9550/0) - see Neoplasm,
    connective tissue, benign
Neurofibromatosis (multiple) (M9540/1) 237.70
  acoustic 237.72
  malignant (M9540/3) - see Neoplasm,
    connective tissue, malignant
  Schwannomatosis 237.73
  specified type NEC 237.79
  type 1 237.71
  type 2 237.72
  von Recklinghausen's 237.71
Neurofibrosarcoma (M9540/3) - see Neoplasm,
  connective tissue, malignant
Neurogenic - see also condition
  bladder (atonic) (automatic) (autonomic)
    (flaccid) (hypertonic) (hypotonic)
    (inertia) (infranuclear) (irritable)
    (motor) (nonreflex) (nuclear)
    (paralysis) (reflex) (sensory) (spastic)
    (supranuclear) (uninhibited) 596.54
    with cauda equina syndrome 344.61
  bowel 564.81
  heart 306.2
Neuroglioma (M9505/1) - see Neoplasm, by
  site, uncertain behavior
Neurolabyrinthitis (of Dix and Hallpike) 386.12
Neurolathyrism 988.2
Neuroleprosy 030.1
Neuroleptic malignant syndrome 333.92
Neurolipomatosis 272.8
Neuroma (M9570/0) - see also Neoplasm,
  connective tissue, benign
  acoustic (nerve) (M9560/0) 225.1
  amputation (traumatic) - see also Injury,
    nerve, by site
    surgical complication (late) 997.61
  appendix 211.3
  auditory nerve 225.1
  digital 355.6
    toe 355.6
  interdigital (toe) 355.6
  intermetatarsal 355.6
  Morton's 355.6
  multiple 237.70
    type 1 237.71
    type 2 237.72
  nonneoplastic 355.9
    arm NEC 354.9
    leg NEC 355.8
    lower extremity NEC 355.8
    specified site NEC - see Mononeuritis, by
      site
    upper extremity NEC 354.9
  optic (nerve) 225.1
  plantar 355.6
  plexiform (M9550/0) - see Neoplasm,
    connective tissue, benign
  surgical (nonneoplastic) 355.9
    arm NEC 354.9
    leg NEC 355.8
    lower extremity NEC 355.8
    upper extremity NEC 354.9
  traumatic - see also Injury, nerve, by site
    old - see Neuroma, nonneoplastic
Neuromyalgia 729.1
Neuromyasthenia (epidemic) 049.8
Neuromyelitis 341.8
  ascending 357.0
  optica 341.0
Neuromyopathy NEC 358.9
Neuromyositis 729.1

Neuronevus (M8725/0) - *see* Neoplasm, skin, benign
Neuronitis 357.0
  ascending (acute) 355.2
  vestibular 386.12
Neuroparalytic - *see* condition
Neuropathy, neuropathic (*see also* Disorder, nerve) 355.9
  acute motor 357.82
  alcoholic 357.5
    with psychosis 291.1
  arm NEC 354.9
  ataxia and retinitis pigmentosa (NARP syndrome) 277.87
  autonomic (peripheral) - *see* Neuropathy, peripheral, autonomic
  axillary nerve 353.0
  brachial plexus 353.0
  cervical plexus 353.2
  chronic
    progressive segmentally demyelinating 357.89
    relapsing demyelinating 357.89
  congenital sensory 356.2
  Déjérine-Sottas 356.0
  diabetic 250.6● [*357.2*]
    autonomic (peripheral) 250.6 [*337.1*]
    due to secondary diabetes 249.6● [*357.2*]
      autonomic (peripheral) 249.6 [*337.1*]
  entrapment 355.9
    iliohypogastric nerve 355.79
    ilioinguinal nerve 355.79
    lateral cutaneous nerve of thigh 355.1
    median nerve 354.0
    obturator nerve 355.79
    peroneal nerve 355.3
    posterior tibial nerve 355.5
    saphenous nerve 355.79
    ulnar nerve 354.2
  facial nerve 351.9
  hereditary 356.9
    peripheral 356.0
    sensory (radicular) 356.2
  hypertrophic
    Charcôt-Marie-Tooth 356.1
    Déjérine-Sottas 356.0
    interstitial 356.9
    Refsum 356.3
  intercostal nerve 354.8
  ischemic - *see* Disorder, nerve
  Jamaican (ginger) 357.7
  leg NEC 355.8
  lower extremity NEC 355.8
  lumbar plexus 353.1
  median nerve 354.1
  motor
    acute 357.82
  multiple (acute) (chronic) (*see also* Polyneuropathy) 356.9
  optic 377.39
    ischemic 377.41
    nutritional 377.33
    toxic 377.34
  peripheral (nerve) (*see also* Polyneuropathy) 356.9
    arm NEC 354.9
    autonomic 337.9
      amyloid 277.39 [*337.1*]
      idiopathic 337.00
      in
        amyloidosis 277.39 [*337.1*]
        diabetes (mellitus) 250.6● [*337.1*]
          due to secondary diabetes 249.6● [*337.1*]
        diseases classified elsewhere 337.1
        gout 274.89 [*337.1*]
        hyperthyroidism 242.9● [*337.1*]
    due to
      antitetanus serum 357.6
      arsenic 357.7
      drugs 357.6

Neuropathy, neuropathic (*Continued*)
  peripheral (*Continued*)
    due to (*Continued*)
      lead 357.7
      organophosphate compounds 357.7
      toxic agent NEC 357.7
    hereditary 356.0
    idiopathic 356.9
      progressive 356.4
      specified type NEC 356.8
    in diseases classified elsewhere - *see* Polyneuropathy, in
    leg NEC 355.8
    lower extremity NEC 355.8
    upper extremity NEC 354.9
  plantar nerves 355.6
  progressive
    hypertrophic interstitial 356.9
    inflammatory 357.89
  radicular NEC 729.2
    brachial 723.4
    cervical NEC 723.4
    hereditary sensory 356.2
    lumbar 724.4
    lumbosacral 724.4
    thoracic NEC 724.4
  sacral plexus 353.1
  sciatic 355.0
  spinal nerve NEC 355.9
    root (*see also* Radiculitis) 729.2
  toxic 357.7
  trigeminal sensory 350.8
  ulnar nerve 354.2
  upper extremity NEC 354.9
  uremic 585.9 [*357.4*]
  vitamin B₁₂ 266.2 [*357.4*]
    with anemia (pernicious) 281.0 [*357.4*]
      due to dietary deficiency 281.1 [*357.4*]
Neurophthisis - *see also* Disorder, nerve
  peripheral 356.9
  diabetic 250.6● [*357.2*]
    due to secondary diabetes 249.6● [*357.2*]
Neuropraxia - *see* Injury, nerve
Neuroretinitis 363.05
  syphilitic 094.85
Neurosarcoma (M9540/3) - *see* Neoplasm, connective tissue, malignant
Neurosclerosis - *see* Disorder, nerve
Neurosis, neurotic 300.9
  accident 300.16
  anancastic, anankastic 300.3
  anxiety (state) 300.00
    generalized 300.02
    panic type 300.01
  asthenic 300.5
  bladder 306.53
  cardiac (reflex) 306.2
  cardiovascular 306.2
  climacteric, unspecified type 627.2
  colon 306.4
  compensation 300.16
  compulsive, compulsion 300.3
  conversion 300.11
  craft 300.89
  cutaneous 306.3
  depersonalization 300.6
  depressive (reaction) (type) 300.4
  endocrine 306.6
  environmental 300.89
  fatigue 300.5
  functional (*see also* Disorder, psychosomatic) 306.9
  gastric 306.4
  gastrointestinal 306.4
  genitourinary 306.50
  heart 306.2
  hypochondriacal 300.7
  hysterical 300.10
    conversion type 300.11
    dissociative type 300.15
  impulsive 300.3

Neurosis, neurotic (*Continued*)
  incoordination 306.0
    larynx 306.1
    vocal cord 306.1
  intestine 306.4
  larynx 306.1
    hysterical 300.11
    sensory 306.1
  menopause, unspecified type 627.2
  mixed NEC 300.89
  musculoskeletal 306.0
  obsessional 300.3
    phobia 300.3
  obsessive-compulsive 300.3
  occupational 300.89
  ocular 306.7
  oral (*see also* Disorder, fluency) 315.35
  organ (*see also* Disorder, psychosomatic) 306.9
  pharynx 306.1
  phobic 300.20
  posttraumatic (acute) (situational) 309.81
    chronic 309.81
  psychasthenic (type) 300.89
  railroad 300.16
  rectum 306.4
  respiratory 306.1
  rumination 306.4
  senile 300.89
  sexual 302.70
  situational 300.89
  specified type NEC 300.89
  state 300.9
    with depersonalization episode 300.6
  stomach 306.4
  vasomotor 306.2
  visceral 306.4
  war 300.16
Neurospongioblastosis diffusa 759.5
Neurosyphilis (arrested) (early) (inactive) (late) (latent) (recurrent) 094.9
  with ataxia (cerebellar) (locomotor) (spastic) (spinal) 094.0
  acute meningitis 094.2
  aneurysm 094.89
  arachnoid (adhesive) 094.2
  arteritis (any artery) 094.89
  asymptomatic 094.3
  congenital 090.40
  dura (mater) 094.89
  general paresis 094.1
  gumma 094.9
  hemorrhagic 094.9
  juvenile (asymptomatic) (meningeal) 090.40
  leptomeninges (aseptic) 094.2
  meningeal 094.2
  meninges (adhesive) 094.2
  meningovascular (diffuse) 094.2
  optic atrophy 094.84
  parenchymatous (degenerative) 094.1
  paresis (*see also* Paresis, general) 094.1
  paretic (*see also* Paresis, general) 094.1
  relapse 094.9
  remission in (sustained) 094.9
  serological 094.3
  specified nature or site NEC 094.89
  tabes (dorsalis) 094.0
    juvenile 090.40
  tabetic 094.0
    juvenile 090.40
  taboparesis 094.1
    juvenile 090.40
  thrombosis 094.89
  vascular 094.89
Neurotic (*see also* Neurosis) 300.9
  excoriation 698.4
    psychogenic 306.3
Neurotmesis - *see* Injury, nerve, by site
Neurotoxemia - *see* Toxemia
Neuro-occlusion 524.21

Neutropenia, neutropenic (idiopathic) (pernicious) (primary) 288.00
  chronic 288.09
    hypoplastic 288.09
  congenital (nontransient) 288.01
  cyclic 288.02
  drug induced 288.03
  due to infection 288.04
  fever 288.00
  genetic 288.01
  immune 288.09
  infantile 288.01
  malignant 288.09
  neonatal, transitory (isoimmune) (maternal transfer) 776.7
  periodic 288.02
  splenic 289.53
  splenomegaly 289.53
  toxic 288.09
Neutrophilia, hereditary giant 288.2
Nevocarcinoma (M8720/3) - see Melanoma
Nevus (M8720/0) - see also Neoplasm, skin, benign

> Note: Except where otherwise indicated, varieties of nevus in the list below that are followed by a morphology code number (M----/0) should be coded by site as for "Neoplasm, skin, benign."

  acanthotic 702.8
  achromic (M8730/0)
  amelanotic (M8730/0)
  anemic, anemicus 709.09
  angiomatous (M9120/0) (see also Hemangioma) 228.00
  araneus 448.1
  avasculosus 709.09
  balloon cell (M8722/0)
  bathing trunk (M8761/1) 238.2
  blue (M8780/0)
    cellular (M8790/0)
    giant (M8790/0)
    Jadassohn's (M8780/0)
    malignant (M8780/3) - see Melanoma
  capillary (M9131/0) (see also Hemangioma) 228.00
  cavernous (M9121/0) (see also Hemangioma) 228.00
  cellular (M8720/0)
    blue (M8790/0)
  comedonicus 757.33
  compound (M8760/0)
  conjunctiva (M8720/0) 224.3
  dermal (M8750/0)
    and epidermal (M8760/0)
  epithelioid cell (and spindle cell) (M8770/0)
  flammeus 757.32
    osteohypertrophic 759.89
  hairy (M8720/0)
  halo (M8723/0)
  hemangiomatous (M9120/0) (see also Hemangioma) 228.00
  intradermal (M8750/0)
  intraepidermal (M8740/0)
  involuting (M8724/0)
  Jadassohn's (blue) (M8780/0)
  junction, junctional (M8740/0)
    malignant melanoma in (M8740/3) - see Melanoma
  juvenile (M8770/0)
  lymphatic (M9170/0) 228.1
  magnocellular (M8726/0)
    specified site - see Neoplasm, by site, benign
    unspecified site 224.0
  malignant (M8720/3) - see Melanoma
  meaning hemangioma (M9120/0) (see also Hemangioma) 228.00
  melanotic (pigmented) (M8720/0)
  multiplex 759.5

Nevus (Continued)
  nonneoplastic 448.1
  nonpigmented (M8730/0)
  nonvascular (M8720/0)
  oral mucosa, white sponge 750.26
  osteohypertrophic, flammeus 759.89
  papillaris (M8720/0)
  papillomatosus (M8720/0)
  pigmented (M8720/0)
    giant (M8761/1) - see also Neoplasm, skin, uncertain behavior
    malignant melanoma in (M8761/3) - see Melanoma
  systematicus 757.33
  pilosus (M8720/0)
  port wine 757.32
  sanguineous 757.32
  sebaceous (senile) 702.8
  senile 448.1
  spider 448.1
  spindle cell (and epithelioid cell) (M8770/0)
  stellar 448.1
  strawberry 757.32
  syringocystadenomatous papilliferous (M8406/0)
  unius lateris 757.33
  Unna's 757.32
  vascular 757.32
  verrucous 757.33
  white sponge (oral mucosa) 750.26
Newborn (infant) (liveborn)
  abstinence syndrome 779.5
  affected by
    amniocentesis 760.61
    maternal abuse of drugs (gestational) (via placenta) (via breast milk) (see also Noxious, substances transmitted through placenta or breast milk (affecting fetus or newborn)) 760.70
      methamphetamine(s) 760.72
    procedure
      amniocentesis 760.61
      in utero NEC 760.62
      surgical on mother
        during pregnancy NEC 760.63
        previous not associated with pregnancy 760.64
  apnea 770.81
    obstructive 770.82
    specified NEC 770.82
  breast buds 779.89
  cardiomyopathy 425.4
    congenital 425.3
  convulsion 779.0
  electrolyte imbalance NEC (transitory) 775.5
  fever (environmentally-induced) 778.4
  gestation
    24 completed weeks 765.22
    25–26 completed weeks 765.23
    27–28 completed weeks 765.24
    29–30 completed weeks 765.25
    31–32 completed weeks 765.26
    33–34 completed weeks 765.27
    35–36 completed weeks 765.28
    37 or more completed weeks 765.29
    less than 24 completed weeks 765.21
    unspecified completed weeks 765.20
  infection 771.89
    candida 771.7
    mastitis 771.5
    specified NEC 771.89
    urinary tract 771.82
  mastitis 771.5
  multiple NEC
    born in hospital (without mention of cesarean delivery or section) V37.00
      with cesarean delivery or section V37.01
    born outside hospital
      hospitalized V37.1●
      not hospitalized V37.2●

Newborn (Continued)
  multiple NEC (Continued)
    mates all liveborn
      born in hospital (without mention of cesarean delivery or section) V34.00
        with cesarean delivery or section V34.01
      born outside hospital
        hospitalized V34.1●
        not hospitalized V34.2●
    mates all stillborn
      born in hospital (without mention of cesarean delivery or section) V35.00
        with cesarean delivery or section V35.01
      born outside hospital
        hospitalized V35.1●
        not hospitalized V35.2●
    mates liveborn and stillborn
      born in hospital (without mention of cesarean delivery or section) V36.00
        with cesarean delivery or section V36.01
      born outside hospital
        hospitalized V36.1●
        not hospitalized V36.2●
  omphalitis 771.4
  seizure 779.0
  sepsis 771.81
  single
    born in hospital (without mention of cesarean delivery or section) V30.00
      with cesarean delivery or section V30.01
    born outside hospital
      hospitalized V30.1●
      not hospitalized V30.2●
  specified condition NEC 779.89
  twin NEC
    born in hospital (without mention of cesarean delivery or section) V33.00
      with cesarean delivery or section V33.01
    born outside hospital
      hospitalized V33.1●
      not hospitalized V33.2●
    mate liveborn
      born in hospital V31.0●
      born outside hospital
        hospitalized V31.1●
        not hospitalized V31.2●
    mate stillborn
      born in hospital V32.0●
      born outside hospital
        hospitalized V32.1●
        not hospitalized V32.2●
  unspecified as to single or multiple birth
    born in hospital (without mention of cesarean delivery or section) V39.00
      with cesarean delivery or section V39.01
    born outside hospital
      hospitalized V39.1●
      not hospitalized V39.2●
  weight check V20.32
Newcastle's conjunctivitis or disease 077.8
Nezelof's syndrome (pure alymphocytosis) 279.13
Niacin (amide) deficiency 265.2
Nicolas-Durand-Favre disease (climatic bubo) 099.1
Nicolas-Favre disease (climatic bubo) 099.1
Nicotinic acid (amide) deficiency 265.2
Niemann-Pick disease (lipid histiocytosis) (splenomegaly) 272.7

Night
blindness (*see also* Blindness, night) 368.60
congenital 368.61
vitamin A deficiency 264.5
cramps 729.82
sweats 780.8
terrors, child 307.46
Nightmare 307.47
REM-sleep type 307.47
Nipple - *see* condition
Nisbet's chancre 099.0
Nishimoto (-Takeuchi) disease 437.5
Nitritoid crisis or reaction - *see* Crisis, nitritoid
Nitrogen retention, extrarenal 788.99
Nitrosohemoglobinemia 289.89
Njovera 104.0
No
diagnosis 799.9
disease (found) V71.9
room at the inn V65.0
Nocardiasis - *see* Nocardiosis
Nocardiosis 039.9
with pneumonia 039.1
lung 039.1
specified type NEC 039.8
Nocturia 788.43
psychogenic 306.53
Nocturnal - *see also* condition
dyspnea (paroxysmal) 786.09
emissions 608.89
enuresis 788.36
psychogenic 307.6
frequency (micturition) 788.43
psychogenic 306.53
Nodal rhythm disorder 427.89
Nodding of head 781.0
Node(s) - *see also* Nodules
Heberden's 715.04
larynx 478.79
lymph - *see* condition
milkers' 051.1
Osler's 421.0
rheumatic 729.89
Schmorl's 722.30
lumbar, lumbosacral 722.32
specified region NEC 722.39
thoracic, thoracolumbar 722.31
singers' 478.5
skin NEC 782.2
tuberculous - *see* Tuberculosis, lymph gland
vocal cords 478.5
Nodosities, Haygarth's 715.04
Nodule(s), nodular
actinomycotic (*see also* Actinomycosis) 039.9
arthritic - *see* Arthritis, nodosa
breast 793.89
cutaneous 782.2
Haygarth's 715.04
inflammatory - *see* Inflammation
juxta-articular 102.7
syphilitic 095.7
yaws 102.7
larynx 478.79
lung
emphysematous 492.8
solitary 793.11
milkers' 051.1
prostate 600.10
with
urinary
obstruction 600.11
retention 600.11
pulmonary, solitary (subsegmental branch of
the bronchial tree) 793.11
multiple 793.19
retrocardiac 785.9
rheumatic 729.89
rheumatoid - *see* Arthritis rheumatoid
scrotum (inflammatory) 608.4
singers' 478.5
skin NEC 782.2

Nodule(s), nodular (*Continued*)
solitary, lung 518.89
emphysematous 492.8
subcutaneous 782.2
thyroid (gland) (nontoxic) (uninodular) 241.0
with
hyperthyroidism 242.1●
thyrotoxicosis 242.1●
toxic or with hyperthyroidism 242.1●
vocal cords 478.5
Noma (gangrenous) (hospital) (infective) 528.1
auricle (*see also* Gangrene) 785.4
mouth 528.1
pudendi (*see also* Vulvitis) 616.10
vulvae (*see also* Vulvitis) 616.10
Nomadism V60.0
Non-adherence
artificial skin graft 996.55
decellularized allodermis graft 996.55
Non-autoimmune hemolytic anemia NEC
283.10
Nonclosure - *see also* Imperfect, closure
ductus
arteriosus 747.0
Botalli 747.0
Eustachian valve 746.89
foramen
Botalli 745.5
ovale 745.5
Noncompliance with medical treatment V15.81
renal dialysis V45.12
Nondescent (congenital) - *see also* Malposition,
congenital
cecum 751.4
colon 751.4
testis 752.51
Nondevelopment
brain 742.1
specified part 742.2
heart 746.89
organ or site, congenital NEC - *see*
Hypoplasia
Nonengagement
head NEC 652.5●
in labor 660.1●
affecting fetus or newborn 763.1
Nonexanthematous tick fever 066.1
Nonexpansion, lung (newborn) NEC 770.4
Nonfunctioning
cystic duct (*see also* Disease, gallbladder)
575.8
gallbladder (*see also* Disease, gallbladder)
575.8
kidney (*see also* Disease, renal) 593.9
labyrinth 386.58
Nonhealing
stump (surgical) 997.69
wound, surgical 998.83
Nonimplantation of ovum, causing infertility
628.3
Noninsufflation, fallopian tube 628.2
Nonne-Milroy-Meige syndrome (chronic
hereditary edema) 757.0
Nonovulation 628.0
Nonpatent fallopian tube 628.2
Nonpneumatization, lung NEC 770.4
Nonreflex bladder 596.54
with cauda equina 344.61
Nonretention of food - *see* Vomiting
Nonrotation - *see* Malrotation
Nonsecretion, urine (*see also* Anuria) 788.5
newborn 753.3
Nonunion
fracture 733.82
organ or site, congenital NEC - *see* Imperfect,
closure
symphysis pubis, congenital 755.69
top sacrum, congenital 756.19
Nonviability 765.0●
Nonvisualization, gallbladder 793.3
Nonvitalized tooth 522.9

Non-working side interference 524.56
Normal
delivery - *see* category 650
menses V65.5
state (feared complaint unfounded) V65.5
Normoblastosis 289.89
Normocytic anemia (infectional) 285.9
due to blood loss (chronic) 280.0
acute 285.1
Norrie's disease (congenital) (progressive
oculoacousticocerebral degeneration)
743.8
North American blastomycosis 116.0
Norwegian itch 133.0
Nose, nasal - *see* condition
Nosebleed 784.7
Nosomania 298.9
Nosophobia 300.29
Nostalgia 309.89
Notch of iris 743.46
Notched lip, congenital (*see also* Cleft, lip)
749.10
Notching nose, congenital (tip) 748.1
Nothnagel's
syndrome 378.52
vasomotor acroparesthesia 443.89
Novy's relapsing fever (American) 087.1
Noxious
foodstuffs, poisoning by
fish 988.0
fungi 988.1
mushrooms 988.1
plants (food) 988.2
shellfish 988.0
specified type NEC 988.8
toadstool 988.1
substances transmitted through placenta or
breast milk (affecting fetus or
newborn) 760.70
acetretin 760.78
alcohol 760.71
aminopterin 760.78
antiandrogens 760.79
anticonvulsant 760.77
antifungal 760.74
anti-infective agents 760.74
antimetabolic 760.78
atorvastatin 760.78
carbamazepine 760.77
cocaine 760.75
"crack" 760.75
diethylstilbestrol (DES) 760.76
divalproex sodium 760.77
endocrine disrupting chemicals 760.79
estrogens 760.79
etretinate 760.78
fluconazole 760.74
fluvastatin 760.78
hallucinogenic agents NEC 760.73
hormones 760.79
lithium 760.79
lovastatin 760.78
medicinal agents NEC 760.79
methotrexate 760.78
misoprostil 760.79
narcotics 760.72
obstetric anesthetic or analgesic 763.5
phenobarbital 760.77
phenytoin 760.77
pravastatin 760.78
progestins 760.79
retinoic acid 760.78
simvastatin 760.78
solvents 760.79
specified agent NEC 760.79
statins 760.78
suspected, affecting management of
pregnancy 655.5●
tetracycline 760.74
thalidomide 760.79
trimethadione 760.77

◀ New   ◀ Revised   ~~deleted~~ Deleted   ● Use Additional Digit(s)   ▓ Omit code   **403**

Noxious *(Continued)*
   substances transmitted through placenta or
      breast milk *(Continued)*
      valproate 760.77
      valproic acid 760.77
      vitamin A 760.78
NPDH (new persistent daily headache)
   339.42
Nuchal hitch (arm) 652.8●
Nucleus pulposus - *see* condition
Numbness 782.0
Nuns' knee 727.2
Nursemaid's
   elbow 832.2
   shoulder 831.0●
Nutmeg liver 573.8

Nutrition, deficient or insufficient (particular
   kind of food) 269.9
   due to
      insufficient food 994.2
      lack of
         care (child) (infant) 995.52
            adult 995.84
         food 994.2
Nyctalopia (*see also* Blindness, night) 368.60
   vitamin A deficiency 264.5
Nycturia 788.43
   psychogenic 306.53
Nymphomania 302.89
Nystagmus 379.50
   associated with vestibular system disorders
      379.54

Nystagmus *(Continued)*
   benign paroxysmal positional
      386.11
   central positional 386.2
   congenital 379.51
   deprivation 379.53
   dissociated 379.55
   latent 379.52
   miners' 300.89
   positional
      benign paroxysmal 386.11
      central 386.2
   specified NEC 379.56
   vestibular 379.54
   visual deprivation 379.53

◀ New   ◀▥ Revised   ~~deleted~~ Deleted   ● Use Additional Digit(s)   ▢ Omit code

O

Oasthouse urine disease 270.2
Obermeyer's relapsing fever (European) 087.0
Obesity (constitutional) (exogenous) (familial) (nutritional) (simple) 278.00
  adrenal 255.8
  complicating pregnancy, childbirth, or puerperium 649.1●
  due to hyperalimentation 278.00
  endocrine NEC 259.9
  endogenous 259.9
  Fröhlich's (adiposogenital dystrophy) 253.8
  glandular NEC 259.9
  hypothyroid (see also Hypothyroidism) 244.9
  hypoventilation syndrome 278.03
  morbid 278.01
  of pregnancy 649.1●
  pituitary 253.8
  severe 278.01
  thyroid (see also Hypothyroidism) 244.9
Oblique - see also condition
  lie before labor, affecting fetus or newborn 761.7
Obliquity, pelvis 738.6
Obliteration
  abdominal aorta 446.7
  appendix (lumen) 543.9
  artery 447.1
  ascending aorta 446.7
  bile ducts 576.8
    with calculus, choledocholithiasis, or stones - see Choledocholithiasis
    congenital 751.61
      jaundice from 751.61 [774.5]
  common duct 576.8
    with calculus, choledocholithiasis, or stones - see Choledocholithiasis
    congenital 751.61
  cystic duct 575.8
    with calculus, choledocholithiasis, or stones - see Choledocholithiasis
  disease, arteriolar 447.1
  endometrium 621.8
  eye, anterior chamber 360.34
  fallopian tube 628.2
  lymphatic vessel 457.1
    postmastectomy 457.0
  organ or site, congenital NEC - see Atresia
  placental blood vessels - see Placenta, abnormal
  supra-aortic branches 446.7
  ureter 593.89
  urethra 599.84
  vein 459.9
  vestibule (oral) 525.8
Observation (for) V71.9
  without need for further medical care V71.9
  accident NEC V71.4
    at work V71.3
  criminal assault V71.6
  deleterious agent ingestion V71.89
  disease V71.9
    cardiovascular V71.7
    heart V71.7
    mental V71.09
    specified condition NEC V71.89
  foreign body ingestion V71.89
  growth and development variations V21.8
  injuries (accidental) V71.4
    inflicted NEC V71.6
      during alleged rape or seduction V71.5
  malignant neoplasm, suspected V71.1
  postpartum
    immediately after delivery V24.0
    routine follow-up V24.2
  pregnancy
    high-risk V23.9
      inconclusive fetal viability V23.87
      specified problem NEC V23.89

Observation (Continued)
  pregnancy (Continued)
    normal (without complication) V22.1
      with nonobstetric complication V22.2
      first V22.0
  rape or seduction, alleged V71.5
    injury during V71.5
  suicide attempt, alleged V71.89
  suspected (undiagnosed) (unproven)
    abuse V71.81
    cardiovascular disease V71.7
    child or wife battering victim V71.6
    concussion (cerebral) V71.6
    condition NEC V71.89
      infant - see Observation, suspected, condition, newborn
      maternal and fetal
        amniotic cavity and membrane problem V89.01
        cervical shortening V89.05
        fetal anomaly V89.03
        fetal growth problem V89.04
        oligohydramnios V89.01
        other specified problem NEC V89.09
        placental problem V89.02
        polyhydramnios V89.01
      newborn V29.9
        cardiovascular disease V29.8
        congenital anomaly V29.8
        genetic V29.3
        infectious V29.0
        ingestion foreign object V29.8
        injury V29.8
        metabolic V29.3
        neoplasm V29.8
        neurological V29.1
        poison, poisoning V29.8
        respiratory V29.2
        specified NEC V29.8
    exposure
      anthrax V71.82
      biologic agent NEC V71.83
      SARS V71.83
    infectious disease not requiring isolation V71.89
    malignant neoplasm V71.1
    mental disorder V71.09
    neglect V71.81
    neoplasm
      benign V71.89
      malignant V71.1
    specified condition NEC V71.89
    tuberculosis V71.2
  tuberculosis, suspected V71.2
Obsession, obsessional 300.3
  ideas and mental images 300.3
  impulses 300.3
  neurosis 300.3
  phobia 300.3
  psychasthenia 300.3
  ruminations 300.3
  state 300.3
  syndrome 300.3
Obsessive-compulsive 300.3
  neurosis 300.3
  personality 301.4
  reaction 300.3
Obstetrical trauma NEC (complicating delivery) 665.9●
  with
    abortion - see Abortion, by type, with damage to pelvic organs
    ectopic pregnancy (see also categories 633.0-633.9) 639.2
    molar pregnancy (see also categories 630-632) 639.2
  affecting fetus or newborn 763.89
  following
    abortion 639.2
    ectopic or molar pregnancy 639.2

Obstipation (see also Constipation) 564.00
  psychogenic 306.4
Obstruction, obstructed, obstructive
  airway NEC 519.8
    with
      allergic alveolitis NEC 495.9
      asthma NEC (see also Asthma) 493.9●
      bronchiectasis 494.0
        with acute exacerbation 494.1
      bronchitis (see also Bronchitis, with, obstruction) 491.20
      emphysema NEC 492.8
    chronic 496
      with
        allergic alveolitis NEC 495.5
        asthma NEC (see also Asthma) 493.2●
        bronchiectasis 494.0
          with acute exacerbation 494.1
        bronchitis (chronic) (see also Bronchitis, chronic, obstructive) 491.20
        emphysema NEC 492.8
    due to
      bronchospasm 519.11
      foreign body 934.9
      inhalation of fumes or vapors 506.9
      laryngospasm 478.75
  alimentary canal (see also Obstruction, intestine) 560.9
  ampulla of Vater 576.2
    with calculus, cholelithiasis, or stones - see Choledocholithiasis
  aortic (heart) (valve) (see also Stenosis, aortic) 424.1
    rheumatic (see also Stenosis, aortic, rheumatic) 395.0
  aortoiliac 444.09
  aqueduct of Sylvius 331.4
    congenital 742.3
      with spina bifida (see also Spina bifida) 741.0●
  Arnold-Chiari (see also Spina bifida) 741.0●
  artery (see also Embolism, artery) 444.9
    basilar (complete) (partial) (see also Occlusion, artery, basilar) 433.0●
    carotid (complete) (partial) (see also Occlusion, artery, carotid) 433.1●
    precerebral - see Occlusion, artery, precerebral NEC
    retinal (central) (see also Occlusion, retina) 362.30
    vertebral (complete) (partial) (see also Occlusion, artery, vertebral) 433.2●
  asthma (chronic) (with obstructive pulmonary disease) 493.2●
  band (intestinal) 560.81
  bile duct or passage (see also Obstruction, biliary) 576.2
    congenital 751.61
      jaundice from 751.61 [774.5]
  biliary (duct) (tract) 576.2
    with calculus 574.51
      with cholecystitis (chronic) 574.41
        acute 574.31
    congenital 751.61
      jaundice from 751.61 [774.5]
    gallbladder 575.2
      with calculus 574.21
        with cholecystitis (chronic) 574.11
          acute 574.01
  bladder neck (acquired) 596.0
    congenital 753.6
  bowel (see also Obstruction, intestine) 560.9
  bronchus 519.19
  canal, ear (see also Stricture, ear canal, acquired) 380.50
  cardia 537.89
  caval veins (inferior) (superior) 459.2
  cecum (see also Obstruction, intestine) 560.9
  circulatory 459.9

Obstruction, obstructed, obstructive
(Continued)
colon (*see also* Obstruction, intestine)
560.9
sympathicotonic 560.89
common duct (*see also* Obstruction, biliary)
576.2
congenital 751.61
coronary (artery) (heart) - (*see also*
Arteriosclerosis, coronary)
acute (*see also* Infarct, myocardium)
410.9●
without myocardial infarction 411.81
cystic duct (*see also* Obstruction, gallbladder)
575.2
congenital 751.61
device, implant, or graft - *see* Complications,
due to (presence of) any device,
implant, or graft classified to
996.0–996.5 NEC
due to foreign body accidentally left in
operation wound 998.4
duodenum 537.3
congenital 751.1
due to
compression NEC 537.3
cyst 537.3
intrinsic lesion or disease NEC
537.3
scarring 537.3
torsion 537.3
ulcer 532.91
volvulus 537.3
ejaculatory duct 608.89
endocardium 424.90
arteriosclerotic 424.99
specified cause, except rheumatic
424.99
esophagus 530.3
Eustachian tube (complete) (partial)
381.60
cartilaginous
extrinsic 381.63
intrinsic 381.62
due to
cholesteatoma 381.61
osseous lesion NEC 381.61
polyp 381.61
osseous 381.61
fallopian tube (bilateral) 628.2
fecal 560.32
with hernia - *see also* Hernia, by site, with
obstruction
gangrenous - *see* Hernia, by site, with
gangrene
foramen of Monro (congenital) 742.3
with spina bifida (*see also* Spina bifida)
741.0●
foreign body - *see* Foreign body
gallbladder 575.2
with calculus, cholelithiasis, or stones
574.21
with cholecystitis (chronic) 574.11
acute 574.01
congenital 751.69
jaundice from 751.69 [774.5]
gastric outlet 537.0
gastrointestinal (*see also* Obstruction,
intestine) 560.9
glottis 478.79
hepatic 573.8
duct (*see also* Obstruction, biliary) 576.2
congenital 751.61
icterus (*see also* Obstruction, biliary) 576.8
congenital 751.61
ileocecal coil (*see also* Obstruction, intestine)
560.9
ileum (*see also* Obstruction, intestine) 560.9
iliofemoral (artery) 444.81
internal anastomosis - *see* Complications,
mechanical, graft

Obstruction, obstructed, obstructive
(Continued)
intestine (mechanical) (neurogenic)
(paroxysmal) (postinfectional) (reflex)
560.9
with
adhesions (intestinal) (peritoneal)
560.81
hernia - *see also* Hernia, by site, with
obstruction
gangrenous - *see* Hernia, by site,
with gangrene
adynamic (*see also* Ileus) 560.1
by gallstone 560.31
congenital or infantile (small) 751.1
large 751.2
due to
Ascaris lumbricoides 127.0
mural thickening 560.89
procedure 997.49
involving urinary tract 997.5
impaction 560.32
infantile - *see* Obstruction, intestine,
congenital
newborn
due to
fecaliths 777.1
inspissated milk 777.2
meconium (plug) 777.1
in mucoviscidosis 277.01
transitory 777.4
specified cause NEC 560.89
transitory, newborn 777.4
volvulus 560.2
intracardiac ball valve prosthesis 996.02
jaundice (*see also* Obstruction, biliary) 576.8
congenital 751.61
jejunum (*see also* Obstruction, intestine)
560.9
kidney 593.89
labor 660.9●
affecting fetus or newborn 763.1
by
bony pelvis (conditions classifiable to
653.0–653.9) 660.1●
deep transverse arrest 660.3●
impacted shoulder 660.4●
locked twins 660.5●
malposition (fetus) (conditions
classifiable to 652.0–652.9)
660.0●
head during labor 660.3●
persistent occipitoposterior position
660.3●
soft tissue, pelvic (conditions
classifiable to 654.0–654.9)
660.2●
lacrimal
canaliculi 375.53
congenital 743.65
punctum 375.52
sac 375.54
lacrimonasal duct 375.56
congenital 743.65
neonatal 375.55
lacteal, with steatorrhea 579.2
laryngitis (*see also* Laryngitis) 464.01
larynx 478.79
congenital 748.3
liver 573.8
cirrhotic (*see also* Cirrhosis, liver) 571.5
lung 518.89
with
asthma - *see* Asthma
bronchitis (chronic) 491.20
emphysema NEC 492.8
airway, chronic 496
chronic NEC 496
with
asthma (chronic) (obstructive)
493.2●

Obstruction, obstructed, obstructive
(Continued)
lung *(Continued)*
disease, chronic 496
with
asthma (chronic) (obstructive)
493.2●
emphysematous 492.8
lymphatic 457.1
meconium
fetus or newborn 777.1
in mucoviscidosis 277.01
newborn due to fecaliths 777.1
mediastinum 519.3
mitral (rheumatic) - *see* Stenosis, mitral
nasal 478.19
duct 375.56
neonatal 375.55
sinus - *see* Sinusitis
nasolacrimal duct 375.56
congenital 743.65
neonatal 375.55
nasopharynx 478.29
nose 478.19
organ or site, congenital NEC - *see* Atresia
pancreatic duct 577.8
parotid gland 527.8
pelviureteral junction (*see also* Obstruction,
ureter) 593.4
pharynx 478.29
portal (circulation) (vein) 452
prostate 600.90
with
other lower urinary tract symptoms
(LUTS) 600.91
urinary
obstruction 600.91
retention 600.91
valve (urinary) 596.0
pulmonary
valve (heart) (*see also* Endocarditis,
pulmonary) 424.3
vein, isolated 747.49
pyemic - *see* Septicemia
pylorus (acquired) 537.0
congenital 750.5
infantile 750.5
rectosigmoid (*see also* Obstruction, intestine)
560.9
rectum 569.49
renal 593.89
respiratory 519.8
chronic 496
retinal (artery) (vein) (central) (*see also*
Occlusion, retina) 362.30
salivary duct (any) 527.8
with calculus 527.5
sigmoid (*see also* Obstruction, intestine)
560.9
sinus (accessory) (nasal) (*see also* Sinusitis)
473.9
Stensen's duct 527.8
stomach 537.89
acute 536.1
congenital 750.7
submaxillary gland 527.8
with calculus 527.5
thoracic duct 457.1
thrombotic - *see* Thrombosis
tooth eruption 520.6
trachea 519.19
tracheostomy airway 519.09
tricuspid - *see* Endocarditis, tricuspid
upper respiratory, congenital 748.8
ureter (functional) 593.4
congenital 753.20
due to calculus 592.1
ureteropelvic junction, congenital 753.21
ureterovesical junction, congenital 753.22
urethra 599.60
congenital 753.6

◄ New ◄▬ Revised ~~deleted~~ Deleted ● Use Additional Digit(s) ▨ Omit code

Obstruction, obstructed, obstructive
(Continued)
  urinary (moderate) 599.60
    organ or tract (lower) 599.60
      due to
        benign prostatic hypertrophy
          (BPH) - *see* category 600
        specified NEC 599.69
          due to
            benign prostatic hypertrophy
              (BPH) - *see* category 600
      prostatic valve 596.0
      specified NEC 599.69
        due to
          benign prostatic hypertrophy
            (BPH) - *see* category 600
  uropathy 599.60
  uterus 621.8
  vagina 623.2
  valvular - *see* Endocarditis
  vascular graft or shunt 996.1
    atherosclerosis - *see* Arteriosclerosis,
      coronary
    embolism 996.74
    occlusion NEC 996.74
    thrombus 996.74
  vein, venous 459.2
    caval (inferior) (superior) 459.2
    thrombotic - *see* Thrombosis
  vena cava (inferior) (superior) 459.2
  ventricular shunt 996.2
  vesical 596.0
  vesicourethral orifice 596.0
  vessel NEC 459.9
Obturator - *see* condition
Occlusal
  plane deviation 524.76
  wear, teeth 521.10
Occlusion
  anus 569.49
    congenital 751.2
    infantile 751.2
  aortoiliac (chronic) 444.09
  aqueduct of Sylvius 331.4
    congenital 742.3
      with spina bifida (*see also* Spina bifida)
        741.0●
  arteries of extremities, lower 444.22
    without thrombus or embolus (*see also*
      Arteriosclerosis, extremities)
        440.20
    due to stricture or stenosis 447.1
    upper 444.21
      without thrombus or embolus (*see also*
        Arteriosclerosis, extremities)
          440.20
      due to stricture or stenosis 447.1
  artery NEC (*see also* Embolism, artery)
    444.9
    auditory, internal 433.8●
    basilar 433.0●
      with other precerebral artery
        433.3●
      bilateral 433.3●
    brain or cerebral (*see also* Infarct, brain)
      434.9●
    carotid 433.1●
      with other precerebral artery
        433.3●
      bilateral 433.3●
    cerebellar (anterior inferior) (posterior
      inferior) (superior) 433.8●
    cerebral (*see also* Infarct, brain) 434.9●
    choroidal (anterior) 433.8●
    chronic total
      coronary 414.2
      extremity(ies) 440.4
    communicating posterior 433.8●
    complete
      coronary 414.2
      extremity(ies) 440.4

Occlusion *(Continued)*
  artery NEC *(Continued)*
    coronary (thrombotic) (*see also* Infarct,
      myocardium) 410.9●
      acute 410.9●
        without myocardial infarction
          411.81
      chronic total 414.2
      complete 414.2
      healed or old 412
      total 414.2
    extremity(ies)
      chronic total 440.4
      complete 440.4
      total 440.4
    hypophyseal 433.8●
    iliac 444.81
    mesenteric (embolic) (thrombotic) (with
      gangrene) 557.0
    pontine 433.8●
    precerebral NEC 433.9●
      late effect - *see* Late effect(s) (of)
        cerebrovascular disease
      multiple or bilateral 433.3●
      puerperal, postpartum, childbirth
        674.0●
      specified NEC 433.8●
    renal 593.81
    retinal - *see* Occlusion, retina, artery
    spinal 433.8●
    vertebral 433.2●
      with other precerebral artery 433.3●
      bilateral 433.3●
  basilar (artery) - *see* Occlusion, artery, basilar
  bile duct (any) (*see also* Obstruction, biliary)
    576.2
  bowel (*see also* Obstruction, intestine) 560.9
  brain (artery) (vascular) (*see also* Infarct,
    brain) 434.9●
  breast (duct) 611.89
  carotid (artery) (common) (internal) - *see*
    Occlusion, artery, carotid
  cerebellar (anterior inferior) (artery)
    (posterior inferior) (superior) 433.8●
  cerebral (artery) (*see also* Infarct, brain)
    434.9●
  cerebrovascular (*see also* Infarct, brain)
    434.9●
    diffuse 437.0
  cervical canal (*see also* Stricture, cervix) 622.4
    by falciparum malaria 084.0
  cervix (uteri) (*see also* Stricture, cervix) 622.4
  choanal 748.0
  choroidal (artery) 433.8●
  colon (*see also* Obstruction, intestine) 560.9
  communicating posterior artery 433.8●
  coronary (artery) (thrombotic) (*see also*
    Infarct, myocardium) 410.9●
    acute 410.9●
      without myocardial infarction 411.81
    healed or old 412
  cystic duct (*see also* Obstruction, gallbladder)
    575.2
    congenital 751.69
  disto
    division I 524.22
    division II 524.22
  embolic - *see* Embolism
  fallopian tube 628.2
    congenital 752.19
  gallbladder (*see also* Obstruction,
    gallbladder) 575.2
    congenital 751.69
      jaundice from 751.69 [744.5]
  gingiva, traumatic 523.8
  hymen 623.3
    congenital 752.42
  hypophyseal (artery) 433.8●
  iliac (artery) 444.81
  intestine (*see also* Obstruction, intestine) 560.9
  kidney 593.89

Occlusion *(Continued)*
  lacrimal apparatus - *see* Stenosis, lacrimal
  lung 518.89
  lymph or lymphatic channel 457.1
  mammary duct 611.89
  mesenteric artery (embolic) (thrombotic)
    (with gangrene) 557.0
  nose 478.19
    congenital 748.0
  organ or site, congenital NEC - *see* Atresia
  oviduct 628.2
    congenital 752.19
  periodontal, traumatic 523.8
  peripheral arteries (lower extremity) 444.22
    without thrombus or embolus (*see also*
      Arteriosclerosis, extremities) 440.20
    due to stricture or stenosis 447.1
    upper extremity 444.21
      without thrombus or embolus (*see also*
        Arteriosclerosis, extremities)
          440.20
      due to stricture or stenosis 447.1
  pontine (artery) 433.8●
  posterior lingual, of mandibular teeth 524.29
  precerebral artery - *see* Occlusion, artery,
    precerebral NEC
  puncta lacrimalia 375.52
  pupil 364.74
  pylorus (*see also* Stricture, pylorus) 537.0
  renal artery 593.81
  retina, retinal (vascular) 362.30
    artery, arterial 362.30
      branch 362.32
      central (total) 362.31
      partial 362.33
      transient 362.34
      tributary 362.32
    vein 362.30
      branch 362.36
      central (total) 362.35
      incipient 362.37
      partial 362.37
      tributary 362.36
  spinal artery 433.8●
  stent
    coronary 996.72
  teeth (mandibular) (posterior lingual) 524.29
  thoracic duct 457.1
  tubal 628.2
  ureter (complete) (partial) 593.4
    congenital 753.29
  urethra (*see also* Stricture, urethra) 598.9
    congenital 753.6
  uterus 621.8
  vagina 623.2
  vascular NEC 459.9
  vein - *see* Thrombosis
  vena cava
    inferior 453.2
    superior (acute) 453.87
      chronic 453.77
  ventricle (brain) NEC 331.4
  vertebral (artery) - *see* Occlusion, artery,
    vertebral
  vessel (blood) NEC 459.9
  vulva 624.8
Occlusio pupillae 364.74
Occupational
  problems NEC V62.29
  therapy V57.21
Ochlophobia 300.29
Ochronosis (alkaptonuric) (congenital)
  (endogenous) 270.2
  with chloasma of eyelid 270.2
Ocular muscle - *see also* condition
  myopathy 359.1
  torticollis 781.93
Oculoauriculovertebral dysplasia 756.0
Oculogyric
  crisis or disturbance 378.87
    psychogenic 306.7

Oculomotor syndrome 378.81
Oddi's sphincter spasm 576.5
Odelberg's disease (juvenile osteochondrosis) 732.1
Odontalgia 525.9
Odontoameloblastoma (M9311/0) 213.1
    upper jaw (bone) 213.0
Odontoclasia 521.05
Odontoclasis 873.63
    complicated 873.73
Odontodysplasia, regional 520.4
Odontogenesis imperfecta 520.5
Odontoma (M9280/0) 213.1
    ameloblastic (M9311/0) 213.1
        upper jaw (bone) 213.0
    calcified (M9280/0) 213.1
        upper jaw (bone) 213.0
    complex (M9282/0) 213.1
        upper jaw (bone) 213.0
    compound (M9281/0) 213.1
        upper jaw (bone) 213.0
    fibroameloblastic (M9290/0) 213.1
        upper jaw (bone) 213.0
    follicular 526.0
        upper jaw (bone) 213.0
Odontomyelitis (closed) (open) 522.0
Odontonecrosis 521.09
Odontorrhagia 525.8
Odontosarcoma, ameloblastic (M9290/3) 170.1
    upper jaw (bone) 170.0
Odynophagia 787.20
Oesophagostomiasis 127.7
Oesophagostomum infestation 127.7
Oestriasis 134.0
Ogilvie's syndrome (sympathicotonic colon obstruction) 560.89
Oguchi's disease (retina) 368.61
Ohara's disease (see also Tularemia) 021.9
Oidiomycosis (see also Candidiasis) 112.9
Oidiomycotic meningitis 112.83
Oidium albicans infection (see also Candidiasis) 112.9
Old age 797
    dementia (of) 290.0
Olfactory - see condition
Oligemia 285.9
Oligergasia (see also Disability, intellectual) 319
Oligoamnios 658.0●
    affecting fetus or newborn 761.2
Oligoastrocytoma, mixed (M9382/3)
    specified site - see Neoplasm, by site, malignant
    unspecified site 191.9
Oligocythemia 285.9
Oligodendroblastoma (M9460/3)
    specified site - see Neoplasm, by site, malignant
    unspecified site 191.9
Oligodendroglioma (M9450/3)
    anaplastic type (M9451/3)
        specified site - see Neoplasm, by site, malignant
        unspecified site 191.9
    specified site - see Neoplasm, by site, malignant
    unspecified site 191.9
Oligodendroma - see Oligodendroglioma
Oligodontia (see also Anodontia) 520.0
Oligoencephalon 742.1
Oligohydramnios 658.0●
    affecting fetus or newborn 761.2
    due to premature rupture of membranes 658.1●
        affecting fetus or newborn 761.2
Oligohydrosis 705.0
Oligomenorrhea 626.1
Oligophrenia (see also Disability, intellectual) 319
    phenylpyruvic 270.1
Oligospermia 606.1

Oligotrichia 704.09
    congenita 757.4
Oliguria 788.5
    with
        abortion - see Abortion, by type, with renal failure
        ectopic pregnancy (see also categories 633.0–633.9) 639.3
        molar pregnancy (see also categories 630–632) 639.3
    complicating
        abortion 639.3
        ectopic or molar pregnancy 639.3
        pregnancy 646.2●
            with hypertension - see Toxemia, of pregnancy
    due to a procedure 997.5
    following labor and delivery 669.3●
    heart or cardiac - see Failure, heart
    puerperal, postpartum 669.3●
    specified due to a procedure 997.5
Ollier's disease (chondrodysplasia) 756.4
Omentitis (see also Peritonitis) 567.9
Omentocele (see also Hernia, omental) 553.8
Omentum, omental - see condition
Omphalitis (congenital) (newborn) 771.4
    not of newborn 686.9
    tetanus 771.3
Omphalocele 756.72
Omphalomesenteric duct, persistent 751.0
Omphalorrhagia, newborn 772.3
Omsk hemorrhagic fever 065.1
Onanism 307.9
Onchocerciasis 125.3
    eye 125.3 [360.13]
Onchocercosis 125.3
Oncocytoma (M8290/0) - see Neoplasm, by site, benign '
Ondine's curse 348.89
Oneirophrenia (see also Schizophrenia) 295.4●
Onychauxis 703.8
    congenital 757.5
Onychia (with lymphangitis) 681.9
    dermatophytic 110.1
    finger 681.02
    toe 681.11
Onychitis (with lymphangitis) 681.9
    finger 681.02
    toe 681.11
Onychocryptosis 703.0
Onychodystrophy 703.8
    congenital 757.5
Onychogryphosis 703.8
Onychogryposis 703.8
Onycholysis 703.8
Onychomadesis 703.8
Onychomalacia 703.8
Onychomycosis 110.1
    finger 110.1
    toe 110.1
Onycho-osteodysplasia 756.89
Onychophagy 307.9
Onychoptosis 703.8
Onychorrhexis 703.8
    congenital 757.5
Onychoschizia 703.8
Onychotrophia (see also Atrophy, nail) 703.8
O'Nyong Nyong fever 066.3
Onyxis (finger) (toe) 703.0
Onyxitis (with lymphangitis) 681.9
    finger 681.02
    toe 681.11
Oocyte (egg) (ovum)
    donor V59.70
        over age 35 V59.73
            anonymous recipient V59.73
            designated recipient V59.74
        under age 35 V59.71
            anonymous recipient V59.71
            designated recipient V59.72

Oophoritis (cystic) (infectional) (interstitial) (see also Salpingo-oophoritis) 614.2
    complicating pregnancy 646.6●
    fetal (acute) 752.0
    gonococcal (acute) 098.19
        chronic or duration of 2 months or over 098.39
    tuberculous (see also Tuberculosis) 016.6●
Opacity, opacities
    cornea 371.00
        central 371.03
        congenital 743.43
            interfering with vision 743.42
        degenerative (see also Degeneration, cornea) 371.40
        hereditary (see also Dystrophy, cornea) 371.50
        inflammatory (see also Keratitis) 370.9
        late effect of trachoma (healed) 139.1
        minor 371.01
        peripheral 371.02
    enamel (fluoride) (nonfluoride) (teeth) 520.3
    lens (see also Cataract) 366.9
    snowball 379.22
    vitreous (humor) 379.24
        congenital 743.51
Opalescent dentin (hereditary) 520.5
Open, opening
    abnormal, organ or site, congenital - see Imperfect, closure
    angle
        with
            borderline findings
                high risk 365.05
                intraocular pressure 365.01
                low risk 365.01
            cupping of discs 365.01
        high risk 365.05
        low risk 365.01
    bite
        anterior 524.24
        posterior 524.25
    false - see Imperfect, closure
    margin on tooth restoration 525.61
    restoration margins 525.61
    wound - see Wound, open, by site
Operation
    causing mutilation of fetus 763.89
    destructive, on live fetus, to facilitate birth 763.89
    for delivery, fetus or newborn 763.89
    maternal, unrelated to current delivery, affecting fetus or newborn (see also Newborn, affected by) 760.64
Operational fatigue 300.89
Operative - see condition
Operculitis (chronic) 523.40
    acute 523.30
Operculum, retina 361.32
    with detachment 361.01
Ophiasis 704.01
Ophthalmia (see also Conjunctivitis) 372.30
    actinic rays 370.24
    allergic (acute) 372.05
        chronic 372.14
    blennorrhagic (neonatorum) 098.40
    catarrhal 372.03
    diphtheritic 032.81
    Egyptian 076.1
    electric, electrica 370.24
    gonococcal (neonatorum) 098.40
    metastatic 360.11
    migraine 346.8●
    neonatorum, newborn 771.6
        gonococcal 098.40
    nodosa 360.14
    phlyctenular 370.31
        with ulcer (see also Ulcer, cornea) 370.00
    sympathetic 360.11
Ophthalmitis - see Ophthalmia
Ophthalmocele (congenital) 743.66

◀ New   ◀▥ Revised   ~~deleted~~ Deleted   ● Use Additional Digit(s)   ▨ Omit code

Ophthalmoneuromyelitis 341.0
Ophthalmopathy, infiltrative with
    thyrotoxicosis 242.0 ●
Ophthalmoplegia (*see also* Strabismus) 378.9
    anterior internuclear 378.86
    ataxia-areflexia syndrome 357.0
    bilateral 378.9
    diabetic 250.5 ● [378.86]
        due to secondary diabetes 249.5 ● [378.86]
    exophthalmic 242.0 ● [376.22]
    external 378.55
        progressive 378.72
        total 378.56
    internal (complete) (total) 367.52
    internuclear 378.86
    migraine 346.2 ●
    painful 378.55
    Parinaud's 378.81
    progressive external 378.72
    supranuclear, progressive 333.0
    total (external) 378.56
        internal 367.52
    unilateral 378.9
Opisthognathism 524.00
Opisthorchiasis (felineus) (tenuicollis)
    (viverrini) 121.0
Opisthotonos, opisthotonus 781.0
Opitz's disease (congestive splenomegaly)
    289.51
Opiumism (*see also* Dependence) 304.0 ●
Oppenheim's disease 358.8
Oppenheim-Urbach disease or syndrome
    (necrobiosis lipoidica diabeticorum)
    250.8 ● [709.3]
    due to secondary diabetes 249.8 ● [709.3]
Opsoclonia 379.59
Optic nerve - *see* condition
Orbit - *see* condition
Orchioblastoma (M9071/3) 186.9
Orchitis (nonspecific) (septic) 604.90
    with abscess 604.0
    blennorrhagic (acute) 098.13
        chronic or duration of 2 months or over
        098.33
    diphtheritic 032.89 [604.91]
    filarial 125.9 [604.91]
    gangrenous 604.99
    gonococcal (acute) 098.13
        chronic or duration of 2 months or over
        098.33
    mumps 072.0
    parotidea 072.0
    suppurative 604.99
    syphilitic 095.8 [604.91]
    tuberculous (*see also* Tuberculosis) 016.5 ●
        [608.81]
Orf 051.2
Organic - *see also* condition
    heart - *see* Disease, heart
    insufficiency 799.89
Oriental
    bilharziasis 120.2
    schistosomiasis 120.2
    sore 085.1
Orientation
    ego-dystonic sexual 302.0
Orifice - *see* condition
Origin, both great vessels from right ventricle
    745.11
Ormond's disease or syndrome 593.4
Ornithosis 073.9
    with
        complication 073.8
            specified NEC 073.7
        pneumonia 073.0
        pneumonitis (lobular) 073.0
Orodigitofacial dysostosis 759.89
Oropouche fever 066.3
Orotaciduria, oroticacciduria (congenital)
    (hereditary) (pyrimidine deficiency) 281.4
Oroya fever 088.0

Orthodontics V58.5
    adjustment V53.4
    aftercare V58.5
    fitting V53.4
Orthopnea 786.02
Os, uterus - *see* condition
Osgood-Schlatter
    disease 732.4
    osteochondrosis 732.4
Osler's
    disease (M9950/1) (polycythemia vera) 238.4
    nodes 421.0
Osler-Rendu disease (familial hemorrhagic
    telangiectasia) 448.0
Osler-Vaquez disease (M9950/1) (polycythemia
    vera) 238.4
Osler-Weber-Rendu syndrome (familial
    hemorrhagic telangiectasia) 448.0
Osmidrosis 705.89
Osseous - *see* condition
Ossification
    artery - *see* Arteriosclerosis
    auricle (ear) 380.39
    bronchus 519.19
    cardiac (*see also* Degeneration, myocardial)
        429.1
    cartilage (senile) 733.99
    coronary - *see* Arteriosclerosis, coronary
    diaphragm 728.10
    ear 380.39
        middle (*see also* Otosclerosis) 387.9
    falx cerebri 349.2
    fascia 728.10
    fontanel
        defective or delayed 756.0
        premature 756.0
    heart (*see also* Degeneration, myocardial)
        429.1
        valve - *see* Endocarditis
    larynx 478.79
    ligament
        posterior longitudinal 724.8
            cervical 723.7
    meninges (cerebral) 349.2
        spinal 336.8
    multiple, eccentric centers 733.99
    muscle 728.10
        heterotopic, postoperative 728.13
    myocardium, myocardial (*see also*
        Degeneration, myocardial) 429.1
    penis 607.81
    periarticular 728.89
    sclera 379.16
    tendon 727.82
    trachea 519.19
    tympanic membrane (*see also*
        Tympanosclerosis) 385.00
    vitreous (humor) 360.44
Osteitis (*see also* Osteomyelitis) 730.2 ●
    acute 730.0 ●
    alveolar 526.5
    chronic 730.1 ●
    condensans (ilii) 733.5
    deformans (Paget's) 731.0
        due to or associated with malignant
            neoplasm (*see also* Neoplasm, bone,
            malignant) 170.9 [731.1]
    due to yaws 102.6
    fibrosa NEC 733.29
        cystica (generalisata) 252.01
        disseminata 756.59
        osteoplastica 252.01
    fragilitans 756.51
    Garré's (sclerosing) 730.1 ●
    infectious (acute) (subacute) 730.0 ●
        chronic or old 730.1 ●
    jaw (acute) (chronic) (lower) (neonatal)
        (suppurative) (upper) 526.4
    parathyroid 252.01
    petrous bone (*see also* Petrositis) 383.20
    pubis 733.5

Osteitis (*Continued*)
    sclerotic, nonsuppurative 730.1 ●
    syphilitic 095.5
    tuberculosa
        cystica (of Jüngling) 135
        multiplex cystoides 135
Osteoarthritica spondylitis (spine) (*see also*
    Spondylosis) 721.90
Osteoarthritis (*see also* Osteoarthrosis) 715.9 ●
    distal interphalangeal 715.9 ●
    hyperplastic 731.2
    interspinalis (*see also* Spondylosis) 721.90
    spine, spinal NEC (*see also* Spondylosis)
        721.90
Osteoarthropathy (*see also* Osteoarthrosis)
    715.9 ●
    chronic idiopathic hypertrophic 757.39
    familial idiopathic 757.39
    hypertrophic pulmonary 731.2
        secondary 731.2
    idiopathic hypertrophic 757.39
    primary hypertrophic 731.2
    pulmonary hypertrophic 731.2
    secondary hypertrophic 731.2
Osteoarthrosis (degenerative) (hypertrophic)
    (rheumatoid) 715.9 ●

+---+
| Note: Use the following fifth-digit |
| subclassification with category 715: |
| |
| 0   site unspecified |
| 1   shoulder region |
| 2   upper arm |
| 3   forearm |
| 4   hand |
| 5   pelvic region and thigh |
| 6   lower leg |
| 7   ankle and foot |
| 8   other specified sites except spine |
| 9   multiple sites |
+---+

    Deformans alkaptonurica 270.2
    generalized 715.09
    juvenilis (Köhler's) 732.5
    localized 715.3 ●
        idiopathic 715.1 ●
        primary 715.1 ●
        secondary 715.2 ●
    multiple sites, not specified as generalized
        715.89
    polyarticular 715.09
    spine (*see also* Spondylosis) 721.90
    temporomandibular joint 524.69
Osteoblastoma (M9200/0) - *see* Neoplasm,
    bone, benign
Osteochondritis (*see also* Osteochondrosis) 732.9
    dissecans 732.7
        hip 732.7
    ischiopubica 732.1
    multiple 756.59
    syphilitic (congenital) 090.0
Osteochondrodermodysplasia 756.59
Osteochondrodystrophy 277.5
    deformans 277.5
    familial 277.5
    fetalis 756.4
Osteochondrolysis 732.7
Osteochondroma (M9210/0) - *see also*
    Neoplasm, bone, benign
    multiple, congenital 756.4
Osteochondromatosis (M9210/1) 238.0
    synovial 727.82
Osteochondromyxosarcoma (M9180/3) - *see*
    Neoplasm, bone, malignant
Osteochondropathy NEC 732.9
Osteochondrosarcoma (M9180/3) - *see*
    Neoplasm, bone, malignant
Osteochondrosis 732.9
    acetabulum 732.1
    adult spine 732.8
    astragalus 732.5
    Blount's 732.4

Osteochondrosis (Continued)
  Buchanan's (juvenile osteochondrosis of iliac crest) 732.1
  Buchman's (juvenile osteochondrosis) 732.1
  Burns' 732.3
  calcaneus 732.5
  capitular epiphysis (femur) 732.1
  carpal
    lunate (wrist) 732.3
    scaphoid 732.3
  coxae juvenilis 732.1
  deformans juvenilis (coxae) (hip) 732.1
    Scheuermann's 732.0
    spine 732.0
    tibia 732.4
    vertebra 732.0
  Diaz's (astragalus) 732.5
  dissecans (knee) (shoulder) 732.7
  femoral capital epiphysis 732.1
  femur (head) (juvenile) 732.1
  foot (juvenile) 732.5
  Freiberg's (disease) (second metatarsal) 732.5
  Haas' 732.3
  Haglund's (os tibiale externum) 732.5
  hand (juvenile) 732.3
  head of
    femur 732.1
    humerus (juvenile) 732.3
  hip (juvenile) 732.1
  humerus (juvenile) 732.3
  iliac crest (juvenile) 732.1
  ilium (juvenile) 732.1
  ischiopubic synchondrosis 732.1
  Iselin's (osteochondrosis fifth metatarsal) 732.5
  juvenile, juvenilis 732.6
    arm 732.3
    capital femoral epiphysis 732.1
    capitellum humeri 732.3
    capitular epiphysis 732.1
    carpal scaphoid 732.3
    clavicle, sternal epiphysis 732.6
    coxae 732.1
    deformans 732.1
    foot 732.5
    hand 732.3
    hip and pelvis 732.1
    lower extremity, except foot 732.4
    lunate, wrist 732.3
    medial cuneiform bone 732.5
    metatarsal (head) 732.5
    metatarsophalangeal 732.5
    navicular, ankle 732.5
    patella 732.4
    primary patellar center (of Köhler) 732.4
    specified site NEC 732.6
    spine 732.0
    tarsal scaphoid 732.5
    tibia (epiphysis) (tuberosity) 732.4
    upper extremity 732.3
    vertebra (body) (Calvé) 732.0
      epiphyseal plates (of Scheuermann) 732.0
  Kienböck's (disease) 732.3
  Köhler's (disease) (navicular, ankle) 732.5
    patellar 732.4
    tarsal navicular 732.5
  Legg-Calvé-Perthes (disease) 732.1
  lower extremity (juvenile) 732.4
  lunate bone 732.3
  Mauclaire's 732.3
  metacarpal heads (of Mauclaire) 732.3
  metatarsal (fifth) (head) (second) 732.5
  navicular, ankle 732.5
  os calcis 732.5
  Osgood-Schlatter 732.4
  os tibiale externum 732.5
  Panner's 732.3
  patella (juvenile) 732.4

Osteochondrosis (Continued)
  patellar center
    primary (of Köhler) 732.4
    secondary (of Sinding-Larsen) 732.4
  pelvis (juvenile) 732.1
  Pierson's 732.1
  radial head (juvenile) 732.3
  Scheuermann's 732.0
  Sever's (calcaneum) 732.5
  Sinding-Larsen (secondary patellar center) 732.4
  spine (juvenile) 732.0
    adult 732.8
  symphysis pubis (of Pierson) (juvenile) 732.1
  syphilitic (congenital) 090.0
  tarsal (navicular) (scaphoid) 732.5
  tibia (proximal) (tubercle) 732.4
  tuberculous - see Tuberculosis, bone
  ulna 732.3
  upper extremity (juvenile) 732.3
  van Neck's (juvenile osteochondrosis) 732.1
  vertebral (juvenile) 732.0
    adult 732.8
Osteoclastoma (M9250/1) 238.0
  malignant (M9250/3) - see Neoplasm, bone, malignant
Osteocopic pain 733.90
Osteodynia 733.90
Osteodystrophy
  azotemic 588.0
  chronica deformans hypertrophica 731.0
  congenital 756.50
    specified type NEC 756.59
  deformans 731.0
  fibrosa localisata 731.0
  parathyroid 252.01
  renal 588.0
Osteofibroma (M9262/0) - see Neoplasm, bone, benign
Osteofibrosarcoma (M9182/3) - see Neoplasm, bone, malignant
Osteogenesis imperfecta 756.51
Osteogenic - see condition
Osteoma (M9180/0) - see also Neoplasm, bone, benign
  osteoid (M9191/0) - see also Neoplasm, bone, benign
    giant (M9200/0) - see Neoplasm, bone, benign
Osteomalacia 268.2
  chronica deformans hypertrophica 731.0
  due to vitamin D deficiency 268.2
  infantile (see also Rickets) 268.0
  juvenile (see also Rickets) 268.0
  oncogenic 275.8
  pelvis 268.2
  vitamin D-resistant 275.3
Osteomalacic bone 268.2
Osteomalacosis 268.2
Osteomyelitis (general) (infective) (localized) (neonatal) (purulent) (pyogenic) (septic) (staphylococcal) (streptococcal) (suppurative) (with periostitis) 730.2●

> Note: Use the following fifth-digit subclassification with category 730:
>
> 0   site unspecified
> 1   shoulder region
> 2   upper arm
> 3   forearm
> 4   hand
> 5   pelvic region and thigh
> 6   lower leg
> 7   ankle and foot
> 8   other specified sites
> 9   multiple sites

  acute or subacute 730.0●
  chronic or old 730.1●

Osteomyelitis (Continued)
  due to or associated with
    diabetes mellitus 250.8● [731.8]
      due to secondary diabetes 249.8● [731.8]
    tuberculosis (see also Tuberculosis, bone) 015.9● [730.8]●
      limb bones 015.5● [730.8]●
      specified bones NEC 015.7● [730.8]●
      spine 015.0● [730.8]●
    typhoid 002.0 [730.8]●
  Garré's 730.1●
  jaw (acute) (chronic) (lower) (neonatal) (suppurative) (upper) 526.4
  nonsuppurating 730.1●
  orbital 376.03
  petrous bone (see also Petrositis) 383.20
  Salmonella 003.24
  sclerosing, nonsuppurative 730.1●
  sicca 730.1●
  syphilitic 095.5
    congenital 090.0 [730.8]●
  tuberculous - see Tuberculosis, bone
  typhoid 002.0 [730.8]●
Osteomyelofibrosis 289.89
Osteomyelosclerosis 289.89
Osteonecrosis 733.40
  meaning osteomyelitis 730.1●
Osteo-onycho-arthro dysplasia 756.89
Osteo-onychodysplasia, hereditary 756.89
Osteopathia
  condensans disseminata 756.53
  hyperostotica multiplex infantilis 756.59
  hypertrophica toxica 731.2
  striata 756.4
Osteopathy resulting from poliomyelitis (see also Poliomyelitis) 045.9● [730.7]
  familial dysplastic 731.2
Osteopecilia 756.53
Osteopenia 733.90
  borderline 733.90
Osteoperiostitis (see also Osteomyelitis) 730.2●
  ossificans toxica 731.2
  toxica ossificans 731.2
Osteopetrosis (familial) 756.52
Osteophyte - see Exostosis
Osteophytosis - see Exostosis
Osteopoikilosis 756.53
Osteoporosis (generalized) 733.00
  circumscripta 731.0
  disuse 733.03
  drug-induced 733.09
  idiopathic 733.02
  postmenopausal 733.01
  posttraumatic 733.7
  screening V82.81
  senile 733.01
  specified type NEC 733.09
Osteoporosis-osteomalacia syndrome 268.2
Osteopsathyrosis 756.51
Osteoradionecrosis, jaw 526.89
Osteosarcoma (M9180/3) - see also Neoplasm, bone, malignant
  chondroblastic (M9181/3) - see Neoplasm, bone, malignant
  fibroblastic (M9182/3) - see Neoplasm, bone, malignant
  in Paget's disease of bone (M9184/3) - see Neoplasm, bone, malignant
  juxtacortical (M9190/3) - see Neoplasm, bone malignant
  parosteal (M9190/3) - see Neoplasm, bone, malignant
  telangiectatic (M9183/3) - see Neoplasm, bone, malignant
Osteosclerosis 756.52
  fragilis (generalisata) 756.52
Osteosclerotic anemia 289.89
Osteosis
  acromegaloid 757.39
  cutis 709.3

◄ New   ◄═ Revised   d̶e̶l̶e̶t̶e̶d̶ Deleted   ● Use Additional Digit(s)   ▨ Omit code

Osteosis *(Continued)*
  parathyroid 252.01
  renal fibrocystic 588.0
Österreicher-Turner syndrome 756.89
Ostium
  atrioventriculare commune 745.69
  primum (arteriosum) (defect) (persistent) 745.61
  secundum (arteriosum) (defect) (patent) (persistent) 745.5
Ostrum-Furst syndrome 756.59
Otalgia 388.70
  otogenic 388.71
  referred 388.72
Othematoma 380.31
Otitic hydrocephalus 348.2
Otitis 382.9
  with effusion 381.4
    purulent 382.4
    secretory 381.4
    serous 381.4
    suppurative 382.4
  acute 382.9
  adhesive *(see also* Adhesions, middle ear) 385.10
  chronic 382.9
    with effusion 381.3
    mucoid, mucous (simple) 381.20
    purulent 382.3
    secretory 381.3
    serous 381.10
    suppurative 382.3
  diffuse parasitic 136.8
  externa (acute) (diffuse) (hemorrhagica) 380.10
    actinic 380.22
    candidal 112.82
    chemical 380.22
    chronic 380.23
      mycotic - *see* Otitis, externa, mycotic
      specified type NEC 380.23
    circumscribed 380.10
    contact 380.22
    due to
      erysipelas 035 *[380.13]*
      impetigo 684 *[380.13]*
      seborrheic dermatitis 690.10 *[380.13]*
    eczematoid 380.22
    furuncular 680.0 *[380.13]*
    infective 380.10
      chronic 380.16
    malignant 380.14
    mycotic (chronic) 380.15
      due to
        aspergillosis 117.3 *[380.15]*
        moniliasis 112.82
        otomycosis 111.8 *[380.15]*
    reactive 380.22
    specified type NEC 380.22
    tropical 111.8 *[380.15]*
  insidiosa *(see also* Otosclerosis) 387.9
  interna *(see also* Labyrinthitis) 386.30
  media (hemorrhagic) (staphylococcal) (streptococcal) 382.9
    acute 382.9
      with effusion 381.00
      allergic 381.04
        mucoid 381.05
        sanguineous 381.06
        serous 381.04
      catarrhal 381.00
      exudative 381.00
      mucoid 381.02
        allergic 381.05
      necrotizing 382.00
        with spontaneous rupture of ear drum 382.01
        in
          influenza *(see also* Influenza) 487.8 *[382.02]*
          measles 055.2
          scarlet fever 034.1 *[382.02]*

Otitis *(Continued)*
  media *(Continued)*
    acute *(Continued)*
      nonsuppurative 381.00
      purulent 382.00
        with spontaneous rupture of ear drum 382.01
      sanguineous 381.03
        allergic 381.06
      secretory 381.01
      seromucinous 381.02
      serous 381.01
        allergic 381.04
      suppurative 382.00
        with spontaneous rupture of ear drum 382.01
        due to
          influenza *(see also* Influenza) 487.8 *[382.02]*
          scarlet fever 034.1 *[382.02]*
      transudative 381.00
    adhesive *(see also* Adhesions, middle ear) 385.10
    allergic 381.4
      acute 381.04
        mucoid 381.05
        sanguineous 381.06
        serous 381.04
      chronic 381.3
    catarrhal 381.4
      acute 381.00
      chronic (simple) 381.10
    chronic 382.9
      with effusion 381.3
      adhesive *(see also* Adhesions, middle ear) 385.10
      allergic 381.3
      atticoantral, suppurative (with posterior or superior marginal perforation of ear drum) 382.2
      benign suppurative (with anterior perforation of ear drum) 382.1
      catarrhal 381.10
      exudative 381.3
      mucinous 381.20
      mucoid, mucous (simple) 381.20
      mucosanguineous 381.29
      nonsuppurative 381.3
      purulent 382.3
      secretory 381.3
      seromucinous 381.3
      serosanguineous 381.19
      serous (simple) 381.10
      suppurative 382.3
        atticoantral (with posterior or superior marginal perforation of ear drum) 382.2
        benign (with anterior perforation of ear drum) 382.1
        tuberculous *(see also* Tuberculosis) 017.4●
        tubotympanic 382.1
      transudative 381.3
    exudative 381.4
      acute 381.00
      chronic 381.3
    fibrotic *(see also* Adhesions, middle ear) 385.10
    mucoid, mucous 381.4
      acute 381.02
      chronic (simple) 381.20
    mucosanguineous, chronic 381.29
    nonsuppurative 381.4
      acute 381.00
      chronic 381.3
    postmeasles 055.2
    purulent 382.4
      acute 382.00
        with spontaneous rupture of ear drum 382.01
      chronic 382.3

Otitis *(Continued)*
  media *(Continued)*
    sanguineous, acute 381.03
      allergic 381.06
    secretory 381.4
      acute or subacute 381.01
      chronic 381.3
    seromucinous 381.4
      acute or subacute 381.02
      chronic 381.3
    serosanguineous, chronic 381.19
    serous 381.4
      acute or subacute 381.01
      chronic (simple) 381.10
    subacute - *see* Otitis, media, acute
    suppurative 382.4
      acute 382.00
        with spontaneous rupture of ear drum 382.01
      chronic 382.3
        atticoantral 382.2
        benign 382.1
        tuberculous *(see also* Tuberculosis) 017.4●
        tubotympanic 382.1
    transudative 381.4
      acute 381.00
      chronic 381.3
    tuberculous *(see also* Tuberculosis) 017.4●
  postmeasles 055.2
Otoconia 386.8
Otolith syndrome 386.19
Otomycosis 111.8 *[380.15]*
  in
    aspergillosis 117.3 *[380.15]*
    moniliasis 112.82
Otopathy 388.9
Otoporosis *(see also* Otosclerosis) 387.9
Otorrhagia 388.69
  traumatic - *see* nature of injury
Otorrhea 388.60
  blood 388.69
  cerebrospinal (fluid) 388.61
Otosclerosis (general) 387.9
  cochlear (endosteal) 387.2
  involving
    otic capsule 387.2
    oval window
      nonobliterative 387.0
      obliterative 387.1
    round window 387.2
  nonobliterative 387.0
  obliterative 387.1
  specified type NEC 387.8
Otospongiosis *(see also* Otosclerosis) 387.9
Otto's disease or pelvis 715.35
Outburst, aggressive *(see also* Disturbance, conduct) 312.0●
  in children or adolescents 313.9
Outcome of delivery
  multiple birth NEC V27.9
    all liveborn V27.5
    all stillborn V27.7
    some liveborn V27.6
    unspecified V27.9
  single V27.9
    liveborn V27.0
    stillborn V27.1
  twins V27.9
    both liveborn V27.2
    both stillborn V27.4
    one liveborn, one stillborn V27.3
Outlet - *see also* condition
  syndrome (thoracic) 353.0
Outstanding ears (bilateral) 744.29
Ovalocytosis (congenital) (hereditary) *(see also* Elliptocytosis) 282.1
Ovarian - *see also* condition
  pregnancy - *see* Pregnancy, ovarian
  remnant syndrome 620.8
  vein syndrome 593.4

Ovaritis (cystic) (*see also* Salpingo-oophoritis) 614.2

Ovary, ovarian - *see* condition

Overactive - *see also* Hyperfunction
  bladder 596.51
  eye muscle (*see also* Strabismus) 378.9
  hypothalamus 253.8
  thyroid (*see also* Thyrotoxicosis) 242.9●

Overactivity, child 314.01

Overbite (deep) (excessive) (horizontal) (vertical) 524.29

Overbreathing (*see also* Hyperventilation) 786.01

Overconscientious personality 301.4

Overdevelopment - *see also* Hypertrophy
  breast (female) (male) 611.1
  nasal bones 738.0
  prostate, congenital 752.89

Overdistention - *see* Distention

Overdose, overdosage (drug) 977.9
  specified drug or substance - *see* Table of Drugs and Chemicals

Overeating 783.6
  nonorganic origin 307.51

Overexertion (effects) (exhaustion) 994.5

Overexposure (effects) 994.9
  exhaustion 994.4

Overfeeding (*see also* Overeating) 783.6

Overfill, endodontic 526.62

Overgrowth, bone NEC 733.99

Overhanging
  tooth restoration 525.62
  unrepairable, dental restorative materials 525.62

Overheated (effects) (places) - *see* Heat

Overinhibited child 313.0

Overjet 524.29
  excessive horizontal 524.26

Overlaid, overlying (suffocation) 994.7

Overlap
  excessive horizontal 524.26

Overlapping toe (acquired) 735.8
  congenital (fifth toe) 755.66

Overload
  fluid 276.69
    due to transfusion (blood) (blood components) 276.61
  iron, due to repeated red blood cell transfusions 275.02
  potassium (K) 276.7
  sodium (Na) 276.0
  transfusion associated circulatory (TACO) 276.61

Overnutrition (*see also* Hyperalimentation) 783.6

Overproduction - *see also* Hypersecretion
  ACTH 255.3
  cortisol 255.0
  growth hormone 253.0
  thyroid-stimulating hormone (TSH) 242.8●

Overriding
  aorta 747.21
  finger (acquired) 736.29
    congenital 755.59
  toe (acquired) 735.8
    congenital 755.66

Oversize
  fetus (weight of 4500 grams or more) 766.0
    affecting management of pregnancy 656.6●

Oversize (*Continued*)
  fetus (*Continued*)
    causing disproportion 653.5●
      with obstructed labor 660.1●
      affecting fetus or newborn 763.1

Overstimulation, ovarian 256.1

Overstrained 780.79
  heart - *see* Hypertrophy, cardiac

Overweight (*see also* Obesity) 278.02

Overwork 780.79

Oviduct - *see* condition

Ovotestis 752.7

Ovulation (cycle)
  failure or lack of 628.0
  pain 625.2

Ovum
  blighted 631.8
  donor V59.70
    over age 35 V59.73
      anonymous recipient V59.73
      designated recipient V59.74
    under age 35 V59.71
      anonymous recipient V59.71
      designated recipient V59.72
  dropsical 631.8
  pathologic 631.8

Owren's disease or syndrome (parahemophilia) (*see also* Defect, coagulation) 286.3

Oxalosis 271.8

Oxaluria 271.8

Ox heart - *see* Hypertrophy, cardiac

OX syndrome 758.6

Oxycephaly, oxycephalic 756.0
  syphilitic, congenital 090.0

Oxyuriasis 127.4

Oxyuris vermicularis (infestation) 127.4

Ozena 472.0

◀ New　◀꜒ Revised　~~deleted~~ Deleted　● Use Additional Digit(s)　▨ Omit code

P

Pacemaker syndrome 429.4
Pachyderma, pachydermia 701.8
 laryngis 478.5
 laryngitis 478.79
 larynx (verrucosa) 478.79
Pachydermatitis 701.8
Pachydermatocele (congenital) 757.39
 acquired 701.8
Pachydermatosis 701.8
Pachydermoperiostitis
 secondary 731.2
Pachydermoperiostosis
 primary idiopathic 757.39
 secondary 731.2
Pachymeningitis (adhesive) (basal) (brain)
  (cerebral) (cervical) (chronic)
  (circumscribed) (external) (fibrous)
  (hemorrhagic) (hypertrophic) (internal)
  (purulent) (spinal) (suppurative) (see also
  Meningitis) 322.9
 gonococcal 098.82
Pachyonychia (congenital) 757.5
 acquired 703.8
Pachyperiosteodermia
 primary or idiopathic 757.39
 secondary 731.2
Pachyperiostosis
 primary or idiopathic 757.39
 secondary 731.2
Pacinian tumor (M9507/0) - see Neoplasm, skin,
 benign
Pads, knuckle or Garrod's 728.79
Paget's disease (osteitis deformans) 731.0
 with infiltrating duct carcinoma of the breast
  (M8541/3) - see Neoplasm, breast,
  malignant
 bone 731.0
  osteosarcoma in (M9184/3) - see
   Neoplasm, bone, malignant
 breast (M8540/3) 174.0
 extramammary (M8542/3) - see also
  Neoplasm, skin, malignant
  anus 154.3
   skin 173.59
 malignant (M8540/3)
  breast 174.0
  specified site NEC (M8542/3) - see
   Neoplasm, skin, malignant
  unspecified site 174.0
 mammary (M8540/3) 174.0
 necrosis of bone 731.0
 nipple (M8540/3) 174.0
 osteitis deformans 731.0
Paget-Schroetter syndrome (intermittent
 venous claudication) 453.89
Pain(s) (see also Painful) 780.96
 abdominal 789.0●
 acute 338.19
  due to trauma 338.11
  postoperative 338.18
   post-thoracotomy 338.12
 adnexa (uteri) 625.9
 alimentary, due to vascular insufficiency
  557.9
 anginoid (see also Pain, precordial) 786.51
 anus 569.42
 arch 729.5
 arm 729.5
 axillary 729.5
 back (postural) 724.5
  low 724.2
  psychogenic 307.89
 bile duct 576.9
 bladder 788.99
 bone 733.90
 breast 611.71
  psychogenic 307.89
 broad ligament 625.9
 cancer associated 338.3

Pain(s) (Continued)
 cartilage NEC 733.90
 cecum 789.0●
 cervicobrachial 723.3
 chest (central) 786.50
  atypical 786.59
  midsternal 786.51
  musculoskeletal 786.59
  noncardiac 786.59
  substernal 786.51
  wall (anterior) 786.52
 chronic 338.29
  associated with significant psychosocial
   dysfunction 338.4
  due to trauma 338.21
  postoperative 338.28
   post-thoracotomy 338.22
  syndrome 338.4
 coccyx 724.79
 colon 789.0●
 common duct 576.9
 coronary - see Angina
 costochondral 786.52
 diaphragm 786.52
 due to (presence of) any device, implant, or
  graft classifiable to 996.0–996.5 - see
  Complications, due to (presence of)
  any device, implant, or graft classified
  to 996.0–996.5 NEC
 malignancy (primary) (secondary) 338.3
 ear (see also Otalgia) 388.70
 epigastric, epigastrium 789.06
 extremity (lower) (upper) 729.5
 eye 379.91
 face, facial 784.0
  atypical 350.2
  nerve 351.8
 false (labor) 644.1●
 female genital organ NEC 625.9
  psychogenic 307.89
 finger 729.5
 flank 789.0●
 foot 729.5
 gallbladder 575.9
 gas (intestinal) 787.3
 gastric 536.8
 generalized 780.96
 genital organ
  female 625.9
  male 608.9
  psychogenic 307.89
 groin 789.0●
 growing 781.99
 hand 729.5
 head (see also Headache) 784.0
 heart (see also Pain, precordial) 786.51
 infraorbital (see also Neuralgia, trigeminal)
  350.1
 intermenstrual 625.2
 jaw 784.92
 joint 719.40
  ankle 719.47
  elbow 719.42
  foot 719.47
  hand 719.44
  hip 719.45
  knee 719.46
  multiple sites 719.49
  pelvic region 719.45
  psychogenic 307.89
  shoulder (region) 719.41
  specified site NEC 719.48
  wrist 719.43
 kidney 788.0
 labor, false or spurious 644.1●
 laryngeal 784.1
 leg 729.5
 limb 729.5
 low back 724.2
 lumbar region 724.2
 mandible, mandibular 784.92

Pain(s) (Continued)
 mastoid (see also Otalgia) 388.70
 maxilla 784.92
 menstrual 625.3
 metacarpophalangeal (joint) 719.44
 metatarsophalangeal (joint) 719.47
 mouth 528.9
 muscle 729.1
  intercostal 786.59
 musculoskeletal (see also Pain, by site) 729.1
 nasal 478.19
 nasopharynx 478.29
 neck NEC 723.1
  psychogenic 307.89
 neoplasm related (acute) (chronic) 338.3
 nerve NEC 729.2
 neuromuscular 729.1
 nose 478.19
 ocular 379.91
 ophthalmic 379.91
 orbital region 379.91
 osteocopic 733.90
 ovary 625.9
  psychogenic 307.89
 over heart (see also Pain, precordial) 786.51
 ovulation 625.2
 pelvic (female) 625.9
  male NEC 789.0●
   psychogenic 307.89
  psychogenic 307.89
 penis 607.9
  psychogenic 307.89
 pericardial (see also Pain, precordial) 786.51
 perineum
  female 625.9
  male 608.9
 pharynx 478.29
 pleura, pleural, pleuritic 786.52
 postoperative 338.18
  acute 338.18
  chronic 338.28
 post-thoracotomy 338.12
  acute 338.12
  chronic 338.22
 preauricular 388.70
 precordial (region) 786.51
  psychogenic 307.89
 premenstrual 625.4
 psychogenic 307.80
  cardiovascular system 307.89
  gastrointestinal system 307.89
  genitourinary system 307.89
  heart 307.89
  musculoskeletal system 307.89
  respiratory system 307.89
  skin 306.3
 radicular (spinal) (see also Radiculitis)
  729.2
 rectum 569.42
 respiration 786.52
 retrosternal 786.51
 rheumatic NEC 729.0
  muscular 729.1
 rib 786.50
 root (spinal) (see also Radiculitis) 729.2
 round ligament (stretch) 625.9
 sacroiliac 724.6
 sciatic 724.3
 scrotum 608.9
  psychogenic 307.89
 seminal vesicle 608.9
 sinus 478.19
 skin 782.0
 spermatic cord 608.9
 spinal root (see also Radiculitis) 729.2
 stomach 536.8
  psychogenic 307.89
 substernal 786.51
 temporomandibular (joint) 524.62
 testis 608.9
  psychogenic 307.89

Pain(s) *(Continued)*
  thoracic spine 724.1
    with radicular and visceral pain
      724.4
  throat 784.1
  tibia 733.90
  toe 729.5
  tongue 529.6
  tooth 525.9
  trigeminal *(see also* Neuralgia, trigeminal)
    350.1
  tumor associated 338.3
  umbilicus 789.05
  ureter 788.0
  urinary (organ) (system) 788.0
  uterus 625.9
    psychogenic 307.89
  vagina 625.9
  vertebrogenic (syndrome) 724.5
  vesical 788.99
  vulva 625.9
  xiphoid 733.90
Painful - *see also* Pain
  arc syndrome 726.19
  coitus
    female 625.0
    male 608.89
    psychogenic 302.76
  ejaculation (semen) 608.89
    psychogenic 302.79
  erection 607.3
  feet syndrome 266.2
  menstruation 625.3
    psychogenic 306.52
  micturition 788.1
  ophthalmoplegia 378.55
  respiration 786.52
  scar NEC 709.2
  total hip replacement 996.77
  total knee replacement 996.77
  urination 788.1
  wire sutures 998.89
Painters' colic 984.9
  specified type of lead - *see* Table of Drugs
    and Chemicals
Palate - *see* condition
Palatoplegia 528.9
Palatoschisis *(see also* Cleft, palate) 749.00
Palilalia 784.69
Palindromic arthritis *(see also* Rheumatism,
  palindromic) 719.3●
Palliative care V66.7
Pallor 782.61
  temporal, optic disc 377.15
Palmar - *see also* condition
  fascia - *see* condition
Palpable
  cecum 569.89
  kidney 593.89
  liver 573.9
  lymph nodes 785.6
  ovary 620.8
  prostate 602.9
  spleen *(see also* Splenomegaly) 789.2
  uterus 625.8
Palpitation (heart) 785.1
  psychogenic 306.2
Palsy *(see also* Paralysis) 344.9
  atrophic diffuse 335.20
  Bell's 351.0
    newborn 767.5
  birth 767.7
  brachial plexus 353.0
    fetus or newborn 767.6
  brain - *see also* Palsy, cerebral
    noncongenital or noninfantile
      344.89
      late effect - *see* Late effect(s) (of)
        cerebrovascular disease
    syphilitic 094.89
      congenital 090.49

Palsy *(Continued)*
  bulbar (chronic) (progressive) 335.22
    pseudo NEC 335.23
    supranuclear NEC 344.89
  cerebral (congenital) (infantile) (spastic)
    343.9
    athetoid 333.71
    diplegic 343.0
      late effect - *see* Late effect(s) (of)
        cerebrovascular disease
    hemiplegic 343.1
    monoplegic 343.3
    noncongenital or noninfantile 437.8
      late effect - *see* Late effect(s) (of)
        cerebrovascular disease
    paraplegic 343.0
    quadriplegic 343.2
    spastic, not congenital or infantile 344.89
    syphilitic 094.89
      congenital 090.49
    tetraplegic 343.2
  cranial nerve - *see also* Disorder, nerve,
    cranial
    multiple 352.6
  creeping 335.21
  divers' 993.3
  Erb's (birth injury) 767.6
  facial 351.0
    newborn 767.5
  glossopharyngeal 352.2
  Klumpke (-Déjérine) 767.6
  lead 984.9
    specified type of lead - *see* Table of Drugs
      and Chemicals
  median nerve (tardy) 354.0
  peroneal nerve (acute) (tardy) 355.3
  progressive supranuclear 333.0
  pseudobulbar NEC 335.23
  radial nerve (acute) 354.3
  seventh nerve 351.0
    newborn 767.5
  shaking *(see also* Parkinsonism) 332.0
  spastic (cerebral) (spinal) 343.9
    hemiplegic 343.1
  specified nerve NEC - *see* Disorder, nerve
  supranuclear NEC 356.8
    progressive 333.0
  ulnar nerve (tardy) 354.2
  wasting 335.21
Paltauf-Sternberg disease 201.9●
Paludism - *see* Malaria
Panama fever 084.0
Panaris (with lymphangitis) 681.9
  finger 681.02
  toe 681.11
Panaritium (with lymphangitis) 681.9
  finger 681.02
  toe 681.11
Panarteritis (nodosa) 446.0
  brain or cerebral 437.4
Pancake heart 793.2
  with cor pulmonale (chronic) 416.9
Pancarditis (acute) (chronic) 429.89
  with
    rheumatic
      fever (active) (acute) (chronic)
        (subacute) 391.8
      inactive or quiescent 398.99
  rheumatic, acute 391.8
    chronic or inactive 398.99
Pancoast's syndrome or tumor (carcinoma,
  pulmonary apex) (M8010/3) 162.3
Pancoast-Tobias syndrome (M8010/3)
  (carcinoma, pulmonary apex) 162.3
Pancolitis 556.6
Pancreas, pancreatic - *see* condition
Pancreatitis 577.0
  acute (edematous) (hemorrhagic) (recurrent)
    577.0
  annular 577.0
  apoplectic 577.0

Pancreatitis *(Continued)*
  calcereous 577.0
  chronic (infectious) 577.1
    recurrent 577.1
  cystic 577.2
  fibrous 577.8
  gangrenous 577.0
  hemorrhagic (acute) 577.0
  interstitial (chronic) 577.1
    acute 577.0
  malignant 577.0
  mumps 072.3
  painless 577.1
  recurrent 577.1
  relapsing 577.1
  subacute 577.0
  suppurative 577.0
  syphilitic 095.8
Pancreatolithiasis 577.8
Pancytolysis 289.9
Pancytopenia (acquired) 284.19
  with
    malformations 284.09
    myelodysplastic syndrome - *see*
      Syndrome, myelodysplastic
  congenital 284.09
  due to
    antineoplastic chemotherapy 284.11
    drug, specified NEC 284.12
  specified NEC 284.19
Panencephalitis - *see also* Encephalitis
  subacute, sclerosing 046.2
Panhematopenia 284.81
  congenital 284.09
  constitutional 284.09
  splenic, primary 289.4
Panhemocytopenia 284.81
  congenital 284.09
  constitutional 284.09
Panhypogonadism 257.2
Panhypopituitarism 253.2
  prepubertal 253.3
Panic (attack) (state) 300.01
  reaction to exceptional stress (transient) 308.0
Panmyelopathy, familial constitutional 284.09
Panmyelophthisis 284.2
  acquired (secondary) 284.81
  congenital 284.2
  idiopathic 284.9
Panmyelosis (acute) (M9951/1) 238.79
Panner's disease 732.3
  capitellum humeri 732.3
  head of humerus 732.3
  tarsal navicular (bone) (osteochondrosis)
    732.5
Panneuritis endemica 265.0 *[357.4]*
Panniculitis 729.30
  back 724.8
  knee 729.31
  mesenteric 567.82
  neck 723.6
  nodular, nonsuppurative 729.30
  sacral 724.8
  specified site NEC 729.39
Panniculus adiposus (abdominal) 278.1
Pannus (corneal) 370.62
  abdominal (symptomatic) 278.1
  allergic eczematous 370.62
  degenerativus 370.62
  keratic 370.62
  rheumatoid - *see* Arthritis, rheumatoid
  trachomatosus, trachomatous (active) 076.1
    [370.62]
    late effect 139.1
Panophthalmitis 360.02
Panotitis - *see* Otitis media
Pansinusitis (chronic) (hyperplastic)
  (nonpurulent) (purulent) 473.8
  acute 461.8
  due to fungus NEC 117.9
  tuberculous *(see also* Tuberculosis) 012.8●

◀ New   ◀▦ Revised   ~~deleted~~ Deleted   ● Use Additional Digit(s)   Omit code

Panuveitis 360.12
  sympathetic 360.11
Panvalvular disease - see Endocarditis, mitral
Papageienkrankheit 073.9
Papanicolaou smear
  anus 796.70
    with
      atypical squamous cells
        cannot exclude high grade
          squamous intraepithelial
          lesion (ASC-H) 796.72
        of undetermined significance
          (ASC-US) 796.71
      cytologic evidence of malignancy
        796.76
      high grade squamous intraepithelial
        lesion (HGSIL) 796.74
      low grade squamous intraepithelial
        lesion (LGSIL) 796.73
    glandular 796.70
    specified finding NEC 796.79
    unsatisfactory cytology 796.78
  cervix (screening test) V76.2
    as part of gynecological examination
      V72.31
    for suspected malignant neoplasm V76.2
      no disease found V71.1
    inadequate cytology sample 795.08
    nonspecific abnormal finding 795.00
      with
        atypical squamous cells
          cannot exclude high grade
            squamous intraepithelial
            lesion (ASC-H) 795.02
          of undetermined significance
            (ASC-US) 795.01
        cytologic evidence of malignancy
          795.06
        high grade squamous
          intraepithelial lesion (HGSIL)
          795.04
        low grade squamous intraepithelial
          lesion (LGSIL) 795.03
      nonspecific finding NEC 795.09
    to confirm findings of recent normal
      smear following initial abnormal
      smear V72.32
    satisfactory smear but lacking
      transformation zone 795.07
    unsatisfactory cervical cytology 795.08
  other specified site - see also Screening,
    malignant neoplasm
    for suspected malignant neoplasm - see
      also Screening, malignant neoplasm
      no disease found V71.1
    nonspecific abnormal finding 796.9
  vagina V76.47
    with
      atypical squamous cells
        cannot exclude high grade
          squamous intraepithelial
          lesion (ASC-H) 795.12
        of undetermined significance
          (ASC-US) 795.11
      cytologic evidence of malignancy
        795.16
      high grade squamous
        intraepithelial lesion (HGSIL)
        795.14
      low grade squamous intraepithelial
        lesion (LGSIL) 795.13
    abnormal NEC 795.19
    following hysterectomy for malignant
      condition V67.01
    inadequate cytology sample 795.18
    unsatisfactory cytology 795.18
Papilledema 377.00
  associated with
    decreased ocular pressure 377.02
    increased intracranial pressure 377.01
    retinal disorder 377.03

Papilledema (Continued)
    choked disc 377.00
    infectional 377.00
Papillitis 377.31
    anus 569.49
    chronic lingual 529.4
    necrotizing, kidney 584.7
    optic 377.31
    rectum 569.49
    renal, necrotizing 584.7
    tongue 529.0
Papilloma (M8050/0) - see also Neoplasm, by
    site, benign

Note: Except where otherwise indicated,
the morphological varieties of papilloma in
the list below should be coded by site as for
"Neoplasm, benign".

    acuminatum (female) (male) 078.11
    bladder (urinary) (transitional cell)
      (M8120/1) 236.7
      benign (M8120/0) 223.3
    choroid plexus (M9390/0) 225.0
      anaplastic type (M9390/3) 191.5
      malignant (M9390/3) 191.5
    ductal (M8503/0)
    dyskeratotic (M8052/0)
    epidermoid (M8052/0)
    hyperkeratotic (M8052/0)
    intracystic (M8504/0)
    intraductal (M8503/0)
    inverted (M8053/0)
    keratotic (M8052/0)
    parakeratotic (M8052/0)
    pinta (primary) 103.0
    renal pelvis (transitional cell) (M8120/1)
      236.99
      benign (M8120/0) 223.1
    Schneiderian (M8121/0)
      specified site - see Neoplasm, by site,
        benign
      unspecified site 212.0
    serous surface (M8461/0)
      borderline malignancy (M8461/1)
        specified site - see Neoplasm, by site,
          uncertain behavior
        unspecified site 236.2
      specified site - see Neoplasm, by site,
        benign
      unspecified site 220
    squamous (cell) (M8052/0)
    transitional (cell) (M8120/0)
      bladder (urinary) (M8120/1) 236.7
      inverted type (M8121/1) - see Neoplasm,
        by site, uncertain behavior
      renal pelvis (M8120/1) 236.91
      ureter (M8120/1) 236.91
    ureter (transitional cell) (M8120/1)
      236.91
      benign (M8120/0) 223.2
    urothelial (M8120/1) - see Neoplasm, by site,
      uncertain behavior
    verrucous (M8051/0)
    villous (M8261/1) - see Neoplasm, by site,
      uncertain behavior
    yaws, plantar or palmar 102.1
Papillomata, multiple, of yaws 102.1
Papillomatosis (M8060/0) - see also Neoplasm,
    by site, benign
    confluent and reticulate 701.8
    cutaneous 701.8
    ductal, breast 610.1
    Gougerot-Carteaud (confluent reticulate)
      701.8
    intraductal (diffuse) (M8505/0) - see
      Neoplasm, by site, benign
    subareolar duct (M8506/0) 217
Papillon-Léage and Psaume syndrome
    (orodigitofacial dysostosis)
    759.89

Papule 709.8
  carate (primary) 103.0
  fibrous, of nose (M8724/0) 216.3
  pinta (primary) 103.0
Papulosis
  lymphomatoid 709.8
  malignant 447.8
Papyraceous fetus 779.89
  complicating pregnancy 646.0●
Paracephalus 759.7
Parachute mitral valve 746.5
Paracoccidioidomycosis 116.1
  mucocutaneous-lymphangitic 116.1
  pulmonary 116.1
  visceral 116.1
Paracoccidiomycosis - see
    Paracoccidioidomycosis
Paracusis 388.40
Paradentosis 523.5
Paradoxical facial movements 374.43
Paraffinoma 999.9
Paraganglioma (M8680/1)
  adrenal (M8700/0) 227.0
    malignant (M8700/3) 194.0
  aortic body (M8691/1) 237.3
    malignant (M8691/3) 194.6
  carotid body (M8692/1) 237.3
    malignant (M8692/3) 194.5
  chromaffin (M8700/0) - see also Neoplasm,
    by site, benign
    malignant (M8700/3) - see Neoplasm, by
      site, malignant
  extra-adrenal (M8693/1)
    malignant (M8693/3)
      specified site - see Neoplasm, by site,
        malignant
      unspecified site 194.6
    specified site - see Neoplasm, by site,
      uncertain behavior
    unspecified site 237.3
  glomus jugulare (M8690/1) 237.3
    malignant (M8690/3) 194.6
  jugular (M8690/1) 237.3
  malignant (M8680/3)
    specified site - see Neoplasm, by site,
      malignant
    unspecified site 194.6
  nonchromaffin (M8693/1)
    malignant (M8693/3)
      specified site - see Neoplasm, by site,
        malignant
      unspecified site 194.6
    specified site - see Neoplasm, by site,
      uncertain behavior
    unspecified site 237.3
  parasympathetic (M8682/1)
    specified site - see Neoplasm, by site,
      uncertain behavior
    unspecified site 237.3
  specified site - see Neoplasm, by site,
    uncertain behavior
  sympathetic (M8681/1)
    specified site - see Neoplasm, by site,
      uncertain behavior
    unspecified site 237.3
  unspecified site 237.3
Parageusia 781.1
  psychogenic 306.7
Paragonimiasis 121.2
Paragranuloma, Hodgkin's (M9660/3) 201.0●
Parahemophilia (see also Defect, coagulation)
    286.3
Parakeratosis 690.8
  psoriasiformis 696.2
  variegata 696.2
Paralysis, paralytic (complete) (incomplete)
    344.9
  with
    broken
      back - see Fracture, vertebra, by site,
        with spinal cord injury

Paralysis, paralytic (Continued)
  with (Continued)
    broken (Continued)
      neck - see Fracture, vertebra, cervical,
          with spinal cord injury
      fracture, vertebra - see Fracture, vertebra,
          by site, with spinal cord injury
    syphilis 094.89
  abdomen and back muscles 355.9
  abdominal muscles 355.9
  abducens (nerve) 378.54
  abductor 355.9
    lower extremity 355.8
    upper extremity 354.9
  accessory nerve 352.4
  accommodation 367.51
    hysterical 300.11
  acoustic nerve 388.5
  agitans 332.0
    arteriosclerotic 332.0
  alternating 344.89
    oculomotor 344.89
  amyotrophic 335.20
  ankle 355.8
  anterior serratus 355.9
  anus (sphincter) 569.49
  apoplectic (current episode) (see also Disease,
      cerebrovascular, acute) 436
    late effect - see Late effect(s) (of)
        cerebrovascular disease
  arm 344.40
    affecting
      dominant side 344.41
      nondominant side 344.42
    both 344.2
    hysterical 300.11
    late effect - see Late effect(s) (of)
        cerebrovascular disease
    psychogenic 306.0
    transient 781.4
      traumatic NEC (see also Injury, nerve,
          upper limb) 955.9
  arteriosclerotic (current episode) 437.0
    late effect - see Late effect(s) (of)
        cerebrovascular disease
  ascending (spinal), acute 357.0
  associated, nuclear 344.89
  asthenic bulbar 358.00
  ataxic NEC 334.9
    general 094.1
  athetoid 333.71
  atrophic 356.9
    infantile, acute (see also Poliomyelitis, with
        paralysis) 045.1●
    muscle NEC 355.9
    progressive 335.21
    spinal (acute) (see also Poliomyelitis, with
        paralysis) 045.1●
  attack (see also Disease, cerebrovascular,
      acute) 436
  axillary 353.0
  Babinski-Nageotte's 344.89
  Bell's 351.0
    newborn 767.5
  Benedikt's 344.89
  birth (injury) 767.7
    brain 767.0
    intracranial 767.0
    spinal cord 767.4
  bladder (sphincter) 596.53
    neurogenic 596.54
      with cauda equina syndrome 344.61
    puerperal, postpartum, childbirth 665.5●
    sensory 596.54
      with cauda equina 344.61
    spastic 596.54
      with cauda equina 344.61
  bowel, colon, or intestine (see also Ileus) 560.1
  brachial plexus 353.0
    due to birth injury 767.6
    newborn 767.6

Paralysis, paralytic (Continued)
  brain
    congenital - see Palsy, cerebral
    current episode 437.8
    diplegia 344.2
      late effect - see Late effect(s) (of)
          cerebrovascular disease
    hemiplegia 342.9●
      late effect - see Late effect(s) (of)
          cerebrovascular disease
    infantile - see Palsy, cerebral
    monoplegia - see Monoplegia
      late effect - see Late effect(s) (of)
          cerebrovascular disease
    paraplegia 344.1
    quadriplegia - see Quadriplegia
    syphilitic, congenital 090.49
    triplegia 344.89
  bronchi 519.19
  Brown-Séquard's 344.89
  bulbar (chronic) (progressive) 335.22
    infantile (see also Poliomyelitis, bulbar)
        045.0●
    poliomyelitic (see also Poliomyelitis,
        bulbar) 045.0●
    pseudo 335.23
    supranuclear 344.89
  bulbospinal 358.00
  cardiac (see also Failure, heart) 428.9
  cerebral
    current episode 437.8
    spastic, infantile - see Palsy,
        cerebral
  cerebrocerebellar 437.8
    diplegic infantile 343.0
  cervical
    plexus 353.2
    sympathetic NEC 337.09
  Céstan-Chenais 344.89
  Charcôt-Marie-Tooth type 356.1
  childhood - see Palsy, cerebral
  Clark's 343.9
  colon (see also Ileus) 560.1
  compressed air 993.3
  compression
    arm NEC 354.9
    cerebral - see Paralysis, brain
    leg NEC 355.8
    lower extremity NEC 355.8
    upper extremity NEC 354.9
  congenital (cerebral) (spastic) (spinal) - see
      Palsy, cerebral
  conjugate movement (of eye) 378.81
    cortical (nuclear) (supranuclear)
        378.81
  convergence 378.83
  cordis (see also Failure, heart) 428.9
  cortical (see also Paralysis, brain) 437.8
  cranial or cerebral nerve (see also Disorder,
      nerve, cranial) 352.9
  creeping 335.21
  crossed leg 344.89
  crutch 953.4
  deglutition 784.99
    hysterical 300.11
  dementia 094.1
  descending (spinal) NEC 335.9
  diaphragm (flaccid) 519.4
    due to accidental section of phrenic nerve
        during procedure 998.2
  digestive organs NEC 564.89
  diplegic - see Diplegia
  divergence (nuclear) 378.85
  divers' 993.3
  Duchenne's 335.22
  due to intracranial or spinal birth injury - see
      Palsy, cerebral
  embolic (current episode) (see also Embolism,
      brain) 434.1●
    late effect - see Late effect(s) (of)
        cerebrovascular disease

Paralysis, paralytic (Continued)
  enteric (see also Ileus) 560.1
    with hernia - see Hernia, by site, with
        obstruction
  Erb's syphilitic spastic spinal 094.89
  Erb (-Duchenne) (birth) (newborn) 767.6
  esophagus 530.89
  essential, infancy (see also Poliomyelitis)
      045.9●
  extremity
    lower - see Paralysis, leg
    spastic (hereditary) 343.3
      noncongenital or noninfantile 344.1
    transient (cause unknown) 781.4
    upper - see Paralysis, arm
  eye muscle (extrinsic) 378.55
    intrinsic 367.51
  facial (nerve) 351.0
    birth injury 767.5
    congenital 767.5
    following operation NEC 998.2
    newborn 767.5
  familial 359.3
    periodic 359.3
    spastic 334.1
  fauces 478.29
  finger NEC 354.9
  foot NEC 355.8
  gait 781.2
  gastric nerve 352.3
  gaze 378.81
  general 094.1
    ataxic 094.1
    insane 094.1
    juvenile 090.40
    progressive 094.1
    tabetic 094.1
  glossopharyngeal (nerve) 352.2
  glottis (see also Paralysis, vocal cord) 478.30
  gluteal 353.4
  Gubler (-Millard) 344.89
  hand 354.9
    hysterical 300.11
    psychogenic 306.0
  heart (see also Failure, heart) 428.9
  hemifacial, progressive 349.89
  hemiplegic - see Hemiplegia
  hyperkalemic periodic (familial) 359.3
  hypertensive (current episode) 437.8
  hypoglossal (nerve) 352.5
  hypokalemic periodic 359.3
  Hyrtl's sphincter (rectum) 569.49
  hysterical 300.11
  ileus (see also Ileus) 560.1
  infantile (see also Poliomyelitis) 045.9●
    atrophic acute 045.1●
    bulbar 045.0●
    cerebral - see Palsy, cerebral
    paralytic 045.1●
    progressive acute 045.9●
    spastic - see Palsy, cerebral
    spinal 045.9●
  infective (see also Poliomyelitis) 045.9●
  inferior nuclear 344.9
  insane, general or progressive 094.1
  internuclear 378.86
  interosseous 355.9
  intestine (see also Ileus) 560.1
  intracranial (current episode) (see also
      Paralysis, brain) 437.8
    due to birth injury 767.0
  iris 379.49
    due to diphtheria (toxin) 032.81 [379.49]
  ischemic, Volkmann's (complicating trauma)
      958.6
  isolated sleep, recurrent 327.43
  Jackson's 344.89
  jake 357.7
  Jamaica ginger (jake) 357.7
  juvenile general 090.40
  Klumpke (-Déjérine) (birth) (newborn) 767.6

◀ New   ◀▥ Revised   ~~deleted~~ Deleted   ● Use Additional Digit(s)   ▨ Omit code

Paralysis, paralytic (Continued)
  labioglossal (laryngeal) (pharyngeal) 335.22
  Landry's 357.0
  laryngeal nerve (recurrent) (superior) (see also Paralysis, vocal cord) 478.30
  larynx (see also Paralysis, vocal cord) 478.30
    due to diphtheria (toxin) 032.3
  late effect
    due to
      birth injury, brain or spinal (cord) - see Palsy, cerebral
      edema, brain or cerebral - see Paralysis, brain
      lesion
        late effect - see Late effect(s) (of) cerebrovascular disease
      spinal (cord) - see Paralysis, spinal
  lateral 335.24
  lead 984.9
    specified type of lead - see Table of Drugs and Chemicals
  left side - see Hemiplegia
  leg 344.30
    affecting
      dominant side 344.31
      nondominant side 344.32
    both (see also Paraplegia) 344.1
    crossed 344.89
    hysterical 300.11
    psychogenic 306.0
    transient or transitory 781.4
      traumatic NEC (see also Injury, nerve, lower limb) 956.9
  levator palpebrae superioris 374.31
  limb NEC 344.5
    all four - see Quadriplegia
    quadriplegia - see Quadriplegia
  lip 528.5
  Lissauer's 094.1
  local 355.9
  lower limb - see also Paralysis, leg
    both (see also Paraplegia) 344.1
  lung 518.89
    newborn 770.89
  median nerve 354.1
  medullary (tegmental) 344.89
  mesencephalic NEC 344.89
    tegmental 344.89
  middle alternating 344.89
  Millard-Gubler-Foville 344.89
  monoplegic - see Monoplegia
  motor NEC 344.9
    cerebral - see Paralysis, brain
    spinal - see Paralysis, spinal
  multiple
    cerebral - see Paralysis, brain
    spinal - see Paralysis, spinal
  muscle (flaccid) 359.9
    due to nerve lesion NEC 355.9
    eye (extrinsic) 378.55
      intrinsic 367.51
      oblique 378.51
    iris sphincter 364.89
    ischemic (complicating trauma) (Volkmann's) 958.6
    pseudohypertrophic 359.1
  muscular (atrophic) 359.9
    progressive 335.21
  musculocutaneous nerve 354.9
  musculospiral 354.9
  nerve - see also Disorder, nerve
    third or oculomotor (partial) 378.51
      total 378.52
    fourth or trochlear 378.53
    sixth or abducens 378.54
    seventh or facial 351.0
      birth injury 767.5
      due to
        injection NEC 999.9
        operation NEC 997.09
      newborn 767.5

Paralysis, paralytic (Continued)
  nerve (Continued)
    accessory 352.4
    auditory 388.5
    birth injury 767.7
    cranial or cerebral (see also Disorder, nerve, cranial) 352.9
    facial 351.0
      birth injury 767.5
      newborn 767.5
    laryngeal (see also Paralysis, vocal cord) 478.30
    newborn 767.7
    phrenic 354.8
      newborn 767.7
    radial 354.3
      birth injury 767.6
      newborn 767.6
    syphilitic 094.89
    traumatic NEC (see also Injury, nerve, by site) 957.9
    trigeminal 350.9
    ulnar 354.2
  newborn NEC 767.0
  normokalemic periodic 359.3
  obstetrical, newborn 767.7
  ocular 378.9
  oculofacial, congenital 352.6
  oculomotor (nerve) (partial) 378.51
    alternating 344.89
    external bilateral 378.55
    total 378.52
  olfactory nerve 352.0
  palate 528.9
  palatopharyngolaryngeal 352.6
  paratrigeminal 350.9
  periodic (familial) (hyperkalemic) (hypokalemic) (normokalemic) (potassium sensitive) (secondary) 359.3
  peripheral
    autonomic nervous system - see Neuropathy, peripheral, autonomic
    nerve NEC 355.9
  peroneal (nerve) 355.3
  pharynx 478.29
  phrenic nerve 354.8
  plantar nerves 355.6
  pneumogastric nerve 352.3
  poliomyelitis (current) (see also Poliomyelitis, with paralysis) 045.1●
    bulbar 045.0●
  popliteal nerve 355.3
  pressure (see also Neuropathy, entrapment) 355.9
  progressive 335.21
    atrophic 335.21
    bulbar 335.22
    general 094.1
    hemifacial 349.89
    infantile, acute (see also Poliomyelitis) 045.9●
    multiple 335.20
  pseudobulbar 335.23
  pseudohypertrophic 359.1
    muscle 359.1
  psychogenic 306.0
  pupil, pupillary 379.49
  quadriceps 355.8
  quadriplegic (see also Quadriplegia) 344.0
  radial nerve 354.3
    birth injury 767.6
  rectum (sphincter) 569.49
  rectus muscle (eye) 378.55
  recurrent
    isolated sleep 327.43
    laryngeal nerve (see also Paralysis, vocal cord) 478.30

Paralysis, paralytic (Continued)
  respiratory (muscle) (system) (tract) 786.09
    center NEC 344.89
      fetus or newborn 770.87
    congenital 768.9
    newborn 768.9
  right side - see Hemiplegia
  Saturday night 354.3
  saturnine 984.9
    specified type of lead - see Table of Drugs and Chemicals
  sciatic nerve 355.0
  secondary - see Paralysis, late effect
  seizure (cerebral) (current episode) (see also Disease, cerebrovascular, acute) 436
    late effect - see Late effect(s) (of) cerebrovascular disease
  senile NEC 344.9
  serratus magnus 355.9
  shaking (see also Parkinsonism) 332.0
  shock (see also Disease, cerebrovascular, acute) 436
    late effect - see Late effect(s) (of) cerebrovascular disease
  shoulder 354.9
  soft palate 528.9
  spasmodic - see Paralysis, spastic
  spastic 344.9
    cerebral infantile - see Palsy, cerebral
    congenital (cerebral) - see Palsy, cerebral
    familial 334.1
    hereditary 334.1
    infantile 343.9
    noncongenital or noninfantile, cerebral 344.9
    syphilitic 094.0
      spinal 094.89
  sphincter, bladder (see also Paralysis, bladder) 596.53
  spinal (cord) NEC 344.1
    accessory nerve 352.4
    acute (see also Poliomyelitis) 045.9●
    ascending acute 357.0
    atrophic (acute) (see also Poliomyelitis, with paralysis) 045.1●
      spastic, syphilitic 094.89
    congenital NEC 343.9
    hemiplegic - see Hemiplegia
    hereditary 336.8
    infantile (see also Poliomyelitis) 045.9●
    late effect NEC 344.89
    monoplegic - see Monoplegia
    nerve 355.9
    progressive 335.10
    quadriplegic - see Quadriplegia
    spastic NEC 343.9
    traumatic - see Injury, spinal, by site
  sternomastoid 352.4
  stomach 536.3
    diabetic 250.6● [536.3]
      due to secondary diabetes 249.6● [536.3]
    nerve (nondiabetic) 352.3
  stroke (current episode) - see Infarct, brain
    late effect - see Late effect(s) (of) cerebrovascular disease
  subscapularis 354.8
  superior nuclear NEC 334.9
  supranuclear 356.8
  sympathetic
    cervical NEC 337.09
    nerve NEC (see also Neuropathy, peripheral, autonomic) 337.9
    nervous system - see Neuropathy, peripheral, autonomic
  syndrome 344.9
    specified NEC 344.89
  syphilitic spastic spinal (Erb's) 094.89
  tabetic general 094.1
  thigh 355.8

Paralysis, paralytic *(Continued)*
  throat 478.29
    diphtheritic 032.0
    muscle 478.29
  thrombotic (current episode) *(see also* Thrombosis, brain) 434.0●
    late effect - *see* Late effect(s) (of) cerebrovascular disease
  thumb NEC 354.9
  tick (-bite) 989.5
  Todd's (postepileptic transitory paralysis) 344.89
  toe 355.6
  tongue 529.8
  transient
    arm or leg NEC 781.4
      traumatic NEC *(see also* Injury, nerve, by site) 957.9
  trapezius 352.4
  traumatic, transient NEC *(see also* Injury, nerve, by site) 957.9
  trembling *(see also* Parkinsonism) 332.0
  triceps brachii 354.9
  trigeminal nerve 350.9
  trochlear nerve 378.53
  ulnar nerve 354.2
  upper limb - *see also* Paralysis, arm
    both *(see also* Diplegia) 344.2
  uremic - *see* Uremia
  uveoparotitic 135
  uvula 528.9
    hysterical 300.11
    postdiphtheritic 032.0
  vagus nerve 352.3
  vasomotor NEC 337.9
  velum palati 528.9
  vesical *(see also* Paralysis, bladder) 596.53
  vestibular nerve 388.5
  visual field, psychic 368.16
  vocal cord 478.30
    bilateral (partial) 478.33
      complete 478.34
    complete (bilateral) 478.34
    unilateral (partial) 478.31
      complete 478.32
  Volkmann's (complicating trauma) 958.6
  wasting 335.21
  Weber's 344.89
  wrist NEC 354.9
Paramedial orifice, urethrovesical 753.8
Paramenia 626.9
Parametritis (chronic) *(see also* Disease, pelvis, inflammatory) 614.4
  acute 614.3
  puerperal, postpartum, childbirth 670.8●
Parametrium, parametric - *see* condition
Paramnesia *(see also* Amnesia) 780.93
Paramolar 520.1
  causing crowding 524.31
Paramyloidosis 277.30
Paramyoclonus multiplex 333.2
Paramyotonia 359.29
  congenita (of von Eulenburg) 359.29
Paraneoplastic syndrome - *see* condition
Parangi *(see also* Yaws) 102.9
Paranoia 297.1
  alcoholic 291.5
  querulans 297.8
  senile 290.20
Paranoid
  dementia *(see also* Schizophrenia) 295.3●
    praecox (acute) 295.3●
    senile 290.20
  personality 301.0
  psychosis 297.9
    alcoholic 291.5
    climacteric 297.2
    drug-induced 292.11
    involutional 297.2
    menopausal 297.2
    protracted reactive 298.4

Paranoid *(Continued)*
  psychosis *(Continued)*
    psychogenic 298.4
      acute 298.3
    senile 290.20
  reaction (chronic) 297.9
    acute 298.3
  schizophrenia (acute) *(see also* Schizophrenia) 295.3●
  state 297.9
    alcohol-induced 291.5
    climacteric 297.2
    drug-induced 292.11
    due to or associated with
      arteriosclerosis (cerebrovascular) 290.42
      presenile brain disease 290.12
      senile brain disease 290.20
    involutional 297.2
    menopausal 297.2
    senile 290.20
    simple 297.0
    specified type NEC 297.8
  tendencies 301.0
  traits 301.0
  trends 301.0
  type, psychopathic personality 301.0
Paraparesis *(see also* Paraplegia) 344.1
Paraphasia 784.3
Paraphilia *(see also* Deviation, sexual) 302.9
Paraphimosis (congenital) 605
  chancroidal 099.0
Paraphrenia, paraphrenic (late) 297.2
  climacteric 297.2
  dementia *(see also* Schizophrenia) 295.3●
  involutional 297.2
  menopausal 297.2
  schizophrenia (acute) *(see also* Schizophrenia) 295.3●
Paraplegia 344.1
  with
    broken back - *see* Fracture, vertebra, by site, with spinal cord injury
    fracture, vertebra - *see* Fracture, vertebra, by site, with spinal cord injury
  ataxic - *see* Degeneration, combined, spinal cord
  brain (current episode) *(see also* Paralysis, brain) 437.8
  cerebral (current episode) *(see also* Paralysis, brain) 437.8
  congenital or infantile (cerebral) (spastic) (spinal) 343.0
  cortical - *see* Paralysis, brain
  familial spastic 334.1
  functional (hysterical) 300.11
  hysterical 300.11
  infantile 343.0
  late effect 344.1
  Pott's *(see also* Tuberculosis) 015.0● *[730.88]*
  psychogenic 306.0
  spastic
    Erb's spinal 094.89
    hereditary 334.1
    not infantile or congenital 344.1
  spinal (cord)
    traumatic NEC - *see* Injury, spinal, by site
  syphilitic (spastic) 094.89
  traumatic NEC - *see* Injury, spinal, by site
Paraproteinemia 273.2
  benign (familial) 273.1
  monoclonal 273.1
  secondary to malignant or inflammatory disease 273.1
Parapsoriasis 696.2
  en plaques 696.2
  guttata 696.2
  lichenoides chronica 696.2
  retiformis 696.2
  varioliformis (acuta) 696.2
Parascarlatina 057.8

Parasitic - *see also* condition
  disease NEC *(see also* Infestation, parasitic) 136.9
    contact V01.89
    exposure to V01.89
    intestinal NEC 129
    skin NEC 134.9
  stomatitis 112.0
  sycosis 110.0
    beard 110.0
    scalp 110.0
  twin 759.4
Parasitism NEC 136.9
  intestinal NEC 129
  skin NEC 134.9
  specified - *see* Infestation
Parasitophobia 300.29
Parasomnia 307.47
  alcohol induced 291.82
  drug induced 292.85
  nonorganic origin 307.47
  organic 327.40
    in conditions classified elsewhere 327.44
    other 327.49
Paraspadias 752.69
Paraspasm facialis 351.8
Parathyroid gland - *see* condition
Parathyroiditis (autoimmune) 252.1
Parathyroprival tetany 252.1
Paratrachoma 077.0
Paratyphilitis *(see also* Appendicitis) 541
Paratyphoid (fever) - *see* Fever, paratyphoid
Paratyphus - *see* Fever, paratyphoid
Paraurethral duct 753.8
Para-urethritis 597.89
  gonococcal (acute) 098.0
    chronic or duration of 2 months or over 098.2
Paravaccinia NEC 051.9
  milkers' node 051.1
Paravaginitis *(see also* Vaginitis) 616.10
Parencephalitis *(see also* Encephalitis) 323.9
  late effect - *see* category 326
Parergasia 298.9
Paresis *(see also* Paralysis) 344.9
  accommodation 367.51
  bladder (spastic) (sphincter) *(see also* Paralysis, bladder) 596.53
    tabetic 094.0
  bowel, colon, or intestine *(see also* Ileus) 560.1
  brain or cerebral - *see* Paralysis, brain
  extrinsic muscle, eye 378.55
  general 094.1
    arrested 094.1
    brain 094.1
    cerebral 094.1
    insane 094.1
    juvenile 090.40
      remission 090.49
    progressive 094.1
    remission (sustained) 094.1
    tabetic 094.1
  heart *(see also* Failure, heart) 428.9
  infantile *(see also* Poliomyelitis) 045.9●
  insane 094.1
  juvenile 090.40
  late effect - *see* Paralysis, late effect
  luetic (general) 094.1
  peripheral progressive 356.9
  pseudohypertrophic 359.1
  senile NEC 344.9
  stomach 536.3
    diabetic 250.6● *[536.3]*
      due to secondary diabetes 249.6● *[536.3]*
  syphilitic (general) 094.1
    congenital 090.40
  transient, limb 781.4
  vesical (sphincter) NEC 596.53

◀ New   ◀▦ Revised   ~~deleted~~ Deleted   ● Use Additional Digit(s)   ▨ Omit code

Paresthesia (*see also* Disturbance, sensation) 782.0
  Berger's (paresthesia of lower limb) 782.0
  Bernhardt 355.1
  Magnan's 782.0
Paretic - *see* condition
Parinaud's
  conjunctivitis 372.02
  oculoglandular syndrome 372.02
  ophthalmoplegia 378.81
  syndrome (paralysis of conjugate upward gaze) 378.81
Parkes Weber and Dimitri syndrome (encephalocutaneous angiomatosis) 759.6
Parkinson's disease, syndrome, or tremor - *see* Parkinsonism
Parkinsonism (arteriosclerotic) (idiopathic) (primary) 332.0
  associated with orthostatic hypotension (idiopathic) (symptomatic) 333.0
  due to drugs 332.1
  neuroleptic-induced 332.1
  secondary 332.1
  syphilitic 094.82
Parodontitis 523.40
Parodontosis 523.5
Paronychia (with lymphangitis) 681.9
  candidal (chronic) 112.3
  chronic 681.9
    candidal 112.3
    finger 681.02
    toe 681.11
  finger 681.02
  toe 681.11
  tuberculous (primary) (*see also* Tuberculosis) 017.0●
Parorexia NEC 307.52
  hysterical 300.11
Parosmia 781.1
  psychogenic 306.7
Parotid gland - *see* condition
Parotiditis (*see also* Parotitis) 527.2
  epidemic 072.9
  infectious 072.9
Parotitis 527.2
  allergic 527.2
  chronic 527.2
  epidemic (*see also* Mumps) 072.9
  infectious (*see also* Mumps) 072.9
  noninfectious 527.2
  nonspecific toxic 527.2
  not mumps 527.2
  postoperative 527.2
  purulent 527.2
  septic 527.2
  suppurative (acute) 527.2
  surgical 527.2
  toxic 527.2
Paroxysmal - *see also* condition
  dyspnea (nocturnal) 786.09
Parrot's disease (syphilitic osteochondritis) 090.0
Parrot fever 073.9
Parry's disease or syndrome (exophthalmic goiter) 242.0●
Parry-Romberg syndrome 349.89
Parson's disease (exophthalmic goiter) 242.0●
Parsonage-Aldren-Turner syndrome 353.5
Parsonage-Turner syndrome 353.5
Pars planitis 363.21
Particolored infant 757.39
Parturition - *see* Delivery
Parvovirus 079.83
  B19 079.83
  human 079.83
Passage
  false, urethra 599.4
  meconium noted during delivery 763.84
  of sounds or bougies (*see also* Attention to artificial opening) V55.9

Passive - *see* condition
Pasteurella septica 027.2
Pasteurellosis (*see also* Infection, Pasteurella) 027.2
PAT (paroxysmal atrial tachycardia) 427.0
Patau's syndrome (trisomy D1) 758.1
Patch
  herald 696.3
Patches
  mucous (syphilitic) 091.3
    congenital 090.0
  smokers' (mouth) 528.6
Patellar - *see* condition
Patellofemoral syndrome 719.46
Patent - *see also* Imperfect closure
  atrioventricular ostium 745.69
  canal of Nuck 752.41
  cervix 622.5
    complicating pregnancy 654.5●
      affecting fetus or newborn 761.0
  ductus arteriosus or Botalli 747.0
  Eustachian
    tube 381.7
    valve 746.89
  foramen
    Botalli 745.5
    ovale 745.5
  interauricular septum 745.5
  interventricular septum 745.4
  omphalomesenteric duct 751.0
  os (uteri) - *see* Patent, cervix
  ostium secundum 745.5
  urachus 753.7
  vitelline duct 751.0
Paternity testing V70.4
Paterson's syndrome (sideropenic dysphagia) 280.8
Paterson (-Brown) (-Kelly) syndrome (sideropenic dysphagia) 280.8
Paterson-Kelly syndrome or web (sideropenic dysphagia) 280.8
Pathologic, pathological - *see also* condition
  asphyxia 799.01
  drunkenness 291.4
  emotionality 301.3
  fracture - *see* Fracture, pathologic
  liar 301.7
  personality 301.9
  resorption, tooth 521.40
    external 521.42
    internal 521.41
    specified NEC 521.49
  sexuality (*see also* Deviation, sexual) 302.9
Pathology (of) - *see also* Disease
  periradicular, associated with previous endodontic treatment 526.69
Patterned motor discharge, idiopathic (*see also* Epilepsy) 345.5●
Patulous - *see also* Patent
  anus 569.49
  Eustachian tube 381.7
Pause, sinoatrial 427.81
Pavor nocturnus 307.46
Pavy's disease 593.6
Paxton's disease (white piedra) 111.2
Payr's disease or syndrome (splenic flexure syndrome) 569.89
PBA (pseudobulbar affect) 310.81
Pearls
  Elschnig 366.51
  enamel 520.2
Pearl-workers' disease (chronic osteomyelitis) (*see also* Osteomyelitis) 730.1●
Pectenitis 569.49
Pectenosis 569.49
Pectoral - *see* condition
Pectus
  carinatum (congenital) 754.82
    acquired 738.3
    rachitic (*see also* Rickets) 268.0

Pectus (*Continued*)
  excavatum (congenital) 754.81
    acquired 738.3
    rachitic (*see also* Rickets) 268.0
  recurvatum (congenital) 754.81
    acquired 738.3
Pedatrophia 261
Pederosis 302.2
Pediculosis (infestation) 132.9
  capitis (head louse) (any site) 132.0
  corporis (body louse) (any site) 132.1
  eyelid 132.0 *[373.6]*
  mixed (classifiable to more than one category in 132.0–132.2) 132.3
  pubis (pubic louse) (any site) 132.2
  vestimenti 132.1
  vulvae 132.2
Pediculus (infestation) - *see* Pediculosis
Pedophilia 302.2
Peg-shaped teeth 520.2
Pel's crisis 094.0
Pel-Ebstein disease - *see* Disease, Hodgkin's
Pelade 704.01
Pelger-Huët anomaly or syndrome (hereditary hyposegmentation) 288.2
Peliosis (rheumatica) 287.0
Pelizaeus-Merzbacher
  disease 330.0
  sclerosis, diffuse cerebral 330.0
Pellagra (alcoholic or with alcoholism) 265.2
  with polyneuropathy 265.2 *[357.4]*
Pellagra-cerebellar-ataxia-renal aminoaciduria syndrome 270.0
Pellegrini's disease (calcification, knee joint) 726.62
Pellegrini (-Stieda) disease or syndrome (calcification, knee joint) 726.62
Pellizzi's syndrome (pineal) 259.8
Pelvic - *see also* condition
  congestion-fibrosis syndrome 625.5
  kidney 753.3
Pelvioectasis 591
Pelviolithiasis 592.0
Pelviperitonitis
  female (*see also* Peritonitis, pelvic, female) 614.5
  male (*see also* Peritonitis) 567.21
Pelvis, pelvic - *see also* condition or type
  infantile 738.6
  Nägele's 738.6
  obliquity 738.6
  Robert's 755.69
Pemphigoid 694.5
  benign, mucous membrane 694.60
    with ocular involvement 694.61
  bullous 694.5
  cicatricial 694.60
    with ocular involvement 694.61
  juvenile 694.2
Pemphigus 694.4
  benign 694.5
    chronic familial 757.39
  Brazilian 694.4
  circinatus 694.0
  congenital, traumatic 757.39
  conjunctiva 694.61
  contagiosus 684
  erythematodes 694.4
  erythematosus 694.4
  foliaceus 694.4
  frambesiodes 694.4
  gangrenous (*see also* Gangrene) 785.4
  malignant 694.4
  neonatorum, newborn 684
  ocular 694.61
  papillaris 694.4
  seborrheic 694.4
  South American 694.4
  syphilitic (congenital) 090.0
  vegetans 694.4

P

Pemphigus (Continued)
vulgaris 694.4
wildfire 694.4
Pendred's syndrome (familial goiter with deaf-mutism) 243
Pendulous
abdomen 701.9
in pregnancy or childbirth 654.4●
affecting fetus or newborn 763.89
breast 611.89
Penetrating wound - see also Wound, open, by site
with internal injury - see Injury, internal, by site, with open wound
eyeball 871.7
with foreign body (nonmagnetic) 871.6
magnetic 871.5
ocular (see also Penetrating wound, eyeball) 871.7
adnexa 870.3
with foreign body 870.4
orbit 870.3
with foreign body 870.4
Penetration, pregnant uterus by instrument
with
abortion - see Abortion, by type, with damage to pelvic organs
ectopic pregnancy (see also categories 633.0–633.9) 639.2
molar pregnancy (see also categories 630–632) 639.2
complication of delivery 665.1●
affecting fetus or newborn 763.89
following
abortion 639.2
ectopic or molar pregnancy 639.2
Penfield's syndrome (see also Epilepsy) 345.5●
Penicilliosis of lung 117.3
Penis - see condition
Penitis 607.2
Penta X syndrome 758.81
Pentalogy (of Fallot) 745.2
Pentosuria (benign) (essential) 271.8
Peptic acid disease 536.8
Peregrinating patient V65.2
Perforated - see Perforation
Perforation, perforative (nontraumatic)
antrum (see also Sinusitis, maxillary) 473.0
appendix 540.0
with peritoneal abscess 540.1
atrial septum, multiple 745.5
attic, ear 384.22
healed 384.81
bile duct, except cystic (see also Disease, biliary) 576.3
cystic 575.4
bladder (urinary) 596.6
with
abortion - see Abortion, by type, with damage to pelvic organs
ectopic pregnancy (see also categories 633.0–633.9) 639.2
molar pregnancy (see also categories 630–632) 639.2
following
abortion 639.2
ectopic or molar pregnancy 639.2
obstetrical trauma 665.5●
bowel 569.83
with
abortion - see Abortion, by type, with damage to pelvic organs
ectopic pregnancy (see also categories 633.0–633.9) 639.2
molar pregnancy (see also categories 630–632) 639.2
fetus or newborn 777.6
following
abortion 639.2
ectopic or molar pregnancy 639.2
obstetrical trauma 665.5●

Perforation, perforative (Continued)
broad ligament
with
abortion - see Abortion, by type, with damage to pelvic organs
ectopic pregnancy (see also categories 633.0–633.9) 639.2
molar pregnancy (see also categories 630–632) 639.2
following
abortion 639.2
ectopic or molar pregnancy 639.2
obstetrical trauma 665.6●
by
device, implant, or graft - see Complications, mechanical
foreign body left accidentally in operation wound 998.4
instrument (any) during a procedure, accidental 998.2
cecum 540.0
with peritoneal abscess 540.1
cervix (uteri) - see also Injury, internal, cervix
with
abortion - see Abortion, by type, with damage to pelvic organs
ectopic pregnancy (see also categories 633.0–633.9) 639.2
molar pregnancy (see also categories 630–632) 639.2
following
abortion 639.2
ectopic or molar pregnancy 639.2
obstetrical trauma 665.3●
colon 569.83
common duct (bile) 576.3
cornea (see also Ulcer, cornea) 370.00
due to ulceration 370.06
cystic duct 575.4
diverticulum (see also Diverticula) 562.10
small intestine 562.00
duodenum, duodenal (ulcer) - see Ulcer, duodenum, with perforation
ear drum - see Perforation, tympanum
enteritis - see Enteritis
esophagus 530.4
ethmoidal sinus (see also Sinusitis, ethmoidal) 473.2
foreign body (external site) - see also Wound, open, by site, complicated
internal site, by ingested object - see Foreign body
frontal sinus (see also Sinusitis, frontal) 473.1
gallbladder or duct (see also Disease, gallbladder) 575.4
gastric (ulcer) - see Ulcer, stomach, with perforation
heart valve - see Endocarditis
ileum (see also Perforation, intestine) 569.83
instrumental
external - see Wound, open, by site
pregnant uterus, complicating delivery 665.9●
surgical (accidental) (blood vessel) (nerve) (organ) 998.2
intestine 569.83
with
abortion - see Abortion, by type, with damage to pelvic organs
ectopic pregnancy (see also categories 633.0–633.9) 639.2
molar pregnancy (see also categories 630–632) 639.2
fetus or newborn 777.6
obstetrical trauma 665.5●
ulcerative NEC 569.83
jejunum, jejunal 569.83
ulcer - see Ulcer, gastrojejunal, with perforation
mastoid (antrum) (cell) 383.89

Perforation, perforative (Continued)
maxillary sinus (see also Sinusitis, maxillary) 473.0
membrana tympani - see Perforation, tympanum
nasal
septum 478.19
congenital 748.1
syphilitic 095.8
sinus (see also Sinusitis) 473.9
congenital 748.1
palate (hard) 526.89
soft 528.9
syphilitic 095.8
syphilitic 095.8
palatine vault 526.89
syphilitic 095.8
congenital 090.5
pelvic
floor
with
abortion - see Abortion, by type, with damage to pelvic organs
ectopic pregnancy (see also categories 633.0–633.9) 639.2
molar pregnancy (see also categories 630–632) 639.2
obstetrical trauma 664.1●
organ
with
abortion - see Abortion, by type, with damage to pelvic organs
ectopic pregnancy (see also categories 633.0–633.9) 639.2
molar pregnancy (see also categories 630–632) 639.2
following
abortion 639.2
ectopic or molar pregnancy 639.2
obstetrical trauma 665.5●
perineum - see Laceration, perineum
periurethral tissue
with
abortion - see Abortion, by type, with damage to pelvic organs
ectopic pregnancy (see also categories 630–632) 639.2
molar pregnancy (see also categories 630–632) 639.2
pharynx 478.29
pylorus, pyloric (ulcer) - see Ulcer, stomach, with perforation
rectum 569.49
root canal space 526.61
sigmoid 569.83
sinus (accessory) (chronic) (nasal) (see also Sinusitis) 473.9
sphenoidal sinus (see also Sinusitis, sphenoidal) 473.3
stomach (due to ulcer) - see Ulcer, stomach, with perforation
surgical (accidental) (by instrument) (blood vessel) (nerve) (organ) 998.2
traumatic
external - see Wound, open, by site
eye (see also Penetrating wound, ocular) 871.7
internal organ - see Injury, internal, by site
tympanum (membrane) (persistent posttraumatic) (postinflammatory) 384.20
with
otitis media - see Otitis media
attic 384.22
central 384.21
healed 384.81
marginal NEC 384.23
multiple 384.24
pars flaccida 384.22
total 384.25
traumatic - see Wound, open, ear, drum

◄ New ◄▬ Revised ~~deleted~~ Deleted ● Use Additional Digit(s) ▓ Omit code

Perforation, perforative *(Continued)*
typhoid, gastrointestinal 002.0
ulcer - *see* Ulcer, by site, with perforation
ureter 593.89
urethra
  with
    abortion - *see* Abortion, by type, with
      damage to pelvic organs
    ectopic pregnancy (*see also* categories
      633.0–633.9) 639.2
    molar pregnancy (*see also* categories
      630–632) 639.2
  following
    abortion 639.2
    ectopic or molar pregnancy 639.2
  obstetrical trauma 665.5●
uterus - *see also* Injury, internal, uterus
  with
    abortion - *see* Abortion, by type, with
      damage to pelvic organs
    ectopic pregnancy (*see also* categories
      633.0–633.9) 639.2
    molar pregnancy (*see also* categories
      630–632) 639.2
  by intrauterine contraceptive device
    996.32
  following
    abortion 639.2
    ectopic or molar pregnancy 639.2
  obstetrical trauma - *see* Injury, internal,
    uterus, obstetrical trauma
uvula 528.9
  syphilitic 095.8
vagina - *see* Laceration, vagina
viscus NEC 799.89
  traumatic 868.00
    with open wound into cavity 868.10
Periadenitis mucosa necrotica recurrens
  528.2
Periangiitis 446.0
Periantritis 535.4●
Periappendicitis (acute) (*see also* Appendicitis)
  541
Periarteritis (disseminated) (infectious)
  (necrotizing) (nodosa) 446.0
Periarthritis (joint) 726.90
  Duplay's 726.2
  gonococcal 098.50
  humeroscapularis 726.2
  scapulohumeral 726.2
  shoulder 726.2
  wrist 726.4
Periarthrosis (angioneural) - *see* Periarthritis
Peribronchitis 491.9
  tuberculous (*see also* Tuberculosis)
    011.3●
Pericapsulitis, adhesive (shoulder)
  726.0
Pericarditis (granular) (with decompensation)
  (with effusion) 423.9
  with
    rheumatic fever (conditions classifiable to
      390)
      active (*see also* Pericarditis, rheumatic)
        391.0
      inactive or quiescent 393
  actinomycotic 039.8 *[420.0]*
  acute (nonrheumatic) 420.90
    with chorea (acute) (rheumatic)
      (Sydenham's) 392.0
    bacterial 420.99
    benign 420.91
    hemorrhagic 420.90
    idiopathic 420.91
    infective 420.90
    nonspecific 420.91
    rheumatic 391.0
      with chorea (acute) (rheumatic)
        (Sydenham's) 392.0
  sicca 420.90
  viral 420.91

Pericarditis *(Continued)*
adhesive or adherent (external) (internal)
  423.1
  acute - *see* Pericarditis, acute
  rheumatic (external) (internal) 393
amebic 006.8 *[420.0]*
bacterial (acute) (subacute) (with serous or
  seropurulent effusion) 420.99
calcareous 423.2
cholesterol (chronic) 423.8
  acute 420.90
chronic (nonrheumatic) 423.8
  rheumatic 393
constrictive 423.2
Coxsackie 074.21
due to
  actinomycosis 039.8 *[420.0]*
  amebiasis 006.8 *[420.0]*
  Coxsackie (virus) 074.21
  histoplasmosis (*see also* Histoplasmosis)
    115.93
  nocardiosis 039.8 *[420.0]*
  tuberculosis (*see also* Tuberculosis) 017.9●
    [420.0]
fibrinocaseous (*see also* Tuberculosis) 017.9●
  [420.0]
fibrinopurulent 420.99
fibrinous - *see* Pericarditis, rheumatic
fibropurulent 420.99
fibrous 423.1
gonococcal 098.83
hemorrhagic 423.0
idiopathic (acute) 420.91
infective (acute) 420.90
meningococcal 036.41
neoplastic (chronic) 423.8
  acute 420.90
nonspecific 420.91
obliterans, obliterating 423.1
plastic 423.1
pneumococcal (acute) 420.99
postinfarction 411.0
purulent (acute) 420.99
rheumatic (active) (acute) (with effusion)
  (with pneumonia) 391.0
  with chorea (acute) (rheumatic)
    (Sydenham's) 392.0
  chronic or inactive (with chorea) 393
septic (acute) 420.99
serofibrinous - *see* Pericarditis, rheumatic
staphylococcal (acute) 420.99
streptococcal (acute) 420.99
suppurative (acute) 420.99
syphilitic 093.81
tuberculous (acute) (chronic) (*see also*
  Tuberculosis) 017.9● *[420.0]*
uremic 585.9 *[420.0]*
viral (acute) 420.91
Pericardium, pericardial - *see* condition
Pericellulitis (*see also* Cellulitis) 682.9
Pericementitis 523.40
  acute 523.30
  chronic (suppurative) 523.40
Pericholecystitis (*see also* Cholecystitis)
  575.10
Perichondritis
  auricle 380.00
    acute 380.01
    chronic 380.02
  bronchus 491.9
  ear (external) 380.00
    acute 380.01
    chronic 380.02
  larynx 478.71
    syphilitic 095.8
    typhoid 002.0 *[478.71]*
  nose 478.19
  pinna 380.00
    acute 380.01
    chronic 380.02
  trachea 478.9

Periclasia 523.5
Pericolitis 569.89
Pericoronitis (chronic) 523.40
  acute 523.33
Pericystitis (*see also* Cystitis) 595.9
Pericytoma (M9150/1) - *see also* Neoplasm,
  connective tissue, uncertain behavior
  benign (M9150/0) - *see* Neoplasm,
    connective tissue, benign
  malignant (M9150/3) - *see* Neoplasm,
    connective tissue, malignant
Peridacryocystitis, acute 375.32
Peridiverticulitis (*see also* Diverticulitis)
  562.11
Periduodenitis 535.6●
Periendocarditis (*see also* Endocarditis)
  424.90
  acute or subacute 421.9
Periepididymitis (*see also* Epididymitis)
  604.90
Perifolliculitis (abscedens) 704.8
  capitis, abscedens et suffodiens 704.8
  dissecting, scalp 704.8
  scalp 704.8
  superficial pustular 704.8
Perigastritis (acute) 535.0●
Perigastrojejunitis (acute) 535.0●
Perihepatitis (acute) 573.3
  chlamydial 099.56
  gonococcal 098.86
Peri-ileitis (subacute) 569.89
Perilabyrinthitis (acute) - *see* Labyrinthitis
Perimeningitis - *see* Meningitis
Perimetritis (*see also* Endometritis) 615.9
Perimetrosalpingitis (*see also* Salpingo-
  oophoritis) 614.2
Perineocele 618.05
Perinephric - *see* condition
Perinephritic - *see* condition
Perinephritis (*see also* Infection, kidney)
  590.9
  purulent (*see also* Abscess, kidney) 590.2
Perineum, perineal - *see* condition
Perineuritis NEC 729.2
Periodic - *see also* condition
  disease (familial) 277.31
  edema 995.1
    hereditary 277.6
  fever 277.31
  headache syndromes in child or adolescent
    346.2●
  limb movement disorder 327.51
  paralysis (familial) 359.3
  peritonitis 277.31
  polyserositis 277.31
  somnolence (*see also* Narcolepsy) 347.00
Periodontal
  cyst 522.8
  pocket 523.8
Periodontitis (chronic) (complex) (compound)
  (simplex) 523.40
  acute 523.33
  aggressive 523.30
    generalized 523.32
    localized 523.31
  apical 522.6
    acute (pulpal origin) 522.4
  generalized 523.42
  localized 523.41
Periodontoclasia 523.5
Periodontosis 523.5
Periods - *see also* Menstruation
  heavy 626.2
  irregular 626.4
Perionychia (with lymphangitis) 681.9
  finger 681.02
  toe 681.11
Perioophoritis (*see also* Salpingo-oophoritis)
  614.2
Periorchitis (*see also* Orchitis) 604.90
Periosteum, periosteal - *see* condition

Periostitis (circumscribed) (diffuse) (infective) 730.3 ●

> Note: Use the following fifth-digit subclassification with category 730:
>
> 0   site unspecified
> 1   shoulder region
> 2   upper arm
> 3   forearm
> 4   hand
> 5   pelvic region and thigh
> 6   lower leg
> 7   ankle and foot
> 8   other specified sites
> 9   multiple sites

   with osteomyelitis (*see also* Osteomyelitis) 730.2 ●
     acute or subacute 730.0 ●
     chronic or old 730.1 ●
   albuminosa, albuminosus 730.3 ●
   alveolar 526.5
   alveolodental 526.5
   dental 526.5
   gonorrheal 098.89
   hyperplastica, generalized 731.2
   jaw (lower) (upper) 526.4
   monomelic 733.99
   orbital 376.02
   syphilitic 095.5
     congenital 090.0 [730.8] ●
     secondary 091.61
   tuberculous (*see also* Tuberculosis, bone) 015.9 ● [730.8] ●
   yaws (early) (hypertrophic) (late) 102.6
Periostosis (*see also* Periostitis) 730.3 ●
   with osteomyelitis (*see also* Osteomyelitis) 730.2 ●
     acute or subacute 730.0 ●
     chronic or old 730.1 ●
   hyperplastic 756.59
Peripartum cardiomyopathy 674.5 ●
Periphlebitis (*see also* Phlebitis) 451.9
   lower extremity 451.2
     deep (vessels) 451.19
     superficial (vessels) 451.0
   portal 572.1
   retina 362.18
   superficial (vessels) 451.0
   tuberculous (*see also* Tuberculosis) 017.9 ●
     retina 017.3 ● [362.18]
Peripneumonia - *see* Pneumonia
Periproctitis 569.49
Periprostatitis (*see also* Prostatitis) 601.9
Perirectal - *see* condition
Perirenal - *see* condition
Perisalpingitis (*see also* Salpingo-oophoritis) 614.2
Perisigmoiditis 569.89
Perisplenitis (infectional) 289.59
Perispondylitis - *see* Spondylitis
Peristalsis reversed or visible 787.4
Peritendinitis (*see also* Tenosynovitis) 726.90
   adhesive (shoulder) 726.0
Perithelioma (M9150/1) - *see* Pericytoma
Peritoneum, peritoneal - *see also* condition
   equilibration test V56.32
Peritonitis (acute) (adhesive) (fibrinous) (hemorrhagic) (idiopathic) (localized) (perforative) (primary) (with adhesions) (with effusion) 567.9
   with or following
     abortion - *see* Abortion, by type, with sepsis
     abscess 567.21
     appendicitis 540.0
       with peritoneal abscess 540.1
     ectopic pregnancy (*see also* categories 633.0–633.9) 639.0
     molar pregnancy (*see also* categories 630–632) 639.0

Peritonitis (*Continued*)
   aseptic 998.7
   bacterial 567.29
     spontaneous 567.23
   bile, biliary 567.81
   chemical 998.7
   chlamydial 099.56
   chronic proliferative 567.89
   congenital NEC 777.6
   diaphragmatic 567.22
   diffuse NEC 567.29
   diphtheritic 032.83
   disseminated NEC 567.29
   due to
     bile 567.81
     foreign
       body or object accidentally left during a procedure (instrument) (sponge) (swab) 998.4
       substance accidentally left during a procedure (chemical) (powder) (talc) 998.7
     talc 998.7
     urine 567.89
   fibrinopurulent 567.29
   fibrinous 567.29
   fibrocaseous (*see also* Tuberculosis) 014.0 ●
   fibropurulent 567.29
   general, generalized (acute) 567.21
   gonococcal 098.86
   in infective disease NEC 136.9 [567.0]
   meconium (newborn) 777.6
   pancreatic 577.8
   paroxysmal, benign 277.31
   pelvic
     female (acute) 614.5
       chronic NEC 614.7
         with adhesions 614.6
       puerperal, postpartum, childbirth 670.8 ●
     male (acute) 567.21
   periodic (familial) 277.31
   phlegmonous 567.29
   pneumococcal 567.1
   postabortal 639.0
   proliferative, chronic 567.89
   puerperal, postpartum, childbirth 670.8 ●
   purulent 567.29
   septic 567.29
   spontaneous bacterial 567.23
   staphylococcal 567.29
   streptococcal 567.29
   subdiaphragmatic 567.29
   subphrenic 567.29
   suppurative 567.29
   syphilitic 095.2
     congenital 090.0 [567.0]
   talc 998.7
   tuberculous (*see also* Tuberculosis) 014.0 ●
   urine 567.89
Peritonsillar - *see* condition
Peritonsillitis 475
Perityphlitis (*see also* Appendicitis) 541
Periureteritis 593.89
Periurethral - *see* condition
Periurethritis (gangrenous) 597.89
Periuterine - *see* condition
Perivaginitis (*see also* Vaginitis) 616.10
Perivasculitis, retinal 362.18
Perivasitis (chronic) 608.4
Periventricular leukomalacia 779.7
Perivesiculitis (seminal) (*see also* Vesiculitis) 608.0
Perlèche 686.8
   due to
     moniliasis 112.0
     riboflavin deficiency 266.0
Pernicious - *see* condition
Pernio, perniosis 991.5

Persecution
   delusion 297.9
   social V62.4
Perseveration (tonic) 784.69
Persistence, persistent (congenital) 759.89
   anal membrane 751.2
   arteria stapedia 744.04
   atrioventricular canal 745.69
   bloody ejaculate 792.2
   branchial cleft 744.41
   bulbus cordis in left ventricle 745.8
   canal of Cloquet 743.51
   capsule (opaque) 743.51
   cilioretinal artery or vein 743.51
   cloaca 751.5
   communication - *see* Fistula, congenital
   convolutions
     aortic arch 747.21
     fallopian tube 752.19
     oviduct 752.19
     uterine tube 752.19
   double aortic arch 747.21
   ductus
     arteriosus 747.0
     Botalli 747.0
   fetal
     circulation 747.83
     form of cervix (uteri) 752.49
     hemoglobin (hereditary) ("Swiss variety") 282.7
     pulmonary hypertension 747.83
   foramen
     Botalli 745.5
     ovale 745.5
   Gartner's duct 752.41
   hemoglobin, fetal (hereditary) (HPFH) 282.7
   hyaloid
     artery (generally incomplete) 743.51
     system 743.51
   hymen (tag)
     in pregnancy or childbirth 654.8 ●
       causing obstructed labor 660.2 ●
   lanugo 757.4
   left
     posterior cardinal vein 747.49
     root with right arch of aorta 747.21
     superior vena cava 747.49
   Meckel's diverticulum 751.0
   mesonephric duct 752.89
     fallopian tube 752.11
   mucosal disease (middle ear) (with posterior or superior marginal perforation of ear drum) 382.2
   nail(s), anomalous 757.5
   occiput, anterior or posterior 660.3 ●
     fetus or newborn 763.1
   omphalomesenteric duct 751.0
   organ or site NEC - *see* Anomaly, specified type NEC
   ostium
     atrioventriculare commune 745.69
     primum 745.61
     secundum 745.5
   ovarian rests in fallopian tube 752.19
   pancreatic tissue in intestinal tract 751.5
   primary (deciduous)
     teeth 520.6
     vitreous hyperplasia 743.51
   pulmonary hypertension 747.83
   pupillary membrane 743.46
     iris 743.46
   Rhesus (Rh) titer (*see also* Complications, transfusion) 999.70
   right aortic arch 747.21
   sinus
     urogenitalis 752.89
     venosus with imperfect incorporation in right auricle 747.49
   thymus (gland) 254.8
     hyperplasia 254.0
   thyroglossal duct 759.2

◀ New   ◀◀ Revised   ~~deleted~~ Deleted   ● Use Additional Digit(s)   ▨ Omit code

Persistence, persistent (Continued)
thyrolingual duct 759.2
truncus arteriosus or communis 745.0
tunica vasculosa lentis 743.39
umbilical sinus 753.7
urachus 753.7
vegetative state 780.03
vitelline duct 751.0
wolffian duct 752.89
Person (with)
admitted for clinical research, as participant or control subject V70.7
affected by
family member
currently on deployment (military) V61.01
returned from deployment (military) (current or past conflict) V61.02
awaiting admission to adequate facility elsewhere V63.2
undergoing social agency investigation V63.8
concern (normal) about sick person in family V61.49
consulting on behalf of another V65.19
pediatric
pre-adoption visit for adoptive parents V65.11
pre-birth visit for expectant parents V65.11
currently deployed in theater or in support of military war, peacekeeping and humanitarian operations V62.21
feared
complaint in whom no diagnosis was made V65.5
condition not demonstrated V65.5
feigning illness V65.2
healthy, accompanying sick person V65.0
history of military war, peacekeeping and humanitarian deployment (current or past conflict) V62.22
living (in)
alone V60.3
boarding school V60.6
residence remote from hospital or medical care facility V63.0
residential institution V60.6
without
adequate
financial resources V60.2
housing (heating) (space) V60.1
housing (permanent) (temporary) V60.0
material resources V60.2
person able to render necessary care V60.4
shelter V60.0
medical services in home not available V63.1
on waiting list V63.2
undergoing social agency investigation V63.8
sick or handicapped in family V61.49
"worried well" V65.5
Personality
affective 301.10
aggressive 301.3
amoral 301.7
anancastic, anankastic 301.4
antisocial 301.7
asocial 301.7
asthenic 301.6
avoidant 301.82
borderline 301.83
change 310.1
compulsive 301.4
cycloid 301.13
cyclothymic 301.13
dependent 301.6
depressive (chronic) 301.12

Personality (Continued)
disorder, disturbance NEC 301.9
with
antisocial disturbance 301.7
pattern disturbance NEC 301.9
sociopathic disturbance 301.7
trait disturbance 301.9
dual 300.14
dyssocial 301.7
eccentric 301.89
"haltlose" type 301.89
emotionally unstable 301.59
epileptoid 301.3
explosive 301.3
fanatic 301.0
histrionic 301.50
hyperthymic 301.11
hypomanic 301.11
hypothymic 301.12
hysterical 301.50
immature 301.89
inadequate 301.6
labile 301.59
masochistic 301.89
morally defective 301.7
multiple 300.14
narcissistic 301.81
obsessional 301.4
obsessive-compulsive 301.4
overconscientious 301.4
paranoid 301.0
passive (-dependent) 301.6
passive-aggressive 301.84
pathologic NEC 301.9
pattern defect or disturbance 301.9
pseudosocial 301.7
psychoinfantile 301.59
psychoneurotic NEC 301.89
psychopathic 301.9
with
amoral trend 301.7
antisocial trend 301.7
asocial trend 301.7
pathologic sexuality (see also Deviation, sexual) 302.9
mixed types 301.9
schizoid 301.20
introverted 301.21
schizotypal 301.22
type A 301.4
unstable (emotional) 301.59
Perthes' disease (capital femoral osteochondrosis) 732.1
Pertussis (see also Whooping cough) 033.9
vaccination, prophylactic (against) V03.6
Peruvian wart 088.0
Perversion, perverted
appetite 307.52
hysterical 300.11
function
pineal gland 259.8
pituitary gland 253.9
anterior lobe
deficient 253.2
excessive 253.1
posterior lobe 253.6
placenta - see Placenta, abnormal
sense of smell or taste 781.1
psychogenic 306.7
sexual (see also Deviation, sexual) 302.9
Pervious, congenital - see also Imperfect, closure
ductus arteriosus 747.0
Pes (congenital) (see also Talipes) 754.70
abductus (congenital) 754.60
acquired 736.79
acquired NEC 736.79
planus 734
adductus (congenital) 754.79
acquired 736.79
cavus 754.71
acquired 736.73

Pes (Continued)
planovalgus (congenital) 754.69
acquired 736.79
planus (acquired) (any degree) 734
congenital 754.61
rachitic 268.1
valgus (congenital) 754.61
acquired 736.79
varus (congenital) 754.50
acquired 736.79
Pest (see also Plague) 020.9
Pestis (see also Plague) 020.9
bubonica 020.0
fulminans 020.0
minor 020.8
pneumonica - see Plague, pneumonic
Petechia, petechiae 782.7
fetus or newborn 772.6
Petechial
fever 036.0
typhus 081.9
Petges-Cléjat or Petges-Clégat syndrome (poikilodermatomyositis) 710.3
Petit's
disease (see also Hernia, lumbar) 553.8
Petit mal (idiopathic) (see also Epilepsy) 345.0●
status 345.2
Petrellidosis 117.6
Petrositis 383.20
acute 383.21
chronic 383.22
Peutz-Jeghers disease or syndrome 759.6
Peyronie's disease 607.85
Pfeiffer's disease 075
Phacentocele 379.32
traumatic 921.3
Phacoanaphylaxis 360.19
Phacocele (old) 379.32
traumatic 921.3
Phaehyphomycosis 117.8
Phagedena (dry) (moist) (see also Gangrene) 785.4
arteriosclerotic 440.24
geometric 686.09
penis 607.89
senile 440.24
sloughing 785.4
tropical (see also Ulcer, skin) 707.9
vulva 616.50
Phagedenic - see also condition
abscess - see also Abscess
chancroid 099.0
bubo NEC 099.8
chancre 099.0
ulcer (tropical) (see also Ulcer, skin) 707.9
Phagomania 307.52
Phakoma 362.89
Phantom limb (syndrome) 353.6
Pharyngeal - see also condition
arch remnant 744.41
pouch syndrome 279.11
Pharyngitis (acute) (catarrhal) (gangrenous) (infective) (malignant) (membranous) (phlegmonous) (pneumococcal) (pseudomembranous) (simple) (staphylococcal) (subacute) (suppurative) (ulcerative) (viral) 462
with influenza, flu, or grippe (see also Influenza) 487.1
aphthous 074.0
atrophic 472.1
chlamydial 099.51
chronic 472.1
Coxsackie virus 074.0
diphtheritic (membranous) 032.0
follicular 472.1
fusospirochetal 101
gonococcal 098.6
granular (chronic) 472.1
herpetic 054.79
hypertrophic 472.1

Pharyngitis (*Continued*)
infectional, chronic 472.1
influenzal (*see also* Influenza) 487.1
lymphonodular, acute 074.8
septic 034.0
streptococcal 034.0
tuberculous (*see also* Tuberculosis) 012.8 ●
vesicular 074.0
Pharyngoconjunctival fever 077.2
Pharyngoconjunctivitis, viral 077.2
Pharyngolaryngitis (acute) 465.0
chronic 478.9
septic 034.0
Pharyngoplegia 478.29
Pharyngotonsillitis 465.8
tuberculous 012.8 ●
Pharyngotracheitis (acute) 465.8
chronic 478.9
Pharynx, pharyngeal - *see* condition
Phase of life problem NEC V62.89
Phenomenon
Arthus 995.21
flashback (drug) 292.89
jaw-winking 742.8
Jod-Basedow 242.8 ●
L. E. cell 710.0
lupus erythematosus cell 710.0
Pelger-Huët (hereditary hyposegmentation) 288.2
Raynaud's (paroxysmal digital cyanosis) (secondary) 443.0
Reilly's (*see also* Neuropathy, peripheral, autonomic) 337.9
vasomotor 780.2
vasospastic 443.9
vasovagal 780.2
Wenckebach's, heart block (second degree) 426.13
Phenylketonuria (PKU) 270.1
Phenylpyruvicaciduria 270.1
Pheochromoblastoma (M8700/3)
specified site - *see* Neoplasm, by site, malignant
unspecified site 194.0
Pheochromocytoma (M8700/0)
malignant (M8700/3)
specified site - *see* Neoplasm, by site, malignant
unspecified site 194.0
specified site - *see* Neoplasm, by site, benign
unspecified site 227.0
Phimosis (congenital) 605
chancroidal 099.0
due to infection 605
Phlebectasia (*see also* Varicose, vein) 454.9
congenital NEC 747.60
esophagus (*see also* Varix, esophagus) 456.1
with hemorrhage (*see also* Varix, esophagus, bleeding) 456.0
Phlebitis (infective) (pyemic) (septic) (suppurative) 451.9
antecubital vein 451.82
arm NEC 451.84
axillary vein 451.89
basilic vein 451.82
deep 451.83
superficial 451.82
axillary vein 451.89
basilic vein 451.82
blue 451.9
brachial vein 451.83
breast, superficial 451.89
cavernous (venous) sinus - *see* Phlebitis, intracranial sinus
cephalic vein 451.82
cerebral (venous) sinus - *see* Phlebitis, intracranial sinus
chest wall, superficial 451.89
complicating pregnancy or puerperium 671.2 ●
affecting fetus or newborn 760.3

Phlebitis (*Continued*)
cranial (venous) sinus - *see* Phlebitis, intracranial sinus
deep (vessels) 451.19
femoral vein 451.11
specified vessel NEC 451.19
due to implanted device - *see* Complications, due to (presence of) any device, implant, or graft classified to 996.0–996.5 NEC
during or resulting from a procedure 997.2
femoral vein (deep) (superficial) 451.11
femoropopliteal 451.19
following infusion, perfusion, or transfusion 999.2
gouty 274.89 [451.9]
hepatic veins 451.89
iliac vein 451.81
iliofemoral 451.11
intracranial sinus (any) (venous) 325
late effect - *see* category 326
nonpyogenic 437.6
in pregnancy or puerperium 671.5 ●
jugular vein 451.89
lateral (venous) sinus - *see* Phlebitis, intracranial sinus
leg 451.2
deep (vessels) 451.19
specified vessel NEC 451.19
superficial (vessels) 451.0
femoral vein 451.11
longitudinal sinus - *see* Phlebitis, intracranial sinus
lower extremity 451.2
deep (vessels) 451.19
specified vessel NEC 451.19
superficial (vessels) 451.0
femoral vein 451.11
migrans, migrating (superficial) 453.1
pelvic
with
abortion - *see* Abortion, by type, with sepsis
ectopic pregnancy (*see also* categories 633.0–633.9) 639.0
molar pregnancy (*see also* categories 630–632) 639.0
following
abortion 639.0
ectopic or molar pregnancy 639.0
puerperal, postpartum 671.4 ●
popliteal vein 451.19
portal (vein) 572.1
postoperative 997.2
pregnancy 671.2 ●
deep 671.3 ●
specified type NEC 671.5 ●
superficial 671.2 ●
puerperal, postpartum, childbirth 671.2 ●
deep 671.4 ●
lower extremities 671.2 ●
pelvis 671.4 ●
specified site NEC 671.5 ●
superficial 671.2 ●
radial vein 451.83
retina 362.18
saphenous (great) (long) 451.0
accessory or small 451.0
sinus (meninges) - *see* Phlebitis, intracranial sinus
specified site NEC 451.89
subclavian vein 451.89
syphilitic 093.89
tibial vein 451.19
ulcer, ulcerative 451.9
leg 451.2
deep (vessels) 451.19
specified vessel NEC 451.19
superficial (vessels) 451.0
femoral vein 451.11

Phlebitis (*Continued*)
ulcer, ulcerative (*Continued*)
lower extremity 451.2
deep (vessels) 451.19
femoral vein 451.11
specified vessel NEC 451.19
superficial (vessels) 451.0
ulnar vein 451.83
umbilicus 451.89
upper extremity - *see* Phlebitis, arm
deep (veins) 451.83
brachial vein 451.83
radial vein 451.83
ulnar vein 451.83
superficial (veins) 451.82
antecubital vein 451.82
basilic vein 451.82
cephalic vein 451.82
uterus (septic) (*see also* Endometritis) 615.9
varicose (leg) (lower extremity) (*see also* Varicose, vein) 454.1
Phlebofibrosis 459.89
Phleboliths 459.89
Phlebosclerosis 459.89
Phlebothrombosis - *see* Thrombosis
Phlebotomus fever 066.0
Phlegm, choked on 933.1
Phlegmasia
alba dolens (deep vessels) 451.19
complicating pregnancy 671.3 ●
nonpuerperal 451.19
puerperal, postpartum, childbirth 671.4 ●
cerulea dolens 451.19
Phlegmon (*see also* Abscess) 682.9
erysipelatous (*see also* Erysipelas) 035
iliac 682.2
fossa 540.1
throat 478.29
Phlegmonous - *see* condition
Phlyctenulosis (allergic) (keratoconjunctivitis) (nontuberculous) 370.31
cornea 370.31
with ulcer (*see also* Ulcer, cornea) 370.00
tuberculous (*see also* Tuberculosis) 017.3 ● [370.31]
Phobia, phobic (reaction) 300.20
animal 300.29
isolated NEC 300.29
obsessional 300.3
simple NEC 300.29
social 300.23
specified NEC 300.29
state 300.20
Phocas' disease 610.1
Phocomelia 755.4
lower limb 755.32
complete 755.33
distal 755.35
proximal 755.34
upper limb 755.22
complete 755.23
distal 755.25
proximal 755.24
Phoria (*see also* Heterophoria) 378.40
Phosphate-losing tubular disorder 588.0
Phosphatemia 275.3
Phosphaturia 275.3
Photoallergic response 692.72
Photocoproporphyria 277.1
Photodermatitis (sun) 692.72
light other than sun 692.82
Photokeratitis 370.24
Photo-ophthalmia 370.24
Photophobia 368.13
Photopsia 368.15
Photoretinitis 363.31
Photoretinopathy 363.31
Photosensitiveness (sun) 692.72
light other than sun 692.82

◀ New   ◀║ Revised   ~~deleted~~ Deleted   ● Use Additional Digit(s)   ▨ Omit code

Photosensitization skin (sun) 692.72
  light other than sun 692.82
Phototoxic response 692.72
Phrenitis 323.9
Phrynoderma 264.8
Phthiriasis (pubis) (any site) 132.2
  with any infestation classifiable to 132.0 and
    132.1 132.3
Phthirus infestation - see Phthiriasis
Phthisis (see also Tuberculosis) 011.9●
  bulbi (infectional) 360.41
  colliers' 011.4●
  cornea 371.05
  eyeball (due to infection) 360.41
  millstone makers' 011.4●
  miners' 011.4●
  potters' 011.4●
  sandblasters' 011.4●
  stonemasons' 011.4●
Phycomycosis 117.7
Physalopteriasis 127.7
Physical therapy NEC V57.1
  breathing exercises V57.0
Physiological cup, optic papilla
  borderline, glaucoma suspect 365.00
  enlarged 377.14
  glaucomatous 377.14
Phytobezoar 938
  intestine 936
  stomach 935.2
Pian (see also Yaws) 102.9
Pianoma 102.1
Piarhemia, piarrhemia (see also Hyperlipemia)
    272.4
  bilharziasis 120.9
Pica 307.52
  hysterical 300.11
Pick's
  cerebral atrophy 331.11
    with dementia
      with behavioral disturbance 331.11
        [294.11]
      without behavioral disturbance 331.11
        [294.10]
  disease
    brain 331.11
      dementia in
        with behavioral disturbance 331.11
          [294.11]
        without behavioral disturbance
          331.11 [294.10]
    lipid histiocytosis 272.7
    liver (pericardial pseudocirrhosis of liver)
      423.2
    pericardium (pericardial pseudocirrhosis
      of liver) 423.2
    polyserositis (pericardial pseudocirrhosis of
      liver) 423.2
  syndrome
    heart (pericardial pseudocirrhosis of liver)
      423.2
    liver (pericardial pseudocirrhosis of liver)
      423.2
  tubular adenoma (M8640/0)
    specified site - see Neoplasm, by site,
      benign
    unspecified site
      female 220
      male 222.0
Pick-Herxheimer syndrome (diffuse idiopathic
    cutaneous atrophy) 701.8
Pick-Niemann disease (lipid histiocytosis)
    272.7
Pickwickian syndrome (cardiopulmonary
    obesity) 278.03
Piebaldism, classic 709.09
Piedra 111.2
  beard 111.2
    black 111.3
    white 111.2
  black 111.3

Piedra (Continued)
  scalp 111.3
    black 111.3
    white 111.2
  white 111.2
Pierre Marie's syndrome (pulmonary
    hypertrophic osteoarthropathy) 731.2
Pierre Marie-Bamberger syndrome
    (hypertrophic pulmonary
    osteoarthropathy) 731.2
Pierre Mauriac's syndrome (diabetes-
    dwarfism-obesity) 258.1
Pierre Robin deformity or syndrome
    (congenital) 756.0
Pierson's disease or osteochondrosis 732.1
Pigeon
  breast or chest (acquired) 738.3
    congenital 754.82
    rachitic (see also Rickets) 268.0
  breeders' disease or lung 495.2
  fanciers' disease or lung 495.2
  toe 735.8
Pigmentation (abnormal) 709.00
  anomalies NEC 709.00
    congenital 757.33
    specified NEC 709.09
  conjunctiva 372.55
  cornea 371.10
    anterior 371.11
    posterior 371.13
    stromal 371.12
  lids (congenital) 757.33
    acquired 374.52
  limbus corneae 371.10
  metals 709.00
  optic papilla, congenital 743.57
  retina (congenital) (grouped) (nevoid)
    743.53
    acquired 362.74
  scrotum, congenital 757.33
Piles - see Hemorrhoids
Pili
  annulati or torti (congenital) 757.4
  incarnati 704.8
Pill roller hand (intrinsic) 736.09
Pilomatrixoma (M8110/0) - see Neoplasm, skin,
    benign
Pilonidal - see condition
Pimple 709.8
PIN I (prostatic intraepithelial neoplasia I)
    602.3
PIN II (prostatic intraepithelial neoplasia II)
    602.3
PIN III (prostatic intraepithelial neoplasia III)
    233.4
Pinched nerve - see Neuropathy, entrapment
Pineal body or gland - see condition
Pinealoblastoma (M9362/3) 194.4
Pinealoma (M9360/1) 237.1
  malignant (M9360/3) 194.4
Pineoblastoma (M9362/3) 194.4
Pineocytoma (M9361/1) 237.1
Pinguecula 372.51
Pingueculitis 372.34
Pinhole meatus (see also Stricture, urethra)
    598.9
Pink
  disease 985.0
  eye 372.03
  puffer 492.8
Pinkus' disease (lichen nitidus) 697.1
Pinpoint
  meatus (see also Stricture, urethra) 598.9
  os (uteri) (see also Stricture, cervix) 622.4
Pinselhaare (congenital) 757.4
Pinta 103.9
  cardiovascular lesions 103.2
  chancre (primary) 103.0
  erythematous plaques 103.1
  hyperchromic lesions 103.1
  hyperkeratosis 103.1

Pinta (Continued)
  lesions 103.9
    cardiovascular 103.2
    hyperchromic 103.1
    intermediate 103.1
    late 103.2
    mixed 103.3
    primary 103.0
    skin (achromic) (cicatricial) (dyschromic)
      103.2
      hyperchromic 103.1
      mixed (achromic and hyperchromic)
        103.3
  papule (primary) 103.0
  skin lesions (achromic) (cicatricial)
      (dyschromic) 103.2
    hyperchromic 103.1
    mixed (achromic and hyperchromic) 103.3
  vitiligo 103.2
Pintid 103.0
Pinworms (disease) (infection) (infestation)
    127.4
Piry fever 066.8
Pistol wound - see Gunshot wound
Pit, lip (mucus), congenital 750.25
Pitchers' elbow 718.82
Pithecoid pelvis 755.69
  with disproportion (fetopelvic) 653.2●
    affecting fetus or newborn 763.1
    causing obstructed labor 660.1●
Pithiatism 300.11
Pitted - see also Pitting
  teeth 520.4
Pitting (edema) (see also Edema) 782.3
  lip 782.3
  nail 703.8
    congenital 757.5
Pituitary gland - see condition
Pituitary snuff-takers' disease 495.8
Pityriasis 696.5
  alba 696.5
  capitis 690.11
  circinata (et maculata) 696.3
  Hebra's (exfoliative dermatitis) 695.89
  lichenoides et varioliformis 696.2
  maculata (et circinata) 696.3
  nigra 111.1
  pilaris 757.39
    acquired 701.1
    Hebra's 696.4
  rosea 696.3
  rotunda 696.3
  rubra (Hebra) 695.89
    pilaris 696.4
  sicca 690.18
  simplex 690.18
  specified type NEC 696.5
  streptogenes 696.5
  versicolor 111.0
  scrotal 111.0
Placenta, placental
  ablatio 641.2●
    affecting fetus or newborn 762.1
  abnormal, abnormality 656.7●
    with hemorrhage 641.8●
      affecting fetus or newborn 762.1
    affecting fetus or newborn 762.2
  abruptio 641.2●
    affecting fetus or newborn 762.1
  accessory lobe - see Placenta, abnormal
  accreta (without hemorrhage) 667.0●
    with hemorrhage 666.0●
  adherent (without hemorrhage) 667.0●
    with hemorrhage 666.0●
  apoplexy - see Placenta, separation
  battledore - see Placenta, abnormal
  bilobate - see Placenta, abnormal
  bipartita - see Placenta, abnormal
  carneous mole 631.8
  centralis - see Placenta, previa
  circumvallata - see Placenta, abnormal

Placenta, placental *(Continued)*
cyst (amniotic) - *see* Placenta, abnormal
deficiency - *see* Placenta, insufficiency
degeneration - *see* Placenta, insufficiency
detachment (partial) (premature) (with hemorrhage) 641.2 ●
affecting fetus or newborn 762.1
dimidiata - *see* Placenta, abnormal
disease 656.7 ●
affecting fetus or newborn 762.2
duplex - *see* Placenta, abnormal
dysfunction - *see* Placenta, insufficiency
fenestrata - *see* Placenta, abnormal
fibrosis - *see* Placenta, abnormal
fleshy mole 631.8
hematoma - *see* Placenta, abnormal
hemorrhage NEC - *see* Placenta, separation
hormone disturbance or malfunction - *see* Placenta, abnormal
hyperplasia - *see* Placenta, abnormal
increta (without hemorrhage) 667.0 ●
with hemorrhage 666.0 ●
infarction 656.7 ●
affecting fetus or newborn 762.2
insertion, vicious - *see* Placenta, previa
insufficiency
affecting
fetus or newborn 762.2
management of pregnancy 656.5 ●
lateral - *see* Placenta, previa
low implantation or insertion - *see* Placenta, previa
low-lying - *see* Placenta, previa
malformation - *see* Placenta, abnormal
malposition - *see* Placenta, previa
marginalis, marginata - *see* Placenta, previa
marginal sinus (hemorrhage) (rupture) 641.2 ●
affecting fetus or newborn 762.1
membranacea - *see* Placenta, abnormal
multilobed - *see* Placenta, abnormal
multipartita - *see* Placenta, abnormal
necrosis - *see* Placenta, abnormal
percreta (without hemorrhage) 667.0 ●
with hemorrhage 666.0 ●
polyp 674.4 ●
previa (central) (centralis) (complete) (lateral) (marginal) (marginalis) (partial) (partialis) (total) (with hemorrhage) 641.1 ●
affecting fetus or newborn 762.0
noted
before labor, without hemorrhage (with cesarean delivery) 641.0 ●
during pregnancy (without hemorrhage) 641.0 ●
without hemorrhage (before labor and delivery) (during pregnancy) 641.0 ●
retention (with hemorrhage) 666.0 ●
fragments, complicating puerperium (delayed hemorrhage) 666.2 ●
without hemorrhage 667.1 ●
postpartum, puerperal 666.2 ●
without hemorrhage 667.0 ●
separation (normally implanted) (partial) (premature) (with hemorrhage) 641.2 ●
affecting fetus or newborn 762.1
septuplex - *see* Placenta, abnormal
small - *see* Placenta, insufficiency
softening (premature) - *see* Placenta, abnormal
spuria - *see* Placenta, abnormal
succenturiata - *see* Placenta, abnormal
syphilitic 095.8
transfusion syndromes 762.3
transmission of chemical substance - *see* Absorption, chemical, through placenta
trapped (with hemorrhage) 666.0 ●
without hemorrhage 667.0 ●

Placenta, placental *(Continued)*
trilobate - *see* Placenta, abnormal
tripartita - *see* Placenta, abnormal
triplex - *see* Placenta, abnormal
varicose vessel - *see* Placenta, abnormal
vicious insertion - *see* Placenta, previa
Placentitis
affecting fetus or newborn 762.7
complicating pregnancy 658.4 ●
Plagiocephaly (skull) 754.0
Plague 020.9
abortive 020.8
ambulatory 020.8
bubonic 020.0
cellulocutaneous 020.1
lymphatic gland 020.0
pneumonic 020.5
primary 020.3
secondary 020.4
pulmonary - *see* Plague, pneumonic
pulmonic - *see* Plague, pneumonic
septicemic 020.2
tonsillar 020.9
septicemic 020.2
vaccination, prophylactic (against) V03.3
Planning, family V25.09
contraception V25.9
natural
procreative V26.41
to avoid pregnancy V25.04
procreation V26.49
natural V26.41
Plaque
artery, arterial - *see* Arteriosclerosis
calcareous - *see* Calcification
Hollenhorst's (retinal) 362.33
tongue 528.6
Plasma cell myeloma 203.0 ●
Plasmacytoma, plasmocytoma (solitary) (M9731/1) 238.6
benign (M9731/0) - *see* Neoplasm, by site, benign
malignant (M9731/3) 203.8 ●
Plasmacytopenia 288.59
Plasmacytosis 288.64
Plaster ulcer (*see also* Ulcer, pressure) 707.00
Plateau iris syndrome (without glaucoma) 364.82
with glaucoma 365.23
Platybasia 756.0
Platyonychia (congenital) 757.5
acquired 703.8
Platypelloid pelvis 738.6
with disproportion (fetopelvic) 653.2 ●
affecting fetus or newborn 763.1
causing obstructed labor 660.1 ●
affecting fetus or newborn 763.1
congenital 755.69
Platyspondylia 756.19
Plethora 782.62
newborn 776.4
Pleura, pleural - *see* condition
Pleuralgia 786.52
Pleurisy (acute) (adhesive) (chronic) (costal) (diaphragmatic) (double) (dry) (fetid) (fibrinous) (fibrous) (interlobar) (latent) (lung) (old) (plastic) (primary) (residual) (sicca) (sterile) (subacute) (unresolved) (with adherent pleura) 511.0
with
effusion (without mention of cause) 511.9
bacterial, nontuberculous 511.1
nontuberculous NEC 511.9
bacterial 511.1
pneumococcal 511.1
specified type NEC 511.89
staphylococcal 511.1
streptococcal 511.1
tuberculous (*see also* Tuberculosis, pleura) 012.0 ●
primary, progressive 010.1 ●

Pleurisy *(Continued)*
with *(Continued)*
influenza, flu, or grippe (*see also* Influenza) 487.1
tuberculosis - *see* Pleurisy, tuberculous
encysted 511.89
exudative (*see also* Pleurisy, with effusion) 511.9
bacterial, nontuberculous 511.1
fibrinopurulent 510.9
with fistula 510.0
fibropurulent 510.9
with fistula 510.0
hemorrhagic 511.89
influenzal (*see also* Influenza) 487.1
pneumococcal 511.0
with effusion 511.1
purulent 510.9
with fistula 510.0
septic 510.9
with fistula 510.0
serofibrinous (*see also* Pleurisy, with effusion) 511.9
bacterial, nontuberculous 511.1
seropurulent 510.9
with fistula 510.0
serous (*see also* Pleurisy, with effusion) 511.9
bacterial, nontuberculous 511.1
staphylococcal 511.0
with effusion 511.1
streptococcal 511.0
with effusion 511.1
suppurative 510.9
with fistula 510.0
traumatic (post) (current) 862.29
with open wound into cavity 862.39
tuberculous (with effusion) (*see also* Tuberculosis, pleura) 012.0 ●
primary, progressive 010.1 ●
Pleuritis sicca - *see* Pleurisy
Pleurobronchopneumonia (*see also* Pneumonia, broncho-) 485
Pleurodynia 786.52
epidemic 074.1
viral 074.1
Pleurohepatitis 573.8
Pleuropericarditis (*see also* Pericarditis) 423.9
acute 420.90
Pleuropneumonia (acute) (bilateral) (double) (septic) (*see also* Pneumonia) 486
chronic (*see also* Fibrosis, lung) 515
Pleurorrhea (*see also* Hydrothorax) 511.89
Plexitis, brachial 353.0
Plica
knee 727.83
polonica 132.0
tonsil 474.8
Plicae dysphonia ventricularis 784.49
Plicated tongue 529.5
congenital 750.13
Plug
bronchus NEC 519.19
meconium (newborn) NEC 777.1
mucus - *see* Mucus, plug
Plumbism 984.9
specified type of lead - *see* Table of Drugs and Chemicals
Plummer's disease (toxic nodular goiter) 242.3 ●
Plummer-Vinson syndrome (sideropenic dysphagia) 280.8
Pluricarential syndrome of infancy 260
Plurideficiency syndrome of infancy 260
Plus (and minus) hand (intrinsic) 736.09
PMDD (premenstrual dysphoric disorder) 625.4
PMS 625.4
Pneumathemia - *see* Air, embolism, by type
Pneumatic drill or hammer disease 994.9
Pneumatocele (lung) 518.89
intracranial 348.89
tension 492.0

◀ New   ◀═ Revised   ~~deleted~~ Deleted   ● Use Additional Digit(s)   ▨ Omit code

Pneumatosis
cystoides intestinalis 569.89
peritonei 568.89
pulmonum 492.8
Pneumaturia 599.84
Pneumoblastoma (M8981/3) - *see* Neoplasm, lung, malignant
Pneumocephalus 348.89
Pneumococcemia 038.2
Pneumococcus, pneumococcal - *see* condition
Pneumoconiosis (due to) (inhalation of) 505
aluminum 503
asbestos 501
bagasse 495.1
bauxite 503
beryllium 503
carbon electrode makers' 503
coal
miners' (simple) 500
workers' (simple) 500
cotton dust 504
diatomite fibrosis 502
dust NEC 504
inorganic 503
lime 502
marble 502
organic NEC 504
fumes or vapors (from silo) 506.9
graphite 503
hard metal 503
mica 502
moldy hay 495.0
rheumatoid 714.81
silica NEC 502
and carbon 500
silicate NEC 502
talc 502
Pneumocystis carinii pneumonia 136.3
Pneumocystis jiroveci pneumonia 136.3
Pneumocystosis 136.3
with pneumonia 136.3
Pneumoenteritis 025
Pneumohemopericardium (*see also* Pericarditis) 423.9
Pneumohemothorax (*see also* Hemothorax) 511.89
traumatic 860.4
with open wound into thorax 860.5
Pneumohydropericardium (*see also* Pericarditis) 423.9
Pneumohydrothorax (*see also* Hydrothorax) 511.89
Pneumomediastinum 518.1
congenital 770.2
fetus or newborn 770.2
Pneumomycosis 117.9
Pneumonia (acute) (Alpenstich) (benign) (bilateral) (brain) (cerebral) (circumscribed) (congestive) (creeping) (delayed resolution) (double) (epidemic) (fever) (flash) (fulminant) (fungoid) (granulomatous) (hemorrhagic) (incipient) (infantile) (infectious) (infiltration) (insular) (intermittent) (latent) (lobe) (migratory) (newborn) (organized) (overwhelming) (primary) (progressive) (pseudolobar) (purulent) (resolved) (secondary) (senile) (septic) (suppurative) (terminal) (true) (unresolved) (vesicular) 486
with influenza, flu, or grippe 487.0
due to
identified (virus)
avian 488.01
(novel) 2009 H1N1 488.11
novel influenza A 488.81
adenoviral 480.0
adynamic 514
alba 090.0
allergic 518.3
alveolar - *see* Pneumonia, lobar

Pneumonia (*Continued*)
anaerobes 482.81
anthrax 022.1 [484.5]
apex, apical - *see* Pneumonia, lobar
ascaris 127.0 [484.8]
aspiration 507.0
due to
aspiration of microorganisms
bacterial 482.9
specified type NEC 482.89
specified organism NEC 483.8
bacterial NEC 482.89
viral 480.9
specified type NEC 480.8
food (regurgitated) 507.0
gastric secretions 507.0
milk 507.0
oils, essences 507.1
solids, liquids NEC 507.8
vomitus 507.0
fetal 770.18
due to
blood 770.16
clear amniotic fluid 770.14
meconium 770.12
postnatal stomach contents 770.86
newborn 770.18
due to
blood 770.16
clear amniotic fluid 770.14
meconium 770.12
postnatal stomach contents 770.86
asthenic 514
atypical (disseminated) (focal) (primary) 486
with influenza (*see also* Influenza) 487.0
bacillus 482.9
specified type NEC 482.89
bacterial 482.9
specified type NEC 482.89
Bacteroides (fragilis) (oralis) (melaninogenicus) 482.81
basal, basic, basilar - *see* Pneumonia, by type
bronchiolitis obliterans organized (BOOP) 516.8
broncho-, bronchial (confluent) (croupous) (diffuse) (disseminated) (hemorrhagic) (involving lobes) (lobar) (terminal) 485
with influenza 487.0
due to
identified (virus)
avian 488.01
(novel) 2009 H1N1 488.11
novel influenza A 488.81
allergic 518.3
aspiration (*see also* Pneumonia, aspiration) 507.0
bacterial 482.9
specified type NEC 482.89
capillary 466.19
with bronchospasm or obstruction 466.19
chronic (*see also* Fibrosis, lung) 515
congenital (infective) 770.0
diplococcal 481
Eaton's agent 483.0
Escherichia coli (E. coli) 482.82
Friedländer's bacillus 482.0
Hemophilus influenzae 482.2
hiberno-vernal 083.0 [484.8]
hypostatic 514
influenzal (*see also* Influenza) 487.0
inhalation (*see also* Pneumonia, aspiration) 507.0
due to fumes or vapors (chemical) 506.0
Klebsiella 482.0
lipid 507.1
endogenous 516.8
Mycoplasma (pneumoniae) 483.0
ornithosis 073.0

Pneumonia (*Continued*)
broncho-, bronchial (*Continued*)
pleuropneumonia-like organisms (PPLO) 483.0
pneumococcal 481
Proteus 482.83
Pseudomonas 482.1
specified organism NEC 483.8
bacterial NEC 482.89
staphylococcal 482.40
aureus 482.41
methicillin
resistant (MRSA) 482.42
susceptible (MSSA) 482.41
specified type NEC 482.49
streptococcal - *see* Pneumonia, streptococcal
typhoid 002.0 [484.8]
viral, virus (*see also* Pneumonia, viral) 480.9
Butyrivibrio (fibrisolvens) 482.81
Candida 112.4
capillary 466.19
with bronchospasm or obstruction 466.19
caseous (*see also* Tuberculosis) 011.6●
catarrhal - *see* Pneumonia, broncho-
central - *see* Pneumonia, lobar
Chlamydia, chlamydial 483.1
pneumoniae 483.1
psittaci 073.0
specified type NEC 483.1
trachomatis 483.1
cholesterol 516.8
chronic (*see also* Fibrosis, lung) 515
cirrhotic (chronic) (*see also* Fibrosis, lung) 515
Clostridium (haemolyticum) (novyi) NEC 482.81
confluent - *see* Pneumonia, broncho-
congenital (infective) 770.0
aspiration 770.18
croupous - *see* Pneumonia, lobar
cryptogenic organizing 516.36
cytomegalic inclusion 078.5 [484.1]
deglutition (*see also* Pneumonia, aspiration) 507.0
desquamative interstitial 516.37
diffuse - *see* Pneumonia, broncho-
diplococcal, diplococcus (broncho-) (lobar) 481
disseminated (focal) - *see* Pneumonia, broncho-
due to
adenovirus 480.0
anaerobes 482.81
Bacterium anitratum 482.83
Chlamydia, chlamydial 483.1
pneumoniae 483.1
psittaci 073.0
specified type NEC 483.1
trachomatis 483.1
coccidioidomycosis 114.0
Diplococcus (pneumoniae) 481
Eaton's agent 483.0
Escherichia coli (E. coli) 482.82
Friedländer's bacillus 482.0
fumes or vapors (chemical) (inhalation) 506.0
fungus NEC 117.9 [484.7]
coccidioidomycosis 114.0
Hemophilus influenzae (H. influenzae) 482.2
Herellea 482.83
influenza (*see also* Influenza) 487.0
Klebsiella pneumoniae 482.0
Mycoplasma (pneumoniae) 483.0
parainfluenza virus 480.2
pleuropneumonia-like organism (PPLO) 483.0
Pneumococcus 481

Pneumonia (Continued)
  due to (Continued)
    Pneumocystis carinii 136.3
    Pneumocystis jiroveci 136.3
    Proteus 482.83
    Pseudomonas 482.1
    respiratory syncytial virus 480.1
    rickettsia 083.9 [484.8]
    SARS-associated coronavirus 480.3
    specified
      bacteria NEC 482.89
      organism NEC 483.8
      virus NEC 480.8
    Staphylococcus 482.40
      aureus 482.41
        methicillin
          resistant (MRSA) 482.42
          susceptible (MSSA) 482.41
      specified type NEC 482.49
    Streptococcus - see also Pneumonia,
        streptococcal
      pneumoniae 481
    virus (see also Pneumonia, viral)
        480.9
      SARS-associated coronavirus
          480.3
  Eaton's agent 483.0
  embolic, embolism (see Embolism,
      pulmonary)
  eosinophilic 518.3
  Escherichia coli (E. coli) 482.82
  Eubacterium 482.81
  fibrinous - see Pneumonia, lobar
  fibroid (chronic) (see also Fibrosis, lung)
      515
  fibrous (see also Fibrosis, lung) 515
  Friedländer's bacillus 482.0
  fusobacterium (nucleatum) 482.81
  gangrenous 513.0
  giant cell (see also Pneumonia, viral)
      480.9
  gram-negative bacteria NEC 482.83
    anaerobic 482.81
  grippal (see also Influenza) 487.0
  Hemophilus influenzae (bronchial) (lobar)
      482.2
  hypostatic (broncho-) (lobar) 514
  in
    actinomycosis 039.1
    anthrax 022.1 [484.5]
    aspergillosis 117.3 [484.6]
    candidiasis 112.4
    coccidioidomycosis 114.0
    cytomegalic inclusion disease 078.5
        [484.1]
    histoplasmosis (see also Histoplasmosis)
        115.95
    infectious disease NEC 136.9
        [484.8]
    measles 055.1
    mycosis, systemic NEC 117.9
        [484.7]
    nocardiasis, nocardiosis 039.1
    ornithosis 073.0
    pneumocystosis 136.3
    psittacosis 073.0
    Q fever 083.0 [484.8]
    salmonellosis 003.22
    toxoplasmosis 130.4
    tularemia 021.2
    typhoid (fever) 002.0 [484.8]
    varicella 052.1
    whooping cough (see also Whooping
        cough) 033.9 [484.3]
  infective, acquired prenatally 770.0
  influenzal (broncho) (lobar) (virus) (see also
      Influenza) 487.0
  inhalation (see also Pneumonia, aspiration)
      507.0
    fumes or vapors (chemical)
        506.0

Pneumonia (Continued)
  interstitial 516.8
    with influenzal (see also Influenza) 487.0
    acute
      due to Pneumocystis (carinii) (jiroveci)
          136.3
      meaning:
        acute interstitial pneumonitis
            516.33
        atypical pneumonia - see
            Pneumonia, atypical
        bacterial pneumonia - see
            Pneumonia, bacterial
    chronic (see also Fibrosis, lung) 515
    desquamative 516.37
    hypostatic 514
    idiopathic 516.30
      lymphoid 516.35
    lipoid 507.1
    lymphoid (due to known underlying
        cause) 516.8
    non-specific (due to known underlying
        cause) 516.8
    organizing (due to known underlying
        cause) 516.8
    plasma cell 136.3
    Pseudomonas 482.1
  intrauterine (infective) 770.0
    aspiration 770.18
    blood 770.16
    clear amniotic fluid 770.14
    meconium 770.12
    postnatal stomach contents 770.86
  Klebsiella pneumoniae 482.0
  Legionnaires' 482.84
  lipid, lipoid (exogenous) (interstitial) 507.1
    endogenous 516.8
  lobar (diplococcal) (disseminated) (double)
      (interstitial) (pneumococcal, any type)
      481
    with influenza (see also Influenza) 487.0
    bacterial 482.9
      specified type NEC 482.89
    chronic (see also Fibrosis, lung) 515
    Escherichia coli (E. coli) 482.82
    Friedländer's bacillus 482.0
    Hemophilus influenzae (H. influenzae)
        482.2
    hypostatic 514
    influenzal (see also Influenza) 487.0
    Klebsiella 482.0
    ornithosis 073.0
    Proteus 482.83
    Pseudomonas 482.1
    psittacosis 073.0
    specified organism NEC 483.8
      bacterial NEC 482.89
    staphylococcal 482.40
      aureus 482.41
        methicillin
          resistant (MRSA) 482.42
          susceptible (MSSA) 482.41
      specified type NEC 482.49
    streptococcal - see Pneumonia,
        streptococcal
    viral, virus (see also Pneumonia, viral)
        480.9
  lobular (confluent) - see Pneumonia,
      broncho-
  Löffler's 518.3
  massive - see Pneumonia, lobar
  meconium aspiration 770.12
  metastatic NEC 038.8 [484.8]
  methicillin resistant Staphylococcus aureus
      (MRSA) 482.42
  methicillin susceptible Staphylococcus
      aureus (MSSA) 482.41
  MRSA (methicillin resistant Staphylococcus
      aureus) 482.42
  MSSA (methicillin susceptible
      Staphylococcus aureus) 482.41

Pneumonia (Continued)
  multilobar - see Pneumonia, by type
  Mycoplasma (pneumoniae) 483.0
  necrotic 513.0
  nitrogen dioxide 506.9
  orthostatic 514
  parainfluenza virus 480.2
  parenchymatous (see also Fibrosis, lung) 515
  passive 514
  patchy - see Pneumonia, broncho
  Peptococcus 482.81
  Peptostreptococcus 482.81
  plasma cell 136.3
  pleurolobar - see Pneumonia, lobar
  pleuropneumonia-like organism (PPLO)
      483.0
  pneumococcal (broncho) (lobar) 481
  Pneumocystis (carinii) (jiroveci) 136.3
  postinfectional NEC 136.9 [484.8]
  postmeasles 055.1
  postoperative 997.39
    aspiration 997.32
  primary atypical 486
  Proprionibacterium 482.81
  Proteus 482.83
  Pseudomonas 482.1
  psittacosis 073.0
  radiation 508.0
  respiratory syncytial virus 480.1
  resulting from a procedure 997.39
    aspiration 997.32
  rheumatic 390 [517.1]
  Salmonella 003.22
  SARS-associated coronavirus 480.3
  segmented, segmental - see Pneumonia,
      broncho-
  Serratia (marcascens) 482.83
  specified
    bacteria NEC 482.89
    organism NEC 483.8
    virus NEC 480.8
  spirochetal 104.8 [484]
  staphylococcal (broncho) (lobar) 482.40
    aureus 482.41
      methicillin
        resistant (MRSA) 482.42
        susceptible (MSSA) 482.41
    specified type NEC 482.49
  static, stasis 514
  streptococcal (broncho) (lobar) NEC 482.30
    Group
      A 482.31
      B 482.32
      specified NEC 482.39
    pneumoniae 481
    specified type NEC 482.39
  Streptococcus pneumoniae 481
  traumatic (complication) (early) (secondary)
      958.8
  tuberculous (any) (see also Tuberculosis)
      011.6●
  tularemic 021.2
  TWAR agent 483.1
  varicella 052.1
  Veillonella 482.81
  ventilator associated 997.31
  viral, virus (broncho) (interstitial) (lobar)
      480.9
    with influenza, flu, or grippe (see also
        Influenza) 487.0
    adenoviral 480.0
    parainfluenza 480.2
    respiratory syncytial 480.1
    SARS-associated coronavirus 480.3
    specified type NEC 480.8
  white (congenital) 090.0
Pneumonic - see condition
Pneumonitis (acute) (primary) (see also
    Pneumonia) 486
  allergic 495.9
    specified type NEC 495.8

◀ New   ◀‖‖ Revised   deleted Deleted   ● Use Additional Digit(s)   ▨ Omit code

Pneumonitis *(Continued)*
  aspiration 507.0
    due to fumes or gases 506.0
    fetal 770.18
      due to
        blood 770.16
        clear amniotic fluid 770.14
        meconium 770.12
        postnatal stomach contents 770.86
    newborn 770.18
      due to
        blood 770.16
        clear amniotic fluid 770.14
        meconium 770.12
        postnatal stomach contents 770.86
    obstetric 668.0●
  chemical 506.0
    due to fumes or gases 506.0
    resulting from a procedure 997.32
  cholesterol 516.8
  chronic *(see also* Fibrosis, lung) 515
  congenital rubella 771.0
  crack 506.0
  due to
    crack (cocaine) 506.0
    fumes or vapors 506.0
    inhalation
      food (regurgitated), milk, vomitus 507.0
      oils, essences 507.1
      saliva 507.0
      solids, liquids NEC 507.8
    toxoplasmosis (acquired) 130.4
      congenital (active) 771.2 *[484.8]*
  eosinophilic 518.3
  fetal aspiration 770.18
    due to
      blood 770.16
      clear amniotic fluid 770.14
      meconium 770.12
      postnatal stomach contents 770.86
  hypersensitivity 495.9
  interstitial (chronic) *(see also* Fibrosis, lung) 515
    acute 516.33
    idiopathic
      lymphocytic 516.35
      non-specific 516.32
    lymphoid 516.8
  lymphoid, interstitial 516.8
  meconium aspiration 770.12
  postanesthetic
    correct substance properly administered 507.0
    obstetric 668.0●
    overdose or wrong substance given 968.4
      specified anesthetic - *see* Table of Drugs and Chemicals
  postoperative 997.39
    aspiration 997.32
    obstetric 668.0●
  radiation 508.0
  rubella, congenital 771.0
  "ventilation" 495.7
  ventilator associated 997.31
  wood-dust 495.8
Pneumonoconiosis - *see* Pneumoconiosis
Pneumoparotid 527.8
Pneumopathy NEC 518.89
  alveolar 516.9
    specified NEC 516.8
  due to dust NEC 504
  parietoalveolar 516.9
  specified condition NEC 516.8
Pneumopericarditis *(see also* Pericarditis) 423.9
  acute 420.90
Pneumopericardium - *see also* Pericarditis
  congenital 770.2
  fetus or newborn 770.2
  traumatic (post) *(see also* Pneumothorax, traumatic) 860.0
    with open wound into thorax 860.1

Pneumoperitoneum 568.89
  fetus or newborn 770.2
Pneumophagia (psychogenic) 306.4
Pneumopleurisy, pneumopleuritis *(see also* Pneumonia) 486
Pneumopyopericardium 420.99
Pneumopyothorax *(see also* Pyopneumothorax) 510.9
  with fistula 510.0
Pneumorrhagia 786.30
  newborn 770.3
  tuberculous *(see also* Tuberculosis, pulmonary) 011.9●
Pneumosiderosis (occupational) 503
Pneumothorax 512.89
  acute 512.89
  chronic 512.83
  congenital 770.2
  due to operative injury of chest wall or lung 512.1
    accidental puncture or laceration 512.1
  fetus or newborn 770.2
  iatrogenic 512.1
  postoperative 512.1
  specified type NEC 512.89
  spontaneous 512.89
    fetus or newborn 770.2
    primary 512.81
    secondary 512.82
    tension 512.0
  sucking 512.89
    iatrogenic 512.1
    postoperative 512.1
  tense valvular, infectional 512.0
  tension 512.0
    iatrogenic 512.1
    postoperative 512.1
    spontaneous 512.0
  traumatic 860.0
    with
      hemothorax 860.4
        with open wound into thorax 860.5
      open wound into thorax 860.1
  tuberculous *(see also* Tuberculosis) 011.7●
Pocket(s)
  endocardial *(see also* Endocarditis) 424.90
  periodontal 523.8
Podagra 274.01
Podencephalus 759.89
Poikilocytosis 790.09
Poikiloderma 709.09
  Civatte's 709.09
  congenital 757.33
  vasculare atrophicans 696.2
Poikilodermatomyositis 710.3
Pointed ear 744.29
Poise imperfect 729.90
Poisoned - *see* Poisoning
Poisoning (acute) - *see also* Table of Drugs and Chemicals
  Bacillus, B.
    aertrycke *(see also* Infection, Salmonella) 003.9
    botulinus 005.1
    cholerae (suis) *(see also* Infection, Salmonella) 003.9
    paratyphosus *(see also* Infection, Salmonella) 003.9
    suipestifer *(see also* Infection, Salmonella) 003.9
  bacterial toxins NEC 005.9
  berries, noxious 988.2
  blood (general) - *see* Septicemia
  botulism 005.1
  bread, moldy, mouldy - *see* Poisoning, food
  Ciguatera 988.0
  damaged meat - *see* Poisoning, food
  death-cap (Amanita phalloides) (Amanita verna) 988.1
  decomposed food - *see* Poisoning, food
  diseased food - *see* Poisoning, food

Poisoning *(Continued)*
  drug - *see* Table of Drugs and Chemicals
  epidemic, fish, meat, or other food - *see* Poisoning, food
  fava bean 282.2
  fish (bacterial) - *see also* Poisoning, food
    noxious 988.0
  food (acute) (bacterial) (diseased) (infected) NEC 005.9
    due to
      bacillus
        aertrycke *(see also* Poisoning, food, due to Salmonella) 003.9
        botulinus 005.1
        cereus 005.89
        choleraesuis *(see also* Poisoning, food, due to Salmonella) 003.9
        paratyphosus *(see also* Poisoning, food, due to Salmonella) 003.9
        suipestifer *(see also* Poisoning, food, due to Salmonella) 003.9
      Clostridium 005.3
        botulinum 005.1
        perfringens 005.2
        welchii 005.2
      Salmonella (aertrycke) (callinarum) (choleraesuis) (enteritidis) (paratyphi) (suipestifer) 003.9
        with
          gastroenteritis 003.0
          localized infection(s) *(see also* Infection, Salmonella) 003.20
          septicemia 003.1
          specified manifestation NEC 003.8
      specified bacterium NEC 005.89
      Staphylococcus 005.0
      Streptococcus 005.89
      Vibrio parahaemolyticus 005.4
      Vibrio vulnificus 005.81
    noxious or naturally toxic 988.0
      berries 988.2
      fish 988.0
      mushroom 988.1
      plants NEC 988.2
  ice cream - *see* Poisoning, food
  ichthyotoxism (bacterial) 005.9
  kreotoxism, food 005.9
  malarial - *see* Malaria
  meat - *see* Poisoning, food
  mushroom (noxious) 988.1
  mussel - *see also* Poisoning, food
    noxious 988.0
  noxious foodstuffs *(see also* Poisoning, food, noxious) 988.9
    specified type NEC 988.8
  plants, noxious 988.2
  pork - *see also* Poisoning, food
    specified NEC 988.8
    Trichinosis 124
  ptomaine - *see* Poisoning, food
  putrefaction, food - *see* Poisoning, food
  radiation 508.0
  Salmonella *(see also* Infection, Salmonella) 003.9
  sausage - *see also* Poisoning, food
    Trichinosis 124
  saxitoxin 988.0
  shellfish - *see also* Poisoning, food
    noxious (amnesic) (azaspiracid) (diarrheic) (neurotoxic) (paralytic) 988.0
  Staphylococcus, food 005.0
  toxic, from disease NEC 799.89
  truffles - *see* Poisoning, food
  uremic - *see* Uremia
  uric acid 274.9
  water 276.69
Poison ivy, oak, sumac or other plant dermatitis 692.6

Poker spine 720.0
Policeman's disease 729.2
Polioencephalitis (acute) (bulbar) (see also
    Poliomyelitis, bulbar) 045.0●
    inferior 335.22
    influenzal (see also Influenza) 487.8
    superior hemorrhagic (acute) (Wernicke's)
        265.1
    Wernicke's (superior hemorrhagic) 265.1
Polioencephalomyelitis (acute) (anterior)
    (bulbar) (see also Polioencephalitis)
    045.0●
Polioencephalopathy, superior hemorrhagic
    265.1
    with
        beriberi 265.0
        pellagra 265.2
Poliomeningoencephalitis - see
    Meningoencephalitis
Poliomyelitis (acute) (anterior) (epidemic)
    045.9●

Note: Use the following fifth-digit
subclassification with category 045:

    0   poliovirus, unspecified type
    1   poliovirus, type I
    2   poliovirus, type II
    3   poliovirus, type III

    with
        paralysis 045.1●
            bulbar 045.0●
        abortive 045.2●
        ascending 045.9●
            progressive 045.9●
        bulbar 045.0●
        cerebral 045.0●
        chronic 335.21
        congenital 771.2
        contact V01.2
        deformities 138
        exposure to V01.2
        late effect 138
        nonepidemic 045.9●
        nonparalytic 045.2●
        old with deformity 138
        posterior, acute 053.19
        residual 138
        sequelae 138
        spinal, acute 045.9●
        syphilitic (chronic) 094.89
        vaccination, prophylactic (against) V04.0
Poliosis (eyebrow) (eyelashes) 704.3
    circumscripta (congenital) 757.4
        acquired 704.3
    congenital 757.4
Pollakiuria 788.41
    psychogenic 306.53
Pollinosis 477.0
Pollitzer's disease (hidradenitis suppurativa)
    705.83
Polyadenitis (see also Adenitis) 289.3
    malignant 020.0
Polyalgia 729.99
Polyangiitis (essential) 446.0
Polyarteritis (nodosa) (renal) 446.0
Polyarthralgia 719.49
    psychogenic 306.0
Polyarthritis, polyarthropathy NEC 716.59
    due to or associated with other specified
        conditions - see Arthritis, due to or
        associated with
    endemic (see also Disease, Kaschin-Beck)
        716.0●
    inflammatory 714.9
        specified type NEC 714.89
    juvenile (chronic) 714.30
        acute 714.31
    migratory - see Fever, rheumatic
    rheumatic 714.0
        fever (acute) - see Fever, rheumatic

Polycarential syndrome of infancy 260
Polychondritis (atrophic) (chronic) (relapsing)
    733.99
Polycoria 743.46
Polycystic (congenital) (disease) 759.89
    degeneration, kidney - see Polycystic, kidney
    kidney (congenital) 753.12
        adult type (APKD) 753.13
        autosomal dominant 753.13
        autosomal recessive 753.14
        childhood type (CPKD) 753.14
        infantile type 753.14
    liver 751.62
    lung 518.89
        congenital 748.4
    ovary, ovaries 256.4
    spleen 759.0
Polycythemia (primary) (rubra) (vera)
    (M9950/1) 238.4
    acquired 289.0
    benign 289.0
        familial 289.6
    due to
        donor twin 776.4
        fall in plasma volume 289.0
        high altitude 289.0
        maternal-fetal transfusion 776.4
        stress 289.0
    emotional 289.0
    erythropoietin 289.0
    familial (benign) 289.6
    Gaisböck's (hypertonica) 289.0
    high altitude 289.0
    hypertonica 289.0
    hypoxemic 289.0
    neonatorum 776.4
    nephrogenous 289.0
    relative 289.0
    secondary 289.0
    spurious 289.0
    stress 289.0
Polycytosis cryptogenica 289.0
Polydactylism, polydactyly 755.00
    fingers 755.01
    toes 755.02
Polydipsia 783.5
Polydystrophic oligophrenia 277.5
Polyembryoma (M9072/3) - see Neoplasm, by
    site, malignant
Polygalactia 676.6●
Polyglandular
    deficiency 258.9
    dyscrasia 258.9
    dysfunction 258.9
    syndrome 258.8
Polyhydramnios (see also Hydramnios) 657●
Polymastia 757.6
Polymenorrhea 626.2
Polymicrogyria 742.2
Polymyalgia 725
    arteritica 446.5
    rheumatica 725
Polymyositis (acute) (chronic) (hemorrhagic)
    710.4
    with involvement of
        lung 710.4 [517.8]
        skin 710.3
    ossificans (generalisata) (progressiva) 728.19
    Wagner's (dermatomyositis) 710.3
Polyneuritis, polyneuritic (see also
    Polyneuropathy) 356.9
    alcoholic 357.5
        with psychosis 291.1
    cranialis 352.6
    demyelinating, chronic inflammatory (CIDP)
        357.81
    diabetic 250.6● [357.2]
        due to secondary diabetes 249.6● [357.2]
    due to lack of vitamin NEC 269.2 [357.4]
    endemic 265.0 [357.4]
    erythredema 985.0

Polyneuritis, polyneuritic (Continued)
    febrile 357.0
    hereditary ataxic 356.3
    idiopathic, acute 357.0
    infective (acute) 357.0
    nutritional 269.9 [357.4]
    postinfectious 357.0
Polyneuropathy (peripheral) 356.9
    alcoholic 357.5
    amyloid 277.39 [357.4]
    arsenical 357.7
    critical illness 357.82
    demyelinating, chronic inflammatory (CIDP)
        357.81
    diabetic 250.6● [357.2]
        due to secondary diabetes 249.6● [357.2]
    due to
        antitetanus serum 357.6
        arsenic 357.7
        drug or medicinal substance 357.6
            correct substance properly
                administered 357.6
            overdose or wrong substance given or
                taken 977.9
            specified drug - see Table of Drugs
                and Chemicals
        lack of vitamin NEC 269.2 [357.4]
        lead 357.7
        organophosphate compounds 357.7
        pellagra 265.2 [357.4]
        porphyria 277.1 [357.4]
        serum 357.6
        toxic agent NEC 357.7
    hereditary 356.0
    idiopathic 356.9
        progressive 356.4
    in
        amyloidosis 277.39 [357.4]
        avitaminosis 269.2 [357.4]
            specified NEC 269.1 [357.4]
        beriberi 265.0 [357.4]
        collagen vascular disease NEC 710.9
            [357.1]
        deficiency
            B-complex NEC 266.2 [357.4]
            vitamin B 266.9 [357.4]
            vitamin B₆ 266.1 [357.4]
        diabetes 250.6● [357.2]
            due to secondary diabetes 249.6●
                [357.2]
        diphtheria (see also Diphtheria) 032.89
            [357.4]
        disseminated lupus erythematosus 710.0
            [357.1]
        herpes zoster 053.13
        hypoglycemia 251.2 [357.4]
        malignant neoplasm (M8000/3) NEC
            199.1 [357.3]
        mumps 072.72
        pellagra 265.2 [357.4]
        polyarteritis nodosa 446.0 [357.1]
        porphyria 277.1 [357.4]
        rheumatoid arthritis 714.0 [357.1]
        sarcoidosis 135 [357.4]
        uremia 585.9 [357.4]
    lead 357.7
    nutritional 269.9 [357.4]
        specified NEC 269.8 [357.4]
    postherpetic 053.13
    progressive 356.4
    sensory (hereditary) 356.2
    specified NEC 356.8
Polyonychia 757.5
Polyopia 368.2
    refractive 368.15
Polyorchism, polyorchidism (three testes)
    752.89
Polyrrhymenitis (peritoneal) (see also
    Polyserositis) 568.82
    pericardial 423.2
Polyostotic fibrous dysplasia 756.54

Polyotia 744.1
Polyp, polypus

> Note: Polyps of organs or sites that do not appear in the list below should be coded to the residual category for diseases of the organ or site concerned.

accessory sinus 471.8
adenoid tissue 471.0
adenomatous (M8210/0) - *see also* Neoplasm, by site, benign
   adenocarcinoma in (M8210/3) - *see* Neoplasm, by site, malignant
   carcinoma in (M8210/3) - *see* Neoplasm, by site, malignant
   multiple (M8221/0) - *see* Neoplasm, by site, benign
antrum 471.8
anus, anal (canal) (nonadenomatous) 569.0
   adenomatous 211.4
Bartholin's gland 624.6
bladder (M8120/1) 236.7
broad ligament 620.8
cervix (uteri) 622.7
   adenomatous 219.0
   in pregnancy or childbirth 654.6●
     affecting fetus or newborn 763.89
     causing obstructed labor 660.2●
   mucous 622.7
   nonneoplastic 622.7
choanal 471.0
cholesterol 575.6
clitoris 624.6
colon (M8210/0) (*see also* Polyp, adenomatous) 211.3
corpus uteri 621.0
dental 522.0
ear (middle) 385.30
endometrium 621.0
ethmoidal (sinus) 471.8
fallopian tube 620.8
female genital organs NEC 624.8
frontal (sinus) 471.8
gallbladder 575.6
gingiva 523.8
gum 523.8
labia 624.6
larynx (mucous) 478.4
malignant (M8000/3) - *see* Neoplasm, by site, malignant
maxillary (sinus) 471.8
middle ear 385.30
myometrium 621.0
nares
   anterior 471.9
   posterior 471.0
nasal (mucous) 471.9
   cavity 471.0
   septum 471.9
nasopharyngeal 471.0
neoplastic (M8210/0) - *see* Neoplasm, by site, benign
nose (mucous) 471.9
oviduct 620.8
paratubal 620.8
pharynx 478.29
   congenital 750.29
placenta, placental 674.4●
prostate 600.20
   with
     other lower urinary tract symptoms (LUTS) 600.21
     urinary
       obstruction 600.21
       retention 600.21
pudenda 624.6
pulp (dental) 522.0
rectosigmoid 211.4
rectum (nonadenomatous) 569.0
   adenomatous 211.4

Polyp, polypus (*Continued*)
septum (nasal) 471.9
sinus (accessory) (ethmoidal) (frontal) (maxillary) (sphenoidal) 471.8
sphenoidal (sinus) 471.8
stomach (M8210/0) 211.1
tube, fallopian 620.8
turbinate, mucous membrane 471.8
ureter 593.89
urethra 599.3
uterine
   ligament 620.8
   tube 620.8
uterus (body) (corpus) (mucous) 621.0
   in pregnancy or childbirth 654.1●
     affecting fetus or newborn 763.89
     causing obstructed labor 660.2●
vagina 623.7
vocal cord (mucous) 478.4
vulva 624.6
Polyphagia 783.6
Polypoid - *see* condition
Polyposis - *see also* Polyp
coli (adenomatous) (M8220/0) 211.3
   adenocarcinoma in (M8220/3) 153.9
   carcinoma in (M8220/3) 153.9
familial (M8220/0) 211.3
intestinal (adenomatous) (M8220/0) 211.3
multiple (M8221/0) - *see* Neoplasm, by site, benign
Polyradiculitis (acute) 357.0
Polyradiculoneuropathy (acute) (segmentally demyelinating) 357.0
Polysarcia 278.00
Polyserositis (peritoneal) 568.82
due to pericarditis 423.2
paroxysmal (familial) 277.31
pericardial 423.2
periodic (familial) 277.31
pleural - *see* Pleurisy
recurrent 277.31
tuberculous (*see also* Tuberculosis, polyserositis) 018.9●
Polysialia 527.7
Polysplenia syndrome 759.0
Polythelia 757.6
Polytrichia (*see also* Hypertrichosis) 704.1
Polyunguia (congenital) 757.5
acquired 703.8
Polyuria 788.42
Pompe's disease (glycogenosis II) 271.0
Pompholyx 705.81
Poncet's disease (tuberculous rheumatism) (*see also* Tuberculosis) 015.9●
Pond fracture - *see* Fracture, skull, vault
Ponos 085.0
Pons, pontine - *see* condition
Poor
aesthetics of existing restoration of tooth 525.67
contractions, labor 661.2●
   affecting fetus or newborn 763.7
fetal growth NEC 764.9●
   affecting management of pregnancy 656.5●
incorporation
   artificial skin graft 996.55
   decellularized allodermis graft 996.55
obstetrical history V13.29
   affecting management of current pregnancy V23.49
     ectopic pregnancy V23.42
     pre-term labor V23.41
   pre-term labor V13.21
sucking reflex (newborn) 796.1
vision NEC 369.9
Poradenitis, nostras 099.1
Porencephaly (congenital) (developmental) (true) 742.4
acquired 348.0
nondevelopmental 348.0
traumatic (post) 310.2

Porocephaliasis 134.1
Porokeratosis 757.39
disseminated superficial actinic (DSAP) 692.75
Poroma, eccrine (M8402/0) - *see* Neoplasm, skin, benign
Porphyria (acute) (congenital) (constitutional) (erythropoietic) (familial) (hepatica) (idiopathic) (idiosyncratic) (intermittent) (latent) (mixed hepatic) (photosensitive) (South African genetic) (Swedish) 277.1
acquired 277.1
cutaneatarda
   hereditaria 277.1
   symptomatica 277.1
due to drugs
   correct substance properly administered 277.1
   overdose or wrong substance given or taken 977.9
     specified drug - *see* Table of Drugs and Chemicals
secondary 277.1
toxic NEC 277.1
variegata 277.1
Porphyrinuria (acquired) (congenital) (secondary) 277.1
Porphyruria (acquired) (congenital) 277.1
Portal - *see* condition
Port wine nevus or mark 757.32
Posadas-Wernicke disease 114.9
Position
fetus, abnormal (*see also* Presentation, fetal) 652.9●
teeth, faulty (*see also* Anomaly, position tooth) 524.30
Positive
culture (nonspecific) 795.39
   AIDS virus V08
   blood 790.7
   HIV V08
   human immunodeficiency virus V08
   nose 795.39
     Staphylococcus - *see* Carrier (suspected) of, Staphylococcus
   skin lesion NEC 795.39
   spinal fluid 792.0
   sputum 795.39
   stool 792.1
   throat 795.39
   urine 791.9
   wound 795.39
findings, anthrax 795.31
HIV V08
human immunodeficiency virus (HIV) V08
PPD 795.51
serology
   AIDS virus V08
     inconclusive 795.71
   HIV V08
     inconclusive 795.71
   human immunodeficiency virus V08
     inconclusive 795.71
   syphilis 097.1
     with signs or symptoms - *see* Syphilis, by site and stage
     false 795.6
skin test 795.7
   tuberculin (without active tuberculosis) 795.51
VDRL 097.1
   with signs or symptoms - *see* Syphilis, by site and stage
   false 795.6
Wassermann reaction 097.1
   false 795.6
Postcardiotomy syndrome 429.4
Postcaval ureter 753.4
Postcholecystectomy syndrome 576.0
Postclimacteric bleeding 627.1
Postcommissurotomy syndrome 429.4

◀ New   ◀▌▌▌ Revised   ~~deleted~~ Deleted   ● Use Additional Digit(s)   ▨ Omit code

Postconcussional syndrome 310.2
Postcontusional syndrome 310.2
Postcricoid region - *see* condition
Post-dates (pregnancy) - *see* Pregnancy
Postencephalitic - *see also* condition
    syndrome 310.89
Posterior - *see* condition
Posterolateral sclerosis (spinal cord) - *see*
    Degeneration, combined
Postexanthematous - *see* condition
Postfebrile - *see* condition
Postgastrectomy dumping syndrome 564.2
Posthemiplegic chorea 344.89
Posthemorrhagic anemia (chronic) 280.0
    acute 285.1
    newborn 776.5
Posthepatitis syndrome 780.79
Postherpetic neuralgia (intercostal) (syndrome)
    (zoster) 053.19
    geniculate ganglion 053.11
    ophthalmica 053.19
    trigeminal 053.12
Posthitis 607.1
Postimmunization complication or reaction -
    see Complications, vaccination
Postinfectious - *see* condition
Postinfluenzal syndrome 780.79
Postlaminectomy syndrome 722.80
    cervical, cervicothoracic 722.81
    kyphosis 737.12
    lumbar, lumbosacral 722.83
    thoracic, thoracolumbar 722.82
Postleukotomy syndrome 310.0
Postlobectomy syndrome 310.0
Postmastectomy lymphedema (syndrome)
    457.0
Postmaturity, postmature (fetus or newborn)
    (gestation period over 42 completed
    weeks) 766.22
    affecting management of pregnancy
        post-term pregnancy 645.1●
        prolonged pregnancy 645.2●
    syndrome 766.22
Postmeasles - *see also* condition
    complication 055.8
        specified NEC 055.79
Postmenopausal
    endometrium (atrophic) 627.8
        suppurative (*see also* Endometritis) 615.9
    hormone replacement therapy V07.4
    status (age related) (natural) V49.81
Postnasal drip 784.91
Postnatal - *see* condition
Postoperative - *see also* condition
    confusion state 293.9
    psychosis 293.9
    status NEC (*see also* Status (post)) V45.89
Postpancreatectomy hyperglycemia 251.3
Postpartum - *see also* condition
    anemia 648.2●
        cardiomyopathy 674.5●
    observation
        immediately after delivery V24.0
        routine follow-up V24.2
Postperfusion syndrome NEC 999.89
    bone marrow 996.85
Postpoliomyelitic - *see* condition
Postsurgery status NEC (*see also* Status (post))
    V45.89
Post-term (pregnancy) 645.1●
    infant (gestation period over 40 completed
        weeks to 42 completed weeks) 766.21
Post-transplant lymphoproliferative disorder
    (PTLD) 238.77
Posttraumatic - *see* condition
Posttraumatic brain syndrome, nonpsychotic
    310.2
Post-Traumatic Stress Disorder (PTSD)
    309.81
Post-typhoid abscess 002.0
Postures, hysterical 300.11

Postvaccinal reaction or complication - *see*
    Complications, vaccination
Postvagotomy syndrome 564.2
Postvalvulotomy syndrome 429.4
Postvasectomy sperm count V25.8
Potain's disease (pulmonary edema) 514
Potain's syndrome (gastrectasis with
    dyspepsia) 536.1
Pott's
    curvature (spinal) (*see also* Tuberculosis)
        015.0● [737.43]
    disease or paraplegia (*see also* Tuberculosis)
        015.0● [730.88]
    fracture (closed) 824.4
        open 824.5
    gangrene 440.24
    osteomyelitis (*see also* Tuberculosis) 015.0●
        [730.88]
    spinal curvature (*see also* Tuberculosis)
        015.0● [737.43]
    tumor, puffy (*see also* Osteomyelitis) 730.2●
Potter's
    asthma 502
    disease 753.0
    facies 754.0
    lung 502
    syndrome (with renal agenesis) 753.0
Pouch
    bronchus 748.3
    Douglas' - *see* condition
    esophagus, esophageal (congenital) 750.4
        acquired 530.6
    gastric 537.1
    Hartmann's (abnormal sacculation of
        gallbladder neck) 575.8
        of intestine V44.3
            attention to V55.3
    pharynx, pharyngeal (congenital) 750.27
Pouchitis 569.71
Poulet's disease 714.2
Poultrymen's itch 133.8
Poverty V60.2
PPE (palmar plantar erythrodysesthesia)
    693.0
Prader-Labhart-Willi-Fanconi syndrome
    (hypogenital dystrophy with diabetic
    tendency) 759.81
Prader-Willi syndrome (hypogenital dystrophy
    with diabetic tendency) 759.81
Preachers' voice 784.49
Pre-AIDS - *see* Human immunodeficiency virus
    (disease) (illness) (infection)
Preauricular appendage 744.1
Prebetalipoproteinemia (acquired) (essential)
    (familial) (hereditary) (primary)
    (secondary) 272.1
    with chylomicronemia 272.3
Precipitate labor 661.3●
    affecting fetus or newborn 763.6
Preclimacteric bleeding 627.0
    menorrhagia 627.0
Precocious
    adrenarche 259.1
    menarche 259.1
    menstruation 259.1
    pubarche 259.1
    puberty NEC 259.1
    sexual development NEC 259.1
    thelarche 259.1
Precocity, sexual (constitutional) (cryptogenic)
    (female) (idiopathic) (male) NEC 259.1
    with adrenal hyperplasia 255.2
Precordial pain 786.51
    psychogenic 307.89
Predeciduous teeth 520.2
Prediabetes, prediabetic 790.29
    complicating pregnancy, childbirth, or
        puerperium 648.8●
    fetus or newborn 775.89
Predislocation status of hip, at birth (*see also*
    Subluxation, congenital, hip) 754.32

Pre-eclampsia (mild) 642.4●
    with pre-existing hypertension 642.7●
    affecting fetus or newborn 760.0
    severe 642.5●
    superimposed on pre-existing hypertensive
        disease 642.7●
Preeruptive color change, teeth, tooth
    520.8
Preexcitation 426.7
    atrioventricular conduction 426.7
    ventricular 426.7
Preglaucoma 365.00
Pregnancy (single) (uterine) (without sickness)
    V22.2

> Note: Use the following fifth-digit
> subclassification with categories 640–649,
> 651–679:
>
>   0   unspecified as to episode of care
>   1   delivered, with or without mention of
>   antepartum condition
>   2   delivered, with mention of
>   postpartum complication
>   3   antepartum condition or complication
>   4   postpartum condition or
>   complication

    abdominal (ectopic) 633.00
        with intrauterine pregnancy 633.01
        affecting fetus or newborn 761.4
    abnormal NEC 646.9●
    ampullar - *see* Pregnancy, tubal
    biochemical 631.0
    broad ligament - *see* Pregnancy, cornual
    cervical - *see* Pregnancy, cornual
    chemical 631.0
    combined (extrauterine and intrauterine) -
        see Pregnancy, cornual
    complicated (by) 646.9●
        abnormal, abnormality NEC 646.9●
            cervix 654.6●
            cord (umbilical) 663.9●
            glucose tolerance (conditions
                classifiable to 790.21–790.29)
                648.8●
            pelvic organs or tissues NEC 654.9●
            pelvis (bony) 653.0●
            perineum or vulva 654.8●
            placenta, placental (vessel) 656.7●
            position
                cervix 654.4●
                placenta 641.1●
                    without hemorrhage 641.0●
                uterus 654.4●
            size, fetus 653.5●
            uterus (congenital) 654.0●
        abscess or cellulitis
            bladder 646.6●
            genitourinary tract (conditions
                classifiable to 590, 595, 597, 599.0,
                614.0–614.5, 614.7–614.9, 615)
                646.6●
            kidney 646.6●
            urinary tract NEC 646.6●
        adhesion, pelvic peritoneal 648.9●
        air embolism 673.0●
        albuminuria 646.2●
            with hypertension - *see* Toxemia, of
                pregnancy
        amnionitis 658.4●
        amniotic fluid embolism 673.1●
        anemia (conditions classifiable to
            280–285) 648.2●
        appendicitis 648.9●
        atrophy, yellow (acute) (liver) (subacute)
            646.7●
        bacilluria, asymptomatic 646.5●
        bacteriuria, asymptomatic 646.5●
        bariatric surgery status 649.2●
        bicornis or bicornuate uterus 654.0●
        biliary problems 646.8●

◀ New   ◀ Revised   ~~deleted~~ Deleted   ● Use Additional Digit(s)   ▨ Omit code

Pregnancy *(Continued)*
  complicated *(Continued)*
    bone and joint disorders (conditions
        classifiable to 720–724 or conditions
        affecting lower limbs classifiable to
        711–719, 725–738) 648.7 ●
    breech presentation (buttocks) (complete)
        (frank) 652.2 ●
      with successful version 652.1 ●
    cardiovascular disease (conditions
        classifiable to 390–398, 410–429)
        648.6 ●
      congenital (conditions classifiable to
          745–747) 648.5 ●
    cerebrovascular disorders (conditions
        classifiable to 430–434, 436–437)
        674.0 ●
    cervicitis (conditions classifiable to 616.0)
        646.6 ●
    chloasma (gravidarum) 646.8 ●
    cholelithiasis 646.8 ●
    cholestasis 646.7 ●
    chorea (gravidarum) - *see* Eclampsia,
        pregnancy
    coagulation defect 649.3 ●
    conjoined twins 678.1 ●
    contraction, pelvis (general) 653.1 ●
      inlet 653.2 ●
      outlet 653.3 ●
    convulsions (eclamptic) (uremic) 642.6 ●
      with pre-existing hypertension 642.7 ●
    current disease or condition
        (nonobstetric)
      abnormal glucose tolerance 648.8 ●
      anemia 648.2 ●
      biliary tract 646.7 ●
      bone and joint (lower limb) 648.7 ●
      cardiovascular 648.6 ●
        congenital 648.5 ●
      cerebrovascular 674.0 ●
      diabetes (conditions classifiable to 249
          and 250) 648.0 ●
      drug dependence 648.3 ●
      female genital mutilation 648.9 ●
      genital organ or tract 646.6 ●
      gonorrheal 647.1 ●
      hypertensive 642.2 ●
        chronic kidney 642.2 ●
        renal 642.1 ●
      infectious 647.9 ●
        specified type NEC 647.8 ●
      liver 646.7 ●
      malarial 647.4 ●
      nutritional deficiency 648.9 ●
      parasitic NEC 647.8 ●
      periodontal disease 648.9 ●
      renal 646.2 ●
        hypertensive 642.1 ●
      rubella 647.5 ●
      specified condition NEC 648.9 ●
      syphilitic 647.0 ●
      thyroid 648.1 ●
      tuberculous 647.3 ●
      urinary 646.6 ●
      venereal 647.2 ●
      viral NEC 647.6 ●
    cystitis 646.6 ●
    cystocele 654.4 ●
    death of fetus (near term) 656.4 ●
      early pregnancy (before 22 completed
          weeks' gestation) 632
    deciduitis 646.6 ●
    decreased fetal movements 655.7 ●
    diabetes (mellitus) (conditions classifiable
        to 249 and 250) 648.0 ●
    disorders of liver and biliary tract 646.7 ●
    displacement, uterus NEC 654.4 ●
    disproportion - *see* Disproportion
    double uterus 654.0 ●
    drug dependence (conditions classifiable
        to 304) 648.3 ●

Pregnancy *(Continued)*
  complicated *(Continued)*
    dysplasia, cervix 654.6 ●
    early onset of delivery (spontaneous)
        644.2 ●
    eclampsia, eclamptic (coma) (convulsions)
        (delirium) (nephritis) (uremia)
        642.6 ●
      with pre-existing hypertension
          642.7 ●
    edema 646.1 ●
      with hypertension - *see* Toxemia, of
          pregnancy
    effusion, amniotic fluid 658.1 ●
      delayed delivery following
          658.2 ●
    embolism
      air 673.0 ●
      amniotic fluid 673.1 ●
      blood-clot 673.2 ●
      cerebral 674.0 ●
      pulmonary NEC 673.2 ●
      pyemic 673.3 ●
      septic 673.3 ●
    emesis (gravidarum) - *see* Pregnancy,
        complicated, vomiting
    endometritis (conditions classifiable to
        615.0–615.9) 670.1 ●
    decidual 646.6 ●
    epilepsy 649.4 ●
    excessive weight gain NEC 646.1 ●
    face presentation 652.4 ●
    failure, fetal head to enter pelvic brim
        652.5 ●
    false labor (pains) 644.1 ●
    fatigue 646.8 ●
    fatty metamorphosis of liver 646.7 ●
    female genital mutilation 648.9 ●
    fetal
      anemia 678.0 ●
      complications from in utero procedure
          679.1 ●
      conjoined twins 678.1 ●
      death (near term) 656.4 ●
        early (before 22 completed weeks'
            gestation) 632
      deformity 653.7 ●
      distress 656.8 ●
      hematologic conditions 678.0 ●
      reduction of multiple fetuses reduced
          to single fetus 651.7 ●
      thrombocytopenia 678.0 ●
      twin to twin transfusion 678.0 ●
    fibroid (tumor) (uterus) 654.1 ●
    footling presentation 652.8 ●
      with successful version 652.1 ●
    gallbladder disease 646.8 ●
    gastric banding status 649.2 ●
    gastric bypass status for obesity 649.2 ●
    genital herpes (asymptomatic) (history of)
        (inactive) 647.6
    goiter 648.1 ●
    gonococcal infection (conditions
        classifiable to 098) 647.1 ●
    gonorrhea (conditions classifiable to 098)
        647.1 ●
    hemorrhage 641.9 ●
      accidental 641.2 ●
      before 22 completed weeks' gestation
          NEC 640.9 ●
      cerebrovascular 674.0 ●
      due to
        afibrinogenemia or other
            coagulation defect (conditions
            classifiable to 286.0–286.9)
            641.3 ●
        leiomyoma, uterine 641.8 ●
        marginal sinus (rupture) 641.2 ●
        premature separation, placenta
            641.2 ●
        trauma 641.8 ●

Pregnancy *(Continued)*
  complicated *(Continued)*
    hemorrhage *(Continued)*
      early (before 22 completed weeks'
          gestation) 640.9 ●
        threatened abortion 640.0 ●
        unavoidable 641.1 ●
    hepatitis (acute) (malignant) (subacute)
        646.7 ●
      viral 647.6 ●
    herniation of uterus 654.4 ●
    high head at term 652.5 ●
    hydatidiform mole (delivered)
        (undelivered) 630
    hydramnios 657 ●
    hydrocephalic fetus 653.6 ●
    hydrops amnii 657 ●
    hydrorrhea 658.1 ●
    hyperemesis (gravidarum) - *see*
        Hyperemesis, gravidarum
    hypertension - *see* Hypertension,
        complicating pregnancy
    hypertensive
      chronic kidney disease 642.2 ●
      heart and chronic kidney disease
          642.2 ●
      heart and renal disease 642.2 ●
      heart disease 642.2 ●
      renal disease 642.2 ●
    hypertensive heart and chronic kidney
        disease 642.2 ●
    hyperthyroidism 648.1 ●
    hypothyroidism 648.1 ●
    hysteralgia 646.8 ●
    icterus gravis 646.7 ●
    incarceration, uterus 654.3 ●
    incompetent cervix (os) 654.5 ●
    infection 647.9 ●
      amniotic fluid 658.4 ●
      bladder 646.6 ●
      genital organ (conditions classifiable to
          614.0– 614.5, 614.7–614.9, 615)
          646.6 ●
      kidney (conditions classifiable to
          590.0–590.9) 646.6 ●
      urinary (tract) 646.6 ●
        asymptomatic 646.5 ●
    infective and parasitic diseases NEC
        647.8 ●
    inflammation
      bladder 646.6 ●
      genital organ (conditions classifiable to
          614.0) 646.6 ●
      urinary tract NEC 646.6 ●
    injury 648.9 ●
      obstetrical NEC 665.9 ●
    insufficient weight gain 646.8 ●
    insulin resistance 648.8 ●
    intrauterine fetal death (near term) NEC
        656.4 ●
      early (before 22 completed weeks'
          gestation) 632
    malaria (conditions classifiable to 084)
        647.4 ●
    malformation, uterus (congenital) 654.0 ●
    malnutrition (conditions classifiable to
        260–269) 648.9 ●
    malposition
      fetus - *see* Pregnancy, complicated,
          malpresentation
      uterus or cervix 654.4 ●
    malpresentation 652.9 ●
      with successful version 652.1 ●
      in multiple gestation 652.6 ●
      specified type NEC 652.8 ●
    marginal sinus hemorrhage or rupture
        641.2 ●
    maternal complications from in utero
        procedure 679.0 ●
    maternal drug abuse 648.4 ●
    maternal obesity syndrome 646.1 ●

Pregnancy *(Continued)*
  complicated *(Continued)*
    menstruation 640.8 ●
    mental disorders (conditions classifiable
      to 290–303, 305.0, 305.2–305.9,
      306–316, 317–319) 648.4 ●
    mentum presentation 652.4 ●
    missed
      abortion 632
      delivery (at or near term) 656.4 ●
      labor (at or near term) 656.4 ●
    necrosis
      genital organ or tract (conditions
        classifiable to 614.0–614.5,
        614.7–614.9, 615) 646.6 ●
      liver (conditions classifiable to 570)
        646.7 ●
      renal, cortical 646.2 ●
    nephritis or nephrosis (conditions
      classifiable to 580–589) 646.2 ●
      with hypertension 642.1 ●
    nephropathy NEC 646.2 ●
    neuritis (peripheral) 646.4 ●
    nutritional deficiency (conditions
      classifiable to 260–269) 648.9 ●
    obesity 649.1 ●
      surgery status 649.2 ●
    oblique lie or presentation 652.3 ●
      with successful version 652.1 ●
    obstetrical trauma NEC 665.9 ●
    oligohydramnios NEC 658.0 ●
    onset of contractions before 37 weeks
      644.0 ■
    oversize fetus 653.5 ●
    papyraceous fetus 646.0 ●
    patent cervix 654.5 ●
    pelvic inflammatory disease (conditions
      classifiable to 614.0–614.5,
      614.7–614.9, 615) 646.6 ●
    pelvic peritoneal adhesion 648.9 ●
    placenta, placental
      abnormality 656.7 ●
      abruptio or ablatio 641.2 ●
      detachment 641.2 ●
      disease 656.7 ●
      infarct 656.7 ●
      low implantation 641.1 ●
        without hemorrhage 641.0 ●
      malformation 656.7 ●
      malposition 641.1 ●
        without hemorrhage 641.0 ●
      marginal sinus hemorrhage 641.2 ●
      previa 641.1 ●
        without hemorrhage 641.0 ●
      separation (premature) (undelivered)
        641.2 ●
    placentitis 658.4 ●
    pneumonia 648.9
    polyhydramnios 657 ●
    postmaturity
      post-term 645.1 ●
      prolonged 645.2 ●
    prediabetes 648.8 ●
    pre-eclampsia (mild) 642.4 ●
      severe 642.5 ●
      superimposed on pre-existing
        hypertensive disease 642.7 ●
    premature rupture of membranes
      658.1 ●
      with delayed delivery 658.2 ●
    previous
      ectopic pregnancy V23.42
      infertility V23.0
      in utero procedure during previous
        pregnancy V23.86
      nonobstetric condition V23.89
      poor obstetrical history V23.49
      premature delivery V23.41
      trophoblastic disease (conditions
        classifiable to 630) V23.1
    prolapse, uterus 654.4 ●

Pregnancy *(Continued)*
  complicated *(Continued)*
    proteinuria (gestational) 646.2 ●
      with hypertension - *see* Toxemia, of
        pregnancy
    pruritus (neurogenic) 646.8 ●
    psychosis or psychoneurosis 648.4 ●
    ptyalism 646.8 ●
    pyelitis (conditions classifiable to
      590.0–590.9) 646.6 ●
    renal disease or failure NEC 646.2 ●
      with secondary hypertension
        642.1 ●
      hypertensive 642.2 ●
    retention, retained dead ovum 631.8
    retroversion, uterus 654.3 ●
    Rh immunization, incompatibility, or
      sensitization 656.1 ●
    rubella (conditions classifiable to 056)
      647.5 ●
    rupture
      amnion (premature) 658.1 ●
        with delayed delivery 658.2 ●
      marginal sinus (hemorrhage) 641.2 ●
      membranes (premature) 658.1 ●
        with delayed delivery 658.2 ●
      uterus (before onset of labor) 665.0 ●
    salivation (excessive) 646.8 ●
    salpingo-oophoritis (conditions
      classifiable to 614.0–614.2)
      646.6 ●
    septicemia (conditions classifiable to
      038.0–038.9) 647.8 ●
      postpartum 670.2 ●
      puerperal 670.2 ●
      smoking 649.0 ●
    spasms, uterus (abnormal) 646.8 ●
    specified condition NEC 646.8 ●
    spotting 649.5 ●
    spurious labor pains 644.1 ●
    status post
      bariatric surgery 649.2 ●
      gastric banding 649.2 ●
      gastric bypass for obesity 649.2 ●
      obesity surgery 649.2 ●
    superfecundation 651.9 ●
    superfetation 651.9 ●
    syphilis (conditions classifiable to
      090–097) 647.0 ●
    threatened
      abortion 640.0 ●
      premature delivery 644.2 ●
      premature labor 644.0 ●
    thrombophlebitis (superficial) 671.2 ●
      deep 671.3 ●
      septic 670.3 ●
    thrombosis 671.2 ●
      venous (superficial) 671.2 ●
      deep 671.3 ●
    thyroid dysfunction (conditions
      classifiable to 240–246) 648.1 ●
    thyroiditis 648.1 ●
    thyrotoxicosis 648.1 ●
    tobacco use disorder 649.0 ●
    torsion of uterus 654.4 ●
    toxemia - *see* Toxemia, of pregnancy
    transverse lie or presentation 652.3 ●
      with successful version 652.1 ●
    trauma 648.9 ●
      obstetrical 665.9 ●
    tuberculosis (conditions classifiable to
      010–018) 647.3 ●
    tumor
      cervix 654.6 ●
      ovary 654.4 ●
      pelvic organs or tissue NEC 654.4 ●
      uterus (body) 654.1 ●
        cervix 654.6 ●
      vagina 654.7 ●
      vulva 654.8 ●
    unstable lie 652.0 ●

Pregnancy *(Continued)*
  complicated *(Continued)*
    uremia - *see* Pregnancy, complicated, renal
      disease
    urethritis 646.6 ●
    vaginitis or vulvitis (conditions
      classifiable to 616.1) 646.6 ●
    varicose
      placental vessels 656.7 ●
      veins (legs) 671.0 ●
        perineum 671.1 ●
        vulva 671.1 ●
    varicosity, labia or vulva 671.1 ●
    venereal disease NEC (conditions
      classifiable to 099) 647.2 ●
    venous complication 671.9 ●
    viral disease NEC (conditions classifiable
      to 042, 050–055, 057–079, 795.05,
      795.15, 796.75) 647.6 ●
    vomiting (incoercible) (pernicious)
      (persistent) (uncontrollable)
      (vicious) 643.9 ●
      due to organic disease or other cause
        643.8 ●
      early - *see* Hyperemesis, gravidarum
      late (after 22 completed weeks
        gestation) 643.2 ●
    young maternal age 659.8 ●
  complications NEC 646.9 ●
  cornual 633.80
    with intrauterine pregnancy 633.81
    affecting fetus or newborn 761.4
  death, maternal NEC 646.9 ●
  delivered - *see* Delivery
  ectopic (ruptured) NEC 633.90
    with intrauterine pregnancy 633.91
    abdominal - *see* Pregnancy, abdominal
    affecting fetus or newborn 761.4
    combined (extrauterine and intrauterine) -
      see Pregnancy, cornual
    ovarian - *see* Pregnancy, ovarian
    specified type NEC 633.80
      with intrauterine pregnancy
        633.81
      affecting fetus or newborn 761.4
    tubal - *see* Pregnancy, tubal
  examination, pregnancy
    negative result V72.41
    not confirmed V72.40
    positive result V72.42
  extrauterine - *see* Pregnancy, ectopic
  fallopian - *see* Pregnancy, tubal
  false 300.11
    labor (pains) 644.1 ●
  fatigue 646.8 ●
  illegitimate V61.6
  incidental finding V22.2
  in double uterus 654.0 ●
  interstitial - *see* Pregnancy, cornual
  intraligamentous - *see* Pregnancy, cornual
  intramural - *see* Pregnancy, cornual
  intraperitoneal - *see* Pregnancy, abdominal
  isthmian - *see* Pregnancy, tubal
  management affected by
    abnormal, abnormality
      fetus (suspected) 655.9 ●
        specified NEC 655.8 ●
      placenta 656.7 ●
    advanced maternal age NEC 659.6 ●
      multigravida 659.6 ●
      primigravida 659.5 ●
    antibodies (maternal)
      anti-c 656.1 ●
      anti-d 656.1 ●
      anti-e 656.1 ●
      blood group (ABO) 656.2 ●
        Rh(esus) 656.1 ●
    appendicitis 648.9 ●
    bariatric surgery status 649.2 ●
    coagulation defect 649.3 ●
    elderly multigravida 659.6 ●

◄ New   ◄ Revised   ~~deleted~~ Deleted   ● Use Additional Digit(s)   ▨ Omit code

Pregnancy *(Continued)*
  management affected by *(Continued)*
    elderly primigravida 659.5●
    epilepsy 649.4●
    fetal (suspected)
      abnormality 655.9●
        abdominal 655.8●
        acid-base balance 656.8●
        cardiovascular 655.8●
        facial 655.8●
        gastrointestinal 655.8●
        genitourinary 655.8●
        heart rate or rhythm 659.7●
        limb 655.8●
        specified NEC 655.8●
      acidemia 656.3●
      anencephaly 655.0●
      aneuploidy 655.1●
      bradycardia 659.7●
      central nervous system malformation 655.0●
      chromosomal abnormalities (conditions classifiable to 758.0–758.9) 655.1●
      damage from
        drugs 655.5●
          obstetric, anesthetic, or sedative 655.5●
        environmental toxins 655.8●
        intrauterine contraceptive device 655.8●
        maternal
          alcohol addiction 655.4●
          disease NEC 655.4●
          drug use 655.5●
          listeriosis 655.4●
          rubella 655.3●
          toxoplasmosis 655.4●
          viral infection 655.3●
        radiation 655.6●
      death (near term) 656.4●
        early (before 22 completed weeks' gestation) 632
      distress 656.8●
      excessive growth 656.6●
      growth retardation 656.5●
      hereditary disease 655.2●
      hydrocephalus 655.0●
      intrauterine death 656.4●
      poor growth 656.5●
      spina bifida (with myelomeningocele) 655.0●
    fetal-maternal hemorrhage 656.0●
    gastric banding status 649.2●
    gastric bypass status for obesity 649.2●
    hereditary disease in family (possibly) affecting fetus 655.2●
    incompatibility, blood groups (ABO) 656.2●
      Rh(esus) 656.1●
    insufficient prenatal care V23.7
    insulin resistance 648.8●
    intrauterine death 656.4●
    isoimmunization (ABO) 656.2●
      Rh(esus) 656.1●
    large-for-dates fetus 656.6●
    light-for-dates fetus 656.5●
    meconium in liquor 656.8●
    mental disorder (conditions classifiable to 290–303, 305.0, 305.2–305.9, 306–316, 317–319) 648.4●
    multiparity (grand) 659.4●
    obesity 649.1●
      surgery status 649.2●
    poor obstetric history V23.49
      pre-term labor V23.41
    postmaturity
      post-term 645.1●
      prolonged 645.2●
    post-term pregnancy 645.1●

Pregnancy *(Continued)*
  management affected by *(Continued)*
    previous
      abortion V23.2
        habitual 646.3●
      cesarean delivery 654.2●
      difficult delivery V23.49
      ectopic pregnancy V23.42
      forceps delivery V23.49
      habitual abortions 646.3●
      hemorrhage, antepartum or postpartum V23.49
      hydatidiform mole V23.1
      infertility V23.0
      in utero procedure during previous pregnancy V23.86
      malignancy NEC V23.89
      nonobstetrical conditions V23.89
      premature delivery V23.41
      recurrent pregnancy loss 646.3
      trophoblastic disease (conditions in 630) V23.1
      vesicular mole V23.1
    prolonged pregnancy 645.2●
    recurrent pregnancy loss 646.3
    small-for-dates fetus 656.5●
    smoking 649.0●
    spotting 649.5●
    suspected conditions not found
      amniotic cavity and membrane problem V89.01
      cervical shortening V89.05
      fetal anomaly V89.03
      fetal growth problem V89.04
      oligohydramnios V89.01
      other specified problem NEC V89.09
      placental problem V89.02
      polyhydramnios V89.01
    tobacco use disorder 649.0●
    venous complication 671.9●
    young maternal age 659.8●
  maternal death NEC 646.9●
  mesometric (mural) - *see* Pregnancy, cornual
  molar 631.8●
    hydatidiform *(see also* Hydatidiform mole) 630
      previous, affecting management of pregnancy V23.1
    previous, affecting management of pregnancy V23.49
  multiple NEC 651.9●
    with fetal loss and retention of one or more fetus(es) 651.6●
    affecting fetus or newborn 761.5
    following (elective) fetal reduction 651.7●
    specified type NEC 651.8●
      with fetal loss and retention of one or more fetus(es) 651.6●
      following (elective) fetal reduction 651.7●
  mural - *see* Pregnancy, cornual
  observation NEC V22.1
    first pregnancy V22.0
    high-risk V23.9
      inconclusive fetal viability V23.87
      specified problem NEC V23.89
  ovarian 633.20
    with intrauterine pregnancy 633.21
    affecting fetus or newborn 761.4
  possible, not (yet) confirmed V72.40
  postmature
    post-term 645.1●
    prolonged 645.2●
  post-term 645.1●
  prenatal care only V22.1
    first pregnancy V22.0
    high-risk V23.9
      inconclusive fetal viability V23.87
      specified problem NEC V23.89
  prolonged 645.2●

Pregnancy *(Continued)*
  quadruplet NEC 651.2●
    with fetal loss and retention of one or more fetus(es) 651.5●
    affecting fetus or newborn 761.5
    following (elective) fetal reduction 651.7●
  quintuplet NEC 651.8●
    with fetal loss and retention of one or more fetus(es) 651.6●
    affecting fetus or newborn 761.5
    following (elective) fetal reduction 651.7●
  resulting from
    assisted reproductive technology V23.85
    in vitro fertilization V23.85
  sextuplet NEC 651.8●
    with fetal loss and retention of one or more fetus(es) 651.6●
    affecting fetus or newborn 761.5
    following (elective) fetal reduction 651.7●
  spurious 300.11
  superfecundation NEC 651.9●
    with fetal loss and retention of one or more fetus(es) 651.6●
    following (elective) fetal reduction 651.7●
  superfetation NEC 651.9●
    with fetal loss and retention of one or more fetus(es) 651.6●
    following (elective) fetal reduction 651.7●
  supervision (of) (for) - *see also* Pregnancy, management affected by
    elderly
      multigravida V23.82
      primigravida V23.81
    high-risk V23.9
      inconclusive fetal viability V23.87
      insufficient prenatal care V23.7
      specified problem NEC V23.89
    inconclusive fetal viability V23.87
    multiparity V23.3
    normal NEC V22.1
      first V22.0
    poor
      obstetric history V23.49
        ectopic pregnancy V23.42
        pre-term labor V23.41
      reproductive history V23.5
    previous
      abortion V23.2
      hydatidiform mole V23.1
      infertility V23.0
      neonatal death V23.5
      stillbirth V23.5
      trophoblastic disease V23.1
      vesicular mole V23.1
    specified problem NEC V23.89
    young
      multigravida V23.84
      primigravida V23.83
  triplet NEC 651.1●
    with fetal loss and retention of one or more fetus(es) 651.4●
    affecting fetus or newborn 761.5
    following (elective) fetal reduction 651.7●
  tubal (with rupture) 633.10
    with intrauterine pregnancy 633.11
    affecting fetus or newborn 761.4
  twin NEC 651.0●
    with fetal loss and retention of one fetus 651.3●
    affecting fetus or newborn 761.5
    conjoined 678.1●
    following (elective) fetal reduction 651.7●
  unconfirmed V72.40
  undelivered (no other diagnosis) V22.2
    with false labor 644.1●
    high-risk V23.9
      specified problem NEC V23.89
  unwanted NEC V61.7
Pregnant uterus - *see* condition
Preiser's disease (osteoporosis) 733.09
Prekwashiorkor 260

Preleukemia 238.75

Preluxation of hip, congenital (*see also* Subluxation, congenital, hip) 754.32

Premature - *see also* condition
  beats (nodal) 427.60
    atrial 427.61
    auricular 427.61
    postoperative 997.1
    specified type NEC 427.69
    supraventricular 427.61
    ventricular 427.69
  birth NEC 765.1●
  closure
    cranial suture 756.0
    fontanel 756.0
    foramen ovale 745.8
  contractions 427.60
    atrial 427.61
    auricular 427.61
    auriculoventricular 427.61
    heart (extrasystole) 427.60
    junctional 427.60
    nodal 427.60
    postoperative 997.1
    ventricular 427.69
  ejaculation 302.75
  infant NEC 765.1●
    excessive 765.0●
    light-for-dates - *see* Light-for-dates
  labor 644.2●
    threatened 644.0●
  lungs 770.4
  menopause 256.31
  puberty 259.1
  rupture of membranes or amnion 658.1●
    affecting fetus or newborn 761.1
    delayed delivery following 658.2●
  senility (syndrome) 259.8
  separation, placenta (partial) - *see* Placenta, separation
  ventricular systole 427.69

Prematurity NEC 765.1●
  extreme 765.0●

Premenstrual syndrome 625.4

Premenstrual tension 625.4

Premolarization, cuspids 520.2

Premyeloma 273.1

Prenatal
  care, normal pregnancy V22.1
    first V22.0
  death, cause unknown - *see* Death, fetus
  screening - *see* Antenatal, screening
  teeth 520.6

Prepartum - *see* condition

Preponderance, left or right ventricular 429.3

Prepuce - *see* condition

PRES (posterior reversible encephalopathy syndrome) 348.39

Presbycardia 797
  hypertensive (*see also* Hypertension, heart) 402.90

Presbycusis 388.01

Presbyesophagus 530.89

Presbyophrenia 310.1

Presbyopia 367.4

Prescription of contraceptives NEC V25.02
  diaphragm V25.02
  oral (pill) V25.01
    emergency V25.03
    postcoital V25.03
    repeat V25.41
  repeat V25.40
    oral (pill) V25.41

Presenile - *see also* condition
  aging 259.8
  dementia (*see also* Dementia, presenile) 290.10

Presenility 259.8

Presentation, fetal
  abnormal 652.9●
    with successful version 652.1●
    before labor, affecting fetus or newborn 761.7
    causing obstructed labor 660.0●
      affecting fetus or newborn, any, except breech 763.1
    in multiple gestation (one or more) 652.6●
    specified NEC 652.8●
  arm 652.7●
    causing obstructed labor 660.0●
  breech (buttocks) (complete) (frank) 652.2●
    with successful version 652.1●
      before labor, affecting fetus or newborn 761.7
    before labor, affecting fetus or newborn 761.7
  brow 652.4●
    causing obstructed labor 660.0●
  buttocks 652.2●
  chin 652.4●
  complete 652.2●
  compound 652.8●
  cord 663.0●
  extended head 652.4●
  face 652.4●
    to pubes 652.8●
  footling 652.8●
  frank 652.2●
  hand, leg, or foot NEC 652.8●
  incomplete 652.8●
  mentum 652.4●
  multiple gestation (one fetus or more) 652.6●
  oblique 652.3●
    with successful version 652.1●
  shoulder 652.8●
    affecting fetus or newborn 763.1
  transverse 652.3●
    with successful version 652.1●
  umbilical cord 663.0●
  unstable 652.0●

Prespondylolisthesis (congenital) (lumbosacral) 756.11

Pressure
  area, skin ulcer (*see also* Ulcer, pressure) 707.00
  atrophy, spine 733.99
  birth, fetus or newborn NEC 767.9
  brachial plexus 353.0
  brain 348.4
    injury at birth 767.0
  cerebral - *see* Pressure, brain
  chest 786.59
  cone, tentorial 348.4
    injury at birth 767.0
  funis - *see* Compression, umbilical cord
  hyposystolic (*see also* Hypotension) 458.9
  increased
    intracranial 781.99
      due to
        benign intracranial hypertension 348.2
        hydrocephalus - *see* hydrocephalus
        injury at birth 767.8
    intraocular 365.00
  lumbosacral plexus 353.1
  mediastinum 519.3
  necrosis (chronic) (skin) (*see also* Decubitus) 707.00
  nerve - *see* Compression, nerve
  paralysis (*see also* Neuropathy, entrapment) 355.9
  pre-ulcer skin changes limited to persistent focal erythema (*see also* Ulcer, pressure) 707.21
  sore (chronic) (*see also* Ulcer, pressure) 707.00
  spinal cord 336.9
  ulcer (chronic) (*see also* Ulcer, pressure) 707.00

Pressure (*Continued*)
  umbilical cord - *see* Compression, umbilical cord
  venous, increased 459.89

Pre-syncope 780.2

Preterm infant NEC 765.1●
  extreme 765.0●

Priapism (penis) 607.3

Prickling sensation (*see also* Disturbance, sensation) 782.0

Prickly heat 705.1

Primary - *see also* condition
  angle closure suspect 365.02

Primigravida, elderly
  affecting
    fetus or newborn 763.89
    management of pregnancy, labor, and delivery 659.5●

Primipara, old
  affecting
    fetus or newborn 763.89
    management of pregnancy, labor, and delivery 659.5●

Primula dermatitis 692.6

Primus varus (bilateral) (metatarsus) 754.52

PRIND (prolonged reversible ischemic neurologic deficit) 434.91
  history of (personal) V12.54

Pringle's disease (tuberous sclerosis) 759.5

Prinzmetal's angina 413.1

Prinzmetal-Massumi syndrome (anterior chest wall) 786.52

Prizefighter ear 738.7

Problem (with) V49.9
  academic V62.3
  acculturation V62.4
  adopted child V61.24
  aged
    in-law V61.3
    parent V61.3
    person NEC V61.8
  alcoholism in family V61.41
  anger reaction (*see also* Disturbance, conduct) 312.0●
  behavior, child 312.9
  behavioral V40.9
    specified NEC V40.39
  betting V69.3
  biological child V61.23
  cardiorespiratory NEC V47.2
  care of sick or handicapped person in family or household V61.49
  career choice V62.29
  communication V40.1
  conscience regarding medical care V62.6
  delinquency (juvenile) 312.9
  diet, inappropriate V69.1
  digestive NEC V47.3
  ear NEC V41.3
  eating habits, inappropriate V69.1
  economic V60.2
    affecting care V60.9
      specified type NEC V60.89
  educational V62.3
  enuresis, child 307.6
  exercise, lack of V69.0
  eye NEC V41.1
  family V61.9
    specified circumstance NEC V61.8
  fear reaction, child 313.0
  feeding (elderly) (infant) 783.3
    newborn 779.31
    nonorganic 307.59
  fetal, affecting management of pregnancy 656.9●
    specified type NEC 656.8●
  financial V60.2
  foster child V61.25
  functional V41.9
    specified type NEC V41.8
  gambling V69.3

◀ New   ◀┅ Revised   ~~deleted~~ Deleted   ● Use Additional Digit(s)   ▨ Omit code

Problem *(Continued)*
  genital NEC V47.5
  head V48.9
    deficiency V48.0
    disfigurement V48.6
    mechanical V48.2
    motor V48.2
    movement of V48.2
    sensory V48.4
    specified condition NEC V48.8
  hearing V41.2
  high-risk sexual behavior V69.2
  identity 313.82
  influencing health status NEC V49.89
  internal organ NEC V47.9
    deficiency V47.0
    mechanical or motor V47.1
  interpersonal NEC V62.81
  jealousy, child 313.3
  learning V40.0
  legal V62.5
  life circumstance NEC V62.89
  lifestyle V69.9
    specified NEC V69.8
  limb V49.9
    deficiency V49.0
    disfigurement V49.4
    mechanical V49.1
    motor V49.2
    movement, involving
      musculoskeletal system V49.1
      nervous system V49.2
    sensory V49.3
    specified condition NEC V49.5
  litigation V62.5
  living alone V60.3
  loneliness NEC V62.89
  marital V61.10
    involving
      divorce V61.03
      estrangement V61.09
      psychosexual disorder 302.9
      sexual function V41.7
    relationship V61.10
  mastication V41.6
  medical care, within family V61.49
  mental V40.9
    specified NEC V40.2
  mental hygiene, adult V40.9
  multiparity V61.5
  nail biting, child 307.9
  neck V48.9
    deficiency V48.1
    disfigurement V48.7
    mechanical V48.3
    motor V48.3
    movement V48.3
    sensory V48.5
    specified condition NEC V48.8
  neurological NEC 781.99
  none (feared complaint unfounded) V65.5
  occupational V62.29
  parent-child V61.20
    adopted child V61.24
    biological child V61.23
    foster child V61.25
    relationship V61.20
  partner V61.10
    relationship V61.10
  personal NEC V62.89
    interpersonal conflict NEC V62.81
  personality *(see also* Disorder, personality)
      301.9
  phase of life V62.89
  placenta, affecting management of
      pregnancy 656.9●
    specified type NEC 656.8●
  poverty V60.2
  presence of sick or handicapped person in
      family or household V61.49
  psychiatric 300.9

Problem *(Continued)*
  psychosocial V62.9
    specified type NEC V62.89
  relational NEC V62.81
  relationship, childhood 313.3
  religious or spiritual belief
    other than medical care V62.89
    regarding medical care V62.6
  self-damaging behavior V69.8
  sexual
    behavior, high-risk V69.2
    function NEC V41.7
  sibling
    relational V61.8
    relationship V61.8
  sight V41.0
  sleep, lack of V69.4
  sleep disorder, child 307.40
  smell V41.5
  speech V40.1
  spite reaction, child *(see also* Disturbance,
      conduct) 312.0●
  spoiled child reaction *(see also* Disturbance,
      conduct) 312.1●
  substance abuse in family V61.42
  swallowing V41.6
  tantrum, child *(see also* Disturbance, conduct)
      312.1●
  taste V41.5
  thumb sucking, child 307.9
  tic (child) 307.21
  trunk V48.9
    deficiency V48.1
    disfigurement V48.7
    mechanical V48.3
    motor V48.3
    movement V48.3
    sensory V48.5
    specified condition NEC V48.8
  unemployment V62.0
  urinary NEC V47.4
  voice production V41.4
Procedure (surgical) not done NEC V64.3
  because of
    contraindication V64.1
    patient's decision V64.2
      for reasons of conscience or religion
          V62.6
    specified reason NEC V64.3
Procidentia
  anus (sphincter) 569.1
  rectum (sphincter) 569.1
  stomach 537.89
  uteri 618.1
Proctalgia 569.42
  fugax 564.6
  spasmodic 564.6
    psychogenic 307.89
Proctitis 569.49
  amebic 006.8
  chlamydial 099.52
  gonococcal 098.7
  granulomatous 555.1
  idiopathic 556.2
    with ulcerative sigmoiditis 556.3
  tuberculous *(see also* Tuberculosis) 014.8●
  ulcerative (chronic) (nonspecific) 556.2
    with ulcerative sigmoiditis 556.3
Proctocele
  female (without uterine prolapse) 618.04
    with uterine prolapse 618.4
      complete 618.3
      incomplete 618.2
  male 569.49
Proctocolitis, idiopathic 556.2
  with ulcerative sigmoiditis 556.3
Proctoptosis 569.1
Proctosigmoiditis 569.89
  ulcerative (chronic) 556.3
Proctospasm 564.6
  psychogenic 306.4

Prodromal-AIDS - *see* Human
    immunodeficiency virus (disease) (illness)
    (infection)
Profichet's disease or syndrome 729.90
Progeria (adultorum) (syndrome) 259.8
Prognathism (mandibular) (maxillary) 524.10
Progonoma (melanotic) (M9363/0) - *see*
    Neoplasm, by site, benign
Progressive - *see* condition
Prolapse, prolapsed
  anus, anal (canal) (sphincter) 569.1
  arm or hand, complicating delivery 652.7●
    causing obstructed labor 660.0●
      affecting fetus or newborn 763.1
    fetus or newborn 763.1
  bladder (acquired) (mucosa) (sphincter)
    congenital (female) (male) 756.71
    female *(see also* Cystocele, female) 618.01
    male 596.89
  breast implant (prosthetic) 996.54
  cecostomy 569.69
  cecum 569.89
  cervix, cervical (hypertrophied) 618.1
    anterior lip, obstructing labor 660.2●
      affecting fetus or newborn 763.1
    congenital 752.49
    postpartal (old) 618.1
    stump 618.84
  ciliary body 871.1
  colon (pedunculated) 569.89
  colostomy 569.69
  conjunctiva 372.73
  cord - *see* Prolapse, umbilical cord
  cystostomy 596.83
  disc (intervertebral) - *see* Displacement,
      intervertebral disc
  duodenum 537.89
  eye implant (orbital) 996.59
    lens (ocular) 996.53
  fallopian tube 620.4
  fetal extremity, complicating delivery
      652.8●
    causing obstructed labor 660.0●
    fetus or newborn 763.1
  funis - *see* Prolapse, umbilical cord
  gastric (mucosa) 537.89
  genital, female 618.9
    specified NEC 618.89
  globe 360.81
  ileostomy bud 569.69
  intervertebral disc - *see* Displacement,
      intervertebral disc
  intestine (small) 569.89
  iris 364.89
    traumatic 871.1
  kidney *(see also* Disease, renal) 593.0
    congenital 753.3
  laryngeal muscles or ventricle 478.79
  leg, complicating delivery 652.8●
    causing obstructed labor 660.0●
    fetus or newborn 763.1
  liver 573.8
  meatus urinarius 599.5
  mitral valve 424.0
  ocular lens implant 996.53
  organ or site, congenital NEC - *see*
      Malposition, congenital
  ovary 620.4
  pelvic (floor), female 618.89
  perineum, female 618.89
  pregnant uterus 654.4●
  rectum (mucosa) (sphincter) 569.1
    due to Trichuris trichiuria 127.3
  spleen 289.59
  stomach 537.89
  umbilical cord
    affecting fetus or newborn 762.4
    complicating delivery 663.0●
  ureter 593.89
    with obstruction 593.4
  ureterovesical orifice 593.89

Prolapse, prolapsed *(Continued)*
  urethra (acquired) (infected) (mucosa) 599.5
    congenital 753.8
  uterovaginal 618.4
    complete 618.3
    incomplete 618.2
    specified NEC 618.89
  uterus (first degree) (second degree) (third
        degree) (complete) (without vaginal
        wall prolapse) 618.1
    with mention of vaginal wall prolapse -
        see Prolapse, uterovaginal
    congenital 752.39
    in pregnancy or childbirth 654.4●
      affecting fetus or newborn 763.1
      causing obstructed labor 660.2●
        affecting fetus or newborn 763.1
    postpartal (old) 618.1
  uveal 871.1
  vagina (anterior) (posterior) (vault) (wall)
        (without uterine prolapse) 618.00
    with uterine prolapse 618.4
      complete 618.3
      incomplete 618.2
    paravaginal 618.02
    posthysterectomy 618.5
    specified NEC 618.09
  vitreous (humor) 379.26
    traumatic 871.1
  womb - *see* Prolapse, uterus
Prolapsus, female 618.9
Proliferative - *see* condition
Prolinemia 270.8
Prolinuria 270.8
Prolonged, prolongation
  bleeding time (*see also* Defect, coagulation)
        790.92
  "idiopathic" (in von Willebrand's disease)
        286.4
  coagulation time (*see also* Defect,
        coagulation) 790.92
  gestation syndrome 766.22
  labor 662.1●
    affecting fetus or newborn 763.89
    first stage 662.0●
    second stage 662.2●
  PR interval 426.11
  pregnancy 645.2●
  prothrombin time (*see also* Defect,
        coagulation) 790.92
  QT interval 794.31
    syndrome 426.82
  rupture of membranes (24 hours or more
        prior to onset of labor) 658.2●
  uterine contractions in labor 661.4●
    affecting fetus or newborn 763.7
Prominauris 744.29
Prominence
  auricle (ear) (congenital) 744.29
    acquired 380.32
  ischial spine or sacral promontory
    with disproportion (fetopelvic) 653.3●
      affecting fetus or newborn 763.1
      causing obstructed labor 660.1●
        affecting fetus or newborn 763.1
  nose (congenital) 748.1
    acquired 738.0
PROMM (proximal myotonic myotonia)
      359.21
Pronation
  ankle 736.79
  foot 736.79
    congenital 755.67
Prophylactic
  administration of
    antibiotics, long-term V58.62
      short-term - *omit code*
    antitoxin, any V07.2
    antivenin V07.2
    chemotherapeutic agent NEC V07.39
      fluoride V07.31

Prophylactic *(Continued)*
  administration of *(Continued)*
    diphtheria antitoxin V07.2
    drug V07.39
    gamma globulin V07.2
    immune sera (gamma globulin) V07.2
    RhoGAM V07.2
    tetanus antitoxin V07.2
  chemotherapy NEC V07.39
    fluoride V07.31
  hormone replacement (postmenopausal)
        V07.4
  immunotherapy V07.2
  measure V07.9
    specified type NEC V07.8
  medication V07.39
  postmenopausal hormone replacement
        V07.4
  sterilization V25.2
Proptosis (ocular) (*see also* Exophthalmos)
      376.30
  thyroid 242.0●
Propulsion
  eyeball 360.81
Prosecution, anxiety concerning V62.5
Prosopagnosia 368.16
Prostate, prostatic - *see* condition
Prostatism 600.90
  with
    other lower urinary tract symptoms
        (LUTS) 600.91
    urinary
      obstruction 600.91
      retention 600.91
Prostatitis (congestive) (suppurative) 601.9
  acute 601.0
  cavitary 601.8
  chlamydial 099.54
  chronic 601.1
  diverticular 601.8
  due to Trichomonas (vaginalis) 131.03
  fibrous 600.90
    with
      other lower urinary tract symptoms
          (LUTS) 600.91
      urinary
        obstruction 600.91
        retention 600.91
  gonococcal (acute) 098.12
    chronic or duration of 2 months or over
        098.32
  granulomatous 601.8
  hypertrophic 600.00
    with
      other lower urinary tract symptoms
          (LUTS) 600.01
      urinary
        obstruction 600.01
        retention 600.01
  specified type NEC 601.8
  subacute 601.1
  trichomonal 131.03
  tuberculous (*see also* Tuberculosis) 016.5●
        [601.4]
Prostatocystitis 601.3
Prostatorrhea 602.8
Prostatoseminovesiculitis, trichomonal
      131.03
Prostration 780.79
  heat 992.5
    anhydrotic 992.3
    due to
      salt (and water) depletion 992.4
      water depletion 992.3
  nervous 300.5
  newborn 779.89
  senile 797
Protanomaly 368.51
Protanopia (anomalous trichromat) (complete)
      (incomplete) 368.51
Protection (against) (from) - *see* Prophylactic

Protein
  deficiency 260
  malnutrition 260
  sickness (prophylactic) (therapeutic) 999.59
Proteinemia 790.99
Proteinosis
  alveolar, lung or pulmonary 516.0
  lipid 272.8
  lipoid (of Urbach) 272.8
Proteinuria (*see also* Albuminuria) 791.0
  Bence-Jones NEC 791.0
  gestational 646.2●
    with hypertension - *see* Toxemia, of
        pregnancy
  orthostatic 593.6
  postural 593.6
Proteolysis, pathologic 286.6
Protocoproporphyria 277.1
Protoporphyria (erythrohepatic)
      (erythropoietic) 277.1
Protrusio acetabuli 718.65
Protrusion
  acetabulum (into pelvis) 718.65
  device, implant, or graft - *see* Complications,
        mechanical
  ear, congenital 744.29
  intervertebral disc - *see* Displacement,
        intervertebral disc
  nucleus pulposus - *see* Displacement,
        intervertebral disc
Proud flesh 701.5
Prune belly (syndrome) 756.71
Prurigo (ferox) (gravis) (Hebra's) (hebrae)
      (mitis) (simplex) 698.2
  agria 698.3
  asthma syndrome 691.8
  Besnier's (atopic dermatitis) (infantile
        eczema) 691.8
  eczematodes allergicum 691.8
  estivalis (Hutchinson's) 692.72
  Hutchinson's 692.72
  nodularis 698.3
  psychogenic 306.3
Pruritus, pruritic 698.9
  ani 698.0
    psychogenic 306.3
  conditions NEC 698.9
    psychogenic 306.3
  due to Onchocerca volvulus 125.3
  ear 698.9
  essential 698.9
  genital organ(s) 698.1
    psychogenic 306.3
  gravidarum 646.8●
  hiemalis 698.8
  neurogenic (any site) 306.3
  perianal 698.0
  psychogenic (any site) 306.3
  scrotum 698.1
    psychogenic 306.3
  senile, senilis 698.8
  Trichomonas 131.9
  vulva, vulvae 698.1
    psychogenic 306.3
Psammocarcinoma (M8140/3) - *see* Neoplasm,
      by site, malignant
Pseudarthrosis, pseudoarthrosis (bone) 733.82
  joint following fusion V45.4
Pseudoacanthosis
  nigricans 701.8
Pseudoaneurysm - *see* Aneurysm
Pseudoangina (pectoris) - *see* Angina
Pseudoangioma 452
Pseudo-Argyll-Robertson pupil 379.45
Pseudoarteriosus 747.89
Pseudoarthrosis - *see* Pseudarthrosis
Pseudoataxia 799.89
Pseudobulbar affect (PBA) 310.81
Pseudobursa 727.89
Pseudocholera 025
Pseudochromidrosis 705.89

◄ New ◄ Revised ~~deleted~~ Deleted ● Use Additional Digit(s) ▨ Omit code

Pseudocirrhosis, liver, pericardial 423.2
Pseudocoarctation 747.21
Pseudocowpox 051.1
Pseudocoxalgia 732.1
Pseudocroup 478.75
Pseudocyesis 300.11
Pseudocyst
    lung 518.89
    pancreas 577.2
    retina 361.19
Pseudodementia 300.16
Pseudoelephantiasis neuroarthritica 757.0
Pseudoemphysema 518.89
Pseudoencephalitis
    superior (acute) hemorrhagic 265.1
Pseudoerosion cervix, congenital 752.49
Pseudoexfoliation, lens capsule 366.11
Pseudofracture (idiopathic) (multiple)
    (spontaneous) (symmetrical) 268.2
Pseudoglanders 025
Pseudoglioma 360.44
Pseudogout - see Chondrocalcinosis
Pseudohallucination 780.1
Pseudohemianesthesia 782.0
Pseudohemophilia (Bernuth's) (hereditary)
    (type B) 286.4
    type A 287.8
    vascular 287.8
Pseudohermaphroditism 752.7
    with chromosomal anomaly - see Anomaly,
        chromosomal
    adrenal 255.2
    female (without adrenocortical disorder)
        752.7
        with adrenocortical disorder 255.2
        adrenal 255.2
    male (without gonadal disorder) 752.7
        with
            adrenocortical disorder 255.2
            cleft scrotum 752.7
            feminizing testis 259.51
            gonadal disorder 257.9
            adrenal 255.2
Pseudohole, macula 362.54
Pseudo-Hurler's disease (mucolipidosis III)
    272.7
Pseudohydrocephalus 348.2
Pseudohypertrophic muscular dystrophy
    (Erb's) 359.1
Pseudohypertrophy, muscle 359.1
Pseudohypoparathyroidism 275.49
Pseudoinfluenza (see also Influenza) 487.1
Pseudoinsomnia 307.49
Pseudoleukemia 288.8
    infantile 285.8
Pseudomembranous - see condition
Pseudomeningocele (cerebral) (infective) 349.2
    postprocedural 997.01
    spinal 349.2
Pseudomenstruation 626.8
Pseudomucinous
    cyst (ovary) (M8470/0) 220
    peritoneum 568.89
Pseudomyeloma 273.1
Pseudomyxoma peritonei (M8480/6) 197.6
Pseudoneuritis optic (nerve) 377.24
    papilla 377.24
        congenital 743.57
Pseudoneuroma - see Injury, nerve, by site
Pseudo-obstruction
    intestine (chronic) (idiopathic) (intermittent
        secondary) (primary) 564.89
        acute 560.89
Pseudopapilledema 377.24
Pseudoparalysis
    arm or leg 781.4
    atonic, congenital 358.8
Pseudopelade 704.09
Pseudophakia V43.1
Pseudopolycythemia 289.0
Pseudopolyposis, colon 556.4

Pseudoporencephaly 348.0
Pseudopseudohypoparathyroidism 275.49
Pseudopsychosis 300.16
Pseudopterygium 372.52
Pseudoptosis (eyelid) 374.34
Pseudorabies 078.89
Pseudoretinitis, pigmentosa 362.65
Pseudorickets 588.0
    senile (Pozzi's) 731.0
Pseudorubella 057.8
Pseudoscarlatina 057.8
Pseudosclerema 778.1
Pseudosclerosis (brain)
    Jakob's 046.19
    of Westphal (-Strümpell) (hepatolenticular
        degeneration) 275.1
    spastic 046.19
        with dementia
            with behavioral disturbance 046.19
                [294.11]
            without behavioral disturbance 046.19
                [294.10]
Pseudoseizure 780.39
    non-psychiatric 780.39
    psychiatric 300.11
Pseudotabes 799.89
    diabetic 250.6 ● [337.1]
        due to secondary diabetes 249.6 ● [337.1]
Pseudotetanus (see also Convulsions) 780.39
Pseudotetany 781.7
    hysterical 300.11
Pseudothalassemia 285.0
Pseudotrichinosis 710.3
Pseudotruncus arteriosus 747.29
Pseudotuberculosis, pasteurella (infection)
    027.2
Pseudotumor
    cerebri 348.2
    orbit (inflammatory) 376.11
Pseudo-Turner's syndrome 759.89
Pseudoxanthoma elasticum 757.39
Psilosis (sprue) (tropical) 579.1
    Monilia 112.89
    nontropical 579.0
    not sprue 704.00
Psittacosis 073.9
Psoitis 728.89
Psora NEC 696.1
Psoriasis 696.1
    any type, except arthropathic 696.1
    arthritic, arthropathic 696.0
    buccal 528.6
    flexural 696.1
    follicularis 696.1
    guttate 696.1
    inverse 696.1
    mouth 528.6
    nummularis 696.1
    psychogenic 316 [696.1]
    punctata 696.1
    pustular 696.1
    rupioides 696.1
    vulgaris 696.1
Psorospermiasis 136.4
Psorospermosis 136.4
    follicularis (vegetans) 757.39
Psychalgia 307.80
Psychasthenia 300.89
    compulsive 300.3
    mixed compulsive states 300.3
    obsession 300.3
Psychiatric disorder or problem NEC 300.9
Psychogenic - see also condition
    factors associated with physical conditions
        316
Psychoneurosis, psychoneurotic (see also
    Neurosis) 300.9
    anxiety (state) 300.00
    climacteric 627.2
    compensation 300.16
    compulsion 300.3

Psychoneurosis, psychoneurotic (Continued)
    conversion hysteria 300.11
    depersonalization 300.6
    depressive type 300.4
    dissociative hysteria 300.15
    hypochondriacal 300.7
    hysteria 300.10
        conversion type 300.11
        dissociative type 300.15
    mixed NEC 300.89
    neurasthenic 300.5
    obsessional 300.3
    obsessive-compulsive 300.3
    occupational 300.89
    personality NEC 301.89
    phobia 300.20
    senile NEC 300.89
Psychopathic - see also condition
    constitution, posttraumatic 310.2
        with psychosis 293.9
    personality 301.9
        amoral trends 301.7
        antisocial trends 301.7
        asocial trends 301.7
        mixed types 301.7
    state 301.9
Psychopathy, sexual (see also Deviation, sexual)
    302.9
Psychophysiologic, psychophysiological
    condition - see Reaction,
        psychophysiologic
Psychose passionelle 297.8
Psychosexual identity disorder 302.6
    adult-life 302.85
    childhood 302.6
Psychosis 298.9
    acute hysterical 298.1
    affecting management of pregnancy,
        childbirth, or puerperium 648.4 ●
    affective (see also Disorder, mood) 296.90

> Note: Use the following fifth-digit
> subclassification with categories 296.0–296.6:
>
> 0   unspecified
> 1   mild
> 2   moderate
> 3   severe, without mention of psychotic
>   behavior
> 4   severe, specified as with psychotic
>   behavior
> 5   in partial or unspecified remission
> 6   in full remission

    drug-induced 292.84
    due to or associated with physical
        condition 293.9
    involutional 293.83
        recurrent episode 296.3 ●
        single episode 296.2 ●
    manic-depressive 296.80
        circular (alternating) 296.7
            currently depressed 296.5 ●
            currently manic 296.4 ●
        depressed type 296.2 ●
            atypical 296.82
            recurrent episode 296.3 ●
            single episode 296.2 ●
        manic 296.0 ●
            atypical 296.81
            recurrent episode 296.1 ●
            single episode 296.0 ●
        mixed type NEC 296.89
        specified type NEC 296.89
        senile 290.21
        specified type NEC 296.99
    alcoholic 291.9
        with
            anxiety 291.89
            delirium tremens 291.0
            delusions 291.5
            dementia 291.2

Psychosis (Continued)
   alcoholic (Continued)
      with (Continued)
         hallucinosis 291.3
         jealousy 291.5
         mood disturbance 291.89
         paranoia 291.5
         persisting amnesia 291.1
         sexual dysfunction 291.89
         sleep disturbance 291.89
      amnestic confabulatory 291.1
      delirium tremens 291.0
      hallucinosis 291.3
      Korsakoff's, Korsakov's, Korsakow's 291.1
      paranoid type 291.5
      pathological intoxication 291.4
      polyneuritic 291.1
      specified type NEC 291.89
   alternating (see also Psychosis, manic-depressive, circular) 296.7
   anergastic (see also Psychosis, organic) 294.9
   arteriosclerotic 290.40
      with
         acute confusional state 290.41
         delirium 290.41
         delusions 290.42
         depressed mood 290.43
      depressed type 290.43
      paranoid type 290.42
      simple type 290.40
      uncomplicated 290.40
   atypical 298.9
      depressive 296.82
      manic 296.81
   borderline (schizophrenia) (see also Schizophrenia) 295.5●
      of childhood (see also Psychosis, childhood) 299.8●
         prepubertal 299.8●
   brief reactive 298.8
   childhood, with origin specific to 299.9●

> Note: Use the following fifth-digit subclassification with category 299:
>
> 0   current or active state
> 1   residual state

      atypical 299.8●
      specified type NEC 299.8●
   circular (see also Psychosis, manic-depressive, circular) 296.7
   climacteric (see also Psychosis, involutional) 298.8
   confusional 298.9
      acute 293.0
      reactive 298.2
      subacute 293.1
   depressive (see also Psychosis, affective) 296.2●
      atypical 296.82
      involutional 296.2●
         with hypomania (bipolar II) 296.89
         recurrent episode 296.3●
         single episode 296.2●
      psychogenic 298.0
      reactive (emotional stress) (psychological trauma) 298.0
      recurrent episode 296.3●
         with hypomania (bipolar II) 296.89
      single episode 296.2●
   disintegrative, childhood (see also Psychosis, childhood) 299.1●
   drug 292.9
      with
         affective syndrome 292.84
         amnestic syndrome 292.83
         anxiety 292.89
         delirium 292.81
            withdrawal 292.0
         delusions 292.11

Psychosis (Continued)
   drug (Continued)
      with (Continued)
         dementia 292.82
         depressive state 292.84
         hallucinations 292.12
         hallucinosis 292.12
         mood disorder 292.84
         mood disturbance 292.84
         organic personality syndrome NEC 292.89
         sexual dysfunction 292.89
         sleep disturbance 292.89
         withdrawal syndrome (and delirium) 292.0
      affective syndrome 292.84
      delusions 292.11
      hallucinatory state 292.12
      hallucinosis 292.12
      paranoid state 292.11
      specified type NEC 292.89
      withdrawal syndrome (and delirium) 292.0
   due to or associated with physical condition (see also Psychosis, organic) 294.9
   epileptic NEC 293.9
   excitation (psychogenic) (reactive) 298.1
   exhaustive (see also Reaction, stress, acute) 308.9
   hypomanic (see also Psychosis, affective) 296.0●
      recurrent episode 296.1●
      single episode 296.0●
   hysterical 298.8
      acute 298.1
   incipient 298.8
      schizophrenic (see also Schizophrenia) 295.5●
   induced 297.3
   infantile (see also Psychosis, childhood) 299.0●
   infective 293.9
      acute 293.0
      subacute 293.1
   in
      conditions classified elsewhere
         with
            delusions 293.81
            hallucinations 293.82
      pregnancy, childbirth, or puerperium 648.4●
   interactional (childhood) (see also Psychosis, childhood) 299.1●
   involutional 298.8
      depressive (see also Psychosis, affective) 296.2●
         recurrent episode 296.3●
         single episode 296.2●
      melancholic 296.2●
         recurrent episode 296.3●
         single episode 296.2●
      paranoid state 297.2
      paraphrenia 297.2
   Korsakoff's, Korakov's, Korsakow's (nonalcoholic) 294.0
      alcoholic 291.1
   mania (phase) (see also Psychosis, affective) 296.0●
      recurrent episode 296.1●
      single episode 296.0●
   manic (see also Psychosis, affective) 296.0●
      atypical 296.81
      recurrent episode 296.1●
      single episode 296.0●
   manic-depressive 296.80
      circular 296.7
         currently
            depressed 296.5●
            manic 296.4●
         mixed 296.6●

Psychosis (Continued)
   manic-depressive (Continued)
      depressive 296.2●
         recurrent episode 296.3●
            with hypomania (bipolar II) 296.89
         single episode 296.2●
      hypomanic 296.0●
         recurrent episode 296.1●
         single episode 296.0●
      manic 296.0●
         atypical 296.81
         recurrent episode 296.1●
         single episode 296.0●
      mixed NEC 296.89
      perplexed 296.89
      stuporous 296.89
   menopausal (see also Psychosis, involutional) 298.8
   mixed schizophrenic and affective (see also Schizophrenia) 295.7●
   multi-infarct (cerebrovascular) (see also Psychosis, arteriosclerotic) 290.40
   organic NEC 294.9
      due to or associated with
         addiction
            alcohol (see also Psychosis, alcoholic) 291.9
            drug (see also Psychosis, drug) 292.9
         alcohol intoxication, acute (see also Psychosis, alcoholic) 291.9
         alcoholism (see also Psychosis, alcoholic) 291.9
         arteriosclerosis (cerebral) (see also Psychosis, arteriosclerotic) 290.40
         cerebrovascular disease
            acute (psychosis) 293.0
            arteriosclerotic (see also Psychosis, arteriosclerotic) 290.40
         childbirth - see Psychosis, puerperal
         dependence
            alcohol (see also Psychosis, alcoholic) 291.9
            drug 292.9
         disease
            alcoholic liver (see also Psychosis, alcoholic) 291.9
            brain
               arteriosclerotic (see also Psychosis, arteriosclerotic) 290.40
            cerebrovascular
               acute (psychosis) 293.0
               arteriosclerotic (see also Psychosis, arteriosclerotic) 290.40
            endocrine or metabolic 293.9
               acute (psychosis) 293.0
               subacute (psychosis) 293.1
            Jakob-Creutzfeldt 046.19
               with behavioral disturbance 046.19 [294.11]
               without behavioral disturbance 046.19 [294.10]
               familial 046.19
               iatrogenic 046.19
               specified NEC 046.19
               sporadic 046.19
               variant 046.11
                  with dementia
                     with behavioral disturbance 046.11 [294.11]
                     without behavioral disturbance 046.11 [294.10]
            liver, alcoholic (see also Psychosis, alcoholic) 291.9

◀ New   ◀▦ Revised   ~~deleted~~ Deleted   ● Use Additional Digit(s)   ▦ Omit code

Psychosis *(Continued)*
  organic NEC *(Continued)*
    due to or associated with *(Continued)*
      disorder
        cerebrovascular
          acute (psychosis) 293.0
        endocrine or metabolic 293.9
          acute (psychosis) 293.0
          subacute (psychosis) 293.1
      epilepsy
        with behavioral disturbance 345.9 *[294.11]*●
        without behavioral disturbance 345.9 *[294.10]*●
        transient (acute) 293.0
      Huntington's chorea
        with behavioral disturbance 333.4 *[294.11]*
        without behavioral disturbance 333.4 *[294.10]*
      infection
        brain 293.9
          acute (psychosis) 293.0
          chronic 294.8
          subacute (psychosis) 293.1
        intracranial NEC 293.9
          acute (psychosis) 293.0
          chronic 294.8
          subacute (psychosis) 293.1
      intoxication
        alcoholic (acute) *(see also* Psychosis, alcoholic) 291.9
          pathological 291.4
        drug *(see also* Psychosis, drug) 292.9
      ischemia
        cerebrovascular (generalized) *(see also* Psychosis, arteriosclerotic) 290.40
      Jakob-Creutzfeldt disease (syndrome) 046.19
        with behavioral disturbance 046.19 *[294.11]*
        without behavioral disturbance 046.19 *[294.10]*
        variant 046.11
          with dementia
            with behavioral disturbance 046.11 *[294.11]*
            without behavioral disturbance 046.11 *[294.10]*
      multiple sclerosis
        with behavioral disturbance 340 *[294.11]*
        without behavioral disturbance 340 *[294.10]*
      physical condition NEC 293.9
        with
          delusions 293.81
          hallucinations 293.82
      presenility 290.10
      puerperium - *see* Psychosis, puerperal
      sclerosis, multiple
        with behavioral disturbance 340 *[294.11]*
        without behavioral disturbance 340 *[294.10]*
      senility 290.20
      status epilepticus
        with behavioral disturbance 345.3 *[294.11]*
        without behavioral disturbance 345.3 *[294.10]*
      trauma
        brain (birth) (from electrical current) (surgical) 293.9
          acute (psychosis) 293.0
          chronic 294.8
          subacute (psychosis) 293.1

Psychosis *(Continued)*
  organic NEC *(Continued)*
    due to or associated with *(Continued)*
      unspecified physical condition 293.9
        with
          delusions 293.81
          hallucinations 293.82
      infective 293.9
        acute (psychosis) 293.0
        subacute 293.1
      posttraumatic 293.9
        acute 293.0
        subacute 293.1
      specified type NEC 294.8
      transient 293.9
        with
          anxiety 293.84
          delusions 293.81
          depression 293.83
          hallucinations 293.82
        depressive type 293.83
        hallucinatory type 293.82
        paranoid type 293.81
        specified type NEC 293.89
  paranoic 297.1
  paranoid (chronic) 297.9
    alcoholic 291.5
    chronic 297.1
    climacteric 297.2
    involutional 297.2
    menopausal 297.2
    protracted reactive 298.4
    psychogenic 298.4
      acute 298.3
    schizophrenic *(see also* Schizophrenia) 295.3●
    senile 290.20
  paroxysmal 298.9
    senile 290.20
  polyneuritic, alcoholic 291.1
  postoperative 293.9
  postpartum - *see* Psychosis, puerperal
  prepsychotic *(see also* Schizophrenia) 295.5●
  presbyophrenic (type) 290.8
  presenile *(see also* Dementia, presenile) 290.10
  prison 300.16
  psychogenic 298.8
    depressive 298.0
    paranoid 298.4
      acute 298.3
  puerperal
    specified type - *see* categories 295–298
    unspecified type 293.89
      acute 293.0
      chronic 293.89
      subacute 293.1
  reactive (emotional stress) (psychological trauma) 298.8
    brief 298.8
    confusion 298.2
    depressive 298.0
    excitation 298.1
  schizo-affective (depressed) (excited) *(see also* Schizophrenia) 295.7●
  schizophrenia, schizophrenic *(see also* Schizophrenia) 295.9●
    borderline type 295.5●
      of childhood *(see also* Psychosis, childhood) 299.8●
    catatonic (excited) (withdrawn) 295.2●
    childhood type *(see also* Psychosis, childhood) 299.9●
    hebephrenic 295.1●
    incipient 295.5●
    latent 295.5●
    paranoid 295.3●
    prepsychotic 295.5●
    prodromal 295.5●
    pseudoneurotic 295.5●
    pseudopsychopathic 295.5●
    schizophreniform 295.4●

Psychosis *(Continued)*
  schizophrenia, schizophrenic *(Continued)*
    simple 295.0●
    undifferentiated type 295.9●
  schizophreniform 295.4●
  senile NEC 290.20
    with
      delusional features 290.20
      depressive features 290.21
    depressed type 290.21
    paranoid type 290.20
    simple deterioration 290.20
    specified type - *see* categories 295–298
  shared 297.3
  situational (reactive) 298.8
  symbiotic (childhood) *(see also* Psychosis, childhood) 299.1●
  toxic (acute) 293.9
Psychotic *(see also* condition) 298.9
  episode 298.9
    due to or associated with physical conditions *(see also* Psychosis, organic) 293.9
Pterygium (eye) 372.40
  central 372.43
  colli 744.5
  double 372.44
  peripheral (stationary) 372.41
    progressive 372.42
  recurrent 372.45
Ptilosis 374.55
PTLD (post-transplant lymphoproliferative disorder) 238.77
Ptomaine (poisoning) *(see also* Poisoning, food) 005.9
Ptosis (adiposa) 374.30
  breast 611.81
  cecum 569.89
  colon 569.89
  congenital (eyelid) 743.61
    specified site NEC - *see* Anomaly, specified type NEC
  epicanthus syndrome 270.2
  eyelid 374.30
    congenital 743.61
    mechanical 374.33
    myogenic 374.32
    paralytic 374.31
  gastric 537.5
  intestine 569.89
  kidney *(see also* Disease, renal) 593.0
    congenital 753.3
  liver 573.8
  renal *(see also* Disease, renal) 593.0
    congenital 753.3
  splanchnic 569.89
  spleen 289.59
  stomach 537.5
  viscera 569.89
PTP (posttransfusion purpura) 287.41
PTSD (Post-Traumatic Stress Disorder) 309.81
Ptyalism 527.7
  hysterical 300.11
  periodic 527.2
  pregnancy 646.8●
  psychogenic 306.4
Ptyalolithiasis 527.5
Pubalgia 848.8
Pubarche, precocious 259.1
Pubertas praecox 259.1
Puberty V21.1
  abnormal 259.9
  bleeding 626.3
  delayed 259.0
  precocious (constitutional) (cryptogenic) (idiopathic) NEC 259.1
    due to
      adrenal
        cortical hyperfunction 255.2
        hyperplasia 255.2
      cortical hyperfunction 255.2

Puberty (Continued)
  precocious NEC (Continued)
    due to (Continued)
      ovarian hyperfunction 256.1
        estrogen 256.0
      pineal tumor 259.8
      testicular hyperfunction 257.0
    premature 259.1
      due to
        adrenal cortical hyperfunction
          255.2
        pineal tumor 259.8
        pituitary (anterior) hyperfunction
          253.1
Puckering, macula 362.56
Pudenda, pudendum - see condition
Puente's disease (simple glandular cheilitis)
  528.5
Puerperal
  abscess
    areola 675.1●
    Bartholin's gland 646.6●
    breast 675.1●
    cervix (uteri) 670.8●
    fallopian tube 670.8●
    genital organ 670.8●
    kidney 646.6●
    mammary 675.1●
    mesosalpinx 670.8●
    nabothian 646.6●
    nipple 675.0●
    ovary, ovarian 670.8●
    oviduct 670.8●
    parametric 670.8●
    para-uterine 670.8●
    pelvic 670.8●
    perimetric 670.8●
    periuterine 670.8●
    retro-uterine 670.8●
    subareolar 675.1●
    suprapelvic 670.8●
    tubal (ruptured) 670.8●
    tubo-ovarian 670.8●
    urinary tract NEC 646.6●
    uterine, uterus 670.8●
    vagina (wall) 646.6●
    vaginorectal 646.6●
    vulvovaginal gland 646.6●
  accident 674.9●
  adnexitis 670.8●
  afibrinogenemia, or other coagulation defect
    666.3●
  albuminuria (acute) (subacute) 646.2●
    pre-eclamptic 642.4●
  anemia (conditions classifiable to 280–285)
    648.2●
  anuria 669.3●
  apoplexy 674.0●
  asymptomatic bacteriuria 646.5●
  atrophy, breast 676.3●
  blood dyscrasia 666.3●
  caked breast 676.2●
  cardiomyopathy 674.5●
  cellulitis - see Puerperal, abscess
  cerebrovascular disorder (conditions
    classifiable to 430–434, 436–437)
    674.0●
  cervicitis (conditions classifiable to 616.0)
    646.6●
  coagulopathy (any) 666.3●
  complications 674.9●
    specified type NEC 674.8●
  convulsions (eclamptic) (uremic) 642.6●
    with pre-existing hypertension 642.7●
  cracked nipple 676.1●
  cystitis 646.6●
  cystopyelitis 646.6●
  deciduitis (acute) 670.8●
  delirium NEC 293.9
  diabetes (mellitus) (conditions classifiable to
    249 and 250) 648.0●

Puerperal (Continued)
  disease 674.9●
    breast NEC 676.3●
    cerebrovascular (acute) 674.0●
    nonobstetric NEC (see also Pregnancy,
      complicated, current disease or
      condition) 648.9●
    pelvis inflammatory 670.8●
    renal NEC 646.2●
    tubo-ovarian 670.8●
    Valsuani's (progressive pernicious
      anemia) 648.2●
  disorder
    lactation 676.9●
      specified type NEC 676.8●
    nonobstetric NEC (see also Pregnancy,
      complicated, current disease or
      condition) 648.9●
  disruption
    cesarean wound 674.1●
    episiotomy wound 674.2●
    perineal laceration wound 674.2●
  drug dependence (conditions classifiable to
    304) 648.3●
  eclampsia 642.6●
    with pre-existing hypertension 642.7●
  embolism (pulmonary) 673.2●
    air 673.0●
    amniotic fluid 673.1●
    blood clot 673.2●
    brain or cerebral 674.0●
    cardiac 674.8●
    fat 673.8●
    intracranial sinus (venous) 671.5●
    pyemic 673.3●
    septic 673.3●
    spinal cord 671.5●
  endometritis (conditions classifiable to
    615.0–615.9) 670.1●
  endophlebitis - see Puerperal, phlebitis
  endotrachelitis 646.6●
  engorgement, breasts 676.2●
  erysipelas 670.8●
  failure
    lactation 676.4●
    renal, acute 669.3●
  fever 672●
    meaning pyrexia (of unknown origin)
      672●
    meaning sepsis 670.2●
    fissure, nipple 676.1●
  fistula
    breast 675.1●
    mammary gland 675.1●
    nipple 675.0●
  galactophoritis 675.2●
  galactorrhea 676.6●
  gangrene
    gas 670.8●
      with sepsis 670.2●
    uterus 670.8●
  gonorrhea (conditions classifiable to 098)
    647.1●
  hematoma, subdural 674.0●
  hematosalpinx, infectional 670.8●
  hemiplegia, cerebral 674.0●
  hemorrhage 666.1●
    brain 674.0●
    bulbar 674.0●
    cerebellar 674.0●
    cerebral 674.0●
    cortical 674.0●
    delayed (after 24 hours) (uterine) 666.2●
    extradural 674.0●
    internal capsule 674.0●
    intracranial 674.0●
    intrapontine 674.0●
    meningeal 674.0●
    pontine 674.0●
    subarachnoid 674.0●
    subcortical 674.0●

Puerperal (Continued)
  hemorrhage (Continued)
    subdural 674.0●
    uterine, delayed 666.2●
    ventricular 674.0●
  hemorrhoids 671.8●
  hepatorenal syndrome 674.8●
  hypertrophy
    breast 676.3●
    mammary gland 676.3●
  induration breast (fibrous) 676.3●
  infarction
    lung - see Puerperal, embolism
    pulmonary - see Puerperal, embolism
  infection
    Bartholin's gland 646.6●
    breast 675.2●
      with nipple 675.9●
        specified type NEC 675.8●
    cervix 646.6●
    endocervix 646.6●
    fallopian tube 670.8●
    generalized 670.0●
    genital tract (major) 670.0●
      minor or localized 646.6●
    kidney (bacillus coli) 646.6●
    mammary gland 675.2●
      with nipple 675.9●
        specified type NEC 675.8●
    nipple 675.0●
      with breast 675.9●
        specified type NEC 675.8●
    ovary 670.8●
    pelvic 670.8●
    peritoneum 670.8●
    renal 646.6●
    tubo-ovarian 670.8●
    urinary (tract) NEC 646.6●
      asymptomatic 646.5●
    uterus, uterine 670.8●
    vagina 646.6●
  inflammation - see also Puerperal, infection
    areola 675.1●
    Bartholin's gland 646.6●
    breast 675.2●
    broad ligament 670.8●
    cervix (uteri) 646.6●
    fallopian tube 670.8●
    genital organs 670.8●
      localized 646.6●
    mammary gland 675.2●
    nipple 675.0●
    ovary 670.8●
    oviduct 670.8●
    pelvis 670.8●
    periuterine 670.8●
    tubal 670.8●
    vagina 646.6●
    vein - see Puerperal, phlebitis
  inversion, nipple 676.3●
  ischemia, cerebral 674.0●
  lymphangitis 670.8●
    breast 675.2●
  malaria (conditions classifiable to 084)
    647.4●
  malnutrition 648.9●
  mammillitis 675.0●
  mammitis 675.2●
  mania 296.0●
    recurrent episode 296.1●
    single episode 296.0●
  mastitis 675.2●
    purulent 675.1●
    retromammary 675.1●
    submammary 675.1●
  melancholia 296.2●
    recurrent episode 296.3●
    single episode 296.2●
  mental disorder (conditions classifiable to
    290–303, 305.0, 305.2–305.9, 306–316,
    317–319) 648.4●

◀ New   ◀▥ Revised   deleted Deleted   ● Use Additional Digit(s)   ▨▨▨ Omit code

Puerperal *(Continued)*
  metritis (suppurative) 670.1●
    septic 670.2●
  metroperitonitis 670.8●
  metrorrhagia 666.2●
  metrosalpingitis 670.8●
  metrovaginitis 670.8●
  milk leg 671.4●
  monoplegia, cerebral 674.0●
  necrosis
    kidney, tubular 669.3●
    liver (acute) (subacute) (conditions
      classifiable to 570) 674.8●
    ovary 670.8●
    renal cortex 669.3●
  nephritis or nephrosis (conditions classifiable
    to 580–589) 646.2●
    with hypertension 642.1●
  nutritional deficiency (conditions classifiable
    to 260–269) 648.9●
  occlusion, precerebral artery 674.0●
  oliguria 669.3●
  oophoritis 670.8●
  ovaritis 670.8●
  paralysis●
    bladder (sphincter) 665.5●
    cerebral 674.0●
  paralytic stroke 674.0●
  parametritis 670.8●
  paravaginitis 646.6●
  pelviperitonitis 670.8●
  perimetritis 670.8●
  perimetrosalpingitis 670.8●
  perinephritis 646.6●
  perioophoritis 670.8●
  periphlebitis - *see* Puerperal, phlebitis
  perisalpingitis 670.8●
  peritoneal infection 670.8●
  peritonitis (pelvic) 670.8●
  perivaginitis 646.6●
  phlebitis 671.2●
    deep 671.4●
    intracranial sinus (venous) 671.5●
    pelvic 671.4●
    specified site NEC 671.5●
    superficial 671.2●
  phlegmasia alba dolens 671.4●
  placental polyp 674.4●
  pneumonia, embolic - *see* Puerperal,
    embolism
  prediabetes 648.8●
  pre-eclampsia (mild) 642.4●
    with pre-existing hypertension 642.7●
    severe 642.5●
  psychosis, unspecified *(see also* Psychosis,
    puerperal) 293.89
  pyelitis 646.6●
  pyelocystitis 646.6●
  pyelohydronephrosis 646.6●
  pyelonephritis 646.6●
  pyelonephrosis 646.6●
  pyemia 670.2●
  pyocystitis 646.6●
  pyohemia 670.2●
  pyometra 670.8●
  pyonephritis 646.6●
  pyonephrosis 646.6●
  pyo-oophoritis 670.8●
  pyosalpingitis 670.8●
  pyosalpinx 670.8●
  pyrexia (of unknown origin) 672●
  renal
    disease NEC 646.2●
    failure, acute 669.3●
  retention
    decidua (fragments) (with delayed
      hemorrhage) 666.2●
      without hemorrhage 667.1●
    placenta (fragments) (with delayed
      hemorrhage) 666.2●
      without hemorrhage 667.1●

Puerperal *(Continued)*
  retention *(Continued)*
    secundines (fragments) (with delayed
      hemorrhage) 666.2●
      without hemorrhage 667.1●
  retracted nipple 676.0●
  rubella (conditions classifiable to 056) 647.5●
  salpingitis 670.8●
  salpingo-oophoritis 670.8●
  salpingo-ovaritis 670.8●
  salpingoperitonitis 670.8●
  sapremia 670.2●
  secondary perineal tear 674.2●
  sepsis (pelvic) 670.2●
  septicemia 670.2●
  subinvolution (uterus) 674.8●
  sudden death (cause unknown) 674.9●
  suppuration - *see* Puerperal, abscess
  syphilis (conditions classifiable to 090–097)
    647.0●
  tetanus 670.8●
  thelitis 675.0●
  thrombocytopenia 666.3●
  thrombophlebitis (superficial) 671.2●
    deep 671.4●
    pelvic 671.4●
    septic 670.3●
    specified site NEC 671.5●
  thrombosis (venous) - *see* Thrombosis,
    puerperal
  thyroid dysfunction (conditions classifiable
    to 240–246) 648.1●
  toxemia *(see also* Toxemia, of pregnancy)
    642.4●
    eclamptic 642.6●
      with pre-existing hypertension
        642.7●
    pre-eclamptic (mild) 642.4●
      with
        convulsions 642.6●
        pre-existing hypertension 642.7●
      severe 642.5●
  tuberculosis (conditions classifiable to
    010–018) 647.3●
  uremia 669.3●
  vaginitis (conditions classifiable to 616.1)
    646.6●
  varicose veins (legs) 671.0●
    vulva or perineum 671.1●
  venous complication 671.9●
  vulvitis (conditions classifiable to 616.1)
    646.6●
  vulvovaginitis (conditions classifiable to
    616.1) 646.6●
  white leg 671.4●
Pulled muscle - *see* Sprain, by site
Pulmolithiasis 518.89
Pulmonary - *see* condition
Pulmonitis (unknown etiology) 486
Pulpitis (acute) (anachoretic) (chronic)
    (hyperplastic) (putrescent) (suppurative)
    (ulcerative) 522.0
Pulpless tooth 522.9
Pulse
  alternating 427.89
    psychogenic 306.2
  bigeminal 427.89
  fast 785.0
  feeble, rapid, due to shock following injury
    958.4
  rapid 785.0
  slow 427.89
  strong 785.9
  trigeminal 427.89
  water-hammer *(see also* Insufficiency, aortic)
    424.1
  weak 785.9
Pulseless disease 446.7
Pulsus
  alternans or trigeminy 427.89
    psychogenic 306.2

Punch drunk 310.2
Puncta lacrimalia occlusion 375.52
Punctiform hymen 752.49
Puncture (traumatic) - *see also* Wound, open, by
    site
  accidental, complicating surgery 998.2
  bladder, nontraumatic 596.6
  by
    device, implant, or graft - *see*
      Complications, mechanical
    foreign body
      internal organs - *see also* Injury,
        internal, by site
      by ingested object - *see* Foreign
        body
      left accidentally in operation wound
        998.4
    instrument (any) during a procedure,
      accidental 998.2
  internal organs, abdomen, chest, or
    pelvis - *see* Injury, internal, by site
  kidney, nontraumatic 593.89
Pupil - *see* condition
Pupillary membrane 364.74
  persistent 743.46
Pupillotonia 379.46
  pseudotabetic 379.46
Purpura 287.2
  abdominal 287.0
  allergic 287.0
  anaphylactoid 287.0
  annularis telangiectodes 709.1
  arthritic 287.0
  autoerythrocyte sensitization 287.2
  autoimmune 287.0
  bacterial 287.0
  Bateman's (senile) 287.2
  capillary fragility (hereditary) (idiopathic)
    287.8
  cryoglobulinemic 273.2
  devil's pinches 287.2
  fibrinolytic *(see also* Fibrinolysis) 286.6
  fulminans, fulminous 286.6
  gangrenous 287.0
  hemorrhagic *(see also* Purpura,
    thrombocytopenic) 287.39
    nodular 272.7
    nonthrombocytopenic 287.0
    thrombocytopenic 287.39
  Henoch's (purpura nervosa) 287.0
  Henoch-Schönlein (allergic) 287.0
  hypergammaglobulinemic (benign primary)
    (Waldenström's) 273.0
  idiopathic 287.31
    nonthrombocytopenic 287.0
    thrombocytopenic 287.31
  immune thrombocytopenic 287.31
  infectious 287.0
  malignant 287.0
  neonatorum 772.6
  nervosa 287.0
  newborn NEC 772.6
  nonthrombocytopenic 287.2
    hemorrhagic 287.0
    idiopathic 287.0
  nonthrombopenic 287.2
  peliosis rheumatica 287.0
  pigmentaria, progressiva 709.09
  posttransfusion (PTP) 287.41
    from whole blood (fresh) or blood
      products 287.41
  primary 287.0
  primitive 287.0
  red cell membrane sensitivity 287.2
  rheumatica 287.0
  Schönlein (-Henoch) (allergic) 287.0
  scorbutic 267
  senile 287.2
  simplex 287.2
  symptomatica 287.0
  telangiectasia annularis 709.1

P

Purpura (Continued)
  thrombocytopenic (see also
      Thrombocytopenia) 287.30
    congenital 287.33
    essential 287.30
    hereditary 287.31
    idiopathic 287.31
    immune 287.31
    neonatal, transitory (see also
      Thrombocytopenia, neonatal
      transitory) 776.1
    primary 287.30
    puerperal, postpartum 666.3●
    thrombotic 446.6
  thrombohemolytic (see also Fibrinolysis)
    286.6
  thrombopenic (see also Thrombocytopenia)
    287.30
    congenital 287.33
    essential 287.30
  thrombotic 446.6
    thrombocytic 446.6
    thrombocytopenic 446.6
  toxic 287.0
  variolosa 050.0
  vascular 287.0
  visceral symptoms 287.0
  Werlhof's (see also Purpura,
    thrombocytopenic) 287.39
Purpuric spots 782.7
Purulent - see condition
Pus
  absorption, general - see Septicemia
  in
    stool 792.1
    urine 791.9
  tube (rupture) (see also Salpingo-oophoritis)
    614.2
Pustular rash 782.1
Pustule 686.9
  malignant 022.0
  nonmalignant 686.9
Putnam's disease (subacute combined sclerosis
  with pernicious anemia) 281.0 [336.2]
Putnam-Dana syndrome (subacute combined
  sclerosis with pernicious anemia) 281.0
  [336.2]
Putrefaction, intestinal 569.89
Putrescent pulp (dental) 522.1
Pyarthritis - see Pyarthrosis
Pyarthrosis (see also Arthritis, pyogenic) 711.0●
  tuberculous - see Tuberculosis, joint
Pycnoepilepsy, pycnolepsy (idiopathic) (see also
  Epilepsy) 345.0●
Pyelectasia 593.89
Pyelectasis 593.89
Pyelitis (congenital) (uremic) 590.80
  with
    abortion - see Abortion, by type, with
      specified complication NEC
    contracted kidney 590.00
    ectopic pregnancy (see also categories
      633.0–633.9) 639.8
    molar pregnancy (see also categories
      630–632) 639.8
  acute 590.10
    with renal medullary necrosis 590.11
  chronic 590.00
    with
      renal medullary necrosis 590.01
  complicating pregnancy, childbirth, or
    puerperium 646.6●
    affecting fetus or newborn 760.1

Pyelitis (Continued)
  cystica 590.3
  following
    abortion 639.8
    ectopic or molar pregnancy 639.8
  gonococcal 098.19
    chronic or duration of 2 months or over
      098.39
  tuberculous (see also Tuberculosis) 016.0●
    [590.81]
Pyelocaliectasis 593.89
Pyelocystitis (see also Pyelitis) 590.80
Pyelohydronephrosis 591
Pyelonephritis (see also Pyelitis) 590.80
  acute 590.10
    with renal medullary necrosis 590.11
  chronic 590.00
  syphilitic (late) 095.4
  tuberculous (see also Tuberculosis) 016.0●
    [590.81]
Pyelonephrosis (see also Pyelitis) 590.80
  chronic 590.00
Pyelophlebitis 451.89
Pyelo-ureteritis cystica 590.3
Pyemia, pyemic (purulent) (see also Septicemia)
  038.9
  abscess - see Abscess
  arthritis (see also Arthritis, pyogenic)
    711.0●
  Bacillus coli 038.42
  embolism (see also Septicemia) 415.12
  fever 038.9
  infection 038.9
  joint (see also Arthritis, pyogenic) 711.0●
  liver 572.1
  meningococcal 036.2
  newborn 771.81
  phlebitis - see Phlebitis
  pneumococcal 038.2
  portal 572.1
  postvaccinal 999.39
  puerperal 670.2●
  specified organism NEC 038.8
  staphylococcal 038.10
    aureus 038.11
      methicillin
        resistant 038.12
        susceptible 038.11
    specified organism NEC 038.19
  streptococcal 038.0
  tuberculous - see Tuberculosis, miliary
Pygopagus 759.4
Pykno-epilepsy, pyknolepsy (idiopathic) (see
  also Epilepsy) 345.0●
Pyle (-Cohn) disease (craniometaphyseal
  dysplasia) 756.89
Pylephlebitis (suppurative) 572.1
Pylethrombophlebitis 572.1
Pylethrombosis 572.1
Pyloritis (see also Gastritis) 535.5●
Pylorospasm (reflex) 537.81
  congenital or infantile 750.5
  neurotic 306.4
  newborn 750.5
  psychogenic 306.4
Pylorus, pyloric - see condition
Pyoarthrosis - see Pyarthrosis
Pyocele
  mastoid 383.00
  sinus (accessory) (nasal) (see also Sinusitis)
    473.9
  turbinate (bone) 473.9
  urethra (see also Urethritis) 597.0

Pyococcal dermatitis 686.00
Pyococcide, skin 686.00
Pyocolpos (see also Vaginitis) 616.10
Pyocyaneus dermatitis 686.09
Pyocystitis (see also Cystitis) 595.9
Pyoderma, pyodermia 686.00
  gangrenosum 686.01
  specified type NEC 686.09
  vegetans 686.8
Pyodermatitis 686.00
  vegetans 686.8
Pyogenic - see condition
Pyohemia - see Septicemia
Pyohydronephrosis (see also Pyelitis)
  590.80
Pyometra 615.9
Pyometritis (see also Endometritis) 615.9
Pyometrium (see also Endometritis) 615.9
Pyomyositis 728.0
  ossificans 728.19
  tropical (bungpagga) 040.81
Pyonephritis (see also Pyelitis) 590.80
  chronic 590.00
Pyonephrosis (congenital) (see also Pyelitis)
  590.80
  acute 590.10
Pyo-oophoritis (see also Salpingo-oophoritis)
  614.2
Pyo-ovarium (see also Salpingo-oophoritis)
  614.2
Pyopericarditis 420.99
Pyopericardium 420.99
Pyophlebitis - see Phlebitis
Pyopneumopericardium 420.99
Pyopneumothorax (infectional) 510.9
  with fistula 510.0
  subdiaphragmatic (see also Peritonitis)
    567.29
  subphrenic (see also Peritonitis) 567.29
  tuberculous (see also Tuberculosis, pleura)
    012.0●
Pyorrhea (alveolar) (alveolaris) 523.40
  degenerative 523.5
Pyosalpingitis (see also Salpingo-oophoritis)
  614.2
Pyosalpinx (see also Salpingo-oophoritis)
  614.2
Pyosepticemia - see Septicemia
Pyosis
  Corlett's (impetigo) 684
  Manson's (pemphigus contagiosus)
    684
Pyothorax 510.9
  with fistula 510.0
  tuberculous (see also Tuberculosis, pleura)
    012.0●
Pyoureter 593.89
  tuberculous (see also Tuberculosis) 016.2●
Pyramidopallidonigral syndrome 332.0
Pyrexia (of unknown origin) (P.U.O.) 780.60
  atmospheric 992.0
  during labor 659.2●
  environmentally-induced newborn
    778.4
  heat 992.0
  newborn, environmentally-induced
    778.4
  puerperal 672●
Pyroglobulinemia 273.8
Pyromania 312.33
Pyrosis 787.1
Pyrroloporphyria 277.1
Pyuria (bacterial) 791.9

◀ New   ◀━ Revised   ~~deleted~~ Deleted   ● Use Additional Digit(s)   � Omit code

Q

Q fever 083.0
with pneumonia 083.0 *[484.8]*
Quadricuspid aortic valve 746.89
Quadrilateral fever 083.0
Quadriparesis - *see* Quadriplegia
meaning muscle weakness 728.87
Quadriplegia 344.00
with fracture, vertebra (process) - *see*
Fracture, vertebra, cervical, with spinal
cord injury
brain (current episode) 437.8
C₁–C₄
complete 344.01
incomplete 344.02
C₅–C₇
complete 344.03
incomplete 344.04
cerebral (current episode) 437.8
congenital or infantile (cerebral) (spastic)
(spinal) 343.2
cortical 437.8
embolic (current episode) (*see also* Embolism,
brain) 434.1●

Quadriplegia *(Continued)*
functional 780.72
infantile (cerebral) (spastic) (spinal)
343.2
newborn NEC 767.0
specified NEC 344.09
thrombotic (current episode) (*see also*
Thrombosis, brain) 434.0●
traumatic - *see* Injury, spinal, cervical
Quadruplet
affected by maternal complications of
pregnancy 761.5
healthy liveborn - *see* Newborn, multiple
pregnancy (complicating delivery) NEC
651.8●
with fetal loss and retention of one or
more fetus(es) 651.5●
following (elective) fetal reduction
651.7●
Quarrelsomeness 301.3
Quartan
fever 084.2
malaria (fever) 084.2
Queensland fever 083.0
coastal 083.0
seven-day 100.89

Quervain's disease 727.04
thyroid (subacute granulomatous thyroiditis)
245.1
Queyrat's erythroplasia (M8080/2)
specified site - *see* Neoplasm, skin, in situ
unspecified site 233.5
Quincke's disease or edema - *see* Edema,
angioneurotic
Quinquaud's disease (acne decalvans)
704.09
Quinsy (gangrenous) 475
Quintan fever 083.1
Quintuplet
affected by maternal complications of
pregnancy 761.5
healthy liveborn - *see* Newborn, multiple
pregnancy (complicating delivery) NEC
651.2●
with fetal loss and retention of one or
more fetus(es) 651.6●
following (elective) fetal reduction
651.7●
Quotidian
fever 084.0
malaria (fever) 084.0

R

Rabbia 071
Rabbit fever (see also Tularemia) 021.9
Rabies 071
  contact V01.5
  exposure to V01.5
  inoculation V04.5
    reaction - see Complications, vaccination
  vaccination, prophylactic (against) V04.5
Rachischisis (see also Spina bifida) 741.9●
Rachitic - see also condition
  deformities of spine 268.1
  pelvis 268.1
    with disproportion (fetopelvic) 653.2●
      affecting fetus or newborn 763.1
      causing obstructed labor 660.1●
        affecting fetus or newborn 763.1
Rachitis, rachitism - see also Rickets
  acute 268.0
  fetalis 756.4
  renalis 588.0
  tarda 268.0
Racket nail 757.5
Radial nerve - see condition
Radiation effects or sickness - see also Effect,
    adverse, radiation
  cataract 366.46
  dermatitis 692.82
    sunburn (see also Sunburn) 692.71
Radiculitis (pressure) (vertebrogenic) 729.2
  accessory nerve 723.4
  anterior crural 724.4
  arm 723.4
  brachial 723.4
  cervical NEC 723.4
  due to displacement of intervertebral
      disc - see Neuritis, due to, displacement
      intervertebral disc
  leg 724.4
  lumbar NEC 724.4
  lumbosacral 724.4
  rheumatic 729.2
  syphilitic 094.89
  thoracic (with visceral pain) 724.4
Radiculomyelitis 357.0
  toxic, due to
    Clostridium tetani 037
    corynebacterium diphtheriae 032.89
Radiculopathy (see also Radiculitis) 729.2
Radioactive substances, adverse effect - see
    Effect, adverse, radioactive substance
Radiodermal burns (acute) (chronic)
    (occupational) - see Burn, by site
Radiodermatitis 692.82
Radionecrosis - see Effect, adverse, radiation
Radiotherapy session V58.0
Radium, adverse effect - see Effect, adverse,
    radioactive substance
Raeder-Harbitz syndrome (pulseless disease)
    446.7
Rage (see also Disturbance, conduct)
    312.0●
  meaning rabies 071
Rag sorters' disease 022.1
Raillietiniasis 123.8
Railroad neurosis 300.16
Railway spine 300.16
Raised - see Elevation
Raiva 071
Rake teeth, tooth 524.39
Rales 786.7
Ramifying renal pelvis 753.3
Ramsay Hunt syndrome (herpetic geniculate
    ganglionitis) 053.11
  meaning dyssynergia cerebellaris
    myoclonica 334.2
Ranke's primary infiltration (see also
    Tuberculosis) 010.0●
Ranula 527.6
  congenital 750.26

Rape
  adult 995.83
  alleged, observation or examination
    V71.5
  child 995.53
Rapid
  feeble pulse, due to shock, following injury
    958.4
  heart (beat) 785.0
    psychogenic 306.2
  respiration 786.06
    psychogenic 306.1
  second stage (delivery) 661.3●
    affecting fetus or newborn 763.6
  time-zone change syndrome 327.35
Rarefaction, bone 733.99
Rash 782.1
  canker 034.1
  diaper 691.0
  drug (internal use) 693.0
    contact 692.3
  ECHO 9 virus 078.89
  enema 692.89
  food (see also Allergy, food) 693.1
  heat 705.1
  napkin 691.0
  nettle 708.8
  pustular 782.1
  rose 782.1
    epidemic 056.9
    of infants 057.8
  scarlet 034.1
  serum (prophylactic) (therapeutic)
    999.59
  toxic 782.1
  wandering tongue 529.1
Rasmussen's aneurysm (see also Tuberculosis)
    011.2●
Rat-bite fever 026.9
  due to Streptobacillus moniliformis
    026.1
  spirochetal (morsus muris) 026.0
Rathke's pouch tumor (M9350/1) 237.0
Raymond (-Céstan) syndrome 433.8●
Raynaud's
  disease or syndrome (paroxysmal digital
    cyanosis) 443.0
  gangrene (symmetric) 443.0 [785.4]
  phenomenon (paroxysmal digital cyanosis)
    (secondary) 443.0
RDS 769
Reaction
  acute situational maladjustment (see also
    Reaction, adjustment) 309.9
  adaptation (see also Reaction, adjustment)
    309.9
  adjustment 309.9
    with
      anxious mood 309.24
        with depressed mood 309.28
      conduct disturbance 309.3
        combined with disturbance of
          emotions 309.4
      depressed mood 309.0
        brief 309.0
          with anxious mood 309.28
        prolonged 309.1
      elective mutism 309.83
      mixed emotions and conduct 309.4
      mutism, elective 309.83
      physical symptoms 309.82
      predominant disturbance (of)
        conduct 309.3
        emotions NEC 309.29
          mixed 309.28
        mixed, emotions and conduct
          309.4
        specified type NEC 309.89
      specific academic or work inhibition
        309.23
      withdrawal 309.83

Reaction (Continued)
  adjustment (Continued)
    depressive 309.0
      with conduct disturbance 309.4
      brief 309.0
      prolonged 309.1
    specified type NEC 309.89
  adverse food NEC 995.7
  affective (see also Psychosis, affective) 296.90
    specified type NEC 296.99
  aggressive 301.3
    unsocialized (see also Disturbance,
      conduct) 312.0●
  allergic (see also Allergy) 995.3
    drug, medicinal substance, and
      biological - see Allergy, drug
    due to correct medical substance properly
      administered 995.27
    food - see Allergy, food
    serum 999.59
  anaphylactic - see Anaphylactic reaction
  anesthesia - see Anesthesia, complication
  anger 312.0●
  antisocial 301.7
  antitoxin (prophylactic) (therapeutic) - see
    Complications, vaccination
  anxiety 300.00
  Arthus 995.21
  asthenic 300.5
  compulsive 300.3
  conversion (anesthetic) (autonomic)
    (hyperkinetic) (mixed paralytic)
    (paresthetic) 300.11
  deoxyribonuclease (DNA) (DNase)
    hypersensitivity NEC 287.2
  depressive 300.4
    acute 309.0
    affective (see also Psychosis, affective)
      296.2●
      recurrent episode 296.3●
      single episode 296.2●
    brief 309.0
    manic (see also Psychosis, affective)
      296.80
    neurotic 300.4
    psychoneurotic 300.4
    psychotic 298.0
  dissociative 300.15
  drug NEC (see also Table of Drugs and
    Chemicals) 995.20
    allergic - see also Allergy, drug 995.27
    correct substance properly administered
      995.20
    obstetric anesthetic or analgesic NEC
      668.9●
      affecting fetus or newborn 763.5
      specified drug - see Table of Drugs and
        Chemicals
    overdose or poisoning 977.9
      specified drug - see Table of Drugs and
        Chemicals
    specific to newborn 779.4
    transmitted via placenta or breast
      milk - see Absorption, drug, through
        placenta
    withdrawal NEC 292.0
      infant of dependent mother 779.5
    wrong substance given or taken in error
      977.9
      specified drug - see Table of Drugs and
        Chemicals
  dyssocial 301.7
  dystonic, acute, due to drugs 333.72
  erysipeloid 027.1
  fear 300.20
    child 313.0
  fluid loss, cerebrospinal 349.0
  food - see also Allergy, food
    adverse NEC 995.7
    anaphylactic shock - see Anaphylactic
      reaction or shock, due to, food

◀ New   ◀|||| Revised   ~~deleted~~ Deleted   ● Use Additional Digit(s)   ▨ Omit code

Reaction (Continued)
  foreign
    body NEC 728.82
      in operative wound (inadvertently left)
        998.4
        due to surgical material
          intentionally left - see
          Complications, due to
          (presence of) any device,
          implant, or graft classified to
          996.0–996.5 NEC
      substance accidentally left during a
        procedure (chemical) (powder)
        (talc) 998.7
        body or object (instrument) (sponge)
          (swab) 998.4
  graft-versus-host (GVH) 279.50
  grief (acute) (brief) 309.0
    prolonged 309.1
  gross stress (see also Reaction, stress, acute)
    308.9
  group delinquent (see also Disturbance,
    conduct) 312.2●
  Herxheimer's 995.91
  hyperkinetic (see also Hyperkinesia) 314.9
  hypochondriacal 300.7
  hypoglycemic, due to insulin 251.0
    therapeutic misadventure 962.3
  hypomanic (see also Psychosis, affective)
    296.0●
    recurrent episode 296.1●
    single episode 296.0●
  hysterical 300.10
    conversion type 300.11
    dissociative 300.15
  id (bacterial cause) 692.89
  immaturity NEC 301.89
    aggressive 301.3
    emotional instability 301.59
  immunization - see Complications,
    vaccination
  incompatibility
    blood group (see also Complications,
      transfusion) 999.80
      ABO (due to transfusion of blood or
        blood products) (see also
        Complications, transfusion)
        999.60
      minor blood group 999.89
      non-ABO (see also Complications,
        transfusion) 999.75
    ABO 999.6
    minor blood group 999.89
    Rh antigen (C) (c) (D) (E) (e) (factor)
      (infusion) (transfusion) (see also
      Complications, transfusion) 999.70
  inflammatory - see Infection
  infusion - see Complications, infusion
  inoculation (immune serum) - see
    Complications, vaccination
  insulin 995.23
  involutional
    paranoid 297.2
    psychotic (see also Psychosis, affective,
      depressive) 296.2●
  leukemoid (basophilic) (lymphocytic)
    (monocytic) (myelocytic) (neutrophilic)
    288.62
  LSD (see also Abuse, drugs, nondependent)
    305.3●
  lumbar puncture 349.0
  manic-depressive (see also Psychosis,
    affective) 296.80
    depressed 296.2●
      recurrent episode 296.3●
      single episode 296.2●
    hypomanic 296.0●
  neurasthenic 300.5
  neurogenic (see also Neurosis) 300.9
  neurotic NEC 300.9
  neurotic-depressive 300.4

Reaction (Continued)
  nitritoid - see Crisis, nitritoid
  nonspecific
    to
      cell mediated immunity measurement
        of gamma interferon antigen
        response without active
        tuberculosis 795.52
      QuantiFERON-TB test (QFT) without
        active tuberculosis 795.52
      tuberculin test (see also Reaction,
        tuberculin skin test) 795.51
  obsessive-compulsive 300.3
  organic 293.9
    acute 293.0
    subacute 293.1
  overanxious, child or adolescent 313.0
  paranoid (chronic) 297.9
    acute 298.3
    climacteric 297.2
    involutional 297.2
    menopausal 297.2
    senile 290.20
    simple 297.0
  passive
    aggressive 301.84
    dependency 301.6
  personality (see also Disorder, personality)
    301.9
  phobic 300.20
  postradiation - see Effect, adverse, radiation
  psychogenic NEC 300.9
  psychoneurotic (see also Neurosis) 300.9
    anxiety 300.00
    compulsive 300.3
    conversion 300.11
    depersonalization 300.6
    depressive 300.4
    dissociative 300.15
    hypochondriacal 300.7
    hysterical 300.10
      conversion type 300.11
      dissociative type 300.15
    neurasthenic 300.5
    obsessive 300.3
    obsessive-compulsive 300.3
    phobic 300.20
    tension state 300.9
  psychophysiologic NEC (see also Disorder,
    psychosomatic) 306.9
    cardiovascular 306.2
    digestive 306.4
    endocrine 306.6
    gastrointestinal 306.4
    genitourinary 306.50
    heart 306.2
    hemic 306.8
    intestinal (large) (small) 306.4
    laryngeal 306.1
    lymphatic 306.8
    musculoskeletal 306.0
    pharyngeal 306.1
    respiratory 306.1
    skin 306.3
    special sense organs 306.7
  psychosomatic (see also Disorder,
    psychosomatic) 306.9
  psychotic (see also Psychosis) 298.9
    depressive 298.0
    due to or associated with physical
      condition (see also Psychosis,
      organic) 293.9
    involutional (see also Psychosis, affective)
      296.2●
      recurrent episode 296.3●
      single episode 296.2●
  pupillary (myotonic) (tonic) 379.46
  radiation - see Effect, adverse, radiation
  runaway - see also Disturbance, conduct
    socialized 312.2●
    undersocialized, unsocialized 312.1●

Reaction (Continued)
  scarlet fever toxin - see Complications,
    vaccination
  schizophrenic (see also Schizophrenia) 295.9●
    latent 295.5●
  serological for syphilis - see Serology for
    syphilis
  serum (prophylactic) (therapeutic) 999.59
    anaphylactic 999.49
    due to
      administration of blood and blood
        products 999.51
        anaphylactic 999.41
      vaccination 999.52
        anaphylactic 999.41
    immediate 999.49
  situational (see also Reaction, adjustment)
    309.9
    acute, to stress 308.3
    adjustment (see also Reaction, adjustment)
      309.9
  somatization (see also Disorder,
    psychosomatic) 306.9
  spinal puncture 349.0
  spite, child (see also Disturbance, conduct)
    312.0●
  stress, acute 308.9
    with predominant disturbance (of)
      consciousness 308.1
      emotions 308.0
      mixed 308.4
      psychomotor 308.2
      specified type NEC 308.3
    bone or cartilage - see Fracture, stress
  surgical procedure - see Complications,
    surgical procedure
  tetanus antitoxin - see Complications,
    vaccination
  toxin-antitoxin - see Complications,
    vaccination
  transfusion (blood) (bone marrow)
    (lymphocytes) (allergic) (see also
    Complications, transfusion) 999.80
  tuberculin skin test, nonspecific (without
    active tuberculosis) 795.51
    positive (without active tuberculosis)
      795.51
  ultraviolet - see Effect, adverse, ultraviolet
  undersocialized, unsocialized - see also
    Disturbance, conduct
    aggressive (type) 312.0●
    unaggressive (type) 312.1●
  vaccination (any) - see Complications,
    vaccination
  white graft (skin) 996.52
  withdrawing, child or adolescent 313.22
  x-ray - see Effect, adverse, x-rays
Reactive depression (see also Reaction,
    depressive) 300.4
  neurotic 300.4
  psychoneurotic 300.4
  psychotic 298.0
Rebound tenderness 789.6●
Recalcitrant patient V15.81
Recanalization, thrombus - see Thrombosis
Recession, receding
  chamber angle (eye) 364.77
  chin 524.06
  gingival (postinfective) (postoperative)
    523.20
    generalized 523.25
    localized 523.24
    minimal 523.21
    moderate 523.22
    severe 523.23
Recklinghausen's disease (M9540/1) 237.71
  bones (osteitis fibrosa cystica) 252.01
Recklinghausen-Applebaum disease
    (hemochromatosis) 275.03
Reclus' disease (cystic) 610.1
Recrudescent typhus (fever) 081.1

Recruitment, auditory 388.44
Rectalgia 569.42
Rectitis 569.49
Rectocele
 female (without uterine prolapse) 618.04
  with uterine prolapse 618.4
   complete 618.3
   incomplete 618.2
 in pregnancy or childbirth 654.4●
  causing obstructed labor 660.2●
   affecting fetus or newborn 763.1
 male 569.49
 vagina, vaginal (outlet) 618.04
Rectosigmoiditis 569.89
 ulcerative (chronic) 556.3
Rectosigmoid junction - see condition
Rectourethral - see condition
Rectovaginal - see condition
Rectovesical - see condition
Rectum, rectal - see condition
Recurrent - see condition
 pregnancy loss - see Pregnancy, management
  affected by, abortion, habitual
Red bugs 133.8
Red cedar asthma 495.8
Redness
 conjunctiva 379.93
 eye 379.93
 nose 478.19
Reduced ventilatory or vital capacity 794.2
Reduction
 function
  kidney (see also Disease, renal) 593.9
  liver 573.8
 ventilatory capacity 794.2
 vital capacity 794.2
Redundant, redundancy
 abdomen 701.9
 anus 751.5
 cardia 537.89
 clitoris 624.2
 colon (congenital) 751.5
 foreskin (congenital) 605
 intestine 751.5
 labia 624.3
 organ or site, congenital NEC - see Accessory
 panniculus (abdominal) 278.1
 prepuce (congenital) 605
 pylorus 537.89
 rectum 751.5
 scrotum 608.89
 sigmoid 751.5
 skin (of face) 701.9
  eyelids 374.30
 stomach 537.89
 uvula 528.9
 vagina 623.8
Reduplication - see Duplication
Referral
 adoption (agency) V68.89
 nursing care V63.8
 patient without examination or treatment
  V68.81
 social services V63.8
Reflex - see also condition
 blink, deficient 374.45
 hyperactive gag 478.29
 neurogenic bladder NEC 596.54
  atonic 596.54
   with cauda equina syndrome
    344.61
 vasoconstriction 443.9
 vasovagal 780.2
Reflux 530.81
 acid 530.81
 esophageal 530.81
  with esophagitis 530.11
 esophagitis 530.11
 gastroesophageal 530.81
 mitral - see Insufficiency, mitral
 ureteral - see Reflux, vesicoureteral

Reflux (Continued)
 vesicoureteral 593.70
  with
   reflux nephropathy 593.73
    bilateral 593.72
    unilateral 593.71
Reformed gallbladder 576.0
Reforming, artificial openings (see also
  Attention to, artificial, opening) V55.9
Refractive error (see also Error, refractive) 367.9
Refsum's disease or syndrome (heredopathia
  atactica polyneuritiformis) 356.3
Refusal of
 food 307.59
  hysterical 300.11
 treatment because of, due to
  patient's decision NEC V64.2
  reason of conscience or religion V62.6
Regaud
 tumor (M8082/3) - see Neoplasm,
  nasopharynx, malignant
 type carcinoma (M8082/3) - see Neoplasm,
  nasopharynx, malignant
Regional - see condition
Regulation feeding (elderly) (infant) 783.3
 newborn 779.31
Regurgitated
 food, choked on 933.1
 stomach contents, choked on 933.1
Regurgitation 787.03
 aortic (valve) (see also Insufficiency, aortic)
  424.1
  congenital 746.4
  syphilitic 093.22
 food - see also Vomiting
  with reswallowing - see Rumination
  newborn 779.33
 gastric contents - see Vomiting
 heart - see Endocarditis
 mitral (valve) - see also Insufficiency, mitral
  congenital 746.6
 myocardial - see Endocarditis
 pulmonary (heart) (valve) (see also
  Endocarditis, pulmonary) 424.3
 stomach - see Vomiting
 tricuspid - see Endocarditis, tricuspid
 valve, valvular - see Endocarditis
 vesicoureteral - see Reflux, vesicoureteral
Rehabilitation V57.9
 multiple types V57.89
 occupational V57.21
 specified type NEC V57.89
 speech (-language) V57.3
 vocational V57.22
Reichmann's disease or syndrome
  (gastrosuccorrhea) 536.8
Reifenstein's syndrome (hereditary familial
  hypogonadism, male) 259.52
Reilly's syndrome or phenomenon (see also
  Neuropathy, peripheral, autonomic)
  337.9
Reimann's periodic disease 277.31
Reinsertion, contraceptive device V25.42
 intrauterine V25.13
Reiter's disease, syndrome, or urethritis 099.3
 [711.1]●
Rejection
 food, hysterical 300.11
 transplant 996.80
  bone marrow 996.85
  corneal 996.51
  organ (immune or nonimmune cause)
   996.80
   bone marrow 996.85
   heart 996.83
   intestines 996.87
   kidney 996.81
   liver 996.82
   lung 996.84
   pancreas 996.86
   specified NEC 996.89

Rejection (Continued)
 transplant (Continued)
  skin 996.52
   artificial 996.55
   decellularized allodermis
    996.55
  stem cell(s) 996.88
   from
    peripheral blood 996.88
    umbilical cord 996.88
Relapsing fever 087.9
 Carter's (Asiatic) 087.0
 Dutton's (West African) 087.1
 Koch's 087.9
 louse-borne (epidemic) 087.0
 Novy's (American) 087.1
 Obermeyer's (European) 087.0
 Spirillum 087.9
 tick-borne (endemic) 087.1
Relaxation
 anus (sphincter) 569.49
  due to hysteria 300.11
 arch (foot) 734
  congenital 754.61
 back ligaments 728.4
 bladder (sphincter) 596.59
 cardio-esophageal 530.89
 cervix (see also Incompetency, cervix)
  622.5
 diaphragm 519.4
 inguinal rings - see Hernia, inguinal
 joint (capsule) (ligament) (paralytic)
  (see also Derangement, joint)
  718.90
  congenital 755.8
 lumbosacral joint 724.6
 pelvic floor 618.89
 pelvis 618.89
 perineum 618.89
 posture 729.90
 rectum (sphincter) 569.49
 sacroiliac (joint) 724.6
 scrotum 608.89
 urethra (sphincter) 599.84
 uterus (outlet) 618.89
 vagina (outlet) 618.89
 vesical 596.59
Remains
 canal of Cloquet 743.51
 capsule (opaque) 743.51
Remittent fever (malarial) 084.6
Remnant
 canal of Cloquet 743.51
 capsule (opaque) 743.51
 cervix, cervical stump (acquired)
  (postoperative) 622.8
 cystic duct, postcholecystectomy 576.0
 fingernail 703.8
  congenital 757.5
 meniscus, knee 717.5
 thyroglossal duct 759.2
 tonsil 474.8
  infected 474.00
 urachus 753.7
Remote effect of cancer - see condition
Removal (of)
 catheter (urinary) (indwelling) V53.6
  from artificial opening - see Attention to,
   artificial, opening
  non-vascular V58.82
  vascular V58.81
 cerebral ventricle (communicating) shunt
  V53.01
 device - see also Fitting (of)
  contraceptive V25.12
   with reinsertion V25.13
  fixation
   external V54.89
   internal V54.01
  traction V54.89
 drains V58.49

◀ New   ◀▥ Revised   d̶e̶l̶e̶t̶e̶d̶ Deleted   ● Use Additional Digit(s)   ▨ Omit code

Removal (Continued)
  dressing
    wound V58.30
      nonsurgical V58.30
      surgical V58.31
  ileostomy V55.2
  Kirschner wire V54.89
  non-vascular catheter V58.82
  pin V54.01
  plaster cast V54.89
  plate (fracture) V54.01
  rod V54.01
  screw V54.01
  splint, external V54.89
  staples V58.32
  subdermal implantable contraceptive V25.43
  sutures V58.32
  traction device, external V54.89
  vascular catheter V58.81
  wound packing V58.30
    nonsurgical V58.30
    surgical V58.31
Ren
  arcuatus 753.3
  mobile, mobilis (see also Disease, renal) 593.0
    congenital 753.3
  unguliformis 753.3
Renal - see also condition
  glomerulohyalinosis-diabetic syndrome
    250.4● [581.81]
    due to secondary diabetes 249.4● [581.81]

Rendu-Osler-Weber disease or syndrome
  (familial hemorrhagic telangiectasia)
  448.0
Reninoma (M8361/1) 236.91
Rénon-Delille syndrome 253.8
Repair
  pelvic floor, previous, in pregnancy or
    childbirth 654.4●
    affecting fetus or newborn 763.89
  scarred tissue V51.8
Replacement by artificial or mechanical device
  or prosthesis of (see also Fitting (of))
  artificial skin V43.83
  bladder V43.5
  blood vessel V43.4
  breast V43.82
  eye globe V43.0
  heart
    with
      assist device V43.21
      fully implantable artificial heart
      V43.22
    valve V43.3
  intestine V43.89
  joint V43.60
    ankle V43.66
    elbow V43.62
    finger V43.69
    hip (partial) (total) V43.64
    knee V43.65
    shoulder V43.61
    specified NEC V43.69
    wrist V43.63
  kidney V43.89
  larynx V43.81
  lens V43.1
  limb(s) V43.7
  liver V43.89
  lung V43.89
  organ NEC V43.89
  pancreas V43.89
  skin (artificial) V43.83
  tissue NEC V43.89
Reprogramming
  cardiac pacemaker V53.31
Request for expert evidence V68.2
Reserve, decreased or low
  cardiac - see Disease, heart
    kidney (see also Disease, renal) 593.9

Residual - see also condition
  bladder 596.89
  foreign body - see Retention, foreign body
  state, schizophrenic (see also Schizophrenia)
    295.6●
  urine 788.69
Resistance, resistant (to)
  activated protein C 289.81

> Note: Use the following subclassification
> for categories V09.5, V09.7, V09.8, V09.9
>
> 0   without mention of resistance to
>   multiple drugs
> 1   with resistance to multiple drugs
>   V09.5 quinolones and
>   fluoro-quinolones
>   V09.7 antimycobacterial agents
>   V09.8 specified drugs NEC
>   V09.9 unspecified drugs

  drugs by microorganisms V09.90
    amikacin V09.4
    aminoglycosides V09.4
    amodiaquine V09.5●
    amoxicillin V09.0
    ampicillin V09.0
    antimycobacterial agents V09.7●
    azithromycin V09.2
    azlocillin V09.0
    aztreonam V09.1
    B-lactam antibiotics V09.1
    bacampicillin V09.0
    bacitracin V09.8●
    benznidazole V09.8●
    capreomycin V09.7●
    carbenicillin V09.0
    cefaclor V09.1
    cefadroxil V09.1
    cefamandole V09.1
    cefatetan V09.1
    cefazolin V09.1
    cefixime V09.1
    cefonicid V09.1
    cefoperazone V09.1
    ceforanide V09.1
    cefotaxime V09.1
    cefoxitin V09.1
    ceftazidine V09.1
    ceftizoxime V09.1
    ceftriaxone V09.1
    cefuroxime V09.1
    cephalexin V09.1
    cephaloglycin V09.1
    cephaloridine V09.1
    cephalosporins V09.1
    cephalothin V09.1
    cephapirin V09.1
    cephradine V09.1
    chloramphenicol V09.8●
    chloraquine V09.5●
    chlorguanide V09.8●
    chlorproguanil V09.8●
    chlortetracycline V09.3
    cinoxacin V09.5●
    ciprofloxacin V09.5●
    clarithromycin V09.2
    clindamycin V09.8●
    clioquinol V09.5●
    clofazimine V09.7●
    cloxacillin V09.0
    cyclacillin V09.0
    cycloserine V09.7●
    dapsone [Dz] V09.7●
    demeclocycline V09.3
    dicloxacillin V09.0
    doxycycline V09.3
    enoxacin V09.5●
    erythromycin V09.2
    ethambutol [EMB] V09.7●
    ethionamide [ETA] V09.7●
    fluoroquinolones NEC V09.5●

Resistance, resistant (Continued)
  drugs by microorganisms (Continued)
    gentamicin V09.4
    halofantrine V09.8●
    imipenem V09.1
    iodoquinol V09.5●
    isoniazid [INH] V09.7●
    kanamycin V09.4
    macrolides V09.2
    mafenide V09.6
    MDRO (multiple drug resistant
      organisms) NOS V09.91
    mefloquine V09.8●
    melarsoprol V09.8●
    methicillin - see Infection, Methicillin
    methacycline V09.3
    methenamine V09.8●
    metronidazole V09.8●
    mezlocillin V09.0
    minocycline V09.3
    multiple drug resistant organisms NOS
      V09.91
    nafcillin V09.0
    nalidixic acid V09.5●
    natamycin V09.2
    neomycin V09.4
    netilmicin V09.4
    nimorazole V09.8●
    nitrofurantoin V09.8●
    norfloxacin V09.5●
    nystatin V09.2
    ofloxacin V09.5●
    oleandomycin V09.2
    oxacillin V09.0
    oxytetracycline V09.3
    para-amino salicyclic acid [PAS]
      V09.7●
    paromomycin V09.4
    penicillin (G) (V) (Vk) V09.0
    penicillins V09.0
    pentamidine V09.8●
    piperacillin V09.0
    primaquine V09.5●
    proguanil V09.8●
    pyrazinamide [PZA] V09.7●
    pyrimethamine/sulfalene V09.8●
    pyrimethamine/sulfodoxine V09.8●
    quinacrine V09.5●
    quinidine V09.8●
    quinine V09.8●
    quinolones V09.5●
    rifabutin V09.7●
    rifampin [Rif] V09.7●
    rifamycin V09.7●
    rolitetracycline V09.3
    specified drugs NEC V09.8●
    spectinomycin V09.8●
    spiramycin V09.2
    streptomycin [Sm] V09.4
    sulfacetamide V09.6
    sulfacytine V09.6
    sulfadiazine V09.6
    sulfadoxine V09.6
    sulfamethoxazole V09.6
    sulfapyridine V09.6
    sulfasalizine V09.6
    sulfasoxazone V09.6
    sulfonamides V09.6
    sulfoxone V09.7●
    tetracycline V09.3
    tetracyclines V09.3
    thiamphenicol V09.8●
    ticarcillin V09.0
    tinidazole V09.8●
    tobramycin V09.4
    triamphenicol V09.8●
    trimethoprim V09.8●
    vancomycin V09.8●
  insulin 277.7
    complicating pregnancy 648.8●
  thyroid hormone 246.8

◀ New   ⬅ Revised   ~~deleted~~ Deleted   ● Use Additional Digit(s)   ▒ Omit code

Resorption
  biliary 576.8
    purulent or putrid (*see also* Cholecystitis)
        576.8
  dental (roots) 521.40
    alveoli 525.8
    pathological
        external 521.42
        internal 521.41
        specified NEC 521.49
    septic - *see* Septicemia
  teeth (roots) 521.40
    pathological
        external 521.42
        internal 521.41
        specified NEC 521.49
Respiration
  asymmetrical 786.09
  bronchial 786.09
  Cheyne-Stokes (periodic respiration) 786.04
  decreased, due to shock following injury
      958.4
  disorder of 786.00
    psychogenic 306.1
    specified NEC 786.09
  failure 518.81
    acute 518.81
        following trauma and surgery 518.51
    acute and chronic 518.84
        following trauma and surgery 518.53
    chronic 518.83
    following trauma and surgery 518.51
    newborn 770.84
  insufficiency 786.09
    acute 518.82
    newborn NEC 770.89
  Kussmaul (air hunger) 786.09
  painful 786.52
  periodic 786.09
  high altitude 327.22
  poor 786.09
    newborn NEC 770.89
  sighing 786.7
    psychogenic 306.1
  wheezing 786.07
Respiratory - *see also* condition
  distress 786.09
    acute 518.82
    fetus or newborn NEC 770.89
    syndrome (newborn) 769
        adult (following trauma and surgery)
            518.52
        specified NEC 518.82
  failure 518.81
    acute 518.81
        following trauma and surgery 518.51
    acute and chronic 518.84
        following trauma and surgery 518.53
    chronic 518.83
    following trauma and surgery 518.51
Respiratory syncytial virus (RSV) 079.6
  bronchiolitis 466.11
  pneumonia 480.1
  vaccination, prophylactic (against) V04.82
Response
  photoallergic 692.72
  phototoxic 692.72
Rest, rests
  mesonephric duct 752.89
    fallopian tube 752.11
  ovarian, in fallopian tubes 752.19
  wolffian duct 752.89
Restless legs syndrome (RLS) 333.94
Restlessness 799.29
Restoration of organ continuity from previous
    sterilization (tuboplasty) (vasoplasty)
    V26.0
Restriction of housing space V60.1
Restzustand, schizophrenic (*see also*
    Schizophrenia) 295.6●
Retained - *see* Retention

Retardation
  development, developmental, specific (*see
      also* Disorder, development, specific)
      315.9
  learning, specific 315.2
    arithmetical 315.1
    language (skills) 315.31
        expressive 315.31
        mixed receptive-expressive
            315.32
    mathematics 315.1
    reading 315.00
        phonological 315.39
    written expression 315.2
  motor 315.4
  endochondral bone growth 733.91
  growth (physical) in childhood 783.43
    due to malnutrition 263.2
    fetal (intrauterine) 764.9●
        affecting management of pregnancy
            656.5●
  intrauterine growth 764.9●
    affecting management of pregnancy
        656.5●
  mental - *see* Disability, intellectual
  motor, specific 315.4
  physical 783.43
    child 783.43
    due to malnutrition 263.2
    fetus (intrauterine) 764.9●
        affecting management of pregnancy
            656.5●
  psychomotor NEC 307.9
  reading 315.00
Retching - *see* Vomiting
Retention, retained
  bladder (*see also* Retention, urine) 788.20
    psychogenic 306.53
  carbon dioxide 276.2
  cholelithisis, following cholecystectomy
      997.41
  cyst - *see* Cyst
  dead
    fetus (after 22 completed weeks'
        gestation) 656.4●
    early fetal death (before 22 completed
        weeks' gestation) 632
  ovum 631.8
  decidua (following delivery) (fragments)
      (with hemorrhage) 666.2●
    without hemorrhage 667.1●
  deciduous tooth 520.6
  dental root 525.3
  fecal (*see also* Constipation) 564.00
  fluid 276.69
  foreign body - *see also* Foreign body,
      retained
    bone 733.99
    current trauma - *see* Foreign body, by site
        or type
    middle ear 385.83
    muscle 729.6
    soft tissue NEC 729.6
  gallstones, following cholecystectomy
      997.41
  gastric 536.8
  membranes (following delivery) (with
      hemorrhage) 666.2●
    with abortion - *see* Abortion, by type
    without hemorrhage 667.1●
  menses 626.8
  milk (puerperal) 676.2●
  nitrogen, extrarenal 788.99
  placenta (total) (with hemorrhage) 666.0●
    with abortion - *see* Abortion, by type
    portions or fragments 666.2●
        without hemorrhage 667.1●
    without hemorrhage 667.0●
  products of conception
    early pregnancy (fetal death before 22
        completed weeks' gestation) 632

Retention, retained (*Continued*)
  products of conception (*Continued*)
    following
        abortion - *see* Abortion, by type
        delivery 666.2●
            with hemorrhage 666.2●
            without hemorrhage 667.1●
    secundines (following delivery) (with
        hemorrhage) 666.2●
    with abortion - *see* Abortion, by type
    complicating puerperium (delayed
        hemorrhage) 666.2●
    without hemorrhage 667.1●
  smegma, clitoris 624.8
  urine NEC 788.20
    bladder, incomplete emptying 788.21
    due to
        benign prostatic hypertrophy
            (BPH) - *see* category 600
    due to
        benign prostatic hypertrophy
            (BPH) - *see* category 600
    psychogenic 306.53
    specified NEC 788.29
  water (in tissue) (*see also* Edema) 782.3
Reticulation, dust (occupational) 504
Reticulocytosis NEC 790.99
Reticuloendotheliosis
  acute infantile (M9722/3) 202.5●
  leukemic (M9940/3) 202.4●
  malignant (M9720/3) 202.3●
  nonlipid (M9722/3) 202.5●
Reticulohistiocytoma (giant cell) 277.89
Reticulohistiocytosis, multicentric 272.8
Reticulolymphosarcoma (diffuse) (M9613/3)
    200.8●
  follicular (M9691/3) 202.0●
  nodular (M9691/3) 202.0●
Reticulosarcoma (M9640/3) 200.0●
  nodular (M9642/3) 200.0●
  pleomorphic cell type (M9641/3) 200.0●
Reticulosis (skin)
  acute of infancy (M9722/3) 202.5●
  familial hemophagocytic 288.4
  histiocytic medullary (M9721/3) 202.3●
  lipomelanotic 695.89
  malignant (M9720/3) 202.3●
  Sézary's (M9701/3) 202.2●
Retina, retinal - *see* condition
Retinitis (*see also* Chorioretinitis) 363.20
  albuminurica 585.9 [363.10]
  arteriosclerotic 440.8 [362.13]
  central angiospastic 362.41
  Coat's 362.12
  diabetic 250.5● [362.01]
    due to secondary diabetes 249.5● [362.01]
  disciformis 362.52
  disseminated 363.10
    metastatic 363.14
    neurosyphilitic 094.83
    pigment epitheliopathy 363.15
  exudative 362.12
  focal 363.00
    in histoplasmosis 115.92
        capsulatum 115.02
        duboisii 115.12
    juxtapapillary 363.05
    macular 363.06
    paramacular 363.06
    peripheral 363.08
    posterior pole NEC 363.07
  gravidarum 646.8●
  hemorrhagica externa 362.12
  juxtapapillary (Jensen's) 363.05
  luetic - *see* Retinitis, syphilitic
  metastatic 363.14
  pigmentosa 362.74
  proliferans 362.29
  proliferating 362.29
  punctata albescens 362.76
  renal 585.9 [363.13]

◄ New   ◄▥ Revised   ~~deleted~~ Deleted   ● Use Additional Digit(s)   ▨ Omit code

Retinitis (Continued)
  syphilitic (secondary) 091.51
    congenital 090.0 [363.13]
    early 091.51
    late 095.8 [363.13]
  syphilitica, central, recurrent 095.8 [363.13]
  tuberculous (see also Tuberculous) 017.3●
    [363.13]
Retinoblastoma (M9510/3) 190.5
  differentiated type (M9511/3) 190.5
  undifferentiated type (M9512/3) 190.5
Retinochoroiditis (see also Chorioretinitis)
    363.20
  central angiospastic 362.41
  disseminated 363.10
    metastatic 363.14
    neurosyphilitic 094.83
    pigment epitheliopathy 363.15
    syphilitic 094.83
  due to toxoplasmosis (acquired) (focal)
    130.2
  focal 363.00
    in histoplasmosis 115.92
      capsulatum 115.02
      duboisii 115.12
    juxtapapillary (Jensen's) 363.05
    macular 363.06
    paramacular 363.06
    peripheral 363.08
    posterior pole NEC 363.07
  juxtapapillaris 363.05
  syphilitic (disseminated) 094.83
Retinopathy (background) 362.10
  arteriosclerotic 440.8 [362.13]
  atherosclerotic 440.8 [362.13]
  central serous 362.41
  circinate 362.10
  Coat's 362.12
  diabetic 250.5● [362.01]
    due to secondary diabetes 249.5●
      [362.01]
    nonproliferative 250.5● [362.03]
      due to secondary diabetes 249.5●
        [362.03]
      mild 250.5● [362.04]
        due to secondary diabetes 249.5●
          [362.04]
      moderate 250.5● [362.05]
        due to secondary diabetes 249.5●
          [362.05]
      severe 250.5● [362.06]
        due to secondary diabetes 249.5●
          [362.06]
    proliferative 250.5● [362.02]
      due to secondary diabetes 249.5●
        [362.02]
  exudative 362.12
  hypertensive 362.11
  nonproliferative
    diabetic 250.5● [362.03]
      due to secondary diabetes 249.5●
        [362.03]
      mild 250.5● [362.04]
        due to secondary diabetes 249.5●
          [362.04]
      moderate 250.5● [362.05]
        due to secondary diabetes 249.5●
          [362.05]
      severe 250.5● [362.06]
        due to secondary diabetes 249.5●
          [362.06]
  of prematurity 362.20
    cicatricial 362.21
    stage
      0 362.22
      1 362.23
      2 362.24
      3 362.25
      4 362.26
      5 362.27
  pigmentary, congenital 362.74

Retinopathy (Continued)
  proliferative 362.29
    diabetic 250.5● [362.02]
      due to secondary diabetes 249.5●
        [362.02]
    sickle-cell 282.60 [362.29]
  solar 363.31
Retinoschisis 361.10
  bullous 361.12
  congenital 743.56
  flat 361.11
  juvenile 362.73
Retractile testis 752.52
Retraction
  cervix see Retraction, uterus
  drum (membrane) 384.82
  eyelid 374.41
  finger 736.29
  head 781.0
  lid 374.41
  lung 518.89
  mediastinum 519.3
  nipple 611.79
    congenital 757.6
    puerperal, postpartum 676.0●
  palmar fascia 728.6
  pleura (see also Pleurisy) 511.0
  ring, uterus (Bandl's) (pathological) 661.4●
    affecting fetus or newborn 763.7
  sternum (congenital) 756.3
    acquired 738.3
    during respiration 786.9
  substernal 738.3
  supraclavicular 738.8
  syndrome (Duane's) 378.71
  uterus 621.6
  valve (heart) - see Endocarditis
Retrobulbar - see condition
Retrocaval ureter 753.4
Retrocecal - see also condition
  appendix (congenital) 751.5
Retrocession - see Retroversion
Retrodisplacement - see Retroversion
Retroflection, retroflexion - see Retroversion
Retrognathia, retrognathism (mandibular)
    (maxillary) 524.10
Retrograde
  ejaculation 608.87
  menstruation 626.8
Retroiliac ureter 753.4
Retroperineal - see condition
Retroperitoneal - see condition
Retroperitonitis 567.39
Retropharyngeal - see condition
Retroplacental - see condition
Retroposition - see Retroversion
Retroprosthetic membrane 996.51
Retrosternal thyroid (congenital) 759.2
Retroversion, retroverted
  cervix - see Retroversion, uterus
  female NEC (see also Retroversion, uterus)
    621.6
  iris 364.70
  testis (congenital) 752.51
  uterus, uterine (acquired) (acute) (adherent)
    (any degree) (asymptomatic) (cervix)
    (postinfectional) (postpartal, old)
    621.6
    congenital 752.39
    in pregnancy or childbirth 654.3●
      affecting fetus or newborn 763.89
      causing obstructed labor 660.2●
        affecting fetus or newborn 763.1
Retrusion, premaxilla (developmental)
    524.04
Rett's syndrome 330.8
Reverse, reversed
  peristalsis 787.4
Reye's syndrome 331.81
Reye-Sheehan syndrome (postpartum pituitary
    necrosis) 253.2

Rh antigen (C) (c) (D) (E) (e) (factor)
  hemolytic disease 773.0
  incompatibility, immunization, or
    sensitization
    affecting management of pregnancy
      656.1●
    fetus or newborn 773.0
    transfusion reaction (see also
      Complications, transfusion) 999.70
  negative mother, affecting fetus or newborn
    773.0
  titer elevated (see also Complications,
    transfusion) 999.70
  transfusion reaction (see also Complications,
    transfusion) 999.70
Rhabdomyolysis (idiopathic) 728.88
Rhabdomyoma (M8900/0) - see also Neoplasm,
    connective tissue, benign
  adult (M8904/0) - see Neoplasm, connective
    tissue, benign
  fetal (M8903/0) - see Neoplasm, connective
    tissue, benign
  glycogenic (M8904/0) - see Neoplasm,
    connective tissue, benign
Rhabdomyosarcoma (M8900/3) - see also
    Neoplasm, connective tissue, malignant
  alveolar (M8920/3) - see Neoplasm,
    connective tissue, malignant
  embryonal (M8910/3) - see Neoplasm,
    connective tissue, malignant
  mixed type (M8902/3) - see Neoplasm,
    connective tissue, malignant
  pleomorphic (M8901/3) - see Neoplasm,
    connective tissue, malignant
Rhabdosarcoma (M8900/3) - see
    Rhabdomyosarcoma
Rhesus (factor) (Rh) incompatibility - see Rh,
    incompatibility
Rheumaticosis - see Rheumatism
Rheumatism, rheumatic (acute NEC) 729.0
  adherent pericardium 393
  arthritis
    acute or subacute - see Fever, rheumatic
    chronic 714.0
      spine 720.0
  articular (chronic) NEC (see also Arthritis)
    716.9●
    acute or subacute - see Fever, rheumatic
  back 724.9
  blennorrhagic 098.59
  carditis - see Disease, heart, rheumatic
  cerebral - see Fever, rheumatic
  chorea (acute) - see Chorea, rheumatic
  chronic NEC 729.0
  coronary arteritis 391.9
    chronic 398.99
  degeneration, myocardium (see also
    Degeneration, myocardium, with
    rheumatic fever) 398.0
  desert 114.0
  febrile - see Fever, rheumatic
  fever - see Fever, rheumatic
  gonococcal 098.59
  gout 714.0
  heart
    disease (see also Disease, heart, rheumatic)
      398.90
    failure (chronic) (congestive) (inactive)
      398.91
  hemopericardium - see Rheumatic,
    pericarditis
  hydropericardium - see Rheumatic,
    pericarditis
  inflammatory (acute) (chronic) (subacute) -
    see Fever, rheumatic
  intercostal 729.0
    meaning Tietze's disease 733.6
  joint (chronic) NEC (see also Arthritis) 716.9●
    acute - see Fever, rheumatic
  mediastinopericarditis - see Rheumatic,
    pericarditis

Rheumatism, rheumatic (Continued)
  muscular 729.0
  myocardial degeneration (see also
      Degeneration, myocardium, with
      rheumatic fever) 398.0
  myocarditis (chronic) (inactive) (with chorea)
      398.0
    active or acute 391.2
      with chorea (acute) (rheumatic)
          (Sydenham's) 392.0
  myositis 729.1
  neck 724.9
  neuralgic 729.0
  neuritis (acute) (chronic) 729.2
  neuromuscular 729.0
  nodose - see Arthritis, nodosa
  nonarticular 729.0
  palindromic 719.30
    ankle 719.37
    elbow 719.32
    foot 719.37
    hand 719.34
    hip 719.35
    knee 719.36
    multiple sites 719.39
    pelvic region 719.35
    shoulder (region) 719.31
    specified site NEC 719.38
    wrist 719.33
  pancarditis, acute 391.8
    with chorea (acute) (rheumatic)
        (Sydenham's) 392.0
    chronic or inactive 398.99
  pericarditis (active) (acute) (with effusion)
      (with pneumonia) 391.0
    with chorea (acute) (rheumatic)
        (Sydenham's) 392.0
    chronic or inactive 393
  pericardium - see Rheumatic, pericarditis
  pleuropericarditis - see Rheumatic,
      pericarditis
  pneumonia 390 [517.1]
  pneumonitis 390 [517.1]
  pneumopericarditis - see Rheumatic,
      pericarditis
  polyarthritis
    acute or subacute - see Fever, rheumatic
    chronic 714.0
  polyarticular NEC (see also Arthritis) 716.9●
  psychogenic 306.0
  radiculitis 729.2
  sciatic 724.3
  septic - see Fever, rheumatic
  spine 724.9
  subacute NEC 729.0
  torticollis 723.5
  tuberculous NEC (see also Tuberculosis) 015.9●
  typhoid fever 002.0
Rheumatoid - see also condition
  lungs 714.81
Rhinitis (atrophic) (catarrhal) (chronic)
    (croupous) (fibrinous) (hyperplastic)
    (hypertrophic) (membranous) (purulent)
    (suppurative) (ulcerative) 472.0
  with
    hay fever (see also Fever, hay) 477.9
      with asthma (bronchial) 493.0●
    sore throat - see Nasopharyngitis
  acute 460
  allergic (nonseasonal) (seasonal) (see also
      Fever, hay) 477.9
    with asthma (see also Asthma) 493.0●
    due to food 477.1
  granulomatous 472.0
  infective 460
  obstructive 472.0
  pneumococcal 460
  syphilitic 095.8
    congenital 090.0
  tuberculous (see also Tuberculosis) 012.8●
  vasomotor (see also Fever, hay) 477.9

Rhinoantritis (chronic) 473.0
  acute 461.0
Rhinodacryolith 375.57
Rhinolalia (aperta) (clausa) (open) 784.43
Rhinolith 478.19
  nasal sinus (see also Sinusitis) 473.9
Rhinomegaly 478.19
Rhinopharyngitis (acute) (subacute) (see also
    Nasopharyngitis) 460
  chronic 472.2
  destructive ulcerating 102.5
  mutilans 102.5
Rhinophyma 695.3
Rhinorrhea 478.19
  cerebrospinal (fluid) 349.81
  paroxysmal (see also Fever, hay) 477.9
  spasmodic (see also Fever, hay) 477.9
Rhinosalpingitis 381.50
  acute 381.51
  chronic 381.52
Rhinoscleroma 040.1
Rhinosporidiosis 117.0
Rhinovirus infection 079.3
Rhizomelic chrondrodysplasia punctata
    277.86
Rhizomelique, pseudopolyarthritic 446.5
Rhoads and Bomford anemia (refractory)
    238.72
Rhus
  diversiloba dermatitis 692.6
  radicans dermatitis 692.6
  toxicodendron dermatitis 692.6
  venenata dermatitis 692.6
  verniciflua dermatitis 692.6
Rhythm
  atrioventricular nodal 427.89
  disorder 427.9
    coronary sinus 427.89
    ectopic 427.89
    nodal 427.89
  escape 427.89
  heart, abnormal 427.9
    fetus or newborn - see Abnormal, heart
        rate
  idioventricular 426.89
    accelerated 427.89
  nodal 427.89
  sleep, inversion 327.39
    nonorganic origin 307.45
Rhytidosis facialis 701.8
Rib - see also condition
  cervical 756.2
Riboflavin deficiency 266.0
Rice bodies (see also Loose, body, joint) 718.1●
  knee 717.6
Richter's hernia - see Hernia, Richter's
Ricinism 988.2
Rickets (active) (acute) (adolescent) (adult)
    (chest wall) (congenital) (current)
    (infantile) (intestinal) 268.0
  celiac 579.0
  fetal 756.4
  hemorrhagic 267
  hypophosphatemic with nephrotic-
      glycosuric dwarfism 270.0
  kidney 588.0
  late effect 268.1
  renal 588.0
  scurvy 267
  vitamin D-resistant 275.3
Rickettsial disease 083.9
  specified type NEC 083.8
Rickettsialpox 083.2
Rickettsiosis NEC 083.9
  specified type NEC 083.8
  tick-borne 082.9
    specified type NEC 082.8
  vesicular 083.2
Ricord's chancre 091.0
Riddoch's syndrome (visual disorientation)
    368.16

Rider's
  bone 733.99
  chancre 091.0
Ridge, alveolus - see also condition
  edentulous
    atrophy 525.20
      mandible 525.20
        minimal 525.21
        moderate 525.22
        severe 525.23
      maxilla 525.20
        minimal 525.24
        moderate 525.25
        severe 525.26
    flabby 525.20
Ridged ear 744.29
Riedel's
  disease (ligneous thyroiditis) 245.3
  lobe, liver 751.69
  struma (ligneous thyroiditis) 245.3
  thyroiditis (ligneous) 245.3
Rieger's anomaly or syndrome (mesodermal
    dysgenesis, anterior ocular segment)
    743.44
Riehl's melanosis 709.09
Rietti-Greppi-Micheli anemia or syndrome
    282.46
Rieux's hernia - see Hernia, Rieux's
Rift Valley fever 066.3
Riga's disease (cachectic aphthae) 529.0
Riga-Fede disease (cachectic aphthae) 529.0
Riggs' disease (compound periodontitis) 523.40
Right middle lobe syndrome 518.0
Rigid, rigidity - see also condition
  abdominal 789.4●
  articular, multiple congenital 754.89
  back 724.8
  cervix uteri
    in pregnancy or childbirth 654.6●
      affecting fetus or newborn 763.89
      causing obstructed labor 660.2●
        affecting fetus or newborn 763.1
  hymen (acquired) (congenital) 623.3
  nuchal 781.6
  pelvic floor
    in pregnancy or childbirth 654.4●
      affecting fetus or newborn 763.89
      causing obstructed labor 660.2●
        affecting fetus or newborn 763.1
  perineum or vulva
    in pregnancy or childbirth 654.8●
      affecting fetus or newborn 763.89
      causing obstructed labor 660.2●
        affecting fetus or newborn 763.1
  spine 724.8
  vagina
    in pregnancy or childbirth 654.7●
      affecting fetus or newborn 763.89
      causing obstructed labor 660.2●
        affecting fetus or newborn 763.1
Rigors 780.99
Riley-Day syndrome (familial dysautonomia)
    742.8
RIND (reversible ischemic neurological deficit)
    434.91
  history of (personal) V12.54
Ring(s)
  aorta 747.21
  Bandl's, complicating delivery 661.4●
    affecting fetus or newborn 763.7
  contraction, complicating delivery 661.4●
    affecting fetus or newborn 763.7
  esophageal (congenital) 750.3
  Fleischer (-Kayser) (cornea) 275.1 [371.14]
  hymenal, tight (acquired) (congenital) 623.3
  Kayser-Fleischer (cornea) 275.1 [371.14]
  retraction, uterus, pathological 661.4●
    affecting fetus or newborn 763.7
  Schatzki's (esophagus) (congenital) (lower)
      750.3
    acquired 530.3

◀ New   ◀▬ Revised   ~~deleted~~ Deleted   ● Use Additional Digit(s)   ▭ Omit code

Ring(s) (Continued)
    Soemmering's 366.51
    trachea, abnormal 748.3
    vascular (congenital) 747.21
    Vossius' 921.3
        late effect 366.21
Ringed hair (congenital) 757.4
Ringing in the ear (see also Tinnitus) 388.30
Ringworm 110.9
    beard 110.0
    body 110.5
    Burmese 110.9
    corporeal 110.5
    foot 110.4
    groin 110.3
    hand 110.2
    honeycomb 110.0
    nails 110.1
    perianal (area) 110.3
    scalp 110.0
    specified site NEC 110.8
    Tokelau 110.5
Rise, venous pressure 459.89
Risk
    factor - see Problem
    falling V15.88
    suicidal 300.9
Ritter's disease (dermatitis exfoliativa
    neonatorum) 695.81
Rivalry, sibling 313.3
Rivalta's disease (cervicofacial actinomycosis)
    039.3
River blindness 125.3 [360.13]
Robert's pelvis 755.69
    with disproportion (fetopelvic) 653.0●
        affecting fetus or newborn 763.1
        causing obstructed labor 660.1●
            affecting fetus or newborn 763.1
Robin's syndrome 756.0
Robinson's (hidrotic) ectodermal dysplasia
    757.31
Robles' disease (onchocerciasis) 125.3 [360.13]
Rochalimea - see Rickettsial disease
Rocky Mountain fever (spotted) 082.0
Rodent ulcer (M8090/3) - see also Neoplasm,
    skin, malignant
    cornea 370.07
Roentgen ray, adverse effect - see Effect,
    adverse, x-ray
Roetheln 056.9
Roger's disease (congenital interventricular
    septal defect) 745.4
Rokitansky's
    disease (see also Necrosis, liver) 570
    tumor 620.2
Rokitansky-Aschoff sinuses (mucosal
    outpouching of gallbladder) (see also
    Disease, gallbladder) 575.8
Rokitansky-Kuster-Hauser syndrome
    (congenital absence vagina) 752.45
Rollet's chancre (syphilitic) 091.0
Rolling of head 781.0
Romano-Ward syndrome (prolonged QT
    interval syndrome) 426.82
Romanus lesion 720.1
Romberg's disease or syndrome 349.89
Roof, mouth - see condition
Rosacea 695.3
    acne 695.3
    keratitis 695.3 [370.49]
Rosary, rachitic 268.0
Rose
    cold 477.0
    fever 477.0
    rash 782.1
        epidemic 056.9
        of infants 057.8
Rosen-Castleman-Liebow syndrome
    (pulmonary proteinosis) 516.0
Rosenbach's erysipelatoid or erysipeloid 027.1
Rosenthal's disease (factor XI deficiency) 286.2

Roseola 057.8
    infantum, infantilis (see also Exanthem
        subitum) 058.10
Rossbach's disease (hyperchlorhydria) 536.8
    psychogenic 306.4
Rossle-Urbach-Wiethe lipoproteinosis 272.8
Ross river fever 066.3
Rostan's asthma (cardiac) (see also Failure,
    ventricular, left) 428.1
Rot
    Barcoo (see also Ulcer, skin) 707.9
    knife-grinders' (see also Tuberculosis) 011.4●
Rot-Bernhardt disease 355.1
Rotation
    anomalous, incomplete or insufficient - see
        Malrotation
    cecum (congenital) 751.4
    colon (congenital) 751.4
    manual, affecting fetus or newborn 763.89
    spine, incomplete or insufficient 737.8
    tooth, teeth 524.35
    vertebra, incomplete or insufficient 737.8
Röteln 056.9
Roth's disease or meralgia 355.1
Roth-Bernhardt disease or syndrome 355.1
Rothmund (-Thomson) syndrome 757.33
Rotor's disease or syndrome (idiopathic
    hyperbilirubinemia) 277.4
Rotundum ulcus - see Ulcer, stomach
Round
    back (with wedging of vertebrae) 737.10
        late effect of rickets 268.1
    hole, retina 361.31
        with detachment 361.01
    ulcer (stomach) - see Ulcer, stomach
    worms (infestation) (large) NEC 127.0
Roussy-Lévy syndrome 334.3
Routine postpartum follow-up V24.2
Roy (-Jutras) syndrome (acropachyderma) 757.39
Rubella (German measles) 056.9
    complicating pregnancy, childbirth, or
        puerperium 647.5●
    complication 056.8
        neurological 056.00
            encephalomyelitis 056.01
            specified type NEC 056.09
        specified type NEC 056.79
    congenital 771.0
    contact V01.4
    exposure to V01.4
    maternal
        with suspected fetal damage affecting
            management of pregnancy 655.3●
        affecting fetus or newborn 760.2
        manifest rubella in infant 771.0
    specified complications NEC 056.79
    vaccination, prophylactic (against) V04.3
Rubeola (measles) (see also Measles) 055.9
    complicated 055.8
    meaning rubella (see also Rubella) 056.9
    scarlatinosis 057.8
Rubeosis iridis 364.42
    diabetica 250.5● [364.42]
    due to secondary diabetes 249.5● [364.42]
Rubinstein-Taybi's syndrome (brachydactylia,
    short stature and intellectual disabilities)
    759.89
Rud's syndrome (mental deficiency, epilepsy,
    and infantilism) 759.89
Rudimentary (congenital) - see also Agenesis
    arm 755.22
    bone 756.9
    cervix uteri 752.43
    eye (see also Microphthalmos) 743.10
    fallopian tube 752.19
    leg 755.32
    lobule of ear 744.21
    patella 755.64
    respiratory organs in thoracopagus 759.4
    tracheal bronchus 748.3
    uterine horn 752.39

Rudimentary (Continued)
    uterus 752.39
        in male 752.7
        solid or with cavity 752.39
    vagina 752.45
Ruiter-Pompen (-Wyers) syndrome
    (angiokeratoma corporis diffusum) 272.7
Ruled out condition (see also Observation,
    suspected) V71.9
Rumination - see also Vomiting
    disorder 307.53
    neurotic 300.3
    obsessional 300.3
    psychogenic 307.53
Runaway reaction - see also Disturbance,
    conduct
    socialized 312.2●
    undersocialized, unsocialized 312.1●
Runeberg's disease (progressive pernicious
    anemia) 281.0
Runge's syndrome (postmaturity) 766.22
Runny nose 784.99
Rupia 091.3
    congenital 090.0
    tertiary 095.9
Rupture, ruptured 553.9
    abdominal viscera NEC 799.89
        obstetrical trauma 665.5●
    abscess (spontaneous) - see Abscess, by site
    amnion - see Rupture, membranes
    aneurysm - see Aneurysm
    anus (sphincter) - see Laceration, anus
    aorta, aortic 441.5
        abdominal 441.3
        arch 441.1
        ascending 441.1
        descending 441.5
            abdominal 441.3
            thoracic 441.1
        syphilitic 093.0
        thoracoabdominal 441.6
        thorax, thoracic 441.1
        transverse 441.1
        traumatic (thoracic) 901.0
            abdominal 902.0
        valve or cusp (see also Endocarditis, aortic)
            424.1
    appendix (with peritonitis) 540.0
        with peritoneal abscess 540.1
        traumatic - see Injury, internal,
            gastrointestinal tract
    arteriovenous fistula, brain (congenital) 430
    artery 447.2
        brain (see also Hemorrhage, brain) 431
        coronary (see also Infarct, myocardium)
            410.9●
        heart (see also Infarct, myocardium)
            410.9●
        pulmonary 417.8
        traumatic (complication) (see also Injury,
            blood vessel, by site) 904.9
    bile duct, except cystic (see also Disease,
        biliary) 576.3
        cystic 575.4
        traumatic - see Injury, internal, intra-
            abdominal
    bladder (sphincter) 596.6
        with
            abortion - see Abortion, by type, with
                damage to pelvic organs
            ectopic pregnancy (see also categories
                633.0–633.9) 639.2
            molar pregnancy (see also categories
                630–632) 639.2
        following
            abortion 639.2
            ectopic or molar pregnancy 639.2
        nontraumatic 596.6
        obstetrical trauma 665.5●
        spontaneous 596.6
        traumatic - see Injury, internal, bladder

Rupture, ruptured *(Continued)*
  blood vessel *(see also* Hemorrhage) 459.0
    brain *(see also* Hemorrhage, brain) 431
    heart *(see also* Infarct, myocardium)
        410.9●
    traumatic (complication) *(see also* Injury,
        blood vessel, by site) 904.9
  bone - *see* Fracture, by site
  bowel 569.89
    traumatic - *see* Injury, internal, intestine
  Bowman's membrane 371.31
  brain
    aneurysm (congenital) *(see also*
        Hemorrhage, subarachnoid) 430
      late effect - *see* Late effect(s) (of)
          cerebrovascular disease
      syphilitic 094.87
    hemorrhagic *(see also* Hemorrhage, brain)
        431
    injury at birth 767.0
    syphilitic 094.89
  capillaries 448.9
  cardiac *(see also* Infarct, myocardium) 410.9●
  cartilage (articular) (current) - *see also* Sprain,
      by site
    knee - *see* Tear, meniscus
    semilunar - *see* Tear, meniscus
  cecum (with peritonitis) 540.0
    with peritoneal abscess 540.1
    traumatic 863.89
      with open wound into cavity 863.99
  cerebral aneurysm (congenital) *(see also*
      Hemorrhage, subarachnoid) 430
    late effect - *see* Late effect(s) (of)
        cerebrovascular disease
  cervix (uteri)
    with
      abortion - *see* Abortion, by type, with
          damage to pelvic organs
      ectopic pregnancy *(see also* categories
          633.0–633.9) 639.2
      molar pregnancy *(see also* categories
          630–632) 639.2
    following
      abortion 639.2
      ectopic or molar pregnancy 639.2
    obstetrical trauma 665.3●
    traumatic - *see* Injury, internal, cervix
  chordae tendineae 429.5
  choroid (direct) (indirect) (traumatic)
      363.63
  circle of Willis *(see also* Hemorrhage,
      subarachnoid) 430
    late effect - *see* Late effect(s) (of)
        cerebrovascular disease
  colon 569.89
    traumatic - *see* Injury, internal, colon
  cornea (traumatic) - *see also* Rupture, eye
    due to ulcer 370.00
  coronary (artery) (thrombotic) *(see also*
      Infarct, myocardium) 410.9●
  corpus luteum (infected) (ovary) 620.1
  cyst - *see* Cyst
  cystic duct *(see also* Disease, gallbladder)
      575.4
  Descemet's membrane 371.33
    traumatic - *see* Rupture, eye
  diaphragm - *see also* Hernia, diaphragm
    traumatic - *see* Injury, internal, diaphragm
  diverticulum
    bladder 596.3
    intestine (large) *(see also* Diverticula)
        562.10
      small 562.00
  duodenal stump 537.89
  duodenum (ulcer) - *see* Ulcer, duodenum,
      with perforation
  ear drum *(see also* Perforation, tympanum)
      384.20
    with otitis media - *see* Otitis media
    traumatic - *see* Wound, open, ear

Rupture, ruptured *(Continued)*
  esophagus 530.4
    traumatic 862.22
      with open wound into cavity 862.32
      cervical region - *see* Wound, open,
          esophagus
  eye (without prolapse of intraocular tissue)
      871.0
    with
      exposure of intraocular tissue 871.1
      partial loss of intraocular tissue 871.2
      prolapse of intraocular tissue 871.1
    due to burn 940.5
  fallopian tube 620.8
    due to pregnancy - *see* Pregnancy, tubal
    traumatic - *see* Injury, internal, fallopian
        tube
  fontanel 767.3
  free wall (ventricle) *(see also* Infarct,
      myocardium) 410.9●
  gallbladder or duct *(see also* Disease,
      gallbladder) 575.4
    traumatic - *see* Injury, internal, gallbladder
  gastric *(see also* Rupture, stomach) 537.89
    vessel 459.0
  globe (eye) (traumatic) - *see* Rupture, eye
  graafian follicle (hematoma) 620.0
  heart (auricle) (ventricle) *(see also* Infarct,
      myocardium) 410.9●
    infectional 422.90
    traumatic - *see* Rupture, myocardium,
        traumatic
  hymen 623.8
  internal
    organ, traumatic - *see also* Injury, internal,
        by site
      heart - *see* Rupture, myocardium,
          traumatic
      kidney - *see* Rupture, kidney
      liver - *see* Rupture, liver
      spleen - *see* Rupture, spleen, traumatic
    semilunar cartilage - *see* Tear, meniscus
  intervertebral disc - *see* Displacement,
      intervertebral disc
    traumatic (current) - *see* Dislocation,
        vertebra
  intestine 569.89
    traumatic - *see* Injury, internal, intestine
  intracranial, birth injury 767.0
  iris 364.76
    traumatic - *see* Rupture, eye
  joint capsule - *see* Sprain, by site
  kidney (traumatic) 866.03
    with open wound into cavity 866.13
    due to birth injury 767.8
    nontraumatic 593.89
  lacrimal apparatus (traumatic) 870.2
  lens (traumatic) 366.20
  ligament - *see also* Sprain, by site
    with open wound - *see* Wound, open, by
        site
    old *(see also* Disorder, cartilage, articular)
        718.0●
  liver (traumatic) 864.04
    with open wound into cavity 864.14
    due to birth injury 767.8
    nontraumatic 573.8
  lymphatic (node) (vessel) 457.8
  marginal sinus (placental) (with
      hemorrhage) 641.2●
    affecting fetus or newborn 762.1
  meaning hernia - *see* Hernia
  membrana tympani *(see also* Perforation,
      tympanum) 384.20
    with otitis media - *see* Otitis media
    traumatic - *see* Wound, open, ear
  membranes (spontaneous)
    artificial
      delayed delivery following 658.3●
        affecting fetus or newborn 761.1
      fetus or newborn 761.1

Rupture, ruptured *(Continued)*
  membranes *(Continued)*
    delayed delivery following 658.2●
      affecting fetus or newborn 761.1
    premature (less than 24 hours prior to
        onset of labor) 658.1●
      affecting fetus or newborn 761.1
      delayed delivery following 658.2●
        affecting fetus or newborn 761.1
  meningeal artery *(see also* Hemorrhage,
      subarachnoid) 430
    late effect - *see* Late effect(s) (of)
        cerebrovascular disease
  meniscus (knee) - *see also* Tear, meniscus
    old *(see also* Derangement, meniscus)
        717.5
    site other than knee - *see* Disorder,
        cartilage, articular
    site other than knee - *see* Sprain, by site
  mesentery 568.89
    traumatic - *see* Injury, internal, mesentery
  mitral - *see* Insufficiency, mitral
  muscle (traumatic) NEC - *see also* Sprain, by
      site
    with open wound - *see* Wound, open, by
        site
    nontraumatic 728.83
  musculotendinous cuff (nontraumatic)
      (shoulder) 840.4
  mycotic aneurysm, causing cerebral
      hemorrhage *(see also* Hemorrhage,
      subarachnoid) 430
    late effect - *see* Late effect(s) (of)
        cerebrovascular disease
  myocardium, myocardial *(see also* Infarct,
      myocardium) 410.9●
    traumatic 861.03
      with open wound into thorax 861.13
  nontraumatic (meaning hernia) *(see also*
      Hernia, by site) 553.9
  obstructed *(see also* Hernia, by site, with
      obstruction) 552.9
    gangrenous *(see also* Hernia, by site, with
        gangrene) 551.9
  operation wound *(see also* Dehiscence) 998.32
    internal 998.31
  ovary, ovarian 620.8
    corpus luteum 620.1
    follicle (graafian) 620.0
  oviduct 620.8
    due to pregnancy - *see* Pregnancy, tubal
  pancreas 577.8
    traumatic - *see* Injury, internal, pancreas
  papillary muscle (ventricular) 429.6
  pelvic
    floor, complicating delivery 664.1●
    organ NEC - *see* Injury, pelvic, organs
  penis (traumatic) - *see* Wound, open, penis
  perineum 624.8
    during delivery *(see also* Laceration,
        perineum, complicating delivery)
        664.4●
  pharynx (nontraumatic) (spontaneous)
      478.29
  pregnant uterus (before onset of labor)
      665.0●
  prostate (traumatic) - *see* Injury, internal,
      prostate
  pulmonary
    artery 417.8
    valve (heart) *(see also* Endocarditis,
        pulmonary) 424.3
    vein 417.8
    vessel 417.8
  pupil, sphincter 364.75
  pus tube *(see also* Salpingo-oophoritis)
      614.2
  pyosalpinx *(see also* Salpingo-oophoritis)
      614.2
  rectum 569.49
    traumatic - *see* Injury, internal, rectum

◀ New   ◀▪ Revised   ~~deleted~~ Deleted   ● Use Additional Digit(s)   ▩ Omit code

Rupture, ruptured *(Continued)*
  retina, retinal (traumatic) (without detachment) 361.30
    with detachment *(see also* Detachment, retina, with retinal defect) 361.00
  rotator cuff (capsule) (traumatic) 840.4
    nontraumatic (complete) 727.61
      partial 726.13
  sclera 871.0
  semilunar cartilage, knee *(see also* Tear, meniscus) 836.2
    old *(see also* Derangement, meniscus) 717.5
  septum (cardiac) 410.8●
  sigmoid 569.89
    traumatic - *see* Injury, internal, colon, sigmoid
  sinus of Valsalva 747.29
  spinal cord - *see also* Injury, spinal, by site
    due to injury at birth 767.4
    fetus or newborn 767.4
    syphilitic 094.89
    traumatic - *see also* Injury, spinal, by site
      with fracture - *see* Fracture, vertebra, by site, with spinal cord injury
  spleen 289.59
    congenital 767.8
    due to injury at birth 767.8
    malarial 084.9
    nontraumatic 289.59
    spontaneous 289.59
    traumatic 865.04
      with open wound into cavity 865.14
  splenic vein 459.0
  stomach 537.89
    due to injury at birth 767.8
    traumatic - *see* Injury, internal, stomach
    ulcer - *see* Ulcer, stomach, with perforation
  synovium 727.50
    specified site NEC 727.59
  tendon (traumatic) - *see also* Sprain, by site
    with open wound - *see* Wound, open, by site
    Achilles 845.09
      nontraumatic 727.67
    ankle 845.09
      nontraumatic 727.68
    biceps (long bead) 840.8
      nontraumatic 727.62
    foot 845.10
      interphalangeal (joint) 845.13
      metatarsophalangeal (joint) 845.12
      nontraumatic 727.68
      specified site NEC 845.19
      tarsometatarsal (joint) 845.11
    hand 842.10
      carpometacarpal (joint) 842.11
      interphalangeal (joint) 842.13
      metacarpophalangeal (joint) 842.12

Rupture, ruptured *(Continued)*
  tendon *(Continued)*
    hand *(Continued)*
      nontraumatic 727.63
        extensors 727.63
        flexors 727.64
      specified site NEC 842.19
    nontraumatic 727.60
      specified site NEC 727.69
    patellar 844.8
      nontraumatic 727.66
    quadriceps 844.8
      nontraumatic 727.65
    rotator cuff (capsule) 840.4
      nontraumatic (complete) 727.61
        partial 726.13
    wrist 842.00
      carpal (joint) 842.01
      nontraumatic 727.63
        extensors 727.63
        flexors 727.64
      radiocarpal (joint) (ligament) 842.02
      radioulnar (joint), distal 842.09
      specified site NEC 842.09
  testis (traumatic) 878.2
    complicated 878.3
    due to syphilis 095.8
  thoracic duct 457.8
  tonsil 474.8
  traumatic
    with open wound - *see* Wound, open, by site
    aorta - *see* Rupture, aorta, traumatic
    ear drum - *see* Wound, open, ear, drum
    external site - *see* Wound, open, by site
    eye 871.2
    globe (eye) - *see* Wound, open, eyeball
    internal organ (abdomen, chest, or pelvis) - *see also* Injury, internal, by site
      heart - *see* Rupture, myocardium, traumatic
      kidney - *see* Rupture, kidney
      liver - *see* Rupture, liver
      spleen - *see* Rupture, spleen, traumatic
    ligament, muscle, or tendon - *see also* Sprain, by site
      with open wound - *see* Wound, open, by site
    meaning hernia - *see* Hernia
  tricuspid (heart) (valve) - *see* Endocarditis, tricuspid
  tube, tubal 620.8
    abscess *(see also* Salpingo-oophoritis) 614.2
    due to pregnancy - *see* Pregnancy, tubal
  tympanum, tympanic (membrane) *(see also* Perforation, tympanum) 384.20
    with otitis media - *see* Otitis media
    traumatic - *see* Wound, open, ear, drum

Rupture, ruptured *(Continued)*
  umbilical cord 663.8●
    fetus or newborn 772.0
  ureter (traumatic) *(see also* Injury, internal, ureter) 867.2
    nontraumatic 593.89
  urethra 599.84
    with
      abortion - *see* Abortion, by type, with damage to pelvic organs
      ectopic pregnancy *(see also* categories 633.0–633.9) 639.2
      molar pregnancy *(see also* categories 630–632) 639.2
    following
      abortion 639.2
      ectopic or molar pregnancy 639.2
    obstetrical trauma 665.5●
    traumatic - *see* Injury, internal urethra
  uterosacral ligament 620.8
  uterus (traumatic) - *see also* Injury, internal uterus
    affecting fetus or newborn 763.89
    during labor 665.1●
    nonpuerperal, nontraumatic 621.8
    nontraumatic 621.8
    pregnant (during labor) 665.1●
      before labor 665.0●
  vagina 878.6
    complicated 878.7
    complicating delivery - *see* Laceration, vagina, complicating delivery
  valve, valvular (heart) - *see* Endocarditis
  varicose vein - *see* Varicose, vein
  varix - *see* Varix
  vena cava 459.0
  ventricle (free wall) (left) *(see also* Infarct, myocardium) 410.9●
  vesical (urinary) 596.6
    traumatic - *see* Injury, internal, bladder
  vessel (blood) 459.0
    pulmonary 417.8
  viscus 799.89
  vulva 878.4
    complicated 878.5
    complicating delivery 664.0●
Russell's dwarf (uterine dwarfism and craniofacial dysostosis) 759.89
Russell's dysentery 004.8
Russell (-Silver) syndrome (congenital hemihypertrophy and short stature) 759.89
Russian spring-summer type encephalitis 063.0
Rust's disease (tuberculous spondylitis) 015.0● [720.81]
Rustitskii's disease (multiple myeloma) (M9730/3) 203.0●
Ruysch's disease (Hirschsprung's disease) 751.3
Rytand-Lipsitch syndrome (complete atrioventricular block) 426.0

S

Saber
 shin 090.5
 tibia 090.5
Sac, lacrimal - *see* condition
Saccharomyces infection (*see also* Candidiasis)
 112.9
Saccharopinuria 270.7
Saccular - *see* condition
Sacculation
 aorta (nonsyphilitic) (*see also* Aneurysm,
  aorta) 441.9
  ruptured 441.5
  syphilitic 093.0
 bladder 596.3
 colon 569.89
 intralaryngeal (congenital) (ventricular)
  748.3
 larynx (congenital) (ventricular) 748.3
 organ or site, congenital - *see* Distortion
 pregnant uterus, complicating delivery
  654.4●
   affecting fetus or newborn 763.1
    causing obstructed labor 660.2●
     affecting fetus or newborn 763.1
 rectosigmoid 569.89
 sigmoid 569.89
 ureter 593.89
 urethra 599.2
 vesical 596.3
Sachs (-Tay) disease (amaurotic familial idiocy)
 330.1
Sacks-Libman disease 710.0 [424.91]
Sacralgia 724.6
Sacralization
 fifth lumbar vertebra 756.15
 incomplete (vertebra) 756.15
Sacrodynia 724.6
Sacroiliac joint - *see* condition
Sacroiliitis NEC 720.2
Sacrum - *see* condition
Saddle
 back 737.8
 embolus
  abdominal aorta 444.01
  pulmonary artery 415.13
 injury - code to condition
 nose 738.0
  congenital 754.0
  due to syphilis 090.5
Sadism (sexual) 302.84
Saemisch's ulcer 370.04
Saenger's syndrome 379.46
Sago spleen 277.39
Sailors' skin 692.74
Saint
 Anthony's fire (*see also* Erysipelas) 035
 Guy's dance - *see* Chorea
 Louis-type encephalitis 062.3
 triad (*see also* Hernia, diaphragm) 553.3
 Vitus' dance - *see* Chorea
Salicylism
 correct substance properly administered
  535.4●
 overdose or wrong substance given or taken
  965.1
Salivary duct or gland - *see also* condition
 virus disease 078.5
Salivation (excessive) (*see also* Ptyalism)
 527.7
Salmonella (aertrycke) (choleraesuis)
  (enteritidis) (gallinarum) (suipestifer)
  (typhimurium) (*see also* Infection,
  Salmonella) 003.9
 arthritis 003.23
 carrier (suspected) of V02.3
 meningitis 003.21
 osteomyelitis 003.24
 pneumonia 003.22
 septicemia 003.1

Salmonella (*Continued*)
 typhosa 002.0
  carrier (suspected) of V02.1
Salmonellosis 003.0
 with pneumonia 003.22
Salpingitis (catarrhal) (fallopian tube) (nodular)
  (pseudofollicular) (purulent) (septic) (*see
  also* Salpingo-oophoritis) 614.2
 ear 381.50
  acute 381.51
  chronic 381.52
 Eustachian (tube) 381.50
  acute 381.51
  chronic 381.52
 follicularis 614.1
 gonococcal (chronic) 098.37
  acute 098.17
 interstitial, chronic 614.1
 isthmica nodosa 614.1
 old - *see* Salpingo-oophoritis, chronic
 puerperal, postpartum, childbirth 670.8●
 specific (chronic) 098.37
  acute 098.17
 tuberculous (acute) (chronic) (*see also*
  Tuberculosis) 016.6●
 venereal (chronic) 098.37
  acute 098.17
Salpingocele 620.4
Salpingo-oophoritis (catarrhal) (purulent)
  (ruptured) (septic) (suppurative) 614.2
 acute 614.0
  with
   abortion - *see* Abortion, by type, with
    sepsis
   ectopic pregnancy (*see also* categories
    633.0–633.9) 639.0
   molar pregnancy (*see also* categories
    630–632) 639.0
  following
   abortion 639.0
   ectopic or molar pregnancy 639.0
  gonococcal 098.17
  puerperal, postpartum, childbirth 670.8●
  tuberculous (*see also* Tuberculosis) 016.6●
 chronic 614.1
  gonococcal 098.37
  tuberculous (*see also* Tuberculosis) 016.6●
 complicating pregnancy 646.6●
  affecting fetus or newborn 760.8
 gonococcal (chronic) 098.37
  acute 098.17
 old - *see* Salpingo-oophoritis, chronic
 puerperal 670.8●
 specific - *see* Salpingo-oophoritis, gonococcal
 subacute (*see also* Salpingo-oophoritis, acute)
  614.0
 tuberculous (acute) (chronic) (*see also*
  Tuberculosis) 016.6●
 venereal - *see* Salpingo-oophoritis,
  gonococcal
Salpingo-ovaritis (*see also* Salpingo-oophoritis)
  614.2
Salpingoperitonitis (*see also* Salpingo-
  oophoritis) 614.2
Salt-losing
 nephritis (*see also* Disease, renal) 593.9
 syndrome (*see also* Disease, renal) 593.9
Salt-rheum (*see also* Eczema) 692.9
Salzmann's nodular dystrophy 371.46
Sampling
 chorionic villus V28.89
Sampson's cyst or tumor 617.1
Sandblasters'
 asthma 502
 lung 502
Sander's disease (paranoia) 297.1
Sandfly fever 066.0
Sandhoff's disease 330.1
Sanfilippo's syndrome
  (mucopolysaccharidosis III) 277.5
Sanger-Brown's ataxia 334.2

San Joaquin Valley fever 114.0
Sao Paulo fever or typhus 082.0
Saponification, mesenteric 567.89
Sapremia - *see* Septicemia
Sarcocele (benign)
 syphilitic 095.8
  congenital 090.5
Sarcoepiplocele (*see also* Hernia) 553.9
Sarcoepiplomphalocele (*see also* Hernia,
  umbilicus) 553.1
Sarcoid (any site) 135
 with lung involvement 135 [517.8]
 Boeck's 135
 Darier-Roussy 135
 Spiegler-Fendt 686.8
Sarcoidosis 135
 cardiac 135 [425.8]
 lung 135 [517.8]
Sarcoma (M8800/3) - *see also* Neoplasm,
  connective tissue, malignant
 alveolar soft part (M9581/3) - *see* Neoplasm,
  connective tissue, malignant
 ameloblastic (M9330/3) 170.1
  upper jaw (bone) 170.0
 botryoid (M8910/3) - *see* Neoplasm,
  connective tissue, malignant
 botryoides (M8910/3) - *see* Neoplasm,
  connective tissue, malignant
 cerebellar (M9480/3) 191.6
  circumscribed (arachnoidal) (M9471/3)
   191.6
 circumscribed (arachnoidal) cerebellar
  (M9471/3) 191.6
 clear cell, of tendons and aponeuroses
  (M9044/3) - *see* Neoplasm, connective
  tissue, malignant
 embryonal (M8991/3) - *see* Neoplasm,
  connective tissue, malignant
 endometrial (stromal) (M8930/3) 182.0
  isthmus 182.1
 endothelial (M9130/3) - *see also* Neoplasm,
  connective tissue, malignant
  bone (M9260/3) - *see* Neoplasm, bone,
   malignant
 epithelioid cell (M8804/3) - *see* Neoplasm,
  connective tissue, malignant
 Ewing's (M9260/3) - *see* Neoplasm, bone,
  malignant
 follicular dendritic cell 202.9●
 germinoblastic (diffuse) (M9632/3)
  202.8●
  follicular (M9697/3) 202.0●
 giant cell (M8802/3) - *see also* Neoplasm,
  connective tissue, malignant
  bone (M9250/3) - *see* Neoplasm, bone,
   malignant
 glomoid (M8710/3) - *see* Neoplasm,
  connective tissue, malignant
 granulocytic (M9930/3) 205.3●
 hemangioendothelial (M9130/3) - *see*
  Neoplasm, connective tissue,
  malignant
 hemorrhagic, multiple (M9140/3) - *see*
  Kaposi's, sarcoma
 Hodgkin's (M9662/3) 201.2●
 immunoblastic (M9612/3) 200.8●
 interdigitating dendritic cell 202.9●
 Kaposi's (M9140/3) - *see* Kaposi's, sarcoma
 Kupffer cell (M9124/3) 155.0
 Langerhans cell 202.9●
 leptomeningeal (M9530/3) - *see* Neoplasm,
  meninges, malignant
 lymphangioendothelial (M9170/3) - *see*
  Neoplasm, connective tissue,
  malignant
 lymphoblastic (M9630/3) 200.1●
 lymphocytic (M9620/3) 200.1●
 mast cell (M9740/3) 202.6●
 melanotic (M8720/3) - *see* Melanoma
 meningeal (M9530/3) - *see* Neoplasm,
  meninges, malignant

◀ New   ◀◀ Revised   ~~deleted~~ Deleted   ● Use Additional Digit(s)   ▨ Omit code

Sarcoma *(Continued)*
    meningothelial (M9530/3) - *see* Neoplasm, meninges, malignant
    mesenchymal (M8800/3) - *see also* Neoplasm, connective tissue, malignant
        mixed (M8990/3) - *see* Neoplasm, connective tissue, malignant
    mesothelial (M9050/3) - *see* Neoplasm, by site, malignant
    monstrocellular (M9481/3)
        specified site - *see* Neoplasm, by site, malignant
        unspecified site 191.9
    myeloid (M9930/3) 205.3●
    neurogenic (M9540/3) - *see* Neoplasm, connective tissue, malignant
    odontogenic (M9270/3) 170.1
        upper jaw (bone) 170.0
    osteoblastic (M9180/3) - *see* Neoplasm, bone, malignant
    osteogenic (M9180/3) - *see also* Neoplasm, bone, malignant
        juxtacortical (M9190/3) - *see* Neoplasm, bone, malignant
        periosteal (M9190/3) - *see* Neoplasm, bone, malignant
    periosteal (M8812/3) - *see also* Neoplasm, bone, malignant
        osteogenic (M9190/3) - *see* Neoplasm, bone, malignant
    plasma cell (M9731/3) 203.8●
    pleomorphic cell (M8802/3) - *see* Neoplasm, connective tissue, malignant
    reticuloendothelial (M9720/3) 202.3●
    reticulum cell (M9640/3) 200.0●
        nodular (M9642/3) 200.0●
        pleomorphic cell type (M9641/3) 200.0●
    round cell (M8803/3) - *see* Neoplasm, connective tissue, malignant
    small cell (M8803/3) - *see* Neoplasm, connective tissue, malignant
    spindle cell (M8801/3) - *see* Neoplasm, connective tissue, malignant
    stromal (endometrial) (M8930/3) 182.0
        isthmus 182.1
    synovial (M9040/3) - *see also* Neoplasm, connective tissue, malignant
        biphasic type (M9043/3) - *see* Neoplasm, connective tissue, malignant
        epithelioid cell type (M9042/3) - *see* Neoplasm, connective tissue, malignant
        spindle cell type (M9041/3) - *see* Neoplasm, connective tissue, malignant
Sarcomatosis
    meningeal (M9539/3) - *see* Neoplasm, meninges, malignant
    specified site NEC (M8800/3) - *see* Neoplasm, connective tissue, malignant
    unspecified site (M8800/6) 171.9
Sarcosinemia 270.8
Sarcosporidiosis 136.5
Satiety, early 780.94
Satisfactory smear but lacking transformation zone
    anal 796.77
    cervical 795.07
Saturnine - *see* condition
Saturnism 984.9
    specified type of lead - *see* Table of Drugs and Chemicals
Satyriasis 302.89
Sauriasis - *see* Ichthyosis
Sauriderma 757.39
Sauriosis - *see* Ichthyosis
Savill's disease (epidemic exfoliative dermatitis) 695.89
SBE (subacute bacterial endocarditis) 421.0

Scabies (any site) 133.0
Scabs 782.8
Scaglietti-Dagnini syndrome (acromegalic macrospondylitis) 253.0
Scald, scalded - *see also* Burn, by site
    skin syndrome 695.81
Scalenus anticus (anterior) syndrome 353.0
Scales 782.8
Scalp - *see* condition
Scaphocephaly 756.0
Scaphoiditis, tarsal 732.5
Scapulalgia 733.90
Scapulohumeral myopathy 359.1
Scar, scarring (*see also* Cicatrix) 709.2
    adherent 709.2
    atrophic 709.2
    cervix
        in pregnancy or childbirth 654.6●
            affecting fetus or newborn 763.89
            causing obstructed labor 660.2●
                affecting fetus or newborn 763.1
    cheloid 701.4
    chorioretinal 363.30
        disseminated 363.35
        macular 363.32
        peripheral 363.34
        posterior pole NEC 363.33
    choroid (*see also* Scar, chorioretinal) 363.30
    compression, pericardial 423.9
    congenital 757.39
    conjunctiva 372.64
    cornea 371.00
        xerophthalmic 264.6
    due to previous cesarean delivery, complicating pregnancy or childbirth 654.2●
        affecting fetus or newborn 763.89
    duodenal (bulb) (cap) 537.3
    hypertrophic 701.4
    keloid 701.4
    labia 624.4
    lung (base) 518.89
    macula 363.32
        disseminated 363.35
        peripheral 363.34
    muscle 728.89
    myocardium, myocardial 412
    painful 709.2
    papillary muscle 429.81
    posterior pole NEC 363.33
        macular - *see* Scar, macula
    postnecrotic (hepatic) (liver) 571.9
    psychic V15.49
    retina (*see also* Scar, chorioretinal) 363.30
    trachea 478.9
    uterus 621.8
        in pregnancy or childbirth NEC 654.9●
            affecting fetus or newborn 763.89
            from previous cesarean delivery 654.2●
    vulva 624.4
Scarabiasis 134.1
Scarlatina 034.1
    anginosa 034.1
    maligna 034.1
    myocarditis, acute 034.1 *[422.0]*
        old (*see also* Myocarditis) 429.0
    otitis media 034.1 *[382.02]*
    ulcerosa 034.1
Scarlatinella 057.8
Scarlet fever (albuminuria) (angina) (convulsions) (lesions of lid) (rash) 034.1
Schamberg's disease, dermatitis, or dermatosis (progressive pigmentary dermatosis) 709.09
Schatzki's ring (esophagus) (lower) (congenital) 750.3
    acquired 530.3
Schaufenster krankheit 413.9

Schaumann's
    benign lymphogranulomatosis 135
    disease (sarcoidosis) 135
    syndrome (sarcoidosis) 135
Scheie's syndrome (mucopolysaccharidosis IS) 277.5
Schenck's disease (sporotrichosis) 117.1
Scheuermann's disease or osteochondrosis 732.0
Scheuthauer-Marie-Sainton syndrome (cleidocranialis dysostosis) 755.59
Schilder (-Flatau) disease 341.1
Schilling-type monocytic leukemia (M9890/3) 206.9●
Schimmelbusch's disease, cystic mastitis, or hyperplasia 610.1
Schirmer's syndrome (encephalocutaneous angiomatosis) 759.6
Schistocelia 756.79
Schistoglossia 750.13
Schistosoma infestation - *see* Infestation, Schistosoma
Schistosomiasis 120.9
    Asiatic 120.2
    bladder 120.0
    chestermani 120.8
    colon 120.1
    cutaneous 120.3
    due to
        S. hematobium 120.0
        S. japonicum 120.2
        S. mansoni 120.1
        S. mattheii 120.8
    eastern 120.2
    genitourinary tract 120.0
    intestinal 120.1
    lung 120.2
    Manson's (intestinal) 120.1
    Oriental 120.2
    pulmonary 120.2
    specified type NEC 120.8
    vesical 120.0
Schizencephaly 742.4
Schizo-affective psychosis (*see also* Schizophrenia) 295.7●
Schizodontia 520.2
Schizoid personality 301.20
    introverted 301.21
    schizotypal 301.22
Schizophrenia, schizophrenic (reaction) 295.9●

> Note: Use the following fifth-digit subclassification with category 295:
>
> 0   unspecified
> 1   subchronic
> 2   chronic
> 3   subchronic with acute exacerbation
> 4   chronic with acute exacerbation
> 5   in remission

    acute (attack) NEC 295.8●
        episode 295.4●
    atypical form 295.8●
    borderline 295.5●
    catalepsy 295.2●
    catatonic (type) (acute) (excited) (withdrawn) 295.2●
    childhood (type) (*see also* Psychosis, childhood) 299.9●
    chronic NEC 295.6●
    coenesthesiopathic 295.8●
    cyclic (type) 295.7●
    disorganized (type) 295.1●
    flexibilitas cerea 295.2●
    hebephrenic (type) (acute) 295.1●
    incipient 295.5●
    latent 295.5●
    paranoid (type) (acute) 295.3●
    paraphrenic (acute) 295.3●
    prepsychotic 295.5●
    primary (acute) 295.0●

Schizophrenia, schizophrenic (Continued)
  prodromal 295.5 ●
  pseudoneurotic 295.5 ●
  pseudopsychopathic 295.5 ●
  reaction 295.9 ●
  residual type (state) 295.6 ●
  restzustand 295.6 ●
  schizo-affective (type) (depressed) (excited)
      295.7 ●
  schizophreniform type 295.4 ●
  simple (type) (acute) 295.0 ●
  simplex (acute) 295.0 ●
  specified type NEC 295.8 ●
  syndrome of childhood NEC (see also
      Psychosis, childhood) 299.9 ●
  undifferentiated type 295.9 ●
    acute 295.8 ●
    chronic 295.6 ●
Schizothymia 301.20
  introverted 301.21
  schizotypal 301.22
Schlafkrankheit 086.5
Schlatter's tibia (osteochondrosis) 732.4
Schlatter-Osgood disease (osteochondrosis,
    tibial tubercle) 732.4
Schloffer's tumor (see also Peritonitis) 567.29
Schmidt's syndrome
  sphallo-pharyngo-laryngeal hemiplegia
      352.6
  thyroid-adrenocortical insufficiency 258.1
  vagoaccessory 352.6
Schmincke
  carcinoma (M8082/3) - see Neoplasm,
      nasopharynx, malignant
  tumor (M8082/3) - see Neoplasm,
      nasopharynx, malignant
Schmitz (-Stutzer) dysentery 004.0
Schmorl's disease or nodes 722.30
  lumbar, lumbosacral 722.32
  specified region NEC 722.39
  thoracic, thoracolumbar 722.31
Schneider's syndrome 047.9
Schneiderian
  carcinoma (M8121/3)
    specified site - see Neoplasm, by site,
        malignant
    unspecified site 160.0
  papilloma (M8121/0)
    specified site - see Neoplasm, by site,
        benign
    unspecified site 212.0
Schnitzler syndrome 273.1
Schoffer's tumor (see also Peritonitis) 567.29
Scholte's syndrome (malignant carcinoid) 259.2
Scholz's disease 330.0
Scholz (-Bielschowsky-Henneberg) syndrome
    330.0
Schönlein (-Henoch) disease (primary)
    (purpura) (rheumatic) 287.0
School examination V70.3
  following surgery V67.09
Schottmüller's disease (see also Fever,
    paratyphoid) 002.9
Schroeder's syndrome (endocrine-
    hypertensive) 255.3
Schüller-Christian disease or syndrome
    (chronic histiocytosis X) 277.89
Schultz's disease or syndrome
    (agranulocytosis) 288.09
Schultze's acroparesthesia, simple 443.89
Schwalbe-Ziehen-Oppenheimer disease 333.6
Schwannoma (M9560/0) - see also Neoplasm,
    connective tissues, benign
  malignant (M9560/3) - see Neoplasm,
      connective tissue, malignant
Schwannomatosis 237.73
Schwartz (-Jampel) syndrome 359.23
Schwartz-Bartter syndrome (inappropriate
    secretion of antidiuretic hormone) 253.6
Schweninger-Buzzi disease (macular atrophy)
    701.3

Sciatic - see condition
Sciatica (infectional) 724.3
  due to
    displacement of intervertebral disc 722.10
    herniation, nucleus pulposus 722.10
  wallet 724.3
Scimitar syndrome (anomalous venous
    drainage, right lung to inferior vena cava)
    747.42
Sclera - see condition
Sclerectasia 379.11
Scleredema
  adultorum 710.1
  Buschke's 710.1
  newborn 778.1
Sclerema
  adiposum (newborn) 778.1
  adultorum 710.1
  edematosum (newborn) 778.1
  neonatorum 778.1
  newborn 778.1
Scleriasis - see Scleroderma
Scleritis 379.00
  with corneal involvement 379.05
  anterior (annular) (localized) 379.03
  brawny 379.06
  granulomatous 379.09
  posterior 379.07
  specified NEC 379.09
  suppurative 379.09
  syphilitic 095.0
  tuberculous (nodular) (see also Tuberculosis)
      017.3 ● [379.09]
Sclerochoroiditis (see also Scleritis) 379.00
Scleroconjunctivitis (see also Scleritis) 379.00
Sclerocystic ovary (syndrome) 256.4
Sclerodactylia 701.0
Scleroderma, sclerodermia (acrosclerotic)
    (diffuse) (generalized) (progressive)
    (pulmonary) 710.1
  circumscribed 701.0
  linear 701.0
  localized (linear) 701.0
  newborn 778.1
Sclerokeratitis 379.05
  meaning sclerosing keratitis 370.54
  tuberculous (see also Tuberculosis) 017.3 ●
      [379.09]
Scleroma, trachea 040.1
Scleromalacia
  multiple 731.0
  perforans 379.04
Scleromyxedema 701.8
Scleroperikeratitis 379.05
Sclerose en plaques 340
Sclerosis, sclerotic
  adrenal (gland) 255.8
  Alzheimer's 331.0
    with dementia - see Alzheimer's,
        dementia
  amyotrophic (lateral) 335.20
  annularis fibrosi
    aortic 424.1
    mitral 424.0
  aorta, aortic 440.0
    valve (see also Endocarditis, aortic) 424.1
  artery, arterial, arteriolar, arteriovascular - see
      Arteriosclerosis
  ascending multiple 340
  Baló's (concentric) 341.1
  basilar - see Sclerosis, brain
  bone (localized) NEC 733.99
  brain (general) (lobular) 348.89
    Alzheimer's - see Alzheimer's, dementia
    artery, arterial 437.0
    atrophic lobar 331.0
      with dementia
        with behavioral disturbance 331.0
            [294.11]
        without behavioral disturbance
            331.0 [294.10]

Sclerosis, sclerotic (Continued)
  brain (Continued)
    diffuse 341.1
      familial (chronic) (infantile) 330.0
      infantile (chronic) (familial) 330.0
      Pelizaeus-Merzbacher type 330.0
    disseminated 340
    hereditary 334.2
    hippocampal 348.81
    infantile (degenerative) (diffuse) 330.0
    insular 340
    Krabbe's 330.0
    mesial temporal 348.81
    miliary 340
    multiple 340
    Pelizaeus-Merzbacher 330.0
    progressive familial 330.0
    senile 437.0
    temporal 348.81
      mesial 348.81
    tuberous 759.5
  bulbar, progressive 340
  bundle of His 426.50
    left 426.3
    right 426.4
  cardiac - see Arteriosclerosis, coronary
  cardiorenal (see also Hypertension,
      cardiorenal) 404.90
  cardiovascular (see also Disease,
      cardiovascular) 429.2
    renal (see also Hypertension, cardiorenal)
        404.90
  centrolobar, familial 330.0
  cerebellar - see Sclerosis, brain
  cerebral - see Sclerosis, brain
  cerebrospinal 340
    disseminated 340
    multiple 340
  cerebrovascular 437.0
  choroid 363.40
    diffuse 363.56
  combined (spinal cord) - see also
      Degeneration, combined
    multiple 340
  concentric, Baló's 341.1
  cornea 370.54
  coronary (artery) - see Arteriosclerosis,
      coronary
  corpus cavernosum
    female 624.8
    male 607.89
  Dewitzky's
    aortic 424.1
    mitral 424.0
  diffuse NEC 341.1
  disease, heart - see Arteriosclerosis, coronary
  disseminated 340
  dorsal 340
  dorsolateral (spinal cord) - see Degeneration,
      combined
  endometrium 621.8
  extrapyramidal 333.90
  eye, nuclear (senile) 366.16
  Friedreich's (spinal cord) 334.0
  funicular (spermatic cord) 608.89
  gastritis 535.4 ●
  general (vascular) - see Arteriosclerosis
  gland (lymphatic) 457.8
  hepatic 571.9
  hereditary
    cerebellar 334.2
    spinal 334.0
  hippocampal 348.81
  idiopathic cortical (Garre's) (see also
      Osteomyelitis) 730.1 ●
  ilium, piriform 733.5
  insular 340
    pancreas 251.8
  Islands of Langerhans 251.8
  kidney - see Sclerosis, renal
  larynx 478.79

◀ New   ◀⁞⁞ Revised   ~~deleted~~ Deleted   ● Use Additional Digit(s)   ▨ Omit code

Sclerosis, sclerotic *(Continued)*
 lateral 335.24
  amyotrophic 335.20
  descending 335.24
  primary 335.24
  spinal 335.24
 liver 571.9
 lobar, atrophic (of brain) 331.0
  with dementia
   with behavioral disturbance 331.0
    [294.11]
   without behavioral disturbance 331.0
    [294.10]
 lung *(see also* Fibrosis, lung) 515
 mastoid 383.1
 mesial temporal 348.81
 mitral - *see* Endocarditis, mitral
 Mönckeberg's (medial) *(see also*
   Arteriosclerosis, extremities) 440.20
 multiple (brain stem) (cerebral) (generalized)
   (spinal cord) 340
 myocardium, myocardial - *see*
   Arteriosclerosis, coronary
 nuclear (senile), eye 366.16
 ovary 620.8
 pancreas 577.8
 penis 607.89
 peripheral arteries *(see also* Arteriosclerosis,
   extremities) 440.20
 plaques 340
 pluriglandular 258.8
 polyglandular 258.8
 posterior (spinal cord) (syphilitic) 094.0
 posterolateral (spinal cord) - *see*
   Degeneration, combined
 prepuce 607.89
 primary lateral 335.24
 progressive systemic 710.1
 pulmonary *(see also* Fibrosis, lung) 515
  artery 416.0
  valve (heart) *(see also* Endocarditis,
    pulmonary) 424.3
 renal 587
  with
   cystine storage disease 270.0
   hypertension *(see also* Hypertension,
     kidney) 403.90
   hypertensive heart disease (conditions
     classifiable to 402) *(see also*
     Hypertension, cardiorenal)
     404.90
   arteriolar (hyaline) *(see also* Hypertension,
     kidney) 403.90
   hyperplastic *(see also* Hypertension,
     kidney) 403.90
 retina (senile) (vascular) 362.17
 rheumatic
  aortic valve 395.9
  mitral valve 394.9
 Schilder's 341.1
 senile - *see* Arteriosclerosis
 spinal (cord) (general) (progressive)
   (transverse) 336.8
  ascending 357.0
  combined - *see also* Degeneration,
    combined
   multiple 340
   syphilitic 094.89
  disseminated 340
  dorsolateral - *see* Degeneration, combined
  hereditary (Friedreich's) (mixed form)
    334.0
  lateral (amyotrophic) 335.24
  multiple 340
  posterior (syphilitic) 094.0
 stomach 537.89
 subendocardial, congenital 425.3
 systemic (progressive) 710.1
  with lung involvement 710.1 *[517.2]*
 temporal 348.81
  mesial 348.81

Sclerosis, sclerotic *(Continued)*
 tricuspid (heart) (valve) - *see* Endocarditis,
   tricuspid
 tuberous (brain) 759.5
 tympanic membrane *(see also*
   Tympanosclerosis) 385.00
 valve, valvular (heart) - *see* Endocarditis
 vascular - *see* Arteriosclerosis
 vein 459.89
Sclerotenonitis 379.07
Sclerotitis *(see also* Scleritis) 379.00
 syphilitic 095.0
 tuberculous *(see also* Tuberculosis) 017.3●
   [379.09]
Scoliosis (acquired) (postural) 737.30
 congenital 754.2
 due to or associated with
  Charcôt-Marie-Tooth disease 356.1
    [737.43]
  mucopolysaccharidosis 277.5 *[737.43]*
  neurofibromatosis 237.71 *[737.43]*
  osteitis
   deformans 731.0 *[737.43]*
   fibrosa cystica 252.01 *[737.43]*
  osteoporosis *(see also* Osteoporosis) 733.00
    [737.43]
  poliomyelitis 138 *[737.43]*
  radiation 737.33
  tuberculosis *(see also* Tuberculosis) 015.0●
    [737.43]
 idiopathic 737.30
  infantile
   progressive 737.32
   resolving 737.31
 paralytic 737.39
 rachitic 268.1
 sciatic 724.3
 specified NEC 737.39
 thoracogenic 737.34
 tuberculous *(see also* Tuberculosis) 015.0●
   [737.43]
Scoliotic pelvis 738.6
 with disproportion (fetopelvic) 653.0●
  affecting fetus or newborn 763.1
  causing obstructed labor 660.1●
   affecting fetus or newborn 763.1
Scorbutus, scorbutic 267
 anemia 281.8
Scotoma (ring) 368.44
 arcuate 368.43
 Bjerrum 368.43
 blind spot area 368.42
 central 368.41
 centrocecal 368.41
 paracecal 368.42
 paracentral 368.41
 scintillating 368.12
 Seidel 368.43
Scratch - *see* Injury, superficial, by site
Scratchy throat 784.99
Screening (for) V82.9
 alcoholism V79.1
 anemia, deficiency NEC V78.1
  iron V78.0
 anomaly, congenital V82.89
 antenatal, of mother V28.9
  alphafetoprotein levels, raised V28.1
  based on amniocentesis V28.2
   chromosomal anomalies V28.0
   raised alphafetoprotein levels V28.1
  fetal growth retardation using ultrasonics
    V28.4
  genomic V28.89
  isoimmunization V28.5
  malformations using ultrasonics V28.3
  proteomic V28.89
  raised alphafetoprotein levels V28.1
  risk
   pre-term labor V28.82
  specified condition NEC V28.89
  Streptococcus B V28.6

Screening *(Continued)*
 arterial hypertension V81.1
 arthropod-borne viral disease NEC V73.5
 asymptomatic bacteriuria V81.5
 bacterial
  and spirochetal sexually transmitted
    diseases V74.5
  conjunctivitis V74.4
  disease V74.9
   sexually transmitted V74.5
   specified condition NEC V74.8
 bacteriuria, asymptomatic V81.5
 blood disorder NEC V78.9
  specified type NEC V78.8
 bronchitis, chronic V81.3
 brucellosis V74.8
 cancer - *see* Screening, malignant neoplasm
 cardiovascular disease NEC V81.2
 cataract V80.2
 Chagas' disease V75.3
 chemical poisoning V82.5
 cholera V74.0
 cholesterol level V77.91
 chromosomal
  anomalies
   by amniocentesis, antenatal V28.0
   maternal postnatal V82.4
  athletes V70.3
 colonoscopy V76.51
 condition
  cardiovascular NEC V81.2
  eye NEC V80.2
  genitourinary NEC V81.6
  neurological NEC V80.09
  respiratory NEC V81.4
  skin V82.0
  specified NEC V82.89
 congenital
  anomaly V82.89
   eye V80.2
  dislocation of hip V82.3
  eye condition or disease V80.2
 conjunctivitis, bacterial V74.4
 contamination NEC *(see also* Poisoning)
   V82.5
 coronary artery disease V81.0
 cystic fibrosis V77.6
 deficiency anemia NEC V78.1
  iron V78.0
 dengue fever V73.5
 depression V79.0
 developmental handicap V79.9
  in early childhood V79.3
  specified type NEC V79.8
 diabetes mellitus V77.1
 diphtheria V74.3
 disease or disorder V82.9
  bacterial V74.9
   specified NEC V74.8
  blood V78.9
   specified type NEC V78.8
  blood-forming organ V78.9
   specified type NEC V78.8
  cardiovascular NEC V81.2
   hypertensive V81.1
   ischemic V81.0
  Chagas' V75.3
  chlamydial V73.98
   specified NEC V73.88
  ear NEC V80.3
  endocrine NEC V77.99
  eye NEC V80.2
  genitourinary NEC V81.6
  heart NEC V81.2
   hypertensive V81.1
   ischemic V81.0
  HPV (human papillomavirus) V73.81
  human papillomavirus (HPV) V73.81
  immunity NEC V77.99
  infectious NEC V75.9
  lipoid NEC V77.91

Screening *(Continued)*
    disease or disorder *(Continued)*
        mental V79.9
            specified type NEC V79.8
        metabolic NEC V77.99
            inborn NEC V77.7
        neurological NEC V80.09
        nutritional NEC V77.99
        rheumatic NEC V82.2
        rickettsial V75.0
        sexually transmitted V74.5
            bacterial V74.5
            spirochetal V74.5
        sickle-cell V78.2
            trait V78.2
        specified type NEC V82.89
        thyroid V77.0
        vascular NEC V81.2
            ischemic V81.0
        venereal V74.5
        viral V73.99
            arthropod-borne NEC V73.5
            specified type NEC V73.89
    dislocation of hip, congenital V82.3
    drugs in athletes V70.3
    elevated titer V82.9
    emphysema (chronic) V81.3
    encephalitis, viral (mosquito or tick borne)
        V73.5
    endocrine disorder NEC V77.99
    eye disorder NEC V80.2
        congenital V80.2
    fever
        dengue V73.5
        hemorrhagic V73.5
        yellow V73.4
    filariasis V75.6
    galactosemia V77.4
    genetic V82.79
        disease carrier status V82.71
    genitourinary condition NEC V81.6
    glaucoma V80.1
    gonorrhea V74.5
    gout V77.5
    Hansen's disease V74.2
    heart disease NEC V81.2
        hypertensive V81.1
        ischemic V81.0
    heavy metal poisoning V82.5
    helminthiasis, intestinal V75.7
    hematopoietic malignancy V76.89
    hemoglobinopathies NEC V78.3
    hemorrhagic fever V73.5
    Hodgkin's disease V76.89
    hormones in athletes V70.3
    HPV (human papillomavirus) V73.81
    human papillomavirus (HPV) V73.81
    hypercholesterolemia V77.91
    hyperlipidemia V77.91
    hypertension V81.1
    immunity disorder NEC V77.99
    inborn errors of metabolism NEC V77.7
    infection
        bacterial V74.9
            specified type NEC V74.8
        mycotic V75.4
        parasitic NEC V75.8
    infectious disease V75.9
        specified type NEC V75.8
    ingestion of radioactive substance V82.5
    intellectual disabilities V79.2
    intestinal helminthiasis V75.7
    iron deficiency anemia V78.0
    ischemic heart disease V81.0
    lead poisoning V82.5
    leishmaniasis V75.2
    leprosy V74.2
    leptospirosis V74.8
    leukemia V76.89
    lipoid disorder NEC V77.91
    lymphoma V76.89

Screening *(Continued)*
    malaria V75.1
    malignant neoplasm (of) V76.9
        bladder V76.3
        blood V76.89
        breast V76.10
            mammogram NEC V76.12
                for high-risk patient V76.11
            specified type NEC V76.19
        cervix V76.2
        colon V76.51
        colorectal V76.51
        hematopoietic system V76.89
        intestine V76.50
            colon V76.51
            small V76.52
        lung V76.0
        lymph (glands) V76.89
        nervous system V76.81
        oral cavity V76.42
        other specified neoplasm NEC V76.89
        ovary V76.46
        prostate V76.44
        rectum V76.41
        respiratory organs V76.0
        skin V76.43
        specified sites NEC V76.49
        testis V76.45
        vagina V76.47
            following hysterectomy for malignant
                condition V67.01
    malnutrition V77.2
    mammogram NEC V76.12
        for high-risk patient V76.11
    maternal postnatal chromosomal anomalies
        V82.4
    measles V73.2
    mental
        disorder V79.9
            specified type NEC V79.8
        retardation - *see* Screening, intellectual
            disabilities
    metabolic disorder NEC V77.99
    metabolic errors, inborn V77.7
    mucoviscidosis V77.6
    multiphasic V82.6
    mycosis V75.4
    mycotic infection V75.4
    nephropathy V81.5
    neurological condition NEC V80.09
    nutritional disorder NEC V77.99
    obesity V77.8
    osteoporosis V82.81
    parasitic infection NEC V75.8
    phenylketonuria V77.3
    plague V74.8
    poisoning
        chemical NEC V82.5
            contaminated water supply V82.5
        heavy metal V82.5
    poliomyelitis V73.0
    postnatal chromosomal anomalies, maternal
        V82.4
    prenatal - *see* Screening, antenatal
    pulmonary tuberculosis V74.1
    radiation exposure V82.5
    renal disease V81.5
    respiratory condition NEC V81.4
    rheumatic disorder NEC V82.2
    rheumatoid arthritis V82.1
    rickettsial disease V75.0
    rubella V73.3
    schistosomiasis V75.5
    senile macular lesions of eye V80.2
    sexually transmitted diseases V74.5
        bacterial V74.5
        spirochetal V74.5
    sickle-cell anemia, disease, or trait V78.2
    skin condition V82.0
    sleeping sickness V75.3
    smallpox V73.1

Screening *(Continued)*
    special V82.9
        specified condition NEC V82.89
    specified type NEC V82.89
    spirochetal disease V74.9
        sexually transmitted V74.5
        specified type NEC V74.8
    stimulants in athletes V70.3
    syphilis V74.5
    tetanus V74.8
    thyroid disorder V77.0
    trachoma V73.6
    traumatic brain injury V80.01
    trypanosomiasis V75.3
    tuberculosis, pulmonary V74.1
    venereal disease V74.5
    viral encephalitis
        mosquito-borne V73.5
        tick-borne V73.5
    whooping cough V74.8
    worms, intestinal V75.7
    yaws V74.6
    yellow fever V73.4
Scrofula (*see also* Tuberculosis) 017.2●
Scrofulide (primary) (*see also* Tuberculosis)
    017.0●
Scrofuloderma, scrofulodermia (any site)
    (primary) (*see also* Tuberculosis)
    017.0●
Scrofulosis (universal) (*see also* Tuberculosis)
    017.2●
Scrofulosis lichen (primary) (*see also*
    Tuberculosis) 017.0●
Scrofulous - *see* condition
Scrotal tongue 529.5
    congenital 750.13
Scrotum - *see* condition
Scurvy (gum) (infantile) (rickets) (scorbutic)
    267
Sea-blue histiocyte syndrome 272.7
Seabright-Bantam syndrome
    (pseudohypoparathyroidism) 275.49
Sealpox 059.12
Seasickness 994.6
Seatworm 127.4
Sebaceous
    cyst (*see also* Cyst, sebaceous) 706.2
    gland disease NEC 706.9
Sebocystomatosis 706.2
Seborrhea, seborrheic 706.3
    adiposa 706.3
    capitis 690.11
    congestiva 695.4
    corporis 706.3
    dermatitis 690.10
        infantile 690.12
    diathesis in infants 695.89
    eczema 690.18
        infantile 690.12
    keratosis 702.19
        inflamed 702.11
    nigricans 759.89
    sicca 690.18
    wart 702.19
        inflamed 702.11
Seckel's syndrome 759.89
Seclusion pupil 364.74
Seclusiveness, child 313.22
Secondary - *see also* condition
    neoplasm - *see* Neoplasm, by site, malignant,
        secondary
Secretan's disease or syndrome (posttraumatic
    edema) 782.3
Secretion
    antidiuretic hormone, inappropriate
        (syndrome) 253.6
    catecholamine, by pheochromocytoma
        255.6
    hormone
        antidiuretic, inappropriate (syndrome)
            253.6

Secretion (*Continued*)
  hormone (*Continued*)
    by
      carcinoid tumor 259.2
      pheochromocytoma 255.6
    ectopic NEC 259.3
  urinary
    excessive 788.42
    suppression 788.5
Section
  cesarean
    affecting fetus or newborn 763.4
    post mortem, affecting fetus or newborn
      761.6
    previous, in pregnancy or childbirth
      654.2●
      affecting fetus or newborn 763.89
  nerve, traumatic - *see* Injury, nerve,
    by site
Seeligmann's syndrome (ichthyosis congenita)
  757.1
Segmentation, incomplete (congenital) - *see also*
  Fusion
  bone NEC 756.9
  lumbosacral (joint) 756.15
  vertebra 756.15
    lumbosacral 756.15
Seizure(s) 780.39
  akinetic (idiopathic) (*see also* Epilepsy)
    345.0●
    psychomotor 345.4●
  apoplexy, apoplectic (*see also* Disease,
    cerebrovascular, acute) 436
  atonic (*see also* Epilepsy) 345.0●
  autonomic 300.11
  brain or cerebral (*see also* Disease,
    cerebrovascular, acute) 436
  convulsive (*see also* Convulsions) 780.39
  cortical (focal) (motor) (*see also* Epilepsy)
    345.5●
  disorder (*see also* Epilepsy) 345.9●
  due to stroke 438.89
  epilepsy, epileptic (cryptogenic) (*see also*
    Epilepsy) 345.9●
  epileptiform, epileptoid 780.39
    focal (*see also* Epilepsy) 345.5●
  febrile (simple) 780.31
    with status epilepticus 345.3
    atypical 780.32
    complex 780.32
    complicated 780.32
  heart - *see* Disease, heart
  hysterical 300.11
  Jacksonian (focal) (*see also* Epilepsy)
    345.5●
    motor type 345.5●
    sensory type 345.5●
  migraine triggered 346.0●
  newborn 779.0
  paralysis (*see also* Disease, cerebrovascular,
    acute) 436
  post traumatic 780.33
  recurrent 345.8●
    epileptic - *see* Epilepsy
  repetitive 780.39
    epileptic - *see* Epilepsy
  salaam (*see also* Epilepsy) 345.6●
  uncinate (*see also* Epilepsy) 345.4●
Self-mutilation 300.9
Semicoma 780.09
Semiconsciousness 780.09
Seminal
  vesicle - *see* condition
  vesiculitis (*see also* Vesiculitis) 608.0
Seminoma (M9061/3)
  anaplastic type (M9062/3)
    specified site - *see* Neoplasm, by site,
      malignant
    unspecified site 186.9
  specified site - *see* Neoplasm, by site,
    malignant

Seminoma (*Continued*)
  spermatocytic (M9063/3)
    specified site - *see* Neoplasm, by site,
      malignant
    unspecified site 186.9
  unspecified site 186.9
Semliki Forest encephalitis 062.8
Senear-Usher disease or syndrome (pemphigus
  erythematosus) 694.4
Senecio jacobae dermatitis 692.6
Senectus 797
Senescence 797
Senile (*see also* condition) 797
  cervix (atrophic) 622.8
  degenerative atrophy, skin 701.3
  endometrium (atrophic) 621.8
  fallopian tube (atrophic) 620.3
  heart (failure) 797
  lung 492.8
  ovary (atrophic) 620.3
  syndrome 259.8
  vagina, vaginitis (atrophic) 627.3
  wart 702.0
Senility 797
  with
    acute confusional state 290.3
    delirium 290.3
    mental changes 290.9
    psychosis NEC (*see also* Psychosis, senile)
      290.20
  premature (syndrome) 259.8
Sensation
  burning (*see also* Disturbance, sensation)
    782.0
    tongue 529.6
  choking 784.99
  loss of (*see also* Disturbance, sensation) 782.0
  prickling (*see also* Disturbance, sensation)
    782.0
  tingling (*see also* Disturbance, sensation)
    782.0
Sense loss (touch) (*see also* Disturbance,
  sensation) 782.0
  smell 781.1
  taste 781.1
Sensibility disturbance NEC (cortical) (deep)
  (vibratory) (*see also* Disturbance,
  sensation) 782.0
Sensitive dentine 521.89
Sensitiver Beziehungswahn 297.8
Sensitivity, sensitization - *see also* Allergy
  autoerythrocyte 287.2
  carotid sinus 337.01
  child (excessive) 313.21
  cold, autoimmune 283.0
  methemoglobin 289.7
  suxamethonium 289.89
  tuberculin, without clinical or radiological
    symptoms 795.51
Sensory
  extinction 781.8
  neglect 781.8
Separation
  acromioclavicular - *see* Dislocation,
    acromioclavicular
  anxiety, abnormal 309.21
  apophysis, traumatic - *see* Fracture, by site
  choroid 363.70
    hemorrhagic 363.72
    serous 363.71
  costochondral (simple) (traumatic) - *see*
    Dislocation, costochondral
  delayed
    umbilical cord 779.83
  epiphysis, epiphyseal
    nontraumatic 732.9
      upper femoral 732.2
    traumatic - *see* Fracture, by site
  fracture - *see* Fracture, by site
  infundibulum cardiac from right ventricle by
    a partition 746.83

Separation (*Continued*)
  joint (current) (traumatic) - *see* Dislocation,
    by site
  placenta (normally implanted) - *see* Placenta,
    separation
  pubic bone, obstetrical trauma 665.6●
  retina, retinal (*see also* Detachment, retina)
    361.9
    layers 362.40
      sensory (*see also* Retinoschisis) 361.10
      pigment epithelium (exudative) 362.42
        hemorrhagic 362.43
  sternoclavicular (traumatic) - *see* Dislocation,
    sternoclavicular
  symphysis pubis, obstetrical trauma 665.6●
  tracheal ring, incomplete (congenital) 748.3
Sepsis (generalized) 995.91
  with
    abortion - *see* Abortion, by type, with
      sepsis
    acute organ dysfunction 995.92
    ectopic pregnancy (*see also* categories
      633.0–633.9) 639.0
    molar pregnancy (*see also* categories
      630–632) 639.0
    multiple organ dysfunction (MOD) 995.92
  buccal 528.3
  complicating labor 659.3●
  dental (pulpal origin) 522.4
  female genital organ NEC 614.9
  fetus (intrauterine) 771.81
  following
    abortion 639.0
    ectopic or molar pregnancy 639.0
    infusion, perfusion, or transfusion 999.39
  Friedländer's 038.49
  intra-abdominal 567.22
  intraocular 360.00
  localized - code to specific localized infection
    in operation wound 998.59
    skin (*see also* Abscess) 682.9
  malleus 024
  nadir 038.9
  newborn (organism unspecified) NEC 771.81
  oral 528.3
  puerperal, postpartum, childbirth (pelvic)
    670.2●
  resulting from infusion, injection,
    transfusion, or vaccination 999.39
  severe 995.92
  skin, localized (*see also* Abscess) 682.9
  umbilical (newborn) (organism unspecified)
    771.89
    tetanus 771.3
  urinary 599.0
    meaning sepsis 995.91
    meaning urinary tract infection 599.0
Septate - *see also* Septum
Septic - *see also* condition
  adenoids 474.01
    and tonsils 474.02
  arm (with lymphangitis) 682.3
  embolus - *see* Embolism
  finger (with lymphangitis) 681.00
  foot (with lymphangitis) 682.7
  gallbladder (*see also* Cholecystitis) 575.8
  hand (with lymphangitis) 682.4
  joint (*see also* Arthritis, septic) 711.0●
  kidney (*see also* Infection, kidney) 590.9
  leg (with lymphangitis) 682.6
  mouth 528.3
  nail 681.9
    finger 681.02
    toe 681.11
  shock (endotoxic) 785.52
  postoperative 998.02
  sore (*see also* Abscess) 682.9
    throat 034.0
      milk-borne 034.0
      streptococcal 034.0
  spleen (acute) 289.59

Septic *(Continued)*
  teeth (pulpal origin) 522.4
  throat 034.0
  thrombus - *see* Thrombosis
  toe (with lymphangitis) 681.10
  tonsils 474.00
    and adenoids 474.02
  umbilical cord (newborn) (organism
      unspecified) 771.89
  uterus *(see also* Endometritis) 615.9
Septicemia, septicemic (generalized)
      (suppurative) 038.9
  with
    abortion - *see* Abortion, by type, with
        sepsis
    ectopic pregnancy *(see also* categories
        633.0–633.9) 639.0
    molar pregnancy *(see also* categories
        630–632) 639.0
  Aerobacter aerogenes 038.49
  anaerobic 038.3
  anthrax 022.3
  Bacillus coli 038.42
  Bacteroides 038.3
  Clostridium 038.3
  complicating labor 659.3●
  cryptogenic 038.9
  enteric gram-negative bacilli 038.40
  Enterobacter aerogenes 038.49
  Erysipelothrix (insidiosa) (rhusiopathiae)
      027.1
  Escherichia coli 038.42
  following
    abortion 639.0
    ectopic or molar pregnancy 639.0
    infusion, injection, transfusion, or
        vaccination 999.39
  Friedländer's (bacillus) 038.49
  gangrenous 038.9
  gonococcal 098.89
  gram-negative (organism) 038.40
    anaerobic 038.3
  Hemophilus influenzae 038.41
  herpes (simplex) 054.5
  herpetic 054.5
  Listeria monocytogenes 027.0
  meningeal - *see* Meningitis
  meningococcal (chronic) (fulminating) 036.2
  methicillin
    resistant Staphylococcus aureus (MRSA)
        038.12
    susceptible Staphylococcus aureus
        (MSSA) 038.11
  MRSA (methicillin resistant Staphylococcus
      aureus) 038.12
  MSSA (methicillin susceptible
      Staphylococcus aureus) 038.11
  navel, newborn (organism unspecified)
      771.89
  newborn (organism unspecified) 771.81
  plague 020.2
  pneumococcal 038.2
  postabortal 639.0
  postoperative 998.59
  Proteus vulgaris 038.49
  Pseudomonas (aeruginosa) 038.43
  puerperal, postpartum 670.2●
  Salmonella (aertrycke) (callinarum)
      (choleraesuis) (enteritidis) (suipestifer)
      003.1
  Serratia 038.44
  Shigella *(see also* Dysentery, bacillary) 004.9
  specified organism NEC 038.8
  staphylococcal 038.10
    aureus 038.11
      methicillin
        resistant (MRSA) 038.12
        susceptible (MSSA) 038.11
    specified organism NEC 038.19
  streptococcal (anaerobic) 038.0
  Streptococcus pneumoniae 038.2

Septicemia, septicemic *(Continued)*
  suipestifer 003.1
  umbilicus, newborn (organism unspecified)
      771.89
  viral 079.99
  Yersinia enterocolitica 038.49
Septum, septate (congenital) - *see also* Anomaly,
      specified type NEC
  anal 751.2
  aqueduct of Sylvius 742.3
    with spina bifida *(see also* Spina bifida)
        741.0●
  hymen 752.49
  uterus (complete) (partial) 752.35
  vagina
    in pregnancy or childbirth 654.7●
      affecting fetus or newborn 763.89
      causing obstructed labor 660.2●
        affecting fetus or newborn 763.1
    longitudinal (with or without obstruction)
        752.47
    transverse 752.46
Sequestration
  lung (congenital) (extralobar) (intralobar)
      748.5
  orbit 376.10
  pulmonary artery (congenital) 747.39
  splenic 289.52
Sequestrum
  bone *(see also* Osteomyelitis) 730.1●
    jaw 526.4
  dental 525.8
  jaw bone 526.4
  sinus (accessory) (nasal) *(see also* Sinusitis)
      473.9
    maxillary 473.0
Sequoiosis asthma 495.8
Serology for syphilis
  doubtful
    with signs or symptoms - *see* Syphilis, by
        site and stage
    follow-up of latent syphilis - *see* Syphilis,
        latent
  false positive 795.6
  negative, with signs or symptoms - *see*
      Syphilis, by site and stage
  positive 097.1
    with signs or symptoms - *see* Syphilis, by
        site and stage
    false 795.6
    follow-up of latent syphilis - *see* Syphilis,
        latent
    only finding - *see* Syphilis, latent
  reactivated 097.1
Seroma - (postoperative) (non-infected)
      998.13
  infected 998.51
  post-traumatic 729.91
Seropurulent - *see* condition
Serositis, multiple 569.89
  pericardial 423.2
  peritoneal 568.82
  pleural - *see* Pleurisy
Serotonin syndrome 333.99
Serous - *see* condition
Sertoli cell
  adenoma (M8640/0)
    specified site - *see* Neoplasm, by site,
        benign
    unspecified site
      female 220
      male 222.0
  carcinoma (M8640/3)
    specified site - *see* Neoplasm, by site,
        malignant
    unspecified site 186.9
  syndrome (germinal aplasia) 606.0
  tumor (M8640/0)
    with lipid storage (M8641/0)
      specified site - *see* Neoplasm, by site,
          benign

Sertoli cell *(Continued)*
  tumor *(Continued)*
    with lipid storage *(Continued)*
      unspecified site
        female 220
        male 222.0
    specified site - *see* Neoplasm, by site,
        benign
    unspecified site
      female 220
      male 222.0
Sertoli-Leydig cell tumor (M8631/0)
  specified site - *see* Neoplasm, by site, benign
  unspecified site
    female 220
    male 222.0
Serum
  allergy, allergic reaction 999.59
    shock 999.49
  arthritis 999.59 *[713.6]*
  complication or reaction NEC 999.59
  disease NEC 999.59
  hepatitis 070.3●
  intoxication 999.59
  jaundice (homologous) - *see* Hepatitis, viral,
      type B
  neuritis 999.59
  poisoning NEC 999.59
  rash NEC 999.59
  reaction NEC 999.59
  sickness NEC 999.59
Sesamoiditis 733.99
Seven-day fever 061
  of
    Japan 100.89
    Queensland 100.89
Sever's disease or osteochondrosis (calcaneum)
      732.5
Sex chromosome mosaics 758.81
Sex reassignment surgery status *(see also*
      Trans-sexualism) 302.50
Sextuplet
  affected by maternal complication of
      pregnancy 761.5
  healthy liveborn - *see* Newborn, multiple
  pregnancy (complicating delivery) NEC
      651.8●
    with fetal loss and retention of one or
        more fetus(es) 651.6●
    following (elective) fetal reduction 651.7●
Sexual
  anesthesia 302.72
  deviation *(see also* Deviation, sexual) 302.9
  disorder *(see also* Deviation, sexual) 302.9
  frigidity (female) 302.72
  function, disorder of (psychogenic) 302.70
    specified type NEC 302.79
  immaturity (female) (male) 259.0
  impotence 607.84
    organic origin NEC 607.84
    psychogenic 302.72
  precocity (constitutional) (cryptogenic)
      (female) (idiopathic) (male) NEC 259.1
    with adrenal hyperplasia 255.2
  sadism 302.84
Sexuality, pathological *(see also* Deviation,
      sexual) 302.9
Sézary's disease, reticulosis, or syndrome
      (M9701/3) 202.2●
Shadow, lung 793.19
Shaken infant syndrome 995.55
Shaking
  head (tremor) 781.0
  palsy or paralysis *(see also* Parkinsonism)
      332.0
Shallowness, acetabulum 736.39
Shaver's disease or syndrome (bauxite
      pneumoconiosis) 503
Shearing
  artificial skin graft 996.55
  decellularized allodermis graft 996.55

◄ New   ◀◀ Revised   ~~deleted~~ Deleted   ● Use Additional Digit(s)   ▓ Omit code

Sheath (tendon) - *see* condition
Shedding
    nail 703.8
    teeth, premature, primary (deciduous) 520.6
Sheehan's disease or syndrome (postpartum
        pituitary necrosis) 253.2
Shelf, rectal 569.49
Shell
    shock (current) (*see also* Reaction, stress,
        acute) 308.9
        lasting state 300.16
    teeth 520.5
Shield kidney 753.3
Shift, mediastinal 793.2
Shifting
    pacemaker 427.89
    sleep-work schedule (affecting sleep) 327.36
Shiga's
    bacillus 004.0
    dysentery 004.0
Shigella (dysentery) (*see also* Dysentery,
        bacillary) 004.9
    carrier (suspected) of V02.3
Shigellosis (*see also* Dysentery, bacillary) 004.9
Shingles (*see also* Herpes, zoster) 053.9
    eye NEC 053.29
Shin splints 844.9
Shipyard eye or disease 077.1
Shirodkar suture, in pregnancy 654.5●
Shock 785.50
    with
        abortion - *see* Abortion, by type, with
            shock
        ectopic pregnancy (*see also* categories
            633.0–633.9) 639.5
        molar pregnancy (*see also* categories
            630–632) 639.5
    allergic - *see* Anaphylactic reaction or shock
    anaclitic 309.21
    anaphylactic *see also* Anaphylactic reaction or
        shock
        due to administration of blood and blood
            products 999.41
    anaphylactoid - *see* Anaphylactic reaction or
        shock
    anesthetic
        correct substance properly administered
            995.4
        overdose or wrong substance given 968.4
            specified anesthetic - *see* Table of Drugs
                and Chemicals
    birth, fetus or newborn NEC 779.89
    cardiogenic 785.51
    chemical substance - *see* Table of Drugs and
        Chemicals
    circulatory 785.59
    complicating
        abortion - *see* Abortion, by type, with
            shock
        ectopic pregnancy - (*see also* categories
            633.0–633.9) 639.5
        labor and delivery 669.1●
        molar pregnancy (*see also* categories
            630–632) 639.5
    culture 309.29
    due to
        drug 995.0
            correct substance properly
                administered 995.0
            overdose or wrong substance given or
                taken 977.9
            specified drug - *see* Table of Drugs and
                Chemicals
        food - *see* Anaphylactic shock, due to,
            food
    during labor and delivery 669.1●
    electric 994.8
        from electroshock gun (taser) 994.8
    endotoxic 785.52
        due to surgical procedure 998.02
        postoperative 998.02

Shock (*Continued*)
    following
        abortion 639.5
        ectopic or molar pregnancy 639.5
        injury (immediate) (delayed) 958.4
        labor and delivery 669.1●
    gram-negative 785.52
        postoperative 998.02
    hematogenic 785.59
    hemorrhagic
        due to
            disease 785.59
            surgery (intraoperative)
                (postoperative) 998.09
            trauma 958.4
    hypovolemic NEC 785.59
        surgical 998.09
        traumatic 958.4
    insulin 251.0
        therapeutic misadventure 962.3
    kidney 584.5
        traumatic (following crushing) 958.5
    lightning 994.0
    lung 518.82
        related to trauma and surgery 518.52
    nervous (*see also* Reaction, stress, acute) 308.9
    obstetric 669.1●
        with
            abortion - *see* Abortion, by type, with
                shock
            ectopic pregnancy (*see also* categories
                633.0–633.9) 639.5
            molar pregnancy (*see also* categories
                630–632) 639.5
        following
            abortion 639.5
            ectopic or molar pregnancy 639.5
    paralysis, paralytic (*see also* Disease,
        cerebrovascular, acute) 436
        late effect - *see* Late effect(s) (of)
            cerebrovascular disease
    pleural (surgical) 998.09
        due to trauma 958.4
    postoperative 998.00
        with
            abortion - *see* Abortion, by type, with
                shock
            ectopic pregnancy (*see also* categories
                633.0–633.9) 639.5
            molar pregnancy (*see also* categories
                630–632) 639.5
        cardiogenic 998.01
        following
            abortion 639.5
            ectopic or molar pregnancy 639.5
        hypovolemic 998.09
        specified NEC 998.09
        septic (endotoxic) (gram-negative) 998.02
    psychic (*see also* Reaction, stress, acute) 308.9
        past history (of) V15.49
    psychogenic (*see also* Reaction, stress, acute)
        308.9
    septic 785.52
        with
            abortion - *see* Abortion, by type, with
                shock
            ectopic pregnancy (*see also* categories
                633.0–633.9) 639.5
            molar pregnancy (*see also* categories
                630–632) 639.5
        due to
            surgical procedure 998.02
            transfusion NEC 999.89
                bone marrow 996.85
        following
            abortion 639.5
            ectopic or molar pregnancy 639.5
            surgical procedure 998.02
            transfusion NEC 999.89
                bone marrow 996.85
        postoperative 998.02

Shock (*Continued*)
    spinal - *see also* Injury, spinal, by site
        with spinal bone injury - *see* Fracture,
            vertebra, by site, with spinal cord
            injury
    surgical 998.00
    therapeutic misadventure NEC (*see also*
        Complications) 998.89
    thyroxin 962.7
    toxic 040.82
    transfusion - *see* Complications, transfusion
    traumatic (immediate) (delayed) 958.4
Shoemakers' chest 738.3
Short, shortening, shortness
    Achilles tendon (acquired) 727.81
    arm 736.89
        congenital 755.20
    back 737.9
    bowel syndrome 579.3
    breath 786.05
    cervical, cervix 649.7●
        gravid uterus 649.7●
        non-gravid uterus 622.5
            acquired 622.5
            congenital 752.49
    chain acyl CoA dehydrogenase deficiency
        (SCAD) 277.85
    common bile duct, congenital 751.69
    cord (umbilical) 663.4●
        affecting fetus or newborn 762.6
    cystic duct, congenital 751.69
    esophagus (congenital) 750.4
    femur (acquired) 736.81
        congenital 755.34
    frenulum linguae 750.0
    frenum, lingual 750.0
    hamstrings 727.81
    hip (acquired) 736.39
        congenital 755.63
    leg (acquired) 736.81
        congenital 755.30
    metatarsus (congenital) 754.79
        acquired 736.79
    organ or site, congenital NEC - *see* Distortion
    palate (congenital) 750.26
    P-R interval syndrome 426.81
    radius (acquired) 736.09
        congenital 755.26
    round ligament 629.89
    sleeper 307.49
    stature, constitutional (hereditary)
        (idiopathic) 783.43
    tendon 727.81
        Achilles (acquired) 727.81
            congenital 754.79
        congenital 756.89
    thigh (acquired) 736.81
        congenital 755.34
    tibialis anticus 727.81
    umbilical cord 663.4●
        affecting fetus or newborn 762.6
    urethra 599.84
    uvula (congenital) 750.26
    vagina 623.8
Shortsightedness 367.1
Shoshin (acute fulminating beriberi) 265.0
Shoulder - *see* condition
Shovel-shaped incisors 520.2
Shower, thromboembolic - *see* Embolism
Shunt (status)
    aortocoronary bypass V45.81
    arterial-venous (dialysis) V45.11
    arteriovenous, pulmonary (acquired) 417.0
        congenital 747.39
        traumatic (complication) 901.40
    cerebral ventricle (communicating) in situ
        V45.2
    coronary artery bypass V45.81
    surgical, prosthetic, with complications - *see*
        Complications, shunt
    vascular NEC V45.89

Shutdown
　renal 586
　　with
　　　abortion - *see* Abortion, by type, with
　　　　renal failure
　　　ectopic pregnancy (*see also* categories
　　　　633.0–633.9) 639.3
　　　molar pregnancy (*see also* categories
　　　　630–632) 639.3
　　complicating
　　　abortion 639.3
　　　ectopic or molar pregnancy 639.3
　　　following labor and delivery 669.3●
Shwachman's syndrome 288.02
Shy-Drager syndrome (orthostatic hypotension
　with multisystem degeneration) 333.0
Sialadenitis (any gland) (chronic) (supportive)
　527.2
　epidemic - *see* Mumps
Sialadenosis, periodic 527.2
Sialaporia 527.7
Sialectasia 527.8
Sialitis 527.2
Sialoadenitis (*see also* Sialadenitis) 527.2
Sialoangitis 527.2
Sialodochitis (fibrinosa) 527.2
Sialodocholithiasis 527.5
Sialolithiasis 527.5
Sialorrhea (*see also* Ptyalism) 527.7
　periodic 527.2
Sialosis 527.8
　rheumatic 710.2
Siamese twin 759.4
　complicating pregnancy 678.1●
Sicard's syndrome 352.6
Sicca syndrome (keratoconjunctivitis) 710.2
Sick 799.9
　cilia syndrome 759.89
　or handicapped person in family V61.49
Sickle-cell
　anemia (*see also* Disease, sickle-cell) 282.60
　disease (*see also* Disease, sickle-cell) 282.60
　hemoglobin
　　C disease (without crisis) 282.63
　　　with
　　　　crisis 282.64
　　　　　vaso-occlusive pain 282.64
　　D disease (without crisis) 282.68
　　　with crisis 282.69
　　E disease (without crisis) 282.68
　　　with crisis 282.69
　thalassemia (without crisis) 282.41
　　with
　　　crisis 282.42
　　　　vaso-occlusive pain 282.42
　trait 282.5
Sicklemia (*see also* Disease, sickle-cell) 282.60
　trait 282.5
Sickness
　air (travel) 994.6
　airplane 994.6
　alpine 993.2
　altitude 993.2
　Andes 993.2
　aviators' 993.2
　balloon 993.2
　car 994.6
　compressed air 993.3
　decompression 993.3
　green 280.9
　harvest 100.89
　milk 988.8
　morning 643.0●
　motion 994.6
　mountain 993.2
　　acute 289.0
　protein (*see also* Complications, vaccination)
　　999.59
　radiation NEC 990
　roundabout (motion) 994.6
　sea 994.6

Sickness (*Continued*)
　serum NEC 999.59
　sleeping (African) 086.5
　　by Trypanosoma 086.5
　　　gambiense 086.3
　　　rhodesiense 086.4
　　Gambian 086.3
　　late effect 139.8
　　Rhodesian 086.4
　sweating 078.2
　swing (motion) 994.6
　train (railway) (travel) 994.6
　travel (any vehicle) 994.6
Sick sinus syndrome 427.81
Sideropenia (*see also* Anemia, iron deficiency)
　280.9
Siderosis (lung) (occupational) 503
　central nervous system (CNS) 437.8
　cornea 371.15
　eye (bulbi) (vitreous) 360.23
　lens 360.23
Siegal-Cattan-Mamou disease (periodic) 277.31
Siemens' syndrome
　ectodermal dysplasia 757.31
　keratosis follicularis spinulosa (decalvans)
　　757.39
Sighing respiration 786.7
Sigmoid
　flexure - *see* condition
　kidney 753.3
Sigmoiditis - *see* Enteritis
Silfverskiöld's syndrome 756.50
Silicosis, silicotic (complicated) (occupational)
　(simple) 502
　fibrosis, lung (confluent) (massive)
　　(occupational) 502
　non-nodular 503
　pulmonum 502
Silicotuberculosis (*see also* Tuberculosis) 011.4●
Silo fillers' disease 506.9
Silver's syndrome (congenital
　hemihypertrophy and short stature)
　759.89
Silver wire arteries, retina 362.13
Silvestroni-Bianco syndrome (thalassemia
　minima) 282.49
Simian crease 757.2
Simmonds' cachexia or disease (pituitary
　cachexia) 253.2
Simons' disease or syndrome (progressive
　lipodystrophy) 272.6
Simple, simplex - *see* condition
Sinding-Larsen disease (juvenile osteopathia
　patellae) 732.4
Singapore hemorrhagic fever 065.4
Singers' node or nodule 478.5
Single
　atrium 745.69
　coronary artery 746.85
　umbilical artery 747.5
　ventricle 745.3
Singultus 786.8
　epidemicus 078.89
Sinus - *see also* Fistula
　abdominal 569.81
　arrest 426.6
　arrhythmia 427.89
　bradycardia 427.89
　　chronic 427.81
　branchial cleft (external) (internal) 744.41
　coccygeal (infected) 685.1
　　with abscess 685.0
　dental 522.7
　dermal (congenital) 685.1
　　with abscess 685.0
　draining - *see* Fistula
　infected, skin NEC 686.9
　marginal, rupture or bleeding 641.2●
　　affecting fetus or newborn 762.1
　pause 426.6
　pericranii 742.0

Sinus (*Continued*)
　pilonidal (infected) (rectum) 685.1
　　with abscess 685.0
　preauricular 744.46
　rectovaginal 619.1
　sacrococcygeal (dermoid) (infected) 685.1
　　with abscess 685.0
　skin
　　infected NEC 686.9
　　noninfected- *see* Ulcer, skin
　tachycardia 427.89
　tarsi syndrome 726.79
　testis 608.89
　tract (postinfectional) - *see* Fistula
　urachus 753.7
Sinuses, Rokitansky-Aschoff (*see also* Disease,
　gallbladder) 575.8
Sinusitis (accessory) (chronic) (hyperplastic)
　(nasal) (nonpurulent) (purulent) 473.9
　with influenza, flu, or grippe (*see also*
　　Influenza) 487.1
　acute 461.9
　　ethmoidal 461.2
　　frontal 461.1
　　maxillary 461.0
　　specified type NEC 461.8
　　sphenoidal 461.3
　allergic (*see also* Fever, hay) 477.9
　antrum - *see* Sinusitis, maxillary
　due to
　　fungus, any sinus 117.9
　　high altitude 993.1
　ethmoidal 473.2
　　acute 461.2
　frontal 473.1
　　acute 461.1
　influenzal (*see also* Influenza) 487.1
　maxillary 473.0
　　acute 461.0
　specified site NEC 473.8
　sphenoidal 473.3
　　acute 461.3
　syphilitic, any sinus 095.8
　tuberculous, any sinus (*see also* Tuberculosis)
　　012.8●
Sinusitis-bronchiectasis-situs inversus
　(syndrome) (triad) 759.3
Sipple's syndrome (medullary thyroid
　carcinoma-pheochromocytoma) 258.02
Sirenomelia 759.89
Siriasis 992.0
Sirkari's disease 085.0
SIRS (systemic inflammatory response
　syndrome) 995.90
　due to
　　infectious process 995.91
　　　with acute organ dysfunction 995.92
　　non-infectious process 995.93
　　　with acute organ dysfunction 995.94
Siti 104.0
Sitophobia 300.29
Situation, psychiatric 300.9
Situational
　disturbance (transient) (*see also* Reaction,
　　adjustment) 309.9
　　acute 308.3
　maladjustment, acute (*see also* Reaction,
　　adjustment) 309.9
　reaction (*see also* Reaction, adjustment)
　　309.9
　　acute 308.3
Situs inversus or transversus 759.3
　abdominalis 759.3
　thoracis 759.3
Sixth disease
　due to
　　human herpesvirus 6 058.11
　　human herpesvirus 7 058.12
Sjögren (-Gougerot) syndrome or disease
　(keratoconjunctivitis sicca) 710.2
　with lung involvement 710.2 [*517.8*]

◀ New　◀▇ Revised　~~deleted~~ Deleted　● Use Additional Digit(s)　▨ Omit code

Sjögren-Larsson syndrome (ichthyosis congenita) 757.1
SJS-TEN (Stevens-Johnson syndrome-toxic epidermal necrolysis overlap syndrome) 695.14
Skeletal - see condition
Skene's gland - see condition
Skenitis (see also Urethritis) 597.89
   gonorrheal (acute) 098.0
      chronic or duration of 2 months or over 098.2
Skerljevo 104.0
Skevas-Zerfus disease 989.5
Skin - see also condition
   donor V59.1
   hidebound 710.9
SLAP lesion (superior glenoid labrum) 840.7
Slate-dressers' lung 502
Slate-miners' lung 502
Sleep
   deprivation V69.4
   disorder 780.50
      with apnea - see Apnea, sleep
      child 307.40
      movement, unspecified 780.58
      nonorganic origin 307.40
         specified type NEC 307.49
   disturbance 780.50
      with apnea - see Apnea, sleep
      nonorganic origin 307.40
         specified type NEC 307.49
   drunkenness 307.47
   movement disorder, unspecified 780.58
   paroxysmal (see also Narcolepsy) 347.00
   related movement disorder, unspecified 780.58
   rhythm inversion 327.39
      nonorganic origin 307.45
   walking 307.46
      hysterical 300.13
Sleeping sickness 086.5
   late effect 139.8
Sleeplessness (see also Insomnia) 780.52
   menopausal 627.2
   nonorganic origin 307.41
Slipped, slipping
   epiphysis (postinfectional) 732.9
      traumatic (old) 732.9
         current - see Fracture, by site
      upper femoral (nontraumatic) 732.2
   intervertebral disc - see Displacement, intervertebral disc
   ligature, umbilical 772.3
   patella 717.89
   rib 733.99
   sacroiliac joint 724.6
   tendon 727.9
   ulnar nerve, nontraumatic 354.2
   vertebra NEC (see also Spondylolisthesis) 756.12
Slocumb's syndrome 255.3
Sloughing (multiple) (skin) 686.9
   abscess - see Abscess, by site
   appendix 543.9
   bladder 596.89
   fascia 728.9
   graft - see Complications, graft
   phagedena (see also Gangrene) 785.4
   reattached extremity (see also Complications, reattached extremity) 996.90
   rectum 569.49
   scrotum 608.89
   tendon 727.9
   transplanted organ (see also Rejection, transplant, organ, by site) 996.80
   ulcer (see also Ulcer, skin) 707.9
Slow
   feeding newborn 779.31
   fetal, growth NEC 764.9●
      affecting management of pregnancy 656.5●

Slowing
   heart 427.89
   urinary stream 788.62
Sluder's neuralgia or syndrome 337.09
Slurred, slurring, speech 784.59
Small, smallness
   cardia reserve - see Disease, heart
   for dates
      fetus or newborn 764.0●
         with malnutrition 764.1●
         affecting management of pregnancy 656.5●
      infant, term 764.0●
         with malnutrition 764.1●
         affecting management of pregnancy 656.5●
   introitus, vagina 623.3
   kidney, unknown cause 589.9
      bilateral 589.1
      unilateral 589.0
   ovary 620.8
   pelvis
      with disproportion (fetopelvic) 653.1●
         affecting fetus or newborn 763.1
      causing obstructed labor 660.1●
         affecting fetus or newborn 763.1
   placenta - see Placenta, insufficiency
   uterus 621.8
   white kidney 582.9
Small-for-dates (see also Light-for-dates) 764.0●
   affecting management of pregnancy 656.5●
Smallpox 050.9
   contact V01.3
   exposure to V01.3
   hemorrhagic (pustular) 050.0
   malignant 050.0
   modified 050.2
   vaccination
      complications - see Complications, vaccination
      prophylactic (against) V04.1
Smearing, fecal 787.62
Smith's fracture (separation) (closed) 813.41
   open 813.51
Smith-Lemli-Opitz syndrome (cerebrohepatorenal syndrome) 759.89
Smith-Magenis syndrome 758.33
Smith-Strang disease (oasthouse urine) 270.2
Smokers'
   bronchitis 491.0
   cough 491.0
   syndrome (see also Abuse, drugs, nondependent) 305.1
   throat 472.1
   tongue 528.6
Smoking complicating pregnancy, childbirth, or the puerperium 649.0●
Smothering spells 786.09
Snaggle teeth, tooth 524.39
Snapping
   finger 727.05
   hip 719.65
   jaw 524.69
      temporomandibular joint sounds on opening or closing 524.64
   knee 717.9
   thumb 727.05
Sneddon-Wilkinson disease or syndrome (subcorneal pustular dermatosis) 694.1
Sneezing 784.99
   intractable 478.19
Sniffing
   cocaine (see also Dependence) 304.2●
   either (see also Dependence) 304.6●
   glue (airplane) (see also Dependence) 304.6●
Snoring 786.09
Snow blindness 370.24
Snuffles (nonsyphilitic) 460
   syphilitic (infant) 090.0
Social migrant V60.0
Sodoku 026.0

Soemmering's ring 366.51
Soft - see also condition
   enlarged prostate 600.00
      with
         other lower urinary tract symptoms (LUTS) 600.01
         urinary
            obstruction 600.01
            retention 600.01
   nails 703.8
Softening
   bone 268.2
   brain (necrotic) (progressive) 348.89
      arteriosclerotic 437.0
      congenital 742.4
      due to cerebrovascular accident 438.89
      embolic (see also Embolism, brain) 434.1●
      hemorrhagic (see also Hemorrhage, brain) 431
      occlusive 434.9●
      thrombotic (see also Thrombosis, brain) 434.0●
   cartilage 733.92
   cerebellar - see Softening, brain
   cerebral - see Softening, brain
   cerebrospinal - see Softening, brain
   myocardial, heart (see also Degeneration, myocardial) 429.1
   nails 703.8
   spinal cord 336.8
   stomach 537.89
Soiling, fecal 787.62
Solar fever 061
Soldier's
   heart 306.2
   patches 423.1
Solitary
   cyst
      bone 733.21
      kidney 593.2
   kidney (congenital) 753.0
   tubercle, brain (see also Tuberculosis, brain) 013.2●
   ulcer, bladder 596.89
Somatization reaction, somatic reaction (see also Disorder, psychosomatic) 306.9
   disorder 300.81
Somatoform disorder 300.82
   atypical 300.82
   severe 300.81
   undifferentiated 300.82
Somnambulism 307.46
   hysterical 300.13
Somnolence 780.09
   nonorganic origin 307.43
   periodic 349.89
Sonne dysentery 004.3
Soor 112.0
Sore
   Delhi 085.1
   desert (see also Ulcer, skin) 707.9
   eye 379.99
   Lahore 085.1
   mouth 528.9
      canker 528.2
      due to dentures 528.9
   muscle 729.1
   naga (see also Ulcer, skin) 707.9
   oriental 085.1
   pressure (see also Ulcer, pressure) 707.00
      with gangrene (see also Ulcer, pressure) 707.00 [785.4]
   skin NEC 709.9
   soft 099.0
   throat 462
      with influenza, flu, or grippe (see also Influenza) 487.1
      acute 462
      chronic 472.1
      clergyman's 784.49
      Coxsackie (virus) 074.0

Sore *(Continued)*
 throat *(Continued)*
  diphtheritic 032.0
  epidemic 034.0
  gangrenous 462
  herpetic 054.79
  influenzal *(see also* Influenza) 487.1
  malignant 462
  purulent 462
  putrid 462
  septic 034.0
  streptococcal (ulcerative) 034.0
  ulcerated 462
  viral NEC 462
   Coxsackie 074.0
 tropical *(see also* Ulcer, skin) 707.9
 veldt *(see also* Ulcer, skin) 707.9
Sotos' syndrome (cerebral gigantism) 253.0
Sounds
 friction, pleural 786.7
 succussion, chest 786.7
 temporomandibular joint
  on opening or closing 524.64
South African cardiomyopathy syndrome 425.2
South American
 blastomycosis 116.1
 trypanosomiasis - *see* Trypanosomiasis
Southeast Asian hemorrhagic fever 065.4
Spacing, teeth, abnormal 524.30
 excessive 524.32
Spade-like hand (congenital) 754.89
Spading nail 703.8
 congenital 757.5
Spanemia 285.9
Spanish collar 605
Sparganosis 123.5
Spasm, spastic, spasticity *(see also* condition) 781.0
 accommodation 367.53
 ampulla of Vater *(see also* Disease, gallbladder) 576.8
 anus, ani (sphincter) (reflex) 564.6
  psychogenic 306.4
 artery NEC 443.9
  basilar 435.0
  carotid 435.8
  cerebral 435.9
   specified artery NEC 435.8
  retinal *(see also* Occlusion, retinal, artery) 362.30
  vertebral 435.1
  vertebrobasilar 435.3
 Bell's 351.0
 bladder (sphincter, external or internal) 596.89
 bowel 564.9
  psychogenic 306.4
 bronchus, bronchiole 519.11
 cardia 530.0
 cardiac - *see* Angina
 carpopedal *(see also* Tetany) 781.7
 cecum 564.9
  psychogenic 306.4
 cerebral (arteries) (vascular) 435.9
  specified artery NEC 435.8
 cerebrovascular 435.9
 cervix, complicating delivery 661.4●
  affecting fetus or newborn 763.7
 ciliary body (of accommodation) 367.53
 colon 564.1
  psychogenic 306.4
 common duct *(see also* Disease, biliary) 576.8
 compulsive 307.22
 conjugate 378.82
 convergence 378.84
 coronary (artery) - *see* Angina
 diaphragm (reflex) 786.8
  psychogenic 306.1
 duodenum, duodenal (bulb) 564.89

Spasm, spastic, spasticity *(Continued)*
 esophagus (diffuse) 530.5
  psychogenic 306.4
 facial 351.8
 fallopian tube 620.8
 gait 781.2
 gastrointestinal (tract) 536.8
  psychogenic 306.4
 glottis 478.75
  hysterical 300.11
  psychogenic 306.1
   specified as conversion reaction 300.11
  reflex through recurrent laryngeal nerve 478.75
 habit 307.20
  chronic 307.22
  transient (of childhood) 307.21
 heart - *see* Angina
 hourglass - *see* Contraction, hourglass
 hysterical 300.11
 infantile *(see also* Epilepsy) 345.6●
 internal oblique, eye 378.51
 intestinal 564.9
  psychogenic 306.4
 larynx, laryngeal 478.75
  hysterical 300.11
  psychogenic 306.1
   specified as conversion reaction 300.11
 levator palpebrae superioris 333.81
 lightning *(see also* Epilepsy) 345.6●
 mobile 781.0
 muscle 728.85
  back 724.8
  psychogenic 306.0
 nerve, trigeminal 350.1
 nervous 306.0
 nodding 307.3
  infantile *(see also* Epilepsy) 345.6●
 occupational 300.89
 oculogyric 378.87
 ophthalmic artery 362.30
 orbicularis 781.0
 perineal 625.8
 peroneo-extensor *(see also* Flat, foot) 734
 pharynx (reflex) 478.29
  hysterical 300.11
  psychogenic 306.1
   specified as conversion reaction 300.11
 pregnant uterus, complicating delivery 661.4●
 psychogenic 306.0
 pylorus 537.81
  adult hypertrophic 537.0
  congenital or infantile 750.5
  psychogenic 306.4
 rectum (sphincter) 564.6
  psychogenic 306.4
 retinal artery NEC *(see also* Occlusion, retina, artery) 362.30
 sacroiliac 724.6
 salaam (infantile) *(see also* Epilepsy) 345.6●
 saltatory 781.0
 sigmoid 564.9
  psychogenic 306.4
 sphincter of Oddi *(see also* Disease, gallbladder) 576.5
 stomach 536.8
  neurotic 306.4
 throat 478.29
  hysterical 300.11
  psychogenic 306.1
   specified as conversion reaction 300.11
 tic 307.20
  chronic 307.22
  transient (of childhood) 307.21
 tongue 529.8
 torsion 333.6
 trigeminal nerve 350.1
  postherpetic 053.12
 ureter 593.89
 urethra (sphincter) 599.84

Spasm, spastic, spasticity *(Continued)*
 uterus 625.8
  complicating labor 661.4●
   affecting fetus or newborn 763.7
 vagina 625.1
  psychogenic 306.51
 vascular NEC 443.9
 vasomotor NEC 443.9
 vein NEC 459.89
 vesical (sphincter, external or internal) 596.89
 viscera 789.0●
Spasmodic - *see* condition
Spasmophilia *(see also* Tetany) 781.7
Spasmus nutans 307.3
Spastic - *see also* Spasm
 child 343.9
Spasticity - *see also* Spasm
 cerebral, child 343.9
Speakers' throat 784.49
Specific, specified - *see* condition
Speech
 defect, disorder, disturbance, impediment NEC 784.59
  psychogenic 307.9
 (language) therapy V57.3
Spells 780.39
 breath-holding 786.9
Spencer's disease (epidemic vomiting) 078.82
Spens' syndrome (syncope with heart block) 426.9
Spermatic cord - *see* condition
Spermatocele 608.1
 congenital 752.89
Spermatocystitis 608.4
Spermatocytoma (M9063/3)
 specified site - *see* Neoplasm, by site, malignant
 unspecified site 186.9
Spermatorrhea 608.89
Sperm counts
 fertility testing V26.21
 following sterilization reversal V26.22
 postvasectomy V25.8
Sphacelus *(see also* Gangrene) 785.4
Sphenoidal - *see* condition
Sphenoiditis (chronic) *(see also* Sinusitis, sphenoidal) 473.3
Sphenopalatine ganglion neuralgia 337.09
Sphericity, increased, lens 743.36
Spherocytosis (congenital) (familial) (hereditary) 282.0
 hemoglobin disease 282.7
 sickle-cell (disease) 282.60
Spherophakia 743.36
Sphincter - *see* condition
Sphincteritis, sphincter of Oddi *(see also* Cholecystitis) 576.8
Sphingolipidosis 272.7
Sphingolipodystrophy 272.7
Sphingomyelinosis 272.7
Spicule tooth 520.2
Spider
 finger 755.59
 nevus 448.1
 vascular 448.1
Spiegler-Fendt sarcoid 686.8
Spielmeyer-Stock disease 330.1
Spielmeyer-Vogt disease 330.1
Spina bifida (aperta) 741.9●

Note: Use the following fifth-digit subclassification with category 741:

0 unspecified region
1 cervical region
2 dorsal [thoracic] region
3 lumbar region

 with hydrocephalus 741.0●
  fetal (suspected), affecting management of pregnancy 655.0●
 occulta 756.17

New   Revised   ~~deleted~~ Deleted   ● Use Additional Digit(s)   Omit code

Spindle, Krukenberg's 371.13
Spine, spinal - *see* condition
Spiradenoma (eccrine) (M8403/0) - *see*
    Neoplasm, skin, benign
Spirillosis NEC (*see also* Fever, relapsing) 087.9
Spirillum minus 026.0
Spirillum obermeieri infection 087.0
Spirochetal - *see* condition
Spirochetosis 104.9
    arthritic, arthritica 104.9 *[711.8]*●
    bronchopulmonary 104.8
    icterohemorrhagica 100.0
    lung 104.8
Spitting blood (*see also* Hemoptysis) 786.30
Splanchnomegaly 569.89
Splanchnoptosis 569.89
Spleen, splenic - *see also* condition
    agenesis 759.0
    flexure syndrome 569.89
    neutropenia syndrome 289.53
    sequestration syndrome 289.52
Splenectasis (*see also* Splenomegaly) 789.2
Splenitis (interstitial) (malignant) (nonspecific)
    289.59
    malarial (*see also* Malaria) 084.6
    tuberculous (*see also* Tuberculosis) 017.7●
Splenocele 289.59
Splenomegalia - *see* Splenomegaly
Splenomegalic - *see* condition
Splenomegaly 789.2
    Bengal 789.2
    cirrhotic 289.51
    congenital 759.0
    congestive, chronic 289.51
    cryptogenic 789.2
    Egyptian 120.1
    Gaucher's (cerebroside lipidosis) 272.7
    idiopathic 789.2
    malarial (*see also* Malaria) 084.6
    neutropenic 289.53
    Niemann-Pick (lipid histiocytosis) 272.7
    siderotic 289.51
    syphilitic 095.8
        congenital 090.0
    tropical (Bengal) (idiopathic) 789.2
Splenopathy 289.50
Splenopneumonia - *see* Pneumonia
Splenoptosis 289.59
Splinter - *see* Injury, superficial, by site
Split, splitting
    heart sounds 427.89
    lip, congenital (*see also* Cleft, lip) 749.10
    nails 703.8
    urinary stream 788.61
Spoiled child reaction (*see also* Disturbance,
    conduct) 312.1●
Spondylarthritis (*see also* Spondylosis) 721.90
Spondylarthrosis (*see also* Spondylosis) 721.90
Spondylitis 720.9
    ankylopoietica 720.0
    ankylosing (chronic) 720.0
    atrophic 720.9
        ligamentous 720.9
    chronic (traumatic) (*see also* Spondylosis)
        721.90
    deformans (chronic) (*see also* Spondylosis)
        721.90
    gonococcal 098.53
    gouty 274.00
    hypertrophic (*see also* Spondylosis) 721.90
    infectious NEC 720.9
    juvenile (adolescent) 720.0
    Kummell's 721.7
    Marie-Strümpell (ankylosing) 720.0
    muscularis 720.9
    ossificans ligamentosa 721.6
    osteoarthritica (*see also* Spondylosis) 721.90
    posttraumatic 721.7
    proliferative 720.0
    rheumatoid 720.0
    rhizomelica 720.0

Spondylitis (*Continued*)
    sacroiliac NEC 720.2
    senescent (*see also* Spondylosis) 721.90
    senile (*see also* Spondylosis) 721.90
    static (*see also* Spondylosis) 721.90
    traumatic (chronic) (*see also* Spondylosis)
        721.90
    tuberculous (*see also* Tuberculosis) 015.0●
        [720.81]
    typhosa 002.0 *[720.81]*
Spondyloarthrosis (*see also* Spondylosis) 721.90
Spondylolisthesis (congenital) (lumbosacral)
    756.12
    with disproportion (fetopelvic) 653.3●
        affecting fetus or newborn 763.1
        causing obstructed labor 660.1●
            affecting fetus or newborn 763.1
    acquired 738.4
    degenerative 738.4
    traumatic 738.4
        acute (lumbar) - *see* Fracture, vertebra,
            lumbar
        site other than lumbosacral - *see*
            Fracture, vertebra, by site
Spondylolysis (congenital) 756.11
    acquired 738.4
    cervical 756.19
    lumbosacral region 756.11
        with disproportion (fetopelvic) 653.3●
            affecting fetus or newborn 763.1
            causing obstructed labor 660.1●
                affecting fetus or newborn 763.1
Spondylopathy
    inflammatory 720.9
        specified type NEC 720.89
    traumatic 721.7
Spondylose rhizomelique 720.0
Spondylosis 721.90
    with
        disproportion 653.3●
            affecting fetus or newborn 763.1
            causing obstructed labor 660.1●
                affecting fetus or newborn 763.1
        myelopathy NEC 721.91
    cervical, cervicodorsal 721.0
        with myelopathy 721.1
    inflammatory 720.9
    lumbar, lumbosacral 721.3
        with myelopathy 721.42
    sacral 721.3
        with myelopathy 721.42
    thoracic 721.2
        with myelopathy 721.41
    traumatic 721.7
Sponge
    divers' disease 989.5
    inadvertently left in operation wound
        998.4
    kidney (medullary) 753.17
Spongioblastoma (M9422/3)
    multiforme (M9440/3)
        specified site - *see* Neoplasm, by site,
            malignant
        unspecified site 191.9
    polare (M9423/3)
        specified site - *see* Neoplasm, by site,
            malignant
        unspecified site 191.9
    primitive polar (M9443/3)
        specified site - *see* Neoplasm, by site,
            malignant
        unspecified site 191.9
    specified site - *see* Neoplasm, by site,
        malignant
    unspecified site 191.9
Spongiocytoma (M9400/3)
    specified site - *see* Neoplasm, by site,
        malignant
    unspecified site 191.9
Spongioneuroblastoma (M9504/3) - *see*
    Neoplasm, by site, malignant

Spontaneous - *see also* condition
    fracture - *see* Fracture, pathologic
Spoon nail 703.8
    congenital 757.5
Sporadic - *see* condition
Sporotrichosis (bones) (cutaneous)
    (disseminated) (epidermal) (lymphatic)
    (lymphocutaneous) (mucous membranes)
    (pulmonary) (skeletal) (visceral) 117.1
Sporotrichum schenckii infection 117.1
Spots, spotting
    atrophic (skin) 701.3
    Bitôt's (in the young child) 264.1
    café au lait 709.09
    cayenne pepper 448.1
    complicating pregnancy 649.5●
    cotton wool (retina) 362.83
    de Morgan's (senile angiomas) 448.1
    Fúchs' black (myopic) 360.21
    intermenstrual
        irregular 626.6
        regular 626.5
    interpalpebral 372.53
    Koplik's 055.9
    liver 709.09
    Mongolian (pigmented) 757.33
    of pregnancy 649.5●
    purpuric 782.7
    ruby 448.1
Spotted fever - *see* Fever, spotted
Sprain, strain (joint) (ligament) (muscle)
    (tendon) 848.9
    abdominal wall (muscle) 848.8
    Achilles tendon 845.09
    acromioclavicular 840.0
    ankle 845.00
        and foot 845.00
    anterior longitudinal, cervical 847.0
    arm 840.9
        upper 840.9
            and shoulder 840.9
    astragalus 845.00
    atlanto-axial 847.0
    atlanto-occipital 847.0
    atlas 847.0
    axis 847.0
    back (*see also* Sprain, spine) 847.9
    breast bone 848.40
    broad ligaments - *see* Injury, internal, broad
        ligament
    calcaneofibular 845.02
    carpal 842.01
    carpometacarpal 842.11
    cartilage
        costal, without mention of injury to
            sternum 848.3
            involving sternum 848.42
        ear 848.8
        knee 844.9
            with current tear (*see also* Tear,
                meniscus) 836.2
            semilunar (knee) 844.8
                with current tear (*see also* Tear,
                     meniscus) 836.2
        septal, nose 848.0
        thyroid region 848.2
        xiphoid 848.49
    cervical, cervicodorsal, cervicothoracic 847.0
    chondrocostal, without mention of injury to
        sternum 848.3
        involving sternum 848.42
    chondrosternal 848.42
    chronic (joint) - *see* Derangement, joint
    clavicle 840.9
    coccyx 847.4
    collar bone 840.9
    collateral, knee (medial) (tibial) 844.1
        lateral (fibular) 844.0
        recurrent or old 717.89
            lateral 717.81
            medial 717.82

Sprain, strain (Continued)
  coracoacromial 840.8
  coracoclavicular 840.1
  coracohumeral 840.2
  coracoid (process) 840.9
  coronary, knee 844.8
  costal cartilage, without mention of injury to
    sternum 848.3
    involving sternum 848.42
  cricoarytenoid articulation 848.2
  cricothyroid articulation 848.2
  cruciate
    knee 844.2
    old 717.89
      anterior 717.83
      posterior 717.84
  deltoid
    ankle 845.01
    shoulder 840.8
  dorsal (spine) 847.1
  ear cartilage 848.8
  elbow 841.9
    and forearm 841.9
    specified site NEC 841.8
  femur (proximal end) 843.9
    distal end 844.9
  fibula (proximal end) 844.9
    distal end 845.00
  fibulocalcaneal 845.02
  finger(s) 842.10
  foot 845.10
    and ankle 845.00
  forearm 841.9
    and elbow 841.9
    specified site NEC 841.8
  glenoid (shoulder) - (see also SLAP lesion)
    840.8
  hand 842.10
  hip 843.9
    and thigh 843.9
  humerus (proximal end) 840.9
    distal end 841.9
  iliofemoral 843.0
  infraspinatus 840.3
  innominate
    acetabulum 843.9
    pubic junction 848.5
    sacral junction 846.1
  internal
    collateral, ankle 845.01
    semilunar cartilage 844.8
      with current tear (see also Tear,
        meniscus) 836.2
      old 717.5
  interphalangeal
    finger 842.13
    toe 845.13
  ischiocapsular 843.1
  jaw (cartilage) (meniscus) 848.1
    old 524.69
  knee 844.9
    and leg 844.9
    old 717.5
      collateral
        lateral 717.81
        medial 717.82
      cruciate
        anterior 717.83
        posterior 717.84
  late effect - see Late, effects (of), sprain
  lateral collateral, knee 844.0
    old 717.81
  leg 844.9
    and knee 844.9
  ligamentum teres femoris 843.8
  low back 846.9
  lumbar (spine) 847.2
  lumbosacral 846.0
    chronic or old 724.6
  mandible 848.1
    old 524.69

Sprain, strain (Continued)
  maxilla 848.1
  medial collateral, knee 844.1
    old 717.82
  meniscus
    jaw 848.1
      old 524.69
    knee 844.8
      with current tear (see also Tear,
        meniscus) 836.2
      old 717.5
    mandible 848.1
      old 524.69
    specified site NEC 848.8
  metacarpal 842.10
    distal 842.12
    proximal 842.11
  metacarpophalangeal 842.12
  metatarsal 845.10
  metatarsophalangeal 845.12
  midcarpal 842.19
  midtarsal 845.19
  multiple sites, except fingers alone or toes
    alone 848.8
  neck 847.0
  nose (septal cartilage) 848.0
  occiput from atlas 847.0
  old - see Derangement, joint
  orbicular, hip 843.8
  patella(r) 844.8
    old 717.89
  pelvis 848.5
  phalanx
    finger 842.10
    toe 845.10
  radiocarpal 842.02
  radiohumeral 841.2
  radioulnar 841.9
    distal 842.09
  radius, radial (proximal end)
    841.9
    and ulna 841.9
      distal 842.09
    collateral 841.0
    distal end 842.00
  recurrent - see Sprain, by site
  rib (cage), without mention of injury to
    sternum 848.3
    involving sternum 848.42
  rotator cuff (capsule) 840.4
  round ligament - see also Injury, internal,
    round ligament
    femur 843.8
  sacral (spine) 847.3
  sacrococcygeal 847.3
  sacroiliac (region) 846.9
    chronic or old 724.6
    ligament 846.1
    specified site NEC 846.8
  sacrospinatus 846.2
  sacrospinous 846.2
  sacrotuberous 846.3
  scaphoid bone, ankle 845.00
  scapula(r) 840.9
  semilunar cartilage (knee) 844.8
    with current tear (see also Tear, meniscus)
      836.2
    old 717.5
  septal cartilage (nose) 848.0
  shoulder 840.9
    and arm, upper 840.9
    blade 840.9
  specified site NEC 848.8
  spine 847.9
    cervical 847.0
    coccyx 847.4
    dorsal 847.1
    lumbar 847.2
    lumbosacral 846.0
      chronic or old 724.6
    sacral 847.3

Sprain, strain (Continued)
  spine (Continued)
    sacroiliac (see also Sprain, sacroiliac) 846.9
      chronic or old 724.6
    thoracic 847.1
  sternoclavicular 848.41
  sternum 848.40
  subglenoid - (see also SLAP lesion) 840.8
  subscapularis 840.5
  supraspinatus 840.6
  symphysis
    jaw 848.1
      old 524.69
    mandibular 848.1
      old 524.69
    pubis 848.5
  talofibular 845.09
  tarsal 845.10
  tarsometatarsal 845.11
  temporomandibular 848.1
    old 524.69
  teres
    ligamentum femoris 843.8
    major or minor 840.8
  thigh (proximal end) 843.9
    and hip 843.9
    distal end 844.9
  thoracic (spine) 847.1
  thorax 848.8
  thumb 842.10
  thyroid cartilage or region 848.2
  tibia (proximal end) 844.9
    distal end 845.00
  tibiofibular
    distal 845.03
    superior 844.3
  toe(s) 845.10
  trachea 848.8
  trapezoid 840.8
  ulna, ulnar (proximal end) 841.9
    collateral 841.1
    distal end 842.00
  ulnohumeral 841.3
  vertebrae (see also Sprain, spine) 847.9
    cervical, cervicodorsal, cervicothoracic
      847.0
  wrist (cuneiform) (scaphoid) (semilunar)
    842.00
  xiphoid cartilage 848.49
Sprengel's deformity (congenital) 755.52
Spring fever 309.23
Sprue 579.1
  celiac 579.0
  idiopathic 579.0
  meaning thrush 112.0
  nontropical 579.0
  tropical 579.1
Spur - see also Exostosis
  bone 726.91
    calcaneal 726.73
  calcaneal 726.73
  iliac crest 726.5
  nose (septum) 478.19
    bone 726.91
  septal 478.19
Spuria placenta - see Placenta, abnormal
Spurway's syndrome (brittle bones and blue
    sclera) 756.51
Sputum, abnormal (amount) (color) (excessive)
    (odor) (purulent) 786.4
  bloody 786.30
Squamous - see also condition
  cell metaplasia
    bladder 596.89
    cervix - see condition
  epithelium in
    cervical canal (congenital) 752.49
    uterine mucosa (congenital) 752.39
  metaplasia
    bladder 596.89
    cervix - see condition

◄ New   ◄▓ Revised   ~~deleted~~ Deleted   ● Use Additional Digit(s)   ▓ Omit code

Squashed nose 738.0
  congenital 754.0
Squeeze, divers' 993.3
Squint (see also Strabismus) 378.9
  accommodative (see also Esotropia) 378.00
  concomitant (see also Heterotropia) 378.30
Stab - see also Wound, open, by site
  internal organs - see Injury, internal, by site,
    with open wound
Staggering gait 781.2
  hysterical 300.11
Staghorn calculus 592.0
Stähl's
  ear 744.29
  pigment line (cornea) 371.11
Stähli's pigment lines (cornea) 371.11
Stain, staining
  meconium 779.84
  port wine 757.32
  tooth, teeth (hard tissues) 521.7
    due to
      accretions 523.6
      deposits (betel) (black) (green) (materia
        alba) (orange) (tobacco) 523.6
      metals (copper) (silver) 521.7
      nicotine 523.6
      pulpal bleeding 521.7
      tobacco 523.6
Stammering (see also Disorder, fluency) 315.35
Standstill
  atrial 426.6
  auricular 426.6
  cardiac (see also Arrest, cardiac) 427.5
  sinoatrial 426.6
  sinus 426.6
  ventricular (see also Arrest, cardiac) 427.5
Stannosis 503
Stanton's disease (melioidosis) 025
Staphylitis (acute) (catarrhal) (chronic)
  (gangrenous) (membranous)
  (suppurative) (ulcerative) 528.3
Staphylococcemia 038.10
  aureus 038.11
  specified organism NEC 038.19
Staphylococcus, staphylococcal - see condition
Staphyloderma (skin) 686.00
Staphyloma 379.11
  anterior, localized 379.14
  ciliary 379.11
  cornea 371.73
  equatorial 379.13
  posterior 379.12
  posticum 379.12
  ring 379.15
  sclera NEC 379.11
Starch eating 307.52
Stargardt's disease 362.75
Starvation (inanition) (due to lack of food) 994.2
  edema 262
  voluntary NEC 307.1
Stasis
  bile (duct) (see also Disease, biliary) 576.8
  bronchus (see also Bronchitis) 490
  cardiac (see also Failure, heart) 428.0
  cecum 564.89
  colon 564.89
  dermatitis (see also Varix, with stasis
    dermatitis) 454.1
  duodenal 536.8
  eczema (see also Varix, with stasis dermatitis)
    454.1
  edema (see also Hypertension, venous) 459.30
  foot 991.4
  gastric 536.3
  ileocecal coil 564.89
  ileum 564.89
  intestinal 564.89
  jejunum 564.89
  kidney 586
  liver 571.9
    cirrhotic - see Cirrhosis, liver

Stasis (Continued)
  lymphatic 457.8
  pneumonia 514
  portal 571.9
  pulmonary 514
  rectal 564.89
  renal 586
    tubular 584.5
  stomach 536.3
  ulcer
    with varicose veins 454.0
    without varicose veins 459.81
  urine NEC (see also Retention, urine)
    788.20
  venous 459.81
State
  affective and paranoid, mixed, organic
    psychotic 294.8
  agitated 307.9
    acute reaction to stress 308.2
  anxiety (neurotic) (see also Anxiety) 300.00
    specified type NEC 300.09
  apprehension (see also Anxiety) 300.00
    specified type NEC 300.09
  climacteric, female 627.2
    following induced menopause 627.4
  clouded
    epileptic (see also Epilepsy) 345.9 ●
    paroxysmal (idiopathic) (see also Epilepsy)
      345.9 ●
  compulsive (mixed) (with obsession)
    300.3
  confusional 298.9
    acute 293.0
      with
        arteriosclerotic dementia 290.41
        presenile brain disease 290.11
        senility 290.3
      alcoholic 291.0
      drug-induced 292.81
    epileptic 293.0
    postoperative 293.9
    reactive (emotional stress) (psychological
      trauma) 298.2
    subacute 293.1
  constitutional psychopathic 301.9
  convulsive (see also Convulsions) 780.39
  depressive NEC 311
    induced by drug 292.84
    neurotic 300.4
  dissociative 300.15
  hallucinatory 780.1
    induced by drug 292.12
  hypercoagulable (primary) 289.81
    secondary 289.82
  hyperdynamic beta-adrenergic circulatory
    429.82
  locked-in 344.81
  menopausal 627.2
    artificial 627.4
    following induced menopause 627.4
  neurotic NEC 300.9
    with depersonalization episode 300.6
  obsessional 300.3
  oneiroid (see also Schizophrenia) 295.4 ●
  panic 300.01
  paranoid 297.9
    alcohol-induced 291.5
    arteriosclerotic 290.42
    climacteric 297.2
    drug-induced 292.11
    in
      presenile brain disease 290.12
      senile brain disease 290.20
    involutional 297.2
    menopausal 297.2
    senile 290.20
    simple 297.0
  postleukotomy 310.0
  pregnant (see also Pregnancy) V22.2
  psychogenic, twilight 298.2

State (Continued)
  psychotic, organic (see also Psychosis,
    organic) 294.9
    mixed paranoid and affective 294.8
    senile or presenile NEC 290.9
    transient NEC 293.9
      with
        anxiety 293.84
        delusions 293.81
        depression 293.83
        hallucinations 293.82
  residual schizophrenic (see also
    Schizophrenia) 295.6 ●
  tension (see also Anxiety) 300.9
  transient organic psychotic 293.9
    anxiety type 293.84
    depressive type 293.83
    hallucinatory type 293.83
    paranoid type 293.81
    specified type NEC 293.89
  twilight
    epileptic 293.0
    psychogenic 298.2
  vegetative (persistent) 780.03
Status (post)
  absence
    epileptic (see also Epilepsy) 345.2
    of organ, acquired (postsurgical) - see
      Absence, by site, acquired
  administration of tPA (rtPA) in a different
    institution within the last 24 hours
    prior to admission to facility V45.88
  anastomosis of intestine (for bypass) V45.3
  anginosus 413.9
  angioplasty, percutaneous transluminal
    coronary V45.82
  ankle prosthesis V43.66
  aortocoronary bypass or shunt V45.81
  arthrodesis V45.4
  artificially induced condition NEC V45.89
  artificial opening (of) V44.9
    gastrointestinal tract NEC V44.4
    specified site NEC V44.8
    urinary tract NEC V44.6
    vagina V44.7
  aspirator V46.0
  asthmaticus (see also Asthma) 493.9 ●
  awaiting organ transplant V49.83
  bariatric surgery V45.86
    complicating pregnancy, childbirth, or the
      puerperium 649.2 ●
  bed confinement V49.84
  breast
    correction V43.82
    implant removal V45.83
    reconstruction V43.82
  cardiac
    device (in situ) V45.00
      carotid sinus V45.09
        fitting or adjustment V53.39
      defibrillator, automatic implantable
        (with synchronous cardiac
        pacemaker) V45.02
      pacemaker V45.01
        fitting or adjustment V53.31
  carotid sinus stimulator V45.09
  cataract extraction V45.61
  chemotherapy V66.2
    current V58.69
  circumcision, female 629.20
  clitorectomy (female genital mutilation type
    I) 629.21
    with excision of labia minora (female
      genital mutilation type II) 629.22
  colonization - see Carrier (suspected) of
  colostomy V44.3
  contraceptive device V45.59
    intrauterine V45.51
    subdermal V45.52
  convulsivus idiopathicus (see also Epilepsy)
    345.3

Status *(Continued)*
    coronary artery bypass or shunt V45.81
    cutting
        female genital 629.20
            specified NEC 629.29
            type I 629.21
            type II 629.22
            type III 629.23
            type IV 629.29
    cystostomy V44.50
        appendico-vesicostomy V44.52
        cutaneous-vesicostomy V44.51
        specifed type NEC V44.59
    defibrillator, automatic implantable cardiac
        (with synchronous cardiac pacemaker)
        V45.02
    delinquent immunization V15.83
    dental crowns V45.84
    dental fillings V45.84
    dental restoration V45.84
    dental sealant V49.82
    dialysis (hemo) (peritoneal) V45.11
    donor V59.9
    do not resuscitate V49.86
    drug therapy or regimen V67.59
        high-risk medication NEC V67.51
    elbow prosthesis V43.62
    embedded
        fragment - *see* Foreign body, retained
        splinter - *see* Foreign body, retained
    enterostomy V44.4
    epileptic, epilepticus (absence) (grand mal)
        (see also Epilepsy) 345.3
        focal motor 345.7●
        partial 345.7●
        petit mal 345.2
        psychomotor 345.7●
        temporal lobe 345.7●
    estrogen receptor
        negative [ER-] V86.1
        positive [ER+] V86.0
    explantation of joint prosthesis NEC V88.29
        hip V88.21
        knee V88.22
    eye (adnexa) surgery V45.69
    female genital
        cutting 629.20
            specified NEC 629.29
            type I 629.21
            type II 629.22
            type III 629.23
            type IV 629.29
        mutilation 629.20
            type I 629.21
            type II 629.22
            type III 629.23
            type IV 629.29
    filtering bleb (eye) (postglaucoma) V45.69
        with rupture or complication 997.99
        postcataract extraction (complication)
            997.99
    finger joint prosthesis V43.69
    foster care V60.81
    gastric
        banding V45.86
            complicating pregnancy, childbirth, or
                the puerperium 649.2●
        bypass for obesity V45.86
            complicating pregnancy, childbirth, or
                the puerperium 649.2●
    gastrostomy V44.1
    grand mal 345.3
    heart valve prosthesis V43.3
    hemodialysis V45.11
    hip prosthesis (joint) (partial) (total) V43.64
        explantation V88.21
    hysterectomy V88.01
        partial with remaining cervical stump
            V88.02
        total V88.01
    ileostomy V44.2

Status *(Continued)*
    infibulation (female genital mutilation type
        III) 629.23
    insulin pump V45.85
    intestinal bypass V45.3
    intrauterine contraceptive device V45.51
    jejunostomy V44.4
    joint prosthesis NEC V43.69
        explantation V88.29
    knee joint prosthesis V43.65
        explantation V88.22
    lacunaris 437.8
    lacunosis 437.8
    lapsed immunization schedule
        V15.83
    low birth weight V21.30
        less than 500 grams V21.31
        500–999 grams V21.32
        1000–1499 grams V21.33
        1500–1999 grams V21.34
        2000–2500 grams V21.35
    lymphaticus 254.8
    malignant neoplasm, ablated or excised - *see*
        History, malignant neoplasm
    marmoratus 333.79
    military deployment V62.22
    mutilation, female 629.20
        type I 629.21
        type II 629.22
        type III 629.23
        type IV 629.29
    nephrostomy V44.6
    neuropacemaker NEC V45.89
        brain V45.89
        carotid sinus V45.09
        neurologic NEC V45.89
    obesity surgery V45.86
        complicating pregnancy, childbirth, or the
            puerperium 649.2●
    organ replacement
        by artificial or mechanical device or
                prosthesis of
            artery V43.4
            artificial skin V43.83
            bladder V43.5
            blood vessel V43.4
            breast V43.82
            eye globe V43.0
            heart
                assist device V43.21
                fully implantable artificial heart
                    V43.22
                valve V43.3
            intestine V43.89
            joint V43.60
                ankle V43.66
                elbow V43.62
                finger V43.69
                hip (partial) (total) V43.64
                knee V43.65
                shoulder V43.61
                specified NEC V43.69
                wrist V43.63
            kidney V43.89
            larynx V43.81
            lens V43.1
            limb(s) V43.7
            liver V43.89
            lung V43.89
            organ NEC V43.89
            pancreas V43.89
            skin (artificial) V43.83
            tissue NEC V43.89
            vein V43.4
        by organ transplant (heterologous)
            (homologous) - *see* Status,
            transplant
    pacemaker
        brain V45.89
        cardiac V45.01
        carotid sinus V45.09

Status *(Continued)*
    pacemaker *(Continued)*
        neurologic NEC V45.89
        specified site NEC V45.89
    percutaneous transluminal coronary
        angioplasty V45.82
    peritoneal dialysis V45.11
    petit mal 345.2
    physical restraints V49.87
    postcommotio cerebri 310.2
    postmenopausal (age related) (natural)
        V49.81
    postoperative NEC V45.89
    postpartum NEC V24.2
        care immediately following delivery
            V24.0
        routine follow-up V24.2
    postsurgical NEC V45.89
    renal dialysis V45.11
        noncompliance V45.12
    respirator [ventilator] V46.11
        encounter
            during
                mechanical failure V46.14
                power failure V46.12
            for weaning V46.13
    retained foreign body - *see* Foreign body,
        retained
    reversed jejunal transposition (for bypass)
        V45.3
    sex reassignment surgery *(see also* Trans-
        sexualism) 302.50
    shoulder prosthesis V43.61
    shunt
        aortocoronary bypass V45.81
        arteriovenous (for dialysis) V45.11
        cerebrospinal fluid V45.2
        vascular NEC V45.89
            aortocoronary (bypass) V45.81
            ventricular (communicating) (for
                drainage) V45.2
    sterilization
        tubal ligation V26.51
        vasectomy V26.52
    subdermal contraceptive device V45.52
    thymicolymphaticus 254.8
    thymicus 254.8
    thymolymphaticus 254.8
    tooth extraction 525.10
    tracheostomy V44.0
    transplant
        blood vessel V42.89
        bone V42.4
            marrow V42.81
        cornea V42.5
        heart V42.1
            valve V42.2
        intestine V42.84
        kidney V42.0
        liver V42.7
        lung V42.6
        organ V42.9
            removal (due to complication,
                failure, rejection or infection)
                V45.87
            specified site NEC V42.89
        pancreas V42.83
        peripheral stem cells V42.82
        skin V42.3
        stem cells, peripheral V42.82
        tissue V42.9
            specified type NEC V42.89
        vessel, blood V42.89
    tubal ligation V26.51
    underimmunization V15.83
    ureterostomy V44.6
    urethrostomy V44.6
    vagina, artificial V44.7
    vascular shunt NEC V45.89
        aortocoronary (bypass) V45.81
    vasectomy V26.52

◄ New   ◄◧ Revised   ~~deleted~~ Deleted   ● Use Additional Digit(s)   ▨ Omit code

Status *(Continued)*
  ventilator [respirator] V46.11
    encounter
      during
        mechanical failure V46.14
        power failure V46.12
      for weaning V46.13
  wheelchair confinement V46.3
  wrist prosthesis V43.63
Stave fracture - *see* Fracture, metacarpus,
  metacarpal bone(s)
Steal
  subclavian artery 435.2
  vertebral artery 435.1
Stealing, solitary, child problem *(see also*
  Disturbance, conduct) 312.1●
Steam burn - *see* Burn, by site
Steatocystoma multiplex 706.2
Steatoma (infected) 706.2
  eyelid (cystic) 374.84
  infected 373.13
Steatorrhea (chronic) 579.8
  with lacteal obstruction 579.2
  idiopathic 579.0
    adult 579.0
    infantile 579.0
  pancreatic 579.4
  primary 579.0
  secondary 579.8
  specified cause NEC 579.8
  tropical 579.1
Steatosis 272.8
  heart *(see also* Degeneration, myocardial)
    429.1
  kidney 593.89
  liver 571.8
Steele-Richardson (-Olszewski) syndrome 333.0
Stein's syndrome (polycystic ovary) 256.4
Stein-Leventhal syndrome (polycystic ovary)
  256.4
Steinbrocker's syndrome *(see also* Neuropathy,
  peripheral, autonomic) 337.9
Steinert's disease 359.21
STEMI (ST elevation myocardial infarction) *(see
  also* - Infarct, myocardium, ST elevation)
  410.9●
Stenocardia *(see also* Angina) 413.9
Stenocephaly 756.0
Stenosis (cicatricial) - *see also* Stricture
  ampulla of Vater 576.2
    with calculus, cholelithiasis, or stones - *see*
      Choledocholithiasis
  anus, anal (canal) (sphincter) 569.2
    congenital 751.2
  aorta (ascending) 747.22
    arch 747.10
    arteriosclerotic 440.0
    calcified 440.0
  aortic (valve) 424.1
    with
      mitral (valve)
        insufficiency or incompetence 396.2
        stenosis or obstruction 396.0
    atypical 396.0
    congenital 746.3
    rheumatic 395.0
      with
        insufficiency, incompetency or
          regurgitation 395.2
          with mitral (valve) disease 396.8
        mitral (valve)
          disease (stenosis) 396.0
          insufficiency or incompetence
            396.2
          stenosis or obstruction 396.0
    specified cause, except rheumatic 424.1
    syphilitic 093.22
  aqueduct of Sylvius (congenital) 742.3
    with spina bifida *(see also* Spina bifida)
      741.0●
    acquired 331.4

Stenosis *(Continued)*
  artery NEC *(see also* Arteriosclerosis*)* 447.1
    basilar - *see* Narrowing, artery, basilar
    carotid (common) (internal) - *see*
      Narrowing, artery, carotid
    celiac 447.4
    cerebral 437.0
      due to
        embolism *(see also* Embolism, brain)
          434.1●
        thrombus *(see also* Thrombosis,
          brain) 434.0●
    extremities 440.20
    precerebral - *see* Narrowing, artery,
      precerebral
    pulmonary (congenital) 747.31
      acquired 417.8
    renal 440.1
    vertebral - *see* Narrowing, artery, vertebral
  bile duct or biliary passage *(see also*
    Obstruction, biliary) 576.2
    congenital 751.61
  bladder neck (acquired) 596.0
    congenital 753.6
  brain 348.89
  bronchus 519.19
    syphilitic 095.8
  cardia (stomach) 537.89
    congenital 750.7
  cardiovascular *(see also* Disease,
    cardiovascular) 429.2
  carotid artery - *see* Narrowing, artery, carotid
  cervix, cervical (canal) 622.4
    congenital 752.49
    in pregnancy or childbirth 654.6●
      affecting fetus or newborn 763.89
      causing obstructed labor 660.2●
        affecting fetus or newborn 763.1
  colon *(see also* Obstruction, intestine) 560.9
    congenital 751.2
  colostomy 569.62
  common bile duct *(see also* Obstruction,
    biliary) 576.2
    congenital 751.61
  coronary (artery) - *see* Arteriosclerosis,
    coronary
  cystic duct *(see also* Obstruction, gallbladder)
    575.2
    congenital 751.61
  due to (presence of) any device, implant, or
    graft classifiable to 996.0–996.5 - *see*
    Complications, due to (presence of)
    any device, implant, or graft classified
    to 996.0–996.5 NEC
  duodenum 537.3
    congenital 751.1
  ejaculatory duct NEC 608.89
  endocervical os - *see* Stenosis, cervix
  enterostomy 569.62
  esophagostomy 530.87
  esophagus 530.3
    congenital 750.3
    syphilitic 095.8
      congenital 090.5
  external ear canal 380.50
    secondary to
      inflammation 380.53
      surgery 380.52
      trauma 380.51
  gallbladder *(see also* Obstruction,
    gallbladder) 575.2
  glottis 478.74
  heart valve (acquired) - *see also* Endocarditis
    congenital NEC 746.89
      aortic 746.3
      mitral 746.5
      pulmonary 746.02
      tricuspid 746.1
  hepatic duct *(see also* Obstruction, biliary)
    576.2
  hymen 623.3

Stenosis *(Continued)*
  hypertrophic subaortic (idiopathic) 425.11
  infundibulum cardiac 746.83
  intestine *(see also* Obstruction, intestine)
    560.9
    congenital (small) 751.1
      large 751.2
  lacrimal
    canaliculi 375.53
    duct 375.56
      congenital 743.65
    punctum 375.52
      congenital 743.65
    sac 375.54
      congenital 743.65
  lacrimonasal duct 375.56
    congenital 743.65
    neonatal 375.55
  larynx 478.74
    congenital 748.3
    syphilitic 095.8
      congenital 090.5
  mitral (valve) (chronic) (inactive) 394.0
    with
      aortic (valve)
        disease (insufficiency) 396.1
        insufficiency or incompetence
          396.1
        stenosis or obstruction 396.0
      incompetency, insufficiency or
        regurgitation 394.2
        with aortic valve disease 396.8
    active or acute 391.1
      with chorea (acute) (rheumatic)
        (Sydenham's) 392.0
    congenital 746.5
    specified cause, except rheumatic 424.0
    syphilitic 093.21
  myocardium, myocardial *(see also*
    Degeneration, myocardial) 429.1
    hypertrophic subaortic (idiopathic)
      425.11
  nares (anterior) (posterior) 478.19
    congenital 748.0
  nasal duct 375.56
    congenital 743.65
  nasolacrimal duct 375.56
    congenital 743.65
    neonatal 375.55
  organ or site, congenital NEC - *see* Atresia
  papilla of Vater 576.2
    with calculus, cholelithiasis, or stones - *see*
      Choledocholithiasis
  pulmonary (artery) (congenital) 747.31
    with ventricular septal defect,
      dextraposition of aorta and
      hypertrophy of right ventricle
      745.2
    acquired 417.8
    infundibular 746.83
    in tetralogy of Fallot 745.2
    subvalvular 746.83
    valve *(see also* Endocarditis, pulmonary)
      424.3
      congenital 746.02
    vein 747.49
      acquired 417.8
    vessel NEC 417.8
  pulmonic (congenital) 746.02
    infundibular 746.83
    subvalvular 746.83
  pylorus (hypertrophic) 537.0
    adult 537.0
    congenital 750.5
    infantile 750.5
  rectum (sphincter) *(see also* Stricture, rectum)
    569.2
  renal artery 440.1
  salivary duct (any) 527.8
  sphincter of Oddi *(see also* Obstruction,
    biliary) 576.2

Stenosis (*Continued*)
spinal 724.00
cervical 723.0
lumbar, lumbosacral (without neurogenic claudication) 724.02
with neurogenic claudication 724.03
nerve (root) NEC 724.9
specified region NEC 724.09
thoracic, thoracolumbar 724.01
stomach, hourglass 537.6
subaortic 746.81
hypertrophic (idiopathic) 425.11
supra (valvular)-aortic 747.22
trachea 519.19
congenital 748.3
syphilitic 095.8
tuberculous (*see also* Tuberculosis) 012.8●
tracheostomy 519.02
tricuspid (valve) (*see also* Endocarditis, tricuspid) 397.0
congenital 746.1
nonrheumatic 424.2
tubal 628.2
ureter (*see also* Stricture, ureter) 593.3
congenital 753.29
urethra (*see also* Stricture, urethra) 598.9
vagina 623.2
congenital 752.49
in pregnancy or childbirth 654.7●
affecting fetus or newborn 763.89
causing obstructed labor 660.2●
affecting fetus or newborn 763.1
valve (cardiac) (heart) (*see also* Endocarditis) 424.90
congenital NEC 746.89
aortic 746.3
mitral 746.5
pulmonary 746.02
tricuspid 746.1
urethra 753.6
valvular (*see also* Endocarditis) 424.90
congenital NEC 746.89
urethra 753.6
vascular graft or shunt 996.1
atherosclerosis - *see* Arteriosclerosis, extremities
embolism 996.74
occlusion NEC 996.74
thrombus 996.74
vena cava (inferior) (superior) 459.2
congenital 747.49
ventricular shunt 996.2
vulva 624.8
Stent jail 996.72
Stercolith (*see also* Fecalith) 560.32
appendix 543.9
Stercoraceous, stercoral ulcer 569.82
anus or rectum 569.41
Stereopsis, defective
with fusion 368.33
without fusion 368.32
Stereotypies NEC 307.3
Sterility
female - *see* Infertility, female
male (*see also* Infertility, male) 606.9
Sterilization, admission for V25.2
status
tubal ligation V26.51
vasectomy V26.52
Sternalgia (*see also* Angina) 413.9
Sternopagus 759.4
Sternum bifidum 756.3
Sternutation 784.99
Steroid
effects (adverse) (iatrogenic)
cushingoid
correct substance properly administered 255.0
overdose or wrong substance given or taken 962.0

Steroid (*Continued*)
effects (*Continued*)
diabetes - *see* Diabetes, secondary
correct substance properly administered 251.8
overdose or wrong substance given or taken 962.0
due to
correct substance properly administered 255.8
overdose or wrong substance given or taken 962.0
fever
correct substance properly administered 780.60
overdose or wrong substance given or taken 962.0
withdrawal
correct substance properly administered 255.41
overdose or wrong substance given or taken 962.0
responder 365.03
Stevens-Johnson disease or syndrome (erythema multiforme exudativum) 695.13
toxic epidermal necrolysis overlap (SJS-TEN overlap syndrome) 695.14
Stewart-Morel syndrome (hyperostosis frontalis interna) 733.3
Sticker's disease (erythema infectiosum) 057.0
Stickler syndrome 759.89
Sticky eye 372.03
Stieda's disease (calcification, knee joint) 726.62
Stiff
back 724.8
neck (*see also* Torticollis) 723.5
Stiff-baby 759.89
Stiff-man syndrome 333.91
Stiffness, joint NEC 719.50
ankle 719.57
back 724.8
elbow 719.52
finger 719.54
hip 719.55
knee 719.56
multiple sites 719.59
sacroiliac 724.6
shoulder 719.51
specified site NEC 719.58
spine 724.9
surgical fusion V45.4
wrist 719.53
Stigmata, congenital syphilis 090.5
Still's disease or syndrome 714.30
adult onset 714.2
Still-Felty syndrome (rheumatoid arthritis with splenomegaly and leukopenia) 714.1
Stillbirth, stillborn NEC 779.9
Stiller's disease (asthenia) 780.79
Stilling-Türk-Duane syndrome (ocular retraction syndrome) 378.71
Stimulation, ovary 256.1
Sting (animal) (bee) (fish) (insect) (jellyfish) (Portuguese man-o-war) (wasp) (venomous) 989.5
anaphylactic shock or reaction 989.5
plant 692.6
Stippled epiphyses 756.59
Stitch
abscess 998.59
burst (in external operation wound) (*see also* Dehiscence) 998.32
internal 998.31
in back 724.5
Stojano's (subcostal) syndrome 098.86
Stokes' disease (exophthalmic goiter) 242.0●
Stokes-Adams syndrome (syncope with heart block) 426.9
Stokvis' (-Talma) disease (enterogenous cyanosis) 289.7

Stomach - *see* condition
Stoma malfunction
colostomy 569.62
cystostomy 596.82
infection 596.81
mechanical 596.82
specified complication NEC 596.83
enterostomy 569.62
esophagostomy 530.87
gastrostomy 536.42
ileostomy 569.62
nephrostomy 997.5
tracheostomy 519.02
ureterostomy 997.5
Stomatitis 528.00
angular 528.5
due to dietary or vitamin deficiency 266.0
aphthous 528.2
bovine 059.11
candidal 112.0
catarrhal 528.00
denture 528.9
diphtheritic (membranous) 032.0
due to
dietary deficiency 266.0
thrush 112.0
vitamin deficiency 266.0
epidemic 078.4
epizootic 078.4
follicular 528.00
gangrenous 528.1
herpetic 054.2
herpetiformis 528.2
malignant 528.00
membranous acute 528.00
monilial 112.0
mycotic 112.0
necrotic 528.1
ulcerative 101
necrotizing ulcerative 101
parasitic 112.0
septic 528.00
specified NEC 528.09
spirochetal 101
suppurative (acute) 528.00
ulcerative 528.00
necrotizing 101
ulceromembranous 101
vesicular 528.00
with exanthem 074.3
Vincent's 101
Stomatocytosis 282.8
Stomatomycosis 112.0
Stomatorrhagia 528.9
Stone(s) - *see also* Calculus
bladder 594.1
diverticulum 594.0
cystine 270.0
heart syndrome (*see also* Failure, ventricular, left) 428.1
kidney 592.0
prostate 602.0
pulp (dental) 522.2
renal 592.0
salivary duct or gland (any) 527.5
ureter 592.1
urethra (impacted) 594.2
urinary (duct) (impacted) (passage) 592.9
bladder 594.1
diverticulum 594.0
lower tract NEC 594.9
specified site 594.8
xanthine 277.2
Stonecutters' lung 502
tuberculous (*see also* Tuberculosis) 011.4●
Stonemasons'
asthma, disease, or lung 502
tuberculous (*see also* Tuberculosis) 011.4●
phthisis (*see also* Tuberculosis) 011.4●

Stoppage
  bowel (*see also* Obstruction, intestine) 560.9
  heart (*see also* Arrest, cardiac) 427.5
  intestine (*see also* Obstruction, intestine) 560.9
  urine NEC (*see also* Retention, urine) 788.20
Storm, thyroid (apathetic) (*see also*
    Thyrotoxicosis) 242.9●
Strabismus (alternating) (congenital)
    (nonparalytic) 378.9
  concomitant (*see also* Heterotropia) 378.30
    convergent (*see also* Esotropia) 378.00
    divergent (*see also* Exotropia) 378.10
  convergent (*see also* Esotropia) 378.00
  divergent (*see also* Exotropia) 378.10
  due to adhesions, scars - *see* Strabismus,
    mechanical
  in neuromuscular disorder NEC 378.73
    intermittent 378.20
      vertical 378.31
  latent 378.40
    convergent (esophoria) 378.41
    divergent (exophoria) 378.42
    vertical 378.43
  mechanical 378.60
    due to
      Brown's tendon sheath syndrome
        378.61
      specified musculofascial disorder NEC
        378.62
  paralytic 378.50
    third or oculomotor nerve (partial) 378.51
      total 378.52
    fourth or trochlear nerve 378.53
    sixth or abducens nerve 378.54
  specified type NEC 378.73
  vertical (hypertropia) 378.31
Strain - *see also* Sprain, by site
  eye NEC 368.13
  heart - *see* Disease, heart
  meaning gonorrhea - *see* Gonorrhea
  on urination 788.65
  physical NEC V62.89
  postural 729.90
  psychological NEC V62.89
Strands
  conjunctiva 372.62
  vitreous humor 379.25
Strangulation, strangulated 994.7
  appendix 543.9
  asphyxiation or suffocation by 994.7
  bladder neck 596.0
  bowel - *see* Strangulation, intestine
  colon - *see* Strangulation, intestine
  cord (umbilical) - *see* Compression, umbilical
    cord
  due to birth injury 767.8
  food or foreign body (*see also* Asphyxia,
    food) 933.1
  hemorrhoids 455.8
    external 455.5
    internal 455.2
  hernia - *see also* Hernia, by site, with
    obstruction
    gangrenous - *see* Hernia, by site, with
      gangrene
  intestine (large) (small) 560.2
    with hernia - *see also* Hernia, by site, with
      obstruction
      gangrenous - *see* Hernia, by site, with
        gangrene
    congenital (small) 751.1
      large 751.2
  mesentery 560.2
  mucus (*see also* Asphyxia, mucus) 933.1
    newborn 770.18
  omentum 560.2
  organ or site, congenital NEC - *see* Atresia
  ovary 620.8
    due to hernia 620.4
  penis 607.89
    foreign body 939.3

Strangulation, strangulated (*Continued*)
  rupture (*see also* Hernia, by site, with
      obstruction) 552.9
    gangrenous (*see also* Hernia, by site, with
      gangrene) 551.9
  stomach, due to hernia (*see also* Hernia, by
    site, with obstruction) 552.9
    with gangrene (*see also* Hernia, by site,
      with gangrene) 551.9
  umbilical cord - *see* Compression, umbilical
    cord
  vesicourethral orifice 596.0
Strangury 788.1
Strawberry
  gallbladder (*see also* Disease, gallbladder)
    575.6
  mark 757.32
  tongue (red) (white) 529.3
Straw itch 133.8
Streak, ovarian 752.0
Strephosymbolia 315.01
  secondary to organic lesion 784.69
Streptobacillary fever 026.1
Streptobacillus moniliformis 026.1
Streptococcemia 038.0
Streptococcicosis - *see* Infection, streptococcal
Streptococcus, streptococcal - *see* condition
Streptoderma 686.00
Streptomycosis - *see* Actinomycosis
Streptothricosis - *see* Actinomycosis
Streptothrix - *see* Actinomycosis
Streptotrichosis - *see* Actinomycosis
Stress 308.9
  fracture - *see* Fracture, stress
  polycythemia 289.0
  reaction (gross) (*see also* Reaction, stress,
    acute) 308.9
Stretching, nerve - *see* Injury, nerve, by site
Striae (albicantes) (atrophicae) (cutis distensae)
    (distensae) 701.3
Striations of nails 703.8
Stricture (*see also* Stenosis) 799.89
  ampulla of Vater 576.2
    with calculus, cholelithiasis, or stones - *see*
      Choledocholithiasis
  anus (sphincter) 569.2
    congenital 751.2
    infantile 751.2
  aorta (ascending) 747.22
    arch 747.10
    arteriosclerotic 440.0
    calcified 440.0
  aortic (valve) (*see also* Stenosis, aortic) 424.1
    congenital 746.3
  aqueduct of Sylvius (congenital) 742.3
    with spina bifida (*see also* Spina bifida)
      741.0●
    acquired 331.4
  artery 447.1
    basilar - *see* Narrowing, artery, basilar
    carotid (common) (internal) - *see*
      Narrowing, artery, carotid
    celiac 447.4
    cerebral 437.0
      congenital 747.81
      due to
        embolism (*see also* Embolism, brain)
          434.1●
        thrombus (*see also* Thrombosis,
          brain) 434.0●
    congenital (peripheral) 747.60
      cerebral 747.81
      coronary 746.85
      gastrointestinal 747.61
      lower limb 747.64
      renal 747.62
      retinal 743.58
      specified NEC 747.69
      spinal 747.82
      umbilical 747.5
      upper limb 747.63

Stricture (*Continued*)
  artery (*Continued*)
    coronary - *see* Arteriosclerosis, coronary
      congenital 746.85
    precerebral - *see* Narrowing, artery,
      precerebral NEC
    pulmonary (congenital) 747.31
      acquired 417.8
    renal 440.1
    vertebral - *see* Narrowing, artery, vertebral
  auditory canal (congenital) (external) 744.02
    acquired (*see also* Stricture, ear canal,
      acquired) 380.50
  bile duct or passage (any) (postoperative)
    (*see also* Obstruction, biliary) 576.2
    congenital 751.61
  bladder 596.89
    congenital 753.6
    neck 596.0
      congenital 753.6
  bowel (*see also* Obstruction, intestine) 560.9
  brain 348.89
  bronchus 519.19
    syphilitic 095.8
  cardia (stomach) 537.89
    congenital 750.7
  cardiac - *see* Disease, heart orifice
    (stomach) 537.89
  cardiovascular (*see also* Disease,
    cardiovascular) 429.2
  carotid artery - *see* Narrowing, artery,
    carotid
  cecum (*see also* Obstruction, intestine) 560.9
  cervix, cervical (canal) 622.4
    congenital 752.49
    in pregnancy or childbirth 654.6●
      affecting fetus or newborn 763.89
      causing obstructed labor 660.2●
        affecting fetus or newborn 763.1
  colon (*see also* Obstruction, intestine)
    560.9
    congenital 751.2
  colostomy 569.62
  common bile duct (*see also* Obstruction,
    biliary) 576.2
    congenital 751.61
  coronary (artery) - *see* Arteriosclerosis,
    coronary
    congenital 746.85
  cystic duct (*see also* Obstruction, gallbladder)
    575.2
    congenital 751.61
  cystostomy 596.83
  digestive organs NEC, congenital 751.8
  duodenum 537.3
    congenital 751.1
  ear canal (external) (congenital) 744.02
    acquired 380.50
      secondary to
        inflammation 380.53
        surgery 380.52
        trauma 380.51
  ejaculatory duct 608.85
  enterostomy 569.62
  esophagostomy 530.87
  esophagus (corrosive) (peptic) 530.3
    congenital 750.3
    syphilitic 095.8
      congenital 090.5
  Eustachian tube (*see also* Obstruction,
    Eustachian tube) 381.60
    congenital 744.24
  fallopian tube 628.2
    gonococcal (chronic) 098.37
      acute 098.17
    tuberculous (*see also* Tuberculosis)
      016.6●
  gallbladder (*see also* Obstruction,
    gallbladder) 575.2
    congenital 751.69
  glottis 478.74

Stricture *(Continued)*
  heart - *see also* Disease, heart
    congenital NEC 746.89
    valve - *see also* Endocarditis
      congenital NEC 746.89
        aortic 746.3
        mitral 746.5
        pulmonary 746.02
        tricuspid 746.1
  hepatic duct *(see also* Obstruction, biliary)
      576.2
  hourglass, of stomach 537.6
  hymen 623.3
  hypopharynx 478.29
  intestine *(see also* Obstruction, intestine) 560.9
    congenital (small) 751.1
      large 751.2
    ischemic 557.1
  lacrimal
    canaliculi 375.53
      congenital 743.65
    punctum 375.52
      congenital 743.65
    sac 375.54
      congenital 743.65
  lacrimonasal duct 375.56
    congenital 743.65
    neonatal 375.55
  larynx 478.79
    congenital 748.3
    syphilitic 095.8
      congenital 090.5
  lung 518.89
  meatus
    ear (congenital) 744.02
      acquired *(see also* Stricture, ear canal,
          acquired) 380.50
      osseous (congenital) (ear) 744.03
        acquired *(see also* Stricture, ear canal,
            acquired) 380.50
    urinarius *(see also* Stricture, urethra) 598.9
      congenital 753.6
  mitral (valve) *(see also* Stenosis, mitral) 394.0
    congenital 746.5
    specified cause, except rheumatic 424.0
  myocardium, myocardial *(see also*
      Degeneration, myocardial) 429.1
    hypertrophic subaortic (idiopathic)
        425.11
  nares (anterior) (posterior) 478.19
    congenital 748.0
  nasal duct 375.56
    congenital 743.65
    neonatal 375.55
  nasolacrimal duct 375.56
    congenital 743.65
    neonatal 375.55
  nasopharynx 478.29
    syphilitic 095.8
  nephrostomy 997.5
  nose 478.19
    congenital 748.0
  nostril (anterior) (posterior) 478.19
    congenital 748.0
  organ or site, congenital NEC - *see* Atresia
  osseous meatus (congenital) (ear) 744.03
    acquired *(see also* Stricture, ear canal,
        acquired) 380.50
  os uteri *(see also* Stricture, cervix) 622.4
  oviduct - *see* Stricture, fallopian tube
  pelviureteric junction 593.3
  pharynx (dilation) 478.29
  prostate 602.8
  pulmonary, pulmonic
    artery (congenital) 747.31
      acquired 417.8
      noncongenital 417.8
    infundibulum (congenital) 746.83
    valve *(see also* Endocarditis, pulmonary)
        424.3
      congenital 746.02

Stricture *(Continued)*
  pulmonary, pulmonic *(Continued)*
    vein (congenital) 747.49
      acquired 417.8
    vessel NEC 417.8
  punctum lacrimale 375.52
    congenital 743.65
  pylorus (hypertrophic) 537.0
    adult 537.0
    congenital 750.5
    infantile 750.5
  rectosigmoid 569.89
  rectum (sphincter) 569.2
    congenital 751.2
    due to
      chemical burn 947.3
      irradiation 569.2
      lymphogranuloma venereum 099.1
    gonococcal 098.7
    inflammatory 099.1
    syphilitic 095.8
    tuberculous *(see also* Tuberculosis) 014.8●
  renal artery 440.1
  salivary duct or gland (any) 527.8
  sigmoid (flexure) *(see also* Obstruction,
      intestine) 560.9
  spermatic cord 608.85
  stoma (following) (of)
    colostomy 569.62
    cystostomy 596.83
    enterostomy 569.62
    esophagostomy 530.87
    gastrostomy 536.42
    ileostomy 569.62
    nephrostomy 997.5
    tracheostomy 519.02
    ureterostomy 997.5
  stomach 537.89
    congenital 750.7
    hourglass 537.6
  subaortic 746.81
    hypertrophic (acquired) (idiopathic)
        425.11
  subglottic 478.74
  syphilitic NEC 095.8
  tendon (sheath) 727.81
  trachea 519.19
    congenital 748.3
    syphilitic 095.8
    tuberculous *(see also* Tuberculosis) 012.8●
  tracheostomy 519.02
  tricuspid (valve) *(see also* Endocarditis,
      tricuspid) 397.0
    congenital 746.1
    nonrheumatic 424.2
  tunica vaginalis 608.85
  ureter (postoperative) 593.3
    congenital 753.29
    tuberculous *(see also* Tuberculosis) 016.2●
  ureteropelvic junction 593.3
    congenital 753.21
  ureterovesical orifice 593.3
    congenital 753.22
  urethra (anterior) (meatal) (organic)
      (posterior) (spasmodic) 598.9
    associated with schistosomiasis *(see also*
        Schistosomiasis) 120.9 *[598.01]*
    congenital (valvular) 753.6
    due to
      infection 598.00
        syphilis 095.8 *[598.01]*
      trauma 598.1
    gonococcal 098.2 *[598.01]*
    gonorrheal 098.2 *[598.01]*
    infective 598.00
    late effect of injury 598.1
    postcatheterization 598.2
    postobstetric 598.1
    postoperative 598.2
    specified cause NEC 598.8
    syphilitic 095.8 *[598.01]*

Stricture *(Continued)*
  urethra *(Continued)*
    traumatic 598.1
    valvular, congenital 753.6
  urinary meatus *(see also* Stricture, urethra)
      598.9
    congenital 753.6
  uterus, uterine 621.5
    os (external) (internal) - *see* Stricture,
        cervix
  vagina (outlet) 623.2
    congenital 752.49
  valve (cardiac) (heart) *(see also* Endocarditis)
      424.90
    congenital (cardiac) (heart) NEC 746.89
      aortic 746.3
      mitral 746.5
      pulmonary 746.02
      tricuspid 746.1
      urethra 753.6
  valvular *(see also* Endocarditis) 424.90
  vascular graft or shunt 996.1
    atherosclerosis - *see* Arteriosclerosis,
        extremities
    embolism 996.74
    occlusion NEC 996.74
    thrombus 996.74
  vas deferens 608.85
    congenital 752.89
  vein 459.2
  vena cava (inferior) (superior) NEC 459.2
    congenital 747.49
  ventricular shunt 996.2
  vesicourethral orifice 596.0
    congenital 753.6
  vulva (acquired) 624.8
Stridor 786.1
  congenital (larynx) 748.3
Stridulous - *see* condition
Strippling of nails 703.8
Stroke 434.91
  apoplectic *(see also* Disease, cerebrovascular,
      acute) 436
  brain - *see* Infarct, brain
  embolic 434.11
  epileptic - *see* Epilepsy
  healed or old V12.54
  heart - *see* Disease, heart
  heat 992.0
  hemorrhagic - *see* Hemorrhage, brain
  iatrogenic 997.02
  in evolution 434.91
  ischemic 434.91
  late effect - *see* Late effect(s) (of)
      cerebrovascular disease
  lightning 994.0
  paralytic - *see* Infarct, brain
  postoperative 997.02
  progressive 435.9
  thrombotic 434.01
Stromatosis, endometrial (M8931/1) 236.0
Strong pulse 785.9
Strongyloides stercoralis infestation 127.2
Strongyloidiasis 127.2
Strongyloidosis 127.2
Strongylus (gibsoni) infestation 127.7
Strophulus (newborn) 779.89
  pruriginosus 698.2
Struck by lighting 994.0
Struma *(see also* Goiter) 240.9
  fibrosa 245.3
  Hashimoto (struma lymphomatosa)
      245.2
  lymphomatosa 245.2
  nodosa (simplex) 241.9
    endemic 241.9
    multinodular 241.1
    sporadic 241.9
    toxic or with hyperthyroidism 242.3●
      multinodular 242.2●
      uninodular 242.1●

◄ New   ◄━ Revised   ~~deleted~~ Deleted   ● Use Additional Digit(s)   ▨ Omit code

Struma *(Continued)*
  nodosa *(Continued)*
    toxicosa 242.3●
      multinodular 242.2●
      uninodular 242.1●
    uninodular 241.0
    ovarii (M9090/0) 220
      and carcinoid (M9091/1) 236.2
      malignant (M9090/3) 183.0
    Riedel's (ligneous thyroiditis) 245.3
    scrofulous *(see also* Tuberculosis) 017.2●
    tuberculous *(see also* Tuberculosis) 017.2●
      abscess 017.2●
      adenitis 017.2●
      lymphangitis 017.2●
      ulcer 017.2●
Strumipriva cachexia *(see also* Hypothyroidism) 244.9
Strümpell-Marie disease or spine (ankylosing spondylitis) 720.0
Strümpell-Westphal pseudosclerosis (hepatolenticular degeneration) 275.1
Stuart's disease (congenital factor X deficiency) *(see also* Defect, coagulation) 286.3
Stuart-Prower factor deficiency (congenital factor X deficiency) *(see also* Defect, coagulation) 286.3
Students' elbow 727.2
Stuffy nose 478.19
Stump - *see also* Amputation
  cervix, cervical (healed) 622.8
Stupor 780.09
  catatonic *(see also* Schizophrenia) 295.2●
  circular *(see also* Psychosis, manic-depressive, circular) 296.7
  manic 296.89
  manic-depressive *(see also* Psychosis, affective) 296.89
  mental (anergic) (delusional) 298.9
  psychogenic 298.8
  reaction to exceptional stress (transient) 308.2
  traumatic NEC - *see also* Injury, intracranial
    with spinal (cord)
      lesion - *see* Injury, spinal, by site
      shock - *see* Injury, spinal, by site
Sturge (-Weber) (-Dimitri) disease or syndrome (encephalocutaneous angiomatosis) 759.6
Sturge-Kalischer-Weber syndrome (encephalocutaneous angiomatosis) 759.6
Stuttering 315.35
  adult onset 307.0
  childhood onset 315.35
  due to late effect of cerebrovascular disease *(see also* Late effect(s) (of) cerebrovascular disease) 438.14
  in conditions classified elsewhere 784.52
Sty, stye 373.11
  external 373.11
  internal 373.12
  meibomian 373.12
Subacidity, gastric 536.8
  psychogenic 306.4
Subacute - *see* condition
Subarachnoid - *see* condition
Subclavian steal syndrome 435.2
Subcortical - *see* condition
Subcostal syndrome 098.86
  nerve compression 354.8
Subcutaneous, subcuticular - *see* condition
Subdelirium 293.1
Subdural - *see* condition
Subendocardium - *see* condition
Subependymoma (M9383/1) 237.5
Suberosis 495.3
Subglossitis - *see* Glossitis
Subhemophilia 286.0
Subinvolution (uterus) 621.1
  breast (postlactational) (postpartum) 611.89
  chronic 621.1
  puerperal, postpartum 674.8●

Sublingual - *see* condition
Sublinguitis 527.2
Subluxation - *see also* Dislocation, by site
  congenital NEC - *see also* Malposition, congenital
    hip (unilateral) 754.32
      with dislocation of other hip 754.35
      bilateral 754.33
    joint
      lower limb 755.69
      shoulder 755.59
      upper limb 755.59
    lower limb (joint) 755.69
    shoulder (joint) 755.59
    upper limb (joint) 755.59
  lens 379.32
    anterior 379.33
    posterior 379.34
  radial head 832.2
  rotary, cervical region of spine - *see* Fracture, vertebra, cervical
Submaxillary - *see* condition
Submersion (fatal) (nonfatal) 994.1
Submissiveness (undue), in child 313.0
Submucous - *see* condition
Subnormal, subnormality
  accommodation *(see also* Disorder, accommodation) 367.9
  mental *(see also* Disability, intellectual) 319
    mild 317
    moderate 318.0
    profound 318.2
    severe 318.1
  temperature (accidental) 991.6
    not associated with low environmental temperature 780.99
Subphrenic - *see* condition
Subscapular nerve - *see* condition
Subseptus uterus 752.35
Subsiding appendicitis 542
Substance abuse in family V61.42
Substernal thyroid *(see also* Goiter) 240.9
  congenital 759.2
Substitution disorder 300.11
Subtentorial - *see* condition
Subtertian
  fever 084.0
  malaria (fever) 084.0
Subthyroidism (acquired) *(see also* Hypothyroidism) 244.9
  congenital 243
Succenturiata placenta - *see* Placenta, abnormal
Succussion sounds, chest 786.7
Sucking thumb, child 307.9
Sudamen 705.1
Sudamina 705.1
Sudanese kala-azar 085.0
Sudden
  death, cause unknown (less than 24 hours) 798.1
    cardiac (SCD)
      family history of V17.41
      personal history of, successfully resuscitated V12.53
    during childbirth 669.9●
    infant 798.0
    puerperal, postpartum 674.9●
  hearing loss NEC 388.2
  heart failure *(see also* Failure, heart) 428.9
  infant death syndrome 798.0
Sudeck's atrophy, disease, or syndrome 733.7
SUDS (Sudden unexplained death) 798.2
Suffocation *(see also* Asphyxia) 799.01
  by
    bed clothes 994.7
    bunny bag 994.7
    cave-in 994.7
    constriction 994.7
    drowning 994.1

Suffocation *(Continued)*
  by *(Continued)*
    inhalation
      food or foreign body *(see also* Asphyxia, food or foreign body) 933.1
      oil or gasoline *(see also* Asphyxia, food or foreign body) 933.1
    overlying 994.7
    plastic bag 994.7
    pressure 994.7
    strangulation 994.7
  during birth 768.1
  mechanical 994.7
Sugar
  blood
    high 790.29
    low 251.2
  in urine 791.5
Suicide, suicidal (attempted)
  by poisoning - *see* Table of Drugs and Chemicals
  ideation V62.84
  risk 300.9
  tendencies 300.9
  trauma NEC *(see also* nature and site of injury) 959.9
Suipestifer infection *(see also* Infection, Salmonella) 003.9
Sulfatidosis 330.0
Sulfhemoglobinemia, sulphemoglobinemia (acquired) (congenital) 289.7
Sumatran mite fever 081.2
Summer - *see* condition
Sunburn 692.71
  dermatitis 692.71
  due to
    other ultraviolet radiation 692.82
    tanning bed 692.82
  first degree 692.71
  second degree 692.76
  third degree 692.77
SUNCT (short lasting unilateral neuralgiform headache with conjunctival injection and tearing) 339.05
Sunken
  acetabulum 718.85
  fontanels 756.0
Sunstroke 992.0
Superfecundation 651.9●
  with fetal loss and retention of one or more fetus(es) 651.6●
  following (elective) fetal reduction 651.7●
Superfetation 651.9●
  with fetal loss and retention of one or more fetus(es) 651.6●
  following (elective) fetal reduction 651.7●
Superinvolution uterus 621.8
Supernumerary (congenital)
  aortic cusps 746.89
  auditory ossicles 744.04
  bone 756.9
  breast 757.6
  carpal bones 755.56
  cusps, heart valve NEC 746.89
    mitral 746.5
    pulmonary 746.09
  digit(s) 755.00
    finger 755.01
    toe 755.02
  ear (lobule) 744.1
  fallopian tube 752.19
  finger 755.01
  hymen 752.49
  kidney 753.3
  lacrimal glands 743.64
  lacrimonasal duct 743.65
  lobule (ear) 744.1
  mitral cusps 746.5
  muscle 756.82
  nipples 757.6

◀ New   ◀◀ Revised   ~~deleted~~ Deleted   ● Use Additional Digit(s)   ▨ Omit code

Supernumerary (Continued)
organ or site NEC - *see* Accessory
ossicles, auditory 744.04
ovary 752.0
oviduct 752.19
pulmonic cusps 746.09
rib 756.3
cervical or first 756.2
syndrome 756.2
roots (of teeth) 520.2
spinal vertebra 756.19
spleen 759.0
tarsal bones 755.67
teeth 520.1
causing crowding 524.31
testis 752.89
thumb 755.01
toe 755.02
uterus 752.2
vagina 752.49
vertebra 756.19
Supervision (of)
contraceptive method previously prescribed
V25.40
intrauterine device V25.42
oral contraceptive (pill) V25.41
specified type NEC V25.49
subdermal implantable contraceptive
V25.43
dietary (for) V65.3
allergy (food) V65.3
colitis V65.3
diabetes mellitus V65.3
food allergy intolerance V65.3
gastritis V65.3
hypercholesterolemia V65.3
hypoglycemia V65.3
intolerance (food) V65.3
obesity V65.3
specified NEC V65.3
lactation V24.1
newborn health
8 to 28 days old V20.32
under 8 days old V20.31
pregnancy - *see* Pregnancy, supervision of
Supplemental teeth 520.1
causing crowding 524.31
Suppression
binocular vision 368.31
lactation 676.5●
menstruation 626.8
ovarian secretion 256.39
renal 586
urinary secretion 788.5
urine 788.5
Suppuration, suppurative - *see also* condition
accessory sinus (chronic) (*see also* Sinusitis)
473.9
adrenal gland 255.8
antrum (chronic) (*see also* Sinusitis,
maxillary) 473.0
bladder (*see also* Cystitis) 595.89
bowel 569.89
brain 324.0
late effect 326
breast 611.0
puerperal, postpartum 675.1●
dental periosteum 526.5
diffuse (skin) 686.00
ear (middle) (*see also* Otitis media) 382.4
external (*see also* Otitis, externa) 380.10
internal 386.33
ethmoidal (sinus) (chronic) (*see also* Sinusitis,
ethmoidal) 473.2
fallopian tube (*see also* Salpingo-oophoritis)
614.2
frontal (sinus) (chronic) (*see also* Sinusitis,
frontal) 473.1
gallbladder (*see also* Cholecystitis, acute)
575.0
gum 523.30

Suppuration, suppurative (Continued)
hernial sac - *see* Hernia, by site
intestine 569.89
joint (*see also* Arthritis, suppurative) 711.0●
labyrinthine 386.33
lung 513.0
mammary gland 611.0
puerperal, postpartum 675.1●
maxilla, maxillary 526.4
sinus (chronic) (*see also* Sinusitis,
maxillary) 473.0
muscle 728.0
nasal sinus (chronic) (*see also* Sinusitis)
473.9
pancreas 577.0
parotid gland 527.2
pelvis, pelvic
female (*see also* Disease, pelvis,
inflammatory) 614.4
acute 614.3
male (*see also* Peritonitis) 567.21
pericranial (*see also* Osteomyelitis) 730.2●
salivary duct or gland (any) 527.2
sinus (nasal) (*see also* Sinusitis) 473.9
sphenoidal (sinus) (chronic) (*see also*
Sinusitis, sphenoidal) 473.3
thymus (gland) 254.1
thyroid (gland) 245.0
tonsil 474.8
uterus (*see also* Endometritis) 615.9
vagina 616.10
wound - *see also* Wound, open, by site,
complicated
dislocation - *see* Dislocation, by site,
compound
fracture - *see* Fracture, by site, open
scratch or other superficial injury - *see*
Injury, superficial, by site
Supraeruption, teeth 524.34
Supraglottitis 464.50
with obstruction 464.51
Suprapubic drainage 596.89
Suprarenal (gland) - *see* condition
Suprascapular nerve - *see* condition
Suprasellar - *see* condition
Supraspinatus syndrome 726.10
Surfer knots 919.8
infected 919.9
Surgery
cosmetic NEC V50.1
breast reconstruction following
mastectomy V51.0
following healed injury or operation
V51.8
hair transplant V50.0
elective V50.9
breast
augmentation or reduction V50.1
reconstruction following mastectomy
V51.0
circumcision, ritual or routine (in absence
of medical indication) V50.2
cosmetic NEC V50.1
ear piercing V50.3
face-lift V50.1
following healed injury or operation
V51.8
hair transplant V50.0
not done because of
contraindication V64.1
patient's decision V64.2
specified reason NEC V64.3
plastic
breast
augmentation or reduction V50.1
reconstruction following mastectomy
V51.0
cosmetic V50.1
face-lift V50.1
following healed injury or operation
V51.8

Surgery (Continued)
plastic (Continued)
repair of scarred tissue (following healed
injury or operation) V51.8
specified type NEC V50.8
previous, in pregnancy or childbirth
cervix 654.6●
affecting fetus or newborn (*see also*
Newborn, affected by) 760.63
causing obstructed labor 660.2●
affecting fetus or newborn 763.1
pelvic soft tissues NEC 654.9●
affecting fetus or newborn (*see also*
Newborn, affected by) 760.63
causing obstructed labor 660.2●
affecting fetus or newborn 763.1
perineum or vulva 654.8●
uterus NEC 654.9●
affecting fetus or newborn (*see also*
Newborn, affected by) 760.63
causing obstructed labor 660.2●
affecting fetus or newborn 763.1
from previous cesarean delivery
654.2●
vagina 654.7●
Surgical
abortion - *see* Abortion, legal
emphysema 998.81
kidney (*see also* Pyelitis) 590.80
operation NEC 799.9
procedures, complication or misadventure -
see Complications, surgical procedure
shock 998.00
Survey
fetal anatomic V28.81
Susceptibility
genetic
to
MEN (multiple endocrine neoplasia)
V84.81
neoplasia
multiple endocrine (MEN) V84.81
neoplasm
malignant, of
breast V84.01
endometrium V84.04
other V84.09
ovary V84.02
prostate V84.03
specified disease NEC V84.89
Suspected condition, ruled out (*see also*
Observation, suspected) V71.9
specified condition NEC V71.89
Suspended uterus, in pregnancy or childbirth
654.4●
affecting fetus or newborn 763.89
causing obstructed labor 660.2●
affecting fetus or newborn 763.1
Sutton's disease 709.09
Sutton and Gull's disease (arteriolar
nephrosclerosis) (*see also* Hypertension,
kidney) 403.90
Suture
burst (in external operation wound) (*see also*
Dehiscence) 998.32
internal 998.31
inadvertently left in operation wound 998.4
removal V58.32
Shirodkar, in pregnancy (with or without
cervical incompetence) 654.5●
Swab inadvertently left in operation wound
998.4
Swallowed, swallowing
difficulty (*see also* Dysphagia) 787.20
foreign body NEC (*see also* Foreign body)
938
Swamp fever 100.89
Swan neck hand (intrinsic) 736.09
Sweat(s), sweating
disease or sickness 078.2
excessive (*see also* Hyperhidrosis) 780.8

◄ New   ◄■ Revised   deleted Deleted   ● Use Additional Digit(s)   Omit code

Sweat(s), sweating *(Continued)*
    fetid 705.89
    fever 078.2
    gland disease 705.9
        specified type NEC 705.89
    miliary 078.2
    night 780.8
Sweeley-Klionsky disease (angiokeratoma
        corporis diffusum) 272.7
Sweet's syndrome (acute febrile neutrophilic
        dermatosis) 695.89
Swelling 782.3
    abdominal (not referable to specific organ)
        789.3●
    adrenal gland, cloudy 255.8
    ankle 719.07
    anus 787.99
    arm 729.81
    breast 611.72
    Calabar 125.2
    cervical gland 785.6
    cheek 784.2
    chest 786.6
    ear 388.8
    epigastric 789.3●
    extremity (lower) (upper) 729.81
    eye 379.92
    female genital organ 625.8
    finger 729.81
    foot 729.81
    glands 785.6
    gum 784.2
    hand 729.81
    head 784.2
    inflammatory - *see* Inflammation
    joint (*see also* Effusion, joint) 719.0●
        tuberculous - *see* Tuberculosis, joint
    kidney, cloudy 593.89
    leg 729.81
    limb 729.81
    liver 573.8
    lung 786.6
    lymph nodes 785.6
    mediastinal 786.6
    mouth 784.2
    muscle (limb) 729.81
    neck 784.2
    nose or sinus 784.2
    palate 784.2
    pelvis 789.3●
    penis 607.83
    perineum 625.8
    rectum 787.99
    scrotum 608.86
    skin 782.2
    splenic (*see also* Splenomegaly) 789.2
    substernal 786.6
    superficial, localized (skin) 782.2
    testicle 608.86
    throat 784.2
    toe 729.81
    tongue 784.2
    tubular (*see also* Disease, renal) 593.9
    umbilicus 789.3●
    uterus 625.8
    vagina 625.8
    vulva 625.8
    wandering, due to Gnathostoma
        (spinigerum) 128.1
    white - *see* Tuberculosis, arthritis
Swift's disease 985.0
Swimmers'
    ear (acute) 380.12
    itch 120.3
Swimming in the head 780.4
Swollen - *see also* Swelling
    glands 785.6
Swyer-James syndrome (unilateral hyperlucent
        lung) 492.8
Swyer's syndrome (XY pure gonadal
        dysgenesis) 752.7

Sycosis 704.8
    barbae (not parasitic) 704.8
    contagiosa 110.0
    lupoid 704.8
    mycotic 110.0
    parasitic 110.0
    vulgaris 704.8
Sydenham's chorea - *see* Chorea, Sydenham's
Sylvatic yellow fever 060.0
Sylvest's disease (epidemic pleurodynia) 074.1
Symblepharon 372.63
    congenital 743.62
Symonds' syndrome 348.2
Sympathetic - *see* condition
Sympatheticotonia (*see also* Neuropathy,
        peripheral, autonomic) 337.9
Sympathicoblastoma (M9500/3)
    specified site - *see* Neoplasm, by site,
        malignant
    unspecified site 194.0
Sympathicogonioma (M9500/3) - *see*
        Sympathicoblastoma
Sympathoblastoma (M9500/3) - *see*
        Sympathicoblastoma
Sympathogonioma (M9500/3) - *see*
        Sympathicoblastoma
Symphalangy (*see also* Syndactylism) 755.10
Symptoms, specified (general) NEC 780.99
    abdomen NEC 789.9
    bone NEC 733.90
    breast NEC 611.79
    cardiac NEC 785.9
    cardiovascular NEC 785.9
    chest NEC 786.9
    cognition 799.59
    development NEC 783.9
    digestive system NEC 787.99
    emotional state NEC 799.29
    eye NEC 379.99
    gastrointestinal tract NEC 787.99
    genital organs NEC
        female 625.9
        male 608.9
    head and neck NEC 784.99
    heart NEC 785.9
    jaw 784.92
    joint NEC 719.60
        ankle 719.67
        elbow 719.62
        foot 719.67
        hand 719.64
        hip 719.65
        knee 719.66
        multiple sites 719.69
        pelvic region 719.65
        shoulder (region) 719.61
        specified site NEC 719.68
        temporomandibular 524.69
        wrist 719.63
    larynx NEC 784.99
    limbs NEC 729.89
    lymphatic system NEC 785.9
    maxilla 784.92
    menopausal 627.2
    metabolism NEC 783.9
    mouth NEC 528.9
    muscle NEC 728.9
    musculoskeletal NEC 781.99
        limbs NEC 729.89
    nervous system NEC 781.99
    neurotic NEC 300.9
    nutrition, metabolism, and development
        NEC 783.9
    pelvis NEC 789.9
        female 625.9
    peritoneum NEC 789.9
    respiratory system NEC 786.9
    skin and integument NEC 782.9
    subcutaneous tissue NEC 782.9
    throat NEC 784.99
    tonsil NEC 784.99

Symptoms, specified *(Continued)*
    urinary system NEC 788.99
    vascular NEC 785.9
Sympus 759.89
Synarthrosis 719.80
    ankle 719.87
    elbow 719.82
    foot 719.87
    hand 719.84
    hip 719.85
    knee 719.86
    multiple sites 719.89
    pelvic region 719.85
    shoulder (region) 719.81
    specified site NEC 719.88
    wrist 719.83
Syncephalus 759.4
Synchondrosis 756.9
    abnormal (congenital) 756.9
    ischiopubic (van Neck's) 732.1
Synchysis (senile) (vitreous humor)
        379.21
    scintillans 379.22
Syncope (near) (pre-) 780.2
    anginosa 413.9
    bradycardia 427.89
    cardiac 780.2
    carotid sinus 337.01
    complicating delivery 669.2●
    due to lumbar puncture 349.0
    fatal 798.1
    heart 780.2
    heat 992.1
    laryngeal 786.2
    tussive 786.2
    vasoconstriction 780.2
    vasodepressor 780.2
    vasomotor 780.2
    vasovagal 780.2
Syncytial infarct - *see* Placenta, abnormal
Syndactylism, syndactyly (multiple sites)
        755.10
    fingers (without fusion of bone) 755.11
        with fusion of bone 755.12
    toes (without fusion of bone) 755.13
        with fusion of bone 755.14
Syndrome - *see also* Disease
    5q minus 238.74
    abdominal
        acute 789.0●
        migraine 346.2●
        muscle deficiency 756.79
    Abercrombie's (amyloid degeneration)
        277.39
    abnormal innervation 374.43
    abstinence
        alcohol 291.81
        drug 292.0
        neonatal 779.5
    Abt-Letterer-Siwe (acute histiocytosis X)
        (M9722/3) 202.5●
    Achard-Thiers (adrenogenital) 255.2
    acid pulmonary aspiration 997.39
        obstetric (Mendelson's) 668.0●
    acquired immune deficiency 042
    acquired immunodeficiency 042
    acrocephalosyndactylism 755.55
    acute abdominal 789.0●
    acute chest 517.3
    acute coronary 411.1
    Adair-Dighton (brittle bones and blue sclera,
        deafness) 756.51
    Adams-Stokes (-Morgagni) (syncope with
        heart block) 426.9
    Addisonian 255.41
    Adie (-Holmes) (pupil) 379.46
    adiposogenital 253.8
    adrenal
        hemorrhage 036.3
        meningococcic 036.3
    adrenocortical 255.3

Syndrome *(Continued)*
  adrenogenital (acquired) (congenital) 255.2
    feminizing 255.2
    iatrogenic 760.79
    virilism (acquired) (congenital) 255.2
  affective organic NEC 293.89
    drug-induced 292.84
  afferent loop NEC 537.89
  African macroglobulinemia 273.3
  Ahumada-Del Castillo (nonpuerperal
      galactorrhea and amenorrhea) 253.1
  air blast concussion - *see* Injury, internal, by
      site
  Alagille 759.89
  Albright (-Martin)
      (pseudohypoparathyroidism) 275.49
  Albright-McCune-Sternberg (osteitis fibrosa
      disseminata) 756.59
  alcohol withdrawal 291.81
  Alder's (leukocyte granulation anomaly)
      288.2
  Aldrich (-Wiskott) (eczema-
      thrombocytopenia) 279.12
  Alibert-Bazin (mycosis fungoides)
      (M9700/3) 202.1●
  Alice in Wonderland 293.89
  alien hand 781.8
  Allen-Masters 620.6
  Alligator baby (ichthyosis congenita) 757.1
  Alport's (hereditary hematuria-nephropathy-
      deafness) 759.89
  Alvarez (transient cerebral ischemia)
      435.9
  alveolar capillary block 516.8
  Alzheimer's 331.0
    with dementia - *see* Alzheimer's,
        dementia
  amnestic (confabulatory) 294.0
    alcohol-induced persisting 291.1
    drug-induced 292.83
    posttraumatic 294.0
  amotivational 292.89
  amyostatic 275.1
  amyotrophic lateral sclerosis 335.20
  androgen insensitivity 259.51
    partial 259.52
  Angelman 759.89
  angina (*see also* Angina) 413.9
  ankyloglossia superior 750.0
  anterior
    chest wall 786.52
    compartment (tibial) 958.8
    spinal artery 433.8●
        compression 721.1
    tibial (compartment) 958.8
  antibody deficiency 279.00
    agammaglobulinemic 279.00
    congenital 279.04
    hypogammaglobulinemic 279.00
  anticardiolipin antibody 289.81
  antimongolism 758.39
  antiphospholipid antibody 289.81
  Anton (-Babinski) (hemiasomatognosia)
      307.9
  anxiety (*see also* Anxiety) 300.00
    organic 293.84
  aortic
    arch 446.7
    bifurcation (occlusion) 444.09
    ring 747.21
  Apert's (acrocephalosyndactyly) 755.55
  Apert-Gallais (adrenogenital) 255.2
  aphasia-apraxia-alexia 784.69
  apical ballooning 429.83
  "approximate answers" 300.16
  arcuate ligament (-celiac axis) 447.4
  arcus aortae 446.7
  arc welders' 370.24
  argentaffin, argentaffinoma 259.2
  Argonz-Del Castillo (nonpuerperal
      galactorrhea and amenorrhea) 253.1

Syndrome *(Continued)*
  Argyll Robertson's (syphilitic) 094.89
    nonsyphilitic 379.45
  Armenian 277.31
  arm-shoulder (*see also* Neuropathy,
      peripheral, autonomic) 337.9
  Arnold-Chiari (*see also* Spina bifida) 741.0●
    type I 348.4
    type II 741.0●
    type III 742.0
    type IV 742.2
  Arrillaga-Ayerza (pulmonary artery sclerosis
      with pulmonary hypertension) 416.0
  arteriomesenteric duodenum occlusion
      537.89
  arteriovenous steal 996.73
  arteritis, young female (obliterative
      brachiocephalic) 446.7
  aseptic meningitis - *see* Meningitis, aseptic
  Asherman's 621.5
  Asperger's 299.8●
  asphyctic (*see also* Anxiety) 300.00
  aspiration, of newborn (massive 770.18)
    meconium 770.12
  ataxia-telangiectasia 334.8
  Audry's (acropachyderma) 757.39
  auriculotemporal 350.8
  autoimmune lymphoproliferative (ALPS)
      279.41
  autosomal - *see also* Abnormal, autosomes
      NEC
    deletion 758.39
      5p 758.31
      22q11.2 758.32
  Avellis' 344.89
  Axenfeld's 743.44
  Ayerza (-Arrillaga) (pulmonary artery
      sclerosis with pulmonary
      hypertension) 416.0
  Baader's (erythema multiforme exudativum)
      695.19
  Baastrup's 721.5
  Babinski (-Vaquez) (cardiovascular syphilis)
      093.89
  Babinski-Fröhlich (adiposogenital
      dystrophy) 253.8
  Babinski-Nageotte 344.89
  Bagratuni's (temporal arteritis) 446.5
  Bakwin-Krida (craniometaphyseal dysplasia)
      756.89
  Balint's (psychic paralysis of visual
      disorientation) 368.16
  Ballantyne (-Runge) (postmaturity) 766.22
  ballooning posterior leaflet 424.0
  Banti's - *see* Cirrhosis, liver
  Bard-Pic's (carcinoma, head of pancreas)
      157.0
  Bardet-Biedl (obesity, polydactyly, and
      intellectual disabilities) 759.89
  Barlow's (mitral valve prolapse) 424.0
  Barlow (-Möller) (infantile scurvy) 267
  Baron Munchausen's 301.51
  Barré-Guillain 357.0
  Barré-Liéou (posterior cervical sympathetic)
      723.2
  Barrett's (chronic peptic ulcer of esophagus)
      530.85
  Bársony-Pólgar (corkscrew esophagus) 530.5
  Bársony-Teschendorf (corkscrew esophagus)
      530.5
  Barth 759.89
  Bartter's (secondary hyperaldosteronism
      with juxtaglomerular hyperplasia)
      255.13
  basal cell nevus 759.89
  Basedow's (exophthalmic goiter) 242.0●
  basilar artery 435.0
  basofrontal 377.04
  Bassen-Kornzweig (abetalipoproteinemia)
      272.5
  Batten-Steinert 359.21

Syndrome *(Continued)*
  battered
    adult 995.81
    baby or child 995.54
    spouse 995.81
  Baumgarten-Cruveilhier (cirrhosis of liver)
      571.5
  Beals 759.82
  Bearn-Kunkel (-Slater) (lupoid hepatitis)
      571.49
  Beau's (*see also* Degeneration, myocardial)
      429.1
  Bechterew-Strümpell-Marie (ankylosing
      spondylitis) 720.0
  Beck's (anterior spinal artery occlusion)
      433.8●
  Beckwith (-Wiedemann) 759.89
  Behçet's 136.1
  Bekhterev-Strümpell-Marie (ankylosing
      spondylitis) 720.0
  Benedikt's 344.89
  Béquez César (-Steinbrinck-Chédiak-
      Higashi) (congenital gigantism of
      peroxidase granules) 288.2
  Bernard-Horner (*see also* Neuropathy,
      peripheral, autonomic) 337.9
  Bernard-Sergent (acute adrenocortical
      insufficiency) 255.41
  Bernhardt-Roth 355.1
  Bernheim's (*see also* Failure, heart) 428.0
  Bertolotti's (sacralization of fifth lumbar
      vertebra) 756.15
  Besnier-Boeck-Schaumann (sarcoidosis) 135
  Bianchi's (aphasia-apraxia-alexia syndrome)
      784.69
  Biedl-Bardet (obesity, polydactyly, and
      intellectual disabilities) 759.89
  Biemond's (obesity, polydactyly, and
      intellectual disabilities) 759.89
  big spleen 289.4
  bilateral polycystic ovarian 256.4
  Bing-Horton's 339.00
  Biörck (-Thorson) (malignant carcinoid)
      259.2
  Birt-Hogg-Dube 759.89
  Blackfan-Diamond (congenital hypoplastic
      anemia) 284.01
  black lung 500
  black widow spider bite 989.5
  bladder neck (*see also* Incontinence, urine)
      788.30
  blast (concussion) - *see* Blast, injury
  blind loop (postoperative) 579.2
  Block-Siemens (incontinentia pigmenti)
      757.33
  Bloch-Sulzberger (incontinentia pigmenti)
      757.33
  Bloom (-Machacek) (-Torre) 757.39
  Blount-Barber (tibia vara) 732.4
  blue
    bloater 491.20
      with
        acute bronchitis 491.22
        exacerbation (acute) 491.21
    diaper 270.0
    drum 381.02
    sclera 756.51
    toe 445.02
  Boder-Sedgwick (ataxia-telangiectasia)
      334.8
  Boerhaave's (spontaneous esophageal
      rupture) 530.4
  Bonnevie-Ullrich 758.6
  Bonnier's 386.19
  Borjeson-Forssman-Lehmann 759.89
  Bouillaud's (rheumatic heart disease) 391.9
  Bourneville (-Pringle) (tuberous sclerosis)
      759.5
  Bouveret (-Hoffmann) (paroxysmal
      tachycardia) 427.2
  brachial plexus 353.0

◀ New   ◀▥ Revised   ~~deleted~~ Deleted   ● Use Additional Digit(s)   ▨ Omit code

Syndrome (Continued)
Brachman-de Lange (Amsterdam dwarf, intellectual disabilities, and brachycephaly) 759.89
bradycardia-tachycardia 427.81
Brailsford-Morquio (dystrophy) (mucopolysaccharidosis IV) 277.5
brain (acute) (chronic) (nonpsychotic) (organic) (with behavioral reaction) (with neurotic reaction) 310.9
with
presenile brain disease (see also Dementia, presenile) 290.10
psychosis, psychotic reaction (see also Psychosis, organic) 294.9
chronic alcoholic 291.2
congenital (see also Disability, intellectual) 319
postcontusional 310.2
posttraumatic
nonpsychotic 310.2
psychotic 293.9
acute 293.0
chronic (see also Psychosis, organic) 294.8
subacute 293.1
psycho-organic (see also Syndrome, psycho-organic) 310.9
psychotic (see also Psychosis, organic) 294.9
senile (see also Dementia, senile) 290.0
branchial arch 744.41
Brandt's (acrodermatitis enteropathica) 686.8
Brennemann's 289.2
Briquet's 300.81
Brissaud-Meige (infantile myxedema) 244.9
broad ligament laceration 620.6
Brock's (atelectasis due to enlarged lymph nodes) 518.0
broken heart 429.83
Brown's tendon sheath 378.61
Brown-Séquard 344.89
brown spot 756.59
Brugada 746.89
Brugsch's (acropachyderma) 757.39
bubbly lung 770.7
Buchem's (hyperostosis corticalis) 733.3
Budd-Chiari (hepatic vein thrombosis) 453.0
Büdinger-Ludloff-Läwen 717.89
bulbar 335.22
lateral (see also Disease, cerebrovascular, acute) 436
Bullis fever 082.8
bundle of Kent (anomalous atrioventricular excitation) 426.7
Bürger-Grutz (essential familial hyperlipemia) 272.3
Burke's (pancreatic insufficiency and chronic neutropenia) 577.8
Burnett's (milk-alkali) 275.42
Burnier's (hypophyseal dwarfism) 253.3
burning feet 266.2
Bywaters' 958.5
Caffey's (infantile cortical hyperostosis) 756.59
Calvé-Legg-Perthes (osteochrondrosis, femoral capital) 732.1
Caplan (-Colinet) syndrome 714.81
capsular thrombosis (see also Thrombosis, brain) 434.0●
carbohydrate-deficient glycoprotein (CDGS) 271.8
carcinogenic thrombophlebitis 453.1
carcinoid 259.2
cardiac asthma (see also Failure, ventricular, left) 428.1
cardiacos negros 416.0
cardiofaciocutaneous 759.89
cardiopulmonary obesity 278.03
cardiorenal (see also Hypertension, cardiorenal) 404.90

Syndrome (Continued)
cardiorespiratory distress (idiopathic), newborn 769
cardiovascular renal (see also Hypertension, cardiorenal) 404.90
cardiovasorenal 272.7
Carini's (ichthyosis congenita) 757.1
carotid
artery (internal) 435.8
body or sinus 337.01
carpal tunnel 354.0
Carpenter's 759.89
Cassidy (-Scholte) (malignant carcinoid) 259.2
cat-cry 758.31
cauda equina 344.60
causalgia 355.9
lower limb 355.71
upper limb 354.4
cavernous sinus 437.6
celiac 579.0
artery compression 447.4
axis 447.4
central pain 338.0
cerebellomedullary malformation (see also Spina bifida) 741.0●
cerebral gigantism 253.0
cerebrohepatorenal 759.89
cervical (root) (spine) NEC 723.8
disc 722.71
posterior, sympathetic 723.2
rib 353.0
sympathetic paralysis 337.09
traumatic (acute) NEC 847.0
cervicobrachial (diffuse) 723.3
cervicocranial 723.2
cervicodorsal outlet 353.2
Céstan's 344.89
Céstan (-Raymond) 433.8●
Céstan-Chenais 344.89
chancriform 114.1
Charcôt's (intermittent claudication) 443.9
angina cruris 443.9
due to atherosclerosis 440.21
Charcôt-Marie-Tooth 356.1
Charcôt-Weiss-Baker 337.01
CHARGE association 759.89
Cheadle (-Möller) (-Barlow) (infantile scurvy) 267
Chédiak-Higashi (-Steinbrinck) (congenital gigantism of peroxidase granules) 288.2
chest wall 786.52
Chiari's (hepatic vein thrombosis) 453.0
Chiari-Frommel 676.6●
chiasmatic 368.41
Chilaiditi's (subphrenic displacement, colon) 751.4
chondroectodermal dysplasia 756.55
chorea-athetosis-agitans 275.1
Christian's (chronic histiocytosis X) 277.89
chromosome 4 short arm deletion 758.39
chronic pain 338.4
Churg-Strauss 446.4
Clarke-Hadfield (pancreatic infantilism) 577.8
Claude's 352.6
Claude Bernard-Horner (see also Neuropathy, peripheral, autonomic) 337.9
Clérambault's
automatism 348.89
erotomania 297.8
Clifford's (postmaturity) 766.22
climacteric 627.2
Clouston's (hidrotic ectodermal dysplasia) 757.31
clumsiness 315.4
Cockayne's (microencephaly and dwarfism) 759.89
Cockayne-Weber (epidermolysis bullosa) 757.39

Syndrome (Continued)
Coffin-Lowry 759.89
Cogan's (nonsyphilitic interstitial keratitis) 370.52
cold injury (newborn) 778.2
Collet (-Sicard) 352.6
combined immunity deficiency 279.2
compartment(al) (anterior) (deep) (posterior) 958.8
nontraumatic
abdomen 729.73
arm 729.71
buttock 729.72
fingers 729.71
foot 729.72
forearm 729.71
hand 729.71
hip 729.72
leg 729.72
lower extremity 729.72
shoulder 729.71
specified site NEC 729.79
thigh 729.72
toes 729.72
upper extremity 729.71
wrist 729.71
post-surgical (see also Syndrome, compartment, non-traumatic) 998.89
traumatic 958.90
abdomen 958.93
arm 958.91
buttock 958.92
fingers 958.91
foot 958.92
forearm 958.91
hand 958.91
hip 958.92
leg 958.92
lower extremity 958.92
shoulder 958.91
specified site NEC 958.99
thigh 958.92
tibial 958.92
toes 958.92
upper extremity 958.91
wrist 958.91
complex regional pain - see also Dystrophy, sympathetic
type I - see Dystrophy, sympathetic (posttraumatic) (reflex)
type II - see Causalgia
compression 958.5
cauda equina 344.60
with neurogenic bladder 344.61
concussion 310.2
congenital
affecting more than one system 759.7
specified type NEC 759.89
congenital central alveolar hypoventilation 327.25
facial diplegia 352.6
muscular hypertrophy-cerebral 759.89
congestion-fibrosis (pelvic) 625.5
conjunctivourethrosynovial 099.3
Conn (-Louis) (primary aldosteronism) 255.12
Conradi (-Hünermann) (chondrodysplasia calcificans congenita) 756.59
conus medullaris 336.8
Cooke-Apert-Gallais (adrenogenital) 255.2
Cornelia de Lange's (Amsterdam dwarf, intellectual disabilities, and brachycephaly) 759.8
coronary insufficiency or intermediate 411.1
cor pulmonale 416.9
corticosexual 255.2
Costen's (complex) 524.60
costochondral junction 733.6
costoclavicular 353.0
costovertebral 253.0

Syndrome *(Continued)*
  Cotard's (paranoia) 297.1
  Cowden 759.6
  craniovertebral 723.2
  Creutzfeldt-Jakob 046.19
    with dementia
      with behavioral disturbance 046.19
        [294.11]
      without behavioral disturbance 046.19
        [294.10]
    variant 046.11
      with dementia
        with behavioral disturbance 046.11
          [294.11]
        without behavioral disturbance
          046.11 *[294.10]*
  crib death 798.0
  cricopharyngeal 787.20
  cri-du-chat 758.31
  Crigler-Najjar (congenital
    hyperbilirubinemia) 277.4
  crocodile tears 351.8
  Cronkhite-Canada 211.3
  croup 464.4
  CRST (cutaneous systemic sclerosis) 710.1
  crush 958.5
  crushed lung *(see also* Injury, internal, lung)
    861.20
  Cruveilhier-Baumgarten (cirrhosis of liver)
    571.5
  cubital tunnel 354.2
  Cuiffini-Pancoast (M8010/3) (carcinoma,
    pulmonary apex) 162.3
  Curschmann (-Batten) (-Steinert) 359.21
  Cushing's (iatrogenic) (idiopathic) (pituitary
    basophilism) (pituitary-dependent)
    255.0
    overdose or wrong substance given or
      taken 962.0
  Cyriax's (slipping rib) 733.99
  cystic duct stump 576.0
  Da Costa's (neurocirculatory asthenia) 306.2
  Dameshek's (erythroblastic anemia) 282.49
  Dana-Putnam (subacute combined sclerosis
    with pernicious anemia) 281.0 *[336.2]*
  Danbolt (-Closs) (acrodermatitis
    enteropathica) 686.8
  Dandy-Walker (atresia, foramen of
    Magendie) 742.3
    with spina bifida *(see also* Spina bifida)
      741.0●
  Danlos' 756.83
  Davies-Colley (slipping rib) 733.99
  dead fetus 641.3●
  defeminization 255.2
  defibrination *(see also* Fibrinolysis) 286.6
  Degos' 447.8
  Deiters' nucleus 386.19
  Déjérine-Roussy 338.0
  Déjérine-Thomas 333.0
  de Lange's (Amsterdam dwarf, intellectual
    disabilities, and brachycephaly)
    (Cornelia) 759.89
  Del Castillo's (germinal aplasia) 606.0
  deletion chromosomes 758.39
  delusional
    induced by drug 292.11
  dementia-aphonia, of childhood *(see also*
    Psychosis, childhood) 299.1●
  demyelinating NEC 341.9
  denial visual hallucination 307.9
  depersonalization 300.6
  de Quervain's 259.51
  Dercum's (adiposis dolorosa) 272.8
  de Toni-Fanconi (-Debre) (cystinosis) 270.0
  diabetes-dwarfism-obesity (juvenile) 258.1
  diabetes mellitus-hypertension-nephrosis
    250.4● *[581.81]*
    due to secondary diabetes 249.4●
      [581.81]
  diabetes mellitus in newborn infant 775.1

Syndrome *(Continued)*
  diabetes-nephrosis 250.4● *[581.81]*
    due to secondary diabetes 249.4● *[581.81]*
  diabetic amyotrophy 250.6● *[353.5]*
    due to secondary diabetes 249.6● *[353.5]*
  Diamond-Blackfan (congenital hypoplastic
    anemia) 284.01
  Diamond-Gardner (autoerythrocyte
    sensitization) 287.2
  DIC (diffuse or disseminated intravascular
    coagulopathy) *(see also* Fibrinolysis)
    286.6
  diencephalohypophyseal NEC 253.8
  diffuse cervicobrachial 723.3
  diffuse obstructive pulmonary 496
  DiGeorge's (thymic hypoplasia) 279.11
  Dighton's 756.51
  Di Guglielmo's (erythremic myelosis)
    (M9841/3) 207.0●
  disequilibrium 276.9
  disseminated platelet thrombosis 446.6
  Ditthomska 307.81
  Doan-Wiseman (primary splenic
    neutropenia) 289.53
  Döhle body-panmyelopathic 288.2
  Donohue's (leprechaunism) 259.8
  dorsolateral medullary *(see also* Disease,
    cerebrovascular, acute) 436
  double athetosis 333.71
  double whammy 360.81
  Down's (mongolism) 758.0
  Dresbach's (elliptocytosis) 282.1
  Dressler's (postmyocardial infarction) 411.0
    hemoglobinuria 283.2
    postcardiotomy 429.4
  drug withdrawal, infant, of dependent
    mother 779.5
  dry skin 701.1
    eye 375.15
  DSAP (disseminated superficial actinic
    porokeratosis) 692.75
  Duane's (retraction) 378.71
  Duane-Stilling-Türk (ocular retraction
    syndrome) 378.71
  Dubin-Johnson (constitutional
    hyperbilirubinemia) 277.4
  Dubin-Sprinz (constitutional
    hyperbilirubinemia) 277.4
  Duchenne's 335.22
  due to abnormality
    autosomal NEC *(see also* Abnormal,
      autosomes NEC) 758.5
      13 758.1
      18 758.2
      21 or 22 758.0
      D_1 758.1
      E_3 758.2
      G 758.0
    chromosomal 758.89
      sex 758.81
  dumping 564.2
    nonsurgical 536.8
  Duplay's 726.2
  Dupré's (meningism) 781.6
  Dyke-Young (acquired macrocytic hemolytic
    anemia) 283.9
  dyspraxia 315.4
  dystocia, dystrophia 654.9●
  Eagle-Barret 756.71
  Eales' 362.18
  Eaton-Lambert *(see also* Syndrome,
    Lambert-Eaton) 358.30
  Ebstein's (downward displacement,
    tricuspid valve into right ventricle)
    746.2
  ectopic ACTH secretion 255.0
  eczema-thrombocytopenia 279.12
  Eddowes' (brittle bones and blue sclera)
    756.51
  Edwards' 758.2
  efferent loop 537.89

Syndrome *(Continued)*
  effort (aviators') (psychogenic) 306.2
  Ehlers-Danlos 756.83
  Eisenmenger's (ventricular septal defect)
    745.4
  Ekbom's (restless legs) 333.94
  Ekman's (brittle bones and blue sclera)
    756.51
  electric feet 266.2
  Elephant man 237.71
  Ellison-Zollinger (gastric hypersecretion
    with pancreatic islet cell tumor) 251.5
  Ellis-van Creveld (chondroectodermal
    dysplasia) 756.55
  embryonic fixation 270.2
  empty sella (turcica) 253.8
  endocrine-hypertensive 255.3
  Engel-von Recklinghausen (osteitis fibrosa
    cystica) 252.01
  enteroarticular 099.3
  entrapment - *see* Neuropathy, entrapment
  eosinophilia myalgia 710.5
  epidemic vomiting 078.82
  Epstein's - *see* Nephrosis
  Erb (-Oppenheim)-Goldflam 358.00
  Erdheim-Chester 277.89
  Erdheim's (acromegalic macrospondylitis)
    253.0
  Erlacher-Blount (tibia vara) 732.4
  erythrocyte fragmentation 283.19
  euthyroid sick 790.94
  Evans' (thrombocytopenic purpura) 287.32
  excess cortisol, iatrogenic 255.0
  exhaustion 300.5
  extrapyramidal 333.90
  eyelid-malar-mandible 756.0
  eye retraction 378.71
  Faber's (achlorhydric anemia) 280.9
  Fabry (-Anderson) (angiokeratoma corporis
    diffusum) 272.7
  facet 724.8
  Fallot's 745.2
  falx *(see also* Hemorrhage, brain) 431
  familial eczema-thrombocytopenia 279.12
  Fanconi's (anemia) (congenital
    pancytopenia) 284.09
  Fanconi (-de Toni) (-Debré) (cystinosis) 270.0
  Farber (-Uzman) (disseminated
    lipogranulomatosis) 272.8
  fatigue NEC 300.5
    chronic 780.71
  faulty bowel habit (idiopathic megacolon)
    564.7
  FDH (focal dermal hypoplasia) 757.39
  fecal reservoir 560.39
  Feil-Klippel (brevicollis) 756.16
  Felty's (rheumatoid arthritis with
    splenomegaly and leukopenia) 714.1
  fertile eunuch 257.2
  fetal alcohol 760.71
    late effect 760.71
  fibrillation-flutter 427.32
  fibrositis (periarticular) 729.0
  Fiedler's (acute isolated myocarditis) 422.91
  Fiessinger-Leroy (-Reiter) 099.3
  Fiessinger-Rendu (erythema multiforme
    exudativum) 695.19
  first arch 756.0
  Fisher's 357.0
  fish odor 270.8
  Fitz's (acute hemorrhagic pancreatitis) 577.0
  Fitz-Hugh and Curtis 098.86
    due to
      Chlamydia trachomatis 099.56
      Neisseria gonorrhoeae (gonococcal
        peritonitis) 098.86
  Flajani (-Basedow) (exophthalmic goiter)
    242.0●
  flat back
    acquired 737.29
    postprocedural 738.5

◀ New   ◀▥ Revised   ~~deleted~~ Deleted   ● Use Additional Digit(s)   ▨ Omit code

Syndrome *(Continued)*
floppy
  infant 781.99
  iris 364.81
  valve (mitral) 424.0
flush 259.2
Foix-Alajouanine 336.1
Fong's (hereditary osteo-onychodysplasia)
  756.89
foramen magnum 348.4
Forbes-Albright (nonpuerperal amenorrhea
  and lactation associated with pituitary
  tumor) 253.1
Foster-Kennedy 377.04
Foville's (peduncular) 344.89
fragile X 759.83
Franceschetti's (mandibulofacial dysostosis)
  756.0
Fraser's 759.89
Freeman-Sheldon 759.89
Frey's (auriculotemporal) 705.22
Friderichsen-Waterhouse 036.3
Friedrich-Erb-Arnold (acropachyderma)
  757.39
Fröhlich's (adiposogenital dystrophy) 253.8
Froin's 336.8
Frommel-Chiari 676.6●
frontal lobe 310.0
Fukuhara 277.87
Fuller Albright's (osteitis fibrosa
  disseminata) 756.59
functional
  bowel 564.9
  prepubertal castrate 752.89
Gaisböck's (polycythemia hypertonica)
  289.0
ganglion (basal, brain) 333.90
  geniculi 351.1
Ganser's, hysterical 300.16
Gardner-Diamond (autoerythrocyte
  sensitization) 287.2
gastroesophageal junction 530.0
gastroesophageal laceration-hemorrhage
  530.7
gastrojejunal loop obstruction 537.89
Gayet-Wernicke's (superior hemorrhagic
  polioencephalitis) 265.1
Gee-Herter-Heubner (nontropical sprue)
  579.0
Gélineau's *(see also* Narcolepsy) 347.00
genito-anorectal 099.1
Gerhardt's (vocal cord paralysis) 478.30
Gerstmann's (finger agnosia) 784.69
Gerstmann-Sträussler-Scheinker (GSS) 046.71
Gianotti Crosti 057.8
  due to known virus - *see* Infection, virus
  due to unknown virus 057.8
Gilbert's 277.4
Gilford (-Hutchinson) (progeria) 259.8
Gilles de la Tourette's 307.23
Gillespie's (dysplasia oculodentodigitalis)
  759.89
Glénard's (enteroptosis) 569.89
Glinski-Simmonds (pituitary cachexia) 253.2
glucuronyl transferase 277.4
glue ear 381.20
Goldberg (-Maxwell) (-Morris) (testicular
  feminization) 259.51
Goldenhar's (oculoauriculovertebral
  dysplasia) 756.0
Goldflam-Erb 358.00
Goltz-Gorlin (dermal hypoplasia) 757.39
Goodpasture's (pneumorenal) 446.21
Good's 279.06
Gopalan's (burning feet) 266.2
Gorlin-Chaudhry-Moss 759.89
Gorlin's 759.89
Gougerot (-Houwer)-Sjögren
  (keratoconjunctivitis sicca) 710.2
Gougerot-Blum (pigmented purpuric
  lichenoid dermatitis) 709.1

Syndrome *(Continued)*
Gougerot-Carteaud (confluent reticulate
  papillomatosis) 701.8
Gouley's (constrictive pericarditis) 423.2
Gowers' (vasovagal attack) 780.2
Gowers-Paton-Kennedy 377.04
Gradenigo's 383.02
Gray or grey (chloramphenicol) (newborn)
  779.4
Greig's (hypertelorism) 756.0
GSS (Gerstmann-Sträussler-Scheinker) 046.71
Gubler-Millard 344.89
Guérin-Stern (arthrogryposis multiplex
  congenita) 754.89
Guillain-Barré (-Strohl) 357.0
Gunn's (jaw-winking syndrome) 742.8
Günther's (congenital erythropoietic
  porphyria) 277.1
gustatory sweating 350.8
H₃O 759.81
Hadfield-Clarke (pancreatic infantilism)
  577.8
Haglund-Läwen-Fründ 717.89
hair tourniquet - *see also* Injury, superficial,
  by site
  finger 915.8
    infected 915.9
  penis 911.8
    infected 911.9
  toe 917.8
    infected 917.9
hairless women 257.8
Hallermann-Strieff 756.0
Hallervorden-Spatz 333.0
Hamman's (spontaneous mediastinal
  emphysema) 518.1
Hamman-Rich (diffuse interstitial
  pulmonary fibrosis) 516.33
Hand-Schüller-Christian (chronic
  histiocytosis X) 277.89
hand-foot 693.0
Hanot-Chauffard (-Troisier) (bronze
  diabetes) 275.01
Harada's 363.22
Hare's (M8010/3) (carcinoma, pulmonary
  apex) 162.3
Harkavy's 446.0
harlequin color change 779.89
Harris' (organic hyperinsulinism) 251.1
Hart's (pellagra-cerebellar ataxia-renal
  aminoaciduria) 270.0
Hayem-Faber (achlorhydric anemia) 280.9
Hayem-Widal (acquired hemolytic jaundice)
  283.9
headache - *see* Headache, syndrome
Heberden's (angina pectoris) 413.9
Hedinger's (malignant carcinoid) 259.2
Hegglin's 288.2
Heller's (infantile psychosis) *(see also*
  Psychosis, childhood) 299.1●
H.E.L.L.P. 642.5●
hemolytic-uremic (adult) (child) 283.11
hemophagocytic 288.4
  infection-associated 288.4
Hench-Rosenberg (palindromic arthritis) *(see
  also* Rheumatism, palindromic) 719.3●
Henoch-Schönlein (allergic purpura) 287.0
hepatic flexure 569.89
hepatopulmonary 573.5
hepatorenal 572.4
  due to a procedure 997.49
  following delivery 674.8●
hepatourologic 572.4
Herrick's (hemoglobin S disease) 282.61
Herter (-Gee) (nontropical sprue) 579.0
Heubner-Herter (nontropical sprue) 579.0
Heyd's (hepatorenal) 572.4
HHHO 759.81
high grade myelodysplastic 238.73
  with 5q deletion 238.73
Hilger's 337.09

Syndrome *(Continued)*
histiocytic 288.4
Hoffa (-Kastert) (liposynovitis prepatellaris)
  272.8
Hoffmann's 244.9 [359.5]
Hoffmann-Bouveret (paroxysmal
  tachycardia) 427.2
Hoffmann-Werdnig 335.0
Holländer-Simons (progressive
  lipodystrophy) 272.6
Holmes' (visual disorientation) 368.16
Holmes-Adie 379.46
Hoppe-Goldflam 358.00
Horner's *(see also* Neuropathy, peripheral,
  autonomic) 337.9
  traumatic - *see* Injury, nerve, cervical
    sympathetic
hospital addiction 301.51
hungry bone 275.5
Hunt's (herpetic geniculate ganglionitis)
  053.11
  dyssynergia cerebellaris myoclonica 334.2
Hunter (-Hurler) (mucopolysaccharidosis II)
  277.5
hunterian glossitis 529.4
Hurler (-Hunter) (mucopolysaccharidosis II)
  277.5
Hutchinson's incisors or teeth 090.5
Hutchinson-Boeck (sarcoidosis) 135
Hutchinson-Gilford (progeria) 259.8
hydralazine
  correct substance properly administered
    695.4
  overdose or wrong substance given or
    taken 972.6
hydraulic concussion (abdomen) *(see also*
  Injury, internal, abdomen) 868.00
hyperabduction 447.8
hyperactive bowel 564.9
hyperaldosteronism with hypokalemic
  alkalosis (Bartter's) 255.13
hypercalcemic 275.42
hypercoagulation NEC 289.89
hypereosinophilic (idiopathic) 288.3
hyperkalemic 276.7
hyperkinetic - *see also* Hyperkinesia, heart
  429.82
hyperlipemia-hemolytic anemia-icterus
  571.1
hypermobility 728.5
hypernatremia 276.0
hyperosmolarity 276.0
hyperperfusion 997.01
hypersomnia-bulimia 349.89
hypersplenic 289.4
hypersympathetic *(see also* Neuropathy,
  peripheral, autonomic) 337.9
hypertransfusion, newborn 776.4
hyperventilation, psychogenic 306.1
hyperviscosity (of serum) NEC 273.3
  polycythemic 289.0
  sclerothymic 282.8
hypoglycemic (familial) (neonatal) 251.2
  functional 251.1
hypokalemic 276.8
hypophyseal 253.8
hypophyseothalamic 253.8
hypopituitarism 253.2
hypoplastic left heart 746.7
hypopotassemia 276.8
hyposmolality 276.1
hypotension, maternal 669.2●
hypothenar hammer 443.89
hypotonia-hypomentia-hypogonadism-
  obesity 759.81
ICF (intravascular coagulation-fibrinolysis)
  (see also Fibrinolysis) 286.6
idiopathic cardiorespiratory distress,
  newborn 769
idiopathic nephrotic (infantile) 581.9
iliotibial band 728.89

◄ New ◄▥ Revised ~~deleted~~ Deleted ● Use Additional Digit(s) ▥ Omit code **481**

Syndrome (Continued)

Imerslund (-Gräsbeck) (anemia due to familial selective vitamin B_{12} malabsorption) 281.1
immobility (paraplegic) 728.3
immune reconstitution inflammatory (IRIS) 995.90
immunity deficiency, combined 279.2
impending coronary 411.1
impingement
    shoulder 726.2
    vertebral bodies 724.4
inappropriate secretion of antidiuretic hormone (ADH) 253.6
incomplete
    mandibulofacial 756.0
infant
    death, sudden (SIDS) 798.0
    Hercules 255.2
    of diabetic mother 775.0
    shaken 995.55
infantilism 253.3
inferior vena cava 459.2
influenza-like (see also Influenza) 487.1
inspissated bile, newborn 774.4
insufficient sleep 307.44
intermediate coronary (artery) 411.1
internal carotid artery (see also Occlusion, artery, carotid) 433.1●
interspinous ligament 724.8
intestinal
    carcinoid 259.2
    gas 787.3
    knot 560.2
intraoperative floppy iris (IFIS) 364.81
intravascular
    coagulation-fibrinolysis (ICF) (see also Fibrinolysis) 286.6
    coagulopathy (see also Fibrinolysis) 286.6
inverted Marfan's 759.89
IRDS (idiopathic respiratory distress, newborn) 769
irritable
    bowel 564.1
    heart 306.2
    weakness 300.5
ischemic bowel (transient) 557.9
    chronic 557.1
    due to mesenteric artery insufficiency 557.1
Itsenko-Cushing (pituitary basophilism) 255.0
IVC (intravascular coagulopathy) (see also Fibrinolysis) 286.6
Ivemark's (asplenia with congenital heart disease) 759.0
Jaccoud's 714.4
Jackson's 344.89
Jadassohn-Lewandowski (pachyonchia congenita) 757.5
Jaffe-Lichtenstein (-Uehlinger) 252.01
Jahnke's (encephalocutaneous angiomatosis) 759.6
Jakob-Creutzfeldt 046.19
    with dementia
        with behavioral disturbance 046.19 [294.11]
        without behavioral disturbance 046.19 [294.10]
    variant 046.11
        with dementia
            with behavioral disturbance 046.11 [294.11]
            without behavioral disturbance 046.11 [294.10]
Jaksch's (pseudoleukemia infantum) 285.8
Jaksch-Hayem (-Luzet) (pseudoleukemia infantum) 285.8
jaw-winking 742.8
jejunal 564.2
Jervell-Lange-Nielsen 426.82

Syndrome (Continued)

jet lag 327.35
Jeune's (asphyxiating thoracic dystrophy of newborn) 756.4
Job's (chronic granulomatous disease) 288.1
Jordan's 288.2
Joseph-Diamond-Blackfan (congenital hypoplastic anemia) 284.01
Joubert 759.89
jugular foramen 352.6
Kabuki 759.89
Kahler's (multiple myeloma) (M9730/3) 203.0●
Kalischer's (encephalocutaneous angiomatosis) 759.6
Kallmann's (hypogonadotropic hypogonadism with anosmia) 253.4
Kanner's (autism) (see also Psychosis, childhood) 299.0●
Kartagener's (sinusitis, bronchiectasis, situs inversus) 759.3
Kasabach-Merritt (capillary hemangioma associated with thrombocytopenic purpura) 287.39
Kast's (dyschondroplasia with hemangiomas) 756.4
Kaznelson's (congenital hypoplastic anemia) 284.01
Kearns-Sayre 277.87
Kelly's (sideropenic dysphagia) 280.8
Kimmelstiel-Wilson (intercapillary glomerulosclerosis) 250.4● [581.81]
    due to secondary diabetes 249.4● [581.81]
Klauder's (erythema multiforme exudativum) 695.19
Klein-Waardenburg (ptosis-epicanthus) 270.2
Kleine-Levin 327.13
Klinefelter's 758.7
Klippel-Feil (brevicollis) 756.16
Klippel-Trenaunay 759.89
Klumpke (-Déjérine) (injury to brachial plexus at birth) 767.6
Klüver-Bucy (-Terzian) 310.0
Köhler-Pelligrini-Stieda (calcification, knee joint) 726.62
König's 564.89
Korsakoff's (nonalcoholic) 294.0
    alcoholic 291.1
Korsakoff (-Wernicke) (nonalcoholic) 294.0
    alcoholic 291.1
Kostmann's (infantile genetic agranulocytosis) 288.01
Krabbe's
    congenital muscle hypoplasia 756.89
    cutaneocerebral angioma 759.6
Kunkel (lupoid hepatitis) 571.49
labyrinthine 386.50
laceration, broad ligament 620.6
Lambert-Eaton 358.30
    in
        diseases classified elsewhere 358.39
        neoplastic disease 358.31
Landau-Kleffner 345.8●
Langdon Down (mongolism) 758.0
Larsen's (flattened facies and multiple congenital dislocations) 755.8
lateral
    cutaneous nerve of thigh 355.1
    medullary (see also Disease, cerebrovascular, acute) 436
Launois' (pituitary gigantism) 253.0
Launois-Cléret (adiposogenital dystrophy) 253.8
Laurence-Moon (-Bardet)-Biedl (obesity, polydactyly, and intellectual disabilities) 759.89
Lawford's (encephalocutaneous angiomatosis) 759.6
lazy
    leukocyte 288.09
    posture 728.3

Syndrome (Continued)

Lederer-Brill (acquired infectious hemolytic anemia) 283.19
Legg-Calvé-Perthes (osteochondrosis capital femoral) 732.1
Lemiere 451.89
Lennox-Gastaut syndrome 345.0● with tonic seizures 345.1●
Lennox's (see also Epilepsy) 345.0●
lenticular 275.1
Léopold-Lévi's (paroxysmal thyroid instability) 242.9●
Lepore hemoglobin 282.45
Léri-Weill 756.59
Leriche's (aortic bifurcation occlusion) 444.09
Lermoyez's (see also Disease, Ménière's) 386.00
Lesch-Nyhan (hypoxanthine-guanine-phosphoribosyltransferase deficiency) 277.2
leukoencephalopathy, reversible, posterior 348.5
Lev's (acquired complete heart block) 426.0
Levi's (pituitary dwarfism) 253.3
Lévy-Roussy 334.3
Lichtheim's (subacute combined sclerosis with pernicious anemia) 281.0 [336.2]
Li-Fraumeni V84.01
Lightwood's (renal tubular acidosis) 588.89
Lignac (-de Toni) (-Fanconi) (-Debré) (cystinosis) 270.0
Likoff's (angina in menopausal women) 413.9
liver-kidney 572.4
Lloyd's 258.1
lobotomy 310.0
Löffler's (eosinophilic pneumonitis) 518.3
Löfgren's (sarcoidosis) 135
long arm 18 or 21 deletion 758.39
Looser (-Debray)-Milkman (osteomalacia with pseudofractures) 268.2
Lorain-Levi (pituitary dwarfism) 253.3
Louis-Bar (ataxia-telangiectasia) 334.8
low
    atmospheric pressure 993.2
    back 724.2
        psychogenic 306.0
    output (cardiac) (see also Failure, heart) 428.9
Lowe's (oculocerebrorenal dystrophy) 270.8
Lowe-Terrey-MacLachlan (oculocerebrorenal dystrophy) 270.8
lower radicular, newborn 767.4
Lown (-Ganong)-Levine (short P-R internal, normal QRS complex, and supraventricular tachycardia) 426.81
Lucey-Driscoll (jaundice due to delayed conjugation) 774.30
Luetscher's (dehydration) 276.51
lumbar vertebral 724.4
Lutembacher's (atrial septal defect with mitral stenosis) 745.5
Lyell's (toxic epidermal necrolysis) 695.15
    due to drug
        correct substance properly administered 695.15
        overdose or wrong substance given or taken 977.9
        specified drug - see Table of Drugs and Chemicals
MacLeod's 492.8
macrogenitosomia praecox 259.8
macroglobulinemia 273.3
macrophage activation 288.4
Maffucci's (dyschondroplasia with hemangiomas) 756.4
Magenblase 306.4
magnesium-deficiency 781.7

◀ New   ◀▦ Revised   ~~deleted~~ Deleted   ● Use Additional Digit(s)   ▨ Omit code

Syndrome *(Continued)*
  malabsorption 579.9
    postsurgical 579.3
    spinal fluid 331.3
  Mal de Debarquement 780.4
  malignant carcinoid 259.2
  Mallory-Weiss 530.7
  mandibulofacial dysostosis 756.0
  manic-depressive *(see also* Psychosis,
      affective) 296.80
  Mankowsky's (familial dysplastic
      osteopathy) 731.2
  maple syrup (urine) 270.3
  Marable's (celiac artery compression) 447.4
  Marchesani (-Weill) (brachymorphism and
      ectopia lentis) 759.89
  Marchiafava-Bignami 341.8
  Marchiafava-Micheli (paroxysmal nocturnal
      hemoglobinuria) 283.2
  Marcus Gunn's (jaw-winking syndrome)
      742.8
  Marfan's (arachnodactyly) 759.82
    meaning congenital syphilis 090.49
      with luxation of lens 090.49 *[379.32]*
  Marie's (acromegaly) 253.0
    primary or idiopathic (acropachyderma)
      757.39
    secondary (hypertrophic pulmonary
      osteoarthropathy) 731.2
  Markus-Adie 379.46
  Maroteaux-Lamy (mucopolysaccharidosis
      VI) 277.5
  Martin's 715.27
  Martin-Albright
      (pseudohypoparathyroidism) 275.49
  Martorell-Fabré (pulseless disease) 446.7
  massive aspiration of newborn 770.18
  Masters-Allen 620.6
  mastocytosis 757.33
  maternal hypotension 669.2●
  maternal obesity 646.1●
  May (-Hegglin) 288.2
  McArdle (-Schmid) (-Pearson) (glycogenosis
      V) 271.0
  McCune-Albright (osteitis fibrosa
      disseminata) 756.59
  McQuarrie's (idiopathic familial
      hypoglycemia) 251.2
  meconium
    aspiration 770.12
    plug (newborn) NEC 777.1
  median arcuate ligament 447.4
  mediastinal fibrosis 519.3
  Meekeren-Ehlers-Danlos 756.83
  Meige (blepharospasm-oromandibular
      dystonia) 333.82
    -Milroy (chronic hereditary edema) 757.0
  MELAS (mitochondrial encephalopathy,
      lactic acidosis and stroke-like episodes)
      277.87
  Melkersson (-Rosenthal) 351.8
  MEN (multiple endocrine neoplasia)
    type I 258.01
    type IIA 258.02
    type IIB 258.03
  Mende's (ptosis-epicanthus) 270.2
  Mendelson's (resulting from a procedure)
      997.32
    during labor 668.0●
    obstetric 668.0●
  Ménétrier's (hypertrophic gastritis) 535.2●
  Ménière's *(see also* Disease, Ménière's) 386.00
  meningo-eruptive 047.1
  Menkes' 759.89
    glutamic acid 759.89
    maple syrup (urine) disease 270.3
  menopause 627.2
    postartificial 627.4
  menstruation 625.4
  MERRF (myoclonus with epilepsy and with
      ragged red fibers) 277.87

Syndrome *(Continued)*
  mesenteric
    artery, superior 557.1
    vascular insufficiency (with gangrene)
      557.1
  metabolic 277.7
  metastatic carcinoid 259.2
  Meyenburg-Altherr-Uehlinger 733.99
  Meyer-Schwickerath and Weyers (dysplasia
      oculodentodigitalis) 759.89
  Micheli-Rietti (thalassemia minor) 282.46
  Michotte's 721.5
  micrognathia-glossoptosis 756.0
  microphthalmos (congenital) 759.89
  midbrain 348.89
  middle
    lobe (lung) (right) 518.0
    radicular 353.0
  Miescher's
    familial acanthosis nigricans 701.2
    granulomatosis disciformis 709.3
  Mieten's 759.89
  migraine 346.0●
  Mikity-Wilson (pulmonary dysmaturity)
      770.7
  Mikulicz's (dryness of mouth, absent or
      decreased lacrimation) 527.1
  milk alkali (milk drinkers') 275.42
  Milkman (-Looser) (osteomalacia with
      pseudofractures) 268.2
  Millard-Gubler 344.89
  Miller-Dieker 758.33
  Miller Fisher's 357.0
  Milles' (encephalocutaneous angiomatosis)
      759.6
  Minkowski-Chauffard *(see also*
      Spherocytosis) 282.0
  Mirizzi's (hepatic duct stenosis) 576.2
    with calculus, cholelithiasis, or stones - *see*
      Choledocholithiasis
  mitochondrial neurogastrointestinal
      encephalopathy (MNGIE) 277.87
  mitral
    click (-murmur) 785.2
    valve prolapse 424.0
  MNGIE (mitochondrial neurogastrointestinal
      encephalopathy) 277.87
  Möbius'
    congenital oculofacial paralysis 352.6
    ophthalmoplegic migraine 346.2●
  Mohr's (types I and II) 759.89
  monofixation 378.34
  Moore's *(see also* Epilepsy) 345.5●
  Morel-Moore (hyperostosis frontalis interna)
      733.3
  Morel-Morgagni (hyperostosis frontalis
      interna) 733.3
  Morgagni (-Stewart-Morel) (hyperostosis
      frontalis interna) 733.3
  Morgagni-Adams-Stokes (syncope with
      heart block) 426.9
  Morquio (-Brailsford) (-Ullrich)
      (mucopolysaccharidosis IV) 277.5
  Morris (testicular feminization) 259.51
  Morton's (foot) (metatarsalgia) (metatarsal
      neuralgia) (neuralgia) (neuroma) (toe)
      355.6
  Moschcowitz (-Singer-Symmers) (thrombotic
      thrombocytopenic purpura) 446.6
  Mounier-Kuhn 748.3
    with
      acute exacerbation 494.1
      bronchiectasis 494.0
        with (acute) exacerbation 494.1
    acquired 519.19
      with bronchiectasis 494.0
        with (acute) exacerbation 494.1
  Mucha-Haberman (acute parapsoriasis
      varioliformis) 696.2
  mucocutaneous lymph node (acute) (febrile)
      (infantile) (MCLS) 446.1

Syndrome *(Continued)*
  multiple
    deficiency 260
    endocrine neoplasia (MEN)
      type I 258.01
      type IIA 258.02
      type IIB 258.03
    operations 301.51
  Munchausen's 301.51
  Munchmeyer's (exostosis luxurians) 728.11
  Murchison-Sanderson - *see* Disease,
      Hodgkin's
  myasthenic - *see* Myasthenia, syndrome
  myelodysplastic 238.75
    with 5q deletion 238.74
    high grade with 5q deletion 238.73
    lesions, low grade 238.72
    therapy-related 289.83
  myeloproliferative (chronic) (M9960/1)
      238.79
  myofascial pain NEC 729.1
  Naffziger's 353.0
  Nager-de Reynier (dysostosis mandibularis)
      756.0
  nail-patella (hereditary osteo-
      onychodysplasia) 756.89
  NARP (neuropathy, ataxia and retinitis
      pigmentosa) 277.87
  Nebécourt's 253.3
  Neill Dingwall (microencephaly and
      dwarfism) 759.89
  nephrotic *(see also* Nephrosis) 581.9
    diabetic 250.4● *[581.81]*
      due to secondary diabetes 249.4●
        [581.81]
  Netherton's (ichthyosiform erythroderma)
      757.1
  neurocutaneous 759.6
  neuroleptic malignant 333.92
  Nezelof's (pure alymphocytosis) 279.13
  Niemann-Pick (lipid histiocytosis) 272.7
  Nonne-Milroy-Meige (chronic hereditary
      edema) 757.0
  nonsense 300.16
  Noonan's 759.89
  Nothnagel's
    ophthalmoplegia-cerebellar ataxia
      378.52
    vasomotor acroparesthesia 443.89
  nucleus ambiguous-hypoglossal 352.6
  OAV (oculoauriculovertebral dysplasia)
      756.0
  obesity hypoventilation 278.03
  obsessional 300.3
  oculocutaneous 364.24
  oculomotor 378.81
  oculourethroarticular 099.3
  Ogilvie's (sympathicotonic colon
      obstruction) 560.89
  ophthalmoplegia-cerebellar ataxia 378.52
  Oppenheim-Urbach (necrobiosis lipoidica
      diabeticorum) 250.8● *[709.3]*
    due to secondary diabetes 249.8● *[709.3]*
  oral-facial-digital 759.89
  organic
    affective NEC 293.83
      drug-induced 292.84
    anxiety 293.84
    delusional 293.81
      alcohol-induced 291.5
      drug-induced 292.11
      due to or associated with
        arteriosclerosis 290.42
        presenile brain disease 290.12
        senility 290.20
    depressive 293.83
      drug-induced 292.84
      due to or associated with
        arteriosclerosis 290.43
        presenile brain disease 290.13
        senile brain disease 290.21

Syndrome *(Continued)*
  organic *(Continued)*
    hallucinosis 293.82
      drug-induced 292.84
    organic affective 293.83
      induced by drug 292.84
    organic personality 310.1
      induced by drug 292.89
  Ormond's 593.4
  orodigitofacial 759.89
  orthostatic hypotensive-dysautonomic-dyskinetic 333.0
  Osler-Weber-Rendu (familial hemmorrhagic telangiectasia) 448.0
  osteodermopathic hyperostosis 757.39
  osteoporosis-osteomalacia 268.2
  Österreicher-Turner (hereditary osteo-onychodysplasia) 756.89
  os trigonum 755.69
  Ostrum-Furst 756.59
  otolith 386.19
  otopalatodigital 759.89
  outlet (thoracic) 353.0
  ovarian remnant 620.8
  Owren's *(see also* Defect, coagulation) 286.3
  OX 758.6
  pacemaker 429.4
  Paget-Schroetter (intermittent venous claudication) 453.89
  pain - *see also* Pain
    central 338.0
    chronic 338.4
    complex regional 355.9
      type I 337.20
        lower limb 337.22
        specified site NEC 337.29
        upper limb 337.21
      type II
        lower limb 355.71
        upper limb 354.4
    myelopathic 338.0
    thalamic (hyperesthetic) 338.0
  painful
    apicocostal vertebral (M8010/3) 162.3
    arc 726.19
    bruising 287.2
    feet 266.2
  Pancoast's (carcinoma, pulmonary apex) (M8010/3) 162.3
  panhypopituitary (postpartum) 253.2
  papillary muscle 429.81
    with myocardial infarction 410.8●
  Papillon-Léage and Psaume (orodigitofacial dysostosis) 759.89
  parabiotic (transfusion)
    donor (twin) 772.0
    recipient (twin) 776.4
  paralysis agitans 332.0
  paralytic 344.9
    specified type NEC 344.89
  paraneoplastic - *see* Condition
  Parinaud's (paralysis of conjugate upward gaze) 378.81
    oculoglandular 372.02
  Parkes Weber and Dimitri (encephalocutaneous angiomatosis) 759.6
  Parkinson's *(see also* Parkinsonism) 332.0
  parkinsonian *(see also* Parkinsonism) 332.0
  Parry's (exophthalmic goiter) 242.0●
  Parry-Romberg 349.89
  Parsonage-Aldren-Turner 353.5
  Parsonage-Turner 353.5
  Patau's (trisomy D₁) 758.1
  patella clunk 719.66
  patellofemoral 719.46
  Paterson (-Brown) (-Kelly) (sideropenic dysphagia) 280.8
  Payr's (splenic flexure syndrome) 569.89
  pectoral girdle 447.8
  pectoralis minor 447.8

Syndrome *(Continued)*
  Pelger-Huët (hereditary hyposegmentation) 288.2
  pellagra-cerebellar ataxia-renal aminoaciduria 270.0
  Pellegrini-Stieda 726.62
  pellagroid 265.2
  Pellizzi's (pineal) 259.8
  pelvic congestion (-fibrosis) 625.5
  Pendred's (familial goiter with deaf-mutism) 243
  Penfield's *(see also* Epilepsy) 345.5●
  Penta X 758.81
  peptic ulcer - *see* Ulcer, peptic 533.9
  perabduction 447.8
  periodic 277.31
  periurethral fibrosis 593.4
  persistent fetal circulation 747.83
  Petges-Cléjat (poikilodermatomyositis) 710.3
  Peutz-Jeghers 759.6
  Pfeiffer (acrocephalosyndactyly) 755.55
  phantom limb 353.6
  pharyngeal pouch 279.11
  Pick's (pericardial pseudocirrhosis of liver) 423.2
    heart 423.2
    liver 423.2
  Pick-Herxheimer (diffuse idiopathic cutaneous atrophy) 701.8
  Pickwickian (cardiopulmonary obesity) 278.03
  PIE (pulmonary infiltration with eosinophilia) 518.3
  Pierre Marie-Bamberger (hypertrophic pulmonary osteoarthropathy) 731.2
  Pierre Mauriac's (diabetes-dwarfism-obesity) 258.1
  Pierre Robin 756.0
  pigment dispersion, iris 364.53
  pineal 259.8
  pink puffer 492.8
  pituitary 253.0
  placental
    dysfunction 762.2
    insufficiency 762.2
    transfusion 762.3
  plantar fascia 728.71
  plateau iris (without glaucoma) 364.82
    with glaucoma 365.23
  plica knee 727.83
  Plummer-Vinson (sideropenic dysphagia) 280.8
  pluricarential of infancy 260
  plurideficiency of infancy 260
  pluriglandular (compensatory) 258.8
  Poland 756.81
  polycarential of infancy 260
  polyglandular 258.8
  polysplenia 759.0
  pontine 433.8●
  popliteal
    artery entrapment 447.8
    web 756.89
  post chemoembolization - code to associated conditions
  postartificial menopause 627.4
  postcardiac injury
    postcardiotomy 429.4
    postmyocardial infarction 411.0
  postcardiotomy 429.4
  postcholecystectomy 576.0
  postcommissurotomy 429.4
  postconcussional 310.2
  postcontusional 310.2
  postencephalitic 310.89
  posterior
    cervical sympathetic 723.2
    fossa compression 348.4
    inferior cerebellar artery *(see also* Disease, cerebrovascular, acute) 436
    reversible encephalopathy (PRES) 348.39

Syndrome *(Continued)*
  postgastrectomy (dumping) 564.2
  post-gastric surgery 564.2
  posthepatitis 780.79
  posttherpetic (neuralgia) (zoster) 053.19
    geniculate ganglion 053.11
    ophthalmica 053.19
  postimmunization - *see* Complications, vaccination
  postinfarction 411.0
  postinfluenza (asthenia) 780.79
  postirradiation 990
  postlaminectomy 722.80
    cervical, cervicothoracic 722.81
    lumbar, lumbosacral 722.83
    thoracic, thoracolumbar 722.82
  postleukotomy 310.0
  postlobotomy 310.0
  postmastectomy lymphedema 457.0
  postmature (of newborn) 766.22
  postmyocardial infarction 411.0
  postoperative NEC 998.9
    blind loop 579.2
  postpartum panhypopituitary 253.2
  postperfusion NEC 999.89
    bone marrow 996.85
  postpericardiotomy 429.4
  postphlebitic (asymptomatic) 459.10
    with
      complications NEC 459.19
      inflammation 459.12
        and ulcer 459.13
      stasis dermatitis 459.12
        with ulcer 459.13
      ulcer 459.11
        with inflammation 459.13
  postpolio (myelitis) 138
  postvagotomy 564.2
  postvalvulotomy 429.4
  postviral (asthenia) NEC 780.79
  Potain's (gastrectasis with dyspepsia) 536.1
  potassium intoxication 276.7
  Potter's 753.0
  Prader (-Labhart)-Willi (-Fanconi) 759.81
  preinfarction 411.1
  preleukemic 238.75
  premature senility 259.8
  premenstrual 625.4
  premenstrual tension 625.4
  pre ulcer 536.9
  Prinzmetal-Massumi (anterior chest wall syndrome) 786.52
  Profichet's 729.90
  progeria 259.8
  progressive pallidal degeneration 333.0
  prolonged gestation 766.22
  Proteus (dermal hypoplasia) 757.39
  prune belly 756.71
  prurigo-asthma 691.8
  pseudocarpal tunnel (sublimis) 354.0
  pseudohermaphroditism-virilism hirsutism 255.2
  pseudoparalytica 358.00
  pseudo-Turner's 759.89
  psycho-organic 293.9
    acute 293.0
    anxiety type 293.84
    depressive type 293.83
    hallucinatory type 293.82
    nonpsychotic severity 310.1
      specified focal (partial) NEC 310.89
    paranoid type 293.81
    specified type NEC 293.89
    subacute 293.1
  pterygolymphangiectasia 758.6
  ptosis-epicanthus 270.2
  pulmonary
    arteriosclerosis 416.0
    hypoperfusion (idiopathic) 769
    renal (hemorrhagic) 446.21
  pulseless 446.7

◀ New   ⬅ Revised   ~~deleted~~ Deleted   ● Use Additional Digit(s)   ▨ Omit code

Syndrome *(Continued)*
  Putnam-Dana (subacute combined sclerosis with pernicious anemia) 281.0 *[336.2]*
  pyloroduodenal 537.89
  pyramidopallidonigral 332.0
  pyriformis 355.0
  QT interval prolongation 426.82
  radicular NEC 729.2
    lower limbs 724.4
    upper limbs 723.4
    newborn 767.4
  Raeder-Harbitz (pulseless disease) 446.7
  Ramsay Hunt's
    dyssynergia cerebellaris myoclonica 334.2
    herpetic geniculate ganglionitis 053.11
  rapid time-zone change 327.35
  Raymond (-Céstan) 433.8●
  Raynaud's (paroxysmal digital cyanosis) 443.0
  RDS (respiratory distress syndrome, newborn) 769
  Refsum's (heredopathia atactica polyneuritiformis) 356.3
  Reichmann's (gastrosuccorrhea) 536.8
  Reifenstein's (hereditary familial hypogonadism, male) 259.52
  Reilly's (*see also* Neuropathy, peripheral, autonomic) 337.9
  Reiter's 099.3
  renal glomerulohyalinosis-diabetic 250.4● *[581.81]*
    due to secondary diabetes 249.4● *[581.81]*
  Rendu-Osler-Weber (familial hemorrhagic telangiectasia) 448.0
  renofacial (congenital biliary fibroangiomatosis) 753.0
  Rénon-Delille 253.8
  respiratory distress (idiopathic) (newborn) 769
    adult (following trauma and surgery) 518.52
      specified NEC 518.82
    type II 770.6
  restless legs (RLS) 333.94
  retinoblastoma (familial) 190.5
  retraction (Duane's) 378.71
  retroperitoneal fibrosis 593.4
  retroviral seroconversion (acute) V08
  Rett's 330.8
  Reye's 331.81
  Reye-Sheehan (postpartum pituitary necrosis) 253.2
  Riddoch's (visual disorientation) 368.16
  Ridley's (*see also* Failure, ventricular, left) 428.1
  Rieger's (mesodermal dysgenesis, anterior ocular segment) 743.44
  Rietti-Greppi-Micheli (thalassemia minor) 282.46
  right ventricular obstruction - *see* Failure, heart
  Riley-Day (familial dysautonomia) 742.8
  Robin's 756.0
  Rokitansky-Kuster-Hauser (congenital absence, vagina) 752.45
  Romano-Ward (prolonged QT interval syndrome) 426.82
  Romberg's 349.89
  Rosen-Castleman-Liebow (pulmonary proteinosis) 516.0
  rotator cuff, shoulder 726.10
  Roth's 355.1
  Rothmund's (congenital poikiloderma) 757.33
  Rotor's (idiopathic hyperbilirubinemia) 277.4
  Roussy-Lévy 334.3
  Roy (-Jutras) (acropachyderma) 757.39
  rubella (congenital) 771.0
  Rubinstein-Taybi's (brachydactylia, short stature, and intellectual disabilities) 759.89

Syndrome *(Continued)*
  Rud's (mental deficiency, epilepsy, and infantilism) 759.89
  Ruiter-Pompen (-Wyers) (angiokeratoma corporis diffusum) 272.7
  Runge's (postmaturity) 766.22
  Russell (-Silver) (congenital hemihypertrophy and short stature) 759.89
  Rytand-Lipsitch (complete atrioventricular block) 426.0
  sacralization-scoliosis-sciatica 756.15
  sacroiliac 724.6
  Saenger's 379.46
  salt
    depletion (*see also* Disease, renal) 593.9
      due to heat NEC 992.8
        causing heat exhaustion or prostration 992.4
    low (*see also* Disease, renal) 593.9
  salt-losing (*see also* Disease, renal) 593.9
  Sanfilippo's (mucopolysaccharidosis III) 277.5
  Scaglietti-Dagnini (acromegalic macrospondylitis) 253.0
  scalded skin 695.81
  scalenus anticus (anterior) 353.0
  scapulocostal 354.8
  scapuloperoneal 359.1
  scapulovertebral 723.4
  Schaumann's (sarcoidosis) 135
  Scheie's (mucopolysaccharidosis IS) 277.5
  Scheuthauer-Marie-Sainton (cleidocranialis dysostosis) 755.59
  Schirmer's (encephalocutaneous angiomatosis) 759.6
  schizophrenic, of childhood NEC (*see also* Psychosis, childhood) 299.9●
  Schmidt's
    sphallo-pharyngo-laryngeal hemiplegia 352.6
    thyroid-adrenocortical insufficiency 258.1
    vagoaccessory 352.6
  Schneider's 047.9
  Schnitzler 273.1
  Scholte's (malignant carcinoid) 259.2
  Scholz (-Bielschowsky-Henneberg) 330.0
  Schroeder's (endocrine-hypertensive) 255.3
  Schüller-Christian (chronic histiocytosis X) 277.89
  Schultz's (agranulocytosis) 288.09
  Schwachman's - *see* Syndrome, Shwachman's
  Schwartz (-Jampel) 359.23
  Schwartz-Bartter (inappropriate secretion of antidiuretic hormone) 253.6
  Scimitar (anomalous venous drainage, right lung to inferior vena cava) 747.49
  sclerocystic ovary 256.4
  sea-blue histiocyte 272.7
  Seabright-Bantam (pseudohypoparathyroidism) 275.49
  Seckel's 759.89
  Secretan's (posttraumatic edema) 782.3
  secretoinhibitor (keratoconjunctivitis sicca) 710.2
  Seeligmann's (ichthyosis congenita) 757.1
  Senear-Usher (pemphigus erythematosus) 694.4
  senilism 259.8
  seroconversion, retroviral (acute) V08
  serotonin 333.99
  serous meningitis 348.2
  Sertoli cell (germinal aplasia) 606.0
  sex chromosome mosaic 758.81
  Sézary's (reticulosis) (M9701/3) 202.2●
  shaken infant 995.55
  Shaver's (bauxite pneumoconiosis) 503
  Sheehan's (postpartum pituitary necrosis) 253.2

Syndrome *(Continued)*
  shock (traumatic) 958.4
    kidney 584.5
      following crush injury 958.5
    lung 518.82
      related to trauma and surgery 518.52
    neurogenic 308.9
    psychic 308.9
  Shone's 746.84
  short
    bowel 579.3
    P-R interval 426.81
  shoulder-arm (*see also* Neuropathy, peripheral, autonomic) 337.9
  shoulder-girdle 723.4
  shoulder-hand (*see also* Neuropathy, peripheral, autonomic) 337.9
  Shwachman's 288.02
  Shy-Drager (orthostatic hypotension with multisystem degeneration) 333.0
  Sicard's 352.6
  sicca (keratoconjunctivitis) 710.2
  sick
    cell 276.1
    cilia 759.89
    sinus 427.81
  sideropenic 280.8
  Siemens'
    ectodermal dysplasia 757.31
    keratosis follicularis spinulosa (decalvans) 757.39
  Silfverskiöld's (osteochondrodystrophy, extremities) 756.50
  Silver's (congenital hemihypertrophy and short stature) 759.89
  Silvestroni-Bianco (thalassemia minima) 282.46
  Simons' (progressive lipodystrophy) 272.6
  sinus tarsi 726.79
  sinusitis-bronchiectasis-situs inversus 759.3
  Sipple's (medullary thyroid carcinoma-pheochromocytoma) 258.02
  Sjögren (-Gougerot) (keratoconjunctivitis sicca) 710.2
    with lung involvement 710.2 *[517.8]*
  Sjögren-Larsson (ichthyosis congenita) 757.1
  SJS-TEN (Stevens-Johnson syndrome-toxic epidermal necrolysis overlap) 695.14
  Slocumb's 255.3
  Sluder's 337.09
  Smith-Lemli-Opitz (cerebrohepatorenal syndrome) 759.89
  Smith-Magenis 758.33
  smokers' 305.1
  Sneddon-Wilkinson (subcorneal pustular dermatosis) 694.1
  Sotos' (cerebral gigantism) 253.0
  South African cardiomyopathy 425.2
  spasmodic
    upward movement, eye(s) 378.82
    winking 307.20
  Spens' (syncope with heart block) 426.9
  spherophakia-brachymorphia 759.89
  spinal cord injury - *see also* Injury, spinal, by site
    with fracture, vertebra - *see* Fracture, vertebra, by site, with spinal cord injury
    cervical - *see* Injury, spinal, cervical
    fluid malabsorption (acquired) 331.3
  splenic
    agenesis 759.0
    flexure 569.89
    neutropenia 289.53
    sequestration 289.52
  Spurway's (brittle bones and blue sclera) 756.51
  staphylococcal scalded skin 695.81
  Stein's (polycystic ovary) 256.4
  Stein-Leventhal (polycystic ovary) 256.4

Syndrome *(Continued)*
  Steinbrocker's *(see also* Neuropathy, peripheral, autonomic) 337.9
  Stevens-Johnson (erythema multiforme exudativum) 695.13
    toxic epidermal necrolysis overlap (SJS-TEN overlap syndrome) 695.14
  Stewart-Morel (hyperostosis frontalis interna) 733.3
  Stickler 759.89
  stiff-baby 759.89
  stiff-man 333.91
  Still's (juvenile rheumatoid arthritis) 714.30
  Still-Felty (rheumatoid arthritis with splenomegaly and leukopenia) 714.1
  Stilling-Türk-Duane (ocular retraction syndrome) 378.71
  Stojano's (subcostal) 098.86
  Stokes (-Adams) (syncope with heart block) 426.0
  Stokvis-Talma (enterogenous cyanosis) 289.7
  stone heart *(see also* Failure, ventricular, left) 428.1
  straight-back 756.19
  stroke *(see also* Disease, cerebrovascular, acute) 436
    little 435.9
  Sturge-Kalischer-Weber (encephalotrigeminal angiomatosis) 759.6
  Sturge-Weber (-Dimitri) (encephalocutaneous angiomatosis) 759.6
  subclavian-carotid obstruction (chronic) 446.7
  subclavian steal 435.2
  subcoracoid-pectoralis minor 447.8
  subcostal 098.86
    nerve compression 354.8
  subperiosteal hematoma 267
  subphrenic interposition 751.4
  sudden infant death (SIDS) 798.0
  Sudeck's 733.7
  Sudeck-Leriche 733.7
  superior
    cerebellar artery *(see also* Disease, cerebrovascular, acute) 436
    mesenteric artery 557.1
    pulmonary sulcus (tumor) (M8010/3) 162.3
    semi-circular canal dehiscence 386.8
    vena cava 459.2
  suprarenal cortical 255.3
  supraspinatus 726.10
  Susac 348.39
  swallowed blood 777.3
  sweat retention 705.1
  Sweet's (acute febrile neutrophilic dermatosis) 695.89
  Swyer-James (unilateral hyperlucent lung) 492.8
  Swyer's (XY pure gonadal dysgenesis) 752.7
  Symonds' 348.2
  sympathetic
    cervical paralysis 337.09
    pelvic 625.5
  syndactylic oxycephaly 755.55
  syphilitic-cardiovascular 093.89
  systemic
    fibrosclerosing 710.8
    inflammatory response (SIRS) 995.90
      due to
        infectious process 995.91
          with acute organ dysfunction 995.92
        non-infectious process 995.93
          with acute organ dysfunction 995.94
  systolic click (-murmur) 785.2
  Tabagism 305.1
  tachycardia-bradycardia 427.81

Syndrome *(Continued)*
  Takayasu (-Onishi) (pulseless disease) 446.7
  Takotsubo 429.83
  Tapia's 352.6
  tarsal tunnel 355.5
  Taussig-Bing (transposition, aorta and overriding pulmonary artery) 745.11
  Taybi's (otopalatodigital) 759.89
  Taylor's 625.5
  teething 520.7
  tegmental 344.89
  telangiectasis-pigmentation-cataract 757.33
  temporal 383.02
    lobectomy behavior 310.0
  temporomandibular joint-pain-dysfunction [TMJ] NEC 524.60
    specified NEC 524.69
  Terry's *(see also* Retinopathy of prematurity) 362.21
  testicular feminization 259.51
  testis, nonvirilizing 257.8
  tethered (spinal) cord 742.59
  thalamic 338.0
  Thibierge-Weissenbach (cutaneous systemic sclerosis) 710.1
  Thiele 724.6
  thoracic outlet (compression) 353.0
  thoracogenous rheumatic (hypertrophic pulmonary osteoarthropathy) 731.2
  Thorn's *(see also* Disease, renal) 593.9
  Thorson-Biörck (malignant carcinoid) 259.2
  thrombopenia-hemangioma 287.39
  thyroid-adrenocortical insufficiency 258.1
  Tietze's 733.6
  time-zone (rapid) 327.35
  Tobias' (carcinoma, pulmonary apex) (M8010/3) 162.3
  toilet seat 926.0
  Tolosa-Hunt 378.55
  Toni-Fanconi (cystinosis) 270.0
  Touraine's (hereditary osteo-onychodysplasia) 756.89
  Touraine-Solente-Golé (acropachyderma) 757.39
  toxic
    oil 710.5
    shock 040.82
  transfusion
    fetal-maternal 772.0
    twin
      donor (infant) 772.0
      recipient (infant) 776.4
  transient left ventricular apical ballooning 429.83
  Treacher Collins' (incomplete mandibulofacial dysostosis) 756.0
  trigeminal plate 259.8
  triplex X female 758.81
  trisomy NEC 758.5
    13 or D$_1$ 758.1
    16–18 or E 758.2
    18 or E$_3$ 758.2
    20 758.5
    21 or G (mongolism) 758.0
    22 or G (mongolism) 758.0
    G 758.0
  Troisier-Hanot-Chauffard (bronze diabetes) 275.01
  tropical wet feet 991.4
  Trousseau's (thrombophlebitis migrans visceral cancer) 453.1
  tumor lysis (following antineoplastic drug therapy) (spontaneous) 277.88
  Türk's (ocular retraction syndrome) 378.71
  Turner's 758.6
  Turner-Varny 758.6
  Twiddler's (due to)
    automatic implantable defibrillator 996.04
    pacemaker 996.01
  twin-to-twin transfusion 762.3
    recipient twin 776.4

Syndrome *(Continued)*
  Uehlinger's (acropachyderma) 757.39
  Ullrich (-Bonnevie) (-Turner) 758.6
  Ullrich-Feichtiger 759.89
  underwater blast injury (abdominal) *(see also* Injury, internal, abdomen) 868.00
  universal joint, cervix 620.6
  Unverricht (-Lundborg) 345.1●
  Unverricht-Wagner (dermatomyositis) 710.3
  upward gaze 378.81
  Urbach-Oppenheim (necrobiosis lipoidica diabeticorum) 250.8● *[709.3]*
    due to secondary diabetes 249.8● *[709.3]*
  Urbach-Wiethe (lipoid proteinosis) 272.8
  uremia, chronic 585.9
  urethral 597.81
  urethro-oculoarticular 099.3
  urethro-oculosynovial 099.3
  urohepatic 572.4
  uveocutaneous 364.24
  uveomeningeal, uveomeningitis 363.22
  vagohypoglossal 352.6
  vagovagal 780.2
  van Buchem's (hyperostosis corticalis) 733.3
  van der Hoeve's (brittle bones and blue sclera, deafness) 756.51
  van der Hoeve-Halbertsma-Waardenburg (ptosis-epicanthus) 270.2
  van der Hoeve-Waarderburg-Gualdi (ptosis-epicanthus) 270.2
  vanishing twin 651.33
  van Neck-Odelberg (juvenile osteochondrosis) 732.1
  vascular splanchnic 557.0
  vasomotor 443.9
  vasovagal 780.2
  VATER 759.89
  Velo-cardio-facial 758.32
  vena cava (inferior) (superior) (obstruction) 459.2
  Verbiest's (claudicatio intermittens spinalis) 435.1
  Vernet's 352.6
  vertebral
    artery 435.1
      compression 721.1
    lumbar 724.4
    steal 435.1
  vertebrogenic (pain) 724.5
  vertiginous NEC 386.9
  video display tube 723.8
  Villaret's 352.6
  Vinson-Plummer (sideropenic dysphagia) 280.8
  virilizing adrenocortical hyperplasia, congenital 255.2
  virus, viral 079.99
  visceral larval migrans 128.0
  visual disorientation 368.16
  vitamin B$_6$ deficiency 266.1
  vitreous touch 997.99
  Vogt's (corpus striatum) 333.71
  Vogt-Koyanagi 364.24
  Volkmann's 958.6
  von Bechterew-Stumpell (ankylosing spondylitis) 720.0
  von Graefe's 378.72
  von Hippel-Lindau (angiomatosis retinocerebellosa) 759.6
  von Schroetter's (intermittent venous claudication) 453.89
  von Willebrand (-Jürgens) (angiohemophilia) 286.4
  Waardenburg-Klein (ptosis epicanthus) 270.2
  Wagner (-Unverricht) (dermatomyositis) 710.3
  Waldenström's (macroglobulinemia) 273.3
  Waldenström-Kjellberg (sideropenic dysphagia) 280.8

◀ New   ◀▦ Revised   ~~deleted~~ Deleted   ● Use Additional Digit(s)   ▦ Omit code

Syndrome *(Continued)*
  Wallenberg's (posterior inferior cerebellar
    artery) *(see also* Disease,
    cerebrovascular, acute) 436
  Waterhouse (-Friderichsen) 036.3
  water retention 276.69
  Weber's 344.89
  Weber-Christian (nodular nonsuppurative
    panniculitis) 729.30
  Weber-Cockayne (epidermolysis bullosa)
    757.39
  Weber-Dimitri (encephalocutaneous
    angiomatosis) 759.6
  Weber-Gubler 344.89
  Weber-Leyden 344.89
  Weber-Osler (familial hemorrhagic
    telangiectasia) 448.0
  Wegener's (necrotizing respiratory
    granulomatosis) 446.4
  Weill-Marchesani (brachymorphism and
    ectopia lentis) 759.89
  Weingarten's (tropical eosinophilia) 518.3
  Weiss-Baker (carotid sinus syncope) 337.01
  Weissenbach-Thibierge (cutaneous systemic
    sclerosis) 710.1
  Werdnig-Hoffmann 335.0
  Werlhof-Wichmann *(see also* Purpura,
    thrombocytopenic) 287.39
  Wermer's (polyendocrine adenomatosis)
    258.01
  Werner's (progeria adultorum) 259.8
  Wernicke's (nonalcoholic) (superior
    hemorrhagic polioencephalitis) 265.1
  Wernicke-Korsakoff (nonalcoholic) 294.0
    alcoholic 291.1
  Westphal-Strümpell (hepatolenticular
    degeneration) 275.1
  wet
    brain (alcoholic) 303.9●
    feet (maceration) (tropical) 991.4
    lung
      adult 518.52
      newborn 770.6
  whiplash 847.0
  Whipple's (intestinal lipodystrophy) 040.2
  "whistling face" (craniocarpotarsal
    dystrophy) 759.89
  Widal (-Abrami) (acquired hemolytic
    jaundice) 283.9
  Wilkie's 557.1
  Wilkinson-Sneddon (subcorneal pustular
    dermatosis) 694.1
  Willan-Plumbe (psoriasis) 696.1
  Willebrand (-Jürgens) (angiohemophilia)
    286.4
  Willi-Prader (hypogenital dystrophy with
    diabetic tendency) 759.81
  Wilson's (hepatolenticular degeneration)
    275.1
  Wilson-Mikity 770.7
  Wiskott-Aldrich (eczema-thrombocytopenia)
    279.12
  withdrawal
    alcohol 291.81
    drug 292.0
      infant of dependent mother 779.5
  Woakes' (ethmoiditis) 471.1
  Wolff-Parkinson-White (anomalous
    atrioventricular excitation) 426.7
  Wright's (hyperabduction) 447.8
  X
    cardiac 413.9
    dysmetabolic 277.7
  xiphoidalgia 733.99
  XO 758.6
  XXX 758.81
  XXXXY 758.81
  XXY 758.7
  yellow vernix (placental dysfunction) 762.2
  Zahorsky's 074.0
  Zellweger 277.86

Syndrome *(Continued)*
  Zieve's (jaundice, hyperlipemia and
    hemolytic anemia) 571.1
  Zollinger-Ellison (gastric hypersecretion
    with pancreatic islet cell tumor) 251.5
  Zuelzer-Ogden (nutritional megaloblastic
    anemia) 281.2
Synechia (iris) (pupil) 364.70
  anterior 364.72
    peripheral 364.73
  intrauterine (traumatic) 621.5
  posterior 364.71
  vulvae, congenital 752.49
Synesthesia *(see also* Disturbance, sensation)
  782.0
Synodontia 520.2
Synophthalmus 759.89
Synorchidism 752.89
Synorchism 752.89
Synostosis (congenital) 756.59
  astragaloscaphoid 755.67
  radioulnar 755.53
  talonavicular (bar) 755.67
  tarsal 755.67
Synovial - *see* condition
Synovioma (M9040/3) - *see also* Neoplasm,
  connective tissue, malignant
  benign (M9040/0) - *see* Neoplasm,
    connective tissue, benign
Synoviosarcoma (M9040/3) - *see* Neoplasm,
  connective tissue, malignant
Synovitis *(see also* Tenosynovitis) 727.00
  chronic crepitant, wrist 727.2
  due to crystals - *see* Arthritis, due to crystals
  gonococcal 098.51
  gouty 274.00
  specified NEC 727.09
  syphilitic 095.7
    congenital 090.0
  traumatic, current - *see* Sprain, by site
  tuberculous - *see* Tuberculosis, synovitis
  villonodular 719.20
    ankle 719.27
    elbow 719.22
    foot 719.27
    hand 719.24
    hip 719.25
    knee 719.26
    multiple sites 719.29
    pelvic region 719.25
    shoulder (region) 719.21
    specified site NEC 719.28
    wrist 719.23
Syphilide 091.3
  congenital 090.0
  newborn 090.0
  tubercular 095.8
    congenital 090.0
Syphilis, syphilitic (acquired) 097.9
  with lung involvement 095.1
  abdomen (late) 095.2
  acoustic nerve 094.86
  adenopathy (secondary) 091.4
  adrenal (gland) 095.8
    with cortical hypofunction 095.8
  age under 2 years NEC *(see also* Syphilis,
    congenital) 090.9
    acquired 097.9
  alopecia (secondary) 091.82
  anemia 095.8
  aneurysm (artery) (ruptured) 093.89
    aorta 093.0
    central nervous system 094.89
    congenital 090.5
  anus 095.8
    primary 091.1
    secondary 091.3
  aorta, aortic (arch) (abdominal) (insufficiency)
    (pulmonary) (regurgitation) (stenosis)
    (thoracic) 093.89
    aneurysm 093.0

Syphilis, syphilitic *(Continued)*
  arachnoid (adhesive) 094.2
  artery 093.89
    cerebral 094.89
    spinal 094.89
  arthropathy (neurogenic) (tabetic) 094.0
    [713.5]
  asymptomatic - *see* Syphilis, latent
  ataxia, locomotor (progressive) 094.0
  atrophoderma maculatum 091.3
  auricular fibrillation 093.89
  Bell's palsy 094.89
  bladder 095.8
  bone 095.5
    secondary 091.61
  brain 094.89
  breast 095.8
  bronchus 095.8
  bubo 091.0
  bulbar palsy 094.89
  bursa (late) 095.7
  cardiac decompensation 093.89
  cardiovascular (early) (late) (primary)
    (secondary) (tertiary) 093.9
    specified type and site NEC 093.89
  causing death under 2 years of age *(see also*
    Syphilis, congenital) 090.9
    stated to be acquired NEC 097.9
  central nervous system (any site) (early)
    (late) (latent) (primary) (recurrent)
    (relapse) (secondary) (tertiary) 094.9
    with
      ataxia 094.0
      paralysis, general 094.1
        juvenile 090.40
      paresis (general) 094.1
        juvenile 090.40
      tabes (dorsalis) 094.0
        juvenile 090.40
      taboparesis 094.1
        juvenile 090.40
    aneurysm (ruptured) 094.87
    congenital 090.40
    juvenile 090.40
    remission in (sustained) 094.9
    serology doubtful, negative, or positive
      094.9
    specified nature or site NEC 094.89
    vascular 094.89
  cerebral 094.89
    meningovascular 094.2
    nerves 094.89
    sclerosis 094.89
    thrombosis 094.89
  cerebrospinal 094.89
    tabetic 094.0
  cerebrovascular 094.89
  cervix 095.8
  chancre (multiple) 091.0
    extragenital 091.2
    Rollet's 091.2
  Charcôt's joint 094.0 [713.5]
  choked disc 094.89 [377.00]
  chorioretinitis 091.51
    congenital 090.0 [363.13]
    late 094.83
  choroiditis 091.51
    congenital 090.0 [363.13]
    late 094.83
    prenatal 090.0 [363.13]
  choroidoretinitis (secondary) 091.51
    congenital 090.0 [363.13]
    late 094.83
  ciliary body (secondary) 091.52
    late 095.8 [364.11]
  colon (late) 095.8
  combined sclerosis 094.89
  complicating pregnancy, childbirth, or
    puerperium 647.0●
    affecting fetus or newborn 760.2
  condyloma (latum) 091.3

Syphilis, syphilitic (Continued)
  congenital 090.9
    with
      encephalitis 090.41
      paresis (general) 090.40
      tabes (dorsalis) 090.40
      taborparesis 090.40
    chorioretinitis, choroiditis 090.0 [363.13]
    early or less than 2 years after birth NEC
        090.2
      with manifestations 090.0
      latent (without manifestations)
          090.1
        negative spinal fluid test 090.1
        serology, positive 090.1
      symptomatic 090.0
    interstitial keratitis 090.3
    juvenile neurosyphilis 090.40
    late or 2 years or more after birth NEC
        090.7
      chorioretinitis, choroiditis 090.5
          [363.13]
      interstitial keratitis 090.3
      juvenile neurosyphilis NEC 090.40
      latent (without manifestations) 090.6
        negative spinal fluid test 090.6
        serology, positive 090.6
      symptomatic or with manifestations
          NEC 090.5
        interstitial keratitis 090.3
  conjugal 097.9
    tabes 094.0
  conjunctiva 095.8 [372.10]
  contact V01.6
  cord, bladder 094.0
  cornea, late 095.8 [370.59]
  coronary (artery) 093.89
    sclerosis 093.89
  coryza 095.8
    congenital 090.0
  cranial nerve 094.89
  cutaneous - see Syphilis, skin
  dacryocystitis 095.8
  degeneration, spinal cord 094.89
  d'emblée 095.8
  dementia 094.1
    paralytica 094.1
      juvenilis 090.40
  destruction of bone 095.5
  dilatation, aorta 093.0
  due to blood transfusion 097.9
  dura mater 094.89
  ear 095.8
    inner 095.8
      nerve (eighth) 094.86
      neurorecurrence 094.86
  early NEC 091.0
    cardiovascular 093.9
    central nervous system 094.9
      paresis 094.1
      tabes 094.0
    latent (without manifestations) (less than
        2 years after infection) 092.9
      negative spinal fluid test 092.9
      serological relapse following treatment
          092.0
      serology positive 092.9
    paresis 094.1
    relapse (treated, untreated) 091.7
    skin 091.3
    symptomatic NEC 091.89
      extragenital chancre 091.2
      primary, except extragenital chancre
          091.0
      secondary (see also Syphilis, secondary)
          091.3
        relapse (treated, untreated) 091.7
    tabes 094.0
    ulcer 091.3
  eighth nerve 094.86
  endemic, nonveneral 104.0

Syphilis, syphilitic (Continued)
  endocarditis 093.20
    aortic 093.22
    mitral 093.21
    pulmonary 093.24
    tricuspid 093.23
  epididymis (late) 095.8
  epiglottis 095.8
  epiphysitis (congenital) 090.0
  esophagus 095.8
  Eustachian tube 095.8
  exposure to V01.6
  eye 095.8 [363.13]
    neuromuscular mechanism 094.85
  eyelid 095.8 [373.5]
    with gumma 095.8 [373.5]
    ptosis 094.89
  fallopian tube 095.8
  fracture 095.5
  gallbladder (late) 095.8
  gastric 095.8
    crisis 094.0
    polyposis 095.8
  general 097.9
    paralysis 094.1
      juvenile 090.40
  genital (primary) 091.0
  glaucoma 095.8
  gumma (late) NEC 095.9
    cardiovascular system 093.9
    central nervous system 094.9
    congenital 090.5
    heart or artery 093.89
  heart 093.89
    block 093.89
    decompensation 093.89
    disease 093.89
    failure 093.89
    valve (see also Syphilis, endocarditis)
        093.20
  hemianesthesia 094.89
  hemianopsia 095.8
  hemiparesis 094.89
  hemiplegia 094.89
  hepatic artery 093.89
  hepatitis 095.3
  hepatomegaly 095.3
    congenital 090.0
  hereditaria tarda (see also Syphilis,
      congenital, late) 090.7
  hereditary (see also Syphilis, congenital) 090.9
    interstitial keratitis 090.3
  Hutchinson's teeth 090.5
  hyalitis 095.8
  inactive - see Syphilis, latent
  infantum NEC (see also Syphilis, congenital)
      090.9
  inherited - see Syphilis, congenital
  internal ear 095.8
  intestine (late) 095.8
  iris, iritis (secondary) 091.52
    late 095.8 [364.11]
  joint (late) 095.8
  keratitis (congenital) (early) (interstitial)
      (late) (parenchymatous) (punctata
      profunda) 090.3
  kidney 095.4
  lacrimal apparatus 095.8
  laryngeal paralysis 095.8
  larynx 095.8
  late 097.0
    cardiovascular 093.9
    central nervous system 094.9
    latent or 2 years or more after infection
        (without manifestation) 096
      negative spinal fluid test 096
      serology positive 096
    paresis 094.1
    specified site NEC 095.8
    symptomatic or with symptoms 095.9
    tabes 094.0

Syphilis, syphilitic (Continued)
  latent 097.1
    central nervous system 094.9
    date of infection unspecified 097.1
    early or less than 2 years after infection
        092.9
    late or 2 years or more after infection 096
    serology
      doubtful
        follow-up of latent syphilis 097.1
          central nervous system 094.9
          date of infection unspecified
              097.1
          early or less than 2 years after
              infection 092.9
          late or 2 years or more after
              infection 096
      positive, only finding 097.1
        date of infection unspecified 097.1
        early or less than 2 years after
            infection 097.1
        late or 2 years or more after
            infection 097.1
  lens 095.8
  leukoderma 091.3
    late 095.8
  lienis 095.8
  lip 091.3
    chancre 091.2
    late 095.8
    primary 091.2
  Lissauer's paralysis 094.1
  liver 095.3
    secondary 091.62
  locomotor ataxia 094.0
  lung 095.1
  lymphadenitis (secondary) 091.4
  lymph gland (early) (secondary) 091.4
    late 095.8
  macular atrophy of skin 091.3
    striated 095.8
  maternal, affecting fetus or newborn 760.2
    manifest syphilis in newborn - see
        Syphilis, congenital
  mediastinum (late) 095.8
  meninges (adhesive) (basilar) (brain) (spinal
      cord) 094.2
  meningitis 094.2
    acute 091.81
    congenital 090.42
  meningoencephalitis 094.2
  meningovascular 094.2
    congenital 090.49
  mesarteritis 093.89
    brain 094.89
    spine 094.89
  middle ear 095.8
  mitral stenosis 093.21
  monoplegia 094.89
  mouth (secondary) 091.3
    late 095.8
  mucocutaneous 091.3
    late 095.8
  mucous
    membrane 091.3
      late 095.8
    patches 091.3
      congenital 090.0
  mulberry molars 090.5
  muscle 095.6
  myocardium 093.82
  myositis 095.6
  nasal sinus 095.8
  neonatorum NEC (see also Syphilis,
      congenital) 090.9
  nerve palsy (any cranial nerve) 094.89
  nervous system, central 094.9
  neuritis 095.8
    acoustic nerve 094.86
  neurorecidive of retina 094.83
  neuroretinitis 094.85

◄ New   ◄▪▪ Revised   ~~deleted~~ Deleted   ● Use Additional Digit(s)   ▒ Omit code

Syphilis, syphilitic *(Continued)*
    newborn *(see also* Syphilis, congenital) 090.9
    nodular superficial 095.8
    nonvenereal, endemic 104.0
    nose 095.8
        saddle back deformity 090.5
        septum 095.8
            perforated 095.8
    occlusive arterial disease 093.89
    ophthalmic 095.8 *[363.13]*
    ophthalmoplegia 094.89
    optic nerve (atrophy) (neuritis) (papilla)
        094.84
    orbit (late) 095.8
    orchitis 095.8
    organic 097.9
    osseous (late) 095.5
    osteochondritis (congenital) 090.0
    osteoporosis 095.5
    ovary 095.8
    oviduct 095.8
    palate 095.8
        gumma 095.8
        perforated 090.5
    pancreas (late) 095.8
    pancreatitis 095.8
    paralysis 094.89
        general 094.1
        juvenile 090.40
    paraplegia 094.89
    paresis (general) 094.1
        juvenile 090.40
    paresthesia 094.89
    Parkinson's disease or syndrome 094.82
    paroxysmal tachycardia 093.89
    pemphigus (congenital) 090.0
    penis 091.0
        chancre 091.0
        late 095.8
    pericardium 093.81
    perichondritis, larynx 095.8
    periosteum 095.5
        congenital 090.0
        early 091.61
        secondary 091.61
    peripheral nerve 095.8
    petrous bone (late) 095.5
    pharynx 095.8
        secondary 091.3
    pituitary (gland) 095.8
    placenta 095.8
    pleura (late) 095.8
    pneumonia, white 090.0
    pontine (lesion) 094.89
    portal vein 093.89
    primary NEC 091.2
        anal 091.1
        and secondary *(see also* Syphilis,
            secondary) 091.9
        cardiovascular 093.9
        central nervous system 094.9
        extragenital chancre NEC 091.2
        fingers 091.2
        genital 091.0
        lip 091.2
        specified site NEC 091.2
        tonsils 091.2
    prostate 095.8
    psychosis (intracranial gumma) 094.89
    ptosis (eyelid) 094.89
    pulmonary (late) 095.1
        artery 093.89
    pulmonum 095.1
    pyelonephritis 095.4
    recently acquired, symptomatic NEC 091.89
    rectum 095.8
    respiratory tract 095.8
    retina
        late 094.83
        neurorecidive 094.83
    retrobulbar neuritis 094.85

Syphilis, syphilitic *(Continued)*
    salpingitis 095.8
    sclera (late) 095.0
    sclerosis
        cerebral 094.89
        coronary 093.89
        multiple 094.89
        subacute 094.89
    scotoma (central) 095.8
    scrotum 095.8
    secondary (and primary) 091.9
        adenopathy 091.4
        anus 091.3
        bone 091.61
        cardiovascular 093.9
        central nervous system 094.9
        chorioretinitis, choroiditis 091.51
        hepatitis 091.62
        liver 091.62
        lymphadenitis 091.4
        meningitis, acute 091.81
        mouth 091.3
        mucous membranes 091.3
        periosteum 091.61
        periostitis 091.61
        pharynx 091.3
        relapse (treated) (untreated) 091.7
        skin 091.3
        specified form NEC 091.89
        tonsil 091.3
        ulcer 091.3
        viscera 091.69
        vulva 091.3
    seminal vesicle (late) 095.8
    seronegative
        with signs or symptoms - *see* Syphilis, by
            site and stage
    seropositive
        with signs or symptoms - *see* Syphilis, by
            site or stage
        follow-up of latent syphilis - *see* Syphilis,
            latent
        only finding - *see* Syphilis, latent
    seventh nerve (paralysis) 094.89
    sinus 095.8
    sinusitis 095.8
    skeletal system 095.5
    skin (early) (secondary) (with ulceration)
        091.3
        late or tertiary 095.8
    small intestine 095.8
    spastic spinal paralysis 094.0
    spermatic cord (late) 095.8
    spinal (cord) 094.89
        with
            paresis 094.1
            tabes 094.0
    spleen 095.8
    splenomegaly 095.8
    spondylitis 095.5
    staphyloma 095.8
    stigmata (congenital) 090.5
    stomach 095.8
    synovium (late) 095.7
    tabes dorsalis (early) (late) 094.0
        juvenile 090.40
    tabetic type 094.0
        juvenile 090.40
    taboparesis 094.1
        juvenile 090.40
    tachycardia 093.89
    tendon (late) 095.7
    tertiary 097.0
        with symptoms 095.8
        cardiovascular 093.9
        central nervous system 094.9
        multiple NEC 095.8
        specified site NEC 095.8
    testis 095.8
    thorax 095.8
    throat 095.8

Syphilis, syphilitic *(Continued)*
    thymus (gland) 095.8
    thyroid (late) 095.8
    tongue 095.8
    tonsil (lingual) 095.8
        primary 091.2
        secondary 091.3
    trachea 095.8
    tricuspid valve 093.23
    tumor, brain 094.89
    tunica vaginalis (late) 095.8
    ulcer (any site) (early) (secondary) 091.3
        late 095.9
        perforating 095.9
            foot 094.0
    urethra (stricture) 095.8
    urogenital 095.8
    uterus 095.8
    uveal tract (secondary) 091.50
        late 095.8 *[363.13]*
    uveitis (secondary) 091.50
        late 095.8 *[363.13]*
    uvula (late) 095.8
        perforated 095.8
    vagina 091.0
        late 095.8
    valvulitis NEC 093.20
    vascular 093.89
        brain or cerebral 094.89
    vein 093.89
        cerebral 094.89
    ventriculi 095.8
    vesicae urinariae 095.8
    viscera (abdominal) 095.2
        secondary 091.69
    vitreous (hemorrhage) (opacities) 095.8
    vulva 091.0
        late 095.8
        secondary 091.3
Syphiloma 095.9
    cardiovascular system 093.9
    central nervous system 094.9
    circulatory system 093.9
    congenital 090.5
Syphilophobia 300.29
Syringadenoma (M8400/0) - *see also* Neoplasm,
        skin, benign
    papillary (M8406/0) - *see* Neoplasm, skin,
        benign
Syringobulbia 336.0
Syringocarcinoma (M8400/3) - *see* Neoplasm,
        skin, malignant
Syringocystadenoma (M8400/0) - *see also*
        Neoplasm, skin, benign
    papillary (M8406/0) - *see* Neoplasm, skin,
        benign
Syringocystoma (M8407/0) - *see* Neoplasm,
        skin, benign
Syringoma (M8407/0) - *see also* Neoplasm, skin,
        benign
    chondroid (M8940/0) - *see* Neoplasm, by site,
        benign
Syringomyelia 336.0
Syringomyelitis 323.9
    late effect - *see* category 326
Syringomyelocele *(see also* Spina bifida)
        741.9●
Syringopontia 336.0
System, systemic - *see also* condition
    disease, combined - *see* Degeneration,
        combined
    fibrosclerosing syndrome 710.8
    inflammatory response syndrome (SIRS)
        995.90
        due to
            infectious process 995.91
                with acute organ dysfunction 995.92
            non-infectious process 995.93
                with acute organ dysfunction 995.94
    lupus erythematosus 710.0
        inhibitor 795.79

T

Tab - *see* Tag
Tabacism 989.84
Tabacosis 989.84
Tabardillo 080
  flea-borne 081.0
  louse-borne 080
Tabes, tabetic
  with
    central nervous system syphilis 094.0
    Charcôt's joint 094.0 [713.5]
    cord bladder 094.0
    crisis, viscera (any) 094.0
    paralysis, general 094.1
    paresis (general) 094.1
    perforating ulcer 094.0
  arthropathy 094.0 [713.5]
  bladder 094.0
  bone 094.0
  cerebrospinal 094.0
  congenital 090.40
  conjugal 094.0
  dorsalis 094.0
    neurosyphilis 094.0
  early 094.0
  juvenile 090.40
  latent 094.0
  mesenterica (*see also* Tuberculosis) 014.8 ●
  paralysis insane, general 094.1
  peripheral (nonsyphilitic) 799.89
  spasmodic 094.0
    not dorsal or dorsalis 343.9
  syphilis (cerebrospinal) 094.0
Taboparalysis 094.1
Taboparesis (remission) 094.1
  with
    Charcôt's joint 094.1 [713.5]
    cord bladder 094.1
    perforating ulcer 094.1
  juvenile 090.40
Tache noir 923.20
Tachyalimentation 579.3
Tachyarrhythmia, tachyrhythmia - *see also*
    Tachycardia
  paroxysmal with sinus bradycardia
    427.81
Tachycardia 785.0
  atrial 427.89
  auricular 427.89
  AV nodal re-entry (re-entrant) 427.89
  junctional ectopic 427.0
  newborn 779.82
  nodal 427.89
    nonparoxysmal atrioventricular 426.89
    nonparoxysmal atrioventricular (nodal)
      426.89
  nonsustained 427.2
  paroxysmal 427.2
    with sinus bradycardia 427.81
    atrial (PAT) 427.0
      psychogenic 316 [427.0]
    atrioventricular (AV) 427.0
      psychogenic 316 [427.0]
    essential 427.2
    junctional 427.0
    nodal 427.0
    psychogenic 316 [427.2]
      atrial 316 [427.0]
      supraventricular 316 [427.0]
      ventricular 316 [427.1]
    supraventricular 427.0
      psychogenic 316 [427.0]
    ventricular 427.1
      psychogenic 316 [427.1]
  postoperative 997.1
  psychogenic 306.2
  sick sinus 427.81
  sinoauricular 427.89
  sinus 427.89
  supraventricular 427.89

Tachycardia (*Continued*)
  sustained 427.2
    supraventricular 427.0
    ventricular 427.1
  ventricular (paroxysmal) 427.1
    psychogenic 316 [427.1]
Tachygastria 536.8
Tachypnea 786.06
  hysterical 300.11
  newborn (idiopathic) (transitory) 770.6
  psychogenic 306.1
  transitory, of newborn 770.6
TACO (transfusion associated circulatory
    overload) 276.61
Taenia (infection) (infestation) (*see also*
    Infestation, taenia) 123.3
  diminuta 123.6
  echinococcal infestation (*see also*
    Echinococcus) 122.9
  nana 123.6
  saginata infestation 123.2
  solium (intestinal form) 123.0
    larval form 123.1
Taeniasis (intestine) (*see also* Infestation, taenia)
    123.3
  saginata 123.2
  solium 123.0
Taenzer's disease 757.4
Tag (hypertrophied skin) (infected)
    701.9
  adenoid 474.8
  anus 455.9
  endocardial (*see also* Endocarditis)
    424.90
  hemorrhoidal 455.9
  hymen 623.8
  perineal 624.8
  preauricular 744.1
  rectum 455.9
  sentinel 455.9
  skin 701.9
    accessory 757.39
    anus 455.9
    congenital 757.39
    preauricular 744.1
    rectum 455.9
  tonsil 474.8
  urethra, urethral 599.84
  vulva 624.8
Tahyna fever 062.5
Takayasu (-Onishi) disease or syndrome
    (pulseless disease) 446.7
Takotsubo syndrome 429.83
Talc granuloma 728.82
  in operation wound 998.7
Talcosis 502
Talipes (congenital) 754.70
  acquired NEC 736.79
    planus 734
  asymmetric 754.79
    acquired 736.79
  calcaneovalgus 754.62
    acquired 736.76
  calcaneovarus 754.59
    acquired 736.76
  calcaneus 754.79
    acquired 736.76
  cavovarus 754.59
    acquired 736.75
  cavus 754.71
    acquired 736.73
  equinovalgus 754.69
    acquired 736.72
  equinovarus 754.51
    acquired 736.71
  equinus 754.79
    acquired, NEC 736.72
  percavus 754.71
    acquired 736.73
  planovalgus 754.69
    acquired 736.79

Talipes (*Continued*)
  planus (acquired) (any degree) 734
    congenital 754.61
    due to rickets 268.1
  valgus 754.60
    acquired 736.79
  varus 754.50
    acquired 736.79
Talma's disease 728.85
Talon noir 924.20
  hand 923.20
  heel 924.20
  toe 924.3
Tamponade heart (Rose's) (*see also* Pericarditis)
    423.3
Tanapox 059.21
Tangier disease (familial high-density
    lipoprotein deficiency) 272.5
Tank ear 380.12
Tantrum (childhood) (*see also* Disturbance,
    conduct) 312.1 ●
Tapeworm (infection) (infestation) (*see also*
    Infestation, tapeworm) 123.9
Tapia's syndrome 352.6
Tarantism 297.8
Target-oval cell anemia 285.8
  with thalassemia - *see* Thalassemia
Tarlov's cyst 355.9
Tarral-Besnier disease (pityriasis rubra pilaris)
    696.4
Tarsalgia 729.2
Tarsal tunnel syndrome 355.5
Tarsitis (eyelid) 373.00
  syphilitic 095.8 [373.00]
  tuberculous (*see also* Tuberculosis) 017.0 ●
    [373.4]
Tartar (teeth) 523.6
Tattoo (mark) 709.09
Taurodontism 520.2
Taussig-Bing defect, heart, or syndrome
    (transposition, aorta and overriding
    pulmonary artery) 745.11
Tay's choroiditis 363.41
Tay-Sachs
  amaurotic familial idiocy 330.1
  disease 330.1
Taybi's syndrome (otopalatodigital) 759.89
Taylor's
  disease (diffuse idiopathic cutaneous
    atrophy) 701.8
  syndrome 625.5
TBI (traumatic brain injury) (*see also* Injury,
    intracranial) 854.0 ●
  with skull fracture - *see* Fracture, skull, by
    site
Tear, torn (traumatic) - *see also* Wound, open, by
    site
  annular fibrosis 722.51
  anus, anal (sphincter) 863.89
    with open wound in cavity 863.99
    complicating delivery (healed) (old)
      654.8 ●
      with mucosa 664.3 ●
      not associated with third-degree
        perineal laceration 664.6 ●
    nontraumatic, nonpuerperal (healed)
      (old) 569.43
  articular cartilage, old (*see also* Disorder,
    cartilage, articular) 718.0 ●
  bladder
    with
      abortion - *see* Abortion, by type, with
        damage to pelvic organs
      ectopic pregnancy (*see also* categories
        633.0–633.9) 639.2
      molar pregnancy (*see also* categories
        630–632) 639.2
    following
      abortion 639.2
      ectopic or molar pregnancy 639.2
    obstetrical trauma 665.5 ●

◀ New   ◀▥ Revised   ~~deleted~~ Deleted   ● Use Additional Digit(s)   ▨ Omit code

Tear, torn *(Continued)*
  bowel
    with
      abortion - *see* Abortion, by type, with damage to pelvic organs
      ectopic pregnancy *(see also* categories 633.0–633.9) 639.2
      molar pregnancy *(see also* categories 630–632) 639.2
    following
      abortion 639.2
      ectopic or molar pregnancy 639.2
    obstetrical trauma 665.5●
  broad ligament
    with
      abortion - *see* Abortion, by type, with damage to pelvic organs
      ectopic pregnancy *(see also* categories 633.0–633.9) 639.2
      molar pregnancy *(see also* categories 630–632) 639.2
    following
      abortion 639.2
      ectopic or molar pregnancy 639.2
    obstetrical trauma 665.6●
  bucket handle (knee) (meniscus) - *see* Tear, meniscus
  capsule
    joint - *see* Sprain, by site
    spleen - *see* Laceration, spleen, capsule
  cartilage - *see also* Sprain, by site
    articular, old *(see also* Disorder, cartilage, articular) 718.0●
    knee - *see* Tear, meniscus
    semilunar (knee) (current injury) - *see* Tear, meniscus
  cervix
    with
      abortion - *see* Abortion, by type, with damage to pelvic organs
      ectopic pregnancy *(see also* categories 633.0–633.9) 639.2
      molar pregnancy *(see also* categories 630–632) 639.2
    following
      abortion 639.2
      ectopic or molar pregnancy 639.2
    obstetrical trauma (current) 665.3●
    old 622.3
  dural 349.31
    accidental puncture or laceration during a procedure 349.31
    incidental (inadvertent) 349.31
    nontraumatic NEC 349.39
  internal organ (abdomen, chest, or pelvis) - *see* Injury, internal, by site
  ligament - *see also* Sprain, by site
    with open wound - *see* Wound, open, by site
  meniscus (knee) (current injury) 836.2
    bucket handle 836.0
      old 717.0
    lateral 836.1
      anterior horn 836.1
        old 717.42
      bucket handle 836.1
        old 717.41
      old 717.40
      posterior horn 836.1
        old 717.43
      specified site NEC 836.1
        old 717.49
    medial 836.0
      anterior horn 836.0
        old 717.1
      bucket handle 836.0
        old 717.0
      old 717.3
      posterior horn 836.0
        old 717.2

Tear, torn *(Continued)*
  meniscus *(Continued)*
    old NEC 717.5
    site other than knee - *see* Sprain, by site
  muscle - *see also* Sprain, by site
    with open wound - *see* Wound, open, by site
  pelvic
    floor, complicating delivery 664.1●
    organ NEC
      with
        abortion - *see* Abortion, by type, with damage to pelvic organs
        ectopic pregnancy *(see also* categories 633.0–633.9) 639.2
        molar pregnancy *(see also* categories 630–632) 639.2
      following
        abortion 639.2
        ectopic or molar pregnancy 639.2
      obstetrical trauma 665.5●
  perineum - *see also* Laceration, perineum
    obstetrical trauma 665.5●
  periurethral tissue
    with
      abortion - *see* Abortion, by type, with damage to pelvic organs
      ectopic pregnancy *(see also* categories 633.0–633.9) 639.2
      molar pregnancy *(see also* categories 630–632) 639.2
    following
      abortion 639.2
      ectopic or molar pregnancy 639.2
    obstetrical trauma 664.8●
  rectovaginal septum - *see* Laceration, rectovaginal septum
  retina, retinal (recent) (with detachment) 361.00
    without detachment 361.30
    dialysis (juvenile) (with detachment) 361.04
    giant (with detachment) 361.03
    horseshoe (without detachment) 361.32
    multiple (with detachment) 361.02
      without detachment 361.33
    old
      delimited (partial) 361.06
      partial 361.06
      total or subtotal 361.07
    partial (without detachment)
      giant 361.03
      multiple defects 361.02
      old (delimited) 361.06
      single defect 361.01
    round hole (without detachment) 361.31
    single defect (with detachment) 361.01
    total or subtotal (recent) 361.05
      old 361.07
  rotator cuff (traumatic) 840.4
    current injury 840.4
    degenerative 726.10
    nontraumatic (complete) 727.61
      partial 726.13
  semilunar cartilage, knee *(see also* Tear, meniscus) 836.2
    old 717.5
  tendon - *see also* Sprain, by site
    with open wound - *see* Wound, open, by site
  tentorial, at birth 767.0
  umbilical cord
    affecting fetus or newborn 772.0
    complicating delivery 663.8●
  urethra
    with
      abortion - *see* Abortion, by type, with damage to pelvic organs
      ectopic pregnancy *(see also* categories 633.0–633.9) 639.2
      molar pregnancy *(see also* categories 630–632) 639.2

Tear, torn *(Continued)*
  urethra *(Continued)*
    following
      abortion 639.2
      ectopic or molar pregnancy 639.2
    obstetrical trauma 665.5●
  uterus - *see* Injury, internal, uterus
  vagina - *see* Laceration, vagina
  vessel, from catheter 998.2
  vulva, complicating delivery 664.0●
Tear stone 375.57
Teeth, tooth - *see also* condition
  grinding 306.8
  prenatal 520.6
Teething 520.7
  syndrome 520.7
Tegmental syndrome 344.89
Telangiectasia, telangiectasis (verrucous) 448.9
  ataxic (cerebellar) 334.8
  familial 448.0
  hemorrhagic, hereditary (congenital) (senile) 448.0
  hereditary hemorrhagic 448.0
  retina 362.15
  spider 448.1
Telecanthus (congenital) 743.63
Telescoped bowel or intestine *(see also* Intussusception) 560.0
Teletherapy, adverse effect NEC 990
Telogen effluvium 704.02
Temperature
  body, high (of unknown origin) *(see also* Pyrexia) 780.60
  cold, trauma from 991.9
    newborn 778.2
    specified effect NEC 991.8
  high
    body (of unknown origin) *(see also* Pyrexia) 780.60
    trauma from - *see* Heat
Temper tantrum (childhood) *(see also* Disturbance, conduct) 312.1●
Temple - *see* condition
Temporal - *see also* condition
  lobe syndrome 310.0
Temporomandibular joint-pain-dysfunction syndrome 524.60
Temporosphenoidal - *see* condition
Tendency
  bleeding *(see also* Defect, coagulation) 286.9
  homosexual, ego-dystonic 302.0
  paranoid 301.0
  suicide 300.9
Tenderness
  abdominal (generalized) (localized) 789.6●
  rebound 789.6●
  skin 782.0
Tendinitis, tendonitis *(see also* Tenosynovitis) 726.90
  Achilles 726.71
  adhesive 726.90
    shoulder 726.0
  calcific 727.82
    shoulder 726.11
  gluteal 726.5
  patellar 726.64
  peroneal 726.79
  pes anserinus 726.61
  psoas 726.5
  tibialis (anterior) (posterior) 726.72
  trochanteric 726.5
Tendon - *see* condition
Tendosynovitis - *see* Tenosynovitis
Tendovaginitis - *see* Tenosynovitis
Tenesmus 787.99
  rectal 787.99
  vesical 788.99
Tenia - *see* Taenia
Teniasis - *see* Taeniasis
Tennis elbow 726.32

Tenonitis - *see also* Tenosynovitis
  eye (capsule) 376.04
Tenontosynovitis - *see* Tenosynovitis
Tenontothecitis - *see* Tenosynovitis
Tenophyte 727.9
Tenosynovitis (*see also* Synovitis) 727.00
  adhesive 726.90
    shoulder 726.0
  ankle 727.06
  bicipital (calcifying) 726.12
  buttock 727.09
  due to crystals - *see* Arthritis, due to crystals
  elbow 727.09
  finger 727.05
  foot 727.06
  gonococcal 098.51
  hand 727.05
  hip 727.09
  knee 727.09
  radial styloid 727.04
  shoulder 726.10
    adhesive 726.0
  specified NEC 727.09
  spine 720.1
  supraspinatus 726.10
  toe 727.06
  tuberculous - *see* Tuberculosis, tenosynovitis
  wrist 727.05
Tenovaginitis - *see* Tenosynovitis
Tension
  arterial, high (*see also* Hypertension) 401.9
    without diagnosis of hypertension
      796.2
  headache 307.81
  intraocular (elevated) 365.00
  nervous 799.21
  ocular (elevated) 365.00
  pneumothorax 512.0
    iatrogenic 512.1
    postoperative 512.1
    spontaneous 512.0
  premenstrual 625.4
  state 300.9
Tentorium - *see* condition
Teratencephalus 759.89
Teratism 759.7
Teratoblastoma (malignant) (M9080/3) - *see*
  Neoplasm, by site, malignant
Teratocarcinoma (M9081/3) - *see also* Neoplasm,
  by site, malignant
  liver 155.0
Teratoma (solid) (M9080/1) - *see also* Neoplasm,
  by site, uncertain behavior
  adult (cystic) (M9080/0) - *see* Neoplasm,
    site, benign
  and embryonal carcinoma, mixed
    (M9081/3) - *see* Neoplasm, by site,
    malignant
  benign (M9080/0) - *see* Neoplasm, by site,
    benign
  combined with choriocarcinoma (M9101/3) -
    see Neoplasm, by site, malignant
  cystic (adult) (M9080/0) - *see* Neoplasm, by
    site, benign
  differentiated type (M9080/0) -
    see Neoplasm, by site, benign
  embryonal (M9080/3) - *see also* Neoplasm, by
    site, malignant
    liver 155.0
  fetal
    sacral, causing fetopelvic disproportion
      653.7●
  immature (M9080/3) - *see* Neoplasm, by site,
    malignant
  liver (M9080/3) 155.0
    adult, benign, cystic, differentiated type,
      or mature (M9080/0) 211.5
  malignant (M9080/3) - *see also* Neoplasm, by
    site, malignant
    anaplastic type (M9082/3) - *see* Neoplasm,
      by site, malignant

Teratoma (*Continued*)
  malignant (*Continued*)
    intermediate type (M9083/3) - *see*
      Neoplasm, by site, malignant
    liver (M9080/3) 155.0
    trophoblastic (M9102/3)
      specified site - *see* Neoplasm, by site,
        malignant
      unspecified site 186.9
    undifferentiated type (M9082/3) - *see*
      Neoplasm, by site, malignant
  mature (M9080/0) - *see* Neoplasm, by site,
    benign
    malignant (M9080/3) - *see* Neoplasm, by
      site, malignant
  ovary (M9080/0) 220
    embryonal, immature, or malignant
      (M9080/3) 183.0
  suprasellar (M9080/3) - *see* Neoplasm, by
    site, malignant
  testis (M9080/3) 186.9
    adult, benign, cystic, differentiated type
      or mature (M9080/0) 222.0
    undescended 186.0
Terminal care V66.7
Termination
  anomalous - *see also* Malposition, congenital
    portal vein 747.49
    right pulmonary vein 747.42
  pregnancy (legal) (therapeutic) (*see* Abortion,
    legal) 635.9●
    fetus NEC 779.6
    illegal (*see also* Abortion, illegal) 636.9●
Ternidens diminutus infestation 127.7
Terrors, night (child) 307.46
Terry's syndrome (*see also* Retinopathy of
  prematurity) 362.21
Tertiary - *see* condition
Tessellated fundus, retina (tigroid) 362.89
Test(s)
  adequacy
    hemodialysis V56.31
    peritoneal dialysis V56.32
  AIDS virus V72.69
  allergen V72.7
  bacterial disease NEC (*see also* Screening, by
    name of disease) V74.9
  basal metabolic rate V72.69
  blood
    alcohol V70.4
    drug V70.4
      for therapeutic drug monitoring
        V58.83
      for routine general physical examination
        V72.62
    prior to treatment or procedure V72.63
    typing V72.86
      Rh typing V72.86
  developmental, infant or child V20.2
  Dick V74.8
  fertility V26.21
  genetic
    female V26.32
    for genetic disease carrier status
      female V26.31
      male V26.34
    male V26.39
  hearing V72.19
    following failed hearing screening V72.11
    routine, for infant and child V20.2
  HIV V72.69
  human immunodeficiency virus V72.69
  immunity status V72.61
  Kveim V82.89
  laboratory V72.60
    for medicolegal reason V70.4
    ordered as part of a routine general
      medical examination V72.62
    pre-operative V72.63
    pre-procedural V72.63
    specified NEC V72.69

Test(s) (*Continued*)
  male partner of female with recurrent
    pregnancy loss V26.35
  Mantoux (for tuberculosis) V74.1
  mycotic organism V75.4
  nuchal translucency V28.89
  parasitic agent NEC V75.8
  paternity V70.4
  peritoneal equilibration V56.32
  pregnancy
    negative result V72.41
    positive result V72.42
      first pregnancy V72.42
    unconfirmed V72.40
  preoperative V72.84
    cardiovascular V72.81
    respiratory V72.82
    specified NEC V72.83
  procreative management NEC V26.29
    genetic disease carrier status
      female V26.31
      male V26.34
  Rh typing V72.86
  sarcoidosis V82.89
  Schick V74.3
  Schultz-Charlton V74.8
  skin, diagnostic
    allergy V72.7
    bacterial agent NEC (*see also* Screening, by
      name of disease) V74.9
    Dick V74.8
    hypersensitivity V72.7
    Kveim V82.89
    Mantoux V74.1
    mycotic organism V75.4
    parasitic agent NEC V75.8
    sarcoidosis V82.89
    Schick V74.3
    Schultz-Charlton V74.8
    tuberculin V74.1
  specified type NEC V72.85
  tuberculin V74.1
  vision V72.0
    routine, for infant and child V20.2
  Wassermann
    positive (*see also* Serology for syphilis,
      positive) 097.1
    false 795.6
Testicle, testicular, testis - *see also* condition
  feminization (syndrome) 259.51
Tetanus, tetanic (cephalic) (convulsions) 037
  with
    abortion - *see* Abortion, by type, with
      sepsis
    ectopic pregnancy (*see also* categories
      633.0–633.9) 639.0
    molar pregnancy (*see* categories 630–632)
      639.0
  following
    abortion 639.0
    ectopic or molar pregnancy 639.0
  inoculation V03.7
    reaction (due to serum) - *see*
      Complications, vaccination
  neonatorum 771.3
  puerperal, postpartum, childbirth 670.8●
Tetany, tetanic 781.7
  alkalosis 276.3
  associated with rickets 268.0
  convulsions 781.7
    hysterical 300.11
  functional (hysterical) 300.11
  hyperkinetic 781.7
    hysterical 300.11
  hyperpnea 786.01
    hysterical 300.11
    psychogenic 306.1
  hyperventilation 786.01
    hysterical 300.11
    psychogenic 306.1
  hypocalcemic, neonatal 775.4

Tetany, tetanic *(Continued)*
  hysterical 300.11
  neonatal 775.4
  parathyroid (gland) 252.1
  parathyroprival 252.1
  postoperative 252.1
  postthyroidectomy 252.1
  pseudotetany 781.7
    hysterical 300.11
  psychogenic 306.1
    specified as conversion reaction 300.11
Tetralogy of Fallot 745.2
Tetraplegia - *see* Quadriplegia
Thailand hemorrhagic fever 065.4
Thalassanemia 282.40
Thalassemia (disease) 282.40
  with other hemoglobinopathy 282.49
  alpha (major) (severe) (triple gene defect)
      282.43
    silent carrier 282.46
  beta (homozygous) (major) (severe) 282.44
  delta-beta (homozygous) 282.45
  dominant 282.49
  Hb-S (without crisis) 282.41
    with
        crisis 282.42
        vaso-occlusive pain 282.42
  hemoglobin
    C (Hb-C) 282.49
    D (Hb-D) 282.49
    E (Hb-E) 282.49
    E-beta 282.47
    H (Hb-H) 282.49
    I (Hb-I) 282.49
  high fetal gene (*see also* Thalassemia) 282.40
  high fetal hemoglobin (*see also* Thalassemia)
      282.40
  intermedia 282.44
  major 282.44
  minor (alpha) (beta) 282.46
  mixed 282.49
  sickle-cell (without crisis) 282.41
    with
        crisis 282.42
        vaso-occlusive pain 282.42
  specified NEC 282.49
  trait (alpha) (beta) (delta-beta) 282.46
Thalassemic variants 282.49
Thaysen-Gee disease (nontropical sprue) 579.0
Thecoma (M8600/0) 220
  malignant (M8600/3) 183.0
Thelarche, precocious 259.1
Thelitis 611.0
  puerperal, postpartum 675.0●
Therapeutic - *see* condition
Therapy V57.9
  blood transfusion, without reported
      diagnosis V58.2
  breathing V57.0
  chemotherapy, antineoplastic V58.11
    fluoride V07.31
    prophylactic NEC V07.39
  dialysis (intermittent) (treatment)
    extracorporeal V56.0
    peritoneal V56.8
    renal V56.0
    specified type NEC V56.8
  exercise NEC V57.1
    breathing V57.0
  extracorporeal dialysis (renal) V56.0
  fluoride prophylaxis V07.31
  hemodialysis V56.0
  hormone replacement (postmenopausal)
      V07.4
  immunotherapy antineoplastic V58.12
  long term oxygen therapy V46.2
  occupational V57.21
  orthoptic V57.4
  orthotic V57.81
  peritoneal dialysis V56.8
  physical NEC V57.1

Therapy *(Continued)*
  postmenopausal hormone replacement V07.4
  radiation V58.0
  speech (-language) V57.3
  vocational V57.22
Thermalgesia 782.0
Thermalgia 782.0
Thermanalgesia 782.0
Thermanesthesia 782.0
Thermic - *see* condition
Thermography (abnormal) 793.99
  breast 793.89
Thermoplegia 992.0
Thesaurismosis
  amyloid 277.39
  bilirubin 277.4
  calcium 275.40
  cystine 270.0
  glycogen (*see also* Disease, glycogen storage)
      271.0
  kerasin 272.7
  lipoid 272.7
  melanin 255.41
  phosphatide 272.7
  urate 274.9
Thiaminic deficiency 265.1
  with beriberi 265.0
Thibierge-Weissenbach syndrome (cutaneous
      systemic sclerosis) 710.1
Thickened endometrium 793.5
Thickening
  bone 733.99
    extremity 733.99
  breast 611.79
  hymen 623.3
  larynx 478.79
  nail 703.8
    congenital 757.5
  periosteal 733.99
  pleura (*see also* Pleurisy) 511.0
  skin 782.8
  subepiglottic 478.79
  tongue 529.8
  valve, heart - *see* Endocarditis
Thiele syndrome 724.6
Thigh - *see* condition
Thinning vertebra (*see also* Osteoporosis)
      733.00
Thirst, excessive 783.5
  due to deprivation of water 994.3
Thomsen's disease 359.22
Thomson's disease (congenital poikiloderma)
      757.33
Thoracic - *see also* condition
  kidney 753.3
  outlet syndrome 353.0
  stomach - *see* Hernia, diaphragm
Thoracogastroschisis (congenital) 759.89
Thoracopagus 759.4
Thoracoschisis 756.3
Thoracoscopic surgical procedure converted to
      open procedure V64.42
Thorax - *see* condition
Thorn's syndrome (*see also* Disease, renal) 593.9
Thornwaldt's, Tornwaldt's
  bursitis (pharyngeal) 478.29
  cyst 478.26
  disease (pharyngeal bursitis) 478.29
Thorson-Biörck syndrome (malignant
      carcinoid) 259.2
Threadworm (infection) (infestation) 127.4
Threatened
  abortion or miscarriage 640.0●
    with subsequent abortion (*see also*
        Abortion, spontaneous) 634.9●
    affecting fetus 762.1
  labor 644.1●
    affecting fetus or newborn 761.8
    premature 644.0●
  miscarriage 640.0●
    affecting fetus 762.1

Threatened *(Continued)*
  premature
    delivery 644.2●
      affecting fetus or newborn 761.8
    labor 644.0●
      before 22 completed weeks gestation
          640.0●
Three-day fever 066.0
Threshers' lung 495.0
Thrix annulata (congenital) 757.4
Throat - *see* condition
Thrombasthenia (Glanzmann's) (hemorrhagic)
      (hereditary) 287.1
Thromboangiitis 443.1
  obliterans (general) 443.1
    cerebral 437.1
    vessels
      brain 437.1
      spinal cord 437.1
Thromboarteritis - *see* Arteritis
Thromboasthenia (Glanzmann's)
      (hemorrhagic) (hereditary) 287.1
Thrombocytasthenia (Glanzmann's) 287.1
Thrombocythemia (primary) (M9962/1) 238.71
  essential 238.71
  hemorrhagic 238.71
  idiopathic (hemorrhagic) (M9962/1) 238.71
Thrombocytopathy (dystrophic) (granulopenic)
      287.1
Thrombocytopenia, thrombocytopenic 287.5
  with
    absent radii (TAR) syndrome 287.33
    giant hemangioma 287.39
  amegakaryocytic, congenital 287.33
  congenital 287.33
  cyclic 287.39
  dilutional 287.49
  due to
    drugs 287.49
    extracorporeal circulation of blood 287.49
    massive blood transfusion 287.49
    platelet alloimmunization 287.49
  essential 287.30
  fetal 678.0●
  heparin-induced (HIT) 289.84
  hereditary 287.33
  Kasabach-Merritt 287.39
  neonatal, transitory 776.1
    due to
      exchange transfusion 776.1
      idiopathic maternal thrombocytopenia
          776.1
      isoimmunization 776.1
  primary 287.30
  puerperal, postpartum 666.3●
  purpura (*see also* Purpura,
      thrombocytopenic) 287.30
  thrombotic 446.6
  secondary NEC 287.49
  sex-linked 287.39
Thrombocytosis 238.71
  essential 238.71
  primary 238.71
Thromboembolism - *see* Embolism
Thrombopathy (Bernard-Soulier) 287.1
  constitutional 286.4
  Willebrand-Jürgens (angiohemophilia) 286.4
Thrombopenia (*see also* Thrombocytopenia)
      287.5
Thrombophlebitis 451.9
  antecubital vein 451.82
  antepartum (superficial) 671.2●
    affecting fetus or newborn 760.3
    deep 671.3●
  arm 451.89
    deep 451.83
    superficial 451.82
  breast, superficial 451.89
  cavernous (venous) sinus - *see*
      Thrombophlebitis, intracranial venous
      sinus

Thrombophlebitis (Continued)
cephalic vein 451.82
cerebral (sinus) (vein) 325
late effect - see category 326
nonpyogenic 437.6
in pregnancy or puerperium 671.5●
late effect - see Late effect(s) (of)
cerebrovascular disease
due to implanted device - see Complications,
due to (presence of) any device,
implant, or graft classified to
996.0–996.5 NEC
during or resulting from a procedure NEC
997.2
femoral 451.11
femoropopliteal 451.19
following infusion, perfusion, or transfusion
999.2
hepatic (vein) 451.89
idiopathic, recurrent 453.1
iliac vein 451.81
iliofemoral 451.11
intracranial venous sinus (any) 325
late effect - see category 326
nonpyogenic 437.6
in pregnancy or puerperium 671.5●
late effect - see Late effect(s) (of)
cerebrovascular disease
jugular vein 451.89
lateral (venous) sinus - see Thrombophlebitis,
intracranial venous sinus
leg 451.2
deep (vessels) 451.19
femoral vein 451.11
specified vessel NEC 451.19
superficial (vessels) 451.0
femoral vein 451.11
longitudinal (venous) sinus - see
Thrombophlebitis, intracranial venous
sinus
lower extremity 451.2
deep (vessels) 451.19
femoral vein 451.11
specified vessel NEC 451.19
superficial (vessels) 451.0
migrans, migrating 453.1
pelvic
with
abortion - see Abortion, by type, with
sepsis
ectopic pregnancy (see also categories
633.0–633.9) 639.0
molar pregnancy (see also categories
630–632) 639.0
following
abortion 639.0
ectopic or molar pregnancy 639.0
puerperal 671.4●
popliteal vein 451.19
portal (vein) 572.1
postoperative 997.2
pregnancy (superficial) 671.2●
affecting fetus or newborn 760.3
deep 671.3●
puerperal, postpartum, childbirth
(extremities) (superficial) 671.2●
deep 671.4●
pelvic 671.4●
septic 670.3●
specified site NEC 671.5●
radial vein 451.82
saphenous (greater) (lesser) 451.0
sinus (intracranial) - see Thrombophlebitis,
intracranial venous sinus
specified site NEC 451.89
tibial vein 451.19
Thrombosis, thrombotic (marantic) (multiple)
(progressive) (vein) (vessel) 453.9
with childbirth or during the puerperium -
see Thrombosis, puerperal, postpartum
antepartum - see Thrombosis, pregnancy

Thrombosis, thrombotic (Continued)
aorta, aortic 444.1
abdominal 444.09
saddle 444.01
bifurcation 444.09
saddle 444.01
terminal 444.09
thoracic 444.1
valve - see Endocarditis, aortic
apoplexy (see also Thrombosis, brain) 434.0●
late effect - see Late effect(s) (of)
cerebrovascular disease
appendix, septic - see Appendicitis, acute
arteriolar-capillary platelet, disseminated
446.6
artery, arteries (postinfectional) 444.9
auditory, internal 433.8●
basilar (see also Occlusion, artery, basilar)
433.0●
carotid (common) (internal) (see also
Occlusion, artery, carotid) 433.1●
with other precerebral artery 433.3●
cerebellar (anterior inferior) (posterior
inferior) (superior) 433.8●
cerebral (see also Thrombosis, brain)
434.0●
choroidal (anterior) 433.8●
communicating posterior 433.8●
coronary (see also Infarct, myocardium)
410.9●
without myocardial infarction 411.81
due to syphilis 093.89
healed or specified as old 412
extremities 444.22
lower 444.22
upper 444.21
femoral 444.22
hepatic 444.89
hypophyseal 433.8●
meningeal, anterior or posterior 433.8●
mesenteric (with gangrene) 557.0
ophthalmic (see also Occlusion, retina)
362.30
pontine 433.8●
popliteal 444.22
precerebral - see Occlusion, artery,
precerebral NEC
pulmonary 415.19
iatrogenic 415.11
personal history of V12.55
postoperative 415.11
septic 415.12
renal 593.81
retinal (see also Occlusion, retina) 362.30
specified site NEC 444.89
spinal, anterior or posterior 433.8●
traumatic (complication) (early) (see also
Injury, blood vessel, by site) 904.9
vertebral (see also Occlusion, artery,
vertebral) 433.2●
with other precerebral artery 433.3●
atrial (endocardial) 424.90
without endocarditis 429.89
due to syphilis 093.89
auricular (see also Infarct, myocardium)
410.9●
axillary (acute) (vein) 453.84
chronic 453.74
personal history of V12.51
basilar (artery) (see also Occlusion, artery,
basilar) 433.0●
bland NEC 453.9
brain (artery) (stem) 434.0●
due to syphilis 094.89
iatrogenic 997.02
late effect - see Late effect(s) (of)
cerebrovascular disease
postoperative 997.02
puerperal, postpartum, childbirth 674.0●
sinus (see also Thrombosis, intracranial
venous sinus) 325

Thrombosis, thrombotic (Continued)
capillary 448.9
arteriolar, generalized 446.6
cardiac (see also Infarct, myocardium)
410.9●
due to syphilis 093.89
healed or specified as old 412
valve - see Endocarditis
carotid (artery) (common) (internal) (see also
Occlusion, artery, carotid) 433.1●
with other precerebral artery 433.3●
cavernous sinus (venous) - see Thrombosis,
intracranial venous sinus
cerebellar artery (anterior inferior) (posterior
inferior) (superior) 433.8●
late effect - see Late effect(s) (of)
cerebrovascular disease
cerebral (arteries) (see also Thrombosis, brain)
434.0●
late effect - see Late effect(s) (of)
cerebrovascular disease
coronary (artery) (see also Infarct,
myocardium) 410.9●
without myocardial infarction 411.81
due to syphilis 093.89
healed or specified as old 412
corpus cavernosum 607.82
cortical (see also Thrombosis, brain)
434.0●
due to (presence of) any device, implant, or
graft classifiable to 996.0–996.5 - see
Complications, due to (presence of)
any device, implant, or graft classified
to 996.0–996.5 NEC
effort 453.89
endocardial - see Infarct, myocardium
eye (see also Occlusion, retina) 362.30
femoral (vein) 453.6
with inflammation or phlebitis 451.11
artery 444.22
deep 453.41
personal history of V12.51
genital organ, male 608.83
heart (chamber) (see also Infarct,
myocardium) 410.9●
hepatic (vein) 453.0
artery 444.89
infectional or septic 572.1
iliac (acute) (vein) 453.41
with inflammation or phlebitis 451.81
artery (common) (external) (internal)
444.81
chronic 453.51
personal history of V12.51
inflammation, vein - see Thrombophlebitis
internal carotid artery (see also Occlusion,
artery, carotid) 433.1●
with other precerebral artery 433.3●
intestine (with gangrene) 557.0
intracranial (see also Thrombosis, brain)
434.0●
venous sinus (any) 325
nonpyogenic origin 437.6
in pregnancy or puerperium
671.5●
intramural (see also Infarct, myocardium)
410.9●
without
cardiac condition 429.89
coronary artery disease 429.89
myocardial infarction 429.89
healed or specified as old 412
jugular (bulb)
external (acute) 453.89
chronic 453.79
internal (acute) 453.86
chronic 453.76
kidney 593.81
artery 593.81
lateral sinus (venous) - see Thrombosis,
intracranial venous sinus

◀ New   ◀╫ Revised   ~~deleted~~ Deleted   ● Use Additional Digit(s)   ▨ Omit code

Thrombosis, thrombotic (*Continued*)
  leg (*see also* Thrombosis, lower extremity)
    453.6
    with inflammation or phlebitis - *see*
      Thrombophlebitis
    deep (vessels) 453.40
      acute 453.40
        lower (distal) 453.42
        upper (proximal) 453.41
      chronic 453.50
        lower (distal) 453.52
        upper (proximal) 453.51
      lower (distal) 453.42
      upper (proximal) 453.41
    personal history of V12.51
    superficial (vessels) 453.6
  liver (venous) 453.0
    artery 444.89
    infectional or septic 572.1
    portal vein 452
  longitudinal sinus (venous) - *see* Thrombosis,
    intracranial venous sinus
  lower extremity (superficial) 453.6
    deep vessels 453.40
      acute 453.40
        calf 453.42
        distal (lower leg) 453.42
        femoral 453.41
        iliac 453.41
        lower leg 453.42
        peroneal 453.42
        popliteal 453.41
        proximal (upper leg) 453.41
        thigh 453.41
        tibial 453.42
      chronic 453.50
        calf 453.52
        distal (lower leg) 453.52
        femoral 453.51
        iliac 453.51
        lower leg 453.52
        peroneal 453.52
        popliteal 453.51
        proximal (upper leg) 453.51
        thigh 453.51
        tibial 453.52
    personal history of V12.51
    saphenous (greater) (lesser) 453.6
    superficial 453.6
  lung 415.19
    iatrogenic 415.11
    personal history of V12.55
    postoperative 415.11
    septic 415.12
  marantic, dural sinus 437.6
  meninges (brain) (*see also* Thrombosis, brain)
    434.0●
  mesenteric (artery) (with gangrene) 557.0
    vein (inferior) (superior) 557.0
  mitral - *see* Insufficiency, mitral
  mural (heart chamber) (*see also* Infarct,
    myocardium) 410.9●
    without
      cardiac condition 429.89
      coronary artery disease 429.89
      myocardial infarction 429.89
    due to syphilis 093.89
    following myocardial infarction 429.79
    healed or specified as old 412
  omentum (with gangrene) 557.0
  ophthalmic (artery) (*see also* Occlusion,
    retina) 362.30
  pampiniform plexus (male) 608.83
    female 620.8
  parietal (*see also* Infarct, myocardium)
    410.9●
  penis, penile 607.82
  peripheral arteries 444.22
    lower 444.22
    upper 444.21
  platelet 446.6

Thrombosis, thrombotic (*Continued*)
  portal 452
    due to syphilis 093.89
    infectional or septic 572.1
  precerebral artery - *see also* Occlusion, artery,
    precerebral NEC
  pregnancy 671.2●
    deep (vein) 671.3●
    superficial (vein) 671.2●
  puerperal, postpartum, childbirth
    671.2●
    brain (artery) 674.0●
      venous 671.5●
    cardiac 674.8●
    cerebral (artery) 674.0●
      venous 671.5●
    deep 671.4●
    intracranial sinus (nonpyogenic) (venous)
      671.5●
    pelvic 671.4●
    pulmonary (artery) 673.2●
    specified site NEC 671.5●
    superficial 671.2●
  pulmonary (artery) (vein) 415.19
    iatrogenic 415.11
    personal history of V12.55
    postoperative 415.11
    septic 415.12
  renal (artery) 593.81
    vein 453.3
  resulting from presence of shunt or other
      internal prosthetic device - *see*
      Complications, due to (presence of)
      any device, implant, or graft
      classifiable to 996.0–996.5 NEC
  retina, retinal (artery) 362.30
    arterial branch 362.32
    central 362.31
    partial 362.33
    vein
      central 362.35
      tributary (branch) 362.36
  saphenous vein (greater) (lesser) 453.6
  scrotum 608.83
  seminal vesicle 608.83
  sigmoid (venous) sinus (*see* Thrombosis,
    intracranial venous sinus) 325
  silent NEC 453.9
  sinus, intracranial (venous) (any) (*see also*
    Thrombosis, intracranial venous sinus)
    325
  softening, brain (*see also* Thrombosis, brain)
    434.0●
  specified site NEC (acute) 453.89
    chronic 453.79
  spermatic cord 608.83
  spinal cord 336.1
    due to syphilis 094.89
    in pregnancy or puerperium 671.5●
    pyogenic origin 324.1
      late effect - *see* category 326
  spleen, splenic 289.59
    artery 444.89
  testis 608.83
  traumatic (complication) (early) (*see also*
    Injury, blood vessel, by site) 904.9
  tricuspid - *see* Endocarditis, tricuspid
  tumor - *see* Neoplasm, by site
  tunica vaginalis 608.83
  umbilical cord (vessels) 663.6●
    affecting fetus or newborn 762.6
  upper extremity (acute) 453.83
    deep 453.82
    superficial 453.81
    chronic 453.73
      deep 453.72
      superficial 453.71
  vas deferens 608.83
  vein
    antecubital (acute) 453.81
      chronic 453.71

Thrombosis, thrombotic (*Continued*)
  vein (*Continued*)
    axillary (acute) 453.84
      chronic 453.74
    basilic (acute) 453.81
      chronic 453.71
    brachial (acute) 453.82
      chronic 453.72
    brachiocephalic (innominate) (acute)
      453.87
      chronic 453.77
    cephalic (acute) 453.81
      chronic 453.71
    deep 453.40
      personal history of V12.51
    internal jugular (acute) 453.86
      chronic 453.76
    lower extremity - *see* Thrombosis, lower
      extremity
    personal history of V12.51
    radial (acute) 453.82
      chronic 453.72
    saphenous (greater) (lesser) 453.6
    specified site NEC (acute) 453.89
      chronic 453.79
    subclavian (acute) 453.85
      chronic 453.75
    superior vena cava (acute) 453.87
      chronic 453.77
    thoracic (acute) 453.87
      chronic 453.77
    ulnar (acute) 453.82
      chronic 453.72
    upper extremity - *see* Thrombosis, upper
      extremity
  vena cava
    inferior 453.2
    personal history of V12.51
    superior (acute) 453.87
      chronic 453.77

Thrombus - *see* Thrombosis
Thrush 112.0
  newborn 771.7
Thumb - *see also* condition
  gamekeeper's 842.12
  sucking (child problem) 307.9
Thygeson's superficial punctate keratitis
  370.21
Thymergasia (*see also* Psychosis, affective)
  296.80
Thymitis 254.8
Thymoma (benign) (M8580/0) 212.6
  malignant (M8580/3) 164.0
Thymus, thymic (gland) - *see* condition
Thyrocele (*see also* Goiter) 240.9
Thyroglossal - *see also* condition
  cyst 759.2
  duct, persistent 759.2
Thyroid (body) (gland) - *see also* condition
  hormone resistance 246.8
  lingual 759.2
Thyroiditis 245.9
  acute (pyogenic) (suppurative) 245.0
    nonsuppurative 245.0
  autoimmune 245.2
  chronic (nonspecific) (sclerosing) 245.8
    fibrous 245.3
    lymphadenoid 245.2
    lymphocytic 245.2
    lymphoid 245.2
  complicating pregnancy, childbirth, or
    puerperium 648.1●
  de Quervain's (subacute granulomatous)
    245.1
  fibrous (chronic) 245.3
  giant (cell) (follicular) 245.1
  granulomatous (de Quervain's) (subacute)
    245.1
  Hashimoto's (struma lymphomatosa) 245.2
  iatrogenic 245.4
  invasive (fibrous) 245.3

Thyroiditis (Continued)
ligneous 245.3
lymphocytic (chronic) 245.2
lymphoid 245.2
lymphomatous 245.2
pseudotuberculous 245.1
pyogenic 245.0
radiation 245.4
Riedel's (ligneous) 245.3
subacute 245.1
suppurative 245.0
tuberculous (see also Tuberculosis) 017.5 ●
viral 245.1
woody 245.3
Thyrolingual duct, persistent 759.2
Thyromegaly 240.9
Thyrotoxic
crisis or storm (see also Thyrotoxicosis) 242.9 ●
heart failure (see also Thyrotoxicosis) 242.9 ●
[425.7]
Thyrotoxicosis 242.9 ●

> Note: Use the following fifth-digit subclassification with category 242:
>
> 0 without mention of thyrotoxic crisis or storm
> 1 with mention of thyrotoxic crisis or storm

with
goiter (diffuse) 242.0 ●
adenomatous 242.3 ●
multinodular 242.2 ●
uninodular 242.1 ●
nodular 242.3 ●
multinodular 242.2 ●
uninodular 242.1 ●
infiltrative
dermopathy 242.0 ●
ophthalmopathy 242.0 ●
thyroid acropachy 242.0 ●
complicating pregnancy, childbirth, or
puerperium 648.1 ●
due to
ectopic thyroid nodule 242.4 ●
ingestion of (excessive) thyroid material
242.8 ●
specified cause NEC 242.8 ●
factitia 242.8 ●
heart 242.9 ● [425.7]
neonatal (transient) 775.3
TIA (transient ischemic attack) 435.9
with transient neurologic deficit 435.9
late effect - see Late effect(s) (of)
cerebrovascular disease
Tibia vara 732.4
Tic 307.20
breathing 307.20
child problem 307.21
compulsive 307.22
convulsive 307.20
degenerative (generalized) (localized)
333.3
facial 351.8
douloureux (see also Neuralgia, trigeminal)
350.1
atypical 350.2
habit 307.20
chronic (motor or vocal) 307.22
transient (of childhood) 307.21
lid 307.20
transient (of childhood) 307.21
motor-verbal 307.23
occupational 300.89
orbicularis 307.20
transient (of childhood) 307.21
organic origin 333.3
postchoreic - see Chorea
psychogenic 307.20
compulsive 307.22

Tic (Continued)
salaam 781.0
spasm 307.20
chronic (motor or vocal) 307.22
transient (of childhood) 307.21
Tick (-borne) fever NEC 066.1
American mountain 066.1
Colorado 066.1
hemorrhagic NEC 065.3
Crimean 065.0
Kyasanur Forest 065.2
Omsk 065.1
mountain 066.1
nonexanthematous 066.1
Tick-bite fever NEC 066.1
African 087.1
Colorado (virus) 066.1
Rocky Mountain 082.0
Tick paralysis 989.5
Tics and spasms, compulsive 307.22
Tietze's disease or syndrome 733.6
Tight, tightness
anus 564.89
chest 786.59
fascia (lata) 728.9
foreskin (congenital) 605
hymen 623.3
introitus (acquired) (congenital) 623.3
rectal sphincter 564.89
tendon 727.81
Achilles (heel) 727.81
urethral sphincter 598.9
Tilting vertebra 737.9
Timidity, child 313.21
Tinea (intersecta) (tarsi) 110.9
amiantacea 110.0
asbestina 110.0
barbae 110.0
beard 110.0
black dot 110.0
blanca 111.2
capitis 110.0
corporis 110.5
cruris 110.3
decalvans 704.09
flava 111.0
foot 110.4
furfuracea 111.0
imbricata (Tokelau) 110.5
lepothrix 039.0
manuum 110.2
microsporic (see also Dermatophytosis)
110.9
nigra 111.1
nodosa 111.2
pedis 110.4
scalp 110.0
specified site NEC 110.8
sycosis 110.0
tonsurans 110.0
trichophytic (see also Dermatophytosis)
110.9
unguium 110.1
versicolor 111.0
Tingling sensation (see also Disturbance,
sensation) 782.0
Tin-miners' lung 503
Tinnitus (aurium) 388.30
audible 388.32
objective 388.32
subjective 388.31
Tipped, teeth 524.33
Tipping
pelvis 738.6
with disproportion (fetopelvic) 653.0 ●
affecting fetus or newborn 763.1
causing obstructed labor 660.1 ●
affecting fetus or newborn 763.1
teeth 524.33
Tiredness 780.79
Tissue - see condition

Tobacco
abuse (affecting health) NEC (see also Abuse,
drugs, nondependent) 305.1
heart 989.84
use disorder complicating pregnancy,
childbirth, or the puerperium 649.0 ●
Tobias' syndrome (carcinoma, pulmonary apex)
(M8010/3) 162.3
Tocopherol deficiency 269.1
Todd's
cirrhosis - see Cirrhosis, biliary
paralysis (postepileptic transitory paralysis)
344.89
Toe - see condition
Toilet, artificial opening (see also Attention to,
artificial, opening) V55.9
Tokelau ringworm 110.5
Tollwut 071
Tolosa-Hunt syndrome 378.55
Tommaselli's disease
correct substance properly administered
599.70
overdose or wrong substance given or taken
961.4
Tongue - see also condition
worms 134.1
Tongue tie 750.0
Toni-Fanconi syndrome (cystinosis) 270.0
Tonic pupil 379.46
Tonsil - see condition
Tonsillitis (acute) (catarrhal) (croupous)
(follicular) (gangrenous) (infective)
(lacunar) (lingual) (malignant)
(membranous) (phlegmonous)
(pneumococcal) (pseudomembranous)
(purulent) (septic) (staphylococcal)
(subacute) (suppurative) (toxic)
(ulcerative) (vesicular) (viral) 463
with influenza, flu, or grippe (see also
Influenza) 487.1
chronic 474.00
diphtheritic (membranous) 032.0
hypertrophic 474.00
influenzal (see also Influenza) 487.1
parenchymatous 475
streptococcal 034.0
tuberculous (see also Tuberculosis) 012.8 ●
Vincent's 101
Tonsillopharyngitis 465.8
Tooth, teeth - see condition
Toothache 525.9
Topagnosis 782.0
Tophi (gouty) 274.03
ear 274.81
heart 274.82
specified site NEC 274.82
**TORCH infection - (see also Infection,
congenital)** 760.2
Torn - see Tear, torn
Tornwaldt's bursitis (disease) (pharyngeal
bursitis) 478.29
cyst 478.26
Torpid liver 573.9
Torsion
accessory tube 620.5
adnexa (female) 620.5
aorta (congenital) 747.29
acquired 447.1
appendix
epididymis 608.24
testis 608.23
bile duct 576.8
with calculus, choledocholithiasis or
stones - see Choledocholithiasis
congenital 751.69
bowel, colon, or intestine 560.2
cervix - see Malposition, uterus
duodenum 537.3
dystonia - see Dystonia, torsion
epididymis 608.24
appendix 608.24

◄ New   ◄▥ Revised   ~~deleted~~ Deleted   ● Use Additional Digit(s)   ▨ Omit code

Torsion *(Continued)*
fallopian tube 620.5
gallbladder *(see also* Disease, gallbladder)
575.8
congenital 751.69
gastric 537.89
hydatid of Morgagni (female) 620.5
kidney (pedicle) 593.89
Meckel's diverticulum (congenital) 751.0
mesentery 560.2
omentum 560.2
organ or site, congenital NEC - *see* Anomaly,
specified type NEC
ovary (pedicle) 620.5
congenital 752.0
oviduct 620.5
penis 607.89
congenital 752.69
renal 593.89
spasm - *see* Dystonia, torsion
spermatic cord 608.22
extravaginal 608.21
intravaginal 608.22
spleen 289.59
testicle, testis 608.20
appendix 608.23
tibia 736.89
umbilical cord - *see* Compression, umbilical
cord
uterus *(see also* Malposition, uterus) 621.6
Torticollis (intermittent) (spastic) 723.5
congenital 754.1
sternomastoid 754.1
due to birth injury 767.8
hysterical 300.11
ocular 781.93
psychogenic 306.0
specified as conversion reaction 300.11
rheumatic 723.5
rheumatoid 714.0
spasmodic 333.83
traumatic, current NEC 847.0
Tortuous
artery 447.1
fallopian tube 752.19
organ or site, congenital NEC - *see* Distortion
renal vessel (congenital) 747.62
retina vessel (congenital) 743.58
acquired 362.17
ureter 593.4
urethra 599.84
vein - *see* Varicose, vein
Torula, torular (infection) 117.5
histolytica 117.5
lung 117.5
Torulosis 117.5
Torus
fracture
fibula 823.41
with tibia 823.42
humerus 812.49
radius (alone) 813.45
with ulna 813.47
tibia 823.40
with fibula 823.42
ulna (alone) 813.46
with radius 813.47
mandibularis 526.81
palatinus 526.81
Touch, vitreous 997.99
Touraine's syndrome (hereditary osteo-
onychodysplasia) 756.89
Touraine-Solente-Golé syndrome
(acropachyderma) 757.39
Tourette's disease (motor-verbal tic) 307.23
Tower skull 756.0
with exophthalmos 756.0
Toxemia 799.89
with
abortion - *see* Abortion, by type, with
toxemia

Toxemia *(Continued)*
bacterial - *see* Septicemia
biliary *(see also* Disease, biliary) 576.8
burn - *see* Burn, by site
congenital NEC 779.89
eclamptic 642.6●
with pre-existing hypertension
642.7●
erysipelatous *(see also* Erysipelas) 035
fatigue 799.89
fetus or newborn NEC 779.89
food *(see also* Poisoning, food) 005.9
gastric 537.89
gastrointestinal 558.2
intestinal 558.2
kidney *(see also* Disease, renal) 593.9
lung 518.89
malarial NEC *(see also* Malaria) 084.6
maternal (of pregnancy), affecting fetus or
newborn 760.0
myocardial - *see* Myocarditis, toxic
of pregnancy (mild) (pre-eclamptic)
642.4●
with
convulsions 642.6●
pre-existing hypertension 642.7●
affecting fetus or newborn 760.0
severe 642.5●
pre-eclamptic - *see* Toxemia, of pregnancy
puerperal, postpartum - *see* Toxemia, of
pregnancy
pulmonary 518.89
renal *(see also* Disease, renal) 593.9
septic *(see also* Septicemia) 038.9
small intestine 558.2
staphylococcal 038.10
aureus 038.11
due to food 005.0
specified organism NEC 038.19
stasis 799.89
stomach 537.89
uremic *(see also* Uremia) 586
urinary 586
Toxemica cerebropathia psychica
(nonalcoholic) 294.0
alcoholic 291.1
Toxic (poisoning) - *see also* condition
from drug or poison - *see* Table of Drugs and
Chemicals
oil syndrome 710.5
shock syndrome 040.82
thyroid (gland) *(see also* Thyrotoxicosis)
242.9●
Toxicemia - *see* Toxemia
Toxicity
dilantin
asymptomatic 796.0
symptomatic -*see* Table of Drugs and
Chemicals
drug
asymptomatic 796.0
symptomatic - *see* Table of Drugs and
Chemicals
fava bean 282.2
from drug or poison
asymptomatic 796.0
symptomatic - *see* Table of Drugs and
Chemicals
Toxicosis *(see also* Toxemia) 799.89
capillary, hemorrhagic 287.0
Toxinfection 799.89
gastrointestinal 558.2
Toxocariasis 128.0
Toxoplasma infection, generalized 130.9
Toxoplasmosis (acquired) 130.9
with pneumonia 130.4
congenital, active 771.2
disseminated (multisystemic) 130.8
maternal
with suspected damage to fetus affecting
management of pregnancy 655.4●

Toxoplasmosis *(Continued)*
maternal *(Continued)*
affecting fetus or newborn 760.2
manifest toxoplasmosis in fetus or
newborn 771.2
multiple sites 130.8
multisystemic disseminated 130.8
specified site NEC 130.7
Trabeculation, bladder 596.89
Trachea - *see* condition
Tracheitis (acute) (catarrhal) (infantile)
(membranous) (plastic) (pneumococcal)
(septic) (suppurative) (viral) 464.10
with
bronchitis 490
acute or subacute 466.0
chronic 491.8
tuberculosis - *see* Tuberculosis,
pulmonary
laryngitis (acute) 464.20
with obstruction 464.21
chronic 476.1
tuberculous *(see also* Tuberculosis,
larynx) 012.3●
obstruction 464.11
chronic 491.8
with
bronchitis (chronic) 491.8
laryngitis (chronic) 476.1
due to external agent - *see* Condition,
respiratory, chronic, due to
diphtheritic (membranous) 032.3
due to external agent - *see* Inflammation,
respiratory, upper, due to
edematous 464.11
influenzal *(see also* Influenza) 487.1
streptococcal 034.0
syphilitic 095.8
tuberculous *(see also* Tuberculosis) 012.8●
Trachelitis (nonvenereal) *(see also* Cervicitis)
616.0
trichomonal 131.09
Tracheobronchial - *see* condition
Tracheobronchitis *(see also* Bronchitis) 490
acute or subacute 466.0
with bronchospasm or obstruction
466.0
chronic 491.8
influenzal *(see also* Influenza) 487.1
senile 491.8
Tracheobronchomegaly (congenital) 748.3
with bronchiectasis 494.0
with (acute) exacerbation 494.1
acquired 519.19
with bronchiectasis 494.0
with (acute) exacerbation 494.1
Tracheobronchopneumonitis - *see* Pneumonia,
broncho
Tracheocele (external) (internal) 519.19
congenital 748.3
Tracheomalacia 519.19
congenital 748.3
Tracheopharyngitis (acute) 465.8
chronic 478.9
due to external agent - *see* Condition,
respiratory, chronic, due to
due to external agent - *see* Inflammation,
respiratory, upper, due to
Tracheostenosis 519.19
congenital 748.3
Tracheostomy
attention to V55.0
complication 519.00
granuloma 519.09
hemorrhage 519.09
infection 519.01
malfunctioning 519.02
obstruction 519.09
sepsis 519.01
status V44.0
stenosis 519.02

Trachoma, trachomatous 076.9
  active (stage) 076.1
  contraction of conjunctiva 076.1
  dubium 076.0
  healed or late effect 139.1
  initial (stage) 076.0
  Türck's (chronic catarrhal laryngitis) 476.0
Trachyphonia 784.49
Traction, vitreomacular 379.27
Training
  insulin pump V65.46
  orthoptic V57.4
  orthotic V57.81
Train sickness 994.6
Trait
  hemoglobin
    abnormal NEC 282.7
      with thalassemia 282.46
    C (see also Disease, hemoglobin, C) 282.7
      with elliptocytosis 282.7
    S (Hb-S) 282.5
  Lepore 282.49
    with other abnormal hemoglobin NEC
      282.49
  paranoid 301.0
  sickle-cell 282.5
    with
      elliptocytosis 282.5
      spherocytosis 282.5
  thalassemia (alpha) (beta) (delta-beta) 282.46
Traits, paranoid 301.0
Tramp V60.0
Trance 780.09
  hysterical 300.13
Transaminasemia 790.4
Transfusion, blood
  donor V59.01
    stem cells V59.02
  fetal twin to twin 678.0●
  incompatible (see also Complications,
    transfusion) 999.80
    ABO (see also Complications, transfusion)
      999.60
    minor blood group 999.89
    non-ABO (see also Complications,
      transfusion) 999.75
    Rh (antigen) (C) (c) (D) (E) (e) (see also
      Complications, transfusion) 999.70
  reaction or complication - see Complications,
    transfusion
  related acute lung injury (TRALI) 518.7
  syndrome
    fetomaternal 772.0
    twin-to-twin
      blood loss (donor twin) 772.0
      recipient twin 776.4
    twin to twin fetal 678.0●
  without reported diagnosis V58.2
Transient - see also condition
  alteration of awareness 780.02
  blindness 368.12
  deafness (ischemic) 388.02
  global amnesia 437.7
  hyperglycemia (post-procedural) 790.29
  hypoglycemia (post-procedural) 251.2
  person (homeless) NEC V60.0
Transitional, lumbosacral joint of vertebra
  756.19
Translocation
  autosomes NEC 758.5
    13–15 758.1
    16–18 758.2
    21 or 22 758.0
    balanced in normal individual 758.4
    D₁ 758.1
    E₃ 758.2
    G 758.0
  balanced autosomal in normal individual
    758.4
  chromosomes NEC 758.89
  Down's syndrome 758.0

Translucency, iris 364.53
Transmission of chemical substances through
  the placenta (affecting fetus or newborn)
  760.70
  alcohol 760.71
  anticonvulsants 760.77
  antifungals 760.74
  anti-infective agents 760.74
  antimetabolics 760.78
  cocaine 760.75
  "crack" 760.75
  diethylstilbestrol [DES] 760.76
  hallucinogenic agents 760.73
  medicinal agents NEC 760.79
  narcotics 760.72
  obstetric anesthetic or analgesic drug 763.5
  specified agent NEC 760.79
  suspected, affecting management of
    pregnancy 655.5●
Transplant (ed)
  bone V42.4
    marrow V42.81
  complication - see also Complications, due to
    (presence of) any device, implant, or
    graft classified to 996.0–996.5 NEC
    bone marrow 996.85
    corneal graft NEC 996.79
      infection or inflammation 996.69
      reaction 996.51
      rejection 996.51
    organ (failure) (immune or nonimmune
      cause) (infection) (rejection) 996.80
      bone marrow 996.85
      heart 996.83
      intestines 996.87
      kidney 996.81
      liver 996.82
      lung 996.84
      pancreas 996.86
      specified NEC 996.89
    previously removed due to complication,
      failure, rejection or infection V45.87
    removal status V45.87
    skin NEC 996.79
      infection or inflammation 996.69
      rejection 996.52
      artificial 996.55
        decellularized allodermis 996.55
    stem cell(s) 996.88
      from
        peripheral blood 996.88
        umbilical cord 996.88
  cornea V42.5
  hair V50.0
  heart V42.1
    valve V42.2
  intestine V42.84
  kidney V42.0
  liver V42.7
  lung V42.6
  organ V42.9
    specified NEC V42.89
  pancreas V42.83
  peripheral stem cells V42.82
  skin V42.3
  stem cells, peripheral V42.82
  tissue V42.9
    specified NEC V42.89
Transplants, ovarian, endometrial 617.1
Transposed - see Transposition
Transposition (congenital) - see also
  Malposition, congenital
  abdominal viscera 759.3
  aorta (dextra) 745.11
  appendix 751.5
  arterial trunk 745.10
  colon 751.5
  great vessels (complete) 745.10
    both originating from right ventricle
      745.11
    corrected 745.12

Transposition (Continued)
  great vessels (Continued)
    double outlet right ventricle 745.11
    incomplete 745.11
    partial 745.11
    specified type NEC 745.19
  heart 746.87
    with complete transposition of viscera
      759.3
  intestine (large) (small) 751.5
  pulmonary veins 747.49
  reversed jejunal (for bypass) (status) V45.3
  scrotal 752.81
  stomach 750.7
    with general transposition of viscera
      759.3
  teeth, tooth 524.30
  vessels (complete) 745.10
    partial 745.11
  viscera (abdominal) (thoracic) 759.3
Trans-sexualism 302.50
  with
    asexual history 302.51
    heterosexual history 302.53
    homosexual history 302.52
Transverse - see also condition
  arrest (deep), in labor 660.3●
    affecting fetus or newborn 763.1
  lie 652.3●
    before labor, affecting fetus or newborn
      761.7
    causing obstructed labor 660.0●
      affecting fetus or newborn 763.1
    during labor, affecting fetus or newborn
      763.1
Transvestism, transvestitism (transvestic
  fetishism) 302.3
Trapped placenta (with hemorrhage)
  666.0●
  without hemorrhage 667.0●
Trauma, traumatism (see also Injury, by site)
  959.9
  birth - see Birth, injury NEC
  causing hemorrhage of pregnancy or
    delivery 641.8●
  complicating
    abortion - see Abortion, by type, with
      damage to pelvic organs
    ectopic pregnancy (see also categories
      633.0–633.9) 639.2
    molar pregnancy (see also categories
      630–632) 639.2
  during delivery NEC 665.9●
  following
    abortion 639.2
    ectopic or molar pregnancy 639.2
  maternal, during pregnancy, affecting fetus
    or newborn 760.5
  neuroma - see Injury, nerve, by site
  previous major, affecting management of
    pregnancy, childbirth, or puerperium
    V23.89
  psychic (current) - see also Reaction,
    adjustment
    previous (history) V15.49
  psychologic, previous (affecting health)
    V15.49
  transient paralysis - see Injury, nerve, by site
Traumatic - see also condition
  brain injury (TBI) (see also Injury, intracranial)
    854.0●
    with skull fracture - see Fracture, skull, by
      site
Treacher Collins' syndrome (incomplete facial
  dysostosis) 756.0
Treitz's hernia - see Hernia, Treitz's
Trematode infestation NEC 121.9
Trematodiasis NEC 121.9
Trembles 988.8
Trembling paralysis (see also Parkinsonism)
  332.0

◀ New   ◀▥ Revised   ~~deleted~~ Deleted   ● Use Additional Digit(s)   ▨ Omit code

Tremor 781.0
  essential (benign) 333.1
  familial 333.1
  flapping (liver) 572.8
  hereditary 333.1
  hysterical 300.11
  intention 333.1
  medication-induced postural 333.1
  mercurial 985.0
  muscle 728.85
  Parkinson's (see also Parkinsonism)
      332.0
  psychogenic 306.0
    specified as conversion reaction
        300.11
  senilis 797
  specified type NEC 333.1
Trench
  fever 083.1
  foot 991.4
  mouth 101
  nephritis - see Nephritis, acute
Treponema pallidum infection (see also
      Syphilis) 097.9
Treponematosis 102.9
  due to
    T. pallidum - see Syphilis
    T. pertenue (yaws) (see also Yaws)
        102.9
Triad
  Kartagener's 759.3
  Reiter's (complete) (incomplete) 099.3
  Saint's (see also Hernia, diaphragm)
      553.3
Trichiasis 704.2
  cicatricial 704.2
  eyelid 374.05
    with entropion (see also Entropion)
        374.00
Trichinella spiralis (infection) (infestation)
      124
Trichinelliasis 124
Trichinellosis 124
Trichiniasis 124
Trichinosis 124
Trichobezoar 938
  intestine 936
  stomach 935.2
Trichocephaliasis 127.3
Trichocephalosis 127.3
Trichocephalus infestation 127.3
Trichoclasis 704.2
Trichoepithelioma (M8100/0) - see also
      Neoplasm, skin, benign
  breast 217
  genital organ NEC - see Neoplasm, by site,
      benign
  malignant (M8100/3) - see Neoplasm, skin,
      malignant
Trichofolliculoma (M8101/0) - see Neoplasm,
      skin, benign
Tricholemmoma (M8102/0) - see Neoplasm,
      skin, benign
Trichomatosis 704.2
Trichomoniasis 131.9
  bladder 131.09
  cervix 131.09
  intestinal 007.3
  prostate 131.03
  seminal vesicle 131.09
  specified site NEC 131.8
  urethra 131.02
  urogenitalis 131.00
  vagina 131.01
  vulva 131.01
  vulvovaginal 131.01
Trichomycosis 039.0
  axillaris 039.0
  nodosa 111.2
  nodularis 111.2
  rubra 039.0

Trichonocardiosis (axillaris) (palmellina)
      039.0
Trichonodosis 704.2
Trichophytid, trichophyton infection (see also
      Dermatophytosis) 110.9
Trichophytide - see Dermatophytosis
Trichophytobezoar 938
  intestine 936
  stomach 935.2
Trichophytosis - see Dermatophytosis
Trichoptilosis 704.2
Trichorrhexis (nodosa) 704.2
Trichosporosis nodosa 111.2
Trichostasis spinulosa (congenital) 757.4
Trichostrongyliasis (small intestine) 127.6
Trichostrongylosis 127.6
Trichostrongylus (instabilis) infection 127.6
Trichotillomania 312.39
Trichromat, anomalous (congenital) 368.59
Trichromatopsia, anomalous (congenital)
      368.59
Trichuriasis 127.3
Trichuris trichiura (any site) (infection)
      (infestation) 127.3
Tricuspid (valve) - see condition
Trifid - see also Accessory
  kidney (pelvis) 753.3
  tongue 750.13
Trigeminal neuralgia (see also Neuralgia,
      trigeminal) 350.1
Trigeminoencephaloangiomatosis 759.6
Trigeminy 427.89
  postoperative 997.1
Trigger finger (acquired) 727.03
  congenital 756.89
Trigonitis (bladder) (chronic)
      (pseudomembranous) 595.3
  tuberculous (see also Tuberculosis)
      016.1●
Trigonocephaly 756.0
Trihexosidosis 272.7
Trilobate placenta - see Placenta, abnormal
Trilocular heart 745.8
Trimethylaminuria 270.8
Tripartita placenta - see Placenta, abnormal
Triple - see also Accessory
  kidneys 753.3
  uteri 752.2
  X female 758.81
Triplegia 344.89
  congenital or infantile 343.8
Triplet
  affected by maternal complications of
      pregnancy 761.5
  healthy liveborn - see Newborn, multiple
  pregnancy (complicating delivery) NEC
      651.1●
    with fetal loss and retention of one or
        more fetus(es) 651.4●
    following (elective) fetal reduction
        651.7●
Triplex placenta - see Placenta, abnormal
Triplication - see Accessory
Trismus 781.0
  neonatorum 771.3
  newborn 771.3
Trisomy (syndrome) NEC 758.5
  13 (partial) 758.1
  16–18 758.2
  18 (partial) 758.2
  21 (partial) 758.0
  22 758.0
  autosomes NEC 758.5
  D₁ 758.1
  E₃ 758.2
  G (group) 758.0
  group D₁ 758.1
  group E 758.2
  group G 758.0
Tritanomaly 368.53
Tritanopia 368.53

Troisier-Hanot-Chauffard syndrome (bronze
      diabetes) 275.01
Trombidiosis 133.8
Trophedema (hereditary) 757.0
  congenital 757.0
Trophoblastic disease (see also Hydatidiform
      mole) 630
  previous, affecting management of
      pregnancy V23.1
Tropholymphedema 757.0
Trophoneurosis NEC 356.9
  arm NEC 354.9
  disseminated 710.1
  facial 349.89
  leg NEC 355.8
  lower extremity NEC 355.8
  upper extremity NEC 354.9
Tropical - see also condition
  maceration feet (syndrome) 991.4
  wet foot (syndrome) 991.4
Trouble - see also Disease
  bowel 569.9
  heart - see Disease, heart
  intestine 569.9
  kidney (see also Disease, renal) 593.9
  nervous 799.21
  sinus (see also Sinusitis) 473.9
Trousseau's syndrome (thrombophlebitis
      migrans) 453.1
Truancy, childhood - see also Disturbance,
      conduct
  socialized 312.2●
  undersocialized, unsocialized 312.1●
Truncus
  arteriosus (persistent) 745.0
  common 745.0
  communis 745.0
Trunk - see condition
Trychophytide - see Dermatophytosis
Trypanosoma infestation - see Trypanosomiasis
Trypanosomiasis 086.9
  with meningoencephalitis 086.9 [323.2]
  African 086.5
    due to Trypanosoma 086.5
      gambiense 086.3
      rhodesiense 086.4
  American 086.2
    with
      heart involvement 086.0
      other organ involvement 086.1
    without mention of organ involvement
        086.2
  Brazilian - see Trypanosomiasis, American
  Chagas' - see Trypanosomiasis, American
  due to Trypanosoma
    cruzi - see Trypanosomiasis, American
    gambiense 086.3
    rhodesiense 086.4
  gambiensis, Gambian 086.3
  North American - see Trypanosomiasis,
      American
  rhodesiensis, Rhodesian 086.4
  South American - see Trypanosomiasis,
      American
T-shaped incisors 520.2
Tsutsugamushi fever 081.2
Tube, tubal, tubular - see also condition
  ligation, admission for V25.2
Tubercle - see also Tuberculosis
  brain, solitary 013.2●
  Darwin's 744.29
  epithelioid noncaseating 135
  Ghon, primary infection 010.0●
Tuberculid, tuberculide (indurating)
      (lichenoid) (miliary) (papulonecrotic)
      (primary) (skin) (subcutaneous) (see also
      Tuberculosis) 017.0●
Tuberculoma - see also Tuberculosis
  brain (any part) 013.2●
  meninges (cerebral) (spinal) 013.1●
  spinal cord 013.4●

Tuberculosis, tubercular, tuberculous
(calcification) (calcified) (caseous)
(chromogenic acid-fast bacilli)
(congenital) (degeneration) (disease)
(fibrocaseous) (fistula) (gangrene)
(interstitial) (isolated circumscribed
lesions) (necrosis) (parenchymatous)
(ulcerative) 011.9●

Note: Use the following fifth-digit
subclassification with categories 010–018:

0   unspecified
1   bacteriological or histological
     examination not done
2   bacteriological or histological
     examination unknown (at
     present)
3   tubercle bacilli found (in sputum) by
     microscopy
4   tubercle bacilli not found (in sputum)
     by microscopy, but found by
     bacterial culture
5   tubercle bacilli not found by
     bacteriological examination,
     but tuberculosis confirmed
     histologically
6   tubercle bacilli not found by
     bacteriological or histological
     examination, but tuberculosis
     confirmed by other methods
     [inoculation of animals]

For tuberculous conditions specified as late
effects or sequelae, see category 137.

abdomen 014.8●
    lymph gland 014.8●
abscess 011.9●
    arm 017.9
    bone (see also Osteomyelitis, due to,
        tuberculosis) 015.9● [730.8]●
        hip 015.1● [730.85]
        knee 015.2● [730.86]
        sacrum 015.0● [730.88]
        specified site NEC 015.7● [730.88]
        spinal 015.0● [730.88]
        vertebra 015.0● [730.88]
    brain 013.3●
    breast 017.9●
    Cowper's gland 016.5●
    dura (mater) 013.8●
        brain 013.3●
        spinal cord 013.5●
    epidural 013.8●
        brain 013.3●
        spinal cord 013.5●
    frontal sinus - see Tuberculosis, sinus
    genital organs NEC 016.9●
        female 016.7●
        male 016.5●
    genitourinary NEC 016.9●
    gland (lymphatic) - see Tuberculosis,
        lymph gland
    hip 015.1●
    iliopsoas 015.0● [730.88]
    intestine 014.8●
    ischiorectal 014.8●
    joint 015.9●
        hip 015.1●
        knee 015.2●
        specified joint NEC 015.8●
        vertebral 015.0● [730.88]
    kidney 016.0● [590.81]
    knee 015.2●
    lumbar 015.0● [730.88]
    lung 011.2●
        primary, progressive 010.8●
    meninges (cerebral) (spinal) 013.0●
    pelvic 016.9●
        female 016.7●
        male 016.5●

Tuberculosis, tubercular, tuberculous
(Continued)
abscess (Continued)
    perianal 014.8●
        fistula 014.8●
    perinephritic 016.0● [590.81]
    perineum 017.9●
    perirectal 014.8●
    psoas 015.0● [730.88]
    rectum 014.8●
    retropharyngeal 012.8●
    sacrum 015.0● [730.88]
    scrofulous 017.2●
    scrotum 016.5●
    skin 017.0●
        primary 017.0●
    spinal cord 013.5●
    spine or vertebra (column) 015.0●
        [730.88]
    strumous 017.2●
    subdiaphragmatic 014.8●
    testis 016.5●
    thigh 017.9●
    urinary 016.3●
        kidney 016.0● [590.81]
    uterus 016.7●
accessory sinus - see Tuberculosis, sinus
Addison's disease 017.6●
adenitis (see also Tuberculosis, lymph gland)
    017.2●
adenoids 012.8●
adenopathy (see also Tuberculosis, lymph
    gland) 017.2●
    tracheobronchial 012.1●
        primary progressive 010.8●
adherent pericardium 017.9● [420.0]
adnexa (uteri) 016.7●
adrenal (capsule) (gland) 017.6●
air passage NEC 012.8●
alimentary canal 014.8●
anemia 017.9●
ankle (joint) 015.8●
    bone 015.5● [730.87]
anus 014.8●
apex (see also Tuberculosis, pulmonary)
    011.9●
apical (see also Tuberculosis, pulmonary)
    011.9●
appendicitis 014.8●
appendix 014.8●
arachnoid 013.0●
artery 017.9●
arthritis (chronic) (synovial) 015.9● [711.40]
    ankle 015.8● [730.87]
    hip 015.1● [711.45]
    knee 015.2● [711.46]
    specified site NEC 015.8● [711.48]
    spine or vertebra (column) 015.0●
        [720.81]
    wrist 015.8● [730.83]
articular - see Tuberculosis, joint
ascites 014.0●
asthma (see also Tuberculosis, pulmonary)
    011.9●
axilla, axillary 017.2●
    gland 017.2●
bilateral (see also Tuberculosis, pulmonary)
    011.9●
bladder 016.1●
bone (see also Osteomyelitis, due to,
    tuberculosis) 015.9● [730.8]
    hip 015.1● [730.85]
    knee 015.2● [730.86]
    limb NEC 015.5● [730.88]
    sacrum 015.0● [730.88]
    specified site NEC 015.7● [730.88]
    spinal or vertebral column 015.0● [730.88]
bowel 014.8●
    miliary 018.9●
brain 013.2●
breast 017.9●

Tuberculosis, tubercular, tuberculous
(Continued)
broad ligament 016.7●
bronchi, bronchial, bronchus 011.3●
    ectasia, ectasis 011.5●
    fistula 011.3●
        primary, progressive 010.8●
    gland 012.1●
        primary, progressive 010.8●
    isolated 012.2●
    lymph gland or node 012.1●
        primary, progressive 010.8●
bronchiectasis 011.5●
bronchitis 011.3●
bronchopleural 012.0●
bronchopneumonia, bronchopneumonic
    011.6●
bronchorrhagia 011.3●
bronchotracheal 011.3●
    isolated 012.2●
bronchus - see Tuberculosis, bronchi
bronze disease (Addison's) 017.6●
buccal cavity 017.9●
bulbourethral gland 016.5●
bursa (see also Tuberculosis, joint) 015.9●
cachexia NEC (see also Tuberculosis,
    pulmonary) 011.9●
cardiomyopathy 017.9● [425.8]
caries (see also Tuberculosis, bone) 015.9●
    [730.8]●
cartilage (see also Tuberculosis, bone) 015.9●
    [730.8]●
    intervertebral 015.0● [730.88]
catarrhal (see also Tuberculosis, pulmonary)
    011.9●
cecum 014.8●
cellular tissue (primary) 017.0●
cellulitis (primary) 017.0●
central nervous system 013.9●
    specified site NEC 013.8●
cerebellum (current) 013.2●
cerebral (current) 013.2●
    meninges 013.0●
cerebrospinal 013.6●
    meninges 013.0●
cerebrum (current) 013.2●
cervical 017.2●
    gland 017.2●
    lymph nodes 017.2●
cervicitis (uteri) 016.7●
cervix 016.7●
chest (see also Tuberculosis, pulmonary)
    011.9●
childhood type or first infection 010.0●
choroid 017.3● [363.13]
choroiditis 017.3● [363.13]
ciliary body 017.3● [364.11]
colitis 014.8●
colliers' 011.4●
colliquativa (primary) 017.0●
colon 014.8●
    ulceration 014.8●
complex, primary 010.0●
complicating pregnancy, childbirth, or
    puerperium 647.3●
    affecting fetus or newborn 760.2
congenital 771.2
conjunctiva 017.3● [370.31]
connective tissue 017.9●
    bone - see Tuberculosis, bone
contact V01.1
converter (tuberculin skin test) (without
    disease) 795.51
cornea (ulcer) 017.3● [370.31]
Cowper's gland 016.5●
coxae 015.1● [730.85]
coxalgia 015.1● [730.85]
cul-de-sac of Douglas 014.8●
curvature, spine 015.0● [737.40]
cutis (colliquativa) (primary) 017.0●
cyst, ovary 016.6●

◀ New ◀═ Revised ~~deleted~~ Deleted ● Use Additional Digit(s) ▓ Omit code

Tuberculosis, tubercular, tuberculous
(Continued)
cystitis 016.1 ●
dacryocystitis 017.3 ● [375.32]
dactylitis 015.5 ●
diarrhea 014.8 ●
diffuse (see also Tuberculosis, miliary) 018.9 ●
lung - see Tuberculosis, pulmonary
meninges 013.0 ●
digestive tract 014.8 ●
disseminated (see also Tuberculosis, miliary) 018.9 ●
meninges 013.0 ●
duodenum 014.8 ●
dura (mater) 013.9 ●
abscess 013.8 ●
cerebral 013.3 ●
spinal 013.5 ●
dysentery 014.8 ●
ear (inner) (middle) 017.4 ●
bone 015.6 ●
external (primary) 017.0 ●
skin (primary) 017.0 ●
elbow 015.8 ●
emphysema - see Tuberculosis, pulmonary
empyema 012.0 ●
encephalitis 013.6 ●
endarteritis 017.9 ●
endocarditis (any valve) 017.9 ● [424.91]
endocardium (any valve) 017.9 ● [424.91]
endocrine glands NEC 017.9 ●
endometrium 016.7 ●
enteric, enterica 014.8 ●
enteritis 014.8 ●
enterocolitis 014.8 ●
epididymis 016.4 ●
epididymitis 016.4 ●
epidural abscess 013.8 ●
brain 013.3 ●
spinal cord 013.5 ●
epiglottis 012.3 ●
episcleritis 017.3 ● [379.00]
erythema (induratum) (nodosum) (primary) 017.1 ●
esophagus 017.8 ●
Eustachian tube 017.4 ●
exposure to V01.1
exudative 012.0 ●
primary, progressive 010.1 ●
eye 017.3 ●
eyelid (primary) 017.0 ●
lupus 017.0 ● [373.4]
fallopian tube 016.6 ●
fascia 017.9 ●
fauces 012.8 ●
finger 017.9 ●
first infection 010.0 ●
fistula, perirectal 014.8 ●
Florida 011.6 ●
foot 017.9 ●
funnel pelvis 137.3
gallbladder 017.9 ●
galloping (see also Tuberculosis, pulmonary) 011.9 ●
ganglionic 015.9 ●
gastritis 017.9 ●
gastrocolic fistula 014.8 ●
gastroenteritis 014.8 ●
gastrointestinal tract 014.8 ●
general, generalized 018.9 ●
acute 018.0 ●
chronic 018.8 ●
genital organs NEC 016.9 ●
female 016.7 ●
male 016.5 ●
genitourinary NEC 016.9 ●
genu 015.2 ●
glandulae suprarenalis 017.6 ●
glandular, general 017.2 ●
glottis 012.3 ●
grinders' 011.4 ●

Tuberculosis, tubercular, tuberculous
(Continued)
groin 017.2 ●
gum 017.9 ●
hand 017.9 ●
heart 017.9 [425.8] ●
hematogenous - see Tuberculosis, miliary
hemoptysis (see also Tuberculosis, pulmonary) 011.9 ●
hemorrhage NEC (see also Tuberculosis, pulmonary) 011.9 ●
hemothorax 012.0 ●
hepatitis 017.9 ●
hilar lymph nodes 012.1 ●
primary, progressive 010.8 ●
hip (disease) (joint) 015.1 ●
bone 015.1 ● [730.85]
hydrocephalus 013.8 ●
hydropneumothorax 012.0 ●
hydrothorax 012.0 ●
hypoadrenalism 017.6 ●
hypopharynx 012.8 ●
ileocecal (hyperplastic) 014.8 ●
ileocolitis 014.8 ●
ileum 014.8 ●
iliac spine (superior) 015.0 ● [730.88]
incipient NEC (see also Tuberculosis, pulmonary) 011.9 ●
indurativa (primary) 017.1 ●
infantile 010.0 ●
infection NEC 011.9 ●
without clinical manifestation 010.0 ●
infraclavicular gland 017.2 ●
inguinal gland 017.2 ●
inguinalis 017.2 ●
intestine (any part) 014.8 ●
iris 017.3 ● [364.11]
iritis 017.3 ● [364.11]
ischiorectal 014.8 ●
jaw 015.7 ● [730.88]
jejunum 014.8 ●
joint 015.9 ●
hip 015.1 ●
knee 015.2 ●
specified site NEC 015.8 ●
vertebral 015.0 ● [730.88]
keratitis 017.3 ● [370.31]
interstitial 017.3 ● [370.59]
keratoconjunctivitis 017.3 ● [370.31]
kidney 016.0 ●
knee (joint) 015.2 ●
kyphoscoliosis 015.0 ● [737.43]
kyphosis 015.0 ● [737.41]
lacrimal apparatus, gland 017.3 ●
laryngitis 012.3 ●
larynx 012.3 ●
latent 795.51
leptomeninges, leptomeningitis (cerebral) (spinal) 013.0 ●
lichenoides (primary) 017.0 ●
linguae 017.9 ●
lip 017.9 ●
liver 017.9 ●
lordosis 015.0 ● [737.42]
lung - see Tuberculosis, pulmonary
luposa 017.0 ●
eyelid 017.0 ● [373.4]
lymphadenitis - see Tuberculosis, lymph gland
lymphangitis - see Tuberculosis, lymph gland
lymphatic (gland) (vessel) - see Tuberculosis, lymph gland
lymph gland or node (peripheral) 017.2 ●
abdomen 014.8 ●
bronchial 012.1 ●
primary, progressive 010.8 ●
cervical 017.2 ●
hilar 012.1 ●
primary, progressive 010.8 ●
intrathoracic 012.1 ●
primary, progressive 010.8 ●

Tuberculosis, tubercular, tuberculous
(Continued)
lymph gland or node (Continued)
mediastinal 012.1 ●
primary, progressive 010.8 ●
mesenteric 014.8 ●
peripheral 017.2 ●
retroperitoneal 014.8 ●
tracheobronchial 012.1 ●
primary, progressive 010.8 ●
malignant NEC (see also Tuberculosis, pulmonary) 011.9 ●
mammary gland 017.9 ●
marasmus NEC (see also Tuberculosis, pulmonary) 011.9 ●
mastoiditis 015.6 ●
maternal, affecting fetus or newborn 760.2
mediastinal (lymph) gland or node 012.1 ●
primary, progressive 010.8 ●
mediastinitis 012.8 ●
primary, progressive 010.8 ●
mediastinopericarditis 017.9 ● [420.0]
mediastinum 012.8 ●
primary, progressive 010.8 ●
medulla 013.9 ●
brain 013.2 ●
spinal cord 013.4 ●
melanosis, Addisonian 017.6 ●
membrane, brain 013.0 ●
meninges (cerebral) (spinal) 013.0 ●
meningitis (basilar) (brain) (cerebral) (cerebrospinal) (spinal) 013.0 ●
meningoencephalitis 013.0 ●
mesentery, mesenteric 014.8 ●
lymph gland or node 014.8 ●
miliary (any site) 018.9 ●
acute 018.0 ●
chronic 018.8 ●
specified type NEC 018.8 ●
millstone makers' 011.4 ●
miners' 011.4 ●
moulders' 011.4 ●
mouth 017.9 ●
multiple 018.9 ●
acute 018.0 ●
chronic 018.8 ●
muscle 017.9 ●
myelitis 013.6 ●
myocarditis 017.9 ● [422.0]
myocardium 017.9 ● [422.0]
nasal (passage) (sinus) 012.8 ●
nasopharynx 012.8 ●
neck gland 017.2 ●
nephritis 016.0 ● [583.81]
nerve 017.9 ●
nose (septum) 012.8 ●
ocular 017.3 ●
old NEC 137.0
without residuals V12.01
omentum 014.8 ●
oophoritis (acute) (chronic) 016.6 ●
optic 017.3 ● [377.39]
nerve trunk 017.3 ● [377.39]
papilla, papillae 017.3 ● [377.39]
orbit 017.3 ●
orchitis 016.5 ● [608.81]
organ, specified NEC 017.9 ●
orificialis (primary) 017.0 ●
osseous (see also Tuberculosis, bone) 015.9 ● [730.8]
osteitis (see also Tuberculosis, bone) 015.9 ● [730.8]
osteomyelitis (see also Tuberculosis, bone) 015.9 ● [730.8]
otitis (media) 017.4 ●
ovaritis (acute) (chronic) 016.6 ●
ovary (acute) (chronic) 016.6 ●
oviducts (acute) (chronic) 016.6 ●
pachymeningitis 013.0 ●
palate (soft) 017.9 ●
pancreas 017.9 ●

Tuberculosis, tubercular, tuberculous
(Continued)
papulonecrotic (primary) 017.0●
parathyroid glands 017.9●
paronychia (primary) 017.0●
parotid gland or region 017.9●
pelvic organ NEC 016.9●
    female 016.7●
    male 016.5●
pelvis (bony) 015.7● *[730.85]*
penis 016.5●
peribronchitis 011.3●
pericarditis 017.9● *[420.0]*
pericardium 017.9● *[420.0]*
perichondritis, larynx 012.3●
perineum 017.9●
periostitis *(see also* Tuberculosis, bone) 015.9●
    [730.8]●
periphlebitis 017.9●
    eye vessel 017.3● *[362.18]*
    retina 017.3● *[362.18]*
perirectal fistula 014.8●
peritoneal gland 014.8●
peritoneum 014.0●
peritonitis 014.0●
pernicious NEC *(see also* Tuberculosis,
    pulmonary) 011.9●
pharyngitis 012.8●
pharynx 012.8●
phlyctenulosis (conjunctiva) 017.3●
    [370.31]
phthisis NEC *(see also* Tuberculosis,
    pulmonary) 011.9●
pituitary gland 017.9●
placenta 016.7●
pleura, pleural, pleurisy, pleuritis (fibrinous)
    (obliterative) (purulent) (simple
    plastic) (with effusion) 012.0●
    primary, progressive 010.1●
pneumonia, pneumonic 011.6●
pneumothorax 011.7●
polyserositis 018.9●
    acute 018.0●
    chronic 018.8●
potters' 011.4●
prepuce 016.5●
primary 010.9●
    complex 010.0●
    complicated 010.8●
        with pleurisy or effusion 010.1●
    progressive 010.8●
        with pleurisy or effusion 010.1●
    skin 017.0●
proctitis 014.8●
prostate 016.5● *[601.4]*
prostatitis 016.5● *[601.4]*
pulmonaris *(see also* Tuberculosis,
    pulmonary) 011.9●
pulmonary (artery) (incipient) (malignant)
    (multiple round foci) (pernicious)
    (reinfection stage) 011.9●
    cavitated or with cavitation 011.2●
        primary, progressive 010.8●
    childhood type or first infection 010.0●
    chromogenic acid-fast bacilli 795.39
    fibrosis or fibrotic 011.4●
    infiltrative 011.0●
        primary, progressive 010.9●
    nodular 011.1●
    specified NEC 011.8●
    sputum positive only 795.39●
    status following surgical collapse of lung
        NEC 011.9●
pyelitis 016.0● *[590.81]*
pyelonephritis 016.0● *[590.81]*
pyemia - *see* Tuberculosis, miliary
pyonephrosis 016.0●
pyopneumothorax 012.0●
pyothorax 012.0●
rectum (with abscess) 014.8●
    fistula 014.8●

Tuberculosis, tubercular, tuberculous
(Continued)
reinfection stage *(see also* Tuberculosis,
    pulmonary) 011.9●
renal 016.0●
renis 016.0●
reproductive organ 016.7●
respiratory NEC *(see also* Tuberculosis,
    pulmonary) 011.9●
    specified site NEC 012.8●
retina 017.3● *[363.13]*
retroperitoneal (lymph gland or node)
    014.8●
    gland 014.8●
retropharyngeal abscess 012.8●
rheumatism 015.9●
rhinitis 012.8●
sacroiliac (joint) 015.8●
sacrum 015.0● *[730.88]*
salivary gland 017.9●
salpingitis (acute) (chronic) 016.6●
sandblasters' 011.4●
sclera 017.3● *[379.09]*
scoliosis 015.0● *[737.43]*
scrofulous 017.2●
scrotum 016.5●
seminal tract or vesicle 016.5● *[608.81]*
senile NEC *(see also* Tuberculosis,
    pulmonary) 011.9●
septic NEC *(see also* Tuberculosis, miliary)
    018.9●
shoulder 015.8●
    blade 015.7● *[730.8]* ●
sigmoid 014.8●
sinus (accessory) (nasal) 012.8●
    bone 015.7● *[730.88]*
    epididymis 016.4●
skeletal NEC *(see also* Osteomyelitis, due to
    tuberculosis) 015.9● *[730.8]*●
skin (any site) (primary) 017.0●
small intestine 014.8●
soft palate 017.9●
spermatic cord 016.5●
spinal
    column 015.0● *[730.88]*
    cord 013.4●
    disease 015.0● *[730.88]*
    medulla 013.4●
    membrane 013.0●
    meninges 013.0●
spine 015.0● *[730.88]*
spleen 017.7●
splenitis 017.7●
spondylitis 015.0● *[720.81]*
spontaneous pneumothorax - *see*
    Tuberculosis, pulmonary
sternoclavicular joint 015.8●
stomach 017.9●
stonemasons' 011.4●
struma 017.2●
subcutaneous tissue (cellular) (primary)
    017.0●
subcutis (primary) 017.0●
subdeltoid bursa 017.9●
submaxillary 017.9●
    region 017.9●
supraclavicular gland 017.2●
suprarenal (capsule) (gland) 017.6●
swelling, joint *(see also* Tuberculosis, joint)
    015.9●
symphysis pubis 015.7● *[730.88]*
synovitis 015.9● *[727.01]*
    hip 015.1● *[727.01]*
    knee 015.2● *[727.01]*
    specified site NEC 015.8● *[727.01]*
    spine or vertebra 015.0● *[727.01]*
systemic - *see* Tuberculosis, miliary
tarsitis (eyelid) 017.0● *[373.4]*
    ankle (bone) 015.5● *[730.87]*
tendon (sheath) - *see* Tuberculosis,
    tenosynovitis

Tuberculosis, tubercular, tuberculous
(Continued)
tenosynovitis 015.9● *[727.01]*
    hip 015.1● *[727.01]*
    knee 015.2● *[727.01]*
    specified site NEC 015.8● *[727.01]*
    spine or vertebra 015.0● *[727.01]*
testis 016.5● *[608.81]*
throat 012.8●
thymus gland 017.9●
thyroid gland 017.5●
toe 017.9●
tongue 017.9●
tonsil (lingual) 012.8●
tonsillitis 012.8●
trachea, tracheal 012.8●
    gland 012.1●
        primary, progressive 010.8●
    isolated 012.2●
tracheobronchial 011.3●
    glandular 012.1●
        primary, progressive 010.8●
    isolated 012.2●
    lymph gland or node 012.1●
        primary, progressive 010.8●
tubal 016.6●
tunica vaginalis 016.5●
typhlitis 014.8●
ulcer (primary) (skin) 017.0●
    bowel or intestine 014.8●
    specified site NEC - *see* Tuberculosis, by
        site
unspecified site - *see* Tuberculosis,
    pulmonary
ureter 016.2●
urethra, urethral 016.3●
urinary organ or tract 016.3●
    kidney 016.0●
uterus 016.7●
uveal tract 017.3● *[363.13]*
uvula 017.9●
vaccination, prophylactic (against) V03.2
vagina 016.7●
vas deferens 016.5●
vein 017.9●
verruca (primary) 017.0●
verrucosa (cutis) (primary) 017.0●
vertebra (column) 015.0● *[730.88]*
vesiculitis 016.5● *[608.81]*
viscera NEC 014.8●
vulva 016.7● *[616.51]*
wrist (joint) 015.8●
    bone 015.5● *[730.83]*
Tuberculum
    auriculae 744.29
    occlusal 520.2
    paramolare 520.2
Tuberosity
    jaw, excessive 524.07
    maxillary, entire 524.07
Tuberous sclerosis (brain) 759.5
Tubo-ovarian - *see* condition
Tuboplasty, after previous sterilization V26.0
Tubotympanitis 381.10
Tularemia 021.9
    with
        conjunctivitis 021.3
        pneumonia 021.2
    bronchopneumonic 021.2
    conjunctivitis 021.3
    cryptogenic 021.1
    disseminated 021.8
    enteric 021.1
    generalized 021.8
    glandular 021.8
    intestinal 021.1
    oculoglandular 021.3
    ophthalmic 021.3
    pneumonia 021.2
    pulmonary 021.2
    specified NEC 021.8

Tularemia *(Continued)*
  typhoidal 021.1
  ulceroglandular 021.0
  vaccination, prophylactic (against) V03.4
Tularensis conjunctivitis 021.3
Tumefaction - *see also* Swelling
  liver (*see also* Hypertrophy, liver) 789.1
Tumor (M8000/1) - *see also* Neoplasm, by site,
    unspecified nature
  Abrikossov's (M9580/0) - *see also* Neoplasm,
    connective tissue, benign
    malignant (M9580/3) - *see* Neoplasm,
      connective tissue, malignant
  acinar cell (M8550/1) - *see* Neoplasm, by site,
    uncertain behavior
  acinic cell (M8550/1) - *see* Neoplasm, by site,
    uncertain behavior
  adenomatoid (M9054/0) - *see also* Neoplasm,
    by site, benign
    odontogenic (M9300/0) 213.1
      upper jaw (bone) 213.0
  adnexal (skin) (M8390/0) - *see* Neoplasm,
    skin, benign
  adrenal
    cortical (benign) (M8370/0) 227.0
      malignant (M8370/3) 194.0
    rest (M8671/0) - *see* Neoplasm, by site,
      benign
  alpha cell (M8152/0)
    malignant (M8152/3)
      pancreas 157.4
      specified site NEC - *see* Neoplasm, by
        site, malignant
      unspecified site 157.4
    pancreas 211.7
    specified site NEC - *see* Neoplasm, by site,
      benign
    unspecified site 211.7
  aneurysmal (*see also* Aneurysm) 442.9
  aortic body (M8691/1) 237.3
    malignant (M8691/3) 194.6
  argentaffin (M8241/1) - *see* Neoplasm, by
    site, uncertain behavior
  basal cell (M8090/1) - *see also* Neoplasm,
    skin, uncertain behavior
  benign (M8000/0) - *see* Neoplasm, by site,
    benign
  beta cell (M8151/0)
    malignant (M8151/3)
      pancreas 157.4
      specified site - *see* Neoplasm, by site,
        malignant
      unspecified site 157.4
    pancreas 211.7
    specified site NEC - *see* Neoplasm, by site,
      benign
    unspecified site 211.7
  blood - *see* Hematoma
  brenner (M9000/0) 220
    borderline malignancy (M9000/1) 236.2
    malignant (M9000/3) 183.0
    proliferating (M9000/1) 236.2
  Brooke's (M8100/0) - *see* Neoplasm, skin,
    benign
  brown fat (M8880/0) - *see* Lipoma, by site
  Burkitt's (M9750/3) 200.2●
  calcifying epithelial odontogenic (M9340/0)
    213.1
    upper jaw (bone) 213.0
  carcinoid (M8240/1) 209.60
    benign 209.60
      appendix 209.51
      ascending colon 209.53
      bronchus 209.61
      cecum 209.52
      colon 209.50
      descending colon 209.55
      duodenum 209.41
      foregut 209.65
      hindgut 209.67
      ileum 209.43

Tumor *(Continued)*
  carcinoid *(Continued)*
    benign *(Continued)*
      jejunum 209.42
      kidney 209.64
      large intestine 209.50
      lung 209.61
      midgut 209.66
      rectum 209.57
      sigmoid colon 209.56
      small intestine 209.40
      specified NEC 209.69
      stomach 209.63
      thymus 209.62
      transverse colon 209.54
    malignant (of) 209.20
      appendix 209.11
      ascending colon 209.13
      bronchus 209.21
      cecum 209.12
      colon 209.10
      descending colon 209.15
      duodenum 209.01
      foregut 209.25
      hindgut 209.27
      ileum 209.03
      jejunum 209.02
      kidney 209.24
      large intestine 209.10
      lung 209.21
      midgut 209.26
      rectum 209.17
      sigmoid colon 209.16
      small intestine 209.00
      specified NEC 209.29
      stomach 209.23
      thymus 209.22
      transverse colon 209.14
    secondary - *see* Tumor, neuroendocrine,
      secondary
  carotid body (M8692/1) 237.3
    malignant (M8692/3) 194.5
  Castleman's (mediastinal lymph node
    hyperplasia) 785.6
  cells (M8001/1) - *see also* Neoplasm, by site,
    unspecified nature
    benign (M8001/0) - *see* Neoplasm, by site,
      benign
    malignant (M8001/3) - *see* Neoplasm, by
      site, malignant
    uncertain whether benign or malignant
      (M8001/1) - *see* Neoplasm, by site,
      uncertain nature
  cervix
    in pregnancy or childbirth 654.6●
      affecting fetus or newborn 763.89
      causing obstructed labor 660.2●
        affecting fetus or newborn
          763.1
  chondromatous giant cell (M9230/0) - *see*
    Neoplasm, bone, benign
  chromaffin (M8700/0) - *see also* Neoplasm,
    by site, benign
    malignant (M8700/3) - *see* Neoplasm, by
      site, malignant
  Cock's peculiar 706.2
  Codman's (benign chondroblastoma)
    (M9230/0) - *see* Neoplasm, bone,
    benign
  dentigerous, mixed (M9282/0) 213.1
    upper jaw (bone) 213.0
  dermoid (M9084/0) - *see* Neoplasm, by site,
    benign
    with malignant transformation (M9084/3)
      183.0
  desmoid (extra-abdominal) (M8821/1) - *see*
    also Neoplasm, connective tissue,
    uncertain behavior
    abdominal (M8822/1) - *see* Neoplasm,
      connective tissue, uncertain
      behavior

Tumor *(Continued)*
  embryonal (mixed) (M9080/1) - *see also*
    Neoplasm, by site, uncertain behavior
    liver (M9080/3) 155.0
  endodermal sinus (M9071/3)
    specified site - *see* Neoplasm, by site,
      malignant
    unspecified site
      female 183.0
      male 186.9
  epithelial
    benign (M8010/0) - *see* Neoplasm, by site,
      benign
    malignant (M8010/3) - *see* Neoplasm, by
      site, malignant
  Ewing's (M9260/3) - *see* Neoplasm, bone,
    malignant
  fatty - *see* Lipoma
  fetal, causing disproportion 653.7●
    causing obstructed labor 660.1●
  fibroid (M8890/0) - *see* Leiomyoma
  G cell (M8153/1)
    malignant (M8153/3)
      pancreas 157.4
      specified site NEC - *see* Neoplasm, by
        site, malignant
      unspecified site 157.4
    specified site - *see* Neoplasm, by site,
      uncertain behavior
    unspecified site 235.5
  giant cell (type) (M8003/1) - *see also*
    Neoplasm, by site, unspecified nature
    bone (M9250/1) 238.0
      malignant (M9250/3) - *see* Neoplasm,
        bone, malignant
    chondromatous (M9230/0) - *see*
      Neoplasm, bone, benign
    malignant (M8003/3) - *see* Neoplasm, by
      site, malignant
    peripheral (gingiva) 523.8
    soft parts (M9251/1) - *see also* Neoplasm,
      connective tissue, uncertain
      behavior
      malignant (M9251/3) - *see* Neoplasm,
        connective tissue, malignant
    tendon sheath 727.02
  glomus (M8711/0) - *see also* Hemangioma, by
    site
    jugulare (M8690/1) 237.3
      malignant (M8690/3) 194.6
  gonadal stromal (M8590/1) - *see* Neoplasm,
    by site, uncertain behavior
  granular cell (M9580/0) - *see also* Neoplasm,
    connective tissue, benign
    malignant (M9580/3) - *see* Neoplasm,
      connective tissue, malignant
  granulosa cell (M8620/1) 236.2
    malignant (M8620/3) 183.0
  granulosa cell-theca cell (M8621/1) 236.2
    malignant (M8621/3) 183.0
  Grawitz's (hypernephroma) (M8312/3) 189.0
  hazard-crile (M8350/3) 193
  hemorrhoidal - *see* Hemorrhoids
  hilar cell (M8660/0) 220
  Hürthle cell (benign) (M8290/0) 226
    malignant (M8290/3) 193
  hydatid (*see also* Echinococcus) 122.9
  hypernephroid (M8311/1) - *see also*
    Neoplasm, by site, uncertain behavior
  interstitial cell (M8650/1) - *see also*
    Neoplasm, by site, uncertain behavior
    benign (M8650/0) - *see* Neoplasm, by site,
      benign
    malignant (M8650/3) - *see* Neoplasm, by
      site, malignant
  islet cell (M8150/0)
    malignant (M8150/3)
      pancreas 157.4
      specified site - *see* Neoplasm, by site,
        malignant
      unspecified site 157.4

Tumor *(Continued)*
  islet cell *(Continued)*
    pancreas 211.7
    specified site NEC - *see* Neoplasm, by site, benign
    unspecified site 211.7
  juxtaglomerular (M8361/1) 236.91
  Krukenberg's (M8490/6) 198.6
  Leydig cell (M8650/1)
    benign (M8650/0)
      specified site - *see* Neoplasm, by site, benign
      unspecified site
        female 220
        male 222.0
    malignant (M8650/3)
      specified site - *see* Neoplasm, by site, malignant
      unspecified site
        female 183.0
        male 186.9
    specified site - *see* Neoplasm, by site, uncertain behavior
    unspecified site
      female 236.2
      male 236.4
  lipid cell, ovary (M8670/0) 220
  lipoid cell, ovary (M8670/0) 220
  lymphomatous, benign (M9590/0) - *see also* Neoplasm, by site, benign
  lysis syndrome (following antineoplastic drug therapy) (spontaneous) 277.88
  Malherbe's (M8110/0) - *see* Neoplasm, skin, benign
  malignant (M8000/3) - *see also* Neoplasm, by site, malignant
    fusiform cell (type) (M8004/3) - *see* Neoplasm, by site, malignant
    giant cell (type) (M8003/3) - *see* Neoplasm, by site, malignant
    mixed NEC (M8940/3) - *see* Neoplasm, by site, malignant
    small cell (type) (M8002/3) - *see* Neoplasm, by site, malignant
    spindle cell (type) (M8004/3) - *see* Neoplasm, by site, malignant
  mast cell (M9740/1) 238.5
    malignant (M9740/3) 202.6●
  melanotic, neuroectodermal (M9363/0) - *see* Neoplasm, by site, benign
  Merkel cell - *see* Carcinoma, Merkel cell
  mesenchymal
    malignant (M8800/3) - *see* Neoplasm, connective tissue, malignant
    mixed (M8990/1) - *see* Neoplasm, connective tissue, uncertain behavior
  mesodermal, mixed (M8951/3) - *see also* Neoplasm, by site, malignant
    liver 155.0
  mesonephric (M9110/1) - *see also* Neoplasm, by site, uncertain behavior
    malignant (M9110/3) - *see* Neoplasm, by site, malignant
  metastatic
    from specified site (M8000/3) - *see* Neoplasm, by site, malignant
    to specified site (M8000/6) - *see* Neoplasm, by site, malignant, secondary
  mixed NEC (M8940/0) - *see also* Neoplasm, by site, benign
    malignant (M8940/3) - *see* Neoplasm, by site, malignant
  mucocarcinoid, malignant (M8243/3) - *see* Neoplasm, by site, malignant
  mucoepidermoid (M8430/1) - *see* Neoplasm, by site, uncertain behavior
  Müllerian, mixed (M8950/3) - *see* Neoplasm, by site, malignant

Tumor *(Continued)*
  myoepithelial (M8982/0) - *see* Neoplasm, by site, benign
  neuroendocrine 209.60
    malignant poorly differentiated 209.30
    secondary 209.70
      bone 209.73
      distant lymph nodes 209.71
      liver 209.72
      peritoneum 209.74
      site specified NEC 209.79
  neurogenic olfactory (M9520/3) 160.0
  nonencapsulated sclerosing (M8350/3) 193
  odontogenic (M9270/1) 238.0
    adenomatoid (M9300/0) 213.1
      upper jaw (bone) 213.0
    benign (M9270/0) 213.1
      upper jaw (bone) 213.0
    calcifying epithelial (M9340/0) 213.1
      upper jaw (bone) 213.0
    malignant (M9270/3) 170.1
      upper jaw (bone) 170.0
    squamous (M9312/0) 213.1
      upper jaw (bone) 213.0
  ovarian stromal (M8590/1) 236.2
  ovary
    in pregnancy or childbirth 654.4●
      affecting fetus or newborn 763.89
      causing obstructed labor 660.2●
        affecting fetus or newborn 763.1
  pacinian (M9507/0) - *see* Neoplasm, skin, benign
  Pancoast's (M8010/3) 162.3
  papillary - *see* Papilloma
  pelvic, in pregnancy or childbirth 654.9●
    affecting fetus or newborn 763.89
    causing obstructed labor 660.2●
      affecting fetus or newborn 763.1
  phantom 300.11
  plasma cell (M9731/1) 238.6
    benign (M9731/0) - *see* Neoplasm, by site, benign
    malignant (M9731/3) 203.8●
  polyvesicular vitelline (M9071/3)
    specified site - *see* Neoplasm, by site, malignant
    unspecified site
      female 183.0
      male 186.9
  Pott's puffy (*see also* Osteomyelitis) 730.2●
  Rathke's pouch (M9350/1) 237.0
  regaud's (M8082/3) - *see* Neoplasm, nasopharynx, malignant
  rete cell (M8140/0) 222.0
  retinal anlage (M9363/0) - *see* Neoplasm, by site, benign
  Rokitansky's 620.2
  salivary gland type, mixed (M8940/0) - *see also* Neoplasm, by site, benign
    malignant (M8940/3) - *see* Neoplasm, by site, malignant
  Sampson's 617.1
  Schloffer's (*see also* Peritonitis) 567.29
  Schmincke (M8082/3) - *see* Neoplasm, nasopharynx, malignant
  sebaceous (*see also* Cyst, sebaceous) 706.2
  secondary (M8000/6) - *see* Neoplasm, by site, secondary
    carcinoid - *see* Tumor, neuroendocrine, secondary
    neuroendocrine - *see* Tumor, neuroendocrine, secondary
  Sertoli cell (M8640/0)
    with lipid storage (M8641/0)
      specified site, - *see* Neoplasm, by site, benign
      unspecified site
        female 220
        male 222.0
    specified site - *see* Neoplasm, by site, benign

Tumor *(Continued)*
  Sertoli cell *(Continued)*
    unspecified site
      female 220
      male 222.0
  Sertoli-Leydig cell (M8631/0)
    specified site - *see* Neoplasm, by site, benign
    unspecified site
      female 220
      male 222.0
  sex cord (-stromal) (M8590/1) - *see* Neoplasm, by site, uncertain behavior
  skin appendage (M8390/0) - *see* Neoplasm, skin, benign
  soft tissue
    benign (M8800/0) - *see* Neoplasm, connective tissue, benign
    malignant (M8800/3) - *see* Neoplasm, connective tissue, malignant
  sternomastoid 754.1
  stromal
    abdomen
      benign 215.5
      malignant NEC 171.5
      uncertain behavior 238.1
    digestive system 238.1
      benign 215.5
      malignant NEC 171.5
      uncertain behavior 238.1
    endometrium (endometrial) 236.0
    gastric 238.1
      benign 215.5
      malignant 151.9
      uncertain behavior 238.1
    gastrointestinal 238.1
      benign 215.5
      malignant NEC 171.5
      uncertain behavior 238.1
    intestine (small) 238.1
      benign 215.5
      malignant 152.9
      uncertain behavior 238.1
    stomach 238.1
      benign 215.5
      malignant 151.9
      uncertain behavior 238.1
  superior sulcus (lung) (pulmonary) (syndrome) (M8010/3) 162.3
  suprasulcus (M8010/3) 162.3
  sweat gland (M8400/1) - *see also* Neoplasm, skin, uncertain behavior
    benign (M8400/0) - *see* Neoplasm, skin, benign
    malignant (M8400/3) - *see* Neoplasm, skin, malignant
  syphilitic brain 094.89
    congenital 090.49
  testicular stromal (M8590/1) 236.4
  theca cell (M8600/0) 220
  theca cell-granulosa cell (M8621/1) 236.2
  theca-lutein (M8610/0) 220
  turban (M8200/0) 216.4
  uterus
    in pregnancy or childbirth 654.1●
      affecting fetus or newborn 763.89
      causing obstructed labor 660.2●
        affecting fetus or newborn 763.1
  vagina
    in pregnancy or childbirth 654.7●
      affecting fetus or newborn 763.89
      causing obstructed labor 660.2●
        affecting fetus or newborn 763.1
  varicose (*see also* Varicose, vein) 454.9
  von Recklinghausen's (M9540/1) 237.71
  vulva
    in pregnancy or childbirth 654.8●
      affecting fetus or newborn 763.89
      causing obstructed labor 660.2●
        affecting fetus or newborn 763.1
  Warthin's (salivary gland) (M8561/0) 210.2

◀ New   ◀◾ Revised   ~~deleted~~ Deleted   ● Use Additional Digit(s)   ▨ Omit code

Tumor (*Continued*)
    white - *see also* Tuberculosis, arthritis
    White-Darier 757.39
    Wilms' (nephroblastoma) (M8960/3) 189.0
    yolk sac (M9071/3)
        specified site - *see* Neoplasm, by site,
            malignant
        unspecified site
            female 183.0
            male 186.9
Tumorlet (M8040/1) - *see* Neoplasm, by site,
    uncertain behavior
Tungiasis 134.1
Tunica vasculosa lentis 743.39
Tunnel vision 368.45
Turban tumor (M8200/0) 216.4
Türck's trachoma (chronic catarrhal laryngitis)
    476.0
Türk's syndrome (ocular retraction syndrome)
    378.71
Turner's
    hypoplasia (tooth) 520.4
    syndrome 758.6
    tooth 520.4
Turner-Kieser syndrome (hereditary osteo-
    onychodysplasia) 756.89
Turner-Varny syndrome 758.6
Turricephaly 756.0
Tussis convulsiva (*see also* Whooping cough)
    033.9
Twiddler's syndrome (due to)
    automatic implantable defibrillator 996.04
    pacemaker 996.01
Twin
    affected by maternal complications of
        pregnancy 761.5
    conjoined 759.4
        fetal 678.1●
    healthy liveborn - *see* Newborn, twin
    pregnancy (complicating delivery) NEC
        651.0●
        with fetal loss and retention of one fetus
            651.3●
        conjoined 678.1●
        following (elective) fetal reduction 651.7●
Twinning, teeth 520.2
Twist, twisted
    bowel, colon, or intestine 560.2
    hair (congenital) 757.4
    mesentery 560.2
    omentum 560.2

Twist, twisted (*Continued*)
    organ or site, congenital NEC - *see* Anomaly,
        specified type NEC
    ovarian pedicle 620.5
        congenital 752.0
    umbilical cord - *see* Compression, umbilical
        cord
Twitch 781.0
Tylosis 700
    buccalis 528.6
    gingiva 523.8
    linguae 528.6
    palmaris et plantaris 757.39
Tympanism 787.3
Tympanites (abdominal) (intestine) 787.3
Tympanitis - *see* Myringitis
Tympanosclerosis 385.00
    involving
        combined sites NEC 385.09
            with tympanic membrane 385.03
        tympanic membrane 385.01
            with ossicles 385.02
                and middle ear 385.03
Tympanum - *see* condition
Tympany
    abdomen 787.3
    chest 786.7
Typhlitis (*see also* Appendicitis) 541
Typhoenteritis 002.0
Typhogastric fever 002.0
Typhoid (abortive) (ambulant) (any site) (fever)
        (hemorrhagic) (infection) (intermittent)
        (malignant) (rheumatic) 002.0
    with pneumonia 002.0 [484.8]
    abdominal 002.0
    carrier (suspected) of V02.1
    cholecystitis (current) 002.0
    clinical (Widal and blood test negative)
        002.0
    endocarditis 002.0 [421.1]
    inoculation reaction - *see* Complications,
        vaccination
    meningitis 002.0 [320.7]
    mesenteric lymph nodes 002.0
    myocarditis 002.0 [422.0]
    osteomyelitis (*see also* Osteomyelitis, due to,
        typhoid) 002.0 [730.8]●
    perichondritis, larynx 002.0 [478.71]
    pneumonia 002.0 [484.8]
    spine 002.0 [720.81]
    ulcer (perforating) 002.0

Typhoid (*Continued*)
    vaccination, prophylactic (against) V03.1
    Widal negative 002.0
Typhomalaria (fever) (*see also* Malaria) 084.6
Typhomania 002.0
Typhoperitonitis 002.0
Typhus (fever) 081.9
    abdominal, abdominalis 002.0
    African tick 082.1
    amarillic (*see also* Fever, Yellow) 060.9
    brain 081.9
    cerebral 081.9
    classical 080
    endemic (flea-borne) 081.0
    epidemic (louse-borne) 080
    exanthematic NEC 080
    exanthematicus SAI 080
        brillii SAI 081.1
        Mexicanus SAI 081.0
        pediculo vestimenti causa 080
        typhus murinus 081.0
    flea-borne 081.0
    Indian tick 082.1
    Kenya tick 082.1
    louse-borne 080
    Mexican 081.0
        flea-borne 081.0
        louse-borne 080
        tabardillo 080
    mite-borne 081.2
    murine 081.0
    North Asian tick-borne 082.2
    petechial 081.9
    Queensland tick 082.3
    rat 081.0
    recrudescent 081.1
    recurrent (*see also* Fever, relapsing) 087.9
    Saˉo Paulo 082.0
    scrub (China) (India) (Malaya) (New Guinea)
        081.2
    shop (of Malaya) 081.0
    Siberian tick 082.2
    tick-borne NEC 082.9
    tropical 081.2
    vaccination, prophylactic (against)
        V05.8
Tyrosinemia 270.2
    neonatal 775.89
Tyrosinosis (Medes) (Sakai) 270.2
Tyrosinuria 270.2
Tyrosyluria 270.2

U

Uehlinger's syndrome (acropachyderma) 757.39
Uhl's anomaly or disease (hypoplasia of myocardium, right ventricle) 746.84
Ulcer, ulcerated, ulcerating, ulceration, ulcerative 707.9
  with gangrene 707.9 [785.4]
  abdomen (wall) (see also Ulcer, skin) 707.8
  ala, nose 478.19
  alveolar process 526.5
  amebic (intestine) 006.9
    skin 006.6
  anastomotic - see Ulcer, gastrojejunal
  anorectal 569.41
  antral - see Ulcer, stomach
  anus (sphincter) (solitary) 569.41
    varicose - see Varicose, ulcer, anus
  aorta - see Aneurysm
  aphthous (oral) (recurrent) 528.2
    genital organ(s)
      female 616.50
      male 608.89
    mouth 528.2
  arm (see also Ulcer, skin) 707.8
  arteriosclerotic plaque - see Arteriosclerosis, by site
  artery NEC 447.2
    without rupture 447.8
  atrophic NEC - see Ulcer, skin
  Barrett's (chronic peptic ulcer of esophagus) 530.85
  bile duct 576.8
  bladder (solitary) (sphincter) 596.89
    bilharzial (see also Schistosomiasis) 120.9 [595.4]
    submucosal (see also Cystitis) 595.1
    tuberculous (see also Tuberculosis) 016.1●
  bleeding NEC - see Ulcer, peptic, with hemorrhage
  bone 730.9●
  bowel (see also Ulcer, intestine) 569.82
  breast 611.0
  bronchitis 491.8
  bronchus 519.19
  buccal (cavity) (traumatic) 528.9
  burn (acute) - see Ulcer, duodenum
  Buruli 031.1
  buttock (see also Ulcer, skin) 707.8
    decubitus (see also Ulcer, pressure) 707.00
  cancerous (M8000/3) - see Neoplasm, by site, malignant
  cardia - see Ulcer, stomach
  cardio-esophageal (peptic) 530.20
    with bleeding 530.21
  cecum (see also Ulcer, intestine) 569.82
  cervix (uteri) (trophic) 622.0
    with mention of cervicitis 616.0
  chancroidal 099.0
  chest (wall) (see also Ulcer, skin) 707.8
  Chiclero 085.4
  chin (pyogenic) (see also Ulcer, skin) 707.8
  chronic (cause unknown) - see also Ulcer, skin
    penis 607.89
  Cochin-China 085.1
  colitis - see Colitis, ulcerative
  colon (see also Ulcer, intestine) 569.82
  conjunctiva (acute) (postinfectional) 372.00
  cornea (infectional) 370.00
    with perforation 370.06
    annular 370.02
    catarrhal 370.01
    central 370.03
    dendritic 054.42
    marginal 370.01
    mycotic 370.05
    phlyctenular, tuberculous (see also Tuberculosis) 017.3● [370.31]
    ring 370.02
    rodent 370.07

Ulcer, ulcerated, ulcerating, ulceration, ulcerative (Continued)
  cornea (Continued)
    serpent, serpiginous 370.04
    superficial marginal 370.01
    tuberculous (see also Tuberculosis) 017.3● [370.31]
  corpus cavernosum (chronic) 607.89
  crural - see Ulcer, lower extremity
  Curling's - see Ulcer, duodenum
  Cushing's - see Ulcer, peptic
  cystitis (interstitial) 595.1
  decubitus (unspecified site) (see also Ulcer, pressure) 707.00
    with gangrene 707.00 [785.4]
    ankle 707.06
    back
      lower 707.03
      upper 707.02
    buttock 707.05
    coccyx 707.03
    elbow 707.01
    head 707.09
    heel 707.07
    hip 707.04
    other site 707.09
    sacrum 707.03
    shoulder blades 707.02
  dendritic 054.42
  diabetes, diabetic (mellitus) 250.8● [707.9]
    due to secondary diabetes 249.8● [707.9]
    lower limb 250.8● [707.10]
      due to secondary diabetes 249.8● [707.10]
      ankle 250.8● [707.13]
        due to secondary diabetes 249.8● [707.13]
      calf 250.8● [707.12]
        due to secondary diabetes 249.8● [707.12]
      foot 250.8● [707.15]
        due to secondary diabetes 249.8● [707.15]
      heel 250.8● [707.14]
        due to secondary diabetes 249.8● [707.14]
      knee 250.8● [707.19]
        due to secondary diabetes 249.8● [707.19]
      specified site NEC 250.8● [707.19]
        due to secondary diabetes 249.8● [707.19]
      thigh 250.8● [707.11]
        due to secondary diabetes 249.8● [707.11]
      toes 250.8● [707.15]
        due to secondary diabetes 249.8● [707.15]
    specified site NEC 250.8● [707.8]
      due to secondary diabetes 249.8● [707.8]
  Dieulafoy - see Lesion, Dieulafoy
  due to
    infection NEC - see Ulcer, skin
    radiation, radium - see Ulcer, by site
    trophic disturbance (any region) - see Ulcer, skin
    x-ray - see Ulcer, by site
  duodenum, duodenal (eroded) (peptic) 532.9●

Note: Use the following fifth-digit subclassification with categories 531–534:

0   without mention of obstruction
1   with obstruction

  with
    hemorrhage (chronic) 532.4●
      and perforation 532.6●
    perforation (chronic) 532.5●
      and hemorrhage 532.6●

Ulcer, ulcerated, ulcerating, ulceration, ulcerative (Continued)
  duodenum, duodenal (Continued)
    acute 532.3●
      with
        hemorrhage 532.0●
          and perforation 532.2●
        perforation 532.1●
          and hemorrhage 532.2●
      bleeding (recurrent) - see Ulcer, duodenum, with hemorrhage
    chronic 532.7●
      with
        hemorrhage 532.4●
          and perforation 532.6●
        perforation 532.5●
          and hemorrhage 532.6●
    penetrating - see Ulcer, duodenum, with perforation
    perforating - see Ulcer, duodenum, with perforation
  dysenteric NEC 009.0
  elusive 595.1
  endocarditis (any valve) (acute) (chronic) (subacute) 421.0
  enteritis - see Colitis, ulcerative
  enterocolitis 556.0
  epiglottis 478.79
  esophagus (peptic) 530.20
    with bleeding 530.21
    due to ingestion
      aspirin 530.20
      chemicals 530.20
      medicinal agents 530.20
    fungal 530.20
    infectional 530.20
    varicose (see also Varix, esophagus) 456.1
      bleeding (see also Varix, esophagus, bleeding) 456.0
  eye NEC 360.00
    dendritic 054.42
  eyelid (region) 373.01
  face (see also Ulcer, skin) 707.8
  fauces 478.29
  Fenwick (-Hunner) (solitary) (see also Cystitis) 595.1
  fistulous NEC - see Ulcer, skin
  foot (indolent) (see also Ulcer, lower extremity) 707.15
    perforating 707.15
      leprous 030.1
      syphilitic 094.0
    trophic 707.15
    varicose 454.0
      inflamed or infected 454.2
  frambesial, initial or primary 102.0
  gallbladder or duct 575.8
  gall duct 576.8
  gangrenous (see also Gangrene) 785.4
  gastric - see Ulcer, stomach
  gastrocolic - see Ulcer, gastrojejunal
  gastroduodenal - see Ulcer, peptic
  gastroesophageal - see Ulcer, stomach
  gastrohepatic - see Ulcer, stomach
  gastrointestinal - see Ulcer, gastrojejunal
  gastrojejunal (eroded) (peptic) 534.9

Note: Use the following fifth-digit subclassification with categories 531–534:

0   without mention of obstruction
1   with obstruction

  with
    hemorrhage (chronic) 534.4●
      and perforation 534.6●
    perforation 534.5●
      and hemorrhage 534.6●

◀ New   ◀||| Revised   ~~deleted~~ Deleted   ● Use Additional Digit(s)   ▨ Omit code

Ulcer, ulcerated, ulcerating, ulceration, ulcerative *(Continued)*
gastrojejunal *(Continued)*
  acute 534.3●
    with
      hemorrhage 534.0●
        and perforation 534.2●
      perforation 534.1●
        and hemorrhage 534.2●
  bleeding (recurrent) - *see* Ulcer, gastrojejunal, with hemorrhage
  chronic 534.7●
    with
      hemorrhage 534.4●
        and perforation 534.6●
      perforation 534.5●
        and hemorrhage 534.6●
  penetrating - *see* Ulcer, gastrojejunal, with perforation
  perforating - *see* Ulcer, gastrojejunal, with perforation
gastrojejunocolic - *see* Ulcer, gastrojejunal
genital organ
  female 629.89
  male 608.89
gingiva 523.8
gingivitis 523.10
glottis 478.79
granuloma of pudenda 099.2
groin *(see also* Ulcer, skin) 707.8
gum 523.8
gumma, due to yaws 102.4
hand *(see also* Ulcer, skin) 707.8
hard palate 528.9
heel *(see also* Ulcer, lower extremity) 707.14
  decubitus *(see also* Ulcer, pressure) 707.07
hemorrhoids 455.8
  external 455.5
  internal 455.2
hip *(see also* Ulcer, skin) 707.8
  decubitus *(see also* Ulcer, pressure) 707.04
Hunner's 595.1
hypopharynx 478.29
hypopyon (chronic) (subacute) 370.04
hypostaticum - *see* Ulcer, varicose
ileocolitis 556.1
ileum *(see also* Ulcer, intestine) 569.82
intestine, intestinal 569.82
  with perforation 569.83
  amebic 006.9
  duodenal - *see* Ulcer, duodenum
  granulocytopenic (with hemorrhage) 288.09
  marginal 569.82
  perforating 569.83
  small, primary 569.82
  stercoraceous 569.82
  stercoral 569.82
  tuberculous *(see also* Tuberculosis) 014.8●
  typhoid (fever) 002.0
  varicose 456.8
ischemic 707.9
  lower extremity *(see also* Ulcer, lower extremity) 707.10
    ankle 707.13
    calf 707.12
    foot 707.15
    heel 707.14
    knee 707.19
    specified site NEC 707.19
    thigh 707.11
    toes 707.15
jejunum, jejunal - *see* Ulcer, gastrojejunal
keratitis *(see also* Ulcer, cornea) 370.00
knee - *see* Ulcer, lower extremity
labium (majus) (minus) 616.50
laryngitis *(see also* Laryngitis) 464.00
  with obstruction 464.01
larynx (aphthous) (contact) 478.79
  diphtheritic 032.3
leg - *see* Ulcer, lower extremity

Ulcer, ulcerated, ulcerating, ulceration, ulcerative *(Continued)*
lip 528.5
Lipschütz's 616.50
lower extremity (atrophic) (chronic) (neurogenic) (perforating) (pyogenic) (trophic) (tropical) 707.10
  with gangrene *(see also* Ulcer, lower extremity) 707.10 [785.4]
    arteriosclerotic 440.24
  ankle 707.13
  arteriosclerotic 440.23
    with gangrene 440.24
  calf 707.12
  decubitus *(see also* Ulcer, pressure) 707.00
    with gangrene 707.00 [785.4]
    ankle 707.06
    buttock 707.05
    heel 707.07
    hip 707.04
  foot 707.15
  heel 707.14
  knee 707.19
  specified site NEC 707.19
  thigh 707.11
  toes 707.15
  varicose 454.0
    inflamed or infected 454.2
luetic - *see* Ulcer, syphilitic
lung 518.89
  tuberculous *(see also* Tuberculosis) 011.2●
malignant (M8000/3) - *see* Neoplasm, by site, malignant
marginal NEC - *see* Ulcer, gastrojejunal
meatus (urinarius) 597.89
Meckel's diverticulum 751.0
Meleney's (chronic undermining) 686.09
Mooren's (cornea) 370.07
mouth (traumatic) 528.9
mycobacterial (skin) 031.1
nasopharynx 478.29
navel cord (newborn) 771.4
neck *(see also* Ulcer, skin) 707.8
  uterus 622.0
neurogenic NEC - *see* Ulcer, skin
nose, nasal (infectional) (passage) 478.19
  septum 478.19
    varicose 456.8
  skin - *see* Ulcer, skin
  spirochetal NEC 104.8
oral mucosa (traumatic) 528.9
palate (soft) 528.9
penetrating NEC - *see* Ulcer, peptic, with perforation
penis (chronic) 607.89
peptic (site unspecified) 533.9

Note: Use the following fifth-digit subclassification with categories 531–534:
0   without mention of obstruction
1   with obstruction

  with
    hemorrhage 533.4●
      and perforation 533.6●
    perforation (chronic) 533.5●
      and hemorrhage 533.6●
  acute 533.3●
    with
      hemorrhage 533.0●
        and perforation 533.2●
      perforation 533.1●
        and hemorrhage 533.2●
  bleeding (recurrent) - *see* Ulcer, peptic, with hemorrhage
  chronic 533.7●
    with
      hemorrhage 533.4●
        and perforation 533.6●
      perforation 533.5●
        and hemorrhage 533.6●

Ulcer, ulcerated, ulcerating, ulceration, ulcerative *(Continued)*
peptic *(Continued)*
  penetrating - *see* Ulcer, peptic, with perforation
  perforating NEC *(see also* Ulcer, peptic, with perforation) 533.5●
  skin 707.9
perineum *(see also* Ulcer, skin) 707.8
peritonsillar 474.8
phagedenic (tropical) NEC - *see* Ulcer, skin
pharynx 478.29
phlebitis - *see* Phlebitis
plaster *(see also* Ulcer, pressure) 707.00
popliteal space - *see* Ulcer, lower extremity
postpyloric - *see* Ulcer, duodenum
prepuce 607.89
prepyloric - *see* Ulcer, stomach
pressure 707.00
  with
    abrasion, blister, partial thickness skin loss involving epidermis and/or dermis 707.22
    full thickness skin loss involving damage or necrosis of subcutaneous tissue 707.23
    gangrene 707.00 [785.4]
    necrosis of soft tissues through to underlying muscle, tendon, or bone 707.24
  ankle 707.06
  back
    lower 707.03
    upper 707.02
  buttock 707.05
  coccyx 707.03
  elbow 707.01
  head 707.09
  healed - *omit code*
  healing - *code to* Ulcer, pressure, by stage
  heel 707.07
  hip 707.04
  other site 707.09
  sacrum 707.03
  shoulder blades 707.02
  stage
    I (healing) 707.21
    II (healing) 707.22
    III (healing) 707.23
    IV (healing) 707.24
    unspecified (healing) 707.20
  unstageable 707.25
primary of intestine 569.82
  with perforation 569.83
proctitis 556.2
  with ulcerative sigmoiditis 556.3
prostate 601.8
pseudopeptic - *see* Ulcer, peptic
pyloric - *see* Ulcer, stomach
rectosigmoid 569.82
  with perforation 569.83
rectum (sphincter) (solitary) 569.41
  stercoraceous, stercoral 569.41
  varicose - *see* Varicose, ulcer, anus
retina *(see also* Chorioretinitis) 363.20
rodent (M8090/3) - *see also* Neoplasm, skin, malignant
  cornea 370.07
round - *see* Ulcer, stomach
sacrum (region) *(see also* Ulcer, skin) 707.8
Saemisch's 370.04
scalp *(see also* Ulcer, skin) 707.8
sclera 379.09
scrofulous *(see also* Tuberculosis) 017.2●
scrotum 608.89
  tuberculous *(see also* Tuberculosis) 016.5●
  varicose 456.4
seminal vesicle 608.89
sigmoid 569.82
  with perforation 569.83

Ulcer, ulcerated, ulcerating, ulceration,
   ulcerative (Continued)
  skin (atrophic) (chronic) (neurogenic)
      (non-healing) (perforating) (pyogenic)
      (trophic) 707.9
    with gangrene 707.9 [785.4]
    amebic 006.6
    decubitus (see also Ulcer, pressure)
        707.00
      with gangrene 707.00 [785.4]
    in granulocytopenia 288.09
    lower extremity (see also Ulcer, lower
        extremity) 707.10
      with gangrene 707.10 [785.4]
        arteriosclerotic 440.24
      ankle 707.13
      arteriosclerotic 440.23
        with gangrene 440.24
      calf 707.12
      foot 707.15
      heel 707.14
      knee 707.19
      specified site NEC 707.19
      thigh 707.11
      toes 707.15
    mycobacterial 031.1
    syphilitic (early) (secondary) 091.3
    tuberculous (primary) (see also
        Tuberculosis) 017.0●
    varicose - see Ulcer, varicose
  sloughing NEC - see Ulcer, skin
  soft palate 528.9
  solitary, anus or rectum (sphincter) 569.41
  sore throat 462
    streptococcal 034.0
  spermatic cord 608.89
  spine (tuberculous) 015.0● [730.88]
  stasis (leg) (venous) 454.0
    with varicose veins 454.0
    without varicose veins 459.81
    inflamed or infected 454.2
  stercoral, stercoraceous 569.82
    with perforation 569.83
    anus or rectum 569.41
  stoma, stomal - see Ulcer, gastrojejunal
  stomach (eroded) (peptic) (round) 531.9●

> Note: Use the following fifth-digit
> subclassification with categories 531–534:
>
> 0   without mention of obstruction
> 1   with obstruction

    with
        hemorrhage 531.4●
          and perforation 531.6●
        perforation (chronic) 531.5●
          and hemorrhage 531.6●
      acute 531.3●
        with
          hemorrhage 531.0●
            and perforation 531.2●
          perforation 531.1●
            and hemorrhage 531.2●
      bleeding (recurrent) - see Ulcer, stomach,
          with hemorrhage
      chronic 531.7●
        with
          hemorrhage 531.4●
            and perforation 531.6●
          perforation 531.5●
            and hemorrhage 531.6●
      penetrating - see Ulcer, stomach, with
          perforation
      perforating - see Ulcer, stomach, with
          perforation
    stomatitis 528.00
    stress - see Ulcer, peptic
    strumous (tuberculous) (see also Tuberculosis)
        017.2●
    submental (see also Ulcer, skin) 707.8
    submucosal, bladder 595.1

Ulcer, ulcerated, ulcerating, ulceration,
   ulcerative (Continued)
  syphilitic (any site) (early) (secondary) 091.3
    late 095.9
    perforating 095.9
      foot 094.0
  testis 608.89
  thigh - see Ulcer, lower extremity
  throat 478.29
    diphtheritic 032.0
  toe - see Ulcer, lower extremity
  tongue (traumatic) 529.0
  tonsil 474.8
    diphtheritic 032.0
  trachea 519.19
  trophic - see Ulcer, skin
  tropical NEC (see also Ulcer, skin) 707.9
  tuberculous - see Tuberculosis, ulcer
  tunica vaginalis 608.89
  turbinate 730.9●
  typhoid (fever) 002.0
    perforating 002.0
  umbilicus (newborn) 771.4
  unspecified site NEC - see Ulcer, skin
  urethra (meatus) (see also Urethritis) 597.89
  uterus 621.8
    cervix 622.0
      with mention of cervicitis 616.0
    neck 622.0
      with mention of cervicitis 616.0
  vagina 616.89
  valve, heart 421.0
  varicose (lower extremity, any part) 454.0
    anus - see Varicose, ulcer, anus
    broad ligament 456.5
    esophagus (see also Varix, esophagus)
        456.1
      bleeding (see also Varix, esophagus,
          bleeding) 456.0
    inflamed or infected 454.2
    nasal septum 456.8
    perineum 456.6
    rectum - see Varicose, ulcer, anus
    scrotum 456.4
    specified site NEC 456.8
    sublingual 456.3
    vulva 456.6
  vas deferens 608.89
  vesical (see also Ulcer, bladder) 596.89
  vulva (acute) (infectional) 616.50
    Behçet's syndrome 136.1 [616.51]
    herpetic 054.12
    tuberculous 016.7● [616.51]
  vulvobuccal, recurring 616.50
  x-ray - see Ulcer, by site
  yaws 102.4
Ulcerosa scarlatina 034.1
Ulcus - see also Ulcer
  cutis tuberculosum (see also Tuberculosis)
      017.0●
  duodeni - see Ulcer, duodenum
  durum 091.0
    extragenital 091.2
  gastrojejunale - see Ulcer, gastrojejunal
  hypostaticum - see Ulcer, varicose
  molle (cutis) (skin) 099.0
  serpens corneae (pneumococcal) 370.04
  ventriculi - see Ulcer, stomach
Ulegyria 742.4
Ulerythema
  acneiforma 701.8
  centrifugum 695.4
  ophryogenes 757.4
Ullrich (-Bonnevie) (-Turner) syndrome 758.6
Ullrich-Feichtiger syndrome 759.89
Ulnar - see condition
Ulorrhagia 523.8
Ulorrhea 523.8
Umbilicus, umbilical - see also condition
  cord necrosis, affecting fetus or newborn
      762.6

Unacceptable
  existing dental restoration
    contours 525.65
    morphology 525.65
Unavailability of medical facilities (at) V63.9
  due to
    investigation by social service agency
        V63.8
    lack of services at home V63.1
    remoteness from facility V63.0
    waiting list V63.2
  home V63.1
  outpatient clinic V63.0
  specified reason NEC V63.8
Uncinaria americana infestation 126.1
Uncinariasis (see also Ancylostomiasis) 126.9
Unconscious, unconsciousness 780.09
Underdevelopment - see also Undeveloped
  sexual 259.0
Underfill, endodontic 526.63
Undernourishment 269.9
Undernutrition 269.9
Under observation - see Observation
Underweight 783.22
  for gestational age - see Light-for-dates
Underwood's disease (sclerema neonatorum)
    778.1
Undescended - see also Malposition, congenital
  cecum 751.4
  colon 751.4
  testis 752.51
Undetermined diagnosis or cause 799.9
Undeveloped, undevelopment - see also
    Hypoplasia
  brain (congenital) 742.1
    cerebral (congenital) 742.1
  fetus or newborn 764.9●
  heart 746.89
  lung 748.5
  testis 257.2
  uterus 259.0
Undiagnosed (disease) 799.9
Undulant fever (see also Brucellosis) 023.9
Unemployment, anxiety concerning V62.0
Unequal leg (acquired) (length) 736.81
  congenital 755.30
Unerupted teeth, tooth 520.6
Unextracted dental root 525.3
Unguis incarnatus 703.0
Unicornis uterus 752.33
Unicornuate uterus (with or without a separate
    uterine horn) 752.33
Unicorporeus uterus 752.39
Uniformis uterus 752.39
Unilateral - see also condition
  development, breast 611.89
  organ or site, congenital NEC - see Agenesis
  vagina 752.49
Unilateralis uterus 752.39
Unilocular heart 745.8
Uninhibited bladder 596.54
  with cauda equina syndrome 344.61
  neurogenic (see also Neurogenic, bladder)
      596.54
Union, abnormal - see also Fusion
  divided tendon 727.89
  larynx and trachea 748.3
Universal
  joint, cervix 620.6
  mesentery 751.4
Unknown
  cause of death 799.9
  diagnosis 799.9
Unna's disease (seborrheic dermatitis) 690.10
Unresponsiveness, adrenocorticotropin
    (ACTH) 255.41
Unsatisfactory
  cytology smear
    anal 796.78
    cervical 795.08
    vaginal 795.18

◀ New   ◀▦ Revised   d̶e̶l̶e̶t̶e̶d̶ Deleted   ● Use Additional Digit(s)   ▨ Omit code

Unsatisfactory (*Continued*)
   restoration, tooth (existing) 525.60
      specified NEC 525.69
Unsoundness of mind (*see also* Psychosis) 298.9
Unspecified cause of death 799.9
Unstable
   back NEC 724.9
   colon 569.89
   joint - *see* Instability, joint
   lie 652.0●
      affecting fetus or newborn (before labor)
         761.7
      causing obstructed labor 660.0●
         affecting fetus or newborn 763.1
   lumbosacral joint (congenital) 756.19
      acquired 724.6
   sacroiliac 724.6
   spine NEC 724.9
Untruthfulness, child problem (*see also*
      Disturbance, conduct) 312.0●
Unverricht (-Lundborg) disease, syndrome, or
      epilepsy 345.1●
Unverricht-Wagner syndrome
      (dermatomyositis) 710.3
Upper respiratory - *see* condition
Upset
   gastric 536.8
      psychogenic 306.4
   gastrointestinal 536.8
      psychogenic 306.4
      virus (*see also* Enteritis, viral) 008.8
   intestinal (large) (small) 564.9
      psychogenic 306.4
   menstruation 626.9
   mental 300.9
   stomach 536.8
      psychogenic 306.4
Urachus - *see also* condition
   patent 753.7
   persistent 753.7
Uratic arthritis 274.00
Urbach's lipoid proteinosis 272.8
Urbach-Oppenheim disease or syndrome
      (necrobiosis lipoidica diabeticorum)
      250.8● [709.3]
   due to secondary diabetes 249.8● [709.3]
Urbach-Wiethe disease or syndrome (lipoid
      proteinosis) 272.8
Urban yellow fever 060.1
Urea, blood, high - *see* Uremia
Uremia, uremic (absorption) (amaurosis)
      (amblyopia) (aphasia) (apoplexy) (coma)
      (delirium) (dementia) (dropsy) (dyspnea)
      (fever) (intoxication) (mania) (paralysis)
      (poisoning) (toxemia) (vomiting) 586
   with
      abortion - *see* Abortion, by type, with
         renal failure
      ectopic pregnancy (*see also* categories
         633.0–633.9) 639.3
      hypertension (*see also* Hypertension,
         kidney) 403.91
      molar pregnancy (*see also* categories
         630–632) 639.3
   chronic 585.9
   complicating
      abortion 639.3
      ectopic or molar pregnancy 639.3
      hypertension (*see also* Hypertension,
         kidney) 403.91
      labor and delivery 669.3●
   congenital 779.89
   extrarenal 788.99
   hypertensive (chronic) (*see also*
      Hypertension, kidney) 403.91
   maternal NEC, affecting fetus or newborn
      760.1
   neuropathy 585.9 [357.4]
   pericarditis 585.9 [420.0]
   prerenal 788.99
   pyelitic (*see also* Pyelitis) 590.80

Ureter, ureteral - *see* condition
Ureteralgia 788.0
Ureterectasis 593.89
Ureteritis 593.89
   cystica 590.3
   due to calculus 592.1
   gonococcal (acute) 098.19
      chronic or duration of 2 months or over
         098.39
   nonspecific 593.89
Ureterocele (acquired) 593.89
   congenital 753.23
Ureterolith 592.1
Ureterolithiasis 592.1
Ureterostomy status V44.6
   with complication 997.5
Urethra, urethral - *see* condition
Urethralgia 788.99
Urethritis (abacterial) (acute) (allergic)
      (anterior) (chronic) (nonvenereal)
      (posterior) (recurrent) (simple) (subacute)
      (ulcerative) (undifferentiated) 597.80
   diplococcal (acute) 098.0
      chronic or duration of 2 months or over
         098.2
   due to Trichomonas (vaginalis) 131.02
   gonococcal (acute) 098.0
      chronic or duration of 2 months or over
         098.2
   nongonococcal (sexually transmitted) 099.40
      Chlamydia trachomatis 099.41
      Reiter's 099.3
      specified organism NEC 099.49
   nonspecific (sexually transmitted) (*see also*
         Urethritis, nongonococcal) 099.40
   not sexually transmitted 597.80
   Reiter's 099.3
   trichomonal or due to Trichomonas
         (vaginalis) 131.02
   tuberculous (*see also* Tuberculosis) 016.3●
   venereal NEC (*see also* Urethritis,
         nongonococcal) 099.40
Urethrocele
   female 618.03
      with uterine prolapse 618.4
         complete 618.3
         incomplete 618.2
   male 599.5
Urethrolithiasis 594.2
Urethro-oculoarticular syndrome 099.3
Urethro-oculosynovial syndrome 099.3
Urethrorectal - *see* condition
Urethrorrhagia 599.84
Urethrorrhea 788.7
Urethrostomy status V44.6
   with complication 997.5
Urethrotrigonitis 595.3
Urethrovaginal - *see* condition
Urgency
   fecal 787.63
   hypertensive - *see* Hypertension
Urhidrosis, uridrosis 705.89
Uric acid
   diathesis 274.9
   in blood 790.6
Uricacidemia 790.6
Uricemia 790.6
Uricosuria 791.9
Urination
   frequent 788.41
   painful 788.1
   urgency 788.63
Urine, urinary - *see also* condition
   abnormality NEC 788.69
   blood in (*see also* Hematuria) 599.70
   discharge, excessive 788.42
   enuresis 788.30
      nonorganic origin 307.6
   extravasation 788.8
   frequency 788.41
   hesitancy 788.64

Urine, urinary (*Continued*)
   incontinence 788.30
      active 788.30
      female 788.30
         stress 625.6
            and urge 788.33
      male 788.30
         stress 788.32
            and urge 788.33
      mixed (stress and urge) 788.33
      neurogenic 788.39
      nonorganic origin 307.6
      overflow 788.38
      stress (female) 625.6
         male NEC 788.32
   intermittent stream 788.61
   pus in 791.9
   retention or stasis NEC 788.20
      bladder, incomplete emptying
         788.21
      psychogenic 306.53
      specified NEC 788.29
   secretion
      deficient 788.5
      excessive 788.42
      frequency 788.41
   strain 788.65
   stream
      intermittent 788.61
      slowing 788.62
      splitting 788.61
      weak 788.62
   urgency 788.63
Urinemia - *see* Uremia
Urinoma NEC 599.9
   bladder 596.89
   kidney 593.89
   renal 593.89
   ureter 593.89
   urethra 599.84
Uroarthritis, infectious 099.3
Urodialysis 788.5
Urolithiasis 592.9
Uronephrosis 593.89
Uropathy 599.9
   obstructive 599.60
Urosepsis 599.0
   meaning sepsis 995.91
   meaning urinary tract infection 599.0
Urticaria 708.9
   with angioneurotic edema 995.1
      hereditary 277.6
   allergic 708.0
   cholinergic 708.5
   chronic 708.8
   cold, familial 708.2
   dermatographic 708.3
   due to
      cold or heat 708.2
      drugs 708.0
      food 708.0
      inhalants 708.0
      plants 708.8
      serum 999.59
   factitial 708.3
   giant 995.1
      hereditary 277.6
   gigantea 995.1
      hereditary 277.6
   idiopathic 708.1
   larynx 995.1
      hereditary 277.6
   neonatorum 778.8
   nonallergic 708.1
   papulosa (Hebra) 698.2
   perstans hemorrhagica 757.39
   pigmentosa 757.33
   recurrent periodic 708.8
   serum 999.59
   solare 692.72
   specified type NEC 708.8

Urticaria (*Continued*)
    thermal (cold) (heat) 708.2
    vibratory 708.4
Urticarioides acarodermatitis 133.9
Use of
    agents affecting estrogen receptors and
        estrogen levels NEC V07.59
    anastrozole (Arimidex) V07.52
    aromatase inhibitors V07.52
    estrogen receptor downregulators V07.59
    exemestane (Aromasin) V07.52
    fulvestrant (Faslodex) V07.59
    gonadotropin-releasing hormone (GnRH)
        agonist V07.59
    goserelin acetate (Zoladex) V07.59
    letrozole (Femara) V07.52
    leuprolide acetate (leuprorelin) (Lupron)
        V07.59
    megestrol acetate (Megace) V07.59
    methadone 304.00
    nonprescribed drugs (*see also* Abuse, drugs,
        nondependent) 305.9●
    patent medicines (*see also* Abuse, drugs,
        nondependent) 305.9●
    raloxifene (Evista) V07.51
    selective estrogen receptor modulators
        (SERMs) V07.51
    tamoxifen (Nolvadex) V07.51
    toremifene (Fareston) V07.51

Usher-Senear disease (pemphigus
    erythematosus) 694.4
Uta 085.5
Uterine size-date discrepancy 649.6●
Uteromegaly 621.2
Uterovaginal - *see* condition
Uterovesical - *see* condition
Uterus - *see also* condition
    with only one functioning horn
        752.33
Utriculitis (utriculus prostaticus) 597.89
Uveal - *see* condition
Uveitis (anterior) (*see also* Iridocyclitis)
    364.3
    acute or subacute 364.00
        due to or associated with
            gonococcal infection 098.41
            herpes (simplex) 054.44
            zoster 053.22
        primary 364.01
        recurrent 364.02
        secondary (noninfectious) 364.04
            infectious 364.03
    allergic 360.11
    chronic 364.10
        due to or associated with
            sarcoidosis 135 [364.11]
            tuberculosis (*see also* Tuberculosis)
                017.3● [364.11]

Uveitis (*Continued*)
    due to
        operation 360.11
        toxoplasmosis (acquired) 130.2
            congenital (active) 771.2
    granulomatous 364.10
    heterochromic 364.21
    lens-induced 364.23
    nongranulomatous 364.00
    posterior 363.20
        disseminated - *see* Chorioretinitis,
            disseminated
        focal - *see* Chorioretinitis, focal
    recurrent 364.02
    sympathetic 360.11
    syphilitic (secondary) 091.50
        congenital 090.0 [363.13]
        late 095.8 [363.13]
    tuberculous (*see also* Tuberculosis) 017.3●
        [364.11]
Uveoencephalitis 363.22
Uveokeratitis (*see also* Iridocyclitis)
    364.3
Uveoparotid fever 135
Uveoparotitis 135
Uvula - *see* condition
Uvulitis (acute) (catarrhal) (chronic)
    (gangrenous) (membranous)
    (suppurative) (ulcerative) 528.3

V

Vaccination
  complication or reaction - see Complications, vaccination
  delayed V64.00
  not carried out V64.00
    because of
      acute illness V64.01
      allergy to vaccine or component V64.04
      caregiver refusal V64.05
      chronic illness V64.02
      guardian refusal V64.05
      immune compromised state V64.03
      parent refusal V64.05
      patient had disease being vaccinated against V64.08
      patient refusal V64.06
      reason NEC V64.09
      religious reasons V64.07
  prophylactic (against) V05.9
    arthropod-borne viral
      disease NEC V05.1
      encephalitis V05.0
    chicken pox V05.4
    cholera (alone) V03.0
      with typhoid-paratyphoid (cholera + TAB) V06.0
    common cold V04.7
    diphtheria (alone) V03.5
      with
        poliomyelitis (DTP + polio) V06.3
        tetanus V06.5
          pertussis combined [DTP] (DTaP) V06.1
        typhoid-paratyphoid (DTP + TAB) V06.2
    disease (single) NEC V05.9
      bacterial NEC V03.9
        specified type NEC V03.89
      combination NEC V06.9
        specified type NEC V06.8
      specified type NEC V05.8
    encephalitis, viral, arthropod-borne V05.0
    Hemophilus influenzae, type B [Hib] V03.81
    hepatitis, viral V05.3
    influenza V04.81
      with
        Streptococcus pneumoniae [pneumococcus] V06.6
    leishmaniasis V05.2
    measles (alone) V04.2
      with mumps-rubella (MMR) V06.4
    mumps (alone) V04.6
      with measles and rubella (MMR) V06.4
    pertussis alone V03.6
    plague V03.3
    poliomyelitis V04.0
      with diphtheria-tetanus-pertussis (DTP polio) V06.3
    rabies V04.5
    respiratory syncytial virus (RSV) V04.82
    rubella (alone) V04.3
      with measles and mumps (MMR) V06.4
    smallpox V04.1
    Streptococcus pneumoniae [pneumococcus] V03.82
      with
        influenza V06.6
    tetanus toxoid (alone) V03.7
      with diphtheria [Td] [DT] V06.5
        with
          pertussis (DTP) (DTaP) V06.1
            with poliomyelitis (DTP + polio) V06.3
    tuberculosis (BCG) V03.2
    tularemia V03.4

Vaccination (Continued)
  prophylactic (Continued)
    typhoid-paratyphoid (TAB) (alone) V03.1
      with diphtheria-tetanus-pertussis (TAB + DTP) V06.2
    varicella V05.4
    viral
      disease NEC V04.89
      encephalitis, arthropod-borne V05.0
      hepatitis V05.3
      yellow fever V04.4
Vaccinia (generalized) 999.0
  congenital 771.2
  conjunctiva 999.39
  eyelids 999.0 [373.5]
  localized 999.39
  nose 999.39
  not from vaccination 051.02
    eyelid 051.02 [373.5]
  sine vaccinatione 051.02
  without vaccination 051.02
Vacuum
  extraction of fetus or newborn 763.3
  in sinus (accessory) (nasal) (see also Sinusitis) 473.9
Vagabond V60.0
Vagabondage V60.0
Vagabonds' disease 132.1
Vagina, vaginal - see also condition
  high risk human papillomavirus (HPV) DNA test positive 795.15
  low risk human papillomavirus (HPV) DNA test positive 795.19
Vaginalitis (tunica) 608.4
Vaginismus (reflex) 625.1
  functional 306.51
  hysterical 300.11
  psychogenic 306.51
Vaginitis (acute) (chronic) (circumscribed) (diffuse) (emphysematous) (Hemophilus vaginalis) (nonspecific) (nonvenereal) (ulcerative) 616.10
  with
    abortion - see Abortion, by type, with sepsis
    ectopic pregnancy (see also categories 633.0–633.9) 639.0
    molar pregnancy (see also categories 630–632) 639.0
  adhesive, congenital 752.49
  atrophic, postmenopausal 627.3
  bacterial 616.10
  blennorrhagic (acute) 098.0
    chronic or duration of 2 months or over 098.2
  candidal 112.1
  chlamydial 099.53
  complicating pregnancy or puerperium 646.6●
    affecting fetus or newborn 760.8
  congenital (adhesive) 752.49
  due to
    C. albicans 112.1
    Trichomonas (vaginalis) 131.01
  following
    abortion 639.0
    ectopic or molar pregnancy 639.0
  gonococcal (acute) 098.0
    chronic or duration of 2 months or over 098.2
  granuloma 099.2
  Monilia 112.1
  mycotic 112.1
  pinworm 127.4 [616.11]
  postirradiation 616.10
  postmenopausal atrophic 627.3
  senile (atrophic) 627.3
  syphilitic (early) 091.0
    late 095.8
  trichomonal 131.01

Vaginitis (Continued)
  tuberculous (see also Tuberculosis) 016.7●
  venereal NEC 099.8
Vaginosis - see Vaginitis
Vagotonia 352.3
Vagrancy V60.0
VAIN I (vaginal intraepithelial neoplasia I) 623.0
VAIN II (vaginal intraepithelial neoplasia II) 623.0
VAIN III (vaginal intraepithelial neoplasia III) 233.31
Vallecula - see condition
Valley fever 114.0
Valsuani's disease (progressive pernicious anemia, puerperal) 648.2●
Valve, valvular (formation) - see also condition
  cerebral ventricle (communicating) in situ V45.2
  cervix, internal os 752.49
  colon 751.5
  congenital NEC - see Atresia
  formation congenital NEC - see Atresia
  heart defect - see Anomaly, heart, valve
  ureter 753.29
    pelvic junction 753.21
    vesical orifice 753.22
  urethra 753.6
Valvulitis (chronic) (see also Endocarditis) 424.90
  rheumatic (chronic) (inactive) (with chorea) 397.9
    active or acute (aortic) (mitral) (pulmonary) (tricuspid) 391.1
  syphilitic NEC 093.20
    aortic 093.22
    mitral 093.21
    pulmonary 093.24
    tricuspid 093.23
Valvulopathy - see Endocarditis
van Bogaert's leukoencephalitis (sclerosing) (subacute) 046.2
van Bogaert-Nijssen (-Peiffer) disease 330.0
van Buchem's syndrome (hyperostosis corticalis) 733.3
Vancomycin (glycopeptide)
  intermediate staphylococcus aureus (VISA/GISA) V09.8
  resistant
    enterococcus (VRE) V09.8
    staphylococcus aureus (VRSA/GRSA) V09.8
van Creveld-von Gierke disease (glycogenosis I) 271.0
van den Bergh's disease (enterogenous cyanosis) 289.7
van der Hoeve's syndrome (brittle bones and blue sclera, deafness) 756.51
van der Hoeve-Halbertsma-Waardenburg syndrome (ptosis-epicanthus) 270.2
van der Hoeve-Waardenburg-Gualdi syndrome (ptosis-epicanthus) 270.2
Vanillism 692.89
Vanishing lung 492.0
Vanishing twin 651.33
van Neck (-Odelberg) disease or syndrome (juvenile osteochondrosis) 732.1
Vapor asphyxia or suffocation NEC 987.9
  specified agent - see Table of Drugs and Chemicals
Vaquez's disease (M9950/1) 238.4
Vaquez-Osler disease (polycythemia vera) (M9950/1) 238.4
Variance, lethal ball, prosthetic heart valve 996.02
Variants, thalassemic 282.49
Variations in hair color 704.3

◄ New   ◄▥ Revised   deleted Deleted   ● Use Additional Digit(s)   ▨ Omit code   511

Varicella 052.9
with
complication 052.8
specified NEC 052.7
pneumonia 052.1
exposure to V01.71
vaccination and inoculation (against)
(prophylactic) V05.4
Varices - see Varix
Varicocele (scrotum) (thrombosed)
456.4
ovary 456.5
perineum 456.6
spermatic cord (ulcerated) 456.4
Varicose
aneurysm (ruptured) (see also Aneurysm)
442.9
dermatitis (lower extremity) - see Varicose,
vein, inflamed or infected
eczema - see Varicose, vein
phlebitis - see Varicose, vein, inflamed or
infected
placental vessel - see Placenta, abnormal
tumor - see Varicose, vein
ulcer (lower extremity, any part) 454.0
anus 455.8
external 455.5
internal 455.2
esophagus (see also Varix, esophagus)
456.1
bleeding (see also Varix, esophagus,
bleeding) 456.0
inflamed or infected 454.2
nasal septum 456.8
perineum 456.6
rectum - see Varicose, ulcer, anus
scrotum 456.4
specified site NEC 456.8
vein (lower extremity) (ruptured) (see also
Varix) 454.9
with
complications NEC 454.8
edema 454.8
inflammation or infection 454.1
ulcerated 454.2
pain 454.8
stasis dermatitis 454.1
with ulcer 454.2
swelling 454.8
ulcer 454.0
inflamed or infected 454.2
anus - see Hemorrhoids
broad ligament 456.5
congenital (peripheral) 747.60
gastrointestinal 747.61
lower limb 747.64
renal 747.62
specified NEC 747.69
upper limb 747.63
esophagus (ulcerated (see also Varix,
esophagus) 456.1
bleeding (see also Varix, esophagus,
bleeding) 456.0
inflamed or infected 454.1
with ulcer 454.2
in pregnancy or puerperium 671.0●
vulva or perineum 671.1●
nasal septum (with ulcer) 456.8
pelvis 456.5
perineum 456.6
in pregnancy, childbirth, or
puerperium 671.1●
rectum - see Hemorrhoids
scrotum (ulcerated) 456.4
specified site NEC 456.8
sublingual 456.3
ulcerated 454.0
inflamed or infected 454.2
umbilical cord, affecting fetus or newborn
762.6
urethra 456.8

Varicose (Continued)
vein (Continued)
vulva 456.6
in pregnancy, childbirth, or
puerperium 671.1●
vessel - see also Varix
placenta - see Placenta, abnormal
Varicosis, varicosities, varicosity (see also Varix)
454.9
Variola 050.9
hemorrhagic (pustular) 050.0
major 050.0
minor 050.1
modified 050.2
Varioloid 050.2
Variolosa, purpura 050.0
Varix (lower extremity) (ruptured) 454.9
with
complications NEC 454.8
edema 454.8
inflammation or infection 454.1
with ulcer 454.2
pain 454.8
stasis dermatitis 454.1
with ulcer 454.2
swelling 454.8
ulcer 454.0
with inflammation or infection
454.2
aneurysmal (see also Aneurysm) 442.9
anus - see Hemorrhoids
arteriovenous (congenital) (peripheral) NEC
747.60
gastrointestinal 747.61
lower limb 747.64
renal 747.62
specified NEC 747.69
spinal 747.82
upper limb 747.63
bladder 456.5
broad ligament 456.5
congenital (peripheral) 747.60
esophagus (ulcerated) 456.1
bleeding 456.0
in
cirrhosis of liver 571.5 [456.20]
portal hypertension 572.3 [456.20]
congenital 747.69
in
cirrhosis of liver 571.5 [456.21]
with bleeding 571.5 [456.20]
portal hypertension 572.3 [456.21]
with bleeding 572.3 [456.20]
gastric 456.8
inflamed or infected 454.1
ulcerated 454.2
in pregnancy or puerperium 671.0●
perineum 671.1●
vulva 671.1●
labia (majora) 456.6
orbit 456.8
congenital 747.69
ovary 456.5
papillary 448.1
pelvis 456.5
perineum 456.6
in pregnancy or puerperium 671.1●
pharynx 456.8
placenta - see Placenta, abnormal
prostate 456.8
rectum - see Hemorrhoids
renal papilla 456.8
retina 362.17
scrotum (ulcerated) 456.4
sigmoid colon 456.8
specified site NEC 456.8
spinal (cord) (vessels) 456.8
spleen, splenic (vein) (with phlebolith) 456.8
sublingual 456.3
ulcerated 454.0
inflamed or infected 454.2

Varix (Continued)
umbilical cord, affecting fetus or newborn
762.6
uterine ligament 456.5
vocal cord 456.8
vulva 456.6
in pregnancy, childbirth, or puerperium
671.1●
Vasa previa 663.5●
affecting fetus or newborn 762.6
hemorrhage from, affecting fetus or newborn
772.0
Vascular - see also condition
loop on papilla (optic) 743.57
sheathing, retina 362.13
spasm 443.9
spider 448.1
Vascularity, pulmonary, congenital 747.39
Vascularization
choroid 362.16
cornea 370.60
deep 370.63
localized 370.61
retina 362.16
subretinal 362.16
Vasculitis 447.6
allergic 287.0
cryoglobulinemic 273.2
disseminated 447.6
kidney 447.8
leukocytoclastic 446.29
nodular 695.2
retinal 362.18
rheumatic - see Fever, rheumatic
Vasculopathy
cardiac allograft 996.83
Vas deferens - see condition
Vas deferentitis 608.4
Vasectomy, admission for V25.2
Vasitis 608.4
nodosa 608.4
scrotum 608.4
spermatic cord 608.4
testis 608.4
tuberculous (see also Tuberculosis) 016.5●
tunica vaginalis 608.4
vas deferens 608.4
Vasodilation 443.9
Vasomotor - see condition
Vasoplasty, after previous sterilization V26.0
Vasoplegia, splanchnic (see also Neuropathy,
peripheral, autonomic) 337.9
Vasospasm 443.9
cerebral (artery) 435.9
with transient neurologic deficit 435.9
coronary 413.1
nerve
arm NEC 354.9
autonomic 337.9
brachial plexus 353.0
cervical plexus 353.2
leg NEC 355.8
lower extremity NEC 355.8
peripheral NEC 335.9
spinal NEC 355.9
sympathetic 337.9
upper extremity NEC 354.9
peripheral NEC 443.9
retina (artery) (see also Occlusion, retinal,
artery) 362.30
Vasospastic - see condition
Vasovagal attack (paroxysmal) 780.2
psychogenic 306.2
Vater's ampulla - see condition
VATER syndrome 759.89
vCJD (variant Creutzfeldt-Jakob disease) 046.11
Vegetation, vegetative
adenoid (nasal fossa) 474.2
consciousness (persistent) 780.03
endocarditis (acute) (any valve) (chronic)
(subacute) 421.0

◄ New ◄ Revised deleted Deleted ● Use Additional Digit(s) Omit code

Vegetation, vegetative *(Continued)*
  heart (mycotic) (valve) 421.0
  state (persistent) 780.03
Veil
  Jackson's 751.4
  over face (causing asphyxia) 768.9
Vein, venous - *see* condition
Veldt sore *(see also* Ulcer, skin) 707.9
Velo-cardio-facial syndrome 758.32
Velpeau's hernia - *see* Hernia, femoral
Venereal
  balanitis NEC 099.8
  bubo 099.1
  disease 099.9
    specified nature or type NEC 099.8
  granuloma inguinale 099.2
  lymphogranuloma (Durand-Nicolas-Favre),
    any site 099.1
  salpingitis 098.37
  urethritis *(see also* Urethritis, nongonococcal)
    099.40
  vaginitis NEC 099.8
  warts 078.11
Vengefulness, in child *(see also* Disturbance,
  conduct) 312.0●
Venofibrosis 459.89
Venom, venomous
  bite or sting (animal or insect) 989.5
  poisoning 989.5
Venous - *see* condition
Ventouse delivery NEC 669.5●
  affecting fetus or newborn 763.3
Ventral - *see* condition
Ventricle, ventricular - *see also* condition
  escape 427.69
  standstill *(see also* Arrest, cardiac) 427.5
Ventriculitis, cerebral *(see also* Meningitis)
  322.9
Ventriculostomy status V45.2
Verbiest's syndrome (claudicatio intermittens
  spinalis) 435.1
Vernet's syndrome 352.6
Verneuil's disease (syphilitic bursitis) 095.7
Verruca (filiformis) 078.10
  acuminata (any site) 078.11
  necrogenica (primary) *(see also* Tuberculosis)
    017.0●
  peruana 088.0
  peruviana 088.0
  plana (juvenilis) 078.19
  plantaris 078.12
  seborrheica 702.19
    inflamed 702.11
  senilis 702.0
  tuberculosa (primary) *(see also* Tuberculosis)
    017.0●
  venereal 078.11
  viral 078.10
    specified NEC 078.19
  vulgaris 078.10
Verrucosities *(see also* Verruca) 078.10
Verrucous endocarditis (acute) (any valve)
  (chronic) (subacute) 710.0 *[424.91]*
  nonbacterial 710.0 *[424.91]*
Verruga
  peruana 088.0
  peruviana 088.0
Verse's disease (calcinosis intervertebralis)
  275.49 *[722.90]*
Version
  before labor, affecting fetus or newborn
    761.7
  cephalic (correcting previous malposition)
    652.1●
    affecting fetus or newborn 763.1
  cervix - *see* Version, uterus
  uterus (postinfectional) (postpartal, old) *(see
    also* Malposition, uterus) 621.6
    forward - *see* Anteversion, uterus
    lateral - *see* Lateroversion, uterus
Vertebra, vertebral - *see* condition

Vertigo 780.4
  auditory 386.19
  aural 386.19
  benign paroxysmal positional 386.11
  central origin 386.2
  cerebral 386.2
  Dix and Hallpike (epidemic) 386.12
  endemic paralytic 078.81
  epidemic 078.81
    Dix and Hallpike 386.12
    Gerlier's 078.81
    Pedersen's 386.12
    vestibular neuronitis 386.12
  epileptic - *see* Epilepsy
  Gerlier's (epidemic) 078.81
  hysterical 300.11
  labyrinthine 386.10
  laryngeal 786.2
  malignant positional 386.2
  Ménière's *(see also* Disease, Ménière's) 386.00
  menopausal 627.2
  otogenic 386.19
  paralytic 078.81
  paroxysmal positional, benign 386.11
  Pedersen's (epidemic) 386.12
  peripheral 386.10
    specified type NEC 386.19
  positional
    benign paroxysmal 386.11
    malignant 386.2
Verumontanitis (chronic) *(see also* Urethritis)
  597.89
Vesania *(see also* Psychosis) 298.9
Vesical - *see* condition
Vesicle
  cutaneous 709.8
  seminal - *see* condition
  skin 709.8
Vesicocolic - *see* condition
Vesicoperineal - *see* condition
Vesicorectal - *see* condition
Vesicourethrorectal - *see* condition
Vesicovaginal - *see* condition
Vesicular - *see* condition
Vesiculitis (seminal) 608.0
  amebic 006.8
  gonorrheal (acute) 098.14
    chronic or duration of 2 months or over
      098.34
  trichomonal 131.09
  tuberculous *(see also* Tuberculosis) 016.5●
    [608.81]
Vestibulitis (ear) *(see also* Labyrinthitis) 386.30
  nose (external) 478.19
  vulvar 625.71
Vestibulopathy, acute peripheral (recurrent)
  386.12
Vestige, vestigial - *see also* Persistence
  branchial 744.41
  structures in vitreous 743.51
Vibriosis NEC 027.9
Vidal's disease (lichen simplex chronicus) 698.3
Video display tube syndrome 723.8
Vienna-type encephalitis 049.8
Villaret's syndrome 352.6
Villous - *see* condition
VIN I (vulvar intraepithelial neoplasia I)
  624.01
VIN II (vulvar intraepithelial neoplasia II)
  624.02
VIN III (vulvar intraepithelial neoplasia III)
  233.32
Vincent's
  angina 101
  bronchitis 101
  disease 101
  gingivitis 101
  infection (any site) 101
  laryngitis 101
  stomatitis 101
  tonsillitis 101

Vinson-Plummer syndrome (sideropenic
  dysphagia) 280.8
Viosterol deficiency *(see also* Deficiency,
  calciferol) 268.9
Virchow's disease 733.99
Viremia 790.8
Virilism (adrenal) (female) NEC 255.2
  with
    3-beta-hydroxysteroid dehydrogenase
      defect 255.2
    11-hydroxylase defect 255.2
    21-hydroxylase defect 255.2
    adrenal
      hyperplasia 255.2
      insufficiency (congenital) 255.2
    cortical hyperfunction 255.2
Virilization (female) (suprarenal) *(see also*
  Virilism) 255.2
  isosexual 256.4
Virulent bubo 099.0
Virus, viral - *see also* condition
  infection NEC *(see also* Infection, viral) 079.99
  septicemia 079.99
  yaba monkey tumor 059.22
VISA (vancomycin intermediate
  staphylococcus aureus) V09.8
Viscera, visceral - *see* condition
Visceroptosis 569.89
Visible peristalsis 787.4
Vision, visual
  binocular, suppression 368.31
  blurred, blurring 368.8
    hysterical 300.11
  defect, defective *(see also* Impaired, vision)
    369.9
  disorientation (syndrome) 368.16
  disturbance NEC *(see also* Disturbance,
    vision) 368.9
    hysterical 300.11
  examination V72.0
  field, limitation 368.40
  fusion, with defective steropsis 368.33
  hallucinations 368.16
  halos 368.16
  loss 369.9
    both eyes *(see also* Blindness, both eyes)
      369.3
    complete *(see also* Blindness, both eyes)
      369.00
    one eye 369.8
    sudden 368.16
  low (both eyes) 369.20
    one eye (other eye normal) *(see also*
      Impaired, vision) 369.70
      blindness, other eye 369.10
  perception, simultaneous without fusion
    368.32
  tunnel 368.45
Vitality, lack or want of 780.79
  newborn 779.89
Vitamin deficiency NEC *(see also* Deficiency,
  vitamin) 269.2
Vitelline duct, persistent 751.0
Vitiligo 709.01
  due to pinta (carate) 103.2
  eyelid 374.53
  vulva 624.8
Vitium cordis - *see* Disease, heart
Vitreous - *see also* condition
  touch syndrome 997.99
VLCAD (long chain/very long chain acyl CoA
  dehydrogenase deficiency, LCAD) 277.85
Vocal cord - *see* condition
Vocational rehabilitation V57.22
Vogt's (Cecile) disease or syndrome 333.7
Vogt-Koyanagi syndrome 364.24
Vogt-Spielmeyer disease (amaurotic familial
  idiocy) 330.1
Voice
  change *(see also* Dysphonia) 784.49
  loss *(see also* Aphonia) 784.41

Volhard-Fahr disease (malignant
nephrosclerosis) 403.00
Volhynian fever 083.1
Volkmann's ischemic contracture or paralysis
(complicating trauma) 958.6
Voluntary starvation 307.1
Volvulus (bowel) (colon) (intestine) 560.2
with
hernia - *see also* Hernia, by site, with
obstruction
gangrenous - *see* Hernia, by site, with
gangrene
perforation 560.2
congenital 751.5
duodenum 537.3
fallopian tube 620.5
oviduct 620.5
stomach (due to absence of gastrocolic
ligament) 537.89
Vomiting 787.03
with nausea 787.01
allergic 535.4●
asphyxia 933.1
bilious (cause unknown) 787.04
following gastrointestinal surgery 564.3
newborn 779.32
blood (*see also* Hematemesis) 578.0
causing asphyxia, choking, or suffocation
(*see also* Asphyxia, food) 933.1
cyclical 536.2
associated with migraine 346.2●
psychogenic 306.4
epidemic 078.82
fecal matter 569.87
following gastrointestinal surgery 564.3
functional 536.8
psychogenic 306.4
habit 536.2
hysterical 300.11
nervous 306.4
neurotic 306.4
newborn 779.33
bilious 779.32
of or complicating pregnancy 643.9●
due to
organic disease 643.8●
specific cause NEC 643.8●
early - *see* Hyperemesis, gravidarum
late (after 22 completed weeks of
gestation) 643.2●

Vomiting (*Continued*)
pernicious or persistent 536.2
complicating pregnancy - *see*
Hyperemesis, gravidarum
psychogenic 306.4
physiological 787.03
bilious 787.04
psychic 306.4
psychogenic 307.54
stercoral 569.89
uncontrollable 536.2
psychogenic 306.4
uremic - *see* Uremia
winter 078.82
von Bechterew (-Strümpell) disease or
syndrome (ankylosing spondylitis)
720.0
von Bezold's abscess 383.01
von Economo's disease (encephalitis lethargica)
049.8
von Eulenburg's disease (congenital
paramyotonia) 359.29
von Gierke's disease (glycogenosis I) 271.0
von Gies' joint 095.8
von Graefe's disease or syndrome 378.72
von Hippel (-Lindau) disease or syndrome
(retinocerebral angiomatosis) 759.6
von Jaksch's anemia or disease
(pseudoleukemia infantum) 285.8
von Recklinghausen's
disease or syndrome (nerves) (skin)
(M9540/1) 237.71
bones (osteitis fibrosa cystica) 252.01
tumor (M9540/1) 237.71
von Recklinghausen-Applebaum disease
(hemochromatosis) (*see also*
Hemochromatosis) 275.03
von Schroetter's syndrome (intermittent
venous claudication) 453.89
von Willebrand (-Jürgens) (-Minot) disease or
syndrome (angiohemophilia) 286.4
von Zambusch's disease (lichen sclerosus et
atrophicus) 701.0
Voorhoeve's disease or dyschondroplasia
756.4
Vossius' ring 921.3
late effect 366.21
Voyeurism 302.82
VRE (vancomycin resistant enterococcus)
V09.8

Vrolik's disease (osteogenesis imperfecta)
756.51
VRSA (vancomycin resistant staphylococcus
aureus) V09.8
Vulva - *see* condition
Vulvismus 625.1
Vulvitis (acute) (allergic) (chronic) (gangrenous)
(hypertrophic) (intertriginous) 616.10
with
abortion - *see* Abortion, by type, with
sepsis
ectopic pregnancy (*see also* categories
633.0–633.9) 639.0
molar pregnancy (*see also* categories
630–632) 639.0
adhesive, congenital 752.49
blennorrhagic (acute) 098.0
chronic or duration of 2 months or over
098.2
chlamydial 099.53
complicating pregnancy or puerperium
646.6●
due to Ducrey's bacillus 099.0
following
abortion 639.0
ectopic or molar pregnancy 639.0
gonococcal (acute) 098.0
chronic or duration of 2 months or over
098.2
herpetic 054.11
leukoplakic 624.09
monilial 112.1
puerperal, postpartum, childbirth
646.6●
syphilitic (early) 091.0
late 095.8
trichomonal 131.01
Vulvodynia 625.70
specified NEC 625.79
Vulvorectal - *see* condition
Vulvovaginitis (*see also* Vulvitis) 616.10
amebic 006.8
chlamydial 099.53
gonococcal (acute) 098.0
chronic or duration of 2 months or over
098.2
herpetic 054.11
monilial 112.1
trichomonal (Trichomonas vaginalis)
131.01

◀ New ◀▥ Revised ~~deleted~~ Deleted ● Use Additional Digit(s) ▨ Omit code

W

Waardenburg's syndrome 756.89
  meaning ptosis-epicanthus 270.2
Waardenburg-Klein syndrome (ptosis-
    epicanthus) 270.2
Wagner's disease (colloid milium) 709.3
Wagner (-Unverricht) syndrome
    (dermatomyositis) 710.3
Waiting list, person on V63.2
  undergoing social agency investigation V63.8
Wakefulness disorder (see also Hypersomnia)
    780.54
  nonorganic origin 307.43
Waldenström's
  disease (osteochondrosis, capital femoral)
      732.1
  hepatitis (lupoid hepatitis) 571.49
  hypergammaglobulinemia 273.0
  macroglobulinemia 273.3
  purpura, hypergammaglobulinemic 273.0
  syndrome (macroglobulinemia) 273.3
Waldenström-Kjellberg syndrome (sideropenic
    dysphagia) 280.8
Walking
  difficulty 719.7
    psychogenic 307.9
  sleep 307.46
    hysterical 300.13
Wall, abdominal - see condition
Wallenberg's syndrome (posterior inferior
    cerebellar artery) (see also Disease,
    cerebrovascular, acute) 436
Wallgren's
  disease (obstruction of splenic vein with
      collateral circulation) 459.89
  meningitis (see also Meningitis, aseptic) 047.9
Wandering
  acetabulum 736.39
  gallbladder 751.69
  in diseases classified elsewhere V40.31
  kidney, congenital 753.3
  organ or site, congenital NEC - see
      Malposition, congenital
  pacemaker (atrial) (heart) 427.89
  spleen 289.59
Wardrop's disease (with lymphangitis) 681.9
  finger 681.02
  toe 681.11
War neurosis 300.16
Wart (digitate) (filiform) (infectious) (viral)
    078.10
  common 078.19
  external genital organs (venereal) 078.11
  fig 078.19
  flat 078.19
  genital 078.11
  Hassall-Henle's (of cornea) 371.41
  Henle's (of cornea) 371.41
  juvenile 078.19
  moist 078.10
  Peruvian 088.0
  plantar 078.12
  prosector (see also Tuberculosis) 017.0●
  seborrheic 702.19
    inflamed 702.11
  senile 702.0
  specified NEC 078.19
  syphilitic 091.3
  tuberculous (see also Tuberculosis) 017.0●
  venereal (female) (male) 078.11
Warthin's tumor (salivary gland) (M8561/0)
    210.2
Washerwoman's itch 692.4
Wassilieff's disease (leptospiral jaundice)
    100.0
Wasting
  disease 799.4
    due to malnutrition 261
    extreme (due to malnutrition) 261
  muscular NEC 728.2

Wasting (Continued)
  palsy, paralysis 335.21
  pelvic muscle 618.83
Water
  clefts 366.12
  deprivation of 994.3
  in joint (see also Effusion, joint) 719.0●
  intoxication 276.69
  itch 120.3
  lack of 994.3
  loading 276.69
  on
    brain - see Hydrocephalus
    chest 511.89
  poisoning 276.69
Waterbrash 787.1
Water-hammer pulse (see also Insufficiency,
    aortic) 424.1
Waterhouse (-Friderichsen) disease or
    syndrome 036.3
Water-losing nephritis 588.89
Watermelon stomach 537.82
  with hemorrhage 537.83
  without hemorrhage 537.82
Wax in ear 380.4
Waxy
  degeneration, any site 277.39
  disease 277.39
  kidney 277.39 [583.81]
  liver (large) 277.39
  spleen 277.39
Weak, weakness (generalized) 780.79
  arches (acquired) 734
    congenital 754.61
  bladder sphincter 596.59
  congenital 779.89
  eye muscle - see Strabismus
  facial 781.94
  foot (double) - see Weak, arches
  heart, cardiac (see also Failure, heart) 428.9
    congenital 746.9
  mind 317
  muscle (generalized) 728.87
  myocardium (see also Failure, heart) 428.9
  newborn 779.89
  pelvic fundus
    pubocervical tissue 618.81
    rectovaginal tissue 618.82
  pulse 785.9
  senile 797
  urinary stream 788.62
  valvular - see Endocarditis
Wear, worn, tooth, teeth (approximal) (hard
    tissues) (interproximal) (occlusal) - see also
    Attrition, teeth 521.10
Weather, weathered
  effects of
    cold NEC 991.9
      specified effect NEC 991.8
    hot (see also Heat) 992.9
  skin 692.74
Web, webbed (congenital) - see also Anomaly,
    specified type NEC
  canthus 743.63
  digits (see also Syndactylism) 755.10
  duodenal 751.5
  esophagus 750.3
  fingers (see also Syndactylism, fingers) 755.11
  larynx (glottic) (subglottic) 748.2
  neck (pterygium colli) 744.5
  Paterson-Kelly (sideropenic dysphagia) 280.8
  popliteal syndrome 756.89
  toes (see also Syndactylism, toes) 755.13
Weber's paralysis or syndrome 344.89
Weber-Christian disease or syndrome (nodular
    nonsuppurative panniculitis) 729.30
Weber-Cockayne syndrome (epidermolysis
    bullosa) 757.39
Weber-Dimitri syndrome 759.6
Weber-Gubler syndrome 344.89
Weber-Leyden syndrome 344.89

Weber-Osler syndrome (familial hemorrhagic
    telangiectasia) 448.0
Wedge-shaped or wedging vertebra (see also
    Osteoporosis) 733.00
Wegener's granulomatosis or syndrome 446.4
Wegner's disease (syphilitic osteochondritis)
    090.0
Weight
  gain (abnormal) (excessive) 783.1
    during pregnancy 646.1●
      insufficient 646.8●
  less than 1000 grams at birth 765.0●
  loss (cause unknown) 783.21
Weightlessness 994.9
Weil's disease (leptospiral jaundice) 100.0
Weill-Marchesani syndrome (brachymorphism
    and ectopia lentis) 759.89
Weingarten's syndrome (tropical eosinophilia)
    518.3
Weir Mitchell's disease (erythromelalgia)
    443.82
Weiss-Baker syndrome (carotid sinus syncope)
    337.01
Weissenbach-Thibierge syndrome (cutaneous
    systemic sclerosis) 710.1
Wen (see also Cyst, sebaceous) 706.2
Wenckebach's phenomenon, heart block
    (second degree) 426.13
Werdnig-Hoffmann syndrome (muscular
    atrophy) 335.0
Werlhof's disease (see also Purpura,
    thrombocytopenic) 287.39
Werlhof-Wichmann syndrome (see also
    Purpura, thrombocytopenic) 287.39
Wermer's syndrome or disease (polyendocrine
    adenomatosis) 258.01
Werner's disease or syndrome (progeria
    adultorum) 259.8
Werner-His disease (trench fever) 083.1
Werner-Schultz disease (agranulocytosis)
    288.09
Wernicke's encephalopathy, disease, or
    syndrome (superior hemorrhagic
    polioencephalitis) 265.1
Wernicke-Korsakoff syndrome or psychosis
    (nonalcoholic) 294.0
  alcoholic 291.1
Wernicke-Posadas disease (see also
    Coccidioidomycosis) 114.9
Wesselsbron fever 066.3
West African fever 084.8
West Nile
  encephalitis 066.41
  encephalomyelitis 066.41
  fever 066.40
    with
      cranial nerve disorders 066.42
      encephalitis 066.41
      optic neuritis 066.42
      other complications 066.49
      other neurologic manifestations 066.42
      polyradiculitis 066.42
  virus 066.40
Westphal-Strümpell syndrome
    (hepatolenticular degeneration) 275.1
Wet
  brain (alcoholic) (see also Alcoholism) 303.9●
  feet, tropical (syndrome) (maceration) 991.4
  lung (syndrome)
    adult 518.52
    newborn 770.6
Wharton's duct - see condition
Wheal 709.8
Wheelchair confinement status V46.3
Wheezing 786.07
Whiplash injury or syndrome 847.0
Whipple's disease or syndrome (intestinal
    lipodystrophy) 040.2
Whipworm 127.3
"Whistling face" syndrome (craniocarpotarsal
    dystrophy) 759.89

White - *see also* condition
  kidney
    large - *see* Nephrosis
    small 582.9
  leg, puerperal, postpartum, childbirth 671.4●
    nonpuerperal 451.19
  mouth 112.0
  patches of mouth 528.6
  sponge nevus of oral mucosa 750.26
  spot lesions, teeth 521.01
White's disease (congenital) (keratosis
  follicularis) 757.39
Whitehead 706.2
Whitlow (with lymphangitis) 681.01
  herpetic 054.6
Whitmore's disease or fever (melioidosis) 025
Whooping cough 033.9
  with pneumonia 033.9 *[484.3]*
  due to
    Bordetella
      bronchoseptica 033.8
        with pneumonia 033.8 *[484.3]*
      parapertussis 033.1
        with pneumonia 033.1 *[484.3]*
      pertussis 033.0
        with pneumonia 033.0 *[484.3]*
    specified organism NEC 033.8
      with pneumonia 033.8 *[484.3]*
  vaccination, prophylactic (against) V03.6
Wichmann's asthma (laryngismus stridulus)
  478.75
Widal (-Abrami) syndrome (acquired hemolytic
  jaundice) 283.9
Widening aorta (*see also* Ectasia, aortic) 447.70
  with aneurysm 441.9
  ruptured 441.5
Wilkie's disease or syndrome 557.1
Wilkinson-Sneddon disease or syndrome
  (subcorneal pustular dermatosis) 694.1
Willan's lepra 696.1
Willan-Plumbe syndrome (psoriasis) 696.1
Willebrand (-Jürgens) syndrome or
  thrombopathy (angiohemophilia) 286.4
Willi-Prader syndrome (hypogenital dystrophy
  with diabetic tendency) 759.81
Willis' disease (diabetes mellitus) (*see also*
  Diabetes) 250.0●
  due to secondary diabetes 249.0●
Wilms' tumor or neoplasm (nephroblastoma)
  (M8960/3) 189.0
Wilson's
  disease or syndrome (hepatolenticular
    degeneration) 275.1
  hepatolenticular degeneration 275.1
  lichen ruber 697.0
Wilson-Brocq disease (dermatitis exfoliativa)
  695.89
Wilson-Mikity syndrome 770.7
Window - *see also* Imperfect, closure
  aorticopulmonary 745.0
Winged scapula 736.89
Winter - *see also* condition
  vomiting disease 078.82
Wise's disease 696.2
Wiskott-Aldrich syndrome (eczema-
  thrombocytopenia) 279.12
Withdrawal symptoms, syndrome
  alcohol 291.81
    delirium (acute) 291.0
      chronic 291.1
      newborn 760.71
  drug or narcotic 292.0
  newborn, infant of dependent mother 779.5
  steroid NEC
    correct substance properly administered
      255.41
    overdose or wrong substance given or
      taken 962.0
Withdrawing reaction, child or adolescent
  313.22
Witts' anemia (achlorhydric anemia) 280.9

Witzelsucht 301.9
Woakes' syndrome (ethmoiditis) 471.1
Wohlfart-Kugelberg-Welander disease 335.11
Woillez's disease (acute idiopathic pulmonary
  congestion) 518.52
Wolff-Parkinson-White syndrome (anomalous
  atrioventricular excitation) 426.7
Wolhynian fever 083.1
Wolman's disease (primary familial
  xanthomatosis) 272.7
Wood asthma 495.8
Woolly, wooly hair (congenital) (nevus)
  757.4
Wool-sorters' disease 022.1
Word
  blindness (congenital) (developmental)
    315.01
    secondary to organic lesion 784.61
  deafness (secondary to organic lesion)
    784.69
  developmental 315.31
Worm(s) (colic) (fever) (infection) (infestation)
  (*see also* Infestation) 128.9
  guinea 125.7
  in intestine NEC 127.9
Worm-eaten soles 102.3
Worn out (*see also* Exhaustion) 780.79
  artificial heart valve 996.02
  cardiac defibrillator (with synchronous
    cardiac pacemaker) V53.32
  cardiac pacemaker lead or battery V53.31
  joint prosthesis (*see also* Complications,
    mechanical, device NEC, prosthetic
    NEC, joint) 996.46
"Worried well" V65.5
Wound, open (by cutting or piercing
  instrument) (by firearms) (cut)
  (dissection) (incised) (laceration)
  (penetration) (perforating) (puncture)
  (with initial hemorrhage, not internal)
  879.8

Note: For fracture with open wound, see
Fracture.

For laceration, traumatic rupture, tear, or
penetrating wound of internal organs, such
as heart, lung, liver, kidney, pelvic organs,
etc., whether or not accompanied by open
wound or fracture in the same region, see
Injury, internal. For contused wound, see
Contusion. For crush injury, see Crush. For
abrasion, insect bite (nonvenomous), blister,
or scratch, see Injury, superficial.

Complicated includes wounds with:

  delayed healing
  delayed treatment
  foreign body
  primary infection

For late effect of open wound, see Late,
effect, wound, open, by site.

---

  abdomen, abdominal (external) (muscle)
    879.2
    complicated 879.3
    wall (anterior) 879.2
      complicated 879.3
      lateral 879.4
        complicated 879.5
  alveolar (process) 873.62
    complicated 873.72
  ankle 891.0
    with tendon involvement 891.2
    complicated 891.1
  anterior chamber, eye (*see also* Wound, open,
    intraocular) 871.9
  anus 863.89
  arm 884.0
    with tendon involvement 884.2
    complicated 884.1

Wound, open (*Continued*)
  arm (*Continued*)
    forearm 881.00
      with tendon involvement 881.20
      complicated 881.10
    multiple sites - *see* Wound, open, multiple,
      upper limb
    upper 880.03
      with tendon involvement 880.23
      complicated 880.13
      multiple sites (with axillary or
        shoulder regions) 880.09
        with tendon involvement 880.29
        complicated 880.19
  artery - *see* Injury, blood vessel, by site
  auditory
    canal (external) (meatus) 872.02
      complicated 872.12
    ossicles (incus) (malleus) (stapes) 872.62
      complicated 872.72
  auricle, ear 872.01
    complicated 872.11
  axilla 880.02
    with tendon involvement 880.22
    complicated 880.12
      with tendon involvement 880.29
    involving other sites of upper arm 880.09
      complicated 880.19
  back 876.0
    complicated 876.1
  bladder - *see* Injury, internal, bladder
  blood vessel - *see* Injury, blood vessel, by site
  brain - *see* Injury, intracranial, with open
    intracranial wound
  breast 879.0
    complicated 879.1
  brow 873.42
    complicated 873.52
  buccal mucosa 873.61
    complicated 873.71
  buttock 877.0
    complicated 877.1
  calf 891.0
    with tendon involvement 891.2
    complicated 891.1
  canaliculus lacrimalis 870.8
    with laceration of eyelid 870.2
  canthus, eye 870.8
    laceration - *see* Laceration, eyelid
  cavernous sinus - *see* Injury, intracranial
  cerebellum - *see* Injury, intracranial
  cervical esophagus 874.4
    complicated 874.5
  cervix - *see* Injury, internal, cervix
  cheek(s) (external) 873.41
    complicated 873.51
    internal 873.61
      complicated 873.71
  chest (wall) (external) 875.0
    complicated 875.1
  chin 873.44
    complicated 873.54
  choroid 363.63
  ciliary body (eye) (*see also* Wound, open,
    intraocular) 871.9
  clitoris 878.8
    complicated 878.9
  cochlea 872.64
    complicated 872.74
  complicated 879.9
  conjunctiva - *see* Wound, open, intraocular
  cornea (nonpenetrating) (*see also* Wound,
    open, intraocular) 871.9
  costal region 875.0
    complicated 875.1
  Descemet's membrane (*see also* Wound, open,
    intraocular) 871.9
  digit(s)
    foot 893.0
      with tendon involvement 893.2
      complicated 893.1

◀ New   ◀▬ Revised   ~~deleted~~ Deleted   ● Use Additional Digit(s)   ▨ Omit code

Wound, open *(Continued)*
  digit(s) *(Continued)*
    hand 883.0
      with tendon involvement 883.2
      complicated 883.1
  drumhead, ear 872.61
    complicated 872.71
  ear 872.8
    canal 872.02
      complicated 872.12
    complicated 872.9
    drum 872.61
      complicated 872.71
    external 872.00
      complicated 872.10
    multiple sites 872.69
      complicated 872.79
    ossicles (incus) (malleus) (stapes) 872.62
      complicated 872.72
    specified part NEC 872.69
      complicated 872.79
  elbow 881.01
    with tendon involvement 881.21
    complicated 881.11
  epididymis 878.2
    complicated 878.3
  epigastric region 879.2
    complicated 879.3
  epiglottis 874.01
    complicated 874.11
  esophagus (cervical) 874.4
    complicated 874.5
    thoracic - *see* Injury, internal, esophagus
  Eustachian tube 872.63
    complicated 872.73
  extremity
    lower (multiple) NEC 894.0
      with tendon involvement 894.2
      complicated 894.1
    upper (multiple) NEC 884.0
      with tendon involvement 884.2
      complicated 884.1
  eye(s) (globe) - *see* Wound, open, intraocular
  eyeball NEC 871.9
    laceration (*see also* Laceration, eyeball) 871.4
    penetrating (*see also* Penetrating wound, eyeball) 871.7
  eyebrow 873.42
    complicated 873.52
  eyelid NEC 870.8
    laceration - *see* Laceration, eyelid
  face 873.40
    complicated 873.50
    multiple sites 873.49
      complicated 873.59
    specified part NEC 873.49
      complicated 873.59
  fallopian tube - *see* Injury, internal, fallopian tube
  finger(s) (nail) (subungual) 883.0
    with tendon involvement 883.2
    complicated 883.1
  flank 879.4
    complicated 879.5
  foot (any part, except toe(s) alone) 892.0
    with tendon involvement 892.2
    complicated 892.1
  forearm 881.00
    with tendon involvement 881.20
    complicated 881.10
  forehead 873.42
    complicated 873.52
  genital organs (external) NEC 878.8
    complicated 878.9
    internal - *see* Injury, internal, by site
  globe (eye) (*see also* Wound, open, eyeball) 871.9
  groin 879.4
    complicated 879.5

Wound, open *(Continued)*
  gum(s) 873.62
    complicated 873.72
  hand (except finger(s) alone) 882.0
    with tendon involvement 882.2
    complicated 882.1
  head NEC 873.8
    with intracranial injury - *see* Injury, intracranial
      due to or associated with skull fracture - *see* Fracture, skull
    complicated 873.9
    scalp - *see* Wound, open, scalp
  heel 892.0
    with tendon involvement 892.2
    complicated 892.1
  high-velocity (grease gun) - *see* Wound, open, complicated, by site
  hip 890.0
    with tendon involvement 890.2
    complicated 890.1
  hymen 878.6
    complicated 878.7
  hypochondrium 879.4
    complicated 879.5
  hypogastric region 879.2
    complicated 879.3
  iliac (region) 879.4
    complicated 879.5
  incidental to
    dislocation - *see* Dislocation, open, by site
    fracture - *see* Fracture, open, by site
    intracranial injury - *see* Injury, intracranial, with open intracranial wound
    nerve injury - *see* Injury, nerve, by site
  inguinal region 879.4
    complicated 879.5
  instep 892.0
    with tendon involvement 892.2
    complicated 892.1
  interscapular region 876.0
    complicated 876.1
  intracranial - *see* Injury, intracranial, with open intracranial wound
  intraocular 871.9
    with
      partial loss (of intraocular tissue) 871.2
      prolapse or exposure (of intraocular tissue) 871.1
    laceration (*see also* Laceration, eyeball) 871.4
    penetrating 871.7
      with foreign body (nonmagnetic) 871.6
        magnetic 871.5
    without prolapse (of intraocular tissue) 871.0
  iris (*see also* Wound, open, eyeball) 871.9
  jaw (fracture not involved) 873.44
    with fracture - *see* Fracture, jaw
    complicated 873.54
  knee 891.0
    with tendon involvement 891.2
    complicated 891.1
  labium (majus) (minus) 878.4
    complicated 878.5
  lacrimal apparatus, gland, or sac 870.8
    with laceration of eyelid 870.2
  larynx 874.01
    with trachea 874.00
      complicated 874.10
    complicated 874.11
  leg (multiple) 891.0
    with tendon involvement 891.2
    complicated 891.1
    lower 891.0
      with tendon involvement 891.2
      complicated 891.1
    thigh 890.0
      with tendon involvement 890.2
      complicated 890.1

Wound, open *(Continued)*
  leg *(Continued)*
    upper 890.0
      with tendon involvement 890.2
      complicated 890.1
  lens (eye) (alone) (*see also* Cataract, traumatic) 366.20
    with involvement of other eye structures - *see* Wound, open, eyeball
  limb
    lower (multiple) NEC 894.0
      with tendon involvement 894.2
      complicated 894.1
    upper (multiple) NEC 884.0
      with tendon involvement 884.2
      complicated 884.1
  lip 873.43
    complicated 873.53
  loin 876.0
    complicated 876.1
  lumbar region 876.0
    complicated 876.1
  malar region 873.41
    complicated 873.51
  mastoid region 873.49
    complicated 873.59
  mediastinum - *see* Injury, internal, mediastinum
  midthoracic region 875.0
    complicated 875.1
  mouth 873.60
    complicated 873.70
    floor 873.64
      complicated 873.74
    multiple sites 873.69
      complicated 873.79
    specified site NEC 873.69
      complicated 873.79
  multiple, unspecified site(s) 879.8

> Note: Multiple open wounds of sites classifiable to the same four-digit category should be classified to that category unless they are in different limbs.
>
> Multiple open wounds of sites classifiable to different four-digit categories, or to different limbs, should be coded separately.

    complicated 879.9
  lower limb(s) (one or both) (sites classifiable to more than one three-digit category in 890–893) 894.0
    with tendon involvement 894.2
    complicated 894.1
  upper limb(s) (one or both) (sites classifiable to more than one three-digit category in 880–883) 884.0
    with tendon involvement 884.2
    complicated 884.1
  muscle - *see* Sprain, by site
  nail
    finger(s) 883.0
      complicated 883.1
    thumb 883.0
      complicated 883.1
    toe(s) 893.0
      complicated 893.1
  nape (neck) 874.8
    complicated 874.9
    specified part NEC 874.8
      complicated 874.9
  nasal - *see also* Wound, open, nose
    cavity 873.22
      complicated 873.32
    septum 873.21
      complicated 873.31
    sinuses 873.23
      complicated 873.33

W

Wound, open *(Continued)*
  nasopharynx 873.22
    complicated 873.32
  neck 874.8
    complicated 874.9
    nape 874.8
      complicated 874.9
    specified part NEC 874.8
      complicated 874.9
  nerve - *see* Injury, nerve, by site
  non-healing surgical 998.83
  nose 873.20
    complicated 873.30
    multiple sites 873.29
      complicated 873.39
    septum 873.21
      complicated 873.31
    sinuses 873.23
      complicated 873.33
  occipital region - *see* Wound, open, scalp
  ocular NEC 871.9
    adnexa 870.9
      specified region NEC 870.8
    laceration (*see also* Laceration, ocular)
      871.4
    muscle (extraocular) 870.3
      with foreign body 870.4
      eyelid 870.1
      intraocular - *see* Wound, open,
        eyeball
    penetrating (*see also* Penetrating wound,
      ocular) 871.7
  orbit 870.8
    penetrating 870.3
      with foreign body 870.4
  orbital region 870.9
  ovary - *see* Injury, internal, pelvic organs
  palate 873.65
    complicated 873.75
  palm 882.0
    with tendon involvement 882.2
    complicated 882.1
  parathyroid (gland) 874.2
    complicated 874.3
  parietal region - *see* Wound, open, scalp
  pelvic floor or region 879.6
    complicated 879.7
  penis 878.0
    complicated 878.1
  perineum 879.6
    complicated 879.7
  periocular area 870.8
    laceration of skin 870.0
  pharynx 874.4
    complicated 874.5
  pinna 872.01
    complicated 872.11
  popliteal space 891.0
    with tendon involvement 891.2
    complicated 891.1
  prepuce 878.0
    complicated 878.1
  pubic region 879.2
    complicated 879.3
  pudenda 878.8
    complicated 878.9
  rectovaginal septum 878.8
    complicated 878.9

Wound, open *(Continued)*
  sacral region 877.0
    complicated 877.1
  sacroiliac region 877.0
    complicated 877.1
  salivary (ducts) (glands) 873.69
    complicated 873.79
  scalp 873.0
    complicated 873.1
  scalpel, fetus or newborn 767.8
  scapular region 880.01
    with tendon involvement 880.21
    complicated 880.11
    involving other sites of upper arm 880.09
      with tendon involvement 880.29
      complicated 880.19
  sclera (*see also* Wound, open, intraocular)
    871.9
  scrotum 878.2
    complicated 878.3
  seminal vesicle - *see* Injury, internal, pelvic
    organs
  shin 891.0
    with tendon involvement 891.2
    complicated 891.1
  shoulder 880.00
    with tendon involvement 880.20
    complicated 880.10
    involving other sites of upper arm 880.09
      with tendon involvement 880.29
      complicated 880.19
  skin NEC 879.8
    complicated 879.9
  skull - *see also* Injury, intracranial, with open
      intracranial wound
    with skull fracture - *see* Fracture, skull
  spermatic cord (scrotal) 878.2
    complicated 878.3
    pelvic region - *see* Injury, internal,
      spermatic cord
  spinal cord - *see* Injury, spinal
  sternal region 875.0
    complicated 875.1
  subconjunctival - *see* Wound, open,
      intraocular
  subcutaneous NEC 879.8
    complicated 879.9
  submaxillary region 873.44
    complicated 873.54
  submental region 873.44
    complicated 873.54
  subungual
    finger(s) (thumb) - *see* Wound, open, finger
    toe(s) - *see* Wound, open, toe
  supraclavicular region 874.8
    complicated 874.9
  supraorbital 873.42
    complicated 873.52
  surgical, non-healing 998.83
  temple 873.49
    complicated 873.59
  temporal region 873.49
    complicated 873.59
  testis 878.2
    complicated 878.3
  thigh 890.0
    with tendon involvement 890.2
    complicated 890.1

Wound, open *(Continued)*
  thorax, thoracic (external) 875.0
    complicated 875.1
  throat 874.8
    complicated 874.9
  thumb (nail) (subungual) 883.0
    with tendon involvement 883.2
    complicated 883.1
  thyroid (gland) 874.2
    complicated 874.3
  toe(s) (nail) (subungual) 893.0
    with tendon involvement 893.2
    complicated 893.1
  tongue 873.64
    complicated 873.74
  tonsil - *see* Wound, open, neck
  trachea (cervical region) 874.02
    with larynx 874.00
      complicated 874.10
    complicated 874.12
    intrathoracic - *see* Injury, internal,
      trachea
  trunk (multiple) NEC 879.6
    complicated 879.7
    specified site NEC 879.6
      complicated 879.7
  tunica vaginalis 878.2
    complicated 878.3
  tympanic membrane 872.61
    complicated 872.71
  tympanum 872.61
    complicated 872.71
  umbilical region 879.2
    complicated 879.3
  ureter - *see* Injury, internal, ureter
  urethra - *see* Injury, internal, urethra
  uterus - *see* Injury, internal, uterus
  uvula 873.69
    complicated 873.79
  vagina 878.6
    complicated 878.7
  vas deferens - *see* Injury, internal, vas
      deferens
  vitreous (humor) 871.2
  vulva 878.4
    complicated 878.5
  wrist 881.02
    with tendon involvement 881.22
    complicated 881.12
Wright's syndrome (hyperabduction)
    447.8
  pneumonia 390 [517.1]
Wringer injury - *see* Crush injury, by site
Wrinkling of skin 701.8
Wrist - *see also* condition
  drop (acquired) 736.05
Wrong drug (given in error) NEC 977.9
  specified drug or substance - *see* Table of
      Drugs and Chemicals
Wry neck - *see also* Torticollis
  congenital 754.1
Wuchereria infestation 125.0
  bancrofti 125.0
  Brugia malayi 125.1
  malayi 125.1
Wuchereriasis 125.0
Wuchererioisis 125.0
Wuchernde struma langhans (M8332/3) 193

◀ New   ◀◀ Revised   ~~deleted~~ Deleted   ● Use Additional Digit(s)   ▨ Omit code

X

Xanthelasma 272.2
  eyelid 272.2 *[374.51]*
  palpebrarum 272.2 *[374.51]*
Xanthelasmatosis (essential) 272.2
Xanthelasmoidea 757.33
Xanthine stones 277.2
Xanthinuria 277.2
Xanthofibroma (M8831/0) - *see* Neoplasm,
  connective tissue, benign
Xanthoma(s), xanthomatosis 272.2
  with
    hyperlipoproteinemia
      type I 272.3
      type III 272.2
      type IV 272.1
      type V 272.3
  bone 272.7
  craniohypophyseal 277.89
  cutaneotendinous 272.7
  diabeticorum 250.8● *[272.2]*
    due to secondary diabetes
      249.8● *[272.2]*
  disseminatum 272.7
  eruptive 272.2
  eyelid 272.2 *[374.51]*
  familial 272.7
  hereditary 272.7
  hypercholesterinemic 272.0

Xanthoma(s) *(Continued)*
  hypercholesterolemic 272.0
  hyperlipemic 272.4
  hyperlipidemic 272.4
  infantile 272.7
  joint 272.7
  juvenile 272.7
  multiple 272.7
  multiplex 272.7
  primary familial 272.7
  tendon (sheath) 272.7
  tuberosum 272.2
  tuberous 272.2
  tubo-eruptive 272.2
Xanthosis 709.09
  surgical 998.81
Xenophobia 300.29
Xeroderma (congenital) 757.39
  acquired 701.1
    eyelid 373.33
  eyelid 373.33
  pigmentosum 757.33
  vitamin A deficiency 264.8
Xerophthalmia 372.53
  vitamin A deficiency 264.7
Xerosis
  conjunctiva 372.53
    with Bitôt's spot 372.53
      vitamin A deficiency 264.1
    vitamin A deficiency 264.0

Xerosis *(Continued)*
  cornea 371.40
    with corneal ulceration
      370.00
      vitamin A deficiency
        264.3
    vitamin A deficiency
      264.2
  cutis 706.8
  skin 706.8
Xerostomia 527.7
Xiphodynia 733.90
Xiphoidalgia 733.90
Xiphoiditis 733.99
Xiphopagus 759.4
XO syndrome 758.6
X-ray
  effects, adverse, NEC 990
  of chest
    for suspected tuberculosis
      V71.2
    routine V72.5
XXX syndrome 758.81
XXXXY syndrome 758.81
XXY syndrome 758.7
Xyloketosuria 271.8
Xylosuria 271.8
Xylulosuria 271.8
XYY syndrome 758.81

Y

Yaba monkey tumor virus 059.22
Yawning 786.09
   psychogenic 306.1
Yaws 102.9
   bone or joint lesions 102.6
   butter 102.1
   chancre 102.0
   cutaneous, less than five years after
      infection 102.2
   early (cutaneous) (macular)
      (maculopapular) (micropapular)
      (papular) 102.2
     frambeside 102.2
     skin lesions NEC 102.2
   eyelid 102.9 [373.4]
   ganglion 102.6
   gangosis, gangosa 102.5
   gumma, gummata 102.4
     bone 102.6

Yaws (Continued)
   gummatous
     frambeside 102.4
     osteitis 102.6
     periostitis 102.6
   hydrarthrosis 102.6
   hyperkeratosis (early) (late) (palmar)
     (plantar) 102.3
   initial lesions 102.0
   joint lesions 102.6
   juxta-articular nodules 102.7
   late nodular (ulcerated) 102.4
   latent (without clinical
     manifestations) (with
     positive serology) 102.8
   mother 102.0
   mucosal 102.7
   multiple papillomata 102.1
   nodular, late (ulcerated) 102.4
   osteitis 102.6

Yaws (Continued)
   papilloma, papillomata (palmar) (plantar)
     102.1
   periostitis (hypertrophic) 102.6
   ulcers 102.4
   wet crab 102.1
Yeast infection (see also Candidiasis)
   112.9
Yellow
   atrophy (liver) 570
     chronic 571.8
     resulting from administration of blood,
       plasma, serum, or other biological
       substance (within 8 months of
       administration) - see Hepatitis,
       viral
   fever - see Fever, yellow
   jack (see also Fever, yellow) 060.9
   jaundice (see also Jaundice) 782.4
Yersinia septica 027.8

◀ New   ◀ Revised   deleted Deleted   ● Use Additional Digit(s)   ▨ Omit code

Z

Zagari's disease (xerostomia) 527.7
Zahorsky's disease (exanthema subitum)
    (*see also* Exanthem subitum)
    058.10
  syndrome (herpangina) 074.0
Zellweger syndrome 277.86
Zenker's diverticulum (esophagus) 530.6
Ziehen-Oppenheim disease 333.6

Zieve's syndrome (jaundice,
    hyperlipemia, and hemolytic
    anemia) 571.1
Zika fever 066.3
Zollinger-Ellison syndrome (gastric
    hypersecretion with pancreatic islet cell
    tumor) 251.5
Zona (*see also* Herpes, zoster) 053.9
Zoophilia (erotica) 302.1
Zoophobia 300.29

Zoster (herpes) (*see also* Herpes, zoster)
    053.9
Zuelzer (-Ogden) anemia or syndrome
    (nutritional megaloblastic anemia)
    281.2
Zygodactyly (*see also* Syndactylism)
    755.10
Zygomycosis 117.7
Zymotic - *see* condition

SECTION II TABLE OF DRUGS AND CHEMICALS

ALPHABETIC INDEX TO POISONING AND EXTERNAL CAUSES OF ADVERSE EFFECTS OF DRUGS AND OTHER CHEMICAL SUBSTANCES

This table contains a classification of drugs and other chemical substances to identify poisoning states and external causes of adverse effects.

Each of the listed substances in the table is assigned a code according to the poisoning classification (960–989). These codes are used when there is a statement of poisoning, overdose, wrong substance given or taken, or intoxication.

The table also contains a listing of external causes of adverse effects. An adverse effect is a pathologic manifestation due to ingestion or exposure to drugs or other chemical substances (e.g., dermatitis, hypersensitivity reaction, aspirin gastritis). The adverse effect is to be identified by the appropriate code found in Section I, Index to Diseases and Injuries. An external cause code can then be used to identify the circumstances involved. The table headings pertaining to external causes are defined below:

Accidental poisoning (E850–E869)-accidental overdose of drug, wrong substance given or taken, drug taken inadvertently, accidents in the usage of drugs and biologicals in medical and surgical procedures, and to show external causes of poisonings classifiable to 980–989.

Therapeutic use (E930–E949)-a correct substance properly administered in therapeutic or prophylactic dosage as the external cause of adverse effects.

Suicide attempt (E950–E952)-instances in which self-inflicted injuries or poisonings are involved.

Assault (E961–E962)-injury or poisoning inflicted by another person with the intent to injure or kill.

Undetermined (E980–E982)-to be used when the intent of the poisoning or injury cannot be determined whether it was intentional or accidental.

The American Hospital Formulary Service (AHFS) list numbers are included in the table to help classify new drugs not identified in the table by name. The AHFS list numbers are keyed to the continually revised AHFS (American Hospital Formulary Service, 2 vol. Washington, D.C.: American Society of Hospital Pharmacists, 1959-). These listings are found in the table under the main term **Drug.**

Excluded from the table are radium and other radioactive substances. The classification of adverse effects and complications pertaining to these substances will be found in Index to Diseases and Injuries, and Index to External Causes of Injuries.

Although certain substances are indexed with one or more subentries, the majority are listed according to one use or state. It is recognized that many substances may be used in various ways, in medicine and in industry, and may cause adverse effects whatever the state of the agent (solid, liquid, or fumes arising from a liquid). In cases in which the reported data indicate a use or state not in the table, or which is clearly different from the one listed, an attempt should be made to classify the substance in the form which most nearly expresses the reported facts.

Substance	Poisoning	External Cause (E Code)				
		Accident	Therapeutic Use	Suicide Attempt	Assault	Undetermined
1-propanol	980.3	E860.4	—	E950.9	E962.1	E980.9
2-propanol	980.2	E860.3	—	E950.9	E962.1	E980.9
2,4-D (dichlorophenoxyacetic acid)	989.4	E863.5	—	E950.6	E962.1	E980.7
2,4-toluene diisocyanate	983.0	E864.0	—	E950.7	E962.1	E980.6
2,4,5-T (trichlorophenoxyacetic acid)	989.2	E863.5	—	E950.6	E962.1	E980.7
14-hydroxydihydromorphinone	965.09	E850.2	E935.2	E950.0	E962.0	E980.0
ABOB	961.7	E857	E931.7	E950.4	E962.0	E980.4
Abrus (seed)	988.2	E865.3	—	E950.9	E962.1	E980.9
Absinthe	980.0	E860.1	—	E950.9	E962.1	E980.9
beverage	980.0	E860.0	—	E950.9	E962.1	E980.9
Acenocoumarin, acenocoumarol	964.2	E858.2	E934.2	E950.4	E962.0	E980.4
Acepromazine	969.1	E853.0	E939.1	E950.3	E962.0	E980.3
Acetal	982.8	E862.4	—	E950.9	E962.1	E980.9
Acetaldehyde (vapor)	987.8	E869.8	—	E952.8	E962.2	E982.8
liquid	989.89	E866.8	—	E950.9	E962.1	E980.9
Acetaminophen	965.4	E850.4	E935.4	E950.0	E962.0	E980.0
Acetaminosalol	965.1	E850.3	E935.3	E950.0	E962.0	E980.0
Acetanilid(e)	965.4	E850.4	E935.4	E950.0	E962.0	E980.0
Acetarsol, acetarsone	961.1	E857	E931.1	E950.4	E962.0	E980.4
Acetazolamide	974.2	E858.5	E944.2	E950.4	E962.0	E980.4
Acetic	—	—	—	—	—	—
acid	983.1	E864.1	—	E950.7	E962.1	E980.6
with sodium acetate (ointment)	976.3	E858.7	E946.3	E950.4	E962.0	E980.4
irrigating solution	974.5	E858.5	E944.5	E950.4	E962.0	E980.4
lotion	976.2	E858.7	E946.2	E950.4	E962.0	E980.4
anhydride	983.1	E864.1	—	E950.7	E962.1	E980.6
ether (vapor)	982.8	E862.4	—	E950.9	E962.1	E980.9
Acetohexamide	962.3	E858.0	E932.3	E950.4	E962.0	E980.4
Acetomenaphthone	964.3	E858.2	E934.3	E950.4	E962.0	E980.4
Acetomorphine	965.01	E850.0	E935.0	E950.0	E962.0	E980.0
Acetone (oils) (vapor)	982.8	E862.4	—	E950.9	E962.1	E980.9
Acetophenazine (maleate)	969.1	E853.0	E939.1	E950.3	E962.0	E980.3
Acetophenetidin	965.4	E850.4	E935.4	E950.0	E962.0	E980.0
Acetophenone	982.0	E862.4	—	E950.9	E962.1	E980.9
Acetorphine	965.09	E850.2	E935.2	E950.0	E962.0	E980.0
Acetosulfone (sodium)	961.8	E857	E931.8	E950.4	E962.0	E980.4
Acetrizoate (sodium)	977.8	E858.8	E947.8	E950.4	E962.0	E980.4
Acetylcarbromal	967.3	E852.2	E937.3	E950.2	E962.0	E980.2

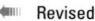

TABLE OF DRUGS AND CHEMICALS

Substance	Poisoning	External Cause (E Code)				
		Accident	Therapeutic Use	Suicide Attempt	Assault	Undetermined
Acetylcholine (chloride)	971.0	E855.3	E941.0	E950.4	E962.0	E980.4
Acetylcysteine	975.5	E858.6	E945.5	E950.4	E962.0	E980.4
Acetyldigitoxin	972.1	E858.3	E942.1	E950.4	E962.0	E980.4
Acetyldihydrocodeine	965.09	E850.2	E935.2	E950.0	E962.0	E980.0
Acetyldihydrocodeinone	965.09	E850.2	E935.2	E950.0	E962.0	E980.0
Acetylene (gas) (industrial)	987.1	E868.1	—	E951.8	E962.2	E981.8
incomplete combustion of - *see* Carbon monoxide, fuel, utility	—	—	—	—	—	—
tetrachloride (vapor)	982.3	E862.4	—	E950.9	E962.1	E980.9
Acetyliodosalicylic acid	965.1	E850.3	E935.3	E950.0	E962.0	E980.0
Acetylphenylhydrazine	965.8	E850.8	E935.8	E950.0	E962.0	E980.0
Acetylsalicylic acid	965.1	E850.3	E935.3	E950.0	E962.0	E980.0
Achromycin	960.4	E856	E930.4	E950.4	E962.0	E980.4
ophthalmic preparation	976.5	E858.7	E946.5	E950.4	E962.0	E980.4
topical NEC	976.0	E858.7	E946.0	E950.4	E962.0	E980.4
Acidifying agents	963.2	E858.1	E933.2	E950.4	E962.0	E980.4
Acids (corrosive) NEC	983.1	E864.1	—	E950.7	E962.1	E980.6
Aconite (wild)	988.2	E865.4	—	E950.9	E962.1	E980.9
Aconitine (liniment)	976.8	E858.7	E946.8	E950.4	E962.0	E980.4
Aconitum ferox	988.2	E865.4	—	E950.9	E962.1	E980.9
Acridine	983.0	E864.0	—	E950.7	E962.1	E980.6
vapor	987.8	E869.8	—	E952.8	E962.2	E982.8
Acriflavine	961.9	E857	E931.9	E950.4	E962.0	E980.4
Acrisorcin	976.0	E858.7	E946.0	E950.4	E962.0	E980.4
Acrolein (gas)	987.8	E869.8	—	E952.8	E962.2	E982.8
liquid	989.89	E866.8	—	E950.9	E962.1	E980.9
Actaea spicata	988.2	E865.4	—	E950.9	E962.1	E980.9
Acterol	961.5	E857	E931.5	E950.4	E962.0	E980.4
ACTH	962.4	E858.0	E932.4	E950.4	E962.0	E980.4
Acthar	962.4	E858.0	E932.4	E950.4	E962.0	E980.4
Actinomycin (C) (D)	960.7	E856	E930.7	E950.4	E962.0	E980.4
Adalin (acetyl)	967.3	E852.2	E937.3	E950.2	E962.0	E980.2
Adenosine (phosphate)	977.8	E858.8	E947.8	E950.4	E962.0	E980.4
Adhesives	989.89	E866.6	—	E950.9	E962.1	E980.9
ADH	962.5	E858.0	E932.5	E950.4	E962.0	E980.4
Adicillin	960.0	E856	E930.0	E950.4	E962.0	E980.4
Adiphenine	975.1	E855.6	E945.1	E950.4	E962.0	E980.4
Adjunct, pharmaceutical	977.4	E858.8	E947.4	E950.4	E962.0	E980.4

◀ New   ◀▬ Revised   ~~deleted~~ Deleted   ● Use Additional Digit(s)

Substance	Poisoning	External Cause (E Code)				
		Accident	Therapeutic Use	Suicide Attempt	Assault	Undetermined
Adrenal (extract, cortex or medulla) (glucocorticoids) (hormones) (mineralocorticoids)	962.0	E858.0	E932.0	E950.4	E962.0	E980.4
ENT agent	976.6	E858.7	E946.6	E950.4	E962.0	E980.4
ophthalmic preparation	976.5	E858.7	E946.5	E950.4	E962.0	E980.4
topical NEC	976.0	E858.7	E946.0	E950.4	E962.0	E980.4
Adrenalin	971.2	E855.5	E941.2	E950.4	E962.0	E980.4
Adrenergic blocking agents	971.3	E855.6	E941.3	E950.4	E962.0	E980.4
Adrenergics	971.2	E855.5	E941.2	E950.4	E962.0	E980.4
Adrenochrome (derivatives)	972.8	E858.3	E942.8	E950.4	E962.0	E980.4
Adrenocorticotropic hormone	962.4	E858.0	E932.4	E950.4	E962.0	E980.4
Adrenocorticotropin	962.4	E858.0	E932.4	E950.4	E962.0	E980.4
Adriamycin	960.7	E856	E930.7	E950.4	E962.0	E980.4
Aerosol spray - *see* Sprays	—	—	—	—	—	—
Aerosporin	960.8	E856	E930.8	E950.4	E962.0	E980.4
ENT agent	976.6	E858.7	E946.6	E950.4	E962.0	E980.4
ophthalmic preparation	976.5	E858.7	E946.5	E950.4	E962.0	E980.4
topical NEC	976.0	E858.7	E946.0	E950.4	E962.0	E980.4
Aethusa cynapium	988.2	E865.4	—	E950.9	E962.1	E980.9
Afghanistan black	969.6	E854.1	E939.6	E950.3	E962.0	E980.3
Aflatoxin	989.7	E865.9	—	E950.9	E962.1	E980.9
African boxwood	988.2	E865.4	—	E950.9	E962.1	E980.9
Agar (-agar)	973.3	E858.4	E943.3	E950.4	E962.0	E980.4
Agricultural agent NEC	989.89	E863.9	—	E950.6	E962.1	E980.7
Agrypnal	967.0	E851	E937.0	E950.1	E962.0	E980.1
Air contaminant(s), source or type not specified	—	—	—	—	—	—
specified type - *see* specific substance	987.9	E869.9	—	E952.9	E962.2	E982.9
Akee	988.2	E865.4	—	E950.9	E962.1	E980.9
Akrinol	976.0	E858.7	E946.0	E950.4	E962.0	E980.4
Alantolactone	961.6	E857	E931.6	E950.4	E962.0	E980.4
Albamycin	960.8	E856	E930.8	E950.4	E962.0	E980.4
Albumin (normal human serum)	964.7	E858.2	E934.7	E950.4	E962.0	E980.4
Albuterol	975.7	E858.6	E945.7	E950.4	E962.0	E980.4
Alcohol	980.9	E860.9	—	E950.9	E962.1	E980.9
absolute	980.0	E860.1	—	E950.9	E962.1	E980.9
beverage	980.0	E860.0	E947.8	E950.9	E962.1	E980.9
amyl	980.3	E860.4	—	E950.9	E962.1	E980.9
antifreeze	980.1	E860.2	—	E950.9	E962.1	E980.9
butyl	980.3	E860.4	—	E950.9	E962.1	E980.9

TABLE OF DRUGS AND CHEMICALS

Substance	Poisoning	External Cause (E Code)				
		Accident	Therapeutic Use	Suicide Attempt	Assault	Undetermined
Alcohol *(Continued)*						
dehydrated	980.0	E860.1	—	E950.9	E862.1	E980.9
beverage	980.0	E860.0	E947.8	E950.9	E962.1	E980.9
denatured	980.0	E860.1	—	E950.9	E962.1	E980.9
deterrents	977.3	E858.8	E947.3	E950.4	E962.0	E980.4
diagnostic (gastric function)	977.8	E858.8	E947.8	E950.4	E962.0	E980.4
ethyl	980.0	E860.1	—	E950.9	E962.1	E980.9
beverage	980.0	E860.0	E947.8	E950.9	E962.1	E980.9
grain	980.0	E860.1	—	E950.9	E962.1	E980.9
beverage	980.0	E860.0	E947.8	E950.9	E962.1	E980.9
industrial	980.9	E860.9	—	E950.9	E962.1	E980.9
isopropyl	980.2	E860.3	—	E950.9	E962.1	E980.9
methyl	980.1	E860.2	—	E950.9	E962.1	E980.9
preparation for consumption	980.0	E860.0	E947.8	E950.9	E962.1	E980.9
propyl	980.3	E860.4	—	E950.9	E962.1	E980.9
secondary	980.2	E860.3	—	E950.9	E962.1	E980.9
radiator	980.1	E860.2	—	E950.9	E962.1	E980.9
rubbing	980.2	E860.3	—	E950.9	E962.1	E980.9
specified type NEC	980.8	E860.8	—	E950.9	E962.1	E980.9
surgical	980.9	E860.9	—	E950.9	E962.1	E980.9
vapor (from any type of alcohol)	987.8	E869.8	—	E952.8	E962.2	E982.8
wood	980.1	E860.2	—	E950.9	E962.1	E980.9
Alcuronium chloride	975.2	E858.6	E945.2	E950.4	E962.0	E980.4
Aldactone	974.4	E858.5	E944.4	E950.4	E962.0	E980.4
Aldicarb	989.3	E863.2	—	E950.6	E962.1	E980.7
Aldomet	972.6	E858.3	E942.6	E950.4	E962.0	E980.4
Aldosterone	962.0	E858.0	E932.0	E950.4	E962.0	E980.4
Aldrin (dust)	989.2	E863.0	—	E950.6	E962.1	E980.7
Aleve - *see* Naproxen	—	—	—	—	—	—
Algeldrate	973.0	E858.4	E943.0	E950.4	E962.0	E980.4
Alidase	963.4	E858.1	E933.4	E950.4	E962.0	E980.4
Aliphatic thiocyanates	989.0	E866.8	—	E950.9	E962.1	E980.9
Alkaline antiseptic solution (aromatic)	976.6	E858.7	E946.6	E950.4	E962.0	E980.4
Alkalinizing agents (medicinal)	963.3	E858.1	E933.3	E950.4	E962.0	E980.4
Alkalis, caustic	983.2	E864.2	—	E950.7	E962.1	E980.6
Alkalizing agents (medicinal)	963.3	E858.1	E933.3	E950.4	E962.0	E980.4
Alka-seltzer	965.1	E850.3	E935.3	E950.0	E962.0	E980.0
Alkavervir	972.6	E858.3	E942.6	E950.4	E962.0	E980.4

◄ New ◄ Revised ~~deleted~~ Deleted ● Use Additional Digit(s)

Substance	Poisoning	External Cause (E Code)				
		Accident	Therapeutic Use	Suicide Attempt	Assault	Undetermined
Allegron	969.05	E854.0	E939.0	E950.3	E962.0	E980.3
Allobarbital, allobarbitone	967.0	E851	E937.0	E950.1	E962.0	E980.1
Allopurinol	974.7	E858.5	E944.7	E950.4	E962.0	E980.4
Allylestrenol	962.2	E858.0	E932.2	E950.4	E962.0	E980.4
Allylisopropylacetylurea	967.8	E852.8	E937.8	E950.2	E962.0	E980.2
Allylisopropylmalonylurea	967.0	E851	E937.0	E950.1	E962.0	E980.1
Allyltribromide	967.3	E852.2	E937.3	E950.2	E962.0	E980.2
Aloe, aloes, aloin	973.1	E858.4	E943.1	E950.4	E962.0	E980.4
Alosetron	973.8	E858.4	E943.8	E950.4	E962.0	E980.4
Aloxidone	966.0	E855.0	E936.0	E950.4	E962.0	E980.4
Aloxiprin	965.1	E850.3	E935.3	E950.0	E962.0	E980.0
Alpha amylase	963.4	E858.1	E933.4	E950.4	E962.0	E980.4
Alpha-1 blockers	971.3	E855.6	E941.3	E950.4	E962.0	E980.4
Alphaprodine (hydrochloride)	965.09	E850.2	E935.2	E950.0	E962.0	E980.0
Alpha tocopherol	963.5	E858.1	E933.5	E950.4	E962.0	E980.4
Alseroxylon	972.6	E858.3	E942.6	E950.4	E962.0	E980.4
Alum (ammonium) (potassium)	983.2	E864.2	—	E950.7	E962.1	E980.6
medicinal (astringent) NEC	976.2	E858.7	E946.2	E950.4	E962.0	E980.4
Aluminium, aluminum (gel) (hydroxide)	973.0	E858.4	E943.0	E950.4	E962.0	E980.4
acetate solution	976.2	E858.7	E946.2	E950.4	E962.0	E980.4
aspirin	965.1	E850.3	E935.3	E950.0	E962.0	E980.0
carbonate	973.0	E858.4	E943.0	E950.4	E962.0	E980.4
glycinate	973.0	E858.4	E943.0	E950.4	E962.0	E980.4
nicotinate	972.2	E858.3	E942.2	E950.4	E962.0	E980.4
ointment (surgical) (topical)	976.3	E858.7	E946.3	E950.4	E962.0	E980.4
phosphate	973.0	E858.4	E943.0	E950.4	E962.0	E980.4
subacetate	976.2	E858.7	E946.2	E950.4	E962.0	E980.4
topical NEC	976.3	E858.7	E946.3	E950.4	E962.0	E980.4
Alurate	967.0	E851	E937.0	E950.1	E962.0	E980.1
Alverine (citrate)	975.1	E858.6	E945.1	E950.4	E962.0	E980.4
Alvodine	965.09	E850.2	E935.2	E950.0	E962.0	E980.0
Amanita phalloides	988.1	E865.5	—	E950.9	E962.1	E980.9
Amantadine (hydrochloride)	966.4	E855.0	E936.4	E950.4	E962.0	E980.4
Ambazone	961.9	E857	E931.9	E950.4	E962.0	E980.4
Ambenonium	971.0	E855.3	E941.0	E950.4	E962.0	E980.4
Ambutonium bromide	971.1	E855.4	E941.1	E950.4	E962.0	E980.4
Ametazole	977.8	E858.8	E947.8	E950.4	E962.0	E980.4
Amethocaine (infiltration) (topical)	968.5	E855.2	E938.5	E950.4	E962.0	E980.4
nerve block (peripheral) (plexus)	968.6	E855.2	E938.6	E950.4	E962.0	E980.4
spinal	968.7	E855.2	E938.7	E950.4	E962.0	E980.4

TABLE OF DRUGS AND CHEMICALS

Substance	Poisoning	External Cause (E Code)				
		Accident	Therapeutic Use	Suicide Attempt	Assault	Undetermined
Amethopterin	963.1	E858.1	E933.1	E950.4	E962.0	E980.4
Amfepramone	977.0	E858.8	E947.0	E950.4	E962.0	E980.4
Amidone	965.02	E850.1	E935.1	E950.0	E962.0	E980.0
Amidopyrine	965.5	E850.5	E935.5	E950.0	E962.0	E980.0
Aminacrine	976.0	E858.7	E946.0	E950.4	E962.0	E980.4
Aminitrozole	961.5	E857	E931.5	E950.4	E962.0	E980.4
Aminoacetic acid	974.5	E858.5	E944.5	E950.4	E962.0	E980.4
Amino acids	974.5	E858.5	E944.5	E950.4	E962.0	E980.4
Aminocaproic acid	964.4	E858.2	E934.4	E950.4	E962.0	E980.4
Aminoethylisothiourium	963.8	E858.1	E933.8	E950.4	E962.0	E980.4
Aminoglutethimide	966.3	E855.0	E936.3	E950.4	E962.0	E980.4
Aminometradine	974.3	E858.5	E944.3	E950.4	E962.0	E980.4
Aminopentamide	971.1	E855.4	E941.1	E950.4	E962.0	E980.4
Aminophenazone	965.5	E850.5	E935.5	E950.0	E962.0	E980.0
Aminophenol	983.0	E864.0	—	E950.7	E962.1	E980.6
Aminophenylpyridone	969.5	E853.8	E939.5	E950.3	E962.0	E980.3
Aminophylline	975.7	E858.6	E945.7	E950.4	E962.0	E980.4
Aminopterin	963.1	E858.1	E933.1	E950.4	E962.0	E980.4
Aminopyrine	965.5	E850.5	E935.5	E950.0	E962.0	E980.0
Aminosalicylic acid	961.8	E857	E931.8	E950.4	E962.0	E980.4
Amiphenazole	970.1	E854.3	E940.1	E950.4	E962.0	E980.4
Amiquinsin	972.6	E858.3	E942.6	E950.4	E962.0	E980.4
Amisometradine	974.3	E858.5	E944.3	E950.4	E962.0	E980.4
Amitriptyline	969.05	E854.0	E939.0	E950.3	E962.0	E980.3
Ammonia (fumes) (gas) (vapor)	987.8	E869.8	—	E952.8	E962.2	E982.8
liquid (household) NEC	983.2	E861.4	—	E950.7	E962.1	E980.6
spirit, aromatic	970.89	E854.3	E940.8	E950.4	E962.0	E980.4
Ammoniated mercury	976.0	E858.7	E946.0	E950.4	E962.0	E980.4
Ammonium	—	—	—	—	—	—
carbonate	983.2	E864.2	—	E950.7	E962.1	E980.6
chloride (acidifying agent)	963.2	E858.1	E933.2	E950.4	E962.0	E980.4
expectorant	975.5	E858.6	E945.5	E950.4	E962.0	E980.4
compounds (household) NEC	983.2	E861.4	—	E950.7	E962.1	E980.6
fumes (any usage)	987.8	E869.8	—	E952.8	E962.2	E982.8
industrial	983.2	E864.2	—	E950.7	E962.1	E980.6
ichthosulfonate	976.4	E858.7	E946.4	E950.4	E962.0	E980.4
mandelate	961.9	E857	E931.9	E950.4	E962.0	E980.4
Amobarbital	967.0	E851	E937.0	E950.1	E962.0	E980.1
Amodiaquin(e)	961.4	E857	E931.4	E950.4	E962.0	E980.4
Amopyroquin(e)	961.4	E857	E931.4	E950.4	E962.0	E980.4

◀ New   ◀▥ Revised   ~~deleted~~ Deleted   ● Use Additional Digit(s)

Substance	External Cause (E Code)					
	Poisoning	Accident	Therapeutic Use	Suicide Attempt	Assault	Undetermined
Amphenidone	969.5	E853.8	E939.5	E950.3	E962.0	E980.3
Amphetamine	969.72	E854.2	E939.7	E950.3	E962.0	E980.3
Amphomycin	960.8	E856	E930.8	E950.4	E962.0	E980.4
Amphotericin B	960.1	E856	E930.1	E950.4	E962.0	E980.4
topical	976.0	E858.7	E946.0	E950.4	E962.0	E980.4
Ampicillin	960.0	E856	E930.0	E950.4	E962.0	E980.4
Amprotropine	971.1	E855.4	E941.1	E950.4	E962.0	E980.4
Amygdalin	977.8	E858.8	E947.8	E950.4	E962.0	E980.4
Amyl	—	—	—	—	—	—
acetate (vapor)	982.8	E862.4	—	E950.9	E962.1	E980.9
alcohol	980.3	E860.4	—	E950.9	E962.1	E980.9
nitrite (medicinal)	972.4	E858.3	E942.4	E950.4	E962.0	E980.4
Amylase (alpha)	963.4	E858.1	E933.4	E950.4	E962.0	E980.4
Amylene hydrate	980.8	E860.8	—	E950.9	E962.1	E980.9
Amylobarbitone	967.0	E851	E937.0	E950.1	E962.0	E980.1
Amylocaine	968.9	E855.2	E938.9	E950.4	E962.0	E980.4
infiltration (subcutaneous)	968.5	E855.2	E938.5	E950.4	E962.0	E980.4
nerve block (peripheral) (plexus)	968.6	E855.2	E938.6	E950.4	E962.0	E980.4
spinal	968.7	E855.2	E938.7	E950.4	E962.0	E980.4
topical (surface)	968.5	E855.2	E938.5	E950.4	E962.0	E980.4
Amytal (sodium)	967.0	E851	E937.0	E950.1	E962.0	E980.1
Analeptics	970.0	E854.3	E940.0	E950.4	E962.0	E980.4
Analgesics	965.9	E850.9	E935.9	E950.0	E962.0	E980.0
aromatic NEC	965.4	E850.4	E935.4	E950.0	E962.0	E980.0
non-narcotic NEC	965.7	E850.7	E935.7	E950.0	E962.0	E980.0
specified NEC	965.8	E850.8	E935.8	E950.0	E962.0	E980.0
Anamirta cocculus	988.2	E865.3	—	E950.9	E962.1	E980.9
Ancillin	960.0	E856	E930.0	E950.4	E962.0	E980.4
Androgens (anabolic congeners)	962.1	E858.0	E932.1	E950.4	E962.0	E980.4
Androstalone	962.1	E858.0	E932.1	E950.4	E962.0	E980.4
Androsterone	962.1	E858.0	E932.1	E950.4	E962.0	E980.4
Anemone pulsatilia	988.2	E865.4	—	E950.9	E962.1	E980.9
Anesthesia, anesthetic (general) NEC	968.4	E855.1	E938.4	E950.4	E962.0	E980.4
block (nerve) (plexus)	968.6	E855.2	E938.6	E950.4	E962.0	E980.4
gaseous NEC	968.2	E855.1	E938.2	E950.4	E962.0	E980.4
halogenated hydrocarbon derivatives NEC	968.2	E855.1	E938.2	E950.4	E962.0	E980.4
infiltration (intradermal) (subcutaneous) (submucosal)	968.5	E855.2	E938.5	E950.4	E962.0	E980.4
intravenous	968.3	E855.1	E938.3	E950.4	E962.0	E980.4
local NEC	968.9	E855.2	E938.9	E950.4	E962.0	E980.4

TABLE OF DRUGS AND CHEMICALS

TABLE OF DRUGS AND CHEMICALS

Substance	Poisoning	External Cause (E Code)				
		Accident	Therapeutic Use	Suicide Attempt	Assault	Undetermined
Anesthesia, anesthetic NEC *(Continued)*						
nerve blocking (peripheral) (plexus)	968.6	E855.2	E938.6	E950.4	E962.0	E980.4
rectal NEC	968.3	E855.1	E938.3	E950.4	E962.0	E980.4
spinal	968.7	E855.2	E938.7	E950.4	E962.0	E980.4
surface	968.5	E855.2	E938.5	E950.4	E962.0	E980.4
topical	968.5	E855.2	E938.5	E950.4	E962.0	E980.4
Aneurine	963.5	E858.1	E933.5	E950.4	E962.0	E980.4
Anginine - *see* Glyceryl trinitrate	971.2	E855.5	E941.2	E950.4	E962.0	E980.4
Angio-Conray	977.8	E858.8	E947.8	E950.4	E962.0	E980.4
Angiotensin	971.2	E855.5	E941.2	E950.4	E962.0	E980.4
Anhydrohydroxyprogesterone	962.2	E858.0	E932.2	E950.4	E962.0	E980.4
Anhydron	974.3	E858.5	E944.3	E950.4	E962.0	E980.4
Anileridine	965.09	E850.2	E935.2	E950.0	E962.0	E980.0
Aniline (dye) (liquid)	983.0	E864.0	—	E950.7	E962.1	E980.6
analgesic	965.4	E850.4	E935.4	E950.0	E962.0	E980.0
derivatives, therapeutic NEC	965.4	E850.4	E935.4	E950.0	E962.0	E980.0
vapor	987.8	E869.8	—	E952.8	E962.2	E982.8
Aniscoropine	971.1	E855.4	E941.1	E950.4	E962.0	E980.4
Anisindione	964.2	E858.2	E934.2	E950.4	E962.0	E980.4
Anorexic agents	977.0	E858.8	E947.0	E950.4	E962.0	E980.4
Ant (bite) (sting)	989.5	E905.5	—	E950.9	E962.1	E980.9
Antabuse	977.3	E858.8	E947.3	E950.4	E962.0	E980.4
Antacids	973.0	E858.4	E943.0	E950.4	E962.0	E980.4
Antazoline	963.0	E858.1	E933.0	E950.4	E962.0	E980.4
Anthelmintics	961.6	E857	E931.6	E950.4	E962.0	E980.4
Anthralin	976.4	E858.7	E946.4	E950.4	E962.0	E980.4
Anthramycin	960.7	E856	E930.7	E950.4	E962.0	E980.4
Antiadrenergics	971.3	E855.6	E941.3	E950.4	E962.0	E980.4
Antiallergic agents	963.0	E858.1	E933.0	E950.4	E962.0	E980.4
Antianemic agents NEC	964.1	E858.2	E934.1	E950.4	E962.0	E980.4
Antiaris toxicaria	988.2	E865.4	—	E950.9	E962.1	E980.9
Antiarteriosclerotic agents	972.2	E858.3	E942.2	E950.4	E962.0	E980.4
Antiasthmatics	975.7	E858.6	E945.7	E950.4	E962.0	E980.4
Antibiotics	960.9	E856	E930.9	E950.4	E962.0	E980.4
antifungal	960.1	E856	E930.1	E950.4	E962.0	E980.4
antimycobacterial	960.6	E856	E930.6	E950.4	E962.0	E980.4
antineoplastic	960.7	E856	E930.7	E950.4	E962.0	E980.4
cephalosporin (group)	960.5	E856	E930.5	E950.4	E962.0	E980.4
chloramphenicol (group)	960.2	E856	E930.2	E950.4	E962.0	E980.4
macrolides	960.3	E856	E930.3	E950.4	E962.0	E980.4

◄ New ◄ⅢⅢ Revised ~~deleted~~ Deleted ● Use Additional Digit(s)

Substance	Poisoning	External Cause (E Code)				
		Accident	Therapeutic Use	Suicide Attempt	Assault	Undetermined
Antibiotics *(Continued)*						
specified NEC	960.8	E856	E930.8	E950.4	E962.0	E980.4
tetracycline (group)	960.4	E856	E930.4	E950.4	E962.0	E980.4
Anticancer agents NEC	963.1	E858.1	E933.1	E950.4	E962.0	E980.4
antibiotics	960.7	E856	E930.7	E950.4	E962.0	E980.4
Anticholinergics	971.1	E855.4	E941.1	E950.4	E962.0	E980.4
Anticholinesterase (organophosphorus) (reversible)	971.0	E855.3	E941.0	E950.4	E962.0	E980.4
Anticoagulants	964.2	E858.2	E934.2	E950.4	E962.0	E980.4
antagonists	964.5	E858.2	E934.5	E950.4	E962.0	E980.4
Anti-common cold agents NEC	975.6	E858.6	E945.6	E950.4	E962.0	E980.4
Anticonvulsants NEC	966.3	E855.0	E936.3	E950.4	E962.0	E980.4
Antidepressants	969.00	E854.0	E939.0	E950.3	E962.0	E980.3
monoamine oxidase inhibitors (MAOI)	969.01	E854.0	E939.0	E950.3	E962.0	E980.3
specified type NEC	969.09	E854.0	E939.0	E950.3	E962.0	E980.3
SSNRI (selective serotonin and norepinephrine reuptake inhibitors)	969.02	E854.0	E939.0	E950.3	E962.0	E980.3
SSRI (selective serotonin reuptake inhibitors)	969.03	E854.0	E939.0	E950.3	E962.0	E980.3
tetracyclic	969.04	E854.0	E939.0	E950.3	E962.0	E980.3
tricyclic	969.05	E854.0	E939.0	E950.3	E962.0	E980.3
Antidiabetic agents	962.3	E858.0	E932.3	E950.4	E962.0	E980.4
Antidiarrheal agents	973.5	E858.4	E943.5	E950.4	E962.0	E980.4
Antidiuretic hormone	962.5	E858.0	E932.5	E950.4	E962.0	E980.4
Antidotes NEC	977.2	E858.8	E947.2	E950.4	E962.0	E980.4
Antiemetic agents	963.0	E858.1	E933.0	E950.4	E962.0	E980.4
Antiepilepsy agent NEC	966.3	E855.0	E936.3	E950.4	E962.0	E980.4
Antifertility pills	962.2	E858.0	E932.2	E950.4	E962.0	E980.4
Antiflatulents	973.8	E858.4	E943.8	E950.4	E962.0	E980.4
Antifreeze	989.89	E866.8	—	E950.9	E962.1	E980.9
alcohol	980.1	E860.2	—	E950.9	E962.1	E980.9
ethylene glycol	982.8	E862.4	—	E950.9	E962.1	E980.9
Antifungals (nonmedicinal) (sprays)	989.4	E863.6	—	E950.6	E962.1	E980.7
medicinal NEC	961.9	E857	E931.9	E950.4	E962.0	E980.4
antibiotic	960.1	E856	E930.1	E950.4	E962.0	E980.4
topical	976.0	E858.7	E946.0	E950.4	E962.0	E980.4
Antigastric secretion agents	973.0	E858.4	E943.0	E950.4	E962.0	E980.4
Antihelmintics	961.6	E857	E931.6	E950.4	E962.0	E980.4
Antihemophilic factor (human)	964.7	E858.2	E934.7	E950.4	E962.0	E980.4
Antihistamine	963.0	E858.1	E933.0	E950.4	E962.0	E980.4
Antihypertensive agents NEC	972.6	E858.3	E942.6	E950.4	E962.0	E980.4

Substance	Poisoning	External Cause (E Code)				
		Accident	Therapeutic Use	Suicide Attempt	Assault	Undetermined
Anti-infectives NEC	961.9	E857	E931.9	E950.4	E962.0	E980.4
antibiotics	960.9	E856	E930.9	E950.4	E962.0	E980.4
specified NEC	960.8	E856	E930.8	E950.4	E962.0	E980.4
anthelmintic	961.6	E857	E931.6	E950.4	E962.0	E980.4
antimalarial	961.4	E857	E931.4	E950.4	E962.0	E980.4
antimycobacterial NEC	961.8	E857	E931.8	E950.4	E962.0	E980.4
antibiotics	960.6	E856	E930.6	E950.4	E962.0	E980.4
antiprotozoal NEC	961.5	E857	E931.5	E950.4	E962.0	E980.4
blood	961.4	E857	E931.4	E950.4	E962.0	E980.4
antiviral	961.7	E857	E931.7	E950.4	E962.0	E980.4
arsenical	961.1	E857	E931.1	E950.4	E962.0	E980.4
ENT agents	976.6	E858.7	E946.6	E950.4	E962.0	E980.4
heavy metals NEC	961.2	E857	E931.2	E950.4	E962.0	E980.4
local	976.0	E858.7	E946.0	E950.4	E962.0	E980.4
ophthalmic preparation	976.5	E858.7	E946.5	E950.4	E962.0	E980.4
topical NEC	976.0	E858.7	E946.0	E950.4	E962.0	E980.4
Anti-inflammatory agents (topical)	976.0	E858.7	E946.0	E950.4	E962.0	E980.4
Antiknock (tetraethyl lead)	984.1	E862.1	—	E950.9	E962.1	E980.9
Antilipemics	972.2	E858.3	E942.2	E950.4	E962.0	E980.4
Antimalarials	961.4	E857	E931.4	E950.4	E962.0	E980.4
Antimony (compounds) (vapor) NEC	985.4	E866.2	—	E950.9	E962.1	E980.9
anti-infectives	961.2	E857	E931.2	E950.4	E962.0	E980.4
pesticides (vapor)	985.4	E863.4	—	E950.6	E962.2	E980.7
potassium tartrate	961.2	E857	E931.2	E950.4	E962.0	E980.4
tartrated	961.2	E857	E931.2	E950.4	E962.0	E980.4
Antimuscarinic agents	971.1	E855.4	E941.1	E950.4	E962.0	E980.4
Antimycobacterials NEC	961.8	E857	E931.8	E950.4	E962.0	E980.4
antibiotics	960.6	E856	E930.6	E950.4	E962.0	E980.4
Antineoplastic agents	963.1	E858.1	E933.1	E950.4	E962.0	E980.4
antibiotics	960.7	E856	E930.7	E950.4	E962.0	E980.4
Anti-Parkinsonism agents	966.4	E855.0	E936.4	E950.4	E962.0	E980.4
Antiphlogistics	965.69	E850.6	E935.6	E950.0	E962.0	E980.0
Antiprotozoals NEC	961.5	E857	E931.5	E950.4	E962.0	E980.4
blood	961.4	E857	E931.4	E950.4	E962.0	E980.4
Antipruritics (local)	976.1	E858.7	E946.1	E950.4	E962.0	E980.4
Antipsychotic agents NEC	969.3	E853.8	E939.3	E950.3	E962.0	E980.3
Antipyretics	965.9	E850.9	E935.9	E950.0	E962.0	E980.0
specified NEC	965.8	E850.8	E935.8	E950.0	E962.0	E980.0
Antipyrine	965.5	E850.5	E935.5	E950.0	E962.0	E980.0
Antirabies serum (equine)	979.9	E858.8	E949.9	E950.4	E962.0	E980.4

◀ New   ◀▦ Revised   ~~deleted~~ Deleted   ● Use Additional Digit(s)

Substance	Poisoning	External Cause (E Code)				
		Accident	Therapeutic Use	Suicide Attempt	Assault	Undetermined
Antirheumatics	965.69	E850.6	E935.6	E950.0	E962.0	E980.0
Antiseborrheics	976.4	E858.7	E946.4	E950.4	E962.0	E980.4
Antiseptics (external) (medicinal)	976.0	E858.7	E946.0	E950.4	E962.0	E980.4
Antistine	963.0	E858.1	E933.0	E950.4	E962.0	E980.4
Antithyroid agents	962.8	E858.0	E932.8	E950.4	E962.0	E980.4
Antitoxin, any	979.9	E858.8	E949.9	E950.4	E962.0	E980.4
Antituberculars	961.8	E857	E931.8	E950.4	E962.0	E980.4
antibiotics	960.6	E856	E930.6	E950.4	E962.0	E980.4
Antitussives	975.4	E858.6	E945.4	E950.4	E962.0	E980.4
Antivaricose agents (sclerosing)	972.7	E858.3	E942.7	E950.4	E962.0	E980.4
Antivenin (crotaline) (spider-bite)	979.9	E858.8	E949.9	E950.4	E962.0	E980.4
Antivert	963.0	E858.1	E933.0	E950.4	E962.0	E980.4
Antivirals NEC	961.7	E857	E931.7	E950.4	E962.0	E980.4
Ant poisons - *see* Pesticides	—	—	—	—	—	—
Antrol	989.4	E863.4	—	E950.6	E962.1	E980.7
fungicide	989.4	E863.6	—	E950.6	E962.1	E980.7
Apomorphine hydrochloride (emetic)	973.6	E858.4	E943.6	E950.4	E962.0	E980.4
Appetite depressants, central	977.0	E858.8	E947.0	E950.4	E962.0	E980.4
Apresoline	972.6	E858.3	E942.6	E950.4	E962.0	E980.4
Aprobarbital, aprobarbitone	967.0	E851	E937.0	E950.1	E962.0	E980.1
Apronalide	967.8	E852.8	E937.8	E950.2	E962.0	E980.2
Aqua fortis	983.1	E864.1	—	E950.7	E962.1	E980.6
Arachis oil (topical)	976.3	E858.7	E946.3	E950.4	E962.0	E980.4
cathartic	973.2	E858.4	E943.2	E950.4	E962.0	E980.4
Aralen	961.4	E857	E931.4	E950.4	E962.0	E980.4
Arginine salts	974.5	E858.5	E944.5	E950.4	E962.0	E980.4
Argyrol	976.0	E858.7	E946.0	E950.4	E962.0	E980.4
ENT agent	976.6	E858.7	E946.6	E950.4	E962.0	E980.4
ophthalmic preparation	976.5	E858.7	E946.5	E950.4	E962.0	E980.4
Aristocort	962.0	E858.0	E932.0	E950.4	E962.0	E980.4
ENT agent	976.6	E858.7	E946.6	E950.4	E962.0	E980.4
ophthalmic preparation	976.5	E858.7	E946.5	E950.4	E962.0	E980.4
topical NEC	976.0	E858.7	E946.0	E950.4	E962.0	E980.4
Aromatics, corrosive	983.0	E864.0	—	E950.7	E962.1	E980.6
disinfectants	983.0	E861.4	—	E950.7	E962.1	E980.6
Arsenate of lead (insecticide)	985.1	E863.4	—	E950.8	E962.1	E980.8
herbicide	985.1	E863.5	—	E950.8	E962.1	E980.8
Arsenic, arsenicals (compounds) (dust) (fumes) (vapor) NEC	985.1	E866.3	—	E950.8	E962.1	E980.8
anti-infectives	961.1	E857	E931.1	E950.4	E962.0	E980.4
pesticide (dust) (fumes)	985.1	E863.4	—	E950.8	E962.1	E980.8

◀ New　◀▥ Revised　d̶e̶l̶e̶t̶e̶d̶ Deleted　● Use Additional Digit(s)

| | External Cause (E Code) | | | | | |
Substance	Poisoning	Accident	Therapeutic Use	Suicide Attempt	Assault	Undetermined
Arsine (gas)	985.1	E866.3	—	E950.8	E962.1	E980.8
Arsphenamine (silver)	961.1	E857	E931.1	E950.4	E962.0	E980.4
Arsthinol	961.1	E857	E931.1	E950.4	E962.0	E980.4
Artane	971.1	E855.4	E941.1	E950.4	E962.0	E980.4
Arthropod (venomous) NEC	989.5	E905.5	—	E950.9	E962.1	E980.9
Asbestos	989.81	E866.8	—	E950.9	E962.1	E980.9
Ascaridole	961.6	E857	E931.6	E950.4	E962.0	E980.4
Ascorbic acid	963.5	E858.1	E933.5	E950.4	E962.0	E980.4
Asiaticoside	976.0	E858.7	E946.0	E950.4	E962.0	E980.4
Aspidium (oleoresin)	961.6	E857	E931.6	E950.4	E962.0	E980.4
Aspirin	965.1	E850.3	E935.3	E950.0	E962.0	E980.0
Astringents (local)	976.2	E858.7	E946.2	E950.4	E962.0	E980.4
Atabrine	961.3	E857	E931.3	E950.4	E962.0	E980.4
Ataractics	969.5	E853.8	E939.5	E950.3	E962.0	E980.3
Atonia drug, intestinal	973.3	E858.4	E943.3	E950.4	E962.0	E980.4
Atophan	974.7	E858.5	E944.7	E950.4	E962.0	E980.4
Atropine	971.1	E855.4	E941.1	E950.4	E962.0	E980.4
Attapulgite	973.5	E858.4	E943.5	E950.4	E962.0	E980.4
Attenuvax	979.4	E858.8	E949.4	E950.4	E962.0	E980.4
Aureomycin	960.4	E856	E930.4	E950.4	E962.0	E980.4
ophthalmic preparation	976.5	E858.7	E946.5	E950.4	E962.0	E980.4
topical NEC	976.0	E858.7	E946.0	E950.4	E962.0	E980.4
Aurothioglucose	965.69	E850.6	E935.6	E950.0	E962.0	E980.0
Aurothioglycanide	965.69	E850.6	E935.6	E950.0	E962.0	E980.0
Aurothiomalate	965.69	E850.6	E935.6	E950.0	E962.0	E980.0
Automobile fuel	981	E862.1	—	E950.9	E962.1	E980.9
Autonomic nervous system agents NEC	971.9	E855.9	E941.9	E950.4	E962.0	E980.4
Avlosulfon	961.8	E857	E931.8	E950.4	E962.0	E980.4
Avomine	967.8	E852.8	E937.8	E950.2	E962.0	E980.2
Azacyclonol	969.5	E853.8	E939.5	E950.3	E962.0	E980.3
Azapetine	971.3	E855.6	E941.3	E950.4	E962.0	E980.4
Azaribine	963.1	E858.1	E933.1	E950.4	E962.0	E980.4
Azaserine	960.7	E856	E930.7	E950.4	E962.0	E980.4
Azathioprine	963.1	E858.1	E933.1	E950.4	E962.0	E980.4
Azosulfamide	961.0	E857	E931.0	E950.4	E962.0	E980.4
Azulfidine	961.0	E857	E931.0	E950.4	E962.0	E980.4
Azuresin	977.8	E858.8	E947.8	E950.4	E962.0	E980.4
Bacimycin	976.0	E858.7	E946.0	E950.4	E962.0	E980.4
ophthalmic preparation	976.5	E858.7	E946.5	E950.4	E962.0	E980.4

◀ New ◀ Revised ~~deleted~~ Deleted ● Use Additional Digit(s)

Substance	Poisoning	External Cause (E Code)				
		Accident	Therapeutic Use	Suicide Attempt	Assault	Undetermined
Bacitracin	960.8	E856	E930.8	E950.4	E962.0	E980.4
ENT agent	976.6	E858.7	E946.6	E950.4	E962.0	E980.4
ophthalmic preparation	976.5	E858.7	E946.5	E950.4	E962.0	E980.4
topical NEC	976.0	E858.7	E946.0	E950.4	E962.0	E980.4
Baking soda	963.3	E858.1	E933.3	E950.4	E962.0	E980.4
BAL	963.8	E858.1	E933.8	E950.4	E962.0	E980.4
Bamethan (sulfate)	972.5	E858.3	E942.5	E950.4	E962.0	E980.4
Bamipine	963.0	E858.1	E933.0	E950.4	E962.0	E980.4
Baneberry	988.2	E865.4	—	E950.9	E962.1	E980.9
Banewort	988.2	E865.4	—	E950.9	E962.1	E980.9
Barbenyl	967.0	E851	E937.0	E950.1	E962.0	E980.1
Barbital, barbitone	967.0	E851	E937.0	E950.1	E962.0	E980.1
Barbiturates, barbituric acid	967.0	E851	E937.0	E950.1	E962.0	E980.1
anesthetic (intravenous)	968.3	E855.1	E938.3	E950.4	E962.0	E980.4
Barium (carbonate) (chloride) (sulfate)	985.8	E866.4	—	E950.9	E962.1	E980.9
diagnostic agent	977.8	E858.8	E947.8	E950.4	E962.0	E980.4
pesticide	985.8	E863.4	—	E950.6	E962.1	E980.7
rodenticide	985.8	E863.7	—	E950.6	E962.1	E980.7
Barrier cream	976.3	E858.7	E946.3	E950.4	E962.0	E980.4
Battery acid or fluid	983.1	E864.1	—	E950.7	E962.1	E980.6
Bay rum	980.8	E860.8	—	E950.9	E962.1	E980.9
BCG vaccine	978.0	E858.8	E948.0	E950.4	E962.0	E980.4
Bearsfoot	988.2	E865.4	—	E950.9	E962.1	E980.9
Beclamide	966.3	E855.0	E936.3	E950.4	E962.0	E980.4
Bee (sting) (venom)	989.5	E905.3	—	E950.9	E962.1	E980.9
Belladonna (alkaloids)	971.1	E855.4	E941.1	E950.4	E962.0	E980.4
Bemegride	970.0	E854.3	E940.0	E950.4	E962.0	E980.4
Benactyzine	969.8	E855.8	E939.8	E950.3	E962.0	E980.3
Benadryl	963.0	E858.1	E933.0	E950.4	E962.0	E980.4
Bendrofluazide	974.3	E858.5	E944.3	E950.4	E962.0	E980.4
Bendroflumethiazide	974.3	E858.5	E944.3	E950.4	E962.0	E980.4
Benemid	974.7	E858.5	E944.7	E950.4	E962.0	E980.4
Benethamine penicillin G	960.0	E856	E930.0	E950.4	E962.0	E980.4
Benisone	976.0	E858.7	E946.0	E950.4	E962.0	E980.4
Benoquin	976.8	E858.7	E946.8	E950.4	E962.0	E980.4
Benoxinate	968.5	E855.2	E938.5	E950.4	E962.0	E980.4
Bentonite	976.3	E858.7	E946.3	E950.4	E962.0	E980.4
Benzalkonium (chloride)	976.0	E858.7	E946.0	E950.4	E962.0	E980.4
ophthalmic preparation	976.5	E858.7	E946.5	E950.4	E962.0	E980.4
Benzamidosalicylate (calcium)	961.8	E857	E931.8	E950.4	E962.0	E980.4

◀ New　◀ Revised　~~deleted~~ Deleted　● Use Additional Digit(s)

TABLE OF DRUGS AND CHEMICALS

Substance	Poisoning	External Cause (E Code)				
		Accident	Therapeutic Use	Suicide Attempt	Assault	Undetermined
Benzathine penicillin	960.0	E856	E930.0	E950.4	E962.0	E980.4
Benzcarbimine	963.1	E858.1	E933.1	E950.4	E962.0	E980.4
Benzedrex	971.2	E855.5	E941.2	E950.4	E962.0	E980.4
Benzedrine (amphetamine)	969.72	E854.2	E939.7	E950.3	E962.0	E980.3
Benzene (acetyl) (dimethyl) (methyl) (solvent) (vapor)	982.0	E862.4	—	E950.9	E962.1	E980.9
hexachloride (gamma) (insecticide) (vapor)	989.2	E863.0	—	E950.6	E962.1	E980.7
Benzethonium	976.0	E858.7	E946.0	E950.4	E962.0	E980.4
Benzhexol (chloride)	966.4	E855.0	E936.4	E950.4	E962.0	E980.4
Benzilonium	971.1	E855.4	E941.1	E950.4	E962.0	E980.4
Benzin(e) - see Ligroin	—	—	—	—	—	—
Benziodarone	972.4	E858.3	E942.4	E950.4	E962.0	E980.4
Benzocaine	968.5	E855.2	E938.5	E950.4	E962.0	E980.4
Benzodiapin	969.4	E853.2	E939.4	E950.3	E962.0	E980.3
Benzodiazepines (tranquilizers) NEC	969.4	E853.2	E939.4	E950.3	E962.0	E980.3
Benzoic acid (with salicylic acid) (anti-infective)	976.0	E858.7	E946.0	E950.4	E962.0	E980.4
Benzoin	976.3	E858.7	E946.3	E950.4	E962.0	E980.4
Benzol (vapor)	982.0	E862.4	—	E950.9	E962.1	E980.9
Benzomorphan	965.09	E850.2	E935.2	E950.0	E962.0	E980.0
Benzonatate	975.4	E858.6	E945.4	E950.4	E962.0	E980.4
Benzothiadiazides	974.3	E858.5	E944.3	E950.4	E962.0	E980.4
Benzoylpas	961.8	E857	E931.8	E950.4	E962.0	E980.4
Benzperidol	969.5	E853.8	E939.5	E950.3	E962.0	E980.3
Benzphetamine	977.0	E858.8	E947.0	E950.4	E962.0	E980.4
Benzpyrinium	971.0	E855.3	E941.0	E950.4	E962.0	E980.4
Benzquinamide	963.0	E858.1	E933.0	E950.4	E962.0	E980.4
Benzthiazide	974.3	E858.5	E944.3	E950.4	E962.0	E980.4
Benztropine	971.1	E855.4	E941.1	E950.4	E962.0	E980.4
Benzyl	—	—	—	—	—	—
acetate	982.8	E862.4	—	E950.9	E962.1	E980.9
benzoate (anti-infective)	976.0	E858.7	E946.0	E950.4	E962.0	E980.4
morphine	965.09	E850.2	E935.2	E950.0	E962.0	E980.0
penicillin	960.0	E856	E930.0	E950.4	E962.0	E980.4
Bephenium	—	—	—	—	—	—
hydroxynapthoate	961.6	E857	E931.6	E950.4	E962.0	E980.4
Bergamot oil	989.89	E866.8	—	E950.9	E962.1	E980.9
Berries, poisonous	988.2	E865.3	—	E950.9	E962.1	E980.9
Beryllium (compounds) (fumes)	985.3	E866.4	—	E950.9	E962.1	E980.9
Beta-carotene	976.3	E858.7	E946.3	E950.4	E962.0	E980.4
Beta-Chlor	967.1	E852.0	E937.1	E950.2	E962.0	E980.2

◄ New ◄ Revised ~~deleted~~ Deleted ● Use Additional Digit(s)

Substance	Poisoning	External Cause (E Code)				
		Accident	Therapeutic Use	Suicide Attempt	Assault	Undetermined
Betamethasone	962.0	E858.0	E932.0	E950.4	E962.0	E980.4
topical	976.0	E858.7	E946.0	E950.4	E962.0	E980.4
Betazole	977.8	E858.8	E947.8	E950.4	E962.0	E980.4
Bethanechol	971.0	E855.3	E941.0	E950.4	E962.0	E980.4
Bethanidine	972.6	E858.3	E942.6	E950.4	E962.0	E980.4
Betula oil	976.3	E858.7	E946.3	E950.4	E962.0	E980.4
Bhang	969.6	E854.1	E939.6	E950.3	E962.0	E980.3
Bialamicol	961.5	E857	E931.5	E950.4	E962.0	E980.4
Bichloride of mercury - see Mercury, chloride	—	—	—	—	—	—
Bichromates (calcium) (crystals) (potassium) (sodium)	983.9	E864.3	—	E950.7	E962.1	E980.6
fumes	987.8	E869.8	—	E952.8	E962.2	E982.8
Biguanide derivatives, oral	962.3	E858.0	E932.3	E950.4	E962.0	E980.4
Biligrafin	977.8	E858.8	E947.8	E950.4	E962.0	E980.4
Bilopaque	977.8	E858.8	E947.8	E950.4	E962.0	E980.4
Bioflavonoids	972.8	E858.3	E942.8	E950.4	E962.0	E980.4
Biological substance NEC	979.9	E858.8	E949.9	E950.4	E962.0	E980.4
Biperiden	966.4	E855.0	E936.4	E950.4	E962.0	E980.4
Bisacodyl	973.1	E858.4	E943.1	E950.4	E962.0	E980.4
Bishydroxycoumarin	964.2	E858.2	E934.2	E950.4	E962.0	E980.4
Bismarsen	961.1	E857	E931.1	E950.4	E962.0	E980.4
Bismuth (compounds) NEC	985.8	E866.4	—	E950.9	E962.1	E980.9
anti-infectives	961.2	E857	E931.2	E950.4	E962.0	E980.4
subcarbonate	973.5	E858.4	E943.5	E950.4	E962.0	E980.4
sulfarsphenamine	961.1	E857	E931.1	E950.4	E962.0	E980.4
Bisphosphonates	—	—	—	—	—	—
intravenous	963.1	E858.1	E933.7	E950.4	E962.0	E980.4
oral	963.1	E858.1	E933.6	E950.4	E962.0	E980.4
Bithionol	961.6	E857	E931.6	E950.4	E962.0	E980.4
Bitter almond oil	989.0	E866.8	—	E950.9	E962.1	E980.9
Bittersweet	988.2	E865.4	—	E950.9	E962.1	E930.9
Black	—	—	—	—	—	—
flag	989.4	E863.4	—	E950.6	E962.1	E980.7
henbane	988.2	E865.4	—	E950.9	E962.1	E980.9
leaf (40)	989.4	E863.4	—	E950.6	E962.1	E980.7
widow spider (bite)	989.5	E905.1	—	E950.9	E962.1	E980.9
antivenin	979.9	E858.8	E949.9	E950.4	E962.0	E980.4
Blast furnace gas (carbon monoxide from)	986	E868.8	—	E952.1	E962.2	E982.1
Bleach NEC	983.9	E864.3	—	E950.7	E962.1	E980.6
Bleaching solutions	983.9	E864.3	—	E950.7	E962.1	E980.6
Bleomycin (sulfate)	960.7	E856	E930.7	E950.4	E962.0	E980.4

◄ New   ◄▦ Revised   deleted Deleted   ● Use Additional Digit(s)

Substance	Poisoning	External Cause (E Code)				
		Accident	Therapeutic Use	Suicide Attempt	Assault	Undetermined
Blockain	968.9	E855.2	E938.9	E950.4	E962.0	E980.4
infiltration (subcutaneous)	968.5	E855.2	E938.5	E950.4	E962.0	E980.4
nerve block (peripheral) (plexus)	968.6	E855.2	E938.6	E950.4	E962.0	E980.4
topical (surface)	968.5	E855.2	E938.5	E950.4	E962.0	E980.4
Blood (derivatives) (natural) (plasma) (whole)	964.7	E858.2	E934.7	E950.4	E962.0	E980.4
affecting agent	964.9	E858.2	E934.9	E950.4	E962.0	E980.4
specified NEC	964.8	E858.2	E934.8	E950.4	E962.0	E980.4
substitute (macromolecular)	964.8	E858.2	E934.8	E950.4	E962.0	E980.4
Blue velvet	965.09	E850.2	E935.2	E950.0	E962.0	E980.0
Bone meal	989.89	E866.5	—	E950.9	E962.1	E980.9
Bonine	963.0	E858.1	E933.0	E950.4	E962.0	E980.4
Boracic acid	976.0	E858.7	E946.0	E950.4	E962.0	E980.4
ENT agent	976.6	E858.7	E946.6	E950.4	E962.0	E980.4
ophthalmic preparation	976.5	E858.7	E946.5	E950.4	E962.0	E980.4
Borate (cleanser) (sodium)	989.6	E861.3	—	E950.9	E962.1	E980.9
Borax (cleanser)	989.6	E861.3	—	E950.9	E962.1	E980.9
Boric acid	976.0	E858.7	E946.0	E950.4	E962.0	E980.4
ENT agent	976.6	E858.7	E946.6	E950.4	E962.0	E980.4
ophthalmic preparation	976.5	E858.7	E946.5	E950.4	E962.0	E980.4
Boron hydride NEC	989.89	E866.8	—	E950.9	E962.1	E980.9
fumes or gas	987.8	E869.8	—	E952.8	E962.2	E982.8
Botox	975.3	E858.6	E945.3	E950.4	E962.0	E980.4
Brake fluid vapor	987.8	E869.8	—	E952.8	E962.2	E982.8
Brass (compounds) (fumes)	985.8	E866.4	—	E950.9	E962.1	E980.9
Brasso	981	E861.3	—	E950.9	E962.1	E980.9
Bretylium (tosylate)	972.6	E858.3	E942.6	E950.4	E962.0	E980.4
Brevital (sodium)	968.3	E855.1	E938.3	E950.4	E962.0	E980.4
British antilewisite	963.8	E858.1	E933.8	E950.4	E962.0	E980.4
Bromal (hydrate)	967.3	E852.2	E937.3	E950.2	E962.0	E980.2
Bromelains	963.4	E858.1	E933.4	E950.4	E962.0	E980.4
Bromides NEC	967.3	E852.2	E937.3	E950.2	E962.0	E980.2
Bromine (vapor)	987.8	E869.8	—	E952.8	E962.2	E982.8
compounds (medicinal)	967.3	E852.2	E937.3	E950.2	E962.0	E980.2
Bromisovalum	967.3	E852.2	E937.3	E950.2	E962.0	E980.2
Bromobenzyl cyanide	987.5	E869.3	—	E952.8	E962.2	E982.8
Bromodiphenhydramine	963.0	E858.1	E933.0	E950.4	E962.0	E980.4
Bromoform	967.3	E852.2	E937.3	E950.2	E962.0	E980.2
Bromophenol blue reagent	977.8	E858.8	E947.8	E950.4	E962.0	E980.4
Bromosalicylhydroxamic acid	961.8	E857	E931.8	E950.4	E962.0	E980.4
Bromo-seltzer	965.4	E850.4	E935.4	E950.0	E962.0	E980.0

◀ New   ◀▥ Revised   ~~deleted~~ Deleted   ● Use Additional Digit(s)

Substance	Poisoning	External Cause (E Code)				
		Accident	Therapeutic Use	Suicide Attempt	Assault	Undetermined
Brompheniramine	963.0	E858.1	E933.0	E950.4	E962.0	E980.4
Bromural	967.3	E852.2	E937.3	E950.2	E962.0	E980.2
Brown spider (bite) (venom)	989.5	E905.1	—	E950.9	E962.1	E980.9
Brucia	988.2	E865.3	—	E950.9	E962.1	E980.9
Brucine	989.1	E863.7	—	E950.6	E962.1	E980.7
Brunswick green - see Copper	—	—	—	—	—	—
Bruten - see Ibuprofen	—	—	—	—	—	—
Bryonia (alba) (dioica)	988.2	E865.4	—	E950.9	E962.1	E980.9
Buclizine	969.5	E853.8	E939.5	E950.3	E962.0	E980.3
Bufferin	965.1	E850.3	E935.3	E950.0	E962.0	E980.0
Bufotenine	969.6	E854.1	E939.6	E950.3	E962.0	E980.3
Buphenine	971.2	E855.5	E941.2	E950.4	E962.0	E980.4
Bupivacaine	968.9	E855.2	E938.9	E950.4	E962.0	E980.4
infiltration (subcutaneous)	968.5	E855.2	E938.5	E950.4	E962.0	E980.4
nerve block (peripheral) (plexus)	968.6	E855.2	E938.6	E950.4	E962.0	E980.4
Busulfan	963.1	E858.1	E933.1	E950.4	E962.0	E980.4
Butabarbital (sodium)	967.0	E851	E937.0	E950.1	E962.0	E980.1
Butabarbitone	967.0	E851	E937.0	E950.1	E962.0	E980.1
Butabarpal	967.0	E851	E937.0	E950.1	E962.0	E980.1
Butacaine	968.5	E855.2	E938.5	E950.4	E962.0	E980.4
Butallylonal	967.0	E851	E937.0	E950.1	E962.0	E980.1
Butane (distributed in mobile container)	987.0	E868.0	—	E951.1	E962.2	E981.1
distributed through pipes	987.0	E867	—	E951.0	E962.2	E981.0
incomplete combustion of - see Carbon monoxide, butane	—	—	—	—	—	—
Butanol	980.3	E860.4	—	E950.9	E962.1	E980.9
Butanone	982.8	E862.4	—	E950.9	E962.1	E980.9
Butaperazine	969.1	E853.0	E939.1	E950.3	E962.0	E980.3
Butazolidin	965.5	E850.5	E935.5	E950.0	E962.0	E980.0
Butethal	967.0	E851	E937.0	E950.1	E962.0	E980.1
Butethamate	971.1	E855.4	E941.1	E950.4	E962.0	E980.4
Buthalitone (sodium)	968.3	E855.1	E938.3	E950.4	E962.0	E980.4
Butisol (sodium)	967.0	E851	E937.0	E950.1	E962.0	E980.1
Butobarbital, butobarbitone	967.0	E851	E937.0	E950.1	E962.0	E980.1
Butriptyline	969.05	E854.0	E939.0	E950.3	E962.0	E980.3
Buttercups	988.2	E865.4	—	E950.9	E962.1	E980.9
Butter of antimony - see Antimony	—	—	—	—	—	—
Butyl	—	—	—	—	—	—
acetate (secondary)	982.8	E862.4	—	E950.9	E962.1	E980.9
alcohol	980.3	E860.4	—	E950.9	E962.1	E980.9

◀ New   ◀▥ Revised   ~~deleted~~ Deleted   ● Use Additional Digit(s)

Substance	Poisoning	External Cause (E Code)				
		Accident	Therapeutic Use	Suicide Attempt	Assault	Undetermined
Butyl *(Continued)*						
carbinol	980.8	E860.8	—	E950.9	E962.1	E980.9
carbitol	982.8	E862.4	—	E950.9	E962.1	E980.9
cellosolve	982.8	E862.4	—	E950.9	E962.1	E980.9
chloral (hydrate)	967.1	E852.0	E937.1	E950.2	E962.0	E980.2
formate	982.8	E862.4	—	E950.9	E962.1	E980.9
scopolammonium bromide	971.1	E855.4	E941.1	E950.4	E962.0	E980.4
Butyn	968.5	E855.2	E938.5	E950.4	E962.0	E980.4
Butyrophenone (-based tranquilizers)	969.2	E853.1	E939.2	E950.3	E962.0	E980.3
Cacodyl, cacodylic acid - *see* Arsenic	—	—	—	—	—	—
Cactinomycin	960.7	E856	E930.7	E950.4	E962.0	E980.4
Cade oil	976.4	E858.7	E946.4	E950.4	E962.0	E980.4
Cadmium (chloride) (compounds) (dust) (fumes) (oxide)	985.5	E866.4	—	E950.9	E962.1	E980.9
sulfide (medicinal) NEC	976.4	E858.7	E946.4	E950.4	E962.0	E980.4
Caffeine	969.71	E854.2	E939.7	E950.3	E962.0	E980.3
Calabar bean	988.2	E865.4	—	E950.9	E962.1	E980.9
Caladium seguinium	988.2	E865.4	—	E950.9	E962.1	E980.9
Calamine (liniment) (lotion)	976.3	E858.7	E946.3	E950.4	E962.0	E980.4
Calciferol	963.5	E858.1	E933.5	E950.4	E962.0	E980.4
Calcium (salts) NEC	974.5	E858.5	E944.5	E950.4	E962.0	E980.4
acetylsalicylate	965.1	E850.3	E935.3	E950.0	E962.0	E980.0
benzamidosalicylate	961.8	E857	E931.8	E950.4	E962.0	E980.4
carbaspirin	965.1	E850.3	E935.3	E950.0	E962.0	E980.0
carbimide (citrated)	977.3	E858.8	E947.3	E950.4	E962.0	E980.4
carbonate (antacid)	973.0	E858.4	E943.0	E950.4	E962.0	E980.4
cyanide (citrated)	977.3	E858.8	E947.3	E950.4	E962.0	E980.4
dioctyl sulfosuccinate	973.2	E858.4	E943.2	E950.4	E962.0	E980.4
disodium edathamil	963.8	E858.1	E933.8	E950.4	E962.0	E980.4
disodium edetate	963.8	E858.1	E933.8	E950.4	E962.0	E980.4
EDTA	963.8	E858.1	E933.8	E950.4	E962.0	E980.4
hydrate, hydroxide	983.2	E864.2	—	E950.7	E962.1	E980.6
mandelate	961.9	E857	E931.9	E950.4	E962.0	E980.4
oxide	983.2	E864.2	—	E950.7	E962.1	E980.6
Calomel - *see* Mercury, chloride	—	—	—	—	—	—
Caloric agents NEC	974.5	E858.5	E944.5	E950.4	E962.0	E980.4
Calusterone	963.1	E858.1	E933.1	E950.4	E962.0	E980.4
Camoquin	961.4	E857	E931.4	E950.4	E962.0	E980.4
Camphor (oil)	976.1	E858.7	E946.1	E950.4	E962.0	E980.4
Candeptin	976.0	E858.7	E946.0	E950.4	E962.0	E980.4

◀ New ◀▪▪ Revised ~~deleted~~ Deleted ● Use Additional Digit(s)

Substance	Poisoning	External Cause (E Code)				
		Accident	Therapeutic Use	Suicide Attempt	Assault	Undetermined
Candicidin	976.0	E858.7	E946.0	E950.4	E962.0	E980.4
Cannabinols	969.6	E854.1	E939.6	E950.3	E962.0	E980.3
Cannabis (derivatives) (indica) (sativa)	969.6	E854.1	E939.6	E950.3	E962.0	E980.3
Canned heat	980.1	E860.2	—	E950.9	E962.1	E980.9
Cantharides, cantharidin, cantharis	976.8	E858.7	E946.8	E950.4	E962.0	E980.4
Capillary agents	972.8	E858.3	E942.8	E950.4	E962.0	E980.4
Capreomycin	960.6	E856	E930.6	E950.4	E962.0	E980.4
Captodiame, captodiamine	969.5	E853.8	E939.5	E950.3	E962.0	E980.3
Caramiphen (hydrochloride)	971.1	E855.4	E941.1	E950.4	E962.0	E980.4
Carbachol	971.0	E855.3	E941.0	E950.4	E962.0	E980.4
Carbacrylamine resins	974.5	E858.5	E944.5	E950.4	E962.0	E980.4
Carbamate (sedative)	967.8	E852.8	E937.8	E950.2	E962.0	E980.2
herbicide	989.3	E863.5	—	E950.6	E962.1	E980.7
insecticide	989.3	E863.2	—	E950.6	E962.1	E980.7
Carbamazepine	966.3	E855.0	E936.3	E950.4	E962.0	E980.4
Carbamic esters	967.8	E852.8	E937.8	E950.2	E962.0	E980.2
Carbamide	974.4	E858.5	E944.4	E950.4	E962.0	E980.4
topical	976.8	E858.7	E946.8	E950.4	E962.0	E980.4
Carbamylcholine chloride	971.0	E855.3	E941.0	E950.4	E962.0	E980.4
Carbarsone	961.1	E857	E931.1	E950.4	E962.0	E980.4
Carbaryl	989.3	E863.2	—	E950.6	E962.1	E980.7
Carbaspirin	965.1	E850.3	E935.3	E950.0	E962.0	E980.0
Carbazochrome	972.8	E858.3	E942.8	E950.4	E962.0	E980.4
Carbenicillin	960.0	E856	E930.0	E950.4	E962.0	E980.4
Carbenoxolone	973.8	E858.4	E943.8	E950.4	E962.0	E980.4
Carbetapentane	975.4	E858.6	E945.4	E950.4	E962.0	E980.4
Carbimazole	962.8	E858.0	E932.8	E950.4	E962.0	E980.4
Carbinol	980.1	E860.2	—	E950.9	E962.1	E980.9
Carbinoxamine	963.0	E858.1	E933.0	E950.4	E962.0	E980.4
Carbitol	982.8	E862.4	—	E950.9	E962.1	E980.9
Carbocaine	968.9	E855.2	E938.9	E950.4	E962.0	E980.4
infiltration (subcutaneous)	968.5	E855.2	E938.5	E950.4	E962.0	E980.4
nerve block (peripheral) (plexus)	968.6	E855.2	E938.6	E950.4	E962.0	E980.4
topical (surface)	968.5	E855.2	E938.5	E950.4	E962.0	E980.4
Carbol-fuchsin solution	976.0	E858.7	E946.0	E950.4	E962.0	E980.4
Carbolic acid (see also Phenol)	983.0	E864.0	—	E950.7	E962.1	E980.6
Carbomycin	960.8	E856	E930.8	E950.4	E962.0	E980.4
Carbon	—	—	—	—	—	—
bisulfide (liquid) (vapor)	982.2	E862.4	—	E950.9	E962.1	E980.9

Substance	Poisoning	External Cause (E Code)				
		Accident	Therapeutic Use	Suicide Attempt	Assault	Undetermined
Carbon *(Continued)*						
dioxide (gas)	987.8	E869.8	—	E952.8	E962.2	E982.8
disulfide (liquid) (vapor)	982.2	E862.4	—	E950.9	E962.1	E980.9
monoxide (from incomplete combustion of) (in) NEC	986	E868.9	—	E952.1	E962.2	E982.1
blast furnace gas	986	E868.8	—	E952.1	E962.2	E982.1
butane (distributed in mobile container)	986	E868.0	—	E951.1	E962.2	E981.1
distributed through pipes	986	E867	—	E951.0	E962.2	E981.0
charcoal fumes	986	E868.3	—	E952.1	E962.2	E982.1
coal						
gas (piped)	986	E867	—	E951.0	E962.2	E981.0
solid (in domestic stoves, fireplaces)	986	E868.3	—	E952.1	E962.2	E982.1
coke (in domestic stoves, fireplaces)	986	E868.3	—	E952.1	E962.2	E982.1
exhaust gas (motor) not in transit	986	E868.2	—	E952.0	E962.2	E982.0
combustion engine, any not in watercraft	986	E868.2	—	E952.0	E962.2	E982.0
farm tractor, not in transit	986	E868.2	—	E952.0	E962.2	E982.0
gas engine	986	E868.2	—	E952.0	E962.2	E982.0
motor pump	986	E868.2	—	E952.0	E962.2	E982.0
motor vehicle, not in transit	986	E868.2	—	E952.0	E962.2	E982.0
fuel (in domestic use)	986	E868.3	—	E952.1	E962.2	E982.1
gas (piped)	986	E867	—	E951.0	E962.2	E981.0
in mobile container	986	E868.0	—	E951.1	E962.2	E981.1
utility	986	E868.1	—	E951.8	E962.2	E981.1
in mobile container	986	E868.0	—	E951.1	E962.2	E981.1
piped (natural)	986	E867	—	E951.0	E962.2	E981.0
illuminating gas	986	E868.1	—	E951.8	E962.2	E981.8
industrial fuels or gases, any	986	E868.8	—	E952.1	E962.2	E982.1
kerosene (in domestic stoves, fireplaces)	986	E868.3	—	E952.1	E962.2	E982.1
kiln gas or vapor	986	E868.8	—	E952.1	E962.2	E982.1
motor exhaust gas, not in transit	986	E868.2	—	E952.0	E962.2	E982.0
piped gas (manufactured) (natural)	986	E867	—	E951.0	E962.2	E981.0
producer gas	986	E868.8	—	E952.1	E962.2	E982.1
propane (distributed in mobile container)	986	E868.0	—	E951.1	E962.2	E981.1
distributed through pipes	986	E867	—	E951.0	E962.2	E981.0
specified source NEC	986	E868.8	—	E952.1	E962.2	E982.1
stove gas	986	E868.1	—	E951.8	E962.2	E981.8
piped	986	E867	—	E951.0	E962.2	E981.0
utility gas	986	E868.1	—	E951.8	E962.2	E981.8
piped	986	E867	—	E951.0	E962.2	E981.0

◀ New ◀ Revised ~~deleted~~ Deleted ● Use Additional Digit(s)

TABLE OF DRUGS AND CHEMICALS

Substance	Poisoning	External Cause (E Code)				
		Accident	Therapeutic Use	Suicide Attempt	Assault	Undetermined
Carbon *(Continued)*						
monoxide (from incomplete combustion of) (in) NEC *(Continued)*						
water gas	986	E868.1	—	E951.8	E962.2	E981.8
wood (in domestic stoves, fireplaces)	986	E868.3	—	E952.1	E962.2	E982.1
tetrachloride (vapor) NEC	987.8	E869.8	—	E952.8	E962.2	E982.8
liquid (cleansing agent) NEC	982.1	E861.3	—	E950.9	E962.1	E980.9
solvent	982.1	E862.4	—	E950.9	E962.1	E980.9
Carbonic acid (gas)	987.8	E869.8	—	E952.8	E962.2	E982.8
anhydrase inhibitors	974.2	E858.5	E944.2	E950.4	E962.0	E980.4
Carbowax	976.3	E858.7	E946.3	E950.4	E962.0	E980.4
Carbrital	967.0	E851	E937.0	E950.1	E962.0	E980.1
Carbromal (derivatives)	967.3	E852.2	E937.3	E950.2	E962.0	E980.2
Cardiac	—	—	—	—	—	—
depressants	972.0	E858.3	E942.0	E950.4	E962.0	E980.4
rhythm regulators	972.0	E858.3	E942.0	E950.4	E962.0	E980.4
Cardiografin	977.8	E858.8	E947.8	E950.4	E962.0	E980.4
Cardio-green	977.8	E858.8	E947.8	E950.4	E962.0	E980.4
Cardiotonic glycosides	972.1	E858.3	E942.1	E950.4	E962.0	E980.4
Cardiovascular agents NEC	972.9	E858.3	E942.9	E950.4	E962.0	E980.4
Cardrase	974.2	E858.5	E944.2	E950.4	E962.0	E980.4
Carfusin	976.0	E858.7	E946.0	E950.4	E962.0	E980.4
Carisoprodol	968.0	E855.1	E938.0	E950.4	E962.0	E980.4
Carmustine	963.1	E858.1	E933.1	E950.4	E962.0	E980.4
Carotene	963.5	E858.1	E933.5	E950.4	E962.0	E980.4
Carphenazine (maleate)	969.1	E853.0	E939.1	E950.3	E962.0	E980.3
Carter's Little Pills	973.1	E858.4	E943.1	E950.4	E962.0	E980.4
Cascara (sagrada)	973.1	E858.4	E943.1	E950.4	E962.0	E980.4
Cassava	988.2	E865.4	—	E950.9	E962.1	E980.9
Castellani's paint	976.0	E858.7	E946.0	E950.4	E962.0	E980.4
Castor	—	—	—	—	—	—
bean	988.2	E865.3	—	E950.9	E962.1	E980.9
oil	973.1	E858.4	E943.1	E950.4	E962.0	E980.4
Caterpillar (sting)	989.5	E905.5	—	E950.9	E962.1	E980.9
Catha (edulis)	970.89	E854.3	E940.8	E950.4	E962.0	E980.4
Cathartics NEC	973.3	E858.4	E943.3	E950.4	E962.0	E980.4
contact	973.1	E858.4	E943.1	E950.4	E962.0	E980.4
emollient	973.2	E858.4	E943.2	E950.4	E962.0	E980.4
intestinal irritants	973.1	E858.4	E943.1	E950.4	E962.0	E980.4
saline	973.3	E858.4	E943.3	E950.4	E962.0	E980.4
Cathomycin	960.8	E856	E930.8	E950.4	E962.0	E980.4

◄ New   ◀‖‖ Revised   ~~deleted~~ Deleted   ● Use Additional Digit(s)

Substance	Poisoning	External Cause (E Code)				
		Accident	Therapeutic Use	Suicide Attempt	Assault	Undetermined
Caustic(s)	983.9	E864.4	—	E950.7	E962.1	E980.6
alkali	983.2	E864.2	—	E950.7	E962.1	E980.6
hydroxide	983.2	E864.2	—	E950.7	E962.1	E980.6
potash	983.2	E864.2	—	E950.7	E962.1	E980.6
soda	983.2	E864.2	—	E950.7	E962.1	E980.6
specified NEC	983.9	E864.3	—	E950.7	E962.1	E980.6
Ceepryn	976.0	E858.7	E946.0	E950.4	E962.0	E980.4
ENT agent	976.6	E858.7	E946.6	E950.4	E962.0	E980.4
lozenges	976.6	E858.7	E946.6	E950.4	E962.0	E980.4
Celestone	962.0	E858.0	E932.0	E950.4	E962.0	E980.4
topical	976.0	E858.7	E946.0	E950.4	E962.0	E980.4
Cellosolve	982.8	E862.4	—	E950.9	E962.1	E980.9
Cell stimulants and proliferants	976.8	E858.7	E946.8	E950.4	E962.0	E980.4
Cellulose derivatives, cathartic	973.3	E858.4	E943.3	E950.4	E962.0	E980.4
nitrates (topical)	976.3	E858.7	E946.3	E950.4	E962.0	E980.4
Centipede (bite)	989.5	E905.4	—	E950.9	E962.1	E980.9
Central nervous system	—	—	—	—	—	—
depressants	968.4	E855.1	E938.4	E950.4	E962.0	E980.4
anesthetic (general) NEC	968.4	E855.1	E938.4	E950.4	E962.0	E980.4
gases NEC	968.2	E855.1	E938.2	E950.4	E962.0	E980.4
intravenous	968.3	E855.1	E938.3	E950.4	E962.0	E980.4
barbiturates	967.0	E851	E937.0	E950.1	E962.0	E980.1
bromides	967.3	E852.2	E937.3	E950.2	E962.0	E980.2
cannabis sativa	969.6	E854.1	E939.6	E950.3	E962.0	E980.3
chloral hydrate	967.1	E852.0	E937.1	E950.2	E962.0	E980.2
hallucinogenics	969.6	E854.1	E939.6	E950.3	E962.0	E980.3
hypnotics	967.9	E852.9	E937.9	E950.2	E962.0	E980.2
specified NEC	967.8	E852.8	E937.8	E950.2	E962.0	E980.2
muscle relaxants	968.0	E855.1	E938.0	E950.4	E962.0	E980.4
paraldehyde	967.2	E852.1	E937.2	E950.2	E962.0	E980.2
sedatives	967.9	E852.9	E937.9	E950.2	E962.0	E980.2
mixed NEC	967.6	E852.5	E937.6	E950.2	E962.0	E980.2
specified NEC	967.8	E852.8	E937.8	E950.2	E962.0	E980.2
muscle-tone depressants	968.0	E855.1	E938.0	E950.4	E962.0	E980.4
stimulants	970.9	E854.3	E940.9	E950.4	E962.0	E980.4
amphetamines	969.72	E854.2	E939.7	E950.3	E962.0	E980.3
analeptics	970.0	E854.3	E940.0	E950.4	E962.0	E980.4
antidepressants	969.00	E854.0	E939.0	E950.3	E962.0	E980.3
opiate antagonists	970.1	E854.3	E940.0	E950.4	E962.0	E980.4
specified NEC	970.89	E854.3	E940.8	E950.4	E962.0	E980.4

◀ New ◀▮▮ Revised ~~deleted~~ Deleted ● Use Additional Digit(s)

Substance	Poisoning	External Cause (E Code)				
		Accident	Therapeutic Use	Suicide Attempt	Assault	Undetermined
Cephalexin	960.5	E856	E930.5	E950.4	E962.0	E980.4
Cephaloglycin	960.5	E856	E930.5	E950.4	E962.0	E980.4
Cephaloridine	960.5	E856	E930.5	E950.4	E962.0	E980.4
Cephalosporins NEC	960.5	E856	E930.5	E950.4	E962.0	E980.4
N (adicillin)	960.0	E856	E930.0	E950.4	E962.0	E980.4
Cephalothin (sodium)	960.5	E856	E930.5	E950.4	E962.0	E980.4
Cerbera (odallam)	988.2	E865.4	—	E950.9	E962.1	E980.9
Cerberin	972.1	E858.3	E942.1	E950.4	E962.0	E980.4
Cerebral stimulants	970.9	E854.3	E940.9	E950.4	E962.0	E980.4
psychotherapeutic	969.79	E854.2	E939.7	E950.3	E962.0	E980.3
specified NEC	970.89	E854.3	E940.8	E950.4	E962.0	E980.4
Cetalkonium (chloride)	976.0	E858.7	E946.0	E950.4	E962.0	E980.4
Cetoxime	963.0	E858.1	E933.0	E950.4	E962.0	E980.4
Cetrimide	976.2	E858.7	E946.2	E950.4	E962.0	E980.4
Cetylpyridinium	976.0	E858.7	E946.0	E950.4	E962.0	E980.4
ENT agent	976.6	E858.7	E946.6	E950.4	E962.0	E980.4
lozenges	976.6	E858.7	E946.6	E950.4	E962.0	E980.4
Cevadilla - see Sabadilla	—	—	—	—	—	—
Cevitamic acid	963.5	E858.1	E933.5	E950.4	E962.0	E980.4
Chalk, precipitated	973.0	E858.4	E943.0	E950.4	E962.0	E980.4
Charcoal	—	—	—	—	—	—
fumes (carbon monoxide)	986	E868.3	—	E952.1	E962.2	E982.1
industrial	986	E868.8	—	E952.1	E962.2	E982.1
medicinal (activated)	973.0	E858.4	E943.0	E950.4	E962.0	E980.4
Chelating agents NEC	977.2	E858.8	E947.2	E950.4	E962.0	E980.4
Chelidonium majus	988.2	E865.4	—	E950.9	E962.1	E980.9
Chemical substance	989.9	E866.9	—	E950.9	E962.1	E980.9
specified NEC	989.89	E866.8	—	E950.9	E962.1	E980.9
Chemotherapy, antineoplastic	963.1	E858.1	E933.1	E950.4	E962.0	E980.4
Chenopodium (oil)	961.6	E857	E931.6	E950.4	E962.0	E980.4
Cherry laurel	988.2	E865.4	—	E950.9	E962.1	E980.9
Chiniofon	961.3	E857	E931.3	E950.4	E962.0	E980.4
Chlophedianol	975.4	E858.6	E945.4	E950.4	E962.0	E980.4
Chloral (betaine) (formamide) (hydrate)	967.1	E852.0	E937.1	E950.2	E962.0	E980.2
Chloralamide	967.1	E852.0	E937.1	E950.2	E962.0	E980.2
Chlorambucil	963.1	E858.1	E933.1	E950.4	E962.0	E980.4
Chloramphenicol	960.2	E856	E930.2	E950.4	E962.0	E980.4
ENT agent	976.6	E858.7	E946.6	E950.4	E962.0	E980.4
ophthalmic preparation	976.5	E858.7	E946.5	E950.4	E962.0	E980.4
topical NEC	976.0	E858.7	E946.0	E950.4	E962.0	E980.4

◀ New ◀ Revised ~~deleted~~ Deleted ● Use Additional Digit(s)

Substance	Poisoning	External Cause (E Code)				
		Accident	Therapeutic Use	Suicide Attempt	Assault	Undetermined
Chlorate(s) (potassium) (sodium) NEC	983.9	E864.3	—	E950.7	E962.1	E980.6
herbicides	989.4	E863.5	—	E950.6	E962.1	E980.7
Chlorcyclizine	963.0	E858.1	E933.0	E950.4	E962.0	E980.4
Chlordan(e) (dust)	989.2	E863.0	—	E950.6	E962.1	E980.7
Chlordantoin	976.0	E858.7	E946.0	E950.4	E962.0	E980.4
Chlordiazepoxide	969.4	E853.2	E939.4	E950.3	E962.0	E980.3
Chloresium	976.8	E858.7	E946.8	E950.4	E962.0	E980.4
Chlorethiazol	967.1	E852.0	E937.1	E950.2	E962.0	E980.2
Chlorethyl - see Ethyl, chloride	—	—	—	—	—	—
Chloretone	967.1	E852.0	E937.1	E950.2	E962.0	E980.2
Chlorex	982.3	E862.4	—	E950.9	E962.1	E980.9
Chlorhexadol	967.1	E852.0	E937.1	E950.2	E962.0	E980.2
Chlorhexidine (hydrochloride)	976.0	E858.7	E946.0	E950.4	E962.0	E980.4
Chlorhydroxyquinolin	976.0	E858.7	E946.0	E950.4	E962.0	E980.4
Chloride of lime (bleach)	983.9	E864.3	—	E950.7	E962.1	E980.6
Chlorinated	—	—	—	—	—	—
camphene	989.2	E863.0	—	E950.6	E962.1	E980.7
diphenyl	989.89	E866.8	—	E950.9	E962.1	E980.9
hydrocarbons NEC	989.2	E863.0	—	E950.6	E962.1	E980.7
solvent	982.3	E862.4	—	E950.9	E962.1	E980.9
lime (bleach)	983.9	E864.3	—	E950.7	E962.1	E980.6
naphthalene - see Naphthalene	—	—	—	—	—	—
pesticides NEC	989.2	E863.0	—	E950.6	E962.1	E980.7
soda - see Sodium, hypochlorite	—	—	—	—	—	—
Chlorine (fumes) (gas)	987.6	E869.8	—	E952.8	E962.2	E982.8
bleach	983.9	E864.3	—	E950.7	E962.1	E980.6
compounds NEC	983.9	E864.3	—	E950.7	E962.1	E980.6
disinfectant	983.9	E861.4	—	E950.7	E962.1	E980.6
releasing agents NEC	983.9	E864.3	—	E950.7	E962.1	E980.6
Chlorisondamine	972.3	E858.3	E942.3	E950.4	E962.0	E980.4
Chlormadinone	962.2	E858.0	E932.2	E950.4	E962.0	E980.4
Chlormerodrin	974.0	E858.5	E944.0	E950.4	E962.0	E980.4
Chlormethiazole	967.1	E852.0	E937.1	E950.2	E962.0	E980.2
Chlormethylenecycline	960.4	E856	E930.4	E950.4	E962.0	E980.4
Chlormezanone	969.5	E853.8	E939.5	E950.3	E962.0	E980.3
Chloroacetophenone	987.5	E869.3	—	E952.8	E962.2	E982.8
Chloroaniline	983.0	E864.0	—	E950.7	E962.1	E980.6
Chlorobenzene, chlorobenzol	982.0	E862.4	—	E950.9	E962.1	E980.9
Chlorobutanol	967.1	E852.0	E937.1	E950.2	E962.0	E980.2

◀ New   ◀◀ Revised   deleted Deleted   ● Use Additional Digit(s)

Substance	Poisoning	External Cause (E Code)				
		Accident	Therapeutic Use	Suicide Attempt	Assault	Undetermined
Chlorodinitrobenzene	983.0	E864.0	—	E950.7	E962.1	E980.6
dust or vapor	987.8	E869.8	—	E952.8	E962.2	E982.8
Chloroethane - *see* Ethyl, chloride	—	—	—	—	—	—
Chloroform (fumes) (vapor)	987.8	E869.8	—	E952.8	E962.2	E982.8
anesthetic (gas)	968.2	E855.1	E938.2	E950.4	E962.0	E980.4
liquid NEC	968.4	E855.1	E938.4	E950.4	E962.0	E980.4
solvent	982.3	E862.4	—	E950.9	E962.1	E980.9
Chloroguanide	961.4	E857	E931.4	E950.4	E962.0	E980.4
Chloromycetin	960.2	E856	E930.2	E950.4	E962.0	E980.4
ENT agent	976.6	E858.7	E946.6	E950.4	E962.0	E980.4
ophthalmic preparation	976.5	E858.7	E946.5	E950.4	E962.0	E980.4
otic solution	976.6	E858.7	E946.6	E950.4	E962.0	E980.4
topical NEC	976.0	E858.7	E946.0	E950.4	E962.0	E980.4
Chloronitrobenzene	983.0	E864.0	—	E950.7	E962.1	E980.6
dust or vapor	987.8	E869.8	—	E952.8	E962.2	E982.8
Chlorophenol	983.0	E864.0	—	E950.7	E962.1	E980.6
Chlorophenothane	989.2	E863.0	—	E950.6	E962.1	E980.7
Chlorophyll (derivatives)	976.8	E858.7	E946.8	E950.4	E962.0	E980.4
Chloropicrin (fumes)	987.8	E869.8	—	E952.8	E962.2	E982.8
fumigant	989.4	E863.8	—	E950.6	E962.1	E980.7
fungicide	989.4	E863.6	—	E950.6	E962.1	E980.7
pesticide (fumes)	989.4	E863.4	—	E950.6	E962.1	E980.7
Chloroprocaine	968.9	E855.2	E938.9	E950.4	E962.0	E980.4
infiltration (subcutaneous)	968.5	E855.2	E938.5	E950.4	E962.0	E980.4
nerve block (peripheral) (plexus)	968.6	E855.2	E938.6	E950.4	E962.0	E980.4
Chloroptic	976.5	E858.7	E946.5	E950.4	E962.0	E980.4
Chloropurine	963.1	E858.1	E933.1	E950.4	E962.0	E980.4
Chloroquine (hydrochloride) (phosphate)	961.4	E857	E931.4	E950.4	E962.0	E980.4
Chlorothen	963.0	E858.1	E933.0	E950.4	E962.0	E980.4
Chlorothiazide	974.3	E858.5	E944.3	E950.4	E962.0	E980.4
Chlorotrianisene	962.2	E858.0	E932.2	E950.4	E962.0	E980.4
Chlorovinyldichloroarsine	985.1	E866.3	—	E950.8	E962.1	E980.8
Chloroxylenol	976.0	E858.7	E946.0	E950.4	E962.0	E980.4
Chlorphenesin (carbamate)	968.0	E855.1	E938.0	E950.4	E962.0	E980.4
topical (antifungal)	976.0	E858.7	E946.0	E950.4	E962.0	E980.4
Chlorpheniramine	963.0	E858.1	E933.0	E950.4	E962.0	E980.4
Chlorphenoxamine	966.4	E855.0	E936.4	E950.4	E962.0	E980.4
Chlorphentermine	977.0	E858.8	E947.0	E950.4	E962.0	E980.4
Chlorproguanil	961.4	E857	E931.4	E950.4	E962.0	E980.4

		External Cause (E Code)				
Substance	Poisoning	Accident	Therapeutic Use	Suicide Attempt	Assault	Undetermined
Chlorpromazine	969.1	E853.0	E939.1	E950.3	E962.0	E980.3
Chlorpropamide	962.3	E858.0	E932.3	E950.4	E962.0	E980.4
Chlorprothixene	969.3	E853.8	E939.3	E950.3	E962.0	E980.3
Chlorquinaldol	976.0	E858.7	E946.0	E950.4	E962.0	E980.4
Chlortetracycline	960.4	E856	E930.4	E950.4	E962.0	E980.4
Chlorthalidone	974.4	E858.5	E944.4	E950.4	E962.0	E980.4
Chlortrianisene	962.2	E858.0	E932.2	E950.4	E962.0	E980.4
Chlor-Trimeton	963.0	E858.1	E933.0	E950.4	E962.0	E980.4
Chlorzoxazone	968.0	E855.1	E938.0	E950.4	E962.0	E980.4
Choke damp	987.8	E869.8	—	E952.8	E962.2	E982.8
Cholebrine	977.8	E858.8	E947.8	E950.4	E962.0	E980.4
Cholera vaccine	978.2	E858.8	E948.2	E950.4	E962.0	E980.4
Cholesterol-lowering agents	972.2	E858.3	E942.2	E950.4	E962.0	E980.4
Cholestyramine (resin)	972.2	E858.3	E942.2	E950.4	E962.0	E980.4
Cholic acid	973.4	E858.4	E943.4	E950.4	E962.0	E980.4
Choline	—	—	—	—	—	—
dihydrogen citrate	977.1	E858.8	E947.1	E950.4	E962.0	E980.4
salicylate	965.1	E850.3	E935.3	E950.0	E962.0	E980.0
theophyllinate	974.1	E858.5	E944.1	E950.4	E962.0	E980.4
Cholinergics	971.0	E855.3	E941.0	E950.4	E962.0	E980.4
Cholografin	977.8	E858.8	E947.8	E950.4	E962.0	E980.4
Chorionic gonadotropin	962.4	E858.0	E932.4	E950.4	E962.0	E980.4
Chromates	983.9	E864.3	—	E950.7	E962.1	E980.6
dust or mist	987.8	E869.8	—	E952.8	E962.2	E982.8
lead	984.0	E866.0	—	E950.9	E962.1	E980.9
paint	984.0	E861.5	—	E950.9	E962.1	E980.9
Chromic acid	983.9	E864.3	—	E950.7	E962.1	E980.6
dust or mist	987.8	E869.8	—	E952.8	E962.2	E982.8
Chromium	985.6	E866.4	—	E950.9	E962.1	E980.9
compounds - see Chromates	—	—	—	—	—	—
Chromonar	972.4	E858.3	E942.4	E950.4	E962.0	E980.4
Chromyl chloride	983.9	E864.3	—	E950.7	E962.1	E980.6
Chrysarobin (ointment)	976.4	E858.7	E946.4	E950.4	E962.0	E980.4
Chrysazin	973.1	E858.4	E943.1	E950.4	E962.0	E980.4
Chymar	963.4	E858.1	E933.4	E950.4	E962.0	E980.4
ophthalmic preparation	976.5	E858.7	E946.5	E950.4	E962.0	E980.4
Chymotrypsin	963.4	E858.1	E933.4	E950.4	E962.0	E980.4
ophthalmic preparation	976.5	E858.7	E946.5	E950.4	E962.0	E980.4
Cicuta maculata or virosa	988.2	E865.4	—	E950.9	E962.1	E980.9

◀ New   ⬅ Revised   ~~deleted~~ Deleted   ● Use Additional Digit(s)

Substance	Poisoning	External Cause (E Code)				
		Accident	Therapeutic Use	Suicide Attempt	Assault	Undetermined
Cigarette lighter fluid	981	E862.1	—	E950.9	E962.1	E980.9
Cinchocaine (spinal)	968.7	E855.2	E938.7	E950.4	E962.0	E980.4
topical (surface)	968.5	E855.2	E938.5	E950.4	E962.0	E980.4
Cinchona	961.4	E857	E931.4	E950.4	E962.0	E980.4
Cinchonine alkaloids	961.4	E857	E931.4	E950.4	E962.0	E980.4
Cinchophen	974.7	E858.5	E944.7	E950.4	E962.0	E980.4
Cinnarizine	963.0	E858.1	E933.0	E950.4	E962.0	E980.4
Citanest	968.9	E855.2	E938.9	E950.4	E962.0	E980.4
infiltration (subcutaneous)	968.5	E855.2	E938.5	E950.4	E962.0	E980.4
nerve block (peripheral) (plexus)	968.6	E855.2	E938.6	E950.4	E962.0	E980.4
Citric acid	989.89	E866.8	—	E950.9	E962.1	E980.9
Citrovorum factor	964.1	E858.2	E934.1	E950.4	E962.0	E980.4
Claviceps purpurea	988.2	E865.4	—	E950.9	E962.1	E980.9
Cleaner, cleansing agent, type not specified	989.89	E861.9	—	E950.9	E962.1	E980.9
of paint or varnish	982.8	E862.9	—	E950.9	E962.1	E980.9
specified type NEC	989.89	E861.3	—	E950.9	E962.1	E980.9
Clematis vitalba	988.2	E865.4	—	E950.9	E962.1	E980.9
Clemizole	963.0	E858.1	E933.0	E950.4	E962.0	E980.4
penicillin	960.0	E856	E930.0	E950.4	E962.0	E980.4
Clidinium	971.1	E855.4	E941.1	E950.4	E962.0	E980.4
Clindamycin	960.8	E856	E930.8	E950.4	E962.0	E980.4
Cliradon	965.09	E850.2	E935.2	E950.0	E962.0	E980.0
Clocortolone	962.0	E858.0	E932.0	E950.4	E962.0	E980.4
Clofedanol	975.4	E858.6	E945.4	E950.4	E962.0	E980.4
Clofibrate	972.2	E858.3	E942.2	E950.4	E962.0	E980.4
Clomethiazole	967.1	E852.0	E937.1	E950.2	E962.0	E980.2
Clomiphene	977.8	E858.8	E947.8	E950.4	E962.0	E980.4
Clonazepam	969.4	E853.2	E939.4	E950.3	E962.0	E980.3
Clonidine	972.6	E858.3	E942.6	E950.4	E962.0	E980.4
Clopamide	974.3	E858.5	E944.3	E950.4	E962.0	E980.4
Clorazepate	969.4	E853.2	E939.4	E950.3	E962.0	E980.3
Clorexolone	974.4	E858.5	E944.4	E950.4	E962.0	E980.4
Clorox (bleach)	983.9	E864.3	—	E950.7	E962.1	E980.6
Clortermine	977.0	E858.8	E947.0	E950.4	E962.0	E980.4
Clotrimazole	976.0	E858.7	E946.0	E950.4	E962.0	E980.4
Cloxacillin	960.0	E856	E930.0	E950.4	E962.0	E980.4
Coagulants NEC	964.5	E858.2	E934.5	E950.4	E962.0	E980.4
Coal (carbon monoxide from) - see also Carbon, monoxide, coal	—	—	—	—	—	—
oil - see Kerosene	—	—	—	—	—	—

◀ New ◀▥ Revised ~~deleted~~ Deleted ● Use Additional Digit(s)

Substance	Poisoning	External Cause (E Code)				
		Accident	Therapeutic Use	Suicide Attempt	Assault	Undetermined
Coal (carbon monoxide from) *(Continued)*						
tar NEC	983.0	E864.0	—	E950.7	E962.1	E980.6
fumes	987.8	E869.8	—	E952.8	E962.2	E982.8
medicinal (ointment)	976.4	E858.7	E946.4	E950.4	E962.0	E980.4
analgesics NEC	965.5	E850.5	E935.5	E950.0	E962.0	E980.0
naphtha (solvent)	981	E862.0	—	E950.9	E962.1	E980.9
Cobalt (fumes) (industrial)	985.8	E866.4	—	E950.9	E962.1	E980.9
Cobra (venom)	989.5	E905.0	—	E950.9	E962.1	E980.9
Coca (leaf)	970.81	E854.3	E940.8	E950.4	E962.0	E980.4
Cocaine (hydrochloride) (salt)	970.81	E854.3	E940.8	E950.4	E962.0	E980.4
topical anesthetic	968.5	E855.2	E938.5	E950.4	E962.0	E980.4
Coccidioidin	977.8	E858.8	E947.8	E950.4	E962.0	E980.4
Cocculus indicus	988.2	E865.3	—	E950.9	E962.1	E980.9
Cochineal	989.89	E866.8	—	E950.9	E962.1	E980.9
medicinal products	977.4	E858.8	E947.4	E950.4	E962.0	E980.4
Codeine	965.09	E850.2	E935.2	E950.0	E962.0	E980.0
Coffee	989.89	E866.8	—	E950.9	E962.1	E980.9
Cogentin	971.1	E855.4	E941.1	E950.4	E962.0	E980.4
Coke fumes or gas (carbon monoxide)	986	E868.3	—	E952.1	E962.2	E982.1
industrial use	986	E868.8	—	E952.1	E962.2	E982.1
Colace	973.2	E858.4	E943.2	E950.4	E962.0	E980.4
Colchicine	974.7	E858.5	E944.7	E950.4	E962.0	E980.4
Colchicum	988.2	E865.3	—	E950.9	E962.1	E980.9
Cold cream	976.3	E858.7	E946.3	E950.4	E962.0	E980.4
Colestipol	972.2	E858.3	E942.2	E950.4	E962.0	E980.4
Colistimethate	960.8	E856	E930.8	E950.4	E962.0	E980.4
Colistin	960.8	E856	E930.8	E950.4	E962.0	E980.4
Collagen	977.8	E866.8	E947.8	E950.9	E962.1	E980.9
Collagenase	976.8	E858.7	E946.8	E950.4	E962.0	E980.4
Collodion (flexible)	976.3	E858.7	E946.3	E950.4	E962.0	E980.4
Colocynth	973.1	E858.4	E943.1	E950.4	E962.0	E980.4
Coloring matter - *see* Dye(s)	—	—	—	—	—	—
Combustion gas - *see* Carbon, monoxide	—	—	—	—	—	—
Compazine	969.1	E853.0	E939.1	E950.3	E962.0	E980.3
Compound	—	—	—	—	—	—
42 (warfarin)	989.4	E863.7	—	E950.6	E962.1	E980.7
269 (endrin)	989.2	E863.0	—	E950.6	E962.1	E980.7
497 (dieldrin)	989.2	E863.0	—	E950.6	E962.1	E980.7

◀ New ◀◀ Revised ~~deleted~~ Deleted ● Use Additional Digit(s)

Substance	Poisoning	External Cause (E Code)				
		Accident	Therapeutic Use	Suicide Attempt	Assault	Undetermined
Compound *(Continued)*						
1080 (sodium fluoroacetate)	989.4	E863.7	—	E950.6	E962.1	E980.7
3422 (parathion)	989.3	E863.1	—	E950.6	E962.1	E980.7
3911 (phorate)	989.3	E863.1	—	E950.6	E962.1	E980.7
3956 (toxaphene)	989.2	E863.0	—	E950.6	E962.1	E980.7
4049 (malathion)	989.3	E863.1	—	E950.6	E962.1	E980.7
4124 (dicapthon)	989.4	E863.4	—	E950.6	E962.1	E980.7
E (cortisone)	962.0	E858.0	E932.0	E950.4	E962.0	E980.4
F (hydrocortisone)	962.0	E858.0	E932.0	E950.4	E962.0	E980.4
Congo red	977.8	E858.8	E947.8	E950.4	E962.0	E980.4
Coniine, conine	965.7	E850.7	E935.7	E950.0	E962.0	E980.0
Conium (maculatum)	988.2	E865.4	—	E950.9	E962.1	E980.9
Conjugated estrogens (equine)	962.2	E858.0	E932.2	E950.4	E962.0	E980.4
Contac	975.6	E858.6	E945.6	E950.4	E962.0	E980.4
Contact lens solution	976.5	E858.7	E946.5	E950.4	E962.0	E980.4
Contraceptives (oral)	962.2	E858.0	E932.2	E950.4	E962.0	E980.4
vaginal	976.8	E858.7	E946.8	E950.4	E962.0	E980.4
Contrast media (roentgenographic)	977.8	E858.8	E947.8	E950.4	E962.0	E980.4
Convallaria majalis	988.2	E865.4	—	E950.9	E962.1	E980.9
Copper (dust) (fumes) (salts) NEC	985.8	E866.4	—	E950.9	E962.1	E980.9
arsenate, arsenite	985.1	E866.3	—	E950.8	E962.1	E980.8
insecticide	985.1	E863.4	—	E950.8	E962.1	E980.8
emetic	973.6	E858.4	E943.6	E950.4	E962.0	E980.4
fungicide	985.8	E863.6	—	E950.6	E962.1	E980.7
insecticide	985.8	E863.4	—	E950.6	E962.1	E980.7
oleate	976.0	E858.7	E946.0	E950.4	E962.0	E980.4
sulfate	983.9	E864.3	—	E950.7	E962.1	E980.6
fungicide	983.9	E863.6	—	E950.7	E962.1	E980.6
cupric	973.6	E858.4	E943.6	E950.4	E962.0	E980.4
cuprous	983.9	E864.3	—	E950.7	E962.1	E980.6
Copperhead snake (bite) (venom)	989.5	E905.0	—	E950.9	E962.1	E980.9
Coral (sting)	989.5	E905.6	—	E950.9	E962.1	E980.9
snake (bite) (venom)	989.5	E905.0	—	E950.9	E962.1	E980.9
Cordran	976.0	E858.7	E946.0	E950.4	E962.0	E980.4
Corn cures	976.4	E858.7	E946.4	E950.4	E962.0	E980.4
Cornhusker's lotion	976.3	E858.7	E946.3	E950.4	E962.0	E980.4
Corn starch	976.3	E858.7	E946.3	E950.4	E962.0	E980.4
Corrosive	983.9	E864.4	—	E950.7	E962.1	E980.6
acids NEC	983.1	E864.1	—	E950.7	E962.1	E980.6

Substance	Poisoning	External Cause (E Code)				
		Accident	Therapeutic Use	Suicide Attempt	Assault	Undetermined
Corrosive *(Continued)*						
aromatics	983.0	E864.0	—	E950.7	E962.1	E980.6
disinfectant	983.0	E861.4	—	E950.7	E962.1	E980.6
fumes NEC	987.9	E869.9	—	E952.9	E962.2	E982.9
specified NEC	983.9	E864.3	—	E950.7	E962.1	E980.6
sublimate - *see* Mercury, chloride	—	—	—	—	—	—
Cortate	962.0	E858.0	E932.0	E950.4	E962.0	E980.4
Cort-Dome	962.0	E858.0	E932.0	E950.4	E962.0	E980.4
ENT agent	976.6	E858.7	E946.6	E950.4	E962.0	E980.4
ophthalmic preparation	976.5	E858.7	E946.5	E950.4	E962.0	E980.4
topical NEC	976.0	E858.7	E946.0	E950.4	E962.0	E980.4
Cortef	962.0	E858.0	E932.0	E950.4	E962.0	E980.4
ENT agent	976.6	E858.7	E946.6	E950.4	E962.0	E980.4
ophthalmic preparation	976.5	E858.7	E946.5	E950.4	E962.0	E980.4
topical NEC	976.0	E858.7	E946.0	E950.4	E962.0	E980.4
Corticosteroids (fluorinated)	962.0	E858.0	E932.0	E950.4	E962.0	E980.4
ENT agent	976.6	E858.7	E946.6	E950.4	E962.0	E980.4
ophthalmic preparation	976.5	E858.7	E946.5	E950.4	E962.0	E980.4
topical NEC	976.0	E858.7	E946.0	E950.4	E962.0	E980.4
Corticotropin	962.4	E858.0	E932.4	E950.4	E962.0	E980.4
Cortisol	962.0	E858.0	E932.0	E950.4	E962.0	E980.4
ENT agent	976.6	E858.7	E946.6	E950.4	E962.0	E980.4
ophthalmic preparation	976.5	E858.7	E946.5	E950.4	E962.0	E980.4
topical NEC	976.0	E858.7	E946.0	E950.4	E962.0	E980.4
Cortisone derivatives (acetate)	962.0	E858.0	E932.0	E950.4	E962.0	E980.4
ENT agent	976.6	E858.7	E946.6	E950.4	E962.0	E980.4
ophthalmic preparation	976.5	E858.7	E946.5	E950.4	E962.0	E980.4
topical NEC	976.0	E858.7	E946.0	E950.4	E962.0	E980.4
Cortogen	962.0	E858.0	E932.0	E950.4	E962.0	E980.4
ENT agent	976.6	E858.7	E946.6	E950.4	E962.0	E980.4
ophthalmic preparation	976.5	E858.7	E946.5	E950.4	E962.0	E980.4
Cortone	962.0	E858.0	E932.0	E950.4	E962.0	E980.4
ENT agent	976.6	E858.7	E946.6	E950.4	E962.0	E980.4
ophthalmic preparation	976.5	E858.7	E946.5	E950.4	E962.0	E980.4
Cortril	962.0	E858.0	E932.0	E950.4	E962.0	E980.4
ENT agent	976.6	E858.7	E946.6	E950.4	E962.0	E980.4
ophthalmic preparation	976.5	E858.7	E946.5	E950.4	E962.0	E980.4
topical NEC	976.0	E858.7	E946.0	E950.4	E962.0	E980.4
Cosmetics	989.89	E866.7	—	E950.9	E962.1	E980.9

◀ New   ◀▥ Revised   ~~deleted~~ Deleted   ● Use Additional Digit(s)

Substance	Poisoning	External Cause (E Code)				
		Accident	Therapeutic Use	Suicide Attempt	Assault	Undetermined
Cosyntropin	977.8	E858.8	E947.8	E950.4	E962.0	E980.4
Cotarnine	964.5	E858.2	E934.5	E950.4	E962.0	E980.4
Cottonseed oil	976.3	E858.7	E946.3	E950.4	E962.0	E980.4
Cough mixtures (antitussives)	975.4	E858.6	E945.4	E950.4	E962.0	E980.4
containing opiates	965.09	E850.2	E935.2	E950.0	E962.0	E980.0
expectorants	975.5	E858.6	E945.5	E950.4	E962.0	E980.4
Coumadin	964.2	E858.2	E934.2	E950.4	E962.0	E980.4
rodenticide	989.4	E863.7	—	E950.6	E962.1	E980.7
Coumarin	964.2	E858.2	E934.2	E950.4	E962.0	E980.4
Coumetarol	964.2	E858.2	E934.2	E950.4	E962.0	E980.4
Cowbane	988.2	E865.4	—	E950.9	E962.1	E980.9
Cozyme	963.5	E858.1	E933.5	E950.4	E962.0	E980.4
Crack	970.81	E854.3	E940.8	E950.4	E962.0	E980.4
Creolin	983.0	E864.0	—	E950.7	E962.1	E980.6
disinfectant	983.0	E861.4	—	E950.7	E962.1	E980.6
Creosol (compound)	983.0	E864.0	—	E950.7	E962.1	E980.6
Creosote (beechwood) (coal tar)	983.0	E864.0	—	E950.7	E962.1	E980.6
medicinal (expectorant)	975.5	E858.6	E945.5	E950.4	E962.0	E980.4
syrup	975.5	E858.6	E945.5	E950.4	E962.0	E980.4
Cresol	983.0	E864.0	—	E950.7	E962.1	E980.6
disinfectant	983.0	E861.4	—	E950.7	E962.1	E980.6
Cresylic acid	983.0	E864.0	—	E950.7	E962.1	E980.6
Cropropamide	965.7	E850.7	E935.7	E950.0	E962.0	E980.0
with crotethamide	970.0	E854.3	E940.0	E950.4	E962.0	E980.4
Crotamiton	976.0	E858.7	E946.0	E950.4	E962.0	E980.4
Crotethamide	965.7	E850.7	E935.7	E950.0	E962.0	E980.0
with cropropamide	970.0	E854.3	E940.0	E950.4	E962.0	E980.4
Croton (oil)	973.1	E858.4	E943.1	E950.4	E962.0	E980.4
chloral	967.1	E852.0	E937.1	E950.2	E962.0	E980.2
Crude oil	981	E862.1	—	E950.9	E962.1	E980.9
Cryogenine	965.8	E850.8	E935.8	E950.0	E962.0	E980.0
Cryolite (pesticide)	989.4	E863.4	—	E950.6	E962.1	E980.7
Cryptenamine	972.6	E858.3	E942.6	E950.4	E962.0	E980.4
Crystal violet	976.0	E858.7	E946.0	E950.4	E962.0	E980.4
Cuckoopint	988.2	E865.4	—	E950.9	E962.1	E980.9
Cumetharol	964.2	E858.2	E934.2	E950.4	E962.0	E980.4
Cupric sulfate	973.6	E858.4	E943.6	E950.4	E962.0	E980.4
Cuprous sulfate	983.9	E864.3	—	E950.7	E962.1	E980.6
Curare, curarine	975.2	E858.6	E945.2	E950.4	E962.0	E980.4

◀ New　◀▥ Revised　~~deleted~~ Deleted　● Use Additional Digit(s)

Substance	Poisoning	External Cause (E Code)				
		Accident	Therapeutic Use	Suicide Attempt	Assault	Undetermined
Cyanic acid - *see* Cyanide(s)	—	—	—	—	—	—
Cyanide(s) (compounds) (hydrogen) (potassium) (sodium) NEC	989.0	E866.8	—	E950.9	E962.1	E980.9
dust or gas (inhalation) NEC	987.7	E869.8	—	E952.8	E962.2	E982.8
fumigant	989.0	E863.8	—	E950.6	E962.1	E980.7
mercuric - *see* Mercury	—	—	—	—	—	—
pesticide (dust) (fumes)	989.0	E863.4	—	E950.6	E962.1	E980.7
Cyanocobalamin	964.1	E858.2	E934.1	E950.4	E962.0	E980.4
Cyanogen (chloride) (gas)	—	—	—	—	—	—
NEC	987.8	E869.8	—	E952.8	E962.2	E982.8
Cyclaine	968.5	E855.2	E938.5	E950.4	E962.0	E980.4
Cyclamen europaeum	988.2	E865.4	—	E950.9	E962.1	E980.9
Cyclandelate	972.5	E858.3	E942.5	E950.4	E962.0	E980.4
Cyclazocine	965.09	E850.2	E935.2	E950.0	E962.0	E980.0
Cyclizine	963.0	E858.1	E933.0	E950.4	E962.0	E980.4
Cyclobarbital, cyclobarbitone	967.0	E851	E937.0	E950.1	E962.0	E980.1
Cycloguanil	961.4	E857	E931.4	E950.4	E962.0	E980.4
Cyclohexane	982.0	E862.4	—	E950.9	E962.1	E980.9
Cyclohexanol	980.8	E860.8	—	E950.9	E962.1	E980.9
Cyclohexanone	982.8	E862.4	—	E950.9	E962.1	E980.9
Cyclomethycaine	968.5	E855.2	E938.5	E950.4	E962.0	E980.4
Cyclopentamine	971.2	E855.5	E941.2	E950.4	E962.0	E980.4
Cyclopenthiazide	974.3	E858.5	E944.3	E950.4	E962.0	E980.4
Cyclopentolate	971.1	E855.4	E941.1	E950.4	E962.0	E980.4
Cyclophosphamide	963.1	E858.1	E933.1	E950.4	E962.0	E980.4
Cyclopropane	968.2	E855.1	E938.2	E950.4	E962.0	E980.4
Cycloserine	960.6	E856	E930.6	E950.4	E962.0	E980.4
Cyclothiazide	974.3	E858.5	E944.3	E950.4	E962.0	E980.4
Cycrimine	966.4	E855.0	E936.4	E950.4	E962.0	E980.4
Cymarin	972.1	E858.3	E942.1	E950.4	E962.0	E980.4
Cyproheptadine	963.0	E858.1	E933.0	E950.4	E962.0	E980.4
Cyprolidol	969.09	E854.0	E939.0	E950.3	E962.0	E980.3
Cytarabine	963.1	E858.1	E933.1	E950.4	E962.0	E980.4
Cytisus	—	—	—	—	—	—
laburnum	988.2	E865.4	—	E950.9	E962.1	E980.9
scoparius	988.2	E865.4	—	E950.9	E962.1	E980.9
Cytomel	962.7	E858.0	E932.7	E950.4	E962.0	E980.4
Cytosine (antineoplastic)	963.1	E858.1	E933.1	E950.4	E962.0	E980.4
Cytoxan	963.1	E858.1	E933.1	E950.4	E962.0	E980.4
Dacarbazine	963.1	E858.1	E933.1	E950.4	E962.0	E980.4

◄ New   ◄ Revised   ~~deleted~~ Deleted   ● Use Additional Digit(s)

TABLE OF DRUGS AND CHEMICALS

Substance	Poisoning	External Cause (E Code)				
		Accident	Therapeutic Use	Suicide Attempt	Assault	Undetermined
Dactinomycin	960.7	E856	E930.7	E950.4	E962.0	E980.4
DADPS	961.8	E857	E931.8	E950.4	E962.0	E980.4
Dakin's solution (external)	976.0	E858.7	E946.0	E950.4	E962.0	E980.4
Dalmane	969.4	E853.2	E939.4	E950.3	E962.0	E980.3
DAM	977.2	E858.8	E947.2	E950.4	E962.0	E980.4
Danilone	964.2	E858.2	E934.2	E950.4	E962.0	E980.4
Danthron	973.1	E858.4	E943.1	E950.4	E962.0	E980.4
Dantrolene	975.2	E858.6	E945.2	E950.4	E962.0	E980.4
Daphne (gnidium) (mezereum)	988.2	E865.4	—	E950.9	E962.1	E980.9
berry	988.2	E865.3	—	E950.9	E962.1	E980.9
Dapsone	961.8	E857	E931.8	E950.4	E962.0	E980.4
Daraprim	961.4	E857	E931.4	E950.4	E962.0	E980.4
Darnel	988.2	E865.3	—	E950.9	E962.1	E980.9
Darvon	965.8	E850.8	E935.8	E950.0	E962.0	E980.0
Daunorubicin	960.7	E856	E930.7	E950.4	E962.0	E980.4
DBI	962.3	E858.0	E932.3	E950.4	E962.0	E980.4
D-Con (rodenticide)	989.4	E863.7	—	E950.6	E962.1	E980.7
DDS	961.8	E857	E931.8	E950.4	E962.0	E980.4
DDT	989.2	E863.0	—	E950.6	E962.1	E980.7
Deadly nightshade	988.2	E865.4	—	E950.9	E962.1	E980.9
berry	988.2	E865.3	—	E950.9	E962.1	E980.9
Deanol	969.79	E854.2	E939.7	E950.3	E962.0	E980.3
Debrisoquine	972.6	E858.3	E942.6	E950.4	E962.0	E980.4
Decaborane	989.89	E866.8	—	E950.9	E962.1	E980.9
fumes	987.8	E869.8	—	E952.8	E962.2	E982.8
Decadron	962.0	E858.0	E932.0	E950.4	E962.0	E980.4
ENT agent	976.6	E858.7	E946.6	E950.4	E962.0	E980.4
ophthalmic preparation	976.5	E858.7	E946.5	E950.4	E962.0	E980.4
topical NEC	976.0	E858.7	E946.0	E950.4	E962.0	E980.4
Decahydronaphthalene	982.0	E862.4	—	E950.9	E962.1	E980.9
Decalin	982.0	E862.4	—	E950.9	E962.1	E980.9
Decamethonium	975.2	E858.6	E945.2	E950.4	E962.0	E980.4
Decholin	973.4	E858.4	E943.4	E950.4	E962.0	E980.4
sodium (diagnostic)	977.8	E858.8	E947.8	E950.4	E962.0	E980.4
Declomycin	960.4	E856	E930.4	E950.4	E962.0	E980.4
Deferoxamine	963.8	E858.1	E933.8	E950.4	E962.0	E980.4
Dehydrocholic acid	973.4	E858.4	E943.4	E950.4	E962.0	E980.4
Dekalin	982.0	E862.4	—	E950.9	E962.1	E980.9
Delalutin	962.2	E858.0	E932.2	E950.4	E962.0	E980.4

◀ New　◀ Revised　deleted Deleted　● Use Additional Digit(s)

Substance	Poisoning	External Cause (E Code)				
		Accident	Therapeutic Use	Suicide Attempt	Assault	Undetermined
Delphinium	988.2	E865.3	—	E950.9	E962.1	E980.9
Deltasone	962.0	E858.0	E932.0	E950.4	E962.0	E980.4
Deltra	962.0	E858.0	E932.0	E950.4	E962.0	E980.4
Delvinal	967.0	E851	E937.0	E950.1	E962.0	E980.1
Demecarium (bromide)	971.0	E855.3	E941.0	E950.4	E962.0	E980.4
Demeclocycline	960.4	E856	E930.4	E950.4	E962.0	E980.4
Demecolcine	963.1	E858.1	E933.1	E950.4	E962.0	E980.4
Demelanizing agents	976.8	E858.7	E946.8	E950.4	E962.0	E980.4
Demerol	965.09	E850.2	E935.2	E950.0	E962.0	E980.0
Demethylchlortetracycline	960.4	E856	E930.4	E950.4	E962.0	E980.4
Demethyltetracycline	960.4	E856	E930.4	E950.4	E962.0	E980.4
Demeton	989.3	E863.1	—	E950.6	E962.1	E980.7
Demulcents	976.3	E858.7	E946.3	E950.4	E962.0	E980.4
Demulen	962.2	E858.0	E932.2	E950.4	E962.0	E980.4
Denatured alcohol	980.0	E860.1	—	E950.9	E962.1	E980.9
Dendrid	976.5	E858.7	E946.5	E950.4	E962.0	E980.4
Dental agents, topical	976.7	E858.7	E946.7	E950.4	E962.0	E980.4
Deodorant spray (feminine hygiene)	976.8	E858.7	E946.8	E950.4	E962.0	E980.4
Deoxyribonuclease	963.4	E858.1	E933.4	E950.4	E962.0	E980.4
Depressants	—	—	—	—	—	—
appetite, central	977.0	E858.8	E947.0	E950.4	E962.0	E980.4
cardiac	972.0	E858.3	E942.0	E950.4	E962.0	E980.4
central nervous system (anesthetic)	968.4	E855.1	E938.4	E950.4	E962.0	E980.4
psychotherapeutic	969.5	E853.9	E939.5	E950.3	E962.0	E980.3
Dequalinium	976.0	E858.7	E946.0	E950.4	E962.0	E980.4
Dermolate	976.2	E858.7	E946.2	E950.4	E962.0	E980.4
DES	962.2	E858.0	E932.2	E950.4	E962.0	E980.4
Desenex	976.0	E858.7	E946.0	E950.4	E962.0	E980.4
Deserpidine	972.6	E858.3	E942.6	E950.4	E962.0	E980.4
Desipramine	969.05	E854.0	E939.0	E950.3	E962.0	E980.3
Deslanoside	972.1	E858.3	E942.1	E950.4	E962.0	E980.4
Desocodeine	965.09	E850.2	E935.2	E950.0	E962.0	E980.0
Desomorphine	965.09	E850.2	E935.2	E950.0	E962.0	E980.0
Desonide	976.0	E858.7	E946.0	E950.4	E962.0	E980.4
Desoxycorticosterone derivatives	962.0	E858.0	E932.0	E950.4	E962.0	E980.4
Desoxyephedrine	969.72	E854.2	E939.7	E950.3	E962.0	E980.3
DET	969.6	E854.1	E939.6	E950.3	E962.0	E980.3
Detergents (ingested) (synthetic)	989.6	E861.0	—	E950.9	E962.1	E980.9
external medication	976.2	E858.7	E946.2	E950.4	E962.0	E980.4

◀ New   ◀≡ Revised   ~~deleted~~ Deleted   ● Use Additional Digit(s)

Substance	Poisoning	External Cause (E Code)				
		Accident	Therapeutic Use	Suicide Attempt	Assault	Undetermined
Deterrent, alcohol	977.3	E858.8	E947.3	E950.4	E962.0	E980.4
Detrothyronine	962.7	E858.0	E932.7	E950.4	E962.0	E980.4
Dettol (external medication)	976.0	E858.7	E946.0	E950.4	E962.0	E980.4
Dexamethasone	962.0	E858.0	E932.0	E950.4	E962.0	E980.4
ENT agent	976.6	E858.7	E946.6	E950.4	E962.0	E980.4
ophthalmic preparation	976.5	E858.7	E946.5	E950.4	E962.0	E980.4
topical NEC	976.0	E858.7	E946.0	E950.4	E962.0	E980.4
Dexamphetamine	969.72	E854.2	E939.7	E950.3	E962.0	E980.3
Dexedrine	969.72	E854.2	E939.7	E950.3	E962.0	E980.3
Dexpanthenol	963.5	E858.1	E933.5	E950.4	E962.0	E980.4
Dextran	964.8	E858.2	E934.8	E950.4	E962.0	E980.4
Dextriferron	964.0	E858.2	E934.0	E950.4	E962.0	E980.4
Dextroamphetamine	969.72	E854.2	E939.7	E950.3	E962.0	E980.3
Dextro calcium pantothenate	963.5	E858.1	E933.5	E950.4	E962.0	E980.4
Dextromethorphan	975.4	E858.6	E945.4	E950.4	E962.0	E980.4
Dextromoramide	965.09	E850.2	E935.2	E950.0	E962.0	E980.0
Dextro pantothenyl alcohol	963.5	E858.1	E933.5	E950.4	E962.0	E980.4
topical	976.8	E858.7	E946.8	E950.4	E962.0	E980.4
Dextropropoxyphene (hydrochloride)	965.8	E850.8	E935.8	E950.0	E962.0	E980.0
Dextrorphan	965.09	E850.2	E935.2	E950.0	E962.0	E980.0
Dextrose NEC	974.5	E858.5	E944.5	E950.4	E962.0	E980.4
Dextrothyroxine	962.7	E858.0	E932.7	E950.4	E962.0	E980.4
DFP	971.0	E855.3	E941.0	E950.4	E962.0	E980.4
DHE-45	972.9	E858.3	E942.9	E950.4	E962.0	E980.4
Diabinese	962.3	E858.0	E932.3	E950.4	E962.0	E980.4
Diacetyl monoxime	977.2	E858.8	E947.2	E950.4	E962.0	E980.4
Diacetylmorphine	965.01	E850.0	E935.0	E950.0	E962.0	E980.0
Diagnostic agents	977.8	E858.8	E947.8	E950.4	E962.0	E980.4
Dial (soap)	976.2	E858.7	E946.2	E950.4	E962.0	E980.4
sedative	967.0	E851	E937.0	E950.1	E962.0	E980.1
Diallylbarbituric acid	967.0	E851	E937.0	E950.1	E962.0	E980.1
Diaminodiphenyisulfone	961.8	E857	E931.8	E950.4	E962.0	E980.4
Diamorphine	965.01	E850.0	E935.0	E950.0	E962.0	E980.0
Diamox	974.2	E858.5	E944.2	E950.4	E962.0	E980.4
Diamthazole	976.0	E858.7	E946.0	E950.4	E962.0	E980.4
Diaphenyisulfone	961.8	E857	E931.8	E950.4	E962.0	E980.4
Diasone (sodium)	961.8	E857	E931.8	E950.4	E962.0	E980.4
Diazepam	969.4	E853.2	E939.4	E950.3	E962.0	E980.3
Diazinon	989.3	E863.1	—	E950.6	E962.1	E980.7

TABLE OF DRUGS AND CHEMICALS

Substance	Poisoning	External Cause (E Code)				
		Accident	Therapeutic Use	Suicide Attempt	Assault	Undetermined
Diazomethane (gas)	987.8	E869.8	—	E952.8	E962.2	E982.8
Diazoxide	972.5	E858.3	E942.5	E950.4	E962.0	E980.4
Dibenamine	971.3	E855.6	E941.3	E950.4	E962.0	E980.4
Dibenzheptropine	963.0	E858.1	E933.0	E950.4	E962.0	E980.4
Dibenzyline	971.3	E855.6	E941.3	E950.4	E962.0	E980.4
Diborane (gas)	987.8	E869.8	—	E952.8	E962.2	E982.8
Dibromomannitol	963.1	E858.1	E933.1	E950.4	E962.0	E980.4
Dibucaine (spinal)	968.7	E855.2	E938.7	E950.4	E962.0	E980.4
topical (surface)	968.5	E855.2	E938.5	E950.4	E962.0	E980.4
Dibunate sodium	975.4	E858.6	E945.4	E950.4	E962.0	E980.4
Dibutoline	971.1	E855.4	E941.1	E950.4	E962.0	E980.4
Dicapthon	989.4	E863.4	—	E950.6	E962.1	E980.7
Dichloralphenazone	967.1	E852.0	E937.1	E950.2	E962.0	E980.2
Dichlorodifluoromethane	987.4	E869.2	—	E952.8	E962.2	E982.8
Dichloroethane	982.3	E862.4	—	E950.9	E961.1	E980.9
Dichloroethylene	982.3	E862.4	—	E950.9	E961.1	E980.9
Dichloroethyl sulfide	987.8	E869.8	—	E952.8	E962.2	E982.8
Dichlorohydrin	982.3	E862.4	—	E950.9	E961.1	E980.9
Dichloromethane (solvent) (vapor)	982.3	E862.4	—	E950.9	E961.1	E980.9
Dichlorophen(e)	961.6	E857	E931.6	E950.4	E962.0	E980.4
Dichlorphenamide	974.2	E858.5	E944.2	E950.4	E962.0	E980.4
Dichlorvos	989.3	E863.1	—	E950.6	E962.1	E980.7
Diclofenac sodium	965.69	E850.6	E935.6	E950.0	E962.0	E980.0
Dicoumarin, dicumarol	964.2	E858.2	E934.2	E950.4	E962.0	E980.4
Dicyanogen (gas)	987.8	E869.8	—	E952.8	E962.2	E982.8
Dicyclomine	971.1	E855.4	E941.1	E950.4	E962.0	E980.4
Dieldrin (vapor)	989.2	E863.0	—	E950.6	E962.1	E980.7
Dienestrol	962.2	E858.0	E932.2	E950.4	E962.0	E980.4
Dietetics	977.0	E858.8	E947.0	E950.4	E962.0	E980.4
Diethazine	966.4	E855.0	E936.4	E950.4	E962.0	E980.4
Diethyl	—	—	—	—	—	—
barbituric acid	967.0	E851	E937.0	E950.1	E962.0	E980.1
carbamazine	961.6	E857	E931.6	E950.4	E962.0	E980.4
carbinol	980.8	E860.8	—	E950.9	E962.1	E980.9
carbonate	982.8	E862.4	—	E950.9	E962.1	E980.9
ether (vapor) - see Ether(s)	—	—	—	—	—	—
propion	977.0	E858.8	E947.0	E950.4	E962.0	E980.4
stilbestrol	962.2	E858.0	E932.2	E950.4	E962.0	E980.4

◄ New ◄▦ Revised ~~deleted~~ Deleted ● Use Additional Digit(s)

Substance	Poisoning	External Cause (E Code)				
		Accident	Therapeutic Use	Suicide Attempt	Assault	Undetermined
Diethylene	—	—	—	—	—	—
dioxide	982.8	E862.4	—	E950.9	E962.1	E980.9
glycol (monoacetate) (monoethyl ether)	982.8	E862.4	—	E950.9	E962.1	E980.9
Diethylsulfone-diethylmethane	967.8	E852.8	E937.8	E950.2	E962.0	E980.2
Difencloxazine	965.09	E850.2	E935.2	E950.0	E962.0	E980.0
Diffusin	963.4	E858.1	E933.4	E950.4	E962.0	E980.4
Diflos	971.0	E855.3	E941.0	E950.4	E962.0	E980.4
Digestants	973.4	E858.4	E943.4	E950.4	E962.0	E980.4
Digitalin(e)	972.1	E858.3	E942.1	E950.4	E962.0	E980.4
Digitalis glycosides	972.1	E858.3	E942.1	E950.4	E962.0	E980.4
Digitoxin	972.1	E858.3	E942.1	E950.4	E962.0	E980.4
Digoxin	972.1	E858.3	E942.1	E950.4	E962.0	E980.4
Dihydrocodeine	965.09	E850.2	E935.2	E950.0	E962.0	E980.0
Dihydrocodeinone	965.09	E850.2	E935.2	E950.0	E962.0	E980.0
Dihydroergocristine	972.9	E858.3	E942.9	E950.4	E962.0	E980.4
Dihydroergotamine	972.9	E858.3	E942.9	E950.4	E962.0	E980.4
Dihydroergotoxine	972.9	E858.3	E942.9	E950.4	E962.0	E980.4
Dihydrohydroxycodeinone	965.09	E850.2	E935.2	E950.0	E962.0	E980.0
Dihydrohydroxymorphinone	965.09	E850.2	E935.2	E950.0	E962.0	E980.0
Dihydroisocodeine	965.09	E850.2	E935.2	E950.0	E962.0	E980.0
Dihydromorphine	965.09	E850.2	E935.2	E950.0	E962.0	E980.0
Dihydromorphinone	965.09	E850.2	E935.2	E950.0	E962.0	E980.0
Dihydrostreptomycin	960.6	E856	E930.6	E950.4	E962.0	E980.4
Dihydrotachysterol	962.6	E858.0	E932.6	E950.4	E962.0	E980.4
Dihydroxyanthraquinone	973.1	E858.4	E943.1	E950.4	E962.0	E980.4
Dihydroxycodeinone	965.09	E850.2	E935.2	E950.0	E962.0	E980.0
Diiodohydroxyquin	961.3	E857	E931.3	E950.4	E962.0	E980.4
topical	976.0	E858.7	E946.0	E950.4	E962.0	E980.4
Diiodohydroxyquinoline	961.3	E857	E931.3	E950.4	E962.0	E980.4
Dilantin	966.1	E855.0	E936.1	E950.4	E962.0	E980.4
Dilaudid	965.09	E850.2	E935.2	E950.0	E962.0	E980.0
Diloxanide	961.5	E857	E931.5	E950.4	E962.0	E980.4
Dimefline	970.0	E854.3	E940.0	E950.4	E962.0	E980.4
Dimenhydrinate	963.0	E858.1	E933.0	E950.4	E962.0	E980.4
Dimercaprol	963.8	E858.1	E933.8	E950.4	E962.0	E980.4
Dimercaptopropanol	963.8	E858.1	E933.8	E950.4	E962.0	E980.4
Dimetane	963.0	E858.1	E933.0	E950.4	E962.0	E980.4
Dimethicone	976.3	E858.7	E946.3	E950.4	E962.0	E980.4
Dimethindene	963.0	E858.1	E933.0	E950.4	E962.0	E980.4

◄ New   ⬅ Revised   ~~deleted~~ Deleted   ● Use Additional Digit(s)

TABLE OF DRUGS AND CHEMICALS

Substance	Poisoning	External Cause (E Code)				
		Accident	Therapeutic Use	Suicide Attempt	Assault	Undetermined
Dimethisoquin	968.5	E855.2	E938.5	E950.4	E962.0	E980.4
Dimethisterone	962.2	E858.0	E932.2	E950.4	E962.0	E980.4
Dimethoxanate	975.4	E858.6	E945.4	E950.4	E962.0	E980.4
Dimethyl	—	—	—	—	—	—
arsine, arsinic acid - *see* Arsenic	—	—	—	—	—	—
carbinol	980.2	E860.3	—	E950.9	E962.1	E980.9
diguanide	962.3	E858.0	E932.3	E950.4	E962.0	E980.4
ketone	982.8	E862.4	—	E950.9	E962.1	E980.9
vapor	987.8	E869.8	—	E952.8	E962.2	E982.8
meperidine	965.09	E850.2	E935.2	E950.0	E962.0	E980.0
parathion	989.3	E863.1	—	E950.6	E962.1	E980.7
polysiloxane	973.8	E858.4	E943.8	E950.4	E962.0	E980.4
sulfate (fumes)	987.8	E869.8	—	E952.8	E962.2	E982.8
liquid	983.9	E864.3	—	E950.7	E962.1	E980.6
sulfoxide NEC	982.8	E862.4	—	E950.9	E962.1	E980.9
medicinal	976.4	E858.7	E946.4	E950.4	E962.0	E980.4
triptamine	969.6	E854.1	E939.6	E950.3	E962.0	E980.3
tubocurarine	975.2	E858.6	E945.2	E950.4	E962.0	E980.4
Dindevan	964.2	E858.2	E934.2	E950.4	E962.0	E980.4
Dinitro (-ortho-) cresol (herbicide) (spray)	989.4	E863.5	—	E950.6	E962.1	E980.7
insecticide	989.4	E863.4	—	E950.6	E962.1	E980.7
Dinitrobenzene	983.0	E864.0	—	E950.7	E962.1	E980.6
vapor	987.8	E869.8	—	E952.8	E962.2	E982.8
Dinitro-orthocresol (herbicide)	989.4	E863.5	—	E950.6	E962.1	E980.7
insecticide	989.4	E863.4	—	E950.6	E962.1	E980.7
Dinitrophenol (herbicide) (spray)	989.4	E863.5	—	E950.6	E962.1	E980.7
insecticide	989.4	E863.4	—	E950.6	E962.1	E980.7
Dinoprost	975.0	E858.6	E945.0	E950.4	E962.0	E980.4
Dioctyl sulfosuccinate (calcium) (sodium)	973.2	E858.4	E943.2	E950.4	E962.0	E980.4
Diodoquin	961.3	E857	E931.3	E950.4	E962.0	E980.4
Dione derivatives NEC	966.3	E855.0	E936.3	E950.4	E962.0	E980.4
Dionin	965.09	E850.2	E935.2	E950.0	E962.0	E980.0
Dioxane	982.8	E862.4	—	E950.9	E962.1	E980.9
Dioxin - *see* herbicide	—	—	—	—	—	—
Dioxyline	972.5	E858.3	E942.5	E950.4	E962.0	E980.4
Dipentene	982.8	E862.4	—	E950.9	E962.1	E980.9
Diphemanil	971.1	E855.4	E941.1	E950.4	E962.0	E980.4
Diphenadione	964.2	E858.2	E934.2	E950.4	E962.0	E980.4
Diphenhydramine	963.0	E858.1	E933.0	E950.4	E962.0	E980.4

◀ New ◀⃒ Revised ~~deleted~~ Deleted ● Use Additional Digit(s)

Substance	Poisoning	External Cause (E Code)				
		Accident	Therapeutic Use	Suicide Attempt	Assault	Undetermined
Diphenidol	963.0	E858.1	E933.0	E950.4	E962.0	E980.4
Diphenoxylate	973.5	E858.4	E943.5	E950.4	E962.0	E980.4
Diphenylchlorarsine	985.1	E866.3	—	E950.8	E962.1	E980.8
Diphenylhydantoin (sodium)	966.1	E855.0	E936.1	E950.4	E962.0	E980.4
Diphenylpyraline	963.0	E858.1	E933.0	E950.4	E962.0	E980.4
Diphtheria	—	—	—	—	—	—
antitoxin	979.9	E858.8	E949.9	E950.4	E962.0	E980.4
toxoid	978.5	E858.8	E948.5	E950.4	E962.0	E980.4
with tetanus toxoid	978.9	E858.8	E948.9	E950.4	E962.0	E980.4
with pertussis component	978.6	E858.8	E948.6	E950.4	E962.0	E980.4
vaccine	978.5	E858.8	E948.5	E950.4	E962.0	E980.4
Dipipanone	965.09	E850.2	E935.2	E950.0	E962.0	E980.0
Diplovax	979.5	E858.8	E949.5	E950.4	E962.0	E980.4
Diprophylline	975.1	E858.6	E945.1	E950.4	E962.0	E980.4
Dipyridamole	972.4	E858.3	E942.4	E950.4	E962.0	E980.4
Dipyrone	965.5	E850.5	E935.5	E950.0	E962.0	E980.0
Diquat	989.4	E863.5	—	E950.6	E962.1	E980.7
Disinfectant NEC	983.9	E861.4	—	E950.7	E962.1	E980.6
alkaline	983.2	E861.4	—	E950.7	E962.1	E980.6
aromatic	983.0	E861.4	—	E950.7	E962.1	E980.6
Disipal	966.4	E855.0	E936.4	E950.4	E962.0	E980.4
Disodium edetate	963.8	E858.1	E933.8	E950.4	E962.0	E980.4
Disulfamide	974.4	E858.5	E944.4	E950.4	E962.0	E980.4
Disulfanilamide	961.0	E857	E931.0	E950.4	E962.0	E980.4
Disulfiram	977.3	E858.8	E947.3	E950.4	E962.0	E980.4
Dithiazanine	961.6	E857	E931.6	E950.4	E962.0	E980.4
Dithioglycerol	963.8	E858.1	E933.8	E950.4	E962.0	E980.4
Dithranol	976.4	E858.7	E946.4	E950.4	E962.0	E980.4
Diucardin	974.3	E858.5	E944.3	E950.4	E962.0	E980.4
Diupres	974.3	E858.5	E944.3	E950.4	E962.0	E980.4
Diuretics NEC	974.4	E858.5	E944.4	E950.4	E962.0	E980.4
carbonic acid anhydrase inhibitors	974.2	E858.5	E944.2	E950.4	E962.0	E980.4
mercurial	974.0	E858.5	E944.0	E950.4	E962.0	E980.4
osmotic	974.4	E858.5	E944.4	E950.4	E962.0	E980.4
purine derivatives	974.1	E858.5	E944.1	E950.4	E962.0	E980.4
saluretic	974.3	E858.5	E944.3	E950.4	E962.0	E980.4
Diuril	974.3	E858.5	E944.3	E950.4	E962.0	E980.4
Divinyl ether	968.2	E855.1	E938.2	E950.4	E962.0	E980.4
D-lysergic acid diethylamide	969.6	E854.1	E939.6	E950.3	E962.0	E980.3

TABLE OF DRUGS AND CHEMICALS

Substance	Poisoning	External Cause (E Code)				
		Accident	Therapeutic Use	Suicide Attempt	Assault	Undetermined
DMCT	960.4	E856	E930.4	E950.4	E962.0	E980.4
DMSO	982.8	E862.4	—	E950.9	E962.1	E980.9
DMT	969.6	E854.1	E939.6	E950.3	E962.0	E980.3
DNOC	989.4	E863.5	—	E950.6	E962.1	E980.7
DOCA	962.0	E858.0	E932.0	E950.4	E962.0	E980.4
Dolophine	965.02	E850.1	E935.1	E950.0	E962.0	E980.0
Doloxene	965.8	E850.8	E935.8	E950.0	E962.0	E980.0
DOM	969.6	E854.1	E939.6	E950.3	E962.0	E980.3
Domestic gas - see Gas, utility	—	—	—	—	—	—
Domiphen (bromide) (lozenges)	976.6	E858.7	E946.6	E950.4	E962.0	E980.4
Dopa (levo)	966.4	E855.0	E936.4	E950.4	E962.0	E980.4
Dopamine	971.2	E855.5	E941.2	E950.4	E962.0	E980.4
Doriden	967.5	E852.4	E937.5	E950.2	E962.0	E980.2
Dormiral	967.0	E851	E937.0	E950.1	E962.0	E980.1
Dormison	967.8	E852.8	E937.8	E950.2	E962.0	E980.2
Dornase	963.4	E858.1	E933.4	E950.4	E962.0	E980.4
Dorsacaine	968.5	E855.2	E938.5	E950.4	E962.0	E980.4
Dothiepin hydrochloride	969.05	E854.0	E939.0	E950.3	E962.0	E980.3
Doxapram	970.0	E854.3	E940.0	E950.4	E962.0	E980.4
Doxepin	969.05	E854.0	E939.0	E950.3	E962.0	E980.3
Doxorubicin	960.7	E856	E930.7	E950.4	E962.0	E980.4
Doxycycline	960.4	E856	E930.4	E950.4	E962.0	E980.4
Doxylamine	963.0	E858.1	E933.0	E950.4	E962.0	E980.4
Dramamine	963.0	E858.1	E933.0	E950.4	E962.0	E980.4
Drano (drain cleaner)	983.2	E864.2	—	E950.7	E962.1	E980.6
Dromoran	965.09	E850.2	E935.2	E950.0	E962.0	E980.0
Dromostanolone	962.1	E858.0	E932.1	E950.4	E962.0	E980.4
Droperidol	969.2	E853.1	E939.2	E950.3	E962.0	E980.3
Drotrecogin alfa	964.2	E858.2	E934.2	E950.4	E962.0	E980.4
Drug	977.9	E858.9	E947.9	E950.5	E962.0	E980.5
specified NEC	977.8	E858.8	E947.8	E950.4	E962.0	E980.4
AHFS List	—	—	—	—	—	—
4:00 antihistamine drugs	963.0	E858.1	E933.0	E950.4	E962.0	E980.4
8:04 amebacides	961.5	E857	E931.5	E950.4	E962.0	E980.4
arsenical anti-infectives	961.1	E857	E931.1	E950.4	E962.0	E980.4
quinoline derivatives	961.3	E857	E931.3	E950.4	E962.0	E980.4
8:08 anthelmintics	961.6	E857	E931.6	E950.4	E962.0	E980.4
quinoline derivatives	961.3	E857	E931.3	E950.4	E962.0	E980.4
8:12.04 antifungal antibiotics	960.1	E856	E930.1	E950.4	E962.0	E980.4

◀ New ◀▥ Revised ~~deleted~~ Deleted ● Use Additional Digit(s)

Substance	Poisoning	External Cause (E Code)				
		Accident	Therapeutic Use	Suicide Attempt	Assault	Undetermined
Drug *(Continued)*						
8:12.06 cephalosporins	960.5	E856	E930.5	E950.4	E962.0	E980.4
8:12.08 chloramphenicol	960.2	E856	E930.2	E950.4	E962.0	E980.4
8:12.12 erythromycins	960.3	E856	E930.3	E950.4	E962.0	E980.4
8:12.16 penicillins	960.0	E856	E930.0	E950.4	E962.0	E980.4
8:12.20 streptomycins	960.6	E856	E930.6	E950.4	E962.0	E980.4
8:12.24 tetracyclines	960.4	E856	E930.4	E950.4	E962.0	E980.4
8:12.28 other antibiotics	960.8	E856	E930.8	E950.4	E962.0	E980.4
antimycobacterial	960.6	E856	E930.6	E950.4	E962.0	E980.4
macrolides	960.3	E856	E930.3	E950.4	E962.0	E980.4
8:16 antituberculars	961.8	E857	E931.8	E950.4	E962.0	E980.4
antibiotics	960.6	E856	E930.6	E950.4	E962.0	E980.4
8:18 antivirals	961.7	E857	E931.7	E950.4	E962.0	E980.4
8:20 plasmodicides (antimalarials)	961.4	E857	E931.4	E950.4	E962.0	E980.4
8:24 sulfonamides	961.0	E857	E931.0	E950.4	E962.0	E980.4
8:26 sulfones	961.8	E857	E931.8	E950.4	E962.0	E980.4
8:28 treponemicides	961.2	E857	E931.2	E950.4	E962.0	E980.4
8:32 trichomonacides	961.5	E857	E931.5	E950.4	E962.0	E980.4
quinoline derivatives	961.3	E857	E931.3	E950.4	E962.0	E980.4
nitrofuran derivatives	961.9	E857	E931.9	E950.4	E962.0	E980.4
8:36 urinary germicides	961.9	E857	E931.9	E950.4	E962.0	E980.4
quinoline derivatives	961.3	E857	E931.3	E950.4	E962.0	E980.4
8:40 other anti-infectives	961.9	E857	E931.9	E950.4	E962.0	E980.4
10:00 antineoplastic agents	963.1	E858.1	E933.1	E950.4	E962.0	E980.4
antibiotics	960.7	E856	E930.7	E950.4	E962.0	E980.4
progestogens	962.2	E858.0	E932.2	E950.4	E962.0	E980.4
12:04 parasympathomimetic (cholinergic) agents	971.0	E855.3	E941.0	E950.4	E962.0	E980.4
12:08 parasympatholytic (cholinergic-blocking) agents	971.1	E855.4	E941.1	E950.4	E962.0	E980.4
12:12 sympathomimetic (adrenergic) agents	971.2	E855.5	E941.2	E950.4	E962.0	E980.4
12:16 sympatholytic (adrenergic-blocking) agents	971.3	E855.6	E941.3	E950.4	E962.0	E980.4
12:20 skeletal muscle relaxants	—	—	—	—	—	—
central nervous system muscle-tone depressants	968.0	E855.1	E938.0	E950.4	E962.0	E980.4
myoneural blocking agents	975.2	E858.6	E945.2	E950.4	E962.0	E980.4
16:00 blood derivatives	964.7	E858.2	E934.7	E950.4	E962.0	E980.4
20:04 antianemia drugs	964.1	E858.2	E934.1	E950.4	E962.0	E980.4
20:04.04 iron preparations	964.0	E858.2	E934.0	E950.4	E962.0	E980.4
20:04.08 liver and stomach preparations	964.1	E858.2	E934.1	E950.4	E962.0	E980.4
20:12.04 anticoagulants	964.2	E858.2	E934.2	E950.4	E962.0	E980.4
20:12.08 antiheparin agents	964.5	E858.2	E934.5	E950.4	E962.0	E980.4

◀ New　◀▥ Revised　~~deleted~~ Deleted　● Use Additional Digit(s)

Substance	Poisoning	External Cause (E Code)				
		Accident	Therapeutic Use	Suicide Attempt	Assault	Undetermined
Drug *(Continued)*						
20:12.12 coagulants	964.5	E858.2	E934.5	E950.4	E962.0	E980.4
20:12.16 hemostatics NEC	964.5	E858.2	E934.5	E950.4	E962.0	E980.4
capillary active drugs	972.8	E858.3	E942.8	E950.4	E962.0	E980.4
24:04 cardiac drugs	972.9	E858.3	E942.9	E950.4	E962.0	E980.4
cardiotonic agents	972.1	E858.3	E942.1	E950.4	E962.0	E980.4
rhythm regulators	972.0	E858.3	E942.0	E950.4	E962.0	E980.4
24:06 antilipemic agents	972.2	E858.3	E942.2	E950.4	E962.0	E980.4
thyroid derivatives	962.7	E858.0	E932.7	E950.4	E962.0	E980.4
24:08 hypotensive agents	972.6	E858.3	E942.6	E950.4	E962.0	E980.4
adrenergic blocking agents	971.3	E855.6	E941.3	E950.4	E962.0	E980.4
ganglion blocking agents	972.3	E858.3	E942.3	E950.4	E962.0	E980.4
vasodilators	972.5	E858.3	E942.5	E950.4	E962.0	E980.4
24:12 vasodilating agents NEC	972.5	E858.3	E942.5	E950.4	E962.0	E980.4
coronary	972.4	E858.3	E942.4	E950.4	E962.0	E980.4
nicotinic acid derivatives	972.2	E858.3	E942.2	E950.4	E962.0	E980.4
24:16 sclerosing agents	972.7	E858.3	E942.7	E950.4	E962.0	E980.4
28:04 general anesthetics	968.4	E855.1	E938.4	E950.4	E962.0	E980.4
gaseous anesthetics	968.2	E855.1	E938.2	E950.4	E962.0	E980.4
halothane	968.1	E855.1	E938.1	E950.4	E962.0	E980.4
intravenous anesthetics	968.3	E855.1	E938.3	E950.4	E962.0	E980.4
28:08 analgesics and antipyretics	965.9	E850.9	E935.9	E950.0	E962.0	E980.0
antirheumatics	965.69	E850.6	E935.6	E950.0	E962.0	E980.0
aromatic analgesics	965.4	E850.4	E935.4	E950.0	E962.0	E980.0
non-narcotic NEC	965.7	E850.7	E935.7	E950.0	E962.0	E980.0
opium alkaloids	965.00	E850.2	E935.2	E950.0	E962.0	E980.0
heroin	965.01	E850.0	E935.0	E950.0	E962.0	E980.0
methadone	965.02	E850.1	E935.1	E950.0	E962.0	E980.0
specified type NEC	965.09	E850.2	E935.2	E950.0	E962.0	E980.0
pyrazole derivatives	965.5	E850.5	E935.5	E950.0	E962.0	E980.0
salicylates	965.1	E850.3	E935.3	E950.0	E962.0	E980.0
specified NEC	965.8	E850.8	E935.8	E950.0	E962.0	E980.0
28:10 narcotic antagonists	970.1	E854.3	E940.1	E950.4	E962.0	E980.4
28:12 anticonvulsants	966.3	E855.0	E936.3	E950.4	E962.0	E980.4
barbiturates	967.0	E851	E937.0	E950.1	E962.0	E980.1
benzodiazepine-based tranquilizers	969.4	E853.2	E939.4	E950.3	E962.0	E980.3
bromides	967.3	E852.2	E937.3	E950.2	E962.0	E980.2
hydantoin derivatives	966.1	E855.0	E936.1	E950.4	E962.0	E980.4
oxazolidine (derivatives)	966.0	E855.0	E936.0	E950.4	E962.0	E980.4
succinimides	966.2	E855.0	E936.2	E950.4	E962.0	E980.4

◀ New   ◀▦ Revised   ~~deleted~~ Deleted   ● Use Additional Digit(s)

Substance	Poisoning	External Cause (E Code)				
		Accident	Therapeutic Use	Suicide Attempt	Assault	Undetermined
Drug *(Continued)*						
28:16.04 antidepressants	969.00	E854.0	E939.0	E950.3	E962.0	E980.3
28:16.08 tranquilizers	969.5	E853.9	E939.5	E950.3	E962.0	E980.3
benzodiazepine-based	969.4	E853.2	E939.4	E950.3	E962.0	E980.3
butyrophenone-based	969.2	E853.1	E939.2	E950.3	E962.0	E980.3
major NEC	969.3	E853.8	E939.3	E950.3	E962.0	E980.3
phenothiazine-based	969.1	E853.0	E939.1	E950.3	E962.0	E980.3
28:16.12 other psychotherapeutic agents	969.8	E855.8	E939.8	E950.3	E962.0	E980.3
28:20 respiratory and cerebral stimulants	970.9	E854.3	E940.9	E950.4	E962.0	E980.4
analeptics	970.0	E854.3	E940.0	E950.4	E962.0	E980.4
anorexigenic agents	977.0	E858.8	E947.0	E950.4	E962.0	E980.4
psychostimulants	969.70	E854.2	E939.7	E950.3	E962.0	E980.3
specified NEC	970.89	E854.3	E940.8	E950.4	E962.0	E980.4
28:24 sedatives and hypnotics	967.9	E852.9	E937.9	E950.2	E962.0	E980.2
barbiturates	967.0	E851	E937.0	E950.1	E962.0	E980.1
benzodiazepine-based tranquilizers	969.4	E853.2	E939.4	E950.3	E962.0	E980.3
chloral hydrate (group)	967.1	E852.0	E937.1	E950.2	E962.0	E980.2
glutethimide group	967.5	E852.4	E937.5	E950.2	E962.0	E980.2
intravenous anesthetics	968.3	E855.1	E938.3	E950.4	E962.0	E980.4
methaqualone (compounds)	967.4	E852.3	E937.4	E950.2	E962.0	E980.2
paraldehyde	967.2	E852.1	E937.2	E950.2	E962.0	E980.2
phenothiazine-based tranquilizers	969.1	E853.0	E939.1	E950.3	E962.0	E980.3
specified NEC	967.8	E852.8	E937.8	E950.2	E962.0	E980.2
thiobarbiturates	968.3	E855.1	E938.3	E950.4	E962.0	E980.4
tranquilizer NEC	969.5	E853.9	E939.5	E950.3	E962.0	E980.3
36:04 to 36:88 diagnostic agents	977.8	E858.8	E947.8	E950.4	E962.0	E980.4
40:00 electrolyte, caloric, and water balance agents NEC	974.5	E858.5	E944.5	E950.4	E962.0	E980.4
40:04 acidifying agents	963.2	E858.1	E933.2	E950.4	E962.0	E980.4
40:08 alkalinizing agents	963.3	E858.1	E933.3	E950.4	E962.0	E980.4
40:10 ammonia detoxicants	974.5	E858.5	E944.5	E950.4	E962.0	E980.4
40:12 replacement solutions	974.5	E858.5	E944.5	E950.4	E962.0	E980.4
plasma expanders	964.8	E858.2	E934.8	E950.4	E962.0	E980.4
40:16 sodium-removing resins	974.5	E858.5	E944.5	E950.4	E962.0	E980.4
40:18 potassium-removing resins	974.5	E858.5	E944.5	E950.4	E962.0	E980.4
40:20 caloric agents	974.5	E858.5	E944.5	E950.4	E962.0	E980.4
40:24 salt and sugar substitutes	974.5	E858.5	E944.5	E950.4	E962.0	E980.4
40:28 diuretics NEC	974.4	E858.5	E944.4	E950.4	E962.0	E980.4
carbonic acid anhydrase inhibitors	974.2	E858.5	E944.2	E950.4	E962.0	E980.4

TABLE OF DRUGS AND CHEMICALS

Substance	External Cause (E Code)					
	Poisoning	Accident	Therapeutic Use	Suicide Attempt	Assault	Undetermined
Drug *(Continued)*						
40:28 diuretics NEC *(Continued)*						
mercurials	974.0	E858.5	E944.0	E950.4	E962.0	E980.4
purine derivatives	974.1	E858.5	E944.1	E950.4	E962.0	E980.4
saluretics	974.3	E858.5	E944.3	E950.4	E962.0	E980.4
thiazides	974.3	E858.5	E944.3	E950.4	E962.0	E980.4
40:36 irrigating solutions	974.5	E858.5	E944.5	E950.4	E962.0	E980.4
40:40 uricosuric agents	974.7	E858.5	E944.7	E950.4	E962.0	E980.4
44:00 enzymes	963.4	E858.1	E933.4	E950.4	E962.0	E980.4
fibrinolysis-affecting agents	964.4	E858.2	E934.4	E950.4	E962.0	E980.4
gastric agents	973.4	E858.4	E943.4	E950.4	E962.0	E980.4
48:00 expectorants and cough preparations	—	—	—	—	—	—
antihistamine agents	963.0	E858.1	E933.0	E950.4	E962.0	E980.4
antitussives	975.4	E858.6	E945.4	E950.4	E962.0	E980.4
codeine derivatives	965.09	E850.2	E935.2	E950.0	E962.0	E980.0
expectorants	975.5	E858.6	E945.5	E950.4	E962.0	E980.4
narcotic agents NEC	965.09	E850.2	E935.2	E950.0	E962.0	E980.0
52:04 anti-infectives (EENT)	—	—	—	—	—	—
ENT agent	976.6	E858.7	E946.6	E950.4	E962.0	E980.4
ophthalmic preparation	976.5	E858.7	E946.5	E950.4	E962.0	E980.4
52:04.04 antibiotics (EENT)	—	—	—	—	—	—
ENT agent	976.6	E858.7	E946.6	E950.4	E962.0	E980.4
ophthalmic preparation	976.5	E858.7	E946.5	E950.4	E962.0	E980.4
52:04.06 antivirals (EENT)	—	—	—	—	—	—
ENT agent	976.6	E858.7	E946.6	E950.4	E962.0	E980.4
ophthalmic preparation	976.5	E858.7	E946.5	E950.4	E962.0	E980.4
52:04.08 sulfonamides (EENT)	—	—	—	—	—	—
ENT agent	976.6	E858.7	E946.6	E950.4	E962.0	E980.4
ophthalmic preparation	976.5	E858.7	E946.5	E950.4	E962.0	E980.4
52:04.12 miscellaneous anti-infectives (EENT)	—	—	—	—	—	—
ENT agent	976.6	E858.7	E946.6	E950.4	E962.0	E980.4
ophthalmic preparation	976.5	E858.7	E946.5	E950.4	E962.0	E980.4
52:08 anti-inflammatory agents (EENT)	—	—	—	—	—	—
ENT agent	976.6	E858.7	E946.6	E950.4	E962.0	E980.4
ophthalmic preparation	976.5	E858.7	E946.5	E950.4	E962.0	E980.4
52:10 carbonic anhydrase inhibitors	974.2	E858.5	E944.2	E950.4	E962.0	E980.4
52:12 contact lens solutions	976.5	E858.7	E946.5	E950.4	E962.0	E980.4
52:16 local anesthetics (EENT)	968.5	E855.2	E938.5	E950.4	E962.0	E980.4

◀ New   ◀▥ Revised   ~~deleted~~ Deleted   ● Use Additional Digit(s)

Substance	Poisoning	External Cause (E Code)				
		Accident	Therapeutic Use	Suicide Attempt	Assault	Undetermined
Drug *(Continued)*						
52:20 miotics	971.0	E855.3	E941.0	E950.4	E962.0	E980.4
52:24 mydriatics	—	—	—	—	—	—
adrenergics	971.2	E855.5	E941.2	E950.4	E962.0	E980.4
anticholinergics	971.1	E855.4	E941.1	E950.4	E962.0	E980.4
antimuscarinics	971.1	E855.4	E941.1	E950.4	E962.0	E980.4
parasympatholytics	971.1	E855.4	E941.1	E950.4	E962.0	E980.4
spasmolytics	971.1	E855.4	E941.1	E950.4	E962.0	E980.4
sympathomimetics	971.2	E855.5	E941.2	E950.4	E962.0	E980.4
52:28 mouth washes and gargles	976.6	E858.7	E946.6	E950.4	E962.0	E980.4
52:32 vasoconstrictors (EENT)	971.2	E855.5	E941.2	E950.4	E962.0	E980.4
52:36 unclassified agents (EENT)	—	—	—	—	—	—
ENT agent	976.6	E858.7	E946.6	E950.4	E962.0	E980.4
ophthalmic preparation	976.5	E858.7	E946.5	E950.4	E962.0	E980.4
56:04 antacids and adsorbents	973.0	E858.4	E943.0	E950.4	E962.0	E980.4
56:08 antidiarrhea agents	973.5	E858.4	E943.5	E950.4	E962.0	E980.4
56:10 antiflatulents	973.8	E858.4	E943.8	E950.4	E962.0	E980.4
56:12 cathartics NEC	973.3	E858.4	E943.3	E950.4	E962.0	E980.4
emollients	973.2	E858.4	E943.2	E950.4	E962.0	E980.4
irritants	973.1	E858.4	E943.1	E950.4	E962.0	E980.4
56:16 digestants	973.4	E858.4	E943.4	E950.4	E962.0	E980.4
56:20 emetics and antiemetics	—	—	—	—	—	—
antiemetics	963.0	E858.1	E933.0	E950.4	E962.0	E980.4
emetics	973.6	E858.4	E943.6	E950.4	E962.0	E980.4
56:24 lipotropic agents	977.1	E858.8	E947.1	E950.4	E962.0	E980.4
56:40 miscellaneous G.I. drugs	973.8	E858.4	E943.8	E950.4	E962.0	E980.4
60:00 gold compounds	965.69	E850.6	E935.6	E950.0	E962.0	E980.0
64:00 heavy metal antagonists	963.8	E858.1	E933.8	E950.4	E962.0	E980.4
68:04 adrenals	962.0	E858.0	E932.0	E950.4	E962.0	E980.4
68:08 androgens	962.1	E858.0	E932.1	E950.4	E962.0	E980.4
68:12 contraceptives, oral	962.2	E858.0	E932.2	E950.4	E962.0	E980.4
68:16 estrogens	962.2	E858.0	E932.2	E950.4	E962.0	E980.4
68:18 gonadotropins	962.4	E858.0	E932.4	E950.4	E962.0	E980.4
68:20 insulins and antidiabetic agents	962.3	E858.0	E932.3	E950.4	E962.0	E980.4
68:20.08 insulins	962.3	E858.0	E932.3	E950.4	E962.0	E980.4
68:24 parathyroid	962.6	E858.0	E932.6	E950.4	E962.0	E980.4
68:28 pituitary (posterior)	962.5	E858.0	E932.5	E950.4	E962.0	E980.4
anterior	962.4	E858.0	E932.4	E950.4	E962.0	E980.4
68:32 progestogens	962.2	E858.0	E932.2	E950.4	E962.0	E980.4

◀ New   ◀◀◀ Revised   ~~deleted~~ Deleted   ● Use Additional Digit(s)

TABLE OF DRUGS AND CHEMICALS

Substance	Poisoning	External Cause (E Code)				
		Accident	Therapeutic Use	Suicide Attempt	Assault	Undetermined
Drug *(Continued)*						
68:34 other corpus luteum hormones NEC	962.2	E858.0	E932.2	E950.4	E962.0	E980.4
68:36 thyroid and antithyroid	—	—	—	—	—	—
antithyroid	962.8	E858.0	E932.8	E950.4	E962.0	E980.4
thyroid (derivatives)	962.7	E858.0	E932.7	E950.4	E962.0	E980.4
72:00 local anesthetics NEC	968.9	E855.2	E938.9	E950.4	E962.0	E980.4
topical (surface)	968.5	E855.2	E938.5	E950.4	E962.0	E980.4
infiltration (intradermal) (subcutaneous) (submucosal)	968.5	E855.2	E938.5	E950.4	E962.0	E980.4
nerve blocking (peripheral) (plexus) (regional)	968.6	E855.2	E938.6	E950.4	E962.0	E980.4
spinal	968.7	E855.2	E938.7	E950.4	E962.0	E980.4
76:00 oxytocics	975.0	E858.6	E945.0	E950.4	E962.0	E980.4
78:00 radioactive agents	990	—	—	—	—	—
80:04 serums NEC	979.9	E858.8	E949.9	E950.4	E962.0	E980.4
immune gamma globulin (human)	964.6	E858.2	E934.6	E950.4	E962.0	E980.4
80:08 toxoids NEC	978.8	E858.8	E948.8	E950.4	E962.0	E980.4
diphtheria	978.5	E858.8	E948.5	E950.4	E962.0	E980.4
and tetanus	978.9	E858.8	E948.9	E950.4	E962.0	E980.4
with pertussis component	978.6	E858.8	E948.6	E950.4	E962.0	E980.4
tetanus	978.4	E858.8	E948.4	E950.4	E962.0	E980.4
and diphtheria	978.9	E858.8	E948.9	E950.4	E962.0	E980.4
with pertussis component	978.6	E858.8	E948.6	E950.4	E962.0	E980.4
80:12 vaccines	979.9	E858.8	E949.9	E950.4	E962.0	E980.4
bacterial NEC	978.8	E858.8	E948.8	E950.4	E962.0	E980.4
with	—	—	—	—	—	—
other bacterial components	978.9	E858.8	E948.9	E950.4	E962.0	E980.4
pertussis component	978.6	E858.8	E948.6	E950.4	E962.0	E980.4
viral and rickettsial components	979.7	E858.8	E949.7	E950.4	E962.0	E980.4
rickettsial NEC	979.6	E858.8	E949.6	E950.4	E962.0	E980.4
with	—	—	—	—	—	—
bacterial component	979.7	E858.8	E949.7	E950.4	E962.0	E980.4
pertussis component	978.6	E858.8	E948.6	E950.4	E962.0	E980.4
viral component	979.7	E858.8	E949.7	E950.4	E962.0	E980.4
viral NEC	979.6	E858.8	E949.6	E950.4	E962.0	E980.4
with	—	—	—	—	—	—
bacterial component	979.7	E858.8	E949.7	E950.4	E962.0	E980.4
pertussis component	978.6	E858.8	E948.6	E950.4	E962.0	E980.4
rickettsial component	979.7	E858.8	E949.7	E950.4	E962.0	E980.4
84:04.04 antibiotics (skin and mucous membrane)	976.0	E858.7	E946.0	E950.4	E962.0	E980.4
84:04.08 fungicides (skin and mucous membrane)	976.0	E858.7	E946.0	E950.4	E962.0	E980.4

◀ New ◀ Revised ~~deleted~~ Deleted ● Use Additional Digit(s)

Substance	Poisoning	External Cause (E Code)				
		Accident	Therapeutic Use	Suicide Attempt	Assault	Undetermined
Drug *(Continued)*						
84:04.12 scabicides and pediculicides (skin and mucous membrane)	976.0	E858.7	E946.0	E950.4	E962.0	E980.4
84:04.16 miscellaneous local anti-infectives (skin and mucous membrane)	976.0	E858.7	E946.0	E950.4	E962.0	E980.4
84:06 anti-inflammatory agents (skin and mucous membrane)	976.0	E858.7	E946.0	E950.4	E962.0	E980.4
84:08 antipruritics and local anesthetics	—	—	—	—	—	—
antipruritics	976.1	E858.7	E946.1	E950.4	E962.0	E980.4
local anesthetics	968.5	E855.2	E938.5	E950.4	E962.0	E980.4
84:12 astringents	976.2	E858.7	E946.2	E950.4	E962.0	E980.4
84:16 cell stimulants and proliferants	976.8	E858.7	E946.8	E950.4	E962.0	E980.4
84:20 detergents	976.2	E858.7	E946.2	E950.4	E962.0	E980.4
84:24 emollients, demulcents, and protectants	976.3	E858.7	E946.3	E950.4	E962.0	E980.4
84:28 keratolytic agents	976.4	E858.7	E946.4	E950.4	E962.0	E980.4
84:32 keratoplastic agents	976.4	E858.7	E946.4	E950.4	E962.0	E980.4
84:36 miscellaneous agents (skin and mucous membrane)	976.8	E858.7	E946.8	E950.4	E962.0	E980.4
86:00 spasmolytic agents	975.1	E858.6	E945.1	E950.4	E962.0	E980.4
antiasthmatics	975.7	E858.6	E945.7	E950.4	E962.0	E980.4
papaverine	972.5	E858.3	E942.5	E950.4	E962.0	E980.4
theophylline	974.1	E858.5	E944.1	E950.4	E962.0	E980.4
88:04 vitamin A	963.5	E858.1	E933.5	E950.4	E962.0	E980.4
88:08 vitamin B complex	963.5	E858.1	E933.5	E950.4	E962.0	E980.4
hematopoietic vitamin	964.1	E858.2	E934.1	E950.4	E962.0	E980.4
nicotinic acid derivatives	972.2	E858.3	E942.2	E950.4	E962.0	E980.4
88:12 vitamin C	963.5	E858.1	E933.5	E950.4	E962.0	E980.4
88:16 vitamin D	963.5	E858.1	E933.5	E950.4	E962.0	E980.4
88:20 vitamin E	963.5	E858.1	E933.5	E950.4	E962.0	E980.4
88:24 vitamin K activity	964.3	E858.2	E934.3	E950.4	E962.0	E980.4
88:28 multivitamin preparations	963.5	E858.1	E933.5	E950.4	E962.0	E980.4
92:00 unclassified therapeutic agents	977.8	E858.8	E947.8	E950.4	E962.0	E980.4
Duboisine	971.1	E855.4	E941.1	E950.4	E962.0	E980.4
Dulcolax	973.1	E858.4	E943.1	E950.4	E962.0	E980.4
Duponol (C) (EP)	976.2	E858.7	E946.2	E950.4	E962.0	E980.4
Durabolin	962.1	E858.0	E932.1	E950.4	E962.0	E980.4
Dyclone	968.5	E855.2	E938.5	E950.4	E962.0	E980.4
Dyclonine	968.5	E855.2	E938.5	E950.4	E962.0	E980.4
Dydrogesterone	962.2	E858.0	E932.2	E950.4	E962.0	E980.4
Dyes NEC	989.89	E866.8	—	E950.9	E962.1	E980.9
diagnostic agents	977.8	E858.8	E947.8	E950.4	E962.0	E980.4
pharmaceutical NEC	977.4	E858.8	E947.4	E950.4	E962.0	E980.4
Dyflos	971.0	E855.3	E941.0	E950.4	E962.0	E980.4

◄ New   ◄▥ Revised   ~~deleted~~ Deleted   ● Use Additional Digit(s)

Substance	Poisoning	External Cause (E Code)				
		Accident	Therapeutic Use	Suicide Attempt	Assault	Undetermined
Dymelor	962.3	E858.0	E932.3	E950.4	E962.0	E980.4
Dynamite	989.89	E866.8	—	E950.9	E962.1	E980.9
fumes	987.8	E869.8	—	E952.8	E962.2	E982.8
Dyphylline	975.1	E858.6	E945.1	E950.4	E962.0	E980.4
Ear preparations	976.6	E858.7	E946.6	E950.4	E962.0	E980.4
Echothiopate, ecothiopate	971.0	E855.3	E941.0	E950.4	E962.0	E980.4
Ecstasy	969.72	E854.2	E939.7	E950.3	E962.0	E980.3
Ectylurea	967.8	E852.8	E937.8	E950.2	E962.0	E980.2
Edathamil disodium	963.8	E858.1	E933.8	E950.4	E962.0	E980.4
Edecrin	974.4	E858.5	E944.4	E950.4	E962.0	E980.4
Edetate, disodium (calcium)	963.8	E858.1	E933.8	E950.4	E962.0	E980.4
Edrophonium	971.0	E855.3	E941.0	E950.4	E962.0	E980.4
Elase	976.8	E858.7	E946.8	E950.4	E962.0	E980.4
Elaterium	973.1	E858.4	E943.1	E950.4	E962.0	E980.4
Elder	988.2	E865.4	—	E950.9	E962.1	E980.9
berry (unripe)	988.2	E865.3	—	E950.9	E962.1	E980.9
Electrolytes NEC	974.5	E858.5	E944.5	E950.4	E962.0	E980.4
Electrolytic agent NEC	974.5	E858.5	E944.5	E950.4	E962.0	E980.4
Embramine	963.0	E858.1	E933.0	E950.4	E962.0	E980.4
Emetics	973.6	E858.4	E943.6	E950.4	E962.0	E980.4
Emetine (hydrochloride)	961.5	E857	E931.5	E950.4	E962.0	E980.4
Emollients	976.3	E858.7	E946.3	E950.4	E962.0	E980.4
Emylcamate	969.5	E853.8	E939.5	E950.3	E962.0	E980.3
Encyprate	969.09	E854.0	E939.0	E950.3	E962.0	E980.3
Endocaine	968.5	E855.2	E938.5	E950.4	E962.0	E980.4
Endrin	989.2	E863.0	—	E950.6	E962.1	E980.7
Enflurane	968.2	E855.1	E938.2	E950.4	E962.0	E980.4
Enovid	962.2	E858.0	E932.2	E950.4	E962.0	E980.4
ENT preparations (anti-infectives)	976.6	E858.7	E946.6	E950.4	E962.0	E980.4
Enzodase	963.4	E858.1	E933.4	E950.4	E962.0	E980.4
Enzymes NEC	963.4	E858.1	E933.4	E950.4	E962.0	E980.4
Epanutin	966.1	E855.0	E936.1	E950.4	E962.0	E980.4
Ephedra (tincture)	971.2	E855.5	E941.2	E950.4	E962.0	E980.4
Ephedrine	971.2	E855.5	E941.2	E950.4	E962.0	E980.4
Epiestriol	962.2	E858.0	E932.2	E950.4	E962.0	E980.4
Epilim - *see* Sodium valproate	—	—	—	—	—	—
Epinephrine	971.2	E855.5	E941.2	E950.4	E962.0	E980.4
Epsom salt	973.3	E858.4	E943.3	E950.4	E962.0	E980.4
Equanil	969.5	E853.8	E939.5	E950.3	E962.0	E980.3

◀ New   ◀ Revised   deleted Deleted   ● Use Additional Digit(s)

Substance	Poisoning	External Cause (E Code)				
		Accident	Therapeutic Use	Suicide Attempt	Assault	Undetermined
Equisetum (diuretic)	974.4	E858.5	E944.4	E950.4	E962.0	E980.4
Ergometrine	975.0	E858.6	E945.0	E950.4	E962.0	E980.4
Ergonovine	975.0	E858.6	E945.0	E950.4	E962.0	E980.4
Ergot NEC	988.2	E865.4	—	E950.9	E962.1	E980.9
medicinal (alkaloids)	975.0	E858.6	E945.0	E950.4	E962.0	E980.4
Ergotamine (tartrate) (for migraine) NEC	972.9	E858.3	E942.9	E950.4	E962.0	E980.4
Ergotrate	975.0	E858.6	E945.0	E950.4	E962.0	E980.4
Erythrityl tetranitrate	972.4	E858.3	E942.4	E950.4	E962.0	E980.4
Erythrol tetranitrate	972.4	E858.3	E942.4	E950.4	E962.0	E980.4
Erythromycin	960.3	E856	E930.3	E950.4	E962.0	E980.4
ophthalmic preparation	976.5	E858.7	E946.5	E950.4	E962.0	E980.4
topical NEC	976.0	E858.7	E946.0	E950.4	E962.0	E980.4
Eserine	971.0	E855.3	E941.0	E950.4	E962.0	E980.4
Eskabarb	967.0	E851	E937.0	E950.1	E962.0	E980.1
Eskalith	969.8	E855.8	E939.8	E950.3	E962.0	E980.3
Estradiol (cypionate) (dipropionate) (valerate)	962.2	E858.0	E932.2	E950.4	E962.0	E980.4
Estriol	962.2	E858.0	E932.2	E950.4	E962.0	E980.4
Estrogens (with progestogens)	962.2	E858.0	E932.2	E950.4	E962.0	E980.4
Estrone	962.2	E858.0	E932.2	E950.4	E962.0	E980.4
Etafedrine	971.2	E855.5	E941.2	E950.4	E962.0	E980.4
Ethacrynate sodium	974.4	E858.5	E944.4	E950.4	E962.0	E980.4
Ethacrynic acid	974.4	E858.5	E944.4	E950.4	E962.0	E980.4
Ethambutol	961.8	E857	E931.8	E950.4	E962.0	E980.4
Ethamide	974.2	E858.5	E944.2	E950.4	E962.0	E980.4
Ethamivan	970.0	E854.3	E940.0	E950.4	E962.0	E980.4
Ethamsylate	964.5	E858.2	E934.5	E950.4	E962.0	E980.4
Ethanol	980.0	E860.1	—	E950.9	E962.1	E980.9
beverage	980.0	E860.0	—	E950.9	E962.1	E980.9
Ethchlorvynol	967.8	E852.8	E937.8	E950.2	E962.0	E980.2
Ethebenecid	974.7	E858.5	E944.7	E950.4	E962.0	E980.4
Ether(s) (diethyl) (ethyl) (vapor)	987.8	E869.8	—	E952.8	E962.2	E982.8
anesthetic	968.2	E855.1	E938.2	E950.4	E962.0	E980.4
petroleum - see Ligroin solvent	982.8	E862.4	—	E950.9	E962.1	E980.9
Ethidine chloride (vapor)	987.8	E869.8	—	E952.8	E962.2	E982.8
liquid (solvent)	982.3	E862.4	—	E950.9	E962.1	E980.9
Ethinamate	967.8	E852.8	E937.8	E950.2	E962.0	E980.2
Ethinylestradiol	962.2	E858.0	E932.2	E950.4	E962.0	E980.4
Ethionamide	961.8	E857	E931.8	E950.4	E962.0	E980.4
Ethisterone	962.2	E858.0	E932.2	E950.4	E962.0	E980.4

◀ New   ◀▥ Revised   ~~deleted~~ Deleted   ● Use Additional Digit(s)

		External Cause (E Code)				
Substance	Poisoning	Accident	Therapeutic Use	Suicide Attempt	Assault	Undetermined
Ethobral	967.0	E851	E937.0	E950.1	E962.0	E980.1
Ethocaine (infiltration) (topical)	968.5	E855.2	E938.5	E950.4	E962.0	E980.4
nerve block (peripheral) (plexus)	968.6	E855.2	E938.6	E950.4	E962.0	E980.4
spinal	968.7	E855.2	E938.7	E950.4	E962.0	E980.4
Ethoheptazine (citrate)	965.7	E850.7	E935.7	E950.0	E962.0	E980.0
Ethopropazine	966.4	E855.0	E936.4	E950.4	E962.0	E980.4
Ethosuximide	966.2	E855.0	E936.2	E950.4	E962.0	E980.4
Ethotoin	966.1	E855.0	E936.1	E950.4	E962.0	E980.4
Ethoxazene	961.9	E857	E931.9	E950.4	E962.0	E980.4
Ethoxzolamide	974.2	E858.5	E944.2	E950.4	E962.0	E980.4
Ethyl	—	—	—	—	—	—
acetate (vapor)	982.8	E862.4	—	E950.9	E962.1	E980.9
alcohol	980.0	E860.1	—	E950.9	E962.1	E980.9
beverage	980.0	E860.0	—	E950.9	E962.1	E980.9
aldehyde (vapor)	987.8	E869.8	—	E952.8	E962.2	E982.8
liquid	989.89	E866.8	—	E950.9	E962.1	E980.9
aminobenzoate	968.5	E855.2	E938.5	E950.4	E962.0	E980.4
biscoumacetate	964.2	E858.2	E934.2	E950.4	E962.0	E980.4
bromide (anesthetic)	968.2	E855.1	E938.2	E950.4	E962.0	E980.4
carbamate (antineoplastic)	963.1	E858.1	E933.1	E950.4	E962.0	E980.4
carbinol	980.3	E860.4	—	E950.9	E962.1	E980.9
chaulmoograte	961.8	E857	E931.8	E950.4	E962.0	E980.4
chloride (vapor)	987.8	E869.8	—	E952.8	E962.2	E982.8
anesthetic (local)	968.5	E855.2	E938.5	E950.4	E962.0	E980.4
inhaled	968.2	E855.1	E938.2	E950.4	E962.0	E980.4
solvent	982.3	E862.4	—	E950.9	E962.1	E980.9
estranol	962.1	E858.0	E932.1	E950.4	E962.0	E980.4
ether - see Ether(s)	—	—	—	—	—	—
formate (solvent) NEC	982.8	E862.4	—	E950.9	E962.1	E980.9
iodoacetate	987.5	E869.3	—	E952.8	E962.2	E982.8
lactate (solvent) NEC	982.8	E862.4	—	E950.9	E962.1	E980.9
methylcarbinol	980.8	E860.8	—	E950.9	E962.1	E980.9
morphine	965.09	E850.2	E935.2	E950.0	E962.0	E980.0
Ethylene (gas)	987.1	E869.8	—	E952.8	E962.2	E982.8
anesthetic (general)	968.2	E855.1	E938.2	E950.4	E962.0	E980.4
chlorohydrin (vapor)	982.3	E862.4	—	E950.9	E962.1	E980.9
dichloride (vapor)	982.3	E862.4	—	E950.9	E962.1	E980.9
glycol(s) (any) (vapor)	982.8	E862.4	—	E950.9	E962.1	E980.9

◀ New   ◀ Revised   ~~deleted~~ Deleted   ● Use Additional Digit(s)

Substance	Poisoning	External Cause (E Code)				
		Accident	Therapeutic Use	Suicide Attempt	Assault	Undetermined
Ethylidene	—	—	—	—	—	—
chloride NEC	982.3	E862.4	—	E950.9	E962.1	E980.9
diethyl ether	982.8	—	E862.4	E950.9	E962.1	E980.9
Ethynodiol	962.2	E858.0	E932.2	E950.4	E962.0	E980.4
Etidocaine	968.9	E855.2	E938.9	E950.4	E962.0	E980.4
infiltration (subcutaneous)	968.5	E855.2	E938.5	E950.4	E962.0	E980.4
nerve (peripheral) (plexus)	968.6	E855.2	E938.6	E950.4	E962.0	E980.4
Etilfen	967.0	E851	E937.0	E950.1	E962.0	E980.1
Etomide	965.7	E850.7	E935.7	E950.0	E962.0	E980.0
Etorphine	965.09	E850.2	E935.2	E950.0	E962.0	E980.0
Etoval	967.0	E851	E937.0	E950.1	E962.0	E980.1
Etryptamine	969.01	E854.0	E939.0	E950.3	E962.0	E980.3
Eucaine	968.5	E855.2	E938.5	E950.4	E962.0	E980.4
Eucalyptus (oil) NEC	975.5	E858.6	E945.5	E950.4	E962.0	E980.4
Eucatropine	971.1	E855.4	E941.1	E950.4	E962.0	E980.4
Eucodal	965.09	E850.2	E935.2	E950.0	E962.0	E980.0
Euneryl	967.0	E851	E937.0	E950.1	E962.0	E980.1
Euphthalmine	971.1	E855.4	E941.1	E950.4	E962.0	E980.4
Eurax	976.0	E858.7	E946.0	E950.4	E962.0	E980.4
Euresol	976.4	E858.7	E946.4	E950.4	E962.0	E980.4
Euthroid	962.7	E858.0	E932.7	E950.4	E962.0	E980.4
Evans blue	977.8	E858.8	E947.8	E950.4	E962.0	E980.4
Evipal	967.0	E851	E937.0	E950.1	E962.0	E980.1
sodium	968.3	E855.1	E938.3	E950.4	E962.0	E980.4
Evipan	967.0	E851	E937.0	E950.1	E962.0	E980.1
sodium	968.3	E855.1	E938.3	E950.4	E962.0	E980.4
Exalgin	965.4	E850.4	E935.4	E950.0	E962.0	E980.0
Excipients, pharmaceutical	977.4	E858.8	E947.4	E950.4	E962.0	E980.4
Exhaust gas - see Carbon, monoxide	—	—	—	—	—	—
Ex-Lax (phenolphthalein)	973.1	E858.4	E943.1	E950.4	E962.0	E980.4
Expectorants	975.5	E858.6	E945.5	E950.4	E962.0	E980.4
External medications (skin) (mucous membrane)	976.9	E858.7	E946.9	E950.4	E962.0	E980.4
dental agent	976.7	E858.7	E946.7	E950.4	E962.0	E980.4
ENT agent	976.6	E858.7	E946.6	E950.4	E962.0	E980.4
ophthalmic preparation	976.5	E858.7	E946.5	E950.4	E962.0	E980.4
specified NEC	976.8	E858.7	E946.8	E950.4	E962.0	E980.4
Eye agents (anti-infective)	976.5	E858.7	E946.5	E950.4	E962.0	E980.4
Factor IX complex (human)	964.5	E858.2	E934.5	E950.4	E962.0	E980.4
Fecal softeners	973.2	E858.4	E943.2	E950.4	E962.0	E980.4

◀ New   ◀▥ Revised   ~~deleted~~ Deleted   ● Use Additional Digit(s)

			External Cause (E Code)			
Substance	**Poisoning**	**Accident**	**Therapeutic Use**	**Suicide Attempt**	**Assault**	**Undetermined**
Fenbutrazate	977.0	E858.8	E947.0	E950.4	E962.0	E980.4
Fencamfamin	970.89	E854.3	E940.8	E950.4	E962.0	E980.4
Fenfluramine	977.0	E858.8	E947.0	E950.4	E962.0	E980.4
Fenoprofen	965.61	E850.6	E935.6	E950.0	E962.0	E980.0
Fentanyl	965.09	E850.2	E935.2	E950.0	E962.0	E980.0
Fentazin	969.1	E853.0	E939.1	E930.3	E962.0	E980.3
Fenticlor, fentichlor	976.0	E858.7	E946.0	E950.4	E962.0	E980.4
Fer de lance (bite) (venom)	989.5	E905.0	—	E950.9	E962.1	E980.9
Ferric - *see* Iron	—	—	—	—	—	—
Ferrocholinate	964.0	E858.2	E934.0	E950.4	E962.0	E980.4
Ferrous fumerate, gluconate, lactate, salt NEC, sulfate (medicinal)	964.0	E858.2	E934.0	E950.4	E962.0	E980.4
Ferrum - *see* Iron	—	—	—	—	—	—
Fertilizers NEC	989.89	E866.5	—	E950.9	E962.1	E980.4
with herbicide mixture	989.4	E863.5	—	E950.6	E962.1	E980.7
Fibrinogen (human)	964.7	E858.2	E934.7	E950.4	E962.0	E980.4
Fibrinolysin	964.4	E858.2	E934.4	E950.4	E962.0	E980.4
Fibrinolysis-affecting agents	964.4	E858.2	E934.4	E950.4	E962.0	E980.4
Filix mas	961.6	E857	E931.6	E950.4	E962.0	E980.4
Fiorinal	965.1	E850.3	E935.3	E950.0	E962.0	E980.0
Fire damp	987.1	E869.8	—	E952.8	E962.2	E982.8
Fish, nonbacterial or noxious	988.0	E865.2	—	E950.9	E962.1	E980.9
shell	988.0	E865.1	—	E950.9	E962.1	E980.9
Flagyl	961.5	E857	E931.5	E950.4	E962.0	E980.4
Flavoxate	975.1	E858.6	E945.1	E950.4	E962.0	E980.4
Flaxedil	975.2	E858.6	E945.2	E950.4	E962.0	E980.4
Flaxseed (medicinal)	976.3	E858.7	E946.3	E950.4	E962.0	E980.4
Flomax	971.3	E855.6	E941.3	E950.4	E962.0	E980.4
Florantyrone	973.4	E858.4	E943.4	E950.4	E962.0	E980.4
Floraquin	961.3	E857	E931.3	E950.4	E962.0	E980.4
Florinef	962.0	E858.0	E932.0	E950.4	E962.0	E980.4
ENT agent	976.6	E858.7	E946.6	E950.4	E962.0	E980.4
ophthalmic preparation	976.5	E858.7	E946.5	E950.4	E962.0	E980.4
topical NEC	976.0	E858.7	E946.0	E950.4	E962.0	E980.4
Flowers of sulfur	976.4	E858.7	E946.4	E950.4	E962.0	E980.4
Floxuridine	963.1	E858.1	E933.1	E950.4	E962.0	E980.4
Flucytosine	961.9	E857	E931.9	E950.4	E962.0	E980.4
Fludrocortisone	962.0	E858.0	E932.0	E950.4	E962.0	E980.4
ENT agent	976.6	E858.7	E946.6	E950.4	E962.0	E980.4
ophthalmic preparation	976.5	E858.7	E946.5	E950.4	E962.0	E980.4

◀ New ◀▦ Revised ~~deleted~~ Deleted ● Use Additional Digit(s)

Substance	Poisoning	External Cause (E Code)				
		Accident	Therapeutic Use	Suicide Attempt	Assault	Undetermined
Fludrocortisone *(Continued)*						
topical NEC	976.0	E858.7	E946.0	E950.4	E962.0	E980.4
Flumethasone	976.0	E858.7	E946.0	E950.4	E962.0	E980.4
Flumethiazide	974.3	E858.5	E944.3	E950.4	E962.0	E980.4
Flumidin	961.7	E857	E931.7	E950.4	E962.0	E980.4
Flunitrazepam	969.4	E853.2	E939.4	E950.3	E962.0	E980.3
Fluocinolone	976.0	E858.7	E946.0	E950.4	E962.0	E980.4
Fluocortolone	962.0	E858.0	E932.0	E950.4	E962.0	E980.4
Fluohydrocortisone	962.0	E858.0	E932.0	E950.4	E962.0	E980.4
ENT agent	976.6	E858.7	E946.6	E950.4	E962.0	E980.4
ophthalmic preparation	976.5	E858.7	E946.5	E950.4	E962.0	E980.4
topical NEC	976.0	E858.7	E946.0	E950.4	E962.0	E980.4
Fluonid	976.0	E858.7	E946.0	E950.4	E962.0	E980.4
Fluopromazine	969.1	E853.0	E939.1	E950.3	E962.0	E980.3
Fluoracetate	989.4	E863.7	—	E950.6	E962.1	E980.7
Fluorescein (sodium)	977.8	E858.8	E947.8	E950.4	E962.0	E980.4
Fluoride(s) (pesticides) (sodium) NEC	989.4	E863.4	—	E950.6	E962.1	E980.7
hydrogen - *see* Hydrofluoric acid	—	—	—	—	—	—
medicinal	976.7	E858.7	E946.7	E950.4	E962.0	E980.4
not pesticide NEC	983.9	E864.4	—	E950.7	E962.1	E980.6
stannous	976.7	E858.7	E946.7	E950.4	E962.0	E980.4
Fluorinated corticosteroids	962.0	E858.0	E932.0	E950.4	E962.0	E980.4
Fluorine (compounds) (gas)	987.8	E869.8	—	E952.8	E962.2	E982.8
salt - *see* Fluoride(s)	—	—	—	—	—	—
Fluoristan	976.7	E858.7	E946.7	E950.4	E962.0	E980.4
Fluoroacetate	989.4	E863.7	—	E950.6	E962.1	E980.7
Fluorodeoxyuridine	963.1	E858.1	E933.1	E950.4	E962.0	E980.4
Fluorometholone (topical) NEC	976.0	E858.7	E946.0	E950.4	E962.0	E980.4
ophthalmic preparation	976.5	E858.7	E946.5	E950.4	E962.0	E980.4
Fluorouracil	963.1	E858.1	E933.1	E950.4	E962.0	E980.4
Fluothane	968.1	E855.1	E938.1	E950.4	E962.0	E980.4
Fluoxetine hydrochloride	969.03	E854.0	E939.0	E950.3	E962.0	E980.3
Fluoxymesterone	962.1	E858.0	E932.1	E950.4	E962.0	E980.4
Fluphenazine	969.1	E853.0	E939.1	E950.3	E962.0	E980.3
Fluprednisolone	962.0	E858.0	E932.0	E950.4	E962.0	E980.4
Flurandrenolide	976.0	E858.7	E946.0	E950.4	E962.0	E980.4
Flurazepam (hydrochloride)	969.4	E853.2	E939.4	E950.3	E962.0	E980.3
Flurbiprofen	965.61	E850.6	E935.6	E950.0	E962.0	E980.0

		External Cause (E Code)				
Substance	Poisoning	Accident	Therapeutic Use	Suicide Attempt	Assault	Undetermined
Flurobate	976.0	E858.7	E946.0	E950.4	E962.0	E980.4
Flurothyl	969.8	E855.8	E939.8	E950.3	E962.0	E980.3
Fluroxene	968.2	E855.1	E938.2	E950.4	E962.0	E980.4
Folacin	964.1	E858.2	E934.1	E950.4	E962.0	E980.4
Folic acid	964.1	E858.2	E934.1	E950.4	E962.0	E980.4
Follicle stimulating hormone	962.4	E858.0	E932.4	E950.4	E962.0	E980.4
Food, foodstuffs, nonbacterial or noxious	988.9	E865.9	—	E950.9	E962.1	E980.9
berries, seeds	988.2	E865.3	—	E950.9	E962.1	E980.9
fish	988.0	E865.2	—	E950.9	E962.1	E980.9
mushrooms	988.1	E865.5	—	E950.9	E962.1	E980.9
plants	988.2	E865.9	—	E950.9	E962.1	E980.9
specified type NEC	988.2	E865.4	—	E950.9	E962.1	E980.9
shellfish	988.0	E865.1	—	E950.9	E962.1	E980.9
specified NEC	988.8	E865.8	—	E950.9	E962.1	E980.9
Fool's parsley	988.2	E865.4	—	E950.9	E962.1	E980.9
Formaldehyde (solution)	989.89	E861.4	—	E950.9	E962.1	E980.9
fungicide	989.4	E863.6	—	E950.6	E962.1	E980.7
gas or vapor	987.8	E869.8	—	E952.8	E962.2	E982.8
Formalin	989.89	E861.4	—	E950.9	E962.1	E980.9
fungicide	989.4	E863.6	—	E950.6	E962.1	E980.7
vapor	987.8	E869.8	—	E952.8	E962.2	E982.8
Formic acid	983.1	E864.1	—	E950.7	E962.1	E980.6
vapor	987.8	E869.8	—	E952.8	E962.2	E982.8
Fowler's solution	985.1	E866.3	—	E950.8	E962.1	E980.8
Foxglove	988.2	E865.4	—	E950.9	E962.1	E980.9
Fox green	977.8	E858.8	E947.8	E950.4	E962.0	E980.4
Framycetin	960.8	E856	E930.8	E950.4	E962.0	E980.4
Frangula (extract)	973.1	E858.4	E943.1	E950.4	E962.0	E980.4
Frei antigen	977.8	E858.8	E947.8	E950.4	E962.0	E980.4
Freons	987.4	E869.2	—	E952.8	E962.2	E982.8
Fructose	974.5	E858.5	E944.5	E950.4	E962.0	E980.4
Frusemide	974.4	E858.5	E944.4	E950.4	E962.0	E980.4
FSH	962.4	E858.0	E932.4	E950.4	E962.0	E980.4
Fuel	—	—	—	—	—	—
automobile	981	E862.1	—	E950.9	E962.1	E980.9
exhaust gas, not in transit	986	E868.2	—	E952.0	E962.2	E982.0
vapor NEC	987.1	E869.8	—	E952.8	E962.2	E982.8

◀ New ◀▦ Revised ~~deleted~~ Deleted ● Use Additional Digit(s)

Substance	Poisoning	External Cause (E Code)				
		Accident	Therapeutic Use	Suicide Attempt	Assault	Undetermined
Fuel *(Continued)*						
gas (domestic use) - *see also* Carbon, monoxide, fuel	—	—	—	—	—	—
utility	987.1	E868.1	—	E951.8	E962.2	E981.8
incomplete combustion of - *see* Carbon, monoxide, fuel, utility	—	—	—	—	—	—
in mobile container	987.0	E868.0	—	E951.1	E962.2	E981.1
piped (natural)	987.1	E867	—	E951.0	E962.2	E981.0
industrial, incomplete combustion	986	E868.3	—	E952.1	E962.2	E982.1
Fugillin	960.8	E856	E930.8	E950.4	E962.0	E980.4
Fulminate of mercury	985.0	E866.1	—	E950.9	E962.1	E980.9
Fulvicin	960.1	E856	E930.1	E950.4	E962.0	E980.4
Fumadil	960.8	E856	E930.8	E950.4	E962.0	E980.4
Fumagillin	960.8	E856	E930.8	E950.4	E962.0	E980.4
Fumes (from)	987.9	E869.9	—	E952.9	E962.2	E982.9
carbon monoxide - *see* Carbon, monoxide	—	—	—	—	—	—
charcoal (domestic use)	986	E868.3	—	E952.1	E962.2	E982.1
chloroform - *see* Chloroform						
coke (in domestic stoves, fireplaces)	986	E868.3	—	E952.1	E962.2	E982.1
corrosive NEC	987.8	E869.8	—	E952.8	E962.2	E982.8
ether - *see* Ether(s)						
freons	987.4	E869.2	—	E952.8	E962.2	E982.8
hydrocarbons	987.1	E869.8	—	E952.8	E962.2	E982.8
petroleum (liquefied)	987.0	E868.0	—	E951.1	E962.2	E981.1
distributed through pipes (pure or mixed with air)	987.0	E867	—	E951.0	E962.2	E981.0
lead - *see* Lead	—	—	—	—	—	—
metals - *see* specified metal	—	—	—	—	—	—
nitrogen dioxide	987.2	E869.0	—	E952.8	E962.2	E982.8
pesticides - *see* Pesticides	—	—	—	—	—	—
petroleum (liquefied)	987.0	E868.0	—	E951.1	E962.2	E981.1
distributed through pipes (pure or mixed with air)	987.0	E867	—	E951.0	E962.2	E981.0
polyester	987.8	E869.8	—	E952.8	E962.2	E982.8
specified source, other (*see also* substance specified)	987.8	E869.8	—	E952.8	E962.2	E982.8
sulfur dioxide	987.3	E869.1	—	E952.8	E962.2	E982.8
Fumigants	989.4	E863.8	—	E950.6	E962.1	E980.7
Fungi, noxious, used as food	988.1	E865.5	—	E950.9	E962.1	E980.9
Fungicides (*see also* Antifungals)	989.4	E863.6	—	E950.6	E962.1	E980.7
Fungizone	960.1	E856	E930.1	E950.4	E962.0	E980.4
topical	976.0	E858.7	E946.0	E950.4	E962.0	E980.4
Furacin	976.0	E858.7	E946.0	E950.4	E962.0	E980.4

◀ New   ◀▥ Revised   ~~deleted~~ Deleted   ● Use Additional Digit(s)

Substance	Poisoning	External Cause (E Code)				
		Accident	Therapeutic Use	Suicide Attempt	Assault	Undetermined
Furadantin	961.9	E857	E931.9	E950.4	E962.0	E980.4
Furazolidone	961.9	E857	E931.9	E950.4	E962.0	E980.4
Furnace (coal burning) (domestic), gas from	986	E868.3	—	E952.1	E962.2	E982.1
industrial	986	E868.8	—	E952.1	E962.2	E982.1
Furniture polish	989.89	E861.2	—	E950.9	E962.1	E980.9
Furosemide	974.4	E858.5	E944.4	E950.4	E962.0	E980.4
Furoxone	961.9	E857	E931.9	E950.4	E962.0	E980.4
Fusel oil (amyl) (butyl) (propyl)	980.3	E860.4	—	E950.9	E962.1	E980.9
Fusidic acid	960.8	E856	E930.8	E950.4	E962.0	E980.4
Gallamine	975.2	E858.6	E945.2	E950.4	E962.0	E980.4
Gallotannic acid	976.2	E858.7	E946.2	E950.4	E962.0	E980.4
Gamboge	973.1	E858.4	E943.1	E950.4	E962.0	E980.4
Gamimune	964.6	E858.2	E934.6	E950.4	E962.0	E980.4
Gamma-benzene hexachloride (vapor)	989.2	E863.0	—	E950.6	E962.1	E980.7
Gamma globulin	964.6	E858.2	E934.6	E950.4	E962.0	E980.4
Gamma hydroxy butyrate (GHB)	968.4	E855.1	E938.4	E950.4	E962.0	E980.4
Gamulin	964.6	E858.2	E934.6	E950.4	E962.0	E980.4
Ganglionic blocking agents	972.3	E858.3	E942.3	E950.4	E962.0	E980.4
Ganja	969.6	E854.1	E939.6	E950.3	E962.0	E980.3
Garamycin	960.8	E856	E930.8	E950.4	E962.0	E980.4
ophthalmic preparation	976.5	E858.7	E946.5	E950.4	E962.0	E980.4
topical NEC	976.0	E858.7	E946.0	E950.4	E962.0	E980.4
Gardenal	967.0	E851	E937.0	E950.1	E962.0	E980.1
Gardepanyl	967.0	E851	E937.0	E950.1	E962.0	E980.1
Gas	987.9	E869.9	—	E952.9	E962.2	E982.9
acetylene	987.1	E868.1	—	E951.8	E962.2	E981.8
incomplete combustion of - see Carbon, monoxide, fuel, utility	—	—	—	—	—	—
air contaminants, source or type not specified	987.9	E869.9	—	E952.9	E962.2	E982.9
anesthetic (general) NEC	968.2	E855.1	E938.2	E950.4	E962.0	E980.4
blast furnace	986	E868.8	—	E952.1	E962.2	E982.1
butane - see Butane	—	—	—	—	—	—
carbon monoxide - see Carbon, monoxide, chlorine	987.6	E869.8	—	E952.8	E962.2	E982.8
coal - see Carbon, monoxide, coal	—	—	—	—	—	—
cyanide	987.7	E869.8	—	E952.8	E962.2	E982.8
dicyanogen	987.8	E869.8	—	E952.8	E962.2	E982.8
domestic - see Gas, utility	—	—	—	—	—	—
exhaust - see Carbon, monoxide, exhaust gas	—	—	—	—	—	—
from wood- or coal-burning stove or fireplace	986	E868.3	—	E952.1	E962.2	E982.1

Substance	Poisoning	External Cause (E Code)				
		Accident	Therapeutic Use	Suicide Attempt	Assault	Undetermined
Gas *(Continued)*						
fuel (domestic use) - *see also* Carbon, monoxide, fuel	—	—	—	—	—	—
industrial use	986	E868.8	—	E952.1	E962.2	E982.1
utility	987.1	E868.1	—	E951.8	E962.2	E981.8
incomplete combustion of - *see* Carbon, monoxide, fuel, utility	—	—	—	—	—	—
in mobile container	987.0	E868.0	—	E951.1	E962.2	E981.1
piped (natural)	987.1	E867	—	E951.0	E962.2	E981.0
garage	986	E868.2	—	E952.0	E962.2	E982.0
hydrocarbon NEC	987.1	E869.8	—	E952.8	E962.2	E982.8
incomplete combustion of - *see* Carbon, monoxide, fuel, utility	—	—	—	—	—	—
liquefied (mobile container)	987.0	E868.0	—	E951.1	E962.2	E981.1
piped	987.0	E867	—	E951.0	E962.2	E981.0
hydrocyanic acid	987.7	E869.8	—	E952.8	E962.2	E982.8
illuminating - *see* Gas, utility	—	—	—	—	—	—
incomplete combustion, any - *see* Carbon, monoxide	—	—	—	—	—	—
kiln	986	E868.8	—	E952.1	E962.2	E982.1
lacrimogenic	987.5	E869.3	—	E952.8	E962.2	E982.8
marsh	987.1	E869.8	—	E952.8	E962.2	E982.8
motor exhaust, not in transit	986	E868.8	—	E952.1	E962.2	E982.1
mustard - *see* Mustard, gas	—	—	—	—	—	—
natural	987.1	E867	—	E951.0	E962.2	E981.0
nerve (war)	987.9	E869.9	—	E952.9	E962.2	E982.9
oils	981	E862.1	—	E950.9	E962.1	E980.9
petroleum (liquefied) (distributed in mobile containers)	987.0	E868.0	—	E951.1	E962.2	E981.1
piped (pure or mixed with air)	987.0	E867	—	E951.1	E962.2	E981.1
piped (manufactured) (natural) NEC	987.1	E867	—	E951.0	E962.2	E981.0
producer	986	E868.8	—	E952.1	E962.2	E982.1
propane - *see* Propane	—	—	—	—	—	—
refrigerant (freon)	987.4	E869.2	—	E952.8	E962.2	E982.8
not freon	987.9	E869.9	—	E952.9	E962.2	E982.9
sewer	987.8	E869.8	—	E952.8	E962.2	E982.8
specified source NEC (*see also* substance specified)	987.8	E869.8	—	E952.8	E962.2	E982.8
stove - *see* Gas, utility	—	—	—	—	—	—
tear	987.5	E869.3	—	E952.8	E962.2	E982.8
utility (for cooking, heating, or lighting) (piped) NEC	987.1	E868.1	—	E951.8	E962.2	E981.8
incomplete combustion of - *see* Carbon, monoxide, fuel, utility	—	—	—	—	—	—
in mobile container	987.0	E868.0	—	E951.1	E962.2	E981.1
piped (natural)	987.1	E867	—	E951.0	E962.2	E981.0
water	987.1	E868.1	—	E951.8	E962.2	E981.8
incomplete combustion of - *see* Carbon, monoxide, fuel, utility	—	—	—	—	—	—

◀ New   ◀‖ Revised   ~~deleted~~ Deleted   ● Use Additional Digit(s)

TABLE OF DRUGS AND CHEMICALS

Substance	Poisoning	External Cause (E Code)				
		Accident	Therapeutic Use	Suicide Attempt	Assault	Undetermined
Gaseous substance - *see* Gas	—	—	—	—	—	—
Gasoline, gasolene	981	E862.1	—	E950.9	E962.1	E980.9
vapor	987.1	E869.8	—	E952.8	E962.2	E982.8
Gastric enzymes	973.4	E858.4	E943.4	E950.4	E962.0	E980.4
Gastrografin	977.8	E858.8	E947.8	E950.4	E962.0	E980.4
Gastrointestinal agents	973.9	E858.4	E943.9	E950.4	E962.0	E980.4
specified NEC	973.8	E858.4	E943.8	E950.4	E962.0	E980.4
Gaultheria procumbens	988.2	E865.4	—	E950.9	E962.1	E980.9
Gelatin (intravenous)	964.8	E858.2	E934.8	E950.4	E962.0	E980.4
absorbable (sponge)	964.5	E858.2	E934.5	E950.4	E962.0	E980.4
Gelfilm	976.8	E858.7	E946.8	E950.4	E962.0	E980.4
Gelfoam	964.5	E858.2	E934.5	E950.4	E962.0	E980.4
Gelsemine	970.89	E854.3	E940.8	E950.4	E962.0	E980.4
Gelsemium (sempervirens)	988.2	E865.4	—	E950.9	E962.1	E980.9
Gemonil	967.0	E851	E937.0	E950.1	E962.0	E980.1
Gentamicin	960.8	E856	E930.8	E950.4	E962.0	E980.4
ophthalmic preparation	976.5	E858.7	E946.5	E950.4	E962.0	E980.4
topical NEC	976.0	E858.7	E946.0	E950.4	E962.0	E980.4
Gentian violet	976.0	E858.7	E946.0	E950.4	E962.0	E980.4
Gexane	976.0	E858.7	E946.0	E950.4	E962.0	E980.4
Gila monster (venom)	989.5	E905.0	—	E950.9	E962.1	E980.9
Ginger, Jamaica	989.89	E866.8	—	E950.9	E962.1	E980.9
Gitalin	972.1	E858.3	E942.1	E950.4	E962.0	E980.4
Gitoxin	972.1	E858.3	E942.1	E950.4	E962.0	E980.4
Glandular extract (medicinal) NEC	977.9	E858.9	E947.9	E950.5	E962.0	E980.5
Glaucarubin	961.5	E857	E931.5	E950.4	E962.0	E980.4
Globin zinc insulin	962.3	E858.0	E932.3	E950.4	E962.0	E980.4
Glucagon	962.3	E858.0	E932.3	E950.4	E962.0	E980.4
Glucochloral	967.1	E852.0	E937.1	E950.2	E962.0	E980.2
Glucocorticoids	962.0	E858.0	E932.0	E950.4	E962.0	E980.4
Glucose	974.5	E858.5	E944.5	E950.4	E962.0	E980.4
oxidase reagent	977.8	E858.8	E947.8	E950.4	E962.0	E980.4
Glucosulfone sodium	961.8	E857	E931.8	E950.4	E962.0	E980.4
Glue(s)	989.89	E866.6	—	E950.9	E962.1	E980.9
Glutamic acid (hydrochloride)	973.4	E858.4	E943.4	E950.4	E962.0	E980.4
Glutaraldehyde	989.89	E861.4	—	E950.9	E962.1	E980.9
Glutathione	963.8	E858.1	E933.8	E950.4	E962.0	E980.4
Glutethimide (group)	967.5	E852.4	E937.5	E950.2	E962.0	E980.2
Glycerin (lotion)	976.3	E858.7	E946.3	E950.4	E962.0	E980.4
Glycerol (topical)	976.3	E858.7	E946.3	E950.4	E962.0	E980.4

◀ New ◀▥ Revised ~~deleted~~ Deleted ● Use Additional Digit(s)

Substance	Poisoning	External Cause (E Code)				
		Accident	Therapeutic Use	Suicide Attempt	Assault	Undetermined
Glyceryl	—	—	—	—	—	—
guaiacolate	975.5	E858.6	E945.5	E950.4	E962.0	E980.4
triacetate (topical)	976.0	E858.7	E946.0	E950.4	E962.0	E980.4
trinitrate	972.4	E858.3	E942.4	E950.4	E962.0	E980.4
Glycine	974.5	E858.5	E944.5	E950.4	E962.0	E980.4
Glycobiarsol	961.1	E857	E931.1	E950.4	E962.0	E980.4
Glycols (ether)	982.8	E862.4	—	E950.9	E962.1	E980.9
Glycopyrrolate	971.1	E855.4	E941.1	E950.4	E962.0	E980.4
Glymidine	962.3	E858.0	E932.3	E950.4	E962.0	E980.4
Gold (compounds) (salts)	965.69	E850.6	E935.6	E950.0	E962.0	E980.0
Golden sulfide of antimony	985.4	E866.2	—	E950.9	E962.1	E980.9
Goldylocks	988.2	E865.4	—	E950.9	E962.1	E980.9
Gonadal tissue extract	962.9	E858.0	E932.9	E950.4	E962.0	E980.4
female	962.2	E858.0	E932.2	E950.4	E962.0	E980.4
male	962.1	E858.0	E932.1	E950.4	E962.0	E980.4
Gonadotropin	962.4	E858.0	E932.4	E950.4	E962.0	E980.4
Grain alcohol	980.0	E860.1	—	E950.9	E962.1	E980.9
beverage	980.0	E860.0	—	E950.9	E962.1	E980.9
Gramicidin	960.8	E856	E930.8	E950.4	E962.0	E980.4
Gratiola officinalis	988.2	E865.4	—	E950.9	E962.1	E980.9
Grease	989.89	E866.8	—	E950.9	E962.1	E980.9
Green hellebore	988.2	E865.4	—	E950.9	E962.1	E980.9
Green soap	976.2	E858.7	E946.2	E950.4	E962.0	E980.4
Grifulvin	960.1	E856	E930.1	E950.4	E962.0	E980.4
Griseofulvin	960.1	E856	E930.1	E950.4	E962.0	E980.4
Growth hormone	962.4	E858.0	E932.4	E950.4	E962.0	E980.4
Guaiacol	975.5	E858.6	E945.5	E950.4	E962.0	E980.4
Givaiac reagent	977.8	E858.8	E947.8	E950.4	E962.0	E980.4
Guaifenesin	975.5	E858.6	E945.5	E950.4	E962.0	E980.4
Guaiphenesin	975.5	E858.6	E945.5	E950.4	E962.0	E980.4
Guanatol	961.4	E857	E931.4	E950.4	E962.0	E980.4
Guanethidine	972.6	E858.3	E942.6	E950.4	E962.0	E980.4
Guano	989.89	E866.5	—	E950.9	E962.1	E980.9
Guanochlor	972.6	E858.3	E942.6	E950.4	E962.0	E980.4
Guanoctine	972.6	E858.3	E942.6	E950.4	E962.0	E980.4
Guanoxan	972.6	E858.3	E942.6	E950.4	E962.0	E980.4
Hair treatment agent NEC	976.4	E858.7	E946.4	E950.4	E962.0	E980.4
Halcinonide	976.0	E858.7	E946.0	E950.4	E962.0	E980.4
Halethazole	976.0	E858.7	E946.0	E950.4	E962.0	E980.4

◀ New   ◀ Revised   ~~deleted~~ Deleted   ● Use Additional Digit(s)

TABLE OF DRUGS AND CHEMICALS

Substance	Poisoning	External Cause (E Code)				
		Accident	Therapeutic Use	Suicide Attempt	Assault	Undetermined
Hallucinogens	969.6	E854.1	E939.6	E950.3	E962.0	E980.3
Haloperidol	969.2	E853.1	E939.2	E950.3	E962.0	E980.3
Haloprogin	976.0	E858.7	E946.0	E950.4	E962.0	E980.4
Halotex	976.0	E858.7	E946.0	E950.4	E962.0	E980.4
Halothane	968.1	E855.1	E938.1	E950.4	E962.0	E980.4
Halquinols	976.0	E858.7	E946.0	E950.4	E962.0	E980.4
Hand sanitizer	976.0	E858.7	E946.0	E950.4	E962.0	E980.4
Harmonyl	972.6	E858.3	E942.6	E950.4	E962.0	E980.4
Hartmann's solution	974.5	E858.5	E944.5	E950.4	E962.0	E980.4
Hashish	969.6	E854.1	E939.6	E950.3	E962.0	E980.3
Hawaiian wood rose seeds	969.6	E854.1	E939.6	E950.3	E962.0	E980.3
Headache cures, drugs, powders NEC	977.9	E858.9	E947.9	E950.5	E962.0	E980.9
Heavenly Blue (morning glory)	969.6	E854.1	E939.6	E950.3	E962.0	E980.3
Heavy metal antagonists	963.8	E858.1	E933.8	E950.4	E962.0	E980.4
anti-infectives	961.2	E857	E931.2	E950.4	E962.0	E980.4
Hedaquinium	976.0	E858.7	E946.0	E950.4	E962.0	E980.4
Hedge hyssop	988.2	E865.4	—	E950.9	E962.1	E980.9
Heet	976.8	E858.7	E946.8	E950.4	E962.0	E980.4
Helenin	961.6	E857	E931.6	E950.4	E962.0	E980.4
Hellebore (black) (green) (white)	988.2	E865.4	—	E950.9	E962.1	E980.9
Hemlock	988.2	E865.4	—	E950.9	E962.1	E980.9
Hemostatics	964.5	E858.2	E934.5	E950.4	E962.0	E980.4
capillary active drugs	972.8	E858.3	E942.8	E950.4	E962.0	E980.4
Henbane	988.2	E865.4	—	E950.9	E962.1	E980.9
Heparin (sodium)	964.2	E858.2	E934.2	E950.4	E962.0	E980.4
Heptabarbital, heptabarbitone	967.0	E851	E937.0	E950.1	E962.0	E980.1
Heptachlor	989.2	E863.0	—	E950.6	E962.1	E980.7
Heptalgin	965.09	E850.2	E935.2	E950.0	E962.0	E980.0
Herbicides	989.4	E863.5	—	E950.6	E962.1	E980.7
Heroin	965.01	E850.0	E935.0	E950.0	E962.0	E980.0
Herplex	976.5	E858.7	E946.5	E950.4	E962.0	E980.4
HES	964.8	E858.2	E934.8	E950.4	E962.0	E980.4
Hetastarch	964.8	E858.2	E934.8	E950.4	E962.0	E980.7
Hexachlorocyclohexane	989.2	E863.0	—	E950.6	E962.1	E980.7
Hexachlorophene	976.2	E858.7	E946.2	E950.4	E962.0	E980.4
Hexadimethrine (bromide)	964.5	E858.2	E934.5	E950.4	E962.0	E980.4
Hexafluorenium	975.2	E858.6	E945.2	E950.4	E962.0	E980.4
Hexa-germ	976.2	E858.7	E946.2	E950.4	E962.0	E980.4
Hexahydrophenol	980.8	E860.8	—	E950.9	E962.1	E980.9

◀ New   ⬅ Revised   deleted Deleted   ● Use Additional Digit(s)

| | External Cause (E Code) | | | | | |
Substance	Poisoning	Accident	Therapeutic Use	Suicide Attempt	Assault	Undetermined
Hexalen	980.8	E860.8	—	E950.9	E962.1	E980.9
Hexamethonium	972.3	E858.3	E942.3	E950.4	E962.0	E980.4
Hexamethylenamine	961.9	E857	E931.9	E950.4	E962.0	E980.4
Hexamine	961.9	E857	E931.9	E950.4	E962.0	E980.4
Hexanone	982.8	E862.4	—	E950.9	E962.1	E980.9
Hexapropymate	967.8	E852.8	E937.8	E950.2	E962.0	E980.2
Hexestrol	962.2	E858.0	E932.2	E950.4	E962.0	E980.4
Hexethal (sodium)	967.0	E851	E937.0	E950.1	E962.0	E980.1
Hexetidine	976.0	E858.7	E946.0	E950.4	E962.0	E980.4
Hexobarbital, hexobarbitone	967.0	E851	E937.0	E950.1	E962.0	E980.1
sodium (anesthetic)	968.3	E855.1	E938.3	E950.4	E962.0	E980.4
soluble	968.3	E855.1	E938.3	E950.4	E962.0	E980.4
Hexocyclium	971.1	E855.4	E941.1	E950.4	E962.0	E980.4
Hexoestrol	962.2	E858.0	E932.2	E950.4	E962.0	E980.4
Hexone	982.8	E862.4	—	E950.9	E962.1	E980.9
Hexylcaine	968.5	E855.2	E938.5	E950.4	E962.0	E980.4
Hexylresorcinol	961.6	E857	E931.6	E950.4	E962.0	E980.4
Hinkle's pills	973.1	E858.4	E943.1	E950.4	E962.0	E980.4
Histalog	977.8	E858.8	E947.8	E950.4	E962.0	E980.4
Histamine (phosphate)	972.5	E858.3	E942.5	E950.4	E962.0	E980.4
Histoplasmin	977.8	E858.8	E947.8	E950.4	E962.0	E980.4
Holly berries	988.2	E865.3	—	E950.9	E962.1	E980.9
Homatropine	971.1	E855.4	E941.1	E950.4	E962.0	E980.4
Homo-tet	964.6	E858.2	E934.6	E950.4	E962.0	E980.4
Hormones (synthetic substitute) NEC	962.9	E858.0	E932.9	E950.4	E962.0	E980.4
adrenal cortical steroids	962.0	E858.0	E932.0	E950.4	E962.0	E980.4
antidiabetic agents	962.3	E858.0	E932.3	E950.4	E962.0	E980.4
follicle stimulating	962.4	E858.0	E932.4	E950.4	E962.0	E980.4
gonadotropic	962.4	E858.0	E932.4	E950.4	E962.0	E980.4
growth	962.4	E858.0	E932.4	E950.4	E962.0	E980.4
ovarian (substitutes)	962.2	E858.0	E932.2	E950.4	E962.0	E980.4
parathyroid (derivatives)	962.6	E858.0	E932.6	E950.4	E962.0	E980.4
pituitary (posterior)	962.5	E858.0	E932.5	E950.4	E962.0	E980.4
anterior	962.4	E858.0	E932.4	E950.4	E962.0	E980.4
thyroid (derivative)	962.7	E858.0	E932.7	E950.4	E962.0	E980.4
Hornet (sting)	989.5	E905.3	—	E950.9	E962.1	E980.9
Horticulture agent NEC	989.4	E863.9	—	E950.6	E962.1	E980.7
Hyaluronidase	963.4	E858.1	E933.4	E950.4	E962.0	E980.4
Hyazyme	963.4	E858.1	E933.4	E950.4	E962.0	E980.4

◀ New   ◀ Revised   ~~deleted~~ Deleted   ● Use Additional Digit(s)

Substance	Poisoning	External Cause (E Code)				
		Accident	Therapeutic Use	Suicide Attempt	Assault	Undetermined
Hycodan	965.09	E850.2	E935.2	E950.0	E962.0	E980.0
Hydantoin derivatives	966.1	E855.0	E936.1	E950.4	E962.0	E980.4
Hydeltra	962.0	E858.0	E932.0	E950.4	E962.0	E980.4
Hydergine	971.3	E855.6	E941.3	E950.4	E962.0	E980.4
Hydrabamine penicillin	960.0	E856	E930.0	E950.4	E962.0	E980.4
Hydralazine, hydrallazine	972.6	E858.3	E942.6	E950.4	E962.0	E980.4
Hydrargaphen	976.0	E858.7	E946.0	E950.4	E962.0	E980.4
Hydrazine	983.9	E864.3	—	E950.7	E962.1	E980.6
Hydriodic acid	975.5	E858.6	E945.5	E950.4	E962.0	E980.4
Hydrocarbon gas	987.1	E869.8	—	E952.8	E962.2	E982.8
incomplete combustion of - see Carbon, monoxide, fuel, utility	—	—	—	—	—	—
liquefied (mobile container)	987.0	E868.0	—	E951.1	E962.2	E981.1
piped (natural)	987.0	E867	—	E951.0	E962.2	E981.0
Hydrochloric acid (liquid)	983.1	E864.1	—	E950.7	E962.1	E980.6
medicinal	973.4	E858.4	E943.4	E950.4	E962.0	E980.4
vapor	987.8	E869.8	—	E952.8	E962.2	E982.8
Hydrochlorothiazide	974.3	E858.5	E944.3	E950.4	E962.0	E980.4
Hydrocodone	965.09	E850.2	E935.2	E950.0	E962.0	E980.0
Hydrocortisone	962.0	E858.0	E932.0	E950.4	E962.0	E980.4
ENT agent	976.6	E858.7	E946.6	E950.4	E962.0	E980.4
ophthalmic preparation	976.5	E858.7	E946.5	E950.4	E962.0	E980.4
topical NEC	976.0	E858.7	E946.0	E950.4	E962.0	E980.4
Hydrocortone	962.0	E858.0	E932.0	E950.4	E962.0	E980.4
ENT agent	976.6	E858.7	E946.6	E950.4	E962.0	E980.4
ophthalmic preparation	976.5	E858.7	E946.5	E950.4	E962.0	E980.4
topical NEC	976.0	E858.7	E946.0	E950.4	E962.0	E980.4
Hydrocyanic acid - see Cyanide(s)	—	—	—	—	—	—
Hydroflumethiazide	974.3	E858.5	E944.3	E950.4	E962.0	E980.4
Hydrofluoric acid (liquid)	983.1	E864.1	—	E950.7	E962.1	E980.6
vapor	987.8	E869.8	—	E952.8	E962.2	E982.8
Hydrogen	987.8	E869.8	—	E952.8	E962.2	E982.8
arsenide	985.1	E866.3	—	E950.8	E962.1	E980.8
arseniurated	985.1	E866.3	—	E950.8	E962.1	E980.8
cyanide (salts)	989.0	E866.8	—	E950.9	E962.1	E980.9
gas	987.7	E869.8	—	E952.8	E962.2	E982.8
fluoride (liquid)	983.1	E864.1	—	E950.7	E962.1	E980.6
vapor	987.8	E869.8	—	E952.8	E962.2	E982.8
peroxide (solution)	976.6	E858.7	E946.6	E950.4	E962.0	E980.4
phosphorated	987.8	E869.8	—	E952.8	E962.2	E982.8

◀ New ◀ Revised ~~deleted~~ Deleted ● Use Additional Digit(s)

Substance	Poisoning	External Cause (E Code)				
		Accident	Therapeutic Use	Suicide Attempt	Assault	Undetermined
Hydrogen *(Continued)*						
sulfide (gas)	987.8	E869.8	—	E952.8	E962.2	E982.8
arseniurated	985.1	E866.3	—	E950.8	E962.1	E980.8
sulfureted	987.8	E869.8	—	E952.8	E962.2	E982.8
Hydromorphinol	965.09	E850.2	E935.2	E950.0	E962.0	E980.0
Hydromorphinone	965.09	E850.2	E935.2	E950.0	E962.0	E980.0
Hydromorphone	965.09	E850.2	E935.2	E950.0	E962.0	E980.0
Hydromox	974.3	E858.5	E944.3	E950.4	E962.0	E980.4
Hydrophilic lotion	976.3	E858.7	E946.3	E950.4	E962.0	E980.4
Hydroquinone	983.0	E864.0	—	E950.7	E962.1	E980.6
vapor	987.8	E869.8	—	E952.8	E962.2	E982.8
Hydrosulfuric acid (gas)	987.8	E869.8	—	E952.8	E962.2	E982.8
Hydrous wool fat (lotion)	976.3	E858.7	E946.3	E950.4	E962.0	E980.4
Hydroxide, caustic	983.2	E864.2	—	E950.7	E962.1	E980.6
Hydroxocobalamin	964.1	E858.2	E934.1	E950.4	E962.0	E980.4
Hydroxyamphetamine	971.2	E858.5	E941.2	E950.4	E962.0	E980.4
Hydroxychloroquine	961.4	E857	E931.4	E950.4	E962.0	E980.4
Hydroxydihydrocodeinone	965.09	E850.2	E935.2	E950.0	E962.0	E980.0
Hydroxyethyl starch	964.8	E858.2	E934.8	E950.4	E962.0	E980.4
Hydroxyphenamate	969.5	E853.8	E939.5	E950.3	E962.0	E980.3
Hydroxyphenylbutazone	965.5	E850.5	E935.5	E950.0	E962.0	E980.0
Hydroxyprogesterone	962.2	E858.0	E932.2	E950.4	E962.0	E980.4
Hydroxyquinoline derivatives	961.3	E857	E931.3	E950.4	E962.0	E980.4
Hydroxystilbamidine	961.5	E857	E931.5	E950.4	E962.0	E980.4
Hydroxyurea	963.1	E858.1	E933.1	E950.4	E962.0	E980.4
Hydroxyzine	969.5	E853.8	E939.5	E950.3	E962.0	E980.3
Hyoscine (hydrobromide)	971.1	E855.4	E941.1	E950.4	E962.0	E980.4
Hyoscyamine	971.1	E855.4	E941.1	E950.4	E962.0	E980.4
Hyoscyamus (albus) (niger)	988.2	E865.4	—	E950.9	E962.1	E980.9
Hypaque	977.8	E858.8	E947.8	E950.4	E962.0	E980.4
Hypertussis	964.6	E858.2	E934.6	E950.4	E962.0	E980.4
Hypnotics NEC	967.9	E852.9	E937.9	E950.2	E962.0	E980.2
Hypochlorites - *see* Sodium, hypochlorite	—	—	—	—	—	—
Hypotensive agents NEC	972.6	E858.3	E942.6	E950.4	E962.0	E980.4
Ibufenac	965.69	E850.6	E935.6	E950.0	E962.0	E980.0
Ibuprofen	965.61	E850.6	E935.6	E950.0	E962.0	E980.0
ICG	977.8	E858.8	E947.8	E950.4	E962.0	E980.4
Ichthammol	976.4	E858.7	E946.4	E950.4	E962.0	E980.4

◀ New ◀▦ Revised ~~deleted~~ Deleted ● Use Additional Digit(s)

Substance	Poisoning	External Cause (E Code)				
		Accident	Therapeutic Use	Suicide Attempt	Assault	Undetermined
Ichthyol	976.4	E858.7	E946.4	E950.4	E962.0	E980.4
Idoxuridine	976.5	E858.7	E946.5	E950.4	E962.0	E980.4
IDU	976.5	E858.7	E946.5	E950.4	E962.0	E980.4
Iletin	962.3	E858.0	E932.3	E950.4	E962.0	E980.4
Ilex	988.2	E865.4	—	E950.9	E962.1	E980.9
Illuminating gas - see Gas, utility	—	—	—	—	—	—
Ilopan	963.5	E858.1	E933.5	E950.4	E962.0	E980.4
Ilotycin	960.3	E856	E930.3	E950.4	E962.0	E980.4
ophthalmic preparation	976.5	E858.7	E946.5	E950.4	E962.0	E980.4
topical NEC	976.0	E858.7	E946.0	E950.4	E962.0	E980.4
Imipramine	969.05	E854.0	E939.0	E950.3	E962.0	E980.3
Immu-G	964.6	E858.2	E934.6	E950.4	E962.0	E980.4
Immuglobin	964.6	E858.2	E934.6	E950.4	E962.0	E980.4
Immune serum globulin	964.6	E858.2	E934.6	E950.4	E962.0	E980.4
Immunosuppressive agents	963.1	E858.1	E933.1	E950.4	E962.0	E980.4
Immu-tetanus	964.6	E858.2	E934.6	E950.4	E962.0	E980.4
Indandione (derivatives)	964.2	E858.2	E934.2	E950.4	E962.0	E980.4
Inderal	972.0	E858.3	E942.0	E950.4	E962.0	E980.4
Indian	—	—	—	—	—	—
hemp	969.6	E854.1	E939.6	E950.3	E962.0	E980.3
tobacco	988.2	E865.4	—	E950.9	E962.1	E980.9
Indigo carmine	977.8	E858.8	E947.8	E950.4	E962.0	E980.4
Indocin	965.69	E850.6	E935.6	E950.0	E962.0	E980.0
Indocyanine green	977.8	E858.8	E947.8	E950.4	E962.0	E980.4
Indomethacin	965.69	E850.6	E935.6	E950.0	E962.0	E980.0
Industrial	—	—	—	—	—	—
alcohol	980.9	E860.9	—	E950.9	E962.1	E980.9
fumes	987.8	E869.8	—	E952.8	E962.2	E982.8
solvents (fumes) (vapors)	982.8	E862.9	—	E950.9	E962.1	E980.9
Influenza vaccine	979.6	E858.8	E949.6	E950.4	E962.0	E982.8
Ingested substances NEC	989.9	E866.9	—	E950.9	E962.1	E980.9
INH (isoniazid)	961.8	E857	E931.8	E950.4	E962.0	E980.4
Inhalation, gas (noxious) - see Gas	—	—	—	—	—	—
Ink	989.89	E866.8	—	E950.9	E962.1	E980.9
Innovar	967.6	E852.5	E937.6	E950.2	E962.0	E980.2
Inositol niacinate	972.2	E858.3	E942.2	E950.4	E962.0	E980.4
Inproquone	963.1	E858.1	E933.1	E950.4	E962.0	E980.4
Insect (sting), venomous	989.5	E905.5		E950.9	E962.1	E980.9

◀ New ◀◀ Revised ~~deleted~~ Deleted ● Use Additional Digit(s)

Substance	Poisoning	External Cause (E Code)				
		Accident	Therapeutic Use	Suicide Attempt	Assault	Undetermined
Insecticides (*see also* Pesticides)	989.4	E863.4	—	E950.6	E962.1	E980.7
chlorinated	989.2	E863.0	—	E950.6	E962.1	E980.7
mixtures	989.4	E863.3	—	E950.6	E962.1	E980.7
organochlorine (compounds)	989.2	E863.0	—	E950.6	E962.1	E980.7
organophosphorus (compounds)	989.3	E863.1	—	E950.6	E962.1	E980.7
Insular tissue extract	962.3	E858.0	E932.3	E950.4	E962.0	E980.4
Insulin (amorphous) (globin) (isophane) (Lente) (NPH) (Protamine) (Semilente) (Ultralente) (zinc)	962.3	E858.0	E932.3	E950.4	E962.0	E980.4
Intranarcon	968.3	E855.1	E938.3	E950.4	E962.0	E980.4
Inulin	977.8	E858.8	E947.8	E950.4	E962.0	E980.4
Invert sugar	974.5	E858.5	E944.5	E950.4	E962.0	E980.4
Inza - see Naproxen	—	—	—	—	—	—
Iodide NEC (*see also* Iodine)	976.0	E858.7	E946.0	E950.4	E962.0	E980.4
mercury (ointment)	976.0	E858.7	E946.0	E950.4	E962.0	E980.4
methylate	976.0	E858.7	E946.0	E950.4	E962.0	E980.4
potassium (expectorant) NEC	975.5	E858.6	E945.5	E950.4	E962.0	E980.4
Iodinated glycerol	975.5	E858.6	E945.5	E950.4	E962.0	E980.4
Iodine (antiseptic, external) (tincture) NEC	976.0	E858.7	E946.0	E950.4	E962.0	E980.4
diagnostic	977.8	E858.8	E947.8	E950.4	E962.0	E980.4
for thyroid conditions (antithyroid)	962.8	E858.0	E932.8	E950.4	E962.0	E980.4
vapor	987.8	E869.8	—	E952.8	E962.2	E982.8
Iodized oil	977.8	E858.8	E947.8	E950.4	E962.0	E980.4
Iodobismitol	961.2	E857	E931.2	E950.4	E962.0	E980.4
Iodochlorhydroxyquin	961.3	E857	E931.3	E950.4	E962.0	E980.4
topical	976.0	E858.7	E946.0	E950.4	E962.0	E980.4
Iodoform	976.0	E858.7	E946.0	E950.4	E962.0	E980.4
Iodopanoic acid	977.8	E858.8	E947.8	E950.4	E962.0	E980.4
Iodophthalein	977.8	E858.8	E947.8	E950.4	E962.0	E980.4
Ion exchange resins	974.5	E858.5	E944.5	E950.4	E962.0	E980.4
Iopanoic acid	977.8	E858.8	E947.8	E950.4	E962.0	E980.4
Iophendylate	977.8	E858.8	E947.8	E950.4	E962.0	E980.4
Iothiouracil	962.8	E858.0	E932.8	E950.4	E962.0	E980.4
Ipecac	973.6	E858.4	E943.6	E950.4	E962.0	E980.4
Ipecacuanha	973.6	E858.4	E943.6	E950.4	E962.0	E980.4
Ipodate	977.8	E858.8	E947.8	E950.4	E962.0	E980.4
Ipral	967.0	E851	E937.0	E950.1	E962.0	E980.1
Ipratropium	975.1	E858.6	E945.1	E950.4	E962.0	E980.4
Iproniazid	969.01	E854.0	E939.0	E950.3	E962.0	E980.3

TABLE OF DRUGS AND CHEMICALS

		External Cause (E Code)				
Substance	Poisoning	Accident	Therapeutic Use	Suicide Attempt	Assault	Undetermined
Iron (compounds) (medicinal) (preparations)	964.0	E858.2	E934.0	E950.4	E962.0	E980.4
dextran	964.0	E858.2	E934.0	E950.4	E962.0	E980.4
nonmedicinal (dust) (fumes) NEC	985.8	E866.4	—	E950.9	E962.1	E980.9
Irritant drug	977.9	E858.9	E947.9	E950.5	E962.0	E980.5
Ismelin	972.6	E858.3	E942.6	E950.4	E962.0	E980.4
Isoamyl nitrite	972.4	E858.3	E942.4	E950.4	E962.0	E980.4
Isobutyl acetate	982.8	E862.4	—	E950.9	E962.1	E980.9
Isocarboxazid	969.01	E854.0	E939.0	E950.3	E962.0	E980.3
Isoephedrine	971.2	E855.5	E941.2	E950.4	E962.0	E980.4
Isoetharine	971.2	E855.5	E941.2	E950.4	E962.0	E980.4
Isofluorophate	971.0	E855.3	E941.0	E950.4	E962.0	E980.4
Isoniazid (INH)	961.8	E857	E931.8	E950.4	E962.0	E980.4
Isopentaquine	961.4	E857	E931.4	E950.4	E962.0	E980.4
Isophane insulin	962.3	E858.0	E932.3	E950.4	E962.0	E980.4
Isopregnenone	962.2	E858.0	E932.2	E950.4	E962.0	E980.4
Isoprenaline	971.2	E855.5	E941.2	E950.4	E962.0	E980.4
Isopropamide	971.1	E855.4	E941.1	E950.4	E962.0	E980.4
Isopropanol	980.2	E860.3	—	E950.9	E962.1	E980.9
topical (germicide)	976.0	E858.7	E946.0	E950.4	E962.0	E980.4
Isopropyl	—	—	—	—	—	—
acetate	982.8	E862.4	—	E950.9	E962.1	E980.9
alcohol	980.2	E860.3	—	E950.9	E962.1	E980.9
topical (germicide)	976.0	E858.7	E946.0	E950.4	E962.0	E980.4
ether	982.8	E862.4	—	E950.9	E962.1	E980.9
Isoproterenol	971.2	E855.5	E941.2	E950.4	E962.0	E980.4
Isosorbide dinitrate	972.4	E858.3	E942.4	E950.4	E962.0	E980.4
Isothipendyl	963.0	E858.1	E933.0	E950.4	E962.0	E980.4
Isoxazolyl penicillin	960.0	E856	E930.0	E950.4	E962.0	E980.4
Isoxsuprine hydrochloride	972.5	E858.3	E942.5	E950.4	E962.0	E980.4
l-thyroxine sodium	962.7	E858.0	E932.7	E950.4	E962.0	E980.4
Jaborandi (pilocarpus) (extract)	971.0	E855.3	E941.0	E950.4	E962.0	E980.4
Jalap	973.1	E858.4	E943.1	E950.4	E962.0	E980.4
Jamaica	—	—	—	—	—	—
dogwood (bark)	965.7	E850.7	E935.7	E950.0	E962.0	E980.0
ginger	989.89	E866.8	—	E950.9	E962.1	E980.9
Jatropha	988.2	E865.4	—	E950.9	E962.1	E980.9
curcas	988.2	E865.3	—	E950.9	E962.1	E980.9
Jectofer	964.0	E858.2	E934.0	E950.4	E962.0	E980.4

◄ New ◄ Revised deleted Deleted ● Use Additional Digit(s)

Substance	Poisoning	External Cause (E Code)				
		Accident	Therapeutic Use	Suicide Attempt	Assault	Undetermined
Jellyfish (sting)	989.5	E905.6	—	E950.9	E962.1	E980.9
Jequirity (bean)	988.2	E865.3	—	E950.9	E962.1	E980.9
Jimson weed	988.2	E865.4	—	E950.9	E962.1	E980.9
seeds	988.2	E865.3	—	E950.9	E962.1	E980.9
Juniper tar (oil) (ointment)	976.4	E858.7	E946.4	E950.4	E962.0	E980.4
Kallikrein	972.5	E858.3	E942.5	E950.4	E962.0	E980.4
Kanamycin	960.6	E856	E930.6	E950.4	E962.0	E980.4
Kantrex	960.6	E856	E930.6	E950.4	E962.0	E980.4
Kaolin	973.5	E858.4	E943.5	E950.4	E962.0	E980.4
Karaya (gum)	973.3	E858.4	E943.3	E950.4	E962.0	E980.4
Kemithal	968.3	E855.1	E938.3	E950.4	E962.0	E980.4
Kenacort	962.0	E858.0	E932.0	E950.4	E962.0	E980.4
Keratolytics	976.4	E858.7	E946.4	E950.4	E962.0	E980.4
Keratoplastics	976.4	E858.7	E946.4	E950.4	E962.0	E980.4
Kerosene, kerosine (fuel) (solvent) NEC	981	E862.1	—	E950.9	E962.1	E980.9
insecticide	981	E863.4	—	E950.6	E962.1	E980.7
vapor	987.1	E869.8	—	E952.8	E962.2	E982.8
Ketamine	968.3	E855.1	E938.3	E950.4	E962.0	E980.4
Ketobemidone	965.09	E850.2	E935.2	E950.0	E962.0	E980.0
Ketols	982.8	E862.4	—	E950.9	E962.1	E980.9
Ketone oils	982.8	E862.4	—	E950.9	E962.1	E980.9
Ketoprofen	965.61	E850.6	E935.6	E950.0	E962.0	E980.0
Kiln gas or vapor (carbon monoxide)	986	E868.8	—	E952.1	E962.2	E982.1
Konsyl	973.3	E858.4	E943.3	E950.4	E962.0	E980.4
Kosam seed	988.2	E865.3	—	E950.9	E962.1	E980.9
Krait (venom)	989.5	E905.0	—	E950.9	E962.1	E980.9
Kwell (insecticide)	989.2	E863.0	—	E950.6	E962.1	E980.7
anti-infective (topical)	976.0	E858.7	E946.0	E950.4	E962.0	E980.4
Laburnum (flowers) (seeds)	988.2	E865.3	—	E950.9	E962.1	E980.9
leaves	988.2	E865.4	—	E950.9	E962.1	E980.9
Lacquers	989.89	E861.6	—	E950.9	E962.1	E980.9
Lacrimogenic gas	987.5	E869.3	—	E952.8	E962.2	E982.8
Lactic acid	983.1	E864.1	—	E950.7	E962.1	E980.6
Lactobacillus acidophilus	973.5	E858.4	E943.5	E950.4	E962.0	E980.4
Lactoflavin	963.5	E858.1	E933.5	E950.4	E962.0	E980.4
Lactuca (virosa) (extract)	967.8	E852.8	E937.8	E950.2	E962.0	E980.2
Lactucarium	967.8	E852.8	E937.8	E950.2	E962.0	E980.2
Laevulose	974.5	E858.5	E944.5	E950.4	E962.0	E980.4
Lanatoside (C)	972.1	E858.3	E942.1	E950.4	E962.0	E980.4
Lanolin (lotion)	976.3	E858.7	E946.3	E950.4	E962.0	E980.4

◀ New   ◀▥ Revised   ~~deleted~~ Deleted   ● Use Additional Digit(s)

Substance	Poisoning	External Cause (E Code)				
		Accident	Therapeutic Use	Suicide Attempt	Assault	Undetermined
Largactil	969.1	E853.0	E939.1	E950.3	E962.0	E980.3
Larkspur	988.2	E865.3	—	E950.9	E962.1	E980.9
Laroxyl	969.05	E854.0	E939.0	E950.3	E962.0	E980.3
Lasix	974.4	E858.5	E944.4	E950.4	E962.0	E980.4
Latex	989.82	E866.8	—	E950.9	E962.1	E980.9
Lathyrus (seed)	988.2	E865.3	—	E950.9	E962.1	E980.9
Laudanum	965.09	E850.2	E935.2	E950.0	E962.0	E980.0
Laudexium	975.2	E858.6	E945.2	E950.4	E962.0	E980.4
Laurel, black or cherry	988.2	E865.4	—	E950.9	E962.1	E980.9
Laurolinium	976.0	E858.7	E946.0	E950.4	E962.0	E980.4
Lauryl sulfoacetate	976.2	E858.7	E946.2	E950.4	E962.0	E980.4
Laxatives NEC	973.3	E858.4	E943.3	E950.4	E962.0	E980.4
emollient	973.2	E858.4	E943.2	E950.4	E962.0	E980.4
L-dopa	966.4	E855.0	E936.4	E950.4	E962.0	E980.4
L-Tryptophan - *see* amino acid	—	—	—	—	—	—
Lead (dust) (fumes) (vapor) NEC	984.9	E866.0	—	E950.9	E962.1	E980.9
acetate (dust)	984.1	E866.0	—	E950.9	E962.1	E980.9
anti-infectives	961.2	E857	E931.2	E950.4	E962.0	E980.4
antiknock compound (tetra-ethyl)	984.1	E862.1	—	E950.9	E962.1	E980.9
arsenate, arsenite (dust) (insecticide) (vapor)	985.1	E863.4	—	E950.8	E962.1	E980.8
herbicide	985.1	E863.5	—	E950.8	E962.1	E980.8
carbonate	984.0	E866.0	—	E950.9	E962.1	E980.9
paint	984.0	E861.5	—	E950.9	E962.1	E980.9
chromate	984.0	E866.0	—	E950.9	E962.1	E980.9
paint	984.0	E861.5	—	E950.9	E962.1	E980.9
dioxide	984.0	E866.0	—	E950.9	E962.1	E980.9
inorganic (compound)	984.0	E866.0	—	E950.9	E962.1	E980.9
paint	984.0	E861.5	—	E950.9	E962.1	E980.9
iodide	984.0	E866.0	—	E950.9	E962.1	E980.9
pigment (paint)	984.0	E861.5	—	E950.9	E962.1	E980.9
monoxide (dust)	984.0	E866.0	—	E950.9	E962.1	E980.9
paint	984.0	E861.5	—	E950.9	E962.1	E980.9
organic	984.1	E866.0	—	E950.9	E962.1	E980.9
oxide	984.0	E866.0	—	E950.9	E962.1	E980.9
paint	984.0	E861.5	—	E950.9	E962.1	E980.9
paint	984.0	E861.5	—	E950.9	E962.1	E980.9
salts	984.0	E866.0	—	E950.9	E962.1	E980.9
specified compound NEC	984.8	E866.0	—	E950.9	E962.1	E980.9
tetra-ethyl	984.1	E862.1	—	E950.9	E962.1	E980.9
Lebanese red	969.6	E854.1	E939.6	E950.3	E962.0	E980.3

◄ New   ◄▬ Revised   ~~deleted~~ Deleted   ● Use Additional Digit(s)

TABLE OF DRUGS AND CHEMICALS

Substance	Poisoning	External Cause (E Code)				
		Accident	Therapeutic Use	Suicide Attempt	Assault	Undetermined
Lente Iletin (insulin)	962.3	E858.0	E932.3	E950.4	E962.0	E980.4
Leptazol	970.0	E854.3	E940.0	E950.4	E962.0	E980.4
Leritine	965.09	E850.2	E935.2	E950.0	E962.0	E980.0
Letter	962.7	E858.0	E932.7	E950.4	E962.0	E980.4
Lettuce opium	967.8	E852.8	E937.8	E950.2	E962.0	E980.2
Leucovorin (factor)	964.1	E858.2	E934.1	E950.4	E962.0	E980.4
Leukeran	963.1	E858.1	E933.1	E950.4	E962.0	E980.4
Levalbuterol	975.7	E858.6	E945.7	E950.4	E962.0	E980.4
Levallorphan	970.1	E854.3	E940.1	E950.4	E962.0	E980.4
Levanil	967.8	E852.8	E937.8	E950.2	E962.0	E980.2
Levarterenol	971.2	E855.5	E941.2	E950.4	E962.0	E980.4
Levodopa	966.4	E855.0	E936.4	E950.4	E962.0	E980.4
Levo-dromoran	965.09	E850.2	E935.2	E950.0	E962.0	E980.0
Levoid	962.7	E858.0	E932.7	E950.4	E962.0	E980.4
Levo-iso-methadone	965.02	E850.1	E935.1	E950.0	E962.0	E980.0
Levomepromazine	967.8	E852.8	E937.8	E950.2	E962.0	E980.2
Levoprome	967.8	E852.8	E937.8	E950.2	E962.0	E980.2
Levopropoxyphene	975.4	E858.6	E945.4	E950.4	E962.0	E980.4
Levorphan, levophanol	965.09	E850.2	E935.2	E950.0	E962.0	E980.0
Levothyroxine (sodium)	962.7	E858.0	E932.7	E950.4	E962.0	E980.4
Levsin	971.1	E855.4	E941.1	E950.4	E962.0	E980.4
Levulose	974.5	E858.5	E944.5	E950.4	E962.0	E980.4
Lewisite (gas)	985.1	E866.3	—	E950.8	E962.1	E980.8
Librium	969.4	E853.2	E939.4	E950.3	E962.0	E980.3
Lidex	976.0	E858.7	E946.0	E950.4	E962.0	E980.4
Lidocaine (infiltration) (topical)	968.5	E855.2	E938.5	E950.4	E962.0	E980.4
nerve block (peripheral) (plexus)	968.6	E855.2	E938.6	E950.4	E962.0	E980.4
spinal	968.7	E855.2	E938.7	E950.4	E962.0	E980.4
Lighter fluid	981	E862.1	—	E950.9	E962.1	E980.9
Lignocaine (infiltration) (topical)	968.5	E855.2	E938.5	E950.4	E962.0	E980.4
nerve block (peripheral) (plexus)	968.6	E855.2	E938.6	E950.4	E962.0	E980.4
spinal	968.7	E855.2	E938.7	E950.4	E962.0	E980.4
Ligroin(e) (solvent)	981	E862.0	—	E950.9	E962.1	E980.9
vapor	987.1	E869.8	—	E952.8	E962.2	E982.8
Ligustrum vulgare	988.2	E865.3	—	E950.9	E962.1	E980.9
Lily of the valley	988.2	E865.4	—	E950.9	E962.1	E980.9
Lime (chloride)	983.2	E864.2	—	E950.7	E962.1	E980.6
solution, sulferated	976.4	E858.7	E946.4	E950.4	E962.0	E980.4
Limonene	982.8	E862.4	—	E950.9	E962.1	E980.9

TABLE OF DRUGS AND CHEMICALS

Substance	Poisoning	External Cause (E Code)				
		Accident	Therapeutic Use	Suicide Attempt	Assault	Undetermined
Lincomycin	960.8	E856	E930.8	E950.4	E962.0	E980.4
Lindane (insecticide) (vapor)	989.2	E863.0	—	E950.6	E962.1	E980.7
anti-infective (topical)	976.0	E858.7	E946.0	E950.4	E962.0	E980.4
Liniments NEC	976.9	E858.7	E946.9	E950.4	E962.0	E980.4
Linoleic acid	972.2	E858.3	E942.2	E950.4	E962.0	E980.4
Liothyronine	962.7	E858.0	E932.7	E950.4	E962.0	E980.4
Liotrix	962.7	E858.0	E932.7	E950.4	E962.0	E980.4
Lipancreatin	973.4	E858.4	E943.4	E950.4	E962.0	E980.4
Lipo-Lutin	962.2	E858.0	E932.2	E950.4	E962.0	E980.4
Lipotropic agents	977.1	E858.8	E947.1	E950.4	E962.0	E980.4
Liquefied petroleum gases	987.0	E868.0	—	E951.1	E962.2	E981.1
piped (pure or mixed with air)	987.0	E867	—	E951.0	E962.2	E981.0
Liquid petrolatum	973.2	E858.4	E943.2	E950.4	E962.0	E980.4
substance	989.9	E866.9	—	E950.9	E962.1	E980.9
specified NEC	989.89	E866.8	—	E950.9	E962.1	E980.9
Lirugen	979.4	E858.8	E949.4	E950.4	E962.0	E980.4
Lithane	969.8	E855.8	E939.8	E950.3	E962.0	E980.3
Lithium	985.8	E866.4	—	E950.9	E962.1	E980.9
carbonate	969.8	E855.8	E939.8	E950.3	E962.0	E980.3
Lithonate	969.8	E855.8	E939.8	E950.3	E962.0	E980.3
Liver (extract) (injection) (preparations)	964.1	E858.2	E934.1	E950.4	E962.0	E980.4
Lizard (bite) (venom)	989.5	E905.0	—	E950.9	E962.1	E980.9
LMD	964.8	E858.2	E934.8	E950.4	E962.0	E980.4
Lobelia	988.2	E865.4	—	E950.9	E962.1	E980.9
Lobeline	970.0	E854.3	E940.0	E950.4	E962.0	E980.4
Locorten	976.0	E858.7	E946.0	E950.4	E962.0	E980.4
Lolium temulentum	988.2	E865.3	—	E950.9	E962.1	E980.9
Lomotil	973.5	E858.4	E943.5	E950.4	E962.0	E980.4
Lomustine	963.1	E858.1	E933.1	E950.4	E962.0	E980.4
Lophophora williamsii	969.6	E854.1	E939.6	E950.3	E962.0	E980.3
Lorazepam	969.4	E853.2	E939.4	E950.3	E962.0	E980.3
Lotions NEC	976.9	E858.7	E946.9	E950.4	E962.0	E980.4
Lotronex	973.8	E858.4	E943.8	E950.4	E962.0	E980.4
Lotusate	967.0	E851	E937.0	E950.1	E962.0	E980.1
Lowila	976.2	E858.7	E946.2	E950.4	E962.0	E980.4
Loxapine	969.3	E853.8	E939.3	E950.3	E962.0	E980.3
Lozenges (throat)	976.6	E858.7	E946.6	E950.4	E962.0	E980.4
LSD (25)	969.6	E854.1	E939.6	E950.3	E962.0	E980.3
Lubricating oil NEC	981	E862.2	—	E950.9	E962.1	E980.9

◀ New ◀ Revised ~~deleted~~ Deleted ● Use Additional Digit(s)

Substance	Poisoning	External Cause (E Code)				
		Accident	Therapeutic Use	Suicide Attempt	Assault	Undetermined
Lucanthone	961.6	E857	E931.6	E950.4	E962.0	E980.4
Luminal	967.0	E851	E937.0	E950.1	E962.0	E980.1
Lung irritant (gas) NEC	987.9	E869.9	—	E952.9	E962.2	E982.9
Lutocylol	962.2	E858.0	E932.2	E950.4	E962.0	E980.4
Lutromone	962.2	E858.0	E932.2	E950.4	E962.0	E980.4
Lututrin	975.0	E858.6	E945.0	E950.4	E962.0	E980.4
Lye (concentrated)	983.2	E864.2	—	E950.7	E962.1	E980.6
Lygranum (skin test)	977.8	E858.8	E947.8	E950.4	E962.0	E980.4
Lymecycline	960.4	E856	E930.4	E950.4	E962.0	E980.4
Lymphogranuloma venereum antigen	977.8	E858.8	E947.8	E950.4	E962.0	E980.4
Lynestrenol	962.2	E858.0	E932.2	E950.4	E962.0	E980.4
Lyovac Sodium Edecrin	974.4	E858.5	E944.4	E950.4	E962.0	E980.4
Lypressin	962.5	E858.0	E932.5	E950.4	E962.0	E980.4
Lysergic acid (amide) (diethylamide)	969.6	E854.1	E939.6	E950.3	E962.0	E980.3
Lysergide	969.6	E854.1	E939.6	E950.3	E962.0	E980.3
Lysine vasopressin	962.5	E858.0	E932.5	E950.4	E962.0	E980.4
Lysol	983.0	E864.0	—	E950.7	E962.1	E980.6
Lytta (vitatta)	976.8	E858.7	E946.8	E950.4	E962.0	E980.4
Mace	987.5	E869.3	—	E952.8	E962.2	E982.8
Macrolides (antibiotics)	960.3	E856	E930.3	E950.4	E962.0	E980.4
Mafenide	976.0	E858.7	E946.0	E950.4	E962.0	E980.4
Magaldrate	973.0	E858.4	E943.0	E950.4	E962.0	E980.4
Magic mushroom	969.6	E854.1	E939.6	E950.3	E962.0	E980.3
Magnamycin	960.8	E856	E930.8	E950.4	E962.0	E980.4
Magnesia magma	973.0	E858.4	E943.0	E950.4	E962.0	E980.4
Magnesium (compounds) (fumes) NEC	985.8	E866.4	—	E950.9	E962.1	E980.9
antacid	973.0	E858.4	E943.0	E950.4	E962.0	E980.4
carbonate	973.0	E858.4	E943.0	E950.4	E962.0	E980.4
cathartic	973.3	E858.4	E943.3	E950.4	E962.0	E980.4
citrate	973.3	E858.4	E943.3	E950.4	E962.0	E980.4
hydroxide	973.0	E858.4	E943.0	E950.4	E962.0	E980.4
oxide	973.0	E858.4	E943.0	E950.4	E962.0	E980.4
sulfate (oral)	973.3	E858.4	E943.3	E950.4	E962.0	E980.4
intravenous	966.3	E855.0	E936.3	E950.4	E962.0	E980.4
trisilicate	973.0	E858.4	E943.0	E950.4	E962.0	E980.4
Malathion (insecticide)	989.3	E863.1	—	E950.6	E962.1	E980.7
Male fern (oleoresin)	961.6	E857	E931.6	E950.4	E962.0	E980.4
Mandelic acid	961.9	E857	E931.9	E950.4	E962.0	E980.4
Manganese compounds (fumes) NEC	985.2	E866.4	—	E950.9	E962.1	E980.9

Substance	Poisoning	External Cause (E Code)				
		Accident	Therapeutic Use	Suicide Attempt	Assault	Undetermined
Mannitol (diuretic) (medicinal) NEC	974.4	E858.5	E944.4	E950.4	E962.0	E980.4
hexanitrate	972.4	E858.3	E942.4	E950.4	E962.0	E980.4
mustard	963.1	E858.1	E933.1	E950.4	E962.0	E980.4
Mannomustine	963.1	E858.1	E933.1	E950.4	E962.0	E980.4
MAO inhibitors	969.01	E854.0	E939.0	E950.3	E962.0	E980.3
Mapharsen	961.1	E857	E931.1	E950.4	E962.0	E980.4
Marcaine	968.9	E855.2	E938.9	E950.4	E962.0	E980.4
infiltration (subcutaneous)	968.5	E855.2	E938.5	E950.4	E962.0	E980.4
nerve block (peripheral) (plexus)	968.6	E855.2	E938.6	E950.4	E962.0	E980.4
Marezine	963.0	E858.1	E933.0	E950.4	E962.0	E980.4
Marihuana, marijuana (derivatives)	969.6	E854.1	E939.6	E950.3	E962.0	E980.3
Marine animals or plants (sting)	989.5	E905.6	—	E950.9	E962.1	E980.9
Marplan	969.01	E854.0	E939.0	E950.3	E962.0	E980.3
Marsh gas	987.1	E869.8	—	E952.8	E962.2	E982.8
Marsilid	969.01	E854.0	E939.0	E950.3	E962.0	E980.3
Matulane	963.1	E858.1	E933.1	E950.4	E962.0	E980.4
Mazindol	977.0	E858.8	E947.0	E950.4	E962.0	E980.4
MDMA	969.72	E854.2	E939.7	E950.3	E962.0	E980.3
Meadow saffron	988.2	E865.3	—	E950.9	E962.1	E980.9
Measles vaccine	979.4	E858.8	E949.4	E950.4	E962.0	E980.4
Meat, noxious or nonbacterial	988.8	E865.0	—	E950.9	E962.1	E980.9
Mebanazine	969.01	E854.0	E939.0	E950.3	E962.0	E980.3
Mebaral	967.0	E851	E937.0	E950.1	E962.0	E980.1
Mebendazole	961.6	E857	E931.6	E950.4	E962.0	E980.4
Mebeverine	975.1	E858.6	E945.1	E950.4	E962.0	E980.4
Mebhydroline	963.0	E858.1	E933.0	E950.4	E962.0	E980.4
Mebrophenhydramine	963.0	E858.1	E933.0	E950.4	E962.0	E980.4
Mebutamate	969.5	E853.8	E939.5	E950.3	E962.0	E980.3
Mecamylamine (chloride)	972.3	E858.3	E942.3	E950.4	E962.0	E980.4
Mechlorethamine hydrochloride	963.1	E858.1	E933.1	E950.4	E962.0	E980.4
Meclizene (hydrochloride)	963.0	E858.1	E933.0	E950.4	E962.0	E980.4
Meclofenoxate	970.0	E854.3	E940.0	E950.4	E962.0	E980.4
Meclozine (hydrochloride)	963.0	E858.1	E933.0	E950.4	E962.0	E980.4
Medazepam	969.4	E853.2	E939.4	E950.3	E962.0	E980.3
Medicine, medicinal substance	977.9	E858.9	E947.9	E950.5	E962.0	E980.5
specified NEC	977.8	E858.8	E947.8	E950.4	E962.0	E980.4
Medinal	967.0	E851	E937.0	E950.1	E962.0	E980.1
Medomin	967.0	E851	E937.0	E950.1	E962.0	E980.1
Medroxyprogesterone	962.2	E858.0	E932.2	E950.4	E962.0	E980.4

◀ New   ◀ Revised   ~~deleted~~ Deleted   ● Use Additional Digit(s)

Substance	Poisoning	External Cause (E Code)				
		Accident	Therapeutic Use	Suicide Attempt	Assault	Undetermined
Medrysone	976.5	E858.7	E946.5	E950.4	E962.0	E980.4
Mefenamic acid	965.7	E850.7	E935.7	E950.0	E962.0	E980.0
Megahallucinogen	969.6	E854.1	E939.6	E950.3	E962.0	E980.3
Megestrol	962.2	E858.0	E932.2	E950.4	E962.0	E980.4
Meglumine	977.8	E858.8	E947.8	E950.4	E962.0	E980.4
Meladinin	976.3	E858.7	E946.3	E950.4	E962.0	E980.4
Melanizing agents	976.3	E858.7	E946.3	E950.4	E962.0	E980.4
Melarsoprol	961.1	E857	E931.1	E950.4	E962.0	E980.4
Melia azedarach	988.2	E865.3	—	E950.9	E962.1	E980.9
Mellaril	969.1	E853.0	E939.1	E950.3	E962.0	E980.3
Meloxine	976.3	E858.7	E946.3	E950.4	E962.0	E980.4
Melphalan	963.1	E858.1	E933.1	E950.4	E962.0	E980.4
Memantine hydrochloride	969.8	E854.8	E939.8	E950.3	E962.0	E980.3
Menadiol sodium diphosphate	964.3	E858.2	E934.3	E950.4	E962.0	E980.4
Menadione (sodium bisulfite)	964.3	E858.2	E934.3	E950.4	E962.0	E980.4
Menaphthone	964.3	E858.2	E934.3	E950.4	E962.0	E980.4
Meningococcal vaccine	978.8	E858.8	E948.8	E950.4	E962.0	E980.4
Menningovax-C	978.8	E858.8	E948.8	E950.4	E962.0	E980.4
Menotropins	962.4	E858.0	E932.4	E950.4	E962.0	E980.4
Menthol NEC	976.1	E858.7	E946.1	E950.4	E962.0	E980.4
Mepacrine	961.3	E857	E931.3	E950.4	E962.0	E980.4
Meparfynol	967.8	E852.8	E937.8	E950.2	E962.0	E980.2
Mepazine	969.1	E853.0	E939.1	E950.3	E962.0	E980.3
Mepenzolate	971.1	E855.4	E941.1	E950.4	E962.0	E980.4
Meperidine	965.09	E850.2	E935.2	E950.0	E962.0	E980.0
Mephenamin(e)	966.4	E855.0	E936.4	E950.4	E962.0	E980.4
Mephenesin (carbamate)	968.0	E855.1	E938.0	E950.4	E962.0	E980.4
Mephenoxalone	969.5	E853.8	E939.5	E950.3	E962.0	E980.3
Mephentermine	971.2	E855.5	E941.2	E950.4	E962.0	E980.4
Mephenytoin	966.1	E855.0	E936.1	E950.4	E962.0	E980.4
Mephobarbital	967.0	E851	E937.0	E950.1	E962.0	E980.1
Mepiperphenidol	971.1	E855.4	E941.1	E950.4	E962.0	E980.4
Mepivacaine	968.9	E855.2	E938.9	E950.4	E962.0	E980.4
infiltration (subcutaneous)	968.5	E855.2	E938.5	E950.4	E962.0	E980.4
nerve block (peripheral) (plexus)	968.6	E855.2	E938.6	E950.4	E962.0	E980.4
topical (surface)	968.5	E855.2	E938.5	E950.4	E962.0	E980.4
Meprednisone	962.0	E858.0	E932.0	E950.4	E962.0	E980.4
Meprobam	969.5	E853.8	E939.5	E950.3	E962.0	E980.3
Meprobamate	969.5	E853.8	E939.5	E950.3	E962.0	E980.3

TABLE OF DRUGS AND CHEMICALS

Substance	Poisoning	External Cause (E Code)				
		Accident	Therapeutic Use	Suicide Attempt	Assault	Undetermined
Mepyramine (maleate)	963.0	E858.1	E933.0	E950.4	E962.0	E980.4
Meralluride	974.0	E858.5	E944.0	E950.4	E962.0	E980.4
Merbaphen	974.0	E858.5	E944.0	E950.4	E962.0	E980.4
Merbromin	976.0	E858.7	E946.0	E950.4	E962.0	E980.4
Mercaptomerin	974.0	E858.5	E944.0	E950.4	E962.0	E980.4
Mercaptopurine	963.1	E858.1	E933.1	E950.4	E962.0	E980.4
Mercumatilin	974.0	E858.5	E944.0	E950.4	E962.0	E980.4
Mercuramide	974.0	E858.5	E944.0	E950.4	E962.0	E980.4
Mercuranin	976.0	E858.7	E946.0	E950.4	E962.0	E980.4
Mercurochrome	976.0	E858.7	E946.0	E950.4	E962.0	E980.4
Mercury, mercuric, mercurous (compounds) (cyanide) (fumes) (nonmedicinal) (vapor) NEC	985.0	E866.1	—	E950.9	E962.1	E980.9
ammoniated	976.0	E858.7	E946.0	E950.4	E962.0	E980.4
anti-infective	961.2	E857	E931.2	E950.4	E962.0	E980.4
topical	976.0	E858.7	E946.0	E950.4	E962.0	E980.4
chloride (antiseptic) NEC	976.0	E858.7	E946.0	E950.4	E962.0	E980.4
fungicide	985.0	E863.6	—	E950.6	E962.1	E980.7
diuretic compounds	974.0	E858.5	E944.0	E950.4	E962.0	E980.4
fungicide	985.0	E863.6	—	E950.6	E962.1	E980.7
organic (fungicide)	985.0	E863.6	—	E950.6	E962.1	E980.7
Merethoxylline	974.0	E858.5	E944.0	E950.4	E962.0	E980.4
Mersalyl	974.0	E858.5	E944.0	E950.4	E962.0	E980.4
Merthiolate (topical)	976.0	E858.7	E946.0	E950.4	E962.0	E980.4
ophthalmic preparation	976.5	E858.7	E946.5	E950.4	E962.0	E980.4
Meruvax	979.4	E858.8	E949.4	E950.4	E962.0	E980.4
Mescal buttons	969.6	E854.1	E939.6	E950.3	E962.0	E980.3
Mescaline (salts)	969.6	E854.1	E939.6	E950.3	E962.0	E980.3
Mesoridazine besylate	969.1	E853.0	E939.1	E950.3	E962.0	E980.3
Mestanolone	962.1	E858.0	E932.1	E950.4	E962.0	E980.4
Mestranol	962.2	E858.0	E932.2	E950.4	E962.0	E980.4
Metactesylacetate	976.0	E858.7	E946.0	E950.4	E962.0	E980.4
Metaldehyde (snail killer) NEC	989.4	E863.4	—	E950.6	E962.1	E980.7
Metals (heavy) (nonmedicinal) NEC	985.9	E866.4	—	E950.9	E962.1	E980.9
dust, fumes, or vapor NEC	985.9	E866.4	—	E950.9	E962.1	E980.9
light NEC	985.9	E866.4	—	E950.9	E962.1	E980.9
dust, fumes, or vapor NEC	985.9	E866.4	—	E950.9	E962.1	E980.9
pesticides (dust) (vapor)	985.9	E863.4	—	E950.6	E962.1	E980.7
Metamucil	973.3	E858.4	E943.3	E950.4	E962.0	E980.4
Metaphen	976.0	E858.7	E946.0	E950.4	E962.0	E980.4

◀ New   ◀◀ Revised   ~~deleted~~ Deleted   ● Use Additional Digit(s)

Substance	Poisoning	External Cause (E Code)				
		Accident	Therapeutic Use	Suicide Attempt	Assault	Undetermined
Metaproterenol	975.1	E858.6	E945.1	E950.4	E962.0	E980.4
Metaraminol	972.8	E858.3	E942.8	E950.4	E962.0	E980.4
Metaxalone	968.0	E855.1	E938.0	E950.4	E962.0	E980.4
Metformin	962.3	E858.0	E932.3	E950.4	E962.0	E980.4
Methacycline	960.4	E856	E930.4	E950.4	E962.0	E980.4
Methadone	965.02	E850.1	E935.1	E950.0	E962.0	E980.0
Methallenestril	962.2	E858.0	E932.2	E950.4	E962.0	E980.4
Methamphetamine	969.72	E854.2	E939.7	E950.3	E962.0	E980.3
Methandienone	962.1	E858.0	E932.1	E950.4	E962.0	E980.4
Methandriol	962.1	E858.0	E932.1	E950.4	E962.0	E980.4
Methandrostenolone	962.1	E858.0	E932.1	E950.4	E962.0	E980.4
Methane gas	987.1	E869.8	—	E952.8	E962.2	E982.8
Methanol	980.1	E860.2	—	E950.9	E962.1	E980.9
vapor	987.8	E869.8	—	E952.8	E962.2	E982.8
Methantheline	971.1	E855.4	E941.1	E950.4	E962.0	E980.4
Methaphenilene	963.0	E858.1	E933.0	E950.4	E962.0	E980.4
Methapyrilene	963.0	E858.1	E933.0	E950.4	E962.0	E980.4
Methaqualone (compounds)	967.4	E852.3	E937.4	E950.2	E962.0	E980.2
Metharbital, metharbitone	967.0	E851	E937.0	E950.1	E962.0	E980.1
Methazolamide	974.2	E858.5	E944.2	E950.4	E962.0	E980.4
Methdilazine	963.0	E858.1	E933.0	E950.4	E962.0	E980.4
Methedrine	969.72	E854.2	E939.7	E950.3	E962.0	E980.3
Methenamine (mandelate)	961.9	E857	E931.9	E950.4	E962.0	E980.4
Methenolone	962.1	E858.0	E932.1	E950.4	E962.0	E980.4
Methergine	975.0	E858.6	E945.0	E950.4	E962.0	E980.4
Methiacil	962.8	E858.0	E932.8	E950.4	E962.0	E980.4
Methicillin (sodium)	960.0	E856	E930.0	E950.4	E962.0	E980.4
Methimazole	962.8	E858.0	E932.8	E950.4	E962.0	E980.4
Methionine	977.1	E858.8	E947.1	E950.4	E962.0	E980.4
Methisazone	961.7	E857	E931.7	E950.4	E962.0	E980.4
Methitural	967.0	E851	E937.0	E950.1	E962.0	E980.1
Methixene	971.1	E855.4	E941.1	E950.4	E962.0	E980.4
Methobarbital, methobarbitone	967.0	E851	E937.0	E950.1	E962.0	E980.1
Methocarbamol	968.0	E855.1	E938.0	E950.4	E962.0	E980.4
Methohexital, methohexitone (sodium)	968.3	E855.1	E938.3	E950.4	E962.0	E980.4
Methoin	966.1	E855.0	E936.1	E950.4	E962.0	E980.4
Methopholine	965.7	E850.7	E935.7	E950.0	E962.0	E980.0
Methorate	975.4	E858.6	E945.4	E950.4	E962.0	E980.4
Methoserpidine	972.6	E858.3	E942.6	E950.4	E962.0	E980.4

TABLE OF DRUGS AND CHEMICALS

Substance	Poisoning	External Cause (E Code)				
		Accident	Therapeutic Use	Suicide Attempt	Assault	Undetermined
Methotrexate	963.1	E858.1	E933.1	E950.4	E962.0	E980.4
Methotrimeprazine	967.8	E852.8	E937.8	E950.2	E962.0	E980.2
Methoxa-Dome	976.3	E858.7	E946.3	E950.4	E962.0	E980.4
Methoxamine	971.2	E855.5	E941.2	E950.4	E962.0	E980.4
Methoxsalen	976.3	E858.7	E946.3	E950.4	E962.0	E980.4
Methoxybenzyl penicillin	960.0	E856	E930.0	E950.4	E962.0	E980.4
Methoxychlor	989.2	E863.0	—	E950.6	E962.1	E980.7
Methoxyflurane	968.2	E855.1	E938.2	E950.4	E962.0	E980.4
Methoxyphenamine	971.2	E855.5	E941.2	E950.4	E962.0	E980.4
Methoxypromazine	969.1	E853.0	E939.1	E950.3	E962.0	E980.3
Methoxypsoralen	976.3	E858.7	E946.3	E950.4	E962.0	E980.4
Methscopolamine (bromide)	971.1	E855.4	E941.1	E950.4	E962.0	E980.4
Methsuximide	966.2	E855.0	E936.2	E950.4	E962.0	E980.4
Methyclothiazide	974.3	E858.5	E944.3	E950.4	E962.0	E980.4
Methyl	—	—	—	—	—	—
acetate	982.8	E862.4	—	E950.9	E962.1	E980.9
acetone II	982.8	E862.4	—	E950.9	E962.1	E980.9
alcohol	980.1	E860.2	—	E950.9	E962.1	E980.9
amphetamine	969.72	E854.2	E939.7	E950.3	E962.0	E980.3
androstanolone	962.1	E858.0	E932.1	E950.4	E962.0	E980.4
atropine	971.1	E855.4	E941.1	E950.4	E962.0	E980.4
benzene	982.0	E862.4	—	E950.9	E962.1	E980.9
bromide (gas)	987.8	E869.8	—	E952.8	E962.2	E982.8
fumigant	987.8	E863.8	—	E950.6	E962.2	E980.7
butanol	980.8	E860.8	—	E950.9	E962.1	E980.9
carbinol	980.1	E860.2	—	E950.9	E962.1	E980.9
cellosolve	982.8	E862.4	—	E950.9	E962.1	E980.9
cellulose	973.3	E858.4	E943.3	E950.4	E962.0	E980.4
chloride (gas)	987.8	E869.8	—	E952.8	E962.2	E982.8
cyclohexane	982.8	E862.4	—	E950.9	E962.1	E980.9
cyclohexanone	982.8	E862.4	—	E950.9	E962.1	E980.9
dihydromorphinone	965.09	E850.2	E935.2	E950.0	E962.0	E980.0
ergometrine	975.0	E858.6	E945.0	E950.4	E962.0	E980.4
ergonovine	975.0	E858.6	E945.0	E950.4	E962.0	E980.4
ethyl ketone	982.8	E862.4	—	E950.9	E962.1	E980.9
hydrazine	983.9	E864.3	—	E950.7	E962.1	E980.6
isobutyl ketone	982.8	E862.4	—	E950.9	E962.1	E980.9
morphine NEC	965.09	E850.2	E935.2	E950.0	E962.0	E980.0
parafynol	967.8	E852.8	E937.8	E950.2	E962.0	E980.2

◀ New ◀▥ Revised ~~deleted~~ Deleted ● Use Additional Digit(s)

Substance	Poisoning	External Cause (E Code)				
		Accident	Therapeutic Use	Suicide Attempt	Assault	Undetermined
Methyl *(Continued)*						
parathion	989.3	E863.1	—	E950.6	E962.1	E980.7
pentynol NEC	967.8	E852.8	E937.8	E950.2	E962.0	E980.2
peridol	969.2	E853.1	E939.2	E950.3	E962.0	E980.3
phenidate	969.73	E854.2	E939.7	E950.3	E962.0	E980.3
prednisolone	962.0	E858.0	E932.0	E950.4	E962.0	E980.4
ENT agent	976.6	E858.7	E946.6	E950.4	E962.0	E980.4
ophthalmic preparation	976.5	E858.7	E946.5	E950.4	E962.0	E980.4
topical NEC	976.0	E858.7	E946.0	E950.4	E962.0	E980.4
propylcarbinol	980.8	E860.8	—	E950.9	E962.1	E980.9
rosaniline NEC	976.0	E858.7	E946.0	E950.4	E962.0	E980.4
salicylate NEC	976.3	E858.7	E946.3	E950.4	E962.0	E980.4
sulfate (fumes)	987.8	E869.8	—	E952.8	E962.2	E982.8
liquid	983.9	E864.3	—	E950.7	E962.1	E980.6
sulfonal	967.8	E852.8	E937.8	E950.2	E962.0	E980.2
testosterone	962.1	E858.0	E932.1	E950.4	E962.0	E980.4
thiouracil	962.8	E858.0	E932.8	E950.4	E962.0	E980.4
Methylated spirit	980.0	E860.1	—	E950.9	E962.1	E980.9
Methyldopa	972.6	E858.3	E942.6	E950.4	E962.0	E980.4
Methylene blue	961.9	E857	E931.9	E950.4	E962.0	E980.4
chloride or dichloride (solvent) NEC	982.3	E862.4	—	E950.9	E962.1	E980.9
Methylhexabital	967.0	E851	E937.0	E950.1	E962.0	E980.1
Methylparaben (ophthalmic)	976.5	E858.7	E946.5	E950.4	E962.0	E980.4
Methyprylon	967.5	E852.4	E937.5	E950.2	E962.0	E980.2
Methysergide	971.3	E855.6	E941.3	E950.4	E962.0	E980.4
Metoclopramide	963.0	E858.1	E933.0	E950.4	E962.0	E980.4
Metofoline	965.7	E850.7	E935.7	E950.0	E962.0	E980.0
Metopon	965.09	E850.2	E935.2	E950.0	E962.0	E980.0
Metronidazole	961.5	E857	E931.5	E950.4	E962.0	E980.4
Metycaine	968.9	E855.2	E938.9	E950.4	E962.0	E980.4
infiltration (subcutaneous)	968.5	E855.2	E938.5	E950.4	E962.0	E980.4
nerve block (peripheral) (plexus)	968.6	E855.2	E938.6	E950.4	E962.0	E980.4
topical (surface)	968.5	E855.2	E938.5	E950.4	E962.0	E980.4
Metyrapone	977.8	E858.8	E947.8	E950.4	E962.0	E980.4
Mevinphos	989.3	E863.1	—	E950.6	E962.1	E980.7
Mezereon (berries)	988.2	E865.3	—	E950.9	E962.1	E980.9
Micatin	976.0	E858.7	E946.0	E950.4	E962.0	E980.4
Miconazole	976.0	E858.7	E946.0	E950.4	E962.0	E980.4
Midol	965.1	E850.3	E935.3	E950.0	E962.0	E980.0

TABLE OF DRUGS AND CHEMICALS

	External Cause (E Code)					
Substance	Poisoning	Accident	Therapeutic Use	Suicide Attempt	Assault	Undetermined
Mifepristone	962.9	E858.0	E932.9	E950.4	E962.0	E980.4
Milk of magnesia	973.0	E858.4	E943.0	E950.4	E962.0	E980.4
Millipede (tropical) (venomous)	989.5	E905.4	—	E950.9	E962.1	E980.9
Miltown	969.5	E853.8	E939.5	E950.3	E962.0	E980.3
Mineral	—	—	—	—	—	—
oil (medicinal)	973.2	E858.4	E943.2	E950.4	E962.0	E980.4
nonmedicinal	981	E862.1	—	E950.9	E962.1	E980.9
topical	976.3	E858.7	E946.3	E950.4	E962.0	E980.4
salts NEC	974.6	E858.5	E944.6	E950.4	E962.0	E980.4
spirits	981	E862.0	—	E950.9	E962.1	E980.9
Minocycline	960.4	E856	E930.4	E950.4	E962.0	E980.4
Mithramycin (antineoplastic)	960.7	E856	E930.7	E950.4	E962.0	E980.4
Mitobronitol	963.1	E858.1	E933.1	E950.4	E962.0	E980.4
Mitomycin (antineoplastic)	960.7	E856	E930.7	E950.4	E962.0	E980.4
Mitotane	963.1	E858.1	E933.1	E950.4	E962.0	E980.4
Moderil	972.6	E858.3	E942.6	E950.4	E962.0	E980.4
Mogadon - *see* Nitrazepam	—	—	—	—	—	—
Molindone	969.3	E853.8	E939.3	E950.3	E962.0	E980.3
Monistat	976.0	E858.7	E946.0	E950.4	E962.0	E980.4
Monkshood	988.2	E865.4	—	E950.9	E962.1	E980.9
Monoamine oxidase inhibitors	969.01	E854.0	E939.0	E950.3	E962.0	E980.3
Monochlorobenzene	982.0	E862.4	—	E950.9	E962.1	E980.9
Monosodium glutamate	989.89	E866.8	—	E950.9	E962.1	E980.9
Monoxide, carbon - *see* Carbon, monoxide	—	—	—	—	—	—
Moperone	969.2	E853.1	E939.2	E950.3	E962.0	E980.3
Morning glory seeds	969.6	E854.1	E939.6	E950.3	E962.0	E980.3
Moroxydine (hydrochloride)	961.7	E857	E931.7	E950.4	E962.0	E980.4
Morphazinamide	961.8	E857	E931.8	E950.4	E962.0	E980.4
Morphinans	965.09	E850.2	E935.2	E950.0	E962.0	E980.0
Morphine NEC	965.09	E850.2	E935.2	E950.0	E962.0	E980.0
antagonists	970.1	E854.3	E940.1	E950.4	E962.0	E980.4
Morpholinylethyl morphine	965.09	E850.2	E935.2	E950.0	E962.0	E980.0
Morrhuate sodium	972.7	E858.3	E942.7	E950.4	E962.0	E980.4
Moth balls (*see also* Pesticides)	989.4	E863.4	—	E950.6	E962.1	E980.7
naphthalene	983.0	E863.4	—	E950.7	E962.1	E980.6
Motor exhaust gas - *see* Carbon, monoxide, exhaust gas	—	—	—	—	—	—
Mouth wash	976.6	E858.7	E946.6	E950.4	E962.0	E980.4
Mucolytic agent	975.5	E858.6	E945.5	E950.4	E962.0	E980.4
Mucomyst	975.5	E858.6	E945.5	E950.4	E962.0	E980.4

◀ New   ◀▥ Revised   ~~deleted~~ Deleted   ● Use Additional Digit(s)

Substance	Poisoning	External Cause (E Code)				
		Accident	Therapeutic Use	Suicide Attempt	Assault	Undetermined
Mucous membrane agents (external)	976.9	E858.7	E946.9	E950.4	E962.0	E980.4
specified NEC	976.8	E858.7	E946.8	E950.4	E962.0	E980.4
Mumps	—	—	—	—	—	—
immune globulin (human)	964.6	E858.2	E934.6	E950.4	E962.0	E980.4
skin test antigen	977.8	E858.8	E947.8	E950.4	E962.0	E980.4
vaccine	979.6	E858.8	E949.6	E950.4	E962.0	E980.4
Mumpsvax	979.6	E858.8	E949.6	E950.4	E962.0	E980.4
Muriatic acid - see Hydrochloric acid	—	—	—	—	—	—
Muscarine	971.0	E855.3	E941.0	E950.4	E962.0	E980.4
Muscle affecting agents NEC	975.3	E858.6	E945.3	E950.4	E962.0	E980.4
oxytocic	975.0	E858.6	E945.0	E950.4	E962.0	E980.4
relaxants	975.3	E858.6	E945.3	E950.4	E962.0	E980.4
central nervous system	968.0	E855.1	E938.0	E950.4	E962.0	E980.4
skeletal	975.2	E858.6	E945.2	E950.4	E962.0	E980.4
smooth	975.1	E858.6	E945.1	E950.4	E962.0	E980.4
Mushrooms, noxious	988.1	E865.5	—	E950.9	E962.1	E980.9
Mussel, noxious	988.0	E865.1	—	E950.9	E962.1	E980.9
Mustard (emetic)	973.6	E858.4	E943.6	E950.4	E962.0	E980.4
gas	987.8	E869.8	—	E952.8	E962.2	E982.8
nitrogen	963.1	E858.1	E933.1	E950.4	E962.0	E980.4
Mustine	963.1	E858.1	E933.1	E950.4	E962.0	E980.4
M-vac	979.4	E858.8	E949.4	E950.4	E962.0	E980.4
Mycifradin	960.8	E856	E930.8	E950.4	E962.0	E980.4
topical	976.0	E858.7	E946.0	E950.4	E962.0	E980.4
Mycitracin	960.8	E856	E930.8	E950.4	E962.0	E980.4
ophthalmic preparation	976.5	E858.7	E946.5	E950.4	E962.0	E980.4
Mycostatin	960.1	E856	E930.1	E950.4	E962.0	E980.4
topical	976.0	E858.7	E946.0	E950.4	E962.0	E980.4
Mydriacyl	971.1	E855.4	E941.1	E950.4	E962.0	E980.4
Myelobromal	963.1	E858.1	E933.1	E950.4	E962.0	E980.4
Myleran	963.1	E858.1	E933.1	E950.4	E962.0	E980.4
Myochrysin(e)	965.69	E850.6	E935.6	E950.0	E962.0	E980.0
Myoneural blocking agents	975.2	E858.6	E945.2	E950.4	E962.0	E980.4
Myristica fragrans	988.2	E865.3	—	E950.9	E962.1	E980.9
Myristicin	988.2	E865.3	—	E950.9	E962.1	E980.9
Mysoline	966.3	E855.0	E936.3	E950.4	E962.0	E980.4
Nafcillin (sodium)	960.0	E856	E930.0	E950.4	E962.0	E980.4
Nail polish remover	982.8	E862.4	—	E950.9	E962.1	E980.9
Nalidixic acid	961.9	E857	E931.9	E950.4	E962.0	E980.4

TABLE OF DRUGS AND CHEMICALS

Substance	Poisoning	External Cause (E Code)				
		Accident	Therapeutic Use	Suicide Attempt	Assault	Undetermined
Nalorphine	970.1	E854.3	E940.1	E950.4	E962.0	E980.4
Naloxone	970.1	E854.3	E940.1	E950.4	E962.0	E980.4
Namenda	969.8	E854.8	E939.8	E950.3	E962.0	E980.3
Nandrolone (decanoate) (phenpropionate)	962.1	E858.0	E932.1	E950.4	E962.0	E980.4
Naphazoline	971.2	E855.5	E941.2	E950.4	E962.0	E980.4
Naphtha (painter's) (petroleum)	981	E862.0	—	E950.9	E962.1	E980.9
solvent	981	E862.0	—	E950.9	E962.1	E980.9
vapor	987.1	E869.8	—	E952.8	E962.2	E982.8
Naphthalene (chlorinated)	983.0	E864.0	—	E950.7	E962.1	E980.6
insecticide or moth repellent	983.0	E863.4	—	E950.7	E962.1	E980.6
vapor	987.8	E869.8	—	E952.8	E962.2	E982.8
Naphthol	983.0	E864.0	—	E950.7	E962.1	E980.6
Naphthylamine	983.0	E864.0	—	E950.7	E962.1	E980.6
Naprosyn - *see* Naproxen	—	—	—	—	—	—
Naproxen	965.61	E850.6	E935.6	E950.0	E962.0	E980.0
Narcotic (drug)	967.9	E852.9	E937.9	E950.2	E962.0	E980.2
analgesic NEC	965.8	E850.8	E935.8	E950.0	E962.0	E980.0
antagonist	970.1	E854.3	E940.1	E950.4	E962.0	E980.4
specified NEC	967.8	E852.8	E937.8	E950.2	E962.0	E980.2
Narcotine	975.4	E858.6	E945.4	E950.4	E962.0	E980.4
Nardil	969.01	E854.0	E939.0	E950.3	E962.0	E980.3
Natrium cyanide - *see* Cyanide(s)	—	—	—	—	—	—
Natural	—	—	—	—	—	—
blood (product)	964.7	E858.2	E934.7	E950.4	E962.0	E980.4
gas (piped)	987.1	E867	—	E951.0	E962.2	E981.0
incomplete combustion	986	E867	—	E951.0	E962.2	E981.0
Nealbarbital, nealbarbitone	967.0	E851	E937.0	E950.1	E962.0	E980.1
Nectadon	975.4	E858.6	E945.4	E950.4	E962.0	E980.4
Nematocyst (sting)	989.5	E905.6	—	E950.9	E962.1	E980.9
Nembutal	967.0	E851	E937.0	E950.1	E962.0	E980.1
Neoarsphenamine	961.1	E857	E931.1	E950.4	E962.0	E980.4
Neocinchophen	974.7	E858.5	E944.7	E950.4	E962.0	E980.4
Neomycin	960.8	E856	E930.8	E950.4	E962.0	E980.4
ENT agent	976.6	E858.7	E946.6	E950.4	E962.0	E980.4
ophthalmic preparation	976.5	E858.7	E946.5	E950.4	E962.0	E980.4
topical NEC	976.0	E858.7	E946.0	E950.4	E962.0	E980.4
Neonal	967.0	E851	E937.0	E950.1	E962.0	E980.1
Neoprontosil	961.0	E857	E931.0	E950.4	E962.0	E980.4
Neosalvarsan	961.1	E857	E931.1	E950.4	E962.0	E980.4

◀ New   ◀▥ Revised   deleted Deleted   ● Use Additional Digit(s)

Substance	Poisoning	External Cause (E Code)				
		Accident	Therapeutic Use	Suicide Attempt	Assault	Undetermined
Neosilversalvarsan	961.1	E857	E931.1	E950.4	E962.0	E980.4
Neosporin	960.8	E856	E930.8	E950.4	E962.0	E980.4
ENT agent	976.6	E858.7	E946.6	E950.4	E962.0	E980.4
ophthalmic preparation	976.5	E858.7	E946.5	E950.4	E962.0	E980.4
topical NEC	976.0	E858.7	E946.0	E950.4	E962.0	E980.4
Neostigmine	971.0	E855.3	E941.0	E950.4	E962.0	E980.4
Neraval	967.0	E851	E937.0	E950.1	E962.0	E980.1
Neravan	967.0	E851	E937.0	E950.1	E962.0	E980.1
Nerium oleander	988.2	E865.4	—	E950.9	E962.1	E980.9
Nerve gases (war)	987.9	E869.9	—	E952.9	E962.2	E982.9
Nesacaine	968.9	E855.2	E938.9	E950.4	E962.0	E980.4
infiltration (subcutaneous)	968.5	E855.2	E938.5	E950.4	E962.0	E980.4
nerve block (peripheral) (plexus)	968.6	E855.2	E938.6	E950.4	E962.0	E980.4
Neurobarb	967.0	E851	E937.0	E950.1	E962.0	E980.1
Neuroleptics NEC	969.3	E853.8	E939.3	E950.3	E962.0	E980.3
Neuroprotective agent	977.8	E858.8	E947.8	E950.4	E962.0	E980.4
Neutral spirits	980.0	E860.1	—	E950.9	E962.1	E980.9
beverage	980.0	E860.0	—	E950.9	E962.1	E980.9
Niacin, niacinamide	972.2	E858.3	E942.2	E950.4	E962.0	E980.4
Nialamide	969.01	E854.0	E939.0	E950.3	E962.0	E980.3
Nickle (carbonyl) (compounds) (fumes) (tetracarbonyl) (vapor)	985.8	E866.4	—	E950.9	E962.1	E980.9
Niclosamide	961.6	E857	E931.6	E950.4	E962.0	E980.4
Nicomorphine	965.09	E850.2	E935.2	E950.0	E962.0	E980.0
Nicotinamide	972.2	E858.3	E942.2	E950.4	E962.0	E980.4
Nicotine (insecticide) (spray) (sulfate) NEC	989.4	E863.4	—	E950.6	E962.1	E980.7
not insecticide	989.89	E866.8	—	E950.9	E962.1	E980.9
Nicotinic acid (derivatives)	972.2	E858.3	E942.2	E950.4	E962.0	E980.4
Nicotinyl alcohol	972.2	E858.3	E942.2	E950.4	E962.0	E980.4
Nicoumalone	964.2	E858.2	E934.2	E950.4	E962.0	E980.4
Nifenazone	965.5	E850.5	E935.5	E950.0	E962.0	E980.0
Nifuraldezone	961.9	E857	E931.9	E950.4	E962.0	E980.4
Nightshade (deadly)	988.2	E865.4	—	E950.9	E962.1	E980.9
Nikethamide	970.0	E854.3	E940.0	E950.4	E962.0	E980.4
Nilstat	960.1	E856	E930.1	E950.4	E962.0	E980.4
topical	976.0	E858.7	E946.0	E950.4	E962.0	E980.4
Nimodipine	977.8	E858.8	E947.8	E950.4	E962.0	E980.4
Niridazole	961.6	E857	E931.6	E950.4	E962.0	E980.4
Nisentil	965.09	E850.2	E935.2	E950.0	E962.0	E980.0
Nitrates	972.4	E858.3	E942.4	E950.4	E962.0	E980.4

TABLE OF DRUGS AND CHEMICALS

Substance	Poisoning	External Cause (E Code)				
		Accident	Therapeutic Use	Suicide Attempt	Assault	Undetermined
Nitrazepam	969.4	E853.2	E939.4	E950.3	E962.0	E980.3
Nitric	—	—	—	—	—	—
acid (liquid)	983.1	E864.1	—	E950.7	E962.1	E980.6
vapor	987.8	E869.8	—	E952.8	E962.2	E982.8
oxide (gas)	987.2	E869.0	—	E952.8	E962.2	E982.8
Nitrite, amyl (medicinal) (vapor)	972.4	E858.3	E942.4	E950.4	E962.0	E980.4
Nitroaniline	983.0	E864.0	—	E950.7	E962.1	E980.6
vapor	987.8	E869.8	—	E952.8	E962.2	E982.8
Nitrobenzene, nitrobenzol	983.0	E864.0	—	E950.7	E962.1	E980.6
vapor	987.8	E869.8	—	E952.8	E962.2	E982.8
Nitrocellulose	976.3	E858.7	E946.3	E950.4	E962.0	E980.4
Nitrofuran derivatives	961.9	E857	E931.9	E950.4	E962.0	E980.4
Nitrofurantoin	961.9	E857	E931.9	E950.4	E962.0	E980.4
Nitrofurazone	976.0	E858.7	E946.0	E950.4	E962.0	E980.4
Nitrogen (dioxide) (gas) (oxide)	987.2	E869.0	—	E952.8	E962.2	E982.8
mustard (antineoplastic)	963.1	E858.1	E933.1	E950.4	E962.0	E980.4
Nitroglycerin, nitroglycerol (medicinal)	972.4	E858.3	E942.4	E950.4	E962.0	E980.4
nonmedicinal	989.89	E866.8	—	E950.9	E962.1	E980.9
fumes	987.8	E869.8	—	E952.8	E962.2	E982.8
Nitrohydrochloric acid	983.1	E864.1	—	E950.7	E962.1	E980.6
Nitromersol	976.0	E858.7	E946.0	E950.4	E962.0	E980.4
Nitronaphthalene	983.0	E864.0	—	E950.7	E962.2	E980.6
Nitrophenol	983.0	E864.0	—	E950.7	E962.2	E980.6
Nitrothiazol	961.6	E857	E931.6	E950.4	E962.0	E980.4
Nitrotoluene, nitrotoluol	983.0	E864.0	—	E950.7	E962.1	E980.6
vapor	987.8	E869.8	—	E952.8	E962.2	E982.8
Nitrous	968.2	E855.1	E938.2	E950.4	E962.0	E980.4
acid (liquid)	983.1	E864.1	—	E950.7	E962.1	E980.6
fumes	987.2	E869.0	—	E952.8	E962.2	E982.8
oxide (anesthetic) NEC	968.2	E855.1	E938.2	E950.4	E962.0	E980.4
Nitrozone	976.0	E858.7	E946.0	E950.4	E962.0	E980.4
Noctec	967.1	E852.0	E937.1	E950.2	E962.0	E980.2
Noludar	967.5	E852.4	E937.5	E950.2	E962.0	E980.2
Noptil	967.0	E851	E937.0	E950.1	E962.0	E980.1
Noradrenalin	971.2	E855.5	E941.2	E950.4	E962.0	E980.4
Noramidopyrine	965.5	E850.5	E935.5	E950.0	E962.0	E980.0
Norepinephrine	971.2	E855.5	E941.2	E950.4	E962.0	E980.4
Norethandrolone	962.1	E858.0	E932.1	E950.4	E962.0	E980.4
Norethindrone	962.2	E858.0	E932.2	E950.4	E962.0	E980.4

◀ New   ◀▥ Revised   deleted Deleted   ● Use Additional Digit(s)

Substance	Poisoning	External Cause (E Code)				
		Accident	Therapeutic Use	Suicide Attempt	Assault	Undetermined
Norethisterone	962.2	E858.0	E932.2	E950.4	E962.0	E980.4
Norethynodrel	962.2	E858.0	E932.2	E950.4	E962.0	E980.4
Norlestrin	962.2	E858.0	E932.2	E950.4	E962.0	E980.4
Norlutin	962.2	E858.0	E932.2	E950.4	E962.0	E980.4
Normison - *see* Benzodiazepines	—	—	—	—	—	—
Normorphine	965.09	E850.2	E935.2	E950.0	E962.0	E980.0
Nortriptyline	969.05	E854.0	E939.0	E950.3	E962.0	E980.3
Noscapine	975.4	E858.6	E945.4	E950.4	E962.0	E980.4
Nose preparations	976.6	E858.7	E946.6	E950.4	E962.0	E980.4
Novobiocin	960.8	E856	E930.8	E950.4	E962.0	E980.4
Novocain (infiltration) (topical)	968.5	E855.2	E938.5	E950.4	E962.0	E980.4
nerve block (peripheral) (plexus)	968.6	E855.2	E938.6	E950.4	E962.0	E980.4
spinal	968.7	E855.2	E938.7	E950.4	E962.0	E980.4
Noxythiolin	961.9	E857	E931.9	E950.4	E962.0	E980.4
NPH Iletin (insulin)	962.3	E858.0	E932.3	E950.4	E962.0	E980.4
Numorphan	965.09	E850.2	E935.2	E950.0	E962.0	E980.0
Nunol	967.0	E851	E937.0	E950.1	E962.0	E980.1
Nupercaine (spinal anesthetic)	968.7	E855.2	E938.7	E950.4	E962.0	E980.4
topical (surface)	968.5	E855.2	E938.5	E950.4	E962.0	E980.4
Nutmeg oil (liniment)	976.3	E858.7	E946.3	E950.4	E962.0	E980.4
Nux vomica	989.1	E863.7	—	E950.6	E962.1	E980.7
Nydrazid	961.8	E857	E931.8	E950.4	E962.0	E980.4
Nylidrin	971.2	E855.5	E941.2	E950.4	E962.0	E980.4
Nystatin	960.1	E856	E930.1	E950.4	E962.0	E980.4
topical	976.0	E858.7	E946.0	E950.4	E962.0	E980.4
Nytol	963.0	E858.1	E933.0	E950.4	E962.0	E980.4
Oblivion	967.8	E852.8	E937.8	E950.2	E962.0	E980.2
Octyl nitrite	972.4	E858.3	E942.4	E950.4	E962.0	E980.4
Oestradiol (cypionate) (dipropionate) (valerate)	962.2	E858.0	E932.2	E950.4	E962.0	E980.4
Oestriol	962.2	E858.0	E932.2	E950.4	E962.0	E980.4
Oestrone	962.2	E858.0	E932.2	E950.4	E962.0	E980.4
Oil (of) NEC	989.89	E866.8	—	E950.9	E962.1	E980.9
bitter almond	989.0	E866.8	—	E950.9	E962.1	E980.9
camphor	976.1	E858.7	E946.1	E950.4	E962.0	E980.4
colors	989.89	E861.6	—	E950.9	E962.1	E980.9
fumes	987.8	E869.8	—	E952.8	E962.2	E982.8
lubricating	981	E862.2	—	E950.9	E962.1	E980.9
specified source, other - *see* substance specified	—	—	—	—	—	—

New   Revised   ~~deleted~~ Deleted   ● Use Additional Digit(s)

Substance	Poisoning	External Cause (E Code)				
		Accident	Therapeutic Use	Suicide Attempt	Assault	Undetermined
Oil (of) NEC *(Continued)*						
vitriol (liquid)	983.1	E864.1	—	E950.7	E962.1	E980.6
fumes	987.8	E869.8	—	E952.8	E962.2	E982.8
wintergreen (bitter) NEC	976.3	E858.7	E946.3	E950.4	E962.0	E980.4
Ointments NEC	976.9	E858.7	E946.9	E950.4	E962.0	E980.4
Oleander	988.2	E865.4	—	E950.9	E962.1	E980.9
Oleandomycin	960.3	E856	E930.3	E950.4	E962.0	E980.4
Oleovitamin A	963.5	E858.1	E933.5	E950.4	E962.0	E980.4
Oleum ricini	973.1	E858.4	E943.1	E950.4	E962.0	E980.4
Olive oil (medicinal) NEC	973.2	E858.4	E943.2	E950.4	E962.0	E980.4
OMPA	989.3	E863.1	—	E950.6	E962.1	E980.7
Oncovin	963.1	E858.1	E933.1	E950.4	E962.0	E980.4
Ophthaine	968.5	E855.2	E938.5	E950.4	E962.0	E980.4
Ophthetic	968.5	E855.2	E938.5	E950.4	E962.0	E980.4
Opiates, opioids, opium NEC	965.00	E850.2	E935.2	E950.0	E962.0	E980.0
antagonists	970.1	E854.3	E940.1	E950.4	E962.0	E980.4
Oracon	962.2	E858.0	E932.2	E950.4	E962.0	E980.4
Oragrafin	977.8	E858.8	E947.8	E950.4	E962.0	E980.4
Oral contraceptives	962.2	E858.0	E932.2	E950.4	E962.0	E980.4
Orciprenaline	975.1	E858.6	E945.1	E950.4	E962.0	E980.4
Organidin	975.5	E858.6	E945.5	E950.4	E962.0	E980.4
Organophosphates	989.3	E863.1	—	E950.6	E962.1	E980.7
Orimune	979.5	E858.8	E949.5	E950.4	E962.0	E980.4
Orinase	962.3	E858.0	E932.3	E950.4	E962.0	E980.4
Orphenadrine	966.4	E855.0	E936.4	E950.4	E962.0	E980.4
Ortal (sodium)	967.0	E851	E937.0	E950.1	E962.0	E980.1
Orthoboric acid	976.0	E858.7	E946.0	E950.4	E962.0	E980.4
ENT agent	976.6	E858.7	E946.6	E950.4	E962.0	E980.4
ophthalmic preparation	976.5	E858.7	E946.5	E950.4	E962.0	E980.4
Orthocaine	968.5	E855.2	E938.5	E950.4	E962.0	E980.4
Ortho-Novum	962.2	E858.0	E932.2	E950.4	E962.0	E980.4
Orthotolidine (reagent)	977.8	E858.8	E947.8	E950.4	E962.0	E980.4
Osmic acid (liquid)	983.1	E864.1	—	E950.7	E962.1	E980.6
fumes	987.8	E869.8	—	E952.8	E962.2	E982.8
Osmotic diuretics	974.4	E858.5	E944.4	E950.4	E962.0	E980.4
Ouabain	972.1	E858.3	E942.1	E950.4	E962.0	E980.4
Ovarian hormones (synthetic substitutes)	962.2	E858.0	E932.2	E950.4	E962.0	E980.4
Ovral	962.2	E858.0	E932.2	E950.4	E962.0	E980.4

◄ New   ◄▥ Revised   ~~deleted~~ Deleted   ● Use Additional Digit(s)

Substance	Poisoning	External Cause (E Code)				
		Accident	Therapeutic Use	Suicide Attempt	Assault	Undetermined
Ovulation suppressants	962.2	E858.0	E932.2	E950.4	E962.0	E980.4
Ovulen	962.2	E858.0	E932.2	E950.4	E962.0	E980.4
Oxacillin (sodium)	960.0	E856	E930.0	E950.4	E962.0	E980.4
Oxalic acid	983.1	E864.1	—	E950.7	E962.1	E980.6
Oxanamide	969.5	E853.8	E939.5	E950.3	E962.0	E980.3
Oxandrolone	962.1	E858.0	E932.1	E950.4	E962.0	E980.4
Oxaprozin	965.61	E850.6	E935.6	E950.0	E962.0	E980.0
Oxazepam	969.4	E853.2	E939.4	E950.3	E962.0	E980.3
Oxazolidine derivatives	966.0	E855.0	E936.0	E950.4	E962.0	E980.4
Ox bile extract	973.4	E858.4	E943.4	E950.4	E962.0	E980.4
Oxedrine	971.2	E855.5	E941.2	E950.4	E962.0	E980.4
Oxeladin	975.4	E858.6	E945.4	E950.4	E962.0	E980.4
Oxethazaine NEC	968.5	E855.2	E938.5	E950.4	E962.0	E980.4
Oxidizing agents NEC	983.9	E864.3	—	E950.7	E962.1	E980.6
Oxolinic acid	961.3	E857	E931.3	E950.4	E962.0	E980.4
Oxophenarsine	961.1	E857	E931.1	E950.4	E962.0	E980.4
Oxsoralen	976.3	E858.7	E946.3	E950.4	E962.0	E980.4
Oxtriphylline	976.7	E858.6	E945.7	E950.4	E962.0	E980.4
Oxybuprocaine	968.5	E855.2	E938.5	E950.4	E962.0	E980.4
Oxybutynin	975.1	E858.6	E945.1	E950.4	E962.0	E980.4
Oxycodone	965.09	E850.2	E935.2	E950.0	E962.0	E980.0
Oxygen	987.8	E869.8	—	E952.8	E962.2	E982.8
Oxylone	976.0	E858.7	E946.0	E950.4	E962.0	E980.4
ophthalmic preparation	976.5	E858.7	E946.5	E950.4	E962.0	E980.4
Oxymesterone	962.1	E858.0	E932.1	E950.4	E962.0	E980.4
Oxymetazoline	971.2	E855.5	E941.2	E950.4	E962.0	E980.4
Oxymetholone	962.1	E858.0	E932.1	E950.4	E962.0	E980.4
Oxymorphone	965.09	E850.2	E935.2	E950.0	E962.0	E980.0
Oxypertine	969.09	E854.0	E939.0	E950.3	E962.0	E980.3
Oxyphenbutazone	965.5	E850.5	E935.5	E950.0	E962.0	E980.0
Oxyphencyclimine	971.1	E855.4	E941.1	E950.4	E962.0	E980.4
Oxyphenisatin	973.1	E858.4	E943.1	E950.4	E962.0	E980.4
Oxyphenonium	971.1	E855.4	E941.1	E950.4	E962.0	E980.4
Oxyquinoline	961.3	E857	E931.3	E950.4	E962.0	E980.4
Oxytetracycline	960.4	E856	E930.4	E950.4	E962.0	E980.4
Oxytocics	975.0	E858.6	E945.0	E950.4	E962.0	E980.4
Oxytocin	975.0	E858.6	E945.0	E950.4	E962.0	E980.4
Ozone	987.8	E869.8	—	E952.8	E962.2	E982.8
PABA	976.3	E858.7	E946.3	E950.4	E962.0	E980.4

TABLE OF DRUGS AND CHEMICALS

◀ New   ◀|||| Revised   ~~deleted~~ Deleted   ● Use Additional Digit(s)

TABLE OF DRUGS AND CHEMICALS

Substance	Poisoning	External Cause (E Code)				
		Accident	Therapeutic Use	Suicide Attempt	Assault	Undetermined
Packed red cells	964.7	E858.2	E934.7	E950.4	E962.0	E980.4
Paint NEC	989.89	E861.6	—	E950.9	E962.1	E980.9
cleaner	982.8	E862.9	—	E950.9	E962.1	E980.9
fumes NEC	987.8	E869.8	—	E952.8	E962.1	E982.8
lead (fumes)	984.0	E861.5	—	E950.9	E962.1	E980.9
solvent NEC	982.8	E862.9	—	E950.9	E962.1	E980.9
stripper	982.8	E862.9	—	E950.9	E962.1	E980.9
Palfium	965.09	E850.2	E935.2	E950.0	E962.0	E980.0
Palivizumab	979.9	E858.8	E949.6	E950.4	E962.0	E980.4
Paludrine	961.4	E857	E931.4	E950.4	E962.0	E980.4
PAM	977.2	E855.8	E947.2	E950.4	E962.0	E980.4
Pamaquine (napthoate)	961.4	E857	E931.4	E950.4	E962.0	E980.4
Pamprin	965.1	E850.3	E935.3	E950.0	E962.0	E980.0
Panadol	965.4	E850.4	E935.4	E950.0	E962.0	E980.0
Pancreatic dornase (mucolytic)	963.4	E858.1	E933.4	E950.4	E962.0	E980.4
Pancreatin	973.4	E858.4	E943.4	E950.4	E962.0	E980.4
Pancrelipase	973.4	E858.4	E943.4	E950.4	E962.0	E980.4
Pangamic acid	963.5	E858.1	E933.5	E950.4	E962.0	E980.4
Panthenol	963.5	E858.1	E933.5	E950.4	E962.0	E980.4
topical	976.8	E858.7	E946.8	E950.4	E962.0	E980.4
Pantopaque	977.8	E858.8	E947.8	E950.4	E962.0	E980.4
Pantopon	965.00	E850.2	E935.2	E950.0	E962.0	E980.0
Pantothenic acid	963.5	E858.1	E933.5	E950.4	E962.0	E980.4
Panwarfin	964.2	E858.2	E934.2	E950.4	E962.0	E980.4
Papain	973.4	E858.4	E943.4	E950.4	E962.0	E980.4
Papaverine	972.5	E858.3	E942.5	E950.4	E962.0	E980.4
Para-aminobenzoic acid	976.3	E858.7	E946.3	E950.4	E962.0	E980.4
Para-aminophenol derivatives	965.4	E850.4	E935.4	E950.0	E962.0	E980.0
Para-aminosalicylic acid (derivatives)	961.8	E857	E931.8	E950.4	E962.0	E980.4
Paracetaldehyde (medicinal)	967.2	E852.1	E937.2	E950.2	E962.0	E980.2
Paracetamol	965.4	E850.4	E935.4	E950.0	E962.0	E980.0
Paracodin	965.09	E850.2	E935.2	E950.0	E962.0	E980.0
Paradione	966.0	E855.0	E936.0	E950.4	E962.0	E980.4
Paraffin(s) (wax)	981	E862.3	—	E950.9	E962.1	E980.9
liquid (medicinal)	973.2	E858.4	E943.2	E950.4	E962.0	E980.4
nonmedicinal (oil)	981	E962.1	—	E950.9	E962.1	E980.9
Paraldehyde (medicinal)	967.2	E852.1	E937.2	E950.2	E962.0	E980.2
Paramethadione	966.0	E855.0	E936.0	E950.4	E962.0	E980.4
Paramethasone	962.0	E858.0	E932.0	E950.4	E962.0	E980.4

◄ New ◄ Revised ~~deleted~~ Deleted ● Use Additional Digit(s)

Substance	Poisoning	External Cause (E Code)				
		Accident	Therapeutic Use	Suicide Attempt	Assault	Undetermined
Paraquat	989.4	E863.5	—	E950.6	E962.1	E980.7
Parasympatholytics	971.1	E855.4	E941.1	E950.4	E962.0	E980.4
Parasympathomimetics	971.0	E855.3	E941.0	E950.4	E962.0	E980.4
Parathion	989.3	E863.1	—	E950.6	E962.1	E980.7
Parathormone	962.6	E858.0	E932.6	E950.4	E962.0	E980.4
Parathyroid (derivatives)	962.6	E858.0	E932.6	E950.4	E962.0	E980.4
Paratyphoid vaccine	978.1	E858.8	E948.1	E950.4	E962.0	E980.4
Paredrine	971.2	E855.5	E941.2	E950.4	E962.0	E980.4
Paregoric	965.00	E850.2	E935.2	E950.0	E962.0	E980.0
Pargyline	972.3	E858.3	E942.3	E950.4	E962.0	E980.4
Paris green	985.1	E866.3	—	E950.8	E962.1	E980.8
insecticide	985.1	E863.4	—	E950.8	E962.1	E980.8
Parnate	969.01	E854.0	E939.0	E950.3	E962.0	E980.3
Paromomycin	960.8	E856	E930.8	E950.4	E962.0	E980.4
Paroxypropione	963.1	E858.1	E933.1	E950.4	E962.0	E980.4
Parzone	965.09	E850.2	E935.2	E950.0	E962.0	E980.0
PAS	961.8	E857	E931.8	E950.4	E962.0	E980.4
PCBs	981	E862.3	—	E950.9	E962.1	E980.9
PCP (pentachlorophenol)	989.4	E863.6	—	E950.6	E962.1	E980.7
herbicide	989.4	E863.5	—	E950.6	E962.1	E980.7
insecticide	989.4	E863.4	—	E950.6	E962.1	E980.7
phencyclidine	968.3	E855.1	E938.3	E950.4	E962.0	E980.4
Peach kernel oil (emulsion)	973.2	E858.4	E943.2	E950.4	E962.0	E980.4
Peanut oil (emulsion) NEC	973.2	E858.4	E943.2	E950.4	E962.0	E980.4
topical	976.3	E858.7	E946.3	E950.4	E962.0	E980.4
Pearly Gates (morning glory seeds)	969.6	E854.1	E939.6	E950.3	E962.0	E980.3
Pecazine	969.1	E853.0	E939.1	E950.3	E962.0	E980.3
Pecilocin	960.1	E856	E930.1	E950.4	E962.0	E980.4
Pectin (with kaolin) NEC	973.5	E858.4	E943.5	E950.4	E962.0	E980.4
Pelletierine tannate	961.6	E857	E931.6	E950.4	E962.0	E980.4
Pemoline	969.79	E854.2	E939.7	E950.3	E962.0	E980.3
Pempidine	972.3	E858.3	E942.3	E950.4	E962.0	E980.4
Penamecillin	960.0	E856	E930.0	E950.4	E962.0	E980.4
Penethamate hydriodide	960.0	E856	E930.0	E950.4	E962.0	E980.4
Penicillamine	963.8	E858.1	E933.8	E950.4	E962.0	E980.4
Penicillin (any type)	960.0	E856	E930.0	E950.4	E962.0	E980.4
Penicillinase	963.4	E858.1	E933.4	E950.4	E962.0	E980.4
Pentachlorophenol (fungicide)	989.4	E863.6	—	E950.6	E962.1	E980.7
herbicide	989.4	E863.5	—	E950.6	E962.1	E980.7
insecticide	989.4	E863.4	—	E950.6	E962.1	E980.7

◄ New   ◄|||| Revised   ~~deleted~~ Deleted   ● Use Additional Digit(s)

Substance	Poisoning	External Cause (E Code)				
		Accident	Therapeutic Use	Suicide Attempt	Assault	Undetermined
Pentaerythritol	972.4	E858.3	E942.4	E950.4	E962.0	E980.4
chloral	967.1	E852.0	E937.1	E950.2	E962.0	E980.2
tetranitrate NEC	972.4	E858.3	E942.4	E950.4	E962.0	E980.4
Pentagastrin	977.8	E858.8	E947.8	E950.4	E962.0	E980.4
Pentalin	982.3	E862.4	—	E950.9	E962.1	E980.9
Pentamethonium (bromide)	972.3	E858.3	E942.3	E950.4	E962.0	E980.4
Pentamidine	961.5	E857	E931.5	E950.4	E962.0	E980.4
Pentanol	980.8	E860.8	—	E950.9	E962.1	E980.9
Pentaquine	961.4	E857	E931.4	E950.4	E962.0	E980.4
Pentazocine	965.8	E850.8	E935.8	E950.0	E962.0	E980.0
Penthienate	971.1	E855.4	E941.1	E950.4	E962.0	E980.4
Pentobarbital, pentobarbitone (sodium)	967.0	E851	E937.0	E950.1	E962.0	E980.1
Pentolinium (tartrate)	972.3	E858.3	E942.3	E950.4	E962.0	E980.4
Pentothal	968.3	E855.1	E938.3	E950.4	E962.0	E980.4
Pentylenetetrazol	970.0	E854.3	E940.0	E950.4	E962.0	E980.4
Pentylsalicylamide	961.8	E857	E931.8	E950.4	E962.0	E980.4
Pepsin	973.4	E858.4	E943.4	E950.4	E962.0	E980.4
Peptavlon	977.8	E858.8	E947.8	E950.4	E962.0	E980.4
Percaine (spinal)	968.7	E855.2	E938.7	E950.4	E962.0	E980.4
topical (surface)	968.5	E855.2	E938.5	E950.4	E962.0	E980.4
Perchloroethylene (vapor)	982.3	E862.4	—	E950.9	E962.1	E980.9
medicinal	961.6	E857	E931.6	E950.4	E962.0	E980.4
Percodan	965.09	E850.2	E935.2	E950.0	E962.0	E980.0
Percogesic	965.09	E850.2	E935.2	E950.0	E962.0	E980.0
Percorten	962.0	E858.0	E932.0	E950.4	E962.0	E980.4
Pergonal	962.4	E858.0	E932.4	E950.4	E962.0	E980.4
Perhexiline	972.4	E858.3	E942.4	E950.4	E962.0	E980.4
Periactin	963.0	E858.1	E933.0	E950.4	E962.0	E980.4
Periclor	967.1	E852.0	E937.1	E950.2	E962.0	E980.2
Pericyazine	969.1	E853.0	E939.1	E950.3	E962.0	E980.3
Peritrate	972.4	E858.3	E942.4	E950.4	E962.0	E980.4
Permanganates NEC	983.9	E864.3	—	E950.7	E962.1	E980.6
potassium (topical)	976.0	E858.7	E946.0	E950.4	E962.0	E980.4
Pernocton	967.0	E851	E937.0	E950.1	E962.0	E980.1
Pernoston	967.0	E851	E937.0	E950.1	E962.0	E980.1
Peronin(e)	965.09	E850.2	E935.2	E950.0	E962.0	E980.0
Perphenazine	969.1	E853.0	E939.1	E950.3	E962.0	E980.3
Pertofrane	969.05	E854	E939.0	E950.3	E962.0	E980.3

◀ New   ◀▥ Revised   d̶e̶l̶e̶t̶e̶d̶ Deleted   ● Use Additional Digit(s)

Substance	Poisoning	External Cause (E Code) Accident	Therapeutic Use	Suicide Attempt	Assault	Undetermined
Pertussis	—	—	—	—	—	—
immune serum (human)	964.6	E858.2	E934.6	E950.4	E962.0	E980.4
vaccine (with diphtheria toxoid) (with tetanus toxoid)	978.6	E858.8	E948.6	E950.4	E962.0	E980.4
Peruvian balsam	976.8	E858.7	E946.8	E950.4	E962.0	E980.4
Pesticides (dust) (fumes) (vapor)	989.4	E863.4	—	E950.6	E962.1	E980.7
arsenic	985.1	E863.4	—	E950.8	E962.1	E980.8
chlorinated	989.2	E863.0	—	E950.6	E962.1	E980.7
cyanide	989.0	E863.4	—	E950.6	E962.1	E980.7
kerosene	981	E863.4	—	E950.6	E962.1	E980.7
mixture (of compounds)	989.4	E863.3	—	E950.6	E962.1	E980.7
naphthalene	983.0	E863.4	—	E950.7	E962.1	E980.6
organochlorine (compounds)	989.2	E863.0	—	E950.6	E962.1	E980.7
petroleum (distillate) (products) NEC	981	E863.4	—	E950.6	E962.1	E980.7
specified ingredient NEC	989.4	E863.4	—	E950.6	E962.1	E980.7
strychnine	989.1	E863.4	—	E950.6	E962.1	E980.7
thallium	985.8	E863.7	—	E950.6	E962.1	E980.7
Pethidine (hydrochloride)	965.09	E850.2	E935.2	E950.0	E962.0	E980.0
Petrichloral	967.1	E852.0	E937.1	E950.2	E962.0	E980.2
Petrol	981	E862.1	—	E950.9	E962.1	E980.9
vapor	987.1	E869.8	—	E952.8	E962.2	E982.8
Petrolatum (jelly) (ointment)	976.3	E858.7	E946.3	E950.4	E962.0	E980.4
hydrophilic	976.3	E858.7	E946.3	E950.4	E962.0	E980.4
liquid	973.2	E858.4	E943.2	E950.4	E962.0	E980.4
topical	976.3	E858.7	E946.3	E950.4	E962.0	E980.4
nonmedicinal	981	E862.1	—	E950.9	E962.1	E980.9
Petroleum (cleaners) (fuels) (products) NEC	981	E862.1	—	E950.9	E962.1	E980.9
benzin(e) - see Ligroin	—	—	—	—	—	—
ether - see Ligroin	—	—	—	—	—	—
jelly - see Petrolatum	—	—	—	—	—	—
aphtha - see Ligroin	—	—	—	—	—	—
pesticide	981	E863.4	—	E950.6	E962.1	E980.7
solids	981	E862.3	—	E950.9	E962.1	E980.9
solvents	981	E862.0	—	E950.9	E962.1	E980.9
vapor	987.1	E869.8	—	E952.8	E962.2	E982.8
Peyote	969.6	E854.1	E939.6	E950.3	E962.0	E980.3
Phanodorm, phanodorn	967.0	E851	E937.0	E950.1	E962.0	E980.1
Phanquinone, phanquone	961.5	E857	E931.5	E950.4	E962.0	E980.4
Pharmaceutical excipient or adjunct	977.4	E858.8	E947.4	E950.4	E962.0	E980.4

◀ New ◀ Revised ~~deleted~~ Deleted ● Use Additional Digit(s)

611

		External Cause (E Code)				
Substance	Poisoning	Accident	Therapeutic Use	Suicide Attempt	Assault	Undetermined
Phenacemide	966.3	E855.0	E936.3	E950.4	E962.0	E980.4
Phenacetin	965.4	E850.4	E935.4	E950.0	E962.0	E980.0
Phenadoxone	965.09	E850.2	E935.2	E950.0	E962.0	E980.0
Phenaglycodol	969.5	E853.8	E939.5	E950.3	E962.0	E980.3
Phenantoin	966.1	E855.0	E936.1	E950.4	E962.0	E980.4
Phenaphthazine reagent	977.8	E858.8	E947.8	E950.4	E962.0	E980.4
Phenazocine	965.09	E850.2	E935.2	E950.0	E962.0	E980.0
Phenazone	965.5	E850.5	E935.5	E950.0	E962.0	E980.0
Phenazopyridine	976.1	E858.7	E946.1	E950.4	E962.0	E980.4
Phenbenicillin	960.0	E856	E930.0	E950.4	E962.0	E980.4
Phenbutrazate	977.0	E858.8	E947.0	E950.4	E962.0	E980.4
Phencyclidine	968.3	E855.1	E938.3	E950.4	E962.0	E980.4
Phendimetrazine	977.0	E858.8	E947.0	E950.4	E962.0	E980.4
Phenelzine	969.01	E854.0	E939.0	E950.3	E962.0	E980.3
Phenergan	967.8	E852.8	E937.8	E950.2	E962.0	E980.2
Phenethicillin (potassium)	960.0	E856	E930.0	E950.4	E962.0	E980.4
Phenetsal	965.1	E850.3	E935.3	E950.0	E962.0	E980.0
Pheneturide	966.3	E855.0	E936.3	E950.4	E962.0	E980.4
Phenformin	962.3	E858.0	E932.3	E950.4	E962.0	E980.4
Phenglutarimide	971.1	E855.4	E941.1	E950.4	E962.0	E980.4
Phenicarbazide	965.8	E850.8	E935.8	E950.0	E962.0	E980.0
Phenindamine (tartrate)	963.0	E858.1	E933.0	E950.4	E962.0	E980.4
Phenindione	964.2	E858.2	E934.2	E950.4	E962.0	E980.4
Pheniprazine	969.01	E854.0	E939.0	E950.3	E962.0	E980.3
Pheniramine (maleate)	963.0	E858.1	E933.0	E950.4	E962.0	E980.4
Phenmetrazine	977.0	E858.8	E947.0	E950.4	E962.0	E980.4
Phenobal	967.0	E851	E937.0	E950.1	E962.0	E980.1
Phenobarbital	967.0	E851	E937.0	E950.1	E962.0	E980.1
Phenobarbitone	967.0	E851	E937.0	E950.1	E962.0	E980.1
Phenoctide	976.0	E858.7	E946.0	E950.4	E962.0	E980.4
Phenol (derivatives) NEC	983.0	E864.0	—	E950.7	E962.1	E980.6
disinfectant	983.0	E864.0	—	E950.7	E962.1	E980.6
pesticide	989.4	E863.4	—	E950.6	E962.1	E980.7
red	977.8	E858.8	E947.8	E950.4	E962.0	E980.4
Phenolphthalein	973.1	E858.4	E943.1	E950.4	E962.0	E980.4
Phenolsulfonphthalein	977.8	E858.8	E947.8	E950.4	E962.0	E980.4
Phenomorphan	965.09	E850.2	E935.2	E950.0	E962.0	E980.0
Phenonyl	967.0	E851	E937.0	E950.1	E962.0	E980.1

◀ New   ◀▬ Revised   ~~deleted~~ Deleted   ● Use Additional Digit(s)

Substance	Poisoning	External Cause (E Code)				
		Accident	Therapeutic Use	Suicide Attempt	Assault	Undetermined
Phenoperidine	965.09	E850.2	E935.2	E950.0	E962.0	E980.0
Phenoquin	974.7	E858.5	E944.7	E950.4	E962.0	E980.4
Phenothiazines (tranquilizers) NEC	969.1	E853.0	E939.1	E950.3	E962.0	E980.3
insecticide	989.3	E863.4	—	E950.6	E962.1	E980.7
Phenoxybenzamine	971.3	E855.6	E941.3	E950.4	E962.0	E980.4
Phenoxymethyl penicillin	960.0	E856	E930.0	E950.4	E962.0	E980.4
Phenprocoumon	964.2	E858.2	E934.2	E950.4	E962.0	E980.4
Phensuximide	966.2	E855.0	E936.2	E950.4	E962.0	E980.4
Phentermine	977.0	E858.8	E947.0	E950.4	E962.0	E980.4
Phentolamine	971.3	E855.6	E941.3	E950.4	E962.0	E980.4
Phenyl	—	—	—	—	—	—
butazone	965.5	E850.5	E935.5	E950.0	E962.0	E980.0
enediamine	983.0	E864.0	—	E950.7	E962.1	E980.6
hydrazine	983.0	E864.0	—	E950.7	E962.1	E980.6
antineoplastic	963.1	E858.1	E933.1	E950.4	E962.0	E980.4
mercuric compounds - see Mercury	—	—	—	—	—	—
salicylate	976.3	E858.7	E946.3	E950.4	E962.0	E980.4
Phenylephrine	971.2	E855.5	E941.2	E950.4	E962.0	E980.4
Phenylethylbiguanide	962.3	E858.0	E932.3	E950.4	E962.0	E980.4
Phenylpropanolamine	971.2	E855.5	E941.2	E950.4	E962.0	E980.4
Phenylsulfthion	989.3	E863.1	—	E950.6	E962.1	E980.7
Phenyramidol, phenyramidon	965.7	E850.7	E935.7	E950.0	E962.0	E980.0
Phenytoin	966.1	E855.0	E936.1	E950.4	E962.0	E980.4
pHisoHex	976.2	E858.7	E946.2	E950.4	E962.0	E980.4
Pholcodine	965.09	E850.2	E935.2	E950.0	E962.0	E980.0
Phorate	989.3	E863.1	—	E950.6	E962.1	E980.7
Phosdrin	989.3	E863.1	—	E950.6	E962.1	E980.7
Phosgene (gas)	987.8	E869.8	—	E952.8	E962.2	E982.8
Phosphate (tricresyl)	989.89	E866.8	—	E950.9	E962.1	E980.9
organic	989.3	E863.1	—	E950.6	E962.1	E980.7
solvent	982.8	E862.4	—	E950.9	E962.1	E980.9
Phosphine	987.8	E869.8	—	E952.8	E962.2	E982.8
fumigant	987.8	E863.8	—	E950.6	E962.2	E980.7
Phospholine	971.0	E855.3	E941.0	E950.4	E962.0	E980.4
Phosphoric acid	983.1	E864.1	—	E950.7	E962.1	E980.6
Phosphorus (compounds) NEC	983.9	E864.3	—	E950.7	E962.1	E980.6
rodenticide	983.9	E863.7	—	E950.7	E962.1	E980.6
Phthalimidoglutarimide	967.8	E852.8	E937.8	E950.2	E962.0	E980.2
Phthalylsulfathiazole	961.0	E857	E931.0	E950.4	E962.0	E980.4
Phylloquinone	964.3	E858.2	E934.3	E950.4	E962.0	E980.4

TABLE OF DRUGS AND CHEMICALS

Substance	Poisoning	External Cause (E Code)				
		Accident	Therapeutic Use	Suicide Attempt	Assault	Undetermined
Physeptone	965.02	E850.1	E935.1	E950.0	E962.0	E980.0
Physostigma venenosum	988.2	E865.4	—	E950.9	E962.1	E980.9
Physostigmine	971.0	E855.3	E941.0	E950.4	E962.0	E980.4
Phytolacca decandra	988.2	E865.4	—	E950.9	E962.1	E980.9
Phytomenadione	964.3	E858.2	E934.3	E950.4	E962.0	E980.4
Phytonadione	964.3	E858.2	E934.3	E950.4	E962.0	E980.4
Picric (acid)	983.0	E864.0	—	E950.7	E962.1	E980.6
Picrotoxin	970.0	E854.3	E940.0	E950.4	E962.0	E980.4
Pilocarpine	971.0	E855.3	E941.0	E950.4	E962.0	E980.4
Pilocarpus (jaborandi) extract	971.0	E855.3	E941.0	E950.4	E962.0	E980.4
Pimaricin	960.1	E856	E930.1	E950.4	E962.0	E980.4
Piminodine	965.09	E850.2	E935.2	E950.0	E962.0	E980.0
Pine oil, pinesol (disinfectant)	983.9	E861.4	—	E950.7	E962.1	E980.6
Pinkroot	961.6	E857	E931.6	E950.4	E962.0	E980.4
Pipadone	965.09	E850.2	E935.2	E950.0	E962.0	E980.0
Pipamazine	963.0	E858.1	E933.0	E950.4	E962.0	E980.4
Pipazethate	975.4	E858.6	E945.4	E950.4	E962.0	E980.4
Pipenzolate	971.1	E855.4	E941.1	E950.4	E962.0	E980.4
Piperacetazine	969.1	E853.0	E939.1	E950.3	E962.0	E980.3
Piperazine NEC	961.6	E857	E931.6	E950.4	E962.0	E980.4
estrone sulfate	962.2	E858.0	E932.2	E950.4	E962.0	E980.4
Piper cubeba	988.2	E865.4	—	E950.9	E962.1	E980.9
Piperidione	975.4	E858.6	E945.4	E950.4	E962.0	E980.4
Piperidolate	971.1	E855.4	E941.1	E950.4	E962.0	E980.4
Piperocaine	968.9	E855.2	E938.9	E950.4	E962.0	E980.4
infiltration (subcutaneous)	968.5	E855.2	E938.5	E950.4	E962.0	E980.4
nerve block (peripheral) (plexus)	968.6	E855.2	E938.6	E950.4	E962.0	E980.4
topical (surface)	968.5	E855.2	E938.5	E950.4	E962.0	E980.4
Pipobroman	963.1	E858.1	E933.1	E950.4	E962.0	E980.4
Pipradrol	970.89	E854.3	E940.8	E950.4	E962.0	E980.4
Piscidia (bark) (erythrina)	965.7	E850.7	E935.7	E950.0	E962.0	E980.0
Pitch	983.0	E864.0	—	E950.7	E962.1	E980.6
Pitkin's solution	968.7	E855.2	E938.7	E950.4	E962.0	E980.4
Pitocin	975.0	E858.6	E945.0	E950.4	E962.0	E980.4
Pitressin (tannate)	962.5	E858.0	E932.5	E950.4	E962.0	E980.4
Pituitary extracts (posterior)	962.5	E858.0	E932.5	E950.4	E962.0	E980.4
anterior	962.4	E858.0	E932.4	E950.4	E962.0	E980.4
Pituitrin	962.5	E858.0	E932.5	E950.4	E962.0	E980.4
Placental extract	962.9	E858.0	E932.9	E950.4	E962.0	E980.4
Placidyl	967.8	E852.8	E937.8	E950.2	E962.0	E980.2

◀ New   ◀▥ Revised   ~~deleted~~ Deleted   ⬤ Use Additional Digit(s)

Substance	Poisoning	External Cause (E Code)				
		Accident	Therapeutic Use	Suicide Attempt	Assault	Undetermined
Plague vaccine	978.3	E858.8	E948.3	E950.4	E962.0	E980.4
Plant foods or fertilizers NEC	989.89	E866.5	—	E950.9	E962.1	E980.9
mixed with herbicides	989.4	E863.5	—	E950.6	E962.1	E930.7
Plants, noxious, used as food	988.2	E865.9	—	E950.9	E962.1	E980.9
berries and seeds	988.2	E865.3	—	E950.9	E962.1	E980.9
specified type NEC	988.2	E865.4	—	E950.9	E962.1	E980.9
Plasma (blood)	964.7	E858.2	E934.7	E950.4	E962.0	E980.4
expanders	964.8	E858.2	E934.8	E950.4	E962.0	E980.4
Plasmanate	964.7	E858.2	E934.7	E950.4	E962.0	E980.4
Plegicil	969.1	E853.0	E939.1	E950.3	E962.0	E980.3
Podophyllin	976.4	E858.7	E946.4	E950.4	E962.0	E980.4
Podophyllum resin	976.4	E858.7	E946.4	E950.4	E962.0	E980.4
Poison NEC	989.9	E866.9	—	E950.9	E962.1	E980.9
Poisonous berries	988.2	E865.3	—	E950.9	E962.1	E980.9
Pokeweed (any part)	988.2	E865.4	—	E950.9	E962.1	E980.9
Poldine	971.1	E855.4	E941.1	E950.4	E962.0	E980.4
Poliomyelitis vaccine	979.5	E858.8	E949.5	E950.4	E962.0	E980.4
Poliovirus vaccine	979.5	E858.8	E949.5	E950.4	E962.0	E980.4
Polish (car) (floor) (furniture) (metal) (silver)	989.89	E861.2	—	E950.9	E962.1	E980.9
abrasive	989.89	E861.3	—	E950.9	E962.1	E980.9
porcelain	989.89	E861.3	—	E950.9	E962.1	E980.9
Poloxalkol	973.2	E858.4	E943.2	E950.4	E962.0	E980.4
Polyaminostyrene resins	974.5	E858.5	E944.5	E950.4	E962.0	E980.4
Polychlorinated biphenyl - *see* PCBs	—	—	—	—	—	—
Polycycline	960.4	E856	E930.4	E950.4	E962.0	E980.4
Polyester resin hardener	982.8	E862.4	—	E950.9	E962.1	E980.9
fumes	987.8	E869.8	—	E952.8	E962.2	E982.8
Polyestradiol (phosphate)	962.2	E858.0	E932.2	E950.4	E962.0	E980.4
Polyethanolamine alkyl sulfate	976.2	E858.7	E946.2	E950.4	E962.0	E980.4
Polyethylene glycol	976.3	E858.7	E946.3	E950.4	E962.0	E980.4
Polyferose	964.0	E858.2	E934.0	E950.4	E962.0	E980.4
Polymyxin B	960.8	E856	E930.8	E950.4	E962.0	E980.4
ENT agent	976.6	E858.7	E946.6	E950.4	E962.0	E980.4
ophthalmic preparation	976.5	E858.7	E946.5	E950.4	E962.0	E980.4
topical NEC	976.0	E858.7	E946.0	E950.4	E962.0	E980.4
Polynoxylin(e)	976.0	E858.7	E946.0	E950.4	E962.0	E980.4
Polyoxymethyleneurea	976.0	E858.7	E946.0	E950.4	E962.0	E980.4
Polytetrafluoroethylene (inhaled)	987.8	E869.8	—	E952.8	E962.2	E982.8
Polythiazide	974.3	E858.5	E944.3	E950.4	E962.0	E980.4

◀ New   ◀║║ Revised   ~~deleted~~ Deleted   ● Use Additional Digit(s)

TABLE OF DRUGS AND CHEMICALS

Substance	Poisoning	External Cause (E Code)				
		Accident	Therapeutic Use	Suicide Attempt	Assault	Undetermined
Polyvinylpyrrolidone	964.8	E858.2	E934.8	E950.4	E962.0	E980.4
Pontocaine (hydrochloride) (infiltration) (topical)	968.5	E855.2	E938.5	E950.4	E962.0	E980.4
nerve block (peripheral) (plexus)	968.6	E855.2	E938.6	E950.4	E962.0	E980.4
spinal	968.7	E855.2	E938.7	E950.4	E962.0	E980.4
Pot	969.6	E854.1	E939.6	E950.3	E962.0	E980.3
Potash (caustic)	983.2	E864.2	—	E950.7	E962.1	E980.6
Potassic saline injection (lactated)	974.5	E858.5	E944.5	E950.4	E962.0	E980.4
Potassium (salts) NEC	974.5	E858.5	E944.5	E950.4	E962.0	E980.4
aminosalicylate	961.8	E857	E931.8	E950.4	E962.0	E980.4
arsenite (solution)	985.1	E866.3	—	E950.8	E962.1	E980.8
bichromate	983.9	E864.3	—	E950.7	E962.1	E980.6
bisulfate	983.9	E864.3	—	E950.7	E962.1	E980.6
bromide (medicinal) NEC	967.3	E852.2	E937.3	E950.2	E962.0	E980.2
carbonate	983.2	E864.2	—	E950.7	E962.1	E980.6
chlorate NEC	983.9	E864.3	—	E950.7	E962.1	E980.6
cyanide - *see* Cyanide	—	—	—	—	—	—
hydroxide	983.2	E864.2	—	E950.7	E962.1	E980.6
iodide (expectorant) NEC	975.5	E858.6	E945.5	E950.4	E962.0	E980.4
nitrate	989.89	E866.8	—	E950.9	E962.1	E980.9
oxalate	983.9	E864.3	—	E950.7	E962.1	E980.6
perchlorate NEC	977.8	E858.8	E947.8	E950.4	E962.0	E980.4
antithyroid	962.8	E858.0	E932.8	E950.4	E962.0	E980.4
permanganate	976.0	E858.7	E946.0	E950.4	E962.0	E980.4
nonmedicinal	983.9	E864.3	—	E950.7	E962.1	E980.6
Povidone-iodine (anti-infective) NEC	976.0	E858.7	E946.0	E950.4	E962.0	E980.4
Practolol	972.0	E858.3	E942.0	E950.4	E962.0	E980.4
Pralidoxime (chloride)	977.2	E858.8	E947.2	E950.4	E962.0	E980.4
Pramoxine	968.5	E855.2	E938.5	E950.4	E962.0	E980.4
Prazosin	972.6	E858.3	E942.6	E950.4	E962.0	E980.4
Prednisolone	962.0	E858.0	E932.0	E950.4	E962.0	E980.4
ENT agent	976.6	E858.7	E946.6	E950.4	E962.0	E980.4
ophthalmic preparation	976.5	E858.7	E946.5	E950.4	E962.0	E980.4
topical NEC	976.0	E858.7	E946.0	E950.4	E962.0	E980.4
Prednisone	962.0	E858.0	E932.0	E950.4	E962.0	E980.4
Pregnanediol	962.2	E858.0	E932.2	E950.4	E962.0	E980.4
Pregneninolone	962.2	E858.0	E932.2	E950.4	E962.0	E980.4
Preludin	977.0	E858.8	E947.0	E950.4	E962.0	E980.4
Premarin	962.2	E858.0	E932.2	E950.4	E962.0	E980.4
Prenylamine	972.4	E858.3	E942.4	E950.4	E962.0	E980.4

◀ New   ◀▥ Revised   ~~deleted~~ Deleted   ● Use Additional Digit(s)

Substance	Poisoning	External Cause (E Code)				
		Accident	Therapeutic Use	Suicide Attempt	Assault	Undetermined
Preparation H	976.8	E858.7	E946.8	E950.4	E962.0	E980.4
Preservatives	989.89	E866.8	—	E950.9	E962.1	E980.9
Pride of China	988.2	E865.3	—	E950.9	E962.1	E980.9
Prilocaine	968.9	E855.2	E938.9	E950.4	E962.0	E980.4
infiltration (subcutaneous)	968.5	E855.2	E938.5	E950.4	E962.0	E980.4
nerve block (peripheral) (plexus)	968.6	E855.2	E938.6	E950.4	E962.0	E980.4
Primaquine	961.4	E857	E931.4	E950.4	E962.0	E980.4
Primidone	966.3	E855.0	E936.3	E950.4	E962.0	E980.4
Primula (veris)	988.2	E865.4	—	E950.9	E962.1	E980.9
Prinodol	965.09	E850.2	E935.2	E950.0	E962.0	E980.0
Priscol, Priscoline	971.3	E855.6	E941.3	E950.4	E962.0	E980.4
Privet	988.2	E865.4	—	E950.9	E962.1	E980.9
Privine	971.2	E855.5	E941.2	E950.4	E962.0	E980.4
Pro-Banthine	971.1	E855.4	E941.1	E950.4	E962.0	E980.4
Probarbital	967.0	E851	E937.0	E950.1	E962.0	E980.1
Probenecid	974.7	E858.5	E944.7	E950.4	E962.0	E980.4
Procainamide (hydrochloride)	972.0	E858.3	E942.0	E950.4	E962.0	E980.4
Procaine (hydrochloride) (infiltration) (topical)	968.5	E855.2	E938.5	E950.4	E962.0	E980.4
nerve block (periphreal) (plexus)	968.6	E855.2	E938.6	E950.4	E962.0	E980.4
penicillin G	960.0	E856	E930.0	E950.4	E962.0	E980.4
spinal	968.7	E855.2	E938.7	E950.4	E962.0	E980.4
Procalmidol	969.5	E853.8	E939.5	E950.3	E962.0	E980.3
Procarbazine	963.1	E858.1	E933.1	E950.4	E962.0	E980.4
Prochlorperazine	969.1	E853.0	E939.1	E950.3	E962.0	E980.3
Procyclidine	966.4	E855.0	E936.4	E950.4	E962.0	E980.4
Producer gas	986	E868.8	—	E952.1	E962.2	E982.1
Profenamine	966.4	E855.0	E936.4	E950.4	E962.0	E980.4
Profenil	975.1	E858.6	E945.1	E950.4	E962.0	E980.4
Progesterones	962.2	E858.0	E932.2	E950.4	E962.0	E980.4
Progestin	962.2	E858.0	E932.2	E950.4	E962.0	E980.4
Progestogens (with estrogens)	962.2	E858.0	E932.2	E950.4	E962.0	E980.4
Progestone	962.2	E858.0	E932.2	E950.4	E962.0	E980.4
Proguanil	961.4	E857	E931.4	E950.4	E962.0	E980.4
Prolactin	962.4	E858.0	E932.4	E950.4	E962.0	E980.4
Proloid	962.7	E858.0	E932.7	E950.4	E962.0	E980.4
Proluton	962.2	E858.0	E932.2	E950.4	E962.0	E980.4
Promacetin	961.8	E857	E931.8	E950.4	E962.0	E980.4
Promazine	969.1	E853.0	E939.1	E950.3	E962.0	E980.3
Promedrol	965.09	E850.2	E935.2	E950.0	E962.0	E980.0

TABLE OF DRUGS AND CHEMICALS

		External Cause (E Code)				
Substance	Poisoning	Accident	Therapeutic Use	Suicide Attempt	Assault	Undetermined
Promethazine	967.8	E852.8	E937.8	E950.2	E962.0	E980.2
Promine	961.8	E857	E931.8	E950.4	E962.0	E980.4
Pronestyl (hydrochloride)	972.0	E858.3	E942.0	E950.4	E962.0	E980.4
Pronetalol, pronethalol	972.0	E858.3	E942.0	E950.4	E962.0	E980.4
Prontosil	961.0	E857	E931.0	E950.4	E962.0	E980.4
Propamidine isethionate	961.5	E857	E931.5	E950.4	E962.0	E980.4
Propanal (medicinal)	967.8	E852.8	E937.8	E950.2	E962.0	E980.2
Propane (gas) (distributed in mobile container)	987.0	E868.0	—	E951.1	E962.2	E981.1
distributed through pipes	987.0	E867	—	E951.0	E962.2	E981.0
incomplete combustion of - *see* Carbon monoxide, Propane	—	—	—	—	—	—
Propanidid	968.3	E855.1	E938.3	E950.4	E962.0	E980.4
Propanol	980.3	E860.4	—	E950.9	E962.1	E980.9
Propantheline	971.1	E855.4	E941.1	E950.4	E962.0	E980.4
Proparacaine	968.5	E855.2	E938.5	E950.4	E962.0	E980.4
Propatyl nitrate	972.4	E858.3	E942.4	E950.4	E962.0	E980.4
Propicillin	960.0	E856	E930.0	E950.4	E962.0	E980.4
Propiolactone (vapor)	987.8	E869.8	—	E952.8	E962.2	E982.8
Propiomazine	967.8	E852.8	E937.8	E950.2	E962.0	E980.2
Propionaldehyde (medicinal)	967.8	E852.8	E937.8	E950.2	E962.0	E980.2
Propionate compound	976.0	E858.7	E946.0	E950.4	E962.0	E980.4
Propion gel	976.0	E858.7	E946.0	E950.4	E962.0	E980.4
Propitocaine	968.9	E855.2	E938.9	E950.4	E962.0	E980.4
infiltration (subcutaneous)	968.5	E855.2	E938.5	E950.4	E962.0	E980.4
nerve block (peripheral) (plexus)	968.6	E855.2	E938.6	E950.4	E962.0	E980.4
Propoxur	989.3	E863.2	—	E950.6	E962.1	E980.7
Propoxycaine	968.9	E855.2	E938.9	E950.4	E962.0	E980.4
infiltration (subcutaneous)	968.5	E855.2	E938.5	E950.4	E962.0	E980.4
nerve block (peripheral) (plexus)	968.6	E855.2	E938.6	E950.4	E962.0	E980.4
topical (surface)	968.5	E855.2	E938.5	E950.4	E962.0	E980.4
Propoxyphene (hydrochloride)	965.8	E850.8	E935.8	E950.0	E962.0	E980.0
Propranolol	972.0	E858.3	E942.0	E950.4	E962.0	E980.4
Propyl	—	—	—	—	—	—
alcohol	980.3	E860.4	—	E950.9	E962.1	E980.9
carbinol	980.3	E860.4	—	E950.9	E962.1	E980.9
hexadrine	971.2	E855.5	E941.2	E950.4	E962.0	E980.4
iodone	977.8	E858.8	E947.8	E950.4	E962.0	E980.4
thiouracil	962.8	E858.0	E932.8	E950.4	E962.0	E980.4
Propylene	987.1	E869.8	—	E952.8	E962.2	E982.8
Propylparaben (ophthalmic)	976.5	E858.7	E946.5	E950.4	E962.0	E980.4

◀ New　◀ Revised　~~deleted~~ Deleted　● Use Additional Digit(s)

Substance	Poisoning	External Cause (E Code)				
		Accident	Therapeutic Use	Suicide Attempt	Assault	Undetermined
Proscillaridin	972.1	E858.3	E942.1	E950.4	E962.0	E980.4
Prostaglandins	975.0	E858.6	E945.0	E950.4	E962.0	E980.4
Prostigmin	971.0	E855.3	E941.0	E950.4	E962.0	E980.4
Protamine (sulfate)	964.5	E858.2	E934.5	E950.4	E962.0	E980.4
zinc insulin	962.3	E858.0	E932.3	E950.4	E962.0	E980.4
Protectants (topical)	976.3	E858.7	E946.3	E950.4	E962.0	E980.4
Protein hydrolysate	974.5	E858.5	E944.5	E950.4	E962.0	E980.4
Prothiaden - *see* Dothiepin hydrochloride	—	—	—	—	—	—
Prothionamide	961.8	E857	E931.8	E950.4	E962.0	E980.4
Prothipendyl	969.5	E853.8	E939.5	E950.3	E962.0	E980.3
Protokylol	971.2	E855.5	E941.2	E950.4	E962.0	E980.4
Protopam	977.2	E858.8	E947.2	E950.4	E962.0	E980.4
Protoveratrine(s) (A) (B)	972.6	E858.3	E942.6	E950.4	E962.0	E980.4
Protriptyline	969.05	E854.0	E939.0	E950.3	E962.0	E980.3
Provera	962.2	E858.0	E932.2	E950.4	E962.0	E980.4
Provitamin A	963.5	E858.1	E933.5	E950.4	E962.0	E980.4
Proxymetacaine	968.5	E855.2	E938.5	E950.4	E962.0	E980.4
Proxyphylline	975.1	E858.6	E945.1	E950.4	E962.0	E980.4
Prozac - *see* Fluoxetine hydrochloride	—	—	—	—	—	—
Prunus	—	—	—	—	—	—
laurocerasus	988.2	E865.4	—	E950.9	E962.1	E980.9
virginiana	988.2	E865.4	—	E950.9	E962.1	E980.9
Prussic acid	989.0	E866.8	—	E950.9	E962.1	E980.9
vapor	987.7	E869.8	—	E952.8	E962.2	E982.8
Pseudoephedrine	971.2	E855.5	E941.2	E950.4	E962.0	E980.4
Psilocin	969.6	E854.1	E939.6	E950.3	E962.0	E980.3
Psilocybin	969.6	E854.1	E939.6	E950.3	E962.0	E980.3
PSP	977.8	E858.8	E947.8	E950.4	E962.0	E980.4
Psychedelic agents	969.6	E854.1	E939.6	E950.3	E962.0	E980.3
Psychodysleptics	969.6	E854.1	E939.6	E950.3	E962.0	E980.3
Psychostimulants	969.70	E854.2	E939.7	E950.3	E962.0	E980.3
Psychotherapeutic agents	969.9	E855.9	E939.9	E950.3	E962.0	E980.3
antidepressants	969.00	E854.0	E939.0	E950.3	E962.0	E980.3
specified NEC	969.8	E855.8	E939.8	E950.3	E962.0	E980.3
tranquilizers NEC	969.5	E853.9	E939.5	E950.3	E962.0	E980.3
Psychotomimetic agents	969.6	E854.1	E939.6	E950.3	E962.0	E980.3
Psychotropic agents	969.9	E854.8	E939.9	E950.3	E962.0	E980.3
specified NEC	969.8	E854.8	E939.8	E950.3	E962.0	E980.3
Psyllium	973.3	E858.4	E943.3	E950.4	E962.0	E980.4

◄ New ◄◄ Revised ~~deleted~~ Deleted ● Use Additional Digit(s)

TABLE OF DRUGS AND CHEMICALS

		External Cause (E Code)				
Substance	Poisoning	Accident	Therapeutic Use	Suicide Attempt	Assault	Undetermined
Pteroylglutamic acid	964.1	E858.2	E934.1	E950.4	E962.0	E980.4
Pteroyltriglutamate	963.1	E858.1	E933.1	E950.4	E962.0	E980.4
PTFE	987.8	E869.8	—	E952.8	E962.2	E982.8
Pulsatilla	988.2	E865.4	—	E950.9	E962.1	E980.9
Purex (bleach)	983.9	E864.3	—	E950.7	E962.1	E980.6
Purine diuretics	974.1	E858.5	E944.1	E950.4	E962.0	E980.4
Purinethol	963.1	E858.1	E933.1	E950.4	E962.0	E980.4
PVP	964.8	E858.2	E934.8	E950.4	E962.0	E980.4
Pyrabital	965.7	E850.7	E935.7	E950.0	E962.0	E980.0
Pyramidon	965.5	E850.5	E935.5	E950.0	E962.0	E980.0
Pyrantel (pamoate)	961.6	E857	E931.6	E950.4	E962.0	E980.4
Pyrathiazine	963.0	E858.1	E933.0	E950.4	E962.0	E980.4
Pyrazinamide	961.8	E857	E931.8	E950.4	E962.0	E980.4
Pyrazinoic acid (amide)	961.8	E857	E931.8	E950.4	E962.0	E980.4
Pyrazole (derivatives)	965.5	E850.5	E935.5	E950.0	E962.0	E980.0
Pyrazolone (analgesics)	965.5	E850.5	E935.5	E950.0	E962.0	E980.0
Pyrethrins, pyrethrum	989.4	E863.4	—	E950.6	E962.1	E980.7
Pyribenzamine	963.0	E858.1	E933.0	E950.4	E962.0	E980.4
Pyridine (liquid) (vapor)	982.0	E862.4	—	E950.9	E962.1	E980.9
aldoxime chloride	977.2	E858.8	E947.2	E950.4	E962.0	E980.4
Pyridium	976.1	E858.7	E946.1	E950.4	E962.0	E980.4
Pyridostigmine	971.0	E855.3	E941.0	E950.4	E962.0	E980.4
Pyridoxine	963.5	E858.1	E933.5	E950.4	E962.0	E980.4
Pyrilamine	963.0	E858.1	E933.0	E950.4	E962.0	E980.4
Pyrimethamine	961.4	E857	E931.4	E950.4	E962.0	E980.4
Pyrogallic acid	983.0	E864.0	—	E950.7	E962.1	E980.6
Pyroxylin	976.3	E858.7	E946.3	E950.4	E962.0	E980.4
Pyrrobutamine	963.0	E858.1	E933.0	E950.4	E962.0	E980.4
Pyrrocitine	968.5	E855.2	E938.5	E950.4	E962.0	E980.4
Pyrvinium (pamoate)	961.6	E857	E931.6	E950.4	E962.0	E980.4
PZI	962.3	E858.0	E932.3	E950.4	E962.0	E980.4
Quaalude	967.4	E852.3	E937.4	E950.2	E962.0	E980.2
Quaternary ammonium derivatives	971.1	E855.4	E941.1	E950.4	E962.0	E980.4
Quicklime	983.2	E864.2	—	E950.7	E962.1	E980.6
Quinacrine	961.3	E857	E931.3	E950.4	E962.0	E980.4
Quinaglute	972.0	E858.3	E942.0	E950.4	E962.0	E980.4
Quinalbarbitone	967.0	E851	E937.0	E950.1	E962.0	E980.1
Quinestradiol	962.2	E858.0	E932.2	E950.4	E962.0	E980.4
Quinethazone	974.3	E858.5	E944.3	E950.4	E962.0	E980.4

Substance	Poisoning	External Cause (E Code)				
		Accident	Therapeutic Use	Suicide Attempt	Assault	Undetermined
Quinidine (gluconate) (polygalacturonate) (salts) (sulfate)	972.0	E858.3	E942.0	E950.4	E962.0	E980.4
Quinine	961.4	E857	E931.4	E950.4	E962.0	E980.4
Quiniobine	961.3	E857	E931.3	E950.4	E962.0	E980.4
Quinolines	961.3	E857	E931.3	E950.4	E962.0	E980.4
Quotane	968.5	E855.2	E938.5	E950.4	E962.0	E980.4
Rabies	—	—	—	—	—	—
immune globulin (human)	964.6	E858.2	E934.6	E950.4	E962.0	E980.4
vaccine	979.1	E858.8	E949.1	E950.4	E962.0	E980.4
Racemoramide	965.09	E850.2	E935.2	E950.0	E962.0	E980.0
Racemorphan	965.09	E850.2	E935.2	E950.0	E962.0	E980.0
Radiator alcohol	980.1	E860.2	—	E950.9	E962.1	E980.9
Radio-opaque (drugs) (materials)	977.8	E858.8	E947.8	E950.4	E962.0	E980.4
Ranunculus	988.2	E865.4	—	E950.9	E962.1	E980.9
Rat poison	989.4	E863.7	—	E950.6	E962.1	E980.7
Rattlesnake (venom)	989.5	E905.0	—	E950.9	E962.1	E980.9
Raudixin	972.6	E858.3	E942.6	E950.4	E962.0	E980.4
Rautensin	972.6	E858.3	E942.6	E950.4	E962.0	E980.4
Rautina	972.6	E858.3	E942.6	E950.4	E962.0	E980.4
Rautotal	972.6	E858.3	E942.6	E950.4	E962.0	E980.4
Rauwiloid	972.6	E858.3	E942.6	E950.4	E962.0	E980.4
Rauwoldin	972.6	E858.3	E942.6	E950.4	E962.0	E980.4
Rauwolfia (alkaloids)	972.6	E858.3	E942.6	E950.4	E962.0	E980.4
Realgar	985.1	E866.3	—	E950.8	E962.1	E980.8
Red cells, packed	964.7	E858.2	E934.7	E950.4	E962.0	E980.4
Reducing agents, industrial NEC	983.9	E864.3	—	E950.7	E962.1	E980.6
Refrigerant gas (freon)	987.4	E869.2	—	E952.8	E962.2	E982.8
not freon	987.9	E869.9	—	E952.9	E962.2	E982.9
Regroton	974.4	E858.5	E944.4	E950.4	E962.0	E980.4
Rela	968.0	E855.1	E938.0	E950.4	E962.0	E980.4
Relaxants, skeletal muscle (autonomic)	975.2	E858.6	E945.2	E950.4	E962.0	E980.4
central nervous system	968.0	E855.1	E938.0	E950.4	E962.0	E980.4
Renese	974.3	E858.5	E944.3	E950.4	E962.0	E980.4
Renografin	977.8	E858.8	E947.8	E950.4	E962.0	E980.4
Replacement solutions	974.5	E858.5	E944.5	E950.4	E962.0	E980.4
Rescinnamine	972.6	E858.3	E942.6	E950.4	E962.0	E980.4
Reserpine	972.6	E858.3	E942.6	E950.4	E962.0	E980.4
Resorcin, resorcinol	976.4	E858.7	E946.4	E950.4	E962.0	E980.4
Respaire	975.5	E858.6	E945.5	E950.4	E962.0	E980.4
Respiratory agents NEC	975.8	E858.6	E945.8	E950.4	E962.0	E980.4

◄ New   ◄ Revised   ~~deleted~~ Deleted   ● Use Additional Digit(s)

Substance	Poisoning	External Cause (E Code)				
		Accident	Therapeutic Use	Suicide Attempt	Assault	Undetermined
Retinoic acid	976.8	E858.7	E946.8	E950.4	E962.0	E980.4
Retinol	963.5	E858.1	E933.5	E950.4	E962.0	E980.4
Rh (D) immune globulin (human)	964.6	E858.2	E934.6	E950.4	E962.0	E980.4
Rhodine	965.1	E850.3	E935.3	E950.0	E962.0	E980.0
RhoGAM	964.6	E858.2	E934.6	E950.4	E962.0	E980.4
Riboflavin	963.5	E858.1	E933.5	E950.4	E962.0	E980.4
Ricin	989.89	E866.8	—	E950.9	E962.1	E980.9
Ricinus communis	988.2	E865.3	—	E950.9	E962.1	E980.9
Rickettsial vaccine NEC	979.6	E858.8	E949.6	E950.4	E962.0	E980.4
with viral and bacterial vaccine	979.7	E858.8	E949.7	E950.4	E962.0	E980.4
Rifampin	960.6	E856	E930.6	E950.4	E962.0	E980.4
Rimifon	961.8	E857	E931.8	E950.4	E962.0	E980.4
Ringer's injection (lactated)	974.5	E858.5	E944.5	E950.4	E962.0	E980.4
Ristocetin	960.8	E856	E930.8	E950.4	E962.0	E980.4
Ritalin	969.73	E854.2	E939.7	E950.3	E962.0	E980.3
Roach killers - see Pesticides	—	—	—	—	—	—
Rocky Mountain spotted fever vaccine	979.6	E858.8	E949.6	E950.4	E962.0	E980.4
Rodenticides	989.4	E863.7	—	E950.6	E962.1	E980.7
Rohypnol	969.4	E853.2	E939.4	E950.3	E962.0	E980.3
Rolaids	973.0	E858.4	E943.0	E950.4	E962.0	E980.4
Rolitetracycline	960.4	E856	E930.4	E950.4	E962.0	E980.4
Romilar	975.4	E858.6	E945.4	E950.4	E962.0	E980.4
Rose water ointment	976.3	E858.7	E946.3	E950.4	E962.0	E980.4
Rotenone	989.4	E863.7	—	E950.6	E962.1	E980.7
Rotoxamine	963.0	E858.1	E933.0	E950.4	E962.0	E980.4
Rough-on-rats	989.4	E863.7	—	E950.6	E962.1	E980.7
RU486	962.9	E858.0	E932.9	E950.4	E962.0	E980.4
Rubbing alcohol	980.2	E860.3	—	E950.9	E962.1	E980.9
Rubella virus vaccine	979.4	E858.8	E949.4	E950.4	E962.0	E980.4
Rubelogen	979.4	E858.8	E949.4	E950.4	E962.0	E980.4
Rubeovax	979.4	E858.8	E949.4	E950.4	E962.0	E980.4
Rubidomycin	960.7	E856	E930.7	E950.4	E962.0	E980.4
Rue	988.2	E865.4	—	E950.9	E962.1	E980.9
Ruta	988.2	E865.4	—	E950.9	E962.1	E980.9
Sabadilla (medicinal)	976.0	E858.7	E946.0	E950.4	E962.0	E980.4
pesticide	989.4	E863.4	—	E950.6	E962.1	E980.7
Sabin oral vaccine	979.5	E858.8	E949.5	E950.4	E962.0	E980.4
Saccharated iron oxide	964.0	E858.2	E934.0	E950.4	E962.0	E980.4
Saccharin	974.5	E858.5	E944.5	E950.4	E962.0	E980.4

◀ New ◀ Revised deleted Deleted ● Use Additional Digit(s)

Substance	Poisoning	External Cause (E Code)				
		Accident	Therapeutic Use	Suicide Attempt	Assault	Undetermined
Safflower oil	972.2	E858.3	E942.2	E950.4	E962.0	E980.4
Salbutamol sulfate	975.7	E858.6	E945.7	E950.4	E962.0	E980.4
Salicylamide	965.1	E850.3	E935.3	E950.0	E962.0	E980.0
Salicylate(s)	965.1	E850.3	E935.3	E950.0	E962.0	E980.0
methyl	976.3	E858.7	E946.3	E950.4	E962.0	E980.4
theobromine calcium	974.1	E858.5	E944.1	E950.4	E962.0	E980.4
Salicylazosulfapyridine	961.0	E857	E931.0	E950.4	E962.0	E980.4
Salicylhydroxamic acid	976.0	E858.7	E946.0	E950.4	E962.0	E980.4
Salicylic acid (keratolytic) NEC	976.4	E858.7	E946.4	E950.4	E962.0	E980.4
congeners	965.1	E850.3	E935.3	E950.0	E962.0	E980.0
salts	965.1	E850.3	E935.3	E950.0	E962.0	E980.0
Saliniazid	961.8	E857	E931.8	E950.4	E962.0	E980.4
Salol	976.3	E858.7	E946.3	E950.4	E962.0	E980.4
Salt (substitute) NEC	974.5	E858.5	E944.5	E950.4	E962.0	E980.4
Saluretics	974.3	E858.5	E944.3	E950.4	E962.0	E980.4
Saluron	974.3	E858.5	E944.3	E950.4	E962.0	E980.4
Salvarsan 606 (neosilver) (silver)	961.1	E857	E931.1	E950.4	E962.0	E980.4
Sambucus canadensis	988.2	E865.4	—	E950.9	E962.1	E980.9
berry	988.2	E865.3	—	E950.9	E962.1	E980.9
Sandril	972.6	E858.3	E942.6	E950.4	E962.0	E980.4
Sanguinaria canadensis	988.2	E865.4	—	E950.9	E962.1	E980.9
Saniflush (cleaner)	983.9	E861.3	—	E950.7	E962.1	E980.6
Santonin	961.6	E857	E931.6	E950.4	E962.0	E980.4
Santyl	976.8	E858.7	E946.8	E950.4	E962.0	E980.4
Sarkomycin	960.7	E856	E930.7	E950.4	E962.0	E980.4
Saroten	969.05	E854.0	E939.0	E950.3	E962.0	E980.3
Saturnine - see Lead	—	—	—	—	—	—
Savin (oil)	976.4	E858.7	E946.4	E950.4	E962.0	E980.4
Scammony	973.1	E858.4	E943.1	E950.4	E962.0	E980.4
Scarlet red	976.8	E858.7	E946.8	E950.4	E962.0	E980.4
Scheele's green	985.1	E866.3	—	E950.8	E962.1	E980.8
insecticide	985.1	E863.4	—	E950.8	E962.1	E980.8
Schradan	989.3	E863.1	—	E950.6	E962.1	E980.7
Schweinfurt(h) green	985.1	E866.3	—	E950.8	E962.1	E980.8
insecticide	985.1	E863.4	—	E950.8	E962.1	E980.8
Scilla - see Squill	—	—	—	—	—	—
Sclerosing agents	972.7	E858.3	E942.7	E950.4	E962.0	E980.4
Scopolamine	971.1	E855.4	E941.1	E950.4	E962.0	E980.4
Scouring powder	989.89	E861.3	—	E950.9	E962.1	E980.9

New ◀ Revised ◀ deleted Deleted ● Use Additional Digit(s)

Substance	Poisoning	External Cause (E Code)				
		Accident	Therapeutic Use	Suicide Attempt	Assault	Undetermined
Sea	—	—	—	—	—	—
anemone (sting)	989.5	E905.6	—	E950.9	E962.1	E980.9
cucumber (sting)	989.5	E905.6	—	E950.9	E962.1	E980.9
snake (bite) (venom)	989.5	E905.0	—	E950.9	E962.1	E980.9
urchin spine (puncture)	989.5	E905.6	—	E950.9	E962.1	E980.9
Secbutabarbital	967.0	E851	E937.0	E950.1	E962.0	E980.1
Secbutabarbitone	967.0	E851	E937.0	E950.1	E962.0	E980.1
Secobarbital	967.0	E851	E937.0	E950.1	E962.0	E980.1
Seconal	967.0	E851	E937.0	E950.1	E962.0	E980.1
Secretin	977.8	E858.8	E947.8	E950.4	E962.0	E980.4
Sedatives, nonbarbiturate	967.9	E852.9	E937.9	E950.2	E962.0	E980.2
specified NEC	967.8	E852.8	E937.8	E950.2	E962.0	E980.2
Sedormid	967.8	E852.8	E937.8	E950.2	E962.0	E980.2
Seed (plant)	988.2	E865.3	—	E950.9	E962.1	E980.9
disinfectant or dressing	989.89	E866.5	—	E950.9	E962.1	E980.9
Selective serotonin and norepinephrine reuptake inhibitors (SSNRI)	969.02	E854.0	E939.0	E950.3	E962.0	E980.3
Selective serotonin reuptake inhibitors (SSRI)	969.03	E854.0	E939.0	E950.3	E962.0	E980.3
Selenium (fumes) NEC	985.8	E866.4	—	E950.9	E962.1	E980.9
disulfide or sulfide	976.4	E858.7	E946.4	E950.4	E962.0	E980.4
Selsun	976.4	E858.7	E946.4	E950.4	E962.0	E980.4
Senna	973.1	E858.4	E943.1	E950.4	E962.0	E980.4
Septisol	976.2	E858.7	E946.2	E950.4	E962.0	E980.4
Serax	969.4	E853.2	E939.4	E950.3	E962.0	E980.3
Serenesil	967.8	E852.8	E937.8	E950.2	E962.0	E980.2
Serenium (hydrochloride)	961.9	E857	E931.9	E950.4	E962.0	E980.4
Serepax - see Oxazepam	—	—	—	—	—	—
Sernyl	968.3	E855.1	E938.3	E950.4	E962.0	E980.4
Serotonin	977.8	E858.8	E947.8	E950.4	E962.0	E980.4
Serpasil	972.6	E858.3	E942.6	E950.4	E962.0	E980.4
Sewer gas	987.8	E869.8	—	E952.8	E962.2	E982.8
Shampoo	989.6	E861.0	—	E950.9	E962.1	E980.9
Shellfish, nonbacterial or noxious	988.0	E865.1	—	E950.9	E962.1	E980.9
Silicones NEC	989.83	E866.8	E947.8	E950.9	E962.1	E980.9
Silvadene	976.0	E858.7	E946.0	E950.4	E962.0	E980.4
Silver (compound) (medicinal) NEC	976.0	E858.7	E946.0	E950.4	E962.0	E980.4
anti-infectives	976.0	E858.7	E946.0	E950.4	E962.0	E980.4
arsphenamine	961.1	E857	E931.1	E950.4	E962.0	E980.4
nitrate	976.0	E858.7	E946.0	E950.4	E962.0	E980.4
ophthalmic preparation	976.5	E858.7	E946.5	E950.4	E962.0	E980.4
toughened (keratolytic)	976.4	E858.7	E946.4	E950.4	E962.0	E980.4

◀ New　◀ Revised　deleted Deleted　● Use Additional Digit(s)

		External Cause (E Code)				
Substance	Poisoning	Accident	Therapeutic Use	Suicide Attempt	Assault	Undetermined
Silver (compound) (medicinal) NEC *(Continued)*						
nonmedicinal (dust)	985.8	E866.4	—	E950.9	E962.1	E980.9
protein (mild) (strong)	976.0	E858.7	E946.0	E950.4	E962.0	E980.4
salvarsan	961.1	E857	E931.1	E950.4	E962.0	E980.4
Simethicone	973.8	E858.4	E943.8	E950.4	E962.0	E980.4
Sinequan	969.05	E854.0	E939.0	E950.3	E962.0	E980.3
Singoserp	972.6	E858.3	E942.6	E950.4	E962.0	E980.4
Sintrom	964.2	E858.2	E934.2	E950.4	E962.0	E980.4
Sitosterols	972.2	E858.3	E942.2	E950.4	E962.0	E980.4
Skeletal muscle relaxants	975.2	E858.6	E945.2	E950.4	E962.0	E980.4
Skin	—	—	—	—	—	—
agents (external)	976.9	E858.7	E946.9	E950.4	E962.0	E980.4
specified NEC	976.8	E858.7	E946.8	E950.4	E962.0	E980.4
test antigen	977.8	E858.8	E947.8	E950.4	E962.0	E980.4
Sleep-eze	963.0	E858.1	E933.0	E950.4	E962.0	E980.4
Sleeping draught (drug) (pill) (tablet)	967.9	E852.9	E937.9	E950.2	E962.0	E980.2
Smallpox vaccine	979.0	E858.8	E949.0	E950.4	E962.0	E980.4
Smelter fumes NEC	985.9	E866.4	—	E950.9	E962.1	E980.9
Smog	987.3	E869.1	—	E952.8	E962.2	E982.8
Smoke NEC	987.9	E869.9	—	E952.9	E962.2	E982.9
Smooth muscle relaxant	975.1	E858.6	E945.1	E950.4	E962.0	E980.4
Snail killer	989.4	E863.4	—	E950.6	E962.1	E980.7
Snake (bite) (venom)	989.5	E905.0	—	E950.9	E962.1	E980.9
Snuff	989.89	E866.8	—	E950.9	E962.1	E980.9
Soap (powder) (product)	989.6	E861.1	—	E950.9	E962.1	E980.9
medicinal, soft	976.2	E858.7	E946.2	E950.4	E962.0	E980.4
Soda (caustic)	983.2	E864.2	—	E950.7	E962.1	E980.6
bicarb	963.3	E858.1	E933.3	E950.4	E962.0	E980.4
chlorinated - *see* Sodium, hypochlorite	—	—	—	—	—	—
Sodium	—	—	—	—	—	—
acetosulfone	961.8	E857	E931.8	E950.4	E962.0	E980.4
acetrizoate	977.8	E858.8	E947.8	E950.4	E962.0	E980.4
amytal	967.0	E851	E937.0	E950.1	E962.0	E980.1
arsenate - *see* Arsenic	—	—	—	—	—	—
bicarbonate	963.3	E858.1	E933.3	E950.4	E962.0	E980.4
bichromate	983.9	E864.3	—	E950.7	E962.1	E980.6
biphosphate	963.2	E858.1	E933.2	E950.4	E962.0	E980.4
bisulfate	983.9	E864.3	—	E950.7	E962.1	E980.6
borate (cleanser)	989.6	E861.3	—	E950.9	E962.1	E980.9
bromide NEC	967.3	E852.2	E937.3	E950.2	E962.0	E980.2

◀ New   ◀▮ Revised   ~~deleted~~ Deleted   ● Use Additional Digit(s)

Substance	Poisoning	External Cause (E Code)				
		Accident	Therapeutic Use	Suicide Attempt	Assault	Undetermined
Sodium *(Continued)*						
cacodylate (nonmedicinal) NEC	978.8	E858.8	E948.8	E950.4	E962.0	E980.4
anti-infective	961.1	E857	E931.1	E950.4	E962.0	E980.4
herbicide	989.4	E863.5	—	E950.6	E962.1	E980.7
calcium edetate	963.8	E858.1	E933.8	E950.4	E962.0	E980.4
carbonate NEC	983.2	E864.2	—	E950.7	E962.1	E980.6
chlorate NEC	983.9	E864.3	—	E950.7	E962.1	E980.6
herbicide	983.9	E863.5	—	E950.7	E962.1	E980.6
chloride NEC	974.5	E858.5	E944.5	E950.4	E962.0	E980.4
chromate	983.9	E864.3	—	E950.7	E962.1	E980.6
citrate	963.3	E858.1	E933.3	E950.4	E962.0	E980.4
cyanide - *see* Cyanide(s)	—	—	—	—	—	—
cyclamate	974.5	E858.5	E944.5	E950.4	E962.0	E980.4
diatrizoate	977.8	E858.8	E947.8	E950.4	E962.0	E980.4
dibunate	975.4	E858.6	E945.4	E950.4	E962.0	E980.4
dioctyl sulfosuccinate	973.2	E858.4	E943.2	E950.4	E962.0	E980.4
edetate	963.8	E858.1	E933.8	E950.4	E962.0	E980.4
ethacrynate	974.4	E858.5	E944.4	E950.4	E962.0	E980.4
fluoracetate (dust) (rodenticide)	989.4	E863.7	—	E950.6	E962.1	E980.7
fluoride - *see* Fluoride(s)	—	—	—	—	—	—
free salt	974.5	E858.5	E944.5	E950.4	E962.0	E980.4
glucosulfone	961.8	E857	E931.8	E950.4	E962.0	E980.4
hydroxide	983.2	E864.2	—	E950.7	E962.1	E980.6
hypochlorite (bleach) NEC	983.9	E864.3	—	E950.7	E962.1	E980.6
disinfectant	983.9	E861.4	—	E950.7	E962.1	E980.6
medicinal (anti-infective) (external)	976.0	E858.7	E946.0	E950.4	E962.0	E980.4
vapor	987.8	E869.8	—	E952.8	E962.2	E982.8
hyposulfite	976.0	E858.7	E946.0	E950.4	E962.0	E980.4
indigotindisulfonate	977.8	E858.8	E947.8	E950.4	E962.0	E980.4
iodide	977.8	E858.8	E947.8	E950.4	E962.0	E980.4
iothalamate	977.8	E858.8	E947.8	E950.4	E962.0	E980.4
iron edetate	964.0	E858.2	E934.0	E950.4	E962.0	E980.4
lactate	963.3	E858.1	E933.3	E950.4	E962.0	E980.4
lauryl sulfate	976.2	E858.7	E946.2	E950.4	E962.0	E980.4
L-triiodothyronine	962.7	E858.0	E932.7	E950.4	E962.0	E980.4
metrizoate	977.8	E858.8	E947.8	E950.4	E962.0	E980.4
monofluoracetate (dust) (rodenticide)	989.4	E863.7	—	E950.6	E962.1	E980.7
morrhuate	972.7	E858.3	E942.7	E950.4	E962.0	E980.4
nafcillin	960.0	E856	E930.0	E950.4	E962.0	E980.4

◀ New ◀◀ Revised ~~deleted~~ Deleted ● Use Additional Digit(s)

Substance	Poisoning	External Cause (E Code)				
		Accident	Therapeutic Use	Suicide Attempt	Assault	Undetermined
Sodium *(Continued)*						
nitrate (oxidizing agent)	983.9	E864.3	—	E950.7	E962.1	E980.6
nitrite (medicinal)	972.4	E858.3	E942.4	E950.4	E962.0	E980.4
nitroferricyanide	972.6	E858.3	E942.6	E950.4	E962.0	E980.4
nitroprusside	972.6	E858.3	E942.6	E950.4	E962.0	E980.4
para-aminohippurate	977.8	E858.8	E947.8	E950.4	E962.0	E980.4
perborate (nonmedicinal) NEC	989.89	E866.8	—	E950.9	E962.1	E980.9
medicinal	976.6	E858.7	E946.6	E950.4	E962.0	E980.4
soap	989.6	E861.1	—	E950.9	E962.1	E980.9
percarbonate - *see* Sodium, perborate	—	—	—	—	—	—
phosphate	973.3	E858.4	E943.3	E950.4	E962.0	E980.4
polystyrene sulfonate	974.5	E858.5	E944.5	E950.4	E962.0	E980.4
propionate	976.0	E858.7	E946.0	E950.4	E962.0	E980.4
psylliate	972.7	E858.3	E942.7	E950.4	E962.0	E980.4
removing resins	974.5	E858.5	E944.5	E950.4	E962.0	E980.4
salicylate	965.1	E850.3	E935.3	E950.0	E962.0	E980.0
sulfate	973.3	E858.4	E943.3	E950.4	E962.0	E980.4
sulfoxone	961.8	E857	E931.8	E950.4	E962.0	E980.4
tetradecyl sulfate	972.7	E858.3	E942.7	E950.4	E962.0	E980.4
thiopental	968.3	E855.1	E938.3	E950.4	E962.0	E980.4
thiosalicylate	965.1	E850.3	E935.3	E950.0	E962.0	E980.0
thiosulfate	976.0	E858.7	E946.0	E950.4	E962.0	E980.4
tolbutamide	977.8	E858.8	E947.8	E950.4	E962.0	E980.4
tyropanoate	977.8	E858.8	E947.8	E950.4	E962.0	E980.4
valproate	966.3	E855.0	E936.3	E950.4	E962.0	E980.4
Solanine	977.8	E858.8	E947.8	E950.4	E962.0	E980.4
Solanum dulcamara	988.2	E865.4	—	E950.9	E962.1	E980.9
Solapsone	961.8	E857	E931.8	E950.4	E962.0	E980.4
Solasulfone	961.8	E857	E931.8	E950.4	E962.0	E980.4
Soldering fluid	983.1	E864.1	—	E950.7	E962.1	E980.6
Solid substance	989.9	E866.9	—	E950.9	E962.1	E980.9
specified NEC	989.9	E866.8	—	E950.9	E962.1	E980.9
Solvents, industrial	982.8	E862.9	—	E950.9	E962.1	E980.9
naphtha	981	E862.0	—	E950.9	E962.1	E980.9
petroleum	981	E862.0	—	E950.9	E962.1	E980.9
specified NEC	982.8	E862.4	—	E950.9	E962.1	E980.9
Soma	968.0	E855.1	E938.0	E950.4	E962.0	E980.4
Somatotropin	962.4	E858.0	E932.4	E950.4	E962.0	E980.4
Sominex	963.0	E858.1	E933.0	E950.4	E962.0	E980.4

◀ New   ◀▭ Revised   ~~deleted~~ Deleted   ● Use Additional Digit(s)

Substance	Poisoning	External Cause (E Code)				
		Accident	Therapeutic Use	Suicide Attempt	Assault	Undetermined
Somnos	967.1	E852.0	E937.1	E950.2	E962.0	E980.2
Somonal	967.0	E851	E937.0	E950.1	E962.0	E980.1
Soneryl	967.0	E851	E937.0	E950.1	E962.0	E980.1
Soothing syrup	977.9	E858.9	E947.9	E950.5	E962.0	E980.5
Sopor	967.4	E852.3	E937.4	E950.2	E962.0	E980.2
Soporific drug	967.9	E852.9	E937.9	E950.2	E962.0	E980.2
specified type NEC	967.8	E852.8	E937.8	E950.2	E962.0	E980.2
Sorbitol NEC	977.4	E858.8	E947.4	E950.4	E962.0	E980.4
Sotradecol	972.7	E858.3	E942.7	E950.4	E962.0	E980.4
Spacoline	975.1	E858.6	E945.1	E950.4	E962.0	E980.4
Spanish fly	976.8	E858.7	E946.8	E950.4	E962.0	E980.4
Sparine	969.1	E853.0	E939.1	E950.3	E962.0	E980.3
Sparteine	975.0	E858.6	E945.0	E950.4	E962.0	E980.4
Spasmolytics	975.1	E858.6	E945.1	E950.4	E962.0	E980.4
anticholinergics	971.1	E855.4	E941.1	E950.4	E962.0	E980.4
Spectinomycin	960.8	E856	E930.8	E950.4	E962.0	E980.4
Speed	969.72	E854.2	E939.7	E950.3	E962.0	E980.3
Spermicides	976.8	E858.7	E946.8	E950.4	E962.0	E980.4
Spider (bite) (venom)	989.5	E905.1	—	E950.9	E962.1	E980.9
antivenin	979.9	E858.8	E949.9	E950.4	E962.0	E980.4
Spigelia (root)	961.6	E857	E931.6	E950.4	E962.0	E980.4
Spiperone	969.2	E853.1	E939.2	E950.3	E962.0	E980.3
Spiramycin	960.3	E856	E930.3	E950.4	E962.0	E980.4
Spirilene	969.5	E853.8	E939.5	E950.3	E962.0	E980.3
Spirit(s) (neutral) NEC	980.0	E860.1	—	E950.9	E962.1	E980.9
beverage	980.0	E860.0	—	E950.9	E962.1	E980.9
industrial	980.9	E860.9	—	E950.9	E962.1	E980.9
mineral	981	E862.0	—	E950.9	E962.1	E980.9
of salt - see Hydrochloric acid	—	—	—	—	—	—
surgical	980.9	E860.9	—	E950.9	E962.1	E980.9
Spironolactone	974.4	E858.5	E944.4	E950.4	E962.0	E980.4
Sponge, absorbable (gelatin)	964.5	E858.2	E934.5	E950.4	E962.0	E980.4
Sporostacin	976.0	E858.7	E946.0	E950.4	E962.0	E980.4
Sprays (aerosol)	989.89	E866.8	—	E950.9	E962.1	E980.9
cosmetic	989.89	E866.7	—	E950.9	E962.1	E980.9
medicinal NEC	977.9	E858.9	E947.9	E950.5	E962.0	E980.5
pesticides - see Pesticides	—	—	—	—	—	—
specified content - see substance specified	—	—	—	—	—	—
Spurge flax	988.2	E865.4	—	E950.9	E962.1	E980.9

◀ New   ◀▥ Revised   ~~deleted~~ Deleted   ● Use Additional Digit(s)

Substance	Poisoning	External Cause (E Code)				
		Accident	Therapeutic Use	Suicide Attempt	Assault	Undetermined
Spurges	988.2	E865.4	—	E950.9	E962.1	E980.9
Squill (expectorant) NEC	975.5	E858.6	E945.5	E950.4	E962.0	E980.4
rat poison	989.4	E863.7	—	E950.6	E962.1	E980.7
Squirting cucumber (cathartic)	973.1	E858.4	E943.1	E950.4	E962.0	E980.4
SSNRI (selective serotonin and norepinephrine reuptake inhibitors)	969.02	E854.0	E939.0	E950.3	E962.0	E980.3
SSRI (selective serotonin reuptake inhibitors)	969.03	E854.0	E939.0	E950.3	E962.0	E980.3
Stains	989.89	E866.8	—	E950.9	E962.1	E980.9
Stannous - see also Tin fluoride	976.7	E858.7	E946.7	E950.4	E962.0	E980.4
Stanolone	962.1	E858.0	E932.1	E950.4	E962.0	E980.4
Stanozolol	962.1	E858.0	E932.1	E950.4	E962.0	E980.4
Staphisagria or stavesacre (pediculicide)	976.0	E858.7	E946.0	E950.4	E962.0	E980.4
Stelazine	969.1	E853.0	E939.1	E950.3	E962.0	E980.3
Stemetil	969.1	E853.0	E939.1	E950.3	E962.0	E980.3
Sterculia (cathartic) (gum)	973.3	E858.4	E943.3	E950.4	E962.0	E980.4
Sternutator gas	987.8	E869.8	—	E952.8	E962.2	E982.8
Steroids NEC	962.0	E858.0	E932.0	E950.4	E962.0	E980.4
ENT agent	976.6	E858.7	E946.6	E950.4	E962.0	E980.4
ophthalmic preparation	976.5	E858.7	E946.5	E950.4	E962.0	E980.4
topical NEC	976.0	E858.7	E946.0	E950.4	E962.0	E980.4
Stibine	985.8	E866.4	—	E950.9	E962.1	E980.9
Stibophen	961.2	E857	E931.2	E950.4	E962.0	E980.4
Stilbamide, stilbamidine	961.5	E857	E931.5	E950.4	E962.0	E980.4
Stilbestrol	962.2	E858.0	E932.2	E950.4	E962.0	E980.4
Stimulants (central nervous system)	970.9	E854.3	E940.9	E950.4	E962.0	E980.4
analeptics	970.0	E854.3	E940.0	E950.4	E962.0	E980.4
opiate antagonist	970.1	E854.3	E940.1	E950.4	E962.0	E980.4
psychotherapeutic NEC	969.09	E854.0	E939.0	E950.3	E962.0	E980.3
specified NEC	970.89	E854.3	E940.8	E950.4	E962.0	E980.4
Storage batteries (acid) (cells)	983.1	E864.1	—	E950.7	E962.1	E980.6
Stovaine	968.9	E855.2	E938.9	E950.4	E962.0	E980.4
infiltration (subcutaneous)	968.5	E855.2	E938.5	E950.4	E962.0	E980.4
nerve block (peripheral) (plexus)	968.6	E855.2	E938.6	E950.4	E962.0	E980.4
spinal	968.7	E855.2	E938.7	E950.4	E962.0	E980.4
topical (surface)	968.5	E855.2	E938.5	E950.4	E962.0	E980.4
Stovarsal	961.1	E857	E931.1	E950.4	E962.0	E980.4
Stove gas - see Gas, utility	—	—	—	—	—	—
Stoxil	976.5	E858.7	E946.5	E950.4	E962.0	E980.4
STP	969.6	E854.1	E939.6	E950.3	E962.0	E980.3
Stramonium (medicinal) NEC	971.1	E855.4	E941.1	E950.4	E962.0	E980.4
natural state	988.2	E865.4	—	E950.9	E962.1	E980.9

◀ New ◀▥ Revised ~~deleted~~ Deleted ● Use Additional Digit(s)

TABLE OF DRUGS AND CHEMICALS

Substance	Poisoning	External Cause (E Code)				
		Accident	Therapeutic Use	Suicide Attempt	Assault	Undetermined
Streptodornase	964.4	E858.2	E934.4	E950.4	E962.0	E980.4
Streptoduocin	960.6	E856	E930.6	E950.4	E962.0	E980.4
Streptokinase	964.4	E858.2	E934.4	E950.4	E962.0	E980.4
Streptomycin	960.6	E856	E930.6	E950.4	E962.0	E980.4
Streptozocin	960.7	E856	E930.7	E950.4	E962.0	E980.4
Stripper (paint) (solvent)	982.8	E862.9	—	E950.9	E962.1	E980.9
Strobane	989.2	E863.0	—	E950.6	E962.1	E980.7
Strophanthin	972.1	E858.3	E942.1	E950.4	E962.0	E980.4
Strophanthus hispidus or kombe	988.2	E865.4	—	E950.9	E962.1	E980.9
Strychnine (rodenticide) (salts)	989.1	E863.7	—	E950.6	E962.1	E980.7
medicinal NEC	970.89	E854.3	E940.8	E950.4	E962.0	E980.4
Strychnos (ignatii) - *see* Strychnine	—	—	—	—	—	—
Styramate	968.0	E855.1	E938.0	E950.4	E962.0	E980.4
Styrene	983.0	E864.0	—	E950.7	E962.1	E980.6
Succinimide (anticonvulsant)	966.2	E855.0	E936.2	E950.4	E962.0	E980.4
mercuric - *see* Mercury	—	—	—	—	—	—
Succinylcholine	975.2	E858.6	E945.2	E950.4	E962.0	E980.4
Succinylsulfathiazole	961.0	E857	E931.0	E950.4	E962.0	E980.4
Sucrose	974.5	E858.5	E944.5	E950.4	E962.0	E980.4
Sulfacetamide	961.0	E857	E931.0	E950.4	E962.0	E980.4
ophthalmic preparation	976.5	E858.7	E946.5	E950.4	E962.0	E980.4
Sulfachlorpyridazine	961.0	E857	E931.0	E950.4	E962.0	E980.4
Sulfacytine	961.0	E857	E931.0	E950.4	E962.0	E980.4
Sulfadiazine	961.0	E857	E931.0	E950.4	E962.0	E980.4
silver (topical)	976.0	E858.7	E946.0	E950.4	E962.0	E980.4
Sulfadimethoxine	961.0	E857	E931.0	E950.4	E962.0	E980.4
Sulfadimidine	961.0	E857	E931.0	E950.4	E962.0	E980.4
Sulfaethidole	961.0	E857	E931.0	E950.4	E962.0	E980.4
Sulfafurazole	961.0	E857	E931.0	E950.4	E962.0	E980.4
Sulfaguanidine	961.0	E857	E931.0	E950.4	E962.0	E980.4
Sulfamerazine	961.0	E857	E931.0	E950.4	E962.0	E980.4
Sulfameter	961.0	E857	E931.0	E950.4	E962.0	E980.4
Sulfamethizole	961.0	E857	E931.0	E950.4	E962.0	E980.4
Sulfamethoxazole	961.0	E857	E931.0	E950.4	E962.0	E980.4
Sulfamethoxydiazine	961.0	E857	E931.0	E950.4	E962.0	E980.4
Sulfamethoxypyridazine	961.0	E857	E931.0	E950.4	E962.0	E980.4
Sulfamethylthiazole	961.0	E857	E931.0	E950.4	E962.0	E980.4
Sulfamylon	976.0	E858.7	E946.0	E950.4	E962.0	E980.4
Sulfan blue (diagnostic dye)	977.8	E858.8	E947.8	E950.4	E962.0	E980.4
Sulfanilamide	961.0	E857	E931.0	E950.4	E962.0	E980.4

◀ New   ◀ Revised   ~~deleted~~ Deleted   ● Use Additional Digit(s)

Substance	Poisoning	External Cause (E Code)				
		Accident	Therapeutic Use	Suicide Attempt	Assault	Undetermined
Sulfanilylguanidine	961.0	E857	E931.0	E950.4	E962.0	E980.4
Sulfaphenazole	961.0	E857	E931.0	E950.4	E962.0	E980.4
Sulfaphenylthiazole	961.0	E857	E931.0	E950.4	E962.0	E980.4
Sulfaproxyline	961.0	E857	E931.0	E950.4	E962.0	E980.4
Sulfapyridine	961.0	E857	E931.0	E950.4	E962.0	E980.4
Sulfapyrimidine	961.0	E857	E931.0	E950.4	E962.0	E980.4
Sulfarsphenamine	961.1	E857	E931.1	E950.4	E962.0	E980.4
Sulfasalazine	961.0	E857	E931.0	E950.4	E962.0	E980.4
Sulfasomizole	961.0	E857	E931.0	E950.4	E962.0	E980.4
Sulfasuxidine	961.0	E857	E931.0	E950.4	E962.0	E980.4
Sulfinpyrazone	974.7	E858.5	E944.7	E950.4	E962.0	E980.4
Sulfisoxazole	961.0	E857	E931.0	E950.4	E962.0	E980.4
ophthalmic preparation	976.5	E858.7	E946.5	E950.4	E962.0	E980.4
Sulfomyxin	960.8	E856	E930.8	E950.4	E962.0	E980.4
Sulfonal	967.8	E852.8	E937.8	E950.2	E962.0	E980.2
Sulfonamides (mixtures)	961.0	E857	E931.0	E950.4	E962.0	E980.4
Sulfones	961.8	E857	E931.8	E950.4	E962.0	E980.4
Sulfonethylmethane	967.8	E852.8	E937.8	E950.2	E962.0	E980.2
Sulfonmethane	967.8	E852.8	E937.8	E950.2	E962.0	E980.2
Sulfonphthal, sulfonphthol	977.8	E858.8	E947.8	E950.4	E962.0	E980.4
Sulfonylurea derivatives, oral	962.3	E858.0	E932.3	E950.4	E962.0	E980.4
Sulfoxone	961.8	E857	E931.8	E950.4	E962.0	E980.4
Sulfur, sulfureted, sulfuric, sulfurous, sulfuryl (compounds) NEC	989.89	E866.8	—	E950.9	E962.1	E980.9
acid	983.1	E864.1	—	E950.7	E962.1	E980.6
dioxide	987.3	E869.1	—	E952.8	E962.2	E982.8
ether - *see* Ether(s)	—	—	—	—	—	—
hydrogen	987.8	E869.8	—	E952.8	E962.2	E982.8
medicinal (keratolytic) (ointment) NEC	976.4	E858.7	E946.4	E950.4	E962.0	E980.4
pesticide (vapor)	989.4	E863.4	—	E950.6	E962.1	E980.7
vapor NEC	987.8	E869.8	—	E952.8	E962.2	E982.8
Sulkowitch's reagent	977.8	E858.8	E947.8	E950.4	E962.0	E980.4
Sulph - *see also* Sulf-	—	—	—	—	—	—
Sulphadione	961.8	E857	E931.8	E950.4	E962.0	E980.4
Sulthiame, sultiame	966.3	E855.0	E936.3	E950.4	E962.0	E980.4
Superinone	975.5	E858.6	E945.5	E950.4	E962.0	E980.4
Suramin	961.5	E857	E931.5	E950.4	E962.0	E980.4
Surfacaine	968.5	E855.2	E938.5	E950.4	E962.0	E980.4
Surital	968.3	E855.1	E938.3	E950.4	E962.0	E980.4
Sutilains	976.8	E858.7	E946.8	E950.4	E962.0	E980.4

TABLE OF DRUGS AND CHEMICALS

◀ New   ◀||| Revised   ~~deleted~~ Deleted   ● Use Additional Digit(s)

Substance	Poisoning	External Cause (E Code)				
		Accident	Therapeutic Use	Suicide Attempt	Assault	Undetermined
Suxamethonium (bromide) (chloride) (iodide)	975.2	E858.6	E945.2	E950.4	E962.0	E980.4
Suxethonium (bromide)	975.2	E858.6	E945.2	E950.4	E962.0	E980.4
Sweet oil (birch)	976.3	E858.7	E946.3	E950.4	E962.0	E980.4
Sym-dichloroethyl ether	982.3	E862.4	—	E950.9	E962.1	E980.9
Sympatholytics	971.3	E855.6	E941.3	E950.4	E962.0	E980.4
Sympathomimetics	971.2	E855.5	E941.2	E950.4	E962.0	E980.4
Synagis	979.6	E858.8	E949.6	E950.4	E962.0	E980.4
Synalar	976.0	E858.7	E946.0	E950.4	E962.0	E980.4
Synthroid	962.7	E858.0	E932.7	E950.4	E962.0	E980.4
Syntocinon	975.0	E858.6	E945.0	E950.4	E962.0	E950.4
Syrosingopine	972.6	E858.3	E942.6	E950.4	E962.0	E980.4
Systemic agents (primarily)	963.9	E858.1	E933.9	E950.4	E962.0	E980.4
specified NEC	963.8	E858.1	E933.8	E950.4	E962.0	E980.4
Tablets (*see also* specified substance)	977.9	E858.9	E947.9	E950.5	E962.0	E980.5
Tace	962.2	E858.0	E932.2	E950.4	E962.0	E980.4
Tacrine	971.0	E855.3	E941.0	E950.4	E962.0	E980.4
Talbutal	967.0	E851	E937.0	E950.1	E962.0	E980.1
Talc	976.3	E858.7	E946.3	E950.4	E962.0	E980.4
Talcum	976.3	E858.7	E946.3	E950.4	E962.0	E980.4
Tamsulosin	971.3	E855.6	E941.3	E950.4	E962.0	E980.4
Tandearil, tanderil	965.5	E850.5	E935.5	E950.0	E962.0	E980.0
Tannic acid	983.1	E864.1	—	E950.7	E962.1	E980.6
medicinal (astringent)	976.2	E858.7	E946.2	E950.4	E962.0	E980.4
Tannin - *see* Tannic acid	—	—	—	—	—	—
Tansy	988.2	E865.4	—	E950.9	E962.1	E980.9
TAO	960.3	E856	E930.3	E950.4	E962.0	E980.4
Tapazole	962.8	E858.0	E932.8	E950.4	E962.0	E980.4
Tar NEC	983.0	E864.0	—	E950.7	E962.1	E980.6
camphor - *see* Naphthalene	—	—	—	—	—	—
fumes	987.8	E869.8	—	E952.8	E962.2	E982.8
Taractan	969.3	E853.8	E939.3	E950.3	E962.0	E980.3
Tarantula (venomous)	989.5	E905.1	—	E950.9	E962.1	E980.9
Tartar emetic (anti-infective)	961.2	E857	E931.2	E950.4	E962.0	E980.4
Tartaric acid	983.1	E864.1	—	E950.7	E962.1	E980.6
Tartrated antimony (anti-infective)	961.2	E857	E931.2	E950.4	E962.0	E980.4
TCA - *see* Trichloroacetic acid	—	—	—	—	—	—
TDI	983.0	E864.0	—	E950.7	E962.1	E980.6
vapor	987.8	E869.8	—	E952.8	E962.2	E982.8
Tear gas	987.5	E869.3	—	E952.8	E962.2	E982.8

◀ New ◀▥ Revised ~~deleted~~ Deleted ● Use Additional Digit(s)

Substance	Poisoning	External Cause (E Code)				
		Accident	Therapeutic Use	Suicide Attempt	Assault	Undetermined
Teclothiazide	974.3	E858.5	E944.3	E950.4	E962.0	E980.4
Tegretol	966.3	E855.0	E936.3	E950.4	E962.0	E980.4
Telepaque	977.8	E858.8	E947.8	E950.4	E962.0	E980.4
Tellurium	985.8	E866.4	—	E950.9	E962.1	E980.9
fumes	985.8	E866.4	—	E950.9	E962.1	E980.9
TEM	963.1	E858.1	E933.1	E950.4	E962.0	E980.4
Temazepam - see Benzodiazepines	—	—	—	—	—	—
TEPA	963.1	E858.1	E933.1	E950.4	E962.0	E980.4
TEPP	989.3	E863.1	—	E950.6	E962.1	E980.7
Terbutaline	971.2	E855.5	E941.2	E950.4	E962.0	E980.4
Teroxalene	961.6	E857	E931.6	E950.4	E962.0	E980.4
Terpin hydrate	975.5	E858.6	E945.5	E950.4	E962.0	E980.4
Terramycin	960.4	E856	E930.4	E950.4	E962.0	E980.4
Tessalon	975.4	E858.6	E945.4	E950.4	E962.0	E980.4
Testosterone	962.1	E858.0	E932.1	E950.4	E962.0	E980.4
Tetanus (vaccine)	978.4	E858.8	E948.4	E950.4	E962.0	E980.4
antitoxin	979.9	E858.8	E949.9	E950.4	E962.0	E980.4
immune globulin (human)	964.6	E858.2	E934.6	E950.4	E962.0	E980.4
toxoid	978.4	E858.8	E948.4	E950.4	E962.0	E980.4
with diphtheria toxoid	978.9	E858.8	E948.9	E950.4	E962.0	E980.4
with pertussis	978.6	E858.8	E948.6	E950.4	E962.0	E980.4
Tetrabenazine	969.5	E853.8	E939.5	E950.3	E962.0	E980.3
Tetracaine (infiltration) (topical)	968.5	E855.2	E938.5	E950.4	E962.0	E980.4
nerve block (peripheral) (plexus)	968.6	E855.2	E938.6	E950.4	E962.0	E980.4
spinal	968.7	E855.2	E938.7	E950.4	E962.0	E980.4
Tetrachlorethylene - see Tetrachloroethylene	—	—	—	—	—	—
Tetrachlormethiazide	974.3	E858.5	E944.3	E950.4	E962.0	E980.4
Tetrachloroethane (liquid) (vapor)	982.3	E862.4	—	E950.9	E962.1	E980.9
paint or varnish	982.3	E861.6	—	E950.9	E962.1	E980.9
Tetrachloroethylene (liquid) (vapor)	982.3	E862.4	—	E950.9	E962.1	E980.9
medicinal	961.6	E857	E931.6	E950.4	E962.0	E980.4
Tetrachloromethane - see Carbon, tetrachloride	—	—	—	—	—	—
Tetracycline	960.4	E856	E930.4	E950.4	E962.0	E980.4
ophthalmic preparation	976.5	E858.7	E946.5	E950.4	E962.0	E980.4
topical NEC	976.0	E858.7	E946.0	E950.4	E962.0	E980.4
Tetraethylammonium chloride	972.3	E858.3	E942.3	E950.4	E962.0	E980.4
Tetraethyl lead (antiknock compound)	984.1	E862.1	—	E950.9	E962.1	E980.9
Tetraethyl pyrophosphate	989.3	E863.1	—	E950.6	E962.1	E980.7
Tetraethylthiuram disulfide	977.3	E858.8	E947.3	E950.4	E962.0	E980.4

Substance	Poisoning	External Cause (E Code)				
		Accident	Therapeutic Use	Suicide Attempt	Assault	Undetermined
Tetrahydroaminoacridine	971.0	E855.3	E941.0	E950.4	E962.0	E980.4
Tetrahydrocannabinol	969.6	E854.1	E939.6	E950.3	E962.0	E980.3
Tetrahydronaphthalene	982.0	E862.4	—	E950.9	E962.1	E980.9
Tetrahydrozoline	971.2	E855.5	E941.2	E950.4	E962.0	E980.4
Tetralin	982.0	E862.4	—	E950.9	E962.1	E980.9
Tetramethylthiuram (disulfide) NEC	989.4	E863.6	—	E950.6	E962.1	E980.7
medicinal	976.2	E858.7	E946.2	E950.4	E962.0	E980.4
Tetronal	967.8	E852.8	E937.8	E950.2	E962.0	E980.2
Tetryl	983.0	E864.0	—	E950.7	E962.1	E980.6
Thalidomide	967.8	E852.8	E937.8	E950.2	E962.0	E980.2
Thallium (compounds) (dust) NEC	985.8	E866.4	—	E950.9	E962.1	E980.9
pesticide (rodenticide)	985.8	E863.7	—	E950.6	E962.1	E980.7
THC	969.6	E854.1	E939.6	E950.3	E962.0	E980.3
Thebacon	965.09	E850.2	E935.2	E950.0	E962.0	E980.0
Thebaine	965.09	E850.2	E935.2	E950.0	E962.0	E980.0
Theobromine (calcium salicylate)	974.1	E858.5	E944.1	E950.4	E962.0	E980.4
Theophylline (diuretic)	974.1	E858.5	E944.1	E950.4	E962.0	E980.4
ethylenediamine	975.7	E858.6	E945.7	E950.4	E962.0	E980.4
Thiabendazole	961.6	E857	E931.6	E950.4	E962.0	E980.4
Thialbarbital, thialbarbitone	968.3	E855.1	E938.3	E950.4	E962.0	E980.4
Thiamine	963.5	E858.1	E933.5	E950.4	E962.0	E980.4
Thiamylal (sodium)	968.3	E855.1	E938.3	E950.4	E962.0	E980.4
Thiazesim	969.09	E854.0	E939.0	E950.3	E962.0	E980.3
Thiazides (diuretics)	974.3	E858.5	E944.3	E950.4	E962.0	E980.4
Thiethylperazine	963.0	E858.1	E933.0	E950.4	E962.0	E980.4
Thimerosal (topical)	976.0	E858.7	E946.0	E950.4	E962.0	E980.4
ophthalmic preparation	976.5	E858.7	E946.5	E950.4	E962.0	E980.4
Thioacetazone	961.8	E857	E931.8	E950.4	E962.0	E980.4
Thiobarbiturates	968.3	E855.1	E938.3	E950.4	E962.0	E980.4
Thiobismol	961.2	E857	E931.2	E950.4	E962.0	E980.4
Thiocarbamide	962.8	E858.0	E932.8	E950.4	E962.0	E980.4
Thiocarbarsone	961.1	E857	E931.1	E950.4	E962.0	E980.4
Thiocarlide	961.8	E857	E931.8	E950.4	E962.0	E980.4
Thioguanine	963.1	E858.1	E933.1	E950.4	E962.0	E980.4
Thiomercaptomerin	974.0	E858.5	E944.0	E950.4	E962.0	E980.4
Thiomerin	974.0	E858.5	E944.0	E950.4	E962.0	E980.4
Thiopental, thiopentone (sodium)	968.3	E855.1	E938.3	E950.4	E962.0	E980.4
Thiopropazate	969.1	E853.0	E939.1	E950.3	E962.0	E980.3
Thioproperazine	969.1	E853.0	E939.1	E950.3	E962.0	E980.3

◀ New ◀ Revised ~~deleted~~ Deleted ● Use Additional Digit(s)

Substance	Poisoning	External Cause (E Code)				
		Accident	Therapeutic Use	Suicide Attempt	Assault	Undetermined
Thioridazine	969.1	E853.0	E939.1	E950.3	E962.0	E980.3
Thio-TEPA, thiotepa	963.1	E858.1	E933.1	E950.4	E962.0	E980.4
Thiothixene	969.3	E853.8	E939.3	E950.3	E962.0	E980.3
Thiouracil	962.8	E858.0	E932.8	E950.4	E962.0	E980.4
Thiourea	962.8	E858.0	E932.8	E950.4	E962.0	E980.4
Thiphenamil	971.1	E855.4	E941.1	E950.4	E962.0	E980.4
Thiram NEC	989.4	E863.6	—	E950.6	E962.1	E980.7
medicinal	976.2	E858.7	E946.2	E950.4	E962.0	E980.4
Thonzylamine	963.0	E858.1	E933.0	E950.4	E962.0	E980.4
Thorazine	969.1	E853.0	E939.1	E950.3	E962.0	E980.3
Thornapple	988.2	E865.4	—	E950.9	E962.1	E980.9
Throat preparation (lozenges) NEC	976.6	E858.7	E946.6	E950.4	E962.0	E980.4
Thrombin	964.5	E858.2	E934.5	E950.4	E962.0	E980.4
Thrombolysin	964.4	E858.2	E934.4	E950.4	E962.0	E980.4
Thymol	983.0	E864.0	—	E950.7	E962.1	E980.6
Thymus extract	962.9	E858.0	E932.9	E950.4	E962.0	E980.4
Thyroglobulin	962.7	E858.0	E932.7	E950.4	E962.0	E980.4
Thyroid (derivatives) (extract)	962.7	E858.0	E932.7	E950.4	E962.0	E980.4
Thyrolar	962.7	E858.0	E932.7	E950.4	E962.0	E980.4
Thyrotrophin, thyrotropin	977.8	E858.8	E947.8	E950.4	E962.0	E980.4
Thyroxin(e)	962.7	E858.0	E932.7	E950.4	E962.0	E980.4
Tigan	963.0	E858.1	E933.0	E950.4	E962.0	E980.4
Tigloidine	968.0	E855.1	E938.0	E950.4	E962.0	E980.4
Tin (chloride) (dust) (oxide) NEC	985.8	E866.4	—	E950.9	E962.1	E980.9
anti-infectives	961.2	E857	E931.2	E950.4	E962.0	E980.4
Tinactin	976.0	E858.7	E946.0	E950.4	E962.0	E980.4
Tincture, iodine - see Iodine	—	—	—	—	—	—
Tindal	969.1	E853.0	E939.1	E950.3	E962.0	E980.3
Titanium (compounds) (vapor)	985.8	E866.4	—	E950.9	E962.1	E980.9
ointment	976.3	E858.7	E946.3	E950.4	E962.0	E980.4
Titroid	962.7	E858.0	E932.7	E950.4	E962.0	E980.4
TMTD - see Tetramethylthiuram disulfide	—	—	—	—	—	—
TNT	989.89	E866.8	—	E950.9	E962.1	E980.9
fumes	987.8	E869.8	—	E952.8	E962.2	E982.8
Toadstool	988.1	E865.5	—	E950.9	E962.1	E980.9
Tobacco NEC	989.84	E866.8	—	E950.9	E962.1	E980.9
Indian	988.2	E865.4	—	E950.9	E962.1	E980.9
smoke, second-hand	987.8	E869.4	—	—	—	—

◀ New ◀◧ Revised ~~deleted~~ Deleted ● Use Additional Digit(s)

Substance	Poisoning	Accident	Therapeutic Use	Suicide Attempt	Assault	Undetermined
Tocopherol	963.5	E858.1	E933.5	E950.4	E962.0	E980.4
Tocosamine	975.0	E858.6	E945.0	E950.4	E962.0	E980.4
Tofranil	969.05	E854.0	E939.0	E950.3	E962.0	E980.3
Toilet deodorizer	989.89	E866.8	—	E950.9	E962.1	E980.9
Tolazamide	962.3	E858.0	E932.3	E950.4	E962.0	E980.4
Tolazoline	971.3	E855.6	E941.3	E950.4	E962.0	E980.4
Tolbutamide	962.3	E858.0	E932.3	E950.4	E962.0	E980.4
sodium	977.8	E858.8	E947.8	E950.4	E962.0	E980.4
Tolmetin	965.69	E850.6	E935.6	E950.0	E962.0	E980.0
Tolnaftate	976.0	E858.7	E946.0	E950.4	E962.0	E980.4
Tolpropamine	976.1	E858.7	E946.1	E950.4	E962.0	E980.4
Tolserol	968.0	E855.1	E938.0	E950.4	E962.0	E980.4
Toluene (liquid) (vapor)	982.0	E862.4	—	E950.9	E962.1	E980.9
diisocyanate	983.0	E864.0	—	E950.7	E962.1	E980.6
Toluidine	983.0	E864.0	—	E950.7	E962.1	E980.6
vapor	987.8	E869.8	—	E952.8	E962.2	E982.8
Toluol (liquid) (vapor)	982.0	E862.4	—	E950.9	E962.1	E980.9
Tolylene-2,4-diisocyanate	983.0	E864.0	—	E950.7	E962.1	E980.6
Tonics, cardiac	972.1	E858.3	E942.1	E950.4	E962.0	E980.4
Toxaphene (dust) (spray)	989.2	E863.0	—	E950.6	E962.1	E980.7
Toxoids NEC	978.8	E858.8	E948.8	E950.4	E962.0	E980.4
Tractor fuel NEC	981	E862.1	—	E950.9	E962.1	E980.9
Tragacanth	973.3	E858.4	E943.3	E950.4	E962.0	E980.4
Tramazoline	971.2	E855.5	E941.2	E950.4	E962.0	E980.4
Tranquilizers	969.5	E853.9	E939.5	E950.3	E962.0	E980.3
benzodiazepine-based	969.4	E853.2	E939.4	E950.3	E962.0	E980.3
butyrophenone-based	969.2	E853.1	E939.2	E950.3	E962.0	E980.3
major NEC	969.3	E853.8	E939.3	E950.3	E962.0	E980.3
phenothiazine-based	969.1	E853.0	E939.1	E950.3	E962.0	E980.3
specified NEC	969.5	E853.8	E939.5	E950.3	E962.0	E980.3
Trantoin	961.9	E857	E931.9	E950.4	E962.0	E980.4
Tranxene	969.4	E853.2	E939.4	E950.3	E962.0	E980.3
Tranylcypromine (sulfate)	969.01	E854.0	E939.0	E950.3	E962.0	E980.3
Trasentine	975.1	E858.6	E945.1	E950.4	E962.0	E980.4
Travert	974.5	E858.5	E944.5	E950.4	E962.0	E980.4
Trecator	961.8	E857	E931.8	E950.4	E962.0	E980.4
Tretinoin	976.8	E858.7	E946.8	E950.4	E962.0	E980.4
Triacetin	976.0	E858.7	E946.0	E950.4	E962.0	E980.4

◄ New ◄ Revised ~~deleted~~ Deleted ● Use Additional Digit(s)

Substance	Poisoning	External Cause (E Code)				
		Accident	Therapeutic Use	Suicide Attempt	Assault	Undetermined
Triacetyloleandomycin	960.3	E856	E930.3	E950.4	E962.0	E980.4
Triamcinolone	962.0	E858.0	E932.0	E950.4	E962.0	E980.4
ENT agent	976.6	E858.7	E946.6	E950.4	E962.0	E980.4
ophthalmic preparation	976.5	E858.7	E946.5	E950.4	E962.0	E980.4
topical NEC	976.0	E858.7	E946.0	E950.4	E962.0	E980.4
Triamterene	974.4	E858.5	E944.4	E950.4	E962.0	E980.4
Triaziquone	963.1	E858.1	E933.1	E950.4	E962.0	E980.4
Tribromacetaldehyde	967.3	E852.2	E937.3	E950.2	E962.0	E980.2
Tribromoethanol	968.2	E855.1	E938.2	E950.4	E962.0	E980.4
Tribromomethane	967.3	E852.2	E937.3	E950.2	E962.0	E980.2
Trichlorethane	982.3	E862.4	—	E950.9	E962.1	E980.9
Trichlormethiazide	974.3	E858.5	E944.3	E950.4	E962.0	E980.4
Trichloroacetic acid	983.1	E864.1	—	E950.7	E962.1	E980.6
medicinal (keratolytic)	976.4	E858.7	E946.4	E950.4	E962.0	E980.4
Trichloroethanol	967.1	E852.0	E937.1	E950.2	E962.0	E980.2
Trichloroethylene (liquid) (vapor)	982.3	E862.4	—	E950.9	E962.1	E980.9
anesthetic (gas)	968.2	E855.1	E938.2	E950.4	E962.0	E980.4
Trichloroethyl phosphate	967.1	E852.0	E937.1	E950.2	E962.0	E980.2
Trichlorofluoromethane NEC	987.4	E869.2	—	E952.8	E962.2	E982.8
Trichlorotriethylamine	963.1	E858.1	E933.1	E950.4	E962.0	E980.4
Trichomonacides NEC	961.5	E857	E931.5	E950.4	E962.0	E980.4
Trichomycin	960.1	E856	E930.1	E950.4	E962.0	E980.4
Triclofos	967.1	E852.0	E937.1	E950.2	E962.0	E980.2
Tricresyl phosphate	989.89	E866.8	—	E950.9	E962.1	E980.9
solvent	982.8	E862.4	—	E950.9	E962.1	E980.9
Tricyclamol	966.4	E855.0	E936.4	E950.4	E962.0	E980.4
Tridesilon	976.0	E858.7	E946.0	E950.4	E962.0	E980.4
Tridihexethyl	971.1	E855.4	E941.1	E950.4	E962.0	E980.4
Tridione	966.0	E855.0	E936.0	E950.4	E962.0	E980.4
Triethanolamine NEC	983.2	E864.2	—	E950.7	E962.1	E980.6
detergent	983.2	E861.0	—	E950.7	E962.1	E980.6
trinitrate	972.4	E858.3	E942.4	E950.4	E962.0	E980.4
Triethanomelamine	963.1	E858.1	E933.1	E950.4	E962.0	E980.4
Triethylene melamine	963.1	E858.1	E933.1	E950.4	E962.0	E980.4
Triethylenephosphoramide	963.1	E858.1	E933.1	E950.4	E962.0	E980.4
Triethylenethiophosphoramide	963.1	E858.1	E933.1	E950.4	E962.0	E980.4
Trifluoperazine	969.1	E853.0	E939.1	E950.3	E962.0	E980.3
Trifluperidol	969.2	E853.1	E939.2	E950.3	E962.0	E980.3
Triflupromazine	969.1	E853.0	E939.1	E950.3	E962.0	E980.3

◀ New ◀ Revised deleted Deleted ● Use Additional Digit(s)

Substance	Poisoning	External Cause (E Code)				
		Accident	Therapeutic Use	Suicide Attempt	Assault	Undetermined
Trihexyphenidyl	971.1	E855.4	E941.1	E950.4	E962.0	E980.4
Triiodothyronine	962.7	E858.0	E932.7	E950.4	E962.0	E980.4
Trilene	968.2	E855.1	E938.2	E950.4	E962.0	E980.4
Trimeprazine	963.0	E858.1	E933.0	E950.4	E962.0	E980.4
Trimetazidine	972.4	E858.3	E942.4	E950.4	E962.0	E980.4
Trimethadione	966.0	E855.0	E936.0	E950.4	E962.0	E980.4
Trimethaphan	972.3	E858.3	E942.3	E950.4	E962.0	E980.4
Trimethidinium	972.3	E858.3	E942.3	E950.4	E962.0	E980.4
Trimethobenzamide	963.0	E858.1	E933.0	E950.4	E962.0	E980.4
Trimethylcarbinol	980.8	E860.8	—	E950.9	E962.1	E980.9
Trimethylpsoralen	976.3	E858.7	E946.3	E950.4	E962.0	E980.4
Trimeton	963.0	E858.1	E933.0	E950.4	E962.0	E980.4
Trimipramine	969.05	E854.0	E939.0	E950.3	E962.0	E980.3
Trimustine	963.1	E858.1	E933.1	E950.4	E962.0	E980.4
Trinitrin	972.4	E858.3	E942.4	E950.4	E962.0	E980.4
Trinitrophenol	983.0	E864.0	—	E950.7	E962.1	E980.6
Trinitrotoluene	989.89	E866.8	—	E950.9	E962.1	E980.9
fumes	987.8	E869.8	—	E952.8	E962.2	E982.8
Trional	967.8	E852.8	E937.8	E950.2	E962.0	E980.2
Trioxide of arsenic - *see* Arsenic	—	—	—	—	—	—
Trioxsalen	976.3	E858.7	E946.3	E950.4	E962.0	E980.4
Tripelennamine	963.0	E858.1	E933.0	E950.4	E962.0	E980.4
Triperidol	969.2	E853.1	E939.2	E950.3	E962.0	E980.3
Triprolidine	963.0	E858.1	E933.0	E950.4	E962.0	E980.4
Trisoralen	976.3	E858.7	E946.3	E950.4	E962.0	E980.4
Troleandomycin	960.3	E856	E930.3	E950.4	E962.0	E980.4
Trolnitrate (phosphate)	972.4	E858.3	E942.4	E950.4	E962.0	E980.4
Trometamol	963.3	E858.1	E933.3	E950.4	E962.0	E980.4
Tromethamine	963.3	E858.1	E933.3	E950.4	E962.0	E980.4
Tronothane	968.5	E855.2	E938.5	E950.4	E962.0	E980.4
Tropicamide	971.1	E855.4	E941.1	E950.4	E962.0	E980.4
Troxidone	966.0	E855.0	E936.0	E950.4	E962.0	E980.4
Tryparsamide	961.1	E857	E931.1	E950.4	E962.0	E980.4
Trypsin	963.4	E858.1	E933.4	E950.4	E962.0	E980.4
Tryptizol	969.05	E854.0	E939.0	E950.3	E962.0	E980.3
Tuaminoheptane	971.2	E855.5	E941.2	E950.4	E962.0	E980.4
Tuberculin (old)	977.8	E858.8	E947.8	E950.4	E962.0	E980.4
Tubocurare	975.2	E858.6	E945.2	E950.4	E962.0	E980.4
Tubocurarine	975.2	E858.6	E945.2	E950.4	E962.0	E980.4

◀ New ◀ Revised ~~deleted~~ Deleted ● Use Additional Digit(s)

Substance	Poisoning	External Cause (E Code)				
		Accident	Therapeutic Use	Suicide Attempt	Assault	Undetermined
Turkish green	969.6	E854.1	E939.6	E950.3	E962.0	E980.3
Turpentine (spirits of) (liquid) (vapor)	982.8	E862.4	—	E950.9	E962.1	E980.9
Tybamate	969.5	E853.8	E939.5	E950.3	E962.0	E980.3
Tyloxapol	975.5	E858.6	E945.5	E950.4	E962.0	E980.4
Tymazoline	971.2	E855.5	E941.2	E950.4	E962.0	E980.4
Typhoid vaccine	978.1	E858.8	E948.1	E950.4	E962.0	E980.4
Typhus vaccine	979.2	E858.8	E949.2	E950.4	E962.0	E980.4
Tyrothricin	976.0	E858.7	E946.0	E950.4	E962.0	E980.4
ENT agent	976.6	E858.7	E946.6	E950.4	E962.0	E980.4
ophthalmic preparation	976.5	E858.7	E946.5	E950.4	E962.0	E980.4
Undecenoic acid	976.0	E858.7	E946.0	E950.4	E962.0	E980.4
Undecylenic acid	976.0	E858.7	E946.0	E950.4	E962.0	E980.4
Unna's boot	976.3	E858.7	E946.3	E950.4	E962.0	E980.4
Uracil mustard	963.1	E858.1	E933.1	E950.4	E962.0	E980.4
Uramustine	963.1	E858.1	E933.1	E950.4	E962.0	E980.4
Urari	975.2	E858.6	E945.2	E950.4	E962.0	E980.4
Urea	974.4	E858.5	E944.4	E950.4	E962.0	E980.4
topical	976.8	E858.7	E946.8	E950.4	E962.0	E980.4
Urethan(e) (antineoplastic)	963.1	E858.1	E933.1	E950.4	E962.0	E980.4
Urginea (maritima) (scilla) - see Squill	—	—	—	—	—	—
Uric acid metabolism agents NEC	974.7	E858.5	E944.7	E950.4	E962.0	E980.4
Urokinase	964.4	E858.2	E934.4	E950.4	E962.0	E980.4
Urokon	977.8	E858.8	E947.8	E950.4	E962.0	E980.4
Urotropin	961.9	E857	E931.9	E950.4	E962.0	E980.4
Urtica	988.2	E865.4	—	E950.9	E962.1	E980.9
Utility gas - see Gas, utility	—	—	—	—	—	—
Vaccine NEC	979.9	E858.8	E949.9	E950.4	E962.0	E980.4
bacterial NEC	978.8	E858.8	E948.8	E950.4	E962.0	E980.4
with	—	—	—	—	—	—
other bacterial component	978.9	E858.8	E948.9	E950.4	E962.0	E980.4
pertussis component	978.6	E858.8	E948.6	E950.4	E962.0	E980.4
viral-rickettsial component	979.7	E858.8	E949.7	E950.4	E962.0	E980.4
mixed NEC	978.9	E858.8	E948.9	E950.4	E962.0	E980.4
BCG	978.0	E858.8	E948.0	E950.4	E962.0	E980.4
cholera	978.2	E858.8	E948.2	E950.4	E962.0	E980.4
diphtheria	978.5	E858.8	E948.5	E950.4	E962.0	E980.4
influenza	979.6	E858.8	E949.6	E950.4	E962.0	E980.4

◀ New ◀▥ Revised ~~deleted~~ Deleted ● Use Additional Digit(s)

Substance	Poisoning	External Cause (E Code)				
		Accident	Therapeutic Use	Suicide Attempt	Assault	Undetermined
Vaccine NEC *(Continued)*						
measles	979.4	E858.8	E949.4	E950.4	E962.0	E980.4
meningococcal	978.8	E858.8	E948.8	E950.4	E962.0	E980.4
mumps	979.6	E858.8	E949.6	E950.4	E962.0	E980.4
paratyphoid	978.1	E858.8	E948.1	E950.4	E962.0	E980.4
pertussis (with diphtheria toxoid) (with tetanus toxoid)	978.6	E858.8	E948.6	E950.4	E962.0	E980.4
plague	978.3	E858.8	E948.3	E950.4	E962.0	E980.4
poliomyelitis	979.5	E858.8	E949.5	E950.4	E962.0	E980.4
poliovirus	979.5	E858.8	E949.5	E950.4	E962.0	E980.4
rabies	979.1	E858.8	E949.1	E950.4	E962.0	E980.4
respiratory syncytial virus	979.6	E858.8	E949.6	E950.4	E962.0	E980.4
rickettsial NEC	979.6	E858.8	E949.6	E950.4	E962.0	E980.4
with	—	—	—	—	—	—
bacterial component	979.7	E858.8	E949.7	E950.4	E962.0	E980.4
pertussis component	978.6	E858.8	E948.6	E950.4	E962.0	E980.4
viral component	979.7	E858.8	E949.7	E950.4	E962.0	E980.4
Rocky Mountain spotted fever	979.6	E858.8	E949.6	E950.4	E962.0	E980.4
rotavirus	979.6	E858.8	E949.6	E950.4	E962.0	E980.4
rubella virus	979.4	E858.8	E949.4	E950.4	E962.0	E980.4
sabin oral	979.5	E858.8	E949.5	E950.4	E962.0	E980.4
smallpox	979.0	E858.8	E949.0	E950.4	E962.0	E980.4
tetanus	978.4	E858.8	E948.4	E950.4	E962.0	E980.4
typhoid	978.1	E858.8	E948.1	E950.4	E962.0	E980.4
typhus	979.2	E858.8	E949.2	E950.4	E962.0	E980.4
viral NEC	979.6	E858.8	E949.6	E950.4	E962.0	E980.4
with	—	—	—	—	—	—
bacterial component	979.7	E858.8	E949.7	E950.4	E962.0	E980.4
pertussis component	978.6	E858.8	E948.6	E950.4	E962.0	E980.4
rickettsial component	979.7	E858.8	E949.7	E950.4	E962.0	E980.4
yellow fever	979.3	E858.8	E949.3	E950.4	E962.0	E980.4
Vaccinia immune globulin (human)	964.6	E858.2	E934.6	E950.4	E962.0	E980.4
Vaginal contraceptives	976.8	E858.7	E946.8	E950.4	E962.0	E980.4
Valethamate	971.1	E855.4	E941.1	E950.4	E962.0	E980.4
Valisone	976.0	E858.7	E946.0	E950.4	E962.0	E980.4
Valium	969.4	E853.2	E939.4	E950.3	E962.0	E980.3
Valmid	967.8	E852.8	E937.8	E950.2	E962.0	E980.2
Vanadium	985.8	E866.4	—	E950.9	E962.1	E980.9
Vancomycin	960.8	E856	E930.8	E950.4	E962.0	E980.4

◀ New   ◀▦ Revised   ~~deleted~~ Deleted   ● Use Additional Digit(s)

Substance	Poisoning	External Cause (E Code)				
		Accident	Therapeutic Use	Suicide Attempt	Assault	Undetermined
Vapor (*see also* Gas)	987.9	E869.9	—	E952.9	E962.2	E982.9
kiln (carbon monoxide)	986	E868.8	—	E952.1	E962.2	E982.1
lead - *see* Lead	—	—	—	—	—	—
specified source NEC - (*see also* specific substance)	987.8	E869.8	—	E952.8	E962.2	E982.8
Varidase	964.4	E858.2	E934.4	E950.4	E962.0	E980.4
Varnish	989.89	E861.6	—	E950.9	E962.1	E980.9
cleaner	982.8	E862.9	—	E950.9	E962.1	E980.9
Vaseline	976.3	E858.7	E946.3	E950.4	E962.0	E980.4
Vasodilan	972.5	E858.3	E942.5	E950.4	E962.0	E980.4
Vasodilators NEC	972.5	E858.3	E942.5	E950.4	E962.0	E980.4
coronary	972.4	E858.3	E942.4	E950.4	E962.0	E980.4
Vasopressin	962.5	E858.0	E932.5	E950.4	E962.0	E980.4
Vasopressor drugs	962.5	E858.0	E932.5	E950.4	E962.0	E980.4
Venom, venomous (bite) (sting)	989.5	E905.9	—	E950.9	E962.1	E980.9
arthropod NEC	989.5	E905.5	—	E950.9	E962.1	E980.9
bee	989.5	E905.3	—	E950.9	E962.1	E980.9
centipede	989.5	E905.4	—	E950.9	E962.1	E980.9
hornet	989.5	E905.3	—	E950.9	E962.1	E980.9
lizard	989.5	E905.0	—	E950.9	E962.1	E980.9
marine animals or plants	989.5	E905.6	—	E950.9	E962.1	E980.9
millipede (tropical)	989.5	E905.4	—	E950.9	E962.1	E980.9
plant NEC	989.5	E905.7	—	E950.9	E962.1	E980.9
marine	989.5	E905.6	—	E950.9	E962.1	E980.9
scorpion	989.5	E905.2	—	E950.9	E962.1	E980.9
snake	989.5	E905.0	—	E950.9	E962.1	E980.9
specified NEC	989.5	E905.8	—	E950.9	E962.1	E980.9
spider	989.5	E905.1	—	E950.9	E962.1	E980.9
wasp	989.5	E905.3	—	E950.9	E962.1	E980.9
Ventolin - *see* Salbutamol sulfate	—	—	—	—	—	—
Veramon	967.0	E851	E937.0	E950.1	E962.0	E980.1
Veratrum	—	—	—	—	—	—
album	988.2	E865.4	—	E950.9	E962.1	E980.9
alkaloids	972.6	E858.3	E942.6	E950.4	E962.0	E980.4
viride	988.2	E865.4	—	E950.9	E962.1	E980.9
Verdigris (*see also* Copper)	985.8	E866.4	—	E950.9	E962.1	E980.9
Veronal	967.0	E851	E937.0	E950.1	E962.0	E980.1
Veroxil	961.6	E857	E931.6	E950.4	E962.0	E980.4
Versidyne	965.7	E850.7	E935.7	E950.0	E962.0	E980.0
Viagra	972.5	E858.3	E942.5	E950.4	E962.0	E980.4

◄ New   ◄IIII Revised   ~~deleted~~ Deleted   ● Use Additional Digit(s)

Substance	Poisoning	Accident	Therapeutic Use	Suicide Attempt	Assault	Undetermined
Vienna	—	—	—	—	—	—
green	985.1	E866.3	—	E950.8	E962.1	E980.8
insecticide	985.1	E863.4	—	E950.6	E962.1	E980.7
red	989.89	E866.8	—	E950.9	E962.1	E980.9
pharmaceutical dye	977.4	E858.8	E947.4	E950.4	E962.0	E980.4
Vinbarbital, vinbarbitone	967.0	E851	E937.0	E950.1	E962.0	E980.1
Vinblastine	963.1	E858.1	E933.1	E950.4	E962.0	E980.4
Vincristine	963.1	E858.1	E933.1	E950.4	E962.0	E980.4
Vinesthene, vinethene	968.2	E855.1	E938.2	E950.4	E962.0	E980.4
Vinyl	—	—	—	—	—	—
bital	967.0	E851	E937.0	E950.1	E962.0	E980.1
ether	968.2	E855.1	E938.2	E950.4	E962.0	E980.4
Vioform	961.3	E857	E931.3	E950.4	E962.0	E980.4
topical	976.0	E858.7	E946.0	E950.4	E962.0	E980.4
Viomycin	960.6	E856	E930.6	E950.4	E962.0	E980.4
Viosterol	963.5	E858.1	E933.5	E950.4	E962.0	E980.4
Viper (venom)	989.5	E905.0	—	E950.9	E962.1	E980.9
Viprynium (embonate)	961.6	E857	E931.6	E950.4	E962.0	E980.4
Virugon	961.7	E857	E931.7	E950.4	E962.0	E980.4
Visine	976.5	E858.7	E946.5	E950.4	E962.0	E980.4
Vitamins NEC	963.5	E858.1	E933.5	E950.4	E962.0	E980.4
B_{12}	964.1	E858.2	E934.1	E950.4	E962.0	E980.4
hematopoietic	964.1	E858.2	E934.1	E950.4	E962.0	E980.4
K	964.3	E858.2	E934.3	E950.4	E962.0	E980.4
Vleminckx's solution	976.4	E858.7	E946.4	E950.4	E962.0	E980.4
Voltaren - *see* Diclofenac sodium	—	—	—	—	—	—
Warfarin (potassium) (sodium)	964.2	E858.2	E934.2	E950.4	E962.0	E980.4
rodenticide	989.4	E863.7	—	E950.6	E962.1	E980.7
Wasp (sting)	989.5	E905.3	—	E950.9	E962.1	E980.9
Water	—	—	—	—	—	—
balance agents NEC	974.5	E858.5	E944.5	E950.4	E962.0	E980.4
gas	987.1	E868.1	—	E951.8	E962.2	E981.8
incomplete combustion of - *see* Carbon, monoxide, fuel, utility	—	—	—	—	—	—
hemlock	988.2	E865.4	—	E950.9	E962.1	E980.9
moccasin (venom)	989.5	E905.0	—	E950.9	E962.1	E980.9
Wax (paraffin) (petroleum)	981	E862.3	—	E950.9	E962.1	E980.9
automobile	989.89	E861.2	—	E950.9	E962.1	E980.9
floor	981	E862.0	—	E950.9	E962.1	E980.9
Weed killers NEC	989.4	E863.5	—	E950.6	E962.1	E980.7

◀ New   ◀▦ Revised   ~~deleted~~ Deleted   ● Use Additional Digit(s)

Substance	Poisoning	External Cause (E Code)				
		Accident	Therapeutic Use	Suicide Attempt	Assault	Undetermined
Welldorm	967.1	E852.0	E937.1	E950.2	E962.0	E980.2
White	—	—	—	—	—	—
arsenic - *see* Arsenic	—	—	—	—	—	—
hellebore	988.2	E865.4	—	E950.9	E962.1	E980.9
lotion (keratolytic)	976.4	E858.7	E946.4	E950.4	E962.0	E980.4
spirit	981	E862.0	—	E950.9	E962.1	E980.9
Whitewashes	989.89	E861.6	—	E950.9	E962.1	E980.9
Whole blood	964.7	E858.2	E934.7	E950.4	E962.0	E980.4
Wild	—	—	—	—	—	—
black cherry	988.2	E865.4	—	E950.9	E962.1	E980.9
poisonous plants NEC	988.2	E865.4	—	E950.9	E962.1	E980.9
Window cleaning fluid	989.89	E861.3	—	E950.9	E962.1	E980.9
Wintergreen (oil)	976.3	E858.7	E946.3	E950.4	E962.0	E980.4
Witch hazel	976.2	E858.7	E946.2	E950.4	E962.0	E980.4
Wood	—	—	—	—	—	—
alcohol	980.1	E860.2	—	E950.9	E962.1	E980.9
spirit	980.1	E860.2	—	E950.9	E962.1	E980.9
Woorali	975.2	E858.6	E945.2	E950.4	E962.0	E980.4
Wormseed, American	961.6	E857	E931.6	E950.4	E962.0	E980.4
Xanthine diuretics	974.1	E858.5	E944.1	E950.4	E962.0	E980.4
Xanthocillin	960.0	E856	E930.0	E950.4	E962.0	E980.4
Xanthotoxin	976.3	E858.7	E946.3	E950.4	E962.0	E980.4
Xigris	964.2	E858.2	E934.2	E950.4	E962.0	E980.4
Xylene (liquid) (vapor)	982.0	E862.4	—	E950.9	E962.1	E980.9
Xylocaine (infiltration) (topical)	968.5	E855.2	E938.5	E950.4	E962.0	E980.4
nerve block (peripheral) (plexus)	968.6	E855.2	E938.6	E950.4	E962.0	E980.4
spinal	968.7	E855.2	E938.7	E950.4	E962.0	E980.4
Xylol (liquid) (vapor)	982.0	E862.4	—	E950.9	E962.1	E980.9
Xylometazoline	971.2	E855.5	E941.2	E950.4	E962.0	E980.4
Yellow	—	—	—	—	—	—
fever vaccine	979.3	E858.8	E949.3	E950.4	E962.0	E980.4
jasmine	988.2	E865.4	—	E950.9	E962.1	E980.9
Yew	988.2	E865.4	—	E950.9	E962.1	E980.9
Zactane	965.7	E850.7	E935.7	E950.0	E962.0	E980.0
Zaroxolyn	974.3	E858.5	E944.3	E950.4	E962.0	E980.4
Zephiran (topical)	976.0	E858.7	E946.0	E950.4	E962.0	E980.4
ophthalmic preparation	976.5	E858.7	E946.5	E950.4	E962.0	E980.4
Zerone	980.1	E860.2	—	E950.9	E962.1	E980.9

TABLE OF DRUGS AND CHEMICALS

		External Cause (E Code)				
Substance	Poisoning	Accident	Therapeutic Use	Suicide Attempt	Assault	Undetermined
Zinc (compounds) (fumes) (salts) (vapor) NEC	985.8	E866.4	—	E950.9	E962.1	E980.9
anti-infectives	976.0	E858.7	E946.0	E950.4	E962.0	E980.4
antivaricose	972.7	E858.3	E942.7	E950.4	E962.0	E980.4
bacitracin	976.0	E858.7	E946.0	E950.4	E962.0	E980.4
chloride	976.2	E858.7	E946.2	E950.4	E962.0	E980.4
gelatin	976.3	E858.7	E946.3	E950.4	E962.0	E980.4
oxide	976.3	E858.7	E946.3	E950.4	E962.0	E980.4
peroxide	976.0	E858.7	E946.0	E950.4	E962.0	E980.4
pesticides	985.8	E863.4	—	E950.6	E962.1	E980.7
phosphide (rodenticide)	985.8	E863.7	—	E950.6	E962.1	E980.7
stearate	976.3	E858.7	E946.3	E950.4	E962.0	E980.4
sulfate (antivaricose)	972.7	E858.3	E942.7	E950.4	E962.0	E980.4
ENT agent	976.6	E858.7	E946.6	E950.4	E962.0	E980.4
ophthalmic solution	976.5	E858.7	E946.5	E950.4	E962.0	E980.4
topical NEC	976.0	E858.7	E946.0	E950.4	E962.0	E980.4
undecylenate	976.0	E858.7	E946.0	E950.4	E962.0	E980.4
Zovant	964.2	E858.2	E934.2	E950.4	E962.0	E980.4
Zoxazolamine	968.0	E855.1	E938.0	E950.4	E962.0	E980.4
Zygadenus (venenosus)	988.2	E865.4	—	E950.9	E962.1	E980.9
Zyprexa	969.3	E853.8	E939.3	E950.3	E962.0	E980.3

◀ New ◀ Revised ~~deleted~~ Deleted ● Use Additional Digit(s)

SECTION III

INDEX TO EXTERNAL CAUSES OF INJURY (E CODE)

This section contains the index to the codes which classify environmental events, circumstances, and other conditions as the cause of injury and other adverse effects. Where a code from the section Supplementary Classification of External Causes of Injury and Poisoning (E800–E998) is applicable, it is intended that the E code shall be used in addition to a code from the main body of the classification, Chapters 1 to 17.

The alphabetic index to the E codes is organized by main terms which describe the accident, circumstance, event, or specific agent which caused the injury or other adverse effect.

Note: Transport accidents (E800–E848) include accidents involving:

> aircraft and spacecraft (E840–E845)
> watercraft (E830–E838)
> motor vehicle (E810–E825)
> railway (E800–E807)
> other road vehicles (E826–E829)

For definitions and examples related to transport accidents - *see* Supplementary Classification of External Causes of Injury and Poisoning (E800–E999).

The fourth-digit subdivisions for use with categories E800–E848 to identify the injured person are found at the end of this section.

For identifying the place in which an accident or poisoning occurred (circumstances classifiable to categories E850–E869 and E880–E928) - *see* the listing in this section under "Accident, occurring."

See the Table of Drugs and Chemicals (Section 2 of this volume) for identifying the specific agent involved in drug overdose or a wrong substance given or taken in error, and for intoxication or poisoning by a drug or other chemical substance.

The specific adverse effect, reaction, or localized toxic effect to a correct drug or substance properly administered in therapeutic or prophylactic dosage should be classified according to the nature of the adverse effect (e.g., allergy, dermatitis, tachycardia) listed in Section I of this volume.

E CODES

A

Abandonment
  causing exposure to weather conditions - *see*
      Exposure
  child, with intent to injure or kill E968.4
  helpless person, infant, newborn E904.0
      with intent to injure or kill E968.4
Abortion, criminal, injury to child E968.8
Abuse (alleged) (suspected)
  adult
      by
          child E967.4
          ex-partner E967.3
          ex-spouse E967.3
          father E967.0
          grandchild E967.7
          grandparent E967.6
          mother E967.2
          non-related caregiver E967.8
          other relative E967.7
          other specified person E967.1
          partner E967.3
          sibling E967.5
          spouse E967.3
          stepfather E967.0
          stepmother E967.2
          unspecified person E967.9
  child
      by
          boyfriend of parent or guardian
              E967.0
          child E967.4
          father E967.0
          female partner of parent or guardian
              E967.2
          girlfriend of parent or guardian E967.2
          grandchild E967.7
          grandparent E967.6
          male partner of parent or guardian
              E967.0
          mother E967.2
          non-related caregiver E967.8
          other relative E967.7
          other specified person(s) E967.1
          sibling E967.5
          stepfather E967.0
          stepmother E967.2
          unspecified person E967.9
Accident (to) E928.9
  aircraft (in transit) (powered) E841 ●
      at landing, take-off E840 ●
      due to, caused by cataclysm - *see*
          categories E908, E909
      late effect of E929.1
      unpowered (*see also* Collision, aircraft,
          unpowered) E842 ●
      while alighting, boarding E843 ●
  amphibious vehicle
      on
          land - *see* Accident, motor vehicle
          water - *see* Accident, watercraft
  animal, ridden NEC E828 ●
  animal-drawn vehicle NEC E827 ●
  balloon (*see also* Collision, aircraft,
      unpowered) E842 ●
  caused by, due to
      abrasive wheel (metalworking) E919.3
      animal NEC E906.9
          being ridden (in sport or transport)
              E828 ●
      avalanche NEC E909.2
      band saw E919.4
      bench saw E919.4
      bore, earth-drilling or mining (land)
          (seabed) E919.1
      bulldozer E919.7
      cataclysmic
          earth surface movement or eruption
              E909.9
          storm E908.9

Accident (*Continued*)
  caused by, due to (*Continued*)
      chain
          hoist E919.2
              agricultural operations E919.0
              mining operations E919.1
          saw E920.1
      circular saw E919.4
      cold (excessive) (*see also* Cold, exposure
          to) E901.9
      combine E919.0
          conflagration - *see* Conflagration
      corrosive liquid, substance NEC
          E924.1
      cotton gin E919.8
      crane E919.2
          agricultural operations E919.0
          mining operations E919.1
      cutting or piercing instrument (*see also*
          Cut) E920.9
      dairy equipment E919.8
      derrick E919.2
          agricultural operations E919.0
          mining operations E919.1
      drill E920.1
          earth (land) (seabed) E919.1
          hand (powered) E920.1
              not powered E920.4
          metalworking E919.3
          woodworking E919.4
      earth(-)
          drilling machine E919.1
          moving machine E919.7
          scraping machine E919.7
      electric
          current (*see also* Electric shock)
              E925.9
          motor - *see also* Accident, machine, by
              type of machine
          current (of) - *see* Electric shock
      elevator (building) (grain) E919.2
          agricultural operations E919.0
          mining operations E919.1
      environmental factors NEC E928.9
      excavating machine E919.7
      explosive material (*see also* Explosion)
          E923.9
      farm machine E919.0
      fire, flames - *see also* Fire
          conflagration - *see* Conflagration
      firearm missile - *see* Shooting
      forging (metalworking) machine
          E919.3
      forklift (truck) E919.2
          agricultural operations E919.0
          mining operations E919.1
      gas turbine E919.5
      harvester E919.0
      hay derrick, mower, or rake E919.0
      heat (excessive) (*see also* Heat) E900.9
      hoist (*see also* Accident, caused by, due to,
          lift) E919.2
          chain - *see* Accident, caused by, due to,
              chain
          shaft E919.1
      hot
          liquid E924.0
              caustic or corrosive E924.1
          object (not producing fire or flames)
              E924.8
          substance E924.9
              caustic or corrosive E924.1
              liquid (metal) NEC E924.0
              specified type NEC E924.8
      human bite E928.3
      ignition - *see* Ignition E919.4
      internal combustion engine E919.5
      landslide NEC E909.2
      lathe (metalworking) E919.3
          turnings E920.8
          woodworking E919.4

Accident (*Continued*)
  caused by, due to (*Continued*)
      lift, lifting (appliances) E919.2
          agricultural operations E919.0
          mining operations E919.1
          shaft E919.1
      lightning NEC E907
      machine, machinery - *see also* Accident,
          machine
          drilling, metal E919.3
          manufacturing, for manufacture of
              steam
              beverages E919.8
              clothing E919.8
              foodstuffs E919.8
              paper E919.8
              textiles E919.8
          milling, metal E919.3
          moulding E919.4
          power press, metal E919.3
          printing E919.8
          rolling mill, metal E919.3
          sawing, metal E919.3
          specified type NEC E919.8
          spinning E919.8
          weaving E919.8
      natural factor NEC E928.9
      overhead plane E919.4
      plane E920.4
          overhead E919.4
      powered
          hand tool NEC E920.1
          saw E919.4
              hand E920.1
      printing machine E919.8
      pulley (block) E919.2
          agricultural operations E919.0
          mining operations E919.1
          transmission E919.6
      radial saw E919.4
      radiation - *see* Radiation
      reaper E919.0
      road scraper E919.7
          when in transport under its own
              power - *see* categories E810–E825
      roller, coaster E919.8
      sander E919.4
      saw E920.4
          band E919.4
          bench E919.4
          chain E920.1
          circular E919.4
          hand E920.4
              powered E920.1
          powered, except hand E919.4
          radial E919.4
      sawing machine, metal E919.3
      shaft
          hoist E919.1
          lift E919.1
          transmission E919.6
      shears E920.4
          hand E920.4
              powered E920.1
          mechanical E919.3
      shovel E920.4
          steam E919.7
      spinning machine E919.8
      steam - *see also* Burning, steam
          engine E919.5
          shovel E919.7
      thresher E919.0
      thunderbolt NEC E907
      tractor E919.0
          when in transport under its own
              power - *see* categories E810–E825
      transmission belt, cable, chain, gear,
          pinion, pulley, shaft E919.6
      turbine (gas) (water driven) E919.5
      under-cutter E919.1
      weaving machine E919.8

◄ New   ◄▭ Revised   ~~deleted~~ Deleted   ● Use Additional Digit(s)   ▭ Omit code

E CODES

Accident *(Continued)*
  caused by, due to *(Continued)*
    winch E919.2
      agricultural operations E919.0
      mining operations E919.1
    diving E883.0
      with insufficient air supply E913.2
    glider (hang) *(see also* Collision, aircraft, unpowered) E842●
    hovercraft
      on
        land - *see* Accident, motor vehicle
        water - *see* Accident, watercraft
    ice yacht *(see also* Accident, vehicle NEC) E848
    in
      medical, surgical procedure
        as, or due to misadventure - *see* Misadventure
        causing an abnormal reaction or later complication without mention of misadventure - *see* Reaction, abnormal
    kite carrying a person *(see also* Collision, involving aircraft, unpowered) E842●
    land yacht *(see also* Accident, vehicle NEC) E848
    late effect of - *see* Late effect
    launching pad E845●
    machine, machinery *(see also* Accident, caused by, due to, by specific type of machine) E919.9
      agricultural including animal-powered premises E919.0
      earth-drilling E919.1
      earth moving or scraping E919.7
      excavating E919.7
      involving transport under own power on highway or transport vehicle - *see* categories E810-E825, E840-E845
      lifting (appliances) E919.2
      metalworking E919.3
      mining E919.1
      prime movers, except electric motors E919.5
        electric motors - *see* Accident, machine, by specific type of machine
      recreational E919.8
      specified type NEC E919.8
      transmission E919.6
      watercraft (deck) (engine room) (galley) (laundry) (loading) E836●
      woodworking or forming E919.4
    motor vehicle (on public highway) (traffic) E819●
      due to cataclysm - *see* categories E908, E909
      involving
        collision *(see also* Collision, motor vehicle) E812●
        nontraffic, not on public highway - *see* categories E820-E825
        not involving collision - *see* categories E816-E819
      nonmotor vehicle NEC E829●
        nonroad - *see* Accident, vehicle NEC
        road, except pedal cycle, animal-drawn vehicle, or animal being ridden E829●
      nonroad vehicle NEC - *see* Accident, vehicle NEC
    not elsewhere classifiable involving
      cable car (not on rails) E847
        on rails E829●
      coal car in mine E846
      hand truck - *see* Accident, vehicle NEC
      logging car E846
      sled(ge), meaning snow or ice vehicle E848
      tram, mine or quarry E846

Accident *(Continued)*
  not elsewhere classifiable involving *(Continued)*
    truck
      mine or quarry E846
      self-propelled, industrial E846
      station baggage E846
    tub, mine or quarry E846
    vehicle NEC E848
      snow and ice E848
      used only on industrial premises E846
    wheelbarrow E848
  occurring (at) (in)
    apartment E849.0
    baseball field, diamond E849.4
    construction site, any E849.3
    dock E849.8
      yard E849.3
    dormitory E849.7
    factory (building) (premises) E849.3
    farm E849.1
      buildings E849.1
      house E849.0
    football field E849.4
    forest E849.8
    garage (place of work) E849.3
      private (home) E849.0
    gravel pit E849.2
    gymnasium E849.4
    highway E849.5
    home (private) (residential) E849.0
      institutional E849.7
    hospital E849.7
    hotel E849.6
    house (private) (residential) E849.0
      movie E849.6
      public E849.6
    institution, residential E849.7
    jail E849.7
    mine E849.2
    motel E849.6
    movie house E849.6
    office (building) E849.6
    orphanage E849.7
    park (public) E849.4
      mobile home E849.8
      trailer E849.8
    parking lot or place E849.8
    place
      industrial NEC E849.3
      parking E849.8
      public E849.8
        specified place NEC E849.5
      recreational NEC E849.4
      sport NEC E849.4
    playground (park) (school) E849.4
    prison E849.6
    public building NEC E849.6
    quarry E849.2
    railway
      line NEC E849.8
      yard E849.3
    residence
      home (private) E849.0
    resort (beach) (lake) (mountain) (seashore) (vacation) E849.4
    restaurant E849.6
    sand pit E849.2
    school (building) (private) (public) (state) E849.6
      reform E849.7
      riding E849.4
    seashore E849.8
      resort E849.4
    shop (place of work) E849.3
      commercial E849.6
    skating rink E849.4
    sports palace E849.4
    stadium E849.4
    store E849.6
    street E849.5

Accident *(Continued)*
  occurring *(Continued)*
    swimming pool (public) E849.4
      private home or garden E849.0
    tennis court E849.4 public
    theatre, theater E849.6
    trailer court E849.8
    tunnel E849.8
      under construction E849.2
    warehouse E849.3
    yard
      dock E849.3
      industrial E849.3
      private (home) E849.0
      railway E849.3
  off-road type motor vehicle (not on public highway) NEC E821●
  on public highway - *see* categories E810-E819
  pedal cycle E826●
  railway E807●
    due to cataclysm - *see* categories E908, E909
    involving
      burning by engine, locomotive, train *(see also* Explosion, railway engine) E803●
      collision *(see also* Collision, railway) E800●
      derailment *(see also* Derailment, railway) E802●
      explosion *(see also* Explosion, railway engine) E803●
      fall *(see also* Fall, from, railway rolling stock) E804●
      fire *(see also* Explosion, railway engine) E803●
      hitting by, being struck by
        object falling in, on, from, rolling stock, train, vehicle E806●
        rolling stock, train, vehicle E805●
      overturning, railway rolling stock, train, vehicle *(see also* Derailment, railway) E802●
      running off rails, railway *(see also* Derailment, railway) E802●
      specified circumstances NEC E806●
      train or vehicle hit by
        avalanche E909.2
        falling object (earth, rock, tree) E806●
          due to cataclysm - *see* categories E908, E909
        landslide E909.2
  roller skate E885.1
  scooter (nonmotorized) E885.0
  skateboard E885.2
  ski(ing) E885.3
    jump E884.9
    lift or tow (with chair or gondola) E847
  snow vehicle, motor driven (not on public highway) E820●
    on public highway - *see* categories E810-E819
  snowboard E885.4
  spacecraft E845●
  specified cause NEC E928.8
  street car E829●
  traffic NEC E819●
  vehicle NEC (with pedestrian) E848
    battery powered
      airport passenger vehicle E846
      truck (baggage) (mail) E846
    powered commercial or industrial (with other vehicle or object within commercial or industrial premises) E846

E CODES

E CODES

Accident (Continued)
watercraft E838 ●
  with
    drowning or submersion resulting
      from
        accident other than to watercraft
          E832 ●
        accident to watercraft E830 ●
    injury, except drowning or
      submersion, resulting from
      accident other than to watercraft -
        see categories E833–E838
      accident to watercraft E831 ●
  due to, caused by cataclysm - *see*
    categories E908, E909
  machinery E836 ●
Acid throwing E961
Acosta syndrome E902.0
Activity (involving) E030
aerobic and step exercise (class)
  E009.2
alpine skiing E003.2
animal care NEC E019.9
arts and handcrafts NEC E012.9
athletics NEC E008.9
  played
    as a team or group NEC E007.9
    individually NEC E006.9
baking E015.2
ballet E005.0
barbells E010.2
BASE (Building, Antenna, Span, Earth)
  jumping E004.2
baseball E007.3
basketball E007.6
bathing (personal) E013.0
beach volleyball E007.7
bike riding E006.4
boogie boarding E002.7
bowling E006.3
boxing E008.0
brass instrument playing E018.3
building and construction E016.2
bungee jumping E004.3
calisthenics E009.1
canoeing (in calm and turbulent water)
  E002.5
capture the flag E007.8
cardiorespiratory exercise NEC E009.9
caregiving (providing) NEC E014.9
  bathing E014.0
  lifting E014.1
cellular
  communication device E011.1
  telephone E011.1
challenge course E009.4
cheerleading E005.4
circuit training E009.3
cleaning
  floor E013.4
climbing NEC E004.9
  mountain E004.0
  rock E004.0
  wall climbing E004.0
combatives E008.4
computer
  keyboarding E011.0
  technology NEC E011.9
confidence course E009.4
construction (building) E016.2
cooking and baking E015.2
cooking and grilling NEC E015.9
cool down exercises E009.1
cricket E007.9
crocheting E012.0
cross country skiing E003.3
dancing (all types) E005.0
digging
  dirt E016.0
dirt digging E016.0
dishwashing E015.0

Activity (Continued)
diving (platform) (springboard) E002.1
  underwater E002.4
dodge ball E007.8
downhill skiing E003.2
drum playing E018.1
dumbbells E010.2
electronic
  devices NEC E011.9
    hand held interactive E011.1
  game playing (using) (with)
    interactive device E011.1
    keyboard or other stationary device
      E011.0
elliptical machine E009.0
exercise(s)
  machines ((primarily) for)
    cardiorespiratory conditioning E009.0
    muscle strengthening E010.0
  muscle strengthening (non-machine) NEC
    E010.9
external motion NEC E017.9
  roller coaster E017.0
field hockey E007.4
figure skating (pairs) (singles) E003.0
flag football E007.1
floor mopping and cleaning E013.4
food preparation and clean up E015.0
football (American) NOS E007.0
  flag E007.1
  tackle E007.0
  touch E007.1
four square E007.8
free weights E010.2
frisbee (ultimate) E008.3
furniture
  building E012.2
  finishing E012.2
  repair E012.2
game playing (electronic)
  using
    interactive device E011.1
    keyboard or other stationary device
      E011.0
gardening E016.1
golf E006.2
grass drills E009.5
grilling and smoking food E015.1
grooming and shearing an animal E019.2
guerilla drills E009.5
gymnastics (rhythmic) E005.2
handball E008.2
handcrafts NEC E012.9
hand held interactive electronic device
  E011.1
hang gliding E004.4
hiking (on level or elevated terrain) E001.0
hockey (ice) E003.1
  field E007.4
horseback riding E006.1
household maintenance NEC E013.9
ice NEC E003.9
  dancing E003.0
  hockey E003.1
  skating E003.0
inline roller skating E006.0
ironing E013.3
judo E008.4
jumping (off) NEC E004.9
  BASE (Building, Antenna, Span, Earth)
    E004.2
  bungee E004.3
  jacks E009.1
  rope E006.5
jumping jacks E009.1
jumping rope E006.5
karate E008.4
kayaking (in calm and turbulent water)
  E002.5
keyboarding (computer) E011.0
kickball E007.8

Activity (Continued)
knitting E012.0
lacrosse E007.4
land maintenance NEC E016.9
landscaping E016.1
laundry E013.1
machines (exercise) primarily for
  cardiorespiratory conditioning E009.0
maintenance
  building E016.9
  household NEC E013.9
  land E016.9
  property E016.9
marching (on level or elevated terrain)
  E001.0
martial arts E008.4
microwave oven E015.2
mopping (floor) E013.4
mountain climbing E004.0
milking an animal E019.1
muscle strengthening
  exercises (non-machine) NEC E010.9
  machines E010.0
musical keyboard (electronic) playing E018.0
nordic skiing E003.3
obstacle course E009.4
oven (microwave) E015.2
packing up and unpacking in moving to a
  new residence E013.5
parasailing E002.9
percussion instrument playing NEC E018.1
personal
  bathing and showering E013.0
  hygiene NEC E013.8
  showering E013.0
physical
  games generally associated with school
    recess, summer camp and children
    007.8
  training NEC E009.9
piano playing E018.0
pilates E010.3
platform diving E002.1
playing musical instrument
  brass instrument E018.3
  drum E018.1
  musical keyboard (electronic) E018.0
  percussion instrument NEC E018.1
  piano E018.0
  string instrument E018.2
  wind instrument E018.3
property maintenance NEC E016.9
pruning (garden and lawn) E016.1
pull-ups E010.1
push-ups E010.1
racquetball E008.2
rafting (in calm and turbulent water) E002.5
raking (leaves) E016.0
rappelling E004.1
refereeing a sports activity E029.0
residential relocation E013.5
rhythmic
  gymnastics E005.2
  movement NEC E005.9
riding
  horseback E006.1
  roller coaster E017.0
rock climbing E004.0
roller coaster riding E017.0
roller skating (inline) E006.0
rough housing and horseplay E029.2
rowing (in calm and turbulent water) E002.5
rugby E007.2
running E001.1
SCUBA diving E002.4
sewing E012.1
shoveling E016.0
  dirt E016.0
  snow E016.0
showering (personal) E013.0
sit-ups E010.1

◀ New   ⬅ Revised   ~~deleted~~ Deleted   ● Use Additional Digit(s)   ▓ Omit code

Activity (*Continued*)
skateboarding E006.0
skating (ice) E003.0
  roller E006.0
skiing (alpine) (downhill) E003.2
  cross country E003.3
  nordic E003.3
sledding (snow) E003.2
smoking and grilling food E015.1
snorkeling E002.4
snow NEC E003.9
  boarding E003.2
  shoveling E016.0
  sledding E003.2
  tubing E003.2
soccer E007.5
softball E007.3
specified NEC E029.9
spectator at an event E029.1
sports NEC E008.9
sports played as a team or group NEC E007.9
sports played individually NEC E006.9
springboard diving E002.1
squash E008.2
stationary bike E009.0
step (stepping) exercise (class) E009.2
stepper machine E009.0
stove E015.2
string instrument playing E018.2
surfing E002.7
swimming E002.0
tackle football E007.0
tap dancing E005.0
tennis E008.2
tobogganing E003.2
touch football E007.1
track and field events (non-running) E006.6
  running E001.1
trampoline E005.3
treadmill E009.0
trimming shrubs E016.1
tubing (in calm and turbulent water) E002.5
  snow E003.2
ultimate frisbee E008.3
underwater diving E002.4
unpacking in moving to a new residence
  E013.5
use of stove, oven and microwave oven
  E015.2
vacuuming E013.2
volleyball (beach) (court) E007.7
wake boarding E002.6
walking an animal E019.0
walking (on level or elevated terrain) E001.0
  an animal E019.0
wall climbing E004.0
warm up and cool down exercises E009.1
water NEC E002.9
  aerobics E002.3
  craft NEC E002.9
  exercise E002.3
  polo E002.2
  skiing E002.6
  sliding E002.8
  survival training and testing E002.9
weeding (garden and lawn) E016.1
wind instrument playing E018.3
windsurfing E002.7
wrestling E008.1
yoga E005.1
Activity status E000.9
child assisting in compensated work of other
  family member E000.8
civilian
  done for
    financial or other compensation E000.0
    pay or income E000.0
family member assisting in compensated
  work of other family member E000.8
for income E000.0
hobby or leisure E000.8

Activity status (*Continued*)
off duty military E000.8
military E000.1
  off duty E000.8
recreation E000.8
specified NEC E000.8
sport not for income E000.8
student E000.8
volunteer E000.2
Aeroneurosis E902.1
Aero-otitis media - *see* Effects of, air pressure
Aerosinusitis - *see* Effects of, air pressure
After-effect, late - *see* Late effect
Air
blast
  in
    terrorism E979.2
    war operations E993.9
embolism (traumatic) NEC E928.9
  in
    infusion or transfusion E874.1
    perfusion E874.2
sickness E903
Alpine sickness E902.0
Altitude sickness - *see* Effects of, air pressure
Anaphylactic shock, anaphylaxis (*see also*
  Table of Drugs and Chemicals)
  E947.9
due to bite or sting (venomous) - *see* Bite,
  venomous
Andes disease E902.0
Apoplexy
heat - *see* Heat
Arachnidism E905.1
Arson E968.0
Asphyxia, asphyxiation
by
  chemical
    in
      terrorism E979.7
      war operations E997.2
  explosion - *see* Explosion E965.8
  food (bone) (regurgitated food) (seed)
    E911
  foreign object, except food E912
  fumes
    in
      terrorism (chemical weapons)
        E979.7
      war operations E997.2
  gas - *see also* Table of Drugs and
    Chemicals
    in
      terrorism E979.7
      war operations E997.2
    legal
      execution E978
      intervention (tear) E972
    tear E972
  mechanical means (*see also* Suffocation)
    E913.9
from
  conflagration - *see* Conflagration
  fire - *see also* Fire E899
    in
      terrorism E979.3
      war operations E990.9
  ignition - *see* Ignition
Aspiration
foreign body - *see* Foreign body, aspiration
mucus, not of newborn (with asphyxia,
  obstruction respiratory passage,
  suffocation) E912
phlegm (with asphyxia, obstruction
  respiratory passage, suffocation)
  E912
vomitus (with asphyxia, obstruction
  respiratory passage, suffocation) (*see
  also* Foreign body, aspiration, food)
  E911
Assassination (attempt) (*see also* Assault) E968.9

Assault (homicidal) (by) (in) E968.9
acid E961
  swallowed E962.1
air gun E968.6
BB gun E968.6
bite NEC E968.8
  of human being E968.7
bomb ((placed in) car or house) E965.8
  antipersonnel E965.5
  letter E965.7
  petrol E965.6
brawl (hand) (fists) (foot) E960.0
burning, burns (by fire) E968.0
  acid E961
    swallowed E962.1
  caustic, corrosive substance E961
    swallowed E962.1
  chemical from swallowing caustic,
    corrosive substance NEC E962.1
  hot liquid E968.3
  scalding E968.3
  vitriol E961
    swallowed E962.1
caustic, corrosive substance E961
  swallowed E962.1
cut, any part of body E966
dagger E966
drowning E964
explosives E965.9
  bomb (*see also* Assault, bomb) E965.8
  dynamite E965.8
fight (hand) (fists) (foot) E960.0
  with weapon E968.9
    blunt or thrown E968.2
    cutting or piercing E966
    firearm - *see* Shooting, homicide
  fire E968.0
  firearm(s) - *see* Shooting, homicide
garrotting E963
gunshot (wound) - *see* Shooting,
  homicide
hanging E963
injury NEC E968.9
knife E966
late effect of E969
ligature E963
poisoning E962.9
  drugs or medicinals E962.0
  gas(es) or vapors, except drugs and
    medicinals E962.2
  solid or liquid substances, except drugs
    and medicinals E962.1
puncture, any part of body E966
pushing
  before moving object, train, vehicle
    E968.5
  from high place E968.1
rape E960.1
scalding E968.3
shooting - *see* Shooting, homicide
sodomy E960.1
stab, any part of body E966
strangulation E963
submersion E964
suffocation E963
transport vehicle E968.5
violence NEC E968.9
vitriol E961
  swallowed E962.1
weapon E968.9
  blunt or thrown E968.2
  cutting or piercing E966
  firearm - *see* Shooting, homicide
wound E968.9
  cutting E966
  gunshot - *see* Shooting, homicide
  knife E966
  piercing E966
  puncture E966
  stab E966
Attack by animal NEC E906.9

E CODES

Avalanche E909.2
  falling on or hitting
    motor vehicle (in motion) (on public
      highway) E909.2
    railway train E909.2
Aviators' disease E902.1

B

Barotitis, barodontalgia, berosinusitis,
  barotrauma (otitic) (sinus) - *see* Effects of,
  air pressure
Battered
  baby or child (syndrome) - *see* Abuse, child;
    category E967
  person other than baby or child - *see* Assault
Bayonet wound (*see also* Cut, by bayonet)
  E920.3
  in
    legal intervention E974
    terrorism E979.8
    war operations E995.2
Bean in nose E912
Bed set on fire NEC E898.0
Beheading (by guillotine)
  homicide E966
  legal execution E978
Bending, injury
  due to
    repetitive movement E927.3
    sudden strenuous movement E927.0
Bends E902.0
Bite
  animal NEC E906.5
    other specified (except arthropod) E906.3
    venomous NEC E905.9
  arthropod (nonvenomous) NEC E906.4
    venomous - *see* Sting
  black widow spider E905.1
  cat E906.3
  centipede E905.4
  cobra E905.0
  copperhead snake E905.0
  coral snake E905.0
  dog E906.0
  fer de lance E905.0
  gila monster E905.0
  human being
    accidental E928.3
    assault E968.7
  insect (nonvenomous) E906.4
    venomous - *see* Sting
  krait E905.0
  late effect of - *see* Late effect
  lizard E906.2
    venomous E905.0
  mamba E905.0
  marine animal
    nonvenomous E906.3
      snake E906.2
    venomous E905.6
      snake E905.0
  millipede E906.4
    venomous E905.4
  moray eel E906.3
  rat E906.1
  rattlesnake E905.0
  rodent, except rat E906.3
  serpent - *see* Bite, snake
  shark E906.3
  snake (venomous) E905.0
    nonvenomous E906.2
    sea E905.0
  spider E905.1
    nonvenomous E906.4
  tarantula (venomous) E905.1
  venomous NEC E905.9
    by specific animal - *see* category E905
  viper E905.0
  water moccasin E905.0

Blast (air)
  in
    terrorism E979.2
      from nuclear explosion E979.5
      underwater E979.0
    war operations E993.9
      from nuclear explosion - *see* War
        operations, injury due to,
        nuclear weapons
      underwater E992.9
Blizzard E908.3
Blow E928.9
  by law-enforcing agent, police (on duty)
    E975
    with blunt object (baton) (nightstick)
      (stave) (truncheon) E973
Blowing up (*see also* Explosion) E923.9
Brawl (hand) (fists) (foot) E960.0
Breakage (accidental)
  cable of cable car not on rails E847
  ladder (causing fall) E881.0
  part (any) of
    animal-drawn vehicle E827●
    ladder (causing fall) E881.0
    motor vehicle
      in motion (on public highway)
        E818●
      not on public highway E825●
    nonmotor road vehicle, except animal-
      drawn vehicle or pedal cycle
      E829●
    off-road type motor vehicle (not on public
      highway) NEC E821●
      on public highway E818●
    pedal cycle E826●
    scaffolding (causing fall) E881.1
    snow vehicle, motor-driven (not on public
      highway) E820●
      on public highway E818●
    vehicle NEC - *see* Accident, vehicle
Broken
  glass
    fall on E888.0
    injury by E920.8
  power line (causing electric shock) E925.1
Bumping against, into (accidentally)
  object (moving) E917.9
    caused by crowd E917.1
      with subsequent fall E917.6
    furniture E917.3
      with subsequent fall E917.7
    in
      running water E917.2
      sports E917.0
        with subsequent fall E917.5
    stationary E917.4
      with subsequent fall E917.8
  person(s) E917.9
    with fall E886.9
      in sports E886.0
    as, or caused by, a crowd E917.1
      with subsequent fall E917.6
    in sports E917.0
      with fall E886.0
Burning, burns (accidental) (by) (from) (on)
  E899
  acid (any kind) E924.1
    swallowed - *see* Table of Drugs and
      Chemicals
  airgun E928.7
  bedclothes (*see also* Fire, specified NEC)
    E898.0
  blowlamp (*see also* Fire, specified NEC)
    E898.1
  blowtorch (*see also* Fire, specified NEC)
    E898.1
  boat, ship, watercraft - *see* categories E830,
    E831, E837
  bonfire (controlled) E897
    uncontrolled E892
  candle (*see also* Fire, specified NEC) E898.1

Burning, burns (*Continued*)
  caustic liquid, substance E924.1
    swallowed - *see* Table of Drugs and
      Chemicals
  chemical E924.1
    from swallowing caustic, corrosive
      substance - *see* Table of Drugs and
      Chemicals
    in
      terrorism E979.7
      war operations E997.2
  cigar(s) or cigarette(s) (*see also* Fire, specified
    NEC) E898.1
  clothes, clothing, nightdress - *see* Ignition,
    clothes
    with conflagration - *see* Conflagration
  conflagration - *see* Conflagration
  corrosive liquid, substance E924.1
    swallowed - *see* Table of Drugs and
      Chemicals
  electric current (*see also* Electric shock)
    E925.9
  fire, flames (*see also* Fire) E899
  firearm E928.7
  flare, Verey pistol E922.8
  heat
    from appliance (electrical) E924.8
    in local application, or packing during
      medical or surgical procedure
      E873.5
  homicide (attempt) (*see also* Assault, burning)
    E968.0
  hot
    liquid E924.0
      caustic or corrosive E924.1
    object (not producing fire or flames)
      E924.8
    substance E924.9
      caustic or corrosive E924.1
      liquid (metal) NEC E924.0
      specified type NEC E924.8
    tap water E924.2
  ignition - *see also* Ignition
    clothes, clothing, nightdress - *see also*
      Ignition, clothes
    with conflagration - *see* Conflagration
    highly inflammable material (benzine)
      (fat) (gasoline) (kerosine) (paraffin)
      (petrol) E894
  inflicted by other person
    stated as
      homicidal, intentional (*see also* Assault,
        burning) E968.0
      undetermined whether accidental or
        intentional (*see also* Burn, stated
        as undetermined whether
        accidental or intentional) E988.1
  internal, from swallowed caustic, corrosive
    liquid, substance - *see* Table of Drugs
    and Chemicals
  in
    terrorism E979.3
      from nuclear explosion E979.5
      petrol bomb E979.3
    war operations (from fire-producing
      device or conventional weapon)
      E990.9
      from nuclear explosion (*see also* War
        operations, injury due to,
        nuclear weapons) E996.2
      incendiary bomb E990.0
      petrol bomb E990.0
  lamp (*see also* Fire, specified NEC) E898.1
  late effect of NEC E929.4
  lighter (cigar) (cigarette) (*see also* Fire,
    specified NEC) E898.1
  lightning E907
  liquid (boiling) (hot) (molten) E924.0
    caustic, corrosive (external) E924.1
      swallowed - *see* Table of Drugs and
        Chemicals

Burning, burns (Continued)

local application of externally applied substance in medical or surgical care E873.5
machinery - *see* Accident, machine
matches (*see also* Fire, specified NEC) E898.1
medicament, externally applied E873.5
metal, molten E924.0
object (hot) E924.8
   producing fire or flames - *see* Fire
oven (electric) (gas) E924.8
pipe (smoking) (*see also* Fire, specified NEC) E898.1
radiation - *see* Radiation
railway engine, locomotive, train (*see also* Explosion, railway engine) E803●
self-inflicted (unspecified whether accidental or intentional) E988.1
   caustic or corrosive substance NEC E988.7
   stated as intentional, purposeful E958.1
      caustic or corrosive substance NEC E958.7
   stated as undetermined whether accidental or intentional E988.1
      caustic or corrosive substance NEC E988.7
steam E924.0
   pipe E924.8
substance (hot) E924.9
   boiling or molten E924.0
   caustic, corrosive (external) E924.1
      swallowed - *see* Table of Drugs and Chemicals
suicidal (attempt) NEC E958.1
   caustic substance E958.7
   late effect of E959
tanning bed E926.2
therapeutic misadventure
   overdose of radiation E873.2
torch, welding (*see also* Fire, specified NEC) E898.1
trash fire (*see also* Burning, bonfire) E897
vapor E924.0
vitriol E924.1
x-rays E926.3
   in medical, surgical procedure - *see* Misadventure, failure, in dosage, radiation operations

Butted by animal E906.8

C

Cachexia, lead or saturnine E866.0
from pesticide NEC (*see also* Table of Drugs and Chemicals) E863.4
Caisson disease E902.2
Capital punishment (any means) E978
Car sickness E903
Casualty (not due to war) NEC E928.9
terrorism E979.8
war (*see also* War operations) E995.9
Cat
bite E906.3
scratch E906.8
Cataclysmic (any injury)
earth surface movement or eruption E909.9
   specified type NEC E909.8
storm or flood resulting from storm E908.9
   specified type NEC E909.8
Catching fire - *see* Ignition
Caught
between
   objects (moving) (stationary and moving) E918
      and machinery - *see* Accident, machine
by cable car, not on rails E847
in
   machinery (moving parts of) - *see* Accident, machine
   object E918

Cave-in (causing asphyxia, suffocation (by pressure)) (*see also* Suffocation, due to, cave-in) E913.3
with injury other than asphyxia or suffocation E916
   with asphyxia or suffocation (*see also* Suffocation, due to, cave-in) E913.3
struck or crushed by E916
   with asphyxia or suffocation (*see also* Suffocation, due to, cave-in) E913.3
Change(s) in air pressure - *see also* Effects of, air pressure
sudden, in aircraft (ascent) (descent) (causing aeroneurosis or aviators' disease) E902.1
Chilblains E901.0
due to manmade conditions E901.1
Choking (on) (any object except food or vomitus) E912
apple E911
bone E911
food, any type (regurgitated) E911
mucus or phlegm E912
seed E911
Civil insurrection - *see* War operations
Cloudburst E908.8
Cold, exposure to (accidental) (excessive) (extreme) (place) E901.9
causing chilblains or immersion foot E901.0
due to
   manmade conditions E901.1
   specified cause NEC E901.8
   weather (conditions) E901.0
late effect of NEC E929.5
self-inflicted (undetermined whether accidental or intentional) E988.3
   suicidal E958.3
suicide E958.3
Colic, lead, painters', or saturnine - *see* category E866
Collapse
building E916
   burning (uncontrolled fire) E891.8
      in terrorism E979.3
      private E890.8
dam E909.3
due to heat - *see* Heat
machinery - *see* Accident, machine or vehicle
man-made structure E909.3
postoperative NEC E878.9
structure
   burning (uncontrolled fire) NEC E891.8
      in terrorism E979.3
Collision (accidental)

> **Note:** In the case of collisions between different types of vehicles, persons and objects, priority in classification is in the following order:
>
> > Aircraft
> > Watercraft
> > Motor vehicle
> > Railway vehicle
> > Pedal cycle
> > Animal-drawn vehicle
> > Animal being ridden
> > Streetcar or other nonmotor road vehicle
> > Other vehicle
> > Pedestrian or person using pedestrian conveyance
> > Object (except where falling from or set in motion by vehicle, etc. listed above)
>
> In the listing below, the combinations are listed only under the vehicle, etc., having priority. For definitions, *see* Supplementary Classification of External Causes of Injury and Poisoning (E800–E999).

Collision (Continued)

aircraft (with object or vehicle) (fixed) (movable) (moving) E841●
   with
      person (while landing, taking off) (without accident to aircraft) E844●
      powered (in transit) (with unpowered aircraft) E841●
      while landing, taking off E840●
   unpowered E842●
   while landing, taking off E840●
animal being ridden (in sport or transport) E828●
   and
      animal (being ridden) (herded) (unattended) E828●
      nonmotor road vehicle, except pedal cycle or animal-drawn vehicle E828●
      object (fallen) (fixed) (movable) (moving) not falling from or set in motion by vehicle of higher priority E828●
      pedestrian (conveyance or vehicle) E828●
animal-drawn vehicle E827●
   and
      animal (being ridden) (herded) (unattended) E827●
      nonmotor road vehicle, except pedal cycle E827●
      object (fallen) (fixed) (movable) (moving) not falling from or set in motion by vehicle of higher priority E827●
      pedestrian (conveyance or vehicle) E827●
      streetcar E827●
motor vehicle (on public highway) (traffic accident) E812●
   after leaving, running off, public highway (without antecedent collision) (without re-entry) E816●
   with antecedent collision on public highway - *see* categories E810–E815
   with re-entrance collision with another motor vehicle E811●
   and
      abutment (bridge) (overpass) E815●
      animal (herded) (unattended) E815●
         carrying person, property E813●
      animal-drawn vehicle E813●
      another motor vehicle (abandoned) (disabled) (parked) (stalled) (stopped) E812●
         with, involving re-entrance (on same roadway) (across median strip) E811●
      any object, person, or vehicle off the public highway resulting from a noncollision motor vehicle nontraffic accident E816●
      avalanche, fallen or not moving E815●
         falling E909.2
      boundary fence E815●
      culvert E815●
      fallen
         stone E815●
         tree E815●
      guard post or guard rail E815●
      inter-highway divider E815●
      landslide, fallen or not moving E815●
         moving E909.2
      machinery (road) E815●
      nonmotor road vehicle NEC E813●

Collision (*Continued*)
  motor vehicle (*Continued*)
    and (*Continued*)
      object (any object, person, or vehicle
        off the public highway resulting
        from a noncollision motor
        vehicle nontraffic accident)
        E815 ●
      off, normally not on, public
        highway resulting from a
        noncollision motor vehicle
        traffic accident E816 ●
      pedal cycle E813 ●
      pedestrian (conveyance) E814 ●
      person (using pedestrian conveyance)
        E814 ●
      post or pole (lamp) (light) (signal)
        (telephone) (utility) E815 ●
      railway rolling stock, train, vehicle
        E810 ●
      safety island E815 ●
      street car E813 ●
      traffic signal, sign, or marker
        (temporary) E815 ●
      tree E815 ●
      tricycle E813 ●
      wall or cut made for road E815 ●
    due to cataclysm - *see* categories E908,
      E909
    not on public highway, nontraffic accident
      E822 ●
    and
      animal (carrying person, property)
        (herded) (unattended) E822 ●
      animal-drawn vehicle E822 ●
      another motor vehicle (moving),
        except off-road motor vehicle
        E822 ●
        stationary E823 ●
      avalanche, fallen, not moving NEC
        E823 ●
        moving E909.2
      landslide, fallen, not moving
        E823 ●
        moving E909.2
      nonmotor vehicle (moving)
        E822 ●
        stationary E823 ●
      object (fallen) ((normally) (fixed)
        (movable but not in motion)
        (stationary) E823 ●
        moving, except when falling
          from, set in motion by,
          aircraft or cataclysm E822 ●
      pedal cycle (moving) E822 ●
        stationary E823 ●
      pedestrian (conveyance) E822 ●
      person (using pedestrian
        conveyance) E822 ●
      railway rolling stock, train, vehicle
        (moving) E822 ●
        stationary E823 ●
      road vehicle (any) (moving) E822 ●
        stationary E823 ●
      tricycle (moving) E822 ●
        stationary E823 ●
  off-road type motor vehicle (not on public
    highway) E821 ●
    and
      animal (being ridden) (-drawn vehicle)
        E821 ●
      another off-road motor vehicle, except
        snow vehicle E821 ●
      other motor vehicle, not on public
        highway E821 ●
      other object or vehicle NEC, fixed or
        movable, not set in motion by
        aircraft, motor vehicle on
        highway, or snow vehicle,
        motor-driven E821 ●
      pedal cycle E821 ●

Collision (*Continued*)
  off-road type motor vehicle (*Continued*)
    and (*Continued*)
      pedestrian (conveyance) E821 ●
      railway train E821 ●
    on public highway - *see* Collision, motor
      vehicle
  pedal cycle E826 ●
    and
      animal (carrying person, property)
        (herded) (unherded) E826 ●
      animal-drawn vehicle E826 ●
      another pedal cycle E826 ●
      nonmotor road vehicle E826 ●
      object (fallen) (fixed) (movable)
        (moving) not falling from or set in
        motion by aircraft, motor vehicle,
        or railway train NEC E826 ●
      pedestrian (conveyance) E826 ●
      person (using pedestrian conveyance)
        E826 ●
      street car E826 ●
  pedestrian(s) (conveyance) E917.9
    with fall E886.9
      in sports E886.0
    and
      crowd, human stampede E917.1
        with subsequent fall E917.6
      furniture E917.3
        with subsequent fall E917.7
      machinery - *see* Accident, machine
      object (fallen) (moving) not falling
        from or set in motion by any
        vehicle classifiable to E800–E848,
        E917.9
        caused by a crowd E917.1
          with subsequent fall E917.6
        furniture E917.3
          with subsequent fall E917.7
        in
          running water E917.2
            with drowning or submersion -
              see Submersion
          sports E917.0
            with subsequent fall E917.5
          stationary E917.4
            with subsequent fall E917.8
      vehicle, nonmotor, nonroad E848
    in
      running water E917.2
        with drowning or submersion - *see*
        Submersion
      sports E917.0
        with fall E886.0
  person(s) (using pedestrian conveyance) (*see
    also* Collision, pedestrian) E917.9
  railway (rolling stock) (train) (vehicle) (with
    (subsequent) derailment, explosion,
    fall or fire) E800 ●
    with antecedent derailment E802 ●
    and
      animal (carrying person) (herded)
        (unattended) E801 ●
      another railway train or vehicle E800 ●
      buffers E801 ●
      fallen tree on railway E801 ●
      farm machinery, nonmotor (in
        transport) (stationary) E801 ●
      gates E801 ●
      nonmotor vehicle E801 ●
      object (fallen) (fixed) (movable)
        (movable) (moving) not falling
        from, set in motion by, aircraft or
        motor vehicle NEC E801 ●
      pedal cycle E801 ●
      pedestrian (conveyance) E805 ●
      person (using pedestrian conveyance)
        E805 ●
      platform E801 ●
      rock on railway E801 ●
      street car E801 ●

Collision (*Continued*)
  snow vehicle, motor-driven (not on public
    highway) E820 ●
    and
      animal (being ridden) (-drawn vehicle)
        E820 ●
      another off-road motor vehicle E820 ●
      other motor vehicle, not on public
        highway E820 ●
      other object or vehicle NEC, fixed or
        movable, not set in motion by
        aircraft or motor vehicle on
        highway E820 ●
      pedal cycle E820 ●
      pedestrian (conveyance) E820 ●
      railway train E820 ●
    on public highway - *see* Collision, motor
      vehicle
  street car(s) E829 ●
    and
      animal, herded, not being ridden,
        unattended E829 ●
      nonmotor road vehicle NEC E829 ●
      object (fallen) (fixed) (movable)
        (moving) not falling from or set
        in motion by aircraft, animal-
        drawn vehicle, animal being
        ridden, motor vehicle, pedal
        cycle, or railway train E829 ●
      pedestrian (conveyance) E829 ●
      person (using pedestrian conveyance)
        E829 ●
  vehicle
    animal-drawn - *see* Collision, animal-
      drawn vehicle
    motor - *see* Collision, motor vehicle
    nonmotor
      nonroad E848
        and
          another nonmotor, nonroad
            vehicle E848
          object (fallen) (fixed) (movable)
            (moving) not falling from
            or set in motion by aircraft,
            animal-drawn vehicle,
            animal being ridden,
            motor vehicle, nonmotor
            road vehicle, pedal cycle,
            railway train, or streetcar
            E848
      road, except animal being ridden,
        animal-drawn vehicle, or pedal
        cycle E829 ●
        and
          animal, herded, not being
            ridden, unattended E829 ●
          another nonmotor road vehicle,
            except animal being ridden,
            animal-drawn vehicle, or
            pedal cycle E829 ●
          object (fallen) (fixed) (movable)
            (moving) not falling from
            or set in motion by,
            aircraft, animal-drawn
            vehicle, animal being
            ridden, motor vehicle,
            pedal cycle, or railway
            train E829 ●
          pedestrian (conveyance) E829 ●
          person (using pedestrian
            conveyance) E829 ●
          vehicle, nonmotor, nonroad
            E829 ●
  watercraft E838 ●
    and
      person swimming or water skiing
        E838 ●
    causing
      drowning, submersion E830 ●
      injury except drowning, submersion
        E831 ●

◄ New   ◄▦ Revised   ~~deleted~~ Deleted   ● Use Additional Digit(s)   ▨ Omit code

E CODES

Combustion, spontaneous - *see* Ignition
Complication of medical or surgical procedure
   or treatment
  as an abnormal reaction - *see* Reaction,
    abnormal
  delayed, without mention of misadventure -
    see Reaction, abnormal
  due to misadventure - *see* Misadventure
Compression
  divers' squeeze E902.2
  trachea by
    food E911
    foreign body, except food E912
Conflagration
  building or structure, except private
      dwelling (barn) (church) (convalescent
      or residential home) (factory) (farm
      outbuilding) (hospital) (hotel) or
      (institution (educational) (dormitory)
      (residential)) (school) (shop) (store)
      (theatre) E891.9
    with or causing (injury due to)
      accident or injury NEC E891.9
        specified circumstance NEC E891.8
      burns, burning E891.3
      carbon monoxide E891.2
      fumes E891.2
      polyvinylchloride (PVC) or similar
        material E891.1
      smoke E891.2
    causing explosion E891.0
    in terrorism E979.3
  not in building or structure E892
  private dwelling (apartment) (boarding
    house) (camping place) (caravan)
    (farmhouse) (home (private)) (house)
    (lodging house) (private garage)
    (rooming house) (tenement) E890.9
    with or causing (injury due to) accident or
      injury NEC E890.9
        specified circumstance NEC E890.8
      burns, burning E890.3
      carbon monoxide E890.2
      fumes E890.2
        polyvinylchloride (PVC) or similar
          material E890.1
      smoke E890.2
    causing explosion E890.0
Constriction, external
  caused by
    hair E928.4
    other object E928.5
Contact with
  dry ice E901.1
  liquid air, hydrogen, nitrogen E901.1
Cramp(s)
  heat - *see* Heat
  swimmers (*see also* category E910) 910.2
    not in recreation or sport E910.3
Cranking (car) (truck) (bus) (engine) injury by
  E917.9
Crash
  aircraft (in transit) (powered) E841●
    at landing, take-off E840●
    in
      terrorism E979.1
      war operations E994.9
    on runway NEC E840●
    stated as
      homicidal E968.8
      suicidal E958.6
      undetermined whether accidental or
        intentional E988.6
    unpowered E842●
  glider E842●
  motor vehicle - *see also* Accident, motor
    vehicle
    homicidal E968.5
    suicidal E958.5
    undetermined whether accidental or
      intentional E988.5

Crushed (accidentally) E928.9
  between
    boat(s), ship(s), watercraft (and dock or
      pier) (without accident to
      watercraft) E838●
      after accident to, or collision,
        watercraft E831●
    objects (moving) (stationary and moving)
      E918
  by
    avalanche NEC E909.2
    boat, ship, watercraft after accident to,
      collision, watercraft E831●
    cave-in E916
      with asphyxiation or suffocation (*see*
        also Suffocation, due to, cave-in)
        E913.3
    crowd, human stampede E917.1
    falling
      aircraft (*see also* Accident, aircraft)
        E841●
        in
          terrorism E979.1
          war operations E994.8
      earth, material E916
        with asphyxiation or suffocation
          (*see also* Suffocation, due to,
          cave-in) E913.3
      object E916
        on ship, watercraft E838●
        while loading, unloading watercraft
          E838●
    firearm E928.7
    landslide NEC E909.2
    lifeboat after abandoning ship E831●
    machinery - *see* Accident, machine
    railway rolling stock, train, vehicle (part
      of) E805●
    slide trigger mechanism, scope or other
      part of gun E928.7
    street car E829●
    vehicle NEC - *see* Accident, vehicle NEC
  in
    machinery - *see* Accident, machine
    object E918
    transport accident - *see*
      categories E800–E848
  late effect of NEC E929.9
Cut, cutting (any part of body) (accidental)
  E920.9
  by
    arrow E920.8
    axe E920.4
    bayonet (*see also* Bayonet wound) E920.3
      in war operations E995.2
    blender E920.2
    broken glass E920.8
      following fall E888.0
    can opener E920.4
      powered E920.2
    chisel E920.4
    circular saw E919.4
    cutting or piercing instrument - *see also*
      category E920
      following fall E888.0
      late effect of E929.8
    dagger E920.3
    dart E920.8
    drill - *see* Accident, caused by drill
    edge of stiff paper E920.8
    electric
      beater E920.2
      fan E920.2
      knife E920.2
      mixer E920.2
    firearm component E928.7
    fork E920.4
    garden fork E920.4
    hand saw or tool (not powered)
      E920.4
      powered E920.1

Cut, cutting (*Continued*)
  by (*Continued*)
    hedge clipper E920.4
      powered E920.1
    hoe E920.4
    ice pick E920.4
    knife E920.3
      electric E920.2
      in war operations E995.2
    lathe turnings E920.8
    lawn mower E920.4
      powered E920.0
      riding E919.8
    machine - *see* Accident, machine
    meat
      grinder E919.8
      slicer E919.8
    nails E920.8
    needle E920.4
      hypodermic E920.5
    object, edged, pointed, sharp - *see*
      category E920
      following fall E888.0
    paper cutter E920.4
    piercing instrument - *see also* category
      E920
      late effect of E929.8
    pitchfork E920.4
    powered
      can opener E920.2
      garden cultivator E920.1
        riding E919.8
      hand saw E920.1
      hand tool NEC E920.1
      hedge clipper E920.1
      household appliance or implement
        E920.2
      lawn mower (hand) E920.0
        riding E919.8
      rivet gun E920.1
      staple gun E920.1
    rake E920.4
    saw
      circular E919.4
      hand E920.4
    scissors E920.4
    screwdriver E920.4
    sewing machine (electric) (powered)
      E920.2
      not powered E920.4
    shears E920.4
    shovel E920.4
    slide trigger mechanism, scope or other
      part of gun E928.7
    spade E920.4
    splinters E920.8
    sword E920.3
      in war operations E995.2
    tin can lid E920.8
    wood slivers E920.8
  homicide (attempt) E966
  inflicted by other person
    stated as
      intentional, homicidal E966
      undetermined whether accidental or
        intentional E986
  late effect of NEC E929.8
  legal
    execution E978
    intervention E974
  self-inflicted (unspecified whether
    accidental or intentional)
    E986
    stated as intentional, purposeful
      E956
  stated as undetermined whether accidental
    or intentional E986
  suicidal (attempt) E956
  terrorism E979.8
  war operations E995.2
Cyclone E908.1

E CODES

D

Death due to injury occurring one year or more previous - *see* Late effect
Decapitation (accidental circumstances) NEC E928.9
  homicidal E966
  legal execution (by guillotine) E978
Deprivation - *see also* Privation action E913.3
  homicidal intent E968.4
Derailment (accidental)
  railway (rolling stock) (train) (vehicle) (with subsequent collision) E802●
    with
      collision (antecedent) (*see also* Collision, railway) E800●
      explosion (subsequent) (without antecedent collision) E802●
        antecedent collision E803●
      fall (without collision (antecedent)) E802●
      fire (without collision (antecedent)) E802●
  street car E829●
Descent
  parachute (voluntary) (without accident to aircraft) E844●
    due to accident to aircraft - *see* categories E840–E842
Desertion
  child, with intent to injure or kill E968.4
  helpless person, infant, newborn E904.0
    with intent to injure or kill E968.4
Destitution - *see* Privation
Dirty bomb (*see also* War operations, injury due to, nuclear weapons) E996.9
Disability, late effect or sequela of injury - *see* Late effect
Disease
  Andes E902.0
  aviators' E902.1
  caisson E902.2
  range E902.0
Divers' disease, palsy, paralysis, squeeze E902.0
Dog bite E906.0
Dragged by
  cable car (not on rails) E847
    on rails E829●
  motor vehicle (on highway) E814●
    not on highway, nontraffic accident E825●
  street car E829●
Drinking poison (accidental) - *see* Table of Drugs and Chemicals
Drowning - *see* Submersion
Dust in eye E914

E

Earth falling (on) (with asphyxia or suffocation (by pressure)) (*see also* Suffocation, due to, cave-in) E913.3
  as, or due to, a cataclysm (involving any transport vehicle) - *see* categories E908, E909
  not due to cataclysmic action E913.3
    motor vehicle (in motion) (on public highway) E813●
      not on public highway E825●
    nonmotor road vehicle NEC E829●
    pedal cycle E826●
    railway rolling stock, train, vehicle E806●
    street car E829●
    struck or crushed by E916
      with asphyxiation or suffocation E913.3
      with injury other than asphyxia, suffocation E916
Earthquake (any injury) E909.0

Effect(s) (adverse) of
  air pressure E902.9
    at high altitude E902.9
      in aircraft E902.1
      residence or prolonged visit (causing conditions classifiable to E902.0) E902.0
    due to
      diving E902.2
      specified cause NEC E902.8
    in aircraft E902.1
  cold, excessive (exposure to) (*see also* Cold, exposure to) E901.9
  heat (excessive) (*see also* Heat) E900.9
  hot
    place - *see* Heat
    weather E900.0
  insulation - *see* Heat
  late - *see* Late effect of
  motion E903
  nuclear explosion or weapon
    in
      terrorism E979.5
      war operations (*see also* War operations, injury due to, nuclear weapons) E996.9
  radiation - *see* Radiation
  terrorism, secondary E979.9
  travel E903
Electric shock, electrocution (accidental) (from exposed wire, faulty appliance, high voltage cable, live rail, open socket) (by) (in) E925.9
  appliance or wiring
    domestic E925.0
    factory E925.2
    farm (building) E925.8
      house E925.0
    home E925.0
    industrial (conductor) (control apparatus) (transformer) E925.2
    outdoors E925.8
    public building E925.8
    residential institution E925.8
    school E925.8
    specified place NEC E925.8
  caused by other person
    stated as
      intentional, homicidal E968.8
      undetermined whether accidental or intentional E988.4
  electric power generating plant, distribution station E925.1
  electroshock gun (taser) (stun gun) E925.8
    caused by other person E968.8
      legal intervention E975
      stated as accidental E925.8
      stated as intentional E968.8
    due to legal intervention E975
    stated as intentional self-harm (suicidal (attempt)) E958.4
    stated as undetermined whether accidental or intentional E988.4
    suicide (attempt) E958.4
  homicidal (attempt) E968.8
  legal execution E978
  lightning E907
  machinery E925.9
    domestic E925.0
    factory E925.2
    farm E925.8
    home E925.0
  misadventure in medical or surgical procedure
    in electroshock therapy E873.4
  self-inflicted (undetermined whether accidental or intentional) E988.4
    stated as intentional E958.4
  stated as undetermined whether accidental or intentional E988.4

Electric shock, electrocution *(Continued)*
  suicidal (attempt) E958.4
  transmission line E925.1
Electrocution - *see* Electric shock
Embolism E921.1
  air (traumatic) NEC - *see* Air, embolism
Encephalitis
  lead or saturnine E866.0
    from pesticide NEC E863.4
Entanglement
  in
    bedclothes, causing suffocation E913.0
    wheel of pedal cycle E826●
Entry of foreign body, material, any - *see* Foreign body
Execution, legal (any method) E978
Exertion, excessive physical, from prolonged activity E927.2
Exhaustion
  cold - *see* Cold, exposure to
  due to excessive exertion E927.2
  heat - *see* Heat
Explosion (accidental) (in) (of) (on) E923.9
  acetylene E923.2
  aerosol can E921.8
  aircraft (in transit) (powered) E841●
    at landing, take-off E840●
    in
      terrorism E979.1
      war operations
        from
          enemy fire or explosive(s) (device placed on aircraft) E994.0
          own onboard explosives E994.1
    unpowered E842●
  air tank (compressed) (in machinery) E921.1
  anesthetic gas in operating theatre E923.2
  automobile tire NEC E921.8
    causing transport accident - *see* categories E810-E825
  blasting (cap) (materials) E923.1
  boiler (machinery), not on transport vehicle E921.0
    steamship - *see* Explosion, watercraft
  bomb E923.8
    in
      terrorism E979.2
      war operations E993.8
        after cessation of hostilities E998.1
        atom, hydrogen or nuclear (*see also* War operations, injury due to, nuclear weapons) E996.9
        injury by fragments from E991.9
          antipersonnel bomb E991.3
  butane E923.2
  caused by
    other person
      stated as
        intentional, homicidal - *see* Assault, explosive
        undetermined whether accidental or homicidal E985.5
  coal gas E923.2
  detonator E923.1
  dynamite E923.1
  explosive (material) NEC E923.9
    gas(es) E923.2
    missile E923.8
      in
        terrorism E979.2
        war operations E993.1
          injury by fragments from E991.9
            antipersonnel bomb E991.3
    used in blasting operations E923.1
  fire-damp E923.2
  fireworks E923.0
  gas E923.2
    cylinder (in machinery) E921.1
    pressure tank (in machinery) E921.1

◀ New   ◀▥ Revised   ~~deleted~~ Deleted   ● Use Additional Digit(s)   ▨ Omit code

Explosion *(Continued)*
gasoline (fumes) (tank) not in moving motor vehicle E923.2
grain store (military) (munitions) E923.8
grenade E923.8
in
terrorism E979.2
war operations E993.8
injury by fragments from E991.4
homicide (attempt) - *see* Assault, explosive
hot water heater, tank (in machinery) E921.0
in mine (of explosive gases) NEC E923.2
late effect of NEC E929.8
machinery - *see also* Accident, machine
pressure vessel - *see* Explosion, pressure vessel
methane E923.2
missile E923.8
in
terrorism E979.2
war operations E993.1
injury by fragments from E991.4
motor vehicle (part of)
in motion (on public highway) E818●
not on public highway E825●
munitions (dump) (factory) E923.8
in
terrorism E979.2
war operations E993.9
of mine E923.8
in
terrorism
at sea or in harbor E979.0
land E979.2
marine E979.0
war operations
after cessation of hostilities E998.0
at sea or in harbor E992.2
land E993.8
after cessation of hostilities E998.0
injury by fragments from E991.4
marine E992.2
own weapons
in
terrorism (*see also* Suicide) E979.2
war operations E993.7
injury by fragments from E991.9
antipersonnel bomb E991.3
pressure
cooker E921.8
gas tank (in machinery) E921.1
vessel (in machinery) E921.9
on transport vehicle - *see* categories E800-E848
specified type NEC E921.8
propane E923.2
railway engine, locomotive, train (boiler) (with subsequent collision, derailment, fall) E803●
with
collision (antecedent) (*see also* Collision, railway) E800●
derailment (antecedent) E802●
fire (without antecedent collision or derailment) E803●
secondary fire resulting from - *see* Fire
self-inflicted (unspecified whether accidental or intentional) E985.5
stated as intentional, purposeful E955.5
shell (artillery) E923.8
in
terrorism E979.2
war operations E993.2
injury by fragments from E991.4
stated as undetermined whether caused accidentally or purposely inflicted E985.5
steam or water lines (in machinery) E921.0
suicide (attempted) E955.5
terrorism - *see* Terrorism, explosion

Explosion *(Continued)*
torpedo E923.8
in
terrorism E979.0
war operations E992.0
transport accident - *see* categories E800–E848
war operations - *see* War operations, explosion
watercraft (boiler) E837●
causing drowning, submersion (after jumping from watercraft) E830●
Exposure (weather) (conditions) (rain) (wind) E904.3
with homicidal intent E968.4
environmental
to
algae bloom E928.6
blue-green algae bloom E928.6
brown tide E928.6
cyanobacteria bloom E928.6
Florida red tide E928.6
harmful algae
and toxins E928.6
bloom E928.6
pfiesteria piscicida E928.6
red tide E928.6
excessive E904.3
cold (*see also* Cold, exposure to) E901.9
self-inflicted - *see* Cold, exposure to, self-inflicted
heat (*see also* Heat) E900.9
helpless person, infant, newborn due to abandonment or neglect E904.0
noise E928.1
prolonged in deep-freeze unit or refrigerator E901.1
radiation - *see* Radiation
resulting from transport accident - *see* categories E800–E848
smoke from, due to
fire - *see* Fire
tobacco, second-hand E869.4
vibration E928.2
External cause status E000.9
child assisting in compensated work of other family member E000.8
civilian
done for
financial or other compensation E000.0
pay or income E000.0
family member assisting in compensated work of other family member E000.8
for income E000.0
hobby or leisure E000.8
off duty military E000.8
military E000.1
off duty E000.8
recreation E000.8
specified NEC E000.8
sport not for income E000.8
student E000.8
volunteer E000.2

F

Fall, falling (accidental) E888.9
building E916
burning E891.8
private E890.8
down
escalator E880.0
ladder E881.0
in boat, ship, watercraft E833●
staircase E880.9
stairs, steps - *see* Fall, from, stairs
earth (with asphyxia or suffocation (by pressure)) (*see also* Earth, falling) E913.3

Fall, falling *(Continued)*
from, off
aircraft (at landing, take-off) (in-transit) (while alighting, boarding) E843●
resulting from accident to aircraft - *see* categories E840–E842
animal (in sport or transport) E828●
animal-drawn vehicle E827●
balcony E882
bed E884.4
bicycle E826●
boat, ship, watercraft (into water) E832●
after accident to, collision, fire on E830●
and subsequently struck by (part of) boat E831●
and subsequently struck by (part of) while alighting, boat E838●
burning, crushed, sinking E830●
and subsequently struck by (part of) boat E831●
bridge E882
building E882
burning (uncontrolled fire) E891.8
in terrorism E979.3
private E890.8
bunk in boat, ship, watercraft E834●
due to accident to watercraft E831●
cable car (not on rails) E847
on rails E829●
car - *see* Fall from motor vehicle E884.9
chair E884.2
cliff E884.1
commode E884.6
curb (sidewalk) E880.1
elevation aboard ship E834●
due to accident to ship E831●
embankment E884.9
escalator E880.0
fire escape E882
flagpole E882
furniture NEC E884.5
gangplank (into water) (*see also* Fall, from, boat) E832●
to deck, dock E834●
hammock on ship E834●
due to accident to watercraft E831●
haystack E884.9
heelies E885.1
high place NEC E884.9
stated as undetermined whether accidental or intentional - *see* Jumping, from, high place
horse (in sport or transport) E828●
in-line skates E885.1
ladder E881.0
in boat, ship, watercraft E833●
due to accident to watercraft E831●
machinery - *see also* Accident, machine
not in operation E884.9
motor vehicle (in motion) (on public highway) E818●
not on public highway E825●
stationary, except while alighting, boarding, entering, leaving E884.9
while alighting, boarding, entering, leaving E824●
stationary, except while alighting, boarding, entering, leaving E884.9
while alighting, boarding, entering, leaving, except off-road type motor vehicle E817●
off-road type - *see* Fall, from, off-road type motor vehicle
motorized
mobility scooter E884.3
wheelchair E884.3

E CODES

Fall, falling *(Continued)*
 from, off *(Continued)*
  nonmotor road vehicle (while alighting, boarding) NEC E829●
  stationary, except while alighting, boarding, entering, leaving E884.9
  off road type motor vehicle (not on public highway) NEC E821●
  on public highway E818●
   while alighting, boarding, entering, leaving E817●
  snow vehicle - *see* Fall from snow vehicle, motor-driven
  one
   deck to another on ship E834●
    due to accident to ship E831●
   level to another NEC E884.9
    boat, ship, or watercraft E834●
     due to accident to watercraft E831●
  pedal cycle E826●
  playground equipment E884.0
  railway rolling stock, train, vehicle (while alighting, boarding) E804●
   with
    collision (*see also* Collision, railway) E800●
    derailment (*see also* Derailment, railway) E802●
    explosion (*see also* Explosion, railway engine) E803●
  rigging (aboard ship) E834●
   due to accident to watercraft E831●
  roller skates E885.1
  scaffolding E881.1
  scooter (nonmotorized) E885.0
   motorized mobility E884.3
  sidewalk (curb) E880.1
   moving E885.9
  skateboard E885.2
  skis E885.3
  snow vehicle, motor-driven (not on public highway) E820●
   on public highway E818●
    while alighting, boarding, entering, leaving E817●
  snowboard E885.4
  stairs, steps E880.9
   boat, ship, watercraft E833●
    due to accident to watercraft E831●
   motor bus, motor vehicle - *see* Fall, from, motor vehicle, while alighting, boarding
   street car E829●
  stationary vehicle NEC E884.9
  stepladder E881.0
  street car (while boarding, alighting) E829●
   stationary, except while boarding or alighting E884.9
  structure NEC E882
   burning (uncontrolled fire) E891.8
    in terrorism E979.3
  table E884.9
  toilet E884.6
  tower E882
  tree E884.9
  turret E882
  vehicle NEC - *see also* Accident, vehicle NEC
   stationary E884.9
  viaduct E882
  wall E882
  wheelchair (electric) (motorized) E884.3
  wheelies E885.1
  window E882

Fall, falling *(Continued)*
 in, on
  aircraft (at landing, take-off) (in-transit) E843●
   resulting from accident to aircraft - *see* categories E840–E842
  boat, ship, watercraft E835●
   due to accident to watercraft E831●
   one level to another NEC E834●
   on ladder, stairs E833●
  cutting or piercing instrument machine E888.0
  deck (of boat, ship, watercraft) E835●
   due to accident to watercraft E831●
  escalator E880.0
  gangplank E835●
  glass, broken E888.0
  knife E888.0
  ladder E881.0
   in boat, ship, watercraft E833●
    due to accident to watercraft E831●
  object
   edged, pointed or sharp E888.0
   other E888.1
  pitchfork E888.0
  railway rolling stock, train, vehicle (while alighting, boarding) E804●
   with
    collision (*see also* Collision, railway) E800●
    derailment (*see also* Derailment, railway) E802●
    explosion (*see also* Explosion, railway engine) E803●
  scaffolding E881.1
  scissors E888.0
  staircase, stairs, steps (*see also* Fall, from, stairs) E880.9
  street car E829●
  water transport (*see also* Fall, in, boat) E835●
 into
  cavity E883.9
  dock E883.9
   from boat, ship, watercraft (*see also* Fall, from, boat) E832●
  hold (of ship) E834●
   due to accident to watercraft E831●
  hole E883.9
  manhole E883.2
  moving part of machinery - *see* Accident, machine
  opening in surface NEC E883.9
  pit E883.9
  quarry E883.9
  shaft E883.9
  storm drain E883.2
  tank E883.9
  water (with drowning or submersion) E910.9
  well E883.1
 late effect of NEC E929.3
 object (*see also* Hit by, object, falling) E916
 other E888.8
 over
  animal E885.9
  cliff E884.1
  embankment E884.9
  small object E885.9
 overboard (*see also* Fall, from, boat) E832●
 resulting in striking against object E888.1
  sharp E888.0
 rock E916
 same level NEC E888.9
  aircraft (any kind) E843●
   resulting from accident to aircraft - *see* categories E840–E842
  boat, ship, watercraft E835●
   due to accident to, collision, watercraft E831●

Fall, falling *(Continued)*
 same level NEC *(Continued)*
  from
   collision, pushing, shoving, by or with other person(s) E886.9
    as, or caused by, a crowd E917.6
    in sports E886.0
   in-line skates E885.1
   roller skates E885.1
   scooter (nonmotorized) E885.0
   skateboard E885.2
   skis E885.3
   slipping, stumbling, tripping E885.9
   snowboard E885.4
  snowslide E916
   as avalanche E909.2
  stone E916
  through
   hatch (on ship) E834●
    due to accident to watercraft E831●
   roof E882
   window E882
  timber E916
  while alighting from, boarding, entering, leaving
   aircraft (any kind) E843●
   motor bus, motor vehicle - *see* Fall, from, motor vehicle, while alighting, boarding
   nonmotor road vehicle NEC E829●
   railway train E804●
   street car E829●
Fallen on by
 animal (horse) (not being ridden) E906.8
 being ridden (in sport or transport) E828●
Fell or jumped from high place, so stated - *see* Jumping, from, high place
Felo-de-se (*see also* Suicide) E958.9
Fever
 heat - *see* Heat
 thermic - *see* Heat
Fight (hand) (fist) (foot) (*see also* Assault, fight) E960.0
Fire (accidental) (caused by great heat from appliance (electrical), hot object, or hot substance) (secondary, resulting from explosion) E899
 conflagration - *see* Conflagration E892
 controlled, normal (in brazier, fireplace, furnace, or stove) (charcoal) (coal) (coke) (electric) (gas) (wood)
  bonfire E897
  brazier, not in building or structure E897
  in building or structure, except private dwelling (barn) (church) (convalescent or residential home) (factory) (farm outbuilding) (hospital) (hotel) (institution (educational) (dormitory) (residential) (private garage) (school) (shop) (store) (theatre) E896
  in private dwelling (apartment) (boarding house) (camping place) (caravan) (farmhouse) (home (private) (house) (lodging house) (rooming house) (tenement) E895
  not in building or structure E897
  trash E897
 forest (uncontrolled) E892
 grass (uncontrolled) E892
 hay (uncontrolled) E892
 homicide (attempt) E968.0
  late effect of E969
 in, of, on, starting in E892
  aircraft (in transit) (powered) E841●
   at landing, take-off E840●
   stationary E892
   unpowered (balloon) (glider) E842●
  balloon E842●
  boat, ship, watercraft - *see* categories E830, E831, E837

Fire (Continued)
in, of, on, starting in (Continued)
building or structure, except private
dwelling (barn) (church)
(convalescent or residential home)
(factory) (farm outbuilding)
(hospital) (hotel) (institution)
(educational) (dormitory)
(residential)) (school) (shop) (store)
(theatre) (see also Conflagration,
building or structure, except private
dwelling) E891.9
forest (uncontrolled) E892
glider E842●
grass (uncontrolled) E892
hay (uncontrolled) E892
lumber (uncontrolled) E892
machinery - see Accident, machine
mine (uncontrolled) E892
motor vehicle (in motion) (on public
highway) E818●
not on public highway E825●
stationary E892
prairie (uncontrolled) E892
private dwelling (apartment) (boarding
house) (camping place) (caravan)
(farmhouse) (home (private))
(house) (lodging house) (private
garage) (rooming house) (tenement)
(see also Conflagration, private
dwelling) E890.9
railway rolling stock, train, vehicle (see also
Explosion, railway engine) E803●
stationary E892
room NEC E898.1
street car (in motion) E829●
stationary E892
terrorism (by fire-producing device)
E979.3
fittings or furniture (burning building)
(uncontrolled fire) E979.3
from nuclear explosion E979.5
transport vehicle, stationary NEC E892
tunnel (uncontrolled) E892
war operations (by fire-producing device
or conventional weapon) E990.9
from nuclear explosion (see also War
operations, injury due to,
nuclear weapons) E996.2
incendiary bomb E990.0
petrol bomb E990.0
late effect of NEC E929.4
lumber (uncontrolled) E892
mine (uncontrolled) E892
prairie (uncontrolled) E892
self-inflicted (unspecified whether accidental
or intentional) E988.1
stated as intentional, purposeful E958.1
specified NEC E898.1
with
conflagration - see Conflagration
ignition (of)
clothing - see Ignition, clothes
highly inflammable material
(benzine) (fat) (gasoline)
(kerosene) (paraffin) (petrol)
E894
started by other person
stated as
with intent to injure or kill E968.0
undetermined whether or not with
intent to injure or kill E988.1
suicide (attempted) E958.1
late effect of E959
tunnel (uncontrolled) E892
Fireball effects from nuclear explosion
in
terrorism E979.5
war operations (see also War operations,
injury due to, nuclear weapons)
E996.2

Fireworks (explosion) E923.0
Flash burns from explosion (see also Explosion)
E923.9
Flood (any injury) (resulting from storm) E908.2
caused by collapse of dam or manmade
structure E909.3
Forced landing (aircraft) E840●
Foreign body, object or material (entrance into
(accidental)
air passage (causing injury) E915
with asphyxia, obstruction, suffocation
E912
food or vomitus E911
nose (with asphyxia, obstruction,
suffocation) E912
causing injury without asphyxia,
obstruction, suffocation E915
alimentary canal (causing injury) (with
obstruction) E915
with asphyxia, obstruction respiratory
passage, suffocation E912
food E911
mouth E915
with asphyxia, obstruction, suffocation
E912
food E911
pharynx E915
with asphyxia, obstruction, suffocation
E912
food E911
aspiration (with asphyxia, obstruction
respiratory passage, suffocation) E912
causing injury without asphyxia,
obstruction respiratory passage,
suffocation E915
food (regurgitated) (vomited) E911
causing injury without asphyxia,
obstruction respiratory passage,
suffocation E915
mucus (not of newborn) E912
phlegm E912
bladder (causing injury or obstruction) E915
bronchus, bronchi - see Foreign body, air
passages
conjunctival sac E914
digestive system - see Foreign body,
alimentary canal
ear (causing injury or obstruction) E915
esophagus (causing injury or obstruction)
(see also Foreign body, alimentary
canal) E915
eye (any part) E914
eyelid E914
hairball (stomach) (with obstruction) E915
ingestion - see Foreign body, alimentary
canal
inhalation - see Foreign body, aspiration
intestine (causing injury or obstruction) E915
iris E914
lacrimal apparatus E914
larynx - see Foreign body, air passage
late effect of NEC E929.8
lung - see Foreign body, air passage
mouth - see Foreign body, alimentary canal,
mouth
nasal passage - see Foreign body, air passage,
nose
nose - see Foreign body, air passage, nose
ocular muscle E914
operation wound (left in) - see Misadventure,
foreign object
orbit E914
pharynx - see Foreign body, alimentary canal,
pharynx
rectum (causing injury or obstruction) E915
stomach (hairball) (causing injury or
obstruction) E915
tear ducts or glands E914
trachea - see Foreign body, air passage
urethra (causing injury or obstruction) E915
vagina (causing injury or obstruction) E915

Found dead, injured
from exposure (to) - see Exposure
on
public highway E819●
railway right of way E807●
Fracture (circumstances unknown or
unspecified) E887
due to specified external means - see manner
of accident
late effect of NEC E929.3
occurring in water transport NEC E835●
Freezing - see Cold, exposure to
Frostbite E901.0
due to manmade conditions E901.1
Frozen - see Cold, exposure to

G

Garrotting, homicidal (attempted) E963
Gored E906.8
Gunshot wound (see also Shooting) E922.9

H

Hailstones, injury by E904.3
Hairball (stomach) (with obstruction) E915
Hanged himself (see also Hanging, self-
inflicted) E983.0
Hang gliding E842●
Hanging (accidental) E913.8
caused by other person
in accidental circumstances E913.8
stated as
intentional, homicidal E963
undetermined whether accidental or
intentional E983.0
homicide (attempt) E963
in bed or cradle E913.0
legal execution E978
self-inflicted (unspecified whether accidental
or intentional) E983.0
in accidental circumstances E913.8
stated as intentional, purposeful E953.0
stated as undetermined whether accidental
or intentional E983.0
suicidal (attempt) E953.0
Heat (apoplexy) (collapse) (cramps) (effects of)
(excessive) (exhaustion) (fever)
(prostration) (stroke) E900.9
due to
manmade conditions (as listed in E900.1,
except boat, ship, watercraft)
E900.1
weather (conditions) E900.0
from
electric heating apparatus causing
burning E924.8
nuclear explosion
in
terrorism E979.5
war operations (see also War
operations, injury due to,
nuclear weapons) E996.2
generated in, boiler, engine, evaporator,
fire room of boat, ship, watercraft
E838●
inappropriate in local application or packing
in medical or surgical procedure
E873.5
late effect of NEC E989
Hemorrhage
delayed following medical or surgical
treatment without mention of
misadventure - see Reaction, abnormal
during medical or surgical treatment as
misadventure - see Misadventure, cut
High
altitude, effects E902.9
level of radioactivity, effects - see Radiation

High *(Continued)*
pressure effects - *see also* Effects of, air
    pressure
    from rapid descent in water (causing
      caisson or divers' disease, palsy, or
      paralysis) E902.2
temperature, effects - *see* Heat
Hit, hitting (accidental) by
aircraft (propeller) (without accident to
    aircraft) E844●
    unpowered E842●
avalanche E909.2
being thrown against object in or part of
    motor vehicle (in motion) (on public
      highway) E818●
      not on public highway E825●
    nonmotor road vehicle NEC E829●
    street car E829●
boat, ship, watercraft
    after fall from watercraft E838●
      damaged, involved in accident
        E831●
    while swimming, water skiing E838●
bullet (*see also* Shooting) E922.9
    from air gun E922.4
    in
      terrorism E979.4
    war operations E991.2
      rubber E991.0
flare, Verey pistol (*see also* Shooting) E922.8
hailstones E904.3
landslide E909.2
law-enforcing agent (on duty) E975
    with blunt object (baton) (night stick)
      (stave) (truncheon) E973
machine - *see* Accident, machine
missile
    firearm (*see also* Shooting) E922.9
    in
      terrorism - *see* Terrorism, missile
      war operations - *see* War operations,
        missile
motor vehicle (on public highway) (traffic
    accident) E814●
    not on public highway, nontraffic accident
      E822●
nonmotor road vehicle NEC E829●
object
    falling E916
      from, in, on
        aircraft E844●
          due to accident to aircraft - *see*
            categories E840–E842
          unpowered E842●
        boat, ship, watercraft E838●
          due to accident to watercraft
            E831●
        building E916
          burning E891.8
            in terrorism E979.3
            private E890.8
        cataclysmic
          earth surface movement or
            eruption E909.9
          storm E908.9
        cave-in E916
          with asphyxiation or suffocation
            (*see also* Suffocation, due
            to, cave-in) E913.3
        earthquake E909.0
        motor vehicle (in motion) (on
          public highway) E818●
          not on public highway E825●
          stationary E916
        nonmotor road vehicle NEC E829●
        pedal cycle E826●
        railway rolling stock, train, vehicle
          E806●
        street car E829●
        structure, burning NEC E891.8
        vehicle, stationary E916

Hit, hitting *(Continued)*
object *(Continued)*
    moving NEC - *see* Striking against,
      object
    projected NEC - *see* Striking against,
      object
    set in motion by
      compressed air or gas, spring, striking,
        throwing - *see* Striking against,
        object
      explosion - *see* Explosion
    thrown into, on, or towards
      motor vehicle (in motion) (on public
        highway) E818●
        not on public highway E825●
      nonmotor road vehicle NEC
        E829●
      pedal cycle E826●
      street car E829●
off-road type motor vehicle (not on public
    highway) E821●
    on public highway E814●
other person(s) E917.9
    with blunt or thrown object E917.9
      in sports E917.0
        with subsequent fall E917.5
      intentionally, homicidal E968.2
    as, or caused by, a crowd E917.1
      with subsequent fall E917.6
    in sports E917.0
pedal cycle E826●
police (on duty) E975
    with blunt object (baton) (nightstick)
      (stave) (truncheon) E973
railway, rolling stock, train, vehicle (part of)
    E805●
shot - *see* Shooting
snow vehicle, motor-driven (not on public
    highway) E820●
    on public highway E814●
street car E829●
vehicle NEC - *see* Accident, vehicle NEC
Homicide, homicidal (attempt) (justifiable) (*see*
    also Assault) E968.9
Hot
liquid, object, substance, accident caused
    by - *see also* Accident, caused by, hot,
    by type of substance
    late effect of E929.8
place, effects - *see* Heat
weather, effects E900.0
Humidity, causing problem E904.3
Hunger E904.1
resulting from
    abandonment or neglect E904.0
    transport accident - *see*
      categories E800–E848
Hurricane (any injury) E908.0
Hypobarism, hypobaropathy - *see* Effects of,
    air pressure
Hypothermia - *see* Cold, exposure to

I

Ictus
caloris - *see* Heat
solaris E900.0
Ignition (accidental)
anesthetic gas in operating theatre
    E923.2
bedclothes
    with
      conflagration - *see* Conflagration
      ignition (of)
        clothing - *see* Ignition, clothes
        highly inflammable material
          obstruction (benzine) (fat)
          (gasoline) (kerosene)
          (paraffin) (petrol) E894
benzine E894

Ignition *(Continued)*
clothes, clothing (from controlled fire) (in
    building) E893.9
    with conflagration - *see* Conflagration
    from
      bonfire E893.2
      highly inflammable material E894
      sources or material as listed in E893.8
      trash fire E893.2
      uncontrolled fire - *see* Conflagration
    in
      private dwelling E893.0
      specified building or structure, except
        of private dwelling E893.1
    not in building or structure E893.2
explosive material - *see* Explosion
fat E894
gasoline E894
kerosene E894
material
    explosive - *see* Explosion
    highly inflammable E894
      with conflagration - *see* Conflagration
      with explosion E923.2
nightdress - *see* Ignition, clothes
paraffin E894
petrol E894
Immersion - *see* Submersion
Implantation of quills of porcupine E906.8
Inanition (from) E904.9
hunger - *see* Lack of, food
resulting from homicidal intent E968.4
thirst - *see* Lack of, water
Inattention after, at birth E904.0
homicidal, infanticidal intent E968.4
Infanticide (*see also* Assault)
Ingestion
foreign body (causing injury) (with
    obstruction) - *see* Foreign body,
    alimentary canal
poisonous substance NEC - *see* Table of
    Drugs and Chemicals
Inhalation
excessively cold substance, manmade E901.1
foreign body - *see* Foreign body, aspiration
liquid air, hydrogen, nitrogen E901.1
mucus, not of newborn (with asphyxia,
    obstruction respiratory passage,
    suffocation) E912
phlegm (with asphyxia, obstruction
    respiratory passage, suffocation) E912
poisonous gas - *see* Table of Drugs and
    Chemicals
smoke from, due to
    fire - *see* Fire
    tobacco, second-hand E869.4
vomitus (with asphyxia, obstruction
    respiratory passage, suffocation) E911
Injury, injured (accidental(ly)) NEC E928.9
by, caused by, from
    air rifle (B-B gun) E922.4
    animal (not being ridden) NEC E906.9
      being ridden (in sport or transport)
        E828●
    assault (*see also* Assault) E968.9
    avalanche E909.2
    bayonet (*see also* Bayonet wound) E920.3
    being thrown against some part of, or
      object in
      motor vehicle (in motion) (on public
        highway) E818●
        not on public highway E825●
      nonmotor road vehicle NEC E829●
      off-road motor vehicle NEC E821●
      railway train E806●
      snow vehicle, motor-driven E820●
      street car E829●
    bending
      due to
        repetitive movement E927.3
        sudden strenuous movement E927.0

Injury, injured *(Continued)*
  by, caused by, from *(Continued)*
    bite, human E928.3
    broken glass E920.8
    bullet - *see* Shooting
    cave-in *(see also* Suffocation, due to,
      cave-in) E913.3
      earth surface movement or eruption
        E909.9
      storm E908.9
      without asphyxiation or suffocation
        E916
    cloudburst E908.8
    component of firearm or air gun E928.7
    cutting or piercing instrument *(see also*
      Cut) E920.9
    cyclone E908.1
    earth surface movement or eruption
      E909.9
    earthquake E909.0
    electric current *(see also* Electric shock)
      E925.9
    explosion *(see also* Explosion) E923.9
      of gun part E928.7
    fire - *see* Fire
    flare, Verey pistol E922.8
    flood E908.2
    foreign body - *see* Foreign body
    gun recoil E928.7
    hailstones E904.3
    hurricane E908.0
    landslide E909.2
    law-enforcing agent, police, in course of
      legal intervention - *see* Legal
      intervention
    lightning E907
    live rail or live wire - *see* Electric shock
    machinery - *see also* Accident, machine
      aircraft, without accident to aircraft
        E844●
      boat, ship, watercraft (deck) (engine
        room) (galley) (laundry)
        (loading) E836●
    mechanism of firearm or air gun E928.7
    missile
      explosive E923.8
      firearm - *see* Shooting
      in
        terrorism - *see* Terrorism, missile
        war operations - *see* War operations,
          missile
    moving part of motor vehicle (in motion)
      (on public highway) E818●
      not on public highway, nontraffic
        accident E825●
      while alighting, boarding, entering,
        leaving - *see* Fall, from, motor
        vehicle, while alighting,
        boarding
    nail E920.8
    needle (sewing) E920.4
      hypodermic E920.5
    noise E928.1
    object
      fallen on
        motor vehicle (in motion) (on
          public highway) E818●
        not on public highway E825●
      falling - *see* Hit by, object, falling
    paintball gun E922.5
    radiation - *see* Radiation
    railway rolling stock, train, vehicle (part
      of) E805●
      door or window E806●
    recoil of firearm E928.7
    rotating propeller, aircraft E844●
    rough landing of off-road type motor
      vehicle (after leaving ground or
      rough terrain) E821●
      snow vehicle E820●
    saber *(see also* Wound, saber) E920.3

Injury, injured *(Continued)*
  by, caused by, from *(Continued)*
    shot - *see* Shooting
    sound waves E928.1
    splinter or sliver, wood E920.8
    straining
      due to
        repetitive movement E927.3
        sudden strenuous movement
          E927.0
    street car (door) E829●
    suicide (attempt) E958.9
    sword E920.3
    terrorism - *see* Terrorism
    third rail - *see* Electric shock
    thunderbolt E907
    tidal wave E909.4
      caused by storm E908.0
    tornado E908.1
    torrential rain E908.2
    twisting
      due to
        repetitive movement E927.3
        sudden strenuous movement
          E927.0
    vehicle NEC - *see* Accident, vehicle
      NEC
    vibration E928.2
    volcanic eruption E909.1
    weapon burst, in war operations
      E993.9
    weightlessness (in spacecraft, real or
      simulated) E928.0
    wood splinter or sliver E920.8
  due to
    civil insurrection - *see* War operations
      occurring after cessation of hostilities
        E993.9
    terrorism - *see* Terrorism
    war operations - *see* War operations
      occurring after cessation of hostilities
        E993.9
      weapon of mass destruction [WMD]
        E997.3
  homicidal *(see also* Assault) E968.9
  in, on
    civil insurrection - *see* War operations
    fight E960.0
    parachute descent (voluntary) (without
      accident to aircraft) E844●
      with accident to aircraft - *see* categories
        E840-E842●
    public highway E819●
    railway right of way E807●
    terrorism - *see* Terrorism
    war operations - *see* War operations
  inflicted (by)
    in course of arrest (attempted),
      suppression of disturbance,
      maintenance of order, by law
      enforcing agents - *see* Legal
      intervention
    law-enforcing agent (on duty) - *see* Legal
      intervention
    other person
      stated as
        accidental E928.9
        homicidal, intentional - *see* Assault
        undetermined whether accidental
          or intentional - *see* Injury,
          stated as undetermined
    police (on duty) - *see* Legal intervention
  late effect of E929.9
  purposely (inflicted) by other person(s) - *see*
    Assault
  self-inflicted (unspecified whether accidental
    or intentional) E988.9
    stated as
      accidental E928.9
      intentionally, purposely E958.9
  specified cause NEC E928.8

Injury, injured *(Continued)*
  stated as
    undetermined whether accidentally or
      purposely inflicted (by) E988.9
      cut (any part of body) E986
      cutting or piercing instrument
        (classifiable to E920) E986
      drowning E984
      explosive(s) (missile) E985.5
      falling from high place E987.9
        manmade structure, except
          residential E987.1
        natural site E987.2
        residential premises E987.0
      hanging E983.0
      knife E986
      late effect of E989
      puncture (any part of body) E986
      shooting - *see* Shooting, stated as
        undetermined whether accidental
        or intentional
      specified means NEC E988.8
      stab (any part of body) E986
      strangulation - *see* Suffocation, stated as
        undetermined whether accidental
        or intentional
      submersion E984
      suffocation - *see* Suffocation, stated as
        undetermined whether accidental
        or intentional
    to child due to criminal abortion E968.8
Insufficient nourishment - *see also* Lack of, food
  homicidal intent E968.4
Insulation, effects - *see* Heat
Interruption of respiration by
  food lodged in esophagus E911
  foreign body, except food, in esophagus E912
Intervention, legal - *see* Legal intervention
Intoxication, drug or poison - *see* Table of
  Drugs and Chemicals
Irradiation - *see* Radiation

J

Jammed (accidentally)
  between objects (moving) (stationary and
    moving) E918
  in object E918
Jumped or fell from high place, so stated - *see*
  Jumping, from, high place, stated as
  in undetermined circumstances
Jumping
  before train, vehicle or other moving object
    (unspecified whether accidental or
    intentional) E988.0
    stated as
      intentional, purposeful E958.0
      suicidal (attempt) E958.0
  from
    aircraft
      by parachute (voluntarily) (without
        accident to aircraft) E844●
      due to accident to aircraft - *see*
        categories E840–E842
    boat, ship, watercraft (into water)
      after accident to, fire on, watercraft
        E830●
      and subsequently struck by (part
        of) boat E831●
      burning, crushed, sinking E830●
      and subsequently struck by (part
        of) boat E831●
      voluntarily, without accident (to boat)
        with injury other than drowning
        or submersion E883.0
    building - *see also* Jumping, from, high
      place
      burning (uncontrolled fire) E891.8
      in terrorism E979.3
      private E890.8

E CODES

E CODES

Jumping (Continued)
  from (Continued)
    cable car (not on rails) E847
      on rails E829●
    high place
      in accidental circumstances or in
        sport - see categories E880–E884
      stated as
        with intent to injure self E957.9
          man-made structures NEC
            E957.1
          natural sites E957.2
          residential premises E957.0
        in undetermined circumstances
          E987.9
          man-made structures NEC
            E987.1
          natural sites E987.2
          residential premises E987.0
        suicidal (attempt) E957.9
          man-made structures NEC
            E957.1
          natural sites E957.1
          residential premises E957.0
    motor vehicle (in motion) (on public
      highway) - see Fall, from, motor
      vehicle
    nonmotor road vehicle NEC E829●
    street car E829●
    structure - see also Jumping, from, high
      place
      burning NEC (uncontrolled fire)
        E891.8
      in terrorism E979.3
  into water
    with injury other than drowning or
      submersion E883.0
      drowning or submersion - see
        Submersion
    from, off, watercraft - see Jumping, from,
      boat
Justifiable homicide - see Assault

K

Kicked by
  animal E906.8
  person(s) (accidentally) E917.9
    with intent to injure or kill E960.0
    as, or caused by a crowd E917.1
      with subsequent fall E917.6
    in fight E960.0
    in sports E917.0
      with subsequent fall E917.5
Kicking against
  object (moving) E917.9
    in sports E917.0
      with subsequent fall E917.5
    stationary E917.4
      with subsequent fall E917.8
  person - see Striking against, person
Killed, killing (accidentally) NEC (see also
    Injury) E928.9
  in
    action - see War operations
    brawl, fight (hand) (fists) (foot) E960.0
      by weapon - see also Assault
        cutting, piercing E966
        firearm - see Shooting, homicide
  self
    stated as
      accident E928.9
      suicide - see Suicide
    unspecified whether accidental or suicidal
      E988.9
Knocked down (accidentally) (by) NEC E928.9
  animal (not being ridden) E906.8
    being ridden (in sport or transport) E828●
  blast from explosion (see also Explosion)
    E923.9

Knocked down NEC (Continued)
  crowd, human stampede E917.6
  late effect of - see Late effect
  person (accidentally) E917.9
    in brawl, fight E960.0
    in sports E917.5
  transport vehicle - see vehicle involved under
    Hit by
  while boxing E917.5

L

Laceration NEC E928.9
Lack of
  air (refrigerator or closed place), suffocation
    by E913.2
  care (helpless person) (infant) (newborn)
    E904.0
    homicidal intent E968.4
  food except as result of transport accident
    E904.1
    helpless person, infant, newborn due to
      abandonment or neglect E904.0
  water except as result of transport accident
    E904.2
    helpless person, infant, newborn due to
      abandonment or neglect E904.0
Landslide E909.2
  falling on, hitting
    motor vehicle (any) (in motion) (on or off
      public highway) E909.2
    railway rolling stock, train, vehicle E909.2
Late effect of
  accident NEC (accident classifiable to E928.9)
    E929.9
    specified NEC (accident classifiable to
      E910–E928.8) E929.8
  assault E969
  fall,
    accidental (accident classifiable to
      E880–E888) E929.3
  fire, accident caused by (accident classifiable
    to E890–E899) E929.4
  homicide, attempt (any means) E969
  injury due to terrorism E999.1
  injury undetermined whether accidentally or
    purposely inflicted (injury classifiable
    to E980–E988) E989
  legal intervention (injury classifiable to
    E970–E976) E977
  medical or surgical procedure, test or
    therapy
    as, or resulting in, or from
      abnormal or delayed reaction or
        complication - see Reaction,
        abnormal
      misadventure - see Misadventure
  motor vehicle accident (accident classifiable
    to E810–E825) E929.0
  natural or environmental factor, accident due
    to (accident classifiable to E900–E909)
    E929.5
  poisoning, accidental (accident classifiable to
    E850–E858, E860–E869) E929.2
  suicide, attempt (any means) E959
  transport accident NEC (accident classifiable
    to E800–E807, E826–E838, E840–E848)
    E929.1
  war operations, injury due to (injury
    classifiable to E990–E998) E999.0
Launching pad accident E845●
Legal
  execution, any method E978
  intervention (by) (injury from) E976
    baton E973
    bayonet E974
    blow E975
    blunt object (baton) (nightstick) (stave)
      (truncheon) E973
    cutting or piercing instrument E974

Legal (Continued)
  intervention (Continued)
    dynamite E971
    execution, any method E973
    explosive(s) (shell) E971
    firearm(s) E970
    gas (asphyxiation) (poisoning) (tear) E972
    grenade E971
    late effect of E977
    machine gun E970
    manhandling E975
    mortar bomb E971
    nightstick E973
    revolver E970
    rifle E970
    specified means NEC E975
    stabbing E974
    stave E973
    truncheon E973
Lifting, injury
  due to
    repetitive movement E927.3
    sudden strenuous movement E927.0
Lightning (shock) (stroke) (struck by) E907
Liquid (noncorrosive) in eye E914
  corrosive E924.1
Loss of control
  motor vehicle (on public highway) (without
    antecedent collision) E816●
    with
      antecedent collision on public
        highway - see Collision, motor
        vehicle
      involving any object, person or
        vehicle not on public
        highway E816●
    on public highway - see Collision,
      motor vehicle
    not on public highway, nontraffic
      accident E825●
      with antecedent collision - see
        Collision, motor vehicle,
        not on public highway
    off-road type motor vehicle (not on public
      highway) E821●
      on public highway - see Loss of control,
        motor vehicle
    snow vehicle, motor-driven (not on public
      highway) E820●
      on public highway - see Loss of control,
        motor vehicle
Lost at sea E832●
  with accident to watercraft E830●
  in war operations E995.8
Low
  pressure, effects - see Effects of, air pressure
  temperature, effects - see Cold exposure to
Lying before train, vehicle or other moving
    object (unspecified whether accidental or
    intentional) E988.0
  stated as intentional, purposeful, suicidal
    (attempt) E958.0
Lynching (see also Assault) E968.9

M

Malfunction, atomic power plant in water
    transport E838●
Mangled (accidentally) NEC E928.9
Manhandling (in brawl, fight) E960.0
  legal intervention E975
Manslaughter (nonaccidental) - see Assault
Marble in nose E912
Mauled by animal E906.8
Medical procedure, complication of
  delayed or as an abnormal reaction without
    mention of misadventure - see
    Reaction, abnormal
  due to or as a result of misadventure - see
    Misadventure

Melting of fittings and furniture in burning
in terrorism E979.3
Minamata disease E865.2
Misadventure(s) to patient(s) during surgical
or medical care E876.9
contaminated blood, fluid, drug or biological
substance (presence of agents and
toxins as listed in E875) E875.9
administered (by) NEC E875.9
infusion E875.0
injection E875.1
specified means NEC E875.2
transfusion E875.0
vaccination E875.1
cut, cutting, puncture, perforation or
hemorrhage (accidental) (inadvertent)
(inappropriate) (during) E870.9
aspiration of fluid or tissue (by puncture
or catheterization, except heart)
E870.5
biopsy E870.8
needle (aspirating) E870.5
blood sampling E870.5
catheterization E870.5
heart E870.6
dialysis (kidney) E870.2
endoscopic examination E870.4
enema E870.7
infusion E870.1
injection E870.3
lumbar puncture E870.5
needle biopsy E870.5
paracentesis, abdominal E870.5
perfusion E870.2
specified procedure NEC E870.8
surgical operation E870.0
thoracentesis E870.5
transfusion E870.1
vaccination E870.3
excessive amount of blood or other fluid
during transfusion or infusion E873.0
failure
in dosage E873.9
electroshock therapy E873.4
inappropriate temperature (too hot or
too cold) in local application and
packing E873.5
infusion
excessive amount of fluid E873.0
incorrect dilution of fluid E873.1
insulin-shock therapy E873.4
nonadministration of necessary drug
or medicinal E873.6
overdose - see also Overdose
radiation, in therapy E873.2
radiation
inadvertent exposure of patient
(receiving radiation for test or
therapy) E873.3
not receiving radiation for test or
therapy - see Radiation
overdose E873.2
specified procedure NEC E873.8
transfusion
excessive amount of blood E873.0
mechanical, of instrument or apparatus
(during procedure) E874.9
aspiration of fluid or tissue (by
puncture or catheterization,
except of heart) E874.4
biopsy E874.8
needle (aspirating) E874.4
blood sampling E874.4
catheterization E874.4
heart E874.5
dialysis (kidney) E874.2
endoscopic examination E874.3
enema E874.8
infusion E874.1
injection E874.8
lumbar puncture E874.4

Misadventure(s) to patient(s) during surgical
or medical care (Continued)
failure (Continued)
mechanical, of instrument or apparatus
(Continued)
needle biopsy E874.4
paracentesis, abdominal E874.4
perfusion E874.2
specified procedure NEC E874.8
surgical operation E874.0
thoracentesis E874.4
transfusion E874.1
vaccination E874.8
sterile precautions (during procedure)
E872.9
aspiration of fluid or tissue (by
puncture or catheterization,
except heart) E872.5
biopsy E872.8
needle (aspirating) E872.5
blood sampling E872.5
catheterization E872.5
heart E872.6
dialysis (kidney) E872.2
endoscopic examination E872.4
enema E872.8
infusion E872.1
injection E872.3
lumbar puncture E872.5
needle biopsy E872.5
paracentesis, abdominal E872.5
perfusion E872.2
removal of catheter or packing E872.8
specified procedure NEC E872.8
surgical operation E872.0
thoracentesis E872.5
transfusion E872.1
vaccination E872.3
suture or ligature during surgical
procedure E872.2
to introduce or to remove tube or
instrument E876.4
foreign object left in body - see
Misadventure, foreign object
foreign object left in body (during procedure)
E871.9
aspiration of fluid or tissue (by puncture
or catheterization, except heart)
E871.5
biopsy E871.8
needle (aspirating) E871.5
blood sampling E871.5
catheterization E871.5
heart E871.6
dialysis (kidney) E871.2
endoscopic examination E871.4
enema E871.8
infusion E871.1
injection E871.3
lumbar puncture E871.5
needle biopsy E871.5
paracentesis, abdominal E871.5
perfusion E871.2
removal of catheter or packing E871.7
specified procedure NEC E871.8
surgical operation E871.0
thoracentesis E871.5
transfusion E871.1
vaccination E871.3
hemorrhage - see Misadventure, cut
inadvertent exposure of patient to radiation
(being received for test or therapy)
E873.3
inappropriate
temperature (too hot or too cold) in local
application or packing E873.5
infusion - see also Misadventure, by specific
type, infusion
excessive amount of fluid E873.0
incorrect dilution of fluid E873.1
wrong fluid E876.1

Misadventure(s) to patient(s) during surgical
or medical care (Continued)
mismatched blood in transfusion E876.0
nonadministration of necessary drug or
medicinal E873.6
overdose - see also Overdose
radiation, in therapy E873.2
perforation - see Misadventure, cut
performance of correct operation (procedure)
on wrong
body part E876.7
side E876.7
site E876.7
performance of operation (procedure)
intended for another patient E876.6
on patient not scheduled for surgery
E876.6
on wrong patient E876.6
performance of wrong operation on correct
patient E876.5
puncture - see Misadventure, cut
specified type NEC E876.8
failure
suture or ligature during surgical
operation E876.2
to introduce or to remove tube or
instrument E876.4
foreign object left in body E871.9
infusion of wrong fluid E876.1
transfusion of mismatched blood
E876.0
wrong
fluid in infusion E876.1
placement of endotracheal tube
during anesthetic procedure
E876.3
transfusion - see also Misadventure, by
specific type, transfusion
excessive amount of blood E873.0
mismatched blood E876.0
wrong
device implanted into correct surgical site
E876.5
drug given in error - see Table of Drugs
and Chemicals
fluid in infusion E876.1
placement of endotracheal tube during
anesthetic procedure E876.3
procedure (operation) performed on the
correct patient E876.5
Motion (effects) E903
sickness E903
Mountain sickness E902.0
Mucus aspiration or inhalation, not of
newborn (with asphyxia, obstruction
respiratory passage, suffocation) E912
Mudslide of cataclysmic nature E909.2
Murder (attempt) (see also Assault) E968.9

N

Nail, injury by E920.8
Needlestick (sewing needle) E920.4
hypodermic E920.5
Neglect - see also Privation
criminal E968.4
homicidal intent E968.4
Noise (causing injury) (pollution) E928.1
Nuclear weapon (see also War operations, injury
due to, nuclear weapons) E996.9

O

Object
falling
from, in, on, hitting
aircraft E844 ●
due to accident to aircraft - see
categories E840–E842

Object *(Continued)*
  falling *(Continued)*
    from, in, on, hitting *(Continued)*
      machinery - *see also* Accident, machine
        not in operation E916
      motor vehicle (in motion) (on public
        highway) E818●
        not on public highway E825●
        stationary E916
      nonmotor road vehicle NEC E829●
      pedal cycle E826●
      person E916
      railway rolling stock, train, vehicle
        E806●
      street car E829●
      watercraft E838●
        due to accident to watercraft
          E831●
  set in motion by
    accidental explosion of pressure
      vessel - *see* category E921
    firearm - *see* category E922
    machine(ry) - *see* Accident, machine
    transport vehicle - *see* categories
      E800–E848
  thrown from, in, on, towards
    aircraft E844●
    cable car (not on rails) E847
      on rails E829●
    motor vehicle (in motion) (on public
      highway) E818●
      not on public highway E825●
    nonmotor road vehicle NEC E829●
    pedal cycle E826●
    street car E829●
    vehicle NEC - *see* Accident, vehicle NEC
Obstruction
  air passages, larynx, respiratory passages
    by
      external means NEC - *see* Suffocation
      food, any type (regurgitated)
        (vomited) E911
      material or object, except food E912
      mucus E912
      phlegm E912
      vomitus E911
  digestive tract, except mouth or pharynx
    by
      food, any type E915
      foreign body (any) E915
  esophagus
    food E911
    foreign body, except food E912
      without asphyxia or obstruction of
        respiratory passage E915
  mouth or pharynx
    by
      food, any type E911
      material or object, except food E912
  respiration - *see* Obstruction, air passages
Oil in eye E914
Overdose
  anesthetic (drug) - *see* Table of Drugs and
    Chemicals
  drug - *see* Table of Drugs and Chemicals
Overexertion E927.9
  from
    lifting
      repetitive movement E927.3
      sudden strenuous movement E927.0
    maintaining prolonged positions E927.1
      holding E927.1
      sitting E927.1
      standing E927.1
    prolonged static position E927.1
    pulling
      repetitive movement E927.3
      sudden strenuous movement E927.0
    pushing
      repetitive movement E927.3
      sudden strenuous movement E927.0

Overexertion *(Continued)*
  from *(Continued)*
    specified NEC E927.8
    sudden strenuous movement E927.0
Overexposure (accidental) (to)
  cold (*see also* Cold, exposure to) E901.9
    due to manmade conditions E901.1
  heat (*see also* Heat) E900.9
  radiation - *see* Radiation
  radioactivity - *see* Radiation
  sun, except sunburn E900.0
  weather - *see* Exposure
  wind - *see* Exposure
Overheated (*see also* Heat) E900.9
Overlaid E913.0
Overturning (accidental)
  animal-drawn vehicle E827●
  boat, ship, watercraft
    causing
      drowning, submersion E830●
      injury except drowning, submersion
        E831●
  machinery - *see* Accident, machine
  motor vehicle (*see also* Loss of control, motor
    vehicle) E816●
    with antecedent collision on public
      highway - *see* Collision, motor
      vehicle
    not on public highway, nontraffic accident
      E825●
      with antecedent collision - *see*
        Collision, motor vehicle, not on
        public highway
  nonmotor road vehicle NEC E829●
  off-road type motor vehicle - *see* Loss of
    control, off-road type motor vehicle
  pedal cycle E826●
  railway rolling stock, train, vehicle (*see also*
    Derailment, railway) E802●
  street car E829●
  vehicle NEC - *see* Accident, vehicle NEC

P

Palsy, divers' E902.2
Parachuting (voluntary) (without accident to
  aircraft) E844●
  due to accident to aircraft - *see* categories
    E840–E842
Paralysis
  divers' E902.2
  lead or saturnine E866.0
    from pesticide NEC E863.4
Pecked by bird E906.8
Performance of correct operation (procedure)
    on wrong
      body part E876.7
      side E876.7
      site E876.7
Performance of operation (procedure)
  intended for another patient E876.6
  on patient not scheduled for surgery
    E876.6
  on wrong patient E876.6
Performance of wrong operation on correct
    patient E876.5
Phlegm aspiration or inhalation (with
  asphyxia, obstruction respiratory
  passage, suffocation) E912
Piercing (*see also* Cut) E920.9
  by slide trigger mechanism, scope or other
    part of gun E928.7
Pinched
  between objects (moving) (stationary and
    moving) E918
  by slide trigger mechanism, scope or other
    part of gun E928.7
  in object E918
Pinned under
  machine(ry) - *see* Accident, machine

Place of occurrence of accident - *see* Accident
  (to), occurring (at) (in)
Plumbism E866.0
  from insecticide NEC E863.4
Poisoning (accidental) (by) - *see also* Table of
  Drugs and Chemicals
  carbon monoxide
    generated by
      aircraft in transit E844●
      motor vehicle
        in motion (on public highway)
          E818●
        not on public highway
          E825●
      watercraft (in transit) (not in transit)
        E838●
  caused by injection of poisons or toxins into
    or through skin by plant thorns,
    spines, or other mechanism E905.7
  marine or sea plants E905.6
  fumes or smoke due to
    conflagration - *see* Conflagration
    explosion or fire - *see* Fire
    ignition - *see* Ignition
  gas
    in legal intervention E972
    legal execution, by E978
    on watercraft E838●
    used as anesthetic - *see* Table of Drugs and
      Chemicals
  in
    terrorism (chemical weapons) E979.7
    war operations E997.2
  late effect of - *see* Late effect
  legal
    execution E978
    intervention
      by gas E972
Pressure, external, causing asphyxia,
  suffocation (*see also* Suffocation)
  E913.9
Privation E904.9
  food (*see also* Lack of, food) E904.1
  helpless person, infant, newborn due to
    abandonment or neglect E904.0
  late effect of NEC E929.5
  resulting from transport accident - *see*
    categories E800–E848
  water (*see also* Lack of, water) E904.2
Projected objects, striking against or struck
  by - *see* Striking against, object
Prolonged stay in
  high altitude (causing conditions as listed in
    E902.0) E902.0
  weightless environment E928.0
Prostration
  heat - *see* Heat
Pulling, injury
  due to
    repetitive movement E927.3
    sudden strenuous movement E927.0
Puncture, puncturing (*see also* Cut) E920.9
  by
    plant thorns or spines E920.8
      toxic reaction E905.7
      marine or sea plants E905.6
    sea-urchin spine E905.6
Pushing (injury in) (overexertion) E927.8
  by other person(s) (accidental) E917.9
    as, or caused by, a crowd, human
      stampede E917.1
      with subsequent fall E917.6
    before moving vehicle or object
      stated as
        intentional, homicidal E968.5
        undetermined whether accidental
          or intentional E988.8
  from
    high place
      in accidental circumstances - *see*
        categories E880–E884

E CODES

Pushing *(Continued)*
  by other person(s) *(Continued)*
    from *(Continued)*
      high place *(Continued)*
        stated as
          intentional, homicidal E968.1
          undetermined whether accidental
            or intentional E987.9
          man-made structure, except
            residential E987.1
          natural site E987.2
          residential E987.0
      motor vehicle *(see also* Fall, from, motor
        vehicle) E818●
        stated as
          intentional, homicidal E968.5
          undetermined whether accidental
            or intentional E988.8
    in sports E917.0
      with fall E886.0
    with fall E886.9
      in sports E886.0
  due to
    repetitive movement E927.3
    sudden strenuous movement E927.0

R

Radiation (exposure to) E926.9
  abnormal reaction to medical test or therapy
    E879.2
  arc lamps E926.2
  atomic power plant (malfunction) NEC
    E926.9
    in water transport E838●
  electromagnetic, ionizing E926.3
  gamma rays E926.3
  in
    terrorism (from or following nuclear
      explosion) (direct) (secondary)
      E979.5
      laser E979.8
    war operations *(see also* War operations,
      injury due to, nuclear weapons)
      E996.3
      laser(s) E997.0
    water transport E838●
  inadvertent exposure of patient (receiving
    test or therapy) E873.3
  infrared (heaters and lamps) E926.1
    excessive heat E900.1
  ionized, ionizing (particles, artificially
    accelerated) E926.8
    electromagnetic E926.3
  isotopes, radioactive - *see* Radiation,
    radioactive isotopes
  laser(s) E926.4
    in
      terrorism E979.8
      war operations E997.0
    misadventure in medical care - *see*
      Misadventure, failure, in dosage,
      radiation
  late effect of NEC E929.8
    excessive heat from - *see* Heat
  light sources (visible) (ultraviolet) E926.2
  misadventure in medical or surgical
    procedure - *see* Misadventure, failure,
    in dosage, radiation
  overdose (in medical or surgical pacemaker
    procedure) E873.2
  radar E926.0
  radioactive isotopes E926.5
    atomic power plant malfunction E926.5
      in water transport E838●
    misadventure in medical or surgical
      treatment - *see* Misadventure,
      failure, in dosage, radiation
  radiobiologicals - *see* Radiation, radioactive
    isotopes

Radiation *(Continued)*
  radiofrequency E926.0
  radiopharmaceuticals - *see* Radiation,
    radioactive isotopes
  radium NEC E926.9
  sun E926.2
    excessive heat from E900.0
  tanning bed E926.2
  welding arc or torch E926.2
    excessive heat from E900.1
  x-rays (hard) (soft) E926.3
    misadventure in medical or surgical
      treatment - *see* Misadventure,
      failure, in dosage, radiation
Rape E960.1
Reaction, abnormal to or following (medical or
  surgical procedure) E879.9
  amputation (of limbs) E878.5
  anastomosis (arteriovenous) (blood vessel)
    (gastrojejunal) (skin) (tendon) (natural,
    artificial material, tissue) E878.2
    external stoma, creation of E878.3
  aspiration (of fluid) E879.4
    tissue E879.8
  biopsy E879.8
  blood
    sampling E879.7
    transfusion
      procedure E879.8
  bypass - *see* Reaction, abnormal, anastomosis
  catheterization
    cardiac E879.0
    urinary E879.6
  colostomy E878.3
  cystostomy E878.3
  dialysis (kidney) E879.1
  drugs or biologicals - *see* Table of Drugs and
    Chemicals
  duodenostomy E878.3
  electroshock therapy E879.3
  formation of external stoma E878.3
  gastrostomy E878.3
  graft - *see* Reaction, abnormal, anastomosis
  hypothermia E879.8
  implant, implantation (of)
    artificial
      internal device (cardiac pacemaker)
        (electrodes in brain) (heart valve
        prosthesis) (orthopedic) E878.1
      material or tissue (for anastomosis or
        bypass) E878.2
        with creation of external stoma
          E878.3
      natural tissues (for anastomosis or
        bypass) E878.2
      as transplantion - *see* Reaction,
        abnormal, transplant
      with creation of external stoma E878.3
  infusion
    procedure E879.8
  injection
    procedure E879.8
  insertion of gastric or duodenal sound E879.5
  insulin-shock therapy E879.3
  lumbar puncture E879.4
  perfusion E879.1
  procedures other than surgical operation *(see
    also* Reaction, abnormal, by specific
    type of procedure) E879.9
    specified procedure NEC E879.8
  radiological procedure or therapy E879.2
  removal of organ (partial) (total) NEC
    E878.6
    with
      anastomosis, bypass or graft E878.2
      formation of external stoma E878.3
      implant of artificial internal device
        E878.1
      transplant(ation)
        partial organ E878.4
        whole organ E878.0

Reaction, abnormal to or following *(Continued)*
  sampling
    blood E879.7
    fluid NEC E879.4
    tissue E879.8
  shock therapy E879.3
  surgical operation *(see also* Reaction,
    abnormal, by specified type of
    operation) E878.9
    restorative NEC E878.4
      with
        anastomosis, bypass or graft E878.2
        formation of external stoma E878.3
        implant(ation) - *see* Reaction,
          abnormal, implant
        transplantation - *see* Reaction,
          abnormal, transplant
    specified operation NEC E878.8
  thoracentesis E879.4
  transfusion
    procedure E879.8
  transplant, transplantation (heart) (kidney)
    (liver) E878.0
    partial organ E878.4
  ureterostomy E878.3
  vaccination E879.8
Reduction in
  atmospheric pressure - *see also* Effects of, air
    pressure
    while surfacing from
      deep water diving causing caisson or
        divers' disease, palsy or
        paralysis E902.2
      underground E902.8
Repetitive movements NEC E927.8
Residual (effect) - *see* Late effect
Rock falling on or hitting (accidentally)
  motor vehicle (in motion) (on public
    highway) E818●
    not on public highway E825●
  nonmotor road vehicle NEC E829●
  pedal cycle E826●
  person E916
  railway rolling stock, train, vehicle
    E806●
Running off, away
  animal (being ridden) (in sport or transport)
    E828●
    not being ridden E906.8
  animal-drawn vehicle E827●
  rails, railway *(see also* Derailment) E802●
  roadway
    motor vehicle (without antecedent
      collision) E816●
    nontraffic accident E825●
      with antecedent collision - *see*
        categories Collision, motor
        vehicle, not on public
        highway
    with
      antecedent collision - *see* Collision
        motor vehicle
      subsequent collision
        involving any object, person or
          vehicle not on public
          highway E816●
        on public highway E811●
    nonmotor road vehicle NEC E829●
    pedal cycle E826●
Run over (accidentally) (by)
  animal (not being ridden) E906.8
    being ridden (in sport or transport)
      E828●
  animal-drawn vehicle E827●
  machinery - *see* Accident, machine
  motor vehicle (on public highway) - *see* Hit
    by, motor vehicle
  nonmotor road vehicle NEC E829●
  railway train E805●
  street car E829●
  vehicle NEC E848

E CODES

E CODES

S

Saturnism E866.0
 from insecticide NEC E863.4
Scald, scalding (accidental) (by) (from) (in)
  E924.0
 acid - *see* Scald, caustic
 boiling tap water E924.2
 caustic or corrosive liquid, substance E924.1
  swallowed - *see* Table of Drugs and
   Chemicals
 homicide (attempt) - *see* Assault, burning
 inflicted by other person
  stated as
   intentional or homicidal E968.3
   undetermined whether accidental or
    intentional E988.2
 late effect of NEC E929.8
 liquid (boiling) (hot) E924.0
 local application of externally applied
   substance in medical or surgical care
   E873.5
 molten metal E924.0
 self-inflicted (unspecified whether accidental
   or intentional) E988.2
  stated as intentional, purposeful E958.2
  stated as undetermined whether accidental
   or intentional E988.2
 steam E924.0
 tap water (boiling) E924.2
 transport accident - *see* categories E800–E848
 vapor E924.0
Scratch, cat E906.8
Sea
 sickness E903
Self-mutilation - *see* Suicide
Sequelae (of)
 in
  terrorism E999.1
  war operations E999.0
Shock
 anaphylactic (*see also* Table of Drugs and
   Chemicals) E947.9
  due to
   bite (venomous) - *see* Bite, venomous
    NEC
   sting - *see* Sting
 electric (*see also* Electric shock) E925.9
 from electric appliance or current (*see also*
   Electric shock) E925.9
Shooting, shot (accidental(ly)) E922.9
 air gun E922.4
 BB gun E922.4
 hand gun (pistol) (revolver) E922.0
 himself (*see also* Shooting, self-inflicted) E985.4
  hand gun (pistol) (revolver) E985.0
  military firearm, except hand gun E985.3
   hand gun (pistol) (revolver) E985.0
  rifle (hunting) E985.2
   military E985.3
  shotgun (automatic) E985.1
  specified firearm NEC E985.4
  Verey pistol E985.4
 homicide (attempt) E965.4
  air gun E968.6
  BB gun E968.6
  hand gun (pistol) (revolver) E965.0
  military firearm, except hand gun E965.3
   hand gun (pistol) (revolver) E965.0
  paintball gun E965.4
  rifle (hunting) E965.2
   military E965.3
  shotgun (automatic) E965.1
  specified firearm NEC E965.4
  Verey pistol E965.4
 inflicted by other person
  in accidental circumstances E922.9
   hand gun (pistol) (revolver) E922.0
   military firearm, except hand gun
    E922.3
    hand gun (pistol) (revolver) E922.0

Shooting, shot (*Continued*)
 inflicted by other person (*Continued*)
  in accidental circumstances (*Continued*)
   rifle (hunting) E922.2
    military E922.3
   shotgun (automatic) E922.1
   specified firearm NEC E922.8
   Verey pistol E922.8
  stated as
   intentional, homicidal E965.4
    hand gun (pistol) (revolver) E965.0
    military firearm, except hand gun
     E965.3
     hand gun (pistol) (revolver)
      E965.0
    paintball gun E965.4
    rifle (hunting) E965.2
     military E965.3
    shotgun (automatic) E965.1
    specified firearm E965.4
    Verey pistol E965.4
   undetermined whether accidental or
    intentional E985.4
    air gun E985.6
    BB gun E985.6
    hand gun (pistol) (revolver) E985.0
    military firearm, except hand gun
     E985.3
     hand gun (pistol) (revolver)
      E985.0
    paintball gun E985.7
    rifle (hunting) E985.2
    shotgun (automatic) E985.1
    specified firearm NEC E985.4
    Verey pistol E985.4
  in
   terrorism - *see* Terrorism, shooting
   war operations - *see* War operations,
    shooting
  legal
   execution E978
   intervention E970
  military firearm, except hand gun E922.3
   hand gun (pistol) (revolver) E922.0
  paintball gun E922.5
  rifle (hunting) E922.2
   military E922.3
  self-inflicted (unspecified whether accidental
    or intentional) E985.4
   air gun E985.6
   BB gun E985.6
   hand gun (pistol) (revolver) E985.0
   military firearm, except hand gun E985.3
    hand gun (pistol) (revolver) E985.0
   paintball gun E985.7
   rifle (hunting) E985.2
    military E985.3
   shotgun (automatic) E985.1
   specified firearm NEC E985.4
   stated as
    accidental E922.9
     hand gun (pistol) (revolver) E922.0
     military firearm, except hand gun
      E922.3
      hand gun (pistol) (revolver)
       E922.0
     paintball gun E922.5
     rifle (hunting) E922.2
      military E922.3
     shotgun (automatic) E922.1
     specified firearm NEC E922.8
     Verey pistol E922.8
    intentional, purposeful E955.4
     hand gun (pistol) (revolver) E955.4
     military firearm, except hand gun
      E955.3
      hand gun (pistol) (revolver)
       E955.0
     paintball gun E955.7
     rifle (hunting) E955.2
      military E955.3

Shooting, shot (*Continued*)
 self-inflicted (*Continued*)
  stated as (*Continued*)
   intentional, purposeful (*Continued*)
    shotgun (automatic) E955.1
    specified firearm NEC E955.4
    Verey pistol E955.4
  shotgun (automatic) E922.1
  specified firearm NEC E922.8
  stated as undetermined whether accidental
    or intentional E985.4
   hand gun (pistol) (revolver) E985.0
   military firearm, except hand gun
    E985.3
    hand gun (pistol) (revolver) E985.0
   paintball gun E985.7
   rifle (hunting) E985.2
    military E985.3
   shotgun (automatic) E985.1
   specified firearm NEC E985.4
   Verey pistol E985.4
  suicidal (attempt) E955.4
   air gun E985.6
   BB gun E985.6
   hand gun (pistol) (revolver) E955.0
   military firearm, except hand gun
    E955.3
    hand gun (pistol) (revolver) E955.0
   paintball gun E955.7
   rifle (hunting) E955.2
    military E955.3
   shotgun (automatic) E955.1
   specified firearm NEC E955.4
   Verey pistol E955.4
  Verey pistol E922.8
Shoving (accidentally) by other person (*see also*
  Pushing by other person) E917.9
Sickness
 air E903
 alpine E902.0
 car E903
 motion E903
 mountain E902.0
 sea E903
 travel E903
Sinking (accidental)
 boat, ship, watercraft (causing drowning,
   submersion) E830●
  causing injury except drowning,
    submersion E831●
Siriasis E900.0
Skydiving E844●
Slashed wrists (*see also* Cut, self-inflicted)
  E986
Slipping (accidental)
 on
  deck (of boat, ship, watercraft) (icy) (oily)
    (wet) E835●
  ice E885.9
  ladder of ship E833●
   due to accident to watercraft E831●
  mud E885.9
  oil E885.9
  snow E885.9
  stairs of ship E833●
   due to accident to watercraft E831●
  surface
   slippery E885.9
   wet E885.9
Sliver, wood, injury by E920.8
Smothering, smothered (*see also* Suffocation)
  E913.9
Smouldering building or structure in
  terrorism E979.3
Sodomy (assault) E960.1
Solid substance in eye (any part) or adnexa
  E914
Sound waves (causing injury) E928.1
Splinter, injury by E920.8
Stab, stabbing E966
 accidental - *see* Cut

◀ New   ◀▥ Revised   ~~deleted~~ Deleted   ● Use Additional Digit(s)   ▨ Omit code

Starvation E904.1
  helpless person, infant, newborn - *see* Lack of
    food
  homicidal intent E968.4
  late effect of NEC E929.5
  resulting from accident connected
    with transport - *see* categories
    E800–E848
Stepped on
  by
    animal (not being ridden) E906.8
      being ridden (in sport or transport)
        E828●
    crowd E917.1
    person E917.9
      in sports E917.0
  in sports E917.0
Stepping on
  object (moving) E917.9
    in sports E917.0
      with subsequent fall E917.5
    stationary E917.4
      with subsequent fall E917.8
  person E917.9
    as, or caused by a crowd E917.1
      with subsequent fall E917.6
    in sports E917.0
Sting E905.9
  ant E905.5
  bee E905.3
  caterpillar E905.5
  coral E905.6
  hornet E905.3
  insect NEC E905.5
  jelly fish E905.6
  marine animal or plant E905.6
  nematocysts E905.6
  scorpion E905.2
  sea anemone E905.6
  sea cucumber E905.6
  wasp E905.3
  yellow jacket E905.3
Storm E908.9
  specified type NEC E908.8
Straining, injury
  due to
    repetitive movement E927.3
    sudden strenuous movement
      E927.0
Strangling - *see* Suffocation
Strangulation - *see* Suffocation
Strenuous movements (in recreational or other
  activities) NEC E927.8
Striking against
  bottom (when jumping or diving into water)
    E883.0
  object (moving) E917.9
    caused by crowd E917.1
      with subsequent fall E917.6
    furniture E917.3
      with subsequent fall E917.7
    in
      running water E917.2
        with drowning or submersion - *see*
          Submersion
      sports E917.0
        with subsequent fall
          E917.5
    stationary E917.4
      with subsequent fall E917.8
  person(s) E917.9
    with fall E886.9
      in sports E886.0
    as, or caused by, a crowd
      E917.1
      with subsequent fall E917.6
      in sports E917.0
        with fall E886.0
Stroke
  heat - *see* Heat
  lightning E907

Struck by - *see also* Hit by
  bullet
    in
      terrorism E979.4
      war operations E991.2
        rubber E991.0
  lightning E907
  missile
    in terrorism - *see* Terrorism, missile
  object
    falling
      from, in, on
        building
          burning (uncontrolled fire)
            in terrorism E979.3
  thunderbolt E907
Stumbling over animal, carpet, curb, rug or
  (small) object (with fall) E885.9
  without fall - *see* Striking against, object
Submersion (accidental) E910.8
  boat, ship, watercraft (causing drowning,
    submersion) E830●
    causing injury except drowning,
      submersion E831●
  by other person
    in accidental circumstances - *see* category
      E910
    intentional, homicidal E964
    stated as undetermined whether
      accidental or intentional E984
  due to
    accident
      machinery - *see* Accident, machine
      to boat, ship, watercraft E830●
      transport - *see* categories E800-E848
    avalanche E909.2
    cataclysmic
      earth surface movement or eruption
        E909.9
      storm E908.9
    cloudburst E908.8
    cyclone E908.1
    fall
      from
        boat, ship, watercraft (not involved
          in accident) E832●
        burning, crushed E830●
        involved in accident, collision
          E830●
        gangplank (into water) E832●
      overboard NEC E832●
    flood E908.2
    hurricane E908.0
    jumping into water E910.8
      from boat, ship, watercraft
        burning, crushed, sinking E830●
        involved in accident, collision
          E830●
        not involved in accident, for swim
          E910.2
      in recreational activity (without diving
        equipment) E910.2
        with or using diving equipment
          E910.1
      to rescue another person E910.3
  homicide (attempt) E964
  in
    bathtub E910.4
    specified activity, not sport, transport or
      recreational E910.3
    sport or recreational activity (without
      diving equipment) E910.2
      with or using diving equipment E910.1
      water skiing E910.0
    swimming pool NEC E910.8
    terrorism E979.8
    war operations E995.4
      intentional E995.3
    water transport E832●
      due to accident to boat, ship,
        watercraft E830●

Submersion (*Continued*)
  landslide E909.2
    overturning boat, ship, watercraft E909.2
    sinking boat, ship, watercraft E909.2
    submersion boat, ship, watercraft E909.2
    tidal wave E909.4
      caused by storm E908.0
    torrential rain E908.2
  late effect of NEC E929.8
  quenching tank E910.8
  self-inflicted (unspecified whether accidental
    or intentional) E984
    in accidental circumstances - *see* category
      E910
    stated as intentional, purposeful E954
  stated as undetermined whether accidental
    or intentional E984
  suicidal (attempted) E954
  while
    attempting rescue of another person
      E910.3
    engaged in
      marine salvage E910.3
      underwater construction or repairs
        E910.3
    fishing, not from boat E910.2
    hunting, not from boat E910.2
    ice skating E910.2
    pearl diving E910.3
    placing fishing nets E910.3
    playing in water E910.2
    scuba diving E910.1
      nonrecreational E910.3
    skin diving E910.1
    snorkel diving E910.2
    spear fishing underwater E910.1
    surfboarding E910.2
    swimming (swimming pool) E910.2
    wading (in water) E910.2
    water skiing E910.0
Sucked
  into
    jet (aircraft) E844●
Suffocation (accidental) (by external means)
  (by pressure) (mechanical) E913.9
  caused by other person
    in accidental circumstances - *see* category
      E913
    stated as
      intentional, homicidal E963
      undetermined whether accidental or
        intentional E983.9
        by, in
          hanging E983.0
          plastic bag E983.1
          specified means NEC E983.8
  due to, by
    avalanche E909.2
    bedclothes E913.0
    bib E913.0
    blanket E913.0
    cave-in E913.3
      caused by cataclysmic earth surface
        movement or eruption E909.9
    conflagration - *see* Conflagration E983.8
    explosion - *see* Explosion
    falling earth, other substance E913.3
    fire - *see* Fire
    food, any type (ingestion) (inhalation)
      (regurgitated) (vomited) E911
    foreign body, except food (ingestion)
      (inhalation) E912
    ignition - *see* Ignition
    landslide E909.2
    machine(ry) - *see* Accident, machine
    material, object except food entering by
      nose or mouth, ingested, inhaled
      E912
    mucus (aspiration) (inhalation), not of
      newborn E912
    phlegm (aspiration) (inhalation) E912

E CODES

Suffocation (*Continued*)
due to, by (*Continued*)
pillow E913.0
plastic bag - *see* Suffocation, in, plastic bag
sheet (plastic) E913.0
specified means NEC E913.8
vomitus (aspiration) (inhalation) E911
homicidal (attempt) E963
in war operations E995.3
in
airtight enclosed place E913.2
baby carriage E913.0
bed E913.0
closed place E913.2
cot, cradle E913.0
perambulator E913.0
plastic bag (in accidental circumstances)
E913.1
homicidal, purposely inflicted by other
person E963
self-inflicted (unspecified whether
accidental or intentional) E983.1
in accidental circumstances E913.1
intentional, suicidal E953.1
stated as undetermined whether
accidentally or purposely
inflicted E983.1
suicidal, purposely self-inflicted E953.1
refrigerator E913.2
war operations E995.3
self-inflicted - *see also* Suffocation, stated as
undetermined whether accidental or
intentional E953.9
in accidental circumstances - *see* category
E913
stated as intentional, purposeful - *see*
Suicide, suffocation
stated as undetermined whether accidental
or intentional E983.9
by, in
hanging E983.0
plastic bag E983.1
specified means NEC E983.8
suicidal - *see* Suicide, suffocation
Suicide, suicidal (attempted) (by) E958.9
burning, burns E958.1
caustic substance E958.7
poisoning E950.7
swallowed E950.7
cold, extreme E958.3
cut (any part of body) E956
cutting or piercing instrument (classifiable to
E920) E956
drowning E954
electrocution E958.4
explosive(s) (classifiable to E923) E955.5
fire E958.1
firearm (classifiable to E922) - *see* Shooting,
suicidal
hanging E953.0
jumping
before moving object, train, vehicle E958.0
from high place - *see* Jumping, from, high
place, stated as, suicidal
knife E956
late effect of E959
motor vehicle, crashing of E958.5
poisoning - *see* Table of Drugs and Chemicals
puncture (any part of body) E956
scald E958.2
shooting - *see* Shooting, suicidal
specified means NEC E958.8
stab (any part of body) E956
strangulation - *see* Suicide, suffocation
submersion E954
suffocation E953.9
by, in
hanging E953.0
plastic bag E953.1
specified means NEC E953.8
wound NEC E958.9

Sunburn E926.2
Sunstroke E900.0
Supersonic waves (causing injury) E928.1
Surgical procedure, complication of
delayed or as an abnormal reaction without
mention of misadventure, *see* Reaction,
abnormal
due to or as a result of misadventure - *see*
Misadventure
Swallowed, swallowing
foreign body - *see* Foreign body, alimentary
canal
poison - *see* Table of Drugs and Chemicals
substance
caustic - *see* Table of Drugs and Chemicals
drugs
corrosive - *see* Table of Drugs and
Chemicals
poisonous - *see* Table of Drugs and
Chemicals
Swimmers' cramp (*see also* category E910)
E910.2
not in recreation or sport E910.3
Syndrome, battered
baby or child - *see* Abuse, child
wife - *see* Assault

T

Tackle in sport E886.0
Terrorism (by) (in) (injury) E979.8
air blast E979.2
aircraft burned, destroyed, exploded, shot
down E979.1
used as a weapon E979.1
anthrax E979.6
asphyxia from
chemical (weapons) E979.7
fire, conflagration (caused by fire-
producing device) E979.3
from nuclear explosion E979.5
gas or fumes E979.7
bayonet E979.8
biological agents E979.6
blast (air) (effects) E979.2
from nuclear explosion E979.5
underwater E979.0
bomb (antipersonnel) (mortar) (explosion)
(fragments) E979.2
bullet(s) (from carbine, machine gun, pistol,
rifle, shotgun) E979.4
burn from
chemical E979.7
fire, conflagration (caused by fire-
producing device) E979.3
from nuclear explosion E979.5
gas E979.7
burning aircraft E979.1
chemical E979.7
cholera E979.6
conflagration E979.3
crushed by falling aircraft E979.1
depth-charge E979.0
destruction of aircraft E979.1
disability, as sequelae one year or more after
injury E999.1
drowning E979.8
effect
of nuclear weapon (direct) (secondary)
E979.5
secondary NEC E979.9
sequelae E999.1
explosion (artillery shell) (breech-block)
(cannon block) E979.2
aircraft E979.1
bomb (antipersonnel) (mortar) E979.2
nuclear (atom) (hydrogen) E979.5
depth-charge E979.0
grenade E979.2
injury by fragments from E979.2

Terrorism (*Continued*)
explosion (*Continued*)
land-mine E979.2
marine weapon E979.0
mine (land) E979.2
at sea or in harbor E979.0
marine E979.0
missile (explosive) NEC E979.2
munitions (dump) (factory) E979.2
nuclear (weapon) E979.5
other direct and secondary effects of
E979.5
sea-based artillery shell E979.0
torpedo E979.0
exposure to ionizing radiation from nuclear
explosion E979.5
falling aircraft E979.1
fire or fire-producing device E979.3
firearms E979.4
fireball effects from nuclear explosion E979.5
fragments from artillery shell, bomb NEC,
grenade, guided missile, land-mine,
rocket, shell, shrapnel E979.2
gas or fumes E979.7
grenade (explosion) (fragments) E979.2
guided missile (explosion) (fragments)
E979.2
nuclear E979.5
heat from nuclear explosion E979.5
hot substances E979.3
hydrogen cyanide E979.7
land-mine (explosion) (fragments) E979.2
laser(s) E979.8
late effect of E999.1
lewisite E979.7
lung irritant (chemical) (fumes) (gas) E979.7
marine mine E979.0
mine E979.2
at sea E979.0
in harbor E979.0
land (explosion) (fragments) E979.2
marine E979.0
missile (explosion) (fragments) (guided)
E979.2
marine E979.0
nuclear weapons E979.5
mortar bomb (explosion) (fragments) E979.2
mustard gas E979.7
nerve gas E979.7
nuclear weapons E979.5
pellets (shotgun) E979.4
petrol bomb E979.3
phosgene E979.7
piercing object E979.8
poisoning (chemical) (fumes) (gas) E979.7
radiation, ionizing from nuclear explosion
E979.5
rocket (explosion) (fragments) E979.2
saber, sabre E979.8
sarin E979.7
screening smoke E979.7
sequelae effect (of) E999.1
shell (aircraft) (artillery) (cannon) (land-
based) (explosion) (fragments) E979.2
sea-based E979.0
shooting E979.4
bullet(s) E979.4
pellet(s) (rifle) (shotgun) E979.4
shrapnel E979.2
smallpox E979.7
stabbing object(s) E979.8
submersion E979.8
torpedo E979.0
underwater blast E979.0
vesicant (chemical) (fumes) (gas) E979.7
weapon burst E979.2
Thermic fever E900.9
Thermoplegia E900.9
Thirst - *see also* Lack of water
resulting from accident connected with
transport - *see* categories E800–E848

◄ New ◄▦ Revised ~~deleted~~ Deleted ● Use Additional Digit(s) ▨ Omit code

Thrown (accidentally)
against object in or part of vehicle
by motion of vehicle
aircraft E844●
boat, ship, watercraft E838●
motor vehicle (on public highway)
E818●
not on public highway E825●
off-road type (not on public
highway) E821●
on public highway E818●
snow vehicle E820●
on public highway E818●
nonmotor road vehicle NEC E829●
railway rolling stock, train, vehicle E806●
street car E829●
from
animal (being ridden) (in sport or
transport) E828●
high place, homicide (attempt) E968.1
machinery - *see* Accident, machine
vehicle NEC - *see* Accident, vehicle NEC
off - *see* Thrown, from
overboard (by motion of boat, ship,
watercraft) E832●
by accident to boat, ship, watercraft E830●
Thunderbolt NEC E907
Tidal wave (any injury) E909.4
caused by storm E908.0
Took
overdose of drug - *see* Table of Drugs and
Chemicals
poison - *see* Table of Drugs and Chemicals
Tornado (any injury) E908.1
Torrential rain (any injury) E908.2
Traffic accident NEC E819●
Trampled by animal E906.8
being ridden (in sport or transport) E828●
Trapped (accidentally)
between
objects (moving) (stationary and moving)
E918
by
door of
elevator E918
motor vehicle (on public highway)
(while alighting, boarding) - *see*
Fall, from, motor vehicle,
while alighting
railway train (underground) E806●
street car E829●
subway train E806●
in object E918
Trauma
cumulative
from
repetitive
impact E927.4
motion or movements E927.3
sudden from strenuous movement E927.0
Travel (effects) E903
sickness E903
Tree
falling on or hitting E916
motor vehicle (in motion) (on public
highway) E818●
not on public highway E825●
nonmotor road vehicle NEC E829●
pedal cycle E826●
person E916
railway rolling stock, train, vehicle E806●
street car E829●
Trench foot E901.0
**Tripping over animal, carpet, curb, rug, or
small object** (with fall) E885.9
without fall - *see* Striking against, object
Tsunami E909.4
Twisting, injury
due to
repetitive movement E927.3
sudden strenuous movement E927.0

V

Violence, nonaccidental (*see also* Assault)
E968.9
Volcanic eruption (any injury) E909.1
Vomitus in air passages (with asphyxia,
obstruction or suffocation) E911

W

War operations (during hostilities) (injury) (by)
(in) E995.9
after cessation of hostilities, injury due to
E998.9
air blast E993.9
aircraft burned, destroyed, exploded, shot
down E991.9
asphyxia from
chemical E997.2
fire, conflagration (caused by fire-
producing device or conventional
weapon) E990.9
from nuclear explosion (*see also*
War operations, injury
due to, nuclear weapons)
E996.8
incendiary bomb E990.0
petrol bomb E990.0
fumes E997.2
gas E997.2
baton (nightstick) E995.1
battle wound NEC E995.8
bayonet E995.2
biological warfare agents E997.1
blast (air) (effects) E993.9
from nuclear explosion - *see* War
operations, injury due to, nuclear
weapons
underwater E992.9
bomb (mortar) (explosion) E993.2
after cessation of hostilities E998.1
fragments, injury by E991.4
antipersonnel E991.3
bullet(s) (from carbine, machine gun, pistol,
rifle, shotgun) E991.2
rubber E991.0
burn from
chemical E997.2
fire, conflagration (caused by fire-
producing device or conventional
weapon) E990.9
from
conventional weapon E990.3
flamethrower E990.1
incendiary bomb E990.0
incendiary bullet E990.2
nuclear explosion E996.2
petrol bomb E990.0
gas E997.2
burning aircraft E994.3
chemical E997.2
chlorine E997.2
conventional warfare, specified form NEC
E995.8
crushing by falling aircraft E994.8
depth charge E992.1
destruction of aircraft E994.9
detonation of own munitions (ammunition)
(artillery) (mortars), unintentional
E993.6
disability as sequela one year or more after
injury E999.0
discharge of own munitions launch device
(autocannons) (automatic grenade
launchers) (missile launchers) (small
arms), unintentional E993.7
drowning E995.4
effect nuclear weapon (*see also* War
operations, injury due to, nuclear
weapons) E996.9

War operations (*Continued*)
explosion (breech block) (cannon shell)
E993.9
after cessation of hostilities
bomb placed in war E998.1
mine placed in war E998.0
aircraft E994.1
due to
enemy fire or explosives E994.0
own onboard explosives E994.1
artillery shell E993.2
bomb (mortar) E993.2
aerial E993.0
atom (*see also* War operations, injury
due to, nuclear weapons) E996.9
hydrogen (*see also* War operations,
injury due to, nuclear weapons)
E996.9
injury by fragments from E991.4
antipersonnel E991.3
nuclear (*see also* War operations, injury
due to, nuclear weapons) E996.9
depth charge E992.1
injury by fragments from E991.4
antipersonnel E991.3
marine weapon NEC E992.8
mine
at sea or in harbor E992.2
land E993.8
injury by fragments from E991.4
marine E992.2
missile, guided E993.1
mortar E993.2
munitions (accidental) (being used in
war) (dump) (factory) E993.9
own E993.7
ammunition (artillery) (mortars)
E993.6
launch device (autocannons)
(automatic grenade
launchers) (missile launchers)
(small arms) E993.7
nuclear (weapon) (*see also* War operations,
injury due to, nuclear weapons)
E996.9
own weapons (accidental) E993.7
injury by fragments from E991.9
antipersonnel E991.3
sea-based artillery shell E992.3
specified NEC E993.8
torpedo E992.0
exposure to ionizing radiation from nuclear
explosion (*see also* War operations,
injury due to, nuclear weapons) E996.3
falling aircraft E994.8
fire or fire-producing device E990.9
flamethrower E990.1
incendiary bomb E990.0
incendiary bullet E990.2
indirectly caused from conventional
weapon E990.3
petrol bomb E990.0
fireball effects from nuclear explosion E996.2
fragments from
antipersonnel bomb E991.3
artillery shell E991.4
bomb NEC E991.4
grenade E991.4
guided missile E991.4
land mine E991.4
rocket E991.4
shell E991.4
shrapnel E991.9
fumes E997.2
gas E997.2
grenade (explosion) E993.8
fragments, injury by E991.4
guided missile (explosion) E993.1
fragments, injury by E991.4
nuclear (*see also* War operations, injury
due to, nuclear weapons) E996.9

E CODES

E CODES

War operations (Continued)
   heat from nuclear explosion E996.2
   injury due to
      aerial bomb E993.0
      air blast E993.9
      aircraft shot down E994.0
      artillery shell E993.2
      blast E993.9
         wave E993.9
         wind E993.9
      bomb E993.8
      but occurring after cessation of hostilities E998.9
         explosion of bombs E998.1
         explosion of mines E998.0
         specified NEC E998.8
      conventional warfare E995.9
         specified form NEC E995.8
      depth charge E992.1
      destruction of aircraft E994.9
         due to
            air to air missile E994.0
            collision with other aircraft E994.2
            enemy fire or explosives E994.0
            on board explosion (explosives) E994.1
            on board fire E994.3
            rocket propelled grenade [RPG] E994.1
            small arms fire E994.0
            surface to air missile E994.0
         specified NEC E994.8
      dirty bomb (see also War operations, injury due to, nuclear weapons) E996.9
      drowning E995.4
      explosion (direct pressure) (indirect pressure) (due to) E993.9
         depth charge E992.1
         improvised explosive device [IED]
            person borne E993.3
            roadside E993.5
            specified NEC E993.5
            transport vehicle (air) (land) (water) borne E993.4
            vehicle (air) (land) (water) borne E993.4
         marine mines (in harbor) (at sea) E992.2
         marine weapons E992.9
            specified NEC E992.8
         sea based artillery shell E992.3
         specified NEC E993.8
         torpedo E992.0
         unintentional (of own)
            autocannons E993.7
            automatic grenade launchers E993.7
            launch device discharge E993.7
            munitions detonation (ammunition) (artillery) (mortars) E993.6
            missile launchers E993.7
            small arms E993.7
      fragments (from) E991.9
         artillery E991.8
         artillery shells E991.4
         autocannons E991.8
         automatic grenade launchers [AGL] E991.8
         bombs E991.4
            antipersonnel E991.3
         detonation of unexploded ordnance [UXO] E991.4
         grenade E991.4
         guided missile E991.4
         improvised explosive device [IED]
            person borne E991.5
            roadside E991.7
            specified NEC E991.7
            transport vehicle (air) (land) (water) borne E991.6
            vehicle (air) (land) (water) borne E991.6

War operations (Continued)
   injury due to (Continued)
      fragments (Continued)
         land mine E991.4
         missile launchers E991.8
         mortars E991.8
         munitions (artillery shells) (bombs) (grenades) (rockets) (shells) E991.4
         rockets E991.4
         shells E991.4
         small arms E991.8
         specified NEC E991.9
         weapons (artillery) (autocannons) (mortars) (small arms) E991.8
      grenade E993.8
      guided missile E993.1
      hand to hand combat, unarmed E995.0
      improvised explosive device [IED]
         person borne E993.3
         roadside E993.5
         specified NEC E993.5
         transport vehicle (air) (land) (water) borne E993.4
         vehicle (air) (land) (water) borne E993.4
      inability to surface or obtain air E995.4
      land mine E993.8
      marine mines (in harbor) (at sea) E992.2
      marine weapons E992.9
         specified NEC E992.8
      mortar E993.2
      nuclear weapons E996.9
         beta burns E996.3
         blast debris E996.1
         blast pressure E996.0
         burns due to thermal radiation E996.2
         direct blast effect E996.0
         fallout exposure E996.3
         fireball effect E996.2
         flash burns E996.2
         heat effect E996.2
         indirect blast effect E996.1
         nuclear radiation effects E996.3
         radiation exposure (acute) E996.3
         radiation sickness E996.3
         secondary effects E996.3
         specified effects NEC E996.8
         thermal radiation effect E996.2
      piercing object E995.2
      restriction of airway, intentional E995.3
      sea based artillery shell E992.3
      shrapnel E991.9
      stave E995.1
      strangulation E995.3
      strike by blunt object (baton) (nightstick) (stave) E995.1
      submersion (accidental) (unintentional) E995.4
         intentional E995.3
      suffocation E995.3
         accidental E995.4
      torpedo E992.0
      underwater blast E992.9
      weapon of mass destruction [WMD] E997.3
   knife E995.2
   lacrimator (gas) (chemical) E997.2
   land mine (explosion) E993.8
      after cessation of hostilities E998.0
      fragments, injury by E991.4
   laser(s) E997.0
   late effect of E999.0
   lewisite E997.2
   lung irritant (chemical) (fumes) (gas) E997.2
   marine mine E992.2
   mine
      after cessation of hostilities E998.0
      at sea E992.2
      in harbor E992.2
      land (explosion) E993.8
         fragments, injury by E991.4
      marine E992.2

War operations (Continued)
   missile (guided) (explosion) E993.1
      fragments, injury by E991.4
      marine E992.8
      nuclear (see also War operations, injury due to, nuclear weapons) E996.9
   mortar bomb (explosion) E993.2
      fragments, injury by E991.4
   mustard gas E997.2
   nerve gas E997.2
   phosgene E997.2
   piercing object E995.2
   poisoning (chemical) (fumes) (gas) E997.2
   radiation, ionizing from nuclear explosion (see also War operations, injury due to, nuclear weapons) E996.3
   rocket (explosion) E993.8
      fragments, injury by E991.4
   saber, sabre E995.2
   screening smoke E997.8
   shell (aircraft) (artillery) (cannon) (land based) (explosion) E993.2
      fragments, injury by E991.4
      sea-based E992.3
   shooting E991.2
      after cessation of hostilities E998.8
      bullet(s) E991.2
         rubber E991.0
      pellet(s) (rifle) E991.1
      shrapnel E991.9
   stave E995.2
   strike by blunt object (baton) (nightstick) (stave) E995.1
   submersion E995.4
      intentional E995.3
   sword E995.2
   torpedo E992.0
   unconventional warfare, except by nuclear weapon E997.9
      biological (warfare) E997.1
      gas, fumes, chemicals E997.2
      laser(s) E997.0
      specified type NEC E997.8
   underwater blast E992.9
   vesicant (chemical) (fumes) (gas) E997.2
   weapon burst E993.9
Washed
   away by flood - see Flood
   away by tidal wave - see Tidal wave
   off road by storm (transport vehicle) E908.9
   overboard E832●
Weapon of mass destruction [WMD] E997.3
Weather exposure - see also Exposure
   cold E901.0
   hot E900.0
Weightlessness (causing injury) (effects of) (in spacecraft, real or simulated) E928.0
Wound (accidental) NEC (see also Injury) E928.9
   battle (see also War operations) E995.9
   bayonet E920.3
      in
         legal intervention E974
         war operations E995.2
   gunshot - see Shooting
   incised - see Cut
   saber, sabre E920.3
      in war operations E995.2
Wrong
   body part, performance of correct operation (procedure) on E876.7
   device implanted into correct surgical site E876.5
   patient, performance of operation (procedure) on E876.6
   procedure (operation) performed on correct patient E876.5
   side, performance of correct operation (procedure) on E876.7
   site, performance of correct operation (procedure) on E876.7

◀ New   ◀|||| Revised   deleted Deleted   ● Use Additional Digit(s)   Omit code

PART III

Diseases: Tabular List Volume 1

1. INFECTIOUS AND PARASITIC DISEASES (001–139)

Note: Categories for "late effects" of infectious and parasitic diseases are to be found at 137–139.

Includes diseases generally recognized as communicable or transmissible as well as a few diseases of unknown but possibly infectious origin

Excludes *acute respiratory infections (460–466)*
carrier or suspected carrier of infectious organism (V02.0–V02.9)
certain localized infections
influenza (487.0–487.8, 488.01–488.19)

INTESTINAL INFECTIOUS DISEASES (001–009)

Excludes *helminthiases (120.0–129)*
Diseases or infestations caused by parasitic worms

● **001 Cholera**
A serious, often deadly, infectious disease of the small intestine

001.0 Due to Vibrio cholerae
(Ex) 001.0-001.9

001.1 Due to Vibrio cholerae el tor
(Ex) 001.0-001.9

001.9 Cholera, unspecified
(Ex) 001.0-001.9

● **002 Typhoid and paratyphoid fevers**
Caused by Salmonella typhi and Salmonella paratyphi A, B, and C bacteria

002.0 Typhoid fever
Typhoid (fever) (infection) [any site]
(Ex) 002.0-002.9

002.1 Paratyphoid fever A
(Ex) 002.0-002.9

002.2 Paratyphoid fever B
(Ex) 002.0-002.9

002.3 Paratyphoid fever C
(Ex) 002.0-002.9

002.9 Paratyphoid fever, unspecified
(Ex) 002.0-002.9

Item 1–1 Salmonella is a bacterium that lives in the intestines of fowl and mammals and can spread to humans through improper food preparation and cooking. Salmonellosis is an infection with the bacterium. Symptoms include diarrhea, fever, and abdominal cramps 12 to 72 hours after infection. The illness usually lasts 4 to 7 days, and most persons recover without treatment. The diarrhea may be so severe that the patient needs to be hospitalized. Patients with immunocompromised systems in chronic, ill health are more likely to have the infection invade their bloodstream with life-threatening results. For example, patients with sickle cell disease are more prone to salmonella osteomyelitis than others.

● **003 Other salmonella infections**

Includes infection or food poisoning by Salmonella [any serotype]

003.0 Salmonella gastroenteritis
Salmonellosis
(Ex) 002.0, 002.9-003.0, 004.9-005.2, 007.5, 008.00-009.0, 040.41-040.42, 536.8, 558.2-558.9, 564.1, 567.21, 567.23, 567.31-567.39, 567.89, 777.50-777.53, 777.8

003.1 Salmonella septicemia
(Ex) 003.1, 020.2, 022.3, 036.2, 038.0-038.9, 040.89-041.85, 041.89-041.9, 054.5, 139.8, 771.81, 771.83-771.89, 995.90-995.94, V09.0-V09.91

● **003.2 Localized salmonella infections**

003.20 Localized salmonella infection, unspecified
Specified in the documentation as localized, but unspecified as to type

003.21 Salmonella meningitis
Specified as localized in the meninges
(Ex) 003.21, 013.00-013.16, 036.0, 047.0-047.9, 049.0-049.1, 072.1, 078.88-078.89, 079.81, 079.88-079.99, 090.42, 091.81, 094.2, 098.89, 100.81, 112.83, 114.2, 115.01, 115.11, 115.91, 130.0, 139.8, 320.0-322.9, 349.89-349.9

003.22 Salmonella pneumonia
Specified as localized in the lungs
(Ex) 003.22, 011.00-012.16, 012.80-012.86, 017.90-017.96, 020.3-020.5, 021.3, 022.1, 031.0, 039.1, 073.0, 115.05, 115.15, 115.95, 122.1, 130.4, 136.3, 480.0-480.2, 480.8-487.1, 488.01-488.02, 488.11-488.12, 488.81-488.82, 495.0-495.7, 500, 502-508.1, 508.8-508.9, 517.1, 517.8, 518.89, 519.8-519.9, 793.11

003.23 Salmonella arthritis 🔎
Specified as localized in the joints
(Ex:) 003.23, 015.80-015.96, 036.82, 056.71, 098.50-098.51, 098.59, 098.89, 711.00-714.0, 715.00, 715.09-715.10, 715.18-716.99, 718.00-718.08, 719.00-719.10, 719.18-719.69, 719.80-719.99

003.24 Salmonella osteomyelitis 🔎
Specified as localized in bone
(Ex:) 003.24, 015.50-015.56, 015.70-015.76, 015.90-015.96, 730.00-730.39, 730.80-730.99

003.29 Other 🔎
Specified as localized (because it is still under localized heading) but does not assign into any of the above codes
(Ex:) 003.29

003.8 Other specified salmonella infections 🔎
Any specified salmonella infection which does NOT assign into any of the above codes (not specified as localized)
(Ex:) 003.8

003.9 Salmonella infection, unspecified 🔎
Unspecified in the documentation as to specific type of salmonella
(Ex:) 003.9

● **004 Shigellosis**
An infectious disease caused by a group of bacteria (Shigella)
Includes bacillary dysentery

004.0 Shigella dysenteriae 🔎
Infection by group A Shigella (Schmitz) (Shiga)
(Ex:) 001.1, 002.0, 002.9-003.0, 004.0, 004.9-005.2, 006.0-006.2, 006.9, 007.1-007.9, 008.1-008.3, 008.5, 008.8-009.0, 014.80-014.86, 040.41-040.42, 112.85, 129, 487.8, 488.00, 488.19, 488.89, 536.3, 536.8, 555.0-557.9, 558.2-558.9, 564.1, 775.0-775.7, 775.9, 777.50-777.53, 777.8

004.1 Shigella flexneri
Infection by group B Shigella

004.2 Shigella boydii
Infection by group C Shigella

004.3 Shigella sonnei
Infection by group D Shigella

004.8 Other specified shigella infections

004.9 Shigellosis, unspecified

● **005 Other food poisoning (bacterial)**
See Table A, Table of Bacterial Food Poisoning, page 1097
Excludes salmonella infections (003.0–003.9)
toxic effect of:
food contaminants (989.7)
noxious foodstuffs (988.0–988.9)

005.0 Staphylococcal food poisoning 🔎
Staphylococcal toxemia specified as due to food
(Ex:) 001.0-009.3, 040.41-040.42

005.1 Botulism food poisoning 🔎
Botulism NOS
Food poisoning due to Clostridium botulinum
Excludes infant botulism (040.41)
wound botulism (040.42)
(Ex:) 005.0-005.2, 008.45-008.46, 040.41-040.42

005.2 Food poisoning due to Clostridium perfringens [C. welchii] 🔎
Enteritis necroticans
(Ex:) 003.0, 004.9-005.2, 007.5, 008.00-009.0, 040.41-040.42, 487.8, 488.09, 488.19, 488.89, 536.3, 536.8, 558.2-558.9, 564.1, 567.21, 567.23, 567.31-567.39, 567.89, 777.50-777.53, 777.8

005.3 Food poisoning due to other Clostridia 🔎
(Ex:) 001.0-009.3, 040.41-040.42

005.4 Food poisoning due to Vibrio parahaemolyticus 🔎
(Ex:) 001.0-009.3, 040.41-040.42

● **005.8 Other bacterial food poisoning**
Excludes salmonella food poisoning (003.0–003.9)

005.81 Food poisoning due to Vibrio vulnificus 🔎
(Ex:) 001.0-009.3, 040.41-040.42

005.89 Other bacterial food poisoning 🔎
Food poisoning due to Bacillus cereus
(Ex:) 001.0-009.3, 040.41-040.42

005.9 Food poisoning, unspecified

● **006 Amebiasis**
An intestinal illness caused by the microscopic parasite Entamoeba histolytica
Includes infection due to Entamoeba histolytica
Excludes amebiasis due to organisms other than Entamoeba histolytica (007.8)

006.0 Acute amebic dysentery without mention of abscess 🔎
Acute amebiasis
(Ex:) 006.0-006.1, 007.5

006.1 Chronic intestinal amebiasis without mention of abscess 🔎
Chronic:
amebiasis
amebic dysentery
(Ex:) 006.0-006.1, 007.5

006.2 Amebic nondysenteric colitis 🔎
(Ex:) 003.0, 004.9-005.0, 005.2, 006.0-006.2, 006.9, 007.1-009.0, 129, 487.8, 488.09, 488.19, 488.89, 536.3, 536.8, 555.0-557.9, 558.2-558.9, 564.1, 777.50-777.53, 777.8

006.3 Amebic liver abscess 🔎
Hepatic amebiasis
(Ex:) 006.3, 572.0

006.4 Amebic lung abscess 🔎
Amebic abscess of lung (and liver)
(Ex:) 006.4, 513.0

006.5 Amebic brain abscess 🔎
Amebic abscess of brain (and liver) (and lung)
(Ex:) 006.5, 324.0

006.6 Amebic skin ulceration
Cutaneous amebiasis

006.8 Amebic infection of other sites 🔎
Amebic:
appendicitis
balanitis
Ameboma
Excludes specific infections by free-living amebae (136.21–136.29)
(Ex:) 006.0-006.5, 006.8

006.9 Amebiasis, unspecified
Amebiasis NOS

● **007 Other protozoal intestinal diseases**
Includes protozoal:
colitis
diarrhea
dysentery

007.0 Balantidiasis
Infection by Balantidium coli

007.1 Giardiasis 🔎
Infection by Giardia lamblia
Lambliasis
(Ex:) 003.0, 004.9-005.0, 005.2, 006.0-006.2, 006.9, 007.1-009.0, 129, 487.8, 488.09, 488.19, 488.89, 536.3, 536.8, 558.2-558.9, 564.1

007.2 Coccidiosis 🔎
Infection by Isospora belli and Isospora hominis
Isosporiasis
(Ex:) 003.0, 004.9-005.0, 005.2, 006.0-006.2, 006.9, 007.1-009.0, 129, 487.8, 488.09, 488.19, 488.89, 536.3, 536.8, 558.2-558.9, 564.1

007.3 Intestinal trichomoniasis

007.4 Cryptosporidiosis 🔎
(Ex:) 003.0, 004.9-005.0, 005.2, 006.0-006.2, 006.9, 007.1-009.0, 129, 487.8, 488.09, 488.19, 488.89, 536.3, 536.8, 558.2-558.9, 564.1
Coding Clinic: 1997, Q4, P30-31

007.5 Cyclosporiasis 🔎
(Ex:) 003.0, 004.9-005.0, 005.2, 006.0-006.2, 006.9, 007.1-009.0, 129, 487.8, 488.09, 488.19, 488.89, 536.3, 536.8, 558.2-558.9, 564.1, 567.21, 567.23, 567.31-567.39, 567.89

007.8 Other specified protozoal intestinal diseases 🔎
Amebiasis due to organisms other than Entamoeba histolytica
(Ex:) 003.0, 004.9-005.0, 005.2, 006.0-006.2, 006.9, 007.1-009.0, 129, 487.8, 488.09, 488.19, 488.89, 536.3, 536.8, 558.2-558.9, 564.1

◀ New   ◀ Revised   ~~deleted~~ Deleted   Excludes   Includes   Use additional   Code first   Omit code
● Unacceptable Principal Diagnosis   ● Use Additional Digit(s)   ▶ Manifestation Code   OGCR Official Guidelines   Coding Clinic

670

007.9 Unspecified protozoal intestinal disease 🔾
Flagellate diarrhea
Protozoal dysentery NOS
Ⓔ 003.0, 004.9-005.0, 005.2, 006.0-006.2, 006.9, 007.1-009.0, 129, 487.8, 488.09, 488.19, 488.89, 536.3, 536.8, 558.2-558.9, 564.1

● **008   Intestinal infections due to other organisms**

⬛ **Includes**   any condition classifiable to 009.0–009.3 with mention of the responsible organisms

⬛ **Excludes**   *food poisoning by these organisms (005.0–005.9)*

● **008.0 Escherichia coli [E. coli]**
Coding Clinic: 1988, Q2, P10

008.00 E. coli, unspecified 🔾
E. coli enteritis NOS
Ⓔ 003.0, 004.9-005.0, 005.2, 007.5, 008.00-009.0, 487.8, 488.09, 488.19, 488.89, 536.3, 536.8, 558.2-558.9, 564.1, 567.21, 567.23, 567.31-567.39, 567.89, 777.50-777.53, 777.8

008.01 Enteropathogenic E. coli 🔾
Ⓔ 003.0, 004.9-005.0, 005.2, 007.5, 008.00-009.0, 487.8, 488.09, 488.19, 488.89, 536.3, 536.8, 558.2-558.9, 564.1, 567.21, 567.23, 567.31-567.39, 567.89, 777.50-777.53, 777.8

008.02 Enterotoxigenic E. coli 🔾
Ⓔ 003.0, 004.9-005.0, 005.2, 007.5, 008.00-009.0, 487.8, 488.09, 488.19, 488.89, 536.3, 536.8, 558.2-558.9, 564.1, 567.21, 567.23, 567.31-567.39, 567.89, 777.50-777.53, 777.8

008.03 Enteroinvasive E. coli 🔾
Ⓔ 003.0, 004.9-005.0, 005.2, 007.5, 008.00-009.0, 487.8, 488.09, 488.19, 488.89, 536.3, 536.8, 558.2-558.9, 564.1, 567.21, 567.23, 567.31-567.39, 567.89, 777.50-777.53, 777.8

008.04 Enterohemorrhagic E. coli 🔾
Ⓔ 003.0, 004.9-005.0, 005.2, 007.5, 008.00-009.0, 487.8, 488.09, 488.19, 488.89, 536.3, 536.8, 558.2-558.9, 564.1, 567.21, 567.23, 567.31-567.39, 567.89, 777.50-777.53, 777.8
Coding Clinic: 2011, Q4, P83

008.09 Other intestinal E. coli infections 🔾
Ⓔ 003.0, 004.9-005.0, 005.2, 007.5, 008.00-009.0, 487.8, 488.09, 488.19, 488.89, 536.3, 536.8, 558.2-558.9, 564.1, 567.21, 567.23, 567.31-567.39, 567.89, 777.50-777.53, 777.8

008.1 Arizona group of paracolon bacilli 🔾
Ⓔ 003.0, 004.9-005.0, 005.2, 007.5, 008.00-009.0, 487.8, 488.09, 488.19, 488.89, 536.3, 536.8, 558.2-558.9, 564.1, 567.21, 567.23, 567.31-567.39, 567.89, 777.50-777.53, 777.8

008.2 Aerobacter aerogenes 🔾
Enterobacter aerogenes
Ⓔ 003.0, 004.9-005.0, 005.2, 007.5, 008.00-009.0, 487.8, 488.09, 488.19, 488.89, 536.3, 536.8, 558.2-558.9, 564.1, 567.21, 567.23, 567.31-567.39, 567.89, 777.50-777.53, 777.8

008.3 Proteus (mirabilis) (morganii) 🔾
Ⓔ 003.0, 004.9-005.0, 005.2, 007.5, 008.00-009.0, 487.8, 488.09, 488.19, 488.89, 536.3, 536.8, 558.2-558.9, 564.1, 567.21, 567.23, 567.31-567.39, 567.89, 777.50-777.53, 777.8

● **008.4 Other specified bacteria**

008.41 Staphylococcus 🔾
Staphylococcal enterocolitis
Ⓔ 001.1, 002.0, 002.9-003.0, 004.9-005.2, 006.0-006.2, 006.9, 007.1-009.0, 014.80-014.86, 040.41-040.42, 112.85, 129, 487.8, 488.09, 488.19, 488.89, 536.3, 536.8, 555.0-557.9, 558.2-558.9, 564.1, 775.0-775.7, 775.9, 777.50-777.53, 777.8

008.42 Pseudomonas 🔾
Ⓔ 001.1, 002.0, 002.9-003.0, 004.9-005.2, 006.0-006.2, 006.9, 007.1-009.0, 014.80-014.86, 040.41-040.42, 112.85, 129, 487.8, 488.09, 488.19, 488.89, 536.3, 536.8, 555.0-557.9, 558.2-558.9, 564.1, 775.0-775.7, 775.9, 777.50-777.53, 777.8
Coding Clinic: 1989, Q2, P10

008.43 Campylobacter 🔾
Ⓔ 001.1, 002.0, 002.9-003.0, 004.9-005.2, 006.0-006.2, 006.9, 007.1-009.0, 014.80-014.86, 040.41-040.42, 112.85, 129, 487.8, 488.09, 488.19, 488.89, 536.3, 536.8, 555.0-557.9, 558.2-558.9, 564.1, 775.0-775.7, 775.9, 777.50-777.53, 777.8

008.44 Yersinia enterocolitica 🔾
Ⓔ 001.1, 002.0, 002.9-003.0, 004.9-005.2, 006.0-006.2, 006.9, 007.1-009.0, 014.80-014.86, 040.41-040.42, 112.85, 129, 487.8, 488.09, 488.19, 488.89, 536.3, 536.8, 555.0-557.9, 558.2-558.9, 564.1, 775.0-775.7, 775.9, 777.50-777.53, 777.8

008.45 Clostridium difficile 🔾
Pseudomembranous colitis
Ⓔ 001.1, 002.0, 002.9-003.0, 004.9-005.2, 006.0-006.2, 006.9, 007.1-009.0, 014.80-014.86, 040.41-040.42, 112.85, 129, 487.8, 488.09, 488.19, 488.89, 536.3, 536.8, 555.0-557.9, 558.2-558.9, 564.1, 775.0-775.7, 775.9, 777.50-777.53, 777.8

008.46 Other anaerobes 🔾
Anaerobic enteritis NOS
Bacteroides (fragilis)
Gram-negative anaerobes
Ⓔ 001.1, 002.0, 002.9-003.0, 004.9-005.2, 006.0-006.2, 006.9, 007.1-009.0, 014.80-014.86, 040.41-040.42, 112.85, 129, 487.8, 488.09, 488.19, 488.89, 536.3, 536.8, 555.0-557.9, 558.2-558.9, 564.1, 775.0-775.7, 775.9, 777.50-777.53, 777.8

008.47 Other gram-negative bacteria 🔾
Gram-negative enteritis NOS
⬛ **Excludes**   *gram-negative anaerobes (008.46)*
Ⓔ 001.1, 002.0, 002.9-003.0, 004.9-005.2, 006.0-006.2, 006.9, 007.1-009.0, 014.80-014.86, 040.41-040.42, 112.85, 129, 487.8, 488.09, 488.19, 488.89, 536.3, 536.8, 555.0-557.9, 558.2-558.9, 564.1, 775.0-775.7, 775.9, 777.50-777.53, 777.8

008.49 Other 🔾
Ⓔ 001.1, 002.0, 002.9-003.0, 004.9-005.2 006.0-006.2, 006.9, 007.1-009.0, 014.80-014.86, 040.41-040.42, 112.85, 129, 487.8, 488.09, 488.19, 488.89, 536.3, 536.8, 555.0-557.9, 558.2-558.9, 564.1, 775.0-775.7, 775.9, 777.50-777.53, 777.8
Coding Clinic: 1989, Q2, P10

008.5 Bacterial enteritis, unspecified 🔾
Ⓔ 001.1, 002.0, 002.9-003.0, 004.9-005.0, 005.2, 006.0-006.2, 006.9, 007.1-009.0 014.80-014.86, 112.85, 129, 487.8, 488.09, 488.19, 488.89, 536.3, 536.8, 558.2-558.9, 564.1, 567.21, 567.23, 567.31-567.39, 567.89, 777.50-777.53, 777.8

● **008.6 Enteritis due to specified virus**

008.61 Rotavirus 🔾
Ⓔ 003.0, 004.9-005.0, 005.2, 006.0-006.2, 006.9, 007.1-009.0, 014.80-014.86, 112.85, 129, 487.8, 488.09, 488.19, 488.89, 536.3, 536.8, 558.2-558.9, 564.1, 567.21, 567.23, 567.31-567.39, 567.89, 777.50-777.53, 777.8

008.62 Adenovirus 🔾
Ⓔ 003.0, 004.9-005.0, 005.2, 006.0-006.2, 006.9, 007.1-009.0, 014.80-014.86, 112.85, 129, 487.8, 488.09, 488.19, 536.3, 536.8, 558.2-558.9, 564.1, 567.21, 567.23, 567.31-567.39, 567.89, 777.50-777.53, 777.8

008.63 Norwalk virus 🔾
Norovirus
Norwalk-like agent
Ⓔ 003.0, 004.9-005.0, 005.2, 006.0-006.2, 006.9, 007.1-009.0, 014.80-014.86, 112.85, 129, 487.8, 488.09, 488.19, 488.89, 536.3, 536.8, 558.2-558.9, 564.1, 567.21, 567.23, 567.31-567.39, 567.89, 777.50-777.53, 777.8

008.64 Other small round viruses [SRV's] 🔾
Small round virus NOS
Ⓔ 003.0, 004.9-005.0, 005.2, 006.0-006.2, 006.9, 007.1-009.0, 014.80-014.86, 112.85, 129, 487.8, 488.09, 488.19, 488.89, 536.3, 536.8, 558.2-558.9, 564.1, 567.21, 567.23, 567.31-567.39, 567.89, 777.50-777.53, 777.8

Figure 1-1   Electron micrograph of escherichia coli *(E. coli)* expressing P fimbriae. (From Mandell, Bennett, & Dolin: Principles and Practice of Infectious Diseases, ed 7, Churchill Livingstone, An Imprint of Elsevier, 2009)

Item 1-2   *Escherichia coli [E. coli]* is a gram-negative bacterium found in the intestinal tracts of humans and animals and is usually nonpathogenic. Pathogenic strains can cause diarrhea or pyogenic (pus-producing) infections. Can be a threat to food safety.

INFECTIOUS AND PARASITIC DISEASES (001–139)

INFECTIOUS AND PARASITIC DISEASES (001–139)

008.65   Calicivirus (Ex)
(Ex) 003.0, 004.9-005.0, 005.2, 006.0-006.2, 006.9, 007.1-009.0,
014.80-014.86, 112.85, 129, 487.8, 488.09, 488.19, 488.89,
536.3, 536.8, 558.2-558.9, 564.1, 567.21, 567.23,
567.31-567.39, 567.89, 777.50-777.53, 777.8

008.66   Astrovirus (Ex)
(Ex) 003.0, 004.9-005.0, 005.2, 006.0-006.2, 006.9, 007.1-009.0,
014.80-014.86, 112.85, 129, 487.8, 488.09, 488.19, 488.89,
536.3, 536.8, 558.2-558.9, 564.1, 567.21, 567.23,
567.31-567.39, 567.89, 777.50-777.53, 777.8

008.67   Enterovirus NEC (Ex)
Coxsackie virus
Echovirus
> **Excludes**   *poliovirus (045.0–045.9)*
(Ex) 003.0, 004.9-005.0, 005.2, 006.0-006.2, 006.9, 007.1-009.0,
014.80-014.86, 112.85, 129, 487.8, 488.09, 488.19, 536.3,
536.8, 558.2-558.9, 564.1, 567.21, 567.23, 567.31-567.39,
567.89, 777.50-777.53, 777.8

008.69   Other viral enteritis (Ex)
Torovirus
(Ex) 003.0, 004.9-005.0, 005.2, 006.0-006.2, 006.9, 007.1-009.0,
014.80-014.86, 112.85, 129, 487.8, 488.09, 488.19, 488.89,
536.3, 536.8, 558.2-558.9, 564.1, 567.21, 567.23,
567.31-567.39, 567.89, 777.50-777.53, 777.8
Coding Clinic: 2003, Q1, P10-11

008.8   Other organism, not elsewhere classified
Viral:
  enteritis NOS
  gastroenteritis
> **Excludes**   *influenza with involvement of gastrointestinal tract (487.8, 488.09, 488.19)*

● **009   Ill-defined intestinal infections**
> **Excludes**   *diarrheal disease or intestinal infection due to specified organism (001.0–008.8)*
> *diarrhea following gastrointestinal surgery (564.4)*
> *intestinal malabsorption (579.0–579.9)*
> *ischemic enteritis (557.0–557.9)*
> *other noninfectious gastroenteritis and colitis (558.1–558.9)*
> *regional enteritis (555.0–555.9)*
> *ulcerative colitis (556)*

009.0   Infectious colitis, enteritis, and gastroenteritis (Ex)
Colitis (septic)   Enteritis (septic)
Dysentery: Gastroenteritis (septic)
  NOS
  catarrhal
  hemorrhagic
(Ex) 001.0-009.3, 040.41-040.42
Coding Clinic: 1988, Q2, P10

009.1   Colitis, enteritis, and gastroenteritis of presumed infectious origin (Ex)
> **Excludes**   *colitis NOS (558.9)*
> *enteritis NOS (558.9)*
> *gastroenteritis NOS (558.9)*
(Ex) 009.1
Coding Clinic: 1999, Q3, P6-7

009.2   Infectious diarrhea (Ex)
Diarrhea:
  dysenteric
  epidemic
Infectious diarrheal disease NOS
(Ex) 001.0-009.3, 040.41-040.42

009.3   Diarrhea of presumed infectious origin (Ex)
> **Excludes**   *diarrhea NOS (787.91)*
(Ex) 009.3
Coding Clinic: 1987, Nov-Dec, P7

TUBERCULOSIS (010–018)

Includes   infection by Mycobacterium tuberculosis (human) (bovine)
Excludes   *congenital tuberculosis (771.2)*
late effects of tuberculosis (137.0–137.4)

The following fifth-digit subclassification is for use with categories 010–018:

> 0   unspecified
> 1   bacteriological or histological examination not done
> 2   bacteriological or histological examination unknown (at present)
> 3   tubercle bacilli found (in sputum) by microscopy
> 4   tubercle bacilli not found (in sputum) by microscopy, but found by bacterial culture
> 5   tubercle bacilli not found by bacteriological examination, but tuberculosis confirmed histologically
> 6   tubercle bacilli not found by bacteriological or histological examination, but tuberculosis confirmed by other methods [inoculation of animals]

● **010   Primary tuberculous infection**
Requires fifth digit. See beginning of section 010–018 for codes and definitions.
● **010.0   Primary tuberculous infection** (Ex)
[0-6]
> **Excludes**   *nonspecific reaction to test for tuberculosis without active tuberculosis (795.51-795.52)*
> *positive PPD (795.51)*
> *positive tuberculin skin test without active tuberculosis (795.51)*
(Ex) 010.00-018.96

● **010.1   Tuberculous pleurisy in primary progressive** (Ex)
[0-6]   **tuberculosis**
(Ex) 010.00-018.96

● **010.8   Other primary progressive tuberculosis** (Ex)
[0-6]
> **Excludes**   *tuberculous erythema nodosum (017.1)*
(Ex) 010.00-018.96

● **010.9   Primary tuberculous infection, unspecified** (Ex)
[0-6]   (Ex) 010.00-018.96

● **011   Pulmonary tuberculosis**
Requires fifth digit. See beginning of section 010–018 for codes and definitions.
Use additional code to identify any associated silicosis (502)
● **011.0   Tuberculosis of lung, infiltrative** (Ex)
[0-6]   (Ex) 011.00-012.86, 017.90-018.96, 031.0, 031.2-031.9, 041.81-041.9, 137.0,
139.8, 480.0-480.2, 480.8-487.1, 488.01-488.02, 488.11-488.12,
488.81-488.82, 494.0-508.1, 508.8-508.9, 517.1, 518.89, 793.11

Figure 1–2   Far advanced bilateral pulmonary tuberculosis before and after 8 months of treatment with streptomycin, PAS, and isoniazid. (From Hinshaw HC, Garland LH: Diseases of the Chest, ed 4, Philadelphia, WB Saunders, 1980)

Item 1–3   Tuberculosis is a common and deadly infectious disease caused by the *Mycobacterium tuberculosis* organism. The first tuberculosis infection is called the **primary infection** and most commonly attacks the lungs but can affect the central nervous system, lymphatic system, circulatory system, genitourinary system, bones, joints, and even the skin. A **Ghon** lesion is the **initial lesion.** A **secondary lesion** occurs when the tubercle bacilli are carried to other areas.

◀ New   ◀ⁱⁱ Revised   ~~deleted~~ Deleted   Excludes   Includes   Use additional   Code first   Omit code
● Unacceptable Principal Diagnosis   ● Use Additional Digit(s)   ▶ Manifestation Code   OGCR Official Guidelines   Coding Clinic

● **011.1 Tuberculosis of lung, nodular**🔴
[0-6]   (Ex:) 011.00-012.86, 017.90-018.96, 031.0, 031.2-031.9, 041.81-041.9, 137.0,
             139.8, 480.0-480.2, 480.8-487.1, 488.01-488.02, 488.11-488.12,
             494.0-508.1, 508.8-508.9, 517.1, 518.89, 793.11

● **011.2 Tuberculosis of lung with cavitation**🔴
[0-6]   *Cavitation = pitting*
             (Ex:) 011.00-012.86, 017.90-018.96, 031.0, 031.2-031.9, 041.81-041.9, 137.0,
             139.8, 480.0-480.2, 480.8-487.1, 488.01-488.02, 488.11-488.12,
             488.81-488.82, 494.0-508.1, 508.8-508.9, 517.1, 518.89, 793.11
           Coding Clinic: 1994, Q4, P36

● **011.3 Tuberculosis of bronchus**🔴
[0-6]   **Excludes**   *isolated bronchial tuberculosis (012.2)*
             (Ex:) 011.00-012.86, 017.90-018.96, 031.0, 031.2-031.9, 041.81-041.9, 137.0,
             139.8, 480.0-480.2, 480.8-487.1, 488.01-488.02, 488.11-488.12,
             488.81-488.82, 494.0-508.1, 508.8-508.9, 517.1, 518.89

● **011.4 Tuberculous fibrosis of lung**🔴
[0-6]   (Ex:) 011.00-012.86, 017.90-018.96, 031.0, 031.2-031.9, 041.81-041.9, 137.0,
             139.8, 480.0-480.2, 480.8-487.1, 488.01-488.02, 488.11-488.12,
             488.81-488.82, 494.0-508.1, 508.8-508.9, 517.1, 518.89, 793.11

● **011.5 Tuberculous bronchiectasis**🔴
[0-6]   (Ex:) 011.00-012.86, 017.90-018.96, 031.0, 031.2-031.9, 041.81-041.9, 137.0,
             139.8, 480.0-480.2, 480.8-487.1, 488.01-488.02, 488.11-488.12,
             488.81-488.82, 494.0-508.1, 508.8-508.9, 517.1, 518.89, 793.11

● **011.6 Tuberculous pneumonia [any form]**🔴
[0-6]   For codes **011.60-011.65:** (Ex:) 011.00-012.86, 017.90-018.96, 031.0,
             031.2-031.9, 041.81-041.9, 137.0, 139.8, 480.0-480.2, 480.8-487.1,
             488.01-488.02, 488.11-488.12, 488.81-488.82, 494.0-508.1, 508.8-508.9,
             517.1, 518.89, 793.11
             For code **011.66:** (Ex:) 011.66, 139.8, 480.0-480.2, 480.8-487.1, 488.01-488.02,
             488.11-488.12, 488.81-488.82, 494.0-508.1, 508.8-508.9, 517.1, 518.89,
             793.11

● **011.7 Tuberculous pneumothorax**🔴
[0-6]   (Ex:) 011.00-012.86, 017.90-018.96, 031.0, 031.2-031.9, 041.81-041.9, 137.0,
             139.8, 480.0-480.2, 480.8-487.1, 488.01-488.02, 488.11-488.12,
             488.81-488.82, 494.0-508.1, 508.8-508.9, 517.1, 518.89, 793.11

● **011.8 Other specified pulmonary tuberculosis**🔴
[0-6]   (Ex:) 011.00-012.86, 017.90-018.96, 031.0, 031.2-031.9, 041.81-041.9, 137.0,
             139.8, 480.0-480.2, 480.8-487.1, 488.01-488.02, 488.11-488.12,
             488.81-488.82, 494.0-508.1, 508.8-508.9, 517.1, 518.89, 793.11

● **011.9 Pulmonary tuberculosis, unspecified**🔴
[0-6]   Respiratory tuberculosis NOS
           Tuberculosis of lung NOS
             (Ex:) 011.00-012.86, 017.90-018.96, 031.0, 031.2-031.9, 041.81-041.9, 137.0,
             139.8, 480.0-480.2, 480.8-487.1, 488.01-488.02, 488.11-488.12,
             488.81-488.82, 494.0-508.1, 508.8-508.9, 517.1, 518.89, 793.11

● **012 Other respiratory tuberculosis**
           Requires fifth digit. See beginning of section 010–018 for codes
           and definitions.
           Excludes   *respiratory tuberculosis, unspecified (011.9)*

● **012.0 Tuberculous pleurisy**🔴
[0-6]   Tuberculosis of pleura
           Tuberculous empyema
           Tuberculous hydrothorax
           Excludes   *pleurisy with effusion without mention of cause
                       (511.9)*
                       *tuberculous pleurisy in primary progressive
                       tuberculosis (010.1)*
             (Ex:) 011.00-012.86, 017.90-018.96, 031.0 031.2-031.9, 041.81-041.9, 137.0,
             139.8, 480.0-480.2, 480.8-487.1, 488.01-488.02, 488.11-488.12,
             488.81-488.82, 494.0-508.1, 508.8-508.9, 517.1, 518.89, 793.11

● **012.1 Tuberculosis of intrathoracic lymph nodes**🔴
[0-6]   Tuberculosis of lymph nodes:
             hilar
             mediastinal
             tracheobronchial
           Tuberculous tracheobronchial adenopathy
           Excludes   *that specified as primary (010.0–010.9)*
             (Ex:) 011.00-012.86, 017.90-018.96, 031.0, 031.2-031.9, 041.81-041.9, 137.0,
             139.8, 480.0-480.2, 480.8-487.1, 488.01-488.02, 488.11-488.12,
             488.81-488.82, 494.0-508.1, 508.8-508.9, 517.1, 518.89, 793.11

● **012.2 Isolated tracheal or bronchial tuberculosis**🔴
[0-6]   (Ex:) 010.00-014.86, 018.00-018.96

● **012.3 Tuberculous laryngitis**🔴
[0-6]   Tuberculosis of glottis
             (Ex:) 010.00-014.86, 018.00-018.96

● **012.8 Other specified respiratory tuberculosis**🔴
[0-6]   Tuberculosis of:
             mediastinum
             nasopharynx
             nose (septum)
             sinus [any nasal]
             (Ex:) 010.00-014.86, 018.00-018.96

● **013 Tuberculosis of meninges and central nervous system**
           Requires fifth digit. See beginning of section 010–018 for codes
           and definitions.

● **013.0 Tuberculous meningitis**🔴
[0-6]   Tuberculosis of meninges (cerebral) (spinal)
           Tuberculous:
             leptomeningitis
             meningoencephalitis
           Excludes   *tuberculoma of meninges (013.1)*
             (Ex:) 003.21, 013.00-013.16, 013.40-013.56, 013.80-013.96, 017.90-017.96,
             031.2-031.9, 036.0, 041.81-041.9, 047.0-047.9, 049.0-049.1, 053.0,
             054.72, 072.1, 090.42, 091.81, 094.2, 098.89, 100.81, 112.83, 114.2,
             115.01, 115.11, 115.91, 130.0, 137.1, 139.8, 320.0-322.9, 349.89-349.9,
             357.0

● **013.1 Tuberculoma of meninges**🔴
[0-6]   (Ex:) 003.21, 013.00-013.16, 013.40-013.56, 013.80-013.96, 017.90-017.96,
             031.2-031.9, 036.0, 041.81-041.9, 047.0-047.9, 049.0-049.1, 053.0,
             054.72, 072.1, 090.42, 091.81, 094.2, 098.89, 100.81, 112.83, 114.2,
             115.01, 115.11, 115.91, 130.0, 137.1, 139.8, 320.0-322.9, 349.89-349.9,
             357.0

● **013.2 Tuberculoma of brain**🔴
[0-6]   Tuberculosis of brain (current disease)
             (Ex:) 013.20-013.36, 013.60-013.96, 017.90-017.96, 031.2-031.9, 041.81-041.9,
             137.1, 139.8

● **013.3 Tuberculous abscess of brain**🔴
[0-6]   (Ex:) 013.20-013.36, 013.60-013.96, 017.90-017.96, 031.2-031.9, 041.81-041.9,
             137.1, 139.8

● **013.4 Tuberculoma of spinal cord**🔴
[0-6]   (Ex:) 013.00-013.16, 013.40-013.56, 013.80-013.96, 017.90-017.96, 031.2-031.9,
             041.81-041.9, 137.1, 139.8

● **013.5 Tuberculous abscess of spinal cord**🔴
[0-6]   (Ex:) 013.00-013.16, 013.40-013.56, 013.80-013.96, 017.90-017.96, 031.2-031.9,
             041.81-041.9, 137.1, 139.8

● **013.6 Tuberculous encephalitis or myelitis**🔴
[0-6]   (Ex:) 013.20-013.36, 013.60-013.96, 017.90-017.96, 031.2-031.9, 041.81-041.9,
             137.1, 139.8

● **013.8 Other specified tuberculosis of central nervous**
[0-6] **system**🔴
             (Ex:) 013.80-013.96, 017.90-017.96, 031.2-031.9, 041.81-041.9, 137.1, 139.8

● **013.9 Unspecified tuberculosis of central nervous**
[0-6] **system**🔴
           Tuberculosis of central nervous system NOS
             (Ex:) 013.80-013.96, 017.90-017.96, 031.2-031.9, 041.81-041.9, 137.1, 139.8

INFECTIOUS AND PARASITIC DISEASES (001–139)

Item 1–4 Although it primarily affects the lungs, the bacteria
Mycobacterium tuberculosis can travel from the pulmonary circulation to
virtually any organ in the body, much as a cancer metastasizes to a secondary
site. If the immune system becomes compromised by age or disease, what
would otherwise be a self-limiting primary tuberculosis in the lungs will develop
in other organs. These are known as extrapulmonary sites.

● **014　Tuberculosis of intestines, peritoneum, and mesenteric glands**
　　Requires fifth digit. See beginning of section 010–018 for codes and definitions.

● **014.0　Tuberculous peritonitis** 🦠
　[0-6]　Tuberculous ascites
　　(Ex) 014.00-014.86, 017.90-017.96, 031.2-031.9, 041.81-041.9, 139.8

● **014.8　Other** 🦠
　[0-6]　Tuberculosis (of):
　　　anus
　　　intestine (large) (small)
　　　mesenteric glands
　　　rectum
　　　retroperitoneal (lymph nodes)
　　Tuberculous enteritis
　　(Ex) 014.00-014.86, 017.90-017.96, 031.2-031.9, 041.81-041.9, 139.8

● **015　Tuberculosis of bones and joints**
　　Requires fifth digit. See beginning of section 010–018 for codes and definitions.
　　Use additional code to identify manifestation, as:
　　tuberculous:
　　　arthropathy (711.4)
　　　necrosis of bone (730.8)
　　　osteitis (730.8)
　　　osteomyelitis (730.8)
　　　synovitis (727.01)
　　　tenosynovitis (727.01)

● **015.0　Vertebral column** 🦠
　[0-6]　Pott's disease
　　Use additional code to identify manifestation, as:
　　　curvature of spine [Pott's] (737.4)
　　　kyphosis (737.4)
　　　spondylitis (720.81)
　　(Ex) 015.00-015.06

● **015.1　Hip** 🦠
　[0-6]　(Ex) 015.10-015.16

● **015.2　Knee** 🦠
　[0-6]　(Ex) 015.20-015.26

● **015.5　Limb bones** 🦠
　[0-6]　Tuberculous dactylitis
　　(Ex) 015.10-015.56

● **015.6　Mastoid** 🦠
　[0-6]　Tuberculous mastoiditis
　　(Ex) 015.60-015.66

● **015.7　Other specified bone** 🦠
　[0-6]　(Ex) 015.00-015.70

● **015.8　Other specified joint** 🦠
　[0-6]　(Ex) 015.80-015.86

● **015.9　Tuberculosis of unspecified bones and joints** 🦠
　[0-6]　(Ex) 015.00-015.66, 015.80-015.96

● **016　Tuberculosis of genitourinary system**
　　Requires fifth digit. See beginning of section 010–018 for codes and definitions.

● **016.0　Kidney** 🦠
　[0-6]　Renal tuberculosis
　　Use additional code to identify manifestation, as:
　　tuberculous:
　　　nephropathy (583.81)
　　　pyelitis (590.81)
　　　pyelonephritis (590.81)
　　(Ex) 016.00-016.36, 016.90-016.96, 017.90-017.96, 031.2-031.9, 041.81-041.9, 137.2, 139.8

● **016.1　Bladder** 🦠
　[0-6]　(Ex) 016.00-016.36, 016.90-016.96, 017.90-017.96, 031.2-031.9, 041.81-041.9, 137.2, 139.8

● **016.2　Ureter** 🦠
　[0-6]　(Ex) 016.00-016.36, 016.90-016.96, 017.90-017.96, 031.2-031.9, 041.81-041.9, 137.2, 139.8

● **016.3　Other urinary organs** 🦠
　[0-6]　(Ex) 016.00-016.36, 016.90-016.96, 017.90-017.96, 031.2-031.9, 041.81-041.9, 137.2, 139.8

● **016.4　Epididymis** ♂ 🦠
　[0-6]　(Ex) 016.40-165.6, 016.90-016.96, 017.90-017.96, 031.2-031.9, 041.81-041.9, 137.2, 139.8

● **016.5　Other male genital organs** ♂ 🦠
　[0-6]　Use additional code to identify manifestation, as:
　　tuberculosis of:
　　　prostate (601.4)
　　　seminal vesicle (608.81)
　　　testis (608.81)
　　(Ex) 016.40-016.56, 016.90-016.96, 017.90-017.96, 031.2-031.9, 041.81-041.9, 137.2, 139.8

● **016.6　Tuberculous oophoritis and salpingitis** ♀ 🦠
　[0-6]　*Oophoritis = inflammation of ovary*
　　Salpingitis = inflammation of fallopian tube
　　(Ex) 016.60-016.96, 017.90-017.96, 031.2-031.9, 041.81-041.9, 137.2, 139.8

● **016.7　Other female genital organs** ♀ 🦠
　[0-6]　Tuberculous:
　　　cervicitis
　　　endometritis
　　(Ex) 016.60-016.96, 017.90-017.96, 031.2-031.9, 041.81-041.9, 137.2, 139.8

● **016.9　Genitourinary tuberculosis, unspecified** 🦠
　[0-6]　(Ex) 016.90-016.96, 017.90-017.96, 031.2-031.9, 041.81-041.9, 137.2, 139.8

● **017　Tuberculosis of other organs**
　　Requires fifth digit. See beginning of section 010–018 for codes and definitions.

● **017.0　Skin and subcutaneous cellular tissue** 🦠
　[0-6]　Lupus:　　　　　　Tuberculosis:
　　　exedens　　　　　　colliquativa
　　　vulgaris　　　　　　cutis
　　Scrofuloderma　　　lichenoides
　　　　　　　　　　　　papulonecrotica
　　　　　　　　　　　　verrucosa cutis
　　Excludes　*lupus erythematosus (695.4)*
　　　　　　　　disseminated (710.0)
　　　　　　lupus NOS (710.0)
　　　　　nonspecific reaction to test for tuberculosis without active tuberculosis (795.51-795.52)
　　　　　positive PPD (795.51)
　　　　　positive tuberculin skin test without active tuberculosis (795.51)
　　(Ex) 010.00-018.96

● **017.1　Erythema nodosum with hypersensitivity reaction in tuberculosis**
　[0-6]　Bazin's disease
　　Erythema:
　　　induratum
　　　nodosum, tuberculous
　　Tuberculosis indurativa
　　Excludes　*erythema nodosum NOS (695.2)*

● **017.2　Peripheral lymph nodes** 🦠
　[0-6]　Scrofula
　　Scrofulous abscess
　　Tuberculous adenitis
　　Excludes　*tuberculosis of lymph nodes:*
　　　　　bronchial and mediastinal (012.1)
　　　　　mesenteric and retroperitoneal (014.8)
　　　　tuberculous tracheobronchial adenopathy (012.1)
　　(Ex) 017.20-017.26, 017.90-017.96, 031.2-031.9, 041.81-041.9, 139.8

● **017.3　Eye** 🦠
　[0-6]　Use additional code to identify manifestation, as:
　　tuberculous:
　　　episcleritis (379.09)
　　　interstitial keratitis (370.59)
　　　iridocyclitis, chronic (364.11)
　　　keratoconjunctivitis (phlyctenular) (370.31)
　　(Ex) 017.30-017.36, 017.90-017.96, 031.2-031.9, 041.81-041.9, 139.8

● **017.4　Ear** 🦠
　[0-6]　Tuberculosis of ear
　　Tuberculous otitis media
　　Excludes　*tuberculous mastoiditis (015.6)*
　　(Ex) 017.40-017.46, 017.90-017.96, 031.2-031.9, 041.81-041.9, 139.8

Item 1–5 Miliary tuberculosis can be a life-threatening condition. If a tuberculous lesion enters a blood vessel, immense dissemination of tuberculous organisms can occur if the immune system is weak. High-risk populations—children under 4 years of age, the elderly, or the immunocompromised—are particularly prone to this type of infection. The lesions will have a millet seed-like appearance on chest x-ray. Bronchial washings and biopsy may aid in diagnosis.

● **017.5 Thyroid gland**
[0-6]   (Ex:) 017.50-017.56, 017.90-017.96, 031.2-031.9, 041.81-041.9, 139.8

● **017.6 Adrenal glands**
[0-6]   Addison's disease, tuberculous
         (Ex:) 017.60-017.66, 017.90-017.96, 031.2-031.9, 041.81-041.9, 139.8

● **017.7 Spleen**
[0-6]   (Ex:) 017.70-017.76, 017.90-017.96, 031.2-031.9, 041.81-041.9, 139.8

● **017.8 Esophagus**
[0-6]   (Ex:) 017.80-017.96, 031.2-031.9, 041.81-041.9, 139.8

● **017.9 Other specified organs**
[0-6]   Use additional code to identify manifestation, as:
         tuberculosis of:
             endocardium [any valve] (424.91)
             myocardium (422.0)
             pericardium (420.0)
         (Ex:) 017.90-017.96, 031.2-031.9, 041.81-041.9, 139.8

● **018 Miliary tuberculosis**
         Requires fifth digit. See beginning of section 010–018 for codes and definitions.
   Includes tuberculosis:
             disseminated
             generalized
             miliary, whether of a single specified site, multiple sites, or unspecified site
             polyserositis

● **018.0 Acute miliary tuberculosis**
[0-6]   (Ex:) 017.90-018.96, 031.2-031.9, 041.81-041.9, 139.8

● **018.8 Other specified miliary tuberculosis**
[0-6]   (Ex:) 017.90-018.96, 031.2-031.9, 041.81-041.9, 139.8

● **018.9 Miliary tuberculosis, unspecified**
[0-6]   (Ex:) 017.90-018.96, 031.2-031.9, 041.81-041.9, 139.8

ZOONOTIC BACTERIAL DISEASES (020–027)

● **020 Plague**
         Infectious disease caused by Yersinia pestis bacterium, transmitted by rodent flea bite or handling infected animal
   Includes infection by Yersinia [Pasteurella] pestis

020.0 Bubonic
         (Ex:) 020.0-020.9

020.1 Cellulocutaneous
         (Ex:) 020.0-020.9

020.2 Septicemic
         (Ex:) 020.0-020.9, 771.81, 771.83-771.89, 995.90-995.94

020.3 Primary pneumonic
         (Ex:) 011.00-012.16, 012.80-012.86, 017.90-017.96, 020.0-020.9, 021.3, 022.1,
         031.0, 039.1, 073.0, 115.05, 115.15, 115.95, 122.1, 130.4, 136.3,
         480.0-487.1, 488.01-488.02, 488.11-488.12, 488.81-488.82, 495.0-495.9,
         500-502

020.4 Secondary pneumonic
         (Ex:) 011.73-011.93, 480.3

020.5 Pneumonic, unspecified
         (Ex:) 020.5, 480.3

020.8 Other specified types of plague
         Abortive plague
         Ambulatory plague
         Pestis minor
         (Ex:) 020.8

020.9 Plague, unspecified
         (Ex:) 020.9

● **021 Tularemia**
         Caused by Francisella tularensis bacterium found in rodents, rabbits, and hares; transmitted by contact with infected animal tissues or ticks, biting flies, and mosquitoes
   Includes deerfly fever
             infection by Francisella [Pasteurella] tularensis
             rabbit fever

021.0 Ulceroglandular tularemia
         (Ex:) 021.0

021.1 Enteric tularemia
         Tularemia:
             cryptogenic
             intestinal
             typhoidal
         (Ex:) 021.1

021.2 Pulmonary tularemia
         Bronchopneumonic tularemia
         (Ex:) 482.49-487.1, 488.01-488.02, 488.11-488.12, 488.81-488.82, 495.0-495.9,
         500-508.1, 508.8-508.9, 517.1, 517.8, 518.89, 519.8-519.9, 793.11

021.3 Oculoglandular tularemia
         (Ex:) 021.3, 480.3

021.8 Other specified tularemia
         Tularemia:
             generalized or disseminated
             glandular
         (Ex:) 021.0-021.9

021.9 Unspecified tularemia
         (Ex:) 021.0-021.9

● **022 Anthrax**
         An acute infectious disease caused by the spore-forming Bacillus anthracis; it may occur in humans exposed to infected animals or tissue from infected animals

022.0 Cutaneous anthrax
         Malignant pustule
         (Ex:) 022.0

022.1 Pulmonary anthrax
         Respiratory anthrax
         Wool-sorters' disease
         (Ex:) 011.00-012.16, 012.80-012.86, 017.90-017.96, 020.3-020.5, 021.3, 022.1,
         031.0, 039.1, 073.0, 115.05, 115.15, 115.95, 122.1, 130.4, 136.3,
         480.0-487.1, 488.01-488.02, 488.11-488.12, 488.81-488.82, 494.0-495.9,
         500-508.1, 508.8-508.9, 517.1, 517.8, 518.89, 519.8-519.9, 793.11

022.2 Gastrointestinal anthrax
         (Ex:) 022.2

022.3 Anthrax septicemia
         (Ex:) 003.1, 020.2, 022.3, 036.2, 038.0-038.9, 040.89-041.9, 054.5, 139.8, 771.81,
         771.83-771.89, 995.90-995.94, V09.0-V09.91

022.8 Other specified manifestations of anthrax
         (Ex:) 022.8

022.9 Anthrax, unspecified
         (Ex:) 022.0-022.9

● **023 Brucellosis**
         Infectious disease caused by bacterium Brucella. Humans are infected by contact with contaminated animals or animal products. Brucellosis symptoms are similar to flu.
   Includes fever:
             Malta
             Mediterranean
             undulant
                 Rising and falling

023.0 Brucella melitensis

023.1 Brucella abortus

023.2 Brucella suis

023.3 Brucella canis

023.8 Other brucellosis
         Infection by more than one organism
         (Ex:) 023.0-023.9

023.9 Brucellosis, unspecified
         (Ex:) 023.0-023.9

INFECTIOUS AND PARASITIC DISEASES (001–139)

N Newborn: 0   **P** Pediatric: 0–17   **M** Maternity: 12–55   **A** Adult: 15–124   ♀ Females Only   ♂ Males Only

(Ex:) CC/MCC Exclusions   Complication\Comorbidity   Major C\C   Present on Admission Requirement   Hospital-Acquired Condition   **675**

024 Glanders 🔍
    Infection by:
        Actinobacillus mallei
        Malleomyces mallei
        Pseudomonas mallei
        Farcy
        Malleus
    (Ex:) 024

025 Melioidosis 🔍
    Infection by:
        Malleomyces pseudomallei
        Pseudomonas pseudomallei
        Whitmore's bacillus
    Pseudoglanders
    (Ex:) 025

● 026 Rat-bite fever
    RBF is an infectious disease caused by Streptobacillus moniliformis or Spirillum minus.
    026.0 Spirillary fever 🔍
        Rat-bite fever due to Spirillum minor [S. minus]
        Sodoku
        (Ex:) 026.0-026.9
    026.1 Streptobacillary fever 🔍
        Epidemic arthritic erythema
        Haverhill fever
        Rat-bite fever due to Streptobacillus moniliformis
        (Ex:) 026.0-026.9
    026.9 Unspecified rat-bite fever 🔍
        (Ex:) 026.0-026.9

● 027 Other zoonotic bacterial diseases
    027.0 Listeriosis 🔍
        Infection by Listeria monocytogenes
        Septicemia by Listeria monocytogenes
        Use additional code to identify manifestations, as
          meningitis (320.7)
        Excludes *congenital listeriosis (771.2)*
        (Ex:) 027.0-027.9
    027.1 Erysipelothrix infection
        Erysipeloid (of Rosenbach)
        Infection by Erysipelothrix insidiosa
          [E. rhusiopathiae]
        Septicemia by Erysipelothrix insidiosa
          [E. rhusiopathiae]
    027.2 Pasteurellosis 🔍
        Pasteurella pseudotuberculosis infection by Pasteurella
          multocida [P. septica]
        Mesenteric adenitis by Pasteurella multocida
          [P. septica]
        Septic infection (cat bite) (dog bite) by Pasteurella
          multocida [P. septica]
        Excludes *infection by:*
          Francisella [Pasteurella] tularensis
            (021.0–021.9)
          Yersinia [Pasteurella] pestis (020.0–020.9)
        (Ex:) 027.0-027.9
        Coding Clinic: 2012, Q3, P14
    027.8 Other specified zoonotic bacterial diseases 🔍
        (Ex:) 027.0-027.9
    027.9 Unspecified zoonotic bacterial disease 🔍
        (Ex:) 027.0-027.9

OTHER BACTERIAL DISEASES (030–041)

    Excludes *bacterial venereal diseases (098.0–099.9)*
        bartonellosis (088.0)

● 030 Leprosy
    Also known as Hansen's disease; chronic infectious disease attacking skin, peripheral nerves, and mucous membranes
    Includes Hansen's disease
        infection by Mycobacterium leprae
    030.0 Lepromatous [type L] 🔍
        Lepromatous leprosy (macular) (diffuse) (infiltrated)
          (nodular) (neuritic)
        (Ex:) 030.0
    030.1 Tuberculoid [type T] 🔍
        Tuberculoid leprosy (macular) (maculoanesthetic)
          (major) (minor) (neuritic)
        (Ex:) 030.1
    030.2 Indeterminate [group I] 🔍
        Indeterminate [uncharacteristic] leprosy (macular)
          (neuritic)
        (Ex:) 030.2
    030.3 Borderline [group B] 🔍
        Borderline or dimorphous leprosy (infiltrated) (neuritic)
        (Ex:) 030.3
    030.8 Other specified leprosy 🔍
        (Ex:) 030.8
    030.9 Leprosy, unspecified 🔍
        (Ex:) 030.9

● 031 Diseases due to other mycobacteria
    031.0 Pulmonary 🔍
        Battey disease
        Infection by Mycobacterium:
          avium
          intracellulare [Battey bacillus]
          kansasii
        (Ex:) 011.00-012.86, 017.90-017.96, 031.0, 031.2-031.9, 041.81-041.9, 137.0,
           139.8, 480.0-480.2, 480.8-487.1, 488.01-488.02, 488.11-488.12,
           488.81-488.82, 494.0-508.1, 508.8-508.9, 517.1, 518.89, 793.11
        Coding Clinic: 2013, Q2, P17
    031.1 Cutaneous 🔍
        Buruli ulcer
        Infection by Mycobacterium:
          marinum [M. balnei]
          ulcerans
        (Ex:) 031.0-031.9
    031.2 Disseminated 🔍
        Disseminated mycobacterium avium-intracellulare
          complex (DMAC)
        Mycobacterium avium-intracellulare complex (MAC)
          bacteremia
        (Ex:) 031.0-031.9
        Coding Clinic: 1997, Q4, P31
    031.8 Other specified mycobacterial diseases 🔍
        (Ex:) 031.0-031.9
    031.9 Unspecified diseases due to mycobacteria 🔍
        Atypical mycobacterium infection NOS
        (Ex:) 031.0-031.9

● 032 Diphtheria
    Highly contagious bacterial disease that results in formation of an adherent membrane in the throat that may lead to suffocation. It may attack the heart and lungs. The exact location is specified in the codes.
    Includes infection by Corynebacterium diphtheriae
    032.0 Faucial diphtheria 🔍
        Membranous angina, diphtheritic
        (Ex:) 032.0-032.9
    032.1 Nasopharyngeal diphtheria 🔍
        (Ex:) 032.0-032.9
    032.2 Anterior nasal diphtheria 🔍
        (Ex:) 032.0-032.9
    032.3 Laryngeal diphtheria 🔍
        Laryngotracheitis, diphtheritic
        (Ex:) 032.0-032.9

◀ New   ◀▨ Revised   ~~deleted~~ Deleted   Excludes   Includes   Use additional   Code first   Omit code

● Unacceptable Principal Diagnosis   ● Use Additional Digit(s)   ▸ Manifestation Code   OGCR Official Guidelines   Coding Clinic

676

● 032.8 **Other specified diphtheria**

    032.81 **Conjunctival diphtheria** 🔲
       Pseudomembranous diphtheritic
       conjunctivitis
       (Ex:) 032.0-032.9

    032.82 **Diphtheritic myocarditis** 🔲
       (Ex:) 032.82, 074.20, 074.22-074.23, 093.82, 390, 391.2-391.9,
       398.0-398.90, 398.99, 422.0-422.99, 429.0, 429.71-429.79,
       459.89-459.9

    032.83 **Diphtheritic peritonitis** 🔲
       (Ex:) 014.00-014.06, 032.83, 090.0, 095.2, 098.86, 099.56,
       540.0-540.1, 567.0-567.1, 567.22, 567.29, 567.81, 567.9,
       569.87-569.9, 577.8, 614.5-614.7, 639.0, 670.00-670.84,
       777.6, 998.7

    032.84 **Diphtheritic cystitis** 🔲
       (Ex:) 032.0-032.9

    032.85 **Cutaneous diphtheria** 🔲
       (Ex:) 032.0-032.9

    032.89 **Other** 🔲
       (Ex:) 032.0-032.9

● 032.9 **Diphtheria, unspecified** 🔲
    (Ex:) 032.0-032.9

● 033 **Whooping cough**
   Pertussis (whooping cough) is a highly contagious disease caused by
   the bacterium Bordetella pertussis and results in a whooping
   sound.

   Includes pertussis

   Use additional code to identify any associated pneumonia
   (484.3)

   033.0 **Bordetella pertussis [B. pertussis]** 🔲
      (Ex:) 033.0-033.9

   033.1 **Bordetella parapertussis [B. parapertussis]** 🔲
      (Ex:) 033.0-033.9

   033.8 **Whooping cough due to other specified organism** 🔲
      Bordetella bronchiseptica [B. bronchiseptica]
      (Ex:) 033.0-033.9

   033.9 **Whooping cough, unspecified organism** 🔲
      (Ex:) 033.0-033.9

● 034 **Streptococcal sore throat and scarlet fever**

   034.0 **Streptococcal sore throat**

     Septic: Streptococcal:
       angina   angina
       sore throat   laryngitis
                    pharyngitis
                    tonsillitis

     Coding Clinic: 1985, Sept-Oct, P9

   034.1 **Scarlet fever** 🔲
      Scarlatina

      Excludes *parascarlatina (057.8)*

      (Ex:) 034.0-035

● 035 **Erysipelas**

   Excludes *postpartum or puerperal erysipelas (670.8)*

● 036 **Meningococcal infection**
   Most commonly caused by bacteria Streptococcus pneumoniae and
   Neisseria meningitidis

   036.0 **Meningococcal meningitis** 🔲
      Cerebrospinal fever (meningococcal)
      Meningitis:
        cerebrospinal
        epidemic
      (Ex:) 003.21, 013.00-013.16, 036.0, 036.89-036.9, 041.81-041.9, 047.0-047.9,
      049.0-049.1, 053.0, 054.72, 072.1, 090.42, 091.81, 094.2, 098.89, 100.81,
      112.83, 114.2, 115.01, 115.11, 115.91, 130.0, 139.8, 320.0-322.9,
      349.89-349.9, 357.0

● 036.1 **Meningococcal encephalitis** 🔲
    (Ex:) 036.1, 036.89-036.9, 041.81-041.9, 139.8

   036.2 **Meningococcemia** 🔲
      Meningococcal septicemia
      (Ex:) 003.1, 020.2, 036.2, 036.89-036.9, 038.0-038.9, 041.81-041.9, 054.5, 139.8,
      995.90-995.94

   036.3 **Waterhouse-Friderichsen syndrome, meningococcal** 🔲
      Meningococcal hemorrhagic adrenalitis
      Meningococcic adrenal syndrome
      Waterhouse-Friderichsen syndrome NOS
      (Ex:) 036.3, 036.89-036.9, 041.81-041.9, 139.8

● 036.4 **Meningococcal carditis**

    036.40 **Meningococcal carditis, unspecified** 🔲
       (Ex:) 036.40, 036.89-036.9, 041.81-041.9, 139.8

    036.41 **Meningococcal pericarditis** 🔲
       (Ex:) 036.41, 036.89-036.9, 041.81-041.9, 139.8

    036.42 **Meningococcal endocarditis** 🔲
       (Ex:) 036.42, 036.89-036.9, 041.81-041.9, 139.8

    036.43 **Meningococcal myocarditis** 🔲
       (Ex:) 036.43, 041.81-041.9, 139.8

● 036.8 **Other specified meningococcal infections**

    036.81 **Meningococcal optic neuritis** 🔲
       (Ex:) 036.81, 036.89-036.9, 041.81-041.9, 139.8

    036.82 **Meningococcal arthropathy** 🔲
       (Ex:) 036.82-036.9, 041.81-041.9, 139.8

    036.89 **Other** 🔲
       (Ex:) 036.89-036.9, 041.81-041.9, 139.8

   036.9 **Meningococcal infection, unspecified** 🔲
      Meningococcal infection NOS
      (Ex:) 036.89-036.9, 041.81-041.9, 139.8

● 037 **Tetanus** 🔲
   Also indexed as "lockjaw." Do not confuse tetanus with tetany, which
   is severe muscle twitches, cramps, and spasms (781.7).

   Excludes *tetanus:*
         complicating:
           abortion (634–638 with .0, 639.0)
           ectopic or molar pregnancy (639.0)
         neonatorum (771.3)
         puerperal (670.8)

   (Ex:) 037, 139.8

● 038 **Septicemia**
   Blood poisoning/bacteremia, often associated with serious illness

   Use additional code for systemic inflammatory response
   syndrome (SIRS) (995.91–995.92).

   Excludes *bacteremia (790.7)*
         septicemia (sepsis) of newborn (771.81)

   Coding Clinic: 2012, Q3, P12; 2010, Q2, P4; 2004, Q2, P16; 1994, Q2, P13;
      1993, Q3, P6; 1988, Q2, P12

   038.0 **Streptococcal septicemia** 🔲
      (Ex:) 003.1, 020.2, 036.2, 038.0-038.9, 040.82-041.9, 054.5, 139.8, 995.90-995.94,
      V09.0-V09.91
      Coding Clinic: 1996, Q2, P5

● 038.1 **Staphylococcal septicemia**

    038.10 **Staphylococcal septicemia, unspecified** 🔲
       (Ex:) 003.1, 020.2, 036.2, 038.0-038.9, 040.82-041.9, 054.5, 139.8,
       995.90-995.94, V09.0-V09.91

    038.11 **Methicillin susceptible Staphylococcus aureus**
       septicemia 🔲
       MSSA septicemia
       Staphylococcus aureus septicemia NOS
       (Ex:) 003.1, 020.2, 036.2, 038.0-038.9, 040.82-041.9, 054.5, 139.8,
       995.90-995.94, V09.0-V09.91
       Coding Clinic: 2008, Q4, P69-73; 1998, Q4, P41-42

    038.12 **Methicillin resistant Staphylococcus aureus**
       septicemia 🔲
       (Ex:) 003.1, 020.2, 036.2, 038.0-038.9, 040.82-041.9, 054.5, 139.8,
       995.90-995.94, V09.0-V09.91
       Coding Clinic: 2011, Q4, P153; Q3, P15; 2008, Q4, P69-73

    038.19 **Other staphylococcal septicemia** 🔲
       (Ex:) 003.1, 020.2, 036.2, 038.0-038.9, 040.82-041.9, 054.5, 139.8,
       995.90-995.94, V09.0-V09.91
       Coding Clinic: 2013, Q2, P21

Item 1–6 034.0 is the common **"strep throat"** (sore throat with strep infection). It is grouped in the same three-digit category with scarlet fever. If a patient has both scarlet fever and the strep throat, use both codes. "Streptococcal" must be indicated on the laboratory report to use 034.0; otherwise use 462 for "sore throat" (pharyngitis).

INFECTIOUS AND PARASITIC DISEASES (001–139)

   N Newborn: 0   P Pediatric: 0–17   M Maternity: 12–55   A Adult: 15–124   ♀ Females Only   ♂ Males Only

(Ex:) CC/MCC Exclusions   🔲 Complication\Comorbidity   🔲 Major C\C   🔲 Present on Admission Requirement   🔲 Hospital-Acquired Condition

INFECTIOUS AND PARASITIC DISEASES (001–139)

038.2 Pneumococcal septicemia [Streptococcus pneumoniae septicemia] 🔍
  (Ex:) 003.1, 020.2, 036.2, 038.0-038.9, 040.82-041.9, 054.5, 139.8, 995.90-995.94, V09.0-V09.91
  Coding Clinic: 1996, Q2, P5; 1991, Q1, P13

038.3 Septicemia due to anaerobes 🔍
  Septicemia due to bacteroides
  Excludes *gas gangrene (040.0)*
            that due to anaerobic streptococci (038.0)
  (Ex:) 003.1, 020.2, 036.2, 038.0-038.9, 040.82-041.9, 054.5, 139.8, 995.90-995.94, V09.0-V09.91

● **038.4 Septicemia due to other gram-negative organisms**
  038.40 Gram-negative organism, unspecified 🔍
    Gram-negative septicemia NOS
    (Ex:) 003.1, 020.2, 036.2, 038.0-038.9, 040.82-041.9, 054.5, 139.8, 995.90-995.94, V09.0-V09.91
    Coding Clinic: 2007, Q4, P84-86

  038.41 Hemophilus influenzae [H. influenzae] 🔍
    (Ex:) 003.1, 020.2, 036.2, 038.0-038.9, 040.82-041.9, 054.5, 139.8, 995.90-995.94, V09.0-V09.91

  038.42 Escherichia coli [E. coli] 🔍
    (Ex:) 003.1, 020.2, 036.2, 038.0-038.9 040.82-041.9, 054.5, 139.8, 995.90-995.94, V09.0-V09.91
    Coding Clinic: 2003, Q4, P73

  038.43 Pseudomonas 🔍
    (Ex:) 003.1, 020.2, 036.2, 038.0-038.9, 040.82-041.9, 054.5, 139.8, 995.90-995.94, V09.0-V09.91

  038.44 Serratia 🔍
    (Ex:) 003.1, 020.2, 036.2, 038.0-038.9, 040.82-041.9, 054.5, 139.8, 995.90-995.94, V09.0-V09.91

  038.49 Other 🔍
    (Ex:) 003.1, 020.2, 036.2, 038.0-038.9, 040.82-041.9, 054.5, 139.8, 995.90-995.94, V09.0-V09.91
    Coding Clinic: 2012, Q3, P14

038.8 Other specified septicemias 🔍
  Excludes *septicemia (due to):*
            anthrax (022.3)
            gonococcal (098.89)
            herpetic (054.5)
            meningococcal (036.2)
            septicemic plague (020.2)
  (Ex:) 003.1, 020.2, 036.2, 038.0-038.9, 040.82-041.9, 054.5, 139.8, 995.90-995.94, V09.0-V09.91

038.9 Unspecified septicemia 🔍
  Septicemia NOS
  Excludes *bacteremia NOS (790.7)*
  (Ex:) 003.1, 020.2, 036.2, 038.0-038.9, 040.82-041.9, 054.5, 139.8, 995.90-995.94, V09.0-V09.91
  Coding Clinic: 2012, Q3, P12, 14; 2010, Q2, P4; 2007, Q4, P96-97; 2005, Q2, P18-20; 2004, Q2, P16; 1999, Q3, P9; Q3, P5-6; 1998, Q1, P5; 1996, Q3, P16; Q2, P6; 1995, Q2, P7

● **039 Actinomycotic infections**
  Includes actinomycotic mycetoma
            infection by Actinomycetales, such as species of Actinomyces, Actinomadura, Nocardia, Streptomyces
            maduromycosis (actinomycotic)
            schizomycetoma (actinomycotic)

  039.0 Cutaneous 🔍
    Erythrasma
    Trichomycosis axillaris
    (Ex:) 039.0, 039.8-039.9

  039.1 Pulmonary 🔍
    Thoracic actinomycosis
    (Ex:) 039.1, 039.8-039.9, 480.3

  039.2 Abdominal 🔍
    (Ex:) 039.2, 039.8-039.9

  039.3 Cervicofacial 🔍
    (Ex:) 039.3, 039.8-039.9

  039.4 Madura foot 🔍
    Excludes *madura foot due to mycotic infection (117.4)*
    (Ex:) 039.4-039.9

Item 1–7 Gas gangrene is a necrotizing subcutaneous infection that will cause tissue death. Patients with poor circulation (e.g., diabetes, peripheral nephropathy) will have low oxygen content in their tissues (hypoxia), which allows the Clostridium bacteria to flourish. Gas gangrene often occurs at the site of a surgical wound or trauma. Onset is sudden and dramatic. Treatment can include debridement, amputation, and/or hyperbaric oxygen treatments.

  039.8 Of other specified sites 🔍
    (Ex:) 039.0-039.9

  039.9 Of unspecified site 🔍
    Actinomycosis NOS
    Maduromycosis NOS
    Nocardiosis NOS
    (Ex:) 039.0-039.9

● **040 Other bacterial diseases**
  Excludes *bacteremia NOS (790.7)*
            bacterial infection NOS (041.9)

  040.0 Gas gangrene 🔍
    Gas bacillus infection or gangrene
    Infection by Clostridium:
        histolyticum
        oedematiens
        perfringens [welchii]
        septicum
        sordellii
    Malignant edema
    Myonecrosis, clostridial
    Myositis, clostridial
    (Ex:) 040.0, 139.8
    Coding Clinic: 1995, Q1, P11

  040.1 Rhinoscleroma

  040.2 Whipple's disease 🔍
    Intestinal lipodystrophy
    (Ex:) 040.2

  040.3 Necrobacillosis 🔍
    (Ex:) No Exclusions
    Coding Clinic: 2007, Q4, P84-86

● **040.4 Other specified botulism**
    Non-foodborne intoxication due to toxins of Clostridium botulinum [C. botulinum]
    Excludes *botulism NOS (005.1)*
            food poisoning due to toxins of Clostridium botulinum (005.1)

  040.41 Infant botulism 🔍   P
    (Ex:) 005.0-005.2, 008.45-008.46, 040.41-040.42
    Coding Clinic: 2007, Q4, P60-61

  040.42 Wound botulism 🔍
    Non-foodborne botulism NOS
    Use additional code to identify complicated open wound
    (Ex:) 005.0-005.2, 008.45-008.46, 040.41-040.42
    Coding Clinic: 2007, Q4, P60-61; 2006, Q2, P7

● **040.8 Other specified bacterial diseases**
  040.81 Tropical pyomyositis 🔍
    (Ex:) 040.81, 040.89

  040.82 Toxic shock syndrome 🔍
    Use additional code to identify the organism
    (Ex:) 040.82, 338.0-338.4, 780.64-780.65, 780.91-780.99, 785.50-785.59, 785.9, 799.81-799.89
    Coding Clinic: 2013, Q2, P21; 2002, Q4, P44

  040.89 Other
    Coding Clinic: 1986, Nov-Dec, P7

● **041 Bacterial infection in conditions classified elsewhere and of unspecified site**

> **Note:** This category is provided to be used as an additional code to identify the bacterial agent in diseases classified elsewhere. This category will also be used to classify bacterial infections of unspecified nature or site.
>
> *Report the disease first, then the bacterium.*

Excludes *septicemia (038.0–038.9)*

Coding Clinic: 2001, Q2, P12; 1984, July-Aug, P19

● **041.0 Streptococcus**
> *Gram-positive bacteria that is the primary cause of strep throat*

041.00 Streptococcus, unspecified
> *Specified in documentation as streptococcus, but unspecified as to Group*

041.01 Group A
> *Specified as Group A*
> Coding Clinic: 2002, Q1, P3-4

041.02 Group B
> *Specified as Group B*

041.03 Group C
> *Specified as Group C*

041.04 Group D [Enterococcus]
> *Specified as Group D*

041.05 Group G
> *Specified as Group G*

041.09 Other Streptococcus
> *Streptococcus that is documented but not specified as Group A, B, C, D, or G*

● **041.1 Staphylococcus**
> *"Staph" infections caused by **Staphylococcus aureus** bacteria and range from common skin infections (pimples and boils) to serious infection of surgical wounds, bloodstream infections, and pneumonia*
> Coding Clinic: 1987, Jan-Feb, P14-15

041.10 Staphylococcus, unspecified
> Coding Clinic: 2006, Q2, P15

041.11 Methicillin susceptible Staphylococcus aureus
> MSSA
> Staphylococcus aureus NOS
> Coding Clinic: 2008, Q4, P69-73; 2006, Q2, P16-17; 2003, Q4, P104-107; 2001, Q2, P11; 1998, Q4, P42-44, 54.55; 1994, Q3, P6

041.12 Methicillin resistant Staphylococcus aureus
> Methicillin-resistant staphylococcus aureus (MRSA)
> Coding Clinic: 2009, Q4, P74; 2008, Q4, P69-73

041.19 Other Staphylococcus
> Coding Clinic: 2008, Q2, P3

041.2 Pneumococcus

041.3 Klebsiella pneumoniae
> Coding Clinic: 2008, Q4, P148-149

● **041.4 Escherichia coli [E. coli]**
> Coding Clinic: 1984, July-Aug, P19

041.41 Shiga toxin-producing Escherichia coli [E. coli] (STEC) O157
> E. coli O157:H- (nonmotile) with confirmation of Shiga toxin
> E. coli O157 with confirmation of Shiga toxin when H antigen is unknown, or is not H7
> O157:H7 Escherichia coli [E.coli] with or without confirmation of Shiga toxin-production
> Shiga toxin-producing Escherichia coli [E.coli] O157:H7 with or without confirmation of Shiga toxin-production
> STEC O157:H7 with or without confirmation of Shiga toxin-production
> Coding Clinic: 2011, Q4, P83

041.42 Other specified Shiga toxin-producing Escherichia coli [E. coli] (STEC)
> Non-O157 Shiga toxin-producing Escherichia coli [E.coli]
> Non-O157 Shiga toxin-producing Escherichia coli [E.coli] with known O group

041.43 Shiga toxin-producing Escherichia coli [E. coli] (STEC), unspecified
> Shiga toxin-producing Escherichia coli [E. coli] with unspecified O group
> STEC NOS

041.49 Other and unspecified Escherichia coli [E. coli]
> Escherichia coli [E. coli] NOS
> Non-Shiga toxin-producing E. coli
> Coding Clinic: 2011, Q4, P155

041.5 Hemophilus influenzae [H. influenzae]

041.6 Proteus (mirabilis) (morganii)

041.7 Pseudomonas
> Coding Clinic: 1988, Q4, P10

● **041.8 Other specified bacterial infections**

041.81 Mycoplasma
> Eaton's agent
> Pleuropneumonia-like organisms [PPLO]

041.82 Bacteroides fragilis

041.83 Clostridium perfringens

041.84 Other anaerobes
> Gram-negative anaerobes
> **Excludes** *Helicobacter pylori (041.86)*

041.85 Other gram-negative organisms
> Aerobacter aerogenes
> Gram-negative bacteria NOS
> Mima polymorpha
> Serratia
> **Excludes** *gram-negative anaerobes (041.84)*
> Coding Clinic: 1994, Q1, P18

041.86 Helicobacter pylori [H. pylori]

041.89 Other specified bacteria
> Coding Clinic: 2006, Q2, P7; 2003, Q2, P7-8

041.9 Bacterial infection, unspecified
> Coding Clinic: 1991, Q2, P9

INFECTIOUS AND PARASITIC DISEASES (001–139)

N Newborn: 0   P Pediatric: 0–17   M Maternity: 12–55   A Adult: 15–124   ♀ Females Only   ♂ Males Only

(Ex) CC/MCC Exclusions   🅒 Complication\Comorbidity   🅜 Major C\C   🅟 Present on Admission Requirement   🅗 Hospital-Acquired Condition   **679**

Item 1–8 **AIDS** (acquired immune deficiency syndrome) is caused by **HIV** (human immunodeficiency virus). HIV affects certain white blood cells (T-4 lymphocytes) and destroys the ability of the cells to fight infections, making patients susceptible to a host of infectious diseases (e.g., ***Pneumocystis carinii* pneumonia (PCP), Kaposi's sarcoma,** and **lymphoma**). **AIDS-related complex (ARC)** is an early stage of AIDS in which tests for HIV are positive but the symptoms are mild.

Figure 1–3 Kaposi's sarcoma. There are large confluent hyperpigmented patch-stage lesions with lymphedema. (From Cohen & Powderly: Infectious Diseases, ed 3, Mosby, An Imprint of Elsevier, 2010)

HUMAN IMMUNODEFICIENCY VIRUS (HIV) INFECTION (042)

042 Human immunodeficiency virus [HIV] disease
Acquired immune deficiency syndrome
Acquired immunodeficiency syndrome
AIDS
AIDS-like syndrome
AIDS-related complex
ARC
HIV infection, symptomatic
Use additional code(s) to identify all manifestations of HIV
Use additional code to identify HIV-2 infection (079.53)

Excludes *asymptomatic HIV infection status (V08)*
exposure to HIV virus (V01.79)
nonspecific serologic evidence of HIV (795.71)

Ex: 042, 139.8

Coding Clinic: 2010, Q3, P14; 2007, Q4, P61-64; 2006, Q3, P14-15; 2004, Q2, P11-12; Q1, P5; 2003, Q1, P10-11,15; 1999, Q1, P14; 1997, Q4, P30-31; 1994, Q4, P35-36x2; 1993, Q3, P9; Q1, P20-22; 1990, Q3, P17; 1989, Q1, P9

OGCR Section I.C.1.a and b

If a patient is admitted for an HIV-related condition, the principal diagnosis should be 042, followed by additional diagnosis codes for all reported HIV-related conditions. If a patient with HIV disease is admitted for an unrelated condition (such as a traumatic injury), the code for the unrelated condition (e.g., the nature of injury code) should be the principal diagnosis. Other diagnoses would be 042 followed by additional diagnosis codes for all reported HIV-related conditions.

POLIOMYELITIS AND OTHER NON-ARTHROPOD-BORNE VIRAL DISEASES AND PRION DISEASES OF CENTRAL NERVOUS SYSTEM (045–049)

045 Acute poliomyelitis
Also called infantile paralysis caused by poliovirus, which enters the body orally and infects the intestinal wall and then enters the bloodstream and central nervous system, causing muscle weakness and paralysis

Excludes *late effects of acute poliomyelitis (138)*

The following fifth-digit subclassification is for use with category 045:

0 poliovirus, unspecified type
1 poliovirus type I
2 poliovirus type II
3 poliovirus type III

045.0 Acute paralytic poliomyelitis specified as bulbar
[0-3] Infantile paralysis (acute) specified as bulbar
Poliomyelitis (acute) (anterior) specified as bulbar
Polioencephalitis (acute) (bulbar)
Polioencephalomyelitis (acute) (anterior) (bulbar)
Ex: 045.00-045.13

045.1 Acute poliomyelitis with other paralysis
[0-3] Paralysis:
acute atrophic, spinal
infantile, paralytic
Poliomyelitis (acute) with paralysis except bulbar
anterior with paralysis except bulbar
epidemic with paralysis except bulbar
Ex: 045.00-045.13

045.2 Acute nonparalytic poliomyelitis
[0-3] Poliomyelitis (acute) specified as nonparalytic
anterior specified as nonparalytic
epidemic specified as nonparalytic

045.9 Acute poliomyelitis, unspecified
[0-3] Infantile paralysis unspecified whether paralytic or nonparalytic
Poliomyelitis (acute) unspecified whether paralytic or nonparalytic
anterior unspecified whether paralytic or nonparalytic
epidemic unspecified whether paralytic or nonparalytic

046 Slow virus infections and prion diseases of central nervous system

046.0 Kuru
Ex: 046.0-046.9

046.1 Jakob-Creutzfeldt disease *(JCD)*
Use additional code to identify dementia:
with behavioral disturbance (294.11)
without behavioral disturbance (294.10)

046.11 Variant Creutzfeldt-Jakob disease
vCJD
Ex: 013.60-013.66, 046.0-046.9, 048-049.0, 049.8, 052.0, 052.2, 054.3, 054.74, 056.01, 057.8-058.29, 059.00-059.9, 062.0-064, 066.2-066.3, 072.2, 073.7, 079.99, 081.9, 083.9, 090.41, 094.81, 117.5, 124, 130.0, 290.12, 323.01-323.9, 341.1, 487.8, 488.09, 488.19, 488.89, 771.2, 984.9

046.19 Other and unspecified Creutzfeldt-Jakob disease
CJD
Familial Creutzfeldt-Jakob disease
Iatrogenic Creutzfeldt-Jakob disease
Jakob-Creutzfeldt disease, unspecified
Sporadic Creutzfeldt-Jakob disease
Subacute spongiform encephalopathy

Excludes *variant Creutzfeldt-Jakob disease (vCJD) (046.11)*

Ex: 013.60-013.66, 046.0-046.9, 048-049.0, 049.8, 052.0, 052.2, 054.3, 054.74, 056.01, 057.8-058.29, 059.00-059.9, 062.0-064, 066.2-066.3, 072.2, 073.7, 079.99, 081.9, 083.9, 090.41, 094.81, 117.5, 124, 130.0, 290.12, 323.01-323.9, 341.1, 487.8, 488.09, 488.19, 488.89, 771.2, 984.9

046.2 Subacute sclerosing panencephalitis
Dawson's inclusion body encephalitis
Van Bogaert's sclerosing leukoencephalitis
Ex: 046.2, 139.8

046.3 Progressive multifocal leukoencephalopathy
Multifocal leukoencephalopathy NOS
Ex: 013.60-013.66, 046.0-046.9, 048-049.0, 049.8, 052.0, 052.2, 054.3, 054.74, 056.01, 057.8-058.29, 059.00-059.9, 062.0-064, 066.2-066.3, 072.2, 073.7, 075, 081.9, 083.9, 090.41, 094.81, 117.5, 124, 130.0, 290.12, 323.01-323.9, 341.1, 487.8, 488.09, 488.19, 488.89, 771.2, 984.9

046.7 Other specified prion diseases of central nervous system

Excludes *Creutzfeldt-Jakob disease (046.11-046.19)*
Jakob-Creutzfeldt disease (046.11-046.19)
kuru (046.0)
variant Creutzfeldt-Jakob disease (vCJD) (046.11)

046.71 Gerstmann-Sträussler-Scheinker syndrome
GSS syndrome
Ex: 046.0-046.9, 066.40-066.49, 079.82

046.72 Fatal familial insomnia
FFI
Ex: 046.0-046.9, 066.40-066.49, 079.82

046.79 Other and unspecified prion disease of central nervous system
Ex: 046.0-046.9, 066.40-066.49, 079.82

◄ New   ◄ Revised   ~~deleted~~ Deleted   Excludes   Includes   Use additional   Code first   Omit code
● Unacceptable Principal Diagnosis   Use Additional Digit(s)   Manifestation Code   OGCR Official Guidelines   Coding Clinic

046.8 **Other specified slow virus infection of central nervous system** 🔒
(Ex) 046.0-046.9, 066.40-066.49, 079.82

046.9 **Unspecified slow virus infection of central nervous system** 🔒
(Ex) 046.0-046.9

● **047** **Meningitis due to enterovirus**

Includes meningitis:
abacterial
aseptic
viral

Excludes meningitis due to:
adenovirus (049.1)
arthropod-borne virus (060.0–066.9)
leptospira (100.81)
virus of:
herpes simplex (054.72)
herpes zoster (053.0)
lymphocytic choriomeningitis (049.0)
mumps (072.1)
poliomyelitis (045.0–045.9)
any other infection specifically classified elsewhere

047.0 **Coxsackie virus** 🔒
(Ex) 003.21, 013.00-013.16, 036.0, 047.0-047.9, 049.0-049.1, 072.1, 078.88-078.89, 079.81, 079.88-079.99, 090.42, 091.81, 094.2, 098.89, 100.81, 112.83, 114.2, 115.01, 115.11, 115.91, 130.0, 139.8, 320.0-322.9, 349.89-349.9, 357.0

047.1 **ECHO virus** 🔒
Meningo-eruptive syndrome
(Ex) 003.21, 013.00-013.16, 036.0, 047.0-047.9, 049.0-049.1, 072.1, 078.88-078.89, 079.81, 079.88-079.99, 090.42, 091.81, 094.2, 098.89, 100.81, 112.83, 114.2, 115.01, 115.11, 115.91, 130.0, 139.8, 320.0-322.9, 349.89-349.9, 357.0

047.8 **Other specified viral meningitis** 🔒
(Ex) 003.21, 013.00-013.16, 036.0, 047.0-047.9, 049.0-049.1, 072.1, 078.88-078.89, 079.81, 079.88-079.99, 090.42, 091.81, 094.2, 098.89, 100.81, 112.83, 114.2, 115.01, 115.11, 115.91, 130.0, 139.8, 320.0-322.9, 349.89-349.9, 357.0

047.9 **Unspecified viral meningitis** 🔒
Viral meningitis NOS
(Ex) 003.21, 013.00-013.16, 036.0, 047.0-047.9, 049.0-049.1, 072.1, 078.88-078.89, 079.81, 079.88-079.99, 090.42, 091.81, 094.2, 098.89, 100.81, 112.83, 114.2, 115.01, 115.11, 115.91, 130.0, 139.8, 320.0-322.9, 349.89-349.9, 357.0

048 **Other enterovirus diseases of central nervous system** 🔒
Boston exanthem
(Ex) 013.60-013.66, 046.2, 046.71-046.8, 048-049.0, 049.8, 052.0, 052.2, 054.3, 054.74, 056.01, 057.8-058.29, 059.00-059.9, 062.0-064, 066.2-066.49, 072.2, 073.7, 075, 079.82, 079.99, 081.9, 083.9, 090.41, 094.81, 117.5, 124, 130.0, 290.12, 323.01-323.9, 341.1, 487.8, 488.09, 488.19, 488.89, 771.2, 984.9

● **049** **Other non-arthropod-borne viral diseases of central nervous system**

Excludes late effects of viral encephalitis (139.0)

049.0 **Lymphocytic choriomeningitis** 🔒
Lymphocytic:
meningitis (serous) (benign)
meningoencephalitis (serous) (benign)
(Ex) 003.21, 013.00-013.16, 036.0, 047.0-047.9, 049.0-049.1, 066.40-066.49, 072.1, 078.88-078.89, 079.81-079.82, 079.88-079.99, 090.42, 091.81, 094.2, 098.89, 100.81, 112.83, 114.2, 115.01, 115.11, 115.91, 130.0, 139.8, 320.0-322.9, 349.89-349.9, 357.0

049.1 **Meningitis due to adenovirus** 🔒
(Ex) 003.21, 013.00-013.16, 036.0, 047.0-047.9, 049.0-049.1, 072.1, 078.88-078.89, 079.81, 079.88-079.99, 090.42, 091.81, 094.2, 098.89, 100.81, 112.83, 114.2, 115.01, 115.11, 115.91, 130.0, 139.8, 320.0-322.9, 349.89-349.9, 357.0

049.8 **Other specified non-arthropod-borne viral diseases of central nervous system** 🔒
Encephalitis:
acute:
inclusion body
necrotizing
epidemic
lethargica
Rio Bravo
von Economo's disease

Excludes human herpesvirus 6 encephalitis (058.21)
other human herpesvirus encephalitis (058.29)
(Ex) 013.60-013.66, 046.2, 046.71-046.8, 048-049.0, 049.8, 052.0, 052.2, 054.3, 054.74, 056.01, 057.8-058.29, 059.00-059.9, 062.0-064, 066.2-066.49, 072.2, 073.7, 075, 079.82, 079.99, 081.9, 083.9, 090.41, 094.81, 117.5, 124, 130.0, 290.12, 323.01-323.9, 341.1, 382.4, 487.8, 488.09, 488.19, 488.89, 710.0, 771.2, 984.9

049.9 **Unspecified non-arthropod-borne viral diseases of central nervous system** 🔒
Viral encephalitis NOS
(Ex) 013.60-013.66, 046.2, 046.71-046.8, 048-049.0, 049.8-049.9, 052.0, 052.2, 054.3, 054.74, 056.01, 057.8-058.29, 059.00-059.9, 062.0-064, 066.2-066.3, 072.2, 073.7, 075, 079.99, 081.9, 083.9, 090.41, 094.81, 117.5, 124, 130.0, 290.12, 323.01-323.9, 341.1, 382.4, 487.8, 488.09, 488.19, 488.89, 710.0, 771.2, 984.9

VIRAL DISEASES GENERALLY ACCOMPANIED BY EXANTHEM (050–059)

Excludes arthropod-borne viral diseases (060.0–066.9)
Boston exanthem (048)

● **050** **Smallpox**
Caused by variola virus and is a serious, contagious, and sometimes fatal infectious disease

050.0 **Variola major** 🔒
Hemorrhagic (pustular) smallpox
Malignant smallpox
Purpura variolosa
(Ex) 050.0-052.9

050.1 **Alastrim**
Variola minor
(Ex) 050.0-052.9

050.2 **Modified smallpox** 🔒
Varioloid
(Ex) 050.0-052.9

050.9 **Smallpox, unspecified** 🔒
(Ex) 050.0-052.9

● **051** **Cowpox and paravaccinia**

● **051.0** **Cowpox and vaccinia not from vaccination**
Coding Clinic: 2008, Q4, P76-78

051.01 **Cowpox**

051.02 **Vaccinia not from vaccination**

Excludes vaccinia (generalized) (from vaccination) (999.0)

051.1 **Pseudocowpox**
Milkers' node

051.2 **Contagious pustular dermatitis**
Ecthyma contagiosum
Orf

051.9 **Paravaccinia, unspecified**

● **052** **Chickenpox**
Very contagious disease caused by varicella zoster virus; results in itchy outbreak of skin blisters (varicella). The same virus causes shingles (zoster). The Varicella zoster virus is a member of the herpes virus family.

052.0 **Postvaricella encephalitis** 🔒
Postchickenpox encephalitis
(Ex) 051.9-052.0, 052.2-052.9, 078.88-078.89, 079.81, 079.88-079.99, 139.8

052.1 **Varicella (hemorrhagic) pneumonitis** 🔒
(Ex) 051.9, 052.1-052.9, 078.88-078.89, 079.81, 079.88-079.99, 139.8

N Newborn: 0   P Pediatric: 0–17   M Maternity: 12–55   A Adult: 15–124   ♀ Females Only   ♂ Males Only

(Ex) CC/MCC Exclusions   🔒 Complication\Comorbidity   🔒 Major C\C   🔒 Present on Admission Requirement   🔒 Hospital-Acquired Condition

681

052.2 Postvaricella myelitis
Postchickenpox myelitis
(Ex:) 051.9, 052.2-052.9, 053.14, 054.74, 078.88-078.89, 079.81, 079.88-079.99,
139.8, 323.01-323.02, 323.41-323.82, 341.20-341.22

052.7 With other specified complications
(Ex:) 051.9, 052.2-052.9, 078.88-078.89, 079.81, 079.88-079.99, 139.8
Coding Clinic: 2002, Q1, P3-4

052.8 With unspecified complication
(Ex:) 051.9, 052.2-052.9, 078.88-078.89, 079.81, 079.88-079.99, 139.8

052.9 Varicella without mention of complication
Chickenpox NOS
Varicella NOS
(Ex:) 051.9, 052.2-052.9, 078.88-078.89, 079.81, 079.88-079.99, 139.8

● **053 Herpes zoster**
*Also known as **shingles,** caused by same virus as chickenpox. After
exposure, the virus lies dormant in nerve tissue and is activated
by factors including aging, stress, suppression of the immune
system, and certain medication. Begins as a unilateral rash that
leads to blisters and sores on skin. Chickenpox NOS is reported
with 052.9.*

Includes shingles
zona

053.0 With meningitis
(Ex:) 003.21, 013.00-013.16, 036.0, 047.0-047.9, 049.0-049.1, 053.0-053.19,
053.79-053.9, 054.72, 054.74-054.9, 058.81-058.89, 072.1,
078.88-078.89, 079.81, 079.88-079.99, 090.42, 091.81, 094.2, 098.89,
100.81, 112.83, 114.2, 115.01, 115.11, 115.91, 130.0, 139.8, 320.0-322.9,
349.89-349.9, 357.0

● **053.1 With other nervous system complications**
053.10 With unspecified nervous system complication
(Ex:) 053.0-053.19, 053.79-053.9, 054.72, 054.74-054.9,
058.81-058.89, 078.88-078.89, 079.81, 079.88-079.99, 139.8

053.11 Geniculate herpes zoster
Herpetic geniculate ganglionitis
(Ex:) 053.0-053.19, 053.79-053.9, 054.72, 054.74-054.9,
058.81-058.89, 078.88-078.89, 079.81, 079.88-079.99, 139.8

053.12 Postherpetic trigeminal neuralgia
(Ex:) 053.0-053.19, 053.79-053.9, 054.72, 054.74-054.9,
058.81-058.89, 078.88-078.89, 079.81, 079.88-079.99, 139.8

053.13 Postherpetic polyneuropathy
(Ex:) 053.0-053.19, 053.79-053.9, 054.72, 054.74-054.9,
058.81-058.89, 078.88-078.89, 079.81, 079.88-079.99, 139.8'

053.14 Herpes zoster myelitis
(Ex:) 052.2, 053.0-053.19, 053.79-053.9, 054.72, 054.74-054.9,
058.81-058.89, 078.88-078.89, 079.81, 079.88-079.99, 139.8,
323.01-323.02, 323.41-323.82, 341.20-341.22

053.19 Other
(Ex:) 053.0-053.19, 053.79-053.9, 054.72, 054.74-054.9,
058.81-058.89, 078.88-078.89, 079.81, 079.88-079.99, 139.8

● **053.2 With ophthalmic complications**
(Ex:) 053.20-053.29
053.20 Herpes zoster dermatitis of eyelid
Herpes zoster ophthalmicus

053.21 Herpes zoster keratoconjunctivitis
(Ex:) 053.20-053.29

053.22 Herpes zoster iridocyclitis
(Ex:) 053.20-053.29

053.29 Other
(Ex:) 053.20-053.29

Figure 1-4 Primary herpes simplex in and
around the mouth. The infection is usually
acquired from siblings or parents and is
readily transmitted to other direct contacts.
(From Forbes, Jackson: Colour Atlas and Text
of Clinical Medicine, International Edition,
Mosby, 2002)

Item 1-9 Herpes is a viral disease for which there is no cure. There are
two types of the herpes simplex virus: **Type I** causes **cold sores** or **fever
blisters,** and **Type II** causes **genital herpes.** The virus can be spread from
a sore on the lips to the genitals or from the genitals to the lips.

● **053.7 With other specified complications**
053.71 Otitis externa due to herpes zoster
(Ex:) 053.71

053.79 Other
(Ex:) 053.0-054.71, 054.73-054.9, 058.21-058.89, 078.88-078.89,
079.81, 079.88-079.99, 139.8

053.8 With unspecified complication
(Ex:) 053.0-054.71, 054.73-054.9, 058.21-058.89, 078.88-078.89, 079.81,
079.88-079.99, 139.8

053.9 Herpes zoster without mention of complication
Herpes zoster NOS

● **054 Herpes simplex**
Excludes *congenital herpes simplex (771.2)*

054.0 Eczema herpeticum
Kaposi's varicelliform eruption

● **054.1 Genital herpes**
054.10 Genital herpes, unspecified
Herpes progenitalis
**Coding Clinic: 2010, Q2, P10; 2007, Q4, P61-64; 1985,
Jan-Feb, P15-16**

054.11 Herpetic vulvovaginitis ♀
054.12 Herpetic ulceration of vulva ♀
054.13 Herpetic infection of penis ♂
054.19 Other

054.2 Herpetic gingivostomatitis
(Ex:) 054.2

054.3 Herpetic meningoencephalitis
Herpes encephalitis   Simian B disease
Excludes *human herpesvirus 6 encephalitis (058.21)*
other human herpesvirus encephalitis (058.29)
(Ex:) 054.3, 054.74-054.9, 058.21-058.89, 139.8

● **054.4 With ophthalmic complications**
054.40 With unspecified ophthalmic complication
(Ex:) 054.40-054.49, 054.79-054.9, 058.81-058.89

054.41 Herpes simplex dermatitis of eyelid
(Ex:) 054.40-054.49, 054.79-054.9, 058.81-058.89

054.42 Dendritic keratitis
(Ex:) 054.40-054.49, 054.79-054.9, 058.81-058.89

054.43 Herpes simplex disciform keratitis
(Ex:) 054.40-054.49, 054.79-054.9, 058.81-058.89

054.44 Herpes simplex iridocyclitis
(Ex:) 054.40-054.49, 054.79-054.9, 058.81-058.89

054.49 Other
(Ex:) 054.40-054.49, 054.79-054.9, 058.81-058.89

054.5 Herpetic septicemia
(Ex:) 003.1, 020.2, 036.2, 038.0-038.9, 054.5, 054.74-054.9, 058.81-058.89, 139.8,
995.90-995.94

054.6 Herpetic whitlow
Herpetic felon

● **054.7 With other specified complications**
054.71 Visceral herpes simplex
(Ex:) 054.71-054.72, 054.74-054.9, 058.81-058.89, 139.8

054.72 Herpes simplex meningitis
(Ex:) 003.21, 013.00-013.16, 036.0, 047.0-047.9, 049.0-049.1, 053.0,
054.72, 054.74-054.9, 058.81-058.89, 072.1, 090.42, 091.81,
094.2, 098.89, 100.81, 112.83, 114.2, 115.01, 115.11, 115.91,
130.0, 139.8, 320.0-322.9, 349.89-349.9, 357.0

054.73 Herpes simplex otitis externa
054.74 Herpes simplex myelitis
(Ex:) 052.2, 053.14, 054.74-054.9, 058.81-058.89, 078.88-078.89,
079.81, 079.88-079.99, 139.8, 323.01-323.02, 323.41-323.82,
341.20-341.22

054.79 Other
(Ex:) 054.74-054.9, 058.81-058.89, 078.88-078.89, 079.81,
079.88-079.99, 139.8

054.8 With unspecified complication
054.9 Herpes simplex without mention of complication

Item 1–10 **Rubeola** (055) and **rubella** (056) are medical terms for two different strains of measles. The MMR (measles, mumps, and rubella) vaccination is an attempt to eradicate these childhood diseases.

● **055 Measles**
  Includes morbilli
              rubeola
  The first four combination codes specify condition(s)/complication(s) manifesting after measles.
  055.0 Postmeasles encephalitis 🔖
    (Ex:) 055.0, 055.79-055.9, 078.88-078.89, 079.81, 079.88-079.99, 139.8
  055.1 Postmeasles pneumonia 🔖
    (Ex:) 055.1, 055.79-055.9, 078.88-078.89, 079.81, 079.88-079.99, 139.8
  055.2 Postmeasles otitis media
  ● **055.7 With other specified complications**
    055.71 Measles keratoconjunctivitis 🔖
            Measles keratitis
      (Ex:) 055.71-055.9, 078.88-078.89, 079.81, 079.88-079.99, 139.8
    055.79 Other 🔖
      (Ex:) 055.79-055.9, 078.88-078.89, 079.81, 079.88-079.99, 139.8
  055.8 With unspecified complication
  055.9 Measles without mention of complication

● **056 Rubella**
  Includes German measles
  Excludes *congenital rubella (771.0)*
  ● **056.0 With neurological complications**
    056.00 With unspecified neurological complication 🔖
      (Ex:) 056.00-056.09, 056.79-056.9, 078.88-078.89, 079.81, 079.88-079.99, 139.8
    056.01 Encephalomyelitis due to rubella 🔖
            Encephalitis due to rubella
            Meningoencephalitis due to rubella
      (Ex:) 056.00-056.09, 056.79-056.9, 078.88-078.89, 079.81, 079.88-079.99, 139.8
    056.09 Other 🔖
      (Ex:) 056.00-056.09, 056.79-056.9, 078.88-078.89, 079.81, 079.88-079.99, 139.8
  ● **056.7 With other specified complications**
    056.71 Arthritis due to rubella 🔖
      (Ex:) 056.71-056.9, 078.88-078.89, 079.81, 079.88-079.99, 139.8
    056.79 Other 🔖
      (Ex:) 056.00-056.09, 056.79-056.9, 078.88-078.89, 079.81, 079.88-079.99, 139.8
  056.8 With unspecified complications
  056.9 Rubella without mention of complication

● **057 Other viral exanthemata**
  057.0 Erythema infectiosum [fifth disease] 🔖
    (Ex:) 057.0, 079.83
  057.8 Other specified viral exanthemata
    Dukes (-Filatow) disease   Parascarlatina
    Fourth disease   Pseudoscarlatina
    Excludes *exanthema subitum [sixth disease] (058.10–058.12)*
                roseola infantum (058.10–058.12)
  057.9 Viral exanthem, unspecified

● **058 Other human herpesvirus**
  Excludes *congenital herpes (771.2)*
              cytomegalovirus (078.5)
              Epstein-Barr virus (075)
              herpes NOS (054.0–054.9)
              herpes simplex (054.0–054.9)
              herpes zoster (053.0–053.9)
              human herpesvirus NOS (054.0–054.9)
              human herpesvirus 1 (054.0–054.9)
              human herpesvirus 2 (054.0–054.9)
              human herpesvirus 3 (052.0–053.9)
              human herpesvirus 4 (075)
              human herpesvirus 5 (078.5)
              varicella (052.0–052.9)
              varicella-zoster virus (052.0–053.9)
  ● **058.1 Roseola infantum**
          Exanthema subitum [sixth disease]
    058.10 Roseola infantum, unspecified   P
            Exanthema subitum [sixth disease], unspecified
    058.11 Roseola infantum due to human herpesvirus 6   P
            Exanthema subitum [sixth disease] due to human herpesvirus 6
    058.12 Roseola infantum due to human herpesvirus 7   P
            Exanthema subitum [sixth disease] due to human herpesvirus 7
  ● **058.2 Other human herpesvirus encephalitis**
    Excludes *herpes encephalitis NOS (054.3)*
                herpes simplex encephalitis (054.3)
                human herpesvirus encephalitis NOS (054.3)
                simian B herpes virus encephalitis (054.3)
    Coding Clinic: 2007, Q4, P61-64
    058.21 Human herpesvirus 6 encephalitis 🔖
      (Ex:) 054.3, 054.74-054.9, 058.21-058.89, 139.8
    058.29 Other human herpesvirus encephalitis 🔖
            Human herpesvirus 7 encephalitis
      (Ex:) 054.3, 054.74-054.9, 058.21-058.89, 139.8
  ● **058.8 Other human herpesvirus infections**
    058.81 Human herpesvirus 6 infection
    058.82 Human herpesvirus 7 infection
    058.89 Other human herpesvirus infection
            Human herpesvirus 8 infection
            Kaposi's sarcoma-associated herpesvirus infection
    Coding Clinic: 2007, Q4, P61-64

● **059 Other poxvirus infections**
  Excludes *contagious pustular dermatitis (051.2)*
              cowpox (051.01)
              ecthyma contagiosum (051.2)
              milker's nodule (051.1)
              orf (051.2)
              paravaccinia NOS (051.9)
              pseudocowpox (051.1)
              smallpox (050.0-050.9)
              vaccinia (generalized) (from vaccination) (999.0)
              vaccinia not from vaccination (051.02)
  Coding Clinic: 2008, Q4, P76-78
  ● **059.0 Other orthopoxvirus infections**
    059.00 Orthopoxvirus infection, unspecified
    059.01 Monkeypox 🔖
      (Ex:) 051.01-051.02, 057.0-057.9, 059.00-059.9
    059.09 Other orthopoxvirus infection
  ● **059.1 Other parapoxvirus infections**
    059.10 Parapoxvirus infection, unspecified
    059.11 Bovine stomatitis
    059.12 Sealpox
    059.19 Other parapoxvirus infections

INFECTIOUS AND PARASITIC DISEASES (001–139)

● **059.2 Yatapoxvirus infections**
  059.20 Yatapoxvirus infection, unspecified
  059.21 Tanapox 🔍
     Ex: 051.01-051.02, 057.0-057.9, 059.00-059.9
  059.22 Yaba monkey tumor virus
 059.8 Other poxvirus infections
 059.9 Poxvirus infections, unspecified

ARTHROPOD-BORNE VIRAL DISEASES (060–066)

Use additional code to identify any associated meningitis (321.2)

Excludes *late effects of viral encephalitis (139.0)*

● **060 Yellow fever**
 060.0 Sylvatic 🔍
     Yellow fever:
        jungle
        sylvan
     Ex: 060.0-060.9
 060.1 Urban 🔍
     Ex: 060.0-060.9
 060.9 Yellow fever, unspecified 🔍
     Ex: 060.0-060.9

● **061 Dengue** 🔍
     Breakbone fever
     Excludes *hemorrhagic fever caused by dengue virus (065.4)*
     Ex: 061

● **062 Mosquito-borne viral encephalitis**
     Inflammation of the brain caused most commonly by Herpes Simplex virus. It may be a complication of Lyme disease and is often transmitted by mosquitoes, ticks, or rabid animals.
 062.0 Japanese encephalitis 🔍
     Japanese B encephalitis
     Ex: 013.60-013.66, 046.2, 046.71-046.8, 048-049.0, 049.8, 052.0, 052.2, 054.3, 054.74, 056.01, 057.8-058.29, 059.00-059.9, 062.0-064, 066.2-066.49, 072.2, 073.7, 075, 079.82, 079.99, 081.9, 083.9, 090.41, 094.81, 117.5, 124, 130.0, 290.12, 323.01-323.9, 341.1, 487.8, 488.09, 488.19, 488.89, 771.2, 984.9
 062.1 Western equine encephalitis 🔍
     Ex: 013.60-013.66, 046.2, 046.71-046.8, 048-049.0, 049.8, 052.0, 052.2, 054.3, 054.74, 056.01, 057.8-058.29, 059.00-059.9, 062.0-064, 066.2-066.49, 072.2, 073.7, 075, 079.99, 081.9, 083.9, 090.41, 094.81, 117.5, 124, 130.0, 290.12, 323.01-323.9, 341.1, 487.8, 488.09, 488.19, 488.89, 771.2, 984.9
 062.2 Eastern equine encephalitis 🔍
     Excludes *Venezuelan equine encephalitis (066.2)*
     Ex: 013.60-013.66, 046.2, 046.71-046.8, 048-049.0, 049.8, 052.0, 052.2, 054.3, 054.74, 056.01, 057.8-058.29, 059.00-059.9, 062.0-064, 066.2-066.49, 072.2, 073.7, 075, 079.82, 079.99, 081.9, 083.9, 090.41, 094.81, 117.5, 124, 130.0, 290.12, 323.01-323.9, 341.1, 487.8, 488.09, 488.19, 488.89, 771.2, 984.9
 062.3 St. Louis encephalitis 🔍
     Ex: 013.60-013.66, 046.2, 046.71-046.8, 048-049.0, 049.8, 052.0, 052.2, 054.3, 054.74, 056.01, 057.8-058.29, 059.00-059.9, 062.0-064, 066.2-066.49, 072.2, 073.7, 075, 079.82, 079.99, 081.9, 083.9, 090.41, 094.81, 117.5, 124, 130.0, 290.12, 323.01-323.9, 341.1, 487.8, 488.09, 488.19, 488.89, 771.2, 984.9
 062.4 Australian encephalitis 🔍
     Australian arboencephalitis
     Australian X disease
     Murray Valley encephalitis
     Ex: 013.60-013.66, 046.2, 046.71-046.8, 048-049.0, 049.8, 052.0, 052.2, 054.3, 054.74, 056.01, 057.8-058.29, 059.00-059.9, 062.0-064, 066.2-066.49, 072.2, 073.7, 075, 079.99, 081.9, 083.9, 090.41, 094.81, 117.5, 124, 130.0, 290.12, 323.01-323.9, 341.1, 487.8, 488.09, 488.19, 488.89, 771.2, 984.9

 062.5 California virus encephalitis 🔍
     Encephalitis: Encephalitis:
        California   Tahyna fever
        La Crosse
     Ex: 013.60-013.66, 046.2, 046.71-046.8, 048-049.0, 049.8, 052.0, 052.2, 054.3, 054.74, 056.01, 057.8-058.29, 059.00-059.9, 062.0-064, 066.2-066.49, 072.2, 073.7, 075, 079.82, 079.99, 081.9, 083.9, 090.41, 094.81, 117.5, 124, 130.0, 290.12, 323.01-323.9, 341.1, 487.8, 488.09, 488.19, 488.89, 771.2, 984.9
 062.8 Other specified mosquito-borne viral encephalitis 🔍
     Encephalitis by Ilheus virus
     Excludes *West Nile virus (066.40–066.49)*
     Ex: 013.60-013.66, 046.2, 046.71-046.8, 048-049.0, 049.8, 052.0, 052.2, 054.3, 054.74, 056.01, 057.8-058.29, 059.00-059.9, 062.0-064, 066.2-066.49, 072.2, 073.7, 075, 079.82, 079.99, 081.9, 083.9, 090.41, 094.81, 117.5, 124, 130.0, 290.12, 323.01-323.9, 341.1, 487.8, 488.09, 488.19, 488.89, 771.2, 984.9
 062.9 Mosquito-borne viral encephalitis, unspecified 🔍
     Ex: 013.60-013.66, 046.2, 046.71-046.8, 048-049.0, 049.8, 052.0, 052.2, 054.3, 054.74, 056.01, 057.8-058.29, 059.00-059.9, 062.0-064, 066.2-066.49, 072.2, 073.7, 075, 079.82, 079.99, 081.9, 083.9, 090.41, 094.81, 117.5, 124, 130.0, 290.12, 323.01-323.9, 341.1, 487.8, 488.09, 488.19, 488.89, 771.2, 984.9

● **063 Tick-borne viral encephalitis**
     Includes diphasic meningoencephalitis
 063.0 Russian spring-summer [taiga] encephalitis 🔍
     Ex: 013.60-013.66, 046.2, 046.71-046.8, 048-049.0, 049.8, 052.0, 052.2, 054.3, 054.74, 056.01, 057.8-058.29, 059.00-059.9, 062.0-064, 066.2-066.49, 072.2, 073.7, 075, 079.99, 081.9, 083.9, 090.41, 094.81, 117.5, 124, 130.0, 290.12, 323.01-323.9, 341.1, 487.8, 488.09, 488.19, 488.89, 771.2, 984.9
 063.1 Louping ill 🔍
     Ex: 013.60-013.66, 046.2, 046.71-046.8, 048-049.0, 049.8, 052.0, 052.2, 054.3, 054.74, 056.01, 057.8-058.29, 059.00-059.9, 062.0-064, 066.2-066.49, 072.2, 073.7, 075, 079.99, 081.9, 083.9, 090.41, 094.81, 117.5, 124, 130.0, 290.12, 323.01-323.9, 341.1, 487.8, 488.09, 488.19, 488.89, 771.2, 984.9
 063.2 Central European encephalitis 🔍
     Ex: 013.60-013.66, 046.2, 046.71-046.8, 048-049.0, 049.8, 052.0, 052.2, 054.3, 054.74, 056.01, 057.8-058.29, 059.00-059.9, 062.0-064, 066.2-066.49, 072.2, 073.7, 075, 079.99, 081.9, 083.9, 090.41, 094.81, 117.5, 124, 130.0, 290.12, 323.01-323.9, 341.1, 487.8, 488.09, 488.19, 488.89, 771.2, 984.9
 063.8 Other specified tick-borne viral encephalitis 🔍
     Langat encephalitis
     Powassan encephalitis
     Ex: 013.60-013.66, 046.2, 046.71-046.8, 048-049.0, 049.8, 052.0, 052.2, 054.3, 054.74, 056.01, 057.8-058.29, 059.00-059.9, 062.0-064, 066.2-066.49, 072.2, 073.7, 075, 079.99, 081.9, 083.9, 090.41, 094.81, 117.5, 124, 130.0, 290.12, 323.01-323.9, 341.1, 487.8, 488.09, 488.19, 488.89, 771.2, 984.9
 063.9 Tick-borne viral encephalitis, unspecified 🔍
     Ex: 013.60-013.66, 046.2, 046.71-046.8, 048-049.0, 049.8, 052.0, 052.2, 054.3, 054.74, 056.01, 057.8-058.29, 059.00-059.9, 062.0-064, 066.2-066.49, 072.2, 073.7, 075, 079.99, 081.9, 083.9, 090.41, 094.81, 117.5, 124, 130.0, 290.12, 323.01-323.9, 341.1, 487.8, 488.09, 488.19, 488.89, 771.2, 984.9

 064 Viral encephalitis transmitted by other and unspecified arthropods 🔍
     Arthropod-borne viral encephalitis, vector unknown
     Negishi virus encephalitis
     Excludes *viral encephalitis NOS (049.9)*
     Ex: 013.60-013.66, 046.2, 046.71-046.8, 048-049.0, 049.8, 052.0, 052.2, 054.3, 054.74, 056.01, 057.8-058.29, 059.00-059.9, 062.0-064, 066.2-066.49, 072.2, 073.7, 075, 079.82, 079.99, 081.9, 083.9, 090.41, 094.81, 117.5, 124, 130.0, 290.12, 323.01-323.9, 341.1, 487.8, 488.09, 488.19, 488.89, 771.2, 984.9

● **065 Arthropod-borne hemorrhagic fever**
 065.0 Crimean hemorrhagic fever [CHF Congo virus] 🔍
     Central Asian hemorrhagic fever
     Ex: 065.0-066.9
 065.1 Omsk hemorrhagic fever 🔍
     Ex: 065.0-066.9

065.2 Kyasanur Forest disease 🔹
    Ⓔ 065.0-066.9

065.3 Other tick-borne hemorrhagic fever 🔹
    Ⓔ 065.0-066.9

065.4 Mosquito-borne hemorrhagic fever 🔹
    Chikungunya hemorrhagic fever
    Dengue hemorrhagic fever

    Excludes   *Chikungunya fever (066.3)*
              dengue (061)
              yellow fever (060.0–060.9)
    Ⓔ 065.0-066.9

065.8 Other specified arthropod-borne hemorrhagic fever 🔹
    Mite-borne hemorrhagic fever
    Ⓔ 065.0-066.9

065.9 Arthropod-borne hemorrhagic fever, unspecified 🔹
    Arbovirus hemorrhagic fever NOS
    Ⓔ 065.0-066.9

⬤ **066 Other arthropod-borne viral diseases**

066.0 Phlebotomus fever 🔹
    Changuinola fever
    Sandfly fever
    Ⓔ 065.0-066.9

066.1 Tick-borne fever 🔹
    Nairobi sheep disease
    Tick fever:
       American mountain
       Colorado
       Kemerovo
       Quaranfil
    Ⓔ 065.0-066.9

066.2 Venezuelan equine fever 🔹
    Venezuelan equine encephalitis
    Ⓔ 013.60-013.66, 046.2, 046.71-046.8, 048-049.0, 049.8, 052.0, 052.2, 054.3,
    054.74, 056.01, 057.8-058.29, 059.00-059.9, 062.0-066.9, 072.2, 073.7,
    075, 079.82, 079.99, 081.9, 083.9, 090.41, 094.81, 117.5, 124, 130.0,
    290.12, 323.01-323.9, 341.1, 487.8, 488.09, 488.19, 488.89, 771.2, 984.9

066.3 Other mosquito-borne fever 🔹
    Fever (viral):   Fever (viral):
       Bunyamwera   Oropouche
       Bwamba   Pixuna
       Chikungunya   Rift valley
       Guama   Ross river
       Mayaro   Wesselsbron
       Mucambo   Zika
       O' Nyong-Nyong

    Excludes   *dengue (061)*
              yellow fever (060.0–060.9)
    Ⓔ 013.60-013.66, 046.2, 046.71-046.8, 048-049.0, 049.8, 052.0, 052.2, 054.3,
    054.74, 056.01, 057.8-058.29, 059.00-059.9, 062.0-066.9, 072.2, 073.7,
    075, 079.82, 079.99, 081.9, 083.9, 090.41, 094.81, 117.5, 124, 130.0,
    290.12, 323.01-323.9, 341.1, 487.8, 488.09, 488.19, 488.89, 771.2, 984.9

⬤ **066.4 West Nile fever**
    Also indexed as West Nile virus
    Coding Clinic: 2004, Q4, P50-52; 2002, Q4, P44

    066.40 West Nile fever, unspecified 🔹
       West Nile fever NOS
       West Nile fever without complications
       West Nile virus NOS
       Ⓔ 013.60-013.66, 046.2, 046.71-046.8, 048-049.0, 049.8, 052.0,
       052.2, 054.3, 054.74, 056.01, 057.8-058.29, 059.00-059.9,
       062.0-066.9, 066.8-066.9, 072.2, 073.7, 075, 079.99, 081.9,
       083.9, 090.41, 094.81, 117.5, 124, 130.0, 323.01-323.9, 341.1,
       487.8, 488.09, 488.19, 488.89, 771.2

    066.41 West Nile fever with encephalitis 🔹
       West Nile encephalitis
       West Nile encephalomyelitis
       Ⓔ 013.60-013.66, 046.2, 046.71-046.8, 048-049.0, 049.8, 052.0,
       052.2, 054.3, 054.74, 056.01, 057.8-058.29, 059.00-059.9,
       062.0-066.3, 066.8-066.9, 072.2, 073.7, 075, 079.99, 081.9,
       083.9, 090.41, 094.81, 117.5, 124, 130.0, 323.01-323.9, 341.1,
       487.8, 488.09, 488.19, 488.89, 771.2

    066.42 West Nile fever with other neurologic manifestation 🔹
       Use additional code to specify the neurologic
       manifestation
       Ⓔ 013.60-013.66, 046.2, 046.71-046.8, 048-049.0, 049.8, 052.0,
       052.2, 054.3, 054.74, 056.01, 057.8-058.29, 059.00-059.9,
       062.0-066.3, 066.8-066.9, 072.2, 073.7, 075, 079.99, 081.9,
       083.9, 090.41, 094.81, 117.5, 124, 130.0, 323.01-323.9, 341.1,
       487.8, 488.09, 488.19, 488.89, 771.2

    066.49 West Nile fever with other complications 🔹
       Use additional code to specify the other
       conditions
       Ⓔ 013.60-013.66, 046.2, 046.71-046.8, 048-049.0, 049.8, 052.0,
       052.2, 054.3, 054.74, 056.01, 057.8-058.29, 059.00-059.9,
       062.0-066.3, 066.8-066.9, 072.2, 073.7, 075, 079.99, 081.9,
       083.9, 090.41, 094.81, 117.5, 124, 130.0, 323.01-323.9, 341.1,
       487.8, 488.09, 488.19, 488.89, 771.2

066.8 Other specified arthropod-borne viral diseases 🔹
    Chandipura fever   Piry fever
    Ⓔ 065.0-066.9

066.9 Arthropod-borne viral disease, unspecified 🔹
    Arbovirus infection NOS
    Ⓔ 065.0-066.9

OTHER DISEASES DUE TO VIRUSES AND CHLAMYDIAE (070–079)

⬤ **070 Viral hepatitis**

    Includes   viral hepatitis (acute) (chronic)

    Excludes   *cytomegalic inclusion virus hepatitis (078.5)*

    The following fifth-digit subclassification is for use with
    categories 070.2 and 070.3:

    0   acute or unspecified, without mention of hepatitis delta
    1   acute or unspecified, with hepatitis delta
    2   chronic, without mention of hepatitis delta
    3   chronic, with hepatitis delta

    Coding Clinic: 2007, Q2, P6-7x3; 2004, Q4, P52-53

070.0 Viral hepatitis A with hepatic coma 🔹
    Ⓔ 070.0-070.9, 078.88-078.89, 079.81, 079.88-079.99, 139.8

070.1 Viral hepatitis A without mention of hepatic coma 🔹
    Infectious hepatitis
    Ⓔ 070.0-070.9, 078.88-078.89, 079.81, 079.88-079.99, 139.8

⬤ **070.2 Viral hepatitis B with hepatic coma** 🔹
    [0-3]   Ⓔ 070.0-070.9, 078.88-078.89, 079.81, 079.88-079.99, 139.8

⬤ **070.3 Viral hepatitis B without mention of hepatic coma** 🔹
    [0-3]   Serum hepatitis
          Ⓔ 070.0-070.9, 078.88-078.89, 079.81, 079.88-079.99, 139.8
          Coding Clinic: 1993, Q1, P28

Figure 1-5   Hepatitis B viral infection. **A.** Liver parenchyma showing hepatocytes with diffuse granular cytoplasm, so-called ground glass hepatocytes (H&E). **B.** Immunoperoxidase stains from the same case, showing cytoplasmic inclusions of viral particles. (From Kumar: Robbins and Cotran: Pathologic Basis of Disease, ed 8, Saunders, An Imprint of Elsevier, 2009)

Item 1-11   Hepatitis A (HAV) was formerly called epidemic, infectious, short-incubation, or acute catarrhal jaundice hepatitis. The primary transmission mode is the oral–fecal route. **Hepatitis B (HBV)** was formerly called long-incubation period, serum, or homologous serum hepatitis. Transmission modes are through blood from infected persons and from body fluids of infected mother to neonate. **Hepatitis C (HCV),** caused by the hepatitis C virus, is primarily transfusion associated. **Hepatitis D (HDV),** also called delta hepatitis, is caused by the hepatitis D virus in patients formerly or currently infected with hepatitis B. **Hepatitis E (HEV)** is also called enterically transmitted non-A, non-B hepatitis. The primary transmission mode is the oral–fecal route, usually through contaminated water.

N   Newborn: 0   **P**   Pediatric: 0–17   **M**   Maternity: 12–55   **A**   Adult: 15–124   ♀   Females Only   ♂   Males Only

Ⓔ   CC/MCC Exclusions   🔹   Complication\Comorbidity   🔹   Major C\C   🔹   Present on Admission Requirement   🔹   Hospital-Acquired Condition   **685**

INFECTIOUS AND PARASITIC DISEASES (001–139)

- **070.4 Other specified viral hepatitis with hepatic coma**
  - **070.41 Acute hepatitis C with hepatic coma** 🔒
    - (Ex:) 070.0-070.9, 078.88-078.89, 079.81, 079.88-079.99, 139.8
  - **070.42 Hepatitis delta without mention of active hepatitis B disease with hepatic coma** 🔒
    - Hepatitis delta with hepatitis B carrier state
    - (Ex:) 070.0-070.9, 078.88-078.89, 079.81, 079.88-079.99, 139.8
  - **070.43 Hepatitis E with hepatic coma** 🔒
    - (Ex:) 070.0-070.9, 078.88-078.89, 079.81, 079.88-079.99, 139.8
  - **070.44 Chronic hepatitis C with hepatic coma** 🔒
    - (Ex:) 070.0-070.9, 078.88-078.89, 079.81, 079.88-079.99, 139.8
  - **070.49 Other specified viral hepatitis with hepatic coma** 🔒
    - (Ex:) 070.0-070.9, 078.88-078.89, 079.81, 079.88-079.99, 139.8
- **070.5 Other specified viral hepatitis without mention of hepatic coma**
  - **070.51 Acute hepatitis C without mention of hepatic coma** 🔒
    - (Ex:) 070.0-070.9, 078.88-078.89, 079.81, 079.88-079.99, 139.8
  - **070.52 Hepatitis delta without mention of active hepatitis B disease or hepatic coma** 🔒
    - (Ex:) 070.0-070.9, 078.88-078.89, 079.81, 079.88-079.99, 139.8
  - **070.53 Hepatitis E without mention of hepatic coma** 🔒
    - (Ex:) 070.0-070.9, 078.88-078.89, 079.81, 079.88-079.99, 139.8
  - **070.54 Chronic hepatitis C without mention of hepatic coma**
    - **Coding Clinic:** 2011, Q1, P23; 2008, Q4, P120; 2007, Q3, P9; 2006, Q2, P13
  - **070.59 Other specified viral hepatitis without mention of hepatic coma** 🔒
    - (Ex:) 070.0-070.9, 078.88-078.89, 079.81, 079.88-079.99, 139.8
  - **070.6 Unspecified viral hepatitis with hepatic coma** 🔒
    - **Excludes** *unspecified viral hepatitis C with hepatic coma (070.71)*
    - (Ex:) 070.0-070.9, 078.88-078.89, 079.81, 079.88-079.99, 139.8
- **070.7 Unspecified viral hepatitis C**
  - **070.70 Unspecified viral hepatitis C without hepatic coma**
    - Unspecified viral hepatitis C NOS
  - **070.71 Unspecified viral hepatitis C with hepatic coma** 🔒
    - (Ex:) 070.0-070.9, 078.88-078.89, 079.81, 079.88-079.99, 139.8
  - **070.9 Unspecified viral hepatitis without mention of hepatic coma** 🔒
    - Viral hepatitis NOS
    - **Excludes** *unspecified viral hepatitis C without hepatic coma (070.70)*
    - (Ex:) 070.0-070.9, 078.88-078.89, 079.81, 079.88-079.99, 139.8

- **071 Rabies** 🔒
  - *Viral disease affecting central nervous system and transmitted from infected mammals*
  - Hydrophobia
  - Lyssa
  - (Ex:) 071

- **072 Mumps**
  - *An acute, contagious, viral disease that causes painful enlargement of the salivary or parotid glands and is spread by respiratory droplets or direct contact. The following combination codes are specific diseases as an existing complication of mumps.*
  - **072.0 Mumps orchitis** ♂ 🔒
    - (Ex:) 072.0, 072.79-072.9, 078.88-078.89, 079.81, 079.88-079.99, 139.8
  - **072.1 Mumps meningitis** 🔒
    - (Ex:) 003.21, 013.00-013.16, 036.0, 047.0-047.9, 049.0-049.1, 053.0, 054.72, 072.1, 072.79-072.9, 078.88-078.89, 079.81, 079.88-079.99, 090.42, 091.81, 094.2, 098.89, 100.81, 112.83, 114.2, 115.01, 115.11, 115.91, 130.0, 139.8, 320.0-322.9, 349.89-349.9, 357.0
  - **072.2 Mumps encephalitis** 🔒
    - Mumps meningoencephalitis
    - (Ex:) 072.2, 072.79-072.9, 078.88-078.89, 079.81, 079.88-079.99, 139.8
  - **072.3 Mumps pancreatitis** 🔒
    - (Ex:) 072.3, 072.79-072.9, 078.88-078.89, 079.81, 079.88-079.99, 139.8

- **072.7 Mumps with other specified complications**
  - **072.71 Mumps hepatitis** 🔒
    - (Ex:) 072.71, 072.79-072.9, 078.88-078.89, 079.81, 079.88-079.99, 139.8
  - **072.72 Mumps polyneuropathy** 🔒
    - (Ex:) 072.72-072.9, 078.88-078.89, 079.81, 079.88-079.99, 139.8
  - **072.79 Other** 🔒
    - (Ex:) 072.79-072.9, 078.88-078.89, 079.81, 079.88-079.99, 139.8
  - **072.8 Mumps with unspecified complication** 🔒
    - (Ex:) 072.79-072.9, 078.88-078.89, 079.81, 079.88-079.99
  - **072.9 Mumps without mention of complication**
    - Epidemic parotitis
    - Infectious parotitis

- **073 Ornithosis**
  - **Includes** parrot fever
    - psittacosis
  - **073.0 With pneumonia** 🔒
    - Lobular pneumonitis due to ornithosis
    - (Ex:) 011.00-012.16, 012.80-012.86, 017.90-017.96, 020.3-020.5, 021.3, 022.1, 031.0, 039.1, 073.0, 073.8-073.9, 115.05, 115.15, 115.95, 122.1, 130.4, 136.3, 480.0-487.1, 488.01-488.02, 488.11-488.12, 488.81-488.82, 494.0-508.1, 495.0-495.9, 508.8-508.9, 517.1, 517.8, 518.89, 519.8-519.9, 793.11
  - **073.7 With other specified complications** 🔒
    - (Ex:) 013.60-013.66, 046.2, 046.71-046.8, 048-049.0, 049.8, 052.0, 052.2, 054.3, 054.74, 056.01, 057.8-058.29, 059.00-059.9, 062.0-064, 066.2-066.49, 072.2, 073.0-073.9, 079.82, 079.99, 081.9, 083.9, 090.41, 094.81, 117.5, 124, 130.0, 290.12, 323.01-323.9, 341.1, 487.8, 488.09, 488.19, 488.89, 771.2, 984.9
  - **073.8 With unspecified complication** 🔒
    - (Ex:) 073.0, 073.8-073.9
  - **073.9 Ornithosis, unspecified** 🔒
    - (Ex:) 073.0, 073.8-073.9

- **074 Specific diseases due to Coxsackie virus**
  - **Excludes** *Coxsackie virus:*
    - *infection NOS (079.2)*
    - *meningitis (047.0)*
  - **074.0 Herpangina**
    - Vesicular pharyngitis
  - **074.1 Epidemic pleurodynia**
    - Bornholm disease   Epidemic:
    - Devil's grip   myalgia
    -                                      myositis
  - **074.2 Coxsackie carditis**
    - **074.20 Coxsackie carditis, unspecified** 🔒
      - (Ex:) 074.20, 074.22-074.23, 093.82, 390, 391.2-391.9, 398.0-398.90, 398.99, 422.0-422.99, 429.0, 429.71-429.79, 459.89-459.9
    - **074.21 Coxsackie pericarditis** 🔒
      - (Ex:) 074.21, 093.81, 391.0, 393, 420.0-420.99, 423.3-423.9, 459.89-459.9
    - **074.22 Coxsackie endocarditis** 🔒
      - (Ex:) 002.0, 036.42, 074.22, 083.0, 093.20-093.24, 098.84, 112.81, 115.94, 116.0, 390, 391.1, 391.8-392.0, 394.0-395.9, 396.9-397.9, 398.90, 398.99, 421.0-421.9, 424.0-424.99, 425.3, 459.89-459.9, 746.09, 746.89, 996.61
    - **074.23 Coxsackie myocarditis** 🔒
      - Aseptic myocarditis of newborn
      - (Ex:) 074.20, 074.22-074.23, 093.82, 390, 391.2-391.9, 398.0-398.90, 398.99, 422.0-422.99, 429.0, 429.71-429.79, 459.89-459.9
  - **074.3 Hand, foot, and mouth disease**
    - Vesicular stomatitis and exanthem
    - *Check your documentation—this code is HAND, foot, and mouth disease. Code 078.4 is foot and mouth disease.*
  - **074.8 Other specified diseases due to Coxsackie virus**
    - Acute lymphonodular pharyngitis

- **075 Infectious mononucleosis**
  - Glandular fever
  - Monocytic angina
  - Pfeiffer's disease
  - **Coding Clinic:** 2001, Q3, P13-14x2

● 076 **Trachoma**
　　Excludes *late effect of trachoma (139.1)*

　　076.0 **Initial stage**
　　　　Trachoma dubium

　　076.1 **Active stage**
　　　　Granular conjunctivitis (trachomatous)
　　　　Trachomatous:
　　　　　follicular conjunctivitis
　　　　　pannus

　　076.9 **Trachoma, unspecified**
　　　　Trachoma NOS

● 077 **Other diseases of conjunctiva due to viruses and Chlamydiae**
　　Excludes *ophthalmic complications of viral diseases classified elsewhere*

　　077.0 **Inclusion conjunctivitis**
　　　　Paratrachoma
　　　　Swimming pool conjunctivitis
　　　　Excludes *inclusion blennorrhea (neonatal) (771.6)*

　　077.1 **Epidemic keratoconjunctivitis**
　　　　Shipyard eye

　　077.2 **Pharyngoconjunctival fever**
　　　　Viral pharyngoconjunctivitis

　　077.3 **Other adenoviral conjunctivitis**
　　　　Acute adenoviral follicular conjunctivitis

　　077.4 **Epidemic hemorrhagic conjunctivitis**
　　　　Apollo:
　　　　　conjunctivitis
　　　　　disease
　　　　Conjunctivitis due to enterovirus type 70
　　　　Hemorrhagic conjunctivitis (acute) (epidemic)

　　077.8 **Other viral conjunctivitis**
　　　　Newcastle conjunctivitis

● 077.9 **Unspecified diseases of conjunctiva due to viruses and Chlamydiae**
　　　　077.98 **Due to Chlamydiae**
　　　　077.99 **Due to viruses**
　　　　　　Viral conjunctivitis NOS

● 078 **Other diseases due to viruses and Chlamydiae**
　　Excludes *viral infection NOS (079.0–079.9)*
　　　　　　　viremia NOS (790.8)

　　078.0 **Molluscum contagiosum**
● 078.1 **Viral warts**
　　　　Viral warts due to human papillomavirus
　　　　Coding Clinic: 1997, Q2, P9

　　　　078.10 **Viral warts, unspecified**
　　　　　　Verruca:
　　　　　　　NOS
　　　　　　　Vulgaris
　　　　　　Warts (infectious)

　　　　078.11 **Condyloma acuminatum**
　　　　　　Condyloma NOS
　　　　　　Genital warts NOS

　　　　078.12 **Plantar wart**
　　　　　　Verruca plantaris
　　　　　　Coding Clinic: 2008, Q4, P78-79

　　　　078.19 **Other specified viral warts**
　　　　　　Common wart
　　　　　　Flat wart
　　　　　　Verruca plana

　　078.2 **Sweating fever**
　　　　Miliary fever
　　　　Sweating disease

　　078.3 **Cat-scratch disease**
　　　　Benign lymphoreticulosis (of inoculation)
　　　　Cat-scratch fever
　　　　(Ex) 078.3, 079.82

　　078.4 **Foot and mouth disease**
　　　　Aphthous fever
　　　　Epizootic:
　　　　　aphthae
　　　　　stomatitis
　　　　Check your documentation. Code 074.3 is for HAND, foot, and mouth disease.

　　078.5 **Cytomegaloviral disease**
　　　　Cytomegalic inclusion disease
　　　　Salivary gland virus disease
　　　　Use additional code to identify manifestation, as:
　　　　　cytomegalic inclusion virus:
　　　　　　hepatitis (573.1)
　　　　　　pneumonia (484.1)
　　　　Excludes *congenital cytomegalovirus infection (771.1)*
　　　　(Ex) 078.5-078.7, 078.89-079.50, 079.59, 079.81-079.82, 079.89, 079.99
　　　　Coding Clinic: 2011, Q3, P5; 2003, Q1, P11; 1993, Q3, P13; Q2, P11; Q1, P24; 1989, Q1, P9

　　078.6 **Hemorrhagic nephrosonephritis**
　　　　Hemorrhagic fever:
　　　　　epidemic
　　　　　Korean
　　　　　Russian with renal syndrome
　　　　(Ex) 016.00-016.06, 016.30-016.36, 016.90-016.96, 017.90-017.96, 078.6, 079.82, 098.10, 098.19, 098.30-098.31, 098.89, 112.2, 131.00, 131.8-131.9, 249.40-249.41, 249.80-249.91, 250.40-250.43, 250.80-250.93, 274.10, 274.19, 580.0-584.9, 586-591, 593.0-593.2, 593.89-593.9, 599.70-599.9

　　078.7 **Arenaviral hemorrhagic fever**
　　　　Hemorrhagic fever:
　　　　　Argentine
　　　　　Bolivian
　　　　　Junin virus
　　　　　Machupo virus
　　　　(Ex) 078.5-079.82, 079.88-079.99

● 078.8 **Other specified diseases due to viruses and Chlamydiae**
　　　　Excludes *epidemic diarrhea (009.2)*
　　　　　　　　lymphogranuloma venereum (099.1)
　　　　078.81 **Epidemic vertigo**
　　　　078.82 **Epidemic vomiting syndrome**
　　　　　　Winter vomiting disease
　　　　078.88 **Other specified diseases due to Chlamydiae**
　　　　078.89 **Other specified diseases due to viruses**
　　　　　　Epidemic cervical myalgia
　　　　　　Marburg disease

● 079 **Viral and chlamydial infection in conditions classified elsewhere and of unspecified site**
　　Note: This category is provided to be used as an additional code to identify the viral agent in diseases classifiable elsewhere. This category will also be used to classify virus infection of unspecified nature or site.

　　079.0 **Adenovirus**
　　079.1 **ECHO virus**
　　079.2 **Coxsackie virus**
　　079.3 **Rhinovirus**
　　079.4 **Human papillomavirus**
　　　　Coding Clinic: 1997, Q2, P9
● 079.5 **Retrovirus**
　　　　Excludes *human immunodeficiency virus, type 1 [HIV-1] (042)*
　　　　　　human T-cell lymphotrophic virus, type III [HTLV-III] (042)
　　　　　　lymphadenopathy-associated virus [LAV] (042)
　　　　079.50 **Retrovirus, unspecified**
　　　　079.51 **Human T-cell lymphotrophic virus, type I [HTLV-I]**
　　　　　　(Ex) 079.51-079.59, 079.81-079.82, 079.88-079.99
　　　　079.52 **Human T-cell lymphotrophic virus, type II [HTLV-II]**
　　　　　　(Ex) 079.50-079.59, 079.81-079.82, 079.88-079.99
　　　　079.53 **Human immunodeficiency virus, type 2 [HIV-2]**
　　　　　　(Ex) 042, 079.50-079.59, 079.81-079.82, 079.88-079.99
　　　　079.59 **Other specified retrovirus**

INFECTIOUS AND PARASITIC DISEASES (001–139)

Item 1–12 **Retrovirus** develops by copying its RNA, genetic materials, into the DNA, which then produces new virus particles. It is from the Retroviridae virus family. **Human T-cell lymphotropic virus, Type I (HTLV-I)** is also called human T-cell leukemia virus, Type I, and is a retrovirus thought to cause T-cell leukemia/lymphoma. **Human T-cell lymphotropic virus, Type II (HTLV-II),** is also called human T-cell leukemia virus, Type II, and is a retrovirus associated with hematologic disorders. **HIV-2** is one of the serotypes of HIV and is usually confined to West Africa, whereas HIV-1 is found worldwide.

079.6 Respiratory syncytial virus (RSV)
Coding Clinic: 1996, Q4, P27-28

● **079.8 Other specified viral and chlamydial infections**
Coding Clinic: 1988, Q1, P12; Q1, P12

079.81 Hantavirus
Ex: 070.70-070.71, 078.5-079.82, 079.88-079.99

079.82 SARS-associated coronavirus
Ex: 011.00-012.16, 012.80-012.86, 017.90-017.96, 021.2, 031.0, 039.1, 079.82-079.89, 115.05, 115.15, 115.95, 122.1, 130.4, 136.3, 480.0-480.2, 480.8-487.1, 488.01-488.02, 488.11-488.12, 488.81-488.82, 494.0-508.1, 508.8-508.9, 517.1, 517.8, 518.89, 519.8-519.9, 748.61, 793.11
Coding Clinic: 2003, Q4, P46-48

079.83 Parvovirus B19
Human parvovirus
Parvovirus NOS
Excludes erythema infectiosum [fifth disease] (057.0)
Ex: 057.0, 079.83
Coding Clinic: 2007, Q4, P64

079.88 Other specified chlamydial infection
079.89 Other specified viral infection
Coding Clinic: 1995, Q1, P7

● **079.9 Unspecified viral and chlamydial infections**
Excludes viremia NOS (790.8)
Coding Clinic: 1988, Q4, P10; 1987, Jan-Feb, P16

079.98 Unspecified chlamydial infection
Chlamydial infection NOS
079.99 Unspecified viral infection
Viral infection NOS
Coding Clinic: 1991, Q2, P8

RICKETTSIOSES AND OTHER ARTHROPOD-BORNE DISEASES (080–088)

Excludes arthropod-borne viral diseases (060.0–066.9)

080 **Louse-borne [epidemic] typhus**
Typhus (fever):   Typhus (fever):
classical   exanthematic NOS
epidemic   louse-borne
Infecting a large number of individuals at the same time
Ex: 080-083.9, 085.0-088.9

●081 **Other typhus**
081.0 Murine [endemic] typhus
Typhus (fever):
endemic
Restricted to a particular region
flea-borne
Ex: 080-083.9, 085.0-088.9

081.1 Brill's disease
Brill-Zinsser disease
Recrudescent typhus (fever)
Ex: 080-083.9, 085.0-088.9

081.2 Scrub typhus
Japanese river fever   Mite-borne typhus
Kedani fever   Tsutsugamushi
Ex: 080-083.9, 085.0-088.9

081.9 Typhus, unspecified
Typhus (fever) NOS
Ex: 013.60-013.66, 046.2, 046.71-046.8, 048-049.0, 049.8, 052.0, 052.2, 054.3, 054.74, 056.01, 057.8-058.29, 059.00-059.9, 062.0-064, 066.2-066.49, 072.2, 073.7, 079.82, 079.99-084.0, 085.0-088.9, 090.41, 094.81, 117.5, 124, 130.0, 290.12, 323.01-323.9, 341.1, 487.8, 488.00, 488.19, 488.89, 771.2, 984.9

Item 1–13 **Rickettsioses** are diseases spread from ticks, lice, fleas, or mites to humans.
Typhus is spread to humans chiefly by the fleas of rats.
Endemic identifies a disease as being present in low numbers of humans at all times, whereas **epidemic** identifies a disease as being present in high numbers of humans at a specific time. Morbidity (death) is higher in epidemic diseases.
Brill's disease, also known as **Brill-Zinsser disease,** is spread from human to human by body lice and also from the lice of flying squirrels. **Scrub typhus** is spread in the same ways as Brill's disease.
Malaria is spread to humans by mosquitoes.

● 082 **Tick-borne rickettsioses**
082.0 Spotted fevers
Rocky mountain spotted fever
Sao Paulo fever
Ex: 080-083.9, 085.0-088.9

082.1 Boutonneuse fever
African tick typhus   Marseilles fever
India tick typhus   Mediterranean tick fever
Kenya tick typhus
Ex: 080-083.9, 085.0-088.9

082.2 North Asian tick fever
Siberian tick typhus
Ex: 080-083.9, 085.0-088.9

082.3 Queensland tick typhus
Ex: 080-083.9, 085.0-088.9

● **082.4 Ehrlichiosis**
082.40 Ehrlichiosis, unspecified
Ex: 080-083.9, 085.0-088.9
082.41 Ehrlichiosis chaffeensis [E. chaffeensis]
Ex: 080-083.9, 085.0-088.9
082.49 Other ehrlichiosis
Ex: 080-083.9, 085.0-088.9

082.8 Other specified tick-borne rickettsioses
Lone star fever
Ex: 080-083.9, 085.0-088.9
Coding Clinic: 1999, Q4, P19

082.9 Tick-borne rickettsiosis, unspecified
Tick-borne typhus NOS
Ex: 080-083.9, 085.0-088.9

● 083 **Other rickettsioses**
083.0 Q fever
Ex: 080-083.9, 085.0-088.9
083.1 Trench fever
Quintan fever
Wolhynian fever
Ex: 080-083.9, 085.0-088.9
083.2 Rickettsialpox
Vesicular rickettsiosis
Ex: 082.0-083.9
083.8 Other specified rickettsioses
Ex: 082.0-083.9
083.9 Rickettsiosis, unspecified
Ex: 082.0-083.9

● 084 **Malaria**
Mosquito-borne disease caused by parasite. Left untreated, severe complications and death may result.
Note: Subcategories 084.0–084.6 exclude the listed conditions with mention of pernicious complications (084.8–084.9).
Excludes congenital malaria (771.2)

084.0 Falciparum malaria [malignant tertian]
Malaria (fever):
by Plasmodium falciparum
subtertian
Ex: 084.0-086.9

084.1 Vivax malaria [benign tertian]
Malaria (fever) by Plasmodium vivax
Ex: 084.0-088.9

084.2 Quartan malaria 🦠
Malaria (fever) by Plasmodium malariae
Malariae malaria
(Ex) 084.0-086.9

084.3 Ovale malaria 🦠
Malaria (fever) by Plasmodium ovale
(Ex) 084.0-086.9

084.4 Other malaria 🦠
Monkey malaria
(Ex) 084.0-086.9

084.5 Mixed malaria 🦠
Malaria (fever) by more than one parasite
(Ex) 084.0-086.9

084.6 Malaria, unspecified 🦠
Malaria (fever) NOS
(Ex) 079.82, 084.0-086.9

084.7 Induced malaria 🦠
Therapeutically induced malaria

Excludes *accidental infection from syringe, blood transfusion, etc. (084.0–084.6, above, according to parasite species)*
transmission from mother to child during delivery (771.2)
(Ex) 084.1-086.9

084.8 Blackwater fever 🦠
Hemoglobinuric:
fever (bilious)
malaria
Malarial hemoglobinuria
(Ex) 084.0-086.9

084.9 Other pernicious complications of malaria 🦠
Algid malaria
Cerebral malaria

Use additional code to identify complication, as:
malarial:
hepatitis (573.2)
nephrosis (581.81)
(Ex) 084.0-086.9

● **085 Leishmaniasis**

085.0 Visceral [kala-azar] 🦠
Dumdum fever
Infection by Leishmania:
donovani
infantum
Leishmaniasis:
dermal, post-kala-azar
Mediterranean
visceral (Indian)
(Ex) 080-088.9

085.1 Cutaneous, urban 🦠
Aleppo boil
Baghdad boil
Delhi boil
Infection by Leishmania tropica (minor)
Leishmaniasis, cutaneous:
dry form
late
recurrent
ulcerating
Oriental sore
(Ex) 080-088.9

085.2 Cutaneous, Asian desert 🦠
Infection by Leishmania tropica major
Leishmaniasis, cutaneous:
acute necrotizing
rural
wet form
zoonotic form
(Ex) 080-088.9

085.3 Cutaneous, Ethiopian 🦠
Infection by Leishmania ethiopica
Leishmaniasis, cutaneous:
diffuse
lepromatous
(Ex) 080-088.9

085.4 Cutaneous, American 🦠
Chiclero ulcer
Infection by Leishmania mexicana
Leishmaniasis tegumentaria diffusa
(Ex) 080-088.9

085.5 Mucocutaneous (American) 🦠
Espundia
Infection by Leishmania braziliensis
Uta
(Ex) 080-088.9

085.9 Leishmaniasis, unspecified 🦠
(Ex) 080-088.9

● **086 Trypanosomiasis**
Human African trypanosomiasis (HAT) is transmitted by fly bites that transmit either Trypanosoma brucei gambiense (causes a chronic infection lasting years) or Trypanosoma brucei rhodesiense (causes acute illness lasting several weeks).

Use additional code to identify manifestations, as:
trypanosomiasis:
encephalitis (323.2)
meningitis (321.3)

086.0 Chagas' disease with heart involvement 🦠
American trypanosomiasis with heart involvement
Infection by Trypanosoma cruzi with heart involvement
Any condition classifiable to 086.2 with heart involvement
(Ex) 086.0, 139.8

086.1 Chagas' disease with other organ involvement 🦠
American trypanosomiasis with involvement of organ other than heart
Infection by Trypanosoma cruzi with involvement of organ other than heart
Any condition classifiable to 086.2 with involvement of organ other than heart
(Ex) 080-088.9

086.2 Chagas' disease without mention of organ involvement 🦠
American trypanosomiasis
Infection by Trypanosoma cruzi
(Ex) 080-088.9

086.3 Gambian trypanosomiasis 🦠
Gambian sleeping sickness
Infection by Trypanosoma gambiense
(Ex) 080-088.9

086.4 Rhodesian trypanosomiasis 🦠
Infection by Trypanosoma rhodesiense
Rhodesian sleeping sickness
(Ex) 080-088.9

086.5 African trypanosomiasis, unspecified 🦠
Sleeping sickness NOS
(Ex) 080-088.9

086.9 Trypanosomiasis, unspecified 🦠
(Ex) 013.60-013.66, 046.2, 046.71-046.8, 048-049.0, 049.8, 052.0, 052.2, 054.3, 054.74, 056.01, 057.8-058.29, 059.00-059.9, 062.0-064, 066.2-066.3, 072.2, 073.7, 075, 078.3, 079.99-088.9, 090.41, 094.81, 117.5, 124, 130.0, 290.12, 323.01-323.9, 341.1, 382.4, 487.8, 488.09, 488.19, 488.89, 771.2, 984.9

● **087 Relapsing fever**
Includes recurrent fever

087.0 Louse-borne 🦠
(Ex) 080-083.9, 085.0-088.9

087.1 Tick-borne 🦠
(Ex) 080-083.9, 085.0-088.9

087.9 Relapsing fever, unspecified 🦠
(Ex) 080-083.9, 085.0-088.9

N Newborn: 0   **P** Pediatric: 0–17   **M** Maternity: 12–55   **A** Adult: 15–124   ♀ Females Only   ♂ Males Only

(Ex) CC/MCC Exclusions   🦠 Complication\Comorbidity   🦠 Major C\C   🦠 Present on Admission Requirement   🦠 Hospital-Acquired Condition   **689**

● **088 Other arthropod-borne diseases**

088.0 Bartonellosis 🔍
Carrión's disease
Oroya fever
Verruga peruana
Ⓔₓ 080-083.9, 085.0-088.9

● **088.8 Other specified arthropod-borne diseases**

088.81 Lyme disease 🔍
Erythema chronicum migrans
Ⓔₓ 080-083.9, 085.0-088.9
Coding Clinic: 1990, Q3, P14; 1989, Q2, P10

088.82 Babesiosis 🔍
Babesiasis
Ⓔₓ 080-088.9

088.89 Other

088.9 Arthropod-borne disease, unspecified

SYPHILIS AND OTHER VENEREAL DISEASES (090–099)

Excludes   *nonvenereal endemic syphilis (104.0)*
urogenital trichomoniasis (131.0)

● **090 Congenital syphilis**

090.0 Early congenital syphilis, symptomatic 🔍
Congenital syphilitic:
choroiditis
coryza (chronic)
hepatomegaly
mucous patches
periostitis
splenomegaly
Syphilitic (congenital):
epiphysitis
osteochondritis
pemphigus
Any congenital syphilitic condition specified as early or
manifest less than two years after birth
Ⓔₓ 090.0-097.9

090.1 Early congenital syphilis, latent
Congenital syphilis without clinical manifestations, with
positive serological reaction and negative spinal
fluid test, less than two years after birth

090.2 Early congenital syphilis, unspecified 🔍
Congenital syphilis NOS, less than two years after birth
Ⓔₓ 090.0-099.9, 139.8

090.3 Syphilitic interstitial keratitis 🔍
Syphilitic keratitis:
parenchymatous
punctata profunda
Excludes *interstitial keratitis NOS (370.50)*
Ⓔₓ 090.0-097.9

Figure 1–6 Chancre of primary syphilis.
(From Mandell, Bennett, & Dolin: Principles
and Practice of Infectious Diseases, ed 7,
Churchill Livingstone, An Imprint of Elsevier,
2009)

Item 1–14 **Syphilis,** also known as lues, is the most serious of the venereal
diseases caused by *Treponema pallidum*. The **primary** stage is characterized
by an ulceration known as **chancre,** which usually appears on the genitals but
can also develop on the anus, lips, tonsils, breasts, or fingers. Syphilis is easy to
cure in its early stages. A single intramuscular injection of penicillin will usually
cure a person who has had syphilis for less than a year.
The **secondary** stage is characterized by a rash that can affect any area of
the body. **Latent** syphilis is divided into **early,** which is diagnosed within
two years of infection, and **late,** which is diagnosed two years or more after
infection. Additional doses of penicillin or another antibiotic are needed to
treat someone who has had syphilis for longer than a year. For those allergic
to penicillin, there are other antibiotic treatments. **Congenital** syphilis is also
labeled **early** or **late** based on the time of diagnosis.

● **090.4 Juvenile neurosyphilis**
Use additional code to identify any associated mental
disorder

090.40 Juvenile neurosyphilis, unspecified 🔍
Congenital neurosyphilis
Dementia paralytica juvenilis
Juvenile:
general paresis
tabes
taboparesis
Ⓔₓ 090.0-097.9, 999.40-099.9, 139.8

090.41 Congenital syphilitic encephalitis 🔍
Ⓔₓ 090.0-097.9, 099.40-099.9, 139.8

090.42 Congenital syphilitic meningitis 🔍
Ⓔₓ 003.21, 013.00-013.16, 036.0, 047.0-047.9, 049.0-049.1, 053.0,
054.72, 072.1, 090.0-097.9, 098.89, 099.40-099.9, 100.81,
112.83, 114.2, 115.01, 115.11, 115.91, 130.0, 139.8,
320.0-322.9, 349.89-349.9, 357.0

090.49 Other 🔍
Ⓔₓ 090.0-097.9, 099.40-099.9, 139.8

090.5 Other late congenital syphilis, symptomatic 🔍
Gumma due to congenital syphilis
Hutchinson's teeth
Syphilitic saddle nose
Any congenital syphilitic condition specified as late or
manifest two years or more after birth
Ⓔₓ 090.0-097.9

090.6 Late congenital syphilis, latent
Congenital syphilis without clinical manifestations, with
positive serological reaction and negative spinal
fluid test, two years or more after birth

090.7 Late congenital syphilis, unspecified
Congenital syphilis NOS, two years or more after birth

090.9 Congenital syphilis, unspecified

● **091 Early syphilis, symptomatic**
Excludes   *early cardiovascular syphilis (093.0–093.9)*
early neurosyphilis (094.0–094.9)

091.0 Genital syphilis (primary)
Genital chancre

091.1 Primary anal syphilis

091.2 Other primary syphilis
Primary syphilis of:
breast
fingers
lip
tonsils

091.3 Secondary syphilis of skin or mucous membranes 🔍
Condyloma latum
Secondary syphilis of:
anus
mouth
pharynx
skin
tonsils
vulva
Ⓔₓ 090.0-097.9

091.4 Adenopathy due to secondary syphilis 🔍
Syphilitic adenopathy (secondary)
Syphilitic lymphadenitis (secondary)
Ⓔₓ 090.0-097.9

● **091.5 Uveitis due to secondary syphilis**

091.50 Syphilitic uveitis, unspecified 🔍
Ⓔₓ 090.0-097.9

091.51 Syphilitic chorioretinitis (secondary) 🔍
Ⓔₓ 090.0-097.9

091.52 Syphilitic iridocyclitis (secondary) 🔍
Ⓔₓ 090.0-097.9

◀ New   ◀═ Revised   ~~deleted~~ Deleted   Excludes   Includes   Use additional   Code first   Omit code

690   ● Unacceptable Principal Diagnosis   ● Use Additional Digit(s)   ▶ Manifestation Code   OGCR Official Guidelines   **Coding Clinic**

Item 1-15 Notice the placement of 091.4 combination code in with the Infectious and Parasitic Disease codes (syphilis). This uveitis does not appear in the eye code section because it is a manifestation of the underlying disease of syphilis.

● **091.6 Secondary syphilis of viscera and bone**

091.61 Secondary syphilitic periostitis 🔖
Ex: 015.90-015.96, 090.0-099.9, 102.6, 730.10-730.19, 730.30-730.39, 733.99

091.62 Secondary syphilitic hepatitis 🔖
Secondary syphilis of liver
Ex: 090.0-099.9, 571.42-571.9, 573.1-573.3, 573.8-573.9

091.69 Other viscera 🔖
Ex: 090.0-099.9, 139.8

091.7 Secondary syphilis, relapse 🔖
Secondary syphilis, relapse (treated) (untreated)
Ex: 090.0-099.9, 139.8

● **091.8 Other forms of secondary syphilis**

091.81 Acute syphilitic meningitis (secondary) 🔖
Ex: 003.21, 013.00-013.16, 036.0, 047.0-047.9, 049.0-049.1, 072.1, 078.88-078.89, 079.81, 079.88-079.99, 090.0-099.9, 100.81, 112.83, 114.2, 115.01, 115.11, 115.91, 130.0, 139.8, 320.0-322.9, 349.89-349.9, 357.0

091.82 Syphilitic alopecia 🔖
Ex: 090.0-099.9

091.89 Other 🔖
Ex: 090.0-099.9, 139.8

091.9 Unspecified secondary syphilis 🔖
Ex: 090.0-099.9, 139.8

● **092 Early syphilis, latent**
Early syphilis is the disease, latent is the characteristic.

Includes syphilis (acquired) without clinical manifestations, with positive serological reaction and negative spinal fluid test, less than two years after infection

092.0 Early syphilis, latent, serological relapse after treatment

092.9 Early syphilis, latent, unspecified

● **093 Cardiovascular syphilis**

093.0 Aneurysm of aorta, specified as syphilitic 🔖
Dilatation of aorta, specified as syphilitic
Ex: 090.0-097.9, 099.40-099.9, 139.8

093.1 Syphilitic aortitis 🔖
Ex: 090.0-097.9, 099.40-099.9, 139.8

● **093.2 Syphilitic endocarditis**
Check documentation for documentation of a specific valve.

093.20 Valve, unspecified 🔖
Syphilitic ostial coronary disease
Ex: 090.0-097.9, 099.40-099.9, 139.8

093.21 Mitral valve 🔖
Ex: 090.0-097.9, 099.40-099.9, 139.8

093.22 Aortic valve 🔖
Syphilitic aortic incompetence or stenosis
Ex: 090.0-097.9, 099.40-099.9, 139.8

093.23 Tricuspid valve 🔖
Ex: 090.0-097.9, 099.40-099.9, 139.8

093.24 Pulmonary valve 🔖
Ex: 090.0-097.9, 099.40-099.9, 139.8

● **093.8 Other specified cardiovascular syphilis**

093.81 Syphilitic pericarditis 🔖
Ex: 090.0-097.9, 099.40-099.9, 139.8

093.82 Syphilitic myocarditis 🔖
Ex: 090.0-097.9, 099.40-099.9, 139.8

093.89 Other 🔖
Ex: 090.0-097.9, 099.40-099.9, 139.8

093.9 Cardiovascular syphilis, unspecified 🔖
Ex: 090.0-097.9, 099.40-099.9, 139.8

● **094 Neurosyphilis**
Use additional code to identify any associated mental disorder

094.0 Tabes dorsalis 🔖
Locomotor ataxia (progressive)
Posterior spinal sclerosis (syphilitic)
Tabetic neurosyphilis
Use additional code to identify manifestation, as: neurogenic arthropathy [Charcot's joint disease] (713.5)
Ex: 090.0-097.9, 099.40-099.9, 139.8
Coding Clinic: 2012, Q3, P4

094.1 General paresis 🔖
Dementia paralytica
General paralysis (of the insane) (progressive)
Paretic neurosyphilis
Taboparesis
Ex: 090.0-097.9, 099.40-099.9, 139.8

094.2 Syphilitic meningitis 🔖
Meningovascular syphilis
Excludes *acute syphilitic meningitis (secondary) (091.81)*
Ex: 003.21, 013.00-013.16, 036.0, 047.0-047.9, 049.0-049.1, 053.0, 054.72, 072.1, 090.0-097.9, 098.89, 099.40-099.9, 100.81, 112.83, 114.2, 115.01, 115.11, 115.91, 130.0, 139.8, 320.0-322.9, 349.89-349.9, 357.0

094.3 Asymptomatic neurosyphilis 🔖
Ex: 090.0-097.9, 099.40-099.9, 139.8

● **094.8 Other specified neurosyphilis**

094.81 Syphilitic encephalitis 🔖
Ex: 090.0-097.9, 099.40-099.9, 139.8

094.82 Syphilitic Parkinsonism 🔖
Ex: 090.0-099.9, 332.0-333.0

094.83 Syphilitic disseminated retinochoroiditis 🔖
Ex: 017.30-017.36, 090.0-099.9, 115.02, 115.12, 362.01, 362.12-362.13, 362.29, 362.41, 362.52, 362.76, 363.00, 363.05-363.10, 363.13-363.15, 646.80-646.84, 679.12, 679.14

094.84 Syphilitic optic atrophy 🔖
Ex: 090.0-099.9

094.85 Syphilitic retrobulbar neuritis 🔖
Ex: 090.0-099.9, 377.32

094.86 Syphilitic acoustic neuritis 🔖
Ex: 090.0-099.9, 388.5

094.87 Syphilitic ruptured cerebral aneurysm 🔖
Ex: 090.0-097.9, 099.40-099.9, 139.8

094.89 Other 🔖
Ex: 090.0-097.9, 099.40-099.9, 139.8

094.9 Neurosyphilis, unspecified 🔖
Gumma (syphilitic) of central nervous system NOS
Syphilis (early) (late) of central nervous system NOS
Syphiloma of central nervous system NOS
Ex: 090.0-097.9, 099.40-099.9, 139.8

● **095 Other forms of late syphilis, with symptoms**
In the late stages, syphilis can damage organs and body systems.

Includes gumma (syphilitic)
Destructive lesions of syphilis
tertiary, or unspecified stage

095.0 Syphilitic episcleritis 🔖
Ex: 017.30-017.36, 090.0-099.9, 379.00-379.02, 379.09

095.1 Syphilis of lung 🔖
Ex: 090.0-099.9

095.2 Syphilitic peritonitis 🔖
Ex: 014.00-014.06, 032.83, 090.0-099.9, 540.0-540.1, 567.0-567.1, 567.22, 567.29, 567.81, 567.9, 569.87-569.9, 577.8, 614.5-614.7, 639.0, 670.00-670.84, 777.6, 998.7

095.3 Syphilis of liver 🔖
Ex: 090.0-099.9

095.4 Syphilis of kidney 🔖
Ex: 090.0-099.9

095.5 Syphilis of bone 🔖
Ex: 090.0-099.9

095.6 Syphilis of muscle 🔖
Syphilitic myositis
Ex: 090.0-099.9

N Newborn: 0   **P** Pediatric: 0-17   **M** Maternity: 12-55   **A** Adult: 15-124   ♀ Females Only   ♂ Males Only

Ex: CC/MCC Exclusions   🔖 Complication\Comorbidity   🔖 Major C\C   🔖 Present on Admission Requirement   🔖 Hospital-Acquired Condition   **691**

INFECTIOUS AND PARASITIC DISEASES (001-139)

095.7 Syphilis of synovium, tendon, and bursa
Syphilitic:
bursitis
synovitis
(Ex) 090.0–099.9

095.8 Other specified forms of late symptomatic syphilis
Excludes *cardiovascular syphilis (093.0–093.9)*
neurosyphilis (094.0–094.9)

095.9 Late symptomatic syphilis, unspecified
(Ex) 090.0–099.9

096 Late syphilis, latent
Syphilis (acquired) without clinical manifestations, with positive serological reaction and negative spinal fluid test, two years or more after infection

● **097 Other and unspecified syphilis**
097.0 Late syphilis, unspecified
097.1 Latent syphilis, unspecified
Positive serological reaction for syphilis
097.9 Syphilis, unspecified
Syphilis (acquired) NOS
Excludes *syphilis NOS causing death under two years of age (090.9)*

● **098 Gonococcal infections**
STD (sexually transmitted disease) caused by Neisseria gonorrhoeae that flourishes in the warm, moist areas of the reproductive tract. Untreated gonorrhea spreads to other parts of the body, causing inflammation of the testes or prostate or pelvic inflammatory disease (PID).
098.0 Acute, of lower genitourinary tract
Gonococcal:
Bartholinitis (acute)
Female only: Bartholin gland
urethritis (acute)
vulvovaginitis (acute)
Gonorrhea (acute):
NOS
genitourinary (tract) NOS
(Ex) 098.0-098.39, 098.89, 099.40-099.9 139.8

● **098.1 Acute, of upper genitourinary tract**
098.10 Gonococcal infection (acute) of upper genitourinary tract, site unspecified
(Ex) 098.0-098.39, 098.89, 099.40-099.9 139.8
098.11 Gonococcal cystitis (acute)
Gonorrhea (acute) of bladder
(Ex) 098.0-098.39, 098.89, 099.40-099.9 139.8
098.12 Gonococcal prostatitis (acute) ♂
(Ex) 098.0-098.39, 098.89, 099.40-099.9 139.8
098.13 Gonococcal epididymo-orchitis (acute) ♂
Gonococcal orchitis (acute)
(Ex) 098.0-098.39, 098.89, 099.40-099.9 139.8
098.14 Gonococcal seminal vesiculitis (acute) ♂
Gonorrhea (acute) of seminal vesicle
(Ex) 098.0-098.39, 098.89, 099.40-099.9 139.8
098.15 Gonococcal cervicitis (acute) ♀
Gonorrhea (acute) of cervix
(Ex) 098.0-098.39, 098.89, 099.40-099.9 139.8
098.16 Gonococcal endometritis (acute) ♀
Gonorrhea (acute) of uterus
(Ex) 098.0-098.39, 098.89, 099.40-099.9 139.8
098.17 Gonococcal salpingitis, specified as acute ♀
(Ex) 098.0-098.39, 098.89, 099.40-099.9 139.8
098.19 Other
(Ex) 098.0-098.39, 098.89, 099.40-099.9 139.8

098.2 Chronic, of lower genitourinary tract
Gonococcal specified as chronic or with duration of two months or more:
Bartholinitis specified as chronic or with duration of two months or more
urethritis specified as chronic or with duration of two months or more
vulvovaginitis specified as chronic or with duration of two months or more
Gonorrhea specified as chronic or with duration of two months or more:
NOS specified as chronic or with duration of two months or more
genitourinary (tract) specified as chronic or with duration of two months or more
Any condition classifiable to 098.0 specified as chronic or with duration of two months or more

● **098.3 Chronic, of upper genitourinary tract**
Any condition classifiable to 098.1 stated as chronic or with a duration of two months or more
098.30 Chronic gonococcal infection of upper genitourinary tract, site unspecified
098.31 Gonococcal cystitis, chronic
Any condition classifiable to 098.11, specified as chronic
Gonorrhea of bladder, chronic
098.32 Gonococcal prostatitis, chronic ♂
Any condition classifiable to 098.12, specified as chronic
098.33 Gonococcal epididymo-orchitis, chronic ♂
Any condition classifiable to 098.13, specified as chronic
Chronic gonococcal orchitis
098.34 Gonococcal seminal vesiculitis, chronic ♂
Any condition classifiable to 098.14, specified as chronic
Gonorrhea of seminal vesicle, chronic
098.35 Gonococcal cervicitis, chronic ♀
Any condition classifiable to 098.15, specified as chronic
Gonorrhea of cervix, chronic
098.36 Gonococcal endometritis, chronic ♀
Any condition classifiable to 098.16, specified as chronic
098.37 Gonococcal salpingitis (chronic) ♀
098.39 Other

● **098.4 Gonococcal infection of eye**
098.40 Gonococcal conjunctivitis (neonatorum)
Neonate = newborn
Gonococcal ophthalmia (neonatorum)
(Ex) 090.0–099.9
098.41 Gonococcal iridocyclitis
(Ex) 090.0–099.9
098.42 Gonococcal endophthalmia
(Ex) 090.0–099.9
098.43 Gonococcal keratitis
(Ex) 090.0–099.9
098.49 Other
(Ex) 090.0–099.9

● **098.5 Gonococcal infection of joint**
098.50 Gonococcal arthritis
Gonococcal infection of joint NOS
(Ex) 003.23, 015.80, 015.96, 017.90-017.96, 036.82, 056.71, 090.0-099.9, 711.00-714.0, 715.00, 715.09-715.10 715.18-716.99, 718.00-718.08, 719.00-719.10, 719.18-719.69, 719.80-719.99
098.51 Gonococcal synovitis and tenosynovitis
(Ex) 003.23, 015.80-015.96, 017.90-017.96, 036.82, 056.71, 090.0-099.9, 711.00-714.0, 715.00, 715.09-715.10, 715.18-716.99, 718.00-718.08, 719.00-719.10, 719.18-719.69, 719.80-719.99

◀ New   ◀▦ Revised   ~~deleted~~ Deleted   Excludes   Includes   Use additional   Code first   Omit code
● Unacceptable Principal Diagnosis   ● Use Additional Digit(s)   ▷ Manifestation Code   OGCR Official Guidelines   Coding Clinic
692

INFECTIOUS AND PARASITIC DISEASES (001–139)

098.52 Gonococcal bursitis 🔗
(Ex:) 003.23, 015.80-015.96, 017.90-017.96, 036.82, 056.71,
090.0-099.9, 711.00-714.0, 715.00, 715.09-715.10,
715.18-716.99, 718.00-718.08, 719.00-719.10, 719.18-719.69,
719.80-719.99

098.53 Gonococcal spondylitis 🔗
(Ex:) 003.23, 015.80-015.96, 017.90-017.96, 036.82, 056.71,
090.0-099.9, 711.00-714.0, 715.00, 715.09-715.10,
715.18-716.99, 718.00-718.08, 719.00-719.10, 719.18-719.69,
719.80-719.99

098.59 Other 🔗
Gonococcal rheumatism
(Ex:) 003.23, 015.80-015.96, 017.90-017.96, 036.82, 056.71,
090.0-099.9, 711.00-714.0, 715.00, 715.09-715.10,
715.18-716.99, 718.00-718.08, 719.00-719.10, 719.18-719.69,
719.80-719.99

098.6 Gonococcal infection of pharynx

098.7 Gonococcal infection of anus and rectum
Gonococcal proctitis

● **098.8 Gonococcal infection of other specified sites**

098.81 Gonococcal keratosis (blennorrhagica) 🔗
(Ex:) 098.40-098.49, 098.81

098.82 Gonococcal meningitis 🔗
(Ex:) 003.21, 013.00-013.16, 036.0, 047.0-047.9, 049.0-049.1, 072.1,
078.88-078.89, 079.81, 079.88-079.99, 090.0-099.9, 100.81,
112.83, 114.2, 115.01, 115.11, 115.91, 130.0, 139.8,
320.0-322.9, 349.89-349.9, 357.0

098.83 Gonococcal pericarditis 🔗
(Ex:) 074.21, 090.0-099.9, 391.0, 393, 420.0-420.99, 423.3-423.9,
459.89-459.9

098.84 Gonococcal endocarditis 🔗
(Ex:) 002.0, 036.42, 074.22, 083.0, 090.0-099.9, 112.81, 115.94, 116.0,
390, 391.1, 391.8-392.0, 394.0-395.9, 396.9-397.9, 398.90,
398.99, 421.0-421.9, 424.0-424.99, 425.3, 459.89-459.9,
711.00, 711.08-711.09, 746.09, 746.89, 996.61

098.85 Other gonococcal heart disease 🔗
(Ex:) 002.0, 036.42, 074.20, 074.22-074.23, 083.0, 090.0-099.9,
112.81, 115.94, 116.0, 390, 391.1-392.0, 394.0-395.9,
396.9-398.90, 398.99, 421.0-422.99, 424.0-424.99, 425.3,
429.0, 429.71-429.79, 459.89-459.9, 711.00, 711.08-711.09,
746.09, 746.89, 996.61

098.86 Gonococcal peritonitis 🔗
(Ex:) 014.00-014.06, 032.83, 090.0-099.9, 540.0-540.1, 567.0-567.1,
567.22, 567.29, 567.81, 567.9, 569.87-569.9, 577.8,
614.5-614.7, 639.0, 670.00-670.84, 777.6, 998.7

098.89 Other 🔗
Gonococcemia
Blood condition
(Ex:) 090.0-099.9, 588.81-588.89

● **099 Other venereal diseases**

099.0 Chancroid
*Sexually transmitted infection caused by bacteria
(Haemophilus ducreyi)*
Bubo (inguinal):
chancroidal
due to Hemophilus ducreyi
Chancre:
Ducrey's simple soft
Ulcus molle (cutis) (skin)

099.1 Lymphogranuloma venereum
Climatic or tropical bubo
(Durand-) Nicolas-Favre disease
Esthiomene
Lymphogranuloma inguinale

099.2 Granuloma inguinale
Donovanosis
Granuloma pudendi (ulcerating)
Granuloma venereum
Pudendal ulcer

099.3 Reiter's disease
Reactive arthritis
Reiter's syndrome
Use additional code for associated:
arthropathy (711.1)
conjunctivitis (372.33)

● **099.4 Other nongonococcal urethritis [NGU]**

099.40 Unspecified
Nonspecific urethritis

099.41 Chlamydia trachomatis

099.49 Other specified organism

● **099.5 Other venereal diseases due to Chlamydia trachomatis**

Excludes *Chlamydia trachomatis infection of conjunctiva
(076.0–076.9, 077.0, 077.9)
Lymphogranuloma venereum (099.1)*

099.50 Unspecified site

099.51 Pharynx

099.52 Anus and rectum

099.53 Lower genitourinary sites
Excludes *urethra (099.41)*
Use additional code to specify site of infection,
such as:
bladder (595.4)
cervix (616.0)
vagina and vulva (616.11)

099.54 Other genitourinary sites
Use additional code to specify site of infection,
such as:
pelvic inflammatory disease NOS (614.9)
testis and epididymis (604.91)

099.55 Unspecified genitourinary site

099.56 Peritoneum 🔗
Perihepatitis
(Ex:) 014.00-014.06, 032.83, 090.0-099.9, 540.0-540.1, 567.0-567.1,
567.22, 567.29, 567.81, 567.9, 569.87-569.9, 577.8,
614.5-614.7, 639.0, 670.00-670.84, 777.6, 998.7

099.59 Other specified site

099.8 Other specified venereal diseases

099.9 Venereal disease, unspecified

OTHER SPIROCHETAL DISEASES (100–104)

● **100 Leptospirosis**

100.0 Leptospirosis icterohemorrhagica 🔗
Leptospiral or spirochetal jaundice (hemorrhagic)
Weil's disease
(Ex:) 100.0-100.9

● **100.8 Other specified leptospiral infections**

100.81 Leptospiral meningitis (aseptic) 🔗
(Ex:) 003.21, 013.00-013.16, 036.0, 047.0-047.9, 049.0-049.1, 072.1
078.88-078.89, 079.81, 079.88-079.99, 090.42, 091.81, 094.2,
098.89, 100.0-100.9, 112.83, 114.2, 115.01, 115.11, 115.91,
130.0, 139.8, 320.0-322.9, 349.89-349.9, 357.0

100.89 Other
Fever:
Fort Bragg
pretibial
swamp
Infection by Leptospira:
australis
bataviae
pyrogenes
(Ex:) 100.0-100.9

100.9 Leptospirosis, unspecified 🔗
(Ex:) 100.0-100.9

INFECTIOUS AND PARASITIC DISEASES (001–139)

101   Vincent's angina 🔎
     Acute necrotizing ulcerative:
         gingivitis
         stomatitis
     Fusospirochetal pharyngitis
     Spirochetal stomatitis
     Trench mouth
     Vincent's:
         gingivitis
         infection [any site]
     (Ex) 101

● **102   Yaws**
     Includes   frambesia
                  pian

   102.0   Initial lesions
     Chancre of yaws
     Frambesia, initial or primary
     Initial frambesial ulcer
     Mother yaw

   102.1   Multiple papillomata and wet crab yaws
     Butter yaws
     Frambesioma
     Pianoma
     Plantar or palmar papilloma of yaws

   102.2   Other early skin lesions
     Cutaneous yaws, less than five years after infection
     Early yaws (cutaneous) (macular) (papular)
         (maculopapular) (micropapular)
     Frambeside of early yaws

   102.3   Hyperkeratosis
     Ghoul hand
     Hyperkeratosis, palmar or plantar (early) (late) due to
         yaws
     Worm-eaten soles

   102.4   Gummata and ulcers
     Nodular late yaws (ulcerated)
     Gummatous frambeside

   102.5   Gangosa
     Rhinopharyngitis mutilans

   102.6   Bone and joint lesions
     Goundou of yaws (late)
     Gumma, bone of yaws (late)
     Gummatous osteitis or periostitis of yaws (late)
     Hydrarthrosis of yaws (early) (late)
     Osteitis of yaws (early) (late)
     Periostitis (hypertrophic) of yaws (early) (late)

   102.7   Other manifestations
     Juxta-articular nodules of yaws
     Mucosal yaws

   102.8   Latent yaws
     Yaws without clinical manifestations, with positive
         serology

   102.9   Yaws, unspecified

● **103   Pinta**
   103.0   Primary lesions
     Chancre (primary) of pinta [carate]
     Papule (primary) of pinta [carate]
     Pintid of pinta [carate]

   103.1   Intermediate lesions
     Erythematous plaques of pinta [carate]
     Hyperchromic lesions of pinta [carate]
     Hyperkeratosis of pinta [carate]

   103.2   Late lesions
     Cardiovascular lesions of pinta [carate]
     Skin lesions of pinta [carate]:
         achromic of pinta [carate]
         cicatricial of pinta [carate]
         dyschromic of pinta [carate]
     Vitiligo of pinta [carate]

   103.3   Mixed lesions
     Achromic and hyperchromic skin lesions of pinta [carate]

   103.9   Pinta, unspecified

● **104   Other spirochetal infection**
   104.0   Nonvenereal endemic syphilis
     Bejel
     Njovera

   104.8   Other specified spirochetal infections
     Excludes   *relapsing fever (087.0–087.9)*
                  syphilis (090.0–097.9)

   104.9   Spirochetal infection, unspecified

MYCOSES (110–118)

   Use additional code to identify manifestation, as:
     arthropathy (711.6)
     meningitis (321.0–321.1)
     otitis externa (380.15)
   Excludes   *infection by Actinomycetales, such as species of*
                 Actinomyces, Actinomadura, Nocardia,
                 Streptomyces (039.0–039.9)

● **110   Dermatophytosis**
     Also known as tinea or ringworm; condition of scalp, glabrous skin,
         and/or nails. Caused by fungi (dermatophytes).
     Includes   infection by species of Epidermophyton,
                  Microsporum, and Trichophyton
                  tinea, any type except those in 111

   110.0   Of scalp and beard
     Kerion
     Sycosis, mycotic
     Trichophytic tinea [black dot tinea], scalp

   110.1   Of nail
     Dermatophytic onychia
     Onychomycosis
     Tinea unguium

   110.2   Of hand
     Tinea manuum

   110.3   Of groin and perianal area
     Dhobie itch
     Eczema marginatum
     Tinea cruris

   110.4   Of foot
     Athlete's foot
     Tinea pedis

   110.5   Of the body
     Herpes circinatus
     Tinea imbricata [Tokelau]

   110.6   Deep seated dermatophytosis
     Granuloma trichophyticum
     Majocchi's granuloma

   110.8   Of other specified sites

   110.9   Of unspecified site
     Favus NOS
     Microsporic tinea NOS
     Ringworm NOS

● **111   Dermatomycosis, other and unspecified**
   111.0   Pityriasis versicolor
     Infection by Malassezia [Pityrosporum] furfur
     Tinea flava
     Tinea versicolor

   111.1   Tinea nigra
     Infection by Cladosporium species
     Keratomycosis nigricans
     Microsporosis nigra
     Pityriasis nigra
     Tinea palmaris nigra

   111.2   Tinea blanca
     Infection by Trichosporon (beigelii) cutaneum
     White piedra

   111.3   Black piedra
     Infection by Piedraia hortai

   111.8   Other specified dermatomycoses

   111.9   Dermatomycosis, unspecified

◀ New   ◀▥ Revised   ~~deleted~~ Deleted   Excludes   Includes   Use additional   Code first   Omit code
● Unacceptable Principal Diagnosis   ● Use Additional Digit(s)   ▷ Manifestation Code   OGCR Official Guidelines   Coding Clinic

694

Figure 1–7 Oral candidiasis (thrush). *(Courtesy of Stephen Raffanti, MD, MPH.)* (From Mandell, Bennett, & Dolin: Principles and Practice of Infectious Diseases, ed 7, Churchill Livingstone, An Imprint of Elsevier, 2009)

Item 1–16 Candidiasis, also called oidiomycosis or moniliasis, is a fungal infection. It most often appears on moist cutaneous areas of the body but can also be responsible for a variety of systemic infections such as endocarditis, meningitis, arthritis, and myositis. Antifungal medications cure most yeast infections.

● **112 Candidiasis**

Includes   infection by Candida species
moniliasis

Excludes   *neonatal monilial infection (771.7)*

112.0 Of mouth
Thrush (oral)
(Ex:) 112.0–112.9, 117.9, 139.8

112.1 Of vulva and vagina ♀
Candidal vulvovaginitis
Monilial vulvovaginitis
Coding Clinic: 1994, Q1, P21

112.2 Of other urogenital sites
Candidal balanitis
Male condition only
HAC: Also excludes the following from acting as a CC/
MCC: 590.10 (CC), 590.11 (MCC),
590.2 (MCC), 590.3 (CC), 590.80 (CC), 590.81
(CC), 595.0 (CC), 597.0 (CC),
599.0 (CC), 996.64 (CC)
(Ex:) 112.2, 112.4–112.9, 588.81–588.89
Coding Clinic: 2012, Q3, P12; 2003, Q4, P105-106; 1996, Q4, P33

112.3 Of skin and nails
Candidal intertrigo
Candidal onychia
Candidal perionyxis [paronychia]

112.4 Of lung
Candidal pneumonia
(Ex:) 112.0–112.9, 117.9, 139.8
Coding Clinic: 1998, Q2, P7

112.5 Disseminated
Systemic candidiasis
(Ex:) 112.0–112.9, 117.9, 139.8
Coding Clinic: 2012, Q3, P12; 1989, Q2, P10

● **112.8 Of other specified sites**

112.81 Candidal endocarditis
(Ex:) 112.0–112.9, 117.9, 139.8

112.82 Candidal otitis externa
Otomycosis in moniliasis
(Ex:) 112.0–112.9, 117.9, 139.8

112.83 Candidal meningitis
(Ex:) 003.21, 013.00–013.16, 036.0, 047.0–047.9, 049.0–049.1, 053.0,
054.72, 072.1, 090.42, 091.81, 094.2, 098.89, 100.81,
112.0–112.9, 114.2, 115.01, 115.11, 115.91, 117.9, 130.0,
139.8, 320.0–322.9, 349.89–349.9, 357.0

112.84 Candidal esophagitis
(Ex:) 112.0–112.9, 117.9, 139.8

112.85 Candidal enteritis
(Ex:) 112.0–112.9, 117.9, 139.8

112.89 Other
(Ex:) 112.4–112.9
Coding Clinic: 1992, Q1, P17; 1991, Q3, P20

112.9 Of unspecified site
Coding Clinic: 1996, Q4, P33

● **114 Coccidioidomycosis**

Includes   infection by Coccidioides (immitis)
Posada-Wernicke disease

114.0 Primary coccidioidomycosis (pulmonary)
Acute pulmonary coccidioidomycosis
Coccidioidomycotic pneumonitis
Desert rheumatism
Pulmonary coccidioidomycosis
San Joaquin Valley fever
(Ex:) 114.0, 114.3–114.9, 117.9, 139.8

114.1 Primary extrapulmonary coccidioidomycosis
Chancriform syndrome
Primary cutaneous coccidioidomycosis
(Ex:) 114.0–114.9

114.2 Coccidioidal meningitis
(Ex:) 003.21, 013.00–013.16, 036.0, 047.0–047.9, 049.0–049.1, 053.0, 054.72,
072.1, 090.42, 091.81, 094.2, 098.89, 100.81, 112.83, 114.2–114.3, 114.9,
115.01, 115.11, 115.91, 117.9, 130.0, 139.8, 320.0–322.9, 349.89–349.9,
357.0

114.3 Other forms of progressive coccidioidomycosis
Coccidioidal granuloma
Disseminated coccidioidomycosis
(Ex:) 114.3, 114.9, 117.9, 139.8

114.4 Chronic pulmonary coccidioidomycosis
(Ex:) 114.0–115.99

114.5 Pulmonary coccidioidomycosis, unspecified
(Ex:) 114.0–115.99

114.9 Coccidioidomycosis, unspecified
(Ex:) 114.3, 114.9, 117.9, 139.8

● **115 Histoplasmosis**

The following fifth-digit subclassification is for use with category 115:

0	**without mention of manifestation**
1	**meningitis**
2	**retinitis**
3	**pericarditis**
4	**endocarditis**
5	**pneumonia**
9	**other**

● **115.0 Infection by Histoplasma capsulatum** 2,9 , 1,3-5
[0-5,9]   American histoplasmosis
Darling's disease
Reticuloendothelial cytomycosis
Small form histoplasmosis
For code **115.01:** (Ex:) 003.21, 013.00–013.16, 036.0, 047.0–047.9, 049.0–049.1,
053.0, 054.72, 072.1, 090.42, 091.81, 094.2, 098.89, 100.81, 112.83,
114.2, 115.00–115.01, 115.09, 115.11, 115.90–115.91, 115.99, 117.9,
130.0, 139.8, 320.0–322.9, 349.89–349.9, 357.0;
For code **115.02:** (Ex:) 115.00, 115.02, 115.09, 115.90, 115.92, 115.99, 117.9,
139.8;
For code **115.03:** (Ex:) 115.00, 115.03, 115.09, 115.90, 115.93, 115.99, 117.9,
139.8;
For code **115.04:** (Ex:) 115.00, 115.04, 115.09, 115.90, 115.94, 115.99, 117.9, 139.8;
For code **115.05:** (Ex:) 115.00, 115.05–115.09, 115.90, 115.95–115.99, 117.9,
139.8, 480.0–480.2, 480.8–487.1, 488.01–488.02, 488.11–488.12,
488.81–488.82, 494.0–508.1, 508.8–508.9, 517.1, 518.89, 793.11;
For code **115.09:** (Ex:) 114.0–115.09

Item 1–17 Bird and bat droppings that fall into the soil give rise to a fungus that can spread airborne spores. When inhaled into the lungs, these spores divide and multiply into lesions. Histoplasmosis capsulatum takes three forms: primary (lodged in the lungs only), chronic (resembles TB), and disseminated (infection has moved to other organs). This is an opportunistic infection in immunosuppressed patients.

N Newborn: 0   **P** Pediatric: 0–17   **M** Maternity: 12–55   **A** Adult: 15–124   ♀ Females Only   ♂ Males Only

(Ex:) CC/MCC Exclusions   Complication\Comorbidity   Major C\C   Present on Admission Requirement   Hospital-Acquired Condition   **695**

INFECTIOUS AND PARASITIC DISEASES (001–139)

● **115.1 Infection by Histoplasma duboisii** 2,9 🔖, 1, 3-5 🔖
[0-5,9]   African histoplasmosis
          Large form histoplasmosis
          For code **115.11:** (Ex) 003.21, 013.00-013.16, 036.0, 047.0-047.9, 049.0-049.1,
          053.0, 054.72, 072.1, 090.42, 091.81, 094.2, 098.89, 100.81, 112.83,
          114.2, 115.01, 115.10-115.11, 115.19-115.91, 115.99, 117.9, 130.0,
          139.8, 320.0-322.9, 349.89-349.9, 357.0;
          For code **115.12:** (Ex) 115.10, 115.12, 115.19-115.90, 115.92, 115.99, 117.9,
          139.8;
          For code **115.13:** (Ex) 115.10, 115.13, 115.19-115.90, 115.93, 115.99, 117.9,
          139.8;
          For code **115.14:** (Ex) 115.10, 115.14, 115.19-115.90, 115.94, 115.99, 117.9,
          139.8;
          For code **115.15:** (Ex) 115.05, 115.10, 115.15-115.90, 115.95-115.99, 117.9,
          139.8, 480.0-480.2, 480.8-487.1, 488.01-488.02, 488.11-488.12, 488.81-
          488.82, 494.0-508.1, 508.8-508.9, 517.1, 518.89, 793.11;
          For code **115.19:** (Ex) 115.10, 115.19-115.90, 115.99, 117.9, 139.8

● **115.9 Histoplasmosis, unspecified** 2 🔖, 1, 3-5 🔖
[0-5,9]   Histoplasmosis NOS
          For code **115.91:** (Ex) 003.21, 013.00-013.16, 036.0, 047.0-047.9, 049.0-049.1,
          053.0, 054.72, 072.1, 090.42, 091.81, 094.2, 098.89, 100.81, 112.83,
          114.2, 115.01, 115.11, 115.91, 115.99, 117.9, 130.0, 139.8, 320.0-322.9,
          349.89-349.9, 357.0;
          For code **115.92:** (Ex) 115.92, 115.99, 117.9, 139.8;
          For code **115.93:** (Ex) 115.93, 115.99, 117.9, 139.8;
          For code **115.94:** (Ex) 115.94, 115.99, 117.9, 139.8;
          For code **115.95:** (Ex) 115.05, 115.15, 115.95-115.99, 117.9, 139.8

● **116 Blastomycotic infection**
      Rare and potentially fatal infections caused by fungus
         B. dermatitidis inhaled and found in moist soil
         in temperate climates

   116.0 Blastomycosis 🔖
            Blastomycotic dermatitis
            Chicago disease
            Cutaneous blastomycosis
            Disseminated blastomycosis
            Gilchrist's disease
            Infection by Blastomyces [Ajellomyces] dermatitidis
            North American blastomycosis
            Primary pulmonary blastomycosis
            (Ex) 116.0, 117.9, 139.8

   116.1 Paracoccidioidomycosis 🔖
            Brazilian blastomycosis
            Infection by Paracoccidioides [Blastomyces] brasiliensis
            Lutz-Splendore-Almeida disease
            Mucocutaneous-lymphangitic paracoccidioidomycosis
            Pulmonary paracoccidioidomycosis
            South American blastomycosis
            Visceral paracoccidioidomycosis
            (Ex) 116.1, 117.9, 139.8

   116.2 Lobomycosis
            Infections by Loboa [Blastomyces] loboi
            Keloidal blastomycosis
            Lobo's disease

● **117 Other mycoses**
   117.0 Rhinosporidiosis
            Infection by Rhinosporidium seeberi

   117.1 Sporotrichosis
            Cutaneous sporotrichosis
            Disseminated sporotrichosis
            Infection by Sporothrix [Sporotrichum] schenckii
            Lymphocutaneous sporotrichosis
            Pulmonary sporotrichosis
            Sporotrichosis of the bones

   117.2 Chromoblastomycosis
            Chromomycosis
            Infection by Cladosporidium carrionii, Fonsecaea
                compactum, Fonsecaea pedrosoi, Phialophora
                verrucosa

   117.3 Aspergillosis 🔖
            Infection by Aspergillus species, mainly A. fumigatus, A.
                flavus group, A. terreus group
            (Ex) 117.3, 117.9, 139.8
            Coding Clinic: 1997, Q4, P40

   117.4 Mycotic mycetomas 🔖
            Infection by various genera and species of Ascomycetes
                and Deuteromycetes, such as Acremonium
                [Cephalosporium] falciforme, Neotestudina
                rosatii, Madurella grisea, Madurella mycetomii,
                Pyrenochaeta romeroi, Zopfia [Leptosphaeria]
                senegalensis
            Madura foot, mycotic
            Maduromycosis, mycotic
            Excludes   *actinomycotic mycetomas (039.0–039.9)*
            (Ex) 117.4, 117.9, 139.8

   117.5 Cryptococcosis 🔖
            Busse-Buschke's disease
            European cryptococcosis
            Infection by Cryptococcus neoformans
            Pulmonary cryptococcosis
            Systemic cryptococcosis
            Torula
            (Ex) 117.5, 117.9, 139.8

   117.6 Allescheriosis [Petriellidosis] 🔖
            Infections by Allescheria [Petriellidium] boydii
                [Monosporium apiospermum]
            Excludes   *mycotic mycetoma (117.4)*
            (Ex) 117.6, 117.9, 139.8

   117.7 Zygomycosis [Phycomycosis or Mucormycosis] 🔖
            Infection by species of Absidia, Basidiobolus,
                Conidiobolus, Cunninghamella, Entomophthora,
                Mucor, Rhizopus, Saksenaea
            (Ex) 117.7, 117.9, 139.8

   **117.8 Infection by dematiacious fungi
            [Phaehyphomycosis]** 🔖
            Infection by dematiacious fungi, such as Cladosporium
                trichoides [bantianum], Dreschlera hawaiiensis,
                Phialophora gougerotii, Phialophora jeanselmi
            (Ex) 117.8-117.9

   117.9 Other and unspecified mycoses 🔖
            (Ex) 117.8-117.9
            Coding Clinic: 1995, Q2, P7

● **118 Opportunistic mycoses** 🔖
      Infection of skin, subcutaneous tissues, and/or organs by
         a wide variety of fungi generally considered to be
         pathogenic to compromised hosts only (e.g., infection by
         species of Alternaria, Dreschlera, Fusarium)
      Use additional code to identify manifestation, such as:
         keratitis (370.8)
      (Ex) 117.9-118, 139.8

HELMINTHIASES (120–129)

● **120 Schistosomiasis [bilharziasis]**
      Parasitic disease (worm induced) that leads to chronic illness

   120.0 Schistosoma haematobium 🔖
            Vesical schistosomiasis NOS
            (Ex) 120.0-120.9

   120.1 Schistosoma mansoni 🔖
            Intestinal schistosomiasis NOS
            (Ex) 120.0-120.9

   120.2 Schistosoma japonicum 🔖
            Asiatic schistosomiasis NOS
            Katayama disease or fever
            (Ex) 120.0-120.9

   120.3 Cutaneous 🔖
            Cercarial dermatitis
            Infection by cercariae of Schistosoma
            Schistosome dermatitis
            Swimmers' itch
            (Ex) 120.0-120.9

◄ New   ◄· Revised   ~~deleted~~ Deleted   Excludes   Includes   Use additional   Code first   Omit code

696   ● Unacceptable Principal Diagnosis   ● Use Additional Digit(s)   ▶ Manifestation Code   OGCR Official Guidelines   Coding Clinic

120.8 Other specified schistosomiasis 🔒
 Infection by Schistosoma:
  bovis
  intercalatum
  mattheii
 Infection by Schistosoma spindale
 Schistosomiasis chestermani
 (Ex) 120.0-120.9

120.9 Schistosomiasis, unspecified 🔒
 Blood flukes NOS   Hemic distomiasis
 (Ex) 120.0-120.9

● **121 Other trematode infections**

121.0 Opisthorchiasis 🔒
 Infection by:
  cat liver fluke
  Opisthorchis (felineus) (tenuicollis) (viverrini)
 (Ex) 121.0-121.9

121.1 Clonorchiasis 🔒
 Biliary cirrhosis due to clonorchiasis
 Chinese liver fluke disease
 Hepatic distomiasis due to Clonorchis sinensis
 Oriental liver fluke disease
 (Ex) 121.0-121.9

121.2 Paragonimiasis 🔒
 Infection by Paragonimus
 Lung fluke disease (oriental)
 Pulmonary distomiasis
 (Ex) 121.0-121.9

121.3 Fascioliasis 🔒
 Infection by Fasciola:
  gigantica
  hepatica
 Liver flukes NOS
 Sheep liver fluke infection
 (Ex) 121.0-121.9

121.4 Fasciolopsiasis 🔒
 Infection by Fasciolopsis (buski)
 Intestinal distomiasis
 (Ex) 121.0-121.9

121.5 Metagonimiasis 🔒
 Infection by Metagonimus yokogawai
 (Ex) 121.0-121.9

121.6 Heterophyiasis 🔒
 Infection by:
  Heterophyes heterophyes
  Stellantchasmus falcatus
 (Ex) 121.0-121.9

121.8 Other specified trematode infections 🔒
 Infection by:
  Dicrocoelium dendriticum
  Echinostoma ilocanum
  Gastrodiscoides hominis
 (Ex) 121.0-121.9

121.9 Trematode infection, unspecified
 Distomiasis NOS
 Fluke disease NOS

● **122 Echinococcosis**
 Also known as hydatid disease; caused by Echinococcus granulosus,
 E. multilocularis, and E. vogeli tapeworms; and is contracted
 from infected food

 Includes echinococciasis
        hydatid disease
        hydatidosis

122.0 Echinococcus granulosus infection of liver 🔒
 (Ex) 122.0, 122.8-122.9

122.1 Echinococcus granulosus infection of lung 🔒
 (Ex) 122.1, 122.8-122.9, 480.3

122.2 Echinococcus granulosus infection of thyroid 🔒
 (Ex) 122.2, 122.8-122.9

122.3 Echinococcus granulosus infection, other 🔒
 (Ex) 122.3, 122.8-122.9

122.4 Echinococcus granulosus infection, unspecified 🔒
 (Ex) 122.4, 122.8-122.9

122.5 Echinococcus multilocularis infection of liver 🔒
 (Ex) 122.5, 122.8-122.9

122.6 Echinococcus multilocularis infection, other 🔒
 (Ex) 122.6, 122.8-122.9

122.7 Echinococcus multilocularis infection, unspecified 🔒
 (Ex) 122.7-122.9

122.8 Echinococcosis, unspecified, of liver 🔒
 (Ex) 122.8-122.9

122.9 Echinococcosis, other and unspecified 🔒
 (Ex) 122.8-122.9

● **123 Other cestode infection**

123.0 Taenia solium infection, intestinal form 🔒
 Pork tapeworm (adult) (infection)
 (Ex) 001.1, 002.0, 002.9-003.0, 004.9-005.2, 006.0-006.2, 006.9, 007.1-009.0,
  014.80-014.86, 040.41-040.42, 112.85, 123.0-123.9, 129, 487.8, 488.09,
  488.19, 488.89, 536.3, 536.8, 558.2-558.9, 564.1, 777.50-777.53, 777.8

123.1 Cysticercosis 🔒
 Cysticerciasis
 Infection by Cysticercus cellulosae [larval form of Taenia
  solium]
 (Ex) 123.0-123.9
 Coding Clinic: 1997, Q2, P8

123.2 Taenia saginata infection 🔒
 Beef tapeworm (infection)
 Infection by Taeniarhynchus saginatus
 (Ex) 123.0-123.9

123.3 Taeniasis, unspecified 🔒
 (Ex) 123.0-123.9

123.4 Diphyllobothriasis, intestinal 🔒
 Diphyllobothrium (adult) (latum) (pacificum) infection
 Fish tapeworm (infection)
 (Ex) 123.0-123.9

123.5 Sparganosis [larval diphyllobothriasis] 🔒
 Infection by:
  Diphyllobothrium larvae
  Sparganum (mansoni) (proliferum)
  Spirometra larvae
 (Ex) 123.0-123.9

123.6 Hymenolepiasis 🔒
 Dwarf tapeworm (infection)
 Hymenolepis (diminuta) (nana) infection
 Rat tapeworm (infection)
 (Ex) 123.0-123.9

123.8 Other specified cestode infection 🔒
 Diplogonoporus (grandis) infection
 Dipylidium (caninum) infection
 Dog tapeworm (infection)
 (Ex) 123.0-123.9

123.9 Cestode infection, unspecified
 Tapeworm (infection) NOS

124 Trichinosis 🔒
 Trichinella spiralis infection
 Trichinellosis
 Trichiniasis
 (Ex) 013.60-013.66, 046.2, 046.71-046.8, 048-049.0, 049.8, 052.0, 052.2, 054.3, 054.74,
  056.01, 057.8-058.29, 059.00-059.9, 062.0-064, 066.2-066.49, 072.2, 073.7,
  079.82, 079.99, 081.9, 083.9, 090.41, 094.81, 117.5, 124, 130.0, 290.12,
  323.01-323.9, 341.1, 487.8, 488.09, 488.19, 488.89, 771.2, 984.9

INFECTIOUS AND PARASITIC DISEASES (001–139)

N Newborn: 0   P Pediatric: 0–17   M Maternity: 12–55   A Adult: 15–124   ♀ Females Only   ♂ Males Only

(Ex) CC/MCC Exclusions   🔒 Complication\Comorbidity   🔒 Major C\C   🔒 Present on Admission Requirement   🔒 Hospital-Acquired Condition   **697**

● **125 Filarial infection and dracontiasis**

125.0 Bancroftian filariasis 🔎
Chyluria due to Wuchereria bancrofti
Elephantiasis due to Wuchereria bancrofti
Infection due to Wuchereria bancrofti
Lymphadenitis due to Wuchereria bancrofti
Lymphangitis due to Wuchereria bancrofti
Wuchereriasis
(Ex) 125.0-125.9

125.1 Malayan filariasis 🔎
Brugia filariasis due to Brugia [Wuchereria] malayi
Chyluria due to Brugia [Wuchereria] malayi
Elephantiasis due to Brugia [Wuchereria] malayi
Infection due to Brugia [Wuchereria] malayi
Lymphadenitis due to Brugia [Wuchereria] malayi
Lymphangitis due to Brugia [Wuchereria] malayi
(Ex) 125.0-125.9

125.2 Loiasis 🔎
Eyeworm disease of Africa
Loa loa infection
(Ex) 125.0-125.9

125.3 Onchocerciasis 🔎
Onchocerca volvulus infection
Onchocercosis
(Ex) 125.0-125.9

125.4 Dipetalonemiasis 🔎
Infection by:
Acanthocheilonema perstans
Dipetalonema perstans
(Ex) 125.0-125.9

125.5 Mansonella ozzardi infection 🔎
Filariasis ozzardi
(Ex) 125.0-125.9

125.6 Other specified filariasis 🔎
Dirofilaria infection
Infection by:
Acanthocheilonema streptocerca
Dipetalonema streptocerca
(Ex) 125.0-125.9

125.7 Dracontiasis 🔎
Guinea-worm infection
Infection by Dracunculus medinensis
(Ex) 125.0-125.9

125.9 Unspecified filariasis 🔎
(Ex) 125.0-125.9

● **126 Ancylostomiasis and necatoriasis**

Includes cutaneous larva migrans due to Ancylostoma
hookworm (disease) (infection)
uncinariasis

126.0 Ancylostoma duodenale 🔎
(Ex) 126.0-126.9

126.1 Necator americanus 🔎
(Ex) 126.0-126.9

126.2 Ancylostoma braziliense 🔎
(Ex) 126.0-126.9

126.3 Ancylostoma ceylanicum 🔎
(Ex) 126.0-126.9

126.8 Other specified Ancylostoma 🔎
(Ex) 126.0-126.9

126.9 Ancylostomiasis and necatoriasis, unspecified 🔎
Creeping eruption NOS
Cutaneous larva migrans NOS
(Ex) 126.0-126.9

● **127 Other intestinal helminthiases**

127.0 Ascariasis 🔎
Ascaridiasis
Infection by Ascaris lumbricoides
Roundworm infection
(Ex) 127.0-127.9

127.1 Anisakiasis 🔎
Infection by Anisakis larva
(Ex) 127.0-127.9

127.2 Strongyloidiasis 🔎
Infection by Strongyloides stercoralis
Excludes trichostrongyliasis (127.6)
(Ex) 127.0-127.9

127.3 Trichuriasis 🔎
Infection by Trichuris trichiuria
Trichocephaliasis
Whipworm (disease) (infection)
(Ex) 127.0-127.9

127.4 Enterobiasis 🔎
Infection by Enterobius vermicularis
Oxyuriasis
Oxyuris vermicularis infection
Pinworm (disease) (infection)
Threadworm infection
(Ex) 127.0-127.9

127.5 Capillariasis 🔎
Infection by Capillaria philippinensis
Excludes infection by Capillaria hepatica (128.8)
(Ex) 127.0-127.9

127.6 Trichostrongyliasis 🔎
Infection by Trichostrongylus species
(Ex) 127.0-127.9

127.7 Other specified intestinal helminthiasis 🔎
Infection by:
Oesophagostomum apiostomum and related species
Ternidens diminutus
other specified intestinal helminth
Physalopteriasis
(Ex) 127.0-129

127.8 Mixed intestinal helminthiasis 🔎
Infection by intestinal helminths classified to more than one of the categories 120.0–127.7
Mixed helminthiasis NOS
(Ex) 127.0-129

127.9 Intestinal helminthiasis, unspecified 🔎
(Ex) 127.0-129

● **128 Other and unspecified helminthiases**

128.0 Toxocariasis
Larva migrans visceralis
Toxocara (canis) (cati) infection
Visceral larva migrans syndrome

128.1 Gnathostomiasis
Infection by Gnathostoma spinigerum and related species

128.8 Other specified helminthiasis
Infection by:
Angiostrongylus cantonensis
Capillaria hepatica
other specified helminth

128.9 Helminth infection, unspecified
Helminthiasis NOS
Worms NOS

129 Intestinal parasitism, unspecified

◀ New   ◀ Revised   ~~deleted~~ Deleted   Excludes   Includes   Use additional   Code first   Omit code
● Unacceptable Principal Diagnosis   ● Use Additional Digit(s)   ▷ Manifestation Code   OGCR Official Guidelines   Coding Clinic

Item 1–18 Toxoplasmosis is caused by the protozoa **Toxoplasma gondii,** of which the house cat can be a host. Human infection occurs when contact is made with materials containing the pathogen, such as feces, contaminated soil, or ingestion of infected lamb, goat, or pork. Of the infected, very few have symptoms because a healthy person's immune system keeps the parasite from causing illness. When the immune system is compromised, symptoms may occur. Clinical symptoms include flu-like symptoms, but the disease progresses to include the eyes and the brain in babies.

OTHER INFECTIOUS AND PARASITIC DISEASES (130–136)

● **130 Toxoplasmosis**

    Includes infection by toxoplasma gondii
              toxoplasmosis (acquired)

    Excludes *congenital toxoplasmosis (771.2)*

  130.0 Meningoencephalitis due to toxoplasmosis
    Encephalitis due to acquired toxoplasmosis
    (Ex:) 130.0, 130.7-130.9, 139.8

  130.1 Conjunctivitis due to toxoplasmosis
    (Ex:) 130.1, 130.7-130.9, 139.8

  130.2 Chorioretinitis due to toxoplasmosis
    Focal retinochoroiditis due to acquired toxoplasmosis
    (Ex:) 130.2, 130.7-130.9, 139.8

  130.3 Myocarditis due to toxoplasmosis
    (Ex:) 130.3, 130.7-130.9, 139.8

  130.4 Pneumonitis due to toxoplasmosis
    (Ex:) 130.4, 130.7-130.9, 139.8, 480.0-480.2, 480.8-487.1, 488.01-488.02, 488.11-488.12, 488.81-488.82, 494.0-508.1, 508.8-508.9, 517.1, 518.89, 793.11

  130.5 Hepatitis due to toxoplasmosis
    (Ex:) 130.5-130.9, 139.8

  130.7 Toxoplasmosis of other specified sites
    (Ex:) 130.7-130.9, 139.8

  130.8 Multisystemic disseminated toxoplasmosis
    Toxoplasmosis of multiple sites
    (Ex:) 130.7-130.9, 139.8

  130.9 Toxoplasmosis, unspecified
    (Ex:) 130.9

● **131 Trichomoniasis**
    A common STD caused by a parasite, Trichomonas vaginalis, affecting both women and men

    Includes infection due to Trichomonas (vaginalis)

● **131.0 Urogenital trichomoniasis**

  131.00 Urogenital trichomoniasis, unspecified
    Fluor (vaginalis) trichomonal or due to Trichomonas (vaginalis)
    Leukorrhea (vaginalis) trichomonal or due to Trichomonas (vaginalis)

  131.01 Trichomonal vulvovaginitis ♀
    Vaginitis, trichomonal or due to Trichomonas (vaginalis)

  131.02 Trichomonal urethritis

  131.03 Trichomonal prostatitis ♂

  131.09 Other

  131.8 Other specified sites
    Excludes *intestinal (007.3)*

  131.9 Trichomoniasis, unspecified

● **132 Pediculosis and phthirus infestation**
    Infestation of lice, Pediculus humanus, specifically capitis infest the head, corporis infest the body-trunk area, and pubis infest the pubic region

  132.0 Pediculus capitis [head louse]

  132.1 Pediculus corporis [body louse]

  132.2 Phthirus pubis [pubic louse]
    Pediculus pubis

  132.3 Mixed infestation
    This is a combination code.
    Infestation classifiable to more than one of the categories 132.0–132.2

  132.9 Pediculosis, unspecified

● **133 Acariasis**

  133.0 Scabies
    Infestation by Sarcoptes scabiei
    Norwegian scabies
    Sarcoptic itch

  133.8 Other acariasis
    Chiggers
    Infestation by:
      Demodex folliculorum
      Trombicula

  133.9 Acariasis, unspecified
    Infestation by mites NOS

● **134 Other infestation**

  134.0 Myiasis
    Infestation by:
      Dermatobia (hominis)
      fly larvae
      Gasterophilus (intestinalis)
      maggots
      Oestrus ovis

  134.1 Other arthropod infestation
    Infestation by:
      chigoe
      Jigger disease
      sand flea
      Scarabiasis
      Tunga penetrans
      Tungiasis

  134.2 Hirudiniasis
    Hirudiniasis (external) (internal)
    Leeches (aquatic) (land)

  134.8 Other specified infestations

  134.9 Infestation, unspecified
    Infestation (skin) NOS
    Skin parasites NOS

  135 Sarcoidosis
    Symptom of an inflammation producing tiny lumps of cells (granulomas) in various organs, most commonly the lungs and lymph nodes, that affect organ function
    Besnier-Boeck-Schaumann disease
    Lupoid (miliary) of Boeck
    Lupus pernio (Besnier)
    Lymphogranulomatosis, benign (Schaumann's)
    Sarcoid (any site):
      NOS
      Boeck
      Darier-Roussy
    Uveoparotid fever

● **136 Other and unspecified infectious and parasitic diseases**

  136.0 Ainhum
    Dactylolysis spontanea

  136.1 Behçet's syndrome

● **136.2 Specific infections by free-living amebae**

  136.21 Specific infection due to acanthamoeba
    Use additional code to identify manifestation, such as:
      keratitis (370.8)
    Coding Clinic: 2008, Q4, P79-81

  136.29 Other specific infections by free-living amebae
    Meningoencephalitis due to Naegleria
    (Ex:) 136.0-136.9
    Coding Clinic: 2008, Q4, P79-81

  136.3 Pneumocystosis
    Pneumonia due to Pneumocystis carinii
    Pneumonia due to Pneumocystis jiroveci
    (Ex:) 136.3, 139.8, 480.0-480.2, 480.8-487.1, 488.01-488.02, 488.11-488.12, 488.81-488.82, 494.0-508.1, 508.8-508.9, 517.1, 518.89, 793.11
    Coding Clinic: 2003, Q1, P15; 1987, Nov-Dec, P5-6

  136.4 Psorospermiasis
    (Ex:) 136.0-136.9

N Newborn: 0   **P** Pediatric: 0–17   **M** Maternity: 12–55   **A** Adult: 15–124   ♀ Females Only   ♂ Males Only

(Ex:) CC/MCC Exclusions   Complication\Comorbidity   Major C\C   Present on Admission Requirement   Hospital-Acquired Condition   **699**

INFECTIOUS AND PARASITIC DISEASES (001–139)

INFECTIOUS AND PARASITIC DISEASES (001-139)

136.5 Sarcosporidiosis 🔖
  Infection by Sarcocystis lindemanni
  (Ex:) 136.0-136.9

136.8 Other specified infectious and parasitic diseases
  Candiru infestation

136.9 Unspecified infectious and parasitic diseases
  Infectious disease NOS
  Parasitic disease NOS
  Coding Clinic: 1991, Q2, P8

LATE EFFECTS OF INFECTIOUS AND PARASITIC DISEASES (137–139)

● **137 Late effects of tuberculosis**
  Note: This category is to be used to indicate conditions
    classifiable to 010–018 as the cause of late effects,
    which are themselves classified elsewhere. The "late
    effects" include those specified as such, as sequelae,
    or as due to old or inactive tuberculosis, without
    evidence of active disease.

137.0 Late effects of respiratory or unspecified tuberculosis 🔖

**137.1 Late effects of central nervous system
    tuberculosis** 🔖

137.2 Late effects of genitourinary tuberculosis 🔖

137.3 Late effects of tuberculosis of bones and joints 🔖

**137.4 Late effects of tuberculosis of other specified
    organs** 🔖

Item 1-19 Before you assign the late code 137.X, check your documentation. The original problem (tuberculosis, TB) that is causing the current late effect (necrosis) must have been attributable to categories 010–018. A patient who originally had TB of a joint (015.2X) now has a late effect (137.3), which is necrosis of bone (730.8). Because there is no active TB, 015.2X is not coded but serves as an authorization to use the late effect code. Remember to code the manifestation of the late effect, which is the current problem (necrosis).

138 Late effects of acute poliomyelitis 🔖
  Note: This category is to be used to indicate conditions
    classifiable to 045 as the cause of late effects, which
    are themselves classified elsewhere. The "late effects"
    include conditions specified as such, or as sequelae,
    or as due to old or inactive poliomyelitis, without
    evidence of active disease.

● **139 Late effects of other infectious and parasitic diseases**
  Note: This category is to be used to indicate conditions
    classifiable to categories 001–009, 020–041, 046–136
    as the cause of late effects, which are themselves
    classified elsewhere. The "late effects" include
    conditions specified as such; they also include sequela
    of diseases classifiable to the above categories if there
    is evidence that the disease itself is no longer present.

139.0 Late effects of viral encephalitis 🔖
  Late effects of conditions classifiable to 049.8–049.9,
    062–064

139.1 Late effects of trachoma 🔖
  Late effects of conditions classifiable to 076

**139.8 Late effects of other and unspecified infectious and
    parasitic diseases** 🔖
  Coding Clinic: 2006, Q2, P17-18; 1990, Q3, P14

Item 2–1 Neoplasm: Neo = new, plasm = growth, development, formation. This new growth (mass, tumor) can be malignant or benign, which is confirmed by the pathology report. Do not assign a code to a neoplasm until you review the pathology report. Certain CPT codes will specify benign or malignant lesion, so be certain the diagnosis code supports the procedure code.

2. NEOPLASMS (140–239)

1. Content:

   This chapter contains the following broad groups:

   140–195   Malignant neoplasms, stated or presumed to be primary, of specified sites, except of lymphatic and hematopoietic tissue

   196–198   Malignant neoplasms, stated or presumed to be secondary, of specified sites

   199   Malignant neoplasms, without specification of site

   200–208   Malignant neoplasms, stated or presumed to be primary, of lymphatic and hematopoietic tissue

   209   Neuroendocrine tumors

   210–229   Benign neoplasms

   230–234   Carcinoma in situ

   235–238   Neoplasms of uncertain behavior [see Note, at beginning of section 235–238]

   239   Neoplasms of unspecified nature

2. Functional activity

   All neoplasms are classified in this chapter, whether or not functionally active. An additional code from Chapter 3 may be used to identify such functional activity associated with any neoplasm, e.g.:

   catecholamine-producing malignant pheochromocytoma of adrenal:

   code 194.0, additional code 255.6

   basophil adenoma of pituitary with Cushing's syndrome:

   code 227.3, additional code 255.0

3. Morphology [Histology]

   For those wishing to identify the histological type of neoplasms, a comprehensive coded nomenclature, which comprises the morphology rubrics of the ICD-Oncology, is given after the E-code chapter.

4. Malignant neoplasms overlapping site boundaries

   Categories 140–195 are for the classification of primary malignant neoplasms according to their point of origin. A malignant neoplasm that overlaps two or more subcategories within a three-digit rubric and whose point of origin cannot be determined should be classified to the subcategory .8 "Other." For example, "carcinoma involving tip and ventral surface of tongue" should be assigned to 141.8. On the other hand, "carcinoma of tip of tongue, extending to involve the ventral surface" should be coded to 141.2, as the point of origin, the tip, is known. Three subcategories (149.8, 159.8, 165.8) have been provided for malignant neoplasms that overlap the boundaries of three-digit rubrics within certain systems. Overlapping malignant neoplasms that cannot be classified as indicated above should be assigned to the appropriate subdivision of category 195 (Malignant neoplasm of other and ill-defined sites).

MALIGNANT NEOPLASM OF LIP, ORAL CAVITY, AND PHARYNX (140–149)

> **Excludes** *carcinoma in situ (230.0)*

● **140 Malignant neoplasm of lip**

> *Malignant neoplasm is a general term used to describe a cancerous growth or tumor.*

> **Excludes** *malignant melanoma of skin of lip (172.0)*
> *malignant neoplasm of skin of lip (173.00-173.09)*

140.0 Upper lip, vermilion border

Upper lip:	Upper lip:
NOS	lipstick area
external	

140.1 Lower lip, vermilion border

Lower lip:	Lower lip:
NOS	lipstick area
external	

140.3 Upper lip, inner aspect

Upper lip:	Upper lip:
buccal aspect	mucosa
frenulum	oral aspect

140.4 Lower lip, inner aspect

Lower lip:	Lower lip:
buccal aspect	mucosa
frenulum	oral aspect

140.5 Lip, unspecified, inner aspect

Lip, not specified whether upper or lower:
buccal aspect
frenulum
mucosa
oral aspect

140.6 Commissure of lip

Labial commissure

140.8 Other sites of lip

Malignant neoplasm of contiguous or overlapping sites of lip whose point of origin cannot be determined

140.9 Lip, unspecified, vermilion border

Lip, not specified as upper or lower:
NOS
external
lipstick area

● **141 Malignant neoplasm of tongue**

141.0 Base of tongue

Dorsal surface of base of tongue
Fixed part of tongue NOS
Coding Clinic: 2006, Q4, P88-91

141.1 Dorsal surface of tongue

Anterior two-thirds of tongue, dorsal surface
Dorsal tongue NOS
Midline of tongue

> **Excludes** *dorsal surface of base of tongue (141.0)*

141.2 Tip and lateral border of tongue

141.3 Ventral surface of tongue

Anterior two-thirds of tongue, ventral surface
Frenulum linguae

141.4 Anterior two-thirds of tongue, part unspecified

Mobile part of tongue NOS

NEOPLASMS (140–239)

Figure 2–1 Anatomical structures of the mouth and lips. **A.** Transitional or vermilion borders. Lips are connected to the gums by frenulum. **B.** Dorsal surface. **C.** Ventral surface.

Transitional or vermilion surfaces

Lips are connected to
A the gums by frenulum

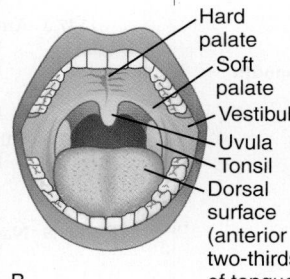

Hard palate
Soft palate
Vestibule
Uvula
Tonsil
Dorsal surface (anterior two-thirds of tongue)

B

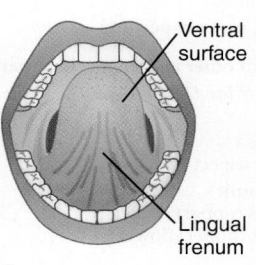

Ventral surface

Lingual frenum

C

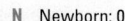

N Newborn: 0   P Pediatric: 0–17   M Maternity: 12–55   A Adult: 15–124   ♀ Females Only   ♂ Males Only

(Ex) CC/MCC Exclusions   🔾 Complication\Comorbidity   🔾 Major C\C   🔾 Present on Admission Requirement   🔾 Hospital-Acquired Condition   **701**

Figure 2–2   Major salivary glands.

Parotid gland
Sublingual gland
Submandibular gland

NEOPLASMS (140–239)

141.5 Junctional zone
Border of tongue at junction of fixed and mobile parts at insertion of anterior tonsillar pillar

141.6 Lingual tonsil

141.8 Other sites of tongue
Malignant neoplasm of contiguous or overlapping sites of tongue whose point of origin cannot be determined

141.9 Tongue, unspecified
Tongue NOS

● **142 Malignant neoplasm of major salivary glands**
Includes salivary ducts
Excludes *malignant neoplasm of minor salivary glands:*
NOS (145.9)
buccal mucosa (145.0)
soft palate (145.3)
tongue (141.0–141.9)
tonsil, palatine (146.0)

142.0 Parotid gland

142.1 Submandibular gland
Submaxillary gland

142.2 Sublingual gland

142.8 Other major salivary glands
Malignant neoplasm of contiguous or overlapping sites of salivary glands and ducts whose point of origin cannot be determined

142.9 Salivary gland, unspecified
Salivary gland (major) NOS

● **143 Malignant neoplasm of gum**
Includes alveolar (ridge) mucosa
gingiva (alveolar) (marginal)
interdental papillae
Excludes *malignant odontogenic neoplasms (170.0–170.1)*

143.0 Upper gum

143.1 Lower gum

143.8 Other sites of gum
Malignant neoplasm of contiguous or overlapping sites of gum whose point of origin cannot be determined

143.9 Gum, unspecified

● **144 Malignant neoplasm of floor of mouth**
144.0 Anterior portion
Anterior to the premolar-canine junction

144.1 Lateral portion

144.8 Other sites of floor of mouth
Malignant neoplasm of contiguous or overlapping sites of floor of mouth whose point of origin cannot be determined

144.9 Floor of mouth, part unspecified

● **145 Malignant neoplasm of other and unspecified parts of mouth**
Excludes *mucosa of lips (140.0–140.9)*

145.0 Cheek mucosa
Buccal mucosa
Cheek, inner aspect

145.1 Vestibule of mouth
Buccal sulcus (upper) (lower)
Labial sulcus (upper) (lower)

145.2 Hard palate

145.3 Soft palate
Excludes *nasopharyngeal [posterior] [superior] surface of soft palate (147.3)*
Coding Clinic: 1993, 5th Issue, P16

145.4 Uvula

145.5 Palate, unspecified
Junction of hard and soft palate
Roof of mouth

145.6 Retromolar area

145.8 Other specified parts of mouth
Malignant neoplasm of contiguous or overlapping sites of mouth whose point of origin cannot be determined

145.9 Mouth, unspecified
Buccal cavity NOS
Minor salivary gland, unspecified site
Oral cavity NOS

● **146 Malignant neoplasm of oropharynx**
146.0 Tonsil
Tonsil: Tonsil:
NOS   palatine
faucial
Excludes *lingual tonsil (141.6)*
pharyngeal tonsil (147.1)
Coding Clinic: 1987, Sept-Oct, P8

146.1 Tonsillar fossa

146.2 Tonsillar pillars (anterior) (posterior)
Faucial pillar
Glossopalatine fold
Palatoglossal arch
Palatopharyngeal arch

146.3 Vallecula
Anterior and medial surface of the pharyngoepiglottic fold

146.4 Anterior aspect of epiglottis
Epiglottis, free border [margin]
Glossoepiglottic fold(s)
Excludes *epiglottis:*
NOS (161.1)
suprahyoid portion (161.1)

146.5 Junctional region
Junction of the free margin of the epiglottis, the aryepiglottic fold, and the pharyngoepiglottic fold

146.6 Lateral wall of oropharynx

146.7 Posterior wall of oropharynx

146.8 Other specified sites of oropharynx
Branchial cleft
Malignant neoplasm of contiguous or overlapping sites of oropharynx whose point of origin cannot be determined

146.9 Oropharynx, unspecified
Coding Clinic: 2002, Q2, P6

● **147 Malignant neoplasm of nasopharynx**
147.0 Superior wall
Roof of nasopharynx

147.1 Posterior wall
Adenoid   Pharyngeal tonsil

147.2 Lateral wall
Fossa of Rosenmüller   Pharyngeal recess
Opening of auditory tube

147.3 Anterior wall
Floor of nasopharynx
Nasopharyngeal [posterior] [superior] surface of soft palate
Posterior margin of nasal septum and choanae

147.8 Other specified sites of nasopharynx
Malignant neoplasm of contiguous or overlapping sites of nasopharynx whose point of origin cannot be determined

147.9 Nasopharynx, unspecified
Nasopharyngeal wall NOS

◀ New   ◀▥ Revised   ~~deleted~~ Deleted   Excludes   Includes   Use additional   Code first   Omit code
● Unacceptable Principal Diagnosis   ● Use Additional Digit(s)   ▶ Manifestation Code   OGCR Official Guidelines   Coding Clinic

● **148 Malignant neoplasm of hypopharynx**

148.0 Postcricoid region
Behind the cricoid cartilage of neck

148.1 Pyriform sinus
Pyriform fossa

148.2 Aryepiglottic fold, hypopharyngeal aspect
Aryepiglottic fold or interarytenoid fold:
NOS
marginal zone
Excludes *aryepiglottic fold or interarytenoid fold, laryngeal aspect (161.1)*

148.3 Posterior hypopharyngeal wall

148.8 Other specified sites of hypopharynx
Malignant neoplasm of contiguous or overlapping sites of hypopharynx whose point of origin cannot be determined

148.9 Hypopharynx, unspecified
Hypopharyngeal wall NOS
Hypopharynx NOS

● **149 Malignant neoplasm of other and ill-defined sites within the lip, oral cavity, and pharynx**

149.0 Pharynx, unspecified

149.1 Waldeyer's ring

149.8 Other
Malignant neoplasms of lip, oral cavity, and pharynx whose point of origin cannot be assigned to any one of the categories 140–148
Excludes *"book leaf" neoplasm [ventral surface of tongue and floor of mouth] (145.8)*

149.9 Ill-defined

MALIGNANT NEOPLASM OF DIGESTIVE ORGANS AND PERITONEUM (150–159)

Excludes *carcinoma in situ (230.1–230.9)*

● **150 Malignant neoplasm of esophagus**

150.0 Cervical esophagus 🅟
(Ex) 150.0-150.9, 159.0, 159.8-159.9, 176.3, 195.8, 199.0-199.2, 209.20, 209.29-209.30, 209.70, 209.75, 239.0, 239.81-239.9

150.1 Thoracic esophagus 🅟
(Ex) 150.0-150.9, 159.0, 159.8-159.9, 176.3, 195.8, 199.0-199.2, 209.20, 209.29-209.30, 209.70, 209.75, 239.0, 239.81-239.9

150.2 Abdominal esophagus 🅟
Excludes *adenocarcinoma (151.0)*
cardio-esophageal junction (151.0)
(Ex) 150.0-150.9, 159.0, 159.8-159.9, 176.3, 195.8, 199.0-199.2, 209.20, 209.29-209.30, 209.70, 209.75, 239.0, 239.81-239.9

150.3 Upper third of esophagus 🅟
Proximal third of esophagus
(Ex) 150.0-150.9, 159.0, 159.8-159.9, 176.3, 195.8, 199.0-199.2, 209.20, 209.29-209.30, 209.70, 209.75, 239.0, 239.81-239.9

Figure 2-3 The esophagus is the muscular tube that connects the pharynx and the stomach. The 10 inch (25 cm) long esophagus is divided into three parts: **cervical, thoracic,** and **abdominal.**

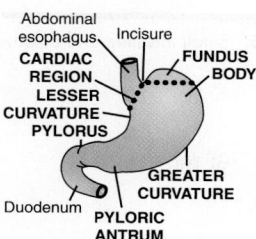

Figure 2-4 Parts of the stomach.

Item 2-2 The esophagus opens into the stomach through the **cardiac orifice,** also called the **cardioesophageal junction.** The **cardia** is adjacent to the cardiac orifice. The stomach widens into the **greater** and **lesser curvatures.** The **pyloric antrum** precedes the **pylorus,** which opens to the duodenum.

150.4 Middle third of esophagus 🅟
(Ex) 150.0-150.9, 159.0, 159.8-159.9, 176.3, 195.8, 199.0-199.2, 209.20, 209.29-209.30, 209.70, 209.75, 239.0, 239.81-239.9

150.5 Lower third of esophagus 🅟
Distal third of esophagus
Excludes *adenocarcinoma (151.0)*
cardio-esophageal junction (151.0)
(Ex) 150.0-150.9, 159.0, 159.8-159.9, 176.3, 195.8, 199.0-199.2, 209.20, 209.29-209.30, 209.70, 209.75, 239.0, 239.81-239.9

150.8 Other specified part 🅟
Malignant neoplasm of contiguous or overlapping sites of esophagus whose point of origin cannot be determined
(Ex) 150.0-150.9, 159.0, 159.8-159.9, 176.3, 195.8, 199.0-199.2, 209.20, 209.29-209.30, 209.70, 209.75, 239.0, 239.81-239.9

150.9 Esophagus, unspecified 🅟
(Ex) 150.0-150.9, 159.0, 159.8-159.9, 176.3, 195.8, 199.0-199.2, 209.20, 209.29-209.30, 209.70, 209.75, 239.0, 239.81-239.9

● **151 Malignant neoplasm of stomach**
Excludes *benign carcinoid tumor of stomach (209.63)*
malignant carcinoid tumor of stomach (209.23)

151.0 Cardia 🅟
Cardiac orifice
Cardio-esophageal junction
Excludes *squamous cell carcinoma (150.2, 150.5)*
(Ex) 151.0-151.9, 159.0, 159.8-159.9, 176.3, 195.8, 199.0-199.2, 209.20, 209.23, 209.25-209.30, 209.70, 209.75, 239.0, 239.81-239.9

151.1 Pylorus 🅟
Prepylorus
Pyloric canal
(Ex) 151.0-151.9, 159.0, 159.8-159.9, 176.3, 195.8, 199.0-199.2, 209.20, 209.23, 209.25-209.30, 209.70, 209.75, 239.0, 239.81-239.9

151.2 Pyloric antrum 🅟
Antrum of stomach NOS
(Ex) 151.0-151.9, 159.0, 159.8-159.9, 176.3, 195.8, 199.0-199.2, 209.20, 209.23, 209.25-209.30, 209.70, 209.75, 239.0, 239.81-239.9

151.3 Fundus of stomach 🅟
(Ex) 151.0-151.9, 159.0, 159.8-159.9, 176.3, 195.8, 199.0-199.2, 209.20, 209.23, 209.25-209.30, 209.70, 209.75, 239.0, 239.81-239.9

151.4 Body of stomach 🅟
(Ex) 151.0-151.9, 159.0, 159.8-159.9, 176.3, 195.8, 199.0-199.2, 209.20, 209.23, 209.25-209.30, 209.70, 209.75, 239.0, 239.81-239.9

151.5 Lesser curvature, unspecified 🅟
Lesser curvature, not classifiable to 151.1–151.4
(Ex) 151.0-151.9, 159.0, 159.8-159.9, 176.3, 195.8, 199.0-199.2, 209.20, 209.23, 209.25-209.30, 209.70, 209.75, 239.0, 239.81-239.9

151.6 Greater curvature, unspecified 🅟
Greater curvature, not classifiable to 151.0–151.4
(Ex) 151.0-151.9, 159.0, 159.8-159.9, 176.3, 195.8, 199.0-199.2, 209.20, 209.23, 209.25-209.30, 209.70, 209.75, 239.0, 239.81-239.9

NEOPLASMS (140–239)

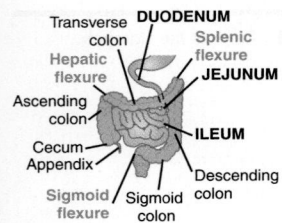

Figure 2–5   Small intestine and colon.

151.8   Other specified sites of stomach
  Anterior wall, not classifiable to 151.0–151.4
  Posterior wall, not classifiable to 151.0–151.4
  Malignant neoplasm of contiguous or overlapping
    sites of stomach whose point of origin cannot be
    determined
  (Ex:) 151.0-151.9, 159.0, 159.8-159.9, 176.3, 195.8, 199.0-199.2, 209.20, 209.23,
       209.25-209.30, 209.70, 209.75, 239.0, 239.81-239.9

151.9   Stomach, unspecified
  Carcinoma ventriculi
  Gastric cancer
  (Ex:) 151.0-151.9, 159.0, 159.8-159.9, 176.3, 195.8, 199.0-199.2, 209.20, 209.23,
       209.25-209.30, 209.70, 209.75, 239.0, 239.81-239.9
  Coding Clinic: 2001, Q2, P17-18; 1988, Q2, P11

●152   **Malignant neoplasm of small intestine, including duodenum**
  Excludes   *benign carcinoid tumor of small intestine and duodenum*
            (209.40-209.43)
            malignant carcinoid tumor of small intestine
            and duodenum (209.00-209.03)

152.0   Duodenum
  (Ex:) 152.0, 152.8-152.9, 159.0, 159.8-159.9, 176.3, 195.8, 199.0-199.2,
       209.00-209.01, 209.20, 209.29-209.30, 209.70, 209.75, 239.0,
       239.81-239.9

152.1   Jejunum
  (Ex:) 152.1, 152.8-152.9, 159.0, 159.8-159.9, 176.3, 195.8, 199.0-199.2, 209.00,
       209.02, 209.20, 209.29-209.30, 209.70, 209.75, 239.0, 239.81-239.9

152.2   Ileum
  Excludes   *ileocecal valve (153.4)*
  (Ex:) 152.2, 152.8-152.9, 159.0, 159.8-159.9 176.3, 195.8, 199.0-199.2, 209.00,
       209.03 209.20, 209.29-209.30, 209.70, 209.75, 239.0, 239.81-239.9

152.3   Meckel's diverticulum
  (Ex:) 152.3-152.9, 159.0, 159.8-159.9, 176.3 195.8, 199.0-199.2, 209.00, 209.20,
       209.29-209.30, 209.70, 209.75, 239.0, 239.81-239.9

152.8   Other specified sites of small intestine
  Duodenojejunal junction
  Malignant neoplasm of contiguous or overlapping sites
    of small intestine whose point of origin cannot be
    determined
  (Ex:) 152.8-152.9, 159.0, 159.8-159.9, 176.3, 195.8, 199.0-199.2, 209.00, 209.20,
       209.29-209.30, 209.70, 209.75, 239.0, 239.81-239.9

152.9   Small intestine, unspecified
  (Ex:) 152.8-152.9, 159.0, 159.8-159.9, 176.3 195.8, 199.0-199.2, 209.00, 209.20,
       209.29-209.30, 209.70, 209.75, 239.0, 239.81-239.9

●153   **Malignant neoplasm of colon**
  Excludes   *benign carcinoid tumor of colon (209.50-*
            209.56)
            malignant carcinoid tumor of colon (209.10-209.16)

153.0   Hepatic flexure
  Flexure is a bending in a structure or organ. Note the three
    flexures illustrated in Figure 2–5. Hepatic = liver,
    sigmoid = colon, splenic = spleen.
  (Ex:) 153.0, 153.8-153.9, 159.0, 159.8-159.9, 176.3, 195.8, 199.0-199.2, 209.10,
       209.20, 209.29-209.30, 209.70, 209.75, 239.0, 239.81-239.9

153.1   Transverse colon
  (Ex:) 153.1, 153.8-153.9, 159.0, 159.8-159.9, 176.3, 195.8, 199.0-199.2, 209.10,
       209.14, 209.20, 209.29-209.30, 209.70, 209.75, 239.0, 239.81-239.9
  Coding Clinic: 2013, Q3, P9

153.2   Descending colon
  Left colon
  (Ex:) 153.2, 153.8-153.9, 159.0, 159.8-159.9, 176.3, 195.8, 199.0-199.2, 209.10,
       209.15, 209.20, 209.29-209.30, 209.70, 209.75, 239.0, 239.81-239.9
  Coding Clinic: 1995, Q1, P4

153.3   Sigmoid colon
  Sigmoid (flexure)
  Excludes   *rectosigmoid junction (154.0)*
  Flexure is a bending in a structure or organ. Note the three
    flexures illustrated in Figure 2–5. Hepatic = liver,
    sigmoid = colon, splenic = spleen.
  (Ex:) 153.3, 153.8-153.9, 159.0, 159.8-159.9, 176.3, 195.8, 199.0-199.2, 209.10,
       209.16, 209.20, 209.29-209.30, 209.70, 209.75, 239.0, 239.81-239.9

153.4   Cecum
  Ileocecal valve
  (Ex:) 153.4, 153.8-153.9, 159.0, 159.8-159.9, 176.3, 195.8, 199.0-199.2, 209.10,
       209.12, 209.20, 209.29-209.30, 209.70, 209.75, 239.0, 239.81-239.9

153.5   Appendix
  (Ex:) 153.5, 153.8-153.9, 159.0, 159.8-159.9, 176.3, 195.8, 199.0-199.2,
       209.10-209.11, 209.20, 209.29-209.30, 209.70, 209.75, 239.0,
       239.81-239.9

153.6   Ascending colon
  Right colon
  (Ex:) 153.6, 153.8-153.9, 159.0, 159.8-159.9, 176.3, 195.8, 199.0-199.2, 209.10,
       209.13, 209.20, 209.29-209.30, 209.70, 209.75, 239.0, 239.81-239.9

153.7   Splenic flexure
  Flexure is a bending in a structure or organ. Note the three
    flexures illustrated in Figure 2–5. Hepatic = liver,
    sigmoid = colon, splenic = spleen.
  (Ex:) 153.7-153.9, 159.0, 159.8-159.9, 176.3, 195.8, 199.0-199.2, 209.10, 209.20,
       209.29-209.30, 209.70, 209.75, 239.0, 239.81-239.9

153.8   Other specified sites of large intestine
  Malignant neoplasm of contiguous or overlapping
    sites of colon whose point of origin cannot be
    determined
  Excludes   *ileocecal valve (153.4)*
            rectosigmoid junction (154.0)
  (Ex:) 153.8-153.9, 159.0, 159.8-159.9, 176.3, 195.8, 199.0-199.2, 209.10, 209.20,
       209.29-209.30, 209.70, 209.75, 239.0, 239.81-239.9

153.9   Colon, unspecified
  Large intestine NOS
  (Ex:) 153.8-153.9, 159.0, 159.8-159.9, 176.3, 195.8, 199.0-199.2, 209.10, 209.20,
       209.29-209.30, 209.70, 209.75, 239.0, 239.81-239.9
  Coding Clinic: 2010, Q2, P12

●154   **Malignant neoplasm of rectum, rectosigmoid junction, and anus**
  Excludes   *benign carcinoid tumor of rectum (209.57)*
            malignant carcinoid tumor of rectum (209.17)

154.0   Rectosigmoid junction
  Colon with rectum
  Rectosigmoid (colon)
  (Ex:) 154.0, 154.8, 159.0, 159.8-159.9, 176.3, 195.8, 199.0-199.2, 209.20,
       209.29-209.30, 209.70, 209.75, 239.0, 239.81-239.9

154.1   Rectum
  Rectal ampulla
  (Ex:) 154.1, 154.8, 159.0, 159.8-159.9, 176.3, 195.8, 199.0-199.2, 209.17-209.20,
       209.29-209.30, 209.70, 209.75, 239.0, 239.81-239.9

154.2   Anal canal
  Anal sphincter
  Excludes   *malignant melanoma of skin of anus*
            (172.5)
            malignant neoplasm of skin of anus
            (173.50-173.59)
  (Ex:) 154.2-154.8, 159.0, 159.8-159.9, 176.3, 195.8, 199.0-199.2, 209.20,
       209.29-209.30, 209.70, 209.75, 239.0, 239.81-239.9
  Coding Clinic: 2001, Q1, P8

154.3   Anus, unspecified
  Excludes   *malignant melanoma of:*
            anus:
              margin (172.5)
              skin (172.5)
            perianal skin (172.5)
            malignant neoplasm of:
            anus:
              margin (173.50-173.59)
              skin (173.50-173.59)
            perianal skin (173.50-173.59)
  (Ex:) 154.2-154.8, 159.0, 159.8-159.9, 176.3, 195.8, 199.0-199.2, 209.20,
       209.29-209.30, 209.70, 209.75, 239.0, 239.81-239.9

◀ New   ◀◀ Revised   ~~deleted~~ Deleted   Excludes   Includes   Use additional   Code first   Omit code
● Unacceptable Principal Diagnosis   ● Use Additional Digit(s)   ▸ Manifestation Code   OGCR Official Guidelines   Coding Clinic

704

NEOPLASMS (140–239)

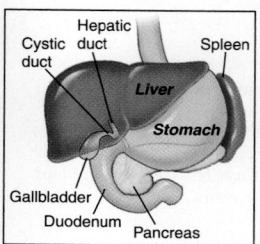

Figure 2-6 Diagram of liver, gallbladder, hepatic duct, pancreas, and spleen. (From Thibodeau and Patton: Anatomy and Physiology, ed 7, Mosby, 2010)

Item 2–3 Islets of Langerhans (endocrine producing cells comprising 1% to 2% of the pancreatic mass) make and secrete hormones that regulate the body's production of insulin, glucagon, and stomach acid. Breakdown of the insulin-producing cells can cause diabetes mellitus.
Islet cell tumors can be benign or malignant and include glucagonomas, insulinomas, gastrinomas, and neuroendocrine tumor. The neoplasm table must be consulted for the correct neoplasm code.

154.8 Other

Anorectum
Cloacogenic zone
Malignant neoplasm of contiguous or overlapping sites of rectum, rectosigmoid junction, and anus whose point of origin cannot be determined
(Ex:) 154.8, 159.0, 159.8-159.9, 176.3, 195.8, 199.0-199.2, 209.20, 209.29-209.30, 209.70, 209.75, 239.0, 239.81-239.9

● 155 Malignant neoplasm of liver and intrahepatic bile ducts

155.0 Liver, primary
Carcinoma:
liver, specified as primary
hepatocellular
liver cell
Hepatoblastoma
(Ex:) 155.0-155.2, 159.0, 159.8-159.9, 176.3, 195.8, 199.0-199.2, 209.20, 209.29-209.30, 209.70, 209.75, 239.0, 239.81-239.9
Coding Clinic: 2008, Q4, P82-83

155.1 Intrahepatic bile ducts
Canaliculi biliferi   Intrahepatic:
Interlobular: biliary passages
  bile ducts   canaliculi
  biliary canals   gall duct
Excludes *hepatic duct (156.1)*
(Ex:) 155.0-155.2, 159.0, 159.8-159.9, 176.3, 195.8, 199.0-199.2, 209.20, 209.29-209.30, 209.70, 209.75, 239.0, 239.81-239.9

155.2 Liver, not specified as primary or secondary
Stated as a liver neoplasm, but not specific as to type
(Ex:) 155.0-155.2, 159.0, 159.8-159.9, 176.3, 195.8, 199.0-199.2, 209.20, 209.29-209.30, 209.70, 209.75, 239.0, 239.81-239.9

● 156 Malignant neoplasm of gallbladder and extrahepatic bile ducts

Extrahepatic = outside the liver

156.0 Gallbladder
(Ex:) 156.0, 156.8-156.9, 159.0, 159.8-159.9, 176.3, 195.8, 199.0-199.2, 209.20, 209.29-209.30, 209.70, 209.75, 239.0, 239.81-239.9

156.1 Extrahepatic bile ducts
Biliary duct or passage   Cystic duct
NOS   Hepatic duct
Common bile duct   Sphincter of Oddi
(Ex:) 156.1, 156.8-156.9, 159.0, 159.8-159.9, 176.3, 195.8, 199.0-199.2, 209.20, 209.29-209.30, 209.70, 209.75, 239.0, 239.81-239.9

156.2 Ampulla of Vater
(Ex:) 156.2-156.9, 159.0, 159.8-159.9, 176.3, 195.8, 199.0-199.2, 209.20, 209.29-209.30, 209.70, 209.75, 239.0, 239.81-239.9

156.8 Other specified sites of gallbladder and extrahepatic bile ducts
Malignant neoplasm of contiguous or overlapping sites of gallbladder and extrahepatic bile ducts whose point of origin cannot be determined
(Ex:) 156.8-156.9, 159.0, 159.8-159.9, 176.3, 195.8, 199.0-199.2, 209.20, 209.29-209.30, 209.70, 209.75, 239.0, 239.81-239.9

156.9 Biliary tract, part unspecified
Malignant neoplasm involving both intrahepatic and extrahepatic bile ducts
Intra = inside; extra = outside
(Ex:) 156.8-156.9, 159.0, 159.8-159.9, 176.3, 195.8, 199.0-199.2, 209.20, 209.29-209.30, 209.70, 209.75, 239.0, 239.81-239.9

● 157 Malignant neoplasm of pancreas

Check documentation for specific site.

157.0 Head of pancreas
(Ex:) 157.0-157.9, 159.0, 159.8-159.9, 176.3, 195.8, 199.0-199.2, 209.20, 209.29-209.30, 209.70, 209.75, 239.0, 239.81-239.9
Coding Clinic: 2005, Q2, P9-10; 2000, Q4, P39-40

157.1 Body of pancreas
(Ex:) 157.0-157.9, 159.0, 159.8-159.9, 176.3, 195.8, 199.0-199.2, 209.20, 209.29-209.30, 209.70, 209.75, 239.0, 239.81-239.9

157.2 Tail of pancreas
(Ex:) 157.0-157.9, 159.0, 159.8-159.9, 176.3, 195.8, 199.0-199.2, 209.20, 209.29-209.30, 209.70, 209.75, 239.0, 239.81-239.9

157.3 Pancreatic duct
Duct of:
Santorini
Wirsung
(Ex:) 157.0-157.9, 159.0, 159.8-159.9, 176.3, 195.8, 199.0-199.2, 209.20, 209.29-209.30, 209.70, 209.75, 239.0, 239.81-289.9

157.4 Islets of Langerhans
Islets of Langerhans, any part of pancreas
Use additional code to identify any functional activity
(Ex:) 157.0-157.9, 159.0, 159.8-159.9, 176.3, 195.8, 199.0-199.2, 209.20, 209.29-209.30, 209.70, 209.75, 239.0, 239.81-239.9
Coding Clinic: 2007, Q4, P70-72

157.8 Other specified sites of pancreas
Ectopic pancreatic tissue
Malignant neoplasm of contiguous or overlapping sites of pancreas whose point of origin cannot be determined
(Ex:) 157.0-157.9, 159.0, 159.8-159.9, 176.3, 195.8, 199.0-199.2, 209.20, 209.29-209.30, 209.70, 209.75, 239.0, 239.81-239.9

157.9 Pancreas, part unspecified
(Ex:) 157.0-157.9, 159.0, 159.8-159.9, 176.3, 195.8, 199.0-199.2, 209.20, 209.29-209.30, 209.70, 209.75, 239.0, 239.81-239.9
Coding Clinic: 1989, Q4, P11

● 158 Malignant neoplasm of retroperitoneum and peritoneum

158.0 Retroperitoneum
Periadrenal tissue   Perirenal tissue
Perinephric tissue   Retrocecal tissue
(Ex:) 158.0, V58.0

158.8 Specified parts of peritoneum
Cul-de-sac (of Douglas)
Mesentery
Mesocolon
Omentum
Peritoneum:
  parietal
  pelvic
Rectouterine pouch
Malignant neoplasm of contiguous or overlapping sites of retroperitoneum and peritoneum whose point of origin cannot be determined
(Ex:) 158.0-158.9, V58.0

158.9 Peritoneum, unspecified
(Ex:) 158.0-158.9, V58.0

NEOPLASMS (140–239)

NEOPLASMS (140–239)

● **159 Malignant neoplasm of other and ill-defined sites within the digestive organs and peritoneum**

    159.0 Intestinal tract, part unspecified
        Intestine NOS

    159.1 Spleen, not elsewhere classified
        Angiosarcoma of spleen
        Fibrosarcoma of spleen
        Excludes *Hodgkin's disease (201.0–201.9)*
                    lymphosarcoma (200.1)
                    reticulosarcoma (200.0)

    159.8 Other sites of digestive system and intra-abdominal organs
        Malignant neoplasm of digestive organs and peritoneum whose point of origin cannot be assigned to any one of the categories 150–158
        Excludes *anus and rectum (154.8)*
                    cardio-esophageal junction (151.0)
                    colon and rectum (154.0)

    159.9 Ill-defined
        Alimentary canal or tract NOS
        Gastrointestinal tract NOS
        Excludes *abdominal NOS (195.2)*
                    intra-abdominal NOS (195.2)

MALIGNANT NEOPLASM OF RESPIRATORY AND INTRATHORACIC ORGANS (160–165)

    Excludes *carcinoma in situ (231.0–231.9)*

● **160 Malignant neoplasm of nasal cavities, middle ear, and accessory sinuses**

    160.0 Nasal cavities
        Cartilage of nose   Septum of nose
        Conchae, nasal   Vestibule of nose
        Internal nose
        Excludes *malignant melanoma of skin of nose (172.3)*
                    malignant neoplasm of skin of nose
                      (173.30-173.39)
                  nasal bone (170.0)
                  nose NOS (195.0)
                  olfactory bulb (192.0)
                  posterior margin of septum and choanae (147.3)
                  turbinates (170.0)

    160.1 Auditory tube, middle ear, and mastoid air cells
        Antrum tympanicum
        Eustachian tube
        Tympanic cavity
        Excludes *bone of ear (meatus) (170.0)*
                    cartilage of ear (171.0)
                  malignant melanoma of:
                    auditory canal (external) (172.2)
                    ear (external) (skin) (172.2)
                  malignant neoplasm of:
                    auditory canal (external) (173.20-173.29)
                    ear (external) (skin) (173.20-173.29)

    160.2 Maxillary sinus
        Antrum (Highmore) (maxillary)

    160.3 Ethmoidal sinus

    160.4 Frontal sinus

    160.5 Sphenoidal sinus

    160.8 Other
        Malignant neoplasm of contiguous or overlapping sites of nasal cavities, middle ear, and accessory sinuses whose point of origin cannot be determined

    160.9 Accessory sinus, unspecified

Figure 2–7 Paranasal sinuses. (From Buck CJ: Step-by-Step Medical Coding, ed 2011, Philadelphia, WB Saunders, 2011)

Frontal sinus
Sphenoidal sinus
Ethmoidal sinus
Maxillary sinus

● **161 Malignant neoplasm of larynx**

    161.0 Glottis
        Intrinsic larynx
        Laryngeal commissure (anterior) (posterior)
        True vocal cord
        True vocal cords (lower vocal folds) produce vocalization when air from lungs passes between them. Check your documentation. Code 161.1 is for malignant neoplasm of false vocal cords.
        Vocal cord NOS

    161.1 Supraglottis
        Aryepiglottic fold or interarytenoid fold, laryngeal aspect
        Epiglottis (suprahyoid portion) NOS
        Extrinsic larynx
        False vocal cords
        False vocal cords (upper vocal folds) are not involved in vocalization. Check your documentation. Code 161.0 is for true vocal cords.
        Posterior (laryngeal) surface of epiglottis
        Ventricular bands
        Excludes *anterior aspect of epiglottis (146.4)*
                    aryepiglottic fold or interarytenoid fold:
                      NOS (148.2)
                      hypopharyngeal aspect (148.2)
                      marginal zone (148.2)

    161.2 Subglottis

    161.3 Laryngeal cartilages
        Cartilage: Cartilage:
          arytenoid   cuneiform
          cricoid   thyroid

    161.8 Other specified sites of larynx
        Malignant neoplasm of contiguous or overlapping sites of larynx whose point of origin cannot be determined
        Coding Clinic: 2007, Q3, P8-9

    161.9 Larynx, unspecified

● **162 Malignant neoplasm of trachea, bronchus, and lung**
    Excludes *benign carcinoid tumor of bronchus (209.61)*
                    malignant carcinoid tumor of bronchus (209.21)
    Coding Clinic: 2006, Q3, P7-8

    162.0 Trachea
        Cartilage of trachea
        Mucosa of trachea
        (Ex) 162.0-162.9, 165.8-165.9, 176.4, 195.1, 195.8, 197.0-197.1, 197.3, 199.0-199.2, 209.20-209.21, 209.29-209.30, 209.70, 209.75, 239.1, 239.81-239.9

    162.2 Main bronchus
        Carina
        Hilus of lung
        (Ex) 162.2, 162.8-162.9, 165.8-165.9, 176.4, 195.8, 199.0-199.2, 209.20-209.21, 209.29- 209.30, 209.70, 209.75, 239.1, 239.81-239.9

    162.3 Upper lobe, bronchus or lung
        (Ex) 162.3, 162.8-162.9, 165.8-165.9, 176.4, 195.8, 199.0-199.2, 209.20-209.21, 209.29-209.30, 209.70, 209.75, 239.1, 239.81-239.9
        Coding Clinic: 2004, Q1, P4-5

    162.4 Middle lobe, bronchus or lung
        (Ex) 162.4, 162.8-162.9, 165.8-165.9, 176.4, 195.8, 199.0-199.2, 209.20-209.21, 209.29-209.30, 209.70, 209.75, 239.1, 239.81-239.9

    162.5 Lower lobe, bronchus or lung
        (Ex) 162.5-162.9, 165.8-165.9, 176.4, 195.8, 199.0-199.2, 209.20-209.21, 209.29-209.30, 209.70, 209.75, 239.1, 239.81-239.9
        Coding Clinic: 2010, Q3, P3

    162.8 Other parts of bronchus or lung
        Malignant neoplasm of contiguous or overlapping sites of bronchus or lung whose point of origin cannot be determined
        (Ex) 162.8-162.9, 165.8-165.9, 176.4, 195.8, 199.0-199.2, 209.20-209.21, 209.29-209.30, 209.70, 209.75, 239.1, 239.81-239.9
        Coding Clinic: 2006, Q3, P7-8

    162.9 Bronchus and lung, unspecified
        (Ex) 162.8-162.9, 165.8-165.9, 176.4, 195.8, 199.0-199.2, 209.20-209.21, 209.29-209.30, 209.70, 209.75, 239.1, 239.81-239.9
        Coding Clinic: 2010, Q2, P14; 2006, Q3, P14-15; 1997, Q2, P3; 1996, Q4, P47-48; 1993, Q4, P36; 1988, Q2, P10; 1984, May-June, P11, 14

◄ New   ◄▥ Revised   ~~deleted~~ Deleted   Excludes   Includes   Use additional   Code first   Omit code

● Unacceptable Principal Diagnosis   ● Use Additional Digit(s)   ▶ Manifestation Code   **OGCR** Official Guidelines   **Coding Clinic**

706

● **163 Malignant neoplasm of pleura**
Pleura are comprised of serous membrane that lines thoracic cavity (parietal) and covers lungs (visceral).

163.0 Parietal pleura 🔖
Ex: 163.0-163.9, 165.8-165.9, 195.8, 199.0-199.2, 209.20, 209.29-209.30, 209.70, 209.75, 239.1, 239.81-239.9

163.1 Visceral pleura 🔖
Ex: 163.0-163.9, 165.8-165.9, 195.8, 199.0-199.2, 209.20, 209.29-209.30, 209.70, 209.75, 239.1, 239.81-239.9

163.8 Other specified sites of pleura 🔖
Malignant neoplasm of contiguous or overlapping sites of pleura whose point of origin cannot be determined
Ex: 163.0-163.9, 165.8-165.9, 195.8, 199.0-199.2, 209.20, 209.29-209.30, 209.70, 209.75, 239.1, 239.81-239.9

163.9 Pleura, unspecified 🔖
Ex: 163.0-163.9, 165.8-165.9, 195.8, 199.0-199.2, 209.20, 209.29-209.30, 209.70, 209.75, 239.1, 239.81-239.9

● **164 Malignant neoplasm of thymus, heart, and mediastinum**

164.0 Thymus 🔖
Excludes *benign carcinoid tumor of the thymus (209.62)*
malignant carcinoid tumor of the thymus (209.22)
Ex: 164.0, 209.22

164.1 Heart 🔖
Endocardium   Myocardium
Epicardium   Pericardium
Excludes *great vessels (171.4)*
Ex: 164.1

164.2 Anterior mediastinum 🔖
Ex: 164.2-164.9, 165.8-165.9, 195.8, 199.0-199.2, 209.20, 209.29-209.30, 209.70, 209.75, 239.1, 239.81-239.9

164.3 Posterior mediastinum 🔖
Ex: 164.2-164.9, 165.8-165.9, 195.8, 199.0-199.2, 209.20, 209.29-209.30, 209.70, 209.75, 239.1, 239.81-239.9

164.8 Other 🔖
Malignant neoplasm of contiguous or overlapping sites of thymus, heart, and mediastinum whose point of origin cannot be determined
Ex: 164.2-164.9, 165.8-165.9, 195.8, 199.0-199.2, 209.20, 209.29-209.30, 209.70, 209.75, 239.1, 239.81-239.9

164.9 Mediastinum, part unspecified 🔖
Ex: 164.2-164.9, 165.8-165.9, 195.8, 199.0-199.2, 209.20, 209.29-209.30, 209.70, 209.75, 239.1, 239.81-239.9

● **165 Malignant neoplasm of other and ill-defined sites within the respiratory system and intrathoracic organs**

165.0 Upper respiratory tract, part unspecified

165.8 Other
Malignant neoplasm of respiratory and intrathoracic organs whose point of origin cannot be assigned to any one of the categories 160–164

165.9 Ill-defined sites within the respiratory system
Respiratory tract NOS
Excludes *intrathoracic NOS (195.1)*
thoracic NOS (195.1)

MALIGNANT NEOPLASM OF BONE, CONNECTIVE TISSUE, SKIN, AND BREAST (170–176)

Excludes *carcinoma in situ:*
breast (233.0)
skin (232.0–232.9)

● **170 Malignant neoplasm of bone and articular cartilage**
Includes cartilage (articular) (joint)
periosteum
Excludes *bone marrow NOS (202.9)*
cartilage:
ear (171.0)
eyelid (171.0)
larynx (161.3)
nose (160.0)
synovia (171.0–171.9)

170.0 Bones of skull and face, except mandible 🔖
Mandible = lower jaw
Bone: Bone:
ethmoid   sphenoid
frontal   temporal
malar   zygomatic
nasal   Maxilla (superior)
occipital   Turbinate
orbital   Upper jaw bone
parietal   Vomer
Excludes *carcinoma, any type except intraosseous or odontogenic:*
maxilla, maxillary (sinus) (160.2)
upper jaw bone (143.0)
jaw bone (lower) (170.1)
Ex: 170.0, 170.9, V58.0

170.1 Mandible 🔖
Inferior maxilla
Jaw bone NOS
Lower jaw bone
Excludes *carcinoma, any type except intraosseous or odontogenic:*
jaw bone NOS (143.9)
lower (143.1)
upper jaw bone (170.0)
Ex: 170.1, 170.9, V58.0

170.2 Vertebral column, excluding sacrum and coccyx 🔖
Spinal column
Spine
Vertebra
Excludes *sacrum and coccyx (170.6)*
Ex: 170.2, 170.9, V58.0

170.3 Ribs, sternum, and clavicle 🔖
Costal cartilage
Costovertebral joint
Xiphoid process
Ex: 170.3, 170.9, V58.0

170.4 Scapula and long bones of upper limb 🔖
Acromion   Radius
Bones NOS of upper limb   Ulna
Humerus
Ex: 170.4, 170.9, V58.0
Coding Clinic: 1999, Q2, P9

170.5 Short bones of upper limb 🔖
Carpal   Scaphoid (of hand)
Cuneiform, wrist   Semilunar or lunate
Metacarpal   Trapezium
Navicular, of hand   Trapezoid
Phalanges of hand   Unciform
Pisiform
Ex: 170.5, 170.9, V58.0

170.6 Pelvic bones, sacrum, and coccyx 🔖
Coccygeal vertebra   Pubic bone
Ilium   Sacral vertebra
Ischium
Ex: 170.6, 170.9, V58.0

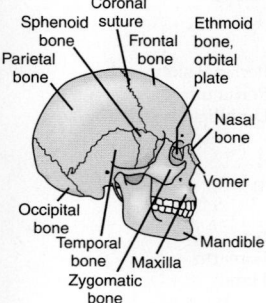

Figure 2–8 Bones of the skull.

Labels: Coronal suture, Sphenoid bone, Frontal bone, Ethmoid bone, orbital plate, Parietal bone, Nasal bone, Vomer, Occipital bone, Temporal bone, Maxilla, Zygomatic bone, Mandible

---

NEOPLASMS (140–239)

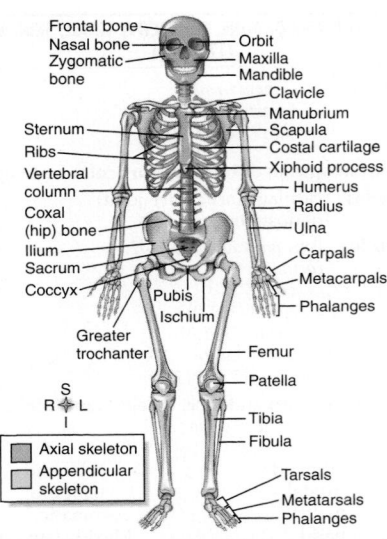

Figure 2–9 Diagram of skeleton of trunk and limbs with bones labeled. (From Thibodeau and Patton: Anatomy and Physiology, ed 7, Mosby, 2010)

170.7 Long bones of lower limb 🔲
  Bones NOS of lower limb   Fibula
  Femur   Tibia
  (Ex:) 170.7, 170.9, V58.0

170.8 Short bones of lower limb 🔲
  Astragalus [talus]   Navicular (of ankle)
  Calcaneus   Patella
  Cuboid   Phalanges of foot
  Cuneiform, ankle   Tarsal
  Metatarsal
  (Ex:) 170.8-170.9, V58.0

170.9 Bone and articular cartilage, site unspecified 🔲
  (Ex:) 170.0-170.9, V58.0

● **171 Malignant neoplasm of connective and other soft tissue**
  Includes   blood vessel
                 bursa
                 fascia
                 fat
                 ligament, except uterine
                 muscle
                 peripheral, sympathetic, and parasympathetic
                     nerves and ganglia
                 synovia
                 tendon (sheath)
  Excludes   *cartilage (of):*
                     articular (170.0–170.9)
                     larynx (161.3)
                     nose (160.0)
                 connective tissue:
                     breast (174.0–175.9)
                     internal organs—code to malignant neoplasm of the
                         site [e.g., leiomyosarcoma of stomach, 151.9]
                     heart (164.1)
                     uterine ligament (183.4)

171.0 Head, face, and neck 🔲
  Cartilage of:
    ear
    eyelid
  (Ex:) V58.0
  Coding Clinic: 1999, Q2, P6-7

171.2 Upper limb, including shoulder 🔲
  Arm   Forearm
  Finger   Hand
  (Ex:) V58.0

171.3 Lower limb, including hip 🔲
  Foot
  Leg
  Popliteal space
    Popliteal space = popliteal cavity, popliteal fossa.
      Depression in posterior aspect of knee (behind knee).
  Thigh
  Toe
  (Ex:) V58.0
  Coding Clinic: 2012, Q3, P8

171.4 Thorax 🔲
  Axilla
  Diaphragm
  Great vessels
  Excludes   *heart (164.1)*
                 mediastinum (164.2–164.9)
                 thymus (164.0)
  (Ex:) V58.0

171.5 Abdomen 🔲
  Abdominal wall
  Hypochondrium
  Excludes   *peritoneum (158.8)*
                 retroperitoneum (158.0)
  (Ex:) V58.0

171.6 Pelvis 🔲
  Buttock   Inguinal region
  Groin Perineum
  Excludes   *pelvic peritoneum (158.8)*
                 retroperitoneum (158.0)
                 uterine ligament, any (183.3–183.5)
  (Ex:) V58.0

171.7 Trunk, unspecified 🔲
  Back NOS
  Flank NOS
  (Ex:) V58.0

171.8 Other specified sites of connective and other soft tissue 🔲
  Malignant neoplasm of contiguous or overlapping sites
      of connective tissue whose point of origin cannot
      be determined
  (Ex:) V58.0

171.9 Connective and other soft tissue, site unspecified 🔲
  (Ex:) V58.0

● **172 Malignant melanoma of skin**
  Includes   melanocarcinoma
                 melanoma in situ of skin
                 melanoma (skin) NOS
  Excludes   *skin of genital organs (184.0–184.9, 187.1–187.9)*
                 sites other than skin - code to malignant neoplasm of the
                     site

172.0 Lip
  Excludes   *vermilion border of lip (140.0–140.1, 140.9)*

172.1 Eyelid, including canthus

172.2 Ear and external auditory canal
  Auricle (ear)
  Auricular canal, external
  External [acoustic] meatus
  Pinna

172.3 Other and unspecified parts of face
  Cheek (external)   Forehead
  Chin   Nose, external
  Eyebrow   Temple

172.4 Scalp and neck

172.5 Trunk, except scrotum
  Axilla   Perianal skin
  Breast   Perineum
  Buttock   Umbilicus
  Groin
  Excludes   *anal canal (154.2)*
                 anus NOS (154.3)
                 scrotum (187.7)

172.6 Upper limb, including shoulder
  Arm   Forearm
  Finger   Hand

172.7 Lower limb, including hip

Ankle	Leg
Foot	Popliteal area
Heel	Thigh
Knee	Toe

172.8 Other specified sites of skin
>   Malignant melanoma of contiguous or overlapping sites of skin whose point of origin cannot be determined

172.9 Melanoma of skin, site unspecified

● **173 Other and unspecified malignant neoplasm of skin**

Includes   malignant neoplasm of:
>   sebaceous glands
>   sudoriferous, sudoriparous glands
>   sweat glands

Excludes   *Kaposi's sarcoma (176.0–176.9)*
>   *malignant melanoma of skin (172.0–172.9)*
>   *Merkel cell carcinoma of skin (209.31-209.36)*
>   *skin of genital organs (184.0–184.9, 187.1–187.9)*

Coding Clinic: 2000, Q1, P8; 1996, Q2, P12

● **173.0 Other and unspecified malignant neoplasm of skin of lip**

Excludes   *vermilion border of lip (140.0–140.1, 140.9)*

173.00 Unspecified malignant neoplasm of skin of lip

173.01 Basal cell carcinoma of skin of lip

173.02 Squamous cell carcinoma of skin of lip

173.09 Other specified malignant neoplasm of skin of lip

● **173.1 Other and unspecified malignant neoplasm of eyelid, including canthus**

Excludes   *cartilage of eyelid (171.0)*

173.10 Unspecified malignant neoplasm of eyelid, including canthus

173.11 Basal cell carcinoma of eyelid, including canthus

173.12 Squamous cell carcinoma of eyelid, including canthus

173.19 Other specified malignant neoplasm of eyelid, including canthus

● **173.2 Other and unspecified malignant neoplasm of skin of ear and external auditory canal**
>   Auricle (ear)
>   Auricular canal, external
>   External meatus
>   Pinna

Excludes   *cartilage of ear (171.0)*

173.20 Unspecified malignant neoplasm of skin of ear and external auditory canal

173.21 Basal cell carcinoma of skin of ear and external auditory canal

173.22 Squamous cell carcinoma of skin of ear and external auditory canal

173.29 Other specified malignant neoplasm of skin of ear and external auditory canal

● **173.3 Other and unspecified malignant neoplasm of skin of other and unspecified parts of face**

Cheek, external	Forehead
Chin	Nose, external
Eyebrow	Temple

Coding Clinic: 2000, Q1, P3

173.30 Unspecified malignant neoplasm of skin of other and unspecified parts of face

173.31 Basal cell carcinoma of skin of other and unspecified parts of face

173.32 Squamous cell carcinoma of skin of other and unspecified parts of face

173.39 Other specified malignant neoplasm of skin of other and unspecified parts of face

● **173.4 Other and unspecified malignant neoplasm of scalp and skin of neck**

173.40 Unspecified malignant neoplasm of scalp and skin of neck

173.41 Basal cell carcinoma of scalp and skin of neck

173.42 Squamous cell carcinoma of scalp and skin of neck

173.49 Other specified malignant neoplasm of scalp and skin of neck

● **173.5 Other and unspecified malignant neoplasm of skin of trunk, except scrotum**
>   Axillary fold
>   Perianal skin
>   Skin of:
>   abdominal wall
>   anus
>   back
>   breast
>   buttock
>   chest wall
>   groin
>   perineum
>   Umbilicus

Excludes   *anal canal (154.2)*
>   *anus NOS (154.3)*
>   *skin of scrotum (187.7)*

Coding Clinic: 2001, Q1, P8

173.50 Unspecified malignant neoplasm of skin of trunk, except scrotum

173.51 Basal cell carcinoma of skin of trunk, except scrotum

173.52 Squamous cell carcinoma of skin of trunk, except scrotum

173.59 Other specified malignant neoplasm of skin of trunk, except scrotum

● **173.6 Other and unspecified malignant neoplasm of skin of upper limb, including shoulder**

Arm	Forearm
Finger	Hand

173.60 Unspecified malignant neoplasm of skin of upper limb, including shoulder

173.61 Basal cell carcinoma of skin of upper limb, including shoulder

173.62 Squamous cell carcinoma of skin of upper limb, including shoulder

173.69 Other specified malignant neoplasm of skin of upper limb, including shoulder

● **173.7 Other and unspecified malignant neoplasm of skin of lower limb, including hip**

Ankle	Leg
Foot	Popliteal area
Heel	Thigh
Knee	Toe

173.70 Unspecified malignant neoplasm of skin of lower limb, including hip

173.71 Basal cell carcinoma of skin of lower limb, including hip

173.72 Squamous cell carcinoma of skin of lower limb, including hip

173.79 Other specified malignant neoplasm of skin of lower limb, including hip

Item 2–4 Malignant melanoma is a serious form of skin cancer that affects the melanocytes (pigment-forming cells) and is caused by ultraviolet (UV) rays from the sun that damage skin. It is most commonly seen in the 40- to 60-year-olds with fair skin, blue or green eyes, and red or blond hair who sunburn easily. Melanoma can spread very rapidly and is the most deadly form of skin cancer. It is less common than other types of skin cancer. The rate of melanoma is increasing and currently is the leading cause of death from skin disease.

Figure 2–10 Malignant melanoma of skin. (From Goldman: Cecil Textbook of Medicine, ed 22, Saunders, 2004)

NEOPLASMS (140–239)

● **173.8** **Other and unspecified malignant neoplasm of other specified sites of skin**
Malignant neoplasm of contiguous or overlapping sites of skin whose point of origin cannot be determined
173.80 Unspecified malignant neoplasm of other specified sites of skin
173.81 Basal cell carcinoma of other specified sites of skin
173.82 Squamous cell carcinoma of other specified sites of skin
173.89 Other specified malignant neoplasm of other specified sites of skin
● **173.9** **Other and unspecified malignant neoplasm of skin, site unspecified**
173.90 Unspecified malignant neoplasm of skin, site unspecified
Malignant neoplasm of skin NOS
173.91 Basal cell carcinoma of skin, site unspecified
173.92 Squamous cell carcinoma of skin, site unspecified
173.99 Other specified malignant neoplasm of skin, site unspecified

● **174** **Malignant neoplasm of female breast**
This code is for female breast; see 175 for male breast.
Includes breast (female)
connective tissue
soft parts
Paget's disease of:
breast
nipple
Use additional code to identify estrogen receptor status (V86.0, V86.1)
Excludes *malignant melanoma of skin of breast (172.5)*
malignant neoplasm of skin of breast (173.50-173.59)
Coding Clinic: 2012, Q1, P11
174.0 Nipple and areola ♀
174.1 Central portion ♀
174.2 Upper-inner quadrant ♀
Coding Clinic: 1989, Q4, P11
174.3 Lower-inner quadrant ♀
Coding Clinic: 1989, Q4, P11
174.4 Upper-outer quadrant ♀
Coding Clinic: 2008, Q4, P152-155; 2004, Q1, P3-4; 1997, Q3, P8; 1984, May-June, P11
174.5 Lower-outer quadrant ♀
174.6 Axillary tail ♀
174.8 Other specified sites of female breast ♀
Ectopic sites
Inner breast
Lower breast
Malignant neoplasm of contiguous or overlapping sites of breast whose point of origin cannot be determined
Midline of breast
Outer breast
Upper breast
Coding Clinic: 1985, July-Aug, P11
174.9 Breast (female), unspecified ♀
Coding Clinic: 2009, Q3, P4; 2005, Q3, P11-12; 1994, Q2, P10x2

Item 2–5 **Kaposi's sarcoma** is a cancer that causes patches of abnormal tissue to grow under the skin; in the lining of the mouth, nose, and throat; or in other organs, often beginning and spreading to other organs. Patients who have had organ transplants or patients with AIDS are at high risk for this malignancy.

● **175** **Malignant neoplasm of male breast**
Use additional code to identify estrogen receptor status (V86.0, V86.1)
Excludes *malignant melanoma of skin of breast (172.5)*
malignant neoplasm of skin of breast (173.50-173.59)
Coding Clinic: 2012, Q1, P11
175.0 Nipple and areola ♂
175.9 Other and unspecified sites of male breast ♂
Ectopic breast tissue, male

● **176** **Kaposi's sarcoma**
176.0 Skin
Ex 176.0, 176.8-176.9, V58.0
Coding Clinic: 2007, Q4, P61-64
176.1 Soft tissue
Blood vessel   Ligament
Connective tissue   Lymphatic(s) NEC
Fascia   Muscle
Excludes *lymph glands and nodes (176.5)*
Ex 176.1, 176.8-176.9, V58.0
176.2 Palate
Ex 176.2, 176.8-176.9, V58.0
176.3 Gastrointestinal sites
Ex 176.3, 176.8-176.9, V58.0
176.4 Lung
Ex 162.8-162.9, 165.8-165.9, 176.4, 195.8, 199.0-199.2, 209.20-209.21, 209.70, 209.75, 209.29-209.30, 239.1, 239.81-239.9
176.5 Lymph nodes
Ex 176.5, 195.8-196.9, 199.0-199.2, 209.20, 209.29-209.30, 209.70-209.71, 209.75, 239.81-239.9
176.8 Other specified sites
Oral cavity NEC
Ex 176.0-176.9, V58.0
176.9 Unspecified
Viscera NOS
Ex 176.0-192.9, 195.0-199.2, 209.20, 209.24, 209.29-209.30, 209.70-209.79, 230.0-237.6, 237.9-238.3, 238.8-239.9, V58.0

MALIGNANT NEOPLASM OF GENITOURINARY ORGANS (179–189)
Excludes *carcinoma in situ (233.1–233.9)*

179 **Malignant neoplasm of uterus, part unspecified** ♀
● **180** **Malignant neoplasm of cervix uteri**
Includes invasive malignancy [carcinoma]
Excludes *carcinoma in situ (233.1)*
180.0 Endocervix ♀
Inside the cervix
Cervical canal NOS
Endocervical canal
Endocervical gland
180.1 Exocervix ♀
Outside the cervix
180.8 Other specified sites of cervix ♀
Cervical stump
Squamocolumnar junction of cervix
Malignant neoplasm of contiguous or overlapping sites of cervix uteri whose point of origin cannot be determined
180.9 Cervix uteri, unspecified ♀

Figure 2–11 Female breast quadrants and axillary tail.

Figure 2–12   Cervix uteri.

Figure 2–13   Penis and other male genital organs.

181   **Malignant neoplasm of placenta** ♀
  Choriocarcinoma NOS
  Chorioepithelioma NOS
   Excludes   *chorioadenoma (destruens) (236.1)*
    hydatidiform mole (630)
     malignant (236.1)
    invasive mole (236.1)
    male choriocarcinoma NOS (186.0–186.9)

● 182   **Malignant neoplasm of body of uterus**
   Excludes   *carcinoma in situ (233.2)*
 182.0   **Corpus uteri, except isthmus** ♀
   Cornu   Fundus
   Endometrium   Myometrium
   Coding Clinic: 2009, Q3, P4
 182.1   **Isthmus** ♀
   Lower uterine segment
 182.8   **Other specified sites of body of uterus** ♀
   Malignant neoplasm of contiguous or overlapping sites
   of body of uterus whose point of origin cannot be
   determined
   Excludes   *uterus NOS (179)*

● 183   **Malignant neoplasm of ovary and other uterine adnexa**
   Excludes   *Douglas' cul-de-sac (158.8)*
 183.0   **Ovary** ♀ 🐾
   Use additional code to identify any functional activity
   (Ex) 183.0-183.9, 195.3, 198.6, 199.0-199.2, 209.20, 209.29-209.30, 209.70,
    209.75
   Coding Clinic: 2007, Q4, P95-96
 183.2   **Fallopian tube** ♀
   Oviduct
   Uterine tube
 183.3   **Broad ligament** ♀
   Mesovarium
   Parovarian region
 183.4   **Parametrium** ♀
   Uterine ligament NOS
   Uterosacral ligament
 183.5   **Round ligament** ♀
 183.8   **Other specified sites of uterine adnexa** ♀
   Tubo-ovarian
   Utero-ovarian
   Malignant neoplasm of contiguous or overlapping sites
   of ovary and other uterine adnexa whose point of
   origin cannot be determined
 183.9   **Uterine adnexa, unspecified** ♀

● 184   **Malignant neoplasm of other and unspecified female genital**
  organs
   Excludes   *carcinoma in situ (233.30–233.39)*
 184.0   **Vagina** ♀
   Gartner's duct   Vaginal vault
 184.1   **Labia majora** ♀
   Greater vestibular [Bartholin's] gland
 184.2   **Labia minora** ♀
 184.3   **Clitoris** ♀
 184.4   **Vulva, unspecified** ♀
   External female genitalia NOS
   Pudendum

 184.8   **Other specified sites of female genital organs** ♀
   Malignant neoplasm of contiguous or overlapping sites
   of female genital organs whose point of origin
   cannot be determined
 184.9   **Female genital organ, site unspecified** ♀
   Female genitourinary tract NOS

185   **Malignant neoplasm of prostate** ♂
   Excludes   *seminal vesicles (187.8)*
   Coding Clinic: 2010, Q2, P3; 2003, Q3, P13; 1999, Q3, P5; 1994, Q1, P20; 1992,
    Q3, P7

● 186   **Malignant neoplasm of testis**
  Use additional code to identify any functional activity
 186.0   **Undescended testis** ♂
   Ectopic testis   Retained testis
 186.9   **Other and unspecified testis** ♂
   Testis: Testis:
    NOS   scrotal
    descended

● 187   **Malignant neoplasm of penis and other male genital organs**
 187.1   **Prepuce** ♂
   Foreskin
 187.2   **Glans penis** ♂
 187.3   **Body of penis** ♂
   Corpus cavernosum
 187.4   **Penis, part unspecified** ♂
   Skin of penis NOS
 187.5   **Epididymis** ♂
 187.6   **Spermatic cord** ♂
   Vas deferens
 187.7   **Scrotum** ♂
   Skin of scrotum
 187.8   **Other specified sites of male genital organs** ♂
   Seminal vesicle
   Tunica vaginalis
   Malignant neoplasm of contiguous or overlapping sites
   of penis and other male genital organs whose point
   of origin cannot be determined
 187.9   **Male genital organ, site unspecified** ♂
   Male genital organ or tract NOS

● 188   **Malignant neoplasm of bladder**
   Excludes   *carcinoma in situ (233.7)*
 188.0   **Trigone of urinary bladder**
 188.1   **Dome of urinary bladder**
 188.2   **Lateral wall of urinary bladder**
 188.3   **Anterior wall of urinary bladder**
 188.4   **Posterior wall of urinary bladder**
 188.5   **Bladder neck**
   Internal urethral orifice
 188.6   **Ureteric orifice**
 188.7   **Urachus**

NEOPLASMS (140–239)

188.8 Other specified sites of bladder
Malignant neoplasm of contiguous or overlapping sites of bladder whose point of origin cannot be determined

188.9 Bladder, part unspecified
Bladder wall NOS
Coding Clinic: 2000, Q1, P5

● **189 Malignant neoplasm of kidney and other and unspecified urinary organs**
Excludes   *benign carcinoid tumor of kidney (209.64)*
malignant carcinoid tumor of kidney (209.24)

189.0 Kidney, except pelvis 🖉
Kidney NOS   Kidney parenchyma
(Ex): 189.0-189.1, 189.8-189.9, 195.8, 199.0-199.2, 209.20, 209.24, 209.29-209.30, 209.70, 209.75, 239.5, 239.81-239.9
Coding Clinic: 2005, Q2, P4-5; 2004, Q2, P4

189.1 Renal pelvis 🖉
Renal calyces   Ureteropelvic junction
(Ex): 189.0-189.1, 189.8-189.9, 195.8, 199.0-199.2, 209.20, 209.24, 209.29-209.30, 209.70, 209.75, 239.5, 239.81-239.9

189.2 Ureter 🖉
Excludes   *ureteric orifice of bladder (188.6)*
(Ex): 189.2, 189.8-189.9, 195.8, 199.0-199.2, 209.20, 209.29-209.30, 209.70, 209.75, 239.5, 239.81-239.9

189.3 Urethra 🖉
Excludes   *urethral orifice of bladder (188.5)*
(Ex): 189.3-189.9, 198.82

189.4 Paraurethral glands 🖉
(Ex): 189.3-189.9, 198.82

189.8 Other specified sites of urinary organs 🖉
Malignant neoplasm of contiguous or overlapping sites of kidney and other urinary organs whose point of origin cannot be determined
(Ex): 189.0-189.9, 195.3, 198.0-198.1, 209.24

189.9 Urinary organ, site unspecified 🖉
Urinary system NOS
Excludes   *carcinoma in situ (234.0–234.9)*
(Ex): 189.0-189.9, 195.3, 198.0-198.1, 209.24

MALIGNANT NEOPLASM OF OTHER AND UNSPECIFIED SITES (190–199)

Excludes   *carcinoma in situ (234.0-234.9)*

● **190 Malignant neoplasm of eye**
Excludes   *carcinoma in situ (234.0)*
dark area on retina and choroid (239.81)
malignant melanoma of eyelid (skin) (172.1)
cartilage (171.0)
malignant neoplasm of eyelid (skin) (173.10-173.19)
optic nerve (192.0)
orbital bone (170.0)
retinal freckle (239.81)

190.0 Eyeball, except conjunctiva, cornea, retina, and choroid
Note the use of "except" in this code.
Ciliary body   Sclera
Crystalline lens   Uveal tract
Iris

190.1 Orbit
Connective tissue of orbit
Extraocular muscle
Retrobulbar
Excludes   *bone of orbit (170.0)*

190.2 Lacrimal gland

190.3 Conjunctiva

190.4 Cornea

190.5 Retina

190.6 Choroid

190.7 Lacrimal duct
Lacrimal sac   Nasolacrimal duct

190.8 Other specified sites of eye
Malignant neoplasm of contiguous or overlapping sites of eye whose point of origin cannot be determined

190.9 Eye, part unspecified

● **191 Malignant neoplasm of brain**
Excludes   *cranial nerves (192.0)*
retrobulbar area (190.1)

191.0 Cerebrum, except lobes and ventricles 🖉
Basal ganglia   Globus pallidus
Cerebral cortex   Hypothalamus
Corpus striatum   Thalamus
(Ex): 191.0-192.1, 192.8-192.9, 195.8, 199.0-199.2, 209.20, 209.29-209.30, 209.70, 209.75, 239.6-239.9

191.1 Frontal lobe 🖉
(Ex): 191.0-192.1, 192.8-192.9, 195.8, 199.0-199.2, 209.20, 209.29-209.30, 209.70, 209.75, 239.6-239.9
Coding Clinic: 2005, Q4, P117-119; 1993, Q4, P33

191.2 Temporal lobe 🖉
Hippocampus   Uncus
(Ex): 191.0-192.1, 192.8-192.9, 195.8, 199.0-199.2, 209.20, 209.29-209.30, 209.70, 209.75, 239.6-239.9
Coding Clinic: 2009, Q3, P4; 2006, Q4, P122-123

191.3 Parietal lobe 🖉
(Ex): 191.0-192.1, 192.8-192.9, 195.8, 199.0-199.2, 209.20, 209.29-209.30, 209.70, 209.75, 239.6-239.9

191.4 Occipital lobe 🖉
(Ex): 191.0-192.1, 192.8-192.9, 195.8, 199.0-199.2, 209.20, 209.29-209.30, 209.70, 209.75, 239.6-239.9

191.5 Ventricles 🖉
Choroid plexus
Floor of ventricle
(Ex): 191.0-192.1, 192.8-192.9, 195.8, 199.0-199.2, 209.20, 209.29-209.30, 209.70, 209.75, 239.6-239.9

191.6 Cerebellum NOS 🖉
Cerebellopontine angle
(Ex): 191.0-192.1, 192.8-192.9, 195.8, 199.0-199.2, 209.20, 209.29-209.30, 209.70, 209.75, 239.6-239.9

191.7 Brain stem 🖉
Cerebral peduncle   Midbrain
Medulla oblongata   Pons
(Ex): 191.0-192.1, 192.8-192.9, 195.8, 199.0-199.2, 209.20, 209.29-209.30, 209.70, 209.75, 239.6-239.9

191.8 Other parts of brain 🖉
Corpus callosum
Tapetum
Malignant neoplasm of contiguous or overlapping sites of brain whose point of origin cannot be determined
(Ex): 191.0-192.1, 192.8-192.9, 195.8, 199.0-199.2, 209.20, 209.29-209.30, 209.70, 209.75, 239.6-239.9
Coding Clinic: 2007, Q4, P103-104

191.9 Brain, unspecified 🖉
Cranial fossa NOS
(Ex): 191.0-192.1, 192.8-192.9, 195.8, 199.0-199.2, 209.20, 209.29-209.30, 209.70, 209.75, 239.6-239.9
Coding Clinic: 2009, Q4, P78; 1994, Q2, P8

FRONTAL LOBE   PARIETAL LOBE
Anterior   Posterior
TEMPORAL LOBE   OCCIPITAL LOBE
CEREBELLUM

Figure 2-14 The brain.

● **192 Malignant neoplasm of other and unspecified parts of nervous system**

> **Excludes** *peripheral, sympathetic, and parasympathetic nerves and ganglia (171.0–171.9)*

192.0 Cranial nerves 🗝
Olfactory bulb
Ⓔ 192.0, 192.8-192.9, 195.8, 199.0-199.2, 209.20, 209.29-209.30, 209.70, 209.75, 239.6-239.9

192.1 Cerebral meninges 🗝
Dura (mater)   Meninges NOS
Falx (cerebelli) (cerebri)   Tentorium
Ⓔ 192.1, 192.8-192.9, 195.8, 199.0-199.2, 209.29-209.30, 209.70, 209.75, 239.6-239.9

192.2 Spinal cord 🗝
Cauda equina
Ⓔ 192.2, 192.8-192.9, 195.8, 199.0-199.2, 209.29-209.30, 209.70, 209.75, 239.6-239.9

192.3 Spinal meninges 🗝
Ⓔ 192.3-192.9, 195.8, 199.0-199.2, 209.20, 209.29-209.30, 209.70, 209.75, 239.6-239.9

192.8 Other specified sites of nervous system 🗝
Malignant neoplasm of contiguous or overlapping sites of other parts of nervous system whose point of origin cannot be determined
Ⓔ 191.0-192.9, 195.8, 199.0-199.2, 209.20, 209.29-209.30, 209.70, 209.75, 239.6-239.9

192.9 Nervous system, part unspecified 🗝
Nervous system (central) NOS

> **Excludes** *meninges NOS (192.1)*

Ⓔ 191.0-192.9, 195.8, 198.3-198.4, 199.0-199.2, 209.20, 209.29-209.30, 209.70, 209.75, 239.6-239.9

193 Malignant neoplasm of thyroid gland
Thyroglossal duct
Use additional code to identify any functional activity

● **194 Malignant neoplasm of other endocrine glands and related structures**

> **Excludes** *islets of Langerhans (157.4)*
> *neuroendocrine tumors (209.00–209.69)*
> *ovary (183.0)*
> *testis (186.0–186.9)*
> *thymus (164.0)*

194.0 Adrenal gland 🗝
Adrenal cortex   Suprarenal gland
Adrenal medulla
Ⓔ 194.0, 194.9, 195.2, 195.8, 198.7, 199.0-199.2, 209.20, 209.29-209.30, 209.70, 209.75

194.1 Parathyroid gland 🗝
Ⓔ 194.1, 194.8-194.9

194.3 Pituitary gland and craniopharyngeal duct 🗝
Craniobuccal pouch   Rathke's pouch
Hypophysis   Sella turcica
Ⓔ 194.3, V58.0
Coding Clinic: 1985, July-Aug, P9

194.4 Pineal gland 🗝
Ⓔ 194.4, V58.0

194.5 Carotid body 🗝
Ⓔ 194.5, 194.8-194.9

194.6 Aortic body and other paraganglia 🗝
Coccygeal body   Para-aortic body
Glomus jugulare
Ⓔ 194.5-194.9

194.8 Other 🗝
Pluriglandular involvement NOS
Note: If the sites of multiple involvements are known, they should be coded separately.
Ⓔ 194.0-194.9

194.9 Endocrine gland, site unspecified 🗝
Ⓔ 194.0-194.9

● **195 Malignant neoplasm of other and ill-defined sites**

> **Includes** malignant neoplasms of contiguous sites, not elsewhere classified, whose point of origin cannot be determined

> **Excludes** *malignant neoplasm:*
> *lymphatic and hematopoietic tissue (200.0–208.9)*
> *secondary sites (196.0–198.8)*
> *unspecified site (199.0–199.1)*

195.0 Head, face, and neck
Cheek NOS
Jaw NOS
Nose NOS
Supraclavicular region NOS
Coding Clinic: 2003, Q4, P107

195.1 Thorax
Axilla   Intrathoracic NOS
Chest (wall) NOS

195.2 Abdomen
Intra-abdominal NOS
Coding Clinic: 1997, Q2, P3

195.3 Pelvis
Groin
Inguinal region NOS
Presacral region
Sacrococcygeal region
Sites overlapping systems within pelvis, as:
rectovaginal (septum)
rectovesical (septum)

195.4 Upper limb

195.5 Lower limb

195.8 Other specified sites
Back NOS   Trunk NOS
Flank NOS

(See Plate 315 on page 53.)

● **196 Secondary and unspecified malignant neoplasm of lymph nodes**

> **Excludes** *any malignant neoplasm of lymph nodes, specified as primary (200.0–202.9)*
> *Hodgkin's disease (201.0–201.9)*
> *lymphosarcoma (200.1)*
> *other forms of lymphoma (202.0–202.9)*
> *reticulosarcoma (200.0)*
> *secondary neuroendocrine tumor of (distant) lymph nodes (209.71)*

Coding Clinic: 1992, Q2, P3-4

196.0 Lymph nodes of head, face, and neck 🗝
Cervical   Scalene
Cervicofacial   Supraclavicular
Ⓔ 176.5, 195.8-196.9, 199.0-199.2, 209.20, 209.29-209.30, 209.70-209.71, 209.75, 239.81-239.9
Coding Clinic: 2007, Q3, P8-9

196.1 Intrathoracic lymph nodes 🗝
Bronchopulmonary   Mediastinal
Intercostal   Tracheobronchial
Ⓔ 176.5, 195.8-196.9, 199.0-199.2, 209.20, 209.29-209.30, 209.70-209.71, 209.75, 239.81-239.9
Coding Clinic: 2006, Q3, P7-8

196.2 Intra-abdominal lymph nodes 🗝
Intestinal   Retroperitoneal
Mesenteric
Ⓔ 176.5, 195.8-196.9, 199.0-199.2, 209.20, 209.29-209.30, 209.70-209.71, 209.75, 239.81-239.9
Coding Clinic: 2003, Q4, P111

196.3 Lymph nodes of axilla and upper limb 🗝
Brachial   Infraclavicular
Epitrochlear   Pectoral
Ⓔ 176.5, 195.8-196.9, 199.0-199.2, 209.20, 209.29-209.30, 209.70-209.71, 209.75, 239.81-239.9

196.5 Lymph nodes of inguinal region and lower limb 🗝
Femoral   Popliteal
Groin Tibial
Ⓔ 176.5, 195.8-196.9, 199.0-199.2, 209.20, 209.29-209.30, 209.70-209.71, 209.75, 239.81-239.9

NEOPLASMS (140–239)

N Newborn: 0   **P** Pediatric: 0–17   **M** Maternity: 12–55   **A** Adult: 15–124   ♀ Females Only   ♂ Males Only

Ⓔ CC/MCC Exclusions   🗝 Complication\Comorbidity   Major C\C   Present on Admission Requirement   Hospital-Acquired Condition   **713**

NEOPLASMS (140–239)

196.6   **Intrapelvic lymph nodes** 🔍
Hypogastric   Obturator
Iliac   Parametrial
Ex: 176.5, 195.8-196.9, 199.0-199.2, 209.20, 209.29-209.30, 209.70-209.71, 209.75, 239.81-239.9
Coding Clinic: 2012, Q2, P9

196.8   **Lymph nodes of multiple sites** 🔍
Ex: 176.5, 195.8-196.9, 199.0-199.2, 209.20, 209.29-209.30, 209.70-209.71, 209.75, 239.81-239.9

196.9   **Site unspecified** 🔍
Lymph nodes NOS
Ex: 176.5, 195.8-196.9, 199.0-199.2, 209.20, 209.29-209.30, 209.70-209.71, 209.75, 239.81-239.9

● **197**   **Secondary malignant neoplasm of respiratory and digestive systems**
   Excludes   *lymph node metastasis (196.0–196.9)*
secondary neuroendocrine tumor of liver (209.72)
secondary neuroendocrine tumor of respiratory organs (209.79)

   197.0   **Lung** 🔍
Bronchus
Ex: 195.8, 197.0, 197.3, 198.89-199.2, 209.20, 209.29-209.30, 209.70, 209.75-209.79, 239.81-239.9
Coding Clinic: 2010, Q3, P3; 2006, Q1, P4-5; 1999, Q2, P9

   197.1   **Mediastinum** 🔍
Ex: 195.8, 197.1, 197.3, 198.89-199.2, 209.20, 209.29-209.30, 209.70, 209.75-209.79, 239.81-239.9
Coding Clinic: 2006, Q3, P7-8

   197.2   **Pleura** 🔍
Ex: 195.8, 197.2-197.3, 198.89-199.2, 209.20, 209.29-209.30, 209.70, 209.75-209.79, 239.81-239.9, 511.81
Coding Clinic: 2008, Q1, P16-17; 2007, Q3, P3; 2003, Q4, P110; 1989, Q4, P11

   197.3   **Other respiratory organs** 🔍
Trachea
Ex: 195.8, 197.0-197.3, 198.89-199.2, 209.20, 209.29-209.30, 209.70, 209.75-209.79, 239.81-239.9

   197.4   **Small intestine, including duodenum** 🔍
Ex: 195.8, 197.4, 197.8, 198.89-199.2, 209.20, 209.29-209.30, 209.70, 209.75-209.79, 239.81-239.9

   197.5   **Large intestine and rectum** 🔍
Ex: 195.8, 197.5, 197.8, 198.89-199.2, 209.20, 209.29-209.30, 209.70, 209.75-209.79, 239.81-239.9

   197.6   **Retroperitoneum and peritoneum** 🔍
Ex: 195.8, 197.6, 197.8, 198.89-199.2, 209.20, 209.29-209.30, 209.70, 209.74-209.79, 239.81-239.9
Coding Clinic: 2011, Q4, P181; 2010, Q3, P3; 2004, Q2, P4; 1989, Q4, P11

   197.7   **Liver, specified as secondary** 🔍
Ex: 195.8, 197.7-197.8, 198.89-199.2, 209.20, 209.29-209.30, 209.70, 209.72, 209.75-209.79, 239.81-239.9
Coding Clinic: 2010, Q3, P3; 2006, Q1, P4-5; 2005, Q2, P9-10; 1984, May-June, P11

   197.8   **Other digestive organs and spleen** 🔍
Ex: 195.8, 197.4-197.8, 198.89-199.2, 209.20, 209.29-209.30, 209.70, 209.72, 209.74-209.79, 239.81-239.9
Coding Clinic: 1997, Q2, P3

● **198**   **Secondary malignant neoplasm of other specified sites**
   Excludes   *lymph node metastasis (196.0–196.9)*
secondary neuroendocrine tumor of other specified sites (209.79)

   198.0   **Kidney** 🔍
Ex: 195.8, 198.0-198.1, 198.89-199.2, 209.20, 209.29-209.30, 209.70, 209.75-209.79, 239.81-239.9

   198.1   **Other urinary organs** 🔍
Ex: 195.8, 198.0-198.1, 198.89-199.2, 209.20, 209.29-209.30, 209.70, 209.75-209.79, 239.81-239.9

   198.2   **Skin** 🔍
Skin of breast
Ex: 195.8, 198.2, 198.89-199.2, 209.20, 209.29- 209.30, 209.70, 209.75-209.79, 239.81-239.9

   198.3   **Brain and spinal cord** 🔍
Ex: 195.8, 198.3, 198.89-199.2, 209.20, 209.29-209.30, 209.70, 209.75-209.79, 239.81-239.9
Coding Clinic: 2007, Q3, P4; 1999, Q3, P7-8; 1984, May-June, P14

   198.4   **Other parts of nervous system** 🔍
Meninges (cerebral) (spinal)
Ex: 195.8, 198.4, 198.89-199.2, 209.20, 209.29-209.30, 209.70, 209.75-209.79, 239.81-239.9

   198.5   **Bone and bone marrow** 🔍
Ex: 195.8, 198.5, 198.89-199.2, 209.20, 209.29-209.30, 209.70, 209.73, 209.75-209.79, 239.81-239.9
Coding Clinic: 2007, Q1, P3-8; 2003, Q4, P110; 1999, Q3, P5; 1989, Q4, P12; 1984, May-June, P14

   198.6   **Ovary** ♀ 🔍
Ex: 195.8, 198.6, 198.89-199.2, 209.20, 209.29-209.30, 209.70, 209.75-209.79, 239.81-239.9

   198.7   **Adrenal gland** 🔍
Suprarenal gland
Ex: 195.8, 198.7, 198.89-199.2, 209.20, 209.29-209.30, 209.70, 209.75-209.79, 239.81-239.9
Coding Clinic: 1988, Q2, P10

● **198.8**   **Other specified sites** 🔍

   198.81   **Breast** 🔍
     Excludes   *skin of breast (198.2)*
Ex: 195.8, 198.81, 198.89-199.2, 209.20, 209.29-209.30, 209.70, 209.75-209.79, 239.81-239.9

   198.82   **Genital organs** 🔍
Ex: 195.8, 198.82-199.2, 209.20, 209.29-209.30, 209.70, 209.75-209.79, 239.81-239.9

   198.89   **Other** 🔍
     Excludes   *retroperitoneal lymph nodes (196.2)*
Ex: 195.8, 198.89-199.2, 209.20, 209.29-209.30, 209.70, 209.75-209.79, 239.81-239.9
Coding Clinic: 2005, Q2, P4-5; 1997, Q2, P4

● **199**   **Malignant neoplasm without specification of site**
   Excludes   *malignant carcinoid tumor of unknown primary site (209.20)*
malignant (poorly differentiated) neuroendocrine carcinoma, any site (209.30)
malignant (poorly differentiated) neuroendocrine tumor, any site (209.30)
neuroendocrine carcinoma (high grade), any site (209.30)

   199.0   **Disseminated** 🔍
Carcinomatosis unspecified site (primary) (secondary)
Generalized:
cancer unspecified site (primary) (secondary)
malignancy unspecified site (primary) (secondary)
Multiple cancer unspecified site (primary) (secondary)
Ex: 195.8, 198.89-199.2, 209.20, 209.29-209.30, 209.70, 209.75-209.79, 239.81-239.9
Coding Clinic: 1989, Q4, P10; 1988, Q2, P11

   199.1   **Other**
Cancer unspecified site (primary) (secondary)
Carcinoma unspecified site (primary) (secondary)
Malignancy unspecified site (primary) (secondary)
Coding Clinic: 2006, Q3, P14-15; Q1, P4-5

● **199.2**   **Malignant neoplasm associated with transplanted organ** 🔍
   Code first complication of transplanted organ *(996.80-996.89)*
   Use additional code for specific malignancy
Ex: 195.8, 198.89-199.2, 209.20, 209.29-209.30, 209.70, 209.75-209.79, 239.81-239.9
Coding Clinic: 2008, Q4, P82-83

Item 2-6 Lymphosarcoma, also known as malignant lymphoma, is a cancer of the lymph system exhibiting abnormal cells encompassing an entire lymph node creating a diffuse pattern without any definite organization. Diffuse pattern lymphoma has a more unfavorable survival outlook than those with a follicular or nodular pattern. Reticulosarcoma is the most common aggressive form of non-Hodgkin's lymphoma.

MALIGNANT NEOPLASM OF LYMPHATIC AND HEMATOPOIETIC TISSUE (200–208)

Excludes *autoimmune lymphoproliferative syndrome (279.41)*
secondary neoplasm of:
bone marrow (198.5)
spleen (197.8)
secondary and unspecified neoplasm of lymph nodes (196.0–196.9)

The following fifth-digit subclassification is for use with categories 200–202:

> 0 unspecified site, extranodal and solid organ sites
> 1 lymph nodes of head, face, and neck
> 2 intrathoracic lymph nodes
> 3 intra-abdominal lymph nodes
> 4 lymph nodes of axilla and upper limb
> 5 lymph nodes of inguinal region and lower limb
> 6 intrapelvic lymph nodes
> 7 spleen
> 8 lymph nodes of multiple sites

● **200 Lymphosarcoma and reticulosarcoma and other specified malignant tumors of lymphatic tissue**

Requires fifth digit. See note before section 200 for codes and definitions.
Coding Clinic: 2007, Q4, P65-67

● **200.0 Reticulosarcoma** 🔾
[0-8]   Lymphoma (malignant):
histiocytic (diffuse):
nodular
pleomorphic cell type
reticulum cell type
Reticulum cell sarcoma:
NOS
pleomorphic cell type
For code **200.00**: (Ex) 200.00-200.08, 239.81-239.9;
For code **200.01**: (Ex) 200.00-200.01, 200.08, 239.81-239.9;
For code **200.02**: (Ex) 200.00, 200.02, 200.08, 239.81-239.9;
For code **200.03**: (Ex) 200.00, 200.03, 200.08, 239.81-239.9;
For code **200.04**: (Ex) 200.00, 200.04, 200.08, 239.81-239.9;
For code **200.05**: (Ex) 200.00, 200.05, 200.08, 239.81-239.9;
For code **200.06**: (Ex) 200.00, 200.06, 200.08, 239.81-239.9;
For code **200.07**: (Ex) 200.00, 200.07-200.08, 239.81-239.9;
For code **200.08**: (Ex) 200.00-200.08, 239.81-239.9
Coding Clinic: 2006, Q4, P135-136; 2001, Q3, P12-13

● **200.1 Lymphosarcoma** 🔾
[0-8]   Lymphoblastoma (diffuse)
Lymphoma (malignant):
lymphoblastic (diffuse)
lymphocytic (cell type) (diffuse)
lymphosarcoma type
Lymphosarcoma:
NOS
diffuse NOS
lymphoblastic (diffuse)
lymphocytic (diffuse)
prolymphocytic

Excludes *lymphosarcoma:*
follicular or nodular (202.0)
mixed cell type (200.8)
lymphosarcoma cell leukemia (207.8)
For code **200.10**: (Ex) 200.10-200.18, 239.81-239.9
For code **200.11**: (Ex) 200.10-200.11, 200.18, 239.81-239.9;
For code **200.12**: (Ex) 200.10, 200.12, 200.18, 239.81-239.9;
For code **200.13**: (Ex) 200.10, 200.13, 200.18, 239.81-239.9;
For code **200.14**: (Ex) 200.10, 200.14, 200.18, 239.81-239.9;
For code **200.15**: (Ex) 200.10, 200.15, 200.18, 239.81-239.9;
For code **200.16**: (Ex) 200.10, 200.16, 200.18, 239.81-239.9;
For code **200.17**: (Ex) 200.10, 200.17-200.18, 239.81-239.9;
For code **200.18**: (Ex) 200.10-200.18, 239.81-239.9

● **200.2 Burkitt's tumor or lymphoma** 🔾
[0-8]   Malignant lymphoma, Burkitt's type
For code **200.20**: (Ex) 200.20-200.28, 239.81-239.9;
For code **200.21**: (Ex) 200.20-200.21, 200.28, 239.81-239.9;
For code **200.22**: (Ex) 200.20, 200.22, 200.28, 239.81-239.9;
For code **200.23**: (Ex) 200.20, 200.23, 200.28, 239.81-239.9;
For code **200.24**: (Ex) 200.20, 200.24, 200.28, 239.81-239.9;
For code **200.25**: (Ex) 200.20, 200.25, 200.28, 239.81-239.9;
For code **200.26**: (Ex) 200.20, 200.26, 200.28, 239.81-239.9;
For code **200.27**: (Ex) 200.20, 200.27-200.28, 239.81-239.9;
For code **200.28**: (Ex) 200.20-200.28, 239.81-239.9

● **200.3 Marginal zone lymphoma** 🔾
[0-8]   Extranodal marginal zone B-cell lymphoma
Mucosa associated lymphoid tissue [MALT]
Nodal marginal zone B-cell lymphoma
Splenic marginal zone B-cell lymphoma
For code **200.30**: (Ex) 200.30-200.78, 202.70-202.90, 239.81-239.9;
For code **200.31**: (Ex) 200.30-200.31, 200.38-200.41, 200.48-200.51, 200.58-200.61, 200.68-200.71, 200.78, 202.70-202.71 202.78-202.81, 202.88, 202.91, 239.81-239.9;
For code **200.32**: (Ex) 200.30, 200.32, 200.38-200.40, 200.42 200.48-200.50, 200.52, 200.58-200.60 200.62, 200.68-200.70, 200.72, 200.78, 202.70, 202.72, 202.78-202.80, 202.82 202.88, 202.92, 239.81-239.9;
For code **200.33**: (Ex) 200.30, 200.33, 200.38-200.40, 200.43, 200.48-200.50, 200.53, 200.58-200.60, 200.63, 200.68-200.70, 200.73, 200.78, 202.70, 202.73, 202.78-202.80, 202.83, 202.88, 202.93, 239.81-239.9;
For code **200.34**: (Ex) 200.30, 200.34, 200.38-200.40, 200.44, 200.48-200.50, 200.54, 200.58-200.60, 200.64, 200.68-200.70, 200.74, 200.78, 202.70, 202.74, 202.78-202.80, 202.84, 202.88, 202.94, 239.81-239.9;
For code **200.35**: (Ex) 200.30, 200.35, 200.38-200.40, 200.45, 200.48-200.50, 200.55, 200.58-200.60, 200.65, 200.68-200.70, 200.75, 200.78, 202.70, 202.75, 202.78-202.80, 202.85, 202.88, 202.95, 239.81-239.9;
For code **200.36**: (Ex) 200.30, 200.36, 200.38-200.40, 200.46, 200.48-200.50, 200.56, 200.58-200.60, 200.66, 200.68-200.70, 200.76, 200.78, 202.70, 202.76, 202.78-202.80, 202.86, 202.88, 202.96, 239.81-239.9;
For code **200.37**: (Ex) 200.30, 200.37-200.40, 200.47-200.50, 200.57-200.60, 200.67-200.70, 200.77-200.78, 202.70, 202.77-202.80, 202.87-202.88, 202.97, 239.81-239.9;
For code **200.38**: (Ex) 200.30-200.78, 202.70-202.88, 202.98, 239.81-239.9

● **200.4 Mantle cell lymphoma** 🔾
[0-8]   For code **200.40**: (Ex) 200.30-200.78, 202.70-202.90, 239.81-239.9;
For code **200.41**: (Ex) 200.30-200.31, 200.38-200.41, 200.48-200.51, 200.58-200.61, 200.68-200.71, 200.78, 202.70-202.71, 202.78-202.81, 202.88, 202.91, 239.81-239.9;
For code **200.42**: (Ex) 200.30, 200.32, 200.38-200.40, 200.42 200.48-200.50, 200.52, 200.58-200.60, 200.62, 200.68-200.70, 200.72, 200.78, 202.70, 202.72, 202.78-202.80, 202.82, 202.88, 202.92, 239.81-239.9;
For code **200.43**: (Ex) 200.30, 200.33, 200.38-200.40, 200.43, 200.48-200.50, 200.53, 200.58-200.60, 200.63, 200.68-200.70, 200.73, 200.78, 202.70, 202.73, 202.78-202.80, 202.83, 202.88, 202.93, 239.81-239.9;
For code **200.44**: (Ex) 200.30, 200.34, 200.38-200.40, 200.44, 200.48-200.50, 200.54, 200.58-200.60, 200.64, 200.68-200.70, 200.74, 200.78, 202.70, 202.74, 202.78-202.80, 202.84, 202.88, 202.94, 239.81-239.9;
For code **200.45**: (Ex) 200.30, 200.35, 200.38-200.40, 200.45, 200.48-200.50, 200.55, 200.58-200.60, 200.65, 200.68-200.70, 200.75, 200.78, 202.70, 202.75, 202.78-202.80, 202.85, 202.88, 202.95, 239.81-239.9;
For code **200.46**: (Ex) 200.30, 200.36, 200.38-200.40, 200.46, 200.48-200.50, 200.56, 200.58-200.60, 200.66, 200.68-200.70, 200.76, 200.78, 202.70, 202.76, 202.78-202.80, 202.86, 202.88, 202.96, 239.81-239.9;
For code **200.47**: (Ex) 200.30, 200.37-200.40, 200.47-200.50, 200.57-200.60, 200.67-200.70, 200.77-200.78, 202 70, 202.77-202.80, 202.87-202.88, 202.97, 239.81-239.9;
For code **200.48**: (Ex) 200.30-200.78, 202.70-202.88, 202.98, 239.81-239.9

NEOPLASMS (140–239)

N Newborn: 0   **P** Pediatric: 0–17   **M** Maternity: 12–55   **A** Adult: 15–124   ♀ Females Only   ♂ Males Only

(Ex) CC/MCC Exclusions   🔾 Complication\Comorbidity   🔾 Major C\C   🔾 Present on Admission Requirement   🔾 Hospital-Acquired Condition   **715**

● **200.5 Primary central nervous system lymphoma** 🔗
[0-8] For code **200.50:** (Ex:) 200.30-200.78, 202.70-202.90, 239.81-239.9;
For code **200.51:** (Ex:) 200.30-200.31, 200.38-200.41, 200.48-200.51,
200.58-200.61, 200.68-200.71, 200.78, 202.70-202.71, 202.78-202.81,
202.88, 202.91, 239.81-239.9;
For code **200.52:** (Ex:) 200.30, 200.32, 200.38-200.40, 200.42, 200.48-200.50,
200.52, 200.58-200.60, 200.62, 200.68-200.70, 200.72, 200.78, 202.70,
202.72, 202.78-202.80, 202.82, 202.88, 202.92, 239.81-239.9;
For code **200.53:** (Ex:) 200.30, 200.33, 200.38-200.40, 200.43, 200.48-200.50,
200.53, 200.58-200.60, 200.63, 200.68-200.70, 200.73, 200.78, 202.70,
202.73, 202.78-202.80, 202.83, 202.88, 202.93, 239.81-239.9;
For code **200.54:** (Ex:) 200.30, 200.34, 200.38-200.40, 200.44, 200.48-200.50,
200.54, 200.58-200.60, 200.64, 200.68-200.70, 200.74, 200.78, 202.70,
202.74, 202.78-202.80, 202.84, 202.88, 202.94, 239.81-239.9;
For code **200.55:** (Ex:) 200.30, 200.35, 200.38-200.40, 200.45, 200.48-200.50,
200.55, 200.58-200.60, 200.65, 200.68-200.70, 200.75, 200.78, 202.70,
202.75, 202.78-202.80, 202.85, 202.88, 202.95, 239.81-239.9;
For code **200.56:** (Ex:) 200.30, 200.36, 200.38-200.40, 200.46, 200.48-200.50,
200.56, 200.58-200.60, 200.66, 200.68-200.70, 200.76, 200.78, 202.70,
202.76, 202.78-202.80, 202.86, 202.88, 202.96, 239.81-239.9;
For code **200.57:** (Ex:) 200.30, 200.37-200.40, 200.47-200.50, 200.57-200.60,
200.67-200.70, 200.77-200.78, 202.70, 202.77-202.80, 202.87-202.88,
202.97, 239.81-239.9;
For code **200.58:** (Ex:) 200.30-200.78, 202.70-202.88, 202.98, 239.81-239.9

Coding Clinic: 2013, Q1, P4

● **200.6 Anaplastic large cell lymphoma** 🔗
[0-8] For code **200.60:** (Ex:) 200.30-200.78, 202.70-202.90, 239.81-239.9;
For code **200.61:** (Ex:) 200.30-200.31, 200.38-200.41, 200.48-200.51,
200.58-200.61, 200.68-200.71, 200.78, 202.70-202.71, 202.78-202.81,
202.88, 202.91, 239.81-239.9;
For code **200.62:** (Ex:) 200.30, 200.32, 200.38-200.40, 200.42, 200.48-200.50,
200.52, 200.58-200.60, 200.62, 200.68-200.70, 200.72, 200.78, 202.70,
202.72, 202.78-202.80, 202.82, 202.88, 202.92, 239.81-239.9;
For code **200.63:** (Ex:) 200.30, 200.33, 200.38-200.40, 200.43, 200.48-200.50,
200.53, 200.58-200.60, 200.63, 200.68-200.70, 200.73, 200.78, 202.70,
202.73, 202.78-202.80, 202.83, 202.88, 202.93, 239.81-239.9;
For code **200.64:** (Ex:) 200.30, 200.34, 200.38-200.40, 200.44, 200.48-200.50,
200.54, 200.58-200.60, 200.64, 200.68- 200.70, 200.74, 200.78, 202.70,
202.74, 202.78-202.80, 202.84, 202.88, 202.94, 239.81-239.9;
For code **200.65:** (Ex:) 200.30, 200.35, 200.38-200.40, 200.45, 200.48-200.50,
200.55, 200.58-200.60, 200.65, 200.68-200.70, 200.75, 200.78, 202.70,
202.75, 202.78-202.80, 202.85, 202.88, 202.95, 239.81-239.9;
For code **200.66:** (Ex:) 200.30, 200.36, 200.38-200.40, 200.46, 200.48-200.50,
200.56, 200.58-200.60, 200.66, 200.68-200.70, 200.76, 200.78, 202.70,
202.76, 202.78-202.80, 202.86, 202.88, 202.96, 239.81-239.9;
For code **200.67:** (Ex:) 200.30, 200.37-200.40, 200.47-200.50, 200.57-200.60,
200.67-200.70, 200.77-200.78, 202.70, 202.77-202.80, 202.87-202.88,
202.97, 239.81-239.9;
For code **200.68:** (Ex:) 200.30-200.78, 202.70-202.88, 202.98, 239.81-239.9

● **200.7 Large cell lymphoma** 🔗
[0-8] For code **200.70:** (Ex:) 200.30-200.78, 202.70-202.90, 239.81-239.9;
For code **200.71:** (Ex:) 200.30-200.31, 200.38-200.41, 200.48-200.51,
200.58-200.61, 200.68-200.71, 200.78, 202.70-202.71, 202.78-202.81,
202.88, 202.91, 239.81-239.9;
For code **200.72:** (Ex:) 200.30, 200.32, 200.38-200.40, 200.42, 200.48-200.50,
200.52, 200.58-200.60, 200.62, 200.68-200.70, 200.72, 200.78, 202.70,
202.72, 202.78-202.80, 202.82, 202.88, 202.92, 239.81-239.9;
For code **200.73:** (Ex:) 200.30, 200.33, 200.38-200.40, 200.43, 200.48-200.50,
200.53, 200.58-200.60, 200.63, 200.68-200.70, 200.73, 200.78, 202.70,
202.73, 202.78-202.80, 202.83, 202.88, 202.93, 239.81-239.9;
For code **200.74:** (Ex:) 200.30, 200.34, 200.38-200.40, 200.44, 200.48-200.50,
200.54, 200.58-200.60, 200.64, 200.68-200.70, 200.74, 200.78, 202.70,
202.74, 202.78-202.80, 202.84, 202.88, 202.94, 239.81-239.9;
For code **200.75:** (Ex:) 200.30, 200.35, 200.38-200.40, 200.45, 200.48-200.50,
200.55, 200.58-200.60, 200.65, 200.68-200.70, 200.75, 200.78, 202.70,
202.75, 202.78-202.80, 202.85, 202.88, 202.95, 239.81-239.9;
For code **200.76:** (Ex:) 200.30, 200.36, 200.38-200.40, 200.46, 200.48-200.50,
200.56, 200.58-200.60, 200.66, 200.68-200.70, 200.76, 200.78, 202.70,
202.76, 202.78-202.80, 202.86, 202.88, 202.96, 239.81-239.9;
For code **200.77:** (Ex:) 200.30, 200.37-200.40, 200.47-200.50, 200.57-200.60,
200.67-200.70, 200.77-200.78, 202.70, 202.77-202.80, 202.87-202.88,
202.97, 239.81-239.9;
For code **200.78:** (Ex:) 200.30-200.78, 202.70-202.88, 202.98, 239.81-239.9

● **200.8 Other named variants** 🔗
[0-8]   Lymphoma (malignant):
                lymphoplasmacytoid type
                mixed lymphocytic-histiocytic (diffuse)
            Lymphosarcoma, mixed cell type (diffuse)
            Reticulolymphosarcoma (diffuse)
For code **200.80:** (Ex:) 200.80-200.88, 239.81-239.9;
For code **200.81:** (Ex:) 200.80-200.81, 200.88, 239.81-239.9;
For code **200.82:** (Ex:) 200.80, 200.82, 200.88, 239.81-239.9;
For code **200.83:** (Ex:) 200.80, 200.83, 200.88, 239.81-239.9;
For code **200.84:** (Ex:) 200.80, 200.84, 200.88, 239.81-239.9;
For code **200.85:** (Ex:) 200.80, 200.85, 200.88, 239.81-239.9;
For code **200.86:** (Ex:) 200.80, 200.86, 200.88, 239.81-239.9;
For code **200.87:** (Ex:) 200.80, 200.87-200.88, 239.81-239.9;
For code **200.88:** (Ex:) 200.80-200.88, 239.81-239.9

● **201 Hodgkin's disease**
*Also known as malignant lymphoma/lymphosarcoma and is cancer
of the lymphatic system including the lymph nodes and related
structures*
Requires fifth digit. See note before section 200 for codes and
definitions.

● **201.0 Hodgkin's paragranuloma** 🔗
[0-8] For code **201.00:** (Ex:) 201.00-201.08, 201.90, 239.81-239.9;
For code **201.01:** (Ex:) 201.00-201.01, 201.08, 201.90-201.91, 239.81-239.9 ;
For code **201.02:** (Ex:) 201.00, 201.02, 201.08, 201.90, 201.92, 239.81-239.9 ;
For code **201.03:** (Ex:) 201.00, 201.03, 201.08, 201.90, 201.93, 239.81-239.9 ;
For code **201.04:** (Ex:) 201.00, 201.04, 201.08, 201.90, 201.94, 239.81-239.9 ;
For code **201.05:** (Ex:) 201.00, 201.05, 201.08, 201.90, 201.95, 239.81-239.9;
For code **201.06:** (Ex:) 201.00, 201.06, 201.08, 201.90, 201.96, 239.81-239.9;
For code **201.07:** (Ex:) 201.00, 201.07-201.08, 201.90, 201.97, 239.81-239.9;
For code **201.08:** (Ex:) 201.00-201.08, 201.90, 201.98, 239.81-239.9

● **201.1 Hodgkin's granuloma** 🔗
[0-8] For code **201.10:** (Ex:) 201.10-201.18, 201.90, 201.98, 239.81-239.9;
For code **201.11:** (Ex:) 201.10-201.11, 201.18, 201.90-201.91, 201.98,
239.81-239.9;
For code **201.12:** (Ex:) 201.10, 201.12, 201.18, 201.90, 201.92, 201.98,
239.81-239.9;
For code **201.13:** (Ex:) 201.10, 201.13, 201.18, 201.90, 201.93, 201.98,
239.81-239.9;
For code **201.14:** (Ex:) 201.10, 201.14, 201.18, 201.90, 201.94, 201.98,
239.81-239.9;
For code **201.15:** (Ex:) 201.10, 201.15, 201.18, 201.90, 201.95, 201.98,
239.81-239.9;
For code **201.16:** (Ex:) 201.10, 201.16, 201.18, 201.90, 201.96, 201.98,
239.81-239.9;
For code **201.17:** (Ex:) 201.10, 201.17-201.18, 201.90, 201.97-201.98,
239.81-239.9;
For code **201.18:** (Ex:) 201.10-201.18, 201.90, 201.98, 239.81-239.9

● **201.2 Hodgkin's sarcoma** 🔗
[0-8] For code **201.20:** (Ex:) 201.20-201.28, 201.90, 201.98, 239.81-239.9;
For code **201.21:** (Ex:) 201.20-201.21, 201.28, 201.90-201.91, 201.98,
239.81-239.9;
For code **201.22:** (Ex:) 201.20, 201.22, 201.28, 201.90, 201.92, 201.98,
239.81-239.9;
For code **201.23:** (Ex:) 201.20, 201.23, 201.28, 201.90, 201.93, 201.98,
239.81-239.9;
For code **201.24:** (Ex:) 201.20, 201.24, 201.28, 201.90, 201.94, 201.98,
239.81-239.9;
For code **201.25:** (Ex:) 201.20, 201.25, 201.28, 201.90, 201.95, 201.98,
239.81-239.9;
For code **201.26:** (Ex:) 201.20, 201.26, 201.28, 201.90, 201.96, 201.98,
239.81-239.9;
For code **201.27:** (Ex:) 201.20, 201.27-201.28, 201.90, 201.97-201.98,
239.81-239.9;
For code **201.28:** (Ex:) 201.20-201.28, 201.90, 201.98, 239.81-239.9

● **201.4 Lymphocytic-histiocytic predominance** 🏷
[0-8]   For code **201.40:** (Ex) 201.40-201.48, 201.90, 201.98, 239.81-239.9;
For code **201.41:** (Ex) 201.40-201.41, 201.48, 201.90-201.91, 201.98, 239.81-239.9;
For code **201.42:** (Ex) 201.40, 201.42, 201.48, 201.90, 201.92, 201.98, 239.81-239.9;
For code **201.43:** (Ex) 201.40, 201.43, 201.48, 201.90, 201.93, 201.98, 239.81-239.9;
For code **201.44:** (Ex) 201.40, 201.44, 201.48, 201.90, 201.94, 201.98, 239.81-239.9;
For code **201.45:** (Ex) 201.40, 201.45, 201.48, 201.90, 201.95, 201.98, 239.81-239.9;
For code **201.46:** (Ex) 201.40, 201.46, 201.48, 201.90, 201.96, 201.98, 239.81-239.9;
For code **201.47:** (Ex) 201.40, 201.47-201.48, 201.90, 201.97-201.98, 239.81-239.9;
For code **201.48:** (Ex) 201.40-201.48, 201.90, 201.98, 239.81-239.9

● **201.5 Nodular sclerosis** 🏷
[0-8]   Hodgkin's disease, nodular sclerosis:
       NOS
       cellular phase
For code **201.50:** (Ex) 201.50-201.58, 201.90, 201.98, 239.81-239.9;
For code **201.51:** (Ex) 201.50-201.51, 201.58, 201.90-201.91, 201.98, 239.81-239.9;
For code **201.52:** (Ex) 201.50, 201.52, 201.58, 201.90, 201.92, 201.98, 239.81-239.9;
For code **201.53:** (Ex) 201.50, 201.53, 201.58, 201.90, 201.93, 201.98, 239.81-239.9;
For code **201.54:** (Ex) 201.50, 201.54, 201.58, 201.90, 201.94, 201.98, 239.81-239.9;
For code **201.55:** (Ex) 201.50, 201.55, 201.58, 201.90, 201.95, 201.98, 239.81-239.9;
For code **201.56:** (Ex) 201.50, 201.56, 201.58, 201.90, 201.96, 201.98, 239.81-239.9;
For code **201.57:** (Ex) 201.50, 201.57-201.58, 201.90, 201.97 -201.98, 239.81-239.9;
For code **201.58:** (Ex) 201.50-201.58, 201.90, 201.98, 239.81-239.9

● **201.6 Mixed cellularity** 🏷
[0-8]   For code **201.60:** (Ex) 201.60-201.68, 201.90, 201.98, 239.81-239.9;
For code **201.61:** (Ex) 201.60-201.61, 201.68, 201.90-201.91, 201.98, 239.81-239.9;
For code **201.62:** (Ex) 201.60, 201.62, 201.68, 201.90, 201.92, 201.98, 239.81-239.9;
For code **201.63:** (Ex) 201.60, 201.63, 201.68, 201.90, 201.93, 201.98, 239.81-239.9;
For code **201.64:** (Ex) 201.60, 201.64, 201.68, 201.90, 201.94, 201.98, 239.81-239.9;
For code **201.65:** (Ex) 201.60, 201.65, 201.68, 201.90, 201.95, 201.98, 239.81-239.9;
For code **201.66:** (Ex) 201.60, 201.66, 201.68, 201.90, 201.96, 201.98, 239.81-239.9;
For code **201.67:** (Ex) 201.60, 201.67-201.68, 201.90, 201.97-201.98, 239.81-239.9;
For code **201.68:** (Ex) 201.60-201.68, 201.90, 201.98, 239.81-239.9

● **201.7 Lymphocytic depletion** 🏷
[0-8]   Hodgkin's disease, lymphocytic depletion:
       NOS
       diffuse fibrosis
       reticular type
For code **201.70:** (Ex) 201.70-201.90, 201.98, 239.81-239.9;
For code **201.71:** (Ex) 201.70-201.71, 201.78, 201.91, 201.98, 239.81-239.9;
For code **201.72:** (Ex) 201.70, 201.72, 201.78, 201.92, 201.98 239.81-239.9;
For code **201.73:** (Ex) 201.70, 201.73, 201.78, 201.93, 201.98, 239.81-239.9;
For code **201.74:** (Ex) 201.70, 201.74, 201.78, 201.94, 201.98, 239.81-239.9;
For code **201.75:** (Ex) 201.70, 201.75, 201.78, 201.95, 201.98, 239.81-239.9;
For code **201.76:** (Ex) 201.70, 201.76, 201.78, 201.96, 201.98, 239.81-239.9;
For code **201.77:** (Ex) 201.70, 201.77-201.78, 201.97-201.98, 239.81-239.9;
For code **201.78:** (Ex) 201.70-201.78, 201.98, 239.81-239.9

● **201.9 Hodgkin's disease, unspecified** 🏷
[0-8]   Hodgkin's:
       disease NOS
       lymphoma NOS
     Malignant:
       lymphogranuloma
       lymphogranulomatosis
For code **201.90:** (Ex) 201.90-201.98, 239.81-239.9;
For code **201.91:** (Ex) 201.90-201.91, 201.98, 239.81-239.9;
For code **201.92:** (Ex) 201.90, 201.92, 201.98, 239.81-239.9;
For code **201.93:** (Ex) 201.90, 201.93, 201.98, 239.81-239.9;
For code **201.94:** (Ex) 201.90, 201.94, 201.98, 239.81-239.9;
For code **201.95:** (Ex) 201.90, 201.95, 201.98, 239.81-239.9;
For code **201.96:** (Ex) 201.90, 201.96, 201.98, 239.81-239.9;
For code **201.97:** (Ex) 201.90, 201.97-201.98, 239.81-239.9;
For code **201.98:** (Ex) 201.90-201.98, 239.81-239.9

● **202 Other malignant neoplasms of lymphoid and histiocytic tissue**
     Requires fifth digit. See note before section 200 for codes and definitions.

● **202.0 Nodular lymphoma** 🏷
[0-8]   Brill-Symmers disease
     Lymphoma:
       follicular (giant) (large cell)
       lymphocytic, nodular
     Lymphosarcoma:
       follicular (giant)
       nodular
For code **202.00:** (Ex) 200.30, 200.40, 200.50, 200.60, 200.70, 202.00-202.08, 202.70, 202.80, 202.90, 239.81-239.9;
For code **202.01:** (Ex) 200.31, 200.41, 200.51, 200.61, 200.71, 202.00-202.01, 202.08, 202.71, 202.81, 202.91, 239.81-239.9;
For code **202.02:** (Ex) 200.32, 200.42, 200.52, 200.62, 200.72, 202.00, 202.02, 202.08, 202.72, 202.82, 202.92, 239.81-239.9;
For code **202.03:** (Ex) 200.33, 200.43, 200.53, 200.63, 200.73, 202.00, 202.03, 202.08, 202.73, 202.83, 202.93, 239.81-239.9;
For code **202.04:** (Ex) 200.34, 200.44, 200.54, 200.64, 200.74, 202.00, 202.04, 202.08, 202.74, 202.84, 202.94, 239.81-239.9;
For code **202.05:** (Ex) 200.35, 200.45, 200.55, 200.65, 200.75, 202.00, 202.05, 202.08, 202.75, 202.85, 202.95, 239.81-239.9;
For code **202.06:** (Ex) 200.36, 200.46, 200.56, 200.66, 200.76, 202.00, 202.06, 202.08, 202.76, 202.86, 202.96, 239.81-239.9;
For code **202.07:** (Ex) 200.37, 200.47, 200.57, 200.67, 200.77, 202.00, 202.07-202.08, 202.77, 202.87, 202.97, 239.81-239.9;
For code **202.08:** (Ex) 200.38, 200.48, 200.58, 200.68, 200.78, 202.00-202.08, 202.78, 202.88, 202.98, 239.81-239.9

Coding Clinic: 2009, Q3, P5x2

● **202.1 Mycosis fungoides** 🏷
[0-8]   **Excludes**   *peripheral T-cell lymphoma (202.7)*
For code **202.10:** (Ex) 200.30, 200.40, 200.50, 200.60, 200.70, 202.10-202.18, 202.70, 202.80, 202.90, 239.81-239.9;
For code **202.11:** (Ex) 200.31, 200.41, 200.51, 200.61, 200.71, 202.10-202.11, 202.18, 202.71, 202.81, 202.91, 239.81-239.9;
For code **202.12:** (Ex) 200.32, 200.42, 200.52, 200.62, 200.72 202.10, 202.12, 202.18, 202.72, 202.82 202.92, 239.81-239.9;
For code **202.13:** (Ex) 200.33, 200.43, 200.53, 200.63, 200.73 202.10, 202.13, 202.18, 202.73, 202.83 202.93, 239.81-239.9;
For code **202.14:** (Ex) 200.34, 200.44, 200.54, 200.64, 200.74 202.10, 202.14, 202.18, 202.74, 202.84 202.94, 239.81-239.9;
For code **202.15:** (Ex) 200.35, 200.45, 200.55, 200.65, 200.75, 202.10, 202.15, 202.18, 202.75, 202.85, 202.95, 239.81-239.9;
For code **202.16:** (Ex) 200.36, 200.46, 200.56, 200.66, 200.76, 202.10, 202.16, 202.18, 202.76, 202.86, 202.96, 239.81-239.9;
For code **202.17:** (Ex) 200.37, 200.47, 200.57, 200.67, 200.77, 202.10, 202.17-202.18, 202.77, 202.87, 202.97, 239.81-239.9;
For code **202.18:** (Ex) 200.38, 200.48, 200.58, 200.68, 200.78, 202.10-202.18, 202.78, 202.88, 202.98, 239.81-239.9

Coding Clinic: 1999, Q2, P7-8; 1992, Q2, P4

NEOPLASMS (140–239)

N Newborn: 0   **P** Pediatric: 0–17   **M** Maternity: 12–55   **A** Adult: 15–124   ♀ Females Only   ♂ Males Only

(Ex) CC/MCC Exclusions   🏷 Complication\Comorbidity   🏷 Major C\C   🏷 Present on Admission Requirement   🏷 Hospital-Acquired Condition   **717**

NEOPLASMS (140–239)

● **202.2 Sézary's disease** 🔎
[0-8]　　For code **202.20:** (Ex) 200.30, 200.40, 200.50, 200.60, 200.70, 202.20-202.28,
　　　　　　　　　202.70, 202.80, 202.90, 239.81-239.9;
　　　　For code **202.21:** (Ex) 200.31, 200.41, 200.51, 200.61, 200.71, 202.20-202.21,
　　　　　　　　　202.28, 202.71, 202.81, 202.91, 239.81-239.9;
　　　　For code **202.22:** (Ex) 200.32, 200.42, 200.52, 200.62, 200.72, 202.20, 202.22,
　　　　　　　　　202.28, 202.72, 202.82, 202.92, 239.81-239.9;
　　　　For code **202.23:** (Ex) 200.33, 200.43, 200.53, 200.63, 200.73, 202.20, 202.23,
　　　　　　　　　202.28, 202.73, 202.83, 202.93, 239.81-239.9;
　　　　For code **202.24:** (Ex) 200.34, 200.44, 200.54, 200.64, 200.74, 202.20, 202.24,
　　　　　　　　　202.28, 202.74, 202.84, 202.94, 239.81-239.9;
　　　　For code **202.25:** (Ex) 200.35, 200.45, 200.55, 200.65, 200.75, 202.20, 202.25,
　　　　　　　　　202.28, 202.75, 202.85, 202.95, 239.81-239.9;
　　　　For code **202.26:** (Ex) 200.36, 200.46, 200.56, 200.66, 200.76, 202.20, 202.26,
　　　　　　　　　202.28, 202.76, 202.86, 202.96, 239.81-239.9;
　　　　For code **202.27:** (Ex) 200.37, 200.47, 200.57, 200.67, 200.77, 202.20,
　　　　　　　　　202.27-202.28, 202.77, 202.87, 202.97, 239.81-239.9;
　　　　For code **202.28:** (Ex) 200.38, 200.48, 200.58, 200.68, 200.78, 202.20-202.28,
　　　　　　　　　202.78, 202.88, 202.98, 239.81-239.9

　　　　Coding Clinic: 1999, Q2, P7-8

● **202.3 Malignant histiocytosis** 🔎
[0-8]　　Histiocytic medullary reticulosis
　　　　Malignant:
　　　　　　reticuloendotheliosis
　　　　　　reticulosis
　　　　For code **202.30:** (Ex) 200.30, 200.40, 200.50, 200.60, 200.70, 202.30-202.38,
　　　　　　　　　202.70, 202.80, 202.90, 239.81-239.9;
　　　　For code **202.31:** (Ex) 200.31, 200.41, 200.51, 200.61, 200.71, 202.30-202.31,
　　　　　　　　　202.38, 202.71, 202.81, 202.91, 239.81-239.9;
　　　　For code **202.32:** (Ex) 200.32, 200.42, 200.52, 200.62, 200.72, 202.30, 202.32,
　　　　　　　　　202.38, 202.72, 202.82, 202.92, 239.81-239.9;
　　　　For code **202.33:** (Ex) 200.33, 200.43, 200.53, 200.63, 200.73, 202.30, 202.33,
　　　　　　　　　202.38, 202.73, 202.83, 202.93, 239.81-239.9;
　　　　For code **202.34:** (Ex) 200.34, 200.44, 200.54, 200.64, 200.74, 202.30, 202.34,
　　　　　　　　　202.38, 202.74, 202.84, 202.94, 239.81-239.9;
　　　　For code **202.35:** (Ex) 200.35, 200.45, 200.55, 200.65, 200.75, 202.30, 202.35,
　　　　　　　　　202.38, 202.75, 202.85, 202.95, 239.81-239.9;
　　　　For code **202.36:** (Ex) 200.36, 200.46, 200.56, 200.66, 200.76, 202.30, 202.36,
　　　　　　　　　202.38, 202.76, 202.86, 202.96, 239.81-239.9;
　　　　For code **202.37:** (Ex) 200.37, 200.47, 200.57, 200.67, 200.77, 202.30,
　　　　　　　　　202.37-202.38, 202.77, 202.87, 202.97, 239.81-239.9;
　　　　For code **202.38:** (Ex) 200.38, 200.48, 200.58, 200.68, 200.78, 202.30-202.38,
　　　　　　　　　202.78, 202.88, 202.98, 239.81-239.9

● **202.4 Leukemic reticuloendotheliosis** 🔎
[0-8]　　Hairy-cell leukemia
　　　　For code **202.40:** (Ex) 200.30, 200.40, 200.50, 200.60, 200.70, 202.40-202.48,
　　　　　　　　　202.70, 202.80, 202.90, 239.81-239.9 ;
　　　　For code **202.41:** (Ex) 200.31, 200.41, 200.51, 200.61, 200.71, 202.40-202.41,
　　　　　　　　　202.48, 202.71, 202.81, 202.91, 239.81-239.9;
　　　　For code **202.42:** (Ex) 200.32, 200.42, 200.52, 200.62, 200.72, 202.40, 202.42,
　　　　　　　　　202.48, 202.72, 202.82, 202.92, 239.81-239.9;
　　　　For code **202.43:** (Ex) 200.33, 200.43, 200.53, 200.63, 200.73, 202.40, 202.43,
　　　　　　　　　202.48, 202.73, 202.83, 202.93, 239.81-239.9;
　　　　For code **202.44:** (Ex) 200.34, 200.44, 200.54, 200.64, 200.74, 202.40, 202.44,
　　　　　　　　　202.48, 202.74, 202.84, 202.94, 239.81-239.9;
　　　　For code **202.45:** (Ex) 200.35, 200.45, 200.55, 200.65, 200.75, 202.40, 202.45,
　　　　　　　　　202.48, 202.75, 202.85, 202.95, 239.81-239.9;
　　　　For code **202.46:** (Ex) 200.36, 200.46, 200.56, 200.66, 200.76, 202.40, 202.46,
　　　　　　　　　202.48, 202.76, 202.86, 202.96, 239.81-239.9;
　　　　For code **202.47:** (Ex) 200.37, 200.47, 200.57, 200.67, 200.77, 202.40,
　　　　　　　　　202.47-202.48, 202.77, 202.87, 202.97, 239.81-239.9;
　　　　For code **202.48:** (Ex) 200.38, 200.48, 200.58, 200.68, 200.78, 202.40-202.48,
　　　　　　　　　202.78, 202.88, 202.98, 239.81-239.9

● **202.5 Letterer-Siwe disease** 🔎
[0-8]　　Acute:
　　　　　　differentiated progressive histiocytosis
　　　　　　histiocytosis X (progressive)
　　　　　　infantile reticuloendotheliosis
　　　　　　reticulosis of infancy
　　　　Excludes　*adult pulmonary Langerhans cell histiocytosis (516.5)*
　　　　　　　　　Hand-Schüller-Christian disease (277.89)
　　　　　　　　　histiocytosis (acute) (chronic) (277.89)
　　　　　　　　　histiocytosis X (chronic) (277.89)
　　　　For code **202.50:** (Ex) 200.30, 200.40, 200.50, 200.60, 200.70, 202.50-202.58,
　　　　　　　　　202.70, 202.80, 202.90, 239.81-239.9;
　　　　For code **202.51:** (Ex) 200.31, 200.41, 200.51, 200.61, 200.71, 202.50-202.51,
　　　　　　　　　202.58, 202.71, 202.81, 202.91, 239.81-239.9;
　　　　For code **202.52:** (Ex) 200.32, 200.42, 200.52, 200.62, 200.72, 202.50, 202.52,
　　　　　　　　　202.58, 202.72, 202.82, 202.92, 239.81-239.9;
　　　　For code **202.53:** (Ex) 200.33, 200.43, 200.53, 200.63, 200.73, 202.50, 202.53,
　　　　　　　　　202.58, 202.73, 202.83, 202.93, 239.81-239.9;
　　　　For code **202.54:** (Ex) 200.34, 200.44, 200.54, 200.64, 200.74, 202.50, 202.54,
　　　　　　　　　202.58, 202.74, 202.84, 202.94, 239.81-239.9;
　　　　For code **202.55:** (Ex) 200.35, 200.45, 200.55, 200.65, 200.75, 202.50, 202.55,
　　　　　　　　　202.58, 202.75, 202.85, 202.95, 239.81-239.9;
　　　　For code **202.56:** (Ex) 200.36, 200.46, 200.56, 200.66, 200.76, 202.50, 202.56,
　　　　　　　　　202.58, 202.76, 202.86, 202.96, 239.81-239.9;
　　　　For code **202.57:** (Ex) 200.37, 200.47, 200.57, 200.67, 200.77, 202.50,
　　　　　　　　　202.57-202.58, 202.77, 202.87, 202.97, 239.81-239.9;
　　　　For code **202.58:** (Ex) 200.38, 200.48, 200.58, 200.68, 200.78, 202.50-202.58,
　　　　　　　　　202.78, 202.88, 202.98, 239.81-239.9

● **202.6 Malignant mast cell tumors** 🔎
[0-8]　　Malignant:
　　　　　　mastocytoma
　　　　　　mastocytosis
　　　　Mast cell sarcoma
　　　　Systemic tissue mast cell disease
　　　　Excludes　*mast cell leukemia (207.8)*
　　　　For code **202.60:** (Ex) 200.30, 200.40, 200.50, 200.60, 200.70, 202.60-202.70,
　　　　　　　　　202.80, 202.90, 239.81-239.9;
　　　　For code **202.61:** (Ex) 200.31, 200.41, 200.51, 200.61, 200.71, 202.60-202.61,
　　　　　　　　　202.68, 202.71, 202.81, 202.91, 239.81-239.9;
　　　　For code **202.62:** (Ex) 200.32, 200.42, 200.52, 200.62, 200.72, 202.60, 202.62,
　　　　　　　　　202.68, 202.72, 202.82, 202.92, 239.81-239.9;
　　　　For code **202.63:** (Ex) 200.33, 200.43, 200.53, 200.63, 200.73, 202.60, 202.63,
　　　　　　　　　202.68, 202.73, 202.83, 202.93, 239.81-239.9;
　　　　For code **202.64:** (Ex) 200.34, 200.44, 200.54, 200.64, 200.74, 202.60, 202.64,
　　　　　　　　　202.68, 202.74, 202.84, 202.94, 239.81-239.9;
　　　　For code **202.65:** (Ex) 200.35, 200.45, 200.55, 200.65, 200.75, 202.60, 202.65,
　　　　　　　　　202.68, 202.75, 202.85, 202.95, 239.81-239.9;
　　　　For code **202.66:** (Ex) 200.36, 200.46, 200.56, 200.66, 200.76, 202.60, 202.66,
　　　　　　　　　202.68, 202.76, 202.86, 202.96, 239.81-239.9;
　　　　For code **202.67:** (Ex) 200.37, 200.47, 200.57, 200.67, 200.77, 202.60,
　　　　　　　　　202.67-202.68, 202.77, 202.87, 202.97, 239.81-239.9;
　　　　For code **202.68:** (Ex) 200.38, 200.48, 200.58, 200.68, 200.78, 202.60-202.68,
　　　　　　　　　202.78, 202.88, 202.98, 239.81-239.9

　　　　Coding Clinic: 2013, Q2, P12

● **202.7 Peripheral T cell lymphoma** 🔎
[0-8]　　For code **202.70:** (Ex) 200.30-200.78, 202.70-202.90, 239.81-239.9;
　　　　For code **202.71:** (Ex) 200.30-200.31, 200.38-200.41, 200.48-200.51,
　　　　　　　　　200.58-200.61, 200.68-200.71, 200.78, 202.70-202.71, 202.78-202.81,
　　　　　　　　　202.88, 202.91, 239.81-239.9;
　　　　For code **202.72:** (Ex) 200.30, 200.32, 200.38-200.40, 200.42, 200.48-200.50,
　　　　　　　　　200.52, 200.58-200.60, 200.62, 200.68-200.70, 200.72, 200.78, 202.70,
　　　　　　　　　202.72, 202.78-202.80, 202.82, 202.88, 202.92, 239.81-239.9;
　　　　For code **202.73:** (Ex) 200.30, 200.33, 200.38-200.40, 200.43, 200.48-200.50,
　　　　　　　　　200.53, 200.58-200.60, 200.63, 200.68-200.70, 200.73, 200.78, 202.70,
　　　　　　　　　202.73, 202.78-202.80, 202.83, 202.88, 202.93, 239.81-239.9;
　　　　For code **202.74:** (Ex) 200.30, 200.34, 200.38-200.40, 200.44, 200.48-200.50,
　　　　　　　　　200.54, 200.58-200.60, 200.64, 200.68-200.70, 200.74, 200.78, 202.70,
　　　　　　　　　202.74, 202.78-202.80, 202.84, 202.88, 202.94, 239.81-239.9;
　　　　For code **202.75:** (Ex) 200.30, 200.35, 200.38-200.40, 200.45, 200.48-200.50,
　　　　　　　　　200.55, 200.58-200.60, 200.65, 200.68-200.70, 200.75, 200.78, 202.70,
　　　　　　　　　202.75, 202.78-202.80, 202.85, 202.88, 202.95, 239.81-239.9;
　　　　For code **202.76:** (Ex) 200.30, 200.36, 200.38-200.40, 200.46, 200.48-200.50,
　　　　　　　　　200.56, 200.58-200.60, 200.66, 200.68-200.70, 200.76, 200.78, 202.70,
　　　　　　　　　202.76, 202.78-202.80, 202.86, 202.88, 202.96, 239.81-239.9;
　　　　For code **202.77:** (Ex) 200.30, 200.37-200.40, 200.47-200.50, 200.57-200.60,
　　　　　　　　　200.67-200.70, 200.77-200.78, 202.70, 202.77-202.80, 202.87-202.88,
　　　　　　　　　202.97, 239.81-239.9;
　　　　For code **202.78:** (Ex) 200.30-200.78, 202.70-202.88, 202.98, 239.81-239.9

● **202.8   Other lymphomas**🔗
[0-8]   Lymphoma (malignant):
                 NOS
                 diffuse
         Excludes *benign lymphoma (229.0)*
         For code **202.80:** (Ex) 200.30-200.78, 202.70-202.90, 239.81-239.9;
         For code **202.81:** (Ex) 200.30-200.31, 200.38-200.41 200.48-200.51,
                 200.58-200.61 200.68-200.71, 200.78, 202.70-202.71 202.78-202.81,
                 202.88, 202.91, 239.81-239.9;
         For code **202.82:** (Ex) 200.30, 200.32, 200.38-200.40, 200.42, 200.48-200.50,
                 200.52, 200.58-200.60 200.62, 200.68-200.70, 200.72, 200.78, 202.70,
                 202.72, 202.78-202.80, 202.82 202.88, 202.92, 239.81-239.9 ;
         For code **202.83:** (Ex) 200.30, 200.33, 200.38-200.40, 200.43 200.48-200.50,
                 200.53, 200.58-200.60 200.63, 200.68-200.70, 200.73, 200.78 202.70,
                 202.73, 202.78-202.80, 202.83 202.88, 202.93, 239.81-239.9 ;
         For code **202.84:** (Ex) 200.30, 200.34, 200.38-200.40, 200.44 200.48-200.50,
                 200.54, 200.58-200.60 200.64, 200.68-200.70, 200.74, 200.78, 202.70,
                 202.74, 202.78-202.80, 202.84, 202.88, 202.94, 239.81-239.9;
         For code **202.85:** (Ex) 200.30, 200.35, 200.38-200.40, 200.45, 200.48-200.50,
                 200.55, 200.58-200.60, 200.65, 200.68-200.70, 200.75, 200.78, 202.70,
                 202.75, 202.78-202.80, 202.85, 202.88, 202.95, 239.81-239.9;
         For code **202.86:** (Ex) 200.30, 200.36, 200.38-200.40, 200.46, 200.48-200.50,
                 200.56, 200.58-200.60, 200.66, 200.68-200.70, 200.76, 200.78, 202.70,
                 202.76, 202.78-202.80, 202.86, 202.88, 202.96, 239.81-239.9;
         For code **202.87:** (Ex) 200.30, 200.37-200.40, 200.47-200.50, 200.57-200.60,
                 200.67-200.70, 200.77-200.78, 202.70, 202.77-202.80, 202.87-202.88,
                 202.97, 239.81-239.9;
         For code **202.88:** (Ex) 200.30-200.78, 202.70-202.88, 202.98, 239.81-239.9
         Coding Clinic: 2008, Q4, P82-83; Q1, P16-17; 2007, Q3, P3; 2006, Q4,
                 P135-136; Q2, P20-22; 1993, Q4, P33; 1992, Q2, P3-4

● **202.9   Other and unspecified malignant neoplasms of**
[0-8] **lymphoid and histiocytic tissue**🔗
                 Follicular dendritic cell sarcoma
                 Interdigitating dendritic cell sarcoma
                 Langerhans cell sarcoma
                 Malignant neoplasm of bone marrow NOS
         For code **202.90:** (Ex) 202.90-202.98, 239.81-239.9;
         For code **202.91:** (Ex) 202.90-202.91, 202.98, 239.81-239.9;
         For code **202.92:** (Ex) 202.90, 202.92, 202.98, 239.81-239.9;
         For code **202.93:** (Ex) 202.90, 202.93, 202.98, 239.81-239.9;
         For code **202.94:** (Ex) 202.90, 202.94, 202.98, 239.81-239.9;
         For code **202.95:** (Ex) 202.90, 202.95, 202.98, 239.81-239.9;
         For code **202.96:** (Ex) 202.90, 202.96, 202.98, 239.81-239.9;
         For code **202.97:** (Ex) 202.90, 202.97-202.98, 239.81-239.9;
         For code **202.98:** (Ex) 202.90-202.98, 239.81-239.9

● **203   Multiple myeloma and immunoproliferative neoplasms**
         *Multiple myeloma is cancer of plasma cell (type of white blood cell)
         and is incurable but treatable disease. Immunoproliferative
         neoplasm is term for diseases (mostly cancers) in which
         immune system cells proliferate.*

         The following fifth-digit subclassification is for use with
         category 203:

0	**without mention of having achieved remission** **failed remission**
1	**in remission**
2	**in relapse**

         Coding Clinic: 2008, Q4, P83-85

● **203.0   Multiple myeloma**🔗
[0-2]   Kahler's disease   Myelomatosis
         Excludes *solitary myeloma (238.6)*
         (Ex) 203.00-208.92, 239.81-239.9
         Coding Clinic: 2012, Q3, P16; 2010, Q2, P6; 2008, Q4, P90-91; 2007,
                 Q2, P9-10; 1999, Q4, P10; 1996, Q1, P16

● **203.1   Plasma cell leukemia**🔗
[0-2]   Plasmacytic leukemia
         (Ex) 203.00-208.92, 239.81-239.9

● **203.8   Other immunoproliferative neoplasms**🔗
[0-2]   (Ex) 203.00-208.92, 239.81-239.9
         Coding Clinic: 1990, Q4, P26

Item 2–7 Leukemia is a cancer (acute or chronic) of the blood-forming
tissues of the bone marrow. Blood cells all start out as stem cells. They mature
and become red cells, white cells, or platelets. There are three main types
of leukocytes (white cells that fight infection): monocytes, lymphocytes, and
granulocytes. **Acute monocytic leukemia** (AML) affects monocytes. **Acute
lymphoid leukemia** (ALL) affects lymphocytes, and **acute myeloid
leukemia** (AML) affects cells that typically develop into white blood cells (not
lymphocytes), though it may develop in other blood cells.

● **204   Lymphoid leukemia**
         Includes   leukemia: leukemia:
                  lymphatic   lymphocytic
                  lymphoblastic   lymphogenous
         The following fifth-digit subclassification is for use with
         category 204:

0	**without mention of having achieved remission** **failed remission**
1	**in remission**
2	**in relapse**

         Coding Clinic: 2008, Q4, P83-85

● **204.0   Acute**🔗
[0-2]   **Excludes** *acute exacerbation of chronic lymphoid leukemia*
                        (204.1)
         (Ex) 203.00-208.92, 239.81-239.9
         Coding Clinic: 2012, Q1, P13-14; 1999, Q3, P4, 6-7; 1993, Q3, P4x2;
                 1985, May-June, P18-19

● **204.1   Chronic**🔗
[0-2]   (Ex) 203.00-208.92, 239.81-239.9

● **204.2   Subacute**🔗
[0-2]   (Ex) 203.00-208.92, 239.81-239.9

● **204.8   Other lymphoid leukemia**🔗
[0-2]   Aleukemic leukemia:
                 lymphatic
                 lymphocytic
                 lymphoid
         (Ex) 203.00-208.92, 239.81-239.9
         Coding Clinic: 2009, Q3, P6

● **204.9   Unspecified lymphoid leukemia**🔗
[0-2]   (Ex) 203.00-208.92, 239.81-239.9

● **205   Myeloid leukemia**
         Includes   leukemia: leukemia:
                  granulocytic   myelomonocytic
                  myeloblastic   myelosclerotic
                  myelocytic   myelosis
                  myelogenous
         The following fifth-digit subclassification is for use with
         category 205:

0	**without mention of having achieved remission** **failed remission**
1	**in remission**
2	**in relapse**

         Coding Clinic: 2008, Q4, P83-85

● **205.0   Acute**🔗
[0-2]   Acute promyelocytic leukemia
         Excludes *acute exacerbation of chronic myeloid leukemia*
                        (205.1)
         (Ex) 203.00-208.92, 239.81-239.9
         Coding Clinic: 2009, Q4, P78; 2006, Q2, P20-22; 2002, Q1, P11-12;
                 1993, Q3, P3-4x2

● **205.1   Chronic**🔗
[0-2]   Eosinophilic leukemia
                 Neutrophilic leukemia
         (Ex) 203.00-208.92, 239.81-239.9
         Coding Clinic: 2012, Q2, P16-17; 2008, Q4, P140-143; 2000, Q1, P6;
                 1995, Q2, P12; 1985, July-Aug, P13

● **205.2   Subacute**🔗
[0-2]   (Ex) 203.00-208.92, 239.81-239.9

NEOPLASMS (140–239)

● **205.3 Myeloid sarcoma** 🔖
[0-2]   Chloroma
          Granulocytic sarcoma
          (Ex) 203.00-208.92, 239.81-239.9

● **205.8 Other myeloid leukemia** 🔖
[0-2]   Aleukemic leukemia:
              granulocytic
              myelogenous
              myeloid
          Aleukemic myelosis
          (Ex) 203.00-208.92, 239.81-239.9

● **205.9 Unspecified myeloid leukemia** 🔖
[0-2]   (Ex) 203.00-208.92, 239.81-239.9
          Coding Clinic: 1985, May-June, P18-19

● **206 Monocytic leukemia**
    Includes   leukemia:
                      histiocytic
                      monoblastic
                      monocytoid

The following fifth-digit subclassification is for use with category 206:

0	without mention of having achieved remission failed remission
1	in remission
2	in relapse

        Coding Clinic: 2008, Q4, P83-85

● **206.0 Acute** 🔖
[0-2]   **Excludes**   acute exacerbation of chronic monocytic leukemia
                        (206.1)
          (Ex) 203.00-208.92, 239.81-239.9

● **206.1 Chronic** 🔖
[0-2]   (Ex) 203.00-208.92, 239.81-239.9

● **206.2 Subacute** 🔖
[0-2]   (Ex) 203.00-208.92, 239.81-239.9

● **206.8 Other monocytic leukemia** 🔖
[0-2]   Aleukemic:
              monocytic leukemia
              monocytoid leukemia
          (Ex) 203.00-208.92, 239.81-239.9

● **206.9 Unspecified monocytic leukemia** 🔖
[0-2]

● **207 Other specified leukemia**
    Excludes   leukemic reticuloendotheliosis (202.4)
                   plasma cell leukemia (203.1)

The following fifth-digit subclassification is for use with category 207:

0	without mention of having achieved remission failed remission
1	in remission
2	in relapse

          (Ex) 203.00-208.92, 239.81-239.9
          Coding Clinic: 2008, Q4, P83-85

● **207.0 Acute erythremia and erythroleukemia** 🔖
[0-2]   Acute erythremic myelosis
          Di Guglielmo's disease
          Erythremic myelosis
          (Ex) 203.00-208.92, 239.81-239.9

● **207.1 Chronic erythremia** 🔖
[0-2]   Heilmeyer-Schöner disease
          (Ex) 203.00-208.92, 239.81-239.9

● **207.2 Megakaryocytic leukemia** 🔖
[0-2]   Megakaryocytic myelosis
          Thrombocytic leukemia
          (Ex) 203.00-208.92, 239.81-239.9

● **207.8 Other specified leukemia** 🔖
[0-2]   Lymphosarcoma cell leukemia
          (Ex) 203.00-208.92, 239.81-239.9

● **208 Leukemia of unspecified cell type**
The following fifth-digit subclassification is for use with category 208:

0	without mention of having achieved remission failed remission
1	in remission
2	in relapse

        Coding Clinic: 2008, Q4, P83-85

● **208.0 Acute** 🔖
[0-2]   Acute leukemia NOS
          Blast cell leukemia
          Stem cell leukemia
          Excludes   acute exacerbation of chronic unspecified
                        leukemia (208.1)
          (Ex) 203.00-208.92, 239.81-239.9
          Coding Clinic: 1987, Mar-April, P12

● **208.1 Chronic** 🔖
[0-2]   Chronic leukemia NOS
          (Ex) 203.00-208.92, 239.81-239.9

● **208.2 Subacute** 🔖
[0-2]   *Somewhat acute, between acute and chronic*
          Subacute leukemia NOS
          (Ex) 203.00-208.92, 239.81-239.9

● **208.8 Other leukemia of unspecified cell type** 🔖
[0-2]   (Ex) 203.00-208.92, 239.81-239.9
          Coding Clinic: 1987, Mar-April, P12

● **208.9 Unspecified leukemia** 🔖
[0-2]   Leukemia NOS
          (Ex) 203.00-208.92, 239.81-239.9
          Coding Clinic: 2011, Q4, P148

NEUROENDOCRINE TUMORS (209)

● **209 Neuroendocrine tumors**
    *Code first any associated multiple endocrine neoplasia syndrome
        (258.01-258.03)*
    Use additional code to identify associated endocrine syndrome,
        such as:
    carcinoid syndrome (259.2)
    Excludes   *benign pancreatic islet cell tumors (211.7)
                   malignant pancreatic islet cell tumors (157.4)*
    Coding Clinic: 2009, Q4, P78; 2008, Q4, P85-90

● **209.0 Malignant carcinoid tumors of the small intestine**
    **209.00 Malignant carcinoid tumor of the small intestine,
              unspecified portion** 🔖
              (Ex) 152.8-152.9, 159.0, 159.8-159.9, 176.3, 195.8, 199.0-199.2,
                   209.00-209.30, 209.70, 209.75, 239.0, 239.81-239.9

    **209.01 Malignant carcinoid tumor of the
              duodenum** 🔖
              (Ex) 152.0, 152.8-152.9, 159.0, 159.8-159.9, 176.3, 195.8,
                   199.0-199.2, 209.00-209.30, 209.70, 209.75, 239.0,
                   239.81-239.9

    **209.02 Malignant carcinoid tumor of the
              jejunum** 🔖
              (Ex) 152.1, 152.8-152.9, 159.0, 159.8-159.9, 176.3, 195.8,
                   199.0-199.2, 209.00-209.30, 209.70, 209.75, 239.0,
                   239.81-239.9

    209.03 Malignant carcinoid tumor of the ileum 🔖
              (Ex) 152.2, 152.8-152.9, 159.0, 159.8-159.9, 176.3, 195.8,
                   199.0-199.2, 209.00-209.30, 209.70, 209.75, 239.0,
                   239.81-239.9

● **209.1 Malignant carcinoid tumors of the appendix,
           large intestine, and rectum**
    **209.10 Malignant carcinoid tumor of the large intestine,
              unspecified portion** 🔖
              Malignant carcinoid tumor of the colon NOS
              (Ex) 153.8-153.9, 159.0, 159.8-159.9, 176.3, 195.8, 199.0-199.2,
                   209.00-209.30, 209.70, 209.75, 239.0, 239.81-239.9

    209.11 Malignant carcinoid tumor of the appendix 🔖
              (Ex) 153.5, 153.8-153.9, 159.0, 159.8-159.9, 176.3, 195.8,
                   199.0-199.2, 209.00-209.30, 209.70, 209.75, 239.0,
                   239.81-239.9

209.12 Malignant carcinoid tumor of the cecum 🅒
   Ex: 153.4, 153.8-153.9, 159.0, 159.8-159.9, 176.3, 195.8, 199.0-199.2, 209.00-209.30, 209.70, 209.75, 239.0, 239.81-239.9

209.13 Malignant carcinoid tumor of the ascending colon 🅒
   Ex: 153.6, 153.8-153.9, 159.0, 159.8-159.9, 176.3, 195.8, 199.0-199.2, 209.00-209.30, 209.70, 209.75, 239.0, 239.81-239.9

209.14 Malignant carcinoid tumor of the transverse colon 🅒
   Ex: 153.1, 153.8-153.9, 159.0, 159.8-159.9, 176.3, 195.8, 199.0-199.2, 209.00, 209.30, 209.70, 209.75, 239.0, 239.81-239.9

209.15 Malignant carcinoid tumor of the descending colon 🅒
   Ex: 153.2, 153.8, 153.9, 159.0, 159.8-159.9, 176.3, 195.8, 199.0-199.2, 209.00-209.30, 209.70, 209.75, 239.0, 239.81-239.9

209.16 Malignant carcinoid tumor of the sigmoid colon 🅒
   Ex: 153.3, 153.8-153.9, 159.0, 159.8-159.9, 176.3, 195.8, 199.0, 199.2, 209.00-209.30, 209.70, 209.75, 239.0, 239.81-239.9

209.17 Malignant carcinoid tumor of the rectum 🅒
   Ex: 154.1, 154.8, 159.0, 159.8-159.9, 176.3, 195.8, 199.0-199.2, 209.00-209.30, 209.70, 209.75, 239.0, 239.81-239.9

● 209.2 **Malignant carcinoid tumors of other and unspecified sites**

209.20 Malignant carcinoid tumor of unknown primary site 🅒
   Ex: 195.8, 198.89-199.2, 209.00-209.30, 209.70, 209.75-209.79, 239.81-239.9

209.21 Malignant carcinoid tumor of the bronchus and lung 🅒
   Ex: 162.8-162.9, 165.8-165.9, 176.4, 195.8, 199.0-199.2, 209.00-209.30, 209.70, 209.75, 239.1, 239.81-239.9

209.22 Malignant carcinoid tumor of the thymus 🅒
   Ex: 164.0, 209.00-209.30

209.23 Malignant carcinoid tumor of the stomach 🅒
   Ex: 151.0-151.9, 159.0, 159.8-159.9, 176.3, 195.8, 199.0-199.2, 209.00-209.30, 209.70, 209.75, 239.0, 239.81-239.9
   Coding Clinic: 2008, Q4, P85-90

209.24 Malignant carcinoid tumor of the kidney 🅒
   Ex: 189.0-189.1, 189.8-189.9, 195.8, 199.0-199.2, 209.00-209.30, 209.70, 209.75, 239.5, 239.81-239.9

209.25 Malignant carcinoid tumor of the foregut NOS 🅒
   Ex: 151.0-151.9, 159.0, 159.8-159.9, 176.3, 195.8, 199.0-199.2, 209.00-209.30, 209.70, 209.75, 239.0, 239.81-239.9

209.26 Malignant carcinoid tumor of the midgut NOS 🅒
   Ex: 151.0-151.9, 159.0, 159.8-159.9, 176.3, 195.8, 199.0-199.2, 209.00-209.30, 209.70, 209.75, 239.0, 239.81-239.9

209.27 Malignant carcinoid tumor of the hindgut NOS 🅒
   Ex: 151.0-151.9, 159.0, 159.8-159.9, 176.3, 195.8, 199.0-199.2, 209.00-209.30, 209.70, 209.75, 239.0, 239.81-239.9

209.29 Malignant carcinoid tumors of other sites 🅒
   Ex: 195.8, 198.89-199.2, 209.00-209.30, 209.70, 209.75-209.79, 239.81-239.9

● 209.3 **Malignant poorly differentiated neuroendocrine tumors**

209.30 Malignant poorly differentiated neuroendocrine carcinoma, any site 🅒
   High grade neuroendocrine carcinoma, any site
   Malignant poorly differentiated neuroendocrine tumor NOS
   Excludes *Merkel cell carcinoma (209.31-209.36)*
   Ex: 195.8, 198.89-199.2, 209.00-209.30, 209.70, 209.75-209.79, 239.81-239.9

209.31 Merkel cell carcinoma of the face
   Merkel cell carcinoma of the ear
   Merkel cell carcinoma of the eyelid, including canthus
   Merkel cell carcinoma of the lip

209.32 Merkel cell carcinoma of the scalp and neck

209.33 Merkel cell carcinoma of the upper limb

209.34 Merkel cell carcinoma of the lower limb

209.35 Merkel cell carcinoma of the trunk

209.36 Merkel cell carcinoma of other sites
   Merkel cell carcinoma of the buttock
   Merkel cell carcinoma of the genitals
   Merkel cell carcinoma NOS
   Coding Clinic: 2009, Q4, P79

● 209.4 **Benign carcinoid tumors of the small intestine**

209.40 Benign carcinoid tumor of the small intestine, unspecified portion

209.41 Benign carcinoid tumor of the duodenum

209.42 Benign carcinoid tumor of the jejunum

209.43 Benign carcinoid tumor of the ileum

● 209.5 **Benign carcinoid tumors of the appendix, large intestine, and rectum**

209.50 Benign carcinoid tumor of the large intestine, unspecified portion
   Benign carcinoid tumor of the colon NOS

209.51 Benign carcinoid tumor of the appendix

209.52 Benign carcinoid tumor of the cecum

209.53 Benign carcinoid tumor of the ascending colon

209.54 Benign carcinoid tumor of the transverse colon

209.55 Benign carcinoid tumor of the descending colon

209.56 Benign carcinoid tumor of the sigmoid colon

209.57 Benign carcinoid tumor of the rectum

● 209.6 **Benign carcinoid tumors of other and unspecified sites**

209.60 Benign carcinoid tumor of unknown primary site
   Carcinoid tumor NOS
   Neuroendocrine tumor NOS

209.61 Benign carcinoid tumor of the bronchus and lung
   Coding Clinic: 2009, Q4, P79

209.62 Benign carcinoid tumor of the thymus

209.63 Benign carcinoid tumor of the stomach

209.64 Benign carcinoid tumor of the kidney

209.65 Benign carcinoid tumor of the foregut NOS

209.66 Benign carcinoid tumor of the midgut NOS

209.67 Benign carcinoid tumor of the hindgut NOS

209.69 Benign carcinoid tumors of other sites

● 209.7 **Secondary neuroendocrine tumors**
   Secondary carcinoid tumors

209.70 Secondary neuroendocrine tumor, unspecified site

209.71 Secondary neuroendocrine tumor of distant lymph nodes 🅒
   Ex: 176.5, 195.8-196.9, 199.0-199.2, 209.20, 209.29-209.30, 209.70-209.79, 239.81-239.9
   Coding Clinic: 2011, Q4, P181

209.72 Secondary neuroendocrine tumor of liver 🅒
   Ex: 195.8, 197.7-197.8, 198.89-199.2, 209.20, 209.29-209.30, 209.70-209.79, 239.81-239.9

209.73 Secondary neuroendocrine tumor of bone 🅒
   Ex: 195.8, 198.5, 198.89-199.2, 209.20, 209.29-209.30, 209.70-209.79, 239.81-239.9

209.74 Secondary neuroendocrine tumor of peritoneum 🅒
   Mesentery metastasis of neuroendocrine tumor
   Ex: 195.8, 197.6, 197.8, 198.89-199.2, 209.20, 209.29-209.30, 209.70-209.79, 239.81-239.9
   Coding Clinic: 2011, Q4, P181-182; 2009, Q4, P79

209.75 Secondary Merkel cell carcinoma
   Merkel cell carcinoma nodal presentation
   Merkel cell carcinoma visceral metastatic presentation
   Secondary Merkel cell carcinoma, any site 🅒

209.79 Secondary neuroendocrine tumor of other sites 🅒
   Ex: 195.8, 198.89-199.2, 209.20, 209.29-209.30, 209.70-209.79, 239.81-239.9

NEOPLASMS (140-239)

NEOPLASMS (140–239)

BENIGN NEOPLASMS (210–229)

Benign neoplasm: Tumor that does not metastasize to other parts of body and is caused by cell overgrowth, differentiating it from cyst or abscess

● **210 Benign neoplasm of lip, oral cavity, and pharynx**

> **Excludes** *cyst (of):*
> *jaw (526.0–526.2, 526.89)*
> *oral soft tissue (528.4)*
> *radicular (522.8)*

210.0 Lip
Frenulum labii
Lip (inner aspect) (mucosa) (vermilion border)

> **Excludes** *labial commissure (210.4)*
> *skin of lip (216.0)*

210.1 Tongue
Lingual tonsil

210.2 Major salivary glands
Gland: Gland:
  parotid   submandibular
  sublingual

> **Excludes** *benign neoplasms of minor salivary glands:*
> *NOS (210.4)*
> *buccal mucosa (210.4)*
> *lips (210.0)*
> *palate (hard) (soft) (210.4)*
> *tongue (210.1)*
> *tonsil, palatine (210.5)*

210.3 Floor of mouth

210.4 Other and unspecified parts of mouth
Gingiva   Oral mucosa
Gum (upper) (lower)   Palate (hard) (soft)
Labial commissure   Uvula
Oral cavity NOS

> **Excludes** *benign odontogenic neoplasms of bone*
> *(213.0–213.1)*
> *developmental odontogenic cysts (526.0)*
> *mucosa of lips (210.0)*
> *nasopharyngeal [posterior] [superior] surface of*
> *soft palate (210.7)*

210.5 Tonsil
Tonsil (faucial) (palatine)

> **Excludes** *lingual tonsil (210.1)*
> *pharyngeal tonsil (210.7)*
> *tonsillar:*
> *fossa (210.6)*
> *pillars (210.6)*

210.6 Other parts of oropharynx
Branchial cleft or vestiges
Epiglottis, anterior aspect
Fauces NOS
Mesopharynx NOS
Tonsillar:
  fossa
  pillars
Vallecula

> **Excludes** *epiglottis:*
> *NOS (212.1)*
> *suprahyoid portion (212.1)*

210.7 Nasopharynx
Adenoid tissue   Pharyngeal tonsil
Lymphadenoid tissue   Posterior nasal septum

210.8 Hypopharynx
Arytenoid fold   Postcricoid region
Laryngopharynx   Pyriform fossa

210.9 Pharynx, unspecified
Throat NOS

● **211 Benign neoplasm of other parts of digestive system**

> **Excludes** *benign stromal tumors of digestive system (215.5)*

211.0 Esophagus

211.1 Stomach
Body of stomach   Cardiac orifice
Cardia of stomach   Pylorus
Fundus of stomach

> **Excludes** *benign carcinoid tumors of the stomach (209.63)*

211.2 Duodenum, jejunum, and ileum
Small intestine NOS

> **Excludes** *ampulla of Vater (211.5)*
> *benign carcinoid tumors of the small intestine*
> *(209.40-209.43)*
> *ileocecal valve (211.3)*

211.3 Colon
Appendix   Ileocecal valve
Cecum   Large intestine NOS

> **Excludes** *benign carcinoid tumors of the large intestine*
> *(209.50-209.56)*
> *rectosigmoid junction (211.4)*
> **Coding Clinic:** 2005, Q3, P17-18; Q2, P16-17; 2001, Q4, P55-56x2;
> 1995, Q1, P4; 1992, Q3, P11

211.4 Rectum and anal canal
Anal canal or sphincter
Anus NOS
Rectosigmoid junction

> **Excludes** *anus:*
> *margin (216.5)*
> *perianal skin (216.5)*
> *skin (216.5)*
> *benign carcinoid tumors of the rectum (209.57)*

211.5 Liver and biliary passages
Ampulla of Vater   Gallbladder
Common bile duct   Hepatic duct
Cystic duct   Sphincter of Oddi

211.6 Pancreas, except islets of Langerhans

211.7 Islets of Langerhans
Islet cell tumor
> Use additional code to identify any functional activity

211.8 Retroperitoneum and peritoneum
Mesentery   Omentum
Mesocolon   Retroperitoneal tissue

211.9 Other and unspecified site
Alimentary tract NOS
Digestive system NOS
Gastrointestinal tract NOS
Intestinal tract NOS
Intestine NOS
Spleen, not elsewhere classified

● **212 Benign neoplasm of respiratory and intrathoracic organs**

212.0 Nasal cavities, middle ear, and accessory sinuses
Cartilage of nose
Eustachian tube
Nares
Septum of nose
Sinus: Sinus:
  ethmoidal   maxillary
  frontal   sphenoidal

> **Excludes** *auditory canal (external) (216.2)*
> *bone of:*
> *ear (213.0)*
> *nose [turbinates] (213.0)*
> *cartilage of ear (215.0)*
> *ear (external) (skin) (216.2)*
> *nose NOS (229.8)*
> *skin (216.3)*
> *olfactory bulb (225.1)*
> *polyp of:*
> *accessory sinus (471.8)*
> *ear (385.30–385.35)*
> *nasal cavity (471.0)*
> *posterior margin of septum and choanae (210.7)*
> **Coding Clinic:** 2000, Q3, P10-11

◀ New   ◀▥ Revised   ~~deleted~~ Deleted   Excludes   Includes   Use additional   Code first   Omit code

722   ● Unacceptable Principal Diagnosis   ● Use Additional Digit(s)   ▶ Manifestation Code   OGCR Official Guidelines   Coding Clinic

212.1 Larynx
    Cartilage:
        arytenoid
        cricoid
        cuneiform
        thyroid
    Epiglottis (suprahyoid portion) NOS
    Glottis
    Vocal cords (false) (true)
        Excludes *epiglottis, anterior aspect (210.6)*
                polyp of vocal cord or larynx (478.4)

212.2 Trachea

212.3 Bronchus and lung
    Carina
    Hilus of lung
        Excludes *benign carcinoid tumors of bronchus and lung*
                (209.61)

212.4 Pleura

212.5 Mediastinum

212.6 Thymus
        Excludes *benign carcinoid tumors of thymus (209.62)*

212.7 Heart
        Excludes *great vessels (215.4)*

212.8 Other specified sites

212.9 Site unspecified
    Respiratory organ NOS
    Upper respiratory tract NOS
        Excludes *intrathoracic NOS (229.8)*
                thoracic NOS (229.8)

● **213 Benign neoplasm of bone and articular cartilage**
    Includes cartilage (articular) (joint)
              periosteum
    Excludes *cartilage of:*
        ear (215.0)
        eyelid (215.0)
        larynx (212.1)
        nose (212.0)
        exostosis NOS (726.91)
        synovia (215.0–215.9)

213.0 Bones of skull and face
        Excludes *lower jaw bone (213.1)*

213.1 Lower jaw bone

213.2 Vertebral column, excluding sacrum and coccyx

213.3 Ribs, sternum, and clavicle

213.4 Scapula and long bones of upper limb

213.5 Short bones of upper limb

213.6 Pelvic bones, sacrum, and coccyx

213.7 Long bones of lower limb

213.8 Short bones of lower limb

213.9 Bone and articular cartilage, site unspecified

● **214 Lipoma**
    Slow growing benign tumors (discrete rubbery masses) of mature fat cells enclosed in a thin fibrous capsule found in subcutaneous tissues of trunk and proximal extremities and in internal organs
    Includes angiolipoma
              fibrolipoma
              hibernoma
              lipoma (fetal) (infiltrating) (intramuscular)
              myelolipoma
              myxolipoma

214.0 Skin and subcutaneous tissue of face

214.1 Other skin and subcutaneous tissue

214.2 Intrathoracic organs

214.3 Intra-abdominal organs

214.4 Spermatic cord ♂

214.8 Other specified sites
    Coding Clinic: 1994, Q3, P7

214.9 Lipoma, unspecified site

● **215 Other benign neoplasm of connective and other soft tissue**
    Includes blood vessel
              bursa
              fascia
              ligament
              muscle
              peripheral, sympathetic, and parasympathetic
                  nerves and ganglia
              synovia
              tendon (sheath)
    Excludes *cartilage:*
        articular (213.0–213.9)
        larynx (212.1)
        nose (212.0)
        connective tissue of:
        breast (217)
        internal organ, except lipoma and hemangioma-code
            to benign neoplasm
            of the site
        lipoma (214.0–214.9)

215.0 Head, face, and neck

215.2 Upper limb, including shoulder

215.3 Lower limb, including hip

215.4 Thorax
        Excludes *heart (212.7)*
                mediastinum (212.5)
                thymus (212.6)

215.5 Abdomen
    Abdominal wall
    Benign stromal tumors of abdomen
    Hypochondrium

215.6 Pelvis
    Buttock   Inguinal region
    Groin Perineum
        Excludes *uterine:*
            leiomyoma (218.0–218.9)
            ligament, any (221.0)

215.7 Trunk, unspecified
    Back NOS
    Flank NOS

215.8 Other specified sites

215.9 Site unspecified

● **216 Benign neoplasm of skin**
    Includes blue nevus
              dermatofibroma
              hydrocystoma
              pigmented nevus
              syringoadenoma
              syringoma
    Excludes *skin of genital organs (221.0–222.9)*
    Coding Clinic: 2000, Q1, P21-22

216.0 Skin of lip
        Excludes *vermilion border of lip (210.0)*

216.1 Eyelid, including canthus
        Excludes *cartilage of eyelid (215.0)*

216.2 Ear and external auditory canal
    Auricle (ear)
    Auricular canal, external
    External meatus
    Pinna
        Excludes *cartilage of ear (215.0)*

216.3 Skin of other and unspecified parts of face
    Cheek, external   Nose, external
    Eyebrow   Temple

216.4 Scalp and skin of neck

NEOPLASMS (140–239)

N Newborn: 0   P Pediatric: 0–17   M Maternity: 12–55   A Adult: 15–124   ♀ Females Only   ♂ Males Only

(Ex) CC/MCC Exclusions   Complication\Comorbidity   Major C\C   Present on Admission Requirement   Hospital-Acquired Condition   **723**

NEOPLASMS (140–239)

216.5　Skin of trunk, except scrotum
　Axillary fold
　Perianal skin
　Skin of:　　　　　　　　　Skin of:
　　abdominal wall　　　　　chest wall
　　anus　　　　　　　　　groin
　　back　　　　　　　　　perineum
　　breast
　　buttock
　Umbilicus

Excludes　*anal canal (211.4)*
　　　　　　anus NOS (211.4)
　　　　　　skin of scrotum (222.4)

216.6　Skin of upper limb, including shoulder
216.7　Skin of lower limb, including hip
216.8　Other specified sites of skin
216.9　Skin, site unspecified

217　Benign neoplasm of breast
　Note no gender difference for this code.
　Breast (male) (female)
　　connective tissue
　　glandular tissue
　　soft parts

Excludes　*adenofibrosis (610.2)*
　　　　　　benign cyst of breast (610.0)
　　　　　　fibrocystic disease (610.1)
　　　　　　skin of breast (216.5)
　Coding Clinic: 2000, Q1, P4

●218　Uterine leiomyoma
　Benign tumors or nodules of the uterine wall

Includes　fibroid (bleeding) (uterine)
　　　　　　uterine:
　　　　　　　fibromyoma
　　　　　　　myoma

218.0　Submucous leiomyoma of uterus ♀
218.1　Intramural leiomyoma of uterus ♀
　Interstitial leiomyoma of uterus
218.2　Subserous leiomyoma of uterus ♀
　Subperitoneal leiomyoma of uterus
218.9　Leiomyoma of uterus, unspecified ♀
　Coding Clinic: 2003, Q1, P4-5; 1995, Q4, P50

●219　Other benign neoplasm of uterus
219.0　Cervix uteri ♀
219.1　Corpus uteri ♀
　Endometrium　　　　Myometrium
　Fundus
219.8　Other specified parts of uterus ♀
219.9　Uterus, part unspecified ♀

220　Benign neoplasm of ovary ♀
　Use additional code to identify any functional activity
　　(256.0–256.1)

Excludes　*cyst:*
　　　　　　corpus albicans (620.2)
　　　　　　corpus luteum (620.1)
　　　　　　endometrial (617.1)
　　　　　　follicular (atretic) (620.0)
　　　　　　graafian follicle (620.0)
　　　　　　ovarian NOS (620.2)
　　　　　　retention (620.2)
　Coding Clinic: 2009, Q4, P79, 82

●221　Benign neoplasm of other female genital organs

Includes　adenomatous polyp
　　　　　　benign teratoma

Excludes　*cyst:*
　　　　　　epoophoron (752.11)
　　　　　　fimbrial (752.11)
　　　　　　Gartner's duct (752.11)
　　　　　　parovarian (752.11)

221.0　Fallopian tube and uterine ligaments ♀
　Oviduct
　Parametrium
　Uterine ligament (broad) (round) (uterosacral)
　Uterine tube
221.1　Vagina ♀
221.2　Vulva ♀
　Clitoris
　External female genitalia NOS
　Greater vestibular [Bartholin's] gland
　Labia (majora) (minora)
　Pudendum

Excludes　*Bartholin's (duct) (gland) cyst (616.2)*
221.8　Other specified sites of female genital organs ♀
221.9　Female genital organ, site unspecified ♀
　Female genitourinary tract NOS

●222　Benign neoplasm of male genital organs
222.0　Testis ♂
　Use additional code to identify any functional activity
222.1　Penis ♂
　Corpus cavernosum
　Glans penis
　Prepuce
222.2　Prostate ♂

Excludes　*adenomatous hyperplasia of prostate*
　　　　　　　(600.20–600.21)
　　　　　　prostatic:
　　　　　　　adenoma (600.20–600.21)
　　　　　　　enlargement (600.00–600.01)
　　　　　　　hypertrophy (600.00–600.01)

222.3　Epididymis ♂
222.4　Scrotum ♂
　Skin of scrotum
222.8　Other specified sites of male genital organs ♂
　Seminal vesicle
　Spermatic cord
222.9　Male genital organ, site unspecified ♂
　Male genitourinary tract NOS

●223　Benign neoplasm of kidney and other urinary organs
223.0　Kidney, except pelvis
　Kidney NOS

Excludes　*benign carcinoid tumors of kidney*
　　　　　　　(209.64)
　　　　　　renal:
　　　　　　　calyces (223.1)
　　　　　　　pelvis (223.1)

223.1　Renal pelvis
223.2　Ureter

Excludes　*ureteric orifice of bladder (223.3)*
223.3　Bladder
●223.8　Other specified sites of urinary organs
223.81　Urethra

Excludes　*urethral orifice of bladder (223.3)*
223.89　Other
　Paraurethral glands
223.9　Urinary organ, site unspecified
　Urinary system NOS

Item 2–8　Teratoma: terat = monster, oma = mass, tumor. Alternate terms: dermoid cyst of the ovary, ovarian teratoma. Teratomas are neoplasms and arise from germ cells (ovaries in female and testes in male) and can be benign or malignant. Teratomas have been known to contain hair, nails, and teeth, giving them a bizarre ("monster") appearance.

● **224** **Benign neoplasm of eye**
　　Excludes *cartilage of eyelid (215.0)*
　　　　　　　eyelid (skin) (216.1)
　　　　　　　optic nerve (225.1)
　　　　　　　orbital bone (213.0)
　　224.0 **Eyeball, except conjunctiva, cornea, retina, and choroid**
　　　　Ciliary body　　　　　Sclera
　　　　Iris　　　　　　　　Uveal tract
　　224.1 **Orbit**
　　　　Excludes *bone of orbit (213.0)*
　　224.2 **Lacrimal gland**
　　224.3 **Conjunctiva**
　　224.4 **Cornea**
　　224.5 **Retina**
　　　　Excludes *hemangioma of retina (228.03)*
　　224.6 **Choroid**
　　224.7 **Lacrimal duct**
　　　　Lacrimal sac
　　　　Nasolacrimal duct
　　224.8 **Other specified parts of eye**
　　224.9 **Eye, part unspecified**

● **225** **Benign neoplasm of brain and other parts of nervous system**
　　Excludes *hemangioma (228.02)*
　　　　　　　neurofibromatosis (237.70–237.79)
　　　　　　　peripheral, sympathetic, and parasympathetic nerves and
　　　　　　　　ganglia (215.0–215.9)
　　　　　　　retrobulbar (224.1)
　　225.0 **Brain**
　　225.1 **Cranial nerves**
　　　　Coding Clinic: 2004, Q4, P111-113
　　225.2 **Cerebral meninges**
　　　　Meninges NOS
　　　　Meningioma (cerebral)
　　225.3 **Spinal cord**
　　　　Cauda equina
　　225.4 **Spinal meninges**
　　　　Spinal meningioma
　　225.8 **Other specified sites of nervous system**
　　225.9 **Nervous system, part unspecified**
　　　　Nervous system (central) NOS
　　　　Excludes *meninges NOS (225.2)*

　226 **Benign neoplasm of thyroid glands**
　　Use additional code to identify any functional activity

● **227** **Benign neoplasm of other endocrine glands and related structures**
　　Use additional code to identify any functional activity
　　Excludes *ovary (220)*
　　　　　　　pancreas (211.6)
　　　　　　　testis (222.0)
　　227.0 **Adrenal gland**
　　　　Suprarenal gland
　　227.1 **Parathyroid gland**
　　227.3 **Pituitary gland and craniopharyngeal duct (pouch)**
　　　　Craniobuccal pouch　　　Rathke's pouch
　　　　Hypophysis　　　　　　Sella turcica
　　227.4 **Pineal gland**
　　　　Pineal body
　　227.5 **Carotid body**
　　227.6 **Aortic body and other paraganglia**
　　　　Coccygeal body
　　　　Glomus jugulare
　　　　Para-aortic body
　　　　Coding Clinic: 1984, Nov-Dec, P17
　　227.8 **Other**
　　227.9 **Endocrine gland, site unspecified**

Item 2-9 **Hemangiomas** are abnormally dense collections of dilated capillaries that occur on the skin or in internal organs. Hemangiomas are both deep and superficial and undergo a rapid growth phase when the size increases rapidly, followed by a rest phase, in which the tumor changes very little, followed by an involutional phase in which the tumor begins to and can disappear altogether. **Lymphangiomas** or cystic hygroma are benign collections of overgrown lymph vessels and, although rare, may occur anywhere but most commonly on the head and neck of children and infants. Visceral organs, lungs, and gastrointestinal tract may also be involved.

Figure 2-15 Hemangioma of skin and subcutaneous tissue. (From Yanoff: Ophthalmology, ed 3, Mosby, Inc., 2008)

● **228** **Hemangioma and lymphangioma, any site**
　　Includes angioma (benign) (cavernous) (congenital) NOS
　　　　　　　cavernous nevus
　　　　　　　glomus tumor
　　　　　　　hemangioma (benign) (congenital)
　　Excludes *benign neoplasm of spleen, except hemangioma and*
　　　　　　　lymphangioma (211.9)
　　　　　　　glomus jugulare (227.6)
　　　　　　　nevus:
　　　　　　　　NOS (216.0–216.9)
　　　　　　　　blue or pigmented (216.0–216.9)
　　　　　　　　vascular (757.32)
● **228.0** **Hemangioma, any site**
　　　　Coding Clinic: 2001, Q1, P18; 1999, Q2, P9
　　228.00 **Of unspecified site**
　　228.01 **Of skin and subcutaneous tissue**
　　　　　Coding Clinic: 2010, Q3, P16; 1988, Q4, P6
　　228.02 **Of intracranial structures**
　　　　　Coding Clinic: 1988, Q4, P6; 1985, Jan-Feb, P15
　　228.03 **Of retina**
　　228.04 **Of intra-abdominal structures**
　　　　　Peritoneum
　　　　　Retroperitoneal tissue
　　　　　Coding Clinic: 1988, Q4, P6
　　228.09 **Of other sites**
　　　　　Systemic angiomatosis
　　　　　Coding Clinic: 1991, Q3, P20
　　228.1 **Lymphangioma, any site**
　　　　Congenital lymphangioma
　　　　Lymphatic nevus

● **229** **Benign neoplasm of other and unspecified sites**
　　229.0 **Lymph nodes**
　　　　Excludes *lymphangioma (228.1)*
　　229.8 **Other specified sites**
　　　　Intrathoracic NOS
　　　　Thoracic NOS
　　229.9 **Site unspecified**

NEOPLASMS (140–239)

CARCINOMA IN SITU (230–234)

Includes   Bowen's disease
erythroplasia
Queyrat's erythroplasia

Excludes   leukoplakia - see Alphabetic Index

● **230   Carcinoma in situ of digestive organs**
Cancer involving cells in localized tissues that has not spread to nearby tissues

230.0   Lip, oral cavity, and pharynx

Gingiva	Oropharynx
Hypopharynx	Salivary gland or duct
Mouth [any part]	Tongue
Nasopharynx	

     Excludes   *aryepiglottic fold or interarytenoid fold, laryngeal aspect (231.0)*
epiglottis:
    NOS (231.0)
    suprahyoid portion (231.0)
skin of lip (232.0)

230.1   Esophagus

230.2   Stomach

Body of stomach	Cardiac orifice
Cardia of stomach	Pylorus
Fundus of stomach	

230.3   Colon

Appendix	Ileocecal valve
Cecum	Large intestine NOS

     Excludes   *rectosigmoid junction (230.4)*

230.4   Rectum
Rectosigmoid junction

230.5   Anal canal
Anal sphincter

230.6   Anus, unspecified

     Excludes   *anus:*
        margin (232.5)
        skin (232.5)
        perianal skin (232.5)

230.7   Other and unspecified parts of intestine

Duodenum	Jejunum
Ileum	Small intestine NOS

     Excludes   *ampulla of Vater (230.8)*

230.8   Liver and biliary system

Ampulla of Vater	Gallbladder
Common bile duct	Hepatic duct
Cystic duct	Sphincter of Oddi

230.9   Other and unspecified digestive organs
Digestive organ NOS
Gastrointestinal tract NOS
Pancreas
Spleen

● **231   Carcinoma in situ of respiratory system**

231.0   Larynx

Cartilage:	Epiglottis:
arytenoid	NOS
cricoid	posterior surface
cuneiform	suprahyoid portion
thyroid	Vocal cords (false) (true)

     Excludes   *aryepiglottic fold or interarytenoid fold:*
        NOS (230.0)
        hypopharyngeal aspect (230.0)
        marginal zone (230.0)

231.1   Trachea

231.2   Bronchus and lung
Carina
Hilus of lung

231.8   Other specified parts of respiratory system

Accessory sinuses	Nasal cavities
Middle ear	Pleura

     Excludes   *ear (external) (skin) (232.2)*
nose NOS (234.8)
skin (232.3)

231.9   Respiratory system, part unspecified
Respiratory organ NOS

● **232   Carcinoma in situ of skin**

Includes   pigment cells

Excludes   *melanoma in situ of skin (172.0-172.9)*

232.0   Skin of lip

     Excludes   *vermilion border of lip (230.0)*

232.1   Eyelid, including canthus

232.2   Ear and external auditory canal

232.3   Skin of other and unspecified parts of face

232.4   Scalp and skin of neck

232.5   Skin of trunk, except scrotum

Anus, margin	Skin of:
Axillary fold	breast
Perianal skin	buttock
Skin of:	chest wall
abdominal wall	groin
anus	perineum
back	Umbilicus

     Excludes   *anal canal (230.5)*
anus NOS (230.6)
skin of genital organs (233.30–233.39, 233.5–233.6)

232.6   Skin of upper limb, including shoulder

232.7   Skin of lower limb, including hip

232.8   Other specified sites of skin

232.9   Skin, site unspecified

● **233   Carcinoma in situ of breast and genitourinary system**
This category incorporates specific male and female genitourinary designations (233.0–233.6), while codes 233.7 and 233.9 apply to either male or female organs.

233.0   Breast

     Excludes   *Paget's disease (174.0–174.9)*
skin of breast (232.5)
     Coding Clinic: 2012, Q1, P11

233.1   Cervix uteri ♀
Adenocarcinoma in situ of cervix
Cervical intraepithelial glandular neoplasia, grade III
Cervical intraepithelial neoplasia III [CIN III]
Severe dysplasia of cervix

     Excludes   *cervical intraepithelial neoplasia II [CIN II] (622.12)*
cytologic evidence of malignancy without histologic confirmation (795.06)
high grade squamous intraepithelial lesion (HGSIL) (795.04)
moderate dysplasia of cervix (622.12)
     Coding Clinic: 1992, Q3, P7-8; 1991, Q1, P11

233.2   Other and unspecified parts of uterus ♀

● **233.3   Other and unspecified female genital organs**
     Coding Clinic: 2007, Q4, P67-68

     233.30   Unspecified female genital organ ♀

     233.31   Vagina ♀
         Severe dysplasia of vagina
         Vaginal intraepithelial neoplasia [VAIN III]

     233.32   Vulva ♀
         Severe dysplasia of vulva
         Vulvar intraepithelial neoplasia [VIN III]
         Coding Clinic: 1995, Q1, P8

     233.39   Other female genital organ ♀

233.4   Prostate ♂

233.5   Penis ♂

233.6   Other and unspecified male genital organs ♂

233.7   Bladder
     Coding Clinic: 2012, Q2, P10

233.9   Other and unspecified urinary organs

◀ New   ◀▥ Revised   ~~deleted~~ Deleted   Excludes   Includes   Use additional   Code first   Omit code

726   ● Unacceptable Principal Diagnosis   ● Use Additional Digit(s)   ▶ Manifestation Code   OGCR Official Guidelines   **Coding Clinic**

● 234 **Carcinoma in situ of other and unspecified sites**
     234.0 **Eye**
          Excludes *cartilage of eyelid (234.8)*
                    eyelid (skin) (232.1)
                    optic nerve (234.8)
                    orbital bone (234.8)

     234.8 **Other specified sites**
          Endocrine gland [any]

     234.9 **Site unspecified**
          Carcinoma in situ NOS

NEOPLASMS OF UNCERTAIN BEHAVIOR (235–238)

Note: Categories 235–238 classify by site certain histo-morphologically well-defined neoplasms, the subsequent behavior of which cannot be predicted from the present appearance.

● 235 **Neoplasm of uncertain behavior of digestive and respiratory systems**
          Excludes *stromal tumors of uncertain behavior of digestive system (238.1)*

     235.0 **Major salivary glands**
          Gland:
               parotid
               sublingual
               submandibular
          Excludes *minor salivary glands (235.1)*

     235.1 **Lip, oral cavity, and pharynx**
          Gingiva   Nasopharynx
          Hypopharynx   Oropharynx
          Minor salivary glands Tongue
          Mouth
          Excludes *aryepiglottic fold or interarytenoid fold, laryngeal*
                    aspect (235.6)
                    epiglottis:
                         NOS (235.6)
                         suprahyoid portion (235.6)
                    skin of lip (238.2)

     235.2 **Stomach, intestines, and rectum**
     235.3 **Liver and biliary passages**
          Ampulla of Vater   Gallbladder
          Bile ducts [any]   Liver

     235.4 **Retroperitoneum and peritoneum**
     235.5 **Other and unspecified digestive organs**
          Anal: Esophagus
               canal   Pancreas
               sphincter   Spleen
          Anus NOS
          Excludes *anus:*
                    margin (238.2)
                    skin (238.2)
                    perianal skin (238.2)

     235.6 **Larynx**
          Excludes *aryepiglottic fold or interarytenoid fold:*
                    NOS (235.1)
                    hypopharyngeal aspect (235.1)
                    marginal zone (235.1)

     235.7 **Trachea, bronchus, and lung**
     235.8 **Pleura, thymus, and mediastinum**
     235.9 **Other and unspecified respiratory organs**
          Accessory sinuses
          Middle ear
          Nasal cavities
          Respiratory organ NOS
          Excludes *ear (external) (skin) (238.2)*
                    nose (238.8)
                    skin (238.2)

● 236 **Neoplasm of uncertain behavior of genitourinary organs**
     236.0 **Uterus ♀**
     236.1 **Placenta ♀**
          Chorioadenoma (destruens)
          Invasive mole
          Malignant hydatid mole
          Malignant hydatidiform mole

     236.2 **Ovary ♀**
          Use additional code to identify any functional activity
     236.3 **Other and unspecified female genital organs ♀**
     236.4 **Testis ♂**
          Use additional code to identify any functional activity
     236.5 **Prostate ♂**
     236.6 **Other and unspecified male genital organs ♂**
     236.7 **Bladder**
● 236.9 **Other and unspecified urinary organs**
          236.90 **Urinary organ, unspecified**
          236.91 **Kidney and ureter**
          236.99 **Other**

● 237 **Neoplasm of uncertain behavior of endocrine glands and nervous system**
     237.0 **Pituitary gland and craniopharyngeal duct**
          Use additional code to identify any functional activity
     237.1 **Pineal gland**
     237.2 **Adrenal gland**
          Suprarenal gland
          Use additional code to identify any functional activity
          Pair of glands situated on top of or above each kidney ("suprarenal") responsible for regulating stress response through corticosteroids
     237.3 **Paraganglia**
          Aortic body   Coccygeal body
          Carotid body   Glomus jugulare
          Coding Clinic: 1984, Nov-Dec, P17
     237.4 **Other and unspecified endocrine glands**
          Parathyroid gland
          Thyroid gland
     237.5 **Brain and spinal cord**
     237.6 **Meninges**
          Meninges:
               NOS
               cerebral
               spinal
● 237.7 **Neurofibromatosis**
          Disorder of nervous system that causes tumors to grow around nerves
          237.70 **Neurofibromatosis, unspecified**
          237.71 **Neurofibromatosis, type 1 [von Recklinghausen's disease]**
          237.72 **Neurofibromatosis, type 2 [acoustic neurofibromatosis]**
          237.73 **Schwannomatosis**
          237.79 **Other neurofibromatosis**
     237.9 **Other and unspecified parts of nervous system**
          Cranial nerves
          Excludes *peripheral, sympathetic, and parasympathetic nerves and ganglia (238.1)*

● 238 **Neoplasm of uncertain behavior of other and unspecified sites and tissues**
     238.0 **Bone and articular cartilage**
          Excludes *cartilage:*
                    ear (238.1)
                    eyelid (238.1)
                    larynx (235.6)
                    nose (235.9)
                    synovia (238.1)
          Coding Clinic: 2004, Q4, P128-129
     238.1 **Connective and other soft tissue**
          Peripheral, sympathetic, and parasympathetic nerves and ganglia
          Stromal tumors of digestive system
          Excludes *cartilage (of):*
                    articular (238.0)
                    larynx (235.6)
                    nose (235.9)
                    connective tissue of breast (238.3)

N Newborn: 0   **P** Pediatric: 0–17   **M** Maternity: 12–55   **A** Adult: 15–124   ♀ Females Only   ♂ Males Only

Ⓔⓧ CC/MCC Exclusions   🔆 Complication\Comorbidity   🔆 Major C\C   🔆 Present on Admission Requirement   🔆 Hospital-Acquired Condition   727

NEOPLASMS (140–239)

238.2　Skin

> **Excludes**　anus NOS (235.5)
> skin of genital organs (236.3, 236.6)
> vermilion border of lip (235.1)

238.3　Breast

> **Excludes**　skin of breast (238.2)

238.4　Polycythemia vera
Primary polycythemia. Secondary polycythemia is 289.0. Check your documentation. Polycythemia is caused by too many red blood cells, which increase thickness of blood (viscosity). This can cause engorgement of the spleen (splenomegaly) with extra RBCs and potential clot formation.

238.5　Histiocytic and mast cells
Mast cell tumor NOS
Mastocytoma NOS
(Ex:) 238.4-238.76, 238.79, 289.83, V58.0

238.6　Plasma cells
Plasmacytoma NOS
Solitary myeloma
(Ex:) 238.4-238.76, 238.79, 289.83, V58.0

● **238.7　Other lymphatic and hematopoietic tissues**

> **Excludes**　acute myelogenous leukemia (205.0)
> chronic myelomonocytic leukemia (205.1)
> myelosclerosis NOS (289.89)
> myelosis:
> NOS (205.9)
> megakaryocytic (207.2)

Coding Clinic: 2006, Q4, P63-66; 2001, Q3, P13-14; 1997, Q1, P5-6

238.71　Essential thrombocythemia
Essential hemorrhagic thrombocythemia
Essential thrombocytosis
Idiopathic (hemorrhagic) thrombocythemia
Primary thrombocytosis
Coding Clinic: 2006, Q4, P64

238.72　Low grade myelodysplastic syndrome lesions
Refractory anemia with excess blasts-1 (RAEB-1)
Refractory anemia (RA)
Refractory anemia with ringed sideroblasts (RARS)
Refractory cytopenia with multilineage dysplasia (RCMD)
Refractory cytopenia with multilineage dysplasia and ringed sideroblasts (RCMD-RS)

238.73　High grade myelodysplastic syndrome lesions
Refractory anemia with excess blasts-2 (RAEB-2)
(Ex:) 202.40-202.48, 203.10-203.11, 203.80-203.81, 204.00-208.92, 238.4-238.76, 238.79-238.9

238.74　Myelodysplastic syndrome with 5q deletion
5q minus syndrome NOS

> **Excludes**　constitutional 5q deletion (758.39)
> high grade myelodysplastic syndrome with 5q deletion (238.73)

(Ex:) 202.40-202.48, 203.10-203.11, 203.80-203.81, 204.00-208.92, 238.4-238.76, 238.79-238.9

238.75　Myelodysplastic syndrome, unspecified

238.76　Myelofibrosis with myeloid metaplasia
Agnogenic myeloid metaplasia
Idiopathic myelofibrosis (chronic)
Myelosclerosis with myeloid metaplasia
Primary myelofibrosis

> **Excludes**　myelofibrosis NOS (289.83)
> myelophthisic anemia (284.2)
> myelophthisis (284.2)
> secondary myelofibrosis (289.83)

(Ex:) 202.40-202.48, 203.10-203.11 203.80-203.81, 204.00-208.92, 238.4-238.76, 238.79-238.9

● **238.77　Post-transplant lymphoproliferative disorder (PTLD)**

> *Code first complications of transplant (996.80-996.89)*
> (Ex:) 238.77, 996.80, 996.87, 997.91-997.99
> **Coding Clinic: 2008, Q4, P90-91**

238.79　Other lymphatic and hematopoietic tissues
Lymphoproliferative disease (chronic) NOS
Megakaryocytic myelosclerosis
Myeloproliferative disease (chronic) NOS
Panmyelosis (acute)
(Ex:) 202.40-202.48, 203.10-203.11, 203.80-203.81, 204.00-208.92, 238.4-238.76, 238.79-238.9

238.8　Other specified sites
Eye
Heart

> **Excludes**　eyelid (skin) (238.2)
> cartilage (238.1)

238.9　Site unspecified

NEOPLASMS OF UNSPECIFIED NATURE (239)

● **239　Neoplasms of unspecified nature**
Note:　Category 239 classifies by site neoplasms of unspecified morphology and behavior. The term "mass," unless otherwise stated, is not to be regarded as a neoplastic growth.

> **Includes**　"growth" NOS
> neoplasm NOS
> new growth NOS
> tumor NOS

239.0　Digestive system

> **Excludes**　anus:
> margin (239.2)
> skin (239.2)
> perianal skin (239.2)

239.1　Respiratory system

239.2　Bone, soft tissue, and skin

> **Excludes**　anal canal (239.0)
> anus NOS (239.0)
> bone marrow (202.9)
> cartilage:
> larynx (239.1)
> nose (239.1)
> connective tissue of breast (239.3)
> skin of genital organs (239.5)
> vermilion border of lip (239.0)

239.3　Breast

> **Excludes**　skin of breast (239.2)

239.4　Bladder

239.5　Other genitourinary organs

239.6　Brain

> **Excludes**　cerebral meninges (239.7)
> cranial nerves (239.7)

239.7　Endocrine glands and other parts of nervous system

> **Excludes**　peripheral, sympathetic, and parasympathetic nerves and ganglia (239.2)

● **239.8　Other specified sites**

> **Excludes**　eyelid (skin) (239.2)
> cartilage (239.2)
> great vessels (239.2)
> optic nerve (239.7)

239.81　Retina and choroid
Dark area on retina
Retinal freckle

239.89　Other specified sites

239.9　Site unspecified

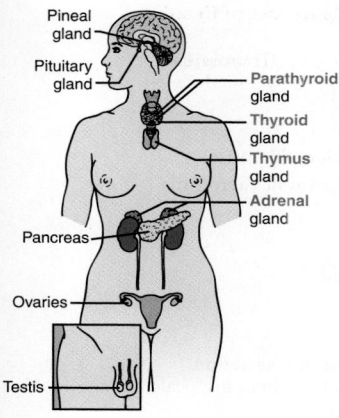

Figure 3-1 The endocrine system. (From Buck CJ: Step-by-Step Medical Coding, ed 2011, Philadelphia, WB Saunders, 2011)

Item 3-1 Simple goiter indicates no nodules are present. The most common type of goiter is a **diffuse colloidal,** also called a **nontoxic** or **endemic** goiter. Goiters classifiable to 240.0 or 240.9 are those goiters without mention of nodules.

Figure 3-2 Goiter is an enlargement of the thyroid gland.

3. ENDOCRINE, NUTRITIONAL AND METABOLIC DISEASES, AND IMMUNITY DISORDERS (240–279)

Excludes *endocrine and metabolic disturbances specific to the fetus and newborn (775.0–775.9)*

Note: All neoplasms, whether functionally active or not, are classified in Chapter 2. Codes in Chapter 3 (i.e., 242.8, 246.0, 251–253, 255–259) may be used to identify such functional activity associated with any neoplasm, or by ectopic endocrine tissue.

DISORDERS OF THYROID GLAND (240–246)

● **240 Simple and unspecified goiter**

240.0 Goiter, specified as simple
Any condition classifiable to 240.9, specified as simple

240.9 Goiter, unspecified
Enlargement of thyroid
Goiter or struma:
  NOS
  diffuse colloid
  endemic
Goiter or struma:
  hyperplastic
  nontoxic (diffuse)
  parenchymatous
  sporadic

Excludes *congenital (dyshormonogenic) goiter (246.1)*

● **241 Nontoxic nodular goiter**

Excludes *adenoma of thyroid (226)*
cystadenoma of thyroid (226)

241.0 Nontoxic uninodular goiter
Thyroid nodule
Uninodular goiter (nontoxic)

241.1 Nontoxic multinodular goiter
Multinodular goiter (nontoxic)

241.9 Unspecified nontoxic nodular goiter
Adenomatous goiter
Nodular goiter (nontoxic) NOS
Struma nodosa (simplex)

Figure 3-3 Graves' disease. In Graves' disease, exophthalmos often looks more pronounced than it actually is because of the extreme lid retraction that may occur. This patient, for instance, had minimal proptosis of the left eye but marked lid retraction.

(Courtesy Dr. HG Scheie. From Yanoff M, Fine BS: Ocular Pathology, ed 6, St. Louis, Mosby, 2008)

Item 3-2 Thyrotoxicosis is a condition caused by excessive amounts of the thyroid hormone thyroxine production or hyperthyroidism. **Graves' disease is associated with hyperthyroidism** (known as **Basedow's disease** in Europe).

● **242 Thyrotoxicosis with or without goiter**
Excludes *neonatal thyrotoxicosis (775.3)*
The following fifth-digit subclassification is for use with category 242:

```
0  without mention of thyrotoxic crisis or storm
1  with mention of thyrotoxic crisis or storm
```

● **242.0 Toxic diffuse goiter** 1
[0-1] Basedow's disease
Exophthalmic or toxic goiter NOS
Graves' disease
Primary thyroid hyperplasia
(Ex) 017.50-017.56, 017.90-017.96, 240.0-246.9, 259.50-259.9

● **242.1 Toxic uninodular goiter** 1
[0-1] Thyroid nodule, toxic or with hyperthyroidism
Uninodular goiter, toxic or with hyperthyroidism
(Ex) 017.50-017.56, 017.90-017.96, 240.0-246.9, 259.50-259.9

● **242.2 Toxic multinodular goiter** 1
[0-1] Secondary thyroid hyperplasia
(Ex) 017.50-017.56, 017.90-017.96, 240.0-246.9, 259.50-259.9

● **242.3 Toxic nodular goiter, unspecified** 1
[0-1] Adenomatous goiter, toxic or with hyperthyroidism
Nodular goiter, toxic or with hyperthyroidism
Struma nodosa, toxic or with hyperthyroidism
Any condition classifiable to 241.9 specified as toxic or with hyperthyroidism
(Ex) 017.50-017.56, 017.90-017.96, 240.0-246.9, 259.50-259.9

● **242.4 Thyrotoxicosis from ectopic thyroid nodule** 1
[0-1] (Ex) 017.50-017.56, 017.90-017.96, 240.0-246.9, 259.50-259.9

● **242.8 Thyrotoxicosis of other specified origin** 1
[0-1] Overproduction of thyroid-stimulating hormone [TSH]
Thyrotoxicosis:
  factitia from ingestion of excessive thyroid material
Use additional E code to identify cause, if drug-induced
(Ex) 017.50-017.56, 017.90-017.96, 240.0-246.9, 259.50-259.9

● **242.9 Thyrotoxicosis without mention of goiter or other**
[0-1] **cause** 1
Hyperthyroidism NOS
Thyrotoxicosis NOS
Thyrotoxicosis is also known as thyroid storm.
(Ex) 017.50-017.56, 017.90-017.96, 240.0-246.9, 259.50-259.9

243 Congenital hypothyroidism
Congenital thyroid insufficiency
Cretinism (athyrotic) (endemic)
Use additional code to identify associated intellectual disabilities
Excludes *congenital (dyshormonogenic) goiter (246.1)*

Figure 3–4 Typical appearance of patients with moderately severe primary hypothyroidism or myxedema. (From Larsen: Williams Textbook of Endocrinology, ed 10, Saunders, An Imprint of Elsevier, 2003)

Item 3–3   Hypothyroidism is a condition in which there are insufficient levels of thyroxine.
Cretinism is congenital hypothyroidism, which can result in mental and physical retardation.

● **244   Acquired hypothyroidism**
> **Includes**   athyroidism (acquired)
> hypothyroidism (acquired)
> myxedema (adult) (juvenile)
> thyroid (gland) insufficiency (acquired)

244.0   Postsurgical hypothyroidism

244.1   Other postablative hypothyroidism
> Hypothyroidism following therapy, such as irradiation

244.2   Iodine hypothyroidism
> Hypothyroidism resulting from administration or ingestion of iodide
> Use additional E code to identify drug
> **Excludes**   hypothyroidism resulting from administration of radioactive iodine (244.1)

244.3   Other iatrogenic hypothyroidism
> Hypothyroidism resulting from:
> P-aminosalicylic acid [PAS]
> Phenylbutazone
> Resorcinol
> Iatrogenic hypothyroidism NOS
> Use additional E code to identify drug

244.8   Other specified acquired hypothyroidism
> Secondary hypothyroidism NEC
> Coding Clinic: 1985, July-Aug, P9

244.9   Unspecified hypothyroidism
> Hypothyroidism, primary or NOS
> Myxedema, primary or NOS
> Coding Clinic: 1999, Q3, P19-20; 1996, Q4, P29

● **245   Thyroiditis**
> *Inflammation of thyroid gland, results in inability to convert iodine into thyroid hormone. Common types are autoimmune or chronic lymphatic thyroiditis.*

245.0   Acute thyroiditis 🔎
> Abscess of thyroid
> Thyroiditis: Thyroiditis:
> nonsuppurative, acute   suppurative
> pyogenic
> Use additional code to identify organism
> Ⓔⓧ 245.0-245.9

245.1   Subacute thyroiditis
> Thyroiditis: Thyroiditis:
> de Quervain's   granulomatous
> giant cell   viral

245.2   Chronic lymphocytic thyroiditis
> Hashimoto's disease   Thyroiditis:
> Struma lymphomatosa   autoimmune
>   lymphocytic (chronic)

245.3   Chronic fibrous thyroiditis
> Struma fibrosa
> Thyroiditis: Thyroiditis:
> invasive (fibrous)   Riedel's
> ligneous

245.4   Iatrogenic thyroiditis
> Use additional E to identify cause

245.8   Other and unspecified chronic thyroiditis
> Chronic thyroiditis:
> NOS
> nonspecific

245.9   Thyroiditis, unspecified
> Thyroiditis NOS

● **246   Other disorders of thyroid**

246.0   Disorders of thyrocalcitonin secretion
> Hypersecretion of calcitonin or thyrocalcitonin

246.1   Dyshormonogenic goiter
> Congenital (dyshormonogenic) goiter
> Goiter due to enzyme defect in synthesis of thyroid hormone
> Goitrous cretinism (sporadic)

246.2   Cyst of thyroid
> **Excludes**   cystadenoma of thyroid (226)

246.3   Hemorrhage and infarction of thyroid 🔎
> Ⓔⓧ 246.3

246.8   Other specified disorders of thyroid
> Abnormality of thyroid-binding globulin
> Atrophy of thyroid
> Hyper-TBG-nemia
> Hypo-TBG-nemia
> Coding Clinic: 2006, Q2, P5

246.9   Unspecified disorder of thyroid

DISEASES OF OTHER ENDOCRINE GLANDS (249–259)

OGCR   Section I.C.3.a.2
> If the type of diabetes mellitus is not documented in the medical record the default is type II.

● **249   Secondary diabetes mellitus**
> **Includes**   diabetes mellitus (due to) (in) (secondary) (with):
> drug-induced or chemical induced
> infection
> **Excludes**   gestational diabetes (648.8)
> *hyperglycemia NOS (790.29)*
> *neonatal diabetes mellitus (775.1)*
> *nonclinical diabetes (790.29)*
> *Type I diabetes – see category 250*
> *Type II diabetes – see category 250*

The following fifth-digit subclassification is for use with category 249:

> **0   not stated as uncontrolled**
> **1   uncontrolled**

> Use additional code to identify any associated insulin use (V58.67)
> Coding Clinic: 2008, Q4, P91-95

● **249.0   Secondary diabetes mellitus without mention of**
  [0-1] **complication**
> Secondary diabetes mellitus without mention of complication or manifestation classifiable to 249.1-249.9
> Secondary diabetes mellitus NOS

● **249.1   Secondary diabetes mellitus with ketoacidosis** 🔎🔎
  [0-1]
> Secondary diabetes mellitus with diabetic acidosis without mention of coma
> Secondary diabetes mellitus with diabetic ketosis without mention of coma
> Ⓔⓧ 249.00-251.3, 259.8-259.9

● **249.2 Secondary diabetes mellitus with**
[0-1] **hyperosmolarity** 🔖 🔖
     Secondary diabetes mellitus with hyperosmolar
     (nonketotic) coma
     (Ex:) 249.00-251.3, 259.8-259.9

● **249.3 Secondary diabetes mellitus with other coma** 🔖
[0-1]   Secondary diabetes mellitus with diabetic coma (with
     ketoacidosis)
     Secondary diabetes mellitus with diabetic hypoglycemic
     coma
     Secondary diabetes mellitus with insulin coma
     NOS

     Excludes *secondary diabetes mellitus with hyperosmolar*
           coma (249.2)
     (Ex:) 249.00-251.3, 259.8-259.9

● **249.4 Secondary diabetes mellitus with renal**
[0-1] **manifestations**
     Use additional code to identify manifestation, as:
       chronic kidney disease (585.1-585.9)
       diabetic nephropathy NOS (583.81)
       diabetic nephrosis (581.81)
       intercapillary glomerulosclerosis (581.81)
       Kimmelstiel-Wilson syndrome (581.81)

● **249.5 Secondary diabetes mellitus with ophthalmic**
[0-1] **manifestations**
     Use additional code to identify manifestation, as:
       diabetic blindness (369.00-369.9)
       diabetic cataract (366.41)
       diabetic glaucoma (365.44)
       diabetic macular edema (362.07)
       diabetic retinal edema (362.07)
       diabetic retinopathy (362.01-362.07)

● **249.6 Secondary diabetes mellitus with neurological**
[0-1] **manifestations**
     Use additional code to identify manifestation, as:
       diabetic amyotrophy (353.5)
       diabetic gastroparalysis (536.3)
       diabetic gastroparesis (536.3)
       diabetic mononeuropathy (354.0-355.9)
       diabetic neurogenic arthropathy (713.5)
       diabetic peripheral autonomic neuropathy
         (337.1)
       diabetic polyneuropathy (357.2)
     Coding Clinic: 2008, Q4, P91-95

● **249.7 Secondary diabetes mellitus with peripheral**
[0-1] **circulatory disorders**
     Use additional code to identify manifestation, as:
       diabetic gangrene (785.4)
       diabetic peripheral angiopathy (443.81)

● **249.8 Secondary diabetes mellitus with other specified**
[0-1] **manifestations**
     Secondary diabetic hypoglycemia in diabetes mellitus
     Secondary hypoglycemic shock in diabetes
     mellitus
     Use additional code to identify manifestation, as:
       any associated ulceration (707.10-707.19, 707.8, 707.9)
       diabetic bone changes (731.8)

● **249.9 Secondary diabetes mellitus with unspecified**
[0-1] **complication**

● **250 Diabetes mellitus**
     Metabolic disease that results in persistent hyperglycemia.
       The three primary forms of diabetes mellitus are differentiated
       by patterns of pancreatic failure—type 1, type 2 and 3.

     Excludes *gestational diabetes (648.8)*
             hyperglycemia NOS (790.29)
             neonatal diabetes mellitus (775.1)
             nonclinical diabetes (790.29)
             secondary diabetes (249.0–249.9)

The following fifth-digit subclassification is for use with
category 250:

> **0 type II or unspecified type, not stated as uncontrolled**
>   Fifth-digit 0 is for use for type II patients, even if the
>   patient requires insulin
>
>   Use additional code, if applicable, for associated
>   long-term (current) insulin use V58.67
> **1 type I [juvenile type], not stated as uncontrolled**
> **2 type II or unspecified type, uncontrolled**
>   Fifth-digit 2 is for use for type II patients, even if the
>   patient requires insulin
>
>   Use additional code, if applicable, for associated
>   long-term (current) insulin use V58.67
>
> **3 type I [juvenile type], uncontrolled**

     Coding Clinic: 2006, Q1, P14; 1996, Q3, P5

OGCR   Section I.C.3.a.3

If the documentation in a medical record does not indicate the
type of diabetes but does indicate that the patient uses insulin,
the appropriate fifth-digit for type II must be used.

An exception to this rule is DKA, which defaults to Type I.

● **250.0 Diabetes mellitus without mention of complication**
[0-3]   Diabetes mellitus without mention of complication or
     manifestation classifiable to 250.1-250.9
     Diabetes (mellitus) NOS
     MCE: Questionable admission, principal diagnosis only
     Coding Clinic: 2013, Q3, P9, P13; 2012, Q2, P19; 2009, Q4, P81-82;
       2005, Q2, P21-22; Q1, P15; 2004, Q2, P17; 2003, Q4,
       P105-106, 108-109, P110; Q2, P6-7, 16; Q1, P5; 2002, Q2,
       P13; Q1, P7-8; 2001, Q2, P16; 1997, Q4, P33; 1994, Q1,
       P16-17, 21; 1993, Q4, P42; 5th Issue, P15; 1992, Q2, P15;
       1990, Q2, P22; 1985, Nov-Dec, P11; Sept-Oct, P11;
       Mar-April, P12

● **250.1 Diabetes with ketoacidosis** 🔖 🔖
[0-3]   Diabetic:
       acidosis without mention of coma
       ketosis without mention of coma
     (Ex:) 249.00-251.3, 259.8-259.9
     Coding Clinic: 2006, Q2, P19-20; 2003, Q4, P81-82; 1987, Jan-Feb, P15

● **250.2 Diabetes with hyperosmolarity** 🔖 🔖
[0-3]   Hyperosmolar (nonketotic) coma
     (Ex:) 249.00-251.3, 259.8-259.9

● **250.3 Diabetes with other coma** 🔖
[0-3]   Diabetic coma (with ketoacidosis)
     Diabetic hypoglycemic coma
     Insulin coma NOS

     Excludes *diabetes with hyperosmolar coma (250.2)*
     (Ex:) 249.00-251.3, 259.8-259.9

● **250.4 Diabetes with renal manifestations**
[0-3]   Use additional code to identify manifestation, as:
       chronic kidney disease (585.1–585.9) diabetic:
         nephropathy NOS (583.81)
         nephrosis (581.81)
       intercapillary glomerulosclerosis (581.81)
       Kimmelstiel-Wilson syndrome (581.81)
     Coding Clinic: 2013, Q2, P6; 2012, Q2, P19; 2003, Q1, P20-21; 1987,
       Sept-Oct, P9

ENDOCRINE, NUTRITIONAL AND METABOLIC DISEASES, AND IMMUNITY DISORDERS (240–279)

N   Newborn: 0   P   Pediatric: 0–17   M   Maternity: 12–55   A   Adult: 15–124   ♀   Females Only   ♂   Males Only

(Ex:) CC/MCC Exclusions   🔖 Complication\Comorbidity   🔖 Major C\C   🔖 Present on Admission Requirement   🔖 Hospital-Acquired Condition   **731**

● **250.5 Diabetes with ophthalmic manifestations**
[0-3]
Use additional code to identify manifestation, as:
diabetic:
blindness (369.00–369.9)
cataract (366.41)
glaucoma (365.44)
macular edema (362.07)
retinal edema (362.07)
retinopathy (362.01–362.07)
Coding Clinic: 2005, Q4, P65-67; 1993, Q4, P38; 1985, Sept-Oct, P11

● **250.6 Diabetes with neurological manifestations**
[0-3]
Use additional code to identify manifestation, as:
diabetic:
amyotrophy (353.5)
gastroparalysis (536.3)
gastroparesis (536.3)
mononeuropathy (354.0–355.9)
neurogenic arthropathy (713.5)
peripheral autonomic neuropathy (337.1)
polyneuropathy (357.2)
Coding Clinic: 2009, Q4, P81; Q2, P13, 15; 2008, Q3, P5-6; 2004, Q2, P7; 2003, Q4, P105; 1993, Q2, P6; 5th Issue, P15; 1984, Nov-Dec, P9

● **250.7 Diabetes with peripheral circulatory disorders**
[0-3]
Use additional code to identify manifestation, as:
diabetic:
gangrene (785.4)
peripheral angiopathy (443.81)
Coding Clinic: 2004, Q1, P14-15; 2002, Q1, P7-8; 1996, Q1, P10; 1994, Q3, P5; Q2, P17; 1990, Q3, P15; 1986, Mar-April, P12

● **250.8 Diabetes with other specified manifestations**
[0-3]
Diabetic hypoglycemia NOS
Hypoglycemic shock NOS
Use additional code to identify manifestation, as:
any associated ulceration (707.10-707.19, 707.8, 707.9)
diabetic bone changes (731.8)
Coding Clinic: 1997, Q4, P43; 1994, Q2, P13

● **250.9 Diabetes with unspecified complication**
[0-3]
Coding Clinic: 2006, Q1, P14; 1993, Q4, P38; 5th Issue, P15; 5th Issue, P11; 1985, Nov-Dec, P11

● **251 Other disorders of pancreatic internal secretion**
251.0 Hypoglycemic coma
Iatrogenic hyperinsulinism
Non-diabetic insulin coma
Use additional E code to identify cause, if drug-induced
Excludes *hypoglycemic coma in diabetes mellitus (249.3, 250.3)*
(Ex) 249.00-251.3, 259.50-259.9
Coding Clinic: 1985, Mar-April, P8-9

251.1 Other specified hypoglycemia
Hyperinsulinism:
NOS
ectopic
functional
Hyperplasia of pancreatic islet beta cells NOS
Excludes *hypoglycemia in diabetes mellitus (249.8, 250.8)*
hypoglycemia in infant of diabetic mother (775.0)
hypoglycemic coma (251.0)
neonatal hypoglycemia (775.6)
Use additional E code to identify cause, if drug-induced
Coding Clinic: 2013, Q3, P12; 2003, Q1, P10

251.2 Hypoglycemia, unspecified
Hypoglycemia:
NOS
reactive
spontaneous
Excludes *hypoglycemia:*
with coma (251.0)
in diabetes mellitus (249.8, 250.8)
leucine-induced (270.3)
Coding Clinic: 1985, Mar-April, P8-9

Figure 3–5 Tetany caused by hypoparathyroidism.

Item 3–4 Hyperparathyroidism is an overactive parathyroid gland that secretes excessive parathormone, causing increased levels of circulating calcium. This results in a loss of calcium in the bone (osteoporosis). **Hypoparathyroidism** is an underactive parathyroid gland that results in decreased levels of circulating calcium. The primary manifestation is **tetany,** a continuous muscle spasm.

251.3 Postsurgical hypoinsulinemia
Hypoinsulinemia following complete or partial pancreatectomy
Postpancreatectomy hyperglycemia
Use additional code to identify (any associated):
acquired absence of pancreas (V88.11-V88.12)
insulin use (V58.67)
secondary diabetes mellitus (249.00-249.91)
Excludes *transient hyperglycemia post procedure (790.29)*
transient hypoglycemia post procedure (251.2)
(Ex) 249.00-251.3, 259.50-259.9

251.4 Abnormality of secretion of glucagon
Hyperplasia of pancreatic islet alpha cells with glucagon excess

251.5 Abnormality of secretion of gastrin
Hyperplasia of pancreatic alpha cells with gastrin excess
Zollinger-Ellison syndrome

251.8 Other specified disorders of pancreatic internal secretion
Coding Clinic: 1998, Q2, P15

251.9 Unspecified disorder of pancreatic internal secretion
Islet cell hyperplasia NOS

● **252 Disorders of parathyroid gland**
Excludes *hungry bone syndrome (275.5)*
● **252.0 Hyperparathyroidism**
Excludes *ectopic hyperparathyroidism (259.3)*
Coding Clinic: 2004, Q4, P57-59

252.00 Hyperparathyroidism, unspecified

252.01 Primary hyperparathyroidism
Hyperplasia of parathyroid

252.02 Secondary hyperparathyroidism, non-renal
Excludes *secondary hyperparathyroidism (of renal origin) (588.81)*

252.08 Other hyperparathyroidism
Tertiary hyperparathyroidism

252.1 Hypoparathyroidism
Parathyroiditis (autoimmune)
Tetany:
parathyroid
parathyroprival
Excludes *pseudohypoparathyroidism (275.49)*
pseudopseudohypoparathyroidism (275.49)
tetany NOS (781.7)
transitory neonatal hypoparathyroidism (775.4)

252.8 Other specified disorders of parathyroid gland
Cyst of parathyroid gland
Hemorrhage of parathyroid gland

252.9 Unspecified disorder of parathyroid gland

● 253 **Disorders of the pituitary gland and its hypothalamic control**

　　Includes　the listed conditions whether the disorder is in the pituitary or the hypothalamus

　　Excludes　*Cushing's syndrome (255.0)*

　253.0 **Acromegaly and gigantism**
　　　　Overproduction of growth hormone

　253.1 **Other and unspecified anterior pituitary hyperfunction** 🔵
　　　　Forbes-Albright syndrome

　　　　Excludes　*overproduction of:*
　　　　　　　　ACTH (255.3)
　　　　　　　　thyroid-stimulating hormone [TSH] (242.8)
　　　　(Ex:) 253.1, 253.4, 253.6
　　　　Coding Clinic: 1985, July-Aug, P9

　253.2 **Panhypopituitarism** 🔵
　　　　Cachexia, pituitary
　　　　Necrosis of pituitary (postpartum)
　　　　Pituitary insufficiency NOS
　　　　Sheehan's syndrome
　　　　Simmonds' disease

　　　　Excludes　*iatrogenic hypopituitarism (253.7)*
　　　　(Ex:) 253.0-253.9, 259.50-259.9

　253.3 **Pituitary dwarfism**
　　　　Isolated deficiency of (human) growth hormone [HGH]
　　　　Lorain-Levi dwarfism

　253.4 **Other anterior pituitary disorders**
　　　　Isolated or partial deficiency of an anterior pituitary hormone, other than growth hormone
　　　　Prolactin deficiency
　　　　Coding Clinic: 1985, July-Aug, P9

　253.5 **Diabetes insipidus** 🔵
　　　　Vasopressin deficiency

　　　　Excludes　*nephrogenic diabetes insipidus (588.1)*
　　　　(Ex:) 253.1-253.2, 253.4-253.9, 259.50-259.9

　253.6 **Other disorders of neurohypophysis** 🔵
　　　　Syndrome of inappropriate secretion of antidiuretic hormone [ADH]

　　　　Excludes　*ectopic antidiuretic hormone secretion (259.3)*
　　　　(Ex:) 253.0-253.9, 259.8-259.9
　　　　Coding Clinic: 1993, 5th Issue, P8

　253.7 **Iatrogenic pituitary disorders**
　　　　Hypopituitarism:
　　　　　　hormone-induced
　　　　　　hypophysectomy-induced
　　　　　　postablative
　　　　　　radiotherapy-induced
　　　　Use additional E code to identify cause

　253.8 **Other disorders of the pituitary and other syndromes of diencephalohypophyseal origin**
　　　　Abscess of pituitary
　　　　Adiposogenital dystrophy
　　　　Cyst of Rathke's pouch
　　　　Fröhlich's syndrome

　　　　Excludes　*craniopharyngioma (237.0)*

　253.9 **Unspecified**
　　　　Dyspituitarism

● 254 **Diseases of thymus gland**

　　Excludes　*aplasia or dysplasia with immunodeficiency (279.2)*
　　　　　　hypoplasia with immunodeficiency (279.2)
　　　　　　myasthenia gravis (358.00–358.01)

　254.0 **Persistent hyperplasia of thymus**
　　　　Hypertrophy of thymus

　254.1 **Abscess of thymus** 🔵
　　　　(Ex:) 254.0-254.9, 259.50-259.9

　254.8 **Other specified diseases of thymus gland**
　　　　Atrophy of thymus
　　　　Cyst of thymus

　　　　Excludes　*thymoma (212.6)*

　254.9 **Unspecified disease of thymus gland**

Figure 3–6　Centripetal and generalized obesity and dorsal kyphosis in a 30-year-old woman with Cushing's disease. (From Larsen: Williams Textbook of Endocrinology, ed 10, Saunders, An Imprint of Elsevier, 2003)

Item 3–5　Hyperadrenalism is overactivity of the adrenal cortex, which secretes corticosterioid hormones. Excessive glucocorticoid hormone results in hyperglycemia **(Cushing's syndrome),** and excessive aldosterone results in **Conn's syndrome. Adrenogenital syndrome** is the result of excessive secretion of androgens, male hormones, which stimulates premature sexual development. **Hypoadrenalism, Addison's disease,** is a condition in which the adrenal glands atrophy.

● 255 **Disorders of adrenal glands**

　　Includes　the listed conditions whether the basic disorder is in the adrenals or is pituitary-induced

　255.0 **Cushing's syndrome** 🔵
　　　　Adrenal hyperplasia due to excess ACTH
　　　　Cushing's syndrome:
　　　　　　NOS
　　　　　　iatrogenic
　　　　　　idiopathic
　　　　　　pituitary-dependent
　　　　Ectopic ACTH syndrome
　　　　Iatrogenic syndrome of excess cortisol
　　　　Overproduction of cortisol

　　　　Use additional E code to identify cause, if drug-induced

　　　　Excludes　*congenital adrenal hyperplasia (255.2)*
　　　　(Ex:) 255.0-255.2, 259.50-259.9

● 255.1 **Hyperaldosteronism**
　　　　Coding Clinic: 2003, Q4, P48-50

　255.10 **Hyperaldosteronism, unspecified**
　　　　Aldosteronism NOS
　　　　Primary aldosteronism, unspecified

　　　　Excludes　*Conn's syndrome (255.12)*

　255.11 **Glucocorticoid-remediable aldosteronism**
　　　　Familial aldosteronism type I

　　　　Excludes　*Conn's syndrome (255.12)*

　255.12 **Conn's syndrome**

　255.13 **Bartter's syndrome**

　255.14 **Other secondary aldosteronism**
　　　　Coding Clinic: 2006, Q3, P24

　255.2 **Adrenogenital disorders**
　　　　Achard-Thiers syndrome
　　　　Adrenogenital syndromes, virilizing or feminizing, whether acquired or associated with congenital adrenal hyperplasia consequent on inborn enzyme defects in hormone synthesis
　　　　Congenital adrenal hyperplasia
　　　　Female adrenal pseudohermaphroditism
　　　　Male:
　　　　　　macrogenitosomia praecox
　　　　　　sexual precocity with adrenal hyperplasia
　　　　Virilization (female) (suprarenal)

　　　　Excludes　*adrenal hyperplasia due to excess ACTH (255.0)*
　　　　　　　isosexual virilization (256.4)

　255.3 **Other corticoadrenal overactivity** 🔵
　　　　Acquired benign adrenal androgenic overactivity
　　　　Overproduction of ACTH
　　　　(Ex:) 017.60-017.66, 017.90-017.96, 255.3-255.9, 259.50-259.9

● **255.4 Corticoadrenal insufficiency**

    Excludes *tuberculous Addison's disease (017.6)*

    Coding Clinic: 2006, Q3, P24; 1985, July-Aug, P8

  255.41 Glucocorticoid deficiency

    Addisonian crisis

    Addison's disease NOS

    Adrenal atrophy (autoimmune)

    Adrenal calcification

    Adrenal crisis

    Adrenal hemorrhage

    Adrenal infarction

    Adrenal insufficiency NOS

    Combined glucocorticoid and mineralocorticoid deficiency

    Corticoadrenal insufficiency NOS

    (Ex) 017.60-017.66, 017.90-017.96, 255.3-255.9, 259.50-259.9

    Coding Clinic: 2007, Q4, P68-70

  255.42 Mineralocorticoid deficiency

    Hypoaldosteronism

    Excludes *combined glucocorticoid and mineralocorticoid deficiency (255.41)*

    (Ex) 017.60-017.66, 017.90-017.96, 255.3-255.9, 259.50-259.9

    Coding Clinic: 2006, Q3, P24

255.5 Other adrenal hypofunction

  Adrenal medullary insufficiency

  Excludes *Waterhouse-Friderichsen syndrome (meningococcal) (036.3)*

  (Ex) 017.60-017.66, 017.90-017.96, 255.3-255.9, 259.50-259.9

255.6 Medulloadrenal hyperfunction

  Catecholamine secretion by pheochromocytoma

  (Ex) 017.60-017.66, 017.90-017.96, 255.3-255.9, 259.50-259.9

255.8 Other specified disorders of adrenal glands

  Abnormality of cortisol-binding globulin

  Coding Clinic: 1985, July-Aug, P8

255.9 Unspecified disorder of adrenal glands

● **256 Ovarian dysfunction**

256.0 Hyperestrogenism ♀

256.1 Other ovarian hyperfunction ♀

  Hypersecretion of ovarian androgens

  Coding Clinic: 1995, Q3, P15

256.2 Postablative ovarian failure ♀

  Ovarian failure:

    iatrogenic

    postirradiation

    postsurgical

  Use additional code for states associated with artificial menopause (627.4)

  Excludes *acquired absence of ovary (V45.77)*
    asymptomatic age-related (natural) postmenopausal status (V49.81)

  Coding Clinic: 2002, Q2, P12-13

● **256.3 Other ovarian failure**

  Use additional code for states associated with natural menopause (627.2)

  Excludes *asymptomatic age-related (natural) postmenopausal status (V49.81)*

  256.31 Premature menopause ♀   A

  256.39 Other ovarian failure ♀

    Delayed menarche

    Ovarian hypofunction

    Primary ovarian failure NOS

256.4 Polycystic ovaries ♀

  Isosexual virilization Stein-Leventhal syndrome

256.8 Other ovarian dysfunction ♀

256.9 Unspecified ovarian dysfunction ♀

● **257 Testicular dysfunction**

257.0 Testicular hyperfunction ♂

  Hypersecretion of testicular hormones

257.1 Postablative testicular hypofunction ♂

  Testicular hypofunction:

    iatrogenic

    postirradiation

    postsurgical

257.2 Other testicular hypofunction

  Defective biosynthesis of testicular androgen

  Eunuchoidism:

    NOS

    hypogonadotropic

  Failure:

    Leydig's cell, adult

    seminiferous tubule, adult

  Testicular hypogonadism

  Excludes *azoospermia (606.0)*

257.8 Other testicular dysfunction

  Excludes *androgen insensitivity syndrome (259.50–259.52)*

257.9 Unspecified testicular dysfunction ♂

● **258 Polyglandular dysfunction and related disorders**

● **258.0 Polyglandular activity in multiple endocrine adenomatosis**

  Multiple endocrine neoplasia [MEN] syndromes

  Use additional codes to identify any malignancies and other conditions associated with the syndromes

  Coding Clinic: 2009, Q4, P84x2

  258.01 Multiple endocrine neoplasia [MEN] type I

    Wermer's syndrome

    Coding Clinic: 2008, Q4, P85-90; 2007, Q4, P70-72

  258.02 Multiple endocrine neoplasia [MEN] type IIA

    Sipple's syndrome

  258.03 Multiple endocrine neoplasia [MEN] type IIB

258.1 Other combinations of endocrine dysfunction

  Lloyd's syndrome

  Schmidt's syndrome

258.8 Other specified polyglandular dysfunction

258.9 Polyglandular dysfunction, unspecified

● **259 Other endocrine disorders**

259.0 Delay in sexual development and puberty, not elsewhere classified

  Delayed puberty

259.1 Precocious sexual development and puberty, not elsewhere classified   P

  Sexual precocity:

    NOS

    constitutional

    cryptogenic

    idiopathic

259.2 Carcinoid syndrome

  Hormone secretion by carcinoid tumors

  (Ex) 259.2-259.3, 259.50-259.9

  Coding Clinic: 2008, Q4, P85-90

259.3 Ectopic hormone secretion, not elsewhere classified

  Ectopic:

    antidiuretic hormone secretion [ADH]

    hyperparathyroidism

  Excludes *ectopic ACTH syndrome (255.0)*

◀ New   ◀▦ Revised   ~~deleted~~ Deleted   Excludes   Includes   Use additional   Code first   Omit code

734   ● Unacceptable Principal Diagnosis   ● Use Additional Digit(s)   ▶ Manifestation Code   OGCR Official Guidelines   Coding Clinic

259.4 Dwarfism, not elsewhere classified
　　Dwarfism:
　　　NOS
　　　constitutional
　　Excludes *dwarfism:*
　　　　　achondroplastic (756.4)
　　　　　intrauterine (759.7)
　　　　　nutritional (263.2)
　　　　　pituitary (253.3)
　　　　　renal (588.0)
　　　　progeria (259.8)

● **259.5 Androgen insensitivity syndrome**
　　Coding Clinic: 2008, Q4, P95-96; 2005, Q4, P53-54

　　259.50 Androgen insensitivity, unspecified

　　259.51 Androgen insensitivity syndrome
　　　　Complete androgen insensitivity
　　　　de Quervain's syndrome
　　　　Goldberg-Maxwell Syndrome

　　259.52 Partial androgen insensitivity
　　　　Partial androgen insensitivity syndrome
　　　　Reifenstein syndrome

259.8 Other specified endocrine disorders
　　Pineal gland dysfunction
　　Progeria
　　Werner's syndrome

259.9 Unspecified endocrine disorder
　　Disturbance:
　　　endocrine NOS
　　　hormone NOS
　　Infantilism NOS

NUTRITIONAL DEFICIENCIES (260–269)

Excludes *deficiency anemias (280.0–281.9)*

260 Kwashiorkor
　　Nutritional edema with dyspigmentation of skin and hair
　　(Ex:) 260-263.9
　　Coding Clinic: 2009, Q3, P6

261 Nutritional marasmus
　　Nutritional atrophy
　　Severe calorie deficiency
　　Severe malnutrition NOS
　　(Ex:) 260-263.9
　　Coding Clinic: 2013, Q1, P13-14; 2012, Q3, P10; 2007, Q4, P96-97; 2006, Q3,
　　　P14-15; Q2, P12

262 Other severe protein-calorie malnutrition
　　Nutritional edema without mention of dyspigmentation of skin
　　　and hair
　　(Ex:) 260-263.9
　　Coding Clinic: 1985, July-Aug, P12-13

● **263 Other and unspecified protein-calorie malnutrition**
　　263.0 Malnutrition of moderate degree
　　　(Ex:) 260-263.9
　　　Coding Clinic: 2012, Q3, P10; 2009, Q3, P6; 1985, July-Aug, P12-13

　　263.1 Malnutrition of mild degree
　　　(Ex:) 260-263.9
　　　Coding Clinic: 1985, July-Aug, P12-13

　　**263.2 Arrested development following protein-calorie
　　　malnutrition**
　　　　Nutritional dwarfism
　　　　Physical retardation due to malnutrition
　　　(Ex:) 260-263.9

　　263.8 Other protein-calorie malnutrition
　　　(Ex:) 260-263.9

　　263.9 Unspecified protein-calorie malnutrition
　　　　Dystrophy due to malnutrition
　　　　Malnutrition (calorie) NOS
　　　Excludes *nutritional deficiency NOS (269.9)*
　　　(Ex:) 260-263.9
　　　Coding Clinic: 2012, Q3, P9; 2006, Q2, P12; 2003, Q4, P109-110;
　　　　1984, Nov-Dec, P19

Figure 3–7 Bitot's spot on the conjunctiva.

Item 3–6 Bitot's spots are the result of a buildup of keratin debris found on the superficial surface the conjunctiva; oval, triangular, or irregular in shape; and a sign of vitamin A deficiency and associated with night blindness. The disease may progress to **keratomalacia,** which can result in eventual prolapse of the iris and loss of the lens.

● **264 Vitamin A deficiency**
　　264.0 With conjunctival xerosis
　　264.1 With conjunctival xerosis and Bitot's spot
　　　　Bitot's spot in the young child
　　264.2 With corneal xerosis
　　264.3 With corneal ulceration and xerosis
　　264.4 With keratomalacia
　　264.5 With night blindness
　　264.6 With xerophthalmic scars of cornea
　　264.7 Other ocular manifestations of vitamin A deficiency
　　　　Xerophthalmia due to vitamin A deficiency
　　264.8 Other manifestations of vitamin A deficiency
　　　　Follicular keratosis due to vitamin A deficiency
　　　　Xeroderma due to vitamin A deficiency
　　264.9 Unspecified vitamin A deficiency
　　　　Hypovitaminosis A NOS

● **265 Thiamine and niacin deficiency states**
　　265.0 Beriberi
　　　(Ex:) 265.0-266.9, 269.1-269.9
　　**265.1 Other and unspecified manifestations of thiamine
　　　deficiency**
　　　　Other vitamin B$_1$ deficiency states
　　　(Ex:) 265.0-266.9, 269.1-269.9
　　265.2 Pellagra
　　　　Deficiency:
　　　　　niacin (-tryptophan)
　　　　　nicotinamide
　　　　　nicotinic acid
　　　　　vitamin PP
　　　　Pellagra (alcoholic)

● **266 Deficiency of B-complex components**
　　266.0 Ariboflavinosis
　　　　Riboflavin [vitamin B$_2$] deficiency
　　　(Ex:) 265.0-266.9, 269.1-269.9
　　　Coding Clinic: 1986, Sept-Oct, P10
　　266.1 Vitamin B$_6$ deficiency
　　　　Deficiency:
　　　　　pyridoxal
　　　　　pyridoxamine
　　　　　pyridoxine
　　　　Vitamin B$_6$ deficiency syndrome
　　　Excludes *vitamin B$_6$-responsive sideroblastic anemia
　　　　(285.0)*

Figure 3–8 The sharply demarcated, characteristic scaling dermatitis of pellagra. (From Kumar: Robbins and Cotran: Pathologic Basis of Disease, ed 8, Saunders, An Imprint of Elsevier, 2009)

Item 3–7 Pellagra is associated with a deficiency of niacin and its precursor, **tryptophan.** Characteristics of the condition include diarrhea, dermatitis on exposed skin surfaces, dementia, and death. It is prevalent in developing countries where nutrition is inadequate. **Beriberi** is associated with thiamine deficiency.

N Newborn: 0　　**P** Pediatric: 0–17　　**M** Maternity: 12–55　　**A** Adult: 15–124　　♀ Females Only　　♂ Males Only

(Ex:) CC/MCC Exclusions　　Complication\Comorbidity　　Major C\C　　Present on Admission Requirement　　Hospital-Acquired Condition　　**735**

ENDOCRINE, NUTRITIONAL AND METABOLIC DISEASES, AND IMMUNITY DISORDERS (240–279)

266.2 Other B-complex deficiencies
Deficiency:
cyanocobalamin
folic acid
vitamin B$_{12}$
   Excludes *combined system disease with anemia*
(281.0–281.1)
deficiency anemias (281.0–281.9)
subacute degeneration of spinal cord with anemia
(281.0–281.1)

266.9 Unspecified vitamin B deficiency

267 Ascorbic acid deficiency
Deficiency of vitamin C
Scurvy
   Excludes *scorbutic anemia (281.8)*

● **268 Vitamin D deficiency**
   Excludes *vitamin D-resistant:*
osteomalacia (275.3)
rickets (275.3)

268.0 Rickets, active
   Excludes *celiac rickets (579.0)*
renal rickets (588.0)
   (Ex) 268.0-269.9

268.1 Rickets, late effect
Any condition specified as due to rickets and stated to be
a late effect or sequela of rickets
Code first the nature of late effect

268.2 Osteomalacia, unspecified
Softening of bone

268.9 Unspecified vitamin D deficiency
Avitaminosis D

● **269 Other nutritional deficiencies**
269.0 Deficiency of vitamin K
   Excludes *deficiency of coagulation factor due to vitamin K*
deficiency (286.7)
vitamin K deficiency of newborn (776.0)

269.1 Deficiency of other vitamins
Deficiency:
vitamin E
vitamin P

269.2 Unspecified vitamin deficiency
Multiple vitamin deficiency NOS

269.3 Mineral deficiency, not elsewhere classified
Deficiency:
calcium, dietary
iodine
   Excludes *deficiency:*
calcium NOS (275.40)
potassium (276.8)
sodium (276.1)

269.8 Other nutritional deficiency
   Excludes *adult failure to thrive (783.7)*
failure to thrive in childhood (783.41)
feeding problems (783.3)
newborn (779.31–779.34)

269.9 Unspecified nutritional deficiency

OTHER METABOLIC AND IMMUNITY DISORDERS (270–279)

Use additional code to identify any associated intellectual
disabilities

● **270 Disorders of amino-acid transport and metabolism**
   Excludes *abnormal findings without manifest disease*
(790.0–796.9)
disorders of purine and pyrimidine metabolism
(277.1–277.2)
gout (274.00–274.9)

270.0 Disturbances of amino-acid transport
Cystinosis
Cystinuria
Fanconi (-de Toni) (-Debré) syndrome
Glycinuria (renal)
Hartnup disease
   (Ex) 270.0-273.3, 273.8-273.9

270.1 Phenylketonuria [PKU]
Hyperphenylalaninemia
   (Ex) 270.0-273.3, 273.8-273.9

270.2 Other disturbances of aromatic amino-acid metabolism
Albinism
Alkaptonuria
Alkaptonuric ochronosis
Disturbances of metabolism of tyrosine and tryptophan
Homogentisic acid defects
Hydroxykynureninuria
Hypertyrosinemia
Indicanuria
Kynureninase defects
Oasthouse urine disease
Ochronosis
Tyrosinosis
Tyrosinuria
Waardenburg syndrome
   Excludes *vitamin B$_6$-deficiency syndrome (266.1)*
   (Ex) 270.0-273.3, 273.8-273.9
   Coding Clinic: 1999, Q3, P20-21

270.3 Disturbances of branched-chain amino-acid metabolism
Disturbances of metabolism of leucine, isoleucine, and
valine
Hypervalinemia
Intermittent branched-chain ketonuria
Leucine-induced hypoglycemia
Leucinosis
Maple syrup urine disease
   (Ex) 270.0-273.3, 273.8-273.9
   Coding Clinic: 2000, Q3, P8

**270.4 Disturbances of sulphur-bearing amino-acid
metabolism**
Cystathioninemia
Cystathioninuria
Disturbances of metabolism of methionine, homocystine,
and cystathionine
Homocystinuria
Hypermethioninemia
Methioninemia
   (Ex) 270.0-273.3, 273.8-273.9
   Coding Clinic: 2007, Q2, P9; 2004, Q1, P6

270.5 Disturbances of histidine metabolism
Carnosinemia   Hyperhistidinemia
Histidinemia   Imidazole
                aminoaciduria
   (Ex) 270.0-273.3, 273.8-273.9

270.6 Disorders of urea cycle metabolism
Argininosuccinic aciduria
Citrullinemia
Disorders of metabolism of ornithine, citrulline,
argininosuccinic acid, arginine, and ammonia
Hyperammonemia
Hyperornithinemia
   (Ex) 270.0-273.3, 273.8-273.9

◀ New   ◀▥ Revised   ~~deleted~~ Deleted   Excludes   Includes   Use additional   Code first   Omit code
● Unacceptable Principal Diagnosis   ● Use Additional Digit(s)   ▶ Manifestation Code   OGCR Official Guidelines   Coding Clinic
736

Item 3–8 Any term ending with "emia" will be a blood condition. Any term ending with "uria" will have to do with urine. A term ending with "opathy" is a disease condition. Check for laboratory work.

270.7 Other disturbances of straight-chain amino-acid metabolism
Glucoglycinuria
Glycinemia (with methylmalonic acidemia)
Hyperglycinemia
Hyperlysinemia
Pipecolic acidemia
Saccharopinuria
Other disturbances of metabolism of glycine, threonine, serine, glutamine, and lysine
(Ex) 270.0-273.3, 273.8-273.9
Coding Clinic: 2000, Q3, P8

270.8 Other specified disorders of amino-acid metabolism
Alaninemia
Ethanolaminuria
Glycoprolinuria
Hydroxyprolinemia
Hyperprolinemia
Iminoacidopathy
Prolinemia
Prolinuria
Sarcosinemia
(Ex) 270.0-273.3, 273.8-273.9

270.9 Unspecified disorder of amino-acid metabolism
(Ex) 270.0-273.3, 273.8-273.9

● **271 Disorders of carbohydrate transport and metabolism**
Excludes abnormality of secretion of glucagon (251.4)
diabetes mellitus (249.0–249.9, 250.0–250.9)
hypoglycemia NOS (251.2)
mucopolysaccharidosis (277.5)

271.0 Glycogenosis
Amylopectinosis
Glucose-6-phosphatase deficiency
Glycogen storage disease
McArdle's disease
Pompe's disease
von Gierke's disease
(Ex) 270.0-273.3, 273.8-273.9
Coding Clinic: 1998, Q1, P5-6

271.1 Galactosemia
Galactose-1-phosphate uridyl transferase deficiency
Galactosuria
(Ex) 270.0-273.3, 273.8-273.9

271.2 Hereditary fructose intolerance
Essential benign fructosuria
Fructosemia

271.3 Intestinal disaccharidase deficiencies and disaccharide malabsorption
Intolerance or malabsorption (congenital) (of):
glucose-galactose
lactose
sucrose-isomaltose

271.4 Renal glycosuria
Renal diabetes

271.8 Other specified disorders of carbohydrate transport and metabolism
Essential benign pentosuria
Fucosidosis
Glycolic aciduria
Hyperoxaluria (primary)
Mannosidosis
Oxalosis
Xylosuria
Xylulosuria
(Ex) 270.0-273.3, 273.8-273.9

271.9 Unspecified disorder of carbohydrate transport and metabolism

● **272 Disorders of lipoid metabolism**
Excludes localized cerebral lipidoses (330.1)

272.0 Pure hypercholesterolemia
Familial hypercholesterolemia
Fredrickson Type IIa hyperlipoproteinemia
Hyperbetalipoproteinemia
Hyperlipidemia, Group A
Low-density-lipoid-type [LDL] hyperlipoproteinemia
Coding Clinic: 2005, Q4, P68-69

272.1 Pure hyperglyceridemia
Endogenous hyperglyceridemia
Fredrickson Type IV hyperlipoproteinemia
Hyperlipidemia, Group B
Hyperprebetalipoproteinemia
Hypertriglyceridemia, essential
Very-low-density-lipoid-type [VLDL] hyperlipoproteinemia
Coding Clinic: 1985, Jan-Feb, P15

272.2 Mixed hyperlipidemia
Broad- or floating-betalipoproteinemia
Combined hyperlipidemia
Elevated cholesterol with elevated triglycerides NEC
Fredrickson Type IIb or III hyperlipoproteinemia
Hypercholesterolemia with endogenous hyperglyceridemia
Hyperbetalipoproteinemia with prebetalipoproteinemia
Tubo-eruptive xanthoma
Xanthoma tuberosum

272.3 Hyperchylomicronemia
Bürger-Grütz syndrome
Fredrickson type I or V hyperlipoproteinemia
Hyperlipidemia, Group D
Mixed hyperglyceridemia

272.4 Other and unspecified hyperlipidemia
Alpha-lipoproteinemia
Hyperlipidemia NOS
Hyperlipoproteinemia NOS
Coding Clinic: 2005, Q1, P17

272.5 Lipoprotein deficiencies
Abetalipoproteinemia
Bassen-Kornzweig syndrome
High-density lipoid deficiency
Hypoalphalipoproteinemia
Hypobetalipoproteinemia (familial)

272.6 Lipodystrophy
Barraquer-Simons disease
Progressive lipodystrophy
Use additional E code to identify cause, if iatrogenic
Excludes intestinal lipodystrophy (040.2)

272.7 Lipidoses
Chemically induced lipidosis
Disease:
Anderson's
Fabry's
Gaucher's
I cell [mucolipidosis I]
lipoid storage NOS
Niemann-Pick
pseudo-Hurler's or mucolipidosis III
triglyceride storage, Type I or II
Wolman's or triglyceride storage, Type III
Mucolipidosis II
Primary familial xanthomatosis
Excludes cerebral lipidoses (330.1)
Tay-Sachs disease (330.1)

272.8 Other disorders of lipoid metabolism
Hoffa's disease or liposynovitis prepatellaris
Launois-Bensaude's lipomatosis
Lipoid dermatoarthritis

272.9 Unspecified disorder of lipoid metabolism

ENDOCRINE, NUTRITIONAL AND METABOLIC DISEASES, AND IMMUNITY DISORDERS (240–279)

● **273   Disorders of plasma protein metabolism**

> **Excludes**   agammaglobulinemia and hypogammaglobulinemia
> (279.0–279.2)
> coagulation defects (286.0–286.9)
> hereditary hemolytic anemias (282.0–282.9)

273.0   Polyclonal hypergammaglobulinemia
Hypergammaglobulinemic purpura:
benign primary
Waldenström's

273.1   Monoclonal paraproteinemia
Benign monoclonal hypergammaglobulinemia [BMH]
Monoclonal gammopathy:
NOS
associated with lymphoplasmacytic dyscrasias
benign
Paraproteinemia:
benign (familial)
secondary to malignant or inflammatory disease

273.2   Other paraproteinemias
Cryoglobulinemic:
purpura
vasculitis
Mixed cryoglobulinemia
Coding Clinic: 2008, Q2, P17

273.3   Macroglobulinemia
Macroglobulinemia (idiopathic) (primary)
Waldenström's macroglobulinemia

273.4   Alpha-1-antitrypsin deficiency
AAT deficiency
Coding Clinic: 2004, Q4, P59-60

273.8   Other disorders of plasma protein metabolism
Abnormality of transport protein
Bisalbuminemia
Coding Clinic: 1998, Q2, P11

273.9   Unspecified disorder of plasma protein metabolism
Coding Clinic: 1998, Q2, P11

● **274   Gout**

> Result of accumulation of uric acid caused by either too much
> production, or insufficient natural removal of uric acid from
> body. Results in swollen, red, hot, painful, stiff joints. Also
> called gouty arthritis.

> **Excludes**   lead gout (984.0–984.9)

● **274.0   Gouty arthropathy**

274.00   Gouty arthropathy, unspecified

274.01   Acute gouty arthropathy
Acute gout   Gout flare
Gout attack   Podagra

**274.02   Chronic gouty arthropathy without mention of
tophus (tophi)**
Chronic gout

274.03   Chronic gouty arthropathy with tophus (tophi)
Chronic tophaceous gout
Gout with tophi NOS
Coding Clinic: 2009, Q4, P84

● **274.1   Gouty nephropathy**

274.10   Gouty nephropathy, unspecified
Coding Clinic: 1985, Nov-Dec, P15

274.11   Uric acid nephrolithiasis 🔷
(Ex) 016.00-016.06, 016.30-016.36, 016.90-016.96, 017.90-017.96,
078.6, 098.10, 098.19, 098.30-098.31, 098.89, 112.2, 131.00,
131.8-131.9, 249.40-249.41, 249.80-249.91, 250.40-250.43,
250.80-250.93, 274.10-274.19, 274.89, 580.0-584.9,
586-588.1, 588.9-591, 593.0-593.2, 593.89-593.9,
599.60-599.9

274.19   Other

● **274.8   Gout with other specified manifestations**

> Tophi = chalky deposit of sodium urate occurring in gout

274.81   Gouty tophi of ear

274.82   Gouty tophi of other sites
Gouty tophi of heart

> **Excludes**   gout with tophi NOS (274.03)
> gouty arthropathy with tophi (274.03)

274.89   Other
Use additional code to identify manifestations,
as:
gouty:
iritis (364.11)
neuritis (357.4)

274.9   Gout, unspecified

● **275   Disorders of mineral metabolism**

> **Excludes**   abnormal findings without manifest disease
> (790.0–796.9)

● **275.0   Disorders of iron metabolism**

> **Excludes**   anemia:
> iron deficiency (280.0–280.9)
> sideroblastic (285.0)

Coding Clinic: 1997, Q2, P11

275.01   Hereditary hemochromatosis
Bronzed diabetes
Pigmentary cirrhosis (of liver)
Primary (hereditary) hemochromatosis

**275.02   Hemochromatosis due to repeated red blood cell
transfusions**
Iron overload due to repeated red blood cell
transfusions
Transfusion (red blood cell) associated
hemochromatosis
Coding Clinic: 2010, Q4, P78-79

275.03   Other hemochromatosis
Hemochromatosis NOS

275.09   Other disorders of iron metabolism

275.1   Disorders of copper metabolism
Hepatolenticular degeneration
Wilson's disease

275.2   Disorders of magnesium metabolism
Hypermagnesemia   Hypomagnesemia
Coding Clinic: 2010, Q1, P3-4; 2009, Q3, P6

275.3   Disorders of phosphorus metabolism
Familial hypophosphatemia
Hypophosphatasia
Vitamin D-resistant:
osteomalacia
rickets

● **275.4   Disorders of calcium metabolism**

> **Excludes**   hungry bone syndrome (275.5)
> parathyroid disorders (252.00–252.9)
> vitamin D deficiency (268.0–268.9)

275.40   Unspecified disorder of calcium metabolism

275.41   Hypocalcemia
Coding Clinic: 2007, Q3, P5-6

275.42   Hypercalcemia
Coding Clinic: 2012, Q3, P16; 2003, Q4, P110

275.49   Other disorders of calcium metabolism
Nephrocalcinosis
Pseudohypoparathyroidism
Pseudopseudohypoparathyroidism

275.5   Hungry bone syndrome
Coding Clinic: 2008, Q4, P96-97

275.8   Other specified disorders of mineral metabolism

275.9   Unspecified disorder of mineral metabolism

Item 3–9 Circulating fluid volume is regulated by the amount of water and sodium ingested, excreted by the kidneys into the urine, and lost through the gastrointestinal tract, lungs, and skin. To maintain blood volume within a normal range, the kidneys regulate the amount of water and sodium lost into the urine. Too much (**fluid overload**) or too little fluid volume (**volume depletion**) will affect blood pressure. Severe cases of vomiting, diarrhea, bleeding, and burns (fluid loss through exposed burn surface area) can contribute to fluid loss. Internal body environment must maintain a precise balance (homeostasis) between too much fluid and too little fluid. This complex balancing mechanism is critical to good health.

● **276 Disorders of fluid, electrolyte, and acid-base balance**

    Excludes *diabetes insipidus (253.5)*
                 familial periodic paralysis (359.3)

  276.0 Hyperosmolality and/or hypernatremia 🔒
    Sodium [Na] excess   Sodium [Na] overload
    Ⓔⓧ 276.0-276.9

  276.1 Hyposmolality and/or hyponatremia 🔒
    Sodium [Na] deficiency
    Ⓔⓧ 276.0-276.9

  276.2 Acidosis 🔒
    Acidosis:
      NOS   metabolic
      lactic   respiratory
    Excludes *diabetic acidosis (249.1, 250.1)*
    Ⓔⓧ 276.0-276.9
    Coding Clinic: 1987, Jan-Feb, P15

  276.3 Alkalosis 🔒
    Alkalosis:
      NOS   respiratory
      metabolic
    Ⓔⓧ 276.0-276.9

  276.4 Mixed acid-base balance disorder 🔒
    Hypercapnia with mixed acid-base disorder
    Ⓔⓧ 276.0-276.9

● **276.5 Volume depletion**
    Excludes *hypovolemic shock:*
                 postoperative (998.09)
                 traumatic (958.4)
    Coding Clinic: 2005, Q4, P54-55; Q2, P9-10; 2003, Q1, P5, 20-22; 2002, Q3, P21x2; 1997, Q4, P30-31; 1993, 5th Issue, P1; 1988, Q2, P9-11; 1984, July-Aug, P19-20

    276.50 Volume depletion, unspecified

    276.51 Dehydration
      Coding Clinic: 2008, Q1, P10-11

    276.52 Hypovolemia
      Depletion of volume of plasma

● **276.6 Fluid overload**
    Excludes *ascites (789.51–789.59)*
                 localized edema (782.3)
    Coding Clinic: 2007, Q3, P11; 2006, Q4, P136; 1987, Sept-Oct, P9

    276.61 Transfusion associated circulatory overload
      Fluid overload due to transfusion (blood) (blood components)
      TACO
      Coding Clinic: 2010, Q4, P80

    276.69 Other fluid overload
      Fluid retention

  276.7 Hyperpotassemia
    Hyperkalemia
    Potassium [K]:   Potassium [K]:
      excess   overload
      intoxication
    Coding Clinic: 2005, Q1, P9-10; 2001, Q2, P12-13

  276.8 Hypopotassemia
    Hypokalemia
    Potassium [K] deficiency

  276.9 Electrolyte and fluid disorders not elsewhere classified
    Electrolyte imbalance
    Hyperchloremia
    Hypochloremia
    Excludes *electrolyte imbalance:*
               associated with hyperemesis gravidarum
                 (643.1)
              complicating labor and delivery (669.0)
              following abortion and ectopic or molar
                 pregnancy (634–638 with .4, 639.4)
    Coding Clinic: 1987, Jan-Feb, P15

● **277 Other and unspecified disorders of metabolism**

● **277.0 Cystic fibrosis**
    Fibrocystic disease of the pancreas
    Mucoviscidosis
    Coding Clinic: 2002, Q4, P45-46; 1994, Q3, P7; 1990, Q3, P18

    277.00 Without mention of meconium ileus 🔒
      Cystic fibrosis NOS
      Ⓔⓧ 277.00-277.09
      Coding Clinic: 2003, Q2, P12

    277.01 With meconium ileus 🔒   N
      Meconium:
        ileus (of newborn)
        obstruction of intestine in mucoviscidosis
      Ⓔⓧ 277.00-277.09

    277.02 With pulmonary manifestations 🔒
      Cystic fibrosis with pulmonary exacerbation
      Use additional code to identify any infectious organism present, such as:
        pseudomonas (041.7)
      Ⓔⓧ 277.00-277.09
      Coding Clinic: 2002, Q4, P46

    277.03 With gastrointestinal manifestations 🔒
      Excludes *with meconium ileus (277.01)*
      Ⓔⓧ 277.00-277.09

    277.09 With other manifestations 🔒
      Ⓔⓧ 277.00-277.09

  277.1 Disorders of porphyrin metabolism 🔒
    Hematoporphyria   Porphyrinuria
    Hematoporphyrinuria   Protocoproporphyria
    Hereditary coproporphyria   Protoporphyria
    Porphyria   Pyrroloporphyria
    Ⓔⓧ 277.1-277.2, 277.4-277.7

  277.2 Other disorders of purine and pyrimidine metabolism 🔒
    Hypoxanthine-guanine-phosphoribosyltransferase deficiency [HG-PRT deficiency]
    Lesch-Nyhan syndrome
    Xanthinuria
    Excludes *gout (274.00–274.9)*
               orotic aciduric anemia (281.4)
    Ⓔⓧ 277.1-277.2, 277.4-277.7

● **277.3 Amyloidosis**
    Disorder resulting from abnormal deposition of particular protein (amyloid) into tissues
    Coding Clinic: 2006, Q4, P66-67; 1997, Q2, P12-13; 1996, Q1, P16; 1985, July-Aug, P9

    277.30 Amyloidosis, unspecified 🔒
      Amyloidosis NOS
      Ⓔⓧ 277.30-277.39, 277.7

    277.31 Familial Mediterranean fever 🔒
      Benign paroxysmal peritonitis
      Hereditary amyloid nephropathy
      Periodic familial polyserositis
      Recurrent polyserositis
      Ⓔⓧ 277.30-277.39, 277.7
      Coding Clinic: 2012, Q2, P18-19

    277.39 Other amyloidosis 🔒
      Hereditary cardiac amyloidosis
      Inherited systemic amyloidosis
      Neuropathic (Portuguese) (Swiss) amyloidosis
      Secondary amyloidosis
      Ⓔⓧ 277.30-277.39, 277.7
      Coding Clinic: 2009, Q1, P17; 2008, Q2, P8-9

ENDOCRINE, NUTRITIONAL AND METABOLIC DISEASES, AND IMMUNITY DISORDERS (240–279)

N   Newborn: 0   P   Pediatric: 0–17   M   Maternity: 12–55   A   Adult: 15–124   ♀   Females Only   ♂   Males Only

Ⓔⓧ   CC/MCC Exclusions   🔒   Complication\Comorbidity   🔒   Major C\C   🔒   Present on Admission Requirement   🔒   Hospital-Acquired Condition

ENDOCRINE, NUTRITIONAL AND METABOLIC DISEASES, AND IMMUNITY DISORDERS (240–279)

277.4 Disorders of bilirubin excretion
   Hyperbilirubinemia: Syndrome:
      congenital   Crigler-Najjar
      constitutional   Dubin-Johnson
                                   Gilbert's
                                   Rotor's

   Excludes *hyperbilirubinemias specific to the perinatal period (774.0–774.7)*

277.5 Mucopolysaccharidosis 🔖
   Gargoylism
   Hunter's syndrome
   Hurler's syndrome
   Lipochondrodystrophy
   Maroteaux-Lamy syndrome
   Morquio-Brailsford disease
   Osteochondrodystrophy
   Sanfilippo's syndrome
   Scheie's syndrome
   (Ex:) 277.1-277.31, 277.4-277.7

277.6 Other deficiencies of circulating enzymes
   Hereditary angioedema
   Coding Clinic: 2010, Q2, P12; 2004, Q4, P59-60

277.7 Dysmetabolic syndrome X
   Use additional code for associated manifestation,
      such as:
      cardiovascular disease (414.00–414.07)
      obesity (278.00–278.03)
   Coding Clinic: 2001, Q4, P42

● **277.8 Other specified disorders of metabolism**
   Coding Clinic: 2003, Q4, P50-51; 2001, Q2, P18-20

   277.81 Primary carnitine deficiency

   277.82 Carnitine deficiency due to inborn errors of metabolism

   277.83 Iatrogenic carnitine deficiency
      Carnitine deficiency due to:
         Hemodialysis
         Valproic acid therapy

   277.84 Other secondary carnitine deficiency

   277.85 Disorders of fatty acid oxidation 🔖
      Carnitine palmitoyltransferase deficiencies
         (CPT1, CPT2)
      Glutaric aciduria type II (type IIA, IIB, IIC)
      Long chain 3-hydroxyacyl CoA dehydrogenase
         deficiency (LCHAD)
      Long chain/very long chain acyl CoA
         dehydrogenase deficiency (LCAD,
         VLCAD)
      Medium chain acyl CoA dehydrogenase
         deficiency (MCAD)
      Short chain acyl CoA dehydrogenase deficiency
         (SCAD)
      Excludes *primary carnitine deficiency (277.81)*
      (Ex:) 277.81-277.84, 277.86-277.87, 277.89
      Coding Clinic: 2004, Q4, P60-61

   277.86 Peroxisomal disorders 🔖
      Adrenomyeloneuropathy
      Neonatal adrenoleukodystrophy
      Rhizomelic chondrodysplasia punctata
      X-linked adrenoleukodystrophy
      Zellweger syndrome
      Excludes *infantile Refsum disease (356.3)*
      (Ex:) 277.4, 277.81-277.85, 277.87-277.89
      Coding Clinic: 2004, Q4, P61-62

277.87 Disorders of mitochondrial metabolism 🔖
   Kearns-Sayre syndrome
   Mitochondrial Encephalopathy, Lactic Acidosis
      and Stroke-like episodes (MELAS
      syndrome)
   Mitochondrial Neurogastrointestinal
      Encephalopathy syndrome (MNGIE)
   Myoclonus with Epilepsy and with Ragged Red
      Fibers (MERRF syndrome)
   Neuropathy, Ataxia and Retinitis Pigmentosa
      (NARP syndrome)
   Use additional code for associated conditions
   Excludes *disorders of pyruvate metabolism (271.8)*
                Leber's optic atrophy (377.16)
                *Leigh's subacute necrotizing
                   encephalopathy (330.8)*
                Reye's syndrome (331.81)
   (Ex:) 277.4, 277.81-277.86, 277.89
   Coding Clinic: 2004, Q4, P62-63

277.88 Tumor lysis syndrome 🔖
   Spontaneous tumor lysis syndrome
   Tumor lysis syndrome following antineoplastic
      drug therapy
   Use additional E code to identify cause,
      if drug-induced
   (Ex:) 277.88, 580.0-581.0, 581.81-581.9, 583.4-584.9
   Coding Clinic: 2009, Q4, P84

277.89 Other specified disorders of metabolism 🔖
   Hand-Schüller-Christian disease
   Histiocytosis (acute) (chronic)
   Histiocytosis X (chronic)
   Excludes *histiocytosis:*
                *acute differentiated progressive
                   (202.5)*
                *adult pulmonary Langerhans cell
                   (516.5)*
                X, acute (progressive) (202.5)
   (Ex:) 277.4, 277.81-277.87

277.9 Unspecified disorder of metabolism
   Enzymopathy NOS
   Coding Clinic: 1987, Sept-Oct, P9

● **278 Overweight, obesity and other hyperalimentation**
   Excludes *hyperalimentation NOS (783.6)*
                poisoning by vitamins NOS (963.5)
                polyphagia (783.6)

● **278.0 Overweight and obesity**
   Excludes *adiposogenital dystrophy (253.8)*
                obesity of endocrine origin NOS (259.9)
   Use additional code to identify Body Mass Index (BMI),
      if known (V85.0–V85.54)
   Coding Clinic: 2005, Q4, P55

   278.00 Obesity, unspecified
      Obesity NOS
      MCE: Questionable admission, principal diagnosis
         only
      Coding Clinic: 2001, Q4, P42; 1999, Q1, P5-6

   278.01 Morbid obesity 🔖
      Severe obesity
      HAC: Principal Diagnosis 278.01, 998.59 (CC),
         and one of the following procedure codes:
         44.38, 44.39, or 44.95
      **Coding Clinic: 2010, Q4, P81; 2009, Q2, P11; 2006, Q2, P5-6;
         2003, Q3, P3-8**

   278.02 Overweight

   278.03 Obesity hypoventilation syndrome 🔖
      Pickwickian syndrome
      (Ex:) 278.03, 416.0-416.1, 416.8-416.9
      Coding Clinic: 2010, Q4, P81

◄ New   ◄▦ Revised   ~~deleted~~ Deleted   Excludes   Includes   Use additional   Code first   Omit code

740   ● Unacceptable Principal Diagnosis   ● Use Additional Digit(s)   ▶ Manifestation Code   OGCR Official Guidelines   Coding Clinic

278.1 Localized adiposity
Fat pad
Coding Clinic: 2006, Q2, P10-11

278.2 Hypervitaminosis A

278.3 Hypercarotinemia

278.4 Hypervitaminosis D

278.8 Other hyperalimentation
Coding Clinic: 2009, Q2, P11

● **279 Disorders involving the immune mechanism**
Use additional code for associated manifestations

● **279.0 Deficiency of humoral immunity**

279.00 Hypogammaglobulinemia, unspecified
Agammaglobulinemia NOS
(Ex) 279.00-279.49, 279.8-279.9

279.01 Selective IgA immunodeficiency
(Ex) 279.00-279.49, 279.8-279.9

279.02 Selective IgM immunodeficiency
(Ex) 279.02-279.49, 279.8-279.9

279.03 Other selective immunoglobulin deficiencies
Selective deficiency of IgG
(Ex) 279.02-279.49, 279.8-279.9

279.04 Congenital hypogammaglobulinemia
Agammaglobulinemia:
Bruton's type
X-linked
(Ex) 279.02-279.49, 279.8-279.9

279.05 Immunodeficiency with increased IgM
Immunodeficiency with hyper-IgM:
autosomal recessive
X-linked
(Ex) 279.02-279.49, 279.8-279.9

279.06 Common variable immunodeficiency
Dysgammaglobulinemia (acquired) (congenital) (primary)
Hypogammaglobulinemia:
acquired primary
congenital non-sex-linked
sporadic
(Ex) 279.02-279.49, 279.8-279.9

279.09 Other
Transient hypogammaglobulinemia of infancy
(Ex) 279.02-279.49, 279.8-279.9

● **279.1 Deficiency of cell-mediated immunity**

279.10 Immunodeficiency with predominant T-cell defect, unspecified
(Ex) 279.02-279.49, 279.8-279.9
Coding Clinic: 1987, Sept-Oct, P10; 1985, Mar-April, P7

279.11 DiGeorge's syndrome
Pharyngeal pouch syndrome
Thymic hypoplasia
(Ex) 279.02-279.49, 279.8-279.9

279.12 Wiskott-Aldrich syndrome
(Ex) 279.02-279.49, 279.8-279.9

279.13 Nezelof's syndrome
Cellular immunodeficiency with abnormal immunoglobulin deficiency
(Ex) 279.02-279.49, 279.8-279.9

279.19 Other
Excludes ataxia-telangiectasia (334.8)
(Ex) 279.02-279.49, 279.8-279.9
Coding Clinic: 1985, Mar-April, P7

279.2 Combined immunity deficiency
Agammaglobulinemia:
autosomal recessive
Swiss-type
X-linked recessive
Severe combined immunodeficiency [SCID]
Thymic:
alymphoplasia
aplasia or dysplasia with immunodeficiency
Excludes thymic hypoplasia (279.11)
(Ex) 279.02-279.49, 279.8-279.9
Coding Clinic: 2011, Q4, P148

279.3 Unspecified immunity deficiency
(Ex) 279.02-279.49, 279.8-279.9

● **279.4 Autoimmune disease, not elsewhere classified**
Excludes transplant failure or rejection (996.80–996.89)
Coding Clinic: 2008, Q3, P5

279.41 Autoimmune lymphoproliferative syndrome
ALPS

279.49 Autoimmune disease, not elsewhere classified
Autoimmune disease NOS
Coding Clinic: 2012, Q3, P8

● **279.5 Graft-versus-host disease**
Code first underlying cause, such as:
complication of blood transfusion (999.89)
complication of transplanted organ (996.80-996.89)
Use additional code to identify associated manifestations, such as:
desquamative dermatitis (695.89)
diarrhea (787.91)
elevated bilirubin (782.4)
hair loss (704.09)
Coding Clinic: 2008, Q4, P97-100

● **279.50 Graft-versus-host disease, unspecified**
(Ex) 279.50-279.53, 996.85, 997.91-997.99

● **279.51 Acute graft-versus-host disease**
(Ex) 279.50-279.53, 996.85, 997.91-997.99
Coding Clinic: 2011, Q4, P148

● **279.52 Chronic graft-versus-host disease**
(Ex) 279.50-279.53, 996.85, 997.91-997.99

● **279.53 Acute on chronic graft-versus-host disease**
(Ex) 279.50-279.53, 996.85, 997.91-997.99

279.8 Other specified disorders involving the immune mechanism
Single complement [C_1-C_9] deficiency or dysfunction

279.9 Unspecified disorder of immune mechanism
Coding Clinic: 1996, Q2, P12; 1992, Q3, P13-14

4. DISEASES OF THE BLOOD AND BLOOD-FORMING ORGANS (280–289)

● **280 Iron deficiency anemias**
Disease characterized by decrease in number of red cells (hemoglobin) in blood, diminishing body's ability to carry adequate amounts of oxygen to cells

Includes anemia:
    asiderotic
    hypochromic-microcytic
    sideropenic

Excludes *familial microcytic anemia (282.49)*

280.0 Secondary to blood loss (chronic)
Normocytic anemia due to blood loss

Excludes *acute posthemorrhagic anemia (285.1)*

Coding Clinic: 2013, Q3, P4; 1993, Q4, P34; 1985, July-Aug, P13

280.1 Secondary to inadequate dietary iron intake

280.8 Other specified iron deficiency anemias
Paterson-Kelly syndrome
Plummer-Vinson syndrome
Sideropenic dysphagia

280.9 Iron deficiency anemia, unspecified
Anemia:
    achlorhydric
    chlorotic
    idiopathic hypochromic
    iron [Fe] deficiency NOS

● **281 Other deficiency anemias**

281.0 Pernicious anemia
Anemia:
    Addison's
    Biermer's
    congenital pernicious
Congenital intrinsic factor [Castle's] deficiency

Excludes *combined system disease without mention of anemia (266.2)*
subacute degeneration of spinal cord without mention of anemia (266.2)

281.1 Other vitamin B$_{12}$ deficiency anemia
Anemia:
    vegan's
    vitamin B$_{12}$ deficiency (dietary)
    due to selective vitamin B$_{12}$ malabsorption with proteinuria
Syndrome:
    Imerslund's
    Imerslund-Gräsbeck

Excludes *combined system disease without mention of anemia (266.2)*
subacute degeneration of spinal cord without mention of anemia (266.2)

281.2 Folate-deficiency anemia
Congenital folate malabsorption
Folate or folic acid deficiency anemia:
    NOS
    dietary
    drug-induced
Goat's milk anemia
Nutritional megaloblastic anemia (of infancy)

Use additional E code to identify drug

281.3 Other specified megaloblastic anemias, not elsewhere classified
Combined B$_{12}$ and folate-deficiency anemia

281.4 Protein-deficiency anemia
Amino-acid-deficiency anemia

281.8 Anemia associated with other specified nutritional deficiency
Scorbutic anemia

281.9 Unspecified deficiency anemia
Anemia:
    dimorphic
    macrocytic
    megaloblastic NOS
    nutritional NOS
    simple chronic
Coding Clinic: 2011, Q1, P16; 1984, Sept-Oct, P16

● **282 Hereditary hemolytic anemias**
Genetic condition in which bone marrow is unable to compensate for premature destruction of red blood cells

282.0 Hereditary spherocytosis
Acholuric (familial) jaundice
Congenital hemolytic anemia (spherocytic)
Congenital spherocytosis
Minkowski-Chauffard syndrome
Spherocytosis (familial)

Excludes *hemolytic anemia of newborn (773.0–773.5)*

282.1 Hereditary elliptocytosis
Elliptocytosis (congenital)
Ovalocytosis (congenital) (hereditary)

282.2 Anemias due to disorders of glutathione metabolism
Anemia:
    6-phosphogluconic dehydrogenase deficiency
    enzyme deficiency, drug-induced
    erythrocytic glutathione deficiency
    glucose-6-phosphate dehydrogenase [G-6-PD] deficiency
    glutathione-reductase deficiency
    hemolytic nonspherocytic (hereditary), type I
Disorder of pentose phosphate pathway
Favism

282.3 Other hemolytic anemias due to enzyme deficiency
Anemia:
    hemolytic nonspherocytic (hereditary), type II
    hexokinase deficiency
    pyruvate kinase [PK] deficiency
    triosephosphate isomerase deficiency

● **282.4 Thalassemias**
Hereditary disorders characterized by low production of hemoglobin or excessive destruction of red blood cells

Excludes *sickle-cell:*
*   disease (282.60–282.69)*
*   trait (282.5)*

Coding Clinic: 2003, Q4, P51-56

282.40 Thalassemia, unspecified
Thalassemia NOS

282.41 Sickle-cell thalassemia without crisis
Microdrepanocytosis
Sickle-cell thalassemia NOS
Thalassemia Hb-S disease without crisis

282.42 Sickle-cell thalassemia with crisis 🖉
Sickle-cell thalassemia with vaso-occlusive pain
Thalassemia Hb-S disease with crisis

Use additional code for type of crisis, such as:
    Acute chest syndrome (517.3)
    Splenic sequestration (289.52)
    Occurs when sickled red blood cells become entrapped in spleen, causing splenomegaly (enlargement) and decreased circulating blood volume
(Ex) 280.0-285.9, 286.53, 289.81-289.83, 289.89-289.9, 517.3

282.43 Alpha thalassemia
Alpha thalassemia major
Hemoglobin H Constant Spring
Hemoglobin H disease
Hydrops fetalis due to alpha thalassemia
Severe alpha thalassemia
Triple gene defect alpha thalassemia

Excludes *alpha thalassemia trait or minor (282.46)*
hydrops fetalis due to isoimmunization (773.3)
hydrops fetalis not due to immune hemolysis (778.0)

◀ New   ◀▥ Revised   ~~deleted~~ Deleted   Excludes   Includes   Use additional   Code first   Omit code
● Unacceptable Principal Diagnosis   ● Use Additional Digit(s)   ▶ Manifestation Code   OGCR Official Guidelines   Coding Clinic
742

282.44 **Beta thalassemia**
Beta thalassemia major
Cooley's anemia
Homozygous beta thalassemia
Severe beta thalassemia
Thalassemia intermedia
Thalassemia major

> **Excludes** *beta thalassemia minor (282.46)*
> *beta thalassemia trait (282.46)*
> *delta-beta thalassemia (282.45)*
> *hemoglobin E beta thalassemia (282.47)*
> *sickle-cell beta thalassemia (282.41, 282.42)*

282.45 **Delta-beta thalassemia**
Homozygous delta-beta thalassemia

> **Excludes** *delta-beta thalassemia trait (282.46)*

282.46 **Thalassemia minor**
Alpha thalassemia minor
Alpha thalassemia silent carrier
Alpha thalassemia trait
Beta thalassemia minor
Beta thalassemia trait
Delta-beta thalassemia trait
Thalassemia trait NOS

> **Excludes** *alpha thalassemia (282.43)*
> *beta thalassemia (282.44)*
> *delta-beta thalassemia (282.45)*
> *hemoglobin E-beta thalassemia (282.47)*
> *sickle-cell trait (282.5)*

282.47 **Hemoglobin E-beta thalassemia**

> **Excludes** *beta thalassemia (282.44)*
> *beta thalassemia minor (282.46)*
> *beta thalassemia trait (282.46)*
> *delta-beta thalassemia (282.45)*
> *delta-beta thalassemia trait (282.46)*
> *hemoglobin E disease (282.7)*
> *other hemoglobinopathies (282.7)*
> *sickle-cell beta thalassemia (282.41, 282.42)*

282.49 **Other thalassemia**
Dominant thalassemia
Hemoglobin C thalassemia
Hereditary leptocytosis
Mediterranean anemia (with other hemoglobinopathy)
Mixed thalassemia
Thalassemia with other hemoglobinopathy

> **Excludes** *hemoglobin C disease (282.7)*
> *hemoglobin E disease (282.7)*
> *other hemoglobinopathies (282.7)*
> *sickle-cell anemias (282.60-282.69)*
> *sickle-cell beta thalassemia (282.41-282.42)*

282.5 **Sickle-cell trait**
Hb-AS genotype
Hemoglobin S [Hb-S] trait
Heterozygous:
hemoglobin S
Hb-S

> **Excludes** *that with other hemoglobinopathy (282.60–282.69)*
> *that with thalassemia (282.41-282.42)*
> **Coding Clinic: 2012, Q3, P5; 2003, Q4, P51-56**

● 282.6 **Sickle-cell disease**
Inherited disease in which red blood cells, normally disc-shaped, become crescent shaped. Small blood clots form, resulting in painful episodes called sickle cell crises.
Sickle-cell anemia

> **Excludes** *sickle-cell thalassemia (282.41–282.42)*
> *sickle-cell trait (282.5)*

282.60 **Sickle-cell disease, unspecified**
Sickle-cell anemia NOS
Coding Clinic: 1997, Q2, P11

282.61 **Hb-SS disease without crisis**
Coding Clinic: 2007, Q2, P9-10

282.62 **Hb-SS disease with crisis** 🖐
Hb-SS disease with vaso-occlusive pain
Sickle-cell crisis NOS

> Use additional code for type of crisis, such as:
> Acute chest syndrome (517.3)
> Splenic sequestration (289.52)
> (Ex) 280.0-285.9, 286.53, 289.81-289.83, 289.89-289.9, 517.3
> **Coding Clinic: 2010, Q4, P78; 2003, Q4, P51-56; 1998, Q2, P8; 1991, Q2, P15**

282.63 **Sickle-cell/Hb-C disease without crisis**
Hb-S/Hb-C disease without crisis

282.64 **Sickle-cell/Hb-C disease with crisis** 🖐
Hb-S/Hb-C disease with crisis
Sickle-cell/Hb-C disease with vaso-occlusive pain

> Use additional code for types of crisis, such as:
> Acute chest syndrome (517.3)
> Splenic sequestration (289.52)
> (Ex) 280.0-285.9, 286.53, 289.81-289.83, 289.89-289.9, 517.3

282.68 **Other sickle-cell disease without crisis**
Hb-S/Hb-D disease without crisis
Hb-S/Hb-E disease without crisis
Sickle-cell/Hb-D disease without crisis
Sickle-cell/Hb-E disease without crisis

282.69 **Other sickle-cell disease with crisis** 🖐
Hb-S/Hb-D disease with crisis
Hb-S/Hb-E disease with crisis
Other sickle-cell disease with vaso-occlusive pain
Sickle-cell/Hb-D disease with crisis
Sickle-cell/Hb-E disease with crisis

> Use additional code for type of crisis, such as:
> Acute chest syndrome (517.3)
> Splenic sequestration (289.52)
> (Ex) 280.0-285.9, 286.53, 289.81-289.83, 289.89-289.9, 517.3

282.7 **Other hemoglobinopathies**
Abnormal hemoglobin NOS
Congenital Heinz-body anemia
Disease:
hemoglobin C [Hb-C]
hemoglobin D [Hb-D]
hemoglobin E [Hb-E]
hemoglobin Zurich [Hb-Zurich]
Hemoglobinopathy NOS
Hereditary persistence of fetal hemoglobin [HPFH]
Unstable hemoglobin hemolytic disease

> **Excludes** *familial polycythemia (289.6)*
> *hemoglobin E-beta thalassemia (282.47)*
> *hemoglobin M [Hb-M] disease (289.7)*
> *high-oxygen-affinity hemoglobin (289.0)*
> *other hemoglobinopathies with thalassemia (282.49)*

282.8 **Other specified hereditary hemolytic anemias** 🖐
Stomatocytosis
(Ex) 280.0-285.9, 289.9, 517.3, 776.5-776.6

282.9 **Hereditary hemolytic anemia, unspecified** 🖐
Hereditary hemolytic anemia NOS
(Ex) 280.0-285.9, 289.9, 517.3, 776.5-776.6

DISEASES OF THE BLOOD AND BLOOD-FORMING ORGANS (280–289)

N Newborn: 0   **P** Pediatric: 0–17   **M** Maternity: 12–55   **A** Adult: 15–124   ♀ Females Only   ♂ Males Only

(Ex) CC/MCC Exclusions   🖐 Complication\Comorbidity   🖐 Major C\C   🖐 Present on Admission Requirement   🖐 Hospital-Acquired Condition   **743**

DISEASES OF THE BLOOD AND BLOOD-FORMING ORGANS (280–289)

● **283   Acquired hemolytic anemias**
> *Also known as autoimmune hemolytic or Coombs positive hemolytic anemia. The red blood cells produced are healthy but are destroyed when trapped in the spleen by infection or certain drugs.*

     283.0   Autoimmune hemolytic anemias 🔖
         Autoimmune hemolytic disease (cold type) (warm type)
         Chronic cold hemagglutinin disease
         Cold agglutinin disease or hemoglobinuria
         Hemolytic anemia:
            cold type (secondary) (symptomatic)
            drug-induced
            warm type (secondary) (symptomatic)
         Use additional E code to identify cause, if drug-induced
         Excludes   *Evans'syndrome (287.32)*
                hemolytic disease of newborn (773.0–773.5)
         (Ex) 280.0-285.9, 286.53, 289.81-289.83, 289.89-289.9, 517.3
         Coding Clinic: 2008, Q3, P5

● **283.1   Non-autoimmune hemolytic anemias**
     283.10   Non-autoimmune hemolytic anemia, unspecified 🔖
         (Ex) 280.0-285.9, 286.53, 289.81-289.83, 289.89-289.9, 517.3

     283.11   Hemolytic-uremic syndrome 🔖
         Use additional code to identify associated:
            E. coli infection (041.41-041.49)
            Pneumococcal pneumonia (481)
            Shigella dysenteriae (004.0)
         (Ex) 280.0-285.9, 286.53, 289.81-289.83, 289.89-289.9, 517.3

     283.19   Other non-autoimmune hemolytic anemias 🔖
         Hemolytic anemia:
            mechanical
            microangiopathic
            toxic
         Use additional E code to identify cause
         (Ex) 280.0-285.9, 286.53, 289.81-289.83, 289.89-289.9, 517.3

     283.2   Hemoglobinuria due to hemolysis from external causes
         Acute intravascular hemolysis
         Hemoglobinuria:
            from exertion
            march
            paroxysmal (cold) (nocturnal)
            due to other hemolysis
         Marchiafava-Micheli syndrome
         Use additional E code to identify cause

     283.9   Acquired hemolytic anemia, unspecified 🔖
         Acquired hemolytic anemia NOS
         Chronic idiopathic hemolytic anemia
         (Ex) 280.0-285.9, 286.53, 289.81-289.83, 289.89-289.9, 517.3

● **284   Aplastic anemia and other bone marrow failure syndromes**
     Coding Clinic: 2006, Q4, P67-69

● **284.0   Constitutional aplastic anemia**
     Coding Clinic: 1991, Q1, P14

     284.01   Constitutional red blood cell aplasia 🔖
         Aplasia, (pure) red cell:
            congenital
            of infants
            primary
         Blackfan-Diamond syndrome
         Familial hypoplastic anemia
         (Ex) 280.0-284.09, 284.81-285.9, 289.9, 776.5-776.6

     284.09   Other constitutional aplastic anemia 🔖
         Fanconi's anemia
         Pancytopenia with malformations
         (Ex) 280.0-284.09, 284.81-285.9, 287.30-287.39, 289.9, 776.5-776.6

● **284.1   Pancytopenia**
> *Marked deficiency of all the blood elements: Red blood cells (erythrocytes), white blood cells (leukocytes), and platelets (thrombocytes). Check laboratory results.*

         Excludes   *pancytopenia (due to) (with):*
            aplastic anemia NOS (284.9)
            bone marrow infiltration (284.2)
            constitutional red blood cell aplasia (284.01)
            hairy cell leukemia (202.4)
            human immunodeficiency virus disease (042)
            leukoerythroblastic anemia (284.2)
            malformations (284.09)
            myelodysplastic syndromes (238.72–238.75)
            myeloproliferative disease (238.79)
            other constitutional aplastic anemia (284.09)
     Coding Clinic: 2011, Q1, P6; 2005, Q3, P11-12

     284.11   Antineoplastic chemotherapy induced pancytopenia 🔖
         Excludes   *aplastic anemia due to antineoplastic chemotherapy (284.89)*
         (Ex) 284.11-285.9, 288.00-288.09, 288.4-288.62, 288.66-288.69, 289.9, 776.6
         Coding Clinic: 2011, Q4, P92

     284.12   Other drug-induced pancytopenia 🔖
         Excludes   *aplastic anemia due to drugs (284.89)*
         (Ex) 284.11-285.9, 288.00-288.09, 288.4-288.62, 288.66-288.69, 289.9, 776.6

     284.19   Other pancytopenia 🔖
         (Ex) 284.11-285.9, 288.00-288.09, 288.4-288.62, 288.66-288.69, 289.9, 776.6

▸ **284.2   *Myelophthisis*** 🔖
         Leukoerythroblastic anemia
         Myelophthisic anemia
         Code first the underlying disorder, such as:
            malignant neoplasm of breast (174.0–174.9, 175.0–175.9)
            tuberculosis (015.0–015.9)
         Excludes   *idiopathic myelofibrosis (238.76)*
                myelofibrosis NOS (289.83)
                myelofibrosis with myeloid metaplasia (238.76)
                primary myelofibrosis (238.76)
                secondary myelofibrosis (289.83)
         (Ex) 284.11-285.9, 288.00-288.09, 288.4-288.62, 288.66-288.69, 289.9, 776.6

● **284.8   Other specified aplastic anemias**
     Coding Clinic: 2007, Q4, P72-73; 2005, Q3, P11-12; 1997, Q1, P5-6; 1991, Q1, P14; 1984, Sept-Oct, P16

     284.81   Red cell aplasia (acquired) (adult) (with thymoma) 🔖
         Red cell aplasia NOS
         (Ex) 280.0-285.9, 286.53, 289.81-289.83, 289.89-289.9, 517.3

     284.89   Other specified aplastic anemias 🔖
         Aplastic anemia (due to):
            chronic systemic disease
            drugs
            infection
            radiation
            toxic (paralytic)
         Use additional E code to identify cause
         (Ex) 280.0-285.9, 286.53, 289.81-289.83, 289.89-289.9, 517.3
         Coding Clinic: 2011, Q1, P6; 2009, Q1, P17; 2008, Q2, P6

● **284.9   Aplastic anemia, unspecified** 🔖
         Anemia:
            aplastic (idiopathic) NOS
            aregenerative
            hypoplastic NOS
            nonregenerative
         Medullary hypoplasia
         Excludes   *refractory anemia (238.72)*
         (Ex) 280.0-285.9, 286.53, 289.81-289.83, 289.89-289.9, 517.3
         Coding Clinic: 2011, Q1, P6

◀ New   ◀◀ Revised   ~~deleted~~ Deleted   Excludes   Includes   Use additional   Code first   Omit code

744   ● Unacceptable Principal Diagnosis   ● Use Additional Digit(s)   ▸ Manifestation Code   **OGCR** Official Guidelines   Coding Clinic

● **285 Other and unspecified anemias**
Coding Clinic: 1990, Q3, P17

285.0 Sideroblastic anemia
Anemia:
hypochromic with iron loading
sideroachrestic
sideroblastic:
acquired
congenital
hereditary
primary
secondary (drug-induced) (due to disease)
sex-linked hypochromic
vitamin B₆-responsive
Pyridoxine-responsive (hypochromic) anemia

Excludes *refractory sideroblastic anemia (238.72)*

Use additional E code to identify cause, if drug-induced

285.1 Acute posthemorrhagic anemia 🍇
Anemia due to acute blood loss

Excludes *anemia due to chronic blood loss (280.0)*
blood loss anemia NOS (280.0)

(Ex) 280.0-285.9, 286.53, 289.81-289.83, 289.89-289.9, 517.3, 958.2
Coding Clinic: 2013, Q3, P9; 2011, Q4, P147; 2007, Q1, P19; 2004, Q3, P4; 1993, Q4, P34; 1992, Q2, P15-16

● **285.2 Anemia of chronic disease**
Anemia in (due to) (with) chronic illness

285.21 Anemia in chronic kidney disease
Anemia in end stage renal disease
Erythropoietin-resistant anemia (EPO resistant anemia)
Coding Clinic: 2000, Q4, P39-40

285.22 Anemia in neoplastic disease

Excludes *anemia due to antineoplastic chemotherapy (285.3)*
aplastic anemia due to antineoplastic chemotherapy (284.89)

Coding Clinic: 2009, Q4, P94x2; 2008, Q2, P6; 2000, Q4, P39-40

285.29 Anemia of other chronic disease
Anemia in other chronic illness

OGCR   Section I.C.4.a.2

When assigning code 285.22, Anemia in neoplastic disease, it is also necessary to assign the neoplasm code that is responsible for the anemia. Code 285.22 is for use for anemia that is due to the malignancy, not for anemia due to antineoplastic chemotherapy drugs. Assign the appropriate code for anemia due to antineoplastic chemotherapy.

285.3 Antineoplastic chemotherapy induced anemia
Anemia due to antineoplastic chemotherapy

Excludes *anemia due to drug NEC – code to type of anemia*
anemia in neoplastic disease (285.22)
aplastic anemia due to antineoplastic chemotherapy (284.89)

Coding Clinic: 2009, Q4, P94x2

285.8 Other specified anemias
Anemia:
dyserythropoietic (congenital)
dyshematopoietic (congenital)
von Jaksch's
Infantile pseudoleukemia

285.9 Anemia, unspecified
Anemia:
NOS
essential
normocytic, not due to blood loss
profound
progressive
secondary
Oligocythemia

Excludes *anemia (due to):*
blood loss:
acute (285.1)
chronic or unspecified (280.0)
iron deficiency (280.0–280.9)

Coding Clinic: 2011, Q1, P16; 2009, Q1, P17x2; 2007, Q1, P19; 2002, Q1, P14; 1992, Q2, P15-16; 1985, Mar-April, P13

● **286 Coagulation defects**
Can be acquired or genetic and results in inability to control blood clotting. Most common genetic coagulation disorder is hemophilia.
Coding Clinic: 2006, Q2, P17; 1992, Q3, P15

286.0 Congenital factor VIII disorder 🍇
Antihemophilic globulin [AHG] deficiency
Factor VIII (functional) deficiency
Hemophilia:
NOS
A
classical
familial
hereditary
Subhemophilia

Excludes *factor VIII deficiency with vascular defect (286.4)*

(Ex) 286.0-287.9, 289.81-289.9

286.1 Congenital factor IX disorder 🍇
Christmas disease
Deficiency:
factor IX (functional)
plasma thromboplastin component [PTC]
Hemophilia B
(Ex) 286.0-287.9, 289.81-289.9

286.2 Congenital factor XI deficiency 🍇
Hemophilia C
Plasma thromboplastin antecedent [PTA] deficiency
Rosenthal's disease
(Ex) 286.0-287.9, 289.81-289.9

286.3 Congenital deficiency of other clotting factors 🍇
Congenital afibrinogenemia
Deficiency:
AC globulin factor:
I [fibrinogen]
II [prothrombin]
V [labile]
VII [stable]
X [Stuart-Prower]
XII [Hageman]
XIII [fibrin stabilizing]
Laki-Lorand factor
proaccelerin
Disease:
Owren's
Stuart-Prower
Dysfibrinogenemia (congenital)
Dysprothrombinemia (constitutional)
Hypoproconvertinemia
Hypoprothrombinemia (hereditary)
Parahemophilia
(Ex) 286.0-287.9, 289.81-289.9

N Newborn: 0   **P** Pediatric: 0–17   **M** Maternity: 12–55   **A** Adult: 15–124   ♀ Females Only   ♂ Males Only

(Ex) CC/MCC Exclusions   🍇 Complication\Comorbidity   🍇 Major C\C   🍇 Present on Admission Requirement   🍇 Hospital-Acquired Condition

745

DISEASES OF THE BLOOD AND BLOOD-FORMING ORGANS (280–289)

286.4 **von Willebrand's disease** 🔗
   Angiohemophilia (A) (B)
   Constitutional thrombopathy
   Factor VIII deficiency with vascular defect
   Pseudohemophilia type B
   Vascular hemophilia
   von Willebrand's (-Jürgens') disease
   Excludes *factor VIII deficiency:*
      NOS (286.0)
      with functional defect (286.0)
      hereditary capillary fragility (287.8)
   Ⓔ 286.0-287.9, 289.81-289.9

● 286.5 **Hemorrhagic disorder due to intrinsic circulating anticoagulants, antibodies, or inhibitors**
   Coding Clinic: 2004, Q3, P7; 1994, Q1, P22; 1993, 5th Issue, P16; 1992, Q3, P15-16; 1990, Q3, P14

286.52 **Acquired hemophilia** 🔗
   Autoimmune hemophilia
   Autoimmune inhibitors to clotting factors
   Secondary hemophilia
   Ⓔ 286.0-287.9, 289.81-289.82, 289.84-289.9

286.53 **Antiphospholipid antibody with hemorrhagic disorder** 🔗
   Lupus anticoagulant (LAC) with hemorrhagic disorder
   Systemic lupus erythematosus [SLE] inhibitor with hemorrhagic disorder
   Excludes *antiphospholipid antibody, finding*
      without diagnosis (795.79)
      antiphospholipid antibody syndrome
      (289.81)
      antiphospholipid antibody with
      hypercoagulable state (289.81)
      lupus anticoagulant (LAC) finding
      without diagnosis (795.79)
      lupus anticoagulant (LAC) with
      hypercoagulable state (289.81)
      systemic lupus erythematosus [SLE]
      inhibitor finding without
      diagnosis (795.79)
      systemic lupus erythematosus [SLE]
      inhibitor with hypercoagulable
      state (289.81)
   Ⓔ 286.0-287.9, 289.81-289.82, 289.84-289.9

286.59 **Other hemorrhagic disorder due to intrinsic circulating anticoagulants, antibodies, or inhibitors** 🔗
   Antithrombinemia
   Antithromboplastinemia
   Antithromboplastinogenemia
   Increase in:
      anti-II (prothrombin)
      anti-VIIIa
      anti-IXa
      anti-XIa
   Ⓔ 286.0-287.9, 289.81-289.82, 289.84-289.9

286.6 **Defibrination syndrome** 🔗
   Afibrinogenemia, acquired
   Consumption coagulopathy
   Diffuse or disseminated intravascular coagulation [DIC syndrome]
   Fibrinolytic hemorrhage, acquired
   Hemorrhagic fibrinogenolysis
   Pathologic fibrinolysis
   Purpura:
      fibrinolytic
      fulminans
   Excludes *that complicating:*
      abortion (634–638 with .1, 639.1)
      pregnancy or the puerperium
      (641.3, 666.3)
      disseminated intravascular coagulation in
      newborn (776.2)
   Ⓔ 286.0-287.9, 289.81-289.9

286.7 **Acquired coagulation factor deficiency** 🔗
   Deficiency of coagulation factor due to:
      liver disease
      vitamin K deficiency
   Hypoprothrombinemia, acquired
   Excludes *vitamin K deficiency of newborn (776.0)*
   Use additional E-code to identify cause, if drug-induced
   Ⓔ 286.0-287.9, 289.81-289.9

286.9 **Other and unspecified coagulation defects** 🔗
   Defective coagulation NOS
   Deficiency, coagulation factor NOS
   Delay, coagulation
   Disorder:
      coagulation
      hemostasis
   Excludes *abnormal coagulation profile (790.92)*
      hemorrhagic disease of newborn (776.0)
      that complicating:
      abortion (634–638 with .1, 639.1)
      pregnancy or the puerperium
      (641.3, 666.3)
   Ⓔ 286.0-287.9, 289.81-289.9
   Coding Clinic: 1999, Q4, P22-23

● 287 **Purpura and other hemorrhagic conditions**
   Excludes *hemorrhagic thrombocythemia (238.79)*
      purpura fulminans (286.6)

287.0 **Allergic purpura** 🔗
   Peliosis rheumatica
   Purpura:
      anaphylactoid
      autoimmune
      Henoch's
      nonthrombocytopenic:
         hemorrhagic
         idiopathic
         rheumatica
      Schönlein-Henoch
      vascular
   Vasculitis, allergic
   Excludes *hemorrhagic purpura (287.39)*
      purpura annularis telangiectodes (709.1)
   Ⓔ 286.0-287.9, 289.81-289.9

287.1 **Qualitative platelet defects**
   Thrombasthenia (hemorrhagic) (hereditary)
   Thrombocytasthenia
   Thrombocytopathy (dystrophic)
   Thrombopathy (Bernard-Soulier)
   Excludes *von Willebrand's disease (286.4)*

287.2 **Other nonthrombocytopenic purpuras**
   Purpura:
      NOS
      senile
      simplex

● 287.3 **Primary thrombocytopenia**
   Also known as idiopathic thrombocytopenia, may be acquired or congenital and is a common cause of coagulation disorders
   Excludes *thrombotic thrombocytopenic purpura (446.6)*
      transient thrombocytopenia of newborn (776.1)
      Thrombo = clot forming, cyto = cell, penia = deficiency of: deficiency of platelets

287.30 **Primary thrombocytopenia unspecified**
   Megakaryocytic hypoplasia

287.31 **Immune thrombocytopenic purpura** 🔗
   Idiopathic thrombocytopenic purpura
   Tidal platelet dysgenesis
   Ⓔ 286.0-287.9, 289.81-289.9
   Coding Clinic: 2005, Q4, P56-57

287.32 **Evans' syndrome** 🔗
   Ⓔ 286.0-287.9, 289.81-289.9

287.33 Congenital and hereditary thrombocytopenic purpura 🔵
Congenital and hereditary thrombocytopenia
Thrombocytopenia with absent radii (TAR) syndrome

Excludes *Wiskott-Aldrich syndrome (279.12)*
(Ex:) 286.0-287.9, 289.81-289.9

287.39 Other primary thrombocytopenia

● **287.4 Secondary thrombocytopenia**
Use additional E code to identify cause

Excludes *heparin-induced thrombocytopenia (HIT) (289.84)*
transient thrombocytopenia of newborn (776.1)
Coding Clinic: 1985, July-Aug, P13; Mar-April, P14

287.41 Posttransfusion purpura
Posttransfusion purpura from whole blood (fresh) or blood products
PTP

287.49 Other secondary thrombocytopenia
Thrombocytopenia (due to):
dilutional
drugs
extracorporeal circulation of blood
massive blood transfusion
platelet alloimmunization
secondary NOS

287.5 Thrombocytopenia, unspecified

287.8 Other specified hemorrhagic conditions
Capillary fragility (hereditary)
Vascular pseudohemophilia
Coding Clinic: 1985, Mar-April, P14

287.9 Unspecified hemorrhagic conditions
Hemorrhagic diathesis (familial)

● **288 Diseases of white blood cells**
Excludes *leukemia (204.0–208.9)*

● **288.0 Neutropenia**
Decreased Absolute Neutrophil Count (ANC)
Use additional code for any associated:
fever (780.61)
mucositis (478.11, 528.00–528.09, 538, 616.81)
Excludes *neutropenic splenomegaly (289.53)*
transitory neonatal neutropenia (776.7)
Coding Clinic: 2005, Q3, P11-12; 1999, Q3, P6-7; 1996, Q3, P16; Q2, P6; 1985, Mar-April, P14

288.00 Neutropenia, unspecified

288.01 Congenital neutropenia
Congenital agranulocytosis
Infantile genetic agranulocytosis
Kostmann's syndrome

288.02 Cyclic neutropenia
Cyclic hematopoiesis
Periodic neutropenia

288.03 Drug induced neutropenia
Use additional E code to identify drug
Coding Clinic: 2006, Q4, P69-73

288.04 Neutropenia due to infection

288.09 Other neutropenia
Agranulocytosis
Neutropenia:
immune
toxic

288.1 Functional disorders of polymorphonuclear neutrophils
Chronic (childhood) granulomatous disease
Congenital dysphagocytosis
Job's syndrome
Lipochrome histiocytosis (familial)
Progressive septic granulomatosis

288.2 Genetic anomalies of leukocytes
Anomaly (granulation) (granulocyte) or syndrome:
Alder's (-Reilly)
Chédiak-Steinbrinck (-Higashi)
Jordan's
May-Hegglin
Pelger-Huet
Hereditary:
hypersegmentation
hyposegmentation
leukomelanopathy

288.3 Eosinophilia
Eosinophilia
allergic
hereditary
idiopathic
secondary
Eosinophilic leukocytosis
Excludes *Löffler's syndrome (518.3)*
pulmonary eosinophilia (518.3)
Coding Clinic: 2010, Q3, P16-17; 2000, Q3, P11

288.4 Hemophagocytic syndromes 🔵
Familial hemophagocytic lymphohistiocytosis
Familial hemophagocytic reticulosis
Hemophagocytic syndrome, infection-associated
Histiocytic syndromes
Macrophage activation syndrome
(Ex:) 284.11-284.9, 286.6, 287.30-288.09, 288.50, 288.59, 289.84, 289.9

● **288.5 Decreased white blood cell count**
Excludes *neutropenia (288.01–288.09)*

288.50 Leukocytopenia, unspecified
Decreased leukocytes, unspecified
Decreased white blood cell count, unspecified
Leukopenia NOS

288.51 Lymphocytopenia
Decreased lymphocytes

288.59 Other decreased white blood cell count
Basophilic leukopenia
Eosinophilic leukopenia
Monocytopenia
Plasmacytopenia

● **288.6 Elevated white blood cell count**
Excludes *eosinophilia (288.3)*

288.60 Leukocytosis, unspecified
Elevated leukocytes, unspecified
Elevated white blood cell count, unspecified

288.61 Lymphocytosis (symptomatic)
Elevated lymphocytes

288.62 Leukemoid reaction
Basophilic leukemoid reaction
Lymphocytic leukemoid reaction
Monocytic leukemoid reaction
Myelocytic leukemoid reaction
Neutrophilic leukemoid reaction

288.63 Monocytosis (symptomatic)
Excludes *infectious mononucleosis (075)*

288.64 Plasmacytosis

288.65 Basophilia

288.66 Bandemia
Bandemia without diagnosis of specific infection
Excludes *confirmed infection – code to infection*
leukemia (204.00–208.9)
Coding Clinic: 2007, Q4, P73-74

288.69 Other elevated white blood cell count

288.8 Other specified disease of white blood cells
Excludes *decreased white blood cell counts (288.50–288.59)*
elevated white blood cell counts (288.60–288.69)
immunity disorders (279.0–279.9)
Coding Clinic: 1987, Mar-April, P12

288.9 Unspecified disease of white blood cells

DISEASES OF THE BLOOD AND BLOOD-FORMING ORGANS (280–289)

● **289 Other diseases of blood and blood-forming organs**

289.0 Polycythemia, secondary

See 238.4 for primary polycythemia (polycythemia vera).

High-oxygen-affinity hemoglobin

Polycythemia:

    acquired

    benign

    due to:

        fall in plasma volume

        high altitude

    emotional

    erythropoietin

    hypoxemic

    nephrogenous

    relative

    spurious

    stress

Excludes   *polycythemia:*
           neonatal (776.4)
           primary (238.4)
           vera (238.4)

289.1 Chronic lymphadenitis

Chronic:

    adenitis any lymph node, except mesenteric

    lymphadenitis any lymph node, except mesenteric

Excludes   *acute lymphadenitis (683)*
           mesenteric (289.2)
           enlarged glands NOS (785.6)

289.2 Nonspecific mesenteric lymphadenitis

Mesenteric lymphadenitis (acute) (chronic)

289.3 Lymphadenitis, unspecified, except mesenteric

Coding Clinic: 2012, Q2, 18-19; 1992, Q2, P8

289.4 Hypersplenism

"Big spleen" syndrome

Dyssplenism

Hypersplenia

Excludes   *primary splenic neutropenia (289.53)*

● **289.5 Other diseases of spleen**

289.50 Disease of spleen, unspecified

289.51 Chronic congestive splenomegaly

▸ **289.52 *Splenic sequestration***

Code first sickle-cell disease in crisis (282.42, 282.62, 282.64, 282.69)

Coding Clinic: 2003, Q4, P51-56

289.53 Neutropenic splenomegaly

289.59 Other

Lien migrans   Splenic:

Perisplenitis   fibrosis

Splenic: infarction

    abscess   rupture, nontraumatic

    atrophy   Splenitis

    cyst   Wandering spleen

Excludes   *bilharzial splenic fibrosis
              (120.0–120.9)*
           hepatolienal fibrosis (571.5)
           splenomegaly NOS (789.2)

289.6 Familial polycythemia

Familial:

    benign polycythemia

    erythrocytosis

289.7 Methemoglobinemia 🔗

Congenital NADH [DPNH]-methemoglobin-reductase
    deficiency

Hemoglobin M [Hb-M] disease

Methemoglobinemia:

    NOS

    acquired (with sulfhemoglobinemia)

    hereditary

    toxic

Stokvis' disease

Sulfhemoglobinemia

Use additional E code to identify cause

Ⓔⓧ 282.7-283.10, 283.19-283.9, 285.3-285.9, 289.7, 289.9

● **289.8 Other specified diseases of blood and blood-forming organs**

Coding Clinic: 2003, Q4, P56-57; 2002, Q1, P16-17; 1987, Mar-April, P12

289.81 Primary hypercoagulable state 🔗

Activated protein C resistance

Antiphospholipid antibody syndrome

Antithrombin III deficiency

Factor V Leiden mutation

Lupus anticoagulant with hypercoagulable state

Protein C deficiency

Protein S deficiency

Prothrombin gene mutation

Systemic lupus erythematosus [SLE] inhibitor
    with hypercoagulable state

Excludes   *anti-phospholipid antibody, finding
              without diagnosis (795.79)*
           *anti-phospholipid antibody with
              hemorrhagic disorder (286.53)*
           *lupus anticoagulant (LAC) finding
              without diagnosis (795.79)*
           *lupus anticoagulant (LAC) with
              hemorrhagic disorder (286.53)*
           *secondary activated protein C resistance
              (289.82)*
           *secondary antiphospholipid antibody
              syndrome (289.82)*
           *secondary lupus anticoagulant with
              hypercoagulable state (289.82)*
           *secondary systemic lupus erythematosus
              [SLE] inhibitor with
              hypercoagulable state (289.82)*
           *systemic lupus erythematosus [SLE]
              inhibitor finding without
              diagnosis (795.79)*
           *systemic lupus erythematosus [SLE]
              inhibitor with hemorrhagic
              disorder (286.53)*

Ⓔⓧ 286.53, 288.00-288.9, 289.53, 289.81-289.83, 289.89-289.9

Coding Clinic: 2008, Q3, P16-17

289.82 Secondary hypercoagulable state 🔗

Excludes   *heparin-induced thrombocytopenia
              (HIT) (289.84)*

Ⓔⓧ 286.53, 288.00-288.9, 289.53, 289.81-289.83, 289.89-289.9

Coding Clinic: 2008, Q3, P16-17

▸ **289.83 *Myelofibrosis*** 🔗

Myelofibrosis NOS

Secondary myelofibrosis

Code first the underlying disorder, such as:
    malignant neoplasm of breast (174.0–174.9,
    175.0–175.9)

Excludes   *idiopathic myelofibrosis (238.76)*
           leukoerythroblastic anemia (284.2)
           *myelofibrosis with myeloid metaplasia
              (238.76)*
           myelophthisic anemia (284.2)
           myelophthisis (284.2)
           primary myelofibrosis (238.76)

Use additional code for associated
    therapy-related myelodysplastic syndrome,
    if applicable (238.72,
    238.73)

Use additional external cause code if
    due to anti-neoplastic chemotherapy
    (E933.1)

Ⓔⓧ 202.40-202.48, 203.10-203.11, 203.80-203.81, 204.00-208.92,
    238.4-238.76, 238.79-238.9

289.84 Heparin-induced thrombocytopenia (HIT)

Coding Clinic: 2008, Q4, P100-101

**289.89 Other specified diseases of blood and
blood-forming organs**

Hypergammaglobulinemia

Pseudocholinesterase deficiency

289.9 Unspecified diseases of blood and blood-forming organs

Blood dyscrasia NOS

Erythroid hyperplasia

Coding Clinic: 1985, Mar-April, P14

◀ New   ⬅ Revised   ~~deleted~~ Deleted   Excludes   Includes   Use additional   Code first   Omit code

748   ● Unacceptable Principal Diagnosis   ● Use Additional Digit(s)   ▸ Manifestation Code   OGCR Official Guidelines   Coding Clinic

Item 5-1 Psychosis was a term formerly applied to any mental disorder but is now restricted to disturbances of a great magnitude in which there is a personality disintegration and loss of contact with reality.

5. MENTAL, BEHAVIORAL AND NEURODEVELOPMENTAL DISORDERS (290-319)

PSYCHOSES (290–299)

Excludes *intellectual disabilities (317–319)*

ORGANIC PSYCHOTIC CONDITIONS (290–294)

Includes psychotic organic brain syndrome

Excludes *nonpsychotic syndromes of organic etiology (310.0–310.9)*

psychoses classifiable to 295–298 and without impairment of orientation, comprehension, calculation, learning capacity, and judgment, but associated with physical disease, injury, or condition affecting the brain [e.g., following childbirth] (295.0–298.8)

● **290 Dementias**

Progressive decline in cognition along with a short- and long-term memory loss due to brain damage/disease

Code first the associated neurological condition

Excludes *dementia due to alcohol (291.0–291.2)*
dementia due to drugs (292.82)
dementia not classified as senile, presenile, or arteriosclerotic (294.10–294.11)
psychoses classifiable to 295–298 occurring in the senium without dementia or delirium (295.0–298.8)
senility with mental changes of nonpsychotic severity (310.1)
transient organic psychotic conditions (293.0–293.9)

290.0 Senile dementia, uncomplicated   A
Senile dementia:
NOS
simple type

Excludes *mild memory disturbances, not amounting to dementia, associated with senile brain disease (310.89)*
senile dementia with:
delirium or confusion (290.3)
delusional [paranoid] features (290.20)
depressive features (290.21)

Coding Clinic: 1999, Q4, P4-5; 1994, Q1, P21

● **290.1 Presenile dementia**
Brain syndrome with presenile brain disease

Excludes *arteriosclerotic dementia (290.40–290.43)*
dementia associated with other cerebral conditions (294.10–294.11)

290.10 Presenile dementia, uncomplicated   A
Presenile dementia:
NOS
simple type
Coding Clinic: 1984, Nov-Dec, P20

290.11 Presenile dementia with delirium 🔗   A
Presenile dementia with acute confusional state
(Ex) 290.0-290.12, 290.20-290.3, 290.8-290.9, 292.81, 293.0, V62.84
Coding Clinic: 1984, Nov-Dec, P20

290.12 Presenile dementia with delusional features 🔗   A
Presenile dementia, paranoid type
(Ex) 079.82, 290.0-290.12, 290.20-290.3, 290.8-290.9, 292.81, 293.0
Coding Clinic: 2010, Q3, P16; 1984, Nov-Dec, P20

290.13 Presenile dementia with depressive features 🔗   A
Presenile dementia, depressed type
(Ex) 290.0, 290.13-290.3, 296.21-296.24, 296.30-296.34, 296.43-296.44, 296.53-296.54, 296.63-296.64
Coding Clinic: 1984, Nov-Dec, P20

● **290.2 Senile dementia with delusional or depressive features**

Excludes *senile dementia:*
NOS (290.0)
with delirium and/or confusion (290.3)

290.20 Senile dementia with delusional features 🔗   A
Senile dementia, paranoid type
Senile psychosis NOS
(Ex) 290.0-290.20, 290.3

290.21 Senile dementia with depressive features 🔗   A
(Ex) 290.13, 290.21

290.3 Senile dementia with delirium 🔗   A
Senile dementia with acute confusional state

Excludes *senile:*
dementia NOS (290.0)
psychosis NOS (290.20)

(Ex) 290.10-290.20, 290.3, V62.84
Coding Clinic: 2009, Q3, P6

● **290.4 Vascular dementia**
Multi-infarct dementia or psychosis

Use additional code to identify cerebral atherosclerosis (437.0)

Excludes *suspected cases with no clear evidence of arteriosclerosis (290.9)*

290.40 Vascular dementia, uncomplicated   A
Arteriosclerotic dementia:
NOS
simple type

290.41 Vascular dementia with delirium 🔗   A
Arteriosclerotic dementia with acute confusional state
(Ex) 290.11-290.12, 290.20, 290.3, 290.41

290.42 Vascular dementia with delusions 🔗   A
Arteriosclerotic dementia, paranoid type
(Ex) 290.42

290.43 Vascular dementia with depressed mood 🔗   A
Arteriosclerotic dementia, depressed type
(Ex) 290.43

290.8 Other specified senile psychotic conditions 🔗
Presbyophrenic psychosis
(Ex) 290.8-291.0, 292.11, 292.81-292.82, 295.00-295.04, 295.10-295.14, 295.21-295.24, 295.31, 295.33-295.34, 295.40-295.44, 295.53-295.54, 295.63-295.64, 295.71, 295.73-295.74, 295.80-295.84, 295.91, 295.93-295.94, 296.21-296.24, 296.30-296.34
Coding Clinic: 2012, Q2, P9-10

290.9 Unspecified senile psychotic condition 🔗   A
(Ex) 290.8-291.0, 292.11, 292.81-292.82, 295.00-295.04, 295.10-295.14, 295.21-295.24, 295.31, 295.33-295.34, 295.40-295.44, 295.53-295.54, 295.63-295.64, 295.71, 295.73-295.74, 295.80-295.84, 295.91, 295.93-295.94, 296.21-296.24, 296.30-296.34

● **291 Alcohol-induced mental disorders**
Excludes *alcoholism without psychosis (303.0–303.9)*

291.0 Alcohol withdrawal delirium 🔗
Alcoholic delirium
Delirium tremens

Excludes *alcohol withdrawal (291.81)*

(Ex) 291.0-294.11, 294.8-294.9, 303.00-305.03, 305.20-305.93, 790.3

291.1 Alcohol-induced persisting amnestic disorder
Alcoholic polyneuritic psychosis
Korsakoff's psychosis, alcoholic
Wernicke-Korsakoff syndrome (alcoholic)

N Newborn: 0   P Pediatric: 0–17   M Maternity: 12–55   A Adult: 15–124   ♀ Females Only   ♂ Males Only

(Ex) CC/MCC Exclusions   🔗 Complication\Comorbidity   🔗 Major C\C   🔗 Present on Admission Requirement   🔗 Hospital-Acquired Condition   749

MENTAL, BEHAVIORAL AND NEURODEVELOPMENTAL DISORDERS (290-319)

291.2 Alcohol-induced persisting dementia
Alcoholic dementia NOS
Alcoholism associated with dementia NOS
Chronic alcoholic brain syndrome
Ex: 291.0-294.11, 294.8-294.9, 303.00-305.03, 305.20-305.93, 790.3

291.3 Alcohol-induced psychotic disorder with hallucinations
Alcoholic:
    hallucinosis (acute)
    psychosis with hallucinosis
Excludes alcohol withdrawal with delirium (291.0)
    schizophrenia (295.0–295.9) and paranoid states
        (297.0–297.9) taking the form of chronic
        hallucinosis with clear consciousness in
        an alcoholic
Ex: 291.0-294.11, 294.8-294.9, 303.00-305.03, 305.20-305.93, 790.3

291.4 Idiosyncratic alcohol intoxication
Pathologic:
    alcohol intoxication
    drunkenness
Excludes acute alcohol intoxication (305.0)
    in alcoholism (303.0)
    simple drunkenness (305.0)

291.5 Alcohol-induced psychotic disorder with delusions
Alcoholic:
    paranoia
    psychosis, paranoid type
Excludes nonalcoholic paranoid states (297.0–297.9)
    schizophrenia, paranoid type (295.3)

291.8 Other specified alcohol-induced mental disorders
Coding Clinic: 1989, Q2, P9

291.81 Alcohol withdrawal
Alcohol:
    abstinence syndrome or symptoms
    withdrawal syndrome or symptoms
Excludes alcohol withdrawal:
    delirium (291.0)
    hallucinosis (291.3)
    delirium tremens (291.0)
Ex: 291.0-294.11, 294.8-294.9, 303.00-305.03, 305.20-305.93, 790.3
Coding Clinic: 1985, July-Aug, P10

291.82 Alcohol induced sleep disorders
Alcohol induced circadian rhythm sleep
    disorders
Alcohol induced hypersomnia
Alcohol induced insomnia
Alcohol induced parasomnia

291.89 Other
Alcohol-induced anxiety disorder
Alcohol-induced mood disorder
Alcohol-induced sexual dysfunction
Ex: 291.0-294.11, 294.8-294.9, 303.00-305.03, 305.20-305.93, 790.3

291.9 Unspecified alcohol-induced mental disorders
Alcoholic:
    mania NOS
    psychosis NOS
Alcoholism (chronic) with psychosis
Alcohol-related disorder NOS
Ex: 291.0-294.11, 294.8-294.9, 303.00-305.03, 305.20-305.93, 790.3

292 Drug-induced mental disorders
Includes organic brain syndrome associated with
    consumption of drugs
Use additional code for any associated drug dependence
    (304.0–304.9)
Use additional E code to identify drug
Coding Clinic: 2004, Q3, P8

292.0 Drug withdrawal
Drug:
    abstinence syndrome or symptoms
    withdrawal syndrome or symptoms
Ex: 291.0-294.11, 294.8-294.9, 303.00-305.03, 305.20-305.93, 790.3
Coding Clinic: 1997, Q1, P12-13

292.1 Drug-induced psychotic disorders

292.11 Drug-induced psychotic disorder with delusions
Paranoid state induced by drugs
Ex: 291.0-294.11, 294.8-294.9, 303.00-305.03, 305.20-305.93, 790.3

292.12 Drug-induced psychotic disorder with hallucinations
Hallucinatory state induced by drugs
Excludes states following LSD or other
    hallucinogens, lasting only a few
    days or less ["bad trips"] (305.3)
Ex: 291.0-294.11, 294.8-294.9, 303.00-305.03, 305.20-305.93, 790.3
Coding Clinic: 2004, Q3, P8

292.2 Pathological drug intoxication
Drug reaction resulting in brief psychotic states
    NOS
    idiosyncratic
    pathologic
Excludes expected brief psychotic reactions to
    hallucinogens ["bad trips"] (305.3)
    physiological side-effects of drugs (e.g., dystonias)

292.8 Other specified drug-induced mental disorders

292.81 Drug-induced delirium
Ex: 291.0-294.11, 294.8-294.9, 303.00-305.03, 305.20-305.93, 790.3

292.82 Drug-induced persisting dementia
Ex: 291.0-294.11, 294.8-294.9, 303.00-305.03, 305.20-305.93, 790.3
Coding Clinic: 2004, Q3, P8

292.83 Drug-induced persisting amnestic disorder

292.84 Drug-induced mood disorder
Depressive state induced by drugs

292.85 Drug induced sleep disorders
Drug induced circadian rhythm sleep disorder
Drug induced hypersomnia
Drug induced insomnia
Drug induced parasomnia

292.89 Other
Drug-induced anxiety disorder
Drug-induced organic personality syndrome
Drug-induced sexual dysfunction
Drug intoxication

292.9 Unspecified drug-induced mental disorder
Drug-related disorder NOS
Organic psychosis NOS due to or associated with drugs

● **293 Transient mental disorders due to conditions classified elsewhere**

> **Includes** transient organic mental disorders not associated with alcohol or drugs

> *Code first the associated physical or neurological condition*

> **Excludes** *confusional state or delirium superimposed on senile*
>   *dementia (290.3)*
>   *dementia due to:*
>   *alcohol (291.0–291.9)*
>   *arteriosclerosis (290.40–290.43)*
>   *drugs (292.82)*
>   *senility (290.0)*

> Coding Clinic: 2011, Q1, P12

293.0 Delirium due to conditions classified elsewhere 🔊
> Acute:
>   confusional state
>   infective psychosis
>   organic reaction
>   posttraumatic organic psychosis
>   psycho-organic syndrome
> Acute psychosis associated with endocrine, metabolic, or
>   cerebrovascular disorder
> Epileptic:
>   confusional state
>   twilight state
> (Ex) 290.11, 290.3, 293.0, V62.84
> Coding Clinic: 1993, Q3, P11

293.1 Subacute delirium 🔊
> Subacute:
>   confusional state
>   infective psychosis
>   organic reaction
>   posttraumatic organic psychosis
>   psycho-organic syndrome
>   psychosis associated with endocrine or metabolic
>   disorder
> (Ex) 293.0-293.1, 293.89-293.9

● **293.8 Other specified transient mental disorders due to conditions classified elsewhere**

**293.81 Psychotic disorder with delusions in conditions
         classified elsewhere** 🔊
> Transient organic psychotic condition, paranoid
>   type
> (Ex) 291.0-294.11, 294.8-294.9, 303.00-305.03, 305.20-305.93, 790.3
> Coding Clinic: 2011, Q1, P12-13

**293.82 Psychotic disorder with hallucinations in
         conditions classified elsewhere** 🔊
> Transient organic psychotic condition,
>   hallucinatory type
> (Ex) 291.0-294.11, 294.8-294.9, 303.00-305.03, 305.20-305.93, 790.3

293.83 Mood disorder in conditions classified elsewhere
> Transient organic psychotic condition, depressive
>   type

293.84 Anxiety disorder in conditions classified elsewhere
> Coding Clinic: 1996, Q4, P29

293.89 Other
> Catatonic disorder in conditions classified
>   elsewhere

**293.9 Unspecified transient mental disorder in conditions
       classified elsewhere** 🔊
> Organic psychosis:
>   infective NOS
>   posttraumatic NOS
>   transient NOS
> Psycho-organic syndrome
> (Ex) 291.0-294.9, 303.00-305.03, 305.20-305.93, 790.3

● **294 Persistent mental disorders due to conditions classified
      elsewhere**

> **Includes** organic psychotic brain syndromes (chronic), not
>   elsewhere classified

294.0 Amnestic disorder in conditions classified elsewhere
> Korsakoff's psychosis or syndrome (nonalcoholic)
> *Code first underlying condition*

> **Excludes** *alcoholic:*
>   *amnestic syndrome (291.1)*
>   *Korsakoff's psychosis (291.1)*

● **294.1 Dementia in conditions classified elsewhere**
> Dementia of the Alzheimer's type

> *Code first any underlying physical condition as:*
>   Alzheimer's disease (331.0)
>   cerebral lipidoses (330.1)
>   dementia with Lewy bodies (331.82)
>   dementia with Parkinsonism (331.82)
>   epilepsy (345.0–345.9)
>   frontal dementia (331.19)
>   frontotemporal dementia (331.19)
>   general paresis [syphilis] (094.1)
>   hepatolenticular degeneration (275.1)
>   Huntington's chorea (333.4)
>   Jakob-Creutzfeldt disease (046.11--046.19)
>   multiple sclerosis (340)
>   Parkinson's disease (332.0)
>   Pick's disease of the brain (331.11)
>   polyarteritis nodosa (446.0)
>   syphilis (094.1)

> **Excludes** *dementia:*
>   *arteriosclerotic (290.40–290.43)*
>   *presenile (290.10–290.13)*
>   *senile (290.0)*
>   *epileptic psychosis NOS (294.8)*

> Coding Clinic: 2011, Q4, P96; 1999, Q1, P14; 1985, Sept-Oct, P12

▶ **294.10 *Dementia in conditions classified elsewhere without
          behavioral disturbance***
> Dementia in conditions classified elsewhere NOS

▶ **294.11 *Dementia in conditions classified elsewhere with
          behavioral disturbance*** 🔊
> Aggressive behavior
> Combative behavior
> Violent behavior

> Use additional code, where applicable, to
>   identify:
>   wandering in conditions classified elsewhere
>   (V40.31)
> (Ex) 294.11, 294.21
> Coding Clinic: 2000, Q4, P40-41

● **294.2 Dementia, unspecified**

> **Excludes** *mild memory disturbances, not amounting to*
>   *dementia (310.89)*

**294.20 Dementia, unspecified, without behavioral
         disturbance**
> Dementia NOS

**294.21 Dementia, unspecified, with behavioral
         disturbance** 🔊
> Aggressive behavior
> Combative behavior
> Violent behavior

> Use additional code, where applicable, to
>   identify:
>   wandering in conditions classified elsewhere
>   (V40.31)
> (Ex) 294.11, 294.21

N Newborn: 0   P Pediatric: 0–17   M Maternity: 12–55   A Adult: 15–124   ♀ Females Only   ♂ Males Only

(Ex) CC/MCC Exclusions   🔊 Complication\Comorbidity   🔊 Major C\C   🔊 Present on Admission Requirement   🔊 Hospital-Acquired Condition   **751**

294.8 Other persistent mental disorders due to conditions classified elsewhere
Amnestic disorder NOS
Epileptic psychosis NOS
Mixed paranoid and affective organic psychotic states
Use additional code for associated epilepsy (345.0–345.9)
Excludes *mild memory disturbances, not amounting to dementia (310.89)*
Coding Clinic: 2009, Q3, P6x2; 2003, Q3, P14

294.9 Unspecified persistent mental disorders due to conditions classified elsewhere
Cognitive disorder NOS
Organic psychosis (chronic)
Coding Clinic: 2007, Q2, P5

OTHER PSYCHOSES (295–299)

Use additional code to identify any associated physical disease, injury, or condition affecting the brain with psychoses classifiable to 295–298

● **295 Schizophrenic disorders**
Personality disorders characterized by multiple mental and behavioral irregularities
Includes schizophrenia of the types described in 295.0–295.9 occurring in children
Excludes *childhood type schizophrenia (299.9)*
infantile autism (299.0)

The following fifth-digit subclassification is for use with category 295:

> 0 unspecified
> 1 subchronic
> 2 chronic
> 3 subchronic with acute exacerbation
> 4 chronic with acute exacerbation
> 5 in remission

● **295.0 Simple type** 0-4
[0-5] Schizophrenia simplex
Excludes *latent schizophrenia (295.5)*
For codes **295.00-295.04:** (Ex) 295.00-301.9, 306.0-310.2, 310.9-315.34, 315.39-319, 339.10-339.12, 388.45, 799.23-799.24

● **295.1 Disorganized type** 0-4
[0-5] Hebephrenia
Hebephrenic type schizophrenia
For codes **295.10-295.14:** (Ex) 295.00-301.9, 306.0-310.2, 310.9-315.34, 315.39-319, 339.10-339.12, 388.45, 799.23-799.24

● **295.2 Catatonic type** 0-4
[0-5] Catatonic (schizophrenia):   Schizophrenic:
    agitation   catalepsy
    excitation   catatonia
    excited type   flexibilitas cerea
    stupor
    withdrawn type
For codes **295.20-295.24:** (Ex) 295.00-301.9, 306.0-310.2, 310.9-315.34, 315.39-319, 339.10-339.12, 388.45, 799.23-799.24

● **295.3 Paranoid type** 0-4
[0-5] Paraphrenic schizophrenia
Excludes *involutional paranoid state (297.2)*
paranoia (297.1)
paraphrenia (297.2)
For codes **295.30-295.34:** (Ex) 295.00-301.9, 306.0-310.2, 310.9-315.34, 315.39-319, 339.10-339.12, 388.45, 799.23-799.24

● **295.4 Schizophreniform disorder** 0-4
[0-5] Oneirophrenia
Schizophreniform:
    attack
    psychosis, confusional type
Excludes *acute forms of schizophrenia of:*
catatonic type (295.2)
hebephrenic type (295.1)
paranoid type (295.3)
simple type (295.0)
undifferentiated type (295.8)
For codes **295.40-295.44:** (Ex) 295.00-301.9, 306.0-310.2, 310.9-315.34, 315.39-319, 339.10-339.12, 388.45, 799.23-799.24

● **295.5 Latent schizophrenia** 3-4
[0-5] Latent schizophrenic reaction
Schizophrenia: Schizophrenia:
    borderline   prodromal
    incipient   pseudoneurotic
    prepsychotic   pseudopsychopathic
Excludes *schizoid personality (301.20–301.22)*
For codes **295.53-595.54:** (Ex) 295.00-295.04, 295.10-295.14, 295.21-295.24, 295.31, 295.33-295.34, 295.40-295.44, 295.53-295.54, 295.63-295.64, 295.71, 295.73-295.74, 295.80-295.84, 295.91, 295.93-295.94

● **295.6 Residual type** 0-4
[0-5] Chronic undifferentiated schizophrenia
Restzustand (schizophrenic)
Schizophrenic residual state
For codes **295.60-295.64:** (Ex) 295.00-301.9, 306.0-310.2, 310.9-315.34, 315.39-319, 339.10-339.12, 388.45, 799.23-799.24
Coding Clinic: 2006, Q4, P76-78

● **295.7 Schizoaffective disorder** 1-4
[0-5] Cyclic schizophrenia
Mixed schizophrenic and affective psychosis
Schizo-affective psychosis
Schizophreniform psychosis, affective type
For codes **295.71-295.74:** (Ex) 295.00-301.9, 306.0-310.2, 310.9-315.34, 315.39-319, 339.10-339.12, 388.45, 799.23-799.24

● **295.8 Other specified types of schizophrenia** 0-4
[0-5] Acute (undifferentiated) schizophrenia
Atypical schizophrenia
Cenesthopathic schizophrenia
Excludes *infantile autism (299.0)*
For codes **295.80-295.84:** (Ex) 295.00-301.9, 306.0-310.2, 310.9-315.34, 315.39-319, 339.10-339.12, 388.45, 799.23-799.24

● **295.9 Unspecified schizophrenia** 1-4
[0-5] Schizophrenia: Schizophrenia:
    NOS   undifferentiated NOS
    mixed NOS   undifferentiated type
Schizophrenic reaction NOS
Schizophreniform psychosis NOS
For codes **295.91-295.94:** (Ex) 295.00-301.9, 306.0-310.2, 310.9-315.34, 315.39-319, 339.10-339.12, 388.45, 799.23-799.24
Coding Clinic: 1995, Q3, P6

● **296 Episodic mood disorders**

> **Includes** episodic affective disorders
> **Excludes** *neurotic depression (300.4)*
> *reactive depressive psychosis (298.0)*
> *reactive excitation (298.1)*
> **Coding Clinic: 1985, Mar-April, P14**

The following fifth-digit subclassification is for use with categories 296.0–296.6:

> 0 **unspecified**
> 1 **mild**
> 2 **moderate**
> 3 **severe, without mention of psychotic behavior**
> 4 **severe, specified as with psychotic behavior**
> 5 **in partial or unspecified remission**
> 6 **in full remission**

● **296.0 Bipolar I disorder, single manic episode** 0-4
[0-6] *Manic depressive disorder, characterized by moods that swing between periods of exaggerated euphoria, irritability, or both (manic) and episodes of depression*
Hypomania (mild) NOS single episode or unspecified
Hypomanic psychosis single episode or unspecified
Mania (monopolar) NOS single episode or unspecified
Manic-depressive psychosis or reaction, single episode or unspecified:
hypomanic, single episode or unspecified
manic, single episode or unspecified
> **Excludes** *circular type, if there was a previous attack of depression (296.4)*
> For codes **296.00-296.02:** (Ex) 295.00-301.9, 306.0-310.2, 315.39-319, 339.10-339.12, 388.45, 799.23-799.24;
> For code **296.03:** (Ex) 296.03-296.04, 296.13-296.14, 296.43-296.44, 296.53-296.54, 296.63-296.64;
> For code **296.04:** (Ex) 295.00-301.9, 306.0-310.2, 310.9-315.34, 315.39-319, 339.10-339.12, 388.45, 799.23-799.24

● **296.1 Manic disorder, recurrent episode** 0-4
[0-6] Any condition classifiable to 296.0, stated to be recurrent
> **Excludes** *circular type, if there was a previous attack of depression (296.4)*
> For codes **296.10-296.12 and 296.14:** (Ex) 295.00-301.9, 306.0-310.2, 310.9-315.34, 315.39-319, 339.10-339.12, 388.45, 799.23-799.24;
> For code **296.13:** (Ex) 296.13-296.14, 296.43-296.44, 296.53-296.54, 296.63-296.64

● **296.2 Major depressive disorder, single episode** 0-4
[0-6] Depressive psychosis, single episode or unspecified
Endogenous depression, single episode or unspecified
Involutional melancholia, single episode or unspecified
Manic-depressive psychosis or reaction, depressed type, single episode or unspecified
Monopolar depression, single episode or unspecified
Psychotic depression, single episode or unspecified
> **Excludes** *circular type, if previous attack was of manic type (296.5)*
> *depression NOS (311)*
> *reactive depression (neurotic) (300.4)*
> *psychotic (298.0)*
> For code **296.20:** (Ex) 295.00-301.9, 306.0-310.2, 310.9-315.34, 315.39-319, 339.10-339.12, 388.45, 799.23-799.24;
> For codes **296.21-296.24:** (Ex) 296.21-296.24, 296.30-296.34
> **Coding Clinic: 2009, Q3, P6x2, 7**

● **296.3 Major depressive disorder, recurrent episode** 0-4
[0-6] Any condition classifiable to 296.2, stated to be recurrent
> **Excludes** *circular type, if previous attack was of manic type (296.5)*
> *depression NOS (311)*
> *reactive depression (neurotic) (300.4)*
> *psychotic (298.0)*
> For codes **296.30-296.33:** (Ex) 296.21-296.24, 296.30-296.34;
> For code **296.34:** (Ex) 295.00-301.9, 306.0-310.2, 310.9-315.34, 315.39-319, 339.10-339.12, 388.45, 799.23-799.24

● **296.4 Bipolar I disorder, most recent episode (or current)**
[0-6] **manic** 0-4
Bipolar disorder, now manic
Manic-depressive psychosis, circular type but currently manic
> **Excludes** *brief compensatory or rebound mood swings (296.99)*
> For codes **296.40-296.42 and 296.44:** (Ex) 295.00-301.9, 306.0-310.2, 310.9-315.34, 315.39-319, 339.10-339.12, 388.45, 799.23-799.24;
> For code **296.43:** (Ex) 296.43-296.44, 296.63-296.64

● **296.5 Bipolar I disorder, most recent episode (or current)**
[0-6] **depressed** 0-4
Bipolar disorder, now depressed
Manic-depressive psychosis, circular type but currently depressed
> **Excludes** *brief compensatory or rebound mood swings (296.99)*
> For codes **296.50-296.52 and 293.54:** (Ex) 295.00-301.9, 306.0-310.2, 310.9-315.34, 315.39-319, 339.10-339.12, 388.45, 799.23-799.24;
> For code **296.53:** (Ex) 296.43-296.44, 296.53-296.54, 296.63-296.64
> **Coding Clinic: 2006, Q1, P10**

● **296.6 Bipolar I disorder, most recent episode (or current)**
[0-6] **mixed** 0-4
Manic-depressive psychosis, circular type, mixed
> For codes **296.60-296.62 and 296.64:** (Ex) 295.00-301.9, 306.0-310.2, 310.9-315.34, 315.39-319, 339.10-339.12, 388.45, 799.23-799.24;
> For code **296.63:** (Ex) 296.43-296.44, 296.53-296.54, 296.63-296.64

296.7 Bipolar I disorder, most recent episode (or current) unspecified
Atypical bipolar affective disorder NOS
Manic-depressive psychosis, circular type, current condition not specified as either manic or depressive

● **296.8 Other and unspecified bipolar disorders**

296.80 Bipolar disorder, unspecified
Bipolar disorder NOS
Manic-depressive:
reaction NOS
syndrome NOS

296.81 Atypical manic disorder

296.82 Atypical depressive disorder

296.89 Other
Bipolar II disorder
Manic-depressive psychosis, mixed type
(Ex) 295.00-301.9, 306.0-310.2, 310.9-315.34, 315.39-319, 339.10-339.12, 388.45, 799.23-799.24

● **296.9 Other and unspecified episodic mood disorder**
> **Excludes** *psychogenic affective psychoses (298.0-298.8)*

296.90 Unspecified episodic mood disorder
Affective psychosis NOS
Melancholia NOS
Mood disorder NOS
Coding Clinic: 1985, Mar-April, P14

296.99 Other specified episodic mood disorder
Mood swings:
brief compensatory
rebound
(Ex) 295.00-301.9, 306.0-310.2, 310.9-315.34, 315.39-319, 339.10-339.12, 388.45, 799.23-799.24

● **297 Delusional disorders**
> **Includes** paranoid disorders
> **Excludes** *acute paranoid reaction (298.3)*
> *alcoholic jealousy or paranoid state (291.5)*
> *paranoid schizophrenia (295.3)*

297.0 Paranoid state, simple

297.1 Delusional disorder
Chronic paranoid psychosis
Sander's disease
Systematized delusions
> **Excludes** *paranoid personality disorder (301.0)*

N Newborn: 0   P Pediatric: 0–17   M Maternity: 12–55   A Adult: 15–124   ♀ Females Only   ♂ Males Only
(Ex) CC/MCC Exclusions   Complication\Comorbidity   Major C\C   Present on Admission Requirement   Hospital-Acquired Condition
753

297.2 Paraphrenia
Involutional paranoid state
Late paraphrenia
Paraphrenia (involutional)

297.3 Shared psychotic disorder
Folie à deux
Induced psychosis or paranoid disorder

297.8 Other specified paranoid states
Paranoia querulans
Sensitiver Beziehungswahn

> **Excludes**   *acute paranoid reaction or state (298.3)*
> *senile paranoid state (290.20)*

297.9 Unspecified paranoid state
Paranoid:
disorder NOS
psychosis NOS
reaction NOS
state NOS

● **298 Other nonorganic psychoses**

> **Includes**   psychotic conditions due to or provoked by:
> emotional stress
> environmental factors as major part of etiology

298.0 Depressive type psychosis
Psychogenic depressive psychosis
Psychotic reactive depression
Reactive depressive psychosis

> **Excludes**   *manic-depressive psychosis, depressed type*
> *(296.2–296.3)*
> *neurotic depression (300.4)*
> *reactive depression NOS (300.4)*
> (Ex) 295.00-301.9, 306.0-310.2, 310.9-315.34, 315.39-319, 339.10-339.12,
> 388.45, 799.23-799.24

298.1 Excitative type psychosis
Acute hysterical psychosis
Psychogenic excitation
Reactive excitation

> **Excludes**   *manic-depressive psychosis, manic type*
> *(296.0–296.1)*
> (Ex) 295.00-301.9, 306.0-310.2, 310.9-315.34, 315.39-319, 339.10-339.12,
> 388.45, 799.23-799.24

298.2 Reactive confusion
Psychogenic confusion
Psychogenic twilight state

> **Excludes**   *acute confusional state (293.0)*

298.3 Acute paranoid reaction
Acute psychogenic paranoid psychosis
Bouffée délirante

> **Excludes**   *paranoid states (297.0–297.9)*
> (Ex) 295.00-301.9, 306.0-310.2, 310.9-315.34, 315.39-319, 339.10-339.12,
> 388.45, 799.23-799.24

298.4 Psychogenic paranoid psychosis
Protracted reactive paranoid psychosis
> (Ex) 295.00-301.9, 306.0-310.2, 310.9-315.34, 315.39-319, 339.10-339.12,
> 388.45, 799.23-799.24

298.8 Other and unspecified reactive psychosis
Brief psychotic disorder
Brief reactive psychosis NOS
Hysterical psychosis
Psychogenic psychosis NOS
Psychogenic stupor

> **Excludes**   *acute hysterical psychosis (298.1)*

298.9 Unspecified psychosis
Atypical psychosis
Psychosis NOS
Psychotic disorder NOS
Coding Clinic: 2006, Q3, P22; 1993, Q3, P11

Item 5-2 Anxiety is also known as **generalized disorder** and is evidenced by persistent, excessive, and unrealistic worry about everyday things. **Dissociative disorders** are characterized by a persistent disruption in the integration of memory, consciousness, or identity and a lack of mental connectedness to events. **Somatoform disorders** are characterized by unusual physical symptoms in the absence of any known physical pathology and may lead to unnecessary medical treatments.

● **299 Pervasive developmental disorders**

> **Excludes**   *adult type psychoses occurring in childhood, as:*
> *affective disorders (296.0–296.9)*
> *manic-depressive disorders (296.0–296.9)*
> *schizophrenia (295.0–295.9)*

The following fifth-digit subclassification is for use with category 299:

0 current or active state	**1 residual state**

● **299.0 Autistic disorder**
[0-1]   Childhood autism   Kanner's syndrome
Infantile psychosis

> **Excludes**   *disintegrative psychosis (299.1)*
> *Heller's syndrome (299.1)*
> *schizophrenic syndrome of childhood (299.9)*
> (Ex) 295.00-301.9, 306.0-310.2, 310.9-315.34, 315.39-319, 339.10-339.12,
> 388.45, 799.23-799.24
> **Coding Clinic: 2012, Q3, P19-20**

● **299.1 Childhood disintegrative disorder**
[0-1]   Heller's syndrome
Use additional code to identify any associated
neurological disorder

> **Excludes**   *infantile autism (299.0)*
> *schizophrenic syndrome of childhood (299.9)*
> (Ex) 295.00-301.9, 306.0-310.2, 310.9-315.34, 315.39-319, 339.10-339.12,
> 388.45, 799.23-799.24

● **299.8 Other specified pervasive developmental**
[0-1]   **disorders**
Asperger's disorder
Atypical childhood psychosis
Borderline psychosis of childhood

> **Excludes**   *simple stereotypes without psychotic disturbance*
> *(307.3)*
> (Ex) 295.00-301.9, 306.0-310.2, 310.9-315.34, 315.39-319, 339.10-339.12,
> 388.45, 799.23-799.24

● **299.9 Unspecified pervasive developmental disorder**
[0-1]   Child psychosis NOS
Pervasive developmental disorder NOS
Schizophrenia, childhood type NOS
Schizophrenic syndrome of childhood NOS

> **Excludes**   *schizophrenia of adult type occurring in*
> *childhood (295.0–295.9)*
> (Ex) 295.00-301.9, 306.0-310.2, 310.9-315.34, 315.39-319, 339.10-339.12,
> 388.45, 799.23-799.24

NEUROTIC DISORDERS, PERSONALITY DISORDERS, AND OTHER NONPSYCHOTIC MENTAL DISORDERS (300–316)

● **300 Anxiety, dissociative and somatoform disorders**

● **300.0 Anxiety states**

> **Excludes**   *anxiety in:*
> *acute stress reaction (308.0)*
> *transient adjustment reaction (309.24)*
> *neurasthenia (300.5)*
> *psychophysiological disorders (306.0–306.9)*
> *separation anxiety (309.21)*

300.00 Anxiety state, unspecified
Anxiety:
neurosis
reaction
state (neurotic)
Atypical anxiety disorder
Coding Clinic: 2011, Q3, P6

◄ New   ◄▦ Revised   ~~deleted~~ Deleted   Excludes   Includes   Use additional   Code first   Omit code

754   ● Unacceptable Principal Diagnosis   ● Use Additional Digit(s)   ▷ Manifestation Code   OGCR Official Guidelines   Coding Clinic

300.01 **Panic disorder without agoraphobia**
    Panic:
       attack
       state
       Excludes *panic disorder with agoraphobia (300.21)*

300.02 **Generalized anxiety disorder**

300.09 **Other**

● 300.1 **Dissociative, conversion and factitious disorders**
       Excludes *adjustment reaction (309.0–309.9)*
                anorexia nervosa (307.1)
                gross stress reaction (308.0–308.9)
                hysterical personality (301.50–301.59)
                psychophysiologic disorders (306.0–306.9)

300.10 **Hysteria, unspecified**

300.11 **Conversion disorder**
    Astasia-abasia, hysterical
    Conversion hysteria or reaction
    Hysterical:
       blindness
       deafness
       paralysis
    Coding Clinic: 1985, Nov-Dec, P15

300.12 **Dissociative amnesia**
    Hysterical amnesia

300.13 **Dissociative fugue**
    Hysterical fugue

300.14 **Dissociative identity disorder**

300.15 **Dissociative disorder or reaction, unspecified**

300.16 **Factitious disorder with predominantly psychological signs and symptoms**
    Compensation neurosis
    Ganser's syndrome, hysterical

300.19 **Other and unspecified factitious illness**
    Factitious disorder (with combined psychological and physical signs and symptoms) (with predominantly physical signs and symptoms) NOS
       Excludes *multiple operations or hospital addiction syndrome (301.51)*

● 300.2 **Phobic disorders**
    Irrational fear with avoidance of the feared subject, activity, or situation. Divided into 3 types: specific phobias, social phobias, and agoraphobia.
       Excludes *anxiety state not associated with a specific situation or object (300.00–300.09)*
                obsessional phobias (300.3)

300.20 **Phobia, unspecified**
    Anxiety-hysteria NOS
    Phobia NOS

300.21 **Agoraphobia with panic disorder**
    Fear of:
       open spaces with panic attacks
       streets with panic attacks
       travel with panic attacks
    Panic disorder with agoraphobia
       Excludes *agoraphobia without panic disorder (300.22)*
                panic disorder without agoraphobia (300.01)

300.22 **Agoraphobia without mention of panic attacks**
    Any condition classifiable to 300.21 without mention of panic attacks

300.23 **Social phobia**
    Fear of:
       eating in public
       public speaking
       washing in public

300.29 **Other isolated or specific phobias**
    Acrophobia
       Fear of heights
    Animal phobias
    Claustrophobia
       Fear of closed spaces
    Fear of crowds

300.3 **Obsessive-compulsive disorders** *(OCD)*
    Anancastic neurosis
    Compulsive neurosis
    Obsessional phobia [any]
       Excludes *obsessive-compulsive symptoms occurring in:*
                endogenous depression (296.2–296.3)
                organic states (e.g., encephalitis)
                schizophrenia (295.0–295.9)

300.4 **Dysthymic disorder**
    Anxiety depression
    Depression with anxiety
    Depressive reaction
    Neurotic depressive state
    Reactive depression
       Excludes *adjustment reaction with depressive symptoms (309.0–309.1)*
                depression NOS (311)
                manic-depressive psychosis, depressed type (296.2–296.3)
                reactive depressive psychosis (298.0)
    Coding Clinic: 2011, Q3, P6

300.5 **Neurasthenia**
    Fatigue neurosis   Psychogenic:
    Nervous debility   asthenia
                         general fatigue
    Use additional code to identify any associated physical disorder
       Excludes *anxiety state (300.00–300.09)*
                neurotic depression (300.4)
                psychophysiological disorders (306.0–306.9)
                specific nonpsychotic mental disorders following organic brain damage (310.0–310.9)

300.6 **Depersonalization disorder**
    Derealization (neurotic)
    Neurotic state with depersonalization episode
       Excludes *depersonalization associated with:*
                anxiety (300.00–300.09)
                depression (300.4)
                manic-depressive disorder or psychosis (296.0–296.9)
                schizophrenia (295.0–295.9)

300.7 **Hypochondriasis**
    Hypochondriac
    Body dysmorphic disorder
       Excludes *hypochondriasis in:*
                hysteria (300.10–300.19)
                manic-depressive psychosis, depressed type (296.2–296.3)
                neurasthenia (300.5)
                obsessional disorder (300.3)
                schizophrenia (295.0–295.9)

● 300.8 **Somatoform disorders**

300.81 **Somatization disorder**
    Briquet's disorder
    Severe somatoform disorder

300.82 **Undifferentiated somatoform disorder**
    Atypical somatoform disorder
    Somatoform disorder NOS

300.89 **Other somatoform disorders**
    Occupational neurosis, including writers' cramp
    Psychasthenia
    Psychasthenic neurosis

300.9 **Unspecified nonpsychotic mental disorder**
    Psychoneurosis NOS

MENTAL, BEHAVIORAL AND NEURODEVELOPMENTAL DISORDERS (290–319)

N Newborn: 0   **P** Pediatric: 0–17   **M** Maternity: 12–55   **A** Adult: 15–124   ♀ Females Only   ♂ Males Only

ⒺⓍ CC/MCC Exclusions   Complication\Comorbidity   Major C\C   Present on Admission Requirement   Hospital-Acquired Condition   755

● **301 Personality disorders**
Long-term patterns of thoughts and behaviors causing serious problems with relationships and work

Includes   character neurosis

Use additional code to identify any associated neurosis or psychosis, or physical condition

Excludes   *nonpsychotic personality disorder associated with organic brain syndromes (310.0–310.9)*

301.0 Paranoid personality disorder
Fanatic personality
Paranoid personality (disorder)
Paranoid traits

    Excludes   *acute paranoid reaction (298.3)*
                       alcoholic paranoia (291.5)
                       paranoid schizophrenia (295.3)
                       paranoid states (297.0–297.9)

● **301.1 Affective personality disorder**

    Excludes   *affective psychotic disorders (296.0–296.9)*
                       neurasthenia (300.5)
                       neurotic depression (300.4)

   301.10 Affective personality disorder, unspecified

   301.11 Chronic hypomanic personality disorder
        Chronic hypomanic disorder
        Hypomanic personality

   301.12 Chronic depressive personality disorder
        Chronic depressive disorder
        Depressive character or personality

   301.13 Cyclothymic disorder
        Cycloid personality
        Cyclothymia
        Cyclothymic personality

● **301.2 Schizoid personality disorder**

    Excludes   *schizophrenia (295.0–295.9)*

   301.20 Schizoid personality disorder, unspecified

   301.21 Introverted personality

   301.22 Schizotypal personality disorder

301.3 Explosive personality disorder
Aggressive:
   personality
   reaction
Aggressiveness
Emotional instability (excessive)
Pathological emotionality
Quarrelsomeness

    Excludes   *dyssocial personality (301.7)*
                       hysterical neurosis (300.10–300.19)

301.4 Obsessive-compulsive personality disorder
Anancastic personality
Obsessional personality

    Excludes   *obsessive-compulsive disorder (300.3)*
                       phobic state (300.20–300.29)

● **301.5 Histrionic personality disorder**

    Excludes   *hysterical neurosis (300.10–300.19)*

   301.50 Histrionic personality disorder, unspecified
        Hysterical personality NOS

   301.51 Chronic factitious illness with physical symptoms ⚠
        Hospital addiction syndrome
        Multiple operations syndrome
        Munchausen syndrome
        ⓔⓧ 295.00-301.9, 306.0-310.2, 310.9-315.34, 315.39-319, 339.10-339.12, 388.45, 799.23-799.24

   301.59 Other histrionic personality disorder
        Personality: Personality:
           emotionally unstable   psychoinfantile
           labile

301.6 Dependent personality disorder
Asthenic personality
Inadequate personality
Passive personality

    Excludes   *neurasthenia (300.5)*
                       passive-aggressive personality (301.84)

301.7 Antisocial personality disorder
Amoral personality
Asocial personality
Dyssocial personality
Personality disorder with predominantly sociopathic or asocial manifestation

    Excludes   *disturbance of conduct without specifiable personality disorder (312.0–312.9)*
                       explosive personality (301.3)

    Coding Clinic: 1984, Sept-Oct, P16

● **301.8 Other personality disorders**

   301.81 Narcissistic personality disorder

   301.82 Avoidant personality disorder

   301.83 Borderline personality disorder

   301.84 Passive-aggressive personality

   301.89 Other
        Personality: Personality:
           eccentric   masochistic
           "haltlose" type   psychoneurotic
           immature

      Excludes   *psychoinfantile personality (301.59)*

301.9 Unspecified personality disorder
Pathological personality NOS
Personality disorder NOS
Psychopathic:
   constitutional state
   personality (disorder)

● **302 Sexual and gender identity disorders**

    Excludes   *sexual disorder manifest in:*
                       organic brain syndrome (290.0–294.9, 310.0–310.9)
                       psychosis (295.0–298.9)

302.0 Ego-dystonic sexual orientation
Ego-dystonic lesbianism
Sexual orientation conflict disorder

    Excludes   *homosexual pedophilia (302.2)*

302.1 Zoophilia
Bestiality

302.2 Pedophilia

302.3 Transvestic fetishism

    Excludes   *trans-sexualism (302.5)*

302.4 Exhibitionism

● **302.5 Trans-sexualism**
Sex reassignment surgery status

    Excludes   *transvestism (302.3)*

   302.50 With unspecified sexual history

   302.51 With asexual history

   302.52 With homosexual history

   302.53 With heterosexual history

302.6 Gender identity disorder in children
Check age: adolescents and adults separately classified under 302.85
Feminism in boys
Gender identity disorder NOS

    Excludes   *gender identity disorder in adult (302.85)*
                       trans-sexualism (302.50–302.53)
                       transvestism (302.3)

◀ New   ◀▦ Revised   ~~deleted~~ Deleted   Excludes   Includes   Use additional   Code first   Omit code

756   ● Unacceptable Principal Diagnosis   ● Use Additional Digit(s)   ▷ Manifestation Code   OGCR Official Guidelines   **Coding Clinic**

● **302.7 Psychosexual dysfunction**

> **Excludes** *decreased sexual desire NOS (799.81)*
> *impotence of organic origin (607.84)*
> *normal transient symptoms from ruptured hymen*
> *transient or occasional failures of erection due to fatigue, anxiety, alcohol, or drugs*

302.70 Psychosexual dysfunction, unspecified
Sexual dysfunction NOS

302.71 Hypoactive sexual desire disorder
> **Excludes** *decreased sexual desire NOS (799.81)*

302.72 With inhibited sexual excitement
Female sexual arousal disorder
Frigidity
Impotence
Male erectile disorder

302.73 Female orgasmic disorder ♀

302.74 Male orgasmic disorder ♂

302.75 Premature ejaculation ♂

302.76 Dyspareunia, psychogenic ♀

302.79 With other specified psychosexual dysfunctions
Sexual aversion disorder

● **302.8 Other specified psychosexual disorders**

302.81 Fetishism

302.82 Voyeurism

302.83 Sexual masochism

302.84 Sexual sadism

302.85 Gender identity disorder in adolescents or adults

Use additional code to identify sex reassignment surgery status (302.5)

> **Excludes** *gender identity disorder NOS (302.6)*
> *gender identity disorder in children (302.6)*

302.89 Other
Frotteurism
Nymphomania
Satyriasis

302.9 Unspecified psychosexual disorder
Paraphilia NOS
Pathologic sexuality NOS
Sexual deviation NOS
Sexual disorder NOS

● **303 Alcohol dependence syndrome**

Use additional code to identify any associated condition, as:
alcoholic psychoses (291.0–291.9)
drug dependence (304.0–304.9)
physical complications of alcohol, such as:
cerebral degeneration (331.7)
cirrhosis of liver (571.2)
epilepsy (345.0–345.9)
gastritis (535.3)
hepatitis (571.1)
liver damage NOS (571.3)

> **Excludes** *drunkenness NOS (305.0)*

Coding Clinic: 2010, Q1, P3-4; 1995, Q3, P6

The following fifth-digit subclassification is for use with category 303:

0	unspecified	2	episodic
1	continuous	3	in remission

● **303.0 Acute alcoholic intoxication**
[0-3]   Acute drunkenness in alcoholism
Coding Clinic: 1985, July-Aug, P15

● **303.9 Other and unspecified alcohol dependence**
[0-3]   Chronic alcoholism
Dipsomania
Coding Clinic: 2012, Q2, P9-10; 2002, Q2, P4; Q1, P3-4; 1989, Q2, P9; 1985, Nov-Dec, P14

● **304 Drug dependence**

For some "dependence" codes there is a corresponding "abuse" code. There is a point at which drug use crosses from "dependence" to "abuse." Check documentation or query provider for patient status.

> **Excludes** *nondependent abuse of drugs (305.1–305.9)*

Coding Clinic: 2013, Q2, P14-15; 2010, Q1, P3

The following fifth-digit subclassification is for use with category 304:

0	unspecified	2	episodic
1	continuous	3	in remission

● **304.0 Opioid type dependence** 1 🔍
[0-3]   Heroin
Meperidine
Methadone
Morphine
Opium
Opium alkaloids and their derivatives
Synthetics with morphine-like effects
For code **304.01**: (Ex) 291.0-292.9, 303.00-305.03, 305.20-305.93, 790.3
Coding Clinic: 2013, Q2, P15; 2011, Q1, P15; 2010, Q2, P13; 2006, Q2, P7; 1988, Q4, P8

● **304.1 Sedative, hypnotic or anxiolytic dependence** 1 🔍
[0-3]   Barbiturates
Nonbarbiturate sedatives and tranquilizers with a similar effect:
chlordiazepoxide
diazepam
glutethimide
meprobamate
methaqualone
For code **304.11**: (Ex) 291.0-292.9, 303.00-305.03, 305.20-305.93, 790.3
Coding Clinic: 2013, Q2, P15

● **304.2 Cocaine dependence** 1 🔍
[0-3]   Coca leaves and derivatives
For code **304.21**: (Ex) 291.0-292.9, 303.00-305.03, 305.20-305.93, 790.3

● **304.3 Cannabis dependence**
[0-3]   *Code 305.2 is for abuse of cannabis.*
Hashish
Hemp
Marihuana

● **304.4 Amphetamine and other psychostimulant**
[0-3] **dependence** 1 🔍
Methylphenidate
Phenmetrazine
For code **304.41**: (Ex) 291.0-292.9, 303.00-305.03, 305.20-305.93, 790.3

● **304.5 Hallucinogen dependence** 1 🔍
[0-3]   Dimethyltryptamine [DMT]
Lysergic acid diethylamide [LSD] and derivatives
Mescaline
Psilocybin
For code **304.51**: (Ex) 291.0-292.9, 303.00-305.03, 305.20-305.93, 790.3

● **304.6 Other specified drug dependence** 1 🔍
[0-3]   Absinthe addiction
Glue sniffing
Inhalant dependence
Phencyclidine dependence
> **Excludes** *tobacco dependence (305.1)*
For code **304.61**: (Ex) 291.0-292.9, 303.00-305.03, 305.20-305.93, 790.3

● **304.7 Combinations of opioid type drug with any other** 1 🔍
[0-3]   For code **304.71**: (Ex) 291.0-292.9, 303.00-305.03, 305.20-305.93, 790.3
Coding Clinic: 1986, Mar-April, P12

● **304.8 Combinations of drug dependence excluding opioid**
[0-3] **type drug** 1 🔍
For code **304.81**: (Ex) 291.0-292.9, 303.00-305.03, 305.20-305.93, 790.3
Coding Clinic: 1986, Mar-April, P12

● **304.9 Unspecified drug dependence** 1 🔍
[0-3]   Drug addiction NOS
Drug dependence NOS
For code **304.91**: (Ex) 291.0-292.9, 303.00-305.03, 305.20-305.93, 790.3
Coding Clinic: 2012, Q2, P16-17; 2003, Q4, P103-104

MENTAL, BEHAVIORAL AND NEURODEVELOPMENTAL DISORDERS (290-319)

N Newborn: 0   P Pediatric: 0–17   M Maternity: 12–55   A Adult: 15–124   ♀ Females Only   ♂ Males Only

(Ex) CC/MCC Exclusions   🔍 Complication\Comorbidity   🔍 Major C\C   🔍 Present on Admission Requirement   🔍 Hospital-Acquired Condition   757

● **305 Nondependent abuse of drugs**

Note: Includes cases where a person, for whom no other diagnosis is possible, has come under medical care because of the maladaptive effect of a drug on which he is not dependent and that he has taken on his own initiative (*self-medicating*) to the detriment of his health or social functioning.

Excludes *alcohol dependence syndrome (303.0–303.9)*
drug dependence (304.0–304.9)
drug withdrawal syndrome (292.0)
poisoning by drugs or medicinal substances (960.0–979.9)

Coding Clinic: 2010, Q1, P5

The following fifth-digit subclassification is for use with codes 305.0, 305.2–305.9:

0 unspecified	2 episodic
1 continuous	3 in remission

● **305.0 Alcohol abuse**
[0-3]   Drunkenness NOS
Excessive drinking of alcohol NOS
"Hangover" (alcohol)
Inebriety NOS

Excludes *acute alcohol intoxication in alcoholism (303.0)*
alcoholic psychoses (291.0–291.9)

Coding Clinic: 2009, Q4, P98; Q1, P8; 1996, Q3, P16; 1985, July-Aug, P15

● **305.1 Tobacco use disorder**
Tobacco dependence

Excludes *history of tobacco use (V15.82)*
smoking complicating pregnancy (649.0)
tobacco use disorder complicating pregnancy (649.0)

Coding Clinic: 2009, Q4, P98; Q1, P8; 1996, Q2, P10; 1984, Nov-Dec, P12

● **305.2 Cannabis abuse**
[0-3]   *Code 304.3 is for cannabis dependence.*

● **305.3 Hallucinogen abuse**
[0-3]   Acute intoxication from hallucinogens ["bad trips"]
LSD reaction

● **305.4 Sedative, hypnotic or anxiolytic abuse**
[0-3]

● **305.5 Opioid abuse**
[0-3]

● **305.6 Cocaine abuse**
[0-3]   Coding Clinic: 1993, Q1, P25; Q1, P25; 1988, Q4, P8

● **305.7 Amphetamine or related acting sympathomimetic**
[0-3]   **abuse**
Coding Clinic: 2003, Q2, P10,11x2

● **305.8 Antidepressant type abuse**
[0-3]

● **305.9 Other, mixed, or unspecified drug abuse**
[0-3]   Caffeine intoxication
Inhalant abuse
"Laxative habit"
Misuse of drugs NOS
Nonprescribed use of drugs or patent medicinals
Phencyclidine abuse
Coding Clinic: 1999, Q3, P20; 1994, Q4, P36

● **306 Physiological malfunction arising from mental factors**

Includes psychogenic:
physical symptoms not involving tissue damage
physiological manifestations not involving tissue damage

Excludes *hysteria (300.11–300.19)*
physical symptoms secondary to a psychiatric disorder classified elsewhere
psychic factors associated with physical conditions involving tissue damage classified elsewhere (316)
specific nonpsychotic mental disorders following organic brain damage (310.0–310.9)

306.0 Musculoskeletal
Psychogenic paralysis
Psychogenic torticollis

Excludes *Gilles de la Tourette's syndrome (307.23)*
paralysis as hysterical or conversion reaction (300.11)
tics (307.20–307.22)

306.1 Respiratory

Psychogenic:	Psychogenic:
air hunger	hyperventilation
cough	yawning
hiccough	

Excludes *psychogenic asthma (316 and 493.9)*

306.2 Cardiovascular
Cardiac neurosis
Cardiovascular neurosis
Neurocirculatory asthenia
Psychogenic cardiovascular disorder

Excludes *psychogenic paroxysmal tachycardia (316 and 427.2)*

Coding Clinic: 1985, July-Aug, P14

306.3 Skin
Psychogenic pruritus

Excludes *psychogenic:*
alopecia (316 and 704.00)
dermatitis (316 and 692.9)
eczema (316 and 691.8 or 692.9)
urticaria (316 and 708.0–708.9)

306.4 Gastrointestinal
Aerophagy
Cyclical vomiting, psychogenic
Diarrhea, psychogenic
Nervous gastritis
Psychogenic dyspepsia

Excludes *cyclical vomiting NOS (536.2)*
associated with migraine (346.2)
globus hystericus (300.11)
mucous colitis (316 and 564.9)
psychogenic:
cardiospasm (316 and 530.0)
duodenal ulcer (316 and 532.0–532.9)
gastric ulcer (316 and 531.0–531.9)
peptic ulcer NOS (316 and 533.0–533.9)
vomiting NOS (307.54)

Coding Clinic: 1989, Q2, P11

● **306.5 Genitourinary**

Excludes *enuresis, psychogenic (307.6)*
frigidity (302.72)
impotence (302.72)
psychogenic dyspareunia (302.76)

306.50 Psychogenic genitourinary malfunction, unspecified

306.51 Psychogenic vaginismus ♀
Functional vaginismus

306.52 Psychogenic dysmenorrhea ♀

306.53 Psychogenic dysuria

306.59 Other

◀ New   ◀▥ Revised   ~~deleted~~ Deleted   Excludes   Includes   Use additional   Code first   Omit code
● Unacceptable Principal Diagnosis   ● Use Additional Digit(s)   ▶ Manifestation Code   **OGCR** Official Guidelines   **Coding Clinic**
758

306.6 Endocrine

306.7 Organs of special sense

> **Excludes** *hysterical blindness or deafness (300.11)*
> *psychophysical visual disturbances (368.16)*

306.8 Other specified psychophysiological malfunction
Bruxism
Sleep-related bruxism, 327.53
Teeth grinding

306.9 Unspecified psychophysiological malfunction
Psychophysiologic disorder NOS
Psychosomatic disorder NOS

● **307 Special symptoms or syndromes, not elsewhere classified**

> **Note:** This category is intended for use if the psychopathology is manifested by a single specific symptom or group of symptoms which is not part of an organic illness or other mental disorder classifiable elsewhere.

> **Excludes** *those due to mental disorders classified elsewhere*
> *those of organic origin*

307.0 Adult onset fluency disorder

> **Excludes** *childhood onset fluency disorder (315.35)*
> *dysphasia (784.59)*
> *fluency disorder due to late effect of cerebrovascular accident (438.14)*
> *fluency disorder in conditions classified elsewhere (784.52)*
> *lisping or lalling (307.9)*
> *retarded development of speech (315.31–315.39)*

307.1 Anorexia nervosa 🔷

> **Excludes** *eating disturbance NOS (307.50)*
> *feeding problem (783.3)*
> *of nonorganic origin (307.59)*
> *loss of appetite (783.0)*
> *of nonorganic origin (307.59)*

> (Ex) 306.4, 306.8-306.9, 307.1, 307.50-307.59, 309.22
> **Coding Clinic: 2006, Q2, P12; 1989, Q4, P11**

● **307.2 Tics**

> **Excludes** *nail-biting or thumb-sucking (307.9)*
> *stereotypes occurring in isolation (307.3)*
> *tics of organic origin (333.3)*

307.20 Tic disorder, unspecified
Tic disorder NOS

307.21 Transient tic disorder

307.22 Chronic motor or vocal tic disorder

307.23 Tourette's disorder
Motor-verbal tic disorder

307.3 Stereotypic movement disorder
Body-rocking   Spasmus nutans
Head banging   Stereotypes NOS

> **Excludes** *tics (307.20–307.23)*
> *of organic origin (333.3)*

● **307.4 Specific disorders of sleep of nonorganic origin**

> **Excludes** *narcolepsy (347.00–347.11)*
> *organic hypersomnia (327.10–327.19)*
> *organic insomnia (327.00–327.09)*
> *those of unspecified cause (780.50–780.59)*

307.40 Nonorganic sleep disorder, unspecified

307.41 Transient disorder of initiating or maintaining sleep
Adjustment insomnia
Hyposomnia associated with acute or intermittent emotional reactions or conflicts
Insomnia associated with acute or intermittent emotional reactions or conflicts
Sleeplessness associated with acute or intermittent emotional reactions or conflicts

307.42 Persistent disorder of initiating or maintaining sleep
Hyposomnia, insomnia, or sleeplessness associated with:
anxiety
conditioned arousal
depression (major) (minor)
psychosis
Idiopathic insomnia
Paradoxical insomnia
Primary insomnia
Psychophysiological insomnia

307.43 Transient disorder of initiating or maintaining wakefulness
Hypersomnia associated with acute or intermittent emotional reactions or conflicts

307.44 Persistent disorder of initiating or maintaining wakefulness
Hypersomnia associated with depression (major) (minor)
Insufficient sleep syndrome
Primary hypersomnia

> **Excludes** *sleep deprivation (V69.4)*

307.45 Circadian rhythm sleep disorder of nonorganic origin

307.46 Sleep arousal disorder
Night terror disorder
Night terrors
Sleep terror disorder
Sleepwalking
Somnambulism

307.47 Other dysfunctions of sleep stages or arousal from sleep
Nightmare disorder
Nightmares:
NOS
REM-sleep type
Sleep drunkenness

307.48 Repetitive intrusions of sleep
Repetitive intrusion of sleep with:
atypical polysomnographic features
environmental disturbances
repeated REM-sleep interruptions

307.49 Other
"Short-sleeper"
Subjective insomnia complaint

● **307.5 Other and unspecified disorders of eating**

> **Excludes** *anorexia:*
> *nervosa (307.1)*
> *of unspecified cause (783.0)*
> *overeating, of unspecified cause (783.6)*
> *vomiting:*
> *NOS (787.03)*
> *cyclical (536.2)*
> *associated with migraine (346.2)*
> *psychogenic (306.4)*

307.50 Eating disorder, unspecified
Eating disorder NOS

307.51 Bulimia nervosa 🔷
Overeating of nonorganic origin
> (Ex) 307.1, 307.50-307.51, 307.53-307.59
> **Coding Clinic: 2012, Q3, P9**

307.52 Pica
Perverted appetite of nonorganic origin
Craving and eating substances such as paint, clay, or dirt to replace a nutritional deficit in the body

307.53 Rumination disorder
Regurgitation, of nonorganic origin, of food with reswallowing

> **Excludes** *obsessional rumination (300.3)*

MENTAL, BEHAVIORAL AND NEURODEVELOPMENTAL DISORDERS (290-319)

Item 5–3   **Enuresis**: Bed wetting by children at night. Causes can be either psychological or medical (diabetes, urinary tract infections, or abnormalities). **Encopresis**: Overflow incontinence of bowels sometimes resulting from chronic constipation or fecal impaction. Check the documentation for additional diagnoses.

307.54 **Psychogenic vomiting**

307.59 **Other**
Feeding disorder of infancy or early childhood of nonorganic origin
Infantile feeding disturbances of nonorganic origin
Loss of appetite of nonorganic origin

307.6 **Enuresis**
Enuresis (primary) (secondary) of nonorganic origin
Excludes *enuresis of unspecified cause (788.3)*

307.7 **Encopresis**
Encopresis (continuous) (discontinuous) of nonorganic origin
Excludes *encopresis of unspecified cause (787.60-787.63)*

● 307.8 **Pain disorders related to psychological factors**

307.80 **Psychogenic pain, site unspecified**

307.81 **Tension headache**
Excludes *headache:*
migraine (346.0–346.9)
NOS (784.0)
syndromes (339.00–339.89)
tension type (339.10–339.12)
Coding Clinic: 1985, Nov-Dec, P16

307.89 **Other**
Code first to type or site of pain
Excludes *pain disorder exclusively attributed to psychological factors (307.80)*
psychogenic pain (307.80)

307.9 **Other and unspecified special symptoms or syndromes, not elsewhere classified**
Communication disorder NOS
Hair plucking
Lalling
Lisping
Masturbation
Nail-biting
Thumb-sucking

● 308 **Acute reaction to stress**
Includes catastrophic stress
combat and operational stress reaction
combat fatigue
gross stress reaction (acute)
transient disorders in response to exceptional physical or mental stress which usually subside within hours or days
Excludes *adjustment reaction or disorder (309.0–309.9)*
chronic stress reaction (309.1–309.9)

308.0 **Predominant disturbance of emotions**
Anxiety as acute reaction to exceptional [gross] stress
Emotional crisis as acute reaction to exceptional [gross] stress
Panic state as acute reaction to exceptional [gross] stress

308.1 **Predominant disturbance of consciousness**
Fugues as acute reaction to exceptional [gross] stress

308.2 **Predominant psychomotor disturbance**
Agitation states as acute reaction to exceptional [gross] stress
Stupor as acute reaction to exceptional [gross] stress

308.3 **Other acute reactions to stress**
Acute situational disturbance
Acute stress disorder
Excludes *prolonged posttraumatic emotional disturbance (309.81)*

308.4 **Mixed disorders as reaction to stress**

308.9 **Unspecified acute reaction to stress**

● 309 **Adjustment reaction**
Includes adjustment disorders
reaction (adjustment) to chronic stress
Excludes *acute reaction to major stress (308.0–308.9)*
neurotic disorders (300.0–300.9)

309.0 **Adjustment disorder with depressed mood**
Grief reaction
Excludes *affective psychoses (296.0–296.9)*
neurotic depression (300.4)
prolonged depressive reaction (309.1)
psychogenic depressive psychosis (298.0)

309.1 **Prolonged depressive reaction**
Excludes *affective psychoses (296.0–296.9)*
brief depressive reaction (309.0)
neurotic depression (300.4)
psychogenic depressive psychosis (298.0)

● 309.2 **With predominant disturbance of other emotions**

309.21 **Separation anxiety disorder**

309.22 **Emancipation disorder of adolescence and early adult life**

309.23 **Specific academic or work inhibition**

309.24 **Adjustment disorder with anxiety**

309.28 **Adjustment disorder with mixed anxiety and depressed mood**
Adjustment reaction with anxiety and depression

309.29 **Other**
Culture shock

309.3 **Adjustment disorder with disturbance of conduct**
Conduct disturbance as adjustment reaction
Destructiveness as adjustment reaction
Excludes *destructiveness in child (312.9)*
disturbance of conduct NOS (312.9)
dyssocial behavior without manifest psychiatric disorder (V71.01–V71.02)
personality disorder with predominantly sociopathic or asocial manifestations (301.7)

309.4 **Adjustment disorder with mixed disturbance of emotions and conduct**

● 309.8 **Other specified adjustment reactions**

309.81 **Posttraumatic stress disorder**
Chronic posttraumatic stress disorder
Concentration camp syndrome
Posttraumatic stress disorder NOS
Post-Traumatic Stress Disorder (PTSD)
Excludes *acute stress disorder (308.3)*
posttraumatic brain syndrome:
nonpsychotic (310.2)
psychotic (293.0–293.9)

309.82 **Adjustment reaction with physical symptoms**

309.83 **Adjustment reaction with withdrawal**
Elective mutism as adjustment reaction
Hospitalism (in children) NOS

309.89 **Other**

309.9 **Unspecified adjustment reaction**
Adaptation reaction NOS
Adjustment reaction NOS

◀ New   ◀ Revised   ~~deleted~~ Deleted   Excludes   Includes   Use additional   Code first   Omit code

760   ● Unacceptable Principal Diagnosis   ● Use Additional Digit(s)   ▶ Manifestation Code   OGCR Official Guidelines   **Coding Clinic**

● **310** **Specific nonpsychotic mental disorders due to brain damage**

> **Excludes** *neuroses, personality disorders, or other nonpsychotic conditions occurring in a form similar to that seen with functional disorders but in association with a physical condition (300.0–300.9, 301.0–301.9)*

310.0 **Frontal lobe syndrome**
Lobotomy syndrome
Postleucotomy syndrome [state]

> **Excludes** *postcontusion syndrome (310.2)*

310.1 **Personality change due to conditions classified elsewhere**
Cognitive or personality change of other type, of nonpsychotic severity
Organic psychosyndrome of nonpsychotic severity
Presbyophrenia NOS
Senility with mental changes of nonpsychotic severity

> **Excludes** *mild cognitive impairment (331.83)*
> *postconcussion syndrome (310.2)*
> *signs and symptoms involving emotional state (799.21-799.29)*

Coding Clinic: 2005, Q2, P6-7

310.2 **Postconcussion syndrome**
Postcontusion syndrome or encephalopathy
Posttraumatic brain syndrome, nonpsychotic
Status postcommotio cerebri

> **Excludes** *any organic psychotic conditions following head injury (293.0–294.0)*
> *frontal lobe syndrome (310.0)*
> *postencephalitic syndrome (310.89)*

Use additional code to identify associated post-traumatic headache, if applicable (339.20-339.22)

● **310.8** **Other specified nonpsychotic mental disorders following organic brain damage**

310.81 **Pseudobulbar affect**
Involuntary emotional expression disorder
Code first underlying cause, if known, such as:
amyotrophic lateral sclerosis (335.20)
late effect of cerebrovascular accident (438.89)
late effect of traumatic brain injury (907.0)
multiple sclerosis (340)
Coding Clinic: 2011, Q4, P97

310.89 **Other specified nonpsychotic mental disorders following organic brain damage**
Mild memory disturbance
Other focal (partial) organic psychosyndromes
Postencephalitic syndrome

> **Excludes** *memory loss of unknown cause (780.93)*

310.9 **Unspecified nonpsychotic mental disorder following organic brain damage**
Coding Clinic: 2003, Q4, P103-104

311 **Depressive disorder, not elsewhere classified**
Depressive disorder NOS
Depressive state NOS
Depression NOS

> **Excludes** *acute reaction to major stress with depressive symptoms (308.0)*
> *affective personality disorder (301.10–301.13)*
> *affective psychoses (296.0–296.9)*
> *brief depressive reaction (309.0)*
> *depressive states associated with stressful events (309.0–309.1)*
> *disturbance of emotions specific to childhood and adolescence, with misery and unhappiness (313.1)*
> *mixed adjustment reaction with depressive symptoms (309.4)*
> *neurotic depression (300.4)*
> *prolonged depressive adjustment reaction (309.1)*
> *psychogenic depressive psychosis (298.0)*

Coding Clinic: 2011, Q3, P6; 2003, Q4, P75-76

● **312** **Disturbance of conduct, not elsewhere classified**

> **Excludes** *adjustment reaction with disturbance of conduct (309.3)*
> *drug dependence (304.0–304.9)*
> *dyssocial behavior without manifest psychiatric disorder (V71.01–V71.02)*
> *personality disorder with predominantly sociopathic or asocial manifestations (301.7)*
> *sexual deviations (302.0–302.9)*

The following fifth-digit subclassification is for use with categories 312.0–312.2:

0	unspecified	2	moderate
1	mild	3	severe

● **312.0** **Undersocialized conduct disorder, aggressive type**
[0-3]
Aggressive outburst
Anger reaction
Unsocialized aggressive disorder

● **312.1** **Undersocialized conduct disorder, unaggressive type**
[0-3]
Childhood truancy, unsocialized
Solitary stealing
Tantrums

● **312.2** **Socialized conduct disorder**
[0-3]
Childhood truancy, socialized
Group delinquency

> **Excludes** *gang activity without manifest psychiatric disorder (V71.01)*

● **312.3** **Disorders of impulse control, not elsewhere classified**

312.30 **Impulse control disorder, unspecified**

312.31 **Pathological gambling**

312.32 **Kleptomania** *(stealing)*

312.33 **Pyromania** *(setting fires)*

312.34 **Intermittent explosive disorder**

312.35 **Isolated explosive disorder**

312.39 **Other**
Trichotillomania
Pulling or twisting hair until it falls out

312.4 **Mixed disturbance of conduct and emotions**
Neurotic delinquency

> **Excludes** *compulsive conduct disorder (312.3)*

● **312.8** **Other specified disturbances of conduct, not elsewhere classified**

312.81 **Conduct disorder, childhood onset type**

312.82 **Conduct disorder, adolescent onset type**

312.89 **Other conduct disorder**
Conduct disorder of unspecified onset

312.9 **Unspecified disturbance of conduct**
Delinquency (juvenile)
Disruptive behavior disorder NOS

● **313** **Disturbance of emotions specific to childhood and adolescence**

> **Excludes** *adjustment reaction (309.0–309.9)*
> *emotional disorder of neurotic type (300.0–300.9)*
> *masturbation, nail-biting, thumb-sucking, and other isolated symptoms (307.0–307.9)*

313.0 **Overanxious disorder**
Anxiety and fearfulness of childhood and adolescence
Overanxious disorder of childhood and adolescence

> **Excludes** *abnormal separation anxiety (309.21)*
> *anxiety states (300.00–300.09)*
> *hospitalism in children (309.83)*
> *phobic state (300.20–300.29)*

313.1 **Misery and unhappiness disorder**

> **Excludes** *depressive neurosis (300.4)*

N Newborn: 0   P Pediatric: 0–17   M Maternity: 12–55   A Adult: 15–124   ♀ Females Only   ♂ Males Only

Ex CC/MCC Exclusions   Complication\Comorbidity   Major C\C   Present on Admission Requirement   Hospital-Acquired Condition   **761**

● **313.2   Sensitivity, shyness, and social withdrawal disorder**

> **Excludes**   *infantile autism (299.0)*
> *schizoid personality (301.20–301.22)*
> *schizophrenia (295.0–295.9)*

313.21   Shyness disorder of childhood
Sensitivity reaction of childhood or adolescence

313.22   Introverted disorder of childhood
Social withdrawal of childhood or adolescence
Withdrawal reaction of childhood or adolescence

313.23   Selective mutism

> **Excludes**   *elective mutism as adjustment reaction (309.83)*

313.3   Relationship problems
Sibling jealousy

> **Excludes**   *relationship problems associated with aggression, destruction, or other forms of conduct disturbance (312.0–312.9)*

● **313.8   Other or mixed emotional disturbances of childhood or adolescence**

313.81   Oppositional defiant disorder

313.82   Identity disorder
Identity problem

313.83   Academic underachievement disorder

313.89   Other   P
Reactive attachment disorder of infancy or early childhood

313.9   Unspecified emotional disturbance of childhood or adolescence   P
Mental disorder of infancy, childhood or adolescence NOS

● **314   Hyperkinetic syndrome of childhood**

> **Excludes**   *hyperkinesis as symptom of underlying disorder-code the underlying disorder*

● **314.0   Attention deficit disorder** *(ADD)*
Adult
Child

314.00   Without mention of hyperactivity
Predominantly inattentive type
Coding Clinic: 2012, Q3, P19; 1997, Q1, P8-9

314.01   With hyperactivity
Attention deficit disorder with hyperactivity = ADHD
Combined type
Overactivity NOS
Predominantly hyperactive/impulsive type
Simple disturbance of attention with overactivity
Coding Clinic: 2012, Q3, P19; 1997, Q1, P8-9

314.1   Hyperkinesis with developmental delay
Developmental disorder of hyperkinesis

> Use additional code to identify any associated neurological disorder

314.2   Hyperkinetic conduct disorder
Hyperkinetic conduct disorder without developmental delay

> **Excludes**   *hyperkinesis with significant delays in specific skills (314.1)*

314.8   Other specified manifestations of hyperkinetic syndrome

314.9   Unspecified hyperkinetic syndrome
Hyperkinetic reaction of childhood or adolescence NOS
Hyperkinetic syndrome NOS

● **315   Specific delays in development**

> **Excludes**   *that due to a neurological disorder (320.0–389.9)*

● **315.0   Specific reading disorder**

315.00   Reading disorder, unspecified

315.01   Alexia

315.02   Developmental dyslexia

315.09   Other
Specific spelling difficulty

315.1   Mathematics disorder
Dyscalculia

315.2   Other specific learning difficulties
Disorder of written expression

> **Excludes**   *specific arithmetical disorder (315.1)*
> *specific reading disorder (315.00–315.09)*

● **315.3   Developmental speech or language disorder**

315.31   Expressive language disorder
Developmental aphasia
Word deafness

> **Excludes**   *acquired aphasia (784.3)*
> *elective mutism (309.83, 313.0, 313.23)*

315.32   Mixed receptive-expressive language disorder
Central auditory processing disorder

> **Excludes**   *acquired auditory processing disorder (388.45)*

Coding Clinic: 2005, Q2, P5-6

315.34   Speech and language developmental delay due to hearing loss
Coding Clinic: 2007, Q4, P80-81

315.35   Childhood onset fluency disorder
Cluttering NOS
Stuttering NOS

> **Excludes**   *adult onset fluency disorder (307.0)*
> *fluency disorder due to late effect of cerebrovascular accident (438.14)*
> *fluency disorder in conditions classified elsewhere (784.52)*

315.39   Other
Developmental articulation disorder
Dyslalia
Phonological disorder

> **Excludes**   *lisping and lalling (307.9)*

Coding Clinic: 2007, Q3, P9-10

315.4   Developmental coordination disorder
Clumsiness syndrome
Dyspraxia syndrome
Specific motor development disorder

315.5   Mixed development disorder
Coding Clinic: 2002, Q2, P11

315.8   Other specified delays in development

315.9   Unspecified delay in development
Developmental disorder NOS
Learning disorder NOS

◀ New   ◀▬ Revised   deleted Deleted   Excludes   Includes   Use additional   Code first   Omit code

762   ● Unacceptable Principal Diagnosis   ● Use Additional Digit(s)   ▷ Manifestation Code   OGCR Official Guidelines   Coding Clinic

316 **Psychic factors associated with diseases classified elsewhere**
Psychologic factors in physical conditions classified elsewhere

Use additional code to identify the associated physical
condition, as:
psychogenic:
asthma (493.9)
dermatitis (692.9)
duodenal ulcer (532.0–532.9)
eczema (691.8, 692.9)
gastric ulcer (531.0–531.9)
mucous colitis (564.9)
paroxysmal tachycardia (427.2)
ulcerative colitis (556)
urticaria (708.0–708.9)
psychosocial dwarfism (259.4)

Excludes *physical symptoms and physiological malfunctions,*
not involving tissue damage, of mental origin
(306.0–306.9)

INTELLECTUAL DISABILITIES (317-319)

Use additional code(s) to identify any associated psychiatric or
physical condition(s)

317 **Mild intellectual disabilities**
High-grade defect
IQ 50–70
Mild mental subnormality

● 318 **Other specified intellectual disabilities**

318.0 **Moderate intellectual disabilities**
IQ 35–49
Moderate mental subnormality

318.1 **Severe intellectual disabilities** 🦠
IQ 20–34
Severe mental subnormality
Ⓔˣ 318.1-318.2

318.2 **Profound intellectual disabilities** 🦠
IQ under 20
Profound mental subnormality
Ⓔˣ 318.1-318.2

319 **Unspecified intellectual disabilities**
Mental deficiency NOS
Mental subnormality NOS

MENTAL, BEHAVIORAL AND NEURODEVELOPMENTAL DISORDERS (290-319)

N Newborn: 0   **P** Pediatric: 0–17   **M** Maternity: 12–55   **A** Adult: 15–124   ♀ Females Only   ♂ Males Only

Ⓔˣ CC/MCC Exclusions   🦠 Complication\Comorbidity   🦠 Major C\C   🦠 Present on Admission Requirement   🦠 Hospital-Acquired Condition   763

(See Plate 164 on page 54.)

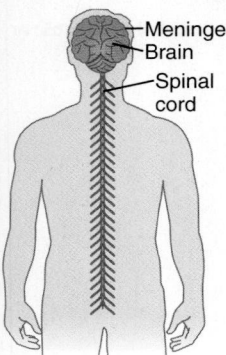

—Meninges
—Brain
—Spinal cord

Figure 6–1 The brain and spinal cord make up the central nervous system.

Item 6–1 The two major classifications of the nervous system are the peripheral nervous system and the central nervous system (CNS). The central nervous system is comprised of the brain and the spinal cord. The peripheral nervous system is comprised of the parasympathetic and sympathetic systems. **Encephalitis** is the swelling of the brain. **Meningitis** is swelling of the covering of the brain, the meninges. Types and causes of brain infections are:

Type	Cause
purulent	bacterial
aseptic/abacterial	viral
chronic meningitis	mycobacterial and fungal

6. DISEASES OF THE NERVOUS SYSTEM AND SENSE ORGANS (320–389)

INFLAMMATORY DISEASES OF THE CENTRAL NERVOUS SYSTEM (320–326)

● **320 Bacterial meningitis**
Infection of cerebrospinal fluid surrounding spinal cord and brain
> **Includes** arachnoiditis bacterial
> leptomeningitis bacterial
> meningitis bacterial
> meningoencephalitis bacterial
> meningomyelitis bacterial
> pachymeningitis bacterial

320.0 Hemophilus meningitis 🔖
Meningitis due to Hemophilus influenzae [H. influenzae]
Ex: 003.21, 013.00-013.16, 036.0, 047.0-047.9, 049.0-049.1, 053.0, 054.72, 072.1, 090.42, 091.81, 094.2, 098.89, 100.81, 112.83, 114.2, 115.01, 115.11, 115.91, 130.0, 249.60-249.61, 249.80-249.91, 250.60-250.63, 250.80-250.93, 320.0-322.9, 349.89-349.9, 357.0

320.1 Pneumococcal meningitis 🔖
Ex: 003.21, 013.00-013.16, 036.0, 047.0-047.9, 049.0-049.1, 053.0, 054.72, 072.1, 090.42, 091.81, 094.2, 098.89, 100.81, 112.83, 114.2, 115.01, 115.11, 115.91, 130.0, 249.60-249.61, 249.80-249.91, 250.60-250.63, 250.80-250.93, 320.0-322.9, 349.89-349.9, 357.0

320.2 Streptococcal meningitis 🔖
Ex: 003.21, 013.00-013.16, 036.0, 047.0-047.9, 049.0-049.1, 053.0, 054.72, 072.1, 090.42, 091.81, 094.2, 098.89, 100.81, 112.83, 114.2, 115.01, 115.11, 115.91, 130.0, 249.60-249.61, 249.80-249.91, 250.60-250.63, 250.80-250.93, 320.0-322.9, 349.89-349.9, 357.0

320.3 Staphylococcal meningitis 🔖
Ex: 003.21, 013.00-013.16, 036.0, 047.0-047.9, 049.0-049.1, 053.0, 054.72, 072.1, 090.42, 091.81, 094.2, 098.89, 100.81, 112.83, 114.2, 115.01, 115.11, 115.91, 130.0, 249.60-249.61, 249.80-249.91, 250.60-250.63, 250.80-250.93, 320.0-322.9, 349.89-349.9, 357.0

▷ **320.7 Meningitis in other bacterial diseases classified elsewhere** 🔖
> *Code first* underlying disease as:
> actinomycosis (039.8)
> listeriosis (027.0)
> typhoid fever (002.0)
> whooping cough (033.0–033.9)
> **Excludes** *meningitis (in):*
> *epidemic (036.0)*
> *gonococcal (098.82)*
> *meningococcal (036.0)*
> *salmonellosis (003.21)*
> *syphilis:*
> *NOS (094.2)*
> *congenital (090.42)*
> *meningovascular (094.2)*
> *secondary (091.81)*
> *tuberculosis (013.0)*
Ex: 003.21, 013.00-013.16, 036.0, 047.0-047.9, 049.0-049.1, 053.0, 054.72, 072.1, 090.42, 091.81, 094.2, 098.89, 100.81, 112.83, 114.2, 115.01, 115.11, 115.91, 130.0, 249.60-249.61, 249.80-249.91, 250.60-250.63, 250.80-250.93, 320.0-322.9, 349.89-349.9, 357.0

● **320.8 Meningitis due to other specified bacteria**
320.81 Anaerobic meningitis 🔖
Bacteroides (fragilis)
Gram-negative anaerobes
Ex: 003.21, 013.00-013.16, 036.0, 047.0-047.9, 049.0-049.1, 053.0, 054.72, 072.1, 090.42, 091.81, 094.2, 098.89, 100.81, 112.83, 114.2, 115.01, 115.11, 115.91, 130.0, 249.60-249.61, 249.80-249.91, 250.60-250.63, 250.80-250.93, 320.0-322.9, 349.89-349.9, 357.0

320.82 Meningitis due to gram-negative bacteria, not elsewhere classified 🔖
Aerobacter aerogenes
Escherichia coli [E. coli]
Friedlander bacillus
Klebsiella pneumoniae
Proteus morganii
Pseudomonas
> **Excludes** *gram-negative anaerobes (320.81)*
Ex: 003.21, 013.00-013.16, 036.0, 047.0-047.9, 049.0-049.1, 053.0, 054.72, 072.1, 090.42, 091.81, 094.2, 098.89, 100.81, 112.83, 114.2, 115.01, 115.11, 115.91, 130.0, 249.60-249.61, 249.80-249.91, 250.60-250.63, 250.80-250.93, 320.0-322.9, 349.89-349.9, 357.0
Coding Clinic: 2011, Q4, P155

320.89 Meningitis due to other specified bacteria 🔖
Bacillus pyocyaneus
Ex: 003.21, 013.00-013.16, 036.0, 047.0-047.9, 049.0-049.1, 053.0, 054.72, 072.1, 090.42, 091.81, 094.2, 098.89, 100.81, 112.83, 114.2, 115.01, 115.11, 115.91, 130.0, 249.60-249.61, 249.80-249.91, 250.60-250.63, 250.80-250.93, 320.0-322.9, 349.89-349.9, 357.0

320.9 Meningitis due to unspecified bacterium 🔖
Meningitis:	Meningitis:
bacterial NOS	pyogenic NOS
purulent NOS	suppurative NOS
Ex: 003.21, 013.00-013.16, 036.0, 047.0-047.9, 049.0-049.1, 053.0, 054.72, 072.1, 090.42, 091.81, 094.2, 098.89, 100.81, 112.83, 114.2, 115.01, 115.11, 115.91, 130.0, 249.60-249.61, 249.80-249.91, 250.60-250.63, 250.80-250.93, 320.0-322.9, 349.89-349.9, 357.0

● 321 **Meningitis due to other organisms**

> **Includes**   arachnoiditis due to organisms other than bacteria
> leptomeningitis due to organisms other than
> bacteria
> meningitis due to organisms other than bacteria
> pachymeningitis due to organisms other than
> bacteria

▶ **321.0   Cryptococcal meningitis** 🔒

> *Code first underlying disease (117.5)*
>
> (Ex) 003.21, 013.00-013.16, 036.0, 047.0-047.9, 049.0-049.1, 053.0, 054.72,
> 072.1, 090.42, 091.81, 094.2, 098.89, 100.81, 112.83, 114.2, 115.01,
> 115.11, 115.91, 130.0, 249.60-249.61, 249.80-249.91, 250.60-250.63,
> 250.80-250.93, 320.0-322.9, 349.89-349.9, 357.0

▶ **321.1   Meningitis in other fungal diseases** 🔒

> *Code first underlying disease (110.0–118)*
>
> **Excludes**   meningitis in:
> candidiasis (112.83)
> coccidioidomycosis (114.2)
> histoplasmosis (115.01, 115.11, 115.91)
>
> (Ex) 003.21, 013.00-013.16, 036.0, 047.0-047.9, 049.0-049.1, 053.0, 054.72,
> 072.1, 090.42, 091.81, 094.2, 098.89, 100.81, 112.83, 114.2, 115.01,
> 115.11, 115.91, 130.0, 249.60-249.61, 249.80-249.91, 250.60-250.63,
> 250.80-250.93, 320.0-322.9, 349.89-349.9, 357.0

▶ **321.2   Meningitis due to viruses not elsewhere classified** 🔒

> *Code first underlying disease, as:*
> meningitis due to arbovirus (060.0–066.9)
>
> **Excludes**   meningitis (due to):
> abacterial (047.0–047.9)
> adenovirus (049.1)
> aseptic NOS (047.9)
> Coxsackie (virus) (047.0)
> ECHO virus (047.1)
> enterovirus (047.0–047.9)
> herpes simplex virus (054.72)
> herpes zoster virus (053.0)
> lymphocytic choriomeningitis virus (049.0)
> mumps (072.1)
> viral NOS (047.9)
> meningo-eruptive syndrome (047.1)
>
> (Ex) 003.21, 013.00-013.16, 036.0, 047.0-047.9, 049.0-049.1, 053.0, 054.72,
> 072.1, 090.42, 091.81, 094.2, 098.89, 100.81, 112.83, 114.2, 115.01,
> 115.11, 115.91, 130.0, 320.0-322.9, 349.89-349.9, 357.0
>
> **Coding Clinic: 2004, Q4, P50-52**

▶ **321.3   Meningitis due to trypanosomiasis** 🔒

> *Code first underlying disease (086.0–086.9)*
>
> (Ex) 003.21, 013.00-013.16, 036.0, 047.0-047.9, 049.0-049.1, 053.0, 054.72,
> 072.1, 090.42, 091.81, 094.2, 098.89, 100.81, 112.83, 114.2, 115.01,
> 115.11, 115.91, 130.0, 249.60-249.61, 249.80-249.91, 250.60-250.63,
> 250.80-250.93, 320.0-322.9, 349.89-349.9, 357.0

▶ **321.4   Meningitis in sarcoidosis** 🔒

> *Code first underlying disease (135)*
>
> (Ex) 003.21, 013.00-013.16, 036.0, 047.0-047.9, 049.0-049.1, 053.0, 054.72,
> 072.1, 090.42, 091.81, 094.2, 098.89, 100.81, 112.83, 114.2, 115.01,
> 115.11, 115.91, 130.0, 249.60-249.61, 249.80-249.91, 250.60-250.63,
> 250.80-250.93, 320.0-322.9, 349.89-349.9, 357.0

▶ **321.8   Meningitis due to other nonbacterial organisms classified elsewhere** 🔒

> *Code first underlying disease*
>
> **Excludes**   leptospiral meningitis (100.81)
>
> (Ex) 003.21, 013.00-013.16, 036.0, 047.0-047.9, 049.0-049.1, 053.0, 054.72,
> 072.1, 090.42, 091.81, 094.2, 098.89, 100.81, 112.83, 114.2, 115.01,
> 115.11, 115.91, 130.0, 249.60-249.61, 249.80-249.91, 250.60-250.63,
> 250.80-250.93, 320.0-322.9, 349.89-349.9, 357.0

● 322 **Meningitis of unspecified cause**

> **Includes**   arachnoiditis with no organism specified as cause
> leptomeningitis with no organism specified as
> cause
> meningitis with no organism specified as cause
> pachymeningitis with no organism specified as
> cause

322.0   Nonpyogenic meningitis 🔒

> Meningitis with clear cerebrospinal fluid
>
> (Ex) 003.21, 013.00-013.16, 036.0, 047.0-047.9, 049.0-049.1, 053.0, 054.72,
> 072.1, 090.42, 091.81, 094.2, 098.89, 100.81, 112.83, 114.2, 115.01,
> 115.11, 115.91, 130.0, 249.60-249.61, 249.80-249.91, 250.60-250.63,
> 250.80-250.93, 320.0-322.9, 349.89-349.9, 357.0

322.1   Eosinophilic meningitis 🔒

> (Ex) 003.21, 013.00-013.16, 036.0, 047.0-047.9, 049.0-049.1, 053.0, 054.72,
> 072.1, 090.42, 091.81, 094.2, 098.89, 100.81, 112.83, 114.2, 115.01,
> 115.11, 115.91, 130.0, 249.60-249.61, 249.80-249.91, 250.60-250.63,
> 250.80-250.93, 320.0-322.9, 349.89-349.9, 357.0

322.2   Chronic meningitis 🔒

> (Ex) 003.21, 013.00-013.16, 036.0, 047.0-047.9, 049.0-049.1, 053.0, 054.72,
> 072.1, 090.42, 091.81, 094.2, 098.89, 100.81, 112.83, 114.2, 115.01,
> 115.11, 115.91, 130.0, 249.60-249.61, 249.80-249.91, 250.60-250.63,
> 250.80-250.93, 320.0-322.9, 349.89-349.9, 357.0

322.9   Meningitis, unspecified 🔒

> (Ex) 003.21, 013.00-013.16, 036.0, 047.0-047.9, 049.0-049.1, 053.0, 054.72,
> 072.1, 090.42, 091.81, 094.2, 098.89, 100.81, 112.83, 114.2, 115.01,
> 115.11, 115.91, 130.0, 249.60-249.61, 249.80-249.91, 250.60-250.63,
> 250.80-250.93, 320.0-322.9, 349.89-349.9, 357.0

● 323 **Encephalitis, myelitis, and encephalomyelitis**

> **Includes**   acute disseminated encephalomyelitis
> meningoencephalitis, except bacterial
> meningomyelitis, except bacterial
> myelitis:
> ascending
> transverse
>
> **Excludes**   acute transverse myelitis NOS (341.20)
> acute transverse myelitis in conditions classified
> elsewhere (341.21)
> bacterial:
> meningoencephalitis (320.0–320.9)
> meningomyelitis (320.0–320.9)
> idiopathic transverse myelitis (341.22)

Coding Clinic: 2006, Q4, P58-63

● **323.0   Encephalitis, myelitis, and encephalomyelitis in viral diseases classified elsewhere**

> *Code first underlying disease, as:*
> cat-scratch disease (078.3)
> human immunodeficiency virus [HIV] disease (042)
> infectious mononucleosis (075)
> ornithosis (073.7)

▶ **323.01   Encephalitis and encephalomyelitis in viral diseases classified elsewhere** 🔒

> **Excludes**   encephalitis (in):
> arthropod-borne viral
> (062.0–064)
> herpes simplex (054.3)
> mumps (072.2)
> other viral diseases of central nervous
> system (049.8–049.9)
> poliomyelitis (045.0–045.9)
> rubella (056.01)
> slow virus infections of central
> nervous system (046.0–046.9)
> viral NOS (049.9)
> West Nile (066.41)
>
> (Ex) 003.21, 013.00-013.16, 013.60-013.66, 036.0, 046.2, 046.71-
> 046.8, 047.0-049.8, 051.9-052.0, 052.7-053.13, 053.19,
> 053.79-053.9, 054.3, 054.72, 054.79-054.9, 056.01,
> 057.8-059.9, 062.0-064, 066.2-066.49, 072.1-072.2, 073.7,
> 075, 078.89, 079.81-079.82, 079.89, 079.99, 090.41-090.42,
> 091.81, 094.2, 094.81, 098.89, 100.81, 112.83, 114.2, 115.01,
> 115.11, 115.91, 130.0, 139.8, 290.12, 320.0-323.9, 341.1,
> 349.89-349.9, 357.0, 487.8, 488.09, 488.19, 488.89, 771.2
>
> **Coding Clinic: 2010, Q3, P14**

N Newborn: 0   **P** Pediatric: 0–17   **M** Maternity: 12–55   **A** Adult: 15–124   ♀ Females Only   ♂ Males Only

(Ex) CC/MCC Exclusions   🔒 Complication\Comorbidity   🔒 Major C\C   🔒 Present on Admission Requirement   🔒 Hospital-Acquired Condition   **765**

Item 6-2   **Encephalitis** is an inflammation of the brain most often caused by a virus but may also be caused by a bacteria and most commonly transmitted by a mosquito. **Myelitis** is an inflammation of the spinal cord that may disrupt CNS function. Untreated myelitis may rapidly lead to permanent damage to the spinal cord. **Encephalomyelitis** is a general term for an inflammation of the brain and spinal cord.

323.02   *Myelitis in viral diseases classified elsewhere* 🔍

    Excludes   *myelitis (in):*
        herpes simplex (054.74)
        herpes zoster (053.14)
        other viral diseases of central nervous
          system (049.8–049.9)
        poliomyelitis (045.0–045.9)
        rubella (056.01)

    Ex: 003.21, 013.00-013.16, 013.60-013.66, 036.0, 046.2, 046.71-046.8, 047.0-049.8, 051.9-052.0, 052.7-053.13, 053.19, 053.79-053.9, 054.3, 054.72, 054.79-054.9, 056.01, 057.8-059.9, 062.0-064, 066.2-066.49, 072.1-072.2, 073.7, 075, 078.89, 079.81-079.82, 079.89, 079.99, 090.41-090.42, 091.81, 094.2, 094.81, 098.89, 100.81, 112.83, 114.2, 115.01, 115.11, 115.91, 130.0, 139.8, 290.12, 320.0-323.9, 341.1, 349.89-349.9, 357, 487.8, 488.09, 488.19, 488.89, 771.2

323.1   *Encephalitis, myelitis, and encephalomyelitis in rickettsial diseases classified elsewhere* 🔍

    Code first underlying disease (080–083.9)

    Ex: 013.60-013.66, 046.2, 046.71-04.68 048-049.0, 049.8, 052.0, 052.2, 054.3 054.74, 056.01, 057.8-058.29, 059.00-059.9, 062.0-064, 066.2-066.49 072.2, 073.7, 079.82, 079.99, 081.9 083.9, 090.41, 094.81, 117.5, 124, 130.0 290.12, 323.01-323.9, 341.1, 487.8, 488.09, 488.19, 488.89, 771.2, 984.9

323.2   *Encephalitis, myelitis, and encephalomyelitis in protozoal diseases classified elsewhere* 🔍

    Code first underlying disease, as:
    malaria (084.0–084.9)
    trypanosomiasis (086.0–086.9)

    Ex: 013.60-013.66, 046.2, 046.71-046.8 048-049.0, 049.8, 052.0, 052.2, 054.3 054.74, 056.01, 057.8-058.29, 059.00-059.9, 062.0-064, 066.2-066.49 072.2, 073.7, 079.82, 079.99, 081.9, 083.9, 084.6, 090.41, 094.81, 117.5, 124, 130.0, 290.12, 323.01-323.9, 341.1, 487.8, 488.09, 488.19, 488.89, 771.2, 984.9

● **323.4**   **Other encephalitis, myelitis, and encephalomyelitis due to other infections classified elsewhere**

    Code first underlying disease

323.41   *Other encephalitis and encephalomyelitis due to other infections classified elsewhere* 🔍

    Excludes   *encephalitis (in):*
        meningococcal (036.1)
        syphilis:
          NOS (094.81)
          congenital (090.41)
        toxoplasmosis (130.0)
        tuberculosis (013.6)
        meningoencephalitis due to free-living
          ameba [Naegleria] (136.29)

    Ex: 003.21, 013.00-013.16, 013.60-013.66 036.0, 046.2, 046.71-046.8, 047.0-049.8 051.9-052.0, 052.7-053.13, 053.19, 053.79-053.9, 054.3, 054.72, 054.79-054.9, 056.01, 057.8-059.9, 062.0-064, 066.2-066.49, 072.1-072.2, 073.7, 075, 078.89, 079.81-079.82, 079.89, 079.99, 090.41-090.42, 091.81, 094.2, 094.81, 098.89, 100.81, 112.83, 114.2, 115.01, 115.11, 115.91, 130.0, 139.8, 290.12, 320.0-323.9, 341.1, 349.89-349.9, 357.0, 487.8, 488.09, 488.19, 488.89, 771.2

323.42   *Other myelitis due to other infections classified elsewhere* 🔍

    Excludes   *myelitis (in):*
        syphilis (094.89)
        tuberculosis (013.6)

    Ex: 003.21, 013.00-013.16, 013.60-013.66, 036.0, 046.2, 046.71-046.8, 047.0-049.8, 051.9-052.0, 052.7-053.13, 053.19, 053.79-053.9, 054.3, 054.72, 054.79-054.9, 056.01, 057.8-059.9, 062.0-064, 066.2-066.49, 072.1-072.2, 073.7, 075, 078.89, 079.81-079.82, 079.89, 079.99, 090.41-090.42, 091.81, 094.2, 094.81, 098.89, 100.81, 112.83, 114.2, 115.01, 115.11, 115.91, 130.0, 139.8, 290.12, 320.0-323.9, 341.1, 349.89-349.9, 357.0, 487.8, 488.09, 488.19, 488.89, 771.2

● **323.5**   **Encephalitis, myelitis, and encephalomyelitis following immunization procedures**

    Use additional E code to identify vaccine

323.51   **Encephalitis and encephalomyelitis following immunization procedures** 🔍
    Encephalitis postimmunization or postvaccinal
    Encephalomyelitis postimmunization or postvaccinal

    Ex: 003.21, 013.00-013.16, 013.60-013.66, 036.0, 046.2, 046.71-046.8, 047.0-049.8, 051.9-052.0, 052.7-053.13, 053.19, 053.79-053.9, 054.3, 054.72, 054.79-054.9, 056.01, 057.8-059.9, 062.0-064, 066.2-066.49, 072.1-072.2, 073.7, 075, 078.89, 079.81-079.82, 079.89, 079.99, 090.41-090.42, 091.81, 094.2, 094.81, 098.89, 100.81, 112.83, 114.2, 115.01, 115.11, 115.91, 130.0, 139.8, 290.12, 320.0-323.9, 341.1, 349.89-349.9, 357, 487.8, 488.09, 488.19, 488.89, 771.2

323.52   **Myelitis following immunization procedures** 🔍
    Myelitis postimmunization or postvaccinal

    Ex: 003.21, 013.00-013.16, 013.60-013.66, 036.0, 046.2, 046.71-046.8, 047.0-049.8, 051.9-052.0, 052.7-053.13, 053.19, 053.79-053.9, 054.3, 054.72, 054.79-054.9, 056.01, 057.8-059.9, 062.0-064, 066.2-066.49, 072.1-072.2, 073.7, 075, 078.89, 079.81-079.82, 079.89, 079.99, 090.41-090.42, 091.81, 094.2, 094.81, 098.89, 100.81, 112.83, 114.2, 115.01, 115.11, 115.91, 130.0, 139.8, 290.12, 320.0-323.9, 341.1, 349.89-349.9, 357, 487.8, 488.09, 488.19, 488.89, 771.2

● **323.6**   **Postinfectious encephalitis, myelitis, and encephalomyelitis**

    Code first underlying disease

323.61   *Infectious acute disseminated encephalomyelitis (ADEM)* 🔍
    Acute necrotizing hemorrhagic encephalopathy

    Excludes   *noninfectious acute disseminated*
        encephalomyelitis (323.81)

    Ex: 003.21, 013.00-013.16, 013.60-013.66, 036.0, 046.2, 046.71-046.8, 047.0-049.8, 051.9-052.0, 052.7-053.13, 053.19, 053.79-053.9, 054.3, 054.72, 054.79-054.9, 056.01, 057.8-059.9, 062.0-064, 066.2-066.49, 072.1-072.2, 073.7, 075, 078.89, 079.81-079.82, 079.89, 079.99, 090.41-090.42, 091.81, 094.2, 094.81, 098.89, 100.81, 112.83, 114.2, 115.01, 115.11, 115.91, 130.0, 139.8, 290.12, 320.0-323.9, 341.1, 349.89-349.9, 357.0, 487.8, 488.09, 488.19, 488.89, 771.2

323.62   *Other postinfectious encephalitis and encephalomyelitis* 🔍

    Excludes   *encephalitis:*
        postchickenpox (052.0)
        postmeasles (055.0)

    Ex: 003.21, 013.00-013.16, 013.60-013.66, 036.0, 046.2, 046.71-046.8, 047.0-049.8, 051.9-052.0, 052.7-053.13, 053.19, 053.79-053.9, 054.3, 054.72, 054.79-054.9, 056.01, 057.8-059.9, 062.0-064, 066.2-066.49, 072.1-072.2, 073.7, 075, 078.89, 079.81-079.82, 079.89, 079.99, 090.41-090.42, 091.81, 094.2, 094.81, 098.89, 100.81, 112.83, 114.2, 115.01, 115.11, 115.91, 130.0, 139.8, 290.12, 320.0-323.9, 341.1, 349.89-349.9, 357.0, 487.8, 488.09, 488.19, 488.89, 771.2

323.63   *Postinfectious myelitis* 🔍

    Ex: 003.21, 013.00-013.16, 013.60-013.66, 036.0, 046.2, 046.71-046.8, 047.0-049.8, 051.9-052.0, 052.7-053.13, 053.19, 053.79-053.9, 054.3, 054.72, 054.79-054.9, 056.01, 057.8-059.9, 062.0-064, 066.2-066.49, 072.1-072.2, 073.7, 075, 078.89, 079.81-079.82, 079.89, 079.99, 090.41-090.42, 091.81, 094.2, 094.81, 098.89, 100.81, 112.83, 114.2, 115.01, 115.11, 115.91, 130.0, 139.8, 290.12, 320.0-323.9, 341.1, 349.89-349.9, 357.0, 487.8, 488.09, 488.19, 771.2

◄ New   ◄ Revised   ~~deleted~~ Deleted   Excludes   Includes   Use additional   Code first   Omit code

● **323.7 Toxic encephalitis, myelitis, and encephalomyelitis**

Code first underlying cause, as:
carbon tetrachloride (982.1)
hydroxyquinoline derivatives (961.3)
lead (984.0–984.9)
mercury (985.0)
thallium (985.8)

▷ **323.71 *Toxic encephalitis and encephalomyelitis*** 🔵
(Ex:) 003.21, 013.00-013.16, 013.60-013.66, 036.0, 046.2,
046.71-046.8, 047.0-049.8, 051.9-052.0, 052.7-053.13,
053.19, 053.79-053.9, 054.3, 054.72, 054.79-054.9, 056.01,
057.8-059.9, 062.0-064, 066.2-066.49, 072.1-072.2, 073.7,
075, 078.89, 079.81-079.82, 079.89, 079.99, 090.41-090.42,
091.81, 094.2, 094.81, 098.89, 100.81, 112.83, 114.2, 115.01,
115.11, 115.91, 130.0, 139.8, 290.12, 320.0-323.9, 341.1,
349.89-349.9, 357.0, 487.8, 488.09, 488.19, 488.89, 771.2

▷ **323.72 *Toxic myelitis*** 🔵
(Ex:) 003.21, 013.00-013.16, 013.60-013.66, 036.0, 046.2,
046.71-046.8, 047.0-049.8, 051.9-052.0, 052.7-053.13,
053.19, 053.79-053.9, 054.3, 054.72, 054.79-054.9, 056.01,
057.8-059.9, 062.0-064, 066.2-066.49, 072.1-072.2, 073.7,
075, 078.89, 079.81-079.82, 079.89, 079.99, 090.41-090.42,
091.81, 094.2, 094.81, 098.89, 100.81, 112.83, 114.2, 115.01,
115.11, 115.91, 130.0, 139.8, 290.12, 320.0-323.9, 341.1,
349.89-349.9, 357.0, 487.8, 488.09, 488.19, 488.89, 771.2

● **323.8 Other causes of encephalitis, myelitis, and encephalomyelitis**
Coding Clinic: 1997, Q2, P8-9

323.81 Other causes of encephalitis and encephalomyelitis 🔵
Noninfectious acute disseminated encephalomyelitis (ADEM)
(Ex:) 003.21, 013.00-013.16, 013.60-013.66, 036.0, 046.2,
046.71-046.8, 047.0-049.8, 051.9-052.0, 052.7-053.13,
053.19, 053.79-053.9, 054.3, 054.72, 054.79-054.9, 056.01,
057.8-059.9, 062.0-064, 066.2-066.49, 072.1-072.2, 073.7,
075, 078.89, 079.81-079.82, 079.89, 079.99, 090.41-090.42,
091.81, 094.2, 094.81, 098.89, 100.81, 112.83, 114.2, 115.01,
115.11, 115.91, 130.0, 139.8, 290.12, 320.0-323.9, 341.1,
349.89-349.9, 357.0, 487.8, 488.09, 488.19, 488.89, 771.2
Coding Clinic: 2011, Q1, P12; 2010, Q3, P16

323.82 Other causes of myelitis 🔵
Transverse myelitis NOS
(Ex:) 003.21, 013.00-013.16, 013.60-013.66, 036.0, 046.2,
046.71-046.8, 047.0-049.8, 051.9-052.0, 052.7-053.13,
053.19, 053.79-053.9, 054.3, 054.72, 054.79-054.9, 056.01,
057.8-059.9, 062.0-064, 066.2-066.49, 072.1-072.2, 073.7,
075, 078.89, 079.81-079.82, 079.89, 079.99, 090.41-090.42,
091.81, 094.2, 094.81, 098.89, 100.81, 112.83, 114.2, 115.01,
115.11, 115.91, 130.0, 139.8, 290.12, 320.0-323.9, 341.1,
349.89-349.9, 357.0, 487.8, 488.09, 488.19, 488.89, 771.2

323.9 Unspecified cause of encephalitis, myelitis, and encephalomyelitis 🔵
(Ex:) 013.60-013.66, 046.2, 046.71-046.8, 048-049.0, 049.8, 052.0, 052.2, 054.3,
054.74, 056.01, 057.8-058.29, 059.00-059.9, 062.0-064, 066.2-066.49,
072.2, 073.7, 075, 078.3, 079.82, 079.99, 081.9, 083.9, 084.6, 090.41,
094.81, 117.5, 124, 130.0, 290.12, 323.01-323.9, 341.1, 382.4, 487.8,
488.09, 488.19, 488.89, 710.0, 771.2, 984.9
Coding Clinic: 2010, Q3, P15; 2006, Q1, P8

● **324 Intracranial and intraspinal abscess**
Accumulation of pus in either brain or spinal cord

324.0 Intracranial abscess 🔵
Abscess (embolic):
cerebellar
cerebral
Abscess (embolic) of brain [any part]:
epidural
extradural
otogenic
subdural

Excludes *tuberculous (013.3)*
(Ex:) 006.5, 013.20-013.36, 249.60-249.61, 249.80-249.91, 250.60-250.63,
250.80-250.93, 324.0-325, 348.81, 348.89-384.9

324.1 Intraspinal abscess 🔵
Abscess (embolic) of spinal cord [any part]:
epidural
extradural
subdural

Excludes *tuberculous (013.5)*
(Ex:) 006.5, 013.20-013.36, 249.60-249.61, 249.80-249.91, 250.60-250.63,
250.80-250.93, 324.1

324.9 Of unspecified site 🔵
Extradural or subdural abscess NOS
(Ex:) 006.5, 013.20-013.36, 249.60-249.61, 249.80-249.91, 250.60-250.63,
250.80-250.93, 324.0-325

325 Phlebitis and thrombophlebitis of intracranial venous sinuses 🔵
Embolism of cavernous, lateral, or other intracranial or unspecified intracranial venous sinus
Endophlebitis of cavernous, lateral, or other intracranial or unspecified intracranial venous sinus
Phlebitis, septic or suppurative of cavernous, lateral, or other intracranial or unspecified intracranial venous sinus
Thrombophlebitis of cavernous, lateral, or other intracranial or unspecified intracranial venous sinus
Thrombosis of cavernous, lateral, or other intracranial or unspecified intracranial venous sinus

Excludes *that specified as:*
complicating pregnancy, childbirth, or the puerperium (671.5)
of nonpyogenic origin (437.6)
(Ex:) 006.5, 013.20-013.36, 249.60-249.61, 249.80-249.91, 250.60-250.63, 250.80-250.93,
324.0-325

326 Late effects of intracranial abscess or pyogenic infection 🔵

Note: This category is to be used to indicate conditions whose primary classification is to 320–325 [excluding 320.7, 321.0–321.8, 323.01–323.42, 323.61–323.72] as the cause of late effects, themselves classifiable elsewhere. The "late effects" include conditions specified as such, or as sequelae, which may occur at any time after the resolution of the causal condition.

Use additional code to identify condition, as:
hydrocephalus (331.4)
paralysis (342.0–342.9, 344.0–344.9)

ORGANIC SLEEP DISORDERS (327)

● **327 Organic sleep disorders**
Involve difficulties of sleep at all levels, including difficulty falling or staying asleep, falling asleep at inappropriate times, excessive total sleep time, or abnormal behaviors associated with sleep

● **327.0 Organic disorders of initiating and maintaining sleep [Organic insomnia]**

Excludes *insomnia NOS (780.52)*
insomnia not due to a substance or known physiological condition (307.41–307.42)
insomnia with sleep apnea NOS (780.51)

327.00 Organic insomnia, unspecified

▷ **327.01 *Insomnia due to medical condition classified elsewhere***
Code first underlying condition
Excludes *insomnia due to mental disorder (327.02)*

▷ **327.02 *Insomnia due to mental disorder***
Code first mental disorder
Excludes *alcohol induced insomnia (291.82)*
drug induced insomnia (292.85)

327.09 Other organic insomnia

DISEASES OF THE NERVOUS SYSTEM AND SENSE ORGANS (320–389)

● **327.1 Organic disorder of excessive somnolence [Organic hypersomnia]**

> **Excludes** *hypersomnia NOS (780.54)*
> *hypersomnia not due to a substance or known physiological condition (307.43–307.44)*
> *hypersomnia with sleep apnea NOS (780.53)*

327.10 Organic hypersomnia, unspecified

327.11 Idiopathic hypersomnia with long sleep time

327.12 Idiopathic hypersomnia without long sleep time

327.13 Recurrent hypersomnia
Kleine-Levin syndrome
Menstrual related hypersomnia

》 **327.14** *Hypersomnia due to medical condition classified elsewhere*
> *Code first underlying condition*
> **Excludes** *hypersomnia due to mental disorder (327.15)*

》 **327.15** *Hypersomnia due to mental disorder*
> *Code first mental disorder*
> **Excludes** *alcohol induced insomnia (291.82)*
> *drug induced insomnia (292.85)*

327.19 Other organic hypersomnia

● **327.2 Organic sleep apnea**
Characterized by episodes in which breathing stops during sleep, resulting in a lack of prolonged deep sleep and excessive daytime sleepiness

> **Excludes** *Cheyne-Stokes breathing (786.04)*
> *hypersomnia with sleep apnea NOS (780.53)*
> *insomnia with sleep apnea NOS (780.51)*
> *sleep apnea in newborn (770.81–770.82)*
> *sleep apnea NOS (780.57)*

327.20 Organic sleep apnea, unspecified

327.21 Primary central sleep apnea

327.22 High altitude periodic breathing

327.23 Obstructive sleep apnea (adult) (pediatric)

327.24 Idiopathic sleep related nonobstructive alveolar hypoventilation
Sleep related hypoxia

327.25 Congenital central alveolar hypoventilation syndrome

》 **327.26** *Sleep related hypoventilation/hypoxemia in conditions classifiable elsewhere*
> *Code first underlying condition*

》 **327.27** *Central sleep apnea in conditions classified elsewhere*
> *Code first underlying condition*

327.29 Other organic sleep apnea

● **327.3 Circadian rhythm sleep disorder**
Involves one of the sleep/wake regulating hormones. The inability to sleep results from a mismatch between the body's internal clock and the external 24-hour schedule.
Organic disorder of sleep wake cycle
Organic disorder of sleep wake schedule

> **Excludes** *alcohol induced circadian rhythm sleep disorder (291.82)*
> *circadian rhythm sleep disorder of nonorganic origin (307.45)*
> *disruption of 24 hour sleep wake cycle NOS (780.55)*
> *drug induced circadian rhythm sleep disorder (292.85)*

327.30 Circadian rhythm sleep disorder, unspecified

327.31 Circadian rhythm sleep disorder, delayed sleep phase type

327.32 Circadian rhythm sleep disorder, advanced sleep phase type

327.33 Circadian rhythm sleep disorder, irregular sleep-wake type

327.34 Circadian rhythm sleep disorder, free-running type

327.35 Circadian rhythm sleep disorder, jet lag type

327.36 Circadian rhythm sleep disorder, shift work type

》 **327.37** *Circadian rhythm sleep disorder in conditions classified elsewhere*
> *Code first underlying condition*

327.39 Other circadian rhythm sleep disorder

● **327.4 Organic parasomnia**

> **Excludes** *alcohol induced parasomnia (291.82)*
> *drug induced parasomnia (292.85)*
> *parasomnia not due to a known physiological condition (307.47)*

327.40 Organic parasomnia, unspecified

327.41 Confusional arousals

327.42 REM sleep behavior disorder

327.43 Recurrent isolated sleep paralysis

》 **327.44** *Parasomnia in conditions classified elsewhere*
> *Code first underlying condition*

327.49 Other organic parasomnia

● **327.5 Organic sleep related movement disorders**

> **Excludes** *restless legs syndrome (333.94)*
> *sleep related movement disorder NOS (780.58)*

327.51 Periodic limb movement disorder
Periodic limb movement sleep disorder

327.52 Sleep related leg cramps

327.53 Sleep related bruxism

327.59 Other organic sleep related movement disorders

327.8 Other organic sleep disorders
Coding Clinic: 2007, Q2, P7-8

HEREDITARY AND DEGENERATIVE DISEASES OF THE CENTRAL NERVOUS SYSTEM (330–337)

> **Excludes** *hepatolenticular degeneration (275.1)*
> *multiple sclerosis (340)*
> *other demyelinating diseases of central nervous system (341.0–341.9)*

● **330 Cerebral degenerations usually manifest in childhood**
Use additional code to identify associated intellectual disabilities

330.0 Leukodystrophy 🔖
Krabbe's disease
Leukodystrophy:
  NOS
  globoid cell
  metachromatic
  sudanophilic
Pelizaeus-Merzbacher disease
Sulfatide lipidosis
(Ex) 330.0-330.9, 331.7, 348.81, 348.89-384.9, 349.89-349.9

330.1 Cerebral lipidoses 🔖
Amaurotic (familial) idiocy
Disease:
  Batten
  Jansky-Bielschowsky
  Kufs'
  Spielmeyer-Vogt
  Tay-Sachs
Gangliosidosis
(Ex) 330.1-331.2, 331.6-331.7, 331.83-331.9

》 **330.2** *Cerebral degeneration in generalized lipidoses* 🔖
> *Code first underlying disease, as:*
> Fabry's disease (272.7)
> Gaucher's disease (272.7)
> Niemann-Pick disease (272.7)
> sphingolipidosis (272.7)
> (Ex) 330.1-331.2, 331.6-331.7, 331.83-331.9

Item 6–3 Leukodystrophy is characterized by degeneration and/or failure of the myelin formation of the central nervous system and sometimes of the peripheral nervous system. The disease is inherited and progressive.

▶ **330.3 Cerebral degeneration of childhood in other diseases classified elsewhere** 🔲
> Code first underlying disease, as:
> Hunter's disease (277.5)
> mucopolysaccharidosis (277.5)
> (Ex) 330.1-331.2, 331.6-331.7, 331.83-331.9

330.8 Other specified cerebral degenerations in childhood 🔲
> Alpers' disease or gray-matter degeneration
> Infantile necrotizing encephalomyelopathy
> Leigh's disease
> Subacute necrotizing encephalopathy or encephalomyelopathy
> (Ex) 330.1-331.2, 331.6-331.7, 331.83-331.9
> **Coding Clinic: 1995, Q1, P9**

330.9 Unspecified cerebral degeneration in childhood 🔲
> (Ex) 330.1-331.2, 331.6-331.7, 331.83-331.9

● **331 Other cerebral degenerations**
> Use additional code, where applicable, to identify dementia:
> with behavioral disturbance (294.11)
> without behavioral disturbance (294.10)

331.0 Alzheimer's disease
> **Coding Clinic: 2000, Q4, P40-41; 1999, Q4, P7; 1994, Q2, P10-11; Q1, P21; 1984, Nov-Dec, P20**

● **331.1 Frontotemporal dementia**
> **331.11 Pick's disease**
> > **Coding Clinic: 2003, Q4, P57-58**
>
> **331.19 Other frontotemporal dementia**
> > Frontal dementia
> > **Coding Clinic: 2003, Q4, P57-58**

331.2 Senile degeneration of brain
> **Excludes** senility NOS (797)

331.3 Communicating hydrocephalus 🔲
> Secondary normal pressure hydrocephalus
> **Excludes** congenital hydrocephalus (742.3)
> idiopathic normal pressure hydrocephalus (331.5)
> normal pressure hydrocephalus (331.5)
> spina bifida with hydrocephalus (741.0)
> (Ex) 331.3-331.5
> **Coding Clinic: 2007, Q4, P74-75; 1985, Sept-Oct, P12**

331.4 Obstructive hydrocephalus 🔲
> Acquired hydrocephalus NOS
> **Excludes** congenital hydrocephalus (742.3)
> idiopathic normal pressure hydrocephalus (331.5)
> normal pressure hydrocephalus (331.5)
> spina bifida with hydrocephalus (741.0)
> (Ex) 249.60-249.61, 249.80-249.91, 250.60-250.63, 250.80-250.93, 331.3-331.7, 331.82-331.9, 348.81, 348.89-348.9, 741.00-741.03, 742.3-742.4, 742.59-742.9
> **Coding Clinic: 2007, Q4, P74-75; 2003, Q4, P106-107; 1999, Q1, P9-10**

331.5 Idiopathic normal pressure hydrocephalus (INPH) 🔲
> Normal pressure hydrocephalus NOS
> **Excludes** congenital hydrocephalus (742.3)
> secondary normal pressure hydrocephalus (331.3)
> spina bifida with hydrocephalus (741.0)
> (Ex) 331.3-331.5
> **Coding Clinic: 2007, Q4, P74-75**

331.6 Corticobasal degeneration

▶ **331.7 Cerebral degeneration in diseases classified elsewhere**
> Code first underlying disease, as:
> alcoholism (303.0–303.9)
> beriberi (265.0)
> cerebrovascular disease (430–438)
> congenital hydrocephalus (741.0, 742.3)
> neoplastic disease (140.0–239.9)
> myxedema (244.0–244.9)
> vitamin B12 deficiency (266.2)
> **Excludes** cerebral degeneration in:
> Jakob-Creutzfeldt disease (046.11–046.19)
> progressive multifocal leukoencephalopathy (046.3)
> subacute spongiform encephalopathy (046.1)

● **331.8 Other cerebral degeneration**
> **331.81 Reye's syndrome** 🔲   P
> > (Ex) 331.81
>
> **331.82 Dementia with Lewy bodies**
> > Dementia with Parkinsonism
> > Lewy body dementia
> > Lewy body disease
> > **Coding Clinic: 2003, Q4, P57-58**
>
> **331.83 Mild cognitive impairment, so stated**
> > **Excludes** altered mental status (780.97)
> > cerebral degeneration (331.0–331.9)
> > change in mental status (780.97)
> > cognitive deficits following (late effects of) cerebral hemorrhage or infarction (438.0)
> > cognitive impairment due to intracranial or head injury (850–854, 959.01)
> > cognitive impairment due to late effect of intracranial injury (907.0)
> > cognitive impairment due to skull fracture (800-801, 803-804)
> > dementia (290.0-290.43, 294.20-294.21)
> > mild memory disturbance (310.89)
> > neurologic neglect syndrome (781.8)
> > personality change, nonpsychotic (310.1)
> > **Coding Clinic: 2006, Q4, P75-76**
>
> **331.89 Other**
> > Cerebral ataxia

331.9 Cerebral degeneration, unspecified

● **332 Parkinson's disease**
> Movement disorder (chronic or progressive); cause unknown, and no cure
> **Excludes** dementia with Parkinsonism (331.82)

332.0 Paralysis agitans
> Parkinsonism or Parkinson's disease:
> NOS
> idiopathic
> primary

332.1 Secondary Parkinsonism 🔲
> Neuroleptic-induced Parkinsonism
> Parkinsonism due to drugs
> Use additional E code to identify drug, if drug-induced
> **Excludes** Parkinsonism (in):
> Huntington's disease (333.4)
> progressive supranuclear palsy (333.0)
> Shy-Drager syndrome (333.0)
> syphilitic (094.82)
> (Ex) 332.0-332.1

DISEASES OF THE NERVOUS SYSTEM AND SENSE ORGANS (320–389)

Item 6–4 Pick's disease is the atrophy of the frontal and temporal lobes, causing dementia; **Alzheimer's** is characterized by a more diffuse cerebral atrophy.

● **333 Other extrapyramidal disease and abnormal movement disorders**

Includes other forms of extrapyramidal, basal ganglia, or striatopallidal disease

Excludes *abnormal movements of head NOS (781.0)*
sleep related movement disorders (327.51–327.59)

333.0 Other degenerative diseases of the basal ganglia 🔖
Atrophy or degeneration:
olivopontocerebellar [Déjérine-Thomas syndrome]
pigmentary pallidal [Hallervorden-Spatz disease]
striatonigral
Parkinsonian syndrome associated with:
idiopathic orthostatic hypotension
symptomatic orthostatic hypotension
Progressive supranuclear ophthalmoplegia
Shy-Drager syndrome
(Ex) 332.0-332.1, 335.23, 337.00-337.09, 348.30-348.39
Coding Clinic: 1996, Q2, P8-9

333.1 Essential and other specified forms of tremor
Benign essential tremor
Familial tremor
Medication-induced postural tremor
Use additional E code to identify drug, if drug-induced
Excludes *tremor NOS (781.0)*

333.2 Myoclonus
Familial essential myoclonus
Palatal myoclonus
Excludes *progressive myoclonic epilepsy (345.1)*
Unverricht-Lundborg disease (345.1)
Use additional E code to identify drug, if drug-induced
Coding Clinic: 1997, Q3, P5; 1987, Mar-April, P12

333.3 Tics of organic origin
Excludes *Gilles de la Tourette's syndrome (307.23)*
habit spasm (307.22)
tic NOS (307.20)
Use additional E code to identify drug, if drug-induced

333.4 Huntington's chorea 🔖
(Ex) 332.0-332.1, 340-341.1, 341.8-341.9, 343.0-344.2, 348.1, 348.30-348.81,
348.89-348.9, 349.1, 349.82-349.9, 780.72

333.5 Other choreas
Hemiballism(us)
Paroxysmal choreo-athetosis
Excludes *Sydenham's or rheumatic chorea
(392.0–392.9)*
Use additional E code to identify drug, if drug-induced

333.6 Genetic torsion dystonia
Dystonia:
deformans progressiva
musculorum deformans
(Schwalbe-) Ziehen-Oppenheim disease
Coding Clinic: 2006, Q4, P76-78

● **333.7 Acquired torsion dystonia**
Coding Clinic: 2006, Q4, P76-78

333.71 Athetoid cerebral palsy 🔖
Double athetosis (syndrome)
Vogt's disease
Excludes *infantile cerebral palsy (343.0–343.9)*
(Ex) 332.0-332.1, 333.71, 333.90, 333.99, 343.0-343.9, 348.30-348.39

333.72 Acute dystonia due to drugs 🔖
Acute dystonic reaction due to drugs
Neuroleptic-induced acute dystonia
Use additional E code to identify drug
Excludes *blepharospasm due to drugs (333.85)*
*orofacial dyskinesia due to drugs
(333.85)*
secondary Parkinsonism (332.1)
*subacute dyskinesia due to drugs
(333.85)*
tardive dyskinesia (333.85)
(Ex) 332.0-332.1, 333.71, 333.90, 333.99, 348.30-348.39

333.79 Other acquired torsion dystonia 🔖
(Ex) 332.0-332.1, 333.71, 333.90, 333.99, 348.30-348.39

● **333.8 Fragments of torsion dystonia**
Use additional E code to identify drug, if drug-induced

333.81 Blepharospasm
Excludes *blepharospasm due to drugs (333.85)*

333.82 Orofacial dyskinesia
Excludes *orofacial dyskinesia due to drugs
(333.85)*

333.83 Spasmodic torticollis
Excludes *torticollis:*
NOS (723.5)
hysterical (300.11)
psychogenic (306.0)

333.84 Organic writers' cramp
Excludes *psychogenic (300.89)*

333.85 Subacute dyskinesia due to drugs
Blepharospasm due to drugs
Orofacial dyskinesia due to drugs
Tardive dyskinesia
Use additional E code to identify drug
Excludes *acute dystonia due to drugs (333.72)*
*acute dystonic reaction due to drugs
(333.72)*
secondary Parkinsonism (332.1)
Coding Clinic: 2006, Q4, P76-78

333.89 Other

● **333.9 Other and unspecified extrapyramidal diseases and abnormal movement disorders**

**333.90 Unspecified extrapyramidal disease and abnormal
movement disorder** 🔖
Medication-induced movement disorders NOS
Use additional E code to identify drug, if
drug-induced
(Ex) 332.0-332.1, 333.1-333.83, 333.85-333.93, 333.99,
335.22-335.23, 340-341.1, 341.8-341.9, 343.0-344.2, 348.1,
348.30-348.81, 348.89-348.9, 349.1, 349.82-349.9, 780.72

333.91 Stiff-man syndrome 🔖
(Ex) 332.0-332.1, 333.1-333.83, 333.85-333.93, 333.99,
335.22-335.23, 340-341.1, 341.8-341.9, 343.0-344.2, 348.1,
348.30-348.81, 348.89-348.9, 349.1, 349.82-349.9, 780.72

333.92 Neuroleptic malignant syndrome 🔖
Use additional E code to identify drug
Excludes *neuroleptic induced Parkinsonism
(332.1)*
(Ex) 333.0-333.93, 333.99, 342.00-342.92, 348.2-348.39

333.93 Benign shuddering attacks

333.94 Restless legs syndrome (RLS)
Coding Clinic: 2006, Q4, P79

333.99 Other
Neuroleptic-induced acute akathisia
Use additional E code to identify drug, if
drug-induced
Coding Clinic: 2004, Q2, P12

Item 6–5 Huntington's chorea is an inherited degenerative disorder of
the central nervous system and is characterized by ceaseless, jerky movements
and progressive cognitive and behavioral deterioration.

● 334 **Spinocerebellar disease**
Group of degenerative disorders in which primary symptom is progressive ataxia (jerky, uncoordinated movements)

> **Excludes** *olivopontocerebellar degeneration (333.0)*
> *peroneal muscular atrophy (356.1)*

334.0 **Friedreich's ataxia** 🔖
(Ex): 334.0-334.9, 348.30-348.39

334.1 **Hereditary spastic paraplegia** 🔖
(Ex): 333.0-333.93, 333.99-337.9, 340-344.9, 348.1, 348.30-348.39, 348.81, 348.89-348.9, 349.82-349.9, 780.72

334.2 **Primary cerebellar degeneration** 🔖
Cerebellar ataxia:
  Marie's
  Sanger-Brown
Dyssynergia cerebellaris myoclonica
Primary cerebellar degeneration:
  NOS
  hereditary
  sporadic
(Ex): 333.0-333.93, 333.99-337.9, 340-344.9, 348.0-348.1, 348.30-348.39, 348.81, 348.89-348.9, 349.82-349.9, 780.72
Coding Clinic: 1987, Mar-April, P9

334.3 **Other cerebellar ataxia** 🔖
Cerebellar ataxia NOS

> Use additional E code to identify drug, if drug-induced

(Ex): 333.0-333.93, 333.99-337.9, 340-344.9, 348.0-348.1, 348.30-348.39, 348.81, 348.89-348.9, 349.82-349.9, 780.72

▶ 334.4 *Cerebellar ataxia in diseases classified elsewhere* 🔖
> *Code first underlying disease, as:*
> alcoholism (303.0–303.9)
> myxedema (244.0–244.9)
> neoplastic disease (140.0–239.9)

(Ex): 333.0-333.93, 333.99-337.9, 340-344.9 348.0-348.1, 348.30-348.39, 348.81, 348.89-348.9, 349.82-349.9, 780.72

334.8 **Other spinocerebellar diseases** 🔖
Ataxia-telangiectasia [Louis-Bar syndrome]
Corticostriatal-spinal degeneration
(Ex): 333.0-333.93, 333.99-337.9, 340-344.9 348.0-348.1, 348.30-348.39, 348.81, 348.89-348.9, 349.82-349.9, 780.72

334.9 **Spinocerebellar disease, unspecified** 🔖
(Ex): 334.0-334.9

● 335 **Anterior horn cell disease**
335.0 **Werdnig-Hoffmann disease** 🔖
Infantile spinal muscular atrophy
Progressive muscular atrophy of infancy
(Ex): 249.60-249.61, 249.80-249.91, 250.60-250.63, 250.80-250.93, 334.8-337.9, 349.89-349.9

● 335.1 **Spinal muscular atrophy**
335.10 **Spinal muscular atrophy, unspecified** 🔖
(Ex): 249.60-249.61, 249.80-249.91, 250.60-250.63, 250.80-250.93, 334.8-337.9, 349.89-349.9

335.11 **Kugelberg-Welander disease** 🔖
Spinal muscular atrophy:
  familial
  juvenile
(Ex): 249.60-249.61, 249.80-249.91, 250.60-250.63, 250.80-250.93, 334.8-337.9, 349.89-349.9

335.19 **Other** 🔖
Adult spinal muscular atrophy
(Ex): 249.60-249.61, 249.80-249.91, 250.60-250.63, 250.80-250.93, 334.8-337.9, 349.89-349.9

● 335.2 **Motor neuron disease**
335.20 **Amyotrophic lateral sclerosis** 🔖   A
Also listed in the Index as "Lou Gehrig's disease" (ALS)
Motor neuron disease (bulbar) (mixed type)
(Ex): 249.60-249.61, 249.80-249.91, 250.60-250.63, 250.80-250.93, 334.8-337.9, 349.89-349.9
Coding Clinic: 1995, Q4, P81

335.21 **Progressive muscular atrophy** 🔖
Duchenne-Aran muscular atrophy
Progressive muscular atrophy (pure)
(Ex): 249.60-249.61, 249.80-249.91, 250.60-250.63, 250.80-250.93, 334.8-337.9, 349.89-349.9

335.22 **Progressive bulbar palsy** 🔖
(Ex): 249.60-249.61, 249.80-249.91, 250.60-250.63, 250.80-250.93, 334.8-337.9, 349.89-349.9

335.23 **Pseudobulbar palsy** 🔖
(Ex): 249.60-249.61, 249.80-249.91, 250.60-250.63, 250.80-250.93, 334.8-337.9, 349.89-349.9

335.24 **Primary lateral sclerosis** 🔖
(Ex): 249.60-249.61, 249.80-249.91, 250.60-250.63, 250.80-250.93, 334.8-337.9, 349.89-349.9

335.29 **Other** 🔖
(Ex): 249.60-249.61, 249.80-249.91, 250.60-250.63, 250.80-250.93, 334.8-337.9, 349.89-349.9

335.8 **Other anterior horn cell diseases** 🔖
(Ex): 249.60-249.61, 249.80-249.91, 250.60-250.63, 250.80-250.93, 334.8-337.9, 349.89-349.9
Coding Clinic: 2006, Q4, P76-78

335.9 **Anterior horn cell disease, unspecified** 🔖
(Ex): 249.60-249.61, 249.80-249.91, 250.60-250.63, 250.80-250.93, 334.8-337.9, 349.89-349.9

● 336 **Other diseases of spinal cord**
336.0 **Syringomyelia and syringobulbia** 🔖
(Ex): 334.8-337.9, 340-344.9, 348.30-348.39, 348.81, 348.89-349.2, 349.89-349.9, 780.72
Coding Clinic: 1989, Q1, P10

336.1 **Vascular myelopathies** 🔖
Acute infarction of spinal cord (embolic) (nonembolic)
Arterial thrombosis of spinal cord
Edema of spinal cord
Hematomyelia
Subacute necrotic myelopathy
(Ex): 249.60-249.61, 250.60-250.63, 334.8-337.9, 340-344.9, 348.1, 348.30-348.39, 349.0-349.2, 349.89-349.9, 780.72

▶ 336.2 *Subacute combined degeneration of spinal cord in diseases classified elsewhere* 🔖
> *Code first underlying disease, as:*
> pernicious anemia (281.0)
> other vitamin B12 deficiency anemia (281.1)
> vitamin B12 deficiency (266.2)

(Ex): 334.8-337.9, 340 -344.9, 348.1, 348.30-348.39, 349.0-349.2, 349.89-349.9, 780.72

▶ 336.3 *Myelopathy in other diseases classified elsewhere* 🔖
> *Code first underlying disease, as:*
> myelopathy in neoplastic disease (140.0–239.9)

> **Excludes** *myelopathy in:*
> *intervertebral disc disorder (722.70–722.73)*
> *spondylosis (721.1, 721.41–721.42, 721.91)*

(Ex): 249.60-249.61, 250.60-250.63, 334.8-337.9, 340-344.9, 348.1, 348.30-348.39, 349.0-349.2, 349.89-349.9, 780.72
Coding Clinic: 1999, Q3, P5

336.8 **Other myelopathy** 🔖
Myelopathy:
  drug-induced
  radiation-induced

> Use additional E code to identify cause

(Ex): 249.60-249.61, 250.60-250.63, 334.8-337.9, 340-344.9, 348.1, 348.30-348.39, 349.0-349.2, 349.89-349.9, 780.72

336.9 **Unspecified disease of spinal cord** 🔖
Cord compression NOS
Myelopathy NOS

> **Excludes** *myelitis (323.02, 323.1, 323.2, 323.42, 323.52, 323.63, 323.72, 323.82, 323.9)*
> *spinal (canal) stenosis (723.0, 724.00–724.09)*

(Ex): 249.60-249.61, 250.60-250.63, 334.1, 334.8-337.9, 340-344.9, 348.1, 348.30-348.39, 349.0-349.2, 349.89-349.9, 780.72

N Newborn: 0   **P** Pediatric: 0–17   **M** Maternity: 12–55   **A** Adult: 15–124   ♀ Females Only   ♂ Males Only

(Ex) CC/MCC Exclusions   🔖 Complication\Comorbidity   Major C\C   Present on Admission Requirement   Hospital-Acquired Condition   771

DISEASES OF THE NERVOUS SYSTEM AND SENSE ORGANS (320–389)

● 337   **Disorders of the autonomic nervous system**

    Includes   disorders of peripheral autonomic, sympathetic, parasympathetic, or vegetative system

    Excludes   *familial dysautonomia [Riley-Day syndrome] (742.8)*

 ● 337.0   **Idiopathic peripheral autonomic neuropathy**

    337.00   **Idiopathic peripheral autonomic neuropathy, unspecified**

    337.01   **Carotid sinus syndrome**
      Carotid sinus syncope
      Coding Clinic: 2008, Q4, P101-102

    337.09   **Other idiopathic peripheral autonomic neuropathy**
      Cervical sympathetic dystrophy or paralysis

 ▷ 337.1   *Peripheral autonomic neuropathy in disorders classified elsewhere*
     Code first underlying disease, as:
      amyloidosis (277.30–277.39)
      diabetes (249.6, 250.6)
      (Ex) 337.00-337.29, 337.9, 348.30-348.39
      Coding Clinic: 2009, Q2, P13; 1993, Q2, P6; 1984, Nov-Dec, P9

 ● 337.2   **Reflex sympathetic dystrophy**

    337.20   **Reflex sympathetic dystrophy, unspecified**
      Complex regional pain syndrome type I, unspecified
      (Ex) 337.20-337.29

    337.21   **Reflex sympathetic dystrophy of the upper limb**
      Complex regional pain syndrome type I of the upper limb
      (Ex) 249.60-249.61, 250.60-250.63, 334.8-337.9, 340-344.9, 348.1, 348.30-348.39, 349.0-349.2, 349.89-349.9, 780.72

    337.22   **Reflex sympathetic dystrophy of the lower limb**
      Complex regional pain syndrome type I of the lower limb
      (Ex) 249.60-249.61, 250.60-250.63, 334.8-337.9, 340-344.9, 348.1, 348.30-348.39, 349.0-349.2, 349.89-349.9, 780.72

    337.29   **Reflex sympathetic dystrophy of other specified site**
      Complex regional pain syndrome type I of other specified site
      (Ex) 249.60-249.61, 250.60-250.63, 334.8-337.9, 340-344.9, 348.1, 348.30-348.39, 349.0-349.2, 349.89-349.9, 780.72

   337.3   **Autonomic dysreflexia**
     Use additional code to identify the cause, such as:
      fecal impaction (560.32)
      pressure ulcer (707.00–707.09)
      urinary tract infection (599.0)
      Coding Clinic: 1998, Q4, P37-38

   337.9   **Unspecified disorder of autonomic nervous system**

PAIN (338)

● 338   **Pain, not elsewhere classified**
    Use additional code to identify:
     pain associated with psychological factors (307.89)

    Excludes   *generalized pain (780.96)*
     headache syndromes (339.00-339.89)
     localized pain, unspecified type - code to pain by site
     migraines (346.0-346.9)
     pain disorder exclusively attributed to psychological factors (307.80)
     vulvar vestibulitis (625.71)
     vulvodynia (625.70-625.79)

   338.0   **Central pain syndrome**
     Déjérine-Roussy syndrome
     Myelopathic pain syndrome
     Thalamic pain syndrome (hyperesthetic)

 ● 338.1   **Acute pain**

    338.11   **Acute pain due to trauma**
      Coding Clinic: 2007, Q1, P3-8

    338.12   **Acute post-thoracotomy pain**
      Post-thoracotomy pain NOS

    338.18   **Other acute postoperative pain**
      Postoperative pain NOS
      Coding Clinic: 2007, Q2, P13-15; 2003, Q1, P4-5, 8

    338.19   **Other acute pain**
      Excludes   *neoplasm related acute pain (338.3)*
      Coding Clinic: 2007, Q2, P13-15

 ● 338.2   **Chronic pain**
     Excludes   *causalgia (355.9)*
      lower limb (355.71)
      upper limb (354.4)
     chronic pain syndrome (338.4)
     myofascial pain syndrome (729.1)
     neoplasm related chronic pain (338.3)
     reflex sympathetic dystrophy (337.20–337.29)
     Coding Clinic: 2008, Q3, P4

    338.21   **Chronic pain due to trauma**

    338.22   **Chronic post-thoracotomy pain**

    338.28   **Other chronic postoperative pain**
      Coding Clinic: 2007, Q2, P13-15

    338.29   **Other chronic pain**
      Coding Clinic: 2007, Q2, P13-15

   338.3   **Neoplasm related pain (acute) (chronic)**
     Cancer associated pain
     Pain due to malignancy (primary) (secondary)
     Tumor associated pain
     Coding Clinic: 2007, Q2, P13-15

   338.4   **Chronic pain syndrome**
     Chronic pain associated with significant psychosocial dysfunction
     Coding Clinic: 2007, Q2, P13-15

OTHER HEADACHE SYNDROMES (339)

● 339   **Other headache syndromes**
    Excludes   *headache:*
     NOS (784.0)
     due to lumbar puncture (349.0)
     migraine (346.0-346.9)
    Coding Clinic: 2008, Q4, P102-109

 ● 339.0   **Cluster headaches and other trigeminal autonomic cephalgias**
     TACS

    339.00   **Cluster headache syndrome, unspecified**
      Ciliary neuralgia
      Cluster headache NOS
      Histamine cephalgia
      Lower half migraine
      Migrainous neuralgia

    339.01   **Episodic cluster headache**

    339.02   **Chronic cluster headache**

    339.03   **Episodic paroxysmal hemicrania**
      Paroxysmal hemicrania NOS

    339.04   **Chronic paroxysmal hemicrania**

    339.05   **Short lasting unilateral neuralgiform headache with conjunctival injection and tearing**
      SUNCT

    339.09   **Other trigeminal autonomic cephalgias**

 ● 339.1   **Tension type headache**
     Excludes   *tension headache NOS (307.81)*
     tension headache related to psychological factors (307.81)

    339.10   **Tension type headache, unspecified**

    339.11   **Episodic tension type headache**

    339.12   **Chronic tension type headache**

 ● 339.2   **Post-traumatic headache**

    339.20   **Post-traumatic headache, unspecified**
      Coding Clinic: 2008, Q4, P102-109

    339.21   **Acute post-traumatic headache**
      Coding Clinic: 2008, Q4, P102-109

    339.22   **Chronic post-traumatic headache**

◀ New   ◀ Revised   ~~deleted~~ Deleted   Excludes   Includes   Use additional   Code first   Omit code

772   ● Unacceptable Principal Diagnosis   ● Use Additional Digit(s)   ▷ Manifestation Code   OGCR Official Guidelines   Coding Clinic

DISEASES OF THE NERVOUS SYSTEM AND SENSE ORGANS (320–389)

339.3 Drug induced headache, not elsewhere classified
Medication overuse headache
Rebound headache

● **339.4 Complicated headache syndromes**

339.41 Hemicrania continua

339.42 New daily persistent headache
NDPH

339.43 Primary thunderclap headache

339.44 Other complicated headache syndrome

● **339.8 Other specified headache syndromes**

339.81 Hypnic headache

339.82 Headache associated with sexual activity
Orgasmic headache
Preorgasmic headache

339.83 Primary cough headache

339.84 Primary exertional headache

339.85 Primary stabbing headache

339.89 Other specified headache syndromes

OTHER DISORDERS OF THE CENTRAL NERVOUS SYSTEM (340–349)

340 Multiple sclerosis *(MS)*
Disseminated or multiple sclerosis:
NOS	cord
brain stem	generalized

● **341 Other demyelinating diseases of central nervous system**

341.0 Neuromyelitis optica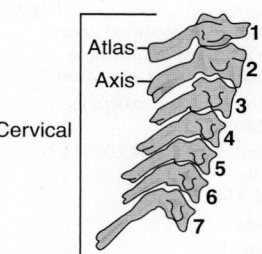
Ex: 341.0, 348.30-348.39

341.1 Schilder's disease
Balo's concentric sclerosis
Encephalitis periaxialis:
concentrica [Balo's]
diffusa [Schilder's]
Ex: 066.40-066.49, 079.82, 348.30-348.39

● **341.2 Acute (transverse) myelitis**

Excludes *acute (transverse) myelitis (in) (due to):*
following immunization procedures (323.52)
infection classified elsewhere (323.42)
postinfectious (323.63)
protozoal diseases classified elsewhere (323.2)
rickettsial diseases classified elsewhere (323.1)
toxic (323.72)
viral diseases classified elsewhere (323.02)
transverse myelitis NOS (323.82)

341.20 Acute (transverse) myelitis NOS
Ex: 003.21, 013.00-013.16, 036.0, 047.0-047.9, 049.0-049.1,
053.0-053.13, 053.19, 053.79-053.9, 054.72, 054.79-054.9,
058.81-058.89, 072.1, 078.89, 079.81, 079.89, 079.99, 090.42,
091.81, 094.2, 098.89, 100.81, 112.83, 114.2, 115.01, 115.11,
115.91, 130.0, 139.8, 249.60-249.61, 250.60-250.63,
320.0-322.9, 334.8-337.9, 340-341.1, 341.8-344.9, 348.1,
348.30-348.39, 349.0-349.2, 349.89-349.9, 357.0, 780.72

▶ **341.21 Acute (transverse) myelitis in conditions classified**
elsewhere
Code first underlying condition
Ex: 003.21, 013.00-013.16, 036.0, 047.0-047.9, 049.0-049.1,
053.0-053.13, 053.19, 053.79-053.9, 054.72, 054.79-054.9,
058.81, 058.89, 072.1, 078.89, 079.81, 079.89, 079.99,
090.42, 091.81, 094.2, 098.89, 100.81, 112.83, 114.2, 115.01,
115.11, 115.91, 130.0, 139.8, 249.60-249.61, 250.60-250.63,
320.0-322.9, 334.8-337.9, 340-341.1, 341.8-344.9, 348.1,
348.30-348.39, 349.0-349.2, 349.89-349.9, 357.0, 780.72

341.22 Idiopathic transverse myelitis
Ex: 003.21, 013.00-013.16, 036.0, 047.0-047.9, 049.0-049.1,
053.0-053.13, 053.19, 053.79-053.9, 054.72, 054.79-054.9,
058.81-058.89, 072.1, 078.89, 079.81, 079.89, 079.99, 090.42,
091.81, 094.2, 098.89, 100.81, 112.83, 114.2, 115.01, 115.11,
115.91, 130.0, 139.8, 249.60-249.61, 250.60-250.63,
320.0-322.9, 334.8-337.9, 340-341.1, 341.8-344.9, 348.1,
348.30-348.39, 349.0-349.2, 349.89-349.9, 357.0, 780.72

341.8 Other demyelinating diseases of central nervous system
Central demyelination of corpus callosum
Central pontine myelinosis
Marchiafava (-Bignami) disease
Ex: 333.1-333.93, 333.99-337.9, 340-344.9, 348.30-348.39, 348.81,
348.89-348.9, 349.82-349.9, 780.72
Coding Clinic: 1987, Nov-Dec, P6

341.9 Demyelinating disease of central nervous system,
unspecified
Ex: 333.1-333.93, 333.99-337.9, 340-344.9, 348.30-348.39, 348.81,
348.89-348.9, 349.82-349.9, 780.72

● **342 Hemiplegia and hemiparesis**
Note: This category is to be used when hemiplegia
(complete) (incomplete) is reported without further
specification, or is stated to be old or long-standing
but of unspecified cause. The category is also for use in
multiple coding to identify these types of hemiplegia
resulting from any cause.

Excludes *congenital (343.1)*
hemiplegia due to late effect of cerebrovascular accident
(438.20–438.22)
infantile NOS (343.4)

The following fifth-digits are for use with codes 342.0–342.9

0	**affecting unspecified side**
1	**affecting dominant side**
2	**affecting nondominant side**

● **342.0 Flaccid hemiplegia**
[0-2] Ex: 334.0-337.9, 340-344.9, 348.30-348.39, 348.81, 348.89-348.9, 349.82-349.9,
780.72

● **342.1 Spastic hemiplegia**
[0-2] Ex: 334.0-337.9, 340-344.9, 348.30-348.39, 348.81, 348.89-348.9, 349.82-349.9,
780.72

Item 6-6 Multiple sclerosis (MS) is a nervous system disease affecting the brain and spinal cord by damaging the myelin sheath surrounding and protecting nerve cells. The damage slows down/blocks messages between the brain and body. Symptoms are: visual disturbances, muscle weakness, coordination and balance issues, numbness, prickling, and thinking and memory problems. The cause is unknown, though it is thought that it may be an autoimmune disease. It affects women more than men, between 20 and 40 years of age. MS can be mild, but it may cause the loss of ability to write, walk, and speak. There is no cure, but medication may slow or control symptoms.

Figure 6–2 Cervical vertebrae.

Item 6–7 Hemiplegia is complete paralysis of one side of the body—arm, leg, and trunk. **Hemiparesis** is a generalized weakness or incomplete paralysis of one side of the body. If most activities (eating, writing) are performed with the right hand, the right is the dominant side, and the left is the nondominant side. **Quadriplegia,** also called tetraplegia, is the complete paralysis of all four limbs. **Quadriparesis** is the incomplete paralysis of all four limbs. Nerve damage in C1–C4 is associated with lower limb paralysis, and C5–C7 damage is associated with upper limb paralysis. **Diplegia** is the paralysis of the upper limbs. **Monoplegia** is the complete paralysis of one limb. There are separate codes for upper (344.4x) and lower (344.3x) limb. Dominant, nondominant, or unspecified side becomes the fifth digit. Dominant side (right/left) is the side that a person leads with for movement, such as in writing and sports.
Cauda equina syndrome is due to pressure on the roots of the spinal nerves and causes paresthesia (abnormal sensations).

DISEASES OF THE NERVOUS SYSTEM AND SENSE ORGANS (320–389)

● 342.8 **Other specified hemiplegia** 🔊
[0-2]   (Ex:) 334.0-337.9, 340-344.9, 348.30-348.39, 348.81, 348.89-348.9, 349.82-349.9, 780.72

● 342.9 **Hemiplegia, unspecified** 🔊
[0-2]   (Ex:) 334.0-337.9, 340-344.9, 348.30-348.39, 348.81, 348.89-348.9, 349.82-349.9, 780.72
Coding Clinic: 2006, Q3, P5; 1998, Q4, P87

● 343 **Infantile cerebral palsy**
Includes   cerebral:
palsy NOS
spastic infantile paralysis
congenital spastic paralysis (cerebral)
Little's disease
paralysis (spastic) due to birth injury:
intracranial
spinal
Excludes   athetoid cerebral palsy (333.71)
hereditary cerebral paralysis, such as:
hereditary spastic paraplegia (334.1)
Vogt's disease (333.71)
spastic paralysis specified as noncongenital or
noninfantile (344.0–344.9)

343.0 **Diplegic** 🔊
Congenital diplegia
Congenital paraplegia
(Ex:) 343.0, 348.30-348.39

343.1 **Hemiplegic** 🔊
Congenital hemiplegia
Excludes   infantile hemiplegia NOS (343.4)
(Ex:) 343.1, 348.30-348.39

343.2 **Quadriplegic** 🔊
Tetraplegic
(Ex:) 249.60-249.61, 249.80-249.91, 250.60-250.63, 250.80-250.93, 342.00-344.9, 348.81, 348.89-348.9, 349.89-349.9, 742.59-742.9, 780.72

343.3 **Monoplegic**

343.4 **Infantile hemiplegia** 🔊
Infantile hemiplegia (postnatal) NOS
(Ex:) 334.0-337.9, 340-344.9, 348.30-348.39, 348.81, 348.89-348.9, 349.82-349.9, 780.72

343.8 **Other specified infantile cerebral palsy**

343.9 **Infantile cerebral palsy, unspecified**
Cerebral palsy NOS
Coding Clinic: 2005, Q4, P89-90

● 344 **Other paralytic syndromes**
Note: This category is to be used when the listed conditions are reported without further specification or are stated to be old or long-standing but of unspecified cause. The category is also for use in multiple coding to identify these conditions resulting from any cause.
Includes   paralysis (complete) (incomplete), except as classifiable to 342 and 343
Excludes   congenital or infantile cerebral palsy (343.0–343.9)
hemiplegia (342.0–342.9)
congenital or infantile (343.1, 343.4)

● 344.0 **Quadriplegia and quadriparesis**
344.00 **Quadriplegia, unspecified** 🔊
(Ex:) 249.60-249.61, 249.80-249.91, 250.60-250.63, 250.80-250.93, 342.00-344.9, 348.81, 348.89-348.9, 349.89-349.9, 742.59-742.9, 780.72
Coding Clinic: 2003, Q4, P103-104; 1998, Q4, P37-38

344.01 **C$_1$-C$_4$, complete** 🔊
(Ex:) 249.60-249.61, 249.80-249.91, 250.60-250.63, 250.80-250.93, 342.00-344.9, 348.81, 348.89-348.9, 349.89-349.9, 742.59-742.9, 780.72

344.02 **C$_1$-C$_4$, incomplete** 🔊
(Ex:) 249.60-249.61, 249.80-249.91, 250.60-250.63, 250.80-250.93, 342.00-344.9, 348.81, 348.89-348.9, 349.89-349.9, 742.59-742.9, 780.72

344.03 **C$_5$-C$_7$, complete** 🔊
(Ex:) 249.60-249.61, 249.80-249.91, 250.60-250.63, 250.80-250.93, 342.00-344.9, 348.81, 348.89-348.9, 349.89-349.9, 742.59-742.9, 780.72

344.04 **C$_5$-C$_7$, incomplete** 🔊
(Ex:) 249.60-249.61, 249.80-249.91, 250.60-250.63, 250.80-250.93, 342.00-344.9, 348.81, 348.89-348.9, 349.89-349.9, 742.59-742.9, 780.72

344.09 **Other** 🔊
(Ex:) 249.60-249.61, 249.80-249.91, 250.60-250.63, 250.80-250.93, 342.00-344.9, 348.81, 348.89-348.9, 349.89-349.9, 742.59-742.9, 780.72
Coding Clinic: 2001, Q1, P12; 1998, Q4, P39-40

344.1 **Paraplegia** 🔊
Paralysis of both lower limbs
Paraplegia (lower)
(Ex:) 334.0-337.9, 340-344.9, 348.30-348.39, 348.81, 348.89-348.9, 349.82-349.9, 780.72
Coding Clinic: 2003, Q4, P110; 1987, Mar-April, P10-11

344.2 **Diplegia of upper limbs** 🔊
Diplegia (upper)
Paralysis of both upper limbs
(Ex:) 344.00-344.09, 344.2, 344.81-344.9, 349.89-349.9, 780.72

● 344.3 **Monoplegia of lower limb**
Paralysis of lower limb
Excludes   monoplegia of lower limb due to late effect of cerebrovascular accident (438.40–438.42)
344.30 **Affecting unspecified side**
344.31 **Affecting dominant side**
344.32 **Affecting nondominant side**

● 344.4 **Monoplegia of upper limb**
Paralysis of upper limb
Excludes   monoplegia of upper limb due to late effect of cerebrovascular accident (438.30–438.32)
344.40 **Affecting unspecified side**
344.41 **Affecting dominant side**
344.42 **Affecting nondominant side**

344.5 **Unspecified monoplegia**

● 344.6 **Cauda equina syndrome**
344.60 **Without mention of neurogenic bladder** 🔊
(Ex:) 344.00-344.1, 344.30-344.32, 344.60-344.9, 349.89-349.9, 780.72
344.61 **With neurogenic bladder** 🔊
Acontractile bladder
Autonomic hyperreflexia of bladder
Cord bladder
Detrusor hyperreflexia
(Ex:) 334.0-337.9, 340-344.9, 348.30-348.39, 348.81, 348.89-348.9, 349.82-349.9, 599.60-599.69, 780.72
Coding Clinic: 1987, Mar-April, P10-11

● 344.8 **Other specified paralytic syndromes**
344.81 **Locked-in state** 🔊
(Ex:) 342.00-344.9, 348.30-348.39, 348.81, 348.89-348.9, 349.82-349.9, 780.72
344.89 **Other specified paralytic syndrome**
Coding Clinic: 1999, Q2, P4

344.9 **Paralysis, unspecified**
Coding Clinic: 1994, Q3, P4

● 345 **Epilepsy and recurrent seizures**

The following fifth-digit subclassification is for use with categories 345.0, .1, .4–.9:

0	**without mention of intractable epilepsy**
1	**with intractable epilepsy**
	pharmacoresistant (pharmacologically resistant)
	poorly controlled
	refractory (medically)
	treatment resistant

> **Excludes** *hippocampal sclerosis (348.81)*
> *mesial temporal sclerosis (348.81)*
> *temporal sclerosis (348.81)*

● **345.0 Generalized nonconvulsive epilepsy** 1
[0-1]

Absences:	Pykno-epilepsy
atonic	Seizures:
typical	akinetic
Minor epilepsy	atonic
Petit mal	

For code **345.01:** (Ex) 249.60-249.61, 250.60-250.63, 345.00-345.91, 348.81, 348.89-348.9, 349.89-349.9, 780.33

Coding Clinic: 2004, Q1, P18; 1992, Q2, P8

● **345.1 Generalized convulsive epilepsy** 1
[0-1]   Epileptic seizures:
clonic
myoclonic
tonic
tonic-clonic
Grand mal
Major epilepsy
Progressive myoclonic epilepsy
Unverricht-Lundborg disease

> **Excludes** *convulsions:*
> *NOS (780.39)*
> *infantile (780.39)*
> *newborn (779.0)*
> *infantile spasms (345.6)*

For code **345.11:** (Ex) 249.60-249.61, 250.60-250.63, 345.00-345.91, 348.81, 348.89-348.9, 349.89-349.9, 780.33

Coding Clinic: 1997, Q3, P5; 1994, Q3, P9

345.2 Petit mal status
Epileptic absence status
Temporary disturbance of brain function caused by abnormal electrical activity

(Ex) 249.60-249.61, 249.80-249.91, 250.60-250.63, 258.80-250.93, 345.00-345.91, 348.81, 348.89-348.9, 349.89-349.9, 780.33

345.3 Grand mal status
Status epilepticus NOS
Grand mal seizure is a generalized tonic-clonic seizure involving the entire body, which involves muscle rigidity, violent muscle contractions, and loss of consciousness.

> **Excludes** *epilepsia partialis continua (345.7) status:*
> *psychomotor (345.7)*
> *temporal lobe (345.7)*

(Ex) 249.60-249.61, 249.80-249.91, 250.60-250.63, 258.80-250.93, 345.00-345.91, 348.81, 348.89-348.9, 349.89-349.9, 780.33

Coding Clinic: 2005, Q3, P12-13

● **345.4 Localization-related (focal) (partial) epilepsy and**
[0-1]   **epileptic syndromes with complex partial seizures**
Epilepsy:
limbic system
partial:
secondarily generalized
with impairment of consciousness
with memory and ideational disturbances
psychomotor
psychosensory
temporal lobe
Epileptic automatism

For code **345.40:** (Ex) 345.00-345.91, 348.30-348.39, 348.9 349.89-349.9, 780.33;

For code **345.41:** (Ex) 249.60-249.61, 250.60-250.63, 345.00-345.91, 348.81, 348.89-348.9, 349.89-349.9, 780.33

Coding Clinic: 2009, Q4, P98

● **345.5 Localization-related (focal) (partial) epilepsy and**
[0-1]   **epileptic syndromes with simple partial seizures**
Epilepsy:
Bravais-Jacksonian NOS
focal (motor) NOS
Jacksonian NOS
motor partial
partial NOS
without mention of impairment of consciousness
sensory-induced
somatomotor
somatosensory
visceral
visual

For code **345.50:** (Ex) 345.00-345.91, 348.30-348.39, 348.9, 349.89-349.9, 780.33;

For code **345.51:** (Ex) 249.60-249.61, 250.60-250.63, 345.00-345.91, 348.81, 348.89-348.9, 349.89-349.9, 780.33

● **345.6 Infantile spasms**
[0-1]   Hypsarrhythmia
Lightning spasms
Salaam attacks

> **Excludes** *salaam tic (781.0)*

For code **345.60:** (Ex) 345.00-345.91, 348.30-348.39, 348.9, 349.89-349.9, 780.33;

For code **345.61:** (Ex) 249.60-249.61, 250.60-250.63, 345.00-345.91, 348.81, 348.89-348.9, 349.89-349.9, 780.33

Coding Clinic: 1984, Nov-Dec, P11

● **345.7 Epilepsia partialis continua** 0 , 1
[0-1]   Kojevnikov's epilepsy

(Ex) 249.60-249.61, 250.60-250.63, 345.00-345.91, 348.81, 348.89-348.9, 349.89-349.9, 780.33

● **345.8 Other forms of epilepsy and recurrent seizures**
[0-1]   Epilepsy:
cursive [running]
gelastic
Recurrent seizures NOS

(Ex) 249.60-249.61, 250.60-250.63, 345.00-345.91, 348.81, 348.89-348.9, 349.89-349.9, 780.33

● **345.9 Epilepsy, unspecified** 1
[0-1]   Epileptic convulsions, fits, or seizures NOS
Seizure disorder NOS

> **Excludes** *convulsion (convulsive) disorder (780.39)*
> *convulsive seizure or fit NOS (780.39)*
> *recurrent convulsions (780.39)*

For code **345.91:** (Ex) 249.60-249.61, 250.60-250.63, 345.00-345.91, 348.81, 348.89-348.9, 349.89-349.9, 780.33

Coding Clinic: 2012, Q2, P9-10; 2009, Q2, P10; 2008, Q1, P17; 1993, Q1, P24; 1987, Nov-Dec, P12

DISEASES OF THE NERVOUS SYSTEM AND SENSE ORGANS (320–389)

N Newborn: 0   **P** Pediatric: 0–17   **M** Maternity: 12–55   **A** Adult: 15–124   ♀ Females Only   ♂ Males Only

(Ex) CC/MCC Exclusions   Complication\Comorbidity   Major C\C   Present on Admission Requirement   Hospital-Acquired Condition   **775**

Item 6-8 Migraine headache is described as an intense pulsing or throbbing pain in one area of the head. It can be accompanied by extreme sensitivity to light (photophoic) and sound and is three times more common in women than in men. Symptoms include nausea and vomiting. Research indicates migraine headaches are caused by inherited abnormalities in genes that control the activities of certain cell populations in the brain.

● 346 **Migraine**
Excludes headache:
NOS (784.0)
syndromes (339.00-339.89)
Coding Clinic: 2008, Q4, P102-109

The following fifth-digit subclassification is for use with category 346:

> 0 without mention of intractable migraine without mention of status migrainosus
> without mention of refractory migraine without mention of status migrainosus
> 1 with intractable migraine, so stated, without mention of status migrainosus
> with refractory migraine, so stated, without mention of status migrainosus
> 2 without mention of intractable migraine with status migrainosus
> without mention of refractory migraine with status migrainosus
> 3 with intractable migraine, so stated, with status migrainosus
> with refractory migraine, so stated, with status migrainosus

Intractable migraine: Not easily cured or managed; relentless pain from a migraine

● 346.0 **Migraine with aura**
[0-3] Basilar migraine
Classic migraine
Migraine preceded or accompanied by transient focal neurological phenomena
Migraine triggered seizures
Migraine with acute-onset aura
Migraine with aura without headache (migraine equivalents)
Migraine with prolonged aura
Migraine with typical aura
Retinal migraine
Excludes persistent migraine aura (346.5, 346.6)

● 346.1 **Migraine without aura**
[0-3] Common migraine

● 346.2 **Variants of migraine, not elsewhere classified**
[0-3] Abdominal migraine
Cyclical vomiting associated with migraine
Ophthalmoplegic migraine
Periodic headache syndromes in child or adolescent
Excludes cyclical vomiting NOS (536.2)
psychogenic cyclical vomiting (306.4)

● 346.3 **Hemiplegic migraine**
[0-3] Familial migraine
Sporadic migraine

● 346.4 **Menstrual migraine** ♀
[0-3] Menstrual headache
Menstrually related migraine
Premenstrual headache
Premenstrual migraine
Pure menstrual migraine

● 346.5 **Persistent migraine aura without cerebral**
[0-3] **infarction**
Persistent migraine aura NOS

● 346.6 **Persistent migraine aura with cerebral**
[0-3] **infarction**
For code 346.60: Ex 346.60-346.63, 433.00-434.91;
For codes 346.61-346.63: Ex 346.60-346.63, 433.00-434.91, 436

● 346.7 **Chronic migraine without aura**
[0-3] Transformed migraine without aura

● 346.8 **Other forms of migraine**
[0-3]

● 346.9 **Migraine, unspecified**
[0-3] Coding Clinic: 1985, Nov-Dec, P16

● 347 **Cataplexy and narcolepsy**
Cataplexy is a disorder evidenced by seizures. Narcolepsy is difficulty remaining awake during daytime.
Coding Clinic: 2004, Q4, P74-75

● 347.0 **Narcolepsy**
347.00 **Without cataplexy**
Narcolepsy NOS
347.01 **With cataplexy**

● 347.1 **Narcolepsy in conditions classified elsewhere**
Code first underlying condition
▸ 347.10 *Without cataplexy*
▸ 347.11 *With cataplexy*

● 348 **Other conditions of brain**
348.0 **Cerebral cysts**
Arachnoid cyst   Porencephaly, acquired
Porencephalic cyst   Pseudoporencephaly

348.1 **Anoxic brain damage**
Brain permanently damaged by lack of oxygen perfusion through brain tissues. This is the result of another problem, so use an additional E code to identify the cause.
Excludes that occurring in:
abortion (634–638 with .7, 639.8)
ectopic or molar pregnancy (639.8)
labor or delivery (668.2, 669.4)
that of newborn (767.0, 768.0–768.9, 772.1–772.2)
Use additional E code to identify cause
Ex: 249.60-249.61, 249.80-249.91, 250.60-250.63, 250.80-250.93, 348.1-348.2, 349.89-349.9
Coding Clinic: 2013, Q3, P11

348.2 **Benign intracranial hypertension**
Pseudotumor cerebri
Excludes hypertensive encephalopathy (437.2)

● 348.3 **Encephalopathy, not elsewhere classified**
A general term for any degenerative brain disease
Coding Clinic: 2003, Q4, P58-59; 1997, Q3, P5
348.30 **Encephalopathy, unspecified**
Ex: 333.92, 344.81, 348.31-348.39
348.31 **Metabolic encephalopathy**
Septic encephalopathy
Excludes toxic metabolic encephalopathy (349.82)
Ex: 333.92, 344.81, 348.30, 348.39
348.39 **Other encephalopathy**
Excludes encephalopathy:
alcoholic (291.2)
hepatic (572.2)
hypertensive (437.2)
toxic (349.82)
Ex: 333.92, 344.81, 348.30-348.31

348.4 **Compression of brain**
Compression brain (stem)
Herniation brain (stem)
Posterior fossa compression syndrome
Ex: 342.90, 348.82
Coding Clinic: 2013, Q2, P9; 2011, Q3, P11

348.5 **Cerebral edema**
Ex: 348.5, 348.82
Coding Clinic: 2011, Q4, P100; 2010, Q1, P6; 2009, Q3, P7

◀ New ◀ Revised deleted Deleted Excludes Includes Use additional Code first Omit code
776 ● Unacceptable Principal Diagnosis ● Use Additional Digit(s) ▸ Manifestation Code OGCR Official Guidelines Coding Clinic

DISEASES OF THE NERVOUS SYSTEM AND SENSE ORGANS (320–389)

● **348.8 Other conditions of brain**
Coding Clinic: 1992, Q3, P8; 1987, Sept-Oct, P9

  348.81 Temporal sclerosis
Hippocampal sclerosis
Mesial temporal sclerosis
Coding Clinic: 2009, Q4, P98

  348.82 Brain death 🔖
(Ex) 070.0-070.9, 249.00-251.3, 338.0-338.4, 348.81-348.9,
349.89-349.9, 430-432.9, 572.2, 780.01-780.09, 780.2, 780.4,
780.64, 780.65, 780.91-780.99, 799.81-799.89, 800.00-801.99,
803.00-804.99, 850.0-854.19
Coding Clinic: 2011, Q4, P100

  348.89 Other conditions of brain
Cerebral:
  calcification
  fungus
  Excludes *brain death (348.82)*

348.9 Unspecified condition of brain

● **349 Other and unspecified disorders of the nervous system**

  349.0 Reaction to spinal or lumbar puncture
Headache following lumbar puncture
Cerebral spinal fluid (CSF) maintains a specific level of
pressure inside brain and spinal cord. If this pressure
does not return to normal after a puncture, headache
will result.
Coding Clinic: 1999, Q2, P9-10; 1990, Q3, P18

  349.1 Nervous system complications from surgically implanted
  device 🔖
  Excludes *immediate postoperative complications*
  (997.00–997.09)
  mechanical complications of nervous system
  device (996.2)
(Ex) 249.60-249.61, 249.80-249.91, 250.60-250.63, 250.80-250.93, 349.1,
349.89-349.9

  349.2 Disorders of meninges, not elsewhere classified
Adhesions, meningeal (cerebral) (spinal)
Cyst, spinal meninges
Meningocele, acquired
Pseudomeningocele, acquired
Coding Clinic: 2006, Q1, P15-16; 1998, Q2, P18; 1994, Q3, P4; Q1,
P22-23

● **349.3 Dural tear**
Coding Clinic: 2008, Q4, P109-110

  349.31 Accidental puncture or laceration of dura during a
  procedure 🔖
Incidental (inadvertent) durotomy
(Ex) 349.31-349.39, 997.91-997.99, 998.2, 998.81, 998.83-998.9

  349.39 Other dural tear 🔖
(Ex) 349.31-349.39, 997.91-997.99, 998.2, 998.81, 998.83-998.9

● **349.8 Other specified disorders of nervous system**

  349.81 Cerebrospinal fluid rhinorrhea 🔖
  Excludes *cerebrospinal fluid otorrhea (388.61)*
(Ex) 249.60-249.61, 249.80-249.91, 250.60-250.63, 250.80-250.93,
349.81, 349.89-349.9

  349.82 Toxic encephalopathy 🔖
Toxic metabolic encephalopathy
Use additional E code to identify cause
(Ex) 013.60-013.66, 017.90-017.96, 036.1, 049.8-049.9, 052.0, 054.3,
058.21-058.29, 062.0-063.9, 072.2, 090.41, 094.81, 130.0,
249.60-249.61, 249.80-249.91, 250.60-250.63, 250.80-250.93,
323.01-323.9, 341.20-341.22, 348.30-348.39, 348.81, 348.89-
348.9, 349.82-349.9

  349.89 Other

  349.9 Unspecified disorders of nervous system
Disorder of nervous system (central) NOS
Coding Clinic: 2012, Q3, P4

Item 6–9 The **peripheral nervous system** consists of 31 pairs of
spinal nerves, 12 pairs of cranial nerves, and the autonomic nerves, which
are divided into the parasympathetic and sympathetic nerves. The cranial
nerves are: olfactory (I), optic (II), oculomotor (III), trochlear (IV), trigeminal (V),
abducens (VI), facial (VII), vestibulocochlear (VIII), glossopharyngeal (IX),
vagus (X), accessory (XI), and hypoglossal (XII).

Item 6-10 Trigeminal neuralgia, tic douloureux, is a pain syndrome
diagnosed from the patient's history alone. The condition is characterized by
pain and a brief facial spasm or tic. Pain is unilateral and follows the sensory
distribution of cranial nerve V, typically radiating to the maxillary (V2) or
mandibular (V3) area.

Item 6-11 The most common facial nerve disorder is **Bell's Palsy,** which
occurs suddenly and results in facial drooping unilaterally. This disorder is the
result of a reaction to a virus that causes the facial nerve in the ear to swell
resulting in pressure in the bony canal.

DISORDERS OF THE PERIPHERAL NERVOUS SYSTEM (350–359)

  Excludes *diseases of:*
  acoustic [8th] nerve (388.5)
  oculomotor [3rd, 4th, 6th] nerves (378.0–378.9)
  optic [2nd] nerve (377.0–377.9)
  peripheral autonomic nerves (337.0–337.9)
  neuralgia NOS or "rheumatic" (729.2)
  neuritis NOS or "rheumatic" (729.2)
  radiculitis NOS or "rheumatic" (729.2)
  peripheral neuritis in pregnancy (646.4)

● **350 Trigeminal nerve disorders**
  Includes disorders of 5th cranial nerve

  350.1 Trigeminal neuralgia
Tic douloureux
Trifacial neuralgia
Trigeminal neuralgia NOS
  Excludes *postherpetic (053.12)*

  350.2 Atypical face pain

  350.8 Other specified trigeminal nerve disorders

  350.9 Trigeminal nerve disorder, unspecified

● **351 Facial nerve disorders**
  Includes disorders of 7th cranial nerve
  Excludes *that in newborn (767.5)*

  351.0 Bell's palsy
Facial palsy

  351.1 Geniculate ganglionitis
Geniculate ganglionitis NOS
  Excludes *herpetic (053.11)*
  Coding Clinic: 2002, Q2, P8

  351.8 Other facial nerve disorders
Facial myokymia
Melkersson's syndrome
Coding Clinic: 2002, Q3, P12-13

  351.9 Facial nerve disorder, unspecified

● **352 Disorders of other cranial nerves**

  352.0 Disorders of olfactory [1st] nerve

  352.1 Glossopharyngeal neuralgia
Coding Clinic: 1987, Jan-Feb, P14

  352.2 Other disorders of glossopharyngeal [9th] nerve

  352.3 Disorders of pneumogastric [10th] nerve
Disorders of vagal nerve
  Excludes *paralysis of vocal cords or larynx*
  (478.30–478.34)

  352.4 Disorders of accessory [11th] nerve

  352.5 Disorders of hypoglossal [12th] nerve

  352.6 Multiple cranial nerve palsies
Collet-Sicard syndrome
Polyneuritis cranialis

  352.9 Unspecified disorder of cranial nerves

● **353 Nerve root and plexus disorders**

> **Excludes** *conditions due to:*
> *intervertebral disc disorders (722.0–722.9)*
> *spondylosis (720.0–721.9)*
> *vertebrogenic disorders (723.0–724.9)*

353.0 Brachial plexus lesions
Cervical rib syndrome
Costoclavicular syndrome
Scalenus anticus syndrome
Thoracic outlet syndrome

> **Excludes** *brachial neuritis or radiculitis NOS (723.4)*
> *that in newborn (767.6)*
> **Coding Clinic: 2006, Q3, P12**

353.1 Lumbosacral plexus lesions

353.2 Cervical root lesions, not elsewhere classified

● **353.3 Thoracic root lesions, not elsewhere classified**

353.4 Lumbosacral root lesions, not elsewhere classified

353.5 Neuralgic amyotrophy
Parsonage-Aldren-Turner syndrome
Phantom limb syndrome: Patients with amputated limbs feel sensations in a limb that no longer exists. There is no separate code for phantom limb pain, and the pain can be part of the syndrome.

> *Code first any associated underlying disease, such as:*
> diabetes mellitus (249.6, 250.6)

353.6 Phantom limb (syndrome)

353.8 Other nerve root and plexus disorders

353.9 Unspecified nerve root and plexus disorder

● **354 Mononeuritis of upper limb and mononeuritis multiplex**

354.0 Carpal tunnel syndrome *(CTS)*
Of the wrist
Median nerve entrapment
Partial thenar atrophy

354.1 Other lesion of median nerve
Median nerve neuritis

354.2 Lesion of ulnar nerve
Cubital tunnel syndrome
Tardy ulnar nerve palsy

354.3 Lesion of radial nerve
Acute radial nerve palsy
Coding Clinic: 1987, Nov-Dec, P6

354.4 Causalgia of upper limb
Complex regional pain syndrome type II of the upper limb

> **Excludes** *causalgia:*
> *NOS (355.9)*
> *lower limb (355.71)*
> *complex regional pain syndrome type II of the lower limb (355.71)*

354.5 Mononeuritis multiplex
Combinations of single conditions classifiable to 354 or 355

354.8 Other mononeuritis of upper limb

354.9 Mononeuritis of upper limb, unspecified

● **355 Mononeuritis of lower limb**
Coding Clinic: 1989, Q2, P12

355.0 Lesion of sciatic nerve

> **Excludes** *sciatica NOS (724.3)*
> **Coding Clinic: 1989, Q2, P12**

355.1 Meralgia paresthetica
Lateral cutaneous femoral nerve of thigh compression or syndrome

355.2 Other lesion of femoral nerve

355.3 Lesion of lateral popliteal nerve
Lesion of common peroneal nerve

355.4 Lesion of medial popliteal nerve

355.5 Tarsal tunnel syndrome
Of the ankle

355.6 Lesion of plantar nerve
Morton's metatarsalgia, neuralgia, or neuroma

● **355.7 Other mononeuritis of lower limb**

355.71 Causalgia of lower limb

> **Excludes** *causalgia:*
> *NOS (355.9)*
> *upper limb (354.4)*
> *complex regional pain syndrome type II of the upper limb (354.4)*

355.79 Other mononeuritis of lower limb

355.8 Mononeuritis of lower limb, unspecified
Coding Clinic: 2013, Q1, P3

355.9 Mononeuritis of unspecified site
Causalgia NOS
Complex regional pain syndrome NOS

> **Excludes** *causalgia:*
> *lower limb (355.71)*
> *upper limb (354.4)*
> *complex regional pain syndrome:*
> *lower limb (355.71)*
> *upper limb (354.4)*
> **Coding Clinic: 2013, Q1, P3-4**

● **356 Hereditary and idiopathic peripheral neuropathy**
Any disease that affects nervous system and of an unknown cause

356.0 Hereditary peripheral neuropathy
Déjérine-Sottas disease

356.1 Peroneal muscular atrophy
Charcot-Marie-Tooth disease
Neuropathic muscular atrophy

356.2 Hereditary sensory neuropathy

356.3 Refsum's disease 🔖
Heredopathia atactica polyneuritiformis
Ⓔⓧ 350.1-357.9

356.4 Idiopathic progressive polyneuropathy

356.8 Other specified idiopathic peripheral neuropathy
Supranuclear paralysis

356.9 Unspecified

● **357 Inflammatory and toxic neuropathy**

357.0 Acute infective polyneuritis 🔖
Guillain-Barre syndrome
Postinfectious polyneuritis
Ⓔⓧ 003.21, 013.00-013.16, 036.0, 036.89-036.9, 041.81-041.9, 047.0-047.9, 049.0-049.1, 053.0, 054.72, 072.1, 090.42, 091.81, 094.2, 098.89, 100.81, 112.83, 114.2, 115.01, 115.11, 115.91, 130.0, 139.8, 320.0-322.9, 349.89-349.9, 357.0
Coding Clinic: 1998, Q2, P12

▷ **357.1 Polyneuropathy in collagen vascular disease**
> *Code first underlying disease, as:*
> disseminated lupus erythematosus (710.0)
> polyarteritis nodosa (446.0)
> rheumatoid arthritis (714.0)

▷ **357.2 Polyneuropathy in diabetes**
> *Code first underlying disease (249.6, 250.6)*
> **Coding Clinic: 2009, Q4, P98; Q2, P13; 2008, Q3, P5-6; 2003, Q4, P105; 1992, Q2, P15**

▷ **357.3 Polyneuropathy in malignant disease**
> *Code first underlying disease (140.0–208.9)*

▷ **357.4 Polyneuropathy in other diseases classified elsewhere**
> *Code first underlying disease, as:*
> amyloidosis (277.30–277.39)
> beriberi (265.0)
> chronic uremia (585.9)
> deficiency of B vitamins (266.0–266.9)
> diphtheria (032.0–032.9)
> hypoglycemia (251.2)
> pellagra (265.2)
> porphyria (277.1)
> sarcoidosis (135)
> uremia NOS (586)

> **Excludes** *polyneuropathy in:*
> *herpes zoster (053.13)*
> *mumps (072.72)*
> **Coding Clinic: 2008, Q2, P8-9; 1998, Q2, P15**

◀ New   ◀≡ Revised   ~~deleted~~ Deleted   Excludes   Includes   Use additional   Code first   Omit code

● Unacceptable Principal Diagnosis   ● Use Additional Digit(s)   ▷ Manifestation Code   OGCR Official Guidelines   **Coding Clinic**

357.5 **Alcoholic polyneuropathy**

357.6 **Polyneuropathy due to drugs**
   Use additional E code to identify drug

357.7 **Polyneuropathy due to other toxic agents**
   Use additional E code to identify toxic agent

● 357.8 **Other**
   Coding Clinic: 2002, Q4, P47-48; 1998, Q2, P12

   357.81 **Chronic inflammatory demyelinating polyneuritis** 🅖
      (Ex) 351.0-353.5, 353.8-356.9, 357.81-357.89

   357.82 **Critical illness polyneuropathy** 🅖
      Acute motor neuropathy
      (Ex) 351.0-353.5, 353.8-356.9, 357.81-357.9
      Coding Clinic: 2003, Q4, P111

   357.89 **Other inflammatory and toxic neuropathy**
      Coding Clinic: 2013, Q1, P3

357.9 **Unspecified**

● 358 **Myoneural disorders**

● 358.0 **Myasthenia gravis**
   *Acquired and results in fatigable muscle weakness exacerbated
   by activity and improved with rest. Caused by
   autoimmune assault against nerve-muscle junction.*
   Coding Clinic: 2003, Q4, P59-60

   358.00 **Myasthenia gravis without (acute) exacerbation**

   358.01 **Myasthenia gravis with acute exacerbation** 🅖
      Myasthenia gravis in crisis
      (Ex) 249.60-249.61, 249.80-249.91, 250.60-250.63, 250.80-250.93,
         349.89-349.9, 358.00-358.1, 358.30-358.39
      Coding Clinic: 2007, Q4, P108-109; 2004, Q4, P139

▷ 358.1 *Myasthenic syndromes in diseases classified elsewhere* 🅖
      Code first underlying disease, as:
         botulism (005.1, 040.41–040.42)
         hypothyroidism (244.0–244.9)
         malignant neoplasm (140.0–208.9)
         pernicious anemia (281.0)
         thyrotoxicosis (242.0–242.9)
      (Ex) 249.60-249.61, 249.80-249.91, 250.60-250.63, 250.80-250.93, 349.89-349.9,
         358.00-358.1, 358.30-358.39

358.2 **Toxic myoneural disorders**
   Use additional E code to identify toxic agent

● 358.3 **Lambert-Eaton syndrome**
      Eaton-Lambert syndrome

   358.30 **Lambert-Eaton syndrome, unspecified** 🅖
      Lambert-Eaton syndrome NOS
      (Ex) 249.60, 249.61, 249.80-249.91, 250.60-250.63, 250.80-250.93,
         349.89, 349.9, 358.00-358.1, 358.30-358.39
      Coding Clinic: 2011, Q4, P101

   ● 358.31 **Lambert-Eaton syndrome in neoplastic disease** 🅖
      Code first the underlying neoplastic disease
      (Ex) 249.60, 249.61, 249.80-249.91, 250.60-250.63, 250.80-250.93,
         349.89, 349.9, 358.00-358.1, 358.30-358.39

   ▷ 358.39 *Lambert-Eaton syndrome in other diseases
      classified elsewhere* 🅖
      Code first the underlying condition
      (Ex) 249.60, 249.61, 249.80-249.91, 250.60-250.63, 250.80-250.93,
         349.89, 349.9, 358.00-358.1, 358.30-358.39

358.8 **Other specified myoneural disorders**

358.9 **Myoneural disorders, unspecified**
   Coding Clinic: 2002, Q2, P16

Item 6-12   Muscular dystrophies (MD) are a group of rare inherited muscle diseases. Voluntary muscles become progressively weaker. In the late stages of MD, fat and connective tissue replace muscle fibers. In some types of muscular dystrophy, heart muscles, other involuntary muscles, and other organs are affected. **Myopathies** is a general term for neuromuscular diseases in which the muscle fibers dysfunction for any one of many reasons, resulting in muscular weakness.

● 359 **Muscular dystrophies and other myopathies**
   Excludes   *idiopathic polymyositis (710.4)*

   359.0 **Congenital hereditary muscular dystrophy** 🅖
      Benign congenital myopathy
      Central core disease
      Centronuclear myopathy
      Myotubular myopathy
      Nemaline body disease
      Excludes   *arthrogryposis multiplex congenita (754.89)*
      (Ex) 249.60-249.61, 249.80-249.91, 250.60-250.63, 250.80-250.93, 349.89-349.9,
         359.0-359.1

   359.1 **Hereditary progressive muscular dystrophy** 🅖
      Muscular dystrophy:
         NOS
         distal
         Duchenne
         Erb's
         fascioscapulohumeral
         Gower's
         Landouzy-Déjérine
         limb-girdle
         ocular
         oculopharyngeal
      (Ex) 249.60-249.61, 249.80-249.91, 250.60-250.63, 250.80-250.93, 349.89-349.9,
         359.0-359.1

● 359.2 **Myotonic disorders**
      Excludes   *periodic paralysis (359.3)*
      Coding Clinic: 2007, Q4, P75-77

   359.21 **Myotonic muscular dystrophy**
      Dystrophia myotonica
      Myotonia atrophica
      Myotonic dystrophy
      Proximal myotonic myopathy (PROMM)
      Steinert's disease

   359.22 **Myotonia congenita**
      Acetazolamide responsive myotonia congenita
      Dominant form (Thomsen's disease)
      Myotonia levior
      Recessive form (Becker's disease)

   359.23 **Myotonic chondrodystrophy**
      Congenital myotonic chondrodystrophy
      Schwartz-Jampel disease

   359.24 **Drug-induced myotonia**
      Use additional E code to identify drug

   359.29 **Other specified myotonic disorder**
      Myotonia fluctuans
      Myotonia permanens
      Paramyotonia congenita (of von Eulenburg)

   359.3 **Periodic paralysis**
      Familial periodic paralysis
      Hyperkalemic periodic paralysis
      Hypokalemic familial periodic paralysis
      Hypokalemic periodic paralysis
      Potassium sensitive periodic paralysis
      Excludes   *paramyotonia congenita (of von Eulenburg)
         (359.29)*

   359.4 **Toxic myopathy** 🅖
      Use additional E code to identify toxic agent
      (Ex) 349.89-349.9, 358.00, 359.6, 359.81-359.9

DISEASES OF THE NERVOUS SYSTEM AND SENSE ORGANS (320–389)

▸ **359.5 Myopathy in endocrine diseases classified elsewhere**

Code first underlying disease, as:
Addison's disease (255.41)
Cushing's syndrome (255.0)
hypopituitarism (253.2)
myxedema (244.0–244.9)
thyrotoxicosis (242.0–242.9)

▸ **359.6 Symptomatic inflammatory myopathy in diseases classified elsewhere** 🔍

Code first underlying disease, as:
amyloidosis (277.30–277.39)
disseminated lupus erythematosus (710.0)
malignant neoplasm (140.0–208.9)
polyarteritis nodosa (446.0)
rheumatoid arthritis (714.0)
sarcoidosis (135)
scleroderma (710.1)
Sjögren's disease (710.2)

Ex: 249.60-249.61, 249.80-249.91, 250.60-250.63, 250.80-250.93, 349.89-349.9, 358.00, 359.6, 359.81-359.9

● **359.7 Inflammatory and immune myopathies, NEC**

359.71 Inclusion body myositis
IBM

359.79 Other inflammatory and immune myopathies, NEC
Inflammatory myopathy NOS

● **359.8 Other myopathies**
Coding Clinic: 2002, Q4, P47-48; 1990, Q3, P17

359.81 Critical illness myopathy 🔍
Acute necrotizing myopathy
Acute quadriplegic myopathy
Intensive care (ICU) myopathy
Myopathy of critical illness
Ex: 358.1, 359.6, 359.81-359.9

359.89 Other myopathies

359.9 Myopathy, unspecified

DISORDERS OF THE EYE AND ADNEXA (360–379)

Use additional external cause code, if applicable, to identify the cause of the eye condition

● **360 Disorders of the globe**
Includes disorders affecting multiple structures of eye

● **360.0 Purulent endophthalmitis**
Excludes bleb associated endophthalmitis (379.63)

360.00 Purulent endophthalmitis, unspecified 🔍
Ex: 360.00-360.04, 360.13, 360.19, 364.05

360.01 Acute endophthalmitis 🔍
Ex: 360.00-360.04, 360.13, 360.19, 364.05

360.02 Panophthalmitis 🔍
Ex: 360.00-360.04, 360.13, 360.19, 364.05

360.03 Chronic endophthalmitis

360.04 Vitreous abscess 🔍
Ex: 360.00-360.19

● **360.1 Other endophthalmitis**
Excludes bleb associated endophthalmitis (379.63)

360.11 Sympathetic uveitis 🔍
Ex: 360.11-360.12

360.12 Panuveitis 🔍
Ex: 360.11-360.12

360.13 Parasitic endophthalmitis NOS 🔍
Ex: 360.00-360.04, 360.13, 360.19, 364.05

360.14 Ophthalmia nodosa

360.19 Other 🔍
Phacoanaphylactic endophthalmitis
Ex: 360.00-360.04, 360.13, 360.19, 364.05

● **360.2 Degenerative disorders of globe**

360.20 Degenerative disorder of globe, unspecified

360.21 Progressive high (degenerative) myopia
Malignant myopia

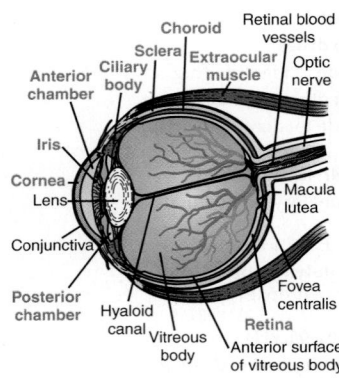

Figure 6–3 Eye and ocular adnexa. (From Buck CJ: Step-by-Step Medical Coding, ed 2011, Philadelphia, WB Saunders, 2011)

360.23 Siderosis

360.24 Other metallosis
Chalcosis

360.29 Other
Excludes xerophthalmia (264.7)

● **360.3 Hypotony of eye**

360.30 Hypotony, unspecified

360.31 Primary hypotony

360.32 Ocular fistula causing hypotony

360.33 Hypotony associated with other ocular disorders

360.34 Flat anterior chamber

● **360.4 Degenerated conditions of globe**

360.40 Degenerated globe or eye, unspecified

360.41 Blind hypotensive eye
Atrophy of globe   Phthisis bulbi

360.42 Blind hypertensive eye
Absolute glaucoma

360.43 Hemophthalmos, except current injury
Excludes traumatic (871.0–871.9, 921.0–921.9)

360.44 Leucocoria

● **360.5 Retained (old) intraocular foreign body, magnetic**
Use additional code to identify foreign body (V90.11)
Excludes current penetrating injury with magnetic foreign body (871.5)
retained (old) foreign body of orbit (376.6)

360.50 Foreign body, magnetic, intraocular, unspecified

360.51 Foreign body, magnetic, in anterior chamber

360.52 Foreign body, magnetic, in iris or ciliary body

360.53 Foreign body, magnetic, in lens

360.54 Foreign body, magnetic, in vitreous

360.55 Foreign body, magnetic, in posterior wall

360.59 Foreign body, magnetic, in other or multiple sites

● **360.6 Retained (old) intraocular foreign body, nonmagnetic**
Retained (old) foreign body:
NOS
nonmagnetic
Use additional code to identify foreign body (V90.01-V90.10, V90.12, V90.2-V90.9)
Excludes current penetrating injury with (nonmagnetic) foreign body (871.6)
retained (old) foreign body in orbit (376.6)

360.60 Foreign body, intraocular, unspecified

360.61 Foreign body in anterior chamber

360.62 Foreign body in iris or ciliary body

360.63 Foreign body in lens

360.64 Foreign body in vitreous

360.65 Foreign body in posterior wall

360.69 Foreign body in other or multiple sites

● **360.8 Other disorders of globe**

360.81 Luxation of globe

360.89 Other

360.9 Unspecified disorder of globe

Item 6-13 Retinal detachments and defects are conditions of the eye in which the retina separates from the underlying tissue. Initial detachment may be localized, requiring rapid treatment (medical emergency) to avoid the entire retina from detaching, which leads to vision loss and blindness.

● **361 Retinal detachments and defects**

● **361.0 Retinal detachment with retinal defect**
Rhegmatogenous retinal detachment

> **Excludes** *detachment of retinal pigment epithelium*
> *(362.42–362.43)*
> *retinal detachment (serous) (without defect)*
> *(361.2)*

Coding Clinic: 1994, Q1, P17

361.00 Retinal detachment with retinal defect, unspecified

361.01 Recent detachment, partial, with single defect

361.02 Recent detachment, partial, with multiple defects

361.03 Recent detachment, partial, with giant tear

361.04 Recent detachment, partial, with retinal dialysis
Dialysis (juvenile) of retina (with detachment)

361.05 Recent detachment, total or subtotal

361.06 Old detachment, partial
Delimited old retinal detachment

361.07 Old detachment, total or subtotal

● **361.1 Retinoschisis and retinal cysts**

> **Excludes** *juvenile retinoschisis (362.73)*
> *microcystoid degeneration of retina (362.62)*
> *parasitic cyst of retina (360.13)*

361.10 Retinoschisis, unspecified

361.11 Flat retinoschisis

361.12 Bullous retinoschisis

361.13 Primary retinal cysts

361.14 Secondary retinal cysts

361.19 Other
Pseudocyst of retina

● **361.2 Serous retinal detachment** 🖐
Retinal detachment without retinal defect

> **Excludes** *central serous retinopathy (362.41)*
> *retinal pigment epithelium detachment*
> *(362.42–362.43)*

(Ex) 361.00-361.9, 362.40-362.43

● **361.3 Retinal defects without detachment**

> **Excludes** *chorioretinal scars after surgery for detachment*
> *(363.30–363.35)*
> *peripheral retinal degeneration without defect*
> *(362.60–362.66)*

361.30 Retinal defect, unspecified
Retinal break(s) NOS

361.31 Round hole of retina without detachment

361.32 Horseshoe tear of retina without detachment
Operculum of retina without mention of detachment

361.33 Multiple defects of retina without detachment

● **361.8 Other forms of retinal detachment**

361.81 Traction detachment of retina 🖐
(Ex) 361.00-361.9, 362.40-362.43
Traction detachment with vitreoretinal organization

361.89 Other 🖐
(Ex) 361.00-361.9, 362.40-362.43
Coding Clinic: 1999, Q3, P12

361.9 Unspecified retinal detachment 🖐
(Ex) 361.00-361.9, 362.40-362.43
Coding Clinic: 1987, Nov-Dec, P10

● **362 Other retinal disorders**

> **Excludes** *chorioretinal scars (363.30–363.35)*
> *chorioretinitis (363.0–363.2)*

● **362.0 Diabetic retinopathy**

Code first diabetes (249.5, 250.5)

Most common diabetic eye disease and leading cause of blindness in adults. Caused by changes in the blood vessels of retina in which the blood vessels swell and leak fluid into retinal surface.

▷ **362.01 Background diabetic retinopathy**
Diabetic retinal microaneurysms
Diabetic retinopathy NOS

▷ **362.02 Proliferative diabetic retinopathy**
Coding Clinic: 1996, Q3, P5

▷ **362.03 Nonproliferative diabetic retinopathy NOS**

▷ **362.04 Mild nonproliferative diabetic retinopathy**

▷ **362.05 Moderate nonproliferative diabetic retinopathy**

▷ **362.06 Severe nonproliferative diabetic retinopathy**
Coding Clinic: 2005, Q4, P65-67

▷ **362.07 Diabetic macular edema**
Diabetic retinal edema

> **Note:** Code 362.07 must be used with a code for diabetic retinopathy (362.01–362.06)

● **362.1 Other background retinopathy and retinal vascular changes**

362.10 Background retinopathy, unspecified
Coding Clinic: 2006, Q1, P12

362.11 Hypertensive retinopathy

OGCR Section I.C.7.a.6

> Two codes are necessary to identify the condition. First assign the code from subcategory 362.11, Hypertensive retinopathy, then the appropriate code from categories 401–405 to indicate the type of hypertension.

362.12 Exudative retinopathy
Coats' syndrome
Coding Clinic: 1999, Q3, P12

362.13 Changes in vascular appearance
Vascular sheathing of retina
> Use additional code for any associated atherosclerosis (440.8)

362.14 Retinal microaneurysms NOS

362.15 Retinal telangiectasia

362.16 Retinal neovascularization NOS
Neovascularization:
choroidal
subretinal

362.17 Other intraretinal microvascular abnormalities
Retinal varices

362.18 Retinal vasculitis
Eales' disease
Retinal:
arteritis
endarteritis
perivasculitis
phlebitis

● **362.2 Other proliferative retinopathy**

362.20 Retinopathy of prematurity, unspecified
Retinopathy of prematurity NOS
Coding Clinic: 2008, Q4, P110-111

362.21 Retrolental fibroplasia
Cicatricial retinopathy of prematurity

362.22 Retinopathy of prematurity, stage 0

362.23 Retinopathy of prematurity, stage 1

362.24 Retinopathy of prematurity, stage 2

362.25 Retinopathy of prematurity, stage 3

362.26 Retinopathy of prematurity, stage 4

362.27 Retinopathy of prematurity, stage 5

362.29 Other nondiabetic proliferative retinopathy
Coding Clinic: 1996, Q3, P5

DISEASES OF THE NERVOUS SYSTEM AND SENSE ORGANS (320–389)

N Newborn: 0   P Pediatric: 0–17   M Maternity: 12–55   A Adult: 15–124   ♀ Females Only   ♂ Males Only

(Ex) CC/MCC Exclusions   🖐 Complication\Comorbidity   🖐 Major C\C   🖐 Present on Admission Requirement   🖐 Hospital-Acquired Condition   781

● **362.3 Retinal vascular occlusion**
Blockage in vessel of the retina

    362.30 Retinal vascular occlusion, unspecified 🔖
        (Ex:) 362.30-362.37

    362.31 Central retinal artery occlusion 🔖
        (Ex:) 362.30-362.37

    362.32 Arterial branch occlusion 🔖
        (Ex:) 362.30-362.37

    362.33 Partial arterial occlusion 🔖
        Hollenhorst plaque
        Retinal microembolism
        (Ex:) 362.30-362.37

    362.34 Transient arterial occlusion 🔖
        Amaurosis fugax
        (Ex:) 362.30-362.37
        Coding Clinic: 2000, Q1, P16

    362.35 Central retinal vein occlusion 🔖
        (Ex:) 362.30-362.37
        Coding Clinic: 1993, Q2, P6

    362.36 Venous tributary (branch) occlusion

    362.37 Venous engorgement
        Occlusion:
            of retinal vein
            incipient of retinal vein
            partial of retinal vein

● **362.4 Separation of retinal layers**

    Excludes *retinal detachment (serous) (361.2)*
                 rhegmatogenous (361.00–361.07)

    362.40 Retinal layer separation, unspecified 🔖
        (Ex:) 361.00-361.9, 362.40-362.43

    362.41 Central serous retinopathy

    362.42 Serous detachment of retinal pigment epithelium 🔖
        Exudative detachment of retinal pigment
            epithelium
        (Ex:) 361.00-361.9, 362.40-362.43

    362.43 Hemorrhagic detachment of retinal pigment epithelium 🔖
        (Ex:) 361.00-361.9, 362.40-362.43

● **362.5 Degeneration of macula and posterior pole**

    Excludes *degeneration of optic disc (377.21–377.24)*
                 hereditary retinal degeneration [dystrophy]
                    (362.70–362.77)

    362.50 Macular degeneration (senile), unspecified

    362.51 Nonexudative senile macular degeneration
        Senile macular degeneration:
            atrophic
            dry

    362.52 Exudative senile macular degeneration
        Kuhnt-Junius degeneration
        Senile macular degeneration:
            disciform
            wet

    362.53 Cystoid macular degeneration
        Cystoid macular edema

    362.54 Macular cyst, hole, or pseudohole
        Coding Clinic: 2011, Q4, P106

    362.55 Toxic maculopathy
        Use additional E code to identify drug, if drug
            induced

    362.56 Macular puckering
        Preretinal fibrosis

    362.57 Drusen (degenerative)

● **362.6 Peripheral retinal degenerations**

    Excludes *hereditary retinal degeneration [dystrophy]*
                    (362.70–362.77)
                 retinal degeneration with retinal defect
                    (361.00–361.07)

    362.60 Peripheral retinal degeneration, unspecified

    362.61 Paving stone degeneration

    362.62 Microcystoid degeneration
        Blessig's cysts
        Iwanoff's cysts

    362.63 Lattice degeneration
        Palisade degeneration of retina

    362.64 Senile reticular degeneration

    362.65 Secondary pigmentary degeneration
        Pseudoretinitis pigmentosa

    362.66 Secondary vitreoretinal degenerations

● **362.7 Hereditary retinal dystrophies**

    362.70 Hereditary retinal dystrophy, unspecified

    ▶ **362.71 *Retinal dystrophy in systemic or cerebroretinal lipidoses***
        Code first underlying disease, as:
            cerebroretinal lipidoses (330.1)
            systemic lipidoses (272.7)

    ▶ **362.72 *Retinal dystrophy in other systemic disorders and syndromes***
        Code first underlying disease, as:
            Bassen-Kornzweig syndrome (272.5)
            Refsum's disease (356.3)

    362.73 Vitreoretinal dystrophies
        Juvenile retinoschisis

    362.74 Pigmentary retinal dystrophy
        Retinal dystrophy, albipunctate
        Retinitis pigmentosa

    362.75 Other dystrophies primarily involving the sensory retina
        Progressive cone (-rod) dystrophy
        Stargardt's disease

    362.76 Dystrophies primarily involving the retinal pigment epithelium
        Fundus flavimaculatus
        Vitelliform dystrophy

    362.77 Dystrophies primarily involving Bruch's membrane
        Dystrophy:
            hyaline
            pseudoinflammatory foveal
        Hereditary drusen

● **362.8 Other retinal disorders**

    Excludes *chorioretinal inflammations (363.0–363.2)*
                 chorioretinal scars (363.30–363.35)

    362.81 Retinal hemorrhage
        Hemorrhage:
            preretinal
            retinal (deep) (superficial)
            subretinal
         Coding Clinic: 1996, Q4, P43-44

    362.82 Retinal exudates and deposits

    362.83 Retinal edema
        Retinal:
            cotton wool spots
            edema (localized) (macular) (peripheral)

    362.84 Retinal ischemia 🔖
        (Ex:) 362.81-362.89

    362.85 Retinal nerve fiber bundle defects

    362.89 Other retinal disorders

362.9 Unspecified retinal disorder

Item 6-14 Macular degeneration is typically age-related, chronic, and is evidenced by deterioration of the macula (the part of the retina that provides for central field vision), resulting in blurred vision or a blind spot in the center of visual field while not affecting peripheral vision.

◀ New   ◀║║║ Revised   ~~deleted~~ Deleted   Excludes   Includes   Use additional   Code first   Omit code

782   ● Unacceptable Principal Diagnosis   ● Use Additional Digit(s)   ▶ Manifestation Code   OGCR Official Guidelines   **Coding Clinic**

● **363 Chorioretinal inflammations, scars, and other disorders of choroid**

● **363.0 Focal chorioretinitis and focal retinochoroiditis**

> **Excludes** *focal chorioretinitis or retinochoroiditis in:*
> *histoplasmosis (115.02, 115.12, 115.92)*
> *toxoplasmosis (130.2)*
> *congenital infection (771.2)*

363.00 Focal chorioretinitis, unspecified
Focal:
  choroiditis or chorioretinitis NOS
  retinitis or retinochoroiditis NOS

363.01 Focal choroiditis and chorioretinitis, juxtapapillary

363.03 Focal choroiditis and chorioretinitis of other posterior pole

363.04 Focal choroiditis and chorioretinitis, peripheral

363.05 Focal retinitis and retinochoroiditis, juxtapapillary
Neuroretinitis

363.06 Focal retinitis and retinochoroiditis, macular or paramacular

363.07 Focal retinitis and retinochoroiditis of other posterior pole

363.08 Focal retinitis and retinochoroiditis, peripheral

● **363.1 Disseminated chorioretinitis and disseminated retinochoroiditis**

> **Excludes** *disseminated choroiditis or chorioretinitis in:*
> *secondary syphilis (091.51)*
> *neurosyphilitic disseminated retinitis or*
> *retinochoroiditis (094.83)*
> *retinal (peri) vasculitis (362.18)*

363.10 Disseminated chorioretinitis, unspecified
Disseminated:
  choroiditis or chorioretinitis NOS
  retinitis or retinochoroiditis NOS
  (Ex) 363.00-363.22

363.11 Disseminated choroiditis and chorioretinitis, posterior pole
(Ex) 363.00-363.22

363.12 Disseminated choroiditis and chorioretinitis, peripheral
(Ex) 363.00-363.22

363.13 Disseminated choroiditis and chorioretinitis, generalized

> *Code first* any underlying disease, as:
> tuberculosis (017.3)
> (Ex) 363.00-363.22

363.14 Disseminated retinitis and retinochoroiditis, metastatic
(Ex) 363.00-363.22

363.15 Disseminated retinitis and retinochoroiditis, pigment epitheliopathy
Acute posterior multifocal placoid pigment epitheliopathy
(Ex) 363.00-363.22

● **363.2 Other and unspecified forms of chorioretinitis and retinochoroiditis**

> **Excludes** *panophthalmitis (360.02)*
> *sympathetic uveitis (360.11)*
> *uveitis NOS (364.3)*

363.20 Chorioretinitis, unspecified
Choroiditis NOS
Retinitis NOS
Uveitis, posterior NOS
(Ex) 363.00-363.22

363.21 Pars planitis
Posterior cyclitis

363.22 Harada's disease

● **363.3 Chorioretinal scars**
Scar (postinflammatory) (postsurgical) (posttraumatic):
  choroid
  retina

363.30 Chorioretinal scar, unspecified

363.31 Solar retinopathy

363.32 Other macular scars

363.33 Other scars of posterior pole

363.34 Peripheral scars

363.35 Disseminated scars

● **363.4 Choroidal degenerations**

363.40 Choroidal degeneration, unspecified
Choroidal sclerosis NOS

363.41 Senile atrophy of choroid

363.42 Diffuse secondary atrophy of choroid

363.43 Angioid streaks of choroid

● **363.5 Hereditary choroidal dystrophies**
Hereditary choroidal atrophy:
  partial [choriocapillaris]
  total [all vessels]

363.50 Hereditary choroidal dystrophy or atrophy, unspecified

363.51 Circumpapillary dystrophy of choroid, partial

363.52 Circumpapillary dystrophy of choroid, total
Helicoid dystrophy of choroid

363.53 Central dystrophy of choroid, partial
Dystrophy, choroidal:
  central areolar
  circinate

363.54 Central choroidal atrophy, total
Dystrophy, choroidal:
  central gyrate
  serpiginous

363.55 Choroideremia

363.56 Other diffuse or generalized dystrophy, partial
Diffuse choroidal sclerosis

363.57 Other diffuse or generalized dystrophy, total
Generalized gyrate atrophy, choroid

● **363.6 Choroidal hemorrhage and rupture**

363.61 Choroidal hemorrhage, unspecified

363.62 Expulsive choroidal hemorrhage

363.63 Choroidal rupture
(Ex) 363.61-363.9

● **363.7 Choroidal detachment**

363.70 Choroidal detachment, unspecified
(Ex) 363.61-363.9

363.71 Serous choroidal detachment
(Ex) 363.61-363.9

363.72 Hemorrhagic choroidal detachment
(Ex) 363.61-363.9

363.8 Other disorders of choroid
Coding Clinic: 2006, Q1, P12

363.9 Unspecified disorder of choroid

● **364 Disorders of iris and ciliary body**

● **364.0 Acute and subacute iridocyclitis**
Anterior uveitis, acute, subacute
Cyclitis, acute, subacute
Iridocyclitis, acute, subacute
Iritis, acute, subacute

> **Excludes** *gonococcal (098.41)*
> *herpes simplex (054.44)*
> *herpes zoster (053.22)*

364.00 Acute and subacute iridocyclitis, unspecified
(Ex) 364.00-364.3

364.01 Primary iridocyclitis
(Ex) 364.00-364.3

364.02 Recurrent iridocyclitis
(Ex) 364.00-364.3

364.03 Secondary iridocyclitis, infectious
(Ex) 364.00-364.3

364.04 Secondary iridocyclitis, noninfectious
Aqueous:
  cells
  fibrin
  flare

364.05 Hypopyon

DISEASES OF THE NERVOUS SYSTEM AND SENSE ORGANS (320-389)

N Newborn: 0   **P** Pediatric: 0–17   **M** Maternity: 12–55   **A** Adult: 15–124   ♀ Females Only   ♂ Males Only

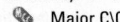 CC/MCC Exclusions   Complication\Comorbidity   Major C\C   Present on Admission Requirement   Hospital-Acquired Condition   **783**

DISEASES OF THE NERVOUS SYSTEM AND SENSE ORGANS (320–389)

● **364.1 Chronic iridocyclitis**
  Excludes *posterior cyclitis (363.21)*
  364.10 Chronic iridocyclitis, unspecified
  ▷ **364.11 Chronic iridocyclitis in diseases classified elsewhere**
    Code first underlying disease, as:
      sarcoidosis (135)
      tuberculosis (017.3)
    Excludes *syphilitic iridocyclitis (091.52)*
● **364.2 Certain types of iridocyclitis**
  Excludes *posterior cyclitis (363.21)*
    sympathetic uveitis (360.11)
  364.21 Fuchs' heterochromic cyclitis
  364.22 Glaucomatocyclitic crises 🔖
    (Ex) 364.00-364.3
  364.23 Lens-induced iridocyclitis
  364.24 Vogt-Koyanagi syndrome
  364.3 Unspecified iridocyclitis 🔖
    Uveitis NOS
    (Ex) 364.00-364.3
● **364.4 Vascular disorders of iris and ciliary body**
  364.41 Hyphema
    Hemorrhage of iris or ciliary body
  364.42 Rubeosis iridis
    Neovascularization of iris or ciliary body
● **364.5 Degenerations of iris and ciliary body**
  364.51 Essential or progressive iris atrophy
  364.52 Iridoschisis
  364.53 Pigmentary iris degeneration
    Acquired heterochromia of iris
    Pigment dispersion syndrome of iris
    Translucency of iris
  364.54 Degeneration of pupillary margin
    Atrophy of sphincter of iris
    Ectropion of pigment epithelium of iris
  364.55 Miotic cysts of pupillary margin
  364.56 Degenerative changes of chamber angle
  364.57 Degenerative changes of ciliary body
  364.59 Other iris atrophy
    Iris atrophy (generalized) (sector shaped)
● **364.6 Cysts of iris, ciliary body, and anterior chamber**
  Excludes *miotic pupillary cyst (364.55)*
    parasitic cyst (360.13)
  364.60 Idiopathic cysts
  364.61 Implantation cysts
    Epithelial down-growth, anterior chamber
    Implantation cysts (surgical) (traumatic)
  364.62 Exudative cysts of iris or anterior chamber
  364.63 Primary cyst of pars plana
  364.64 Exudative cyst of pars plana
● **364.7 Adhesions and disruptions of iris and ciliary body**
  Excludes *flat anterior chamber (360.34)*
  364.70 Adhesions of iris, unspecified
    Synechiae (iris) NOS
  364.71 Posterior synechiae
  364.72 Anterior synechiae
  364.73 Goniosynechiae
    Peripheral anterior synechiae
  364.74 Pupillary membranes
    Iris bombé
    Pupillary:
      occlusion
      seclusion
  364.75 Pupillary abnormalities
    Deformed pupil
    Ectopic pupil
    Rupture of sphincter, pupil
  364.76 Iridodialysis
    Coding Clinic: 1985, July-Aug, P16
  364.77 Recession of chamber angle

● **364.8 Other disorders of iris and ciliary body**
  Coding Clinic: 2007, Q2, P11
  364.81 Floppy iris syndrome
    Intraoperative floppy iris syndrome (IFIS)
    Use additional E code to identify cause, such as:
      sympatholytics [antiadrenergics] causing
      adverse effect in therapeutic use
      (E941.3)
    Coding Clinic: 2007, Q4, P77-79
  364.82 Plateau iris syndrome
    Coding Clinic: 2008, Q4, P112
  364.89 Other disorders of iris and ciliary body
    Prolapse of iris NOS
    Excludes *prolapse of iris in recent wound (871.1)*
  364.9 Unspecified disorder of iris and ciliary body
● **365 Glaucoma**
  Intraocular pressure (IOP) is too high. IOP is the result of too much aqueous humor because of excess production or inadequate drainage. Leads to optic nerve damage and vision loss.
  Excludes *blind hypertensive eye [absolute glaucoma] (360.42)*
    congenital glaucoma (743.20–743.22)
● **365.0 Borderline glaucoma [glaucoma suspect]**
  365.00 Preglaucoma, unspecified
    Coding Clinic: 1990, Q1, P8
  365.01 Open angle with borderline findings, low risk
    Open angle, low risk
  365.02 Anatomical narrow angle
    Primary angle closure suspect
  365.03 Steroid responders
  365.04 Ocular hypertension
  365.05 Open angle with borderline findings, high risk
    Open angle, high risk
  365.06 Primary angle closure without glaucoma damage
● **365.1 Open-angle glaucoma**
  365.10 Open-angle glaucoma, unspecified
    Wide-angle glaucoma NOS
    Use additional code to identify glaucoma stage (365.70-365.74)
  365.11 Primary open angle glaucoma
    Chronic simple glaucoma
    Use additional code to identify glaucoma stage (365.70-365.74)
  365.12 Low tension glaucoma
    Use additional code to identify glaucoma stage (365.70-365.74)
  365.13 Pigmentary glaucoma
    Use additional code to identify glaucoma stage (365.70-365.74)
  365.14 Glaucoma of childhood
    Infantile or juvenile glaucoma
  365.15 Residual stage of open angle glaucoma
● **365.2 Primary angle-closure glaucoma**
  365.20 Primary angle-closure glaucoma, unspecified
    Use additional code to identify glaucoma stage (365.70-365.74)
  365.21 Intermittent angle-closure glaucoma
    Angle-closure glaucoma:
      interval   subacute
  365.22 Acute angle-closure glaucoma 🔖
    Acute angle-closure glaucoma attack
    Acute angle-closure glaucoma crisis
    (Ex) 365.22
  365.23 Chronic angle-closure glaucoma
    Chronic primary angle closure glaucoma
    Use additional code to identify glaucoma stage (365.70-365.74)
    Coding Clinic: 1998, Q2, P16
  365.24 Residual stage of angle-closure glaucoma

● 365.3 Corticosteroid-induced glaucoma
    365.31 Glaucomatous stage
        Use additional code to identify glaucoma stage
        (365.70-365.74)
    365.32 Residual stage
● 365.4 Glaucoma associated with congenital anomalies, dystrophies, and systemic syndromes
    365.41 Glaucoma associated with chamber angle anomalies
    365.42 Glaucoma associated with anomalies of iris
    365.43 Glaucoma associated with other anterior segment anomalies
    365.44 *Glaucoma associated with systemic syndromes*
        Code first associated disease, as:
          neurofibromatosis (237.70-237.79)
          Sturge-Weber (-Dimitri) syndrome (759.6)
● 365.5 Glaucoma associated with disorders of the lens
    365.51 Phacolytic glaucoma
    365.52 Pseudoexfoliation glaucoma
        Use additional code to identify glaucoma stage
        (365.70-365.74)
    365.59 Glaucoma associated with other lens disorders
● 365.6 Glaucoma associated with other ocular disorders
    365.60 Glaucoma associated with unspecified ocular disorder
    365.61 Glaucoma associated with pupillary block
    365.62 Glaucoma associated with ocular inflammations
        Use additional code to identify glaucoma stage
        (365.70-365.74)
    365.63 Glaucoma associated with vascular disorders
        Use additional code to identify glaucoma stage
        (365.70-365.74)
    365.64 Glaucoma associated with tumors or cysts
    365.65 Glaucoma associated with ocular trauma
        Use additional code to identify glaucoma stage
        (365.70-365.74)
● 365.7 Glaucoma stage
    Code first associated type of glaucoma (365.10-365.13, 365.20, 365.23, 365.31, 365.52, 365.62-365.63, 365.65)
  ● 365.70 Glaucoma stage, unspecified
        Glaucoma stage NOS
  ● 365.71 Mild stage glaucoma
        Early stage glaucoma
  ● 365.72 Moderate stage glaucoma
  ● 365.73 Severe stage glaucoma
        Advanced stage glaucoma
        End-stage glaucoma
  ● 365.74 Indeterminate stage glaucoma
● 365.8 Other specified forms of glaucoma
    365.81 Hypersecretion glaucoma
    365.82 Glaucoma with increased episcleral venous pressure
    365.83 Aqueous misdirection
        Malignant glaucoma
        Coding Clinic: 2002, Q4, P48
    365.89 Other specified glaucoma
        Coding Clinic: 1998, Q2, P16
365.9 Unspecified glaucoma
    Coding Clinic: 2003, Q3, P14; 2001, Q2, P16-17

Figure 6-4   Age-related cataract.
Nuclear sclerosis and cortical lens opacities are present. (From Yanoff: Ophthalmology, ed 3, Mosby, Inc., 2008)

Item 6-15   Senile cataracts are linked to the aging process. The most common area for the formation of a cataract is the cortical area of the lens. **Polar cataracts** can be either anterior or posterior. **Anterior polar cataracts** are more common and are small, white, capsular cataracts located on the anterior portion of the lens. **Total cataracts,** also called **complete** or **mature,** cause an opacity of all fibers of the lens. **Hypermature** describes a mature cataract with a swollen, milky cortex that covers the entire lens. **Immature,** also called **incipient,** cataracts have a clear cortex and are only slightly opaque. Treatment for all cataracts is the removal of the lens.

● 366 Cataract
    Excludes *congenital cataract (743.30–743.34)*
  ● 366.0 Infantile, juvenile, and presenile cataract
    366.00 Nonsenile cataract, unspecified
        Coding Clinic: 1987, Mar-April, P9
    366.01 Anterior subcapsular polar cataract
    366.02 Posterior subcapsular polar cataract
    366.03 Cortical, lamellar, or zonular cataract
    366.04 Nuclear cataract
    366.09 Other and combined forms of nonsenile cataract
  ● 366.1 Senile cataract
    366.10 Senile cataract, unspecified   A
        Coding Clinic: 2003, Q1, P5
    366.11 Pseudoexfoliation of lens capsule   A
    366.12 Incipient cataract   A
        Cataract:
          coronary
          immature NOS
          punctate
        Water clefts
    366.13 Anterior subcapsular polar senile cataract   A
    366.14 Posterior subcapsular polar senile cataract   A
    366.15 Cortical senile cataract   A
    366.16 Nuclear sclerosis   A
        Cataracta brunescens
        Nuclear cataract
        Coding Clinic: 2007, Q4, P77-79; 1985, Sept-Oct, P11
    366.17 Total or mature cataract   A
    366.18 Hypermature cataract   A
        Morgagni cataract
    366.19 Other and combined forms of senile cataract   A
  ● 366.2 Traumatic cataract
    366.20 Traumatic cataract, unspecified
    366.21 Localized traumatic opacities
        Vossius' ring
    366.22 Total traumatic cataract
    366.23 Partially resolved traumatic cataract
  ● 366.3 Cataract secondary to ocular disorders
    366.30 Cataracta complicata, unspecified
    366.31 Glaucomatous flecks (subcapsular)
        Code first underlying glaucoma (365.0–365.9)
    366.32 Cataract in inflammatory disorders
        Code first underlying condition, as:
          chronic choroiditis (363.0–363.2)

DISEASES OF THE NERVOUS SYSTEM AND SENSE ORGANS (320–389)

N Newborn: 0   P Pediatric: 0–17   M Maternity: 12–55   A Adult: 15–124   ♀ Females Only   ♂ Males Only

(Ex) CC/MCC Exclusions   Complication\Comorbidity   Major C\C   Present on Admission Requirement   Hospital-Acquired Condition   **785**

DISEASES OF THE NERVOUS SYSTEM AND SENSE ORGANS (320–389)

Figure 6–5　Corneal perforation.
Preoperative appearance of a patient who has a small, 1.5 mm corneal perforation at the 10 o'clock limbus. *(Courtesy of Dr RK Forster.)* (From Yanoff: Ophthalmology, ed 3, Mosby, Inc., 2008)

Item 6–16　Vossius' ring is the result of contusion-type traumatic injury and results in a ring of iris pigment pressed onto the anterior lens capsule.

366.33　Cataract with neovascularization
　　Code first underlying condition, as:
　　　chronic iridocyclitis (364.10)

366.34　Cataract in degenerative disorders
　　Sunflower cataract
　　Code first underlying condition, as:
　　　chalcosis (360.24)
　　　degenerative myopia (360.21)
　　　pigmentary retinal dystrophy (362.74)

●**366.4　Cataract associated with other disorders**
▷**366.41　*Diabetic cataract***
　　Code first diabetes (249.5, 250.5)
　　Coding Clinic: 1985, Sept-Oct, P11

▷**366.42　*Tetanic cataract***
　　Code first underlying disease as:
　　　calcinosis (275.40)
　　　hypoparathyroidism (252.1)

▷**366.43　*Myotonic cataract***
　　Code first underlying disorder (359.21, 359.23)

▷**366.44　*Cataract associated with other syndromes***
　　Code first underlying condition, as:
　　　craniofacial dysostosis (756.0)
　　　galactosemia (271.1)

366.45　Toxic cataract
　　Drug-induced cataract
　　Use additional E code to identify drug or other
　　　toxic substance
　　Coding Clinic: 1995, Q4, P51

366.46　Cataract associated with radiation and other physical influences
　　Use additional E code to identify cause

●**366.5　After-cataract**
366.50　After-cataract, unspecified
　　Secondary cataract NOS
366.51　Soemmering's ring
366.52　Other after-cataract, not obscuring vision
366.53　After-cataract, obscuring vision

366.8　Other cataract
　　Calcification of lens
　　Coding Clinic: 1994, Q1, P16

366.9　Unspecified cataract
　　Coding Clinic: 2009, Q4, P101; 1985, Sept-Oct, P10

●**367　Disorders of refraction and accommodation**
367.0　Hypermetropia
　　Far-sightedness
　　Hyperopia
367.1　Myopia
　　Near-sightedness
●**367.2　Astigmatism**
367.20　Astigmatism, unspecified
367.21　Regular astigmatism
367.22　Irregular astigmatism
●**367.3　Anisometropia and aniseikonia**
367.31　Anisometropia
367.32　Aniseikonia
367.4　Presbyopia

Item 6-17　Disorders of refraction: **Hypermetropia**, or far-sightedness, means focus at a distance is adequate but not on close objects. **Myopia** is near-sightedness or short-sightedness and means the focus on nearby objects is clear but distant objects appear blurred. **Astigmatism** is warping of the curvature of the cornea so light rays entering do not meet a single focal point, resulting in a distorted image. **Anisometropia** is unequal refractive power in which one eye may be myopic (near-sighted) and the other hyperopic (far-sighted). **Presbyopia** is the loss of focus on near objects, which occurs with age because the lens loses elasticity.

●**367.5　Disorders of accommodation**
367.51　Paresis of accommodation
　　Cycloplegia
367.52　Total or complete internal ophthalmoplegia
367.53　Spasm of accommodation
●**367.8　Other disorders of refraction and accommodation**
367.81　Transient refractive change
367.89　Other
　　Drug-induced disorders of refraction and
　　　accommodation
　　Toxic disorders of refraction and accommodation
367.9　Unspecified disorder of refraction and accommodation

●**368　Visual disturbances**
　　Excludes　*electrophysiological disturbances (794.11–794.14)*
●**368.0　Amblyopia ex anopsia**
368.00　Amblyopia, unspecified
368.01　Strabismic amblyopia
　　Suppression amblyopia
368.02　Deprivation amblyopia
368.03　Refractive amblyopia
●**368.1　Subjective visual disturbances**
368.10　Subjective visual disturbance, unspecified
368.11　Sudden visual loss 📎
　　(Ex:) 368.10-368.12, 368.16
368.12　Transient visual loss 📎
　　Concentric fading
　　Scintillating scotoma
　　(Ex:) 368.10-368.12, 368.16
368.13　Visual discomfort
　　Asthenopia　　　　　Photophobia
　　Eye strain
368.14　Visual distortions of shape and size
　　Macropsia　　　　　Micropsia
　　Metamorphopsia
368.15　Other visual distortions and entoptic phenomena
　　Photopsia
　　Refractive:
　　　diplopia
　　　polyopia
　　Visual halos
368.16　Psychophysical visual disturbances
　　Prosopagnosia
　　Visual:
　　　agnosia
　　　disorientation syndrome
　　　hallucinations
　　　object agnosia

368.2　Diplopia
　　Double vision
●**368.3　Other disorders of binocular vision**
368.30　Binocular vision disorder, unspecified
368.31　Suppression of binocular vision
368.32　Simultaneous visual perception without fusion
368.33　Fusion with defective stereopsis
368.34　Abnormal retinal correspondence

● 368.4 **Visual field defects**

  368.40 **Visual field defect, unspecified**

  368.41 **Scotoma involving central area**
    Scotoma:
      central
      centrocecal
      paracentral

  368.42 **Scotoma of blind spot area**
    Enlarged:
      angioscotoma
      blind spot
    Paracecal scotoma

  368.43 **Sector or arcuate defects**
    Scotoma:
      arcuate
      Bjerrum
      Seidel

  368.44 **Other localized visual field defect**
    Scotoma: Visual field defect:
      NOS   nasal step
      ring   peripheral

  368.45 **Generalized contraction or constriction**

  368.46 **Homonymous bilateral field defects**
    Hemianopsia (altitudinal) (homonymous)
    Quadrant anopia

  368.47 **Heteronymous bilateral field defects**
    Hemianopsia:
      binasal
      bitemporal

● 368.5 **Color vision deficiencies**
    Color blindness

  368.51 **Protan defect**
    Protanomaly
    Protanopia

  368.52 **Deutan defect**
    Deuteranomaly
    Deuteranopia

  368.53 **Tritan defect**
    Tritanomaly
    Tritanopia

  368.54 **Achromatopsia**
    Monochromatism (cone) (rod)

  368.55 **Acquired color vision deficiencies**

  368.59 **Other color vision deficiencies**

● 368.6 **Night blindness**

  368.60 **Night blindness, unspecified**

  368.61 **Congenital night blindness**
    Hereditary night blindness
    Oguchi's disease

  368.62 **Acquired night blindness**
    Excludes *that due to vitamin A deficiency (264.5)*

  368.63 **Abnormal dark adaptation curve**
    Abnormal threshold of cones or rods
    Delayed adaptation of cones or rods

  368.69 **Other night blindness**

368.8 **Other specified visual disturbances**
    Blurred vision NOS
    Coding Clinic: 2002, Q4, P56

368.9 **Unspecified visual disturbance**
    Coding Clinic: 2006, Q3, P22

● 369 **Blindness and low vision**

  Excludes *correctable impaired vision due to refractive errors (367.0–367.9)*

  Note: Visual impairment refers to a functional limitation of the eye (e.g., limited visual acuity or visual field). It should be distinguished from visual disability, indicating a limitation of the abilities of the individual (e.g., limited reading skills, vocational skills), and from visual handicap, indicating a limitation of personal and socioeconomic independence (e.g., limited mobility, limited employability).

  The levels of impairment defined in the table after 369.9 are based on the recommendations of the WHO Study Group on Prevention of Blindness (Geneva, November 6–10, 1972; WHO Technical Report Series 518), and of the International Council of Ophthalmology (1976).

  Note that definitions of blindness vary in different settings.

  For international reporting, WHO defines blindness as profound impairment. This definition can be applied to blindness of one eye (369.1, 369.6) and to blindness of the individual (369.0).

  For determination of benefits in the U.S.A., the definition of legal blindness as severe impairment is often used. This definition applies to blindness of the individual only.

● 369.0 **Profound impairment, both eyes**

  369.00 **Impairment level not further specified**
    Blindness:
      NOS according to WHO definition
      both eyes

  369.01 **Better eye: total impairment; lesser eye: total impairment**

  369.02 **Better eye: near-total impairment; lesser eye: not further specified**

  369.03 **Better eye: near-total impairment; lesser eye: total impairment**

  369.04 **Better eye: near-total impairment; lesser eye: near-total impairment**

  369.05 **Better eye: profound impairment; lesser eye: not further specified**

  369.06 **Better eye: profound impairment; lesser eye: total impairment**

  369.07 **Better eye: profound impairment; lesser eye: near-total impairment**

  369.08 **Better eye: profound impairment; lesser eye: profound impairment**

● 369.1 **Moderate or severe impairment, better eye, profound impairment lesser eye**

  369.10 **Impairment level not further specified**
    Blindness, one eye, low vision other eye

  369.11 **Better eye: severe impairment; lesser eye: blind, not further specified**

  369.12 **Better eye: severe impairment; lesser eye: total impairment**

  369.13 **Better eye: severe impairment; lesser eye: near-total impairment**

  369.14 **Better eye: severe impairment; lesser eye: profound impairment**

  369.15 **Better eye: moderate impairment; lesser eye: blind, not further specified**

  369.16 **Better eye: moderate impairment; lesser eye: total impairment**

  369.17 **Better eye: moderate impairment; lesser eye: near-total impairment**

  369.18 **Better eye: moderate impairment; lesser eye: profound impairment**

DISEASES OF THE NERVOUS SYSTEM AND SENSE ORGANS (320–389)

- **369.2** **Moderate or severe impairment, both eyes**
  - **369.20** **Impairment level not further specified**
    Low vision, both eyes NOS
  - **369.21** **Better eye: severe impairment; lesser eye: not further specified**
  - **369.22** **Better eye: severe impairment; lesser eye: severe impairment**
  - **369.23** **Better eye: moderate impairment; lesser eye: not further specified**
  - **369.24** **Better eye: moderate impairment; lesser eye: severe impairment**
  - **369.25** **Better eye: moderate impairment; lesser eye: moderate impairment**
- **369.3** **Unqualified visual loss, both eyes**
  - **Excludes** *blindness NOS:*
    legal [U.S.A. definition] (369.4)
    WHO definition (369.00)
- **369.4** **Legal blindness, as defined in U.S.A.**
  Blindness NOS according to U.S.A. definition
  - **Excludes** *legal blindness with specification of impairment level (369.01–369.08, 369.11–369.14, 369.21–369.22)*
- ● **369.6** **Profound impairment, one eye**
  Coding Clinic: 2002, Q3, P20-21
  - **369.60** **Impairment level not further specified**
    Blindness, one eye
  - **369.61** **One eye: total impairment; other eye: not specified**
  - **369.62** **One eye: total impairment; other eye: near-normal vision**
  - **369.63** **One eye: total impairment; other eye: normal vision**
  - **369.64** **One eye: near-total impairment; other eye: not specified**
  - **369.65** **One eye: near-total impairment; other eye: near-normal vision**
  - **369.66** **One eye: near-total impairment; other eye: normal vision**
  - **369.67** **One eye: profound impairment; other eye: not specified**
  - **369.68** **One eye: profound impairment; other eye: near-normal vision**
  - **369.69** **One eye: profound impairment; other eye: normal vision**
- ● **369.7** **Moderate or severe impairment, one eye**
  - **369.70** **Impairment level not further specified**
    Low vision, one eye
  - **369.71** **One eye: severe impairment; other eye: not specified**
  - **369.72** **One eye: severe impairment; other eye: near-normal vision**
  - **369.73** **One eye: severe impairment; other eye: normal vision**
  - **369.74** **One eye: moderate impairment; other eye: not specified**
  - **369.75** **One eye: moderate impairment; other eye: near-normal vision**
  - **369.76** **One eye: moderate impairment; other eye: normal vision**
- **369.8** **Unqualified visual loss, one eye**
- **369.9** **Unspecified visual loss**

Classification		Levels of Visual Impairment	Additional Descriptors Which May Be Encountered
"Legal"	**WHO**	**Visual Acuity and/or Visual Field Limitation (Whichever Is Worse)**	
	(Near-) normal vision	**Range of Normal Vision** 20/10 20/13 20/16 20/20 20/25 2.0 1.6 1.25 1.0 0.8	
		Near-Normal Vision 20/30 20/40 20/50 20/60 0.7 0.6 0.5 0.4 0.3	
	Low vision	**Moderate Visual Impairment** 20/70 20/80 20/100 20/125 20/160 0.25 0.20 0.16 0.12	Moderate low vision
Legal Blindness (U.S.A.) both eyes		**Severe Visual Impairment** 20/200 20/250 20/320 20/400 0.10 0.08 0.06 0.05 Visual field: 20 degrees or less	Severe low vision, "Legal" blindness
	Blindness (WHO) one or both eyes	**Profound Visual Impairment** 20/500 20/630 20/800 20/1000 0.04 0.03 0.025 0.02 Count fingers at: less than 3 m (10 ft) Visual field: 10 degrees or less	Profound low vision, Moderate blindness
		Near-Total Visual Impairment Visual acuity: less than 0.02 (20/1000) Count fingers: 1 m (3 ft) or less Hand movements: 5 m (15 ft) or less Light projection, light perception Visual field: 5 degrees or less	Severe blindness, Near-total blindness
		Total Visual Impairment No light perception (NLP)	Total blindness

Visual acuity refers to best achievable acuity with correction.
Non-listed Snellen fractions may be classified by converting to the nearest decimal equivalent, e.g., 10/200 = 0.05, 6/30 = 0.20.
CF (count fingers) without designation of distance, may be classified to profound impairment.
HM (hand motion) without designation of distance, may be classified to near-total impairment.
Visual field measurements refer to the largest field diameter for a 1/100 white test object.

Marginal (catarrhal) ulcer   Ring ulcer   Central corneal ulcer   Rosacea ulcer   Mooren's (rodent) ulcer

Figure 6–6 Corneal ulcers: marginal, ring, central corneal, rosacea, and Mooren's.

Item 6–18 An infected ulcer is usually called a **serpiginous** or **hypopyon** ulcer which is a pus sac in the anterior chamber of the eye.
Marginal ulcers are usually asymptomatic, not primary, and are often superficial and simple. More severe marginal ulcers spread to form a ring ulcer.
Ring ulcers can extend around the entire corneal periphery.
Central corneal ulcers develop when there is an abrasion to the epithelium and an infection develops in the eroded area.
The **pyocyaneal** ulcer is the most serious corneal infection, which, if left untreated, can lead to loss of the eye.

◀ New   ◀ Revised   ~~deleted~~ Deleted   Excludes   Includes   Use additional   Code first   Omit code
● Unacceptable Principal Diagnosis   ● Use Additional Digit(s)   ▶ Manifestation Code   OGCR Official Guidelines   **Coding Clinic**
788

370 Keratitis
- **370.0 Corneal ulcer**
  - **Excludes** *that due to vitamin A deficiency (264.3)*
  - 370.00 Corneal ulcer, unspecified
  - 370.01 Marginal corneal ulcer
  - 370.02 Ring corneal ulcer
  - 370.03 Central corneal ulcer
  - 370.04 Hypopyon ulcer
    - Serpiginous ulcer
  - 370.05 Mycotic corneal ulcer
  - 370.06 Perforated corneal ulcer
  - 370.07 Mooren's ulcer
- **370.2 Superficial keratitis without conjunctivitis**
  - **Excludes** *dendritic [herpes simplex] keratitis (054.42)*
  - 370.20 Superficial keratitis, unspecified
  - 370.21 Punctate keratitis
    - Thygeson's superficial punctate keratitis
  - 370.22 Macular keratitis
    - Keratitis: areolar, nummular
    - Keratitis: stellate, striate
  - 370.23 Filamentary keratitis
  - 370.24 Photokeratitis
    - Snow blindness
    - Welders' keratitis
    - Coding Clinic: 1996, Q3, P6
- **370.3 Certain types of keratoconjunctivitis**
  - 370.31 Phlyctenular keratoconjunctivitis
    - Phlyctenulosis
    - Use additional code for any associated tuberculosis (017.3)
  - 370.32 Limbal and corneal involvement in vernal conjunctivitis
    - Use additional code for vernal conjunctivitis (372.13)
  - 370.33 Keratoconjunctivitis sicca, not specified as Sjögren's
    - **Excludes** *Sjögren's syndrome (710.2)*
  - 370.34 Exposure keratoconjunctivitis
    - Coding Clinic: 1996, Q3, P6
  - 370.35 Neurotrophic keratoconjunctivitis
- **370.4 Other and unspecified keratoconjunctivitis**
  - 370.40 Keratoconjunctivitis, unspecified
    - Superficial keratitis with conjunctivitis NOS
  - 370.44 *Keratitis or keratoconjunctivitis in exanthema*
    - *Code first underlying condition (050.0–052.9)*
    - **Excludes** *herpes simplex (054.43)*
      herpes zoster (053.21)
      measles (055.71)
  - 370.49 Other
    - **Excludes** *epidemic keratoconjunctivitis (077.1)*
- **370.5 Interstitial and deep keratitis**
  - 370.50 Interstitial keratitis, unspecified
  - 370.52 Diffuse interstitial keratitis
    - Cogan's syndrome
  - 370.54 Sclerosing keratitis
  - 370.55 Corneal abscess
  - 370.59 Other
    - **Excludes** *disciform herpes simplex keratitis (054.43)*
      syphilitic keratitis (090.3)
- **370.6 Corneal neovascularization**
  - 370.60 Corneal neovascularization, unspecified
  - 370.61 Localized vascularization of cornea
  - 370.62 Pannus (corneal)
    - Coding Clinic: 2002, Q3, P20-21
  - 370.63 Deep vascularization of cornea
  - 370.64 Ghost vessels (corneal)

- **370.8 Other forms of keratitis**
  - *Code first underlying condition, such as:*
    - Acanthamoeba (136.21)
    - Fusarium (118)
  - Coding Clinic: 2008, Q4, P79-81; 1994, Q3, P5
- **370.9 Unspecified keratitis**
- **371 Corneal opacity and other disorders of cornea**
  - **371.0 Corneal scars and opacities**
    - **Excludes** *that due to vitamin A deficiency (264.6)*
    - 371.00 Corneal opacity, unspecified
      - Corneal scar NOS
    - 371.01 Minor opacity of cornea
      - Corneal nebula
    - 371.02 Peripheral opacity of cornea
      - Corneal macula not interfering with central vision
    - 371.03 Central opacity of cornea
      - Corneal: leucoma interfering with central vision
        macula interfering with central vision
    - 371.04 Adherent leucoma
    - 371.05 *Phthisical cornea*
      - *Code first underlying tuberculosis (017.3)*
  - **371.1 Corneal pigmentations and deposits**
    - 371.10 Corneal deposit, unspecified
    - 371.11 Anterior pigmentations
      - Stähli's lines
    - 371.12 Stromal pigmentations
      - Hematocornea
    - 371.13 Posterior pigmentations
      - Krukenberg spindle
    - 371.14 Kayser-Fleischer ring
    - 371.15 Other deposits associated with metabolic disorders
    - 371.16 Argentous deposits
  - **371.2 Corneal edema**
    - 371.20 Corneal edema, unspecified
    - 371.21 Idiopathic corneal edema
    - 371.22 Secondary corneal edema
    - 371.23 Bullous keratopathy
    - 371.24 Corneal edema due to wearing of contact lenses
  - **371.3 Changes of corneal membranes**
    - 371.30 Corneal membrane change, unspecified
    - 371.31 Folds and rupture of Bowman's membrane
    - 371.32 Folds in Descemet's membrane
    - 371.33 Rupture in Descemet's membrane
  - **371.4 Corneal degenerations**
    - 371.40 Corneal degeneration, unspecified
    - 371.41 Senile corneal changes
      - Arcus senilis   Hassall-Henle bodies
    - 371.42 Recurrent erosion of cornea
      - **Excludes** *Mooren's ulcer (370.07)*
    - 371.43 Band-shaped keratopathy
    - 371.44 Other calcerous degenerations of cornea
    - 371.45 Keratomalacia NOS
      - **Excludes** *that due to vitamin A deficiency (264.4)*
    - 371.46 Nodular degeneration of cornea
      - Salzmann's nodular dystrophy
    - 371.48 Peripheral degenerations of cornea
      - Marginal degeneration of cornea [Terrien's]
    - 371.49 Other
      - Discrete colliquative keratopathy

DISEASES OF THE NERVOUS SYSTEM AND SENSE ORGANS (320–389)

Figure 6-7 Lateral view of the displacement of the cone apex in keratoconus. (From Yanoff: Ophthalmology, ed 3, Mosby, Inc., 2008)

Item 6-19 Keratoconus results in corneal degeneration that begins in childhood, gradually changes the cornea from a round to cone shape, decreasing visual acuity. Treatment includes contact lenses. In severe cases the need for corneal transplant may be the treatment of choice; however, newer technologies may use high frequency radio energy to shrink the edges of the cornea, pulling the central area back to a more normal shape. It can help delay or avoid the need for a corneal transplantation.

● **371.5 Hereditary corneal dystrophies**
  371.50 Corneal dystrophy, unspecified
  371.51 Juvenile epithelial corneal dystrophy
  371.52 Other anterior corneal dystrophies
      Corneal dystrophy:
        microscopic cystic
        ring-like
  371.53 Granular corneal dystrophy
  371.54 Lattice corneal dystrophy
  371.55 Macular corneal dystrophy
  371.56 Other stromal corneal dystrophies
      Crystalline corneal dystrophy
  371.57 Endothelial corneal dystrophy
      Combined corneal dystrophy
      Cornea guttata
      Fuchs' endothelial dystrophy
  371.58 Other posterior corneal dystrophies
      Polymorphous corneal dystrophy
● **371.6 Keratoconus**
  371.60 Keratoconus, unspecified
  371.61 Keratoconus, stable condition
  371.62 Keratoconus, acute hydrops
● **371.7 Other corneal deformities**
  371.70 Corneal deformity, unspecified
  371.71 Corneal ectasia
  371.72 Descemetocele
  371.73 Corneal staphyloma
● **371.8 Other corneal disorders**
  371.81 Corneal anesthesia and hypoesthesia
  371.82 Corneal disorder due to contact lens
      Excludes corneal edema due to contact lens (371.24)
  371.89 Other
      Coding Clinic: 1999, Q3, P12
  371.9 Unspecified corneal disorder
● **372 Disorders of conjunctiva**
    Excludes keratoconjunctivitis (370.3-370.4)
● **372.0 Acute conjunctivitis**
  372.00 Acute conjunctivitis, unspecified
  372.01 Serous conjunctivitis, except viral
      Excludes viral conjunctivitis NOS (077.9)
      Coding Clinic: 2008, Q3, P6-7
  372.02 Acute follicular conjunctivitis
      Conjunctival folliculosis NOS
      Excludes conjunctivitis:
        adenoviral (acute follicular) (077.3)
        epidemic hemorrhagic (077.4)
        inclusion (077.0)
        Newcastle (077.8)
      epidemic keratoconjunctivitis (077.1)
      pharyngoconjunctival fever (077.2)

  372.03 Other mucopurulent conjunctivitis
      Catarrhal conjunctivitis
      Excludes blennorrhea neonatorum (gonococcal) (098.40)
        neonatal conjunctivitis (771.6)
        ophthalmia neonatorum NOS (771.6)
  372.04 Pseudomembranous conjunctivitis
      Membranous conjunctivitis
      Excludes diphtheritic conjunctivitis (032.81)
  372.05 Acute atopic conjunctivitis
  372.06 Acute chemical conjunctivitis
      Acute toxic conjunctivitis
      Use additional E code to identify the chemical or toxic agent
      Excludes burn of eye and adnexa (940.0-940.9)
        chemical corrosion injury of eye (940.2-940.3)
● **372.1 Chronic conjunctivitis**
  372.10 Chronic conjunctivitis, unspecified
  372.11 Simple chronic conjunctivitis
  372.12 Chronic follicular conjunctivitis
  372.13 Vernal conjunctivitis
      Coding Clinic: 1996, Q3, P8
  372.14 Other chronic allergic conjunctivitis
      Coding Clinic: 1996, Q3, P8
  372.15 *Parasitic conjunctivitis*
      Code first underlying disease as:
        filariasis (125.0-125.9)
        mucocutaneous leishmaniasis (085.5)
● **372.2 Blepharoconjunctivitis**
  372.20 Blepharoconjunctivitis, unspecified
  372.21 Angular blepharoconjunctivitis
  372.22 Contact blepharoconjunctivitis
● **372.3 Other and unspecified conjunctivitis**
  372.30 Conjunctivitis, unspecified
  372.31 *Rosacea conjunctivitis*
      Code first underlying rosacea dermatitis (695.3)
  372.33 *Conjunctivitis in mucocutaneous disease*
      Code first underlying disease as:
        erythema multiforme (695.10-695.19)
        Reiter's disease (099.3)
      Excludes ocular pemphigoid (694.61)
  372.34 Pingueculitis
      Excludes pinguecula (372.51)
      Coding Clinic: 2008, Q4, P112-113
  372.39 Other
      Coding Clinic: 2007, Q2, P11
● **372.4 Pterygium**
    Excludes pseudopterygium (372.52)
  372.40 Pterygium, unspecified
  372.41 Peripheral pterygium, stationary
  372.42 Peripheral pterygium, progressive
  372.43 Central pterygium
  372.44 Double pterygium
  372.45 Recurrent pterygium

Figure 6-8 Double pterygium. Note both nasal and temporal pterygia in a 57-year-old farmer. (From Yanoff: Ophthalmology, ed 3, Mosby, Inc., 2008)

Item 6-20 Pterygium is Greek for batlike. The condition is characterized by a membrane that extends from the limbus to the center of the cornea and resembles a wing.

● **372.5 Conjunctival degenerations and deposits**
  372.50 Conjunctival degeneration, unspecified
  372.51 Pinguecula
     Excludes *pingueculitis (372.34)*
  372.52 Pseudopterygium
  372.53 Conjunctival xerosis
     Excludes *conjunctival xerosis due to vitamin A deficiency (264.0, 264.1, 264.7)*
  372.54 Conjunctival concretions
  372.55 Conjunctival pigmentations
    Conjunctival argyrosis
  372.56 Conjunctival deposits
● **372.6 Conjunctival scars**
  372.61 Granuloma of conjunctiva
  372.62 Localized adhesions and strands of conjunctiva
  372.63 Symblepharon
    Extensive adhesions of conjunctiva
  372.64 Scarring of conjunctiva
    Contraction of eye socket (after enucleation)
● **372.7 Conjunctival vascular disorders and cysts**
  372.71 Hyperemia of conjunctiva
  372.72 Conjunctival hemorrhage
    Hyposphagma
    Subconjunctival hemorrhage
  372.73 Conjunctival edema
    Chemosis of conjunctiva
    Subconjunctival edema
  372.74 Vascular abnormalities of conjunctiva
    Aneurysm(ata) of conjunctiva
  372.75 Conjunctival cysts
● **372.8 Other disorders of conjunctiva**
  372.81 Conjunctivochalasis
    Coding Clinic: 2000, Q4, P41
  372.89 Other disorders of conjunctiva
372.9 Unspecified disorder of conjunctiva
● **373 Inflammation of eyelids**
● **373.0 Blepharitis**
     Excludes *blepharoconjunctivitis (372.20–372.22)*
  373.00 Blepharitis, unspecified
  373.01 Ulcerative blepharitis
  373.02 Squamous blepharitis
● **373.1 Hordeolum and other deep inflammation of eyelid**
  Bacterial infection (staphylococcus) of sebaceous gland of eyelid (stye)
  373.11 Hordeolum externum
    Hordeolum NOS
    Stye
  373.12 Hordeolum internum
    Infection of meibomian gland
  373.13 Abscess of eyelid
    Furuncle of eyelid
373.2 Chalazion
  Most often caused by accumulation of meibomian gland secretions resulting from blockage of duct
  Meibomian (gland) cyst
  Excludes *infected meibomian gland (373.12)*

373.3 Noninfectious dermatoses of eyelid
  373.31 Eczematous dermatitis of eyelid
  373.32 Contact and allergic dermatitis of eyelid
  373.33 Xeroderma of eyelid
  373.34 Discoid lupus erythematosus of eyelid
▶ **373.4 *Infective dermatitis of eyelid of types resulting in deformity***
  Code first underlying disease, as:
    leprosy (030.0–030.9)
    lupus vulgaris (tuberculous) (017.0)
    yaws (102.0–102.9)
▶ **373.5 *Other infective dermatitis of eyelid***
  Code first underlying disease, as:
    actinomycosis (039.3)
    impetigo (684)
    mycotic dermatitis (110.0–111.9)
    vaccinia (051.0)
    postvaccination (999.0)
  Excludes *herpes:*
    simplex (054.41)
    zoster (053.20)
▶ **373.6 *Parasitic infestation of eyelid***
  Code first underlying disease, as:
    leishmaniasis (085.0–085.9)
    loiasis (125.2)
    onchocerciasis (125.3)
    pediculosis (132.0)
373.8 Other inflammations of eyelids
373.9 Unspecified inflammation of eyelid
● **374 Other disorders of eyelids**
● **374.0 Entropion and trichiasis of eyelid**
  374.00 Entropion, unspecified
  374.01 Senile entropion   A
  374.02 Mechanical entropion
  374.03 Spastic entropion
  374.04 Cicatricial entropion
  374.05 Trichiasis without entropion
● **374.1 Ectropion**
  374.10 Ectropion, unspecified
  374.11 Senile ectropion   A
  374.12 Mechanical ectropion
  374.13 Spastic ectropion
  374.14 Cicatricial ectropion
● **374.2 Lagophthalmos**
  374.20 Lagophthalmos, unspecified
  374.21 Paralytic lagophthalmos
  374.22 Mechanical lagophthalmos
  374.23 Cicatricial lagophthalmos
● **374.3 Ptosis of eyelid**
  Falling forward, drooping, sagging of eyelid
  374.30 Ptosis of eyelid, unspecified
    Coding Clinic: 1996, Q2, P11
  374.31 Paralytic ptosis
  374.32 Myogenic ptosis
  374.33 Mechanical ptosis
  374.34 Blepharochalasis
    Pseudoptosis

Figure 6–9 Photograph of eyelids with marginal blepharitis. (From Mandell, Bennett, & Dolin: Principles and Practice of Infectious Diseases, ed 7, Churchill Livingstone, An Imprint of Elsevier, 2009)

Item 6–21 Blepharitis is a common condition in which the eyelid is swollen and yellow scaling and conjunctivitis develop. Usually the hair on the scalp and brow is involved.

Figure 6–10 Right lower eyelid entropion. Note the inward rotation of the tarsal plate about the horizontal axis and the resultant contact between the mucocutaneous junction and ocular surface. (From Yanoff: Ophthalmology, ed 3, Mosby, Inc., 2008)

Item 6-22 Ptosis of eyelid is drooping of the upper eyelid over the pupil when the eyes are fully opened resulting from nerve or muscle damage, which may require surgical correction.

Figure 6-11 Ptosis of eyelid. (From Yanoff: Ophthalmology, ed 3, Mosby, Inc., 2008)

● **374.4   Other disorders affecting eyelid function**

> **Excludes**   *blepharoclonus (333.81)*
> *blepharospasm (333.81)*
> *facial nerve palsy (351.0)*
> *third nerve palsy or paralysis (378.51–378.52)*
> *tic (psychogenic) (307.20–307.23)*
> *organic (333.3)*

374.41   **Lid retraction or lag**

374.43   **Abnormal innervation syndrome**
Jaw-blinking
Paradoxical facial movements

374.44   **Sensory disorders**

374.45   **Other sensorimotor disorders**
Deficient blink reflex

374.46   **Blepharophimosis**
Ankyloblepharon

● **374.5   Degenerative disorders of eyelid and periocular area**

374.50   **Degenerative disorder of eyelid, unspecified**

▷ 374.51   *Xanthelasma*
Xanthoma (planum) (tuberosum) of eyelid
Code first underlying condition (272.0–272.9)

374.52   **Hyperpigmentation of eyelid**
Chloasma   Dyspigmentation

374.53   **Hypopigmentation of eyelid**
Vitiligo of eyelid

374.54   **Hypertrichosis of eyelid**

374.55   **Hypotrichosis of eyelid**
Madarosis of eyelid

374.56   **Other degenerative disorders of skin affecting eyelid**

● **374.8   Other disorders of eyelid**

374.81   **Hemorrhage of eyelid**
> **Excludes**   *black eye (921.0)*

374.82   **Edema of eyelid**
Hyperemia of eyelid
Coding Clinic: 2008, Q4, P128-131

374.83   **Elephantiasis of eyelid**

374.84   **Cysts of eyelids**
Sebaceous cyst of eyelid

374.85   **Vascular anomalies of eyelid**

374.86   **Retained foreign body of eyelid**
Use additional code to identify foreign body
(V90.01-V90.9)

374.87   **Dermatochalasis**

374.89   **Other disorders of eyelid**

374.9   **Unspecified disorder of eyelid**

● **375   Disorders of lacrimal system**

● **375.0   Dacryoadenitis**

375.00   **Dacryoadenitis, unspecified**

375.01   **Acute dacryoadenitis**

375.02   **Chronic dacryoadenitis**

375.03   **Chronic enlargement of lacrimal gland**

● **375.1   Other disorders of lacrimal gland**

375.11   **Dacryops**

375.12   **Other lacrimal cysts and cystic degeneration**

375.13   **Primary lacrimal atrophy**

375.14   **Secondary lacrimal atrophy**

375.15   **Tear film insufficiency, unspecified**
Dry eye syndrome
Coding Clinic: 1996, Q3, P6

375.16   **Dislocation of lacrimal gland**

● **375.2   Epiphora**

375.20   **Epiphora, unspecified as to cause**

375.21   **Epiphora due to excess lacrimation**

375.22   **Epiphora due to insufficient drainage**

● **375.3   Acute and unspecified inflammation of lacrimal passages**

> **Excludes**   *neonatal dacryocystitis (771.6)*

375.30   **Dacryocystitis, unspecified**

375.31   **Acute canaliculitis, lacrimal**

375.32   **Acute dacryocystitis**
Acute peridacryocystitis

375.33   **Phlegmonous dacryocystitis**

● **375.4   Chronic inflammation of lacrimal passages**

375.41   **Chronic canaliculitis**

375.42   **Chronic dacryocystitis**

375.43   **Lacrimal mucocele**

● **375.5   Stenosis and insufficiency of lacrimal passages**

375.51   **Eversion of lacrimal punctum**

375.52   **Stenosis of lacrimal punctum**

375.53   **Stenosis of lacrimal canaliculi**

375.54   **Stenosis of lacrimal sac**

375.55   **Obstruction of nasolacrimal duct, neonatal**
> **Excludes**   *congenital anomaly of nasolacrimal duct (743.65)*

375.56   **Stenosis of nasolacrimal duct, acquired**

375.57   **Dacryolith**

● **375.6   Other changes of lacrimal passages**

375.61   **Lacrimal fistula**

375.69   **Other**

● **375.8   Other disorders of lacrimal system**

375.81   **Granuloma of lacrimal passages**

375.89   **Other**

375.9   **Unspecified disorder of lacrimal system**

● **376   Disorders of the orbit**

● **376.0   Acute inflammation of orbit**

376.00   **Acute inflammation of orbit, unspecified**

376.01   **Orbital cellulitis** 🔲
Abscess of orbit
Ⓔⓧ 376.00-376.04

376.02   **Orbital periostitis** 🔲
Ⓔⓧ 003.24, 015.50-015.56, 015.70-015.76, 015.90-015.96,
017.90-017.96, 376.02, 730.00-730.39, 730.80-730.99

376.03   **Orbital osteomyelitis** 🔲
Ⓔⓧ 003.24, 015.50-015.56, 015.70-015.76, 015.90-015.96,
017.90-017.96, 376.03, 730.00-730.39, 730.80-730.99

376.04   **Tenonitis**

● **376.1   Chronic inflammatory disorders of orbit**

376.10   **Chronic inflammation of orbit, unspecified**

376.11   **Orbital granuloma**
Pseudotumor (inflammatory) of orbit

376.12   **Orbital myositis**

▷ 376.13   *Parasitic infestation of orbit*
Code first underlying disease, as:
hydatid infestation of orbit (122.3, 122.6, 122.9)
myiasis of orbit (134.0)

Iris
Lacrimal sac
Nasolacrimal duct
Lacrimal glands
Eyelid
Sclera
Pupil
Lacrimal duct

Figure 6-12 Lacrimal apparatus. (From Buck CJ: Step-by-Step Medical Coding. Philadelphia, WB Saunders, 2006, p 302)

● **376.2 Endocrine exophthalmos**
    Code first underlying thyroid disorder (242.0–242.9)
  ◗ **376.21 *Thyrotoxic exophthalmos***
  ◗ **376.22 *Exophthalmic ophthalmoplegia***
● **376.3 Other exophthalmic conditions**
    376.30 Exophthalmos, unspecified
    376.31 Constant exophthalmos
    376.32 Orbital hemorrhage
    376.33 Orbital edema or congestion
    376.34 Intermittent exophthalmos
    376.35 Pulsating exophthalmos
    376.36 Lateral displacement of globe
● **376.4 Deformity of orbit**
    376.40 Deformity of orbit, unspecified
    376.41 Hypertelorism of orbit
    376.42 Exostosis of orbit
    376.43 Local deformities due to bone disease
    376.44 Orbital deformities associated with craniofacial deformities
    376.45 Atrophy of orbit
    376.46 Enlargement of orbit
    376.47 Deformity due to trauma or surgery
● **376.5 Enophthalmos**
    376.50 Enophthalmos, unspecified as to cause
    376.51 Enophthalmos due to atrophy of orbital tissue
    376.52 Enophthalmos due to trauma or surgery
  376.6 Retained (old) foreign body following penetrating wound of orbit
    Retrobulbar foreign body
    Use additional code to identify foreign body (V90.01-V90.9)
● **376.8 Other orbital disorders**
    376.81 Orbital cysts
      Encephalocele of orbit
      Coding Clinic: 1999, Q3, P13
    376.82 Myopathy of extraocular muscles
    376.89 Other
  376.9 Unspecified disorder of orbit
● **377 Disorders of optic nerve and visual pathways**
● **377.0 Papilledema**
    377.00 Papilledema, unspecified 🔖
      (Ex) 017.30-017.36, 017.90-017.96, 036.81, 249.50-249.51,
        249.80-249.91, 250.50-250.53, 250.80-250.93, 377.00-377.03,
        377.14, 377.24, 379.60-379.90, 379.99, 743.8-743.9
    377.01 Papilledema associated with increased intracranial pressure 🔖
      (Ex) 017.30-017.36, 017.90-017.96, 036.81, 249.50-249.51,
        249.80-249.91, 250.50-250.53, 250.80-250.93, 377.00-377.03,
        377.14, 377.24, 379.60-379.90, 379.99, 743.8-743.9
    377.02 Papilledema associated with decreased ocular pressure
    377.03 Papilledema associated with retinal disorder
    377.04 Foster-Kennedy syndrome
● **377.1 Optic atrophy**
    377.10 Optic atrophy, unspecified
    377.11 Primary optic atrophy
      Excludes *neurosyphilitic optic atrophy (094.84)*
    377.12 Postinflammatory optic atrophy
    377.13 Optic atrophy associated with retinal dystrophies
    377.14 Glaucomatous atrophy [cupping] of optic disc

    377.15 Partial optic atrophy
      Temporal pallor of optic disc
    377.16 Hereditary optic atrophy
      Optic atrophy:
        dominant hereditary
        Leber's
● **377.2 Other disorders of optic disc**
    377.21 Drusen of optic disc
    377.22 Crater-like holes of optic disc
    377.23 Coloboma of optic disc
    377.24 Pseudopapilledema
● **377.3 Optic neuritis**
    Excludes *meningococcal optic neuritis (036.81)*
    377.30 Optic neuritis, unspecified 🔖
      (Ex) 377.30-377.39
    377.31 Optic papillitis 🔖
      (Ex) 377.30-377.39
    377.32 Retrobulbar neuritis (acute) 🔖
      Excludes *syphilitic retrobulbar neuritis (094.85)*
      (Ex) 377.30-377.39
    377.33 Nutritional optic neuropathy
    377.34 Toxic optic neuropathy
      Toxic amblyopia
    377.39 Other 🔖
      Excludes *ischemic optic neuropathy (377.41)*
      (Ex) 377.30-377.39
● **377.4 Other disorders of optic nerve**
    377.41 Ischemic optic neuropathy
    377.42 Hemorrhage in optic nerve sheaths
    377.43 Optic nerve hypoplasia
      Coding Clinic: 2006, Q4, P81-82
    377.49 Other
      Compression of optic nerve
● **377.5 Disorders of optic chiasm**
    377.51 Associated with pituitary neoplasms and disorders 🔖
      (Ex) 377.51-377.63
    377.52 Associated with other neoplasms 🔖
      (Ex) 377.51-377.63
    377.53 Associated with vascular disorders 🔖
      (Ex) 377.51-377.63
    377.54 Associated with inflammatory disorders 🔖
      (Ex) 377.51-377.63
● **377.6 Disorders of other visual pathways**
    377.61 Associated with neoplasms 🔖
      (Ex) 377.51-377.63
    377.62 Associated with vascular disorders 🔖
      (Ex) 377.51-377.63
    377.63 Associated with inflammatory disorders 🔖
      (Ex) 377.51-377.63
● **377.7 Disorders of visual cortex**
    Excludes *visual:*
        agnosia (368.16)
        hallucinations (368.16)
        halos (368.15)
    377.71 Associated with neoplasms 🔖
      (Ex) 377.71-377.9
    377.72 Associated with vascular disorders 🔖
      (Ex) 377.71-377.9
    377.73 Associated with inflammatory disorders 🔖
      (Ex) 377.71-377.9
    377.75 Cortical blindness
  377.9 Unspecified disorder of optic nerve and visual pathways

Item 6-23 Papilledema is swelling of the optic disc caused by increased intracranial pressure. It is most often bilateral and occurs quickly (hours) or over weeks of time. It is a common symptom of a brain tumor. The term should not be used to describe optic disc swelling with underlying infectious, infiltrative, or inflammatory etiologies.

DISEASES OF THE NERVOUS SYSTEM AND SENSE ORGANS (320–389)

DISEASES OF THE NERVOUS SYSTEM AND SENSE ORGANS (320–389)

Item 6-24 Strabismus or esotropia (crossed eyes) is a condition of the extraocular eye muscles, resulting in an inability of the eyes to focus and also affects depth perception.

A

B

Figure 6-13 A. Image of strabismus. **B.** Exotropia. (**A** from Yanoff: Ophthalmology, ed 3, Mosby, Inc., 2008. **B** from Rakel: Textbook of Family Practice, ed 7, Saunders, 2007)

● **378 Strabismus and other disorders of binocular eye movements**
     Excludes *nystagmus and other irregular eye movements (379.50–379.59)*

● **378.0 Esotropia**
     Convergent concomitant strabismus
       Excludes *intermittent esotropia (378.20–378.22)*
     378.00 Esotropia, unspecified
     378.01 Monocular esotropia
     378.02 Monocular esotropia with A pattern
     378.03 Monocular esotropia with V pattern
     378.04 Monocular esotropia with other noncomitancies
       Monocular esotropia with X or Y pattern
     378.05 Alternating esotropia
     378.06 Alternating esotropia with A pattern
     378.07 Alternating esotropia with V pattern
     378.08 Alternating esotropia with other noncomitancies
       Alternating esotropia with X or Y pattern

● **378.1 Exotropia**
     Misalignment in which one eye deviates outward (away from nose) while other fixates normally
     Divergent concomitant strabismus
       Excludes *intermittent exotropia (378.20, 378.23–378.24)*
     378.10 Exotropia, unspecified
     378.11 Monocular exotropia
     378.12 Monocular exotropia with A pattern
     378.13 Monocular exotropia with V pattern
     378.14 Monocular exotropia with other noncomitancies
       Monocular exotropia with X or Y pattern
     378.15 Alternating exotropia
     378.16 Alternating exotropia with A pattern
     378.17 Alternating exotropia with V pattern
     378.18 Alternating exotropia with other noncomitancies
       Alternating exotropia with X or Y pattern

● **378.2 Intermittent heterotropia**
     Displacement of an organ or part of an organ from normal position
       Excludes *vertical heterotropia (intermittent) (378.31)*
     378.20 Intermittent heterotropia, unspecified
       Intermittent:
         esotropia NOS
         exotropia NOS
     378.21 Intermittent esotropia, monocular
     378.22 Intermittent esotropia, alternating
     378.23 Intermittent exotropia, monocular
     378.24 Intermittent exotropia, alternating

● **378.3 Other and unspecified heterotropia**
     378.30 Heterotropia, unspecified
     378.31 Hypertropia
       Vertical heterotropia (constant) (intermittent)
     378.32 Hypotropia
     378.33 Cyclotropia

     378.34 Monofixation syndrome
       Microtropia
     378.35 Accommodative component in esotropia

● **378.4 Heterophoria**
     Condition in which one or both eyes wander away from position where both eyes are looking
     378.40 Heterophoria, unspecified
     378.41 Esophoria
       Eye deviates inward (toward nose)
     378.42 Exophoria
       Eye deviates outward (toward ear)
     378.43 Vertical heterophoria
     378.44 Cyclophoria
     378.45 Alternating hyperphoria

● **378.5 Paralytic strabismus**
     378.50 Paralytic strabismus, unspecified
     378.51 Third or oculomotor nerve palsy, partial
     378.52 Third or oculomotor nerve palsy, total
     378.53 Fourth or trochlear nerve palsy
       Coding Clinic: 2001, Q2, P21
     378.54 Sixth or abducens nerve palsy
     378.55 External ophthalmoplegia
       Coding Clinic: 1989, Q2, P12
     378.56 Total ophthalmoplegia

● **378.6 Mechanical strabismus**
     378.60 Mechanical strabismus, unspecified
     378.61 Brown's (tendon) sheath syndrome
     378.62 Mechanical strabismus from other musculofascial disorders
     378.63 Limited duction associated with other conditions

● **378.7 Other specified strabismus**
     378.71 Duane's syndrome
     378.72 Progressive external ophthalmoplegia
     378.73 Strabismus in other neuromuscular disorders

● **378.8 Other disorders of binocular eye movements**
       Excludes *nystagmus (379.50–379.56)*
     378.81 Palsy of conjugate gaze
     378.82 Spasm of conjugate gaze
     378.83 Convergence insufficiency or palsy
     378.84 Convergence excess or spasm
     378.85 Anomalies of divergence
     378.86 Internuclear ophthalmoplegia
     378.87 Other dissociated deviation of eye movements
       Skew deviation

     378.9 Unspecified disorder of eye movements
       Ophthalmoplegia NOS
       Strabismus NOS
       Coding Clinic: 2001, Q2, P21

● **379 Other disorders of eye**
● **379.0 Scleritis and episcleritis**
     Inflammation of white (sclera and episclera) of eye.
       Autoimmune disorders are most common cause.
       Excludes *syphilitic episcleritis (095.0)*
     379.00 Scleritis, unspecified
       Episcleritis NOS
     379.01 Episcleritis periodica fugax
     379.02 Nodular episcleritis
     379.03 Anterior scleritis
     379.04 Scleromalacia perforans
     379.05 Scleritis with corneal involvement
       Scleroperikeratitis
     379.06 Brawny scleritis
     379.07 Posterior scleritis
       Sclerotenonitis
     379.09 Other
       Scleral abscess

● **379.1 Other disorders of sclera**
  Excludes *blue sclera (743.47)*
  379.11 Scleral ectasia
      Scleral staphyloma NOS
  379.12 Staphyloma posticum
  379.13 Equatorial staphyloma
  379.14 Anterior staphyloma, localized
  379.15 Ring staphyloma
  379.16 Other degenerative disorders of sclera
  379.19 Other
● **379.2 Disorders of vitreous body**
  379.21 Vitreous degeneration
      Vitreous:
        cavitation
        detachment
        liquefaction
  379.22 Crystalline deposits in vitreous
      Asteroid hyalitis
      Synchysis scintillans
  379.23 Vitreous hemorrhage
      Coding Clinic: 1991, Q3, P15-16
  379.24 Other vitreous opacities
      Vitreous floaters
      *Small clumps of cells that float in vitreous of the eye,
        appearing as black specks or dots in field of
        vision*
      Coding Clinic: 1994, Q1, P16
  379.25 Vitreous membranes and strands
  379.26 Vitreous prolapse
  379.27 Vitreomacular adhesion   A
      Vitreomacular traction
      Excludes *traction detachment with vitreoretinal
                      organization (361.81)*
      Coding Clinic: 2011, Q4, P106
  379.29 Other disorders of vitreous
      Excludes *vitreous abscess (360.04)*
      Coding Clinic: 1999, Q1, P11
● **379.3 Aphakia and other disorders of lens**
  Excludes *after-cataract (366.50–366.53)*
  379.31 Aphakia
      Excludes *cataract extraction status (V45.61)*
  379.32 Subluxation of lens
      Coding Clinic: 1994, Q1, P16-17
  379.33 Anterior dislocation of lens
  379.34 Posterior dislocation of lens
  379.39 Other disorders of lens
● **379.4 Anomalies of pupillary function**
  379.40 Abnormal pupillary function, unspecified
  379.41 Anisocoria
  379.42 Miosis (persistent), not due to miotics
  379.43 Mydriasis (persistent), not due to mydriatics
  379.45 Argyll Robertson pupil, atypical
      Argyll Robertson phenomenon or pupil,
        nonsyphilitic
      Excludes *Argyll Robertson pupil (syphilitic)
                      (094.89)*
  379.46 Tonic pupillary reaction
      Adie's pupil or syndrome
  379.49 Other
      Hippus
      Pupillary paralysis
● **379.5 Nystagmus and other irregular eye movements**
      *Nystagmus is rapid, involuntary movements of eyes in
        horizontal or vertical direction.*
  379.50 Nystagmus, unspecified
      Coding Clinic: 2002, Q4, P68; 2001, Q2, P21
  379.51 Congenital nystagmus
  379.52 Latent nystagmus

  379.53 Visual deprivation nystagmus
  **379.54 Nystagmus associated with disorders of the
            vestibular system**
  379.55 Dissociated nystagmus
  379.56 Other forms of nystagmus
  379.57 Deficiencies of saccadic eye movements
      Abnormal optokinetic response
  379.58 Deficiencies of smooth pursuit movements
  379.59 Other irregularities of eye movements
      Opsoclonus
● **379.6 Inflammation (infection) of postprocedural bleb**
      Postprocedural blebitis
  **379.60 Inflammation (infection) of postprocedural bleb,
            unspecified**
  **379.61 Inflammation (infection) of postprocedural bleb,
            stage 1**
  **379.62 Inflammation (infection) of postprocedural bleb,
            stage 2**
      Coding Clinic: 2006, Q4, P82-83
  **379.63 Inflammation (infection) of postprocedural bleb,
            stage 3**
      Bleb associated endophthalmitis
  379.8 Other specified disorders of eye and adnexa
● **379.9 Unspecified disorder of eye and adnexa**
  379.90 Disorder of eye, unspecified
  379.91 Pain in or around eye
  379.92 Swelling or mass of eye
  379.93 Redness or discharge of eye
  379.99 Other ill-defined disorders of eye
      Excludes *blurred vision NOS (368.8)*

DISEASES OF THE EAR AND MASTOID PROCESS (380–389)

Use additional external cause code, if applicable, to identify the
cause of the ear condition

● **380 Disorders of external ear**
● **380.0 Perichondritis and chondritis of pinna**
      Chondritis of auricle
      Perichondritis of auricle
  380.00 Perichondritis of pinna, unspecified
  380.01 Acute perichondritis of pinna
  380.02 Chronic perichondritis of pinna
  380.03 Chondritis of pinna
      Coding Clinic: 2004, Q4, P75-76
● **380.1 Infective otitis externa**
  380.10 Infective otitis externa, unspecified
      Otitis externa (acute):
        NOS
        circumscribed
        diffuse
        hemorrhagica
        infective NOS
  380.11 Acute infection of pinna
      Excludes *furuncular otitis externa (680.0)*
  380.12 Acute swimmers' ear
      Beach ear
      Tank ear
  ▶ **380.13 Other acute infections of external ear**
      Code first underlying disease, as:
        erysipelas (035)
        impetigo (684)
        seborrheic dermatitis (690.10–690.18)
      Excludes *herpes simplex (054.73)
                      herpes zoster (053.71)*
  380.14 Malignant otitis externa 🔖
      (Ex:) 380.14, 383.00-383.1

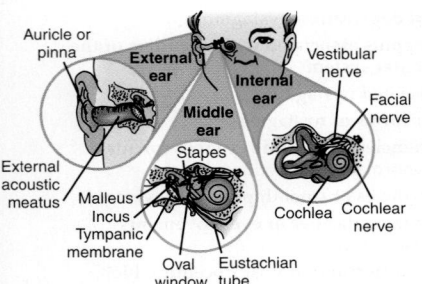

Figure 6–14
Auditory system. (From Buck CJ: Step-by-Step Medical Coding, ed 2010, Philadelphia, WB Saunders, 2010)

▷ 380.15 *Chronic mycotic otitis externa*
Code first underlying disease, as:
aspergillosis (117.3)
otomycosis NOS (111.9)

  Excludes *candidal otitis externa (112.82)*

380.16 **Other chronic infective otitis externa**
Chronic infective otitis externa NOS

● 380.2 **Other otitis externa**

380.21 **Cholesteatoma of external ear**
Keratosis obturans of external ear (canal)

  Excludes *cholesteatoma NOS (385.30–385.35)*
postmastoidectomy (383.32)

380.22 **Other acute otitis externa**
Acute otitis externa:
actinic
chemical
contact
eczematoid
reactive

380.23 **Other chronic otitis externa**
Chronic otitis externa NOS

● 380.3 **Noninfectious disorders of pinna**

380.30 **Disorder of pinna, unspecified**

380.31 **Hematoma of auricle or pinna**

380.32 **Acquired deformities of auricle or pinna**

  Excludes *cauliflower ear (738.7)*
  Coding Clinic: 2003, Q3, P12-13

380.39 **Other**

  Excludes *gouty tophi of ear (274.81)*

● 380.4 **Impacted cerumen**
Wax in ear
MCE: Questionable admission, principal diagnosis only

● 380.5 **Acquired stenosis of external ear canal**
Collapse of external ear canal

380.50 **Acquired stenosis of external ear canal, unspecified as to cause**

380.51 **Secondary to trauma**

380.52 **Secondary to surgery**

380.53 **Secondary to inflammation**

● 380.8 **Other disorders of external ear**

380.81 **Exostosis of external ear canal**

380.89 **Other**

380.9 **Unspecified disorder of external ear**

● 381 **Nonsuppurative otitis media and Eustachian tube disorders**
Nonsuppurative: not producing pus

● 381.0 **Acute nonsuppurative otitis media**
Acute tubotympanic catarrh
Otitis media, acute or subacute:
catarrhal
exudative
transudative
with effusion

  Excludes *otitic barotrauma (993.0)*

381.00 **Acute nonsuppurative otitis media, unspecified**

381.01 **Acute serous otitis media**
Acute or subacute secretory otitis media

381.02 **Acute mucoid otitis media**
Acute or subacute seromucinous otitis media
Blue drum syndrome

381.03 **Acute sanguinous otitis media**

381.04 **Acute allergic serous otitis media**

381.05 **Acute allergic mucoid otitis media**

381.06 **Acute allergic sanguinous otitis media**

● 381.1 **Chronic serous otitis media**
Chronic tubotympanic catarrh

381.10 **Chronic serous otitis media, simple or unspecified**

381.19 **Other**
Serosanguinous chronic otitis media

● 381.2 **Chronic mucoid otitis media**
Glue ear

  Excludes *adhesive middle ear disease (385.10–385.19)*

381.20 **Chronic mucoid otitis media, simple or unspecified**

381.29 **Other**
Mucosanguinous chronic otitis media

381.3 **Other and unspecified chronic nonsuppurative otitis media**
Otitis media, chronic: Otitis media, chronic:
allergic   seromucinous
exudative   transudative
secretory   with effusion

381.4 **Nonsuppurative otitis media, not specified as acute or chronic**
Otitis media: Otitis media:
allergic   seromucinous
catarrhal   serous
exudative   transudative
mucoid   with effusion
secretory

● 381.5 **Eustachian salpingitis**

381.50 **Eustachian salpingitis, unspecified**

381.51 **Acute Eustachian salpingitis**

381.52 **Chronic Eustachian salpingitis**

● 381.6 **Obstruction of Eustachian tube**
Stenosis of Eustachian tube
Stricture of Eustachian tube

381.60 **Obstruction of Eustachian tube, unspecified**

381.61 **Osseous obstruction of Eustachian tube**
Obstruction of Eustachian tube from cholesteatoma, polyp, or other osseous lesion

381.62 **Intrinsic cartilaginous obstruction of Eustachian tube**

381.63 **Extrinsic cartilaginous obstruction of Eustachian tube**
Compression of Eustachian tube

381.7 **Patulous Eustachian tube**

● 381.8 **Other disorders of Eustachian tube**

381.81 **Dysfunction of Eustachian tube**

381.89 **Other**

381.9 **Unspecified Eustachian tube disorder**

● 382 **Suppurative and unspecified otitis media**

● 382.0 **Acute suppurative otitis media**
Suppurative: Discharging pus
Otitis media, acute:
necrotizing NOS
purulent
pus-filled

382.00 **Acute suppurative otitis media without spontaneous rupture of ear drum**

382.01 **Acute suppurative otitis media with spontaneous rupture of ear drum**

▶ **382.02** *Acute suppurative otitis media in diseases classified elsewhere*
> *Code first underlying disease, as:*
> influenza (487.8, 488.09, 488.19)
> scarlet fever (034.1)
>
> **Excludes** *postmeasles otitis (055.2)*

382.1 Chronic tubotympanic suppurative otitis media
Benign chronic suppurative otitis media (with anterior perforation of ear drum)
Chronic tubotympanic disease (with anterior perforation of ear drum)

382.2 Chronic atticoantral suppurative otitis media
Chronic atticoantral disease (with posterior or superior marginal perforation of ear drum)
Persistent mucosal disease (with posterior or superior marginal perforation of ear drum)

382.3 Unspecified chronic suppurative otitis media
Chronic purulent otitis media
> **Excludes** *tuberculous otitis media (017.4)*

382.4 Unspecified suppurative otitis media
Purulent otitis media NOS

382.9 Unspecified otitis media
Otitis media:
NOS
acute NOS
chronic NOS

● **383 Mastoiditis and related conditions**
● **383.0 Acute mastoiditis**
Abscess of mastoid
Empyema of mastoid

383.00 Acute mastoiditis without complications
(Ex) 015.60-015.66, 017.40-017.46, 017.90-017.96, 383.00-383.9, 388.71-388.9, 744.00, 744.02, 744.09 744.29-744.3

383.01 Subperiosteal abscess of mastoid
(Ex) 015.60-015.66, 017.40-017.46, 017.90-017.96, 383.00-383.9, 388.71-388.9, 744.00, 744.02, 744.09 744.29-744.3

383.02 Acute mastoiditis with other complications
Gradenigo's syndrome
(Ex) 015.60-015.66, 017.40-017.46, 017.90-017.96, 383.00-383.9, 388.71-388.9, 744.00, 744.02, 744.09, 744.29-744.3

383.1 Chronic mastoiditis
Caries of mastoid
Fistula of mastoid
> **Excludes** *tuberculous mastoiditis (015.6)*

● **383.2 Petrositis**
Coalescing osteitis of petrous bone
Inflammation of petrous bone
Osteomyelitis of petrous bone

383.20 Petrositis, unspecified
383.21 Acute petrositis
383.22 Chronic petrositis

● **383.3 Complications following mastoidectomy**
383.30 Postmastoidectomy complication, unspecified
383.31 Mucosal cyst of postmastoidectomy cavity
383.32 Recurrent cholesteatoma of postmastoidectomy cavity
383.33 Granulations of postmastoidectomy cavity
Chronic inflammation of postmastoidectomy cavity

● **383.8 Other disorders of mastoid**
383.81 Postauricular fistula
383.89 Other

383.9 Unspecified mastoiditis

● **384 Other disorders of tympanic membrane**
● **384.0 Acute myringitis without mention of otitis media**
384.00 Acute myringitis, unspecified
Acute tympanitis NOS
384.01 Bullous myringitis
Myringitis bullosa hemorrhagica
384.09 Other

384.1 Chronic myringitis without mention of otitis media
Chronic tympanitis

● **384.2 Perforation of tympanic membrane**
Perforation of ear drum:
NOS
persistent posttraumatic
postinflammatory
> **Excludes** *otitis media with perforation of tympanic membrane (382.00–382.9)*
> *traumatic perforation [current injury] (872.61)*

384.20 Perforation of tympanic membrane, unspecified
384.21 Central perforation of tympanic membrane
384.22 Attic perforation of tympanic membrane
Pars flaccida
384.23 Other marginal perforation of tympanic membrane
384.24 Multiple perforations of tympanic membrane
384.25 Total perforation of tympanic membrane

● **384.8 Other specified disorders of tympanic membrane**
384.81 Atrophic flaccid tympanic membrane
Healed perforation of ear drum
384.82 Atrophic nonflaccid tympanic membrane

384.9 Unspecified disorder of tympanic membrane

● **385 Other disorders of middle ear and mastoid**
> **Excludes** *mastoiditis (383.0–383.9)*

● **385.0 Tympanosclerosis**
385.00 Tympanosclerosis, unspecified as to involvement
385.01 Tympanosclerosis involving tympanic membrane only
385.02 Tympanosclerosis involving tympanic membrane and ear ossicles
385.03 Tympanosclerosis involving tympanic membrane, ear ossicles, and middle ear
385.09 Tympanosclerosis involving other combination of structures

● **385.1 Adhesive middle ear disease**
Adhesive otitis
Otitis media: Otitis media:
chronic adhesive   fibrotic
> **Excludes** *glue ear (381.20–381.29)*

385.10 Adhesive middle ear disease, unspecified as to involvement
385.11 Adhesions of drum head to incus
385.12 Adhesions of drum head to stapes
385.13 Adhesions of drum head to promontorium
385.19 Other adhesions and combinations

● **385.2 Other acquired abnormality of ear ossicles**
385.21 Impaired mobility of malleus
Ankylosis of malleus
385.22 Impaired mobility of other ear ossicles
Ankylosis of ear ossicles, except malleus
385.23 Discontinuity or dislocation of ear ossicles
385.24 Partial loss or necrosis of ear ossicles

Item 6-25 Mastoiditis is an infection of the portion of the temporal bone of the skull that is behind the ear (mastoid process) caused by an untreated otitis media, leading to an infection of the surrounding structures which may include the brain.

DISEASES OF THE NERVOUS SYSTEM AND SENSE ORGANS (320–389)

N Newborn: 0   P Pediatric: 0–17   M Maternity: 12–55   A Adult: 15–124   ♀ Females Only   ♂ Males Only
(Ex) CC/MCC Exclusions   Complication\Comorbidity   Major C\C   Present on Admission Requirement   Hospital-Acquired Condition   797

● 385.3 **Cholesteatoma of middle ear and mastoid**
Cholesterosis of (middle) ear
Epidermosis of (middle) ear
Keratosis of (middle) ear
Polyp of (middle) ear

> **Excludes**   *cholesteatoma:*
>   *external ear canal (380.21)*
>   *recurrent of postmastoidectomy cavity*
>   *(383.32)*

   385.30 **Cholesteatoma, unspecified**

   385.31 **Cholesteatoma of attic**

   385.32 **Cholesteatoma of middle ear**

   385.33 **Cholesteatoma of middle ear and mastoid**
     Coding Clinic: 2000, Q3, P10-11

   385.35 **Diffuse cholesteatosis**

● 385.8 **Other disorders of middle ear and mastoid**

   385.82 **Cholesterin granuloma**

   385.83 **Retained foreign body of middle ear**
     Use additional code to identify foreign body
     (V90.01-V90.9)
     Coding Clinic: 1987, Nov-Dec, P9

   385.89 **Other**

   385.9 **Unspecified disorder of middle ear and mastoid**

● 386 **Vertiginous syndromes and other disorders of vestibular system**
> **Excludes**   *vertigo NOS (780.4)*

Coding Clinic: 1985, Mar-April, P12

● 386.0 **Méniére's disease**
*Vestibular disorder that produces recurring symptoms
   including severe and intermittent hearing loss including
   feeling of ear pressure or pain*
Endolymphatic hydrops
Lermoyez's syndrome
Méniére's syndrome or vertigo

   386.00 **Méniére's disease, unspecified**
     Méniére's disease (active)
     Coding Clinic: 1985, Mar-April, P12

   386.01 **Active Méniére's disease, cochleovestibular**

   386.02 **Active Méniére's disease, cochlear**

   386.03 **Active Méniére's disease, vestibular**

   386.04 **Inactive Méniére's disease**
     Méniére's disease in remission

● 386.1 **Other and unspecified peripheral vertigo**
> **Excludes**   *epidemic vertigo (078.81)*

   386.10 **Peripheral vertigo, unspecified**

   386.11 **Benign paroxysmal positional vertigo**
     Benign paroxysmal positional nystagmus

   386.12 **Vestibular neuronitis**
     Acute (and recurrent) peripheral vestibulopathy

   386.19 **Other**
     Aural vertigo   Otogenic vertigo

   386.2 **Vertigo of central origin**
     Central positional nystagmus
     Malignant positional vertigo

● 386.3 **Labyrinthitis**
*Balance disorder that follows a URI or head injury. The
   inflammatory process affects the labyrinth that houses
   vestibular system (senses changes in head position) of
   inner ear.*

   386.30 **Labyrinthitis, unspecified**

   386.31 **Serous labyrinthitis**
     Diffuse labyrinthitis

   386.32 **Circumscribed labyrinthitis**
     Focal labyrinthitis

   386.33 **Suppurative labyrinthitis**
     Purulent labyrinthitis

   386.34 **Toxic labyrinthitis**

   386.35 **Viral labyrinthitis**

● 386.4 **Labyrinthine fistula**

   386.40 **Labyrinthine fistula, unspecified**

   386.41 **Round window fistula**

   386.42 **Oval window fistula**

   386.43 **Semicircular canal fistula**

   386.48 **Labyrinthine fistula of combined sites**

● 386.5 **Labyrinthine dysfunction**

   386.50 **Labyrinthine dysfunction, unspecified**

   386.51 **Hyperactive labyrinth, unilateral**

   386.52 **Hyperactive labyrinth, bilateral**

   386.53 **Hypoactive labyrinth, unilateral**

   386.54 **Hypoactive labyrinth, bilateral**

   386.55 **Loss of labyrinthine reactivity, unilateral**

   386.56 **Loss of labyrinthine reactivity, bilateral**

   386.58 **Other forms and combinations**

   386.8 **Other disorders of labyrinth**
     Coding Clinic: 2011, Q1, P7

   386.9 **Unspecified vertiginous syndromes and labyrinthine disorders**

● 387 **Otosclerosis**
*Inherited middle ear spongelike bone growth causing hearing loss
   because growth prevents vibration from sound waves required
   for hearing*

> **Includes**   *otospongiosis*

   387.0 **Otosclerosis involving oval window, nonobliterative**

   387.1 **Otosclerosis involving oval window, obliterative**

   387.2 **Cochlear otosclerosis**
     Otosclerosis involving:
       otic capsule
       round window

   387.8 **Other otosclerosis**

   387.9 **Otosclerosis, unspecified**

● 388 **Other disorders of ear**

● 388.0 **Degenerative and vascular disorders of ear**

   388.00 **Degenerative and vascular disorders, unspecified**

   388.01 **Presbyacusis**

   388.02 **Transient ischemic deafness**

● 388.1 **Noise effects on inner ear**

   388.10 **Noise effects on inner ear, unspecified**

   388.11 **Acoustic trauma (explosive) to ear**
     Otitic blast injury

   388.12 **Noise-induced hearing loss**

   388.2 **Sudden hearing loss, unspecified**

● 388.3 **Tinnitus**
*Perception of sound in absence of external noise and may affect
   one or both ears and/or head*

   388.30 **Tinnitus, unspecified**

   388.31 **Subjective tinnitus**

   388.32 **Objective tinnitus**

● 388.4 **Other abnormal auditory perception**

   388.40 **Abnormal auditory perception, unspecified**

   388.41 **Diplacusis**

   388.42 **Hyperacusis**

   388.43 **Impairment of auditory discrimination**

   388.44 **Recruitment**

   388.45 **Acquired auditory processing disorder**
     Auditory processing disorder NOS

>   **Excludes**   *central auditory processing disorder*
>   *(315.32)*
>   **Coding Clinic: 2007, Q4, P79**

   388.5 **Disorders of acoustic nerve**
     Acoustic neuritis
     Degeneration of acoustic or eighth nerve
     Disorder of acoustic or eighth nerve

>   **Excludes**   *acoustic neuroma (225.1)*
>   *syphilitic acoustic neuritis (094.86)*
>   **Coding Clinic: 1987, Mar-April, P8**

◀ New   ◀ Revised   ~~deleted~~ Deleted   Excludes   Includes   Use additional   Code first   Omit code

● 388.6 **Otorrhea**
    388.60 **Otorrhea, unspecified**
        Discharging ear NOS
    388.61 **Cerebrospinal fluid otorrhea**
            Excludes *cerebrospinal fluid rhinorrhea (349.81)*
            (Ex) 388.61-388.69
            Coding Clinic: 2013, Q2, P9
    388.69 **Other**
        Otorrhagia
● 388.7 **Otalgia**
    388.70 **Otalgia, unspecified**
        Earache NOS
    388.71 **Otogenic pain**
    388.72 **Referred pain**
        Pain from a diseased area of the body that is not felt directly in that area, but in another part of the body
● 388.8 **Other disorders of ear**
● 388.9 **Unspecified disorder of ear**
● 389 **Hearing loss**
● 389.0 **Conductive hearing loss**
    Conductive deafness
    Excludes *mixed conductive and sensorineural hearing loss (389.20–389.22)*
    389.00 **Conductive hearing loss, unspecified**
        Coding Clinic: 2013, Q2, P9
    389.01 **Conductive hearing loss, external ear**
    389.02 **Conductive hearing loss, tympanic membrane**
    389.03 **Conductive hearing loss, middle ear**
    389.04 **Conductive hearing loss, inner ear**
    389.05 **Conductive hearing loss, unilateral**
    389.06 **Conductive hearing loss, bilateral**
        Coding Clinic: 2007, Q4, P80-81
    389.08 **Conductive hearing loss of combined types**

● 389.1 **Sensorineural hearing loss**
    Perceptive hearing loss or deafness
    Excludes *abnormal auditory perception (388.40–388.44)*
        mixed conductive and sensorineural hearing loss (389.20–389.22)
        psychogenic deafness (306.7)
    Coding Clinic: 2007, Q4, P80-81; 2006, Q4, P84
    389.10 **Sensorineural hearing loss, unspecified**
        Coding Clinic: 1993, Q1, P29
    389.11 **Sensory hearing loss, bilateral**
    389.12 **Neural hearing loss, bilateral**
    389.13 **Neural hearing loss, unilateral**
    389.14 **Central hearing loss**
    389.15 **Sensorineural hearing loss, unilateral**
    389.16 **Sensorineural hearing loss, asymmetrical**
    389.17 **Sensory hearing loss, unilateral**
    389.18 **Sensorineural hearing loss, bilateral**
● 389.2 **Mixed conductive and sensorineural hearing loss**
    Deafness or hearing loss of type classifiable to 389.00–389.08 with type classifiable to 389.10–389.18
    Coding Clinic: 2007, Q4, P80-81
    389.20 **Mixed hearing loss, unspecified**
    389.21 **Mixed hearing loss, unilateral**
    389.22 **Mixed hearing loss, bilateral**
● 389.7 **Deaf nonspeaking, not elsewhere classifiable**
● 389.8 **Other specified forms of hearing loss**
● 389.9 **Unspecified hearing loss**
    Deafness NOS
    Coding Clinic: 2004, Q1, P15-16

DISEASES OF THE NERVOUS SYSTEM AND SENSE ORGANS (320–389)

Pulmonary valve
Aortic valve
Mitral valve
Tricuspid valve
RA
LA
RV

Figure 7-1 Cardiovascular valves.

Item 7-1 Rheumatic fever is the inflammation of the valve(s) of the heart, usually the mitral or aortic, which leads to valve damage. Rheumatic heart inflammations are usually **pericarditis** (sac surrounding heart), **endocarditis** (heart cavity), or **myocarditis** (heart muscle).

7. DISEASES OF THE CIRCULATORY SYSTEM (390–459)

ACUTE RHEUMATIC FEVER (390–392)

390 Rheumatic fever without mention of heart involvement
Arthritis, rheumatic, acute or subacute
Rheumatic fever (active) (acute)
Rheumatism, articular, acute or subacute
> **Excludes** *that with heart involvement (391.0–391.9)*

● **391 Rheumatic fever with heart involvement**
> **Excludes** *chronic heart diseases of rheumatic origin (393–398.99) unless rheumatic fever is also present or there is evidence of recrudescence or activity of the rheumatic process*

  391.0 Acute rheumatic pericarditis🔗
Rheumatic:
    fever (active) (acute) with pericarditis
    pericarditis (acute)
Any condition classifiable to 390 with pericarditis
> **Excludes** *that not specified as rheumatic (420.0–420.9)*
  Ex) 074.21, 093.81, 391.0, 393, 420.0-420.99, 423.3-423.9, 459.89-459.9

  391.1 Acute rheumatic endocarditis🔗
Rheumatic:
    endocarditis, acute
    fever (active) (acute) with endocarditis or valvulitis
    valvulitis acute
Any condition classifiable to 390 with endocarditis or valvulitis
  Ex) 002.0, 036.42, 074.22, 083.0, 093.20-093.24, 098.84, 112.81, 115.94, 390, 391.1, 391.8-392.0, 394.0-395.9, 396.9-397.9, 398.90, 398.99, 421.0-421.9, 424.0-424.99, 425.3, 459.89-459.9, 746.09, 746.89, 996.61

  391.2 Acute rheumatic myocarditis🔗
Rheumatic fever (active) (acute) with myocarditis
Any condition classifiable to 390 with myocarditis
  Ex) 074.20, 074.22-074.23, 093.82, 390, 391.2-391.9, 398.0-398.90, 398.99, 422.0-422.99, 429.0, 429.71-429.79, 459.89-459.9

  391.8 Other acute rheumatic heart disease🔗
Rheumatic:
    fever (active) (acute) with other or multiple types of heart involvement
    pancarditis, acute
Any condition classifiable to 390 with other or multiple types of heart involvement
  Ex) 391.0-398.99, 428.20-428.43

  391.9 Acute rheumatic heart disease, unspecified🔗
Rheumatic:
    carditis, acute
    fever (active) (acute) with unspecified type of heart involvement
    heart disease, active or acute
Any condition classifiable to 390 with unspecified type of heart involvement
  Ex) 391.0-398.99

Item 7-2 Rheumatic chorea, also called Sydenham's, juvenile, minor, simple, or St. Vitus' dance, is a major symptom of rheumatic fever and is characterized by ceaseless, involuntary, jerky, purposeless movements.

● **392 Rheumatic chorea**
> **Includes** Sydenham's chorea
> **Excludes** *chorea:*
>   *NOS (333.5)*
>   *Huntington's (333.4)*

  392.0 With heart involvement🔗
Rheumatic chorea with heart involvement of any type classifiable to 391
  Ex) 391.0-398.99, 428.20-428.43

  392.9 Without mention of heart involvement🔗
  Ex) 391.0-398.99

CHRONIC RHEUMATIC HEART DISEASE (393–398)

393 Chronic rheumatic pericarditis🔗
Adherent pericardium, rheumatic
Chronic rheumatic:
    mediastinopericarditis
    myopericarditis
> **Excludes** *pericarditis NOS or not specified as rheumatic (423.0–423.9)*
  Ex) 074.21, 093.81, 391.0, 393, 420.0-420.99, 423.3-423.9, 459.89-459.9

● **394 Diseases of mitral valve**
> **Excludes** *that with aortic valve involvement (396.0–396.9)*

  394.0 Mitral stenosis
Mitral (valve):
    obstruction (rheumatic)
    stenosis NOS

  394.1 Rheumatic mitral insufficiency
Rheumatic mitral:
    incompetence
    regurgitation
> **Excludes** *that not specified as rheumatic (424.0)*
  Coding Clinic: 2005, Q2, P14-15

  394.2 Mitral stenosis with insufficiency
Mitral stenosis with incompetence or regurgitation
  Coding Clinic: 2007, Q2, P11-12

  394.9 Other and unspecified mitral valve diseases
Mitral (valve):
    disease (chronic)
    failure

● **395 Diseases of aortic valve**
> **Excludes** *that not specified as rheumatic (424.1)*
>   *that with mitral valve involvement (396.0–396.9)*

  395.0 Rheumatic aortic stenosis
Rheumatic aortic (valve) obstruction
  Coding Clinic: 1988, Q4, P8

  395.1 Rheumatic aortic insufficiency
Rheumatic aortic:
    incompetence
    regurgitation

  395.2 Rheumatic aortic stenosis with insufficiency
Rheumatic aortic stenosis with incompetence or regurgitation

  395.9 Other and unspecified rheumatic aortic diseases
Rheumatic aortic (valve) disease

Item 7-3 Mitral stenosis is the narrowing of the mitral valve separating the left atrium from the left ventricle. **Mitral insufficiency** is the improper closure of the mitral valve which may lead to enlargement (hypertrophy) of the left atrium.

Item 7-4 Aortic stenosis is the narrowing of the aortic valve located between the left ventricle and the aorta. **Aortic insufficiency** is the improper closure of the aortic valve which may lead to enlargement (hypertrophy) of the left ventricle.

◀ New   ◀◀ Revised   ~~deleted~~ Deleted   Excludes   Includes   Use additional   Code first   Omit code

800   ● Unacceptable Principal Diagnosis   🔗 Use Additional Digit(s)   ▸ Manifestation Code   **OGCR** Official Guidelines   **Coding Clinic**

Item 7–5 Mitral and aortic valve stenosis is the narrowing of these valves, which leads to enlargement (hypertrophy) of the left atrium and left ventricle respectively, while **mitral and aortic insufficiency** is the improper closure of the mitral and aortic valves resulting in the same outcome as stenosis.

● **396 Diseases of mitral and aortic valves**

  Includes   involvement of both mitral and aortic valves, whether specified as rheumatic or not

  396.0 Mitral valve stenosis and aortic valve stenosis
  Atypical aortic (valve) stenosis
  Mitral and aortic (valve) obstruction (rheumatic)

  396.1 Mitral valve stenosis and aortic valve insufficiency

  396.2 Mitral valve insufficiency and aortic valve stenosis
  Coding Clinic: 2009, Q2, P11; 2000, Q2, P16-17; 1987, Nov-Dec, P8

  396.3 Mitral valve insufficiency and aortic valve insufficiency
  Mitral and aortic (valve):
      incompetence
      regurgitation
  Coding Clinic: 2009, Q2, P11; Q1, P8; 1995, Q1, P6

  396.8 Multiple involvement of mitral and aortic valves
  Stenosis and insufficiency of mitral or aortic valve with stenosis or insufficiency, or both, of the other valve

  396.9 Mitral and aortic valve diseases, unspecified

● **397 Diseases of other endocardial structures**
  Affects thin serous endothelial tissue that lines inside of heart

  397.0 Diseases of tricuspid valve
  Tricuspid (valve) (rheumatic):
      disease
      insufficiency
      obstruction
      regurgitation
      stenosis
  Coding Clinic: 2006, Q3, P7; 2000, Q2, P16-17

  397.1 Rheumatic diseases of pulmonary valve
      Excludes   *that not specified as rheumatic (424.3)*

  397.9 Rheumatic diseases of endocardium, valve unspecified
  Rheumatic:
      endocarditis (chronic)
      valvulitis (chronic)
      Excludes   *that not specified as rheumatic (424.90–424.99)*

● **398 Other rheumatic heart disease**

  398.0 Rheumatic myocarditis 🔎
  Rheumatic degeneration of myocardium
      Excludes   *myocarditis not specified as rheumatic (429.0)*
      (Ex:) 390, 391.2-391.9, 398.0-398.90, 398.99, 422.0-422.99, 429.0, 429.71-429.79, 459.89-459.9

● **398.9 Other and unspecified rheumatic heart diseases**

  398.90 Rheumatic heart disease, unspecified
  Rheumatic:
      carditis
      heart disease NOS
      Excludes   *carditis not specified as rheumatic (429.89)*
      heart disease NOS not specified as rheumatic (429.9)

  398.91 Rheumatic heart failure (congestive) 🔎
  Rheumatic left ventricular failure
      (Ex:) 398.90-398.99, 402.01, 402.11, 402.91, 428.0-428.9, 459.89-459.9
  Coding Clinic: 2005, Q2, P14-15; 1995, Q1, P6

  398.99 Other

Item 7–6 Hypertension is caused by high arterial blood pressure in the arteries. **Essential, primary,** or **idiopathic** hypertension occurs without identifiable organic cause.
Secondary hypertension is that which has an organic cause. **Malignant** hypertension is severely elevated blood pressure. **Benign** hypertension is mildly elevated blood pressure.

HYPERTENSIVE DISEASE (401–405)

  Excludes   *that complicating pregnancy, childbirth, or the puerperium (642.0–642.9)*
  that involving coronary vessels (410.00–414.9)

● **401 Essential hypertension**

  Includes   high blood pressure
  hyperpiesia
  hyperpiesis
  hypertension (arterial) (essential) (primary) (systemic)
  hypertensive vascular:
      degeneration
      disease

  Excludes   *elevated blood pressure without diagnosis of hypertension (796.2)*
  pulmonary hypertension (416.0–416.9)
  that involving vessels of:
      brain (430–438)
      eye (362.11)
  Coding Clinic: 1992, Q2, P5

  401.0 Malignant 🔎
      (Ex:) 401.0-405.99, 459.89-459.9
  Coding Clinic: 1993, Q4, P37; 5th Issue, P9-10

  401.1 Benign
  MCE: Questionable admission, principal diagnosis only

  401.9 Unspecified
  Coding Clinic: 2012, Q1, P14; 2010, Q4, P124-125, 135; 2009, Q4, P101-102; Q1, P6; 2008, Q2, P16; 2005, Q4, P68-69; Q3, P3-9; 2004, Q4, P77-78; 2003, Q4, P105-106, 108, 111; Q3, P14-15; Q2, P16; 1997, Q4, P35-37; 1989, Q2, P12; 1987, Sept-Oct, P11

  OGCR   Section I.C.7.a.2
  Heart conditions (425.8, 429.0-429.3, 429.8, 429.9) are assigned to a code from category 402 when a causal relationship is stated (due to hypertension) or implied (hypertensive). Use an additional code from category 428 to identify the type of heart failure in those patients with heart failure. More than one code from category 428 may be assigned if the patient has systolic or diastolic failure and congestive heart failure. The same heart conditions (425.8, 429.0-429.3, 429.8, 429.9) with hypertension, but without a stated causal relationship, are coded separately. Sequence according to the circumstances of the admission/ encounter.

● **402 Hypertensive heart disease**

  Includes   hypertensive:
      cardiomegaly
      cardiopathy
      cardiovascular disease
      heart (disease) (failure)
      any condition classifiable to 429.0–429.3, 429.8, 429.9 due to hypertension
  Use additional code to specify type of heart failure (428.0–428.43), if known
  Coding Clinic: 1993, Q2, P9; 1987, Nov-Dec, P9

● **402.0 Malignant**

  402.00 Without heart failure 🔎
      (Ex:) 401.0-405.99, 459.89-459.9
  Coding Clinic: 2008, Q4, P177-180

  402.01 With heart failure 🔎
      (Ex:) 398.91, 401.0-405.99, 428.0-428.9, 459.89-459.9

N Newborn: 0   **P** Pediatric: 0–17   **M** Maternity: 12–55   **A** Adult: 15–124   ♀ Females Only   ♂ Males Only

(Ex:) CC/MCC Exclusions   🔎 Complication\Comorbidity   🔎 Major C\C   🔎 Present on Admission Requirement   🔎 Hospital-Acquired Condition   801

● 402.1 **Benign**
  402.10 **Without heart failure**
  402.11 **With heart failure**

● 402.9 **Unspecified**
  Coding Clinic: 1993, Q2, P9
  402.90 **Without heart failure**
  402.91 **With heart failure**
      Coding Clinic: 2002, Q4, P52; 1993, Q1, P19-20; 1989, Q2,
      P12; 1984, Nov-Dec, P18

OGCR Section I.C.7.a.3

Assign codes from category 403, Hypertensive chronic kidney disease, when conditions classified to category 585 or code 587 are present with hypertension. Unlike hypertension with heart disease, ICD-9-CM presumes a cause-and-effect relationship and classifies chronic kidney disease (CKD) with hypertension as hypertensive chronic kidney disease.

● 403 **Hypertensive chronic kidney disease**
  Includes   arteriolar nephritis
      arteriosclerosis of:
          kidney
          renal arterioles
      arteriosclerotic nephritis (chronic) (interstitial)
      hypertensive:
          nephropathy
          renal failure
          uremia (chronic)
      nephrosclerosis
      renal sclerosis with hypertension
      any condition classifiable to 585 and 587 with any
          condition classifiable to 401
  Excludes   *acute kidney failure (584.5–584.9)*
      renal disease stated as not due to hypertension
      renovascular hypertension (405.0–405.9 with
          fifth-digit 1)
  Coding Clinic: 2010, Q3, P13; 2003, Q1, P20-21; 1992, Q2, P5

The following fifth-digit subclassification is for use with category 403:

> 0 **with chronic kidney disease stage I through stage IV, or unspecified**
>   Use additional code to identify the stage of chronic kidney disease (585.1–585.4, 585.9)
> 1 **with chronic kidney disease stage V or end stage renal disease**
>   Use additional code to identify the stage of chronic kidney disease (585.5, 585.6)

● 403.0 **Malignant**🔖
  [0-1]   (Ex:) 401.0-405.99, 459.89-459.9
● 403.1 **Benign** 1🔖
  [0-1]   For code **403.11:** (Ex:) 401.0-405.99, 459.89-459.9
      Coding Clinic: 2010, Q3, P13
● 403.9 **Unspecified** 1🔖
  [0-1]   For code **403.91:** (Ex:) 401.0-405.99, 459.89-459.9, 585.6
      Coding Clinic: 2010, Q4, P137; 2008, Q1, P7-8, 10-11; 2007, Q2, P3;
      2006, Q4, P84-86; 2005, Q4, P68-69; 2004, Q1, P14-15; 2001,
      Q2, P11; 1987, Sept-Oct, P9, 11; 1985, Nov-Dec, P15

OGCR Section I.C.7.a.4

Assign codes from combination category 404, Hypertensive heart and chronic kidney disease, when both hypertensive kidney disease and hypertensive heart disease are stated in the diagnosis. Assume a relationship between the hypertension and the chronic kidney disease, whether or not the condition is so designated. Assign an additional code from category 428, to identify the type of heart failure. More than one code from category 428 may be assigned if the patient has systolic or diastolic failure and congestive heart failure.

● 404 **Hypertensive heart and chronic kidney disease**
  Includes   disease:
          cardiorenal
          cardiovascular renal
      any condition classifiable to 402 with any condition
          classifiable to 403
  Use additional code to specify type of heart failure
      (428.0–428.43), if known
  Coding Clinic: 2006, Q4, P84-86; 2005, Q4, P68-69

The following fifth-digit subclassification is for use with category 404:

> 0 **without heart failure and with chronic kidney disease stage I through stage IV, or unspecified**
>   Use additional code to identify the stage of chronic kidney disease (585.1–585.4, 585.9)
> 1 **with heart failure and with chronic kidney disease stage I through stage IV, or unspecified**
>   Use additional code to identify the stage of chronic kidney disease (585.1–585.4, 585.9)
> 2 **without heart failure and with chronic kidney disease stage V or end stage renal disease**
>   Use additional code to identify the stage of chronic kidney disease (585.5, 585.6)
> 3 **with heart failure and chronic kidney disease stage V or end stage renal disease**
>   Use additional code to identify the stage of chronic kidney disease (585.5, 585.6)

● 404.0 **Malignant**🔖
  [0-3]   (Ex:) 401.0-405.99, 459.89-459.9
● 404.1 **Benign** 1-3🔖
  [0-3]   For codes **404.11-404.13:** (Ex:) 401.0-405.99, 459.89-459.9
● 404.9 **Unspecified** 1-3🔖
  [0-3]   For codes **404.91-404.93:** (Ex:) 401.0-405.99, 459.89-459.9

● 405 **Secondary hypertension**
  ● 405.0 **Malignant**
      405.01 **Renovascular**🔖
          (Ex:) 401.0-405.99, 459.89-459.9
      405.09 **Other**
          (Ex:) 401.0-405.99, 459.89-459.9
  ● 405.1 **Benign**
      405.11 **Renovascular**
      405.19 **Other**
  ● 405.9 **Unspecified**
      405.91 **Renovascular**
      405.99 **Other**
          Coding Clinic: 2000, Q3, P4-5; 1987, Sept-Oct, P9, 11

◀ New   ◀▬ Revised   ~~deleted~~ Deleted   Excludes   Includes   Use additional   Code first   Omit code
● Unacceptable Principal Diagnosis   ● Use Additional Digit(s)   ▶ Manifestation Code   OGCR Official Guidelines   Coding Clinic

Zone of
injury
Zone of
infarction
Zone of
ischemia

Figure 7-2 Myocardial infarction.

Item 7-7   Myocardial infarction is a sudden decrease in the coronary artery blood flow that results in death of the heart muscle. Classifications are based on the affected heart tissue.

ISCHEMIC HEART DISEASE (410–414)

Includes   that with mention of hypertension

Use additional code to identify presence of hypertension (401.0–405.9)

● **410   Acute myocardial infarction**

Includes   cardiac infarction
coronary (artery):
embolism
occlusion
rupture
thrombosis
infarction of heart, myocardium, or ventricle
rupture of heart, myocardium, or ventricle
ST elevation (STEMI) and non-ST elevation
(NSTEMI) myocardial infarction
any condition classifiable to 414.1–414.9 specified as acute or with a stated duration of 8 weeks or less

Coding Clinic: 2006, Q2, P9; 1997, Q4, P37; 1994, Q4, P55; 1993, Q4, P39-41; 1992, Q1, P10; 1991, Q3, P18; 1986, Nov-Dec, P12

The following fifth-digit subclassification is for use with category 410:

> **0   episode of care unspecified**
> Use when the source document does not contain sufficient information for the assignment of fifth-digit 1 or 2.
> **1   initial episode of care**
> Use fifth-digit 1 to designate the first episode of care (regardless of facility site) for a newly diagnosed myocardial infarction. The fifth-digit 1 is assigned regardless of the number of times a patient may be transferred during the initial episode of care.
> **2   subsequent episode of care**
> Use fifth-digit 2 to designate an episode of care following the initial episode when the patient is admitted for further observation, evaluation or treatment for a myocardial infarction that has received initial treatment, but is still less than 8 weeks old.

● **410.0   Of anterolateral wall** 1
[0-2]   ST elevation myocardial infarction (STEMI) of anterolateral wall
For code **410.01:** (Ex) 410.00-410.92, 459.89-459.9
Coding Clinic: 2009, Q4, P102; 2008, Q4, P69-73; 2001, Q3, P21; 1998, Q3, P15; 1993, 5th Issue, P14, 17-24

● **410.1   Of other anterior wall** 1
[0-2]   Infarction:
anterior (wall) NOS (with contiguous portion of intraventricular septum)
anteroapical (with contiguous portion of intraventricular septum)
anteroseptal (with contiguous portion of intraventricular septum)
ST elevation myocardial infarction (STEMI) of other anterior wall
For code **410.11:** (Ex) 410.00-410.92, 459.89-459.9
Coding Clinic: 2003, Q3, P10-11

● **410.2   Of inferolateral wall** 1
[0-2]   ST elevation myocardial infarction (STEMI) of inferolateral wall
For code **410.31:** (Ex) 410.00-410.92, 459.89-459.9
Coding Clinic: 1993, 5th Issue, P17-24

● **410.3   Of inferoposterior wall** 1
[0-2]   ST elevation myocardial infarction (STEMI) of inferoposterior wall
For code **410.31:** (Ex) 410.00-410.92, 459.89-459.9

● **410.4   Of other inferior wall** 1
[0-2]   Infarction:
diaphragmatic wall NOS (with contiguous portion of intraventricular septum)
inferior (wall) NOS (with contiguous portion of intraventricular septum)
ST elevation myocardial infarction (STEMI) of other inferior wall
For code **410.41:** (Ex) 410.00-410.92, 459.89-459.9
Coding Clinic: 2009, Q3, P10; 2006, Q3, P8-9; 2001, Q2, P8-9; 2000, Q1, P7; 1997, Q3, P10; 1993, 5th Issue, P13-14x2

● **410.5   Of other lateral wall** 1
[0-2]   Infarction:
apical-lateral
basal-lateral
high lateral
posterolateral
ST elevation myocardial infarction (STEMI) of other lateral wall
For code **410.51:** (Ex) 410.00-410.92, 459.89-459.9
Coding Clinic: 2009, Q3, P7

● **410.6   True posterior wall infarction** 1
[0-2]   Infarction:
posterobasal
strictly posterior
ST elevation myocardial infarction (STEMI) of true posterior wall
For code **410.61:** (Ex) 410.00-410.92, 459.89-459.9

● **410.7   Subendocardial infarction** 1
[0-2]   Non-ST elevation myocardial infarction (NSTEMI)
Nontransmural infarction
For code **410.71:** (Ex) 410.00-410.92, 459.89-459.9
Coding Clinic: 2010, Q2, P9; 2005, Q4, P69-72; Q2, P19-20; 2000, Q1, P7

OGCR   Section I.C.7.e.1

> The ICD-9-CM codes for acute myocardial infarction (AMI) identify the site, such as anterolateral wall or true posterior wall. Subcategories 410.0–410.6 and 410.8 are used for ST elevation myocardial infarction (STEMI). Subcategory 410.7, Subendocardial infarction, is used for non ST elevation myocardial infarction (NSTEMI) and nontransmural MIs.

● **410.8   Of other specified sites** 1
[0-2]   Infarction of:
atrium
papillary muscle
septum alone
ST elevation myocardial infarction (STEMI) of other specified sites
For code **410.81:** (Ex) 410.00-410.92, 459.89-459.9

● **410.9   Unspecified site** 1
[0-2]   Acute myocardial infarction NOS
Coronary occlusion NOS
Myocardial infarction NOS
For code **410.91:** (Ex) 410.00-410.92, 459.89-459.9
Coding Clinic: 2005, Q2, P18-19; 2002, Q3, P5; 1999, Q4, P9; 1993, 5th Issue, P13

OGCR   Section I.C.7.e.2

> Subcategory 410.9 is the default for the unspecified term acute myocardial infarction. If only STEMI or transmural MI without the site is documented, query the provider as to the site, or assign a code from subcategory 410.9.

DISEASES OF THE CIRCULATORY SYSTEM (390–459)

N Newborn: 0   P Pediatric: 0–17   M Maternity: 12–55   A Adult: 15–124   ♀ Females Only   ♂ Males Only

(Ex) CC/MCC Exclusions   Complication\Comorbidity   Major C\C   Present on Admission Requirement   Hospital-Acquired Condition   **803**

Item 7–8   "Old" (healed) myocardial infarction: Code 412 cannot be used if the patient is experiencing current ischemic heart disease symptoms. Recent infarctions still under care cannot be coded to 412. This code is only assigned if infarction has some impact on the current episode of care—essentially, it is a history of (H/O) a past, healed MI. (There is no V code for this status/post MI.)

●411   **Other acute and subacute forms of ischemic heart disease**
    Coding Clinic: 1994, Q4, P55

    411.0   **Postmyocardial infarction syndrome** 🔍
        Dressler's syndrome
        (Ex) 411.0, 411.81-411.89, 459.89-459.9

    411.1   **Intermediate coronary syndrome** 🔍
        Impending infarction
        Preinfarction angina
        Preinfarction syndrome
        Unstable angina
            Excludes   *angina (pectoris) (413.9)*
                            decubitus (413.0)
        (Ex) 398.91, 402.01, 402.11, 402.91, 404.01, 404.03, 404.11, 404.13, 404.91, 404.93, 410.00-410.92, 411.1-411.89, 413.0-414.00, 414.2-414.3, 414.8-414.9, 428.0-428.1, 428.9, 459.89-459.9, 785.50-785.51
        Coding Clinic: 2005, Q4, P103-106; 2004, Q2, P3-4; 2003, Q1, P12-13; 2001, Q3, P15; Q2, P7-9; 1998, Q4, P85-86; 1996, Q2, P10; 1995, Q2, P18-19; 1993, Q4, P39-40; 5th Issue, P17-24; 1991, Q1, P14; 1989, Q4, P10

●411.8   **Other**
    411.81   **Acute coronary occlusion without myocardial infarction** 🔍
        Acute coronary (artery):
            embolism without or not resulting in myocardial infarction
            obstruction without or not resulting in myocardial infarction
            occlusion without or not resulting in myocardial infarction
            thrombosis without or not resulting in myocardial infarction
                Excludes   *obstruction without infarction due to atherosclerosis (414.00–414.07)*
                                occlusion without infarction due to atherosclerosis (414.00–414.07)
            (Ex) 410.00-411.89, 413.0-413.9, 414.8-414.9, 459.89-459.9
            Coding Clinic: 2001, Q2, P7-8; 1991, Q3, P18; Q1, P14

    411.89   **Other** 🔍
        Coronary insufficiency (acute)
        Subendocardial ischemia
        (Ex) 410.00-411.89, 413.0-413.9, 414.8-414.9, 459.89-459.9
        Coding Clinic: 2001, Q3, P14; 1992, Q1, P9-10; 1991, Q3, P18

412   **Old myocardial infarction** 🔍
    Healed myocardial infarction
    Past myocardial infarction diagnosed on ECG [EKG] or other special investigation, but currently presenting no symptoms
    Coding Clinic: 2003, Q2, P10; 2001, Q3, P21; Q2, P9; 1998, Q3, P15; 1993, 5th Issue, P17-24

●413   **Angina pectoris**
    Chest pain/discomfort due to lack of oxygen to heart muscle. Principal symptom of myocardial infarction.

    413.0   **Angina decubitus** 🔍
        Nocturnal angina
        (Ex) 410.00-410.92, 411.1-411.89, 413.0-413.9, 414.8-414.9, 459.89-459.9

    413.1   **Prinzmetal angina** 🔍
        Variant angina pectoris
        (Ex) 410.00-410.92, 411.1-411.89, 413.0-413.9, 414.8-414.9, 459.89-459.9
        Coding Clinic: 2006, Q3, P23

    413.9   **Other and unspecified angina pectoris**
        Angina: Anginal syndrome
            NOS   Status anginosus
            cardiac   Stenocardia
            equivalent   Syncope anginosa
            of effort
            Excludes   *preinfarction angina (411.1)*
        Use additional code(s) for symptoms associated with angina equivalent
        Coding Clinic: 2008, Q2, P16, 2003, Q1, P12-13; 2002, Q3, P4-5; 1995, Q2, P18; 1993, 5th Issue, P17-24; 1991, Q3, P16; 1985, Sept-Oct, P9

●414   **Other forms of chronic ischemic heart disease**
    Excludes   *arteriosclerotic cardiovascular disease [ASCVD] (429.2)*
                    cardiovascular:
                        arteriosclerosis or sclerosis (429.2)
                        degeneration or disease (429.2)

●414.0   **Coronary atherosclerosis**
    Arteriosclerotic heart disease [ASHD]
    Atherosclerotic heart disease
    Coronary (artery):
        arteriosclerosis
        arteritis or endarteritis
        atheroma
        sclerosis
        stricture
    Use additional code, if applicable, to identify chronic total occlusion of coronary artery (414.2)
        Excludes   *embolism of graft (996.72)*
                        occlusion NOS of graft (996.72)
                        thrombus of graft (996.72)
    Coding Clinic: 2002, Q3, P3-9; 1994, Q2, P13, 15; Q1, P6-7; 1993, Q1, P20; 5th Issue, P17-24; 5th Issue, P14; 1984, Nov-Dec, P18

    414.00   **Of unspecified type of vessel, native or graft**   A
        Coding Clinic: 2003, Q2, P16; 2001, Q3, P15; 1997, Q3, P15; 1996, Q4, P31

    414.01   **Of native coronary artery**   A
        Coding Clinic: 2012, Q3, P17; 2009, Q3, P8; 2008, Q3, P10-11; Q2, P16; 2006, Q3, P25; 2005, Q4, P68-69; 2004, Q2, P3-4; 2003, Q4, P105-106, 108-109; Q3, P9.10, 14; 2001, Q3, P15-16; Q2, P8-9; 1997, Q3, P15; 1996, Q2, P10; 1995, Q2, P17-19

    414.02   **Of autologous biological bypass graft** 🔍   A
        (Ex) 414.00-414.05, 414.07, 414.2-414.3-414.4
        Coding Clinic: 2010, Q2, P9; 1995, Q2, P18-19

    414.03   **Of nonautologous biological bypass graft** 🔍   A
        (Ex) 414.00-414.05, 414.07, 414.2-414.3-414.4

    414.04   **Of artery bypass graft** 🔍   A
        Internal mammary artery
        (Ex) 414.00-414.05, 414.07, 414.2-414.3-414.4

    414.05   **Of unspecified type of bypass graft**   A
        Bypass graft NOS
        Coding Clinic: 1997, Q3, P15; 1996, Q4, P31

    414.06   **Of native coronary artery of transplanted heart** 🔍   A
        (Ex) 414.00-414.07, 414.2-414.3-414.4
        Coding Clinic: 2003, Q4, P60; 2002, Q4, P53-54; Q4, P53-54

    414.07   **Of bypass graft (artery) (vein) of transplanted heart** 🔍   A
        (Ex) 414.00-414.06, 414.2-414.3-414.4
        Coding Clinic: 2003, Q4, P60

Figure 7–3 Atherosclerosis. (From Buck CJ: Step-by-Step Medical Coding, ed 2008, Philadelphia, WB Saunders, 2008)

Item 7–9 Classification is based on the location of the atherosclerosis. **"Of native coronary artery"** indicates the atherosclerosis is within an original heart artery. **"Of autologous vein bypass graft"** indicates that the atherosclerosis is within a vein graft that was taken from within the patient. **"Of nonautologous biological bypass graft"** indicates the atherosclerosis is within a vessel grafted from other than the patient. **"Of artery bypass graft"** indicates the atherosclerosis is within an artery that was grafted from within the patient.

- **414.1 Aneurysm and dissection of heart**
    - **414.10 Aneurysm of heart (wall)**🔹
      Aneurysm (arteriovenous):
        mural
        ventricular
      Ⓔₓ 414.10-414.11, 414.19
    - **414.11 Aneurysm of coronary vessels**
      Aneurysm (arteriovenous) of coronary vessels
      Coding Clinic: 2010, Q2, P9; 1999, Q1, P17-18
    - **414.12 Dissection of coronary artery**🔹
      Ⓔₓ 414.12, 443.29, 447.2, 447.5-447.6, 447.8-447.9
      Coding Clinic: 2011, Q1, P3-4; 2002, Q4, P54-55
    - **414.19 Other aneurysm of heart**🔹
      Arteriovenous fistula, acquired, of heart
      Ⓔₓ 414.10-414.11, 414.19
- **414.2 Chronic total occlusion of coronary artery**
    Complete occlusion of coronary artery
    Total occlusion of coronary artery
    Code first coronary atherosclerosis (414.00–414.07)
    Excludes *acute coronary occlusion with myocardial infarction (410.00–410.92)*
    acute coronary occlusion without myocardial infarction (411.81)
    Coding Clinic: 2007, Q4, P82
- **414.3 Coronary atherosclerosis due to lipid rich plaque**   A
    Code first coronary atherosclerosis (414.00–414.07)
    Coding Clinic: 2008, Q4, P113
- **414.4 Coronary atherosclerosis due to calcified coronary lesion**
    Coronary atherosclerosis due to severely calcified coronary lesion
    Code first coronary atherosclerosis (414.00–414.07)
- **414.8 Other specified forms of chronic ischemic heart disease**
    Chronic coronary insufficiency
    Ischemia, myocardial (chronic)
    Any condition classifiable to 410 specified as chronic, or presenting with symptoms after 8 weeks from date of infarction
    Excludes *coronary insufficiency (acute) (411.89)*
    Coding Clinic: 2003, Q2, P10; 2001, Q3, P15-16; 1992, Q1, P10; 1990, Q3, P15; Q2, P19; 1986, Nov-Dec, P12
- **414.9 Chronic ischemic heart disease, unspecified**
    Ischemic heart disease NOS
    Coding Clinic: 2001, Q3, P15-16

Item 7–10 Pulmonary heart disease or cor pulmonale is right ventricle hypertrophy or RVH as a result of a respiratory disorder increasing back flow pressure to the right ventricle. Left untreated, cor pulmonale leads to right-heart failure and death.

DISEASES OF PULMONARY CIRCULATION (415–417)

- **415 Acute pulmonary heart disease**
    - **415.0 Acute cor pulmonale**🔹
      Excludes *cor pulmonale NOS (416.9)*
      Ⓔₓ 415.0, 416.8-416.9, 459.89-459.9
    - **415.1 Pulmonary embolism and infarction**
      Pulmonary (artery) (vein):
        apoplexy   infarction (hemorrhagic)
        embolism   thrombosis
      Excludes *chronic pulmonary embolism (416.2)*
        personal history of pulmonary embolism (V12.55)
        that complicating:
          abortion (634–638 with .6, 639.6)
          ectopic or molar pregnancy (639.6)
          pregnancy, childbirth, or the puerperium (673.0–673.8)
        - **415.11 Iatrogenic pulmonary embolism and infarction**🔹
          Use additional code for associated septic pulmonary embolism, if applicable, 415.12
          HAC: And one of the following procedure codes:
          00.85-00.87, 81.51-81.52, 81.54
          Ⓔₓ 415.11-415.19, 416.2, 444.01-444.09,459.89-459.9
          Coding Clinic: 1990, Q4, P25
        - **415.12 Septic pulmonary embolism**🔹
          Septic embolism NOS
          Code first underlying infection, such as:
            septicemia (038.0–038.9)
          Excludes *septic arterial embolism (449)*
          Ⓔₓ 415.11-415.19, 416.2, 444.01-444.09, 459.89-459.9
          Coding Clinic: 2007, Q4, P84-86
        - **415.13 Saddle embolus of pulmonary artery**🔹🔹
          Ⓔₓ 415.11-415.19, 416.2, 444.01-444.09, 459.89-459.9
        - **415.19 Other**🔹🔹
          HAC: And one of the following procedure codes:
          00.85-00.87, 81.51-81.52, 81.54
          Ⓔₓ 415.11-415.19, 416.2, 444.01-444.09, 459.89-459.9
          Coding Clinic: 2010, Q3, P11; 1998, Q2, P8
- **416 Chronic pulmonary heart disease**
    - **416.0 Primary pulmonary hypertension**🔹
      Idiopathic pulmonary arteriosclerosis
      Pulmonary hypertension (essential) (idiopathic) (primary)
      Excludes *pulmonary hypertension NOS (416.8)*
        secondary pulmonary hypertension (416.8)
      Ⓔₓ 278.03, 416.0, 416.8-416.9, 417.8-417.9, 459.89-459.9
      Coding Clinic: 2010, Q2, P11
    - **416.1 Kyphoscoliotic heart disease**🔹
      Ⓔₓ 278.03, 416.0, 416.1, 416.8-416.9
    - **416.2 Chronic pulmonary embolism**🔹
      Use additional code, if applicable, for associated long-term (current) use of anticoagulants (V58.61)
      Excludes *personal history of pulmonary embolism (V12.55)*
      Ⓔₓ 415.11-415.19, 416.2, 444.01-444.09, 459.89-459.9
    - **416.8 Other chronic pulmonary heart diseases**
      Pulmonary hypertension NOS
      Pulmonary hypertension, secondary
      Coding Clinic: 2012, Q1, P17; 2011, Q1, P10; 2010, Q3, P13; Q2, P10-11
    - **416.9 Chronic pulmonary heart disease, unspecified**
      Chronic cardiopulmonary disease
      Cor pulmonale (chronic) NOS

DISEASES OF THE CIRCULATORY SYSTEM (390–459)

| N | Newborn: 0 | P | Pediatric: 0–17 | M | Maternity: 12–55 | A | Adult: 15–124 | ♀ | Females Only | ♂ | Males Only |

Ⓔₓ CC/MCC Exclusions   🔹 Complication\Comorbidity   🔹 Major C\C   🔹 Present on Admission Requirement   🔹 Hospital-Acquired Condition   **805**

DISEASES OF THE CIRCULATORY SYSTEM (390–459)

●417   **Other diseases of pulmonary circulation**

     417.0   **Arteriovenous fistula of pulmonary vessels** 🔍

         Excludes   *congenital arteriovenous fistula (747.32)*

         Ex: 417.0-417.9

     417.1   **Aneurysm of pulmonary artery** 🔍

         Excludes   *congenital aneurysm (747.39)*

                      congenital arteriovenous aneurysm (747.32)

         Ex: 417.0-417.9

     417.8   **Other specified diseases of pulmonary circulation**

         Pulmonary:

            arteritis

            endarteritis

         Rupture of pulmonary vessel

         Stricture of pulmonary vessel

     417.9   **Unspecified disease of pulmonary circulation**

OTHER FORMS OF HEART DISEASE (420–429)

●420   **Acute pericarditis**

     Inflammation of the sac surrounding the heart caused by infection. The chest pain is significant on inspiration, and onset is sudden and worst when lying down.

     Includes   acute:

            mediastinopericarditis

            myopericarditis

            pericardial effusion

            pleuropericarditis

            pneumopericarditis

     Excludes   *acute rheumatic pericarditis (391.0)*

                    postmyocardial infarction syndrome [Dressler's] (411.0)

  ▷ 420.0   ***Acute pericarditis in diseases classified elsewhere*** 🔍

         Code first underlying disease, as:

            actinomycosis (039.8)

            amebiasis (006.8)

            chronic uremia (585.9)

            nocardiosis (039.8)

            tuberculosis (017.9)

            uremia NOS (586)

         Excludes   *pericarditis (acute) (in):*

                    Coxsackie (virus) (074.21)

                    gonococcal (098.83)

                    histoplasmosis (115.0–115.9 with fifth-digit 3)

                    meningococcal infection (036.41)

                    syphilitic (093.81)

         Ex: 391.0, 393, 420.0-420.99, 423.3-423.9, 459.89-459.9

●420.9   **Other and unspecified acute pericarditis**

     420.90   **Acute pericarditis, unspecified** 🔍

         Pericarditis (acute):

            NOS

            infective NOS

            sicca

         Ex: 391.0, 393, 420.0-420.99, 423.3-423.9, 459.89-459.9

         Coding Clinic: 1989, Q2, P12

     420.91   **Acute idiopathic pericarditis** 🔍

         Pericarditis, acute:

            benign

            nonspecific

            viral

         Ex: 391.0, 393, 420.0-420.99, 423.3-423.9, 459.89-459.9

     420.99   **Other** 🔍

         Pericarditis (acute):

            pneumococcal

            purulent

            staphylococcal

            streptococcal

            suppurative

         Pneumopyopericardium

         Pyopericardium

         Excludes   *pericarditis in diseases classified elsewhere (420.0)*

         Ex: 391.0, 393, 420.0-420.99, 423.3-423.9, 459.89-459.9

●421   **Acute and subacute endocarditis**

     Inflammation/infection of lining of heart, affecting heart valves, usually caused by bacterial infection

     421.0   **Acute and subacute bacterial endocarditis** 🔍

         Endocarditis (acute) (chronic) (subacute):

            bacterial

            infective NOS

            lenta

            malignant

            purulent

            septic

            ulcerative

            vegetative

         Infective aneurysm

         Subacute bacterial endocarditis [SBE]

         Use additional code, if desired, to identify infectious organism [e.g., Streptococcus 041.0, Staphylococcus 041.1]

         Ex: 391.1, 397.9, 421.0-421.9, 424.90-424.99, 459.89-459.9

         Coding Clinic: 2008, Q4, P69-73; 2006, Q2, P16-17; 1999, Q1, P12; 1991, Q1, P15

  ▷ 421.1   ***Acute and subacute infective endocarditis in diseases classified elsewhere*** 🔍

         Code first underlying disease, as:

            blastomycosis (116.0)

            Q fever (083.0)

            typhoid (fever) (002.0)

         Excludes   *endocarditis (in):*

                    Coxsackie (virus) (074.22)

                    gonococcal (098.84)

                    histoplasmosis (115.0–115.9 with fifth-digit 4)

                    meningococcal infection (036.42)

                    monilial (112.81)

         Ex: 391.1, 397.9, 421.0-421.9, 424.90-424.99, 459.89-459.9

     421.9   **Acute endocarditis, unspecified** 🔍

         Endocarditis, acute or subacute

         Myoendocarditis, acute or subacute

         Periendocarditis, acute or subacute

         Excludes   *acute rheumatic endocarditis (391.1)*

         Ex: 391.1, 397.9, 421.0-421.9, 424.90-424.99, 459.89-459.9

●422   **Acute myocarditis**

     An inflammation of the heart muscle due to an infection (viral/ bacterial)

     Excludes   *acute rheumatic myocarditis (391.2)*

  ▷ 422.0   ***Acute myocarditis in diseases classified elsewhere*** 🔍

         Code first underlying disease, as:

         myocarditis (acute):

            influenzal (487.8, 488.09, 488.19)

            tuberculous (017.9)

         Excludes   *myocarditis (acute) (due to):*

                    aseptic, of newborn (074.23)

                    Coxsackie (virus) (074.23)

                    diphtheritic (032.82)

                    meningococcal infection (036.43)

                    syphilitic (093.82)

                    toxoplasmosis (130.3)

         Ex: 391.2, 398.0, 422.0-422.99, 429.0, 429.71-429.79, 459.89-459.9

●422.9   **Other and unspecified acute myocarditis**

     422.90   **Acute myocarditis, unspecified** 🔍

         Acute or subacute (interstitial) myocarditis

         Ex: 391.2, 398.0, 422.0-422.99, 429.0, 429.71-429.79, 459.89-459.9

     422.91   **Idiopathic myocarditis** 🔍

         Myocarditis (acute or subacute):

            Fiedler's

            giant cell

            isolated (diffuse) (granulomatous)

            nonspecific granulomatous

         Ex: 391.2, 398.0, 422.0-422.99, 429.0, 429.71-429.79, 459.89-459.9

◀ New   ◀◀ Revised   ~~deleted~~ Deleted   Excludes   Includes   Use additional   Code first   Omit code

● Unacceptable Principal Diagnosis   ● Use Additional Digit(s)   ▷ Manifestation Code   **OGCR** Official Guidelines   **Coding Clinic**

806

422.92 **Septic myocarditis** 🔖
Myocarditis, acute or subacute:
pneumococcal
staphylococcal
Use additional code to identify infectious
organism [e.g., Staphylococcus 041.1]
Excludes *myocarditis, acute or subacute:*
in bacterial diseases classified
elsewhere (422.0)
streptococcal (391.2)
(Ex:) 391.2, 398.0, 422.0-422.99, 429.0, 429.71-429.79, 459.89-459.9

422.93 **Toxic myocarditis** 🔖
(Ex:) 391.2, 398.0, 422.0-422.99, 429.0, 429.71-429.79, 459.89-459.9

422.99 **Other** 🔖
(Ex:) 391.2, 398.0, 422.0-422.99, 429.0, 429.71-429.79, 459.89-459.9

● 423 **Other diseases of pericardium**
Excludes *that specified as rheumatic (393)*

423.0 **Hemopericardium** 🔖
(Ex:) 423.0-423.9, 459.89-459.9

423.1 **Adhesive pericarditis** 🔖
Adherent pericardium
Fibrosis of pericardium
Milk spots
Pericarditis:
adhesive
obliterative
Soldiers' patches
(Ex:) 423.0-423.9, 459.89-459.9

423.2 **Constrictive pericarditis** 🔖
Concato's disease
Pick's disease of heart (and liver)
(Ex:) 423.0-423.9, 459.89-459.9

● 423.3 **Cardiac tamponade** 🔖
Code first the underlying cause
(Ex:) 074.21, 093.81, 391.0, 393, 420.0-420.99, 423.3-423.9, 459.89-459.9
Coding Clinic: 2007, Q4, P86-87; 2007, Q2, P11-12

423.8 **Other specified diseases of pericardium** 🔖
Calcification of pericardium
Fistula of pericardium
(Ex:) 074.21, 093.81, 391.0, 393, 420.0-420.99, 423.3-423.9, 459.89-459.9
Coding Clinic: 1989, Q2, P12

423.9 **Unspecified disease of pericardium** 🔖
(Ex:) 074.21, 093.81, 391.0, 393, 420.0-420.99, 423.3-423.9, 459.89-459.9
Coding Clinic: 2007, Q2, P11-12

● 424 **Other diseases of endocardium**
Excludes *bacterial endocarditis (421.0–421.9)*
rheumatic endocarditis (391.1, 394.0–397.9)
syphilitic endocarditis (093.20–093.24)

424.0 **Mitral valve disorders**
Mitral (valve):
incompetence NOS of specified cause, except
rheumatic
insufficiency NOS of specified cause, except
rheumatic
regurgitation NOS of specified cause, except
rheumatic
Excludes *mitral (valve):*
disease (394.9)
failure (394.9)
stenosis (394.0)
the listed conditions:
specified as rheumatic (394.1)
unspecified as to cause but with mention of:
diseases of aortic valve (396.0–396.9)
mitral stenosis or obstruction (394.2)
Coding Clinic: 2006, Q3, P7; 2000, Q2, P16-17; 1998, Q3, P11; 1987,
Nov-Dec, P8

424.1 **Aortic valve disorders** 🔖
Aortic (valve):
incompetence NOS of specified cause, except
rheumatic
insufficiency NOS of specified cause, except
rheumatic
regurgitation NOS of specified cause, except
rheumatic
stenosis NOS of specified cause, except rheumatic
Excludes *hypertrophic subaortic stenosis (425.11)*
that specified as rheumatic (395.0–395.9)
that of unspecified cause but with mention of
diseases of mitral valve (396.0–396.9)
Coding Clinic: 2011, Q4, P152; 2008, Q4, P177-180; 1988, Q4, P8;
1987, Nov-Dec, P8

424.2 **Tricuspid valve disorders, specified as nonrheumatic**
Tricuspid valve:
incompetence of specified cause, except rheumatic
insufficiency of specified cause, except rheumatic
regurgitation of specified cause, except rheumatic
stenosis of specified cause, except rheumatic
Excludes *rheumatic or of unspecified cause (397.0)*

424.3 **Pulmonary valve disorders**
Pulmonic:
incompetence NOS
insufficiency NOS
regurgitation NOS
stenosis NOS
Excludes *that specified as rheumatic (397.1)*

● 424.9 **Endocarditis, valve unspecified**

424.90 **Endocarditis, valve unspecified, unspecified**
cause 🔖
Endocarditis (chronic):
NOS
nonbacterial thrombotic
Valvular:
incompetence of unspecified valve,
unspecified cause
insufficiency of unspecified valve, unspecified
cause
regurgitation of unspecified valve, unspecified
cause
stenosis of unspecified valve, unspecified
cause
Valvulitis (chronic)
(Ex:) 424.90-424.99, 459.89-459.9

▷ 424.91 *Endocarditis in diseases classified elsewhere* 🔖
Code first underlying disease, as:
atypical verrucous endocarditis
[Libman-Sacks] (710.0)
disseminated lupus erythematosus (710.0)
tuberculosis (017.9)
Excludes *syphilitic (093.20–093.24)*
(Ex:) 424.90-424.99, 459.89-459.9

424.99 **Other** 🔖
Any condition classifiable to 424.90 with
specified cause, except rheumatic
Excludes *endocardial fibroelastosis (425.3)*
that specified as rheumatic (397.9)
(Ex:) 424.90-424.99, 459.89-459.9

DISEASES OF THE CIRCULATORY SYSTEM (390–459)

N Newborn: 0   P Pediatric: 0–17   M Maternity: 12–55   A Adult: 15–124   ♀ Females Only   ♂ Males Only

(Ex:) CC/MCC Exclusions   🔖 Complication\Comorbidity   Major C\C   Present on Admission Requirement   Hospital-Acquired Condition   **807**

● 425 **Cardiomyopathy**
Disease of the heart muscle resulting in abnormally enlarged, weakened, thickened, and/or stiffened muscle causing an inability to pump blood normally and leads to CHF

Includes myocardiopathy

425.0 **Endomyocardial fibrosis**
(Ex:) 398.91, 402.01, 402.11, 402.91, 404.01, 404.03, 404.11, 404.13, 404.91, 404.93, 414.00-414.07, 414.2-414.9, 425.0-425.9, 426.10-426.13, 426.50-426.54, 426.81-426.89, 427.31-427.42, 427.60-427.89, 428.0-428.1, 428.9, 459.89-459.9, 746.86, 785.0-785.1, 785.50-785.51

● 425.1 **Hypertrophic cardiomyopathy**
Excludes ventricular hypertrophy (429.3)

425.11 **Hypertrophic obstructive cardiomyopathy**
Hypertrophic subaortic stenosis (idiopathic)
(Ex:) 398.91, 402.01, 402.11, 402.91, 404.01, 404.03, 404.11, 404.13, 404.91, 404.93, 414.00-414.07, 414.2-414.9, 425.0-425.9, 426.10-426.13, 426.50-425.54, 426.81-426.89, 427.31-427.42, 427.60-427.89, 428.0-428.1, 428.9, 459.89-459.9, 746.86, 785.0-785.1, 785.50-785.51
Coding Clinic: 2013, Q3, P10

425.18 **Other hypertrophic cardiomyopathy**
Nonobstructive hypertrophic cardiomyopathy
(Ex:) 398.91, 402.01, 402.11, 402.91, 404.01, 404.03, 404.11, 404.13, 404.91, 404.93, 414.00-414.07, 414.2-414.9, 425.0-425.9, 426.10-426.13, 426.50-425.54, 426.81-426.89, 427.31-427.42, 427.60-427.89, 428.0-428.1, 428.9, 459.89-459.9, 746.86, 785.0-785.1, 785.50-785.51

425.2 **Obscure cardiomyopathy of Africa**
Becker's disease
Idiopathic mural endomyocardial disease
(Ex:) 398.91, 402.01, 402.11, 402.91, 404.01, 404.03, 404.11, 404.13, 404.91, 404.93, 414.00-414.07, 414.2-414.9, 425.0-425.9, 426.10-426.13, 426.50-426.54, 426.81-426.89, 427.31-427.42, 427.60-427.89, 428.0-428.1, 428.9, 459.89-459.9, 746.86, 785.0-785.1, 785.50-785.51

425.3 **Endocardial fibroelastosis**
Elastomyofibrosis
(Ex:) 398.91, 402.01, 402.11, 402.91, 404.01, 404.03, 404.11, 404.13, 404.91, 404.93, 414.00-414.07, 414.2-414.9, 425.0-425.9, 426.10-426.13, 426.50-426.54, 426.81-426.89, 427.31-427.42, 427.60-427.89, 428.0-428.1, 428.9, 459.89-459.9, 746.86, 785.0-785.1, 785.50-785.51

425.4 **Other primary cardiomyopathies**
Cardiomyopathy:
  NOS
  congestive
  constrictive
  familial
  idiopathic
  obstructive
  restrictive
Cardiovascular collagenosis
(Ex:) 398.91, 402.01, 402.11, 402.91, 404.01, 404.03, 404.11, 404.13, 404.91, 404.93, 414.00-414.07, 414.2-414.9, 425.0-425.9, 426.10-426.13, 426.50-426.54, 426.81-426.89, 427.31-427.42, 427.60-427.89, 428.0-428.1, 428.9, 459.89-459.9, 746.86, 785.0-785.1, 785.50-785.51
Coding Clinic: 2009, Q4, P102; 2007, Q1, P20; 2005, Q2, P14-15; 2000, Q1, P22; 1997, Q4, P54-55; 1990, Q2, P19; 1985, Sept-Oct, P15

425.5 **Alcoholic cardiomyopathy**
(Ex:) 398.91, 402.01, 402.11, 402.91, 404.01, 404.03, 404.11, 404.13, 404.91, 404.93, 414.00-414.07, 414.2-414.9, 425.0-425.9 426.10-426.13, 426.50-426.54, 426.81-426.89, 427.31-427.42, 427.60-427.89, 428.0-428.1, 428.9, 459.89-459.9, 746.86, 785.0-785.1, 785.50-785.51
Coding Clinic: 1985, Sept-Oct, P15; July-Aug, P15

▷ 425.7 **Nutritional and metabolic cardiomyopathy**
Code first underlying disease, as:
  amyloidosis (277.30–277.39)
  beriberi (265.0)
  cardiac glycogenosis (271.0)
  mucopolysaccharidosis (277.5)
  thyrotoxicosis (242.0–242.9)
Excludes gouty tophi of heart (274.82)
(Ex:) 398.91, 402.01, 402.11, 402.91, 404.01, 404.03, 404.11, 404.13, 404.91, 404.93, 414.00-414.07, 414.2-414.9, 425.0-425.9, 426.10-426.13, 426.50-426.54, 426.81-426.89, 427.31-427.42, 427.60-427.89, 428.0-428.1, 428.9, 459.89-459.9, 746.86, 785.0-785.1, 785.50-785.51

▷ 425.8 **Cardiomyopathy in other diseases classified elsewhere**
Code first underlying disease, as:
  Friedreich's ataxia (334.0)
  myotonia atrophica (359.21)
  progressive muscular dystrophy (359.1)
  sarcoidosis (135)
Excludes cardiomyopathy in Chagas' disease (086.0)
(Ex:) 398.91, 402.01, 402.11, 402.91, 404.01, 404.03, 404.11, 404.13, 404.91, 404.93, 414.00-414.07, 414.2-414.9, 425.0-425.9, 426.10-426.13, 426.50-426.54, 426.81-426.89, 427.31-427.42, 427.60-427.89, 428.0-428.1, 428.9, 459.89-459.9, 746.86, 785.0-785.1, 785.50-785.51
Coding Clinic: 1993, Q2, P9

425.9 **Secondary cardiomyopathy, unspecified**
(Ex:) 398.91, 402.01, 402.11, 402.91, 404.01, 404.03, 404.11, 404.13, 404.91, 404.93, 414.00-414.07, 414.2-414.9, 425.0-425.9, 426.10-426.13, 426.50-426.54, 426.81-426.89, 427.31-427.42, 427.60-427.89, 428.0-428.1, 428.9, 459.89-459.9, 746.86, 785.0-785.1, 785.50-785.51

● 426 **Conduction disorders**
Heart block or atrioventricular block (AV block) caused by conduction problem resulting in arrhythmias/dysrhythmias due to lack of electrical impulses being transmitted normally through heart

426.0 **Atrioventricular block, complete**
Third degree atrioventricular block
(Ex:) 426.0-427.5, 427.89, 459.89-459.9
Coding Clinic: 2006, Q2, P14

● 426.1 **Atrioventricular block, other and unspecified**

426.10 **Atrioventricular block, unspecified**
Atrioventricular [AV] block (incomplete) (partial)

426.11 **First degree atrioventricular block**
Incomplete atrioventricular block, first degree
Prolonged P-R interval NOS
Coding Clinic: 2006, Q2, P14

426.12 **Mobitz (type) II atrioventricular block**
Incomplete atrioventricular block:
  Mobitz (type) II
  second degree, Mobitz (type) II
(Ex:) 426.0-427.5, 427.89, 459.89-459.9
Coding Clinic: 2006, Q2, P14

426.13 **Other second degree atrioventricular block**
Incomplete atrioventricular block:
  Mobitz (type) I [Wenckebach's]
  second degree:
    NOS
    Mobitz (type) I
  with 2:1 atrioventricular response [block]
Wenckebach's phenomenon

426.2 **Left bundle branch hemiblock**
Block:
  left anterior fascicular
  left posterior fascicular
MCE: Questionable admission, principal diagnosis only

426.3 **Other left bundle branch block**
Left bundle branch block:
  NOS
  anterior fascicular with posterior fascicular
  complete
  main stem
MCE: Questionable admission, principal diagnosis only

426.4 **Right bundle branch block**
MCE: Questionable admission, principal diagnosis only
Coding Clinic: 2000, Q3, P3

● 426.5 **Bundle branch block, other and unspecified**

426.50 **Bundle branch block, unspecified**

426.51 **Right bundle branch block and left posterior fascicular block**

426.52 **Right bundle branch block and left anterior fascicular block**

◀ New   ◀ Revised   ~~deleted~~ Deleted   Excludes   Includes   Use additional   Code first   Omit code
● Unacceptable Principal Diagnosis   ● Use Additional Digit(s)   ▷ Manifestation Code   OGCR Official Guidelines   Coding Clinic

426.53 Other bilateral bundle branch block 🔖
    Bifascicular block NOS
    Bilateral bundle branch block NOS
    Right bundle branch with left bundle branch
        block (incomplete) (main stem)
    (Ex) 426.0–427.5, 427.89, 459.89–459.9

426.54 Trifascicular block 🔖
    (Ex) 426.0–427.5, 427.89, 459.89–459.9

426.6 Other heart block
    Intraventricular block: Sinoatrial block
      NOS   Sinoauricular block
      diffuse
      myofibrillar

426.7 Anomalous atrioventricular excitation
    Atrioventricular conduction:
      accelerated
      accessory
      pre-excitation
    Ventricular pre-excitation
    Wolff-Parkinson-White syndrome

● **426.8 Other specified conduction disorders**

426.81 Lown-Ganong-Levine syndrome
    Syndrome of short P-R interval, normal
        QRS complexes, and supraventricular
        tachycardias

426.82 Long QT syndrome
    Coding Clinic: 2005, Q4, P72-73

426.89 Other 🔖
    Dissociation:
      atrioventricular [AV]
      interference
      isorhythmic
    Nonparoxysmal AV nodal tachycardia
    (Ex) 426.0–427.5, 427.89, 459.89–459.9
    Coding Clinic: 2013, Q2, P26

426.9 Conduction disorder, unspecified
    Heart block NOS
    Stokes-Adams syndrome

● **427 Cardiac dysrhythmias**
Abnormality in rate, regularity, or sequence of cardiac activation

    Excludes *that complicating:*
      abortion (634–638 with .7, 639.8)
      ectopic or molar pregnancy (639.8)
      labor or delivery (668.1, 669.4)

427.0 Paroxysmal supraventricular tachycardia 🔖
    Paroxysmal tachycardia:
      atrial [PAT]   junctional
      atrioventricular [AV]   nodal
    (Ex) 426.0–427.5, 427.89, 459.89–459.9

427.1 Paroxysmal ventricular tachycardia 🔖
    Ventricular tachycardia (paroxysmal)
    (Ex) 426.0–427.5, 427.89, 459.89–459.9
    Coding Clinic: 2013, Q3, P6, Q1, P11; 2008, Q1, P14-15; 2006, Q2,
      P15-16; 1995, Q3, P9; Q1, P8; 1986, Mar-April, P11-12; 1985,
      July-Aug, P15

427.2 Paroxysmal tachycardia, unspecified
    Bouveret-Hoffmann syndrome
    Paroxysmal tachycardia:
      NOS
      essential

● **427.3 Atrial fibrillation and flutter**

427.31 Atrial fibrillation
*Most common abnormal heart rhythm (arrhythmia)
presenting as irregular, rapid beating
(tachycardia) of the heart's upper chamber*
    Coding Clinic: 2008, Q4, P134-136; 2005, Q3, P3-9; 2004,
      Q4, P77-78, 121-122; Q3, P7; 2003, Q4, P93-95,
      105-106; Q1, P8; 1999, Q2, P17; 1996, Q2, P7x2;
      1995, Q3, P8; 1994, Q1, P22; 1985, July-Aug, P15

427.32 Atrial flutter 🔖
*Rapid contractions of the upper heart chamber, but
regular, rather than irregular, beats*
    (Ex) 426.0–427.5, 427.89, 459.89–459.9
    Coding Clinic: 2003, Q4, P93-95

● **427.4 Ventricular fibrillation and flutter**

427.41 Ventricular fibrillation 🔖
MCC only for patients discharged alive
    (Ex) 426.0–427.5, 427.89, 459.89–459.9
    Coding Clinic: 2002, Q3, P5

427.42 Ventricular flutter 🔖
    (Ex) 426.0–427.5, 427.89, 459.89–459.9

427.5 Cardiac arrest 🔖
    Cardiorespiratory arrest
MCC only for patients discharged alive
    (Ex) 427.0–427.5, 459.89–459.9
    Coding Clinic: 2013, Q1, P9-11; 2002, Q3, P5; 2000, Q2, P12;
      1995, Q3, P9

● **427.6 Premature beats**

427.60 Premature beats, unspecified
    Ectopic beats
    Extrasystoles
    Extrasystolic arrhythmia
    Premature contractions or systoles NOS

427.61 Supraventricular premature beats
    Atrial premature beats, contractions, or systoles
    Coding Clinic: 1994, Q1, P20

427.69 Other
    Ventricular premature beats, contractions, or
      systoles
    Coding Clinic: 1993, Q4, P42-43

● **427.8 Other specified cardiac dysrhythmias**

427.81 Sinoatrial node dysfunction
    Sinus bradycardia:
      persistent
      severe
    Syndrome:
      sick sinus
      tachycardia-bradycardia
    Excludes *sinus bradycardia NOS (427.89)*
    Coding Clinic: 2011, Q4, P168

427.89 Other
    Rhythm disorder:
      coronary sinus
      ectopic
      nodal
    Wandering (atrial) pacemaker
    Excludes *carotid sinus syncope (337.0)*
      neonatal bradycardia (779.81)
      neonatal tachycardia (779.82)
      reflex bradycardia (337.0)
      tachycardia NOS (785.0)
    Coding Clinic: 2012, Q3, P9; 2000, Q3, P8-9;
      1985, July-Aug, P15

427.9 Cardiac dysrhythmia, unspecified
    Arrhythmia (cardiac) NOS
    Coding Clinic: 1989, Q2, P10

● **428 Heart failure**
    Code, if applicable, heart failure due to hypertension first
      (402.0–402.9, with fifth-digit 1 or 404.0–404.9 with
      fifth-digit 1 or 3)
    Excludes *rheumatic (398.91)*
      that complicating:
        abortion (634–638 with .7, 639.8)
        ectopic or molar pregnancy (639.8)
        labor or delivery (668.1, 669.4)
    Coding Clinic: 2005, Q2, P14-15; 2002, Q4, P49-53

428.0 Congestive heart failure, unspecified
    Congestive heart disease
    Right heart failure (secondary to left heart failure)
    Excludes *fluid overload NOS (276.69)*
    Coding Clinic: 2012, Q3, P10; 2009, Q4, P106x2; Q1, P6x2; 2008, Q4,
      P69-73, 177-182; Q3, P12-13x2; 2007, Q3, P11; Q1, P20;
      2006, Q3, P7; 2005, Q4, P119-120; Q3, P3-9; Q1, P9; 2004, Q4,
      P140; Q3, P7; 2003, Q4, P109-110; Q1, P9; 2002, Q4, P52-53;
      2001, Q2, P13; 2000, Q4, P47-48; Q2, P16-17; Q1, P22; 1999,
      Q4, P13-14; Q1, P11; 1998, Q3, P5; 1997, Q4, P54-55; Q3, P10;
      1996, Q3, P9; 1991, Q3, P18-20; 1990, Q2, P19; 1989, Q2,
      P12; 1987, Sept-Oct, P11; 1985, Sept-Oct, P15; Nov-Dec, P14

DISEASES OF THE CIRCULATORY SYSTEM (390–459)

N Newborn: 0   **P** Pediatric: 0–17   **M** Maternity: 12–55   **A** Adult: 15–124   ♀ Females Only   ♂ Males Only

(Ex) CC/MCC Exclusions   🔖 Complication\Comorbidity   🔖 Major C\C   🔖 Present on Admission Requirement   🔖 Hospital-Acquired Condition   **809**

Item 7-11   Congestive heart failure (CHF) is a condition in which the left ventricle of the heart cannot pump enough blood to the body. The blood flow from the heart slows or returns to the heart from the venous system back flow resulting in congestion (fluid accumulation) particularly in the abdomen. Most commonly, fluid collects in the lungs and results in shortness of breath, especially when in a reclining position.

428.1   Left heart failure
Acute edema of lung with heart disease NOS or heart failure
Acute pulmonary edema with heart disease NOS or heart failure
Cardiac asthma
Left ventricular failure
Ex: 398.91, 402.01, 402.11, 402.91, 428.0-428.9, 459.89-459.9
Coding Clinic: 1990, Q2, P19

428.2   Systolic heart failure
Excludes   *combined systolic and diastolic heart failure (428.40–428.43)*

   428.20   Unspecified
   Ex: 398.91, 402.01, 402.11, 402.91, 428.0-428.9, 459.89-459.9, 518.4

   428.21   Acute
   Presenting a short and relatively severe episode
   Ex: 398.91, 402.01, 402.11, 402.91, 428.0-428.9, 459.89-459.9, 518.4

   428.22   Chronic
   Long-lasting, presenting over time
   Ex: 398.91, 402.01, 402.11, 402.91, 428.0-428.9, 459.89-459.9, 518.4
   Coding Clinic: 2005, Q4, P119-120

   428.23   Acute on chronic
   Combination code. What was a chronic condition now has an acute exacerbation (to make more severe). Because two conditions are now present, the combination code reports both.
   Ex: 398.91, 402.01, 402.11, 402.91, 428.0-428.9, 459.89-459.9, 518.4
   Coding Clinic: 2009, Q1, P10; 2003, Q1, P9

428.3   Diastolic heart failure
Excludes   *combined systolic and diastolic heart failure (428.40–428.43)*

   428.30   Unspecified
   Ex: 398.91, 402.01, 402.11, 402.91, 428.0-428.9, 459.89-459.9, 518.4
   Coding Clinic: 2002, Q4, P52

   428.31   Acute
   Ex: 398.91, 402.01, 402.11, 402.91, 428.0-428.9, 459.89-459.9, 518.4

   428.32   Chronic
   Ex: 398.91, 402.01, 402.11, 402.91, 428.0-428.9, 459.89-459.9, 518.4
   Coding Clinic: 2008, Q3, P12-13

   428.33   Acute on chronic
   Ex: 398.91, 402.01, 402.11, 402.91, 428.0-428.9, 459.89-459.9, 518.4
   Coding Clinic: 2009, Q1, P106; 2008, Q3, P12; 2007, Q1, P20

428.4   Combined systolic and diastolic heart failure
   428.40   Unspecified
   Ex: 398.91, 402.01, 402.11, 402.91, 428.0-428.9, 459.89-459.9, 518.4

   428.41   Acute
   Ex: 398.91, 402.01, 402.11, 402.91, 428.0-428.9, 459.89-459.9, 518.4
   Coding Clinic: 2004, Q4, P140

   428.42   Chronic
   Ex: 398.91, 402.01, 402.11, 402.91, 428.0-428.9, 459.89-459.9, 518.4

   428.43   Acute on chronic
   Ex: 398.91, 402.01, 402.11, 402.91, 428.0-428.9, 459.89-459.9, 518.4
   Coding Clinic: 2006, Q3, P7; 2002, Q4, P52-53

428.9   Heart failure, unspecified
Cardiac failure NOS
Heart failure NOS
Myocardial failure NOS
Weak heart
Coding Clinic: 1989, Q2, P10; 1985, Nov-Dec, P14

429   Ill-defined descriptions and complications of heart disease
   429.0   Myocarditis, unspecified
   Myocarditis (with mention of arteriosclerosis):
      NOS (with mention of arteriosclerosis)
      chronic (interstitial) (with mention of arteriosclerosis)
      fibroid (with mention of arteriosclerosis)
      senile (with mention of arteriosclerosis)
   Use additional code to identify presence of arteriosclerosis
   Excludes   *acute or subacute (422.0–422.9)*
      rheumatic (398.0)
         acute (391.2)
      that due to hypertension (402.0–402.9)

   429.1   Myocardial degeneration
   Degeneration of heart or myocardium (with mention of arteriosclerosis):
      fatty (with mention of arteriosclerosis)
      mural (with mention of arteriosclerosis)
      muscular (with mention of arteriosclerosis)
   Myocardial (with mention of arteriosclerosis):
      degeneration (with mention of arteriosclerosis)
      disease (with mention of arteriosclerosis)
   Use additional code to identify presence of arteriosclerosis
   Excludes   *that due to hypertension (402.0–402.9)*

   429.2   Cardiovascular disease, unspecified
   Arteriosclerotic cardiovascular disease [ASCVD]
   Cardiovascular arteriosclerosis
   Cardiovascular:
      degeneration (with mention of arteriosclerosis)
      disease (with mention of arteriosclerosis)
      sclerosis (with mention of arteriosclerosis)
   Use additional code to identify presence of arteriosclerosis
   Excludes   *that due to hypertension (402.0–402.9)*
   Coding Clinic: 2012, Q3, P17

   429.3   Cardiomegaly
   Cardiac:
      dilatation
      hypertrophy
   Ventricular dilatation
   Excludes   *that due to hypertension (402.0–402.9)*

   429.4   Functional disturbances following cardiac surgery
   Cardiac insufficiency following cardiac surgery or due to prosthesis
   Heart failure following cardiac surgery or due to prosthesis
   Postcardiotomy syndrome
   Postvalvulotomy syndrome
   Excludes   *cardiac failure in the immediate postoperative period (997.1)*
   Coding Clinic: 2002, Q2, P12-13

   429.5   Rupture of chordae tendineae
   Ex: 429.5, 429.71-429.79, 459.89-459.9

   429.6   Rupture of papillary muscle
   Ex: 429.6-429.81, 459.89-459.9

   429.7   Certain sequelae of myocardial infarction, not elsewhere classified
   Use additional code to identify the associated myocardial infarction:
      with onset of 8 weeks or less (410.00–410.92)
      with onset of more than 8 weeks (414.8)
   Excludes   *congenital defects of heart (745, 746)*
      coronary aneurysm (414.11)
      disorders of papillary muscle (429.6, 429.81)
      postmyocardial infarction syndrome (411.0)
      rupture of chordae tendineae (429.5)

      429.71   Acquired cardiac septal defect   A
      Excludes   *acute septal infarction (410.00–410.92)*
      Ex: 422.0-422.99, 429.0, 429.4-429.82, 459.89-459.9, 745.0-745.9, 746.89-746.9, 747.83-747.9, 759.7-759.89

429.79 Other 🔵
Mural thrombus (atrial) (ventricular) acquired, following myocardial infarction
Ⓔ 422.0-422.99, 429.0, 429.4-429.82, 459.89-459.9, 745.0-745.9, 746.89-746.9, 747.83-747.9, 759.7-759.89
Coding Clinic: 1992, Q1, P10

● **429.8 Other ill-defined heart diseases**

429.81 Other disorders of papillary muscle 🔵
Papillary muscle:
atrophy
degeneration
dysfunction
incompetence
incoordination
scarring
Ⓔ 429.6-429.81, 459.89-459.9

429.82 Hyperkinetic heart disease 🔵
Ⓔ 429.71-429.79, 429.82, 459.89-459.9

429.83 Takotsubo syndrome 🔵
Broken heart syndrome
Reversible left ventricular dysfunction following sudden emotional stress
Stress induced cardiomyopathy
Transient left ventricular apical ballooning syndrome
Ⓔ 398.91, 402.01, 402.11, 402.91, 428.0-428.9, 429.83, 429.9, 459.89-459.9
Coding Clinic: 2006, Q4, P87

429.89 Other
Carditis
Excludes *that due to hypertension (402.0–402.9)*
Coding Clinic: 2006, Q2, P18-19; 2005, Q3, P14; 1992, Q1, P10

429.9 Heart disease, unspecified
Heart disease (organic) NOS
Morbus cordis NOS
Excludes *that due to hypertension (402.0–402.9)*
Coding Clinic: 2009, Q1, P10x2; 1993, Q1, P19-20

CEREBROVASCULAR DISEASE (430–438)

Includes with mention of hypertension (conditions classifiable to 401–405)

Use additional code to identify presence of hypertension

Excludes *any condition classifiable to 430–434, 436, 437 occurring during pregnancy, childbirth, or the puerperium, or specified as puerperal (674.0) iatrogenic cerebrovascular infarction or hemorrhage (997.02)*

OGCR Section I.C.7.a.5

First assign codes from 430-438, Cerebrovascular disease, then the appropriate hypertension code from categories 401-405.

430 Subarachnoid hemorrhage 🔵
Meningeal hemorrhage
Ruptured:
berry aneurysm
(congenital) cerebral aneurysm NOS
Excludes *berry aneurysm, nonruptured (437.3) syphilitic ruptured cerebral aneurysm (094.87)*
Ⓔ 348.82, 430-432.9, 459.89-459.9, 780.01-780.09, 800.00-801.99, 803.00-804.96, 850.0-852.19, 852.21-854.19
Coding Clinic: 2000, Q3, P16; 1991, Q3, P15-16

431 Intracerebral hemorrhage 🔵
Hemorrhage (of):
basilar
bulbar
cerebellar
cerebral
cerebromeningeal
cortical
internal capsule
intrapontine
pontine
subcortical
ventricular
Rupture of blood vessel in brain
Ⓔ 348.82, 430-432.9, 459.89-459.9, 780.01-780.09, 800.00-801.99, 803.00-804.96, 850.0-852.19, 852.21-854.19
Coding Clinic: 2013, Q2, P10; 2012, Q1, P14; 2010, Q3, P5-6; Q1, P7; 2007, Q3, P4; 1997, Q3, P11

● **432 Other and unspecified intracranial hemorrhage**

432.0 Nontraumatic extradural hemorrhage 🔵
Nontraumatic epidural hemorrhage
Ⓔ 348.82, 430-432.9, 459.89-459.9, 780.01-780.09, 800.00-801.99, 803.00-804.96, 850.0-852.19, 852.21-854.19

432.1 Subdural hemorrhage 🔵
Subdural hematoma, nontraumatic
Ⓔ 348.82, 430-432.9, 459.89-459.9, 780.01-780.09, 800.00-801.99, 803.00-804.96, 850.0-852.19, 852.21-854.19

432.9 Unspecified intracranial hemorrhage 🔵
Intracranial hemorrhage NOS
Ⓔ 348.82, 430-432.9, 459.89-459.9, 780.01-780.09, 800.00-801.99, 803.00-804.96, 850.0-852.19, 852.21-854.19

● **433 Occlusion and stenosis of precerebral arteries**
The following fifth-digit subclassification is for use with category 433:

0	without mention of cerebral infarction
1	with cerebral infarction

Includes embolism of basilar, carotid, and vertebral arteries
narrowing of basilar, carotid, and vertebral arteries
obstruction of basilar, carotid, and vertebral arteries
thrombosis of basilar, carotid, and vertebral arteries
Excludes *insufficiency NOS of precerebral arteries (435.0–435.9)*
Use additional code, if applicable, to identify status post administration of tPA (rtPA) in a different facility within the last 24 hours prior to admission to current facility (V45.88)
Coding Clinic: 1995, Q2, P16; 1993, Q4, P38-39

● **433.0 Basilar artery 1** 🔵
[0-1] For code **433.01:** Ⓔ 249.70-249.91, 250.70-250.93, 346.60-346.63, 433.00-433.91, 435.0, 459.89-459.9

● **433.1 Carotid artery 1** 🔵
[0-1] For code **433.11:** Ⓔ 249.70-249.91, 250.70-250.93, 346.60-346.63, 433.00-433.91, 459.89-459.9
Coding Clinic: 2006, Q1, P17; 2002, Q1, P7-8, 10-11; 2000, Q1, P16; 1995, Q2, P16

● **433.2 Vertebral artery 1** 🔵
[0-1] For code **433.21:** Ⓔ 249.70-249.91, 250.70-250.93, 346.60-346.63, 433.00-433.91, 435.1, 459.89-459.9

● **433.3 Multiple and bilateral 1** 🔵
[0-1] For code **433.31:** Ⓔ 249.70-249.91, 250.70-250.93, 346.60-346.63, 433.00-433.91, 459.89-459.9
Coding Clinic: 2006, Q1, P17; 2002, Q1, P10-11

OGCR Section I.C.7.b

The terms stroke and CVA are often used interchangeably to refer to a cerebral vascular infarction. The terms stroke, CVA, and cerebral infarction NOS are all indexed to the default code 434.91, Cerebral artery occlusion, unspecified, with infarction. Additional code(s) should be assigned for any neurologic deficits associated with the acute CVA, regardless of whether or not the neurologic deficit resolves prior to discharge.

● **433.8 Other specified precerebral artery 1**
[0-1]   For code **433.81**: (Ex) 249.70-249.91, 250.70-250.93, 346.60-346.63, 433.00-433.91, 435.0, 459.89-459.9

● **433.9 Unspecified precerebral artery 1**
[0-1]   Precerebral artery NOS
For code **433.91**: (Ex) 249.70-249.91, 250.70-250.93, 346.60-346.63, 433.00-433.91, 435.0, 459.89-459.9

● **434 Occlusion of cerebral arteries**
The following fifth-digit subclassification is for use with category 434:

> 0   without mention of cerebral infarction
> 1   with cerebral infarction

Use additional code, if applicable, to identify status post administration of tPA (rtPA) in a different facility within the last 24 hours prior to admission to current facility (V45.88)
Coding Clinic: 2007, Q3, P12; 1995, Q2, P16; 1993, Q4, P38-39

● **434.0 Cerebral thrombosis 1**
[0-1]   Thrombosis of cerebral arteries
For code **434.01**: (Ex) 249.70-249.91, 250.70-250.93, 346.60-346.63, 434.00-434.91, 436, 459.89-459.9

● **434.1 Cerebral embolism 1**
[0-1]   For code **434.11**: (Ex) 249.70-249.91, 250.70-250.93, 346.60-346.63, 434.00-434.91, 436, 459.89-459.9
Coding Clinic: 1997, Q3, P11

● **434.9 Cerebral artery occlusion, unspecified 1**
[0-1]   For code **434.91**: (Ex) 249.70-249.91, 250.70-250.93, 346.60-346.63, 434.00-434.91, 436, 459.89-459.9
Coding Clinic: 2013, Q2, P10; 2010, Q3, P5-6; 2008, Q4, P102-109; 2007, Q1, P23-24; 2004, Q4, P77-78; 1998, Q4, P87; 1996, Q2, P5

● **435 Transient cerebral ischemia**
Includes   cerebrovascular insufficiency (acute) with transient focal neurological signs and symptoms
insufficiency of basilar, carotid, and vertebral arteries
spasm of cerebral arteries
Excludes   *acute cerebrovascular insufficiency NOS (437.1)*
that due to any condition classifiable to 433 (433.0–433.9)

435.0 Basilar artery syndrome
(Ex) 249.70-249.91, 250.70-250.93, 433.00-433.91, 435.0-435.9, 459.89-459.9

435.1 Vertebral artery syndrome
(Ex) 249.70-249.91, 250.70-250.93, 433.00-433.91, 435.0-435.9, 459.89-459.9

435.2 Subclavian steal syndrome
(Ex) 249.70-249.91, 250.70-250.93, 433.00-433.91, 435.0-435.9, 459.89-459.9

435.3 Vertebrobasilar artery syndrome
(Ex) 249.70-249.91, 250.70-250.93, 433.00-433.91, 435.0-435.9, 459.89-459.9

435.8 Other specified transient cerebral ischemias
(Ex) 249.70-249.91, 250.70-250.93, 433.00-433.91, 435.0-435.9, 459.89-459.9

435.9 Unspecified transient cerebral ischemia
Impending cerebrovascular accident
Intermittent cerebral ischemia
Transient ischemic attack [TIA]
(Ex) 249.70-249.91, 250.70-250.93, 433.00-433.91, 435.0-435.9, 459.89-459.9
Coding Clinic: 1985, Nov-Dec, P12

● **436 Acute, but ill-defined, cerebrovascular disease**
Apoplexy, apoplectic:
NOS
attack
cerebral
seizure
Cerebral seizure
Excludes   *any condition classifiable to categories 430–435*
cerebrovascular accident (434.91)
CVA (ischemic) (434.91)
   embolic (434.11)
   hemorrhagic (430, 431, 432.0–432.9)
   thrombotic (434.01)
postoperative cerebrovascular accident (997.02)
stroke (ischemic) (434.91)
   embolic (434.11)
   hemorrhagic (430, 431, 432.0–432.9)
   thrombotic (434.01)
(Ex) 249.70-249.91, 250.70-250.93, 346.60-346.63, 348.82, 430-432.9, 434.00-434.91, 436, 459.89-459.9, 780.01-780.09, 800.00-801.99, 803.00-804.96, 850.0-852.19, 852.21-854.19
Coding Clinic: 2004, Q4, P77-78; 1999, Q4, P3-4; 1993, Q4, P38-39; Q1, P27

● **437 Other and ill-defined cerebrovascular disease**
437.0 Cerebral atherosclerosis   A
Atheroma of cerebral arteries
Cerebral arteriosclerosis
Coding Clinic: 2010, Q3, P16

437.1 Other generalized ischemic cerebrovascular disease
Acute cerebrovascular insufficiency NOS
Cerebral ischemia (chronic)
(Ex) 249.70-249.91, 250.70-250.93, 430-432.9, 434.00-436, 437.1, 459.89-459.9
Coding Clinic: 2009, Q1, P10

437.2 Hypertensive encephalopathy
(Ex) 249.70-249.91, 250.70-250.93, 437.2, 459.89-459.9

437.3 Cerebral aneurysm, nonruptured
Internal carotid artery, intracranial portion
Internal carotid artery NOS
Excludes   *congenital cerebral aneurysm, nonruptured (747.81)*
internal carotid artery, extracranial portion (442.81)
Coding Clinic: 2009, Q2, P12

437.4 Cerebral arteritis
(Ex) 249.70-249.91, 250.70-250.93, 437.4, 459.89-459.9
Coding Clinic: 1999, Q4, P21-22

437.5 Moyamoya disease
(Ex) 249.70-249.91, 250.70-250.93, 437.5, 459.89-459.9

437.6 Nonpyogenic thrombosis of intracranial venous sinus
Excludes   *pyogenic (325)*
(Ex) 249.70-249.91, 250.70-250.93, 437.6, 459.89-459.9

437.7 Transient global amnesia

437.8 Other
Coding Clinic: 2013, Q2, P10

437.9 Unspecified
Cerebrovascular disease or lesion NOS
Coding Clinic: 2009, Q1, P16; 1986, Nov-Dec, P12

◄ New   ◄ Revised   deleted Deleted   Excludes   Includes   Use additional   Code first   Omit code
● Unacceptable Principal Diagnosis   ● Use Additional Digit(s)   ▶ Manifestation Code   OGCR Official Guidelines   Coding Clinic
812

Assign code V12.54, Transient ischemic attack (TIA), and cerebral infarction without residual deficits (and not a code from category 438) as an additional code for history of cerebrovascular disease when no neurologic deficits are present.

● **438 Late effects of cerebrovascular disease**

> **Note:** This category is to be used to indicate conditions in 430–437 as the cause of late effects. The "late effects" include conditions specified as such, or as sequelae, which may occur at any time after the onset of the causal condition.

> **Excludes** *personal history of:*
> *cerebral infarction without residual deficits (V12.54)*
> *PRIND (Prolonged reversible ischemic neurologic deficit) (V12.54)*
> *RIND (Reversible ischemic neurological deficit) (V12.54)*
> *transient ischemic attack (TIA) (V12.54)*

> Coding Clinic: 2006, Q3, P3-4, 6; 1999, Q4, P6-8x2; Q4, P4-5; 1994, Q1, P22-23; 1993, Q1, P27

438.0 **Cognitive deficits** 🔒
> Coding Clinic: 2007, Q2, P5

● 438.1 **Speech and language deficits**

438.10 **Speech and language deficit, unspecified** 🔒

438.11 **Aphasia** 🔒
> Coding Clinic: 2003, Q4, P105-106; 1997, Q4, P35-37

438.12 **Dysphasia** 🔒
> Coding Clinic: 1999, Q4, P9; Q4, P3-4

438.13 **Dysarthria** 🔒

438.14 **Fluency disorder** 🔒
> Stuttering due to late effect of cerebrovascular accident

438.19 **Other speech and language deficits** 🔒

● 438.2 **Hemiplegia/hemiparesis**
> Coding Clinic: 2005, Q1, P13

438.20 **Hemiplegia affecting unspecified side** 🔒 🔒
> (Ex) 438.20
> Coding Clinic: 2007, Q4, P92-95; 2003, Q4, P105-106; 1999, Q4, P9; Q4, P3-4

438.21 **Hemiplegia affecting dominant side** 🔒 🔒
> (Ex) 438.21

438.22 **Hemiplegia affecting nondominant side** 🔒 🔒
> (Ex) 438.22
> Coding Clinic: 2003, Q4, P105; 2002, Q1, P16

● 438.3 **Monoplegia of upper limb**

438.30 **Monoplegia of upper limb affecting unspecified side** 🔒

438.31 **Monoplegia of upper limb affecting dominant side** 🔒

438.32 **Monoplegia of upper limb affecting nondominant side** 🔒

● 438.4 **Monoplegia of lower limb**

438.40 **Monoplegia of lower limb affecting unspecified side** 🔒

438.41 **Monoplegia of lower limb affecting dominant side** 🔒

438.42 **Monoplegia of lower limb affecting nondominant side** 🔒

● 438.5 **Other paralytic syndrome**
> Use additional code to identify type of paralytic syndrome, such as:
> locked-in state (344.81)
> quadriplegia (344.00–344.09)

> **Excludes** *late effects of cerebrovascular accident with:*
> *hemiplegia/hemiparesis (438.20–438.22)*
> *monoplegia of lower limb (438.40–438.42)*
> *monoplegia of upper limb (438.40–438.42)*

438.50 **Other paralytic syndrome affecting unspecified side** 🔒

438.51 **Other paralytic syndrome affecting dominant side** 🔒

438.52 **Other paralytic syndrome affecting nondominant side** 🔒

438.53 **Other paralytic syndrome, bilateral** 🔒
> Coding Clinic: 1998, Q4, P39-40

438.6 **Alterations of sensations** 🔒
> Use additional code to identify the altered sensation
> Coding Clinic: 2002, Q4, P56

438.7 **Disturbances of vision** 🔒
> Use additional code to identify the visual disturbance
> Coding Clinic: 2002, Q4, P56

● 438.8 **Other late effects of cerebrovascular disease**
> Coding Clinic: 2005, Q1, P13; 2002, Q4, P56

438.81 **Apraxia** 🔒

438.82 **Dysphagia** 🔒
> Use additional code to identify the type of dysphagia, if known (787.20–787.29)
> Coding Clinic: 2007, Q4, P92-95

438.83 **Facial weakness** 🔒
> Facial droop

438.84 **Ataxia** 🔒

438.85 **Vertigo** 🔒
> Coding Clinic: 2002, Q4, P56

438.89 **Other late effects of cerebrovascular disease** 🔒
> Use additional code to identify the late effect
> Coding Clinic: 2009, Q2, P10; 2005, Q1, P13; 1998, Q4, P39-40

438.9 **Unspecified late effects of cerebrovascular disease** 🔒

DISEASES OF ARTERIES, ARTERIOLES, AND CAPILLARIES (440–449)

● **440 Atherosclerosis**
> *Disease in which fatty deposits form on walls of arteries*

> **Includes** arteriolosclerosis
> arteriosclerosis (obliterans) (senile)
> arteriosclerotic vascular disease
> atheroma
> degeneration:
> arterial
> arteriovascular
> vascular
> endarteritis deformans or obliterans
> senile:
> arteritis
> endarteritis

> **Excludes** *atheroembolism (445.01–445.89)*
> *atherosclerosis of bypass graft of the extremities (440.30–440.32)*

440.0 **Of aorta** A
> Coding Clinic: 1993, Q2, P7-8; 1988, Q4, P8

440.1 **Of renal artery** A
> **Excludes** *atherosclerosis of renal arterioles (403.00–403.91)*

N Newborn: 0 **P** Pediatric: 0–17 **M** Maternity: 12–55 **A** Adult: 15–124 ♀ Females Only ♂ Males Only

(Ex) CC/MCC Exclusions 🔒 Complication\Comorbidity 🔒 Major C\C 🔒 Present on Admission Requirement 🔒 Hospital-Acquired Condition 813

Figure 7-4 Atherosclerotic plaque.

Atherosclerotic
plaque
(atheromas)

● **440.2 Of native arteries of the extremities**
Use additional code, if applicable, to identify chronic
total occlusion of artery of the extremities (440.4)

Excludes *atherosclerosis of bypass graft of the extremities (440.30–440.32)*

Coding Clinic: 1994, Q3, P5; 1990, Q3, P15

440.20 Atherosclerosis of the extremities, unspecified A
440.21 Atherosclerosis of the extremities with intermittent claudication A
440.22 Atherosclerosis of the extremities with rest pain A
Any condition classifiable to 440.21
440.23 Atherosclerosis of the extremities with ulceration A
Any condition classifiable to 440.21–440.22
Use additional code for any associated ulceration (707.10-707.19, 707.8, 707.9)
440.24 Atherosclerosis of the extremities with gangrene
Any condition classifiable to 440.21, 440.22, and 440.23 with ischemic gangrene 785.4
Use additional code for any associated ulceration (707.10-707.19, 707.8, 707.9)
Excludes *gas gangrene 040.0*
(Ex) 338.0-338.4, 440.24, 780.64-780.65, 780.91-780.99, 785.4, 799.81-799.89
Coding Clinic: 2003, Q4, P109-110; Q3, P14x2; 1995, Q1, P11; 1994, Q3, P5
440.29 Other A
Coding Clinic: 1995, Q1, P11

● **440.3 Of bypass graft of the extremities**
Excludes *atherosclerosis of native artery of the extremity (440.21–440.24)*
embolism [occlusion NOS] [thrombus] of graft (996.74)
440.30 Of unspecified graft A
440.31 Of autologous vein bypass graft A
440.32 Of nonautologous vein bypass graft A

● **440.4 Chronic total occlusion of artery of the extremities**
Complete occlusion of artery of the extremities
Total occlusion of artery of the extremities
Code first atherosclerosis of arteries of the extremities (440.20–440.29, 440.30–440.32)
Excludes *acute occlusion of artery of extremity (444.21–444.22)*
(Ex) 440.4, 443.81-445.89, 447.0-447.2, 447.5-447.73, 449
Coding Clinic: 2007, Q4, P82-83

440.8 Of other specified arteries A
Excludes *basilar (433.0)*
carotid (433.1)
cerebral (437.0)
coronary (414.00–414.07)
mesenteric (557.1)
precerebral (433.0–433.9)
pulmonary (416.0)
vertebral (433.2)
Coding Clinic: 2009, Q3, P9

440.9 Generalized and unspecified atherosclerosis A
Arteriosclerotic vascular disease NOS
Excludes *arteriosclerotic cardiovascular disease [ASCVD] (429.2)*

● **441 Aortic aneurysm and dissection**
Excludes *aortic ectasia (447.70-447.73)*
syphilitic aortic aneurysm (093.0)
traumatic aortic aneurysm (901.0, 902.0)
● **441.0 Dissection of aorta**
Coding Clinic: 1989, Q4, P10
441.00 Unspecified site
(Ex) 249.70-249.91, 250.70-250.93, 441.00-441.9, 447.70-447.73, 459.89-459.9
441.01 Thoracic
(Ex) 249.70-249.91, 250.70-250.93, 441.00-441.9, 447.70-447.73, 459.89-459.9
Coding Clinic: 2009, Q1, P16; 2007, Q4, P86-87
441.02 Abdominal
(Ex) 249.70-249.91, 250.70-250.93, 441.00-441.9, 447.70-447.73, 459.89-459.9
441.03 Thoracoabdominal
(Ex) 249.70-249.91, 250.70-250.93, 441.00-441.9, 447.70-447.73, 459.89-459.9

441.1 Thoracic aneurysm, ruptured
(Ex) 249.70-249.91, 250.70-250.93, 441.00-441.9, 447.70-447.73, 459.89-459.9
Coding Clinic: 1994, Q2, P15
441.2 Thoracic aneurysm without mention of rupture
Coding Clinic: 1992, Q3, P10-11
441.3 Abdominal aneurysm, ruptured
(Ex) 249.70-249.91, 250.70-250.93, 441.00-441.9, 447.70-447.73, 459.89-459.9
441.4 Abdominal aneurysm without mention of rupture
Coding Clinic: 2000, Q4, P63-64; 1999, Q1, P15-17x2; 1992, Q3, P10-11
441.5 Aortic aneurysm of unspecified site, ruptured
Rupture of aorta NOS
(Ex) 249.70-249.91, 250.70-250.93, 441.00-441.9, 447.70-447.73, 459.89-459.9
441.6 Thoracoabdominal aneurysm, ruptured
(Ex) 249.70-249.91, 250.70-250.93, 441.00-441.9, 447.70-447.73, 459.89-459.9
441.7 Thoracoabdominal aneurysm, without mention of rupture
Coding Clinic: 2006, Q2, P16-17
441.9 Aortic aneurysm of unspecified site without mention of rupture
Aneurysm
Dilatation of aorta
Hyaline necrosis of aorta
Coding Clinic: 1992, Q3, P10-11

● **442 Other aneurysm**
Includes aneurysm (ruptured) (cirsoid) (false) (varicose)
aneurysmal varix
Excludes *arteriovenous aneurysm or fistula:*
acquired (447.0)
congenital (747.60–747.69)
traumatic (900.0–904.9)
442.0 Of artery of upper extremity
442.1 Of renal artery
442.2 Of iliac artery
Coding Clinic: 1999, Q1, P16-17
442.3 Of artery of lower extremity
Aneurysm:
femoral artery
popliteal artery
Coding Clinic: 2008, Q2, P13; 2002, Q3, P24-27; 1999, Q1, P16

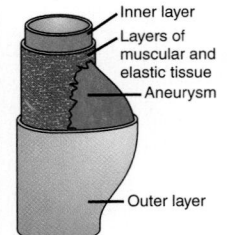

Inner layer
Layers of muscular and elastic tissue
Aneurysm
Outer layer

Figure 7-5 An aneurysm is an enclosed swelling on the wall of the vessel.

Item 7-12 **Rupture** is the tearing of the aneurysm.

● **442.8 Of other specified artery**

442.81 Artery of neck

Aneurysm of carotid artery (common) (external)
(internal, extracranial portion)

> **Excludes** *internal carotid artery, intracranial*
> *portion (437.3)*

442.82 Subclavian artery

442.83 Splenic artery

442.84 Other visceral artery

Aneurysm:
celiac artery
gastroduodenal artery
gastroepiploic artery
hepatic artery
pancreaticoduodenal artery
superior mesenteric artery

442.89 Other

Aneurysm: Aneurysm:
mediastinal artery   spinal artery

> **Excludes** *cerebral (nonruptured) (437.3)*
> *congenital (747.81)*
> *ruptured (430)*
> *coronary (414.11)*
> *heart (414.10)*
> *pulmonary (417.1)*

442.9 Of unspecified site

● **443 Other peripheral vascular disease**

443.0 Raynaud's syndrome

Resulting from a diminishing oxygen supply to fingers, toes,
nose, and ears when exposed to temperature changes or
stress with symptoms of pallor, numbness, and feeling
cold

Raynaud's:
disease
phenomenon (secondary)

> Use additional code to identify gangrene (785.4)

443.1 Thromboangiitis obliterans [Buerger's disease]

Inflammatory occlusive disease resulting in poor circulation
to legs, feet, and sometimes hands due to progressive
inflammatory narrowing of the small arteries

Presenile gangrene

● **443.2 Other arterial dissection**

> **Excludes** *dissection of aorta (441.00–441.03)*
> *dissection of coronary arteries (414.12)*
> Coding Clinic: 2002, Q4, P54-55

443.21 Dissection of carotid artery 🗲
Ⓔⓧ 447.2, 447.5-447.6, 447.8-447.9

443.22 Dissection of iliac artery 🗲
Ⓔⓧ 447.2, 447.5-447.6, 447.8-447.9

443.23 Dissection of renal artery 🗲
Ⓔⓧ 447.2, 447.5-447.6, 447.8-447.9

443.24 Dissection of vertebral artery 🗲
Ⓔⓧ 447.2, 447.5-447.6, 447.8-447.9

443.29 Dissection of other artery 🗲
Ⓔⓧ 447.2, 447.5-447.6, 447.8-447.9

● **443.8 Other specified peripheral vascular diseases**

▷ *443.81 Peripheral angiopathy in diseases classified*
elsewhere

> *Code first* underlying disease, as:
> diabetes mellitus (249.7, 250.7)
> Coding Clinic: 2004, Q1, P14-15; 1996, Q1, P10

443.82 Erythromelalgia
Coding Clinic: 2005, Q4, P73-74

443.89 Other

Acrocyanosis
Acroparesthesia:
simple [Schultze's type]
vasomotor [Nothnagel's type]
Erythrocyanosis

> **Excludes** *chilblains (991.5)*
> *frostbite (991.0–991.3)*
> *immersion foot (991.4)*
> Coding Clinic: 2007, Q4, P124

443.9 Peripheral vascular disease, unspecified

Intermittent claudication NOS
Peripheral:
angiopathy NOS
vascular disease NOS
Spasm of artery

> **Excludes** *atherosclerosis of the arteries of the extremities*
> *(440.20–440.22)*
> *spasm of cerebral artery (435.0–435.9)*

● **444 Arterial embolism and thrombosis**

> **Includes** infarction:
> embolic
> thrombotic
> occlusion

> **Excludes** *atheroembolism (445.01–445.89)*
> *septic arterial embolism (449)*
> *that complicating:*
> *abortion (634–638 with .6, 639.6)*
> *ectopic or molar pregnancy (639.6)*
> *pregnancy, childbirth, or the puerperium*
> *(673.0–673.8)*
> Coding Clinic: 2003, Q1, P16-18x2; 1992, Q2, P10-11

● **444.0 Of abdominal aorta**
Coding Clinic: 1990, Q4, P27

444.01 Saddle embolus of abdominal aorta 🗲
Ⓔⓧ 415.11-415.19, 416.2, 444.01-444.09, 459.89, 459.9
Coding Clinic: 2011, Q4, P109

444.09 Other arterial embolism and thrombosis of
abdominal aorta 🗲

Aortic bifurcation syndrome
Aortoiliac obstruction
Leriche's syndrome
Ⓔⓧ 415.11-415.19, 416.2, 444.01-444.09, 459.89-459.9

444.1 Of thoracic aorta 🗲

Embolism or thrombosis of aorta (thoracic)
Ⓔⓧ 249.70-249.91, 250.70-250.93, 444.1, 444.89-444.9, 449, 459.89-459.9

● **444.2 Of arteries of the extremities**

444.21 Upper extremity 🗲
Ⓔⓧ 249.70-249.91, 250.70-250.93, 444.21, 444.89-444.9, 449,
459.89-459.9
Coding Clinic: 1990, Q3, P16

444.22 Lower extremity 🗲

Arterial embolism or thrombosis:
femoral   popliteal
peripheral NOS

> **Excludes** *iliofemoral (444.81)*
> Ⓔⓧ 249.70-249.91, 250.70-250.93, 444.22, 444.89-444.9, 449,
> 459.89-459.9
> Coding Clinic: 2007, Q4, P84-86; 2003, Q3, P10

Embolus

Figure 7–6 An arterial embolus.

Item 7–13 An **embolus** is a mass of undissolved matter present in the
blood that is transported by the blood current. A **thrombus** is a blood clot
that occludes or shuts off a vessel. When a thrombus is dislodged, it becomes
an embolus.

N Newborn: 0   **P** Pediatric: 0–17   **M** Maternity: 12–55   **A** Adult: 15–124   ♀ Females Only   ♂ Males Only

Ⓔⓧ CC/MCC Exclusions   🗲 Complication\Comorbidity   🗲 Major C\C   🗲 Present on Admission Requirement   🗲 Hospital-Acquired Condition   815

DISEASES OF THE CIRCULATORY SYSTEM (390–459)

DISEASES OF THE CIRCULATORY SYSTEM (390–459)

● 444.8 **Of other specified artery**
  444.81 **Iliac artery** 🗨
    Ex: 249.70-249.91, 250.70-250.93, 444.81-444.9, 449, 459.89-459.9
    Coding Clinic: 2003, Q1, P16-17

  444.89 **Other** 🗨
    Excludes   basilar (433.0)
      carotid (433.1)
      cerebral (434.0–434.9)
      coronary (410.00–410.92)
      mesenteric (557.0)
      ophthalmic (362.30–362.34)
      precerebral (433.0–433.9)
      pulmonary (415.11-415.19)
      renal (593.81)
      retinal (362.30–362.34)
      vertebral (433.2)
    Ex: 249.70-249.91, 250.70-250.93, 444.89-444.9, 449, 459.89-459.9

● 444.9 **Of unspecified artery** 🗨
  Ex: 249.70-249.91, 250.70-250.93, 444.89-444.9, 449, 459.89-459.9

● 445 **Atheroembolism**
  Includes   Atherothrombotic microembolism
    Cholesterol embolism
  Coding Clinic: 2002, Q4, P57-58

● 445.0 **Of extremities**
  445.01 **Upper extremity** 🗨
    Ex: 249.70-249.91, 250.70-250.93, 444.89-445.01, 449, 459.89-459.9
  445.02 **Lower extremity** 🗨
    Ex: 249.70-249.91, 250.70-250.93, 444.89-444.9, 445.02, 449, 459.89-459.9

● 445.8 **Of other sites**
  445.81 **Kidney** 🗨
    Use additional code for any associated acute kidney failure or chronic kidney disease (584, 585)
    Ex: 249.70-249.91, 250.70-250.93, 444.89-444.9, 445.81, 449, 459.89-459.9
  445.89 **Other site** 🗨
    Ex: 249.70-249.91, 250.70-250.93, 444.89-444.9, 445.89, 449, 459.89-459.9

● 446 **Polyarteritis nodosa and allied conditions**
  446.0 **Polyarteritis nodosa** 🗨
    Disseminated necrotizing periarteritis
    Necrotizing angiitis
    Panarteritis (nodosa)
    Periarteritis (nodosa)
    Ex: 249.70-249.91, 250.70-250.93, 446.0-446.7, 459.89-459.9

  446.1 **Acute febrile mucocutaneous lymph node syndrome [MCLS]** 🗨
    Kawasaki disease
    Ex: 446.0-446.29, 446.4-446.7, 459.89-459.9

● 446.2 **Hypersensitivity angiitis**
  Excludes   antiglomerular basement membrane disease without pulmonary hemorrhage (583.89)
  446.20 **Hypersensitivity angiitis, unspecified** 🗨
    Ex: 249.70-249.91, 250.70-250.93, 446.0-446.7, 459.89-459.9
  446.21 **Goodpasture's syndrome** 🗨
    Antiglomerular basement membrane antibody-mediated nephritis with pulmonary hemorrhage
    Use additional code to identify renal disease (583.81)
    Ex: 249.70-249.91, 250.70-250.93, 446.0-446.7, 459.89-459.9
  446.29 **Other specified hypersensitivity angiitis** 🗨
    Ex: 249.70-249.91, 250.70-250.93, 446.0-446.7, 459.89-459.9
    Coding Clinic: 1995, Q1, P3

  446.3 **Lethal midline granuloma** 🗨
    Malignant granuloma of face
    Ex: 249.70-249.91, 250.70-250.93, 446.0-446.7, 459.89-459.9

  446.4 **Wegener's granulomatosis** 🗨
    Necrotizing respiratory granulomatosis
    Wegener's syndrome
    Ex: 249.70-249.91, 250.70-250.93, 446.0-446.7, 459.89-459.9
    Coding Clinic: 2000, Q3, P11

  446.5 **Giant cell arteritis**
    Cranial arteritis
    Horton's disease
    Temporal arteritis

  446.6 **Thrombotic microangiopathy** 🗨
    Moschcowitz's syndrome
    Thrombotic thrombocytopenic purpura
    Ex: 249.70-249.91, 250.70-250.93, 446.0-446.7, 459.89-459.9

  446.7 **Takayasu's disease** 🗨
    Aortic arch arteritis
    Pulseless disease
    Ex: 249.70-249.91, 250.70-250.93, 446.0-446.7, 459.89-459.9

● 447 **Other disorders of arteries and arterioles**
  447.0 **Arteriovenous fistula, acquired**
    Arteriovenous aneurysm, acquired
    Excludes   cerebrovascular (437.3)
      coronary (414.19)
      pulmonary (417.0)
      surgically created arteriovenous shunt or fistula:
        complication (996.1, 996.61–996.62)
        status or presence (V45.11)
      traumatic (900.0–904.9)

  447.1 **Stricture of artery**
    Coding Clinic: 1993, Q2, P8; 1987, Jan-Feb, P14

  447.2 **Rupture of artery** 🗨
    Erosion of artery
    Fistula, except arteriovenous of artery
    Ulcer of artery
    Excludes   traumatic rupture of artery (900.0–904.9)
    Ex: 414.12, 443.22-443.29, 447.2

  447.3 **Hyperplasia of renal artery**
    Fibromuscular hyperplasia of renal artery

  447.4 **Celiac artery compression syndrome** 🗨
    Celiac axis syndrome
    Marable's syndrome
    Ex: 447.4

  447.5 **Necrosis of artery** 🗨
    Ex: 447.5

  447.6 **Arteritis, unspecified**
    Aortitis NOS
    Endarteritis NOS
    Excludes   arteritis, endarteritis:
      aortic arch (446.7)
      cerebral (437.4)
      coronary (414.00–414.07)
      deformans (440.0–440.9)
      obliterans (440.0–440.9)
      pulmonary (417.8)
      senile (440.0–440.9)
      polyarteritis NOS (446.0)
      syphilitic aortitis (093.1)
    Coding Clinic: 1999, Q4, P21-22

● 447.7 **Aortic ectasia**
    Ectasis aorta
    Excludes   aortic aneurysm and dissection (441.00-441.9)
  447.70 **Aortic ectasia, unspecified site**
  447.71 **Thoracic aortic ectasia**
  447.72 **Abdominal aortic ectasia**
  447.73 **Thoracoabdominal aortic ectasia**

  447.8 **Other specified disorders of arteries and arterioles**
    Fibromuscular hyperplasia of arteries, except renal

  447.9 **Unspecified disorders of arteries and arterioles**

● 448 **Disease of capillaries**

   448.0 Hereditary hemorrhagic telangiectasia
     Rendu-Osler-Weber disease

   448.1 Nevus, non-neoplastic
     Nevus:
       araneus
       senile
       spider
       stellar

     Excludes *neoplastic (216.0–216.9)*
             port wine (757.32)
             strawberry (757.32)

   448.9 Other and unspecified capillary diseases
     Capillary:
       hemorrhage
       hyperpermeability
       thrombosis

     Excludes *capillary fragility (hereditary) (287.8)*

● 449 **Septic arterial embolism** 🔒

   Code first underlying infection, such as:
     infective endocarditis (421.0)
     lung abscess (513.0)

   Use additional code to identify the site of the embolism
     (433.0–433.9, 444.01–444.9)

     Excludes *septic pulmonary embolism (415.12)*

   (Ex) 249.70-249.91, 250.70-250.93, 444.89-444.9, 449, 459.89-459.9
   Coding Clinic: 2007, Q4, P84-86

**DISEASES OF VEINS AND LYMPHATICS, AND OTHER DISEASES
OF CIRCULATORY SYSTEM (451–459)**

● 451 **Phlebitis and thrombophlebitis**
   *Inflammation of vein with infiltration of walls (phlebitis) and, usually,
   formation of clot (thrombus) in vein (**thrombophlebitis**)*

   Includes endophlebitis
         inflammation, vein
         periphlebitis
         suppurative phlebitis

   Use additional E code to identify drug if drug-induced

     Excludes *that complicating:*
         abortion (634–638 with .7, 639.8)
         ectopic or molar pregnancy (639.8)
         pregnancy, childbirth, or the puerperium
           (671.0–671.9)
        that due to or following:
         implant or catheter device (996.61–996.62)
         infusion, perfusion, or transfusion (999.2)

   **Coding Clinic: 2013, Q2, P4; 2011, Q1, P19; 2004, Q4, P78-80; 1993, Q1, P26;
   1992, Q1, P15-16**

   451.0 Of superficial vessels of lower extremities
     Saphenous vein (greater) (lesser)

  ● **451.1 Of deep vessels of lower extremities**
     Coding Clinic: 1991, Q3, P16

     451.11 Femoral vein (deep) (superficial) 🔒
       (Ex) 249.70-249.91, 250.70-250.93, 451.0-451.9, 459.89-459.9

     451.19 Other 🔒
       Femoropopliteal vein
       Popliteal vein
       Tibial vein
       (Ex) 249.70-249.91, 250.70-250.93, 451.0-451.9, 459.89-459.9

   451.2 Of lower extremities, unspecified
     Coding Clinic: 2004, Q4, P78-80

  ● **451.8 Of other sites**

     Excludes *intracranial venous sinus (325)*
          nonpyogenic (437.6)
          portal (vein) (572.1)

     451.81 Iliac vein 🔒
       (Ex) 249.70-249.91, 250.70-250.93, 451.0-451.9, 459.89-459.9

     451.82 Of superficial veins of upper extremities
       Antecubital vein
       Basilic vein
       Cephalic vein

     451.83 Of deep veins of upper extremities 🔒
       Brachial vein
       Radial vein
       Ulnar vein
       (Ex) 451.0-451.2, 451.83, 451.89-451.9

     451.84 Of upper extremities, unspecified

     451.89 Other 🔒
       Axillary vein
       Jugular vein
       Subclavian vein
       Thrombophlebitis of breast (Mondor's disease)
       (Ex) 451.0-451.2, 451.89-451.9

   451.9 Of unspecified site

 452 **Portal vein thrombosis** 🔒
   Portal (vein) obstruction

     Excludes *hepatic vein thrombosis (453.0)*
         phlebitis of portal vein (572.1)
     (Ex) 249.70-249.91, 250.70-250.93, 452, 453.40-453.9, 459.89-459.9

● 453 **Other venous embolism and thrombosis**

     Excludes *that complicating:*
         abortion (634–638 with .7, 639.8)
         ectopic or molar pregnancy (639.8)
         pregnancy, childbirth, or the puerperium
          (671.0–671.9)
   Coding Clinic: 2011, Q1, P19-20; 2004, Q4, P78-80; 1992, Q1, P15-16

   453.0 Budd-Chiari syndrome 🔒
     Hepatic vein thrombosis
     (Ex) 249.70-249.91, 250.70-250.93, 453.0, 453.40-453.9, 459.89-459.9

   453.1 Thrombophlebitis migrans 🔒
     *"White leg" is the other term used to describe a migrating
      thrombus.*
     (Ex) 249.70-249.91, 250.70-250.93, 453.1, 453.40-453.9, 459.89-459.9

   453.2 Of inferior vena cava 🔒
     (Ex) 249.70-249.91, 250.70-250.93, 453.2, 453.40-453.9, 459.89-459.9

   453.3 Of renal vein 🔒
     (Ex) 249.70-249.91, 250.70-250.93, 453.3-453.9, 459.89-459.9

  ● **453.4 Acute venous embolism and thrombosis of deep vessels of
     lower extremity**

     **453.40 Acute venous embolism and thrombosis of
       unspecified deep vessels of lower extremity** 🔒 🔒
       Deep vein thrombosis NOS
       DVT NOS
       HAC: And one of the following procedure codes:
         00.85-00.87, 81.51-81.52, 81.54
       (Ex) 249.70-249.91, 250.70-250.93, 453.40-453.9, 459.89-459.9
       Coding Clinic: 2012, Q1, P18

     **453.41 Acute venous embolism and thrombosis of deep
       vessels of proximal lower extremity** 🔒 🔒
       Femoral   Thigh
       Iliac   Upper leg NOS
       Popliteal
       HAC: And one of the following procedure codes:
         00.85-00.87, 81.51-81.52, 81.54
       (Ex) 249.70-249.91, 250.70-250.93, 453.40-453.9, 459.89-459.9
       Coding Clinic: 2004, Q4, P78-80

     **453.42 Acute venous embolism and thrombosis of deep
       vessels of distal lower extremity** 🔒 🔒
       Calf   Peroneal
       Lower leg NOS   Tibial
       HAC: And one of the following procedure codes:
         00.85-00.87, 81.51-81.52, 81.54
       (Ex) 249.70-249.91, 250.70-250.93, 453.40-453.9, 459.89-459.9

N Newborn: 0   P Pediatric: 0–17   M Maternity: 12–55   A Adult: 15–124   ♀ Females Only   ♂ Males Only

(Ex) CC/MCC Exclusions   🔒 Complication\Comorbidity   🔒 Major C\C   🔒 Present on Admission Requirement   🔒 Hospital-Acquired Condition

● **453.5 Chronic venous embolism and thrombosis of deep vessels of lower extremity**

Use additional code, if applicable, for associated long-term (current) use of anticoagulants (V58.61)

Excludes *personal history of venous thrombosis and embolism (V12.51)*

453.50 Chronic venous embolism and thrombosis of unspecified deep vessels of lower extremity 🔎
(Ex) 249.70-249.91, 250.70-250.93, 453.40-453.9, 459.89-459.9

453.51 Chronic venous embolism and thrombosis of deep vessels of proximal lower extremity 🔎
Femoral   Thigh
Iliac   Upper leg NOS
Popliteal
(Ex) 249.70-249.91, 250.70-250.93, 453.40-453.9, 459.89-459.9

453.52 Chronic venous embolism and thrombosis of deep vessels of distal lower extremity 🔎
Calf
Lower leg NOS
Peroneal
Tibial
(Ex) 249.70-249.91, 250.70-250.93, 453.40-453.9, 459.89-459.9

453.6 Venous embolism and thrombosis of superficial vessels of lower extremity 🔎
Saphenous vein (greater) (lesser)

Use additional code, if applicable, for associated long-term (current) use of anticoagulants (V58.61)
(Ex) 249.70-249.91, 250.70-250.93, 453.40-453.9, 459.89-459.9

● **453.7 Chronic venous embolism and thrombosis of other specified vessels**

Use additional code, if applicable, for associated long-term (current) use of anticoagulants (V58.61)

Excludes *personal history of venous thrombosis and embolism (V12.51)*

453.71 Chronic venous embolism and thrombosis of superficial veins of upper extremity 🔎
Antecubital vein   Cephalic vein
Basilic vein
(Ex) 249.70-249.91, 250.70-250.93, 453.40-453.9, 459.89-459.9

453.72 Chronic venous embolism and thrombosis of deep veins of upper extremity 🔎
Brachial vein   Ulnar vein
Radial vein
(Ex) 249.70-249.91, 250.70-250.93, 453.40-453.9, 459.89-459.9

453.73 Chronic venous embolism and thrombosis of upper extremity, unspecified 🔎
(Ex) 249.70-249.91, 250.70-250.93, 453.40-453.9, 459.89-459.9

453.74 Chronic venous embolism and thrombosis of axillary veins 🔎
(Ex) 249.70-249.91, 250.70-250.93, 453.40-453.9, 459.89-459.9

453.75 Chronic venous embolism and thrombosis of subclavian veins 🔎
(Ex) 249.70-249.91, 250.70-250.93, 453.40-453.9, 459.89-459.9

453.76 Chronic venous embolism and thrombosis of internal jugular veins 🔎
(Ex) 249.70-249.91, 250.70-250.93, 453.40-453.9, 459.89-459.9

453.77 Chronic venous embolism and thrombosis of other thoracic veins 🔎
Brachiocephalic (innominate)
Superior vena cava
(Ex) 249.70-249.91, 250.70-250.93, 453.40-453.9, 459.89-459.9

453.79 Chronic venous embolism and thrombosis of other specified veins 🔎
(Ex) 249.70-249.91, 250.70-250.93, 453.40-453.9, 459.89-459.9

● **453.8 Acute venous embolism and thrombosis of other specified veins**

Excludes *cerebral (434.0–434.9)*
coronary (410.00–410.92)
intracranial venous sinus (325)
   nonpyogenic (437.6)
mesenteric (557.0)
portal (452)
precerebral (433.0–433.9)
pulmonary (415.19)
(Ex) 249.70-249.91, 250.70-250.93, 453.40-453.9, 459.89-459.9
Coding Clinic: 2004, Q4, P78-80; 1992, Q1, P15-16

453.81 Acute venous embolism and thrombosis of superficial veins of upper extremity 🔎
Antecubital vein   Cephalic vein
Basilic vein
(Ex) 249.70-249.91, 250.70-250.93, 453.40-453.9, 459.89-459.9

453.82 Acute venous embolism and thrombosis of deep veins of upper extremity 🔎
Brachial vein   Ulnar vein
Radial vein
(Ex) 249.70-249.91, 250.70-250.93, 453.40-453.9, 459.89-459.9

453.83 Acute venous embolism and thrombosis of upper extremity, unspecified 🔎
(Ex) 249.70-249.91, 250.70-250.93, 453.40-453.9, 459.89-459.9

453.84 Acute venous embolism and thrombosis of axillary veins 🔎
(Ex) 249.70-249.91, 250.70-250.93, 453.40-453.9, 459.89-459.9

453.85 Acute venous embolism and thrombosis of subclavian veins 🔎
(Ex) 249.70-249.91, 250.70-250.93, 453.40-453.9, 459.89-459.9

453.86 Acute venous embolism and thrombosis of internal jugular veins 🔎
(Ex) 249.70-249.91, 250.70-250.93, 453.40-453.9, 459.89-459.9

453.87 Acute venous embolism and thrombosis of other thoracic veins 🔎
Brachiocephalic (innominate)
Superior vena cava
(Ex) 249.70-249.91, 250.70-250.93, 453.40-453.9, 459.89-459.9

453.89 Acute venous embolism and thrombosis of other specified veins 🔎
(Ex) 249.70-249.91, 250.70-250.93, 453.40-453.9, 459.89-459.9

453.9 Of unspecified site 🔎
Embolism of vein   Thrombosis (vein)
(Ex) 249.70-249.91, 250.70-250.93, 453.40-453.9, 459.89-459.9
Coding Clinic: 2012, Q1, P18; 2011, Q1, P21

● **454 Varicose veins of lower extremities**

Excludes *that complicating pregnancy, childbirth, or the puerperium (671.0)*

454.0 With ulcer   A
Varicose ulcer (lower extremity, any part)
Varicose veins with ulcer of lower extremity [any part] or of unspecified site
Any condition classifiable to 454.9 with ulcer or specified as ulcerated
Coding Clinic: 1999, Q4, P18

454.1 With inflammation   A
Stasis dermatitis
Varicose veins with inflammation of lower extremity [any part] or of unspecified site
Any condition classifiable to 454.9 with inflammation or specified as inflamed
Coding Clinic: 1991, Q2, P20

454.2 With ulcer and inflammation 🔎   A
Varicose veins with ulcer and inflammation of lower extremity [any part] or of unspecified site
Any condition classifiable to 454.9 with ulcer and inflammation
(Ex) 454.0-454.2, 454.9
Coding Clinic: 2004, Q3, P5-6; 1991, Q2, P20

◀ New   ◀ Revised   ~~deleted~~ Deleted   Excludes   Includes   Use additional   Code first   Omit code
● Unacceptable Principal Diagnosis   ● Use Additional Digit(s)   ▷ Manifestation Code   OGCR Official Guidelines   Coding Clinic
818

Item 7–14 Varicose/Varicosities (varix = singular, varices = plural): Enlarged, engorged, tortuous, twisted vascular vessels (veins, arteries, lymphatics). As such, the condition can present in various parts of the body, although the most familiar locations are the lower extremities. A common complication of varices is thrombophlebitis. Varicosities of the anus and rectum are called hemorrhoids. There are additional codes for esophageal, sublingual (under the tongue), scrotal, pelvic, vulval, and nasal varices as well.

Figure 7–7 Varicose veins of the legs. (From Goldman: Cecil Medicine, ed 23, Saunders, 2008)

454.8 With other complications
Edema
Pain
Swelling
Coding Clinic: 2002, Q4, P58-60

454.9 Asymptomatic varicose veins   A
Phlebectasia of lower extremity [any part] or of
unspecified site
Varicose veins NOS
Varicose veins of lower extremity [any part] or of
unspecified site
Varix of lower extremity [any part] or of unspecified site

● **455 Hemorrhoids**
Includes   hemorrhoids (anus) (rectum)
piles
varicose veins, anus or rectum

Excludes   *that complicating pregnancy, childbirth, or the*
puerperium (671.8)

455.0 Internal hemorrhoids without mention of complication
Coding Clinic: 2005, Q3, P17

455.1 Internal thrombosed hemorrhoids

455.2 Internal hemorrhoids with other complication
Internal hemorrhoids:
bleeding
prolapsed
strangulated
ulcerated
Coding Clinic: 2005, Q3, P17; 2003, Q1, P8

455.3 External hemorrhoids without mention of complication
Coding Clinic: 2007, Q1, P13

455.4 External thrombosed hemorrhoids

455.5 External hemorrhoids with other complication
External hemorrhoids:
bleeding
prolapsed
strangulated
ulcerated
Coding Clinic: 2005, Q3, P17; 2003, Q1, P8

455.6 Unspecified hemorrhoids without mention of complication
Hemorrhoids NOS

455.7 Unspecified thrombosed hemorrhoids
Thrombosed hemorrhoids, unspecified whether internal
or external

455.8 Unspecified hemorrhoids with other complication
Hemorrhoids, unspecified whether internal or external:
bleeding
prolapsed
strangulated
ulcerated

455.9 Residual hemorrhoidal skin tags
Skin tags, anus or rectum

● **456 Varicose veins of other sites**
456.0 Esophageal varices with bleeding 🔾
(Ex) 251.5, 456.0, 456.20, 459.89-459.9, 530.20-530.21, 530.7, 530.82, 530.85,
531.00-534.91, 535.01, 535.11, 535.21, 535.31, 535.41, 535.51, 535.61,
535.71, 537.83, 562.02-562.03, 562.12-562.13, 569.3, 569.85,
578.0-578.9

456.1 Esophageal varices without mention of bleeding 🔾
(Ex) 251.5, 456.0-456.20, 459.89-459.9, 530.7, 530.82, 531.00-534.91, 535.01,
535.11, 535.21, 535.31, 535.41, 535.51, 535.61, 535.71, 537.83,
578.0-578.9

● **456.2 Esophageal varices in diseases classified elsewhere**
Code first underlying disease, as:
cirrhosis of liver (571.0–571.9)
portal hypertension (572.3)

▶ **456.20 With bleeding** 🔾
(Ex) 456.0, 456.20, 459.89-459.9, 530.82
Coding Clinic: 1985, Nov-Dec, P14

▶ **456.21 Without mention of bleeding** 🔾
(Ex) 251.5, 456.0, 456.20-456.21, 459.89-459.9, 530.7, 530.82,
531.00-534.91, 535.01, 535.11, 535.21, 535.31, 535.41,
535.51, 535.61, 535.71, 537.83, 578.0-578.9
Coding Clinic: 2005, Q3, P15-16; 2002, Q2, P4

456.3 Sublingual varices

456.4 Scrotal varices ♂
Varicocele

456.5 Pelvic varices
Varices of broad ligament

456.6 Vulval varices ♀
Varices of perineum
Excludes   *that complicating pregnancy, childbirth, or the*
puerperium (671.1)

456.8 Varices of other sites
Varicose veins of nasal septum (with ulcer)
Excludes   *placental varices (656.7)*
retinal varices (362.17)
varicose ulcer of unspecified site (454.0)
varicose veins of unspecified site (454.9)
Coding Clinic: 2002, Q2, P4

● **457 Noninfectious disorders of lymphatic channels**
457.0 Postmastectomy lymphedema syndrome   A
Elephantiasis due to mastectomy
Obliteration of lymphatic vessel due to mastectomy
Coding Clinic: 2002, Q2, P12-13

457.1 Other lymphedema
Elephantiasis (nonfilarial) NOS
Lymphangiectasis
Lymphedema:
acquired (chronic)
praecox
secondary
Obliteration, lymphatic vessel
Excludes   *elephantiasis (nonfilarial):*
congenital (757.0)
eyelid (374.83)
vulva (624.8)
Coding Clinic: 2004, Q3, P5-6

457.2 Lymphangitis
Lymphangitis:
NOS
chronic
subacute
Excludes   *acute lymphangitis (682.0–682.9)*

457.8 Other noninfectious disorders of lymphatic channels
Chylocele (nonfilarial)   Lymph node or vessel:
Chylous: fistula
ascites   infarction
cyst   rupture
Excludes   *chylocele:*
filarial (125.0–125.9)
tunica vaginalis (nonfilarial) (608.84)
Coding Clinic: 2004, Q1, P5; 2003, Q3, P16-17

457.9 Unspecified noninfectious disorder of lymphatic channels

DISEASES OF THE CIRCULATORY SYSTEM (390–459)

N Newborn: 0   **P** Pediatric: 0–17   **M** Maternity: 12–55   **A** Adult: 15–124   ♀ Females Only   ♂ Males Only

(Ex) CC/MCC Exclusions   🔾 Complication\Comorbidity   🔾 Major C\C   🔾 Present on Admission Requirement   🔾 Hospital-Acquired Condition   **819**

● 458   **Hypotension**
Subnormal arterial blood pressure
Includes   hypopiesis
Excludes   *cardiovascular collapse (785.50)*
maternal hypotension syndrome (669.2)
shock (785.50–785.59)
Shy-Drager syndrome (333.0)
Coding Clinic: 1994, Q3, P9; 1993, 5th Issue, P6-7

458.0   **Orthostatic hypotension**
Hypotension:
   orthostatic (chronic)
   postural
   Moving from sitting or reclining position to standing
   position precipitates sudden drop in blood
   pressure.
Coding Clinic: 2000, Q3, P8-9

458.1   **Chronic hypotension**
Permanent idiopathic hypotension

● 458.2   **Iatrogenic hypotension**
Coding Clinic: 2002, Q3, P12; 1993, Q4, P41-42

458.21   **Hypotension of hemodialysis**
Intra-dialytic hypotension
Coding Clinic: 2003, Q4, P60-61

458.29   **Other iatrogenic hypotension**
Postoperative hypotension
Coding Clinic: 1993, Q4, P41-42

458.8   **Other specified hypotension**
Coding Clinic: 1997. Q4, P37

458.9   **Hypotension, unspecified**
Hypotension (arterial) NOS

● 459   **Other disorders of circulatory system**

459.0   **Hemorrhage, unspecified**
Rupture of blood vessel NOS
Spontaneous hemorrhage NEC

Excludes   *hemorrhage:*
gastrointestinal NOS (578.9)
in newborn NOS (772.9)
nontraumatic hematoma of soft tissue
(729.92)
secondary or recurrent following trauma
(958.2)
traumatic rupture of blood vessel
(900.0–904.9)
Coding Clinic: 1999, Q4, P18

● 459.1   **Postphlebitic syndrome**
Chronic venous hypertension due to deep vein
   thrombosis
Excludes   *chronic venous hypertension without deep vein*
thrombosis (459.30–459.39)
Coding Clinic: 2002, Q4, P58-60; 1991, Q2, P20

459.10   **Postphlebitic syndrome without complications**
Asymptomatic postphlebitic syndrome
Postphlebitic syndrome NOS

459.11   **Postphlebitic syndrome with ulcer** 🔗
Ⓔⓧ 451.0-451.9

459.12   **Postphlebitic syndrome with inflammation**

459.13   **Postphlebitic syndrome with ulcer and
inflammation** 🔗
Ⓔⓧ 451.0-451.9

459.19   **Postphlebitic syndrome with other complication**

459.2   **Compression of vein** 🔗
Stricture of vein
Vena cava syndrome (inferior) (superior)
Ⓔⓧ 459.2

● 459.3   **Chronic venous hypertension (idiopathic)**
Stasis edema
Excludes   *chronic venous hypertension due to deep vein*
thrombosis (459.10–459.19)
varicose veins (454.0–454.9)
Coding Clinic: 2002, Q4, P58-60

459.30   **Chronic venous hypertension without
complications**
Asymptomatic chronic venous hypertension
Chronic venous hypertension NOS

459.31   **Chronic venous hypertension with ulcer** 🔗
Ⓔⓧ 454.0-454.2, 454.9, 459.81-459.9

459.32   **Chronic venous hypertension with inflammation**

459.33   **Chronic venous hypertension with ulcer and
inflammation** 🔗
Ⓔⓧ 454.0-454.2, 454.9, 459.81-459.9

459.39   **Chronic venous hypertension with other
complication**

● 459.8   **Other specified disorders of circulatory system**

459.81   **Venous (peripheral) insufficiency, unspecified**
Chronic venous insufficiency NOS

Use additional code for any associated
ulceration (707.10-707.19, 707.8, 707.9)
Coding Clinic: 2004, Q3, P5-6; 1991, Q2, P20

459.89   **Other**
Collateral circulation (venous), any site
Phlebosclerosis
Venofibrosis

459.9   **Unspecified circulatory system disorder**
Coding Clinic: 2013, Q1, P7

8. DISEASES OF THE RESPIRATORY SYSTEM (460–519)

Use additional code to identify infectious organism

ACUTE RESPIRATORY INFECTIONS (460–466)

Excludes *pneumonia and influenza (480.0-488.19)*

460 Acute nasopharyngitis [common cold]
Coryza (acute)
Nasal catarrh, acute

Nasopharyngitis:	Rhinitis:
NOS	acute
acute	infective
infective NOS	

Excludes *nasopharyngitis, chronic (472.2)*
 pharyngitis:
  acute or unspecified (462)
  chronic (472.1)
 rhinitis:
  allergic (477.0–477.9)
  chronic or unspecified (472.0)
 sore throat:
  acute or unspecified (462)
  chronic (472.1)

Coding Clinic: 1988, Q1, P12

● **461 Acute sinusitis**
Code to specific sinus if indicated in documentation.

Includes abscess, acute, of sinus (accessory) (nasal)
empyema, acute, of sinus (accessory) (nasal)
infection, acute, of sinus (accessory) (nasal)
inflammation, acute, of sinus (accessory) (nasal)
suppuration, acute, of sinus (accessory) (nasal)

Excludes *chronic or unspecified sinusitis (473.0–473.9)*

461.0 Maxillary
Acute antritis

461.1 Frontal

461.2 Ethmoidal

461.3 Sphenoidal

461.8 Other acute sinusitis
Acute pansinusitis

461.9 Acute sinusitis, unspecified
Acute sinusitis NOS

462 Acute pharyngitis
Acute sore throat NOS
Pharyngitis (acute):
 NOS
 gangrenous
 infective
 phlegmonous
 pneumococcal
 staphylococcal
 suppurative
 ulcerative
Sore throat (viral) NOS
Viral pharyngitis

Excludes *abscess:*
  peritonsillar [quinsy] (475)
  pharyngeal NOS (478.29)
  retropharyngeal (478.24)
 chronic pharyngitis (472.1)
 infectious mononucleosis (075)
 that specified as (due to):
  Coxsackie (virus) (074.0)
  gonococcus (098.6)
  herpes simplex (054.79)
  influenza (487.1, 488.02, 488.12)
  septic (034.0)
  streptococcal (034.0)

Coding Clinic: 2012, Q2, P18-19; 1985, Sept-Oct, P9

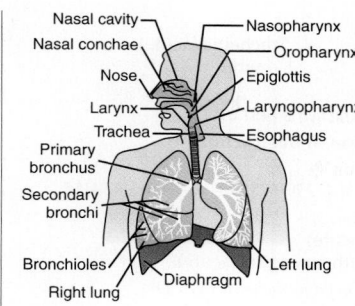

Figure 8–1 Respiratory system. (From Buck CJ: Step-by-Step Medical Coding, ed 2011, Philadelphia, WB Saunders, 2011)

Figure 8–2 Paranasal sinuses. (From Buck CJ: Step-by-Step Medical Coding, ed 2011, Philadelphia, WB Saunders, 2011)

Item 8-1 Pharyngitis is painful inflammation of the pharynx (sore throat). Ninety percent of the infections are caused by a virus with the remaining being bacterial and rarely a fungus (candidiasis). Other irritants such as pollutants, chemicals, or smoke may cause similar symptoms.

463 Acute tonsillitis
Inflammation of pharyngeal tonsils caused by virus/bacteria

Tonsillitis (acute):	Tonsillitis (acute):
NOS	septic
follicular	staphylococcal
gangrenous	suppurative
infective	ulcerative
pneumococcal	viral

Excludes *chronic tonsillitis (474.0)*
 hypertrophy of tonsils (474.1)
 peritonsillar abscess [quinsy] (475)
 sore throat:
  acute or NOS (462)
  septic (034.0)
 streptococcal tonsillitis (034.0)

Coding Clinic: 1984, Nov-Dec, P16

● **464 Acute laryngitis and tracheitis**

Excludes *that associated with influenza (487.1, 488.02, 488.12)*
 that due to Streptococcus (034.0)

● **464.0 Acute laryngitis**
Laryngitis (acute):
 NOS
 edematous
 Hemophilus influenzae [H. influenzae]
 pneumococcal
 septic
 suppurative
 ulcerative

Excludes *chronic laryngitis (476.0–476.1)*
 influenzal laryngitis (487.1, 488.02, 488.12)

464.00 Without mention of obstruction

464.01 With obstruction 🔖
 (Ex) 012.20-012.86, 464.00-464.31, 519.8-519.9

Item 8-2 Laryngitis is an inflammation of the larynx (voice box) resulting in hoarse voice or the complete loss of the voice. **Tracheitis** is an inflammation of the trachea (often following a URI) commonly caused by *staphylococcus aureus* resulting in inspiratory stridor (crowing sound on inspiration) and a croup-like cough.

● **464.1 Acute tracheitis**

Tracheitis (acute):   Tracheitis (acute):
  NOS   viral
  catarrhal

Excludes   *chronic tracheitis (491.8)*

464.10 Without mention of obstruction

464.11 With obstruction
Ex: 012.20-012.86, 017.90-017.96, 464.10-464.31, 519.8-519.9

● **464.2 Acute laryngotracheitis**

Laryngotracheitis (acute)
Tracheitis (acute) with laryngitis (acute)

Excludes   *chronic laryngotracheitis (476.1)*

464.20 Without mention of obstruction

464.21 With obstruction
Ex: 012.20-012.86, 017.90-017.96, 464.10-464.31, 519.8-519.9

● **464.3 Acute epiglottitis**

Viral epiglottitis

Excludes   *epiglottitis, chronic (476.1)*

464.30 Without mention of obstruction
Ex: 464.01, 464.30-464.31, 464.51

464.31 With obstruction
Ex: 012.20-012.86, 017.90-017.96, 464.10-464.31, 519.8-519.9

464.4 Croup

Croup syndrome

● **464.5 Supraglottitis, unspecified**

464.50 Without mention of obstruction
Coding Clinic: 2001, Q4, P42-43

464.51 With obstruction
Ex: 012.20-012.86, 017.90-017.96, 464.00-464.31, 519.8-519.9

● **465 Acute upper respiratory infections of multiple or unspecified sites**

Excludes   *upper respiratory infection due to:*
    influenza (487.1, 488.02, 488.12)
    Streptococcus (034.0)

465.0 Acute laryngopharyngitis

465.8 Other multiple sites
Multiple URI
Coding Clinic: 2007, Q4, P84-86

465.9 Unspecified site
Acute URI NOS
Upper respiratory infection (acute)
Coding Clinic: 1990, Q1, P19

● **466 Acute bronchitis and bronchiolitis**

Includes   that with:
    bronchospasm
    obstruction

466.0 Acute bronchitis
Inflammation/irritation of bronchial tubes lasting 2-3 weeks, which is most commonly caused by a virus

Bronchitis, acute or   Bronchitis, acute or
  subacute: subacute:
  fibrinous   septic
  membranous   viral
  pneumococcal   with tracheitis
  purulent
Croupous bronchitis
Tracheobronchitis, acute

Excludes   *acute bronchitis with chronic obstructive pulmonary disease (491.22)*
Coding Clinic: 2004, Q4, P81-82,137; Q1, P3; 2002, Q4, P46; 1996, Q4, P27-28; 1993, 5th Issue, P4x2; 1991, Q3, P17-18; 1988, Q1, P12

OGCR   Section I.C.8.b.1

Acute bronchitis, 466.0, is due to an infectious organism. When acute bronchitis is documented with COPD, code 491.22, Obstructive chronic bronchitis with acute bronchitis, should be assigned. It is not necessary to also assign code 466.0. If a medical record documents acute bronchitis with COPD with acute exacerbation, only code 491.22 should be assigned. The acute bronchitis included in code 491.22 supersedes the acute exacerbation. If a medical record documents COPD with acute exacerbation without mention of acute bronchitis, only code 491.21 should be assigned.

● **466.1 Acute bronchiolitis**

Bronchiolitis (acute)
Capillary pneumonia

Excludes   *respiratory bronchiolitis interstitial lung disease (516.34)*
Coding Clinic: 1988, Q1, P12

466.11 Acute bronchiolitis due to respiratory syncytial virus (RSV)
Ex: 466.11
Coding Clinic: 2005, Q1, P10; 1996, Q4, P27-28

466.19 Acute bronchiolitis due to other infectious organisms
Use additional code to identify organism
Ex: 466.0-466.19

OTHER DISEASES OF THE UPPER RESPIRATORY TRACT (470–478)

470 Deviated nasal septum
Deflected septum (nasal) (acquired)

Excludes   *congenital (754.0)*

● **471 Nasal polyps**

Excludes   *adenomatous polyps (212.0)*

471.0 Polyp of nasal cavity
Polyp:
  choanal
  nasopharyngeal

471.1 Polypoid sinus degeneration
Woakes' syndrome or ethmoiditis

471.8 Other polyp of sinus
Polyp of sinus:
  accessory
  ethmoidal
  maxillary
  sphenoidal

471.9 Unspecified nasal polyp
Nasal polyp NOS

● **472 Chronic pharyngitis and nasopharyngitis**

472.0 Chronic rhinitis
Ozena
Rhinitis: Rhinitis:
  NOS   obstructive
  atrophic   purulent
  granulomatous   ulcerative
  hypertrophic

Excludes   *allergic rhinitis (477.0–477.9)*

472.1 Chronic pharyngitis
Chronic sore throat
Pharyngitis: Pharyngitis:
  atrophic   hypertrophic
  granular (chronic)

472.2 Chronic nasopharyngitis

Excludes   *acute or unspecified nasopharyngitis (460)*

Deviated septal cartilage

Figure 8–3   Deviated nasal septum.

Item 8–3   A deviated nasal septum is the displacement of the septal cartilage that separates the nares. This displacement causes obstructed air flow through the nasal passages. A child can be born with this displacement (congenital), or the condition may be acquired through trauma, such as a sports injury. Symptoms include nasal block, sinusitis, and related secondary infections. Septoplasty is surgical repair of this condition.

Item 8-4 Nasal polyps are an abnormal growth of tissue (tumor) projecting from a mucous membrane and attached to the surface by a narrow elongated stalk (pedunculated). Nasal polyps usually originate in the ethmoid sinus but also may occur in the maxillary sinus. Symptoms are nasal block, sinusitis, anosmia, and secondary infections.

● **473 Chronic sinusitis**

Includes   abscess (chronic) of sinus (accessory) (nasal)
empyema (chronic) of sinus (accessory) (nasal)
infection (chronic) of sinus (accessory) (nasal)
suppuration (chronic) of sinus (accessory) (nasal)

Excludes   acute sinusitis (461.0–461.9)

473.0 Maxillary
Antritis (chronic)

473.1 Frontal

473.2 Ethmoidal

Excludes Woakes' ethmoiditis (471.1)

473.3 Sphenoidal

473.8 Other chronic sinusitis
Pansinusitis (chronic)

473.9 Unspecified sinusitis (chronic)
Sinusitis (chronic) NOS

● **474 Chronic disease of tonsils and adenoids**

● **474.0 Chronic tonsillitis and adenoiditis**

Excludes acute or unspecified tonsillitis (463)

474.00 Chronic tonsillitis
Coding Clinic: 1984, Nov-Dec, P16

474.01 Chronic adenoiditis

474.02 Chronic tonsillitis and adenoiditis

● **474.1 Hypertrophy of tonsils and adenoids**
Enlargement of tonsils or adenoids
Hyperplasia of tonsils or adenoids
Hypertrophy of tonsils or adenoids

Excludes that with:
adenoiditis (474.01)
adenoiditis and tonsillitis (474.02)
tonsillitis (474.00)

474.10 Tonsils with adenoids
Coding Clinic: 2005, Q2, P16

474.11 Tonsils alone
Coding Clinic: 1984, Nov-Dec, P16

474.12 Adenoids alone

474.2 Adenoid vegetations

474.8 Other chronic disease of tonsils and adenoids
Amygdalolith
Calculus, tonsil
Cicatrix of tonsil (and adenoid)
Tonsillar tag
Ulcer, tonsil

474.9 Unspecified chronic disease of tonsils and adenoids
Disease (chronic) of tonsils (and adenoids)

● **475 Peritonsillar abscess** 🗝
Abscess of tonsil
Peritonsillar cellulitis
Quinsy

Excludes tonsillitis:
acute or NOS (463)
chronic (474.0)

(Ex:) 475, 519.8-519.9

● **476 Chronic laryngitis and laryngotracheitis**

476.0 Chronic laryngitis
Laryngitis: Laryngitis:
catarrhal   sicca
hypertrophic

476.1 Chronic laryngotracheitis
Laryngitis, chronic, with tracheitis (chronic)
Tracheitis, chronic, with laryngitis

Excludes chronic tracheitis (491.8)
laryngitis and tracheitis, acute or unspecified
(464.00–464.51)

● **477 Allergic rhinitis**

Includes   allergic rhinitis (nonseasonal) (seasonal)
hay fever
spasmodic rhinorrhea

Excludes allergic rhinitis with asthma (bronchial) (493.0)

477.0 Due to pollen
Pollinosis

477.1 Due to food

477.2 Due to animal (cat) (dog) hair and dander

477.8 Due to other allergen

477.9 Cause unspecified
Coding Clinic: 1997, Q2, P9-10

● **478 Other diseases of upper respiratory tract**

478.0 Hypertrophy of nasal turbinates

● **478.1 Other diseases of nasal cavity and sinuses**

Excludes varicose ulcer of nasal septum (456.8)
Coding Clinic: 1995, Q4, P50; 1990, Q1, P8

478.11 Nasal mucositis (ulcerative)
Use additional E code to identify adverse effects
of therapy, such as:
antineoplastic and immunosuppressive drugs
(E930.7, E933.1)
radiation therapy (E879.2)
Coding Clinic: 2006, Q4, P88-91

478.19 Other disease of nasal cavity and sinuses
Abscess of nose (septum)
Cyst or mucocele of sinus (nasal)
Necrosis of nose (septum)
Rhinolith
Ulcer of nose (septum)

● **478.2 Other diseases of pharynx, not elsewhere classified**

478.20 Unspecified disease of pharynx

478.21 Cellulitis of pharynx or nasopharynx 🗝
(Ex:) 478.20-478.24, 519.8-519.9

478.22 Parapharyngeal abscess 🗝
(Ex:) 478.20-478.24, 519.8-519.9

478.24 Retropharyngeal abscess 🗝
(Ex:) 478.20-478.24, 519.8-519.9

478.25 Edema of pharynx or nasopharynx

478.26 Cyst of pharynx or nasopharynx

478.29 Other
Abscess of pharynx or nasopharynx

Excludes ulcerative pharyngitis (462)

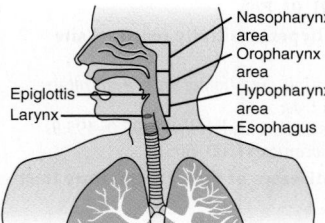

Figure 8-4 The pharynx.

Item 8-5 The **pharynx** is the passage for both food and air between
the mouth and the esophagus and is divided into three areas: nasopharynx,
oropharynx, and hypopharynx. The hypopharynx branches into the esophagus
and the voice box.

DISEASES OF THE RESPIRATORY SYSTEM (460-519)

N Newborn: 0   **P** Pediatric: 0–17   **M** Maternity: 12–55   **A** Adult: 15–124   ♀ Females Only   ♂ Males Only

(Ex:) CC/MCC Exclusions   🗝 Complication\Comorbidity   🗝 Major C\C   🗝 Present on Admission Requirement   🗝 Hospital-Acquired Condition   **823**

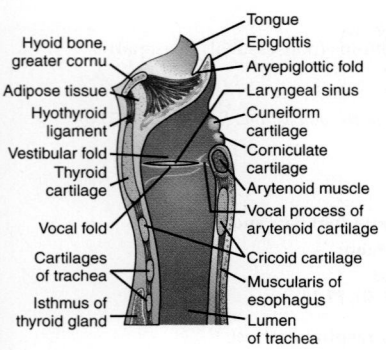

Tongue
Epiglottis
Aryepiglottic fold
Laryngeal sinus
Cuneiform cartilage
Corniculate cartilage
Arytenoid muscle
Vocal process of arytenoid cartilage
Cricoid cartilage
Muscularis of esophagus
Lumen of trachea

Hyoid bone, greater cornu
Adipose tissue
Hyothyroid ligament
Vestibular fold
Thyroid cartilage
Vocal fold
Cartilages of trachea
Isthmus of thyroid gland

Figure 8–5 Coronal section of the larynx.

Item 8–6 The **larynx** extends from the tongue to the trachea and is divided into an upper and lower portion separated by folds. The framework of the larynx is cartilage composed of the single cricoid, thyroid, and epiglottic cartilages, and the paired arytenoid, cuneiform, and corniculate cartilages.

● **478.3 Paralysis of vocal cords or larynx**
    478.30 Paralysis, unspecified
        Laryngoplegia
        Paralysis of glottis
    478.31 Unilateral, partial
    478.32 Unilateral, complete
    478.33 Bilateral, partial
    478.34 Bilateral, complete
        (Ex) 478.30-478.34, 478.5, 478.70, 519.8-519.9

478.4 Polyp of vocal cord or larynx
    Excludes *adenomatous polyps (212.1)*

478.5 Other diseases of vocal cords
    Abscess of vocal cords
    Cellulitis of vocal cords
    Granuloma of vocal cords
    Leukoplakia of vocal cords
    Chorditis (fibrinous) (nodosa) (tuberosa)
    Singers' nodes

478.6 Edema of larynx
    Edema (of):
        glottis
        subglottic
        supraglottic

● **478.7 Other diseases of larynx, not elsewhere classified**
    478.70 Unspecified disease of larynx
    478.71 Cellulitis and perichondritis of larynx
        (Ex) 478.70-478.71, 478.79
    478.74 Stenosis of larynx
    478.75 Laryngeal spasm
        Laryngismus (stridulus)
    478.79 Other
        Abscess of larynx
        Necrosis of larynx
        Obstruction of larynx
        Pachyderma of larynx
        Ulcer of larynx
        Excludes *ulcerative laryngitis (464.00–464.01)*
        Coding Clinic: 1991, Q3, P20

478.8 Upper respiratory tract hypersensitivity reaction, site unspecified
    Excludes *hypersensitivity reaction of lower respiratory tract, as:*
        extrinsic allergic alveolitis (495.0–495.9)
        pneumoconiosis (500–505)

478.9 Other and unspecified diseases of upper respiratory tract
    Abscess of trachea
    Cicatrix of trachea

Item 8–7 Pneumonia is an infection of the lungs, caused by a variety of microorganisms, including viruses, most commonly the *Streptococcus pneumoniae* (pneumococcus) bacteria, fungi, and parasites. Pneumonia occurs when the immune system is weakened, often by a URI or influenza.

PNEUMONIA AND INFLUENZA (480–488)

Excludes *pneumonia:*
    allergic or eosinophilic (518.3)
    aspiration:
        NOS (507.0)
        newborn (770.18)
        solids and liquids (507.0–507.8)
    congenital (770.0)
    lipoid (507.1)
    passive (514)
    rheumatic (390)
    ventilator-associated (997.31)

● **480 Viral pneumonia**
    480.0 Pneumonia due to adenovirus
        (Ex) 011.00-012.16, 012.80-012.86, 017.90-017.96, 020.3-020.5, 021.3, 022.1, 031.0, 039.1, 073.0, 115.05, 115.15, 115.95, 122.1, 130.4, 136.3, 480.0-487.1, 488.01-488.02, 488.11-488.12, 488.81-488.82, 495.0-495.9, 500-508.1, 508.8-508.9, 517.1, 517.8, 518.89, 519.8-519.9, 793.11
    480.1 Pneumonia due to respiratory syncytial virus
        (Ex) 011.00-012.16, 012.80-012.86, 017.90-017.96, 020.3-020.5, 021.3, 022.1, 031.0, 039.1, 073.0, 115.05, 115.15, 115.95, 122.1, 130.4, 136.3, 480.0-487.1, 488.01-488.02, 488.11-488.12, 488.81-488.82, 495.0-495.9, 500-508.1, 508.8-508.9, 517.1, 517.8, 518.89, 519.8-519.9, 793.11
        Coding Clinic: 2010, Q4, P98; 1996, Q4, P27-28; 1988, Q1, P12
    480.2 Pneumonia due to parainfluenza virus
        (Ex) 011.00-012.16, 012.80-012.86, 017.90-017.96, 020.3-020.5, 021.3, 022.1, 031.0, 039.1, 073.0, 115.05, 115.15, 115.95, 122.1, 130.4, 136.3, 480.0-487.1, 488.01-488.02, 488.11-488.12, 488.81-488.82, 495.0-495.9, 500-508.1, 508.8-508.9, 517.1, 517.8, 518.89, 519.8-519.9, 793.11
    480.3 Pneumonia due to SARS-associated coronavirus
        (Ex) 011.00-012.16, 012.80-012.86, 017.90-017.96, 021.2, 031.0, 039.1, 115.05, 115.15, 115.95, 122.1, 130.4, 136.3, 480.0-487.1, 488.01-488.02, 488.11-488.12, 488.81-488.82, 494.0-508.1, 508.8-508.9, 517.1, 517.8, 518.89, 519.8-519.9, 748.61, 793.11
        Coding Clinic: 2003, Q4, P46-48
    480.8 Pneumonia due to other virus not elsewhere classified
        Excludes *congenital rubella pneumonitis (771.0)*
        pneumonia complicating viral diseases classified elsewhere (484.1–484.8)
        (Ex) 011.00-012.16, 012.80-012.86, 017.90-017.96, 020.3-020.5, 021.3, 022.1, 031.0, 039.1, 073.0, 115.05, 115.15, 115.95, 122.1, 130.4, 136.3, 480.0-487.1, 488.01-488.02, 488.11-488.12, 488.81-488.82, 495.0-495.9, 500-508.1, 508.8-508.9, 517.1, 517.8, 518.89, 519.8-519.9, 793.11
    480.9 Viral pneumonia, unspecified
        (Ex) 011.00-012.16, 012.80-012.86, 017.90-017.96, 020.3-020.5, 021.3, 022.1, 031.0, 039.1, 073.0, 115.05, 115.15, 115.95, 122.1, 130.4, 136.3, 480.0-487.1, 488.01-488.02, 488.11-488.12, 488.81-488.82, 495.0-495.9, 500-508.1, 508.8-508.9, 517.1, 517.8, 518.89, 519.8-519.9, 793.11
        Coding Clinic: 2010, Q4, P135; 1998, Q3, P5

481 Pneumococcal pneumonia [Streptococcus pneumoniae pneumonia]
    Lobar pneumonia, organism unspecified
    (Ex) 011.00-012.16, 012.80-012.86, 017.90-017.96, 021.2, 031.0, 039.1, 115.05, 115.15, 115.95, 122.1, 130.4, 136.3, 480.0-480.2, 480.8-487.1, 488.01-488.02, 488.11-488.12, 488.81-488.82, 494.0-508.1, 508.8-508.9, 517.1, 517.8, 518.89, 519.8-519.9, 748.61, 793.11
    Coding Clinic: 2009, Q3, P9; 1998, Q2, P7; 1991, Q1, P13; 1988, Q1, P13; 1985, Mar-April, P6

◄ New   ◄▥ Revised   ~~deleted~~ Deleted   Excludes   Includes   Use additional   Code first   Omit code

824   ● Unacceptable Principal Diagnosis   ● Use Additional Digit(s)   ▷ Manifestation Code   OGCR Official Guidelines   Coding Clinic

● **482 Other bacterial pneumonia**

482.0 Pneumonia due to Klebsiella pneumoniae 🔹
Ex: 011.00-012.16, 012.80-012.86, 017.90-017.96, 021.2, 031.0, 039.1, 115.05, 115.15, 115.95, 122.1, 130.4, 136.3, 480.0-480.2, 480.8-487.1, 488.01-488.02, 488.11-488.12, 488.81-488.82, 494.0-508.1, 508.8-508.9, 517.1, 517.8, 518.89, 519.8-519.9, 748.61, 793.11

482.1 Pneumonia due to Pseudomonas 🔹
Ex: 011.00-012.16, 012.80-012.86, 017.90-017.96, 021.2, 031.0, 039.1, 115.05, 115.15, 115.95, 122.1, 130.4, 136.3, 480.0-480.2, 480.8-487.1, 488.01-488.02, 488.11-488.12, 488.81-488.82, 494.0-508.1, 508.8-508.9, 517.1, 517.8, 518.89, 519.8-519.9, 748.61, 793.11

482.2 Pneumonia due to Hemophilus influenzae [H. influenzae] 🔹
Ex: 011.00-012.16, 012.80-012.86, 017.90-017.96, 021.2, 031.0, 039.1, 115.05, 115.15, 115.95, 122.1, 130.4 136.3, 480.0-480.2, 480.8-487.1, 488.01-488.02, 488.11-488.12, 488.81-488.82, 494.0-508.1, 508.8-508.9, 517.1, 517.8, 518.89, 519.8-519.9, 748.61, 793.11
Coding Clinic: 2005, Q2, P19-20; 1993, Q4, P39

● **482.3 Pneumonia due to Streptococcus**
Excludes Streptococcus pneumoniae pneumonia (481)
Coding Clinic: 1988, Q1, P13

482.30 Streptococcus, unspecified 🔹
Ex: 011.00-012.16, 012.80-012.86, 017.90-017.96, 021.2, 031.0, 039.1, 115.05, 115.15, 115.95, 122.1, 130.4, 136.3, 480.0-480.2, 480.8-487.1, 488.01-488.02, 488.11-488.12, 488.81-488.82, 494.0-508.1, 508.8-508.9, 517.1, 517.8, 518.89, 519.8-519.9, 748.61, 793.11

482.31 Group A 🔹
Ex: 011.00-012.16, 012.80-012.86, 017.90-017.96, 021.2, 031.0, 039.1, 115.05, 115.15, 115.95, 122.1, 130.4, 136.3, 480.0-480.2, 480.8-487.1, 488.01-488.02, 488.11-488.12, 488.81-488.82, 494.0-508.1, 508.8-508.9, 517.1, 517.8, 518.89, 519.8-519.9, 748.61, 793.11

482.32 Group B 🔹
Ex: 011.00-012.16, 012.80-012.86, 017.90-017.96, 021.2, 031.0, 039.1, 115.05, 115.15, 115.95, 122.1, 130.4, 136.3, 480.0-480.2, 480.8-487.1, 488.01-488.02, 488.11-488.12, 488.81-488.82, 494.0-508.1, 508.8-508.9, 517.1, 517.8, 518.89, 519.8-519.9, 748.61, 793.11

482.39 Other Streptococcus 🔹
Ex: 011.00-012.16, 012.80-012.86, 017.90-017.96, 021.2, 031.0, 039.1, 115.05, 115.15, 115.95, 122.1, 130.4, 136.3, 480.0-480.2, 480.8-487.1, 488.01-488.02, 488.11-488.12, 488.81-488.82, 494.0-508.1, 508.8-508.9, 517.1, 517.8, 518.89, 519.8-519.9, 748.61, 793.11

● **482.4 Pneumonia due to Staphylococcus**
Coding Clinic: 1991, Q3, P16-17

482.40 Pneumonia due to Staphylococcus, unspecified 🔹
Ex: 011.00-012.16, 012.80-012.86, 017.90-017.96, 021.2, 031.0, 039.1, 115.05, 115.15, 115.95, 122.1, 130.4, 136.3, 480.0-480.2, 480.8-487.1, 488.01-488.02, 488.11-488.12, 488.81-488.82, 494.0-508.1, 508.8-508.9, 517.1, 517.8, 518.89, 519.8-519.9, 748.61, 793.11

482.41 Methicillin susceptible pneumonia due to Staphylococcus aureus 🔹
MSSA pneumonia
Pneumonia due to Staphylococcus aureus NOS
Ex: 011.00-012.16, 012.80-012.86, 017.90-017.96, 021.2, 031.0, 039.1, 115.05, 115.15, 115.95, 122.1, 130.4, 136.3, 480.0-480.2, 480.8-487.1, 488.01-488.02, 488.11-488.12, 488.81-488.82, 494.0-508.1, 508.8-508.9, 517.1, 517.8, 518.89, 519.8-519.9, 748.61, 793.11
Coding Clinic: 2008, Q4, P69-73

482.42 Methicillin resistant pneumonia due to Staphylococcus aureus 🔹
Ex: 011.00-012.16, 012.80-012.86, 017.90-017.96, 021.2, 031.0, 039.1, 115.05, 115.15, 115.95, 122.1, 130.4, 136.3, 480.0-480.2, 480.8-487.1, 488.01-488.02, 488.11-488.12, 488.81-488.82, 494.0-508.1, 508.8-508.9, 517.1, 517.8, 518.89, 519.8-519.9, 748.61, 793.11
Coding Clinic: 2008, Q4, P69-73

482.49 Other Staphylococcus pneumonia 🔹
Ex: 011.00-012.16, 012.80-012.86, 017.90-017.96, 021.2, 031.0, 039.1, 115.05, 115.15, 115.95, 122.1, 130.4, 136.3, 480.0-480.2, 480.8-487.1, 488.01-488.02, 488.11-488.12, 488.81-488.82, 494.0-508.1, 508.8-508.9, 517.1, 517.8, 518.89, 519.8-519.9, 748.61, 793.11
Coding Clinic: 2013, Q2, P21

● **482.8 Pneumonia due to other specified bacteria**
Excludes pneumonia complicating infectious disease classified elsewhere (484.1-484.8)
Coding Clinic: 1988, Q3, P11

482.81 Anaerobes 🔹
Bacteroides (melaninogenicus)
Gram-negative anaerobes
Ex: 011.00-012.16, 012.80-012.86, 017.90-017.96, 021.2, 031.0, 039.1, 115.05, 115.15, 115.95, 122.1, 130.4, 136.3, 480.0-480.2, 480.8-487.1, 488.01-488.02, 488.11-488.12, 488.81-488.82, 494.0-508.1, 508.8-508.9, 517.1, 517.8, 518.89, 519.8-519.9, 748.61, 793.11

482.82 Escherichia coli [E. coli] 🔹
Ex: 011.00-012.16, 012.80-012.86, 017.90-017.96, 021.2, 031.0, 039.1, 115.05, 115.15, 115.95, 122.1, 130.4, 136.3, 480.0-480.2, 480.8-487.1, 488.01-488.02, 488.11-488.12, 488.81-488.82, 494.0-508.1, 508.8-508.9, 517.1, 517.8, 518.89, 519.8-519.9, 748.61, 793.11

482.83 Other gram-negative bacteria 🔹
Gram-negative pneumonia NOS
Proteus
Serratia marcescens
Excludes gram-negative anaerobes (482.81) Legionnaires' disease (482.84)
Ex: 011.00-012.16, 012.80-012.86, 017.90-017.96, 021.2, 031.0, 039.1, 115.05, 115.15, 115.95, 122.1, 130.4, 136.3, 480.0-480.2, 480.8-487.1, 488.01-488.02, 488.11-488.12, 488.81-488.82, 494.0-508.1, 508.8-508.9, 517.1, 517.8, 518.89, 519.8-519.9, 748.61, 793.11
Coding Clinic: 1998, Q2, P5; 1994, Q3, P9; 1993, Q4, P39

482.84 Legionnaires' disease 🔹
Ex: 011.00-012.16, 012.80-012.86, 017.90-017.96, 021.2, 031.0, 039.1, 115.05, 115.15, 115.95, 122.1, 130.4, 136.3, 480.0-480.2, 480.8-487.1, 488.01-488.02, 488.11-488.12, 488.81-488.82, 494.0-508.1, 508.8-508.9, 517.1, 517.8, 518.89, 519.8-519.9, 748.61, 793.11

482.89 Other specified bacteria 🔹
Ex: 011.00-012.16, 012.80-012.86, 017.90-017.96, 021.2, 031.0, 039.1, 115.05, 115.15, 115.95, 122.1, 130.4, 136.3, 480.0-480.2, 480.8-487.1, 488.01-488.02, 488.11-488.12, 488.81-488.82, 494.0-508.1, 508.8-508.9, 517.1, 517.8, 518.89, 519.8-519.9, 748.61, 793.11
Coding Clinic: 2013, Q2, P13; 1998, Q2, P6; 1997, Q2, P6; 1994, Q1, P17-18

482.9 Bacterial pneumonia unspecified 🔹
Ex: 011.00-012.16, 012.80-012.86, 017.90-017.96, 021.2, 031.0, 039.1, 115.05, 115.15, 115.95, 122.1, 130.4, 136.3, 480.0-480.2, 480.8-487.1, 488.01-488.02, 488.11-488.12, 488.81-488.82, 494.0-508.1, 508.8-508.9, 517.1, 517.8, 518.89, 519.8-519.9, 748.61, 793.11
Coding Clinic: 1998, Q2, P4, 6X2; 1997, Q2, P6; 1994, Q1, P17-18

● **483 Pneumonia due to other specified organism**

483.0 Mycoplasma pneumoniae 🔹
Eaton's agent
Pleuropneumonia-like organisms [PPLO]
Ex: 011.00-012.16, 012.80-012.86, 017.90-017.96, 021.2, 031.0, 039.1, 115.05, 115.15, 115.95, 122.1, 130.4, 136.3, 480.0-480.2, 480.8-487.1, 488.01-488.02, 488.11-488.12, 488.81-488.82, 494.0-508.1, 508.8-508.9, 517.1, 517.8, 518.89, 519.8-519.9, 748.61, 793.11
Coding Clinic: 1987, Nov-Dec, P5-6

483.1 Chlamydia 🔹
Ex: 011.00-012.16, 012.80-012.86, 017.90-017.96, 021.2, 031.0, 039.1, 115.05, 115.15, 115.95, 122.1, 130.4, 136.3, 480.0-480.2, 480.8-487.1, 488.01-488.02, 488.11-488.12, 488.81-488.82, 494.0-508.1, 508.8-508.9, 517.1, 517.8, 518.89, 519.8-519.9, 748.61, 793.11

483.8 Other specified organism 🔹
Ex: 011.00-012.16, 012.80-012.86, 017.90-017.96, 021.2, 031.0, 039.1, 115.05, 115.15, 115.95, 122.1, 130.4, 136.3, 480.0-480.2, 480.8-487.1, 488.01-488.02, 488.11-488.12, 488.81-488.82, 494.0-508.1, 508.8-508.9, 517.1, 517.8, 518.89, 519.8-519.9, 748.61, 793.11

DISEASES OF THE RESPIRATORY SYSTEM (460-519)

N Newborn: 0   P Pediatric: 0-17   M Maternity: 12-55   A Adult: 15-124   ♀ Females Only   ♂ Males Only
Ex: CC/MCC Exclusions   🔹 Complication\Comorbidity   🔹 Major C\C   🔹 Present on Admission Requirement   🔹 Hospital-Acquired Condition

● **484 Pneumonia in infectious diseases classified elsewhere**

▷ **484.1 Pneumonia in cytomegalic inclusion disease** 🔖

Code first underlying disease, as: (078.5)

(Ex:) 011.00-012.16, 012.80-012.86, 017.90-017.96, 021.2, 031.0, 039.1, 115.05, 115.15, 115.95, 122.1, 130.4, 136.3, 480.0-480.2, 480.8-487.1, 488.01-488.02, 488.11-488.12, 488.81-488.82, 494.0-508.1, 508.8-508.9, 517.1, 517.8, 518.89, 519.8-519.9, 748.61, 793.11

▷ **484.3 Pneumonia in whooping cough** 🔖

Code first underlying disease, as: (033.0–033.9)

(Ex:) 011.00-012.16, 012.80-012.86, 017.90-017.96, 021.2, 031.0, 039.1, 115.05, 115.15, 115.95, 122.1, 130.4, 136.3, 480.0-480.2, 480.8-487.1, 488.01-488.02, 488.11-488.12, 488.81-488.82, 494.0-508.1, 508.8-508.9, 517.1, 517.8, 518.89, 519.8-519.9, 748.61, 793.11

▷ **484.5 Pneumonia in anthrax** 🔖

Code first underlying disease (022.1)

(Ex:) 011.00-012.16, 012.80-012.86, 017.90-017.96, 021.2, 031.0, 039.1, 115.05, 115.15, 115.95, 122.1, 130.4, 136.3, 480.0-480.2, 480.8-487.1, 488.01-488.02, 488.11-488.12, 488.81-488.82, 494.0-508.1, 508.8-508.9, 517.1, 517.8, 518.89, 519.8-519.9, 748.61, 793.11

▷ **484.6 Pneumonia in aspergillosis** 🔖

Code first underlying disease (117.3)

(Ex:) 011.00-012.16, 012.80-012.86, 017.90-017.96, 021.2, 031.0, 039.1, 115.05, 115.15, 115.95, 122.1, 130.4, 136.3, 480.0-480.2, 480.8-487.1, 488.01-488.02, 488.11-488.12, 488.81-488.82, 494.0-508.1, 508.8-508.9, 517.1, 517.8, 518.89, 519.8-519.9, 748.61, 793.11

Coding Clinic: 1997, Q4, P40

▷ **484.7 Pneumonia in other systemic mycoses** 🔖

Code first underlying disease

Excludes pneumonia in:
candidiasis (112.4)
coccidioidomycosis (114.0)
histoplasmosis (115.0–115.9 with fifth-digit 5)

(Ex:) 011.00-012.16, 012.80-012.86, 017.90-017.96, 021.2, 031.0, 039.1, 115.05, 115.15, 115.95, 122.1, 130.4, 136.3, 480.0-480.2, 480.8-487.1, 488.01-488.02, 488.11-488.12, 488.81-488.82, 494.0-508.1, 508.8-508.9, 517.1, 517.8, 518.89, 519.8-519.9, 748.61, 793.11

▷ **484.8 Pneumonia in other infectious diseases classified elsewhere** 🔖

Code first underlying disease, as:
Q fever (083.0)
typhoid fever (002.0)

Excludes pneumonia in:
actinomycosis (039.1)
measles (055.1)
nocardiosis (039.1)
ornithosis (073.0)
Pneumocystis carinii (136.3)
salmonellosis (003.22)
toxoplasmosis (130.4)
tuberculosis (011.6)
tularemia (021.2)
varicella (052.1)

(Ex:) 011.00-012.16, 012.80-012.86, 017.90-017.96, 021.2, 031.0, 039.1, 115.05, 115.15, 115.95, 122.1, 130.4, 136.3, 480.0-480.2, 480.8-487.1, 488.01-488.02, 488.11-488.12, 488.81-488.82, 494.0-508.1, 508.8-508.9, 517.1, 517.8, 519.8-519.9, 748.61, 793.11

● **485 Bronchopneumonia, organism unspecified** 🔖

Bronchopneumonia: Pneumonia:
hemorrhagic   lobular
terminal   segmental
Pleurobronchopneumonia

Excludes bronchiolitis (acute) (466.11–466.19)
chronic (491.8)
lipoid pneumonia (507.1)

(Ex:) 011.00-012.16, 012.80-012.86, 017.90-017.96, 021.2, 031.0, 039.1, 115.05, 115.15, 115.95, 122.1, 130.4, 136.3, 480.0-480.2, 480.8-487.1, 488.01-488.02, 488.11-488.12, 488.81-488.82, 494.0-508.1, 508.8-508.9, 517.1, 517.8, 518.89, 519.8-519.9, 748.61, 793.11

● **486 Pneumonia, organism unspecified** 🔖

Excludes hypostatic or passive pneumonia (514)
inhalation or aspiration pneumonia due to foreign materials (507.0–507.8)
pneumonitis due to fumes and vapors (506.0)

(Ex:) 011.00-012.16, 012.80-012.86, 017.90-017.96, 021.2, 031.0, 039.1, 115.05, 115.15, 115.95, 122.1, 130.4, 136.3, 480.0-480.2, 480.8-487.1, 488.01-488.02, 488.11-488.12, 488.81-488.82, 494.0-508.1, 508.8-508.9, 517.1, 517.8, 518.89, 519.8-519.9, 748.61, 793.11

Coding Clinic: 2010, Q4, P137; Q1, P8; 2008, Q4, P140-143; 2006, Q2, P20; 1999, Q4, P6; Q3, P9; 1998, Q3, P7; Q2, P4-5; Q1, P8; 1997, Q3, P9; 1995, Q4, P52; 1994, Q1, P17-18; 1993, Q3, P9; Q1, P21; 1985, Mar-April, P6

● **487 Influenza**

Influenza caused by unspecified influenza virus

Excludes Hemophilus influenzae [H. influenzae]:
infection NOS (041.5)
laryngitis (464.00–464.01)
meningitis (320.0)
influenza due to 2009 H1N1 [swine] influenza virus (488.11-488.19)
influenza due to identified avian influenza virus (488.01-488.09)
influenza due to identified (novel) 2009 H1N1 influenza virus (488.11-488.19)

487.0 With pneumonia 🔖

Influenza with pneumonia, any form
Influenzal:
bronchopneumonia
pneumonia

Use additional code to identify the type of pneumonia (480.0–480.9, 481, 482.0–482.9, 483.0–483.8, 485)

(Ex:) 011.00-012.16, 012.80-012.86, 017.90-017.96, 021.2, 031.0, 039.1, 115.05, 115.15, 115.95, 122.1, 130.4, 136.3, 480.0-480.2, 480.8-487.1, 488.01-488.02, 488.11-488.12, 488.81-488.82, 494.0-508.1, 508.8-508.9, 517.1, 517.8, 518.89, 519.8-519.9, 748.61, 793.11

Coding Clinic: 2010, Q1, P8; 2005, Q2, P18-19

487.1 With other respiratory manifestations

Influenza NEC
Influenza NOS
Influenzal:
laryngitis
pharyngitis
respiratory infection (upper) (acute)

Coding Clinic: 2011, Q4, P114; 2005, Q2, P18-19; 1999, Q4, P26; 1987, Jan-Feb, P16

487.8 With other manifestations

Encephalopathy due to influenza
Influenza with involvement of gastrointestinal tract

Excludes "intestinal flu" [viral gastroenteritis] (008.8)

● **488 Influenza due to certain identified influenza viruses**

Excludes influenza caused by unspecified or seasonal influenza viruses (487.0-487.8)

Coding Clinic: 2007, Q4, P87-88

● **488.0 Influenza due to identified avian influenza virus**

Avian influenza
Bird flu
Influenza A/H5N1

488.01 Influenza due to identified avian influenza virus with pneumonia 🔖

Avian influenzal:
bronchopneumonia
pneumonia
Influenza due to identified avian influenza virus with pneumonia, any form

Use additional code to identify the type of pneumonia (480.0- 480.9, 481, 482.0-482.9, 483.0-483.8, 485)

(Ex:) 011.00-012.16, 012.80-012.86, 017.90-017.96, 021.2, 031.0, 039.1, 115.05, 115.15, 115.95, 122.1, 130.4, 136.3, 480.0-480.2, 480.8-487.1, 488.01-488.82, 491.21-491.22, 493.01-493.02, 493.11-493.12, 493.21-493.22, 493.91-508.1, 508.8-508.9, 517.1, 517.8, 518.89, 519.8-519.9, 748.61, 793.11

488.02 Influenza due to identified avian influenza virus with other respiratory manifestations 🔗
  Avian influenzal:
    laryngitis
    pharyngitis
    respiratory infection (acute) (upper)
  Identified avian influenza NOS
  (Ex) 488.01-488.19, 491.21-491.22, 493.01-493.02, 493.11-493.12, 493.21-493.22, 493.91-493.92, 494.1

488.09 Influenza due to identified avian influenza virus with other manifestations 🔗
  Avian influenza with involvement of gastrointestinal tract
  Encephalopathy due to identified avian influenza
  Excludes "intestinal flu" [viral gastroenteritis] (008.8)
  (Ex) 488.01-488.19, 491.21-491.22, 493.01-493.02, 493.11-493.12, 493.21-493.22, 493.91-493.92, 494.1

● **488.1 Influenza due to identified 2009 H1N1 influenza virus**
  2009 H1N1 swine influenza virus
  (Novel) 2009 influenza H1N1
  Novel H1N1 influenza
  Novel influenza A/H1N1
  Excludes bird influenza virus infection (488.01-488.09)
      influenza A/H5N1 (488.01-488.09)
      other human infection with influenza virus of animal origin (488.81-488.89)
      swine influenza virus infection (488.81-488.89)
  Coding Clinic: 2011, Q4, P114; 2010, Q1, P8

488.11 Influenza due to identified 2009 H1N1 influenza virus with pneumonia 🔗
  Influenza due to identified (novel) 2009 H1N1 with pneumonia, any form
  (Novel) 2009 H1N1 influenzal:
    bronchopneumonia
    pneumonia
  Use additional code to identify the type of pneumonia (480.0-480.9, 481, 482.0-482.9, 483.0-483.8, 485)
  (Ex) 011.00-012.16, 012.80-012.86, 017.90-017.96, 021.2, 031.0, 039.1, 115.05, 115.15, 115.95, 122.1, 130.4, 136.3, 480.0-480.2, 480.8-487.1, 488.01-488.82, 491.21-491.22, 493.01-493.02, 493.11-493.12, 493.21-493.22, 493.91-508.1, 508.8-508.9, 517.1, 517.8, 518.89, 519.8-519.9, 748.61, 793.11

488.12 Influenza due to identified 2009 H1N1 influenza virus with other respiratory manifestations
  (Novel) 2009 H1N1 influenza NOS
  (Novel) 2009 H1N1 influenzal:
    laryngitis
    pharyngitis
    respiratory infection (acute) (upper)

488.19 Influenza due to identified 2009 H1N1 influenza virus with other manifestations
  Encephalopathy due to identified (novel) 2009 H1N1 influenza
  (Novel) 2009 H1N1 influenza with involvement of gastrointestinal tract
  Excludes "intestinal flu" [viral gastroenteritis] (008.8)

● **488.8 Influenza due to novel influenza A**
  Influenza due to animal origin influenza virus
  Infection with influenza viruses occurring in pigs or other animals
  Other novel influenza A viruses not previously found in humans
  Excludes bird influenza virus infection (488.01-488.09)
      influenza A/H5N1 (488.01-488.09)
      influenza due to identified 2009 H1N1 influenza virus (488.11-488.19)
  Coding Clinic: 2011, Q4, P114

488.81 Influenza due to identified novel influenza A virus with pneumonia 🔗
  Influenza due to animal origin influenza virus with pneumonia, any form
  Novel influenza A:
    bronchopneumonia
    pneumonia
  Use additional code to identify the type of pneumonia (480.0-480.9, 481, 482.0-482.9, 483.0-483.8, 485)

488.82 Influenza due to identified novel influenza A virus with other respiratory manifestations
  Influenza due to animal origin influenza A virus with other respiratory manifestations
  Novel influenza A:
    laryngitis
    pharyngitis
    respiratory infection (acute) (upper)

488.89 Influenza due to identified novel influenza A virus with other manifestations
  Encephalopathy due to novel influenza A
  Influenza due to animal origin influenza virus with encephalopathy
  Influenza due to animal origin influenza virus with involvement of gastrointestinal tract
  Novel influenza A with involvement of gastrointestinal tract
  Excludes "intestinal flu" [viral gastroenteritis] (008.8)

CHRONIC OBSTRUCTIVE PULMONARY DISEASE AND ALLIED CONDITIONS (490–496)

490 Bronchitis, not specified as acute or chronic
  Bronchitis NOS: Bronchitis NOS:
    catarrhal   with tracheitis NOS
  Tracheobronchitis NOS
  Excludes bronchitis:
      allergic NOS (493.9)
      asthmatic NOS (493.9)
      due to fumes and vapors (506.0)

● **491 Chronic bronchitis**
  Excludes chronic obstructive asthma (493.2)

491.0 Simple chronic bronchitis
  Catarrhal bronchitis, chronic
  Smokers' cough

491.1 Mucopurulent chronic bronchitis
  Bronchitis (chronic) (recurrent):
    fetid   purulent
    mucopurulent
  Coding Clinic: 1988, Q2, P11

Item 8–8 Chronic bronchitis is usually defined as being present in any patient who has persistent cough with sputum production for at least three months in at least two consecutive years. **Simple chronic bronchitis** is marked by a productive cough but no pathological airflow obstruction. **Chronic obstructive pulmonary disease (COPD)** is a group of conditions—bronchitis, emphysema, asthma, bronchiectasis, allergic alveolitis—marked by dyspnea. **Catarrhal** bronchitis is an acute form of bronchitis marked by profuse mucus and pus production (**mucopurulent** discharge). **Croupous** bronchitis, also known as pseudomembranous, fibrinous, plastic, exudative, or membranous, is marked by a violent cough and dyspnea.

DISEASES OF THE RESPIRATORY SYSTEM (460–519)

N Newborn: 0   P Pediatric: 0–17   M Maternity: 12–55   A Adult: 15–124   ♀ Females Only   ♂ Males Only

(Ex) CC/MCC Exclusions   🔗 Complication\Comorbidity   🔗 Major C\C   🔗 Present on Admission Requirement   🔗 Hospital-Acquired Condition

827

DISEASES OF THE RESPIRATORY SYSTEM (460–519)

● **491.2 Obstructive chronic bronchitis**

Bronchitis: Bronchitis with:
  emphysematous   chronic airway
  obstructive (chronic)   obstruction
  (diffuse)   emphysema

Excludes *asthmatic bronchitis (acute) (NOS) 493.9*
chronic obstructive asthma 493.2

Coding Clinic: 2004, Q4, P81-82; 2002, Q3, P18, 19x2; 1991, Q2, P21; 1984, Nov-Dec, P17

491.20 Without exacerbation
Emphysema with chronic bronchitis
Coding Clinic: 1997, Q3, P9

491.21 With (acute) exacerbation
Acute exacerbation of chronic obstructive pulmonary disease [COPD]
Decompensated chronic obstructive pulmonary disease [COPD]
Decompensated chronic obstructive pulmonary disease [COPD] with exacerbation

Excludes *chronic obstructive asthma with acute exacerbation 493.22*

(Ex) 488.01-488.11, 491.1-491.9, 493.20-493.21
Coding Clinic: 2010, Q1, P9; 2004, Q1, P3; 1996, Q2, P10; 1993, 5th Issue, P5x2

491.22 With acute bronchitis
(Ex) 488.01-488.11, 491.1-491.9, 493.20-493.21
Coding Clinic: 2006, Q3, P20; 2004, Q4, P80-81; Q1, P3

OGCR Section I.C.8.b.1

> When acute bronchitis, 466.0, is documented with COPD, code 491.22 should be assigned. It is not necessary to also assign code 466.0. If a medical record documents acute bronchitis with COPD with acute exacerbation, only code 491.22 should be assigned. The acute bronchitis included in code 491.22 supersedes the acute exacerbation. If a medical record documents COPD with acute exacerbation without mention of acute bronchitis, only code 491.21 should be assigned.

491.8 Other chronic bronchitis
Chronic: Chronic:
  tracheitis   tracheobronchitis

491.9 Unspecified chronic bronchitis
Coding Clinic: 1991, Q3, P17-18

● **492 Emphysema**
Coding Clinic: 1991, Q2, P21; 1984, Nov-Dec, P19

492.0 Emphysematous bleb
Giant bullous emphysema
Ruptured emphysematous bleb
Tension pneumatocele
Vanishing lung

492.8 Other emphysema
Emphysema (lung or pulmonary):
  NOS   panacinar
  centriacinar   panlobular
  centrilobular   unilateral
  obstructive   vesicular
MacLeod's syndrome
Swyer-James syndrome
Unilateral hyperlucent lung

Excludes *emphysema:*
with chronic bronchitis 491.20–491.22)
compensatory (518.2)
due to fumes and vapors (506.4)
interstitial (518.1)
newborn (770.2)
mediastinal (518.1)
surgical (subcutaneous) (998.81)
traumatic (958.7)
Coding Clinic: 2008, Q4, P174-175; 1993, Q4, P41; 5th Issue, P4

Item 8–9 Asthma is a bronchial condition marked by airway obstruction, hyper-responsiveness, and inflammation. **Extrinsic** asthma, also known as allergic asthma, is characterized by the same symptoms that occur with exposure to allergens and is divided into the following types: **atopic, occupational, and allergic bronchopulmonary aspergillosis. Intrinsic** asthma occurs in patients who have no history of allergy or sensitivities to allergens and is divided into the following types: **nonreaginic and pharmacologic. Status asthmaticus** is the most severe form of asthma attack and can last for days or weeks.

● **493 Asthma**

Excludes *wheezing NOS (786.07)*
Coding Clinic: 2003, Q4, P62, 137; 1991, Q1, P13; 1985, July-Aug, P8

The following fifth-digit subclassification is for use with category 493.0–493.2, 493.9:

0 unspecified
1 with status asthmaticus
2 with (acute) exacerbation

● **493.0 Extrinsic asthma** 1-2
[0-2] Asthma:
  allergic with stated cause
  atopic
  childhood
  hay
  platinum
Hay fever with asthma

Excludes *asthma:*
allergic NOS (493.9)
detergent (507.8)
miners' (500)
wood (495.8)

For codes **493.01-493.02:** (Ex) 488.01-488.11, 493.00-493.92, 517.8, 518.89, 519.8-519.9, 793.11
Coding Clinic: 1990, Q2, P20

● **493.1 Intrinsic asthma** 1-2
[0-2] Late-onset asthma
For codes **493.11-493.12:** (Ex) 488.01-488.11, 493.00-493.92, 517.8, 518.89, 519.8-519.9, 793.11
Coding Clinic: 1990, Q2, P20

● **493.2 Chronic obstructive asthma** 1-2
[0-2] Asthma with chronic obstructive pulmonary disease [COPD]
Chronic asthmatic bronchitis

Excludes *acute bronchitis (466.0)*
chronic obstructive bronchitis (491.20–491.22)

For code **493.21:** (Ex) 488.01-488.11, 491.1-493.92, 517.8, 518.89, 519.8-519.9;
For code **493.22:** (Ex) 488.01-488.11, 493.00-493.92, 517.8, 518.89, 519.8-519.9, 793.11
Coding Clinic: 2009, Q1, P16; 2006, Q3, P20; 2003, Q4, P108; 1993, 5th Issue, P4; 1991, Q2, P21; 1990, Q2, P20

● **493.8 Other forms of asthma**

493.81 Exercise induced bronchospasm
Coding Clinic: 2003, Q4, P62

493.82 Cough variant asthma
Coding Clinic: 2003, Q4, P62

● **493.9 Asthma, unspecified** 1-2
[0-2] Asthma (bronchial) (allergic NOS)
Bronchitis:
  allergic
  asthmatic
For codes **493.91-493.92:** (Ex) 488.01-488.11, 493.00-493.92, 517.8, 518.89, 519.8-519.9, 793.11
Coding Clinic: 2004, Q4, P137; 2003, Q4, P108-109; Q1, P9; 1999, Q4, P25; 1997, Q4, P39-40; Q1, P7; 1996, Q3, P20; 1993, Q4, P32; 1992, Q1, P15; 1990, Q2, P20; 1984, Nov-Dec, P17

◀ New   ◀ Revised   ~~deleted~~ Deleted   Excludes   Includes   Use additional   Code first   Omit code

● Unacceptable Principal Diagnosis   ● Use Additional Digit(s)   ▶ Manifestation Code   OGCR Official Guidelines   Coding Clinic

828

● 494 **Bronchiectasis**
Bronchiectasis (fusiform) (postinfectious) (recurrent)
Bronchiolectasis
> **Excludes** *congenital (748.61)*
> *tuberculous bronchiectasis (current disease) (011.5)*

494.0 **Bronchiectasis without acute exacerbation**

494.1 **Bronchiectasis with acute exacerbation** 🔒
(Ex) 017.90-017.96, 487.1, 488.01-488.12, 488.82, 494.1, 496, 506.1,
506.4-506.9, 748.61

● 495 **Extrinsic allergic alveolitis**
> **Includes** allergic alveolitis and pneumonitis due to inhaled
> organic dust particles of fungal, thermophilic
> actinomycete, or other origin

495.0 **Farmers' lung**

495.1 **Bagassosis**

495.2 **Bird-fanciers' lung**
Budgerigar-fanciers' disease or lung
Pigeon-fanciers' disease or lung

495.3 **Suberosis**
Cork-handlers' disease or lung

495.4 **Malt workers' lung**
Alveolitis due to Aspergillus clavatus

495.5 **Mushroom workers' lung**

495.6 **Maple bark-strippers' lung**
Alveolitis due to Cryptostroma corticale

495.7 **"Ventilation" pneumonitis** 🔒
Allergic alveolitis due to fungal, thermophilic
actinomycete, and other organisms growing in
ventilation [air conditioning] systems
(Ex) 011.00-012.16, 012.80-012.86, 017.90-017.96, 021.2, 031.0, 039.1, 115.05,
115.15, 115.95, 122.1, 130.4, 136.3, 480.0-480.2, 480.8-487.1, 488.01-
488.02, 488.11-488.12, 488.81-488.82, 494.0-508.1, 508.8-508.9, 517.1,
517.8, 518.89, 519.8-519.9, 748.61, 793.11

495.8 **Other specified allergic alveolitis and pneumonitis** 🔒
Cheese-washers' lung
Coffee workers' lung
Fish-meal workers' lung
Furriers' lung
Grain-handlers' disease or lung
Pituitary snuff-takers' disease
Sequoiosis or red-cedar asthma
Wood asthma
(Ex) 011.00-012.16, 012.80-012.86, 017.90-017.96, 021.2, 031.0, 039.1, 115.05,
115.15, 115.95, 122.1, 130.4, 136.3, 480.0-480.2, 480.8-487.1, 488.01-
488.02, 488.11-488.12, 488.81-488.82, 494.0-508.1, 508.8-508.9, 517.1,
517.8, 518.89, 519.8-519.9, 748.61, 793.11

495.9 **Unspecified allergic alveolitis and pneumonitis** 🔒
Alveolitis, allergic (extrinsic)
Hypersensitivity pneumonitis
(Ex) 011.00-012.16, 012.80-012.86, 017.90-017.96, 021.2, 031.0, 039.1, 115.05,
115.15, 115.95, 122.1, 130.4, 136.3, 480.0-480.2, 480.8-487.1, 488.01-
488.02, 488.11-488.12, 488.81-488.82, 494.0-508.1, 508.8-508.9, 517.1,
517.8, 518.89, 519.8-519.9, 748.61, 793.11

496 **Chronic airway obstruction, not elsewhere classified**
Chronic:
nonspecific lung disease
obstructive lung disease
obstructive pulmonary disease [COPD] NOS
> **Note:** This code is not to be used with any code from
> categories 491–493.
> **Excludes** *chronic obstructive lung disease [COPD] specified (as)*
> *(with):*
> *allergic alveolitis (495.0–495.9)*
> *asthma (493.2)*
> *bronchiectasis (494.0–494.1)*
> *bronchitis (491.20–491.22)*
> *with emphysema (491.20–491.22)*
> *decompensated (491.21)*
> *emphysema (492.0–492.8)*
Coding Clinic: 2010, Q1, P9; 2009, Q1, P16; 2006, Q3, P20; 2003, Q4, P109-110;
2000, Q2, P15; 1994, Q1, P19; 1993, Q4, P43; 1992, Q2, P16-17; 1991,
Q2, P21; 1988, Q2, P12

Figure 8–6 Progressive massive fibrosis
superimposed on coal workers' pneumoconiosis.
The large, blackened scars are located principally
in the upper lobe. (From Cotran R, Kumar V,
Collins T: Robbins Pathologic Basis of Disease,
ed 8, Philadelphia, WB Saunders, 2009.
Courtesy of Dr. Warner Laquer, Dr. Jerome
Kleinerman, and the National Institute of
Occupational Safety and Health, Morgantown,
WV)

Item 8–10 Pneumoconiosis refers to a lung condition resulting from
exposure to inorganic or organic airborne particles, such as coal dust or
moldy hay, as well as chemical fumes and vapors, such as insecticides. In this
condition, the lungs retain the airborne particles.

OGCR Section I.C.8.a.1
> Code 496, Chronic airway obstruction, not elsewhere classified, is a
> nonspecific code that should only be used when the documentation in
> a medical record does not specify the type of COPD being treated.

PNEUMOCONIOSES AND OTHER LUNG DISEASES DUE TO EXTERNAL AGENTS (500–508)

500 **Coal workers' pneumoconiosis**   A
Anthracosilicosis   Coal workers' lung
Anthracosis   Miners' asthma
Black lung disease

501 **Asbestosis**   A

502 **Pneumoconiosis due to other silica or silicates**
Pneumoconiosis due to talc
Silicotic fibrosis (massive) of lung
Silicosis (simple) (complicated)

503 **Pneumoconiosis due to other inorganic dust**
Aluminosis (of lung) Graphite fibrosis (of lung)
Bauxite fibrosis (of lung)   Siderosis
Berylliosis   Stannosis

504 **Pneumonopathy due to inhalation of other dust**
Byssinosis
Cannabinosis
Flax-dressers' disease
> **Excludes** *allergic alveolitis (495.0–495.9)*
> *asbestosis (501)*
> *bagassosis (495.1)*
> *farmers' lung (495.0)*

505 **Pneumoconiosis, unspecified**

● 506 **Respiratory conditions due to chemical fumes and vapors**
Use additional code to identify associated respiratory
conditions, such as:
acute respiratory failure (518.81)
Use additional E code to identify cause

506.0 **Bronchitis and pneumonitis due to fumes and vapors** 🔒
Chemical bronchitis (acute)
(Ex) 011.00-012.16, 012.80-012.86, 017.90-017.96, 021.2, 031.0, 039.1, 115.05,
115.15, 115.95, 122.1, 130.4, 136.3, 480.0-480.2, 480.8-487.1, 488.01-
488.02, 488.11-488.12, 488.81-488.82, 494.0-508.1, 508.8-508.9, 517.1,
517.8, 518.89, 519.8-519.9, 748.61, 793.11
Coding Clinic: 2010, Q3, P19; 2008, Q3, P6-7

506.1 **Acute pulmonary edema due to fumes and vapors** 🔒
Chemical pulmonary edema (acute)
> **Excludes** *acute pulmonary edema NOS (518.4)*
> *chronic or unspecified pulmonary edema (514)*
(Ex) 011.00-012.16, 012.80-012.86, 017.90-017.96, 021.2, 031.0, 039.1, 115.05,
115.15, 115.95, 122.1, 130.4, 136.3, 480.0-480.2, 480.8-487.1, 488.01-
488.02, 488.11-488.82, 494.0-508.1, 508.8-508.9, 517.1,
517.8, 518.89, 519.8-519.9, 748.61, 793.11

DISEASES OF THE RESPIRATORY SYSTEM (460–519)

DISEASES OF THE RESPIRATORY SYSTEM (460–519)

506.2 Upper respiratory inflammation due to fumes and vapors
Coding Clinic: 2005, Q3, P10

506.3 Other acute and subacute respiratory conditions due to fumes and vapors
Coding Clinic: 2010, Q3, P19

506.4 Chronic respiratory conditions due to fumes and vapors
Emphysema (diffuse) (chronic) due to inhalation of chemical fumes and vapors
Obliterative bronchiolitis (chronic) (subacute) due to inhalation of chemical fumes and vapors
Pulmonary fibrosis (chronic) due to inhalation of chemical fumes and vapors

506.9 Unspecified respiratory conditions due to fumes and vapors
Silo-fillers' disease

● **507 Pneumonitis due to solids and liquids**
Excludes fetal aspiration pneumonitis (770.18)
postprocedural pneumonitis (997.32)
Coding Clinic: 1993, Q2, P9-10

507.0 Due to inhalation of food or vomitus
Aspiration pneumonia (due to):
NOS milk
food (regurgitated) saliva
gastric secretions vomitus
(Ex) 011.00-012.16, 012.80-012.86, 017.90-017.96, 021.2, 031.0, 039.1 115.05, 115.15, 115.95, 122.1, 130.4 136.3, 480.0-480.2, 480.8-487.1, 488.01-488.02, 488.11-488.12, 488.81-488.82, 494.0-508.1, 508.8-508.9, 517.1, 517.8, 518.89, 519.8-519.9, 748.61, 793.11
Coding Clinic: 2011, Q4, P150; Q1, P16; 2008, Q1, P18-19; Q1, P18-19; 1991, Q3, P16-17; 1989, Q1, P10

507.1 Due to inhalation of oils and essences
Lipoid pneumonia (exogenous)
Excludes endogenous lipoid pneumonia (516.8)
(Ex) 011.00-012.16, 012.80-012.86, 017.90-017.96, 021.2, 031.0, 039.1 115.05, 115.15, 115.95, 122.1, 130.4, 136.3, 480.0-480.2, 480.8-487.1, 488.01-488.02, 488.11-488.12, 488.81-488.82, 494.0-508.1, 508.8-508.9, 517.1, 517.8, 518.89, 519.8-519.9, 748.61, 793.11
Coding Clinic: 1991, Q3, P16-17

507.8 Due to other solids and liquids
Detergent asthma
(Ex) 011.00-012.16, 012.80-012.86, 017.90-017.96, 021.2, 031.0, 039.1, 115.05, 115.15, 115.95, 122.1, 130.4, 136.3, 480.0-480.2, 480.8-487.1, 488.01-488.02, 488.11-488.12, 488.81-488.82, 494.0-508.1, 508.8-508.9, 517.1, 517.8, 518.89, 519.8-519.9, 748.61, 793.11
Coding Clinic: 1991, Q3, P16-17

● **508 Respiratory conditions due to other and unspecified external agents**
Use additional code to identify associated respiratory conditions, such as:
acute respiratory failure (518.81)
Use additional E code to identify cause

508.0 Acute pulmonary manifestations due to radiation
Radiation pneumonitis
(Ex) 011.00-012.16, 012.80-012.86, 017.90-017.96, 021.2, 031.0, 039.1, 115.05, 115.15, 115.95, 122.1, 130.4, 136.3, 480.0-480.2, 480.8-487.1, 488.01-488.02, 488.11-488.12, 488.81-488.82, 494.0-508.1, 508.8-508.9, 517.1, 517.8, 518.89, 519.8-519.9, 748.61, 793.11

508.1 Chronic and other pulmonary manifestations due to radiation
Fibrosis of lung following radiation
(Ex) 011.00-012.16, 012.80-012.86, 017.90-017.96, 021.2, 031.0, 039.1, 115.05, 115.15, 115.95, 122.1, 130.4, 136.3, 480.0-480.2, 480.8-487.1, 488.01-488.02, 488.11-488.12, 488.81-488.82, 494.0-508.1, 508.8-508.9, 517.1, 517.8, 518.89, 519.8-519.9, 748.61, 793.11

508.2 Respiratory conditions due to smoke inhalation
Smoke inhalation NOS
Excludes smoke inhalation due to chemical fumes and vapors (506.9)

508.8 Respiratory conditions due to other specified external agents

508.9 Respiratory conditions due to unspecified external agent

Figure 8–7 Bullous emphysema with large subpleural bullae *(upper left)*. (From Kumar: Robbins and Cotran: Pathologic Basis of Disease, ed 8, Saunders, An Imprint of Elsevier, 2009)

Item 8–11 Empyema is a condition in which pus accumulates in a body cavity. Empyema **with fistula** occurs when the pus passes from one cavity to another organ or structure.

OTHER DISEASES OF RESPIRATORY SYSTEM (510–519)

● **510 Empyema**
Use additional code to identify infectious organism (041.0–041.9)
Excludes abscess of lung (513.0)

510.0 With fistula
Fistula:
bronchocutaneous
bronchopleural
hepatopleural
mediastinal
pleural
thoracic
Any condition classifiable to 510.9 with fistula
(Ex) 510.0-510.9, 517.8, 518.89, 519.8-519.9, 793.11

510.9 Without mention of fistula
Abscess:
pleura
thorax
Empyema (chest) (lung) (pleura)
Fibrinopurulent pleurisy
Pleurisy:
purulent
septic
seropurulent
suppurative
Pyopneumothorax
Pyothorax
(Ex) 510.0-510.9, 517.8, 518.89, 519.8-519.9, 793.11
Coding Clinic: 2007, Q4, P109-113; 1994, Q3, P6

● **511 Pleurisy**
Occurs when double membrane (pleura) lining chest cavity and lung surface becomes inflamed causing sharp pain on inspiration and expiration
Excludes pleurisy with mention of tuberculosis, current disease (012.0)

511.0 Without mention of effusion or current tuberculosis
Adhesion, lung or pleura
Calcification of pleura
Pleurisy (acute) (sterile):
diaphragmatic
fibrinous
interlobar
Pleurisy:
NOS
pneumococcal
staphylococcal
streptococcal
Thickening of pleura
Coding Clinic: 1994, Q3, P5

511.1 With effusion, with mention of a bacterial cause other than tuberculosis
Pleurisy with effusion (exudative) (serous):
pneumococcal
staphylococcal
streptococcal
other specified nontuberculous bacterial cause
(Ex) 011.00-012.16, 012.80-012.86, 017.90-017.96, 511.0-511.9, 517.8, 518.89, 519.8-519.9, 793.11

New ◀ Revised ◀ ~~deleted~~ Deleted Excludes Includes Use additional Code first Omit code
● Unacceptable Principal Diagnosis ● Use Additional Digit(s) ▶ Manifestation Code OGCR Official Guidelines Coding Clinic

● **511.8 Other specified forms of effusion, except tuberculous**
Excludes *traumatic (860.2–860.5, 862.29, 862.39)*
Coding Clinic: 2008, Q1, P16-17; 1997, Q1, P10

511.81 Malignant pleural effusion 🗝
Code first malignant neoplasm, if known
(Ex) 195.8, 197.2-197.3, 198.89-199.2, 209.20, 209.29-209.30, 209.70, 209.75-209.79, 239.81-239.9, 511.81-511.89, 793.1
Coding Clinic: 2008, Q4, P113-114

511.89 Other specified forms of effusion, except tuberculous 🗝
Encysted pleurisy
Hemopneumothorax
Hemothorax
Hydropneumothorax
Hydrothorax
(Ex) 011.00-012.16, 012.80-012.86, 017.90-017.96, 511.0-511.9, 517.8, 518.89, 519.8-519.9, 793.11

511.9 Unspecified pleural effusion 🗝
Pleural effusion NOS
Pleurisy:
exudative
serofibrinous
serous
with effusion NOS
(Ex) 011.00-012.16, 012.80-012.86, 017.90-017.96, 511.0-511.9, 517.8, 518.89, 519.8-519.9, 793.11
Coding Clinic: 2003, Q2, P7-8; 1991, Q3, P19-20; 1989, Q4, P11; 1988, Q1, P9

● **512 Pneumothorax and air leak**
Collapsed lung

512.0 Spontaneous tension pneumothorax 🗝
Tension pneumothorax (most serious type) occurs when air (positive pressure) collects in the pleural space
(Ex) 512.0-512.89, 517.8, 518.89, 519.8-519.9, 793.11

512.1 Iatrogenic pneumothorax 🗝
Postoperative pneumothorax
(Ex) 512.0-512.89, 517.8, 518.89, 519.8-519.9, 793.11
Coding Clinic: 2011, Q1, P14; 2003, Q3, P19

512.2 Postoperative air leak
Coding Clinic: 2011, Q4, P117

● **512.8 Other pneumothorax and air leak**
Excludes *pneumothorax:*
congenital (770.2)
traumatic (860.0–860.1, 860.4–860.5)
tuberculous, current disease (011.7)
Coding Clinic: 1993, Q2, P3

512.81 Primary spontaneous pneumothorax 🗝
(Ex) 512.0-512.89, 517.8, 518.89, 519.8-519.9, 793.11

● **512.82 Secondary spontaneous pneumothorax** 🗝
Code first underlying condition, such as:
cancer metastatic to lung (197.0)
catamenial pneumothorax due to endometriosis (617.8)
cystic fibrosis (277.02)
eosinophilic pneumonia (518.3)
lymphangioleiomyomatosis (516.4)
Marfan syndrome (759.82)
pneumocystis carinii pneumonia (136.3)
primary lung cancer (162.3-162.9)
spontaneous rupture of the esophagus (530.4)
(Ex) 512.0-512.89, 517.8, 518.89, 519.8-519.9, 793.11

512.83 Chronic pneumothorax 🗝
(Ex) 512.0-512.89, 517.8, 518.89, 519.8-519.9, 793.11

512.84 Other air leak 🗝
Persistent air leak
(Ex) 512.0-512.89, 517.8, 518.89, 519.8-519.9, 793.11

512.89 Other pneumothorax 🗝
Acute pneumothorax
Pneumothorax NOS
Spontaneous pneumothorax NOS
(Ex) 512.0-512.89, 517.8, 518.89, 519.8-519.9, 793.11

● **513 Abscess of lung and mediastinum**

513.0 Abscess of lung 🗝
Abscess (multiple) of lung
Gangrenous or necrotic pneumonia
Pulmonary gangrene or necrosis
(Ex) 006.4, 011.00-012.16, 012.80-012.86, 017.90-017.96, 513.0, 519.8-519.9
Coding Clinic: 2007, Q4, P84-86; 2005, Q2, P14-15; 1998, Q2, P7

513.1 Abscess of mediastinum 🗝
(Ex) 513.1, 519.8-519.9

514 Pulmonary congestion and hypostasis 🗝
Hypostatic:
bronchopneumonia
pneumonia
Passive pneumonia
Pulmonary congestion (chronic) (passive)
Pulmonary edema:
NOS
chronic
Excludes *acute pulmonary edema:*
NOS (518.4)
with mention of heart disease or failure (428.1)
hypostatic pneumonia due to or specified as a specific type of pneumonia - code to the type of pneumonia (480.0–480.9, 481, 482.0–482.9, 483.0–483.8, 487.0, 488.01, 488.11)
(Ex) 514, 517.8, 518.89, 519.8-519.9, 793.11
Coding Clinic: 1998, Q2, P6-7

515 Postinflammatory pulmonary fibrosis
Cirrhosis of lung chronic or unspecified
Fibrosis of lung (atrophic) (confluent) (massive) (perialveolar) (peribronchial) chronic or unspecified
Induration of lung chronic or unspecified

● **516 Other alveolar and parietoalveolar pneumonopathy**

516.0 Pulmonary alveolar proteinosis 🗝
(Ex) 011.00-012.16, 012.80-012.86, 017.90-017.96, 494.0-508.1, 508.8-508.9, 515-516.5, 516.8-516.9, 517.2, 517.8, 518.89, 519.8-519.9, 748.61, 793.11

▷ **516.1 Idiopathic pulmonary hemosiderosis** 🗝
Essential brown induration of lung
Code first underlying disease (275.01-275.09)
Excludes *acute idiopathic pulmonary hemorrhage in infants [AIPHI] (786.31)*
(Ex) 011.00-012.16, 012.80-012.86, 017.90-017.96, 494.0-508.1, 508.8-508.9, 515-516.5, 516.8-516.9, 517.2, 517.8, 518.89, 519.8-519.9, 748.61, 793.11

516.2 Pulmonary alveolar microlithiasis 🗝
(Ex) 011.00-012.16, 012.80-012.86, 017.90-017.96, 494.0-508.1, 508.8-508.9, 515-516.5, 516.8-516.9, 517.2, 517.8, 518.89, 519.8-519.9, 748.61, 793.11

● **516.3 Idiopathic interstitial pneumonia**

516.30 Idiopathic interstitial pneumonia, not otherwise specified 🗝
Idiopathic fibrosing alveolitis

516.31 Idiopathic pulmonary fibrosis
Cryptogenic fibrosing alveolitis

516.32 Idiopathic non-specific interstitial pneumonitis
Excludes *non-specific interstitial pneumonia NOS, or due to known underlying cause (516.8)*

516.33 Acute interstitial pneumonitis 🗝
Hamman-Rich syndrome
Excludes *pneumocystis pneumonia (136.3)*
(Ex) 011.00-012.16, 012.80-012.86, 017.90-017.96, 494.0-508.1, 508.8-508.9, 515-516.5, 516.8-516.9, 517.2, 517.8, 518.89, 519.8, 519.9, 748.61, 793.11

516.34 Respiratory bronchiolitis interstitial lung disease

DISEASES OF THE RESPIRATORY SYSTEM (460–519)

N Newborn: 0   P Pediatric: 0–17   M Maternity: 12–55   A Adult: 15–124   ♀ Females Only   ♂ Males Only
(Ex) CC/MCC Exclusions   🗝 Complication\Comorbidity   🗝 Major C\C   🗝 Present on Admission Requirement   🗝 Hospital-Acquired Condition

831

DISEASES OF THE RESPIRATORY SYSTEM (460–519)

516.35 Idiopathic lymphoid interstitial pneumonia
Idiopathic lymphocytic interstitial pneumonitis
> **Excludes** *lymphoid interstitial pneumonia NOS, or due to known underlying cause (516.8)*
> *pneumocystis pneumonia (136.3)*
> Ex: 011.00-012.16, 012.80-012.86, 017.90-017.96, 494.0-508.1, 508.8-508.9, 515-516.5, 516.8-516.9, 517.2, 517.8, 518.89, 519.8, 519.9, 748.61, 793.11

516.36 Cryptogenic organizing pneumonia
> **Excludes** *organizing pneumonia NOS, or due to known underlying cause (516.8)*
> Ex: 011.00-012.16, 012.80-012.86, 017.90-017.96, 494.0-508.1, 508.8-508.9, 515-516.5, 516.8-516.9, 517.2, 517.8, 518.89, 519.8, 519.9, 748.61, 793.11

516.37 Desquamative interstitial pneumonia
> Ex: 011.00-012.16, 012.80-012.86, 017.90-017.96, 494.0-508.1, 508.8-508.9, 515-516.5, 516.8-516.9, 517.2, 517.8, 518.89, 519.8, 519.9, 748.61, 793.11

516.4 Lymphangioleiomyomatosis ♀
Lymphangiomyomatosis
> Ex: 011.00-012.16, 012.80-012.86, 017.90-017.96, 494.0-508.1, 508.8-508.9, 515-516.5, 516.8-516.9, 517.2, 517.8, 518.89, 519.8, 519.9, 748.61, 793.11

516.5 Adult pulmonary Langerhans cell histiocytosis   A
Adult PLCH
> Ex: 011.00-012.16, 012.80-012.86, 017.90-017.96, 494.0-508.1, 508.8-508.9, 515-516.5, 516.8-516.9, 517.2, 517.8, 518.89, 519.8, 519.9, 748.61, 793.11

● **516.6 Interstitial lung diseases of childhood**

516.61 Neuroendocrine cell hyperplasia of infancy
> Ex: 515.61-516.69, 768.5, 768.6, 768.9-770.86, 770.89, 770.9, 779.81-779.84, 770.89

516.62 Pulmonary interstitial glycogenosis
> Ex: 515.61-516.69, 768.5, 768.6, 768.9-770.86, 770.89, 770.9, 779.81-779.84, 770.89

516.63 Surfactant mutations of the lung
> Ex: 515.61-516.69, 768.5, 768.6, 768.9-770.86, 770.89, 770.9, 779.81-779.84, 770.89

516.64 Alveolar capillary dysplasia with vein misalignment
> Ex: 515.61-516.69, 768.5, 768.6, 768.9-770.86, 770.89, 770.9, 779.81-779.84, 770.89

516.69 Other interstitial lung diseases of childhood
> Ex: 515.61-516.69, 768.5, 768.6, 768.9-770.86, 770.89, 770.9, 779.81-779.84, 770.89

516.8 Other specified alveolar and parietoalveolar pneumonopathies
Endogenous lipoid pneumonia
Interstitial pneumonia
Lymphoid interstitial pneumonia due to known underlying cause
Lymphoid interstitial pneumonia NOS
Non-specific interstitial pneumonia due to known underlying cause
Non-specific interstitial pneumonia NOS
Organizing pneumonia due to known underlying cause
Organizing pneumonia NOS
> *Code first*, if applicable, underlying cause of pneumonopathy, if known
> Use additional E code, if applicable, for drug-induced or toxic pneumonopathy
> **Excludes** *cryptogenic organizing pneumonia (516.36)*
> *idiopathic lymphoid interstitial pneumonia (516.35)*
> *idiopathic non-specific interstitial pneumonitis (516.32)*
> *lipoid pneumonia, exogenous or unspecified (507.1)*
> Ex: 011.00-012.16, 012.80-012.86, 017.90-017.96, 494.0-508.1, 508.8-508.9, 515-516.5, 516.8-516.9, 517.2, 517.8, 518.89, 519.8-519.9, 748.61, 793.11
> **Coding Clinic: 2011, Q1, P17; 2010, Q1, P9; 2006, Q2, P20; 1992, Q1, P12**

516.9 Unspecified alveolar and parietoalveolar pneumonopathy
> Ex: 011.00-012.16, 012.80-012.86, 017.90-017.96, 494.0-508.1, 508.8-508.9, 515-516.5, 516.8-516.9, 517.2, 517.8, 518.89, 519.8-519.9, 748.61, 793.11

● **517 Lung involvement in conditions classified elsewhere**
> **Excludes** *rheumatoid lung (714.81)*

▷ **517.1 Rheumatic pneumonia**
> *Code first underlying disease (390)*
> Ex: 011.00-012.16, 012.80-012.86, 017.90-017.96, 480.0-480.2, 480.8-487.1, 488.01-488.02, 488.11-488.12, 488.81-488.82, 494.0-508.1, 508.8-508.9, 515-516.5, 516.8-517.2, 517.8, 518.89, 519.8-519.9, 748.61, 793.11

▷ **517.2 Lung involvement in systemic sclerosis**
> *Code first underlying disease (710.1)*
> Ex: 011.00-012.16, 012.80-012.86, 017.90-017.96, 488.81-488.82, 494.0-508.1, 508.8-508.9, 515-516.5, 516.8-516.9, 517.2, 517.8, 518.89, 519.8-519.9, 748.61, 793.11

▷ **517.3 Acute chest syndrome**
> *Code first sickle-cell disease in crisis (282.42, 282.62, 282.64, 282.69)*
> Ex: 280.0-282.3, 282.5-282.63, 282.69-285.9, 289.9, 776.5-776.6
> **Coding Clinic: 2003, Q4, P51-56; 1998, Q2, P8**

▷ **517.8 Lung involvement in other diseases classified elsewhere**
> *Code first underlying disease, as:*
> amyloidosis (277.30–277.39)
> polymyositis (710.4)
> sarcoidosis (135)
> Sjögren's disease (710.2)
> systemic lupus erythematosus (710.0)
> **Excludes** *syphilis (095.1)*
> **Coding Clinic: 2003, Q2, P7-8**

● **518 Other diseases of lung**

518.0 Pulmonary collapse
Atelectasis
Collapse of lung
Middle lobe syndrome
> **Excludes** *atelectasis:*
> *congenital (partial) (770.5)*
> *primary (770.4)*
> *tuberculous, current disease (011.8)*
> Ex: 518.0, 519.8-519.9
> **Coding Clinic: 1990, Q4, P25**

518.1 Interstitial emphysema
Mediastinal emphysema
> **Excludes** *surgical (subcutaneous) emphysema (998.81)*
> *that in fetus or newborn (770.2)*
> *traumatic emphysema (958.7)*

518.2 Compensatory emphysema

518.3 Pulmonary eosinophilia
Eosinophilic asthma
Löffler's syndrome
Pneumonia:
  allergic
  eosinophilic
Tropical eosinophilia
> **Excludes** *pulmonary infiltrate NOS (793.19)*
> Ex: 011.00-012.16, 012.80-012.86, 017.90-017.96, 020.3-020.5, 021.3, 022.1, 031.0, 039.1, 073.0, 115.05, 115.15, 115.95, 122.1, 130.4, 136.3, 480.0-480.2, 480.8-487.1, 488.01-488.02, 488.11-488.12, 488.81-488.82, 494.0-495.9, 500-508.1, 508.8-.508.9, 517.1, 517.8, 518.3, 518.89, 519.8-519.9, 748.61, 793.11

518.4 Acute edema of lung, unspecified
Acute pulmonary edema NOS
Pulmonary edema, postoperative
> **Excludes** *pulmonary edema:*
> *acute, with mention of heart disease or failure (428.1)*
> *chronic or unspecified (514)*
> *due to external agents (506.0–508.9)*
> Ex: 398.91, 428.0-428.9, 518.4, 519.8-519.9

◄ New   ▦ Revised   ~~deleted~~ Deleted   Excludes   Includes   Use additional   Code first   Omit code

● Unacceptable Principal Diagnosis   ● Use Additional Digit(s)   ▷ Manifestation Code   OGCR Official Guidelines   Coding Clinic

832

● **518.5 Pulmonary insufficiency following trauma and surgery**
> **Excludes** *adult respiratory distress syndrome associated*
> *with other conditions (518.82)*
> *pneumonia:*
> *aspiration (507.0)*
> *hypostatic (514)*
> *respiratory failure in other conditions (518.81,*
> *518.83–518.84)*
> Coding Clinic: 2010, Q3, P19; 2004, Q4, P139

518.51 Acute respiratory failure following trauma and surgery 🔖
Respiratory failure, not otherwise specified, following trauma and surgery
> **Excludes** *acute respiratory failure in other*
> *conditions (518.81)*
> (Ex) 518.51-518.53, 519.8, 519.9

518.52 Other pulmonary insufficiency, not elsewhere classified, following trauma and surgery 🔖
Adult respiratory distress syndrome
Pulmonary insufficiency following surgery
Pulmonary insufficiency following trauma
Shock lung related to trauma and surgery
> **Excludes** *adult respiratory distress syndrome*
> *associated with other conditions*
> *(518.82)*
> *aspiration pneumonia (507.0)*
> *hypostatic pneumonia (514)*
> *shock lung, not related to trauma or*
> *surgery (518.82)*
> (Ex) 518.51-518.53, 519.8, 519.9

518.53 Acute and chronic respiratory failure following trauma and surgery 🔖
> **Excludes** *acute and chronic respiratory failure in*
> *other conditions (518.84)*
> (Ex) 518.51-518.53, 519.8, 519.9

518.6 Allergic bronchopulmonary aspergillosis 🔖
> (Ex) 518.6, 519.8-519.9
> Coding Clinic: 1997, Q4, P39-40

518.7 Transfusion related acute lung injury (TRALI) 🔖
> (Ex) 518.7, 997.31-997.39, 997.91-997.99, 998.81, 998.83-998.9
> Coding Clinic: 2006, Q4, P91-92

● **518.8 Other diseases of lung**

518.81 Acute respiratory failure 🔖
Respiratory failure NOS
> **Excludes** *acute and chronic respiratory failure*
> *(518.84)*
> *acute respiratory distress (518.82)*
> *acute respiratory failure following*
> *trauma and surgery (518.51)*
> *chronic respiratory failure (518.83)*
> *respiratory arrest (799.1)*
> *respiratory failure, newborn (770.84)*
> (Ex) 518.81-518.84, 519.8-519.9, 799.1
> Coding Clinic: 2012, Q3, P21-22; 2010, Q4, P81; 2009, Q2,
> P11; 2008, Q1, P18-19; 2007, Q3, P7-8; 2005, Q2,
> P19-20; Q1, P3-8; 2004, Q4, P139; 2003, Q2, P21-22;
> Q1, P15; 1993, Q1, P25; 1991, Q3, P14; 1990, Q4,
> P25; 1987, Nov-Dec, P5-6

518.82 Other pulmonary insufficiency, not elsewhere classified 🔖
Acute respiratory distress
Acute respiratory insufficiency
Adult respiratory distress syndrome NEC
> **Excludes** *acute interstitial pneumonitis (516.33)*
> *adult respiratory distress syndrome*
> *associated with trauma or surgery*
> *(518.52)*
> *pulmonary insufficiency following*
> *trauma or surgery (518.52)*
> *respiratory distress:*
> *NOS (786.09)*
> *newborn (770.89)*
> *syndrome, newborn (769)*
> (Ex) 518.81-518.84, 519.8-519.9, 799.1
> Coding Clinic: 2003, Q4, P105-106; 1995, Q1, P7;
> 1991, Q2, P21

518.83 Chronic respiratory failure 🔖
> (Ex) 518.81-518.84, 519.8-519.9, 799.1
> Coding Clinic: 2003, Q4, P103-104, 111

518.84 Acute and chronic respiratory failure 🔖
Acute on chronic respiratory failure
> **Excludes** *acute and chronic respiratory failure*
> *following trauma or surgery*
> *(518.53)*
> (Ex) 518.81-518.84, 519.8-519.9, 799.1

518.89 Other diseases of lung, not elsewhere classified
Broncholithiasis   Lung disease NOS
Calcification of lung   Pulmolithiasis
> Coding Clinic: 1988, Q4, P6; 1987, Nov-Dec, P8; 1986,
> Sept-Oct, P10

● **519 Other diseases of respiratory system**

● **519.0 Tracheostomy complications**
These complications do not appear in the usual complication range of 996–999.

519.00 Tracheostomy complication, unspecified 🔖
> (Ex) 519.00-519.19, 519.8-519.9

519.01 Infection of tracheostomy 🔖
> Use additional code to identify type of infection,
> such as:
> abscess or cellulitis of neck (682.1)
> septicemia (038.0–038.9)
> Use additional code to identify organism
> (041.00–041.9)
> (Ex) 519.00-519.19, 519.8-519.9
> Coding Clinic: 1998, Q4, P41-42

519.02 Mechanical complication of tracheostomy 🔖
Tracheal stenosis due to tracheostomy
> (Ex) 519.00-519.19, 519.8-519.9

519.09 Other tracheostomy complications 🔖
Hemorrhage due to tracheostomy
Tracheoesophageal fistula due to tracheostomy
> (Ex) 519.00-519.19, 519.8-519.9

● **519.1 Other diseases of trachea and bronchus, not elsewhere classified**
> Coding Clinic: 2002, Q3, P18

519.11 Acute bronchospasm
Bronchospasm NOS
> **Excludes** *acute bronchitis with bronchospasm*
> *(466.0)*
> *asthma (493.00–493.92)*
> *exercise induced bronchospasm (493.81)*
> Coding Clinic: 2006, Q4, P92-93

519.19 Other diseases of trachea and bronchus
Calcification of bronchus or trachea
Stenosis of bronchus or trachea
Ulcer of bronchus or trachea

519.2 Mediastinitis 🔖 🔖
HAC: And one of the following procedure codes:
36.10-36.19
> (Ex) 519.2-519.3, 519.8-519.9

519.3 Other diseases of mediastinum, not elsewhere classified
Fibrosis of mediastinum
Hernia of mediastinum
Retraction of mediastinum

519.4 Disorders of diaphragm
Diaphragmitis
Paralysis of diaphragm
Relaxation of diaphragm
> **Excludes** *congenital defect of diaphragm (756.6)*
> *diaphragmatic hernia (551–553 with .3)*
> *congenital (756.6)*

519.8 Other diseases of respiratory system, not elsewhere classified
> Coding Clinic: 1989, Q4, P12

519.9 Unspecified disease of respiratory system
Respiratory disease (chronic) NOS

N Newborn: 0   **P** Pediatric: 0–17   **M** Maternity: 12–55   **A** Adult: 15–124   ♀ Females Only   ♂ Males Only

(Ex) CC/MCC Exclusions   🔖 Complication\Comorbidity   🔖 Major C\C   🔖 Present on Admission Requirement   🔖 Hospital-Acquired Condition   **833**

DISEASES OF THE RESPIRATORY SYSTEM (460–519)

DISEASES OF THE DIGESTIVE SYSTEM (520–579)

Enamel
Dentin
Pulp
Blood vessels
Periodontal membrane
Mandible
Blood vessels and nerves
Crown
Gingival margin
Root

Figure 9–1 Anatomy of a tooth.

Item 9–1 Anodontia is the congenital absence of teeth. **Hypodontia** is partial anodontia. **Oligodontia** is the congenital absence of some teeth, whereas **supernumerary** is having more teeth than the normal number. **Mesiodens** are small extra teeth that often appear in pairs, although single small teeth are not uncommon.

9. DISEASES OF THE DIGESTIVE SYSTEM (520–579)

DISEASES OF ORAL CAVITY, SALIVARY GLANDS, AND JAWS (520–529)

● **520 Disorders of tooth development and eruption**

520.0 Anodontia
Absence of teeth (complete) (congenital) (partial)
Hypodontia
Oligodontia
Excludes *acquired absence of teeth (525.10–525.19)*

520.1 Supernumerary teeth
Distomolar   Paramolar
Fourth molar   Supplemental teeth
Mesiodens
Excludes *supernumerary roots (520.2)*

520.2 Abnormalities of size and form
Concrescence of teeth   Macrodontia
Fusion of teeth   Microdontia
Gemination of teeth   Peg-shaped [conical] teeth
Dens evaginatus   Supernumerary roots
Dens in dente   Taurodontism
Dens invaginatus   Tuberculum paramolare
Enamel pearls
Excludes *that due to congenital syphilis (090.5)*
tuberculum Carabelli, which is regarded as a normal variation

520.3 Mottled teeth
Dental fluorosis
Mottling of enamel
Nonfluoride enamel opacities

520.4 Disturbances of tooth formation
Aplasia and hypoplasia of cementum
Dilaceration of tooth
Enamel hypoplasia (neonatal) (postnatal) (prenatal)
Horner's teeth
Hypocalcification of teeth
Regional odontodysplasia
Turner's tooth
Excludes *Hutchinson's teeth and mulberry molars in congenital syphilis (090.5)*
mottled teeth (520.3)

520.5 Hereditary disturbances in tooth structure, not elsewhere classified
Amelogenesis imperfecta
Dentinogenesis imperfecta
Odontogenesis imperfecta
Dentinal dysplasia
Shell teeth

520.6 Disturbances in tooth eruption
Teeth:
embedded
impacted
natal
neonatal
prenatal
primary [deciduous]:
persistent
shedding, premature
Tooth eruption:
late
obstructed
premature
Excludes *exfoliation of teeth (attributable to disease of surrounding tissues) (525.0–525.19)*
Coding Clinic: 2006, Q1, P18; 2005, Q2, P15-16; 2004, Q1, P17

520.7 Teething syndrome

520.8 Other specified disorders of tooth development and eruption
Color changes during tooth formation
Pre-eruptive color changes
Excludes *posteruptive color changes (521.7)*

520.9 Unspecified disorder of tooth development and eruption

● **521 Diseases of hard tissues of teeth**

● **521.0 Dental caries**

521.00 Dental caries, unspecified

521.01 Dental caries limited to enamel
Initial caries
White spot lesion

521.02 Dental caries extending into dentin

521.03 Dental caries extending into pulp

521.04 Arrested dental caries

521.05 Odontoclasia
Infantile melanodontia
Melanodontoclasia
Excludes *internal and external resorption of teeth (521.40–521.49)*

521.06 Dental caries pit and fissure
Primary dental caries, pit and fissure origin

521.07 Dental caries of smooth surface
Primary dental caries, smooth surface origin

521.08 Dental caries of root surface
Primary dental caries, root surface

521.09 Other dental caries
Coding Clinic: 2002, Q3, P14

● **521.1 Excessive attrition (approximal wear) (occlusal wear)**

521.10 Excessive attrition, unspecified

521.11 Excessive attrition, limited to enamel

521.12 Excessive attrition, extending into dentine

521.13 Excessive attrition, extending into pulp

521.14 Excessive attrition, localized

521.15 Excessive attrition, generalized

Incisal edge
Medial surface
Distal surface
Occlusal surface
LABIAL (facial)
Median line
Central incisor
Lateral incisor
Cuspid or canine
First premolar
Second premolar
First molar
Second molar
Third molar or wisdom tooth
LINGUAL
BUCCAL (facial)

Figure 9–2 The permanent teeth within the dental arch.

Item 9–2 Each dental arch (jaw) normally contains 16 teeth. Tooth decay or **dental caries** is a disease of the enamel, dentin, and cementum of the tooth and can result in a cavity.

● **521.2 Abrasion**
  Abrasion of teeth:
    dentifrice
    habitual
    occupational
    ritual
    traditional
  Wedge defect NOS of teeth
  521.20 Abrasion, unspecified
  521.21 Abrasion, limited to enamel
  521.22 Abrasion, extending into dentine
  521.23 Abrasion, extending into pulp
  521.24 Abrasion, localized
  521.25 Abrasion, generalized
● **521.3 Erosion**
  Erosion of teeth:
    NOS
    due to:
      medicine
      persistent vomiting
    idiopathic
    occupational
  521.30 Erosion, unspecified
  521.31 Erosion, limited to enamel
  521.32 Erosion, extending into dentine
  521.33 Erosion, extending into pulp
  521.34 Erosion, localized
  521.35 Erosion, generalized
● **521.4 Pathological resorption**
  521.40 Pathological resorption, unspecified
  521.41 Pathological resorption, internal
  521.42 Pathological resorption, external
  521.49 Other pathological resorption
        Internal granuloma of pulp
  521.5 Hypercementosis
        Cementation hyperplasia
  521.6 Ankylosis of teeth
  521.7 Intrinsic posteruptive color changes
        Staining [discoloration] of teeth:
          NOS
          due to:
            drugs
            metals
            pulpal bleeding
        Excludes *accretions [deposits] on teeth (523.6)*
                  extrinsic color changes (523.6)
                  pre-eruptive color changes (520.8)
● **521.8 Other specified diseases of hard tissues of teeth**
  521.81 Cracked tooth
        Excludes *asymptomatic craze lines in enamel -*
                  omit code
                  broken tooth due to trauma
                    (873.63, 873.73)
                  fractured tooth due to trauma
                    (873.63, 873.73)
  521.89 Other specified diseases of hard tissues of teeth
        Irradiated enamel
        Sensitive dentin
  521.9 Unspecified disease of hard tissues of teeth

● **522 Diseases of pulp and periapical tissues**
  522.0 Pulpitis 🔖
        Pulpal:
          abscess
          polyp
        Pulpitis:
          acute
          chronic (hyperplastic) (ulcerative)
          suppurative
        (Ex:) 520.0-525.9
  522.1 Necrosis of the pulp
        Pulp gangrene
  522.2 Pulp degeneration
        Denticles   Pulp calcifications
        Pulp stones
  522.3 Abnormal hard tissue formation in pulp
        Secondary or irregular dentin
  522.4 Acute apical periodontitis of pulpal origin 🔖
        (Ex:) 520.0-525.9
  522.5 Periapical abscess without sinus
        Abscess:
          dental
          dentoalveolar
        Excludes *periapical abscess with sinus (522.7)*
  522.6 Chronic apical periodontitis
        Apical or periapical granuloma
        Apical periodontitis NOS
  522.7 Periapical abscess with sinus
        Fistula:
          alveolar process
          dental
  522.8 Radicular cyst
        Cyst:
          apical (periodontal)
          periapical
          radiculodental
          residual radicular
        Excludes *lateral developmental or lateral periodontal cyst*
                  (526.0)
  522.9 Other and unspecified diseases of pulp and periapical tissues

● **523 Gingival and periodontal diseases**
  ● **523.0 Acute gingivitis**
        Excludes *acute necrotizing ulcerative gingivitis (101)*
                  herpetic gingivostomatitis (054.2)
    523.00 Acute gingivitis, plaque induced
          Acute gingivitis NOS
    523.01 Acute gingivitis, non-plaque induced
  ● **523.1 Chronic gingivitis**
        Gingivitis (chronic):
          desquamative   simple marginal
          hyperplastic   ulcerative
        Excludes *herpetic gingivostomatitis (054.2)*
    523.10 Chronic gingivitis, plaque induced
          Chronic gingivitis NOS
          Gingivitis NOS
    523.11 Chronic gingivitis, non-plaque induced
  ● **523.2 Gingival recession**
        Gingival recession (postinfective) (postoperative)
    523.20 Gingival recession, unspecified
    523.21 Gingival recession, minimal
    523.22 Gingival recession, moderate
    523.23 Gingival recession, severe
    523.24 Gingival recession, localized
    523.25 Gingival recession, generalized

Item 9–3 Acute gingivitis, also known as orilitis or ulitis, is the short-term, severe inflammation of the gums (gingiva) caused by bacteria. **Chronic gingivitis** is persistent inflammation of the gums. When the gingivitis moves into the periodontium it is called periodontitis, also known as paradentitis.

DISEASES OF THE DIGESTIVE SYSTEM (520–579)

DISEASES OF THE DIGESTIVE SYSTEM (520–579)

● **523.3 Aggressive and acute periodontitis**
Acute:
  pericementitis
  pericoronitis

> **Excludes** *acute apical periodontitis (522.4)*
> *periapical abscess (522.5, 522.7)*

  523.30 Aggressive periodontitis, unspecified
  523.31 Aggressive periodontitis, localized
    Periodontal abscess
  523.32 Aggressive periodontitis, generalized
  523.33 Acute periodontitis

● **523.4 Chronic periodontitis**
Chronic pericoronitis
Pericementitis (chronic)
Periodontitis:
  NOS
  complex
  simplex

> **Excludes** *chronic apical periodontitis (522.6)*

  523.40 Chronic periodontitis, unspecified
  523.41 Chronic periodontitis, localized
  523.42 Chronic periodontitis, generalized

  523.5 Periodontosis
  523.6 Accretions on teeth
Dental calculus:
  subgingival
  supragingival
Deposits on teeth:
  betel
  materia alba
  soft
  tartar
  tobacco
Extrinsic discoloration of teeth

> **Excludes** *intrinsic discoloration of teeth (521.7)*

  523.8 Other specified periodontal diseases
Giant cell:
  epulis
  peripheral granuloma
Gingival:
  cysts
  enlargement NOS
  fibromatosis
Gingival polyp
Periodontal lesions due to traumatic occlusion
Peripheral giant cell granuloma

> **Excludes** *leukoplakia of gingiva (528.6)*

  523.9 Unspecified gingival and periodontal disease
    Coding Clinic: 2002, Q3, P14

● **524 Dentofacial anomalies, including malocclusion**
● **524.0 Major anomalies of jaw size**

> **Excludes** *hemifacial atrophy or hypertrophy (754.0)*
> *unilateral condylar hyperplasia or hypoplasia of*
> *mandible*

  524.00 Unspecified anomaly
  524.01 Maxillary hyperplasia
  524.02 Mandibular hyperplasia
  524.03 Maxillary hypoplasia
  524.04 Mandibular hypoplasia
    Coding Clinic: 2012, Q2, P17
  524.05 Macrogenia
  524.06 Microgenia
  524.07 Excessive tuberosity of jaw
    Entire maxillary tuberosity
  524.09 Other specified anomaly
● **524.1 Anomalies of relationship of jaw to cranial base**
  524.10 Unspecified anomaly
    Prognathism   Retrognathism
  524.11 Maxillary asymmetry
  524.12 Other jaw asymmetry
  524.19 Other specified anomaly

Figure 9–3 Dentofacial malocclusion.

Item 9–4 Hyperplasia is a condition of overdevelopment, whereas **hypoplasia** is a condition of underdevelopment. **Macrogenia** is overdevelopment of the chin, whereas microgenia is underdevelopment of the chin.

● **524.2 Anomalies of dental arch relationship**
Anomaly of dental arch

> **Excludes** *hemifacial atrophy or hypertrophy (754.0)*
> *soft tissue impingement (524.81–524.82)*
> *unilateral condylar hyperplasia or hypoplasia of*
> *mandible (526.89)*

  524.20 Unspecified anomaly of dental arch relationship
  524.21 Malocclusion, Angle's class I
    Neutro-occlusion
  524.22 Malocclusion, Angle's class II
    Disto-occlusion Division I
    Disto-occlusion Division II
  524.23 Malocclusion, Angle's class III
    Mesio-occlusion
  524.24 Open anterior occlusal relationship
    Anterior open bite
  524.25 Open posterior occlusal relationship
    Posterior open bite
  524.26 Excessive horizontal overlap
    Excessive horizontal overjet
  524.27 Reverse articulation
    Anterior articulation
    Crossbite
    Posterior articulation
  524.28 Anomalies of interarch distance
    Excessive interarch distance
    Inadequate interarch distance
  524.29 Other anomalies of dental arch relationship
    Other anomalies of dental arch
● **524.3 Anomalies of tooth position of fully erupted teeth**

> **Excludes** *impacted or embedded teeth with abnormal*
> *position of such teeth or adjacent teeth*
> *(520.6)*

    Coding Clinic: 2004, Q1, P17
  524.30 Unspecified anomaly of tooth position
    Diastema of teeth NOS
    Displacement of teeth NOS
    Transposition of teeth NOS
  524.31 Crowding of teeth
  524.32 Excessive spacing of teeth
  524.33 Horizontal displacement of teeth
    Tipped teeth
    Tipping of teeth
  524.34 Vertical displacement of teeth
    Extruded tooth
    Infraeruption of teeth
    Intruded tooth
    Supraeruption of teeth
  524.35 Rotation of tooth/teeth
  524.36 Insufficient interocclusal distance of teeth (ridge)
    Lack of adequate intermaxillary vertical
      dimension
  524.37 Excessive interocclusal distance of teeth
    Excessive intermaxillary vertical dimension
    Loss of occlusal vertical dimension
  524.39 Other anomalies of tooth position
  524.4 Malocclusion, unspecified

◄ New   ◄▦ Revised   ~~deleted~~ Deleted   Excludes   Includes   Use additional   Code first   Omit code

836   ● Unacceptable Principal Diagnosis   ● Use Additional Digit(s)   ▶ Manifestation Code   **OGCR** Official Guidelines   **Coding Clinic**

● **524.5 Dentofacial functional abnormalities**

  524.50 Dentofacial functional abnormality, unspecified

  524.51 Abnormal jaw closure

  524.52 Limited mandibular range of motion

  524.53 Deviation in opening and closing of the mandible

  524.54 Insufficient anterior guidance
      Insufficient anterior occlusal guidance

  524.55 Centric occlusion maximum intercuspation discrepancy
      Centric occlusion of teeth discrepancy

  524.56 Non-working side interference
      Balancing side interference

  524.57 Lack of posterior occlusal support

  524.59 Other dentofacial functional abnormalities
      Abnormal swallowing
      Mouth breathing
      Sleep postures
      Tongue, lip, or finger habits

● **524.6 Temporomandibular joint disorders**

  Excludes current temporomandibular joint:
      dislocation (830.0–830.1)
      strain (848.1)

  524.60 Temporomandibular joint disorders, unspecified
      Temporomandibular joint-pain-dysfunction syndrome [TMJ]

  524.61 Adhesions and ankylosis (bony or fibrous)

  524.62 Arthralgia of temporomandibular joint

  524.63 Articular disc disorder (reducing or nonreducing)

  524.64 Temporomandibular joint sounds on opening and/or closing the jaw

  524.69 Other specified temporomandibular joint disorders

● **524.7 Dental alveolar anomalies**

  524.70 Unspecified alveolar anomaly

  524.71 Alveolar maxillary hyperplasia

  524.72 Alveolar mandibular hyperplasia

  524.73 Alveolar maxillary hypoplasia

  524.74 Alveolar mandibular hypoplasia

  524.75 Vertical displacement of alveolus and teeth
      Extrusion of alveolus and teeth

  524.76 Occlusal plane deviation

  524.79 Other specified alveolar anomaly

● **524.8 Other specified dentofacial anomalies**

  524.81 Anterior soft tissue impingement

  524.82 Posterior soft tissue impingement

  524.89 Other specified dentofacial anomalies

  524.9 Unspecified dentofacial anomalies

● **525 Other diseases and conditions of the teeth and supporting structures**

  525.0 Exfoliation of teeth due to systemic causes

● **525.1 Loss of teeth due to trauma, extraction, or periodontal disease**

      Code first class of edentulism (525.40–525.44, 525.50–525.54)

  ▷ **525.10 Acquired absence of teeth, unspecified**
      Tooth extraction status, NOS

  ▷ **525.11 Loss of teeth due to trauma**
      Check for E code assignment.

  ▷ **525.12 Loss of teeth due to periodontal disease**

  ▷ **525.13 Loss of teeth due to caries**

  ▷ **525.19 Other loss of teeth**

● **525.2 Atrophy of edentulous alveolar ridge**

  525.20 Unspecified atrophy of edentulous alveolar ridge
      Atrophy of the mandible NOS
      Atrophy of the maxilla NOS

  525.21 Minimal atrophy of the mandible

  525.22 Moderate atrophy of the mandible

  525.23 Severe atrophy of the mandible

  525.24 Minimal atrophy of the maxilla

  525.25 Moderate atrophy of the maxilla

  525.26 Severe atrophy of the maxilla

  525.3 Retained dental root

● **525.4 Complete edentulism**

      Use additional code to identify cause of edentulism (525.10–525.19)

  525.40 Complete edentulism, unspecified
      Edentulism NOS

  525.41 Complete edentulism, class I

  525.42 Complete edentulism, class II

  525.43 Complete edentulism, class III

  525.44 Complete edentulism, class IV

● **525.5 Partial edentulism**

      Use additional code to identify cause of edentulism (525.10–525.19)

  525.50 Partial edentulism, unspecified

  525.51 Partial edentulism, class I

  525.52 Partial edentulism, class II

  525.53 Partial edentulism, class III

  525.54 Partial edentulism, class IV

● **525.6 Unsatisfactory restoration of tooth**
      Defective bridge, crown, fillings
      Defective dental restoration

  Excludes dental restoration status (V45.84)
      unsatisfactory endodontic treatment (526.61–526.69)

  525.60 Unspecified unsatisfactory restoration of tooth
      Unspecified defective dental restoration

  525.61 Open restoration margins
      Dental restoration failure of marginal integrity
      Open margin on tooth restoration

  525.62 Unrepairable overhanging of dental restorative materials
      Overhanging of tooth restoration

  525.63 Fractured dental restorative material without loss of material

      Excludes cracked tooth (521.81)
          fractured tooth (873.63, 873.73)

  525.64 Fractured dental restorative material with loss of material

      Excludes cracked tooth (521.81)
          fractured tooth (873.63, 873.73)

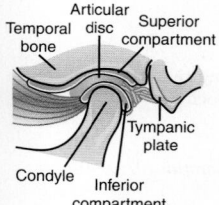

Temporal bone
Articular disc
Superior compartment
Tympanic plate
Condyle
Inferior compartment

Figure 9–4 Temporomandibular joint.

Item 9–5 Dysfunction of the temporomandibular joint is termed **temporomandibular joint (TMJ) syndrome** and is characterized by pain and tenderness/spasm of the muscles of mastication, joint noise, and in the later stages, limited mandibular movement.

DISEASES OF THE DIGESTIVE SYSTEM (520–579)

525.65 Contour of existing restoration of tooth biologically incompatible with oral health
Dental restoration failure of periodontal anatomical integrity
Unacceptable contours of existing restoration
Unacceptable morphology of existing restoration

525.66 Allergy to existing dental restorative material
Use additional code to identify the specific type of allergy

525.67 Poor aesthetics of existing restoration
Dental restoration aesthetically inadequate or displeasing

525.69 Other unsatisfactory restoration of existing tooth

● **525.7 Endosseous dental implant failure**

525.71 Osseointegration failure of dental implant
Failure of dental implant due to infection
Failure of dental implant due to unintentional loading
Failure of dental implant osseointegration due to premature loading
Failure of dental implant to osseointegrate prior to intentional prosthetic loading
Hemorrhagic complications of dental implant placement
Iatrogenic osseointegration failure of dental implant
Osseointegration failure of dental implant due to complications of systemic disease
Osseointegration failure of dental implant due to poor bone quality
Pre-integration failure of dental implant NOS
Pre-osseointegration failure of dental implant

525.72 Post-osseointegration biological failure of dental implant
Failure of dental implant due to lack of attached gingiva
Failure of dental implant due to occlusal trauma (caused by poor prosthetic design)
Failure of dental implant due to parafunctional habits
Failure of dental implant due to periodontal infection (peri-implantitis)
Failure of dental implant due to poor oral hygiene
Failure of dental implant to osseointegrate following intentional prosthetic loading
Iatrogenic post-osseointegration failure of dental implant
Post-osseointegration failure of dental implant due to complications of systemic disease

525.73 Post-osseointegration mechanical failure of dental implant
Failure of dental prosthesis causing loss of dental implant
Fracture of dental implant
Mechanical failure of dental implant NOS

> **Excludes**   *cracked tooth (521.81)*
> *fractured dental restorative material with loss of material (525.64)*
> *fractured dental restorative material without loss of material (525.63)*
> *fractured tooth (873.63, 873.73)*

525.79 Other endosseous dental implant failure
Dental implant failure NOS

525.8 Other specified disorders of the teeth and supporting structures
Enlargement of alveolar ridge NOS
Irregular alveolar process

525.9 Unspecified disorder of the teeth and supporting structures

● **526 Diseases of the jaws**

526.0 Developmental odontogenic cysts
Cyst:
dentigerous
eruption
follicular
lateral developmental
lateral periodontal
primordial
Keratocyst

> **Excludes**   *radicular cyst (522.8)*

526.1 Fissural cysts of jaw
Cyst:
globulomaxillary
incisor canal
median anterior maxillary
median palatal
nasopalatine
palatine of papilla

> **Excludes**   *cysts of oral soft tissues (528.4)*

526.2 Other cysts of jaws
Cyst of jaw: Cyst of jaw:
NOS   hemorrhagic
aneurysmal   traumatic

526.3 Central giant cell (reparative) granuloma

> **Excludes**   *peripheral giant cell granuloma (523.8)*

526.4 Inflammatory conditions
Abscess of jaw (acute) (chronic) (suppurative)
Osteitis of jaw (acute) (chronic) (suppurative)
Osteomyelitis (neonatal) of jaw (acute) (chronic) (suppurative)
Periostitis of jaw (acute) (chronic) (suppurative)
Sequestrum of jaw bone

> **Excludes**   *alveolar osteitis (526.5)*
> *osteonecrosis of jaw (733.45)*

526.5 Alveolitis of jaw
Alveolar osteitis
Dry socket

● **526.6 Periradicular pathology associated with previous endodontic treatment**

526.61 Perforation of root canal space

526.62 Endodontic overfill

526.63 Endodontic underfill

526.69 Other periradicular pathology associated with previous endodontic treatment

● **526.8 Other specified diseases of the jaws**

526.81 Exostosis of jaw
Torus mandibularis
Torus palatinus

526.89 Other
Cherubism
Fibrous dysplasia of jaw(s)
Latent bone cyst of jaw(s)
Osteoradionecrosis of jaw(s)
Unilateral condylar hyperplasia or hypoplasia of mandible

526.9 Unspecified disease of the jaws

● **527 Diseases of the salivary glands**

527.0 Atrophy

527.1 Hypertrophy

527.2 Sialoadenitis
Parotitis: Sialoangitis
NOS   Sialodochitis
allergic
toxic

> **Excludes**   *epidemic or infectious parotitis (072.0–072.9)*
> *uveoparotid fever (135)*

527.3 Abscess 🔗
Ⓔⓧ 527.0-527.9, 537.89-538

527.4 Fistula 🔗

> **Excludes**   *congenital fistula of salivary gland (750.24)*
Ⓔⓧ 527.0-527.9, 537.89-538

◀ New   ◀◀ Revised   ~~deleted~~ Deleted   Excludes   Includes   Use additional   Code first   Omit code
● Unacceptable Principal Diagnosis   ● Use Additional Digit(s)   ▶ Manifestation Code   OGCR Official Guidelines   Coding Clinic

838

Figure 9–5 Major salivary glands.

Parotid gland
Sublingual gland
Submandibular gland

Item 9–6 Atrophy is wasting away of a tissue or organ, whereas **hypertrophy** is overdevelopment or enlargement of a tissue or organ. **Sialoadenitis** is salivary gland inflammation. **Parotitis** is the inflammation of the parotid gland. In the epidemic form, parotitis is also known as mumps. **Sialolithiasis** is the formation of calculus within a salivary gland. **Mucocele** is a polyp composed of mucus.

527.5 Sialolithiasis
Calculus of salivary gland or duct
Stone of salivary gland or duct
Sialodocholithiasis

527.6 Mucocele
Mucous:
extravasation cyst of salivary gland
retention cyst of salivary gland
Ranula

527.7 Disturbance of salivary secretion
Hyposecretion   Sialorrhea
Ptyalism   Xerostomia

527.8 Other specified diseases of the salivary glands
Benign lymphoepithelial lesion of salivary gland
Sialectasia
Sialosis
Stenosis of salivary duct
Stricture of salivary duct

527.9 Unspecified disease of the salivary glands

● **528 Diseases of the oral soft tissues, excluding lesions specific for gingiva and tongue**

● **528.0 Stomatitis and mucositis (ulcerative)**
Excludes *Stevens-Johnson syndrome (695.13)*
stomatitis:
acute necrotizing ulcerative (101)
aphthous (528.2)
cellulitis and abscess of mouth (528.3)
diphtheritic stomatitis (032.0)
epizootic stomatitis (078.4)
gangrenous (528.1)
gingivitis (523.0–523.1)
herpetic (054.2)
oral thrush (112.0)
Vincent's (101)
Coding Clinic: 1999, Q2, P9

528.00 Stomatitis and mucositis, unspecified
Mucositis NOS
Ulcerative mucositis NOS
Ulcerative stomatitis NOS
Vesicular stomatitis NOS

528.01 Mucositis (ulcerative) due to antineoplastic therapy
Use additional E code to identify adverse effects of therapy, such as:
antineoplastic and immunosuppressive drugs (E930.7, E933.1)
radiation therapy (E879.2)
Coding Clinic: 2006, Q4, P88-91

528.02 Mucositis (ulcerative) due to other drugs
Use additional E code to identify drug

528.09 Other stomatitis and mucositis (ulcerative)

Item 9–7 Stomatitis is the inflammation of the oral mucosa. **Cancrum oris,** also known as **noma** or **gangrenous stomatitis,** begins as an ulcer of the gingiva and results in a progressive gangrenous process. Mucositis is the inflammation of the mucous membranes lining the digestive tract from the mouth to the anus. It is a common side effect of chemotherapy and of radiotherapy that involves any part of the digestive tract.

Figure 9–6 Oral leukoplakia and associated squamous carcinoma. (From Feldman: Sleisenger & Fordtran's Gastrointestinal and Liver Disease, ed 8, Saunders, An Imprint of Elsevier, 2006)

528.1 Cancrum oris
Gangrenous stomatitis
Noma

528.2 Oral aphthae
Aphthous stomatitis
Canker sore
Periadenitis mucosa necrotica recurrens
Recurrent aphthous ulcer
Stomatitis herpetiformis
Excludes *herpetic stomatitis (054.2)*
Coding Clinic: 2012, Q2, P18-19

528.3 Cellulitis and abscess 🔵
Cellulitis of mouth (floor)
Ludwig's angina
Oral fistula
Excludes *abscess of tongue (529.0)*
cellulitis or abscess of lip (528.5)
fistula (of):
dental (522.7)
lip (528.5)
gingivitis (523.00–523.11)
(Ex) 528.00-528.09, 528.3, 529.0, 529.2

528.4 Cysts
Dermoid cyst of mouth
Epidermoid cyst of mouth
Epstein's pearl of mouth
Lymphoepithelial cyst of mouth
Nasoalveolar cyst of mouth
Nasolabial cyst of mouth
Excludes *cyst:*
gingiva (523.8)
tongue (529.8)

528.5 Diseases of lips
Abscess of lip(s)   Cheilitis:
Cellulitis of lip(s)   NOS
Fistula of lip(s)   angular
Hypertrophy of lip(s)   Cheilodynia
                           Cheilosis
Excludes *actinic cheilitis (692.79)*
congenital fistula of lip (750.25)
leukoplakia of lips (528.6)
Coding Clinic: 1986, Sept-Oct, P10

528.6 Leukoplakia of oral mucosa, including tongue
Considered precancerous and evidenced by thickened white patches of epithelium on mucous membranes
Leukokeratosis of oral mucosa
Leukoplakia of:
gingiva
lips
tongue
Excludes *carcinoma in situ (230.0, 232.0)*
leukokeratosis nicotina palati (528.79)

● **528.7 Other disturbances of oral epithelium, including tongue**
Excludes *carcinoma in situ (230.0, 232.0)*
leukokeratosis NOS (702.8)

528.71 Minimal keratinized residual ridge mucosa
Minimal keratinization of alveolar ridge mucosa

528.72 Excessive keratinized residual ridge mucosa
Excessive keratinization of alveolar ridge mucosa

528.79 Other disturbances of oral epithelium, including tongue
Erythroplakia of mouth or tongue
Focal epithelial hyperplasia of mouth or tongue
Leukoedema of mouth or tongue
Leukokeratosis nicotina palati
Other oral epithelium disturbances

N Newborn: 0   **P** Pediatric: 0–17   **M** Maternity: 12–55   **A** Adult: 15–124   ♀ Females Only   ♂ Males Only

(Ex) CC/MCC Exclusions   🔵 Complication\Comorbidity   🔵 Major C\C   🔵 Present on Admission Requirement   🔵 Hospital-Acquired Condition

839

528.8   Oral submucosal fibrosis, including of tongue

528.9   Other and unspecified diseases of the oral soft tissues
     Cheek and lip biting
     Denture sore mouth
     Denture stomatitis
     Melanoplakia
     Papillary hyperplasia of palate
     Eosinophilic granuloma of oral mucosa
     Irritative hyperplasia of oral mucosa
     Pyogenic granuloma of oral mucosa
     Ulcer (traumatic) of oral mucosa

● **529   Diseases and other conditions of the tongue**

529.0   Glossitis
     Abscess of tongue
     Ulceration (traumatic) of tongue
     Excludes   *glossitis:*
         benign migratory (529.1)
         Hunter's (529.4)
         median rhomboid (529.2)
         Moeller's (529.4)

529.1   Geographic tongue
     Benign migratory glossitis
     Glossitis areata exfoliativa

529.2   Median rhomboid glossitis

529.3   Hypertrophy of tongue papillae
     Black hairy tongue
     Coated tongue
     Hypertrophy of foliate papillae
     Lingua villosa nigra

529.4   Atrophy of tongue papillae
     Bald tongue   Glossodynia exfoliativa
     Glazed tongue   Smooth atrophic tongue
     Glossitis:
         Hunter's
         Moeller's

529.5   Plicated tongue
     Fissured tongue   Scrotal tongue
     Furrowed tongue
     Excludes   *fissure of tongue, congenital (750.13)*

529.6   Glossodynia
     Glossopyrosis   Painful tongue
     Excludes   *glossodynia exfoliativa (529.4)*

529.8   Other specified conditions of the tongue
     Atrophy (of) tongue
     Crenated (of) tongue
     Enlargement (of) tongue
     Hypertrophy (of) tongue
     Glossocele
     Glossoptosis
     Excludes   *erythroplasia of tongue (528.79)*
         leukoplakia of tongue (528.6)
         macroglossia (congenital) (750.15)
         microglossia (congenital) (750.16)
         oral submucosal fibrosis (528.8)

529.9   Unspecified condition of the tongue

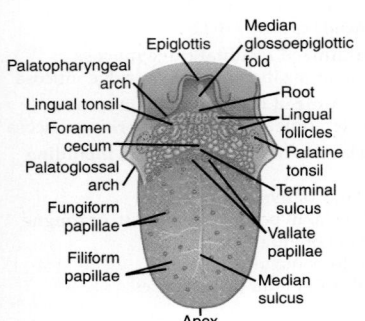

Figure 9–7   Structure of the tongue.

CERVICAL ESOPHAGUS
Left subclavian artery
First rib
Arch of aorta
Diaphragm
THORACIC ESOPHAGUS
ABDOMINAL ESOPHAGUS   Stomach

Figure 9–8   The esophagus is the muscular tube that connects the pharynx and the stomach. The 10 inch (25 cm) long esophagus is divided into three parts: **cervical, thoracic,** and **abdominal.**

Item 9–8 Achalasia is a condition in which the smooth muscle fibers of the esophagus do not relax. Most frequently, this condition occurs at the esophagogastric sphincter. **Cardiospasm,** also known as **megaesophagus,** is achalasia of the thoracic esophagus.

DISEASES OF ESOPHAGUS, STOMACH, AND DUODENUM (530–539)

● **530   Diseases of esophagus**
     Excludes   *esophageal varices (456.0–456.2)*

530.0   Achalasia and cardiospasm
     Achalasia (of cardia)
     Aperistalsis of esophagus
     Megaesophagus
     Excludes   *congenital cardiospasm (750.7)*

● **530.1   Esophagitis**
     Esophagitis: Esophagitis:
       chemical   postoperative
       peptic   regurgitant
     Use additional E code to identify cause, if induced by chemical
     Excludes   *tuberculous esophagitis (017.8)*
     Coding Clinic: 1985, Sept-Oct, P9

     530.10   Esophagitis, unspecified
         Esophagitis NOS
         Coding Clinic: 2005, Q3, P17-18

     530.11   Reflux esophagitis
         Coding Clinic: 1995, Q4, P82

     530.12   Acute esophagitis 🔒
         (Ex) 530.10-530.21, 530.4, 530.7, 530.82, 530.85-530.89

     530.13   Eosinophilic esophagitis
         Coding Clinic: 2008, Q4, P115-116

     530.19   Other esophagitis
         Abscess of esophagus
         Coding Clinic: 2001, Q3, P15

● **530.2   Ulcer of esophagus**
     Ulcer of esophagus
       fungal
       peptic
     Ulcer of esophagus due to ingestion of:
       aspirin
       chemicals
       medicines
     Use additional E code to identify cause, if induced by chemical or drug

     530.20   Ulcer of esophagus without bleeding 🔒
         Ulcer of esophagus NOS
         (Ex) 530.21, 530.89-530.9, 537.84

     530.21   Ulcer of esophagus with bleeding 🔒
         Excludes   *bleeding esophageal varices (456.0, 456.20)*
         (Ex) 251.5, 456.0, 530.20-530.21, 530.7, 530.82, 530.85, 531.00-534.91, 535.01, 535.11, 535.21, 535.31, 535.41, 535.51, 535.61, 535.71, 537.83, 537.89-538, 562.02-562.03, 562.12-562.13, 569.3, 569.85, 578.0-578.9

◀ New   ◀◀ Revised   ~~deleted~~ Deleted   Excludes   Includes   Use additional   Code first   Omit code

840   ● Unacceptable Principal Diagnosis   ● Use Additional Digit(s)   ▶ Manifestation Code   OGCR Official Guidelines   Coding Clinic

Item 9–9 Dyskinesia is difficulty in moving, and **diverticulum** is a sac or pouch.

530.3 Stricture and stenosis of esophagus
Compression of esophagus
Obstruction of esophagus
> **Excludes** *congenital stricture of esophagus (750.3)*

Coding Clinic: 2012, Q1, P15-16; 2001, Q2, P4; 1997, Q2, P3; 1988, Q1, P13

530.4 Perforation of esophagus
Rupture of esophagus
> **Excludes** *traumatic perforation of esophagus (862.22, 862.32, 874.4–874.5)*

(Ex) 530.4, 530.7-530.81, 530.83-530.84, 530.89-530.9

530.5 Dyskinesia of esophagus
Corkscrew esophagus
Curling esophagus
Esophagospasm
Spasm of esophagus
> **Excludes** *cardiospasm (530.0)*

Coding Clinic: 1988, Q1, P13; 1984, Nov-Dec, P19

530.6 Diverticulum of esophagus, acquired
Diverticulum, acquired:
  epiphrenic
  pharyngoesophageal
  pulsion
  subdiaphragmatic
  traction
  Zenker's (hypopharyngeal)
Esophageal pouch, acquired
Esophagocele, acquired
> **Excludes** *congenital diverticulum of esophagus (750.4)*

Coding Clinic: 1985, Mar-April, P15

530.7 Gastroesophageal laceration-hemorrhage syndrome
Mallory-Weiss syndrome
(Ex) 251.5, 456.0, 530.20-530.21, 530.4, 530.7-530.85, 530.89-534.91, 535.01, 535.11, 535.21, 535.31, 535.41, 535.51, 535.61, 535.71, 537.83, 562.02-562.03, 562.12-562.13, 569.3, 569.85, 578.0-578.9

● 530.8 Other specified disorders of esophagus
530.81 Esophageal reflux
Gastroesophageal reflux
> **Excludes** *reflux esophagitis (530.11)*

Coding Clinic: 2010, Q4, P98; 2001, Q2, P4; 1995, Q1, P7

530.82 Esophageal hemorrhage
> **Excludes** *hemorrhage due to esophageal varices (456.0–456.2)*

(Ex) 251.5, 456.0, 456.20, 459.89-459.9, 530.20-530.21, 530.7, 530.82, 530.85, 531.00-534.91, 535.01, 535.11, 535.21, 535.31, 535.41, 535.51, 535.61, 535.71, 537.83, 562.02-562.03, 562.12-562.13, 569.3, 569.85, 578.0-578.9

Coding Clinic: 2005, Q1, P17-18

530.83 Esophageal leukoplakia

Figure 9–9 A. Ulcer. **B.** Perforated ulcer. **C.** Laparoscopic view of a perforated duodenal ulcer *(arrow)* with fibrinous exudate on the adjacent peritoneum. (**C** from Feldman: Sleisenger & Fordtran's Gastrointestinal and Liver Disease, ed 8, Saunders, An Imprint of Elsevier, 2006)

Item 9–10 Gastric ulcers are lesions of the stomach that result in the death of the tissue and a defect of the surface. **Perforated ulcers** are those in which the lesion penetrates the gastric wall, leaving a hole. **Peptic ulcers** are lesions of the stomach or the duodenum.
Peptic refers to the gastric juice, pepsin.

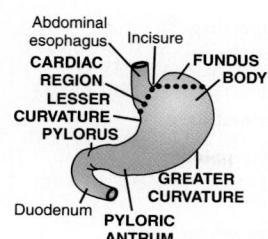

Figure 9–10 Parts of the stomach.

Item 9–11 Esophageal reflux is the return flow of the contents of the stomach to the esophagus and is referred to as GERD and/or "heartburn." **Gastroesophageal reflux** is the return flow of the contents of the stomach and duodenum to the esophagus. **Esophageal leukoplakia** are white areas on the mucous membrane of the esophagus for which no specific cause can be identified.

530.84 Tracheoesophageal fistula
> **Excludes** *congenital tracheoesophageal fistula (750.3)*

(Ex) 530.4, 530.7-530.81, 530.83-530.84, 530.89-530.9

530.85 Barrett's esophagus
Coding Clinic: 2003, Q4, P63

530.86 Infection of esophagostomy
Use additional code to specify infection
(Ex) 530.86-530.87, 536.40-536.49, 539.01-539.89, 569.71-569.79, 997.41-997.49, 997.71, 997.91-997.99, 998.81, 998.83-998.9
Coding Clinic: 2004, Q4, P83

530.87 Mechanical complication of esophagostomy
Malfunction of esophagostomy
(Ex) 530.86-530.87, 536.40-536.49, 539.01-539.89, 569.71-569.79, 997.41-997.49, 997.71, 997.91-997.99, 998.81, 998.83-998.9
Coding Clinic: 2004, Q4, P83

530.89 Other
> **Excludes** *Paterson-Kelly syndrome (280.8)*

530.9 Unspecified disorder of esophagus

● 531 Gastric ulcer
> **Includes** ulcer (peptic):
>   prepyloric
>   pylorus
>   stomach

Use additional E code to identify drug, if drug-induced
> **Excludes** *peptic ulcer NOS (533.0–533.9)*

Coding Clinic: 1990, Q4, P27

The following fifth-digit subclassification is for use with category 531:

0	without mention of obstruction
1	with obstruction

● 531.0 Acute with hemorrhage
[0-1] (Ex) 251.5, 456.0, 530.20-530.21, 530.7, 530.82, 530.85, 531.00-534.91, 535.01, 535.11, 535.21, 535.31, 535.41, 535.51, 535.61, 535.71, 537.83, 537.89-538, 562.02-562.03, 562.12-562.13, 569.3, 569.85, 578.0-578.9
Coding Clinic: 1984, Nov-Dec, P15

● 531.1 Acute with perforation
[0-1] (Ex) 251.5, 456.0, 530.20-530.21, 530.7, 530.82, 530.85, 531.00-534.91, 535.01, 535.11, 535.21, 535.31, 535.41, 535.51, 535.61, 535.71, 537.83, 537.89-538, 562.02-562.03, 562.12-562.13, 569.3, 569.85, 578.0-578.9

● 531.2 Acute with hemorrhage and perforation
[0-1] (Ex) 251.5, 456.0, 530.20-530.21, 530.7, 530.82, 530.85, 531.00-534.91, 535.01, 535.11, 535.21, 535.31, 535.41, 535.51, 535.61, 535.71, 537.83, 537.89-538, 562.02-562.03, 562.12-562.13, 569.3, 569.85, 578.0-578.9

● 531.3 Acute without mention of hemorrhage or
[0-1] **perforation** 0 , 1
(Ex) 251.5, 456.0, 530.20-530.21, 530.7, 530.82, 530.85, 531.00-534.91, 535.01, 535.11, 535.21, 535.31, 535.41, 535.51, 535.61, 535.71, 537.83, 537.89-538, 562.02-562.03, 562.12-562.13, 569.3, 569.85, 578.0-578.9

DISEASES OF THE DIGESTIVE SYSTEM (520–579)

N Newborn: 0 **P** Pediatric: 0–17 **M** Maternity: 12–55 **A** Adult: 15–124 ♀ Females Only ♂ Males Only

(Ex) CC/MCC Exclusions Complication\Comorbidity Major C\C Present on Admission Requirement Hospital-Acquired Condition   841

● **531.4 Chronic or unspecified with hemorrhage** 🚫
[0-1]   (Ex) 251.5, 456.0, 530.20-530.21, 530.7, 530.82, 530.85, 531.00-534.91, 535.01,
535.11, 535.21, 535.31, 535.41, 535.51, 535.61, 535.71, 537.83,
537.89-538, 562.02-562.03, 562.12-562.13, 569.3, 569.85, 578.0-578.9

● **531.5 Chronic or unspecified with perforation** 🚫
[0-1]   (Ex) 251.5, 456.0, 530.20-530.21, 530.82, 530.85, 531.00-534.91, 535.01,
535.11, 535.21, 535.31, 535.41, 535.51, 535.61, 535.71, 537.83,
537.89-538, 562.02-562.03, 562.12-562.13, 569.3, 569.85, 578.0-578.9

Coding Clinic: 2011, Q1, P11-12

● **531.6 Chronic or unspecified with hemorrhage and**
[0-1] **perforation** 🚫
(Ex) 251.5, 456.0, 530.20-530.21, 530.7, 530.82, 530.85, 531.00-534.91, 535.01,
535.11, 535.21, 535.31, 535.41, 535.51, 535.61, 535.71, 537.83,
537.89-538, 562.02-562.03, 562.12-562.13, 569.3, 569.85, 578.0-578.9

● **531.7 Chronic without mention of hemorrhage or**
[0-1] **perforation** 1 🚫
For code **531.71:** (Ex) 251.5, 456.0, 530.20-530.21, 530.7, 530.82, 530.85,
531.00-534.91, 535.01, 535.11, 535.21, 535.31, 535.41, 535.51, 535.61,
535.71, 537.83, 537.89-538, 562.02-562.03, 562.12-562.13, 569.3,
569.85, 578.0-578.9

● **531.9 Unspecified as acute or chronic, without mention of**
[0-1] **hemorrhage or perforation** 1 🚫
For code **531.91:** (Ex) 251.5, 456.0, 530.20-530.21, 530.7, 530.82, 530.85,
531.00-534.91, 535.01, 535.11, 535.21, 535.31, 535.41, 535.51, 535.61,
535.71, 537.83, 537.89-538, 562.02-562.03, 562.12-562.13, 569.3,
569.85, 578.0-578.9

● **532 Duodenal ulcer**

Includes   erosion (acute) of duodenum
ulcer (peptic):
duodenum
postpyloric

Use additional E code to identify drug, if drug-induced

Excludes   peptic ulcer NOS (533.0–533.9)

Coding Clinic: 1990, Q4, P27

The following fifth-digit subclassification is for use with
category 532:

| 0   without mention of obstruction |
| 1   with obstruction |

● **532.0 Acute with hemorrhage** 🚫
[0-1]   (Ex) 251.5, 456.0, 530.20-530.21, 530.7, 530.82, 530.85, 531.00-534.91, 535.01,
535.11, 535.21, 535.31, 535.41, 535.51, 535.61, 535.71, 537.3, 537.83,
537.89-538, 562.02-562.03, 562.12-562.13, 569.3, 569.85, 578.0-578.9

● **532.1 Acute with perforation** 🚫
[0-1]   (Ex) 251.5, 456.0, 530.20-530.21, 530.7, 530.82, 530.85, 531.00-534.91, 535.01,
535.11, 535.21, 535.31, 535.41, 535.51, 535.61, 535.71, 537.3, 537.83,
537.89-538, 562.02-562.03, 562.12-562.13, 569.3, 569.85, 578.0-578.9

● **532.2 Acute with hemorrhage and perforation** 🚫
[0-1]   (Ex) 251.5, 456.0, 530.20-530.21, 530.7, 530.82, 530.85, 531.00-534.91, 535.01,
535.11, 535.21, 535.31, 535.41, 535.51, 535.61, 535.71, 537.3, 537.83,
537.89-538, 562.02-562.03, 562.12-562.13, 569.3, 569.85, 578.0-578.9

● **532.3 Acute without mention of hemorrhage or**
[0-1] **perforation** 0 🚫, 1 🚫
For code **532.30:** (Ex) 251.5, 456.0, 530.7, 530.82, 531.00-534.91, 535.01,
535.11, 535.21, 535.31, 535.41, 535.51, 535.61, 535.71, 537.3,
537.83-538, 562.02-562.03, 562.12-562.13, 569.3, 569.85, 578.0-578.9;
For code **532.31:** (Ex) 251.5, 456.0, 530.20-530.21, 530.7, 530.82, 530.85,
531.00-534.91, 535.01, 535.11, 535.21, 535.31, 535.41, 535.51, 535.61,
535.71, 537.3, 537.83, 537.89-538, 562.02-562.03, 562.12-562.13, 569.3,
569.85, 578.0-578.9

● **532.4 Chronic or unspecified with hemorrhage** 🚫
[0-1]   (Ex) 251.5, 456.0, 530.20-530.21, 530.7, 530.82, 530.85, 531.00-534.91, 535.01,
535.11, 535.21, 535.31, 535.41, 535.51, 535.61, 535.71, 537.3, 537.83,
537.89-538, 562.02-562.03, 562.12-562.13, 569.3, 569.85, 578.0-578.9

● **532.5 Chronic or unspecified with perforation** 🚫
[0-1]   (Ex) 251.5, 456.0, 530.20-530.21, 530.7, 530.82, 530.85, 531.00-534.91, 535.01,
535.11, 535.21, 535.31, 535.41, 535.51, 535.61, 535.71, 537.3, 537.83,
537.89-538, 562.02-562.03, 562.12-562.13, 569.3, 569.85, 578.0-578.9

● **532.6 Chronic or unspecified with hemorrhage and**
[0-1] **perforation** 🚫
(Ex) 251.5, 456.0, 530.20-530.21, 530.7, 530.82, 530.85, 531.00-534.91, 535.01,
535.11, 535.21, 535.31, 535.41, 535.51, 535.61, 535.71, 537.3, 537.83,
537.89-538, 562.02-562.03, 562.12-562.13, 569.3, 569.85, 578.0-578.9

● **532.7 Chronic without mention of hemorrhage or**
[0-1] **perforation** 1 🚫
(Ex) 251.5, 456.0, 530.20-530.21, 530.7, 530.82, 530.85, 531.00-534.91, 535.01,
535.11, 535.21, 535.31, 535.41, 535.51, 535.61, 535.71, 537.3, 537.83,
537.89-538, 562.02-562.03, 562.12-562.13, 569.3, 569.85, 578.0-578.9

● **532.9 Unspecified as acute or chronic, without mention of**
[0-1] **hemorrhage or perforation** 1 🚫
(Ex) 251.5, 456.0, 530.20-530.21, 530.7, 530.82, 530.85, 531.00-534.91, 535.01,
535.11, 535.21, 535.31, 535.41, 535.51, 535.61, 535.71, 537.3, 537.83,
537.89-538, 562.02-562.03, 562.12-562.13, 569.3, 569.85, 578.0-578.9

● **533 Peptic ulcer, site unspecified**

Includes   gastroduodenal ulcer NOS
peptic ulcer NOS
stress ulcer NOS

Use additional E code to identify drug, if drug-induced

Excludes   peptic ulcer:
duodenal (532.0–532.9)
gastric (531.0–531.9)

Coding Clinic: 1990, Q4, P27

The following fifth-digit subclassification is for use with
category 533:

| 0   without mention of obstruction |
| 1   with obstruction |

● **533.0 Acute with hemorrhage** 🚫
[0-1]   (Ex) 251.5, 456.0, 530.20-530.21, 530.7, 530.82, 530.85, 531.00-534.91, 535.01,
535.11, 535.21, 535.31, 535.41, 535.51, 535.61, 535.71, 537.3, 537.83,
537.89-538, 562.02-562.03, 562.12-562.13, 569.3, 569.85, 578.0-578.9

● **533.1 Acute with perforation** 🚫
[0-1]   (Ex) 251.5, 456.0, 530.20-530.21, 530.7, 530.82, 530.85, 531.00-534.91, 535.01,
535.11, 535.21, 535.31, 535.41, 535.51, 535.61, 535.71, 537.3, 537.83,
537.89-538, 562.02-562.03, 562.12-562.13, 569.3, 569.85, 578.0-578.9

● **533.2 Acute with hemorrhage and perforation** 🚫
[0-1]   (Ex) 251.5, 456.0, 530.20-530.21, 530.7, 530.82, 530.85, 531.00-534.91, 535.01,
535.11, 535.21, 535.31, 535.41, 535.51, 535.61, 535.71, 537.3, 537.83,
537.89-538, 562.02-562.03, 562.12-562.13, 569.3, 569.85, 578.0-578.9

● **533.3 Acute without mention of hemorrhage and**
[0-1] **perforation** 0 🚫, 1 🚫
(Ex) 251.5, 456.0, 530.20-530.21, 530.7, 530.82, 530.85, 531.00-534.91, 535.01,
535.11, 535.21, 535.31, 535.41, 535.51, 535.61, 535.71, 537.3, 537.83,
537.89-538, 562.02-562.03, 562.12-562.13, 569.3, 569.85, 578.0-578.9

● **533.4 Chronic or unspecified with hemorrhage** 🚫
[0-1]   (Ex) 251.5, 456.0, 530.20-530.21, 530.7, 530.82, 530.85, 531.00-534.91, 535.01,
535.11, 535.21, 535.31, 535.41, 535.51, 535.61, 535.71, 537.3, 537.83,
537.89-538, 562.02-562.03, 562.12-562.13, 569.3, 569.85, 578.0-578.9

● **533.5 Chronic or unspecified with perforation** 🚫
[0-1]   (Ex) 251.5, 456.0, 530.20-530.21, 530.7 530.82, 530.85, 531.00-534.91, 535.01
535.11, 535.21, 535.31, 535.41, 535.51, 535.61, 535.71, 537.3, 537.83,
537.89-538, 562.02-562.03, 562.12-562.13, 569.3, 569.85, 578.0-578.9

● **533.6 Chronic or unspecified with hemorrhage and**
[0-1] **perforation** 🚫
(Ex) 251.5, 456.0, 530.20-530.21, 530.7, 530.82, 530.85, 531.00-534.91, 535.01
535.11, 535.21, 535.31, 535.41, 535.51, 535.61, 535.71, 537.3, 537.83,
537.89-538, 562.02-562.03, 562.12-562.13, 569.3, 569.85, 578.0-578.9

● **533.7 Chronic without mention of hemorrhage or**
[0-1] **perforation** 1 🚫
For code **533.71:** (Ex) 251.5, 456.0, 530.20-530.21, 530.7, 530.82, 530.85,
531.00-534.91, 535.01, 535.11, 535.21, 535.31, 535.41, 535.51, 535.61,
535.71, 537.3, 537.83, 537.89-538, 562.02-562.03, 562.12-562.13, 569.3,
569.85, 578.0-578.9

Coding Clinic: 1989, Q2, P16

● **533.9 Unspecified as acute or chronic, without mention of**
[0-1] **hemorrhage or perforation** 1 🚫
For code **533.91:** (Ex) 251.5, 456.0, 530.20-530.21, 530.7, 530.82, 530.85,
531.00-534.91, 535.01, 535.11, 535.21, 535.31, 535.41, 535.51, 535.61,
535.71, 537.3, 537.83, 537.89-538, 562.02-562.03, 562.12-562.13, 569.3,
569.85, 578.0-578.9

◄ New   ◄◁◁ Revised   deleted Deleted   Excludes   Includes   Use additional   Code first   Omit code
● Unacceptable Principal Diagnosis   ● Use Additional Digit(s)   ▶ Manifestation Code   OGCR Official Guidelines   Coding Clinic

842

● 534 Gastrojejunal ulcer

Includes   ulcer (peptic) or erosion:
                anastomotic
                gastrocolic
                gastrointestinal
                gastrojejunal
                jejunal
                marginal
                stomal

Excludes *primary ulcer of small intestine (569.82)*
Coding Clinic: 1990, Q4, P27

The following fifth-digit subclassification is for use with category 534:

0	**without mention of obstruction**
1	**with obstruction**

● 534.0 Acute with hemorrhage 🦠
[0-1]   Ex) 251.5, 456.0, 530.20-530.21, 530.7, 530.82, 530.85, 531.00-534.91, 535.01,
535.11, 535.21, 535.31, 535.41, 535.51, 535.61, 535.71, 537.83,
537.89-538, 562.02-562.03, 562.12-562.13, 569.3, 569.85, 578.0-578.9

● 534.1 Acute with perforation 🦠
[0-1]   Ex) 251.5, 456.0, 530.20-530.21, 530.7, 530.82, 530.85, 531.00-534.91, 535.01,
535.11, 535.21, 535.31, 535.41, 535.51, 535.61, 535.71, 537.83,
537.89-538, 562.02-562.03, 562.12-562.13, 569.3, 569.85, 578.0-578.9

● 534.2 Acute with hemorrhage and perforation 🦠
[0-1]   Ex) 251.5, 456.0, 530.20-530.21, 530.7, 530.82, 530.85, 531.00-534.91, 535.01,
535.11, 535.21, 535.31, 535.41, 535.51, 535.61, 535.71, 537.83,
537.89-538, 562.02-562.03, 562.12-562.13, 569.3, 569.85, 578.0-578.9

● 534.3 Acute without mention of hemorrhage or
[0-1] perforation 0 🦠, 1 🦠
Ex) 251.5, 456.0, 530.20-530.21, 530.7, 530.82, 530.85, 531.00-534.91, 535.01,
535.11, 535.21, 535.31, 535.41, 535.51, 535.61, 535.71, 537.83,
537.89-538, 562.02-562.03, 562.12-562.13, 569.3, 569.85, 578.0-578.9

● 534.4 Chronic or unspecified with hemorrhage 🦠
[0-1]   Ex) 251.5, 456.0, 530.20-530.21, 530.7, 530.82, 530.85, 531.00-534.91, 535.01,
535.11, 535.21, 535.31, 535.41, 535.51, 535.61, 535.71, 537.83,
537.89-538, 562.02-562.03, 562.12-562.13, 569.3, 569.85, 578.0-578.9

● 534.5 Chronic or unspecified with perforation 🦠
[0-1]   Ex) 251.5, 456.0, 530.20-530.21, 530.7, 530.82, 530.85, 531.00-534.91, 535.01,
535.11, 535.21, 535.31, 535.41, 535.51, 535.61, 535.71, 537.83,
537.89-538, 562.02-562.03, 562.12-562.13, 569.3, 569.85, 578.0-578.9

● 534.6 Chronic or unspecified with hemorrhage and
[0-1] perforation 🦠
Ex) 251.5, 456.0, 530.20-530.21, 530.7, 530.82, 530.85, 531.00-534.91, 535.01,
535.11, 535.21, 535.31, 535.41, 535.51, 535.61, 535.71, 537.83,
537.89-538, 562.02-562.03, 562.12-562.13, 569.3, 569.85, 578.0-578.9

● 534.7 Chronic without mention of hemorrhage or
[0-1] perforation 1 🦠
For code 534.71: Ex) 251.5, 456.0, 530.20-530.21, 530.7, 530.82, 530.85,
531.00-534.91, 535.01, 535.11, 535.21, 535.31, 535.41, 535.51, 535.61,
535.71, 537.83, 537.89-538, 562.02-562.03, 562.12-562.13, 569.3,
569.85, 578.0-578.9

● 534.9 Unspecified as acute or chronic, without mention of
[0-1] hemorrhage or perforation 1 🦠
For code 534.91: Ex) 251.5, 456.0, 530.20-530.21, 530.7, 530.82, 530.85,
531.00-534.91, 535.01, 535.11, 535.21, 535.31, 535.41, 535.51, 535.61,
535.71, 537.83, 537.89-538, 562.02-562.03, 562.12-562.13, 569.3,
569.85, 578.0-578.9

● 535 Gastritis and duodenitis
Coding Clinic: 2007, Q2, P13; 2005, Q3, P17-18

The following fifth-digit subclassification is for use with category 535:

0	**without mention of hemorrhage**
1	**with hemorrhage**

● 535.0 Acute gastritis 1 🦠
[0-1]   For code 535.01: Ex) 251.5, 456.0, 530.20-530.21, 530.7, 530.82, 530.85,
531.00-534.91, 535.01, 535.11, 535.21, 535.31, 535.41, 535.51,
535.61, 535.71, 537.83, 562.02-562.03, 562.12-562.13, 569.3, 569.85,
578.0-578.9
Coding Clinic: 1992, Q2, P8-9; 1986, Nov-Dec, P9

Item 9–12 Gastritis is a severe inflammation of the stomach. **Atrophic gastritis** is a chronic inflammation of the stomach that results in destruction of the cells of the mucosa of the stomach. Duodenitis is an inflammation of the duodenum, the first section of the small intestine.

● 535.1 Atrophic gastritis 1 🦠
[0-1]   Gastritis:
         atrophic-hyperplastic   chronic (atrophic)
For code 535.11: Ex) 251.5, 456.0, 530.20-530.21, 530.7, 530.82, 530.85,
531.00-534.91, 535.01, 535.11, 535.21, 535.31, 535.41, 535.51, 535.61,
535.71, 537.83, 562.02-562.03, 562.12-562.13, 569.3, 569.85,
578.0-578.9
Coding Clinic: 1994, Q1, P18

● 535.2 Gastric mucosal hypertrophy 1 🦠
[0-1]   Hypertrophic gastritis
For code 535.21: Ex) 251.5, 456.0, 530.20-530.21, 530.7, 530.82, 530.85,
531.00-534.91, 535.01, 535.11, 535.21, 535.31, 535.41, 535.51, 535.61,
535.71, 537.83, 562.02-562.03, 562.12-562.13, 569.3, 569.85,
578.0-578.9

● 535.3 Alcoholic gastritis 1 🦠
[0-1]   For code 535.31: Ex) 251.5, 456.0, 530.20-530.21, 530.7, 530.82, 530.85,
531.00-534.91, 535.01, 535.11, 535.21, 535.31, 535.41, 535.51,
535.61, 535.71, 537.83, 562.02-562.03, 562.12-562.13, 569.3, 569.85,
578.0-578.9

● 535.4 Other specified gastritis 1 🦠
[0-1]   Gastritis:
         allergic
         bile induced
         irritant
         superficial
         toxic
         Excludes *eosinophilic gastritis (535.7)*
For code 535.41: Ex) 251.5, 456.0, 530.20-530.21, 530.7, 530.82, 530.85,
531.00-534.91, 535.01, 535.11, 535.21, 535.31, 535.41, 535.51, 535.61,
535.71, 537.83, 562.02-562.03, 562.12-562.13, 569.3, 569.85,
578.0-578.9
Coding Clinic: 1990, Q4, P27

● 535.5 Unspecified gastritis and gastroduodenitis 1 🦠
[0-1]   For code 535.51: Ex) 251.5, 456.0, 530.20-530.21, 530.7, 530.82, 530.85,
531.00-534.91, 535.01, 535.11, 535.21, 535.31, 535.41, 535.51,
535.61, 535.71, 537.83, 562.02-562.03, 562.12-562.13, 569.3, 569.85,
578.0-578.9
Coding Clinic: 2005, Q3, P17-18; 1999, Q4, P25-26; 1992, Q3, P15

● 535.6 Duodenitis 1 🦠
[0-1]   For code 535.61: Ex) 251.5, 456.0, 530.20-530.21, 530.7, 530.82, 530.85,
531.00-534.91, 535.01, 535.11, 535.21, 535.31, 535.41, 535.51,
535.61, 535.71, 537.83, 562.02-562.03, 562.12-562.13, 569.3, 569.85,
578.0-578.9
Coding Clinic: 2005, Q3, P17-18

● 535.7 Eosinophilic gastritis 1 🦠
[0-1]   For code 535.71: Ex) 251.5, 456.0, 530.20-530.21, 530.7, 530.82, 530.85,
531.00-534.91, 535.01, 535.11, 535.21, 535.31, 535.41, 535.51,
535.61-535.71, 535.81, 558.41, 562.02-562.03, 562.12-562.13, 569.3,
569.85, 578.0-578.9
Coding Clinic: 2008, Q4, P115-116

● 536 Disorders of function of stomach
Excludes *functional disorders of stomach specified as psychogenic (306.4)*

536.0 Achlorhydria

536.1 Acute dilatation of stomach 🦠
      Acute distention of stomach
      Ex) 536.1

536.2 Persistent vomiting
      Cyclical vomiting
      Habit vomiting
      Persistent vomiting [not of pregnancy]
      Uncontrollable vomiting
      Excludes *bilious emesis (vomiting) (787.04)*
               excessive vomiting in pregnancy (643.0–643.9)
               vomiting NOS (787.03)
                  cyclical, associated with migraine (346.2)
               vomiting of fecal matter (569.87)

DISEASES OF THE DIGESTIVE SYSTEM (520–579)

Item 9-13　**Achlorhydria,** also known as gastric anacidity, is the absence of gastric acid. **Gastroparesis** is paralysis of the stomach.

DISEASES OF THE DIGESTIVE SYSTEM (520-579)

536.3　Gastroparesis
Gastroparalysis
Code first underlying disease, if known, such as:
diabetes mellitus (249.6, 250.6)
Coding Clinic: 2004, Q2, P7-8x2; 2001, Q2, P4

●**536.4　Gastrostomy complications**
536.40　Gastrostomy complication, unspecified
536.41　Infection of gastrostomy 🔒
Use additional code to identify type of infection, such as:
abscess or cellulitis of abdomen (682.2)
septicemia (038.0-038.9)
Use additional code to identify organism (041.00-041.9)
(Ex:) 530.86-530.87, 536.40-536.49, 539.01-539.89, 569.71-569.79, 997.41-997.49, 997.71, 997.91-997.99, 998.81, 998.83-998.9
Coding Clinic: 1998, Q4, P42-44
536.42　Mechanical complication of gastrostomy 🔒
(Ex:) 530.86-530.87, 536.40-536.49, 539.01-539.89, 569.71-569.79, 997.41-997.49, 997.71, 997.91-997.99, 998.81, 998.83-998.9
536.49　Other gastrostomy complications
Coding Clinic: 1998, Q4, P42-44

536.8　Dyspepsia and other specified disorders of function of stomach

Achylia gastrica	Hyperchlorhydria
Hourglass contraction of stomach	Hypochlorhydria
	Indigestion
Hyperacidity	Tachygastria

Excludes　*achlorhydria (536.0)*
heartburn (787.1)
Coding Clinic: 1993, Q2, P6; 1989, Q2, P16; 1984, Nov-Dec, P9

536.9　Unspecified functional disorder of stomach
Functional gastrointestinal:
disorder
disturbance
irritation
Coding Clinic: 2007, Q1, P19

●**537　Other disorders of stomach and duodenum**
537.0　Acquired hypertrophic pyloric stenosis 🔒
Constriction of pylorus, acquired or adult
Obstruction of pylorus, acquired or adult
Stricture of pylorus, acquired or adult
Excludes　*congenital or infantile pyloric stenosis (750.5)*
(Ex:) 536.3, 536.8-537.0, 537.3, 750.5, 751.5
Coding Clinic: 2001, Q2, P17-18; 1985, Jan-Feb, P14-15
537.1　Gastric diverticulum
Excludes　*congenital diverticulum of stomach (750.7)*
537.2　Chronic duodenal ileus
537.3　Other obstruction of duodenum 🔒
Cicatrix of duodenum
Cicatrix = scar
Stenosis of duodenum
Stenosis = narrowing
Stricture of duodenum
Stricture = narrowing
Volvulus of duodenum
Volvulus = twisting/knotting
Excludes　*congenital obstruction of duodenum (751.1)*
(Ex:) 537.3, 750.8-750.9, 751.1, 751.5
537.4　Fistula of stomach or duodenum 🔒
Gastrocolic fistula
Gastrojejunocolic fistula
(Ex:) 537.4, 750.8-750.9, 751.5
Coding Clinic: 2012, Q1, P10-11
537.5　Gastroptosis
537.6　Hourglass stricture or stenosis of stomach
Cascade stomach
Excludes　*congenital hourglass stomach (750.7)*
hourglass contraction of stomach (536.8)

●**537.8　Other specified disorders of stomach and duodenum**
537.81　Pylorospasm
Excludes　*congenital pylorospasm (750.5)*
537.82　Angiodysplasia of stomach and duodenum without mention of hemorrhage
Coding Clinic: 2007, Q2, P9; 1996, Q3, P10
537.83　Angiodysplasia of stomach and duodenum with hemorrhage 🔒
(Ex:) 251.5, 456.0, 530.20-530.21, 530.7, 530.82, 530.85, 531.00-534.91, 535.01, 535.11, 535.21, 535.31, 535.41, 535.51, 535.61, 535.71, 537.83, 562.02-562.03, 562.12-562.13, 569.3, 569.85, 578.0-578.9
Coding Clinic: 2007, Q2, P9
537.84　Dieulafoy lesion (hemorrhagic) of stomach and duodenum 🔒
(Ex:) 251.5, 456.0, 530.20-530.21, 530.7, 530.82, 530.85, 531.00-534.91, 535.01, 535.11, 535.21, 535.31, 535.41, 535.51, 535.61, 535.71, 537.83-537.84, 562.02-562.03, 562.12-562.13, 569.3, 569.85, 578.0-578.9
Coding Clinic: 2002, Q4, P60-61
537.89　Other
Gastric or duodenal:
prolapse
rupture
Intestinal metaplasia of gastric mucosa
Passive congestion of stomach
Excludes　*diverticula of duodenum (562.00-562.01)*
gastrointestinal hemorrhage (578.0-578.9)
Coding Clinic: 2011, Q1, P11; 2005, Q3, P15-16
537.9　Unspecified disorder of stomach and duodenum

●**538　Gastrointestinal mucositis (ulcerative)** 🔒
Use additional E code to identify adverse effects of therapy, such as:
antineoplastic and immunosuppressive drugs (E930.7, E933.1)
radiation therapy (E879.2)
Excludes　*mucositis (ulcerative) of mouth and oral soft tissue (528.00-528.09)*
(Ex:) 251.5, 456.0, 530.20-530.21, 530.7, 530.82, 530.85, 531.00-534.91, 535.01, 535.11, 535.21, 535.31, 535.41, 535.51, 535.61, 535.71, 537.83, 537.89-538, 562.02-562.03, 562.12-562.13, 569.3, 569.85, 578.0-578.9

●**539　Complications of bariatric procedures**
●**539.0　Complications of gastric band procedure**
539.01　Infection due to gastric band procedure 🔒🔒
Use additional code to specify type of infection, such as:
abscess or cellulitis of abdomen (682.2)
septicemia (038.0-038.9)
Use additional code to identify organism (041.00-041.9)
(Ex:) 530.86, 530.87, 536.40-536.49, 539.01-539.89, 569.71-569.79, 997.41-997.49, 997.71, 997.91-997.99, 998.81, 998.83-998.9
Coding Clinic: 2011, Q4, P127
539.09　Other complications of gastric band procedure 🔒
Use additional code(s) to further specify complication
(Ex:) 530.86, 530.87, 536.40-536.49, 539.01-539.89, 569.71-569.79, 997.41-997.49, 997.71, 997.91-997.99, 998.81, 998.83-998.9

●**539.8　Complications of other bariatric procedure**
Excludes　*complications of gastric band surgery (539.01-539.09)*
539.81　Infection due to other bariatric procedure 🔒🔒
Use additional code to specify type of infection, such as:
abscess or cellulitis of abdomen (682.2)
septicemia (038.0-038.9)
Use additional code to identify organism (041.00-041.9)
(Ex:) 530.86, 530.87, 536.40-536.49, 539.01-539.89, 569.71-569.79, 997.41-997.49, 997.71-997.91, 997.99, 998.81, 998.83-998.9

539.89   Other complications of other bariatric procedure 🔖
        Use additional code(s) to further specify
        complication
        (Ex:) 530.86, 530.87, 536.40-536.49, 539.01-539.89, 569.71-569.79,
              997.41-997.49, 997.71-997.91, 997.99, 998.81, 998.83-998.9
        Coding Clinic: 2013, Q3, P12

APPENDICITIS (540–543)

● 540   Acute appendicitis
   540.0   With generalized peritonitis 🔖
           Appendicitis (acute) with: perforation, peritonitis
              (generalized), rupture:
              fulminating
              gangrenous
              obstructive
           Cecitis (acute) with: perforation, peritonitis (generalized),
              rupture
           Rupture of appendix
           Excludes   *acute appendicitis with peritoneal abscess (540.1)*
           (Ex:) 537.89-538, 540.0-543.9
           Coding Clinic: 1984, Nov-Dec, P19

   540.1   With peritoneal abscess 🔖
           Abscess of appendix
              With generalized peritonitis
           (Ex:) 537.89-538, 540.0-543.9
           Coding Clinic: 1984, Nov-Dec, P19

   540.9   Without mention of peritonitis 🔖
           Acute:
              appendicitis without mention of perforation,
                 peritonitis, or rupture:
                 fulminating
                 gangrenous
                 inflamed
                 obstructive
              cecitis without mention of perforation, peritonitis, or
                 rupture
           (Ex:) 537.89-538, 540.0-543.9
           Coding Clinic: 2013, Q2, P7; 2001, Q1, P15-16; 1997, Q4, P52

  541   Appendicitis, unqualified
        Coding Clinic: 1990, Q2, P26

  542   Other appendicitis
        Appendicitis:
           chronic
           recurrent
           relapsing
           subacute
        Excludes   *hyperplasia (lymphoid) of appendix (543.0)*
        Coding Clinic: 2001, Q1, P15-16

● 543   Other diseases of appendix
   543.0   Hyperplasia of appendix (lymphoid)
   543.9   Other and unspecified diseases of appendix
           Appendicular or appendiceal:
              colic
              concretion
              fistula
           Diverticulum of appendix
           Fecalith of appendix
           Intussusception of appendix
           Mucocele of appendix
           Stercolith of appendix

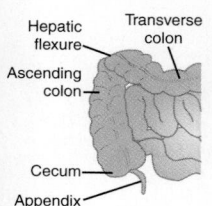

Figure 9–11 Acute appendicitis is the
inflammation of the appendix, usually associated
with obstruction. Most often this is a disease of
adolescents and young adults.

Hepatic flexure
Transverse colon
Ascending colon
Cecum
Appendix

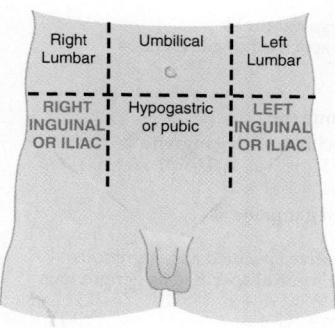

Right Lumbar | Umbilical | Left Lumbar
RIGHT INGUINAL OR ILIAC | Hypogastric or pubic | LEFT INGUINAL OR ILIAC

Figure 9–12 Inguinal hernias
are those that are located in the
inguinal or iliac areas of the
abdomen.

Item 9–14   Hernias of the groin are the most common type, accounting for
80 percent of all hernias. There are two major types of inguinal hernias: indirect
(oblique) affecting men only and direct. **Indirect inguinal hernias** result
when the intestines emerge through the abdominal wall in an indirect fashion
through the inguinal canal. **Direct inguinal hernias** penetrate through the
abdominal wall in a direct fashion. **Femoral hernias** occur at the femoral
ring where the femoral vessels enter the thigh and is most common in women.
An abdominal wall hernia is also called a ventral or epigastric hernia and
occurs in both sexes. Classification is based on location of the hernia and
whether there is obstruction or gangrene.

HERNIA OF ABDOMINAL CAVITY (550–553)

Includes   hernia:
              acquired
              congenital, except diaphragmatic or hiatal

● 550   Inguinal hernia
        Includes   bubonocele
              inguinal hernia (direct) (double) (indirect) (oblique)
                 (sliding)
              scrotal hernia
        The following fifth-digit subclassification is for use with
        category 550:

        0   unilateral or unspecified (not specified as recurrent)
            Unilateral NOS
        1   unilateral or unspecified, recurrent
        2   bilateral (not specified as recurrent)
            Bilateral NOS
        3   bilateral, recurrent

   550.0   Inguinal hernia, with gangrene 🔖
   [0-3]   Inguinal hernia with gangrene (and obstruction)
           (Ex:) 537.89-538, 550.00-550.93, 552.8-552.9, 553.8-553.9

   550.1   Inguinal hernia, with obstruction, without mention
   [0-3]   of gangrene 🔖
           Inguinal hernia with mention of incarceration,
              irreducibility, or strangulation
           (Ex:) 537.89-538, 550.00-550.93, 552.8-552.9, 553.8-553.9

   550.9   Inguinal hernia, without mention of obstruction or
   [0-3]   gangrene
           Inguinal hernia NOS
           Coding Clinic: 2003, Q3, P10-11; 2003, Q1, P4; 1985, Nov-Dec, P12;
           1984, May-June, P11

● 551   Other hernia of abdominal cavity, with gangrene
        Includes   that with gangrene (and obstruction)
   ● 551.0   Femoral hernia with gangrene
        551.00   Unilateral or unspecified (not specified as
                 recurrent) 🔖
                 Femoral hernia NOS with gangrene
                 (Ex:) 537.89-538, 551.00-551.03, 552.8-553.03, 553.8-553.9
        551.01   Unilateral or unspecified, recurrent 🔖
                 (Ex:) 537.89-538, 551.00-551.03, 552.8-553.03, 553.8-553.9
        551.02   Bilateral (not specified as recurrent) 🔖
                 (Ex:) 537.89-538, 551.00-551.03, 552.8-553.03, 553.8-553.9
        551.03   Bilateral, recurrent 🔖
                 (Ex:) 537.89-538, 551.00-551.03, 552.8-553.03, 553.8-553.9

DISEASES OF THE DIGESTIVE SYSTEM (520–579)

551.1 Umbilical hernia with gangrene 🔹
Parumbilical hernia specified as gangrenous
Ⓔⓧ 537.89-538, 551.1-551.29, 552.1-552.29, 552.8-55.29, 553.1-553.29, 553.8-553.9

● **551.2 Ventral hernia with gangrene**

    551.20 Ventral, unspecified, with gangrene 🔹
Ⓔⓧ 537.89-538, 551.1-551.29, 552.1-552.29, 552.8-552.9, 553.1-553.29, 553.8-553.9

    551.21 Incisional, with gangrene 🔹
Hernia:
    postoperative specified as gangrenous
    recurrent, ventral specified as gangrenous
Ⓔⓧ 537.89-538, 551.1-551.29, 552.1-552.29, 552.8-552.9, 553.1-553.29, 553.8-553.9

    551.29 Other 🔹
Epigastric hernia specified as gangrenous
Ⓔⓧ 537.89-538, 551.1-551.29, 552.1-552.29, 552.8-552.9, 553.1-553.29, 553.8-553.9

551.3 Diaphragmatic hernia with gangrene 🔹
Hernia:
    hiatal (esophageal) (sliding) specified as gangrenous
    paraesophageal specified as gangrenous
Thoracic stomach specified as gangrenous

> **Excludes** *congenital diaphragmatic hernia (756.6)*

Ⓔⓧ 551.3, 552.3-552.9, 553.3-553.9

551.8 Hernia of other specified sites, with gangrene 🔹
Any condition classifiable to 553.8 if specified as gangrenous
Ⓔⓧ 537.89-538, 550.00-553.9

551.9 Hernia of unspecified site, with gangrene 🔹
Any condition classifiable to 553.9 if specified as gangrenous
Ⓔⓧ 537.89-538, 550.00-553.9

● **552 Other hernia of abdominal cavity, with obstruction, but without mention of gangrene**

> **Excludes** *that with mention of gangrene (551.0–551.9)*

● **552.0 Femoral hernia with obstruction**
Femoral hernia specified as incarcerated, irreducible, strangulated, or causing obstruction

    552.00 Unilateral or unspecified (not specified as recurrent) 🔹
Ⓔⓧ 537.89-538, 551.00-551.03, 552.00-552.03, 552.8-553.03, 553.8-553.9

    552.01 Unilateral or unspecified, recurrent 🔹
Ⓔⓧ 537.89-538, 551.00-551.03, 552.00-552.03, 552.8-553.03, 553.8-553.9

    552.02 Bilateral (not specified as recurrent) 🔹
Ⓔⓧ 537.89-538, 551.00-551.03, 552.00-552.03, 552.8-553.03, 553.8-553.9

    552.03 Bilateral, recurrent 🔹
Ⓔⓧ 537.89-538, 551.00-551.03, 552.00-552.03, 552.8-553.03, 553.8-553.9

552.1 Umbilical hernia with obstruction 🔹
Ⓔⓧ 551.1-551.29, 552.1-552.29, 552.8-552.9, 553.8-553.9
Parumbilical hernia specified as incarcerated, irreducible, strangulated, or causing obstruction

● **552.2 Ventral hernia with obstruction**
Ventral hernia specified as incarcerated, irreducible, strangulated, or causing obstruction

    552.20 Ventral, unspecified, with obstruction 🔹
Ⓔⓧ 551.1-551.29, 552.1-552.29, 552.8-552.9, 553.8-553.9

    552.21 Incisional, with obstruction 🔹
Hernia:
    postoperative specified as incarcerated, irreducible, strangulated, or causing obstruction
    recurrent, ventral specified as incarcerated, irreducible, strangulated, or causing obstruction
Ⓔⓧ 551.1-551.29, 552.1-552.29, 552.8-552.9, 553.8-553.9
Coding Clinic: 2012, Q1, P8-9; 2003, Q3, P11

Item 9-15 Ventral, epigastric, or incisional hernia occurs on the abdominal surface caused by musculature weakness or a tear at a previous surgical site and is evidenced by a bulge that changes in size, becoming larger with exertion. An **incarcerated** hernia is one in which the intestines become trapped in the hernia. A **strangulated** hernia is one in which the blood supply to the intestines is lost. Hiatal hernia occurs when a loop of the stomach protrudes upward through the small opening in the diaphragm through which the esophagus passes, leaving the abdominal cavity and entering the chest. It occurs in both sexes.

    552.29 Other 🔹
Epigastric hernia specified as incarcerated, irreducible, strangulated, or causing obstruction
Ⓔⓧ 551.1-551.29, 552.1-552.29, 552.8-552.9, 553.8-553.9

552.3 Diaphragmatic hernia with obstruction 🔹
Hernia:
    hiatal (esophageal) (sliding) specified as incarcerated, irreducible, strangulated, or causing obstruction
    paraesophageal specified as incarcerated, irreducible, strangulated, or causing obstruction
Thoracic stomach specified as incarcerated, irreducible, strangulated, or causing obstruction

> **Excludes** *congenital diaphragmatic hernia (756.6)*

Ⓔⓧ 551.3, 552.3-552.9, 553.3-553.9

552.8 Hernia of other specified sites, with obstruction 🔹
Any condition classifiable to 553.8 if specified as incarcerated, irreducible, strangulated, or causing obstruction
Ⓔⓧ 550.00-553.9
Coding Clinic: 2004, Q1, P10-11

552.9 Hernia of unspecified site, with obstruction 🔹
Any condition classifiable to 553.9 if specified as incarcerated, irreducible, strangulated, or causing obstruction
Ⓔⓧ 550.00-553.9

● **553 Other hernia of abdominal cavity without mention of obstruction or gangrene**

> **Excludes** *the listed conditions with mention of:*
> *gangrene (and obstruction) (551.0–551.9)*
> *obstruction (552.0–552.9)*

● **553.0 Femoral hernia**

    553.00 Unilateral or unspecified (not specified as recurrent)
Femoral hernia NOS

    553.01 Unilateral or unspecified, recurrent

    553.02 Bilateral (not specified as recurrent)

    553.03 Bilateral, recurrent

553.1 Umbilical hernia
Parumbilical hernia

● **553.2 Ventral hernia**

    553.20 Ventral, unspecified
Coding Clinic: 2006, Q2, P10-11; 2003, Q3, P6-7; 1996, Q3, P15

    553.21 Incisional
Hernia:
    postoperative
    recurrent, ventral
Coding Clinic: 2003, Q3, P6

    553.29 Other
Hernia:
    epigastric
    spigelian

553.3 Diaphragmatic hernia
Hernia:
    hiatal (esophageal) (sliding)
    paraesophageal
Thoracic stomach

> **Excludes** *congenital:*
> *diaphragmatic hernia (756.6)*
> *hiatal hernia (750.6)*
> *esophagocele (530.6)*

Coding Clinic: 2001, Q2, P6; 2000, Q1, P6

◄ New   ◀▥ Revised   ~~deleted~~ Deleted   Excludes   Includes   Use additional   Code first   Omit code
● Unacceptable Principal Diagnosis   ● Use Additional Digit(s)   ▶ Manifestation Code   OGCR Official Guidelines   Coding Clinic

553.8 Hernia of other specified sites
Hernia:
ischiatic
ischiorectal
lumbar
obturator
pudendal
retroperitoneal
sciatic
Other abdominal hernia of specified site
Excludes *vaginal enterocele (618.6)*

553.9 Hernia of unspecified site
Enterocele
Epiplocele
Hernia:
NOS
interstitial
intestinal
intra-abdominal
Rupture (nontraumatic)
Sarcoepiplocele

NONINFECTIOUS ENTERITIS AND COLITIS (555–558)

● **555 Regional enteritis**
Includes Crohn's disease
Granulomatous enteritis
Excludes *ulcerative colitis (556)*

555.0 Small intestine
Ileitis:
regional
segmental
terminal
Regional enteritis or Crohn's disease of:
duodenum
ileum
jejunum
(Ex:) 555.0-556.9

555.1 Large intestine
Colitis:
granulomatous
regional
transmural
Regional enteritis or Crohn's disease of:
colon
large bowel
rectum
(Ex:) 555.0-556.9
Coding Clinic: 1999, Q3, P8

555.2 Small intestine with large intestine
Regional ileocolitis
(Ex:) 555.0-556.9
Coding Clinic: 2003, Q1, P18

555.9 Unspecified site
Crohn's disease NOS   Regional enteritis NOS
(Ex:) 555.0-555.9
Coding Clinic: 2009, Q1, P20; 2005, Q2, P11-12; 1999, Q3, P8-9; 1997, Q4, P37; Q2, P3; 1996, Q1, P13; 1988, Q2, P9-10

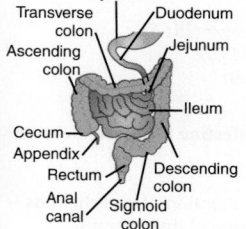

Figure 9–13 Small and large intestines.

Item 9–17 Ulcerative colitis attacks the colonic mucosa and forms abscesses. The disease involves the intestines. Classification is based on the location:
Enterocolitis: large and small intestine
Ileocolitis: ileum and colon
Proctitis: rectum
Proctosigmoiditis: sigmoid colon and rectum

● **556 Ulcerative colitis**
556.0 Ulcerative (chronic) enterocolitis
(Ex:) 555.0-556.9
556.1 Ulcerative (chronic) ileocolitis
(Ex:) 555.0-556.9
556.2 Ulcerative (chronic) proctitis
(Ex:) 555.0-556.9
556.3 Ulcerative (chronic) proctosigmoiditis
(Ex:) 555.0-556.9
556.4 Pseudopolyposis of colon
(Ex:) 555.0-556.9
556.5 Left-sided ulcerative (chronic) colitis
(Ex:) 555.0-556.9
556.6 Universal ulcerative (chronic) colitis
Pancolitis
(Ex:) 555.0-556.9
556.8 Other ulcerative colitis
(Ex:) 555.0-556.9
556.9 Ulcerative colitis, unspecified
Ulcerative enteritis NOS
(Ex:) 556.0-556.9
Coding Clinic: 2003, Q1, P10-11

● **557 Vascular insufficiency of intestine**
Excludes *necrotizing enterocolitis of the newborn (777.50–777.53)*
557.0 Acute vascular insufficiency of intestine
Acute:
hemorrhagic enterocolitis
ischemic colitis, enteritis, or enterocolitis
massive necrosis of intestine
Bowel infarction
Embolism of mesenteric artery
Fulminant enterocolitis
Hemorrhagic necrosis of intestine
Infarction of appendices epiploicae
Intestinal gangrene
Intestinal infarction (acute) (agnogenic) (hemorrhagic) (nonocclusive)
Mesenteric infarction (embolic) (thrombotic)
Necrosis of intestine
Terminal hemorrhagic enteropathy
Thrombosis of mesenteric artery
(Ex:) 557.0-557.1
Coding Clinic: 2011, Q3, P12; 2008, Q2, P15-16
557.1 Chronic vascular insufficiency of intestine
Angina, abdominal
Chronic ischemic colitis, enteritis, or enterocolitis
Ischemic stricture of intestine
Mesenteric:
angina
artery syndrome (superior)
vascular insufficiency
(Ex:) 557.0-557.9
Coding Clinic: 1996, Q3, P9-10; 1986, Nov-Dec, P11; 1985, Sept-Oct, P9
557.9 Unspecified vascular insufficiency of intestine
Alimentary pain due to vascular insufficiency
Ischemic colitis, enteritis, or enterocolitis NOS
(Ex:) 557.0-557.9

Item 9–16 Crohn's disease, also known as **regional enteritis,** is a chronic inflammatory disease of the intestines. Classification is based on location in the small (duodenum, ileum, jejunum) or large (cecum, colon, rectum, anal canal) intestine.

● 558 **Other and unspecified noninfectious gastroenteritis and colitis**

Excludes *infectious:*
  colitis, enteritis, or gastroenteritis (009.0–009.1)
  diarrhea (009.2–009.3)

558.1 **Gastroenteritis and colitis due to radiation** 🔖
  Radiation enterocolitis
  (Ex:) 558.1

558.2 **Toxic gastroenteritis and colitis** 🔖
  Use additional E code to identify cause
  (Ex:) 558.2
  Coding Clinic: 2008, Q2, P10-11

558.3 **Allergic gastroenteritis and colitis**
  Use additional code to identify type of food allergy
  (V15.01–V15.05)
  Coding Clinic: 2008, Q4, P115-116; 2003, Q1, P12

● 558.4 **Eosinophilic gastroenteritis and colitis**

558.41 **Eosinophilic gastroenteritis**
  Eosinophilic enteritis
  Coding Clinic: 2008, Q4, P115-116

558.42 **Eosinophilic colitis**
  Coding Clinic: 2008, Q4, P115-116

558.9 **Other and unspecified noninfectious gastroenteritis and colitis**
  Colitis, NOS, dietetic, or noninfectious
  Enteritis, NOS, dietetic, or noninfectious
  Gastroenteritis, NOS, dietetic, or noninfectious
  Ileitis, NOS, dietetic or noninfectious
  Jejunitis, NOS, dietetic, or noninfectious
  Sigmoiditis, NOS, dietetic, or noninfectious
  Coding Clinic: 2011,Q3, P12; 2008, Q2, P10-11; Q1, P10-12; 1999, Q3, P4-7; 1987, Nov-Dec, P7-8; 1984, July-Aug, P19-20

OTHER DISEASES OF INTESTINES AND PERITONEUM (560–569)

● 560 **Intestinal obstruction without mention of hernia**

Excludes *duodenum (537.2–537.3)*
  inguinal hernia with obstruction (550.1)
  intestinal obstruction complicating hernia (552.0–552.9)
  mesenteric:
    embolism (557.0)
    infarction (557.0)
    thrombosis (557.0)
  neonatal intestinal obstruction (277.01, 777.1–777.2, 777.4)

560.0 **Intussusception** 🔖
  Intussusception (colon) (intestine) (rectum)
  Invagination of intestine or colon
  Excludes *intussusception of appendix (543.9)*
  (Ex:) 560.0-560.31, 560.39-560.9, 569.87-569.9
  Coding Clinic: 1998, Q4, P82-83

Figure 9–14 Types of intussusception.

SIMPLE TYPES   DOUBLE TYPES

Cecum and appendix

Ileum
Ileocecal valve

Ileum Ileocecal valve

ILEOCOLIC

ILEOCECAL

Item 9–18 Intussusception is the prolapse (telescoping) of a part of the intestine into another adjacent part of the intestine. Intussusception may be enteric (ileoileal, jejunoileal, jejunojejunal), colic (colocolic), or intracolic (ileocecal, ileocolic).

Item 9–19 Volvulus is the twisting of a segment of the intestine, resulting in obstruction. Paralytic ileus is paralysis of the intestine. It need not be a complete paralysis, but it must prohibit the passage of food through the intestine and lead to intestinal blockage. It is a common aftermath of some types of surgery.

560.1 **Paralytic ileus** 🔖
  Adynamic ileus
  Ileus (of intestine) (of bowel) (of colon)
  Paralysis of intestine or colon
  Excludes *gallstone ileus (560.31)*
  (Ex:) 560.0-560.31, 560.39-560.9, 569.87-569.9
  Coding Clinic: 2012, Q1, P6-7; 1987, Jan-Feb, P13-14

560.2 **Volvulus** 🔖
  Knotting of intestine, bowel, or colon
  Strangulation of intestine, bowel, or colon
  Torsion of intestine, bowel, or colon
  Twist of intestine, bowel, or colon
  (Ex:) 560.0-560.31, 560.39-560.9, 569.87-569.9

● 560.3 **Impaction of intestine**

560.30 **Impaction of intestine, unspecified** 🔖
  Impaction of colon
  (Ex:) 560.0-560.31, 560.39-560.9, 569.87-569.9

560.31 **Gallstone ileus**
  Obstruction of intestine by gallstone
  (Ex:) 560.0-560.31, 560.39-560.9, 569.87-569.9

560.32 **Fecal impaction**
  Excludes *constipation (564.00-564.09)*
  incomplete defecation (787.61)

560.39 **Other** 🔖
  Concretion of intestine
  Enterolith
  (Ex:) 560.0-560.31, 560.39-560.9, 569.87-569.9
  Coding Clinic: 1998, Q4, P37-38

● 560.8 **Other specified intestinal obstruction**

560.81 **Intestinal or peritoneal adhesions with obstruction (postoperative) (postinfection)** 🔖
  Excludes *adhesions without obstruction (568.0)*
  (Ex:) 560.0-560.31, 560.39-560.9, 569.87-569.9
  Coding Clinic: 2010, Q1, P10-11; 1995, Q3, P6; 1987, Nov-Dec, P9

560.89 **Other** 🔖
  Acute pseudo-obstruction of intestine
  Mural thickening causing obstruction
  Excludes *ischemic stricture of intestine (557.1)*
  (Ex:) 560.0-560.31, 560.39-560.9, 569.87-569.9
  Coding Clinic: 1997, Q2, P3

560.9 **Unspecified intestinal obstruction** 🔖
  Enterostenosis
  Obstruction of intestine or colon
  Occlusion of intestine or colon
  Stenosis of intestine or colon
  Stricture of intestine or colon
  Excludes *congenital stricture or stenosis of intestine (751.1–751.2)*
  (Ex:) 560.0-560.31, 560.39-560.9, 569.87-569.9

● 562 **Diverticula of intestine**
  Use additional code to identify any associated:
  peritonitis (567.0–567.9)
  Excludes *congenital diverticulum of colon (751.5)*
  diverticulum of appendix (543.9)
  Meckel's diverticulum (751.0)

● 562.0 **Small intestine**

562.00 **Diverticulosis of small intestine (without mention of hemorrhage)**
  Diverticulosis:
    duodenum without mention of diverticulitis
    ileum without mention of diverticulitis
    jejunum without mention of diverticulitis

◀ New   ◀▥ Revised   ~~deleted~~ Deleted   Excludes   Includes   Use additional   Code first   Omit code
● Unacceptable Principal Diagnosis   ● Use Additional Digit(s)   ⟩ Manifestation Code   OGCR Official Guidelines   Coding Clinic

848

Item 9–20 Diverticula of the intestines are acquired herniations of the mucosa. Diverticulum (singular): Pocket or pouch that bulges outward through a weak spot (herniation) in the colon. Diverticula (plural). **Diverticulosis** is the condition of having diverticula. **Diverticulitis** is inflammation of these pouches or herniations. Classification is based on location (small intestine or colon) and whether it occurs with or without hemorrhage.

562.01 Diverticulitis of small intestine (without mention of hemorrhage)
Diverticulitis (with diverticulosis):
  duodenum
  ileum
  jejunum
  small intestine
(Ex:) 562.00-562.03

562.02 Diverticulosis of small intestine with hemorrhage
(Ex:) 251.5, 456.0, 530.20-530.21, 530.7, 530.82, 530.85, 531.00-534.91, 535.01, 535.11, 535.21, 535.31, 535.41, 535.51, 535.61, 535.71, 537.83, 562.02-562.03, 562.12-562.13, 569.3, 569.85, 578.0-578.9

562.03 Diverticulitis of small intestine with hemorrhage
(Ex:) 251.5, 456.0, 530.20-530.21, 530.7, 530.82, 530.85, 531.00-534.91, 535.01, 535.11, 535.21, 535.31, 535.41, 535.51, 535.61, 535.71, 537.83, 562.02-562.03, 562.12-562.13, 569.3, 569.85, 578.0-578.9

● 562.1 Colon

562.10 Diverticulosis of colon (without mention of hemorrhage)
Diverticulosis without mention of diverticulitis:
  NOS
  intestine (large) without mention of
    diverticulitis
Diverticular disease (colon) without mention of
  diverticulitis
Coding Clinic: 2005, Q3, P17-18; 2002, Q3, P14-15

562.11 Diverticulitis of colon without mention of hemorrhage
Diverticulitis (with diverticulosis):
  NOS
  colon
  intestine (large)
(Ex:) 562.10-562.13
Coding Clinic: 1996, Q1, P13-14

562.12 Diverticulosis of colon with hemorrhage
(Ex:) 251.5, 456.0, 530.20-530.21, 530.7, 530.82, 530.85, 531.00-534.91, 535.01, 535.11, 535.21, 535.31, 535.41, 535.51, 535.61, 535.71, 537.83, 562.02-562.03, 562.12-562.13, 569.3, 569.85, 578.0-578.9

562.13 Diverticulitis of colon with hemorrhage
(Ex:) 251.5, 456.0, 530.20-530.21, 530.7, 530.82, 530.85, 531.00-534.91, 535.01, 535.11, 535.21, 535.31, 535.41, 535.51, 535.61, 535.71, 537.83, 562.02-562.03, 562.12-562.13, 569.3, 569.85, 578.0-578.9

● 564 Functional digestive disorders, not elsewhere classified
Excludes *functional disorders of stomach (536.0–536.9)*
those specified as psychogenic (306.4)

● 564.0 Constipation
Excludes *fecal impaction (560.32)*
incomplete defecation (787.61)
psychogenic constipation (306.4)

564.00 Constipation, unspecified
564.01 Slow transit constipation
564.02 Outlet dysfunction constipation
564.09 Other constipation
564.1 Irritable bowel syndrome
Irritable colon
Spastic colon

564.2 Postgastric surgery syndromes
Dumping syndrome
Jejunal syndrome
Postgastrectomy syndrome
Postvagotomy syndrome
Excludes *malnutrition following gastrointestinal surgery (579.3)*
postgastrojejunostomy ulcer (534.0–534.9)
Coding Clinic: 1995, Q1, P11

564.3 Vomiting following gastrointestinal surgery
Vomiting (bilious) following gastrointestinal surgery

564.4 Other postoperative functional disorders
Diarrhea following gastrointestinal surgery
Excludes *colostomy and enterostomy complications (569.60–569.69)*

564.5 Functional diarrhea
Excludes *diarrhea:*
  NOS (787.91)
  psychogenic (306.4)
Coding Clinic: 1988, Q2, P9-10

564.6 Anal spasm
Proctalgia fugax

564.7 Megacolon, other than Hirschsprung's
Dilatation of colon
Excludes *megacolon:*
  congenital [Hirschsprung's] (751.3)
  toxic (556)
(Ex:) 564.1-564.9

● 564.8 Other specified functional disorders of intestine
Excludes *malabsorption (579.0–579.9)*

564.81 Neurogenic bowel
(Ex:) 564.1-564.9
Coding Clinic: 2001, Q1, P12

564.89 Other functional disorders of intestine
Atony of colon
Coding Clinic: 2012, Q3, P22

564.9 Unspecified functional disorder of intestine

● 565 Anal fissure and fistula
565.0 Anal fissure
Excludes *anal sphincter tear (healed) (non-traumatic) (old) (569.43)*
traumatic (863.89, 863.99)

565.1 Anal fistula
Fistula:
  anorectal
  rectal
  rectum to skin
Excludes *fistula of rectum to internal organs - see Alphabetic Index*
  ischiorectal fistula (566)
  rectovaginal fistula (619.1)
Coding Clinic: 2007, Q1, P13

566 Abscess of anal and rectal regions
Abscess: Cellulitis:
  ischiorectal   anal
  perianal   perirectal
  perirectal   rectal
                     Ischiorectal fistula
(Ex:) 566
Coding Clinic: 1999, Q3, P8-9

Item 9–21 A **fissure** is a groove in the surface, whereas a **fistula** is an abnormal passage. An abscess is an accumulation of pus in a tissue cavity resulting from a bacterial or parasitic infection.

DISEASES OF THE DIGESTIVE SYSTEM (520–579)

Item 9-22 Peritonitis is an inflammation of the lining (peritoneum) of the abdominal cavity and surface of the intestines. **Retroperitoneal infections** occur between the posterior parietal peritoneum and posterior abdominal wall where the kidneys, adrenal glands, ureters, duodenum, ascending colon, descending colon, pancreas, and the large vessels and nerves are located. Both are caused by bacteria, parasites, injury, bleeding, or diseases such as systemic lupus erythematosus.

● **567 Peritonitis and retroperitoneal infections**

Excludes *peritonitis:*
  benign paroxysmal (277.31)
  pelvic, female (614.5, 614.7)
  periodic familial (277.31)
  puerperal (670.8)
  with or following:
    abortion (634–638 with .0, 639.0)
    appendicitis (540.0–540.1)
    ectopic or molar pregnancy (639.0)

▷ **567.0 Peritonitis in infectious diseases classified elsewhere** 🔎

Code first underlying disease

Excludes *peritonitis:*
  gonococcal (098.86)
  syphilitic (095.2)
  tuberculous (014.0)

Ex: 567.0-567.29, 567.38-567.9, 569.87-569.9

567.1 Pneumococcal peritonitis 🔎
Ex: 567.0-567.29, 567.38-567.9, 569.87-569.9

● **567.2 Other suppurative peritonitis**
Coding Clinic: 2005, Q4, P74-77; 1998, Q2, P19-20; 1996, Q1, P13-14; 1987, Jan-Feb, P14-15

567.21 Peritonitis (acute) generalized 🔎
Pelvic peritonitis, male
Ex: 567.0-567.29, 567.38-56.79, 569.87-569.9

567.22 Peritoneal abscess 🔎
Abscess (of):   Abscess (of):
  abdominopelvic   retrocecal
  mesenteric   subdiaphragmatic
  omentum   subhepatic
  peritoneum   subphrenic
Ex: 567.0-567.29, 567.38-567.9, 569.87-569.9

567.23 Spontaneous bacterial peritonitis 🔎
Excludes *bacterial peritonitis NOS (567.29)*
Ex: 567.0-567.29, 567.38-567.9, 569.87-569.9

567.29 Other suppurative peritonitis 🔎
Subphrenic peritonitis
Ex: 567.0-567.29, 567.38-567.9, 569.87-569.9
Coding Clinic: 2010, Q2, P4; 2001, Q2, P11-12; 1999, Q3, P9; 1995, Q3, P5

● **567.3 Retroperitoneal infections**

567.31 Psoas muscle abscess 🔎
Ex: 567.31, 728.0, 728.11-728.3, 728.81, 728.86

567.38 Other retroperitoneal abscess 🔎
Ex: 567.0-567.29, 567.38-567.9, 569.87-569.9
Coding Clinic: 2005, Q4, P74-77; 1998, Q2, P19-20

567.39 Other retroperitoneal infections 🔎
Ex: 567.0-567.29, 567.38-567.9, 569.87-569.9

● **567.8 Other specified peritonitis**

567.81 Choleperitonitis 🔎
Peritonitis due to bile
Ex: 567.0-567.29, 567.38-567.9, 569.87-569.9

567.82 Sclerosing mesenteritis 🔎
Fat necrosis of peritoneum
(Idiopathic) sclerosing mesenteric fibrosis
Mesenteric lipodystrophy
Mesenteric panniculitis
Retractile mesenteritis
Ex: 567.0-567.29, 567.38-567.9, 569.87-569.9
Coding Clinic: 2005, Q4, P74-77

567.89 Other specified peritonitis 🔎
Chronic proliferative peritonitis
Mesenteric saponification
Peritonitis due to urine
Ex: 567.0-567.29, 567.38-567.9, 569.87-569.9

567.9 Unspecified peritonitis 🔎
Peritonitis: Peritonitis:
  NOS   of unspecified cause
Ex: 567.0-567.29, 567.38-567.9, 569.87-569.9
Coding Clinic: 2013, Q2, P3; 2004, Q1, P10-11

● **568 Other disorders of peritoneum**

568.0 Peritoneal adhesions (postoperative) (postinfection)
Adhesions (of):   Adhesions (of):
  abdominal (wall)   mesenteric
  diaphragm   omentum
  intestine   stomach
  male pelvis
Adhesive bands

Excludes *adhesions:*
  pelvic, female (614.6)
  with obstruction:
    duodenum (537.3)
    intestine (560.81)
Coding Clinic: 2012, Q1, P8-9; 2003, Q3, P7&11; 1995, Q3, P7; 1985, Sept-Oct, P11

● **568.8 Other specified disorders of peritoneum**

568.81 Hemoperitoneum (nontraumatic) 🔎
Ex: 568.81

568.82 Peritoneal effusion (chronic) 🔎
Excludes *ascites NOS (789.51–789.59)*
Ex: 568.82

568.89 Other
Peritoneal: Penitoneal:
  cyst   granuloma

568.9 Unspecified disorder of peritoneum

● **569 Other disorders of intestine**

569.0 Anal and rectal polyp
Anal and rectal polyp NOS
Excludes *adenomatous anal and rectal polyp (211.4)*

569.1 Rectal prolapse
Procidentia: Prolapse:
  anus (sphincter)   anal canal
  rectum (sphincter)   rectal mucosa
Proctoptosis
Excludes *prolapsed hemorrhoids (455.2, 455.5)*

569.2 Stenosis of rectum and anus
Stricture of anus (sphincter)

569.3 Hemorrhage of rectum and anus 🔎
Excludes *gastrointestinal bleeding NOS (578.9)*
  melena (578.1)
Ex: 251.5, 456.0, 530.20-530.21, 530.7, 530.82, 530.85, 531.00-534.91, 535.01, 535.11, 535.21, 535.31, 535.41, 535.51, 535.61, 535.71, 537.83, 562.02-562.03, 562.12-562.13, 569.3, 569.85, 578.0-578.9
Coding Clinic: 2005, Q3, P17

● **569.4 Other specified disorders of rectum and anus**

569.41 Ulcer of anus and rectum 🔎
Solitary ulcer of anus (sphincter) or rectum (sphincter)
Stercoral ulcer of anus (sphincter) or rectum (sphincter)
Ex: 569.41

569.42 Anal or rectal pain
Coding Clinic: 2003, Q1, P8; 1996, Q1, P13

569.43 Anal sphincter tear (healed) (old)
Tear of anus, nontraumatic
Use additional code for any associated fecal incontinence (787.60-787.63)
Excludes *anal fissure (565.0)*
  anal sphincter tear (healed) (old) complicating delivery (654.8)

569.44 **Dysplasia of anus**
Anal intraepithelial neoplasia I and II
(AIN I and II) (histologically confirmed)
Dysplasia of anus NOS
Mild and moderate dysplasia of anus
(histologically confirmed)
Excludes *abnormal results from anal cytologic*
examination without histologic
confirmation (796.70-796.79)
anal intraepithelial neoplasia III (230.5,
230.6)
carcinoma in situ of anus (230.5, 230.6)
HGSIL of anus (796.74)
severe dysplasia of anus (230.5, 230.6)
Coding Clinic: 2008, Q4, P117-119
569.49 **Other**
Granuloma of rectum (sphincter)
Rupture of rectum (sphincter)
Hypertrophy of anal papillae
Proctitis NOS
Use additional code for any associated fecal
incontinence (787.60-787.63)
Excludes *fistula of rectum to:*
internal organs - see Alphabetic Index
skin (565.1)
hemorrhoids (455.0–455.9)
569.5 **Abscess of intestine**
Excludes *appendiceal abscess (540.1)*
(Ex) 569.5
Coding Clinic: 1996, Q1, P13-14
● 569.6 **Colostomy and enterostomy complications**
569.60 **Colostomy and enterostomy complication,**
unspecified
569.61 **Infection of colostomy and enterostomy**
Use additional code to specify type of infection,
such as:
abscess or cellulitis of abdomen (682.2)
septicemia (038.0–038.9)
Use additional code to identify organism
(041.00–041.9)
(Ex) 569.60-569.69
569.62 **Mechanical complication of colostomy and**
enterostomy
Malfunction of colostomy and enterostomy
(Ex) 530.86-530.87, 536.40-536.49, 539.01-539.89, 569.60-569.79,
997.41-997.49, 997.71, 997.91-997.99, 998.81, 998.83-998.9
Coding Clinic: 2005, Q2, P11-12; 2003, Q1, P10
569.69 **Other complication**
Fistula   Prolapse
Hernia
(Ex) 569.60-569.69
● 569.7 **Complications of intestinal pouch**
569.71 **Pouchitis**
Inflammation of internal ileoanal pouch
(Ex) 530.86-530.87, 536.40-536.49, 539.01-539.89, 569.71-569.79,
997.41-997.49, 997.71, 997.91-997.99, 998.81, 998.83-998.9
Coding Clinic: 2009, Q4, P106
569.79 **Other complications of intestinal pouch**
(Ex) 530.86-530.87, 536.40-536.49, 539.01-539.89, 569.71-569.79,
997.41-997.49, 997.71, 997.91-997.99, 998.81, 998.83-998.9
● 569.8 **Other specified disorders of intestine**
569.81 **Fistula of intestine, excluding rectum and anus**
Fistula:
abdominal wall
enterocolic
enteroenteric
ileorectal
Excludes *fistula of intestine to internal organs -*
see Alphabetic Index
persistent postoperative fistula (998.6)
(Ex) 569.81
Coding Clinic: 1999, Q3, P8

569.82 **Ulceration of intestine**
Primary ulcer of intestine
Ulceration of colon
Excludes *that with perforation (569.83)*
(Ex) 569.82
569.83 **Perforation of intestine**
(Ex) 569.83
Coding Clinic: 2012, Q2, P5-6
569.84 **Angiodysplasia of intestine (without mention of**
hemorrhage)
Coding Clinic: 1996, Q3, P9-10
569.85 **Angiodysplasia of intestine with hemorrhage**
(Ex) 251.5, 456.0, 530.20-530.21, 530.7, 530.82, 530.85,
531.00-534.91, 535.01, 535.11, 535.21, 535.31, 535.41,
535.51 535.61, 535.71, 537.83, 562.02-562.03, 562.12-562.13,
569.3, 569.85-569.86, 578.0-578.9
Coding Clinic: 1996, Q3, P9-10
569.86 **Dieulafoy lesion (hemorrhagic) of intestine**
(Ex) 251.5, 456.0, 530.20-530.21, 530.7, 530.82, 530.85,
531.00-534.91, 535.01, 535.11, 535.21, 535.31, 535.41,
535.51 535.61, 535.71, 537.83, 562.02-562.03, 562.12-562.13,
569.3, 569.85-569.86, 578.0-578.9
Coding Clinic: 2002, Q4, P60-61
569.87 **Vomiting of fecal matter**
569.89 **Other**
Enteroptosis   Pericolitis
Granuloma of intestine   Perisigmoiditis
Prolapse of intestine   Visceroptosis
Excludes *gangrene of intestine, mesentery, or*
omentum (557.0)
hemorrhage of intestine NOS (578.9)
obstruction of intestine (560.0–560.9)
Coding Clinic: 2013, Q2, P3
569.9 **Unspecified disorder of intestine**

OTHER DISEASES OF DIGESTIVE SYSTEM (570–579)

570 **Acute and subacute necrosis of liver**
Acute hepatic failure
Acute or subacute hepatitis, not specified as infective
Necrosis of liver (acute) (diffuse) (massive) (subacute)
Parenchymatous degeneration of liver
Yellow atrophy (liver) (acute) (subacute)
Excludes *icterus gravis of newborn (773.0–773.2)*
serum hepatitis (070.2–070.3)
that with:
abortion (634–638 with .7, 639.8)
ectopic or molar pregnancy (639.8)
pregnancy, childbirth, or the puerperium (646.7)
viral hepatitis (070.0–070.9)
(Ex) 570, 573.4, 573.8-573.9
Coding Clinic: 2005, Q2, P9-10; 2000, Q1, P22
● 571 **Chronic liver disease and cirrhosis**
571.0 **Alcoholic fatty liver**   A
571.1 **Acute alcoholic hepatitis**   A
Acute alcoholic liver disease
Coding Clinic: 2002, Q2, P4
571.2 **Alcoholic cirrhosis of liver**   A
Florid cirrhosis
Laennec's cirrhosis (alcoholic)
Coding Clinic: 2011, Q1, P23; 2007, Q3, P9; Q2, P6-7x2; 2002, Q2, P4;
Q1, P3; 1985, Nov-Dec, P14
571.3 **Alcoholic liver damage, unspecified**   A
● 571.4 **Chronic hepatitis**
Excludes *viral hepatitis (acute) (chronic) (070.0–070.9)*
571.40 **Chronic hepatitis, unspecified**
571.41 **Chronic persistent hepatitis**
571.42 **Autoimmune hepatitis**
Coding Clinic: 2008, Q4, P120
571.49 **Other**
Chronic hepatitis:
active
aggressive
Recurrent hepatitis
Coding Clinic: 1999, Q3, P19

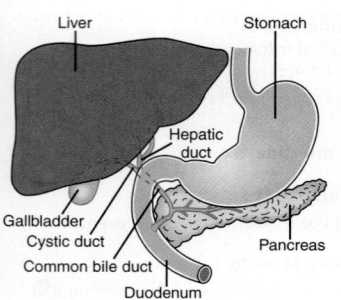

Figure 9–15 Liver and bile ducts.

Item 9–23 Cirrhosis is the progressive fibrosis of the liver resulting in loss of liver function. The main causes of cirrhosis of the liver are alcohol abuse, chronic hepatitis (inflammation of the liver), biliary disease, and excessive amounts of iron. **Alcoholic cirrhosis of the liver** is also called portal, Laënnec's, or fatty nutritional cirrhosis.

571.5 Cirrhosis of liver without mention of alcohol
Cirrhosis of liver:
  NOS
  cryptogenic
  macronodular
Cirrhosis of liver:
  micronodular
  posthepatitic
  postnecrotic
Healed yellow atrophy (liver)
Portal cirrhosis
Code first, if applicable, viral hepatitis (acute) (chronic) (070.0-070.9)
Coding Clinic: 2011, Q1, P23; 2007, Q3, P9

571.6 Biliary cirrhosis
Chronic nonsuppurative destructive cholangitis
Cirrhosis:
  cholangitic
  cholestatic

571.8 Other chronic nonalcoholic liver disease
Chronic yellow atrophy (liver)
Fatty liver, without mention of alcohol
Coding Clinic: 1996, Q2, P12

571.9 Unspecified chronic liver disease without mention of alcohol

● **572 Liver abscess and sequelae of chronic liver disease**
  572.0 Abscess of liver
    Excludes amebic liver abscess (006.3)
    Ex: 006.3, 572.0-572.1, 573.8-573.9

  572.1 Portal pyemia
    Phlebitis of portal vein
    Portal thrombophlebitis
    Pylephlebitis
    Pylethrombophlebitis
    Ex: 006.3, 572.0-572.1, 573.8-573.9

  572.2 Hepatic encephalopathy
    Hepatic coma
    Hepatocerebral intoxication
    Portal-systemic encephalopathy
    Excludes hepatic coma associated with viral hepatitis - see category 070
    Ex: 572.2, 573.8-573.9
    Coding Clinic: 2007, Q2, P6; 2005, Q2, P9-10; 2002, Q1, P3; 1995, Q3, P14

  572.3 Portal hypertension
    Use additional code for any associated complications, such as:
    portal hypertensive gastropathy (537.89)
    Ex: 572.2-572.3, 573.8-573.9
    Coding Clinic: 2005, Q3, P15-16

  572.4 Hepatorenal syndrome
    Excludes that following delivery (674.8)
    Ex: 572.4, 573.8-573.9
    Coding Clinic: 1992, Q3, P15

  572.8 Other sequelae of chronic liver disease
    Excludes hepatopulmonary syndrome (573.5)

● **573 Other disorders of liver**
  Excludes amyloid or lardaceous degeneration of liver (277.39)
    congenital cystic disease of liver (751.62)
    glycogen infiltration of liver (271.0)
    hepatomegaly NOS (789.1)
    portal vein obstruction (452)

  573.0 Chronic passive congestion of liver
  573.1 Hepatitis in viral diseases classified elsewhere
    Code first underlying disease, as:
    Coxsackie virus disease (074.8)
    cytomegalic inclusion virus disease (078.5)
    infectious mononucleosis (075)
    Excludes hepatitis (in):
      mumps (072.71)
      viral (070.0–070.9)
      yellow fever (060.0–060.9)
    Ex: 573.1-573.3, 573.8-573.9

  573.2 Hepatitis in other infectious diseases classified elsewhere
    Code first underlying disease, as:
    malaria (084.9)
    Excludes hepatitis in:
      late syphilis (095.3)
      secondary syphilis (091.62)
      toxoplasmosis (130.5)
    Ex: 573.1-573.3, 573.8-573.9

  573.3 Hepatitis, unspecified
    Toxic (noninfectious) hepatitis
    Use additional E code to identify cause
    Coding Clinic: 1998, Q3, P4; 1990, Q4, P26

  573.4 Hepatic infarction
    Ex: 570, 573.4, 573.8-573.9

  ● **573.5 Hepatopulmonary syndrome**
    Code first underlying liver disease, such as:
    alcoholic cirrhosis of liver (571.2)
    cirrhosis of liver without mention of alcohol (571.5)

  573.8 Other specified disorders of liver
    Hepatoptosis

  573.9 Unspecified disorder of liver

● **574 Cholelithiasis**
  Presence or formation of gallstones
  Excludes retained cholelithiasis following cholecystectomy (997.41)
  Coding Clinic: 1990, Q1, P19

  The following fifth-digit subclassification is for use with category 574:

  | 0 | without mention of obstruction |
  | 1 | with obstruction |

  Check documentation for acute/chronic gallbladder/common bile duct either with or without obstruction.

  ● **574.0 Calculus of gallbladder with acute cholecystitis**
  [0-1] Biliary calculus with acute cholecystitis
    Calculus of cystic duct with acute cholecystitis
    Cholelithiasis with acute cholecystitis
    Any condition classifiable to 574.2 with acute cholecystitis
    For code **574.00:** Ex: 574.00-574.21, 574.40, 574.60-574.61, 574.80-574.81, 575.0-575.12, 575.9, 576.8-576.9;
    For code **574.01:** Ex: 574.00-574.21, 574.60-574.61, 574.80-574.81, 575.0-575.12, 575.9, 576.8-576.9
    Coding Clinic: 1996, Q4, P32; 1984, Nov-Dec, P18

  ● **574.1 Calculus of gallbladder with other cholecystitis**
  [0-1] Biliary calculus with cholecystitis
    Calculus of cystic duct with cholecystitis
    Cholelithiasis with cholecystitis
    Cholecystitis with cholelithiasis NOS
    Any condition classifiable to 574.2 with cholecystitis (chronic)
    Ex: 574.00-574.21, 574.60-574.61, 574.80-574.81, 575.0-575.12, 575.9, 576.8-576.9
    Coding Clinic: 2003, Q1, P5; 1999, Q3, P9; 1996, Q4, P69; Q2, P13-15; Q1, P7

DISEASES OF THE DIGESTIVE SYSTEM (520–579)

◀ New   ◀ Revised   ~~deleted~~ Deleted   Excludes   Includes   Use additional   Code first   Omit code
● Unacceptable Principal Diagnosis   ● Use Additional Digit(s)   Manifestation Code   OGCR Official Guidelines   Coding Clinic

● **574.2 Calculus of gallbladder without mention of**
[0-1] **cholecystitis** 1 🔹
        Biliary:
            calculus NOS
            colic NOS
        Calculus of cystic duct
        Cholelithiasis NOS
        Colic (recurrent) of gallbladder
        Gallstone (impacted)
        For code **574.21**: (Ex) 574.00-574.21, 574.60-574.61, 574.80-574.81,
            575.0-575.12, 575.9, 576.8-576.9
        Coding Clinic: 1995, Q4, P51-52; 1988, Q1, P14

● **574.3 Calculus of bile duct with acute cholecystitis** 🔹
[0-1] Calculus of bile duct [any] with acute cholecystitis
        Choledocholithiasis with acute cholecystitis
        Any condition classifiable to 574.5 with acute
            cholecystitis
        (Ex) 574.30-575.12, 576.8-576.9

● **574.4 Calculus of bile duct with other cholecystitis** 🔹
[0-1] Calculus of bile duct [any] with cholecystitis (chronic)
        Choledocholithiasis with cholecystitis (chronic)
        Any condition classifiable to 574.5 with cholecystitis
            (chronic)
        (Ex) 574.30-575.12, 576.8-576.9
        Coding Clinic: 1996, Q1, P7

● **574.5 Calculus of bile duct without mention of**
[0-1] **cholecystitis** 1 🔹
        Calculus of: Choledocholithiasis
            bile duct [any]   Hepatic:
            common duct   colic (recurrent)
            hepatic duct   lithiasis
        For code **574.51**: (Ex) 574.30-575.12, 576.8-576.9
        Coding Clinic: 1996, Q2, P13-15; 1994, Q3, P11

● **574.6 Calculus of gallbladder and bile duct with acute**
[0-1] **cholecystitis** 🔹
        Any condition classifiable to 574.0 and 574.3
        (Ex) 574.60-574.61, 575.0-575.12, 575.9, 576.8-576.9

● **574.7 Calculus of gallbladder and bile duct with other**
[0-1] **cholecystitis** 🔹
        Any condition classifiable to 574.1 and 574.4
        (Ex) 574.30-575.12, 576.8-576.9

● **574.8 Calculus of gallbladder and bile duct with acute and**
[0-1] **chronic cholecystitis** 0 🔹, 1 🔹
        Any condition classifiable to 574.6 and 574.7
        (Ex) 574.80-574.81, 575.0-575.12, 575.9, 576.8-576.9
        Coding Clinic: 1996, Q4, P32

● **574.9 Calculus of gallbladder and bile duct without**
[0-1] **cholecystitis** 1 🔹
        Any condition classifiable to 574.2 and 574.5
        For code **574.91**: (Ex) 574.30-575.12, 576.8-576.9

● **575 Other disorders of gallbladder**
        Cholecystitis is chronic or acute inflammation of gallbladder.

    575.0 Acute cholecystitis 🔹
        Abscess of gallbladder without mention of calculus
        Angiocholecystitis without mention of calculus
        Cholecystitis without mention of calculus:
            emphysematous (acute)
            gangrenous
            suppurative
        Empyema of gallbladder without mention of calculus
        Gangrene of gallbladder without mention of calculus
        Excludes *that with:*
                    acute and chronic cholecystitis (575.12)
                    choledocholithiasis (574.3)
                    choledocholithiasis and cholelithiasis (574.6)
                    cholelithiasis (574.0)
        (Ex) 574.00, 574.60-574.61, 574.80-574.81, 575.0-575.12, 575.9, 576.8-576.9
        Coding Clinic: 1991, Q3, P17-18

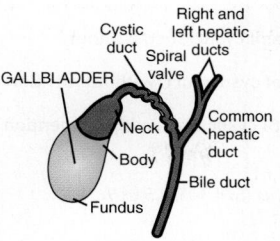

Figure 9-16 Gallbladder and bile ducts.

● **575.1 Other cholecystitis**
        Cholecystitis without mention of calculus:
            NOS without mention of calculus
            chronic without mention of calculus
        Excludes *that with:*
                    choledocholithiasis (574.4)
                    choledocholithiasis and cholelithiasis (574.8)
                    cholelithiasis (574.1)
        Coding Clinic: 1991, Q3, P17-18

    575.10 Cholecystitis, unspecified
            Cholecystitis NOS
    575.11 Chronic cholecystitis
    575.12 Acute and chronic cholecystitis 🔹
            (Ex) 575.0-575.12, 575.9, 576.8-576.9
            Coding Clinic: 1997, Q4, P52; 1996, Q4, P32

    575.2 Obstruction of gallbladder 🔹
        Occlusion of cystic duct or gallbladder without mention
            of calculus
        Stenosis of cystic duct or gallbladder without mention of
            calculus
        Stricture of cystic duct or gallbladder without mention
            of calculus
        (Ex) 575.2-575.9, 576.8-576.9

    575.3 Hydrops of gallbladder 🔹
        Mucocele of gallbladder
        (Ex) 575.2-575.9, 576.8-576.9

    575.4 Perforation of gallbladder 🔹
        Rupture of cystic duct or gallbladder
        (Ex) 575.2-575.9, 576.8-576.9

    575.5 Fistula of gallbladder 🔹
        Fistula: Fistula:
            cholecystoduodenal   cholecystoenteric
        (Ex) 575.2-575.9, 576.8-576.9

    575.6 Cholesterolosis of gallbladder
        Strawberry gallbladder

    575.8 Other specified disorders of gallbladder
        Adhesions (of) cystic duct gallbladder
        Atrophy (of) cystic duct gallbladder
        Cyst (of) cystic duct gallbladder
        Hypertrophy (of) cystic duct gallbladder
        Nonfunctioning (of) cystic duct gallbladder
        Ulcer (of) cystic duct gallbladder
        Biliary dyskinesia
        Excludes *Hartmann's pouch of intestine (V44.3)*
                    nonvisualization of gallbladder (793.3)
        Coding Clinic: 1989, Q2, P13

    575.9 Unspecified disorder of gallbladder

● **576 Other disorders of biliary tract**
        Excludes *that involving the:*
                    cystic duct (575.0–575.9)
                    gallbladder (575.0–575.9)

    576.0 Postcholecystectomy syndrome
        Coding Clinic: 1988, Q1, P10

    576.1 Cholangitis 🔹
        Cholangitis: Cholangitis:
            NOS   recurrent
            acute   sclerosing
            ascending   secondary
            chronic   stenosing
            primary   suppurative
        (Ex) 576.1, 576.8-576.9
        Coding Clinic: 1999, Q2, P13-14; 1995, Q2, P7

DISEASES OF THE DIGESTIVE SYSTEM (520–579)

N Newborn: 0   **P** Pediatric: 0–17   **M** Maternity: 12–55   **A** Adult: 15–124   ♀ Females Only   ♂ Males Only

(Ex) CC/MCC Exclusions   🔹 Complication\Comorbidity   🔹 Major C\C   🔹 Present on Admission Requirement   🔹 Hospital-Acquired Condition   853

576.2 Obstruction of bile duct
  Occlusion of bile duct, except cystic duct, without mention of calculus
  Stenosis of bile duct, except cystic duct, without mention of calculus
  Stricture of bile duct, except cystic duct, without mention of calculus

  Excludes *congenital (751.61)*
  that with calculus (574.3–574.5 with fifth-digit 1)
  Ex: 574.31, 574.41, 574.51, 576.2, 576.8-576.9, 751.61
  Coding Clinic: 2003, Q3, P17-18; 2001, Q1, P8-9; 1999, Q2, P13-14

576.3 Perforation of bile duct
  Rupture of bile duct, except cystic duct
  Ex: 576.3-576.4, 576.8-576.9

576.4 Fistula of bile duct
  Choledochoduodenal fistula
  Ex: 576.3-576.4, 576.8-576.9

576.5 Spasm of sphincter of Oddi

576.8 Other specified disorders of biliary tract
  Adhesions of bile duct [any]
  Atrophy of bile duct [any]
  Cyst of bile duct [any]
  Hypertrophy of bile duct [any]
  Stasis of bile duct [any]
  Ulcer of bile duct [any]

  Excludes *congenital choledochal cyst (751.69)*
  Coding Clinic: 2003, Q3, P17-18; 1999, Q2, P14

576.9 Unspecified disorder of biliary tract

● **577 Diseases of pancreas**
  Pancreatitis is inflammatory process that may be acute or chronic.

  577.0 Acute pancreatitis
  Abscess of pancreas   Pancreatitis:
  Necrosis of pancreas: NOS
    acute   acute (recurrent)
    infective   apoplectic
                                 hemorrhagic
                                 subacute
                                 suppurative

  Excludes *mumps pancreatitis (072.3)*
  Ex: 577.0-577.1, 577.8-577.9
  Coding Clinic: 1999, Q3, P9; 1998, Q2, P19-20; 1996, Q2, P13-15; 1989, Q2, P9

  577.1 Chronic pancreatitis
  Chronic pancreatitis: Pancreatitis:
    NOS   painless
    infectious   recurrent
    interstitial   relapsing
  Ex: 251.8, 577.0-577.9
  Coding Clinic: 2001, Q1, P8-9; 1996, Q2, P13-15; 1994, Q3, P11

  577.2 Cyst and pseudocyst of pancreas
  Ex: 577.2-577.9

  577.8 Other specified diseases of pancreas
  Atrophy of pancreas   Pancreatic:
  Calculus of pancreas   infantilism
  Cirrhosis of pancreas   necrosis:
  Fibrosis of pancreas   NOS
                                  aseptic
                                  fat
                                Pancreatolithiasis

  Excludes *fibrocystic disease of pancreas (277.00–277.09)*
  islet cell tumor of pancreas (211.7)
  pancreatic steatorrhea (579.4)
  Coding Clinic: 2001, Q1, P8-9

  577.9 Unspecified disease of pancreas

Figure 9–17 Pancreatic ductal system.

Pancreatic duct
Common bile duct
Accessory duct
Ampulla of Vater

● **578 Gastrointestinal hemorrhage**
  Excludes *that with mention of:*
  angiodysplasia of stomach and duodenum (537.83)
  angiodysplasia of intestine (569.85)
  diverticulitis, intestine:
    large (562.13)
    small (562.03)
  diverticulosis, intestine:
    large (562.12)
    small (562.02)
  gastritis and duodenitis (535.0–535.6)
  ulcer:
    duodenal, gastric, gastrojejunal, or peptic (531.00–534.91)
  Coding Clinic: 2007, Q2, P13; 1992, Q2, P9-10; Q2, P8-9

  578.0 Hematemesis
  Vomiting of blood
  Ex: 251.5, 456.0, 530.20-530.21, 530.7, 530.82, 530.85, 531.00-534.91, 535.01, 535.11, 535.21, 535.31, 535.41, 535.51, 535.61, 535.71, 537.83, 562.02-562.03, 562.12-562.13, 569.3, 569.85, 578.0-578.9
  Coding Clinic: 2002, Q2, P4

  578.1 Blood in stool
  Melena
  Excludes *melena of the newborn (772.4, 777.3)*
  occult blood (792.1)
  Ex: 251.5, 456.0, 530.20-530.21, 530.7, 530.82, 530.85, 531.00-534.91, 535.01, 535.11, 535.21, 535.31, 535.41, 535.51, 535.61, 535.71, 537.83, 562.02-562.03, 562.12-562.13, 569.3, 569.85, 578.0-578.9
  Coding Clinic: 2013, Q3, P9; 2006, Q2, P17; 1992, Q2, P8-9

  578.9 Hemorrhage of gastrointestinal tract, unspecified
  Gastric hemorrhage   Intestinal hemorrhage
  Ex: 251.5, 456.0, 530.20-530.21, 530.7, 530.82, 530.85, 531.00-534.91, 535.01, 535.11, 535.21, 535.31, 535.41, 535.51, 535.61, 535.71, 537.83, 562.02-562.03, 562.12-562.13, 569.3, 569.85, 578.0-578.9
  Coding Clinic: 2008, Q2, P15-16; 2006, Q4, P91-92; 2005, Q3, P17-18; 1986, Nov-Dec, P9; 1985, Sept-Oct, P9

● **579 Intestinal malabsorption**
  579.0 Celiac disease
  Celiac: Gee (-Herter) disease
    crisis   Gluten enteropathy
    infantilism   Idiopathic steatorrhea
    rickets   Nontropical sprue

  579.1 Tropical sprue
  Sprue:
    NOS
    tropical
  Tropical steatorrhea
  Ex: 277.03, 579.0-579.9

  579.2 Blind loop syndrome
  Postoperative blind loop syndrome
  Ex: 277.03, 579.0-579.9

  579.3 Other and unspecified postsurgical nonabsorption
  Hypoglycemia following gastrointestinal surgery
  Malnutrition following gastrointestinal surgery
  Ex: 579.3-579.9
  Coding Clinic: 2003, Q4, P104-105

  579.4 Pancreatic steatorrhea
  Ex: 277.03, 579.0-579.9

  579.8 Other specified intestinal malabsorption
  Enteropathy:
    exudative
    protein-losing
  Steatorrhea (chronic)
  Ex: 277.03, 579.0-579.9
  Coding Clinic: 2003, Q1, P12

  579.9 Unspecified intestinal malabsorption
  Malabsorption syndrome NOS
  Ex: 277.03, 579.0-579.9
  Coding Clinic: 2004, Q4, P57-59

Figure 10-1 Kidneys within the urinary system.

Item 10-1 Glomerulonephritis is nephritis accompanied by inflammation of the glomeruli of the kidney, resulting in the degeneration of the glomeruli and the nephrons.
Acute glomerulonephritis primarily affects children and young adults and is usually a result of a streptococcal infection.
Proliferative glomerulonephritis is the acute form of the disease resulting from a streptococcal infection.
Rapidly progressive glomerulonephritis, also known as **crescentic** or **malignant glomerulonephritis,** is the acute form of the disease, which leads quickly to rapid and progressive decline in renal function.

10.   DISEASES OF THE GENITOURINARY SYSTEM (580–629)

NEPHRITIS, NEPHROTIC SYNDROME, AND NEPHROSIS (580–589)

> **Excludes** *hypertensive chronic kidney disease (403.00–403.91, 404.00–404.93)*

● **580   Acute glomerulonephritis**

> **Includes**   acute nephritis

580.0   With lesion of proliferative glomerulonephritis🔖
> Acute (diffuse) proliferative glomerulonephritis
> Acute poststreptococcal glomerulonephritis
> (Ex:) 016.00-016.06, 016.30-016.36, 016.90-016.96, 017.90-017.96, 098.10, 098.19, 098.30-098.31, 098.89, 112.2, 131.00, 131.8-131.9, 249.40-249.41, 249.80-249.91, 250.40-250.43, 250.80-250.93, 274.10, 274.19, 277.88, 580.0-591, 593.0-593.2, 593.89-593.9, 599.70-599.9

580.4   With lesion of rapidly progressive glomerulonephritis🔖
> Acute nephritis with lesion of necrotizing glomerulitis
> (Ex:) 016.00-016.06, 016.30-016.36, 016.90-016.96, 017.90-017.96, 098.10, 098.19, 098.30-098.31, 098.89, 112.2, 131.00, 131.8-131.9, 249.40-249.41, 249.80-249.91, 250.40-250.43, 250.80-250.93, 274.10, 274.19, 277.88, 580.0-591, 593.0-593.2, 593.89-593.9, 599.70-599.9

● **580.8   With other specified pathological lesion in kidney**

▷ **580.81   *Acute glomerulonephritis in diseases classified elsewhere***🔖
> *Code first underlying disease, as:*
> infectious hepatitis (070.0–070.9)
> mumps (072.79)
> subacute bacterial endocarditis (421.0)
> typhoid fever (002.0)
> (Ex:) 016.00-016.06, 016.30-016.36, 016.90-016.96, 017.90-017.96, 098.10, 098.19, 098.30-098.31, 098.89, 112.2, 131.00, 131.8-131.9, 249.40-249.41, 249.80-249.91, 250.40-250.43, 250.80-250.93, 274.10, 274.19, 277.88, 580.0-591, 593.0-593.2, 593.89-593.9, 599.70-599.9

580.89   Other🔖
> Glomerulonephritis, acute, with lesion of:
> exudative nephritis
> interstitial (diffuse) (focal) nephritis
> (Ex:) 016.00-016.06, 016.30-016.36, 016.90-016.96, 017.90-017.96, 098.10, 098.19, 098.30-098.31, 098.89, 112.2, 131.00, 131.8-131.9, 274.10, 274.19, 277.88, 580.0-591, 593.0-593.2, 593.89-593.9, 599.70-599.9

580.9   Acute glomerulonephritis with unspecified pathological lesion in kidney🔖
> Glomerulonephritis: specified as acute
> NOS specified as acute
> hemorrhagic specified as acute
> Nephritis specified as acute
> Nephropathy specified as acute
> (Ex:) 016.00-016.06, 016.30-016.36, 016.90-016.96, 017.90-017.96, 098.10, 098.19, 098.30-098.31, 098.89, 112.2, 131.00, 131.8-131.9, 249.40-249.41, 249.80-249.91, 250.40-250.43, 250.80-250.93, 274.10, 274.19, 277.88, 580.0-591, 593.0-593.2, 593.89-593.9, 599.70-599.9

● **581   Nephrotic syndrome**

581.0   With lesion of proliferative glomerulonephritis🔖
> (Ex:) 016.00-016.06, 016.30-016.36, 016.90-016.96, 017.90-017.96, 098.10, 098.19, 098.30-098.31, 098.89, 112.2, 131.00, 131.8-131.9, 249.40-249.41, 249.80-249.91, 250.40-250.43, 250.80-250.93, 274.10, 274.19, 277.88, 580.0-591, 593.0-593.2, 593.89-593.9, 599.70-599.9

581.1   With lesion of membranous glomerulonephritis🔖
> Epimembranous nephritis
> Idiopathic membranous glomerular disease
> Nephrotic syndrome with lesion of:
> focal glomerulosclerosis
> sclerosing membranous glomerulonephritis
> segmental hyalinosis
> (Ex:) 016.00-016.06, 016.30-016.36, 016.90-016.96, 017.90-017.96, 098.10, 098.19, 098.30-098.31, 098.89, 112.2, 131.00, 131.8-131.9, 249.40-249.41, 249.80-249.91, 250.40-250.43, 250.80-250.93, 274.10, 274.19, 277.88, 580.0-591, 593.0-593.2, 593.89-593.9, 599.70-599.9

581.2   With lesion of membranoproliferative glomerulonephritis🔖
> Nephrotic syndrome with lesion (of):
> endothelial glomerulonephritis
> hypocomplementemic glomerulonephritis persistent glomerulonephritis
> lobular glomerulonephritis
> mesangiocapillary glomerulonephritis
> mixed membranous and proliferative glomerulonephritis
> (Ex:) 016.00-016.06, 016.30-016.36, 016.90-016.96, 017.90-017.96, 098.10, 098.19, 098.30-098.31, 098.89, 112.2, 131.00, 131.8-131.9, 249.40-249.41, 249.80-249.91, 250.40-250.43, 250.80-250.93, 274.10, 274.19, 580.0-591, 593.0-593.2, 593.89-593.9, 599.70-599.9

Figure 10-2 Kidney cross section.

Item 10-2 Nephrotic syndrome (NS) is marked by massive proteinuria (protein in the urine) and water retention. Patients with NS are particularly vulnerable to staphylococcal and pneumococcal infections. NS with lesion of proliferative glomerulonephritis results from a streptococcal infection. NS with lesion of membranous glomerulonephritis results in thickening of the capillary walls. NS with lesion of minimal change glomerulonephritis is usually a benign disorder that occurs mostly in children and requires electron microscopy (biopsy) to verify changes in the glomeruli.

N Newborn: 0   **P** Pediatric: 0–17   **M** Maternity: 12–55   **A** Adult: 15–124   ♀ Females Only   ♂ Males Only

(Ex:) CC/MCC Exclusions   🔖 Complication\Comorbidity   🔖 Major C\C   Present on Admission Requirement   🔖 Hospital-Acquired Condition   855

581.3 **With lesion of minimal change glomerulonephritis** 🔖
Foot process disease
Lipoid nephrosis
Minimal change:
  glomerular disease
  glomerulitis
  nephrotic syndrome
(Ex:) 016.00-016.06, 016.30-016.36, 016.90-016.96, 017.90-017.96, 098.10,
    098.19, 098.30-098.31, 098.89, 112.2, 131.00, 131.8-131.9,
    249.40-249.41, 249.80-249.91, 250.40-250.43, 250.80-250.93, 274.10,
    274.19, 580.0-591, 593.0-593.2, 593.89-593.9, 599.70-599.9
Coding Clinic: 2007, Q1, P23

● **581.8** **With other specified pathological lesion in kidney**
▷ **581.81** *Nephrotic syndrome in diseases classified*
      elsewhere 🔖
      Code first underlying disease, as:
          amyloidosis (277.30–277.39)
          diabetes mellitus (249.4, 250.4)
          malaria (084.9)
          polyarteritis (446.0)
          systemic lupus erythematosus (710.0)
      Excludes *nephrosis in epidemic hemorrhagic fever*
          (078.6)
      (Ex:) 016.00-016.06, 016.30-016.36, 016.90-016.96, 017.90-017.96,
          098.10, 098.19, 098.30-098.31, 098.89, 112.2, 131.00,
          131.8-131.9, 249.40-249.41, 249.80-249.91, 250.40-250.43,
          250.80-250.93, 274.10, 274.19, 277.88, 580.0-591,
          593.0-593.2, 593.89-593.9, 599.70-599.9

  581.89 **Other** 🔖
      Glomerulonephritis with edema and lesion of:
          exudative nephritis
          interstitial (diffuse) (focal) nephritis
      (Ex:) 016.00-016.06, 016.30-016.36, 016.90-016.96, 017.90-017.96,
          098.10, 098.19, 098.30-098.31, 098.89, 112.2, 131.00,
          131.8-131.9, 249.40-249.41, 249.80-249.91, 250.40-250.43,
          250.80-250.93, 274.10, 274.19, 277.88, 580.0-591,
          593.0-593.2, 593.89-593.9, 599.70-599.9

581.9 **Nephrotic syndrome with unspecified pathological lesion**
in kidney 🔖
Glomerulonephritis with edema NOS
Nephritis:
  nephrotic NOS
    with edema NOS
Nephrosis NOS
Renal disease with edema NOS
(Ex:) 016.00-016.06, 016.30-016.36, 016.90-016.96, 017.90-017.96, 098.10,
    098.19, 098.30-098.31, 098.89, 112.2, 131.00, 131.8-131.9,
    249.40-249.41, 249.80-249.91, 250.40-250.43, 250.80-250.93, 274.10,
    274.19, 277.88, 580.0-591, 593.0-593.2, 593.89-593.9, 599.70-599.9

● **582** **Chronic glomerulonephritis**
  Includes chronic nephritis

582.0 **With lesion of proliferative glomerulonephritis** 🔖
Chronic (diffuse) proliferative glomerulonephritis
(Ex:) 016.00-016.06, 016.30-016.36, 016.90-016.96, 017.90-017.96, 078.6, 098.10,
    098.19, 098.30-098.31, 098.89, 112.2, 131.00, 131.8-131.9,
    249.40-249.41, 249.80-249.91, 250.40-250.43, 250.80-250.93, 274.10,
    274.19, 580.0-584.9, 586-591, 593.0-593.2, 593.89-593.9, 599.70-599.9

582.1 **With lesion of membranous glomerulonephritis** 🔖
Chronic glomerulonephritis:
  membranous
  sclerosing
Focal glomerulosclerosis
Segmental hyalinosis
(Ex:) 016.00-016.06, 016.30 -016.36, 016.90-016.96, 017.90-017.96, 078.6,
    098.10, 098.19, 098.30-098.31, 098.89, 112.2, 131.00, 131.8-131.9,
    249.40-249.41, 249.80-249.91, 250.40-250.43, 250.80-250.93, 274.10,
    274.19, 580.0-584.9, 586-591, 593.0-593.2, 593.89-593.9, 599.70-599.9
Coding Clinic: 1984, Sept-Oct, P16

Item 10–3 **Chronic glomerulonephritis** (GN) persists over a period of years, with remissions and exacerbation.
Chronic GN with lesion of proliferative glomerulonephritis results from a streptococcal infection.
Chronic GN with lesion of membranous glomerulonephritis, also known as membranous nephropathy, is characterized by deposits along the epithelial side of the basement membrane.
Chronic GN with lesion of membranoproliferative glomerulonephritis (MPGN) is a group of disorders characterized by alterations in the basement membranes of the kidney and the glomerular cells.
Chronic GN with lesion of rapidly progressive glomerulonephritis is characterized by necrosis, endothelial proliferation, and mesangial proliferation. The condition is marked by rapid and progressive decline in renal function.

582.2 **With lesion of membranoproliferative**
glomerulonephritis 🔖
Chronic glomerulonephritis:
  endothelial
  hypocomplementemic persistent
  lobular
  membranoproliferative
  mesangiocapillary
  mixed membranous and proliferative
(Ex:) 016.00-016.06, 016.30-016.36, 016.90-016.96, 017.90-017.96, 078.6, 098.10,
    098.19, 098.30-098.31, 098.89, 112.2, 131.00, 131.8-131.9,
    249.40-249.41, 249.80-249.91, 250.40-250.43, 250.80-250.93, 274.10,
    274.19, 580.0-584.9, 586-591, 593.0-593.2, 593.89-593.9, 599.70-599.9

582.4 **With lesion of rapidly progressive glomerulonephritis** 🔖
Chronic nephritis with lesion of necrotizing glomerulitis
(Ex:) 016.00-016.06, 016.30-016.36, 016.90-016.96, 017.90-017.96, 078.6, 098.10,
    098.19, 098.30-098.31, 098.89, 112.2, 131.00, 131.8-131.9,
    249.40-249.41, 249.80-249.91, 250.40-250.43, 250.80-250.93, 274.10,
    274.19, 580.0-584.9, 586-591, 593.0-593.2, 593.89-593.9, 599.70-599.9

● **582.8** **With other specified pathological lesion in kidney**
▷ **582.81** *Chronic glomerulonephritis in diseases classified*
      elsewhere 🔖
      Code first underlying disease, as:
          amyloidosis (277.30–277.39)
          systemic lupus erythematosus (710.0)
      (Ex:) 016.00-016.06, 016.30-016.36, 016.90-016.96, 017.90-017.96,
          078.6, 098.10, 098.19, 098.30-098.31, 098.89, 112.2, 131.00,
          131.8-131.9, 249.40-249.41, 249.80-249.91, 250.40-250.43,
          250.80-250.93, 274.10, 274.19, 580.0-584.9, 586-591,
          593.0-593.2, 593.89-593.9, 599.70-599.9

  582.89 **Other** 🔖
      Chronic glomerulonephritis with lesion of:
          exudative nephritis
          interstitial (diffuse) (focal) nephritis
      (Ex:) 016.00-016.06, 016.30-016.36, 016.90-016.96, 017.90-017.96,
          078.6, 098.10, 098.19, 098.30-098.31, 098.89, 112.2, 131.00,
          131.8-131.9, 249.40-249.41, 249.80-249.91, 250.40-250.43,
          250.80-250.93, 274.10, 274.19, 580.0-584.9, 586-591,
          593.0-593.2, 593.89-593.9, 599.70-599.9

582.9 **Chronic glomerulonephritis with unspecified pathological**
lesion in kidney 🔖
Glomerulonephritis: specified as chronic
    NOS specified as chronic
    hemorrhagic specified as chronic
Nephritis specified as chronic
Nephropathy specified as chronic
(Ex:) 016.00-016.06, 016.30-016.36, 016.90-016.96, 017.90-017.96, 078.6, 098.10,
    098.19, 098.30-098.31, 098.89, 112.2, 131.00, 131.8-131.9,
    249.40-249.41, 249.80-249.91, 250.40-250.43, 250.80-250.93, 274.10,
    274.19, 580.0-584.9, 586-591, 593.0-593.2, 593.89-593.9, 599.70-599.9
Coding Clinic: 2001, Q2, P12

Item 10–4 **Nephritis** (inflammation) or **nephropathy** (disease) **with lesion of proliferative glomerulonephritis** results from a streptococcal infection.

Nephritis (inflammation) or **nephropathy** (disease) **with lesion of membranous glomerulonephritis** is characterized by deposits along the epithelial side of the basement membrane.

Nephritis (inflammation) or **nephropathy** (disease) **with lesion of membranoproliferative glomerulonephritis** is characterized by alterations in the basement membranes of the kidney and the glomerular cells.

Nephritis (inflammation) or **nephropathy** (disease) **with lesion of rapidly progressive glomerulonephritis** is characterized by rapid and progressive decline in renal function.

Nephritis (inflammation) or **nephropathy** (disease) **with lesion of renal cortical necrosis** is characterized by death of the cortical tissues.

Nephritis (inflammation) or **nephropathy** (disease) **with lesion of renal medullary necrosis** is characterized by death of the tissues that collect urine.

● **583** **Nephritis and nephropathy, not specified as acute or chronic**

> **Includes** "renal disease" so stated, not specified as acute or chronic but with stated pathology or cause

583.0 **With lesion of proliferative glomerulonephritis** 🖑
Proliferative:
glomerulonephritis (diffuse) NOS
nephritis NOS
nephropathy NOS
Ⓔ 016.00-016.06, 016.30-016.36, 016.90-016.96, 017.90-017.96, 078.6, 098.10, 098.19, 098.30-098.31, 098.89, 112.2, 131.00, 131.8-131.9, 249.40-249.41, 249.80-249.91, 250.40-250.43, 250.80-250.93, 274.10, 274.19, 580.0-584.9, 586-591, 593.0-593.2, 593.89-593.9, 599.70-599.9

583.1 **With lesion of membranous glomerulonephritis** 🖑
Membranous:
glomerulonephritis NOS
nephritis NOS
Membranous nephropathy NOS
Ⓔ 016.00-016.06, 016.30-016.36, 016.90-016.96, 017.90-017.96, 078.6, 098.10, 098.19, 098.30-098.31, 098.89, 112.2, 131.00, 131.8-131.9, 249.40-249.41, 249.80-249.91, 250.40-250.43, 250.80-250.93, 274.10, 274.19, 580.0-584.9, 586-591, 593.0-593.2, 593.89-593.9, 599.70-599.9

583.2 **With lesion of membranoproliferative glomerulonephritis** 🖑
Membranoproliferative:
glomerulonephritis NOS
nephritis NOS
nephropathy NOS
Nephritis NOS, with lesion of:
hypocomplementemic persistent glomerulonephritis
lobular glomerulonephritis
mesangiocapillary glomerulonephritis
mixed membranous and proliferative glomerulonephritis
Ⓔ 016.00-016.06, 016.30-016.36, 016.90-016.96, 017.90-017.96, 078.6, 098.10, 098.19, 098.30-098.31, 098.89, 112.2, 131.00, 131.8-131.9, 249.40-249.41, 249.80-249.91, 250.40-250.43, 250.80-250.93, 274.10, 274.19, 580.0-584.9, 586-591, 593.0-593.2, 593.89-593.9, 599.70-599.9

583.4 **With lesion of rapidly progressive glomerulonephritis** 🖑
Necrotizing or rapidly progressive:
glomerulitis NOS
glomerulonephritis NOS
nephritis NOS
nephropathy NOS
Nephritis, unspecified, with lesion of necrotizing glomerulitis
Ⓔ 016.00-016.06, 016.30-016.36, 016.90-016.96, 017.90-017.96, 098.10, 098.19, 098.30-098.31, 098.89, 112.2, 131.00, 131.8-131.9, 249.40-249.41, 249.80-249.91, 250.40-250.43, 250.80-250.93, 274.10, 274.19, 277.88, 580.0-591, 593.0-593.2, 593.89-593.9, 599.70-599.9

583.6 **With lesion of renal cortical necrosis** 🖑
Nephritis NOS with (renal) cortical necrosis
Nephropathy NOS with (renal) cortical necrosis
Renal cortical necrosis NOS
Ⓔ 277.88, 583.6, 588.81 -588.89

583.7 **With lesion of renal medullary necrosis** 🖑
Nephritis NOS with (renal) medullary [papillary] necrosis
Nephropathy NOS with (renal) medullary [papillary] necrosis
Ⓔ 277.88, 583.7, 588.81-588.89

● **583.8** **With other specified pathological lesion in kidney**

▷ **583.81** **Nephritis and nephropathy, not specified as acute or chronic, in diseases classified elsewhere**
Code first underlying disease, as:
amyloidosis (277.30–277.39)
diabetes mellitus (249.4, 250.4)
gonococcal infection (098.19)
Goodpasture's syndrome (446.21)
systemic lupus erythematosus (710.0)
tuberculosis (016.0)
Excludes *gouty nephropathy (274.10)*
syphilitic nephritis (095.4)
Coding Clinic: 2013, Q2, P6; 2012, Q2, P19; 2003, Q2, P7

583.89 **Other**
Glomerulitis with lesion of:
exudative nephritis
interstitial nephritis
Glomerulonephritis with lesion of:
exudative nephritis
interstitial nephritis
Nephritis with lesion of:
exudative nephritis
interstitial nephritis
Nephropathy with lesion of:
exudative nephritis
interstitial nephritis
Renal disease with lesion of:
exudative nephritis
interstitial nephritis

583.9 **With unspecified pathological lesion in kidney**
Glomerulitis NOS   Nephritis NOS
Glomerulonephritis NOS Nephropathy NOS
Excludes *nephropathy complicating pregnancy, labor, or the puerperium (642.0–642.9, 646.2)*
renal disease NOS with no stated cause (593.9)
Coding Clinic: 1994, Q4, P35

● **584** **Acute kidney failure**
Includes Acute renal failure
Excludes *following labor and delivery (669.3)*
posttraumatic (958.5)
that complicating:
abortion (634–638 with .3, 639.3)
ectopic or molar pregnancy (639.3)
Coding Clinic: 2011, Q3, P17; 1992, Q2, P5x2

584.5 **Acute kidney failure with lesion of tubular necrosis** 🖑
Lower nephron nephrosis
Renal failure with (acute) tubular necrosis
Tubular necrosis:
NOS
acute
Ⓔ 249.40-249.41, 249.80-249.91, 250.40-250.43, 250.80-250.93, 274.10, 274.19, 277.88, 580.0-591, 593.0-593.2, 593.89-593.9, 599.70-599.9, 753.0-753.3, 753.9

584.6 **Acute kidney failure with lesion of renal cortical necrosis** 🖑
Ⓔ 249.40-249.41, 249.80-249.91, 250.40-250.43, 250.80-250.93, 274.10, 274.19, 277.88, 580.0-591, 593.0-593.2, 593.89-593.9, 599.70-599.9, 753.0-753.3, 753.9

584.7 **Acute kidney failure with lesion of renal medullary [papillary] necrosis** 🖑
Necrotizing renal papillitis
Ⓔ 249.40-249.41, 249.80-249.91, 250.40-250.43, 250.80-250.93, 274.10, 274.19, 277.88, 580.0-591, 593.0-593.2, 593.89-593.9, 599.70-599.9, 753.0-753.3, 753.9

DISEASES OF THE GENITOURINARY SYSTEM (580–629)

584.8 Acute kidney failure with other specified pathological lesion in kidney 🔵
Ⓔ 249.40-249.41, 249.80-249.91, 250.40-250.43, 250.80-250.93, 274.10, 274.19, 277.88, 580.0-591, 593.0-593.2, 593.89-593.9, 599.70-599.9
Coding Clinic: 2011, Q3, P16-17

584.9 Acute kidney failure, unspecified 🔵
Acute kidney injury (nontraumatic)
Excludes *traumatic kidney injury (866.00-866.13)*
Ⓔ 249.40-249.41, 249.80-249.91, 250.40-250.43, 250.80-250.93, 274.10, 274.19, 277.88, 580.0-591, 593.0-593.2, 593.89-593.9, 599.70-599.9, 753.0-753.3, 753.9
Coding Clinic: 2011, Q3, P16-17; 2009, Q4, P106; 2008, Q4, P192-193; 2007, Q4, P96-97; 2005, Q2, P18-19; 2003, Q2, P7; 2003, Q1, P22; 2002, Q3, P21x2, 28x2; 2001, Q2, P14x2; 2000, Q3, P9; 2000, Q1, P22; 1996, Q3, P9; 1993, Q4, P34

OGCR   Section I.C.10.a.1
The ICD-9-CM classifies CKD based on severity. The severity of CKD is designated by stages I-V. Stage II, code 585.2, equates to mild CKD; stage III, code 585.3, equates to moderate CKD; and stage IV, code 585.4, equates to severe CKD. Code 585.6, End stage renal disease (ESRD), is assigned when the provider has documented end-stage-renal disease (ESRD). If both a stage of CKD and ESRD are documented, assign code 585.6 only.

● **585 Chronic kidney disease (CKD)**
Includes Chronic uremia
Code first hypertensive chronic kidney disease, if applicable, (403.00–403.91, 404.00–404.93)
Use additional code to identify:
kidney transplant status, if applicable (V42.0)
manifestation as:
uremic:
neuropathy (357.4)
pericarditis (420.0)

585.1 Chronic kidney disease, Stage I

585.2 Chronic kidney disease, Stage II (mild)

585.3 Chronic kidney disease, Stage III (moderate)
Coding Clinic: 2013, Q2, P13; 2005, Q4, P68-69

585.4 Chronic kidney disease, Stage IV (severe) 🔵
Ⓔ 249.40-249.41, 249.80-249.91, 250.40-250.43, 250.80-250.93, 274.10, 274.19, 580.0-591, 593.0-593.2, 593.89-593.9, 599.70-599.9, 753.0-753.3, 753.9

585.5 Chronic kidney disease, Stage V 🔵
Excludes *chronic kidney disease, stage V requiring chronic dialysis (585.6)*
Ⓔ 249.40-249.41, 249.80-249.91, 250.40-250.43, 250.80-250.93, 274.10, 274.19, 580.0-591, 593.0-593.2, 593.89-593.9, 599.70-599.9, 753.0-753.3, 753.9
Coding Clinic: 2013, Q2, P6; 2011, Q3, P15; 2010, Q4, P137

585.6 End stage renal disease 🔵
Chronic kidney disease, stage V requiring chronic dialysis
Ⓔ 249.40-249.41, 249.80-249.91, 250.40-250.43, 250.80-250.93, 274.10, 274.19, 403.90, 580.0-591, 593.0-593.2, 593.89-593.9, 599.70-599.9, 753.0-753.3, 753.9
Coding Clinic: 2013, Q2, P5-6; 2010, Q3, P13; 2008, Q4, P193; Q1, P7-8; 2007, Q4, P84-86; Q3, P5-6; Q3, P11; 2006, Q4, P136; 2004, Q1, P5

585.9 Chronic kidney disease, unspecified
Chronic renal disease
Chronic renal failure NOS
Chronic renal insufficiency
Coding Clinic: 2008, Q1, P7-8, 19; 2007, Q2, P3; 2006, Q4, P84-86; 2003, Q4, P60-61,111-112; 2001, Q2, P11-13x2; Q1, P3; 2000, Q4, P39-40; 1998, Q4, P54-55; Q3, P6-7; Q2, P20-21; 1996, Q3, P9; 1995, Q2, P10; 1987, Sept-Oct, P10; 1985, Nov-Dec, P15

586 Renal failure, unspecified
Includes Uremia NOS
Excludes *following labor and delivery (669.3)*
posttraumatic renal failure (958.5)
that complicating:
abortion (634–638 with .3, 639.3)
ectopic or molar pregnancy (639.3)
uremia:
extrarenal (788.9)
prerenal (788.9)
Coding Clinic: 1998, Q3, P6; 1984, Sept-Oct, P16

587 Renal sclerosis, unspecified
Includes Atrophy of kidney
Contracted kidney
Renal:
cirrhosis
fibrosis
Coding Clinic: 2010, Q4, P137

● **588 Disorders resulting from impaired renal function**
588.0 Renal osteodystrophy
Azotemic osteodystrophy
Phosphate-losing tubular disorders
Renal:
dwarfism
infantilism
rickets

588.1 Nephrogenic diabetes insipidus 🔵
Excludes *diabetes insipidus NOS (253.5)*
Ⓔ 016.00-016.06, 016.30-016.36, 016.90 -016.96, 017.90-017.96, 078.6, 098.10, 098.19, 098.30-098.31, 098.89, 112.2, 131.00, 131.8-131.9, 249.40-249.41, 249.80-249.91, 250.40-250.43, 250.80-250.93, 274.10, 274.19, 580.0-584.9, 585.3-585.6, 586-591, 593.0-593.2, 593.89-593.9, 599.70-599.9

● **588.8 Other specified disorders resulting from impaired renal function**
Excludes *secondary hypertension (405.0–405.9)*
Coding Clinic: 2004, Q4, P57-59

588.81 Secondary hyperparathyroidism (of renal origin) 🔵
Secondary hyperparathyroidism NOS
Ⓔ 016.00-016.06, 016.30-016.36, 016.90-016.96, 017.90-017.96, 078.6, 098.10, 098.19, 098.30-098.31, 098.89, 112.2, 131.00, 131.8-131.9, 249.40-249.41, 249.80-249.91, 250.40-250.43, 250.80-250.93, 274.10, 274.19, 580.0-584.9, 586-588.1, 588.89-591, 593.0-593.2, 593.89-593.9, 599.70-599.9

588.89 Other specified disorders resulting from impaired renal function
Hypokalemic nephropathy

588.9 Unspecified disorder resulting from impaired renal function

● **589 Small kidney of unknown cause**
589.0 Unilateral small kidney
589.1 Bilateral small kidneys
589.9 Small kidney, unspecified

OTHER DISEASES OF URINARY SYSTEM (590–599)

● **590 Infections of kidney**
Use additional code to identify organism, such as Escherichia coli [E. coli] (041.41-041.49)

● **590.0 Chronic pyelonephritis**
Chronic pyelitis   Chronic pyonephrosis
Code, if applicable, any causal condition first

590.00 Without lesion of renal medullary necrosis

590.01 With lesion of renal medullary necrosis 🔵
Ⓔ 016.00-016.06, 016.30-016.36, 016.90-016.96, 017.90-017.96, 078.6, 098.10, 098.19, 098.30-098.31, 098.89, 112.2, 131.00, 131.8-131.9, 249.40-249.41, 249.80-249.91, 250.40-250.43, 250.80-250.93, 274.10, 274.19, 580.0-584.9, 586-591, 593.0-593.2, 593.89-593.9, 599.70-599.9, 646.61-646.64

Item 10–5 Decreased blood flow is the usual cause of **acute renal failure** that offers a good prognosis for recovery. **Chronic renal failure** is usually the result of long-standing kidney disease and is a very serious condition that generally results in death.

Figure 10–3 Acute pyelonephritis. Cortical surface exhibits grayish white areas of inflammation and abscess formation. (From Kumar: Robbins and Cotran: Pathologic Basis of Disease, ed 8, Saunders, An Imprint of Elsevier, 2009)

Figure 10–4 Hydronephrosis of the kidney, with marked dilatation of pelvis and calyces and thinning of renal parenchyma. (From Kumar: Robbins and Cotran: Pathologic Basis of Disease, ed 8, Saunders, An Imprint of Elsevier, 2009)

Figure 10–5 Multiple urinary calculi.

Multiple calculi

Item 10-6 Pyelonephritis is an infection of the kidneys and ureters and may be chronic or acute in one or both kidneys.

● **590.1 Acute pyelonephritis**
  Acute pyelitis
  Acute pyonephrosis
  590.10 Without lesion of renal medullary necrosis 🔲 🔲
    HAC: Also excludes the following from acting as a CC/MCC: 112.2 (CC), 590.11 (MCC), 590.2 (MCC), 590.3 (CC), 590.80 (CC), 590.81 (CC), 595.0 (CC), 597.0 (CC), 599.0 (CC), 996.64 (CC)
    (Ex:) 016.00-016.06, 016.30-016.36, 016.90-016.96, 017.90-017.96, 098.10, 098.19, 098.30-098.31, 098.89, 112.2, 131.00, 131.8-131.9, 249.40-249.41, 249.80-249.91, 250.40-250.43, 250.80-250.93, 274.10, 274.19, 580.0-591, 593.0-593.2, 593.89-593.9, 599.0, 599.70-599.9

  590.11 With lesion of renal medullary necrosis 🔲 🔲
    HAC: Also excludes the following from acting as a CC/MCC: 112.2 (CC), 590.10 (CC), 590.2 (MCC), 590.3 (CC), 590.80 (CC), 590.81 (CC), 595.0 (CC), 597.0 (CC), 599.0 (CC), 996.64 (CC)
    (Ex:) 016.00-016.06, 016.30-016.36, 016.90-016.96, 017.90-017.96, 098.10, 098.19, 098.30-098.31, 098.89, 112.2, 131.00, 131.8-131.9, 249.40-249.41, 249.80- 249.91, 250.40-250.43, 250.80-250.93, 274.10, 274.19, 580.0-591, 593.0-593.2, 593.89-593.9, 599.0, 599.70-599.9

  590.2 Renal and perinephric abscess 🔲 🔲
    Abscess:
      kidney
      nephritic
      perirenal
    Carbuncle of kidney
    HAC: Also excludes the following from acting as a CC/MCC: 112.2 (CC), 590.10 (CC), 590.11 (MCC), 590.3 (CC), 590.80 (CC), 590.81 (CC), 595.0 (CC), 597.0 (CC), 599.0 (CC), 996.64 (CC)
    (Ex:) 016.00-016.06, 016.30-016.36, 016.90- 016.96, 017.90-017.96, 098.10, 098.19, 098.30-098.31, 098.89, 112.2, 131.00, 131.8-131.9, 249.40-249.41, 249.80-249.91, 250.40-250.43, 250.80-250.93, 274.10, 274.19, 580.0-591, 593.0-593.2, 593.89-593.9, 599.0, 599.70-599.9

  590.3 Pyeloureteritis cystica 🔲 🔲
    Infection of renal pelvis and ureter
    Ureteritis cystica
    Cystica is an infection of the urinary bladder.
    HAC: Also excludes the following from acting as a CC/MCC: 112.2 (CC), 590.10 (CC), 590.11 (MCC), 590.2 (MCC), 590.80 (CC), 590.81 (CC), 595.0 (CC), 597.0 (CC), 599.0 (CC), 996.64 (CC)
    (Ex:) 016.00-016.06, 016.30-016.36, 016.90-016.96, 017.90-017.96, 098.10, 098.19, 098.30-098.31, 098.89, 112.2, 131.00, 131.8-131.9, 274.10, 274.19, 580.0-591, 593.0-593.2, 593.89-593.9, 599.0, 599.70-599.9

● **590.8 Other pyelonephritis or pyonephrosis, not specified as acute or chronic**
  590.80 Pyelonephritis, unspecified 🔲 🔲
    Pyelitis NOS
    Pyelonephritis NOS
    HAC: Also excludes the following from acting as a CC/MCC: 112.2 (CC), 590.10 (CC), 590.11 (MCC), 590.2 (MCC), 590.3 (CC), 590.81 (CC), 595.0 (CC), 597.0 (CC), 599.0 (CC), 996.64 (CC)
    (Ex:) 016.00-016.06, 016.30-016.36, 016.90-016.96, 017.90-017.96, 098.10, 098.19, 098.30-098.31, 098.89, 112.2, 131.00, 131.8-131.9, 274.10, 274.19, 580.0-591, 593.0-593.2, 593.89-593.9, 599.0, 599.70-599.9
    Coding Clinic: 1997, Q4, P40

▸ **590.81 *Pyelitis or pyelonephritis in diseases classified elsewhere*** 🔲 🔲
    Code first underlying disease, as:
      tuberculosis (016.0)
    HAC: Also excludes the following from acting as a CC/MCC: 112.2 (CC), 590.10 (CC), 590.11 (MCC), 590.2 (MCC), 590.3 (CC), 590.80 (CC), 595.0 (CC), 597.0 (CC), 599.0 (CC), 996.64 (CC)
    (Ex:) 016.00-016.06, 016.30-016.36, 016.90-016.96, 017.90-017.96, 098.10, 098.19, 098.30-098.31, 098.89, 112.2, 131.00, 131.8-131.9, 274.10, 274.19, 580.0-591, 593.0-593.2, 593.89-593.9, 599.0, 599.70-599.9

  590.9 Infection of kidney, unspecified
    Excludes   urinary tract infection NOS (599.0)

591 Hydronephrosis 🔲
  Hydrocalycosis   Hydroureteronephrosis
  Hydronephrosis
  Excludes   congenital hydronephrosis (753.29)
              hydroureter (593.5)
  (Ex:) 016.00-016.06, 016.30-016.36, 016.90-016.96, 017.90-017.96, 098.10, 098.19, 098.30-098.31, 098.89, 112.2, 131.00, 131.8-131.9, 274.10, 274.19, 580.0-591, 593.0-593.2, 593.89-593.9, 599.0, 599.70-599.9
  Coding Clinic: 2012, Q3, P12; 1998, Q2, P9

● **592 Calculus of kidney and ureter**
  Excludes   nephrocalcinosis (275.49)
  592.0 Calculus of kidney
    Nephrolithiasis NOS   Staghorn calculus
    Renal calculus or stone   Stone in kidney
    Excludes   uric acid nephrolithiasis (274.11)
    Coding Clinic: 2012, Q3, P12; 2000, Q1, P4; 1993, Q2, P3

  592.1 Calculus of ureter 🔲
    Ureteric stone   Ureterolithiasis
    (Ex:) 592.0-592.9, 593.3-593.5, 593.89-594.9, 599.60-599.9
    Coding Clinic: 1998, Q2, P9; 1991, Q1, P11

  592.9 Urinary calculus, unspecified
    Coding Clinic: 1997, Q4, P40

● **593 Other disorders of kidney and ureter**
  593.0 Nephroptosis
    Floating kidney   Mobile kidney
  593.1 Hypertrophy of kidney
  593.2 Cyst of kidney, acquired
    Cyst (multiple) (solitary) of kidney, not congenital
    Peripelvic (lymphatic) cyst
    Excludes   calyceal or pyelogenic cyst of kidney (591)
              congenital cyst of kidney (753.1)
              polycystic (disease of) kidney (753.1)

DISEASES OF THE GENITOURINARY SYSTEM (580–629)

593.3   Stricture or kinking of ureter
Angulation of ureter (postoperative)
Constriction of ureter (postoperative)
Stricture of pelviureteric junction
Coding Clinic: 1994, Q3, P8

593.4   Other ureteric obstruction 🔵
Idiopathic retroperitoneal fibrosis
Occlusion NOS of ureter
> **Excludes**   *that due to calculus (592.1)*
> Ⓔ 593.3-593.5, 593.89-593.9, 595.0-595.9, 596.89-596.9, 599.0, 599.60-599.9, 753.4-75.35, 753.9, V45.74
Coding Clinic: 2010, Q1, P10; 1997, Q2, P4

593.5   Hydroureter 🔵
> **Excludes**   *congenital hydroureter (753.22)*
>   *hydroureteronephrosis (591)*
> Ⓔ 593.3-593.5, 593.89-593.9, 595.0-595.9, 596.89-596.9, 599.0, 599.60-599.9, 753.4-753.5, 753.9

593.6   Postural proteinuria
Benign postural proteinuria
Orthostatic proteinuria
> **Excludes**   *proteinuria NOS (791.0)*

🔴 **593.7   Vesicoureteral reflux**
Occurs when urine flows from bladder back into ureters

    593.70   Unspecified or without reflux nephropathy

    593.71   With reflux nephropathy, unilateral

    593.72   With reflux nephropathy, bilateral

    593.73   With reflux nephropathy NOS

🔴 **593.8   Other specified disorders of kidney and ureter**

    593.81   Vascular disorders of kidney 🔵
      Renal (artery):
        embolism
        hemorrhage
        thrombosis
      Renal infarction
      Ⓔ 593.70-593.81, 593.9

    593.82   Ureteral fistula 🔵
      Intestinoureteral fistula
>   **Excludes**   *fistula between ureter and female genital*
>   *tract (619.0)*
      Ⓔ 593.82-593.9

    593.89   Other
      Adhesions, kidney or ureter
      Periureteritis
      Polyp of ureter
      Pyelectasia
      Ureterocele
>   **Excludes**   *tuberculosis of ureter (016.2)*
>   *ureteritis cystica (590.3)*
      Coding Clinic: 1984, Nov-Dec, P17

593.9   Unspecified disorder of kidney and ureter
Acute renal disease
Acute renal insufficiency
Renal disease NOS
Salt-losing nephritis or syndrome
> **Excludes**   *chronic renal insufficiency (585.9)*
>   *cystic kidney disease (753.1)*
>   *nephropathy, so stated (583.0–583.9)*
>   *renal disease:*
>   *arising in pregnancy or the puerperium*
>   *(642.1–642.2, 642.4–642.7, 646.2)*
>   *not specified as acute or chronic, but with*
>   *stated pathology or cause (583.0–583.9)*
Coding Clinic: 2005, Q4, P79-80; 1998, Q2, P9

🔴 **594   Calculus of lower urinary tract**

594.0   Calculus in diverticulum of bladder

594.1   Other calculus in bladder
Urinary bladder stone
> **Excludes**   *staghorn calculus (592.0)*

594.2   Calculus in urethra

594.8   Other lower urinary tract calculus
Coding Clinic: 1985, Jan-Feb, P16

594.9   Calculus of lower urinary tract, unspecified
> **Excludes**   *calculus of urinary tract NOS (592.9)*

🔴 **595   Cystitis**
A general term used to describe an infection of the bladder and
irritations in the lower urinary tract
> **Excludes**   *prostatocystitis (601.3)*
Use additional code to identify organism, such as Escherichia
coli [E. coli] (041.41-041.49)

595.0   Acute cystitis 🔵 🔵
> **Excludes**   *trigonitis (595.3)*
HAC: Also excludes the following from acting as a CC/
MCC: 112.2 (CC), 590.10 (CC), 590.11 (MCC),
590.2 (MCC), 590.3 (CC), 590.80 (CC), 590.81
(CC), 597.0 (CC), 599.0 (CC), 996.64 (CC)
Ⓔ 016.10-016.16, 016.30-016.36, 016.90-016.96, 017.90-017.96, 098.0, 098.11,
098.2, 098.39, 098.89, 112.2, 131.00, 131.8-131.9, 593.3-593.5,
593.89-593.9, 595.0-595.9, 596.89-596.9, 599.0, 599.60-599.9
Coding Clinic: 1999, Q2, P15-16; 1984, Nov-Dec, P15

595.1   Chronic interstitial cystitis
Describes chronic symptomatic inflammation of the
submucosal layers of the bladder
Hunner's ulcer
Panmural fibrosis of bladder
Submucous cystitis

595.2   Other chronic cystitis
Chronic cystitis NOS
Subacute cystitis
> **Excludes**   *trigonitis (595.3)*

595.3   Trigonitis
Inflammation of triangular area of bladder (where ureters and
urethra come together)
Follicular cystitis
Trigonitis (acute) (chronic)
Urethrotrigonitis

▷ **595.4   *Cystitis in diseases classified elsewhere***
Code first underlying disease, as:
  actinomycosis (039.8)
  amebiasis (006.8)
  bilharziasis (120.0–120.9)
  Echinococcus infestation (122.3, 122.6)
> **Excludes**   *cystitis:*
>   *diphtheritic (032.84)*
>   *gonococcal (098.11, 098.31)*
>   *monilial (112.2)*
>   *trichomonal (131.09)*
>   *tuberculous (016.1)*

🔴 **595.8   Other specified types of cystitis**

    595.81   Cystitis cystica

    595.82   Irradiation cystitis 🔵
      Use additional E code to identify cause
      Ⓔ 016.10-016.16, 016.30-016.36, 016.90-016.96, 017.90-017.96,
      098.0, 098.11, 098.2, 098.39, 098.89, 112.2, 131.00,
      131.8-131.9, 593.3-593.5, 593.89-593.9, 595.0-595.9,
      596.89-596.9, 599.0, 599.60-599.9

    595.89   Other
      Abscess of bladder
      Cystitis:
        bullous
        emphysematous
        glandularis

595.9   Cystitis, unspecified

● **596 Other disorders of bladder**

Use additional code to identify urinary incontinence (625.6, 788.30–788.39)

596.0 Bladder neck obstruction

Contracture (acquired) of bladder neck or vesicourethral orifice

Obstruction (acquired) of bladder neck or vesicourethral orifice

Stenosis (acquired) of bladder neck or vesicourethral orifice

Excludes *congenital (753.6)*

Coding Clinic: 2002, Q3, P28; 2001, Q2, P14; 1994, Q3, P12

596.1 Intestinovesical fistula 🔖

Passage between bladder and the intestine

Fistula:	Fistula:
enterovesical	vesicoenteric
vesicocolic	vesicorectal

Ⓔⓧ 098.0, 098.2, 098.39, 098.89, 596.1-596.2, 596.89-596.9, 599.70-599.9, 788.1

596.2 Vesical fistula, not elsewhere classified 🔖

Fistula:	Fistula:
bladder NOS	vesicocutaneous
urethrovesical	vesicoperineal

Excludes *fistula between bladder and female genital tract (619.0)*

Ⓔⓧ 098.0, 098.2, 098.39, 098.89, 596.1-596.2, 596.89-596.9, 599.70-599.9, 788.1

596.3 Diverticulum of bladder

Formation of a sac from a herniation of the wall of the bladder

Diverticulitis of bladder

Diverticulum (acquired) (false) of bladder

Excludes *that with calculus in diverticulum of bladder (594.0)*

596.4 Atony of bladder

Diminished tone of bladder muscle

High compliance bladder

Hypotonicity of bladder

Inertia of bladder

Excludes *neurogenic bladder (596.54)*

● **596.5 Other functional disorders of bladder**

Excludes *cauda equina syndrome with neurogenic bladder (344.61)*

596.51 Hypertonicity of bladder

Hyperactivity   Overactive bladder

596.52 Low bladder compliance

596.53 Paralysis of bladder

596.54 Neurogenic bladder NOS

Coding Clinic: 2001, Q1, P12

596.55 Detrusor sphincter dyssynergia

596.59 Other functional disorder of bladder

Detrusor instability

Coding Clinic: 1995, Q4, P72-73

596.6 Rupture of bladder, nontraumatic 🔖

Ⓔⓧ 596.6-596.7, 596.89-596.9, 599.70-599.9, 788.1

596.7 Hemorrhage into bladder wall 🔖

Hyperemia of bladder

Excludes *acute hemorrhagic cystitis (595.0)*

Ⓔⓧ 596.6-596.7, 596.89-596.9, 599.70-599.9, 788.1

● **596.8 Other specified disorders of bladder**

Excludes *cystocele, female (618.01–618.02, 618.09, 618.2–618.4)*

hernia or prolapse of bladder, female (618.01–618.02, 618.09, 618.2–618.4)

596.81 Infection of cystostomy 🔖

Use additional code to specify type of infection, such as:

abscess or cellulitis of abdomen (682.2)

septicemia (038.0-038.9)

Use additional code to identify organism (041.00-041.9)

Ⓔⓧ 596.81-596.89, 599.0, 996.30, 996.39, 996.56-996.60, 996.64, 996.65, 996.68-996.70, 996.76, 996.79, 997.91-997.99, 998.81, 998.83-998.9

Coding Clinic: 2011, Q4, P129

596.82 Mechanical complication of cystostomy 🔖

Malfunction of cystostomy

Ⓔⓧ 596.81-596.89, 996.39, 996.64, 996.65, 996.76, 997.91-997.99, 998.81, 998.83-998.9

596.83 Other complication of cystostomy 🔖

Fistula

Hernia

Prolapse

Ⓔⓧ 596.81-596.89, 996.30, 996.39, 996.55-996.60, 996.64, 996.65, 996.68-996.70, 996.76, 996.79, 997.91-997.99, 998.81-998.9

596.89 Other specified disorders of bladder

Bladder hemorrhage

Bladder hypertrophy

Calcified bladder

Contracted bladder

Coding Clinic: 2013, Q1, P6

596.9 Unspecified disorder of bladder

● **597 Urethritis, not sexually transmitted, and urethral syndrome**

Inflammation of urethra caused by bacteria or virus

Excludes *nonspecific urethritis, so stated (099.4)*

597.0 Urethral abscess 🔖 🔖

Abscess of:	Abscess:
bulbourethral gland	periurethral
Cowper's gland	urethral (gland)
Littré's gland	Periurethral cellulitis

Excludes *urethral caruncle (599.3)*

HAC: Also excludes the following from acting as a CC/MCC: 112.2 (CC), 590.10 (CC), 590.11 (MCC), 590.2 (MCC), 590.3 (CC), 590.80 (CC), 590.81 (CC), 595.0 (CC), 599.0 (CC), 996.64 (CC)

Ⓔⓧ 098.0, 098.2, 098.39, 098.89, 099.40-099.49, 112.2, 131.00, 131.02 131.8-131.9, 597.0-598.01, 598.8-599.0, 599.60-599.9, 607.1-607.83, 607.85-607.9, 608.4-608.81, 608.85, 608.87-608.89, 752.61-752.69, 752.81-75.29, 753.6-753.9, 788.1

● **597.8 Other urethritis**

597.80 Urethritis, unspecified

597.81 Urethral syndrome NOS

597.89 Other

Adenitis, Skene's glands

Cowperitis

Meatitis, urethral

Ulcer, urethra (meatus)

Verumontanitis

Excludes *trichomonal (131.02)*

| N Newborn: 0 | P Pediatric: 0–17 | M Maternity: 12–55 | A Adult: 15–124 | ♀ Females Only | ♂ Males Only |

Ⓔⓧ CC/MCC Exclusions   🔖 Complication\Comorbidity   🔖 Major C\C   🔖 Present on Admission Requirement   🔖 Hospital-Acquired Condition   **861**

DISEASES OF THE GENITOURINARY SYSTEM (580–629)

● 598   **Urethral stricture**
Narrowing of lumen of urethra caused by scarring from an infection or injury, which results in functional obstruction

> **Includes**   pinhole meatus
>   stricture of urinary meatus

Use additional code to identify urinary incontinence (625.6, 788.30–788.39)

> **Excludes**   *congenital stricture of urethra and urinary meatus (753.6)*

● 598.0   **Urethral stricture due to infection**

     598.00   **Due to unspecified infection**

     ▶ 598.01   *Due to infective diseases classified elsewhere*

         Code first underlying disease, as:
            gonococcal infection (098.2)
            schistosomiasis (120.0–120.9)
            syphilis (095.8)

     598.1   **Traumatic urethral stricture**
         Stricture of urethra:
           late effect of injury
           postobstetric

> **Excludes**   *postoperative following surgery on genitourinary tract (598.2)*

     598.2   **Postoperative urethral stricture**
         Postcatheterization stricture of urethra
         Coding Clinic: 1997, Q3, P6

     598.8   **Other specified causes of urethral stricture**
         Coding Clinic: 1984, Nov-Dec, P9

     598.9   **Urethral stricture, unspecified**

● 599   **Other disorders of urethra and urinary tract**

     599.0   **Urinary tract infection, site not specified** 🔵 🔵

> **Excludes**   *Candidiasis of urinary tract (112.2)*
>   *urinary tract infection of newborn (771.82)*

> Use additional code to identify organism, such as Escherichia coli [E. coli] (041.41-041.49)

HAC/ Also excludes the following from acting as a CC/ MCC: 112.2 (CC), 590.10 (CC), 590.11 (MCC), 590.2 (MCC), 590.3 (CC), 590.80 (CC), 590.81 (CC), 595.0 (CC), 597.0 (CC), 996.64 (CC)

Ⓔⓧ 098.2, 098.39, 098.89, 099.40-099.49, 112.2, 131.00, 131.8-131.9, 590.10-591, 593.89-593.9, 595.0-595.9, 599.0, 596.81, 599.60-599.9, 788.1, 996.64

Coding Clinic: 2012, Q2, P20-21; Q1, P11-12; 2011, Q4, P129; 2010, Q1, P11; 2009, Q3, P10x2; 2005, Q3, P12-13; 2004, Q2, P13; 1999, Q4, P6; Q2, P15-16; 1998, Q1, P5; 1996, Q4, P33; 1995, Q2, P7; 1994, Q1, P21; 1992, Q1, P13; 1988, Q4, P10; 1984, Nov-Dec, P15; July-Aug, P19

     599.1   **Urethral fistula** 🔵
         Fistula: Urinary fistula NOS
           urethroperineal
           urethrorectal

> **Excludes**   *fistula:*
>   *urethroscrotal (608.89)*
>   *urethrovaginal (619.0)*
>   *urethrovesicovaginal (619.0)*

Ⓔⓧ 597.0-598.9, 599.1-599.9, 607.1-607.83 607.85-607.9, 608.4-608.81, 608.85, 608.87-608.89, 752.61-752.69, 752.81-752.9, 753.9, 788.1

Coding Clinic: 1997, Q3, P6

     599.2   **Urethral diverticulum**

     599.3   **Urethral caruncle**
         Polyp of urethra

     599.4   **Urethral false passage**

     599.5   **Prolapsed urethral mucosa**
         Prolapse of urethra   Urethrocele

> **Excludes**   *urethrocele, female (618.03, 618.09, 618.2–618.4)*

● 599.6   **Urinary obstruction**

> Use additional code to identify urinary incontinence (625.6, 788.30–788.39)

> **Excludes**   *obstructive nephropathy NOS (593.89)*

Coding Clinic: 2005, Q4, P80-81

     599.60   **Urinary obstruction, unspecified**
         Obstructive uropathy NOS
         Urinary (tract) obstruction NOS

     599.69   **Urinary obstruction, not elsewhere classified**
         Code, if applicable, any causal condition first, such as:
         hyperplasia of prostate (600.0–600.9 with fifth-digit 1)

● 599.7   **Hematuria**
     Hematuria (benign) (essential)

> **Excludes**   *hemoglobinuria (791.2)*

Coding Clinic: 2008, Q4, P121; 2000, Q1, P5; 1995, Q3, P8; 1993, Q1, P26; 5th Issue, P16; 1985, Nov-Dec, P15

     599.70   **Hematuria, unspecified**

     599.71   **Gross hematuria**
         Coding Clinic: 2010, Q2, P3

     599.72   **Microscopic hematuria**

● 599.8   **Other specified disorders of urethra and urinary tract**

> Use additional code to identify urinary incontinence (625.6, 788.30–788.39)

> **Excludes**   *symptoms and other conditions classifiable to 788.0–788.2, 788.4–788.9, 791.0–791.9*

     599.81   **Urethral hypermobility**

     599.82   **Intrinsic (urethral) sphincter deficiency [ISD]**

     599.83   **Urethral instability**

     599.84   **Other specified disorders of urethra**
         Rupture of urethra (nontraumatic)
         Urethral:
           cyst
           granuloma
         Coding Clinic: 2009, Q1, P20

     599.89   **Other specified disorders of urinary tract**

     599.9   **Unspecified disorder of urethra and urinary tract**

(See Plates 366B and 387 on pages 55 and 57.)

DISEASES OF MALE GENITAL ORGANS (600–608)

● 600   **Hyperplasia of prostate**
Benign prostatic hyperplasia (BPH) and is an enlargement of prostate gland usually occurring with age and causing obstructed urine flow

> **Includes**   Enlarged prostate

Coding Clinic: 2005, Q3, P20; 2003, Q4, P63-64; 2002, Q3, P28; 1994, Q3, P12-13; 1992, Q3, P7; 1986, Sept-Oct, P12; Nov-Dec, P10; 1984, Nov-Dec, P9

● 600.0   **Hypertrophy (benign) of prostate**
     Benign prostatic hypertrophy
     Enlargement of prostate
     Smooth enlarged prostate
     Soft enlarged prostate
     Coding Clinic: 2003, Q1, P6; 2001, Q2, P14

     600.00   **Hypertrophy (benign) of prostate without urinary obstruction and other lower urinary tract symptoms (LUTS)** ♂   A
         Hypertrophy (benign) of prostate NOS

     600.01   **Hypertrophy (benign) of prostate with urinary obstruction and other lower urinary tract symptoms (LUTS)** ♂   A
         Hypertrophy (benign) of prostate with urinary retention

> Use additional code to identify symptoms:
>   incomplete bladder emptying (788.21)
>   nocturia (788.43)
>   straining on urination (788.65)
>   urinary frequency (788.41)
>   urinary hesitancy (788.64)
>   urinary incontinence (788.30–788.39)
>   urinary obstruction (599.69)
>   urinary retention (788.20)
>   urinary urgency (788.63)
>   weak urinary stream (788.62)

         Coding Clinic: 2006, Q4, P93-95

● 600.1   **Nodular prostate**
     Hard, firm prostate
     Multinodular prostate

> **Excludes**   *malignant neoplasm of prostate (185)*

     600.10   **Nodular prostate without urinary obstruction** ♂   A
         Nodular prostate NOS

     600.11   **Nodular prostate with urinary obstruction** ♂   A
         Nodular prostate with urinary retention

◀ New   ◀ Revised   ~~deleted~~ Deleted   Excludes   Includes   Use additional   Code first   Omit code

862   ● Unacceptable Principal Diagnosis   ● Use Additional Digit(s)   ▶ Manifestation Code   OGCR Official Guidelines   Coding Clinic

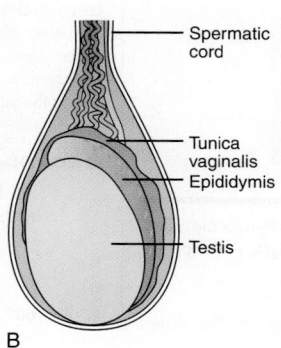

Figure 10–6 **A.** Male genital system. **B.** Testis.

- ● **600.2 Benign localized hyperplasia of prostate**
  Adenofibromatous hypertrophy of prostate
  Adenoma of prostate
  Fibroadenoma of prostate
  Fibroma of prostate
  Myoma of prostate
  Polyp of prostate
  Excludes *benign neoplasms of prostate (222.2)*
  hypertrophy of prostate (600.00–600.01)
  malignant neoplasm of prostate (185)

  600.20 Benign localized hyperplasia of prostate without urinary obstruction and other lower urinary tract symptoms (LUTS) ♂   A
  Benign localized hyperplasia of prostate NOS

  600.21 Benign localized hyperplasia of prostate with urinary obstruction and other lower urinary tract symptoms (LUTS) ♂   A
  Benign localized hyperplasia of prostate with urinary retention
  Use additional code to identify symptoms:
  incomplete bladder emptying (788.21)
  nocturia (788.43)
  straining on urination (788.65)
  urinary frequency (788.41)
  urinary hesitancy (788.64)
  urinary incontinence (788.30–788.39)
  urinary obstruction (599.69)
  urinary retention (788.20)
  urinary urgency (788.63)
  weak urinary stream (788.62)

- **600.3 Cyst of prostate** ♂   A

- ● **600.9 Hyperplasia of prostate, unspecified**
  Median bar
  Prostatic obstruction NOS

  600.90 Hyperplasia of prostate, unspecified, without urinary obstruction and other lower urinary tract symptoms (LUTS) ♂   A
  Hyperplasia of prostate NOS

  600.91 Hyperplasia of prostate, unspecified, with urinary obstruction and other lower urinary tract symptoms (LUTS) ♂   A
  Hyperplasia of prostate, unspecified, with urinary retention
  Use additional code to identify symptoms:
  incomplete bladder emptying (788.21)
  nocturia (788.43)
  straining on urination (788.65)
  urinary frequency (788.41)
  urinary hesitancy (788.64)
  urinary incontinence (788.30–788.39)
  urinary obstruction (599.69)
  urinary retention (788.20)
  urinary urgency (788.63)
  weak urinary stream (788.62)

- ● **601 Inflammatory diseases of prostate**
  Use additional code to identify organism, such as
  Staphylococcus (041.1), or Streptococcus (041.0)

  601.0 Acute prostatitis ♂ 🔴   A
  (Ex) 098.12, 098.32, 098.89, 112.2, 131.00, 131.03, 131.8-131.9, 600.00-602.9

  601.1 Chronic prostatitis ♂   A

  601.2 Abscess of prostate ♂ 🔴   A
  (Ex) 098.12, 098.32, 098.89, 112.2, 131.00, 131.03, 131.8-131.9, 600.00-602.9

  601.3 Prostatocystitis ♂   A

  601.4 *Prostatitis in diseases classified elsewhere* ♂   A
  Code first underlying disease, as:
  actinomycosis (039.8)   syphilis (095.8)
  blastomycosis (116.0)   tuberculosis (016.5)
  Excludes *prostatitis:*
  gonococcal (098.12, 098.32)
  monilial (112.2)
  trichomonal (131.03)

  601.8 Other specified inflammatory diseases of prostate ♂   A
  Prostatitis:
  cavitary
  diverticular
  granulomatous

  601.9 Prostatitis, unspecified ♂   A
  Prostatitis NOS

- ● **602 Other disorders of prostate**
  602.0 Calculus of prostate ♂   A
  Prostatic stone

  602.1 Congestion or hemorrhage of prostate ♂   A

  602.2 Atrophy of prostate ♂   A

  602.3 Dysplasia of prostate ♂
  Prostatic intraepithelial neoplasia I (PIN I)
  Prostatic intraepithelial neoplasia II (PIN II)
  Excludes *prostatic intraepithelial neoplasia III (PIN III)*
  (233.4)

  602.8 Other specified disorders of prostate ♂   A
  Fistula of prostate   Stricture of prostate
  Infarction of prostate   Periprostatic adhesions

  602.9 Unspecified disorder of prostate ♂   A

- ● **603 Hydrocele**
  Includes hydrocele of spermatic cord, testis, or tunica vaginalis
  Excludes *congenital (778.6)*

  603.0 Encysted hydrocele ♂

  603.1 Infected hydrocele ♂ 🔴
  Use additional code to identify organism
  (Ex) 112.2, 131.00, 131.8-131.9, 603.0-603.9

  603.8 Other specified types of hydrocele ♂

  603.9 Hydrocele, unspecified ♂

N Newborn: 0   **P** Pediatric: 0–17   **M** Maternity: 12–55   **A** Adult: 15–124   ♀ Females Only   ♂ Males Only

(Ex) CC/MCC Exclusions   🔴 Complication\Comorbidity   🔴 Major C\C   🔴 Present on Admission Requirement   🔴 Hospital-Acquired Condition   **863**

DISEASES OF THE GENITOURINARY SYSTEM (580–629)

DISEASES OF THE GENITOURINARY SYSTEM (580–629)

Figure 10–7 **A.** Hydrocele. **B.** Newborn with large right hydrocele. (**B** from Behrman: Nelson Textbook of Pediatrics, ed 18, Saunders, An Imprint of Elsevier, 2007)

Item 10–7 Hydrocele is a sac of fluid accumulating in the testes membrane.

● **604 Orchitis and epididymitis**
*An inflammation of one or both testes as a result of mumps or other infection, trauma, or metastasis. **Epididymitis** is an inflammation of the epididymis (the tubular structure that connects testicle with vas deferens).*

Use additional code to identify organism, such as:
Escherichia coli [E. coli] (041.41-041.49)
Staphylococcus (041.10-041.19)
Streptococcus (041.00-041.09)

604.0 Orchitis, epididymitis, and epididymo-orchitis, with abscess ♂ 🔍
Abscess of epididymis or testis
Ex: 072.0, 098.13-098.14, 098.33-098.34, 098.89, 112.2, 131.00, 131.8-131.9, 604.0 -604.99

● **604.9 Other orchitis, epididymitis, and epididymo-orchitis, without mention of abscess**

604.90 Orchitis and epididymitis, unspecified ♂

▸ **604.91 Orchitis and epididymitis in diseases classified elsewhere** ♂
Code first underlying disease, as:
diphtheria (032.89)
filariasis (125.0–125.9)
syphilis (095.8)
Excludes orchitis:
gonococcal (098.13, 098.33)
mumps (072.0)
tuberculous (016.5)
tuberculous epididymitis (016.4)

604.99 Other ♂

605 Redundant prepuce and phimosis ♂
Adherent prepuce   Phimosis (congenital)
Paraphimosis   Tight foreskin
Coding Clinic: 2008, Q3, P9

● **606 Infertility, male**
Coding Clinic: 1996, Q2, P9

606.0 Azoospermia ♂   A
Absolute infertility
Infertility due to:
germinal (cell) aplasia
spermatogenic arrest (complete)

606.1 Oligospermia ♂   A
Infertility due to:
germinal cell desquamation
hypospermatogenesis
incomplete spermatogenic arrest

606.8 Infertility due to extratesticular causes ♂   A
Infertility due to:
drug therapy
infection
obstruction of efferent ducts
radiation
systemic disease

606.9 Male infertility, unspecified ♂   A

Item 10–8 Male infertility is the inability of the female sex partner to conceive after one year of unprotected intercourse. **Azoospermia** is no sperm ejaculated and **oligospermia** is few sperm ejaculated—both resulting in infertility. Extratesticular causes such as injury, infections, radiation, and chemotherapy may also cause male infertility.

● **607 Disorders of penis**
Excludes phimosis (605)

607.0 Leukoplakia of penis ♂
Kraurosis of penis
Excludes carcinoma in situ of penis (233.5)
erythroplasia of Queyrat (233.5)

607.1 Balanoposthitis ♂
Balanitis
Use additional code to identify organism

607.2 Other inflammatory disorders of penis ♂
Abscess of corpus cavernosum or penis
Boil of corpus cavernosum or penis
Carbuncle of corpus cavernosum or penis
Cellulitis of corpus cavernosum or penis
Cavernitis (penis)
Use additional code to identify organism
Excludes herpetic infection (054.13)

607.3 Priapism ♂ 🔍
Painful erection
Ex: 607.0-607.9

● **607.8 Other specified disorders of penis**

607.81 Balanitis xerotica obliterans ♂
Induratio penis plastica

607.82 Vascular disorders of penis ♂ 🔍
Embolism of corpus cavernosum or penis
Hematoma (nontraumatic) of corpus cavernosum or penis
Hemorrhage of corpus cavernosum or penis
Thrombosis of corpus cavernosum or penis
Ex: 607.82-607.83

607.83 Edema of penis ♂

607.84 Impotence of organic origin ♂   A
Excludes nonorganic (302.72)
Coding Clinic: 1985, July-Aug, P9

607.85 Peyronie's disease ♂
Coding Clinic: 2003, Q4, P64-65

607.89 Other ♂
Atrophy of corpus cavernosum or penis
Fibrosis of corpus cavernosum or penis
Hypertrophy of corpus cavernosum or penis
Ulcer (chronic) of corpus cavernosum or penis

607.9 Unspecified disorder of penis ♂

● **608 Other disorders of male genital organs**

608.0 Seminal vesiculitis ♂
Abscess of seminal vesicle
Cellulitis of seminal vesicle
Vesiculitis (seminal)
Use additional code to identify organism
Excludes gonococcal infection (098.14, 098.34)

608.1 Spermatocele ♂

● **608.2 Torsion of testis**
Coding Clinic: 2006, Q4, P95-96

608.20 Torsion of testis, unspecified ♂ 🔍
Ex: 608.20-608.24

608.21 Extravaginal torsion of spermatic cord ♂ 🔍
Ex: 608.20-608.24

608.22 Intravaginal torsion of spermatic cord ♂ 🔍
Torsion of spermatic cord NOS
Ex: 608.20-608.24

608.23 Torsion of appendix testis ♂ 🔍
Ex: 608.20-608.24

608.24 Torsion of appendix epididymis ♂ 🔍
Ex: 608.20-608.24

608.3 Atrophy of testis ♂

◀ New   ◀ Revised   deleted Deleted   Excludes   Includes   Use additional   Code first   Omit code

864   ● Unacceptable Principal Diagnosis   ● Use Additional Digit(s)   ▸ Manifestation Code   OGCR Official Guidelines   **Coding Clinic**

Rotation of spermatic cord

Epididymis

Testis

A   B

Figure 10–8 **A.** Torsion of testis. **B.** Torsion of the testis. (**B** from Kumar: Robbins and Cotran: Pathologic Basis of Disease, ed 8, Saunders, An Imprint of Elsevier, 2009)

Item 10–9 Seminal vesiculitis is an inflammation of the seminal vesicle. Spermatocele is a benign cystic accumulation of sperm arising from the head of the epididymis. Torsion of the testis is a medical emergency occurring most commonly in boys 7 to 12 years of age and results from a congenital abnormality of the covering of the testis allowing the testis to twist within its sac and cutting off the blood supply to the testis.

608.4 **Other inflammatory disorders of male genital organs** ♂
Abscess of scrotum, spermatic cord, testis [except abscess], tunica vaginalis, or vas deferens
Boil of scrotum, spermatic cord, testis [except abscess], tunica vaginalis, or vas deferens
Carbuncle of scrotum, spermatic cord, testis [except abscess], tunica vaginalis, or vas deferens
Cellulitis of scrotum, spermatic cord, testis [except abscess], tunica vaginalis, or vas deferens
Vasitis
Use additional code to identify organism
Excludes *abscess of testis (604.0)*

● **608.8** **Other specified disorders of male genital organs**

▷ *608.81* *Disorders of male genital organs in diseases classified elsewhere* ♂
Code first underlying disease, as:
filariasis (125.0–125.9)
tuberculosis (016.5)

608.82 **Hematospermia** ♂
608.83 **Vascular disorders** ♂
Hematoma (nontraumatic) of seminal vesicle, spermatic cord, testis, scrotum, tunica vaginalis, or vas deferens
Hemorrhage of seminal vesicle, spermatic cord, testis, scrotum, tunica vaginalis, or vas deferens
Thrombosis of seminal vesicle, spermatic cord, testis, scrotum, tunica vaginalis, or vas deferens
Hematocele NOS, male
Coding Clinic: 2003, Q4, P110

608.84 **Chylocele of tunica vaginalis** ♂
608.85 **Stricture** ♂
Stricture of: Stricture of:
spermatic cord   vas deferens
tunica vaginalis

608.86 **Edema** ♂
608.87 **Retrograde ejaculation** ♂
608.89 **Other** ♂
Atrophy of seminal vesicle, spermatic cord, testis, scrotum tunica vaginalis, or vas deferens
Fibrosis of seminal vesicle, spermatic cord, testis, scrotum tunica vaginalis, or vas deferens
Hypertrophy of seminal vesicle, spermatic cord, testis, scrotum tunica vaginalis, or vas deferens
Ulcer of seminal vesicle, spermatic cord, testis, scrotum tunica vaginalis, or vas deferens
Excludes *atrophy of testis (608.3)*

608.9 **Unspecified disorder of male genital organs** ♂

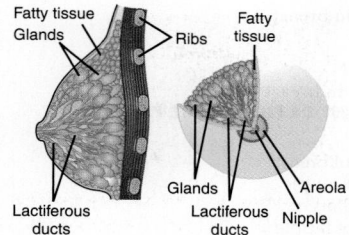
Figure 10–9 Breast.

Fatty tissue
Glands
Ribs
Fatty tissue
Lactiferous ducts
Glands
Lactiferous ducts
Areola
Nipple

DISORDERS OF BREAST (610–612)

● **610** **Benign mammary dysplasias**
Benign lumpiness of the breast

610.0 **Solitary cyst of breast**   A
Cyst (solitary) of breast

610.1 **Diffuse cystic mastopathy**
Chronic cystic mastitis
Cystic breast
Fibrocystic disease of breast
Coding Clinic: 2006, Q2, P10

610.2 **Fibroadenosis of breast**
Fibroadenosis of breast: Fibroadenosis of breast:
NOS   diffuse
chronic   periodic
cystic   segmental

610.3 **Fibrosclerosis of breast**

610.4 **Mammary duct ectasia**
Comedomastitis   Mastitis:
Duct ectasia   periductal
plasma cell

610.8 **Other specified benign mammary dysplasias**
Mazoplasia
Sebaceous cyst of breast
Coding Clinic: 2009, Q2, P9

610.9 **Benign mammary dysplasia, unspecified**

● **611** **Other disorders of breast**
Excludes *that associated with lactation or the puerperium (675.0–676.9)*
Coding Clinic: 2013, Q2, P23

611.0 **Inflammatory disease of breast**
Abscess (acute) (chronic) (nonpuerperal) of:
areola
breast
Mammillary fistula
Mastitis (acute) (subacute) (nonpuerperal):
NOS
infective
retromammary
submammary
Excludes *carbuncle of breast (680.2)*
chronic cystic mastitis (610.1)
neonatal infective mastitis (771.5)
thrombophlebitis of breast [Mondor's disease] (451.89)

611.1 **Hypertrophy of breast**
Gynecomastia
Hypertrophy of breast:
NOS
massive pubertal
Excludes *breast engorgement in newborn (778.7)*
disproportion of reconstructed breast (612.1)

611.2 **Fissure of nipple**
● **611.3** **Fat necrosis of breast**
Fat necrosis (segmental) of breast
Code first breast necrosis due to breast graft (996.79)

611.4 **Atrophy of breast**
611.5 **Galactocele**
611.6 **Galactorrhea not associated with childbirth**
Excessive or spontaneous flow of milk
Coding Clinic: 1985, July-Aug, P9

DISEASES OF THE GENITOURINARY SYSTEM (580–629)

● **611.7 Signs and symptoms in breast**

  611.71 Mastodynia
    Pain in breast

  611.72 Lump or mass in breast
    Coding Clinic: 2009, Q4, P108; 2003, Q2, P3-5

  611.79 Other
    Induration of breast
    Inversion of nipple
    Nipple discharge
    Retraction of nipple

● **611.8 Other specified disorders of breast**
  Coding Clinic: 2008, Q4, P121-122

  611.81 Ptosis of breast   A

    Excludes *ptosis of native breast in relation to*
                reconstructed breast (612.1)

  611.82 Hypoplasia of breast   A
    Micromastia

    Excludes *congenital absence of breast (757.6)*
                hypoplasia of native breast in relation to
                reconstructed breast (612.1)

  611.83 Capsular contracture of breast implant   A

  611.89 Other specified disorders of breast
    Hematoma (nontraumatic) of breast
    Infarction of breast
    Occlusion of breast duct
    Subinvolution of breast (postlactational)
      (postpartum)

  611.9 Unspecified breast disorder

● **612 Deformity and disproportion of reconstructed breast**
  Coding Clinic: 2008, Q4, P123

  612.0 Deformity of reconstructed breast   A
    Contour irregularity in reconstructed breast
    Excess tissue in reconstructed breast
    Misshapen reconstructed breast

  612.1 Disproportion of reconstructed breast   A
    Breast asymmetry between native breast and
      reconstructed breast
    Disproportion between native breast and reconstructed
      breast

(See Plate 366A on page 55.)

INFLAMMATORY DISEASE OF FEMALE PELVIC ORGANS (614–616)

Use additional code to identify organism, such as
  Staphylococcus (041.1), or Streptococcus (041.0)

Excludes *that associated with pregnancy, abortion, childbirth, or*
            the puerperium (630–676.9)

● **614 Inflammatory disease of ovary, fallopian tube, pelvic cellular
tissue, and peritoneum**

  Excludes *endometritis (615.0–615.9)*
              major infection following delivery (670.0-670.8)
              that complicating:
                abortion (634–638 with .0, 639.0)
                ectopic or molar pregnancy (639.0)
                pregnancy or labor (646.6)

  614.0 Acute salpingitis and oophoritis ♀ ◎
    Any condition classifiable to 614.2, specified as acute or
      subacute
    (Ex) 016.60-016.96, 017.90-017.96, 098.15-098.17, 098.35-098.37, 098.89, 112.2,
         131.00, 131.8-131.9, 614.0-615.9, 616.81-616.9, 625.70, 625.79-625.9,
         629.20-629.29, 629.81-629.9, 752.81-752.9

  614.1 Chronic salpingitis and oophoritis ♀
    Hydrosalpinx
    Salpingitis:
      follicularis
      isthmica nodosa
    Any condition classifiable to 614.2, specified as chronic

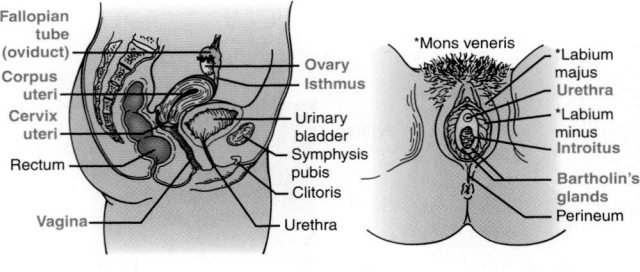

Fallopian
tube
(oviduct)
Corpus
uteri
Cervix
uteri
Rectum
Vagina
Ovary
Isthmus
Urinary
bladder
Symphysis
pubis
Clitoris
Urethra

*Mons veneris
*Labium
majus
Urethra
*Labium
minus
Introitus
Bartholin's
glands
Perineum

A   Female Genital System   B   *The three parts of the vulva

Figure 10–10 A. Female genital system. **B.** External female genital
system. (From Buck CJ: Step-by-Step Medical Coding, ed 2011,
Philadelphia, WB Saunders, 2011)

Item 10-10 Salpingitis is an infection of one or both fallopian tubes.
Oophoritis is an infection of one or both ovaries.

  **614.2 Salpingitis and oophoritis not specified as acute, subacute,
  or chronic ♀**
    Abscess (of):
      fallopian tube
      ovary
      tubo-ovarian
    Oophoritis
    Perioophoritis
    Perisalpingitis
    Pyosalpinx
    Salpingitis
    Salpingo-oophoritis
    Tubo-ovarian inflammatory disease

    Excludes *gonococcal infection (chronic) (098.37)*
                acute (098.17)
                tuberculous (016.6)

  614.3 Acute parametritis and pelvic cellulitis ♀ ◎
    Acute inflammatory pelvic disease
    Any condition classifiable to 614.4, specified as acute
    (Ex) 016.60-016.96, 017.90-017.96, 098.15-098.17, 098.35-098.37, 098.89, 112.2,
         131.00, 131.8-131.9, 614.0-615.9, 616.81-616.9, 625.70, 625.79-625.9,
         629.20-629.29, 629.81-629.9, 752.81-752.9

  614.4 Chronic or unspecified parametritis and pelvic cellulitis ♀
    Abscess (of):
      broad ligament chronic or NOS
      parametrium chronic or NOS
      pelvis, female chronic or NOS
      pouch of Douglas chronic or NOS
    Chronic inflammatory pelvic disease
    Pelvic cellulitis, female

    Excludes *tuberculous (016.7)*

  614.5 Acute or unspecified pelvic peritonitis, female ♀ ◎
    (Ex) 016.60-016.96, 017.90-017.96, 098.15-098.17, 098.35-098.37, 098.89, 112.2,
         131.00, 131.8-131.9, 614.0-615.9, 616.81-616.9, 625.70, 625.79-625.9,
         629.20-629.29, 629.81-629.9, 752.81-752.9

  **614.6 Pelvic peritoneal adhesions, female (postoperative)
  (postinfection) ♀**
    Adhesions:
      peritubal
      tubo-ovarian
    Use additional code to identify any associated infertility
      (628.2)
    Coding Clinic: 2003, Q3, P6-7; Q1, P4-5; 1995, Q3, P7

  614.7 Other chronic pelvic peritonitis, female ♀ ◎

    Excludes *tuberculous (016.7)*
    (Ex) 016.60-016.96, 017.90-017.96, 098.15-098.17, 098.35-098.37, 098.89, 112.2,
         131.00, 131.8-131.9, 614.0-615.9, 616.81-616.9, 625.70, 625.79-625.9,
         629.20-629.29, 629.81-629.9, 752.81-752.9

  **614.8 Other specified inflammatory disease of female pelvic
  organs and tissues ♀**

  **614.9 Unspecified inflammatory disease of female pelvic organs
  and tissues ♀**
    Pelvic infection or inflammation, female NOS
    Pelvic inflammatory disease [PID]

◀ New   ◀▦ Revised   ~~deleted~~ Deleted   Excludes   Includes   Use additional   Code first   Omit code
● Unacceptable Principal Diagnosis   ● Use Additional Digit(s)   ▶ Manifestation Code   OGCR Official Guidelines   Coding Clinic

866

● **615   Inflammatory diseases of uterus, except cervix**
> **Excludes** *following delivery (670.0-670.8)*
> *hyperplastic endometritis (621.30–621.35)*
> *that complicating:*
> *abortion (634–638 with .0, 639.0)*
> *ectopic or molar pregnancy (639.0)*
> *pregnancy or labor (646.6)*

615.0   Acute ♀
> Any condition classifiable to 615.9, specified as acute or subacute
> Ⓔⅹ 016.60-016.96, 017.90-017.96, 098.15-098.17, 098.35-098.37, 098.89, 112.2, 131.00, 131.8-131.9, 614.0-616.0, 616.81-616.9, 621.8-621.9, 625.70, 625.79-625.9, 629.20-629.29, 629.81-629.9, 752.81-752.9

615.1   Chronic ♀
> Any condition classifiable to 615.9, specified as chronic

615.9   Unspecified inflammatory disease of uterus ♀
> Endometritis   Perimetritis
> Endomyometritis   Pyometra
> Metritis   Uterine abscess
> Myometritis

● **616   Inflammatory disease of cervix, vagina, and vulva**
> **Excludes** *that complicating:*
> *abortion (634–638 with .0, 639.0)*
> *ectopic or molar pregnancy (639.0)*
> *pregnancy, childbirth, or the puerperium (646.6)*

616.0   Cervicitis and endocervicitis ♀
> Cervicitis with or without mention of erosion or ectropion
> Endocervicitis with or without mention of erosion or ectropion
> Nabothian (gland) cyst or follicle
> **Excludes** *erosion or ectropion without mention of cervicitis (622.0)*

● **616.1   Vaginitis and vulvovaginitis**
> **Excludes** *vulvar vestibulitis (625.71)*

616.10   Vaginitis and vulvovaginitis, unspecified ♀
> Vaginitis:
> NOS
> postirradiation
> Vulvitis NOS
> Vulvovaginitis NOS
> Use additional code to identify organism, such as:
> Escherichia coli [E. coli] (041.41-041.49)
> Staphylococcus (041.10-041.19)
> Streptococcus (041.00-041.09)
> **Excludes** *noninfective leukorrhea (623.5)*
> *postmenopausal or senile vaginitis (627.3)*

▸ **616.11   Vaginitis and vulvovaginitis in diseases classified elsewhere** ♀
> *Code first* underlying disease, as:
> pinworm vaginitis (127.4)
> **Excludes** *herpetic vulvovaginitis (054.11)*
> *monilial vulvovaginitis (112.1)*
> *trichomonal vaginitis or vulvovaginitis (131.01)*

616.2   Cyst of Bartholin's gland ♀
> *Cysts filled with liquid or semisolid material*
> Bartholin's duct cyst

616.3   Abscess of Bartholin's gland ♀ ⓒ
> *Localized collection of pus*
> Vulvovaginal gland abscess
> Ⓔⅹ 016.70-016.96, 017.90-017.96, 112.1-112.2, 131.00-131.01, 131.8-131.9, 616.10-616.9, 624.3-624.9, 625.70-625.9, 629.20-629.29, 629.81-629.9, 752.81-752.9

616.4   Other abscess of vulva ♀ ⓒ
> Abscess of vulva
> Carbuncle of vulva
> Furuncle of vulva
> Ⓔⅹ 016.70-016.96, 017.90-017.96, 112.1-112.2, 131.00-131.01, 131.8-131.9, 616.10-616.9, 624.3-624.9, 625.70-625.9, 629.20-629.29, 629.81-629.9, 752.81-752.9

616.5   Ulceration of vulva

616.50   Ulceration of vulva, unspecified ♀
> Ulcer NOS of vulva

▸ **616.51   Ulceration of vulva in diseases classified elsewhere** ♀
> *Code first* underlying disease, as:
> Behçet's syndrome (136.1)
> tuberculosis (016.7)
> **Excludes** *vulvar ulcer (in):*
> *gonococcal (098.0)*
> *herpes simplex (054.12)*
> *syphilitic (091.0)*

● **616.8   Other specified inflammatory diseases of cervix, vagina, and vulva**
> **Excludes** *noninflammatory disorders of:*
> *cervix (622.0–622.9)*
> *vagina (623.0–623.9)*
> *vulva (624.0–624.9)*

616.81   Mucositis (ulcerative) of cervix, vagina, and vulva ♀ ⓒ
> Use additional E code to identify adverse effects of therapy, such as:
> antineoplastic and immunosuppressive drugs (E930.7, E933.1)
> radiation therapy (E879.2)
> Ⓔⅹ 616.0, 616.81-616.9

616.89   Other inflammatory disease of cervix, vagina and vulva ♀
> Caruncle, vagina or labium
> Ulcer, vagina

616.9   Unspecified inflammatory disease of cervix, vagina, and vulva ♀

OTHER DISORDERS OF FEMALE GENITAL TRACT (617–629)

● **617   Endometriosis**
Coding Clinic: 1995, Q1, P7

617.0   Endometriosis of uterus ♀
> Adenomyosis
> Endometriosis:
> cervix
> internal
> myometrium
> **Excludes** *stromal endometriosis (236.0)*
> **Coding Clinic: 1992, Q3, P7-8**

617.1   Endometriosis of ovary ♀
> Chocolate cyst of ovary
> Endometrial cystoma of ovary

617.2   Endometriosis of fallopian tube ♀

Intestines   Fallopian tube   Peritoneum
Ovary
Uterus   Vagina

Figure 10–11   Sites of potential endometrial implants.

Item 10–11   Endometriosis is a condition for which no clear cause has been identified. Endometrial tissue is expelled from the uterus into the abdominal cavity and can implant onto a variety of organs. Classification is based on the site of implant of the endometrial tissue.

DISEASES OF THE GENITOURINARY SYSTEM (580–629)

N Newborn: 0   P Pediatric: 0–17   M Maternity: 12–55   A Adult: 15–124   ♀ Females Only   ♂ Males Only
Ⓔⅹ CC/MCC Exclusions   ⓒ Complication\Comorbidity   Major C\C   Present on Admission Requirement   Hospital-Acquired Condition   867

DISEASES OF THE GENITOURINARY SYSTEM (580–629)

617.3 Endometriosis of pelvic peritoneum ♀
   Endometriosis:
      broad ligament
      cul-de-sac (Douglas')
      parametrium
      round ligament

617.4 Endometriosis of rectovaginal septum and vagina ♀

617.5 Endometriosis of intestine ♀
   Endometriosis:
      appendix
      colon
      rectum

617.6 Endometriosis in scar of skin ♀

617.8 Endometriosis of other specified sites ♀
   Endometriosis:
      bladder   umbilicus
      lung   vulva

617.9 Endometriosis, site unspecified ♀

●**618 Genital prolapse**
   Use additional code to identify urinary incontinence (625.6, 788.31, 788.33–788.39)
   Excludes *that complicating pregnancy, labor, or delivery (654.4)*

●**618.0 Prolapse of vaginal walls without mention of uterine prolapse**
   Excludes *that with uterine prolapse (618.2–618.4)*
                enterocele (618.6)
                vaginal vault prolapse following hysterectomy (618.5)
   Coding Clinic: 2004, Q4, P83-85

   618.00 Unspecified prolapse of vaginal walls ♀
      Vaginal prolapse NOS

   618.01 Cystocele, midline ♀
      Cystocele NOS

   618.02 Cystocele, lateral ♀
      Paravaginal

   618.03 Urethrocele ♀

   618.04 Rectocele ♀
      Proctocele
      Use additional code for any associated fecal incontinence (787.60-787.63)

   618.05 Perineocele ♀

   618.09 Other prolapse of vaginal walls without mention of uterine prolapse ♀
      Cystourethrocele

618.1 Uterine prolapse without mention of vaginal wall prolapse ♀
   Descensus uteri
   Uterine prolapse:
      NOS
      complete
      first degree
      second degree
      third degree
   Excludes *that with mention of cystocele, urethrocele, or rectocele (618.2–618.4)*

618.2 Uterovaginal prolapse, incomplete ♀

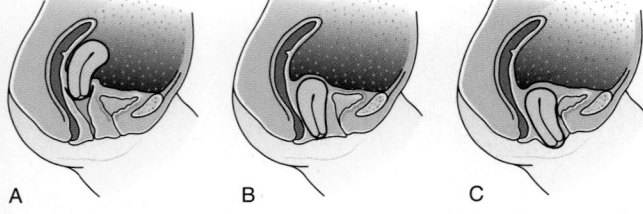

Figure 10–12 Three stages of uterine prolapse. **A.** Uterus is prolapsed. **B.** Vagina and uterus are prolapsed (incomplete uterovaginal prolapse). **C.** Vagina and uterus are completely prolapsed and are exposed through the external genitalia (complete uterovaginal prolapse).

618.3 Uterovaginal prolapse, complete ♀
618.4 Uterovaginal prolapse, unspecified ♀
618.5 Prolapse of vaginal vault after hysterectomy ♀
618.6 Vaginal enterocele, congenital or acquired ♀
   Pelvic enterocele, congenital or acquired
618.7 Old laceration of muscles of pelvic floor ♀
●**618.8 Other specified genital prolapse**
   618.81 Incompetence or weakening of pubocervical tissue ♀
   618.82 Incompetence or weakening of rectovaginal tissue ♀
   618.83 Pelvic muscle wasting ♀
      Disuse atrophy of pelvic muscles and anal sphincter
   618.84 Cervical stump prolapse ♀
   618.89 Other specified genital prolapse ♀
618.9 Unspecified genital prolapse ♀

●**619 Fistula involving female genital tract**
   Excludes *vesicorectal and intestinovesical fistula (596.1)*
619.0 Urinary-genital tract fistula, female ♀ 🔍
   Fistula:
      cervicovesical
      ureterovaginal
      urethrovaginal
      urethrovesicovaginal
      uteroureteric
      uterovesical
      vesicocervicovaginal
      vesicovaginal
   (Ex) 619.0-619.9
619.1 Digestive-genital tract fistula, female ♀ 🔍
   Fistula: Fistula:
      intestinouterine   rectovulval
      intestinovaginal   sigmoidovaginal
      rectovaginal   uterorectal
   (Ex) 619.0-619.9
619.2 Genital tract-skin fistula, female ♀ 🔍
   Fistula:
      uterus to abdominal wall
      vaginoperineal
   (Ex) 619.0-619.9
619.8 Other specified fistulas involving female genital tract ♀ 🔍
   Fistula:
      cervix
      cul-de-sac (Douglas')
      uterus
      vagina
   (Ex) 619.0-619.9
619.9 Unspecified fistula involving female genital tract ♀ 🔍
   (Ex) 619.0-619.9

●**620 Noninflammatory disorders of ovary, fallopian tube, and broad ligament**
   Excludes *hydrosalpinx (614.1)*
620.0 Follicular cyst of ovary ♀
   Cyst of graafian follicle
620.1 Corpus luteum cyst or hematoma ♀
   Corpus luteum hemorrhage or rupture
   Lutein cyst
620.2 Other and unspecified ovarian cyst ♀
   Cyst of ovary:
      NOS
      corpus albicans
      retention NOS
      serous
      theca-lutein
   Simple cystoma of ovary
   Excludes *cystadenoma (benign) (serous) (220)*
                developmental cysts (752.0)
                neoplastic cysts (220)
                polycystic ovaries (256.4)
                Stein-Leventhal syndrome (256.4)

620.3 Acquired atrophy of ovary and fallopian tube ♀
Senile involution of ovary

620.4 Prolapse or hernia of ovary and fallopian tube ♀
Displacement of ovary and fallopian tube
Salpingocele

620.5 Torsion of ovary, ovarian pedicle, or fallopian tube ♀ 🔖
Torsion:
accessory tube
hydatid of Morgagni
Ⓔ 620.0-620.9

620.6 Broad ligament laceration syndrome ♀
Masters-Allen syndrome

620.7 Hematoma of broad ligament ♀
Hematocele, broad ligament

620.8 Other noninflammatory disorders of ovary, fallopian tube, and broad ligament ♀
Cyst of broad ligament or fallopian tube
Polyp of broad ligament or fallopian tube
Infarction of ovary or fallopian tube
Rupture of ovary or fallopian tube
Hematosalpinx of ovary or fallopian tube

> **Excludes** *hematosalpinx in ectopic pregnancy (639.2)*
> *peritubal adhesions (614.6)*
> *torsion of ovary, ovarian pedicle, or fallopian tube (620.5)*

620.9 Unspecified noninflammatory disorder of ovary, fallopian tube, and broad ligament ♀

● **621 Disorders of uterus, not elsewhere classified**

621.0 Polyp of corpus uteri ♀
Polyp:
endometrium
uterus NOS

> **Excludes** *cervical polyp NOS (622.7)*

621.1 Chronic subinvolution of uterus ♀
> **Excludes** *puerperal (674.8)*

621.2 Hypertrophy of uterus ♀
Bulky or enlarged uterus
> **Excludes** *puerperal (674.8)*

● **621.3 Endometrial hyperplasia**
Coding Clinic: 2004, Q4, P85-86

621.30 Endometrial hyperplasia, unspecified ♀
Endometrial hyperplasia NOS
Hyperplasia (adenomatous) (cystic) (glandular) of endometrium
Hyperplastic endometritis

621.31 Simple endometrial hyperplasia without atypia ♀
> **Excludes** *benign endometrial hyperplasia (621.34)*

621.32 Complex endometrial hyperplasia without atypia ♀
> **Excludes** *benign endometrial hyperplasia (621.34)*

621.33 Endometrial hyperplasia with atypia ♀
> **Excludes** *endometrial intraepithelial neoplasia [EIN] (621.35)*

621.34 Benign endometrial hyperplasia ♀

621.35 Endometrial intraepithelial neoplasia [EIN] ♀
> **Excludes** *malignant neoplasm of endometrium with endometrium intraepithelial neoplasia [EIN] (182.0)*

621.4 Hematometra ♀
Hemometra
> **Excludes** *that in congenital anomaly (752.2-752.39)*

621.5 Intrauterine synechiae ♀
Adhesions of uterus   Band(s) of uterus

621.6 Malposition of uterus ♀
Anteversion of uterus
Retroflexion of uterus
Retroversion of uterus

> **Excludes** *malposition complicating pregnancy, labor, or delivery (654.3–654.4)*
> *prolapse of uterus (618.1–618.4)*

621.7 Chronic inversion of uterus ♀
> **Excludes** *current obstetrical trauma (665.2)*
> *prolapse of uterus (618.1–618.4)*

621.8 Other specified disorders of uterus, not elsewhere classified ♀
Atrophy, acquired of uterus
Cyst of uterus
Fibrosis NOS of uterus
Old laceration (postpartum) of uterus
Ulcer of uterus

> **Excludes** *bilharzial fibrosis (120.0–120.9)*
> *endometriosis (617.0)*
> *fistulas (619.0–619.8)*
> *inflammatory diseases (615.0–615.9)*

621.9 Unspecified disorder of uterus ♀

● **622 Noninflammatory disorders of cervix**
> **Excludes** *abnormality of cervix complicating pregnancy, labor, or delivery (654.5–654.6)*
> *fistula (619.0–619.8)*

622.0 Erosion and ectropion of cervix ♀
Eversion of cervix
Ulcer of cervix
> **Excludes** *that in chronic cervicitis (616.0)*

● **622.1 Dysplasia of cervix (uteri)**
> **Excludes** *abnormal results from cervical cytologic examination without histologic confirmation (795.00–795.09)*
> *carcinoma in situ of cervix (233.1)*
> *cervical intraepithelial neoplasia III [CIN III] (233.1)*
> *HGSIL of cervix (795.04)*
Coding Clinic: 2004, Q4, P86-88; 1991, Q1, P11

622.10 Dysplasia of cervix, unspecified ♀
Anaplasia of cervix
Cervical atypism
Cervical dysplasia NOS

622.11 Mild dysplasia of cervix ♀
Cervical intraepithelial neoplasia I [CIN I]

622.12 Moderate dysplasia of cervix ♀
Cervical intraepithelial neoplasia II [CIN II]
> **Excludes** *carcinoma in situ of cervix (233.1)*
> *cervical intraepithelial neoplasia III [CIN III] (233.1)*
> *severe dysplasia (233.1)*

622.2 Leukoplakia of cervix (uteri) ♀
> **Excludes** *carcinoma in situ of cervix (233.1)*

622.3 Old laceration of cervix ♀
Adhesions of cervix
Band(s) of cervix
Cicatrix (postpartum) of cervix
> **Excludes** *current obstetrical trauma (665.3)*

622.4 Stricture and stenosis of cervix ♀
Atresia (acquired) of cervix
Contracture of cervix
Occlusion of cervix
Pinpoint os uteri
> **Excludes** *congenital (752.49)*
> *that complicating labor (654.6)*

DISEASES OF THE GENITOURINARY SYSTEM (580–629)

622.5 Incompetence of cervix ♀
    Excludes *complicating pregnancy (654.5)*
        that affecting fetus or newborn (761.0)

622.6 Hypertrophic elongation of cervix ♀

622.7 Mucous polyp of cervix ♀
    Polyp NOS of cervix
    Excludes *adenomatous polyp of cervix (219.0)*

622.8 Other specified noninflammatory disorders of cervix ♀
    Atrophy (senile) of cervix
    Cyst of cervix
    Fibrosis of cervix
    Hemorrhage of cervix
    Excludes *endometriosis (617.0)*
        fistula (619.0–619.8)
        inflammatory diseases (616.0)

622.9 Unspecified noninflammatory disorder of cervix ♀

● 623 Noninflammatory disorders of vagina
    Excludes *abnormality of vagina complicating pregnancy, labor, or*
        delivery (654.7)
        congenital absence of vagina (752.49)
        congenital diaphragm or bands (752.49)
        fistulas involving vagina (619.0–619.8)

623.0 Dysplasia of vagina ♀
    Mild and moderate dysplasia of vagina
    Vaginal intraepithelial neoplasia I and II [VAIN I and II]
    Excludes *abnormal results from vaginal cytological*
        examination without histologic
        confirmation (795.10-795.19)
        carcinoma in situ of vagina (233.31)
        HGSIL of vagina (795.14)
        severe dysplasia of vagina (233.31)
        vaginal intraepithelial neoplasia III [VAIN III]
        (233.31)

623.1 Leukoplakia of vagina ♀

623.2 Stricture or atresia of vagina ♀
    Adhesions (postoperative) (postradiation) of vagina
    Occlusion of vagina
    Stenosis, vagina
    Use additional E code to identify any external cause
    Excludes *congenital atresia or stricture (752.49)*

623.3 Tight hymenal ring ♀
    Rigid hymen acquired or congenital
    Tight hymenal ring acquired or congenital
    Tight introitus acquired or congenital
    Excludes *imperforate hymen (752.42)*

623.4 Old vaginal laceration ♀
    Excludes *old laceration involving muscles of pelvic floor*
        (618.7)

623.5 Leukorrhea, not specified as infective ♀
    Leukorrhea NOS of vagina
    Vaginal discharge NOS
    Excludes *trichomonal (131.00)*

623.6 Vaginal hematoma ♀
    Excludes *current obstetrical trauma (665.7)*

623.7 Polyp of vagina ♀

623.8 Other specified noninflammatory disorders of vagina ♀
    Cyst of vagina
    Hemorrhage of vagina

623.9 Unspecified noninflammatory disorder of vagina ♀

● 624 Noninflammatory disorders of vulva and perineum
    Excludes *abnormality of vulva and perineum complicating*
        pregnancy, labor, or delivery (654.8)
        condyloma acuminatum (078.11)
        fistulas involving:
        perineum - see Alphabetic Index
        vulva (619.0–619.8)
        vulval varices (456.6)
        vulvar involvement in skin conditions (690–709.9)

● 624.0 Dystrophy of vulva
    Excludes *carcinoma in situ of vulva (233.32)*
        severe dysplasia of vulva (233.32)
        vulvar intraepithelial neoplasia III [VIN III]
        (233.32)

624.01 Vulvar intraepithelial neoplasia I [VIN I] ♀
    Mild dysplasia of vulva

624.02 Vulvar intraepithelial neoplasia II [VIN II] ♀
    Moderate dysplasia of vulva
    Coding Clinic: 2007, Q4, P90-91

624.09 Other dystrophy of vulva ♀
    Kraurosis of vulva
    Leukoplakia of vulva

624.1 Atrophy of vulva ♀

624.2 Hypertrophy of clitoris ♀
    Excludes *that in endocrine disorders (255.2, 256.1)*

624.3 Hypertrophy of labia ♀
    Hypertrophy of vulva NOS

624.4 Old laceration or scarring of vulva ♀

624.5 Hematoma of vulva ♀
    Excludes *that complicating delivery (664.5)*

624.6 Polyp of labia and vulva ♀

624.8 Other specified noninflammatory disorders of vulva and perineum ♀
    Cyst of vulva
    Edema of vulva
    Stricture of vulva
    Coding Clinic: 2003, Q1, P13-14; 1995, Q1, P8

624.9 Unspecified noninflammatory disorder of vulva and perineum ♀

● 625 Pain and other symptoms associated with female genital organs

625.0 Dyspareunia ♀
    Painful intercourse/coitus
    Excludes *psychogenic dyspareunia (302.76)*

625.1 Vaginismus ♀
    Colpospasm
    Vulvismus
    Excludes *psychogenic vaginismus (306.51)*

625.2 Mittelschmerz ♀
    Intermenstrual pain
    Ovulation pain

625.3 Dysmenorrhea ♀
    Painful menstruation
    Excludes *psychogenic dysmenorrhea (306.52)*
    Coding Clinic: 1994, Q2, P12

625.4 Premenstrual tension syndromes ♀
    Menstrual molimen
    Premenstrual dysphoric disorder
    Premenstrual syndrome
    Premenstrual tension NOS
    Excludes *menstrual migraine (346.4)*
    Coding Clinic: 2003, Q4, P116

625.5 Pelvic congestion syndrome ♀
    Congestion-fibrosis syndrome
    Taylor's syndrome

625.6 Stress incontinence, female ♀
    Excludes *mixed incontinence (788.33)*
        stress incontinence, male (788.32)

- **625.7 Vulvodynia**
  - Coding Clinic: 2008, Q4, P124
  - **625.70 Vulvodynia, unspecified ♀**
    - Vulvodynia NOS
  - **625.71 Vulvar vestibulitis ♀**
  - **625.79 Other vulvodynia ♀**
- **625.8 Other specified symptoms associated with female genital organs ♀**
  - Coding Clinic: 1985, Nov-Dec, P16
- **625.9 Unspecified symptom associated with female genital organs ♀**
  - Coding Clinic: 2006, Q4, P109-110; 1994, Q2, P12; 1985, Nov-Dec, P16

- **626 Disorders of menstruation and other abnormal bleeding from female genital tract**
  - **Excludes** *menopausal and premenopausal bleeding (627.0)*
    pain and other symptoms associated with menstrual cycle (625.2–625.4)
    postmenopausal bleeding (627.1)
    precocious puberty (259.1)
  - **626.0 Absence of menstruation ♀**
    - Amenorrhea (primary) (secondary)
    - Coding Clinic: 1985, July-Aug, P9
  - **626.1 Scanty or infrequent menstruation ♀**
    - Hypomenorrhea
    - Oligomenorrhea
  - **626.2 Excessive or frequent menstruation ♀**
    - Heavy periods   Menorrhagia
    - Menometrorrhagia   Polymenorrhea
    - **Excludes** *premenopausal (627.0)*
      that in puberty (626.3)
    - Coding Clinic: 2011, Q4, P147; 2006, Q4, P97-98; 2004, Q4, P88-90; 1994, Q2, P12
  - **626.3 Puberty bleeding ♀**
    - Excessive bleeding associated with onset of menstrual periods
    - Pubertal menorrhagia
  - **626.4 Irregular menstrual cycle ♀**
    - Irregular: Irregular:
    - bleeding NOS   periods
    - menstruation
  - **626.5 Ovulation bleeding ♀**
    - Regular intermenstrual bleeding
  - **626.6 Metrorrhagia ♀**
    - Bleeding unrelated to menstrual cycle
    - Irregular intermenstrual bleeding
  - **626.7 Postcoital bleeding ♀**
  - **626.8 Other ♀**
    - Dysfunctional or functional uterine hemorrhage NOS
    - Menstruation: Menstruation:
    - retained   suppression of
  - **626.9 Unspecified ♀**

- **627 Menopausal and postmenopausal disorders**
  - **Excludes** *asymptomatic age-related (natural) postmenopausal status (V49.81)*
  - **627.0 Premenopausal menorrhagia ♀**
    - Excessive bleeding associated with onset of menopause
    - Menorrhagia: Menorrhagia:
    - climacteric   preclimacteric
    - menopausal
  - **627.1 Postmenopausal bleeding ♀**
  - **627.2 Symptomatic menopausal or female climacteric states ♀**
    - Symptoms, such as flushing, sleeplessness, headache, lack of concentration, associated with the menopause
  - **627.3 Postmenopausal atrophic vaginitis ♀**
    - Senile (atrophic) vaginitis
  - **627.4 Symptomatic states associated with artificial menopause ♀**
    - Postartificial menopause syndromes
    - Any condition classifiable to 627.1, 627.2, or 627.3 which follows induced menopause

- **627.8 Other specified menopausal and postmenopausal disorders ♀**
  - **Excludes** *premature menopause NOS (256.31)*
- **627.9 Unspecified menopausal and postmenopausal disorder ♀**

- **628 Infertility, female**
  - **Includes** primary and secondary sterility
  - Coding Clinic: 1996, Q2, P9; 1995, Q1, P7
  - **628.0 Associated with anovulation**
    - Anovulatory cycle
    - Use additional code for any associated Stein-Leventhal syndrome (256.4)
  - **628.1 *Of pituitary-hypothalamic origin* ♀**
    - *Code first underlying disease, as:*
      - adiposogenital dystrophy (253.8)
      - anterior pituitary disorder (253.0–253.4)
  - **628.2 Of tubal origin ♀**
    - Infertility associated with congenital anomaly of tube
    - Tubal: Tubal:
    - block   stenosis
    - occlusion
    - Use additional code for any associated peritubal adhesions (614.6)
  - **628.3 Of uterine origin ♀**
    - Infertility associated with congenital anomaly of uterus
    - Nonimplantation
    - Use additional code for any associated tuberculous endometritis (016.7)
  - **628.4 Of cervical or vaginal origin ♀**
    - Infertility associated with:
      - anomaly or cervical mucus
      - congenital structural anomaly
      - dysmucorrhea
  - **628.8 Of other specified origin ♀**
  - **628.9 Of unspecified origin ♀**

- **629 Other disorders of female genital organs**
  - **629.0 Hematocele, female, not elsewhere classified ♀**
    - **Excludes** *hematocele or hematoma:*
      broad ligament (620.7)
      fallopian tube (620.8)
      that associated with ectopic pregnancy (633.00–633.91)
      uterus (621.4)
      vagina (623.6)
      vulva (624.5)
  - **629.1 Hydrocele, canal of Nuck ♀**
    - Cyst of canal of Nuck (acquired)
    - **Excludes** *congenital (752.41)*
  - **629.2 Female genital multilation status**
    - Female circumcision status
    - Female genital cutting
    - **629.20 Female genital mutilation status, unspecified ♀**
      - Female genital cutting status, unspecified
      - Female genital mutilation status NOS
    - **629.21 Female genital mutilation Type I status ♀**
      - Clitorectomy status
      - Female genital cutting Type I status
    - **629.22 Female genital mutilation Type II status ♀**
      - Clitorectomy with excision of labia minora status
      - Female genital cutting Type II status
      - Coding Clinic: 2004, Q4, P88-90
    - **629.23 Female genital mutilation Type III status ♀**
      - Female genital cutting Type III status
      - Infibulation status
    - **629.29 Other female genital mutilation status ♀**
      - Female genital cutting Type IV status
      - Female genital mutilation Type IV status
      - Other female genital cutting status

N Newborn: 0   **P** Pediatric: 0–17   **M** Maternity: 12–55   **A** Adult: 15–124   ♀ Females Only   ♂ Males Only

(Ex.) CC/MCC Exclusions   Complication\Comorbidity   Major C\C   Present on Admission Requirement   Hospital-Acquired Condition   **871**

DISEASES OF THE GENITOURINARY SYSTEM (580–629)

● **629.3 Complication of implanted vaginal mesh and other prosthetic materials**

     629.31 Erosion of implanted vaginal mesh and other prosthetic materials to surrounding organ or tissue ♀

         Erosion of implanted vaginal mesh and other prosthetic materials into pelvic floor muscles

     629.32 Exposure of implanted vaginal mesh and other prosthetic materials into vagina ♀

         Exposure of vaginal mesh and other prosthetic materials through vaginal wall

● **629.8 Other specified disorders of female genital organs**

     629.81 Recurrent pregnancy loss without current pregnancy ♀

         Excludes *recurrent pregnancy loss with current pregnancy (646.3)*

         Coding Clinic: 2006, Q4, P98

     629.89 Other specified disorders of female genital organs ♀

629.9 Unspecified disorder of female genital organs ♀

◀ New   ◀▥ Revised   ~~deleted~~ Deleted   Excludes   Includes   Use additional   Code first   Omit code

872   ● Unacceptable Principal Diagnosis   ● Use Additional Digit(s)   ▶ Manifestation Code   OGCR Official Guidelines   Coding Clinic

(See Plate 375 on page 56.)

Figure 11-1 Implantation sites of ectopic pregnancy.

Item 11-1 Ectopic pregnancy most often occurs in the fallopian tube. Pregnancy outside the uterus may end in a life-threatening rupture.

Item 11-2 A hydatidiform mole is a benign tumor of the placenta. The tumor secretes a hormone, chorionic gonadotropic hormone (CGH), that indicates a positive pregnancy test.

OGCR Section I.C.11.a.1

> Obstetric cases require codes from chapter 11, codes in the range 630-679, Complications of Pregnancy, Childbirth, and the Puerperium. Chapter 11 codes have sequencing priority over codes from other chapters. Additional codes from other chapters may be used in conjunction with chapter 11 codes to further specify conditions. Should the provider document that the pregnancy is incidental to the encounter, then code V22.2 should be used in place of any chapter 11 codes. It is the provider's responsibility to state that the condition being treated is not affecting the pregnancy.

11. COMPLICATIONS OF PREGNANCY, CHILDBIRTH, AND THE PUERPERIUM (630–679)

ECTOPIC AND MOLAR PREGNANCY (630–633)

Use additional code from category 639 to identify any complications

630   **Hydatidiform mole** ♀   M
      Trophoblastic disease NOS
      Vesicular mole
      Excludes *chorioadenoma (destruens) (236.1)*
      chorionepithelioma (181)
      malignant hydatidiform mole (236.1)

● 631   **Other abnormal product of conception**
      631.0   **Inappropriate change in quantitative human chorionic gonadotropin (hCG) in early pregnancy** ♀   M
              Biochemical pregnancy
              Chemical pregnancy
              Inappropriate level of quantitative human chorionic gonadotropin (hCG) for gestational age in early pregnancy
              Excludes *blighted ovum (631.8)*
              molar pregnancy (631.8)
      631.8   **Other abnormal products of conception** ♀   M
              Blighted ovum

632   **Missed abortion** ♀   M
      Early fetal death before completion of 22 weeks' gestation with retention of dead fetus
      Retained products of conception, not following spontaneous or induced abortion or delivery
      Excludes *failed induced abortion (638.0–638.9)*
      fetal death (intrauterine) (late) (656.4)
      missed delivery (656.4)
      that with hydatidiform mole (630)
      that with other abnormal products of conception (631.8)
      Coding Clinic: 2001, Q1, P5

● 633   **Ectopic pregnancy**
      Includes   ruptured ectopic pregnancy
      Coding Clinic: 2002, Q4, P61-62
      ● 633.0   **Abdominal pregnancy**
              Intraperitoneal pregnancy
              633.00   **Abdominal pregnancy without intrauterine pregnancy** ♀ 🔖   M
                       Ⓔx 633.01, 633.11-633.91
              633.01   **Abdominal pregnancy with intrauterine pregnancy** ♀ 🔖   M
                       Ⓔx 633.00-633.91
      ● 633.1   **Tubal pregnancy**
              Fallopian pregnancy
              Rupture of (fallopian) tube due to pregnancy
              Tubal abortion
              633.10   **Tubal pregnancy without intrauterine pregnancy** ♀ 🔖   M
                       Ⓔx 633.00-633.91
              633.11   **Tubal pregnancy with intrauterine pregnancy** ♀ 🔖   M
                       Ⓔx 633.00-633.91
      ● 633.2   **Ovarian pregnancy**
              633.20   **Ovarian pregnancy without intrauterine pregnancy** ♀ 🔖   M
                       Ⓔx 633.00-633.91
              633.21   **Ovarian pregnancy with intrauterine pregnancy** ♀ 🔖   M
                       Ⓔx 633.00-633.91
      ● 633.8   **Other ectopic pregnancy**
              Pregnancy:
                cervical
                combined
                cornual
                intraligamentous
                mesometric
                mural
              633.80   **Other ectopic pregnancy without intrauterine pregnancy** ♀ 🔖   M
                       Ⓔx 633.00-633.91
              633.81   **Other ectopic pregnancy with intrauterine pregnancy** ♀ 🔖   M
                       Ⓔx 633.00-633.91
      ● 633.9   **Unspecified ectopic pregnancy**
              633.90   **Unspecified ectopic pregnancy without intrauterine pregnancy** ♀ 🔖   M
                       Ⓔx 633.00-633.91
              633.91   **Unspecified ectopic pregnancy with intrauterine pregnancy** ♀ 🔖   M
                       Ⓔx 633.00-633.91

COMPLICATIONS OF PREGNANCY, CHILDBIRTH, AND THE PUERPERIUM (630–679)

OTHER PREGNANCY WITH ABORTIVE OUTCOME (634–639)

The following fourth digit subdivisions are for use with categories 634–638:

0 Complicated by genital tract and pelvic infection
   Endometritis
   Salpingo-oophoritis
   Sepsis NOS
   Septicemia NOS
   Any condition classifiable to 639.0, with condition classifiable to 634–638
   Excludes *urinary tract infection (634–638 with .7)*

1 Complicated by delayed or excessive hemorrhage
   Afibrinogenemia
   Defibrination syndrome
   Intravascular hemolysis
   Any condition classifiable to 639.1, with condition classifiable to 634–638

2 Complicated by damage to pelvic organs and tissues
   Laceration, perforation, or tear of:
     bladder
     uterus
   Any condition classifiable to 639.2, with condition classifiable to 634–638

3 Complicated by renal failure
   Oliguria
   Uremia
   Any condition classifiable to 639.3, with condition classifiable to 634–638

4 Complicated by metabolic disorder
   Electrolyte imbalance with conditions classifiable to 634–638

5 Complicated by shock
   Circulatory collapse
   Shock (postoperative) (septic)
   Any condition classifiable to 639.5, with condition classifiable to 634–638

6 Complicated by embolism
   Embolism:
     NOS
     amniotic fluid
     pulmonary
   Any condition classifiable to 639.6, with condition classifiable to 634–638

7 With other specified complications
   Cardiac arrest or failure
   Urinary tract infection
   Any condition classifiable to 639.8, with condition classifiable to 634–638

8 With unspecified complications

9 Without mention of complication

OGCR   Section I.C.11.k.1

Fifth-digits are required for abortion categories 634-637. Fifth digit assignment is based on the status of the patient at the beginning (or start) of the encounter. Fifth-digit 1, incomplete, indicates that all of the products of conception have not been expelled from the uterus. Fifth-digit 2, complete, indicates that all products of conception have been expelled from the uterus.

OGCR   Section I.C.11.k.5

Subsequent admissions for retained products of conception following a spontaneous or legally induced abortion are assigned the appropriate code from category 634, Spontaneous abortion, or 635 Legally induced abortion, with a fifth digit of "1" (incomplete). This advice is appropriate even when the patient was discharged previously with a discharge diagnosis of complete abortion.

● **634 Spontaneous abortion**
   Requires fifth digit to identify stage:

> 0   **unspecified**
> 1   **incomplete**
> 2   **complete**

   Includes   miscarriage
               spontaneous abortion

● **634.0 Complicated by genital tract and pelvic infection** ♀   M
[0-2]   (Ex:) 634.00-638.9, 640.00-641.23, 646.80-646.93, 648.90-649.64, 650, 669.40-669.44, 669.80-669.94, 679.00-679.04, 679.12, 679.14

● **634.1 Complicated by delayed or excessive hemorrhage** ♀   M
[0-2]   **Coding Clinic: 2003, Q1, P6**

● **634.2 Complicated by damage to pelvic organs or tissues** ♀   M
[0-2]   (Ex:) 634.00-638.9, 640.00-641.23, 646.80-646.93, 648.90-649.64, 650, 669.40-669.44, 669.80-669.94, 679.00-679.04, 679.12, 679.14

● **634.3 Complicated by renal failure** ♀   M
[0-2]   (Ex:) 634.00-638.9, 640.00-641.23, 646.80-646.93, 648.90-649.64, 650, 669.40-669.44, 669.80-669.94, 679.00-679.04, 679.12, 679.14

● **634.4 Complicated by metabolic disorder** ♀   M
[0-2]   (Ex:) 634.00-638.9, 640.00-641.23, 646.80-646.93, 648.90-649.64, 650, 669.40-669.44, 669.80-669.94, 679.00-679.04, 679.12, 679.14

● **634.5 Complicated by shock** ♀   M
[0-2]   (Ex:) 634.00-638.9, 640.00-641.23, 646.80-646.93, 648.90-649.64, 650, 669.40-669.44, 669.80-669.94, 679.00-679.04, 679.12, 679.14

● **634.6 Complicated by embolism** ♀ 0, 1,2   M
[0-2]   (Ex:) 634.00-638.9, 640.00-641.23, 646.80-646.93, 648.90-649.64, 650, 669.40-669.44, 669.80-669.94, 679.00-679.04, 679.12, 679.14

● **634.7 With other specified complications** ♀   M
[0-2]   (Ex:) 634.00-638.9, 640.00-641.23, 646.80-646.93, 648.90-649.64, 650, 669.40-669.44, 669.80-669.94, 679.00-679.04, 679.12, 679.14

● **634.8 With unspecified complication** ♀   M
[0-2]   (Ex:) 634.00-638.9, 640.00-641.23, 646.80-646.93, 648.90-649.64, 650, 669.40-669.44, 669.80-669.94, 679.00-679.04, 679.12, 679.14

● **634.9 Without mention of complication** ♀   M
[0-2]

● **635 Legally induced abortion**
   Requires fifth digit to identify stage:

> 0   **unspecified**
> 1   **incomplete**
> 2   **complete**

   Includes   abortion or termination of pregnancy:
               elective
               legal
               therapeutic

   Excludes *menstrual extraction or regulation (V25.3)*

● **635.0 Complicated by genital tract and pelvic infection** ♀   M
[0-2]   (Ex:) 634.00-635.02, 635.20-635.22, 635.70-638.9, 640.00-641.23, 646.80-646.93, 648.90-649.64, 650, 669.40-669.44, 669.80-669.94, 679.00-679.04, 679.12, 679.14

● **635.1 Complicated by delayed or excessive hemorrhage** ♀   M
[0-2]

● **635.2 Complicated by damage to pelvic organs or tissues** ♀   M
[0-2]   For code **635.20**: (Ex:) 634.00-638.9, 640.00-641.23, 646.80-646.93, 648.90-649.64, 650, 669.40-669.44, 669.80-669.94, 679.00-679.04, 679.12, 679.14;
     For code **635.21**: (Ex:) 634.00-635.62, 638.5-638.9, 640.00-641.00;
     For code **635.22**: (Ex:) 635.22

● **635.3 Complicated by renal failure** ♀   M
[0-2]   For code **635.30**: (Ex:) 635.30-635.32;
     For code **635.31**: (Ex:) 635.30-635.32, 637.11-638.9, 640.00-641.23, 646.80-646.93, 648.90-649.64, 650, 669.40-669.44, 669.80-669.94, 679.00-679.04, 679.12, 679.14;
     For code **635.32**: (Ex:) 634.00-634.92, 635.30-635.32, 635.70-638.9, 640.00-641.23, 646.80-646.93, 648.90-649.64, 650, 669.40-669.44, 669.80-669.94, 679.00-679.04, 679.12, 679.14

◄ New   ◄ Revised   ~~deleted~~ Deleted   Excludes   Includes   Use additional   Code first   Omit code

874   ● Unacceptable Principal Diagnosis   ● Use Additional Digit(s)   ▷ Manifestation Code   **OGCR** Official Guidelines   **Coding Clinic**

● **635.4 Complicated by metabolic disorder** ♀ 🐾   **M**
[0-2]   (Ex) 634.00-638.9, 640.00-641.23, 646.80-646.93, 648.90-649.64, 650, 669.40-669.44, 669.80-669.94, 679.00-679.04, 679.12, 679.14

● **635.5 Complicated by shock** ♀ 🐾   **M**
[0-2]   (Ex) 634.00 -634.92, 635.50-635.52, 635.70-638.9, 640.00-641.23, 646.80-646.93, 648.90-649.64, 650, 669.40-669.44, 669.80-669.94, 679.00-679.04, 679.12, 679.14

● **635.6 Complicated by embolism** ♀ 🐾   **M**
[0-2]   (Ex) 634.00-634.92, 635.60-638.9, 640.00-641.23, 646.80-646.93, 648.90-649.64, 650, 669.40-669.44, 669.80-669.94, 679.00-679.04, 679.12, 679.14

● **635.7 With other specified complications** ♀   **M**
[0-2]   (Ex) 634.00-638.9, 640.00-641.23, 646.80-646.93, 648.90-649.64, 650, 669.40-669.44, 669.80-669.94, 679.00-679.04, 679.12, 679.14

● **635.8 With unspecified complication** ♀ 🐾   **M**
[0-2]   (Ex) 634.00-638.9, 640.00-641.23, 646.80-646.93, 648.90-649.64, 650, 669.40-669.44, 669.80-669.94, 679.00-679.04, 679.12, 679.14

● **635.9 Without mention of complication** ♀   **M**
[0-2]   **Coding Clinic: 2010, Q2, P7; 1994, Q2, P14**

● **636 Illegally induced abortion**
Requires fifth digit to identify stage:

0	unspecified
1	incomplete
2	complete

   Includes   abortion:
             criminal
             illegal
             self-induced

● **636.0 Complicated by genital tract and pelvic**   **M**
[0-2] **infection** ♀ 🐾
  (Ex) 634.00-636.02, 636.70-638.9, 640.00-641.23, 646.80-646.93, 648.90-649.64, 650, 669.40-669.44, 669.80-669.94, 679.00-679.04, 679.12, 679.14

● **636.1 Complicated by delayed or excessive hemorrhage** ♀   **M**
[0-2]

● **636.2 Complicated by damage to pelvic organs or**   **M**
[0-2] **tissues** ♀ 🐾
  (Ex) 634.00-638.9, 640.00-641.23, 646.80-646.93, 648.90-649.64, 650, 669.40-669.44, 669.80-669.94, 679.00-679.04, 679.12, 679.14

● **636.3 Complicated by renal failure** ♀ 🐾   **M**
[0-2]   (Ex) 634.00-635.92, 636.30-636.32, 636.70-638.9, 640.00-641.23, 646.80-646.93, 648.90-649.64, 650, 669.40-669.44, 669.80-669.94, 679.00-679.04, 679.12, 679.14

● **636.4 Complicated by metabolic disorder** ♀ 🐾   **M**
[0-2]   (Ex) 634.00-638.9, 640.00-641.23, 646.80-646.93, 648.90-649.64, 650, 669.40-669.44, 669.80-669.94, 679.00-679.04, 679.12, 679.14

● **636.5 Complicated by shock** ♀ 🐾   **M**
[0-2]   For codes **635.50-635.51:** (Ex) 634.00-635.92, 636.50-636.52, 636.70-638.9, 640.00-641.23, 646.80-646.93, 648.90-649.64, 650, 669.40-669.44, 669.80-669.94, 679.00-679.04, 679.12, 679.14;
For code **636.52:** (Ex) 634.00-635.92, 636.50-636.52, 636.70-636.92, 637.50-637.52, 637.70-637.92, 638.5, 638.7-638.9, 640.00-641.23, 646.80-646.93, 648.90-649.64, 650, 669.40-669.44, 669.80-669.94, 679.00-679.04, 679.12, 679.14

● **636.6 Complicated by embolism** ♀ 🐾   **M**
[0-2]   (Ex) 634.00-635.92, 636.60-638.9, 640.00-641.23, 646.80-646.93, 648.90-649.64, 650, 669.40-669.44, 669.80-669.94, 679.00-679.04, 679.12, 679.14

● **636.7 With other specified complications** ♀ 🐾   **M**
[0-2]   (Ex) 634.00-638.9, 640.00-641.23, 646.80-646.93, 648.90-649.64, 650, 669.40-669.44, 669.80-669.94, 679.00-679.04, 679.12, 679.14

● **636.8 With unspecified complication** ♀ 🐾   **M**
[0-2]   (Ex) 634.00-638.9, 640.00-641.23, 646.80-646.93, 648.90-649.64, 650, 669.40-669.44, 669.80-669.94, 679.00-679.04, 679.12, 679.14

● **636.9 Without mention of complication** ♀   **M**
[0-2]

● **637 Unspecified abortion**
Requires following fifth digit to identify stage:
Coding Clinic: 1994, Q2, P14

0	unspecified
1	incomplete
2	complete

   Includes   abortion NOS
         retained products of conception following abortion, not classifiable elsewhere

● **637.0 Complicated by genital tract and pelvic**   **M**
[0-2] **infection** ♀ 🐾
  (Ex) 634.00-637.02, 637.70-638.9, 640.00-641.23, 646.80-646.93, 648.90-649.64, 650, 669.40-669.44, 669.80-669.94, 679.00-679.04, 679.12, 679.14

● **637.1 Complicated by delayed or excessive hemorrhage** ♀   **M**
[0-2]

● **637.2 Complicated by damage to pelvic organs or**   **M**
[0-2] **tissues** ♀ 🐾
  (Ex) 634.00-638.9, 640.00-641.23, 646.80-646.93, 648.90-649.64, 650, 669.40-669.44, 669.80-669.94, 679.00-679.04, 679.12, 679.14

● **637.3 Complicated by renal failure** ♀ 🐾   **M**
[0-2]   (Ex) 634.00-636.92, 637.30-637.32, 637.70-638.9, 640.00-641.23, 646.80-646.93, 648.90-649.64, 650, 669.40-669.44, 669.80-669.94, 679.00-679.04, 679.12, 679.14

● **637.4 Complicated by metabolic disorder** ♀ 🐾   **M**
[0-2]   (Ex) 634.00-638.9, 640.00-641.23, 646.80-646.93, 648.90-649.64, 650, 669.40-669.44, 669.80-669.94, 679.00-679.04, 679.12, 679.14

● **637.5 Complicated by shock** ♀ 🐾   **M**
[0-2]   (Ex) 634.00-636.92, 637.50-637.52, 637.70-638.9, 640.00-641.23, 646.80-646.93, 648.90-649.64, 650, 669.40-669.44, 669.80-669.94, 679.00-679.04, 679.12, 679.14

● **637.6 Complicated by embolism** ♀ 🐾   **M**
[0-2]   For codes **637.60-637.61:** (Ex) 634.00-636.92, 637.60-638.9, 640.00-641.23, 646.80-646.93, 648.90-649.64, 650, 669.40-669.44, 669.80-669.94, 679.00-679.04, 679.12, 679.14;
For code **637.62:** (Ex) 634.00-636.02, 636.11-636.92, 637.60-638.9, 640.00-641.23, 646.80-646.93, 648.90-649.64, 650, 669.40-669.44, 669.80-669.94, 679.00-679.04, 679.12, 679.14

● **637.7 With other specified complications** ♀ 🐾   **M**
[0-2]   (Ex) 634.00-638.9, 640.00-641.23, 646.80-646.93, 648.90-649.64, 650, 669.40-669.44, 669.80-669.94, 679.00-679.04, 679.12, 679.14

● **637.8 With unspecified complication** ♀ 🐾   **M**
[0-2]   (Ex) 634.00-638.9, 640.00-641.23, 646.80-646.93, 648.90-649.64, 650, 669.40-669.44, 669.80-669.94, 679.00-679.04, 679.12, 679.14

● **637.9 Without mention of complication** ♀   **M**
[0-2]

● **638 Failed attempted abortion**
   Includes   failure of attempted induction of (legal) abortion
   Excludes   *incomplete abortion (634.0–637.9)*

638.0 Complicated by genital tract and pelvic   **M**
infection ♀ 🐾
  (Ex) 634.00-638.0, 638.7-638.9, 640.00-641.23, 646.80-646.93, 648.90-649.64, 650, 669.40-669.44, 669.80-669.94, 679.00-679.04, 679.12, 679.14

638.1 Complicated by delayed or excessive   **M**
hemorrhage ♀
  (Ex) 634.00-637.92, 638.1, 638.7-638.9, 640.00-641.23, 646.80-646.93, 648.90-649.64, 650, 669.40-669.44, 669.80-669.94, 679.00-679.04, 679.12, 679.14

638.2 Complicated by damage to pelvic organs or   **M**
tissues ♀ 🐾
  (Ex) 634.00-637.92, 638.2, 638.7-638.9, 640.00-641.23, 646.80-646.93, 648.90-649.64, 650, 669.40-669.44, 669.80-669.94, 679.00-679.04, 679.12, 679.14

638.3 Complicated by renal failure ♀ 🐾   **M**
  (Ex) 634.00-637.92, 638.3, 638.7-638.9, 640.00-641.23, 646.80-646.93, 648.90-649.64, 650, 669.40-669.44, 669.80-669.94, 679.00-679.04, 679.12, 679.14

N Newborn: 0   **P** Pediatric: 0–17   **M** Maternity: 12–55   **A** Adult: 15–124   ♀ Females Only   ♂ Males Only

(Ex) CC/MCC Exclusions   🐾 Complication\Comorbidity   🐾 Major C\C   🐾 Present on Admission Requirement   🐾 Hospital-Acquired Condition   **875**

638.4   Complicated by metabolic disorder ♀ 🐾   M
(Ex:) 634.00-638.9, 640.00-641.23, 646.80-646.93, 648.90-649.64, 650, 669.40-669.44, 669.80-669.94, 679.00-679.04, 679.12, 679.14

638.5   Complicated by shock ♀ 🐾   M
(Ex:) 634.00-637.12, 637.21-637.92, 638.4-638.5, 638.7-638.9, 640.00-641.23, 646.80-646.93, 648.90-649.64, 650, 669.40-669.44, 669.80-669.94, 679.00-679.04, 679.12, 679.14

638.6   Complicated by embolism ♀ 🐾   M
(Ex:) 634.00-637.92, 638.6-638.9, 640.00-641.23, 646.80-646.93, 648.90-649.64, 650, 669.40-669.44, 669.80-669.94, 679.00-679.04, 679.12, 679.14

638.7   With other specified complications ♀ 🐾   M
(Ex:) 634.00-638.9, 640.00-641.23, 646.80-646.93, 648.90-649.64, 650, 669.40-669.44, 669.80-669.94, 679.00-679.04, 679.12, 679.14

638.8   With unspecified complication ♀ 🐾   M
(Ex:) 634.00-638.9, 640.00-641.23, 646.80-646.93, 648.90-649.64, 650, 669.40-669.44, 669.80-669.94, 679.00-679.04, 679.12, 679.14

638.9   Without mention of complication ♀   M

● **639   Complications following abortion and ectopic and molar pregnancies**

> **Note:** This category is provided for use when it is required to classify separately the complications classifiable to the fourth digit level in categories 634–638; for example:
> a) when the complication itself was responsible for an episode of medical care, the abortion, ectopic or molar pregnancy itself having been dealt with at a previous episode
> b) when these conditions are immediate complications of ectopic or molar pregnancies classifiable to 630–633 where they cannot be identified at fourth digit level.

> **OGCR   Section I.C.11.k.3**
> Code 639 is to be used for all complications following abortion. Code 639 cannot be assigned with codes from categories 634-638.

639.0   Genital tract and pelvic infection ♀ 🐾   M
Endometritis following conditions classifiable to 630–638
Parametritis following conditions classifiable to 630–638
Pelvic peritonitis following conditions classifiable to 630–638
Salpingitis following conditions classifiable to 630–638
Salpingo-oophoritis following conditions classifiable to 630–638
Sepsis NOS following conditions classifiable to 630–638
Septicemia NOS following conditions classifiable to 630–638

> **Excludes**   *urinary tract infection (639.8)*

(Ex:) 639.0, 639.2-641.23, 646.80-646.93, 648.90-649.64, 650, 669.40-669.44, 669.80-669.94, 679.00-679.04, 679.12, 679.14

639.1   Delayed or excessive hemorrhage ♀ 🐾   M
Afibrinogenemia following conditions classifiable to 630–638
Defibrination syndrome following conditions classifiable to 630–638
Intravascular hemolysis following conditions classifiable to 630–638

(Ex:) 639.1-641.23, 646.80-646.93, 648.90-649.64, 650, 669.40-669.44, 669.80-669.94, 679.00-679.04, 679.12, 679.14

639.2   Damage to pelvic organs and tissues ♀ 🐾   M
Laceration, perforation, or tear of:
bladder following conditions classifiable to 630–638
bowel following conditions classifiable to 630–638
broad ligament following conditions classifiable to 630–638
cervix following conditions classifiable to 630–638
periurethral tissue following conditions classifiable to 630–638
uterus following conditions classifiable to 630–638
vagina following conditions classifiable to 630–638

(Ex:) 639.2-641.23, 646.80-646.93, 648.90-649.64, 650, 669.40-669.44, 669.80-669.94, 679.00-679.04, 679.12, 679.14

639.3   Kidney failure ♀ 🐾   M
Oliguria following conditions classifiable to 630–638
Renal (kidney):
failure (acute) following conditions classifiable to 630–638
shutdown following conditions classifiable to 630–638
tubular necrosis following conditions classifiable to 630–638
Uremia following conditions classifiable to 630–638

(Ex:) 639.2-641.23, 646.80-646.93, 648.90-649.64, 650, 669.40-669.44, 669.80-669.94, 679.00-679.04, 679.12, 679.14

639.4   Metabolic disorders ♀ 🐾   M
Electrolyte imbalance following conditions classifiable to 630–638

(Ex:) 639.2-641.23, 646.80-646.93, 648.90-649.64, 650, 669.40-669.44, 669.80-669.94, 679.00-679.04, 679.12, 679.14

639.5   Shock ♀ 🐾   M
Circulatory collapse following conditions classifiable to 630–638
Shock (postoperative) (septic) following conditions classifiable to 630–638

(Ex:) 639.2-641.23, 646.80-646.93, 648.90-649.64, 650, 669.40-669.44, 669.80-669.94, 679.00-679.04, 679.12, 679.14

639.6   Embolism ♀ 🐾   M
Embolism:
NOS following conditions classifiable to 630–638
air following conditions classifiable to 630–638
amniotic fluid following conditions classifiable to 630–638
blood-clot following conditions classifiable to 630–638
fat following conditions classifiable to 630–638
pulmonary following conditions classifiable to 630–638
pyemic following conditions classifiable to 630–638
septic following conditions classifiable to 630–638
soap following conditions classifiable to 630–638

(Ex:) 639.2-641.23, 646.80-646.93, 648.90-649.64, 650, 669.40-669.44, 669.80-669.94, 679.00-679.04, 679.12, 679.14

639.8   Other specified complications following abortion or ectopic and molar pregnancy ♀ 🐾   M
Acute yellow atrophy or necrosis of liver following conditions classifiable to 630–638
Cardiac arrest or failure following conditions classifiable to 630–638
Cerebral anoxia following conditions classifiable to 630–638
Urinary tract infection following conditions classifiable to 630–638

(Ex:) 639.2-641.23, 646.80-646.93, 648.90-649.64, 650, 669.40-669.44, 669.80-669.94, 679.00-679.04, 679.12, 679.14

639.9   Unspecified complication following abortion or ectopic and molar pregnancy ♀ 🐾   M
Complication(s) not further specified following conditions classifiable to 630–638

(Ex:) 639.2-641.23, 646.80-646.93, 648.90-649.64, 650, 669.40-669.44, 669.80-669.94, 679.00-679.04, 679.12, 679.14

OGCR Section I.C.11.k.2

A code from categories 640-649 and 651-659 may be used as additional codes with an abortion code to indicate the complication leading to the abortion. Fifth digit 3 is assigned with codes from these categories when used with an abortion code because the other fifth digits will not apply. Codes from the 660-669 series are not to be used for complications of abortion.

COMPLICATIONS MAINLY RELATED TO PREGNANCY (640–649)

Includes the listed conditions even if they arose or were present during labor, delivery, or the puerperium

The following fifth-digit subclassification is for use with categories 640–649 to denote the current episode of care:

0   unspecified as to episode of care or not applicable
1   delivered, with or without mention of antepartum condition
    Antepartum condition with delivery
      Delivery NOS (with mention of antepartum complication during current episode of care)
    Intrapartum
      obstetric condition (with mention of antepartum complication during current episode of care)
    Pregnancy, delivered (with mention of antepartum complication during current episode of care)
2   delivered, with mention of postpartum complication
    Delivery with mention of puerperal complication during current episode of care
3   antepartum condition or complication
    Antepartum obstetric condition, not delivered during the current episode of care
4   postpartum condition or complication
    Postpartum or puerperal obstetric condition or complication following delivery that occurred:
      during previous episode of care
      outside hospital, with subsequent admission for observation or care

● **640 Hemorrhage in early pregnancy**
Requires fifth digit; valid digits are in [brackets] under each code. See beginning of section 640–649 for definitions.
    Includes hemorrhage before completion of 22 weeks' gestation

● **640.0 Threatened abortion** ♀ 1,3   M
[0,1,3]   For codes **640.01 and 640.03:** 640.00-641.13, 646.80-646.93, 648.90-649.64, 650, 669.40-669.94, 669.80-669.94, 679.00-679.04, 679.12, 679.14

● **640.8 Other specified hemorrhage in early pregnancy** ♀   M
[0,1,3]

● **640.9 Unspecified hemorrhage in early pregnancy** ♀ 3   M
[0,1,3]   For code **640.93:** 640.00-641.13, 646.80-646.93, 648.90-649.64, 650, 669.40-669.44, 669.80-669.94, 679.00-679.04, 679.12, 679.14

● **641 Antepartum hemorrhage, abruptio placentae, and placenta previa**
Requires fifth digit; valid digits are in [brackets] under each code. See beginning of section 640–649 for definitions.

● **641.0 Placenta previa without hemorrhage** ♀ 1,3   M
[0,1,3]   Low implantation of placenta without hemorrhage
Placenta previa noted:
    during pregnancy without hemorrhage
    before labor (and delivered by cesarean delivery) without hemorrhage
For codes **641.01 and 641.03:** 640.00-641.13, 646.80-646.93, 648.90-649.64, 650, 669.40-669.44, 669.80-669.94, 679.00-679.04, 679.12, 679.14

Item 11–3 Placenta previa is a condition in which the opening of the cervix is obstructed by the displaced placenta. The three types, marginal, partial, and total, are varying degrees of placenta displacement. Placenta abruption is the premature breaking away of the placenta from the site of the uterine implant before the delivery of the fetus.

Figure 11–2 Abruptio placentae is classified according to the grade of separation of the placenta from the uterine wall. **A.** Mild separation in which hemorrhage is internal. **B.** Moderate separation in which there is external hemorrhage. **C.** Severe separation in which there is external hemorrhage and extreme separation.

● **641.1 Hemorrhage from placenta previa** ♀ 1,3   M
[0,1,3]   Low-lying placenta NOS or with hemorrhage (intrapartum)
Placenta previa:
    incomplete NOS or with hemorrhage (intrapartum)
    marginal NOS or with hemorrhage (intrapartum)
    partial NOS or with hemorrhage (intrapartum)
    total NOS or with hemorrhage (intrapartum)
Excludes hemorrhage from vasa previa (663.5)
For codes **641.11 and 641.13:** 640.00-641.13, 646.80-646.93, 648.90-649.64, 650, 669.40-669.44, 669.80-669.94, 679.00-679.04, 679.12, 679.14

● **641.2 Premature separation of placenta** ♀ 3, 1   M
[0,1,3]   Ablatio placentae
Abruptio placentae
Accidental antepartum hemorrhage
Couvelaire uterus
Detachment of placenta (premature)
Premature separation of normally implanted placenta
For codes **641.21 and 641.23:** 640.00-641.13, 641.21, 646.80-646.93, 648.90-649.64, 650, 669.40-669.44, 669.80-669.94, 679.00-679.04, 679.12, 679.14

● **641.3 Antepartum hemorrhage associated with coagulation defects** ♀ 1,3   M
[0,1,3]   Antepartum or intrapartum hemorrhage associated with:
    afibrinogenemia
    hyperfibrinolysis
    hypofibrinogenemia
Excludes coagulation defects not associated with antepartum hemorrhage (649.3)
For codes **641.31 and 641.33:** 641.30-641.93, 646.80-646.93, 648.90-649.64, 650, 669.40-669.44, 669.80-669.94, 679.00-679.04, 679.12, 679.14

● **641.8 Other antepartum hemorrhage** ♀   M
[0,1,3]   Antepartum or intrapartum hemorrhage associated with:
    trauma
    uterine leiomyoma

● **641.9 Unspecified antepartum hemorrhage** ♀   M
[0,1,3]   Hemorrhage:
    antepartum NOS
    intrapartum NOS
    of pregnancy NOS

N Newborn: 0   P Pediatric: 0–17   M Maternity: 12–55   A Adult: 15–124   ♀ Females Only   ♂ Males Only

Ex CC/MCC Exclusions   Complication\Comorbidity   Major C\C   Present on Admission Requirement   Hospital-Acquired Condition   877

● 642   **Hypertension complicating pregnancy, childbirth, and the puerperium**

> Requires fifth digit; valid digits are in [brackets] under each code. See beginning of section 640–649 for definitions.

● 642.0   **Benign essential hypertension complicating**
[0-4]   **pregnancy, childbirth, and the puerperium** ♀ 1-3 🔖   M

> Hypertension:
>> benign essential specified as complicating, or as a reason for obstetric care during pregnancy, childbirth, or the puerperium
>> chronic NOS specified as complicating, or as a reason for obstetric care during pregnancy, childbirth, or the puerperium
>> essential specified as complicating, or as a reason for obstetric care during pregnancy, childbirth, or the puerperium
>> pre-existing NOS specified as complicating, or as a reason for obstetric care during pregnancy, childbirth, or the puerperium

> For codes **642.01-642.03**: (Ex) 642.00-642.94, 646.10-646.14, 646.80-646.93, 648.90-649.64, 650, 669.40-669.44, 669.80-669.94, 679.00-679.04, 679.12, 679.14

● 642.1   **Hypertension secondary to renal disease,**
[0-4]   **complicating pregnancy, childbirth, and the**
     puerperium ♀ 3,4 🔖, 1,2 🔖   M

> Hypertension secondary to renal disease, specified as complicating, or as a reason for obstetric care during pregnancy, childbirth, or the puerperium

> For codes **641.11-642.14**: (Ex) 642.00-642.94, 646.10-646.14, 646.80-646.93, 648.90-649.64, 650, 669.40-669.44, 669.80-669.94, 679.00-679.04, 679.12, 679.14

● 642.2   **Other pre-existing hypertension complicating**
[0-4]   **pregnancy, childbirth, and the puerperium** ♀   M

> Hypertensive:
>> chronic kidney disease specified as complicating, or as a reason for obstetric care during pregnancy, childbirth, or the puerperium
>> heart and chronic kidney disease specified as complicating, or as a reason for obstetric care during pregnancy, childbirth, or the puerperium
>> heart disease specified as complicating, or as a reason for obstetric care during pregnancy, childbirth, or the puerperium
> Malignant hypertension specified as complicating, or as a reason for obstetric care during pregnancy, childbirth, or the puerperium

● 642.3   **Transient hypertension of pregnancy** ♀ 1,2 🔖   M
[0-4]

> Gestational hypertension
> Transient hypertension, so described, in pregnancy, childbirth, or the puerperium

> For codes **642.31-642.32**: (Ex) 642.00-642.94, 646.10-646.14, 646.80-646.93, 648.90-649.64, 650, 669.40-669.44, 669.80-669.94, 679.00-679.04, 679.12, 679.14

> **OGCR**   Section I.C.7.a.8

> Assign code 796.2, Elevated blood pressure reading without diagnosis of hypertension, unless patient has an established diagnosis of hypertension. Assign code 642.3x for transient hypertension of pregnancy.

● 642.4   **Mild or unspecified pre-eclampsia** ♀ 1,3,4 🔖, 2 🔖   M
[0-4]

> Hypertension in pregnancy, childbirth, or the puerperium, not specified as pre-existing, with either albuminuria or edema, or both; mild or unspecified
> Pre-eclampsia:
>> NOS
>> mild
> Toxemia (pre-eclamptic):
>> NOS
>> mild

> **Excludes**   albuminuria in pregnancy, without mention of hypertension (646.2)
> edema in pregnancy, without mention of hypertension (646.1)

> For codes **642.41-642.44**: (Ex) 642.00-642.94, 646.10-646.14, 646.80-646.93, 648.90-649.64, 650, 669.40-669.44, 669.80-669.94, 679.00-679.04, 679.12, 679.14

> **Coding Clinic: 2009, Q4, P108**

● 642.5   **Severe pre-eclampsia** ♀ 1-4 🔖   M
[0-4]

> Hypertension in pregnancy, childbirth, or the puerperium, not specified as pre-existing, with either albuminuria or edema, or both; specified as severe
> Pre-eclampsia, severe
> Toxemia (pre-eclamptic), severe

> For codes **642.51-642.54**: (Ex) 642.00-642.94, 646.10-646.14, 646.80-646.93, 648.90-649.64, 650, 669.40-669.44, 669.80-669.94, 679.00-679.04, 679.12, 679.14

● 642.6   **Eclampsia** ♀ 1-4 🔖   M
[0-4]

> Toxemia:
>> eclamptic
>> with convulsions

> For codes **642.61-642.64**: (Ex) 642.00-642.94, 646.10-646.14, 646.80-646.93, 648.90-649.64, 650, 669.40-669.44, 669.80-669.94, 679.00-679.04, 679.12, 679.14

● 642.7   **Pre-eclampsia or eclampsia superimposed on pre-**
[0-4]   **existing hypertension** ♀ 1-4 🔖   M

> Conditions classifiable to 642.4–642.6, with conditions classifiable to 642.0–642.2

> For codes **642.71-642.74**: (Ex) 642.00-642.94, 646.10-646.14, 646.80-646.93, 648.90-649.64, 650, 669.40-669.44, 669.80-669.94, 679.00-679.04, 679.12, 679.14

● 642.9   **Unspecified hypertension complicating pregnancy,**
[0-4]   **childbirth, or the puerperium** ♀ 1-4 🔖   M

> Hypertension NOS, without mention of albuminuria or edema, complicating pregnancy, childbirth, or the puerperium

> For codes **642.91-642.92**: (Ex) 642.00-642.94, 646.10-646.14, 646.80-646.93, 648.90-649.64, 650, 669.40-669.44, 669.80-669.94, 679.00-679.04, 679.12, 679.14;

> For codes **642.93-642.94**: (Ex) 642.01-642.44, 642.61-642.94

> **Coding Clinic: 2009, Q1, P18**

● 643   **Excessive vomiting in pregnancy**

> Requires fifth digit; valid digits are in [brackets] under each code. See beginning of section 640–649 for definitions.

> **Includes**   hyperemesis arising during pregnancy
> vomiting:
>> persistent arising during pregnancy
>> vicious arising during pregnancy
>> hyperemesis gravidarum

● 643.0   **Mild hyperemesis gravidarum** ♀   M
[0,1,3]

> Hyperemesis gravidarum, mild or unspecified, starting before the end of the 22nd week of gestation

● 643.1   **Hyperemesis gravidarum with metabolic**
[0,1,3]   **disturbance** ♀   M

> Hyperemesis gravidarum, starting before the end of the 22nd week of gestation, with metabolic disturbance, such as:
>> carbohydrate depletion
>> dehydration
>> electrolyte imbalance

● 643.2   **Late vomiting of pregnancy** ♀   M
[0,1,3]

> Excessive vomiting starting after 22 completed weeks of gestation

● 643.8   **Other vomiting complicating pregnancy** ♀   M
[0,1,3]

> Vomiting due to organic disease or other cause, specified as complicating pregnancy, or as a reason for obstetric care during pregnancy

> Use additional code to specify cause

● 643.9   **Unspecified vomiting of pregnancy** ♀   M
[0,1,3]

> Vomiting as a reason for care during pregnancy, length of gestation unspecified

◀ New   ◀▥ Revised   ~~deleted~~ Deleted   Excludes   Includes   Use additional   Code first   Omit code

878   ● Unacceptable Principal Diagnosis   ● Use Additional Digit(s)   ▷ Manifestation Code   OGCR Official Guidelines   **Coding Clinic**

644   Early or threatened labor

Requires fifth digit; valid digits are in [brackets] under each code. See beginning of section 640–649 for definitions.

● **644.0   Threatened premature labor** ♀ 3 🔖   M
[0,3]   Premature labor after 22 weeks, but before 37 completed weeks of gestation without delivery

Excludes   *that occurring before 22 completed weeks of gestation (640.0)*

For code **644.03:** Ⓔⓧ 644.00-644.21, 646.80-646.93, 648.90-649.64, 650, 669.40-669.44, 669.80-669.94, 679.00-679.04, 679.12, 679.14

● **644.1   Other threatened labor** ♀ 3 🔖   M
[0,3]   False labor:
           NOS without delivery
           after 37 completed weeks of gestation without delivery
           Threatened labor NOS without delivery

For code **644.13:** Ⓔⓧ 644.00-644.21, 646.80-646.93, 648.90-649.64, 650, 669.40-669.44, 669.80-669.94, 679.00-679.04, 679.12, 679.14

● **644.2   Early onset of delivery** ♀ 0 🔖, 1 🔖   M
[0-1]   Onset (spontaneous) of delivery before 37 completed weeks of gestation
           Premature labor with onset of delivery before 37 completed weeks of gestation

Ⓔⓧ 644.00-644.21, 646.80-646.93, 648.90-649.64, 650, 669.40-669.44, 669.80-669.94, 679.00-679.04, 679.12, 679.14

Coding Clinic: 2011, Q3, P3; 1991, Q2, P16

OGCR   Section I.C.11.k.4

When an attempted termination of pregnancy results in a liveborn fetus assign code 644.21, Early onset of delivery, with an appropriate code from category V27, Outcome of Delivery. The procedure code for the attempted termination of pregnancy should also be assigned.

● **645   Late pregnancy**

Requires fifth digit; valid digits are in [brackets] under each code. See beginning of section 640–649 for definitions.

Coding Clinic: 2000, Q1, P17-18

● **645.1   Post term pregnancy** ♀   M
[0,1,3]   Pregnancy over 40 completed weeks to 42 completed weeks gestation

● **645.2   Prolonged pregnancy** ♀   M
[0,1,3]   Pregnancy which has advanced beyond 42 completed weeks of gestation

● **646   Other complications of pregnancy, not elsewhere classified**

Use additional code(s) to further specify complication

Requires fifth digit; valid digits are in [brackets] under each code. See beginning of section 640–649 for definitions.

● **646.0   Papyraceous fetus** ♀   M
[0,1,3]

● **646.1   Edema or excessive weight gain in pregnancy,**
[0-4]   **without mention of hypertension** ♀   M
           Gestational edema
           Maternal obesity syndrome

Excludes   *that with mention of hypertension (642.0–642.9)*

● **646.2   Unspecified renal disease in pregnancy, without**
[0-4]   **mention of hypertension** ♀ 1-4 🔖   M
           Albuminuria in pregnancy or the puerperium, without mention of hypertension
           Nephropathy NOS in pregnancy or the puerperium, without mention of hypertension
           Renal disease NOS in pregnancy or the puerperium, without mention of hypertension
           Uremia in pregnancy or the puerperium, without mention of hypertension
           Gestational proteinuria in pregnancy or the puerperium, without mention of hypertension

Excludes   *that with mention of hypertension (642.0–642.9)*

For codes **646.21-646.24:** Ⓔⓧ 646.21-646.24

● **646.3   Recurrent pregnancy loss** ♀ 1 🔖   M
[0,1,3]

Excludes   *with current abortion (634.0–634.9)*
              without current pregnancy (629.81)

For code **646.31:** Ⓔⓧ 646.31

● **646.4   Peripheral neuritis in pregnancy** ♀   M
[0-4]

● **646.5   Asymptomatic bacteriuria in pregnancy** ♀   M
[0-4]

● **646.6   Infections of genitourinary tract in**
[0-4]   **pregnancy** ♀ 1-4 🔖   M
           Conditions classifiable to 590, 595, 597, 599.0, 616 complicating pregnancy, childbirth, or the puerperium
           Conditions classifiable to 614.0–614.5, 614.7–614.9, 615 complicating pregnancy or labor

Excludes   *major puerperal infection (670.0-670.8)*

For codes **646.61-646.64:** Ⓔⓧ 646.60-646.64, 646.80-646.93, 648.90-649.64, 650, 669.40-669.44, 669.80-669.94, 679.00-679.04, 679.12, 679.14

Coding Clinic: 2004, Q4, P88-90

OGCR   Section I.C.2.g.

During pregnancy, childbirth or the puerperium, a patient admitted (or presenting for a health care encounter) because of an HIV-related illness should receive a principal diagnosis code of 647.6X, Other specified infectious and parasitic diseases in the mother classifiable elsewhere, but complicating the pregnancy, childbirth or the puerperium, followed by 042 and the code(s) for the HIV-related illness(es). Codes from Chapter 15 always take sequencing priority. Patients with asymptomatic HIV infection status admitted (or presenting for a health care encounter) during pregnancy, childbirth, or the puerperium should receive codes of 647.6X and V08.

● **646.7   Liver and biliary tract disorders in**
[0,1,3]   **pregnancy** ♀ 1,3 🔖   M
           Acute yellow atrophy of liver (obstetric) (true) of pregnancy
           Icterus gravis of pregnancy
           Necrosis of liver of pregnancy

Excludes   *hepatorenal syndrome following delivery (674.8)*
              viral hepatitis (647.6)

For codes **646.71 and 646.73:** Ⓔⓧ 646.70-646.93, 648.90-649.64, 650, 669.40-669.44, 669.80-669.94, 679.00-679.04, 679.12, 679.14

● **646.8   Other specified complications of pregnancy** ♀   M
[0-4]   Fatigue during pregnancy
           Herpes gestationis
           Insufficient weight gain of pregnancy
           Coding Clinic: 1998, Q3, P16; 1985, Jan-Feb, P15-16

● **646.9   Unspecified complication of pregnancy** ♀   M
[0,1,3]

● **647   Infectious and parasitic conditions in the mother classifiable elsewhere, but complicating pregnancy, childbirth, or the puerperium**

Use additional code(s) to further specify complication

Requires fifth digit; valid digits are in [brackets] under each code. See beginning of section 640–649 for definitions.

Includes   the listed conditions when complicating the pregnant state, aggravated by the pregnancy, or when a main reason for obstetric care

Excludes   *those conditions in the mother known or suspected to have affected the fetus (655.0–655.9)*

● **647.0   Syphilis** ♀ 1-4 🔖   M
[0-4]   Conditions classifiable to 090–097

For codes **647.01-647.04:** Ⓔⓧ 646.81-647.24, 679.12, 679.14

● **647.1   Gonorrhea** ♀ 1-4 🔖   M
[0-4]   Conditions classifiable to 098

For codes **647.11-647.14:** Ⓔⓧ 646.81-647.24, 679.12, 679.14

● **647.2   Other venereal diseases** ♀ 1-4 🔖   M
[0-4]   Conditions classifiable to 099

For codes **647.21-647.24:** Ⓔⓧ 646.81-647.24, 679.12, 679.14

COMPLICATIONS OF PREGNANCY, CHILDBIRTH, AND THE PUERPERIUM (630–679)

N Newborn: 0   **P** Pediatric: 0–17   **M** Maternity: 12–55   **A** Adult: 15–124   ♀ Females Only   ♂ Males Only

Ⓔⓧ CC/MCC Exclusions   🔖 Complication\Comorbidity   🔖 Major C\C   🔖 Present on Admission Requirement   🔖 Hospital-Acquired Condition   879

● **647.3 Tuberculosis** ♀ 1-4 🔄   M
[0-4]   Conditions classifiable to 010–018
For codes **647.31-647.34:** (Ex:) 646.80-646.93, 647.30-647.34, 648.90-649.64, 650, 669.40-669.44, 669.80-669.94, 679.00-679.04, 679.12 679.14

● **647.4 Malaria** ♀ 1-4 🔄   M
[0-4]   Conditions classifiable to 084
For codes **647.41-647.44:** (Ex:) 646.80-646.93, 647.40-647.44, 648.90-649.64, 650, 669.40-669.44, 669.80-669.94, 679.00-679.04, 679.12, 679.14

● **647.5 Rubella** ♀ 1-4 🔄   M
[0-4]   Conditions classifiable to 056
For codes **647.51-647.54:** (Ex:) 647.51-647.94

● **647.6 Other viral diseases** ♀ 1-4 🔄   M
[0-4]   Conditions classifiable to 042, 050-055, 057-079, 795.05, 795.15, 796.75
For codes **647.61-647.64:** (Ex:) 647.51-647.94
Coding Clinic: 2010, Q2, P10; 1985, Jan-Feb, P15-16

● **647.8 Other specified infectious and parasitic**   M
[0-4]   **diseases** ♀ 1-4 🔄
For codes **647.81-647.84:** (Ex:) 647.51-647.94

● **647.9 Unspecified infection or infestation** ♀ 1-4 🔄   M
[0-4]   For codes **647.91-647.94:** (Ex:) 647.51-647.94

● **648 Other current conditions in the mother classifiable elsewhere, but complicating pregnancy, childbirth, or the puerperium**
Use additional code(s) to identify the condition
Requires fifth digit; valid digits are in [brackets] under each code. See beginning of section 640–649 for definitions.
Includes   the listed conditions when complicating the pregnant state, aggravated by the pregnancy, or when a main reason for obstetric care
Excludes   *those conditions in the mother known or suspected to have affected the fetus (655.0–655.9)*

● **648.0 Diabetes mellitus** ♀ 0,3,4 🔄 1-2 🔄   M
[0-4]   Conditions classifiable to 249, 250
Excludes   *gestational diabetes (648.8)*
(Ex:) 646.80-646.93, 648.00-648.04, 648.90-649.64, 650, 669.40-669.44, 669.80-669.94, 679.00-679.04, 679.12, 679.14

● **648.1 Thyroid dysfunction** ♀   M
[0-4]   Conditions classifiable to 240–246

● **648.2 Anemia** ♀   M
[0-4]   Conditions classifiable to 280–285
Coding Clinic: 2002, Q1, P14

● **648.3 Drug dependence** ♀ 1-4 🔄   M
[0-4]   Conditions classifiable to 304
For codes **648.31-648.34:** (Ex:) 646.80-646.93, 648.30-648.34, 648.90-649.64, 650, 669.40-669.44, 669.80-669.94, 679.00-679.04, 679.12, 679.14
Coding Clinic: 1998, Q2, P13-14; 1988, Q4, P8

● **648.4 Mental disorders** ♀   M
[0-4]   Conditions classifiable to 290–303, 305.0, 305.2–305.9, 306–316, 317–319
Coding Clinic: 1998, Q2, P13-14

● **648.5 Congenital cardiovascular disorders** ♀ 1-4 🔄   M
[0-4]   Conditions classifiable to 745–747
For codes **648.51-648.54:** (Ex:) 646.80-646.93, 648.50-648.64, 648.90-649.64, 650, 669.40-669.44, 669.80-669.94, 679.00-679.04, 679.12, 679.14

● **648.6 Other cardiovascular diseases** ♀ 1-4 🔄   M
[0-4]   Conditions classifiable to 390–398, 410–429
Excludes   *cerebrovascular disorders in the puerperium (674.0)*
peripartum cardiomyopathy (674.5)
venous complications (671.0–671.9)
For codes **648.61-648.64:** (Ex:) 646.80-646.93, 648.50-648.64, 648.90-649.64, 650, 669.40-669.44, 669.80-669.94, 679.00-679.04, 679.12, 679.14
Coding Clinic: 2012, Q3, P10; 1998, Q3, P11

● **648.7 Bone and joint disorders of back, pelvis, and lower**   M
[0-4]   **limbs** ♀ 1-4 🔄
Conditions classifiable to 720–724, and those classifiable to 711–719 or 725–738, specified as affecting the lower limbs
For codes **648.71-648.74:** (Ex:) 648.71-648.74

● **648.8 Abnormal glucose tolerance** ♀   M
[0-4]   Conditions classifiable to 790.21–790.29
Gestational diabetes
Use additional code, if applicable, for associated long-term (current) insulin use V58.67
Coding Clinic: 2004, Q4, P53-56

● **648.9 Other current conditions classifiable elsewhere** ♀   M
[0-4]   Conditions classifiable to 440–459, 795.01–795.04, 795.06, 795.10–795.14, 795.16, 796.70–796.74, 796.76
Nutritional deficiencies [conditions classifiable to 260–269]
Coding Clinic: 2009, Q1, P17; 2006, Q3, P14; 2004, Q4, P88-90; 2002, Q1, P14-15; 1984, Nov-Dec, P18

● **649 Other conditions or status of the mother complicating pregnancy, childbirth, or the puerperium**
Requires fifth digit; valid digits are in [brackets] under each code. See beginning of section 640-649 for definitions.

● **649.0 Tobacco use disorder complicating pregnancy,**   M
[0-4]   **childbirth, or the puerperium** ♀
Smoking complicating pregnancy, childbirth, or the puerperium

● **649.1 Obesity complicating pregnancy, childbirth, or the**   M
[0-4]   **puerperium** ♀
Use additional code to identify the obesity (278.00-278.03)

● **649.2 Bariatric surgery status complicating pregnancy,**   M
[0-4]   **childbirth, or the puerperium** ♀
Gastric banding status complicating pregnancy, childbirth, or the puerperium
Gastric bypass status for obesity complicating pregnancy, childbirth, or the puerperium
Obesity surgery status complicating pregnancy, childbirth, or the puerperium

● **649.3 Coagulation defects complicating pregnancy,**   M
[0-4]   **childbirth, or the puerperium** ♀ 🔄
Conditions classifiable to 286, 287, 289
Use additional code to identify the specific coagulation defect (286.0–286.9, 287.0–287.9, 289.0–289.9)
Excludes   *coagulation defects causing antepartum hemorrhage (641.3)*
(Ex:) 648.90

● **649.4 Epilepsy complicating pregnancy, childbirth, or the**   M
[0-4]   **puerperium** ♀ 1-4 🔄
Conditions classifiable to 345
Use additional code to identify the specific type of epilepsy (345.00–345.91)
Excludes   *eclampsia (642.6)*
For codes **649.41-649.44:** (Ex:) 648.91-648.94

● **649.5 Spotting complicating pregnancy** ♀   M
[0,1,3]   **Excludes**   *antepartum hemorrhage (641.0–641.9)*
hemorrhage in early pregnancy (640.0–640.9)

● **649.6 Uterine size date discrepancy** ♀   M
[0-4]   **Excludes**   *suspected problem with fetal growth not found (V89.04)*

● **649.7 Cervical shortening** ♀ 🔄   M
[0,1,3]   **Excludes**   *suspected cervical shortening not found (V89.05)*
For codes **649.70, 649.71, and 649.73:** (Ex:) 649.70-649.73, 654.51-654.54
Coding Clinic: 2008, Q4, P124-125

● **649.8 Onset (spontaneous) of labor after 37 completed weeks of**   M
[1-2]   **gestation but before 39 completed weeks gestation, with delivery by (planned) cesarean section** ♀
Delivery by (planned) cesarean section occurring after 37 completed weeks of gestation but before 39 completed weeks gestation due to (spontaneous) onset of labor
Use additional code to specify reason for planned cesarean section such as:
cephalopelvic disproportion (normally formed fetus) (653.4)
previous cesarean delivery (654.2)
Coding Clinic: 2011, Q4, P133

OGCR Section I.C.11.h.1

Code 650 is for use in cases when a woman is admitted for a full-term normal delivery and delivers a single, healthy infant without any complications antepartum, during the delivery, or postpartum during the delivery episode. Code 650 is always a principal diagnosis. It is not to be used if any other code from chapter 11 is needed to describe a current complication of the antenatal, delivery, or perinatal period. Additional codes from other chapters may be used with code 650 if they are not related to or are in any way complicating the pregnancy.

OGCR Section I.C.11.h.2

Code 650 may be used if the patient had a complication at some point during her pregnancy, but the complication is not present at the time of the admission for delivery.

OGCR Section I.C.11.h.3

V27.0, Single liveborn, is the only outcome of delivery code appropriate for use with 650.

OGCR Section I.C.11.i.1

The postpartum period begins immediately after delivery and continues for six weeks following delivery. The peripartum period is defined as the last month of pregnancy to five months postpartum.

NORMAL DELIVERY, AND OTHER INDICATIONS FOR CARE IN PREGNANCY, LABOR, AND DELIVERY (650–659)

The following fifth-digit subclassification is for use with categories 651–659 to denote the current episode of care:

> 0 unspecified as to episode of care or not applicable
> 1 delivered, with or without mention of antepartum condition
> 2 delivered, with mention of postpartum complication
> 3 antepartum condition or complication
> 4 postpartum condition or complication

● 650 **Normal delivery** ♀ 🌐   M

Delivery requiring minimal or no assistance, with or without episiotomy, without fetal manipulation [e.g., rotation version] or instrumentation [forceps] of a spontaneous, cephalic, vaginal, full-term, single, live-born infant. This code is for use as a single diagnosis code and is not to be used with any other code in the range 630–676.

Use additional code to indicate outcome of delivery (V27.0)

Excludes breech delivery (assisted) (spontaneous) NOS (652.2)
delivery by vacuum extractor, forceps, cesarean section, or breech extraction, without specified complication (669.5–669.7)

Coding Clinic: 2002, Q2, P10; 2001, Q3, P12; 2000, Q3, P5

● 651 **Multiple gestation**

Requires fifth digit; valid digits are in [brackets] under each code. See beginning of section 650–659 for definitions.

Use additional code to specify placenta status (V91.00-V91.99)

Excludes fetal conjoined twins (678.1)

● 651.0 **Twin pregnancy** ♀ 1 🌐   M
[0,1,3]
　　　Excludes fetal conjoined twins (678.1)
　　　For code **651.01:** (Ex:) 650-651.63, 651.71-652.20, 652.23-652.93
　　　Coding Clinic: 2006, Q3, P16-18; 1992, Q3, P10

● 651.1 **Triplet pregnancy** ♀ 1,3 🌐   M
[0,1,3]   For codes **651.11** and **651.13:** (Ex:) 650-651.63, 651.71-652.93

● 651.2 **Quadruplet pregnancy** ♀ 1,3 🌐   M
[0,1,3]   For codes **651.21** and **651.23:** (Ex:) 650-651.63, 651.71-652.93

● 651.3 **Twin pregnancy with fetal loss and retention of one**   M
[0,1,3] **fetus** ♀

OGCR Section I.C.11.k.2

A code from categories 640-649 and 651-659 may be used as additional codes with an abortion code to indicate the complication leading to the abortion. Fifth digit 3 is assigned with codes from these categories when used with an abortion code because the other fifth digits will not apply. Codes from the 660-669 series are not to be used for complications of abortion.

● 651.4 **Triplet pregnancy with fetal loss and retention of**   M
[0,1,3] **one or more fetus(es)** ♀ 1,3 🌐
　　　For codes **654.41** and **651.43:** (Ex:) 650-651.63, 651.71-652.93

● 651.5 **Quadruplet pregnancy with fetal loss and retention**   M
[0,1,3] **of one or more fetus(es)** ♀ 1,3 🌐
　　　For codes **651.51** and **651.53:** (Ex:) 650-651.63, 651.71-652.93

● 651.6 **Other multiple pregnancy with fetal loss and**   M
[0,1,3] **retention of one or more fetus(es)** ♀

● 651.7 **Multiple gestation following (elective) fetal**   M
[0,1,3] **reduction** ♀
　　　Fetal reduction of multiple fetuses reduced to single fetus
　　　Coding Clinic: 2006, Q3, P16-18; 2005, Q4, P81

● 651.8 **Other specified multiple gestation** ♀ 1,3 🌐   M
[0,1,3]   For codes **651.81** and **651.83:** (Ex:) 650-651.63, 651.71-652.93

● 651.9 **Unspecified multiple gestation** ♀   M
[0,1,3]

● 652 **Malposition and malpresentation of fetus**

Requires fifth digit; valid digits are in [brackets] under each code. See beginning of section 650–659 for definitions.

Code first any associated obstructed labor (660.0)

Coding Clinic: 1995, Q3, P10

● 652.0 **Unstable lie** ♀   M
[0,1,3]

● 652.1 **Breech or other malpresentation successfully**   M
[0,1,3] **converted to cephalic presentation** ♀
　　　Cephalic version NOS

● 652.2 **Breech presentation without mention of version** ♀   M
[0,1,3] 　　Breech delivery (assisted) (spontaneous) NOS
　　　Buttocks presentation
　　　Complete breech
　　　Frank breech

　　　Excludes footling presentation (652.8)
　　　　　　　incomplete breech (652.8)
　　　Coding Clinic: 2013, Q3, P7

● 652.3 **Transverse or oblique presentation** ♀   M
[0,1,3] 　　Oblique lie
　　　Transverse lie

　　　Excludes transverse arrest of fetal head (660.3)

● 652.4 **Face or brow presentation** ♀   M
[0,1,3] 　　Mentum presentation

● 652.5 **High head at term** ♀   M
[0,1,3] 　　Failure of head to enter pelvic brim
　　　Coding Clinic: 2013, Q3, P8

● 652.6 **Multiple gestation with malpresentation of one**   M
[0,1,3] **fetus or more** ♀

Figure 11-3 Five types of malposition and malpresentation of the fetus: **A.** Breech. **B.** Vertex. **C.** Face. **D.** Brow. **E.** Shoulder.

N Newborn: 0   P Pediatric: 0–17   M Maternity: 12–55   A Adult: 15–124   ♀ Females Only   ♂ Males Only
(Ex:) CC/MCC Exclusions   🌐 Complication\Comorbidity   🌐 Major C\C   🌐 Present on Admission Requirement   🌐 Hospital-Acquired Condition

Figure 11-4 Hydrocephalic fetus causing disproportion.

COMPLICATIONS OF PREGNANCY, CHILDBIRTH, AND THE PUERPERIUM (630–679)

● **652.7 Prolapsed arm** ♀   M
[0,1,3]

● **652.8 Other specified malposition or malpresentation** ♀   M
[0,1,3]   Compound presentation

● **652.9 Unspecified malposition or malpresentation** ♀   M
[0,1,3]

● **653 Disproportion**

Requires fifth digit; valid digits are in [brackets] under each code. See beginning of section 650–659 for definitions.
Code first any associated obstructed labor (660.1)
Coding Clinic: 2013, Q3, P8; 1995, Q3, P10

● **653.0 Major abnormality of bony pelvis, not further**
[0,1,3] **specified** ♀   M
Pelvic deformity NOS

● **653.1 Generally contracted pelvis** ♀   M
[0,1,3]   Contracted pelvis NOS

● **653.2 Inlet contraction of pelvis** ♀   M
[0,1,3]   Inlet contraction (pelvis)

● **653.3 Outlet contraction of pelvis** ♀   M
[0,1,3]   Outlet contraction (pelvis)

● **653.4 Fetopelvic disproportion** ♀   M
[0,1,3]   Cephalopelvic disproportion NOS
Disproportion of mixed maternal and fetal origin, with normally formed fetus

● **653.5 Unusually large fetus causing disproportion** ♀   M
[0,1,3]   Disproportion of fetal origin with normally formed fetus
Fetal disproportion NOS
Excludes   *that when the reason for medical care was concern for the fetus (656.6)*

● **653.6 Hydrocephalic fetus causing disproportion** ♀   M
[0,1,3]
Excludes   *that when the reason for medical care was concern for the fetus (655.0)*

● **653.7 Other fetal abnormality causing disproportion** ♀   M
[0,1,3]   Fetal: Fetal:
ascites   sacral teratoma
hydrops   tumor
myelomeningocele
Excludes   *conjoined twins causing disproportion (678.1)*

● **653.8 Disproportion of other origin** ♀   M
[0,1,3]
Excludes   *shoulder (girdle) dystocia (660.4)*

● **653.9 Unspecified disproportion** ♀   M
[0,1,3]

● **654 Abnormality of organs and soft tissues of pelvis**

Requires fifth digit; valid digits are in [brackets] under each code. See beginning of section 650–659 for definitions.
Includes   the listed conditions during pregnancy, childbirth, or the puerperium
Code first any associated obstructed labor (660.2)
Excludes   *trauma to perineum and vulva complicating current delivery (664.0–664.9)*
Coding Clinic: 2013, Q3, P8; 1995, Q3, P10

● **654.0 Congenital abnormalities of uterus** ♀   M
[0-4]   Double uterus
Uterus bicornis

● **654.1 Tumors of body of uterus** ♀   M
[0-4]   Uterine fibroids
Coding Clinic: 1994, Q2, P14

● **654.2 Previous cesarean delivery** ♀   M
[0,1,3]   Uterine scar from previous cesarean delivery
Coding Clinic: 2013, Q3, P7; 2011, Q4, P133

● **654.3 Retroverted and incarcerated gravid uterus** ♀   M
[0-4]

● **654.4 Other abnormalities in shape or position of**
[0-4] **gravid uterus and of neighboring structures** ♀   M
Cystocele
Pelvic floor repair
Pendulous abdomen
Prolapse of gravid uterus
Rectocele
Rigid pelvic floor

● **654.5 Cervical incompetence** ♀ 1-4 🔖   M
[0-4]   Presence of Shirodkar suture with or without mention of cervical incompetence
For codes **654.51-654.54:** (Ex) 649.70-649.73, 654.51-654.54

● **654.6 Other congenital or acquired abnormality of**
[0-4] **cervix** ♀   M
Cicatricial cervix
Polyp of cervix
Previous surgery to cervix
Rigid cervix (uteri)
Stenosis or stricture of cervix
Tumor of cervix

● **654.7 Congenital or acquired abnormality of vagina** ♀   M
[0-4]   Previous surgery to vagina
Septate vagina
Stenosis of vagina (acquired) (congenital)
Stricture of vagina
Tumor of vagina

● **654.8 Congenital or acquired abnormality of vulva** ♀   M
[0-4]   Anal sphincter tear (healed) (old) complicating delivery
Fibrosis of perineum
Persistent hymen
Previous surgery to perineum or vulva
Rigid perineum
Tumor of vulva
Excludes   *anal sphincter tear (healed) (old) not associated with delivery (569.43)*
varicose veins of vulva (671.1)
Coding Clinic: 2003, Q1, P14

● **654.9 Other and unspecified** ♀   M
[0-4]   Uterine scar NEC

OGCR   Section I.C.11.c.2

In cases when in utero surgery is performed on the fetus, a diagnosis code from category 655, Known or suspected fetal abnormalities affecting management of the mother, should be assigned identifying the fetal condition. Procedure code 75.36, Correction of fetal defect, should be assigned on the hospital inpatient record. No code from Chapter 15, the perinatal codes, should be used on the mother's record to identify fetal conditions. Surgery performed in utero on a fetus is still to be coded as an obstetric encounter.

● **655 Known or suspected fetal abnormality affecting management of mother**

Requires fifth digit; valid digits are in [brackets] under each code. See beginning of section 650–659 for definitions.
Includes   the listed conditions in the fetus as a reason for observation or obstetrical care of the mother, or for termination of pregnancy

● **655.0 Central nervous system malformation in fetus** ♀   M
[0,1,3]   Fetal or suspected fetal:
anencephaly
hydrocephalus
spina bifida (with myelomeningocele)

● **655.1 Chromosomal abnormality in fetus** ♀   M
[0,1,3]

● **655.2 Hereditary disease in family possibly affecting**
[0,1,3] **fetus** ♀   M

● **655.3 Suspected damage to fetus from viral disease in the**
[0,1,3] **mother** ♀   M
Suspected damage to fetus from maternal rubella

● **655.4 Suspected damage to fetus from other disease in the**
[0,1,3] **mother** ♀   M
Suspected damage to fetus from maternal:
alcohol addiction
listeriosis
toxoplasmosis

● **655.5 Suspected damage to fetus from drugs** ♀   M
[0,1,3]

● **655.6 Suspected damage to fetus from radiation** ♀   M
[0,1,3]

● **655.7 Decreased fetal movements** ♀   M
[0,1,3]   Coding Clinic: 1997, Q4, P41

● **655.8 Other known or suspected fetal abnormality, not   M
elsewhere classified** ♀
[0,1,3]   Suspected damage to fetus from:
               environmental toxins
               intrauterine contraceptive device
            Coding Clinic: 2006, Q3, P16-18x2

● **655.9 Unspecified** ♀   M
[0,1,3]   Coding Clinic: 2010, Q2, P7

● 656 **Other known or suspected fetal and placental problems affecting
       management of mother**
            Requires fifth digit; valid digits are in [brackets] under each
               code. See beginning of section 650–659 for definitions.
            Excludes *fetal hematologic conditions (678.0)*
                          suspected placental problems not found (V89.02)

● **656.0 Fetal-maternal hemorrhage** ♀   M
[0,1,3]   Leakage (microscopic) of fetal blood into maternal
               circulation

● **656.1 Rhesus isoimmunization** ♀ 3 🌀   M
[0,1,3]   Anti-D [Rh] antibodies
            Rh incompatibility
            For code **656.13**: (Ex) 656.11-656.13

● **656.2 Isoimmunization from other and unspecified blood-   M
       group incompatibility** ♀
[0,1,3]   ABO isoimmunization
            Coding Clinic: 2006, Q4, P135

● **656.3 Fetal distress** ♀ 1 🌀   M
[0,1,3]   Fetal metabolic acidemia
            Excludes *abnormal fetal acid-base balance (656.8)*
                          abnormality in fetal heart rate or rhythm (659.7)
                          fetal bradycardia (659.7)
                          fetal tachycardia (659.7)
                          meconium in liquor (656.8)
            For code **656.31**: (Ex) 656.31-656.33, 659.71, 763.82
            Coding Clinic: 2010, Q2, P7

● **656.4 Intrauterine death** ♀ 1,3 🌀   M
[0,1,3]   Fetal death:
               NOS
               after completion of 22 weeks' gestation
               late
            Missed delivery
            Excludes *missed abortion (632)*
            For codes **656.41 and 656.43**: (Ex) 656.41-656.43
            Coding Clinic: 2010, Q2, P7

● **656.5 Poor fetal growth** ♀ 1 🌀   M
[0,1,3]   "Light-for-dates"
            "Placental insufficiency"
            "Small-for-dates"
            For code **656.51**: (Ex) 656.51-656.53

● **656.6 Excessive fetal growth** ♀   M
[0,1,3]   "Large-for-dates"

● **656.7 Other placental conditions** ♀   M
[0,1,3]   Abnormal placenta
            Placental infarct
            Excludes *placental polyp (674.4)*
                          placentitis (658.4)

● **656.8 Other specified fetal and placental problems** ♀   M
[0,1,3]   Abnormal acid-base balance
            Intrauterine acidosis
            Lithopedian
            Meconium in liquor
            Subchorionic hematoma

● **656.9 Unspecified fetal and placental problem** ♀   M
[0,1,3]

● **657 Polyhydramnios** ♀ 1 🌀   M
[0,1,3]   Hydramnios
            Requires fifth digit; valid digits are in [brackets] under each
               code. See beginning of section 650–659 for definitions.
            Use 0 as fourth digit for category 657
            Excludes *suspected polyhydramnios not found (V89.01)*
            For code **657.01**: (Ex) 657.01-657.03
            Coding Clinic: 2006, Q3, P16-18

● **658 Other problems associated with amniotic cavity and membranes**
            Requires fifth digit; valid digits are in [brackets] under each
               code. See beginning of section 650–659 for definitions.
            Excludes *amniotic fluid embolism (673.1)*
                          *suspected problems with amniotic cavity and membranes
                          not found (V89.01)*

● **658.0 Oligohydramnios** ♀ 1,3 🌀   M
[0,1,3]   Oligohydramnios without mention of rupture of
               membranes
            For codes **658.01 and 658.03**: (Ex) 658.01-658.03
            Coding Clinic: 2006, Q3, P16-18

● **658.1 Premature rupture of membranes** ♀   M
[0,1,3]   Rupture of amniotic sac less than 24 hours prior to the
               onset of labor
            Coding Clinic: 2001, Q1, P5; 1998, Q4, P76-77

● **658.2 Delayed delivery after spontaneous or unspecified   M
       rupture of membranes** ♀
[0,1,3]   Prolonged rupture of membranes NOS
            Rupture of amniotic sac 24 hours or more prior to the
               onset of labor

● **658.3 Delayed delivery after artificial rupture of   M
       membranes** ♀
[0,1,3]

● **658.4 Infection of amniotic cavity** ♀ 1,3 🌀   M
[0,1,3]   Amnionitis   Membranitis
            Chorioamnionitis   Placentitis
            For codes **658.41 and 658.43**: (Ex) 658.41-658.43

● **658.8 Other** ♀ 1 🌀   M
[0,1,3]   Amnion nodosum
            Amniotic cyst
            For code **658.81**: (Ex) 658.81

● **658.9 Unspecified** ♀   M
[0,1,3]

● **659 Other indications for care or intervention related to labor and
       delivery, not elsewhere classified**
            Requires fifth digit; valid digits are in [brackets] under each
               code. See beginning of section 650–659 for definitions.

● **659.0 Failed mechanical induction** ♀   M
[0,1,3]   Failure of induction of labor by surgical or other
               instrumental methods

● **659.1 Failed medical or unspecified induction** ♀   M
[0,1,3]   Failed induction NOS
            Failure of induction of labor by medical methods, such as
               oxytocic drugs

● **659.2 Maternal pyrexia during labor, unspecified** ♀ 1 🌀   M
[0,1,3]   For code **659.21**: (Ex) 659.21-659.23

● **659.3 Generalized infection during labor** ♀ 1,3 🌀   M
[0,1,3]   Septicemia during labor
            For codes **659.31 and 659.33**: (Ex) 646.80-646.93, 648.90-649.64, 650,
               659.30-659.33, 669.40-669.44, 669.80-669.94, 679.00-679.04, 679.12,
               679.14

● **659.4 Grand multiparity** ♀   M
[0,1,3]   **Excludes** *supervision only, in pregnancy (V23.3)*
                          without current pregnancy (V61.5)

● **659.5 Elderly primigravida** ♀   M
[0,1,3]   First pregnancy in a woman who will be 35 years of age
               or older at expected date of delivery
            Excludes *supervision only, in pregnancy (V23.81)*
            Coding Clinic: 2001, Q3, P12

N Newborn: 0   **P** Pediatric: 0–17   **M** Maternity: 12–55   **A** Adult: 15–124   ♀ Females Only   ♂ Males Only

(Ex) CC/MCC Exclusions   🌀 Complication\Comorbidity   🌀 Major C\C   🌀 Present on Admission Requirement   🌀 Hospital-Acquired Condition   883

COMPLICATIONS OF PREGNANCY, CHILDBIRTH, AND THE PUERPERIUM (630–679)

COMPLICATIONS OF PREGNANCY, CHILDBIRTH, AND THE PUERPERIUM (630–679)

● **659.6　Elderly multigravida** ♀ .... M
[0,1,3]　　Second or more pregnancy in a woman who will be 35 years of age or older at expected date of delivery
　　　　Excludes　*elderly primigravida (659.5)*
　　　　　　　　　supervision only, in pregnancy (V23.82)
　　　　Coding Clinic: 2013, Q1, P19; 2001, Q3, P12

● **659.7　Abnormality in fetal heart rate or rhythm** ♀ .... M
[0,1,3]　　Depressed fetal heart tones
　　　　Fetal:
　　　　　　bradycardia
　　　　　　tachycardia
　　　　Fetal heart rate decelerations
　　　　Non-reassuring fetal heart rate or rhythm
　　　　Coding Clinic: 1998, Q4, P47-48

● **659.8　Other specified indications for care or intervention**
[0,1,3]　**related to labor and delivery** ♀ .... M
　　　　Pregnancy in a female less than 16 years of age at expected date of delivery
　　　　Very young maternal age
　　　　Coding Clinic: 2001, Q3, P12

● **659.9　Unspecified indication for care or intervention**
[0,1,3]　**related to labor and delivery** ♀ .... M
　　OGCR　Section I.C.11.k.2
　　　　Codes from the 660-669 series are not to be used for complications of abortion.

COMPLICATIONS OCCURRING MAINLY IN THE COURSE OF LABOR AND DELIVERY (660–669)

The following fifth-digit subclassification is for use with categories 660–669 to denote the current episode of care:

> 0　unspecified as to episode of care or not applicable
> 1　delivered, with or without mention of antepartum condition
> 2　delivered, with mention of postpartum complication
> 3　antepartum condition or complication
> 4　postpartum condition or complication

● **660　Obstructed labor**
　　　Requires fifth digit; valid digits are in [brackets] under each code. See beginning of section 660–669 for definitions.
　　　Coding Clinic: 1995, Q3, P10

● **660.0　Obstruction caused by malposition of fetus at onset**
[0,1,3]　**of labor** ♀ 3 🔖 .... M
　　　　Any condition classifiable to 652, causing obstruction during labor
　　　　Use additional code from 652.0–652.9 to identify condition
　　　　For code 660.03: Ⓔx 646.80-646.93, 648.90-649.64, 650 655.70-655.73, 660.03, 665.00-665.11 665.50-665.54, 665.80-665.94, 669.40-669.44, 669.80-669.94, 679.00-679.04, 679.12, 679.14
　　　　Coding Clinic: 1995, Q3, P10

● **660.1　Obstruction by bony pelvis** ♀ .... M
[0,1,3]　　Any condition classifiable to 653, causing obstruction during labor
　　　　Use additional code from 653.0–653.9 to identify condition
　　　　Coding Clinic: 1995, Q3, P10

● **660.2　Obstruction by abnormal pelvic soft tissues** ♀ ...... M
[0,1,3]　　Prolapse of anterior lip of cervix
　　　　Any condition classifiable to 654, causing obstruction during labor
　　　　Use additional code from 654.0–654.9 to identify condition
　　　　Coding Clinic: 1995, Q3, P10

● **660.3　Deep transverse arrest and persistent occipito-**
[0,1,3]　**posterior position** ♀ .... M

● **660.4　Shoulder (girdle) dystocia** ♀ .... M
[0,1,3]　　Impacted shoulders

● **660.5　Locked twins** ♀ .... M
[0,1,3]

● **660.6　Failed trial of labor, unspecified** ♀ .... M
[0,1,3]　　Failed trial of labor, without mention of condition or suspected condition

● **660.7　Failed forceps or vacuum extractor, unspecified** ♀ 🔖 ... M
[0,1,3]　　Application of ventouse or forceps, without mention of condition

● **660.8　Other causes of obstructed labor** ♀ .... M
[0,1,3]　　Use additional code to identify condition

● **660.9　Unspecified obstructed labor** ♀ .... M
[0,1,3]　　Dystocia:
　　　　　　NOS
　　　　　　fetal NOS
　　　　　　maternal NOS

● **661　Abnormality of forces of labor**
　　　Requires fifth digit; valid digits are in [brackets] under each code. See beginning of section 660–669 for definitions.

● **661.0　Primary uterine inertia** ♀ .... M
[0,1,3]　　Failure of cervical dilation
　　　　Hypotonic uterine dysfunction, primary
　　　　Prolonged latent phase of labor
　　　　Coding Clinic: 1985, July-Aug, P11

● **661.1　Secondary uterine inertia** ♀ .... M
[0,1,3]　　Arrested active phase of labor
　　　　Hypotonic uterine dysfunction, secondary
　　　　Coding Clinic: 1985, July-Aug, P11

● **661.2　Other and unspecified uterine inertia** ♀ .... M
[0,1,3]　　Atony of uterus without hemorrhage
　　　　Desultory labor
　　　　Irregular labor
　　　　Poor contractions
　　　　Slow slope active phase of labor
　　　　Excludes　*atony of uterus with hemorrhage (666.1)*
　　　　　　　　　postpartum atony of uterus without hemorrhage (669.8)
　　　　Coding Clinic: 1985, July-Aug, P11

● **661.3　Precipitate labor** ♀ .... M
[0,1,3]

● **661.4　Hypertonic, incoordinate, or prolonged uterine**
[0,1,3]　**contractions** ♀ .... M
　　　　Cervical spasm
　　　　Contraction ring (dystocia)
　　　　Dyscoordinate labor
　　　　Hourglass contraction of uterus
　　　　Hypertonic uterine dysfunction
　　　　Incoordinate uterine action
　　　　Retraction ring (Bandl's) (pathological)
　　　　Tetanic contractions
　　　　Uterine dystocia NOS
　　　　Uterine spasm

● **661.9　Unspecified abnormality of labor** ♀ .... M
[0,1,3]

● **662　Long labor**
　　　Requires fifth digit; valid digits are in [brackets] under each code. See beginning of section 660–669 for definitions.

● **662.0　Prolonged first stage** ♀ .... M
[0,1,3]

● **662.1　Prolonged labor, unspecified** ♀ 1 🔖 .... M
[0,1,3]　　For code 662.11: Ⓔx 646.80-646.93, 648.90-649.64, 650, 655.70-655.73, 662.11, 665.00-665.11 665.50-665.54, 665.80-665.94, 669.40-669.44, 669.80-669.94, 679.00-679.04, 679.12, 679.14

● **662.2　Prolonged second stage** ♀ .... M
[0,1,3]

● **662.3　Delayed delivery of second twin, triplet, etc.** ♀ .... M
[0,1,3]

663 Umbilical cord complications

Requires fifth digit; valid digits are in [brackets] under each code. See beginning of section 660–669 for definitions.

663.0 Prolapse of cord ♀   M
[0,1,3]   Presentation of cord

663.1 Cord around neck, with compression ♀   M
[0,1,3]   Cord tightly around neck

663.2 Other and unspecified cord entanglement, with   M
[0,1,3] **compression ♀**
    Entanglement of cords of twins in mono-amniotic sac
    Knot in cord (with compression)

663.3 Other and unspecified cord entanglement, without   M
[0,1,3] **mention of compression ♀**
    Coding Clinic: 2003, Q2, P9

663.4 Short cord ♀   M
[0,1,3]

663.5 Vasa previa ♀   M
[0,1,3]

663.6 Vascular lesions of cord ♀   M
[0,1,3]   Bruising of cord
    Hematoma of cord
    Thrombosis of vessels of cord

663.8 Other umbilical cord complications ♀   M
[0,1,3]   Velamentous insertion of umbilical cord

663.9 Unspecified umbilical cord complication ♀   M
[0,1,3]

664 Trauma to perineum and vulva during delivery

Requires fifth digit; valid digits are in [brackets] under each code. See beginning of section 660–669 for definitions.

Includes damage from instruments
    that from extension of episiotomy
Coding Clinic: 2008, Q4, P192; 1992, Q1, P10-11

664.0 First-degree perineal laceration ♀   M
[0,1,4]   Perineal laceration, rupture, or tear involving:
    fourchette
    hymen
    labia vulva
    skin
    vagina
    Coding Clinic: 1984, Nov-Dec, P10

664.1 Second-degree perineal laceration ♀   M
[0,1,4]   Perineal laceration, rupture, or tear (following
    episiotomy) involving:
    pelvic floor
    perineal muscles
    vaginal muscles

    Excludes that involving anal sphincter (664.2)
    Coding Clinic: 2008, Q4, P192; 1984, Nov-Dec, P10

664.2 Third-degree perineal laceration ♀ 1 🦠   M
[0,1,4]   Perineal laceration, rupture, or tear (following
    episiotomy) involving:
    anal sphincter
    rectovaginal septum
    sphincter NOS

    Excludes anal sphincter tear during delivery not associated
    with third-degree perineal laceration
    (664.6)
    that with anal or rectal mucosal laceration
    (664.3)
    For code **664.21:** (Ex) 646.80-646.93, 648.90-649.64, 650, 655.70-655.73,
    664.21, 664.61, 665.00-665.11, 665.50-665.54, 665.80-665.94,
    669.40-669.44, 669.80-669.94, 679.00-679.04, 679.12, 679.14
    Coding Clinic: 1984, Nov-Dec, P10

664.3 Fourth-degree perineal laceration ♀ 1 🦠   M
[0,1,4]   Perineal laceration, rupture, or tear as classifiable to 664.2
    and involving also:
    anal mucosa
    rectal mucosa
    For code **664.31:** (Ex) 646.80-646.93, 648.90-649.64, 650, 655.70-655.73,
    664.31, 665.00-665.11, 665.50-665.54, 665.80-665.94, 669.40-669.44,
    669.80-669.94, 679.00-679.04, 679.12, 679.14
    Coding Clinic: 1984, Nov-Dec, P10

Figure 11–5 Perineal lacerations:
A. First-degree is laceration of superficial tissues.
B. Second-degree is limited to the pelvic floor and may involve the perineal or vaginal muscles.
C. Third-degree involves the anal sphincter.
D. Fourth-degree involves anal or rectal mucosa.

664.4 Unspecified perineal laceration ♀   M
[0,1,4]   Central laceration

664.5 Vulval and perineal hematoma ♀   M
[0,1,4]   Coding Clinic: 1984, Nov-Dec, P10

664.6 Anal sphincter tear complicating delivery,   M
[0,1,4] **not associated with third-degree perineal**
  laceration ♀ 1,4 🦠

    Excludes third-degree perineal laceration (664.2)

    For codes **664.61 and 664.64:** (Ex) 646.80-646.93, 648.90-649.64, 650,
    655.70-655.73, 664.21, 664.60-664.64, 665.00-665.11, 665.50-665.54,
    665.80-665.94, 669.40-669.44, 669.80-669.94, 679.00-679.04, 679.12,
    679.14
    Coding Clinic: 2007, Q4, P88-90

664.8 Other specified trauma to perineum and vulva ♀   M
[0,1,4]   Periurethral trauma
    Coding Clinic: 2007, Q4, P125

664.9 Unspecified trauma to perineum and vulva ♀   M
[0,1,4]

665 Other obstetrical trauma

Requires fifth digit; valid digits are in [brackets] under each code. See beginning of section 660–669 for definitions.

Includes damage from instruments

665.0 Rupture of uterus before onset of labor ♀ 1,3 🦠   M
[0,1,3]   For codes **665.01 and 665.03:** (Ex) 646.80-646.93, 648.90-649.64, 650,
    655.70-655.73, 665.00-665.11, 665.50-665.54, 665.80-665.94,
    669.40-669.44, 669.80-669.94, 679.00-679.04, 679.12, 679.14

665.1 Rupture of uterus during labor ♀ 1 🦠   M
[0,1]   Rupture of uterus NOS
    For code **665.11:** (Ex) 646.80-646.93, 648.90-649.64, 650, 655.70-655.73,
    665.00-665.11, 665.50-665.54, 665.80-665.94, 669.40-669.44,
    669.80-669.94, 679.00-679.04, 679.12, 679.14

665.2 Inversion of uterus ♀ 2 🦠   M
[0,2,4]   For code **665.22:** (Ex) 646.80-646.93, 648.90-649.64, 650, 655.70-655.73,
    665.00-665.11, 665.22, 665.50-665.54, 665.80-665.94, 669.40-669.44,
    669.80-669.94, 679.00-679.04, 679.12, 679.14

665.3 Laceration of cervix ♀ 1 🦠   M
[0,1,4]   For code **665.31:** (Ex) 646.80-646.93, 648.90-649.64, 650, 655.70-655.73,
    665.00-665.11, 665.31, 665.50-665.54, 665.80-665.94, 669.40-669.44,
    669.80-669.94, 679.00-679.04, 679.12, 679.14

    Coding Clinic: 1984, Nov-Dec, P10

665.4 High vaginal laceration ♀ 1 🦠   M
[0,1,4]   Laceration of vaginal wall or sulcus without mention of
    perineal laceration
    For code **664.41:** (Ex) 646.80-646.93, 648.90-649.64, 650, 655.70-655.73,
    665.00-665.11, 665.41, 665.50-665.54, 665.80-665.94, 669.40-669.44,
    669.80-669.94, 679.00-679.04, 679.12, 679.14

    Coding Clinic: 1984, Nov-Dec, P10

665.5 Other injury to pelvic organs ♀ 1 🦠   M
[0,1,4]   Injury to:
    bladder
    urethra

    Excludes periurethral trauma (664.8)

    For code **665.51:** (Ex) 646.80-646.93, 648.90-649.64, 650, 655.70-655.73,
    665.00-665.11, 665.50-665.54, 665.80-665.94, 669.40-669.44,
    669.80-669.94, 679.00-679.04, 679.12, 679.14

    Coding Clinic: 1984, Nov-Dec, P10, 12

N Newborn: 0   P Pediatric: 0–17   M Maternity: 12–55   A Adult: 15–124   ♀ Females Only   ♂ Males Only

(Ex) CC/MCC Exclusions   🦠 Complication\Comorbidity   🦠 Major C\C   🦠 Present on Admission Requirement   🦠 Hospital-Acquired Condition   885

COMPLICATIONS OF PREGNANCY, CHILDBIRTH, AND THE PUERPERIUM (630–679)

● **665.6 Damage to pelvic joints and ligaments** ♀ 1 🔖   M
[0,1,4]   Avulsion of inner symphyseal cartilage
Damage to coccyx
Separation of symphysis (pubis)
For code **665.61:** (Ex:) 646.80-646.93, 648.90-649.64, 650, 655.70-655.73, 665.00-665.11, 665.50-665.54, 665.61, 665.80-665.94, 669.40-669.44, 669.80-669.94, 679.00-679.04, 679.12, 679.14

● **665.7 Pelvic hematoma** ♀ 1,2 🔖   M
[0-2,4]   Hematoma of vagina
For codes **665.71-665.72:** (Ex:) 646.80-646.93, 648.90-649.64, 650, 655.70-655.73, 665.00-665.11, 665.50-665.54, 665.71, 665.80-665.94, 669.40-669.44, 669.80-669.94, 679.00-679.04, 679.12, 679.14
Coding Clinic: 1984, Nov-Dec, P10

● **665.8 Other specified obstetrical trauma** ♀   M
[0-4]

● **665.9 Unspecified obstetrical trauma** ♀   M
[0-4]

● **666 Postpartum hemorrhage**
Requires fifth digit; valid digits are in [brackets] under each code. See beginning of section 660–669 for definitions.

● **666.0 Third-stage hemorrhage** ♀ 2,4 🔖   M
[0,2,4]   Hemorrhage associated with retained, trapped, or adherent placenta
Retained placenta NOS
For codes **666.02 and 666.04:** (Ex:) 646.80-646.93, 648.90-649.64, 650, 655.70-655.73, 665.00-665.11, 665.50-665.54, 665.80-665.94, 666.02, 669.40-669.44, 669.80-669.94, 679.00-679.04, 679.12, 679.14
Coding Clinic: 1988, Q1, P14

● **666.1 Other immediate postpartum hemorrhage** ♀ 2,4 🔖   M
[0,2,4]   Atony of uterus with hemorrhage
Hemorrhage within the first 24 hours following delivery of placenta
Postpartum atony of uterus with hemorrhage
Postpartum hemorrhage (atonic) NOS

Excludes   *atony of uterus without hemorrhage (661.2)*
postpartum atony of uterus without hemorrhage (669.8)
For code **666.12:** (Ex:) 646.80-646.93, 648.90-649.64, 650, 655.70-655.73, 665.00-665.11, 665.50-665.54, 665.80-665.94, 666.12, 669.40-669.44, 669.80-669.94, 679.00-679.04, 679.12, 679.14;
For code **666.14:** (Ex:) 666.10-666.14
Coding Clinic: 1988, Q1, P14

● **666.2 Delayed and secondary postpartum**
[0,2,4] **hemorrhage** ♀ 2,4 🔖   M
Hemorrhage:
after the first 24 hours following delivery
associated with retained portions of placenta or membranes
Postpartum hemorrhage specified as delayed or secondary
Retained products of conception NOS, following delivery
For code **666.22:** (Ex:) 646.80-646.93, 648.90-649.64, 650, 655.70-655.73, 665.00-665.11, 665.50-665.54, 665.80-665.94, 666.22, 669.40-669.44, 669.80-669.94, 679.00-679.04, 679.12, 679.14;
For code **666.24:** (Ex:) 666.20-666.24
Coding Clinic: 1988, Q1, P14

● **666.3 Postpartum coagulation defects** ♀ 2 🔖   M
[0,2,4]   Postpartum:
afibrinogenemia
fibrinolysis
For code **666.32:** (Ex:) 646.80-646.93, 648.90-649.64, 650, 666.00-666.34, 669.40-669.44, 669.80-669.94, 679.00-679.04, 679.12, 679.14

● **667 Retained placenta without hemorrhage**
Requires fifth digit; valid digits are in [brackets] under each code. See beginning of section 660–669 for definitions.

● **667.0 Retained placenta without hemorrhage** ♀   M
[0,2,4]   Placenta accreta without hemorrhage
Retained placenta:
NOS without hemorrhage
total without hemorrhage
Coding Clinic: 1988, Q1, P14

● **667.1 Retained portions of placenta or membranes,**
[0,2,4] **without hemorrhage** ♀   M
Retained products of conception following delivery, without hemorrhage
Coding Clinic: 1988, Q1, P14

● **668 Complications of the administration of anesthetic or other sedation in labor and delivery**
Use additional code(s) to further specify complication
Requires fifth digit; valid digits are in [brackets] under each code. See beginning of section 660–669 for definitions.

Includes   complications arising from the administration of a general or local anesthetic, analgesic, or other sedation in labor and delivery

Excludes   *reaction to spinal or lumbar puncture (349.0)*
spinal headache (349.0)

● **668.0 Pulmonary complications** ♀   M
[0-4]   Inhalation [aspiration] of stomach contents or secretions following anesthesia or other sedation in labor or delivery
Mendelson's syndrome following anesthesia or other sedation in labor or delivery
Pressure collapse of lung following anesthesia or other sedation in labor or delivery

● **668.1 Cardiac complications** ♀   M
[0-4]   Cardiac arrest or failure following anesthesia or other sedation in labor and delivery

● **668.2 Central nervous system complications** ♀   M
[0-4]   Cerebral anoxia following anesthesia or other sedation in labor and delivery

● **668.8 Other complications of anesthesia or other sedation**
[0-4] **in labor and delivery** ♀   M
Coding Clinic: 1999, Q2, P9-10

● **668.9 Unspecified complication of anesthesia and other**
[0-4] **sedation** ♀   M

● **669 Other complications of labor and delivery, not elsewhere classified**
Requires fifth digit; valid digits are in [brackets] under each code. See beginning of section 660–669 for definitions.

● **669.0 Maternal distress** ♀   M
[0-4]   Metabolic disturbance in labor and delivery

● **669.1 Shock during or following labor and**
[0-4] **delivery** ♀ 1-4 🔖   M
Obstetric shock
For codes **669.11-669.14:** (Ex:) 646.80-646.93, 648.90-649.64, 650, 669.10-669.14, 669.40-669.44, 669.80-669.94, 679.00-679.04, 679.12, 679.14

● **669.2 Maternal hypotension syndrome** ♀ 4 🔖, 1,2 🔖   M
[0-4]   For codes **669.21, 669.22, and 669.24:** (Ex:) 646.80-646.93, 648.90-649.64, 650, 669.10-669.14, 669.21, 669.40-669.44, 669.80-669.94, 679.00-679.04, 679.12, 679.14

● **669.3 Acute kidney failure following labor and**
[0,2,4] **delivery** ♀ 2,4 🔖   M
For codes **669.32 and 669.34:** (Ex:) 646.80-646.93, 648.90-649.64, 650, 669.30-669.44, 669.80-669.94, 679.00-679.04, 679.12, 679.14

● **669.4** **Other complications of obstetrical surgery and** **M**
[0-4] **procedures** ♀
    Cardiac:
        arrest following cesarean or other obstetrical surgery
          or procedure, including delivery NOS
        failure following cesarean or other obstetrical surgery
          or procedure, including delivery NOS
    Cerebral anoxia following cesarean or other obstetrical
        surgery or procedure, including delivery NOS

    Excludes *complications of obstetrical surgical wounds*
        (674.1–674.3)

● **669.5** **Forceps or vacuum extractor delivery without** **M**
[0,1] **mention of indication** ♀
    Delivery by ventouse, without mention of indication

● **669.6** **Breech extraction, without mention of indication** ♀ **M**
[0,1]
    Excludes *breech delivery NOS (652.2)*

● **669.7** **Cesarean delivery, without mention of indication** ♀ **M**
[0,1]   **Coding Clinic: 2001, Q1, P11-12**

● **669.8** **Other complications of labor and delivery** ♀ **M**
[0-4]   **Coding Clinic: 2006, Q4, P135**

● **669.9** **Unspecified complication of labor and delivery** ♀ **M**
[0-4]

COMPLICATIONS OF THE PUERPERIUM (670–677)

Note: Categories 671 and 673–676 include the listed
      conditions even if they occur during pregnancy or
      childbirth.

The following fifth-digit subclassification is for use with
categories 670–676 to denote the current episode of care:

  0 **unspecified as to episode of care or not applicable**
  1 **delivered, with or without mention of antepartum**
      condition
  2 **delivered, with mention of postpartum complication**
  3 **antepartum condition or complication**
  4 **postpartum condition or complication**

● **670** **Major puerperal infection**
    Requires fifth digit; valid digits are in [brackets] under each
      code. See beginning of section 670–676 for definitions.

    Excludes *infection following abortion (639.0)*
        minor genital tract infection following delivery (646.6)
        puerperal fever NOS (672)
        puerperal pyrexia NOS (672)
        puerperal pyrexia of unknown origin (672)
        urinary tract infection following delivery (646.6)
    For codes 670.02 and 670.04: (Ex) 646.80-646.93, 648.90-649.64, 650, 669.40-669.44,
      669.80-670.04, 679.00-679.04, 679.12, 679.14
    Coding Clinic: 2007, Q3, P10

● **670.0** **Major puerpal infection, unspecified** ♀ 2,4 🔖 **M**
[0,2,4] For codes 670.02 and 670.04: (Ex) 646.80-646.93, 648.90-649.64, 650,
      669.40-669.44, 669.80-670.84, 679.00-679.04, 679.12, 679.14

● **670.1** **Puerpal endometritis** ♀ 0,2,4 🔖 **M**
[0,2,4] For codes 670.10, 670.12, and 670.14: (Ex) 646.80-646.93, 648.90-649.64,
      650, 669.40-669.44, 669.80-670.84, 679.00-679.04, 679.12, 679.14

● **670.2** **Puerpal sepsis** ♀ 0 🔖, 2,4 🔖 **M**
[0,2,4] Puerpal pyemia
    Use additional code to identify severe sepsis (995.92)
      and any associated acute organ dysfunction, if
      applicable
    For codes 670.20, 670.22, and 670.24: (Ex) 646.80-646.93, 648.90-649.64,
      650, 669.40-669.44, 669.80-670.84, 679.00-679.04, 679.12, 679.14
    Coding Clinic: 2009, Q4, P108

● **670.3** **Puerpal septic thrombophlebitis** ♀ 0 🔖, 2,4 🔖 **M**
[0,2,4] For codes 670.30, 670.32, and 670.34: (Ex) 646.80-646.93, 648.90-649.64,
      650, 669.40-669.44, 669.80-670.84, 679.00-679.04, 679.12, 679.14

● **670.8** **Other major puerpal infection** ♀ 🔖 **M**
[0,2,4] Puerpal:
      pelvic cellulitis
      peritonitis
      salpingitis
    For codes 670.80, 670.82, and 670.84: (Ex) 646.80-646.93, 648.90-649.64,
      650, 669.40-669.44, 669.80-670.84, 679.00-679.04, 679.12, 679.14

● **671** **Venous complications in pregnancy and the puerperium**
    Excludes *personal history of venous complications prior to*
        pregnancy, such as:
        thrombophlebitis (V12.52)
        thrombosis and embolism (V12.51)
    Requires fifth digit; valid digits are in [brackets] under each
      code. See beginning of section 670–676 for definitions.

● **671.0** **Varicose veins of legs** ♀ **M**
[0-4] Varicose veins NOS

● **671.1** **Varicose veins of vulva and perineum** ♀ **M**
[0-4]

● **671.2** **Superficial thrombophlebitis** ♀ 🔖 **M**
[0-4] Phlebitis NOS
    Thrombophlebitis (superficial)
    Thrombosis NOS

    Use additional code to identify the superficial
      thrombophlebitis (453.6, 453.71, 453.81)
    (Ex) 646.80-646.93, 648.90-649.64, 650, 669.40-669.44, 669.80-669.94,
      671.20-671.94, 679.00-679.04, 679.12, 679.14

● **671.3** **Deep phlebothrombosis, antepartum** ♀ 0 🔖, 1,3 🔖 **M**
[0,1,3] Deep-vein thrombosis, antepartum
    Use additional code to identify the deep vein thrombosis
      (453.40-453.42, 453.50-453.52, 453.72-453.79,
      453.82-453.89)
    Use additional code for long-term (current) use of
      anticoagulants if applicable (V58.61)
    For codes 671.30, 671.31, and 671.33: (Ex) 646.80-646.93, 648.90-649.64,
      650, 669.40-669.44, 669.80-669.94, 671.20-671.94, 679.00-679.04,
      679.12, 679.14

● **671.4** **Deep phlebothrombosis, postpartum** ♀ 0 🔖, 2,4 🔖 **M**
[0,2,4] Deep-vein thrombosis, postpartum
    Pelvic thrombophlebitis, postpartum
    Phlegmasia alba dolens (puerperal)
    Use additional code to identify the deep vein thrombosis
      (453.40-453.42, 453.50-453.52, 453.72-453.79,
      453.82-453.89)
    Use additional code for long-term (current) use of
      anticoagulants if applicable (V58.61)
    For codes 671.40, 671.42, and 671.44: (Ex) 646.80-646.93, 648.90-649.64,
      650, 669.40-669.44, 669.80-669.94, 671.20-671.94, 679.00-679.04,
      679.12, 679.14

● **671.5** **Other phlebitis and thrombosis** ♀ 🔖 **M**
[0-4] Cerebral venous thrombosis
    Thrombosis of intracranial venous sinus
    (Ex) 646.80-646.93, 648.90-649.64, 650, 669.40-669.44, 669.80-669.94,
      671.20-671.94, 679.00-679.04, 679.12, 679.14

● **671.8** **Other venous complications** ♀ 🔖 **M**
[0-4] Hemorrhoids
    For codes 671.80-671.83: (Ex) 646.80-646.93, 648.90-649.64, 650,
      669.40-669.44, 669.80-669.94, 671.20-671.94, 679.00-679.04, 679.12,
      679.14;
    For code 671.84: (Ex) 671.80-671.84

● **671.9** **Unspecified venous complication** ♀ 0-2 🔖 **M**
[0-4] For codes 671.90-671.92: (Ex) 646.80-646.93, 648.90-649.64, 650,
      669.40-669.44, 669.80-669.94, 671.20-671.94, 679.00-679.04, 679.12,
      679.14

● **672** **Pyrexia of unknown origin during the**
[0,2,4] **puerperium** ♀ 2,4 🔖 **M**
    Postpartum fever NOS
    Puerperal fever NOS
    Puerperal pyrexia NOS
    Requires fifth digit; valid digits are in [brackets] under each
      code. See beginning of section 670–676 for definitions.
    Use 0 as fourth digit for category 672
    For code 672.02: (Ex) 646.80-646.93, 648.90-649.64, 650, 669.40-669.44, 669.80-669.94,
      671.20, 671.23-671.30, 671.33-671.40, 671.50, 671.53-671.80, 671.83-671.90,
      671.93-671.94, 672.02, 679.00-679.04, 679.12, 679.14;
    For code 672.04: (Ex) 672.02-672.04

COMPLICATIONS OF PREGNANCY, CHILDBIRTH, AND THE PUERPERIUM (630–679)

● 673 **Obstetrical pulmonary embolism**

Requires fifth digit; valid digits are in [brackets] under each code. See beginning of section 670–676 for definitions.

Includes pulmonary emboli in pregnancy, childbirth, or the puerperium, or specified as puerperal

Excludes *embolism following abortion (639.6)*

● 673.0 **Obstetrical air embolism** ♀ 1-4 M
[0-4] For codes 673.01-673.04: (Ex:) 646.80-646.93, 648.90-649.64, 650, 669.40-669.44, 669.80-669.94, 673.00-673.84, 679.00-679.04, 679.12, 679.14

● 673.1 **Amniotic fluid embolism** ♀ 1-4 M
[0-4] For codes 673.11-673.14: (Ex:) 646.80-646.93, 648.90-649.64, 650, 669.40-669.44, 669.80-669.94, 673.00-673.84, 679.00-679.04, 679.12, 679.14

● 673.2 **Obstetrical blood-clot embolism** ♀ 1-4 M
[0-4] Puerperal pulmonary embolism NOS
For codes 673.21-673.24: (Ex:) 646.80-646.93, 648.90-649.64, 650, 669.40-669.44, 669.80-669.94, 673.00-673.84, 679.00-679.04, 679.12, 679.14

● 673.3 **Obstetrical pyemic and septic**
[0-4] **embolism** ♀ 0, 1-4 M
(Ex:) 646.80-646.93, 648.90-649.64, 650, 669.40-669.44, 669.80-669.94, 673.00-673.84, 679.00-679.04, 679.12, 679.14

● 673.8 **Other pulmonary embolism** ♀ 1-4 M
[0-4] Fat embolism
For codes 673.81-673.84: (Ex:) 646.80-646.93, 648.90-649.64, 650, 669.40-669.44, 669.80-669.94, 673.00-673.84, 679.00-679.04, 679.12, 679.14

● 674 **Other and unspecified complications of the puerperium, not elsewhere classified**

Requires fifth digit; valid digits are in [brackets] under each code. See beginning of section 670–676 for definitions.

● 674.0 **Cerebrovascular disorders in the**
[0-4] **puerperium** ♀ 2-4, 1 M
Any condition classifiable to 430–434, 436–437 occurring during pregnancy, childbirth, or the puerperium, or specified as puerperal

Excludes *intracranial venous sinus thrombosis (671.5)*
For codes 674.01-674.04: (Ex:) 646.80-646.93, 648.90-649.64, 650, 669.40-669.44, 669.80-669.94, 674.00-674.04, 674.50-674.54, 679.00-679.04, 679.12, 679.14

● 674.1 **Disruption of cesarean wound** ♀ M
[0,2,4] Dehiscence or disruption of uterine wound

Excludes *uterine rupture before onset of labor (665.0)*
uterine rupture during labor (665.1)

● 674.2 **Disruption of perineal wound** ♀ M
[0,2,4] Breakdown of perineum
Disruption of wound of:
episiotomy
perineal laceration
Secondary perineal tear
Coding Clinic: 1997, Q1, P9-10

● 674.3 **Other complications of obstetrical surgical**
[0,2,4] **wounds** ♀ M
Hematoma of cesarean section or perineal wound
Hemorrhage of cesarean section or perineal wound
Infection of cesarean section or perineal wound

Excludes *damage from instruments in delivery (664.0–665.9)*

Coding Clinic: 2009, Q4, P108

● 674.4 **Placental polyp** ♀ M
[0,2,4]

● 674.5 **Peripartum cardiomyopathy** ♀ M
[0-4] Postpartum cardiomyopathy
(Ex:) 646.80-646.93, 648.90-649.64, 650, 669.40-669.44, 669.80-669.94, 674.00-674.04, 674.50-674.54, 679.00-679.04, 679.12, 679.14
Coding Clinic: 2012, Q3, P10; 2003, Q4, P65

● 674.8 **Other** ♀ M
[0,2,4] Hepatorenal syndrome, following delivery
Postpartum:
subinvolution of uterus
uterine hypertrophy
Coding Clinic: 1998, Q3, P16

● 674.9 **Unspecified** ♀ M
[0,2,4] Sudden death of unknown cause during the puerperium

● 675 **Infections of the breast and nipple associated with childbirth**

Requires fifth digit; valid digits are in [brackets] under each code. See beginning of section 670–676 for definitions.

Includes the listed conditions during pregnancy, childbirth, or the puerperium

● 675.0 **Infections of nipple** ♀ M
[0-4] Abscess of nipple

● 675.1 **Abscess of breast** ♀ 1,2 M
[0-4] Abscess: Mastitis:
mammary   purulent
subareolar   retromammary
submammary   submammary
For codes 675.11-675.12: (Ex:) 646.80-646.93, 648.90-649.64, 650, 669.40-669.44, 669.80-669.94, 675.00-675.94, 679.00-679.04, 679.12, 679.14

● 675.2 **Nonpurulent mastitis** ♀ M
[0-4] Lymphangitis of breast
Mastitis:
NOS
interstitial
parenchymatous

● 675.8 **Other specified infections of the breast and**
[0-4] **nipple** ♀ M

● 675.9 **Unspecified infection of the breast and nipple** ♀ M
[0-4]

● 676 **Other disorders of the breast associated with childbirth and disorders of lactation**

Requires fifth digit; valid digits are in [brackets] under each code. See beginning of section 670–676 for definitions.

Includes the listed conditions during pregnancy, the puerperium, or lactation

● 676.0 **Retracted nipple** ♀ M
[0-4]

● 676.1 **Cracked nipple** ♀ M
[0-4] Fissure of nipple

● 676.2 **Engorgement of breasts** ♀ M
[0-4]

● 676.3 **Other and unspecified disorder of breast** ♀ M
[0-4]

● 676.4 **Failure of lactation** ♀ M
[0-4] Agalactia

● 676.5 **Suppressed lactation** ♀ M
[0-4]

● 676.6 **Galactorrhea** ♀ M
[0-4] Excludes *galactorrhea not associated with childbirth (611.6)*
Coding Clinic: 1985, July-Aug, P9

● 676.8 **Other disorders of lactation** ♀ M
[0-4] Galactocele
Coding Clinic: 2012, Q3, P7

● 676.9 **Unspecified disorder of lactation** ♀ M
[0-4]

OGCR   Section I.C.11.j.1-3

1) **Code 677**
Code 677, Late effect of complication of pregnancy, childbirth, and the puerperium is for use in those cases when an initial complication of a pregnancy develops a sequelae requiring care or treatment at a future date.

2) **After the initial postpartum period**
This code may be used at any time after the initial postpartum period.

3) **Sequencing of Code 677**
This code, like all late effect codes, is to be sequenced following the code describing the sequelae of the complication.

677   **Late effect of complication of pregnancy, childbirth, and the puerperium** ♀ 🐾

> **Note:** This category is to be used to indicate conditions in 632–648.9 and 651–676.9 as the cause of the late effect, themselves classifiable elsewhere. The "late effects " include conditions specified as such, or as sequelae, which may occur at any time after the puerperium.

> *Code first* any sequelae

> Coding Clinic: 2013, Q3, P7; 1997, Q1, P9-10

OTHER MATERNAL AND FETAL COMPLICATIONS (678-679)

The following fifth-digit subclassification is for use with categories 678-679 to denote the current episode of care:

> 0   unspecified as to episode of care or not applicable
> 1   delivered, with or without mention of antepartum condition
> 2   delivered, with mention of postpartum complication
> 3   antepartum condition or complication
> 4   postpartum condition or complication

● 678   **Other fetal conditions**

> Requires fifth digit; valid digits are in [brackets] under each code. See beginning of section 678-679 for definitions.
> Coding Clinic: 2008, Q4, P125-127

● 678.0   **Fetal hematologic conditions** ♀   M
[0,1,3]   Fetal anemia
             Fetal thrombocytopenia
             Fetal twin to twin transfusion

> **Excludes** *fetal and neonatal hemorrhage (772.0-772.9)*
>   *fetal hematologic disorders affecting newborn (776.0-776.9)*
>   *fetal-maternal hemorrhage (656.00-656.03)*
>   *isoimmunization incompatibility (656.10-656.13, 656.20-656.23)*

● 678.1   **Fetal conjoined twins** ♀   M
[0,1,3]

● 679   **Complications of in utero procedures**

> Requires fifth digit; valid digits are in [brackets] under each code. See beginning of section 678-679 for definitions.
> Coding Clinic: 2008, Q4, P127-128

● 679.0   **Maternal complications from in utero procedure** ♀   M
[0-4]   **Excludes** *maternal history of in utero procedure during previous pregnancy (V23.86)*

● 679.1   **Fetal complications from in utero procedure** ♀   M
[0-4]   Fetal complications from amniocentesis
           Excludes *newborn affected by in utero procedure (760.61-760.64)*

COMPLICATIONS OF PREGNANCY, CHILDBIRTH, AND THE PUERPERIUM (630—679)

N Newborn: 0   P Pediatric: 0–17   M Maternity: 12–55   A Adult: 15–124   ♀ Females Only   ♂ Males Only

Ex CC/MCC Exclusions   🐾 Complication\Comorbidity   🐾 Major C\C   🐾 Present on Admission Requirement   🐾 Hospital-Acquired Condition

889

A   B

Figure 12–1   Furuncle, also known as a boil, is a staphylococcal infection. The organism enters the body through a hair follicle and so furuncles usually appear in hairy areas of the body. A cluster of furuncles is known as a carbuncle and involves infection into the deep subcutaneous fascia. These usually appear on the back and neck. (**B** from Habif: Clinical Dermatology, ed 5, Mosby, 2009)

12. DISEASES OF THE SKIN AND SUBCUTANEOUS TISSUE (680–709)

INFECTIONS OF SKIN AND SUBCUTANEOUS TISSUE (680–686)

Excludes   *certain infections of skin classified under "Infectious and Parasitic Diseases," such as:*
erysipelas (035)
erysipeloid of Rosenbach (027.1)
herpes:
    simplex (054.0–054.9)
    zoster (053.0–053.9)
molluscum contagiosum (078.0)
viral warts (078.10-078.19)

● 680 **Carbuncle and furuncle**
    Includes   boil
                 furunculosis

    680.0 Face
         Ear [any part]   Nose (septum)
         Face [any part, except eye]   Temple (region)
         Excludes   *eyelid (373.13)*
                          lacrimal apparatus (375.31)
                          orbit (376.01)

    680.1 Neck

    680.2 Trunk
         Abdominal wall
         Back [any part, except buttocks]
         Breast
         Chest wall
         Flank
         Groin
         Pectoral region
         Perineum
         Umbilicus
         Excludes   *buttocks (680.5)*
                          external genital organs:
                            female (616.4)
                            male (607.2, 608.4)

    680.3 Upper arm and forearm
         Arm [any part, except hand]
         Axilla
         Shoulder

    680.4 Hand
         Finger [any]   Wrist
         Thumb

    680.5 Buttock
         Anus   Gluteal region

    680.6 Leg, except foot
         Ankle   Knee
         Hip   Thigh

    680.7 Foot
         Heel
         Toe

    680.8 Other specified sites
         Head [any part, except face]
         Scalp
         Excludes   *external genital organs:*
                          female (616.4)
                          male (607.2, 608.4)

    680.9 Unspecified site
         Boil NOS   Furuncle NOS
         Carbuncle NOS

● 681 **Cellulitis and abscess of finger and toe**
    Includes   that with lymphangitis
    Use additional code to identify organism, such as:
         Staphylococcus (041.1)

  ● **681.0 Finger**
      681.00 Cellulitis and abscess, unspecified
      681.01 Felon
          Pulp abscess   Whitlow
          Excludes   *herpetic whitlow (054.6)*
      681.02 Onychia and paronychia of finger
          Panaritium of finger
          Perionychia of finger

  ● **681.1 Toe**
      681.10 Cellulitis and abscess, unspecified
          Coding Clinic: 2005, Q1, P14
      681.11 Onychia and paronychia of toe
          Panaritium of toe
          Perionychia of toe

    681.9 Cellulitis and abscess of unspecified digit
         Infection of nail NOS

● 682 **Other cellulitis and abscess**
    Includes   abscess (acute) (with lymphangitis) except of finger
                 or toe
               cellulitis (diffuse) (with lymphangitis) except of
                 finger or toe
              lymphangitis, acute (with lymphangitis) except of
                 finger or toe
    Use additional code to identify organism, such as:
         Staphylococcus (041.1)
    Excludes   *lymphangitis (chronic) (subacute) (457.2)*

    682.0 Face 🔖
         This code reports forehead but not head (682.8).
         Cheek, external   Nose, external
         Chin   Submandibular
         Forehead   Temple (region)
         Excludes   *ear [any part] (380.10–380.16)*
                          eyelid (373.13)
                          lacrimal apparatus (375.31)
                          lip (528.5)
                          mouth (528.3)
                          nose (internal) (478.1)
                          orbit (376.01)
         (Ex:) 017.00-017.06, 017.90-017.96, 040.82-041.9, 682.0, 682.8-682.9,
              686.00-686.9, 705.83, 709.8, V09.0-V09.91

    682.1 Neck 🔖
         (Ex:) 017.00-017.06, 017.90-017.96, 040.82-041.9, 682.1, 682.8-682.9,
              686.00-686.9, 705.83, 709.8, V09.0-V09.91

Item 12-1   **Cellulitis** is an acute spreading bacterial infection below the surface of the skin characterized by redness (erythema), warmth, swelling, pain, fever, chills, and enlarged lymph nodes ("swollen glands"). **Abscess** is a localized collection of pus in tissues or organs and is a sign of infection resulting in swelling and inflammation. **Onychia** is an inflammation of the tissue surrounding the nail with pus accumulation and loss of the nail, resulting from microscopic pathogens entering through small wounds. **Paronychia** is a nail disease also known as felon or whitlow and is a bacterial or fungal infection.

◀ New   ◀▦ Revised   ~~deleted~~ Deleted   Excludes   Includes   Use additional   Code first   Omit code
● Unacceptable Principal Diagnosis   ● Use Additional Digit(s)   ▶ Manifestation Code   OGCR Official Guidelines   **Coding Clinic**

890

682.2 Trunk 🔵
Abdominal wall
Back [any part, except buttock]
Buttocks see 682.5
Chest wall
Flank
Groin
Pectoral region
Perineum
Umbilicus, except newborn

Excludes *anal and rectal regions (566)*
breast:
NOS (611.0)
puerperal (675.1)
external genital organs:
female (616.3–616.4)
male (604.0, 607.2, 608.4)
umbilicus, newborn (771.4)

Ⓔ 017.00-017.06, 017.90-017.96, 040.82-041.9, 682.2, 682.8-682.9, 686-686.9, 705.83, 709.8, V09.0-V09.91

Coding Clinic: 1993, Q1, P26

682.3 Upper arm and forearm 🔵
Arm [any part, except hand]
Axilla
Shoulder

Excludes *hand (682.4)*

Ⓔ 017.00-017.06, 017.90-017.96, 040.82-041.9, 682.3, 682.8-682.9, 686.00-686.9, 705.83, 709.8, V09.0-V09.91

Coding Clinic: 2003, Q2, P7-8; 1998, Q4, P42-44

682.4 Hand, except fingers and thumb 🔵
Wrist

Excludes *finger and thumb (681.00–681.02)*

Ⓔ 017.00-017.06, 017.90-017.96, 040.82-041.9, 682.4, 682.8-682.9, 686.00-686.9, 705.83, 709.8, V09.0-V09.91

682.5 Buttock 🔵
Gluteal region

Excludes *anal and rectal regions (566)*

Ⓔ 017.00-017.06, 017.90-017.96, 040.82-041.9, 682.5, 682.8-682.9, 686.00-686.9, 705.83, 709.8, V09.0-V09.91

682.6 Leg, except foot 🔵
Ankle   Knee
Hip   Thigh

Ⓔ 017.00-017.06, 017.90-017.96, 040.82-041.9, 682.6, 682.8-682.9, 686.00-686.9, 705.83, 709.8, V09.0-V09.91

Coding Clinic: 2012, Q3, P14; 2009, Q1, P18x2; 2004, Q3, P5-6; 2003, Q4, P108; 1995, Q1, P3

682.7 Foot, except toes 🔵
Heel

Excludes *toe (681.10–681.11)*

Ⓔ 017.00-017.06, 017.90-017.96, 040.82-041.9, 682.7-682.9, 686.00-686.9, 705.83, 709.8, V09.0-V09.91

682.8 Other specified sites 🔵
Head [except face]
Scalp

Excludes *face (682.0)*

Ⓔ 017.00-017.06, 017.90-017.96, 040.82-041.9, 682.8-682.9, 686.00-686.9 705.83, 709.8, V09.0-V09.91

682.9 Unspecified site 🔵
Abscess NOS
Cellulitis NOS
Lymphangitis, acute NOS

Excludes *lymphangitis NOS (457.2)*

Ⓔ 017.00-017.06, 017.90-017.96, 040.82-041.9, 682.8-682.9, 686.00-686.9 705.83, 709.8, V09.0-V09.91

Figure 12–2 Impetigo. A thick, honey-yellow adherent crust covers the entire eroded surface. (From Habif: Clinical Dermatology, ed 4, Mosby, Inc., 2004)

Item 12–2 Pilonidal cyst, also called a coccygeal cyst, is the result of a disorder called pilonidal disease. The cyst usually contains hair and pus.

683 Acute lymphadenitis
Short term inflammation of lymph nodes which can be regionalized to involve a given area of lymph system or systemic involvement
Abscess (acute) lymph gland or node, except mesenteric
Adenitis, acute lymph gland or node, except mesenteric
Lymphadenitis, acute lymph gland or node, except mesenteric

Use additional code to identify organism such as Staphylococcus (041.1)

Excludes *enlarged glands NOS (785.6)*
lymphadenitis:
chronic or subacute, except mesenteric (289.1)
mesenteric (acute) (chronic) (subacute) (289.2)
unspecified (289.3)

684 Impetigo
Contagious skin infection caused by streptococcus or staphylococcus aureus that produces blisters or sores on the face and hands
Impetiginization of other dermatoses
Impetigo (contagiosa) [any site] [any organism]:
bullousneonatorum   simplex
circinate
Pemphigus neonatorum

Excludes *impetigo herpetiformis (694.3)*

⬤**685 Pilonidal cyst**
Includes fistula, coccygeal or pilonidal
sinus, coccygeal or pilonidal

685.0 With abscess 🔵
Ⓔ 685.0-685.1, 709.8

685.1 Without mention of abscess
Coding Clinic: 2011, Q3, P9

⬤**686 Other local infections of skin and subcutaneous tissue**
Use additional code to identify any infectious organism (041.0–041.8)

⬤**686.0 Pyoderma**
Dermatitis:
purulent   suppurative
septic

686.00 Pyoderma, unspecified

686.01 Pyoderma gangrenosum 🔵
Ⓔ 686.00-686.09
Coding Clinic: 1997, Q4, P42

686.09 Other pyoderma

686.1 Pyogenic granuloma
Granuloma:
septic   telangiectaticum
suppurative

Excludes *pyogenic granuloma of oral mucosa (528.9)*

686.8 Other specified local infections of skin and subcutaneous tissue
Bacterid (pustular)   Ecthyma
Dermatitis vegetans   Perlèche

Excludes *dermatitis infectiosa eczematoides (690.8)*
panniculitis (729.30–729.39)

686.9 Unspecified local infection of skin and subcutaneous tissue
Fistula of skin NOS   Skin infection NOS

Excludes *fistula to skin from internal organs—see Alphabetic Index*

DISEASES OF THE SKIN AND SUBCUTANEOUS TISSUE (680–709)

N Newborn: 0   **P** Pediatric: 0–17   **M** Maternity: 12–55   **A** Adult: 15–124   ♀ Females Only   ♂ Males Only

Ⓔ CC/MCC Exclusions   🔵 Complication\Comorbidity   🔵 Major C\C   🔵 Present on Admission Requirement   🔵 Hospital-Acquired Condition   891

Figure 12-3 Seborrheic dermatitis. (From Cohen BA: Atlas of Pediatric Dermatology. St. Louis, Mosby, 1993)

Item 12-3 Seborrheic dermatitis is characterized by greasy, scaly, red patches and is associated with oily skin and scalp.

OTHER INFLAMMATORY CONDITIONS OF SKIN AND SUBCUTANEOUS TISSUE (690–698)

Excludes *panniculitis (729.30–729.39)*

690 Erythematosquamous dermatosis

Excludes *eczematous dermatitis of eyelid (373.31)*
parakeratosis variegata (696.2)
psoriasis (696.0–696.1)
seborrheic keratosis (702.11–702.19)

690.1 Seborrheic dermatitis

690.10 Seborrheic dermatitis, unspecified
Seborrheic dermatitis NOS

690.11 Seborrhea capitis   P
Cradle cap

690.12 Seborrheic infantile dermatitis   P

690.18 Other seborrheic dermatitis

690.8 Other erythematosquamous dermatosis

691 Atopic dermatitis and related conditions

691.0 Diaper or napkin rash
Ammonia dermatitis
Diaper or napkin:
dermatitis
erythema
rash
Psoriasiform napkin eruption

691.8 Other atopic dermatitis and related conditions
Atopic dermatitis
Besnier's prurigo
Eczema:
atopic
flexural
intrinsic (allergic)
Neurodermatitis:
atopic
diffuse (of Brocq)

Figure 12-4 Atopic dermatitis. (From Moschella SL, Hurley HJ: Dermatology, ed 3, Philadelphia, WB Saunders, 1993)

Item 12-4 Atopic dermatitis, also known as atopic eczema, infantile eczema, disseminated neurodermatitis, flexural eczema, and *prurigo diathesique* (Besnier), is characterized by intense itching and is often hereditary.

692 Contact dermatitis and other eczema

Includes dermatitis:
NOS
contact
occupational
venenata
eczema (acute) (chronic):
NOS
allergic
erythematous
occupational

Excludes *allergy NOS (995.3)*
contact dermatitis of eyelids (373.32)
dermatitis due to substances taken internally (693.0–693.9)
eczema of external ear (380.22)
perioral dermatitis (695.3)
urticarial reactions (708.0–708.9, 995.1)

692.0 Due to detergents

692.1 Due to oils and greases

692.2 Due to solvents
Dermatitis due to solvents of:
chlorocompound group
cyclohexane group
ester group
glycol group
hydrocarbon group
ketone group

692.3 Due to drugs and medicines in contact with skin
Dermatitis (allergic) (contact) due to:
arnica
fungicides
iodine
keratolytics
mercurials
neomycin
pediculocides
phenols
scabicides
any drug applied to skin
Dermatitis medicamentosa due to drug applied to skin
Use additional E code to identify drug

Excludes *allergy NOS due to drugs (995.27)*
dermatitis due to ingested drugs (693.0)
dermatitis medicamentosa NOS (693.0)

692.4 Due to other chemical products

Dermatitis due to:	Dermatitis due to:
acids	insecticide
adhesive plaster	nylon
alkalis	plastic
caustics	rubber
dichromate	

Coding Clinic: 2008, Q3, P6-7; 1989, Q2, P16

692.5 Due to food in contact with skin
Dermatitis, contact, due to:
cereals
fish
flour
fruit
meat
milk

Excludes *dermatitis due to:*
dyes (692.89)
ingested foods (693.1)
preservatives (692.89)

692.6 Due to plants [except food]
Dermatitis due to:
lacquer tree [Rhus verniciflua]
poison:
 ivy [Rhus toxicodendron]
 oak [Rhus diversiloba]
 sumac [Rhus venenata]
 vine [Rhus radicans]
primrose [Primula]
ragweed [Senecio jacobae]
other plants in contact with the skin

> **Excludes** *allergy NOS due to pollen (477.0)*
> *nettle rash (708.8)*

● 692.7 Due to solar radiation

> **Excludes** *sunburn due to other ultraviolet radiation exposure (692.82)*

692.70 Unspecified dermatitis due to sun

692.71 Sunburn
First degree sunburn
See codes 692.76 and 692.77 for second and third degrees.
Sunburn NOS

692.72 Acute dermatitis due to solar radiation
Berloque dermatitis
Photoallergic response
Phototoxic response
Polymorphous light eruption
Acute solar skin damage NOS

> **Excludes** *sunburn (692.71, 692.76–692.77)*

Use additional E code to identify drug, if drug induced

692.73 Actinic reticuloid and actinic granuloma

692.74 Other chronic dermatitis due to solar radiation
Chronic solar skin damage NOS
Solar elastosis

> **Excludes** *actinic [solar] keratosis (702.0)*

692.75 Disseminated superficial actinic porokeratosis (DSAP)

692.76 Sunburn of second degree

692.77 Sunburn of third degree

692.79 Other dermatitis due to solar radiation
Hydroa aestivale
Photodermatitis (due to sun)
Photosensitiveness (due to sun)
Solar skin damage NOS

● 692.8 Due to other specified agents

692.81 Dermatitis due to cosmetics

692.82 Dermatitis due to other radiation
Infrared rays
Light, except from sun
Radiation NOS
Tanning bed
Ultraviolet rays, except from sun
X-rays

> **Excludes** *that due to solar radiation (692.70–692.79)*

Coding Clinic: 2000, Q3, P5

692.83 Dermatitis due to metals
Jewelry

692.84 Due to animal (cat) (dog) dander
Due to animal (cat) (dog) hair
Coding Clinic: 2004, Q4, P90-91

692.89 Other
Dermatitis due to:
 cold weather
 dyes
 hot weather
 preservatives

> **Excludes** *allergy (NOS) (rhinitis) due to animal hair or dander (477.2)*
> *allergy to dust (477.8)*
> *sunburn (692.71, 692.76–692.77)*

692.9 Unspecified cause
Dermatitis:
 NOS
  contact NOS
  venenata NOS
Eczema NOS

● 693 Dermatitis due to substances taken internally

> **Excludes** *adverse effect NOS of drugs and medicines (995.20)*
> *allergy NOS (995.3)*
> *contact dermatitis (692.0–692.9)*
> *urticarial reactions (708.0–708.9, 995.1)*

693.0 Due to drugs and medicines
Dermatitis medicamentosa NOS
Use additional E code to identify drug

> **Excludes** *that due to drugs in contact with skin (692.3)*

Coding Clinic: 2007, Q2, P9-10

693.1 Due to food

693.8 Due to other specified substances taken internally

693.9 Due to unspecified substance taken internally

> **Excludes** *dermatitis NOS (692.9)*

● 694 Bullous dermatoses

694.0 Dermatitis herpetiformis
Dermatosis herpetiformis
Duhring's disease
Hydroa herpetiformis

> **Excludes** *herpes gestationis (646.8)*
> *dermatitis herpetiformis:*
> *juvenile (694.2)*
> *senile (694.5)*

694.1 Subcorneal pustular dermatosis
Sneddon-Wilkinson disease or syndrome

694.2 Juvenile dermatitis herpetiformis
Juvenile pemphigoid

694.3 Impetigo herpetiformis

694.4 Pemphigus 🖐
Pemphigus:
 NOS
 erythematosus
 foliaceus
 malignant
 vegetans
 vulgaris

> **Excludes** *pemphigus neonatorum (684)*

Ⓔⓧ 694.4-694.9, 709.8

694.5 Pemphigoid 🖐
Benign pemphigus NOS
Bullous pemphigoid
Herpes circinatus bullosus
Senile dermatitis herpetiformis
Ⓔⓧ 694.4-694.9, 709.8

Figure 12–5 Dermatitis herpetiformis. (From Arnold HL, Odom RB, James WD: Andrews' Diseases of the Skin, Clinical Dermatology, ed 8, Philadelphia, WB Saunders, 1990)

Item 12–5 Dermatitis herpetiformis, also known as Duhring's disease, is a systemic disease characterized by small blisters (3 to 5 mm) and occasionally large bullae (+5 mm).

DISEASES OF THE SKIN AND SUBCUTANEOUS TISSUE (680–709)

N Newborn: 0   P Pediatric: 0–17   M Maternity: 12–55   A Adult: 15–124   ♀ Females Only   ♂ Males Only

Ⓔⓧ CC/MCC Exclusions   🖐 Complication\Comorbidity   🖐 Major C\C   🖐 Present on Admission Requirement   🖐 Hospital-Acquired Condition   **893**

● **694.6 Benign mucous membrane pemphigoid**
     Cicatricial pemphigoid
     Mucosynechial atrophic bullous dermatitis

     694.60 Without mention of ocular involvement

     694.61 With ocular involvement
         Ocular pemphigus

     694.8 Other specified bullous dermatoses
         Excludes *herpes gestationis (646.8)*

     694.9 Unspecified bullous dermatoses

● **695 Erythematous conditions**

     695.0 Toxic erythema 🔍
         Erythema venenatum
         (Ex:) 695.0-695.4, 709.8

● **695.1 Erythema multiforme**
     Use additional code to identify associated
         manifestations, such as:
         arthropathy associated with dermatological disorders
             (713.3)
         conjunctival edema (372.73)
         conjunctivitis (372.04, 372.33)
         corneal scars and opacities (371.00-371.05)
         corneal ulcer (370.00-370.07)
         edema of eyelid (374.82)
         inflammation of eyelid (373.8)
         keratoconjunctivitis sicca (370.33)
         mechanical lagophthalmos (374.22)
         mucositis (478.11, 528.00, 538, 616.81)
         stomatitis (528.00)
         symblepharon (372.63)

     Use additional E-code to identify drug, if drug-induced
     Use additional code to identify percentage of skin
         exfoliation (695.50–695.59)

     Excludes *(staphylococcal) scalded skin syndrome (695.81)*
     Coding Clinic: 2008, Q4, P128-131

     695.10 Erythema multiforme, unspecified
         Erythema iris
         Herpes iris

     695.11 Erythema multiforme minor

     695.12 Erythema multiforme major 🔍
         (Ex:) 695.0-695.4, 695.81-695.9, 709.8

     695.13 Stevens-Johnson syndrome 🔍
         (Ex:) 695.0-695.4, 695.81-695.9, 709.8

     695.14 Stevens-Johnson syndrome-toxic epidermal
         necrolysis overlap syndrome 🔍
         SJS-TEN overlap syndrome
         (Ex:) 695.0-695.4, 695.81-695.9, 709.8
         Coding Clinic: 2008, Q4, P128-131

     695.15 Toxic epidermal necrolysis 🔍
         Lyell's syndrome
         (Ex:) 695.0-695.4, 695.81-695.9, 709.8

     695.19 Other erythema multiforme

     695.2 Erythema nodosum
         Excludes *tuberculous erythema nodosum (017.1)*

     695.3 Rosacea
         Acne: Perioral dermatitis
         erythematosa   Rhinophyma
         rosacea

     695.4 Lupus erythematosus
         See 710.0 for designated as systemic lupus erythematosus
         (SLE).
         Lupus:
             erythematodes (discoid)
             erythematosus (discoid), not disseminated
         Excludes *lupus (vulgaris) NOS (017.0)*
                   systemic [disseminated] lupus erythematosus
                     (710.0)

● **695.5 Exfoliation due to erythematous conditions according to extent of body surface involved**
     Code first erythematous condition causing exfoliation,
         such as:
     Ritter's disease (695.81)
     (Staphylococcal) scalded skin syndrome (695.81)
     Stevens-Johnson syndrome (695.13)
     Stevens-Johnson syndrome-toxic epidermal necrolysis
         overlap syndrome (695.14)
     toxic epidermal necrolysis (695.15)

● **695.50 Exfoliation due to erythematous condition involving less than 10 percent of body surface**
     Exfoliation due to erythematous condition NOS

● **695.51 Exfoliation due to erythematous condition involving 10-19 percent of body surface**

● **695.52 Exfoliation due to erythematous condition involving 20-29 percent of body surface**

● **695.53 Exfoliation due to erythematous condition involving 30-39 percent of body surface** 🔍
     (Ex:) 695.53
     Coding Clinic: 2008, Q4, P128-131

● **695.54 Exfoliation due to erythematous condition involving 40-49 percent of body surface** 🔍
     (Ex:) 695.54

● **695.55 Exfoliation due to erythematous condition involving 50-59 percent of body surface** 🔍
     (Ex:) 695.55

● **695.56 Exfoliation due to erythematous condition involving 60-69 percent of body surface** 🔍
     (Ex:) 695.56

● **695.57 Exfoliation due to erythematous condition involving 70-79 percent of body surface** 🔍
     (Ex:) 695.57

● **695.58 Exfoliation due to erythematous condition involving 80-89 percent of body surface** 🔍
     (Ex:) 695.58

● **695.59 Exfoliation due to erythematous condition involving 90 percent or more of body surface** 🔍
     (Ex:) 695.59

● **695.8 Other specified erythematous conditions**

     695.81 Ritter's disease
         Dermatitis exfoliativa neonatorum
         (Staphylococcal) Scalded skin syndrome
         Use additional code to identify percentage of
             skin exfoliation (695.50-695.59)

     695.89 Other
         Erythema intertrigo
         Intertrigo
         Pityriasis rubra (Hebra)
         Excludes *mycotic intertrigo (111.0–111.9)*
         Coding Clinic: 1986, Sept-Oct, P10

     695.9 Unspecified erythematous condition
         Erythema NOS
         Erythroderma (secondary)

● **696 Psoriasis and similar disorders**

     696.0 Psoriatic arthropathy

     696.1 Other psoriasis
         Acrodermatitis continua
         Dermatitis repens
         Psoriasis:
             NOS
         any type, except arthropathic
         Excludes *psoriatic arthropathy (696.0)*
         Coding Clinic: 1996, Q2, P12

     696.2 Parapsoriasis
         Parakeratosis variegata
         Parapsoriasis lichenoides chronica
         Pityriasis lichenoides et varioliformis

     696.3 Pityriasis rosea
         Pityriasis circinata (et maculata)

◀ New   ◀|||| Revised   ~~deleted~~ Deleted   Excludes   Includes   Use additional   Code first   Omit code

894   ● Unacceptable Principal Diagnosis   ● Use Additional Digit(s)   ▶ Manifestation Code   **OGCR** Official Guidelines   **Coding Clinic**

Figure 12-6 Erythematous plaques with silvery scales in a patient with psoriasis. (From Goldman: Cecil Textbook of Medicine, ed 22, Saunders, 2004)

Item 12-6 Psoriasis is a chronic, recurrent inflammatory skin disease characterized by small patches covered with thick silvery scales. **Parapsoriasis** is a treatment-resistant erythroderma. **Pityriasis rosea** is characterized by a herald patch that is a single large lesion and that usually appears on the trunk and is followed by scattered, smaller lesions.

696.4 Pityriasis rubra pilaris
Devergie's disease
Lichen ruber acuminatus

Excludes *pityriasis rubra (Hebra) (695.89)*

696.5 Other and unspecified pityriasis
Pityriasis:
NOS
alba
streptogenes

Excludes *pityriasis:*
simplex (690.18)
versicolor (111.0)

696.8 Other

● **697 Lichen**
Excludes *lichen:*
obtusus corneus (698.3)
pilaris (congenital) (757.39)
ruber acuminatus (696.4)
sclerosus et atrophicus (701.0)
scrofulosus (017.0)
simplex chronicus (698.3)
spinulosus (congenital) (757.39)
urticatus (698.2)

697.0 Lichen planus
Lichen:
planopilaris
ruber planus

697.1 Lichen nitidus
Pinkus' disease

697.8 Other lichen, not elsewhere classified
Lichen:
ruber moniliforme
striata

697.9 Lichen, unspecified

● **698 Pruritus and related conditions**
Excludes *pruritus specified as psychogenic (306.3)*

698.0 Pruritus ani
Perianal itch

698.1 Pruritus of genital organs

698.2 Prurigo
Lichen urticatus
Prurigo: Prurigo:
NOS   mitis
Hebra's   simplex
Urticaria papulosa (Hebra)

Excludes *prurigo nodularis (698.3)*

698.3 Lichenification and lichen simplex chronicus
Hyde's disease
Neurodermatitis (circumscripta) (local)
Prurigo nodularis

Excludes *neurodermatitis, diffuse (of Brocq) (691.8)*

698.4 Dermatitis factitia [artefacta]
Dermatitis ficta
Neurotic excoriation

Use additional code to identify any associated mental disorder

698.8 Other specified pruritic conditions
Pruritus:
hiemalis
senilis
Winter itch

698.9 Unspecified pruritic disorder
Itch NOS
Pruritus NOS

OTHER DISEASES OF SKIN AND SUBCUTANEOUS TISSUE (700–709)

Excludes *conditions confined to eyelids (373.0–374.9)*
congenital conditions of skin, hair, and nails (757.0–757.9)

700 Corns and callosities
Callus
Clavus

● **701 Other hypertrophic and atrophic conditions of skin**
Excludes *dermatomyositis (710.3)*
hereditary edema of legs (757.0)
scleroderma (generalized) (710.1)

701.0 Circumscribed scleroderma
Addison's keloid
Dermatosclerosis, localized
Lichen sclerosus et atrophicus
Morphea
Scleroderma, circumscribed or localized

701.1 Keratoderma, acquired
Acquired:
ichthyosis
keratoderma palmaris et plantaris
Elastosis perforans serpiginosa
Hyperkeratosis:
NOS
follicularis in cutem penetrans
palmoplantaris climacterica
Keratoderma:
climactericum
tylodes, progressive
Keratosis (blennorrhagica)

Excludes *Darier's disease [keratosis follicularis]*
(congenital) (757.39)
keratosis:
arsenical (692.4)
gonococcal (098.81)

701.2 Acquired acanthosis nigricans
Keratosis nigricans

701.3 Striae atrophicae
Atrophic spots of skin
Atrophoderma maculatum
Atrophy blanche (of Milian)
Degenerative colloid atrophy
Senile degenerative atrophy
Striae distensae

701.4 Keloid scar
Cheloid
Hypertrophic scar
Keloid
Coding Clinic: 1995, Q3, P14

Item 12-7 Scleroderma means hard skin. It is a group of diseases that causes abnormal growth of connective tissues that support the skin and organs. There are two types: localized scleroderma affecting the skin and systemic scleroderma affecting blood vessels and internal organs and the skin. **Keratoderma** is characterized by firm horny papules that have a cobblestone appearance. **Keratoderma climactericum,** also known as endocrine keratoderma, is hyperkeratosis located on the palms and soles.

DISEASES OF THE SKIN AND SUBCUTANEOUS TISSUE (680–709)

701.5 Other abnormal granulation tissue
Excessive granulation

701.8 Other specified hypertrophic and atrophic conditions of skin
Acrodermatitis atrophicans chronica
Atrophia cutis senilis
Atrophoderma neuriticum
Confluent and reticulate papillomatosis
Cutis laxa senilis
Elastosis senilis
Folliculitis ulerythematosa reticulata
Gougerot-Carteaud syndrome or disease
Coding Clinic: 2008, Q1, P7-8

701.9 Unspecified hypertrophic and atrophic conditions of skin
Atrophoderma

● **702 Other dermatoses**
Excludes *carcinoma in situ (232.0–232.9)*

702.0 Actinic keratosis

● **702.1 Seborrheic keratosis**

702.11 Inflamed seborrheic keratosis

702.19 Other seborrheic keratosis
Seborrheic keratosis NOS

702.8 Other specified dermatoses

● **703 Diseases of nail**
Excludes *congenital anomalies (757.5)*
onychia and paronychia (681.02, 681.11)

703.0 Ingrowing nail
Ingrowing nail with infection
Unguis incarnatus
Excludes *infection, nail NOS (681.9)*

703.8 Other specified diseases of nail
Dystrophia unguium
Hypertrophy of nail
Koilonychia
Leukonychia (punctata) (striata)
Onychauxis
Onychogryposis
Onycholysis

703.9 Unspecified disease of nail

● **704 Diseases of hair and hair follicles**
Excludes *congenital anomalies (757.4)*

● **704.0 Alopecia**
Excludes *madarosis (374.55)*
syphilitic alopecia (091.82)

704.00 Alopecia, unspecified
Baldness   Loss of hair

704.01 Alopecia areata
Ophiasis

704.02 Telogen effluvium

704.09 Other
Folliculitis decalvans
Hypotrichosis:
NOS
postinfectional NOS
Pseudopelade

Item 12–8 Alopecia is lack of hair and takes many forms. The most common is male pattern alopecia, also known as **androgenetic alopecia.** **Telogen effluvium** is early and excessive loss of hair resulting from a trauma to the hair follicle (fever, drugs, surgery, etc.).

Figure 12–7 Male pattern alopecia.

704.1 Hirsutism
Excessive growth of hair
Hypertrichosis:
NOS
lanuginosa, acquired
Polytrichia
Excludes *hypertrichosis of eyelid (374.54)*

704.2 Abnormalities of the hair
Atrophic hair   Trichiasis:
Clastothrix   NOS
Fragilitas crinium   cicatrical
                              Trichorrhexis (nodosa)
Excludes *trichiasis of eyelid (374.05)*
Coding Clinic: 2004, Q4, P91-92

704.3 Variations in hair color
Canities (premature)
Grayness, hair (premature)
Heterochromia of hair
Poliosis:
NOS
circumscripta, acquired

● **704.4 Pilar and trichilemmal cysts**
704.41 Pilar cyst
704.42 Trichilemmal cyst
Trichilemmal proliferating cyst
Coding Clinic: 2011, Q4, P135

704.8 Other specified diseases of hair and hair follicles
Folliculitis:
NOS
abscedens et suffodiens
pustular
Perifolliculitis:
NOS
capitis abscedens et suffodiens
scalp
Sycosis:
NOS
barbae [not parasitic]
lupoid
vulgaris
Coding Clinic: 2011, Q1, P8

704.9 Unspecified disease of hair and hair follicles

● **705 Disorders of sweat glands**
705.0 Anhidrosis
Hypohidrosis   Oligohidrosis

705.1 Prickly heat
Heat rash   Sudamina
Miliaria rubra (tropicalis)

● **705.2 Focal hyperhidrosis**
Excludes *generalized (secondary) hyperhidrosis (780.8)*

705.21 Primary focal hyperhidrosis
Focal hyperhidrosis NOS
Hyperhidrosis NOS
Hyperhidrosis of:
axilla   palms
face   soles

705.22 Secondary focal hyperhidrosis
Frey's syndrome

● **705.8 Other specified disorders of sweat glands**
705.81 Dyshidrosis
Cheiropompholyx
Pompholyx

705.82 Fox-Fordyce disease

705.83 Hidradenitis
Hidradenitis suppurativa

705.89 Other
Bromhidrosis   Granulosis rubra nasi
Chromhidrosis   Urhidrosis
Excludes *hidrocystoma (216.0–216.9)*
generalized hyperhidrosis (780.8)

705.9 Unspecified disorder of sweat glands
Disorder of sweat glands NOS

● 706   Diseases of sebaceous glands

706.0   Acne varioliformis
Acne:
  frontalis
  necrotica

706.1   Other acne
Acne:
  NOS
  conglobata
  cystic
  pustular
  vulgaris
Blackhead
Comedo
Excludes *acne rosacea (695.3)*

706.2   Sebaceous cyst
Atheroma, skin   Wen
Keratin cyst
Excludes *pilar cyst (704.41)*
     trichilemmal (proliferating) cyst (704.42)

706.3   Seborrhea
Excludes *seborrhea:*
     capitis (690.11)
     sicca (690.18)
     seborrheic
       dermatitis (690.10)
       keratosis (702.11–702.19)

706.8   Other specified diseases of sebaceous glands
Asteatosis (cutis)
Xerosis cutis

706.9   Unspecified disease of sebaceous glands

● 707   Chronic ulcer of skin
Includes   non-infected sinus of skin
     non-healing ulcer
Excludes *varicose ulcer (454.0, 454.2)*

● 707.0   Pressure ulcer
Bed sore
Decubitus ulcer
Plaster ulcer
Use additional code to identify pressure ulcer stage (707.20–707.25)
Coding Clinic: 2004, Q4, P92-93; Q1, P14-15; 2003, Q4, P110; 1999, Q4, P20; 1996, Q1, P15; 1990, Q3, P15; 1987, Nov-Dec, P9

707.00   Unspecified site
Coding Clinic: 2012, Q2, P3

707.01   Elbow

707.02   Upper back
Shoulder blades

707.03   Lower back
Coccyx
Sacrum
Coding Clinic: 2008, Q3, P17; 2005, Q1, P16

707.04   Hip

707.05   Buttock
Coding Clinic: 2012, Q2, P3

707.06   Ankle

707.07   Heel
Coding Clinic: 2009, Q4, P108; 2005, Q1, P16

707.09   Other site
Head
Coding Clinic: 2008, Q3, P17

● 707.1   Ulcer of lower limbs, except pressure ulcer
Ulcer, chronic, of lower limb:
  neurogenic of lower limb
  trophic of lower limb
Code if applicable, any causal condition first:
  atherosclerosis of the extremities with ulceration (440.23)
  chronic venous hypertension with ulcer (459.31)
  chronic venous hypertension with ulcer and inflammation (459.33)
  diabetes mellitus (249.80–249.81, 250.80–250.83)
  postphlebitic syndrome with ulcer (459.11)
  postphlebitic syndrome with ulcer and inflammation (459.13)
Coding Clinic: 2004, Q1, P14-15; 1999, Q4, P15; 1996, Q1, P10

707.10   Ulcer of lower limb, unspecified
(Ex) 440.23, 707.10-707.19, 707.8-707.9, 709.8
Coding Clinic: 2004, Q3, P5-6

707.11   Ulcer of thigh
(Ex) 440.23, 707.10-707.19, 707.8-707.9, 709.8

707.12   Ulcer of calf
(Ex) 440.23, 707.10-707.19, 707.8-707.9, 709.8

707.13   Ulcer of ankle
(Ex) 440.23, 707.10-707.19, 707.8-707.9, 709.8

707.14   Ulcer of heel and midfoot
Plantar surface of midfoot
(Ex) 440.23, 707.10-707.19, 707.8-707.9, 709.8

707.15   Ulcer of other part of foot
Toes

707.19   Ulcer of other part of lower limb
(Ex) 440.23, 707.10-707.19, 707.8-707.9, 709.8

● 707.2   Pressure ulcer stages
Code first site of pressure ulcer (707.00-707.09)
Coding Clinic: 2008, Q4, P132-134

707.20   Pressure ulcer, unspecified stage
Healing pressure ulcer NOS
Healing pressure ulcer, unspecified stage

707.21   Pressure ulcer stage I
Healing pressure ulcer, stage I
Pressure pre-ulcer skin changes limited to persistent focal erythema

707.22   Pressure ulcer stage II
Healing pressure ulcer, stage II
Pressure ulcer with abrasion, blister, partial thickness skin loss involving epidermis and/or dermis

707.23   Pressure ulcer stage III
Healing pressure ulcer, stage III
Pressure ulcer with full thickness skin loss involving damage or necrosis of subcutaneous tissue
(Ex) 707.10-707.9
Coding Clinic: 2009, Q4, P113

707.24   Pressure ulcer stage IV
Healing pressure ulcer, stage IV
Pressure ulcer with necrosis of soft tissues through to underlying muscle, tendon, or bone
(Ex) 707.10-707.9
Coding Clinic: 2010, Q2, P18

707.25   Pressure ulcer, unstageable

707.8   Chronic ulcer of other specified sites
Ulcer, chronic, of other specified sites:
  neurogenic of other specified sites
  trophic of other specified sites

707.9   Chronic ulcer of unspecified site
Chronic ulcer NOS   Tropical ulcer NOS
Trophic ulcer NOS   Ulcer of skin NOS

DISEASES OF THE SKIN AND SUBCUTANEOUS TISSUE (680–709)

Figure 12–8   Urticaria (hives). *(Courtesy of David Effron, MD.)* (From Marx: Rosen's Emergency Medicine: Concepts and Clinical Practice, ed 6, Mosby, Inc., 2006)

Item 12–9   Urticaria is a vascular reaction in which wheals surrounded by a red halo appear and cause severe itching. The causes of urticaria or hives are extensive and varied (e.g., food, heat, cold, drugs, stress, infections). Dyschromia is any disorder of the pigmentation of the skin or hair.

● **708   Urticaria**

     Excludes   *edema:*
                angioneurotic (995.1)
                Quincke's (995.1)
            hereditary angioedema (277.6)
            urticaria:
                giant (995.1)
                papulosa (Hebra) (698.2)
                pigmentosa (juvenile) (congenital) (757.33)

     708.0   Allergic urticaria
         Coding Clinic: 1984, May-June, P11

     708.1   Idiopathic urticaria

     708.2   Urticaria due to cold and heat
         Thermal urticaria

     708.3   Dermatographic urticaria
         Dermatographia   Factitial urticaria

     708.4   Vibratory urticaria

     708.5   Cholinergic urticaria
         Coding Clinic: 1995, Q4, P50

     708.8   Other specified urticaria
         Nettle rash
         Urticaria:
            chronic
            recurrent periodic

     708.9   Urticaria, unspecified
         Hives NOS

● **709   Other disorders of skin and subcutaneous tissue**

   ● **709.0   Dyschromia**

     Excludes   *albinism (270.2)*
                   pigmented nevus (216.0–216.9)
                   that of eyelid (374.52–374.53)

     709.00   Dyschromia, unspecified

     709.01   Vitiligo

     709.09   Other

     709.1   Vascular disorders of skin
         Angioma serpiginosum
         Purpura (primary) annularis telangiectodes

     709.2   Scar conditions and fibrosis of skin
         Adherent scar (skin)
         Cicatrix
         Disfigurement (due to scar)
         Fibrosis, skin NOS
         Scar NOS

     Excludes   *keloid scar (701.4)*
     Coding Clinic: 1984, Nov-Dec, P19

     709.3   Degenerative skin disorders
         Calcinosis:
            circumscripta
            cutis
         Colloid milium
         Degeneration, skin
         Deposits, skin
         Senile dermatosis NOS
         Subcutaneous calcification

     709.4   Foreign body granuloma of skin and subcutaneous tissue
         Use additional code to identify foreign body
            (V90.01-V90.9)

     Excludes   *residual foreign body without granuloma of skin*
                   and subcutaneous tissue (729.6)
                   that of muscle (728.82)

     709.8   Other specified disorders of skin
         Epithelial hyperplasia
         Menstrual dermatosis
         Vesicular eruption
         Coding Clinic: 2013, Q2, P9; 1987, Nov-Dec, P6

     709.9   Unspecified disorder of skin and subcutaneous tissue
         Dermatosis NOS

◄ New   ◄III Revised   ~~deleted~~ Deleted   Excludes   Includes   Use additional   Code first   Omit code

898   ● Unacceptable Principal Diagnosis   ● Use Additional Digit(s)   ▶ Manifestation Code   OGCR Official Guidelines   Coding Clinic

13. DISEASES OF THE MUSCULOSKELETAL SYSTEM AND CONNECTIVE TISSUE (710–739)

Use additional external cause code, if applicable, to identify the cause of the musculoskeletal condition

The following fifth-digit subclassification is for use with categories 711–712, 715–716, 718–719, and 730:

0 **site unspecified**	6 **lower leg**
1 **shoulder region**	Fibula
Acromioclavicular	Knee joint
joint(s)	Patella
Clavicle	Tibia
Glenohumeral joint(s)	7 **ankle and foot**
Scapula	Ankle joint
Sternoclavicular	Digits [toes]
joint(s)	Metatarsus
2 **upper arm**	Phalanges, foot
Elbow joint	Tarsus
Humerus	Other joints in foot
3 **forearm**	8 **other specified sites**
Radius	Head
Ulna	Neck
Wrist joint	Ribs
4 **hand**	Skull
Carpus	Trunk
Metacarpus	Vertebral column
Phalanges [fingers]	9 **multiple sites**
5 **pelvic region and thigh**	
Buttock	
Femur	
Hip (joint)	

ARTHROPATHIES AND RELATED DISORDERS (710–719)

Excludes   *disorders of spine (720.0–724.9)*

● **710 Diffuse diseases of connective tissue**

   Includes   all collagen diseases whose effects are not mainly confined to a single system

   Excludes   *those affecting mainly the cardiovascular system, i.e., polyarteritis nodosa and allied conditions (446.0–446.7)*

710.0 Systemic lupus erythematosus

   Autoimmune inflammatory connective tissue disease of unknown cause that occurs most often in women. See 695.4 for nonsystemic.

   Disseminated lupus erythematosus

   Libman-Sacks disease

   Use additional code to identify manifestation, as:
      endocarditis (424.91)
      nephritis (583.81)
         chronic (582.81)
      nephrotic syndrome (581.81)

   Excludes   *lupus erythematosus (discoid) NOS (695.4)*

   Coding Clinic: 2003, Q2, P7x2; 1997, Q2, P8-9; 1987, Sept-Oct, P8

710.1 Systemic sclerosis

   Acrosclerosis

   CRST syndrome

   Progressive systemic sclerosis

   Scleroderma

   Use additional code to identify manifestation, as:
      lung involvement (517.2)
      myopathy (359.6)

   Excludes   *circumscribed scleroderma (701.0)*

710.2 Sicca syndrome

   Keratoconjunctivitis sicca

   Sjögren's disease

710.3 Dermatomyositis 🔖

   Poikilodermatomyositis

   Polymyositis with skin involvement

   (Ex) 710.3

710.4 Polymyositis 🔖

   (Ex) 710.4

710.5 Eosinophilia myalgia syndrome 🔖

   Toxic oil syndrome

   Use additional E code to identify drug, if drug induced

   (Ex) 292.0-293.9, 710.5

710.8 Other specified diffuse diseases of connective tissue 🔖

   Multifocal fibrosclerosis (idiopathic) NEC

   Systemic fibrosclerosing syndrome

   (Ex) 359.71-359.79, 710.8

   Coding Clinic: 1987, Mar-April, P12

710.9 Unspecified diffuse connective tissue disease

   Collagen disease NOS

● **711 Arthropathy associated with infections**

   Abnormality of a joint

   Includes   arthritis associated with conditions classifiable below

      arthropathy associated with conditions classifiable below

      polyarthritis associated with conditions classifiable below

      polyarthropathy associated with conditions classifiable below

   Excludes   *rheumatic fever (390)*

   Coding Clinic: 1992, Q1, P16-17

The following fifth-digit subclassification is for use with category 711; valid digits are in [brackets] under each code. See list at beginning of chapter for definitions:

0 **site unspecified**	5 **pelvic region and thigh**
1 **shoulder region**	6 **lower leg**
2 **upper arm**	7 **ankle and foot**
3 **forearm**	8 **other specified sites**
4 **hand**	9 **multiple sites**

N Newborn: 0   P Pediatric: 0–17   M Maternity: 12–55   A Adult: 15–124   ♀ Females Only   ♂ Males Only

(Ex) CC/MCC Exclusions   🔖 Complication\Comorbidity   🔖 Major C\C   🔖 Present on Admission Requirement   🔖 Hospital-Acquired Condition   **899**

● **711.0 Pyogenic arthritis** 🔎
[0-9]   Arthritis or polyarthritis (due to):
           coliform [Escherichia coli]
           Hemophilus influenzae [H. influenzae]
           pneumococcal
           Pseudomonas
           staphylococcal
           streptococcal
        Pyarthrosis
        Use additional code to identify infectious organism
           (041.0–041.8)
        For codes **711.00, 711.08-711.09:** (Ex) 015.80-015.96, 017.90-017.96, 036.82,
           056.71, 098.50-098.51, 098.59, 098.89, 711.00-714.0, 715.00,
           715.09-715.10, 715.18-716.99, 718.00-718.08, 719.00-719.10,
           719.18-719.99;
        For code **711.01:** (Ex) 015.80-015.96, 017.90-017.96, 036.82, 056.71,
           098.50-098.51, 098.59, 098.89, 711.00-711.01, 711.08-711.11,
           711.18-711.21, 711.28-711.31, 711.38-711.41, 711.48-711.51,
           711.58-711.61, 711.68-711.71, 711.78-711.81, 711.88-711.91,
           711.98-712.11, 712.18-712.21, 712.28-712.31, 712.38-712.81,
           712.88-712.91, 712.98-714.0, 715.00, 715.09-715.11, 715.18-715.21,
           715.28-715.31, 715.38-715.91, 715.98-716.01, 716.08-716.11,
           716.18-716.21, 716.28-716.31, 716.38-716.41, 716.48-716.51,
           716.58-716.61, 716.68-716.81, 716.88-716.91, 716.98-716.99,
           718.00-718.01, 718.08, 719.00-719.01, 719.08-719.11, 719.18-719.21,
           719.28-719.31, 719.38-719.41, 719.48-719.51, 719.58-719.61,
           719.68-719.81, 719.88-719.91, 719.98-719.99;
        For code **711.02:** (Ex) 015.80-015.96, 017.90-017.96, 036.82, 056.71,
           098.50-098.51, 098.59, 098.89, 711.00, 711.02, 711.08-711.10, 711.12,
           711.18-711.20, 711.22, 711.28-711.30, 711.32, 711.38-711.40, 711.42,
           711.48-711.50, 711.52, 711.58-711.60, 711.62, 711.68-711.70, 711.72,
           711.78-711.80, 711.82, 711.88-711.90, 711.92, 711.98-712.10, 712.12,
           712.18-712.20, 712.22, 712.28-712.30, 712.32, 712.38-712.80, 712.82,
           712.88-712.90, 712.92, 712.98-714.0, 715.00, 715.09-715.10, 715.12,
           715.18-715.20, 715.22, 715.28-715.30, 715.32, 715.38-715.90, 715.92,
           715.98-716.00, 716.02, 716.08-716.10, 716.12, 716.18-716.20, 716.22,
           716.28-716.30, 716.32, 716.38-716.40, 716.42, 716.48-716.50, 716.52,
           716.58-716.60, 716.62, 716.68-716.80, 716.82, 716.88-716.90, 716.92,
           716.98-716.99, 718.00, 718.02, 718.08, 719.00, 719.02, 719.08-719.10,
           719.12, 719.18-719.20, 719.22, 719.28-719.30, 719.32, 719.38-719.40,
           719.42, 719.48-719.50, 719.52, 719.58-719.60, 719.62, 719.68-719.80,
           719.82, 719.88-719.90, 719.92, 719.98-719.99;
        For code **711.03:** (Ex) 015.80-015.96, 017.90-017.96, 036.82, 056.71,
           098.50-098.51, 098.59, 098.89, 711.00, 711.03, 711.08-711.10, 711.13,
           711.18-711.20, 711.23, 711.28-711.30, 711.33, 711.38-711.40, 711.43,
           711.48-711.50, 711.53, 711.58-711.60, 711.63, 711.68-711.70, 711.73,
           711.78-711.80, 711.83, 711.88-711.90, 711.93, 711.98-712.10, 712.13,
           712.18-712.20, 712.23, 712.28-712.30, 712.33, 712.38-712.80, 712.83,
           712.88-712.90, 712.93, 712.98-714.0, 715.00, 715.09-715.10, 715.13,
           715.18-715.20, 715.23, 715.28-715.30, 715.33, 715.38-715.90, 715.93,
           715.98-716.00, 716.03, 716.08-716.10, 716.13, 716.18-716.20, 716.23,
           716.28-716.30, 716.33, 716.38-716.40, 716.43, 716.48-716.50, 716.53,
           716.58-716.60, 716.63, 716.68-716.80, 716.83, 716.88-716.90, 716.93,
           716.98-716.99, 718.00, 718.03, 718.08, 719.00, 719.03, 719.08-719.10,
           719.13, 719.18-719.20, 719.23, 719.28-719.30, 719.33, 719.38-719.40,
           719.43, 719.48-719.50, 719.53, 719.58-719.60, 719.63, 719.68-719.80,
           719.83, 719.88-719.90, 719.93, 719.98-719.99;
        For code **711.04:** (Ex) 015.80-015.96, 017.90-017.96, 036.82, 056.71,
           098.50-098.51, 098.59, 098.89, 711.00, 711.04, 711.08-711.10, 711.14,
           711.18-711.20, 711.24, 711.28-711.30, 711.34, 711.38-711.40, 711.44,
           711.48-711.50, 711.54, 711.58-711.60, 711.64, 711.68-711.70, 711.74,
           711.78-711.80, 711.84, 711.88-711.90, 711.94, 711.98-712.10, 712.14,
           712.18-712.20, 712.24, 712.28-712.30, 712.34, 712.38-712.80, 712.84,
           712.88-712.90, 712.94, 712.98-714.0, 715.00-715.10, 715.14,
           715.18-715.20, 715.24, 715.28-715.30, 715.34, 715.38-715.90, 715.94,
           715.98-716.00, 716.04, 716.08-716.10, 716.14, 716.18-716.20, 716.24,
           716.28-716.30, 716.34, 716.38-716.40, 716.44, 716.48-716.50, 716.54,
           716.58-716.60, 716.64, 716.68-716.80, 716.84, 716.88-716.90, 716.94,
           716.98-716.99, 718.00, 718.04, 718.08, 719.00, 719.04, 719.08-719.10,
           719.14, 719.18-719.20, 719.24, 719.28-719.30, 719.34, 719.38-719.40,
           719.44, 719.48-719.50, 719.54, 719.58-719.60, 719.64, 719.68-719.80,
           719.84, 719.88-719.90, 719.94, 719.98-719.99;

For code **711.05:** (Ex) 015.80-015.96, 017.90-017.96, 036.82, 056.71,
   098.50-098.51, 098.59, 098.89, 711.00, 711.05, 711.08-711.10, 711.15,
   711.18-711.20, 711.25, 711.28-711.30, 711.35, 711.38-711.40, 711.45,
   711.48-711.50, 711.55, 711.58-711.60, 711.65, 711.68-711.70, 711.75,
   711.78-711.80, 711.85, 711.88-711.90, 711.95, 711.98-712.10, 712.15,
   712.18-712.20, 712.25, 712.28-712.30, 712.35, 712.38-712.80, 712.85,
   712.88-712.90, 712.95, 712.98-714.0, 715.00, 715.09-715.10, 715.15,
   715.18-715.20, 715.25, 715.28-715.30, 715.35, 715.38-715.90, 715.95,
   715.98-716.00, 716.05, 716.08-716.10, 716.15, 716.18-716.20, 716.25,
   716.28-716.30, 716.35, 716.38-716.40, 716.45, 716.48-716.50, 716.55,
   716.58-716.60, 716.65, 716.68-716.80, 716.85, 716.88-716.90, 716.95,
   716.98-716.99, 718.00, 718.05, 718.08, 719.00, 719.05, 719.08-719.10,
   719.15, 719.18-719.20, 719.25, 719.28-719.30, 719.35, 719.38-719.40,
   719.45, 719.48-719.50, 719.55, 719.58-719.60, 719.65, 719.68-719.80,
   719.85, 719.88-719.90, 719.95, 719.98-719.99;
For code **711.06:** (Ex) 015.80-015.96, 017.90-017.96, 036.82, 056.71,
   098.50-098.51, 098.59, 098.89, 711.00, 711.06, 711.08-711.10, 711.16,
   711.18-711.20, 711.26, 711.28-711.30, 711.36, 711.38-711.40, 711.46,
   711.48-711.50, 711.56, 711.58-711.60, 711.66, 711.68-711.70, 711.76,
   711.78-711.80, 711.86, 711.88-711.90, 711.96, 711.98-712.10, 712.16,
   712.18-712.20, 712.26, 712.28-712.30, 712.36, 712.38-712.80, 712.86,
   712.88-712.90, 712.96, 712.98-714.0, 715.00, 715.09-715.10, 715.16,
   715.18-715.20, 715.26, 715.28-715.30, 715.36, 715.38-715.90, 715.96,
   715.98-716.00, 716.06, 716.08-716.10, 716.16, 716.18-716.20, 716.26,
   716.28-716.30, 716.36, 716.38-716.40, 716.46, 716.48-716.50, 716.56,
   716.58-716.60, 716.66, 716.68-716.80, 716.86, 716.88-716.90, 716.96,
   716.98-716.99, 718.00, 718.08, 719.00, 719.06, 719.08-719.10, 719.16,
   719.18-719.20, 719.26, 719.28-719.30, 719.36, 719.38-719.40, 719.46,
   719.48-719.50, 719.56, 719.58-719.60, 719.66, 719.68-719.80, 719.86,
   719.88-719.90, 719.96, 719.98-719.99;

Coding Clinic: 1992, Q1, P16-17; 1991, Q1, P15
For code **711.07:** (Ex) 015.80-015.96, 017.90-017.96, 036.82, 056.71,
   098.50-098.51, 098.59, 098.89, 711.00, 711.07-711.10, 711.17-711.20,
   711.27-711.30, 711.37-711.40, 711.47-711.50, 711.57-711.60,
   711.67-711.70, 711.77-711.80, 711.87-711.90, 711.97-712.10,
   712.17-712.20, 712.27-712.30, 712.37-712.80, 712.87-712.90,
   712.97-714.0, 715.00, 715.09-715.10, 715.17-715.20, 715.27-715.30,
   715.37-715.90, 715.97-716.00, 716.07-716.10, 716.17-716.20,
   716.27-716.30, 716.37-716.40, 716.47-716.50, 716.57-716.60,
   716.67-716.80, 716.87-716.90, 716.97-716.99, 718.00, 718.07-718.08,
   719.00, 719.07-719.10, 719.17-719.20, 719.27-719.30, 719.37-719.40,
   719.47-719.50, 719.57-719.60, 719.67-719.80, 719.87-719.90,
   719.97-719.99

● ▌ **711.1 Arthropathy associated with Reiter's disease and**
[0-9] **nonspecific urethritis** 🔎
        Code first underlying disease, as:
           nonspecific urethritis (099.4)
           Reiter's disease (099.3)
        (Ex) 003.23, 015.80-015.96, 017.90-017.96, 036.82, 056.71, 098.50-098.51,
           098.59, 098.89, 711.00-714.0, 715.00, 715.09-715.10, 715.18-716.99,
           718.00-718.08, 719.00-719.10, 719.18-719.69, 719.80-719.99

● ▌ **711.2 Arthropathy in Behçet's syndrome** 🔎
[0-9]   *Code first underlying disease (136.1)*
        (Ex) 003.23, 015.80-015.96, 017.90-017.96, 036.82, 056.71, 098.50-098.51,
           098.59, 098.89, 711.00-714.0, 715.00, 715.09-715.10, 715.18-716.99,
           718.00-718.08, 719.00-719.10, 719.18-719.69, 719.80-719.99

● ▌ **711.3 Postdysenteric arthropathy** 🔎
[0-9]   *Code first underlying disease, as:*
           dysentery (009.0)
           enteritis, infectious (008.0–009.3)
           paratyphoid fever (002.1–002.9)
           typhoid fever (002.0)
        Excludes *salmonella arthritis (003.23)*
        For codes **711.30-711.35, 711.37, and 711.39:** (Ex) 003.23, 015.80-015.96,
           017.90-017.96, 036.82, 056.71, 098.50-098.51, 098.59, 098.89,
           711.00-714.0, 715.00, 715.09-715.10, 715.18-716.99, 718.00-718.08,
           719.00-719.10, 719.18-719.69, 719.80-719.99;
        For code **711.36:** (Ex) 003.23, 015.80-015.96, 017.90-017.96, 036.82, 056.71,
           098.50-098.51, 098.59, 098.89, 711.00-714.0, 715.00, 715.09-715.10,
           715.18-716.07, 716.09-716.99, 718.00-718.08, 719.00-719.10,
           719.18-719.69, 719.80-719.99;
        For code **711.38:** (Ex) 003.23, 015.80-015.96, 017.90-017.96, 036.82, 056.71,
           098.50-098.51, 098.59, 098.89, 711.00-714.0, 715.00, 715.09-715.10,
           715.18-716.57, 716.59-716.99, 718.00-718.08, 719.00-719.10,
           719.18-719.69, 719.80-719.99

◄ New   ◄▥ Revised   ~~deleted~~ Deleted   Excludes   Includes   Use additional   Code first   Omit code
● Unacceptable Principal Diagnosis   ● Use Additional Digit(s)   ▌ Manifestation Code   OGCR Official Guidelines   Coding Clinic

● ▶ **711.4** **Arthropathy associated with other bacterial**
[0-9] *diseases* 🔖

> *Code first* underlying disease, as:
> diseases classifiable to 010–040, 090–099, except as in
> 711.1, 711.3, and 713.5
> leprosy (030.0–030.9)
> tuberculosis (015.0–015.9)
>
> **Excludes** *gonococcal arthritis (098.50)*
> *meningococcal arthritis (036.82)*
>
> For codes **711.40, 711.42-711.49:** (Ex) 003.23, 015.80-015.96, 017.90-017.96,
> 036.82, 056.71, 098.50-098.51, 098.59, 098.89, 711.00-714.0, 715.00,
> 715.09-715.10, 715.18-716.99, 718.00-718.08, 719.00-719.10,
> 719.18-719.69, 719.80-719.99;
>
> For code **711.41:** (Ex) 003.23, 015.80-015.96, 017.90-017.96, 036.82, 056.71,
> 098.50-098.51, 098.59, 098.89, 711.00-714.0, 715.00, 715.09-715.10,
> 715.18-716.99, 718.00-718.08, 719.00-719.10, 719.18-719.39,
> 719.41-719.69, 719.80-719.99

● ▶ **711.5** **Arthropathy associated with other viral diseases** 🔖
[0-9]
> *Code first* underlying disease, as:
> diseases classifiable to 045–049, 050–079, 480, 487
> O'nyong-nyong (066.3)
>
> **Excludes** *that due to rubella (056.71)*
>
> (Ex) 003.23, 015.80-015.96, 017.90-017.96, 036.82, 056.71, 098.50-098.51,
> 098.59, 098.89, 711.00-714.0, 715.00, 715.09-715.10, 715.18-716.99,
> 718.00-718.08, 719.00-719.10, 719.18-719.69, 719.80-719.99

● ▶ **711.6** **Arthropathy associated with mycoses** 🔖
[0-9]
> *Code first* underlying disease (110.0–118)
>
> For codes **711.60, 711.68-711.69:** (Ex) 015.80-015.96, 017.90-017.96, 036.82,
> 056.71, 098.50-098.51, 098.59, 098.89, 711.00-714.0, 715.00,
> 715.09-715.10, 715.18-716.99, 718.00-718.08, 719.00-719.10,
> 719.18-719.99;
>
> For code **711.61:** (Ex) 015.80-015.96, 017.90-017.96, 036.82, 056.71,
> 098.50-098.51, 098.59, 098.89, 711.00-711.01, 711.08-711.11,
> 711.18-711.21, 711.28-711.31, 711.38-711.41, 711.48-711.51,
> 711.58-711.61, 711.68-711.71, 711.78-711.81, 711.88-711.91,
> 711.98-712.11, 712.18-712.21, 712.28-712.31, 712.38-712.81,
> 712.88-712.91, 712.98-714.0, 715.00, 715.09-715.11, 715.18-715.21,
> 715.28-715.31, 715.38-715.91, 715.98-716.01, 716.08-716.11,
> 716.18-716.21, 716.28-716.31, 716.38-716.41, 716.48-716.51,
> 716.58-716.61, 716.68-716.81, 716.88-716.91, 716.98-716.99,
> 718.00-718.01, 718.08, 719.00-719.01, 719.08-719.11, 719.18-719.21,
> 719.28-719.31, 719.38-719.41, 719.48-719.51, 719.58-719.61,
> 719.68-719.81, 719.88-719.91, 719.98-719.99;
>
> For code **711.62:** (Ex) 015.80-015.96, 017.90-017.96, 036.82, 056.71,
> 098.50-098.51, 098.59, 098.89, 711.00, 711.02, 711.08-711.10, 711.12,
> 711.18-711.20, 711.22, 711.28-711.30, 711.32, 711.38-711.40, 711.42,
> 711.48-711.50, 711.52, 711.58-711.60, 711.62, 711.68-711.70, 711.72,
> 711.78-711.80, 711.82, 711.88-711.90, 711.92, 711.98-712.10, 712.12,
> 712.18-712.20, 712.22, 712.28-712.30, 712.32, 712.38-712.80, 712.82,
> 712.88-712.90, 712.92, 712.98-714.0, 715.00, 715.09-715.10, 715.12,
> 715.18-715.20, 715.22, 715.28-715.30, 715.32, 715.38-715.90, 715.92,
> 715.98-716.00, 716.02, 716.08-716.10, 716.12, 716.18-716.20, 716.22,
> 716.28-716.30, 716.32, 716.38-716.40, 716.42, 716.48-716.50, 716.52,
> 716.58-716.60, 716.62, 716.68-716.80, 716.82, 716.88-716.90, 716.92,
> 716.98-716.99, 718.00, 718.02, 718.08, 719.00, 719.02, 719.08-719.10,
> 719.12, 719.18-719.20, 719.22, 719.28-719.30, 719.32, 719.38-719.40,
> 719.42, 719.48-719.50, 719.52, 719.58-719.60, 719.62, 719.68-719.80,
> 719.82, 719.88-719.90, 719.92, 719.98-719.99;
>
> For code **711.63:** (Ex) 015.80-015.96, 017.90-017.96, 036.82, 056.71,
> 098.50-098.51, 098.59, 098.89, 711.00, 711.03, 711.08-711.10, 711.13,
> 711.18-711.20, 711.23, 711.28-711.30, 711.33, 711.38-711.40, 711.43,
> 711.48-711.50, 711.53, 711.58-711.60, 711.63, 711.68-711.70, 711.73,
> 711.78-711.80, 711.83, 711.88-711.90, 711.93, 711.98-712.10, 712.13,
> 712.18-712.20, 712.23, 712.28-712.30, 712.33, 712.38-712.80, 712.83,
> 712.88-712.90, 712.93, 712.98-714.0, 715.00, 715.09-715.10, 715.13,
> 715.18-715.20, 715.23, 715.28-715.30, 715.33, 715.38-715.90, 715.93,
> 715.98-716.00, 716.03, 716.08-716.10, 716.13, 716.18-716.20, 716.23,
> 716.28-716.30, 716.33, 716.38-716.40, 716.43, 716.48-716.50, 716.53,
> 716.58-716.60, 716.63, 716.68-716.80, 716.83, 716.88-716.90, 716.93,
> 716.98-716.99, 718.00, 718.03, 718.08, 719.00, 719.03, 719.08-719.10,
> 719.13, 719.18-719.20, 719.23, 719.28-719.30, 719.33, 719.38-719.40,
> 719.43, 719.48-719.50, 719.53, 719.58-719.60, 719.63, 719.68-719.80,
> 719.83, 719.88-719.90, 719.93, 719.98-719.99;
>
> For code **711.64:** (Ex) 015.80-015.96, 017.90-017.96, 036.82, 056.71,
> 098.50-098.51, 098.59, 098.89, 711.00, 711.04, 711.08-711.10, 711.14,
> 711.18-711.20, 711.24, 711.28-711.30, 711.34, 711.38-711.40, 711.44,
> 711.48-711.50, 711.54, 711.58-711.60, 711.64, 711.68-711.70, 711.74,

711.78-711.80, 711.84, 711.88-711.90, 711.94, 711.98-712.10, 712.14,
712.18-712.20, 712.24, 712.28-712.30, 712.34, 712.38-712.80, 712.84,
712.88-712.90, 712.94, 712.98-714.0, 715.00-715.10, 715.14,
715.18-715.20, 715.24, 715.28-715.30, 715.34, 715.38-715.90, 715.94,
715.98-716.00, 716.04, 716.08-716.10, 716.14, 716.18-716.20, 716.24,
716.28-716.30, 716.34, 716.38-716.40, 716.44, 716.48-716.50, 716.54,
716.58-716.60, 716.64, 716.68-716.80, 716.84, 716.88-716.90, 716.94,
716.98-716.99, 718.00, 718.04, 718.08, 719.00, 719.04, 719.08-719.10,
719.14, 719.18-719.20, 719.24, 719.28-719.30, 719.34, 719.38-719.40,
719.44, 719.48-719.50, 719.54, 719.58-719.60, 719.64, 719.68-719.80,
719.84, 719.88-719.90, 719.94, 719.98-719.99;

For code **711.65:** (Ex) 015.80-015.96, 017.90-017.96, 036.82, 056.71,
098.50-098.51, 098.59, 098.89, 711.00, 711.05, 711.08-711.10, 711.15,
711.18-711.20, 711.25, 711.28-711.30, 711.35, 711.38-711.40, 711.45,
711.48-711.50, 711.55, 711.58-711.60, 711.65, 711.68-711.70, 711.75,
711.78-711.80, 711.85, 711.88-711.90 711.95, 711.98-712.10, 712.15,
712.18-712.20, 712.25, 712.28-712.30 712.35, 712.38-712.80, 712.85,
712.88-712.90, 712.95, 712.98-714.0 715.00, 715.09-715.10, 715.15,
715.18-715.20, 715.25, 715.28-715.30, 715.35, 715.38-715.90, 715.95,
715.98-716.00, 716.05, 716.08-716.10, 716.15, 716.18-716.20, 716.25,
716.28-716.30, 716.35, 716.38-716.40, 716.45, 716.48-716.50, 716.55,
716.58-716.60, 716.65, 716.68-716.80, 716.85, 716.88-716.90, 716.95,
716.98-716.99, 718.00, 718.05, 718.08, 719.00, 719.05, 719.08-719.10,
719.15, 719.18-719.20, 719.25, 719.28-719.30, 719.35, 719.38-719.40,
719.45, 719.48-719.50, 719.55, 719.58-719.60, 719.65, 719.68-719.80,
719.85, 719.88-719.90, 719.95, 719.98-719.99;

For code **711.66:** (Ex) 015.80-015.96, 017.90-017.96, 036.82, 056.71,
098.50-098.51, 098.59, 098.89, 711.00, 711.06, 711.08-711.10, 711.16,
711.18-711.20, 711.26, 711.28-711.30, 711.36, 711.38-711.40, 711.46,
711.48-711.50, 711.56, 711.58-711.60, 711.66, 711.68-711.70, 711.76,
711.78-711.80, 711.86, 711.88-711.90, 711.96, 711.98-712.10, 712.16,
712.18-712.20, 712.26, 712.28-712.30, 712.36, 712.38-712.80, 712.86,
712.88-712.90, 712.96, 712.98-714.0, 715.00, 715.09-715.10, 715.16,
715.18-715.20, 715.26, 715.28-715.30, 715.36, 715.38-715.90, 715.96,
715.98-716.00, 716.06, 716.08-716.10, 716.16, 716.18-716.20, 716.26,
716.28-716.30, 716.36, 716.38-716.40, 716.46, 716.48-716.50, 716.56,
716.58-716.60, 716.66, 716.68-716.80, 716.86, 716.88-716.90, 716.96,
716.98-716.99, 718.00, 718.08, 719.00, 719.06, 719.08-719.10, 719.16,
719.18-719.20, 719.26, 719.28-719.30, 719.36, 719.38-719.40, 719.46,
719.48-719.50, 719.56, 719.58-719.60, 719.66, 719.68-719.80, 719.86,
719.88-719.90, 719.96, 719.98-719.99;

For code **711.67:** (Ex) 015.80-015.96, 017.90-017.96, 036.82, 056.71,
098.50-098.51, 098.59, 098.89, 711.00, 711.07-711.10, 711.17-711.20,
711.27-711.30, 711.37-711.40, 711.47-711.50, 711.57-711.60,
711.67-711.70, 711.77-711.80, 711.87-711.90, 711.97-712.10,
712.17-712.20, 712.27-712.30, 712.37-712.80, 712.87-712.90,
712.97-714.0, 715.00, 715.09-715.10, 715.17-715.20, 715.27-715.30,
715.37-715.90, 715.97-716.00, 716.07-716.10, 716.17-716.20,
716.27-716.30, 716.37-716.40, 716.47-716.50, 716.57-716.60,
716.67-716.80, 716.87-716.90, 716.97-716.99, 718.00, 718.07-718.08,
719.00, 719.07-719.10, 719.17-719.20, 719.27-719.30, 719.37-719.40,
719.47-719.50, 719.57-719.60, 719.67-719.80, 719.87-719.90,
719.97-719.99

● ▶ **711.7** **Arthropathy associated with helminthiasis** 🔖
[0-9]
> *Code first* underlying disease, as:
> filariasis (125.0–125.9)
>
> For codes **711.70-711.14, 711.76, 711.78-711.79:** (Ex) 003.23,
> 015.80-015.96, 017.90-017.96, 036.82, 056.71, 098.50-098.51, 098.59,
> 098.89, 711.00-714.0, 715.00, 715.09-715.10, 715.18-716.99,
> 718.00-718.08, 719.00-719.10, 719.18-719.69, 719.80-719.99;
>
> For code **711.75:** (Ex) 003.23, 015.80-015.96, 017.90-017.96, 036.82, 056.71,
> 098.50-098.51, 098.59, 098.89, 711.00-714.0, 715.00, 715.09-715.10,
> 715.18-716.99, 718.00-718.08, 719.00-719.10, 719.18-719.43,
> 719.45-719.69, 719.80-719.99;
>
> For code **711.77:** (Ex) 003.23, 015.80-015.96, 017.90-017.96, 036.82, 056.71,
> 098.50-098.51, 098.59, 098.89, 711.00-714.0, 715.00, 715.09-715.10,
> 715.18-716.99, 718.00-718.08, 719.00-719.10, 719.18-719.69,
> 719.80-719.97, 719.99

N Newborn: 0 **P** Pediatric: 0–17 **M** Maternity: 12–55 **A** Adult: 15–124 ♀ Females Only ♂ Males Only

(Ex) CC/MCC Exclusions 🔖 Complication\Comorbidity 🔖 Major C\C 🔖 Present on Admission Requirement 🔖 Hospital-Acquired Condition

901

● ▶ **711.8** *Arthropathy associated with other infectious and*
[0-9] *parasitic diseases*
> *Code first* underlying disease, as:
>> diseases classifiable to 080–088, 100–104, 130–136
>
> **Excludes** *arthropathy associated with sarcoidosis (713.7)*
>
> For codes: **711.80, 711.82-711.89:** (Ex) 003.23, 015.80-015.96, 017.90-017.96,
> 036.82, 056.71, 098.50-098.51, 098.59, 098.89, 711.00-714.0, 715.00,
> 715.09-715.10, 715.18-716.99, 718.00-718.08, 719.00-719.10,
> 719.18-719.69, 719.80-719.99;
> For code **711.81:** (Ex) 003.23, 015.80-015.96, 017.90-017.96, 036.82, 056.71,
> 098.50-098.51, 098.59, 098.89, 711.00-711.41, 711.43-714.0, 715.00,
> 715.09-715.10, 715.18-716.99, 718.00-718.08, 719.00-719.10,
> 719.18-719.69, 719.80-719.99
>
> **Coding Clinic: 1990, Q3, P14**

● **711.9** **Unspecified infective arthritis**
[0-9] Infective arthritis or polyarthritis (acute) (chronic)
(subacute) NOS
> (Ex) 003.23, 015.80-015.96, 017.90-017.96, 036.82, 056.71, 098.50-098.51,
> 098.59, 098.89, 711.00-714.0, 715.00, 715.09-715.10, 715.18-716.99,
> 718.00-718.08, 719.00-719.10, 719.18-719.69, 719.80-719.99

● **712** **Crystal arthropathies**
> **Includes** crystal-induced arthritis and synovitis
>
> **Excludes** *gouty arthropathy (274.00-274.03)*

The following fifth-digit subclassification is for use with
category 712; valid digits are in [brackets] under each code. See list
at beginning of chapter for definitions:

0	site unspecified	5	pelvic region and thigh
1	shoulder region	6	lower leg
2	upper arm	7	ankle and foot
3	forearm	8	other specified sites
4	hand	9	multiple sites

● ▶ **712.1** *Chondrocalcinosis due to dicalcium phosphate*
[0-9] *crystals*
> Chondrocalcinosis due to dicalcium phosphate crystals
> (with other crystals)
>
> *Code first* underlying disease (275.49)

● ▶ **712.2** *Chondrocalcinosis due to pyrophosphate crystals*
[0-9]
> *Code first* underlying disease (275.49)

● ▶ **712.3** *Chondrocalcinosis, unspecified*
[0-9]
> *Code first* underlying disease (275.49)

● **712.8** **Other specified crystal arthropathies**
[0-9]

● **712.9** **Unspecified crystal arthropathy**
[0-9]

● **713** **Arthropathy associated with other disorders classified elsewhere**
> **Includes** arthritis associated with conditions classifiable
> below
> arthropathy associated with conditions classifiable
> below
> polyarthritis associated with conditions classifiable
> below
> polyarthropathy associated with conditions
> classifiable below

▶ **713.0** *Arthropathy associated with other endocrine and metabolic
disorders*
> *Code first* underlying disease, as:
>> acromegaly (253.0)
>> hemochromatosis (275.01-275.09)
>> hyperparathyroidism (252.00–252.08)
>> hypogammaglobulinemia (279.00–279.09)
>> hypothyroidism (243–244.9)
>> lipoid metabolism disorder (272.0–272.9)
>> ochronosis (270.2)
>
> **Excludes** *arthropathy associated with:*
>> *amyloidosis (713.7)*
>> *crystal deposition disorders, except gout
>> (712.1–712.9)*
>> *diabetic neuropathy (713.5)*
>> *gout (274.00-274.03)*

▶ **713.1** *Arthropathy associated with gastrointestinal conditions
other than infections*
> *Code first* underlying disease, as:
>> regional enteritis (555.0–555.9)
>> ulcerative colitis (556)

▶ **713.2** *Arthropathy associated with hematological disorders*
> *Code first* underlying disease, as:
>> hemoglobinopathy (282.4–282.7)
>> hemophilia (286.0–286.2)
>> leukemia (204.0–208.9)
>> malignant reticulosis (202.3)
>> multiple myelomatosis (203.0)
>
> **Excludes** *arthropathy associated with Henoch-Schönlein
>> purpura (713.6)*

▶ **713.3** *Arthropathy associated with dermatological disorders*
> *Code first* underlying disease, as:
>> erythema multiforme (695.10–695.19)
>> erythema nodosum (695.2)
>
> **Excludes** *psoriatic arthropathy (696.0)*

▶ **713.4** *Arthropathy associated with respiratory disorders*
> *Code first* underlying disease, as:
>> diseases classifiable to 490–519
>
> **Excludes** *arthropathy associated with respiratory infections
>> (711.0, 711.4–711.8)*

▶ **713.5** *Arthropathy associated with neurological disorders*
> Charcot's arthropathy associated with diseases
> classifiable elsewhere
> Neuropathic arthritis associated with diseases classifiable
> elsewhere
>
> *Code first* underlying disease, as:
>> neuropathic joint disease [Charcot's joints]:
>>> NOS (094.0)
>>> diabetic (249.6, 250.6)
>>> syringomyelic (336.0)
>>> tabetic [syphilitic] (094.0)
>
> **Coding Clinic: 2012, Q3, P4**

▶ **713.6** *Arthropathy associated with hypersensitivity reaction*
> *Code first* underlying disease, as:
>> Henoch-Schönlein purpura (287.0)
>> serum sickness (999.51-999.59)
>
> **Excludes** *allergic arthritis NOS (716.2)*

▶ **713.7** *Other general diseases with articular involvement*
> *Code first* underlying disease, as:
>> amyloidosis (277.30–277.39)
>> familial Mediterranean fever (277.31)
>> sarcoidosis (135)
>
> **Coding Clinic: 1997, Q2, P12-13**

▶ **713.8** *Arthropathy associated with other conditions classifiable
elsewhere*
> *Code first* underlying disease, as:
>> conditions classifiable elsewhere except as in
>> 711.1–711.8, 712, and 713.0–713.7

● **714** **Rheumatoid arthritis and other inflammatory polyarthropathies**
> **Excludes** *rheumatic fever (390)*
>> *rheumatoid arthritis of spine NOS (720.0)*

714.0 **Rheumatoid arthritis**
> Arthritis or polyarthritis:
>> atrophic
>> rheumatic (chronic)
>
> Use additional code to identify manifestation, as:
>> myopathy (359.6)
>> polyneuropathy (357.1)
>
> **Excludes** *juvenile rheumatoid arthritis NOS (714.30)*
>
> **Coding Clinic: 2006, Q2, P20; 1995, Q4, P51**

714.1 **Felty's syndrome**
> Rheumatoid arthritis with splenoadenomegaly and
> leukopenia

714.2 **Other rheumatoid arthritis with visceral or systemic
involvement**
> Rheumatoid carditis

◀ New   ◀ⁿⁿ Revised   ~~deleted~~ Deleted   Excludes   Includes   Use additional   Code first   Omit code

902   ● Unacceptable Principal Diagnosis   ● Use Additional Digit(s)   ▶ Manifestation Code   OGCR Official Guidelines   Coding Clinic

Item 13-1   Rheumatoid arthritis (RA) is a chronic systemic inflammatory disease of undetermined etiology involving primarily the synovial membranes and articular structures of multiple joints. The disease is often progressive and results in pain, stiffness, and swelling of joints. In late stages, deformity, ankylosis, and other **inflammatory polyarthropathies** develop.

● **714.3   Juvenile chronic polyarthritis**

    714.30   Polyarticular juvenile rheumatoid arthritis, chronic or unspecified
        Juvenile rheumatoid arthritis NOS
        Still's disease

    714.31   Polyarticular juvenile rheumatoid arthritis, acute 🗲
        (Ex): 036.82, 056.71, 711.00-714.4, 715.00, 715.09-715.10, 715.18-716.99, 718.00-718.08, 719.00-719.10, 719.18-719.99

    714.32   Pauciarticular juvenile rheumatoid arthritis

    714.33   Monoarticular juvenile rheumatoid arthritis

  714.4   Chronic postrheumatic arthropathy
    Chronic rheumatoid nodular fibrositis
    Jaccoud's syndrome

● **714.8   Other specified inflammatory polyarthropathies**

    714.81   Rheumatoid lung
        Caplan's syndrome
        Diffuse interstitial rheumatoid disease of lung
        Fibrosing alveolitis, rheumatoid

    714.89   Other

  714.9   Unspecified inflammatory polyarthropathy
    Inflammatory polyarthropathy or polyarthritis NOS
    Excludes   *polyarthropathy NOS (716.5)*

● **715   Osteoarthrosis and allied disorders**
    Degenerative joint disease with breaking down the cartilage causing pain, swelling, and reduced motion in the joints, affecting any joint

    Note: Localized, in the subcategories below, includes bilateral involvement of the same site.

    Includes   arthritis or polyarthritis:
        degenerative
        hypertrophic
        degenerative joint disease
        osteoarthritis

    Excludes   *Marie-Strümpell spondylitis (720.0)*
        osteoarthrosis [osteoarthritis] of spine (721.0–721.9)

The following fifth-digit subclassification is for use with category 715; valid digits are in [brackets] under each code. See list at beginning of chapter for definitions:

0	site unspecified	5	pelvic region and thigh
1	shoulder region	6	lower leg
2	upper arm	7	ankle and foot
3	forearm	8	other specified sites
4	hand	9	multiple sites

● **715.0   Osteoarthrosis, generalized**
  [0,4,9] Degenerative joint disease, involving multiple joints
        Primary generalized hypertrophic osteoarthrosis
        Coding Clinic: 1995, Q2, P5

● **715.1   Osteoarthrosis, localized, primary**
  [0-8] Localized osteoarthropathy, idiopathic

● **715.2   Osteoarthrosis, localized, secondary**
  [0-8] Coxae malum senilis

● **715.3   Osteoarthrosis, localized, not specified whether**
  [0-8] **primary or secondary**
        Otto's pelvis
        Coding Clinic: 2004, Q2, P15; 2003, Q2, P18; 1995, Q2, P5

● **715.8   Osteoarthrosis involving, or with mention of more**
  [0,9] **than one site, but not specified as generalized**
        Coding Clinic: 1995, Q2, P5

● **715.9   Osteoarthrosis, unspecified whether generalized or**
  [0-8] **localized**
        Coding Clinic: 2003, Q2, P18; 1997, Q2, P12-13; 1996, Q1, P16; 1995, Q2, P5

● **716   Other and unspecified arthropathies**
    Excludes   *cricoarytenoid arthropathy (478.79)*

The following fifth-digit subclassification is for use with category 716; valid digits are in [brackets] under each code. See list at beginning of chapter for definitions:

0	site unspecified	5	pelvic region and thigh
1	shoulder region	6	lower leg
2	upper arm	7	ankle and foot
3	forearm	8	other specified sites
4	hand	9	multiple sites

● **716.0   Kaschin-Beck disease**
  [0-9] Endemic polyarthritis

● **716.1   Traumatic arthropathy**
  [0-9] **Coding Clinic: 2009, Q2, P11; 2002, Q1, P9-10**

● **716.2   Allergic arthritis**
  [0-9] **Excludes**   *arthritis associated with Henoch-Schönlein purpura or serum sickness (713.6)*

● **716.3   Climacteric arthritis** ♀
  [0-9] Menopausal arthritis

● **716.4   Transient arthropathy**
  [0-9] **Excludes**   *palindromic rheumatism (719.3)*

● **716.5   Unspecified polyarthropathy or polyarthritis**
  [0-9]

● **716.6   Unspecified monoarthritis**
  [0-8] Coxitis

● **716.8   Other specified arthropathy**
  [0-9]

● **716.9   Arthropathy, unspecified**
  [0-9] Arthritis (acute) (chronic) (subacute)
        Arthropathy (acute) (chronic) (subacute)
        Articular rheumatism (chronic)
        Inflammation of joint NOS

● **717   Internal derangement of knee**
    Includes   degeneration of articular cartilage or meniscus of knee
        rupture, old of articular cartilage or meniscus of knee
        tear, old of articular cartilage or meniscus of knee

    Excludes   *acute derangement of knee (836.0–836.6)*
        ankylosis (718.5)
        contracture (718.4)
        current injury (836.0–836.6)
        deformity (736.4–736.6)
        recurrent dislocation (718.3)

  717.0   Old bucket handle tear of medial meniscus
    Old bucket handle tear of unspecified cartilage

  717.1   Derangement of anterior horn of medial meniscus

  717.2   Derangement of posterior horn of medial meniscus

  717.3   Other and unspecified derangement of medial meniscus
    Degeneration of internal semilunar cartilage

● **717.4   Derangement of lateral meniscus**

    717.40   Derangement of lateral meniscus, unspecified

    717.41   Bucket handle tear of lateral meniscus

    717.42   Derangement of anterior horn of lateral meniscus

    717.43   Derangement of posterior horn of lateral meniscus

    717.49   Other

  717.5   Derangement of meniscus, not elsewhere classified
    Congenital discoid meniscus
    Cyst of semilunar cartilage
    Derangement of semilunar cartilage NOS

  717.6   Loose body in knee
    Joint mice, knee
    Rice bodies, knee (joint)

  717.7   Chondromalacia of patella
    Chondromalacia patellae
    Degeneration [softening] of articular cartilage of patella
    Coding Clinic: 1985, July-Aug, P14; 1984, Nov-Dec, P9

N Newborn: 0   **P** Pediatric: 0–17   **M** Maternity: 12–55   **A** Adult: 15–124   ♀ Females Only   ♂ Males Only

(Ex) CC/MCC Exclusions   🗲 Complication\Comorbidity   Major C\C   Present on Admission Requirement   Hospital-Acquired Condition

903

Figure 13–1 Collateral and cruciate ligament of knee. (From DeLee: DeLee and Drez's Orthopaedic Sports Medicine, ed 3, Saunders, 2009)

Fibular collateral ligament
Lateral capsular ligament
Fibular
Plate
Tibial collateral ligament
Medial capsular ligament
Tibial

● **717.8 Other internal derangement of knee**

     717.81 Old disruption of lateral collateral ligament

     717.82 Old disruption of medial collateral ligament

     717.83 Old disruption of anterior cruciate ligament

     717.84 Old disruption of posterior cruciate ligament

     717.85 Old disruption of other ligaments of knee
         Capsular ligament of knee

     717.89 Other
         Old disruption of ligaments of knee NOS

     717.9 Unspecified internal derangement of knee
         Derangement NOS of knee

● **718 Other derangement of joint**

     Excludes   *current injury (830.0–848.9)*
                  jaw (524.60–524.69)

The following fifth-digit subclassification is for use with category 718; valid digits are in [brackets] under each code. See list at beginning of chapter for definitions:

0	site unspecified	5	pelvic region and thigh
1	shoulder region	6	lower leg
2	upper arm	7	ankle and foot
3	forearm	8	other specified sites
4	hand	9	multiple sites

● **718.0 Articular cartilage disorder**
[0-5,7-9]   Meniscus:
         disorder
         rupture, old
         tear, old
     Old rupture of ligament(s) of joint NOS

     Excludes   *articular cartilage disorder:*
                in ochronosis (270.2)
                knee (717.0–717.9)
             chondrocalcinosis (275.49)
             metastatic calcification (275.40)

● **718.1 Loose body in joint**
[0-5,7-9]   Joint mice

     Excludes   *knee (717.6)*

     Coding Clinic: 2001, Q2, P14-15

● **718.2 Pathological dislocation**
[0-9]   Dislocation or displacement of joint, not recurrent and
         not current

● **718.3 Recurrent dislocation of joint**
[0-9]   **Coding Clinic: 1987, Nov-Dec, P7**

● **718.4 Contracture of joint**
[0-9]   **Coding Clinic: 1998, Q4, P39-40**

● **718.5 Ankylosis of joint**
[0-9]   Ankylosis of joint (fibrous) (osseous)

     Excludes   *spine (724.9)*
                stiffness of joint without mention of ankylosis
                  (719.5)

     Coding Clinic: 1995, Q1, P10

● **718.6 Unspecified intrapelvic protrusion of acetabulum**
[5]   Protrusio acetabuli, unspecified

● **718.7 Developmental dislocation of joint**
[0-9]   **Excludes**   *congenital dislocation of joint (754.0–755.8)*
                traumatic dislocation of joint (830–839)

● **718.8 Other joint derangement, not elsewhere classified**
[0-9]   Flail joint (paralytic)
     Instability of joint

     Excludes   *deformities classifiable to 736 (736.0–736.9)*

     Coding Clinic: 2000, Q2, P14-15

● **718.9 Unspecified derangement of joint**
[0-5,7-9]   **Excludes**   *knee (717.9)*

● **719 Other and unspecified disorders of joint**

     Excludes   *jaw (524.60–524.69)*

The following fifth-digit subclassification is for use with codes 719.0–719.6, 719.8–719.9; valid digits are in [brackets] under each code. See list at beginning of chapter for definitions:

0	site unspecified	5	pelvic region and thigh
1	shoulder region	6	lower leg
2	upper arm	7	ankle and foot
3	forearm	8	other specified sites
4	hand	9	multiple sites

● **719.0 Effusion of joint**
[0-9]   Hydrarthrosis
     Swelling of joint, with or without pain

     Excludes   *intermittent hydrarthrosis (719.3)*

● **719.1 Hemarthrosis**
[0-9]   **Excludes**   *current injury (840.0–848.9)*

     For codes **719.10, 719.15, 719.18-719.19:** (Ex) 719.10-719.19,
         958.91-958.92;
     For code **719.11:** (Ex) 719.10-719.13, 719.18-719.19, 958.91;
     For code **719.12:** (Ex) 719.10-719.12, 719.18-719.19, 958.91;
     For code **719.13:** (Ex) 719.10, 719.12-719.14, 719.18-719.19, 958.91;
     For code **719.14:** (Ex) 719.10, 719.13-719.14, 719.18-719.19, 958.91;
     For codes **719.16-719.17:** (Ex) 719.10, 719.16-719.19, 958.92

● **719.2 Villonodular synovitis**
[0-9]

● **719.3 Palindromic rheumatism**
[0-9]   Hench-Rosenberg syndrome
     Intermittent hydrarthrosis

● **719.4 Pain in joint**
[0-9]   Arthralgia
     Coding Clinic: 2001, Q1, P3-4

● **719.5 Stiffness of joint, not elsewhere classified**
[0-9]

● **719.6 Other symptoms referable to joint**
[0-9]   Joint crepitus
     Snapping hip
     Coding Clinic: 2007, Q2, P7; 1984, Sept-Oct, P15-16

     719.7 Difficulty in walking

     Excludes   *abnormality of gait (781.2)*

     Coding Clinic: 2004, Q2, P15

● **719.8 Other specified disorders of joint**
[0-9]   Calcification of joint
     Fistula of joint

     Excludes   *temporomandibular joint-pain-dysfunction*
                  syndrome [Costen's syndrome] (524.60)

● **719.9 Unspecified disorder of joint**
[0-9]

DORSOPATHIES (720–724)

     Excludes   *curvature of spine (737.0–737.9)*
                osteochondrosis of spine (juvenile) (732.0) adult (732.8)

● **720 Ankylosing spondylitis and other inflammatory spondylopathies**

     720.0 Ankylosing spondylitis
         Rheumatoid arthritis of spine NOS
         Spondylitis:
             Marie-Strümpell
             rheumatoid

     720.1 Spinal enthesopathy
         Disorder of peripheral ligamentous or muscular
             attachments of spine
         Romanus lesion

     720.2 Sacroiliitis, not elsewhere classified
         Inflammation of sacroiliac joint NOS

Item 13-2 Ankylosis or arthrokleisis is a consolidation of a joint due to disease, injury, or surgical procedure. **Spondylosis** is the degeneration of the vertebral processes and formation of osteophytes and commonly occurs with age. **Spondylitis** or ankylosing spondylitis is a type of arthritis that affects the spine or backbone causing back pain and stiffness.

◄ New   ◄◄ Revised   ~~deleted~~ Deleted   Excludes   Includes   Use additional   Code first   Omit code

904   ● Unacceptable Principal Diagnosis   ● Use Additional Digit(s)   ▶ Manifestation Code   **OGCR** Official Guidelines   **Coding Clinic**

● 720.8 **Other inflammatory spondylopathies**

▷ 720.81 *Inflammatory spondylopathies in diseases classified elsewhere*

Code first underlying disease, as:
tuberculosis (015.0)

720.89 **Other**

720.9 **Unspecified inflammatory spondylopathy**
Spondylitis NOS

● 721 **Spondylosis and allied disorders**
Coding Clinic: 1989, Q2, P14

721.0 **Cervical spondylosis without myelopathy**
Cervical or cervicodorsal:
arthritis
osteoarthritis
spondylarthritis

721.1 **Cervical spondylosis with myelopathy** 🔗
Anterior spinal artery compression syndrome
Spondylogenic compression of cervical spinal cord
Vertebral artery compression syndrome
(Ex) 721.0-721.1

721.2 **Thoracic spondylosis without myelopathy**
Thoracic:
arthritis
osteoarthritis
spondylarthritis

721.3 **Lumbosacral spondylosis without myelopathy**
Lumbar or lumbosacral:
arthritis
osteoarthritis
spondylarthritis
Coding Clinic: 2002, Q4, P107-108

● 721.4 **Thoracic or lumbar spondylosis with myelopathy**

721.41 **Thoracic region** 🔗
Spondylogenic compression of thoracic spinal cord
(Ex) 721.41

721.42 **Lumbar region** 🔗
(Ex) 721.3, 721.42, 722.10, 722.2, 722.32, 722.52-722.70, 722.73, 722.83-722.90, 722.93

721.5 **Kissing spine**
Baastrup's syndrome

721.6 **Ankylosing vertebral hyperostosis**

721.7 **Traumatic spondylopathy** 🔗
Kümmell's disease or spondylitis
(Ex) 721.7

721.8 **Other allied disorders of spine**

● 721.9 **Spondylosis of unspecified site**

721.90 **Without mention of myelopathy**
Spinal:
arthritis (deformans) (degenerative) (hypertrophic)
osteoarthritis NOS
Spondylarthrosis NOS

721.91 **With myelopathy** 🔗
Spondylogenic compression of spinal cord NOS
(Ex) 721.0-721.91, 724.03

● 722 **Intervertebral disc disorders**
Coding Clinic: 1989, Q2, P14

722.0 **Displacement of cervical intervertebral disc without myelopathy**
Neuritis (brachial) or radiculitis due to displacement or rupture of cervical intervertebral disc
Any condition classifiable to 722.2 of the cervical or cervicothoracic intervertebral disc
Coding Clinic: 1988, Q1, P10

● 722.1 **Displacement of thoracic or lumbar intervertebral disc without myelopathy**

722.10 **Lumbar intervertebral disc without myelopathy**
Lumbago or sciatica due to displacement of intervertebral disc
Neuritis or radiculitis due to displacement or rupture of lumbar intervertebral disc
Any condition classifiable to 722.2 of the lumbar or lumbosacral intervertebral disc
Coding Clinic: 2008, Q4, P183-184; 2007, Q1, P9; 2003, Q3, P12; Q1, P7; 2002, Q4, P107-108; 1994, Q3, P14

722.11 **Thoracic intervertebral disc without myelopathy**
Any condition classifiable to 722.2 of thoracic intervertebral disc

722.2 **Displacement of intervertebral disc, site unspecified, without myelopathy**
Discogenic syndrome NOS
Herniation of nucleus pulposus NOS
Intervertebral disc NOS:
extrusion
prolapse
protrusion
rupture
Neuritis or radiculitis due to displacement or rupture of intervertebral disc
Coding Clinic: 1988, Q1, P10

● 722.3 **Schmorl's nodes**

722.30 **Unspecified region**

722.31 **Thoracic region**

722.32 **Lumbar region**

722.39 **Other**

● 722.4 **Degeneration of cervical intervertebral disc**
Degeneration of cervicothoracic intervertebral disc

● 722.5 **Degeneration of thoracic or lumbar intervertebral disc**

722.51 **Thoracic or thoracolumbar intervertebral disc**

722.52 **Lumbar or lumbosacral intervertebral disc**
Coding Clinic: 2006, Q2, P18; 2004, Q4, P129-133

722.6 **Degeneration of intervertebral disc, site unspecified**
Degenerative disc disease NOS
Narrowing of intervertebral disc or space NOS

● 722.7 **Intervertebral disc disorder with myelopathy**

722.70 **Unspecified region**

722.71 **Cervical region** 🔗
(Ex) 722.0, 722.71

722.72 **Thoracic region** 🔗
(Ex) 722.11, 722.72

722.73 **Lumbar region** 🔗
(Ex) 722.11, 722.73, 724.03

● 722.8 **Postlaminectomy syndrome**

722.80 **Unspecified region**

722.81 **Cervical region**

722.82 **Thoracic region**

722.83 **Lumbar region**
Coding Clinic: 1997, Q2, P15x2

● 722.9 **Other and unspecified disc disorder**
Calcification of intervertebral cartilage or disc
Discitis

722.90 **Unspecified region**
Coding Clinic: 1984, Nov-Dec, P19

722.91 **Cervical region**

722.92 **Thoracic region**

722.93 **Lumbar region**

N Newborn: 0   P Pediatric: 0–17   M Maternity: 12–55   A Adult: 15–124   ♀ Females Only   ♂ Males Only

(Ex) CC/MCC Exclusions   🔗 Complication\Comorbidity   🔗 Major C\C   🔗 Present on Admission Requirement   🔗 Hospital-Acquired Condition

905

● **723 Other disorders of cervical region**
> **Excludes** conditions due to:
>> *intervertebral disc disorders (722.0–722.9)*
>> *spondylosis (721.0–721.9)*
>
> Coding Clinic: 1989, Q2, P14

723.0 Spinal stenosis of cervical region
> Coding Clinic: 2003, Q4, P99-101

723.1 Cervicalgia
> Pain in neck

723.2 Cervicocranial syndrome
> Barré-Liéou syndrome
> Posterior cervical sympathetic syndrome

723.3 Cervicobrachial syndrome (diffuse)
> Coding Clinic: 1985, Nov-Dec, P12

723.4 Brachia neuritis or radiculitis NOS
> Cervical radiculitis
> Radicular syndrome of upper limbs

723.5 Torticollis, unspecified
> Contracture of neck
>> **Excludes** *congenital (754.1)*
>>> *due to birth injury (767.8)*
>>> *hysterical (300.11)*
>>> *ocular torticollis (781.93)*
>>> *psychogenic (306.0)*
>>> *spasmodic (333.83)*
>>> *traumatic, current (847.0)*
>> Coding Clinic: 2001, Q2, P21; 1995, Q1, P7

723.6 Panniculitis specified as affecting neck

723.7 Ossification of posterior longitudinal ligament in cervical region

723.8 Other syndromes affecting cervical region
> Cervical syndrome NEC
> Klippel's disease
> Occipital neuralgia
> Coding Clinic: 2000, Q1, P7-8

723.9 Unspecified musculoskeletal disorders and symptoms referable to neck
> Cervical (region) disorder NOS

● **724 Other and unspecified disorders of back**
> **Excludes** collapsed vertebra (code to cause, e.g., osteoporosis, 733.00–733.09)
>> conditions due to:
>>> *intervertebral disc disorders (722.0–722.9)*
>>> *spondylosis (721.0–721.9)*
>
> Coding Clinic: 1989, Q2, P14

● **724.0 Spinal stenosis, other than cervical**

724.00 Spinal stenosis, unspecified region

724.01 Thoracic region

724.02 Lumbar region, without neurogenic claudication
> Lumbar region NOS
> Coding Clinic: 2008, Q4, P109-110; 2007, Q4, P116-120; Q1, P20-21; 1999, Q4, P13-14; 1994, Q3, P14

724.03 Lumbar region, with neurogenic claudication

724.09 Other

724.1 Pain in thoracic spine

724.2 Lumbago
> Low back pain   Lumbalgia
> Low back syndrome
> Coding Clinic: 2007, Q2, P13-15; 1985, Nov-Dec, P12

724.3 Sciatica
> Neuralgia or neuritis of sciatic nerve
>> **Excludes** *specified lesion of sciatic nerve (355.0)*
>> Coding Clinic: 1989, Q2, P12

724.4 Thoracic or lumbosacral neuritis or radiculitis, unspecified
> Radicular syndrome of lower limbs
> Coding Clinic: 1999, Q2, P3-4

724.5 Backache, unspecified
> Vertebrogenic (pain) syndrome NOS

724.6 Disorders of sacrum
> Ankylosis, lumbosacral or sacroiliac (joint)
> Instability, lumbosacral or sacroiliac (joint)

724.7 Disorders of coccyx

724.70 Unspecified disorder of coccyx

724.71 Hypermobility of coccyx

724.79 Other
> Coccygodynia

724.8 Other symptoms referable to back
> Ossification of posterior longitudinal ligament NOS
> Panniculitis specified as sacral or affecting back

724.9 Other unspecified back disorders
> Ankylosis of spine NOS
> Compression of spinal nerve root NEC
> Spinal disorder NOS
>> **Excludes** *sacroiliitis (720.2)*

RHEUMATISM, EXCLUDING THE BACK (725–729)

> **Includes** disorders of muscles and tendons and their attachments, and of other soft tissues

725 Polymyalgia rheumatica

● **726 Peripheral enthesopathies and allied syndromes**
> **Note:** Enthesopathies are disorders of peripheral ligamentous or muscular attachments.
>> **Excludes** *spinal enthesopathy (720.1)*

726.0 Adhesive capsulitis of shoulder

● **726.1 Rotator cuff syndrome of shoulder and allied disorders**

726.10 Disorders of bursae and tendons in shoulder region, unspecified
> Rotator cuff syndrome NOS
> Supraspinatus syndrome NOS
> Coding Clinic: 2001, Q2, P12

726.11 Calcifying tendinitis of shoulder

726.12 Bicipital tenosynovitis

726.13 Partial tear of rotator cuff
>> **Excludes** *complete rupture of rotator cuff, nontraumatic (727.61)*
>> Coding Clinic: 2011, Q4, P136

726.19 Other specified disorders
>> **Excludes** *complete rupture of rotator cuff, nontraumatic (727.61)*
>> Coding Clinic: 2002, Q1, P9-10

726.2 Other affections of shoulder region, not elsewhere classified
> Periarthritis of shoulder
> Scapulohumeral fibrositis

● **726.3 Enthesopathy of elbow region**

726.30 Enthesopathy of elbow, unspecified

726.31 Medial epicondylitis

726.32 Lateral epicondylitis
> Epicondylitis NOS   Tennis elbow
> Golfers' elbow

726.33 Olecranon bursitis
> Bursitis of elbow

726.39 Other

726.4 Enthesopathy of wrist and carpus
> Bursitis of hand or wrist
> Periarthritis of wrist

726.5 Enthesopathy of hip region
> Bursitis of hip   Psoas tendinitis
> Gluteal tendinitis   Trochanteric tendinitis
> Iliac crest spur

● **726.6 Enthesopathy of knee**

726.60 Enthesopathy of knee, unspecified
> Bursitis of knee NOS

726.61 Pes anserinus tendinitis or bursitis

726.62 Tibial collateral ligament bursitis
> Pellegrini-Stieda syndrome

726.63 Fibular collateral ligament bursitis

Item 13–3 Polymyalgia rheumatica is a syndrome characterized by aching and morning stiffness and is related to aging and hereditary predisposition.

◀ New   ◀ Revised   ~~deleted~~ Deleted   Excludes   Includes   Use additional   Code first   Omit code
● Unacceptable Principal Diagnosis   ● Use Additional Digit(s)   ▶ Manifestation Code   OGCR Official Guidelines   Coding Clinic

906

726.64 **Patellar tendinitis**

726.65 **Prepatellar bursitis**
Coding Clinic: 2006, Q2, P15

726.69 **Other**
Bursitis:
infrapatellar
subpatellar

● 726.7 **Enthesopathy of ankle and tarsus**

726.70 **Enthesopathy of ankle and tarsus, unspecified**
Metatarsalgia NOS

Excludes *Morton's metatarsalgia (355.6)*

726.71 **Achilles bursitis or tendinitis**

726.72 **Tibialis tendinitis**
Tibialis (anterior) (posterior) tendinitis

726.73 **Calcaneal spur**

726.79 **Other**
Peroneal tendinitis

726.8 **Other peripheral enthesopathies**

● 726.9 **Unspecified enthesopathy**

726.90 **Enthesopathy of unspecified site**
Capsulitis NOS   Tendinitis NOS
Periarthritis NOS

726.91 **Exostosis of unspecified site**
Bone spur NOS
Coding Clinic: 2001, Q2, P13-15

● 727 **Other disorders of synovium, tendon, and bursa**

● 727.0 **Synovitis and tenosynovitis**

727.00 **Synovitis and tenosynovitis, unspecified**
Synovitis NOS   Tenosynovitis NOS

727.01 *Synovitis and tenosynovitis in diseases classified elsewhere*
Code first underlying disease, as:
tuberculosis (015.0–015.9)

Excludes *crystal-induced (275.49)*
gonococcal (098.51)
gout (274.00-274.03)
syphilitic (095.7)

727.02 **Giant cell tumor of tendon sheath**

727.03 **Trigger finger (acquired)**

727.04 **Radial styloid tenosynovitis**
de Quervain's disease

727.05 **Other tenosynovitis of hand and wrist**

727.06 **Tenosynovitis of foot and ankle**

727.09 **Other**

727.1 **Bunion**

727.2 **Specific bursitides often of occupational origin**
Beat:
elbow
hand
knee
Chronic crepitant synovitis of wrist
Miners':
elbow
knee

727.3 **Other bursitis**
Bursitis NOS

Excludes *bursitis:*
gonococcal (098.52)
subacromial (726.19)
subcoracoid (726.19)
subdeltoid (726.19)
syphilitic (095.7)
"frozen shoulder" (726.0)

Item 13-4   Synovitis is an inflammation of a synovial membrane resulting in pain on motion and is characterized by fluctuating swelling due to effusion in a synovial sac. **Tenosynovitis** is an inflammation of a tendon sheath and occurs most commonly in the wrists, hands, and feet. Bursitis is inflammation of a bursa (fluid filled sac) caused by repetitive use, trauma, infection, or systemic inflammatory disease. Bursae act as protectors and facilitate movement between bones and overlapping muscles (deep bursae) or between bones and tendons/skin (superficial bursae).

● 727.4 **Ganglion and cyst of synovium, tendon, and bursa**

727.40 **Synovial cyst, unspecified**

Excludes *that of popliteal space (727.51)*
Coding Clinic: 1997, Q2, P6

727.41 **Ganglion of joint**

727.42 **Ganglion of tendon sheath**

727.43 **Ganglion, unspecified**

727.49 **Other**
Cyst of bursa

● 727.5 **Rupture of synovium**

727.50 **Rupture of synovium, unspecified**

727.51 **Synovial cyst of popliteal space**
Baker's cyst (knee)

727.59 **Other**

● 727.6 **Rupture of tendon, nontraumatic**

727.60 **Nontraumatic rupture of unspecified tendon**

727.61 **Complete rupture of rotator cuff**

Excludes *partial tear of rotator cuff (726.13)*

727.62 **Tendons of biceps (long head)**

727.63 **Extensor tendons of hand and wrist**

727.64 **Flexor tendons of hand and wrist**

727.65 **Quadriceps tendon**

727.66 **Patellar tendon**

727.67 **Achilles tendon**

727.68 **Other tendons of foot and ankle**

727.69 **Other**

● 727.8 **Other disorders of synovium, tendon, and bursa**

727.81 **Contracture of tendon (sheath)**
Short Achilles tendon (acquired)

727.82 **Calcium deposits in tendon and bursa**
Calcification of tendon NOS
Calcific tendinitis NOS

Excludes *peripheral ligamentous or muscular attachments (726.0–726.9)*

727.83 **Plica syndrome**
Plica knee

727.89 **Other**
Abscess of bursa or tendon

Excludes *xanthomatosis localized to tendons (272.7)*
Coding Clinic: 1989, Q2, P15; 1985, July-Aug, P14; 1984, Nov-Dec, P9

727.9 **Unspecified disorder of synovium, tendon, and bursa**

● 728 **Disorders of muscle, ligament, and fascia**

Excludes *enthesopathies (726.0–726.9)*
muscular dystrophies (359.0–359.1)
myoneural disorders (358.00–358.9)
myopathies (359.2–359.9)
nontraumatic hematoma of muscle (729.92)
old disruption of ligaments of knee (717.81–717.89)

728.0 **Infective myositis** 🔵
Myositis:
purulent   suppurative

Excludes *myositis:*
epidemic (074.1)
interstitial (728.81)
myoneural disorder (358.00–358.9)
syphilitic (095.6)
tropical (040.81)
(Ex) 567.31, 728.0, 728.11-728.3, 728.81, 728.86

● 728.1 **Muscular calcification and ossification**

728.10 **Calcification and ossification, unspecified**
Massive calcification (paraplegic)

728.11 **Progressive myositis ossificans**

728.12 **Traumatic myositis ossifications**
Myositis ossificans (circumscripta)

728.13 **Postoperative heterotopic calcification**

728.19 **Other**
Polymyositis ossificans

N Newborn: 0   P Pediatric: 0–17   M Maternity: 12–55   A Adult: 15–124   ♀ Females Only   ♂ Males Only

(Ex) CC/MCC Exclusions   🔵 Complication\Comorbidity   🔵 Major C\C   🔵 Present on Admission Requirement   🔵 Hospital-Acquired Condition   **907**

728.2 Muscular wasting and disuse atrophy, not elsewhere classified

Amyotrophia NOS   Myofibrosis

> **Excludes** *neuralgic amyotrophy (353.5)*
> *pelvic muscle wasting and disuse atrophy (618.83)*
> *progressive muscular atrophy (335.0–335.9)*

728.3 Other specific muscle disorders

Arthrogryposis

Immobility syndrome (paraplegic)

> **Excludes** *arthrogryposis multiplex congenita (754.89)*
> *stiff-man syndrome (333.91)*

728.4 Laxity of ligament

728.5 Hypermobility syndrome

728.6 Contracture of palmar fascia

Dupuytren's contracture   A

● **728.7 Other fibromatoses**

728.71 Plantar fascial fibromatosis

Contracture of plantar fascia

Plantar fasciitis (traumatic)

728.79 Other

Garrod's or knuckle pads

Nodular fasciitis

Pseudosarcomatous Fibromatosis (proliferative) (subcutaneous)

● **728.8 Other disorders of muscle, ligament, and fascia**

728.81 Interstitial myositis

728.82 Foreign body granuloma of muscle

Talc granuloma of muscle

> Use additional code to identify foreign body (V90.01-V90.9)

728.83 Rupture of muscle, nontraumatic

728.84 Diastasis of muscle

Diastasis recti (abdomen)

> **Excludes** *diastasis recti complicating pregnancy, labor, and delivery (665.8)*

728.85 Spasm of muscle

728.86 Necrotizing fasciitis 🔒

> Use additional code to identify:
> infectious organism (041.00–041.89)
> gangrene (785.4), if applicable
> (Ex) 567.31, 728.0, 728.11-728.3, 728.81, 728.86

728.87 Muscle weakness (generalized)

> **Excludes** *generalized weakness (780.79)*
> **Coding Clinic: 2005, Q1, P13**

728.88 Rhabdomyolysis 🔒

> (Ex) 567.31, 728.0, 728.11-728.3, 728.81, 728.86, 728.88
> **Coding Clinic: 2003, Q4, P66-67; 2001, Q2, P14**

728.89 Other

Eosinophilic fasciitis

> Use additional E code to identify drug, if drug induced
> **Coding Clinic: 2006, Q3, P13; 2002, Q3, P28; 2001, Q2, P15**

728.9 Unspecified disorder of muscle, ligament, and fascia

● **729 Other disorders of soft tissues**

> **Excludes** *acroparesthesia (443.89)*
> *carpal tunnel syndrome (354.0)*
> *disorders of the back (720.0–724.9)*
> *entrapment syndromes (354.0–355.9)*
> *palindromic rheumatism (719.3)*
> *periarthritis (726.0–726.9)*
> *psychogenic rheumatism (306.0)*
> **Coding Clinic: 1984, Nov-Dec, P17**

729.0 Rheumatism, unspecified and fibrositis

729.1 Myalgia and myositis, unspecified

Fibromyositis NOS

Coding Clinic: 1984, Nov-Dec, P17

729.2 Neuralgia, neuritis, and radiculitis, unspecified

> **Excludes** *brachia radiculitis (723.4)*
> *cervical radiculitis (723.4)*
> *lumbosacral radiculitis (724.4)*
> *mononeuritis (354.0–355.9)*
> *radiculitis due to intervertebral disc involvement (722.0–722.2, 722.7)*
> *sciatica (724.3)*

● **729.3 Panniculitis, unspecified**

Inflammation of adipose tissue of heel pad

729.30 Panniculitis, unspecified site

Weber-Christian disease

729.31 Hypertrophy of fat pad, knee

Hypertrophy of infrapatellar fat pad

729.39 Other site

> **Excludes** *panniculitis specified as (affecting):*
> *back (724.8)*
> *neck (723.6)*
> *sacral (724.8)*

729.4 Fasciitis, unspecified

> **Excludes** *necrotizing fasciitis (728.86)*
> *nodular fasciitis (728.79)*
> **Coding Clinic: 1994, Q2, P13**

729.5 Pain in limb

Coding Clinic: 2007, Q2, P13-15

729.6 Residual foreign body in soft tissue

> Use additional code to identify foreign body (V90.01-V90.9)
>
> **Excludes** *foreign body granuloma:*
> *muscle (728.82)*
> *skin and subcutaneous tissue (709.4)*

● **729.7 Nontraumatic compartment syndrome**

> **Excludes** *compartment syndrome NOS (958.90)*
> *traumatic compartment syndrome (958.90–958.99)*
>
> *Code first, if applicable, postprocedural complication (998.89)*

729.71 Nontraumatic compartment syndrome of upper extremity 🔒

Nontraumatic compartment syndrome of shoulder, arm, forearm, wrist, hand and fingers

> (Ex) 729.81, 729.89-729.99, 903.8, 904.9
> **Coding Clinic: 2006, Q4, P100-102**

729.72 Nontraumatic compartment syndrome of lower extremity 🔒

Nontraumatic compartment syndrome of hip, buttock, thigh, leg, foot and toes

> (Ex) 729.81, 729.89-729.99, 904.7, 904.9

729.73 Nontraumatic compartment syndrome of abdomen 🔒

> (Ex) 863.0-867.3, 867.5-868.14, 869.0-869.1, 879.2-879.9, 929.0-929.9, 958.8, 959.8-959.9

729.79 Nontraumatic compartment syndrome of other sites 🔒

> (Ex) 868.03-868.10, 868.13-869.1

● **729.8 Other musculoskeletal symptoms referable to limbs**

729.81 Swelling of limb

Coding Clinic: 1988, Q4, P6

729.82 Cramp

729.89 Other

> **Excludes** *abnormality of gait (781.2)*
> *tetany (781.7)*
> *transient paralysis of limb (781.4)*
> **Coding Clinic: 1988, Q4, P12**

● **729.9 Other and unspecified disorders of soft tissue**

Coding Clinic: 2008, Q4, P134-136

729.90 Disorders of soft tissue, unspecified

729.91 Post-traumatic seroma

> **Excludes** *seroma complicating a procedure (998.13)*

729.92 Nontraumatic hematoma of soft tissue

Nontraumatic hematoma of muscle

Coding Clinic: 2013, Q2, P8

729.99 Other disorders of soft tissue

Polyalgia

Figure 13-2 Osteomyelitis of the spine. A lateral view of the lower thoracic spine demonstrates destruction of the disk space *(arrow)* as well as destruction of the adjoining vertebral bodies. (From Mettler: Essentials of Radiology, ed 2, Saunders, An Imprint of Elsevier, 2005)

OSTEOPATHIES, CHONDROPATHIES, AND ACQUIRED MUSCULOSKELETAL DEFORMITIES (730–739)

● **730 Osteomyelitis, periostitis, and other infections involving bone**

> **Excludes** jaw (526.4–526.5)
>   petrous bone (383.2)

Use additional code to identify organism, such as:
Staphylococcus (041.1)
Coding Clinic: 1997, Q4, P43; 1993, 5th Issue, P3

The following fifth-digit subclassification is for use with category 730; valid digits are in [brackets] under each code. See list at beginning of chapter for definitions:

0	site unspecified	5	pelvic region and thigh
1	shoulder region	6	lower leg
2	upper arm	7	ankle and foot
3	forearm	8	other specified sites
4	hand	9	multiple sites

● **730.0 Acute osteomyelitis**🔍
[0-9]   Abscess of any bone except accessory sinus, jaw, or mastoid
Acute or subacute osteomyelitis, with or without mention of periostitis

> Use additional code to identify major osseous defect, if applicable (731.3)

For code **730.00:** (Ex) 015.50-015.56, 015.70-015.76, 015.90-015.96, 017.90-017.96, 730.80-730.99;
For code **730.01:** (Ex) 015.50-015.56, 015.70-015.76, 015.90-015.96, 017.90-017.96, 730.00, 730.08-730.11, 730.18-730.21, 730.28-730.31, 730.38-730.39, 730.80-730.81, 730.88-730.91, 730.98-730.99;
For code **730.02:** (Ex) 015.50-015.56, 015.70-015.76, 015.90-015.96, 017.90-017.96, 730.00, 730.08-730.10, 730.12, 730.18-730.20, 730.22, 730.28-730.30, 730.32, 730.38-730.39, 730.80, 730.82, 730.88-730.90, 730.92, 730.98-730.99;
For code **730.03:** (Ex) 015.50-015.56, 015.70-015.76, 015.90-015.96, 017.90-017.96, 730.00, 730.08-730.10, 730.13, 730.18-730.20, 730.23, 730.28-730.30, 730.33, 730.38-730.39, 730.80, 730.83, 730.88-730.90, 730.93, 730.98-730.99;
For code **730.04:** (Ex) 015.50-015.56, 015.70-015.76, 015.90-015.96, 017.90-017.96, 730.00, 730.08-730.10, 730.14, 730.18-730.20, 730.24, 730.28-730.30, 730.34, 730.38-730.39, 730.80, 730.84, 730.88-730.90, 730.94, 730.98-730.99;
For code **730.05:** (Ex) 015.10-015.16, 015.50-015.56, 015.70-015.76, 015.90-015.96, 017.90-017.96, 730.00, 730.08-730.10, 730.15, 730.18-730.20, 730.25, 730.28-730.30, 730.35, 730.38-730.39, 730.80, 730.85, 730.88-730.90, 730.95, 730.98-730.99;
For code **730.06:** (Ex) 015.20-015.26, 015.50-015.56, 015.70-015.76, 015.90-015.96, 017.90-017.96, 730.00, 730.08-730.10, 730.16, 730.18-730.20, 730.26, 730.28-730.30, 730.36, 730.38-730.39, 730.80, 730.86, 730.88-730.90, 730.96, 730.98-730.99;
For code **730.07:** (Ex) 015.50-015.56, 015.70-015.76, 015.90-015.96, 017.90-017.96, 730.00, 730.08-730.10, 730.17-730.20, 730.27-730.30, 730.37-730.39, 730.80, 730.87-730.90, 730.97-730.99;
For code **730.08:** (Ex) 015.00-015.06, 015.50-015.56, 015.70-015.76, 015.90-015.96, 017.90-017.96, 730.00-730.39, 730.80-730.99;
For code **730.09:** (Ex) 015.50-015.56, 015.70-015.76, 015.90-015.96, 017.90-017.96, 730.00-730.39, 730.80-730.99
Coding Clinic: 2004, Q1, P14-15; 2002, Q1, P3-4

Item 13-5 Osteomyelitis is an inflammation of the bone. **Acute osteomyelitis** is a rapidly destructive, pus-producing infection capable of causing severe bone destruction. **Chronic osteomyelitis** can remain long after the initial acute episode has passed and may lead to a recurrence of the acute phase. **Brodie's abscess** is an encapsulated focal abscess that must be surgically drained. Periostitis is an inflammation of the periosteum, a dense membrane composed of fibrous connective tissue that closely wraps all bone, except those with articulating surfaces in joints, which are covered by synovial membranes.

● **730.1 Chronic osteomyelitis**🔍
[0-9]   Brodie's abscess
Chronic or old osteomyelitis, with or without mention of periostitis
Sequestrum
Sclerosing osteomyelitis of Garré

> Use additional code to identify major osseous defect, if applicable (731.3)

> **Excludes** aseptic necrosis of bone (733.40–733.49)

For code **730.10:** (Ex) 730.10-730.39, 730.80-731.1;
For codes **730.11-730.19:** (Ex) 003.24, 015.50-015.56, 015.70-015.76, 015.90-015.96, 017.90-017.96, 730.00-730.39, 730.80-730.99
Coding Clinic: 2011, Q3, P15; 2000, Q3, P4

● **730.2 Unspecified osteomyelitis**🔍
[0-9]   Osteitis or osteomyelitis NOS, with or without mention of periostitis

> Use additional code to identify major osseous defect, if applicable (731.3)

For code **730.20:** (Ex) 730.10-730.39, 730.80-731.1;
For codes **730.21-730.29:** (Ex) 003.24, 015.50-015.56, 015.70-015.76, 015.90-015.96, 017.90-017.96, 730.00-730.39, 730.80-730.99

● **730.3 Periostitis without mention of osteomyelitis**
[0-9]   Abscess of periosteum, without mention of osteomyelitis
Periostosis, without mention of osteomyelitis

> **Excludes** that in secondary syphilis (091.61)

●》**730.7 Osteopathy resulting from poliomyelitis**
[0-9]   Code first underlying disease (045.0–045.9)

●》**730.8 Other infections involving bone in disease classified**
[0-9]   **elsewhere**🔍

> Code first underlying disease, as:
>   tuberculosis (015.0–015.9)
>   typhoid fever (002.0)

> **Excludes** syphilitis of bone NOS (095.5)

For codes **730.80, 730.89:** (Ex) 015.50-015.56, 015.70-015.76, 015.90-015.96, 017.90-017.96, 730.00-730.39, 730.80-730.99;
For code **730.81:** (Ex) 015.50-015.56, 015.70-015.76, 015.90-015.96, 017.90-017.96, 730.00-730.01, 730.08-730.11, 730.18-730.21, 730.28-730.31, 730.38-730.39, 730.80, 730.88-730.91 730.98-730.99;
For code **730.82:** (Ex) 015.50-015.56, 015.70-015.76, 015.90-015.96, 017.90-017.96, 730.00, 730.02, 730.08-730.10, 730.12, 730.18-730.20, 730.22, 730.28-730.30 730.32, 730.38-730.39, 730.80 730.88-730.90, 730.92, 730.98-730.99;
For code **730.83:** (Ex) 015.50-015.56, 015.70-015.76, 015.90-015.96, 017.90-017.96, 730.00, 730.03, 730.08-730.10, 730.13, 730.18-730.20, 730.23, 730.28-730.30, 730.33, 730.38-730.39, 730.80, 730.88-730.90, 730.93, 730.98-730.99;
For code **730.84:** (Ex) 015.50-015.56, 015.70-015.76, 015.90-015.96, 017.90-017.96, 730.00, 730.04, 730.08-730.10, 730.14, 730.18-730.20, 730.24, 730.28-730.30, 730.34, 730.38-730.39, 730.80, 730.88-730.90, 730.94, 730.98-730.99;
For code **730.85:** (Ex) 015.10-015.16, 015.50-015.56, 015.70-015.76, 015.90-015.96, 017.90-017.96, 730.00, 730.05, 730.08-730.10, 730.15, 730.18-730.20, 730.25, 730.28-730.30, 730.35, 730.38-730.39, 730.80, 730.88-730.90, 730.95, 730.98-730.99;
For code **730.86:** (Ex) 015.20-015.26, 015.70-015.76, 015.90-015.96, 017.90-017.96, 730.00, 730.06, 730.08-730.10, 730.16, 730.18-730.20, 730.26, 730.28-730.30, 730.36, 730.38-730.39, 730.80, 730.88-730.90, 730.96, 730.98-730.99;
For code **730.87:** (Ex) 015.50-015.56, 015.70-015.76, 015.90-015.96, 017.90-017.96, 730.00, 730.07-730.10, 730.17-730.20, 730.27-730.30, 730.37-730.39, 730.80, 730.88-730.90, 730.97-730.99;
For code **730.88:** (Ex) 015.00-015.06, 015.50-015.56, 015.70-015.76, 015.90-015.96, 017.90-017.96, 730.00-730.39, 730.80-730.99

● **730.9 Unspecified infection of bone** 🔍
  [0-9]   For codes **730.90, 730.99:** (Ex) 015.50-015.56, 015.70-015.76, 015.90-015.96,
              017.90-017.96, 730.00-730.39, 730.80-730.99;
           For code **730.91:** (Ex) 015.50-015.56, 015.70-015.76, 015.90-015.96,
              017.90-017.96, 730.00-730.01, 730.08-730.11, 730.18-730.21,
              730.28-730.31, 730.38-730.39, 730.80-730.81, 730.88-730.90,
              730.98-730.99;
           For code **730.92:** (Ex) 015.50-015.56, 015.70-015.76, 015.90-015.96,
              017.90-017.96, 730.00, 730.02, 730.08-730.10, 730.12, 730.18-730.20,
              730.22, 730.28-730.30, 730.32, 730.38-730.39, 730.80, 730.82,
              730.88-730.90, 730.98-730.99;
           For code **730.93:** (Ex) 015.50-015.56, 015.70-015.76, 015.90-015.96,
              017.90-017.96, 730.00, 730.03, 730.08-730.10, 730.13, 730.18-730.20,
              730.23, 730.28-730.30, 730.33, 730.38-730.39, 730.80, 730.83,
              730.88-730.90, 730.98-730.99;
           For code **730.94:** (Ex) 015.50-015.56, 015.70-015.76, 015.90-015.96,
              017.90-017.96, 730.00, 730.04, 730.08-730.10, 730.14, 730.18-730.20,
              730.24, 730.28-730.30, 730.34, 730.38-730.39, 730.80, 730.84,
              730.88-730.90, 730.98-730.99;
           For code **730.95:** (Ex) 015.10-015.16, 015.50-015.56, 015.70-015.76,
              015.90-015.96, 017.90-017.96, 730.00, 730.05, 730.08-730.10, 730.15,
              730.18-730.20, 730.25, 730.28-730.30, 730.35, 730.38-730.39, 730.80,
              730.85, 730.88-730.90, 730.98-730.99;
           For code **730.96:** (Ex) 015.20-015.56, 015.70-015.76, 015.90-015.96,
              017.90-017.96, 730.00, 730.06, 730.08-730.10, 730.16, 730.18-730.20,
              730.26, 730.28-730.30, 730.36, 730.38-730.39, 730.80, 730.86,
              730.88-730.90, 730.98-730.99;
           For code **730.97:** (Ex) 015.50-015.56, 015.70-015.76, 015.90-015.96,
              017.90-017.96, 730.00, 730.07-730.10, 730.17-730.20, 730.27-730.30,
              730.37-730.39, 730.80, 730.87-730.90, 730.98-730.99;
           For code **730.98:** (Ex) 015.00-015.06, 015.50-015.56, 015.70-015.76,
              015.90-015.96, 017.90-017.96, 730.00-730.39, 730.80-730.99

● **731 Osteitis deformans and osteopathies associated with other
      disorders classified elsewhere**
    *Also known as Paget's Disease; chronic disorder that results in
    enlarged and deformed bones. The excessive breakdown and
    formation of bone tissue causes bones to weaken and results in
    bone pain, arthritis, deformities, and fractures.*

  731.0 Osteitis deformans without mention of bone tumor
          Paget's disease of bone
          Coding Clinic: 1994, Q2, P6-7

  ▷ **731.1 *Osteitis deformans in diseases classified elsewhere***
          Code first *underlying disease, as:*
            malignant neoplasm of bone (170.0–170.9)

  731.2 Hypertrophic pulmonary osteoarthropathy
          Bamberger-Marie disease

  731.3 Major osseous defects
          Code first *underlying disease, if known, such as:*
            aseptic necrosis (733.40–733.49)
            malignant neoplasm of bone (170.0–170.9)
            osteomyelitis (730.00–730.29)
            osteoporosis (733.00–733.09)
            peri-prosthetic osteolysis (996.45)
          Coding Clinic: 2006, Q4, P103-104

  ▷ **731.8 *Other bone involvement in diseases classified elsewhere***
          Code first *underlying disease, as:*
            diabetes mellitus (249.8, 250.8)
          Use additional *code to specify bone condition, such as:*
            acute osteomyelitis (730.00–730.09)
          Coding Clinic: 2010, Q2, P6; 2004, Q1, P14-15; 1997, Q4, P43

● **732 Osteochondropathies**

  732.0 Juvenile osteochondrosis of spine
          Juvenile osteochondrosis (of):
            marginal or vertebral ephiphysis (of Scheuermann)
            spine NOS
          Vertebral epiphysitis
          Excludes *adolescent postural kyphosis (737.0)*

  732.1 Juvenile osteochondrosis of hip and pelvis
          Coxa plana
          Ischiopubic synchondrosis (of van Neck)
          Osteochondrosis (juvenile) of:
            acetabulum
            head of femur (of Legg-Calvé-Perthes)
            iliac crest (of Buchanan)
            symphysis pubis (of Pierson)
          Pseudocoxalgia

  732.2 Nontraumatic slipped upper femoral epiphysis
          Slipped upper femoral epiphysis NOS

  732.3 Juvenile osteochondrosis of upper extremity
          Osteochondrosis (juvenile) of:
            capitulum of humerus (of Panner)
            carpal lunate (of Kienbock)
            hand NOS
            head of humerus (of Haas)
            heads of metacarpals (of Mauclaire)
            lower ulna (of Burns)
            radial head (of Brailsford)
            upper extremity NOS

  **732.4 Juvenile osteochondrosis of lower extremity, excluding
        foot**
          Osteochondrosis (juvenile) of:
            lower extremity NOS
            primary patellar center (of Köhler)
            proximal tibia (of Blount)
            secondary patellar center (of Sinding-Larsen)
            tibial tubercle (of Osgood-Schlatter)
          Tibia vara

  732.5 Juvenile osteochondrosis of foot
          Calcaneal apophysitis
          Epiphysitis, os calcis
          Osteochondrosis (juvenile) of:
            astragalus (of Diaz)
            calcaneum (of Sever)
            foot NOS
            metatarsal:
              second (of Freiberg)
              fifth (of Iselin)
            os tibiale externum (of Haglund)
            tarsal navicular (of Köhler)

  732.6 Other juvenile osteochondrosis
          Apophysitis specified as juvenile, of other site, or site
            NOS
          Epiphysitis specified as juvenile, of other site, or site
            NOS
          Osteochondritis specified as juvenile, of other site, or site
            NOS
          Osteochondrosis specified as juvenile, of other site, or
            site NOS

  732.7 Osteochondritis dissecans

  732.8 Other specified forms of osteochondropathy
          Adult osteochondrosis of spine

  732.9 Unspecified osteochondropathy
          Apophysitis
            NOS
            not specified as adult or juvenile, of unspecified site
          Epiphysitis
            NOS
            not specified as adult or juvenile, of unspecified site
          Osteochondritis
            NOS
            not specified as adult or juvenile, of unspecified site
          Osteochondrosis
            NOS
            not specified as adult or juvenile, of unspecified site

● 733 **Other disorders of bone and cartilage**

Excludes *bone spur (726.91)*
cartilage of, or loose body in, joint (717.0–717.9, 718.0–718.9)
giant cell granuloma of jaw (526.3)
osteitis fibrosa cystica generalisata (252.01)
osteomalacia (268.2)
polyostotic fibrous dysplasia of bone (756.54)
prognathism, retrognathism (524.1)
xanthomatosis localized to bone (272.7)

● 733.0 **Osteoporosis**
Condition of excessive skeletal fragility (porous bone) resulting in bone fractures
Use additional code to identify:
major osseous defect, if applicable (731.3)
personal history of pathologic (healed) fracture (V13.51)
Coding Clinic: 1993, Q4, P25-26

733.00 **Osteoporosis, unspecified**
Wedging of vertebra NOS
Coding Clinic: 2007, Q4, P91-92; Q1, P22; 2001, Q3, P19; 1998, Q2, P12

733.01 **Senile osteoporosis**
Postmenopausal osteoporosis
Coding Clinic: 2007, Q1, P3-8

733.02 **Idiopathic osteoporosis**

733.03 **Disuse osteoporosis**

733.09 **Other**
Drug-induced osteoporosis
Use additional E code to identify drug
Coding Clinic: 2003, Q4, P108-109

● 733.1 **Pathologic fracture**
Chronic fracture
Spontaneous fracture
Excludes *stress fracture (733.93–733.95)*
traumatic fractures (800–829)
Coding Clinic: 1986, Nov-Dec, P10; 1985, Nov-Dec, P16

733.10 **Pathologic fracture, unspecified site**
Ⓔ 733.10-733.19, 733.93-733.98

733.11 **Pathologic fracture of humerus**
Ⓔ 733.10-733.19, 733.93-733.98
Coding Clinic: 2010, Q2, P6

733.12 **Pathologic fracture of distal radius and ulna**
Wrist NOS
Ⓔ 733.10-733.19, 733.93-733.98

733.13 **Pathologic fracture of vertebrae**
Collapse of vertebra NOS
Ⓔ 733.10-733.19, 733.93-733.98
Coding Clinic: 2008, Q3, P4; 2007, Q1, P3-8,22; 1999, Q3, P5

733.14 **Pathologic fracture of neck of femur**
Femur NOS
Hip NOS
Ⓔ 733.10-733.19, 733.93-733.98
Coding Clinic: 2001, Q1, P10-11; 1996, Q1, P16; 1993, Q4, P25-26

733.15 **Pathologic fracture of other specified part of femur**
Ⓔ 733.10-733.19, 733.93-733.98
Coding Clinic: 2010, Q2, P6; 1998, Q2, P12; 1994, Q2, P6-7

733.16 **Pathologic fracture of tibia and fibula**
Ankle NOS
Ⓔ 733.10-733.19, 733.93-733.98

733.19 **Pathologic fracture of other specified site**
Ⓔ 733.10-733.19, 733.93-733.98

● 733.2 **Cyst of bone**
733.20 **Cyst of bone (localized), unspecified**

733.21 **Solitary bone cyst**
Unicameral bone cyst

733.22 **Aneurysmal bone cyst**

733.29 **Other**
Fibrous dysplasia (monostotic)
Excludes *cyst of jaw (526.0–526.2, 526.89)*
osteitis fibrosa cystica (252.01)
polyostotic fibrous dysplasia of bone (756.54)

733.3 **Hyperostosis of skull**
Hyperostosis interna frontalis
Leontiasis ossium

● 733.4 **Aseptic necrosis of bone**
Use additional code to identify major osseous defect, if applicable (731.3)
Excludes *osteochondropathies (732.0–732.9)*
Coding Clinic: 2007, Q4, P116-120

733.40 **Aseptic necrosis of bone, site unspecified**
Ⓔ 733.40-733.49

733.41 **Head of humerus**
Ⓔ 733.40-733.41, 733.45-733.49

733.42 **Head and neck of femur**
Femur NOS
Excludes *Legg-Calvé-Perthes disease (732.1)*
Ⓔ 733.40, 733.42, 733.45-733.49

733.43 **Medial femoral condyle**
Ⓔ 733.40, 733.43, 733.45-733.49

733.44 **Talus**
Ⓔ 733.40, 733.44-733.49

733.45 **Jaw**
Use additional E code to identify drug, if drug-induced
Excludes *osteoradionecrosis of jaw (526.89)*
Ⓔ 733.40-733.49
Coding Clinic: 2007, Q4, P91-92

733.49 **Other**
Ⓔ 733.40-733.49

733.5 **Osteitis condensans**
Piriform sclerosis of ilium

733.6 **Tietze's disease**
Costochondral junction syndrome
Costochondritis

733.7 **Algoneurodystrophy**
Disuse atrophy of bone
Sudeck's atrophy

● 733.8 **Malunion and nonunion of fracture**
733.81 **Malunion of fracture**
Fracture ends do not heal together correctly.
Ⓔ 733.81-733.82

733.82 **Nonunion of fracture**
Total failure of fracture healing
Pseudoarthrosis (bone)
Ⓔ 733.81-733.82
Coding Clinic: 1994, Q2, P7; 1987, Jan-Feb, P13; 1984, Nov-Dec, P18

● 733.9 **Other and unspecified disorders of bone and cartilage**
Coding Clinic: 2008, Q4, P136-137

733.90 **Disorder of bone and cartilage, unspecified**

733.91 **Arrest of bone development or growth**
Epiphyseal arrest

733.92 **Chondromalacia**
Chondromalacia:
NOS
localized, except patella
systemic
tibial plateau
Excludes *chondromalacia of patella (717.7)*

DISEASES OF THE MUSCULOSKELETAL SYSTEM AND CONNECTIVE TISSUE (710–739)

733.93 Stress fracture of tibia or fibula
Stress reaction of tibia or fibula
Use additional external cause code(s) to identify the cause of the stress fracture

733.94 Stress fracture of the metatarsals
Stress reaction of metatarsals
Use additional external cause code(s) to identify the cause of the stress fracture
Coding Clinic: 2001, Q4, P48-49

733.95 Stress fracture of other bone
Stress reaction of other bone
Use additional external cause code(s) to identify the cause of the stress fracture
Excludes *stress fracture of:*
femoral neck (733.96)
fibula (733.93)
metatarsals (733.94)
pelvis (733.98)
shaft of femur (733.97)
tibia (733.93)

733.96 Stress fracture of femoral neck
Stress reaction of femoral neck
Use additional external cause code(s) to identify the cause of the stress fracture

733.97 Stress fracture of shaft of femur
Stress reaction of shaft of femur
Use additional external cause code(s) to identify the cause of the stress fracture

733.98 Stress fracture of pelvis
Stress reaction of pelvis
Use additional external cause code(s) to identify the cause of the stress fracture

733.99 Other
Diaphysitis
Hypertrophy of bone
Relapsing polychondritis
Coding Clinic: 2011, Q1, P7; 2000, Q3, P4; 1987, Jan-Feb, P14

734 Flat foot
Pes planus (acquired)
Talipes planus (acquired)
Excludes *congenital (754.61)*
rigid flat foot (754.61)
spastic (everted) flat foot (754.61)

●**735 Acquired deformities of toe**
Excludes *congenital (754.60–754.69, 755.65–755.66)*
735.0 Hallux valgus (acquired)
735.1 Hallux varus (acquired)
735.2 Hallux rigidus
735.3 Hallux malleus
735.4 Other hammer toe (acquired)
735.5 Claw toe (acquired)
Coding Clinic: 2007, Q4, P123
735.8 Other acquired deformities of toe
735.9 Unspecified acquired deformity of toe

Figure 13–3   A. Claw toes, right foot, secondary to medial and lateral plantar nerve laceration. **B.** Metatarsophalangeal joints of second and third toes could not be flexed to neutral position and none could be flexed past neutral. **C.** Extension posture of claw toes increases plantar pressure on metatarsal heads. (From Canale: Campbell's Operative Orthopaedics, ed 11, Mosby, Inc., 2007)

Item 13–6 Claw toe is caused by a contraction of the flexor tendon producing a flexion deformity characterized by hyperextension of the big toe.

Figure 13–4   Hallux valgus or bunion.

Item 13–7 Hallux valgus, or bunion, is a bursa usually found along the medial aspect of the big toe. It is most often attributed to heredity or poorly fitted shoes.

Item 13-8 Hallux valgus or bunion is a sometimes painful structural deformity caused by an inflammation of the bursal sac at the base of the metatarsophalangeal joint (big toe). **Hallus varus** is a deviation of the great toe to the inner side of the foot or away from the next toe.

Item 13-9 Cubitus valgus is a deformity of the elbow resulting in an increased carrying angle in which the arm extends at the side and the palm faces forward, which results in the forearm and hand extended at greater than 15 degrees. **Cubitus varus** is a deformity of the elbow resulting in the arm extended at the side and the palm facing forward so that the forearm and hand are held at less than 5 degrees.

●**736 Other acquired deformities of limbs**
Excludes *congenital (754.3–755.9)*
●**736.0 Acquired deformities of forearm, excluding fingers**
736.00 Unspecified deformity
Deformity of elbow, forearm, hand, or wrist (acquired) NOS
736.01 Cubitus valgus (acquired)
736.02 Cubitus varus (acquired)
736.03 Valgus deformity of wrist (acquired)
736.04 Varus deformity of wrist (acquired)
736.05 Wrist drop (acquired)
736.06 Claw hand (acquired)
736.07 Club hand (acquired)
736.09 Other
736.1 Mallet finger
●**736.2 Other acquired deformities of finger**
736.20 Unspecified deformity
Deformity of finger (acquired) NOS
736.21 Boutonniere deformity
736.22 Swan-neck deformity
736.29 Other
Excludes *trigger finger (727.03)*
Coding Clinic: 2005, Q2, P7; 1989, Q2, P13
●**736.3 Acquired deformities of hip**
Coding Clinic: 2008, Q2, P3-4
736.30 Unspecified deformity
Deformity of hip (acquired) NOS
736.31 Coxa valga (acquired)
736.32 Coxa vara (acquired)
736.39 Other
●**736.4 Genu valgum or varum (acquired)**
736.41 Genu valgum (acquired)
736.42 Genu varum (acquired)
736.5 Genu recurvatum (acquired)

Figure 13–5 Supination and cavus deformity of forefoot. *(Courtesy Jay Cummings, MD.)* (From Canale: Campbell's Operative Orthopaedics, ed 11, Mosby, Inc., 2007)

Item 13–10 **Equinus foot** is a term referring to the hoof of a horse. The deformity is usually congenital or spastic. Talipes equinovarus is referred to as clubfoot. The foot tends to be smaller than normal, with the heel pointing downward and the forefoot turning inward. The heel cord (Achilles tendon) is tight, causing the heel to be drawn up toward the leg.

736.6 **Other acquired deformities of knee**
Deformity of knee (acquired) NOS

● 736.7 **Other acquired deformities of ankle and foot**
Excludes *deformities of toe (acquired) (735.0–735.9)*
pes planus (acquired) (734)

736.70 **Unspecified deformity of ankle and foot, acquired**
736.71 **Acquired equinovarus deformity**
Clubfoot, acquired
Excludes *clubfoot not specified as acquired (754.5–754.7)*

736.72 **Equinus deformity of foot, acquired**
736.73 **Cavus deformity of foot**
Excludes *that with claw foot (736.74)*
736.74 **Claw foot, acquired**
736.75 **Cavovarus deformity of foot, acquired**
736.76 **Other calcaneus deformity**
736.79 **Other**
Acquired:
pes not elsewhere classified
talipes not elsewhere classified

● 736.8 **Acquired deformities of other parts of limbs**
736.81 **Unequal leg length (acquired)**
Coding Clinic: 1995, Q1, P10
736.89 **Other**
Deformity (acquired):
arm or leg, not elsewhere classified
shoulder
Coding Clinic: 2008, Q2, P5-6

736.9 **Acquired deformity of limb, site unspecified**
Coding Clinic: 2008, Q2, P3-4

● 737 **Curvature of spine**
Excludes *congenital (754.2)*
737.0 **Adolescent postural kyphosis**
Excludes *osteochondrosis of spine (juvenile) (732.0)*
adult (732.8)

● 737.1 **Kyphosis (acquired)**
737.10 **Kyphosis (acquired) (postural)**
737.11 **Kyphosis due to radiation**
737.12 **Kyphosis, postlaminectomy**
737.19 **Other**
Excludes *that associated with conditions classifiable elsewhere (737.41)*
Coding Clinic: 2007, Q1, P20-21

● 737.2 **Lordosis (acquired)**
Abnormal increase in normal curvature of lumbar spine (sway back)
737.20 **Lordosis (acquired) (postural)**
737.21 **Lordosis, postlaminectomy**
737.22 **Other postsurgical lordosis**
737.29 **Other**
Excludes *that associated with conditions classifiable elsewhere (737.42)*

Item 13–11 **Kyphosis** is an abnormal curvature of the spine. **Senile kyphosis** is a result of disc degeneration causing ossification (turning to bone). **Adolescent** or **juvenile kyphosis** is also known as **Scheuermann's disease**, a condition in which the discs of the lower thoracic spine herniate, causing the disc space to narrow and the spine to tilt forward. This condition is attributed to poor posture. Lordosis or swayback is an abnormal curvature of the spine resulting in an inward curve of the lumbar spine just above the buttocks. Scoliosis causes a sideways curve to the spine. The curves are S- or C-shaped, and it is most commonly acquired in late childhood and early teen years, when growth is fast.

Item 13–12 **Spondylolisthesis** is a condition caused by the slipping forward of one disc over another.

Figure 13–6 Scoliosis is a lateral curvature of the spine.

● 737.3 **Kyphoscoliosis and scoliosis**
737.30 **Scoliosis [and kyphoscoliosis], idiopathic**
Coding Clinic: 2003, Q3, P19x2
737.31 **Resolving infantile idiopathic scoliosis**
737.32 **Progressive infantile idiopathic scoliosis**
Coding Clinic: 2002, Q3, P12
737.33 **Scoliosis due to radiation**
737.34 **Thoracogenic scoliosis**
737.39 **Other**
Excludes *that associated with conditions classifiable elsewhere (737.43)*
that in kyphoscoliotic heart disease (416.1)
Coding Clinic: 2002, Q2, P16

● 737.4 **Curvature of spine associated with other conditions**
Code first associated condition, as:
Charcot-Marie-Tooth disease (356.1)
mucopolysaccharidosis (277.5)
neurofibromatosis (237.70-237.79)
osteitis deformans (731.0)
osteitis fibrosa cystica (252.01)
osteoporosis (733.00–733.09)
poliomyelitis (138)
tuberculosis [Pott's curvature] (015.0)
▶ 737.40 *Curvature of spine, unspecified*
▶ 737.41 *Kyphosis*
▶ 737.42 *Lordosis*
▶ 737.43 *Scoliosis*
737.8 **Other curvatures of spine**
737.9 **Unspecified curvature of spine**
Curvature of spine (acquired) (idiopathic) NOS
Hunchback, acquired
Excludes *deformity of spine NOS (738.5)*

● 738 Other acquired deformity
  Excludes   congenital (754.0–756.9, 758.0–759.9)
              dentofacial anomalies (524.0–524.9)

  738.0 Acquired deformity of nose
          Deformity of nose (acquired)
          Overdevelopment of nasal bones
          Excludes   deflected or deviated nasal septum (470)

● 738.1 Other acquired deformity of head
    738.10 Unspecified deformity
    738.11 Zygomatic hyperplasia
    738.12 Zygomatic hypoplasia
    738.19 Other specified deformity
            Coding Clinic: 2006, Q1, P6-7; 2003, Q2, P13

  738.2 Acquired deformity of neck

  738.3 Acquired deformity of chest and rib
          Deformity:
            chest (acquired)
            rib (acquired)
          Pectus:
            carinatum, acquired
            excavatum, acquired

  738.4 Acquired spondylolisthesis
          Degenerative spondylolisthesis
          Spondylolysis, acquired
          Excludes   congenital (756.12)
          Coding Clinic: 2007, Q4, P116-120

  738.5 Other acquired deformity of back or spine
          Deformity of spine NOS
          Excludes   curvature of spine (737.0–737.9)
          Coding Clinic: 2007, Q4, P116-120

  738.6 Acquired deformity of pelvis
          Pelvic obliquity
          Excludes   intrapelvic protrusion of acetabulum (718.6)
                      that in relation to labor and delivery
                      (653.0–653.4, 653.8–653.9)

  738.7 Cauliflower ear

  738.8 Acquired deformity of other specified site
          Deformity of clavicle
          Coding Clinic: 2001, Q2, P14-15

  738.9 Acquired deformity of unspecified site

● 739 Nonallopathic lesions, not elsewhere classified
  Includes   segmental dysfunction
              somatic dysfunction
          Coding Clinic: 1995, Q4, P51; 1990, Q1, P18

  739.0 Head region
          Occipitocervical region

  739.1 Cervical region
          Cervicothoracic region

  739.2 Thoracic region
          Thoracolumbar region

  739.3 Lumbar region
          Lumbosacral region

  739.4 Sacral region
          Sacrococcygeal region
          Sacroiliac region

  739.5 Pelvic region
          Hip region
          Pubic region

  739.6 Lower extremities

  739.7 Upper extremities
          Acromioclavicular region
          Sternoclavicular region

  739.8 Rib cage
          Costochondral region
          Costovertebral region
          Sternochondral region

  739.9 Abdomen and other

Figure 14–1 Generalized craniosynostosis in a 4-year-old girl without symptoms or signs of increased intracranial pressure. (From Bell WE, McCormick WF: Increased Intracranial Pressure in Children, ed 2, Philadelphia, WB Saunders, 1978)

Item 14–1 **Anencephalus** is a congenital deformity of the cranial vault. **Craniosynostosis**, also known as craniostenosis and stenocephaly, signifies any form of congenital deformity of the skull that results from the premature closing of the sutures of the skull. **Iniencephaly** is a deformity in which the head and neck are flexed backward to a great extent and the head is very large in comparison to the shortened body.

14. CONGENITAL ANOMALIES (740–759)

● **740 Anencephalus and similar anomalies**

740.0 Anencephalus 🖐🖐
Acrania
Amyelencephalus
Hemianencephaly
Hemicephaly
(Ex) 740.0-740.2

740.1 Craniorachischisis 🖐🖐
(Ex) 740.0-740.2

740.2 Iniencephaly 🖐🖐
(Ex) 740.0-740.2

● **741 Spina bifida**

Excludes *spina bifida occulta (756.17)*
Coding Clinic: 1994, Q3, P7

The following fifth-digit subclassification is for use with category 741:

| 0 | unspecified region | 2 | dorsal (thoracic) region |
| 1 | cervical region | 3 | lumbar region |

● **741.0 With hydrocephalus** 🖐🖐
[0-3] Arnold-Chiari syndrome, type II
Any condition classifiable to 741.9 with any condition classifiable to 742.3
Chiari malformation, type II
(Ex) 741.00-741.93, 742.59-742.9, 759.7-759.89
Coding Clinic: 1997, Q4, P51; 1987, Sept-Oct, P10

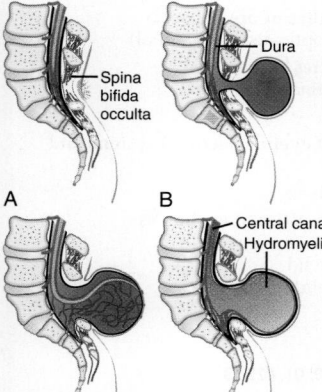

A B C D

Figure 14–2
A. Spina bifida occulta.
B. Meningocele.
C. Myelomeningocele.
D. Myelocystocele (syringomyelocele) or hydromyelia.

Item 14–2 **Spina bifida** is a midline spinal defect in which one or more vertebrae fail to fuse, leaving an opening in the vertebral canal. When the defect is not visible, it is called spina bifida occulta, and when it is visible, it is called spina bifida cystica.

● **741.9 Without mention of hydrocephalus** 🖐
[0-3] Hydromeningocele (spinal)
Hydromyelocele
Meningocele (spinal)
Meningomyelocele
Myelocele
Myelocystocele
Rachischisis
Spina bifida (aperta)
Syringomyelocele
Coding Clinic: 1987, Sept-Oct, P10

● **742 Other congenital anomalies of nervous system**

Excludes *congenital central alveolar hypoventilation syndrome (327.25)*

742.0 Encephalocele 🖐🖐
Sac-like protrusions of brain and membranes visible through an opening in various locations in skull
Encephalocystocele
Encephalomyelocele
Hydroencephalocele
Hydromeningocele, cranial
Meningocele, cerebral
Meningoencephalocele
(Ex) 742.0-742.2, 742.4

742.1 Microcephalus 🖐
Describes head size that measures significantly below normal based on standardized charts for age and sex
Hydromicrocephaly
Micrencephaly

742.2 Reduction deformities of brain 🖐🖐
Absence of part of brain
Agenesis of part of brain
Agyria
Aplasia of part of brain
Arhinencephaly
Holoprosencephaly
Hypoplasia of part of brain
Microgyria
(Ex) 742.0-742.2, 742.4
Coding Clinic: 2003, Q3, P15-16

742.3 Congenital hydrocephalus 🖐
An accumulation of cerebrospinal fluid in ventricles resulting in swelling and enlargement
Aqueduct of Sylvius:
anomaly
obstruction, congenital
stenosis
Atresia of foramina of Magendie and Luschka
Hydrocephalus in newborn
Excludes *hydrocephalus:*
acquired (331.3–331.4)
due to congenital toxoplasmosis (771.2)
with any condition classifiable to 741.9 (741.0)
Coding Clinic: 2005, Q4, P82-83

742.4 Other specified anomalies of brain 🖐🖐
Congenital cerebral cyst
Macroencephaly
Macrogyria
Megalencephaly
Multiple anomalies of brain NOS
Porencephaly
Ulegyria
(Ex) 742.4
Coding Clinic: 1999, Q1, P9-10; 1992, Q3, P12

Figure 14–3 An infant with a large occipital encephalocele. The large skin-covered encephalocele is visible. (From Townsend: Sabiston Textbook of Surgery, ed 19, Saunders, An Imprint of Elsevier, 2012)

CONGENITAL ANOMALIES (740–759)

CONGENITAL ANOMALIES (740–759)

●742.5 **Other specified anomalies of spinal cord**

    742.51 **Diastematomyelia** 🔍

    742.53 **Hydromyelia** 🔍
        Hydrorhachis

    742.59 **Other** 🔍
        Amyelia
        Atelomyelia
        Congenital anomaly of spinal meninges
        Defective development of cauda equina
        Hypoplasia of spinal cord
        Myelatelia
        Myelodysplasia
        Coding Clinic: 1991, Q2, P14; 1989, Q1, P10

  742.8 **Other specified anomalies of nervous system** 🔍
      Agenesis of nerve
      Displacement of brachial plexus
      Familial dysautonomia
      Jaw-winking syndrome
      Marcus-Gunn syndrome
      Riley-Day syndrome

      Excludes *neurofibromatosis (237.70-237.79)*

  742.9 **Unspecified anomaly of brain, spinal cord, and nervous system** 🔍
      Anomaly of brain, nervous system, and spinal cord
      Congenital, of brain, nervous system, and spinal cord:
        disease of brain, nervous system, and spinal cord
        lesion of brain, nervous system, and spinal cord
      Deformity of brain, nervous system, and spinal cord

●743 **Congenital anomalies of eye**

●743.0 **Anophthalmos**
    Absence of eye and optic pit

    743.00 **Clinical anophthalmos, unspecified** 🔍
        Agenesis
        Congenital absence of eye
        Anophthalmos NOS

    743.03 **Cystic eyeball, congenital** 🔍

    743.06 **Cryptophthalmos** 🔍

●743.1 **Microphthalmos**
    Partial absence of eye and optic pit
    Dysplasia of eye
    Hypoplasia of eye
    Rudimentary eye

    743.10 **Microphthalmos, unspecified** 🔍

    743.11 **Simple microphthalmos** 🔍

    743.12 **Microphthalmos associated with other anomalies of eye and adnexa** 🔍

●743.2 **Buphthalmos**
    Also known as Sturge-Weber Syndrome and is congenital syndrome characterized by a port-wine nevus covering portions of face and cranium
    Glaucoma:
      congenital
      newborn
    Hydrophthalmos

    Excludes *glaucoma of childhood (365.14)*
             traumatic glaucoma due to birth injury (767.8)

    743.20 **Buphthalmos, unspecified** 🔍

    743.21 **Simple buphthalmos** 🔍

    743.22 **Buphthalmos associated with other ocular anomalies** 🔍
        Keratoglobus, congenital, associated with buphthalmos
        Megalocornea associated with buphthalmos

Figure 14–4 Bilateral congenital **hydrophthalmia,** in which the eyes are very large in comparison to the other facial features due to glaucoma.

●743.3 **Congenital cataract and lens anomalies**

    Excludes *infantile cataract (366.00–366.09)*

    743.30 **Congenital cataract, unspecified** 🔍

    743.31 **Capsular and subcapsular cataract** 🔍

    743.32 **Cortical and zonular cataract** 🔍

    743.33 **Nuclear cataract** 🔍

    743.34 **Total and subtotal cataract, congenital** 🔍

    743.35 **Congenital aphakia** 🔍
        Congenital absence of lens

    743.36 **Anomalies of lens shape** 🔍
        Microphakia   Spherophakia

    743.37 **Congenital ectopic lens** 🔍

    743.39 **Other** 🔍

●743.4 **Coloboma and other anomalies of anterior segment**

    743.41 **Anomalies of corneal size and shape** 🔍
        Microcornea

      Excludes *that associated with buphthalmos (743.22)*

    743.42 **Corneal opacities, interfering with vision, congenital** 🔍

    743.43 **Other corneal opacities, congenital** 🔍

    743.44 **Specified anomalies of anterior chamber, chamber angle, and related structures** 🔍
        Anomaly:
          Axenfeld's
          Peters'
          Rieger's

    743.45 **Aniridia** 🔍
        Coding Clinic: 2010, Q2, P5; 2002, Q3, P20-21

    743.46 **Other specified anomalies of iris and ciliary body** 🔍
        Anisocoria, congenital
        Atresia of pupil
        Coloboma of iris
        Corectopia

    743.47 **Specified anomalies of sclera** 🔍

    743.48 **Multiple and combined anomalies of anterior segment** 🔍

    743.49 **Other** 🔍

●743.5 **Congenital anomalies of posterior segment**

    743.51 **Vitreous anomalies** 🔍
        Congenital vitreous opacity

    743.52 **Fundus coloboma** 🔍

    743.53 **Chorioretinal degeneration, congenital** 🔍

    743.54 **Congenital folds and cysts of posterior segment** 🔍

    743.55 **Congenital macular changes** 🔍

    743.56 **Other retinal changes, congenital** 🔍
        Coding Clinic: 1999, Q3, P12

    743.57 **Specified anomalies of optic disc** 🔍
        Coloboma of optic disc (congenital)

    743.58 **Vascular anomalies** 🔍
        Congenital retinal aneurysm

    743.59 **Other** 🔍

●743.6 **Congenital anomalies of eyelids, lacrimal system, and orbit**

    743.61 **Congenital ptosis** 🔍

    743.62 **Congenital deformities of eyelids** 🔍
        Ablepharon
        Absence of eyelid
        Accessory eyelid
        Congenital:
          ectropion
          entropion
        Coding Clinic: 2000, Q1, P22-23

    743.63 **Other specified congenital anomalies of eyelid** 🔍
        Absence, agenesis, of cilia

    743.64 **Specified congenital anomalies of lacrimal gland** 🔍

New ◀   Revised ◀   ~~deleted~~ Deleted   Excludes   Includes   Use additional   Code first   Omit code

916   ● Unacceptable Principal Diagnosis   ● Use Additional Digit(s)   ▶ Manifestation Code   OGCR Official Guidelines   Coding Clinic

743.65 **Specified congenital anomalies of lacrimal passages** 🔖
    Absence, agenesis of:
        lacrimal apparatus
        punctum lacrimale
        Accessory lacrimal canal

743.66 **Specified congenital anomalies of orbit** 🔖

743.69 **Other** 🔖
    Accessory eye muscles

743.8 **Other specified anomalies of eye** 🔖
> **Excludes** *congenital nystagmus (379.51)*
> *ocular albinism (270.2)*
> *optic nerve hypoplasia (377.43)*
> *retinitis pigmentosa (362.74)*

743.9 **Unspecified anomaly of eye** 🔖
    Congenital:
        anomaly NOS of eye [any part]
        deformity NOS of eye [any part]

● **744 Congenital anomalies of ear, face, and neck**
> **Excludes** *anomaly of:*
> *cervical spine (754.2, 756.10–756.19)*
> *larynx (748.2–748.3)*
> *nose (748.0–748.1)*
> *parathyroid gland (759.2)*
> *thyroid gland (759.2)*
> *cleft lip (749.10–749.25)*

● **744.0 Anomalies of ear causing impairment of hearing**
> **Excludes** *congenital deafness without mention of cause*
> *(380.0–389.9)*

744.00 **Unspecified anomaly of ear with impairment of hearing** 🔖

744.01 **Absence of external ear** 🔖
    Absence of:
        auditory canal (external)
        auricle (ear) (with stenosis or atresia of
          auditory canal)

744.02 **Other anomalies of external ear with impairment of hearing** 🔖
    Atresia or stricture of auditory canal (external)

744.03 **Anomaly of middle ear, except ossicles** 🔖
    Atresia or stricture of osseous meatus (ear)

744.04 **Anomalies of ear ossicles** 🔖
    Fusion of ear ossicles

744.05 **Anomalies of inner ear** 🔖
    Congenital anomaly of:
        membranous labyrinth
        organ of Corti

744.09 **Other** 🔖
    Absence of ear, congenital

744.1 **Accessory auricle** 🔖
    Accessory tragus   Supernumerary:
    Polyotia   ear
    Preauricular appendage   lobule

● **744.2 Other specified anomalies of ear**
> **Excludes** *that with impairment of hearing (744.00–744.09)*

744.21 **Absence of ear lobe, congenital** 🔖

744.22 **Macrotia** 🔖
    Enlarged ear

744.23 **Microtia** 🔖
    Abnormally small ear

744.24 **Specified anomalies of Eustachian tube** 🔖
    Absence of Eustachian tube

744.29 **Other** 🔖
    Bat ear
    Darwin's tubercle
    Pointed ear
    Prominence of auricle
    Ridge ear
> **Excludes** *preauricular sinus (744.46)*

744.3 **Unspecified anomaly of ear** 🔖
    Congenital:
        anomaly NOS of ear, NEC
        deformity NOS of ear, NEC

● **744.4 Branchial cleft cyst or fistula; preauricular sinus**

744.41 **Branchial cleft sinus or fistula** 🔖
    Branchial:
        sinus (external) (internal)
        vestige

744.42 **Branchial cleft cyst** 🔖

744.43 **Cervical auricle** 🔖

744.46 **Preauricular sinus or fistula** 🔖

744.47 **Preauricular cyst** 🔖

744.49 **Other** 🔖
    Fistula (of):
        auricle, congenital
        cervicoaural

744.5 **Webbing of neck** 🔖
    Pterygium colli

● **744.8 Other specified anomalies of face and neck**

744.81 **Macrocheilia** 🔖
    Hypertrophy of lip, congenital

744.82 **Microcheilia** 🔖

744.83 **Macrostomia** 🔖
    Abnormally large mouth

744.84 **Microstomia** 🔖

744.89 **Other** 🔖
> **Excludes** *congenital fistula of lip (750.25)*
> *musculoskeletal anomalies*
> *(754.0–754.1, 756.0)*

744.9 **Unspecified anomalies of face and neck** 🔖
    Congenital:
        anomaly NOS of face [any part] or neck [any part]
        deformity NOS of face [any part] or neck [any part]

● **745 Bulbus cordis anomalies and anomalies of cardiac septal closure**

● **745.0 Common truncus** 🔖 🔖
    Absent septum between aorta and pulmonary artery
    Communication (abnormal) between aorta and
        pulmonary artery
    Aortic septal defect
    Common aortopulmonary trunk
    Persistent truncus arteriosus
    (Ex) 429.71-429.79, 745.0-745.9, 746.89-746.9, 747.83-747.9, 759.7-759.89

● **745.1 Transposition of great vessels**

745.10 **Complete transposition of great vessels** 🔖 🔖
    Transposition of great vessels:
        NOS
        classical
    (Ex) 429.71-429.79, 745.0-745.9, 746.89-746.9, 747.83-747.9,
    759.7-759.89

745.11 **Double outlet right ventricle** 🔖 🔖
    Dextrotransposition of aorta
    Incomplete transposition of great vessels
    Origin of both great vessels from right ventricle
    Taussig-Bing syndrome or defect
    (Ex) 429.71-429.79, 745.0-745.9, 746.89-746.9, 747.83-747.9,
    759.7-759.89

745.12 **Corrected transposition of great vessels** 🔖 🔖
    (Ex) 429.71-429.79, 745.0-745.9, 746.89-746.9, 747.83-747.9,
    759.7-759.89

745.19 **Other** 🔖 🔖
    (Ex) 429.71-429.79, 745.0-745.9, 746.89-746.9, 747.83-747.9,
    759.7-759.89

745.2 **Tetralogy of Fallot** 🔖 🔖
    Fallot's pentalogy
    Ventricular septal defect with pulmonary stenosis or
        atresia, dextroposition of aorta, and hypertrophy of
        right ventricle
> **Excludes** *Fallot's triad (746.09)*
    (Ex) 429.71-429.79, 745.0-745.9, 746.89-746.9, 747.83-747.9, 759.7-759.89

CONGENITAL ANOMALIES (740–759)

745.3　Common ventricle 🔖🔖
Cor triloculare biatriatum
Single ventricle
(Ex:) 429.71-429.79, 745.0-745.9, 746.89-746.9, 747.83-747.9, 759.7-759.89

745.4　Ventricular septal defect 🔖🔖
Eisenmenger's defect or complex
Gerbode defect
Interventricular septal defect
Left ventricular-right atrial communication
Roger's disease

> **Excludes**　*common atrioventricular canal type (745.69)*
> *single ventricle (745.3)*

(Ex:) 429.71-429.79, 745.0-745.9, 746.89-746.9, 747.83-747.9, 759.7-759.89

745.5　Ostium secundum type atrial septal defect 🔖🔖
Defect:　　　　　　　　Patent or persistent:
　atrium secundum　　　　foramen ovale
　fossa ovalis　　　　　　ostium secundum
Lutembacher's syndrome
(Ex:) 429.71-429.79, 745.0-745.3, 745.5-745.9, 746.89-746.9, 747.89-747.9, 759.7, 759.89

Coding Clinic: 2012, Q2, P3-4; 2009, Q3, P10

● **745.6　Endocardial cushion defects**

745.60　Endocardial cushion defect, unspecified type 🔖🔖
(Ex:) 429.71-429.79, 745.0-745.9, 746.89-746.9, 747.83-747.9, 759.7-759.89

745.61　Ostium primum defect 🔖🔖
Persistent ostium primum
(Ex:) 429.71-429.79, 745.0-745.3, 745.5-745.9, 746.89-746.9, 747.89-747.9, 759.7, 759.89

745.69　Other 🔖🔖
Absence of atrial septum
Atrioventricular canal type ventricular septal defect
Common atrioventricular canal
Common atrium
(Ex:) 429.71-429.79, 745.0-745.9, 746.89-746.9, 747.83-747.9, 759.7-759.89

745.7　Cor biloculare 🔖🔖
Absence of atrial and ventricular septa
(Ex:) 429.71-429.79, 745.0-745.9, 746.89-746.9, 747.83-747.9, 759.7-759.89

745.8　Other 🔖

745.9　Unspecified defect of septal closure 🔖
Septal defect NOS

● **746　Other congenital anomalies of heart**

> **Excludes**　*endocardial fibroelastosis (425.3)*

Coding Clinic: 2004, Q3, P4-5

● **746.0　Anomalies of pulmonary valve**

> **Excludes**　*infundibular or subvalvular pulmonic stenosis (746.83)*
> *tetralogy of Fallot (745.2)*

746.00　Pulmonary valve anomaly, unspecified 🔖🔖
(Ex:) 746.00-746.09, 746.89-746.9, 747.89-747.9, 759.7, 759.89

746.01　Atresia, congenital 🔖🔖
Congenital absence of pulmonary valve
(Ex:) 746.00-746.09, 746.89-746.9, 747.83-747.9, 759.7-759.89

746.02　Stenosis, congenital 🔖🔖
(Ex:) 746.00-746.09, 746.89-746.9, 747.83-747.9, 759.7-759.89

Coding Clinic: 2004, Q1, P16-17

746.09　Other 🔖🔖
Congenital insufficiency of pulmonary valve
Fallot's triad or trilogy
(Ex:) 746.00-746.09, 746.89-746.9, 747.89-747.9, 759.7, 759.89

746.1　Tricuspid atresia and stenosis, congenital 🔖🔖
Absence of tricuspid valve
(Ex:) 746.1-746.7, 746.89-746.9, 747.83-747.9, 759.7-759.89

746.2　Ebstein's anomaly 🔖🔖
(Ex:) 746.1-746.7, 746.89-746.9, 747.83-747.9, 759.7-759.89

746.3　Congenital stenosis of aortic valve 🔖🔖
Congenital aortic stenosis

> **Excludes**　*congenital:*
> *subaortic stenosis (746.81)*
> *supravalvular aortic stenosis (747.22)*

(Ex:) 746.1-746.7, 746.89-746.9, 747.83-747.9, 759.7-759.89

Coding Clinic: 1988, Q4, P8

746.4　Congenital insufficiency of aortic valve 🔖🔖
Bicuspid aortic valve
Congenital aortic insufficiency
(Ex:) 746.1-746.7, 746.89-746.9, 747.83-747.9, 759.7-759.89

746.5　Congenital mitral stenosis 🔖🔖
Fused commissure of mitral valve
Parachute deformity of mitral valve
Supernumerary cusps of mitral valve
(Ex:) 746.1-746.7, 746.89-746.9, 747.83-747.9, 759.7-759.89

Coding Clinic: 2007, Q3, P3

746.6　Congenital mitral insufficiency 🔖🔖
(Ex:) 746.1-746.7, 746.89-746.9, 747.83-747.9, 759.7-759.89

746.7　Hypoplastic left heart syndrome 🔖🔖
Atresia, or marked hypoplasia, of aortic orifice or valve,
with hypoplasia of ascending aorta and defective
development of left ventricle (with mitral valve
atresia)
(Ex:) 746.1-746.7, 746.89-746.9, 747.83-747.9, 759.7-759.89

● **746.8　Other specified anomalies of heart**

746.81　Subaortic stenosis 🔖🔖
(Ex:) 746.81-746.84, 746.89-746.9, 747.83-747.9, 759.7-759.89

Coding Clinic: 2007, Q3, P3

746.82　Cor triatriatum 🔖🔖
(Ex:) 746.81-746.84, 746.89-746.9, 747.83-747.9, 759.7-759.89

746.83　Infundibular pulmonic stenosis 🔖🔖
Subvalvular pulmonic stenosis
(Ex:) 746.81-746.84, 746.89-746.9, 747.83-747.9, 759.7-759.89

746.84　Obstructive anomalies of heart, NEC 🔖🔖
Shone's syndrome
Uhl's disease

> Use additional code for associated anomalies, such as:
> coarctation of aorta (747.10)
> congenital mitral stenosis (746.5)
> subaortic stenosis (746.81)

(Ex:) 746.81-746.84, 746.89-746.9, 747.83-747.9, 759.7-759.89

Coding Clinic: 2012, Q2, P3-4

746.85　Coronary artery anomaly 🔖🔖
Anomalous origin or communication of coronary
artery
Arteriovenous malformation of coronary artery
Coronary artery:
absence
arising from aorta or pulmonary trunk
single
(Ex:) 746.85, 746.89-746.9

746.86　Congenital heart block 🔖🔖
Complete or incomplete atrioventricular [AV]
block
(Ex:) 746.86, 746.89-746.9, 747.83-747.9, 759.7-759.89

746.87　Malposition of heart and cardiac apex 🔖🔖
Abdominal heart　　　Levocardia (isolated)
Dextrocardia　　　　Mesocardia
Ectopia cordis

> **Excludes**　*dextrocardia with complete transposition of viscera (759.3)*

(Ex:) 746.81-746.84, 746.87-746.9, 747.89-747.9, 759.7, 759.89

746.89　Other 🔖
Atresia of cardiac vein
Hypoplasia of cardiac vein
Congenital:
cardiomegaly
diverticulum, left ventricle
pericardial defect

Coding Clinic: 2000, Q3, P3; 1999, Q1, P11; 1995, Q1, P8

746.9　Unspecified anomaly of heart 🔖
Congenital:
anomaly of heart NOS
heart disease NOS

● **747 Other congenital anomalies of circulatory system**

    747.0 Patent ductus arteriosus *(PDA)* 🅒🅟
        Patent ductus Botalli
        Persistent ductus arteriosus
        (Ex) 747.0, 747.89
        Coding Clinic: 2009, Q3, P10-11x2

    ● **747.1 Coarctation of aorta**

        747.10 Coarctation of aorta (preductal) (postductal) 🅒🅟
            Hypoplasia of aortic arch
            (Ex) 747.10-747.22, 747.89-747.9, 759.7, 759.89
            Coding Clinic: 2007, Q3, P3; 1999, Q1, P11; 1988, Q4, P8

        747.11 Interruption of aortic arch 🅒🅟
            (Ex) 747.10-747.22, 747.83-747.9, 759.7-759.89

    ● **747.2 Other anomalies of aorta**

        747.20 Anomaly of aorta, unspecified 🅒🅟
            (Ex) 747.10-747.22, 747.89-747.9, 759.7, 759.89

        747.21 Anomalies of aortic arch 🅒🅟
            Anomalous origin, right subclavian artery
            Dextroposition of aorta
            Double aortic arch
            Kommerell's diverticulum
            Overriding aorta
            Persistent:
                convolutions, aortic arch
                right aortic arch
            Vascular ring
               Excludes *hypoplasia of aortic arch (747.10)*
            (Ex) 747.10-747.22, 747.89-747.9, 759.7, 759.89
            Coding Clinic: 2003, Q1, P15-16

        747.22 Atresia and stenosis of aorta 🅒🅟
            Absence of aorta
            Aplasia of aorta
            Hypoplasia of aorta
            Stricture of aorta
            Supra (valvular)-aortic stenosis
             Excludes *congenital aortic (valvular) stenosis or*
                      stricture, so stated (746.3)
                     hypoplasia of aorta in hypoplastic left
                      heart syndrome (746.7)
            (Ex) 747.10-747.22, 747.83-747.9, 759.7-759.89
            Coding Clinic: 1988, Q4, P8

        747.29 Other 🅒🅟
            Aneurysm of sinus of Valsalva
            Congenital: Congenital:
              aneurysm of aorta   dilation of aorta
            (Ex) 747.10-747.29, 747.89-747.9, 759.7, 759.89

    ● **747.3 Anomalies of pulmonary artery**
        Coding Clinic: 2010, Q3, P9; 2009, Q3, P10x2; 2004, Q1, P16-17; 1994,
        Q1, P15

        747.31 Pulmonary artery coarctation and atresia 🅒🅟🅜
            Agenesis of pulmonary artery
            Atresia of pulmonary artery
            Coarctation of pulmonary artery
            Hypoplasia of pulmonary artery
            Stenosis of pulmonary artery
            (Ex) 747.31-747.39, 747.89, 747.9
            Coding Clinic: 2012, Q2, P3-4

        747.32 Pulmonary arteriovenous malformation 🅒🅟🅜
            Pulmonary arteriovenous aneurysm
             Excludes *acquired pulmonary arteriovenous*
                      fistula (417.0)
            (Ex) 747.31-747.39, 747.89, 747.9
            Coding Clinic: 2011, Q4, P138

        747.39 Other anomalies of pulmonary artery and
            pulmonary circulation 🅒🅟🅜
            Anomaly of pulmonary artery
            (Ex) 747.31-747.39, 747.89, 747.9

    ● **747.4 Anomalies of great veins**

        747.40 Anomaly of great veins, unspecified 🅒🅟
            Anomaly NOS of: Anomaly NOS of:
              pulmonary veins   vena cava
            (Ex) 747.40, 747.89-747.9

        747.41 Total anomalous pulmonary venous
            connection 🅒🅟
            Total anomalous pulmonary venous return
              [TAPVR]:
                subdiaphragmatic
                supradiaphragmatic
            (Ex) 747.41, 747.89-747.9

        747.42 Partial anomalous pulmonary venous
            connection 🅒🅟
            Partial anomalous pulmonary venous return
            (Ex) 747.42, 747.89-747.9

        747.49 Other anomalies of great veins 🅒🅟
            Absence of vena cava (inferior) (superior)
            Congenital stenosis of vena cava (inferior)
              (superior)
            Persistent:
              left posterior cardinal vein
              left superior vena cava
            Scimitar syndrome
            Transposition of pulmonary veins NOS
            (Ex) 747.49, 747.89-747.9

    747.5 Absence or hypoplasia of umbilical artery 🅟
        Single umbilical artery

    ● **747.6 Other anomalies of peripheral vascular system**
        Absence of artery or vein, NEC
        Anomaly of artery or vein, NEC
        Atresia of artery or vein, NEC
        Arteriovenous aneurysm (peripheral)
        Arteriovenous malformation of the peripheral vascular
            system
        Congenital: Congenital:
           aneurysm (peripheral)   stricture, artery
           phlebectasia   varix
        Multiple renal arteries
           Excludes *anomalies of:*
                 cerebral vessels (747.81)
                 pulmonary artery (747.39)
                 congenital retinal aneurysm (743.58)
                 hemangioma (228.00–228.09)
                 lymphangioma (228.1)

        747.60 Anomaly of the peripheral vascular system,
            unspecified site 🅟

        747.61 Gastrointestinal vessel anomaly 🅟
            Coding Clinic: 1996, Q3, P10

        747.62 Renal vessel anomaly 🅟

        747.63 Upper limb vessel anomaly 🅟

        747.64 Lower limb vessel anomaly 🅟

        747.69 Anomalies of other specified sites of peripheral
            vascular system 🅟
            Coding Clinic: 2010, Q3, P9

    ● **747.8 Other specified anomalies of circulatory system**

        747.81 Anomalies of cerebrovascular system 🅒🅟
            Arteriovenous malformation of brain
            Cerebral arteriovenous aneurysm, congenital
            Congenital anomalies of cerebral vessels
             Excludes *ruptured cerebral (arteriovenous)*
                      aneurysm (430)
            (Ex) 747.81, 747.89-747.9
            Coding Clinic: 1985, Jan-Feb, P15

        747.82 Spinal vessel anomaly 🅒🅟
            Arteriovenous malformation of spinal vessel
            (Ex) 747.82, 747.89-747.9
            Coding Clinic: 1995, Q3, P5-6

CONGENITAL ANOMALIES (740–759)

N Newborn: 0   P Pediatric: 0–17   M Maternity: 12–55   A Adult: 15–124   ♀ Females Only   ♂ Males Only

(Ex) CC/MCC Exclusions 🅒 Complication\Comorbidity 🅜 Major C\C 🅟 Present on Admission Requirement 🅗 Hospital-Acquired Condition   **919**

CONGENITAL ANOMALIES (740–759)

747.83 Persistent fetal circulation 🔸🔸   N
    Persistent pulmonary hypertension
    Primary pulmonary hypertension of newborn
    (Ex:) 416.0, 416.8-416.9
    Coding Clinic: 2002, Q4, P62-63

747.89 Other 🔸🔸
    Aneurysm, congenital, specified site not
       elsewhere classified
    Excludes *congenital aneurysm:*
        coronary (746.85)
        peripheral (747.6)
        pulmonary (747.39)
         arteriovenous (747.32)
        retinal (743.58)
    (Ex:) 745.0-745.9, 747.89

747.9 Unspecified anomaly of circulatory system 🔸🔸
    (Ex:) 745.0-747.82, 747.89-747.9

● **748 Congenital anomalies of respiratory system**
    Excludes *congenital central alveolar hypoventilation syndrome*
        (327.25)
       congenital defect of diaphragm (756.6)

748.0 Choanal atresia 🔸
    Atresia of nares (anterior) (posterior)
    Congenital stenosis of nares (anterior) (posterior)

748.1 Other anomalies of nose 🔸
    Absent nose
    Accessory nose
    Cleft nose
    Deformity of wall of nasal sinus
    Congenital:
       deformity of nose
       notching of tip of nose
       perforation of wall of nasal sinus
    Excludes *congenital deviation of nasal septum (754.0)*

748.2 Web of larynx 🔸
    Web of larynx: Web of larynx:
       NOS   subglottic
       glottic

748.3 Other anomalies of larynx, trachea, and bronchus 🔸🔸
    Absence or agenesis of:
       bronchus
       larynx
       trachea
    Anomaly (of):   Anomaly (of):
       cricoid cartilage   thyroid cartilage
       epiglottis   tracheal cartilage
    Atresia (of):   Atresia (of):
       epiglottis   larynx
       glottis   trachea
    Cleft thyroid, cartilage, congenital
    Congenital:
       dilation, trachea
       stenosis:
          larynx
          trachea
       tracheocele
    Diverticulum:
       bronchus
       trachea
    Fissure of epiglottis
    Laryngocele
    Posterior cleft of cricoid cartilage (congenital)
    Rudimentary tracheal bronchus
    Stridor, laryngeal, congenital
    (Ex:) 493.81, 519.19, 748.3, 748.8-748.9
    Coding Clinic: 1999, Q1, P14

748.4 Congenital cystic lung 🔸🔸
    Disease, lung:
       cystic, congenital
       polycystic, congenital
    Honeycomb lung, congenital
    Excludes *acquired or unspecified cystic lung (518.89)*
    (Ex:) 748.4-748.9

748.5 Agenesis, hypoplasia, and dysplasia of lung 🔸🔸
    Absence of lung (fissures) (lobe)
    Aplasia of lung
    Hypoplasia of lung (lobe)
    Sequestration of lung
    (Ex:) 748.4-748.9

● **748.6 Other anomalies of lung**
    748.60 Anomaly of lung, unspecified 🔸
    748.61 Congenital bronchiectasis 🔸🔸
       (Ex:) 494.0-494.1, 496, 506.1, 506.4-506.9, 748.61
    748.69 Other 🔸
       Accessory lung (lobe)
       Azygos lobe (fissure), lung

748.8 Other specified anomalies of respiratory system 🔸
    Abnormal communication between pericardial and
       pleural sacs
    Anomaly, pleural folds
    Atresia of nasopharynx
    Congenital cyst of mediastinum

748.9 Unspecified anomaly of respiratory system 🔸
    Anomaly of respiratory system NOS

● **749 Cleft palate and cleft lip**
    Coding Clinic: 2012, Q2, P17

● **749.0 Cleft palate**
    749.00 Cleft palate, unspecified 🔸
    749.01 Unilateral, complete 🔸
    749.02 Unilateral, incomplete 🔸
       Cleft uvula
    749.03 Bilateral, complete 🔸
    749.04 Bilateral, incomplete 🔸

● **749.1 Cleft lip**
    Cheiloschisis   Harelip
    Congenital fissure of lip   Labium leporinum
    749.10 Cleft lip, unspecified 🔸
    749.11 Unilateral, complete 🔸
    749.12 Unilateral, incomplete 🔸
    749.13 Bilateral, complete 🔸
    749.14 Bilateral, incomplete 🔸

● **749.2 Cleft palate with cleft lip**
    Cheilopalatoschisis
    749.20 Cleft palate with cleft lip, unspecified 🔸
    749.21 Unilateral, complete 🔸
    749.22 Unilateral, incomplete 🔸
    749.23 Bilateral, complete 🔸
       Coding Clinic: 1996, Q1, P14
    749.24 Bilateral, incomplete 🔸
    749.25 Other combinations 🔸

Figure 14–5 Cleft palate.

◀ New   ◀▥ Revised   ~~deleted~~ Deleted   Excludes   Includes   Use additional   Code first   Omit code

● Unacceptable Principal Diagnosis   ● Use Additional Digit(s)   ▶ Manifestation Code   OGCR Official Guidelines   Coding Clinic

920

750 Other congenital anomalies of upper alimentary tract

Excludes *dentofacial anomalies (524.0–524.9)*

750.0 Tongue tie 🔖
Ankyloglossia

●**750.1 Other anomalies of tongue**

750.10 Anomaly of tongue, unspecified 🔖

750.11 Aglossia 🔖

750.12 Congenital adhesions of tongue 🔖

750.13 Fissure of tongue 🔖
Bifid tongue
Double tongue

750.15 Macroglossia 🔖
Congenital hypertrophy of tongue

750.16 Microglossia 🔖
Hypoplasia of tongue

750.19 Other 🔖

●**750.2 Other specified anomalies of mouth and pharynx**

750.21 Absence of salivary gland 🔖

750.22 Accessory salivary gland 🔖

750.23 Atresia, salivary gland 🔖
Imperforate salivary duct

750.24 Congenital fistula of salivary gland 🔖

750.25 Congenital fistula of lip 🔖
Congenital (mucus) lip pits

750.26 Other specified anomalies of mouth 🔖
Absence of uvula

750.27 Diverticulum of pharynx 🔖
Pharyngeal pouch

750.29 Other specified anomalies of pharynx 🔖
Imperforate pharynx

750.3 Tracheoesophageal fistula, esophageal atresia and stenosis 🔖 🔖
Absent esophagus
Atresia of esophagus
Congenital:
esophageal ring
stenosis of esophagus
stricture of esophagus
Congenital fistula:
esophagobronchial
esophagotracheal
Imperforate esophagus
Webbed esophagus
ⓔ 530.84, 750.3-750.4, 751.8-751.9
Coding Clinic: 2012, Q1, P15-16

750.4 Other specified anomalies of esophagus 🔖 🔖
Dilatation, congenital, of esophagus
Displacement, congenital, of esophagus
Diverticulum of esophagus
Duplication of esophagus
Esophageal pouch
Giant esophagus
Excludes *congenital hiatus hernia (750.6)*
ⓔ 750.4, 751.8-751.9

750.5 Congenital hypertrophic pyloric stenosis 🔖
Congenital or infantile:
constriction of pylorus
hypertrophy of pylorus
spasm of pylorus
stenosis of pylorus
stricture of pylorus

750.6 Congenital hiatus hernia 🔖
Displacement of cardia through esophageal hiatus
Excludes *congenital diaphragmatic hernia (756.6)*

Item 14-3 A muscle thickening and pyloric stenosis overgrows the pyloric sphincter, resulting in a narrowing of the outlet between the stomach and small intestine. Infants with pyloric stenosis have projectile vomiting, leading to dehydration and electrolyte imbalance.

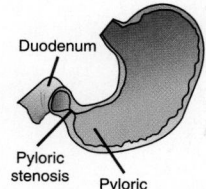

Figure 14–6 Pyloric stenosis.

750.7 Other specified anomalies of stomach 🔖
Congenital:
cardiospasm
hourglass stomach
Displacement of stomach
Diverticulum of stomach, congenital
Duplication of stomach
Megalogastria
Microgastria
Transposition of stomach

750.8 Other specified anomalies of upper alimentary tract 🔖

750.9 Unspecified anomaly of upper alimentary tract 🔖
Congenital:
anomaly NOS of upper alimentary tract [any part, except tongue]
deformity NOS of upper alimentary tract [any part, except tongue]

●**751 Other congenital anomalies of digestive system**

751.0 Meckel's diverticulum 🔖
Meckel's diverticulum (displaced) (hypertrophic)
Persistent:
omphalomesenteric duct
vitelline duct
Coding Clinic: 2004, Q1, P10-11

751.1 Atresia and stenosis of small intestine 🔖 🔖
Atresia of:
duodenum
ileum
intestine NOS
Congenital:
absence of small intestine or intestine NOS
obstruction of small intestine or intestine NOS
stenosis of small intestine or intestine NOS
stricture of small intestine or intestine NOS
Imperforate jejunum
ⓔ 751.1, 751.8-751.9

751.2 Atresia and stenosis of large intestine, rectum, and anal canal 🔖 🔖
Absence:
anus (congenital)
appendix, congenital
large intestine, congenital
rectum
Atresia of:
anus
colon
rectum
Congenital or infantile:
obstruction of large intestine
occlusion of anus
stricture of anus
Imperforate:
anus
rectum
Stricture of rectum, congenital
ⓔ 751.2, 751.8-751.9
Coding Clinic: 1998, Q2, P16-17

CONGENITAL ANOMALIES (740–759)

N Newborn: 0   **P** Pediatric: 0–17   **M** Maternity: 12–55   **A** Adult: 15–124   ♀ Females Only   ♂ Males Only

ⓔ CC/MCC Exclusions   🔖 Complication\Comorbidity   Major C\C   🔖 Present on Admission Requirement   🔖 Hospital-Acquired Condition   **921**

751.3   Hirschsprung's disease and other congenital functional disorders of colon 🅖 🅖
Absence of ganglion cells in distal colon resulting in functional obstruction
Aganglionosis
Congenital dilation of colon
Congenital megacolon
Macrocolon
(Ex:) 751.3, 751.8-751.9

751.4   Anomalies of intestinal fixation 🅖 🅖
Congenital adhesions:
    omental, anomalous
    peritoneal
Jackson's membrane
Malrotation of colon
Rotation of cecum or colon:
    failure of
    incomplete
    insufficient
Universal mesentery
(Ex:) 751.4-751.5
Coding Clinic: 1985, Sept-Oct, P11

751.5   Other anomalies of intestine 🅖 🅖
Congenital diverticulum,   Megaloappendix
    colon   Megaloduodenum
Dolichocolon   Microcolon
Duplication of: Persistent cloaca
    anus   Transposition of:
    appendix   appendix
    cecum   colon
    intestine   intestine
Ectopic anus
(Ex:) 751.0-751.5
Coding Clinic: 2013, Q2, P3; 2010, Q2, P12; 2002, Q3, P11; 2001, Q3, P8-9

● **751.6   Anomalies of gallbladder, bile ducts, and liver**

751.60   Unspecified anomaly of gallbladder, bile ducts, and liver 🅖 🅖
(Ex:) 751.60

751.61   Biliary atresia 🅖 🅖
Congenital:
    absence of bile duct (common) or passage
    hypoplasia of bile duct (common) or passage
    obstruction of bile duct (common) or passage
    stricture of bile duct (common) or passage
(Ex:) 751.61, 751.8-751.9
Coding Clinic: 1987, Sept-Oct, P8

751.62   Congenital cystic disease of liver 🅖 🅖
Congenital polycystic disease of liver
Fibrocystic disease of liver
(Ex:) 751.62-751.69

751.69   Other anomalies of gallbladder, bile ducts, and liver 🅖 🅖
Absence of:
    gallbladder, congenital
    liver (lobe)
Accessory:
    hepatic ducts
    liver
Congenital:
    choledochal cyst
    hepatomegaly
Duplication of: Duplication of:
    biliary duct   gallbladder
    cystic duct   liver
Floating: Floating:
    gallbladder   liver
Intrahepatic gallbladder
(Ex:) 751.60-751.69
Coding Clinic: 1987, Sept-Oct, P8

751.7   Anomalies of pancreas 🅖 🅖
Absence of pancreas
Accessory pancreas
Agenesis of pancreas
Annular pancreas
Ectopic pancreatic tissue
Hypoplasia of pancreas
Pancreatic heterotopia
Excludes *diabetes mellitus (249.0–249.9, (250.0–250.9)*
        fibrocystic disease of pancreas (277.00–277.09)
        neonatal diabetes mellitus (775.1)
(Ex:) 751.7-751.9

751.8   Other specified anomalies of digestive system 🅖
Absence (complete) (partial) of alimentary tract NOS
Duplication of digestive organs NOS
Malposition, congenital of digestive organs NOS
Excludes *congenital diaphragmatic hernia (756.6)*
        congenital hiatus hernia (750.6)

751.9   Unspecified anomaly of digestive system 🅖
Congenital:
    anomaly NOS of digestive system NOS
    deformity NOS of digestive system NOS

● **752   Congenital anomalies of genital organs**
Excludes *syndromes associated with anomalies in the number and form of chromosomes (758.0–758.9)*

752.0   Anomalies of ovaries ♀ 🅖
Absence, congenital, of ovary
Accessory ovary
Ectopic ovary
Streak of ovary

● **752.1   Anomalies of fallopian tubes and broad ligaments**

752.10   Unspecified anomaly of fallopian tubes and broad ligaments ♀ 🅖

752.11   Embryonic cyst of fallopian tubes and broad ligaments ♀ 🅖
Cyst:
    epoophoron
    fimbrial
    parovarian
Coding Clinic: 1985, Sept-Oct, P13

752.19   Other ♀ 🅖
Absence of fallopian tube or broad ligament
Accessory fallopian tube or broad ligament
Atresia of fallopian tube or broad ligament

752.2   Doubling of uterus ♀ 🅖
Didelphic uterus
Doubling of uterus [any degree] (associated with doubling of cervix and vagina)

● **752.3   Other anomalies of uterus**
Coding Clinic: 2006, Q3, P18-19

752.31   Agenesis of uterus ♀ 🅖
Congenital absence of uterus

752.32   Hypoplasia of uterus ♀ 🅖

752.33   Unicornuate uterus ♀ 🅖
Unicornate uterus with or without a separate uterine horn
Uterus with only one functioning horn

752.34   Bicornuate uterus ♀ 🅖
Bicornuate uterus, complete or partial

752.35   Septate uterus ♀ 🅖
Septate uterus, complete or partial

752.36   Arcuate uterus ♀ 🅖

752.39   Other anomalies of uterus ♀ 🅖
Aplasia of uterus NOS
Müllerian anomaly of the uterus, NEC
Excludes *anomaly of uterus due to exposure to diethylstilbestrol [DES] in utero (760.76)*
        didelphic uterus (752.2)
        doubling of uterus (752.2)

● **752.4 Anomalies of cervix, vagina, and external female genitalia**

    752.40 Unspecified anomaly of cervix, vagina, and external female genitalia ♀ 🦠

    752.41 Embryonic cyst of cervix, vagina, and external female genitalia ♀ 🦠
        Cyst of:
          canal of Nuck, congenital
          Gartner's duct
          vagina, embryonal
          vulva, congenital

    752.42 Imperforate hymen ♀ 🦠

    752.43 Cervical agenesis ♀ 🦠
        Cervical hypoplasia

    752.44 Cervical duplication ♀ 🦠

    752.45 Vaginal agenesis ♀ 🦠
        Agenesis of vagina, total or partial

    752.46 Transverse vaginal septum ♀ 🦠

    752.47 Longitudinal vaginal septum ♀ 🦠
        Longitudinal vaginal septum with or without obstruction

    752.49 Other anomalies of cervix, vagina, and external female genitalia ♀ 🦠
        Absence of clitoris or vulva
        Agenesis of clitoris or vulva
        Anomalies of cervix, NEC
        Anomalies of hymen, NEC
        Congenital stenosis or stricture of:
          cervical canal
          vagina
        Müllerian anomalies of the cervix and vagina, NEC
        Excludes *double vagina associated with total duplication (752.2)*
        Coding Clinic: 2006, Q3, P18-19

● **752.5 Undescended and retractile testicle**

    752.51 Undescended testis ♂ 🦠
        Cryptorchism
        Ectopic testis

    752.52 Retractile testis ♂ 🦠

● **752.6 Hypospadias and epispadias and other penile anomalies**

    752.61 Hypospadias ♂ 🦠
        Coding Clinic: 2003, Q4, P67-68; 1997, Q3, P6; Q3, P6; 1996, Q4, P34-35

    752.62 Epispadias ♂ 🦠
        Anaspadias

    752.63 Congenital chordee ♂ 🦠
        Coding Clinic: 1996, Q4, P34-35

    752.64 Micropenis ♂ 🦠

    752.65 Hidden penis ♂ 🦠

    752.69 Other penile anomalies ♂ 🦠

752.7 Indeterminate sex and pseudohermaphroditism 🦠
Condition in which internal reproductive organs are opposite external physical characteristics
Gynandrism
Hermaphroditism
Ovotestis
Pseudohermaphroditism (male) (female)
Pure gonadal dysgenesis
    Excludes *androgen insensitivity (259.50–259.52)*
        pseudohermaphroditism:
          female, with adrenocortical disorder (255.2)
          male, with gonadal disorder (257.8)
          with specified chromosomal anomaly (758.0–758.9)
        testicular feminization syndrome (259.50–259.52)

● **752.8 Other specified anomalies of genital organs**
    Excludes *congenital hydrocele (778.6)*
        penile anomalies (752.61–752.69)
        phimosis or paraphimosis (605)

    752.81 Scrotal transposition ♂ 🦠
        Coding Clinic: 2003, Q4, P67-68

    752.89 Other specified anomalies of genital organs 🦠
        Absence of:
        Check Index for V codes for acquired or congenital.
          prostate
          spermatic cord
          vas deferens
        Anorchism
        Aplasia (congenital) of:
          prostate
          round ligament
          testicle
        Atresia of:
          ejaculatory duct
          vas deferens
        Fusion of testes
        Hypoplasia of testis
        Monorchism
        Polyorchism

752.9 Unspecified anomaly of genital organs 🦠
    Congenital:
        anomaly NOS of genital organ, NEC
        deformity NOS of genital organ, NEC

● **753 Congenital anomalies of urinary system**

    753.0 Renal agenesis and dysgenesis 🦠 🦠
        Atrophy of kidney:
          congenital
          infantile
        Congenital absence of kidney(s)
        Hypoplasia of kidney(s)
        (Ex) 599.60-599.69, 753.0

● **753.1 Cystic kidney disease**
    Excludes *acquired cyst of kidney (593.2)*

    753.10 Cystic kidney disease, unspecified 🦠 🦠
        (Ex) 599.60-599.69, 753.10

    753.11 Congenital single renal cyst 🦠 🦠
        (Ex) 599.60-599.69, 753.11

    753.12 Polycystic kidney, unspecified type 🦠 🦠
        PKD (polycystic kidney disease)
        (Ex) 599.60-599.69, 753.12-753.14
        Coding Clinic: 2013, Q3, P6

    753.13 Polycystic kidney, autosomal dominant 🦠 🦠
        (Ex) 599.60-599.69, 753.12-753.14

    753.14 Polycystic kidney, autosomal recessive 🦠 🦠
        (Ex) 599.60-599.69, 753.12-753.14

    753.15 Renal dysplasia 🦠 🦠
        (Ex) 599.60-599.69, 753.15

    753.16 Medullary cystic kidney 🦠 🦠
        Nephronophthisis
        (Ex) 599.60-599.69, 753.16-753.19

    753.17 Medullary sponge kidney 🦠 🦠
        (Ex) 599.60-599.69, 753.16-753.19

    753.19 Other specified cystic kidney disease 🦠 🦠
        Multicystic kidney
        (Ex) 599.60-599.69, 753.16-753.19

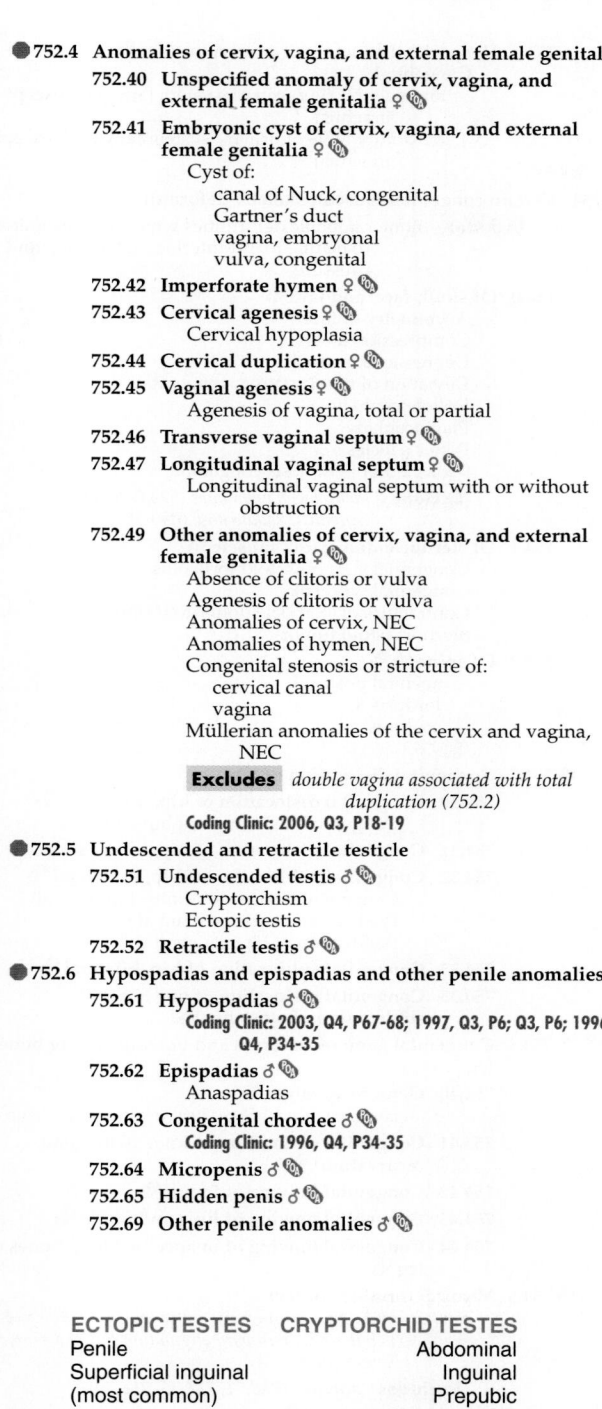

ECTOPIC TESTES	CRYPTORCHID TESTES
Penile	Abdominal
Superficial inguinal (most common)	Inguinal
	Prepubic
Femoral	(most common)

Penile — Internal inguinal ring — Superficial inguinal (most common) — Femoral — Abdominal — Inguinal — External inguinal ring — Prepubic (most common)

Figure 14–7 Undescended testes and the positions of the testes in various types of cryptorchidism or abnormal paths of descent.

Item 14-4 Testes form in the abdomen of the male and only descend into the scrotum during normal embryonic development. "Ectopic" testes are out of their normal place or "retained" (left behind) in the abdomen. Crypto (hidden) orchism (testicle) is a major risk factor for testicular cancer.

CONGENITAL ANOMALIES (740–759)

N Newborn: 0   P Pediatric: 0–17   M Maternity: 12–55   A Adult: 15–124   ♀ Females Only   ♂ Males Only

(Ex) CC/MCC Exclusions   🦠 Complication\Comorbidity   🦠 Major C\C   🦠 Present on Admission Requirement   🦠 Hospital-Acquired Condition   **923**

- **753.2 Obstructive defects of renal pelvis and ureter**
  - **753.20 Unspecified obstructive defect of renal pelvis and ureter** 🔖🔖
    - (Ex) 599.60-599.69, 753.20-753.22, 753.29
  - **753.21 Congenital obstruction of ureteropelvic junction** 🔖🔖
    - (Ex) 599.60-599.69, 753.20-753.22, 753.29
  - **753.22 Congenital obstruction of ureterovesical junction** 🔖🔖
    - Adynamic ureter
    - Congenital hydroureter
    - (Ex) 599.60-599.69, 753.20-753.22, 753.29
  - **753.23 Congenital ureterocele** 🔖🔖
    - (Ex) 599.60-599.69, 753.20-753.22, 753.29
  - **753.29 Other** 🔖🔖
    - (Ex) 599.60-599.69, 753.20-753.22, 753.29
- **753.3 Other specified anomalies of kidney** 🔖
  - Accessory kidney
  - Congenital:
    - calculus of kidney
    - displaced kidney
  - Discoid kidney
  - Double kidney with double pelvis
  - Ectopic kidney
  - Fusion of kidneys
  - Giant kidney
  - Horseshoe kidney
  - Hyperplasia of kidney
  - Lobulation of kidney
  - Malrotation of kidney
  - Trifid kidney (pelvis)
  - **Coding Clinic: 2007, Q1, P23**
- **753.4 Other specified anomalies of ureter** 🔖
  - Absent ureter
  - Accessory ureter
  - Deviation of ureter
  - Displaced ureteric orifice
  - Double ureter
  - Ectopic ureter
  - Implantation, anomalous, of ureter
- **753.5 Exstrophy of urinary bladder** 🔖🔖
  - Ectopia vesicae   Extroversion of bladder
  - (Ex) 599.60-599.69, 753.5, 753.9
- **753.6 Atresia and stenosis of urethra and bladder neck** 🔖🔖
  - Congenital obstruction:
    - bladder neck
    - urethra
  - Congenital stricture of:
    - urethra (valvular)
    - urinary meatus
    - vesicourethral orifice
  - Imperforate urinary meatus
  - Impervious urethra
  - Urethral valve formation
  - (Ex) 599.60-599.69, 753.6, 753.9
- **753.7 Anomalies of urachus** 🔖
  - Cyst (of) urachus   Patent (of) urachus
  - Fistula (of) urachus   Persistent umbilical sinus
- **753.8 Other specified anomalies of bladder and urethra** 🔖
  - Absence, congenital of:
    - bladder
    - urethra
  - Accessory:
    - bladder
    - urethra
  - Congenital:
    - diverticulum of bladder
    - hernia of bladder
  - Congenital urethrorectal fistula
  - Congenital prolapse of:
    - bladder (mucosa)
    - urethra
  - Double:
    - urethra
    - urinary meatus

- **753.9 Unspecified anomaly of urinary system** 🔖
  - Congenital:
    - anomaly NOS of urinary system [any part, except urachus]
    - deformity NOS of urinary system [any part, except urachus]
- **754 Certain congenital musculoskeletal deformities**
  - **Includes** nonteratogenic deformities which are considered to be due to intrauterine malposition and pressure
  - **754.0 Of skull, face, and jaw** 🔖
    - Asymmetry of face
    - Compression facies
    - Depressions in skull
    - Deviation of nasal septum, congenital
    - Dolichocephaly
    - Plagiocephaly
    - Potter's facies
    - Squashed or bent nose, congenital
    - **Excludes** *dentofacial anomalies (524.0–524.9)*
      - *syphilitic saddle nose (090.5)*
  - **754.1 Of sternocleidomastoid muscle** 🔖
    - Congenital sternomastoid torticollis
    - Congenital wryneck
    - Contracture of sternocleidomastoid (muscle)
    - Sternomastoid tumor
  - **754.2 Of spine** 🔖🔖
    - Congenital postural:
      - lordosis
      - scoliosis
    - (Ex) 754.2
  - **754.3 Congenital dislocation of hip**
    - **754.30 Congenital dislocation of hip, unilateral** 🔖
      - Congenital dislocation of hip NOS
    - **754.31 Congenital dislocation of hip, bilateral** 🔖
    - **754.32 Congenital subluxation of hip, unilateral** 🔖
      - Congenital flexion deformity, hip or thigh
      - Predislocation status of hip at birth
      - Preluxation of hip, congenital
    - **754.33 Congenital subluxation of hip, bilateral** 🔖
    - **754.35 Congenital dislocation of one hip with subluxation of other hip** 🔖
  - **754.4 Congenital genu recurvatum and bowing of long bones of leg**
    - **754.40 Genu recurvatum** 🔖
      - *Hyperextension of knee resulting from hypermobility*
    - **754.41 Congenital dislocation of knee (with genu recurvatum)** 🔖
    - **754.42 Congenital bowing of femur** 🔖
    - **754.43 Congenital bowing of tibia and fibula** 🔖
    - **754.44 Congenital bowing of unspecified long bones of leg** 🔖
  - **754.5 Varus deformities of feet**
    - *Foot deformity (pes equino varus) also known as club foot in which there is an inward angulation of distal segment of a bone or joint*
    - **Excludes** *acquired (736.71, 736.75, 736.79)*
    - **754.50 Talipes varus** 🔖
      - Congenital varus deformity of foot, unspecified
      - Pes varus
    - **754.51 Talipes equinovarus** 🔖
      - Equinovarus (congenital)

Figure 14–8 Mild to moderate inbowing of the lower leg. (From Jones KL: Smith's Recognizable Patterns of Human Malformation, ed 6, Philadelphia, Saunders, 2005)

CONGENITAL ANOMALIES (740–759)

754.52 **Metatarsus primus varus** 🔖
754.53 **Metatarsus varus** 🔖
754.59 **Other** 🔖
         Talipes calcaneovarus
● 754.6 **Valgus deformities of feet**
         Inward angulation
         Excludes *valgus deformity of foot (acquired) (736.79)*
754.60 **Talipes valgus** 🔖
         Congenital valgus deformity of foot, unspecified
754.61 **Congenital pes planus** 🔖
         Congenital rocker bottom flat foot
         Flat foot, congenital
         Excludes *pes planus (acquired) (734)*
754.62 **Talipes calcaneovalgus** 🔖
754.69 **Other** 🔖
         Talipes:
             equinovalgus
             planovalgus
● 754.7 **Other deformities of feet**
         Excludes *acquired (736.70–736.79)*
754.70 **Talipes, unspecified** 🔖
         Congenital deformity of foot NOS
754.71 **Talipes cavus** 🔖
         Cavus foot (congenital)
754.79 **Other** 🔖
         Asymmetric talipes
         Talipes:
             calcaneus
             equinus
● 754.8 **Other specified nonteratogenic anomalies**
754.81 **Pectus excavatum** 🔖
         Congenital funnel chest
754.82 **Pectus carinatum** 🔖
         Congenital pigeon chest [breast]
754.89 **Other** 🔖🔖
         Club hand (congenital)
         Congenital:
             deformity of chest wall
             dislocation of elbow
         Generalized flexion contractures of lower limb
             joints, congenital
         Spade-like hand (congenital)
         (Ex) 754.81-754.89
● 755 **Other congenital anomalies of limbs**
         Excludes *those deformities classifiable to 754.0–754.8*
● 755.0 **Polydactyly**
         *Also known as hyperdactyly, consists of duplicate fingers or
             toes*
755.00 **Polydactyly, unspecified digits** 🔖
         Supernumerary digits
755.01 **Of fingers** 🔖
         Accessory fingers
755.02 **Of toes** 🔖
         Accessory toes
● 755.1 **Syndactyly**
         Symphalangy
         Webbing of digits
755.10 **Of multiple and unspecified sites** 🔖
755.11 **Of fingers without fusion of bone** 🔖
755.12 **Of fingers with fusion of bone** 🔖
755.13 **Of toes without fusion of bone** 🔖
755.14 **Of toes with fusion of bone** 🔖

● 755.2 **Reduction deformities of upper limb**
755.20 **Unspecified reduction deformity of upper limb** 🔖
         Ectromelia NOS of upper limb
             *Gross hypoplasia or aplasia of one or more long
                 bones of one or more limbs*
         Hemimelia NOS of upper limb
             Absence of one-half of long bone
         Shortening of arm, congenital
755.21 **Transverse deficiency of upper limb** 🔖
         Amelia of upper limb
         Congenital absence of:
             fingers, all (complete or partial)
             forearm, including hand and fingers
             upper limb, complete
         Congenital amputation of upper limb
         Transverse hemimelia of upper limb
755.22 **Longitudinal deficiency of upper limb, NEC** 🔖
         Phocomelia NOS of upper limb
             *Absence/shortening of long bones primarily as a
                 result of thalidomide*
         Rudimentary arm
755.23 **Longitudinal deficiency, combined, involving
         humerus, radius, and ulna (complete or
         incomplete)** 🔖
         Congenital absence of arm and forearm
             (complete or incomplete) with or without
             metacarpal deficiency and/or phalangeal
             deficiency, incomplete
         Phocomelia, complete, of upper limb
755.24 **Longitudinal deficiency, humeral, complete or
         partial (with or without distal deficiencies,
         incomplete)** 🔖
         Congenital absence of humerus (with or without
             absence of some [but not all] distal
             elements)
         Proximal phocomelia of upper limb
755.25 **Longitudinal deficiency, radioulnar, complete or
         partial (with or without distal deficiencies,
         incomplete)** 🔖
         Congenital absence of radius and ulna (with or
             without absence of some [but not all] distal
             elements)
         Distal phocomelia of upper limb
755.26 **Longitudinal deficiency, radial, complete or partial
         (with or without distal deficiencies, incomplete)** 🔖
         Agenesis of radius
         Congenital absence of radius (with or without
             absence of some [but not all] distal
             elements)
755.27 **Longitudinal deficiency, ulnar, complete or partial
         (with or without distal deficiencies, incomplete)** 🔖
         Agenesis of ulna
         Congenital absence of ulna (with or without
             absence of some [but not all] distal
             elements)
755.28 **Longitudinal deficiency, carpals or metacarpals,
         complete or partial (with or without incomplete
         phalangeal deficiency)** 🔖
755.29 **Longitudinal deficiency, phalanges, complete or
         partial** 🔖
         Absence of finger, congenital
         Aphalangia of upper limb, terminal, complete or
             partial
         Excludes *terminal deficiency of all five digits
                 (755.21)*
                 *transverse deficiency of phalanges
                 (755.21)*

Figure 14–9 Polydactyly, congenital
duplicated thumb. (From DeLee: DeLee and
Drez's Orthopaedic Sports Medicine, ed 3,
Saunders, An Imprint of Elsevier, 2009)

CONGENITAL ANOMALIES (740–759)

● **755.3 Reduction deformities of lower limb**

  755.30 **Unspecified reduction deformity of lower limb** 🔍
      Ectromelia NOS of lower limb
      Hemimelia NOS of lower limb
      Shortening of leg, congenital

  755.31 **Transverse deficiency of lower limb** 🔍
      Amelia of lower limb
      Congenital absence of:
        foot
        leg, including foot and toes
        lower limb, complete
        toes, all, complete
      Transverse hemimelia of lower limb

  755.32 **Longitudinal deficiency of lower limb, NEC** 🔍
      Phocomelia NOS of lower limb

  755.33 **Longitudinal deficiency, combined, involving femur, tibia, and fibula (complete or incomplete)** 🔍
      Congenital absence of thigh and (lower) leg (complete or incomplete) with or without metacarpal deficiency and/or phalangeal deficiency, incomplete
      Phocomelia, complete, of lower limb

  755.34 **Longitudinal deficiency, femoral, complete or partial (with or without distal deficiencies, incomplete)** 🔍
      Congenital absence of femur (with or without absence of some [but not all] distal elements)
      Proximal phocomelia of lower limb

  755.35 **Longitudinal deficiency, tibiofibular, complete or partial (with or without distal deficiencies, incomplete)** 🔍
      Congenital absence of tibia and fibula (with or without absence of some [but not all] distal elements)
      Distal phocomelia of lower limb

  755.36 **Longitudinal deficiency, tibia, complete or partial (with or without distal deficiencies, incomplete)** 🔍
      Agenesis of tibia
      Congenital absence of tibia (with or without absence of some [but not all] distal elements)

  755.37 **Longitudinal deficiency, fibular, complete or partial (with or without distal deficiencies, incomplete)** 🔍
      Agenesis of fibula
      Congenital absence of fibula (with or without absence of some [but not all] distal elements)

  755.38 **Longitudinal deficiency, tarsals or metatarsals, complete or partial (with or without incomplete phalangeal deficiency)** 🔍

  755.39 **Longitudinal deficiency, phalanges, complete or partial** 🔍
      Absence of toe, congenital
      Aphalangia of lower limb, terminal, complete or partial
      Excludes *terminal deficiency of all five digits (755.31)*
      transverse deficiency of phalanges (755.31)

755.4 **Reduction deformities, unspecified limb** 🔍
    Absence, congenital (complete or partial) of limb NOS
    Amelia of unspecified limb
    Ectromelia of unspecified limb
    Hemimelia of unspecified limb
    Phocomelia of unspecified limb

● **755.5 Other anomalies of upper limb, including shoulder girdle**

  755.50 **Unspecified anomaly of upper limb** 🔍

  755.51 **Congenital deformity of clavicle** 🔍

  755.52 **Congenital elevation of scapula** 🔍
      Sprengel's deformity

  755.53 **Radioulnar synostosis** 🔍

  755.54 **Madelung's deformity** 🔍

  755.55 **Acrocephalosyndactyly** 🔍 🔍
      Apert's syndrome
      Ⓔⓧ 755.50, 755.55, 755.59

  755.56 **Accessory carpal bones** 🔍

  755.57 **Macrodactylia (fingers)** 🔍

  755.58 **Cleft hand, congenital** 🔍
      Lobster-claw hand

  755.59 **Other** 🔍
      Cleidocranial dysostosis
      Cubitus:
        valgus, congenital
        varus, congenital
      Excludes *club hand (congenital) (754.89)*
      congenital dislocation of elbow (754.89)

● **755.6 Other anomalies of lower limb, including pelvic girdle**

  755.60 **Unspecified anomaly of lower limb** 🔍

  755.61 **Coxa valga, congenital** 🔍

  755.62 **Coxa vara, congenital** 🔍

  755.63 **Other congenital deformity of hip (joint)** 🔍
      Congenital anteversion of femur (neck)
      Excludes *congenital dislocation of hip (754.30–754.35)*

  755.64 **Congenital deformity of knee (joint)** 🔍
      Congenital:
        absence of patella
        genu valgum [knock-knee]
        genu varum [bowleg]
      Rudimentary patella
      Coding Clinic: 1985, July-Aug, P14; 1984, Nov-Dec, P9

  755.65 **Macrodactylia of toes** 🔍

  755.66 **Other anomalies of toes** 🔍
      Congenital:
        hallux valgus
        hallux varus
        hammer toe

  755.67 **Anomalies of foot, NEC** 🔍
      Astragaloscaphoid synostosis
      Calcaneonavicular bar
      Coalition of calcaneus
      Talonavicular synostosis
      Tarsal coalitions

  755.69 **Other** 🔍
      Congenital:
        angulation of tibia
        deformity (of):
          ankle (joint)
          sacroiliac (joint)
        fusion of sacroiliac joint

755.8 **Other specified anomalies of unspecified limb** 🔍

755.9 **Unspecified anomaly of unspecified limb** 🔍
    Congenital:
      anomaly NOS of unspecified limb
      deformity NOS of unspecified limb
    Excludes *reduction deformity of unspecified limb (755.4)*

● **756 Other congenital musculoskeletal anomalies**

> **Excludes** *congenital myotonic chondrodystrophy (359.23)*
> *those deformities classifiable to 754.0–754.8*

756.0 Anomalies of skull and face bones 🅟
> Absence of skull bones
> Acrocephaly
> Congenital deformity of forehead
> Craniosynostosis
> Crouzon's disease
> Hypertelorism
> Imperfect fusion of skull
> Oxycephaly
> Platybasia
> Premature closure of cranial sutures
> Tower skull
> Trigonocephaly
>
> > **Excludes** *acrocephalosyndactyly [Apert's syndrome]*
> > *(755.55)*
> > *dentofacial anomalies (524.0–524.9)*
> > *skull defects associated with brain anomalies,*
> > *such as:*
> > *anencephalus (740.0)*
> > *encephalocele (742.0)*
> > *hydrocephalus (742.3)*
> > *microcephalus (742.1)*
>
> Coding Clinic: 2012, Q2, P17; 1998, Q3, P9-10; 1996, Q3, P15

● **756.1 Anomalies of spine**

756.10 Anomaly of spine, unspecified 🅟

756.11 Spondylolysis, lumbosacral region 🅟
> Prespondylolisthesis (lumbosacral)

756.12 Spondylolisthesis 🅟

756.13 Absence of vertebra, congenital 🅟 🅟
> (Ex) 756.10-756.19

756.14 Hemivertebra 🅟

756.15 Fusion of spine [vertebra], congenital 🅟

756.16 Klippel-Feil syndrome 🅟

756.17 Spina bifida occulta 🅟
> > **Excludes** *spina bifida (aperta) (741.0–741.9)*

756.19 Other 🅟
> Platyspondylia
> Supernumerary vertebra

756.2 Cervical rib 🅟
> Supernumerary rib in the cervical region

756.3 Other anomalies of ribs and sternum 🅟 🅟
> Congenital absence of:
> rib
> sternum
> Congenital:
> fissure of sternum
> fusion of ribs
> Sternum bifidum
>
> > **Excludes** *nonteratogenic deformity of chest wall*
> > *(754.81–754.89)*
>
> (Ex) 756.2-756.3

756.4 Chondrodystrophy 🅟
> *Skeletal dysplasia (dwarfism) is caused by genetic mutations*
> *affecting hyaline cartilage capping long bones and*
> *vertebrae*
>
> Achondroplasia   Enchondromatosis
> Chondrodystrophia (fetalis)   Ollier's disease
> Dyschondroplasia
>
> > **Excludes** *congenital myotonic chondrodystrophy (359.23)*
> > *lipochondrodystrophy [Hurler's syndrome]*
> > *(277.5)*
> > *Morquio's disease (277.5)*
> Coding Clinic: 2002, Q2, P16-17; 1987, Sept-Oct, P10

● **756.5 Osteodystrophies**
> *Defective bone development; most commonly caused by renal*
> *disease or disturbances in calcium and phosphorus*
> *metabolism*

756.50 Osteodystrophy, unspecified 🅟

756.51 Osteogenesis imperfecta 🅟 🅟
> Fragilitas ossium
> Osteopsathyrosis
> (Ex) 756.50-756.59

756.52 Osteopetrosis 🅟 🅟
> (Ex) 756.50-756.59

756.53 Osteopoikilosis 🅟

756.54 Polyostotic fibrous dysplasia of bone 🅟

756.55 Chondroectodermal dysplasia 🅟
> Ellis-van Creveld syndrome

756.56 Multiple epiphyseal dysplasia 🅟

756.59 Other 🅟
> Albright (-McCune)-Sternberg syndrome

756.6 Anomalies of diaphragm 🅟 🅟
> Absence of diaphragm
> Congenital hernia:
> diaphragmatic
> foramen of Morgagni
> Eventration of diaphragm
>
> > **Excludes** *congenital hiatus hernia (750.6)*
>
> (Ex) 750.6, 756.6

● **756.7 Anomalies of abdominal wall**

756.70 Anomaly of abdominal wall, unspecified 🅟 🅟
> (Ex) 756.70-756.79

756.71 Prune belly syndrome 🅟 🅟
> Eagle-Barrett syndrome
> Prolapse of bladder mucosa
> (Ex) 756.70-756.79

756.72 Omphalocele 🅟 🅟
> Exomphalos
> (Ex) 756.70-756.79

756.73 Gastroschisis 🅟 🅟
> (Ex) 756.70-756.79

756.79 Other congenital anomalies of abdominal wall 🅟 🅟
> > **Excludes** *umbilical hernia (551–553 with .1)*
> (Ex) 756.70-756.79

● **756.8 Other specified anomalies of muscle, tendon, fascia, and connective tissue**

756.81 Absence of muscle and tendon 🅟
> Absence of muscle (pectoral)
> Coding Clinic: 2010, Q1, P11

756.82 Accessory muscle 🅟

756.83 Ehlers-Danlos syndrome 🅟 🅟
> (Ex) 756.83-756.89

756.89 Other 🅟
> Amyotrophia congenita
> Congenital shortening of tendon
> Coding Clinic: 1999, Q3, P16-17

756.9 Other and unspecified anomalies of musculoskeletal system 🅟
> Congenital:
> anomaly NOS of musculoskeletal system, NEC
> deformity NOS of musculoskeletal system, NEC

CONGENITAL ANOMALIES (740–759)

N Newborn: 0   P Pediatric: 0–17   M Maternity: 12–55   A Adult: 15–124   ♀ Females Only   ♂ Males Only

(Ex) CC/MCC Exclusions   🅟 Complication\Comorbidity   Major C\C   Present on Admission Requirement   Hospital-Acquired Condition   **927**

● **757 Congenital anomalies of the integument**

> **Includes** anomalies of skin, subcutaneous tissue, hair, nails, and breast

> **Excludes** *hemangioma (228.00–228.09)*
> *pigmented nevus (216.0–216.9)*

757.0 Hereditary edema of legs 🔍
Congenital lymphedema
Hereditary trophedema
Milroy's disease

757.1 Ichthyosis congenita 🔍
Congenital ichthyosis
Harlequin fetus
Ichthyosiform erythroderma

757.2 Dermatoglyphic anomalies 🔍
Abnormal palmar creases

● **757.3 Other specified anomalies of skin**

757.31 Congenital ectodermal dysplasia 🔍

757.32 Vascular hamartomas 🔍
Birthmarks
Port-wine stain
Strawberry nevus
Coding Clinic: 2012, Q2, P7

757.33 Congenital pigmentary anomalies of skin 🔍
Congenital poikiloderma
Urticaria pigmentosa
Xeroderma pigmentosum

> **Excludes** *albinism (270.2)*

Coding Clinic: 2013, Q1, P14

757.39 Other 🔍
Accessory skin tags, congenital
Congenital scar
Epidermolysis bullosa
Keratoderma (congenital)

> **Excludes** *pilonidal cyst (685.0–685.1)*

Coding Clinic: 2013, Q1, P15

757.4 Specified anomalies of hair 🔍
Congenital:
alopecia
atrichosis
beaded hair
hypertrichosis
monilethrix
Persistent lanugo

757.5 Specified anomalies of nails 🔍
Anonychia
Congenital:
clubnail
koilonychia
leukonychia
onychauxis
pachyonychia

757.6 Specified congenital anomalies of breast 🔍
Congenital absent breast or nipple
Accessory breast or nipple
Supernumerary breast or nipple

> **Excludes** *absence of pectoral muscle (756.81)*
> *hypoplasia of breast (611.82)*
> *micromastia (611.82)*

757.8 Other specified anomalies of the integument 🔍

757.9 Unspecified anomaly of the integument 🔍
Congenital:
anomaly NOS of integument
deformity NOS of integument

● **758 Chromosomal anomalies**

> **Includes** syndromes associated with anomalies in the number and form of chromosomes

Use additional codes for conditions associated with the chromosomal anomalies

758.0 Down's syndrome 🔍
Mongolism
Translocation Down's syndrome
Trisomy:
21 or 22
G

758.1 Patau's syndrome 🔍 🔍
Trisomy:
13
D_1
(Ex:) 758.0-758.9

758.2 Edward's syndrome 🔍 🔍
Trisomy:
18
E_3
(Ex:) 758.0-758.9

● **758.3 Autosomal deletion syndromes**
Coding Clinic: 2004, Q4, P93-95; 1995, Q2, P6-7, 11

758.31 Cri-du-chat syndrome 🔍 🔍
Deletion 5p
(Ex:) 758.0-758.2, 758.32-758.9

758.32 Velo-cardio-facial syndrome 🔍 🔍
Deletion 22q11.2
(Ex:) 758.0-758.31, 758.33-758.9

758.33 Other microdeletions 🔍 🔍
Miller-Dieker syndrome
Smith-Magenis syndrome
(Ex:) 758.0-758.32, 758.39-758.9

758.39 Other autosomal deletions 🔍 🔍
(Ex:) 758.0-758.33, 758.4-758.9

758.4 Balanced autosomal translocation in normal individual 🔍

758.5 Other conditions due to autosomal anomalies 🔍
Accessory autosomes NEC

758.6 Gonadal dysgenesis 🔍
Ovarian dysgenesis
Turner's syndrome
XO syndrome

> **Excludes** *pure gonadal dysgenesis (752.7)*

758.7 Klinefelter's syndrome ♂ 🔍
XXY syndrome

● **758.8 Other conditions due to chromosome anomalies**

758.81 Other conditions due to sex chromosome anomalies 🔍

758.89 Other 🔍

758.9 Conditions due to anomaly of unspecified chromosome 🔍

● **759 Other and unspecified congenital anomalies**

759.0 Anomalies of spleen 🔍 🔍
Aberrant spleen   Congenital splenomegaly
Absent spleen   Ectopic spleen
Accessory spleen   Lobulation of spleen
(Ex:) 759.0, 759.9

759.1 Anomalies of adrenal gland 🔍
Aberrant adrenal gland
Absent adrenal gland
Accessory adrenal gland

> **Excludes** *adrenogenital disorders (255.2)*
> *congenital disorders of steroid metabolism (255.2)*

759.2 Anomalies of other endocrine glands 🌢
    Absent parathyroid gland
    Accessory thyroid gland
    Persistent thyroglossal or thyrolingual duct
    Thyroglossal (duct) cyst
    Excludes *congenital:*
        goiter (246.1)
        hypothyroidism (243)

759.3 Situs inversus 🌢 🌢
    Situs inversus or transversus:
        abdominalis
        thoracis
    Transposition of viscera:
        abdominal
        thoracic
    Excludes *dextrocardia without mention of complete*
        transposition (746.87)
    (Ex) 759.3, 759.7, 759.9

759.4 Conjoined twins 🌢 🌢
    Craniopagus   Thoracopagus
    Dicephalus   Xiphopagus
    Pygopagus
    (Ex) 759.4, 759.7, 759.9

759.5 Tuberous sclerosis 🌢 🌢
    Bourneville's disease
    Epiloia
    (Ex) 759.5-759.7, 759.9

759.6 Other hamartoses, NEC 🌢 🌢
    Syndrome:
        Peutz-Jeghers
        Sturge-Weber (-Dimitri)
        von Hippel-Lindau
    Excludes *neurofibromatosis (237.70-237.79)*
    (Ex) 759.6, 759.9
    Coding Clinic: 1992, Q3, P11

759.7 Multiple congenital anomalies, so described 🌢 🌢
    Congenital:
        anomaly, multiple NOS
        deformity, multiple NOS
    (Ex) 759.3, 759.7, 759.9

● **759.8 Other specified anomalies**
    759.81 Prader-Willi syndrome 🌢 🌢
        (Ex) 759.6-759.9
    759.82 Marfan syndrome 🌢 🌢
        (Ex) 759.6-759.9
        Coding Clinic: 1993, Q3, P11
    759.83 Fragile X syndrome 🌢
    759.89 Other 🌢 🌢
        Index directs coder to this code for Noonan's
        syndrome.
        Congenital malformation syndromes affecting
        multiple systems, NEC
        Laurence-Moon-Biedl syndrome
        (Ex) 759.81-759.89
        Coding Clinic: 2012, Q2, P3-4; 2008, Q3, P3-4; 2006, Q3, P21;
        2005, Q2, P17; 2004, Q2, P12; 2001, Q1, P3; 1999,
        Q3, P17-19x2; 1998, Q3, P8; 1987, Sept-Oct, P9;
        1985, Sept-Oct, P11

759.9 Congenital anomaly, unspecified 🌢

OGCR   Section I.C.15.a

For coding and reporting purposes the perinatal period is defined as before birth through the 28th day following birth. The following guidelines are provided for reporting purposes. Hospitals may record other diagnoses as needed for internal data use.

1) **Chapter 15 Codes**
They are <u>never</u> for use on the maternal record. Codes from Chapter 11, the obstetric chapter, are never permitted on the newborn record. Chapter 15 code may be used throughout the life of the patient if the condition is still present.

2) **Sequencing of perinatal codes**
Generally, codes from Chapter 15 should be sequenced as the principal/first-listed diagnosis on the newborn record, with the exception of the appropriate V30 code for the birth episode, followed by codes from any other chapter that provide additional detail. The "use additional code" note at the beginning of the chapter supports this guideline. If the index does not provide a specific code for a perinatal condition, assign code 779.89, Other specified conditions originating in the perinatal period, followed by the code from another chapter that specifies the condition. Codes for signs and symptoms may be assigned when a definitive diagnosis has not been established.

3) **Birth process or community acquired conditions**
If a newborn has a condition that may be either due to the birth process or community acquired and the documentation does not indicate which it is, the default is due to the birth process and the code from Chapter 15 should be used. If the condition is community-acquired, a code from Chapter 15 should not be assigned.

15.   CERTAIN CONDITIONS ORIGINATING IN THE PERINATAL PERIOD (760–779)

> **Includes**   conditions which have their origin in the perinatal period, before birth through the first 28 days after birth, even though death or morbidity occurs later
>
> Use additional code(s) to further specify condition

MATERNAL CAUSES OF PERINATAL MORBIDITY AND MORTALITY (760–763)

● **760**   **Fetus or newborn affected by maternal conditions which may be unrelated to present pregnancy**
> **Includes**   the listed maternal conditions only when specified as a cause of mortality or morbidity of the fetus or newborn
>
> **Excludes**   *maternal endocrine and metabolic disorders affecting fetus or newborn (775.0–775.9)*
>
> Coding Clinic: 1992, Q2, P12

760.0   **Maternal hypertensive disorders**
Fetus or newborn affected by maternal conditions classifiable to 642

760.1   **Maternal renal and urinary tract diseases**
Fetus or newborn affected by maternal conditions classifiable to 580–599

760.2   **Maternal infections**
Fetus or newborn affected by maternal infectious disease classifiable to 001–136 and 487, but fetus or newborn not manifesting that disease
> **Excludes**   *congenital infectious diseases (771.0–771.8)*
> *maternal genital tract and other localized infections (760.8)*

760.3   **Other chronic maternal circulatory and respiratory diseases**
Fetus or newborn affected by chronic maternal conditions classifiable to 390–459, 490–519, 745–748

760.4   **Maternal nutritional disorders**
Fetus or newborn affected by:
maternal disorders classifiable to 260–269
maternal malnutrition NOS
> **Excludes**   *fetal malnutrition (764.10–764.29)*

760.5   **Maternal injury**
Fetus or newborn affected by maternal conditions classifiable to 800–995

● **760.6**   **Surgical operation on mother and fetus**
> **Excludes**   *cesarean section for present delivery (763.4)*
> *damage to placenta from amniocentesis, cesarean section, or surgical induction (762.1)*
>
> Coding Clinic: 2008, Q4, P137-138

760.61   **Newborn affected by amniocentesis**
> **Excludes**   *fetal complications from amniocentesis (679.1)*

760.62   **Newborn affected by other in utero procedure**
> **Excludes**   *fetal complications of in utero procedure (679.1)*

760.63   **Newborn affected by other surgical operations on mother during pregnancy**
> **Excludes**   *newborn affected by previous surgical procedure on mother not associated with pregnancy (760.64)*

760.64   **Newborn affected by previous surgical procedure on mother not associated with pregnancy**

● **760.7**   **Noxious influences affecting fetus or newborn via placenta or breast milk**
Fetus or newborn affected by noxious substance transmitted via placenta or breast milk
> **Excludes**   *anesthetic and analgesic drugs administered during labor and delivery (763.5)*
> *drug withdrawal syndrome in newborn (779.5)*
>
> Coding Clinic: 1991, Q3, P21

760.70   **Unspecified noxious substance**
Fetus or newborn affected by:
drug NEC

760.71   **Alcohol**
Fetal alcohol syndrome

760.72   **Narcotics**

760.73   **Hallucinogenic agents**

760.74   **Anti-infectives**
Antibiotics
Antifungals

760.75   **Cocaine**
Coding Clinic: 1994, Q3, P6; 1992, Q2, P12

760.76   **Diethylstilbestrol [DES]**

760.77   **Anticonvulsants**   N
Carbamazepine   Phenytoin
Phenobarbital   Valproic acid
Coding Clinic: 2005, Q4, P82-83

760.78   **Antimetabolic agents**   N
Methotrexate
Retinoic acid
Statins
Coding Clinic: 2005, Q4, P82-83

760.79   **Other**
Fetus or newborn affected by:
immune sera transmitted via placenta or breast milk
medicinal agents NEC transmitted via placenta or breast milk
toxic substance NEC transmitted via placenta or breast milk
Coding Clinic: 2010, Q1, P12; 2009, Q3, P12x3

760.8   **Other specified maternal conditions affecting fetus or newborn**
Maternal genital tract and other localized infection affecting fetus or newborn, but fetus or newborn not manifesting that disease
> **Excludes**   *maternal urinary tract infection affecting fetus or newborn (760.1)*

760.9   **Unspecified maternal condition affecting fetus or newborn**

◀ New   ◀▬ Revised   ~~deleted~~ Deleted   Excludes   Includes   Use additional   Code first   Omit code

930   ● Unacceptable Principal Diagnosis   ● Use Additional Digit(s)   ▶ Manifestation Code   **OGCR** Official Guidelines   **Coding Clinic**

● **761 Fetus or newborn affected by maternal complications of pregnancy**

> **Includes** the listed maternal conditions only when specified as a cause of mortality or morbidity of the fetus or newborn

761.0 Incompetent cervix

761.1 Premature rupture of membranes

761.2 Oligohydramnios
> *Scant volume of amniotic fluid*

> **Excludes** *that due to premature rupture of membranes (761.1)*

761.3 Polyhydramnios
> *Overabundance of amniotic fluid*
> Hydramnios (acute) (chronic)

761.4 Ectopic pregnancy
> Pregnancy:
>> abdominal
>> intraperitoneal
>> tubal

761.5 Multiple pregnancy
> Triplet (pregnancy)
> Twin (pregnancy)

761.6 Maternal death

761.7 Malpresentation before labor
> Breech presentation before labor
> External version before labor
> Oblique lie before labor
> Transverse lie before labor
> Unstable lie before labor

761.8 Other specified maternal complications of pregnancy affecting fetus or newborn
> Spontaneous abortion, fetus

761.9 Unspecified maternal complication of pregnancy affecting fetus or newborn

● **762 Fetus or newborn affected by complications of placenta, cord, and membranes**

> **Includes** the listed maternal conditions only when specified as a cause of mortality or morbidity in the fetus or newborn

762.0 Placenta previa N

762.1 Other forms of placental separation and hemorrhage N
> Abruptio placentae
> Antepartum hemorrhage
> Damage to placenta from amniocentesis, cesarean section, or surgical induction
> Maternal blood loss
> Premature separation of placenta
> Rupture of marginal sinus

762.2 Other and unspecified morphological and functional abnormalities of placenta N
> Placental:
>> dysfunction
>> infarction
>> insufficiency

762.3 Placental transfusion syndromes N
> Placental and cord abnormality resulting in twin-to-twin or other transplacental transfusion

> Use additional code to indicate resultant condition in newborn:
>> fetal blood loss (772.0)
>> polycythemia neonatorum (776.4)

762.4 Prolapsed cord N
> Cord presentation

762.5 Other compression of umbilical cord N
> Cord around neck   Knot in cord
> Entanglement of cord   Torsion of cord
> **Coding Clinic: 2003, Q2, P9**

762.6 Other and unspecified conditions of umbilical cord N
> Short cord
> Thrombosis of umbilical cord
> Varices of umbilical cord
> Velamentous insertion of umbilical cord
> Vasa previa

> **Excludes** *infection of umbilical cord (771.4)*
>> *single umbilical artery (747.5)*

762.7 Chorioamnionitis N
> Amnionitis
> Membranitis
> Placentitis

762.8 Other specified abnormalities of chorion and amnion N

762.9 Unspecified abnormality of chorion and amnion N

● **763 Fetus or newborn affected by other complications of labor and delivery**

> **Includes** the listed conditions only when specified as a cause of mortality or morbidity in the fetus or newborn

> **Excludes** *newborn affected by surgical procedures on mother (760.61-760.64)*

763.0 Breech delivery and extraction N

763.1 Other malpresentation, malposition, and disproportion during labor and delivery N
> Fetus or newborn affected by:
>> abnormality of bony pelvis
>> contracted pelvis
>> persistent occipitoposterior position
>> shoulder presentation
>> transverse lie
>> conditions classifiable to 652, 653, and 660

763.2 Forceps delivery N
> Fetus or newborn affected by forceps extraction

763.3 Delivery by vacuum extractor N

763.4 Cesarean delivery N

> **Excludes** *placental separation or hemorrhage from cesarean section (762.1)*

763.5 Maternal anesthesia and analgesia N
> Reactions and intoxications from maternal opiates and tranquilizers during labor and delivery

> **Excludes** *drug withdrawal syndrome in newborn (779.5)*

763.6 Precipitate delivery N
> Rapid second stage

763.7 Abnormal uterine contractions N
> Fetus or newborn affected by:
>> contraction ring
>> hypertonic labor
>> hypotonic uterine dysfunction
>> uterine inertia or dysfunction
>> conditions classifiable to 661, except 661.3

● **763.8 Other specified complications of labor and delivery affecting fetus or newborn**

763.81 Abnormality in fetal heart rate or rhythm before the onset of labor N

763.82 Abnormality in fetal heart rate or rhythm during labor N
> **Coding Clinic: 1998, Q4, P46-47**

763.83 Abnormality in fetal heart rate or rhythm, unspecified as to time of onset N

763.84 Meconium passage during delivery N

> **Excludes** *meconium aspiration (770.11, 770.12)*
>> *meconium staining (779.84)*
> **Coding Clinic: 2005, Q4, P83-89**

763.89 Other specified complications of labor and delivery affecting fetus or newborn N
> Fetus or newborn affected by:
>> abnormality of maternal soft tissues
>> destructive operation on live fetus to facilitate delivery
>> induction of labor (medical)
>> other conditions classifiable to 650–669
>> other procedures used in labor and delivery

763.9 Unspecified complication of labor and delivery affecting fetus or newborn N

N Newborn: 0   **P** Pediatric: 0–17   **M** Maternity: 12–55   **A** Adult: 15–124   ♀ Females Only   ♂ Males Only

ⓧ CC/MCC Exclusions   🔍 Complication\Comorbidity   🔍 Major C\C   🔍 Present on Admission Requirement   🔍 Hospital-Acquired Condition

931

CERTAIN CONDITIONS ORIGINATING IN THE PERINATAL PERIOD (760–779)

OTHER CONDITIONS ORIGINATING IN THE PERINATAL PERIOD (764–779)

The following fifth-digit subclassification is for use with category 764 and codes 765.0 and 765.1 to denote birthweight:

0	unspecified [weight]	5	1,250–1,499 grams
1	less than 500 grams	6	1,500–1,749 grams
2	500–749 grams	7	1,750–1,999 grams
3	750–999 grams	8	2,000–2,499 grams
4	1,000–1,249 grams	9	2,500 grams and over

● **764 Slow fetal growth and fetal malnutrition**
Requires fifth digit. See beginning of section 764–779 for codes and definitions.
Coding Clinic: 2009, Q1, P7; 2004, Q3, P4-5; 1994, Q1, P15; 1989, Q2, P15

OGCR   Section I.C.15.i
Providers utilize different criteria in determining prematurity. A code for prematurity should not be assigned unless it is documented. The 5th digit assignment for codes from category 764 and subcategories 765.0 and 765.1 should be based on the recorded birth weight and estimated gestational age.

● **764.0 "Light-for-dates" without mention of fetal**   N
[0-9] **malnutrition**
Infants underweight for gestational age
"Small-for-dates"

● **764.1 "Light-for-dates" with signs of fetal malnutrition**   N
[0-9] Infants "light-for-dates" classifiable to 764.0, who in addition show signs of fetal malnutrition, such as dry peeling skin and loss of subcutaneous tissue

● **764.2 Fetal malnutrition without mention of**   N
[0-9] **"light-for-dates"**
Infants, not underweight for gestational age, showing signs of fetal malnutrition, such as dry peeling skin and loss of subcutaneous tissue
Intrauterine malnutrition

● **764.9 Fetal growth retardation, unspecified**   N
[0-9] Intrauterine growth retardation
Coding Clinic: 1997, Q1, P6

● **765 Disorders relating to short gestation and low birthweight**
Requires fifth digit. See beginning of section 764–779 for codes and definitions.
Includes the listed conditions, without further specification, as causes of mortality, morbidity, or additional care, in fetus or newborn
Coding Clinic: 2002, Q4, P63-64; 1994, Q1, P15; 1991, Q2, P19, 1989, Q2, P15

● **765.0 Extreme immaturity**   N
[0-9] **Note:** Usually implies a birthweight of less than 1,000 grams
Use additional code for weeks of gestation (765.20–765.29)
Coding Clinic: 2009, Q1, P12; 2004, Q3, P4-5; 2001, Q4, P50-51

OGCR   Section I.C.15.i
Providers utilize different criteria in determining prematurity. A code for prematurity should not be assigned unless it is documented. The 5th digit assignment for codes from subcategory 765.0 should be based on the recorded birth weight and estimated gestational age.

● **765.1 Other preterm infants**   N
[0-9] Prematurity NOS
Prematurity or small size, not classifiable to 765.0 or as "light-for-dates" in 764
Note: Usually implies birthweight of 1,000–2,499 grams
Use additional code for weeks of gestation (765.20–765.29)
Coding Clinic: 2009, Q1, P12; 2008, Q4, P138-140; 2004, Q3, P4-5; 2002, Q4, P64; 1997, Q1, P6; 1994, Q1, P14

OGCR   Section I.C.15.i
Providers utilize different criteria in determining prematurity. A code for prematurity should not be assigned unless it is documented. The 5th digit assignment for codes from category 764 and subcategories 765.0 and 765.1 should be based on the recorded birth weight and estimated gestational age.

● **765.2 Weeks of gestation**
Coding Clinic: 2004, Q3, P4-5

OGCR   Section I.C.15.i
A code from subcategory 765.2, Weeks of gestation, should be assigned as an additional code with category 764 and codes from 765.0 and 765.1 to specify weeks of gestation as documented by the provider in the record.

765.20 **Unspecified weeks of gestation**   N
765.21 **Less than 24 completed weeks of gestation**   N
765.22 **24 weeks of gestation**   N
765.23 **25–26 weeks of gestation**   N
Coding Clinic: 2009, Q1, P6
765.24 **27–28 weeks of gestation**   N
765.25 **29–30 weeks of gestation**   N
765.26 **31–32 weeks of gestation**   N
Coding Clinic: 2009, Q1, P6; 2008, Q4, P138-140
765.27 **33–34 weeks of gestation**   N
Coding Clinic: 2010, Q4, P98
765.28 **35–36 weeks of gestation**   N
Coding Clinic: 2002, Q4, P64
765.29 **37 or more weeks of gestation**   N

● **766 Disorders relating to long gestation and high birthweight**
Includes the listed conditions, without further specification, as causes of mortality, morbidity, or additional care, in fetus or newborn

766.0 **Exceptionally large baby**   N
Note: Usually implies a birthweight of 4,500 grams or more.

766.1 **Other "heavy-for-dates" infants**   N
Other fetus or infant "heavy-" or "large-for-dates" regardless of period of gestation

● **766.2 Late infant, not "heavy-for-dates"**
Coding Clinic: 2006, Q2, P12-13; 2003, Q4, P69

766.21 **Post-term infant**   N
Infant with gestation period over 40 completed weeks to 42 completed weeks
Coding Clinic: 2009, Q1, P6; 2006, Q2, P12-13

766.22 **Prolonged gestation of infant**   N
Infant with gestation period over 42 completed weeks
Postmaturity NOS
Coding Clinic: 2009, Q1, P6; 2006, Q2, P12-13

● **767 Birth trauma**
767.0 **Subdural and cerebral hemorrhage**
Subdural and cerebral hemorrhage, whether described as due to birth trauma or to intrapartum anoxia or hypoxia
Subdural hematoma (localized)
Tentorial tear
Use additional code to identify cause
Excludes *intraventricular hemorrhage (772.10–772.14)*
subarachnoid hemorrhage (772.2)
Ex) 767.0, 767.8-767.9, 779.81-779.84, 779.89

767.1 **Injuries to scalp**
Coding Clinic: 2003, Q4, P69-70

767.11 **Epicranial subaponeurotic hemorrhage (massive)**   N
Subgaleal hemorrhage
Ex) 767.0-767.11, 767.8-767.9, 779.81-779.84, 779.89

767.19 **Other injuries to scalp**   N
Caput succedaneum
Cephalhematoma
Chignon (from vacuum extraction)

◄ New   ◄■■■ Revised   ~~deleted~~ Deleted   Excludes   Includes   Use additional   Code first   Omit code
● Unacceptable Principal Diagnosis   ● Use Additional Digit(s)   ▶ Manifestation Code   OGCR Official Guidelines   Coding Clinic

767.2 **Fracture of clavicle** N

767.3 **Other injuries to skeleton** N
Fracture of:
  long bones
  skull
  Excludes *congenital dislocation of hip (754.30–754.35)*
  fracture of spine, congenital (767.4)

767.4 **Injury to spine and spinal cord** N
Dislocation of spine or spinal cord due to birth trauma
Fracture of spine or spinal cord due to birth trauma
Laceration of spine or spinal cord due to birth trauma
Rupture of spine or spinal cord due to birth trauma

767.5 **Facial nerve injury** N
Facial palsy

767.6 **Injury to brachial plexus** N
Palsy or paralysis:
  brachial
  Erb (-Duchenne)
  Klumpke (-Déjérine)

767.7 **Other cranial and peripheral nerve injuries** N
Phrenic nerve paralysis

767.8 **Other specified birth trauma** N
Eye damage   Rupture of:
Hematoma of: liver
  liver (subcapsular)   spleen
  testes   Scalpel wound
  vulva Traumatic glaucoma
  Excludes *hemorrhage classifiable to 772.0–772.9*

767.9 **Birth trauma, unspecified** N
Birth injury NOS

● 768 **Intrauterine hypoxia and birth asphyxia**
Use only when associated with newborn morbidity classifiable elsewhere
  Excludes *acidemia NOS of newborn (775.81)*
  acidosis NOS of newborn (775.81)
  cerebral ischemia NOS (779.2)
  hypoxia NOS of newborn (770.88)
  mixed metabolic and respiratory acidosis of newborn (775.81)
  respiratory arrest of newborn (770.87)

768.0 **Fetal death from asphyxia or anoxia before onset of labor or at unspecified time** N

768.1 **Fetal death from asphyxia or anoxia during labor** N

768.2 **Fetal distress before onset of labor, in liveborn infant** N
Fetal metabolic acidemia before onset of labor, in liveborn infant

768.3 **Fetal distress first noted during labor and delivery, in liveborn infant** N
Fetal metabolic acidemia first noted during labor and delivery, in liveborn infant

768.4 **Fetal distress, unspecified as to time of onset, in liveborn infant** N
Fetal metabolic acidemia unspecified as to time of onset, in liveborn infant
Coding Clinic: 1986, Nov-Dec, P10

768.5 **Severe birth asphyxia** ✎ N
Birth asphyxia with neurologic involvement
  Excludes *hypoxic-ischemic encephalopathy (HIE) (768.70-768.73)*
  (Ex) 516.61-516.69, 768.5-768.6, 768.9-770.86, 770.89-770.9, 779.81-779.84, 779.89

768.6 **Mild or moderate birth asphyxia** N
Other specified birth asphyxia (without mention of neurologic involvement)
  Excludes *hypoxic-ischemic encephalopathy (HIE) (768.70-768.73)*

● 768.7 **Hypoxic-ischemic encephalopathy (HIE)**
  (Ex) 768.5-768.6, 768.9
  Coding Clinic: 2006, Q4, P104-106

768.70 **Hypoxic-ischemic encephalopathy, unspecified** ✎ N
  (Ex) 768.5-768.9

768.71 **Mild hypoxic-ischemic encephalopathy** ✎ N
  (Ex) 768.5-768.9

768.72 **Moderate hypoxic-ischemic encephalopathy** ✎ N
  (Ex) 768.5-768.9
  Coding Clinic: 2009, Q4, P113

768.73 **Severe hypoxic-ischemic encephalopathy** ✎ N
  (Ex) 768.5-768.9

768.9 **Unspecified birth asphyxia in liveborn infant** N
Anoxia NOS, in liveborn infant
Asphyxia NOS, in liveborn infant

769 **Respiratory distress syndrome** ✎ N
Cardiorespiratory distress syndrome of newborn
Hyaline membrane disease (pulmonary)
Idiopathic respiratory distress syndrome [IRDS or RDS] of newborn
Pulmonary hypoperfusion syndrome
  Excludes *transient tachypnea of newborn (770.6)*
  (Ex) 516.61-516.69, 768.5-768.6, 768.9-770.86, 770.89-770.9, 779.81-779.84, 779.89
  Coding Clinic: 2009, Q3, P12; 1989, Q1, P10

● 770 **Other respiratory conditions of fetus and newborn**
770.0 **Congenital pneumonia** ✎ N
Infective pneumonia acquired prenatally
  Excludes *pneumonia from infection acquired after birth (480.0–486)*
  (Ex) 516.61-516.69, 768.5-768.6, 768.9-770.86, 770.89-770.9, 779.81-779.84, 779.89
  Coding Clinic: 2005, Q1, P10-11

● 770.1 **Fetal and newborn aspiration**
  Excludes *aspiration of postnatal stomach contents (770.85, 770.86)*
  meconium passage during delivery (763.84)
  meconium staining (779.84)
  Coding Clinic: 2005, Q4, P83-89

770.10 **Fetal and newborn aspiration, unspecified** N

770.11 **Meconium aspiration without respiratory symptoms** N
Meconium aspiration NOS

770.12 **Meconium aspiration with respiratory symptoms** ✎ N
Meconium aspiration pneumonia
Meconium aspiration pneumonitis
Meconium aspiration syndrome NOS
  Use additional code to identify any secondary pulmonary hypertension (416.8), if applicable
  (Ex) 516.61-516.69, 768.5-768.6, 768.9-770.86, 770.89-770.9, 779.81-779.84, 779.89

770.13 **Aspiration of clear amniotic fluid without respiratory symptoms** N
Aspiration of clear amniotic fluid NOS

770.14 **Aspiration of clear amniotic fluid with respiratory symptoms** ✎ N
Aspiration of clear amniotic fluid with pneumonia
Aspiration of clear amniotic fluid with pneumonitis
  Use additional code to identify any secondary pulmonary hypertension (416.8), if applicable
  (Ex) 516.61-516.69, 768.5-768.6, 768.9-770.86, 770.89-770.9, 779.81-779.84, 779.89

770.15 **Aspiration of blood without respiratory symptoms** N
Aspiration of blood NOS

N Newborn: 0   **P** Pediatric: 0–17   **M** Maternity: 12–55   **A** Adult: 15–124   ♀ Females Only   ♂ Males Only
(Ex) CC/MCC Exclusions   ✎ Complication\Comorbidity   ◆ Major C\C   Present on Admission Requirement   Hospital-Acquired Condition

933

770.16 Aspiration of blood with respiratory symptoms N
Aspiration of blood with pneumonia
Aspiration of blood with pneumonitis
Use additional code to identify any secondary pulmonary hypertension (416.8), if applicable
(Ex:) 516.61-516.69, 768.5-768.6, 768.9-770.86, 770.89-770.9, 779.81-779.84, 779.89

770.17 Other fetal and newborn aspiration without respiratory symptoms N

770.18 Other fetal and newborn aspiration with respiratory symptoms N
Other aspiration pneumonia
Other aspiration pneumonitis
Use additional code to identify any secondary pulmonary hypertension (416.8), if applicable
(Ex:) 516.61-516.69, 768.5-768.6, 768.9-770.86, 770.89-770.9, 779.81-779.84, 779.89

770.2 Interstitial emphysema and related conditions N
Pneumomediastinum originating in the perinatal period
Pneumopericardium originating in the perinatal period
Pneumothorax originating in the perinatal period
(Ex:) 516.61-516.69, 768.5-768.6, 768.9-770.86, 770.89-770.9, 779.81-779.84, 779.89

770.3 Pulmonary hemorrhage N
Hemorrhage:
alveolar (lung) originating in the perinatal period
intra-alveolar (lung) originating in the perinatal period
massive pulmonary originating in the perinatal period
(Ex:) 516.61-516.69, 768.5-768.6, 768.9-770.86, 770.89-770.9, 779.81-779.84, 779.89

770.4 Primary atelectasis N
Failure of lungs to expand properly at birth
Pulmonary immaturity NOS
(Ex:) 516.61-516.69, 768.5-768.6, 768.9-770.86, 770.89-770.9, 779.81-779.84, 779.89

770.5 Other and unspecified atelectasis N
Atelectasis:
NOS originating in the perinatal period
partial originating in the perinatal period
secondary originating in the perinatal period
Pulmonary collapse originating in the perinatal period
(Ex:) 516.61-516.69, 768.5-768.6, 768.9-770.86, 770.89-770.9, 779.81-779.84, 779.89

770.6 Transitory tachypnea of newborn N
Idiopathic tachypnea of newborn
Wet lung syndrome
Excludes *respiratory distress syndrome (769)*
Coding Clinic: 2009, Q3, P17x2; 1993, Q3, P7x2; 1989, Q1, P10

770.7 Chronic respiratory disease arising in the perinatal period
Bronchopulmonary dysplasia
Interstitial pulmonary fibrosis of prematurity
Wilson-Mikity syndrome
(Ex:) 516.61-516.69, 768.5-768.6, 768.9-770.86, 770.89-770.9, 779.81-779.84, 779.89
Coding Clinic: 2011, Q1, P17; 1991, Q2, P19; 1986, Nov-Dec, P11-12

770.8 Other respiratory problems after birth
Excludes *mixed metabolic and respiratory acidosis of newborn (775.81)*
Coding Clinic: 2005, Q4, P83-89; 2002, Q4, P65-66; 1998, Q2, P10; 1996, Q2, P10-11

770.81 Primary apnea of newborn N
Apneic spells of newborn NOS
Essential apnea of newborn
Sleep apnea of newborn
(Ex:) 770.82-770.83, 770.87-770.9, 786.03

770.82 Other apnea of newborn N
Obstructive apnea of newborn
(Ex:) 770.81-770.83, 770.87-770.9, 786.03
Coding Clinic: 2010, Q4, P98

770.83 Cyanotic attacks of newborn N
(Ex:) 770.81-770.83, 770.87-770.9, 782.5, 786.03

770.84 Respiratory failure of newborn N
Excludes *respiratory distress syndrome (769)*
(Ex:) 516.61-516.69, 768.5-768.6, 768.9-770.86, 770.89-770.9, 779.81-779.84, 779.89

770.85 Aspiration of postnatal stomach contents without respiratory symptoms N
Aspiration of postnatal stomach contents NOS

770.86 Aspiration of postnatal stomach contents with respiratory symptoms N
Aspiration of postnatal stomach contents with pneumonia
Aspiration of postnatal stomach contents with pneumonitis
Use additional code to identify any secondary pulmonary hypertension (416.8), if applicable
(Ex:) 768.5-768.6, 768.9-770.86, 770.89-770.9, 779.81-779.84, 779.89

770.87 Respiratory arrest of newborn N
(Ex:) 770.11, 770.13, 770.15, 770.17, 770.6, 770.81-770.85, 770.88-770.9, 779.85, 786.03, 799.1

770.88 Hypoxemia of newborn N
Hypoxia NOS, in liveborn infant

770.89 Other respiratory problems after birth N
Coding Clinic: 2009, Q3, P17

770.9 Unspecified respiratory condition of fetus and newborn N

771 Infections specific to the perinatal period
Includes infections acquired before or during birth or via the umbilicus or during the first 28 days after birth
Excludes *congenital pneumonia (770.0)*
congenital syphilis (090.0–090.9)
infant botulism (040.41)
maternal infectious disease as a cause of mortality or morbidity in fetus or newborn, but fetus or newborn not manifesting the disease (760.2)
ophthalmia neonatorum due to gonococcus (098.40)
other infections not specifically classified to this category
Coding Clinic: 2005, Q1, P10

771.0 Congenital rubella N
Congenital rubella pneumonitis
(Ex:) 771.0-771.2, 779.81-779.84, 779.89

771.1 Congenital cytomegalovirus infection N
Congenital cytomegalic inclusion disease
(Ex:) 771.0-771.2, 779.81-779.84, 779.89

771.2 Other congenital infections N
Congenital: herpes simplex, listeriosis, malaria
Congenital: toxoplasmosis, tuberculosis
(Ex:) 013.60-013.66, 046.2, 046.71-046.8, 048-049.0, 049.8, 052.0, 052.2, 054.3, 054.74, 056.01, 057.8-058.29, 059.00-059.9, 062.0-064, 066.2-066.49, 072.2, 073.7, 075, 078.3, 079.82, 079.99, 081.9, 083.9, 084.6, 090.41, 094.81, 117.5, 124, 130.0, 290.12, 323.01-323.9, 341.1, 382.4, 487.8, 488.09, 488.19, 488.89, 710.0, 771.2, 984.9

771.3 Tetanus neonatorum N
Tetanus omphalitis
Excludes *hypocalcemic tetany (775.4)*
(Ex:) 771.3, 779.81-779.84, 779.89

771.4 Omphalitis of the newborn N
Infection: navel cord
Infection: umbilical stump
Excludes *tetanus omphalitis (771.3)*
(Ex:) 771.89
Coding Clinic: 2009, Q4, P113

771.5 Neonatal infective mastitis N
Excludes *noninfective neonatal mastitis (778.7)*
(Ex:) 771.89

771.6 Neonatal conjunctivitis and dacryocystitis   N
Ophthalmia neonatorum NOS

> **Excludes** *ophthalmia neonatorum due to gonococcus (098.40)*

771.7 Neonatal Candida infection   N
Neonatal moniliasis
Thrush in newborn

● **771.8 Other infections specific to the perinatal period**
Use additional code to identify organism or specific
infection

771.81 Septicemia [sepsis] of newborn 🔍   N
Use additional code to identify severe sepsis
(995.92) and any associated acute organ
dysfunction, if applicable
(Ex:) 771.4-771.89, 776.0-776.9, 779.81-779.84, 779.89

OGCR Section I.C.15.j

> 771.81, Septicemia [sepsis] of newborn, should
> be assigned with a secondary code from
> category 041, Bacterial infections in conditions
> classified elsewhere and of unspecified site, to
> identify the organism.

771.82 Urinary tract infection of newborn 🔍   N
(Ex:) 041.9, 590.00-590.9, 593.89-593.9, 595.0-595.81, 595.89-595.9,
599.0, 596.81, 599.9 771.89, 788.1, 996.64

771.83 Bacteremia of newborn 🔍   N
(Ex:) 771.4-771.89, 776.0-776.9, 779.81-779.84, 779.89

771.89 Other infections specific to the perinatal period 🔍🔍N
Intra-amniotic infection of fetus NOS
Infection of newborn NOS
(Ex:) 003.1, 020.2, 022.3, 036.2, 038.0-038.9, 040.89-041.9, 054.5,
139.8, 771.82-771.89, 779.9, 790.7
Coding Clinic: 2005, Q1, P10

● **772 Fetal and neonatal hemorrhage**

> **Excludes** *fetal hematologic conditions complicating pregnancy*
> *(678.0)*
> *hematological disorders of fetus and newborn*
> *(776.0–776.9)*

772.0 Fetal blood loss affecting newborn   N
Fetal blood loss from:
cut end of co-twin's cord
placenta
ruptured cord
vasa previa
Fetal exsanguination
Fetal hemorrhage into:
co-twin
mother's circulation

● **772.1 Intraventricular hemorrhage**
Intraventricular hemorrhage from any perinatal cause
Coding Clinic: 1992, Q3, P8; 1988, Q4, P8

772.10 Unspecified grade 🔍   N
(Ex:) 772.0-772.2, 772.8-772.9, 776.0-776.9, 779.81-779.84, 779.89

772.11 Grade I 🔍   N
Bleeding into germinal matrix
(Ex:) 772.0-772.2, 772.8-772.9, 776.0-776.9, 779.81-779.84, 779.89

772.12 Grade II 🔍   N
Bleeding into ventricle
(Ex:) 772.0-772.2, 772.8-772.9, 776.0-776.9, 779.81-779.84, 779.89

772.13 Grade III 🔍   N
Bleeding with enlargement of ventricle
(Ex:) 772.0-772.2, 772.8-772.9, 776.0-776.9, 779.81-779.84, 779.89
Coding Clinic: 2001, Q4, P50-51

772.14 Grade IV 🔍   N
Bleeding into cerebral cortex
(Ex:) 772.0-772.2, 772.8-772.9, 776.0-776.9, 779.81-779.84, 779.89

772.2 Subarachnoid hemorrhage 🔍   N
Subarachnoid hemorrhage from any perinatal cause

> **Excludes** *subdural and cerebral hemorrhage (767.0)*

(Ex:) 772.0-772.2, 772.8-772.9, 776.0-776.9, 779.7-779.84, 779.89

772.3 Umbilical hemorrhage after birth   N
Slipped umbilical ligature

772.4 Gastrointestinal hemorrhage 🔍   N

> **Excludes** *swallowed maternal blood (777.3)*

(Ex:) 772.0, 772.4-772.5, 772.8-772.9, 776.0-776.9, 779.81-779.84, 779.89

772.5 Adrenal hemorrhage 🔍   N
(Ex:) 772.0, 772.4-772.5, 772.8-772.9, 776.0-776.9, 779.81-779.84, 779.89

772.6 Cutaneous hemorrhage   N
Bruising in fetus or newborn
Ecchymoses in fetus or newborn
Petechiae in fetus or newborn
Superficial hematoma in fetus or newborn

772.8 Other specified hemorrhage of fetus or newborn   N

> **Excludes** *hemorrhagic disease of newborn (776.0)*
> *pulmonary hemorrhage (770.3)*

772.9 Unspecified hemorrhage of newborn   N

● **773 Hemolytic disease of fetus or newborn, due to isoimmunization**
Also known as erythroblastosis fetalis as a result of Rh blood factor
incompatibilities between mother (Rh negative) and fetus (Rh
positive)

773.0 Hemolytic disease due to Rh isoimmunization   N
Anemia due to RH:
antibodies
isoimmunization
maternal/fetal incompatibility
Erythroblastosis (fetalis) due to RH:
antibodies
isoimmunization
maternal/fetal incompatibility
Hemolytic disease (fetus) (newborn) due to RH:
antibodies
isoimmunization
maternal/fetal incompatibility
Jaundice due to RH:
antibodies
isoimmunization
maternal/fetal incompatibility
Rh hemolytic disease
Rh isoimmunization

773.1 Hemolytic disease due to ABO isoimmunization   N
ABO hemolytic disease
ABO isoimmunization
Anemia due to ABO:
antibodies
isoimmunization
maternal/fetal incompatibility
Erythroblastosis (fetalis) due to ABO:
antibodies
isoimmunization
maternal/fetal incompatibility
Hemolytic disease (fetus) (newborn) due to ABO:
antibodies
isoimmunization
maternal/fetal incompatibility
Jaundice due to ABO:
antibodies
isoimmunization
maternal/fetal incompatibility
Coding Clinic: 2003, Q2, P14-15; 1992, Q3, P8-9

773.2 Hemolytic disease due to other and unspecified
isoimmunization   N
Erythroblastosis (fetalis) (neonatorum) NOS
Hemolytic disease (fetus) (newborn) NOS
Jaundice or anemia due to other and unspecified
blood-group incompatibility
Coding Clinic: 1994, Q1, P13

773.3 Hydrops fetalis due to isoimmunization 🔍   N

> Use additional code, if desired, to identify type of
> isoimmunization (773.0–773.2)

(Ex:) 773.0-773.5, 779.81-779.84, 779.89

773.4 Kernicterus due to isoimmunization 🔍   N

> Use additional code, if desired, to identify type of
> isoimmunization (773.0–773.2)

(Ex:) 773.0-773.5, 779.81-779.84, 779.89

773.5 Late anemia due to isoimmunization   N

N Newborn: 0   P Pediatric: 0–17   M Maternity: 12–55   A Adult: 15–124   ♀ Females Only   ♂ Males Only

(Ex:) CC/MCC Exclusions   🔍 Complication\Comorbidity   🔍 Major C\C   🔍 Present on Admission Requirement   🔍 Hospital-Acquired Condition   935

● **774   Other perinatal jaundice**

▷ *774.0   Perinatal jaundice from hereditary hemolytic anemias*   N
   Code first underlying disease (282.0–282.9)

774.1   Perinatal jaundice from other excessive hemolysis   N
   Fetal or neonatal jaundice from:
      bruising
      drugs or toxins transmitted from mother
      infection
      polycythemia
      swallowed maternal blood
   Use additional code to identify cause
   Excludes   jaundice due to isoimmunization (773.0–773.2)

774.2   Neonatal jaundice associated with preterm delivery   N
   Hyperbilirubinemia of prematurity
   Jaundice due to delayed conjugation associated with
      preterm delivery
   Coding Clinic: 1994, Q1, P13; 1991, Q3, P21

● **774.3   Neonatal jaundice due to delayed conjugation from other causes**
   774.30   Neonatal jaundice due to delayed conjugation, cause unspecified   N

▷ **774.31   *Neonatal jaundice due to delayed conjugation in diseases classified elsewhere***   N
      Code first underlying diseases, as:
         congenital hypothyroidism (243)
         Crigler-Najjar syndrome (277.4)
         Gilbert's syndrome (277.4)

   774.39   Other   N
      Jaundice due to delayed conjugation from causes,
         such as:
         breast milk inhibitors
         delayed development of conjugating system

774.4   Perinatal jaundice due to hepatocellular damage 🔖   N
   Fetal or neonatal hepatitis
   Giant cell hepatitis
   Inspissated bile syndrome
   Ⓔⓧ 774.0-774.7, 779.81-779.84, 779.89

▷ *774.5   Perinatal jaundice from other causes*   N
   Code first underlying cause, as:
      congenital obstruction of bile duct (751.61)
      galactosemia (271.1)
      mucoviscidosis (277.00–277.09)

774.6   Unspecified fetal and neonatal jaundice   N
   Icterus neonatorum
   Neonatal hyperbilirubinemia (transient)
   Physiologic jaundice NOS in newborn
   Excludes   that in preterm infants (774.2)
   Coding Clinic: 1994, Q1, P13

774.7   Kernicterus not due to isoimmunization 🔖   N
   Bilirubin encephalopathy
   Kernicterus of newborn NOS
   Excludes   kernicterus due to isoimmunization (773.4)
   Ⓔⓧ 774.0-774.7, 779.81-779.84, 779.89

● **775   Endocrine and metabolic disturbances specific to the fetus and newborn**
   Includes   transitory endocrine and metabolic disturbances
      caused by the infant's response to maternal
      endocrine and metabolic factors, its removal
      from them, or its adjustment to extrauterine
      existence

775.0   Syndrome of "infant of a diabetic mother"   N
   Maternal diabetes mellitus affecting fetus or newborn
      (with hypoglycemia)
   Coding Clinic: 2004, Q1, P7-8x3

775.1   Neonatal diabetes mellitus 🔖   N
   Diabetes mellitus syndrome in newborn infant
   Ⓔⓧ 775.0-775.7, 775.9, 779.81-779.84, 779.89

775.2   Neonatal myasthenia gravis 🔖   N
   Ⓔⓧ 775.0-775.7, 775.9, 779.81-779.84, 779.89

775.3   Neonatal thyrotoxicosis 🔖   N
   Neonatal hyperthyroidism (transient)
   Ⓔⓧ 775.0-775.7, 775.9, 779.81-779.84, 779.89

775.4   Hypocalcemia and hypomagnesemia of newborn 🔖   N
   Cow's milk hypocalcemia
   Hypocalcemic tetany, neonatal
   Neonatal hypoparathyroidism
   Phosphate-loading hypocalcemia
   Ⓔⓧ 775.0-775.7, 775.9, 779.81-779.84, 779.89

775.5   Other transitory neonatal electrolyte disturbances   N
   Dehydration, neonatal
   Coding Clinic: 2010, Q1, P12; 2009, Q3, P18; 2008, Q4, P139-140;
      2005, Q1, P9-10

775.6   Neonatal hypoglycemia   N
   Excludes   infant of mother with diabetes mellitus (775.0)

775.7   Late metabolic acidosis of newborn 🔖   N
   Ⓔⓧ 775.0-775.7, 775.9, 779.81-779.84, 779.89

● **775.8   Other neonatal endocrine and metabolic disturbances**
   775.81   Other acidosis of newborn 🔖   N
      Acidemia NOS of newborn
      Acidosis of newborn NOS
      Mixed metabolic and respiratory acidosis of
         newborn
      Ⓔⓧ 775.5, 775.7, 775.9

   775.89   Other neonatal endocrine and metabolic disturbances 🔖   N
      Amino-acid metabolic disorders described as
         transitory
      Ⓔⓧ 775.0-775.7, 775.9

775.9   Unspecified endocrine and metabolic disturbances specific to the fetus and newborn   N

● **776   Hematological disorders of newborn**
   Includes   disorders specific to the newborn though possibly
      originating in utero
   Excludes   fetal hematologic conditions (678.0)

776.0   Hemorrhagic disease of newborn 🔖   N
   Hemorrhagic diathesis of newborn
   Vitamin K deficiency of newborn
   Excludes   fetal or neonatal hemorrhage (772.0–772.9)
   Ⓔⓧ 776.0-776.9, 779.81-779.84, 779.89

776.1   Transient neonatal thrombocytopenia 🔖   N
   *Lack of sufficient numbers of circulating thrombocytes
      (platelets)*
   Neonatal thrombocytopenia due to:
      exchange transfusion
      idiopathic maternal thrombocytopenia
      isoimmunization
   Ⓔⓧ 776.0-776.9, 779.81-779.84, 779.89

776.2   Disseminated intravascular coagulation in newborn 🔖   N
   Ⓔⓧ 776.0-776.9, 779.81-779.84, 779.89

776.3   Other transient neonatal disorders of coagulation 🔖   N
   Transient coagulation defect, newborn
   Ⓔⓧ 776.0-776.9, 779.81-779.84, 779.89

776.4   Polycythemia neonatorum   N
   Excess number of thrombocytes (platelets)
   Plethora of newborn
   Polycythemia due to:
      donor twin transfusion
      maternal-fetal transfusion

776.5   Congenital anemia 🔖   N
   Anemia following fetal blood loss
   Excludes   anemia due to isoimmunization
      (773.0–773.2, 773.5)
      hereditary hemolytic anemias (282.0–282.9)
   Ⓔⓧ 280.0-282.3, 282.5-285.9, 289.9, 517.3, 776.5-776.6

776.6   Anemia of prematurity 🔖   N
   Ⓔⓧ 280.0-282.3, 282.5-285.9, 289.9, 517.3, 776.5-776.6

776.7   Transient neonatal neutropenia 🔖   N
   Isoimmune neutropenia
   Low levels of white blood cells
   Maternal transfer neutropenia
   Excludes   congenital neutropenia (nontransient) (288.01)
   Ⓔⓧ 280.1-281.9, 282.5-282.63, 282.69-282.7, 283.0, 283.11, 284.01-285.0,
      285.21-285.9, 289.9, 776.7-776.9

776.8   Other specified transient hematological disorders   N

776.9   Unspecified hematological disorder specific to newborn   N

◀ New   ◀▥ Revised   ~~deleted~~ Deleted   Excludes   Includes   Use additional   Code first   Omit code
● Unacceptable Principal Diagnosis   ● Use Additional Digit(s)   ▷ Manifestation Code   OGCR Official Guidelines   Coding Clinic

936

● **777** **Perinatal disorders of digestive system**

   Includes   disorders specific to the fetus and newborn

   Excludes   *intestinal obstruction classifiable to 560.0–560.9*

  777.1 **Meconium obstruction**   N

       Congenital fecaliths

        Stoney feces formations

       Delayed passage of meconium

       Meconium ileus NOS

       Meconium plug syndrome

       Excludes *meconium ileus in cystic fibrosis (277.01)*

  777.2 **Intestinal obstruction due to inspissated milk**   N

       Being thickened, dried, or made less fluid

  777.3 **Hematemesis and melena due to swallowed maternal blood**   N

       Swallowed blood syndrome in newborn

       Excludes *that not due to swallowed maternal blood (772.4)*

  777.4 **Transitory ileus of newborn** 🔒   N

       Excludes *Hirschsprung's disease (751.3)*

       Ⓔⓧ 777.1-777.9

● **777.5** **Necrotizing enterocolitis in newborn**

  777.50 **Necrotizing enterocolitis in newborn, unspecified** 🔒   N

       Necrotizing enterocolitis in newborn, NOS

       Ⓔⓧ 777.1-777.9, 779.81-779.84, 779.89

  777.51 **Stage I necrotizing enterocolitis in newborn** 🔒   N

       Necrotizing enterocolitis without pneumatosis, without perforation

       Ⓔⓧ 777.1-777.9, 779.81-779.84, 779.89

  777.52 **Stage II necrotizing enterocolitis in newborn** 🔒   N

       Necrotizing enterocolitis with pneumatosis, without perforation

       Ⓔⓧ 777.1-777.9, 779.81-779.84, 779.89

  777.53 **Stage III necrotizing enterocolitis in newborn** 🔒   N

       Necrotizing enterocolitis with perforation

       Necrotizing enterocolitis with pneumatosis and perforation

       Ⓔⓧ 777.1-777.9, 779.81-779.84, 779.89

       Coding Clinic: 2008, Q4, P138-140

  777.6 **Perinatal intestinal perforation** 🔒   N

       Meconium peritonitis

       Ⓔⓧ 777.1-777.9, 779.81-779.84, 779.89

  777.8 **Other specified perinatal disorders of digestive system**   N

       Coding Clinic: 2010, Q4, P98

  777.9 **Unspecified perinatal disorder of digestive system**   N

● **778** **Conditions involving the integument and temperature regulation of fetus and newborn**

  778.0 **Hydrops fetalis not due to isoimmunization** 🔒   N

       Idiopathic hydrops

       Severe, life-threatening problem of edema (swelling) in fetus and newborn

       Excludes *hydrops fetalis due to isoimmunization (773.3)*

       Ⓔⓧ 778.0, 779.81-779.84, 779.89

  778.1 **Sclerema neonatorum** 🔒   N

       Ⓔⓧ 778.1, 778.5

  778.2 **Cold injury syndrome of newborn**   N

  778.3 **Other hypothermia of newborn**   N

  778.4 **Other disturbances of temperature regulation of newborn**   N

       Dehydration fever in newborn

       Environmentally induced pyrexia

       Hyperthermia in newborn

       Transitory fever of newborn

  778.5 **Other and unspecified edema of newborn** 🔒   N

       Edema neonatorum

       Ⓔⓧ 778.1-778.5

  778.6 **Congenital hydrocele**

       Congenital hydrocele of tunica vaginalis

  778.7 **Breast engorgement in newborn**   N

       Noninfective mastitis of newborn

       Excludes *infective mastitis of newborn (771.5)*

  778.8 **Other specified conditions involving the integument of fetus and newborn**   N

       Urticaria neonatorum

       Skin rash

       Excludes *impetigo neonatorum (684)*

                  pemphigus neonatorum (684)

  778.9 **Unspecified condition involving the integument and temperature regulation of fetus and newborn**   N

● **779** **Other and ill-defined conditions originating in the perinatal period**

  779.0 **Convulsions in newborn** 🔒   N

       Fits in newborn

       Seizures in newborn

       Ⓔⓧ 779.0-779.1, 779.81-779.84, 779.89

       Coding Clinic: 1984, Nov-Dec, P11

  779.1 **Other and unspecified cerebral irritability in newborn**   N

  779.2 **Cerebral depression, coma, and other abnormal cerebral signs** 🔒   N

       Cerebral ischemia NOS of newborn

       CNS dysfunction in newborn NOS

       Excludes *cerebral ischemia due to birth trauma (767.0)*

                  intrauterine cerebral ischemia (768.2–768.9)

                  intraventricular hemorrhage (772.10–772.14)

       Ⓔⓧ 779.0-779.2

● **779.3** **Disorder of stomach function and feeding problems in newborn**

       Coding Clinic: 1989, Q2, P15

  779.31 **Feeding problems in newborn**   N

       Slow feeding in newborn

       Excludes *feeding problem in child over 28 days old (783.3)*

       Coding Clinic: 2012, Q3, P7; 2009, Q4, P113

  779.32 **Bilious vomiting in newborn** 🔒   N

       Excludes *bilious vomiting in child over 28 days old (787.04)*

       Ⓔⓧ 779.32-779.33

  779.33 **Other vomiting in newborn**   N

       Regurgitation of food in newborn

       Excludes *vomiting in child over 28 days old (536.2, 787.01-787.03, 787.04)*

  779.34 **Failure to thrive in newborn**   N

       Excludes *failure to thrive in child over 28 days old (783.41)*

  779.4 **Drug reactions and intoxications specific to newborn** 🔒   N

       Gray syndrome from chloramphenicol administration in newborn

       Excludes *fetal alcohol syndrome (760.71)*

                  reactions and intoxications from maternal opiates and tranquilizers (763.5)

       Ⓔⓧ 779.4-779.5

  779.5 **Drug withdrawal syndrome in newborn** 🔒   N

       Drug withdrawal syndrome in infant of dependent mother

       Excludes *fetal alcohol syndrome (760.71)*

       Ⓔⓧ 779.4-779.5

       Coding Clinic: 1994, Q3, P6

  779.6 **Termination of pregnancy (fetus)**   N

       Fetal death due to:

         induced abortion

         termination of pregnancy

       Excludes *spontaneous abortion (fetus) (761.8)*

  779.7 **Periventricular leukomalacia** 🔒   N

       Ⓔⓧ 772.0-772.2, 772.8-772.9, 776.0-776.9, 779.7-779.84, 779.89

       Coding Clinic: 2001, Q4, P50-51

(side tab) **CERTAIN CONDITIONS ORIGINATING IN THE PERINATAL PERIOD (760–779)**

N Newborn: 0   **P** Pediatric: 0–17   **M** Maternity: 12–55   **A** Adult: 15–124   ♀ Females Only   ♂ Males Only

Ⓔⓧ CC/MCC Exclusions   🔒 Complication\Comorbidity   🔒 Major C\C   🔒 Present on Admission Requirement   🔒 Hospital-Acquired Condition   **937**

● **779.8**   **Other specified conditions originating in the perinatal period**
Coding Clinic: 2006, Q1, P18; 2002, Q4, P67; 1994, Q1, P15

     779.81   **Neonatal bradycardia**   N

         Excludes   *abnormality in fetal heart rate or rhythm complicating labor and delivery (763.81–763.83)*
                bradycardia due to birth asphyxia (768.5–768.9)

     779.82   **Neonatal tachycardia**   N

         Excludes   *abnormality in fetal heart rate or rhythm complicating labor and delivery (763.81–763.83)*

     779.83   **Delayed separation of umbilical cord**   N
         Coding Clinic: 2003, Q4, P71

     779.84   **Meconium staining**   N

         Excludes   *meconium aspiration (770.11, 770.12)*
                meconium passage during delivery (763.84)
         Coding Clinic: 2005, Q4, P83-89x2

     779.85   **Cardiac arrest of newborn**   N
         (Ex) 779.85

     779.89   **Other specified conditions originating in the perinatal period**   N

         Use additional code to specify condition

         Coding Clinic: 2012, Q3, P5; 2011, Q3, P3-4; 2005, Q2, P15-16; Q1, P9

         OGCR   Section I.C.15.a.2

         If the index does not provide a specific code for a perinatal condition, assign code 779.89 followed by the code from another chapter that specifies the condition.

779.9   **Unspecified condition originating in the perinatal period**   N
     Congenital debility NOS
     Stillbirth NEC

◀ New   ◀|||| Revised   ~~deleted~~ Deleted   Excludes   Includes   Use additional   Code first   Omit code
● Unacceptable Principal Diagnosis   ● Use Additional Digit(s)   ▷ Manifestation Code   OGCR Official Guidelines   Coding Clinic

16. SYMPTOMS, SIGNS, AND ILL-DEFINED CONDITIONS (780–799)

This section includes symptoms, signs, abnormal results of laboratory or other investigative procedures, and ill-defined conditions regarding which no diagnosis classifiable elsewhere is recorded.

Signs and symptoms that point rather definitely to a given diagnosis are assigned to some category in the preceding part of the classification. In general, categories 780–796 include the more ill-defined conditions and symptoms that point with perhaps equal suspicion to two or more diseases or to two or more systems of the body, and without the necessary study of the case to make a final diagnosis. Practically all categories in this group could be designated as "not otherwise specified," or as "unknown etiology," or as "transient." The Alphabetic Index should be consulted to determine which symptoms and signs are to be allocated here and which to more specific sections of the classification; the residual subcategories numbered .9 are provided for other relevant symptoms which cannot be allocated elsewhere in the classification.

The conditions and signs or symptoms included in categories 780–796 consist of: (a) cases for which no more specific diagnosis can be made even after all facts bearing on the case have been investigated; (b) signs or symptoms existing at the time of initial encounter that proved to be transient and whose causes could not be determined; (c) provisional diagnoses in a patient who failed to return for further investigation or care; (d) cases referred elsewhere for investigation or treatment before the diagnosis was made; (e) cases in which a more precise diagnosis was not available for any other reason; (f) certain symptoms which represent important problems in medical care and which it might be desired to classify in addition to a known cause.

SYMPTOMS (780–789)

● **780 General symptoms**

● **780.0 Alteration of consciousness**

> **Excludes** *alteration of consciousness due to:*
> *intracranial injuries (850.0-854.19)*
> *skull fractures (800.00-801.99,*
> *803.00-804.99)*
> *coma:*
> *diabetic (249.2–249.3, 250.2–250.3)*
> *hepatic (572.2)*
> *originating in the perinatal period (779.2)*

780.01 Coma 🔗
> Ex: 070.0-070.9, 249.00-251.3, 338.0-338.4, 348.81-348.9, 349.89-349.9, 430-432.9, 572.2, 780.01-780.09, 780.2, 780.4, 780.64-780.65, 780.91-780.99, 799.81-799.89, 800.00-801.99, 803.00-804.96, 850.0-852.19, 852.21-854.19
> Coding Clinic: 2013, Q3, P11; 2012, Q1, P14; 1996, Q3, P16

780.02 Transient alteration of awareness

780.03 Persistent vegetative state 🔗
> Ex: 070.0-070.9, 249.00-251.3, 338.0-338.4, 348.81-348.9, 349.89-349.9, 430-432.9, 572.2, 780.01-780.09, 780.2, 780.4, 780.64-780.65, 780.91-780.99, 799.81-799.89, 800.00-801.99, 803.00-804.96, 850.0-852.19, 852.21-854.19

780.09 Other

Drowsiness	Somnolence
Semicoma	Stupor
	Unconsciousness

780.1 Hallucinations 🔗
Hallucinations:
> NOS
> auditory
> gustatory
> olfactory
> tactile

> **Excludes** *those associated with mental disorders, as*
> *functional psychoses (295.0–298.9)*
> *organic brain syndromes (290.0–294.9,*
> *310.0–310.9)*
> *visual hallucinations (368.16)*
> Ex: 338.0-338.4, 780.1, 780.4, 780.64-780.65, 780.91-780.99, 799.81-799.89

780.2 Syncope and collapse

Blackout	(Near) (Pre)syncope
Fainting	Vasovagal attack

> **Excludes** *carotid sinus syncope (337.0)*
> *heat syncope (992.1)*
> *neurocirculatory asthenia (306.2)*
> *orthostatic hypotension (458.0)*
> *shock NOS (785.50)*
> Coding Clinic: 2002, Q1, P6; 2000, Q3, P12; 1995, Q4, P50-51; Q3, P14; 1992, Q3, P16; 1990, Q1, P9; 1985, Nov-Dec, P12

● **780.3 Convulsions**

> **Excludes** *convulsions:*
> *epileptic (345.10–345.91)*
> *in newborn (779.0)*
> Coding Clinic: 2012, Q2, P9-10; 1984, Nov-Dec, P11

780.31 Febrile convulsions (simple), unspecified 🔗
Febrile seizures NOS
> Ex: 338.0-338.4, 345.00-345.91, 348.81, 348.89-348.9, 349.89-349.9, 779.0-779.1, 780.31-780.39, 780.64-780.65, 780.91-780.99, 799.81-799.89
> Coding Clinic: 2005, Q3, P12-13; 1987, Nov-Dec, P11

780.32 Complex febrile convulsions 🔗
Febrile seizure:
> atypical
> complex
> complicated

> **Excludes** *status epilepticus (345.3)*
> Ex: 338.0-338.4, 345.00-345.91, 348.81, 348.89-348.9, 349.89-349.9, 779.0-779.1, 780.31-780.39, 780.64-780.65, 780.91-780.99, 799.81-799.89
> Coding Clinic: 2006, Q4, P106-107

780.33 Post traumatic seizures 🔗
> **Excludes** *post traumatic epilepsy (345.00-345.91)*
> Ex: 249.60-249.61, 250.60-250.63, 345.00-345.91, 348.81, 348.89-348.9, 349.89-349.9, 780.33
> Coding Clinic: 2010, Q4, P93

780.39 Other convulsions
Convulsive disorder NOS
Fits NOS
Recurrent convulsions NOS
Seizure NOS
Seizures NOS
> Coding Clinic: 2012, Q2, P9-10; 2008, Q1, P17; 2006, Q3, P22; 2004, Q4, P50-52; 2003, Q1, P7; 1998, Q4, P39-40; 1997, Q2, P8; Q1, P12-13; 1994, Q3, P9; 1993, Q1, P24; 1987, Nov-Dec, P12; 1985, July-Aug, P10; 1984, May-June, P14

780.4 Dizziness and giddiness
Light-headedness
Vertigo NOS

> **Excludes** *Méniére's disease and other specified vertiginous*
> *syndromes (386.0–386.9)*
> Coding Clinic: 2003, Q2, P11; 2000, Q3, P12; 1997, Q2, P9-10; 1991, Q2, P17

● **780.5 Sleep disturbances**

> **Excludes** *circadian rhythm sleep disorders (327.30–327.39)*
> *organic hypersomnia (327.10–327.19)*
> *organic insomnia (327.00–327.09)*
> *organic sleep apnea (327.20–327.29)*
> *organic sleep related movement disorders*
> *(327.51–327.59)*
> *parasomnias (327.40–327.49)*
> *that of nonorganic origin (307.40–307.49)*

780.50 Sleep disturbance, unspecified

780.51 Insomnia with sleep apnea, unspecified
> Coding Clinic: 1993, Q1, P28-29

780.52 Insomnia, unspecified

780.53 Hypersomnia with sleep apnea, unspecified
> Coding Clinic: 1993, Q1, P28-29

780.54 Hypersomnia, unspecified

780.55 Disruptions of 24 hour sleep wake cycle, unspecified

N Newborn: 0	**P** Pediatric: 0–17	**M** Maternity: 12–55	**A** Adult: 15–124	♀ Females Only	♂ Males Only
Ex CC/MCC Exclusions	🔗 Complication\Comorbidity	Major C\C	🔗 Present on Admission Requirement		🔗 Hospital-Acquired Condition

780.56 Dysfunctions associated with sleep stages or arousal from sleep

780.57 Unspecified sleep apnea
Coding Clinic: 2001, Q1, P6-7; 1997, Q1, P5; 1993, Q1, P28-29

780.58 Sleep related movement disorder, unspecified
Excludes restless legs syndrome (333.94)
Coding Clinic: 2004, Q4, P95-96

780.59 Other

● **780.6 Fever and other physiologic disturbances of temperature regulation**
Excludes effects of reduced environmental temperature (991.0-991.9)
effects of heat and light (992.0-992.9)
fever, chills or hypothermia associated with confirmed infection – code to infection
Coding Clinic: 2008, Q4, P140-143; 2005, Q3, P16-17; 2000, Q3, P13; 1991, Q2, P8x2; 1990, Q1, P8; 1985, July-Aug, P13

780.60 Fever, unspecified
Chills with fever
Fever NOS
Fever of unknown origin (FUO)
Hyperpyrexia NOS
Pyrexia NOS
Pyrexia of unknown origin
Excludes chills without fever (780.64)
neonatal fever (778.4)
pyrexia of unknown origin (during):
in newborn (778.4)
labor (659.2)
the puerperium (672)

▷ **780.61 Fever presenting with conditions classified elsewhere**
Code first underlying condition when associated fever is present, such as with:
leukemia (conditions classifiable to 204-208)
neutropenia (288.00-288.09)
sickle-cell disease (282.60-282.69)
Coding Clinic: 2012, Q2, P18-19; 2008, Q4, P140-143

780.62 Postprocedural fever
Excludes posttransfusion fever (780.66)
postvaccination fever (780.63)

780.63 Postvaccination fever
Postimmunization fever

780.64 Chills (without fever)
Chills NOS
Excludes chills with fever (780.60)

780.65 Hypothermia not associated with low environmental temperature
Excludes hypothermia:
associated with low environmental temperature (991.6)
due to anesthesia (995.89)
of newborn (778.2, 778.3)

780.66 Febrile nonhemolytic transfusion reaction
FNHTR   Posttransfusion fever

● **780.7 Malaise and fatigue**
Excludes debility, unspecified (799.3)
fatigue (during):
combat (308.0–308.9)
heat (992.6)
pregnancy (646.8)
neurasthenia (300.5)
senile asthenia (797)

780.71 Chronic fatigue syndrome
Coding Clinic: 1998, Q4, P48-49

780.72 Functional quadriplegia 🔒
Complete immobility due to severe physical disability or frailty
Excludes hysterical paralysis (300.11)
immobility syndrome (728.3)
neurologic quadriplegia (344.00-344.09)
quadriplegia NOS (344.00)
Ⓔⓧ 249.60-249.61, 249.80-249.91, 250.60-250.63, 250.80-250.93, 342.00-344.9, 348.81, 348.89-348.9, 349.89-349.9, 742.59-742.9, 780.72
Coding Clinic: 2008, Q4, P143

780.79 Other malaise and fatigue
Asthenia NOS
Lethargy
Postviral (asthenic) syndrome
Tiredness
Coding Clinic: 2004, Q4, P77-78; 2000, Q1, P6

780.8 Generalized hyperhidrosis
Diaphoresis   Secondary hyperhidrosis
Excessive sweating
Excludes focal (localized) (primary) (secondary) hyperhidrosis (705.21–705.22)
Frey's syndrome (705.22)

● **780.9 Other general symptoms**
Excludes hypothermia:
NOS (accidental) (991.6)
due to anesthesia (995.89)
memory disturbance as part of a pattern of mental disorder
of newborn (778.2–778.3)
Coding Clinic: 2002, Q4, P67-68

780.91 Fussy infant (baby)   P

780.92 Excessive crying of infant (baby)   N
Excludes excessive crying of child, adolescent or adult (780.95)
Coding Clinic: 2005, Q4, P89-90

780.93 Memory loss
Amnesia (retrograde)
Memory loss NOS
Excludes memory loss due to:
intracranial injuries (850.0-854.19)
skull fractures (800.00-801.99, 803.00-804.99)
mild memory disturbance due to organic brain damage (310.89)
transient global amnesia (437.7)
Coding Clinic: 2003, Q4, P71

780.94 Early satiety
Coding Clinic: 2003, Q4, P72

780.95 Excessive crying of child, adolescent, or adult
Excludes excessive crying of infant (baby) (780.92)
Coding Clinic: 2005, Q4, P89-90

780.96 Generalized pain
Pain NOS

780.97 Altered mental status
Change in mental status
Excludes altered level of consciousness (780.01–780.09)
altered mental status due to known condition - code to condition
delirium NOS (780.09)
Coding Clinic: 2006, Q4, P107-108; 1993, Q3, P11

780.99 Other general symptoms
Coding Clinic: 2003, Q4, P103-104; 1999, Q4, P10; 1985, Nov-Dec, P12

● **781** **Symptoms involving nervous and musculoskeletal systems**

    Excludes *depression NOS (311)*
        disorders specifically relating to:
          back (724.0–724.9)
          hearing (388.0–389.9)
          joint (718.0–719.9)
          limb (729.0–729.9)
          neck (723.0–723.9)
          vision (368.0–369.9)
        pain in limb (729.5)

  781.0 **Abnormal involuntary movements**
    Abnormal head movements
    Fasciculation
    Spasms NOS
    Tremor NOS

    Excludes *abnormal reflex (796.1)*
        chorea NOS (333.5)
        infantile spasms (345.60–345.61)
        spastic paralysis (342.1, 343.0–344.9)
        specified movement disorders classifiable to 333
          (333.0–333.9)
        that of nonorganic origin (307.2–307.3)

  781.1 **Disturbances of sensation of smell and taste**
    Anosmia   Parosmia
    Parageusia

  781.2 **Abnormality of gait**
    Gait:
      ataxic
      paralytic
      spastic
      staggering

    Excludes *ataxia:*
        NOS (781.3)
        difficulty in walking (719.7)
        locomotor (progressive) (094.0)
    Coding Clinic: 2011, Q1, P9; 2005, Q2, P6-7; 2004, Q2, P15

  781.3 **Lack of coordination**
    Ataxia NOS
    Muscular incoordination

    Excludes *ataxic gait (781.2)*
        cerebellar ataxia (334.0–334.9)
        difficulty in walking (719.7)
        vertigo NOS (780.4)
    Coding Clinic: 2004, Q4, P50-52; 1997, Q3, P12-13

  781.4 **Transient paralysis of limb** 🔖
    Monoplegia, transient NOS

    Excludes *paralysis (342.0–344.9)*
    (Ex) 781.4, 781.94

  781.5 **Clubbing of fingers**

  781.6 **Meningismus** 🔖
    Dupre's syndrome   Meningism
    (Ex) 781.6, 781.94
    Coding Clinic: 2000, Q3, P13

  781.7 **Tetany** 🔖
    Carpopedal spasm

    Excludes *tetanus neonatorum (771.3)*
        tetany:
        hysterical (300.11)
        newborn (hypocalcemic) (775.4)
        parathyroid (252.1)
        psychogenic (306.0)
    (Ex) 037, 332.0-333.93, 333.99-334.4, 338.0-338.4, 342.10-342.12, 771.3,
        780.64-780.65, 780.91-780.99, 781.7, 799.81-799.89

  781.8 **Neurologic neglect syndrome** 🔖
    Asomatognosia   Left-sided neglect
    Hemi-akinesia   Sensory extinction
    Hemi-inattention   Sensory neglect
    Hemispatial neglect   Visuospatial neglect

    Excludes *visuospatial deficit (799.53)*
    (Ex) 781.8-781.92, 781.94-781.99

● **781.9** **Other symptoms involving nervous and musculoskeletal systems**

  781.91 **Loss of height**
    Excludes *osteoporosis (733.00–733.09)*

  781.92 **Abnormal posture**

  781.93 **Ocular torticollis**
    Coding Clinic: 2002, Q4, P68; Q4, P68

  781.94 **Facial weakness**
    Facial droop

    Excludes *facial weakness due to late effect of*
          cerebrovascular accident (438.83)
    Coding Clinic: 2003, Q4, P72

  781.99 **Other symptoms involving nervous and musculoskeletal systems**

● **782** **Symptoms involving skin and other integumentary tissue**

    Excludes *symptoms relating to breast (611.71–611.79)*

  782.0 **Disturbance of skin sensation**
    Anesthesia of skin
    Burning or prickling sensation
    Hyperesthesia
    Hypoesthesia
    Numbness
    Paresthesia
    Tingling
    Coding Clinic: 2009, Q4, P113

  782.1 **Rash and other nonspecific skin eruption**
    Exanthem
    Excludes *vesicular eruption (709.8)*

  782.2 **Localized superficial swelling, mass, or lump**
    Subcutaneous nodules
    Excludes *localized adiposity (278.1)*

  782.3 **Edema**
    Anasarca
    Dropsy
    Localized edema NOS

    Excludes *ascites (789.51–789.59)*
        edema of:
        newborn NOS (778.5)
        pregnancy (642.0–642.9, 646.1)
        fluid retention (276.69)
        hydrops fetalis (773.3, 778.0)
        hydrothorax (511.81–511.89)
        nutritional edema (260, 262)
    Coding Clinic: 2000, Q2, P18

  782.4 **Jaundice, unspecified, not of newborn** 🔖
    Cholemia NOS   Icterus NOS

    Excludes *due to isoimmunization (773.0–773.2, 773.4)*
        jaundice in newborn (774.0–774.7)
    (Ex) 774.0-774.7, 782.4, 782.9

  782.5 **Cyanosis**
    Excludes *newborn (770.83)*

● **782.6** **Pallor and flushing**

  782.61 **Pallor**

  782.62 **Flushing**
    Excessive blushing

  782.7 **Spontaneous ecchymoses**
    Petechiae

    Excludes *ecchymosis in fetus or newborn (772.6)*
        purpura (287.0–287.9)

  782.8 **Changes in skin texture**
    Induration of skin   Thickening of skin

  782.9 **Other symptoms involving skin and integumentary tissues**

N Newborn: 0   **P** Pediatric: 0–17   **M** Maternity: 12–55   **A** Adult: 15–124   ♀ Females Only   ♂ Males Only

(Ex) CC/MCC Exclusions   🔖 Complication\Comorbidity   🔖 Major C\C   🔖 Present on Admission Requirement   🔖 Hospital-Acquired Condition   **941**

SYMPTOMS, SIGNS, AND ILL-DEFINED CONDITIONS (780–799)

● **783 Symptoms concerning nutrition, metabolism, and development**

    783.0 Anorexia

        Loss of appetite

        Excludes *anorexia nervosa (307.1)*
                    loss of appetite of nonorganic origin (307.59)

    783.1 Abnormal weight gain

        Excludes *excessive weight gain in pregnancy (646.1)*
                    obesity (278.00)
                    morbid (278.01)

● **783.2 Abnormal loss of weight and underweight**

        Use additional code to identify Body Mass Index (BMI), if known (V85.0–V85.54)

        783.21 Loss of weight

        783.22 Underweight

    783.3 Feeding difficulties and mismanagement

        Feeding problem (elderly) (infant)

        Excludes *feeding disturbance or problems:*
                    in newborn (779.31-779.34)
                    of nonorganic origin (307.50–307.59)

        Coding Clinic: 1997, Q3, P12-13; 1994, Q2, P10-11

● **783.4 Lack of expected normal physiological development in childhood**

        Excludes *delay in sexual development and puberty (259.0)*
                    gonadal dysgenesis (758.6)
                    pituitary dwarfism (253.3)
                    slow fetal growth and fetal malnutrition (764.00–764.99)
                    specific delays in mental development (315.0–315.9)

        Coding Clinic: 1997, Q3, P5

        783.40 Lack of normal physiological development, unspecified

           Inadequate development
           Lack of development

        783.41 Failure to thrive   P

           Failure to gain weight

           Excludes *failure to thrive in newborn (779.34)*

           Coding Clinic: 2003, Q1, P12

        783.42 Delayed milestones   P

           Late talker   Late walker

        783.43 Short stature

           Growth failure   Lack of growth
           Growth retardation   Physical retardation

           Coding Clinic: 2004, Q2, P3

    783.5 Polydipsia

        Excessive thirst

    783.6 Polyphagia

        Excessive eating
        Hyperalimentation NOS

        Excludes *disorders of eating of nonorganic origin (307.50–307.59)*

    783.7 Adult failure to thrive   A

    783.9 Other symptoms concerning nutrition, metabolism, and development

        Hypometabolism

        Excludes *abnormal basal metabolic rate (794.7)*
                    dehydration (276.51)
                    other disorders of fluid, electrolyte, and acid-base balance (276.0–276.9)

        Coding Clinic: 2004, Q2, P3

● **784 Symptoms involving head and neck**

     Excludes *encephalopathy NOS (348.30)*
                specific symptoms involving neck classifiable to 723 (723.0–723.9)

    784.0 Headache

        Facial pain   Pain in head NOS

        Excludes *atypical face pain (350.2)*
                    migraine (346.0–346.9)
                    tension headache (307.81)

        Coding Clinic: 2006, Q3, P22; Q2, P17-18; 2000, Q3, P13; 1992, Q3, P14; 1990, Q1, P9

    784.1 Throat pain

        Excludes *dysphagia (787.20–787.29)*
                    neck pain (723.1)
                    sore throat (462)
                    chronic (472.1)

    784.2 Swelling, mass, or lump in head and neck

        Space-occupying lesion, intracranial NOS

        Coding Clinic: 2003, Q1, P8

    784.3 Aphasia ◐

        Excludes *aphasia due to late effects of cerebrovascular disease (438.11)*
                    developmental aphasia (315.31)

        (Ex): 315.31, 315.35, 432.0-434.91, 436, 784.3-784.59

        Coding Clinic: 2010, Q3, P5; 2004, Q4, P77-78; 1998, Q4, P87; 1997, Q3, P12-13

● **784.4 Voice and resonance disorders**

        784.40 Voice and resonance disorder, unspecified

        784.41 Aphonia

           Loss of voice

        784.42 Dysphonia

           Hoarseness

        784.43 Hypernasality

        784.44 Hyponasality

        784.49 Other voice and resonance disorders

           Change in voice

● **784.5 Other speech disturbance**

        Excludes *speech disorder due to late effect of cerebrovascular accident (438.10-438.19)*
                    stuttering (315.35)

        784.51 Dysarthria

           Excludes *dysarthria due to late effect of cerebrovascular accident (438.13)*

        ▷ **784.52 Fluency disorder in conditions classified elsewhere**

           Stuttering in conditions classified elsewhere

           Code first underlying disease or condition, such as:
           Parkinson's disease (332.0)

           Excludes *adult onset fluency disorder (307.0)*
                    childhood onset fluency disorder (315.35)
                    fluency disorder due to late effect of cerebrovascular accident (438.14)

        784.59 Other speech disturbance

           Dysphasia   Speech disturbance NOS
           Slurred speech

● **784.6 Other symbolic dysfunction**

        Excludes *developmental learning delays (315.0–315.9)*

        784.60 Symbolic dysfunction, unspecified

        784.61 Alexia and dyslexia

           Alexia (with agraphia)
           Loss of ability to read

        784.69 Other

           Acalculia
           Difficulty performing simple mathematical tasks
           Agnosia
           Loss of ability to recognize objects, persons, sounds, shapes, or smells
           Agraphia NOS
           Apraxia
           Loss of the ability to execute or carry out movements

◀ New   ⬴ Revised   ~~deleted~~ Deleted   Excludes   Includes   Use additional   Code first   Omit code
● Unacceptable Principal Diagnosis   ● Use Additional Digit(s)   ▷ Manifestation Code   OGCR Official Guidelines   Coding Clinic

942

784.7 Epistaxis
Hemorrhage from nose
Nosebleed
Coding Clinic: 2004, Q3, P7; 1995, Q1, P5

784.8 Hemorrhage from throat
Excludes *hemoptysis (786.30-786.39)*
Spitting blood

● **784.9 Other symptoms involving head and neck**

784.91 Postnasal drip

784.92 Jaw pain
Mandibular pain   Maxilla pain
Excludes *temporomandibular joint arthralgia
(524.62)*
Coding Clinic: 2010, Q4, P94

784.99 Other symptoms involving head and neck
Choking sensation
Feeling of foreign body in throat
Halitosis
Bad breath
Mouth breathing
Sneezing
Excludes *foreign body in throat (933.0)*

● **785 Symptoms involving cardiovascular system**
Excludes *heart failure NOS (428.9)*

785.0 Tachycardia, unspecified
Rapid heart beat
Excludes *neonatal tachycardia (779.82)
paroxysmal tachycardia (427.0–427.2)*
Coding Clinic: 2003, Q2, P11

785.1 Palpitations
Awareness of heart beat
Excludes *specified dysrhythmias (427.0–427.9)*

785.2 Undiagnosed cardiac murmurs
Heart murmur NOS

785.3 Other abnormal heart sounds
Cardiac dullness, increased or decreased
Friction fremitus, cardiac
Precordial friction

785.4 Gangrene 🔖
Gangrene: Gangrene:
  NOS   Gangrenous cellulitis
  spreading cutaneous Phagedena
Rapidly spreading destructive ulceration of soft tissue
Code first any associated underlying condition
Excludes *gangrene of certain sites-see Alphabetic Index
gangrene with atherosclerosis of the extremities
(440.24)
gas gangrene (040.0)*
(Ex:) 338.0-338.4, 440.24, 780.64-780.65, 780.91-780.99, 785.4, 799.81-799.89
Coding Clinic: 2004, Q1, P14-15; 1994, Q3, P5; 1990, Q3, P15; 1986, Mar-April, P12

● **785.5 Shock without mention of trauma**

785.50 Shock, unspecified 🔖
Failure of peripheral circulation
Resulting in significant blood pressure drop
(Ex:) 338.0-338.4, 780.64-780.65, 780.91-780.99, 785.50-785.59, 785.9, 799.81-799.89

785.51 Cardiogenic shock 🔖
MCC only for patients discharged alive
(Ex:) 338.0-338.4, 780.64-780.65, 780.91-780.99, 785.50-785.59, 785.9, 799.81-799.89
Coding Clinic: 2008, Q4, P180-182; 2005, Q3, P14

▷ **785.52 Septic shock** 🔖
Endotoxic   Gram-negative
Code first underlying infection
Use additional code, if applicable, to identify
systemic inflammatory response syndrome
due to infectious process with organ
dysfunction (995.92)
(Ex:) 338.0-338.4, 780.64-780.65, 780.91-780.99, 785.50-785.59, 785.9, 799.81-799.89
Coding Clinic: 2013, Q2, P21; 2010, Q2, P4; 2005, Q3, P23; Q2, P18-20x2; 2003, Q4, P73, 79-81

785.59 Other 🔖
Shock:
hypovolemic
Decreased blood volume
Excludes *shock (due to):
anesthetic (995.4)
anaphylactic (995.0)
due to serum (999.41-999.49)
electric (994.8)
following abortion (639.5)
lightning (994.0)
obstetrical (669.1)
postoperative (998.00-998.09)
traumatic (958.4)*
MCC only for patients discharged alive
(Ex:) 338.0-338.4, 780.64-780.65, 780.91-780.99, 785.50-785.59, 785.9, 799.81-799.89
Coding Clinic: 2008, Q4, P97-100

785.6 Enlargement of lymph nodes
Lymphadenopathy   "Swollen glands"
Excludes *lymphadenitis (chronic) (289.1–289.3)
acute (683)*

785.9 Other symptoms involving cardiovascular system
Bruit (arterial)   Weak pulse

● **786 Symptoms involving respiratory system and other chest symptoms**

● **786.0 Dyspnea and respiratory abnormalities**

786.00 Respiratory abnormality, unspecified

786.01 Hyperventilation
Excludes *hyperventilation, psychogenic (306.1)*

786.02 Orthopnea

786.03 Apnea
Excludes *apnea of newborn (770.81, 770.82)
sleep apnea (780.51, 780.53, 780.57)*
Coding Clinic: 1998, Q2, P10

786.04 Cheyne-Stokes respiration 🔖
*Abnormal pattern of breathing with gradually
increasing and decreasing tidal volume with
some periods of apnea*
(Ex:) 518.81-518.84, 519.8-519.9, 786.03-786.04, 799.1

786.05 Shortness of breath
Coding Clinic: 1999, Q4, P25; Q1, P6

786.06 Tachypnea
Excludes *transitory tachypnea of newborn (770.6)*
Coding Clinic: 2011, Q1, P17

786.07 Wheezing
Excludes *asthma (493.00–493.92)*

786.09 Other
Respiratory:
distress
insufficiency
Excludes *respiratory distress:
following trauma and surgery
(518.52)
newborn (770.89)
respiratory failure (518.81,
518.83–518.84)
newborn (770.84)
syndrome (newborn) (769)
adult (518.52)*
Coding Clinic: 1990, Q1, P9

786.1 Stridor
Excludes *congenital laryngeal stridor (748.3)*

786.2 Cough
Excludes *cough:
psychogenic (306.1)
smokers' (491.0)
with hemorrhage (786.39)*
Coding Clinic: 1995, Q4, P50; 1990, Q1, P8

SYMPTOMS, SIGNS, AND ILL-DEFINED CONDITIONS (780–799)

● **786.3 Hemoptysis**
    Coding Clinic: 2006, Q2, P17

    786.30 Hemoptysis, unspecified 🔁
        Pulmonary hemorrhage NOS
        (Ex) 786.30-786.4, 799.82

    786.31 Acute idiopathic pulmonary hemorrhage in   P
            infants [AIPHI] 🔁
        Acute idiopathic pulmonary hemorrhage in
            infant over 28 days old

        Excludes *pulmonary hemorrhage of newborn*
                      under 28 days old (770.3)
                      von Willebrand's disease (286.4)
        (Ex) 786.30-786.4, 799.82

    786.39 Other hemoptysis 🔁
        Cough with hemorrhage
        (Ex) 786.30-786.4, 799.82

786.4 Abnormal sputum
    Abnormal:
        amount of sputum
        color of sputum
        odor of sputum
    Excessive sputum

● **786.5 Chest pain**

    786.50 Chest pain, unspecified
        Coding Clinic: 2007, Q1, P19; 2006, Q2, P7-8; 2003, Q1, P6-7;
            2002, Q1, P4-5; 1999, Q4, P25-26; 1993, Q1, P25

    786.51 Precordial pain
        Coding Clinic: 1984, May-June, P11

    786.52 Painful respiration
        Pain:
            anterior chest wall
            pleuritic
            Pleurodynia

        Excludes *epidemic pleurodynia (074.1)*
        Coding Clinic: 1984, Nov-Dec, P17

    786.59 Other
        Discomfort in chest
        Pressure in chest
        Tightness in chest

        Excludes *pain in breast (611.71)*
        Coding Clinic: 2007, Q1, P19; 2002, Q1, P6

786.6 Swelling, mass, or lump in chest
    Excludes *lump in breast (611.72)*

786.7 Abnormal chest sounds
    Abnormal percussion, chest
    Friction sounds, chest
    Rales
        Wet rattling, clicking, crackling sounds on auscultation
    Tympany, chest
    Excludes *wheezing (786.07)*

786.8 Hiccough
    Excludes *psychogenic hiccough (306.1)*

786.9 Other symptoms involving respiratory system and chest
    Breath-holding spell

● **787 Symptoms involving digestive system**
    Excludes *constipation (564.0–564.9)*
                  pylorospasm (537.81)
                  congenital (750.5)

● **787.0 Nausea and vomiting**
    Emesis
    Excludes *hematemesis NOS (578.0)*
                  vomiting:
                      bilious, following gastrointestinal surgery
                          (564.3)
                      cyclical (536.2)
                          associated with migraine (346.2)
                          psychogenic (306.4)
                      excessive, in pregnancy (643.0–643.9)
                      fecal matter (569.87)
                      habit (536.2)
                      of newborn (779.32, 779.33)
                      persistent (536.2)
                      psychogenic NOS (307.54)

787.01 Nausea with vomiting
    Concurrent conditions
    Coding Clinic: 2003, Q1, P5

787.02 Nausea alone
    Separate condition
    Coding Clinic: 2000, Q3, P12; 1997, Q2, P9-10

787.03 Vomiting alone
    Separate condition
    Coding Clinic: 1985, Mar-April, P11

787.04 Bilious emesis
    Bilious vomiting
    Excludes *bilious emesis (vomiting) in newborn*
                  (779.32)

787.1 Heartburn
    Pyrosis   Waterbrash
    Excludes *dyspepsia or indigestion (536.8)*
    Coding Clinic: 2001, Q2, P6

● **787.2 Dysphagia**
    Code first, *if applicable, dysphagia due to late effect of*
        cerebrovascular accident (438.82)
    Coding Clinic: 2007, Q3, P8-9; 2003, Q4, P103-104, 109-110; 2001, Q2,
        P4-6; 1993, 5th Issue, P16; 1986, Nov-Dec, P10

    787.20 Dysphagia, unspecified
        Difficulty in swallowing NOS

    787.21 Dysphagia, oral phase

    787.22 Dysphagia, oropharyngeal phase
        Coding Clinic: 2007, Q4, P92-95

    787.23 Dysphagia, pharyngeal phase

    787.24 Dysphagia, pharyngoesophageal phase

    787.29 Other dysphagia
        Cervical dysphagia
        Neurogenic dysphagia

787.3 Flatulence, eructation, and gas pain
    Abdominal distention (gaseous)
    Bloating
    Tympanites (abdominal) (intestinal)
    Excludes *aerophagy (306.4)*

787.4 Visible peristalsis
    Hyperperistalsis

787.5 Abnormal bowel sounds
    Absent bowel sounds
    Hyperactive bowel sounds

● **787.6 Incontinence of feces**
    Encopresis NOS
    Incontinence of sphincter ani
    Excludes *that of nonorganic origin (307.7)*
    Coding Clinic: 1997, Q1, P9-10

    787.60 Full incontinence of feces
        Fecal incontinence NOS

    787.61 Incomplete defecation
        Excludes *constipation (564.00-564.09)*
                      fecal impaction (560.32)

    787.62 Fecal smearing
        Fecal soiling

    787.63 Fecal urgency

787.7 Abnormal feces
    Bulky stools
    Excludes *abnormal stool content (792.1)*
                  melena:
                      NOS (578.1)
                      newborn (772.4, 777.3)

◄ New   ◄▦ Revised   ~~deleted~~ Deleted   Excludes   Includes   Use additional   Code first   Omit code

● Unacceptable Principal Diagnosis ● Use Additional Digit(s) ▶ Manifestation Code   OGCR Official Guidelines   Coding Clinic

● **787.9 Other symptoms involving digestive system**

Excludes *gastrointestinal hemorrhage (578.0–578.9)*
intestinal obstruction (560.0–560.9)
specific functional digestive disorders:
esophagus (530.0–530.9)
stomach and duodenum (536.0–536.9)
those not elsewhere classified (564.0–564.9)

787.91 Diarrhea
Diarrhea NOS
Coding Clinic: 2010, Q2, P12; 2008, Q4, P97-100

787.99 Other
Change in bowel habits
Tenesmus (rectal)

● **788 Symptoms involving urinary system**

Excludes *hematuria (599.70–599.72)*
nonspecific findings on examination of the urine
(791.0–791.9)
small kidney of unknown cause (589.0–589.9)
uremia NOS (586)
urinary obstruction (599.60, 599.69)

788.0 Renal colic
Colic (recurrent) of:
kidney
ureter
Coding Clinic: 2004, Q3, P8

788.1 Dysuria
Painful urination   Strangury

● **788.2 Retention of urine**
Code first, if applicable, hyperplasia of prostate (600.0–600.9
with fifth-digit 1)
Coding Clinic: 2003, Q3, P13; 1994, Q1, P20; 1986, Sept-Oct, P12

788.20 Retention of urine, unspecified
Coding Clinic: 2013, Q1, P6; 2006, Q4, P93-95; 2004, Q2,
P18; 2003, Q3, P12; Q1, P6; 1996, Q3, P10-11; 1994,
Q3, P13

788.21 Incomplete bladder emptying

788.29 Other specified retention of urine

● **788.3 Urinary incontinence**

Excludes *functional urinary incontinence (788.91)*
that of nonorganic origin (307.6)
urinary incontinence associated with cognitive
impairment (788.91)
Code, if applicable, any causal condition first, such as:
congenital ureterocele (753.23)
genital prolapse (618.00–618.9)
hyperplasia of prostate (600.0–600.9 with fifth-digit 1)
Coding Clinic: 2005, Q3, P20

788.30 Urinary incontinence, unspecified
Enuresis NOS
Coding Clinic: 2009, Q1, P18; 1995, Q4, P72-73

788.31 Urge incontinence
Coding Clinic: 2000, Q1, P19-20

788.32 Stress incontinence, male ♂

Excludes *stress incontinence, female (625.6)*
Coding Clinic: 1995, Q4, P72-73

788.33 Mixed incontinence (female) (male)
Urge and stress

788.34 Incontinence without sensory awareness

788.35 Post-void dribbling

788.36 Nocturnal enuresis

788.37 Continuous leakage

788.38 Overflow incontinence
Coding Clinic: 2004, Q4, P96

788.39 Other urinary incontinence

● **788.4 Frequency of urination and polyuria**
Code first, if applicable, hyperplasia of prostate (600.0–600.9
with fifth-digit 1)

788.41 Urinary frequency
Frequency of micturition

788.42 Polyuria

788.43 Nocturia

788.5 Oliguria and anuria
Deficient secretion of urine
Suppression of urinary secretion

Excludes *that complicating:*
abortion (634–638 with .3, 639.3)
ectopic or molar pregnancy (639.3)
pregnancy, childbirth, or the puerperium
(642.0–642.9, 646.2)

● **788.6 Other abnormality of urination**
Code first, if applicable, hyperplasia of prostate (600.0–600.9
with fifth-digit 1)

788.61 Splitting of urinary stream
Intermittent urinary stream

788.62 Slowing of urinary stream
Weak stream

788.63 Urgency of urination

Excludes *urge incontinence (788.31, 788.33)*
Coding Clinic: 2003, Q4, P74

788.64 Urinary hesitancy

788.65 Straining on urination

788.69 Other

788.7 Urethral discharge
Penile discharge   Urethrorrhea

788.8 Extravasation of urine 🔗
Leakage, discharge
Ⓔ 788.8-788.99

● **788.9 Other symptoms involving urinary system**
Coding Clinic: 2005, Q1, P12-13

788.91 Functional urinary incontinence
Urinary incontinence due to cognitive
impairment, or severe physical disability or
immobility

Excludes *urinary incontinence due to physiologic*
condition (788.30-788.39)
Coding Clinic: 2008, Q4, P144-145

788.99 Other symptoms involving urinary system
Extrarenal uremia
Vesical:
pain
tenesmus

● **789 Other symptoms involving abdomen and pelvis**
The following fifth-digit subclassification is to be used for codes
789.0, 789.3, 789.4, 789.6

0	unspecified site	5	periumbilic
1	right upper quadrant	6	epigastric
2	left upper quadrant	7	generalized
3	right lower quadrant	9	other specified site
4	left lower quadrant		multiple sites

Excludes *symptoms referable to genital organs:*
female (625.0–625.9)
male (607.0–608.9)
psychogenic (302.70–302.79)

● **789.0 Abdominal pain**
[0-7,9]   Cramps, abdominal
Coding Clinic: 2002, Q1, P5; 1995, Q1, P3; 1990, Q2, P26

789.1 Hepatomegaly
Enlargement of liver

789.2 Splenomegaly
Enlargement of spleen

● **789.3 Abdominal or pelvic swelling, mass, or lump**
[0-7,9]   Diffuse or generalized swelling or mass:
abdominal NOS
umbilical

Excludes *abdominal distention (gaseous) (787.3)*
ascites (789.51–789.59)

● **789.4 Abdominal rigidity**
[0-7,9]

SYMPTOMS, SIGNS, AND ILL-DEFINED CONDITIONS (780–799)

N Newborn: 0   P Pediatric: 0–17   M Maternity: 12–55   A Adult: 15–124   ♀ Females Only   ♂ Males Only

Ⓔ CC/MCC Exclusions   🔗 Complication\Comorbidity   ⬥ Major C\C   Ⓟ Present on Admission Requirement   🔗 Hospital-Acquired Condition   **945**

SYMPTOMS, SIGNS, AND ILL-DEFINED CONDITIONS (780–799)

● **789.5 Ascites**
Fluid in peritoneal cavity
Coding Clinic: 2008, Q1, P16-18; 2007, Q4, P95-96; 2005, Q2, P8; 1989, Q4, P11

● **789.51 Malignant ascites** ℗
Code first malignancy, such as:
malignant neoplasm of ovary (183.0)
secondary malignant neoplasm of
retroperitoneum and peritoneum (197.6)
Ⓔ 338.0-338.4, 780.64-780.65, 780.91-780.99, 789.30-789.59, 789.9, 799.81-799.89
Coding Clinic: 2008, Q1, P16-17

789.59 Other ascites ℗
Ⓔ 338.0-338.4, 780.64-780.65, 780.91-780.99, 789.30-789.59, 789.9, 799.81-799.89

● **789.6 Abdominal tenderness**
[0-7,9] Rebound tenderness

789.7 Colic   P
Colic NOS   Infantile colic
Excludes colic in adult and child over 12 months old
(789.0)
renal colic (788.0)

789.9 Other symptoms involving abdomen and pelvis
Umbilical: Umbilical:
bleeding   discharge

NONSPECIFIC ABNORMAL FINDINGS (790–796)

● **790 Nonspecific findings on examination of blood**
Excludes abnormality of:
platelets (287.0–287.9)
thrombocytes (287.0–287.9)
white blood cells (288.00–288.9)

● **790.0 Abnormality of red blood cells**
Excludes anemia:
congenital (776.5)
newborn, due to isoimmunization
(773.0–773.2, 773.5)
of premature infant (776.6)
other specified types (280.0–285.9)
hemoglobin disorders (282.5–282.7)
polycythemia:
familial (289.6)
neonatorum (776.4)
secondary (289.0)
vera (238.4)

790.01 Precipitous drop in hematocrit ℗
Drop in hematocrit
Drop in hemoglobin
Decrease in red blood cells
Ⓔ 285.1, 285.3-285.9

790.09 Other abnormality of red blood cells
Abnormal red cell morphology NOS
Abnormal red cell volume NOS
Anisocytosis
Red blood cells of unequal size
Poikilocytosis
Red blood cells of abnormal shape

● **790.1 Elevated sedimentation rate**

● **790.2 Abnormal glucose**
Excludes diabetes mellitus (249.00–249.91,
250.00–250.93)
dysmetabolic syndrome X (277.7)
gestational diabetes (648.8)
glycosuria (791.5)
hypoglycemia (251.2)
that complicating pregnancy, childbirth, or the
puerperium (648.8)
Coding Clinic: 2012, Q1, P17; 2011, Q1, P10; 2003, Q4, P74-75

790.21 Impaired fasting glucose
Elevated fasting glucose

790.22 Impaired glucose tolerance test (oral)
Elevated glucose tolerance test

790.29 Other abnormal glucose
Abnormal glucose NOS
Abnormal non-fasting glucose
Hyperglycemia NOS
Pre-diabetes NOS
Coding Clinic: 2009, Q3, P18; 2005, Q2, P21-22; 2004, Q4, P53-56

790.3 Excessive blood level of alcohol
Elevated blood-alcohol

**790.4 Nonspecific elevation of levels of transaminase or lactic
acid dehydrogenase [LDH]**

790.5 Other nonspecific abnormal serum enzyme levels
Abnormal serum level of:
acid phosphatase
alkaline phosphatase
amylase
lipase
Excludes deficiency of circulating enzymes (277.6)

790.6 Other abnormal blood chemistry
Abnormal blood levels of:
cobalt
copper
iron
lead
lithium
magnesium
mineral
zinc
Excludes abnormality of electrolyte or acid-base balance
(276.0–276.9)
hypoglycemia NOS (251.2)
lead poisoning (984.0–984.9)
specific finding indicating abnormality of:
amino-acid transport and metabolism
(270.0–270.9)
carbohydrate transport and metabolism
(271.0–271.9)
lipid metabolism (272.0–272.9)
uremia NOS (586)
Coding Clinic: 2013, Q2, P13

790.7 Bacteremia ℗
Excludes bacteremia of newborn (771.83)
septicemia (038)
Use additional code to identify organism (041)
Ⓔ 338.0-338.4, 780.64-780.65, 780.91-780.99, 790.7-790.99, 799.81-799.89
Coding Clinic: 2003, Q2, P7-8

790.8 Viremia, unspecified
Coding Clinic: 1988, Q4, P10

● **790.9 Other nonspecific findings on examination of blood**

790.91 Abnormal arterial blood gases

790.92 Abnormal coagulation profile
Abnormal or prolonged:
bleeding time
coagulation time
partial thromboplastin time [PTT]
prothrombin time [PT]
Excludes coagulation (hemorrhagic) disorders
(286.0–286.9)
Coding Clinic: 1994, Q1, P22

790.93 Elevated prostate specific antigen [PSA] ♂   A
MCE: Questionable admission, principal diagnosis
only

790.94 Euthyroid sick syndrome

790.95 Elevated C-reactive protein (CRP)
Coding Clinic: 2004, Q4, P96-97

790.99 Other
Coding Clinic: 2012, Q3, P18; 2011, Q3, P4

● **791 Nonspecific findings on examination of urine**

> **Excludes** *hematuria NOS (599.70–599.72)*
> *specific findings indicating abnormality of:*
> *amino-acid transport and metabolism (270.0–270.9)*
> *carbohydrate transport and metabolism*
> *(271.0–271.9)*

791.0 Proteinuria
  Albuminuria
  Bence-Jones proteinuria

> **Excludes** *postural proteinuria (593.6)*
> *that arising during pregnancy or the puerperium*
> *(642.0–642.9, 646.2)*

  Coding Clinic: 2012, Q2, P19

791.1 Chyluria 🔓
  White milky urine

> **Excludes** *filarial (125.0–125.9)*

  (Ex) 338.0–338.4, 780.64–780.65, 780.91–780.99, 791.1, 791.9, 799.81–799.89

791.2 Hemoglobinuria

791.3 Myoglobinuria 🔓
  (Ex) 338.0–338.4, 780.64–780.65, 780.91–780.99, 791.2–791.3, 791.9,
  799.81–799.89

791.4 Biliuria

791.5 Glycosuria

> **Excludes** *renal glycosuria (271.4)*

791.6 Acetonuria
  Ketonuria

791.7 Other cells and casts in urine

791.9 Other nonspecific findings on examination of urine
  Crystalluria
  Elevated urine levels of:
    17-ketosteroids
    catecholamines
    indolacetic acid
    vanillylmandelic acid [VMA]
  Melanuria
  Coding Clinic: 2005, Q1, P12

● **792 Nonspecific abnormal findings in other body substances**

> **Excludes** *that in chromosomal analysis (795.2)*

792.0 Cerebrospinal fluid

792.1 Stool contents
  Abnormal stool color   Occult blood
  Fat in stool   Pus in stool
  Mucus in stool

> **Excludes** *blood in stool [melena] (578.1)*
> *newborn (772.4, 777.3)*

  Coding Clinic: 1992, Q2, P9-10; Q2, P9

792.2 Semen ♂
  Abnormal spermatozoa

> **Excludes** *azoospermia (606.0)*
> *oligospermia (606.1)*

792.3 Amniotic fluid ♀   M

792.4 Saliva

> **Excludes** *that in chromosomal analysis (795.2)*

792.5 Cloudy (hemodialysis) (peritoneal) dialysis effluent

792.9 Other nonspecific abnormal findings in body substances
  Peritoneal fluid   Synovial fluid
  Pleural fluid   Vaginal fluids

● **793 Nonspecific (abnormal) findings on radiological and other examination of body structure**

> **Includes** nonspecific abnormal findings of:
> thermography
> ultrasound examination [echogram]
> x-ray examination

> **Excludes** *abnormal results of function studies and radioisotope*
> *scans (794.0–794.9)*

793.0 Skull and head

> **Excludes** *nonspecific abnormal echoencephalogram*
> *(794.01)*

  Coding Clinic: 2006, Q3, P22

● **793.1 Lung field**

793.11 Solitary pulmonary nodule
  Coin lesion lung
  Solitary pulmonary nodule, subsegmental branch
    of the bronchial tree

793.19 Other nonspecific abnormal finding of lung field
  Pulmonary infiltrate NOS
  Shadow, lung
  Coding Clinic: 2011, Q4, P139

793.2 Other intrathoracic organ
  Abnormal:
    echocardiogram
    heart shadow
    ultrasound cardiogram
  Mediastinal shift
  Coding Clinic: 2012, Q1, P17

793.3 Biliary tract
  Nonvisualization of gallbladder

793.4 Gastrointestinal tract

793.5 Genitourinary organs
  Filling defect:
    bladder
    kidney
    ureter

793.6 Abdominal area, including retroperitoneum

793.7 Musculoskeletal system

● **793.8 Breast**

793.80 Abnormal mammogram, unspecified

793.81 Mammographic microcalcification

> **Excludes** *mammographic calcification (793.89)*
> *mammographic calculus (793.89)*

793.82 Inconclusive mammogram
  Dense breasts NOS
  Inconclusive mammogram NEC
  Inconclusive mammography due to dense breasts
  Inconclusive mammography NEC
  Coding Clinic: 2009, Q4, P113

793.89 Other (abnormal) findings on radiological examination of breast
  Mammographic calcification
  Mammographic calculus

● **793.9 Other**

> **Excludes** *abnormal finding by radioisotope localization of*
> *placenta (794.9)*

793.91 Image test inconclusive due to excess body fat
  Use additional code to identify Body Mass Index
    (BMI), if known (V85.0–V85.54)
  Coding Clinic: 2006, Q4, P109-110

793.99 Other nonspecific (abnormal) findings on radiological and other examinations of body structure
  Abnormal:
    placental finding by x-ray or ultrasound
      method
    radiological findings in skin and
      subcutaneous tissue

SYMPTOMS, SIGNS, AND ILL-DEFINED CONDITIONS (780–799)

N Newborn: 0   **P** Pediatric: 0–17   **M** Maternity: 12–55   **A** Adult: 15–124   ♀ Females Only   ♂ Males Only

(Ex) CC/MCC Exclusions   🔓 Complication\Comorbidity   🔓 Major C\C   🔓 Present on Admission Requirement   🔓 Hospital-Acquired Condition   **947**

● **794   Nonspecific abnormal results of function studies**

  Includes   radioisotope:
                 scans
                 uptake studies
             scintiphotography

● **794.0   Brain and central nervous system**

  794.00   Abnormal function study, unspecified

  794.01   Abnormal echoencephalogram

  794.02   Abnormal electroencephalogram [EEG]

  794.09   Other
             Abnormal brain scan

● **794.1   Peripheral nervous system and special senses**

  794.10   Abnormal response to nerve stimulation, unspecified

  794.11   Abnormal retinal function studies
             Abnormal electroretinogram [ERG]

  794.12   Abnormal electro-oculogram [EOG]

  794.13   Abnormal visually evoked potential

  794.14   Abnormal oculomotor studies

  794.15   Abnormal auditory function studies
             Coding Clinic: 2011, Q3, P3; 2004, Q1, P15-16

  794.16   Abnormal vestibular function studies

  794.17   Abnormal electromyogram [EMG]

          Excludes   *that of eye (794.14)*

  794.19   Other

● **794.2   Pulmonary**
          Abnormal lung scan
          Reduced:
             ventilatory capacity
             vital capacity

● **794.3   Cardiovascular**

  794.30   Abnormal function study, unspecified

  794.31   Abnormal electrocardiogram [ECG] [EKG]

          Excludes   *long QT syndrome (426.82)*

             Coding Clinic: 1985, Mar-April, P13

  794.39   Other
             Abnormal:
                ballistocardiogram
                phonocardiogram
                vectorcardiogram

794.4   Kidney
          Abnormal renal function test
          Coding Clinic: 2013, Q2, P13

794.5   Thyroid
          Abnormal thyroid:
             scan
             uptake

794.6   Other endocrine function study

794.7   Basal metabolism
          Abnormal basal metabolic rate [BMR]

794.8   Liver
          Abnormal liver scan

794.9   Other
          Bladder   Placenta
          Pancreas   Spleen

● **795   Other and nonspecific abnormal cytological, histological, immunological, and DNA test findings**

  Excludes   *abnormal cytologic smear of anus and anal HPV (796.70-796.79)*
               nonspecific abnormalities of red blood cells (790.01–790.09)

     Coding Clinic: 2002, Q4, P69-70

● **795.0   Abnormal Papanicolaou smear of cervix and cervical HPV**
          Abnormal thin preparation smear of cervix
          Abnormal cervical cytology

  Excludes   *abnormal cytologic smear of vagina and vaginal HPV (795.10-795.19)*
               carcinoma in situ of cervix (233.1)
               cervical intraepithelial neoplasia I (CIN I) (622.11)
               cervical intraepithelial neoplasia II (CIN II) (622.12)
               cervical intraepithelial neoplasia III (CIN III) (233.1)
               dysplasia (histologically confirmed) of cervix (uteri) NOS (622.10)
               mild cervical dysplasia (histologically confirmed) (622.11)
               moderate cervical dysplasia (histologically confirmed) (622.12)
               severe cervical dysplasia (histologically confirmed) (233.1)

     Coding Clinic: 2008, Q4, P145-148; 2004, Q4, P97-99

  795.00   Abnormal glandular Papanicolaou smear of cervix ♀
             Atypical endocervical cells NOS
             Atypical endometrial cells NOS
             Atypical cervical glandular cells NOS

  795.01   Papanicolaou smear of cervix with atypical squamous cells of undetermined significance (ASC-US) ♀
             Coding Clinic: 2006, Q2, P3,4

  795.02   Papanicolaou smear of cervix with atypical squamous cells cannot exclude high grade squamous intraepithelial lesion (ASC-H) ♀

  795.03   Papanicolaou smear of cervix with low grade squamous intraepithelial lesion (LGSIL) ♀

  795.04   Papanicolaou smear of cervix with high grade squamous intraepithelial lesion (HGSIL) ♀

  795.05   Cervical high risk human papillomavirus (HPV) DNA test positive ♀

  795.06   Papanicolaou smear of cervix with cytologic evidence of malignancy ♀

  795.07   Satisfactory cervical smear but lacking transformation zone ♀

  795.08   Unsatisfactory cervical cytology smear ♀
             Inadequate cervical cytology sample
             Coding Clinic: 2006, Q2, P3,4

  795.09   Other abnormal Papanicolaou smear of cervix and cervical HPV ♀
             Cervical low risk human papillomavirus (HPV) DNA test positive

          Use additional code for associated human papillomavirus (079.4)

          Excludes   *encounter for Papanicolaou cervical smear to confirm findings of recent normal smear following initial abnormal smear (V72.32)*

◀ New   ◀▥ Revised   ~~deleted~~ Deleted   Excludes   Includes   Use additional   Code first   Omit code
● Unacceptable Principal Diagnosis   ● Use Additional Digit(s)   ▶ Manifestation Code   OGCR Official Guidelines   Coding Clinic

948

● **795.1 Abnormal Papanicolaou smear of vagina and vaginal HPV**
Abnormal thin preparation smear of vagina NOS
Abnormal vaginal cytology NOS

Use additional code to identify acquired absence of uterus and cervix, if applicable (V88.01–V88.03)

Excludes *abnormal cytologic smear of cervix and cervical HPV (795.00–795.09)*
carcinoma in situ of vagina (233.31)
carcinoma in situ of vulva (233.32)
dysplasia (histologically confirmed) of vagina NOS (623.0, 233.31)
dysplasia (histologically confirmed) of vulva NOS (624.01, 624.02, 233.32)
mild vaginal dysplasia (histologically confirmed) (623.0)
mild vulvar dysplasia (histologically confirmed) (624.01)
moderate vaginal dysplasia (histologically confirmed) (623.0)
moderate vulvar dysplasia (histologically confirmed) (624.02)
severe vaginal dysplasia (histologically confirmed) (233.31)
severe vulvar dysplasia (histologically confirmed) (233.32)
vaginal intraepithelial neoplasia I (VAIN I) (623.0)
vaginal intraepithelial neoplasia II (VAIN II) (623.0)
vaginal intraepithelial neoplasia III (VAIN III) (233.31)
vulvar intraepithelial neoplasia I (VIN I) (624.01)
vulvar intraepithelial neoplasia II (VIN II) (624.02)
vulvar intraepithelial neoplasia III (VIN III) (233.32)
Coding Clinic: 2008, Q4, P145-148

795.10 Abnormal glandular Papanicolaou smear of vagina ♀
Atypical vaginal glandular cells NOS

795.11 Papanicolaou smear of vagina with atypical squamous cells of undetermined significance (ASC-US) ♀

795.12 Papanicolaou smear of vagina with atypical squamous cells cannot exclude high grade squamous intraepithelial lesion (ASC-H) ♀

795.13 Papanicolaou smear of vagina with low grade squamous intraepithelial lesion (LGSIL) ♀

795.14 Papanicolaou smear of vagina with high grade squamous intraepithelial lesion (HGSIL) ♀

795.15 Vaginal high risk human papillomavirus (HPV) DNA test positive ♀
Excludes *condyloma acuminatum (078.11)*
genital warts (078.11)

795.16 Papanicolaou smear of vagina with cytologic evidence of malignancy ♀
Coding Clinic: 2004, Q2, P11

795.18 Unsatisfactory vaginal cytology smear ♀
Inadequate vaginal cytology sample

795.19 Other abnormal Papanicolaou smear of vagina and vaginal HPV ♀
Vaginal low risk human papillomavirus (HPV) DNA test positive
Use additional code for associated human papillomavirus (079.4)

795.2 Nonspecific abnormal findings on chromosomal analysis
Abnormal karyotype

● **795.3 Nonspecific positive culture findings**
Positive culture findings in:
nose
sputum
throat
wound
Excludes *that of:*
blood (790.7–790.8)
urine (791.9)

795.31 Nonspecific positive findings for anthrax
Positive findings by nasal swab
Coding Clinic: 2002, Q4, P70

795.39 Other nonspecific positive culture findings
Excludes *colonization status (V02.0–V02.9)*

795.4 Other nonspecific abnormal histological findings

● **795.5 Nonspecific reaction to test for tuberculosis**

795.51 Nonspecific reaction to tuberculin skin test without active tuberculosis
Abnormal result of Mantoux test
PPD positive
Tuberculin (skin test) positive
Tuberculin (skin test) reactor
Excludes *nonspecific reaction to cell mediated immunity measurement of gamma interferon antigen response without active tuberculosis (795.52)*
Coding Clinic: 2011, Q4, P183

795.52 Nonspecific reaction to cell mediated immunity measurement of gamma interferon antigen response without active tuberculosis
Nonspecific reaction to QuantiFERON-TB test (QFT) without active tuberculosis
Excludes *nonspecific reaction to tuberculin skin test without active tuberculosis (795.51)*
positive tuberculin skin test (795.51)

795.6 False positive serological test for syphilis
False positive Wassermann reaction

● **795.7 Other nonspecific immunological findings**
Excludes *abnormal tumor markers (795.81–795.89)*
elevated prostate specific antigen [PSA] (790.93)
elevated tumor associated antigens (795.81–795.89)
isoimmunization, in pregnancy (656.1–656.2)
affecting fetus or newborn (773.0–773.2)

795.71 Nonspecific serologic evidence of human immunodeficiency virus [HIV]
Inconclusive human immunodeficiency virus [HIV] test (adult) (infant)
Note: This code is ONLY to be used when a test finding is reported as nonspecific. Asymptomatic positive findings are coded to V08. If any HIV infection symptom or condition is present, see code 042. Negative findings are not coded.
Excludes *acquired immunodeficiency syndrome [AIDS] (042)*
asymptomatic human immunodeficiency virus [HIV] infection status (V08)
HIV infection, symptomatic (042)
human immunodeficiency virus [HIV] disease (042)
positive (status) NOS (V08)

OGCR Section I.C.1.a.2.e
Patients with inconclusive HIV serology, but no definitive diagnosis or manifestations of the illness, may be assigned code 795.71, Inconclusive serologic test for Human Immunodeficiency Virus [HIV].

795.79 Other and unspecified nonspecific immunological findings
Raised antibody titer
Raised level of immunoglobulins
Coding Clinic: 1993, Q2, P6

N Newborn: 0   **P** Pediatric: 0–17   **M** Maternity: 12–55   **A** Adult: 15–124   ♀ Females Only   ♂ Males Only

(Ex) CC/MCC Exclusions   Complication\Comorbidity   Major C\C   Present on Admission Requirement   Hospital-Acquired Condition   **949**

SYMPTOMS, SIGNS, AND ILL-DEFINED CONDITIONS (780–799)

● **795.8 Abnormal tumor markers**
Elevated tumor associated antigens [TAA]
Elevated tumor specific antigens [TSA]

> **Excludes** *elevated prostate specific antigen [PSA] (790.93)*

> Coding Clinic: 2006, Q4, P111-112; 1993, Q1, P21-22; 1992, Q2, P11

     795.81 Elevated carcinoembryonic antigen [CEA]

     795.82 Elevated cancer antigen 125 [CA 125] ♀

     795.89 Other abnormal tumor markers

● **796 Other nonspecific abnormal findings**

     796.0 Nonspecific abnormal toxicological findings
Abnormal levels of heavy metals or drugs in blood, urine, or other tissue

> Use additional code for retained foreign body, if applicable, (V90.01-V90.9)

> **Excludes** *excessive blood level of alcohol (790.3)*

> Coding Clinic: 1997, Q1, P16

     796.1 Abnormal reflex

     796.2 Elevated blood pressure reading without diagnosis of hypertension

> **Note:** This category is to be used to record an episode of elevated blood pressure in a patient in whom no formal diagnosis of hypertension has been made, or as an incidental finding.

> MCE: Questionable admission, principal diagnosis only

> Coding Clinic: 2003, Q2, P11; 1993, 5th Issue, P6-7

> OGCR   Section I.C.7.a.8

> Assign code 796.2, Elevated blood pressure reading without diagnosis of hypertension, unless patient has an established diagnosis of hypertension. Assign code 642.3x for transient hypertension of pregnancy.

     796.3 Nonspecific low blood pressure reading

     796.4 Other abnormal clinical findings

> Coding Clinic: 1995, Q3, P13

     796.5 Abnormal finding on antenatal screening ♀   M

     796.6 Abnormal findings on neonatal screening   N

> **Excludes** *nonspecific serologic evidence of human immunodeficiency virus [HIV] (795.71)*

> Coding Clinic: 2004, Q4, P99-100

● **796.7 Abnormal cytologic smear of anus and anal HPV**

> **Excludes** *abnormal cytologic smear of cervix and cervical HPV (795.00-795.09)*
> *abnormal cytologic smear of vagina and vaginal HPV (795.10-795.19)*
> *anal intraepithelial neoplasia I (AIN I) (569.44)*
> *anal intraepithelial neoplasia II (AIN II) (569.44)*
> *anal intraepithelial neoplasia III (AIN III) (230.5, 230.6)*
> *carcinoma in situ of anus (230.5, 230.6)*
> *dysplasia (histologically confirmed) of anus NOS (569.44)*
> *mild anal dysplasia (histologically confirmed) (569.44)*
> *moderate anal dysplasia (histologically confirmed) (569.44)*
> *severe anal dysplasia (histologically confirmed) (230.5, 230.6)*

> Coding Clinic: 2008, Q4, P117-119

     796.70 Abnormal glandular Papanicolaou smear of anus
Atypical anal glandular cells NOS

     796.71 Papanicolaou smear of anus with atypical squamous cells of undetermined significance (ASC-US)

     796.72 Papanicolaou smear of anus with atypical squamous cells cannot exclude high grade squamous intraepithelial lesion (ASC-H)

     796.73 Papanicolaou smear of anus with low grade squamous intraepithelial lesion (LGSIL)

     796.74 Papanicolaou smear of anus with high grade squamous intraepithelial lesion (HGSIL)

     796.75 Anal high risk human papillomavirus (HPV) DNA test positive

     796.76 Papanicolaou smear of anus with cytologic evidence of malignancy

     796.77 Satisfactory anal smear but lacking transformation zone

     796.78 Unsatisfactory anal cytology smear
Inadequate anal cytology sample

     796.79 Other abnormal Papanicolaou smear of anus and anal HPV
Anal low risk human papillomavirus (HPV) DNA test positive

> Use additional code for associated human papillomavirus (079.4)

     796.9 Other

ILL-DEFINED AND UNKNOWN CAUSES OF MORBIDITY AND MORTALITY (797–799)

797 Senility without mention of psychosis

Frailty	Senile:
Old age	debility
Senescence	exhaustion
Senile asthenia	

> **Excludes** *senile psychoses (290.0–290.9)*

● **798 Sudden death, cause unknown**

     798.0 Sudden infant death syndrome *(SIDS)*   P
Cot death
Crib death
Sudden death of nonspecific cause in infancy

● **798.1 Instantaneous death**

● **798.2 Death occurring in less than 24 hours from onset of symptoms, not otherwise explained**
Death known not to be violent or instantaneous, for which no cause could be discovered
Died without sign of disease

● **798.9 Unattended death**
Death in circumstances where the body of the deceased was found and no cause could be discovered
Found dead

● **799 Other ill-defined and unknown causes of morbidity and mortality**

● **799.0 Asphyxia and hypoxemia**

> **Excludes** *asphyxia and hypoxemia (due to):*
> *carbon monoxide (986)*
> *hypercapnia (786.09)*
> *inhalation of food or foreign body (932–934.9)*
> *newborn (768.0–768.9)*
> *traumatic (994.7)*

> Coding Clinic: 2005, Q4, P90; 1990, Q1, P20

     799.01 Asphyxia
> (Ex:) 338.0-338.4, 518.81-518.84, 780.64-780.65, 780.91-780.99, 798.0, 799.01-799.1, 799.81-799.89

     799.02 Hypoxemia
> Coding Clinic: 2009, Q3, P18; 2006, Q2, P24,25

     799.1 Respiratory arrest
Cardiorespiratory failure

> **Excludes** *cardiac arrest (427.5)*
> *failure of peripheral circulation (785.50)*
> *respiratory distress:*
> *NOS (786.09)*
> *acute (518.82)*
> *following trauma or surgery (518.52)*
> *newborn (770.89)*
> *syndrome (newborn) (769)*
> *adult (following trauma or surgery) (518.52)*
> *other (518.82)*
> *respiratory failure (518.81, 518.83–518.84)*
> *newborn (770.84)*
> *respiratory insufficiency (786.09)*
> *acute (518.82)*

> MCC only for patients discharged alive

> (Ex:) 338.0-338.4, 518.81-518.84, 780.64-780.65, 780.91-780.99, 798.0, 799.01-799.1, 799.81-799.89

● **799.2 Signs and symptoms involving emotional state**

    Excludes *anxiety (293.84, 300.00-300.09)*
                     depression (311)

  799.21 Nervousness
    Nervous
    Coding Clinic: 2009, Q4, P120

  799.22 Irritability
    Irritable
    Coding Clinic: 2009, Q4, P120

  799.23 Impulsiveness
    Impulsive
    Excludes *impulsive neurosis (300.3)*

  799.24 Emotional lability

  799.25 Demoralization and apathy
    Apathetic

  799.29 Other signs and symptoms involving emotional state

799.3 Debility, unspecified

    Excludes *asthenia (780.79)*
                     nervous debility (300.5)
                     neurasthenia (300.5)
                     senile asthenia (797)
    Coding Clinic: 1997, Q3, P11-12

799.4 Cachexia 🔗
  Wasting disease

  Code first underlying condition, if known

  (Ex) 338.0-338.4, 780.64-780.65, 780.91-780.99, 799.3-799.4, 799.81-799.89
  Coding Clinic: 2013, Q1, P14; 2006, Q3, P14-15x2; 1990, Q3, P17

● **799.5 Signs and symptoms involving cognition**

    Excludes *amnesia (780.93)*
                     amnestic syndrome (294.0)
                     attention deficit disorder (314.00-314.01)
                     late effects of cerebrovascular disease (438)
                     memory loss (780.93)
                     mild cognitive impairment, so stated (331.83)
                     specific problems in developmental delay (315.00-315.9)
                     transient global amnesia (437.7)
                     visuospatial neglect 781.8
    Coding Clinic: 2012, Q3, P19

  799.51 Attention or concentration deficit
    Coding Clinic: 2012, Q3, P20

  799.52 Cognitive communication deficit
    Coding Clinic: 2012, Q3, P19-21

  799.53 Visuospatial deficit

  799.54 Psychomotor deficit
    Coding Clinic: 2010, Q4, P97

  799.55 Frontal lobe and executive function deficit
    Coding Clinic: 2012, Q3, P20

  799.59 Other signs and symptoms involving cognition

● **799.8 Other ill-defined conditions**

  799.81 Decreased libido   A
    Decreased sexual desire

    Excludes *psychosexual dysfunction with inhibited sexual desire (302.71)*
    Coding Clinic: 2003, Q4, P75-76; Q4, P75-76

  799.82 Apparent life threatening event in infant   P
    ALTE
    Apparent life threatening event in newborn and infant

    Code first confirmed diagnosis, if known

    Use additional code(s) for associated signs and symptoms if no confirmed diagnosis established, or if signs and symptoms are not associated routinely with confirmed diagnosis, or provide additional information for cause of ALTE
    Coding Clinic: 2010, Q4, P98

  799.89 Other ill-defined conditions

799.9 Other unknown and unspecified cause
  Undiagnosed disease, not specified as to site or system involved
  Unknown cause of morbidity or mortality
  Coding Clinic: 1998, Q1, P4; 1990, Q1, P22

SYMPTOMS, SIGNS, AND ILL-DEFINED CONDITIONS (780–799)

N   Newborn: 0   P   Pediatric: 0–17   M   Maternity: 12–55   A   Adult: 15–124   ♀   Females Only   ♂   Males Only

(Ex) CC/MCC Exclusions   🔗 Complication\Comorbidity   🔗 Major C\C   🔗 Present on Admission Requirement   🔗 Hospital-Acquired Condition   **951**

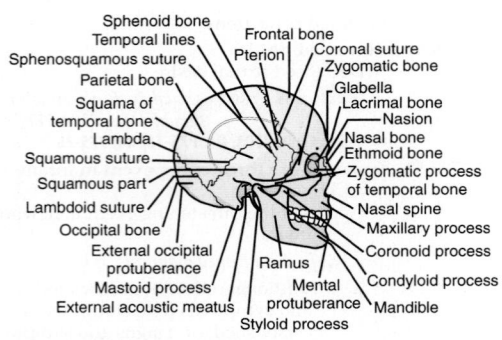

Figure 17-1 Lateral view of skull.

Figure 17-2 Frontal view of skull.

Figure 17-3 Anterior view of vertebral column.

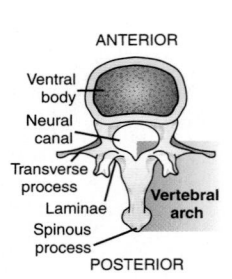

Figure 17-4 Vertebra viewed from above.

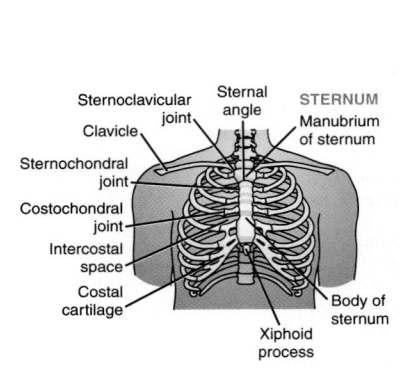

Figure 17-5 Anterior view of rib cage.

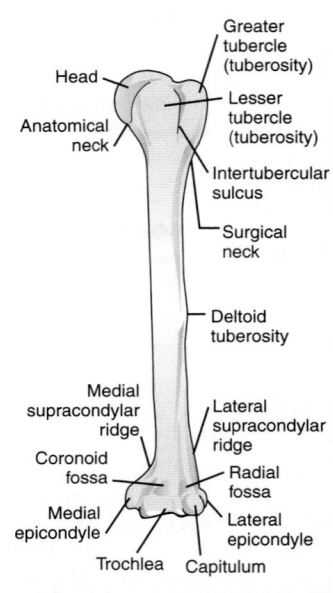

Figure 17-6 Anterior aspect of left humerus.

Figure 17-7 Anterior aspect of left radius and ulna.

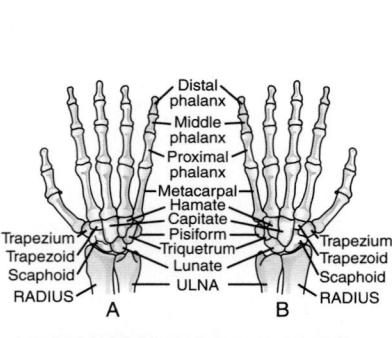

Figure 17-8 Right hand and wrist: **A.** Dorsal surface. **B.** Palmar surface.

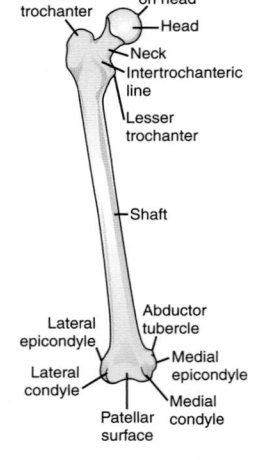

Figure 17-9 Anterior aspect of right femur.

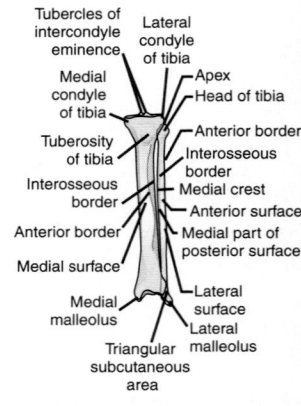

Figure 17-10 Anterior aspect of left tibia and fibula.

◀ New   ◀ Revised   ~~deleted~~ Deleted   Excludes   Includes   Use additional   Code first   Omit code

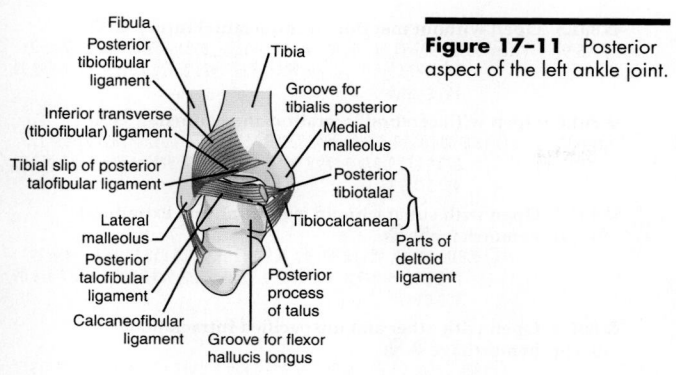

Figure 17-11 Posterior aspect of the left ankle joint.

Figure 17-12 Right foot viewed from above.

OGCR Section I.C.17.a

When coding injuries, assign separate codes for each injury unless a combination code is provided, in which case the combination code is assigned. Multiple injury codes are provided in ICD-9-CM, but should not be assigned unless information for a more specific code is not available. These traumatic injury codes are not to be used for normal, healing surgical wounds or to identify complications of surgical wounds.

The code for the most serious injury, as determined by the provider and the focus of treatment, is sequenced first.

1) **Superficial injuries:** Superficial injuries such as abrasions or contusions are not coded when associated with more severe injuries of the same site.

2) **Primary injury with damage to nerves/blood vessels:** When a primary injury results in minor damage to peripheral nerves or blood vessels, the primary injury is sequenced first with additional code(s) from categories 950-957, Injury to nerves and spinal cord, and/or 900-904, Injury to blood vessels. When the primary injury is to the blood vessels or nerves, that injury should be sequenced first.

17. INJURY AND POISONING (800–999)

Use additional code for retained foreign body, if applicable, V90.01-V90.9)

Use E code(s) to identify the cause and intent of the injury or poisoning (E800-E999)

Note:

1. The principle of multiple coding of injuries should be followed wherever possible. Combination categories for multiple injuries are provided for use when there is insufficient detail as to the nature of the individual conditions, or for primary tabulation purposes when it is more convenient to record a single code; otherwise, the component injuries should be coded separately.
   Where multiple sites of injury are specified in the titles, the word "with" indicates involvement of both sites, and the word "and" indicates involvement of either or both sites. The word "finger" includes thumb.
2. Categories for "late effect" of injuries are to be found at 905–909.

FRACTURES (800–829)

Excludes *malunion (733.81)*
nonunion (733.82)
pathologic or spontaneous fracture (733.10–733.19)
stress fracture (733.93–733.95)

The terms "condyle," "coronoid process," "ramus," and "symphysis" indicate the portion of the bone fractured, not the name of the bone involved.

The descriptions "closed" and "open" used in the fourth-digit subdivisions include the following terms:
   closed (with or without delayed healing):
      comminuted
      depressed
      elevated
      fissured
      fracture NOS
      greenstick
      impacted
      linear
      simple
      slipped epiphysis
      spiral
   open (with or without delayed healing):
      compound
      infected
      missile
      puncture
      with foreign body

Note: A fracture not indicated as closed or open should be classified as closed.

FRACTURE OF SKULL (800–804)

Includes   *traumatic brain injury due to fracture of skull*

The following fifth-digit subclassification is for use with the appropriate codes in categories 800, 801, 803, and 804:

```
0   unspecified state of consciousness
1   with no loss of consciousness
2   with brief [less than one hour] loss of consciousness
3   with moderate [1–24 hours] loss of consciousness
4   with prolonged [more than 24 hours] loss of
    consciousness and return to pre-existing conscious level
5   with prolonged [more than 24 hours] loss of
    consciousness, without return to pre-existing conscious
    level
       Use fifth-digit 5 to designate when a patient is
       unconscious and dies before regaining
       consciousness, regardless of the duration of the
       loss of consciousness
6   with loss of consciousness of unspecified duration
9   with concussion, unspecified
```

● **800 Fracture of vault of skull**

Requires fifth digit. See beginning of section 800–804 for codes and definitions.

Includes   frontal bone
parietal bone

● **800.0 Closed without mention of intracranial injury**
[0-6,9] 0-2,6,9 🔖 🔖 3-5 🔖 🔖
   (Ex) 800.00-801.99, 803.00-804.99, 829.0-829.1, 850.0-852.19, 852.21-854.19,
   873.8-873.9, 879.8-879.9, 905.0, 925.1-925.2, 929.0-929.9, 958.8-959.09,
   959.8-959.9

● **800.1 Closed with cerebral laceration and contusion** 🔖 🔖
[0-6,9]   (Ex) 800.00-801.99, 803.00-804.99, 829.0-829.1, 850.0-852.19, 852.21-854.19,
   873.8-873.9, 879.8-879.9, 905.0, 925.1-925.2, 929.0-929.9, 958.8-959.09,
   959.8-959.9

● **800.2 Closed with subarachnoid, subdural, and extradural**
[0-6,9] **hemorrhage** 🔖 🔖
   (Ex) 800.00-801.99, 803.00-804.99, 829.0-829.1, 850.0-852.19, 852.21-854.19,
   873.8-873.9, 879.8-879.9, 905.0, 925.1-925.2, 929.0-929.9, 958.8-959.09,
   959.8-959.9

● **800.3** **Closed with other and unspecified intracranial**
[0-6,9] **hemorrhage** 🔎 🔎
   ⒺⓍ 800.00-801.99, 803.00-804.99, 829.0-829.1, 850.0-852.19, 852.21-854.19, 873.8-873.9, 879.8-879.9, 905.0, 925.1-925.2, 929.0-929.9, 958.8-959.09, 959.8-959.9

● **800.4** **Closed with intracranial injury of other and**
[0-6,9] **unspecified nature** 0-2,6,9 🔎 🔎, 3-5 🔎 🔎
   ⒺⓍ 800.00-801.99, 803.00-804.99, 829.0-829.9, 850.0-852.19, 852.21-854.19, 873.8-873.9, 879.8-879.9, 905.0, 925.1-925.2, 929.0-929.9, 958.8-959.09, 959.8-959.9

● **800.5** **Open without mention of intracranial injury** 🔎 🔎
[0-6,9]
   ⒺⓍ 800.00-801.99, 803.00-804.99, 850.0-852.19, 852.21-854.19, 873.8-873.9, 879.8-879.9, 905.0, 925.1-925.2, 929.0-929.9, 958.8-959.09, 959.8-959.9

● **800.6** **Open with cerebral laceration and contusion** 🔎 🔎
[0-6,9]
   ⒺⓍ 800.00-801.99, 803.00-804.99, 829.0-829.1, 850.0-852.19, 852.21-854.19, 873.8-873.9, 879.8-879.9, 905.0, 925.1-925.2, 929.0-929.9, 958.8-959.09, 959.8-959.9

● **800.7** **Open with subarachnoid, subdural, and extradural**
[0-6,9] **hemorrhage** 🔎 🔎
   ⒺⓍ 800.00-801.99, 803.00-804.99, 829.0-829.1, 850.0-852.19, 852.21-854.19, 873.8-873.9, 879.8-879.9, 905.0, 925.1-925.2, 929.0-929.9, 958.8-959.09, 959.8-959.9

● **800.8** **Open with other and unspecified intracranial**
[0-6,9] **hemorrhage** 🔎 🔎
   ⒺⓍ 800.00-801.99, 803.00-804.99, 829.0-829.1, 850.0-852.19, 852.21-854.19, 873.8-873.9, 879.8-879.9, 905.0, 925.1-925.2, 929.0-929.9, 958.8-959.09, 959.8-959.9

● **800.9** **Open with intracranial injury of other and**
[0-6,9] **unspecified nature** 🔎 🔎
   ⒺⓍ 800.00-801.99, 803.00-804.99, 829.0-829.1, 850.0-852.19, 852.21-854.19, 873.8-873.9, 879.8-879.9, 905.0, 925.1-925.2, 929.0-929.9, 958.8-959.09, 959.8-959.9

● **801** **Fracture of base of skull**
   Requires fifth digit. See beginning of section 800–804 for codes and definitions.

   Includes   fossa:
         anterior
         middle
         posterior
      occiput bone
      orbital roof
      sinus:
         ethmoid
         frontal
      sphenoid bone
      temporal bone

● **801.0** **Closed without mention of intracranial**
[0-6,9] **injury** 0-2,6,9 🔎 🔎, 3-5 🔎 🔎
   ⒺⓍ 800.00-801.99, 803.00-804.99, 829.0-829.1, 850.0-852.19, 852.21-854.19, 873.8-873.9, 879.8-879.9, 905.0, 925.1-925.2, 929.0-929.9, 958.8-959.09, 959.8-959.9

● **801.1** **Closed with cerebral laceration and contusion** 🔎 🔎
[0-6,9]
   ⒺⓍ 800.00-801.99, 803.00-804.99, 829.0-829.1, 850.0-852.19, 852.21-854.19, 873.8-873.9, 879.8-879.9, 905.0, 925.1-925.2, 929.0-929.9, 958.8-959.09, 959.8-959.9

   Coding Clinic: 1996, Q4, P36.37

● **801.2** **Closed with subarachnoid, subdural, and extradural**
[0-6,9] **hemorrhage** 🔎 🔎
   ⒺⓍ 800.00-801.99, 803.00-804.99, 829.0-829.1, 850.0-852.19, 852.21-854.19, 873.8-873.9, 879.8-879.9, 905.0, 925.1-925.2, 929.0-929.9, 958.8-959.09, 959.8-959.9

● **801.3** **Closed with other and unspecified intracranial**
[0-6,9] **hemorrhage** 🔎 🔎
   ⒺⓍ 800.00-801.99, 803.00-804.99, 829.0-829.1, 850.0-852.19, 852.21-854.19, 873.8-873.9, 879.8-879.9, 905.0, 925.1-925.2, 929.0-929.9, 958.8-959.09, 959.8-959.9

● **801.4** **Closed with intracranial injury of other and**
[0-6,9] **unspecified nature** 0-2,6,9 🔎 🔎, 3-5 🔎 🔎
   ⒺⓍ 800.00-801.99, 803.00-804.99, 829.0-829.1, 850.0-852.19, 852.21-854.19, 873.8-873.9, 879.8-879.9, 905.0, 925.1-925.2, 929.0-929.9, 958.8-959.09, 959.8-959.9

● **801.5** **Open without mention of intracranial injury** 🔎 🔎
[0-6,9]
   ⒺⓍ 800.00-801.99, 803.00-804.99, 829.0-829.1, 850.0-852.19, 852.21-854.19, 873.8-873.9, 879.8-879.9, 905.0, 925.1-925.2, 929.0-929.9, 958.8-959.09, 959.8-959.9

● **801.6** **Open with cerebral laceration and contusion** 🔎 🔎
[0-6,9]
   ⒺⓍ 800.00-801.99, 803.00-804.99, 829.0-829.1, 850.0-852.19, 852.21-854.19, 873.8-873.9, 879.8-879.9, 905.0, 925.1-925.2, 929.0-929.9, 958.8-959.09, 959.8-959.9

● **801.7** **Open with subarachnoid, subdural, and extradural**
[0-6,9] **hemorrhage** 🔎 🔎
   ⒺⓍ 800.00-801.99, 803.00-804.99, 829.0-829.1, 850.0-852.19, 852.21-854.19, 873.8-873.9, 879.8-879.9, 905.0, 925.1-925.2, 929.0-929.9, 958.8-959.09, 959.8-959.9

● **801.8** **Open with other and unspecified intracranial**
[0-6,9] **hemorrhage** 🔎 🔎
   ⒺⓍ 800.00-801.99, 803.00-804.99, 829.0-829.1, 850.0-852.19, 852.21-854.19, 873.8-873.9, 879.8-879.9, 905.0, 925.1-925.2, 929.0-929.9, 958.8-959.09, 959.8-959.9

● **801.9** **Open with intracranial injury of other and**
[0-6,9] **unspecified nature** 🔎 🔎
   ⒺⓍ 800.00-801.99, 803.00-804.99, 829.0-829.1, 850.0-852.19, 852.21-854.19, 873.8-873.9, 879.8-879.9, 905.0, 925.1-925.2, 929.0-929.9, 958.8-959.09, 959.8-959.9

● **802** **Fracture of face bones**

   802.0 **Nasal bones, closed**

   802.1 **Nasal bones, open** 🔎 🔎
   ⒺⓍ 800.00-802.1, 803.00-804.99, 829.0-829.1, 850.0-852.19, 852.21-854.19, 873.8-873.9, 879.8-879.9, 905.0, 925.1-925.2, 929.0-929.9, 958.8-959.09, 959.8-959.9

● **802.2** **Mandible, closed**
   Inferior maxilla
   Lower jaw (bone)

   802.20 **Unspecified site** 🔎 🔎
   ⒺⓍ 800.00-801.99, 802.20-802.5, 803.00-804.99, 829.0-830.1, 850.0-852.19, 852.21-854.19, 873.8-873.9, 879.8-879.9, 905.0, 925.1-925.2, 929.0-929.9, 958.8-959.09, 959.8-959.9

   802.21 **Condylar process** 🔎 🔎
   ⒺⓍ 800.00-801.99, 802.20-802.5, 803.00-804.99, 829.0-830.1, 850.0-852.19, 852.21-854.19, 873.8-873.9, 879.8-879.9, 905.0, 925.1-925.2, 929.0-929.9, 958.8-959.09, 959.8-959.9

   802.22 **Subcondylar** 🔎 🔎
   ⒺⓍ 800.00-801.99, 802.20-802.5, 803.00-804.99, 829.0-830.1, 850.0-852.19, 852.21-854.19, 873.8-873.9, 879.8-879.9, 905.0, 925.1-925.2, 929.0-929.9, 958.8-959.09, 959.8-959.9

   802.23 **Coronoid process** 🔎 🔎
   ⒺⓍ 800.00-801.99, 802.20-802.5, 803.00-804.99, 829.0-830.1, 850.0-852.19, 852.21-854.19, 873.8-873.9, 879.8-879.9, 905.0, 925.1-925.2, 929.0-929.9, 958.8-959.09, 959.8-959.9

   802.24 **Ramus, unspecified** 🔎 🔎
   ⒺⓍ 800.00-801.99, 802.20-802.5, 803.00-804.99, 829.0-830.1, 850.0-852.19, 852.21-854.19, 873.8-873.9, 879.8-879.9, 905.0, 925.1-925.2, 929.0-929.9, 958.8-959.09, 959.8-959.9

   802.25 **Angle of jaw** 🔎 🔎
   ⒺⓍ 800.00-801.99, 802.20-802.5, 803.00-804.99, 829.0-830.1, 850.0-852.19, 852.21-854.19, 873.8-873.9, 879.8-879.9, 905.0, 925.1-925.2, 929.0-929.9, 958.8-959.09, 959.8-959.9

   802.26 **Symphysis of body** 🔎 🔎
   ⒺⓍ 800.00-801.99, 802.20-802.5, 803.00-804.99, 829.0-830.1, 850.0-852.19, 852.21-854.19, 873.8-873.9, 879.8-879.9, 905.0, 925.1-925.2, 929.0-929.9, 958.8-959.09, 959.8-959.9

   802.27 **Alveolar border of body** 🔎 🔎
   ⒺⓍ 800.00-801.99, 802.20-802.5, 803.00-804.99, 829.0-830.1, 850.0-852.19, 852.21-854.19, 873.8-873.9, 879.8-879.9, 905.0, 925.1-925.2, 929.0-929.9, 958.8-959.09, 959.8-959.9

   802.28 **Body, other and unspecified** 🔎 🔎
   ⒺⓍ 800.00-801.99, 802.20-802.5, 803.00-804.99, 829.0-830.1, 850.0-852.19, 852.21-854.19, 873.8-873.9, 879.8-879.9, 905.0, 925.1-925.2, 929.0-929.9, 958.8-959.09, 959.8-959.9

   802.29 **Multiple sites** 🔎 🔎
   ⒺⓍ 800.00-801.99, 802.20-802.5, 803.00-804.99, 829.0-830.1, 850.0-852.19, 852.21-854.19, 873.8-873.9, 879.8-879.9, 905.0, 925.1-925.2, 929.0-929.9, 958.8-959.09, 959.8-959.9

◀ New   ◀▦ Revised   ~~deleted~~ Deleted   Excludes   Includes   Use additional   Code first   Omit code

954   ● Unacceptable Principal Diagnosis   ● Use Additional Digit(s)   ▸ Manifestation Code   OGCR Official Guidelines   **Coding Clinic**

● 802.3 **Mandible, open**

    802.30 **Unspecified site** 🕯️ 🕯️
       (Ex) 800.00-801.99, 802.20-802.5, 803.00-804.99, 829.0-830.1,
       850.0-852.19, 852.21-854.19, 873.8-873.9, 879.8-879.9,
       905.0, 925.1-925.2, 929.0-929.9, 958.8-959.09, 959.8-959.9

    802.31 **Condylar process** 🕯️ 🕯️
       (Ex) 800.00-801.99, 802.20-802.5, 803.00-804.99, 829.0-830.1,
       850.0-852.19, 852.21-854.19, 873.8-873.9, 879.8-879.9,
       905.0, 925.1-925.2, 929.0-929.9, 958.8-959.09, 959.8-959.9

    802.32 **Subcondylar** 🕯️ 🕯️
       (Ex) 800.00-801.99, 802.20-802.5, 803.00-804.99, 829.0-830.1,
       850.0-852.19, 852.21-854.19, 873.8-873.9, 879.8-879.9,
       905.0, 925.1-925.2, 929.0-929.9, 958.8-959.09, 959.8-959.9

    802.33 **Coronoid process** 🕯️ 🕯️
       (Ex) 800.00-801.99, 802.20-802.5, 803.00-804.99, 829.0-830.1,
       850.0-852.19, 852.21-854.19, 873.8-873.9, 879.8-879.9,
       905.0, 925.1-925.2, 929.0-929.9, 958.8-959.09, 959.8-959.9

    802.34 **Ramus, unspecified** 🕯️ 🕯️
       (Ex) 800.00-801.99, 802.20-802.5, 803.00-804.99, 829.0-830.1,
       850.0-852.19, 852.21-854.19, 873.8-873.9, 879.8-879.9,
       905.0, 925.1-925.2, 929.0-929.9, 958.8-959.09, 959.8-959.9

    802.35 **Angle of jaw** 🕯️ 🕯️
       (Ex) 800.00-801.99, 802.20-802.5, 803.00-804.99, 829.0-830.1,
       850.0-852.19, 852.21-854.19, 873.8-873.9, 879.8-879.9,
       905.0, 925.1-925.2, 929.0-929.9, 958.8-959.09, 959.8-959.9

    802.36 **Symphysis of body** 🕯️ 🕯️
       (Ex) 800.00-801.99, 802.20-802.5, 803.00-804.99, 829.0-830.1,
       850.0-852.19, 852.21-854.19, 873.8-873.9, 879.8-879.9,
       905.0, 925.1-925.2, 929.0-929.9, 958.8-959.09, 959.8-959.9

    802.37 **Alveolar border of body** 🕯️ 🕯️
       (Ex) 800.00-801.99, 802.20-802.5, 803.00-804.99, 829.0-830.1,
       850.0-852.19, 852.21-854.19, 873.8-873.9, 879.8-879.9,
       905.0, 925.1-925.2, 929.0-929.9, 958.8-959.09, 959.8-959.9

    802.38 **Body, other and unspecified** 🕯️ 🕯️
       (Ex) 800.00-801.99, 802.20-802.5, 803.00-804.99, 829.0-830.1,
       850.0-852.19, 852.21-854.19, 873.8-873.9, 879.8-879.9,
       905.0, 925.1-925.2, 929.0-929.9, 958.8-959.09, 959.8-959.9

    802.39 **Multiple sites** 🕯️ 🕯️
       (Ex) 800.00-801.99, 802.20-802.5, 803.00-804.99, 829.0-830.1,
       850.0-852.19, 852.21-854.19, 873.8-873.9, 879.8-879.9,
       905.0, 925.1-925.2, 929.0-929.9, 958.8-959.09, 959.8-959.9

● 802.4 **Malar and maxillary bones, closed** 🕯️ 🕯️
    Superior maxilla   Zygoma
    Upper jaw (bone)   Zygomatic arch
    (Ex) 800.00-801.99, 802.20-802.5, 803.00-804.99, 829.0-830.1, 850.0-852.19,
    852.21-854.19, 873.8-873.9, 879.8-879.9, 905.0, 925.1-925.2,
    929.0-929.9, 958.8-959.09, 959.8-959.9

● 802.5 **Malar and maxillary bones, open** 🕯️ 🕯️
    (Ex) 800.00-801.99, 802.20-802.5, 803.00-804.99, 829.0-830.1, 850.0-852.19,
    852.21-854.19, 873.8-873.9, 879.8-879.9, 905.0, 925.1-925.2,
    929.0-929.9, 958.8-959.09, 959.8-959.9

● 802.6 **Orbital floor (blow-out), closed** 🕯️ 🕯️
    (Ex) 800.00-801.99, 802.6-804.99, 829.0-829.1, 850.0-852.19, 852.21-854.19,
    873.8-873.9, 879.8-879.9, 905.0, 925.1-925.2, 929.0-929.9, 958.8-959.09,
    959.8-959.9

● 802.7 **Orbital floor (blow-out), open** 🕯️ 🕯️
    (Ex) 800.00-801.99, 802.6-804.99, 829.0-829.1, 850.0-852.19, 852.21-854.19,
    873.8-873.9, 879.8-879.9, 905.0, 925.1-925.2, 929.0-929.9, 958.8-959.09,
    959.8-959.9

● 802.8 **Other facial bones, closed** 🕯️ 🕯️
    Alveolus
    Orbit:
      NOS
      part other than roof or floor
    Palate
    Excludes *orbital:*
       floor (802.6)
       roof (801.0–801.9)
    (Ex) 800.00-801.99, 802.6-804.99, 829.0-829.1, 850.0-852.19, 852.21-854.19,
    873.8-873.9, 879.8-879.9, 905.0, 925.1-925.2, 929.0-929.9, 958.8-959.09,
    959.8-959.9

● 802.9 **Other facial bones, open** 🕯️ 🕯️
    (Ex) 800.00-801.99, 802.6-804.99, 829.0-829.1, 850.0-852.19, 852.21-854.19,
    873.8-873.9, 879.8-879.9, 905.0, 925.1-925.2, 929.0-929.9, 958.8-959.09,
    959.8-959.9

● 803 **Other and unqualified skull fractures**

    Requires fifth digit. See beginning of section 800–804 for codes
    and definitions.

    Includes   skull NOS
               skull multiple NOS

● 803.0 **Closed without mention of intracranial injury**
[0-6,9] 0-2,6,9 🕯️ 🕯️, 3-5 🕯️ 🕯️
    (Ex) 800.00-801.99, 803.00-804.99, 829.0-829.1, 850.0-852.19, 852.21-854.19,
    873.8-873.9, 879.8-879.9, 905.0, 925.1-925.2, 929.0-929.9, 958.8-959.09,
    959.8-959.9

● 803.1 **Closed with cerebral laceration and contusion** 🕯️ 🕯️
[0-6,9] (Ex) 800.00-801.99, 803.00-804.99, 829.0-829.1, 850.0-852.19, 852.21-854.19,
    873.8-873.9, 879.8-879.9, 905.0, 925.1-925.2, 929.0-929.9, 958.8-959.09,
    959.8-959.9

● 803.2 **Closed with subarachnoid, subdural, and extradural**
[0-6,9] **hemorrhage** 🕯️ 🕯️
    (Ex) 800.00-801.99, 803.00-804.99, 829.0-829.1, 850.0-852.19, 852.21-854.19,
    873.8-873.9, 879.8-879.9, 905.0, 925.1-925.2, 929.0-929.9, 958.8-959.09,
    959.8-959.9

● 803.3 **Closed with other and unspecified intracranial**
[0-6,9] **hemorrhage** 🕯️ 🕯️
    (Ex) 800.00-801.99, 803.00-804.99, 829.0-829.1, 850.0-852.19, 852.21-854.19,
    873.8-873.9, 879.8-879.9, 905.0, 925.1-925.2, 929.0-929.9, 958.8-959.09,
    959.8-959.9

● 803.4 **Closed with intracranial injury of other and**
[0-6,9] **unspecified nature** 0-2,6,9 🕯️ 🕯️, 3-5 🕯️ 🕯️
    (Ex) 800.00-801.99, 803.00-804.99, 829.0-829.1, 850.0-852.19, 852.21-854.19,
    873.8-873.9, 879.8-879.9, 905.0, 925.1-925.2, 929.0-929.9, 958.8-959.09,
    959.8-959.9

● 803.5 **Open without mention of intracranial injury** 🕯️ 🕯️
[0-6,9] (Ex) 800.00-801.99, 803.00-804.99, 829.0-829.1, 850.0-852.19, 852.21-854.19,
    873.8-873.9, 879.8-879.9, 905.0, 925.1-925.2, 929.0-929.9, 958.8-959.09,
    959.8-959.9

● 803.6 **Open with cerebral laceration and contusion** 🕯️ 🕯️
[0-6,9] (Ex) 800.00-801.99, 803.00-804.99, 829.0-829.1, 850.0-852.19, 852.21-854.19,
    873.8-873.9, 879.8-879.9, 905.0, 925.1-925.2, 929.0-929.9, 958.8-959.09,
    959.8-959.9

● 803.7 **Open with subarachnoid, subdural, and extradural**
[0-6,9] **hemorrhage** 🕯️ 🕯️
    (Ex) 800.00-801.99, 803.00-804.99, 829.0-829.1, 850.0-852.19, 852.21-854.19,
    873.8-873.9, 879.8-879.9, 905.0, 925.1-925.2, 929.0-929.9, 958.8-959.09,
    959.8-959.9

● 803.8 **Open with other and unspecified intracranial**
[0-6,9] **hemorrhage** 🕯️ 🕯️
    (Ex) 800.00-801.99, 803.00-804.99, 829.0-829.1, 850.0-852.19, 852.21-854.19,
    873.8-873.9, 879.8-879.9, 905.0, 925.1-925.2, 929.0-929.9, 958.8-959.09,
    959.8-959.9

● 803.9 **Open with intracranial injury of other and**
[0-6,9] **unspecified nature** 🕯️ 🕯️
    (Ex) 800.00-801.99, 803.00-804.99, 829.0-829.1, 850.0-852.19, 852.21-854.19,
    873.8-873.9, 879.8-879.9, 905.0, 925.1-925.2, 929.0-929.9, 958.8-959.09,
    959.8-959.9

● 804 **Multiple fractures involving skull or face with other bones**

    Requires fifth digit. See beginning of section 800–804 for codes
    and definitions.

● 804.0 **Closed without mention of intracranial injury**
[0-6,9] 0-2,6,9 🕯️ 🕯️, 3-5 🕯️ 🕯️
    (Ex) 800.00-801.99, 803.00-804.99, 829.0-829.1, 850.0-852.19, 852.21-854.19,
    873.8-873.9, 879.8-879.9, 905.0, 925.1-925.2, 929.0-929.9, 958.8-959.09,
    959.8-959.9

● 804.1 **Closed with cerebral laceration and contusion** 🕯️ 🕯️
[0-6,9] (Ex) 800.00-801.99, 803.00-804.99, 829.0-829.1, 850.0-852.19, 852.21-854.19,
    873.8-873.9, 879.8-879.9, 905.0, 925.1-925.2, 929.0-929.9, 958.8-959.09,
    959.8-959.9

    Coding Clinic: 2006, Q1, P6-7

● 804.2 **Closed with subarachnoid, subdural, and extradural**
[0-6,9] **hemorrhage** 🕯️ 🕯️
    (Ex) 800.00-801.99, 803.00-804.99, 829.0-829.1, 850.0-852.19, 852.21-854.19,
    873.8-873.9, 879.8-879.9, 905.0, 925.1-925.2, 929.0-929.9, 958.8-959.09,
    959.8-959.9

N Newborn: 0   **P** Pediatric: 0–17   **M** Maternity: 12–55   **A** Adult: 15–124   ♀ Females Only   ♂ Males Only

(Ex) CC/MCC Exclusions   🕯️ Complication\Comorbidity   🕯️ Major C\C   🕯️ Present on Admission Requirement   🕯️ Hospital-Acquired Condition   **955**

● **804.3** Closed with other and unspecified intracranial
[0-6,9] hemorrhage 🔖 🔖
  (Ex:) 800.00-801.99, 803.00-804.99, 829.0-829.1, 850.0-852.19, 852.21-854.19,
  873.8-873.9, 879.8-879.9, 905.0, 925.1-925.2, 929.0-929.9, 958.8-959.09,
  959.8-959.9

● **804.4** Closed with intracranial injury of other and
[0-6,9] unspecified nature 0-2,6,9 🔖 🔖, 3-5 🔖 🔖
  (Ex:) 800.00-801.99, 803.00-804.99, 829.0-829.1, 850.0-852.19, 852.21-854.19,
  873.8-873.9, 879.8-879.9, 905.0, 925.1-925.2, 929.0-929.9, 958.8-959.09,
  959.8-959.9

● **804.5** Open without mention of intracranial injury
[0-6,9] 0-2,6,9 🔖 🔖, 3-5 🔖 🔖
  (Ex:) 800.00-801.99, 803.00-804.99, 829.0-829.1, 850.0-852.19, 852.21-854.19,
  873.8-873.9, 879.8-879.9, 905.0, 925.1-925.2, 929.0-929.9, 958.8-959.09,
  959.8-959.9

● **804.6** Open with cerebral laceration and contusion 🔖 🔖
[0-6,9]
  (Ex:) 800.00-801.99, 803.00-804.99, 829.0-829.1, 850.0-852.19, 852.21-854.19,
  873.8-873.9, 879.8-879.9, 905.0, 925.1-925.2, 929.0-929.9, 958.8-959.09,
  959.8-959.9

● **804.7** Open with subarachnoid, subdural, and extradural
[0-6,9] hemorrhage 🔖 🔖
  (Ex:) 800.00-801.99, 803.00-804.99, 829.0-829.1, 850.0-852.19, 852.21-854.19,
  873.8-873.9, 879.8-879.9, 905.0, 925.1-925.2, 929.0-929.9, 958.8-959.09,
  959.8-959.9

● **804.8** Open with other and unspecified intracranial
[0-6,9] hemorrhage 🔖 🔖
  (Ex:) 800.00-801.99, 803.00-804.99, 829.0-829.1, 850.0-852.19, 852.21-854.19,
  873.8-873.9, 879.8-879.9, 905.0, 925.1-925.2, 929.0-929.9, 958.8-959.09,
  959.8-959.9

● **804.9** Open with intracranial injury of other and
[0-6,9] unspecified nature 0-2,6,9 🔖 🔖, 3-5 🔖 🔖
  (Ex:) 800.00-801.99, 803.00-804.99, 829.0-829.1, 850.0-852.19, 852.21-854.19,
  873.8-873.9, 879.8-879.9, 905.0, 925.1-925.2, 929.0-929.9, 958.8-959.09,
  959.8-959.9

FRACTURE OF NECK AND TRUNK (805–809)

● **805** **Fracture of vertebral column without mention of spinal cord
injury**

  Includes   neural arch
  spine
  spinous process
  transverse process
  vertebra

  Coding Clinic: 1985, Nov-Dec, P16

  The following fifth-digit subclassification is for use with codes
  805.0–805.1:

  > 0   cervical vertebra, unspecified level
  > 1   first cervical vertebra
  > 2   second cervical vertebra
  > 3   third cervical vertebra
  > 4   fourth cervical vertebra
  > 5   fifth cervical vertebra
  > 6   sixth cervical vertebra
  > 7   seventh cervical vertebra
  > 8   multiple cervical vertebrae

● **805.0** Cervical, closed 🔖 🔖
[0-8]   Atlas
   Axis
  (Ex:) 805.00-805.18, 805.8-806.19, 806.8-806.9, 829.0-829.1, 839.00-839.18,
  839.40, 839.49-839.50, 839.59, 839.69, 839.79-839.9, 847.0, 847.9,
  848.8-848.9, 879.8-879.9, 905.1, 926.11, 929.0-929.9, 952.00-952.09,
  952.8-952.9, 958.8-958.99, 959.11-959.19, 959.8-959.9

● **805.1** Cervical, open 🔖 🔖
[0-8]
  (Ex:) 805.00-805.18, 805.8-806.19, 806.8-806.9, 829.0-829.1, 839.00-839.18,
  839.40, 839.49-839.50, 839.59, 839.69, 839.79-839.9, 847.0, 847.9,
  848.8-848.9, 879.8-879.9, 905.1, 926.11, 929.0-929.9, 952.00-952.09,
  952.8-952.9, 958.8-958.99, 959.11-959.19, 959.8-959.9

  805.2 Dorsal [thoracic], closed 🔖 🔖
  (Ex:) 805.2-805.3, 805.8-805.9, 806.20-806.39, 806.8-806.9, 829.0-829.1, 839.21,
  839.31-839.40, 839.49-839.50, 839.59, 839.69, 839.79-839.9, 847.1,
  847.9, 848.8-848.9, 879.8-879.9, 905.1, 926.11, 929.0-929.9,
  952.10-952.19, 952.8-952.9, 958.8-958.99, 959.11-959.19, 959.8-959.9

  805.3 Dorsal [thoracic], open 🔖 🔖
  (Ex:) 805.2-805.3, 805.8-805.9, 806.20-806.39, 806.8-806.9, 829.0-829.1, 839.21,
  839.31-839.40, 839.49-839.50, 839.59, 839.69, 839.79-839.9, 847.1,
  847.9, 848.8-848.9, 879.8-879.9, 905.1, 926.11, 929.0-929.9,
  952.10-952.19, 952.8-952.9, 958.8-958.99, 959.11-959.19, 959.8-959.9

  805.4 Lumbar, closed 🔖 🔖
  (Ex:) 805.4-805.5, 805.8-805.9, 806.4-806.5, 806.8-806.9, 829.0-829.1, 839.20,
  839.30, 839.40, 839.49-839.50, 839.59, 839.69, 839.79-839.9, 847.2,
  847.9, 848.8-848.9, 879.8-879.9, 905.1, 926.11, 929.0-929.9, 952.2,
  952.8-952.9, 958.8-958.99, 959.11-959.19, 959.8-959.9

  Coding Clinic: 2007, Q1, P3-8

  805.5 Lumbar, open 🔖 🔖
  (Ex:) 805.4-805.5, 805.8-805.9, 806.4-806.5, 806.8-806.9, 829.0-829.1, 839.20,
  839.30, 839.40, 839.49-839.50, 839.59, 839.69, 839.79-839.9, 847.2,
  847.9, 848.8-848.9, 879.8-879.9, 905.1, 926.11, 929.0-929.9, 952.2,
  952.8-952.9, 958.8-958.99, 959.11-959.19, 959.8-959.9

  805.6 Sacrum and coccyx, closed 🔖 🔖
  (Ex:) 805.6-805.9, 806.60-806.9, 829.0-829.1, 839.40-839.59, 839.69,
  839.79-839.9, 846.0-846.9, 847.3-847.9, 848.5-848.9, 879.8-879.9, 905.1,
  926.11, 929.0-929.9, 952.3-952.9, 958.8-958.99, 959.11-959.19,
  959.8-959.9

  805.7 Sacrum and coccyx, open 🔖 🔖
  (Ex:) 805.6-805.9, 806.60-806.9, 829.0-829.1, 839.40-839.59, 839.69,
  839.79-839.9, 846.0-846.9, 847.3-847.9, 848.5-848.9, 879.8-879.9, 905.1,
  926.11, 929.0-929.9, 952.3-952.9, 958.8-958.99, 959.11-959.19,
  959.8-959.9

  805.8 Unspecified, closed 🔖 🔖
  (Ex:) 733.10-733.19, 733.93-733.98, 805.00-806.9, 829.0-829.1, 839.00-839.59,
  839.69, 839.79-839.9, 846.0-847.9, 848.5-848.9, 879.8-879.9, 905.1,
  926.11, 929.0-929.9, 952.00-952.9, 958.8-958.99, 959.11-959.19,
  959.8-959.9

  805.9 Unspecified, open 🔖 🔖
  (Ex:) 733.10-733.19, 733.93-733.98, 805.00-806.9, 829.0-829.1, 839.00-839.59,
  839.69, 839.79-839.9, 846.0-847.9, 848.5-848.9, 879.8-879.9, 905.1,
  926.11, 929.0-929.9, 952.00-952.9, 958.8-958.99, 959.11-959.19,
  959.8-959.9

● **806** **Fracture of vertebral column with spinal cord injury**

  Includes   any condition classifiable to 805 with:
  complete or incomplete transverse lesion (of cord)
  hematomyelia
  injury to:
     cauda equina
     nerve
  paralysis
  paraplegia
  quadriplegia
  spinal concussion

● **806.0** Cervical, closed

  806.00 C_1-C_4 level with unspecified spinal cord
  injury 🔖 🔖
  Cervical region NOS with spinal cord injury NOS
  (Ex:) 733.10-733.19, 733.93-733.98, 805.00-805.18, 805.8-806.19,
  806.8-806.9, 829.0-829.1, 839.00-839.18, 839.40,
  839.49-839.50, 839.59, 839.69, 839.79-839.9, 847.9,
  848.8-848.9, 879.8-879.9, 905.1, 926.11, 929.0-929.9,
  952.00-952.09, 952.8-952.9, 958.8-958.99, 959.11-959.19,
  959.8-959.9

  806.01 C_1-C_4 level with complete lesion of cord 🔖 🔖
  (Ex:) 733.10-733.19, 733.93-733.98, 805.00-805.18, 805.8-806.19,
  806.8-806.9, 829.0-829.1, 839.00-839.18, 839.40,
  839.49-839.50, 839.59, 839.69, 839.79-839.9, 847.9,
  848.8-848.9, 879.8-879.9, 905.1, 926.11, 929.0-929.9,
  952.00-952.09, 952.8-952.9, 958.8-958.99, 959.11-959.19,
  959.8-959.9

  806.02 C_1-C_4 level with anterior cord syndrome 🔖 🔖
  (Ex:) 733.10-733.19, 733.93-733.98, 805.00-805.18, 805.8-806.19,
  806.8-806.9, 829.0-829.1, 839.00-839.18, 839.40,
  839.49-839.50, 839.59, 839.69, 839.79-839.9, 847.9,
  848.8-848.9, 879.8-879.9, 905.1, 926.11, 929.0-929.9,
  952.00-952.09, 952.8-952.9, 958.8-958.99, 959.11-959.19,
  959.8-959.9

806.03 C_1-C_4 level with central cord syndrome 🏵 🏵
ⒺⓍ 733.10-733.19, 733.93-733.98, 805.00-805.18, 805.8-806.19, 806.8-806.9, 829.0-829.1, 839.00-839.18, 839.40, 839.49-839.50, 839.59, 839.69, 839.79-839.9, 847.9, 848.8-848.9, 879.8-879.9, 905.1, 926.11, 929.0-929.9, 952.00-952.09, 952.8-952.9, 958.8-958.99, 959.11-959.19, 959.8-959.9

806.04 C_1-C_4 level with other specified spinal cord injury 🏵 🏵
     C_1-C_4 level with:
       incomplete spinal cord lesion NOS
       posterior cord syndrome
ⒺⓍ 733.10-733.19, 733.93-733.98, 805.00-805.18, 805.8-806.19, 806.8-806.9, 829.0-829.1, 839.00-839.18, 839.40, 839.49-839.50, 839.59, 839.69, 839.79-839.9, 847.9, 848.8-848.9, 879.8-879.9, 905.1, 926.11, 929.0-929.9, 952.00-952.09, 952.8-952.9, 958.8-958.99, 959.11-959.19, 959.8-959.9

806.05 C_5-C_7 level with unspecified spinal cord injury 🏵 🏵
ⒺⓍ 733.10-733.19, 733.93-733.98, 805.00-805.18, 805.8-806.19, 806.8-806.9, 829.0-829.1, 839.00-839.18, 839.40, 839.49-839.50, 839.59, 839.69, 839.79-839.9, 847.9, 848.8-848.9, 879.8-879.9, 905.1, 926.11, 929.0-929.9, 952.00-952.09, 952.8-952.9, 958.8-958.99, 959.11-959.19, 959.8-959.9

806.06 C_5-C_7 level with complete lesion of cord 🏵 🏵
ⒺⓍ 733.10-733.19, 733.93-733.98, 805.00-805.18, 805.8-806.19, 806.8-806.9, 829.0-829.1, 839.00-839.18, 839.40, 839.49-839.50, 839.59, 839.69, 839.79-839.9, 847.9, 848.8-848.9, 879.8-879.9, 905.1, 926.11, 929.0-929.9, 952.00-952.09, 952.8-952.9, 958.8-958.99, 959.11-959.19, 959.8-959.9

806.07 C_5-C_7 level with anterior cord syndrome 🏵 🏵
ⒺⓍ 733.10-733.19, 733.93-733.98, 805.00-805.18, 805.8-806.19, 806.8-806.9, 829.0-829.1, 839.00-839.18, 839.40, 839.49-839.50, 839.59, 839.69, 839.79-839.9, 847.9, 848.8-848.9, 879.8-879.9, 905.1, 926.11, 929.0-929.9, 952.00-952.09, 952.8-952.9, 958.8-958.99, 959.11-959.19, 959.8-959.9

806.08 C_5-C_7 level with central cord syndrome 🏵 🏵
ⒺⓍ 733.10-733.19, 733.93-733.98, 805.00-805.18, 805.8-806.19, 806.8-806.9, 829.0-829.1, 839.00-839.18, 839.40, 839.49-839.50, 839.59, 839.69, 839.79-839.9, 847.9, 848.8-848.9, 879.8-879.9, 905.1, 926.11, 929.0-929.9, 952.00-952.09, 952.8-952.9, 958.8-958.99, 959.11-959.19, 959.8-959.9

806.09 C_5-C_7 level with other specified spinal cord injury 🏵 🏵
     C_5-C_7 level with:
       incomplete spinal cord lesion NOS
       posterior cord syndrome
ⒺⓍ 733.10-733.19, 733.93-733.98, 805.00-805.18, 805.8-806.19, 806.8-806.9, 829.0-829.1, 839.00-839.18, 839.40, 839.49-839.50, 839.59, 839.69, 839.79-839.9, 847.9, 848.8-848.9, 879.8-879.9, 905.1, 926.11, 929.0-929.9, 952.00-952.09, 952.8-952.9, 958.8-958.99, 959.11-959.19, 959.8-959.9

● **806.1   Cervical, open**

806.10 C_1-C_4 level with unspecified spinal cord injury 🏵 🏵
ⒺⓍ 733.10-733.19, 733.93-733.98, 805.00-805.18, 805.8-806.19, 806.8-806.9, 829.0-829.1, 839.00-839.18, 839.40, 839.49-839.50, 839.59, 839.69, 839.79-839.9, 847.9, 848.8-848.9, 879.8-879.9, 905.1, 926.11, 929.0-929.9, 952.00-952.09, 952.8-952.9, 958.8-958.99, 959.11-959.19, 959.8-959.9

806.11 C_1-C_4 level with complete lesion of cord 🏵 🏵
ⒺⓍ 733.10-733.19, 733.93-733.98, 805.00-805.18, 805.8-806.19, 806.8-806.9, 829.0-829.1, 839.00-839.18, 839.40, 839.49-839.50, 839.59, 839.69, 839.79-839.9, 847.9, 848.8-848.9, 879.8-879.9, 905.1, 926.11, 929.0-929.9, 952.00-952.09, 952.8-952.9, 958.8-958.99, 959.11-959.19, 959.8-959.9

806.12 C_1-C_4 level with anterior cord syndrome 🏵 🏵
ⒺⓍ 733.10-733.19, 733.93-733.98, 805.00-805.18, 805.8-806.19, 806.8-806.9, 829.0-829.1, 839.00-839.18, 839.40, 839.49-839.50, 839.59, 839.69, 839.79-839.9, 847.9, 848.8-848.9, 879.8-879.9, 905.1, 926.11, 929.0-929.9, 952.00-952.09, 952.8-952.9, 958.8-958.99, 959.11-959.19, 959.8-959.9

806.13 C_1-C_4 level with central cord syndrome 🏵 🏵
ⒺⓍ 733.10-733.19, 733.93-733.98, 805.00-805.18, 805.8-806.19, 806.8-806.9, 829.0-829.1, 839.00-839.18, 839.40, 839.49-839.50, 839.59, 839.69, 839.79-839.9, 847.9, 848.8-848.9, 879.8-879.9, 905.1, 926.11, 929.0-929.9, 952.00-952.09, 952.8-952.9, 958.8-958.99, 959.11-959.19, 959.8-959.9

806.14 C_1-C_4 level with other specified spinal cord injury 🏵 🏵
     C_1-C_4 level with:
       incomplete spinal cord lesion NOS
       posterior cord syndrome
ⒺⓍ 733.10-733.19, 733.93-733.98, 805.00-805.18, 805.8-806.19, 806.8-806.9, 829.0-829.1, 839.00-839.18, 839.40, 839.49-839.50, 839.59, 839.69, 839.79-839.9, 847.9, 848.8-848.9, 879.8-879.9, 905.1, 926.11, 929.0-929.9, 952.00-952.09, 952.8-952.9, 958.8-958.99, 959.11-959.19, 959.8-959.9

806.15 C_5-C_7 level with unspecified spinal cord injury 🏵 🏵
ⒺⓍ 733.10-733.19, 733.93-733.98, 805.00-805.18, 805.8-806.19, 806.8-806.9, 829.0-829.1, 839.00-839.18, 839.40, 839.49-839.50, 839.59, 839.69, 839.79-839.9, 847.9, 848.8-848.9, 879.8-879.9, 905.1, 926.11, 929.0-929.9, 952.00-952.09, 952.8-952.9, 958.8-958.99, 959.11-959.19, 959.8-959.9

806.16 C_5-C_7 level with complete lesion of cord 🏵 🏵
ⒺⓍ 733.10-733.19, 733.93-733.98, 805.00-805.18, 805.8-806.19, 806.8-806.9, 829.0-829.1, 839.00-839.18, 839.40, 839.49-839.50, 839.59, 839.69, 839.79-839.9, 847.9, 848.8-848.9, 879.8-879.9, 905.1, 926.11, 929.0-929.9, 952.00-952.09, 952.8-952.9, 958.8-958.99, 959.11-959.19, 959.8-959.9

806.17 C_5-C_7 level with anterior cord syndrome 🏵 🏵
ⒺⓍ 733.10-733.19, 733.93-733.98, 805.00-805.18, 805.8-806.19, 806.8-806.9, 829.0-829.1, 839.00-839.18, 839.40, 839.49-839.50, 839.59, 839.69, 839.79-839.9, 847.9, 848.8-848.9, 879.8-879.9, 905.1, 926.11, 929.0-929.9, 952.00-952.09, 952.8-952.9, 958.8-958.99, 959.11-959.19, 959.8-959.9

806.18 C_5-C_7 level with central cord syndrome 🏵 🏵
ⒺⓍ 733.10-733.19, 733.93-733.98, 805.00-805.18, 805.8-806.19, 806.8-806.9, 829.0-829.1, 839.00-839.18, 839.40, 839.49-839.50, 839.59, 839.69, 839.79-839.9, 847.9, 848.8-848.9, 879.8-879.9, 905.1, 926.11, 929.0-929.9, 952.00-952.09, 952.8-952.9, 958.8-958.99, 959.11-959.19, 959.8-959.9

806.19 C_5-C_7 level with other specified spinal cord injury 🏵 🏵
     C_5-C_7 level with:
       incomplete spinal cord lesion NOS
       posterior cord syndrome
ⒺⓍ 733.10-733.19, 733.93-733.98, 805.00-805.18, 805.8-806.19, 806.8-806.9, 829.0-829.1, 839.00-839.18, 839.40, 839.49-839.50, 839.59, 839.69, 839.79-839.9, 847.9, 848.8-848.9, 879.8-879.9, 905.1, 926.11, 929.0-929.9, 952.00-952.09, 952.8-952.9, 958.8-958.99, 959.11-959.19, 959.8-959.9

INJURY AND POISONING (800–999)

N Newborn: 0   **P** Pediatric: 0–17   **M** Maternity: 12–55   **A** Adult: 15–124   ♀ Females Only   ♂ Males Only

ⒺⓍ CC/MCC Exclusions   🏵 Complication\Comorbidity   🏵 Major C\C   🏵 Present on Admission Requirement   🏵 Hospital-Acquired Condition   **957**

INJURY AND POISONING (800–999)

● 806.2　Dorsal [thoracic], closed

806.20　T_1-T_6 level with unspecified spinal cord injury 🅠 🅠

Thoracic region NOS with spinal cord injury NOS

Ex: 733.10-733.19, 733.93-733.98, 805.2-805.3, 805.8-805.9, 806.20-806.39, 806.8-806.9, 829.0-829.1, 839.21, 839.31-839.40, 839.49-839.50, 839.59, 839.69, 839.79-839.9, 847.1, 847.9, 848.8-848.9, 879.8-879.9, 905.1, 926.11, 929.0-929.9, 952.10-952.19, 952.8-952.9, 958.8-958.99, 959.11-959.19, 959.8-959.9

806.21　T_1-T_6 level with complete lesion of cord 🅠 🅠

Ex: 733.10-733.19, 733.93-733.98, 805.2-805.3, 805.8-805.9, 806.20-806.39, 806.8-806.9, 829.0-829.1, 839.21, 839.31-839.40, 839.49-839.50, 839.59, 839.69, 839.79-839.9, 847.1, 847.9, 848.8-848.9, 879.8-879.9, 905.1, 926.11, 929.0-929.9, 952.10-952.19, 952.8-952.9, 958.8-958.99, 959.11-959.19, 959.8-959.9

806.22　T_1-T_6 level with anterior cord syndrome 🅠 🅠

Ex: 733.10-733.19, 733.93-733.98, 805.2-805.3, 805.8-805.9, 806.20-806.39, 806.8-806.9, 829.0-829.1, 839.21, 839.31-839.40, 839.49-839.50, 839.59, 839.69, 839.79-839.9, 847.1, 847.9, 848.8-848.9, 879.8-879.9, 905.1, 926.11, 929.0-929.9, 952.10-952.19, 952.8-952.9, 958.8-958.99, 959.11-959.19, 959.8-959.9

806.23　T_1-T_6 level with central cord syndrome 🅠 🅠

Ex: 733.10-733.19, 733.93-733.98, 805.2-805.3, 805.8-805.9, 806.20-806.39, 806.8-806.9, 829.0-829.1, 839.21, 839.31-839.40, 839.49-839.50, 839.59, 839.69, 839.79-839.9, 847.1, 847.9, 848.8-848.9, 879.8-879.9, 905.1, 926.11, 929.0-929.9, 952.10-952.19, 952.8-952.9, 958.8-958.99, 959.11-959.19, 959.8-959.9

806.24　T_1-T_6 level with other specified spinal cord injury 🅠 🅠

T_1-T_6 level with:
incomplete spinal cord lesion NOS
posterior cord syndrome

Ex: 733.10-733.19, 733.93-733.98, 805.2-805.3, 805.8-805.9, 806.20-806.39, 806.8-806.9, 829.0-829.1, 839.21, 839.31-839.40, 839.49-839.50, 839.59, 839.69, 839.79-839.9, 847.1, 847.9, 848.8-848.9, 879.8-879.9, 905.1, 926.11, 929.0-929.9, 952.10-952.19, 952.8-952.9, 958.8-958.99, 959.11-959.19, 959.8-959.9

806.25　T_7-T_{12} level with unspecified spinal cord injury 🅠 🅠

Ex: 733.10-733.19, 733.93-733.98, 805.2-805.3, 805.8-805.9, 806.20-806.39, 806.8-806.9, 829.0-829.1, 839.21, 839.31-839.40, 839.49-839.50, 839.59, 839.69, 839.79-839.9, 847.1, 847.9, 848.8-848.9, 879.8-879.9, 905.1, 926.11, 929.0-929.9, 952.10-952.19, 952.8-952.9, 958.8-958.99, 959.11-959.19, 959.8-959.9

806.26　T_7-T_{12} level with complete lesion of cord 🅠 🅠

Ex: 733.10-733.19, 733.93-733.98, 805.2-805.3, 805.8-805.9, 806.20-806.39, 806.8-806.9, 829.0-829.1, 839.21, 839.31-839.40, 839.49-839.50, 839.59, 839.69, 839.79-839.9, 847.1, 847.9, 848.8-848.9, 879.8-879.9, 905.1, 926.11, 929.0-929.9, 952.10-952.19, 952.8-952.9, 958.8-958.99, 959.11-959.19, 959.8-959.9

806.27　T_7-T_{12} level with anterior cord syndrome 🅠 🅠

Ex: 733.10-733.19, 733.93-733.98, 805.2-805.3, 805.8-805.9, 806.20-806.39, 806.8-806.9, 829.0-829.1, 839.21, 839.31-839.40, 839.49-839.50, 839.59, 839.69, 839.79-839.9, 847.1, 847.9, 848.8-848.9, 879.8-879.9, 905.1, 926.11, 929.0-929.9, 952.10-952.19, 952.8-952.9, 958.8-958.99, 959.11-959.19, 959.8-959.9

806.28　T_7-T_{12} level with central cord syndrome 🅠 🅠

Ex: 733.10-733.19, 733.93-733.98, 805.2-805.3, 805.8-805.9, 806.20-806.39, 806.8-806.9, 829.0-829.1, 839.21, 839.31-839.40, 839.49-839.50, 839.59, 839.69, 839.79-839.9, 847.1, 847.9, 848.8-848.9, 879.8-879.9, 905.1, 926.11, 929.0-929.9, 952.10-952.19, 952.8-952.9, 958.8-958.99, 959.11-959.19, 959.8-959.9

806.29　T_7-T_{12} level with other specified spinal cord injury 🅠 🅠

T_7-T_{12} level with:
incomplete spinal cord lesion NOS
posterior cord syndrome

Ex: 733.10-733.19, 733.93-733.98, 805.2-805.3, 805.8-805.9, 806.20-806.39, 806.8-806.9, 829.0-829.1, 839.21, 839.31-839.40, 839.49-839.50, 839.59, 839.69, 839.79-839.9, 847.1, 847.9, 848.8-848.9, 879.8-879.9, 905.1, 926.11, 929.0-929.9, 952.10-952.19, 952.8-952.9, 958.8-958.99, 959.11-959.19, 959.8-959.9

● 806.3　Dorsal [thoracic], open

806.30　T_1-T_6 level with unspecified spinal cord injury 🅠 🅠

Ex: 733.10-733.19, 733.93-733.98, 805.2-805.3, 805.8-805.9, 806.20-806.39, 806.8-806.9, 829.0-829.1, 839.21, 839.31-839.40, 839.49-839.50, 839.59, 839.69, 839.79-839.9, 847.1, 847.9, 848.8-848.9, 879.8-879.9, 905.1, 926.11, 929.0-929.9, 952.10-952.19, 952.8-952.9, 958.8-958.99, 959.11-959.19, 959.8-959.9

806.31　T_1-T_6 level with complete lesion of cord 🅠 🅠

Ex: 733.10-733.19, 733.93-733.98, 805.2-805.3, 805.8-805.9, 806.20-806.39, 806.8-806.9, 829.0-829.1, 839.21, 839.31-839.40, 839.49-839.50, 839.59, 839.69, 839.79-839.9, 847.1, 847.9, 848.8-848.9, 879.8-879.9, 905.1, 926.11, 929.0-929.9, 952.10-952.19, 952.8-952.9, 958.8-958.99, 959.11-959.19, 959.8-959.9

806.32　T_1-T_6 level with anterior cord syndrome 🅠 🅠

Ex: 733.10-733.19, 733.93-733.98, 805.2-805.3, 805.8-805.9, 806.20-806.39, 806.8-806.9, 829.0-829.1, 839.21, 839.31-839.40, 839.49-839.50, 839.59, 839.69, 839.79-839.9, 847.1, 847.9, 848.8-848.9, 879.8-879.9, 905.1, 926.11, 929.0-929.9, 952.10-952.19, 952.8-952.9, 958.8-958.99, 959.11-959.19, 959.8-959.9

806.33　T_1-T_6 level with central cord syndrome 🅠 🅠

Ex: 733.10-733.19, 733.93-733.98, 805.2-805.3, 805.8-805.9, 806.20-806.39, 806.8-806.9, 829.0-829.1, 839.21, 839.31-839.40, 839.49-839.50, 839.59, 839.69, 839.79-839.9, 847.1, 847.9, 848.8-848.9, 879.8-879.9, 905.1, 926.11, 929.0-929.9, 952.10-952.19, 952.8-952.9, 958.8-958.99, 959.11-959.19, 959.8-959.9

806.34　T_1-T_6 level with other specified spinal cord injury 🅠 🅠

T_1-T_6 level with:
incomplete spinal cord lesion NOS
posterior cord syndrome

Ex: 733.10-733.19, 733.93-733.98, 805.2-805.3, 805.8-805.9, 806.20-806.39, 806.8-806.9, 829.0-829.1, 839.21, 839.31-839.40, 839.49-839.50, 839.59, 839.69, 839.79-839.9, 847.1, 847.9, 848.8-848.9, 879.8-879.9, 905.1, 926.11, 929.0-929.9, 952.10-952.19, 952.8-952.9, 958.8-958.99, 959.11-959.19, 959.8-959.9

806.35　T_7-T_{12} level with unspecified spinal cord injury 🅠 🅠

Ex: 733.10-733.19, 733.93-733.98, 805.2-805.3, 805.8-805.9, 806.20-806.39, 806.8-806.9, 829.0-829.1, 839.21, 839.31-839.40, 839.49-839.50, 839.59, 839.69, 839.79-839.9, 847.1, 847.9, 848.8-848.9, 879.8-879.9, 905.1, 926.11, 929.0-929.9, 952.10-952.19, 952.8-952.9, 958.8-958.99, 959.11-959.19, 959.8-959.9

806.36　T_7-T_{12} level with complete lesion of cord 🅠 🅠

Ex: 733.10-733.19, 733.93-733.98, 805.2-805.3, 805.8-805.9, 806.20-806.39, 806.8-806.9, 829.0-829.1, 839.21, 839.31-839.40, 839.49-839.50, 839.59, 839.69, 839.79-839.9, 847.1, 847.9, 848.8-848.9, 879.8-879.9, 905.1, 926.11, 929.0-929.9, 952.10-952.19, 952.8-952.9, 958.8-958.99, 959.11-959.19, 959.8-959.9

806.37　T_7-T_{12} level with anterior cord syndrome 🅠 🅠

Ex: 733.10-733.19, 733.93-733.98, 805.2-805.3, 805.8-805.9, 806.20-806.39, 806.8-806.9, 829.0-829.1, 839.21, 839.31-839.40, 839.49-839.50, 839.59, 839.69, 839.79-839.9, 847.1, 847.9, 848.8-848.9, 879.8-879.9, 905.1, 926.11, 929.0-929.9, 952.10-952.19, 952.8-952.9, 958.8-958.99, 959.11-959.19, 959.8-959.9

806.38 T₇-T₁₂ level with central cord syndrome 🗫 🗫
(Ex) 733.10-733.19, 733.93-733.98, 805.2-805.3, 805.8-805.9,
806.20-806.39, 806.8-806.9, 829.0-829.1, 839.21,
839.31-839.40, 839.49-839.50, 839.59, 839.69, 839.79-839.9,
847.1, 847.9, 848.8-848.9, 879.8-879.9, 905.1, 926.11,
929.0-929.9, 952.10-952.19, 952.8-952.9, 958.8-958.99,
959.11-959.19, 959.8-959.9

806.39 T₇-T₁₂ level with other specified spinal cord
injury 🗫 🗫
T₇-T₁₂ level with:
incomplete spinal cord lesion NOS
posterior cord syndrome
(Ex) 733.10-733.19, 733.93-733.98, 805.2-805.3, 805.8-805.9,
806.20-806.39, 806.8-806.9, 829.0-829.1, 839.21,
839.31-839.40, 839.49-839.50, 839.59, 839.69, 839.79-839.9,
847.1, 847.9, 848.8-848.9, 879.8-879.9, 905.1, 926.11,
929.0-929.9, 952.10-952.19, 952.8-952.9, 958.8-958.99,
959.11-959.19, 959.8-959.9

806.4 Lumbar, closed 🗫 🗫
(Ex) 733.10-733.19, 733.93-733.98, 805.4-805.5, 805.8-805.9, 806.4-806.5,
806.8-806.9, 829.0-829.1, 839.20, 839.30, 839.40, 839.49-839.50, 839.59,
839.69, 839.79-839.9, 847.2, 847.9, 848.8-848.9, 879.8-879.9, 905.1,
926.11, 929.0-929.9, 952.2, 952.8-952.9, 958.8-958.99, 959.11-959.19,
959.8-959.9

Coding Clinic: 1999, Q4, P11-13

806.5 Lumbar, open 🗫 🗫
(Ex) 733.10-733.19, 733.93-733.98, 805.4-805.5, 805.8-805.9, 806.4-806.5,
806.8-806.9, 829.0-829.1, 839.20, 839.30, 839.40, 839.49-839.50, 839.59,
839.69, 839.79-839.9, 847.2, 847.9, 848.8-848.9, 879.8-879.9, 905.1,
926.11, 929.0-929.9, 952.2, 952.8-952.9, 958.8-958.99, 959.11-959.19,
959.8-959.9

● 806.6 Sacrum and coccyx, closed
806.60 With unspecified spinal cord injury 🗫 🗫
(Ex) 733.10-733.19, 733.93-733.98, 805.6-805.9, 806.60-806.9,
829.0-829.1, 839.40-839.59, 839.69, 839.79-839.9,
846.0-847.0, 847.3-847.9, 848.5-848.9, 879.8-879.9, 905.1,
926.11, 929.0-929.9, 952.3-952.9, 958.8-958.99,
959.11-959.19, 959.8-959.9

806.61 With complete cauda equina lesion 🗫 🗫
(Ex) 733.10-733.19, 733.93-733.98, 805.6-805.9, 806.60-806.9,
829.0-829.1, 839.40-839.59, 839.69, 839.79-839.9,
846.0-847.0, 847.3-847.9, 848.5-848.9, 879.8-879.9, 905.1,
926.11, 929.0-929.9, 952.3-952.9, 958.8-958.99,
959.11-959.19, 959.8-959.9

806.62 With other cauda equina injury 🗫 🗫
(Ex) 733.10-733.19, 733.93-733.98, 805.6-805.9, 806.60-806.9,
829.0-829.1, 839.40-839.59, 839.69, 839.79-839.9,
846.0-847.0, 847.3-847.9, 848.5-848.9, 879.8-879.9, 905.1,
926.11, 929.0-929.9, 952.3-952.9, 958.8-958.99,
959.11-959.19, 959.8-959.9

806.69 With other spinal cord injury 🗫 🗫
(Ex) 733.10-733.19, 733.93-733.98, 805.6-805.9, 806.60-806.9,
829.0-829.1, 839.40-839.59, 839.69, 839.79-839.9,
846.0-847.0, 847.3-847.9, 848.5-848.9, 879.8-879.9, 905.1,
926.11, 929.0-929.9, 952.3-952.9, 958.8-958.99,
959.11-959.19, 959.8-959.9

● 806.7 Sacrum and coccyx, open
806.70 With unspecified spinal cord injury 🗫 🗫
(Ex) 733.10-733.19, 733.93-733.98, 805.6-805.9, 806.60-806.9,
829.0-829.1, 839.40-839.59, 839.69, 839.79-839.9,
846.0-847.0, 847.3-847.9, 848.5-848.9, 879.8-879.9, 905.1,
926.11, 929.0-929.9, 952.3-952.9, 958.8-958.99,
959.11-959.19, 959.8-959.9

806.71 With complete cauda equina lesion 🗫 🗫
(Ex) 733.10-733.19, 733.93-733.98, 805.6-805.9, 806.60-806.9,
829.0-829.1, 839.40-839.59, 839.69, 839.79-839.9,
846.0-847.0, 847.3-847.9, 848.5-848.9, 879.8-879.9, 905.1,
926.11, 929.0-929.9, 952.3-952.9, 958.8-958.99,
959.11-959.19, 959.8-959.9

806.72 With other cauda equina injury 🗫 🗫
(Ex) 733.10-733.19, 733.93-733.98, 805.6-805.9, 806.60-806.9,
829.0-829.1, 839.40-839.59, 839.69, 839.79-839.9,
846.0-847.0, 847.3-847.9, 848.5-848.9, 879.8-879.9, 905.1,
926.11, 929.0-929.9, 952.3-952.9, 958.8-958.99,
959.11-959.19, 959.8-959.9

806.79 With other spinal cord injury 🗫 🗫
(Ex) 733.10-733.19, 733.93-733.98, 805.6-805.9, 806.60-806.9,
829.0-829.1, 839.40-839.59, 839.69, 839.79-839.9,
846.0-847.0, 847.3-847.9, 848.5-848.9, 879.8-879.9, 905.1,
926.11, 929.0-929.9, 952.3-952.9, 958.8-958.99,
959.11-959.19, 959.8-959.9

806.8 Unspecified, closed 🗫 🗫
(Ex) 733.10-733.19, 733.93-733.98, 805.00-806.9, 829.0-829.1, 839.00-839.59,
839.69, 839.79-839.9, 846.0-847.0, 848.5-848.9, 879.8-879.9, 905.1,
926.11, 929.0-929.9, 952.00-952.9, 958.8-958.99, 959.11-959.19,
959.8-959.9

806.9 Unspecified, open 🗫 🗫
(Ex) 733.10-733.19, 733.93-733.98, 805.00-806.9, 829.0-829.1, 839.00-839.59,
839.69, 839.79-839.9, 846.0-847.0, 848.5-848.9, 879.8-879.9, 905.1,
926.11, 929.0-929.9, 952.00-952.9, 958.8-958.99, 959.11-959.19,
959.8-959.9

● 807 Fracture of rib(s), sternum, larynx, and trachea
The following fifth-digit subclassification is for use with codes
807.0–807.1:

0	rib(s), unspecified	5	five ribs
1	one rib	6	six ribs
2	two ribs	7	seven ribs
3	three ribs	8	eight or more ribs
4	four ribs	9	multiple ribs, unspecified

● 807.0 Rib(s), closed 🗫 🗫
[0-9] For codes **807.00-807.02:** (Ex) 807.00-807.4, 819.0-819.1, 828.0-829.1,
848.8-848.9, 879.8-879.9, 929.0-929.9, 958.8-958.99, 959.8-959.9;
For code **807.03:** (Ex) 807.00-807.19, 807.4, 819.0-819.1, 828.0-829.1,
848.8-848.9, 879.8-879.9, 929.0-929.9, 958.8, 959.8-959.9;
For codes **807.04-807.09:** (Ex) 807.00-807.19, 807.4, 819.0-819.1, 828.0-829.1,
848.8-848.9, 879.8-879.9, 929.0-929.9, 958.8-958.99, 959.8-959.9

Coding Clinic: 2013, Q1, P15

● 807.1 Rib(s), open 🗫 🗫
[0-9] (Ex) 807.00-807.19, 807.4, 819.0-819.1, 828.0-829.1, 848.8-848.9, 879.8-879.9,
929.0-929.9, 958.8-958.99, 959.8-959.9

807.2 Sternum, closed 🗫 🗫
(Ex) 807.2-807.4, 829.0-829.1, 848.8-848.9, 879.8-879.9, 929.0-929.9,
958.8-958.99, 959.8-959.9

807.3 Sternum, open 🗫 🗫
(Ex) 807.2-807.4, 829.0-829.1, 848.8-848.9, 879.8-879.9, 929.0-929.9,
958.8-958.99, 959.8-959.9

807.4 Flail chest 🗫 🗫
Unstable chest due to sternum and/or rib fracture
(Ex) 807.00-807.4, 829.0-829.1, 848.8-848.9, 879.8-879.9, 929.0-929.9,
958.8-958.99, 959.8-9599

807.5 Larynx and trachea, closed 🗫 🗫
Hyoid bone
Thyroid cartilage
Trachea
(Ex) 807.5-807.6, 829.0-829.1, 848.8-848.9, 879.8-879.9, 929.0-929.9,
958.8-958.99, 959.8-959.9

807.6 Larynx and trachea, open 🗫 🗫
(Ex) 807.5-807.6, 829.0-829.1, 848.8-848.9, 879.8-879.9, 929.0-929.9,
958.8-958.99, 959.8-959.9

● 808 Fracture of pelvis
808.0 Acetabulum, closed 🗫 🗫
(Ex) 733.10-733.19, 733.93-733.98, 808.0-808.1, 808.43-808.49, 808.53,
808.59-809.1, 829.0-829.1, 835.00-835.13, 843.0-843.9, 846.0-846.9,
848.5-848.9, 879.8-879.9, 929.0-929.9, 958.8-958.99, 959.6, 959.8-959.9

808.1 Acetabulum, open 🗫 🗫
(Ex) 808.0-808.1, 808.43-808.49, 808.53, 808.59-809.1, 829.0-829.1,
835.00-835.13, 843.0-843.9, 846.0-846.9, 848.5-848.9, 879.8-879.9,
929.0-929.9, 958.8-958.99, 959.6, 959.8-959.9

808.2 Pubis, closed 🗫 🗫
(Ex) 733.10-733.19, 733.93-733.98, 808.2-808.3, 808.43-808.49, 808.53,
808.59-809.1, 829.0-829.1, 835.00-835.13, 843.0-843.9, 846.0-846.9,
848.5-848.9, 879.8-879.9, 929.0-929.9, 958.8-958.99, 959.6, 959.8-959.9

Coding Clinic: 2008, Q1, P9-10

808.3 Pubis, open 🗫 🗫
(Ex) 733.10-733.19, 733.93-733.98, 808.2-808.3, 808.43-808.49, 808.53,
808.59-809.1, 829.0-829.1, 835.00-835.13, 843.0-843.9, 846.0-846.9,
848.5-848.9, 879.8-879.9, 929.0-929.9, 958.8-958.99, 959.6, 959.8-959.9

N Newborn: 0   P Pediatric: 0–17   M Maternity: 12–55   A Adult: 15–124   ♀ Females Only   ♂ Males Only

(Ex) CC/MCC Exclusions   🗫 Complication\Comorbidity   🗫 Major C\C   🗫 Present on Admission Requirement   🗫 Hospital-Acquired Condition

● 808.4 **Other specified part, closed**
   808.41 **Ilium** 🔖 🔖
   (Ex:) 733.10, 733.19, 808.0-808.43, 808.49-808.53, 808.59-809.1,
   829.0-829.1, 835.00-835.13, 843.0-843.9, 846.0-846.9,
   848.5-848.9, 879.8-879.9, 929.0-929.9, 958.8, 958.99, 959.6,
   959.8-959.9

   808.42 **Ischium** 🔖 🔖
   (Ex:) 808.42

   808.43 **Multiple closed pelvic fractures with disruption of
   pelvic circle** 🔖 🔖
   Multiple closed pelvic fractures with disruption
   of pelvic ring
   (Ex:) 733.10-733.19, 733.93-733.98, 808.0-808.43, 808.49-808.53,
   808.59-809.1, 829.0-829.1, 835.00-835.13, 843.0-843.9,
   846.0-846.9, 848.5-848.9, 879.8-879.9, 929.0-929.9,
   958.8-958.99, 959.6, 959.8-959.9

   Coding Clinic: 2008, Q1, P9-10

   808.44 **Multiple closed pelvic fractures without
   disruption of pelvic circle** 🔖 🔖
   Multiple closed pelvic fractures without
   disruption of pelvic ring
   (Ex:) 808.49

   808.49 **Other** 🔖 🔖
   Innominate bone
   Pelvic rim
   (Ex:) 733.10-733.19, 733.93-733.98, 808.0-809.1, 829.0-829.1,
   835.00-835.13, 843.0-843.9, 846.0-846.9, 848.5-848.9,
   879.8-879.9, 929.0-929.9, 958.8-958.99, 959.6, 959.8-959.9

● 808.5 **Other specified part, open**
   808.51 **Ilium** 🔖 🔖
   (Ex:) 733.10-733.19, 733.93-733.98, 808.41, 808.43, 808.49-808.51,
   808.53, 808.59-809.1, 829.0-829.1, 835.00-835.13,
   843.0-843.9, 846.0-846.9, 848.5-848.9, 879.8-879.9,
   929.0-929.9, 958.8-958.99, 959.6, 959.8-959.9

   808.52 **Ischium** 🔖 🔖
   (Ex:) 733.10-733.19, 733.93-733.98, 808.42-808.43, 808.49,
   808.52-808.53, 808.59-809.1, 829.0-829.1, 835.00-835.13,
   843.0-843.9, 846.0-846.9, 848.5-848.9, 879.8-879.9,
   929.0-929.9, 958.8-958.99, 959.6, 959.8-959.9

   808.53 **Multiple open pelvic fractures with disruption of
   pelvic circle** 🔖 🔖
   Multiple open pelvic fractures with disruption of
   pelvic ring
   (Ex:) 733.10-733.19, 733.93-733.98, 808.0-808.43, 808.49-808.53,
   808.59-809.1, 829.0-829.1, 835.00-835.13, 843.0-843.9,
   846.0-846.9, 848.5-848.9, 879.8-879.9, 929.0-929.9,
   958.8-958.99, 959.6, 959.8-959.9

   808.54 **Multiple open pelvic fractures without disruption
   of pelvic circle** 🔖 🔖
   Multiple open pelvic fractures without
   disruption of pelvic ring
   (Ex:) 808.49

   808.59 **Other** 🔖 🔖
   (Ex:) 733.10-733.19, 733.93-733.98, 808.0-809.1, 829.0-829.1,
   835.00-835.13, 843.0-843.9, 846.0-846.9, 848.5-848.9,
   879.8-879.9, 929.0-929.9, 958.8-958.99, 959.6, 959.8-959.9

   808.8 **Unspecified, closed** 🔖 🔖
   (Ex:) 733.10-733.19, 733.93-733.98, 808.0-808.43, 808.49-808.53, 808.59-809.1,
   829.0-829.1, 835.00-835.13, 843.0-843.9, 846.0-846.9, 848.5-848.9,
   879.8-879.9, 929.0-929.9, 958.8-958.99, 959.6, 959.8-959.9

   808.9 **Unspecified, open** 🔖 🔖
   (Ex:) 733.10-733.19, 733.93-733.98, 808.0-808.43, 808.49-808.53, 808.59-809.1,
   829.0-829.1, 835.00-835.13, 843.0-843.9, 846.0-846.9, 848.5-848.9,
   879.8-879.9, 929.0-929.9, 958.8-958.99, 959.6, 959.8-959.9

● 809 **Ill-defined fractures of bones of trunk**
   Includes bones of trunk with other bones except those of
   skull and face
   multiple bones of trunk
   Excludes *multiple fractures of:*
   pelvic bones alone (808.0–808.9)
   ribs alone (807.0–807.1, 807.4)
   *ribs or sternum with limb bones (819.0–819.1,
   828.0–828.1)*
   skull or face with other bones (804.0–804.9)

   809.0 **Fracture of bones of trunk, closed** 🔖 🔖
   (Ex:) 733.10, 733.19, 808.0-808.43, 808.49-808.53, 808.59-809.1, 829.0-829.1,
   835.00-835.13, 843.0-843.9, 846.0-846.9, 848.5-848.9, 879.8-879.9,
   929.0-929.9, 958.8, 958.99, 959.6, 959.8-959.9

   809.1 **Fracture of bones of trunk, open** 🔖 🔖
   (Ex:) 733.10, 733.19, 808.0-808.43, 808.49-808.53, 808.59-809.1, 829.0-829.1,
   835.00-835.13, 843.0-843.9, 846.0-846.9, 848.5-848.9, 879.8-879.9,
   929.0-929.9, 958.8, 958.99, 959.6, 959.8-959.9

FRACTURE OF UPPER LIMB (810–819)

● 810 **Fracture of clavicle**
   Includes collar bone
   interligamentous part of clavicle
   The following fifth-digit subclassification is for use with
   category 810:

0 unspecified part
Clavicle NOS
1 sternal end of clavicle
2 shaft of clavicle
3 acromial end of clavicle

● 810.0 **Closed**
   [0-3]
● 810.1 **Open** 🔖 🔖
   [0-3]   (Ex:) 810.00-810.13, 818.0-819.1

● 811 **Fracture of scapula**
   Includes shoulder blade
   The following fifth-digit subclassification is for use with
   category 811:

0 unspecified part
1 acromial process
Acromion (process)
2 coracoid process
3 glenoid cavity and neck of scapula
9 other

● 811.0 **Closed**
   [0-3,9]
● 811.1 **Open** 🔖 🔖
   [0-3,9]   (Ex:) 811.00-811.19, 818.0-819.1

● 812 **Fracture of humerus**
   ● 812.0 **Upper end, closed**
      812.00 **Upper end, unspecified part** 🔖 🔖
      Proximal end   Shoulder
      (Ex:) 812.00-812.59, 819.0-819.1

      812.01 **Surgical neck** 🔖 🔖
      Neck of humerus NOS
      (Ex:) 812.00-812.59, 819.0-819.1

      812.02 **Anatomical neck** 🔖 🔖
      (Ex:) 812.00-812.59, 819.0-819.1

      812.03 **Greater tuberosity** 🔖 🔖
      (Ex:) 812.00-812.59, 819.0-819.1

      812.09 **Other** 🔖 🔖
      Head   Upper epiphysis
      (Ex:) 812.00-812.59, 819.0-819.1

◀ New   ◀◀ Revised   deleted Deleted   Excludes   Includes   Use additional   Code first   Omit code
● Unacceptable Principal Diagnosis   ● Use Additional Digit(s)   ▷ Manifestation Code   OGCR Official Guidelines   Coding Clinic

● 812.1 **Upper end, open**

812.10 **Upper end, unspecified part** 🐾 🐾
(Ex) 812.10-812.59, 818.0-819.1

812.11 **Surgical neck** 🐾 🐾
(Ex) 812.10-812.59, 818.0-819.1

812.12 **Anatomical neck** 🐾 🐾
(Ex) 812.10-812.59, 818.0-819.1

812.13 **Greater tuberosity** 🐾 🐾
(Ex) 812.10-812.59, 818.0-819.1

812.19 **Other** 🐾 🐾
(Ex) 812.10-812.59, 818.0-819.1

● 812.2 **Shaft or unspecified part, closed**

812.20 **Unspecified part of humerus** 🐾 🐾
Humerus NOS   Upper arm NOS

812.21 **Shaft of humerus** 🐾 🐾
(Ex) 812.21
Coding Clinic: 2005, Q4, P127-129; 1999, Q3, P14-15

● 812.3 **Shaft or unspecified part, open**

812.30 **Unspecified part of humerus** 🐾 🐾
(Ex) 812.10-812.59, 818.0-819.1

812.31 **Shaft of humerus** 🐾 🐾
(Ex) 812.10-812.59, 818.0-819.1

● 812.4 **Lower end, closed**
Distal end of humerus   Elbow

812.40 **Lower end, unspecified part** 🐾 🐾
(Ex) 812.00-812.59, 819.0-819.1

812.41 **Supracondylar fracture of humerus** 🐾 🐾
(Ex) 812.00-812.59, 818.0-819.1

812.42 **Lateral condyle** 🐾 🐾
External condyle
(Ex) 812.00-812.59, 819.0-819.1

812.43 **Medial condyle** 🐾 🐾
Internal epicondyle
(Ex) 812.00-812.59, 819.0-819.1

812.44 **Condyle(s), unspecified** 🐾 🐾
Articular process NOS
Lower epiphysis
(Ex) 812.00-812.59, 819.0-819.1

812.49 **Other** 🐾 🐾
Multiple fractures of lower end
Trochlea
(Ex) 812.00-812.59, 819.0-819.1

● 812.5 **Lower end, open**

812.50 **Lower end, unspecified part** 🐾 🐾
(Ex) 812.00-812.59, 819.0-819.1

812.51 **Supracondylar fracture of humerus** 🐾 🐾
(Ex) 812.10-812.59, 818.0-819.1

812.52 **Lateral condyle** 🐾 🐾
(Ex) 812.10-812.59, 818.0-819.1

812.53 **Medial condyle** 🐾 🐾
(Ex) 812.10-812.59, 818.0-819.1

812.54 **Condyle(s), unspecified** 🐾 🐾
(Ex) 812.10-812.59, 818.0-819.1

812.59 **Other** 🐾 🐾
(Ex) 812.10-812.59, 818.0-819.1

● 813 **Fracture of radius and ulna**

● 813.0 **Upper end, closed**
Proximal end

813.00 **Upper end of forearm, unspecified**

813.01 **Olecranon process of ulna**

813.02 **Coronoid process of ulna**

813.03 **Monteggia's fracture**

813.04 **Other and unspecified fractures of proximal end of ulna (alone)**
Multiple fractures of ulna, upper end

813.05 **Head of radius**

813.06 **Neck of radius**

813.07 **Other and unspecified fractures of proximal end of radius (alone)**
Multiple fractures of radius, upper end

813.08 **Radius with ulna, upper end [any part]**

● 813.1 **Upper end, open**

813.10 **Upper end of forearm, unspecified** 🐾 🐾
(Ex) 813.10-813.44, 813.50-813.93, 818.0-819.1

813.11 **Olecranon process of ulna** 🐾 🐾
(Ex) 813.10-813.40, 813.42-813.44, 813.50-813.93, 818.0-819.1

813.12 **Coronoid process of ulna** 🐾 🐾
(Ex) 813.10-813.44, 813.50-813.93, 818.0-819.1

813.13 **Monteggia's fracture** 🐾 🐾
(Ex) 813.10-813.44, 813.50-813.93, 818.0-819.1

813.14 **Other and unspecified fractures of proximal end of ulna (alone)** 🐾 🐾
(Ex) 813.10-813.44, 813.50-813.93, 818.0-819.1

813.15 **Head of radius** 🐾 🐾
(Ex) 813.10-813.44, 813.50-813.93, 818.0-819.1

813.16 **Neck of radius** 🐾 🐾
(Ex) 813.10-813.44, 813.50-813.93, 818.0-819.1

813.17 **Other and unspecified fractures of proximal end of radius (alone)** 🐾 🐾
(Ex) 813.10-813.44, 813.50-813.93, 818.0-819.1

813.18 **Radius with ulna, upper end [any part]** 🐾 🐾
(Ex) 813.10-813.44, 813.50-813.93, 818.0-819.1

● 813.2 **Shaft, closed**

813.20 **Shaft, unspecified** 🐾 🐾
(Ex) 813.00-813.93, 819.0-819.1

813.21 **Radius (alone)** 🐾 🐾
(Ex) 813.00-813.93, 819.0-819.1

813.22 **Ulna (alone)** 🐾 🐾
(Ex) 813.00-813.93, 819.0-819.1

813.23 **Radius with ulna** 🐾 🐾
(Ex) 813.00-813.93, 819.0-819.1
Coding Clinic: 2009, Q4, P120

● 813.3 **Shaft, open**

813.30 **Shaft, unspecified** 🐾 🐾
(Ex) 813.10-813.44, 813.50-813.93, 818.0-819.1

813.31 **Radius (alone)** 🐾 🐾
(Ex) 813.10-813.44, 813.50-813.93, 818.0-819.1

813.32 **Ulna (alone)** 🐾 🐾
(Ex) 813.10-813.44, 813.50-813.93, 818.0-819.1

813.33 **Radius with ulna** 🐾 🐾
(Ex) 813.10-813.44, 813.50-813.93, 818.0-819.1

● 813.4 **Lower end, closed**
Distal end

813.40 **Lower end of forearm, unspecified** 🐾 🐾
(Ex) 813.00-813.93, 819.0-819.1

813.41 **Colles' fracture** 🐾 🐾
Smith's fracture
(Ex) 813.00-813.93, 819.0-819.1

813.42 **Other fractures of distal end of radius (alone)** 🐾 🐾
Dupuytren's fracture, radius
Radius, lower end
(Ex) 813.00-813.93, 819.0-819.1

813.43 **Distal end of ulna (alone)** 🐾 🐾
Ulna: Ulna:
head   lower epiphysis
lower end   styloid process
(Ex) 813.00-813.93, 819.0-819.1

813.44 **Radius with ulna, lower end** 🐾 🐾
(Ex) 813.00-813.93, 819.0-819.1
Coding Clinic: 2007, Q1, P3-8

813.45 **Torus fracture of radius (alone)** 🐾 🐾
Excludes *torus fracture of radius and ulna (813.47)*
(Ex) 813.00-813.93, 819.0-819.1
Coding Clinic: 2002, Q4, P70-71

N Newborn: 0   P Pediatric: 0–17   M Maternity: 12–55   A Adult: 15–124   ♀ Females Only   ♂ Males Only

(Ex) CC/MCC Exclusions   🐾 Complication\Comorbidity   🐾 Major C\C   🐾 Present on Admission Requirement   🐾 Hospital-Acquired Condition   961

INJURY AND POISONING (800–999)

813.46   Torus fracture of ulna (alone) 🔲🔲
     Excludes   *torus fracture of radius and ulna (813.47)*
     (Ex) 813.00-813.93, 819.0-819.1

813.47 Torus fracture of radius and ulna 🔲🔲
     (Ex) 813.00-813.93, 819.0-819.1

● **813.5**   Lower end, open

813.50   Lower end of forearm, unspecified 🔲🔲
     (Ex) 813.10-813.44, 813.50-813.93, 818.0-819.1

813.51   Colles' fracture 🔲🔲
     (Ex) 813.10-813.44, 813.50-813.93, 818.0-819.1

813.52   Other fractures of distal end of radius (alone) 🔲🔲
     (Ex) 813.10-813.44, 813.50-813.93, 818.0-819.1

813.53   Distal end of ulna (alone) 🔲🔲
     (Ex) 813.10-813.44, 813.50-813.93, 818.0-819.1

813.54   Radius with ulna, lower end 🔲🔲
     (Ex) 813.10-813.44, 813.50-813.93, 818.0-819.1

● **813.8**   Unspecified part, closed

813.80   Forearm, unspecified 🔲🔲
     (Ex) 813.00-813.93, 819.0-819.1

813.81   Radius (alone)
     Coding Clinic: 1998, Q2, P19

813.82   Ulna (alone) 🔲🔲
     (Ex) 813.00-813.93, 819.0-819.1

813.83   Radius with ulna 🔲🔲
     (Ex) 813.00-813.93, 819.0-819.1

● **813.9**   Unspecified part, open

813.90   Forearm, unspecified 🔲🔲
     (Ex) 813.10-813.44, 813.50-813.93, 818.0-819.1

813.91   Radius (alone) 🔲🔲
     (Ex) 813.10-813.44, 813.50-813.93, 818.0-819.1

813.92   Ulna (alone) 🔲🔲
     (Ex) 813.10-813.44, 813.50-813.93, 818.0-819.1

813.93   Radius with ulna 🔲🔲
     (Ex) 813.10-813.44, 813.50-813.93, 818.0-819.1

● **814**   **Fracture of carpal bone(s)**
The following fifth-digit subclassification is for use with category 814:

> 0   carpal bone, unspecified
>   Wrist NOS
> 1   navicular [scaphoid] of wrist
> 2   lunate [semilunar] bone of wrist
> 3   triquetral [cuneiform] bone of wrist
> 4   pisiform
> 5   trapezium bone [larger multangular]
> 6   trapezoid bone [smaller multangular]
> 7   capitate bone [os magnum]
> 8   hamate [unciform] bone
> 9   other

● **814.0**   Closed
[0-9]

● **814.1**   Open 🔲🔲
[0-9]   (Ex) 814.00-814.19, 819.0-819.1

● **815**   **Fracture of metacarpal bone(s)**
    Includes   hand [except finger]
                  metacarpus
The following fifth-digit subclassification is for use with category 815:

> 0   metacarpal bone(s), site unspecified
> 1   base of thumb [first] metacarpal
>   Bennett's fracture
> 2   base of other metacarpal bone(s)
> 3   shaft of metacarpal bone(s)
> 4   neck of metacarpal bone(s)
> 9   multiple sites of metacarpus

● **815.0**   Closed
[0-4,9]   **Coding Clinic: 1994, Q2, P6**

● **815.1**   Open 🔲🔲
[0-4,9]   (Ex) 815.00-815.19, 817.0-817.1

● **816**   **Fracture of one or more phalanges of hand**
    Includes   finger(s)
                  thumb
The following fifth-digit subclassification is for use with category 816:

> 0   phalanx or phalanges, unspecified
> 1   middle or proximal phalanx or phalanges
> 2   distal phalanx or phalanges
> 3   multiple sites

● **816.0**   Closed
[0-3]

● **816.1**   Open 🔲🔲
[0-3]   For codes **816.10-816.12:** (Ex) 816.00-817.1;
        For code **816.13:** (Ex) 816.00-816.13, 818.0-819.1
        Coding Clinic: 2003, Q4, P76-78

● **817**   **Multiple fractures of hand bones**
    Includes   metacarpal bone(s) with phalanx or phalanges of
                  same hand

817.0   Closed

817.1   Open 🔲🔲
     (Ex) 814.00-819.1

● **818**   **Ill-defined fractures of upper limb**
    Includes   arm NOS
                  multiple bones of same upper limb
    Excludes   *multiple fractures of:*
                  metacarpal bone(s) with phalanx or phalanges
                     (817.0–817.1)
                  phalanges of hand alone (816.0–816.1)
                  radius with ulna (813.0–813.9)

818.0   Closed

818.1   Open 🔲🔲
     (Ex) 812.00-813.44, 813.50-819.1

OGCR   Section I.C.17.b.4

Multiple fracture categories 819 and 828 classify bilateral fractures of both upper limbs (819) and both lower limbs (828), but without any detail at the fourth-digit level other than open and closed type of fractures.

● **819**   **Multiple fractures involving both upper limbs, and upper limb with rib(s) and sternum**
    Includes   arm(s) with rib(s) or sternum
                  both arms [any bones]

819.0   Closed
     (Ex) 807.00-807.4, 812.00-813.44, 813.50-819.1

819.1   Open 🔲🔲
     (Ex) 807.00-807.4, 812.00-813.44, 813.50-819.1

FRACTURE OF LOWER LIMB (820–829)

● **820**   **Fracture of neck of femur**

● **820.0**   Transcervical fracture, closed

820.00   Intracapsular section, unspecified 🔲🔲
     (Ex) 733.10-733.19, 733.93-733.98, 820.00-821.39, 827.0-829.1,
         843.0-843.9, 848.8-848.9, 879.8-879.9, 929.0-929.9,
         958.8-958.99, 959.6, 959.8-959.9

820.01   Epiphysis (separation) (upper) 🔲🔲
     Transepiphyseal
     Fracture and separation across growth plate
     (Ex) 733.10-733.19, 733.93-733.98, 820.00-821.39, 827.0-829.1,
         843.0-843.9, 848.8-848.9, 879.8-879.9, 929.0-929.9,
         958.8-958.99, 959.6, 959.8-959.9

820.02   Midcervical section 🔲🔲
     Transcervical NOS
     (Ex) 733.10-733.19, 733.93-733.98, 820.00-821.39, 827.0-829.1,
         843.0-843.9, 848.8-848.9, 879.8-879.9, 929.0-929.9,
         958.8-958.99, 959.6, 959.8-959.9
     Coding Clinic: 2003, Q3, P12-13

◀ New   ◀▥ Revised   ~~deleted~~ Deleted   Excludes   Includes   Use additional   Code first   Omit code
● Unacceptable Principal Diagnosis   ● Use Additional Digit(s)   ▷ Manifestation Code   **OGCR** Official Guidelines   **Coding Clinic**

962

820.03   **Base of neck** 🏵️ 🏵️
     Cervicotrochanteric section
     (Ex:) 733.10-733.19, 733.93-733.98, 820.00-821.39, 827.0-829.1, 843.0-843.9, 848.8-848.9, 879.8-879.9, 929.0-929.9, 958.8-958.99, 959.6, 959.8-959.9

820.09   **Other** 🏵️ 🏵️
     Head of femur   Subcapital
     (Ex:) 733.10-733.19, 733.93-733.98, 820.00-821.39, 827.0-829.1, 843.0-843.9, 848.8-848.9, 879.8-879.9, 929.0-929.9, 958.8-958.99, 959.6, 959.8-959.9

● **820.1**   **Transcervical fracture, open**

820.10   **Intracapsular section, unspecified** 🏵️ 🏵️
     (Ex:) 733.10-733.19, 733.93-733.98, 820.00-821.39, 827.0-829.1, 843.0-843.9, 848.8-848.9, 879.8-879.9, 929.0-929.9, 958.8-958.99, 959.6, 959.8-959.9

820.11   **Epiphysis (separation) (upper)** 🏵️ 🏵️
     (Ex:) 733.10-733.19, 733.93-733.98, 820.00-821.39, 827.0-829.1, 843.0-843.9, 848.8-848.9, 879.8-879.9, 929.0-929.9, 958.8-958.99, 959.6, 959.8-959.9

820.12   **Midcervical section** 🏵️ 🏵️
     (Ex:) 733.10-733.19, 733.93-733.98, 820.00-821.39, 827.0-829.1, 843.0-843.9, 848.8-848.9, 879.8-879.9, 929.0-929.9, 958.8-958.99, 959.6, 959.8-959.9

820.13   **Base of neck** 🏵️ 🏵️
     (Ex:) 733.10-733.19, 733.93-733.98, 820.00-821.39, 827.0-829.1, 843.0-843.9, 848.8-848.9, 879.8-879.9, 929.0-929.9, 958.8-958.99, 959.6, 959.8-959.9

820.19   **Other** 🏵️ 🏵️
     (Ex:) 733.10-733.19, 733.93-733.98, 820.00-821.39, 827.0-829.1, 843.0-843.9, 848.8-848.9, 879.8-879.9, 929.0-929.9, 958.8-958.99, 959.6, 959.8-959.9

● **820.2**   **Pertrochanteric fracture, closed**

820.20   **Trochanteric section, unspecified** 🏵️ 🏵️
     Trochanter:
      NOS
      greater
      lesser
     (Ex:) 733.10-733.19, 733.93-733.98, 820.00-821.39, 827.0-829.1, 843.0-843.9, 848.8-848.9, 879.8-879.9, 929.0-929.9, 958.8-958.99, 959.6, 959.8-959.9

820.21   **Intertrochanteric section** 🏵️ 🏵️
     (Ex:) 733.10-733.19, 733.93-733.98, 820.00-821.39, 827.0-829.1, 843.0-843.9, 848.8-848.9, 879.8-879.9, 929.0-929.9, 958.8-958.99, 959.6, 959.8-959.9
     Coding Clinic: 1994, Q2, P6; 1984, May-June, P11

820.22   **Subtrochanteric section** 🏵️ 🏵️
     (Ex:) 733.10-733.19, 733.93-733.98, 820.00-821.39, 827.0-829.1, 843.0-843.9, 848.8-848.9, 879.8-879.9, 929.0-929.9, 958.8-958.99, 959.6, 959.8-959.9

● **820.3**   **Pertrochanteric fracture, open**

820.30   **Trochanteric section, unspecified** 🏵️ 🏵️
     (Ex:) 733.10-733.19, 733.93-733.98, 820.00-821.39, 827.0-829.1, 843.0-843.9, 848.8-848.9, 879.8-879.9, 929.0-929.9, 958.8-958.99, 959.6, 959.8-959.9

820.31   **Intertrochanteric section** 🏵️ 🏵️
     (Ex:) 733.10-733.19, 733.93-733.98, 820.00-821.39, 827.0-829.1, 843.0-843.9, 848.8-848.9, 879.8-879.9, 929.0-929.9, 958.8-958.99, 959.6, 959.8-959.9

820.32   **Subtrochanteric section** 🏵️ 🏵️
     (Ex:) 733.10-733.19, 733.93-733.98, 820.00-821.39, 827.0-829.1, 843.0-843.9, 848.8-848.9, 879.8-879.9, 929.0-929.9, 958.8-958.99, 959.6, 959.8-959.9

820.8   **Unspecified part of neck of femur, closed** 🏵️ 🏵️
     Hip NOS   Neck of femur NOS
     (Ex:) 733.10-733.19, 733.93-733.98, 820.00-821.39, 827.0-829.1, 843.0-843.9, 848.8-848.9, 879.8-879.9, 929.0-929.9, 958.8-958.99, 959.6, 959.8-959.9
     Coding Clinic: 1994, Q2, P9; 1985, Nov-Dec, P16

820.9   **Unspecified part of neck of femur, open** 🏵️ 🏵️
     (Ex:) 733.10-733.19, 733.93-733.98, 820.00-821.39, 827.0-829.1, 843.0-843.9, 848.8-848.9, 879.8-879.9, 929.0-929.9, 958.8-958.99, 959.6, 959.8-959.9

● **821**   **Fracture of other and unspecified parts of femur**

● **821.0**   **Shaft or unspecified part, closed**

821.00   **Unspecified part of femur** 🏵️ 🏵️
     ThighUpper leg
     Excludes   *hip NOS (820.8)*
     (Ex:) 733.10-733.19, 733.93-733.98, 820.00-821.39, 827.0-829.1, 843.0-843.9, 848.8-848.9, 879.8-879.9, 929.0-929.9, 958.8-958.99, 959.6, 959.8-959.9

821.01   **Shaft** 🏵️ 🏵️
     (Ex:) 733.10-733.19, 733.93-733.98, 820.00-821.39, 827.0-829.1, 843.0-843.9, 848.8-848.9, 879.8-879.9, 929.0-929.9, 958.8-958.99, 959.6, 959.8-959.9
     Coding Clinic: 2007, Q1, P3-8; 1999, Q1, P5

● **821.1**   **Shaft or unspecified part, open**

821.10   **Unspecified part of femur** 🏵️ 🏵️
     (Ex:) 733.10-733.19, 733.93-733.98, 820.00-821.39, 827.0-829.1, 843.0-843.9, 848.8-848.9, 879.8-879.9, 929.0-929.9, 958.8-958.99, 959.6, 959.8-959.9

821.11   **Shaft** 🏵️ 🏵️
     (Ex:) 733.10-733.19, 733.93-733.98, 820.00-821.39, 827.0-829.1, 843.0-843.9, 848.8-848.9, 879.8-879.9, 929.0-929.9, 958.8-958.99, 959.6, 959.8-959.9

● **821.2**   **Lower end, closed**
     Distal end

821.20   **Lower end, unspecified part** 🏵️ 🏵️
     (Ex:) 733.10, 733.14-733.15, 733.19, 820.00-821.39, 827.0-829.1, 843.0-843.9, 848.8-848.9, 879.8-879.9, 929.0-929.9, 958.8, 958.99, 959.6, 959.8-959.9

821.21   **Condyle, femoral** 🏵️ 🏵️
     (Ex:) 733.10, 733.14-733.15, 733.19, 820.00-821.39, 827.0-829.1, 843.0-843.9, 848.8-848.9, 879.8-879.9, 929.0-929.9, 958.8, 958.99, 959.6, 959.8-959.9

821.22   **Epiphysis, lower (separation)** 🏵️ 🏵️
     (Ex:) 733.10, 733.14-733.15, 733.19, 820.00-821.39, 827.0-829.1, 843.0-843.9, 848.8-848.9, 879.8-879.9, 929.0-929.9, 958.8, 958.99, 959.6, 959.8-959.9

821.23   **Supracondylar fracture of femur** 🏵️ 🏵️
     (Ex:) 733.10, 733.14-733.15, 733.19, 820.00-821.39, 827.0-829.1, 843.0-843.9, 848.8-848.9, 879.8-879.9, 929.0-929.9, 958.8, 958.99, 959.6, 959.8-959.9

821.29   **Other** 🏵️ 🏵️
     Multiple fractures of lower end
     (Ex:) 733.10, 733.14-733.15, 733.19, 820.00-821.39, 827.0-829.1, 843.0-843.9, 848.8-848.9, 879.8-879.9, 929.0-929.9, 958.8, 958.99, 959.6, 959.8-959.9

● **821.3**   **Lower end, open**

821.30   **Lower end, unspecified part** 🏵️ 🏵️
     (Ex:) 733.10, 733.14-733.15, 733.19, 820.00-821.39, 827.0-829.1, 843.0-843.9, 848.8-848.9, 879.8-879.9, 929.0-929.9, 958.8, 958.99, 959.6, 959.8-959.9

821.31   **Condyle, femoral** 🏵️ 🏵️
     (Ex:) 733.10, 733.14-733.15, 733.19, 820.00-821.39, 827.0-829.1, 843.0-843.9, 848.8-848.9, 879.8-879.9, 929.0-929.9, 958.8, 959.6, 959.8-959.9

821.32   **Epiphysis, lower (separation)** 🏵️ 🏵️
     (Ex:) 733.10, 733.14-733.15, 733.19, 820.00-821.39, 827.0-829.1, 843.0-843.9, 848.8-848.9, 879.8-879.9, 929.0-929.9, 958.8, 958.99, 959.6, 959.8-959.9

821.33   **Supracondylar fracture of femur** 🏵️ 🏵️
     (Ex:) 733.10, 733.14-733.15, 733.19, 820.00-821.39, 827.0-829.1, 843.0-843.9, 848.8-848.9, 879.8-879.9, 929.0-929.9, 958.8, 959.6, 959.8-959.9

821.39   **Other** 🏵️ 🏵️
     (Ex:) 733.10, 733.14-733.15, 733.19, 821.39-822.1, 827.0-829.1, 843.0-843.9, 848.8-848.9, 879.8-879.9, 929.0-929.9, 958.8, 958.99, 959.6, 959.8-959.9

● **822**   **Fracture of patella**

822.0   **Closed** 🏵️ 🏵️
     (Ex:) 822.0-822.1, 828.0-828.1

822.1   **Open** 🏵️ 🏵️
     (Ex:) 733.10, 733.19, 822.1-823.32, 823.80-823.92, 827.0-829.1, 843.0-843.9, 848.8-848.9, 879.8-879.9, 929.0-929.9, 958.8, 958.99, 959.6, 959.8-959.9

INJURY AND POISONING (800–999)

N   Newborn: 0   **P**   Pediatric: 0–17   **M**   Maternity: 12–55   **A**   Adult: 15–124   ♀   Females Only   ♂   Males Only

(Ex:)   CC/MCC Exclusions   🏵️   Complication\Comorbidity   🏵️   Major C\C   Present on Admission Requirement   🏵️   Hospital-Acquired Condition   **963**

● 823 **Fracture of tibia and fibula**

Excludes   *Dupuytren's fracture (824.4–824.5)*
                ankle (824.4–824.5)
                radius (813.42, 813.52)
                Pott's fracture (824.4–824.5)
                that involving ankle (824.0–824.9)

The following fifth-digit subclassification is for use with category 823:

> 0   tibia alone
> 1   fibula alone
> 2   fibula with tibia

● 823.0 **Upper end, closed** 0,2 , 0,2
[0-2]   Head   Tibia:
             Proximal end   condyles
                                          tuberosity
        For codes **823.00 and 823.02:** (Ex) 733.10, 733.16-733.19, 823.00-823.32,
        823.80-823.92, 827.0-829.1, 843.0-843.9, 848.8-848.9, 879.8-879.9,
        929.0-929.9, 958.8, 958.99, 959.6, 959.8-959.9

● 823.1 **Upper end, open**
[0-2]   (Ex) 733.10, 733.16-733.19, 823.00-823.32, 823.80-823.92, 827.0-829.1,
             843.0-843.9, 848.8-848.9, 879.8-879.9, 929.0-929.9, 958.8, 958.99,
             959.6, 959.8-959.9

● 823.2 **Shaft, closed** 0,2 , 0,2
[0-2]   For codes **823.20 and 823.22:** (Ex) 733.10, 733.16-733.19, 823.00-823.32,
             823.80-823.92, 827.0-829.1, 843.0-843.9, 848.8-848.9, 879.8-879.9,
             929.0-929.9, 958.8, 958.99, 959.6, 959.8-959.9

● 823.3 **Shaft, open**
[0-2]   (Ex) 733.10, 733.16-733.19, 823.00-823.32, 823.80-823.92, 827.0-829.1,
             843.0-843.9, 848.8-848.9, 879.8-879.9, 929.0-929.9, 958.8, 958.99,
             959.6, 959.8-959.9

● 823.4 **Torus fracture** 0,2 , 0,2
[0-2]   For code **823.40 and 823.42:** (Ex) 823.00-823.92
        Coding Clinic: 2002, Q4, P70-71

● 823.8 **Unspecified part, closed** 0,2 , 0,2
[0-2]   Lower leg NOS
             For code **823.80:** (Ex) 823.00-823.92;
             For code **823.82:** (Ex) 733.10, 733.16-733.19, 823.00-823.32, 823.80-823.92,
             827.0-829.1, 843.0-843.9, 848.8-848.9, 879.8-879.9, 929.0-929.9, 958.8,
             958.99, 959.6, 959.8-959.9
        Coding Clinic: 1997, Q1, P8

● 823.9 **Unspecified part, open**
[0-2]   (Ex) 733.10, 733.16-733.19, 823.00-823.32, 823.80-823.92, 827.0-829.1,
             843.0-843.9, 848.8-848.9, 879.8-879.9, 929.0-929.9, 958.8, 958.99,
             959.6, 959.8-959.9

● 824 **Fracture of ankle**

824.0 **Medial malleolus, closed**
        Tibia involving:
          ankle   malleolus
        Coding Clinic: 2004, Q1, P9

824.1 **Medial malleolus, open**
        (Ex) 733.10, 733.16-733.19, 824.1-824.9, 827.0-829.1, 843.0-843.9, 848.8-848.9,
        879.8-879.9, 929.0-929.9, 958.8, 958.99, 959.6, 959.8-959.9

824.2 **Lateral malleolus, closed**
        Fibula involving:
          ankle   malleolus
        Coding Clinic: 2002, Q2, P3

824.3 **Lateral malleolus, open**
        (Ex) 733.10, 733.16-733.19, 824.1-824.9, 827.0-829.1, 843.0-843.9, 848.8-848.9,
        879.8-879.9, 929.0-929.9, 958.8, 958.99, 959.6, 959.8-959.9

824.4 **Bimalleolar, closed**
        Dupuytren's fracture, fibula
        Pott's fracture
        Coding Clinic: 2012, Q2, P11

824.5 **Bimalleolar, open**
        (Ex) 733.10, 733.16-733.19, 824.1-824.9, 827.0-829.1, 843.0-843.9, 848.8-848.9,
        879.8-879.9, 929.0-929.9, 958.8, 958.99, 959.6, 959.8-959.9

824.6 **Trimalleolar, closed**
        Lateral and medial malleolus with anterior or posterior
        lip of tibia

824.7 **Trimalleolar, open**
        (Ex) 733.10, 733.16-733.19, 824.1-824.9, 827.0-829.1, 843.0-843.9, 848.8-848.9,
        879.8-879.9, 929.0-929.9, 958.8, 958.99, 959.6, 959.8-959.9

824.8 **Unspecified, closed**
        Ankle NOS
        Coding Clinic: 2000, Q3, P12; 1994, Q2, P7

824.9 **Unspecified, open**
        (Ex) 733.10, 733.16-733.19, 824.1-824.9, 827.0-829.1, 843.0-843.9, 848.8-848.9,
        879.8-879.9, 929.0-929.9, 958.8, 958.99, 959.6, 959.8-959.9

● 825 **Fracture of one or more tarsal and metatarsal bones**

825.0 **Fracture of calcaneus, closed**
        Heel bone   Os calcis

825.1 **Fracture of calcaneus, open**
        (Ex) 733.10, 733.16-733.19, 825.1-825.39, 827.0-829.1, 843.0-843.9, 848.8-848.9,
        879.8-879.9, 929.0-929.9, 958.8, 958.99, 959.6, 959.8-959.9

● 825.2 **Fracture of other tarsal and metatarsal bones, closed**

825.20 **Unspecified bone(s) of foot [except toes]**
         Instep

825.21 **Astragalus**
         Talus

825.22 **Navicular [scaphoid], foot**

825.23 **Cuboid**

825.24 **Cuneiform, foot**

825.25 **Metatarsal bone(s)**

825.29 **Other**
         Tarsal with metatarsal bone(s) only
         Excludes   *calcaneus (825.0)*
         Coding Clinic: 1994, Q2, P5

● 825.3 **Fracture of other tarsal and metatarsal bones, open**

825.30 **Unspecified bone(s) of foot [except toes]**
         (Ex) 825.0-826.1

825.31 **Astragalus**
         (Ex) 733.10, 733.19, 825.1-825.39, 827.0-829.1, 843.0-843.9,
         848.8-848.9, 879.8-879.9, 929.0-929.9, 958.8, 958.99, 959.6,
         959.8-959.9

825.32 **Navicular [scaphoid], foot**
         (Ex) 733.10, 733.19, 825.1-825.39, 827.0-829.1, 843.0-843.9,
         848.8-848.9, 879.8-879.9, 929.0-929.9, 958.8, 958.99, 959.6,
         959.8-959.9

825.33 **Cuboid**
         (Ex) 733.10, 733.19, 825.1-825.39, 827.0-829.1, 843.0-843.9,
         848.8-848.9, 879.8-879.9, 929.0-929.9, 958.8, 958.99, 959.6,
         959.8-959.9

825.34 **Cuneiform, foot**
         (Ex) 733.10, 733.19, 825.1-825.39, 827.0-829.1, 843.0-843.9,
         848.8-848.9, 879.8-879.9, 929.0-929.9, 958.8, 958.99, 959.6,
         959.8-959.9

825.35 **Metatarsal bone(s)**
         (Ex) 733.10, 733.19, 825.1-825.39, 827.0-829.1, 843.0-843.9,
         848.8-848.9, 879.8-879.9, 929.0-929.9, 958.8, 958.99, 959.6,
         959.8-959.9

825.39 **Other**
         (Ex) 825.0-826.1

● 826 **Fracture of one or more phalanges of foot**
        Includes   toe(s)

826.0 **Closed**

826.1 **Open**

● 827 **Other, multiple, and ill-defined fractures of lower limb**
        Includes   leg NOS
                       multiple bones of same lower limb
        Excludes   *multiple fractures of:*
                       ankle bones alone (824.4–824.9)
                       phalanges of foot alone (826.0–826.1)
                       tarsal with metatarsal bones (825.29, 825.39)
                       tibia with fibula (823.0–823.9 with fifth-digit 2)

827.0 **Closed**

827.1 **Open**
        (Ex) 820.00-823.32, 823.80-829.1

▲ New   ◀▥ Revised   ~~deleted~~ Deleted   Excludes   Includes   Use additional   Code first   Omit code

964   ● Unacceptable Principal Diagnosis   ● Use Additional Digit(s)   ▷ Manifestation Code   **OGCR** Official Guidelines   **Coding Clinic**

● **828 Multiple fractures involving both lower limbs, lower with upper limb, and lower limb(s) with rib(s) and sternum**

　　Includes　arm(s) with leg(s) [any bones]
　　　　　　　both legs [any bones]
　　　　　　　leg(s) with rib(s) or sternum

　　OGCR　Section I.C.17.b.4

　　Multiple fracture categories 819 and 828 classify bilateral fractures of both upper limbs (819) and both lower limbs (828), but without any detail at the fourth-digit level other than open and closed type of fractures.

　　828.0 Closed 🔹 🔹
　　　　(Ex) 820.00-823.32, 823.80-829.1

　　828.1 Open 🔹 🔹
　　　　(Ex) 820.00-823.32, 823.80-829.1

● **829 Fracture of unspecified bones**

　　829.0 Unspecified bone, closed

　　829.1 Unspecified bone, open

DISLOCATION (830–839)

　　Includes　displacement
　　　　　　　subluxation
　　　　　　　　Out of position

　　Excludes　*congenital dislocation (754.0–755.8)*
　　　　　　　pathological dislocation (718.2)
　　　　　　　recurrent dislocation (718.3)

The descriptions "closed" and "open," used in the fourth-digit subdivisions, include the following terms:

closed:	open:
complete	compound
dislocation NOS	infected
partial	with foreign body
simple	
uncomplicated	

Note:　A dislocation not indicated as closed or open should be classified as closed.

● **830 Dislocation of jaw**

　　Includes　jaw (cartilage) (meniscus)
　　　　　　　mandible
　　　　　　　maxilla (inferior)
　　　　　　　temporomandibular (joint)

　　830.0 Closed dislocation

　　830.1 Open dislocation 🔹 🔹
　　　　(Ex) 830.0-830.1, 839.69, 839.79-839.9

● **831 Dislocation of shoulder**

　　Excludes　*sternoclavicular joint (839.61, 839.71)*
　　　　　　　sternum (839.61, 839.71)

The following fifth-digit subclassification is for use with category 831:

```
0  shoulder, unspecified
     Humerus NOS
1  anterior dislocation of humerus
2  posterior dislocation of humerus
3  inferior dislocation of humerus
4  acromioclavicular (joint)
     Clavicle
9  other
     Scapula
```

● **831.0 Closed dislocation**
　　[0-4,9]　**Coding Clinic: 1987, Nov-Dec, P7**

● **831.1 Open dislocation** 🔹 🔹
　　[0-4,9]　For code **831.10:** (Ex) 831.10, 839.69, 839.79-839.9;
　　　　　　For code **831.11:** (Ex) 831.11, 839.69, 839.79-839.9;
　　　　　　For code **831.12:** (Ex) 831.12, 839.69, 839.79-839.9;
　　　　　　For code **831.13:** (Ex) 831.13, 839.69, 839.79-839.9;
　　　　　　For code **831.14:** (Ex) 831.14, 839.69, 839.79-839.9;
　　　　　　For code **831.19:** (Ex) 831.19, 839.69, 839.79-839.9

Figure 17–13　Dislocation including displacement and subluxation. (From Grainger & Allison's Diagnostic Radiology: A Textbook of Medical Imaging, ed 4, Churchill Livingstone, 2001)

A　　B

● **832 Dislocation of elbow**

The following fifth-digit subclassification is for use with subcategories 832.0 and 832.1:

```
0  elbow unspecified
1  anterior dislocation of elbow
2  posterior dislocation of elbow
3  medial dislocation of elbow
4  lateral dislocation of elbow
9  other
```

● **832.0 Closed dislocation**
　　[0-4,9]

● **832.1 Open dislocation** 🔹 🔹
　　[0-4,9]　For code **832.10:** (Ex) 832.10;
　　　　　　For code **832.11:** (Ex) 832.11;
　　　　　　For code **832.12:** (Ex) 832.12;
　　　　　　For code **832.13:** (Ex) 832.13;
　　　　　　For code **832.14:** (Ex) 832.14;
　　　　　　For code **832.19:** (Ex) 832.19

　　832.2 Nursemaid's elbow
　　　　Subluxation of radial head

● **833 Dislocation of wrist**

The following fifth-digit subclassification is for use with category 833:

```
0  wrist, unspecified part
     Carpal (bone)
     Radius, distal end
1  radioulnar (joint), distal
2  radiocarpal (joint)
3  midcarpal (joint)
4  carpometacarpal (joint)
5  metacarpal (bone), proximal end
9  other
     Ulna, distal end
```

● **833.0 Closed dislocation**
　　[0-5,9]

● **833.1 Open dislocation** 🔹 🔹
　　[0-5,9]　For codes **833.10, 833.13-833.19:** (Ex) 833.00-833.19;
　　　　　　For code **833.11:** (Ex) 833.11;
　　　　　　For code **833.12:** (Ex) 833.12

● **834 Dislocation of finger**

　　Includes　finger(s)
　　　　　　　phalanx of hand
　　　　　　　thumb

The following fifth-digit subclassification is for use with category 834:

```
0  finger, unspecified part
1  metacarpophalangeal (joint)
     Metacarpal (bone), distal end
2  interphalangeal (joint), hand
```

● **834.0 Closed dislocation**
　　[0-2]

● **834.1 Open dislocation**
　　[0-2]

N Newborn: 0　**P** Pediatric: 0–17　**M** Maternity: 12–55　**A** Adult: 15–124　♀ Females Only　♂ Males Only

(Ex) CC/MCC Exclusions　🔹 Complication\Comorbidity　🔹 Major C\C　🔹 Present on Admission Requirement　🔹 Hospital-Acquired Condition　**965**

● 835 **Dislocation of hip**
The following fifth-digit subclassification is for use with category 835:

> 0 dislocation of hip, unspecified
> 1 posterior dislocation
> 2 obturator dislocation
> 3 other anterior dislocation

● 835.0 **Closed dislocation** 🔍 🔍
[0-3]   For code **835.00:** (Ex:) 835.00, 839.69, 839.79-839.9;
        For code **835.01:** (Ex:) 835.01, 839.69, 839.79-839.9;
        For code **835.02:** (Ex:) 835.02, 839.69, 839.79-839.9;
        For code **835.03:** (Ex:) 835.03, 839.69, 839.79-839.9

● 835.1 **Open dislocation** 🔍 🔍
[0-3]   For code **835.10:** (Ex:) 835.10, 839.69, 839.79-839.9;
        For code **835.11:** (Ex:) 835.11, 839.69, 839.79-839.9;
        For code **835.12:** (Ex:) 835.12, 839.69, 839.79-839.9;
        For code **835.13:** (Ex:) 835.13, 839.69, 839.79-839.9

● 836 **Dislocation of knee**

> **Excludes** dislocation of knee:
> old or pathological (718.2)
> recurrent (718.3)
> internal derangement of knee joint (717.0–717.5, 717.8–717.9)
> old tear of cartilage or meniscus of knee (717.0–717.5, 717.8–717.9)

836.0 **Tear of medial cartilage or meniscus of knee, current**
Bucket handle tear:
NOS current injury
medial meniscus current injury

836.1 **Tear of lateral cartilage or meniscus of knee, current**

836.2 **Other tear of cartilage or meniscus of knee, current**
Tear of:
cartilage (semilunar) current injury, not specified as medial or lateral
meniscus current injury, not specified as medial or lateral

836.3 **Dislocation of patella, closed**

836.4 **Dislocation of patella, open** 🔍 🔍
(Ex:) 836.3-836.4

● 836.5 **Other dislocation of knee, closed**

836.50 **Dislocation of knee, unspecified**

836.51 **Anterior dislocation of tibia, proximal end**
Posterior dislocation of femur, distal end, closed

836.52 **Posterior dislocation of tibia, proximal end**
Anterior dislocation of femur, distal end, closed

836.53 **Medial dislocation of tibia, proximal end**

836.54 **Lateral dislocation of tibia, proximal end**

836.59 **Other**

● 836.6 **Other dislocation of knee, open**

836.60 **Dislocation of knee, unspecified** 🔍 🔍
(Ex:) 717.0-717.9, 718.26, 718.36, 836.60, 839.69, 839.79-839.9

836.61 **Anterior dislocation of tibia, proximal end** 🔍 🔍
Posterior dislocation of femur, distal end, open
(Ex:) 836.61, 839.69, 839.79-839.9

836.62 **Posterior dislocation of tibia, proximal end** 🔍 🔍
Anterior dislocation of femur, distal end, open
(Ex:) 836.62, 839.69, 839.79-839.9

836.63 **Medial dislocation of tibia, proximal end** 🔍 🔍
(Ex:) 836.63, 839.69, 839.79-839.9

836.64 **Lateral dislocation of tibia, proximal end** 🔍 🔍
(Ex:) 836.64, 839.69, 839.79-839.9

836.69 **Other** 🔍 🔍
(Ex:) 836.69, 839.69, 839.79-839.9

● 837 **Dislocation of ankle**

> **Includes** astragalus   scaphoid, foot
> fibula, distal end   tibia, distal end
> navicular, foot

837.0 **Closed dislocation**

837.1 **Open dislocation** 🔍 🔍
(Ex:) 837.1, 839.69, 839.79-839.9

● 838 **Dislocation of foot**
The following fifth-digit subclassification is for use with category 838:

> 0 foot, unspecified
> 1 tarsal (bone), joint unspecified
> 2 midtarsal (joint)
> 3 tarsometatarsal (joint)
> 4 metatarsal (bone), joint unspecified
> 5 metatarsophalangeal (joint)
> 6 interphalangeal (joint), foot
> 9 other
>   Phalanx of foot
>   Toe(s)

● 838.0 **Closed dislocation**
[0-6,9]

● 838.1 **Open dislocation**
[0-6,9]

● 839 **Other, multiple, and ill-defined dislocations**
Coding Clinic: 1995, Q4, P51

● 839.0 **Cervical vertebra, closed**
Cervical spine
Neck

839.00 **Cervical vertebra, unspecified** 🔍 🔍
(Ex:) 805.00-805.18, 806.00-806.19, 806.8-806.9, 839.00-839.18, 847.0, 848.8-848.9, 879.8-879.9, 929.0-929.9, 952.00-952.09, 958.8-958.99, 959.8-959.9

839.01 **First cervical vertebra** 🔍 🔍
(Ex:) 805.00-805.18, 806.00-806.19, 806.8-806.9, 839.00-839.18, 847.0, 848.8-848.9, 879.8-879.9, 929.0-929.9, 952.00-952.09, 958.8-958.99, 959.8-959.9

839.02 **Second cervical vertebra** 🔍 🔍
(Ex:) 805.00-805.18, 806.00-806.19, 806.8-806.9, 839.00-839.18, 847.0, 848.8-848.9, 879.8-879.9, 929.0-929.9, 952.00-952.09, 958.8-958.99, 959.8-959.9

839.03 **Third cervical vertebra** 🔍 🔍
(Ex:) 805.00-805.18, 806.00-806.19, 806.8-806.9, 839.00-839.18, 847.0, 848.8-848.9, 879.8-879.9, 929.0-929.9, 952.00-952.09, 958.8-958.99, 959.8-959.9

839.04 **Fourth cervical vertebra** 🔍 🔍
(Ex:) 805.00-805.18, 806.00-806.19, 806.8-806.9, 839.00-839.18, 847.0, 848.8-848.9, 879.8-879.9, 929.0-929.9, 952.00-952.09, 958.8-958.99, 959.8-959.9

839.05 **Fifth cervical vertebra** 🔍 🔍
(Ex:) 805.00-805.18, 806.00-806.19, 806.8-806.9, 839.00-839.18, 847.0, 848.8-848.9, 879.8-879.9, 929.0-929.9, 952.00-952.09, 958.8-958.99, 959.8-959.9

839.06 **Sixth cervical vertebra** 🔍 🔍
(Ex:) 805.00-805.18, 806.00-806.19, 806.8-806.9, 839.00-839.18, 847.0, 848.8-848.9, 879.8-879.9, 929.0-929.9, 952.00-952.09, 958.8-958.99, 959.8-959.9

839.07 **Seventh cervical vertebra** 🔍 🔍
(Ex:) 805.00-805.18, 806.00-806.19, 806.8-806.9, 839.00-839.18, 847.0, 848.8-848.9, 879.8-879.9, 929.0-929.9, 952.00-952.09, 958.8-958.99, 959.8-959.9

839.08 **Multiple cervical vertebrae** 🔍 🔍
(Ex:) 805.00-805.18, 806.00-806.19, 806.8-806.9, 839.00-839.18, 847.0, 848.8-848.9, 879.8-879.9, 929.0-929.9, 952.00-952.09, 958.8-958.99, 959.8-959.9

◀ New ◀▥ Revised ~~deleted~~ Deleted Excludes Includes Use additional Code first Omit code
● Unacceptable Principal Diagnosis ● Use Additional Digit(s) ▶ Manifestation Code OGCR Official Guidelines Coding Clinic

● **839.1 Cervical vertebra, open**

   839.10 Cervical vertebra, unspecified 🔹 🔹
     Ex: 805.00-805.18, 806.00-806.19, 806.8-806.9, 839.00-839.18, 847.0, 848.8-848.9, 879.8-879.9, 929.0-929.9, 952.00-952.09, 958.8-958.99, 959.8-959.9

   839.11 First cervical vertebra 🔹 🔹
     Ex: 805.00-805.18, 806.00-806.19, 806.8-806.9, 839.00-839.18, 847.0, 848.8-848.9, 879.8-879.9, 929.0-929.9, 952.00-952.09, 958.8-958.99, 959.8-959.9

   839.12 Second cervical vertebra 🔹 🔹
     Ex: 805.00-805.18, 806.00-806.19, 806.8-806.9, 839.00-839.18, 847.0, 848.8-848.9, 879.8-879.9, 929.0-929.9, 952.00-952.09, 958.8-958.99, 959.8-959.9

   839.13 Third cervical vertebra 🔹 🔹
     Ex: 805.00-805.18, 806.00-806.19, 806.8-806.9, 839.00-839.18, 847.0, 848.8-848.9, 879.8-879.9, 929.0-929.9, 952.00-952.09, 958.8-958.99, 959.8-959.9

   839.14 Fourth cervical vertebra 🔹 🔹
     Ex: 805.00-805.18, 806.00-806.19, 806.8-806.9, 839.00-839.18, 847.0, 848.8-848.9, 879.8-879.9, 929.0-929.9, 952.00-952.09, 958.8-958.99, 959.8-959.9

   839.15 Fifth cervical vertebra 🔹 🔹
     Ex: 805.00-805.18, 806.00-806.19, 806.8-806.9, 839.00-839.18, 847.0, 848.8-848.9, 879.8-879.9, 929.0-929.9, 952.00-952.09, 958.8-958.99, 959.8-959.9

   839.16 Sixth cervical vertebra 🔹 🔹
     Ex: 805.00-805.18, 806.00-806.19, 806.8-806.9, 839.00-839.18, 847.0, 848.8-848.9, 879.8-879.9, 929.0-929.9, 952.00-952.09, 958.8-958.99, 959.8-959.9

   839.17 Seventh cervical vertebra 🔹 🔹
     Ex: 805.00-805.18, 806.00-806.19, 806.8-806.9, 839.00-839.18, 847.0, 848.8-848.9, 879.8-879.9, 929.0-929.9, 952.00-952.09, 958.8-958.99, 959.8-959.9

   839.18 Multiple cervical vertebrae 🔹 🔹
     Ex: 805.00-805.18, 806.00-806.19, 806.8-806.9, 839.00-839.18, 847.0, 848.8-848.9, 879.8-879.9, 929.0-929.9, 952.00-952.09, 958.8-958.99, 959.8-959.9

● **839.2 Thoracic and lumbar vertebra, closed**

   839.20 Lumbar vertebra

   839.21 Thoracic vertebra
     Dorsal [thoracic] vertebra

● **839.3 Thoracic and lumbar vertebra, open**

   839.30 Lumbar vertebra 🔹 🔹
     Ex: 839.30

   839.31 Thoracic vertebra 🔹 🔹
     Ex: 839.21, 839.31

● **839.4 Other vertebra, closed**

   839.40 Vertebra, unspecified site
     Spine NOS

   839.41 Coccyx

   839.42 Sacrum
     Sacroiliac (joint)

   839.49 Other

● **839.5 Other vertebra, open**

   839.50 Vertebra, unspecified site 🔹 🔹
     Ex: 839.10-839.18, 839.30-839.31, 839.50-839.59, 839.79, 839.9

   839.51 Coccyx 🔹 🔹
     Ex: 839.51

   839.52 Sacrum 🔹 🔹
     Ex: 839.52

   839.59 Other 🔹 🔹
     Ex: 839.10-839.18, 839.30-839.31, 839.50-839.59, 839.79, 839.9

● **839.6 Other location, closed**

   839.61 Sternum 🔹 🔹
     Sternoclavicular joint
     Ex: 839.61, 839.71

   839.69 Other
     Pelvis

● **839.7 Other location, open**

   839.71 Sternum 🔹 🔹
     Ex: 839.61, 839.71

   839.79 Other 🔹 🔹
     Ex: 830.1, 831.10-831.19, 832.10-832.19, 833.10-833.19, 834.10-834.12, 835.10-835.13, 836.4, 836.60-836.69, 837.1, 838.10-838.19, 839.10-839.18, 839.30-839.31, 839.50-839.59, 839.71-839.79, 839.9

● **839.8 Multiple and ill-defined, closed**
     Arm
     Back
     Hand
     Multiple locations, except fingers or toes alone
     Other ill-defined locations
     Unspecified location

● **839.9 Multiple and ill-defined, open** 🔹 🔹
     Ex: 830.1, 831.10-831.19, 832.10-832.19, 833.10-833.19, 834.10-834.12, 835.10-835.13, 836.4, 836.60-836.69, 837.1, 838.10-838.19, 839.10-839.18, 839.30-839.31, 839.50-839.59, 839.71-839.79, 839.9

SPRAINS AND STRAINS OF JOINTS AND ADJACENT MUSCLES (840–848)

Includes	avulsion of joint capsule, ligament, muscle, tendon
	hemarthrosis of joint capsule, ligament, muscle, tendon
	Bleeding into joint space
	laceration of joint capsule, ligament, muscle, tendon
	rupture of joint capsule, ligament, muscle, tendon
	sprain of joint capsule, ligament, muscle, tendon
	strain of joint capsule, ligament, muscle, tendon
	tear of joint capsule, ligament, muscle, tendon
Excludes	*laceration of tendon in open wounds (880–884 and 890–894 with .2)*

● **840 Sprains and strains of shoulder and upper arm**
   Sprains are an injury to ligaments when one or more is stretched/torn and *strains* are caused by twisting or pulling a muscle(s) or tendon.

   840.0 Acromioclavicular (joint) (ligament)

   840.1 Coracoclavicular (ligament)

   840.2 Coracohumeral (ligament)

   840.3 Infraspinatus (muscle) (tendon)

   840.4 Rotator cuff (capsule)

     | **Excludes** | *complete rupture of rotator cuff, nontraumatic (727.61)* |

   840.5 Subscapularis (muscle)

   840.6 Supraspinatus (muscle) (tendon)

   840.7 Superior glenoid labrum lesion
     SLAP lesion
     Coding Clinic: 2012, Q2, P15; 2001, Q4, P52

   840.8 Other specified sites of shoulder and upper arm

   840.9 Unspecified site of shoulder and upper arm
     Arm NOS   Shoulder NOS

● **841 Sprains and strains of elbow and forearm**

   841.0 Radial collateral ligament

   841.1 Ulnar collateral ligament

   841.2 Radiohumeral (joint)

   841.3 Ulnohumeral (joint)

   841.8 Other specified sites of elbow and forearm

   841.9 Unspecified site of elbow and forearm
     Elbow NOS

● **842 Sprains and strains of wrist and hand**

  ● **842.0 Wrist**

     842.00 Unspecified site

     842.01 Carpal (joint)

     842.02 Radiocarpal (joint) (ligament)

     842.09 Other
       Radioulnar joint, distal

INJURY AND POISONING (800–999)

N Newborn: 0   **P** Pediatric: 0–17   **M** Maternity: 12–55   **A** Adult: 15–124   ♀ Females Only   ♂ Males Only

Ex: CC/MCC Exclusions   🔹 Complication\Comorbidity   🔹 Major C\C   🔹 Present on Admission Requirement   🔹 Hospital-Acquired Condition   **967**

● **842.1 Hand**
　　842.10 Unspecified site
　　842.11 Carpometacarpal (joint)
　　842.12 Metacarpophalangeal (joint)
　　842.13 Interphalangeal (joint)
　　842.19 Other
　　　　Midcarpal (joint)

● **843 Sprains and strains of hip and thigh**
　　843.0 Iliofemoral (ligament)
　　843.1 Ischiocapsular (ligament)
　　843.8 Other specified sites of hip and thigh
　　843.9 Unspecified site of hip and thigh
　　　　Hip NOS　　　　　Thigh NOS

● **844 Sprains and strains of knee and leg**
　　844.0 Lateral collateral ligament of knee
　　844.1 Medial collateral ligament of knee
　　844.2 Cruciate ligament of knee
　　844.3 Tibiofibular (joint) (ligament), superior
　　844.8 Other specified sites of knee and leg
　　844.9 Unspecified site of knee and leg
　　　　Knee NOS　　　　　Leg NOS

● **845 Sprains and strains of ankle and foot**
　● **845.0 Ankle**
　　　845.00 Unspecified site
　　　　　Coding Clinic: 2002, Q2, P3
　　　845.01 Deltoid (ligament), ankle
　　　　　Internal collateral (ligament), ankle
　　　845.02 Calcaneofibular (ligament)
　　　845.03 Tibiofibular (ligament), distal
　　　　　Coding Clinic: 2004, Q1, P9
　　　845.09 Other
　　　　　Achilles tendon
　● **845.1 Foot**
　　　845.10 Unspecified site
　　　845.11 Tarsometatarsal (joint) (ligament)
　　　845.12 Metatarsophalangeal (joint)
　　　845.13 Interphalangeal (joint), toe
　　　845.19 Other

● **846 Sprains and strains of sacroiliac region**
　　846.0 Lumbosacral (joint) (ligament)
　　846.1 Sacroiliac ligament
　　846.2 Sacrospinatus (ligament)
　　846.3 Sacrotuberous (ligament)
　　846.8 Other specified sites of sacroiliac region
　　846.9 Unspecified site of sacroiliac region

● **847 Sprains and strains of other and unspecified parts of back**
　　Excludes *lumbosacral (846.0)*
　　847.0 Neck
　　　　Anterior longitudinal (ligament), cervical
　　　　Atlanto-axial (joints)
　　　　Atlanto-occipital (joints)
　　　　Whiplash injury
　　　　Excludes *neck injury NOS (959.09)*
　　　　　　　　thyroid region (848.2)
　　847.1 Thoracic
　　847.2 Lumbar
　　847.3 Sacrum
　　　　Sacrococcygeal (ligament)
　　847.4 Coccyx
　　847.9 Unspecified site of back
　　　　Back NOS

● **848 Other and ill-defined sprains and strains**
　　848.0 Septal cartilage of nose
　　848.1 Jaw
　　　　Temporomandibular (joint) (ligament)
　　848.2 Thyroid region
　　　　Cricoarytenoid (joint) (ligament)
　　　　Cricothyroid (joint) (ligament)
　　　　Thyroid cartilage
　　848.3 Ribs
　　　　Chondrocostal (joint) without mention of injury to sternum
　　　　Costal cartilage without mention of injury to sternum
　● **848.4 Sternum**
　　　848.40 Unspecified site
　　　848.41 Sternoclavicular (joint) (ligament)
　　　848.42 Chondrosternal (joint)
　　　848.49 Other
　　　　　Xiphoid cartilage
　　848.5 Pelvis
　　　　Symphysis pubis
　　　　Excludes *that in childbirth (665.6)*
　　848.8 Other specified sites of sprains and strains
　　848.9 Unspecified site of sprain and strain

INTRACRANIAL INJURY, EXCLUDING THOSE WITH SKULL FRACTURE (850–854)

　Includes traumatic brain injury without skull fracture
　Excludes *intracranial injury with skull fracture (800–801 and 803–804, except .0 and .5)*
　　　　open wound of head without intracranial injury (870.0–873.9)
　　　　skull fracture alone (800–801 and 803–804 with .0, .5)

Note: The description "with open intracranial wound," used in the fourth-digit subdivisions, includes those specified as open or with mention of infection or foreign body.

The following fifth-digit subclassification is for use with categories 851–854:

> **0** unspecified state of consciousness
> **1** with no loss of consciousness
> **2** with brief [less than one hour] loss of consciousness
> **3** with moderate [1–24 hours] loss of consciousness
> **4** with prolonged [more than 24 hours] loss of consciousness and return to pre-existing conscious level
> **5** with prolonged [more than 24 hours] loss of consciousness without return to pre-existing conscious level
> 　　Use fifth-digit 5 to designate when a patient is unconscious and dies before regaining consciousness, regardless of the duration of the loss of consciousness
> **6** with loss of consciousness of unspecified duration
> **9** with concussion, unspecified

● **850 Concussion**
　　Includes commotio cerebri
　　Excludes *concussion with:*
　　　　cerebral laceration or contusion (851.0–851.9)
　　　　cerebral hemorrhage (852–853)
　　　　head injury NOS (959.01)
　　Coding Clinic: 1993, Q1, P22-23
　　850.0 With no loss of consciousness
　　　　Concussion with mental confusion or disorientation, without loss of consciousness
　　　　Coding Clinic: 1992, Q2, P5-6
● **850.1 With brief loss of consciousness**
　　　　Loss of consciousness for less than one hour
　　　　Coding Clinic: 2003, Q4, P76; 1999, Q1, P10; 1992, Q2, P5-6
　　850.11 With loss of consciousness of 30 minutes or less
　　　　(Ex) 800.00-801.99, 803.00-804.99, 850.0-852.19, 852.21-854.19, 873.8-873.9, 879.8-879.9, 905.0, 925.1-925.2, 929.0-929.9, 958.8-959.09, 959.8-959.9

850.12 With loss of consciousness from 31 to 59 minutes 🔵 🔵
(Ex:) 800.00-801.99, 803.00-804.99, 850.0-852.19, 852.21-854.19, 873.8-873.9, 879.8-879.9, 905.0, 925.1-925.2, 929.0-929.9, 958.8-959.09, 959.8-959.9
Coding Clinic: 2010, Q4, P111

850.2 With moderate loss of consciousness 🔵 🔵
Loss of consciousness for 1–24 hours
(Ex:) 800.00-801.99, 803.00-804.99, 850.0-852.19, 852.21-854.19, 873.8-873.9, 879.8-879.9, 905.0, 925.1-925.2, 929.0-929.9, 958.8-959.09, 959.8-959.9

850.3 With prolonged loss of consciousness and return to pre-existing conscious level 🔵 🔵
Loss of consciousness for more than 24 hours with complete recovery
(Ex:) 800.00-801.99, 803.00-804.99, 850.0-852.19, 852.21-854.19, 873.8-873.9, 879.8-879.9, 905.0, 925.1-925.2, 929.0-929.9, 958.8-959.09, 959.8-959.9

850.4 With prolonged loss of consciousness, without return to pre-existing conscious level 🔵 🔵
(Ex:) 800.00-801.99, 803.00-804.99, 850.0-852.19, 852.21-854.19, 873.8-873.9, 879.8-879.9, 905.0, 925.1-925.2, 929.0-929.9, 958.8-959.09, 959.8-959.9

850.5 With loss of consciousness of unspecified duration 🔵 🔵
(Ex:) 800.00-801.99, 803.00-804.99, 850.0-852.19, 852.21-854.19, 873.8-873.9, 879.8-879.9, 905.0, 925.1-925.2, 929.0-929.9, 958.8-959.09, 959.8-959.9

850.9 Concussion, unspecified

● **851 Cerebral laceration and contusion**
Cerebral lacerations are tears in brain tissue. Cerebral contusions are bruises on brain.
Requires fifth digit. See beginning of section 850–854 for codes and definitions.
Coding Clinic: 1993, Q1, P22-23

● **851.0 Cortex (cerebral) contusion without mention of open**
[0-6,9] **intracranial wound** 2-4,6 🔵 🔵, 5 🔵 🔵
For codes **851.02-851.06:** (Ex:) 800.00-801.99, 803.00-804.99, 850.0-852.19, 852.21-854.19, 873.8-873.9, 879.8-879.9, 905.0, 925.1-925.2, 929.0-929.9, 958.8-959.09, 959.8-959.9
Coding Clinic: 2010, Q4, P93

● **851.1 Cortex (cerebral) contusion with open intracranial**
[0-6,9] **wound** 🔵 🔵
(Ex:) 800.00-801.99, 803.00-804.99, 850.0-852.19, 852.21-854.19, 873.8-873.9, 879.8-879.9, 905.0, 925.1-925.2, 929.0-929.9, 958.8-959.09, 959.8-959.9

● **851.2 Cortex (cerebral) laceration without mention of open**
[0-6,9] **intracranial wound** 🔵 🔵
(Ex:) 800.00-801.99, 803.00-804.99, 850.0-852.19, 852.21-854.19, 873.8-873.9, 879.8-879.9, 905.0, 925.1-925.2, 929.0-929.9, 958.8-959.09, 959.8-959.9

● **851.3 Cortex (cerebral) laceration with open intracranial**
[0-6,9] **wound** 🔵 🔵
(Ex:) 800.00-801.99, 803.00-804.99, 850.0-852.19, 852.21-854.19, 873.8-873.9, 879.8-879.9, 905.0, 925.1-925.2, 929.0-929.9, 958.8-959.09, 959.8-959.9

● **851.4 Cerebellar or brain stem contusion without mention of**
[0-6,9] **open intracranial wound** 2-4,6 🔵 🔵, 5 🔵 🔵
For codes **851.42-851.46:** (Ex:) 800.00-801.99, 803.00-804.99, 850.0-852.19, 852.21-854.19, 873.8-873.9, 879.8-879.9, 905.0, 925.1-925.2, 929.0-929.9, 958.8-959.09, 959.8-959.9

● **851.5 Cerebellar or brain stem contusion with open intracranial**
[0-6,9] **wound** 🔵 🔵
(Ex:) 800.00-801.99, 803.00-804.99, 850.0-852.19, 852.21-854.19, 873.8-873.9, 879.8-879.9, 905.0, 925.1-925.2, 929.0-929.9, 958.8-959.09, 959.8-959.9

● **851.6 Cerebellar or brain stem laceration without mention of**
[0-6,9] **open intracranial wound** 🔵 🔵
(Ex:) 800.00-801.99, 803.00-804.99, 850.0-852.19, 852.21-854.19, 873.8-873.9, 879.8-879.9, 905.0, 925.1-925.2, 929.0-929.9, 958.8-959.09, 959.8-959.9

● **851.7 Cerebellar or brain stem laceration with open intracranial**
[0-6,9] **wound** 🔵 🔵
(Ex:) 800.00-801.99, 803.00-804.99, 850.0-852.19, 852.21-854.19, 873.8-873.9, 879.8-879.9, 905.0, 925.1-925.2, 929.0-929.9, 958.8-959.09, 959.8-959.9

● **851.8 Other and unspecified cerebral laceration and contusion,**
[0-6,9] **without mention of open intracranial wound** 🔵 🔵
Brain (membrane) NOS
(Ex:) 800.00-801.99, 803.00-804.99, 850.0-852.19, 852.21-854.19, 873.8-873.9, 879.8-879.9, 905.0, 925.1-925.2, 929.0-929.9, 958.8-959.09, 959.8-959.9
Coding Clinic: 1996, Q4, P36.37

● **851.9 Other and unspecified cerebral laceration and**
[0-6,9] **contusion, with open intracranial wound** 🔵 🔵
(Ex:) 800.00-801.99, 803.00-804.99, 850.0-852.19, 852.21-854.19, 873.8-873.9, 879.8-879.9, 905.0, 925.1-925.2, 929.0-929.9, 958.8-959.09, 959.8-959.9

● **852 Subarachnoid, subdural, and extradural hemorrhage, following injury**
Requires fifth digit. See beginning of section 850–854 for codes and definitions.
Excludes *cerebral contusion or laceration (with hemorrhage) (851.0–851.9)*

● **852.0 Subarachnoid hemorrhage following injury without**
[0-6,9] **mention of open intracranial wound** 🔵 🔵
Middle meningeal hemorrhage following injury
(Ex:) 800.00-801.99, 803.00-804.99, 850.0-852.19, 852.21-854.19, 873.8-873.9, 879.8-879.9, 905.0, 925.1-925.2, 929.0-929.9, 958.8-959.09, 959.8-959.9
Coding Clinic: 2010, Q2, P17; 1991, Q3, P15-16

● **852.1 Subarachnoid hemorrhage following injury with**
[0-6,9] **open intracranial wound** 🔵 🔵
(Ex:) 800.00-801.99, 803.00-804.99, 850.0-852.19, 852.21-854.19, 873.8-873.9, 879.8-879.9, 905.0, 925.1-925.2, 929.0-929.9, 958.8-959.09, 959.8-959.9
Coding Clinic: 1991, Q3, P15-16

● **852.2 Subdural hemorrhage following injury without**
[0-6,9] **mention of open intracranial wound** 🔵 🔵
For codes **852.20:** (Ex:) 800.00-801.99, 803.00-804.99, 850.0-854.19, 873.8-873.9, 879.8-879.9, 905.0, 925.1-925.2, 929.0-929.9, 958.8-959.09, 959.8-959.9;
For codes **852.21-852.29:** (Ex:) 800.00-801.99, 803.00-804.99, 850.0-852.19, 852.21-854.19, 873.8-873.9, 879.8-879.9, 905.0, 925.1-925.2, 929.0-929.9, 958.8-959.09, 959.8-959.9
Coding Clinic: 2011, Q4, P100; 2007, Q4, P105-107; 1996, Q4, P43-44

● **852.3 Subdural hemorrhage following injury with open**
[0-6,9] **intracranial wound** 🔵 🔵
(Ex:) 800.00-801.99, 803.00-804.99, 850.0-852.19, 852.21-854.19, 873.8-873.9, 879.8-879.9, 905.0, 925.1-925.2, 929.0-929.9, 958.8-959.09, 959.8-959.9

● **852.4 Extradural hemorrhage following injury without**
[0-6,9] **mention of open intracranial wound** 🔵 🔵
Epidural hematoma following injury
(Ex:) 800.00-801.99, 803.00-804.99, 850.0-852.19, 852.21-854.19, 873.8-873.9, 879.8-879.9, 905.0, 925.1-925.2, 929.0-929.9, 958.8-959.09, 959.8-959.9

● **852.5 Extradural hemorrhage following injury with open**
[0-6,9] **intracranial wound** 🔵 🔵
(Ex:) 800.00-801.99, 803.00-804.99, 850.0-852.19, 852.21-854.19, 873.8-873.9, 879.8-879.9, 905.0, 925.1-925.2, 929.0-929.9, 958.8-959.09, 959.8-959.9

● **853 Other and unspecified intracranial hemorrhage following injury**
Requires fifth digit. See beginning of section 850–854 for codes and definitions.

● **853.0 Without mention of open intracranial wound** 🔵 🔵
[0-6,9] Cerebral compression due to injury
Intracranial hematoma following injury
Traumatic cerebral hemorrhage
(Ex:) 800.00-801.99, 803.00-804.99, 850.0-852.19, 852.21-854.19, 873.8-873.9, 879.8-879.9, 905.0, 925.1-925.2, 929.0-929.9, 958.8-959.09, 959.8-959.9
Coding Clinic: 1990, Q3, P14

● **853.1 With open intracranial wound** 🔵 🔵
[0-6,9] (Ex:) 800.00-801.99, 803.00-804.99, 850.0-852.19, 852.21-854.19, 873.8-873.9, 879.8-879.9, 905.0, 925.1-925.2, 929.0-929.9, 958.8-959.09, 959.8-959.9

● **854 Intracranial injury of other and unspecified nature**
Requires fifth digit. See beginning of section 850-854 for codes and definitions.
Includes injury:
brain NOS
cavernous sinus
intracranial
traumatic brain NOS
Excludes *any condition classifiable to 850–853*
head injury NOS (959.01)
Coding Clinic: 1999, Q1, P10; 1992, Q2, P5-6

● **854.0 Without mention of open intracranial wound**
[0-6,9] 2-4,6 🔵 🔵, 5 🔵 🔵
For codes **854.02-854.06:** (Ex:) 800.00-801.99, 803.00-804.99, 850.0-852.19, 852.21-854.19, 873.8-873.9, 879.8-879.9, 905.0, 925.1-925.2, 929.0-929.9, 958.8-959.09, 959.8-959.9
Coding Clinic: 2009, Q4, P120; 2005, Q2, P6-7

● **854.1 With open intracranial wound** 🔵 🔵
[0-6,9] (Ex:) 800.00-801.99, 803.00-804.99, 850.0-852.19, 852.21-854.19, 873.8-873.9, 879.8-879.9, 905.0, 925.1-925.2, 929.0-929.9, 958.8-959.09, 959.8-959.9

INJURY AND POISONING (800–999)

N Newborn: 0 P Pediatric: 0–17 M Maternity: 12–55 A Adult: 15–124 ♀ Females Only ♂ Males Only
(Ex:) CC/MCC Exclusions 🔵 Complication\Comorbidity 🔵 Major C\C 🔵 Present on Admission Requirement 🔵 Hospital-Acquired Condition

969

INJURY AND POISONING (800-999)

Item 17-1   Pneumothorax is a collection of gas (positive air pressure) in the pleural space resulting in the lung collapsing. A tension pneumothorax is life-threatening and is a result of air in the pleural space causing a displacement in the mediastinal structures and cardiopulmonary function compromise. A traumatic pneumothorax results from blunt or penetrating injury that disrupts the parietal/visceral pleura. **Hemothorax** is blood or bloody fluid in the pleural cavity as a result of traumatic blood vessel rupture or inflammation of the lungs from pneumonia.

INTERNAL INJURY OF THORAX, ABDOMEN, AND PELVIS (860–869)

Includes   blast injuries of internal organs
blunt trauma of internal organs
bruise of internal organs
concussion injuries (except cerebral) of internal organs
crushing of internal organs
hematoma of internal organs
laceration of internal organs
puncture of internal organs
tear of internal organs
traumatic rupture of internal organs

Excludes   *concussion NOS (850.0–850.9)*
flail chest (807.4)
foreign body entering through orifice (930.0–939.9)
injury to blood vessels (901.0–902.9)

Note: The description "with open wound," used in the fourth-digit subdivisions, includes those with mention of infection or foreign body.

● **860   Traumatic pneumothorax and hemothorax**

860.0   **Pneumothorax without mention of open wound into thorax**
Ex: 860.0-860.5, 861.20-861.32, 862.29, 862.39-862.9, 875.0-875.1, 879.8-879.9, 929.0-929.9, 958.7-958.99, 959.8-959.9
Coding Clinic: 1993, Q2, P4-5

860.1   **Pneumothorax with open wound into thorax**
Ex: 860.0-860.5, 861.20-861.32, 862.29, 862.39-862.9, 875.0-875.1, 879.8-879.9, 929.0-929.9, 958.7-958.99, 959.8-959.9
Coding Clinic: 1995, Q3, P17; 1993, Q2, P4-5

860.2   **Hemothorax without mention of open wound into thorax**
Ex: 860.0-860.5, 861.20-861.32, 862.29, 862.39-862.9, 875.0-875.1, 879.8-879.9, 929.0-929.9, 958.7-958.99, 959.8-959.9

860.3   **Hemothorax with open wound into thorax**
Ex: 860.0-860.5, 861.20-861.32, 862.29, 862.39-862.9, 875.0-875.1, 879.8-879.9, 929.0-929.9, 958.7-958.99, 959.8-959.9
Coding Clinic: 1995, Q3, P17

860.4   **Pneumohemothorax without mention of open wound into thorax**
Ex: 860.0-860.5, 861.20-861.32, 862.29, 862.39-862.9, 875.0-875.1, 879.8-879.9, 929.0-929.9, 958.7-958.99, 959.8-959.9

860.5   **Pneumohemothorax with open wound into thorax**
Ex: 860.0-860.5, 861.20-861.32, 862.29, 862.39-862.9, 875.0-875.1, 879.8-879.9, 929.0-929.9, 958.7-958.99, 959.8-959.9
Coding Clinic: 1995, Q3, P17

● **861   Injury to heart and lung**
Excludes   *injury to blood vessels of thorax (901.0–901.9)*
Coding Clinic: 1992, Q1, P9-10

● 861.0   **Heart, without mention of open wound into thorax**
861.00   **Unspecified injury**
Ex: 861.00-861.13, 862.29, 862.39-862.9, 959.9

861.01   **Contusion**
Cardiac contusion
Myocardial contusion
Ex: 861.00-861.13, 862.29, 862.39-862.9, 875.0-875.1, 879.8-879.9, 929.0-929.9, 958.7-958.99, 959.8-959.9

861.02   **Laceration without penetration of heart chambers**
Ex: 861.00-861.13, 862.29, 862.39-862.9, 875.0-875.1, 879.8-879.9, 929.0-929.9, 958.7-958.99, 959.8-959.9

861.03   **Laceration with penetration of heart chambers**
Ex: 861.00-861.13, 862.29, 862.39-862.9, 875.0-875.1, 879.8-879.9, 929.0-929.9, 958.7-958.99, 959.8-959.9

● 861.1   **Heart, with open wound into thorax**
861.10   **Unspecified injury**
Ex: 861.00-861.13, 862.29, 862.39-862.9, 875.0-875.1, 879.8-879.9, 929.0-929.9, 958.7-958.99, 959.8-959.9

861.11   **Contusion**
Ex: 861.00-861.13, 862.29, 862.39-862.9, 875.0-875.1, 879.8-879.9, 929.0-929.9, 958.7-958.99, 959.8-959.9

861.12   **Laceration without penetration of heart chambers**
Ex: 861.00-861.13, 862.29, 862.39-862.9, 875.0-875.1, 879.8-879.9, 929.0-929.9, 958.7-958.99, 959.8-959.9

861.13   **Laceration with penetration of heart chambers**
Ex: 861.00-861.13, 862.29, 862.39-862.9, 875.0-875.1, 879.8-879.9, 929.0-929.9, 958.7-958.99, 959.8-959.9

● 861.2   **Lung, without mention of open wound into thorax**
861.20   **Unspecified injury**
Ex: 861.00-861.13, 862.29, 862.39-862.9, 875.0-875.1, 879.8-879.9, 929.0-929.9, 958.7-958.99, 959.8-959.9

861.21   **Contusion**
Ex: 861.00-861.13, 862.29, 862.39-862.9, 875.0-875.1, 879.8-879.9, 929.0-929.9, 958.7-958.99, 959.8-959.9

861.22   **Laceration**
Ex: 861.00-861.13, 862.29, 862.39-862.9, 875.0-875.1, 879.8-879.9, 929.0-929.9, 958.7-958.99, 959.8-959.9

● 861.3   **Lung, with open wound into thorax**
861.30   **Unspecified injury**
Ex: 861.00-861.13, 862.29, 862.39-862.9, 875.0-875.1, 879.8-879.9, 929.0-929.9, 958.7-958.99, 959.8-959.9

861.31   **Contusion**
Ex: 861.00-861.13, 862.29, 862.39-862.9, 875.0-875.1, 879.8-879.9, 929.0-929.9, 958.7-958.99, 959.8-959.9

861.32   **Laceration**
Ex: 861.00-861.13, 862.29, 862.39-862.9, 875.0-875.1, 879.8-879.9, 929.0-929.9, 958.7-958.99, 959.8-959.9

● **862   Injury to other and unspecified intrathoracic organs**
Excludes   *injury to blood vessels of thorax (901.0–901.9)*

862.0   **Diaphragm, without mention of open wound into cavity**
Ex: 862.0-862.1, 862.29, 862.39-862.9, 875.0-875.1, 879.8-879.9, 929.0-929.9 958.7-958.8, 958.99, 959.8-959.9

862.1   **Diaphragm, with open wound into cavity**
Ex: 862.0-862.1, 862.29, 862.39-862.9, 875.0-875.1, 879.8-879.9, 929.0-929.9, 958.7-958.99, 959.8-959.9

● 862.2   **Other specified intrathoracic organs, without mention of open wound into cavity**
862.21   **Bronchus**
Ex: 862.0-862.1, 862.29, 862.39-862.9, 875.0-875.1, 879.8-879.9, 929.0-929.9 958.7-958.8, 958.99, 959.8-959.9

862.22   **Esophagus**
Ex: 862.0-862.1, 862.29, 862.39-862.9, 875.0-875.1, 879.8-879.9, 929.0-929.9 958.7-958.8, 958.99, 959.8-959.9

862.29   **Other**
Pleura
Thymus gland
Ex: 862.29, 862.39-862.9, 875.0-875.1, 879.8-879.9, 929.0-929.9, 958.7-958.99, 959.8-959.9

● 862.3   **Other specified intrathoracic organs, with open wound into cavity**
862.31   **Bronchus**
Ex: 862.0-862.1, 862.29, 862.39-862.9, 875.0-875.1, 879.8-879.9, 929.0-929.9 958.7-958.8, 958.99, 959.8-959.9

862.32   **Esophagus**
Ex: 862.22-862.29, 862.32-862.9, 875.0-875.1, 879.8-879.9, 929.0-929.9, 958.7-958.99, 959.8-959.9

862.39   **Other**
Ex: 862.29, 862.39-862.9, 875.0-875.1, 879.8-879.9, 929.0-929.9, 958.7-958.99, 959.8-959.9

◄ New   ◄■■ Revised   ~~deleted~~ Deleted   Excludes   Includes   Use additional   Code first   Omit code
● Unacceptable Principal Diagnosis   ● Use Additional Digit(s)   ▶ Manifestation Code   **OGCR** Official Guidelines   **Coding Clinic**

862.8 Multiple and unspecified intrathoracic organs, without mention of open wound into cavity 🗘
    Crushed chest
    Multiple intrathoracic organs
    (Ex:) 862.29, 862.39-862.9, 875.0-875.1, 879.8-879.9, 929.0-929.9, 958.7-958.8, 958.93-958.99, 959.8-959.9

862.9 Multiple and unspecified intrathoracic organs, with open wound into cavity 🗘
    (Ex:) 862.29, 862.39-862.9, 875.0-875.1, 879.8-879.9, 929.0-929.9, 958.7-958.8, 959.8-959.9

● **863 Injury to gastrointestinal tract**
    Trauma to any structure from the stomach to the anus
    Excludes *anal sphincter laceration during delivery (664.2)*
        bile duct (868.0–868.1 with fifth-digit 2)
        gallbladder (868.0–868.1 with fifth-digit 2)

863.0 Stomach, without mention of open wound into cavity 🗘
    (Ex:) 729.73, 863.0-863.1, 863.80, 863.89-863.90, 863.99, 868.00, 868.03-868.10, 868.13-869.1, 879.2-879.9, 929.0-929.9, 958.8, 958.93-958.99, 959.8-959.9

863.1 Stomach, with open wound into cavity 🗘
    (Ex:) 863.0-863.1, 863.80, 863.89-863.90, 863.99, 868.00, 868.03-868.10, 868.13-869.1, 879.2-879.9, 929.0-929.9, 958.8-958.99, 959.8-959.9

● **863.2 Small intestine, without mention of open wound into cavity**

   863.20 Small intestine, unspecified site 🗘
      (Ex:) 729.73, 863.0-863.1, 863.80, 863.89-863.90, 863.99, 868.00, 868.03-868.10, 868.13-869.1, 879.2-879.9, 929.0-929.9, 958.8, 958.93-958.99, 959.8-959.9

   863.21 Duodenum 🗘
      (Ex:) 729.73, 863.20-863.39, 863.80, 863.89-863.90, 863.99, 868.00, 868.03-868.10, 868.13-869.1, 879.2-879.9, 929.0-929.9, 958.8, 958.93-958.99, 959.8-959.9

   863.29 Other 🗘
      (Ex:) 729.73, 863.20-863.39, 863.80, 863.89-863.90, 863.99, 868.00, 868.03-868.10, 868.13-869.1, 879.2-879.9, 929.0-929.9, 958.8, 958.93-958.99, 959.8-959.9

● **863.3 Small intestine, with open wound into cavity**

   863.30 Small intestine, unspecified site 🗘
      (Ex:) 863.20-863.39, 863.80, 863.89-863.90, 863.99, 868.00, 868.03-868.10, 868.13-869.1, 879.2-879.9, 929.0-929.9, 958.8-958.99, 959.8-959.9

   863.31 Duodenum 🗘
      (Ex:) 863.21, 863.31-863.39, 863.80, 863.89-863.90, 863.99, 868.00, 868.03-868.10, 868.13-869.1, 879.2-879.9, 929.0-929.9, 958.8-958.99, 959.8-959.9

   863.39 Other 🗘
      (Ex:) 863.20-863.39, 863.80, 863.89-863.90, 863.99, 868.00, 868.03-868.10, 868.13-869.1, 879.2-879.9, 929.0-929.9, 958.8-958.99, 959.8-959.9

● **863.4 Colon or rectum, without mention of open wound into cavity**

   863.40 Colon, unspecified site 🗘
      (Ex:) 729.73, 863.40-863.80, 863.89-863.90, 863.99, 868.00, 868.03-868.10, 868.13-869.1, 879.2-879.9, 929.0-929.9, 958.8, 958.93-958.99, 959.8-959.9

   863.41 Ascending [right] colon 🗘
      (Ex:) 729.73, 863.40-863.80, 863.89-863.90, 863.99, 868.00, 868.03-868.10, 868.13-869.1, 879.2-879.9, 929.0-929.9, 958.8, 958.93-958.99, 959.8-959.9

   863.42 Transverse colon 🗘
      (Ex:) 729.73, 863.40-863.80, 863.89-863.90, 863.99, 868.00, 868.03-868.10, 868.13-869.1, 879.2-879.9, 929.0-929.9, 958.8, 958.93-958.99, 959.8-959.9

   863.43 Descending [left] colon 🗘
      (Ex:) 729.73, 863.40-863.80, 863.89-863.90, 863.99, 868.00, 868.03-868.10, 868.13-869.1, 879.2-879.9, 929.0-929.9, 958.8, 958.93-958.99, 959.8-959.9

   863.44 Sigmoid colon 🗘
      (Ex:) 729.73, 863.40-863.80, 863.89-863.90, 863.99, 868.00, 868.03-868.10, 868.13-869.1, 879.2-879.9, 929.0-929.9, 958.8, 958.93-958.99, 959.8-959.9

   863.45 Rectum 🗘
      (Ex:) 729.73, 863.40-863.80, 863.89-863.90, 863.99, 868.00, 868.03-868.10, 868.13-869.1, 879.2-879.9, 929.0-929.9, 958.8, 958.93-958.99, 959.8-959.9

   863.46 Multiple sites in colon and rectum 🗘
      (Ex:) 729.73, 863.40-863.80, 863.89-863.90, 863.99, 868.00, 868.03-868.10, 868.13-869.1, 879.2-879.9, 929.0-929.9, 958.8, 958.93-958.99, 959.8-959.9

   863.49 Other 🗘
      (Ex:) 729.73, 863.40-863.80, 863.89-863.90, 863.99, 868.00, 868.03-868.10, 868.13-869.1, 879.2-879.9, 929.0-929.9, 958.8, 958.93-958.99, 959.8-959.9

● **863.5 Colon or rectum, with open wound into cavity**

   863.50 Colon, unspecified site 🗘
      (Ex:) 863.40-863.80, 863.89-863.90, 863.99, 868.00, 868.03-868.10, 868.13-869.1, 879.2-879.9, 929.0-929.9, 958.8-958.99, 959.8-959.9

   863.51 Ascending [right] colon 🗘
      (Ex:) 863.40-863.80, 863.89-863.90, 863.99, 868.00, 868.03-868.10, 868.13-869.1, 879.2-879.9, 929.0-929.9, 958.8-958.99, 959.8-959.9

   863.52 Transverse colon 🗘
      (Ex:) 863.40-863.80, 863.89-863.90, 863.99, 868.00, 868.03-868.10, 868.13-869.1, 879.2-879.9, 929.0-929.9, 958.8-958.99, 959.8-959.9

   863.53 Descending [left] colon 🗘
      (Ex:) 863.40-863.80, 863.89-863.90, 863.99, 868.00, 868.03-868.10, 868.13-869.1, 879.2-879.9, 929.0-929.9, 958.8-958.99, 959.8-959.9

   863.54 Sigmoid colon 🗘
      (Ex:) 863.40-863.80, 863.89-863.90, 863.99, 868.00, 868.03-868.10, 868.13-869.1, 879.2-879.9, 929.0-929.9, 958.8-958.99, 959.8-959.9

   863.55 Rectum 🗘
      (Ex:) 863.40-863.80, 863.89-863.90, 863.99, 868.00, 868.03-868.10, 868.13-869.1, 879.2-879.9, 929.0-929.9, 958.8-958.99, 959.8-959.9

   863.56 Multiple sites in colon and rectum 🗘
      (Ex:) 863.40-863.80, 863.89-863.90, 863.99, 868.00, 868.03-868.10, 868.13-869.1, 879.2-879.9, 929.0-929.9, 958.8-958.99, 959.8-959.9

   863.59 Other 🗘
      (Ex:) 863.40-863.80, 863.89-863.90, 863.99, 868.00, 868.03-868.10, 868.13-869.1, 879.2-879.9, 929.0-929.9, 958.8-958.99, 959.8-959.9

● **863.8 Other and unspecified gastrointestinal sites, without mention of open wound into cavity**

   863.80 Gastrointestinal tract, unspecified site 🗘
      (Ex:) 729.73, 863.0-863.80, 863.89-863.90, 863.99, 868.00, 868.03-868.10, 868.13-869.1, 879.2-879.9, 929.0-929.9, 958.8, 958.93-958.99, 959.8-959.9

   863.81 Pancreas, head 🗘
      (Ex:) 729.73, 863.80-863.84, 863.91-863.94, 863.99, 868.00, 868.03-868.10, 868.13-869.1, 879.2-879.9, 929.0-929.9, 958.8, 958.93-958.99, 959.8-959.9

   863.82 Pancreas, body 🗘
      (Ex:) 729.73, 863.80-863.84, 863.91-863.94, 863.99, 868.00, 868.03-868.10, 868.13-869.1, 879.2-879.9, 929.0-929.9, 958.8, 958.93-958.99, 959.8-959.9

   863.83 Pancreas, tail 🗘
      (Ex:) 729.73, 863.80-863.84, 863.91-863.94, 863.99, 868.00, 868.03-868.10, 868.13-869.1, 879.2-879.9, 929.0-929.9, 958.8, 958.93-958.99, 959.8-959.9

   863.84 Pancreas, multiple and unspecified sites 🗘
      (Ex:) 729.73, 863.80-863.84, 863.91-863.94, 863.99, 868.00, 868.03-868.10, 868.13-869.1, 879.2-879.9, 929.0-929.9, 958.8, 958.93-958.99, 959.8-959.9

   863.85 Appendix 🗘
      (Ex:) 729.73, 863.80-863.84, 863.91-863.94, 863.99, 868.00, 868.03-868.10, 868.13-869.1, 879.2-879.9, 929.0-929.9, 958.8, 958.93-958.99, 959.8-959.9

   863.89 Other 🗘
      Intestine NOS
      (Ex:) 729.73, 863.80-863.84, 863.91-863.94, 863.99, 868.00, 868.03-868.10, 868.13-869.1, 879.2-879.9, 929.0-929.9, 958.8, 958.93-958.99, 959.8-959.9

● **863.9 Other and unspecified gastrointestinal sites, with open wound into cavity**

863.90 Gastrointestinal tract, unspecified site 🔹
(Ex:) 863.80-863.84, 863.89-863.94, 863.99, 868.00, 868.03-868.10, 868.13-869.1, 879.2-879.9, 929.0-929.9, 958.8-958.99, 959.8-959.9

863.91 Pancreas, head 🔹
(Ex:) 863.80-863.84, 863.89-863.94, 863.99, 868.00, 868.03-868.10, 868.13-869.1, 879.2-879.9, 929.0-929.9, 958.8-958.99, 959.8-959.9

863.92 Pancreas, body 🔹
(Ex:) 863.80-863.84, 863.89-863.94, 863.99, 868.00, 868.03-868.10, 868.13-869.1, 879.2-879.9, 929.0-929.9, 958.8-958.99, 959.8-959.9

863.93 Pancreas, tail 🔹
(Ex:) 863.80-863.84, 863.89-863.94, 863.99, 868.00, 868.03-868.10, 868.13-869.1, 879.2-879.9, 929.0-929.9, 958.8-958.99, 959.8-959.9

863.94 Pancreas, multiple and unspecified sites 🔹
(Ex:) 863.80-863.84, 863.89-863.94, 863.99, 868.00, 868.03-868.10, 868.13-869.1, 879.2-879.9, 929.0-929.9, 958.8-958.99, 959.8-959.9

863.95 Appendix 🔹
(Ex:) 863.80, 863.85, 863.95-863.99, 868.00, 868.03-868.10, 868.13-869.1, 879.2-879.9, 929.0-929.9, 958.8-958.99, 959.8-959.9

863.99 Other 🔹
(Ex:) 863.80, 863.99, 868.00, 868.03-868.10, 868.13-869.1, 879.2-879.9, 929.0-929.9, 958.8-958.99, 959.8-959.9

● **864 Injury to liver**

The following fifth-digit subclassification is for use with category 864:

0	unspecified injury
1	hematoma and contusion
2	laceration, minor
	Laceration involving capsule only, or without significant involvement of hepatic parenchyma [i.e., less than 1 cm deep]
3	laceration, moderate
	Laceration involving parenchyma but without major disruption of parenchyma [i.e., less than 10 cm long and less than 3 cm deep]
4	laceration, major
	Laceration with significant disruption of hepatic parenchyma [i.e., 10 cm long and 3 cm deep]
	Multiple moderate lacerations, with or without hematoma
	Stellate lacerations of liver
5	laceration, unspecified
9	other

● **864.0 Without mention of open wound into**
[0-5,9] **cavity** 0-2,5,9 🔹, 3,4 🔹
(Ex:) 863.80, 863.99-864.19, 868.00, 868.03-868.10, 868.13-869.1, 879.2-879.9, 929.0-929.9, 958.8-958.99, 959.8-959.9

● **864.1 With open wound into cavity** 🔹
[0-5,9] (Ex:) 863.80, 863.99-864.19, 868.00, 868.03-868.10, 868.13-869.1, 879.2-879.9, 929.0-929.9, 958.8-959.9

● **865 Injury to spleen**

The following fifth-digit subclassification is for use with category 865:

0	unspecified injury
1	hematoma without rupture of capsule
2	capsular tears, without major disruption of parenchyma
3	laceration extending into parenchyma
4	massive parenchymal disruption
9	other

● **865.0 Without mention of open wound into**
[0-4,9] **cavity** 0-2,9 🔹, 3,4 🔹
(Ex:) 865.00-865.19, 868.00, 868.03-868.10, 868.13-869.1, 879.2-879.9, 929.0-929.9, 958.8-958.99, 959.8-959.9

● **865.1 With open wound into cavity** 🔹
[0-4,9] (Ex:) 865.00-865.19, 868.00, 868.03-868.10, 868.13-869.1, 879.2-879.9, 929.0-929.9, 958.8-958.99, 959.8-959.9

● **866 Injury to kidney**

The following fifth-digit subclassification is for use with category 866:

0	unspecified injury
1	hematoma without rupture of capsule
2	laceration
3	complete disruption of kidney parenchyma

Excludes *acute kidney injury (nontraumatic) (584.9)*

● **866.0 Without mention of open wound into cavity** 0-2 🔹, 3 🔹
[0-3] (Ex:) 866.00-866.13, 868.00, 868.03-868.10, 868.13-869.1, 879.2-879.9, 929.0-929.9, 958.8-958.99, 959.8-959.9

Coding Clinic: 2008, Q4, P192-193

● **866.1 With open wound into cavity** 🔹
[0-3] (Ex:) 866.00-866.13, 868.00, 868.03-868.10, 868.13-869.1, 879.2-879.9, 929.0-929.9, 958.8-958.99, 959.8-959.9

● **867 Injury to pelvic organs**

Excludes *injury during delivery (664.0–665.9)*

867.0 Bladder and urethra, without mention of open wound into cavity 🔹
(Ex:) 867.0-867.1, 867.6-868.00, 868.03-868.10, 868.13-869.1, 879.2-879.9, 929.0-929.9, 958.8-958.99, 959.8-959.9

Coding Clinic: 2009, Q1, P8; 1985, Nov-Dec, P15; 1984, Nov-Dec, P15

867.1 Bladder and urethra, with open wound into cavity 🔹
(Ex:) 867.0-867.1, 867.6-868.00, 868.03-868.10, 868.13-869.1, 879.2-879.9, 929.0-929.9, 958.8-958.99, 959.8-959.9

Coding Clinic: 1984, Nov-Dec, P12

867.2 Ureter, without mention of open wound into cavity 🔹
(Ex:) 867.2-867.3, 867.6-868.00, 868.03-868.10, 868.13-86.91, 879.2-879.9, 929.0-929.9, 958.8-958.99, 959.8-959.9

867.3 Ureter, with open wound into cavity 🔹
(Ex:) 867.2-867.3, 867.6-868.00, 868.03-868.10, 868.13-869.1, 879.2-879.9, 929.0-929.9, 958.8-958.99, 959.8-959.9

867.4 Uterus, without mention of open wound into cavity ♀ 🔹
(Ex:) 867.4-868.00, 868.03-868.10, 868.13-869.1, 879.2-879.9, 929.0-929.9, 958.8-958.99, 959.8-959.9

867.5 Uterus, with open wound into cavity ♀ 🔹
(Ex:) 867.4-868.00, 868.03-868.10, 868.13-869.1, 879.2-879.9, 929.0-929.9, 958.8-958.99, 959.8-959.9

867.6 Other specified pelvic organs, without mention of open wound into cavity 🔹

Fallopian tube	Seminal vesicle
Ovary	Vas deferens
Prostate	

(Ex:) 867.6-868.00, 868.03-868.10, 868.13-869.1, 879.2-879.9, 929.0-929.9, 958.8-958.99, 959.8-959.9

867.7 Other specified pelvic organs, with open wound into cavity 🔹
(Ex:) 867.6-868.00, 868.03-868.10, 868.13-869.1, 879.2-879.9, 929.0-929.9, 958.8-958.99, 959.8-959.9

867.8 Unspecified pelvic organ, without mention of open wound into cavity 🔹
(Ex:) 867.6-868.00, 868.03-868.10, 868.13-869.1, 879.2-879.9, 929.0-929.9, 958.8-958.99, 959.8-959.9

867.9 Unspecified pelvic organ, with open wound into cavity 🔹
(Ex:) 867.6-868.00, 868.03-868.10, 868.13-869.1, 879.2-879.9, 929.0-929.9, 958.8-958.99, 959.8-959.9

● **868 Injury to other intra-abdominal organs**

The following fifth-digit subclassification is for use with category 868:

0	unspecified intra-abdominal organ
1	adrenal gland
2	bile duct and gallbladder
3	peritoneum
4	retroperitoneum
9	other and multiple intra-abdominal organs

● **868.0 Without mention of open wound into cavity** 🔹
[0-4,9] For codes **868.00, 868.03-868.09:** (Ex:) 868.00, 868.03-868.10, 868.13-869.1, 879.2-879.9, 929.0-929.9, 958.8-958.99, 959.8-959.9;
For code **868.01:** (Ex:) 868.00-868.01, 868.03-868.11, 868.13-869.1, 879.2-879.9, 929.0-929.9, 958.8-958.99, 959.8-959.9;
For code **868.02:** (Ex:) 868.00, 868.02-868.10, 868.13-869.1, 879.2-879.9, 929.0-929.9, 958.8-958.99, 959.8-959.9

● 868.1 With open wound into cavity 🔲
[0-4,9]   For codes **868.10, 868.13-868.19:** (Ex) 868.00, 868.03-868.10, 868.13-869.1,
879.2-879.9, 929.0-929.9, 958.8-958.99, 959.8-959.9;
For code **868.11:** (Ex) 868.00-868.01, 868.03-868.11, 868.13-86.91, 879.2-879.9,
929.0-929.9, 958.8-958.99, 959.8-959.9;
For code **868.12:** (Ex) 868.00, 868.03-868.10, 868.12-86.91, 879.2-879.9,
929.0-929.9, 958.8-958.99, 959.8-959.9

● 869 Internal injury to unspecified or ill-defined organs
Includes   internal injury NOS
multiple internal injury NOS

869.0 **Without mention of open wound into cavity** 🔲
(Ex) 868.00, 868.03-868.10, 868.13-869.1, 879.2-879.9, 929.0-929.9,
958.8-958.99, 959.8-959.9

869.1 **With open wound into cavity** 🔲
(Ex) 868.00, 868.03-868.10, 868.13-869.1, 879.2-879.9, 929.0-929.9,
958.8-958.99, 959.8-959.9

OPEN WOUNDS (870–897)

Includes   animal bite
avulsion
cut
laceration
puncture wound
traumatic amputation

Excludes   *burn (940.0–949.5)*
crushing (925–929.9)
puncture of internal organs (860.0–869.1)
superficial injury (910.0–919.9)
that incidental to:
dislocation (830.0–839.9)
fracture (800.0–829.1)
internal injury (860.0–869.1)
intracranial injury (851.0–854.1)

Note: The description "complicated" used in the fourth-digit
subdivisions includes those with mention of delayed
healing, delayed treatment, foreign body, or infection.

OPEN WOUND OF HEAD, NECK, AND TRUNK (870–879)

● 870 Open wound of ocular adnexa
870.0 Laceration of skin of eyelid and periocular area
870.1 Laceration of eyelid, full-thickness, not involving lacrimal
passages
870.2 Laceration of eyelid involving lacrimal passages 🔲
(Ex) 870.0-871.9, 879.8-879.9, 929.0-929.9, 958.8, 959.8-959.9
870.3 Penetrating wound of orbit, without mention of foreign
body 🔲
(Ex) 870.0-871.9, 879.8-879.9, 929.0-929.9, 958.8-958.99, 959.8-959.9
870.4 Penetrating wound of orbit with foreign body 🔲
Excludes   *retained (old) foreign body in orbit (376.6)*
(Ex) 870.0-871.9, 879.8-879.9, 929.0-929.9, 958.8-958.99, 959.8-959.9
870.8 Other specified open wounds of ocular adnexa 🔲
(Ex) 870.0-871.9, 879.8-879.9, 929.0-929.9, 958.8-958.99, 959.8-959.9
870.9 Unspecified open wound of ocular adnexa 🔲
(Ex) 870.0-871.9, 879.8-879.9, 929.0-929.9, 958.8-958.99, 959.8-959.9

● 871 Open wound of eyeball
Excludes   *2nd cranial nerve [optic] injury (950.0–950.9)*
3rd cranial nerve [oculomotor] injury (951.0)
871.0 Ocular laceration without prolapse of intraocular tissue 🔲
(Ex) 870.0-871.9, 879.8-879.9, 929.0-929.9, 958.8-958.99, 959.8-959.9
Coding Clinic: 1996, Q3, P7
871.1 Ocular laceration with prolapse or exposure of intraocular
tissue 🔲
(Ex) 870.0-871.9, 879.8-879.9, 929.0-929.9, 958.8-958.99, 959.8-959.9
871.2 Rupture of eye with partial loss of intraocular tissue 🔲
(Ex) 870.0-871.9, 879.8-879.9, 929.0-929.9, 958.8-958.99, 959.8-959.9
871.3 Avulsion of eye 🔲
Traumatic enucleation
(Ex) 870.0-871.9, 879.8-879.9, 929.0-929.9, 958.8-958.99, 959.8-959.9

871.4 Unspecified laceration of eye
871.5 Penetration of eyeball with magnetic foreign body 🔲
Excludes   *retained (old) magnetic foreign body in globe*
(360.50–360.59)
(Ex) 870.0-871.9, 879.8-879.9, 929.0-929.9, 958.8, 959.8-959.9
871.6 Penetration of eyeball with (nonmagnetic) foreign body 🔲
Excludes   *retained (old) (nonmagnetic) foreign body in*
globe (360.60–360.69)
(Ex) 870.0-871.9, 879.8-879.9, 929.0-929.9, 958.8, 959.8-959.9
871.7 Unspecified ocular penetration
871.9 Unspecified open wound of eyeball 🔲
(Ex) 870.0-871.9, 879.8-879.9, 929.0-929.9, 958.8, 959.8-959.9

● 872 Open wound of ear
● 872.0 External ear, without mention of complication
872.00 External ear, unspecified site
872.01 Auricle, ear
Pinna
872.02 Auditory canal
● 872.1 External ear, complicated
872.10 External ear, unspecified site
872.11 Auricle, ear
872.12 Auditory canal 🔲
(Ex) 872.00-872.9, 879.8-879.9, 929.0-929.9, 958.8, 959.8-959.9
● 872.6 Other specified parts of ear, without mention of
complication
872.61 Ear drum 🔲
Drumhead
Tympanic membrane
(Ex) 872.00-872.9, 879.8-879.9, 929.0-929.9, 958.8, 959.8-959.9
872.62 Ossicles 🔲
(Ex) 872.00-872.9, 879.8-879.9, 929.0-929.9, 958.8, 959.8-959.9
872.63 Eustachian tube 🔲
(Ex) 872.00-872.9, 879.8-879.9, 929.0-929.9, 958.8, 959.8-959.9
872.64 Cochlea 🔲
(Ex) 872.00-872.9, 879.8-879.9, 929.0-929.9, 958.8, 959.8-959.9
872.69 Other and multiple sites 🔲
(Ex) 872.00-872.9, 879.8-879.9, 929.0-929.9, 958.8, 959.8-959.9
● 872.7 Other specified parts of ear, complicated
872.71 Ear drum 🔲
(Ex) 872.00-872.9, 879.8-879.9, 929.0-929.9, 958.8, 959.8-959.9
872.72 Ossicles 🔲
(Ex) 872.00-872.9, 879.8-879.9, 929.0-929.9, 958.8-958.99,
959.8-959.9
872.73 Eustachian tube 🔲
(Ex) 872.00-872.9, 879.8-879.9, 929.0-929.9, 958.8-958.99,
959.8-959.9
872.74 Cochlea 🔲
(Ex) 872.00-872.9, 879.8-879.9, 929.0-929.9, 958.8-958.99,
959.8-959.9
872.79 Other and multiple sites 🔲
(Ex) 872.00-872.9, 879.8-879.9, 929.0-929.9, 958.8, 959.8-959.9
872.8 Ear, part unspecified, without mention of complication
Ear NOS
872.9 Ear, part unspecified, complicated

● 873 Other open wound of head
873.0 Scalp, without mention of complication
873.1 Scalp, complicated
● 873.2 Nose, without mention of complication
873.20 Nose, unspecified site
873.21 Nasal septum
873.22 Nasal cavity
873.23 Nasal sinus 🔲
(Ex) 873.20-873.39, 879.8-879.9, 929.0-929.9, 958.8, 959.8-959.9
873.29 Multiple sites

N Newborn: 0   **P** Pediatric: 0–17   **M** Maternity: 12–55   **A** Adult: 15–124   ♀ Females Only   ♂ Males Only
(Ex) CC/MCC Exclusions   🔲 Complication\Comorbidity   🔲 Major C\C   🔲 Present on Admission Requirement   🔲 Hospital-Acquired Condition

● **873.3 Nose, complicated**
   873.30 Nose, unspecified site
   873.31 Nasal septum
   873.32 Nasal cavity
   873.33 Nasal sinus
     (Ex) 873.20-873.39, 879.8-879.9, 929.0-929.9, 958.8-958.99, 959.8-959.9
   873.39 Multiple sites

● **873.4 Face, without mention of complication**
   873.40 Face, unspecified site
   873.41 Cheek
   873.42 Forehead
     Eyebrow
     Coding Clinic: 1996, Q4, P43-44
   873.43 Lip
   873.44 Jaw
   873.49 Other and multiple sites

● **873.5 Face, complicated**
   873.50 Face, unspecified site
   873.51 Cheek
   873.52 Forehead
   873.53 Lip
   873.54 Jaw
   873.59 Other and multiple sites

● **873.6 Internal structures of mouth, without mention of complication**
   873.60 Mouth, unspecified site
   873.61 Buccal mucosa
   873.62 Gum (alveolar process)
   873.63 Tooth (broken) (fractured) (due to trauma)
     Excludes cracked tooth (521.81)
     Coding Clinic: 2004, Q1, P17
   873.64 Tongue and floor of mouth
   873.65 Palate
   873.69 Other and multiple sites

● **873.7 Internal structures of mouth, complicated**
   873.70 Mouth, unspecified site
   873.71 Buccal mucosa
   873.72 Gum (alveolar process)
   873.73 Tooth (broken) (fractured) (due to trauma)
     Excludes cracked tooth (521.81)
     Coding Clinic: 2004, Q1, P17
   873.74 Tongue and floor of mouth
   873.75 Palate
   873.79 Other and multiple sites

873.8 Other and unspecified open wound of head without mention of complication
   Head NOS
873.9 Other and unspecified open wound of head, complicated

● **874 Open wound of neck**
● **874.0 Larynx and trachea, without mention of complication**
   874.00 Larynx with trachea
     (Ex) 847.0, 874.00-874.12, 874.8-874.9, 879.8-879.9, 929.0-929.9, 958.8-958.99, 959.8-959.9
   874.01 Larynx
     (Ex) 847.0, 874.00-874.12, 874.8-874.9, 879.8-879.9, 929.0-929.9, 958.8-958.99, 959.8-959.9
   874.02 Trachea
     (Ex) 847.0, 874.00-874.12, 874.8-874.9, 879.8-879.9, 929.0-929.9, 958.8-958.99, 959.8-959.9

● **874.1 Larynx and trachea, complicated**
   874.10 Larynx with trachea
     (Ex) 847.0, 874.00-874.12, 874.8-874.9, 879.8-879.9, 929.0-929.9, 958.8-958.99, 959.8-959.9
   874.11 Larynx
     (Ex) 847.0, 874.00-874.12, 874.8-874.9, 879.8-879.9, 929.0-929.9, 958.8-958.99, 959.8-959.9
   874.12 Trachea
     (Ex) 847.0, 874.00-874.12, 874.8-874.9, 879.8-879.9, 929.0-929.9, 958.8-958.99, 959.8-959.9

874.2 Thyroid gland, without mention of complication
   (Ex) 847.0, 874.2-874.3, 874.8-874.9, 879.8-879.9, 929.0-929.9, 958.8, 959.8-959.9
874.3 Thyroid gland, complicated
   (Ex) 847.0, 874.2-874.3, 874.8-874.9, 879.8-879.9, 929.0-929.9, 958.8-958.99, 959.8-959.9
874.4 Pharynx, without mention of complication
   Cervical esophagus
   (Ex) 847.0, 874.4-874.9, 879.8-879.9, 929.0-929.9, 958.8, 959.8-959.9
874.5 Pharynx, complicated
   (Ex) 847.0, 874.4-874.9, 879.8-879.9, 929.0-929.9, 958.8-958.99, 959.8-959.9
874.8 Other and unspecified parts, without mention of complication
   Nape of neck   Throat NOS
   Supraclavicular region
874.9 Other and unspecified parts, complicated

● **875 Open wound of chest (wall)**
   Excludes open wound into thoracic cavity (860.0–862.9)
     traumatic pneumothorax and hemothorax (860.1, 860.3, 860.5)
   Coding Clinic: 1995, Q3, P17
875.0 Without mention of complication
   (Ex) 847.1, 862.29, 862.39-862.9, 875.0-875.1, 879.8-879.9, 929.0-929.9, 958.7-958.99, 959.8-959.9
875.1 Complicated
   (Ex) 847.1, 862.29, 862.39-862.9, 875.0-875.1, 879.8-879.9, 929.0-929.9, 958.7-958.99, 959.8-959.9

● **876 Open wound of back**
   Includes loin
     lumbar region
   Excludes open wound into thoracic cavity (860.0–862.9)
     traumatic pneumothorax and hemothorax (860.1, 860.3, 860.5)
   Coding Clinic: 1995, Q3, P17
876.0 Without mention of complication
   Coding Clinic: 1993, Q2, P4-5
876.1 Complicated

● **877 Open wound of buttock**
   Includes sacroiliac region
877.0 Without mention of complication
877.1 Complicated

● **878 Open wound of genital organs (external), including traumatic amputation**
   Excludes injury during delivery (664.0–665.9)
     internal genital organs (867.0–867.9)
878.0 Penis, without mention of complication ♂
878.1 Penis, complicated ♂
878.2 Scrotum and testes, without mention of complication ♂
878.3 Scrotum and testes, complicated ♂
878.4 Vulva, without mention of complication ♀
   Labium (majus) (minus)
878.5 Vulva, complicated ♀
878.6 Vagina, without mention of complication ♀
878.7 Vagina, complicated ♀
878.8 Other and unspecified parts, without mention of complication
878.9 Other and unspecified parts, complicated

● 879 Open wound of other and unspecified sites, except limbs

879.0 Breast, without mention of complication

879.1 Breast, complicated

879.2 Abdominal wall, anterior, without mention of complication

Abdominal wall NOS	Pubic region
Epigastric region	Umbilical region
Hypogastric region	

879.3 Abdominal wall, anterior, complicated

879.4 Abdominal wall, lateral, without mention of complication

Flank	Iliac (region)
Groin Inguinal region	
Hypochondrium	

879.5 Abdominal wall, lateral, complicated

879.6 Other and unspecified parts of trunk, without mention of complication

| Pelvic region | Trunk NOS |
| Perineum | |

879.7 Other and unspecified parts of trunk, complicated

879.8 Open wound(s) (multiple) of unspecified site(s) without mention of complication

Multiple open wounds NOS
Open wound NOS

879.9 Open wound(s) (multiple) of unspecified site(s), complicated

OPEN WOUND OF UPPER LIMB (880–887)

● 880 Open wound of shoulder and upper arm

The following fifth-digit subclassification is for use with category 880:

0	shoulder region
1	scapular region
2	axillary region
3	upper arm
9	multiple sites

● 880.0 Without mention of complication
[0-3,9]

● 880.1 Complicated
[0-3,9]   Coding Clinic: 2006, Q2, P7

● 880.2 With tendon involvement 🔖
[0-3,9]   Ex: 880.00-880.29

● 881 Open wound of elbow, forearm, and wrist

The following fifth-digit subclassification is for use with category 881:

0	forearm
1	elbow
2	wrist

● 881.0 Without mention of complication
[0-2]

● 881.1 Complicated
[0-2]

● 881.2 With tendon involvement 🔖
[0-2]   Ex: 881.00-881.22

● 882 Open wound of hand except finger(s) alone

882.0 Without mention of complication

882.1 Complicated
Coding Clinic: 2008, Q4, P149-152

882.2 With tendon involvement 🔖
Ex: 882.0-882.2

● 883 Open wound of finger(s)

Includes   fingernail
            thumb (nail)

883.0 Without mention of complication
Avulsion of fingernail reported with this code

883.1 Complicated

883.2 With tendon involvement 🔖
Ex: 883.0-883.2

● 884 Multiple and unspecified open wound of upper limb

Includes   arm NOS
            multiple sites of one upper limb
            upper limb NOS

884.0 Without mention of complication

884.1 Complicated

884.2 With tendon involvement 🔖
Ex: 884.0-884.2

● 885 Traumatic amputation of thumb (complete) (partial)

Includes   thumb(s) (with finger(s) of either hand)

885.0 Without mention of complication
Coding Clinic: 2003, Q1, P7

885.1 Complicated

● 886 Traumatic amputation of other finger(s) (complete) (partial)

Includes   finger(s) of one or both hands, without mention of thumb(s)

886.0 Without mention of complication

886.1 Complicated

● 887 Traumatic amputation of arm and hand (complete) (partial)

887.0 Unilateral, below elbow, without mention of complication 🔖
Ex: 880.00-887.7, 929.0-929.9, 958.8-958.99, 959.8-959.9

887.1 Unilateral, below elbow, complicated 🔖
Ex: 880.00-887.7, 929.0-929.9, 958.8-958.99, 959.8-959.9

887.2 Unilateral, at or above elbow, without mention of complication 🔖
Ex: 880.00-887.7, 929.0-929.9, 958.8-958.99, 959.8-959.9

887.3 Unilateral, at or above elbow, complicated 🔖
Ex: 880.00-887.7, 929.0-929.9, 958.8-958.99, 959.8-959.9

887.4 Unilateral, level not specified, without mention of complication 🔖
Ex: 880.00-887.7, 929.0-929.9, 958.8-958.99, 959.8-959.9

887.5 Unilateral, level not specified, complicated 🔖
Ex: 880.00-887.7, 929.0-929.9, 958.8-958.99, 959.8-959.9

887.6 Bilateral [any level], without mention of complication 🔖
One hand and other arm
Ex: 880.00-887.7, 929.0-929.9, 958.8-958.99, 959.8-959.9

887.7 Bilateral [any level], complicated 🔖
Ex: 880.00-887.7, 929.0-929.9, 958.8-958.99, 959.8-959.9,

OPEN WOUND OF LOWER LIMB (890–897)

● 890 Open wound of hip and thigh

890.0 Without mention of complication

890.1 Complicated

890.2 With tendon involvement 🔖
Ex: 890.0-890.2

● 891 Open wound of knee, leg [except thigh], and ankle

Includes   leg NOS
            multiple sites of leg, except thigh

Excludes   *that of thigh (890.0–890.2)*
            with multiple sites of lower limb (894.0–894.2)

891.0 Without mention of complication

891.1 Complicated

891.2 With tendon involvement 🔖
Ex: 891.0-891.2

N Newborn: 0   P Pediatric: 0–17   M Maternity: 12–55   A Adult: 15–124   ♀ Females Only   ♂ Males Only

Ex: CC/MCC Exclusions   🔖 Complication\Comorbidity   🔖 Major C\C   🔖 Present on Admission Requirement   🔖 Hospital-Acquired Condition   975

INJURY AND POISONING (800–999)

● **892   Open wound of foot except toe(s) alone**
Includes   heel
892.0   Without mention of complication
892.1   Complicated
Coding Clinic: 1985, Sept-Oct, P10
892.2   With tendon involvement 🔖
Ⓔ 892.0-892.2

● **893   Open wound of toe(s)**
Includes   toenail
893.0   Without mention of complication
893.1   Complicated
Coding Clinic: 2008, Q4, P69-73
893.2   With tendon involvement 🔖
Ⓔ 893.0-893.2

● **894   Multiple and unspecified open wound of lower limb**
Includes   lower limb NOS
multiple sites of one lower limb, with thigh
894.0   Without mention of complication
894.1   Complicated
894.2   With tendon involvement 🔖
Ⓔ 894.0-894.2

● **895   Traumatic amputation of toe(s) (complete) (partial)**
Includes   toe(s) of one or both feet
895.0   Without mention of complication
895.1   Complicated

● **896   Traumatic amputation of foot (complete) (partial)**
896.0   Unilateral, without mention of complication 🔖
Ⓔ 890.0-897.7, 929.0-929.9, 958.8-958.99, 959.8-959.9
896.1   Unilateral, complicated 🔖
Ⓔ 890.0-897.7, 929.0-929.9, 958.8-958.99, 959.8-959.9
896.2   Bilateral, without mention of complication 🔖
Excludes   one foot and other leg (897.6–897.7)
Ⓔ 890.0-897.7, 929.0-929.9, 958.8-958.99, 959.8-959.9
896.3   Bilateral, complicated 🔖
Ⓔ 890.0-897.7, 929.0-929.9, 958.8-958.99, 959.8-959.9

● **897   Traumatic amputation of leg(s) (complete) (partial)**
897.0   Unilateral, below knee, without mention of complication 🔖
Ⓔ 890.0-897.7, 929.0-929.9, 958.8-958.99, 959.8-959.9
897.1   Unilateral, below knee, complicated 🔖
Ⓔ 890.0-897.7, 929.0-929.9, 958.8-958.99, 959.8-959.9
897.2   Unilateral, at or above knee, without mention of complication 🔖
Ⓔ 890.0-897.7, 929.0-929.9, 958.8-958.99, 959.8-959.9
897.3   Unilateral, at or above knee, complicated 🔖
Ⓔ 890.0-897.7, 929.0-929.9, 958.8-958.99, 959.8-959.9
897.4   Unilateral, level not specified, without mention of complication 🔖
Ⓔ 890.0-897.7, 929.0-929.9, 958.8-958.99, 959.8-959.9
897.5   Unilateral, level not specified, complicated 🔖
Ⓔ 890.0-897.7, 929.0-929.9, 958.8-958.99, 959.8-959.9
897.6   Bilateral [any level], without mention of complication 🔖
One foot and other leg
Ⓔ 890.0-897.7, 929.0-929.9, 958.8-958.99, 959.8-959.9
897.7   Bilateral [any level], complicated 🔖
Ⓔ 890.0-897.7, 929.0-929.9, 958.8-958.99, 959.8-959.9

Includes   arterial hematoma of blood vessel, secondary to other injuries, e.g., fracture or open wound
avulsion of blood vessel, secondary to other injuries, e.g., fracture or open wound
cut of blood vessel, secondary to other injuries, e.g., fracture or open wound
laceration of blood vessel, secondary to other injuries, e.g., fracture or open wound
rupture of blood vessel, secondary to other injuries, e.g., fracture or open wound
traumatic aneurysm or fistula (arteriovenous) of blood vessel, secondary to other injuries, e.g., fracture or open wound
Excludes   *accidental puncture or laceration during medical procedure (998.2)*
intracranial hemorrhage following injury (851.0–854.1)

● **900   Injury to blood vessels of head and neck**
● **900.0   Carotid artery**
900.00   Carotid artery, unspecified 🔖
Ⓔ 900.00, 900.82-900.9, 904.9, 929.0-929.9, 958.8-958.99, 959.8-959.9
900.01   Common carotid artery 🔖
Ⓔ 900.00, 900.82-900.9, 904.9, 929.0-929.9, 958.8-958.99, 959.8-959.9
900.02   External carotid artery 🔖
Ⓔ 900.00, 900.82-900.9, 904.9, 929.0-929.9, 958.8-958.99, 959.8-959.9
900.03   Internal carotid artery 🔖
Ⓔ 900.00, 900.82-900.9, 904.9, 929.0-929.9, 958.8-958.99, 959.8-959.9
900.1   Internal jugular vein 🔖
Ⓔ 900.82-900.9, 904.9, 929.0-929.9, 958.8-958.99, 959.8-959.9
● **900.8   Other specified blood vessels of head and neck**
900.81   External jugular vein 🔖
Jugular vein NOS
Ⓔ 900.82-900.9, 904.9, 929.0-929.9, 958.8-958.99, 959.8-959.9
900.82   Multiple blood vessels of head and neck 🔖
Ⓔ 900.82-900.9, 904.9, 929.0-929.9, 958.8-958.99, 959.8-959.9
900.89   Other 🔖
Ⓔ 900.82-900.9, 904.9, 929.0-929.9, 958.8-958.99, 959.8-959.9
900.9   Unspecified blood vessel of head and neck 🔖
Ⓔ 900.82-900.9, 904.9, 929.0-929.9, 958.8-958.99, 959.8-959.9

● **901   Injury to blood vessels of thorax**
Excludes   *traumatic hemothorax (860.2–860.5)*
901.0   Thoracic aorta 🔖
Ⓔ 901.0, 904.9, 929.0-929.9, 958.8-958.99, 959.8-959.9
901.1   Innominate and subclavian arteries 🔖
Ⓔ 901.1, 904.9, 929.0-929.9, 958.8-958.99, 959.8-959.9
901.2   Superior vena cava 🔖
Ⓔ 901.2, 904.9, 929.0-929.9, 958.8-958.99, 959.8-959.9
901.3   Innominate and subclavian veins 🔖
Ⓔ 901.3, 904.9, 929.0-929.9, 958.8-958.99, 959.8-959.9
● **901.4   Pulmonary blood vessels**
901.40   Pulmonary vessel(s), unspecified 🔖
Ⓔ 901.40-901.41, 904.9, 929.0-929.9, 958.8-958.90, 958.99, 959.8-959.9
901.41   Pulmonary artery 🔖
Ⓔ 901.40-901.41, 904.9, 929.0-929.9, 958.8-958.99, 959.8-959.9
901.42   Pulmonary vein 🔖
Ⓔ 901.40, 901.42, 904.9, 929.0-929.9, 958.8-958.99, 959.8-959.9

◀ New   ◀ Revised   ~~deleted~~ Deleted   Excludes   Includes   Use additional   Code first   Omit code
● Unacceptable Principal Diagnosis   ● Use Additional Digit(s)   ▶ Manifestation Code   OGCR Official Guidelines   Coding Clinic

● **901.8   Other specified blood vessels of thorax**

    901.81   Intercostal artery or vein 🖓
        Ⓔ 901.81, 901.83-901.89

    901.82   Internal mammary artery or vein 🖓
        Ⓔ 901.82-901.89

    901.83   Multiple blood vessels of thorax 🖓
        Ⓔ 904.9, 929.0-929.9, 958.8-958.99, 959.8-959.9

    901.89   Other 🖓
        Azygos vein
        Hemiazygos vein
        Ⓔ 901.0-901.9

  901.9   Unspecified blood vessel of thorax 🖓
      Ⓔ 901.0-901.9

● **902   Injury to blood vessels of abdomen and pelvis**

  902.0   Abdominal aorta 🖓
      Ⓔ 902.0, 902.87-902.9, 904.9, 929.0-929.9, 958.8-958.99, 959.8-959.9

● **902.1   Inferior vena cava**

    902.10   Inferior vena cava, unspecified 🖓
        Ⓔ 902.10, 902.87-902.9, 904.9, 929.0-929.9 958.8-958.99, 959.8-959.9

    902.11   Hepatic veins 🖓
        Ⓔ 902.11, 902.87-902.9, 904.9, 929.0-929.9 958.8-958.99, 959.8-959.9

    902.19   Other 🖓
        Ⓔ 902.19, 902.87-902.9, 904.9, 929.0-929.9 958.8-958.99, 959.8-959.9

● **902.2   Celiac and mesenteric arteries**

    902.20   Celiac and mesenteric arteries, unspecified 🖓
        Ⓔ 902.20, 902.87-902.9, 904.9, 929.0-929.9 958.8-958.99, 959.8-959.9

    902.21   Gastric artery 🖓
        Ⓔ 902.21, 902.87-902.9, 904.9, 929.0-929.9, 958.8-958.90, 958.93-958.99, 959.8-959.9

    902.22   Hepatic artery 🖓
        Ⓔ 902.22, 902.87-902.9, 904.9, 929.0-929.9, 958.8-958.99, 959.8-959.9

    902.23   Splenic artery 🖓
        Ⓔ 902.23, 902.87-902.9, 904.9, 929.0-929.9, 958.8-958.99, 959.8-959.9

    902.24   Other specified branches of celiac axis 🖓
        Ⓔ 902.24, 902.87-902.9, 904.9, 929.0-929.9, 958.8-958.99, 959.8-959.9

    902.25   Superior mesenteric artery (trunk) 🖓
        Ⓔ 902.25, 902.87-902.9, 904.9, 929.0-929.9, 958.8-958.99, 959.8-959.9

    902.26   Primary branches of superior mesenteric artery 🖓
        Ileo-colic artery
        Ⓔ 902.26, 902.87-902.9, 904.9, 929.0-929.9, 958.8-958.99, 959.8-959.9

    902.27   Inferior mesenteric artery 🖓
        Ⓔ 902.27, 902.87-902.9, 904.9, 929.0-929.9, 958.8-958.99, 959.8-959.9

    902.29   Other 🖓
        Ⓔ 902.29, 902.87-902.9, 904.9, 929.0-929.9, 958.8-958.99, 959.8-959.9

● **902.3   Portal and splenic veins**

    902.31   Superior mesenteric vein and primary subdivisions 🖓
        Ileo-colic vein
        Ⓔ 902.31, 902.87-902.9, 904.9, 929.0-929.9, 958.8-958.99, 959.8-959.9

    902.32   Inferior mesenteric vein 🖓
        Ⓔ 902.32, 902.87-902.9, 904.9, 929.0-929.9, 958.8-958.99, 959.8-959.9

    902.33   Portal vein 🖓
        Ⓔ 902.33, 902.87-902.9, 904.9, 929.0-929.9, 958.8-958.99, 959.8-959.9

    902.34   Splenic vein 🖓
        Ⓔ 902.34, 902.87-902.9, 904.9, 929.0-929.9, 958.8-958.99, 959.8-959.9

    902.39   Other 🖓
        Cystic vein
        Gastric vein
        Ⓔ 902.39, 902.87-902.9, 904.9, 929.0-929.9, 958.8-958.99, 959.8-959.9

● **902.4   Renal blood vessels**

    902.40   Renal vessel(s), unspecified 🖓
        Ⓔ 902.40, 902.87-902.9, 904.9, 929.0-929.9, 958.8-958.99, 959.8-959.9

    902.41   Renal artery 🖓
        Ⓔ 902.41, 902.87-902.9, 904.9, 929.0-929.9, 958.8-958.99, 959.8-959.9

    902.42   Renal vein 🖓
        Ⓔ 902.42, 902.87-902.9, 904.9, 929.0-929.9, 958.8-958.99, 959.8-959.9

    902.49   Other 🖓
        Suprarenal arteries
        Ⓔ 902.49, 902.87-902.9, 904.9, 929.0-929.9, 958.8-958.99, 959.8-959.9

● **902.5   Iliac blood vessels**

    902.50   Iliac vessel(s), unspecified 🖓
        Ⓔ 902.50, 902.53-902.54, 902.59, 902.87-902.9, 904.9, 929.0-929.9, 958.8-958.99, 959.8-959.9

    902.51   Hypogastric artery 🖓
        Ⓔ 902.51, 902.87-902.9, 904.9, 929.0-929.9, 958.8-958.99, 959.8-959.9

    902.52   Hypogastric vein 🖓
        Ⓔ 902.52, 902.87-902.9, 904.9, 929.0-929.9, 958.8-958.99, 959.8-959.9

    902.53   Iliac artery 🖓
        Ⓔ 902.50, 902.53, 902.59, 902.87-902.9, 904.9, 929.0-929.9, 958.8-958.99, 959.8-959.9

    902.54   Iliac vein 🖓
        Ⓔ 902.50, 902.54, 902.59, 902.87-902.9, 904.9, 929.0-929.9, 958.8-958.99, 959.8-959.9

    902.55   Uterine artery ♀ 🖓
        Ⓔ 902.55, 902.59, 902.87-902.9, 904.9, 929.0-929.9, 958.8-958.90, 958.93-958.99, 959.8-959.9

    902.56   Uterine vein ♀ 🖓
        Ⓔ 902.56-902.59, 902.87-902.9, 904.9, 929.0-929.9, 958.8-958.90, 958.93-958.99, 959.8-959.9

    902.59   Other 🖓
        Ⓔ 902.50, 902.53-902.54, 902.59, 902.87-902.9, 904.9, 929.0-929.9, 958.8-958.99, 959.8-959.9

● **902.8   Other specified blood vessels of abdomen and pelvis**

    902.81   Ovarian artery ♀ 🖓
        Ⓔ 902.81, 902.87-902.9, 904.9, 929.0-929.9, 958.8-958.90, 958.93-958.99, 959.8-959.9

    902.82   Ovarian vein ♀ 🖓
        Ⓔ 902.82-902.9, 904.9, 929.0-929.9, 958.8-958.90, 958.93-958.99, 959.8-959.9

    902.87   Multiple blood vessels of abdomen and pelvis 🖓
        Ⓔ 902.87-902.9, 904.9, 929.0-929.9, 958.8-958.99, 959.8-959.9

    902.89   Other 🖓
        Ⓔ 902.87-902.9, 904.9, 929.0-929.9, 958.8-958.90, 958.93-958.99, 959.8-959.9

  902.9   Unspecified blood vessel of abdomen and pelvis 🖓
      Ⓔ 902.0-902.9, 904.9, 929.0-929.9, 958.8-958.90, 958.93-958.99, 959.8-959.9

N Newborn: 0   **P** Pediatric: 0–17   **M** Maternity: 12–55   **A** Adult: 15–124   ♀ Females Only   ♂ Males Only

Ⓔ CC/MCC Exclusions 🖓 Complication\Comorbidity 🖓 Major C\C 🖓 Present on Admission Requirement 🖓 Hospital-Acquired Condition   **977**

INJURY AND POISONING (800–999)

INJURY AND POISONING (800–999)

● 903　Injury to blood vessels of upper extremity
　　● 903.0　Axillary blood vessels
　　　　　903.00　Axillary vessel(s), unspecified 🔖
　　　　　　　　(Ex:) 903.00-903.02, 903.8-903.9, 904.9
　　　　　903.01　Axillary artery 🔖
　　　　　　　　(Ex:) 903.00-903.01, 903.8-903.9, 904.9
　　　　　903.02　Axillary vein 🔖
　　　　　　　　(Ex:) 903.00, 903.02, 903.8-903.9, 904.9
　　● 903.1　Brachial blood vessels 🔖
　　　　　(Ex:) 903.1, 903.8-903.9, 904.9
　　● 903.2　Radial blood vessels 🔖
　　　　　(Ex:) 903.2, 903.8-903.9, 904.9
　　● 903.3　Ulnar blood vessels 🔖
　　　　　(Ex:) 903.3, 903.8-903.9, 904.9
　　● 903.4　Palmar artery 🔖
　　　　　(Ex:) 903.4, 903.8-903.9, 904.9
　　● 903.5　Digital blood vessels 🔖
　　　　　(Ex:) 903.5-903.9, 904.9
　　● 903.8　Other specified blood vessels of upper extremity 🔖
　　　　　Multiple blood vessels of upper extremity
　　　　　(Ex:) 903.3-903.9, 904.9
　　● 903.9　Unspecified blood vessel of upper extremity 🔖
　　　　　(Ex:) 903.3-903.9, 904.9

● 904　Injury to blood vessels of lower extremity and unspecified sites
　　● 904.0　Common femoral artery
　　　　　Femoral artery above profunda origin
　　　　　Profunda = deep and posterior
　　　　　(Ex:) 904.0, 904.7-904.9
　　● 904.1　Superficial femoral artery 🔖
　　　　　(Ex:) 904.1, 904.7-904.9
　　● 904.2　Femoral veins 🔖
　　　　　(Ex:) 904.2, 904.7-904.9
　　● 904.3　Saphenous veins 🔖
　　　　　Saphenous vein (greater) (lesser)
　　　　　(Ex:) 904.3, 904.7-904.9
　　● 904.4　Popliteal blood vessels
　　　　　904.40　Popliteal vessel(s), unspecified 🔖
　　　　　　　　(Ex:) 904.40, 904.7-904.9
　　　　　904.41　Popliteal artery 🔖
　　　　　　　　(Ex:) 904.41, 904.7-904.9
　　　　　904.42　Popliteal vein 🔖
　　　　　　　　(Ex:) 904.42, 904.7-904.9
　　● 904.5　Tibial blood vessels
　　　　　904.50　Tibial vessel(s), unspecified 🔖
　　　　　　　　(Ex:) 904.50, 904.7-904.9
　　　　　904.51　Anterior tibial artery 🔖
　　　　　　　　(Ex:) 904.51, 904.7-904.9
　　　　　904.52　Anterior tibial vein 🔖
　　　　　　　　(Ex:) 904.52, 904.7-904.9
　　　　　904.53　Posterior tibial artery 🔖
　　　　　　　　(Ex:) 904.53, 904.7-904.9
　　　　　904.54　Posterior tibial vein 🔖
　　　　　　　　(Ex:) 904.54, 904.7-904.9
　　● 904.6　Deep plantar blood vessels 🔖
　　　　　(Ex:) 904.6-904.9
　　● 904.7　Other specified blood vessels of lower extremity 🔖
　　　　　Multiple blood vessels of lower extremity
　　　　　(Ex:) 729.72, 904.0-904.9
　　● 904.8　Unspecified blood vessel of lower extremity 🔖
　　　　　(Ex:) 729.72, 904.0-904.9
　　● 904.9　Unspecified site 🔖
　　　　　Injury to blood vessel NOS
　　　　　(Ex:) 729.71-729.72, 900.00-904.9

LATE EFFECTS OF INJURIES, POISONINGS, TOXIC EFFECTS, AND OTHER EXTERNAL CAUSES (905–909)

Note:　These categories are to be used to indicate conditions classifiable to 800–999 as the cause of late effects, which are themselves classified elsewhere. The "late effects" include those specified as such, or as sequelae, which may occur at any time after the acute injury.

● 905　Late effects of musculoskeletal and connective tissue injuries
　　905.0　Late effect of fracture of skull and face bones 🔖
　　　　Late effect of injury classifiable to 800–804
　　　　Coding Clinic: 2013, Q2, P9; 1997, Q3, P12-13
　　905.1　Late effect of fracture of spine and trunk without mention of spinal cord lesion 🔖
　　　　Late effects of injury classifiable to 805, 807–809
　　　　Coding Clinic: 2007, Q1, P20-21
　　905.2　Late effect of fracture of upper extremities 🔖
　　　　Late effect of injury classifiable to 810–819
　　905.3　Late effect of fracture of neck of femur 🔖
　　　　Late effect of injury classifiable to 820
　　905.4　Late effect of fracture of lower extremities 🔖
　　　　Late effect of injury classifiable to 821–827
　　　　Coding Clinic: 1995, Q1, P10; 1994, Q2, P7
　　905.5　Late effect of fracture of multiple and unspecified bones 🔖
　　　　Late effect of injury classifiable to 828–829
　　905.6　Late effect of dislocation 🔖
　　　　Late effect of injury classifiable to 830–839
　　905.7　Late effect of sprain and strain without mention of tendon injury 🔖
　　　　Late effect of injury classifiable to 840–848, except tendon injury
　　905.8　Late effect of tendon injury 🔖
　　　　Late effect of tendon injury due to:
　　　　　open wound [injury classifiable to 880–884 with .2, 890–894 with .2]
　　　　　sprain and strain [injury classifiable to 840–848]
　　　　Coding Clinic: 1989, Q2, P15; Q2, P13
　　905.9　Late effect of traumatic amputation 🔖
　　　　Late effect of injury classifiable to 885–887, 895–897
　　　　Excludes　late amputation stump complication (997.60–997.69)

● 906　Late effects of injuries to skin and subcutaneous tissues
　　906.0　Late effect of open wound of head, neck, and trunk 🔖
　　　　Late effect of injury classifiable to 870–879
　　906.1　Late effect of open wound of extremities without mention of tendon injury 🔖
　　　　Late effect of injury classifiable to 880–884, 890–894 except .2
　　　　Coding Clinic: 1993, 5th Issue, P3
　　906.2　Late effect of superficial injury 🔖
　　　　Late effect of injury classifiable to 910–919
　　906.3　Late effect of contusion 🔖
　　　　Late effect of injury classifiable to 920–924
　　906.4　Late effect of crushing 🔖
　　　　Late effect of injury classifiable to 925–929
　　906.5　Late effect of burn of eye, face, head, and neck 🔖
　　　　Late effect of injury classifiable to 940–941
　　　　Coding Clinic: 2004, Q4, P75-76
　　906.6　Late effect of burn of wrist and hand 🔖
　　　　Late effect of injury classifiable to 944
　　906.7　Late effect of burn of other extremities 🔖
　　　　Late effect of injury classifiable to 943 or 945
　　906.8　Late effect of burns of other specified sites 🔖
　　　　Late effect of injury classifiable to 942, 946–947
　　906.9　Late effect of burn of unspecified site 🔖
　　　　Late effect of injury classifiable to 948–949

OGCR　Section I.C.17.c.7

Encounters for the treatment of the late effects of burns (i.e., scars or joint contractures) should be coded to the residual condition (sequelae) followed by the appropriate late effect code (906.5-906.9). A late effect E code may also be used, if desired.

◀ New　◀ Revised　~~deleted~~ Deleted　Excludes　Includes　Use additional　Code first　Omit code

978　● Unacceptable Principal Diagnosis　● Use Additional Digit(s)　▷ Manifestation Code　OGCR Official Guidelines　Coding Clinic

● **907 Late effects of injuries to the nervous system**

907.0 Late effect of intracranial injury without mention of skull fracture 🕲
Late effect of injury classifiable to 850–854
Coding Clinic: 2012, Q3, P20; 2011, Q4, P97; 2010, Q4, P97; 2009, Q4, P120; 2008, Q4, P102-109; 2003, Q4, P103-104; 1987, Nov-Dec, P12

907.1 Late effect of injury to cranial nerve 🕲
Late effect of injury classifiable to 950–951

907.2 Late effect of spinal cord injury 🕲
Late effect of injury classifiable to 806, 952
Coding Clinic: 2003, Q4, P103-104; 1998, Q4, P37-38; 1994, Q3, P4

907.3 Late effect of injury to nerve root(s), spinal plexus(es), and other nerves of trunk 🕲
Late effect of injury classifiable to 953–954
Coding Clinic: 2007, Q2, P13-15

907.4 Late effect of injury to peripheral nerve of shoulder girdle and upper limb 🕲
Late effect of injury classifiable to 955

907.5 Late effect of injury to peripheral nerve of pelvic girdle and lower limb 🕲
Late effect of injury classifiable to 956

907.9 Late effect of injury to other and unspecified nerve 🕲
Late effect of injury classifiable to 957

● **908 Late effects of other and unspecified injuries**

908.0 Late effect of internal injury to chest 🕲
Late effect of injury classifiable to 860–862

908.1 Late effect of internal injury to intra-abdominal organs 🕲
Late effect of injury classifiable to 863–866, 868

908.2 Late effect of internal injury to other internal organs 🕲
Late effect of injury classifiable to 867 or 869

908.3 Late effect of injury to blood vessel of head, neck, and extremities 🕲
Late effect of injury classifiable to 900, 903–904

908.4 Late effect of injury to blood vessel of thorax, abdomen, and pelvis 🕲
Late effect of injury classifiable to 901–902

908.5 Late effect of foreign body in orifice 🕲
Late effect of injury classifiable to 930–939

908.6 Late effect of certain complications of trauma 🕲
Late effect of complications classifiable to 958

908.9 Late effect of unspecified injury 🕲
Late effect of injury classifiable to 959
Coding Clinic: 2000, Q3, P4

● **909 Late effects of other and unspecified external causes**

909.0 Late effect of poisoning due to drug, medicinal or biological substance 🕲
Late effect of conditions classifiable to 960–979

Excludes Late effect of adverse effect of drug, medicinal or biological substance (909.5)
Coding Clinic: 2003, Q4, P103-104; 1984, Sept-Oct, P16

909.1 Late effect of toxic effects of nonmedical substances 🕲
Late effect of conditions classifiable to 980–989

909.2 Late effect of radiation 🕲
Late effect of conditions classifiable to 990
Coding Clinic: 1984, Nov-Dec, P19

909.3 Late effect of complications of surgical and medical care 🕲
Late effect of conditions classifiable to 996–999
Coding Clinic: 1993, Q1, P29

909.4 Late effect of certain other external causes 🕲
Late effect of conditions classifiable to 991–994

909.5 Late effect of adverse effect of drug, medicinal or biological substance 🕲

Excludes late effect of poisoning due to drug, medicinal or biological substances (909.0)

909.9 Late effect of other and unspecified external causes 🕲

SUPERFICIAL INJURY (910–919)

Excludes burn (blisters) (940.0–949.5)
contusion (920–924.9)
foreign body:
   granuloma (728.82)
   inadvertently left in operative wound (998.4)
   residual, in soft tissue (729.6)
   insect bite, venomous (989.5)
   open wound with incidental foreign body
     (870.0–897.7)

● **910 Superficial injury of face, neck, and scalp except eye**

Includes cheek lip
       ear   nose
       gum   throat

Excludes eye and adnexa (918.0–918.9)

910.0 Abrasion or friction burn without mention of infection

910.1 Abrasion or friction burn, infected

910.2 Blister without mention of infection

910.3 Blister, infected

910.4 Insect bite, nonvenomous, without mention of infection

910.5 Insect bite, nonvenomous, infected

910.6 Superficial foreign body (splinter) without major open wound and without mention of infection

910.7 Superficial foreign body (splinter) without major open wound, infected

910.8 Other and unspecified superficial injury of face, neck, and scalp without mention of infection

910.9 Other and unspecified superficial injury of face, neck, and scalp, infected

● **911 Superficial injury of trunk**

Includes abdominal wall   interscapular region
       anus   labium (majus) (minus)
       back   penis
       breastperineum
       buttock   scrotum
       chest wall   testis
       flank   vagina
       groin   vulva

Excludes hip (916.0–916.9)
scapular region (912.0–912.9)

911.0 Abrasion or friction burn without mention of infection
Coding Clinic: 2001, Q3, P10

911.1 Abrasion or friction burn, infected

911.2 Blister without mention of infection

911.3 Blister, infected

911.4 Insect bite, nonvenomous, without mention of infection

911.5 Insect bite, nonvenomous, infected

911.6 Superficial foreign body (splinter) without major open wound and without mention of infection

911.7 Superficial foreign body (splinter) without major open wound, infected

911.8 Other and unspecified superficial injury of trunk without mention of infection

911.9 Other and unspecified superficial injury of trunk, infected

● **912 Superficial injury of shoulder and upper arm**

Includes axilla
       scapular region

912.0 Abrasion or friction burn without mention of infection

912.1 Abrasion or friction burn, infected

912.2 Blister without mention of infection

912.3 Blister, infected

912.4 Insect bite, nonvenomous, without mention of infection

912.5 Insect bite, nonvenomous, infected

INJURY AND POISONING (800–999)

N Newborn: 0   P Pediatric: 0–17   M Maternity: 12–55   A Adult: 15–124   ♀ Females Only   ♂ Males Only

Ⓔⓧ CC/MCC Exclusions   🕲 Complication\Comorbidity   🕲 Major C\C   🕲 Present on Admission Requirement   🕲 Hospital-Acquired Condition

979

912.6 Superficial foreign body (splinter) without major open wound and without mention of infection

912.7 Superficial foreign body (splinter) without major open wound, infected

912.8 Other and unspecified superficial injury of shoulder and upper arm without mention of infection

912.9 Other and unspecified superficial injury of shoulder and upper arm, infected

● 913 Superficial injury of elbow, forearm, and wrist

913.0 Abrasion or friction burn without mention of infection

913.1 Abrasion or friction burn, infected

913.2 Blister without mention of infection

913.3 Blister, infected

913.4 Insect bite, nonvenomous, without mention of infection

913.5 Insect bite, nonvenomous, infected

913.6 Superficial foreign body (splinter) without major open wound and without mention of infection

913.7 Superficial foreign body (splinter) without major open wound, infected

913.8 Other and unspecified superficial injury of elbow, forearm, and wrist without mention of infection

913.9 Other and unspecified superficial injury of elbow, forearm, and wrist, infected

● 914 Superficial injury of hand(s) except finger(s) alone

914.0 Abrasion or friction burn without mention of infection

914.1 Abrasion or friction burn, infected

914.2 Blister without mention of infection

914.3 Blister, infected

914.4 Insect bite, nonvenomous, without mention of infection

914.5 Insect bite, nonvenomous, infected

914.6 Superficial foreign body (splinter) without major open wound and without mention of infection

914.7 Superficial foreign body (splinter) without major open wound, infected

914.8 Other and unspecified superficial injury of hand without mention of infection

914.9 Other and unspecified superficial injury of hand, infected

● 915 Superficial injury of finger(s)

Includes   fingernail
             thumb (nail)

915.0 Abrasion or friction burn without mention of infection

915.1 Abrasion or friction burn, infected

915.2 Blister without mention of infection

915.3 Blister, infected

915.4 Insect bite, nonvenomous, without mention of infection

915.5 Insect bite, nonvenomous, infected

915.6 Superficial foreign body (splinter) without major open wound and without mention of infection

915.7 Superficial foreign body (splinter) without major open wound, infected

915.8 Other and unspecified superficial injury of fingers without mention of infection
       Coding Clinic: 2001, Q3, P10

915.9 Other and unspecified superficial injury of fingers, infected

● 916 Superficial injury of hip, thigh, leg, and ankle

916.0 Abrasion or friction burn without mention of infection
       Coding Clinic: 2000, Q4, P61

916.1 Abrasion or friction burn, infected

916.2 Blister without mention of infection

916.3 Blister, infected

916.4 Insect bite, nonvenomous, without mention of infection

916.5 Insect bite, nonvenomous, infected

916.6 Superficial foreign body (splinter) without major open wound and without mention of infection

916.7 Superficial foreign body (splinter) without major open wound, infected

916.8 Other and unspecified superficial injury of hip, thigh, leg, and ankle without mention of infection

916.9 Other and unspecified superficial injury of hip, thigh, leg, and ankle, infected

● 917 Superficial injury of foot and toe(s)

Includes   heel
             toenail

917.0 Abrasion or friction burn without mention of infection

917.1 Abrasion or friction burn, infected

917.2 Blister without mention of infection

917.3 Blister, infected

917.4 Insect bite, nonvenomous, without mention of infection

917.5 Insect bite, nonvenomous, infected

917.6 Superficial foreign body (splinter) without major open wound and without mention of infection

917.7 Superficial foreign body (splinter) without major open wound, infected

917.8 Other and unspecified superficial injury of foot and toes without mention of infection
       Coding Clinic: 2003, Q1, P13

917.9 Other and unspecified superficial injury of foot and toes, infected
       Coding Clinic: 2003, Q1, P13

● 918 Superficial injury of eye and adnexa

Excludes   burn (940.0–940.9)
             foreign body on external eye (930.0–930.9)

918.0 Eyelids and periocular area
       Abrasion
       Insect bite
       Superficial foreign body (splinter)

918.1 Cornea
       Corneal abrasion
       Superficial laceration
       Excludes   corneal injury due to contact lens (371.82)

918.2 Conjunctiva

918.9 Other and unspecified superficial injuries of eye
       Eye (ball) NOS

● 919 Superficial injury of other, multiple, and unspecified sites

Excludes   multiple sites classifiable to the same three-digit category (910.0–918.9)

919.0 Abrasion or friction burn without mention of infection

919.1 Abrasion or friction burn, infected

919.2 Blister without mention of infection

919.3 Blister, infected

919.4 Insect bite, nonvenomous, without mention of infection

919.5 Insect bite, nonvenomous, infected

919.6 Superficial foreign body (splinter) without major open wound and without mention of infection

919.7 Superficial foreign body (splinter) without major open wound, infected

919.8 Other and unspecified superficial injury without mention of infection

919.9 Other and unspecified superficial injury, infected

◀ New   ◀▥ Revised   ~~deleted~~ Deleted   Excludes   Includes   Use additional   Code first   Omit code

980   ● Unacceptable Principal Diagnosis   ● Use Additional Digit(s)   ▸ Manifestation Code   OGCR Official Guidelines   **Coding Clinic**

CONTUSION WITH INTACT SKIN SURFACE (920–924)

Includes bruise without fracture or open wound
hematoma without fracture or open wound

Excludes *concussion (850.0–850.9)*
hemarthrosis (840.0–848.9)
internal organs (860.0–869.1)
that incidental to:
  crushing injury (925–929.9)
  dislocation (830.0–839.9)
  fracture (800.0–829.1)
  internal injury (860.0–869.1)
  intracranial injury (850.0–854.1)
  nerve injury (950.0–957.9)
  open wound (870.0–897.7)

920 Contusion of face, scalp, and neck except eye(s)
Cheek   Mandibular joint area
Ear (auricle)   Nose
Gum   Throat
Lip

● **921 Contusion of eye and adnexa**
921.0 Black eye, NOS
921.1 Contusion of eyelids and periocular area
921.2 Contusion of orbital tissues
921.3 Contusion of eyeball
Coding Clinic: 1985, July-Aug, P16
921.9 Unspecified contusion of eye
Injury of eye NOS

● **922 Contusion of trunk**
922.0 Breast
922.1 Chest wall
922.2 Abdominal wall
Flank
Groin
● **922.3 Back**
922.31 Back
Excludes *interscapular region (922.33)*
Coding Clinic: 1999, Q3, P14-15
922.32 Buttock
922.33 Interscapular region
Excludes *scapular region (923.01)*
922.4 Genital organs
Labium (majus) (minus)   Testis
Penis   Vagina
Perineum   Vulva
Scrotum
922.8 Multiple sites of trunk
922.9 Unspecified part
Trunk NOS

● **923 Contusion of upper limb**
● **923.0 Shoulder and upper arm**
923.00 Shoulder region
923.01 Scapular region
923.02 Axillary region
923.03 Upper arm
923.09 Multiple sites
● **923.1 Elbow and forearm**
923.10 Forearm
923.11 Elbow
● **923.2 Wrist and hand(s), except finger(s) alone**
923.20 Hand(s)
923.21 Wrist
923.3 Finger
Fingernail
Thumb (nail)
923.8 Multiple sites of upper limb
923.9 Unspecified part of upper limb
Arm NOS

● **924 Contusion of lower limb and of other and unspecified sites**
● **924.0 Hip and thigh**
924.00 Thigh
Coding Clinic: 2009, Q1, P10x2
924.01 Hip
● **924.1 Knee and lower leg**
924.10 Lower leg
924.11 Knee
● **924.2 Ankle and foot, excluding toe(s)**
924.20 Foot
Heel
924.21 Ankle
924.3 Toe
Toenail
924.4 Multiple sites of lower limb
924.5 Unspecified part of lower limb
Leg NOS
924.8 Multiple sites, not elsewhere classified
Coding Clinic: 2003, Q1, P7
924.9 Unspecified site

CRUSHING INJURY (925–929)

Use additional code to identify any associated injuries, such as:
fractures (800–829)
internal injuries (860.0–869.1)
intracranial injury (850.0–854.1)

● **925 Crushing injury of face, scalp, and neck**
Cheek   Pharynx
Ear   Throat
Larynx
Coding Clinic: 2003, Q4, P76-78
925.1 Crushing injury of face and scalp 🔹 🔹
Cheek
Ear
(Ex) 873.8-873.9, 905.0, 925.1-925.2, 929.0-929.9, 958.8-959.09, 959.8-959.9
925.2 Crushing injury of neck 🔹 🔹
Larynx
Throat
Pharynx
(Ex) 873.8-873.9, 905.0, 925.1-925.2, 929.0-929.9, 958.8-959.09, 959.8-959.9

● **926 Crushing injury of trunk**
Coding Clinic: 2003, Q4, P76-78
926.0 External genitalia
Labium (majus) (minus)
Penis
Scrotum
Testis
Vulva
● **926.1 Other specified sites**
926.11 Back
926.12 Buttock
926.19 Other
Breast
926.8 Multiple sites of trunk
926.9 Unspecified site
Trunk NOS

● **927 Crushing injury of upper limb**
● **927.0 Shoulder and upper arm**
927.00 Shoulder region
927.01 Scapular region
927.02 Axillary region
927.03 Upper arm
927.09 Multiple sites
● **927.1 Elbow and forearm**
927.10 Forearm
927.11 Elbow

INJURY AND POISONING (800–999)

INJURY AND POISONING (800–999)

● 927.2 **Wrist and hand(s), except finger(s) alone**
　　927.20 **Hand(s)**
　　927.21 **Wrist**
　927.3 **Finger(s)**
　　　Coding Clinic: 2003, Q4, P76-78
　927.8 **Multiple sites of upper limb**
　927.9 **Unspecified site**
　　　Arm NOS

● 928 **Crushing injury of lower limb**
　　Coding Clinic: 2003, Q4, P76-78
　● 928.0 **Hip and thigh**
　　928.00 **Thigh** ☒ ☒
　　　(Ex) 928.00, 928.8-929.9
　　928.01 **Hip** ☒ ☒
　　　(Ex) 928.01, 928.8-929.9
　928.1 **Knee and lower leg**
　　928.10 **Lower leg**
　　928.11 **Knee**
　● 928.2 **Ankle and foot, excluding toe(s) alone**
　　928.20 **Foot**
　　　Heel
　　928.21 **Ankle**
　928.3 **Toe(s)**
　928.8 **Multiple sites of lower limb**
　928.9 **Unspecified site**
　　　Leg NOS

● 929 **Crushing injury of multiple and unspecified sites**
　　Coding Clinic: 2003, Q4, P76-78
　929.0 **Multiple sites, not elsewhere classified**
　929.9 **Unspecified site**

EFFECTS OF FOREIGN BODY ENTERING THROUGH ORIFICE (930–939)

Excludes *foreign body:*
　granuloma (728.82)
　inadvertently left in operative wound (998.4, 998.7)
　in open wound (800–839, 851–897)
　residual, in soft tissues (729.6)
　superficial without major open wound (910–919 with .6 or .7)

● 930 **Foreign body on external eye**
　Excludes *foreign body in penetrating wound of:*
　　eyeball (871.5–871.6)
　　　retained (old) (360.5–360.6)
　　ocular adnexa (870.4)
　　　retained (old) (376.6)
　930.0 **Corneal foreign body**
　930.1 **Foreign body in conjunctival sac**
　930.2 **Foreign body in lacrimal punctum**
　930.8 **Other and combined sites**
　930.9 **Unspecified site**
　　　External eye NOS

931 **Foreign body in ear**
　Auditory canal
　Auricle

932 **Foreign body in nose**
　Nasal sinus
　Nostril

● 933 **Foreign body in pharynx and larynx**
　933.0 **Pharynx**
　　　Nasopharynx
　　　Throat NOS
　933.1 **Larynx**
　　　Asphyxia due to foreign body
　　　Choking due to:
　　　　food (regurgitated)
　　　　phlegm

● 934 **Foreign body in trachea, bronchus, and lung**
　934.0 **Trachea** ☒
　　　(Ex) 934.0
　934.1 **Main bronchus** ☒
　　　(Ex) 934.0-934.9
　934.8 **Other specified parts** ☒
　　　Bronchioles
　　　Lung
　　　(Ex) 934.0-934.9
　934.9 **Respiratory tree, unspecified**
　　　Inhalation of liquid or vomitus, lower respiratory tract NOS

● 935 **Foreign body in mouth, esophagus, and stomach**
　935.0 **Mouth**
　935.1 **Esophagus**
　　　Coding Clinic: 1988, Q1, P13
　935.2 **Stomach**
　　　Coding Clinic: 1985, Jan-Feb, P14-15

936 **Foreign body in intestine and colon**

937 **Foreign body in anus and rectum**
　Rectosigmoid (junction)

938 **Foreign body in digestive system, unspecified**
　Alimentary tract NOS
　Swallowed foreign body

● 939 **Foreign body in genitourinary tract**
　939.0 **Bladder and urethra**
　939.1 **Uterus, any part** ♀
　　　Excludes *intrauterine contraceptive device: complications from (996.32, 996.65) presence of (V45.51)*
　939.2 **Vulva and vagina** ♀
　939.3 **Penis** ♂
　939.9 **Unspecified site**

OGCR Section I.C.17.c

Current burns (940-948) are classified by depth, extent and by agent (E code). Burns are classified by depth as first degree (erythema), second degree (blistering), and third degree (full-thickness involvement).

OGCR Section I.C.17.c.1

Sequence first the code that reflects the highest degree of burn when more than one burn is present.

OGCR Section I.C.17.c.2

Classify burns of the same local site (three-digit category level, 940-947) but of different degrees to the subcategory identifying the highest degree recorded in the diagnosis.

Figure 17–14 A. Second-degree burn. **B.** Third-degree burn. (From Cummings: Otolaryngology: Head & Neck Surgery, ed 4, Mosby, 2005)

BURNS (940–949)

Includes   burns from:
        electrical heating appliance
        electricity
        flame
        hot object
        lightning
        radiation
    chemical burns (external) (internal)
    scalds

Excludes   *friction burns (910–919 with .0, .1)*
        sunburn (692.71, 692.76–692.77)

● **940   Burn confined to eye and adnexa**

940.0   Chemical burn of eyelids and periocular area

940.1   Other burns of eyelids and periocular area

940.2   Alkaline chemical burn of cornea and conjunctival sac

940.3   Acid chemical burn of cornea and conjunctival sac

940.4   Other burn of cornea and conjunctival sac

940.5   Burn with resulting rupture and destruction of eyeball 🔵 🔵
      (Ex) No Exclusions

940.9   Unspecified burn of eye and adnexa

● **941   Burn of face, head, and neck**

Excludes   *mouth (947.0)*

The following fifth-digit subclassification is for use with category 941:

0	face and head, unspecified site
1	ear [any part]
2	eye (with other parts of face, head, and neck)
3	lip(s)
4	chin
5	nose (septum)
6	scalp [any part]
	Temple (region)
7	forehead and cheek
8	neck
9	multiple sites [except with eye] of face, head, and neck

● **941.0   Unspecified degree**
[0-9]

● **941.1   Erythema [first degree]**
[0-9]   Coding Clinic: 2010, Q3, P19; 2005, Q3, P10-11

● **941.2   Blisters, epidermal loss [second degree]**
[0-9]

● **941.3   Full-thickness skin loss [third degree NOS]** 🔵 🔵
[0-9]   For code **941.30:** (Ex) 941.30, 941.39;
    For code **941.31:** (Ex) 941.31, 941.39;
    For code **941.32:** (Ex) 941.32, 941.39;
    For code **941.33:** (Ex) 941.33, 941.39;
    For code **941.34:** (Ex) 941.34, 941.39;
    For code **941.35:** (Ex) 941.35, 941.39;
    For code **941.36:** (Ex) 941.36, 941.39;
    For code **941.37:** (Ex) 941.37, 941.39;
    For code **941.38:** (Ex) 941.38-941.39;
    For code **941.39:** (Ex) 941.30-941.39

● **941.4   Deep necrosis of underlying tissues [deep third**
[0-9]   **degree] without mention of loss of a body part** 🔵 🔵
    For codes **941.40, 941.49:** (Ex) 941.40, 941.49;
    For code **941.41:** (Ex) 941.40-941.41, 941.49;
    For code **941.42:** (Ex) 941.40, 941.42, 941.49;
    For code **941.43:** (Ex) 941.40, 941.43, 941.49;
    For code **941.44:** (Ex) 941.40, 941.44, 941.49;
    For code **941.45:** (Ex) 941.40, 941.45, 941.49;
    For code **941.46:** (Ex) 941.40, 941.46, 941.49;
    For code **941.47:** (Ex) 941.40, 941.47, 941.49;
    For code **941.48:** (Ex) 941.40, 941.48-941.49

● **941.5   Deep necrosis of underlying tissues [deep third**
[0-9]   **degree] with loss of a body part** 🔵 🔵
    For codes **941.50, 941.59:** (Ex) 941.50, 941.59;
    For code **941.51:** (Ex) 941.50-941.51, 941.59;
    For code **941.52:** (Ex) 941.50, 941.52, 941.59;
    For code **941.53:** (Ex) 941.50, 941.53, 941.59;
    For code **941.54:** (Ex) 941.50, 941.54, 941.59;
    For code **941.55:** (Ex) 941.50, 941.55, 941.59;
    For code **941.56:** (Ex) 941.50, 941.56, 941.59;
    For code **941.57:** (Ex) 941.50, 941.57, 941.59;
    For code **941.58:** (Ex) 941.50, 941.58-941.59

● **942   Burn of trunk**

Excludes   *scapular region (943.0–943.5 with fifth-digit 6)*

The following fifth-digit subclassification is for use with category 942:

0	trunk, unspecified site	
1	breast	
2	chest wall, excluding breast and nipple	
3	abdominal wall	
	Flank	
	Groin	
4	back [any part]	
	Buttock	
	Interscapular region	
5	genitalia	
	Labium (majus) (minus)	Scrotum
	Penis	Testis
	Perineum	Vulva
9	other and multiple sites of trunk	

● **942.0   Unspecified degree**
[0-5,9]

● **942.1   Erythema [first degree]**
[0-5,9]

● **942.2   Blisters, epidermal loss [second degree]**
[0-5,9]   Coding Clinic: 1984, Nov-Dec, P13

● **942.3   Full-thickness skin loss [third degree NOS]** 🔵 🔵
[0-5,9]   For codes **942.30, 942.39:** (Ex) 942.30, 942.39;
    For code **942.31:** (Ex) 942.30-942.31, 942.39;
    For code **942.32:** (Ex) 942.30, 942.32, 942.39;
    For code **942.33:** (Ex) 942.30, 942.33, 942.39;
    For code **942.34:** (Ex) 942.30, 942.34, 942.39;
    For code **942.35:** (Ex) 942.30, 942.35-942.39

● **942.4   Deep necrosis of underlying tissues [deep third**
[0-5,9]   **degree] without mention of loss of a body part** 🔵 🔵
    For code **942.40:** (Ex) 942.40, 942.49;
    For code **942.41:** (Ex) 942.40-942.41, 942.49;
    For code **942.42:** (Ex) 942.40, 942.42, 942.49;
    For code **942.43:** (Ex) 942.40, 942.43, 942.49;
    For code **942.44:** (Ex) 942.40, 942.44, 942.49;
    For code **942.45:** (Ex) 942.40, 942.45-942.49;
    For code **942.49:** (Ex) 942.40-942.49

● **942.5   Deep necrosis of underlying tissues [deep third**
[0-5,9]   **degree] with loss of a body part** 🔵 🔵
    For code **942.50:** (Ex) 942.50-942.59;
    For code **942.51:** (Ex) 942.50-942.51, 942.59;
    For code **942.52:** (Ex) 942.50, 942.52, 942.59;
    For code **942.53:** (Ex) 942.50, 942.53, 942.59;
    For code **942.54:** (Ex) 942.50, 942.54, 942.59;
    For code **942.55:** (Ex) 942.50, 942.55-942.59;
    For code **942.59:** (Ex) 942.50, 942.59

INJURY AND POISONING (800–999)

N Newborn: 0   P Pediatric: 0–17   M Maternity: 12–55   A Adult: 15–124   ♀ Females Only   ♂ Males Only

(Ex) CC/MCC Exclusions   🔵 Complication\Comorbidity   🔵 Major C\C   🔵 Present on Admission Requirement   🔵 Hospital-Acquired Condition   **983**

● 943 Burn of upper limb, except wrist and hand

The following fifth-digit subclassification is for use with category 943:

> 0 upper limb, unspecified site
> 1 forearm
> 2 elbow
> 3 upper arm
> 4 axilla
> 5 shoulder
> 6 scapular region
> 9 multiple sites of upper limb, except wrist and hand

● 943.0 Unspecified degree
[0-6,9]   Coding Clinic: 2010, Q3, P19

● 943.1 Erythema [first degree]
[0-6,9]

● 943.2 Blisters, epidermal loss [second degree]
[0-6,9]

● 943.3 Full-thickness skin loss [third degree NOS] 🅐 🅑
[0-6,9]   For codes **943.30, 943.39:** (Ex:) 943.30, 943.39;
             For code **943.31:** (Ex:) 943.30-943.31, 943.39;
             For code **943.32:** (Ex:) 943.30, 943.32, 943.39;
             For code **943.33:** (Ex:) 943.30, 943.33, 943.39;
             For code **943.34:** (Ex:) 943.30, 943.34, 943.39;
             For code **943.35:** (Ex:) 943.30, 943.35, 943.39;
             For code **943.36:** (Ex:) 943.30, 943.36-943.39

● 943.4 Deep necrosis of underlying tissues [deep third degree] without mention of loss of a body part 🅐 🅑
[0-6,9]   For codes **943.40, 943.49:** (Ex:) 943.40, 943.49;
             For code **943.41:** (Ex:) 943.40-943.41, 943.49;
             For code **943.42:** (Ex:) 943.40, 943.42, 943.49;
             For code **943.43:** (Ex:) 943.40, 943.43, 943.49;
             For code **943.44:** (Ex:) 943.40, 943.44, 943.49;
             For code **943.45:** (Ex:) 943.40, 943.45, 943.49;
             For code **943.46:** (Ex:) 943.40, 943.46-943.49

● 943.5 Deep necrosis of underlying tissues [deep third degree] with loss of a body part 🅐 🅑
[0-6,9]   For codes **943.50, 943.59:** (Ex:) 943.50, 943.59;
             For code **943.51:** (Ex:) 943.50-943.51, 943.59;
             For code **943.52:** (Ex:) 943.50, 943.52, 943.59;
             For code **943.53:** (Ex:) 943.50, 943.53, 943.59;
             For code **943.54:** (Ex:) 943.50, 943.54, 943.59;
             For code **943.55:** (Ex:) 943.50, 943.55, 943.59;
             For code **943.56:** (Ex:) 843.50, 943.56-943.59

● 944 Burn of wrist(s) and hand(s)

The following fifth-digit subclassification is for use with category 944:

> 0 hand, unspecified site
> 1 single digit [finger (nail)] other than thumb
> 2 thumb (nail)
> 3 two or more digits, not including thumb
> 4 two or more digits including thumb
> 5 palm
> 6 back of hand
> 7 wrist
> 8 multiple sites of wrist(s) and hand(s)

● 944.0 Unspecified degree
[0-8]

● 944.1 Erythema [first degree]
[0-8]

● 944.2 Blisters, epidermal loss [second degree]
[0-8]

● 944.3 Full-thickness skin loss [third degree NOS] 🅐 🅑
[0-8]   For codes **944.30, 944.38:** (Ex:) 944.30, 944.38;
            For code **944.31:** (Ex:) 944.30-944.31, 944.38;
            For code **944.32:** (Ex:) 944.30, 944.32, 944.38;
            For code **944.33:** (Ex:) 944.30, 944.33, 944.38;
            For code **944.34:** (Ex:) 944.30, 944.34, 944.38;
            For code **944.35:** (Ex:) 944.30, 944.35, 944.38;
            For code **944.36:** (Ex:) 944.30, 944.36, 944.38;
            For code **944.37:** (Ex:) 944.30, 944.37-944.38

● 944.4 Deep necrosis of underlying tissues [deep third degree] without mention of loss of a body part 🅐 🅑
[0-8]   For codes **944.40, 944.48:** (Ex:) 944.40, 944.48;
            For code **944.41:** (Ex:) 944.40-944.41, 944.48;
            For code **944.42:** (Ex:) 944.40, 944.42, 944.48;
            For code **944.43:** (Ex:) 944.40, 944.43, 944.48;
            For code **944.44:** (Ex:) 944.40, 944.44, 944.48;
            For code **944.45:** (Ex:) 944.40, 944.45, 944.48;
            For code **944.46:** (Ex:) 944.40, 944.46, 944.48;
            For code **944.47:** (Ex:) 944.40, 944.47-944.48

● 944.5 Deep necrosis of underlying tissues [deep third degree] with loss of a body part 🅐 🅑
[0-8]   For codes **944.50, 944.58:** (Ex:) 944.50, 944.58;
            For code **944.51:** (Ex:) 944.50-944.51, 944.58;
            For code **944.52:** (Ex:) 944.50, 944.52, 944.58;
            For code **944.53:** (Ex:) 944.50, 944.53, 944.58;
            For code **944.54:** (Ex:) 944.50, 944.54, 944.58;
            For code **944.55:** (Ex:) 944.50, 944.55, 944.58;
            For code **944.56:** (Ex:) 944.50, 944.56, 944.58;
            For code **944.57:** (Ex:) 944.50, 944.57-944.58

● 945 Burn of lower limb(s)

The following fifth-digit subclassification is for use with category 945:

> 0 lower limb [leg], unspecified site
> 1 toe(s) (nail)
> 2 foot
> 3 ankle
> 4 lower leg
> 5 knee
> 6 thigh [any part]
> 9 multiple sites of lower limb(s)

● 945.0 Unspecified degree
[0-6,9]

● 945.1 Erythema [first degree]
[0-6,9]

● 945.2 Blisters, epidermal loss [second degree]
[0-6,9]

● 945.3 Full-thickness skin loss [third degree NOS] 🅐 🅑
[0-6,9]   For codes **945.30, 945.39:** (Ex:) 945.30, 945.39;
             For code **945.31:** (Ex:) 945.30-945.31, 945.39;
             For code **945.32:** (Ex:) 945.30, 945.32, 945.39;
             For code **945.33:** (Ex:) 945.30, 945.33, 945.39;
             For code **945.34:** (Ex:) 945.30, 945.34, 945.39;
             For code **945.35:** (Ex:) 945.30, 945.35, 945.39;
             For code **945.36:** (Ex:) 945.30, 945.36-945.39

● 945.4 Deep necrosis of underlying tissues [deep third degree] without mention of loss of a body part 🅐 🅑
[0-6,9]   For codes **945.40, 945.49:** (Ex:) 945.40, 945.49;
             For code **945.41:** (Ex:) 945.40-945.41, 945.49;
             For code **945.42:** (Ex:) 945.40, 945.42, 945.49;
             For code **945.43:** (Ex:) 945.40, 945.43, 945.49;
             For code **945.44:** (Ex:) 945.40, 945.44, 945.49;
             For code **945.45:** (Ex:) 945.40, 945.45, 945.49;
             For code **945.46:** (Ex:) 945.40, 945.46-945.49

● 945.5 Deep necrosis of underlying tissues [deep third degree] with loss of a body part 🅐 🅑
[0-6,9]   For codes **945.50, 945.59:** (Ex:) 945.50, 945.59;
             For code **945.51:** (Ex:) 945.50-945.51, 945.59;
             For code **945.52:** (Ex:) 945.50, 945.52, 945.59;
             For code **945.53:** (Ex:) 945.50, 945.53, 945.59;
             For code **945.54:** (Ex:) 945.50, 945.54, 945.59;
             For code **945.55:** (Ex:) 945.50, 945.55, 945.59;
             For code **945.56:** (Ex:) 945.50, 945.56-945.59

INJURY AND POISONING (800–999)

OGCR   Section I.C.17.c.5

When coding burns, assign separate codes for each burn site. Category 946 should only be used if the location of the burns are not documented.

● **946   Burns of multiple specified sites**
     Documented as multiple sites but not specified as to location
     Includes   burns of sites classifiable to more than one
                    three-digit category in 940–945
     Excludes   *multiple burns NOS (949.0–949.5)*
     946.0   Unspecified degree
     946.1   Erythema [first degree]
     946.2   Blisters, epidermal loss [second degree]
     946.3   Full-thickness skin loss [third degree NOS] 🏷️ 🏷️
            (Ex) 946.3
     **946.4   Deep necrosis of underlying tissues [deep third degree]
            without mention of loss of a body part** 🏷️ 🏷️
            (Ex) 946.4
     **946.5   Deep necrosis of underlying tissues [deep third degree]
            with loss of a body part** 🏷️ 🏷️
            (Ex) 946.5

● **947   Burn of internal organs**
     Includes   burns from chemical agents (ingested)
     947.0   Mouth and pharynx
            Gum
            Tongue
     947.1   Larynx, trachea, and lung 🏷️ 🏷️
            (Ex) 947.1, 947.8-947.9
     947.2   Esophagus 🏷️ 🏷️
            (Ex) 947.2, 947.8-947.9
     947.3   Gastrointestinal tract 🏷️ 🏷️
            Colon
            Rectum
            Small intestine
            Stomach
            (Ex) 947.3, 947.8-947.9
            Coding Clinic: 2012, Q2, P8
     947.4   Vagina and uterus ♀ 🏷️ 🏷️
            (Ex) 947.4-947.9
     947.8   Other specified sites
     947.9   Unspecified site

OGCR   Section I.C.17.c.6

Fourth-digit identifies percentage of **total body surface** involved in a burn (all degrees). **Fifth-digit** identifies the percentage of body surface involved in **third-degree burn.** Fifth-digit zero (0) assigned when less than 10 percent or when no body surface is involved in a third-degree burn.

Category 948 is based on the classic "rule of nines" in estimating body surface involved: head and neck are assigned nine percent, each arm nine percent, each leg 18 percent, the anterior trunk 18 percent, posterior trunk 18 percent, and genitalia one percent. Providers may change these percentage assignments where necessary to accommodate infants and children who have proportionately larger heads than adults and patients who have large buttocks, thighs, or abdomen that involve burns.

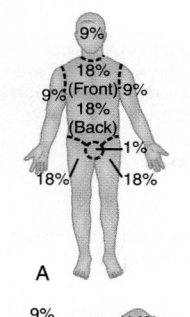

Figure 17–15   Rule of nines: percentages of total body area. (From Marx: Rosen's Emergency Medicine: Concepts and Clinical Practice, ed 6, Mosby, 2006)

● **948   Burns classified according to extent of body surface involved**
     Excludes   *sunburn (692.71, 692.76–692.77)*
     Note: This category is to be used when the site of the burn is
                unspecified, or with categories 940–947 when the site
                is specified.
     Coding Clinic: 1984, Nov-Dec, P13
     The following fifth-digit subclassification is for use with category 948 to indicate the percent of body surface with third degree burn; valid digits are in [brackets] under each code:

0	less than 10 percent or unspecified
1	10–19%
2	20–29%
3	30–39%
4	40–49%
5	50–59%
6	60–69%
7	70–79%
8	80–89%
9	90% or more of body surface

● **948.0   Burn [any degree] involving less than 10 percent of**
  [0]   **body surface**
● **948.1   10–19 percent of body surface** 🏷️ 🏷️
  [0-1]   (Ex) 948.00-948.99
           Coding Clinic: 1984, Nov-Dec, P13
● **948.2   20–29 percent of body surface** 0 🏷️ 🏷️, 1,2 🏷️ 🏷️
  [0-2]   (Ex) 948.00-948.99
           Coding Clinic: 1984, Nov-Dec, P13
● **948.3   30–39 percent of body surface** 0 🏷️ 🏷️, 1-3 🏷️ 🏷️
  [0-3]   (Ex) 948.00-948.99
● **948.4   40–49 percent of body surface** 0 🏷️ 🏷️, 1-4 🏷️ 🏷️
  [0-4]   (Ex) 948.00-948.99
● **948.5   50–59 percent of body surface** 0 🏷️ 🏷️, 1-5 🏷️ 🏷️
  [0-5]   (Ex) 948.00-948.99
● **948.6   60–69 percent of body surface** 0 🏷️ 🏷️, 1-6 🏷️ 🏷️
  [0-6]   (Ex) 948.00-948.99
● **948.7   70–79 percent of body surface** 0 🏷️ 🏷️, 1-7 🏷️ 🏷️
  [0-7]   (Ex) 948.00-948.99
● **948.8   80–89 percent of body surface** 0 🏷️ 🏷️, 1-8 🏷️ 🏷️
  [0-8]   (Ex) 948.00-948.99
● **948.9   90 percent or more of body surface** 0 🏷️ 🏷️, 1-9 🏷️ 🏷️
  [0-9]   (Ex) 948.00-948.99

INJURY AND POISONING (800–999)

OGCR   Section I.C.17.c.5

When coding burns, assign separate codes for each burn site. Category 946 Burns of Multiple specified sites, should only be used if the location of the burns are not documented. Category 949, Burn, unspecified, is extremely vague and should rarely be used.

● 949   **Burn, unspecified**

Includes   burn NOS
multiple burns NOS

Excludes   *burn of unspecified site but with statement of the extent of body surface involved (948.0–948.9)*

949.0   **Unspecified degree**

949.1   **Erythema [first degree]**

949.2   **Blisters, epidermal loss [second degree]**

949.3   **Full-thickness skin loss [third degree NOS]** 🔖 🔖
(Ex) 941.30-941.39, 942.30-942.39, 944.30-944.38, 945.30-945.39, 946.3, 949.3

949.4   **Deep necrosis of underlying tissues [deep third degree] without mention of loss of a body part** 🔖 🔖
(Ex) 941.40-941.49, 942.40-942.49, 944.40-944.48, 945.40-945.49, 946.4, 949.4

949.5   **Deep necrosis of underlying tissues [deep third degree] with loss of a body part** 🔖 🔖

Includes   division of nerve
lesion in continuity (with open wound)
traumatic neuroma (with open wound)
traumatic transient paralysis (with open wound)

Excludes   *accidental puncture or laceration during medical procedure (998.2)*

(Ex) 946.5, 949.5

INJURY TO NERVES AND SPINAL CORD (950–957)

● 950   **Injury to optic nerve and pathways**

950.0   **Optic nerve injury** 🔖
Second cranial nerve
(Ex) 950.0-950.9, 951.8-951.9

950.1   **Injury to optic chiasm** 🔖
(Ex) 950.0-950.9, 951.8-951.9

950.2   **Injury to optic pathways** 🔖
(Ex) 950.0-950.9, 951.8-951.9

950.3   **Injury to visual cortex** 🔖
(Ex) 950.0-950.9, 951.8-951.9

950.9   **Unspecified** 🔖
Traumatic blindness NOS
(Ex) 950.0-950.9, 951.8-951.9

● 951   **Injury to other cranial nerve(s)**

951.0   **Injury to oculomotor nerve** 🔖
Third cranial nerve
(Ex) 951.0, 951.8-951.9

951.1   **Injury to trochlear nerve** 🔖
Fourth cranial nerve
(Ex) 951.1, 951.8-951.9

951.2   **Injury to trigeminal nerve** 🔖
Fifth cranial nerve
(Ex) 951.2, 951.8-951.9

951.3   **Injury to abducens nerve** 🔖
Sixth cranial nerve
(Ex) 951.3, 951.8-951.9

951.4   **Injury to facial nerve** 🔖
Seventh cranial nerve
(Ex) 951.4, 951.8-951.9

951.5   **Injury to acoustic nerve** 🔖
Auditory nerve
Eighth cranial nerve
Traumatic deafness NOS
(Ex) 951.5, 951.8-951.9

951.6   **Injury to accessory nerve** 🔖
Eleventh cranial nerve
(Ex) 951.6, 951.8-951.9

951.7   **Injury to hypoglossal nerve** 🔖
Twelfth cranial nerve
(Ex) 951.7-951.9

951.8   **Injury to other specified cranial nerves** 🔖
Glossopharyngeal [9th cranial] nerve
Olfactory [1st cranial] nerve
Pneumogastric [10th cranial] nerve
Traumatic anosmia NOS
Vagus [10th cranial] nerve
(Ex) 951.8-951.9

951.9   **Injury to unspecified cranial nerve** 🔖
(Ex) 951.8-951.9

● 952   **Spinal cord injury without evidence of spinal bone injury**

● 952.0   **Cervical**

952.00   **C_1-C_4 level with unspecified spinal cord injury** 🔖
Spinal cord injury, cervical region NOS
(Ex) 805.00-805.18, 805.8-806.19, 806.8-806.9, 839.00-839.18, 839.40, 839.49-839.50, 839.59, 839.69, 839.79-839.9, 847.9, 905.1, 926.11, 952.00-952.09, 952.8-952.9, 958.8-958.99, 959.11-959.19, 959.8-959.9

952.01   **C_1-C_4 level with complete lesion of spinal cord** 🔖
(Ex) 805.00-805.18, 805.8-806.19, 806.8-806.9, 839.00-839.18, 839.40, 839.49-839.50, 839.59, 839.69, 839.79-839.9, 847.9, 905.1, 926.11, 952.00-952.09, 952.8-952.9, 958.8-958.99, 959.11-959.19, 959.8-959.9

952.02   **C_1-C_4 level with anterior cord syndrome** 🔖
(Ex) 805.00-805.18, 805.8-806.19, 806.8-806.9, 839.00-839.18, 839.40, 839.49-839.50, 839.59, 839.69, 839.79-839.9, 847.9, 905.1, 926.11, 952.00-952.09, 952.8-952.9, 958.8-958.99, 959.11-959.19, 959.8-959.9

952.03   **C_1-C_4 level with central cord syndrome** 🔖
(Ex) 805.00-805.18, 805.8-806.19, 806.8-806.9, 839.00-839.18, 839.40, 839.49-839.50, 839.59, 839.69, 839.79-839.9, 847.9, 905.1, 926.11, 952.00-952.09, 952.8-952.9, 958.8-958.99, 959.11-959.19, 959.8-959.9

952.04   **C_1-C_4 level with other specified spinal cord injury** 🔖
Incomplete spinal cord lesion at C_1-C_4 level:
NOS
with posterior cord syndrome
(Ex) 805.00-805.18, 805.8-806.19, 806.8-806.9, 839.00-839.18, 839.40, 839.49-839.50, 839.59, 839.69, 839.79-839.9, 847.9, 905.1, 926.11, 952.00-952.09, 952.8-952.9, 958.8-958.99, 959.11-959.19, 959.8-959.9

952.05   **C_5-C_7 level with unspecified spinal cord injury** 🔖
(Ex) 805.00-805.18, 805.8-806.19, 806.8-806.9, 839.00-839.18, 839.40, 839.49-839.50, 839.59, 839.69, 839.79-839.9, 847.9, 905.1, 926.11, 952.00-952.09, 952.8-952.9, 958.8-958.99, 959.11-959.19, 959.8-959.9

952.06   **C_5-C_7 level with complete lesion of spinal cord** 🔖
(Ex) 805.00-805.18, 805.8-806.19, 806.8-806.9, 839.00-839.18, 839.40, 839.49-839.50, 839.59, 839.69, 839.79-839.9, 847.9, 905.1, 926.11, 952.00-952.09, 952.8-952.9, 958.8-958.99, 959.11-959.19, 959.8-959.9

952.07   **C_5-C_7 level with anterior cord syndrome** 🔖
(Ex) 805.00-805.18, 805.8-806.19, 806.8-806.9, 839.00-839.18, 839.40, 839.49-839.50, 839.59, 839.69, 839.79-839.9, 847.9, 905.1, 926.11, 952.00-952.09, 952.8-952.9, 958.8-958.99, 959.11-959.19, 959.8-959.9

952.08   **C_5-C_7 level with central cord syndrome** 🔖
(Ex) 805.00-805.18, 805.8-806.19, 806.8-806.9, 839.00-839.18, 839.40, 839.49-839.50, 839.59, 839.69, 839.79-839.9, 847.9, 905.1, 926.11, 952.00-952.09, 952.8-952.9, 958.8-958.99, 959.11-959.19, 959.8-959.9

952.09   **C_5-C_7 level with other specified spinal cord injury** 🔖
Incomplete spinal cord lesion at C_5-C_7 level:
NOS
with posterior cord syndrome
(Ex) 805.00-805.18, 805.8-806.19, 806.8-806.9, 839.00-839.18, 839.40, 839.49-839.50, 839.59, 839.69, 839.79-839.9, 847.9, 905.1, 926.11, 952.00-952.09, 952.8-952.9, 958.8-958.99, 959.11-959.19, 959.8-959.9

● 952.1   **Dorsal [thoracic]**

952.10 T_1-T_6 **level with unspecified spinal cord injury** 🔖
Spinal cord injury, thoracic region NOS
(Ex) 805.8-805.9, 806.20-806.39, 839.40, 839.49-839.50, 839.59, 839.69, 839.79-839.9, 847.9, 905.1, 926.11, 952.10-952.19, 952.8-952.9, 958.8-958.99, 959.11-959.19, 959.8-959.9

952.11 T_1-T_6 **level with complete lesion of spinal cord** 🔖
(Ex) 805.8-805.9, 806.20-806.39, 839.40, 839.49-839.50, 839.59, 839.69, 839.79-839.9, 847.9, 905.1, 926.11, 952.10-952.19, 952.8-952.9, 958.8-958.99, 959.11-959.19, 959.8-959.9

952.12 T_1-T_6 **level with anterior cord syndrome** 🔖
(Ex) 805.8-805.9, 806.20-806.39, 839.40, 839.49-839.50, 839.59, 839.69, 839.79-839.9, 847.9, 905.1, 926.11, 952.10-952.19, 952.8-952.9, 958.8-958.99, 959.11-959.19, 959.8-959.9

952.13 T_1-T_6 **level with central cord syndrome** 🔖
(Ex) 805.8-805.9, 806.20-806.39, 839.40, 839.49-839.50, 839.59, 839.69, 839.79-839.9, 847.9, 905.1, 926.11, 952.10-952.19, 952.8-952.9, 958.8-958.99, 959.11-959.19, 959.8-959.9

952.14 T_1-T_6 **level with other specified spinal cord injury** 🔖
Incomplete spinal cord lesion at T_1-T_6 level:
NOS
with posterior cord syndrome
(Ex) 805.8-805.9, 806.20-806.39, 839.40, 839.49-839.50, 839.59, 839.69, 839.79-839.9, 847.9, 905.1, 926.11, 952.10-952.19, 952.8-952.9, 958.8-958.99, 959.11-959.19, 959.8-959.9

952.15 T_7-T_{12} **level with unspecified spinal cord injury** 🔖
(Ex) 805.8-805.9, 806.20-806.39, 839.40, 839.49-839.50, 839.59, 839.69, 839.79-839.9, 847.9, 905.1, 926.11, 952.10-952.19, 952.8-952.9, 958.8-958.99, 959.11-959.19, 959.8-959.9

952.16 T_7-T_{12} **level with complete lesion of spinal cord** 🔖
(Ex) 805.8-805.9, 806.20-806.39, 839.40, 839.49-839.50, 839.59, 839.69, 839.79-839.9, 847.9, 905.1, 926.11, 952.10-952.19, 952.8-952.9, 958.8-958.99, 959.11-959.19, 959.8-959.9

952.17 T_7-T_{12} **level with anterior cord syndrome** 🔖
(Ex) 805.8-805.9, 806.20-806.39, 839.40, 839.49-839.50, 839.59, 839.69, 839.79-839.9, 847.9, 905.1, 926.11, 952.10-952.19, 952.8-952.9, 958.8-958.99, 959.11-959.19, 959.8-959.9

952.18 T_7-T_{12} **level with central cord syndrome** 🔖
(Ex) 805.8-805.9, 806.20-806.39, 839.40, 839.49-839.50, 839.59, 839.69, 839.79-839.9, 847.9, 905.1, 926.11, 952.10-952.19, 952.8-952.9, 958.8-958.99, 959.11-959.19, 959.8-959.9

952.19 T_7-T_{12} **level with other specified spinal cord injury** 🔖
Incomplete spinal cord lesion at T_7-T_{12} level:
NOS
with posterior cord syndrome
(Ex) 805.8-805.9, 806.20-806.39, 839.40, 839.49-839.50, 839.59, 839.69, 839.79-839.9, 847.9, 905.1, 926.11, 952.10-952.19, 952.8-952.9, 958.8-958.99, 959.11-959.19, 959.8-959.9

952.2   **Lumbar** 🔖
(Ex) 805.8-805.9, 806.4-806.5, 839.40, 839.49-839.50, 839.59, 839.69, 839.79-839.9, 847.9, 905.1, 926.11, 952.2, 952.8-952.9, 958.8-958.99, 959.11-959.19, 959.8-959.9

952.3   **Sacral** 🔖
(Ex) 805.8-805.9, 806.60-806.79, 839.40, 839.49-839.50, 839.59, 839.69, 839.79-839.9, 847.9, 905.1, 926.11, 952.3-952.9, 958.8-958.99, 959.11-959.19, 959.8-959.9

952.4   **Cauda equina** 🔖
(Ex) 805.8-805.9, 806.60-806.79, 839.40, 839.49-839.50, 839.59, 839.69, 839.79-839.9, 847.9, 905.1, 926.11, 952.3-952.9, 958.8-958.99, 959.11-959.19, 959.8-959.9

952.8   **Multiple sites of spinal cord** 🔖
(Ex) 805.8-805.9, 839.40, 839.49-839.50, 839.59, 839.69, 839.79-839.9, 847.9, 905.1, 926.11, 952.8-952.9, 958.8-958.99, 959.11-959.19, 959.8-959.9

952.9   **Unspecified site of spinal cord**

● 953   **Injury to nerve roots and spinal plexus**

953.0   **Cervical root**

953.1   **Dorsal root**

953.2   **Lumbar root**

953.3   **Sacral root**

953.4   **Brachial plexus**

953.5   **Lumbosacral plexus**

953.8   **Multiple sites**

953.9   **Unspecified site**

● 954   **Injury to other nerve(s) of trunk, excluding shoulder and pelvic girdles**

954.0   **Cervical sympathetic**

954.1   **Other sympathetic**
Celiac ganglion or plexus   Splanchnic nerve(s)
Inferior mesenteric plexus   Stellate ganglion

954.8   **Other specified nerve(s) of trunk**

954.9   **Unspecified nerve of trunk**

● 955   **Injury to peripheral nerve(s) of shoulder girdle and upper limb**

955.0   **Axillary nerve**

955.1   **Median nerve**

955.2   **Ulnar nerve**

955.3   **Radial nerve**

955.4   **Musculocutaneous nerve**

955.5   **Cutaneous sensory nerve, upper limb**

955.6   **Digital nerve**

955.7   **Other specified nerve(s) of shoulder girdle and upper limb**

955.8   **Multiple nerves of shoulder girdle and upper limb**

955.9   **Unspecified nerve of shoulder girdle and upper limb**

● 956   **Injury to peripheral nerve(s) of pelvic girdle and lower limb**

956.0   **Sciatic nerve**

956.1   **Femoral nerve**

956.2   **Posterior tibial nerve**

956.3   **Peroneal nerve**

956.4   **Cutaneous sensory nerve, lower limb**

956.5   **Other specified nerve(s) of pelvic girdle and lower limb**

956.8   **Multiple nerves of pelvic girdle and lower limb**

956.9   **Unspecified nerve of pelvic girdle and lower limb**

● 957   **Injury to other and unspecified nerves**

957.0   **Superficial nerves of head and neck**

957.1   **Other specified nerve(s)**

957.8   **Multiple nerves in several parts**
Multiple nerve injury NOS

957.9   **Unspecified site**
Nerve injury NOS

CERTAIN TRAUMATIC COMPLICATIONS AND UNSPECIFIED INJURIES (958–959)

● 958   **Certain early complications of trauma**

Excludes *adult respiratory distress syndrome (518.52)*
flail chest (807.4)
post-traumatic seroma (729.91)
shock lung related to trauma and surgery (518.52)
that occurring during or following medical procedures (996.0–999.9)

958.0   **Air embolism** 🔖
Pneumathemia
Excludes *that complicating:*
abortion (634–638 with .6, 639.6)
ectopic or molar pregnancy (639.6)
pregnancy, childbirth, or the puerperium (673.0)
(Ex) 958.0, 958.8-958.99, 959.8-959.9, 997.91-997.99, 998.81, 998.83-998.9, 999.1

958.1   **Fat embolism** 🔖
Excludes *that complicating:*
abortion (634–638 with .6, 639.6)
pregnancy, childbirth, or the puerperium (673.8)
(Ex) 958.1, 958.8-958.99, 959.8-959.9, 997.91-997.99, 998.81, 998.83-998.9

958.2   **Secondary and recurrent hemorrhage** 🔖
(Ex) 958.2, 958.8-958.99, 959.8-959.9, 997.91-997.99, 998.81, 998.83-998.9

N Newborn: 0   **P** Pediatric: 0–17   **M** Maternity: 12–55   **A** Adult: 15–124   ♀ Females Only   ♂ Males Only

(Ex) CC/MCC Exclusions   🔖 Complication\Comorbidity   Major C\C   Present on Admission Requirement   Hospital-Acquired Condition   **987**

INJURY AND POISONING (800–999)

958.3 Posttraumatic wound infection, not elsewhere classified 🔖

　　Excludes *infected open wounds - code to complicated open wound of site*

　　Ex) 958.3, 958.8-958.99, 959.8-959.9, 997.91-997.99, 998.81, 998.83-998.9

　　Coding Clinic: 1993, 5th Issue, P3; 1985, Sept-Oct, P10; 1984, Nov-Dec, P20

　　OGCR Section I.C.17.c.4

　　Assign code 958.3, Posttraumatic wound infection, not elsewhere classified, as an additional code for any documented infected burn site.

958.4 Traumatic shock 🔖
Shock (immediate) (delayed) following injury

　　Excludes *shock:*
　　　　anaphylactic (995.0)
　　　　　due to serum (999.41-999.49)
　　　　anesthetic (995.4)
　　　　electric (994.8)
　　　　following abortion (639.5)
　　　　lightning (994.0)
　　　　nontraumatic NOS (785.50)
　　　　obstetric (669.1)
　　　　postoperative (998.00-998.09)

　　Ex) 958.4, 958.8-958.99, 959.8-959.9, 997.91-997.99, 998.81, 998.83-998.9

958.5 Traumatic anuria 🔖
Crush syndrome
Renal failure following crushing

　　Excludes *that due to a medical procedure (997.5)*

　　Ex) 958.5, 958.8-958.99, 959.8-959.9, 995.4, 997.91-998.13, 998.81, 998.83-998.9

958.6 Volkmann's ischemic contracture
Posttraumatic muscle contracture

958.7 Traumatic subcutaneous emphysema 🔖

　　Excludes *subcutaneous emphysema resulting from a procedure (998.81)*

　　Ex) 860.0-860.5, 861.20-862.1, 862.29-862.9, 875.0-875.1, 958.7-958.99, 959.8-959.9, 997.91-997.99, 998.81, 998.83-998.9

958.8 Other early complications of trauma
　　Coding Clinic: 1992, Q2, P13

● **958.9 Traumatic compartment syndrome**

　　Excludes *nontraumatic compartment syndrome (729.71-729.79)*

958.90 Compartment syndrome, unspecified 🔖
　　Ex) 868.03-868.10, 868.13-869.1

958.91 Traumatic compartment syndrome of upper extremity 🔖
Traumatic compartment syndrome of shoulder, arm, forearm, wrist, hand, and fingers
　　Ex) 729.81, 729.89-729.99

958.92 Traumatic compartment syndrome of lower extremity 🔖
Traumatic compartment syndrome of hip, buttock, thigh, leg, foot, and toes
　　Ex) 729.81, 729.89-729.99

958.93 Traumatic compartment syndrome of abdomen 🔖
　　Ex) 863.0-867.3, 867.5-869.1, 879.2-879.9, 929.0-929.9, 958.8, 959.8-959.9
　　Coding Clinic: 2006, Q4, P100-102

958.99 Traumatic compartment syndrome of other sites 🔖
　　Ex) 868.03-868.10, 868.13-869.1

● **959 Injury, other and unspecified**
　　Includes injury NOS
　　Excludes *injury NOS of:*
　　　　blood vessels (900.0–904.9)
　　　　eye (921.0–921.9)
　　　　internal organs (860.0–869.1)
　　　　intracranial sites (854.0–854.1)
　　　　nerves (950.0–951.9, 953.0–957.9)
　　　　spinal cord (952.0–952.9)
　　Coding Clinic: 1984, Nov-Dec, P9

● **959.0 Head, face, and neck**

959.01 Head injury, unspecified

　　Excludes *concussion (850.0–850.9)*
　　　　　with head injury NOS (850.0–850.9)
　　　　head injury NOS with loss of consciousness (850.1–850.5)
　　　　specified head injuries (850.0–854.1)
　　　　Coding Clinic: 2008, Q4, P102-109; 1999, Q1, P10

959.09 Injury of face and neck

● **959.1 Trunk**

　　Excludes *scapular region (959.2)*

959.11 Other injury of chest wall

959.12 Other injury of abdomen

959.13 Fracture of corpus cavernosum penis ♂

959.14 Other injury of external genitals

959.19 Other injury of other sites of trunk
Injury of trunk NOS

959.2 Shoulder and upper arm
Axilla
Scapular region

959.3 Elbow, forearm, and wrist
　　Coding Clinic: 1997, Q1, P8

959.4 Hand, except finger

959.5 Finger
Fingernail
Thumb (nail)

959.6 Hip and thigh
Upper leg

959.7 Knee, leg, ankle, and foot

959.8 Other specified sites, including multiple

　　Excludes *multiple sites classifiable to the same four-digit category (959.0–959.7)*

959.9 Unspecified site
　　Coding Clinic: 1984, Nov-Dec, P9

POISONING BY DRUGS, MEDICINAL AND BIOLOGICAL SUBSTANCES (960–979)

　　Includes overdose of these substances
　　　　wrong substance given or taken in error
　　Excludes *adverse effects ["hypersensitivity," "reaction," etc.] of correct substance properly administered. Such cases are to be classified according to the nature of the adverse effect, such as:*
　　　　adverse effect NOS (995.20)
　　　　allergic lymphadenitis (289.3)
　　　　aspirin gastritis (535.4)
　　　　blood disorders (280.0–289.9)
　　　　dermatitis:
　　　　　contact (692.0–692.9)
　　　　　due to ingestion (693.0–693.9)
　　　　nephropathy (583.9)
　　　　[The drug giving rise to the adverse effect may be identified by use of categories E930–E949.]
　　　　drug dependence (304.0–304.9)
　　　　drug reaction and poisoning affecting the newborn (760.0–779.9)
　　　　nondependent abuse of drugs (305.0–305.9)
　　　　pathological drug intoxication (292.2)

　　Use additional code to specify the effects of the poisoning

◀ New　◀▥ Revised　~~deleted~~ Deleted　Excludes　Includes　Use additional　Code first　Omit code

988　● Unacceptable Principal Diagnosis　● Use Additional Digit(s)　▶ Manifestation Code　OGCR Official Guidelines　Coding Clinic

● **960   Poisoning by antibiotics**

Excludes *antibiotics:*
ear, nose, and throat (976.6)
eye (976.5)
local (976.0)

960.0   Penicillins
Ampicillin   Cloxacillin
Carbenicillin   Penicillin G

OGCR   Section I.C.17.e.2

Poisoning. Errors made in drug prescription or in the administration of the drug by provider, nurse, patient, or other person, use the appropriate poisoning code from the 960-979 series. If an overdose of a drug was **intentionally** taken or administered and resulted in drug toxicity, it would be coded as a poisoning (960-979 series). If a **nonprescribed** drug or medicinal agent was taken in combination with a correctly prescribed and properly administered drug, any drug toxicity or other reaction resulting from the interaction of the two drugs would be classified as a poisoning.

When a reaction results from the interaction of a drug(s) and alcohol, this would be classified as poisoning.

Sequencing of poisoning: When coding a poisoning or reaction to the improper use of a medication (e.g., wrong dose, wrong substance, wrong route of administration) the poisoning code is sequenced first, followed by a code for the manifestation. If there is also a diagnosis of drug abuse or dependence to the substance, the abuse or dependence is coded as an additional code.

See Section I.C.3.a.6.b. if poisoning is the result of insulin pump malfunctions and Section I.C.19 for general use of E-codes.

960.1   Antifungal antibiotics
Amphotericin B   Nystatin
Griseofulvin   Trichomycin
Excludes *preparations intended for topical use (976.0–976.9)*

960.2   Chloramphenicol group
Chloramphenicol
Thiamphenicol

960.3   Erythromycin and other macrolides
Oleandomycin
Spiramycin

960.4   Tetracycline group
Doxycycline
Minocycline
Oxytetracycline

960.5   Cephalosporin group
Cephalexin   Cephaloridine
Cephaloglycin   Cephalothin

960.6   Antimycobacterial antibiotics
Cycloserine   Rifampin
Kanamycin   Streptomycin

960.7   Antineoplastic antibiotics
Actinomycin such as:
Bleomycin   Dactinomycin
Cactinomycin   Daunorubicin
          Mitomycin

960.8   Other specified antibiotics

960.9   Unspecified antibiotic

● **961   Poisoning by other anti-infectives**
Excludes *anti-infectives:*
ear, nose, and throat (976.6)
eye (976.5)
local (976.0)

961.0   Sulfonamides
Sulfadiazine
Sulfafurazole
Sulfamethoxazole

961.1   Arsenical anti-infectives

961.2   Heavy metal anti-infectives
Compounds of: Compounds of:
antimony   lead
bismuth   mercury
Excludes *mercurial diuretics (974.0)*

961.3   Quinoline and hydroxyquinoline derivatives
Chiniofon
Diiodohydroxyquin
Excludes *antimalarial drugs (961.4)*

961.4   Antimalarials and drugs acting on other blood protozoa
Chloroquine
Cycloguanil
Primaquine
Proguanil [chloroguanide]
Pyrimethamine
Quinine

961.5   Other antiprotozoal drugs
Emetine

961.6   Anthelmintics
Hexylresorcinol   Thiabendazole
Piperazine

961.7   Antiviral drugs
Methisazone
Excludes *amantadine (966.4)*
cytarabine (963.1)
idoxuridine (976.5)

961.8   Other antimycobacterial drugs
Ethambutol
Ethionamide
Isoniazid
Para-aminosalicylic acid derivatives
Sulfones

961.9   Other and unspecified anti-infectives
Flucytosine
Nitrofuran derivatives

● **962   Poisoning by hormones and synthetic substitutes**
Excludes *oxytocic hormones (975.0)*

962.0   Adrenal cortical steroids
Cortisone derivatives
Desoxycorticosterone derivatives
Fluorinated corticosteroids

962.1   Androgens and anabolic congeners
Methandriol   Oxymetholone
Nandrolone   Testosterone

962.2   Ovarian hormones and synthetic substitutes
Contraceptives, oral
Estrogens
Estrogens and progestogens, combined
Progestogens

962.3   Insulins and antidiabetic agents
Acetohexamide
Biguanide derivatives, oral
Chlorpropamide
Glucagon
Insulin
Phenformin
Sulfonylurea derivatives, oral
Tolbutamide

962.4   Anterior pituitary hormones
Corticotropin
Gonadotropin
Somatotropin [growth hormone]

962.5   Posterior pituitary hormones
Vasopressin
Excludes *oxytocic hormones (975.0)*

962.6   Parathyroid and parathyroid derivatives

962.7   Thyroid and thyroid derivatives
Dextrothyroxin
Levothyroxine sodium
Liothyronine
Thyroglobulin

962.8 Antithyroid agents
Iodides
Thiouracil
Thiourea

962.9 Other and unspecified hormones and synthetic substitutes

● **963 Poisoning by primarily systemic agents**
963.0 Antiallergic and antiemetic drugs
Antihistamines   Diphenylpyraline
Chlorpheniramine   Thonzylamine
Diphenhydramine   Tripelennamine
Excludes *phenothiazine-based tranquilizers (969.1)*

963.1 Antineoplastic and immunosuppressive drugs
Azathioprine   Cytarabine
Busulfan   Fluorouracil
Chlorambucil   Mercaptopurine
Cyclophosphamide   thio-TEPA
Excludes *antineoplastic antibiotics (960.7)*

963.2 Acidifying agents
963.3 Alkalizing agents
963.4 Enzymes, not elsewhere classified
Penicillinase
963.5 Vitamins, not elsewhere classified
Vitamin A
Vitamin D
Excludes *nicotinic acid (972.2)*
vitamin K (964.3)
963.8 Other specified systemic agents
Heavy metal antagonists
963.9 Unspecified systemic agent

● **964 Poisoning by agents primarily affecting blood constituents**
964.0 Iron and its compounds
Ferric salts
Ferrous sulfate and other ferrous salts
964.1 Liver preparations and other antianemic agents
Folic acid
964.2 Anticoagulants
Coumarin   Phenindione
Heparin   Warfarin sodium
Coding Clinic: 1994, Q1, P22
964.3 Vitamin K [phytonadione]
964.4 Fibrinolysis-affecting drugs
Aminocaproic acid   Streptokinase
Streptodornase   Urokinase
964.5 Anticoagulant antagonists and other coagulants
Hexadimethrine
Protamine sulfate
964.6 Gamma globulin
964.7 Natural blood and blood products
Blood plasma   Packed red cells
Human fibrinogen   Whole blood
Excludes *transfusion reactions (999.41-999.8)*
964.8 Other specified agents affecting blood constituents
Macromolecular blood substitutes
Plasma expanders
964.9 Unspecified agents affecting blood constituents

● **965 Poisoning by analgesics, antipyretics, and antirheumatics**
Use additional code to identify:
drug dependence (304.0–304.9)
nondependent abuse (305.0–305.9)
● **965.0 Opiates and related narcotics**
965.00 Opium (alkaloids), unspecified
Coding Clinic: 2007, Q3, P7-8
965.01 Heroin
Diacetylmorphine
965.02 Methadone
965.09 Other
Codeine [methylmorphine]
Meperidine [pethidine]
Morphine
Coding Clinic: 2007, Q3, P7-8

965.1 Salicylates
Acetylsalicylic acid [aspirin]
Salicylic acid salts
Coding Clinic: 1984, Nov-Dec, P15
965.4 Aromatic analgesics, not elsewhere classified
Acetanilid
Paracetamol [acetaminophen]
Phenacetin [acetophenetidin]
965.5 Pyrazole derivatives
Aminophenazone [aminopyrine]
Phenylbutazone
● **965.6 Antirheumatics [antiphlogistics]**
Excludes *salicylates (965.1)*
steroids (962.0–962.9)
965.61 Propionic acid derivatives
Fenoprofen   Ketoprofen
Flurbiprofen   Naproxen
Ibuprofen   Oxaprozin
Coding Clinic: 1998, Q4, P42-44
965.69 Other antirheumatics
Gold salts
Indomethacin
965.7 Other non-narcotic analgesics
Pyrabital
965.8 Other specified analgesics and antipyretics
Pentazocine
965.9 Unspecified analgesic and antipyretic

● **966 Poisoning by anticonvulsants and anti-Parkinsonism drugs**
966.0 Oxazolidine derivatives
Paramethadione
Trimethadione
966.1 Hydantoin derivatives
Phenytoin
966.2 Succinimides
Ethosuximide
Phensuximide
966.3 Other and unspecified anticonvulsants
Primidone
Excludes *barbiturates (967.0)*
sulfonamides (961.0)
966.4 Anti-Parkinsonism drugs
Amantadine
Ethopropazine [profenamine]
Levodopa [L-dopa]

● **967 Poisoning by sedatives and hypnotics**
Use additional code to identify:
drug dependence (304.0–304.9)
nondependent abuse (305.0–305.9)
967.0 Barbiturates
Amobarbital [amylobarbitone]
Barbital [barbitone]
Butabarbital [butabarbitone]
Pentobarbital [pentobarbitone]
Phenobarbital [phenobarbitone]
Secobarbital [quinalbarbitone]
Excludes *thiobarbiturate anesthetics (968.3)*
967.1 Chloral hydrate group
967.2 Paraldehyde
967.3 Bromine compounds
Bromide
Carbromal (derivatives)
967.4 Methaqualone compounds
967.5 Glutethimide group
967.6 Mixed sedatives, not elsewhere classified
967.8 Other sedatives and hypnotics
967.9 Unspecified sedative or hypnotic
Sleeping: Sleeping:
drug NOS   tablet NOS
pill NOS

● **968 Poisoning by other central nervous system depressants and anesthetics**

     Use additional code to identify:
         drug dependence (304.0–304.9)
         nondependent abuse (305.0–305.9)

     968.0 Central nervous system muscle-tone depressants
         Chlorphenesin (carbamate)
         Mephenesin
         Methocarbamol

     968.1 Halothane

     968.2 Other gaseous anesthetics
         Ether
         Halogenated hydrocarbon derivatives, except halothane
         Nitrous oxide

     968.3 Intravenous anesthetics
         Ketamine
         Methohexital [methohexitone]
         Thiobarbiturates, such as thiopental sodium

     968.4 Other and unspecified general anesthetics

     968.5 Surface (topical) and infiltration anesthetics
         Cocaine (topical)   Procaine
         Lidocaine [lignocaine]   Tetracaine

         Excludes *poisoning by cocaine used as a central nervous system stimulant (970.81)*
         Coding Clinic: 1993, Q1, P25

     968.6 Peripheral nerve- and plexus-blocking anesthetics

     968.7 Spinal anesthetics

     968.9 Other and unspecified local anesthetics

● **969 Poisoning by psychotropic agents**

     Use additional code to identify:
         drug dependence (304.0–304.9)
         nondependent abuse (305.0–305.9)

     ● **969.0 Antidepressants**
         Coding Clinic: 2007, Q3, P7-8; 1991, Q3, P14

         969.00 Antidepressant, unspecified

         969.01 Monoamine oxidase inhibitors
            MAOI

         969.02 Selective serotonin and norepinephrine reuptake inhibitors
            SSNRI antidepressants

         969.03 Selective serotonin reuptake inhibitors
            SSRI antidepressants

         969.04 Tetracyclic antidepressants

         969.05 Tricyclic antidepressants
            Coding Clinic: 2009, Q4, P129

         969.09 Other antidepressants

     969.1 Phenothiazine-based tranquilizers
         Chlorpromazine   Prochlorperazine
         Fluphenazine   Promazine

     969.2 Butyrophenone-based tranquilizers
         Haloperidol   Trifluperidol
         Spiperone

     969.3 Other antipsychotics, neuroleptics, and major tranquilizers

     969.4 Benzodiazepine-based tranquilizers
         Chlordiazepoxide   Lorazepam
         Diazepam   Medazepam
         Flurazepam   Nitrazepam
         Coding Clinic: 2009, Q4, P129; 1991, Q3, P14

     969.5 Other tranquilizers
         Hydroxyzine
         Meprobamate

     969.6 Psychodysleptics [hallucinogens]
         Cannabis (derivatives)
         Lysergide [LSD]
         Marihuana (derivatives)
           Marijuana
         Mescaline
         Psilocin
         Psilocybin
         Coding Clinic: 2013, Q2, P16

     969.7 Psychostimulants

         Excludes *central appetite depressants (977.0)*
         Coding Clinic: 2003, Q2, P11

         969.70 Psychostimulant, unspecified

         969.71 Caffeine

         969.72 Amphetamines
            Methamphetamines

         969.73 Methylphenidate

         969.79 Other psychostimulants

     969.8 Other specified psychotropic agents

     969.9 Unspecified psychotropic agent

● **970 Poisoning by central nervous system stimulants**

     970.0 Analeptics
         Lobeline
         Nikethamide

     970.1 Opiate antagonists
         Levallorphan
         Nalorphine
         Naloxone

     ● **970.8 Other specified central nervous system stimulants**

         970.81 Cocaine
            Crack

         970.89 Other central nervous system stimulants
            Coding Clinic: 2013, Q2, P16

     970.9 Unspecified central nervous system stimulant

● **971 Poisoning by drugs primarily affecting the autonomic nervous system**

     971.0 Parasympathomimetics [cholinergics]
         Acetylcholine
         Anticholinesterase:
           organophosphorus
           reversible
         Pilocarpine

     971.1 Parasympatholytics [anticholinergics and antimuscarinics] and spasmolytics
         Atropine
         Homatropine
         Hyoscine [scopolamine]
         Quaternary ammonium derivatives

         Excludes *papaverine (972.5)*

     971.2 Sympathomimetics [adrenergics]
         Epinephrine [adrenalin]
         Levarterenol [noradrenalin]

     971.3 Sympatholytics [antiadrenergics]
         Phenoxybenzamine
         Tolazoline hydrochloride

     971.9 Unspecified drug primarily affecting autonomic nervous system

● **972 Poisoning by agents primarily affecting the cardiovascular system**

     972.0 Cardiac rhythm regulators
         Practolol   Propranolol
         Procainamide   Quinidine

         Excludes *lidocaine (968.5)*

     972.1 Cardiotonic glycosides and drugs of similar action
         Digitalis glycosides   Strophanthins
         Digoxin

     972.2 Antilipemic and antiarteriosclerotic drugs
         Clofibrate
         Nicotinic acid derivatives

     972.3 Ganglion-blocking agents
         Pentamethonium bromide

     972.4 Coronary vasodilators
         Dipyridamole
         Nitrates [nitroglycerin]
         Nitrites

INJURY AND POISONING (800–999)

N Newborn: 0   P Pediatric: 0–17   M Maternity: 12–55   A Adult: 15–124   ♀ Females Only   ♂ Males Only

(Ex) CC/MCC Exclusions   Complication\Comorbidity   Major C\C   Present on Admission Requirement   Hospital-Acquired Condition   **991**

972.5 Other vasodilators
Cyclandelate
Diazoxide
Papaverine
> **Excludes** *nicotinic acid (972.2)*

972.6 Other antihypertensive agents
Clonidine　　　　　　　Rauwolfia alkaloids
Guanethidine　　　　　Reserpine

972.7 Antivaricose drugs, including sclerosing agents
Sodium morrhuate
Zinc salts

972.8 Capillary-active drugs
Adrenochrome derivatives
Metaraminol

972.9 Other and unspecified agents primarily affecting the cardiovascular system

● **973 Poisoning by agents primarily affecting the gastrointestinal system**

973.0 Antacids and antigastric secretion drugs
Aluminum hydroxide
Magnesium trisilicate
Coding Clinic: 2003, Q1, P19

973.1 Irritant cathartics
Bisacodyl
Castor oil
Phenolphthalein

973.2 Emollient cathartics
Dioctyl sulfosuccinates

973.3 Other cathartics, including intestinal atonia drugs
Magnesium sulfate

973.4 Digestants
Pancreatin　　　　　　Pepsin
Papain

973.5 Antidiarrheal drugs
Kaolin
Pectin
> **Excludes** *anti-infectives (960.0–961.9)*

973.6 Emetics

973.8 Other specified agents primarily affecting the gastrointestinal system

973.9 Unspecified agent primarily affecting the gastrointestinal system

● **974 Poisoning by water, mineral, and uric acid metabolism drugs**

974.0 Mercurial diuretics
Chlormerodrin
Mercaptomerin
Mersalyl

974.1 Purine derivative diuretics
Theobromine
Theophylline
> **Excludes** *aminophylline [theophylline ethylenediamine] (975.7)*
> *caffeine (969.71)*

974.2 Carbonic acid anhydrase inhibitors
Acetazolamide

974.3 Saluretics
Benzothiadiazides
Chlorothiazide group

974.4 Other diuretics
Ethacrynic acid
Furosemide

974.5 Electrolytic, caloric, and water-balance agents

974.6 Other mineral salts, not elsewhere classified

974.7 Uric acid metabolism drugs
Allopurinol
Colchicine
Probenecid

● **975 Poisoning by agents primarily acting on the smooth and skeletal muscles and respiratory system**

975.0 Oxytocic agents
Ergot alkaloids
Oxytocin
Prostaglandins

975.1 Smooth muscle relaxants
Adiphenine
Metaproterenol [orciprenaline]
> **Excludes** *papaverine (972.5)*

975.2 Skeletal muscle relaxants

975.3 Other and unspecified drugs acting on muscles

975.4 Antitussives
Dextromethorphan
Pipazethate

975.5 Expectorants
Acetylcysteine
Guaifenesin
Terpin hydrate

975.6 Anti-common cold drugs

975.7 Antiasthmatics
Aminophylline [theophylline ethylenediamine]

975.8 Other and unspecified respiratory drugs

● **976 Poisoning by agents primarily affecting skin and mucous membrane, ophthalmological, otorhinolaryngological, and dental drugs**

976.0 Local anti-infectives and anti-inflammatory drugs

976.1 Antipruritics

976.2 Local astringents and local detergents

976.3 Emollients, demulcents, and protectants

976.4 Keratolytics, keratoplastics, other hair treatment drugs and preparations

976.5 Eye anti-infectives and other eye drugs
Idoxuridine

976.6 Anti-infectives and other drugs and preparations for ear, nose, and throat

976.7 Dental drugs topically applied
> **Excludes** *anti-infectives (976.0)*
> *local anesthetics (968.5)*

976.8 Other agents primarily affecting skin and mucous membrane
Spermicides [vaginal contraceptives]

976.9 Unspecified agent primarily affecting skin and mucous membrane

● **977 Poisoning by other and unspecified drugs and medicinal substances**

977.0 Dietetics
Central appetite depressants

977.1 Lipotropic drugs

977.2 Antidotes and chelating agents, not elsewhere classified

977.3 Alcohol deterrents

977.4 Pharmaceutical excipients
Pharmaceutical adjuncts

977.8 Other specified drugs and medicinal substances
Contrast media used for diagnostic x-ray procedures
Diagnostic agents and kits

977.9 Unspecified drug or medicinal substance
Coding Clinic: 1986, Mar-April, P12

● **978 Poisoning by bacterial vaccines**

978.0 BCG

978.1 Typhoid and paratyphoid

978.2 Cholera

978.3 Plague

978.4 Tetanus

978.5 Diphtheria

978.6 Pertussis vaccine, including combinations with a pertussis component

978.8 Other and unspecified bacterial vaccines

978.9 Mixed bacterial vaccines, except combinations with a pertussis component

● 979 Poisoning by other vaccines and biological substances

> **Excludes** *gamma globulin (964.6)*

979.0 Smallpox vaccine

979.1 Rabies vaccine

979.2 Typhus vaccine

979.3 Yellow fever vaccine

979.4 Measles vaccine

979.5 Poliomyelitis vaccine

979.6 Other and unspecified viral and rickettsial vaccines
        Mumps vaccine

979.7 Mixed viral-rickettsial and bacterial vaccines, except combinations with a pertussis component

> **Excludes** *combinations with a pertussis component (978.6)*

979.9 Other and unspecified vaccines and biological substances

OGCR Section I.C.17.e.3

> When a harmful substance is ingested or comes in contact with a person, this is classified as a toxic effect. The toxic effect codes are in categories 980-989. A toxic effect code should be sequenced first, followed by the code(s) that identify the result of the toxic effect. An external cause code from categories E860-E869 for accidental exposure, codes E950.6 or E950.7 for intentional self-harm, category E962 for assault, or categories E980-E982, for undetermined, should also be assigned to indicate intent.

TOXIC EFFECTS OF SUBSTANCES CHIEFLY NONMEDICINAL AS TO SOURCE (980–989)

> **Excludes** *burns from chemical agents (ingested) (947.0–947.9)*
> *localized toxic effects indexed elsewhere (001.0–799.9)*
> *respiratory conditions due to external agents (506.0–508.9)*
> *respiratory conditions due to smoke inhalation NOS (508.2)*

Use additional code to identify:
    personal history of retained foreign body fully removed (V15.53)
    retained foreign body status, if applicable (V90.01-V90.9)
Use additional code to specify the nature of the toxic effect

● 980 Toxic effect of alcohol

980.0 Ethyl alcohol
        Denatured alcohol
        Ethanol
        Grain alcohol

        Use additional code to identify any associated:
            acute alcohol intoxication (305.0)
            in alcoholism (303.0)
            drunkenness (simple) (305.0)
            pathological (291.4)
        Coding Clinic: 2009, Q4, P129; 1996, Q3, P16; 1991, Q3, P14

980.1 Methyl alcohol
        Methanol
        Wood alcohol

980.2 Isopropyl alcohol
        Dimethyl carbinol
        Isopropanol
        Rubbing alcohol

980.3 Fusel oil
        Alcohol:
            amyl
            butyl
            propyl

980.8 Other specified alcohols

980.9 Unspecified alcohol

981 Toxic effect of petroleum products
        Benzine   Petroleum:
        Gasoline   ether
        Kerosene   naphtha
        Paraffin wax   spirit

● 982 Toxic effect of solvents other than petroleum based

982.0 Benzene and homologues

982.1 Carbon tetrachloride

982.2 Carbon disulfide
        Carbon bisulfide

982.3 Other chlorinated hydrocarbon solvents
        Tetrachloroethylene
        Trichloroethylene

> **Excludes** *chlorinated hydrocarbon preparations other than solvents (989.2)*
> Coding Clinic: 2008, Q3, P6, 7x2

982.4 Nitroglycol

982.8 Other nonpetroleum-based solvents
        Acetone

● 983 Toxic effect of corrosive aromatics, acids, and caustic alkalis

983.0 Corrosive aromatics
        Carbolic acid or phenol
        Cresol

983.1 Acids
        Acid:
            hydrochloric
            nitric
            sulfuric

983.2 Caustic alkalis
        Lye
        Potassium hydroxide
        Sodium hydroxide

983.9 Caustic, unspecified

● 984 Toxic effect of lead and its compounds (including fumes)

> **Includes** that from all sources except medicinal substances

984.0 Inorganic lead compounds
        Lead dioxide
        Lead salts

984.1 Organic lead compounds
        Lead acetate
        Tetraethyl lead

984.8 Other lead compounds

984.9 Unspecified lead compound

● 985 Toxic effect of other metals

> **Includes** that from all sources except medicinal substances

985.0 Mercury and its compounds
        Minamata disease

985.1 Arsenic and its compounds

985.2 Manganese and its compounds

985.3 Beryllium and its compounds

985.4 Antimony and its compounds

985.5 Cadmium and its compounds

985.6 Chromium

985.8 Other specified metals
        Brass fumes   Iron compounds
        Copper salts   Nickel compounds

985.9 Unspecified metal

986 Toxic effect of carbon monoxide

● 987 Toxic effect of other gases, fumes, or vapors

987.0 Liquefied petroleum gases
        Butane
        Propane

987.1 Other hydrocarbon gas

987.2 Nitrogen oxides
        Nitrogen dioxide
        Nitrous fumes

987.3 Sulfur dioxide

987.4 Freon
        Dichloromonofluoromethane

INJURY AND POISONING (800–999)

N Newborn: 0   P Pediatric: 0–17   M Maternity: 12–55   A Adult: 15–124   ♀ Females Only   ♂ Males Only

Ex: CC/MCC Exclusions   Complication\Comorbidity   Major C\C   Present on Admission Requirement   Hospital-Acquired Condition   **993**

987.5 Lacrimogenic gas
Bromobenzyl cyanide
Chloroacetophenone
Ethyliodoacetate

987.6 Chlorine gas

987.7 Hydrocyanic acid gas

987.8 Other specified gases, fumes, or vapors
Phosgene
Polyester fumes

987.9 Unspecified gas, fume, or vapor
Coding Clinic: 2005, Q3, P10-11

● **988 Toxic effect of noxious substances eaten as food**
Excludes allergic reaction to food, such as:
gastroenteritis (558.3)
rash (692.5, 693.1)
food poisoning (bacterial) (005.0–005.9)
toxic effects of food contaminants, such as:
aflatoxin and other mycotoxin (989.7)
mercury (985.0)

988.0 Fish and shellfish

988.1 Mushrooms

988.2 Berries and other plants

988.8 Other specified noxious substances eaten as food

988.9 Unspecified noxious substance eaten as food

● **989 Toxic effect of other substances, chiefly nonmedicinal as to source**

989.0 Hydrocyanic acid and cyanides
Potassium cyanide   Sodium cyanide
Excludes gas and fumes (987.7)

989.1 Strychnine and salts

989.2 Chlorinated hydrocarbons
Aldrin   DDT
Chlordane   Dieldrin
Excludes chlorinated hydrocarbon solvents (982.0–982.3)

989.3 Organophosphate and carbamate
Carbaryl   Parathion
Dichlorvos   Phorate
Malathion   Phosdrin

989.4 Other pesticides, not elsewhere classified
Mixtures of insecticides

989.5 Venom
Bites of venomous snakes, lizards, and spiders
Tick paralysis

989.6 Soaps and detergents

989.7 Aflatoxin and other mycotoxin [food contaminants]

● **989.8 Other substances, chiefly nonmedicinal as to source**
989.81 Asbestos
Excludes asbestosis (501)
exposure to asbestos (V15.84)
989.82 Latex
989.83 Silicone
Excludes silicone used in medical devices, implants and grafts (996.00–996.79)
989.84 Tobacco
989.89 Other

989.9 Unspecified substance, chiefly nonmedicinal as to source

OTHER AND UNSPECIFIED EFFECTS OF EXTERNAL CAUSES (990–995)

990 Effects of radiation, unspecified
Complication of:
phototherapy
radiation therapy
Radiation sickness
Excludes specified adverse effects of radiation. Such conditions are to be classified according to the nature of the adverse effect, as:
burns (940.0–949.5)
dermatitis (692.7–692.8)
leukemia (204.0–208.9)
pneumonia (508.0)
sunburn (692.71, 692.76–692.77)
[The type of radiation giving rise to the adverse effect may be identified by use of the E codes.]

● **991 Effects of reduced temperature**
991.0 Frostbite of face
(Ex:) 991.6, 991.3
991.1 Frostbite of hand
(Ex:) 991.1, 991.3
991.2 Frostbite of foot
(Ex:) 991.2-991.3
991.3 Frostbite of other and unspecified sites
(Ex:) 991.0-991.4
991.4 Immersion foot
Trench foot
(Ex:) 991.3-991.4
991.5 Chilblains
Erythema pernio   Perniosis
991.6 Hypothermia
Hypothermia (accidental)
Excludes hypothermia following anesthesia (995.89)
hypothermia not associated with low environmental temperature (780.65)
991.8 Other specified effects of reduced temperature
991.9 Unspecified effect of reduced temperature
Effects of freezing or excessive cold NOS

● **992 Effects of heat and light**
Excludes burns (940.0–949.5)
diseases of sweat glands due to heat (705.0–705.9)
malignant hyperpyrexia following anesthesia (995.86)
sunburn (692.71, 692.76–692.77)
992.0 Heat stroke and sunstroke
Heat apoplexy   Siriasis
Heat pyrexia   Thermoplegia
Ictus solaris
Use additional code(s) to identify any associated complication of heat stroke, such as:
alterations of consciousness (780.01-780.09)
systemic inflammatory response syndrome (995.93-995.94)
(Ex:) 992.0-992.9
992.1 Heat syncope
Heat collapse
992.2 Heat cramps
992.3 Heat exhaustion, anhydrotic
Heat prostration due to water depletion
Excludes that associated with salt depletion (992.4)
992.4 Heat exhaustion due to salt depletion
Heat prostration due to salt (and water) depletion
992.5 Heat exhaustion, unspecified
Heat prostration NOS
992.6 Heat fatigue, transient
992.7 Heat edema
992.8 Other specified heat effects
992.9 Unspecified

INJURY AND POISONING (800–999)

994

◀ New   ◀▦ Revised   d̶e̶l̶e̶t̶e̶d̶ Deleted   Excludes   Includes   Use additional   Code first   Omit code
● Unacceptable Principal Diagnosis   ● Use Additional Digit(s)   ▷ Manifestation Code   OGCR Official Guidelines   Coding Clinic

● **993 Effects of air pressure**

  993.0 Barotrauma, otitic
    Aero-otitis media
    Effects of high altitude on ears

  993.1 Barotrauma, sinus
    Aerosinusitis
    Effects of high altitude on sinuses

  993.2 Other and unspecified effects of high altitude
    Alpine sickness
    Andes disease
    Anoxia due to high altitude
    Hypobaropathy
    Mountain sickness

  993.3 Caisson disease 🔗 🔗
    Bends
    Compressed-air disease
    Decompression sickness
    Divers' palsy or paralysis
    Ⓔx 993.3-993.9

  993.4 Effects of air pressure caused by explosion

  993.8 Other specified effects of air pressure

  993.9 Unspecified effect of air pressure

● **994 Effects of other external causes**

  Excludes *certain adverse effects not elsewhere classified (995.0–995.8)*

  994.0 Effects of lightning
    Shock from lightning
    Struck by lightning NOS
    Excludes *burns (940.0–949.5)*

  994.1 Drowning and nonfatal submersion 🔗 🔗
    Bathing cramp
    Immersion
    Ⓔx 994.1
    Coding Clinic: 2013, Q3, P11

  994.2 Effects of hunger
    Deprivation of food
    Starvation

  994.3 Effects of thirst
    Deprivation of water

  994.4 Exhaustion due to exposure

  994.5 Exhaustion due to excessive exertion
    Exhaustion due to overexertion

  994.6 Motion sickness
    Air sickness
    Seasickness
    Travel sickness

  994.7 Asphyxiation and strangulation 🔗 🔗
    Suffocation (by):
      bedclothes
      cave-in
      constriction
      mechanical
      plastic bag
      pressure
      strangulation
    Excludes *asphyxia from:*
      carbon monoxide (986)
      inhalation of food or foreign body (932–934.9)
      other gases, fumes, and vapors (987.0–987.9)
    Ⓔx 994.7

  994.8 Electrocution and nonfatal effects of electric current
    Shock from electric current
    Shock from electroshock gun (taser)
    Excludes *electric burns (940.0–949.5)*

  994.9 Other effects of external causes
    Effects of:
      abnormal gravitational [G] forces or states
      weightlessness

● **995 Certain adverse effects not elsewhere classified**

  Excludes *complications of surgical and medical care (996.0–999.9)*
  Coding Clinic: 2008, Q1, P12-13

  995.0 Other anaphylactic reaction 🔗
    Allergic shock NOS or due to adverse effect of correct medicinal substance properly administered
    Anaphylactic reaction NOS or due to adverse effect of correct medicinal substance properly administered
    Anaphylactic shock NOS or due to adverse effect of correct medicinal substance properly administered
    Anaphylactoid reaction NOS
    Anaphylaxis NOS or due to adverse effect of correct medicinal substance properly administered
    Excludes *anaphylactic reaction to serum (999.41-999.49)*
      anaphylactic shock or reaction due to adverse food reaction (995.60-995.69)
    Use additional E code to identify external cause, such as: adverse effects of correct medicinal substance properly administered [E930–E949]
    Ⓔx 995.60-995.69
    Coding Clinic: 2013, Q2, P12

  995.1 Angioneurotic edema
    Allergic angioedema
    Giant urticaria
    Excludes *urticaria:*
      due to serum (999.51-999.59)
      other specified (698.2, 708.0–708.9, 757.33)

● **995.2 Other and unspecified adverse effect of drug, medicinal and biological substance**
    Excludes *pathological drug intoxication (292.2)*
    Coding Clinic: 2010, Q2, P4; 2006, Q4, P112-113; 1997, Q2, P12; 1995, Q3, P13; 1992, Q3, P16-17

  995.20 Unspecified adverse effect of unspecified drug, medicinal and biological substance
    Unspecified adverse effect of unspecified medicinal substance properly administered

  995.21 Arthus phenomenon
    Arthus reaction
    Hypersensitivity reaction resulting from immune complex reactions

  995.22 Unspecified adverse effect of anesthesia

  995.23 Unspecified adverse effect of insulin

  995.24 Failed moderate sedation during procedure
    Failed conscious sedation during procedure

  995.27 Other drug allergy
    Allergic reaction NEC (due) to correct medical substance properly administered
    Drug allergy NOS
    Drug hypersensitivity NOS
    Hypersensitivity (due) to correct medical substance properly administered

  995.29 Unspecified adverse effect of other drug, medicinal and biological substance
    Unspecified adverse effect of medicinal substance NEC properly administered

  995.3 Allergy, unspecified
    Allergic reaction NOS
    Hypersensitivity NOS
    Idiosyncrasy NOS
    Excludes *allergic reaction NOS to correct medicinal substance properly administered (995.27)*
      allergy to existing dental restorative materials (525.66)
      specific types of allergic reaction, such as:
        allergic diarrhea (558.3)
        dermatitis (691.0–693.9)
        hayfever (477.0–477.9)

INJURY AND POISONING (800–999)

    N Newborn: 0   P Pediatric: 0–17   M Maternity: 12–55   A Adult: 15–124   ♀ Females Only   ♂ Males Only

Ⓔx CC/MCC Exclusions   🔗 Complication\Comorbidity   🔗 Major C\C   🔗 Present on Admission Requirement   🔗 Hospital-Acquired Condition   **995**

ICD-9-CM

995.4 Shock due to anesthesia 🏷
Shock due to anesthesia in which the correct substance was properly administered

Excludes *complications of anesthesia in labor or delivery (668.0–668.9)*
overdose or wrong substance given (968.0–969.9)
postoperative shock NOS (998.00)
specified adverse effects of anesthesia classified elsewhere, such as:
anoxic brain damage (348.1)
hepatitis (070.0–070.9), etc.
unspecified adverse effect of anesthesia (995.22)
(Ex) 958.4, 995.4, 997.91-998.13, 998.81, 998.83-998.9

● **995.5 Child maltreatment syndrome**
Use additional code(s), if applicable, to identify any associated injuries
Use additional E code to identify:
nature of abuse (E960–E968)
perpetrator (E967.0–E967.9)
Coding Clinic: 1998, Q1, P11; 1984, Sept-Oct, P16; 1984, Nov-Dec, P9

995.50 Child abuse, unspecified 🏷 P
(Ex) 995.50-995.59, 995.80-995.85
Coding Clinic: 2012, Q2, P12-13

995.51 Child emotional/psychological abuse 🏷 P
(Ex) 995.50-995.59, 995.80-995.85
Coding Clinic: 2012, Q2, P12-13

995.52 Child neglect (nutritional) 🏷 P
Use additional code to identify intent of neglect (E904.0,E968.4)
(Ex) 995.50-995.59, 995.80-995.85
Coding Clinic: 2012, Q2, P12-13

995.53 Child sexual abuse 🏷 P
(Ex) 995.50-995.59, 995.80-995.85
Coding Clinic: 2012, Q2, P12-13

995.54 Child physical abuse 🏷 P
Battered baby or child syndrome
Excludes *Shaken infant syndrome (995.55)*
(Ex) 995.50-995.59, 995.80-995.85
Coding Clinic: 2012, Q2, P12-13; 1999, Q3, P14-15

995.55 Shaken infant syndrome 🏷 P
Use additional code(s) to identify any associated injuries
(Ex) 995.50-995.59, 995.80-995.85
Coding Clinic: 2012, Q2, P12-13; 1996, Q4, P43-44

995.59 Other child abuse and neglect 🏷 P
Multiple forms of abuse
Use additional code to identify intent of neglect (E904.0,E968.4)
(Ex) 995.50-995.59, 995.80-995.85
Coding Clinic: 2012, Q2, P12-13

● **995.6 Anaphylactic reaction due to food**
Anaphylactic reaction due to adverse food reaction
Anaphylactic shock or reaction due to nonpoisonous foods
Anaphylactoid reaction due to food

995.60 Anaphylactic reaction due to unspecified food 🏷
(Ex) 995.60-995.69

995.61 Anaphylactic reaction due to peanuts 🏷
(Ex) 995.60-995.69

995.62 Anaphylactic reaction due to crustaceans 🏷
(Ex) 995.60-995.69

995.63 Anaphylactic reaction due to fruits and vegetables 🏷
(Ex) 995.60-995.69

995.64 Anaphylactic reaction due to tree nuts and seeds 🏷
(Ex) 995.60-995.69
Coding Clinic: 2008, Q1, P12-13

995.65 Anaphylactic reaction due to fish 🏷
(Ex) 995.60-995.69

995.66 Anaphylactic reaction due to food additives 🏷
(Ex) 995.60-995.69

995.67 Anaphylactic reaction due to milk products 🏷
(Ex) 995.60-995.69

995.68 Anaphylactic reaction due to eggs 🏷
(Ex) 995.60-995.69

995.69 Anaphylactic reaction due to other specified food 🏷
(Ex) 995.60-995.69

995.7 Other adverse food reactions, not elsewhere classified
Use additional code to identify the type of reaction, such as:
hives (708.0)
wheezing (786.07)
Excludes *anaphylactic reaction or shock due to adverse food reaction (995.60-995.69)*
asthma (493.0, 493.9)
dermatitis due to food (693.1)
in contact with the skin (692.5)
gastroenteritis and colitis due to food (558.3)
rhinitis due to food (477.1)

● **995.8 Other specified adverse effects, not elsewhere classified**

995.80 Adult maltreatment, unspecified 🏷 A
Abused person NOS
Use additional code to identify:
any associated injury
nature of abuse (E960–E968)
perpetrator (E967.0–E967.9)
(Ex) 995.80
Coding Clinic: 2012, Q2, P12-13

995.81 Adult physical abuse 🏷 A
Battered:
person syndrome NEC
man
spouse
woman
Use additional code to identify:
any associated injury
nature of abuse (E960–E968)
perpetrator (E967.0–E967.9)
(Ex) 995.50-995.59, 995.80-995.85
Coding Clinic: 2012, Q2, P12-13; 1996, Q4, P43-44; 1984, Sept-Oct, P16

995.82 Adult emotional/psychological abuse A
Use additional E code to identify perpetrator (E967.0–E967.9)
Coding Clinic: 2012, Q2, P12-13

995.83 Adult sexual abuse 🏷 A
Use additional code to identify:
any associated injury
perpetrator (E967.0–E967.9)
(Ex) 995.50-995.59, 995.80-995.85
Coding Clinic: 2012, Q2, P12-13

◄ New ⬅ Revised ~~deleted~~ Deleted Excludes Includes Use additional Code first Omit code
● Unacceptable Principal Diagnosis ● Use Additional Digit(s) ▶ Manifestation Code OGCR Official Guidelines Coding Clinic

INJURY AND POISONING (800–999)

995.84 Adult neglect (nutritional) 🔖   A

  Use additional code to identify:
    intent of neglect (E904.0–E968.4)
    perpetrator (E967.0–E967.9)
  (Ex) 995.50-995.59, 995.80-995.85
  Coding Clinic: 2012, Q2, P12-13

995.85 Other adult abuse and neglect 🔖   A

  Multiple forms of abuse and neglect
  Use additional code to identify:
    any associated injury
    intent of neglect (E904.0, E968.4)
    nature of abuse (E960–E968)
    perpetrator (E967.0–E967.9)
  (Ex) 995.50-995.59, 995.80-995.85
  Coding Clinic: 2012, Q2, P12-13

995.86 Malignant hyperthermia 🔖

  Malignant hyperpyrexia due to anesthesia
  *Extremely high body temperature—greater than
    106° F or 41.1° C*
  (Ex) 958.4, 995.4, 995.86, 997.91-998.13, 998.81, 998.83-998.9
  Coding Clinic: 2012, Q2, P12-13

995.89 Other

  Hypothermia due to anesthesia
  **Coding Clinic: 2012, Q2, P12-13; 2004, Q2, P18;
    2003, Q3, P12**

● **995.9 Systemic inflammatory response syndrome (SIRS)**
  **Coding Clinic: 2010, Q1, P12; 2006, Q4, P113-116; 2005, Q3, P23;
    2004, Q2, P16; 2002, Q4, P71-73**

**995.90 Systemic inflammatory response syndrome,
    unspecified SIRS NOS** 🔖
  (Ex) 003.1, 020.2, 036.2, 038.0-038.9, 040.82-041.9, 054.5, 139.8,
    995.90-995.94, V09.0-V09.91

● **995.91 Sepsis** 🔖

  Systemic inflammatory response syndrome due
    to infectious process without acute organ
    dysfunction
  Code first underlying infection
  Excludes *sepsis with acute organ dysfunction
      (995.92)*
      *sepsis with multiple organ dysfunction
      (995.92)*
      severe sepsis (995.92)
  (Ex) 003.1, 020.2, 036.2, 038.0-038.9, 040.82-041.9, 054.5, 139.8,
    995.90-995.94, V09.0-V09.91
  **Coding Clinic: 2012, Q3, P12, 14; 2011, Q3, P15; 2008, Q4,
    P69-73; 2007, Q4, P84-86; 2004, Q2, P16**

995.92 Severe sepsis 🔖

  Sepsis with acute organ dysfunction
  Sepsis with multiple organ dysfunction (MOD)
  Systemic inflammatory response syndrome due
    to infectious process with acute organ
    dysfunction
  Code first underlying infection
  Use additional code to specify acute organ
    dysfunction, such as:
    acute kidney failure (584.5–584.9)
    acute respiratory failure (518.81)
    critical illness myopathy (359.81)
    critical illness polyneuropathy (357.82)
    disseminated intravascular coagulopathy
      (DIC) syndrome (286.6)
    encephalopathy (348.31)
    hepatic failure (570)
    septic shock (785.52)
  (Ex) 003.1, 020.2, 036.2, 038.0-038.9, 040.82-041.9, 054.5, 139.8,
    995.90-995.94, V09.0-V09.91
  **Coding Clinic: 2013, Q2, P21; 2012, Q3, P12; 2011, Q4, P153;
    Q3, P15; 2010, Q2, P4; 2009, Q4, P129; 2007, Q4,
    P96-97; 2005, Q2, P18-20x2; 2004, Q2, P16; 2003,
    Q4, P73, 79-81**

**995.93 Systemic inflammatory response syndrome due to
    noninfectious process without acute organ
    dysfunction** 🔖

  Code first underlying conditions, such as:
    acute pancreatitis (577.0)
    trauma
  Excludes *systemic inflammatory response
      syndrome due to noninfectious
      process with acute organ
      dysfunction (995.94)*
  (Ex) 003.1, 020.2, 036.2, 038.0-038.9, 040.82-041.9, 054.5, 139.8,
    995.90-995.94, V09.0-V09.91
  Coding Clinic: 2011, Q1, P22; 2010, Q1, P12

**995.94 Systemic inflammatory response syndrome due to
    non-infectious process with acute organ
    dysfunction** 🔖

  Code first underlying conditions, such as:
    acute pancreatitis (577.0)
    heat stroke (992.0)
    trauma
  Use additional code to specify acute organ
    dysfunction, such as:
    acute kidney failure (584.5–584.9)
    acute respiratory failure (518.81)
    critical illness myopathy (359.81)
    critical illness polyneuropathy (357.82)
    disseminated intravascular coagulopathy
      (DIC) syndrome (286.6)
    encephalopathy (348.31)
    hepatic failure (570)
  Excludes *severe sepsis (995.92)*
  (Ex) 003.1, 020.2, 036.2, 038.0-038.9, 040.82-041.9, 054.5, 139.8,
    995.90-995.94, V09.0-V09.91
  Coding Clinic: 2010, Q1, P12; 2005, Q2, P19-20

OGCR   Section I.C.1.b.2.12

Only one code from subcategory 995.9 should be assigned. Therefore,
when a non-infectious condition leads to an infection resulting in sepsis
or severe sepsis, assign either code 995.91 or 995.92. Do not additionally
assign code 995.93, Systemic inflammatory response syndrome
due to noninfectious process without acute organ dysfunctiion, or
995.94, Systemic inflammatory response syndrome with acute organ
dysfunction.

OGCR   Section I.C.19.a.7

An external cause code is not appropriate with a code from subcategory
995.9, unless the patient also has another condition for which an E code
would be appropriate (such as an injury, poisoning, or adverse effect of
drugs).

N Newborn: 0   **P** Pediatric: 0–17   **M** Maternity: 12–55   **A** Adult: 15–124   ♀ Females Only   ♂ Males Only

(Ex) CC/MCC Exclusions   🔖 Complication\Comorbidity   🔖 Major C\C   🔖 Present on Admission Requirement   🔖 Hospital-Acquired Condition   **997**

INJURY AND POISONING (800–999)

COMPLICATIONS OF SURGICAL AND MEDICAL CARE, NOT ELSEWHERE CLASSIFIED (996–999)

Excludes *adverse effects of medicinal agents (001.0–799.9,*
           995.0–995.8)
           burns from local applications and irradiation
           (940.0–949.5)
           complications of:
             conditions for which the procedure was performed
             surgical procedures during abortion, labor, and
               delivery (630–676.9)
           poisoning and toxic effects of drugs and chemicals
             (960.0–989.9)
           postoperative conditions in which no complications
             are present, such as:
               artificial opening status (V44.0–V44.9)
               closure of external stoma (V55.0–V55.9)
               fitting of prosthetic device (V52.0–V52.9)
           specified complications classified elsewhere:
             anesthetic shock (995.4)
             electrolyte imbalance (276.0–276.9)
             postlaminectomy syndrome (722.80–722.83)
             postmastectomy lymphedema syndrome (457.0)
             postoperative psychosis (293.0–293.9)
           any other condition classified elsewhere in the
             Alphabetic Index when described as due to a
             procedure

● **996 Complications peculiar to certain specified procedures**

Includes complications, not elsewhere classified, in the use
          of artificial substitutes [e.g., Dacron, metal,
          Silastic, Teflon] or natural sources [e.g., bone]
            involving:
              anastomosis (internal)
              graft (bypass) (patch)
              implant
              internal device:
                catheter
                electronic
                fixation
                prosthetic
              reimplant
              transplant

Excludes *accidental puncture or laceration during procedure*
           (998.2)
           capsular contracture of breast implant (611.83)
           complications of internal anastomosis of:
             gastrointestinal tract (997.49)
             urinary tract (997.5)
           endosseous dental implant failures (525.71–525.79)
           intraoperative floppy iris syndrome (IFIS) (364.81)
           mechanical complication of respirator (V46.14)
           other specified complications classified elsewhere, such
             as:
               hemolytic anemia (283.1)
               functional cardiac disturbances (429.4)
               serum hepatitis (070.2–070.3)

● **996.0 Mechanical complication of cardiac device, implant, and graft**

Breakdown (mechanical)   Obstruction, mechanical
Displacement   Perforation
Leakage   Protrusion
Coding Clinic: 2007, Q3, P7-8

996.00 Unspecified device, implant, and graft 🐾
         (Ex:) 996.00, 996.04, 996.61-996.62, 996.70-996.74, 997.91-997.99,
               998.81, 998.83-998.9

996.01 Due to cardiac pacemaker (electrode) 🐾
         (Ex:) 996.01, 997.91-997.99, 998.81, 998.83-998.9
         Coding Clinic: 2006, Q2, P15-16; 1999, Q2, P11-12

996.02 Due to heart valve prosthesis 🐾
         (Ex:) 996.02, 997.91-997.99, 998.81, 998.83-998.9
         Coding Clinic: 1999, Q2, P4

996.03 Due to coronary bypass graft 🐾
         Excludes *atherosclerosis of graft (414.02, 414.03)*
                    embolism [occlusion NOS] [thrombus] of
                    graft (996.72)
         (Ex:) 996.03, 997.91-997.99, 998.81, 998.83-998.9
         Coding Clinic: 1993, Q4, P40-41

996.04 Due to automatic implantable cardiac defibrillator 🐾
         (Ex:) 996.04, 997.91-997.99, 998.81, 998.83-998.9
         Coding Clinic: 2005, Q2, P3

996.09 Other 🐾
         (Ex:) 996.09, 997.91-997.99, 998.81, 998.83-998.9
         Coding Clinic: 2013, Q1, P5; 1993, Q2, P9

996.1 Mechanical complication of other vascular device, implant, and graft
         Mechanical complications involving:
           aortic (bifurcation) graft (replacement)
           arteriovenous:
             dialysis catheter
             fistula surgically created
             shunt surgically created
           balloon (counterpulsation) device, intra-aortic
           carotid artery bypass graft
           femoral-popliteal bypass graft
           umbrella device, vena cava
         Excludes *atherosclerosis of biological graft (440.30–440.32)*
                    embolism [occlusion NOS] [thrombus] of
                    (biological) (synthetic) graft (996.74)
                    peritoneal dialysis catheter (996.56)
         (Ex:) 996.1, 997.91-997.99, 998.81, 998.83-998.9
         Coding Clinic: 2012, Q1, P18; 2011, Q1, P6; 2006, Q1, P10-11; 2005,
               Q2, P8; 2002, Q1, P13; 1995, Q1, P3

996.2 Mechanical complication of nervous system device, implant, and graft 🐾
         Mechanical complications involving:
           dorsal column stimulator
           electrodes implanted in brain [brain "pacemaker"]
           peripheral nerve graft
           ventricular (communicating) shunt
         (Ex:) 996.2, 996.63, 996.75, 997.91-997.99, 998.81, 998.83-998.9
         Coding Clinic: 1987, Sept-Oct, P10

● **996.3 Mechanical complication of genitourinary device, implant, and graft**

996.30 Unspecified device, implant, and graft 🐾
         (Ex:) 596.81, 596.83, 996.30, 996.64-996.65, 996.76, 997.91-997.99,
               998.81, 998.83-998.9

996.31 Due to urethral [indwelling] catheter

996.32 Due to intrauterine contraceptive device ♀

996.39 Other 🐾
         Prosthetic reconstruction of vas deferens
         Repair (graft) of ureter without mention of
           resection
         Excludes *complications due to:*
                    external stoma of urinary tract
                    (596.81-596.83)
                    internal anastomosis of urinary tract
                    (997.5)
         (Ex:) 596.81-596.83, 996.39, 996.64-996.65, 996.76, 997.91-997.99,
               998.81, 998.83-998.9

◄ New   ◄|||| Revised   ~~deleted~~ Deleted   Excludes   Includes   Use additional   Code first   Omit code

998   ● Unacceptable Principal Diagnosis   ● Use Additional Digit(s)   ▶ Manifestation Code   OGCR Official Guidelines   Coding Clinic

● **996.4 Mechanical complication of internal orthopedic device, implant, and graft**
    Mechanical complications involving:
        external (fixation) device utilizing internal screw(s), pin(s) or other methods of fixation
        grafts of bone, cartilage, muscle, or tendon
        internal (fixation) device such as nail, plate, rod, etc.

    Use additional code to identify prosthetic joint with mechanical complication (V43.60–V43.69)

    Excludes *complications of external orthopedic device, such as:*
        pressure ulcer due to cast (707.00–707.09)
    Coding Clinic: 2005, Q4, P91-93, 110-112; 1999, Q2, P10-11; 1998, Q2, P19; 1996, Q2, P11; 1985, Nov-Dec, P11; 1984, Nov-Dec, P18

    996.40 Unspecified mechanical complication of internal orthopedic device, implant, and graft 🔧
        (Ex) 996.40-996.49, 996.66-996.67, 996.77-996.78, 997.91-997.99, 998.81, 998.83-998.9

    996.41 Mechanical loosening of prosthetic joint 🔧
        Aseptic loosening
        (Ex) 996.40-996.49, 996.66-996.67, 996.77-996.78, 997.91-997.99, 998.81, 998.83-998.9
        Coding Clinic: 2005, Q4, P91-93

    996.42 Dislocation of prosthetic joint 🔧
        Instability of prosthetic joint
        Subluxation of prosthetic joint
        (Ex) 996.40-996.49, 996.66-996.67, 996.77-996.78, 997.91-997.99, 998.81, 998.83-998.9

    996.43 Broken prosthetic joint implant 🔧
        Breakage (fracture) of prosthetic joint
        (Ex) 996.40-996.49, 996.66-996.67, 996.77-996.78, 997.91-997.99, 998.81, 998.83-998.9
        Coding Clinic: 2005, Q4, P91-93

    996.44 Peri-prosthetic fracture around prosthetic joint 🔧
        (Ex) 996.40-996.49, 996.66-996.67, 996.77-996.78, 997.91-997.99, 998.81, 998.83-998.9
        Coding Clinic: 2005, Q4, P91-93

    996.45 Peri-prosthetic osteolysis 🔧
        Use additional code to identify major osseous defect, if applicable (731.3)
        (Ex) 996.40-996.49, 996.66-996.67, 996.77-996.78, 997.91-997.99, 998.81, 998.83-998.9
        Coding Clinic: 2006, Q4, P103-104

    996.46 Articular bearing surface wear of prosthetic joint 🔧
        (Ex) 996.40-996.49, 996.66-996.67, 996.77-996.78, 997.91-997.99, 998.81, 998.83-998.9

    996.47 Other mechanical complication of prosthetic joint implant 🔧
        Mechanical complication of prosthetic joint NOS
        · Prosthetic joint implant failure NOS
        (Ex) 996.40-996.49, 996.66-996.67, 996.77-996.78, 997.91-997.99, 998.81, 998.83-998.9

    996.49 Other mechanical complication of other internal orthopedic device, implant, and graft 🔧
        Breakage of internal fixation device in bone
        Dislocation of internal fixation device in bone
        Excludes *mechanical complication of prosthetic joint implant (996.41–996.46)*
        (Ex) 996.40-996.49, 996.66-996.67, 996.77-996.78, 997.91-997.99, 998.81, 998.83-998.9
        Coding Clinic: 2013, Q2, P22; 2010, Q1, P13

● **996.5 Mechanical complication of other specified prosthetic device, implant, and graft**
    Mechanical complications involving:
        prosthetic implant in:
            bile duct
            breast
            chin
            orbit of eye
        nonabsorbable surgical material NOS
        other graft, implant, and internal device, not elsewhere classified

    996.51 Due to corneal graft 🔧
        (Ex) 996.51, 997.91-997.99
        Coding Clinic: 2010, Q2, P5

    996.52 Due to graft of other tissue, not elsewhere classified 🔧
        Skin graft failure or rejection
        Excludes *failure of artificial skin graft (996.55)*
            failure of decellularized allodermis (996.55)
            sloughing of temporary skin allografts or xenografts (pigskin)- omit code
        (Ex) 996.52, 996.55, 997.91-99.799
        Coding Clinic: 2012, Q3, P6-7; 1996, Q1, P10; 1990, Q3, P15

    996.53 Due to ocular lens prosthesis 🔧
        Excludes *contact lenses—code to condition*
        (Ex) 996.53, 997.91-997.99
        Coding Clinic: 2000, Q1, P9-10

    996.54 Due to breast prosthesis 🔧
        Breast capsule (prosthesis)
        Mammary implant
        (Ex) 996.54, 997.91-997.99
        Coding Clinic: 1998, Q2, P14; 1992, Q3, P4-5

    996.55 Due to artificial skin graft and decellularized allodermis 🔧
        Dislodgement   Non-adherence
        Displacement   Poor incorporation
        Failure   Shearing
        (Ex) 996.52, 996.55-996.60, 996.68-996.70, 996.79, 997.91-997.99
        Coding Clinic: 2012, Q3, P6; 1998, Q4, P52-53

    996.56 Due to peritoneal dialysis catheter 🔧
        Excludes *mechanical complication of arteriovenous dialysis catheter (996.1)*
        (Ex) 996.56-996.60, 996.68-996.70, 996.79, 997.91-997.99
        Coding Clinic: 1998, Q4, P54

    996.57 Due to insulin pump 🔧
        (Ex) 596.81-596.83, 996.00-996.30, 996.39-996.79, 997.91-997.99, 998.81, 998.83-998.9
        Coding Clinic: 2003, Q4, P81-82

OGCR   **Section I.C.3.a.6.a**

An underdose of insulin due to an insulin pump failure should be assigned 996.57, Mechanical complication due to insulin pump, as the principal or first listed code, followed by the appropriate diabetes mellitus code based on documentation.

OGCR   **Section I.C.3.a.6.b**

The principal or first listed code for an encounter due to an insulin pump malfunction resulting in an overdose of insulin, should also be 996.57, Mechanical complication due to insulin pump, followed by 962.3, Poisoning by insulins and antidiabetic agents, and the appropriate diabetes mellitus code based on documentation.

INJURY AND POISONING (800–999)

N Newborn: 0   **P** Pediatric: 0–17   **M** Maternity: 12–55   **A** Adult: 15–124   ♀ Females Only   ♂ Males Only

(Ex) CC/MCC Exclusions   🔧 Complication\Comorbidity   Major C\C   Present on Admission Requirement   Hospital-Acquired Condition   **999**

INJURY AND POISONING (800–999)

996.59 Due to other implant and internal device, not elsewhere classified 🔖
Nonabsorbable surgical material NOS
Prosthetic implant in:
bile duct
chin
orbit of eye
(Ex) 996.56-996.60, 996.68-996.70, 996.79, 997.91-997.99
Coding Clinic: 2013, Q2, P11; 2011, Q1, P11; 1999, Q2, P13-14; 1997, Q3, P7; 1994, Q3, P7x2

● **996.6 Infection and inflammatory reaction due to internal prosthetic device, implant, and graft**
Infection (causing obstruction) due to (presence of) any device, implant, and graft classifiable to 996.0–996.5
Inflammation due to (presence of) any device, implant, and graft classifiable to 996.0–996.5
Use additional code to identify specified infections
Coding Clinic: 2008, Q2, P9-10; 1987, Jan-Feb, P14-15

996.60 Due to unspecified device, implant and graft 🔖
(Ex) 596.81-596.83, 996.00-996.30, 996.39-996.79, 997.91-997.99, 998.81, 998.83-998.9

996.61 Due to cardiac device, implant and graft 🔖
Cardiac pacemaker or defibrillator:
electrode(s), lead(s)
pulse generator
subcutaneous pocket
Coronary artery bypass graft
Heart valve prosthesis
(Ex) 996.00-996.1, 996.52, 996.55-996.62, 996.68-996.74, 996.79, 997.91-997.99, 998.81, 998.83-998.9

996.62 Due to vascular device, implant and graft 🔖
Arterial graft
Arteriovenous fistula or shunt
Infusion pump
Vascular catheter (arterial) (dialysis) (peripheral venous)

     Excludes *infection due to:*
central venous catheter (999.31-999.32)
Hickman catheter (999.31-999.32)
peripherally inserted central catheter (PICC) (999.31-999.32)
portacath (port-a-cath) (999.31-999.32)
triple lumen catheter (999.31-999.32)
umbilical venous catheter (999.31-999.32)
(Ex) 996.00-996.1, 996.52, 996.55-996.62, 996.68-996.74, 996.79, 997.91-997.99, 998.81, 998.83-998.9
Coding Clinic: 2010, Q2, P8; 2007, Q4, P84-86; 2004, Q2, P16; Q1, P5; 2003, Q4, P111-112; Q2, P7-8; 1994, Q2, P13

996.63 Due to nervous system device, implant and graft 🔖
Electrodes implanted in brain
Peripheral nerve graft
Spinal canal catheter
Ventricular (communicating) shunt (catheter)
(Ex) 996.2, 996.52, 996.55-996.60, 996.63, 996.68-996.70, 996.75, 996.79, 997.91-997.99, 998.81, 998.83-998.9

996.64 Due to indwelling urinary catheter 🔖 🔖
Use additional code to identify specified infections, such as:
cystitis (595.0–595.9)
sepsis (038.0–038.9)
     Excludes *complications due to:*
external stoma of urinary tract (596.81-596.83)
HAC: Also excludes the following from acting as a CC/MCC:112.2 (CC), 590.10 (CC), 590.11 (MCC), 590.2 (MCC), 590.3 (CC), 590.80 (CC), 590.81 (CC), 595.0 (CC), 597.0 (CC), 599.0 (CC)
(Ex) 596.81-596.83, 599.0, 996.30, 996.39, 996.56-996.60, 996.64-996.65, 996.68-996.70, 996.76, 996.79, 997.91-997.99, 998.81, 998.83-998.9
Coding Clinic: 2012, Q2, P20-21; Q1, P11-12; 2009, Q3, P18-19; 1993, Q3, P6

996.65 Due to other genitourinary device, implant and graft 🔖
Intrauterine contraceptive device
(Ex) 596.81-596.83, 996.30, 996.39, 996.52, 996.55-996.60, 996.64-996.65, 996.68-996.70, 996.76, 996.79, 997.91-997.99, 998.81, 998.83-998.9
Coding Clinic: 2000, Q1, P15-16

996.66 Due to internal joint prosthesis 🔖
Use additional code to identify infected prosthetic joint (V43.60–V43.69)
(Ex) 996.40-996.49, 996.52, 996.55-996.60, 996.66-996.70, 996.77-996.79, 997.91-997.99, 998.81, 998.83-998.9
Coding Clinic: 2008, Q2, P3-5x3; 2007, Q2, P8-9; 2005, Q4, P110-112; 1991, Q2, P18

996.67 Due to other internal orthopedic device, implant and graft 🔖 🔖
Bone growth stimulator (electrode)
Internal fixation device (pin) (rod) (screw)
HAC: And one of the following procedure codes: 81.01-81.08, 81.23, 81.24, 81.31-81.38, 81.83, 81.85
(Ex) 996.40-996.49, 996.52, 996.55-996.60, 996.66-996.70, 996.77-996.79, 997.91-997.99, 998.81, 998.83-998.9

996.68 Due to peritoneal dialysis catheter 🔖
Exit-site infection or inflammation
(Ex) 996.56-996.60, 996.68-996.70, 996.79, 997.91-997.99
Coding Clinic: 2001, Q2, P11; 1998, Q4, P55

996.69 Due to other internal prosthetic device, implant, and graft 🔖
Breast prosthesis
Ocular lens prosthesis
Prosthetic orbital implant
(Ex) 596.81-596.83, 996.00-996.30, 996.39-996.79, 997.91-997.99, 998.81, 998.83-998.9
Coding Clinic: 2011, Q1, P11; 2008, Q2, P9-11; 2003, Q4, P108; 1998, Q4, P52-53

● **996.7 Other complications of internal (biological) (synthetic) prosthetic device, implant, and graft**
Complication NOS due to (presence of) any device, implant, and graft classifiable to 996.0–996.5
occlusion NOS
Embolism due to (presence of) any device, implant, and graft classifiable to 996.0–996.5
Fibrosis due to (presence of) any device, implant, and graft classifiable to 996.0–996.5
Hemorrhage due to (presence of) any device, implant, and graft classifiable to 996.0–996.5
Pain due to (presence of) any device, implant, and graft classifiable to 996.0–996.5
Stenosis due to (presence of) any device, implant, and graft classifiable to 996.0–996.5
Thrombus due to (presence of) any device, implant, and graft classifiable to 996.0–996.5
Use additional code to identify complication, such as:
pain due to presence of device, implant or graft (338.18–338.19, 338.28–338.29)
venous embolism and thrombosis (453.2-453.9)
     Excludes *disruption (dehiscence) of internal suture material (998.31)*
transplant rejection (996.80-996.89)
Coding Clinic: 2012, Q2, P5; Q1, P18; 2010, Q2, P9; 2007, Q2, P13-15; 2004, Q2, P7-8; 1989, Q1, P9&10; 1984, Nov-Dec, P18

996.70 Due to unspecified device, implant, and graft

996.71 Due to heart valve prosthesis 🔖
(Ex) 996.00, 996.02, 996.09-996.1, 996.52, 996.55-996.62, 996.68-996.74, 996.79, 997.91-997.99, 998.81, 998.83-998.9
Coding Clinic: 2008, Q2, P9-10

◀ New   ◀‖‖ Revised   ~~deleted~~ Deleted   Excludes   Includes   Use additional   Code first   Omit code
● Unacceptable Principal Diagnosis   ● Use Additional Digit(s)   ▶ Manifestation Code   OGCR Official Guidelines   Coding Clinic
1000

996.72 Due to other cardiac device, implant, and graft
Cardiac pacemaker or defibrillator:
electrode(s), lead(s)
subcutaneous pocket
Coronary artery bypass (graft)

Excludes *occlusion due to atherosclerosis*
(414.00–414.07)

(Ex) 996.00-996.02, 996.04-996.1, 996.52, 996.55-996.62,
996.68-996.74, 996.79, 997.91-997.99, 998.81, 998.83-998.9
Coding Clinic: 2010, Q2, P9; 2008, Q3, P10-11; 2006, Q3,
P8-9, 25; 2001, Q3, P20

996.73 Due to renal dialysis device, implant, and graft
(Ex) 996.1, 996.52, 996.55-996.60, 996.68-996.70, 996.73, 996.79,
997.91-997.99, 998.81, 998.83-998.9
Coding Clinic: 1991, Q2, P18

996.74 Due to vascular device, implant, and graft
Excludes *occlusion of biological graft due to*
atherosclerosis (440.30–440.32)
(Ex) 996.00-996.1, 996.52, 996.55-996.62, 996.68-996.74, 996.79,
997.91-997.99, 998.81, 998.83-998.9
Coding Clinic: 2013, Q2, P4; 2012, Q1, P18; 2003, Q1,
P16-18x2; 2000, Q1, P10

996.75 Due to nervous system device, implant, and graft
(Ex) 996.2, 996.52, 996.55-996.60, 996.63, 996.68-996.70, 996.75,
996.79, 997.91-997.99, 998.81, 998.83-998.9

996.76 Due to genitourinary device, implant, and graft
Excludes *complications of implanted vaginal mesh*
(629.31-629.32)
(Ex) 596.81-596.83, 996.30, 996.39, 996.52, 996.55-996.60,
996.64-996.65, 996.68-996.70, 996.76, 996.79, 997.91-997.99,
998.81, 998.83-998.9
Coding Clinic: 2009, Q1, P13; 2000, Q1, P15-16

996.77 Due to internal joint prosthesis
Use additional code to identify prosthetic joint
(V43.60–V43.69)
(Ex) 996.40-996.49, 996.52, 996.55-996.60, 996.66-996.70,
996.77-996.79, 997.91-997.99, 998.81, 998.83-998.9

996.78 Due to other internal orthopedic device, implant, and graft
(Ex) 996.40-996.49, 996.52, 996.55-996.60, 996.66-996.70,
996.77-996.79, 997.91-997.99, 998.81, 998.83-998.9
Coding Clinic: 2003, Q2, P14

996.79 Due to other internal prosthetic device, implant, and graft
(Ex) 596.81-596.83, 996.00-996.30, 996.39-996.79, 997.91-997.99,
998.81, 998.83-998.9
Coding Clinic: 2004, Q2, P7; 2001, Q1, P8-9; 1995, Q3, P14;
1992, Q3, P4-5

● **996.8 Complications of transplanted organ**
Transplant failure or rejection
Use additional code to identify nature of complication,
such as:
cytomegalovirus [CMV] infection (078.5)
graft-versus-host disease (279.50–279.53)
malignancy associated with organ transplant (199.2)
post-transplant lymphoproliferative disorder (PTLD)
(238.77)
Coding Clinic: 2003, Q1, P11; 2002, Q4, P53-54; 2001, Q3, P12-13;
1993, Q2, P11; Q1, P24

996.80 Transplanted organ, unspecified
(Ex) 238.77, 996.80, 996.87, 997.91-997.99

996.81 Kidney
(Ex) 996.81, 997.91-997.99
Coding Clinic: 2012, Q2, P6-7; 2010, Q1, P15; 2008, Q4, P82-
83; 2003, Q3, P16-17; 1998, Q3, P6x2&7; 1994, Q3,
P8; Q2, P9; 1993, Q4, P32-33; Q1, P24-25

996.82 Liver
(Ex) 996.82, 997.91-997.99
Coding Clinic: 2008, Q4, P82-83, 97-100; 2003, Q3,
P16x2&17; 1998, Q3, P4

996.83 Heart
(Ex) 996.83, 997.91-997.99
Coding Clinic: 2003, Q3, P16; 2002, Q4, P53-54; 2001, Q3,
P13-14x2; 1998, Q3, P5; 1993, Q3, P13

996.84 Lung
(Ex) 996.84, 997.91-997.99
Coding Clinic: 2003, Q2, P12; 1998, Q3, P5

996.85 Bone marrow
(Ex) 279.50-279.53, 996.85, 997.91-997.99
Coding Clinic: 2012, Q1, P13-14; 2011, Q1, P9; 2008, Q4,
P90-91

996.86 Pancreas
(Ex) 996.86, 997.91-997.99

996.87 Intestine
(Ex) 238.77, 996.80, 996.87, 997.91-997.99
Coding Clinic: 2000, Q4, P47-48

996.88 Stem cell
Complications from stem cells from:
peripheral blood
umbilical cord
(Ex) 996.88-996.89, 997.91-997.99
Coding Clinic: 2011, Q4, P148

996.89 Other specified transplanted organ
(Ex) 996.88-996.89, 997.91-997.99
Coding Clinic: 2011, Q1, P9; 1994, Q3, P5

● **996.9 Complications of reattached extremity or body part**

996.90 Unspecified extremity
(Ex) 996.90, 997.91-997.99, 998.81, 998.83-998.9

996.91 Forearm
(Ex) 996.91, 997.91-997.99, 998.81, 998.83-998.9

996.92 Hand
(Ex) 996.92, 997.91-997.99, 998.81, 998.83-998.9

996.93 Finger(s)
(Ex) 996.93, 997.91-997.99, 998.81, 998.83-998.9

996.94 Upper extremity, other and unspecified
(Ex) 996.94, 997.91-997.99, 998.81, 998.83-998.9

996.95 Foot and toe(s)
(Ex) 996.95, 997.91-997.99, 998.81, 998.83-998.9

996.96 Lower extremity, other and unspecified
(Ex) 996.96, 997.91-997.99, 998.81, 998.83-998.9

996.99 Other specified body part
(Ex) 996.99, 997.91-997.99, 998.81, 998.83-998.9

OGCR Section I.C.17.f.2.a

Transplant complications other than kidney: Codes under subcategory
996.8, Complications of transplanted organ, are for use for both
complications and rejection of transplanted organs. A transplant
complication code is only assigned if the complication affects
the function of the transplanted organ. Two codes are required
to fully describe a transplant complication, the appropriate code
from subcategory 996.8 and a secondary code that identifies the
complication.

Pre-existing conditions or conditions that develop after the transplant
are not coded as complications unless they affect the function of the
transplanted organs.

See I.C.18.d.3 for transplant organ removal status

See I.C.2.i for malignant neoplasm associated with transplanted organ.

INJURY AND POISONING (800–999)

INJURY AND POISONING (800–999)

● **997 Complications affecting specified body systems, not elsewhere classified**

Use additional code to identify complication

Excludes *the listed conditions when specified as:*
causing shock (998.00–998.09)
complications of:
anesthesia:
adverse effect (001.0–799.9, 995.0–995.8)
in labor or delivery (668.0–668.9)
poisoning (968.0–969.9)
implanted device or graft (996.0–996.9)
obstetrical procedures (669.0–669.4)
reattached extremity (996.90–996.96)
transplanted organ (996.80–996.89)

Coding Clinic: 2011, Q4, P150; Q1, P16; 1995, Q2, P7; 1993, Q2, P9-10; 1992, Q1, P13

● **997.0 Nervous system complications**

997.00 Nervous system complication, unspecified

997.01 Central nervous system complication 🖢
Anoxic brain damage
Cerebral hypoxia

Excludes *Cerebrovascular hemorrhage or infarction (997.02)*

(Ex) 997.00-997.09, 997.91-997.99, 998.81, 998.83-998.9
Coding Clinic: 2007, Q1, P22-23; 2006, Q1, P15-16

997.02 Iatrogenic cerebrovascular infarction or hemorrhage 🖢
Postoperative stroke
(Ex) 997.00-997.09, 997.91-997.99, 998.81, 998.83-998.9
Coding Clinic: 2010, Q3, P5; 2006, Q3, P6; 2004, Q2, P8-9

OGCR Section I.C.7.c

A cerebrovascular hemorrhage or infarction that occurs as a result of medical intervention is coded to 997.02. Documentation should clearly specify cause-and-effect relationship between the medical intervention and the cerebrovascular accident in order to assign this code. A secondary code from the code range 430-432 or from a code from subcategories 433 or 434 with a fifth digit of "1" should also be used to identify the type of hemorrhage or infarct.

997.09 Other nervous system complications 🖢
(Ex) 997.00-997.09, 997.91-997.99, 998.81, 998.83-998.9

997.1 Cardiac complications 🖢
Cardiac:
arrest during or resulting from a procedure
insufficiency during or resulting from a procedure
Cardiorespiratory failure during or resulting from a procedure
Heart failure during or resulting from a procedure

Excludes *the listed conditions as long-term effects of cardiac surgery or due to the presence of cardiac prosthetic device (429.4)*
(Ex) 997.1, 997.91-997.99, 998.81, 998.83-998.9
Coding Clinic: 2013, Q1, P11; 2011, Q1, P3-4; 2008, Q4, P177-180; 2000, Q2, P12; 1994, Q3, P9; Q1, P20; 1993, Q4, P37, 39-43; 5th Issue, P6-7

997.2 Peripheral vascular complications 🖢
Phlebitis or thrombophlebitis during or resulting from a procedure

Excludes *the listed conditions due to:*
implant or catheter device (996.62)
infusion, perfusion, or transfusion (999.2)
complications affecting blood vessels (997.71–997.79)
(Ex) 997.2, 997.79-997.99, 998.81, 998.83-998.9
Coding Clinic: 2003, Q1, P6-7; 2002, Q3, P24-27; 1993, Q1, P26

● **997.3 Respiratory complications**

Excludes *iatrogenic [postoperative] pneumothorax (512.1)*
iatrogenic pulmonary embolism (415.11)
specified complications classified elsewhere, such as:
adult respiratory distress syndrome (518.52)
pulmonary edema, postoperative (518.4)
respiratory insufficiency, acute, postoperative (518.52)
shock lung related to trauma and surgery (518.52)
tracheostomy complications (519.00–519.09)
transfusion related acute lung injury (TRALI) (518.7)

Coding Clinic: 1997, Q1, P10; 1993, Q4, P43; Q2, P9-10; Q2, P3-4; 1990, Q4, P25x2; 1989, Q1, P10

997.31 Ventilator associated pneumonia 🖢
Ventilator associated pneumonitis

Use additional code to identify organism
(Ex) 518.7, 997.31-997.39, 997.91-997.99, 998.81, 998.83-998.9
Coding Clinic: 2008, Q4, P148-149; 2006, Q2, P25

997.32 Postprocedural aspiration pneumonia 🖢
Chemical pneumonitis resulting from a procedure
Mendelson's syndrome resulting from a procedure

Excludes *aspiration pneumonia during labor and delivery (668.0)*
(Ex) 518.7, 997.31-997.39, 997.91-997.99, 998.81, 998.83-998.9
Coding Clinic: 2011, Q4, P150

997.39 Other respiratory complications 🖢
(Ex) 518.7, 997.31-997.39, 997.91-997.99, 998.81, 998.83-998.9
Coding Clinic: 2011, Q1, P16

● **997.4 Digestive system complications**
Complications of:
intestinal (internal) anastomosis and bypass, not elsewhere classified, except that involving urinary tract
Hepatic failure specified as due to a procedure
Hepatorenal syndrome specified as due to a procedure
Acute renal failure occurring along with cirrhosis or fulminant liver failure associated with portal hypertension
Intestinal obstruction NOS specified as due to a procedure

Excludes *complications of gastric band procedure (539.01-539.09)*
complications of other bariatric procedure (539.81-539.89)
specified gastrointestinal complications classified elsewhere, such as:
blind loop syndrome (579.2)
colostomy or enterostomy complications (569.60–569.69)
complications of intestinal pouch (569.71–569.79)
gastrojejunal ulcer (534.0–534.9)
gastrostomy complications (536.40–536.49)
infection of esophagostomy (530.86)
infection of external stoma (569.61)
mechanical complication of esophagostomy (530.87)
pelvic peritoneal adhesions, female (614.6)
peritoneal adhesions (568.0)
peritoneal adhesions with obstruction (560.81)
postcholecystectomy syndrome (576.0)
postgastric surgery syndromes (564.2)
pouchitis (569.71)
vomiting following gastrointestinal surgery (564.3)

Coding Clinic: 2009, Q4, P129; 2003, Q1, P18; 2001, Q2, P4-6x2; 1999, Q3, P4-5; Q2, P14; 1997, Q3, P7; Q1, P11; 1995, Q3, P7, 16; Q2, P7; 1993, Q1, P26; 1992, Q3, P15; 1989, Q2, P15; 1988, Q1, P14; 1987, Nov-Dec, P9; 1985, Sept-Oct, P11; Mar-April, P11

997.41 **Retained cholelithiasis following cholecystectomy** 🔍
  Ex: 530.86, 530.87, 536.40-536.49, 539.01-539.89, 569.71-569.79, 997.41-997.49, 997.71, 997.91, 997.99, 998.81, 998.83-998.9

997.49 **Other digestive system complications** 🔍
  Ex: 530.86, 530.87, 536.40-536.49, 539.01-539.89, 569.71-569.79, 997.41-997.49, 997.71, 997.91, 997.99, 998.81, 998.83-998.9
  Coding Clinic: 2012, Q1, P6-7

997.5 **Urinary complications**
  Complications of:
    internal anastomosis and bypass of urinary tract, including that involving intestinal tract
  Oliguria or anuria specified as due to procedure
  Renal (kidney):
    failure (acute) specified as due to procedure
    insufficiency (acute) specified as due to procedure
  Tubular necrosis (acute) specified as due to procedure
  Excludes *complications of cystostomy (596.81-596.83)*
    complications of external stoma of urinary tract (596.81-596.83)
    specified complications classified elsewhere, such as:
      postoperative stricture of:
        ureter (593.3)
        urethra (598.2)
  Coding Clinic: 2012, Q1, P11-12; 2003, Q3, P13; 1996, Q3, P10-11,15; 1995, Q4, P72-73; 1994, Q1, P20; 1992, Q1, P13; 1989, Q2, P16

●997.6 **Amputation stump complication**
  Excludes *admission for treatment for a current traumatic amputation - code to complicated traumatic amputation*
    phantom limb (syndrome) (353.6)
  Coding Clinic: 1996, Q4, P45-46

997.60 **Unspecified complication**

997.61 **Neuroma of amputation stump**

997.62 **Infection (chronic)** 🔍
  Use additional code to identify the organism
  Ex: 997.60, 997.62-997.69, 997.91-997.99, 998.81, 998.83-998.9
  Coding Clinic: 2005, Q1, P14-15; 2003, Q3, P14; 1996, Q4, P45-46

997.69 **Other**
  Coding Clinic: 2005, Q1, P15

●997.7 **Vascular complications of other vessels**
  Excludes *peripheral vascular complications (997.2)*

997.71 **Vascular complications of mesenteric artery** 🔍
  Ex: 997.2, 997.71-997.99, 998.81, 998.83-998.9
  Coding Clinic: 2001, Q4, P53

997.72 **Vascular complications of renal artery** 🔍
  Ex: 997.2, 997.71-997.99, 998.81, 998.83-998.9

997.79 **Vascular complications of other vessels** 🔍
  Ex: 997.2, 997.71-997.99, 998.81, 998.83-998.9

●997.9 **Complications affecting other specified body systems, not elsewhere classified**
  Excludes *specified complications classified elsewhere, such as:*
    broad ligament laceration syndrome (620.6)
    postartificial menopause syndrome (627.4)
    postoperative stricture of vagina (623.2)
  Coding Clinic: 1994, Q1, P16; 1993, Q4, P41-42

997.91 **Hypertension**
  Excludes *Essential hypertension (401.0–401.9)*

997.99 **Other** 🔍
  Vitreous touch syndrome
  Ex: 997.91-997.99, 998.81, 998.83-998.9
  Coding Clinic: 1994, Q2, P12; Q1, P17; Q1, P16-17

●998 **Other complications of procedures, NEC**
  Excludes *fluid overload due to transfusion (blood) (276.61)*
    TACO (276.61)
    transfusion associated circulatory overload (276.61)

●998.0 **Postoperative shock**
  Shock during or resulting from a surgical procedure
  Excludes *shock:*
    anaphylactic due to serum (999.41-999.49)
    anesthetic (995.4)
    electric (994.8)
    following abortion (639.5)
    obstetric (669.1)
    traumatic (958.4)

998.00 **Postoperative shock, unspecified** 🔍
  Collapse, not otherwise specified, during or resulting from a surgical procedure
  Failure of peripheral circulation, postoperative

998.01 **Postoperative shock, cardiogenic** 🔍
  Ex: 958.4, 995.4, 997.91-998.13, 998.81, 998.83-998.9
  Coding Clinic: 2011, Q4, P152

●998.02 **Postoperative shock, septic** 🔍
  Postoperative endotoxic shock
  Postoperative gram-negative shock
  Code first underlying infection
    Use additional code, to identify severe sepsis (995.92) and any associated acute organ dysfunction, if applicable
  Ex: 958.4, 995.4, 997.91-998.13, 998.81, 998.83-998.9
  Coding Clinic: 2011, Q4, P152

998.09 **Postoperative shock, other** 🔍
  Postoperative hypovolemic shock
  Ex: 958.4, 995.4, 997.91-998.13, 998.81, 998.83-998.9

●998.1 **Hemorrhage or hematoma or seroma complicating a procedure**
  Excludes *hemorrhage, hematoma or seroma:*
    complicating cesarean section or puerperal perineal wound (674.3)
    due to implanted device or graft (996.70–996.79)
  Coding Clinic: 2003, Q3, P13; 1993, Q1, P26; 1992, Q2, P15-16; 1987, Sept-Oct, P8

998.11 **Hemorrhage complicating a procedure** 🔍
  Ex: 456.0, 456.20, 530.81-530.83, 530.89, 531.00-531.01, 531.20-531.21, 531.40-531.41, 531.60-531.61, 532.00-532.01, 532.20-532.21, 532.40-532.41, 532.60-532.61, 533.00-533.01, 533.20-533.21, 533.40-533.41, 533.60-533.61, 534.00-534.01, 534.20-534.21, 534.40-534.41, 534.60-534.61, 535.01, 535.11, 535.21, 535.31, 535.41, 535.51, 535.61, 535.71, 537.83, 562.02-562.03, 562.12-562.13, 569.3, 569.85, 578.0-578.9, 772.4, 997.91-998.13, 998.81, 998.89-998.9
  Coding Clinic: 2003, Q3, P13; Q1, P4; 1997, Q4, P52; Q1, P10; 1994, Q1, P19-20

998.12 **Hematoma complicating a procedure** 🔍
  Ex: 456.0, 456.20, 530.81-530.83, 530.89, 531.00-531.01, 531.20-531.21, 531.40-531.41, 531.60-531.61, 532.00-532.01, 532.20-532.21, 532.40-532.41, 532.60-532.61, 533.00-533.01, 533.20-533.21, 533.40-533.41, 533.60-533.61, 534.00-534.01, 534.20-534.21, 534.40-534.41, 534.60-534.61, 535.01, 535.11, 535.21, 535.31, 535.41, 535.51, 535.61, 535.71, 537.83, 562.02-562.03, 562.12-562.13, 569.3, 569.85, 578.0-578.9, 772.4, 997.91-998.13, 998.81, 998.89-998.9
  Coding Clinic: 2006, Q3, P12; 2003, Q1, P6-7; 2002, Q3, P24-25; 1994, Q1, P20

998.13 **Seroma complicating a procedure** 🔍
  Pocket of clear serous fluid that sometimes develops in the body after surgery
  Ex: 456.0, 456.20, 530.81-530.83, 530.89, 531.00-531.01, 531.20-531.21, 531.40-531.41, 531.60-531.61, 532.00-532.01, 532.20-532.21, 532.40-532.41, 532.60-532.61, 533.00-533.01, 533.20-533.21, 533.40-533.41, 533.60-533.61, 534.00-534.01, 534.20-534.21, 534.40-534.41, 534.60-534.61, 535.01, 535.11, 535.21, 535.31, 535.41, 535.51, 535.61, 535.71, 537.83, 562.02-562.03, 562.12-562.13, 569.3, 569.85, 578.0-578.9, 772.4, 997.91-998.13, 998.81, 998.89-998.9
  Coding Clinic: 1996, Q4, P46

INJURY AND POISONING (800–999)

998.2   Accidental puncture or laceration during a procedure 🔲
    Accidental perforation by catheter or other instrument during a procedure on:
      blood vessel
      nerve
      organ

    Excludes *iatrogenic [postoperative] pneumothorax (512.1)*
        puncture or laceration caused by implanted device intentionally left in operation wound (996.0–996.5)
        specified complications classified elsewhere, such as:
          broad ligament laceration syndrome (620.6)
          dural tear (349.31)
          incidental durotomy (349.31)
          trauma from instruments during delivery (664.0–665.9)

    (Ex:) 349.31-349.39, 997.91-997.99, 998.2, 998.81, 998.83-998.9
    Coding Clinic: 2012, Q2, P5-6, 8; 2011, Q1, P3-4; 2010, Q1, P15; 2007, Q2, P11-12; 2006, Q1, P15; 2002, Q3, P24-27; 1994, Q3, P6; 1994, Q1, P17; 1990, Q3, P17-18; 1984, Nov-Dec, P12

● **998.3   Disruption of wound**
    Dehiscence of operation wound
      Splitting open
    Disruption of any suture materials or other closure method
    Rupture of operation wound

    Excludes *disruption of:*
        amputation of stump (997.69)
        cesarean wound (674.1)
        perineal wound, puerperal (674.2)
    Coding Clinic: 2008, Q4, P149-152; 2002, Q4, P73; 1993, Q1, P19

    998.30   Disruption of wound, unspecified 🔲
      Disruption of wound NOS
      (Ex:) 997.91-997.99, 998.30-998.33, 998.81, 998.83-998.9

    998.31   Disruption of internal operation surgical wound 🔲
      Disruption or dehiscence of closure of:
        fascia, superficial or muscular
        internal organ
        muscle or muscle flap
        ribs or rib cage
        skull or craniotomy
        sternum or sternotomy
        tendon or ligament
      Deep disruption or dehiscence of operation wound NOS

      Excludes *complications of internal anastomosis of:*
          gastrointestinal tract (997.49)
          urinary tract (997.5)
      (Ex:) 997.91-997.99, 998.30-998.33, 998.81, 998.83-998.9
      Coding Clinic: 2010, Q4, P131

    998.32   Disruption of external operation (surgical) wound 🔲
      Disruption or dehiscence of closure of:
        cornea
        mucosa
        skin
        subcutaneous tissue
      Full-thickness skin disruption or dehiscence
      Superficial disruption or dehiscence of operation wound
      (Ex:) 997.91-997.99, 998.30-998.33, 998.81, 998.83-998.9
      Coding Clinic: 2006, Q1, P8; 2005, Q1, P11; 2003, Q4, P104-107

    998.33   Disruption of traumatic injury wound repair 🔲
      Disruption or dehiscence of closure of traumatic laceration (external) (internal)
      (Ex:) 997.91-997.99, 998.30-998.33, 998.81, 998.83-998.9

998.4   Foreign body accidentally left during a procedure 🔲 🔲
    Adhesions due to foreign body accidentally left in operative wound or body cavity during a procedure
    Obstruction due to foreign body accidentally left in operative wound or body cavity during a procedure
    Perforation due to foreign body accidentally left in operative wound or body cavity during a procedure

    Excludes *obstruction or perforation caused by implanted device intentionally left in body (996.0–996.5)*
    (Ex:) 997.91-997.99, 998.4, 998.81, 998.83-998.9
    Coding Clinic: 2012, Q1, P12-13; 2011, Q1, P5-6; 2009, Q1, P13; 1989, Q1, P9

● **998.5   Postoperative infection**
    Excludes *bleb associated endophthalmitis (379.63)*
        infection due to:
          implanted device (996.60–996.69)
          infusion, perfusion, or transfusion (999.31–999.39)
        postoperative obstetrical wound infection (674.3)
    Coding Clinic: 1996, Q4, P45-46; 1995, Q2, P7; 1994, Q3, P6; 1987, Jan-Feb, P13-14

    998.51   Infected postoperative seroma 🔲
      Use additional code to identify organism
      (Ex:) 997.91-997.99, 998.51-998.59, 998.81, 998.89-998.9
      Coding Clinic: 1996, Q4, P46

    998.59   Other postoperative infection 🔲 🔲
      Abscess: postoperative
        intra-abdominal postoperative
        stitch postoperative
        subphrenic postoperative
        wound postoperative
      Septicemia postoperative
      Use additional code to identify infection
      HAC: And one of the following procedure codes: 81.01-81.08, 81.23, 81.24, 81.31-81.38, 81.83, 81.85
      HAC: Principal Diagnosis 278.01, 998.59 (CC), and one of the following procedure codes: 44.38, 44.39, or 44.95
      (Ex:) 997.91-997.99, 998.51-998.59, 998.81, 998.89-998.9
      Coding Clinic: 2011, Q4, P153; 2006, Q2, P23-24; 2004, Q4, P75-76; 2003, Q4, P104-107; 1995, Q3, P5; Q2, P7, 11; 1993, Q1, P19

      OGCR Section I.C.1.b.10.b

      Sepsis due to postprocedural infection: In cases of postprocedural sepsis, the complication code, such as code 998.59, Other postoperative infection, or 674.3x, Other complications of obstetrical surgical wounds should be coded first followed by the appropriate sepsis codes (systemic infection code and either code 995.91 or 995.92). An additional code(s) for any acute organ dysfunction should also be assigned for cases of severe sepsis.

998.6   Persistent postoperative fistula 🔲
    (Ex:) 997.91-997.99, 998.6, 998.81, 998.83-998.9
    Coding Clinic: 1987, Jan-Feb, P14

998.7   Acute reaction to foreign substance accidentally left during a procedure 🔲 🔲
    Peritonitis:
      aseptic
      chemical
    (Ex:) 997.91-997.99, 998.7-998.81, 998.83-998.9

◀ New   ◀ Revised   deleted Deleted   Excludes Excludes   Includes Includes   Use additional   Code first   Omit code
● Unacceptable Principal Diagnosis   ● Use Additional Digit(s)   ▶ Manifestation Code   OGCR Official Guidelines   Coding Clinic

1004

● **998.8 Other specified complications of procedures, not elsewhere classified**
Coding Clinic: 1993, 5th Issue, P8, 15; 1989, Q1, P9; 1987, Jan-Feb, P13

998.81 Emphysema (subcutaneous) (surgical) resulting from a procedure

998.82 Cataract fragments in eye following cataract surgery

998.83 Non-healing surgical wound 🕭
(Ex) 997.91-997.99, 998.81, 998.83-998.9
Coding Clinic: 1996, Q4, P47

998.89 Other specified complications
Coding Clinic: 2009, Q2, P11; 2006, Q3, P9-10; 2005, Q3, P16-17; 1999, Q3, P13; 1998, Q2, P16

998.9 Unspecified complication of procedure, not elsewhere classified
Postoperative complication NOS
Excludes *complication NOS of obstetrical surgery or procedure (669.4)*
Coding Clinic: 1993, Q4, P41-42

● **999 Complications of medical care, not elsewhere classified**
Includes complications, not elsewhere classified, of:
dialysis (hemodialysis) (peritoneal) (renal)
extracorporeal circulation
hyperalimentation therapy
immunization
infusion
inhalation therapy
injection
inoculation
perfusion
transfusion
vaccination
ventilation therapy
Use additional code, where applicable, to identify specific complication
Excludes *specified complications classified elsewhere such as:*
complications of implanted device (996.0–996.9)
contact dermatitis due to drugs (692.3)
dementia dialysis (294.8)
transient (293.9)
dialysis disequilibrium syndrome (276.0–276.9)
poisoning and toxic effects of drugs and chemicals (960.0–989.9)
postvaccinal encephalitis (323.51)
water and electrolyte imbalance (276.0–276.9)

999.0 Generalized vaccinia 🕭
Excludes *vaccinia not from vaccine (051.02)*
(Ex) 999.0

999.1 Air embolism 🕭 🕭
Air embolism to any site following infusion, perfusion, or transfusion
Excludes *embolism specified as:*
complicating:
abortion (634–638 with .6, 639.6)
ectopic or molar pregnancy (639.6)
pregnancy, childbirth, or the puerperium (673.0)
due to implanted device (996.7)
traumatic (958.0)
(Ex) 958.0, 999.1

999.2 Other vascular complications 🕭
Phlebitis following infusion, perfusion, or transfusion
Thromboembolism following infusion, perfusion, or transfusion
Thrombophlebitis following infusion, perfusion, or transfusion
Excludes *extravasation of vesicant drugs (999.81, 999.82)*
the listed conditions when specified as:
due to implanted device (996.61–996.62, 996.72–996.74)
postoperative NOS (997.2, 997.71–997.79)
(Ex) 999.2, 999.81-999.82, 999.88
Coding Clinic: 1997, Q2, P5

● **999.3 Other infection**
Infection following infusion, injection, transfusion, or vaccination
Sepsis following infusion, injection, transfusion, or vaccination
Septicemia following infusion, injection, transfusion, or vaccination
Use additional code to identify the specified infection, such as:
septicemia (038.0–038.9)
Excludes *the listed conditions when specified as:*
due to implanted device (996.60–996.69)
postoperative NOS (998.51–998.59)
Coding Clinic: 2001, Q2, P11-12; 1987, Jan-Feb, P14-15

999.31 Other and unspecified infection due to central venous catheter 🕭 🕭
Central line-associated infection
Infection due to:
central venous catheter NOS
Hickman catheter
peripherally inserted central catheter (PICC)
triple lumen catheter
umbilical venous catheter
Excludes *infection due to:*
arterial catheter (996.62)
catheter NOS (996.69)
peripheral venous catheter (996.62)
urinary catheter (996.64)
(Ex) 996.62, 999.31-999.39
Coding Clinic: 2013, Q2, P4; 2012, Q2, P16-17; 2010, Q2, P8; 2008, Q4, P69-73, 192-193; 2007, Q4, P96-97

999.32 Bloodstream infection due to central venous catheter 🕭 🕭
Bloodstream infection due to:
Hickman catheter
peripherally inserted central catheter (PICC)
portacath (port-a-cath)
triple lumen catheter
umbilical venous catheter
Catheter-related bloodstream infection (CRBSI) NOS
Central line-associated bloodstream infection (CLABSI)
(Ex) 996.62, 999.31-999.39

999.33 Local infection due to central venous catheter 🕭 🕭
Exit or insertion site infection
Local infection due to:
Hickman catheter
peripherally inserted central catheter (PICC)
portacath (port-a-cath)
triple lumen catheter
umbilical venous catheter
Port or reservoir infection
Tunnel infection
(Ex) 996.62, 999.31-999.39

999.34 Acute infection following transfusion, infusion, or injection of blood and blood products 🕭 🕭
(Ex) 996.62, 999.31-999.39
Coding Clinic: 2011, Q4, P155

999.39 Infection following other infusion, injection, transfusion, or vaccination 🕭
(Ex) 996.62, 999.31-999.39

INJURY AND POISONING (800–999)

N Newborn: 0   **P** Pediatric: 0–17   **M** Maternity: 12–55   **A** Adult: 15–124   ♀ Females Only   ♂ Males Only
(Ex) CC/MCC Exclusions   🕭 Complication\Comorbidity   🕭 Major C\C   🕭 Present on Admission Requirement   🕭 Hospital-Acquired Condition

1005

● **999.4 Anaphylactic reaction due to serum**
    Allergic shock
    Anaphylactic shock due to serum
    Anaphylactoid reaction due to serum
    Anaphylaxis

    Excludes   *ABO incompatibility reaction due to transfusion*
                of blood or blood products (999.60-999.69)
              reaction:
                allergic NOS (995.0)
                anaphylactic:
                   due to drugs and chemicals (995.0)
                   NOS (995.0)
                other serum (999.51-999.59)
              shock:
                allergic NOS (995.0)
                anaphylactic:
                   due to drugs and chemicals (995.0)
                   NOS (995.0)

    999.41 Anaphylactic reaction due to administration of blood and blood products
        (Ex:) 999.41-999.59
        Coding Clinic: 2011, Q4, P147

    999.42 Anaphylactic reaction due to vaccination
        (Ex:) 999.41-999.59

    999.49 Anaphylactic reaction due to other serum
        (Ex:) 999.41-999.59

● **999.5 Other serum reaction**
    Intoxication by serum   Serum sickness
    Protein sickness   Urticaria due to serum
    Serum rash

    Excludes   *serum hepatitis (070.2–070.3)*

    999.51 Other serum reaction due to administration of blood and blood products
        (Ex:) 999.41-999.59

    999.52 Other serum reaction due to vaccination
        (Ex:) 999.41-999.59

    999.59 Other serum reaction
        (Ex:) 991.51-999.59

● **999.6 ABO incompatibility reaction due to transfusion of blood or blood products**

    Excludes   *minor blood group antigens reactions (Duffy)*
                (E) (K(ell)) (Kidd) (Lewis) (M) (N) (P) (S)
                (999.75-999.79)

    999.60 ABO incompatibility reaction, unspecified
        ABO incompatible blood transfusion NOS
        Reaction to ABO incompatibility from
            transfusion NOS
        (Ex:) 999.60-999.80, 999.83-999.85, 999.89

    999.61 ABO incompatibility with hemolytic transfusion reaction not specified as acute or delayed
        ABO incompatibility with hemolytic transfusion
            reaction at unspecified time after
            transfusion
        Hemolytic transfusion reaction (HTR) due to
            ABO incompatibility
        (Ex:) 999.60-999.80, 999.83-999.85, 999.89

    999.62 ABO incompatibility with acute hemolytic transfusion reaction
        ABO incompatibility with hemolytic transfusion
            reaction less than 24 hours after transfusion
        Acute hemolytic transfusion reaction (AHTR)
            due to ABO incompatibility
        (Ex:) 999.60-999.80, 999.83-999.85, 999.89

    999.63 ABO incompatibility with delayed hemolytic transfusion reaction
        ABO incompatibility with hemolytic transfusion
            reaction 24 hours or more after transfusion
        Delayed hemolytic transfusion reaction (DHTR)
            due to ABO incompatibility
        (Ex:) 999.60-999.80, 999.83-999.85, 999.89

    999.69 Other ABO incompatibility reaction
        Delayed serologic transfusion reaction (DSTR)
            from ABO incompatibility
        Other ABO incompatible blood transfusion
        Other reaction to ABO incompatibility from
            transfusion
        (Ex:) 999.60-999.80, 999.83-999.85, 999.89

● **999.7 Rh and other non-ABO incompatibility reaction due to transfusion of blood or blood products**

    999.70 Rh incompatibility reaction, unspecified
        Reaction due to Rh factor in transfusion NOS
        Rh incompatible blood transfusion NOS
        Unspecified reaction due to incompatibility
            related to Rh antigens (C) (c) (D) (E) (e)
        Unspecified reaction to Rh incompatibility
        (Ex:) 999.60-999.80, 999.83-999.85, 999.89

    999.71 Rh incompatibility with hemolytic transfusion reaction not specified as acute or delayed
        Hemolytic transfusion reaction (HTR) due to Rh
            incompatibility
        HTR due to incompatibility related to Rh
            antigens (C) (c) (D) (E) (e), not specified as
            acute or delayed
        Rh incompatibility with hemolytic transfusion
            reaction at unspecified time after
            transfusion
        (Ex:) 999.60-999.80, 999.83-999.85, 999.89

    999.72 Rh incompatibility with acute hemolytic transfusion reaction
        Acute hemolytic transfusion reaction (AHTR)
            due to Rh incompatibility
        AHTR due to incompatibility related to Rh
            antigens (C) (c) (D) (E) (e)
        Rh incompatibility with hemolytic transfusion
            reaction less than 24 hours after transfusion
        (Ex:) 999.60-999.80, 999.83-999.85, 999.89

    999.73 Rh incompatibility with delayed hemolytic transfusion reaction
        Delayed hemolytic transfusion reaction (DHTR)
            due to Rh incompatibility
        DHTR due to incompatibility related to Rh
            antigens (C) (c) (D) (E) (e)
        Rh incompatibility with hemolytic transfusion
            reaction 24 hours or more after transfusion
        (Ex:) 999.60-999.80, 999.83-999.85, 999.89

    999.74 Other Rh incompatibility reaction
        Delayed serologic transfusion reaction (DSTR)
            from Rh incompatibility
        Other reaction due to incompatibility related to
            Rh antigens (C) (c) (D) (E) (e)
        Other reaction to Rh incompatible blood
            transfusion
        (Ex:) 999.60-999.73, 999.79-999.80, 999.83-999.85, 999.89

    999.75 Non-ABO incompatibility reaction, unspecified
        Non-ABO incompatible blood transfusion NOS
        Reaction to non-ABO antigen incompatibility
            from transfusion NOS
        Unspecified reaction due to incompatibility
            related to minor antigens (Duffy) (Kell)
            (Kidd) (Lewis) (M) (N) (P) (S)
        (Ex:) 999.60-999.73, 999.79-999.80, 999.83-999.85, 999.89

    999.76 Non-ABO incompatibility with hemolytic transfusion reaction not specified as acute or delayed
        Hemolytic transfusion reaction (HTR) due to
            non-ABO incompatibility
        HTR from incompatibility related to minor
            antigens (Duffy) (Kell) (Kidd) (Lewis) (M)
            (N) (P) (S)
        Non-ABO incompatibility with hemolytic
            transfusion reaction at unspecified time
            after transfusion
        (Ex:) 999.60-999.73, 999.79-999.80, 999.83-999.85, 999.89

◄ New   ◄▥ Revised   ~~deleted~~ Deleted   Excludes   Includes   Use additional   Code first   Omit code
● Unacceptable Principal Diagnosis   ● Use Additional Digit(s)   ▶ Manifestation Code   OGCR Official Guidelines   Coding Clinic

1006

999.77 **Non-ABO incompatibility with acute hemolytic transfusion reaction**🔲
  Acute hemolytic transfusion reaction (AHTR) due to non-ABO incompatibility
  AHTR from incompatibility related to minor antigens (Duffy) (Kell) (Kidd) (Lewis) (M) (N) (P) (S)
  Non-ABO incompatibility with hemolytic transfusion reaction less than 24 hours after transfusion
  (Ex) 999.60-999.73, 999.79-999.80, 999.83-999.85, 999.89

999.78 **Non-ABO incompatibility with delayed hemolytic transfusion reaction**🔲
  Delayed hemolytic transfusion reaction (DHTR) due to non-ABO incompatibility
  DHTR from incompatibility related to minor antigens (Duffy) (Kell) (Kidd) (Lewis) (M) (N) (P) (S)
  Non-ABO incompatibility with hemolytic transfusion reaction 24 hours or more after transfusion
  (Ex) 999.60-999.73, 999.79-999.80, 999.83-999.85, 999.89

999.79 **Other non-ABO incompatibility reaction**🔲
  Delayed serologic transfusion reaction (DSTR) from non-ABO incompatibility
  Other non-ABO incompatible blood transfusion
  Other reaction due to incompatibility related to minor antigens (Duffy) (Kell) (Kidd) (Lewis) (M) (N) (P) (S)
  Other reaction to non-ABO incompatibility from transfusion
  (Ex) 999.60-999.80, 999.83-999.85, 999.89

● **999.8** **Other and unspecified infusion and transfusion reaction**
  Excludes *ABO incompatibility reactions (999.60-999.69)*
    febrile nonhemolytic transfusion reaction (FNHTR) (780.66)
    hemochromatosis due to repeated red blood cell transfusions (275.02)
    non-ABO incompatibility reactions (999.70-999.79)
    postoperative shock (998.00-998.09)
    posttransfusion purpura (287.41)
    Rh incompatibility reactions (999.70-999.74)
    transfusion associated circulatory overload (TACO) (276.61)
    transfusion related acute lung injury (TRALI) (518.7)
  Coding Clinic: 2008, Q4, P152-155; 2000, Q3, P9

999.80 **Transfusion reaction, unspecified**
  Incompatible blood transfusion NOS
  Reaction to blood group incompatibility in infusion or transfusion NOS

999.81 **Extravasation of vesicant chemotherapy**🔲
  Infiltration of vesicant chemotherapy
  (Ex) 999.2, 999.81-999.82, 999.88
  Coding Clinic: 2008, Q4, P152-155

999.82 **Extravasation of other vesicant agent**🔲
  Infiltration of other vesicant agent
  (Ex) 999.2, 999.81-999.82, 999.88

999.83 **Hemolytic transfusion reaction, incompatibility unspecified**🔲
  Hemolytic transfusion reaction (HTR) with antigen incompatibility unspecified, not specified as acute or delayed
  HTR with incompatibility unspecified at unspecified time after transfusion
  (Ex) 999.60-999.80, 999.83-999.85, 999.89

999.84 **Acute hemolytic transfusion reaction, incompatibility unspecified**🔲
  Acute hemolytic transfusion reaction (AHTR) with antigen incompatibility unspecified
  AHTR, incompatibility unspecified
  (Ex) 999.60-999.80, 999.83-999.85, 999.89

999.85 **Delayed hemolytic transfusion reaction, incompatibility unspecified**🔲
  Delayed hemolytic transfusion reaction (DHTR) with antigen incompatibility unspecified
  DHTR, incompatibility unspecified
  (Ex) 999.60-999.80, 999.83-999.85, 999.89

999.88 **Other infusion reaction**

999.89 **Other transfusion reaction**
  Delayed serologic transfusion reaction (DSTR), incompatibility unspecified
  Use additional code to identify graft-versus-host reaction (279.5)

999.9 **Other and unspecified complications of medical care, not elsewhere classified**
  Complications, not elsewhere classified, of:
    electroshock therapy   ultrasound therapy
    inhalation therapy   ventilation therapy
  Unspecified misadventure of medical care
  Excludes *unspecified complication of:*
    phototherapy (990)
    radiation therapy (990)
    ventilator associated pneumonia (997.31)
  MCE: Questionable admission, principal diagnosis only
  Coding Clinic: 2006, Q2, P25; 2003, Q1, P19; 1997, Q2, P5; 1994, Q3, P9

INJURY AND POISONING (800–999)

SUPPLEMENTARY CLASSIFICATION OF FACTORS INFLUENCING HEALTH STATUS AND CONTACT WITH HEALTH SERVICES (V01–V91)

This classification is provided to deal with occasions when circumstances other than a disease or injury classifiable to categories 001–999 (the main part of ICD) are recorded as "diagnoses" or "problems." This can arise mainly in three ways:

a) When a person who is not currently sick encounters the health services for some specific purpose, such as to act as a donor of an organ or tissue, to receive prophylactic vaccination, or to discuss a problem which is in itself not a disease or injury. This will be a fairly rare occurrence among hospital inpatients, but will be relatively more common among hospital outpatients and patients of family practitioners, health clinics, etc.

b) When a person with a known disease or injury, whether it is current or resolving, encounters the health care system for a specific treatment of that disease or injury (e.g., dialysis for renal disease; chemotherapy for malignancy; cast change).

c) When some circumstance or problem is present which influences the person's health status but is not in itself a current illness or injury. Such factors may be elicited during population surveys, when the person may or may not be currently sick, or be recorded as an additional factor to be borne in mind when the person is receiving care for some current illness or injury classifiable to categories 001–999.

In the latter circumstances the V code should be used only as a supplementary code and should not be the one selected for use in primary, single cause tabulations. Examples of these circumstances are a personal history of certain diseases, or a person with an artificial heart valve in situ.

OGCR   Section I.C.18.b

V codes use in any healthcare setting
V codes are for use in any healthcare setting. V codes may be used as either a first listed (principal diagnosis code in the inpatient setting) or secondary code, depending on the circumstances of the encounter. Certain V codes may only be used as first listed, others only as secondary codes.
See Section I.C.18.e, **V Codes That May Only be Principal/First-Listed Diagnosis.**

OGCR   Section I.C.18.d.1

Category V01 indicates contact with or exposure to communicable diseases. These codes are for patients who do not show any sign or symptom of a disease but have been exposed to it by close personal contact with an infected individual or are in an area where a disease is epidemic. These codes may be used as a first listed code to explain an encounter for testing, or, more commonly, as a secondary code to identify a potential risk.

PERSONS WITH POTENTIAL HEALTH HAZARDS RELATED TO COMMUNICABLE DISEASES (V01–V06)

Excludes *family history of infectious and parasitic diseases (V18.8)*
personal history of infectious and parasitic diseases (V12.0)

● **V01   Contact with or exposure to communicable diseases**
   Coding Clinic: 2001, Q1, P10
   ● **V01.0   Cholera**
     Conditions classifiable to 001
   ● **V01.1   Tuberculosis**
     Conditions classifiable to 010–018
   ● **V01.2   Poliomyelitis**
     Conditions classifiable to 045
   ● **V01.3   Smallpox**
     Conditions classifiable to 050
   ● **V01.4   Rubella**
     Conditions classifiable to 056
   ● **V01.5   Rabies**
     Conditions classifiable to 071
   ● **V01.6   Venereal diseases**
     Conditions classifiable to 090–099
     Coding Clinic: 2007, Q4, P124-125x2

● **V01.7   Other viral diseases**
     Conditions classifiable to 042–078, and V08, except as above
   V01.71   Varicella
   V01.79   Other viral diseases
     Coding Clinic: 1992, Q2, P11
● **V01.8   Other communicable diseases**
     Conditions classifiable to 001–136, except as above
   ● **V01.81   Anthrax**
   V01.82   Exposure to SARS-associated coronavirus
     Coding Clinic: 2003, Q4, P46-48
   V01.83   Escherichia coli (E. coli)
   V01.84   Meningococcus
   ● **V01.89   Other communicable diseases**
● **V01.9   Unspecified communicable disease**

● **V02   Carrier or suspected carrier of infectious diseases**
   Includes   Colonization status
   ● **V02.0   Cholera**
   ● **V02.1   Typhoid**
   ● **V02.2   Amebiasis**
   ● **V02.3   Other gastrointestinal pathogens**
   ● **V02.4   Diphtheria**
   ● **V02.5   Other specified bacterial diseases**
     ● **V02.51   Group B streptococcus**
      Coding Clinic: 2006, Q3, P14; 2002, Q1, P14-15; 1998, Q4, P56; 1994, Q3, P4
     ● **V02.52   Other streptococcus**
     ● **V02.53   Methicillin susceptible Staphylococcus aureus**
      MSSA colonization
      Coding Clinic: 2008, Q4, P69-73
     ● **V02.54   Methicillin resistant Staphylococcus aureus**
      MRSA colonization
      Coding Clinic: 2008, Q4, P69-73
     ● **V02.59   Other specified bacterial diseases**
      Meningococcal
      Staphylococcal
   ● **V02.6   Viral hepatitis**
     ● **V02.60   Viral hepatitis carrier, unspecified**
     ● **V02.61   Hepatitis B carrier**
     ● **V02.62   Hepatitis C carrier**
     ● **V02.69   Other viral hepatitis carrier**
   ● **V02.7   Gonorrhea**
   ● **V02.8   Other venereal diseases**
   ● **V02.9   Other specified infectious organism**
     Coding Clinic: 1994, Q4, P36; 1993, Q1, P22

OGCR   Section I.C.18.d.2

Categories V03-V06 are for encounters for inoculations and vaccinations. They indicate that a patient is being seen to receive a prophylactic inoculation against a disease. The injection itself must be represented by the appropriate procedure code. A code from V03-V06 may be used as a secondary code if the inoculation is given as a routine part of preventive health care, such as a well-baby visit.

● **V03   Need for prophylactic vaccination and inoculation against bacterial diseases**
   Excludes *vaccination not carried out (V64.00–V64.09)*
     vaccines against combinations of diseases (V06.0–V06.9)
   ● **V03.0   Cholera alone**
   ● **V03.1   Typhoid-paratyphoid alone [TAB]**
   ● **V03.2   Tuberculosis [BCG]**
   ● **V03.3   Plague**
   ● **V03.4   Tularemia**
   ● **V03.5   Diphtheria alone**
   ● **V03.6   Pertussis alone**
   ● **V03.7   Tetanus toxoid alone**

◀ New   ◀ Revised   ~~deleted~~ Deleted   Excludes   Includes   Use additional   Code first   ● Use Additional Digit(s)   Manifestation Code   OGCR Official Guidelines   Coding Clinic   Ex CC/MCC Exclusions

● **V03.8** **Other specified vaccinations against single bacterial diseases**
- ● **V03.81** Hemophilus influenza, type B [Hib] 🔍
- ● **V03.82** Streptococcus pneumoniae [pneumococcus] 🔍
- ● **V03.89** Other specified vaccination 🔍
  - Coding Clinic: 2000, Q2, P9
● **V03.9** Unspecified single bacterial disease 🔍

● **V04** **Need for prophylactic vaccination and inoculation against certain diseases**
- **Excludes** *vaccines against combinations of diseases (V06.0–V06.9)*
- ● **V04.0** Poliomyelitis 🔍
- ● **V04.1** Smallpox 🔍
- ● **V04.2** Measles alone 🔍
- ● **V04.3** Rubella alone 🔍
- ● **V04.4** Yellow fever 🔍
- ● **V04.5** Rabies 🔍
- ● **V04.6** Mumps alone 🔍
- ● **V04.7** Common cold 🔍
- ● **V04.8** Other viral diseases
  - ● **V04.81** Influenza 🔍
  - ● **V04.82** Respiratory syncytial virus (RSV) 🔍
    - Coding Clinic: 2009, Q1, P5; 2001, Q1, P4
  - ● **V04.89** Other viral diseases 🔍
    - Coding Clinic: 2007, Q2, P11

● **V05** **Need for prophylactic vaccination and inoculation against single diseases**
- **Excludes** *vaccines against combinations of diseases (V06.0–V06.9)*
- ● **V05.0** Arthropod-borne viral encephalitis 🔍
- ● **V05.1** Other arthropod-borne viral diseases 🔍
- ● **V05.2** Leishmaniasis 🔍
- ● **V05.3** Viral hepatitis 🔍
- ● **V05.4** Varicella 🔍
  - Chicken pox
- ● **V05.8** Other specified disease 🔍
  - Coding Clinic: 2001, Q1, P4; 1991, Q3, P20-21
- ● **V05.9** Unspecified single disease 🔍

● **V06** **Need for prophylactic vaccination and inoculation against combinations of diseases**
- **Note:** Use additional single vaccination codes from categories V03–V05 to identify any vaccinations not included in a combination code.
- Coding Clinic: 2012, Q1, P11
- ● **V06.0** Cholera with typhoid-paratyphoid [cholera TAB] 🔍
- ● **V06.1** Diphtheria-tetanus-pertussis, combined [DTP] [DTaP] 🔍
  - Coding Clinic: 1998, Q3, P13-14
- ● **V06.2** Diphtheria-tetanus-pertussis with typhoid-paratyphoid [DTP TAB] 🔍
- ● **V06.3** Diphtheria-tetanus-pertussis with poliomyelitis [DTP+polio] 🔍
- ● **V06.4** Measles-mumps-rubella [MMR] 🔍
- ● **V06.5** Tetanus-diphtheria [Td] [DT] 🔍
- ● **V06.6** Streptococcus pneumoniae [pneumococcus] and influenza 🔍
- ● **V06.8** Other combinations 🔍
  - **Excludes** *multiple single vaccination codes (V03.0–V05.9)*
  - Coding Clinic: 2012, Q1, P11; 1994, Q1, P19
- ● **V06.9** Unspecified combined vaccine 🔍

PERSONS WITH NEED FOR ISOLATION, OTHER POTENTIAL HEALTH HAZARDS AND PROPHYLACTIC MEASURES (V07–V09)

● **V07** **Need for isolation and other prophylactic or treatment measures**
- **Excludes** *long-term (current) (prophylactic) use of certain specific drugs (V58.61-V58.69)*
  - *prophylactic organ removal (V50.41–V50.49)*
- ● **V07.0** Isolation 🔍
  - Admission to protect the individual from his surroundings or for isolation of individual after contact with infectious diseases
- ● **V07.1** Desensitization to allergens 🔍
- ● **V07.2** Prophylactic immunotherapy 🔍
  - Administration of:
    - antivenin
    - immune sera [gamma globulin]
    - RhoGAM
    - tetanus antitoxin
- ● **V07.3** Other prophylactic chemotherapy
  - ● **V07.31** Prophylactic fluoride administration 🔍
  - **V07.39** Other prophylactic chemotherapy 🔍
    - **Excludes** *maintenance chemotherapy following disease (V58.11)*
- ● **V07.4** Hormone replacement therapy (postmenopausal) ♀ 🔍
- ● **V07.5** Use of agents affecting estrogen receptors and estrogen levels
  - *Code first, if applicable:*
    - malignant neoplasm of breast (174.0-174.9, 175.0-175.9)
    - malignant neoplasm of prostate (185)
  - Use additional code, if applicable, to identify:
    - estrogen receptor positive status (V86.0)
    - family history of breast cancer (V16.3)
    - genetic susceptibility to cancer (V84.01-V84.09)
    - personal history of breast cancer (V10.3)
    - personal history of prostate cancer (V10.46)
    - postmenopausal status (V49.81)
  - **Excludes** *hormone replacement therapy (postmenopausal) (V07.4)*
  - ● **V07.51** Use of selective estrogen receptor modulators (SERMs) 🔍
    - Use of:
      - raloxifene (Evista)
      - tamoxifen (Nolvadex)
      - toremifene (Fareston)
  - ● **V07.52** Use of aromatase inhibitors 🔍
    - Use of:
      - anastrozole (Arimidex)
      - exemestane (Aromasin)
      - letrozole (Femara)
  - ● **V07.59** Use of other agents affecting estrogen receptors and estrogen levels 🔍
    - Use of:
      - estrogen receptor downregulators
      - fulvestrant (Faslodex)
      - gonadotropin-releasing hormone (GnRH) agonist
      - goserelin acetate (Zoladex)
      - leuprolide acetate (leuprorelin) (Lupron)
      - megestrol acetate (Megace)
- ● **V07.8** Other specified prophylactic or treatment measure 🔍
  - Coding Clinic: 2013, Q1, P9; 2010, Q2, P6, 14; 1992, Q1, P11
- ● **V07.9** Unspecified prophylactic or treatment measure 🔍

V01-V91

N   Newborn: 0   P   Pediatric: 0–17   M   Maternity: 12–55   A   Adult: 15–124   ♀ Females Only   ♂ Males Only

● Unacceptable Principal Diagnosis   🔍 Complication\Comorbidity   🔍 Major C\C   🔍 Present on Admission Requirement   🔍 Hospital Acquired Condition   **1009**

OGCR Section I.C.1.d
V08, Asymptomatic human immunodeficiency virus [HIV] infection, is to be applied when the patient without any documentation of symptoms is listed as being "HIV positive," "known HIV," "HIV test positive," or similar terminology. Do not use this code if the term "AIDS" is used or if the patient is treated for any HIV-related illness or is described as having any condition(s) resulting from HIV positive status; use 042 in these cases.

● **V08 Asymptomatic human immunodeficiency virus [HIV] infection status**
    HIV positive NOS
    Note: This code is ONLY to be used when NO HIV infection symptoms or conditions are present. If any HIV infection symptoms or conditions are present, see code 042.
    Excludes *AIDS (042)*
        human immunodeficiency virus [HIV] disease (042)
        exposure to HIV (V01.79)
        nonspecific serologic evidence of HIV (795.71)
        symptomatic human immunodeficiency virus [HIV] infection (042)
    MCE: Questionable admission, principal diagnosis only
    Coding Clinic: 2004, Q2, P11; 1999, Q2, P8

● **V09 Infection with drug-resistant microorganisms**
    Note: This category is intended for use as an additional code for infectious conditions classified elsewhere to indicate the presence of drug-resistance of the infectious organism.
    Coding Clinic: 2008, Q4, P69-73

    ● **V09.0 Infection with microorganisms resistant to penicillins**
        Coding Clinic: 2006, Q2, P16-17; 2003, Q4, P104-107; 1994, Q3, P4

    ● **V09.1 Infection with microorganisms resistant to cephalosporins and other B-lactam antibiotics**

    ● **V09.2 Infection with microorganisms resistant to macrolides**

    ● **V09.3 Infection with microorganisms resistant to tetracyclines**

    ● **V09.4 Infection with microorganisms resistant to aminoglycosides**

    ● **V09.5 Infection with microorganisms resistant to quinolones and fluoroquinolones**

        ● **V09.50 Without mention of resistance to multiple quinolones and fluoroquinoles**

        ● **V09.51 With resistance to multiple quinolones and fluoroquinoles**

    ● **V09.6 Infection with microorganisms resistant to sulfonamides**

    ● **V09.7 Infection with microorganisms resistant to other specified antimycobacterial agents**
        Excludes *Amikacin (V09.4)*
            Kanamycin (V09.4)
            Streptomycin [SM] (V09.4)

        ● **V09.70 Without mention of resistance to multiple antimycobacterial agents**

        ● **V09.71 With resistance to multiple antimycobacterial agents**

    ● **V09.8 Infection with microorganisms resistant to other specified drugs**
        Vancomycin (glycopeptide) intermediate staphylococcus aureus (VISA/GISA)
        Vancomycin (glycopeptide) resistant enterococcus (VRE)
        Vancomycin (glycopeptide) resistant staphylococcus aureus (VRSA/GRSA)

        ● **V09.80 Without mention of resistance to multiple drugs**

        ● **V09.81 With resistance to multiple drugs**

    ● **V09.9 Infection with drug-resistant microorganisms, unspecified**
        Drug resistance NOS

        ● **V09.90 Without mention of multiple drug resistance**

        ● **V09.91 With multiple drug resistance**
            Multiple drug resistance NOS

OGCR Section I.C.2.d
When a primary malignancy has been previously excised or eradicated from its site and there is no further treatment directed to that site and there is no evidence of any existing primary malignancy, a code from category V10 should be used to indicate the former site of the malignancy. Any mention of extension, invasion, or metastasis to another site is coded as a secondary malignant neoplasm to that site. The secondary site may be the principal or first-listed with the V10 code used as a secondary code.

OGCR Section I.C.18.d.4
Personal history codes explain a patient's past medical condition that no longer exists and is not receiving any treatment, but that has the potential for recurrence, and therefore may require continued monitoring. The exceptions to this general rule are category V14, Personal history of allergy to medicinal agents, and subcategory V15.0, Allergy, other than to medicinal agents. A person who has had an allergic episode to a substance or food in the past should always be considered allergic to the substance.

PERSONS WITH POTENTIAL HEALTH HAZARDS RELATED TO PERSONAL AND FAMILY HISTORY (V10–V19)

Excludes *obstetric patients where the possibility that the fetus might be affected is the reason for observation or management during pregnancy (655.0–655.9)*

● **V10 Personal history of malignant neoplasm**
    Coding Clinic: 1994, Q2, P8

    ● **V10.0 Gastrointestinal tract**
        History of conditions classifiable to 140–159
        Excludes *personal history of malignant carcinoid tumor (V10.91)*
            personal history of malignant neuroendocrine tumor (V10.91)

        ● **V10.00 Gastrointestinal tract, unspecified** ⊕

        ● **V10.01 Tongue** ⊕

        ● **V10.02 Other and unspecified oral cavity and pharynx** ⊕

        ● **V10.03 Esophagus** ⊕

        ● **V10.04 Stomach** ⊕

        ● **V10.05 Large intestine** ⊕
            Coding Clinic: 1999, Q3, P7-8; 1995, Q1, P3-4

        ● **V10.06 Rectum, rectosigmoid junction, and anus** ⊕

        ● **V10.07 Liver** ⊕

        ● **V10.09 Other** ⊕
            Coding Clinic: 2003, Q4, P111

    ● **V10.1 Trachea, bronchus, and lung**
        History of conditions classifiable to 162
        Excludes *personal history of malignant carcinoid tumor (V10.91)*
            personal history of malignant neuroendocrine tumor (V10.91)

        ● **V10.11 Bronchus and lung** ⊕
            Coding Clinic: 2013, Q1, P8

        ● **V10.12 Trachea** ⊕

    ● **V10.2 Other respiratory and intrathoracic organs**
        History of conditions classifiable to 160, 161, 163–165

        ● **V10.20 Respiratory organ, unspecified** ⊕

        ● **V10.21 Larynx** ⊕
            Coding Clinic: 2003, Q4, P108,110

        ● **V10.22 Nasal cavities, middle ear, and accessory sinuses** ⊕

        ● **V10.29 Other** ⊕

    ● **V10.3 Breast** ⊕
        History of conditions classifiable to 174 and 175
        Coding Clinic: 2012, Q1, P11; 2007, Q3, P4; Q1, P3-8; 2003, Q2, P3-5; 2001, Q4, P66; 1997, Q4, P50; 1995, Q4, P53; 1990, Q1, P21

● **V10.4 Genital organs**
    History of conditions classifiable to 179–187
    ● **V10.40 Female genital organ, unspecified** ♀ 🔍
    ● **V10.41 Cervix uteri** ♀ 🔍
        Coding Clinic: 2007, Q4, P99-101
    ● **V10.42 Other parts of uterus** ♀ 🔍
    ● **V10.43 Ovary** ♀ 🔍
    ● **V10.44 Other female genital organs** ♀ 🔍
    ● **V10.45 Male genital organ, unspecified** ♂ 🔍
    ● **V10.46 Prostate** ♂ 🔍
        Coding Clinic: 2009, Q1, P5; 1994, Q2, P12; 1984, May-June, P10
    ● **V10.47 Testis** ♂ 🔍
    ● **V10.48 Epididymis** ♂ 🔍
    ● **V10.49 Other male genital organs** ♂ 🔍
● **V10.5 Urinary organs**
    History of conditions classifiable to 188 and 189
    Excludes *personal history of malignant carcinoid tumor (V10.91)*
          personal history of malignant neuroendocrine tumor (V10.91)
    Coding Clinic: 1995, Q2, P8
    ● **V10.50 Urinary organ, unspecified** 🔍
    ● **V10.51 Bladder** 🔍
        Coding Clinic: 1995, Q2, P8;1985, July-Aug, P16
    ● **V10.52 Kidney** 🔍
        Excludes *renal pelvis (V10.53)*
        Coding Clinic: 2004, Q2, P4
    ● **V10.53 Renal pelvis** 🔍
    ● **V10.59 Other** 🔍
● **V10.6 Leukemia**
    Conditions classifiable to 204–208
    Excludes *leukemia in remission (204–208)*
    Coding Clinic: 1992, Q2, P13; 1985, May-June, P8-9
    ● **V10.60 Leukemia, unspecified** 🔍
    ● **V10.61 Lymphoid leukemia** 🔍
    ● **V10.62 Myeloid leukemia** 🔍
    ● **V10.63 Monocytic leukemia** 🔍
    ● **V10.69 Other** 🔍
● **V10.7 Other lymphatic and hematopoietic neoplasms**
    Conditions classifiable to 200–203
    Excludes *listed conditions in 200–203 in remission*
    Coding Clinic: 1985, May-June, P8-9
    ● **V10.71 Lymphosarcoma and reticulosarcoma** 🔍
    ● **V10.72 Hodgkin's disease** 🔍
    ● **V10.79 Other** 🔍
● **V10.8 Personal history of malignant neoplasm of other sites**
    History of conditions classifiable to 170–173, 190–195
    Excludes *personal history of malignant carcinoid tumor (V10.91)*
          personal history of malignant neuroendocrine tumor (V10.91)
    ● **V10.81 Bone** 🔍
        Coding Clinic: 2003, Q2, P13
    ● **V10.82 Malignant melanoma of skin** 🔍
    ● **V10.83 Other malignant neoplasm of skin** 🔍
    ● **V10.84 Eye** 🔍
    ● **V10.85 Brain** 🔍
        Coding Clinic: 2001, Q1, P6-7
    ● **V10.86 Other parts of nervous system** 🔍
        Excludes *peripheral, sympathetic, and parasympathetic nerves (V10.89)*
    ● **V10.87 Thyroid** 🔍
    ● **V10.88 Other endocrine glands and related structures** 🔍
    ● **V10.89 Other** 🔍

● **V10.9 Other and unspecified personal history of malignant neoplasm**
    ● **V10.90 Personal history of unspecified malignant neoplasm** 🔍
        Personal history of malignant neoplasm NOS
        Excludes *personal history of malignant carcinoid tumor (V10.91)*
            personal history of malignant neuroendocrine tumor (V10.91)
            personal history of Merkel cell carcinoma (V10.91)
    ● **V10.91 Personal history of malignant neuroendocrine tumor** 🔍
        Personal history of malignant carcinoid tumor NOS
        Personal history of malignant neuroendocrine tumor NOS
        Personal history of Merkel cell carcinoma NOS
        Code first any continuing functional activity, such as:
          carcinoid syndrome (259.2)

● **V11 Personal history of mental disorder**
    ● **V11.0 Schizophrenia** 🔍
        Excludes *that in remission (295.0–295.9 with fifth-digit 5)*
        Coding Clinic: 1995, Q3, P6
    ● **V11.1 Affective disorders** 🔍
        Personal history of manic-depressive psychosis
        Excludes *that in remission (296.0–296.6 with fifth-digit 5, 6)*
    ● **V11.2 Neurosis** 🔍
    ● **V11.3 Alcoholism** 🔍
    ● **V11.4 Combat and operational stress reaction** 🔍   A
    ● **V11.8 Other mental disorders** 🔍
    ● **V11.9 Unspecified mental disorder** 🔍

● **V12 Personal history of certain other diseases**
    Coding Clinic: 2005, Q4, P94-100; 1992, Q3, P11
    ● **V12.0 Infectious and parasitic diseases**
        Excludes *personal history of infectious diseases specific to a body system*
        ● **V12.00 Unspecified infectious and parasitic disease** 🔍
        ● **V12.01 Tuberculosis** 🔍
        ● **V12.02 Poliomyelitis** 🔍
        ● **V12.03 Malaria** 🔍
        ● **V12.04 Methicillin resistant Staphylococcus aureus** 🔍
          MRSA
          Coding Clinic: 2008, Q4, P69-73
        ● **V12.09 Other** 🔍
    ● **V12.1 Nutritional deficiency** 🔍
    ● **V12.2 Personal history endocrine, metabolic, and immunity disorders**
        Excludes *history of allergy (V14.0–V14.9, V15.01–V15.09)*
        Coding Clinic: 2007, Q3, P5-6
        ● **V12.21 Gestational diabetes** ♀ 🔍
        ● **V12.29 Other endocrine, metabolic, and immunity disorders** 🔍
    ● **V12.3 Diseases of blood and blood-forming organs** 🔍

V01-V91

V01-V91

- ● **V12.4 Disorders of nervous system and sense organs**
  - ● **V12.40 Unspecified disorder of nervous system and sense organs** ✎
  - ● **V12.41 Benign neoplasm of the brain** ✎
  - ● **V12.42 Infections of the central nervous system** ✎
    Encephalitis
    Meningitis
  - ● **V12.49 Other disorders of nervous system and sense organs** ✎
    Coding Clinic: 1998, Q4, P59-60
- ● **V12.5 Diseases of circulatory system**
  - **Excludes** *history of anaphylactic shock (V13.81)*
    old myocardial infarction (412)
    postmyocardial infarction syndrome (411.0)
  - ● **V12.50 Unspecified circulatory disease** ✎
  - ● **V12.51 Venous thrombosis and embolism** ✎
    - **Excludes** *pulmonary embolism (V12.55)*
    Coding Clinic: 2011, Q1, P20; 2006, Q3, P12; 2003, Q4, P108; 2002, Q1, P15-16
  - ● **V12.52 Thrombophlebitis** ✎
  - ● **V12.53 Sudden cardiac arrest** ✎
    Sudden cardiac death successfully resuscitated
    Coding Clinic: 2007, Q4, P99-101
  - ● **V12.54 Transient ischemic attack (TIA), and cerebral infarction without residual deficits** ✎
    Prolonged reversible ischemic neurological deficit (PRIND)
    Reversible ischemic neurologic deficit (RIND)
    Stroke NOS without residual deficits
    - **Excludes** *history of traumatic brain injury (V15.52)*
      late effects of cerebrovascular disease (438.0–438.9)
    Coding Clinic: 2007, Q4, P99-101; 2007, Q2, P3
    OGCR Section I.C.7.d.3
    Assign code V12.54, Transient ischemic attack (TIA), and cerebral infarction without residual deficits (and not a code from category 438) as an additional code for history of cerebrovascular disease when no neurologic deficits are present.
  - ● **V12.55 Pulmonary embolism** ✎
  - ● **V12.59 Other** ✎
    Coding Clinic: 2007, Q2, P3; 1997, Q4, P35-37
- ● **V12.6 Diseases of respiratory system**
  - **Excludes** *tuberculosis (V12.01)*
  - ● **V12.60 Unspecified disease of respiratory system** ✎
  - ● **V12.61 Pneumonia (recurrent)** ✎
  - ● **V12.69 Other diseases of respiratory system** ✎
- ● **V12.7 Diseases of digestive system**
    Coding Clinic: 1995, Q1, P3; 1992, Q3, P11; 1989, Q2, P16
  - ● **V12.70 Unspecified digestive disease** ✎
  - ● **V12.71 Peptic ulcer disease** ✎
  - ● **V12.72 Colonic polyps** ✎
    Coding Clinic: 2002, Q3, P14-15
  - ● **V12.79 Other** ✎
- ● **V13 Personal history of other diseases**
  - ● **V13.0 Disorders of urinary system**
    - ● **V13.00 Unspecified urinary disorder** ✎
    - ● **V13.01 Urinary calculi** ✎
    - ● **V13.02 Urinary (tract) infection** ✎
    - ● **V13.03 Nephrotic syndrome** ✎
    - ● **V13.09 Other** ✎
      Coding Clinic: 1996, Q2, P7x2
  - ● **V13.1 Trophoblastic disease** ♀ ✎
    - **Excludes** *supervision during a current pregnancy (V23.1)*

- ● **V13.2 Other genital system and obstetric disorders**
  - **Excludes** *supervision during a current pregnancy of a woman with poor obstetric history (V23.0–V23.9)*
    recurrent pregnancy loss (646.3)
    without current pregnancy (629.81)
  - ● **V13.21 Personal history of pre-term labor** ♀ ✎
    - **Excludes** *current pregnancy with history of pre-term labor (V23.41)*
  - ● **V13.22 Personal history of cervical dysplasia** ♀ ✎
    Personal history of conditions classifiable to 622.10–622.12
    - **Excludes** *personal history of malignant neoplasm of cervix uteri (V10.41)*
    Coding Clinic: 2007, Q4, P99-101
  - ● **V13.23 Personal history of vaginal dysplasia** ♀ ✎
    Personal history of conditions classifiable to 623.0
    - **Excludes** *personal history of malignant neoplasm of vagina (V10.44)*
  - ● **V13.24 Personal history of vulvar dysplasia** ♀ ✎
    Personal history of conditions classifiable to 624.01-624.02
    - **Excludes** *personal history of malignant neoplasm of vulva (V10.44)*
  - ● **V13.29 Other genital system and obstetric disorders** ♀ ✎
- ● **V13.3 Diseases of skin and subcutaneous tissue** ✎
- ● **V13.4 Arthritis** ✎
- ● **V13.5 Other musculoskeletal disorders**
  - ● **V13.51 Pathologic fracture** ✎
    Healed pathologic fracture
    - **Excludes** *personal history of traumatic fracture (V15.51)*
  - ● **V13.52 Stress fracture** ✎
    Healed stress fracture
    - **Excludes** *personal history of traumatic fracture (V15.51)*
  - ● **V13.59 Other musculoskeletal disorders** ✎
- ● **V13.6 Congenital (corrected) malformations**
  - ● **V13.61 Personal history of (corrected) hypospadias** ♂ ✎
  - ● **V13.62 Personal history of other (corrected) congenital malformations of genitourinary system** ✎
  - ● **V13.63 Personal history of (corrected) congenital malformations of nervous system** ✎
  - ● **V13.64 Personal history of (corrected) congenital malformations of eye, ear, face and neck** ✎
    Corrected cleft lip and palate
  - ● **V13.65 Personal history of (corrected) congenital malformations of heart and circulatory system** ✎
    Coding Clinic: 2010, Q4, P137
  - ● **V13.66 Personal history of (corrected) congenital malformations of respiratory system** ✎
  - ● **V13.67 Personal history of (corrected) congenital malformations of digestive system** ✎
  - ● **V13.68 Personal history of (corrected) congenital malformations of integument, limbs, and musculoskeletal systems** ✎
  - ● **V13.69 Personal history of other (corrected) congenital malformations** ✎
    Coding Clinic: 2004, Q1, P16-17
- ● **V13.7 Perinatal problems** ✎
  - **Excludes** *low birth weight status (V21.30–V21.35)*

◀ New   ◀▦ Revised   ~~deleted~~ Deleted   Excludes   Includes   Use additional   Code first
● Use Additional Digit(s)   ▶ Manifestation Code   OGCR Official Guidelines   **Coding Clinic**   (Ex) CC/MCC Exclusions

● **V13.8 Other specified diseases**
    Coding Clinic: 2012, Q1, P11
  ● **V13.81 Anaphylaxis** 🔍
  ● **V13.89 Other specified diseases** 🔍
● **V13.9 Unspecified disease** 🔍

● **V14 Personal history of allergy to medicinal agents**
  ● **V14.0 Penicillin** 🔍
  ● **V14.1 Other antibiotic agent** 🔍
  ● **V14.2 Sulfonamides** 🔍
  ● **V14.3 Other anti-infective agent** 🔍
  ● **V14.4 Anesthetic agent** 🔍
  ● **V14.5 Narcotic agent** 🔍
  ● **V14.6 Analgesic agent** 🔍
  ● **V14.7 Serum or vaccine** 🔍
  ● **V14.8 Other specified medicinal agents** 🔍
  ● **V14.9 Unspecified medicinal agent** 🔍

● **V15 Other personal history presenting hazards to health**
    Excludes *personal history of drug therapy (V87.41–V87.49)*
  ● **V15.0 Allergy, other than to medicinal agents**
     Excludes *allergy to food substance used as base for medicinal agent (V14.0– V14.9)*
   ● **V15.01 Allergy to peanuts** 🔍
   ● **V15.02 Allergy to milk products** 🔍
     Excludes *lactose intolerance (271.3)*
     Coding Clinic: 2003, Q1, P12
   ● **V15.03 Allergy to eggs** 🔍
   ● **V15.04 Allergy to seafood** 🔍
     Seafood (octopus) (squid) ink
     Shellfish
   ● **V15.05 Allergy to other foods** 🔍
     Food additives
     Nuts other than peanuts
   ● **V15.06 Allergy to insects and arachnids** 🔍
     Bugs
     Insect bites and stings
     Spiders
   ● **V15.07 Allergy to latex** 🔍
     Latex sensitivity
   ● **V15.08 Allergy to radiographic dye** 🔍
     Contrast media used for diagnostic x-ray procedures
   ● **V15.09 Other allergy, other than to medicinal agents** 🔍
  ● **V15.1 Surgery to heart and great vessels** 🔍
     Excludes *replacement by transplant or other means (V42.1–V42.2, V43.2–V43.4)*
     Coding Clinic: 2004, Q1, P16-17
  ● **V15.2 Surgery to other organs** 🔍
     Excludes *replacement by transplant or other means (V42.0–V43.8)*
   ● **V15.21 Personal history of undergoing in utero procedure during pregnancy** ♀
   ● **V15.22 Personal history of undergoing in utero procedure while a fetus** 🔍
   ● **V15.29 Surgery to other organs** 🔍
  ● **V15.3 Irradiation** 🔍
     Previous exposure to therapeutic or other ionizing radiation
  ● **V15.4 Psychological trauma**
     Excludes *history of condition classifiable to 290–316 (V11.0–V11.9)*
   ● **V15.41 History of physical abuse** 🔍
     Rape
     Coding Clinic: 1999, Q3, P15
   ● **V15.42 History of emotional abuse** 🔍
     Neglect
     Coding Clinic: 1999, Q3, P15
   ● **V15.49 Other** 🔍
     Coding Clinic: 1999, Q3, P15

● **V15.5 Injury**
  ● **V15.51 Traumatic fracture** 🔍
     Healed traumatic fracture
     Excludes *personal history of pathologic and stress fracture (V13.51, V13.52)*
  ● **V15.52 History of traumatic brain injury** 🔍
     Excludes *personal history of cerebrovascular accident (cerebral infarction) without residual deficits (V12.54)*
  ● **V15.53 Personal history of retained foreign body fully removed** 🔍
  ● **V15.59 Other injury** 🔍
● **V15.6 Poisoning** 🔍
● **V15.7 Contraception** 🔍
     Excludes *current contraceptive management (V25.0–V25.4)*
     presence of intrauterine contraceptive device as incidental finding (V45.5)
● **V15.8 Other specified personal history presenting hazards to health**
     Excludes *contact with and (suspected) exposure to:*
      aromatic compounds and dyes (V87.11-V87.19)
      arsenic and other metals (V87.01-V87.09)
      molds (V87.31)
  ● **V15.80 History of failed moderate sedation** 🔍
     History of failed conscious sedation
  ● **V15.81 Noncompliance with medical treatment** 🔍
     Excludes *noncompliance with renal dialysis (V45.12)*
     Coding Clinic: 2012, Q2, P16-17; 2007, Q3, P11; 2006, Q4, P136; 2003, Q2, P7-8; 2001, Q2, P13; 1999, Q2, P17; Q1, P13-14; 1997, Q2, P11; 1996, Q3, P9
  ● **V15.82 History of tobacco use** 🔍
     Excludes *tobacco dependence (305.1)*
     Coding Clinic: 2009, Q1, P15
  ● **V15.83 Underimmunization status** 🔍
     Delinquent immunization status
     Lapsed immunization schedule status
  ● **V15.84 Contact with and (suspected) exposure to asbestos** 🔍
  ● **V15.85 Contact with and (suspected) exposure to potentially hazardous body fluids** 🔍
  ● **V15.86 Contact with and (suspected) exposure to lead** 🔍
  ● **V15.87 History of extracorporeal membrane oxygenation [ECMO]** 🔍
  ● **V15.88 History of fall** 🔍
     At risk for falling
     Coding Clinic: 2005, Q4, P94-100
  ● **V15.89 Other** 🔍
     Excludes *contact with and (suspected) exposure to other potentially hazardous chemicals (V87.2)*
     contact with and (suspected) exposure to other potentially hazardous substances (V87.39)
     Coding Clinic: 2008, Q3, P6-7; 2007, Q3, P6; 1990, Q1, P21
● **V15.9 Unspecified personal history presenting hazards to health** 🔍

OGCR Section I.C.18.d.3

> Family history codes are for use when a patient has a family member(s) who has had a particular disease that causes the patient to be at higher risk of also contracting the disease.

● **V16 Family history of malignant neoplasm**
    Coding Clinic: 1985, Nov-Dec, P13

  ● **V16.0 Gastrointestinal tract** 🔍
      Family history of condition classifiable to 140–159
      Coding Clinic: 1999, Q1, P4

  ● **V16.1 Trachea, bronchus, and lung** 🔍
      Family history of condition classifiable to 162

  ● **V16.2 Other respiratory and intrathoracic organs** 🔍
      Family history of condition classifiable to 160–161, 163–165

  ● **V16.3 Breast** 🔍
      Family history of condition classifiable to 174
      Coding Clinic: 2004, Q4, P106-107; 2003, Q2, P3-5; 2000, Q2, P8-9; 1995, Q4, P61; 1992, Q1, P11; 1990, Q1, P21

  ● **V16.4 Genital organs**
      Family history of condition classifiable to 179–187

    ● **V16.40 Genital organ, unspecified** 🔍

    ● **V16.41 Ovary** 🔍
        Coding Clinic: 2009, Q3, P21

    ● **V16.42 Prostate** 🔍

    ● **V16.43 Testis** 🔍

    ● **V16.49 Other** 🔍
        Coding Clinic: 2006, Q2, P3,4

  ● **V16.5 Urinary organs**
      Family history of condition classifiable to 188–189

    ● **V16.51 Kidney** 🔍

    ● **V16.52 Bladder** 🔍

    ● **V16.59 Other** 🔍

  ● **V16.6 Leukemia** 🔍
      Family history of condition classifiable to 204–208

  ● **V16.7 Other lymphatic and hematopoietic neoplasms** 🔍
      Family history of condition classifiable to 200–203

  ● **V16.8 Other specified malignant neoplasm** 🔍
      Family history of other condition classifiable to 140–199

  ● **V16.9 Unspecified malignant neoplasm** 🔍

● **V17 Family history of certain chronic disabling diseases**
    Coding Clinic: 1985, Nov-Dec, P13

  ● **V17.0 Psychiatric condition** 🔍
      Excludes *family history of intellectual disabilities (V18.4)*

  ● **V17.1 Stroke (cerebrovascular)** 🔍

  ● **V17.2 Other neurological diseases** 🔍
      Epilepsy   Huntington's chorea

  ● **V17.3 Ischemic heart disease** 🔍

  ● **V17.4 Other cardiovascular diseases**
      Coding Clinic: 2004, Q1, P6-7

    ● **V17.41 Family history of sudden cardiac death (SCD)** 🔍
        Excludes *family history of ischemic heart disease (V17.3)*
                 family history of myocardial infarction (V17.3)

    ● **V17.49 Family history of other cardiovascular diseases** 🔍
        Family history of cardiovascular disease NOS

  ● **V17.5 Asthma** 🔍

  ● **V17.6 Other chronic respiratory conditions** 🔍

  ● **V17.7 Arthritis** 🔍

  ● **V17.8 Other musculoskeletal diseases**

    ● **V17.81 Osteoporosis** 🔍

    ● **V17.89 Other musculoskeletal diseases** 🔍

● **V18 Family history of certain other specific conditions**
    Coding Clinic: 1985, Nov-Dec, P13

  ● **V18.0 Diabetes mellitus** 🔍
      Coding Clinic: 2005, Q2, P21; 2004, Q1, P8

  ● **V18.1 Other endocrine and metabolic diseases**

    ● **V18.11 Multiple endocrine neoplasia [MEN] syndrome**

    ● **V18.19 Other endocrine and metabolic diseases** 🔍

  ● **V18.2 Anemia** 🔍

  ● **V18.3 Other blood disorders** 🔍

  ● **V18.4 Intellectual disabilities** 🔍

  ● **V18.5 Digestive disorders**

    ● **V18.51 Colonic polyps** 🔍
        Excludes *family history of malignant neoplasm of gastrointestinal tract (V16.0)*

    ● **V18.59 Other digestive disorders** 🔍

  ● **V18.6 Kidney diseases**

    ● **V18.61 Polycystic kidney** 🔍

    ● **V18.69 Other kidney diseases** 🔍

  ● **V18.7 Other genitourinary diseases** 🔍

  ● **V18.8 Infectious and parasitic diseases** 🔍

  ● **V18.9 Genetic disease carrier** 🔍

● **V19 Family history of other conditions**
    Coding Clinic: 1985, Nov-Dec, P13

  ● **V19.0 Blindness or visual loss** 🔍

  ● **V19.1 Other eye disorders**

    ● **V19.11 Glaucoma** 🔍

    ● **V19.19 Other specified eye disorder** 🔍

  ● **V19.2 Deafness or hearing loss** 🔍

  ● **V19.3 Other ear disorders** 🔍

  ● **V19.4 Skin conditions** 🔍

  ● **V19.5 Congenital anomalies** 🔍

  ● **V19.6 Allergic disorders** 🔍

  ● **V19.7 Consanguinity** 🔍

  ● **V19.8 Other condition** 🔍

PERSONS ENCOUNTERING HEALTH SERVICES IN CIRCUMSTANCES RELATED TO REPRODUCTION AND DEVELOPMENT (V20–V29)

● **V20 Health supervision of infant or child**

  V20.0 Foundling 🔍   P

  ● **V20.1 Other healthy infant or child receiving care** 🔍   P
      Medical or nursing care supervision of healthy infant in cases of:
        maternal illness, physical or psychiatric
        socioeconomic adverse condition at home
        too many children at home preventing or interfering with normal care
      Coding Clinic: 2000, Q1, P25; 1993, Q4, P36; 1989, Q3, P14

  ● **V20.2 Routine infant or child health check** 🔍   P
      Developmental testing of infant or child
      Health check for child over 28 days old
      Immunizations appropriate for age
      Routine vision and hearing testing
      Excludes *health check for child under 29 days old (V20.31-V20.32)*
                 newborn health supervision (V20.31-V20.32)
                 special screening for developmental handicaps (V79.3)
      Use additional code(s) to identify:
        Special screening examination(s) performed (V73.0–V82.9)
      Coding Clinic: 2009, Q1, P15; 2004, Q1, P15-16x2

New   ◀━ Revised   ~~deleted~~ Deleted   Excludes   Includes   Use additional   Code first

1014   ● Use Additional Digit(s)   ▶ Manifestation Code   **OGCR** Official Guidelines   **Coding Clinic**   (Ex) CC/MCC Exclusions

● **V20.3 Newborn health supervision**
Health check for child under 29 days old
Excludes *health check for child over 28 days old (V20.2)*

　● **V20.31 Health supervision for newborn under 8 days old** 🐾 　　　　　　N
Health check for newborn under 8 days old

　● **V20.32 Health supervision for newborn 8 to 28 days old** 🐾 　　　　　N
Health check for newborn 8 to 28 days old
Newborn weight check

● **V21 Constitutional states in development**
● **V21.0 Period of rapid growth in childhood** 🐾
● **V21.1 Puberty** 🐾
● **V21.2 Other adolescence** 🐾
● **V21.3 Low birth weight status**
Excludes *history of perinatal problems (V13.7)*

　● **V21.30 Low birth weight status, unspecified** 🐾
　● **V21.31 Low birth weight status, less than 500 grams** 🐾
　● **V21.32 Low birth weight status, 500–999 grams** 🐾
Coding Clinic: 2009, Q4, P151
　● **V21.33 Low birth weight status, 1000–1499 grams** 🐾
　● **V21.34 Low birth weight status, 1500–1999 grams** 🐾
　● **V21.35 Low birth weight status, 2000–2500 grams** 🐾

● **V21.8 Other specified constitutional states in development** 🐾
● **V21.9 Unspecified constitutional state in development** 🐾

● **V22 Normal pregnancy**
Excludes *pregnancy examination or test, pregnancy unconfirmed (V72.40)*
Coding Clinic: 2012, Q1, P10; 2007, Q4, P124-125

OGCR　Section I.C.11.b.1
For routine outpatient prenatal visits when no complications are present codes V22.0, Supervision of normal first pregnancy, and V22.1, Supervision of other normal pregnancy, should be used as the first-listed diagnoses. These codes should not be used in conjunction with chapter 11 codes.

● **V22.0 Supervision of normal first pregnancy** ♀ 🐾
Coding Clinic: 1999, Q3, P16; 1990, Q1, P10; 1984, Nov-Dec, P18
● **V22.1 Supervision of other normal pregnancy** ♀ 🐾
Coding Clinic: 1999, Q3, P16; 1990, Q1, P10
● **V22.2 Pregnant state, incidental** ♀ 🐾
Pregnant state NOS
Coding Clinic: 1998, Q2, P13-14; 1994, Q2, P14

OGCR　Section I.C.11.b.2
For routine prenatal outpatient visits for patients with high-risk pregnancies, a code from category V23, Supervision of high-risk pregnancy, should be used as the first-listed diagnosis. Secondary chapter 11 codes may be used in conjunction with these codes if appropriate.

● **V23 Supervision of high-risk pregnancy**
Coding Clinic: 2012, Q1, P10; 1990, Q1, P10
● **V23.0 Pregnancy with history of infertility** ♀ 🐾　M
● **V23.1 Pregnancy with history of trophoblastic disease** ♀ 🐾 M
Pregnancy with history of:
hydatidiform mole
vesicular mole
Excludes *that without current pregnancy (V13.1)*
● **V23.2 Pregnancy with history of abortion** ♀ 🐾　M
Pregnancy with history of conditions classifiable to 634–638
Excludes *recurrent pregnancy loss:*
care during pregnancy (646.3)
that without current pregnancy (629.81)
● **V23.3 Grand multiparity** ♀ 🐾　M
Excludes *care in relation to labor and delivery (659.4)*
that without current pregnancy (V61.5)

● **V23.4 Pregnancy with other poor obstetric history**
Pregnancy with history of other conditions classifiable to 630–676
　● **V23.41 Pregnancy with history of pre-term labor** ♀ 🐾　　　　　M
　● **V23.42 Pregnancy with history of ectopic pregnancy** ♀ 🐾　　　　M
　● **V23.49 Pregnancy with other poor obstetric history** ♀ 🐾　　　　M
● **V23.5 Pregnancy with other poor reproductive history** ♀ 🐾 M
Pregnancy with history of stillbirth or neonatal death
● **V23.7 Insufficient prenatal care** ♀ 🐾　M
History of little or no prenatal care
● **V23.8 Other high-risk pregnancy**
Coding Clinic: 1998, Q4, P50-51
　● **V23.81 Elderly primigravida** ♀ 🐾　　M
First pregnancy in a woman who will be 35 years of age or older at expected date of delivery
Excludes *elderly primigravida complicating pregnancy (659.5)*
Coding Clinic: 1998, Q4, P58
　● **V23.82 Elderly multigravida** ♀ 🐾　　M
Second or more pregnancy in a woman who will be 35 years of age or older at expected date of delivery
Excludes *elderly multigravida complicating pregnancy (659.6)*
Coding Clinic: 2013, Q1, P19; 2011, Q4, P133
　● **V23.83 Young primigravida** ♀ 🐾　　M
First pregnancy in a female less than 16 years old at expected date of delivery
Excludes *young primigravida complicating pregnancy (659.8)*
　● **V23.84 Young multigravida** ♀ 🐾　　M
Second or more pregnancy in a female less than 16 years old at expected date of delivery
Excludes *young multigravida complicating pregnancy (659.8)*
　● **V23.85 Pregnancy resulting from assisted reproductive technology** ♀ 🐾　M A
Pregnancy resulting from in vitro fertilization
　● **V23.86 Pregnancy with history of in utero procedure during previous pregnancy** ♀ 🐾　M
Excludes *management of pregnancy affected by in utero procedure during current pregnancy (679.0–679.1)*
　● **V23.87 Pregnancy with inconclusive fetal viability** ♀ 🐾　　M
Encounter to determine fetal viability of pregnancy
　● **V23.89 Other high-risk pregnancy** ♀ 🐾　　M
Coding Clinic: 2006, Q3, P14
● **V23.9 Unspecified high-risk pregnancy** ♀ 🐾　M

OGCR Section I.C.18.d.8

The follow-up codes (V24, V67 and V89), are used to explain continuing surveillance following completed treatment of a disease, condition, or injury. They imply that the condition has been fully treated and no longer exists. They should not be confused with aftercare codes that explain current treatment for a healing condition or its sequelae. Follow-up codes may be used in conjunction with history codes to provide the full picture of the healed condition and its treatment. The follow-up code is sequenced first, followed by the history code. A follow-up code may be used to explain repeated visits. Should a condition be found to have recurred on the follow-up visit, then the diagnosis code should be used in place of the follow-up code.

● **V24 Postpartum care and examination**
  V24.0 Immediately after delivery ♀ ◐   **M**
      Care and observation in uncomplicated cases
      Coding Clinic: 2006, Q3, P11

    OGCR Section I.C.10.i.5
      When the mother delivers outside the hospital prior to admission and is admitted for routine postpartum care and no complications are noted, code V24.0, Postpartum care and examination immediately after delivery, should be assigned as the principal diagnosis.

  ● **V24.1 Lactating mother** ♀ ◐
      Supervision of lactation
      Coding Clinic: 2012, Q3, P7

  ● **V24.2 Routine postpartum follow-up** ♀ ◐

● **V25 Encounter for contraceptive management**
  ● **V25.0 General counseling and advice**
    ● **V25.01 Prescription of oral contraceptives** ♀ ◐
    ● **V25.02 Initiation of other contraceptive measures** ◐
        Fitting of diaphragm
        Prescription of foams, creams, or other agents
        Coding Clinic: 1997, Q3, P7
    ● **V25.03 Encounter for emergency contraceptive counseling and prescription** ◐
        Encounter for postcoital contraceptive counseling and prescription
    ● **V25.04 Counseling and instruction in natural family planning to avoid pregnancy** ◐
        Coding Clinic: 2007, Q4, P99-101
    ● **V25.09 Other** ◐
        Family planning advice
  ● **V25.1 Encounter for insertion or removal of intrauterine contraceptive device**
      Excludes *encounter for routine checking of intrauterine contraceptive device (V25.42)*
    ● **V25.11 Encounter for insertion of intrauterine contraceptive device** ♀ ◐
    ● **V25.12 Encounter for removal of intrauterine contraceptive device** ♀ ◐
    ● **V25.13 Encounter for removal and reinsertion of intrauterine contraceptive device** ♀ ◐
        Encounter for replacement of intrauterine contraceptive device
  V25.2 Sterilization ◐
      Admission for interruption of fallopian tubes or vas deferens
  V25.3 Menstrual extraction ♀ ◐
      Menstrual regulation

  ● **V25.4 Surveillance of previously prescribed contraceptive methods**
      Checking, reinsertion, or removal of contraceptive device
      Repeat prescription for contraceptive method
      Routine examination in connection with contraceptive maintenance
    ● **V25.40 Contraceptive surveillance, unspecified** ◐
    ● **V25.41 Contraceptive pill** ♀ ◐
    ● **V25.42 Intrauterine contraceptive device** ♀ ◐
        Checking of intrauterine contraceptive device
        Excludes *insertion or removal of intrauterine contraceptive device (V25.11-V25.13)*
                    presence of intrauterine contraceptive device as incidental finding (V45.5)
    ● **V25.43 Implantable subdermal contraceptive** ♀ ◐
    ● **V25.49 Other contraceptive method** ◐
        Coding Clinic: 1997, Q3, P7
  ● **V25.5 Insertion of implantable subdermal contraceptive** ♀ ◐
  ● **V25.8 Other specified contraceptive management** ◐
      Postvasectomy sperm count
      Excludes *sperm count following sterilization reversal (V26.22)*
                  sperm count for fertility testing (V26.21)
      Coding Clinic: 1996, Q3, P9
  ● **V25.9 Unspecified contraceptive management** ◐

● **V26 Procreative management**
  V26.0 Tuboplasty or vasoplasty after previous sterilization ◐
      Coding Clinic: 1995, Q2, P10
  ● **V26.1 Artificial insemination** ♀ ◐
  ● **V26.2 Investigation and testing**
      Excludes *postvasectomy sperm count (V25.8)*
      Coding Clinic: 1996, Q2, P9; 1985, Nov-Dec, P15
    ● **V26.21 Fertility testing** ◐
        Fallopian insufflation
        Sperm count for fertility testing
        Excludes *genetic counseling and testing (V26.31–V26.39)*
    ● **V26.22 Aftercare following sterilization reversal** ◐
        Fallopian insufflation following sterilization reversal
        Sperm count following sterilization reversal
    ● **V26.29 Other investigation and testing** ◐

    OGCR Section I.C.18.d.3
      If the purpose of the encounter is genetic counseling associated with procreative management, a code from subcategory V26.3 should be assigned as the first-listed code, followed by a code from category V84, Genetic susceptibility to disease. Additional codes should be assigned for any applicable family or personal history.

  ● **V26.3 Genetic counseling and testing**
      Excludes *fertility testing (V26.21)*
                  nonprocreative genetic screening (V82.71, V82.79)
      Coding Clinic: 2006, Q4, P117; 2005, Q4, P94-100
    ● **V26.31 Testing of female genetic disease carrier status** ♀ ◐
    ● **V26.32 Other genetic testing of female** ♀ ◐
        Use additional code to identify recurrent pregnancy loss (629.81, 646.3)
    ● **V26.33 Genetic counseling** ◐
    ● **V26.34 Testing of male for genetic disease carrier status** ♂ ◐
    ● **V26.35 Encounter for testing of male partner of female with recurrent pregnancy loss** ♂ ◐
    ● **V26.39 Other genetic testing of male** ♂ ◐

● **V26.4   General counseling and advice**
   ● **V26.41   Procreative counseling and advice using natural family planning** 🔖
      Coding Clinic: 2007, Q4, P99-101
   ● **V26.42   Encounter for fertility preservation counseling**
      Encounter for fertility preservation counseling prior to cancer therapy
      Encounter for fertility preservation counseling prior to surgical removal of gonads
   ● **V26.49   Other procreative management counseling and advice** 🔖
● **V26.5   Sterilization status**
   ● **V26.51   Tubal ligation status** ♀ 🔖
      Excludes   *infertility not due to previous tubal ligation (628.0–628.9)*
   ● **V26.52   Vasectomy status** ♂ 🔖
● **V26.8   Other specified procreative management**
   ● **V26.81   Encounter for assisted reproductive fertility procedure cycle** ♀ 🔖
      Patient undergoing in vitro fertilization cycle
      Use additional code to identify the type of infertility
      Excludes   *pre-cycle diagnosis and testing - code to reason for encounter*
      Coding Clinic: 2007, Q4, P99-101
   ● **V26.82   Encounter for fertility preservation procedure** 🔖
      Encounter for fertility preservation counseling prior to cancer therapy
      Encounter for fertility preservation procedure prior to surgical removal of gonads
   ● **V26.89   Other specified procreative management** 🔖
● **V26.9   Unspecified procreative management** 🔖

OGCR   Section I.C.11.h.3
V27.0, Single liveborn, is the only outcome of delivery code appropriate for use with 650.

OGCR   Section I.C.11.k.4
When an attempted termination of pregnancy results in a liveborn fetus assign code 644.21 with an appropriate code from category V27, Outcome of Delivery. The procedure code for the attempted termination of pregnancy should also be assigned.

OGCR   Section I.C.11.b.5
An outcome of delivery code, V27.0-V27.9, should be included on every maternal record when a delivery has occurred. These codes are not to be used on subsequent records or on the newborn record.

● **V27   Outcome of delivery**
   Note: This category is intended for the coding of the outcome of delivery on the mother's record.
   Coding Clinic: 1991, Q2, P16
   ● **V27.0   Single liveborn** ♀ 🔖   M
      Coding Clinic: 2011, Q4, P133; 2008, Q4, P192; 2005, Q4, P81; 2003, Q2, P9; 2002, Q2, P10; 2000, Q3, P5; 1998, Q4, P76-77
   ● **V27.1   Single stillborn** ♀ 🔖   M
      Coding Clinic: 2001, Q1, P11-12
   ● **V27.2   Twins, both liveborn** ♀ 🔖   M
      Coding Clinic: 1992, Q3, P10
   ● **V27.3   Twins, one liveborn and one stillborn** ♀ 🔖   M
   ● **V27.4   Twins, both stillborn** ♀ 🔖   M
   ● **V27.5   Other multiple birth, all liveborn** ♀ 🔖   M
   ● **V27.6   Other multiple birth, some liveborn** ♀ 🔖   M
   ● **V27.7   Other multiple birth, all stillborn** ♀ 🔖   M
   ● **V27.9   Unspecified outcome of delivery** ♀ 🔖   M
      Routine prenatal care (V22.0–V23.9)

● **V28   Encounter for antenatal screening of mother**
   Excludes   *abnormal findings on screening - code to findings*
      suspected fetal conditions affecting management of pregnancy (655.00–655.93, 656.00–656.93, 657.00–657.03, 658.00–658.93)
      suspected fetal conditions not found (V89.01-V89.09)

   OGCR   Section I.C.18.d.5
   See V28, Antenatal screening; V73-V82 to report special screening examinations.

   ● **V28.0   Screening for chromosomal anomalies by amniocentesis** ♀ 🔖   M
   ● **V28.1   Screening for raised alpha-fetoprotein levels in amniotic fluid** ♀ 🔖   M
   ● **V28.2   Other screening based on amniocentesis** ♀ 🔖   M
   ● **V28.3   Encounter for routine screening for malformation using ultrasonics** ♀ 🔖
      Encounter for routine fetal ultrasound NOS
      Excludes   *encounter for fetal anatomic survey (V28.81) genetic counseling and testing (V26.31–V26.39)*
   ● **V28.4   Screening for fetal growth retardation using ultrasonics** ♀ 🔖
   ● **V28.5   Screening for isoimmunization** ♀ 🔖
   ● **V28.6   Screening for Streptococcus B** ♀ 🔖   M
   ● **V28.8   Other specified antenatal screening**
      Coding Clinic: 1999, Q3, P16
      ● **V28.81   Encounter for fetal anatomic survey** ♀ 🔖   M
      ● **V28.82   Encounter for screening for risk of pre-term labor** ♀ 🔖   M
      ● **V28.89   Other specified antenatal screening** ♀ 🔖   M
         Chorionic villus sampling
         Genomic screening
         Nuchal translucency testing
         Proteomic screening
   ● **V28.9   Unspecified antenatal screening** ♀ 🔖

● **V29   Observation and evaluation of newborns for suspected condition not found**
   Note: This category is to be used for newborns, within the neonatal period (the first 28 days of life), who are suspected of having an abnormal condition resulting from exposure from the mother or the birth process, but without signs or symptoms, and which, after examination and observation, is found not to exist.
   Excludes   *suspected fetal conditions not found (V89.01–V89.09)*
   Coding Clinic: 2000, Q1, P25-26

   V29.0   Observation for suspected infectious condition 🔖   N
      Coding Clinic: 2001, Q1, P10
   V29.1   Observation for suspected neurological condition 🔖   N
   V29.2   Observation for suspected respiratory condition 🔖   N
   ● **V29.3   Observation for suspected genetic or metabolic condition** 🔖   N
      Coding Clinic: 2005, Q2, P21; 2004, Q1, P8; 1998, Q4, P59
   V29.8   Observation for other specified suspected condition 🔖   N
      Coding Clinic: 2003, Q2, P15-16
   ● **V29.9   Observation for unspecified suspected condition** 🔖   N
      Coding Clinic: 2002, Q1, P6-7

OGCR Section I.C.15.d.1
Assign a code from category V29, Observation and evaluation of newborns and infants for suspected conditions not found, to identify those instances when a healthy newborn is evaluated for a suspected condition that is determined after study not to be present. Do not use a code from category V29 when the patient has identified signs or symptoms of a suspected problem; in such cases, code the sign or symptom. A code from category V29 may also be assigned as a principal code for readmissions or encounters when the V30 code no longer applies. Codes from category V29 are for use only for healthy newborns and infants for which no condition after study is found to be present.

OGCR   Section I.C.15.d.2
A V29 code is to be used as a secondary code after the V30.

N   Newborn: 0   P   Pediatric: 0–17   M   Maternity: 12–55   A   Adult: 15–124   ♀ Females Only   ♂ Males Only
● Unacceptable Principal Diagnosis   🔖 Complication\Comorbidity   🔖 Major C\C   🔖 Present on Admission Requirement   🔖 Hospital Acquired Condition   **1017**

OGCR   Section I.C.18.d.6

There are three observation V code categories. They are for use in very limited circumstances when a person is being observed for a suspected condition that is ruled out. The observation codes are not for use if an injury or illness or any signs or symptoms related to the suspected condition are present. In such cases the diagnosis/symptom code is used with the corresponding E code to identify any external cause. The observation codes are to be used as principal diagnosis only. The only exception to this is when the principal diagnosis is required to be a code from the V30, Live born infant, category. Then the V29 observation code is sequenced after the V30 code. Additional codes may be used in addition to the observation code but only if they are unrelated to the suspected condition being observed.

OGCR   Section I.C.15.b

When coding the birth of an infant, assign a code from categories V30-V39, according to the type of birth. A code from this series is assigned as a principal diagnosis, and assigned only once to a newborn at the time of birth.

OGCR   Section I.C.15.c

If the newborn is transferred to another institution, the V30 series is not used at the receiving hospital.

LIVEBORN INFANTS ACCORDING TO TYPE OF BIRTH (V30–V39)

Note: These categories are intended for the coding of liveborn infants who are consuming health care [e.g., crib or bassinet occupancy].

The following fourth-digit subdivisions are for use with categories V30–V39:

> 0   Born in hospital
> ● 1   Born before admission to hospital
> ● 2   Born outside hospital and not hospitalized

The following two fifths-digits are for use with the fourth-digit .0, Born in hospital:

> 0   delivered without mention of cesarean delivery
> 1   delivered by cesarean delivery

● V30   Single liveborn 🔖   N
   Coding Clinic: 2012, Q3, P5; Q2, P17; 2009, Q4, P151x2; 2006, Q3, P10-11;
      2005, Q4, P83-89; Q2, P21; 2004, Q1, P8, 16; 2003, Q4, P67-68;
      Q2, P9; 2001, Q4, P50-51; 2000, Q1, P25-26; 1998, Q4, P46-47, 59;
      1994, Q3, P4; 1993, Q4, P36

● V31   Twin, mate liveborn 🔖   N
   Coding Clinic: 1992, Q3, P10

● V32   Twin, mate stillborn 🔖   N

● V33   Twin, unspecified 🔖   N

● V34   Other multiple, mates all liveborn 🔖   N

● V35   Other multiple, mates all stillborn 🔖   N

● V36   Other multiple, mates live- and stillborn 🔖   N

● V37   Other multiple, unspecified 🔖   N

● V39   Unspecified 🔖   N
         MCE: V39.1 and V39.2 are unacceptable PDx

PERSONS WITH A CONDITION INFLUENCING THEIR HEALTH STATUS (V40–V49)

Note: These categories are intended for use when these conditions are recorded as "diagnoses" or "problems."

● V40   Mental and behavioral problems
   ● V40.0   Problems with learning
   ● V40.1   Problems with communication [including speech]
   ● V40.2   Other mental problems
   ● V40.3   Other behavioral problems
      ▷ V40.31   *Wandering in diseases classified elsewhere*
                  Code first underlying disorder such as:
                     Alzheimer's disease (331.0)
                     autism or pervasive developmental
                        disorder (299.0-299.9)
                     dementia, unspecified, with behavioral
                        disturbance (294.21)
                     intellectual disabilities (317-319)
      ● V40.39   Other specified behavioral problem
   ● V40.9   Unspecified mental or behavioral problem

● V41   Problems with special senses and other special functions
   ● V41.0   Problems with sight
   ● V41.1   Other eye problems
   ● V41.2   Problems with hearing
   ● V41.3   Other ear problems
   ● V41.4   Problems with voice production
   ● V41.5   Problems with smell and taste
   ● V41.6   Problems with swallowing and mastication
   ● V41.7   Problems with sexual function
            Excludes   *marital problems (V61.10)*
                           psychosexual disorders (302.0–302.9)
   ● V41.8   Other problems with special functions
   ● V41.9   Unspecified problem with special functions

● V42   Organ or tissue replaced by transplant
         Includes   homologous or heterologous (animal) (human)
                        transplant organ status
         Coding Clinic: 1998, Q3, P5
   OGCR   Section I.C.17.f.2.a

   Transplant complications other than kidney: Codes under subcategory 996.8, Complications of transplanted organ, are for use for both complications and rejection of transplanted organs. A transplant complication code is only assigned if the complication affects the function of the transplanted organ. Two codes are required to fully describe a transplant complication, the appropriate code from subcategory 996.8 and a secondary code that identifies the complication.
      Pre-existing conditions or conditions that develop after the transplant are not coded as complications unless they affect the function of the transplanted organs.
   See I.C.18.d.3) for transplant organ removal status.
   See I.C.2.i for malignant neoplasm associated with transplanted organ.

   ● V42.0   Kidney 🔖🔖
            Ⓔ 238.77, 996.80-996.81, 996.87, V42.0, V42.89-V42.9
            Coding Clinic: 2013, Q3, P6; 2008, Q1, P10-13; 2003, Q1, P10-11;
               2001, Q3, P12-13; 1994, Q2, P9x2
   ● V42.1   Heart 🔖🔖
            Ⓔ 238.77, 996.80, 996.83, 996.87, V42.1, V42.89-V42.9
            Coding Clinic: 2011, Q3, P5; 2003, Q3, P16; 2001, Q3, P13-14x2;
               1994, Q2, P13
   ● V42.2   Heart valve 🔖
   ● V42.3   Skin 🔖
   ● V42.4   Bone 🔖
   ● V42.5   Cornea 🔖
   ● V42.6   Lung 🔖🔖
            Ⓔ 238.77, 999.80, 996.84, 996.87, V42.6, V42.89-V42.9
   ● V42.7   Liver 🔖🔖
            Ⓔ 238.77, 996.80, 996.82, 996.87, V42.7, V42.89-V42.9
            Coding Clinic: 2011, Q3, P6

V01-V91

OGCR　Section I.C.17.f.2.b

Patients who have undergone kidney transplant may still have some form of chronic kidney disease (CKD) because the kidney transplant may not fully restore kidney function. Code 996.81 should be assigned for documented complications of a kidney transplant, such as transplant failure or rejection or other transplant complication. Code 996.81 should not be assigned for post kidney transplant patients who have chronic kidney (CKD) unless a transplant complication such as transplant failure or rejection is documented. If the documentation is unclear as to whether the patient has a complication of the transplant, query the provider. For patients with CKD following a kidney transplant, but who do not have a complication such as failure or rejection, *see section I.C.10.a.2, Chronic kidney disease and kidney transplant status*.

● **V42.8　Other specified organ or tissue**
  ● **V42.81　Bone marrow** 🔹
    (Ex:) 238.77, 279.50-279.53, 996.80, 996.85, 996.87, V42.9
    Coding Clinic: 2012, Q1, P13-14
  ● **V42.82　Peripheral stem cells** 🔹🔹
    (Ex:) 238.77, 996.80, 996.87, V42.9
  ● **V42.83　Pancreas** 🔹🔹
    (Ex:) 238.77, 996.80, 996.86-996.87, V42.83, V42.9
    Coding Clinic: 2003, Q1, P10-11; 2001, Q2, P16
  ● **V42.84　Intestines** 🔹🔹
    (Ex:) 238.77, 996.80, 996.89, V42.84-V42.9
    Coding Clinic: 2000, Q4, P47-48
  ● **V42.89　Other** 🔹
● **V42.9　Unspecified organ or tissue** 🔹

● **V43　Organ or tissue replaced by other means**
Includes	organ or tissue assisted by other means replacement of organ by:

  　　　　　artificial device
  　　　　　mechanical device
  　　　　　prosthesis
Excludes	*cardiac pacemaker in situ (V45.01)*

  　　　　　fitting and adjustment of prosthetic device (V52.0–V52.9)
  　　　　　renal dialysis status (V45.11)
  ● **V43.0　Eye globe** 🔹
  ● **V43.1　Lens** 🔹
    　　Pseudophakos
  ● **V43.2　Heart**
    ● **V43.21　Heart assist device** 🔹🔹
      (Ex:) 238.77, 996.80, 996.83, 996.87, V42.1, V43.21-V43.22
    ● **V43.22　Fully implantable artificial heart** 🔹🔹🔹
      (Ex:) 238.77, 996.80, 996.83, 996.87, V42.1, V43.21-V43.22
  ● **V43.3　Heart valve** 🔹
    Coding Clinic: 2006, Q3, P7; 2002, Q3, P13-15
  ● **V43.4　Blood vessel** 🔹
  ● **V43.5　Bladder** 🔹
  ● **V43.6　Joint**
    Coding Clinic: 1991, Q1, P15
    ● **V43.60　Unspecified joint** 🔹
    ● **V43.61　Shoulder** 🔹
    ● **V43.62　Elbow** 🔹
    ● **V43.63　Wrist** 🔹
    ● **V43.64　Hip** 🔹
      Coding Clinic: 2009, Q1, P15; 2008, Q2, P3-5; 2006, Q3, P4-5; 2005, Q4, P83-89, 110-112; 2004, Q2, P15
    ● **V43.65　Knee** 🔹
      Coding Clinic: 2006, Q3, P5
    ● **V43.66　Ankle** 🔹
    ● **V43.69　Other** 🔹
  ● **V43.7　Limb** 🔹
  ● **V43.8　Other organ or tissue**
    ● **V43.81　Larynx** 🔹
    ● **V43.82　Breast** 🔹
    ● **V43.83　Artificial skin** 🔹
    ● **V43.89　Other** 🔹

● **V44　Artificial opening status**
Excludes	*artificial openings requiring attention or management (V55.0–V55.9)*
  ● **V44.0　Tracheostomy** 🔹
    Coding Clinic: 2003, Q4, P103-104, 107, 111; 2001, Q1, P6-7
  ● **V44.1　Gastrostomy** 🔹
    Coding Clinic: 2003, Q4, P103-104, 107-108, 110; 2001, Q1, P12; 1998, Q4, P42-44; 1997, Q3, P12-13; 1993, Q1, P26
  ● **V44.2　Ileostomy** 🔹
    Coding Clinic: 1988, Q2, P9-10
  ● **V44.3　Colostomy** 🔹
    Coding Clinic: 2003, Q4, P110
  ● **V44.4　Other artificial opening of gastrointestinal tract** 🔹
  ● **V44.5　Cystostomy**
    ● **V44.50　Cystostomy, unspecified** 🔹
    ● **V44.51　Cutaneous-vesicostomy** 🔹
    ● **V44.52　Appendico-vesicostomy** 🔹
    ● **V44.59　Other cystostomy** 🔹
  ● **V44.6　Other artificial opening of urinary tract** 🔹
    　　Nephrostomy
    　　Ureterostomy
    　　Urethrostomy
    Coding Clinic: 2012, Q3, P12
  ● **V44.7　Artificial vagina** 🔹
  ● **V44.8　Other artificial opening status** 🔹
  ● **V44.9　Unspecified artificial opening status** 🔹

● **V45　Other postprocedural states**
Excludes	*aftercare management (V51–V58.9)*

  　　　　　malfunction or other complication-code to condition
  ● **V45.0　Cardiac device in situ**
Excludes	*artificial heart (V43.22)*

    　　　　　heart assist device (V43.21)
    Coding Clinic: 1994, Q2, P10x2; 1993, 5th Issue, P12
    ● **V45.00　Unspecified cardiac device** 🔹
    ● **V45.01　Cardiac pacemaker** 🔹
Excludes	*cardiac defibrillator with synchronous cardiac pacemaker (V45.02)*
    ● **V45.02　Automatic implantable cardiac defibrillator** 🔹
      　　With synchronous cardiac pacemaker
    ● **V45.09　Other specified cardiac device** 🔹
      　　Carotid sinus pacemaker in situ
  ● **V45.1　Renal dialysis status**
Excludes	*admission for dialysis treatment or session (V56.0)*
    Coding Clinic: 2008, Q1, P7-8; 2007, Q4, P84-86; Q3, P11; 2006, Q4, P136; 2004, Q1, P22,23; 2001, Q2, P12-13; 1987, Sept-Oct, P8; Jan-Feb, P15
    ● **V45.11　Renal dialysis status** 🔹
      　　Hemodialysis status
      　　Patient requiring intermittent renal dialysis
      　　Peritoneal dialysis status
      　　Presence of arterial-venous shunt (for dialysis)
      Coding Clinic: 2011, Q3, P15; 2008, Q4, P193; 2004, Q1, P23
    ● **V45.12　Noncompliance with renal dialysis** 🔹
      Coding Clinic: 2006, Q4, P136
  ● **V45.2　Presence of cerebrospinal fluid drainage device** 🔹
    　　Cerebral ventricle (communicating) shunt, valve, or device in situ
Excludes	*malfunction (996.2)*
    Coding Clinic: 2003, Q4, P106-107
  ● **V45.3　Intestinal bypass or anastomosis status** 🔹
Excludes	*bariatric surgery status (V45.86)*

    　　　　　gastric bypass status (V45.86)
    　　　　　obesity surgery status (V45.86)
  ● **V45.4　Arthrodesis status** 🔹
    Coding Clinic: 2013, Q2, P22; 1984, Nov-Dec, P18

V01-V91

N　Newborn: 0　　　P　Pediatric: 0–17　　　M　Maternity: 12–55　　　A　Adult: 15–124　　　♀　Females Only　　　♂　Males Only

- **V45.5   Presence of contraceptive device**
  - **V45.51   Intrauterine contraceptive device ♀** 🔍
    - Excludes   *checking of device (V25.42)*
      complication from device (996.32)
      insertion and removal of device
      (V25.11–V25.13)
  - **V45.52   Subdermal contraceptive implant** 🔍
    - Coding Clinic: 1995, Q3, P14
  - **V45.59   Other** 🔍
- **V45.6   States following surgery of eye and adnexa**
  - Excludes   *aphakia (379.31)*
    artificial:
    eye globe (V43.0)
  - **V45.61   Cataract extraction status** 🔍
    - Use additional code for associated artificial lens status (V43.1)
  - **V45.69   Other states following surgery of eye and adnexa** 🔍
    - Coding Clinic: 2001, Q2, P16-17
- **V45.7   Acquired absence of organ**
  - **V45.71   Acquired absence of breast and nipple** 🔍
    - Excludes   *congenital absence of breast and nipple (757.6)*
    - Coding Clinic: 2001, Q4, P66; 1997, Q4, P50
  - **V45.72   Acquired absence of intestine (large) (small)** 🔍
  - **V45.73   Acquired absence of kidney** 🔍
  - **V45.74   Other parts of urinary tract** 🔍
    - Bladder
  - **V45.75   Stomach** 🔍
  - **V45.76   Lung** 🔍
  - **V45.77   Genital organs** 🔍
    - Excludes   *acquired absence of cervix and uterus (V88.01–V88.03)*
      female genital mutilation status (629.20–629.29)
    - Coding Clinic: 2003, Q1, P13-14x2
  - **V45.78   Eye** 🔍
  - **V45.79   Other acquired absence of organ** 🔍
    - Excludes   *acquired absence of pancreas (V88.11-V88.12)*
- **V45.8   Other postprocedural status**
  - **V45.81   Aortocoronary bypass status** 🔍
    - Coding Clinic: 2011, Q4, P153; 2010, Q4, P131; 2003, Q4, P105-106; 2001, Q3, P15; 1997, Q3, P16
  - **V45.82   Percutaneous transluminal coronary angioplasty status** 🔍
    - Coding Clinic: 1995, Q2, P18
  - **V45.83   Breast implant removal status** 🔍
  - **V45.84   Dental restoration status** 🔍
    - Dental crowns status
    - Dental fillings status
  - **V45.85   Insulin pump status** 🔍
  - **V45.86   Bariatric surgery status** 🔍
    - Gastric banding status
    - Gastric bypass status for obesity
    - Obesity surgery status
    - Excludes   *bariatric surgery status complicating pregnancy, childbirth or the puerperium (649.2)*
      intestinal bypass or anastomosis status (V45.3)
    - Coding Clinic: 2009, Q2, P10

- **V45.87   Transplanted organ removal status** 🔍
  - Transplanted organ previously removed due to complication, failure, rejection or infection
  - Excludes   *encounter for removal of transplanted organ – code to complication of transplanted organ (996.80–996.89)*
- **V45.88   Status post administration of tPA (rtPA) in a different facility within the last 24 hours prior to admission to the current facility** 🔍
  - *Code first* condition requiring tPA administration, such as:
    - acute cerebral infarction (433.0–433.9 with fifth-digit 1, 434.0–434.9 with fifth digit 1)
    - acute myocardial infarction (410.00–410.92)
- **V45.89   Other** 🔍
  - Presence of neuropacemaker or other electronic device
  - Excludes   *artificial heart valve in situ (V43.3)*
    vascular prosthesis in situ (V43.4)
  - Coding Clinic: 1995, Q1, P11

- **V46   Other dependence on machines and devices**
  - **V46.0   Aspirator** 🔍
  - **V46.1   Respirator [Ventilator]**
    - Iron lung
    - Coding Clinic: 2005, Q4, P94-100; 2004, Q4, P100-101
    - **V46.11   Dependence on respirator, status** 🔍🔍
      - Ex V46.0-V46.2, V46.8-V46.9
      - Coding Clinic: 2013, Q2, P25; 2003, Q4, P104-105; 2001, Q1, P12
    - **V46.12   Encounter for respirator dependence during power failure** 🔍🔍
      - Ex V46.0-V46.2, V46.8-V46.9
    - **V46.13   Encounter for weaning from respirator [ventilator]** 🔍🔍
      - Ex V46.0-V46.2, V46.8-V46.9
    - **V46.14   Mechanical complication of respirator [ventilator]** 🔍🔍
      - Mechanical failure of respirator [ventilator]
      - Ex V46.0-V46.2, V46.8-V46.9
  - **V46.2   Supplemental oxygen** 🔍
    - Long-term oxygen therapy
  - **V46.3   Wheelchair dependence** 🔍
    - Wheelchair confinement status
    - *Code first* cause of dependence, such as:
      - muscular dystrophy (359.1)
      - obesity (278.00-278.03)
  - **V46.8   Other enabling machines** 🔍
    - Hyperbaric chamber
    - Possum [Patient-Operated-Selector-Mechanism]
    - Excludes   *cardiac pacemaker (V45.0)*
      kidney dialysis machine (V45.11)
  - **V46.9   Unspecified machine dependence** 🔍

- **V47   Other problems with internal organs**
  - **V47.0   Deficiencies of internal organs**
  - **V47.1   Mechanical and motor problems with internal organs**
  - **V47.2   Other cardiorespiratory problems**
    - Cardiovascular exercise intolerance with pain (with):
      - at rest
      - less than ordinary activity
      - ordinary activity
  - **V47.3   Other digestive problems**
  - **V47.4   Other urinary problems**
  - **V47.5   Other genital problems**
  - **V47.9   Unspecified**

- V48 **Problems with head, neck, and trunk**
  - V48.0 **Deficiencies of head**
    - **Excludes** *deficiencies of ears, eyelids, and nose (V48.8)*
  - V48.1 **Deficiencies of neck and trunk**
  - V48.2 **Mechanical and motor problems with head**
  - V48.3 **Mechanical and motor problems with neck and trunk**
  - V48.4 **Sensory problem with head**
  - V48.5 **Sensory problem with neck and trunk**
  - V48.6 **Disfigurements of head**
  - V48.7 **Disfigurements of neck and trunk**
  - V48.8 **Other problems with head, neck, and trunk**
  - V48.9 **Unspecified problem with head, neck, or trunk**
- V49 **Other conditions influencing health status**
  - V49.0 **Deficiencies of limbs**
  - V49.1 **Mechanical problems with limbs**
  - V49.2 **Motor problems with limbs**
  - V49.3 **Sensory problems with limbs**
  - V49.4 **Disfigurements of limbs**
  - V49.5 **Other problems of limbs**
  - V49.6 **Upper limb amputation status**
    - Coding Clinic: 1998, Q4, P42-44
    - V49.60 **Unspecified level**
    - V49.61 **Thumb**
    - V49.62 **Other finger(s)**
      - Coding Clinic: 2005, Q2, P7
    - V49.63 **Hand**
    - V49.64 **Wrist**
      - Disarticulation of wrist
    - V49.65 **Below elbow**
    - V49.66 **Above elbow**
      - Disarticulation of elbow
    - V49.67 **Shoulder**
      - Disarticulation of shoulder
  - V49.7 **Lower limb amputation status**
    - Coding Clinic: 2006, Q3, P5; 1998, Q4, P42-44
    - V49.70 **Unspecified level**
    - V49.71 **Great toe**
    - V49.72 **Other toe(s)**
    - V49.73 **Foot**
    - V49.74 **Ankle**
      - Disarticulation of ankle
    - V49.75 **Below knee**
    - V49.76 **Above knee**
      - Disarticulation of knee
      - Coding Clinic: 2005, Q2, P14
    - V49.77 **Hip**
      - Disarticulation of hip
  - V49.8 **Other specified conditions influencing health status**
    - V49.81 **Asymptomatic postmenopausal status (age-related) (natural)** ♀   A
      - **Excludes** *menopausal and premenopausal disorders (627.0–627.9)*
        postsurgical menopause (256.2)
        premature menopause (256.31)
        symptomatic menopause (627.0–627.9)
      - Coding Clinic: 2009, Q4, P151; 2000, Q4, P53-54
    - V49.82 **Dental sealant status**
    - V49.83 **Awaiting organ transplant status**
      - Coding Clinic: 2004, Q4, P101
    - V49.84 **Bed confinement status**
      - Coding Clinic: 2005, Q4, P94-100

- V49.85 **Dual sensory impairment**
  - Blindness with deafness
  - Combined visual hearing impairment
  - *Code first:*
    - hearing impairment (389.00–389.9)
    - visual impairment (369.00–369.9)
  - Coding Clinic: 2007, Q4, P99-101
- V49.86 **Do not resuscitate status**
  - Coding Clinic: 2012, Q1, P14
- V49.87 **Physical restraints status**
  - **Excludes** *restraint due to a procedure – omit code*
- V49.89 **Other specified conditions influencing health status**
- V49.9 **Unspecified**

PERSONS ENCOUNTERING HEALTH SERVICES FOR SPECIFIC PROCEDURES AND AFTERCARE (V50–V59)

Note: Categories V51–V58 are intended for use to indicate a reason for care in patients who may have already been treated for some disease or injury not now present, or who are receiving care to consolidate the treatment, to deal with residual states, or to prevent recurrence.

Excludes *follow-up examination for medical surveillance following treatment (V67.0–V67.9)*

- V50 **Elective surgery for purposes other than remedying health states**
  - V50.0 **Hair transplant**
  - V50.1 **Other plastic surgery for unacceptable cosmetic appearance**
    - Breast augmentation or reduction
    - Face-lift
    - **Excludes** *encounter for breast reduction (611.1)*
      plastic surgery following healed injury or operation (V51.0–V51.8)
  - V50.2 **Routine or ritual circumcision** ♂
    - Circumcision in the absence of significant medical indication
  - V50.3 **Ear piercing**
    - OGCR Section I.C.18.d.14
    - For encounters specifically for prophylactic removal of breasts, ovaries, or another organ due to a genetic susceptibility to cancer or a family history of cancer, the principal or first listed code should be a code from subcategory V50.4, Prophylactic organ removal, followed by the appropriate genetic susceptibility code and the appropriate family history code.
  - V50.4 **Prophylactic organ removal**
    - **Excludes** *organ donations (V59.0–V59.9)*
      therapeutic organ removal-code to condition
    - Coding Clinic: 2009, Q3, P21
    - V50.41 **Breast**
      - Coding Clinic: 2004, Q4, P106-107
    - V50.42 **Ovary** ♀
      - Coding Clinic: 2009, Q3, P21x2
    - V50.49 **Other**
      - Coding Clinic: 2009, Q3, P21
  - V50.8 **Other**
  - V50.9 **Unspecified**

N Newborn: 0   **P** Pediatric: 0–17   **M** Maternity: 12–55   **A** Adult: 15–124   ♀ Females Only   ♂ Males Only

● Unacceptable Principal Diagnosis   Complication\Comorbidity   Major C\C   Present on Admission Requirement   Hospital Acquired Condition   **1021**

V01-V91

V01-V91

● **V51 Aftercare involving the use of plastic surgery**
  Includes plastic surgery following healed injury or operation
  Excludes *cosmetic plastic surgery (V50.1)*
       plastic surgery as treatment for current condition or injury - code to condition or injury
       repair of scar tissue - code to scar

  V51.0 Encounter for breast reconstruction following mastectomy 🔍   A
      Excludes *deformity and disproportion of reconstructed breast (612.0–612.1)*

  V51.8 Other aftercare involving the use of plastic surgery 🔍

● **V52 Fitting and adjustment of prosthetic device and implant**
  Includes removal of device
  Excludes *malfunction or complication of prosthetic device (996.0–996.7)*
       status only, without need for care (V43.0–V43.8)

  V52.0 Artificial arm (complete) (partial) 🔍
  V52.1 Artificial leg (complete) (partial) 🔍
  V52.2 Artificial eye 🔍
  V52.3 Dental prosthetic device 🔍
  V52.4 Breast prosthesis and implant ♀ 🔍
      Elective implant exchange (different material) (different size)
      Removal of tissue expander without synchronous insertion of permanent implant
      Excludes *admission for initial breast implant insertion for breast augmentation (V50.1)*
           complications of breast implant (996.54, 996.69, 996.79)
           encounter for breast reconstruction following mastectomy (V51.0)
      Coding Clinic: 1995, Q4, P80.81
  V52.8 Other specified prosthetic device 🔍
      Coding Clinic: 2002, Q3, P12; Q2, P16-17
  ● **V52.9 Unspecified prosthetic device** 🔍

● **V53 Fitting and adjustment of other device**
  Includes removal of device
       replacement of device
  Excludes *status only, without need for care (V45.0–V45.8)*

  ● **V53.0 Devices related to nervous system and special senses**
      V53.01 Fitting and adjustment of cerebral ventricle (communicating) shunt 🔍
          Coding Clinic: 1997, Q4, P51
      V53.02 Neuropacemaker (brain) (peripheral nerve) (spinal cord) 🔍
      V53.09 Fitting and adjustment of other devices related to nervous system and special senses 🔍
          Auditory substitution device
          Visual substitution device
          Coding Clinic: 1999, Q2, P3-4
  ● **V53.1 Spectacles and contact lenses** 🔍
  ● **V53.2 Hearing aid** 🔍
  ● **V53.3 Cardiac device**
      Reprogramming
      Coding Clinic: 1992, Q3, P3
      V53.31 Cardiac pacemaker 🔍
          Excludes *automatic implantable cardiac defibrillator with synchronous cardiac pacemaker (V53.32)*
               mechanical complication of cardiac pacemaker (996.01)
          MCE: Questionable admission, principal diagnosis only
          Coding Clinic: 2010, Q3, P10; 2002, Q1, P3; 1984, Nov-Dec, P18

V53.32 Automatic implantable cardiac defibrillator 🔍
    With synchronous cardiac pacemaker
    MCE: Questionable admission, principal diagnosis only
    Coding Clinic: 2005, Q3, P3-9

V53.39 Other cardiac device 🔍
    MCE: Questionable admission, principal diagnosis only
    Coding Clinic: 2010, Q4, P124-125; 2008, Q2, P9-10; 2007, Q1, P20

● **V53.4 Orthodontic devices** 🔍

● **V53.5 Other gastrointestinal appliance and device**
    Excludes *colostomy (V55.3)*
         ileostomy (V55.2)
         other artifical opening of digestive tract (V55.4)
  ● **V53.50 Fitting and adjustment of intestinal appliance and device** 🔍
  ● **V53.51 Fitting and adjustment of gastric lap band** 🔍
  ● **V53.59 Fitting and adjustment of other gastrointestinal appliance and device** 🔍

● **V53.6 Urinary devices** 🔍
    Urinary catheter
    Excludes *cystostomy (V55.5)*
         nephrostomy (V55.6)
         ureterostomy (V55.6)
         urethrostomy (V55.6)

● **V53.7 Orthopedic devices** 🔍
    Orthopedic:
      brace
      cast
      corset
      shoes
    Excludes *other orthopedic aftercare (V54)*

● **V53.8 Wheelchair** 🔍

● **V53.9 Other and unspecified device**
    Coding Clinic: 2003, Q2, P6-7
  ● **V53.90 Unspecified device** 🔍
  ● **V53.91 Fitting and adjustment of insulin pump** 🔍
      Insulin pump titration
  ● **V53.99 Other device** 🔍
      Coding Clinic: 2009, Q2, P10

● **V54 Other orthopedic aftercare**
    Excludes *fitting and adjustment of orthopedic devices (V53.7)*
         malfunction of internal orthopedic device (996.40–996.49)
         other complication of nonmechanical nature (996.60–996.79)

  ● **V54.0 Aftercare involving internal fixation device**
      Excludes *malfunction of internal orthopedic device (996.40–996.49)*
           other complication of nonmechanical nature (996.60–996.79)
           removal of external fixation device (V54.89)
      V54.01 Encounter for removal of internal fixation device 🔍
      V54.02 Encounter for lengthening/adjustment of growth rod 🔍
      V54.09 Other aftercare involving internal fixation device 🔍
          Coding Clinic: 2009, Q1, P15

  ● **V54.1 Aftercare for healing traumatic fracture**
      Excludes *aftercare following joint replacement (V54.81)*
           aftercare for amputation stump (V54.89)
      V54.10 Aftercare for healing traumatic fracture of arm, unspecified 🔍
      V54.11 Aftercare for healing traumatic fracture of upper arm 🔍

◀ New   ◀▥ Revised   ~~deleted~~ Deleted   Excludes   Includes   Use additional   Code first
● Use Additional Digit(s)   ▶ Manifestation Code   OGCR Official Guidelines   Coding Clinic   🔍 CC/MCC Exclusions

V54.12　**Aftercare for healing traumatic fracture of lower arm** 🔖
　Coding Clinic: 2007, Q1, P3-8

V54.13　**Aftercare for healing traumatic fracture of hip** 🔖
　Coding Clinic: 2009, Q1, P15; 2007, Q1, P3-8; 2003, Q4, P103-105

V54.14　**Aftercare for healing traumatic fracture of leg, unspecified** 🔖

V54.15　**Aftercare for healing traumatic fracture of upper leg** 🔖
　Excludes *aftercare for healing traumatic fracture of hip (V54.13)*
　Coding Clinic: 2006, Q3, P6

V54.16　**Aftercare for healing traumatic fracture of lower leg** 🔖
　Coding Clinic: 2009, Q1, P14

V54.17　**Aftercare for healing traumatic fracture of vertebrae** 🔖

V54.19　**Aftercare for healing traumatic fracture of other bone** 🔖
　Coding Clinic: 2005, Q1, P13

● V54.2　**Aftercare for healing pathologic fracture**
　Excludes *aftercare following joint replacement (V54.81)*

V54.20　**Aftercare for healing pathologic fracture of arm, unspecified** 🔖

V54.21　**Aftercare for healing pathologic fracture of upper arm** 🔖

V54.22　**Aftercare for healing pathologic fracture of lower arm** 🔖

V54.23　**Aftercare for healing pathologic fracture of hip** 🔖

V54.24　**Aftercare for healing pathologic fracture of leg, unspecified** 🔖

V54.25　**Aftercare for healing pathologic fracture of upper leg** 🔖
　Excludes *aftercare for healing pathologic fracture of hip (V54.23)*

V54.26　**Aftercare for healing pathologic fracture of lower leg** 🔖

V54.27　**Aftercare for healing pathologic fracture of vertebrae** 🔖
　Coding Clinic: 2008, Q3, P4; 2003, Q4, P108-109

V54.29　**Aftercare for healing pathologic fracture of other bone** 🔖

● V54.8　**Other orthopedic aftercare**
　Coding Clinic: 2001, Q3, P19; 1999, Q4, P5x2; 1990, Q1, P10, 20

V54.81　**Aftercare following joint replacement** 🔖
　Use additional code to identify joint replacement site (V43.60–V43.69)
　Coding Clinic: 2011, Q1, P9; 2009, Q1, P14; 2006, Q3, P4; 2004, Q3, P12; Q2, P15

V54.82　**Aftercare following explantation of joint prosthesis** 🔖
　Aftercare following explantation of joint prosthesis, staged procedure
　Encounter for joint prosthesis insertion following prior explantation of joint prosthesis

V54.89　**Other orthopedic aftercare** 🔖
　Aftercare for healing fracture NOS
　Coding Clinic: 2007, Q2, P8-9

● V54.9　**Unspecified orthopedic aftercare** 🔖

● V55　**Attention to artificial openings**
　Includes adjustment or repositioning of catheter
　　closure
　　passage of sounds or bougies
　　reforming
　　removal or replacement of catheter
　　toilet or cleansing
　Excludes *complications of external stoma (519.00-519.09, 569.60-569.69, 596.81-596.83, 997.49)*
　　status only, without need for care (V44.0–V44.9)
　Coding Clinic: 1995, Q3, P13

V55.0　**Tracheostomy** 🔖

V55.1　**Gastrostomy** 🔖🔖
　(Ex) V55.1
　Coding Clinic: 1999, Q4, P9; 1997, Q3, P7-8; 1996, Q1, P14; 1995, Q3, P13

V55.2　**Ileostomy** 🔖

V55.3　**Colostomy** 🔖
　Coding Clinic: 2009, Q1, P14; 2005, Q2, P4-5; 1997, Q3, P9-10

V55.4　**Other artificial opening of digestive tract** 🔖
　Coding Clinic: 2005, Q2, P14; 2003, Q1, P10

V55.5　**Cystostomy** 🔖

V55.6　**Other artificial opening of urinary tract** 🔖
　Nephrostomy　　　　Urethrostomy
　Ureterostomy

V55.7　**Artificial vagina** 🔖

V55.8　**Other specified artificial opening** 🔖

● V55.9　**Unspecified artificial opening** 🔖

● V56　**Encounter for dialysis and dialysis catheter care**
　Use additional code to identify the associated condition
　Excludes *dialysis preparation-code to condition*
　Coding Clinic: 1993, Q1, P29

V56.0　**Extracorporeal dialysis** 🔖
　Dialysis (renal) NOS
　Excludes *dialysis status (V45.11)*
　Coding Clinic: 2005, Q4, P77-79; 2004, Q1, P23; 2000, Q4, P39-40; 1998, Q3, P6; Q2, P20-21; 1993, Q4, P34

V56.1　**Fitting and adjustment of extracorporeal dialysis catheter** 🔖
　Removal or replacement of catheter
　Toilet or cleansing
　Use additional code for any concurrent extracorporeal dialysis (V56.0)
　Coding Clinic: 1998, Q2, P20-21

● V56.2　**Fitting and adjustment of peritoneal dialysis catheter** 🔖
　Use additional code for any concurrent peritoneal dialysis (V56.8)
　Coding Clinic: 1998, Q4, P55

● V56.3　**Encounter for adequacy testing for dialysis**
　● V56.31　**Encounter for adequacy testing for hemodialysis** 🔖
　● V56.32　**Encounter for adequacy testing for peritoneal dialysis** 🔖
　　Peritoneal equilibration test

V56.8　**Other dialysis** 🔖
　Peritoneal dialysis
　Coding Clinic: 1998, Q4, P55

V01-V91

● **V57 Care involving use of rehabilitation procedures**
    Use additional code to identify underlying condition
    Coding Clinic: 2002, Q1, P18-19; 1997, Q3, P12

● **V57.0 Breathing exercises** ⊚

● **V57.1 Other physical therapy** ⊚
        Therapeutic and remedial exercises, except breathing
        MCE: Secondary DX may qualify codes as acceptable
            PDX
        Coding Clinic: 2006, Q3, P4; 2004, Q2, P15; 2002, Q4, P56; 1999,
            Q4, P5

● **V57.2 Occupational therapy and vocational rehabilitation**
    ● **V57.21 Encounter for occupational therapy** ⊚
            MCE: Secondary DX may qualify codes as
                acceptable PDX
            Coding Clinic: 1999, Q4, P7

    ● **V57.22 Encounter for vocational therapy** ⊚
            MCE: Secondary DX may qualify codes as
                acceptable PDX

● **V57.3 Speech-language therapy** ⊚
        MCE: Secondary DX may qualify codes as acceptable
            PDX
        Coding Clinic: 1997, Q4, P35-37

● **V57.4 Orthoptic training** ⊚

● **V57.8 Other specified rehabilitation procedure**
    ● **V57.81 Orthotic training** ⊚
            Gait training in the use of artificial limbs

    ● **V57.89 Other** ⊚
            Multiple training or therapy
            MCE: Secondary DX may qualify codes as
                acceptable PDX
            Coding Clinic: 2007, Q4, P92-95; 2006, Q3, P6; 2003,
                Q4, P105-106, 108-109; Q2, P16; 2002, Q1,
                P16; 2001, Q3, P21; 1997, Q3, P11-13

● **V57.9 Unspecified rehabilitation procedure** ⊚
        MCE: Secondary DX may qualify codes as acceptable
            PDX

OGCR   Section I.C.2.e.2
    If a patient admission/encounter is solely for the
    administration of chemotherapy, immunotherapy or
    radiation therapy assign code V58.0, Encounter for
    radiation therapy, or V58.11, Encounter for antineoplastic
    chemotherapy, or V58.12, Encounter for antineoplastic
    immunotherapy as the first-listed or principal diagnosis. If
    a patient receives more than one of these therapies during
    the same admission more than one of these codes may be
    assigned, in any sequence.
    The malignancy for which the therapy is being
    administered should be assigned as a secondary diagnosis.

● **V58 Encounter for other and unspecified procedures and aftercare**
    Excludes convalescence and palliative care (V66.0–V66.9)

    V58.0 Radiotherapy ⊚
        Encounter or admission for radiotherapy
        Excludes encounter for radioactive implant-code to
                        condition
                    radioactive iodine therapy-code to condition
        Coding Clinic: 2013, Q1, P8; 1994, Q2, P10x2; 1993, Q4, P36;
            1987, Jan-Feb, P13

● **V58.1 Encounter for chemotherapy and immunotherapy for neoplastic conditions**
        Encounter or admission for chemotherapy
        Excludes chemotherapy and immunotherapy for
                        nonneoplastic conditions-code to
                        condition
        Coding Clinic: 2005, Q4, P94-100; 2004, Q1, P13-14; 2003, Q2,
            P16-17; 2000, Q1, P23; 1993, Q4, P34, 36; Q3, P4x5;
            1992, Q2, P16-17; 1991, Q2, P17; 1987, Sept-Oct, P8

    V58.11 Encounter for antineoplastic chemotherapy ⊚
            Coding Clinic: 2012, Q1, P13-14; 2009, Q4, P152x2;
                2008, Q4, P82-83, 152-155; 2007, Q4,
                P103-104; 2006, Q2, P20-22; 2004, Q1, P13-14

    V58.12 Encounter for antineoplastic immunotherapy ⊚
            Coding Clinic: 2004, Q1, P13-14

● **V58.2 Blood transfusion, without reported diagnosis** ⊚
        Coding Clinic: 1994, Q1, P22

● **V58.3 Attention to dressings and sutures**
        Change or removal of wound packing
        Excludes attention to drains (V58.49)
                    planned postoperative wound closure
                        (V58.41)
        Coding Clinic: 2006, Q4, P117-118; 2005, Q2, P14

    ● **V58.30 Encounter for change or removal of nonsurgical wound dressing** ⊚
            Encounter for change or removal of wound
                dressing NOS
            Coding Clinic: 2009, Q4, P152x2

    ● **V58.31 Encounter for change or removal of surgical wound dressing** ⊚

    ● **V58.32 Encounter for removal of sutures** ⊚
            Encounter for removal of staples

● **V58.4 Other aftercare following surgery**
        Note: Codes from this subcategory should be used in
            conjunction with other aftercare codes
            to fully identify the reason for the aftercare
            encounter.
        Excludes aftercare following sterilization reversal
                        surgery (V26.22)
                    attention to artificial openings
                        (V55.0–V55.9)
                    orthopedic aftercare (V54.0–V54.9)
        Coding Clinic: 1999, Q4, P8-9

    V58.41 Encounter for planned post-operative wound closure ⊚
            Excludes disruption of operative wound
                            (998.31–998.32)
                        encounter for dressings and suture
                            aftercare (V58.30–V58.32)
            Coding Clinic: 1999, Q4, P15

    V58.42 Aftercare following surgery for neoplasm ⊚
            Conditions classifiable to 140–239

    V58.43 Aftercare following surgery for injury and trauma ⊚
            Conditions classifiable to 800–999
            Excludes aftercare for healing traumatic
                            fracture (V54.10–V54.19)
            Coding Clinic: 2007, Q2, P8-9; 1987, Nov-Dec, P9

    V58.44 Aftercare following organ transplant ⊚
            Use additional code to identify the organ
                transplanted (V42.0–V42.9)
            Coding Clinic: 2011, Q3, P5; 2004, Q4, P101

    V58.49 Other specified aftercare following surgery ⊚
            Change or removal of drains
            Coding Clinic: 1996, Q1, P8-9x2

    V58.5 Orthodontics ⊚
            Excludes fitting and adjustment of orthodontic device
                            (V53.4)

● **V58.6 Long-term (current) drug use**
        Long-term (current) prophylactic drug use
        Excludes drug abuse (305.00–305.93)
                    drug abuse and dependence complicating
                        pregnancy (648.3–648.4)
                    drug dependence (304.00–304.93)
                    hormone replacement therapy
                        (postmenopausal) (V07.4)
                    use of agents affecting estrogen receptors and
                        estrogen levels (V07.51–V07.59)
        Coding Clinic: 2011, Q1, P15; 2010, Q2, P13

    V58.61 Long-term (current) use of anticoagulants ⊚
            Excludes long-term (current) use of aspirin
                            (V58.66)
            Coding Clinic: 2008, Q4, P134-136; 2006, Q3, P13;
                2004, Q3, P7; 2003, Q4, P108; 2003, Q1,
                P11-12; 2002, Q3, P13-16; Q1, P16

● **V58.62 Long-term (current) use of antibiotics** ⊚
            Coding Clinic: 1998, Q4, P59-60

◀ New   ◀━ Revised   ~~deleted~~ Deleted   Excludes   Includes   Use additional   Code first
● Use Additional Digit(s)   ▶ Manifestation Code   OGCR Official Guidelines   Coding Clinic   Ⓔ⨯ CC/MCC Exclusions

V01-V91

OGCR Section I.C.18.d.3

Codes from this subcategory (V58) indicate a patient's continuous use of a prescribed drug (including such things as aspirin therapy) for the long-term treatment of a condition or for prophylactic use. It is not for use for patients who have addictions to drugs. This subcategory is not for use of medications for detoxification or maintenance programs to prevent withdrawal symptoms in patients with drug dependence (e.g., methadone maintenance for opiate dependence). Assign the appropriate code for the drug dependence instead.

Assign a code from subcategory V58.6, Long-term (current) drug use, if the patient is receiving a medication for an extended period as a prophylactic measure (such as for the prevention of deep vein thrombosis) or as treatment of a chronic condition (such as arthritis) or a disease requiring a lengthy course of treatment (such as cancer). Do not assign a code from subcategory V58.6 for medication being administered for a brief period of time to treat an acute illness or injury (such as a course of antibiotics to treat acute bronchitis).

● **V58.63** **Long-term (current) use of antiplatelets/ antithrombotics** 🔍

Excludes *long-term (current) use of aspirin (V58.66)*

● **V58.64** **Long-term (current) use of non-steroidal anti-inflammatories (NSAID)** 🔍

Excludes *long-term (current) use of aspirin (V58.66)*

● **V58.65** **Long-term (current) use of steroids** 🔍

V58.66 **Long-term (current) use of aspirin** 🔍
Coding Clinic: 2004, Q4, P102-103; 2003, Q1, P11-12

V58.67 **Long-term (current) use of insulin** 🔍
Coding Clinic: 2013, Q3, P10; 2004, Q4, P53-56

● **V58.68** **Long term (current) use of bisphosphonates** 🔍

V58.69 **Long-term (current) use of other medications** 🔍
Long term current use of methadone for pain control
Long term current use of opiate analgesic
Other high-risk medications

Excludes *methadone maintenance NOS (304.00)*
methadone use NOS (304.00)
Coding Clinic: 2013, Q2, P14-15; 2011, Q1, P15; 2010, Q2, P10, 13; 2009, Q4, P152; Q3, P21; 2004, Q2, P10; Q1, P13-14; 2003, Q1, P11-12; 2000, Q2, P8-9; 1999, Q3, 13-14; 1996, Q3, P20; Q2, P7x2; 1995, Q4, P51, 61

● **V58.7** **Aftercare following surgery to specified body systems, not elsewhere classified**
Note: Codes from this subcategory should be used in conjunction with other aftercare codes to fully identify the reason for the aftercare encounter.

Excludes *aftercare following organ transplant (V58.44)*
aftercare following surgery for neoplasm (V58.42)
Coding Clinic: 2003, Q4, P104-105

V58.71 **Aftercare following surgery of the sense organs, NEC** 🔍
Conditions classifiable to 360–379, 380–389
Coding Clinic: 2013, Q2, P11

V58.72 **Aftercare following surgery of the nervous system, NEC** 🔍
Conditions classifiable to 320–359

Excludes *aftercare following surgery of the sense organs, NEC (V58.71)*

V58.73 **Aftercare following surgery of the circulatory system, NEC** 🔍
Conditions classifiable to 390–459
Coding Clinic: 2009, Q2, P12

V58.74 **Aftercare following surgery of the respiratory system, NEC** 🔍
Conditions classifiable to 460–519

V58.75 **Aftercare following surgery of the teeth, oral cavity and digestive system, NEC** 🔍
Conditions classifiable to 520–579
Coding Clinic: 2005, Q2, P14

V58.76 **Aftercare following surgery of the genitourinary system, NEC** 🔍
Conditions classifiable to 580–629

Excludes *aftercare following sterilization reversal (V26.22)*
Coding Clinic: 2005, Q1, P11,12

V58.77 **Aftercare following surgery of the skin and subcutaneous tissue, NEC** 🔍
Conditions classifiable to 680–709

V58.78 **Aftercare following surgery of the musculoskeletal system, NEC** 🔍
Conditions classifiable to 710–739

Excludes *orthopedic aftercare (V54.01–V54.9)*

● **V58.8** **Other specified procedures and aftercare**
Coding Clinic: 1994, Q2, P8x2

V58.81 **Fitting and adjustment of vascular catheter** 🔍
Removal or replacement of catheter
Toilet or cleansing

Excludes *complications of renal dialysis (996.73)*
complications of vascular catheter (996.74)
dialysis preparation—code to condition
encounter for dialysis (V56.0–V56.8)
fitting and adjustment of dialysis catheter (V56.1)

V58.82 **Fitting and adjustment of non-vascular catheter NEC** 🔍
Removal or replacement of catheter
Toilet or cleansing

Excludes *fitting and adjustment of peritoneal dialysis catheter (V56.2)*
fitting and adjustment of urinary catheter (V53.6)

V58.83 **Encounter for therapeutic drug monitoring** 🔍
Use additional code for any associated long-term (current) drug use (V58.61–V58.69)

Excludes *blood-drug testing for medicolegal reasons (V70.4)*
Coding Clinic: 2004, Q2, P10-11; Q1, P13-14; 2002, Q3, P13-16

V58.89 **Other specified aftercare** 🔍
Coding Clinic: 2003, Q4, P106-107; 1998, Q4, P59-60

● **V58.9** **Unspecified aftercare** 🔍

OGCR Section I.C.18.d.9

Category V59 is the donor codes. They are used for living individuals who are donating blood or other body tissue. These codes are only for individuals donating for others, not for self donations. They are not for use to identify cadaveric donations.

● **V59** **Donors**

Excludes *examination of potential donor (V70.8)*
self-donation of organ or tissue--code to condition
Coding Clinic: 2008, Q2, P8-9; 1995, Q4, P50x2

● **V59.0** **Blood**
Coding Clinic: 1990, Q1, P9-10

● **V59.01** **Whole blood** 🔍

● **V59.02** **Stem cells** 🔍
Coding Clinic: 1995, Q4, P51

● **V59.09** **Other** 🔍

V59.1 **Skin** 🔍

V59.2 **Bone** 🔍

V59.3 **Bone marrow** 🔍
Coding Clinic: 1985, Jan-Feb, P15

V59.4 **Kidney** 🔍

V59.5 **Cornea** 🔍

V59.6 **Liver** 🔍

N Newborn: 0   **P** Pediatric: 0–17   **M** Maternity: 12–55   **A** Adult: 15–124   ♀ Females Only   ♂ Males Only
● Unacceptable Principal Diagnosis   🔍 Complication\Comorbidity   🔍 Major C\C   🔍 Present on Admission Requirement   🔍 Hospital Acquired Condition

1025

V01-V91

● **V59.7 Egg (oocyte) (ovum)**
  ● V59.70 Egg (oocyte) (ovum) donor, unspecified ♀ ⓠ
  ● V59.71 Egg (oocyte) (ovum) donor, under age 35, anonymous recipient ♀ ⓠ
    Egg donor, under age 35 NOS
  ● V59.72 Egg (oocyte) (ovum) donor, under age 35, designated recipient ♀ ⓠ
  ● V59.73 Egg (oocyte) (ovum) donor, age 35 and over, anonymous recipient ♀ ⓠ
    Egg donor, age 35 and over NOS
  ● V59.74 Egg (oocyte) (ovum) donor, age 35 and over, designated recipient ♀ ⓠ
  V59.8 Other specified organ or tissue ⓠ
    Coding Clinic: 2002, Q3, P20-21
  V59.9 Unspecified organ or tissue ⓠ

PERSONS ENCOUNTERING HEALTH SERVICES IN OTHER CIRCUMSTANCES (V60–V69)

● **V60 Housing, household, and economic circumstances**
  ● **V60.0 Lack of housing** ⓠ
    Hobos
    Social migrants
    Tramps
    Transients
    Vagabonds
  ● **V60.1 Inadequate housing** ⓠ
    Lack of heating
    Restriction of space
    Technical defects in home preventing adequate care
  ● **V60.2 Inadequate material resources** ⓠ
    Economic problem
    Poverty NOS
  ● **V60.3 Person living alone** ⓠ
  ● **V60.4 No other household member able to render care** ⓠ
    Person requiring care (has) (is):
      family member too handicapped, ill, or otherwise unsuited to render care
      partner temporarily away from home
      temporarily away from usual place of abode
    Excludes *holiday relief care (V60.5)*
  ● **V60.5 Holiday relief care** ⓠ
    Provision of health care facilities to a person normally cared for at home, to enable relatives to take a vacation
  ● **V60.6 Person living in residential institution** ⓠ
    Boarding school resident
  ● **V60.8 Other specified housing or economic circumstances**
    ● V60.81 Foster care (status) ⓠ
    ● V60.89 Other specified housing or economic circumstances ⓠ
  ● **V60.9 Unspecified housing or economic circumstance** ⓠ

● **V61 Other family circumstances**
  Includes when these circumstances or fear of them, affecting the person directly involved or others, are mentioned as the reason, justified or not, for seeking or receiving medical advice or care
  ● **V61.0 Family disruption**
    ● V61.01 Family disruption due to family member on military deployment ⓠ
      Individual or family affected by other family member being on deployment
      Excludes *family disruption due to family member on non-military extended absence from home (V61.08)*
    ● V61.02 Family disruption due to return of family member from military deployment ⓠ
      Individual or family affected by other family member having returned from deployment (current or past conflict)

● V61.03 Family disruption due to divorce or legal separation ⓠ
● V61.04 Family disruption due to parent-child estrangement ⓠ
    Excludes *other family estrangement (V61.09)*
● V61.05 Family disruption due to child in welfare custody ⓠ
● V61.06 Family disruption due to child in foster care or in care of non-parental family member ⓠ
● V61.07 Family disruption due to death of family member ⓠ
    Excludes *bereavement (V62.82)*
● V61.08 Family disruption due to other extended absence of family member ⓠ
    Excludes *family disruption due to family member on military deployment (V61.01)*
● V61.09 Other family disruption ⓠ
    Family estrangement NOS
● **V61.1 Counseling for marital and partner problems**
    Excludes *problems related to: psychosexual disorders (302.0–302.9) sexual function (V41.7)*
  ● V61.10 Counseling for marital and partner problems, unspecified ⓠ
    Marital conflict
    Marital relationship problem
    Partner conflict
    Partner relationship problem
  ● V61.11 Counseling for victim of spousal and partner abuse ⓠ
    Excludes *encounter for treatment of current injuries due to abuse (995.80–995.85)*
  ● V61.12 Counseling for perpetrator of spousal and partner abuse ⓠ
● **V61.2 Parent-child problems**
  ● V61.20 Counseling for parent-child problem, unspecified ⓠ
    Concern about behavior of child
    Parent-child conflict
    Parent-child relationship problem
  ● V61.21 Counseling for victim of child abuse ⓠ
    Child battering
    Child neglect
    Excludes *current injuries due to abuse (995.50–995.59)*
  ● V61.22 Counseling for perpetrator of parental child abuse ⓠ
    Excludes *counseling for non-parental abuser (V62.83)*
  ● V61.23 Counseling for parent-biological child problem ⓠ
    Concern about behavior of biological child
    Parent-biological child conflict
    Parent-biological child relationship problem
  ● V61.24 Counseling for parent-adopted child problem ⓠ
    Concern about behavior of adopted child
    Parent-adopted child conflict
    Parent-adopted child relationship problem
  ● V61.25 Counseling for parent (guardian)-foster child problem ⓠ
    Concern about behavior of foster child
    Parent (guardian)-foster child conflict
    Parent (guardian)-foster child relationship problem
  ● V61.29 Other parent-child problems ⓠ
    Coding Clinic: 1999, Q3, P16
● **V61.3 Problems with aged parents or in-laws** ⓠ

◀ New　◀▥ Revised　~~deleted~~ Deleted　Excludes　Includes　Use additional　Code first
● Use Additional Digit(s)　▶ Manifestation Code　OGCR Official Guidelines　Coding Clinic　(Ex) CC/MCC Exclusions

● V61.4 **Health problems within family**
  ● V61.41 **Alcoholism in family** 🔖
  ● V61.42 **Substance abuse in family** 🔖
  ● V61.49 **Other** 🔖
      Care of sick or handicapped person in family or household
      Presence of sick or handicapped person in family or household
● V61.5 **Multiparity** 🔖
● V61.6 **Illegitimacy or illegitimate pregnancy** ♀ 🔖   M
● V61.7 **Other unwanted pregnancy** ♀ 🔖   M
● V61.8 **Other specified family circumstances** 🔖
      Problems with family members NEC
      Sibling relationship problem
      Coding Clinic: 1994, Q1, P21
● V61.9 **Unspecified family circumstance** 🔖

● V62 **Other psychosocial circumstances**
  Includes those circumstances or fear of them, affecting the person directly involved or others, mentioned as the reason, justified or not, for seeking or receiving medical advice or care
  Excludes *previous psychological trauma (V15.41–V15.49)*
● V62.0 **Unemployment** 🔖
  Excludes *circumstances when main problem is economic inadequacy or poverty (V60.2)*
● V62.1 **Adverse effects of work environment** 🔖
● V62.2 **Other occupational circumstances or maladjustment**
  ● V62.21 **Personal current military deployment status** 🔖   A
      Individual (civilian or military) currently deployed in theater or in support of military war, peacekeeping and humanitarian operations
  ● V62.22 **Personal history of return from military deployment** 🔖   A
      Individual (civilian or military) with past history of military war, peacekeeping and humanitarian deployment (current or past conflict)
  ● V62.29 **Other occupational circumstances or maladjustment** 🔖   A
      Career choice problem
      Dissatisfaction with employment
      Occupational problem
● V62.3 **Educational circumstances** 🔖
      Academic problem
      Dissatisfaction with school environment
      Educational handicap
● V62.4 **Social maladjustment** 🔖
      Acculturation problem
      Cultural deprivation
      Political, religious, or sex discrimination
      Social:
          isolation
          persecution
● V62.5 **Legal circumstances** 🔖
      Imprisonment   Litigation
      Legal investigation   Prosecution
● V62.6 **Refusal of treatment for reasons of religion or conscience** 🔖
● V62.8 **Other psychological or physical stress, not elsewhere classified**
  ● V62.81 **Interpersonal problems, not elsewhere classified** 🔖
      Relational problem NOS
  ● V62.82 **Bereavement, uncomplicated** 🔖
    Excludes *bereavement as adjustment reaction (309.0)*
          family disruption due to death of family member (V61.07)

● V62.83 **Counseling for perpetrator of physical/sexual abuse** 🔖
  Excludes *counseling for perpetrator of parental child abuse (V61.22)*
         counseling for perpetrator of spousal and partner abuse (V61.12)
● V62.84 **Suicidal ideation** 🔖🔖
  Excludes *suicidal tendencies (300.9)*
  Ⓔⓧ 290.11, 290.3, 293.0
  Coding Clinic: 2005, Q4, P94-100
● V62.85 **Homicidal ideation** 🔖
● V62.89 **Other** 🔖
      Borderline intellectual functioning
      Life circumstance problems
      Phase of life problems
      Religious or spiritual problem
● V62.9 **Unspecified psychosocial circumstance** 🔖

● V63 **Unavailability of other medical facilities for care**
● V63.0 **Residence remote from hospital or other health care facility** 🔖
● V63.1 **Medical services in home not available** 🔖
  Excludes *no other household member able to render care (V60.4)*
  Coding Clinic: 2001, Q4, P67; Q1, P12
● V63.2 **Person awaiting admission to adequate facility elsewhere** 🔖
  Coding Clinic: 1994, Q1, P22-23
● V63.8 **Other specified reasons for unavailability of medical facilities** 🔖
      Person on waiting list undergoing social agency investigation
● V63.9 **Unspecified reason for unavailability of medical facilities** 🔖

● V64 **Persons encountering health services for specific procedures, not carried out**
● V64.0 **Vaccination not carried out**
  ● V64.00 **Vaccination not carried out, unspecified reason** 🔖
  ● V64.01 **Vaccination not carried out because of acute illness** 🔖
  ● V64.02 **Vaccination not carried out because of chronic illness or condition** 🔖
  ● V64.03 **Vaccination not carried out because of immune compromised state** 🔖
  ● V64.04 **Vaccination not carried out because of allergy to vaccine or component** 🔖
  ● V64.05 **Vaccination not carried out because of caregiver refusal** 🔖
      Guardian refusal Parent refusal
    Excludes *vaccination not carried out because of caregiver refusal for religious reasons (V64.07)*
    Coding Clinic: 2013, Q3, P4-5; 2007, Q1, P12
  ● V64.06 **Vaccination not carried out because of patient refusal** 🔖
  ● V64.07 **Vaccination not carried out for religious reasons** 🔖
  ● V64.08 **Vaccination not carried out because patient had disease being vaccinated against** 🔖
  ● V64.09 **Vaccination not carried out for other reason** 🔖
● V64.1 **Surgical or other procedure not carried out because of contraindication** 🔖
  Coding Clinic: 1993, 5th Issue, P9-10; 1985, Mar-April, P13; 1984, May-June, P11
● V64.2 **Surgical or other procedure not carried out because of patient's decision** 🔖
  Coding Clinic: 2001, Q2, P8-9; 1999, Q1, P13-14; 1987, Jan-Feb, P13; 1985, July-Aug, P14

V01-V91

- ● V64.3   Procedure not carried out for other reasons 🔖
- ● V64.4   Closed surgical procedure converted to open procedure
  - ● V64.41   Laparoscopic surgical procedure converted to open procedure 🔖
    - Coding Clinic: 2011, Q1, P14-15; 1997, Q4, P52
  - ● V64.42   Thoracoscopic surgical procedure converted to open procedure 🔖
  - ● V64.43   Arthroscopic surgical procedure converted to open procedure 🔖
- ● V65   Other persons seeking consultation
  - V65.0   Healthy person accompanying sick person 🔖
    - Boarder
    - Coding Clinic: 1993, Q4, P36
  - ● V65.1   Person consulting on behalf of another person
    - Advice or treatment for nonattending third party
    - **Excludes** *concern (normal) about sick person in family (V61.41–V61.49)*
    - ● V65.11   Pediatric pre-birth visit for expectant parent(s)
      - Pre-adoption visit for adoptive parent(s)
    - ● V65.19   Other person consulting on behalf of another person 🔖
  - V65.2   Person feigning illness 🔖
    - Malingerer
    - Peregrinating patient
    - Coding Clinic: 1999, Q3, P20
  - ● V65.3   Dietary surveillance and counseling 🔖
    - Dietary surveillance and counseling (in):
      - NOS
      - colitis
      - diabetes mellitus
      - food allergies or intolerance
      - gastritis
      - hypercholesterolemia
      - hypoglycemia
      - obesity
    - Use additional code to identify Body Mass Index (BMI), if known (V85.0–V85.54)
  - ● V65.4   Other counseling, not elsewhere classified
    - Health:
      - advice
      - education
      - instruction
    - **Excludes** *counseling (for):*
      - *contraception (V25.40–V25.49)*
      - *genetic (V26.31–V26.39)*
      - *on behalf of third party (V65.11–V65.19)*
      - *procreative management (V26.41–V26.49)*
    - ● V65.40   Counseling NOS 🔖
    - ● V65.41   Exercise counseling 🔖
    - ● V65.42   Counseling on substance use and abuse 🔖
    - ● V65.43   Counseling on injury prevention 🔖
    - ● V65.44   Human immunodeficiency virus [HIV] counseling 🔖
      - Coding Clinic: 1994, Q4, P35x3
      - OGCR   Section I.C.1.h
        - When a patient returns to be informed of HIV test results use V65.44 if the results of the test are negative.
    - ● V65.45   Counseling on other sexually transmitted diseases 🔖
    - ● V65.46   Encounter for insulin pump training 🔖
    - ● V65.49   Other specified counseling 🔖
      - Coding Clinic: 2000, Q2, P8-9
  - ● V65.5   Person with feared complaint in whom no diagnosis was made 🔖
    - Feared condition not demonstrated
    - Problem was normal state
    - "Worried well"
    - Coding Clinic: 1984, July-Aug, P20

- ● V65.8   Other reasons for seeking consultation 🔖
  - **Excludes** *specified symptoms*
  - Coding Clinic: 1992, Q3, P4
- ● V65.9   Unspecified reason for consultation 🔖
- ● V66   Convalescence and palliative care
  - V66.0   Following surgery 🔖
  - V66.1   Following radiotherapy 🔖
  - V66.2   Following chemotherapy 🔖
  - V66.3   Following psychotherapy and other treatment for mental disorder 🔖
  - V66.4   Following treatment of fracture 🔖
  - ● V66.5   Following other treatment 🔖
  - ● V66.6   Following combined treatment 🔖
  - ● V66.7   Encounter for palliative care 🔖
    - End-of-life care
    - Hospice care
    - Terminal care
    - *Code first underlying disease*
    - Coding Clinic: 2012, Q1, P14; 2010, Q3, P18; 2008, Q3, P13-14; 2005, Q2, P9-10; 2003, Q4, P107; 1996, Q4, P47-48
  - ● V66.9   Unspecified convalescence 🔖
    - Coding Clinic: 2012, Q3, P16; 1999, Q4, P8
- ● V67   Follow-up examination
  - **Includes**   surveillance only following completed treatment
  - **Excludes**   *surveillance of contraception (V25.40–V25.49)*
  - Coding Clinic: 2009, Q1, P14; 2003, Q2, P5
  - ● V67.0   Following surgery
    - Coding Clinic: 1997, Q4, P50; 1995, Q1, P4; 1992, Q3, P11; 1985, July-Aug, P16
    - V67.00   Following surgery, unspecified 🔖
      - OGCR   Section I.C.18.d.8
        - The follow-up codes are used to explain continuing surveillance following completed treatment of a disease, condition, or injury. They imply that the condition has been fully treated and no longer exists. They should not be confused with aftercare codes that explain current treatment for a healing condition or its sequelae. Follow-up codes may be used in conjunction with history codes to provide the full picture of the healed condition and its treatment. The follow-up code is sequenced first, followed by the history code. A follow-up code may be used to explain repeated visits. Should a condition be found to have recurred on the follow-up visit, then the diagnosis code should be used in place of the follow-up code.
    - V67.01   Follow-up vaginal pap smear ♀ 🔖
      - Vaginal pap smear, status-post hysterectomy for malignant condition
      - Use additional code to identify:
        - acquired absence of uterus (V88.01–V88.03)
        - personal history of malignant neoplasm (V10.40–V10.44)
      - **Excludes** *vaginal pap smear status-post hysterectomy for non-malignant condition (V76.47)*
    - V67.09   Following other surgery 🔖
      - **Excludes** *sperm count following sterilization reversal (V26.22)*
      - *sperm count for fertility testing (V26.21)*
      - Coding Clinic: 2008, Q3, P6; 2003, Q3, P16; 2002, Q3, P14-15; 1995, Q4, P53; Q2, P8; 1993, Q4, P32; 1992, Q3, P11; 1984, May-June, P10

V67.1 Following radiotherapy 🔍
    Coding Clinic: 1985, July-Aug, P16

V67.2 Following chemotherapy 🔍
    Cancer chemotherapy follow-up
    Coding Clinic: 1985, July-Aug, P16

V67.3 Following psychotherapy and other treatment for mental disorder

V67.4 Following treatment of healed fracture 🔍
    Excludes *current (healing) fracture aftercare (V54.0–V54.9)*
    Coding Clinic: 2009, Q1, P14

● **V67.5 Following other treatment**
    V67.51 Following completed treatment with high-risk medication, not elsewhere classified 🔍
        Excludes *long-term (current) drug use (V58.61–V58.69)*
        Coding Clinic: 1999, Q1, P5-6x2; 1990, Q1, P18
    V67.59 Other 🔍

V67.6 Following combined treatment 🔍

● **V67.9 Unspecified follow-up examination** 🔍

● **V68 Encounters for administrative purposes**
  ● **V68.0 Issue of medical certificates**
    Excludes *encounter for general medical examination (V70.0–V70.9)*
    ● **V68.01 Disability examination** 🔍
      Use additional code(s) to identify:
        specific examination(s), screening and testing performed (V72.0–V82.9)
      Coding Clinic: 2007, Q4, P99-101
    ● **V68.09 Other issue of medical certificates** 🔍
  ● **V68.1 Issue of repeat prescriptions** 🔍
    Issue of repeat prescription for:
      appliance
      glasses
      medications
    Excludes *repeat prescription for contraceptives (V25.41–V25.49)*
  ● **V68.2 Request for expert evidence** 🔍
  ● **V68.8 Other specified administrative purpose**
    ● **V68.81 Referral of patient without examination or treatment** 🔍
    ● **V68.89 Other** 🔍
  ● **V68.9 Unspecified administrative purpose** 🔍

● **V69 Problems related to lifestyle**
  ● **V69.0 Lack of physical exercise** 🔍
  ● **V69.1 Inappropriate diet and eating habits** 🔍
    Excludes *anorexia nervosa (307.1)*
             bulimia (783.6)
             malnutrition and other nutritional deficiencies (260–269.9)
             other and unspecified eating disorders (307.50–307.59)
  ● **V69.2 High-risk sexual behavior** 🔍
  ● **V69.3 Gambling and betting** 🔍
    Excludes *pathological gambling (312.31)*
  V69.4 Lack of adequate sleep 🔍
    Sleep deprivation
    Excludes *insomnia (780.52)*
    Coding Clinic: 2004, Q4, P104
  ● **V69.5 Behavioral insomnia of childhood** 🔍   P
  ● **V69.8 Other problems related to lifestyle** 🔍
    Self-damaging behavior
  ● **V69.9 Problem related to lifestyle, unspecified** 🔍

PERSONS WITHOUT REPORTED DIAGNOSIS ENCOUNTERED DURING EXAMINATION AND INVESTIGATION OF INDIVIDUALS AND POPULATIONS (V70–V82)

Note: Nonspecific abnormal findings disclosed at the time of these examinations are classifiable to categories 790–796.

● **V70 General medical examination**
  Use additional code(s) to identify any special screening examination(s) performed (V73.0–V82.9)
  Coding Clinic: 1993, Q1, P28; 1985, Nov-Dec, P13
  ● **V70.0 Routine general medical examination at a health care facility** 🔍
    Health checkup
    Excludes *health checkup of infant or child over 28 days old (V20.2)*
        health supervision of newborn 8 to 28 days old (V20.32)
        health supervision of newborn under 8 days old (V20.31)
        pre-procedural general physical examination (V72.83)
  V70.1 General psychiatric examination, requested by the authority 🔍
  ● **V70.2 General psychiatric examination, other and unspecified** 🔍
  ● **V70.3 Other medical examination for administrative purposes** 🔍
    General medical examination for:
      admission to old age home
      adoption
      camp
      driving license
      immigration and naturalization
      insurance certification
      marriage
      prison
      school admission
      sports competition
    Excludes *attendance for issue of medical certificates (V68.0)*
        pre-employment screening (V70.5)
    Coding Clinic: 2008, Q3, P6
  V70.4 Examination for medicolegal reasons 🔍
    Blood-alcohol tests
    Blood-drug tests
    Paternity testing
    Excludes *examination and observation following:*
        accidents (V71.3, V71.4)
        assault (V71.6)
        rape (V71.5)
  V70.5 Health examination of defined subpopulations 🔍
    Armed forces personnel
    Inhabitants of institutions
    Occupational health examinations
    Pre-employment screening
    Preschool children
    Prisoners
    Prostitutes
    Refugees
    School children
    Students
  ● **V70.6 Health examination in population surveys** 🔍
    Excludes *special screening (V73.0–V82.9)*
  V70.7 Examination of participant in clinical trial 🔍
    Examination of participant or control in clinical research
    Coding Clinic: 2006, Q2, P5-6
  ● **V70.8 Other specified general medical examinations** 🔍
    Examination of potential donor of organ or tissue
  ● **V70.9 Unspecified general medical examination** 🔍

OGCR Section I.C.18.d.6

There are three observation V code categories. They are for use in very limited circumstances when a person is being observed for a suspected condition that is ruled out. The observation codes are not for use if an injury or illness or any signs or symptoms related to the suspected condition are present. In such cases the diagnosis/symptom code is used with the corresponding E code to identify any external cause. The observation codes are to be used as principal diagnosis only. The only exception to this is when the principal diagnosis is required to be a code from the V30, Live born infant, category. Then the V29 observation code is sequenced after the V30 code. Additional codes may be used in addition to the observation code but only if they are unrelated to the suspected condition being observed.

● **V71 Observation and evaluation for suspected conditions not found**

  Note: This category is to be used when persons without a diagnosis are suspected of having an abnormal condition, without signs or symptoms, which requires study, but after examination and observation, is found not to exist. This category is also for use for administrative and legal observation status.

    Excludes *suspected maternal and fetal conditions not found (V89.01–V89.09)*
    Coding Clinic: 1990, Q1, P19; 1985, Nov-Dec, P10, 13

  ● **V71.0 Observation for suspected mental condition**

    V71.01 Adult antisocial behavior 🔍   A
      Dyssocial behavior or gang activity in adult without manifest psychiatric disorder

    V71.02 Childhood or adolescent antisocial behavior 🔍
      Dyssocial behavior or gang activity in child or adolescent without manifest psychiatric disorder

    V71.09 Other suspected mental condition 🔍

  V71.1 Observation for suspected malignant neoplasm 🔍
    Coding Clinic: 1990, Q1, P21

  V71.2 Observation for suspected tuberculosis 🔍

  V71.3 Observation following accident at work 🔍

  V71.4 Observation following other accident 🔍
    Examination of individual involved in motor vehicle traffic accident
    Coding Clinic: 2006, Q1, P9; 2004, Q1, P6-7

  V71.5 Observation following alleged rape or seduction 🔍
    Examination of victim or culprit

  V71.6 Observation following other inflicted injury 🔍
    Examination of victim or culprit

  V71.7 Observation for suspected cardiovascular disease 🔍
    Coding Clinic: 2004, Q1, P6-7; 1993, 5th Issue, P17-24; 1990, Q1, P19; 1987, Sept-Oct, P10

  ● **V71.8 Observation and evaluation for other specified suspected conditions**

    Excludes *contact with and (suspected) exposure to (potentially) hazardous substances (V15.84–V15.86, V87.0–V87.31)*
    Coding Clinic: 1990, Q1, P19

    V71.81 Abuse and neglect 🔍

      Excludes *adult abuse and neglect (995.80–995.85)*
      child abuse and neglect (995.50–995.59)
      Coding Clinic: 2000, Q4, P54–55

    V71.82 Observation and evaluation for suspected exposure to anthrax 🔍

    V71.83 Observation and evaluation for suspected exposure to other biological agent 🔍
      Coding Clinic: 2003, Q4, P46-48

    V71.89 Other specified suspected conditions 🔍
      Coding Clinic: 2008, Q3, P6-7; 2003, Q2, P15-16

  ● **V71.9 Observation for unspecified suspected condition** 🔍
    Coding Clinic: 2002, Q1, P6-7

● **V72 Special investigations and examinations**

  Includes routine examination of specific system

  Excludes *general medical examination (V70.0–70.4)*
    general screening examination of defined population groups (V70.5, V70.6, V70.7)
    health supervision of newborn 8 to 28 days old (V20.32)
    health supervision of newborn under 8 days old (V20.31)
    routine examination of infant or child over 28 days old (V20.2)

  Use additional code(s) to identify any special screening examination(s) performed (V73.0–V82.9)
    Coding Clinic: 2004, Q1, P15-16; 1985, Nov-Dec, P13

  V72.0 Examination of eyes and vision 🔍

  ● **V72.1 Examination of ears and hearing**
    Coding Clinic: 2004, Q1, P15-16

    ● **V72.11 Encounter for hearing examination following failed hearing screening** 🔍
      Coding Clinic: 2011, Q3, P3; 2006, Q4, P118

    ● **V72.12 Encounter for hearing conservation and treatment** 🔍
      Coding Clinic: 2007, Q4, P99-101

    ● **V72.19 Other examination of ears and hearing** 🔍

  ● **V72.2 Dental examination** 🔍

  ● **V72.3 Gynecological examination**

    Excludes *cervical Papanicolaou smear without general gynecological examination (V76.2)*
      routine examination in contraceptive management (V25.40–V25.49)
      Coding Clinic: 2004, Q4, P104-105

    V72.31 Routine gynecological examination ♀ 🔍
      General gynecological examination with or without Papanicolaou cervical smear
      Pelvic examination (annual) (periodic)
      Use additional code to identify:
        human papillomavirus (HPV) screening (V73.81)
        routine vaginal Papanicolaou smear (V76.47)
      Coding Clinic: 2006, Q2, P3,4

    V72.32 Encounter for Papanicolaou cervical smear to confirm findings of recent normal smear following initial abnormal smear ♀ 🔍
      Coding Clinic: 2006, Q2, P3-4

  ● **V72.4 Pregnancy examination or test**
    Coding Clinic: 2005, Q4, P94-100; 2004, Q4, P105

    V72.40 Pregnancy examination or test, pregnancy unconfirmed ♀ 🔍
      Possible pregnancy, not (yet) confirmed

    V72.41 Pregnancy examination or test, negative result ♀ 🔍

    V72.42 Pregnancy examination or test, positive result ♀ 🔍   M

  ● **V72.5 Radiological examination, not elsewhere classified** 🔍
    Routine chest x-ray

    Excludes *radiologic examinations as part of pre-procedural testing (V72.81-V72.84)*
    Coding Clinic: 1990, Q1, P8, 10, 19-21; 1985, Nov-Dec, P13

OGCR Section I.C.18.d.13 (outpatient)

Codes V72.5 and V72.62 may be used if the reason for the patient encounter is for routine laboratory/radiology testing in the absence of any signs, symptoms, or associated diagnosis. If routine testing is performed during the same encounter as a test to evaluate a sign, symptom, or diagnosis, it is appropriate to assign both the V code and the code describing the reason for the non-routine test.

● **V72.6 Laboratory examination**
Encounters for blood and urine testing
Coding Clinic: 2006, Q2, P4; 1994, Q4, P35; 1990, Q1, P22; 1985, Nov-Dec, P13

OGCR   Section I.C.18.d.13 (outpatient)
V72.6 is not to be used if any sign or symptoms, or reason for a test is documented.

● **V72.60 Laboratory examination, unspecified** ◎

● **V72.61 Antibody response examination** ◎
Immunity status testing

Excludes *encounter for allergy testing (V72.7)*

● **V72.62 Laboratory examination ordered as part of a routine general medical examination** ◎
Blood tests for routine general physical examination

● **V72.63 Pre-procedural laboratory examination** ◎
Blood tests prior to treatment or procedure
Pre-operative laboratory examination

● **V72.69 Other laboratory examination** ◎

● **V72.7 Diagnostic skin and sensitization tests** ◎
Allergy tests
Skin tests for hypersensitivity

Excludes *diagnostic skin tests for bacterial diseases (V74.0–V74.9)*

Coding Clinic: 1985, Nov-Dec, P13

● **V72.8 Other specified examinations**

Excludes *pre-procedural laboratory examinations (V72.63)*

Coding Clinic: 1995, Q4, P51-52; 1990, Q1, P10; 1985, Nov-Dec, P13

V72.81 Preoperative cardiovascular examination ◎
Pre-procedural cardiovascular examination
Coding Clinic: 1995, Q4, P51-52

V72.82 Preoperative respiratory examination ◎
Pre-procedural respiratory examination
Coding Clinic: 1996, Q3, P14

V72.83 Other specified preoperative examination ◎
Examination prior to chemotherapy
Other pre-procedural examination
Pre-procedural general physical examination

Excludes *routine general medical examination (V70.0)*

Coding Clinic: 2013, Q2, P11; 1996, Q3, P14; 1995, Q4, P52

● **V72.84 Preoperative examination, unspecified** ◎
Pre-procedural examination, unspecified
Coding Clinic: 1995, Q4, P52

● **V72.85 Other specified examination** ◎
Coding Clinic: 2012, Q1, P10; 2004, Q1, P12-13

● **V72.86 Encounter for blood typing** ◎

● **V72.9 Unspecified examination** ◎

● **V73 Special screening examination for viral and chlamydial diseases**

● **V73.0 Poliomyelitis** ◎

● **V73.1 Smallpox** ◎

● **V73.2 Measles** ◎

● **V73.3 Rubella** ◎

● **V73.4 Yellow fever** ◎

● **V73.5 Other arthropod-borne viral diseases** ◎
Dengue fever
Hemorrhagic fever
Viral encephalitis:
  mosquito-borne
  tick-borne

● **V73.6 Trachoma** ◎

● **V73.8 Other specified viral and chlamydial diseases**

● **V73.81 Human papillomavirus (HPV)** ◎
Coding Clinic: 2007, Q4, P99-101

● **V73.88 Other specified chlamydial diseases** ◎
Coding Clinic: 2007, Q4, P124-125

● **V73.89 Other specified viral diseases** ◎

OGCR   Section I.C.1.h.
If a patient is being seen to determine his/her HIV status, use V73.89, Screening for other specified viral disease. Use V69.8, Other problems related to lifestyle, as a secondary code if an asymptomatic patient is in a known high risk group for HIV. Should a patient with signs or symptoms or illness, or a confirmed HIV related diagnosis be tested for HIV, code the signs and symptoms or the diagnosis. An additional counseling code V65.44 may be used if counseling is provided during the encounter for the test.

● **V73.9 Unspecified viral and chlamydial disease**

● **V73.98 Unspecified chlamydial disease** ◎

● **V73.99 Unspecified viral disease** ◎

● **V74 Special screening examination for bacterial and spirochetal diseases**

Includes diagnostic skin tests for these diseases

● **V74.0 Cholera** ◎

● **V74.1 Pulmonary tuberculosis** ◎

● **V74.2 Leprosy [Hansen's disease]** ◎

● **V74.3 Diphtheria** ◎

● **V74.4 Bacterial conjunctivitis** ◎

● **V74.5 Venereal disease** ◎
Screening for bacterial and spirochetal sexually transmitted diseases
Screening for sexually transmitted diseases NOS

Excludes *special screening for nonbacterial sexually transmitted diseases (V73.81–V73.89, V75.4, V75.8)*

Coding Clinic: 2007, Q4, P124-125

● **V74.6 Yaws** ◎

● **V74.8 Other specified bacterial and spirochetal diseases** ◎
Brucellosis
Leptospirosis
Plague
Tetanus
Whooping cough

● **V74.9 Unspecified bacterial and spirochetal disease** ◎

● **V75 Special screening examination for other infectious diseases**

● **V75.0 Rickettsial diseases** ◎

● **V75.1 Malaria** ◎

● **V75.2 Leishmaniasis** ◎

● **V75.3 Trypanosomiasis** ◎
Chagas' disease   Sleeping sickness

● **V75.4 Mycotic infections** ◎

● **V75.5 Schistosomiasis** ◎

● **V75.6 Filariasis** ◎

● **V75.7 Intestinal helminthiasis** ◎

● **V75.8 Other specified parasitic infections** ◎

● **V75.9 Unspecified infectious disease** ◎

V01-V91

V01-V91

● **V76**   **Special screening for malignant neoplasms**
    ● **V76.0**   **Respiratory organs** 🔍
    ● **V76.1**   **Breast**
       ● **V76.10**   **Breast screening, unspecified** 🔍
       ● **V76.11**   **Screening mammogram for high-risk patient** ♀ 🔍
          Coding Clinic: 2003, Q2, P3-5
       ● **V76.12**   **Other screening mammogram** 🔍
          Coding Clinic: 2009, Q4, P153; 2006, Q2, P10; Q2, P3-5
       ● **V76.19**   **Other screening breast examination** 🔍
    ● **V76.2**   **Cervix** ♀ 🔍
       Routine cervical Papanicolaou smear
       Excludes   *special screening for human papillomavirus (V73.81)*
                  that as part of a general gynecological examination (V72.31)
    ● **V76.3**   **Bladder** 🔍
    ● **V76.4**   **Other sites**
       ● **V76.41**   **Rectum** 🔍
       ● **V76.42**   **Oral cavity** 🔍
       ● **V76.43**   **Skin** 🔍
       V76.44   **Prostate** ♂ 🔍
       ● **V76.45**   **Testis** ♂ 🔍
       ● **V76.46**   **Ovary** ♀ 🔍
       ● **V76.47**   **Vagina** ♀ 🔍
          Vaginal pap smear status-post hysterectomy for non-malignant condition
          Use additional code to identify acquired absence of uterus (V88.01–V88.03)
          Excludes   *vaginal pap smear status-post hysterectomy for malignant condition (V67.01)*
       ● **V76.49**   **Other sites** 🔍
          Coding Clinic: 1999, Q1, P4
    ● **V76.5**   **Intestine**
       ● **V76.50**   **Intestine, unspecified** 🔍
       ● **V76.51**   **Colon** 🔍
          Screening colonoscopy NOS
          Excludes   *rectum (V76.41)*
          Coding Clinic: 2004, Q1, P11-12; 2001, Q4, P55-56x2
       ● **V76.52**   **Small intestine** 🔍
    ● **V76.8**   **Other neoplasm**
       ● **V76.81**   **Nervous system** 🔍
       ● **V76.89**   **Other neoplasm** 🔍
    ● **V76.9**   **Unspecified** 🔍

● **V77**   **Special screening for endocrine, nutritional, metabolic, and immunity disorders**
    ● **V77.0**   **Thyroid disorders** 🔍
    ● **V77.1**   **Diabetes mellitus** 🔍
    ● **V77.2**   **Malnutrition** 🔍
    ● **V77.3**   **Phenylketonuria [PKU]** 🔍
    ● **V77.4**   **Galactosemia** 🔍
    ● **V77.5**   **Gout** 🔍
    ● **V77.6**   **Cystic fibrosis** 🔍
       Screening for mucoviscidosis
    ● **V77.7**   **Other inborn errors of metabolism** 🔍
    ● **V77.8**   **Obesity** 🔍
    ● **V77.9**   **Other and unspecified endocrine, nutritional, metabolic, and immunity disorders**
       ● **V77.91**   **Screening for lipoid disorders** 🔍
          Screening cholesterol level
          Screening for hypercholesterolemia
          Screening for hyperlipidemia
       ● **V77.99**   **Other and unspecified endocrine, nutritional, metabolic, and immunity disorders** 🔍

● **V78**   **Special screening for disorders of blood and blood-forming organs**
    ● **V78.0**   **Iron deficiency anemia** 🔍
    ● **V78.1**   **Other and unspecified deficiency anemia** 🔍
    ● **V78.2**   **Sickle-cell disease or trait** 🔍
    ● **V78.3**   **Other hemoglobinopathies** 🔍
    ● **V78.8**   **Other disorders of blood and blood-forming organs** 🔍
    ● **V78.9**   **Unspecified disorder of blood and blood-forming organs** 🔍

● **V79**   **Special screening for mental disorders and developmental handicaps**
    ● **V79.0**   **Depression** 🔍
    ● **V79.1**   **Alcoholism** 🔍
    ● **V79.2**   **Intellectual disabilities** 🔍
    ● **V79.3**   **Developmental handicaps in early childhood** 🔍
    ● **V79.8**   **Other specified mental disorders and developmental handicaps** 🔍
    ● **V79.9**   **Unspecified mental disorder and developmental handicap** 🔍

● **V80**   **Special screening for neurological, eye, and ear diseases**
    ● **V80.0**   **Neurological conditions**
       ● **V80.01**   **Traumatic brain injury** 🔍
       ● **V80.09**   **Other neurological conditions** 🔍
    ● **V80.1**   **Glaucoma** 🔍
    ● **V80.2**   **Other eye conditions** 🔍
       Screening for:
          cataract
          congenital anomaly of eye
          senile macular lesions
       Excludes   *general vision examination (V72.0)*
    ● **V80.3**   **Ear diseases** 🔍
       Excludes   *general hearing examination (V72.11–V72.19)*

● **V81**   **Special screening for cardiovascular, respiratory, and genitourinary diseases**
    ● **V81.0**   **Ischemic heart disease** 🔍
    ● **V81.1**   **Hypertension** 🔍
    ● **V81.2**   **Other and unspecified cardiovascular conditions** 🔍
    ● **V81.3**   **Chronic bronchitis and emphysema** 🔍
    ● **V81.4**   **Other and unspecified respiratory conditions** 🔍
       Excludes   *screening for:*
          lung neoplasm (V76.0)
          pulmonary tuberculosis (V74.1)
    ● **V81.5**   **Nephropathy** 🔍
       Screening for asymptomatic bacteriuria
    ● **V81.6**   **Other and unspecified genitourinary conditions** 🔍

● **V82**   **Special screening for other conditions**
    ● **V82.0**   **Skin conditions** 🔍
    ● **V82.1**   **Rheumatoid arthritis** 🔍
    ● **V82.2**   **Other rheumatic disorders** 🔍
    ● **V82.3**   **Congenital dislocation of hip** 🔍
    ● **V82.4**   **Maternal postnatal screening for chromosomal anomalies** ♀ 🔍
       Excludes   *antenatal screening by amniocentesis (V28.0)*
    ● **V82.5**   **Chemical poisoning and other contamination** 🔍
       Screening for:
          heavy metal poisoning
          ingestion of radioactive substance
          poisoning from contaminated water supply
          radiation exposure
    ● **V82.6**   **Multiphasic screening** 🔍

- **V82.7 Genetic screening**
  - **Excludes** *genetic testing for procreative management (V26.31–V26.39)*
  - Coding Clinic: 2006, Q4, P118
  - **V82.71 Screening for genetic disease carrier status** 🔗
  - **V82.79 Other genetic screening** 🔗
- **V82.8 Other specified conditions**
  - **V82.81 Osteoporosis** 🔗
    - Use additional code to identify:
      - hormone replacement therapy (postmenopausal) status (V07.4)
      - postmenopausal (natural) status (V49.81)
    - Coding Clinic: 2000, Q4, P53-54
  - **V82.89 Other specified conditions** 🔗
- **V82.9 Unspecified condition** 🔗

GENETICS (V83–V84)

OGCR   Section I.C.18.d.3

Genetic carrier status indicates that a person carries a gene, associated with a particular disease, which may be passed to offspring who may develop that disease. The person does not have the disease and is not at risk of developing the disease.

- **V83 Genetic carrier status**
  - **V83.0 Hemophilia A carrier**
    - **V83.01 Asymptomatic hemophilia A carrier** 🔗
    - **V83.02 Symptomatic hemophilia A carrier** 🔗
  - **V83.8 Other genetic carrier status**
    - **V83.81 Cystic fibrosis gene carrier** 🔗
    - **V83.89 Other genetic carrier status** 🔗

OGCR   Section I.C.18.d.3

Genetic susceptibility indicates that a person has a gene that increases the risk of that person developing the disease. Codes from category V84, Genetic susceptibility to disease, should not be used as principal or first-listed codes.

- **V84 Genetic susceptibility to disease**
  - **Includes** Confirmed abnormal gene
  - Use additional code, if applicable, for any associated family history of the disease (V16–V19)
  - **Excludes** *chromosomal anomalies (758.0-758.9)*
  - **V84.0 Genetic susceptibility to malignant neoplasm**
    - *Code first, if applicable, any current malignant neoplasms (140.0–195.8, 200.0–208.9, 230.0–234.9)*
    - Use additional code, if applicable, for any personal history of malignant neoplasm (V10.0–V10.9)
    - **V84.01 Genetic susceptibility to malignant neoplasm of breast** 🔗
      - Coding Clinic: 2004, Q4, P106-107
    - **V84.02 Genetic susceptibility to malignant neoplasm of ovary** ♀ 🔗
    - **V84.03 Genetic susceptibility to malignant neoplasm of prostate** ♂ 🔗
    - **V84.04 Genetic susceptibility to malignant neoplasm of endometrium** ♀ 🔗
    - **V84.09 Genetic susceptibility to other malignant neoplasm** 🔗
      - Coding Clinic: 2013, Q2, P15
  - **V84.8 Genetic susceptibility to other disease**
    - **V84.81 Genetic susceptibility to multiple endocrine neoplasia [MEN]** 🔗
      - **Excludes** *multiple endocrine neoplasia [MEN] syndromes (258.01-258.03)*
      - Coding Clinic: 2007, Q4, P99-101
    - **V84.89 Genetic susceptibility to other disease** 🔗

BODY MASS INDEX (V85)

- **V85 Body mass index (BMI)**
  - Kilograms per meters squared
  - **Note:** BMI adult codes are for use for persons over 20 years old
  - Coding Clinic: 2012, Q2, P13; 2008, Q4, P191; 2005, Q4, P94-100
  - **V85.0 Body Mass Index less than 19, adult** 🔗 🔗   A
    - (Ex) 278.00-278.01, V77.8, V85.0-V85.54
  - **V85.1 Body Mass Index between 19–24, adult** 🔗   A
  - **V85.2 Body Mass Index between 25–29, adult**
    - **V85.21 Body Mass Index 25.0–25.9, adult** 🔗   A
    - **V85.22 Body Mass Index 26.0–26.9, adult** 🔗   A
    - **V85.23 Body Mass Index 27.0–27.9, adult** 🔗   A
    - **V85.24 Body Mass Index 28.0–28.9, adult** 🔗   A
    - **V85.25 Body Mass Index 29.0–29.9, adult** 🔗   A
  - **V85.3 Body Mass Index between 30–39, adult**
    - **V85.30 Body Mass Index 30.0–30.9, adult** 🔗   A
    - **V85.31 Body Mass Index 31.0–31.9, adult** 🔗   A
    - **V85.32 Body Mass Index 32.0–32.9, adult** 🔗   A
    - **V85.33 Body Mass Index 33.0–33.9, adult** 🔗   A
    - **V85.34 Body Mass Index 34.0–34.9, adult** 🔗   A
    - **V85.35 Body Mass Index 35.0–35.9, adult** 🔗   A
    - **V85.36 Body Mass Index 36.0–36.9, adult** 🔗   A
    - **V85.37 Body Mass Index 37.0–37.9, adult** 🔗   A
    - **V85.38 Body Mass Index 38.0–38.9, adult** 🔗   A
    - **V85.39 Body Mass Index 39.0–39.9, adult** 🔗   A
  - **V85.4 Body Mass Index 40 and over, adult**
    - Coding Clinic: 2010, Q4, P81
    - **V85.41 Body Mass Index 40.0-44.9, adult** 🔗 🔗   A
    - **V85.42 Body Mass Index 45.0-49.9, adult** 🔗 🔗   A
    - **V85.43 Body Mass Index 50.0-59.9, adult** 🔗 🔗   A
    - **V85.44 Body Mass Index 60.0-69.9, adult** 🔗 🔗   A
    - **V85.45 Body Mass Index 70 and over, adult** 🔗 🔗   A
      - (Ex) 278.00-278.01, 278.1, V85.0, V85.54
  - **V85.5 Body Mass Index, pediatric**
    - **Note:** BMI pediatric codes are for use for persons age 2–20 years old. These percentiles are based on the growth charts published by the Centers for Disease Control and Prevention (CDC)
    - **V85.51 Body Mass Index, pediatric, less than 5th percentile for age** 🔗   P
    - **V85.52 Body Mass Index, pediatric, 5th percentile to less than 85th percentile for age** 🔗   P
    - **V85.53 Body Mass Index, pediatric, 85th percentile to less than 95th percentile for age** 🔗   P
    - **V85.54 Body Mass Index, pediatric, greater than or equal to 95th percentile for age** 🔗   P

ESTROGEN RECEPTOR STATUS (V86)

- **V86 Estrogen receptor status**
  - *Code first malignant neoplasm of breast (174.0–174.9, 175.0–175.9)*
  - **V86.0 Estrogen receptor positive status [ER+]** 🔗
  - **V86.1 Estrogen receptor negative status [ER-]** 🔗

N Newborn: 0   P Pediatric: 0–17   M Maternity: 12–55   A Adult: 15–124   ♀ Females Only   ♂ Males Only

● Unacceptable Principal Diagnosis   🔗 Complication\Comorbidity   🔗 Major C\C   🔗 Present on Admission Requirement   🔗 Hospital Acquired Condition   **1033**

OTHER SPECIFIED PERSONAL EXPOSURES AND HISTORY PRESENTING HAZARDS TO HEALTH (V87)

● V87   Other specified personal exposures and history presenting hazards to health

  ● V87.0   Contact with and (suspected) exposure to hazardous metals

    Excludes   *exposure to lead (V15.86)*
      toxic effect of metals (984.0-985.9)

    ● V87.01   **Arsenic**

    ● V87.02   **Contact with and (suspected) exposure to uranium**

      Excludes   *retained depleted uranium fragments (V90.01)*

    ● V87.09   **Other hazardous metals**
      Chromium compounds
      Nickel dust

  ● V87.1   Contact with and (suspected) exposure to hazardous aromatic compounds

    Excludes   *toxic effects of aromatic compounds (982.0, 983.0)*

    ● V87.11   **Aromatic amines**

    ● V87.12   **Benzene**

    ● V87.19   **Other hazardous aromatic compounds**
      Aromatic dyes NOS
      Polycyclic aromatic hydrocarbons

  ● V87.2   Contact with and (suspected) exposure to other potentially hazardous chemicals
    Dyes NOS

    Excludes   *exposure to asbestos (V15.84)*
      toxic effect of chemicals (980–989)

  ● V87.3   Contact with and (suspected) exposure to other potentially hazardous substances

    Excludes   *contact with and (suspected) exposure to potentially hazardous body fluids (V15.85)*
      personal history of retained foreign body fully removed (V15.53)
      toxic effect of substances (980–989)

    ● V87.31   **Exposure to mold**

    ● V87.32   **Contact with and (suspected) exposure to algae bloom** 🔍

    ● V87.39   **Contact with and (suspected) exposure to other potentially hazardous substances**

  ● V87.4   Personal history of drug therapy

    Excludes   *long-term (current) drug use (V58.61-V58.69)*

    ● V87.41   **Personal history of antineoplastic chemotherapy** 🔍

    ● V87.42   **Personal history of monoclonal drug therapy** 🔍

    ● V87.43   **Personal history of estrogen therapy** 🔍

    ● V87.44   **Personal history of inhaled steroid therapy** 🔍

    ● V87.45   **Personal history of systemic steroid therapy** 🔍
      Personal history of steroid therapy NOS

    ● V87.46   **Personal history of immunosuppression therapy** 🔍

      Excludes   *personal history of steroid therapy (V87.44, V87.45)*

    ● V87.49   **Personal history of other drug therapy** 🔍

ACQUIRED ABSENCE OF OTHER ORGANS AND TISSUE (V88)

● V88   Acquired absence of other organs and tissue

  ● V88.0   Acquired absence of cervix and uterus

    ● V88.01   **Acquired absence of both cervix and uterus** ♀ 🔍
      Acquired absence of uterus NOS
      Status post total hysterectomy

    ● V88.02   **Acquired absence of uterus with remaining cervical stump** ♀ 🔍
      Status post partial hysterectomy with remaining cervical stump

    ● V88.03   **Acquired absence of cervix with remaining uterus** ♀ 🔍

  ● V88.1   Acquired absence of pancreas

    Use additional code to identify any associated:
      insulin use (V58.67)
      secondary diabetes mellitus (249.00-249.91)

    ● V88.11   **Acquired total absence of pancreas** 🔍
      Acquired absence of pancreas NOS

    ● V88.12   **Acquired partial absence of pancreas** 🔍

  ● V88.2   Acquired absence of joint
    Acquired absence of joint following prior explantation of joint prosthesis
    Joint prosthesis explantation status

    ● V88.21   **Acquired absence of hip joint** 🔍
      Acquired absence of hip joint following explantation of joint prosthesis, with or without presence of antibiotic-impregnated cement spacer

    ● V88.22   **Acquired absence of knee joint** 🔍
      Acquired absence of knee joint following explantation of joint prosthesis, with or without presence of antibiotic-impregnated cement spacer

    ● V88.29   **Acquired absence of other joint** 🔍
      Acquired absence of other joint following explantation of joint prosthesis, with or without presence of antibiotic-impregnated cement spacer

OTHER SUSPECTED CONDITIONS NOT FOUND (V89)

● V89   Other suspected conditions not found

  ● V89.0   Suspected maternal and fetal conditions not found

    Excludes   *known or suspected fetal anomalies affecting management of mother, not ruled out (655.00 655.93, 656.00–656.93, 657.00–657.03, 658.00–658.93)*
      newborn and perinatal conditions – code to condition

    ● V89.01   **Suspected problem with amniotic cavity and membrane not found** ♀ 🔍   M
      Suspected oligohydramnios not found
      Suspected polyhydramnios not found

    ● V89.02   **Suspected placental problem not found** ♀ 🔍 M

    ● V89.03   **Suspected fetal anomaly not found** ♀ 🔍   M

    ● V89.04   **Suspected problem with fetal growth not found** ♀ 🔍   M

    ● V89.05   **Suspected cervical shortening not found** ♀ 🔍   M

    ● V89.09   **Other suspected maternal and fetal condition not found** ♀ 🔍   M

V01-V91

RETAINED FOREIGN BODY (V90)

● V90   Retained foreign body
　　　　Embedded fragment (status)
　　　　Embedded splinter (status)
　　　　Retained foreign body status

Excludes   *artificial joint prosthesis status (V43.60-V43.69)*
　　　　　　　foreign body accidentally left during a procedure
　　　　　　　　(998.4)
　　　　　　　foreign body entering through orifice (930.0-939.9)
　　　　　　　in situ cardiac devices (V45.00-V45.09)
　　　　　　　organ or tissue replaced by other means
　　　　　　　　(V43.0-V43.89)
　　　　　　　organ or tissue replaced by transplant (V42.0-V42.9)
　　　　　　　personal history of retained foreign body removed
　　　　　　　　(V15.53)
　　　　　　　superficial foreign body (splinter) (categories 910-917
　　　　　　　　and 919 with 4th character 6 or 7, 918.0)

● V90.0   Retained radioactive fragment
　　● V90.01   Retained depleted uranium fragments
　　● V90.09   Other retained radioactive fragments
　　　　　　　Other retained depleted isotope fragments
　　　　　　　Retained nontherapeutic radioactive
　　　　　　　　fragments

● V90.1   Retained metal fragments

Excludes   *retained radioactive metal fragments*
　　　　　　　　(V90.01-V90.09)

　　● V90.10   Retained metal fragments, unspecified
　　　　　　　Retained metal fragment NOS
　　● V90.11   Retained magnetic metal fragments
　　● V90.12   Retained nonmagnetic metal fragments

● V90.2   Retained plastic fragments
　　　　　Acrylics fragments
　　　　　Diethylhexylphthalates fragments
　　　　　Isocyanate fragments

● V90.3   Retained organic fragments
　　● V90.31   Retained animal quills or spines
　　● V90.32   Retained tooth
　　● V90.33   Retained wood fragments
　　● V90.39   Other retained organic fragments

● V90.8   Other specified retained foreign body
　　● V90.81   Retained glass fragments
　　● V90.83   Retained stone or crystalline fragments
　　　　　　　Retained concrete or cement fragments
　　● V90.89   Other specified retained foreign body

● V90.9   Retained foreign body, unspecified material

MULTIPLE GESTATION PLACENTA STATUS (V91)

● V91   Multiple gestation placenta status
　　　　Code first multiple gestation (651.0-651.9)

● V91.0   Twin gestation placenta status
　　● V91.00   Twin gestation, unspecified number of
　　　　　　　placenta, unspecified number of amniotic
　　　　　　　sacs ♀ 🖲　　　　　　　　　　　　　　　M
　　● V91.01   Twin gestation, monochorionic/monoamniotic
　　　　　　　(one placenta, one amniotic sac) ♀ 🖲　　　M
　　● V91.02   Twin gestation, monochorionic/diamniotic
　　　　　　　(one placenta, two amniotic sacs) ♀ 🖲　　M
　　● V91.03   Twin gestation, dichorionic/diamniotic (two
　　　　　　　placentae, two amniotic sacs) ♀ 🖲　　　　M
　　● V91.09   Twin gestation, unable to determine
　　　　　　　number of placenta and number of amniotic
　　　　　　　sacs ♀ 🖲　　　　　　　　　　　　　　　M

● V91.1   Triplet gestation placenta status
　　● V91.10   Triplet gestation, unspecified number of
　　　　　　　placenta and unspecified number of amniotic
　　　　　　　sacs ♀ 🖲　　　　　　　　　　　　　　　M
　　● V91.11   Triplet gestation, with two or more
　　　　　　　monochorionic fetuses ♀ 🖲　　　　　　　M
　　● V91.12   Triplet gestation, with two or more
　　　　　　　monoamniotic fetuses ♀ 🖲　　　　　　　M
　　● V91.19   Triplet gestation, unable to determine
　　　　　　　number of placenta and number of amniotic
　　　　　　　sacs ♀ 🖲　　　　　　　　　　　　　　　M

● V91.2   Quadruplet gestation placenta status
　　● V91.20   Quadruplet gestation, unspecified number of
　　　　　　　placenta and unspecified number of amniotic
　　　　　　　sacs ♀ 🖲　　　　　　　　　　　　　　　M
　　● V91.21   Quadruplet gestation, with two or more
　　　　　　　monochorionic fetuses ♀ 🖲　　　　　　　M
　　● V91.22   Quadruplet gestation, with two or more
　　　　　　　monoamniotic fetuses ♀ 🖲　　　　　　　M
　　● V91.29   Quadruplet gestation, unable to determine
　　　　　　　number of placenta and number of amniotic
　　　　　　　sacs ♀ 🖲　　　　　　　　　　　　　　　M

● V91.9   Other specified multiple gestation placenta status
　　　　　Placenta status for multiple gestations greater than
　　　　　　quadruplets
　　● V91.90   Other specified multiple gestation,
　　　　　　　unspecified number of placenta and
　　　　　　　unspecified number of amniotic sacs ♀ 🖲　M
　　● V91.91   Other specified multiple gestation, with two
　　　　　　　or more monochorionic fetuses ♀ 🖲　　　M
　　● V91.92   Other specified multiple gestation, with two
　　　　　　　or more monoamniotic fetuses ♀ 🖲　　　M
　　● V91.99   Other specified multiple gestation, unable to
　　　　　　　determine number of placenta and number of
　　　　　　　amniotic sacs ♀ 🖲　　　　　　　　　　M

V01-V91

N Newborn: 0   P Pediatric: 0–17   M Maternity: 12–55   A Adult: 15–124   ♀ Females Only   ♂ Males Only

● Unacceptable Principal Diagnosis   🖲 Complication\Comorbidity   🖲 Major C\C   🖲 Present on Admission Requirement   🖲 Hospital Acquired Condition

1035

Medicare Code Edit: E-codes are ICD-9-CM codes beginning with the letter E. They describe the circumstance causing an injury, not the nature of the injury, and therefore should not be used as a principal diagnosis.

SUPPLEMENTARY CLASSIFICATION OF EXTERNAL CAUSES OF INJURY AND POISONING (E000-E999)

This section is provided to permit the classification of environmental events, circumstances, and conditions as the cause of injury, poisoning, and other adverse effects. Where a code from this section is applicable, it is intended that it shall be used in addition to a code from one of the main chapters of ICD-9-CM, indicating the nature of the condition. Certain other conditions which may be stated to be due to external causes are classified in Chapters 1 to 16 of ICD-9-CM. For these, the "E" code classification should be used as an additional code for more detailed analysis.

Machinery accidents [other than those connected with transport] are classifiable to category E919, in which the fourth digit allows a broad classification of the type of machinery involved.

Categories for "late effects" of accidents and other external causes are to be found at E929, E959, E969, E977, E989, and E999.

(a) A transport accident (E800–E848) is any accident involving a device designed primarily for, or being used at the time primarily for, conveying persons or goods from one place to another.

Includes accidents involving:
aircraft and spacecraft (E840–E845)
watercraft (E830–E838)
motor vehicle (E810–E825)
railway (E800–E807)
other road vehicles (E826–E829)

In classifying accidents which involve more than one kind of transport, the above order of precedence of transport accidents should be used.

Accidents involving agricultural and construction machines, such as tractors, cranes, and bulldozers, are regarded as transport accidents only when these vehicles are under their own power on a highway [otherwise the vehicles are regarded as machinery]. Vehicles which can travel on land or water, such as hovercraft and other amphibious vehicles, are regarded as watercraft when on the water, as motor vehicles when on the highway, and as off-road motor vehicles when on land, but off the highway.

Excludes *accidents:*
in sports which involve the use of transport but where the transport vehicle itself was not involved in the accident
involving vehicles which are part of industrial equipment used entirely on industrial premises
occurring during transportation but unrelated to the hazards associated with the means of transportation [e.g., injuries received in a fight on board ship; transport vehicle involved in a cataclysm such as an earthquake]
to persons engaged in the maintenance or repair of transport equipment or vehicle not in motion, unless injured by another vehicle in motion

(b) A railway accident is a transport accident involving a railway train or other railway vehicle operated on rails, whether in motion or not.

Excludes *accidents:*
in repair shops
in roundhouse or on turntable
on railway premises but not involving a train or other railway vehicle

(c) A railway train or railway vehicle is any device with or without cars coupled to it, designed for traffic on a railway.

Includes interurban:
electric car (operated chiefly on its own right-of-way, not open to other traffic)
streetcar (operated chiefly on its own right-of-way, not open to other traffic)
railway train, any power [diesel] [electric] [steam]
funicular
monorail or two-rail
subterranean or elevated
other vehicle designed to run on a railway track

Excludes *interurban electric cars [streetcars] specified to be operating on a right-of-way that forms part of the public street or highway [definition (n)]*

(d) A railway or railroad is a right-of-way designed for traffic on rails, which is used by carriages or wagons transporting passengers or freight, and by other rolling stock, and which is not open to other public vehicular traffic.

(e) A motor vehicle accident is a transport accident involving a motor vehicle. It is defined as a motor vehicle traffic accident or as a motor vehicle nontraffic accident according to whether the accident occurs on a public highway or elsewhere.

Excludes *injury or damage due to cataclysm*
injury or damage while a motor vehicle, not under its own power, is being loaded on, or unloaded from, another conveyance

(f) A motor vehicle traffic accident is any motor vehicle accident occurring on a public highway [i.e., originating, terminating, or involving a vehicle partially on the highway]. A motor vehicle accident is assumed to have occurred on the highway unless another place is specified, except in the case of accidents involving only off-road motor vehicles which are classified as nontraffic accidents unless the contrary is stated.

(g) A motor vehicle nontraffic accident is any motor vehicle accident which occurs entirely in any place other than a public highway.

(h) A public highway [trafficway] or street is the entire width between property lines [or other boundary lines] of every way or place, of which any part is open to the use of the public for purposes of vehicular traffic as a matter of right or custom. A roadway is that part of the public highway designed, improved, and ordinarily used, for vehicular travel.

Includes approaches (public) to:
docks
public building
station

Excludes *driveway (private)*
parking lot
ramp
roads in:
airfield
farm
industrial premises
mine
private grounds
quarry

(i) A motor vehicle is any mechanically or electrically powered device, not operated on rails, upon which any person or property may be transported or drawn upon a highway. Any object such as a trailer, coaster, sled, or wagon being towed by a motor vehicle is considered a part of the motor vehicle.

Includes automobile [any type]
bus
construction machinery, farm and industrial machinery, steam roller, tractor, army tank, highway grader, or similar vehicle on wheels or treads, while in transport under own power
fire engine (motorized)
motorcycle
motorized bicycle [moped] or scooter
trolley bus not operating on rails
truck
van

Excludes *devices used solely to move persons or materials within the confines of a building and its premises, such as:*
building elevator
coal car in mine
electric baggage or mail truck used solely within a railroad station
electric truck used solely within an industrial plant
moving overhead crane

(j) A motorcycle is a two-wheeled motor vehicle having one or two riding saddles and sometimes having a third wheel for the support of a sidecar. The sidecar is considered part of the motorcycle.

Includes motorized:
bicycle [moped]
scooter
tricycle

(k) An off-road motor vehicle is a motor vehicle of special design, to enable it to negotiate rough or soft terrain or snow. Examples of special design are high construction, special wheels and tires, driven by treads, or support on a cushion of air.

Includes all terrain vehicle [ATV]
army tank
hovercraft, on land or swamp
snowmobile

(l) A driver of a motor vehicle is the occupant of the motor vehicle operating it or intending to operate it. A motorcyclist is the driver of a motorcycle. Other authorized occupants of a motor vehicle are passengers.

(m) An other road vehicle is any device, except a motor vehicle, in, on, or by which any person or property may be transported on a highway.

Includes animal carrying a person or goods
animal-drawn vehicle
animal harnessed to conveyance
bicycle [pedal cycle]
streetcar
tricycle (pedal)

Excludes *pedestrian conveyance [definition (q)]*

(n) A streetcar is a device designed and used primarily for transporting persons within a municipality, running on rails, usually subject to normal traffic control signals, and operated principally on a right-of-way that forms part of the traffic way. A trailer being towed by a streetcar is considered a part of the streetcar.

Includes interurban or intraurban electric or streetcar, when specified to be operating on a street or public highway
tram (car)
trolley (car)

(o) A pedal cycle is any road transport vehicle operated solely by pedals.

Includes bicycle
pedal cycle
tricycle

Excludes *motorized bicycle [definition (i)]*

(p) A pedal cyclist is any person riding on a pedal cycle or in a sidecar attached to such a vehicle.

(q) A pedestrian conveyance is any human powered device by which a pedestrian may move other than by walking or by which a walking person may move another pedestrian.

Includes baby carriage
coaster wagon
heelies
ice skates
motorized mobility scooter
perambulator
pushcart
pushchair
roller skates
scooter
skateboard
skis
sled
wheelchair (electric)
wheelies

(r) A pedestrian is any person involved in an accident who was not at the time of the accident riding in or on a motor vehicle, railroad train, streetcar, animal-drawn or other vehicle, or on a bicycle or animal.

Includes person:
changing tire of vehicle
in or operating a pedestrian conveyance
making adjustment to motor of vehicle
on foot

(s) A watercraft is any device for transporting passengers or goods on the water.

(t) A small boat is any watercraft propelled by paddle, oars, or small motor, with a passenger capacity of less than ten.

Includes boat NOS
canoe
coble
dinghy
punt
raft
rowboat
rowing shell
scull
skiff
small motorboat

Excludes *barge*
lifeboat (used after abandoning ship)
raft (anchored) being used as a diving platform
yacht

(u) An aircraft is any device for transporting passengers or goods in the air.

Includes airplane [any type]
balloon
bomber
dirigible
glider (hang)
military aircraft
parachute

(v) A commercial transport aircraft is any device for collective passenger or freight transportation by air, whether run on commercial lines for profit or by government authorities, with the exception of military craft.

E000-E999

N Newborn: 0   P Pediatric: 0–17   M Maternity: 12–55   A Adult: 15–124   ♀ Females Only   ♂ Males Only

Ⓔ CC/MCC Exclusions   Complication\Comorbidity   Major C\C   Present on Admission Requirement   Hospital-Acquired Condition   1037

EXTERNAL CAUSE STATUS (E000)

Note: A code from category E000 should be used in conjunction with the external cause code(s) assigned to a record to indicate the status of the person at the time the event occurred. A single code from category E000 should be assigned for an encounter.

● **E000   External cause status**

● **E000.0   Civilian activity done for income or pay** 🔍
     Civilian activity done for financial or other compensation
     Excludes   *military activity (E000.1)*
     Coding Clinic: 2009, Q4, P130

● **E000.1   Military activity** 🔍
     Excludes   *activity of off duty military personnel (E000.8)*

● **E000.2   Volunteer activity** 🔍
     Excludes   *activity of child or other family member assisting in compensated work of other family member (E000.8)*
     Coding Clinic: 2010, Q4, P111

● **E000.8   Other external cause status** 🔍
     Activity NEC
     Activity of child or other family member assisting in compensated work of other family member
     Hobby not done for income
     Leisure activity
     Off-duty activity of military personnel
     Recreation or sport not for income or while a student
     Student activity
     Excludes   *civilian activity done for income or compensation (E000.0)*
          military activity (E000.1)
     Coding Clinic: 2013, Q3, P11; 2010, Q4, P93; 2009, Q4, P130

● **E000.9   Unspecified external cause status** 🔍

ACTIVITY (E001-E030)

Note: Categories E001 to E030 are provided for use to indicate the activity of the person seeking healthcare for an injury or health condition, such as a heart attack while shoveling snow, which resulted from, or was contributed to, by the activity. These codes are appropriate for use for both acute injuries, such as those from chapter 17, and conditions that are due to the long-term, cumulative effects of an activity, such as those from chapter 13. They are also appropriate for use with external cause codes for cause and intent if identifying the activity provides additional information on the event.

These codes should be used in conjunction with other external cause codes for external cause status (E000) and place of occurrence (E849).

This section contains the following broad activity categories:

     E001   Activities involving walking and running
     E002   Activities involving water and water craft
     E003   Activities involving ice and snow
     E004   Activities involving climbing, rappelling, and jumping off
     E005   Activities involving dancing and other rhythmic movement
     E006   Activities involving other sports and athletics played individually
     E007   Activities involving other sports and athletics played as a team or group
     E008   Activities involving other specified sports and athletics
     E009   Activity involving other cardiorespiratory exercise

     E010   Activity involving other muscle strengthening exercises
     E011   Activities involving computer technology and electronic devices
     E012   Activities involving arts and handcrafts
     E013   Activities involving personal hygiene and household maintenance
     E014   Activities involving person providing caregiving
     E015   Activities involving food preparation, cooking and grilling
     E016   Activities involving property and land maintenance, building and construction
     E017   Activities involving roller coasters and other types of external motion
     E018   Activities involving playing musical instrument
     E019   Activities involving animal care
     E029   Other activity
     E030   Unspecified activity

● **E001   Activities involving walking and running**
     Excludes   *walking an animal (E019.0)*
          walking or running on a treadmill (E009.0)

● **E001.0   Walking, marching and hiking** 🔍
     Walking, marching and hiking on level or elevated terrain
     Excludes   *mountain climbing (E004.0)*
     Coding Clinic: 2009, Q4, P141

● **E001.1   Running** 🔍

● **E002   Activities involving water and water craft**
     Excludes   *activities involving ice (E003.0-E003.9)*
          boating and other watercraft transport accidents (E830-E838)

● **E002.0   Swimming** 🔍

● **E002.1   Springboard and platform diving** 🔍

● **E002.2   Water polo** 🔍

● **E002.3   Water aerobics and water exercise** 🔍

● **E002.4   Underwater diving and snorkeling** 🔍
     SCUBA diving

● **E002.5   Rowing, canoeing, kayaking, rafting and tubing** 🔍
     Canoeing, kayaking, rafting and tubing in calm and turbulent water

● **E002.6   Water skiing and wake boarding** 🔍

● **E002.7   Surfing, windsurfing and boogie boarding** 🔍
     Coding Clinic: 2013, Q3, P11

● **E002.8   Water sliding** 🔍

● **E002.9   Other activity involving water and watercraft** 🔍
     Activity involving water NOS
     Parasailing
     Water survival training and testing
     Coding Clinic: 2010, Q2, P16

● **E003   Activities involving ice and snow**
     Excludes   *shoveling ice and snow (E016.0)*

● **E003.0   Ice skating** 🔍
     Figure skating (singles) (pairs)
     Ice dancing
     Excludes   *ice hockey (E003.1)*

● **E003.1   Ice hockey** 🔍

● **E003.2   Snow (alpine) (downhill) skiing, snow boarding, sledding, tobogganing and snow tubing** 🔍
     Excludes   *cross country skiing (E003.3)*

● **E003.3   Cross country skiing** 🔍
     Nordic skiing

● **E003.9   Other activity involving ice and snow** 🔍
     Activity involving ice and snow NOS

◀ New   ◀ Revised   ~~deleted~~ Deleted   Excludes   Includes   Use additional   Code first   Omit code

1038   ● Unacceptable Principal Diagnosis   ● Use Additional Digit(s)   ▶ Manifestation Code   OGCR Official Guidelines   Coding Clinic

● **E004   Activities involving climbing, rappelling and jumping off**
　　Excludes　 *hiking on level or elevated terrain (E001.0)*
　　　　　　　　 jumping rope (E006.5)
　　　　　　　　 sky diving (E840-E844)
　　　　　　　　 trampoline jumping (E005.3)
　● **E004.0   Mountain climbing, rock climbing and wall climbing** 🖐
　● **E004.1   Rappelling** 🖐
　● **E004.2   BASE jumping** 🖐
　　　　　Building, Antenna, Span, Earth jumping
　● **E004.3   Bungee jumping** 🖐
　● **E004.4   Hang gliding** 🖐
　● **E004.9   Other activity involving climbing, rappelling and jumping off** 🖐

● **E005   Activities involving dancing and other rhythmic movement**
　　Excludes　 *martial arts (E008.4)*
　● **E005.0   Dancing** 🖐
　● **E005.1   Yoga** 🖐
　● **E005.2   Gymnastics** 🖐
　　　　　Rhythmic gymnastics
　　　　Excludes　 *trampoline (E005.3)*
　● **E005.3   Trampoline** 🖐
　● **E005.4   Cheerleading** 🖐
　● **E005.9   Other activity involving dancing and other rhythmic movements** 🖐

● **E006   Activities involving other sports and athletics played individually**
　　Excludes　 *dancing (E005.0)*
　　　　　　　　 gymnastics (E005.2)
　　　　　　　　 trampoline (E005.3)
　　　　　　　　 yoga (E005.1)
　● **E006.0   Roller skating (inline) and skateboarding** 🖐
　　　　　Coding Clinic: 2010, Q4, P93
　● **E006.1   Horseback riding** 🖐
　● **E006.2   Golf** 🖐
　● **E006.3   Bowling** 🖐
　● **E006.4   Bike riding** 🖐
　　　　Excludes　 *transport accident involving bike riding (E800-E829)*
　● **E006.5   Jumping rope** 🖐
　● **E006.6   Non-running track and field events** 🖐
　　　　Excludes　 *running (any form) (E001.1)*
　● **E006.9   Other activity involving other sports and athletics played individually** 🖐
　　　　Excludes　 *activities involving climbing, rappelling, and jumping (E004.0-E004.9)*
　　　　　　　　 activities involving ice and snow (E003.0-E003.9)
　　　　　　　　 activities involving walking and running (E001.0-E001.9)
　　　　　　　　 activities involving water and watercraft (E002.0-E002.9)

● **E007   Activities involving other sports and athletics played as a team or group**
　　Excludes　 *ice hockey (E003.1)*
　　　　　　　　 water polo (E002.2)
　● **E007.0   American tackle football** 🖐
　　　　　Football NOS
　● **E007.1   American flag or touch football** 🖐
　● **E007.2   Rugby** 🖐
　● **E007.3   Baseball** 🖐
　　　　　Softball

　● **E007.4   Lacrosse and field hockey** 🖐
　● **E007.5   Soccer** 🖐
　● **E007.6   Basketball** 🖐
　● **E007.7   Volleyball (beach) (court)** 🖐
　● **E007.8   Physical games generally associated with school recess, summer camp and children** 🖐
　　　　　Capture the flag
　　　　　Dodge ball
　　　　　Four square
　　　　　Kickball
　● **E007.9   Other activity involving other sports and athletics played as a team or group** 🖐
　　　　　Cricket

● **E008   Activities involving other specified sports and athletics**
　● **E008.0   Boxing** 🖐
　● **E008.1   Wrestling** 🖐
　● **E008.2   Racquet and hand sports** 🖐
　　　　　Handball
　　　　　Racquetball
　　　　　Squash
　　　　　Tennis
　● **E008.3   Frisbee** 🖐
　　　　　Ultimate frisbee
　● **E008.4   Martial arts** 🖐
　　　　　Combatives
　● **E008.9   Other specified sports and athletics activity** 🖐
　　　　Excludes　 *sports and athletics activities specified in categories E001-E007*

● **E009   Activity involving other cardiorespiratory exercise**
　　　　Activity involving physical training
　● **E009.0   Exercise machines primarily for cardiorespiratory conditioning** 🖐
　　　　　Elliptical and stepper machines
　　　　　Stationary bike
　　　　　Treadmill
　● **E009.1   Calisthenics** 🖐
　　　　　Jumping jacks
　　　　　Warm up and cool down
　● **E009.2   Aerobic and step exercise** 🖐
　● **E009.3   Circuit training** 🖐
　● **E009.4   Obstacle course** 🖐
　　　　　Challenge course
　　　　　Confidence course
　● **E009.5   Grass drills** 🖐
　　　　　Guerilla drills
　● **E009.9   Other activity involving other cardiorespiratory exercise** 🖐
　　　　Excludes　 *activities involving cardiorespiratory exercise specified in categories E001-E008*

● **E010   Activity involving other muscle strengthening exercises**
　● **E010.0   Exercise machines primarily for muscle strengthening** 🖐
　● **E010.1   Push-ups, pull-ups, sit-ups** 🖐
　● **E010.2   Free weights** 🖐
　　　　　Barbells
　　　　　Dumbbells
　● **E010.3   Pilates** 🖐
　● **E010.9   Other activity involving other muscle strengthening exercises** 🖐
　　　　Excludes　 *activities involving muscle strengthening specified in categories E001-E009*

E000-E999

N Newborn: 0　　**P** Pediatric: 0–17　　**M** Maternity: 12–55　　**A** Adult: 15–124　　♀ Females Only　　♂ Males Only

(Ex) CC/MCC Exclusions　　🖐 Complication\Comorbidity　　Major C\C　　🖐 Present on Admission Requirement　　🖐 Hospital-Acquired Condition

1039

● E011   Activities involving computer technology and electronic devices
> **Excludes**   *electronic musical keyboard or instruments (E018.0)*

● E011.0   Computer keyboarding 🔍
> Electronic game playing using keyboard or other stationary device

● E011.1   Hand held interactive electronic device 🔍
> Cellular telephone and communication device
> Electronic game playing using interactive device
>> **Excludes**   *electronic game playing using keyboard or other stationary device (E011.0)*

● E011.9   Other activity involving computer technology and electronic devices 🔍

● E012   Activities involving arts and handcrafts
> **Excludes**   *activities involving playing musical instrument (E018.0-E018.3)*

● E012.0   Knitting and crocheting 🔍
● E012.1   Sewing 🔍
● E012.2   Furniture building and finishing 🔍
> Furniture repair
● E012.9   Activity involving other arts and handcrafts 🔍

● E013   Activities involving personal hygiene and household maintenance
> **Excludes**   *activities involving cooking and grilling (E015.0-E015.9)*
> *activities involving property and land maintenance, building and construction (E016.0-E016.9)*
> *activity involving persons providing caregiving (E014.0-E014.9)*
> *dishwashing (E015.0)*
> *food preparation (E015.0)*
> *gardening (E016.1)*

● E013.0   Personal bathing and showering 🔍
● E013.1   Laundry 🔍
● E013.2   Vacuuming 🔍
● E013.3   Ironing 🔍
● E013.4   Floor mopping and cleaning 🔍
● E013.5   Residential relocation 🔍
> Packing up and unpacking involved in moving to a new residence
● E013.8   Other personal hygiene activity 🔍
● E013.9   Other household maintenance 🔍

● E014   Activities involving person providing caregiving
● E014.0   Caregiving involving bathing 🔍
● E014.1   Caregiving involving lifting 🔍
● E014.9   Other activity involving person providing caregiving 🔍

● E015   Activities involving food preparation, cooking and grilling
● E015.0   Food preparation and clean up 🔍
> Dishwashing
● E015.1   Grilling and smoking food 🔍
● E015.2   Cooking and baking 🔍
> Use of stove, oven and microwave oven
● E015.9   Other activity involving cooking and grilling 🔍

● E016   Activities involving property and land maintenance, building and construction
● E016.0   Digging, shoveling and raking 🔍
> Dirt digging
> Raking leaves
> Snow shoveling
> **Coding Clinic: 2009, Q4, P141**
● E016.1   Gardening and landscaping 🔍
> Pruning, trimming shrubs, weeding
● E016.2   Building and construction 🔍
● E016.9   Other activity involving property and land maintenance, building and construction 🔍

● E017   Activities involving roller coasters and other types of external motion
● E017.0   Roller coaster riding 🔍
● E017.9   Other activity involving external motion 🔍

● E018   Activities involving playing musical instrument
> Activity involving playing electric musical instrument
● E018.0   Piano playing 🔍
> Musical keyboard (electronic) playing
● E018.1   Drum and other percussion instrument playing 🔍
● E018.2   String instrument playing 🔍
● E018.3   Wind and brass instrument playing 🔍

● E019   Activities involving animal care
> **Excludes**   *horseback riding (E006.1)*
● E019.0   Walking an animal 🔍
● E019.1   Milking an animal 🔍
● E019.2   Grooming and shearing an animal 🔍
● E019.9   Other activity involving animal care 🔍

● E029   Other activity
> **Coding Clinic: 2010, Q4, P111**
● E029.0   Refereeing a sports activity 🔍
● E029.1   Spectator at an event 🔍
● E029.2   Rough housing and horseplay 🔍
● E029.9   Other activity 🔍

● E030   Unspecified activity 🔍

TRANSPORT ACCIDENTS (E800-E848)

Definitions and examples related to transport accidents

(a) A transport accident (E800-E848) is any accident involving a device designed primarily for, or being used at the time primarily for, conveying persons or goods from one place to another.

◀ New   ◀ Revised   ~~deleted~~ Deleted   Excludes   Includes   Use additional   Code first   Omit code
● Unacceptable Principal Diagnosis   ● Use Additional Digit(s)   ▶ Manifestation Code   OGCR Official Guidelines   Coding Clinic

RAILWAY ACCIDENTS (E800-E807)

Note: For definitions of railway accident and related terms see definitions (a) to (d).

Excludes *accidents involving railway train and:*
aircraft (E840.0-E845.9)
motor vehicle (E810.0-E825.9)
watercraft (E830.0-E838.9)

The following fourth-digit subdivisions are for use with categories E800-E807 to identify the injured person:

0 Railway employee
Any person who by virtue of his employment in connection with a railway, whether by the railway company or not, is at increased risk of involvement in a railway accident, such as:
catering staff of train
driver
guard
porter
postal staff on train
railway fireman
shunter
sleeping car attendant
1 Passenger on railway
Any authorized person traveling on a train, except a railway employee.
Excludes *intending passenger waiting at station (8)*
unauthorized rider on railway vehicle (8)
2 Pedestrian
See definition (r)
3 Pedal cyclist
See definition (p)
8 Other specified person
Intending passenger or bystander waiting at station
Unauthorized rider on railway vehicle
9 Unspecified person

● ● **E800 Railway accident involving collision with rolling stock** 🖐
Requires fourth digit. See beginning of section E800-E845 for codes and definitions.
Includes collision between railway trains or railway vehicles, any kind
collision NOS on railway
derailment with antecedent collision with rolling stock or NOS

● ● **E801 Railway accident involving collision with other object** 🖐
Requires fourth digit. See beginning of section E800-E845 for codes and definitions.
Includes collision of railway train with:
buffers
fallen tree on railway
gates
platform
rock on railway
streetcar
other nonmotor vehicle
other object
Excludes *collision with:*
aircraft (E840.0-E842.9)
motor vehicle (E810.0-E810.9, E820.0-E822.9)

● ● **E802 Railway accident involving derailment without antecedent collision** 🖐
Requires fourth digit. See beginning of section E800-E845 for codes and definitions.

● ● **E803 Railway accident involving explosion, fire, or burning** 🖐
Requires fourth digit. See beginning of section E800-E845 for codes and definitions.
Excludes *explosion or fire, with antecedent derailment (E802.0-E802.9)*
explosion or fire, with mention of antecedent collision (E800.0-E801.9)

● ● **E804 Fall in, on, or from railway train** 🖐
Requires fourth digit. See beginning of section E800-E845 for codes and definitions.
Includes fall while alighting from or boarding railway train
Excludes *fall related to collision, derailment, or explosion of railway train (E800.0-E803.9)*

● ● **E805 Hit by rolling stock** 🖐
Requires fourth digit. See beginning of section E800-E845 for codes and definitions.
Includes crushed by railway train or part
injured by railway train or part
killed by railway train or part
knocked down by railway train or part
run over by railway train or part
Excludes *pedestrian hit by object set in motion by railway train (E806.0-E806.9)*

● ● **E806 Other specified railway accident** 🖐
Requires fourth digit. See beginning of section E800-E845 for codes and definitions.
Includes hit by object falling in railway train
injured by door or window on railway train
nonmotor road vehicle or pedestrian hit by object set in motion by railway train
railway train hit by falling:
earth NOS
rock
tree
other object
Excludes *railway accident due to cataclysm (E908-E909)*

● ● **E807 Railway accident of unspecified nature** 🖐
Requires fourth digit. See beginning of section E800-E845 for codes and definitions.
Includes found dead on railway right-of-way NOS
injured on railway right-of-way NOS
railway accident NOS

E000-E999

N Newborn: 0   **P** Pediatric: 0–17   **M** Maternity: 12–55   **A** Adult: 15–124   ♀ Females Only   ♂ Males Only

(Ex) CC/MCC Exclusions   🖐 Complication\Comorbidity   🖐 Major C\C   🖐 Present on Admission Requirement   🖐 Hospital-Acquired Condition   **1041**

MOTOR VEHICLE TRAFFIC ACCIDENTS (E810-E819)

Note: For definitions of motor vehicle traffic accident, and related terms, see definitions (e) to (k).

Excludes *accidents involving motor vehicle and aircraft (E840.0-E845.9)*

The following fourth-digit subdivisions are for use with categories E810-E819 to identify the injured person:

> 0 **Driver of motor vehicle other than motorcycle**
> See definition (l)
> 1 **Passenger in motor vehicle other than motorcycle**
> See definition (l)
> 2 **Motorcyclist**
> See definition (l)
> 3 **Passenger on motorcycle**
> See definition (l)
> 4 **Occupant of streetcar**
> 5 **Rider of animal; occupant of animal-drawn vehicle**
> 6 **Pedal cyclist**
> See definition (p)
> 7 **Pedestrian**
> See definition (r)
> 8 **Other specified person**
> Occupant of vehicle other than above
> Person in railway train involved in accident
> Unauthorized rider of motor vehicle
> 9 **Unspecified person**

E810 Motor vehicle traffic accident involving collision with train 🖉

Requires fourth digit. See beginning of section E800-E845 for codes and definitions.

Excludes *motor vehicle collision with object set in motion by railway train (E815.0-E815.9)*
railway train hit by object set in motion by motor vehicle (E818.0-E818.9)

E811 Motor vehicle traffic accident involving re-entrant collision with another motor vehicle 🖉

Requires fourth digit. See beginning of section E800-E845 for codes and definitions.

Includes collision between motor vehicle which accidentally leaves the roadway then re-enters the same roadway, or the opposite roadway on a divided highway, and another motor vehicle

Excludes *collision on the same roadway when none of the motor vehicles involved have left and re-entered the roadway (E812.0-E812.9)*

E812 Other motor vehicle traffic accident involving collision with motor vehicle 🖉

Requires fourth digit. See beginning of section E800-E845 for codes and definitions.

Includes collision with another motor vehicle parked, stopped, stalled, disabled, or abandoned on the highway
motor vehicle collision NOS

Excludes *collision with object set in motion by another motor vehicle (E815.0-E815.9)*
re-entrant collision with another motor vehicle (E811.0-E811.9)

Coding Clinic: 2011, Q4, P100; 2007, Q4, P105-107; 1996, Q4, P36-37

E813 Motor vehicle traffic accident involving collision with other vehicle 🖉

Requires fourth digit. See beginning of section E800-E845 for codes and definitions.

Includes collision between motor vehicle, any kind, and:
other road (nonmotor transport) vehicle, such as:
animal carrying a person
animal-drawn vehicle
pedal cycle
streetcar

Excludes *collision with:*
object set in motion by nonmotor road vehicle (E815.0-E815.9)
pedestrian (E814.0-E814.9)
nonmotor road vehicle hit by object set in motion by motor vehicle (E818.0-E818.9)

E814 Motor vehicle traffic accident involving collision with pedestrian 🖉

Requires fourth digit. See beginning of section E800-E845 for codes and definitions.

Includes collision between motor vehicle, any kind, and pedestrian
pedestrian dragged, hit, or run over by motor vehicle, any kind

Excludes *pedestrian hit by object set in motion by motor vehicle (E818.0-E818.9)*

Coding Clinic: 2010, Q4, P93; 1996, Q4, P36-37

E815 Other motor vehicle traffic accident involving collision on the highway 🖉

Requires fourth digit. See beginning of section E800-E845 for codes and definitions.

Includes collision (due to loss of control) (on highway) between motor vehicle, any kind, and:
abutment (bridge) (overpass)
animal (herded) (unattended)
fallen stone, traffic sign, tree, utility pole
guard rail or boundary fence
interhighway divider
landslide (not moving)
object set in motion by railway train or road vehicle (motor) (nonmotor)
object thrown in front of motor vehicle
safety island
temporary traffic sign or marker
wall of cut made for road
other object, fixed, movable, or moving

Excludes *collision with:*
any object off the highway (resulting from loss of control) (E816.0-E816.9)
any object which normally would have been off the highway and is not stated to have been on it (E816.0-E816.9)
motor vehicle parked, stopped, stalled, disabled, or abandoned on highway (E812.0-E812.9)
moving landslide (E909.2)
motor vehicle hit by object:
set in motion by railway train or road vehicle (motor) (nonmotor) (E818.0-E818.9)
thrown into or on vehicle (E818.0-E818.9)

● ● **E816 Motor vehicle traffic accident due to loss of control, without collision on the highway** 🔖

> Requires fourth digit. See beginning of section E800-E845 for codes and definitions.

Includes motor vehicle:
> failing to make curve and:
>> colliding with object off the highway
>> overturning
>> stopping abruptly off the highway
> going out of control (due to)
>> blowout and:
>>> colliding with object off the highway
>>> overturning
>>> stopping abruptly off the highway
>> burst tire and:
>>> colliding with object off the highway
>>> overturning
>>> stopping abruptly off the highway
>> driver falling asleep and:
>>> colliding with object off the highway
>>> overturning
>>> stopping abruptly off the highway
>> driver inattention and:
>>> colliding with object off the highway
>>> overturning
>>> stopping abruptly off the highway
>> excessive speed and:
>>> colliding with object off the highway
>>> overturning
>>> stopping abruptly off the highway
>> failure of mechanical part and:
>>> colliding with object off the highway
>>> overturning
>>> stopping abruptly off the highway

Excludes *collision on highway following loss of control (E810.0-E815.9)*
> *loss of control of motor vehicle following collision on the highway (E810.0-E815.9)*

● ● **E817 Noncollision motor vehicle traffic accident while boarding or alighting** 🔖

> Requires fourth digit. See beginning of section E800-E845 for codes and definitions.

Includes fall down stairs of motor bus while boarding or alighting
> fall from car in street while boarding or alighting
> injured by moving part of the vehicle while boarding or alighting
> trapped by door of motor bus boarding or alighting while boarding or alighting

● ● **E818 Other noncollision motor vehicle traffic accident** 🔖

> Requires fourth digit. See beginning of section E800-E845 for codes and definitions.

Includes accidental poisoning from exhaust gas generated by motor vehicle while in motion
> breakage of any part of motor vehicle while in motion
> explosion of any part of motor vehicle while in motion
> fall, jump, or being accidentally pushed from motor vehicle while in motion
> fire starting in motor vehicle while in motion
> hit by object thrown into or on motor vehicle while in motion
> injured by being thrown against some part of, or object in motor vehicle while in motion
> injury from moving part of motor vehicle while in motion
> object falling in or on motor vehicle while in motion
> object thrown on motor vehicle while in motion
> collision of railway train or road vehicle except motor vehicle, with object set in motion by motor vehicle
> motor vehicle hit by object set in motion by railway train or road vehicle (motor) (nonmotor)
> pedestrian, railway train, or road vehicle (motor) (nonmotor) hit by object set in motion by motor vehicle

Excludes *collision between motor vehicle and:*
> *object set in motion by railway train or road vehicle (motor) (nonmotor) (E815.0-E815.9)*
> *object thrown towards the motor vehicle (E815.0-E815.9)*
> *person overcome by carbon monoxide generated by stationary motor vehicle off the roadway with motor running (E868.2)*

● ● **E819 Motor vehicle traffic accident of unspecified nature** 🔖

> Requires fourth digit. See beginning of section E800-E845 for codes and definitions.

Includes motor vehicle traffic accident NOS
> traffic accident NOS

Coding Clinic: 2009, Q4, P141; 2008, Q4, P96-97; 2006, Q4, P100-102; 2003, Q1, P7; 1999, Q4, P11-12; Q1, P10; 1993, Q2, P4-5

E000-E999

N Newborn: 0   **P** Pediatric: 0–17   **M** Maternity: 12–55   **A** Adult: 15–124   ♀ Females Only   ♂ Males Only

(Ex) CC/MCC Exclusions   🔖 Complication\Comorbidity   🔖 Major C\C   🔖 Present on Admission Requirement   🔖 Hospital-Acquired Condition   **1043**

MOTOR VEHICLE NONTRAFFIC ACCIDENTS (E820-E825)

Note: For definitions of motor vehicle nontraffic accident and related terms see definition (a) to (k).

Includes accidents involving motor vehicles being used in recreational or sporting activities off the highway
collision and noncollision motor vehicle accidents occurring entirely off the highway

Excludes *accidents involving motor vehicle and:*
aircraft (E840.0-E845.9)
watercraft (E830.0-E838.9)
accidents, not on the public highway, involving agricultural and construction machinery but not involving another motor vehicle (E919.0, E919.2, E919.7)

The following fourth-digit subdivisions are for use with categories E820-E825 to identify the injured person:

> 0 **Driver of motor vehicle other than motorcycle**
>   See definition (l)
> 1 **Passenger in motor vehicle other than motorcycle**
>   See definition (l)
> 2 **Motorcyclist**
>   See definition (l)
> 3 **Passenger on motorcycle**
>   See definition (l)
> 4 **Occupant of streetcar**
> 5 **Rider of animal; occupant of animal-drawn vehicle**
> 6 **Pedal cyclist**
>   See definition (p)
> 7 **Pedestrian**
>   See definition (r)
> 8 **Other specified person**
>   Occupant of vehicle other than above
>   Person on railway train involved in accident
>   Unauthorized rider of motor vehicle
> 9 **Unspecified person**

E820 **Nontraffic accident involving motor-driven snow vehicle** 🔍
Requires fourth digit. See beginning of section E800-E845 for codes and definitions.

Includes breakage of part of motor-driven snow vehicle (not on public highway)
fall from motor-driven snow vehicle (not on public highway)
hit by motor-driven snow vehicle (not on public highway)
overturning of motor-driven snow vehicle (not on public highway)
run over or dragged by motor-driven snow vehicle (not on public highway)
collision of motor-driven snow vehicle with:
  animal (being ridden) (-drawn vehicle)
  another off-road motor vehicle
  other motor vehicle, not on public highway
  railway train
  other object, fixed or movable
injury caused by rough landing of motor-driven snow vehicle (after leaving ground on rough terrain)

Excludes *accident on the public highway involving motor driven snow vehicle (E810.0-E819.9)*

E821 **Nontraffic accident involving other off-road motor vehicle** 🔍
Requires fourth digit. See beginning of section E800-E845 for codes and definitions.

Includes breakage of part of off-road motor vehicle, except snow vehicle (not on public highway)
fall from off-road motor vehicle, except snow vehicle (not on public highway)
hit by off-road motor vehicle, except snow vehicle (not on public highway)
overturning of off-road motor vehicle, except snow vehicle (not on public highway)
run over or dragged by off-road motor vehicle, except snow vehicle (not on public highway)
thrown against some part of or object in off-road motor vehicle, except snow vehicle (not on public highway)
collision with:
  animal (being ridden) (-drawn vehicle)
  another off-road motor vehicle, except snow vehicle
  other motor vehicle, not on public highway
  other object, fixed or movable

Excludes *accident on public highway involving off-road motor vehicle (E810.0-E819.9)*
collision between motor driven snow vehicle and other off-road motor vehicle (E820.0-E820.9)
hovercraft accident on water (E830.0-E838.9)

E822 **Other motor vehicle nontraffic accident involving collision with moving object** 🔍
Requires fourth digit. See beginning of section E800-E845 for codes and definitions.

Includes collision, not on public highway, between motor vehicle, except off-road motor vehicle and:
  animal
  nonmotor vehicle
  other motor vehicle, except off-road motor vehicle
  pedestrian
  railway train
  other moving object

Excludes *collision with:*
motor-driven snow vehicle (E820.0-E820.9)
other off-road motor vehicle (E821.0-E821.9)

E823 **Other motor vehicle nontraffic accident involving collision with stationary object** 🔍
Requires fourth digit. See beginning of section E800-E845 for codes and definitions.

Includes collision, not on public highway, between motor vehicle, except off-road motor vehicle, and any object, fixed or movable, but not in motion

E824 **Other motor vehicle nontraffic accident while boarding and alighting** 🔍
Requires fourth digit. See beginning of section E800-E845 for codes and definitions.

Includes fall while boarding or alighting from motor vehicle except off-road motor vehicle, not on public highway
injury from moving part of motor vehicle while boarding or alighting from motor vehicle except off-road motor vehicle, not on public highway
trapped by door of motor vehicle while boarding or alighting from motor vehicle except off-road motor vehicle, not on public highway

Coding Clinic: 2010, Q4, P111

E000-E999

● ● **E825** **Other motor vehicle nontraffic accident of other and unspecified nature** 🔲

Requires fourth digit. See beginning of section E800-E845 for codes and definitions.

Includes   accidental poisoning from carbon monoxide generated by motor vehicle while in motion, not on public highway

breakage of any part of motor vehicle while in motion, not on public highway

explosion of any part of motor vehicle while in motion, not on public highway

fall, jump, or being accidentally pushed from motor vehicle while in motion, not on public highway

fire starting in motor vehicle while in motion, not on public highway

hit by object thrown into, towards, or on motor vehicle while in motion, not on public highway

injured by being thrown against some part of, or object in motor vehicle while in motion, not on public highway

injury from moving part of motor vehicle while in motion, not on public highway

object falling in or on motor vehicle while in motion, not on public highway

motor vehicle nontraffic accident NOS

Excludes   *fall from or in stationary motor vehicle (E884.9, E885.9)*

overcome by carbon monoxide or exhaust gas generated by stationary motor vehicle off the roadway with motor running (E868.2)

struck by falling object from or in stationary motor vehicle (E916)

OTHER ROAD VEHICLE ACCIDENTS (E826-E829)

Note: Other road vehicle accidents are transport accidents involving road vehicles other than motor vehicles. For definitions of other road vehicle and related terms see definitions (m) to (o).

Includes   accidents involving other road vehicles being used in recreational or sporting activities

Excludes   *collision of other road vehicle [any] with:*
aircraft (E840.0-E845.9)
motor vehicle (E813.0-E813.9, E820.0-E822.9)
railway train (E801.0-E801.9)

The following fourth-digit subdivisions are for use with categories E826-E829 to identify the injured person:

> 0   **Pedestrian**
>   See definition (r)
> 1   **Pedal cyclist**
>   See definition (p)
> 2   **Rider of animal**
> 3   **Occupant of animal-drawn vehicle**
> 4   **Occupant of streetcar**
> 8   **Other specified person**
> 9   **Unspecified person**

● ● **E826** **Pedal cycle accident** 🔲
[0-9]

Requires fourth digit. See beginning of section E800-E845 for codes and definitions.

Includes   breakage of any part of pedal cycle
collision between pedal cycle and:
animal (being ridden) (herded) (unattended)
another pedal cycle
nonmotor road vehicle, any
pedestrian
other object, fixed, movable, or moving, not set in motion by motor vehicle, railway train, or aircraft
entanglement in wheel of pedal cycle
fall from pedal cycle
hit by object falling or thrown on the pedal cycle
pedal cycle accident NOS
pedal cycle overturned

● ● **E827** **Animal-drawn vehicle accident** 🔲
[0,2-4,8,9]

Requires fourth digit. See beginning of section E800-E845 for codes and definitions.

Includes   breakage of any part of vehicle
collision between animal-drawn vehicle and:
animal (being ridden) (herded) (unattended)
nonmotor road vehicle, except pedal cycle
pedestrian, pedestrian conveyance, or pedestrian vehicle
other object, fixed, movable, or moving, not set in motion by motor vehicle, railway train, or aircraft
fall from animal-drawn vehicle
knocked down by animal-drawn vehicle
overturning of animal-drawn vehicle
run over by animal-drawn vehicle
thrown from animal-drawn vehicle

Excludes   *collision of animal-drawn vehicle with pedal cycle (E826.0-E826.9)*

● ● **E828** **Accident involving animal being ridden** 🔲
[0,2,4,8,9]

Requires fourth digit. See beginning of section E800-E845 for codes and definitions.

Includes   collision between animal being ridden and:
another animal
nonmotor road vehicle, except pedal cycle, and animal-drawn vehicle
pedestrian, pedestrian conveyance, or pedestrian vehicle
other object, fixed, movable, or moving, not set in motion by motor vehicle, railway train, or aircraft
fall from animal being ridden
knocked down by animal being ridden
thrown from animal being ridden
trampled by animal being ridden
ridden animal stumbled and fell

Excludes   *collision of animal being ridden with:*
animal-drawn vehicle (E827.0-E827.9)
pedal cycle (E826.0-E826.9)

E000-E999

N Newborn: 0   **P** Pediatric: 0–17   **M** Maternity: 12–55   **A** Adult: 15–124   ♀ Females Only   ♂ Males Only

(Ex) CC/MCC Exclusions   🔲 Complication\Comorbidity   🔲 Major C\C   🔲 Present on Admission Requirement   🔲 Hospital-Acquired Condition   **1045**

E000-E999

● ● **E829** **Other road vehicle accidents** 🔊
[0,4,8,9]
Requires fourth digit. See beginning of section E800-E845 for codes and definitions.

Includes　accident while boarding or alighting from
　　　　streetcar
　　　　nonmotor road vehicle not classifiable to
　　　　　　E826-E828
　　blow from object in
　　　　streetcar
　　　　nonmotor road vehicle not classifiable to
　　　　　　E826-E828
　　breakage of any part of
　　　　streetcar
　　　　nonmotor road vehicle not classifiable to
　　　　　　E826-E828
　　caught in door of
　　　　streetcar
　　　　nonmotor road vehicle not classifiable to
　　　　　　E826-E828
　　derailment of
　　　　streetcar
　　　　nonmotor road vehicle not classifiable to
　　　　　　E826-E828
　　fall in, on, or from
　　　　streetcar
　　　　nonmotor road vehicle not classifiable to
　　　　　　E826-E828
　　fire in
　　　　streetcar
　　　　nonmotor road vehicle not classifiable to
　　　　　　E826-E828
　　collision between streetcar or nonmotor road
　　　　vehicle, except as in E826-E828, and:
　　　　animal (not being ridden)
　　　　another nonmotor road vehicle not
　　　　　　classifiable to E826-E828
　　　　pedestrian
　　　　other object, fixed, movable, or moving, not
　　　　　　set in motion by motor vehicle, railway
　　　　　　train, or aircraft
　　nonmotor road vehicle accident NOS
　　streetcar accident NOS

Excludes　*collision with:*
　　　　animal being ridden (E828.0-E828.9)
　　　　animal-drawn vehicle (E827.0-E827.9)
　　　　pedal cycle (E826.0-E826.9)

WATER TRANSPORT ACCIDENTS (E830-E838)

Note: For definitions of water transport accident and related terms see definitions (a), (s), and (t).

Includes　watercraft accidents in the course of recreational
　　　　activities

Excludes　*accidents involving both aircraft, including objects*
　　　　set in motion by aircraft, and watercraft
　　　　(E840.0-E845.9)

The following fourth-digit subdivisions are for use with categories E830-E838 to identify the injured person:

0　**Occupant of small boat, unpowered**
1　**Occupant of small boat, powered**
　　See definition (t)
　　Excludes　*water skier (4)*
2　**Occupant of other watercraft-crew**
　　Persons:
　　　　engaged in operation of watercraft
　　　　providing passenger services [cabin attendants,
　　　　　　ship's physician, catering personnel]
　　　　working on ship during voyage in other capacity
　　　　　　[musician in band, operators of shops and
　　　　　　beauty parlors]
3　**Occupant of other watercraft -- other than crew**
　　Passenger
　　Occupant of lifeboat, other than crew, after
　　　　abandoning ship
4　**Water skier**
5　**Swimmer**
6　**Dockers, stevedores**
　　Longshoreman employed on the dock in loading
　　　　and unloading ships
7　**Occupant of military watercraft, any type**
8　**Other specified person**
　　Immigration and custom officials on board ship
　　Person:
　　　　accompanying passenger or member of crew
　　　　visiting boat
　　Pilot (guiding ship into port)
9　**Unspecified person**

● ● **E830** **Accident to watercraft causing submersion** 🔊
Requires fourth digit. See beginning of section E800-E845 for codes and definitions.

Includes　submersion and drowning due to:
　　　　boat overturning
　　　　boat submerging
　　　　falling or jumping from burning ship
　　　　falling or jumping from crushed watercraft
　　　　ship sinking
　　　　other accident to watercraft

● ● **E831** **Accident to watercraft causing other injury** 🔊
Requires fourth digit. See beginning of section E800-E845 for codes and definitions.

Includes　any injury, except submersion and drowning, as
　　　　a result of an accident to watercraft
　　burned while ship on fire
　　crushed between ships in collision
　　crushed by lifeboat after abandoning ship
　　fall due to collision or other accident to
　　　　watercraft
　　hit by falling object due to accident to watercraft
　　injured in watercraft accident involving
　　　　collision
　　struck by boat or part thereof after fall or jump
　　　　from damaged boat

Excludes　*burns from localized fire or explosion on board ship*
　　　　(E837.0-E837.9)

◀ New　◀ Revised　d̶e̶l̶e̶t̶e̶d̶ Deleted　Excludes　Includes　Use additional　Code first　Omit code
● Unacceptable Principal Diagnosis　● Use Additional Digit(s)　▷ Manifestation Code　OGCR Official Guidelines　**Coding Clinic**

● ● **E832 Other accidental submersion or drowning in water transport accident** 🔖

    Requires fourth digit. See beginning of section E800-E845 for codes and definitions.

    Includes   submersion or drowning as a result of an accident other than accident to the watercraft, such as:
        fall:
            from gangplank
            from ship
            overboard
        thrown overboard by motion of ship
        washed overboard

    Excludes   *submersion or drowning of swimmer or diver who voluntarily jumps from boat not involved in an accident (E910.0-E910.9)*

● ● **E833 Fall on stairs or ladders in water transport** 🔖

    Requires fourth digit. See beginning of section E800-E845 for codes and definitions.

    Excludes   *fall due to accident to watercraft (E831.0-E831.9)*

● ● **E834 Other fall from one level to another in water transport** 🔖

    Requires fourth digit. See beginning of section E800-E845 for codes and definitions.

    Excludes   *fall due to accident to watercraft (E831.0-E831.9)*

● ● **E835 Other and unspecified fall in water transport** 🔖

    Requires fourth digit. See beginning of section E800-E845 for codes and definitions.

    Excludes   *fall due to accident to watercraft (E831.0-E831.9)*

● ● **E836 Machinery accident in water transport** 🔖

    Requires fourth digit. See beginning of section E800-E845 for codes and definitions.

    Includes   injuries in water transport caused by:
        deck machinery
        engine room machinery
        galley machinery
        laundry machinery
        loading machinery

● ● **E837 Explosion, fire, or burning in watercraft** 🔖

    Requires fourth digit. See beginning of section E800-E845 for codes and definitions.

    Includes   explosion of boiler on steamship
        localized fire on ship

    Excludes   *burning ship (due to collision or explosion) resulting in:*
        submersion or drowning (E830.0-E830.9)
        other injury (E831.0-E831.9)

● ● **E838 Other and unspecified water transport accident** 🔖

    Requires fourth digit. See beginning of section E800-E845 for codes and definitions.

    Includes   accidental poisoning by gases or fumes on ship
        atomic power plant malfunction in watercraft
        crushed between ship and stationary object [wharf]
        crushed between ships without accident to watercraft
        crushed by falling object on ship or while loading or unloading
        hit by boat while water skiing
        struck by boat or part thereof (after fall from boat)
        watercraft accident NOS

AIR AND SPACE TRANSPORT ACCIDENTS (E840-E845)

Note: For definition of aircraft and related terms see definitions (u) and (v).

The following fourth-digit subdivisions are for use with categories E840-E845 to identify the injured person:

0 Occupant of spacecraft

1 Occupant of military aircraft, any
    Crew in military aircraft [air force] [army] [national guard] [navy]
    Passenger (civilian) (military) in military aircraft [air force] [army] [national guard] [navy]
    Troops in military aircraft [air force] [army] [national guard] [navy]

    Excludes   *occupants of aircraft operated under jurisdiction of police departments (5)*
        parachutist (7)

2 Crew of commercial aircraft (powered) in surface-to-surface transport

3 Other occupant of commercial aircraft (powered) in surface-to-surface transport
    Flight personnel:
        not part of crew
        on familiarization flight
    Passenger on aircraft (powered) NOS

4 Occupant of commercial aircraft (powered) in surface-to-air transport
    Occupant [crew] [passenger] of aircraft (powered) engaged in activities, such as:
        aerial spraying (crops) (fire retardants)
        air drops of emergency supplies
        air drops of parachutists, except from military craft
        crop dusting
        lowering of construction material [bridge or telephone pole]
        sky writing

5 Occupant of other powered aircraft
    Occupant [crew] [passenger] of aircraft [powered] engaged in activities, such as:
        aerobatic flying
        aircraft racing
        rescue operation
        storm surveillance
        traffic surveillance
    Occupant of private plane NOS

6 Occupant of unpowered aircraft, except parachutist
    Occupant of aircraft classifiable to E842

7 Parachutist (military) (other)
    Person making voluntary descent

    Excludes   *person making descent after accident to aircraft (.1-.6)*

8 Ground crew, airline employee
    Persons employed at airfields (civil) (military) or launching pads, not occupants of aircraft

9 Other person

● ● **E840 Accident to powered aircraft at takeoff or landing** 🔖

    Requires fourth digit. See beginning of section E800-E845 for codes and definitions.

    Includes   collision of aircraft with any object, fixed, movable, or moving while taking off or landing
        crash while taking off or landing
        explosion on aircraft while taking off or landing
        fire on aircraft while taking off or landing
        forced landing

E000-E999

N Newborn: 0   **P** Pediatric: 0–17   **M** Maternity: 12–55   **A** Adult: 15–124   ♀ Females Only   ♂ Males Only

(Ex.) CC/MCC Exclusions   🔖 Complication\Comorbidity   🔖 Major C\C   🔖 Present on Admission Requirement   🔖 Hospital-Acquired Condition   **1047**

● ● **E841** **Accident to powered aircraft, other and unspecified** 🕭

Requires fourth digit. See beginning of section E800-E845 for codes and definitions.

Includes   aircraft accident NOS
aircraft crash or wreck NOS
any accident to powered aircraft while in transit or when not specified whether in transit, taking off, or landing
collision of aircraft with another aircraft, bird, or any object, while in transit
explosion on aircraft while in transit
fire on aircraft while in transit

● ● **E842** **Accident to unpowered aircraft** 🕭
[6-9]

Requires fourth digit. See beginning of section E800-E845 for codes and definitions.

Includes   any accident, except collision with powered aircraft, to:
balloon
glider
hang glider
kite carrying a person
hit by object falling from unpowered aircraft

● ● **E843** **Fall in, on, or from aircraft** 🕭
[0-9]

Requires fourth digit. See beginning of section E800-E845 for codes and definitions.

Includes   accident in boarding or alighting from aircraft, any kind
fall in, on, or from aircraft [any kind], while in transit, taking off, or landing, except when as a result of an accident to aircraft

● ● **E844** **Other specified air transport accidents** 🕭
[0-9]

Requires fourth digit. See beginning of section E800-E845 for codes and definitions.

Includes   hit by aircraft without accident to aircraft
hit by object falling from aircraft without accident to aircraft
injury by or from machinery on aircraft without accident to aircraft
injury by or from rotating propeller without accident to aircraft
injury by or from voluntary parachute descent without accident to aircraft
poisoning by carbon monoxide from aircraft while in transit without accident to aircraft
sucked into jet without accident to aircraft
any accident involving other transport vehicle (motor) (nonmotor) due to being hit by object set in motion by aircraft (powered)

Excludes   air sickness (E903)
effects of:
high altitude (E902.0-E902.1)
pressure change (E902.0-E902.1)
injury in parachute descent due to accident to aircraft (E840.0-E842.9)

● ● **E845** **Accident involving spacecraft** 🕭
[0,8,9]

Requires fourth digit. See beginning of section E800-E845 for codes and definitions.

Includes   launching pad accident
Excludes   effects of weightlessness in spacecraft (E928.0)

VEHICLE ACCIDENTS NOT ELSEWHERE CLASSIFIABLE (E846-E848)

● **E846** **Accidents involving powered vehicles used solely within the buildings and premises of industrial or commercial establishment** 🕭

Accident to, on, or involving:
battery-powered airport passenger vehicle
battery-powered trucks (baggage) (mail)
coal car in mine
logging car
self-propelled truck, industrial
station baggage truck (powered)
tram, truck, or tub (powered) in mine or quarry
Breakage of any part of vehicle
Collision with:
pedestrian
other vehicle or object within premises
Explosion of powered vehicle, industrial or commercial
Fall from powered vehicle, industrial or commercial
Overturning of powered vehicle, industrial or commercial
Struck by powered vehicle, industrial or commercial

Excludes   accidental poisoning by exhaust gas from vehicle not elsewhere classifiable (E868.2)
injury by crane, lift (fork), or elevator (E919.2)

● **E847** **Accidents involving cable cars not running on rails** 🕭

Accident to, on, or involving:
cable car, not on rails
ski chair-lift
ski-lift with gondola
teleferique
Breakage of cable
caught or dragged by cable car, not on rails
fall or jump from cable car, not on rails
object thrown from or in cable car not on rails

● **E848** **Accidents involving other vehicles, not elsewhere classifiable** 🕭

Accident to, on, or involving:
ice yacht
land yacht
nonmotor, nonroad vehicle NOS

OGCR   Section I.C.19.b

Use an additional code from category E849 to indicate the Place of Occurrence. The Place of Occurrence describes the place where the event occurred and not the patient's activity at the time of the event. Do not use E849.9 if the place of occurrence is not stated.

PLACE OF OCCURRENCE (E849)

● **E849** **Place of Occurrence**

Note: The following category is for use to denote the place where the injury or poisoning occurred.

● **E849.0** **Home** 🕭
Apartment
Boarding house
Farm house
Home premises
House (residential)
Noninstitutional place of residence
Private:
driveway
garage
garden
home
walk
Swimming pool in private house or garden
Yard of home

Excludes   home under construction but not yet occupied (E849.3)
institutional place of residence (E849.7)

◀ New   ◀▥ Revised   ~~deleted~~ Deleted   Excludes   Includes   Use additional   Code first   Omit code

1048   ● Unacceptable Principal Diagnosis   ◐ Use Additional Digit(s)   ▸ Manifestation Code   OGCR Official Guidelines   Coding Clinic

● **E849.1 Farm** 🔗
    Buildings   Land under cultivation
    Excludes *farm house and home premises of farm*
                 (E849.0)

● **E849.2 Mine and quarry** 🔗
    Gravel pit   Tunnel under
    Sand pit   construction

● **E849.3 Industrial place and premises** 🔗
    Building under construction
    Dockyard
    Dry dock
    Factory
       building
       premises
    Garage (place of work)
    Industrial yard
    Loading platform (factory) (store)
    Plant, industrial
    Railway yard
    Shop (place of work)
    Warehouse
    Workhouse
    Coding Clinic: 2010, Q4, P111; 2003, Q4, P76-78

● **E849.4 Place for recreation and sport** 🔗
    Amusement park   Playground, including
    Baseball field   school playground
    Basketball court   Public park
    Beach resort   Racecourse
    Cricket ground   Resort NOS
    Fives court   Riding school
    Football field   Rifle range
    Golf course   Seashore resort
    Gymnasium   Skating rink
    Hockey field   Sports palace
    Holiday camp   Stadium
    Ice palace   Swimming pool, public
    Lake resort   Tennis court
    Mountain resort   Vacation resort
    Excludes *that in private house or garden (E849.0)*

● **E849.5 Street and highway** 🔗
    **Coding Clinic: 2011, Q4, P100; 2010, Q4, P93; 2009, Q4, P144;
             1995, Q1, P10**

● **E849.6 Public building** 🔗
    Building (including adjacent grounds) used by the
       general public or by a particular group of the
       public, such as:
       airport
       bank
       cafe
       casino
       church
       cinema
       clubhouse
       courthouse
       dance hall
       garage building (for car storage)
       hotel
       market (grocery or other commodity)
       movie house
       music hall
       nightclub
       office
       office building
       opera house
       post office
       public hall
       radio broadcasting station
       restaurant
       school (state) (public) (private)
       shop, commercial
       station (bus) (railway)
       store
       theater
    Excludes *home garage (E849.0)*
                 industrial building or workplace (E849.3)

● **E849.7 Residential institution** 🔗
    Children's home
    Dormitory
    Hospital
    Jail
    Old people's home
    Orphanage
    Prison
    Reform School

● **E849.8 Other specified places** 🔗
    Beach NOS
    Canal
    Caravan site NOS
    Derelict house
    Desert
    Dock
    Forest
    Harbor
    Hill
    Lake NOS
    Mountain
    Parking lot
    Parking place
    Pond or pool (natural)
    Prairie
    Public place NOS
    Railway line
    Reservoir
    River
    Sea
    Seashore NOS
    Stream
    Swamp
    Trailer court
    Woods
    Coding Clinic: 2013, Q3, P11

● **E849.9 Unspecified place** 🔗

ACCIDENTAL POISONING BY DRUGS, MEDICINAL SUBSTANCES, AND BIOLOGICALS (E850-E858)

Includes   accidental overdose of drug, wrong drug
               given or taken in error, and drug taken
               inadvertently
               accidents in the use of drugs and biologicals in
               medical and surgical procedures

Excludes *administration with suicidal or homicidal intent or
               intent to harm, or in circumstances classifiable
               to E980-E989 (E950.0-E950.5, E962.0,
               E980.0-E980.5)*
              *correct drug properly administered in therapeutic or
               prophylactic dosage, as the cause of adverse
               effect (E930.0-E949.9)*

Note: See Alphabetic Index for more complete list of
          specific drugs to be classified under the fourth-digit
          subdivisions. The American Hospital Formulary
          numbers can be used to classify new drugs listed by
          the American Hospital Formulary Service (AHFS).
          See Appendix C.

● **E850 Accidental poisoning by analgesics, antipyretics, and
          antirheumatics**
    Coding Clinic: 2008, Q3, P21

● **E850.0 Heroin**
    Diacetylmorphine

● **E850.1 Methadone**

● **E850.2 Other opiates and related narcotics**
    Codeine [methylmorphine]
    Meperidine [pethidine]
    Morphine
    Opium (alkaloids)

● **E850.3 Salicylates**
    Acetylsalicylic acid [aspirin]
    Amino derivatives of salicylic acid
    Salicylic acid salts

E000-E999

● **E850.4** **Aromatic analgesics, not elsewhere classified**
  Acetanilid
  Paracetamol [acetaminophen]
  Phenacetin [acetophenetidin]

● **E850.5** **Pyrazole derivatives**
  Aminophenazone [amidopyrine]
  Phenylbutazone

● **E850.6** **Antirheumatics [antiphlogistics]**
  Gold salts
  Indomethacin
  > **Excludes** *salicylates (E850.3)*
  >   *steroids (E858.0)*

● **E850.7** **Other non-narcotic analgesics**
  Pyrabital

● **E850.8** **Other specified analgesics and antipyretics**
  Pentazocine

● **E850.9** **Unspecified analgesic or antipyretic**

● **E851** **Accidental poisoning by barbiturates**
  Amobarbital [amylobarbitone]
  Barbital [barbitone]
  Butabarbital [butabarbitone]
  Pentobarbital [pentobarbitone]
  Phenobarbital [phenobarbitone]
  Secobarbital [quinalbarbitone]
  > **Excludes** *thiobarbiturates (E855.1)*

● **E852** **Accidental poisoning by other sedatives and hypnotics**

  ● **E852.0** **Chloral hydrate group**

  ● **E852.1** **Paraldehyde**

  ● **E852.2** **Bromine compounds**
    Bromides
    Carbromal (derivatives)

  ● **E852.3** **Methaqualone compounds**

  ● **E852.4** **Glutethimide group**

  ● **E852.5** **Mixed sedatives, not elsewhere classified**

  ● **E852.8** **Other specified sedatives and hypnotics**

  ● **E852.9** **Unspecified sedative or hypnotic**
    Sleeping:
      drug NOS
      pill NOS
      tablet NOS

● **E853** **Accidental poisoning by tranquilizers**

  ● **E853.0** **Phenothiazine-based tranquilizers**
    Chlorpromazine
    Fluphenazine
    Prochlorperazine
    Promazine

  ● **E853.1** **Butyrophenone-based tranquilizers**
    Haloperidol
    Spiperone
    Trifluperidol

  ● **E853.2** **Benzodiazepine-based tranquilizers**
    Chlordiazepoxide   Lorazepam
    Diazepam   Medazepam
    Flurazepam   Nitrazepam
    Coding Clinic: 2009, Q4, P150; 1991, Q3, P14

  ● **E853.8** **Other specified tranquilizers**
    Hydroxyzine
    Meprobamate

  ● **E853.9** **Unspecified tranquilizer**

● **E854** **Accidental poisoning by other psychotropic agents**

  ● **E854.0** **Antidepressants**
    Amitriptyline
    Imipramine
    Monoamine oxidase [MAO] inhibitors
    Coding Clinic: 2009, Q4, P150; 1991, Q3, P14

  ● **E854.1** **Psychodysleptics [hallucinogens]**
    Cannabis derivatives
    Lysergide [LSD]
    Marihuana (derivatives)
    Mescaline
    Psilocin
    Psilocybin

  ● **E854.2** **Psychostimulants**
    Amphetamine
    Caffeine
    > **Excludes** *central appetite depressants (E858.8)*
    Coding Clinic: 2003, Q2, P11

  ● **E854.3** **Central nervous system stimulants**
    Analeptics
    Opiate antagonists

  ● **E854.8** **Other psychotropic agents**

● **E855** **Accidental poisoning by other drugs acting on central and autonomic nervous system**

  ● **E855.0** **Anticonvulsant and anti-Parkinsonism drugs**
    Amantadine
    Hydantoin derivatives
    Levodopa [L-dopa]
    Oxazolidine derivatives [paramethadione]
        [trimethadione]
    Succinimides

  ● **E855.1** **Other central nervous system depressants**
    Ether
    Gaseous anesthetics
    Halogenated hydrocarbon derivatives
    Intravenous anesthetics
    Thiobarbiturates, such as thiopental sodium

  ● **E855.2** **Local anesthetics**
    Cocaine
    Lidocaine [lignocaine]
    Procaine
    Tetracaine

  ● **E855.3** **Parasympathomimetics [cholinergics]**
    Acetylcholine
    Anticholinesterase:
        organophosphorus
        reversible
    Pilocarpine

  ● **E855.4** **Parasympatholytics [anticholinergics and antimuscarinics] and spasmolytics**
    Atropine
    Homatropine
    Hyoscine [scopolamine]
    Quaternary ammonium derivatives

  ● **E855.5** **Sympathomimetics [adrenergics]**
    Epinephrine [adrenalin]
    Levarterenol [noradrenalin]

  ● **E855.6** **Sympatholytics [antiadrenergics]**
    Phenoxybenzamine
    Tolazoline hydrochloride

  ● **E855.8** **Other specified drugs acting on central and autonomic nervous systems**

  ● **E855.9** **Unspecified drug acting on central and autonomic nervous systems**

● **E856** **Accidental poisoning by antibiotics**

● **E857** **Accidental poisoning by other anti-infectives**

◄ New   ◄▦ Revised   ~~deleted~~ Deleted   Excludes   Includes   Use additional   Code first   Omit code
● Unacceptable Principal Diagnosis   ● Use Additional Digit(s)   ▌ Manifestation Code   OGCR Official Guidelines   Coding Clinic

● **E858 Accidental poisoning by other drugs**
    Coding Clinic: 2008, Q3, P21
  ● **E858.0 Hormones and synthetic substitutes**
  ● **E858.1 Primarily systemic agents**
  ● **E858.2 Agents primarily affecting blood constituents**
  ● **E858.3 Agents primarily affecting cardiovascular system**
  ● **E858.4 Agents primarily affecting gastrointestinal system**
  ● **E858.5 Water, mineral, and uric acid metabolism drugs**
  ● **E858.6 Agents primarily acting on the smooth and skeletal muscles and respiratory system**
  ● **E858.7 Agents primarily affecting skin and mucous membrane, ophthalmological, otorhinolaryngological, and dental drugs**
  ● **E858.8 Other specified drugs**
      Central appetite depressants
  ● **E858.9 Unspecified drug**

ACCIDENTAL POISONING BY OTHER SOLID AND LIQUID SUBSTANCES, GASES, AND VAPORS (E860-E869)

Note: Categories in this section are intended primarily to indicate the external cause of poisoning states classifiable to 980–989. They may also be used to indicate external causes of localized effects classifiable to 001–799.

● **E860 Accidental poisoning by alcohol, not elsewhere classified**
  ● **E860.0 Alcoholic beverages**
      Alcohol in preparations intended for consumption
      Coding Clinic: 2009, Q4, P150; 1996, Q3, P161; 1991, Q3, P14
  ● **E860.1 Other and unspecified ethyl alcohol and its products**
      Denatured alcohol
      Ethanol NOS
      Grain alcohol NOS
      Methylated spirit
  ● **E860.2 Methyl alcohol**
      Methanol
      Wood alcohol
  ● **E860.3 Isopropyl alcohol**
      Dimethyl carbinol
      Isopropanol
      Rubbing alcohol substitute
      Secondary propyl alcohol
  ● **E860.4 Fusel oil**
      Alcohol:
        amyl
        butyl
        propyl
  ● **E860.8 Other specified alcohols**
  ● **E860.9 Unspecified alcohol**

● **E861 Accidental poisoning by cleansing and polishing agents, disinfectants, paints, and varnishes**
  ● **E861.0 Synthetic detergents and shampoos**
  ● **E861.1 Soap products**
  ● **E861.2 Polishes**
  ● **E861.3 Other cleansing and polishing agents**
      Scouring powders
  ● **E861.4 Disinfectants**
      Household and other disinfectants not ordinarily used on the person
      Excludes *carbolic acid or phenol (E864.0)*
  ● **E861.5 Lead paints**
  ● **E861.6 Other paints and varnishes**
      Lacquers
      Oil colors
      Paints, other than lead
      Whitewashes
  ● **E861.9 Unspecified**

● **E862 Accidental poisoning by petroleum products, other solvents and their vapors, not elsewhere classified**
  ● **E862.0 Petroleum solvents**
      Petroleum:
        ether
        benzine
        naphtha
  ● **E862.1 Petroleum fuels and cleaners**
      Antiknock additives to petroleum fuels
      Gas oils
      Gasoline or petrol
      Kerosene
      Excludes *kerosene insecticides (E863.4)*
  ● **E862.2 Lubricating oils**
  ● **E862.3 Petroleum solids**
      Paraffin wax
  ● **E862.4 Other specified solvents**
      Benzene
      Coding Clinic: 2008, Q3, P6-7
  ● **E862.9 Unspecified solvent**

● **E863 Accidental poisoning by agricultural and horticultural chemical and pharmaceutical preparations other than plant foods and fertilizers**
    Excludes *plant foods and fertilizers (E866.5)*
  ● **E863.0 Insecticides of organochlorine compounds**
      Benzene hexachloride   Dieldrin
      Chlordane   Endrine
      DDT   Toxaphene
  ● **E863.1 Insecticides of organophosphorus compounds**
      Demeton   Parathion
      Diazinon   Phenylsulphthion
      Dichlorvos   Phorate
      Malathion   Phosdrin
      Methyl parathion
  ● **E863.2 Carbamates**
      Aldicarb
      Carbaryl
      Propoxur
  ● **E863.3 Mixtures of insecticides**
  ● **E863.4 Other and unspecified insecticides**
      Kerosene insecticides
  ● **E863.5 Herbicides**
      2,4-Dichlorophenoxyacetic acid [2, 4-D]
      2,4,5-Trichlorophenoxyacetic acid [2, 4, 5-T]
      Chlorates
      Diquat
      Mixtures of plant foods and fertilizers with herbicides
      Paraquat
  ● **E863.6 Fungicides**
      Organic mercurials (used in seed dressing)
      Pentachlorophenols
  ● **E863.7 Rodenticides**
      Fluoroacetates   Warfarin
      Squill and derivatives   Zinc phosphide
      Thallium
  ● **E863.8 Fumigants**
      Cyanides   Phosphine
      Methyl bromide
  ● **E863.9 Other and unspecified**

● **E864 Accidental poisoning by corrosives and caustics, not elsewhere classified**
    Excludes *those as components of disinfectants (E861.4)*
  ● **E864.0 Corrosive aromatics**
      Carbolic acid or phenol
  ● **E864.1 Acids**
      Acid:
        hydrochloric
        nitric
        sulfuric

E000-E999

N Newborn: 0   P Pediatric: 0–17   M Maternity: 12–55   A Adult: 15–124   ♀ Females Only   ♂ Males Only

Ⓔ CC/MCC Exclusions   Complication\Comorbidity   Major C\C   Present on Admission Requirement   Hospital-Acquired Condition   **1051**

E000-E999

- E864.2 **Caustic alkalis**
    Lye
- E864.3 **Other specified corrosives and caustics**
- E864.4 **Unspecified corrosives and caustics**

- E865 **Accidental poisoning from poisonous foodstuffs and poisonous plants**
    Includes   any meat, fish, or shellfish
    plants, berries, and fungi eaten as, or in mistake for food, or by a child
    Excludes   *anaphylactic shock due to adverse food reaction (995.60–995.69)*
    food poisoning (bacterial) (005.0–005.9)
    poisoning and toxic reactions to venomous plants (E905.6–E905.7)
- E865.0 **Meat**
- E865.1 **Shellfish**
- E865.2 **Other fish**
- E865.3 **Berries and seeds**
- E865.4 **Other specified plants**
- E865.5 **Mushrooms and other fungi**
- E865.8 **Other specified foods**
- E865.9 **Unspecified foodstuff or poisonous plant**

- E866 **Accidental poisoning by other and unspecified solid and liquid substances**
    Excludes   *these substances as a component of:*
    medicines (E850.0-E858.9)
    paints (E861.5-E861.6)
    pesticides (E863.0-E863.9)
    petroleum fuels (E862.1)
- E866.0 **Lead and its compounds and fumes**
- E866.1 **Mercury and its compounds and fumes**
- E866.2 **Antimony and its compounds and fumes**
- E866.3 **Arsenic and its compounds and fumes**
- E866.4 **Other metals and their compounds and fumes**
    Beryllium (compounds)
    Brass fumes
    Cadmium (compounds)
    Copper salts
    Iron (compounds)
    Manganese (compounds)
    Nickel (compounds)
    Thallium (compounds)
- E866.5 **Plant foods and fertilizers**
    Excludes   *mixtures with herbicides (E863.5)*
- E866.6 **Glues and adhesives**
- E866.7 **Cosmetics**
- E866.8 **Other specified solid or liquid substances**
    Coding Clinic: 1990, Q4, P25
- E866.9 **Unspecified solid or liquid substance**

- E867 **Accidental poisoning by gas distributed by pipeline**
    Carbon monoxide from incomplete combustion of piped gas
    Coal gas NOS
    Liquefied petroleum gas distributed through pipes (pure or mixed with air)
    Piped gas (natural) (manufactured)

- E868 **Accidental poisoning by other utility gas and other carbon monoxide**
- E868.0 **Liquefied petroleum gas distributed in mobile containers**
    Butane or carbon monoxide from incomplete combustion of these gases
    Liquefied hydrocarbon gas NOS or carbon monoxide from incomplete combustion of these gases
    Propane or carbon monoxide from incomplete combustion of these gases
- E868.1 **Other and unspecified utility gas**
    Acetylene or carbon monoxide from incomplete combustion of these gases
    Gas NOS used for lighting, heating, or cooking or carbon monoxide from incomplete combustion of these gases
    Water gas or carbon monoxide from incomplete combustion of these gases
- E868.2 **Motor vehicle exhaust gas**
    Exhaust gas from:
    farm tractor, not in transit
    gas engine
    motor pump
    motor vehicle, not in transit
    any type of combustion engine not in watercraft
    Excludes   *poisoning by carbon monoxide from:*
    aircraft while in transit (E844.0-E844.9)
    motor vehicle while in transit (E818.0-E818.9)
    watercraft whether or not in transit (E838.0-E838.9)
- E868.3 **Carbon monoxide from incomplete combustion of other domestic fuels**
    Carbon monoxide from incomplete combustion of:
    coal in domestic stove or fireplace
    coke in domestic stove or fireplace
    kerosene in domestic stove or fireplace
    wood in domestic stove or fireplace
    Excludes   *carbon monoxide from smoke and fumes due to conflagration (E890.0-E893.9)*
- E868.8 **Carbon monoxide from other sources**
    Carbon monoxide from:
    blast furnace gas
    incomplete combustion of fuels in industrial use
    kiln vapor
- E868.9 **Unspecified carbon monoxide**

- E869 **Accidental poisoning by other gases and vapors**
    Excludes   *effects of gases used as anesthetics (E855.1, E938.2)*
    fumes from heavy metals (E866.0-E866.4)
    smoke and fumes due to conflagration or explosion (E890.0-E899)
- E869.0 **Nitrogen oxides**
- E869.1 **Sulfur dioxide**
- E869.2 **Freon**
- E869.3 **Lacrimogenic gas [tear gas]**
    Bromobenzyl cyanide
    Chloroacetophenone
    Ethyliodoacetate
- E869.4 **Second-hand tobacco smoke**
    Coding Clinic: 1996, Q2, P10
- E869.8 **Other specified gases and vapors**
    Chlorine
    Hydrocyanic acid gas
- E869.9 **Unspecified gases and vapors**

◄ New   ◄▥ Revised   ~~deleted~~ Deleted   Excludes   Includes   Use additional   Code first   Omit code
● Unacceptable Principal Diagnosis   ◉ Use Additional Digit(s)   ▸ Manifestation Code   **OGCR** Official Guidelines   **Coding Clinic**
1052

MISADVENTURES TO PATIENTS DURING SURGICAL AND MEDICAL CARE (E870-E876)

> **Excludes** *accidental overdose of drug and wrong drug given in error (E850.0-E858.9)*
> *surgical and medical procedures as the cause of abnormal reaction by the patient, without mention of misadventure at the time of procedure (E878.0-E879.9)*

OGCR Section I.C.19.h.1
Assign a code in the range of E870-E876 if misadventures are stated by the provider. **When applying the E code guidelines pertaining to sequencing, these E codes are considered causal codes.**

● **E870 Accidental cut, puncture, perforation, or hemorrhage during medical care**
  ● **E870.0 Surgical operation**
    Coding Clinic: 2010, Q1, P20-21
  ● **E870.1 Infusion or transfusion**
  ● **E870.2 Kidney dialysis or other perfusion**
  ● **E870.3 Injection or vaccination**
  ● **E870.4 Endoscopic examination**
  ● **E870.5 Aspiration of fluid or tissue, puncture, and catheterization**
    Abdominal paracentesis
    Aspirating needle biopsy
    Blood sampling
    Lumbar puncture
    Thoracentesis
> **Excludes** *heart catheterization (E870.6)*
  ● **E870.6 Heart catheterization**
  ● **E870.7 Administration of enema**
  ● **E870.8 Other specified medical care**
  ● **E870.9 Unspecified medical care**

● **E871 Foreign object left in body during procedure**
  ● **E871.0 Surgical operation**
  ● **E871.1 Infusion or transfusion**
  ● **E871.2 Kidney dialysis or other perfusion**
  ● **E871.3 Injection or vaccination**
  ● **E871.4 Endoscopic examination**
  ● **E871.5 Aspiration of fluid or tissue, puncture, and catheterization**
    Abdominal paracentesis
    Aspiration needle biopsy
    Blood sampling
    Lumbar puncture
    Thoracentesis
> **Excludes** *heart catheterization (E871.6)*
  ● **E871.6 Heart catheterization**
  ● **E871.7 Removal of catheter or packing**
  ● **E871.8 Other specified procedures**
  ● **E871.9 Unspecified procedure**

● **E872 Failure of sterile precautions during procedure**
  ● **E872.0 Surgical operation**
  ● **E872.1 Infusion or transfusion**
  ● **E872.2 Kidney dialysis and other perfusion**
  ● **E872.3 Injection or vaccination**
  ● **E872.4 Endoscopic examination**
  ● **E872.5 Aspiration of fluid or tissue, puncture, and catheterization**
    Abdominal paracentesis
    Aspirating needle biopsy
    Blood sampling
    Lumbar puncture
    Thoracentesis
> **Excludes** *heart catheterization (E872.6)*

  ● **E872.6 Heart catheterization**
  ● **E872.8 Other specified procedures**
  ● **E872.9 Unspecified procedure**

● **E873 Failure in dosage**
> **Excludes** *accidental overdose of drug, medicinal or biological substance (E850.0-E858.9)*
  ● **E873.0 Excessive amount of blood or other fluid during transfusion or infusion**
  ● **E873.1 Incorrect dilution of fluid during infusion**
  ● **E873.2 Overdose of radiation in therapy**
  ● **E873.3 Inadvertent exposure of patient to radiation during medical care**
  ● **E873.4 Failure in dosage in electroshock or insulin-shock therapy**
  ● **E873.5 Inappropriate [too hot or too cold] temperature in local application and packing**
  ● **E873.6 Nonadministration of necessary drug or medicinal substance**
  ● **E873.8 Other specified failure in dosage**
  ● **E873.9 Unspecified failure in dosage**

● **E874 Mechanical failure of instrument or apparatus during procedure**
  ● **E874.0 Surgical operation**
  ● **E874.1 Infusion and transfusion**
    Air in system
  ● **E874.2 Kidney dialysis and other perfusion**
  ● **E874.3 Endoscopic examination**
  ● **E874.4 Aspiration of fluid or tissue, puncture, and catheterization**
    Abdominal paracentesis
    Aspirating needle biopsy
    Blood sampling
    Lumbar puncture
    Thoracentesis
> **Excludes** *heart catheterization (E874.5)*
  ● **E874.5 Heart catheterization**
    Coding Clinic: 2013, Q1, P5
  ● **E874.8 Other specified procedures**
  ● **E874.9 Unspecified procedure**

● **E875 Contaminated or infected blood, other fluid, drug, or biological substance**
> **Includes** *presence of:*
> *bacterial pyrogens*
> *endotoxin-producing bacteria*
> *serum hepatitis-producing agent*
  ● **E875.0 Contaminated substance transfused or infused**
  ● **E875.1 Contaminated substance injected or used for vaccination**
  ● **E875.2 Contaminated drug or biological substance administered by other means**
  ● **E875.8 Other**
  ● **E875.9 Unspecified**

● **E876 Other and unspecified misadventures during medical care**
  ● **E876.0 Mismatched blood in transfusion**
  ● **E876.1 Wrong fluid in infusion**
  ● **E876.2 Failure in suture and ligature during surgical operation**
  ● **E876.3 Endotracheal tube wrongly placed during anesthetic procedure**
  ● **E876.4 Failure to introduce or to remove other tube or instrument**
> **Excludes** *foreign object left in body during procedure (E871.0-E871.9)*

E000-E999

N Newborn: 0   P Pediatric: 0–17   M Maternity: 12–55   A Adult: 15–124   ♀ Females Only   ♂ Males Only

Ex CC/MCC Exclusions   Complication\Comorbidity   Major C\C   Present on Admission Requirement   Hospital-Acquired Condition   **1053**

● **E876.5 Performance of wrong operation (procedure) on correct patient**
Wrong device implanted into correct surgical site

> **Excludes** *correct operation (procedure) performed on wrong body part (E876.7)*

MCE: Wrong procedure performed
Coding Clinic: 2006, Q3, P9-10

● **E876.6 Performance of operation (procedure) on patient not scheduled for surgery**
Performance of operation (procedure) intended for another patient
Performance of operation (procedure) on wrong patient
MCE: Wrong procedure performed

● **E876.7 Performance of correct operation (procedure) on wrong side/body part**
Performance of correct operation (procedure) on wrong side
Performance of correct operation (procedure) on wrong site
MCE: Wrong procedure performed
Coding Clinic: 2009, Q4, P150-151

● **E876.8 Other specified misadventures during medical care**
Performance of inappropriate treatment, NEC
Coding Clinic: 2012, Q2, P8; 2009, Q2, P11; 2008, Q4, P152-155

● **E876.9 Unspecified misadventure during medical care**

SURGICAL AND MEDICAL PROCEDURES AS THE CAUSE OF ABNORMAL REACTION OF PATIENT OR LATER COMPLICATION, WITHOUT MENTION OF MISADVENTURE AT THE TIME OF PROCEDURE (E878-E879)

> **Includes** procedures as the cause of abnormal reaction, such as:
> displacement or malfunction of prosthetic device
> hepatorenal failure, postoperative
> malfunction of external stoma
> postoperative intestinal obstruction
> rejection of transplanted organ

> **Excludes** *anesthetic management properly carried out as the cause of adverse effect (E937.0-E938.9)*
> *infusion and transfusion, without mention of misadventure in the technique of procedure (E930.0-E949.9)*

OGCR   Section I.C.19.h.2
Assign a code in the range of E878-E879 if the provider attributes an abnormal reaction or later complication to a surgical or medical procedure, but does not mention misadventure at the time of the procedure as the cause of the reaction.

● **E878 Surgical operation and other surgical procedures as the cause of abnormal reaction of patient, or of later complication, without mention of misadventure at the time of operation**

● **E878.0 Surgical operation with transplant of whole organ**
Transplantation of:
heart
kidney
liver

● **E878.1 Surgical operation with implant of artificial internal device**
Cardiac pacemaker
Electrodes implanted in brain
Heart valve prosthesis
Internal orthopedic device

● **E878.2 Surgical operation with anastomosis, bypass, or graft, with natural or artificial tissues used as implant**
Anastomosis:
arteriovenous
gastrojejunal
Graft of blood vessel, tendon, or skin

> **Excludes** *external stoma (E878.3)*

Coding Clinic: 2010, Q2, P9

● **E878.3 Surgical operation with formation of external stoma**
Colostomy
Cystostomy
Duodenostomy
Gastrostomy
Ureterostomy

● **E878.4 Other restorative surgery**

● **E878.5 Amputation of limb(s)**

● **E878.6 Removal of other organ (partial) (total)**

● **E878.8 Other specified surgical operations and procedures**

● **E878.9 Unspecified surgical operations and procedures**

OGCR   Section I.C.19.i.2
Assign a code in the range of E878-E879 if the provider attributes an abnormal reaction or later complication to a surgical or medical procedure, but does not mention misadventure at the time of the procedure as the cause of the reaction.

● **E879 Other procedures, without mention of misadventure at the time of procedure, as the cause of abnormal reaction of patient, or of later complication**

● **E879.0 Cardiac catheterization**

● **E879.1 Kidney dialysis**
Coding Clinic: 2003, Q4, P60-61; 1994, Q3, P9

● **E879.2 Radiological procedure and radiotherapy**

> **Excludes** *radio-opaque dyes for diagnostic x-ray procedures (E947.8)*

Coding Clinic: 2006, Q4, P88-91

● **E879.3 Shock therapy**
Electroshock therapy
Insulin-shock therapy

● **E879.4 Aspiration of fluid**
Lumbar puncture
Thoracentesis

● **E879.5 Insertion of gastric or duodenal sound**

● **E879.6 Urinary catheterization**

● **E879.7 Blood sampling**

● **E879.8 Other specified procedures**
Blood transfusion
Coding Clinic: 2013, Q1, P15; 1993, Q2, P3-4

● **E879.9 Unspecified procedure**

ACCIDENTAL FALLS (E880-E888)

> **Excludes** *falls (in or from):*
> *burning building (E890.8, E891.8)*
> *into fire (E890.0-E899)*
> *into water (with submersion or drowning) (E910.0-E910.9)*
> *machinery (in operation) (E919.0-E919.9)*
> *on edged, pointed, or sharp object (E920.0-E920.9)*
> *transport vehicle (E800.0-E845.9)*
> *vehicle not elsewhere classifiable (E846-E848)*

● **E880 Fall on or from stairs or steps**

● **E880.0 Escalator**

● **E880.1 Fall on or from sidewalk curb**

> **Excludes** *fall from moving sidewalk (E885.9)*

● **E880.9 Other stairs or steps**

● **E881 Fall on or from ladders or scaffolding**

● **E881.0 Fall from ladder**
Coding Clinic: 2007, Q1, P3-8

● **E881.1 Fall from scaffolding**
Coding Clinic: 1999, Q4, P13

● **E882 Fall from or out of building or other structure**
Fall from:
balcony
bridge
building
flagpole
tower
turret
viaduct
wall
window
Fall through roof

Excludes *collapse of a building or structure (E916)*
fall or jump from burning building (E890.8, E891.8)

● **E883 Fall into hole or other opening in surface**
Includes fall into:
cavity
dock
hole
pit
quarry
shaft
swimming pool
tank
well

Excludes *fall into water NOS (E910.9)*
that resulting in drowning or submersion without mention of injury (E910.0-E910.9)

● **E883.0 Accident from diving or jumping into water [swimming pool]**
Strike or hit:
against bottom when jumping or diving into water
wall or board of swimming pool
water surface

Excludes *diving with insufficient air supply (E913.2)*
effects of air pressure from diving (E902.2)

● **E883.1 Accidental fall into well** 🖐
● **E883.2 Accidental fall into storm drain or manhole** 🖐
● **E883.9 Fall into other hole or other opening in surface**

● **E884 Other fall from one level to another**
● **E884.0 Fall from playground equipment** 🖐
Excludes *recreational machinery (E919.8)*
Coding Clinic: 2007, Q1, P3-8
● **E884.1 Fall from cliff** 🖐
● **E884.2 Fall from chair**
● **E884.3 Fall from wheelchair**
Fall from motorized mobility scooter
Fall from motorized wheelchair
Coding Clinic: 2010, Q4, P135
● **E884.4 Fall from bed**
● **E884.5 Fall from other furniture**
● **E884.6 Fall from commode**
Toilet
● **E884.9 Other fall from one level to another**
Fall from:
embankment
haystack
stationary vehicle
tree

● **E885 Fall on same level from slipping, tripping, or stumbling**
● **E885.0 Fall from (nonmotorized) scooter** 🖐
Excludes *fall from motorized mobility scooter (E884.3)*
Coding Clinic: 2002, Q4, P73
● **E885.1 Fall from roller skates** 🖐
Heelies   Wheelies
In-line skates
● **E885.2 Fall from skateboard** 🖐
Coding Clinic: 2000, Q4, P61

● **E885.3 Fall from skis** 🖐
Coding Clinic: 2007, Q2, P3-4
● **E885.4 Fall from snowboard** 🖐
● **E885.9 Fall from other slipping, tripping, or stumbling**
Fall on moving sidewalk
Coding Clinic: 2009, Q4, P150

● **E886 Fall on same level from collision, pushing, or shoving, by or with other person**
Excludes *crushed or pushed by a crowd or human stampede (E917.1, E917.6)*
● **E886.0 In sports** 🖐
Tackles in sports
Excludes *kicked, stepped on, struck by object, in sports (E917.0, E917.5)*
Coding Clinic: 2007, Q2, P3-4
● **E886.9 Other and unspecified**
Fall from collision of pedestrian (conveyance) with another pedestrian (conveyance)

● **E887 Fracture, cause unspecified**

● **E888 Other and unspecified fall**
Accidental fall NOS
Fall on same level NOS
Coding Clinic: 1993, Q4, P25-26
● **E888.0 Fall resulting in striking against sharp object**
Use additional external cause code to identify object (E920)
● **E888.1 Fall resulting in striking against other object**
● **E888.8 Other fall**
● **E888.9 Unspecified fall**
Fall NOS

ACCIDENTS CAUSED BY FIRE AND FLAMES (E890-E899)

Includes asphyxia or poisoning due to conflagration or ignition
burning by fire
secondary fires resulting from explosion

Excludes *arson (E968.0)*
fire in or on:
machinery (in operation) (E919.0-E919.9)
transport vehicle other than stationary vehicle (E800.0-E845.9)
vehicle not elsewhere classifiable (E846-E848)

● **E890 Conflagration in private dwelling**
Includes conflagration in:
apartment   lodging house
boarding house   mobile home
camping place   private garage
caravan   rooming house
farmhouse   tenement
house
conflagration originating from sources classifiable to E893-E898 in the above buildings
● **E890.0 Explosion caused by conflagration** 🖐
● **E890.1 Fumes from combustion of polyvinylchloride [PVC] and similar material in conflagration** 🖐
● **E890.2 Other smoke and fumes from conflagration** 🖐
Carbon monoxide from conflagration in private building
Fumes NOS from conflagration in private building
Smoke NOS from conflagration in private building
Coding Clinic: 2010, Q3, P19; 2005, Q3, P10-11
● **E890.3 Burning caused by conflagration** 🖐
● **E890.8 Other accident resulting from conflagration** 🖐
Collapse of burning private building
Fall from burning private building
Hit by object falling from burning private building
Jump from burning private building
● **E890.9 Unspecified accident resulting from conflagration in private dwelling** 🖐

● **E891 Conflagration in other and unspecified building or structure**
    Conflagration in:
      barn
      church
      convalescent and other residential home
      dormitory of educational institution
      factory
      farm outbuildings
      hospital
      hotel
      school
      store
      theater
    Conflagration originating from sources classifiable to
      E893-E898, in the above buildings

● **E891.0 Explosion caused by conflagration**

● **E891.1 Fumes from combustion of polyvinylchloride [PVC] and similar material in conflagration**

● **E891.2 Other smoke and fumes from conflagration**
    Carbon monoxide from conflagration in building
      or structure
    Fumes NOS from conflagration in building or
      structure
    Smoke NOS from conflagration in building or
      structure

● **E891.3 Burning caused by conflagration**

● **E891.8 Other accident resulting from conflagration**
    Collapse of burning building or structure
    Fall from burning building or structure
    Hit by object falling from burning building or
      structure
    Jump from burning building or structure

● **E891.9 Unspecified accident resulting from conflagration of other and unspecified building or structure**

● **E892 Conflagration not in building or structure**
    Fire (uncontrolled) (in) (of):
      forest
      grass
      hay
      lumber
      mine
      prairie
      transport vehicle [any], except while in transit
      tunnel

● **E893 Accident caused by ignition of clothing**
    Excludes *ignition of clothing:*
        from highly inflammable material (E894)
        with conflagration (E890.0-E892)

● **E893.0 From controlled fire in private dwelling** 🔍
    Ignition of clothing from:
      normal fire (charcoal) (coal) (electric) (gas)
        (wood) in:
        brazier in private dwelling (as listed in E890)
        fireplace in private dwelling (as listed in
          E890)
        furnace in private dwelling (as listed in E890)
        stove in private dwelling (as listed in E890)

● **E893.1 From controlled fire in other building or structure**
    Ignition of clothing from:
      normal fire (charcoal) (coal) (electric) (gas)
        (wood) in:
        brazier in other building or structure (as
          listed in E891)
        fireplace in other building or structure (as
          listed in E891)
        furnace in other building or structure (as
          listed in E891)
        stove in other building or structure (as listed
          in E891)

● **E893.2 From controlled fire not in building or structure** 🔍
    Ignition of clothing from:
      bonfire (controlled)
      brazier fire (controlled), not in building or
        structure
      trash fire (controlled)
    Excludes *conflagration not in building (E892)*
        trash fire out of control (E892)

● **E893.8 From other specified sources**
    Ignition of clothing from:
      blowlamp
      blowtorch
      burning bedspread
      candle
      cigar
      cigarette
      lighter
      matches
      pipe
      welding torch

● **E893.9 Unspecified source**
    Ignition of clothing (from controlled fire NOS) (in
      building NOS) NOS

● **E894 Ignition of highly inflammable material** 🔍
    Ignition of:
      benzine (with ignition of clothing)
      gasoline (with ignition of clothing)
      fat (with ignition of clothing)
      kerosene (with ignition of clothing)
      paraffin (with ignition of clothing)
      petrol (with ignition of clothing)
    Excludes *ignition of highly inflammable material with:*
        conflagration (E890.0-E892)
        explosion (E923.0-E923.9)

● **E895 Accident caused by controlled fire in private dwelling** 🔍
    Burning by (flame of) normal fire (charcoal) (coal) (electric)
      (gas) (wood) in:
      brazier in private dwelling (as listed in E890)
      fireplace in private dwelling (as listed in E890)
      furnace in private dwelling (as listed in E890)
      stove in private dwelling (as listed in E890)
    Excludes *burning by hot objects not producing fire or flames*
        (E924.0-E924.9)
        ignition of clothing from these sources (E893.0)
        poisoning by carbon monoxide from incomplete
          combustion of fuel (E867-E868.9)
        that with conflagration (E890.0-E890.9)

● **E896 Accident caused by controlled fire in other and unspecified building or structure**
    Burning by (flame of) normal fire (charcoal) (coal) (electric)
      (gas) (wood) in:
      brazier in other building or structure (as listed in E891)
      fireplace in other building or structure (as listed in E891)
      furnace in other building or structure (as listed in E891)
      stove in other building or structure (as listed in E891)
    Excludes *burning by hot objects not producing fire or flames*
        (E924.0-E924.9)
        ignition of clothing from these sources (E893.1)
        poisoning by carbon monoxide from incomplete
          combustion of fuel (E867-E868.9)
        that with conflagration (E891.0-E891.9)

E000-E999

◀ New   ◀ Revised   ~~deleted~~ Deleted   Excludes   Includes   Use additional   Code first   Omit code

1056   ● Unacceptable Principal Diagnosis   ● Use Additional Digit(s)   ▶ Manifestation Code   OGCR Official Guidelines   Coding Clinic

- E897   **Accident caused by controlled fire not in building or structure** 🕮
  - Burns from flame of:
    - bonfire (controlled)
    - brazier fire (controlled), not in building or structure
    - trash fire (controlled)
  - **Excludes**   *ignition of clothing from these sources (E893.2)*
    trash fire out of control (E892)
    that with conflagration (E892)

- E898   **Accident caused by other specified fire and flames**
  - **Excludes**   *conflagration (E890.0-E892)*
    that with ignition of:
    clothing (E893.0-E893.9)
    highly inflammable material (E894)
  - E898.0   **Burning bedclothes**
    - Bed set on fire NOS
  - E898.1   **Other**
    - Burning by:
      - blowlamp
      - blowtorch
      - candle
      - cigar
      - cigarette
      - fire in room NOS
    - Burning by:
      - lamp
      - lighter
      - matches
      - pipe
      - welding torch

- E899   **Accident caused by unspecified fire**
  - Burning NOS

ACCIDENTS DUE TO NATURAL AND ENVIRONMENTAL FACTORS (E900-E909)

- E900   **Excessive heat**
  - E900.0   **Due to weather conditions**
    - Excessive heat as the external cause of:
      - ictus solaris
      - siriasis
      - sunstroke
  - E900.1   **Of man-made origin**
    - Heat (in):
      - boiler room
      - drying room
      - factory
      - furnace room
      - generated in transport vehicle
      - kitchen
  - E900.9   **Of unspecified origin**

- E901   **Excessive cold**
  - E901.0   **Due to weather conditions**
    - Excessive cold as the cause of:
      - chilblains NOS
      - immersion foot
  - E901.1   **Of man-made origin**
    - Contact with or inhalation of:
      - dry ice
      - liquid air
      - liquid hydrogen
      - liquid nitrogen
    - Prolonged exposure in:
      - deep freeze unit
      - refrigerator
  - E901.8   **Other specified origin**
  - E901.9   **Of unspecified origin**

- E902   **High and low air pressure and changes in air pressure**
  - E902.0   **Residence or prolonged visit at high altitude**
    - Residence or prolonged visit at high altitude as the cause of:
      - Acosta syndrome
      - Alpine sickness
      - altitude sickness
      - Andes disease
      - anoxia, hypoxia
      - barotitis, barodontalgia, barosinusitis, otitic barotrauma
      - hypobarism, hypobaropathy
      - mountain sickness
      - range disease
  - E902.1   **In aircraft**
    - Sudden change in air pressure in aircraft during ascent or descent as the cause of:
      - aeroneurosis
      - aviators' disease
  - E902.2   **Due to diving**
    - High air pressure from rapid descent in water as the cause of:
      - caisson disease
      - divers' disease
      - divers' palsy or paralysis
    - Reduction in atmospheric pressure while surfacing from deep water diving as the cause of:
      - caisson disease
      - divers' disease
      - divers' palsy or paralysis
  - E902.8   **Due to other specified causes**
    - Reduction in atmospheric pressure while surfacing from under ground
  - E902.9   **Unspecified cause**

- E903   **Travel and motion**

- E904   **Hunger, thirst, exposure, and neglect**
  - **Excludes**   *any condition resulting from homicidal intent (E968.0-E968.9)*
    hunger, thirst, and exposure resulting from accidents connected with transport (E800.0-E848)
  - E904.0   **Abandonment or neglect of infants and helpless persons**
    - Desertion of newborn
    - Exposure to weather conditions resulting from abandonment or neglect
    - Hunger or thirst resulting from abandonment or neglect
    - Inattention at or after birth
    - Lack of care (helpless person) (infant)
    - **Excludes**   *criminal [purposeful] neglect (E968.4)*
    - **OGCR**   Section I.C.19.e.2
      - In cases of neglect when the intent is determined to be accidental E code E904.0 should be the first listed E code.
  - E904.1   **Lack of food**
    - Lack of food as the cause of:
      - inanition
      - insufficient nourishment
      - starvation
    - **Excludes**   *hunger resulting from abandonment or neglect (E904.0)*
  - E904.2   **Lack of water**
    - Lack of water as the cause of:
      - dehydration
      - inanition
    - **Excludes**   *dehydration due to acute fluid loss (276.51)*

N   Newborn: 0   P   Pediatric: 0–17   M   Maternity: 12–55   A   Adult: 15–124   ♀   Females Only   ♂   Males Only

Ex   CC/MCC Exclusions   🕮   Complication\Comorbidity   🕮   Major C\C   🕮   Present on Admission Requirement   🕮   Hospital-Acquired Condition   1057

● **E904.3 Exposure (to weather conditions), not elsewhere classifiable**
  Exposure NOS
  Humidity
  Struck by hailstones
  | **Excludes** | struck by lightning (E907) |

● **E904.9 Privation, unqualified**
  Destitution

● **E905 Venomous animals and plants as the cause of poisoning and toxic reactions**
  | **Includes** | chemical released by animal |
  insects
  release of venom through fangs, hairs, spines, tentacles, and other venom apparatus
  | **Excludes** | eating of poisonous animals or plants (E865.0-E865.9) |

● **E905.0 Venomous snakes and lizards**
  Cobra
  Copperhead snake
  Coral snake
  Fer de lance
  Gila monster
  Krait
  Mamba
  Rattlesnake
  Sea snake
  Snake (venomous)
  Viper
  Water moccasin
  | **Excludes** | bites of snakes and lizards known to be nonvenomous (E906.2) |

● **E905.1 Venomous spiders**
  Black widow spider
  Brown spider
  Tarantula (venomous)

● **E905.2 Scorpion**

● **E905.3 Hornets, wasps, and bees**
  Yellow jacket

● **E905.4 Centipede and venomous millipede (tropical)**

● **E905.5 Other venomous arthropods**
  Sting of:
    ant
    caterpillar

● **E905.6 Venomous marine animals and plants**
  Puncture by sea urchin spine
  Sting of:
    coral
    jelly fish
    nematocysts
    sea anemone
    sea cucumber
    other marine animal or plant
  | **Excludes** | bites and other injuries caused by nonvenomous marine animal (E906.2-E906.8) |
  | | bite of sea snake (venomous) (E905.0) |

● **E905.7 Poisoning and toxic reactions caused by other plants**
  Injection of poisons or toxins into or through skin by plant thorns, spines, or other mechanisms
  | **Excludes** | puncture wound NOS by plant thorns or spines (E920.8) |

● **E905.8 Other specified**

● **E905.9 Unspecified**
  Sting NOS
  Venomous bite NOS

● **E906 Other injury caused by animals**
Excludes	poisoning and toxic reactions caused by venomous animals and insects (E905.0-E905.9)
	road vehicle accident involving animals (E827.0-E828.9)
	tripping or falling over an animal (E885.9)

● **E906.0 Dog bite**
● **E906.1 Rat bite**
● **E906.2 Bite of nonvenomous snakes and lizards**
● **E906.3 Bite of other animal except arthropod**
  Cats
  Moray eel
  Rodents, except rats
  Shark
● **E906.4 Bite of nonvenomous arthropod**
  Insect bite NOS
● **E906.5 Bite by unspecified animal**
  Animal bite NOS
● **E906.8 Other specified injury caused by animal**
  Butted by animal
  Fallen on by horse or other animal, not being ridden
  Gored by animal
  Implantation of quills of porcupine
  Pecked by bird
  Run over by animal, not being ridden
  Stepped on by animal, not being ridden
  | **Excludes** | injury by animal being ridden (E828.0-E828.9) |
● **E906.9 Unspecified injury caused by animal**

● **E907 Lightning**
Excludes	injury from:
	fall of tree or other object caused by lightning (E916)
	fire caused by lightning (E890.0-E892)

● **E908 Cataclysmic storms, and floods resulting from storms**
  | **Excludes** | collapse of dam or man-made structure causing flood (E909.3) |

● **E908.0 Hurricane**
  Storm surge
  "Tidal wave" caused by storm action
  Typhoon
● **E908.1 Tornado**
  Cyclone   Twisters
● **E908.2 Floods**
  Torrential rainfall   Flash flood
  | **Excludes** | collapse of dam or man-made structure causing flood (E909.3) |
● **E908.3 Blizzard (snow) (ice)**
● **E908.4 Dust storm**
● **E908.8 Other cataclysmic storms**
● **E908.9 Unspecified cataclysmic storms, and floods resulting from storms**
  Storm NOS

● **E909 Cataclysmic earth surface movements and eruptions**
● **E909.0 Earthquakes**
● **E909.1 Volcanic eruptions**
  Burns from lava   Ash inhalation
● **E909.2 Avalanche, landslide, or mudslide**
● **E909.3 Collapse of dam or man-made structure**
● **E909.4 Tidal wave caused by earthquake**
  Tidal wave NOS   Tsunami
  | **Excludes** | tidal wave caused by tropical storm (E908.0) |
● **E909.8 Other cataclysmic earth surface movements and eruptions**
● **E909.9 Unspecified cataclysmic earth surface movements and eruptions**

◀ New   ◀▥ Revised   ~~deleted~~ Deleted   Excludes   Includes   Use additional   Code first   Omit code

● Unacceptable Principal Diagnosis   ● Use Additional Digit(s)   ▷ Manifestation Code   OGCR Official Guidelines   Coding Clinic

1058

ACCIDENTS CAUSED BY SUBMERSION, SUFFOCATION, AND FOREIGN BODIES (E910-E915)

● **E910 Accidental drowning and submersion**

Includes   immersion
            swimmers' cramp

Excludes   *diving accident (NOS) (resulting in injury except drowning) (E883.0)*
diving with insufficient air supply (E913.2)
drowning and submersion due to:
  cataclysm (E908-E909)
  machinery accident (E919.0-E919.9)
  transport accident (E800.0-E845.9)
  effect of high and low air pressure (E902.2)
    injury from striking against objects while in running water (E917.2)

● **E910.0   While water-skiing**

Fall from water skis with submersion or drowning

Excludes   *accident to water-skier involving a watercraft and resulting in submersion or other injury (E830.4, E831.4)*

● **E910.1   While engaged in other sport or recreational activity with diving equipment**

Scuba diving NOS
Skin diving NOS
Underwater spear fishing NOS

● **E910.2   While engaged in other sport or recreational activity without diving equipment**

Fishing or hunting, except from boat or with diving equipment
Ice skating
Playing in water
Surfboarding
Swimming NOS
Voluntarily jumping from boat, not involved in accident, for swim NOS
Wading in water

Excludes   *jumping into water to rescue another person (E910.3)*

Coding Clinic: 2013, Q3, P11

● **E910.3   While swimming or diving for purposes other than recreation or sport**

Marine salvage (with diving equipment)
Pearl diving (with diving equipment)
Placement of fishing nets (with diving equipment)
Rescue (attempt) of another person (with diving equipment)
Underwater construction or repairs (with diving equipment)

● **E910.4   In bathtub**

● **E910.8   Other accidental drowning or submersion**

Drowning in:
  quenching tank
  swimming pool

● **E910.9   Unspecified accidental drowning or submersion**

Accidental fall into water NOS
Drowning NOS

● **E911 Inhalation and ingestion of food causing obstruction of respiratory tract or suffocation**

Aspiration and inhalation of food [any] (into respiratory tract) NOS
Asphyxia by food [including bone, seed in food, regurgitated food]
Choked on food [including bone, seed in food, regurgitated food]
Suffocation by food [including bone, seed in food, regurgitated food]
Compression of trachea by food lodged in esophagus
Interruption of respiration by food lodged in esophagus
Obstruction of respiration by food lodged in esophagus
Obstruction of pharynx by food (bolus)

Excludes   *injury, except asphyxia and obstruction of respiratory passage, caused by food (E915)*
obstruction of esophagus by food without mention of asphyxia or obstruction of respiratory passage (E915)

● **E912 Inhalation and ingestion of other object causing obstruction of respiratory tract or suffocation**

Aspiration and inhalation of foreign body except food (into respiratory tract) NOS
Compression by foreign body in esophagus
Foreign object [bean] [marble] in nose
Interruption of respiration by foreign body in esophagus
Obstruction of pharynx by foreign body
Obstruction of respiration by foreign body in esophagus

Excludes   *injury, except asphyxia and obstruction of respiratory passage, caused by foreign body (E915)*
obstruction of esophagus by foreign body without mention of asphyxia or obstruction in respiratory passage (E915)

● **E913 Accidental mechanical suffocation**

Excludes   *mechanical suffocation from or by:*
  accidental inhalation or ingestion of:
    food (E911)
    foreign object (E912)
  cataclysm (E908-E909)
  explosion (E921.0-E921.9, E923.0-E923.9)
  machinery accident (E919.0-E919.9)

● **E913.0   In bed or cradle**

Excludes   *suffocation by plastic bag (E913.1)*

● **E913.1   By plastic bag**

● **E913.2   Due to lack of air (in closed place)**

Accidentally closed up in refrigerator or other airtight enclosed space
Diving with insufficient air supply

Excludes   *suffocation by plastic bag (E913.1)*

● **E913.3   By falling earth or other substance**

Cave-in NOS

Excludes   *cave-in caused by cataclysmic earth surface movements and eruptions (E909.8)*
struck by cave-in without asphyxiation or suffocation (E916)

● **E913.8   Other specified means**

Accidental hanging, except in bed or cradle

● **E913.9   Unspecified means**

Asphyxia, mechanical NOS
Strangulation NOS
Suffocation NOS

● **E914 Foreign body accidentally entering eye and adnexa**

Excludes   *corrosive liquid (E924.1)*

● **E915 Foreign body accidentally entering other orifice**

Excludes   *aspiration and inhalation of foreign body, any, (into respiratory tract) NOS (E911-E912)*

E000-E999

OTHER ACCIDENTS (E916-E928)

● E916 **Struck accidentally by falling object**
Collapse of building, except on fire
Falling:
rock
snowslide NOS
stone
tree
Object falling from:
machine, not in operation
stationary vehicle
Code first collapse of building on fire (E890.0-E891.9)
falling object in:
cataclysm (E908-E909)
machinery accidents (E919.0-E919.9)
transport accidents (E800.0-E845.9)
vehicle accidents not elsewhere classifiable
(E846-E848)
object set in motion by:
explosion (E921.0-E921.9, E923.0-E923.9)
firearm (E922.0-E922.9)
projected object (E917.0-E917.9)

● E917 **Striking against or struck accidentally by objects or persons**
Includes bumping into or against
object (moving) (projected) (stationary)
pedestrian conveyance
person
colliding with
object (moving) (projected) (stationary)
pedestrian conveyance
person
kicking against
object (moving) (projected) (stationary)
pedestrian conveyance
person
stepping on
object (moving) (projected) (stationary)
pedestrian conveyance
person
struck by
object (moving) (projected) (stationary)
pedestrian conveyance
person
Excludes *fall from:*
collision with another person, except when caused
by a crowd (E886.0-E886.9)
stumbling over object (E885.9)
fall resulting in striking against object
(E888.0-E888.1)
injury caused by:
assault (E960.0-E960.1, E967.0-E967.9)
cutting or piercing instrument
(E920.0-E920.9)
explosion (E921.0-E921.9, E923.0-E923.9)
firearm (E922.0-E922.9)
machinery (E919.0-E919.9)
transport vehicle (E800.0-E845.9)
vehicle not elsewhere classifiable (E846-E848)

● E917.0 **In sports without subsequent fall** 🔍
Kicked or stepped on during game (football)
(rugby)
Struck by hit or thrown ball
Struck by hockey stick or puck
Coding Clinic: 2007, Q2, P3-4; 2006, Q1, P8; 2004, Q1, P9

● E917.1 **Caused by a crowd, by collective fear or panic without subsequent fall** 🔍
Crushed by crowd or human stampede
Pushed by crowd or human stampede
Stepped on by crowd or human stampede

● E917.2 **In running water without subsequent fall** 🔍
Excludes *drowning or submersion (E910.0-E910.9)*
that in sports (E917.0, E917.5)

● E917.3 **Furniture without subsequent fall**
Excludes *fall from furniture (E884.2,*
E884.4-E884.5)

● E917.4 **Other stationary object without subsequent fall**
Bath tub
Fence
Lamp-post

● E917.5 **Object in sports with subsequent fall** 🔍
Knocked down while boxing
Coding Clinic: 2007, Q2, P3-4

● E917.6 **Caused by a crowd, by collective fear or panic with subsequent fall** 🔍

● E917.7 **Furniture with subsequent fall**
Excludes *fall from furniture (E884.2,*
E884.4-E884.5)

● E917.8 **Other stationary object with subsequent fall**
Bath tub
Fence
Lamp-post

● E917.9 **Other striking against with or without subsequent fall**

● E918 **Caught accidentally in or between objects**
Caught, crushed, jammed, or pinched in or between moving
or stationary objects, such as:
escalator
folding object
hand tools, appliances, or implements
sliding door and door frame
under packing crate
washing machine wringer
Excludes *injury caused by:*
cutting or piercing instrument (E920.0-E920.9)
machinery (E919.0-E919.9)
mechanism or component of firearm and air gun
(E928.7)
transport vehicle (E800.0-E845.9)
vehicle not elsewhere classifiable (E846-E848)
struck accidentally by:
falling object (E916)
object (moving) (projected) (E917.0-E917.9)

◄ New   ⇇ Revised   ~~deleted~~ Deleted   Excludes   Includes   Use additional   Code first   Omit code
● Unacceptable Principal Diagnosis   ● Use Additional Digit(s)   ▶ Manifestation Code   OGCR Official Guidelines   Coding Clinic

● **E919**   **Accidents caused by machinery**

Includes   burned by machinery (accident)
caught between machinery and other object
caught in (moving parts of) machinery (accident)
collapse of machinery (accident)
crushed by machinery (accident)
cut or pierced by machinery (accident)
drowning or submersion caused by machinery
(accident)
explosion of, on, in machinery (accident)
fall from or into moving part of machinery
(accident)
fire starting in or on machinery (accident)
mechanical suffocation caused by machinery
(accident)
object falling from, on, in motion by machinery
(accident)
overturning of machinery (accident)
pinned under machinery (accident)
run over by machinery (accident)
struck by machinery (accident)
thrown from machinery (accident)
machinery accident NOS

Excludes   *accidents involving machinery, not in operation
(E884.9, E916-E918)
injury caused by:
electric current in connection with machinery
(E925.0-E925.9)
escalator (E880.0, E918)
explosion of pressure vessel in connection with
machinery (E921.0-E921.9)
mechanism or component of firearm and air gun
(E928.7)
moving sidewalk (E885.9)
powered hand tools, appliances, and
implements (E916-E918, E920.0-E921.9,
E923.0-E926.9)
transport vehicle accidents involving machinery
(E800.0-E848.9)
poisoning by carbon monoxide generated by
machine (E868.8)*

● **E919.0**   **Agricultural machines** 🔍
Animal-powered agricultural machine
Combine
Derrick, hay
Farm machinery NOS
Farm tractor
Harvester
Hay mower or rake
Reaper
Thresher

Excludes   *that being towed by another vehicle on
the highway (E810.0-E819.9,
E827.0-E827.9, E829.0-E829.9)
that in transport under own power on the
highway (E810.0-E819.9)
that involved in accident classifiable to
E820-E829 (E820.0-E829.9)*

● **E919.1**   **Mining and earth-drilling machinery** 🔍
Bore or drill (land) (seabed)
Shaft hoist
Shaft lift
Under-cutter

Excludes   *coal car, tram, truck, and tub in mine
(E846)*

● **E919.2**   **Lifting machines and appliances**
Chain hoist except in agricultural or mining
operations
Crane except in agricultural or mining operations
Derrick except in agricultural or mining operations
Elevator (building) (grain) except in agricultural or
mining operations
Forklift truck except in agricultural or mining
operations
Lift except in agricultural or mining operations
Pulley block except in agricultural or mining
operations
Winch except in agricultural or mining operations

Excludes   *that being towed by another vehicle on
the highway (E810.0-E819.9,
E827.0-E827.9, E829.0-E829.9)
that in transport under own power on the
highway (E810.0-E819.9)
that involved in accident classifiable to
E820-E829 (E820.0-E829.9)*

● **E919.3**   **Metalworking machines** 🔍
Abrasive wheel   Metal:
Forging machine   milling machine
Lathe   power press
Mechanical shears   rolling-mill
Metal: sawing machine
drilling machine
Coding Clinic: 2003, Q4, P76-78

● **E919.4**   **Woodworking and forming machines** 🔍
Band saw   Overhead plane
Bench saw   Powered saw
Circular saw   Radial saw
Molding machine   Sander

Excludes   *hand saw (E920.1)*

● **E919.5**   **Prime movers, except electrical motors** 🔍
Gas turbine
Internal combustion engine
Steam engine
Water driven turbine

Excludes   *that being towed by other vehicle on
the highway (E810.0-E819.9,
E827.0-E827.9, E829.0-E829.9)
that in transport under own power on the
highway (E810.0-E819.9)*

● **E919.6**   **Transmission machinery** 🔍
Transmission: Transmission:
belt   pinion
cable   pulley
chain   shaft
gear

● **E919.7**   **Earth moving, scraping, and other excavating
machines** 🔍
Bulldozer   Steam shovel
Road scraper

Excludes   *that being towed by other vehicle on the
highway (E810.0-E819.9)
that in transport under own power on the
highway (E810.0-E819.9)*

● **E919.8**   **Other specified machinery** 🔍
Machines for manufacture of:
clothing
foodstuffs and beverages
paper
Printing machine
Recreational machinery
Spinning, weaving, and textile machines

● **E919.9**   **Unspecified machinery** 🔍

E000-E999

N   Newborn: 0   P   Pediatric: 0–17   M   Maternity: 12–55   A   Adult: 15–124   ♀   Females Only   ♂   Males Only
Ⓔⓧ   CC/MCC Exclusions   🔍 Complication\Comorbidity   🔍 Major C\C   🔍 Present on Admission Requirement   🔍 Hospital-Acquired Condition   **1061**

● **E920 Accidents caused by cutting and piercing instruments or objects**

> **Includes** accidental injury (by) object:
>> edged
>> pointed
>> sharp

> **Excludes** *injury caused by mechanism or component of firearm and air gun (E928.7)*

● **E920.0 Powered lawn mower**

● **E920.1 Other powered hand tools**
> Any powered hand tool [compressed air] [electric] [explosive cartridge] [hydraulic power], such as:
>> drill
>> hand saw
>> hedge clipper
>> rivet gun
>> snow blower
>> staple gun

>> **Excludes** *band saw (E919.4)*
>>> *bench saw (E919.4)*

● **E920.2 Powered household appliances and implements**
> Blender
> Electric:
>> beater or mixer
>> can opener
>> fan
>> knife
>> sewing machine
> Garbage disposal appliance

● **E920.3 Knives, swords, and daggers**

● **E920.4 Other hand tools and implements**
> Axe
> Can opener NOS
> Chisel
> Fork
> Hand saw
> Hoe
> Ice pick
> Needle (sewing)
> Paper cutter
> Pitchfork
> Rake
> Scissors
> Screwdriver
> Sewing machine, not powered
> Shovel

● **E920.5 Hypodermic needle**
> Contaminated needle
> Needle stick

● **E920.8 Other specified cutting and piercing instruments or objects**

Arrow	Nail
Broken glass	Plant thorn
Dart	Splinter
Edge of stiff paper	Tin can lid
Lathe turnings	

>> **Excludes** *animal spines or quills (E906.8)*
>>> *flying glass due to explosion (E921.0-E923.9)*

Coding Clinic: 2001, Q3, P10

● **E920.9 Unspecified cutting and piercing instrument or object**

● **E921 Accident caused by explosion of pressure vessel**

> **Includes** accidental explosion of pressure vessels, whether or not part of machinery

> **Excludes** *explosion of pressure vessel on transport vehicle (E800.0-E845.9)*

● **E921.0 Boilers**
Coding Clinic: 2005, Q3, P10-11

● **E921.1 Gas cylinders**
> Air tank
> Pressure gas tank

● **E921.8 Other specified pressure vessels**
> Aerosol can
> Automobile tire
> Pressure cooker

E921.9 Unspecified pressure vessel

● **E922 Accident caused by firearm and air gun missile**

> **Excludes** *injury caused by mechanism or component of firearm and air gun (E928.7)*

● **E922.0 Handgun**
> Pistol
> Revolver

>> **Excludes** *Verey pistol (E922.8)*

● **E922.1 Shotgun (automatic)**

● **E922.2 Hunting rifle**

● **E922.3 Military firearms**
> Army rifle
> Machine gun

● **E922.4 Air gun**
> BB gun
> Pellet gun

● **E922.5 Paintball gun**
Coding Clinic: 2002, Q4, P74

● **E922.8 Other specified firearm missile**
> Verey pistol [flare]

● **E922.9 Unspecified firearm missile**
> Gunshot wound NOS
> Shot NOS

● **E923 Accident caused by explosive material**

> **Includes** flash burns and other injuries resulting from explosion of explosive material
>> ignition of highly explosive material with explosion

> **Excludes** *explosion:*
>> *in or on machinery (E919.0-E919.9)*
>> *on any transport vehicle, except stationary motor vehicle (E800.0-E848)*
>> *with conflagration (E890.0, E891.0, E892)*
>> *injury caused by mechanism or component of firearm and air gun (E928.7)*
>> *secondary fires resulting from explosion (E890.0-E899)*

● **E923.0 Fireworks**

● **E923.1 Blasting materials**

Blasting cap	Explosive [any]
Detonator	used in blasting
Dynamite	operations

● **E923.2 Explosive gases**
> Acetylene
> Butane
> Coal gas
> Explosion in mine NOS
> Fire damp
> Gasoline fumes
> Methane
> Propane

● **E923.8 Other explosive materials**

Bomb Torpedo	
Explosive missile	Explosion in munitions:
Grenade	dump
Mine	factory
Shell	

● **E923.9 Unspecified explosive material**
> Explosion NOS

E000-E999

● **E924 Accident caused by hot substance or object, caustic or corrosive material, and steam**

> **Excludes** *burning NOS (E899)*
> *chemical burn resulting from swallowing a corrosive substance (E860.0–E864.4)*
> *fire caused by these substances and objects (E890.0–E894)*
> *radiation burns (E926.0–E926.9)*
> *therapeutic misadventures (E870.0–E876.9)*

● **E924.0 Hot liquids and vapors, including steam**
> Burning or scalding by:
> boiling water
> hot or boiling liquids not primarily caustic or corrosive
> liquid metal
> other hot vapor
> steam
>
> > **Excludes** *hot (boiling) tap water (E924.2)*

● **E924.1 Caustic and corrosive substances**
> Burning by:
> acid [any kind]
> ammonia
> caustic oven cleaner or other substance
> corrosive substance
> lye
> vitriol

● **E924.2 Hot (boiling) tap water**

● **E924.8 Other**
> Burning by:
> heat from electric heating appliance
> hot object NOS
> light bulb
> steam pipe

● **E924.9 Unspecified**

● **E925 Accident caused by electric current**

> **Includes** electric current from exposed wire, faulty appliance, high voltage cable, live rail, or open electric socket as the cause of:
> burn
> cardiac fibrillation
> convulsion
> electric shock
> electrocution
> puncture wound
> respiratory paralysis
>
> **Excludes** *burn by heat from electrical appliance (E924.8)*
> *lightning (E907)*

● **E925.0 Domestic wiring and appliances**

● **E925.1 Electric power generating plants, distribution stations, transmission lines**
> Broken power line

● **E925.2 Industrial wiring, appliances, and electrical machinery**
> Conductors
> Control apparatus
> Electrical equipment and machinery
> Transformers

● **E925.8 Other electric current**
> Wiring and appliances in or on:
> farm [not farmhouse]
> outdoors
> public building
> residential institutions
> schools

● **E925.9 Unspecified electric current**
> Burns or other injury from electric current NOS
> Electric shock NOS
> Electrocution NOS

● **E926 Exposure to radiation**

> **Excludes** *abnormal reaction to or complication of treatment without mention of misadventure (E879.2)*
> *atomic power plant malfunction in water transport (E838.0–E838.9)*
> *misadventure to patient in surgical and medical procedures (E873.2–E873.3)*
> *use of radiation in war operations (E996–E997.9)*

● **E926.0 Radiofrequency radiation**
> Overexposure to:
> microwave radiation from:
> high-powered radio and television transmitters
> industrial radiofrequency induction heaters
> radar installations
> radar radiation from:
> high-powered radio and television transmitters
> industrial radiofrequency induction heaters
> radar installations
> radiofrequency from:
> high-powered radio and television transmitters
> industrial radiofrequency induction heaters
> radar installations
> radiofrequency radiation [any] from:
> high-powered radio and television transmitters
> industrial radiofrequency induction heaters
> radar installations

● **E926.1 Infra-red heaters and lamps**
> Exposure to infra-red radiation from heaters and lamps as the cause of:
> blistering   charring
> burning   inflammatory change
>
> > **Excludes** *physical contact with heater or lamp (E924.8)*

● **E926.2 Visible and ultraviolet light sources** 🔲
> Arc lamps
> Black light sources
> Electrical welding arc
> Oxygas welding torch
> Sun rays
> Tanning bed
>
> > **Excludes** *excessive heat from these sources (E900.1–E900.9)*
>
> **Coding Clinic: 1996, Q3, P6**

● **E926.3 X-rays and other electromagnetic ionizing radiation**
> Gamma rays
> X-rays (hard) (soft)

● **E926.4 Lasers**

● **E926.5 Radioactive isotopes**
> Radiobiologicals
> Radiopharmaceuticals

● **E926.8 Other specified radiation**
> Artificially accelerated beams of ionized particles generated by:
> betatrons
> synchrotrons

● **E926.9 Unspecified radiation**
> Radiation NOS

E000–E999

N Newborn: 0   P Pediatric: 0–17   M Maternity: 12–55   A Adult: 15–124   ♀ Females Only   ♂ Males Only

Ex CC/MCC Exclusions   🔲 Complication\Comorbidity   🔲 Major C\C   🔲 Present on Admission Requirement   🔲 Hospital-Acquired Condition   1063

E000-E999

● **E927 Overexertion and strenuous and repetitive movements or loads**

Use additional code to identify activity (E001-E030)
Coding Clinic: 2009, Q3, P18; 2008, Q3, P21

● **E927.0 Overexertion from sudden strenuous movement**
Sudden trauma from strenuous movement

● **E927.1 Overexertion from prolonged static position**
Overexertion from maintaining prolonged
positions, such as:
holding
sitting
standing

● **E927.2 Excessive physical exertion from prolonged activity**

● **E927.3 Cumulative trauma from repetitive motion**
Cumulative trauma from repetitive movements
Coding Clinic: 2009, Q3, P20

● **E927.4 Cumulative trauma from repetitive impact**
Coding Clinic: 2009, Q3, P20x3, 21

● **E927.8 Other overexertion and strenuous and repetitive movements or loads**

● **E927.9 Unspecified overexertion and strenuous and repetitive movements or loads**

● **E928 Other and unspecified environmental and accidental causes**

● **E928.0 Prolonged stay in weightless environment** 🔍
Weightlessness in spacecraft (simulator)

● **E928.1 Exposure to noise** 🔍
Noise (pollution)
Sound waves
Supersonic waves

● **E928.2 Vibration** 🔍

● **E928.3 Human bite** 🔍

● **E928.4 External constriction caused by hair** 🔍

● **E928.5 External constriction caused by other object** 🔍

● **E928.6 Environmental exposure to harmful algae and toxins** 🔍
Algae bloom NOS
Blue-green algae bloom
Brown tide
Cyanobacteria bloom
Florida red tide
Harmful algae bloom
Pfiesteria piscicida
Red tide
Coding Clinic: 2007, Q4, P101-102

● **E928.7 Mechanism or component of firearm and air gun** 🔍
Injury due to:
explosion of gun parts
recoil
Pierced, cut, crushed, or pinched by slide trigger
mechanism, scope or other gun part
Powder burn from firearm or air gun
Excludes *accident caused by firearm and air gun missile (E922.0-E922.9)*

● **E928.8 Other** 🔍

● **E928.9 Unspecified accident**
Accident NOS stated as accidentally inflicted
Blow NOS stated as accidentally inflicted
Casualty (not due to war) stated as accidentally inflicted
Decapitation stated as accidentally inflicted
Injury [any part of body, or unspecified] stated as accidentally inflicted, but not otherwise specified
Killed stated as accidentally inflicted, but not otherwise specified
Knocked down stated as accidentally inflicted, but not otherwise specified
Mangled stated as accidentally inflicted, but not otherwise specified
Wound stated as accidentally inflicted, but not otherwise specified

Excludes *fracture, cause unspecified (E887)*
injuries undetermined whether accidentally or purposely inflicted (E980.0-E989)
Coding Clinic: 1996, Q3, P7; 1985, Nov-Dec, P15; 1984, Nov-Dec, P15

LATE EFFECTS OF ACCIDENTAL INJURY (E929)

Note: This category is to be used to indicate accidental injury as the cause of death or disability from late effects, which are themselves classifiable elsewhere. The "late effects" include conditions reported as such or as sequelae, which may occur at any time after the acute accidental injury.

● **E929 Late effects of accidental injury**
Excludes *late effects of:*
surgical and medical procedures (E870.0-E879.9)
therapeutic use of drugs and medicines (E930.0-E949.9)

● **E929.0 Late effects of motor vehicle accident** 🔍
Late effects of accidents classifiable to E810-E825
Coding Clinic: 2008, Q4, P102-109; 1997, Q3, P12-13; 1995, Q1, P10; 1994, Q3, P4

● **E929.1 Late effects of other transport accident** 🔍
Late effects of accidents classifiable to E800-E807, E826-E838, E840-E848

● **E929.2 Late effects of accidental poisoning** 🔍
Late effects of accidents classifiable to E850-E858, E860-E869

● **E929.3 Late effects of accidental fall** 🔍
Late effects of accidents classifiable to E880-E888

● **E929.4 Late effects of accident caused by fire** 🔍
Late effects of accidents classifiable to E890-E899

● **E929.5 Late effects of accident due to natural and environmental factors** 🔍
Late effects of accidents classifiable to E900-E909

● **E929.8 Late effects of other accidents** 🔍
Late effects of accidents classifiable to E910-E928.8

● **E929.9 Late effects of unspecified accident** 🔍
Late effects of accidents classifiable to E928.9

◄ New   ◄▌ Revised   ~~deleted~~ Deleted   Excludes   Includes   Use additional   Code first   Omit code
● Unacceptable Principal Diagnosis   ● Use Additional Digit(s)   ▶ Manifestation Code   OGCR Official Guidelines   Coding Clinic

OGCR Section I.C.17.e.1

Adverse Effect: When the drug was correctly prescribed and properly administered, code the reaction plus the appropriate code from the E930-E949 series. Codes from the E930-E949 series must be used to identify the causative substance for an adverse effect of drug, medicinal and biological substances, correctly prescribed and properly administered. The effect, such as tachycardia, delirium, gastrointestinal hemorrhaging, vomiting, hypokalemia, hepatitis, renal failure, or respiratory failure, is coded and followed by the appropriate code from the E930-E949 series.

DRUGS, MEDICINAL AND BIOLOGICAL SUBSTANCES CAUSING ADVERSE EFFECTS IN THERAPEUTIC USE (E930-E949)

Includes   correct drug properly administered in therapeutic or prophylactic dosage, as the cause of any adverse effect including allergic or hypersensitivity reactions

Excludes   *accidental overdose of drug and wrong drug given or taken in error (E850.0-E858.9)*
accidents in the technique of administration of drug or biological substance such as accidental puncture during injection, or contamination of drug (E870.0-E876.9)
administration with suicidal or homicidal intent or intent to harm, or in circumstances classifiable to E950.0-E950.5, E962.0, E980.0-E980.5

See Alphabetic Index for more complete list of specific drugs to be classified under the fourth-digit subdivisions. The American Hospital Formulary numbers can be used to classify new drugs listed by the American Hospital Formulary Service (AHFS). See appendix C.

● **E930**   **Antibiotics**

Excludes   *that used as eye, ear, nose, and throat [ENT], and local anti-infectives (E946.0-E946.9)*
Coding Clinic: 2008, Q3, P21

● **E930.0**   **Penicillins**
Natural
Synthetic
Semisynthetic, such as:
ampicillin
cloxacillin
nafcillin
oxacillin
Coding Clinic: 2008, Q4, P128-131

● **E930.1**   **Antifungal antibiotics**
Amphotericin B
Griseofulvin
Hachimycin [trichomycin]
Nystatin

● **E930.2**   **Chloramphenicol group**
Chloramphenicol
Thiamphenicol

● **E930.3**   **Erythromycin and other macrolides**
Oleandomycin
Spiramycin

● **E930.4**   **Tetracycline group**
Doxycycline
Minocycline
Oxytetracycline
Coding Clinic: 1988, Q2, P9-10

● **E930.5**   **Cephalosporin group**
Cephalexin
Cephaloglycin
Cephaloridine
Cephalothin

● **E930.6**   **Antimycobacterial antibiotics**
Cycloserine
Kanamycin
Rifampin
Streptomycin

● **E930.7**   **Antineoplastic antibiotics**
Actinomycins, such as:
bleomycin
cactinomycin
dactinomycin
daunorubicin
mitomycin

Excludes   *other antineoplastic drugs (E933.1)*
Coding Clinic: 2007, Q2, P9-10

● **E930.8**   **Other specified antibiotics**
Coding Clinic: 1993, Q1, P29

● **E930.9**   **Unspecified antibiotic**

● **E931**   **Other anti-infectives**

Excludes   *ENT, and local anti-infectives (E946.0-E946.9)*

● **E931.0**   **Sulfonamides**
Sulfadiazine
Sulfafurazole
Sulfamethoxazole

● **E931.1**   **Arsenical anti-infectives**

● **E931.2**   **Heavy metal anti-infectives**
Compounds of:
antimony
bismuth
lead
mercury

Excludes   *mercurial diuretics (E944.0)*

● **E931.3**   **Quinoline and hydroxyquinoline derivatives**
Chiniofon
Diiodohydroxyquin

Excludes   *antimalarial drugs (E931.4)*

● **E931.4**   **Antimalarials and drugs acting on other blood protozoa**
Chloroquine phosphate
Cycloguanil
Primaquine
Proguanil [chloroguanide]
Pyrimethamine
Quinine (sulphate)

● **E931.5**   **Other antiprotozoal drugs**
Emetine

● **E931.6**   **Anthelmintics**
Hexylresorcinol
Male fern oleoresin
Piperazine
Thiabendazole

● **E931.7**   **Antiviral drugs**
Methisazone

Excludes   *amantadine (E936.4)*
cytarabine (E933.1)
idoxuridine (E946.5)

● **E931.8**   **Other antimycobacterial drugs**
Ethambutol
Ethionamide
Isoniazid
Para-aminosalicylic acid derivatives
Sulfones

● **E931.9**   **Other and unspecified anti-infectives**
Flucytosine
Nitrofuran derivatives

E000-E999

● **E932 Hormones and synthetic substitutes**

   ● **E932.0 Adrenal cortical steroids**
      Cortisone derivatives
      Desoxycorticosterone derivatives
      Fluorinated corticosteroids
      Coding Clinic: 2008, Q4, P91-95; 2003, Q4, P108-109; 2000, Q3, P4-5

   ● **E932.1 Androgens and anabolic congeners**
      Nandrolone phenpropionate
      Oxymetholone
      Testosterone and preparations
      Coding Clinic: 1985, July-Aug, P8

   ● **E932.2 Ovarian hormones and synthetic substitutes**
      Contraceptives, oral
      Estrogens
      Estrogens and progestogens combined
      Progestogens

   ● **E932.3 Insulins and antidiabetic agents**
      Acetohexamide
      Biguanide derivatives, oral
      Chlorpropamide
      Glucagon
      Insulin
      Phenformin
      Sulfonylurea derivatives, oral
      Tolbutamide
      Excludes *adverse effect of insulin administered for shock therapy (E879.3)*

   ● **E932.4 Anterior pituitary hormones**
      Corticotropin
      Gonadotropin
      Somatotropin [growth hormone]
      Coding Clinic: 1995, Q3, P15

   ● **E932.5 Posterior pituitary hormones**
      Vasopressin
      Excludes *oxytocic agents (E945.0)*

   ● **E932.6 Parathyroid and parathyroid derivatives**

   ● **E932.7 Thyroid and thyroid derivatives**
      Dextrothyroxine
      Levothyroxine sodium
      Liothyronine
      Thyroglobulin

   ● **E932.8 Antithyroid agents**
      Iodides
      Thiouracil
      Thiourea

   ● **E932.9 Other and unspecified hormones and synthetic substitutes**

● **E933 Primarily systemic agents**

   ● **E933.0 Antiallergic and antiemetic drugs**
      Antihistamines
      Chlorpheniramine
      Diphenhydramine
      Diphenylpyraline
      Thonzylamine
      Tripelennamine
      Excludes *phenothiazine-based tranquilizers (E939.1)*
      Coding Clinic: 1997, Q2, P9-10

   ● **E933.1 Antineoplastic and immunosuppressive drugs**
      Azathioprine
      Busulfan
      Chlorambucil
      Cyclophosphamide
      Cytarabine
      Fluorouracil
      Mechlorethamine hydrochloride
      Mercaptopurine
      Triethylenethiophosphoramide [thio-TEPA]
      Excludes *antineoplastic antibiotics (E930.7)*
      Coding Clinic: 2011, Q4, P83; 2010, Q2, P12; 2009, Q4, P151; 2008, Q2, P6, 10-11; 2006, Q4, P69-73; Q2, P20; 2005, Q3, P11-12; 1999, Q3, P6-7; Q2, P9; 1996, Q2, P12; 1985, Mar-April, P14

● **E933.2 Acidifying agents**

● **E933.3 Alkalizing agents**

● **E933.4 Enzymes, not elsewhere classified**
      Penicillinase

● **E933.5 Vitamins, not elsewhere classified**
      Vitamin A   Vitamin D
      Excludes *nicotinic acid (E942.2)*
      vitamin K (E934.3)

● **E933.6 Oral bisphosphonates**
      Coding Clinic: 2007, Q4, P91-92, 102

● **E933.7 Intravenous bisphosphonates**
      Coding Clinic: 2007, Q4, P102

● **E933.8 Other systemic agents, not elsewhere classified**
      Heavy metal antagonists

● **E933.9 Unspecified systemic agent**

● **E934 Agents primarily affecting blood constituents**
   Coding Clinic: 1993, 5th Issue, P16

   ● **E934.0 Iron and its compounds**
      Ferric salts
      Ferrous sulphate and other ferrous salts

   ● **E934.1 Liver preparations and other antianemic agents**
      Folic acid

   ● **E934.2 Anticoagulants**
      Coumarin
      Heparin
      Phenindione
      Prothrombin synthesis inhibitor
      Warfarin sodium
      Coding Clinic: 2013, Q2, P8; 2008, Q4, P134-136; 2006, Q3, P12-13; Q2, P17; 2004, Q3, P7; 1994, Q1, P22; 1990, Q3, P14

   ● **E934.3 Vitamin K [phytonadione]**

   ● **E934.4 Fibrinolysis-affecting drugs**
      Aminocaproic acid
      Streptodornase
      Streptokinase
      Urokinase
      Coding Clinic: 2010, Q3, P5

   ● **E934.5 Anticoagulant antagonists and other coagulants**
      Hexadimethrine bromide
      Protamine sulfate

   ● **E934.6 Gamma globulin**

   ● **E934.7 Natural blood and blood products**
      Blood plasma
      Human fibrinogen
      Packed red cells
      Whole blood
      Coding Clinic: 2013, Q2, P8; 2011, Q4, P147; 2010, Q4, P79; 2006, Q4, P91-92; 2000, Q3, P9; 1997, Q2, P11

   ● **E934.8 Other agents affecting blood constituents**
      Macromolecular blood substitutes

   ● **E934.9 Unspecified agent affecting blood constituents**

● **E935 Analgesics, antipyretics, and antirheumatics**

   ● **E935.0 Heroin**
      Diacetylmorphine

   ● **E935.1 Methadone**

   ● **E935.2 Other opiates and related narcotics**
      Codeine [methylmorphine]
      Morphine
      Opium (alkaloids)
      Meperidine [pethidine]

   ● **E935.3 Salicylates**
      Acetylsalicylic acid [aspirin]
      Amino derivatives of salicylic acid
      Salicylic acid salts
      Coding Clinic: 1984, Nov-Dec, P15

   ● **E935.4 Aromatic analgesics, not elsewhere classified**
      Acetanilid
      Paracetamol [acetaminophen]
      Phenacetin [acetophenetidin]

◀ New   ◀ Revised   ~~deleted~~ Deleted   Excludes   Includes   Use additional   Code first   Omit code

1066   ● Unacceptable Principal Diagnosis   ● Use Additional Digit(s)   ▶ Manifestation Code   OGCR Official Guidelines   Coding Clinic

E000-E999

● **E935.5 Pyrazole derivatives**
    Aminophenazone [aminopyrine]
    Phenylbutazone
    Coding Clinic: 1990, Q4, P26

● **E935.6 Antirheumatics [antiphlogistics]**
    Gold salts
    Indomethacin
    Excludes   *salicylates (E935.3)*
              steroids (E932.0)

● **E935.7 Other non-narcotic analgesics**
    Pyrabital

● **E935.8 Other specified analgesics and antipyretics**
    Pentazocine
    Coding Clinic: 1992, Q3, P16-17

● **E935.9 Unspecified analgesic and antipyretic**

● **E936 Anticonvulsants and anti-Parkinsonism drugs**

● **E936.0 Oxazolidine derivatives**
    Paramethadione
    Trimethadione

● **E936.1 Hydantoin derivatives**
    Phenytoin

● **E936.2 Succinimides**
    Ethosuximide
    Phensuximide

● **E936.3 Other and unspecified anticonvulsants**
    Beclamide
    Primidone

● **E936.4 Anti-Parkinsonism drugs**
    Amantadine
    Ethopropazine [profenamine]
    Levodopa [L-dopa]

● **E937 Sedatives and hypnotics**

● **E937.0 Barbiturates**
    Amobarbital [amylobarbitone]
    Barbital [barbitone]
    Butabarbital [butabarbitone]
    Pentobarbital [pentobarbitone]
    Phenobarbital [phenobarbitone]
    Secobarbital [quinalbarbitone]
    Excludes   *thiobarbiturates (E938.3)*

● **E937.1 Chloral hydrate group**
● **E937.2 Paraldehyde**
● **E937.3 Bromine compounds**
    Bromide
    Carbromal (derivatives)

● **E937.4 Methaqualone compounds**
● **E937.5 Glutethimide group**
● **E937.6 Mixed sedatives, not elsewhere classified**
● **E937.8 Other sedatives and hypnotics**
● **E937.9 Unspecified**
    Sleeping:
       drug NOS
       pill NOS
       tablet NOS

● **E938 Other central nervous system depressants and anesthetics**

● **E938.0 Central nervous system muscle-tone depressants**
    Chlorphenesin (carbamate)
    Mephenesin
    Methocarbamol

● **E938.1 Halothane**
● **E938.2 Other gaseous anesthetics**
    Ether
    Halogenated hydrocarbon derivatives, except
       halothane
    Nitrous oxide

● **E938.3 Intravenous anesthetics**
    Ketamine
    Methohexital [methohexitone]
    Thiobarbiturates, such as thiopental sodium

● **E938.4 Other and unspecified general anesthetics**

● **E938.5 Surface and infiltration anesthetics**
    Cocaine
    Lidocaine [lignocaine]
    Procaine
    Tetracaine

● **E938.6 Peripheral nerve- and plexus-blocking anesthetics**

● **E938.7 Spinal anesthetics**
    Coding Clinic: 2004, Q2, P18; 2003, Q3, P12; 1987, Jan-Feb,
       P13-14

● **E938.9 Other and unspecified local anesthetics**

● **E939 Psychotropic agents**

● **E939.0 Antidepressants**
    Amitriptyline
    Imipramine
    Monoamine oxidase [MAO] inhibitors
    Coding Clinic: 2003, Q4, P75-76; 1992, Q3, P16

● **E939.1 Phenothiazine-based tranquilizers**
    Chlorpromazine   Prochlorperazine
    Fluphenazine   Promazine
    Phenothiazine

● **E939.2 Butyrophenone-based tranquilizers**
    Haloperidol
    Spiperone
    Trifluperidol

● **E939.3 Other antipsychotics, neuroleptics, and major tranquilizers**
    Coding Clinic: 2010, Q1, P20-21; 2006, Q4, P76-78

● **E939.4 Benzodiazepine-based tranquilizers**
    Chlordiazepoxide   Lorazepam
    Diazepam   Medazepam
    Flurazepam   Nitrazepam

● **E939.5 Other tranquilizers**
    Hydroxyzine
    Meprobamate

● **E939.6 Psychodysleptics [hallucinogens]**
    Cannabis (derivatives)
    Lysergide [LSD]
    Marihuana (derivatives)
    Mescaline
    Psilocin
    Psilocybin

● **E939.7 Psychostimulants**
    Amphetamine
    Caffeine
    Excludes   *central appetite depressants (E947.0)*

● **E939.8 Other psychotropic agents**
● **E939.9 Unspecified psychotropic agent**

● **E940 Central nervous system stimulants**

● **E940.0 Analeptics**
    Lobeline
    Nikethamide

● **E940.1 Opiate antagonists**
    Levallorphan
    Nalorphine
    Naloxone

● **E940.8 Other specified central nervous system stimulants**
● **E940.9 Unspecified central nervous system stimulant**

E000-E999

N Newborn: 0   **P** Pediatric: 0–17   **M** Maternity: 12–55   **A** Adult: 15–124   ♀ Females Only   ♂ Males Only

(Ex) **CC/MCC Exclusions**   🔮 **Complication\Comorbidity**   🔮 **Major C\C**   🔮 **Present on Admission Requirement**   🔮 **Hospital-Acquired Condition**   **1067**

● **E941 Drugs primarily affecting the autonomic nervous system**

   ● **E941.0 Parasympathomimetics [cholinergics]**
       Acetylcholine
       Anticholinesterase:
          organophosphorus
          reversible
       Pilocarpine

   ● **E941.1 Parasympatholytics [anticholinergics and antimuscarinics] and spasmolytics**
       Atropine
       Homatropine
       Hyoscine [scopolamine]
       Quaternary ammonium derivatives
       Excludes *papaverine (E942.5)*

   ● **E941.2 Sympathomimetics [adrenergics]**
       Epinephrine [adrenalin]
       Levarterenol [noradrenalin]
       Coding Clinic: 2002, Q3, P12

   ● **E941.3 Sympatholytics [antiadrenergics]**
       Phenoxybenzamine
       Tolazoline hydrochloride
       Coding Clinic: 2007, Q4, P77-79

   ● **E941.9 Unspecified drug primarily affecting the autonomic nervous system**

● **E942 Agents primarily affecting the cardiovascular system**

   ● **E942.0 Cardiac rhythm regulators**
       Practolol
       Procainamide
       Propranolol
       Quinidine
       Coding Clinic: 1986, Mar-April, P11-12

   ● **E942.1 Cardiotonic glycosides and drugs of similar action**
       Digitalis glycosides
       Digoxin
       Strophanthins

   ● **E942.2 Antilipemic and antiarteriosclerotic drugs**
       Cholestyramine
       Clofibrate
       Nicotinic acid derivatives
       Sitosterols
       Excludes *dextrothyroxine (E932.7)*

   ● **E942.3 Ganglion-blocking agents**
       Pentamethonium bromide

   ● **E942.4 Coronary vasodilators**
       Dipyridamole
       Nitrates [nitroglycerin]
       Nitrites
       Prenylamine

   ● **E942.5 Other vasodilators**
       Cyclandelate
       Diazoxide
       Hydralazine
       Papaverine

   ● **E942.6 Other antihypertensive agents**
       Clonidine
       Guanethidine
       Rauwolfia alkaloids
       Reserpine

   ● **E942.7 Antivaricose drugs, including sclerosing agents**
       Monoethanolamine
       Zinc salts

   ● **E942.8 Capillary-active drugs**
       Adrenochrome derivatives
       Bioflavonoids
       Metaraminol

   ● **E942.9 Other and unspecified agents primarily affecting the cardiovascular system**

● **E943 Agents primarily affecting gastrointestinal system**

   ● **E943.0 Antacids and antigastric secretion drugs**
       Aluminum hydroxide
       Magnesium trisilicate

   ● **E943.1 Irritant cathartics**
       Bisacodyl
       Castor oil
       Phenolphthalein

   ● **E943.2 Emollient cathartics**
       Sodium dioctyl sulfosuccinate

   ● **E943.3 Other cathartics, including intestinal atonia drugs**
       Magnesium sulfate

   ● **E943.4 Digestants**
       Pancreatin
       Papain
       Pepsin

   ● **E943.5 Antidiarrheal drugs**
       Bismuth subcarbonate
       Kaolin
       Pectin
       Excludes *anti-infectives (E930.0-E931.9)*

   ● **E943.6 Emetics**

   ● **E943.8 Other specified agents primarily affecting the gastrointestinal system**

   ● **E943.9 Unspecified agent primarily affecting the gastrointestinal system**

● **E944 Water, mineral, and uric acid metabolism drugs**

   ● **E944.0 Mercurial diuretics**
       Chlormerodrin
       Mercaptomerin
       Mercurophylline
       Mersalyl

   ● **E944.1 Purine derivative diuretics**
       Theobromine
       Theophylline
       Excludes *aminophylline [theophylline ethylenediamine] (E945.7)*

   ● **E944.2 Carbonic acid anhydrase inhibitors**
       Acetazolamide

   ● **E944.3 Saluretics**
       Benzothiadiazides
       Chlorothiazide group

   ● **E944.4 Other diuretics**
       Ethacrynic acid
       Furosemide

   ● **E944.5 Electrolytic, caloric, and water-balance agents**

   ● **E944.6 Other mineral salts, not elsewhere classified**

   ● **E944.7 Uric acid metabolism drugs**
       Cinchophen and congeners
       Colchicine
       Phenoquin
       Probenecid

● **E945 Agents primarily acting on the smooth and skeletal muscles and respiratory system**

   ● **E945.0 Oxytocic agents**
       Ergot alkaloids
       Prostaglandins

   ● **E945.1 Smooth muscle relaxants**
       Adiphenine
       Metaproterenol [orciprenaline]
       Excludes *papaverine (E942.5)*

   ● **E945.2 Skeletal muscle relaxants**
       Alcuronium chloride
       Suxamethonium chloride

   ● **E945.3 Other and unspecified drugs acting on muscles**

E000-E999

◀ New   ◀═ Revised   ~~deleted~~ Deleted   Excludes   Includes   Use additional   Code first   Omit code

1068   ● Unacceptable Principal Diagnosis   ● Use Additional Digit(s)   ▶ Manifestation Code   OGCR Official Guidelines   **Coding Clinic**

- E945.4 **Antitussives**
  Dextromethorphan
  Pipazethate hydrochloride
- E945.5 **Expectorants**
  Acetylcysteine
  Cocillana
  Guaifenesin [glyceryl guaiacolate]
  Ipecacuanha
  Terpin hydrate
- E945.6 **Anti-common cold drugs**
- E945.7 **Antiasthmatics**
  Aminophylline [theophylline ethylenediamine]
- E945.8 **Other and unspecified respiratory drugs**

- E946 **Agents primarily affecting skin and mucous membrane, ophthalmological, otorhinolaryngological, and dental drugs**
  - E946.0 **Local anti-infectives and anti-inflammatory drugs**
  - E946.1 **Antipruritics**
  - E946.2 **Local astringents and local detergents**
  - E946.3 **Emollients, demulcents, and protectants**
  - E946.4 **Keratolytics, keratoplastics, other hair treatment drugs and preparations**
  - E946.5 **Eye anti-infectives and other eye drugs**
    Idoxuridine
  - E946.6 **Anti-infectives and other drugs and preparations for ear, nose, and throat**
  - E946.7 **Dental drugs topically applied**
  - E946.8 **Other agents primarily affecting skin and mucous membrane**
    Spermicides
  - E946.9 **Unspecified agent primarily affecting skin and mucous membrane**

- E947 **Other and unspecified drugs and medicinal substances**
  - E947.0 **Dietetics**
  - E947.1 **Lipotropic drugs**
  - E947.2 **Antidotes and chelating agents, not elsewhere classified**
  - E947.3 **Alcohol deterrents**
  - E947.4 **Pharmaceutical excipients**
  - E947.8 **Other drugs and medicinal substances**
    Contrast media used for diagnostic x-ray procedures
    Diagnostic agents and kits
  - E947.9 **Unspecified drug or medicinal substance**

- E948 **Bacterial vaccines**
  - E948.0 **BCG vaccine**
  - E948.1 **Typhoid and paratyphoid**
  - E948.2 **Cholera**
  - E948.3 **Plague**
  - E948.4 **Tetanus**
  - E948.5 **Diphtheria**
  - E948.6 **Pertussis vaccine, including combinations with a pertussis component**
  - E948.8 **Other and unspecified bacterial vaccines**
  - E948.9 **Mixed bacterial vaccines, except combinations with a pertussis component**

- E949 **Other vaccines and biological substances**
  Excludes *gamma globulin (E934.6)*
  Coding Clinic: 2008, Q3, P21
  - E949.0 **Smallpox vaccine**
  - E949.1 **Rabies vaccine**
  - E949.2 **Typhus vaccine**
  - E949.3 **Yellow fever vaccine**
  - E949.4 **Measles vaccine**
  - E949.5 **Poliomyelitis vaccine**

- E949.6 **Other and unspecified viral and rickettsial vaccines**
  Mumps vaccine
- E949.7 **Mixed viral-rickettsial and bacterial vaccines, except combinations with a pertussis component**
  Excludes *combinations with a pertussis component (E948.6)*
- E949.9 **Other and unspecified vaccines and biological substances**

SUICIDE AND SELF-INFLICTED INJURY (E950-E959)

Includes injuries in suicide and attempted suicide
self-inflicted injuries specified as intentional

- E950 **Suicide and self-inflicted poisoning by solid or liquid substances**
  - E950.0 **Analgesics, antipyretics, and antirheumatics**
    Coding Clinic: 1998, Q4, P50-51
  - E950.1 **Barbiturates**
  - E950.2 **Other sedatives and hypnotics**
  - E950.3 **Tranquilizers and other psychotropic agents**
  - E950.4 **Other specified drugs and medicinal substances**
  - E950.5 **Unspecified drug or medicinal substance**
  - E950.6 **Agricultural and horticultural chemical and pharmaceutical preparations other than plant foods and fertilizers**
  - E950.7 **Corrosive and caustic substances**
    Suicide and self-inflicted poisoning by substances classifiable to E864
  - E950.8 **Arsenic and its compounds**
  - E950.9 **Other and unspecified solid and liquid substances**

- E951 **Suicide and self-inflicted poisoning by gases in domestic use**
  - E951.0 **Gas distributed by pipeline**
  - E951.1 **Liquefied petroleum gas distributed in mobile containers**
  - E951.8 **Other utility gas**

- E952 **Suicide and self-inflicted poisoning by other gases and vapors**
  - E952.0 **Motor vehicle exhaust gas**
  - E952.1 **Other carbon monoxide**
  - E952.8 **Other specified gases and vapors**
  - E952.9 **Unspecified gases and vapors**

- E953 **Suicide and self-inflicted injury by hanging, strangulation, and suffocation**
  - E953.0 **Hanging**
  - E953.1 **Suffocation by plastic bag**
  - E953.8 **Other specified means**
  - E953.9 **Unspecified means**

- E954 **Suicide and self-inflicted injury by submersion [drowning]**

- E955 **Suicide and self-inflicted injury by firearms, air guns and explosives**
  - E955.0 **Handgun**
  - E955.1 **Shotgun**
  - E955.2 **Hunting rifle**
  - E955.3 **Military firearms**
  - E955.4 **Other and unspecified firearm**
    Gunshot NOS
    Shot NOS
  - E955.5 **Explosives**
  - E955.6 **Air gun**
    BB gun
    Pellet gun
  - E955.7 **Paintball gun**
  - E955.9 **Unspecified**

E000-E999

N Newborn: 0   P Pediatric: 0–17   M Maternity: 12–55   A Adult: 15–124   ♀ Females Only   ♂ Males Only

(Ex) CC/MCC Exclusions   🔖 Complication\Comorbidity   🔖 Major C\C   🔖 Present on Admission Requirement   🔖 Hospital-Acquired Condition

1069

- E956 Suicide and self-inflicted injury by cutting and piercing instrument
- E957 Suicide and self-inflicted injuries by jumping from high place
  - E957.0 Residential premises
  - E957.1 Other man-made structures
  - E957.2 Natural sites
  - E957.9 Unspecified
- E958 Suicide and self-inflicted injury by other and unspecified means
  - E958.0 Jumping or lying before moving object
  - E958.1 Burns, fire
  - E958.2 Scald
  - E958.3 Extremes of cold
  - E958.4 Electrocution
  - E958.5 Crashing of motor vehicle
  - E958.6 Crashing of aircraft
  - E958.7 Caustic substances, except poisoning
    - Excludes *poisoning by caustic substance (E950.7)*
  - E958.8 Other specified means
  - E958.9 Unspecified means
- E959 Late effects of self-inflicted injury
  - **Note:** This category is to be used to indicate circumstances classifiable to E950-E958 as the cause of death or disability from late effects, which are themselves classifiable elsewhere. The "late effects" include conditions reported as such or as sequelae which may occur at any time after the attempted suicide or self-inflicted injury.

    OGCR Section I.C.19.d.1

    When the cause of an injury or neglect is intentional child or adult abuse, the first listed E code should be assigned from categories E960-E968, Homicide and injury purposely inflicted by other persons, (except category E967). An E code from category E967, Child and adult battering and other maltreatment, should be added as an additional code to identify the perpetrator, if known.

HOMICIDE AND INJURY PURPOSELY INFLICTED BY OTHER PERSONS (E960-E969)

Includes injuries inflicted by another person with intent to injure or kill, by any means

Excludes *injuries due to:*
  legal intervention (E970-E978)
  operations of war (E990-E999)
  terrorism (E979)

- E960 Fight, brawl, rape
  - E960.0 Unarmed fight or brawl
    Beatings NOS
    Brawl or fight with hands, fists, feet
    Injured or killed in fight NOS
    - Excludes *homicidal:*
      injury by weapons (E965.0-E966, E969)
      strangulation (E963)
      submersion (E964)
  - E960.1 Rape
    Coding Clinic: 1999, Q3, P15
- E961 Assault by corrosive or caustic substance, except poisoning
  Injury or death purposely caused by corrosive or caustic substance, such as:
    acid [any]
    corrosive substance
    vitriol
  - Excludes *burns from hot liquid (E968.3)*
    chemical burns from swallowing a corrosive substance (E962.0-E962.9)

- E962 Assault by poisoning
  - E962.0 Drugs and medicinal substances
    Homicidal poisoning by any drug or medicinal substance
  - E962.1 Other solid and liquid substances
  - E962.2 Other gases and vapors
  - E962.9 Unspecified poisoning
- E963 Assault by hanging and strangulation
  Homicidal (attempt):
    garrotting or ligature
    hanging
    strangulation
    suffocation
- E964 Assault by submersion [drowning]
- E965 Assault by firearms and explosives
  - E965.0 Handgun
    Pistol
    Revolver
  - E965.1 Shotgun
  - E965.2 Hunting rifle
  - E965.3 Military firearms
  - E965.4 Other and unspecified firearm
  - E965.5 Antipersonnel bomb
  - E965.6 Gasoline bomb
  - E965.7 Letter bomb
  - E965.8 Other specified explosive
    Bomb NOS (placed in):
      car
      house
    Dynamite
  - E965.9 Unspecified explosive
- E966 Assault by cutting and piercing instrument
  Assassination (attempt), homicide (attempt) by any instrument classifiable under E920
  Homicidal:
    cut any part of body
    puncture any part of body
    stab any part of body
  Stabbed any part of body
  Coding Clinic: 1993, Q2, P4-5
- E967 Perpetrator of child and adult abuse
  - **Note:** Selection of the correct perpetrator code is based on the relationship between the perpetrator and the victim.
  - E967.0 By father, stepfather, or boyfriend
    Male partner of child's parent or guardian
  - E967.1 By other specified person
    Coding Clinic: 1999, Q3, P14-15
  - E967.2 By mother, stepmother, or girlfriend
    Female partner of child's parent or guardian
    Coding Clinic: 1996, Q4, P43-44
  - E967.3 By spouse or partner
    Abuse of spouse or partner by ex-spouse or ex-partner
    Coding Clinic: 1996, Q4, P43-44
  - E967.4 By child
  - E967.5 By sibling
  - E967.6 By grandparent
  - E967.7 By other relative
  - E967.8 By non-related caregiver
  - E967.9 By unspecified person

● **E968   Assault by other and unspecified means**

   ● **E968.0   Fire**

       Arson

       Homicidal burns NOS

       Excludes   *burns from hot liquid (E968.3)*

   ● **E968.1   Pushing from a high place**

   ● **E968.2   Striking by blunt or thrown object**

       Coding Clinic: 1996, Q4, P43-44

   ● **E968.3   Hot liquid**

       Homicidal burns by scalding

   ● **E968.4   Criminal neglect**

       Abandonment of child, infant, or other helpless
          person with intent to injure or kill

   ● **E968.5   Transport vehicle**

       Being struck by other vehicle or run down with
          intent to injure

       Pushed in front of, thrown from, or dragged by
          moving vehicle with intent to injure

   ● **E968.6   Air gun**

       BB gun

       Pellet gun

   ● **E968.7   Human bite**

   ● **E968.8   Other specified means**

       Coding Clinic: 1999, Q3, P14-15x2

   ● **E968.9   Unspecified means**

       Assassination (attempt) NOS

       Homicidal (attempt):

          injury NOS

          wound NOS

       Manslaughter (nonaccidental)

       Murder (attempt) NOS

       Violence, non-accidental

● **E969   Late effects of injury purposely inflicted by other person**

     Note: This category is to be used to indicate circumstances
       classifiable to E960-E968 as the cause of death or
       disability from late effects, which are themselves
       classifiable elsewhere. The "late effects" include
       conditions reported as such, or as sequelae which
       may occur at any time after the injury purposely
       inflicted by another person.

LEGAL INTERVENTION (E970-E978)

  Includes   injuries inflicted by the police or other
        law-enforcing agents, including military
        on duty, in the course of arresting
        or attempting to arrest lawbreakers,
        suppressing disturbances, maintaining
        order, and other legal action
        legal execution

  Excludes   *injuries caused by civil insurrections (E990.0-E999)*

● **E970   Injury due to legal intervention by firearms** 🔗

     Gunshot wound

     Injury by:

        machine gun

        revolver

        rifle pellet or rubber bullet

        shot NOS

● **E971   Injury due to legal intervention by explosives** 🔗

     Injury by:

        dynamite

        explosive shell

        grenade

        motor bomb

● **E972   Injury due to legal intervention by gas** 🔗

     Asphyxiation by gas

     Injury by tear gas

     Poisoning by gas

● **E973   Injury due to legal intervention by blunt object** 🔗

     Hit, struck by:

        baton (nightstick)

        blunt object

        stave

● **E974   Injury due to legal intervention by cutting and piercing instrument** 🔗

     Cut

     Incised wound

     Injured by bayonet

     Stab wound

● **E975   Injury due to legal intervention by other specified means** 🔗

     Blow

     Manhandling

● **E976   Injury due to legal intervention by unspecified means** 🔗

● **E977   Late effects of injuries due to legal intervention** 🔗

     Note: This category is to be used to indicate circumstances
       classifiable to E970-E976 as the cause of death or
       disability from late effects, which are themselves
       classifiable elsewhere. The "late effects" include
       conditions reported as such, or as sequelae which
       may occur at any time after the injury due to legal
       intervention.

● **E978   Legal execution** 🔗

     All executions performed at the behest of the judiciary or
       ruling authority [whether permanent or temporary] as:

       asphyxiation by gas

       beheading, decapitation (by guillotine)

       capital punishment

       electrocution

       hanging

       poisoning

       shooting

       other specified means

  OGCR   Section I.C.19.j.1-3

> When the cause of an injury is identified by the Federal
> Government (FBI) as terrorism, the first-listed E-code
> should be a code from category E979, Terrorism. The
> definition of terrorism employed by the FBI is found at the
> inclusion note at E979. The terrorism E-code is the only
> E-code that should be assigned. Additional E codes from
> the assault categories should not be assigned.
>
>   When the cause of an injury is suspected to be the
> result of terrorism a code from category E979 should
> not be assigned. Assign a code in the range of E codes
> based circumstances on the documentation of intent and
> mechanism.
>
>   Assign code E979.9, Terrorism, secondary effects, for
> conditions occurring subsequent to the terrorist event. This
> code should not be assigned for conditions that are due to
> the initial terrorist act.

TERRORISM (E979)

● **E979   Terrorism**

     Injuries resulting from the unlawful use of force or violence
       against persons or property to intimidate or coerce a
       Government, the civilian population, or any segment
       thereof, in furtherance of political or social objective

     Coding Clinic: 2002, Q4, P74-77

   ● **E979.0   Terrorism involving explosion of marine weapons** 🔗

       Depth-charge

       Marine mine

          Mine NOS, at sea or in harbour

       Sea-based artillery shell

       Torpedo

       Underwater blast

   ● **E979.1   Terrorism involving destruction of aircraft** 🔗

       Aircraft:

          burned

          exploded

          shot down

       Aircraft used as a weapon

       Crushed by falling aircraft

E000-E999

N Newborn: 0   P Pediatric: 0–17   M Maternity: 12–55   A Adult: 15–124   ♀ Females Only   ♂ Males Only

(Ex) CC/MCC Exclusions   🔗 Complication\Comorbidity   🔗 Major C\C   🔗 Present on Admission Requirement   🔗 Hospital-Acquired Condition   **1071**

● **E979.2 Terrorism involving other explosions and fragments** 🖐
 Antipersonnel bomb (fragments)
 Blast NOS
 Explosion (of):
  artillery shell
  breech-block
  cannon block
  mortar bomb
  munitions being used in terrorism
  NOS
 Fragments from:
  artillery shell
  bomb
  grenade
  guided missile
  land-mine
  rocket
  shell
  shrapnel
 Mine NOS

● **E979.3 Terrorism involving fires, conflagration and hot substances** 🖐
 Burning building or structure:
  collapse of
  fall from
  hit by falling object in
  jump from
 Conflagration NOS
 Fire (causing):
  asphyxia
  burns
  NOS
  other injury
 Melting of fittings and furniture in burning
 Petrol bomb
 Smouldering building or structure

● **E979.4 Terrorism involving firearms** 🖐
 Bullet:
  carbine
  machine gun
  pistol
  rifle
  rubber (rifle)
 Pellets (shotgun)

● **E979.5 Terrorism involving nuclear weapons** 🖐
 Blast effects
 Exposure to ionizing radiation from nuclear weapon
 Fireball effects
 Heat from nuclear weapon
 Other direct and secondary effects of nuclear weapons

● **E979.6 Terrorism involving biological weapons** 🖐
 Anthrax
 Cholera
 Smallpox

● **E979.7 Terrorism involving chemical weapons** 🖐
 Gases, fumes, chemicals
 Hydrogen cyanide
 Phosgene
 Sarin

● **E979.8 Terrorism involving other means** 🖐
 Drowning and submersion
 Lasers
 Piercing or stabbing instruments
 Terrorism NOS

● **E979.9 Terrorism secondary effects** 🖐
 Note: This code is for use to identify conditions occurring subsequent to a terrorist attack, not those that are due to the initial terrorist attack.
 Excludes *late effect of terrorist attack (E999.1)*

 Note: Categories E980-E989 are for use when it is unspecified or it cannot be determined whether the injuries are accidental (unintentional), suicide (attempted), or assault.

● **E980 Poisoning by solid or liquid substances, undetermined whether accidentally or purposely inflicted**
 ● **E980.0 Analgesics, antipyretics, and antirheumatics**
 ● **E980.1 Barbiturates**
 ● **E980.2 Other sedatives and hypnotics**
 ● **E980.3 Tranquilizers and other psychotropic agents**
 ● **E980.4 Other specified drugs and medicinal substances**
 ● **E980.5 Unspecified drug or medicinal substance**
 ● **E980.6 Corrosive and caustic substances**
  Poisoning, undetermined whether accidental or purposeful, by substances classifiable to E864
 ● **E980.7 Agricultural and horticultural chemical and pharmaceutical preparations other than plant foods and fertilizers**
 ● **E980.8 Arsenic and its compounds**
 ● **E980.9 Other and unspecified solid and liquid substances**

● **E981 Poisoning by gases in domestic use, undetermined whether accidentally or purposely inflicted**
 ● **E981.0 Gas distributed by pipeline** 🖐
 ● **E981.1 Liquefied petroleum gas distributed in mobile containers** 🖐
 ● **E981.8 Other utility gas** 🖐

● **E982 Poisoning by other gases, undetermined whether accidentally or purposely inflicted**
 ● **E982.0 Motor vehicle exhaust gas** 🖐
 ● **E982.1 Other carbon monoxide** 🖐
 ● **E982.8 Other specified gases and vapors** 🖐
 ● **E982.9 Unspecified gases and vapors** 🖐

● **E983 Hanging, strangulation, or suffocation, undetermined whether accidentally or purposely inflicted**
 ● **E983.0 Hanging**
 ● **E983.1 Suffocation by plastic bag**
 ● **E983.8 Other specified means**
 ● **E983.9 Unspecified means**

● **E984 Submersion [drowning], undetermined whether accidentally or purposely inflicted**

● **E985 Injury by firearms, air guns and explosives, undetermined whether accidentally or purposely inflicted**
 ● **E985.0 Handgun** 🖐
 ● **E985.1 Shotgun** 🖐
 ● **E985.2 Hunting rifle** 🖐
 ● **E985.3 Military firearms** 🖐
 ● **E985.4 Other and unspecified firearm** 🖐
 ● **E985.5 Explosives** 🖐
 ● **E985.6 Air gun** 🖐
  BB gun
  Pellet gun
 ● **E985.7 Paintball gun** 🖐

● **E986 Injury by cutting and piercing instruments, undetermined whether accidentally or purposely inflicted**

● **E987 Falling from high place, undetermined whether accidentally or purposely inflicted**
- ● **E987.0 Residential premises** 🗊
- ● **E987.1 Other man-made structures**
- ● **E987.2 Natural sites** 🗊
- ● **E987.9 Unspecified site**

● **E988 Injury by other and unspecified means, undetermined whether accidentally or purposely inflicted**
- ● **E988.0 Jumping or lying before moving object**
- ● **E988.1 Burns, fire**
- ● **E988.2 Scald**
- ● **E988.3 Extremes of cold**
- ● **E988.4 Electrocution**
- ● **E988.5 Crashing of motor vehicle**
- ● **E988.6 Crashing of aircraft**
- ● **E988.7 Caustic substances, except poisoning**
- ● **E988.8 Other specified means**
  Coding Clinic: 2012, Q2, P16-17
- ● **E988.9 Unspecified means**

● **E989 Late effects of injury, undetermined whether accidentally or purposely inflicted** 🗊
- **Note:** This category is to be used to indicate circumstances classifiable to E980-E988 as the cause of death or disability from late effects, which are themselves classifiable elsewhere. The "late effects" include conditions reported as such or as sequelae which may occur at any time after injury, undetermined whether accidentally or purposely inflicted.

INJURY RESULTING FROM OPERATIONS OF WAR (E990-E999)

Includes   injuries to military personnel and civilians caused by war and civil insurrections and occurring during the time of war and insurrection, and peacekeeping missions

Excludes   *accidents during training of military personnel, manufacture of war material and transport, unless attributable to enemy action*

● **E990 Injury due to war operations by fires and conflagrations**
- **Includes**   asphyxia, burns, or other injury originating from fire caused by a fire-producing device or indirectly by any conventional weapon
- ● **E990.0 From gasoline bomb** 🗊
  Incendiary bomb
- ● **E990.1 From flamethrower** 🗊
- ● **E990.2 From incendiary bullet** 🗊
- ● **E990.3 From fire caused indirectly from conventional weapon** 🗊
  - **Excludes**   *fire aboard military aircraft (E994.3)*
- ● **E990.9 From other and unspecified source** 🗊

● **E991 Injury due to war operations by bullets and fragments**
- **Excludes**   *injury due to bullets and fragments due to war operations, but occurring after cessation of hostilities (E998.0)*
  injury due to explosion of artillery shells and mortars (E993.2)
  injury due to explosion of improvised explosive device [IED] (E993.3-E993.5)
  injury due to sea-based artillery shell (E992.3)
- ● **E991.0 Rubber bullets (rifle)** 🗊
- ● **E991.1 Pellets (rifle)** 🗊
- ● **E991.2 Other bullets** 🗊
  Bullet [any, except rubber bullets and pellets]
  carbine
  machine gun
  pistol
  rifle
  shotgun
- ● **E991.3 Antipersonnel bomb (fragments)** 🗊
- ● **E991.4 Fragments from munitions** 🗊
  Fragments from:
  artillery shell
  bombs, except antipersonnel
  detonation of unexploded ordnance [UXO]
  grenade
  guided missile
  land mine
  rockets
  shell
- ● **E991.5 Fragments from person-borne improvised explosive device [IED]** 🗊
- ● **E991.6 Fragments from vehicle-borne improvised explosive device [IED]** 🗊
  IED borne by land, air, or water transport vehicle
- ● **E991.7 Fragments from other improvised explosive device [IED]** 🗊
  Roadside IED
- ● **E991.8 Fragments from weapons** 🗊
  Fragments from:
  artillery
  autocannons
  automatic grenade launchers
  missile launchers
  mortars
  small arms
- ● **E991.9 Other and unspecified fragments** 🗊
  Shrapnel NOS

● **E992 Injury due to war operations by explosion of marine weapons**
- ● **E992.0 Torpedo** 🗊
- ● **E992.1 Depth charge** 🗊
- ● **E992.2 Marine mines** 🗊
  Marine mines at sea or in harbor
- ● **E992.3 Sea-based artillery shell** 🗊
- ● **E992.8 Other by other marine weapons** 🗊
- ● **E992.9 Unspecified marine weapon** 🗊
  Underwater blast NOS

E000-E999

N Newborn: 0   P Pediatric: 0–17   M Maternity: 12–55   A Adult: 15–124   ♀ Females Only   ♂ Males Only

(Ex) CC/MCC Exclusions   🗊 Complication\Comorbidity   🗊 Major C\C   🗊 Present on Admission Requirement   🗊 Hospital-Acquired Condition   **1073**

E000-E999

● **E993 Injury due to war operations by other explosion**
      Injuries due to direct or indirect pressure or air blast of an explosion occurring during war operations

      Excludes *injury due to fragments resulting from an explosion (E991.0-E991.9)*
              injury due to detonation of unexploded ordnance but occurring after cessation of hostilities (E998.0-E998.9)
              injury due to nuclear weapons (E996.0-E996.9)

  ● **E993.0 Aerial bomb** 🔍
  ● **E993.1 Guided missile** 🔍
  ● **E993.2 Mortar** 🔍
        Artillery shell
  ● **E993.3 Person-borne improvised explosive device [IED]** 🔍
  ● **E993.4 Vehicle-borne improvised explosive device [IED]** 🔍
        IED borne by land, air, or water transport vehicle
  ● **E993.5 Other improvised explosive device [IED]** 🔍
        Roadside IED
  ● **E993.6 Unintentional detonation of own munitions** 🔍
        Unintentional detonation of own ammunition (artillery) (mortars)
  ● **E993.7 Unintentional discharge of own munitions launch device** 🔍
        Unintentional explosion of own:
           autocannons
           automatic grenade launchers
           missile launchers
           small arms
  ● **E993.8 Other specified explosion** 🔍
        Bomb
        Grenade
        Land mine
  ● **E993.9 Unspecified explosion** 🔍
        Air blast NOS
        Blast NOS
        Blast wave NOS
        Blast wind NOS
        Explosion NOS

● **E994 Injury due to war operations by destruction of aircraft**
  ● **E994.0 Destruction of aircraft due to enemy fire or explosives** 🔍
        Air to air missile
        Explosive device placed on aircraft
        Rocket propelled grenade [RPG]
        Small arms fire
        Surface to air missile
  ● **E994.1 Unintentional destruction of aircraft due to own onboard explosives** 🔍
  ● **E994.2 Destruction of aircraft due to collision with other aircraft** 🔍
  ● **E994.3 Destruction of aircraft due to onboard fire** 🔍
  ● **E994.8 Other destruction of aircraft** 🔍
  ● **E994.9 Unspecified destruction of aircraft** 🔍

● **E995 Injury due to war operations by other and unspecified forms of conventional warfare**
  ● **E995.0 Unarmed hand-to-hand combat** 🔍
      Excludes *intentional restriction of airway (E995.3)*
  ● **E995.1 Struck by blunt object** 🔍
        Baton (nightstick)
        Stave
  ● **E995.2 Piercing object** 🔍
        Bayonet
        Knife
        Sword
  ● **E995.3 Intentional restriction of air and airway** 🔍
        Intentional submersion
        Strangulation
        Suffocation

  ● **E995.4 Unintentional drowning due to inability to surface or obtain air** 🔍
        Submersion
  ● **E995.8 Other forms of conventional warfare** 🔍
  ● **E995.9 Unspecified form of conventional warfare** 🔍

● **E996 Injury due to war operations by nuclear weapons**
      Dirty bomb NOS

      Excludes *late effects of injury due to nuclear weapons (E999.1, E999.0)*

  ● **E996.0 Direct blast effect of nuclear weapon** 🔍
        Injury to bodily organs due to blast pressure
  ● **E996.1 Indirect blast effect of nuclear weapon** 🔍
        Injury due to being thrown by blast
        Injury due to being struck or crushed by blast debris
  ● **E996.2 Thermal radiation effect of nuclear weapon** 🔍
        Burns due to thermal radiation
        Fireball effects
        Flash burns
        Heat effects
  ● **E996.3 Nuclear radiation effects** 🔍
        Acute radiation exposure
        Beta burns
        Fallout exposure
        Radiation sickness
        Secondary effects of nuclear weapons
  ● **E996.8 Other effects of nuclear weapons** 🔍
  ● **E996.9 Unspecified effect of nuclear weapon** 🔍

● **E997 Injury due to war operations by other forms of unconventional warfare**
  ● **E997.0 Lasers** 🔍
  ● **E997.1 Biological warfare** 🔍
  ● **E997.2 Gases, fumes, and chemicals** 🔍
  ● **E997.3 Weapon of mass destruction [WMD], unspecified** 🔍
  ● **E997.8 Other specified forms of unconventional warfare** 🔍
  ● **E997.9 Unspecified form of unconventional warfare** 🔍

● **E998 Injury due to war operations but occurring after cessation of hostilities**
      Injuries due to operations of war but occurring after cessation of hostilities by any means classifiable under E990-E997
      Injuries by explosion of bombs or mines placed in the course of operations of war, if the explosion occurred after cessation of hostilities
  ● **E998.0 Explosion of mines** 🔍
  ● **E998.1 Explosion of bombs** 🔍
  ● **E998.8 Injury due to other war operations but occurring after cessation of hostilities** 🔍
  ● **E998.9 Injury due to unspecified war operations but occurring after cessation of hostilities** 🔍

● **E999 Late effect of injury due to war operations and terrorism**
      Note: This category is to be used to indicate circumstances classifiable to E979, E990-E998 as the cause of death or disability from late effects, which are themselves classifiable elsewhere. The "late effects" include conditions reported as such or as sequelae which may occur at any time after injury resulting from operations of war or terrorism.
  ● **E999.0 Late effect of injury due to war operations** 🔍
      Coding Clinic: 2012, Q3, P21; 1998, Q1, P4; 1996, Q2, P12
  ● **E999.1 Late effect of injury due to terrorism** 🔍

◀ New   ◀ Revised   ~~deleted~~ Deleted   Excludes   Includes   Use additional   Code first   Omit code

1074   ● Unacceptable Principal Diagnosis   ● Use Additional Digit(s)   ▶ Manifestation Code   OGCR Official Guidelines   Coding Clinic

APPENDIX A
MORPHOLOGY OF NEOPLASMS

The World Health Organization has published an adaptation of the International Classification of Diseases for Oncology (ICD-O). It contains a coded nomenclature for the morphology of neoplasms, which is reproduced here for those who wish to use it in conjunction with Chapter 2 of the International Classification of Diseases, 9th Revision, Clinical Modification.

The morphology code numbers consist of five digits; the first four identify the histological type of the neoplasm and the fifth indicates its behavior. The one-digit behavior code is as follows:

/0   Benign
/1   Uncertain whether benign or malignant
      Borderline malignancy
/2   Carcinoma in situ
      Intraepithelial
      Noninfiltrating
      Noninvasive
/3   Malignant, primary site
/6   Malignant, metastatic site
      Secondary site
/9   Malignant, uncertain whether primary or metastatic site

In the nomenclature below, the morphology code numbers include the behavior code appropriate to the histological type of neoplasm, but this behavior code should be changed if other reported information makes this necessary. For example, "chordoma (M9370/3)" is assumed to be malignant; the term "benign chordoma" should be coded M9370/0. Similarly, "superficial spreading adenocarcinoma (M8143/3)" described as "noninvasive" should be coded M8143/2 and "melanoma (M8720/3)" described as "secondary" should be coded M8720/6.

The following table shows the correspondence between the morphology code and the different sections of Chapter 2:

Morphology Code Histology/Behavior		ICD-9-CM Chapter 2	
Any	0	210-229	Benign neoplasms
M8000-M8004	1	239	Neoplasms of unspecified nature
M8010+	1	235-238	Neoplasms of uncertain behavior
Any	2	230-234	Carcinoma in situ
Any	3	140-195 200-208	Malignant neoplasms, stated or presumed to be primary
Any	6	196-198	Malignant neoplasms, stated or presumed to be secondary

The ICD-O behavior digit /9 is inapplicable in an ICD context, since all malignant neoplasms are presumed to be primary (/3) or secondary (/6) according to other information on the medical record.

Only the first-listed term of the full ICD-O morphology nomenclature appears against each code number in the list below. The ICD-9-CM Alphabetical Index (Volume 2), however, includes all the ICD-O synonyms as well as a number of other morphological names still likely to be encountered on medical records but omitted from ICD-O as outdated or otherwise undesirable.

A coding difficulty sometimes arises where a morphological diagnosis contains two qualifying adjectives that have different code numbers. An example is "transitional cell epidermoid carcinomas." "Transitional cell carcinoma NOS" is M8120/3 and "epidermoid carcinoma NOS" is M8070/3. In such circumstances, the higher number (M8120/3 in this example) should be used, as it is usually more specific.

CODED NOMENCLATURE FOR MORPHOLOGY OF NEOPLASMS

M800	Neoplasms NOS
M8000/0	Neoplasm, benign
M8000/1	Neoplasm, uncertain whether benign or malignant
M8000/3	Neoplasm, malignant
M8000/6	Neoplasm, metastatic
M8000/9	Neoplasm, malignant, uncertain whether primary or metastatic
M8001/0	Tumor cells, benign
M8001/1	Tumor cells, uncertain whether benign or malignant
M8001/3	Tumor cells, malignant
M8002/3	Malignant tumor, small cell type
M8003/3	Malignant tumor, giant cell type
M8004/3	Malignant tumor, fusiform cell type

M801-M804	Epithelial neoplasms NOS
M8010/0	Epithelial tumor, benign
M8010/2	Carcinoma in situ NOS
M8010/3	Carcinoma NOS
M8010/6	Carcinoma, metastatic NOS
M8010/9	Carcinomatosis
M8011/0	Epithelioma, benign
M8011/3	Epithelioma, malignant
M8012/3	Large cell carcinoma NOS
M8020/3	Carcinoma, undifferentiated type NOS
M8021/3	Carcinoma, anaplastic type NOS
M8022/3	Pleomorphic carcinoma
M8030/3	Giant cell and spindle cell carcinoma
M8031/3	Giant cell carcinoma
M8032/3	Spindle cell carcinoma
M8033/3	Pseudosarcomatous carcinoma
M8034/3	Polygonal cell carcinoma
M8035/3	Spheroidal cell carcinoma
M8040/1	Tumorlet
M8041/3	Small cell carcinoma NOS
M8042/3	Oat cell carcinoma
M8043/3	Small cell carcinoma, fusiform cell type

M805-M808	Papillary and squamous cell neoplasms
M8050/0	Papilloma NOS (except Papilloma of urinary bladder M8120/1)
M8050/2	Papillary carcinoma in situ
M8050/3	Papillary carcinoma NOS
M8051/0	Verrucous papilloma
M8051/3	Verrucous carcinoma NOS
M8052/0	Squamous cell papilloma
M8052/3	Papillary squamous cell carcinoma
M8053/0	Inverted papilloma
M8060/0	Papillomatosis NOS
M8070/2	Squamous cell carcinoma in situ NOS
M8070/3	Squamous cell carcinoma NOS
M8070/6	Squamous cell carcinoma, metastatic NOS
M8071/3	Squamous cell carcinoma, keratinizing type NOS
M8072/3	Squamous cell carcinoma, large cell, nonkeratinizing type
M8073/3	Squamous cell carcinoma, small cell, nonkeratinizing type
M8074/3	Squamous cell carcinoma, spindle cell type
M8075/3	Adenoid squamous cell carcinoma
M8076/2	Squamous cell carcinoma in situ with questionable stromal invasion
M8076/3	Squamous cell carcinoma, microinvasive
M8080/2	Queyrat's erythroplasia
M8081/2	Bowen's disease
M8082/3	Lymphoepithelial carcinoma

M809-M811	Basal cell neoplasms
M8090/1	Basal cell tumor
M8090/3	Basal cell carcinoma NOS
M8091/3	Multicentric basal cell carcinoma
M8092/3	Basal cell carcinoma, morphea type
M8093/3	Basal cell carcinoma, fibroepithelial type
M8094/3	Basosquamous carcinoma
M8095/3	Metatypical carcinoma
M8096/3	Intraepidermal epithelioma of Jadassohn
M8100/0	Trichoepithelioma
M8101/0	Trichofolliculoma
M8102/0	Tricholemmoma
M8110/0	Pilomatrixoma

M812-M813	Transitional cell papillomas and carcinomas
M8120/0	Transitional cell papilloma NOS
M8120/1	Urothelial papilloma
M8120/2	Transitional cell carcinoma in situ
M8120/3	Transitional cell carcinoma NOS
M8121/0	Schneiderian papilloma
M8121/1	Transitional cell papilloma, inverted type
M8121/3	Schneiderian carcinoma
M8122/3	Transitional cell carcinoma, spindle cell type
M8123/3	Basaloid carcinoma
M8124/3	Cloacogenic carcinoma
M8130/3	Papillary transitional cell carcinoma

M814-M838	**Adenomas and adenocarcinomas**
M8140/0	Adenoma NOS
M8140/1	Bronchial adenoma NOS
M8140/2	Adenocarcinoma in situ
M8140/3	Adenocarcinoma NOS
M8140/6	Adenocarcinoma, metastatic NOS
M8141/3	Scirrhous adenocarcinoma
M8142/3	Linitis plastica
M8143/3	Superficial spreading adenocarcinoma
M8144/3	Adenocarcinoma, intestinal type
M8145/3	Carcinoma, diffuse type
M8146/0	Monomorphic adenoma
M8147/0	Basal cell adenoma
M8150/0	Islet cell adenoma
M8150/3	Islet cell carcinoma
M8151/0	Insulinoma NOS
M8151/3	Insulinoma, malignant
M8152/0	Glucagonoma NOS
M8152/3	Glucagonoma, malignant
M8153/1	Gastrinoma NOS
M8153/3	Gastrinoma, malignant
M8154/3	Mixed islet cell and exocrine adenocarcinoma
M8160/0	Bile duct adenoma
M8160/3	Cholangiocarcinoma
M8161/0	Bile duct cystadenoma
M8161/3	Bile duct cystadenocarcinoma
M8170/0	Liver cell adenoma
M8170/3	Hepatocellular carcinoma NOS
M8180/0	Hepatocholangioma, benign
M8180/3	Combined hepatocellular carcinoma and cholangiocarcinoma
M8190/0	Trabecular adenoma
M8190/3	Trabecular adenocarcinoma
M8191/0	Embryonal adenoma
M8200/0	Eccrine dermal cylindroma
M8200/3	Adenoid cystic carcinoma
M8201/3	Cribriform carcinoma
M8210/0	Adenomatous polyp NOS
M8210/3	Adenocarcinoma in adenomatous polyp
M8211/0	Tubular adenoma NOS
M8211/3	Tubular adenocarcinoma
M8220/0	Adenomatous polyposis coli
M8220/3	Adenocarcinoma in adenomatous polyposis coli
M8221/0	Multiple adenomatous polyps
M8230/3	Solid carcinoma NOS
M8231/3	Carcinoma simplex
M8240/1	Carcinoid tumor NOS
M8240/3	Carcinoid tumor, malignant
M8241/1	Carcinoid tumor, argentaffin NOS
M8241/3	Carcinoid tumor, argentaffin, malignant
M8242/1	Carcinoid tumor, nonargentaffin NOS
M8242/3	Carcinoid tumor, nonargentaffin, malignant
M8243/3	Mucocarcinoid tumor, malignant
M8244/3	Composite carcinoid
M8250/1	Pulmonary adenomatosis
M8250/3	Bronchiolo-alveolar adenocarcinoma
M8251/0	Alveolar adenoma
M8251/3	Alveolar adenocarcinoma
M8260/0	Papillary adenoma NOS
M8260/3	Papillary adenocarcinoma NOS
M8261/1	Villous adenoma NOS
M8261/3	Adenocarcinoma in villous adenoma
M8262/3	Villous adenocarcinoma
M8263/0	Tubulovillous adenoma
M8270/0	Chromophobe adenoma
M8270/3	Chromophobe carcinoma
M8280/0	Acidophil adenoma
M8280/3	Acidophil carcinoma
M8281/0	Mixed acidophil-basophil adenoma
M8281/3	Mixed acidophil-basophil carcinoma
M8290/0	Oxyphilic adenoma
M8290/3	Oxyphilic adenocarcinoma
M8300/0	Basophil adenoma
M8300/3	Basophil carcinoma
M8310/0	Clear cell adenoma
M8310/3	Clear cell adenocarcinoma NOS
M8311/1	Hypernephroid tumor
M8312/3	Renal cell carcinoma
M8313/0	Clear cell adenofibroma
M8320/3	Granular cell carcinoma

M8321/0	Chief cell adenoma
M8322/0	Water-clear cell adenoma
M8322/3	Water-clear cell adenocarcinoma
M8323/0	Mixed cell adenoma
M8323/3	Mixed cell adenocarcinoma
M8324/0	Lipoadenoma
M8330/0	Follicular adenoma
M8330/3	Follicular adenocarcinoma NOS
M8331/3	Follicular adenocarcinoma, well differentiated type
M8332/3	Follicular adenocarcinoma, trabecular type
M8333/0	Microfollicular adenoma
M8334/0	Macrofollicular adenoma
M8340/3	Papillary and follicular adenocarcinoma
M8350/3	Nonencapsulated sclerosing carcinoma
M8360/1	Multiple endocrine adenomas
M8361/1	Juxtaglomerular tumor
M8370/0	Adrenal cortical adenoma NOS
M8370/3	Adrenal cortical carcinoma
M8371/0	Adrenal cortical adenoma, compact cell type
M8372/0	Adrenal cortical adenoma, heavily pigmented variant
M8373/0	Adrenal cortical adenoma, clear cell type
M8374/0	Adrenal cortical adenoma, glomerulosa cell type
M8375/0	Adrenal cortical adenoma, mixed cell type
M8380/0	Endometrioid adenoma NOS
M8380/1	Endometrioid adenoma, borderline malignancy
M8380/3	Endometrioid carcinoma
M8381/0	Endometrioid adenofibroma NOS
M8381/1	Endometrioid adenofibroma, borderline malignancy
M8381/3	Endometrioid adenofibroma, malignant
M839-M842	**Adnexal and skin appendage neoplasms**
M8390/0	Skin appendage adenoma
M8390/3	Skin appendage carcinoma
M8400/0	Sweat gland adenoma
M8400/1	Sweat gland tumor NOS
M8400/3	Sweat gland adenocarcinoma
M8401/0	Apocrine adenoma
M8401/3	Apocrine adenocarcinoma
M8402/0	Eccrine acrospiroma
M8403/0	Eccrine spiradenoma
M8404/0	Hidrocystoma
M8405/0	Papillary hydradenoma
M8406/0	Papillary syringadenoma
M8407/0	Syringoma NOS
M8410/0	Sebaceous adenoma
M8410/3	Sebaceous adenocarcinoma
M8420/0	Ceruminous adenoma
M8420/3	Ceruminous adenocarcinoma
M843	**Mucoepidermoid neoplasms**
M8430/1	Mucoepidermoid tumor
M8430/3	Mucoepidermoid carcinoma
M844-M849	**Cystic, mucinous, and serous neoplasms**
M8440/0	Cystadenoma NOS
M8440/3	Cystadenocarcinoma NOS
M8441/0	Serous cystadenoma NOS
M8441/1	Serous cystadenoma, borderline malignancy
M8441/3	Serous cystadenocarcinoma NOS
M8450/0	Papillary cystadenoma NOS
M8450/1	Papillary cystadenoma, borderline malignancy
M8450/3	Papillary cystadenocarcinoma NOS
M8460/0	Papillary serous cystadenoma NOS
M8460/1	Papillary serous cystadenoma, borderline malignancy
M8460/3	Papillary serous cystadenocarcinoma
M8461/0	Serous surface papilloma NOS
M8461/1	Serous surface papilloma, borderline malignancy
M8461/3	Serous surface papillary carcinoma
M8470/0	Mucinous cystadenoma NOS
M8470/1	Mucinous cystadenoma, borderline malignancy
M8470/3	Mucinous cystadenocarcinoma NOS
M8471/0	Papillary mucinous cystadenoma NOS
M8471/1	Papillary mucinous cystadenoma, borderline malignancy
M8471/3	Papillary mucinous cystadenocarcinoma
M8480/0	Mucinous adenoma
M8480/3	Mucinous adenocarcinoma
M8480/6	Pseudomyxoma peritonei
M8481/3	Mucin-producing adenocarcinoma
M8490/3	Signet ring cell carcinoma
M8490/6	Metastatic signet ring cell carcinoma

M850-M854	**Ductal, lobular, and medullary neoplasms**
M8500/2	*Intraductal carcinoma, noninfiltrating NOS*
M8500/3	*Infiltrating duct carcinoma*
M8501/2	*Comedocarcinoma, noninfiltrating*
M8501/3	*Comedocarcinoma NOS*
M8502/3	*Juvenile carcinoma of the breast*
M8503/0	*Intraductal papilloma*
M8503/3	*Noninfiltrating intraductal papillary adenocarcinoma*
M8504/0	*Intracystic papillary adenoma*
M8504/2	*Noninfiltrating intracystic carcinoma*
M8505/0	*Intraductal papillomatosis NOS*
M8506/0	*Subareolar duct papillomatosis*
M8510/3	*Medullary carcinoma NOS*
M8511/3	*Medullary carcinoma with amyloid stroma*
M8512/3	*Medullary carcinoma with lymphoid stroma*
M8520/2	*Lobular carcinoma in situ*
M8520/3	*Lobular carcinoma NOS*
M8521/3	*Infiltrating ductular carcinoma*
M8530/3	*Inflammatory carcinoma*
M8540/3	*Paget's disease, mammary*
M8541/3	*Paget's disease and infiltrating duct carcinoma of breast*
M8542/3	*Paget's disease, extramammary (except Paget's disease of bone)*
M855	**Acinar cell neoplasms**
M8550/0	*Acinar cell adenoma*
M8550/1	*Acinar cell tumor*
M8550/3	*Acinar cell carcinoma*
M856-M858	**Complex epithelial neoplasms**
M8560/3	*Adenosquamous carcinoma*
M8561/0	*Adenolymphoma*
M8570/3	*Adenocarcinoma with squamous metaplasia*
M8571/3	*Adenocarcinoma with cartilaginous and osseous metaplasia*
M8572/3	*Adenocarcinoma with spindle cell metaplasia*
M8573/3	*Adenocarcinoma with apocrine metaplasia*
M8580/0	*Thymoma, benign*
M8580/3	*Thymoma, malignant*
M859-M867	**Specialized gonadal neoplasms**
M8590/1	*Sex cord-stromal tumor*
M8600/0	*Thecoma NOS*
M8600/3	*Theca cell carcinoma*
M8610/0	*Luteoma NOS*
M8620/1	*Granulosa cell tumor NOS*
M8620/3	*Granulosa cell tumor, malignant*
M8621/1	*Granulosa cell-theca cell tumor*
M8630/0	*Androblastoma, benign*
M8630/1	*Androblastoma NOS*
M8630/3	*Androblastoma, malignant*
M8631/0	*Sertoli-Leydig cell tumor*
M8632/1	*Gynandroblastoma*
M8640/0	*Tubular androblastoma NOS*
M8640/3	*Sertoli cell carcinoma*
M8641/0	*Tubular androblastoma with lipid storage*
M8650/0	*Leydig cell tumor, benign*
M8650/1	*Leydig cell tumor NOS*
M8650/3	*Leydig cell tumor, malignant*
M8660/0	*Hilar cell tumor*
M8670/0	*Lipid cell tumor of ovary*
M8671/0	*Adrenal rest tumor*
M868-M871	**Paragangliomas and glomus tumors**
M8680/1	*Paraganglioma NOS*
M8680/3	*Paraganglioma, malignant*
M8681/1	*Sympathetic paraganglioma*
M8682/1	*Parasympathetic paraganglioma*
M8690/1	*Glomus jugulare tumor*
M8691/1	*Aortic body tumor*
M8692/1	*Carotid body tumor*
M8693/1	*Extra-adrenal paraganglioma NOS*
M8693/3	*Extra-adrenal paraganglioma, malignant*
M8700/0	*Pheochromocytoma NOS*
M8700/3	*Pheochromocytoma, malignant*
M8710/3	*Glomangiosarcoma*
M8711/0	*Glomus tumor*
M8712/0	*Glomangioma*
M872-M879	**Nevi and melanomas**
M8720/0	*Pigmented nevus NOS*
M8720/3	*Malignant melanoma NOS*
M8721/3	*Nodular melanoma*
M8722/0	*Balloon cell nevus*
M8722/3	*Balloon cell melanoma*

M8723/0	*Halo nevus*
M8724/0	*Fibrous papule of the nose*
M8725/0	*Neuronevus*
M8726/0	*Magnocellular nevus*
M8730/0	*Nonpigmented nevus*
M8730/3	*Amelanotic melanoma*
M8740/0	*Junctional nevus*
M8740/3	*Malignant melanoma in junctional nevus*
M8741/2	*Precancerous melanosis NOS*
M8741/3	*Malignant melanoma in precancerous melanosis*
M8742/2	*Hutchinson's melanotic freckle*
M8742/3	*Malignant melanoma in Hutchinson's melanotic freckle*
M8743/3	*Superficial spreading melanoma*
M8750/0	*Intradermal nevus*
M8760/0	*Compound nevus*
M8761/1	*Giant pigmented nevus*
M8761/3	*Malignant melanoma in giant pigmented nevus*
M8770/0	*Epithelioid and spindle cell nevus*
M8771/3	*Epithelioid cell melanoma*
M8772/3	*Spindle cell melanoma NOS*
M8773/3	*Spindle cell melanoma, type A*
M8774/3	*Spindle cell melanoma, type B*
M8775/3	*Mixed epithelioid and spindle cell melanoma*
M8780/0	*Blue nevus NOS*
M8780/3	*Blue nevus, malignant*
M8790/0	*Cellular blue nevus*
M880	**Soft tissue tumors and sarcomas NOS**
M8800/0	*Soft tissue tumor, benign*
M8800/3	*Sarcoma NOS*
M8800/9	*Sarcomatosis NOS*
M8801/3	*Spindle cell sarcoma*
M8802/3	*Giant cell sarcoma (except of bone M9250/3)*
M8803/3	*Small cell sarcoma*
M8804/3	*Epithelioid cell sarcoma*
M881-M883	**Fibromatous neoplasms**
M8810/0	*Fibroma NOS*
M8810/3	*Fibrosarcoma NOS*
M8811/0	*Fibromyxoma*
M8811/3	*Fibromyxosarcoma*
M8812/0	*Periosteal fibroma*
M8812/3	*Periosteal fibrosarcoma*
M8813/0	*Fascial fibroma*
M8813/3	*Fascial fibrosarcoma*
M8814/3	*Infantile fibrosarcoma*
M8820/0	*Elastofibroma*
M8821/1	*Aggressive fibromatosis*
M8822/1	*Abdominal fibromatosis*
M8823/1	*Desmoplastic fibroma*
M8830/0	*Fibrous histiocytoma NOS*
M8830/1	*Atypical fibrous histiocytoma*
M8830/3	*Fibrous histiocytoma, malignant*
M8831/0	*Fibroxanthoma NOS*
M8831/1	*Atypical fibroxanthoma*
M8831/3	*Fibroxanthoma, malignant*
M8832/0	*Dermatofibroma NOS*
M8832/1	*Dermatofibroma protuberans*
M8832/3	*Dermatofibrosarcoma NOS*
M884	**Myxomatous neoplasms**
M8840/0	*Myxoma NOS*
M8840/3	*Myxosarcoma*
M885-M888	**Lipomatous neoplasms**
M8850/0	*Lipoma NOS*
M8850/3	*Liposarcoma NOS*
M8851/0	*Fibrolipoma*
M8851/3	*Liposarcoma, well differentiated type*
M8852/0	*Fibromyxolipoma*
M8852/3	*Myxoid liposarcoma*
M8853/3	*Round cell liposarcoma*
M8854/3	*Pleomorphic liposarcoma*
M8855/3	*Mixed type liposarcoma*
M8856/0	*Intramuscular lipoma*
M8857/0	*Spindle cell lipoma*
M8860/0	*Angiomyolipoma*
M8860/3	*Angiomyoliposarcoma*
M8861/0	*Angiolipoma NOS*
M8861/1	*Angiolipoma, infiltrating*

M8870/0	*Myelolipoma*
M8880/0	*Hibernoma*
M8881/0	*Lipoblastomatosis*

M889-M892	**Myomatous neoplasms**
M8890/0	*Leiomyoma NOS*
M8890/1	*Intravascular leiomyomatosis*
M8890/3	*Leiomyosarcoma NOS*
M8891/1	*Epithelioid leiomyoma*
M8891/3	*Epithelioid leiomyosarcoma*
M8892/1	*Cellular leiomyoma*
M8893/0	*Bizarre leiomyoma*
M8894/0	*Angiomyoma*
M8894/3	*Angiomyosarcoma*
M8895/0	*Myoma*
M8895/3	*Myosarcoma*
M8900/0	*Rhabdomyoma NOS*
M8900/3	*Rhabdomyosarcoma NOS*
M8901/3	*Pleomorphic rhabdomyosarcoma*
M8902/3	*Mixed type rhabdomyosarcoma*
M8903/0	*Fetal rhabdomyoma*
M8904/0	*Adult rhabdomyoma*
M8910/3	*Embryonal rhabdomyosarcoma*
M8920/3	*Alveolar rhabdomyosarcoma*

M893-M899	**Complex mixed and stromal neoplasms**
M8930/3	*Endometrial stromal sarcoma*
M8931/1	*Endolymphatic stromal myosis*
M8932/0	*Adenomyoma*
M8940/0	*Pleomorphic adenoma*
M8940/3	*Mixed tumor, malignant NOS*
M8950/3	*Mullerian mixed tumor*
M8951/3	*Mesodermal mixed tumor*
M8960/1	*Mesoblastic nephroma*
M8960/3	*Nephroblastoma NOS*
M8961/3	*Epithelial nephroblastoma*
M8962/3	*Mesenchymal nephroblastoma*
M8970/3	*Hepatoblastoma*
M8980/3	*Carcinosarcoma NOS*
M8981/3	*Carcinosarcoma, embryonal type*
M8982/0	*Myoepithelioma*
M8990/0	*Mesenchymoma, benign*
M8990/1	*Mesenchymoma NOS*
M8990/3	*Mesenchymoma, malignant*
M8991/3	*Embryonal sarcoma*

M900-M903	**Fibroepithelial neoplasms**
M9000/0	*Brenner tumor NOS*
M9000/1	*Brenner tumor, borderline malignancy*
M9000/3	*Brenner tumor, malignant*
M9010/0	*Fibroadenoma NOS*
M9011/0	*Intracanalicular fibroadenoma NOS*
M9012/0	*Pericanalicular fibroadenoma*
M9013/0	*Adenofibroma NOS*
M9014/0	*Serous adenofibroma*
M9015/0	*Mucinous adenofibroma*
M9020/0	*Cellular intracanalicular fibroadenoma*
M9020/1	*Cystosarcoma phyllodes NOS*
M9020/3	*Cystosarcoma phyllodes, malignant*
M9030/0	*Juvenile fibroadenoma*

M904	**Synovial neoplasms**
M9040/0	*Synovioma, benign*
M9040/3	*Synovial sarcoma NOS*
M9041/3	*Synovial sarcoma, spindle cell type*
M9042/3	*Synovial sarcoma, epithelioid cell type*
M9043/3	*Synovial sarcoma, biphasic type*
M9044/3	*Clear cell sarcoma of tendons and aponeuroses*

M905	**Mesothelial neoplasms**
M9050/0	*Mesothelioma, benign*
M9050/3	*Mesothelioma, malignant*
M9051/0	*Fibrous mesothelioma, benign*
M9051/3	*Fibrous mesothelioma, malignant*
M9052/0	*Epithelioid mesothelioma, benign*
M9052/3	*Epithelioid mesothelioma, malignant*
M9053/0	*Mesothelioma, biphasic type, benign*
M9053/3	*Mesothelioma, biphasic type, malignant*
M9054/0	*Adenomatoid tumor NOS*

M906-M909	**Germ cell neoplasms**
M9060/3	*Dysgerminoma*
M9061/3	*Seminoma NOS*
M9062/3	*Seminoma, anaplastic type*
M9063/3	*Spermatocytic seminoma*
M9064/3	*Germinoma*
M9070/3	*Embryonal carcinoma NOS*
M9071/3	*Endodermal sinus tumor*
M9072/3	*Polyembryoma*
M9073/1	*Gonadoblastoma*
M9080/0	*Teratoma, benign*
M9080/1	*Teratoma NOS*
M9080/3	*Teratoma, malignant NOS*
M9081/3	*Teratocarcinoma*
M9082/3	*Malignant teratoma, undifferentiated type*
M9083/3	*Malignant teratoma, intermediate type*
M9084/0	*Dermoid cyst*
M9084/3	*Dermoid cyst with malignant transformation*
M9090/0	*Struma ovarii NOS*
M9090/3	*Struma ovarii, malignant*
M9091/1	*Strumal carcinoid*

M910	**Trophoblastic neoplasms**
M9100/0	*Hydatidiform mole NOS*
M9100/1	*Invasive hydatidiform mole*
M9100/3	*Choriocarcinoma*
M9101/3	*Choriocarcinoma combined with teratoma*
M9102/3	*Malignant teratoma, trophoblastic*

M911	**Mesonephromas**
M9110/0	*Mesonephroma, benign*
M9110/1	*Mesonephric tumor*
M9110/3	*Mesonephroma, malignant*
M9111/1	*Endosalpingioma*

M912-M916	**Blood vessel tumors**
M9120/0	*Hemangioma NOS*
M9120/3	*Hemangiosarcoma*
M9121/0	*Cavernous hemangioma*
M9122/0	*Venous hemangioma*
M9123/0	*Racemose hemangioma*
M9124/3	*Kupffer cell sarcoma*
M9130/0	*Hemangioendothelioma, benign*
M9130/1	*Hemangioendothelioma NOS*
M9130/3	*Hemangioendothelioma, malignant*
M9131/0	*Capillary hemangioma*
M9132/0	*Intramuscular hemangioma*
M9140/3	*Kaposi's sarcoma*
M9141/0	*Angiokeratoma*
M9142/0	*Verrucous keratotic hemangioma*
M9150/0	*Hemangiopericytoma, benign*
M9150/1	*Hemangiopericytoma NOS*
M9150/3	*Hemangiopericytoma, malignant*
M9160/0	*Angiofibroma NOS*
M9161/1	*Hemangioblastoma*

M917	**Lymphatic vessel tumors**
M9170/0	*Lymphangioma NOS*
M9170/3	*Lymphangiosarcoma*
M9171/0	*Capillary lymphangioma*
M9172/0	*Cavernous lymphangioma*
M9173/0	*Cystic lymphangioma*
M9174/0	*Lymphangiomyoma*
M9174/1	*Lymphangiomyomatosis*
M9175/0	*Hemolymphangioma*

M918-M920	**Osteomas and osteosarcomas**
M9180/0	*Osteoma NOS*
M9180/3	*Osteosarcoma NOS*
M9181/3	*Chondroblastic osteosarcoma*
M9182/3	*Fibroblastic osteosarcoma*
M9183/3	*Telangiectatic osteosarcoma*
M9184/3	*Osteosarcoma in Paget's disease of bone*
M9190/3	*Juxtacortical osteosarcoma*
M9191/0	*Osteoid osteoma NOS*
M9200/0	*Osteoblastoma*

M921-M924	**Chondromatous neoplasms**
M9210/0	*Osteochondroma*
M9210/1	*Osteochondromatosis NOS*
M9220/0	*Chondroma NOS*
M9220/1	*Chondromatosis NOS*

M9220/3	Chondrosarcoma NOS
M9221/0	Juxtacortical chondroma
M9221/3	Juxtacortical chondrosarcoma
M9230/0	Chondroblastoma NOS
M9230/3	Chondroblastoma, malignant
M9240/3	Mesenchymal chondrosarcoma
M9241/0	Chondromyxoid fibroma

M925 **Giant cell tumors**

M9250/1	Giant cell tumor of bone NOS
M9250/3	Giant cell tumor of bone, malignant
M9251/1	Giant cell tumor of soft parts NOS
M9251/3	Malignant giant cell tumor of soft parts

M926 **Miscellaneous bone tumors**

M9260/3	Ewing's sarcoma
M9261/3	Adamantinoma of long bones
M9262/0	Ossifying fibroma

M927-M934 **Odontogenic tumors**

M9270/0	Odontogenic tumor, benign
M9270/1	Odontogenic tumor NOS
M9270/3	Odontogenic tumor, malignant
M9271/0	Dentinoma
M9272/0	Cementoma NOS
M9273/0	Cementoblastoma, benign
M9274/0	Cementifying fibroma
M9275/0	Gigantiform cementoma
M9280/0	Odontoma NOS
M9281/0	Compound odontoma
M9282/0	Complex odontoma
M9290/0	Ameloblastic fibro-odontoma
M9290/3	Ameloblastic odontosarcoma
M9300/0	Adenomatoid odontogenic tumor
M9301/0	Calcifying odontogenic cyst
M9310/0	Ameloblastoma NOS
M9310/3	Ameloblastoma, malignant
M9311/0	Odontoameloblastoma
M9312/0	Squamous odontogenic tumor
M9320/0	Odontogenic myxoma
M9321/0	Odontogenic fibroma NOS
M9330/0	Ameloblastic fibroma
M9330/3	Ameloblastic fibrosarcoma
M9340/0	Calcifying epithelial odontogenic tumor

M935-M937 **Miscellaneous tumors**

M9350/1	Craniopharyngioma
M9360/1	Pinealoma
M9361/1	Pineocytoma
M9362/3	Pineoblastoma
M9363/0	Melanotic neuroectodermal tumor
M9370/3	Chordoma

M938-M948 **Gliomas**

M9380/3	Glioma, malignant
M9381/3	Gliomatosis cerebri
M9382/3	Mixed glioma
M9383/1	Subependymal glioma
M9384/1	Subependymal giant cell astrocytoma
M9390/0	Choroid plexus papilloma NOS
M9390/3	Choroid plexus papilloma, malignant
M9391/3	Ependymoma NOS
M9392/3	Ependymoma, anaplastic type
M9393/1	Papillary ependymoma
M9394/1	Myxopapillary ependymoma
M9400/3	Astrocytoma NOS
M9401/3	Astrocytoma, anaplastic type
M9410/3	Protoplasmic astrocytoma
M9411/3	Gemistocytic astrocytoma
M9420/3	Fibrillary astrocytoma
M9421/3	Pilocytic astrocytoma
M9422/3	Spongioblastoma NOS
M9423/3	Spongioblastoma polare
M9430/3	Astroblastoma
M9440/3	Glioblastoma NOS
M9441/3	Giant cell glioblastoma
M9442/3	Glioblastoma with sarcomatous component
M9443/3	Primitive polar spongioblastoma
M9450/3	Oligodendroglioma NOS

M9451/3	Oligodendroglioma, anaplastic type
M9460/3	Oligodendroblastoma
M9470/3	Medulloblastoma NOS
M9471/3	Desmoplastic medulloblastoma
M9472/3	Medullomyoblastoma
M9480/3	Cerebellar sarcoma NOS
M9481/3	Monstrocellular sarcoma

M949-M952 **Neuroepitheliomatous neoplasms**

M9490/0	Ganglioneuroma
M9490/3	Ganglioneuroblastoma
M9491/0	Ganglioneuromatosis
M9500/3	Neuroblastoma NOS
M9501/3	Medulloepithelioma NOS
M9502/3	Teratoid medulloepithelioma
M9503/3	Neuroepithelioma NOS
M9504/3	Spongioneuroblastoma
M9505/1	Ganglioglioma
M9506/0	Neurocytoma
M9507/0	Pacinian tumor
M9510/3	Retinoblastoma NOS
M9511/3	Retinoblastoma, differentiated type
M9512/3	Retinoblastoma, undifferentiated type
M9520/3	Olfactory neurogenic tumor
M9521/3	Esthesioneurocytoma
M9522/3	Esthesioneuroblastoma
M9523/3	Esthesioneuroepithelioma

M953 **Meningiomas**

M9530/0	Meningioma NOS
M9530/1	Meningiomatosis NOS
M9530/3	Meningioma, malignant
M9531/0	Meningotheliomatous meningioma
M9532/0	Fibrous meningioma
M9533/0	Psammomatous meningioma
M9534/0	Angiomatous meningioma
M9535/0	Hemangioblastic meningioma
M9536/0	Hemangiopericytic meningioma
M9537/0	Transitional meningioma
M9538/1	Papillary meningioma
M9539/3	Meningeal sarcomatosis

M954-M957 **Nerve sheath tumor**

M9540/0	Neurofibroma NOS
M9540/1	Neurofibromatosis NOS
M9540/3	Neurofibrosarcoma
M9541/0	Melanotic neurofibroma
M9550/0	Plexiform neurofibroma
M9560/0	Neurilemmoma NOS
M9560/1	Neurinomatosis
M9560/3	Neurilemmoma, malignant
M9570/0	Neuroma NOS

M958 **Granular cell tumors and alveolar soft part sarcoma**

M9580/0	Granular cell tumor NOS
M9580/3	Granular cell tumor, malignant
M9581/3	Alveolar soft part sarcoma

M959-M963 **Lymphomas, NOS or diffuse**

M9590/0	Lymphomatous tumor, benign
M9590/3	Malignant lymphoma NOS
M9591/3	Malignant lymphoma, non Hodgkin's type
M9600/3	Malignant lymphoma, undifferentiated cell type NOS
M9601/3	Malignant lymphoma, stem cell type
M9602/3	Malignant lymphoma, convoluted cell type NOS
M9610/3	Lymphosarcoma NOS
M9611/3	Malignant lymphoma, lymphoplasmacytoid type
M9612/3	Malignant lymphoma, immunoblastic type
M9613/3	Malignant lymphoma, mixed lymphocytic-histiocytic NOS
M9614/3	Malignant lymphoma, centroblastic-centrocytic, diffuse
M9615/3	Malignant lymphoma, follicular center cell NOS
M9620/3	Malignant lymphoma, lymphocytic, well differentiated NOS
M9621/3	Malignant lymphoma, lymphocytic, intermediate differentiation NOS
M9622/3	Malignant lymphoma, centrocytic
M9623/3	Malignant lymphoma, follicular center cell, cleaved NOS
M9630/3	Malignant lymphoma, lymphocytic, poorly differentiated NOS
M9631/3	Prolymphocytic lymphosarcoma
M9632/3	Malignant lymphoma, centroblastic type NOS
M9633/3	Malignant lymphoma, follicular center cell, noncleaved NOS

M964		**Reticulosarcomas**
M9640/3		*Reticulosarcoma NOS*
M9641/3		*Reticulosarcoma, pleomorphic cell type*
M9642/3		*Reticulosarcoma, nodular*

M965-M966   **Hodgkin's disease**
M9650/3   *Hodgkin's disease NOS*
M9651/3   *Hodgkin's disease, lymphocytic predominance*
M9652/3   *Hodgkin's disease, mixed cellularity*
M9653/3   *Hodgkin's disease, lymphocytic depletion NOS*
M9654/3   *Hodgkin's disease, lymphocytic depletion, diffuse fibrosis*
M9655/3   *Hodgkin's disease, lymphocytic depletion, reticular type*
M9656/3   *Hodgkin's disease, nodular sclerosis NOS*
M9657/3   *Hodgkin's disease, nodular sclerosis, cellular phase*
M9660/3   *Hodgkin's paragranuloma*
M9661/3   *Hodgkin's granuloma*
M9662/3   *Hodgkin's sarcoma*

M969   **Lymphomas, nodular or follicular**
M9690/3   *Malignant lymphoma, nodular NOS*
M9691/3   *Malignant lymphoma, mixed lymphocytic-histiocytic, nodular*
M9692/3   *Malignant lymphoma, centroblastic-centrocytic, follicular*
M9693/3   *Malignant lymphoma, lymphocytic, well differentiated, nodular*
M9694/3   *Malignant lymphoma, lymphocytic, intermediate differentiation, nodular*
M9695/3   *Malignant lymphoma, follicular center cell, cleaved, follicular*
M9696/3   *Malignant lymphoma, lymphocytic, poorly differentiated, nodular*
M9697/3   *Malignant lymphoma, centroblastic type, follicular*
M9698/3   *Malignant lymphoma, follicular center cell, noncleaved, follicular*

M970   **Mycosis fungoides**
M9700/3   *Mycosis fungoides*
M9701/3   *Sezary's disease*

M971-M972   **Miscellaneous reticuloendothelial neoplasms**
M9710/3   *Microglioma*
M9720/3   *Malignant histiocytosis*
M9721/3   *Histiocytic medullary reticulosis*
M9722/3   *Letterer-Siwe's disease*

M973   **Plasma cell tumors**
M9730/3   *Plasma cell myeloma*
M9731/0   *Plasma cell tumor, benign*
M9731/1   *Plasmacytoma NOS*
M9731/3   *Plasma cell tumor, malignant*

M974   **Mast cell tumors**
M9740/1   *Mastocytoma NOS*
M9740/3   *Mast cell sarcoma*
M9741/3   *Malignant mastocytosis*

M975   **Burkitt's tumor**
M9750/3   *Burkitt's tumor*

M980-M994   **Leukemias**

M980   **Leukemias NOS**
M9800/3   *Leukemia NOS*
M9801/3   *Acute leukemia NOS*
M9802/3   *Subacute leukemia NOS*
M9803/3   *Chronic leukemia NOS*
M9804/3   *Aleukemic leukemia NOS*

M981   **Compound leukemias**
M9810/3   *Compound leukemia*

M982   **Lymphoid leukemias**
M9820/3   *Lymphoid leukemia NOS*
M9821/3   *Acute lymphoid leukemia*
M9822/3   *Subacute lymphoid leukemia*
M9823/3   *Chronic lymphoid leukemia*
M9824/3   *Aleukemic lymphoid leukemia*
M9825/3   *Prolymphocytic leukemia*

M983   **Plasma cell leukemias**
M9830/3   *Plasma cell leukemia*

M984   **Erythroleukemias**
M9840/3   *Erythroleukemia*
M9841/3   *Acute erythremia*
M9842/3   *Chronic erythremia*

M985   **Lymphosarcoma cell leukemias**
M9850/3   *Lymphosarcoma cell leukemia*

M986   **Myeloid leukemias**
M9860/3   *Myeloid leukemia NOS*
M9861/3   *Acute myeloid leukemia*
M9862/3   *Subacute myeloid leukemia*
M9863/3   *Chronic myeloid leukemia*
M9864/3   *Aleukemic myeloid leukemia*
M9865/3   *Neutrophilic leukemia*
M9866/3   *Acute promyelocytic leukemia*

M987   **Basophilic leukemias**
M9870/3   *Basophilic leukemia*

M988   **Eosinophilic leukemias**
M9880/3   *Eosinophilic leukemia*

M989   **Monocytic leukemias**
M9890/3   *Monocytic leukemia NOS*
M9891/3   *Acute monocytic leukemia*
M9892/3   *Subacute monocytic leukemia*
M9893/3   *Chronic monocytic leukemia*
M9894/3   *Aleukemic monocytic leukemia*

M990-M994   **Miscellaneous leukemias**
M9900/3   *Mast cell leukemia*
M9910/3   *Megakaryocytic leukemia*
M9920/3   *Megakaryocytic myelosis*
M9930/3   *Myeloid sarcoma*
M9940/3   *Hairy cell leukemia*

M995-M997   **Miscellaneous myeloproliferative and lymphoproliferative disorders**
M9950/1   *Polycythemia vera*
M9951/1   *Acute panmyelosis*
M9960/1   *Chronic myeloproliferative disease*
M9961/1   *Myelosclerosis with myeloid metaplasia*
M9962/1   *Idiopathic thrombocythemia*
M9970/1   *Chronic lymphoproliferative disease*

Deleted as of October 1, 2004

APPENDIX C

CLASSIFICATION OF DRUGS BY AMERICAN HOSPITAL FORMULARY SERVICES LIST NUMBER AND THEIR ICD-9-CM EQUIVALENTS

The coding of adverse effects of drugs is keyed to the continually revised Hospital Formulary of the American Hospital Formulary Service (AHFS) published under the direction of the American Society of Hospital Pharmacists.

The following section gives the ICD-9-CM diagnosis code for each AHFS list.

AHFS List		ICD-9-CM Diagnosis Code
4:00	**ANTIHISTAMINE DRUGS**	**963.0**
8:00	**ANTI-INFECTIVE AGENTS**	
8:04	Amebicides	961.5
	hydroxyquinoline derivatives	961.3
	arsenical anti-infectives	961.1
8:08	Anthelmintics	961.6
	quinoline derivatives	961.3
8:12.04	Antifungal Antibiotics	960.1
	nonantibiotics	961.9
8:12.06	Cephalosporins	960.5
8:12.08	Chloramphenicol	960.2
8:12.12	The Erythromycins	960.3
8:12.16	The Penicillins	960.0
8:12.20	The Streptomycins	960.6
8:12.24	The Tetracyclines	960.4
8:12.28	Other Antibiotics	960.8
	antimycobacterial antibiotics	960.6
	macrolides	960.3
8:16	Antituberculars	961.8
	antibiotics	960.6
8:18	Antivirals	961.7
8:20	Plasmodicides (antimalarials)	961.4
8:24	Sulfonamides	961.0
8:26	The Sulfones	961.8
8:28	Treponemicides	961.2
8:32	Trichomonacides	961.5
	hydroxyquinoline derivatives	961.3
	nitrofuran derivatives	961.9
8:36	Urinary Germicides	961.9
	quinoline derivatives	961.3
8:40	Other Anti-Infectives	961.9
10:00	**ANTINEOPLASTIC AGENTS**	**963.1**
	antibiotics	960.7
	progestogens	962.2
12:00	**AUTONOMIC DRUGS**	
12:04	Parasympathomimetic (Cholinergic) Agents	971.0
12:08	Parasympatholytic (Cholinergic Blocking) Agents	971.1
12:12	Sympathomimetic (Adrenergic) Agents	971.2
12:16	Sympatholytic (Adrenergic Blocking) Agents	971.3
12:20	Skeletal Muscle Relaxants	975.2
	central nervous system muscle-tone depressants	968.0
16:00	**BLOOD DERIVATIVES**	**964.7**
20:00	**BLOOD FORMATION AND COAGULATION**	
20:04	Antianemia Drugs	964.1
20:04.04	Iron Preparations	964.0
20:04.08	Liver and Stomach Preparations	964.1
20:12.04	Anticoagulants	964.2
20:12.08	Antiheparin agents	964.5
20:12.12	Coagulants	964.5
20:12.16	Hemostatics	964.5
	capillary-active drugs	972.8
	fibrinolysis-affecting agents	964.4
	natural products	964.7
24:00	**CARDIOVASCULAR DRUGS**	
24:04	Cardiac Drugs	972.9
	cardiotonic agents	972.1
	rhythm regulators	972.0

24:06	Antilipemic Agents	972.2
	thyroid derivatives	962.7
24:08	Hypotensive Agents	972.6
	adrenergic blocking agents	971.3
	ganglion-blocking agents	972.3
	vasodilators	972.5
24:12	Vasodilating Agents	972.5
	coronary	972.4
	nicotinic acid derivatives	972.2
24:16	Sclerosing Agents	972.7
28:00	**CENTRAL NERVOUS SYSTEM DRUGS**	
28:04	General Anesthetics	968.4
	gaseous anesthetics	968.2
	halothane	968.1
	intravenous anesthetics	968.3
28:08	Analgesics and Antipyretics	965.9
	antirheumatics	965.6
	aromatic analgesics	965.4
	non-narcotics NEC	965.7
	opium alkaloids	965.00
	heroin	965.01
	methadone	965.02
	specified type NEC	965.09
	pyrazole derivatives	965.5
	salicylates	965.1
	specified type NEC	965.8
28:10	Narcotic Antagonists	970.1
28:12	Anticonvulsants	966.3
	barbiturates	967.0
	benzodiazepine-based tranquilizers	969.4
	bromides	967.3
	hydantoin derivatives	966.1
	oxazolidine derivative	966.0
	succinimides	966.2
28:16.04	Antidepressants	969.0
28:16.08	Tranquilizers	969.5
	benzodiazepine-based	969.4
	butyrophenone-based	969.2
	major NEC	969.3
	phenothiazine-based	969.1
28:16.12	Other Psychotherapeutic Agents	969.8
28:20	Respiratory and Cerebral Stimulants	970.9
	analeptics	970.0
	anorexigenic agents	977.0
	psychostimulants	969.7
	specified type NEC	970.8
28:24	Sedatives and Hypnotics	967.9
	barbiturates	967.0
	benzodiazepine-based tranquilizers	969.4
	chloral hydrate group	967.1
	glutethimide group	967.5
	intravenous anesthetics	968.3
	methaqualone	967.4
	paraldehyde	967.2
	phenothiazine-based tranquilizers	969.1
	specified type NEC	967.8
	thiobarbiturates	968.3
	tranquilizer NEC	969.5
36:00	**DIAGNOSTIC AGENTS**	**977.8**
40:00	**ELECTROLYTE, CALORIC, AND WATER BALANCE AGENTS NEC**	**974.5**
40:04	Acidifying Agents	963.2
40:08	Alkalinizing Agents	963.3
40:10	Ammonia Detoxicants	974.5
40:12	Replacement Solutions NEC	974.5
	plasma volume expanders	964.8
40:16	Sodium-Removing Resins	974.5
40:18	Potassium-Removing Resins	974.5
40:20	Caloric Agents	974.5
40:24	Salt and Sugar Substitutes	974.5

40:28	Diuretics NEC	974.4
	carbonic acid anhydrase inhibitors	974.2
	mercurials	974.0
	purine derivatives	974.1
	saluretics	974.3
40:36	Irrigating Solutions	974.5
40:40	Uricosuric Agents	974.7
44:00	**ENZYMES NEC**	**963.4**
	fibrinolysis-affecting agents	964.4
	gastric agents	973.4
48:00	**EXPECTORANTS AND COUGH PREPARATIONS**	
	antihistamine agents	963.0
	antitussives	975.4
	codeine derivatives	965.09
	expectorants	975.5
	narcotic agents NEC	965.09
52:00	**EYE, EAR, NOSE, AND THROAT PREPARATIONS**	
52:04	Anti-Infectives	
	ENT976.6	
	ophthalmic	976.5
52:04.04	Antibiotics	
	ENT976.6	
	ophthalmic	976.5
52:04.06	Antivirals	
	ENT976.6	
	ophthalmic	976.5
52:04.08	Sulfonamides	
	ENT976.6	
	ophthalmic	976.5
52:04.12	Miscellaneous Anti-Infectives	
	ENT976.6	
	ophthalmic	976.5
52:08	Anti-Inflammatory Agents	
	ENT976.6	
	ophthalmic	976.5
52:10	Carbonic Anhydrase Inhibitors	974.2
52:12	Contact Lens Solutions	976.5
52:16	Local Anesthetics	968.5
52:20	Miotics	971.0
52:24	Mydriatics	
	adrenergics	971.2
	anticholinergics	971.1
	antimuscarinics	971.1
	parasympatholytics	971.1
	spasmolytics	971.1
	sympathomimetics	971.2
52:28	Mouth Washes and Gargles	976.6
52:32	Vasoconstrictors	971.2
52:36	Unclassified Agents	
	ENT976.6	
	ophthalmic	976.5
56:00	**GASTROINTESTINAL DRUGS**	
56:04	Antacids and Absorbents	973.0
56:08	Anti-Diarrhea Agents	973.5
56:10	Antiflatulents	973.8
56:12	Cathartics NEC	973.3
	emollients	973.2
	irritants	973.1
56:16	Digestants	973.4
56:20	Emetics and Antiemetics	
	antiemetics	963.0
	emetics	973.6
56:24	Lipotropic Agents	977.1
60:00	**GOLD COMPOUNDS**	**965.6**
64:00	**HEAVY METAL ANTAGONISTS**	**963.8**
68:00	**HORMONES AND SYNTHETIC SUBSTITUTES**	
68:04	Adrenals	962.0
68:08	Androgens	962.1
68:12	Contraceptives	962.2
68:16	Estrogens	962.2
68:18	Gonadotropins	962.4
68:20	Insulins and Antidiabetic Agents	962.3
68:20.08	Insulins	962.3
68:24	Parathyroid	962.6

68:28	Pituitary	
	anterior	962.4
	posterior	962.5
68:32	Progestogens	962.2
68:34	Other Corpus Luteum Hormones	962.2
68:36	Thyroid and Antithyroid	
	antithyroid	962.8
	thyroid	962.7
72:00	**LOCAL ANESTHETICS NEC**	**968.9**
	topical (surface) agents	968.5
	infiltrating agents (intradermal) (subcutaneous) (submucosal)	968.5
	nerve blocking agents (peripheral) (plexus) (regional)	968.6
	spinal	968.7
76:00	**OXYTOCICS**	**975.0**
78:00	**RADIOACTIVE AGENTS**	**990**
80:00	**SERUMS, TOXOIDS, AND VACCINES**	
80:04	Serums	979.9
	immune globulin (gamma) (human)	964.6
80:08	Toxoids NEC	978.8
	diphtheria	978.5
	and tetanus	978.9
	with pertussis component	978.6
	tetanus	978.4
	and diphtheria	978.9
	with pertussis component	978.6
80:12	Vaccines NEC	979.9
	bacterial NEC	978.8
	with	
	other bacterial component	978.9
	pertussis component	978.6
	viral and rickettsial component	979.7
	rickettsial NEC	979.6
	with	
	bacterial component	979.7
	pertussis component	978.6
	viral component	979.7
	viral NEC	979.6
	with	
	bacterial component	979.7
	pertussis component	978.6
	rickettsial component	979.7
84:00	**SKIN AND MUCOUS MEMBRANE PREPARATIONS**	
84:04	Anti-Infectives	976.0
84:04.04	Antibiotics	976.0
84:04.08	Fungicides	976.0
84:04.12	Scabicides and Pediculicides	976.0
84:04.16	Miscellaneous Local Anti-Infectives	976.0
84:06	Anti-Inflammatory Agents	976.0
84:08	Antipruritics and Local Anesthetics	
	antipruritics	976.1
	local anesthetics	968.5
84:12	Astringents	976.2
84:16	Cell Stimulants and Proliferants	976.8
84:20	Detergents	976.2
84:24	Emollients, Demulcents, and Protectants	976.3
84:28	Keratolytic Agents	976.4
84:32	Keratoplastic Agents	976.4
84:36	Miscellaneous Agents	976.8
86:00	**SPASMOLYTIC AGENTS**	**975.1**
	antiasthmatics	975.7
	papaverine	972.5
	theophylline	974.1
88:00	**VITAMINS**	
88:04	Vitamin A	963.5
88:08	Vitamin B Complex	963.5
	hematopoietic vitamin	964.1
	nicotinic acid derivatives	972.2
88:12	Vitamin C	963.5
88:16	Vitamin D	963.5
88:20	Vitamin E	963.5
88:24	Vitamin K Activity	964.3
88:28	Multivitamin Preparations	963.5
92:00	**UNCLASSIFIED THERAPEUTIC AGENTS**	**977.8**

ICD-9-CM, APPENDIX C

APPENDIX D

CLASSIFICATION OF INDUSTRIAL ACCIDENTS ACCORDING TO AGENCY

Annex B to the Resolution concerning Statistics of Employment Injuries adopted by the Tenth International Conference of Labor Statisticians on 12 October 1962

1 MACHINES

11 Prime-Movers, except Electrical Motors
111 *Steam engines*
112 *Internal combustion engines*
119 *Others*

12 Transmission Machinery
121 *Transmission shafts*
122 *Transmission belts, cables, pulleys, pinions, chains, gears*
129 *Others*

13 Metalworking Machines
131 *Power presses*
132 *Lathes*
133 *Milling machines*
134 *Abrasive wheels*
135 *Mechanical shears*
136 *Forging machines*
137 *Rolling-mills*
139 *Others*

14 Wood and Assimilated Machines
141 *Circular saws*
142 *Other saws*
143 *Molding machines*
144 *Overhand planes*
149 *Others*

15 Agricultural Machines
151 *Reapers (including combine reapers)*
152 *Threshers*
159 *Others*

16 Mining Machinery
161 *Under-cutters*
169 *Others*

19 Other Machines Not Elsewhere Classified
191 *Earth-moving machines, excavating and scraping machines, except means of transport*
192 *Spinning, weaving and other textile machines*
193 *Machines for the manufacture of foodstuffs and beverages*
194 *Machines for the manufacture of paper*
195 *Printing machines*
199 *Others*

2 MEANS OF TRANSPORT AND LIFTING EQUIPMENT

21 Lifting Machines and Appliances
211 *Cranes*
212 *Lifts and elevators*
213 *Winches*
214 *Pulley blocks*
219 *Others*

22 Means of Rail Transport
221 *Inter-urban railways*
222 *Rail transport in mines, tunnels, quarries, industrial establishments, docks, etc.*
229 *Others*

23 Other Wheeled Means of Transport, Excluding Rail Transport
231 *Tractors*
232 *Lorries*
233 *Trucks*
234 *Motor vehicles, not elsewhere classified*
235 *Animal-drawn vehicles*
236 *Hand-drawn vehicles*
239 *Others*

24 Means of Air Transport

25 Means of Water Transport
251 *Motorized means of water transport*
252 *Non-motorized means of water transport*

26 Other Means of Transport
261 *Cable-cars*
262 *Mechanical conveyors, except cable-cars*
269 *Others*

3 OTHER EQUIPMENT

31 Pressure Vessels
311 *Boilers*
312 *Pressurized containers*
313 *Pressurized piping and accessories*
314 *Gas cylinders*
315 *Caissons, diving equipment*
319 *Others*

32 Furnaces, Ovens, Kilns
321 *Blast furnaces*
322 *Refining furnaces*
323 *Other furnaces*
324 *Kilns*
325 *Ovens*

33 Refrigerating Plants

34 Electrical Installations, Including Electric Motors, but Excluding Electric Hand Tools
341 *Rotating machines*
342 *Conductors*
343 *Transformers*
344 *Control apparatus*
349 *Others*

35 Electric Hand Tools

36 Tools, Implements, and Appliances, Except Electric Hand Tools
361 *Power-driven hand tools, except electric hand tools*
362 *Hand tools, not power-driven*
369 *Others*

37 Ladders, Mobile Ramps

38 Scaffolding

39 Other Equipment, Not Elsewhere Classified

4 MATERIALS, SUBSTANCES, AND RADIATIONS

41 Explosives

42 Dusts, Gases, Liquids and Chemicals, Excluding Explosives
421 *Dusts*
422 *Gases, vapors, fumes*
423 *Liquids, not elsewhere classified*
424 *Chemicals, not elsewhere classified*

43 Flying Fragments

44 Radiations
441 *Ionizing radiations*
449 *Others*

49 Other Materials and Substances Not Elsewhere Classified

5 WORKING ENVIRONMENT

51 Outdoor
511 *Weather*
512 *Traffic and working surfaces*
513 *Water*
519 *Others*

52 **Indoor**
    521 *Floors*
    522 *Confined quarters*
    523 *Stairs*
    524 *Other traffic and working surfaces*
    525 *Floor openings and wall openings*
    526 *Environmental factors (lighting, ventilation, temperature, noise, etc.)*
    529 *Others*

53 **Underground**
    531 *Roofs and faces of mine roads and tunnels, etc.*
    532 *Floors of mine roads and tunnels, etc.*
    533 *Working-faces of mines, tunnels, etc.*
    534 *Mine shafts*
    535 *Fire*
    536 *Water*
    539 *Others*

6 OTHER AGENCIES, NOT ELSEWHERE CLASSIFIED

61 **Animals**
    611 *Live animals*
    612 *Animals products*

69 **Other Agencies, Not Elsewhere Classified**

7 AGENCIES NOT CLASSIFIED FOR LACK OF SUFFICIENT DATA

ICD-9-CM, APPENDIX D

1. INFECTIOUS AND PARASITIC DISEASES

Intestinal infectious diseases (001–009)
001 Cholera
002 Typhoid and paratyphoid fevers
003 Other salmonella infections
004 Shigellosis
005 Other food poisoning (bacterial)
006 Amebiasis
007 Other protozoal intestinal diseases
008 Intestinal infections due to other organisms
009 Ill-defined intestinal infections

Tuberculosis (010–018)
010 Primary tuberculous infection
011 Pulmonary tuberculosis
012 Other respiratory tuberculosis
013 Tuberculosis of meninges and central nervous system
014 Tuberculosis of intestines, peritoneum, and mesenteric glands
015 Tuberculosis of bones and joints
016 Tuberculosis of genitourinary system
017 Tuberculosis of other organs
018 Miliary tuberculosis

Zoonotic bacterial diseases (020–027)
020 Plague
021 Tularemia
022 Anthrax
023 Brucellosis
024 Glanders
025 Melioidosis
026 Rat-bite fever
027 Other zoonotic bacterial diseases

Other bacterial diseases (030–041)
030 Leprosy
031 Diseases due to other mycobacteria
032 Diphtheria
033 Whooping cough
034 Streptococcal sore throat and scarlet fever
035 Erysipelas
036 Meningococcal infection
037 Tetanus
038 Septicemia
039 Actinomycotic infections
040 Other bacterial diseases
041 Bacterial infection in conditions classified elsewhere and of unspecified site

Human immunodeficiency virus (042)
042   Human immunodeficiency virus [HIV] disease

Poliomyelitis and other non-arthropod-borne viral diseases of central nervous system (045–049)
045 Acute poliomyelitis
046 Slow virus infection of central nervous system
047 Meningitis due to enterovirus
048 Other enterovirus diseases of central nervous system
049 Other non-arthropod-borne viral diseases of central nervous system

Viral diseases accompanied by exanthem (050–059)
050 Smallpox
051 Cowpox and paravaccinia
052 Chickenpox
053 Herpes zoster
054 Herpes simplex
055 Measles
056 Rubella
057 Other viral exanthemata
058 Other human herpesvirus
059 Other poxvirus infections

Arthropod-borne viral diseases (060–066)
060 Yellow fever
061 Dengue
062 Mosquito-borne viral encephalitis
063 Tick-borne viral encephalitis
064 Viral encephalitis transmitted by other and unspecified arthropods
065 Arthropod-borne hemorrhagic fever
066 Other arthropod-borne viral diseases

Other diseases due to viruses and Chlamydiae (070–079)
070 Viral hepatitis
071 Rabies
072 Mumps
073 Ornithosis
074 Specific diseases due to Coxsackie virus
075 Infectious mononucleosis
076 Trachoma
077 Other diseases of conjunctiva due to viruses and Chlamydiae
078 Other diseases due to viruses and Chlamydiae
079 Viral infection in conditions classified elsewhere and of unspecified site

Rickettsioses and other arthropod-borne diseases (080–088)
080 Louse-borne [epidemic] typhus
081 Other typhus
082 Tick-borne rickettsioses
083 Other rickettsioses
084 Malaria
085 Leishmaniasis
086 Trypanosomiasis
087 Relapsing fever
088 Other arthropod-borne diseases

Syphilis and other venereal diseases (090–099)
090 Congenital syphilis
091 Early syphilis, symptomatic
092 Early syphilis, latent
093 Cardiovascular syphilis
094 Neurosyphilis
095 Other forms of late syphilis, with symptoms
096 Late syphilis, latent
097 Other and unspecified syphilis
098 Gonococcal infections
099 Other venereal diseases

Other spirochetal diseases (100–104)
100 Leptospirosis
101 Vincent's angina
102 Yaws
103 Pinta
104 Other spirochetal infection

Mycoses (110–118)
110 Dermatophytosis
111 Dermatomycosis, other and unspecified
112 Candidiasis
114 Coccidioidomycosis
115 Histoplasmosis
116 Blastomycotic infection
117 Other mycoses
118 Opportunistic mycoses

Helminthiases (120–129)
120 Schistosomiasis [bilharziasis]
121 Other trematode infections
122 Echinococcosis
123 Other cestode infection
124 Trichinosis
125 Filarial infection and dracontiasis
126 Ancylostomiasis and necatoriasis
127 Other intestinal helminthiases
128 Other and unspecified helminthiases
129 Intestinal parasitism, unspecified

Other infectious and parasitic diseases (130–136)
130 Toxoplasmosis
131 Trichomoniasis
132 Pediculosis and phthirus infestation
133 Acariasis
134 Other infestation
135 Sarcoidosis
136 Other and unspecified infectious and parasitic diseases

Late effects of infectious and parasitic diseases (137–139)
137 Late effects of tuberculosis
138 Late effects of acute poliomyelitis
139 Late effects of other infectious and parasitic diseases

2. NEOPLASMS

Malignant neoplasm of lip, oral cavity, and pharynx (140–149)
140   Malignant neoplasm of lip
141   Malignant neoplasm of tongue
142   Malignant neoplasm of major salivary glands
143   Malignant neoplasm of gum
144   Malignant neoplasm of floor of mouth
145   Malignant neoplasm of other and unspecified parts of mouth
146   Malignant neoplasm of oropharynx
147   Malignant neoplasm of nasopharynx
148   Malignant neoplasm of hypopharynx
149   Malignant neoplasm of other and ill-defined sites within the lip, oral cavity, and pharynx

Malignant neoplasm of digestive organs and peritoneum (150–159)
150   Malignant neoplasm of esophagus
151   Malignant neoplasm of stomach
152   Malignant neoplasm of small intestine, including duodenum
153   Malignant neoplasm of colon
154   Malignant neoplasm of rectum, rectosigmoid junction, and anus
155   Malignant neoplasm of liver and intrahepatic bile ducts
156   Malignant neoplasm of gallbladder and extrahepatic bile ducts
157   Malignant neoplasm of pancreas
158   Malignant neoplasm of retroperitoneum and peritoneum
159   Malignant neoplasm of other and ill-defined sites within the digestive organs and peritoneum

Malignant neoplasm of respiratory and intrathoracic organs (160–165)
160   Malignant neoplasm of nasal cavities, middle ear, and accessory sinuses
161   Malignant neoplasm of larynx
162   Malignant neoplasm of trachea, bronchus, and lung
163   Malignant neoplasm of pleura
164   Malignant neoplasm of thymus, heart, and mediastinum
165   Malignant neoplasm of other and ill-defined sites within the respiratory system and intrathoracic organs

Malignant neoplasm of bone, connective tissue, skin, and breast (170–176)
170   Malignant neoplasm of bone and articular cartilage
171   Malignant neoplasm of connective and other soft tissue
172   Malignant melanoma of skin
173   Other malignant neoplasm of skin
174   Malignant neoplasm of female breast
175   Malignant neoplasm of male breast

Kaposi's sarcoma (176)
176   Kaposi's sarcoma

Malignant neoplasm of genitourinary organs (179–189)
179   Malignant neoplasm of uterus, part unspecified
180   Malignant neoplasm of cervix uteri
181   Malignant neoplasm of placenta
182   Malignant neoplasm of body of uterus
183   Malignant neoplasm of ovary and other uterine adnexa
184   Malignant neoplasm of other and unspecified female genital organs
185   Malignant neoplasm of prostate
186   Malignant neoplasm of testis
187   Malignant neoplasm of penis and other male genital organs
188   Malignant neoplasm of bladder
189   Malignant neoplasm of kidney and other and unspecified urinary organs

Malignant neoplasm of other and unspecified sites (190–199)
190   Malignant neoplasm of eye
191   Malignant neoplasm of brain
192   Malignant neoplasm of other and unspecified parts of nervous system
193   Malignant neoplasm of thyroid gland
194   Malignant neoplasm of other endocrine glands and related structures
195   Malignant neoplasm of other and ill-defined sites
196   Secondary and unspecified malignant neoplasm of lymph nodes
197   Secondary malignant neoplasm of respiratory and digestive systems
198   Secondary malignant neoplasm of other specified sites
199   Malignant neoplasm without specification of site

Malignant neoplasm of lymphatic and hematopoietic tissue (200–208)
200   Lymphosarcoma and reticulosarcoma
201   Hodgkin's disease
202   Other malignant neoplasm of lymphoid and histiocytic tissue
203   Multiple myeloma and immunoproliferative neoplasms
204   Lymphoid leukemia
205   Myeloid leukemia
206   Monocytic leukemia
207   Other specified leukemia
208   Leukemia of unspecified cell type

Neuroendocrine tumors (209)
209   Neuroendocrine tumors

Benign neoplasms (210–229)
210   Benign neoplasm of lip, oral cavity, and pharynx
211   Benign neoplasm of other parts of digestive system
212   Benign neoplasm of respiratory and intrathoracic organs
213   Benign neoplasm of bone and articular cartilage
214   Lipoma
215   Other benign neoplasm of connective and other soft tissue
216   Benign neoplasm of skin
217   Benign neoplasm of breast
218   Uterine leiomyoma
219   Other benign neoplasm of uterus
220   Benign neoplasm of ovary
221   Benign neoplasm of other female genital organs
222   Benign neoplasm of male genital organs
223   Benign neoplasm of kidney and other urinary organs
224   Benign neoplasm of eye
225   Benign neoplasm of brain and other parts of nervous system
226   Benign neoplasm of thyroid gland
227   Benign neoplasm of other endocrine glands and related structures
228   Hemangioma and lymphangioma, any site
229   Benign neoplasm of other and unspecified sites

Carcinoma in situ (230–234)
230   Carcinoma in situ of digestive organs
231   Carcinoma in situ of respiratory system
232   Carcinoma in situ of skin
233   Carcinoma in situ of breast and genitourinary system
234   Carcinoma in situ of other and unspecified sites

Neoplasms of uncertain behavior (235–238)
235   Neoplasm of uncertain behavior of digestive and respiratory systems
236   Neoplasm of uncertain behavior of genitourinary organs
237   Neoplasm of uncertain behavior of endocrine glands and nervous system
238   Neoplasm of uncertain behavior of other and unspecified sites and tissues

Neoplasms of unspecified nature (239)
239   Neoplasm of unspecified nature

3. ENDOCRINE, NUTRITIONAL AND METABOLIC DISEASES, AND IMMUNITY DISORDERS

Disorders of thyroid gland (240–246)
240   Simple and unspecified goiter
241   Nontoxic nodular goiter
242   Thyrotoxicosis with or without goiter
243   Congenital hypothyroidism
244   Acquired hypothyroidism
245   Thyroiditis
246   Other disorders of thyroid

Diseases of other endocrine glands (249–259)
249   Secondary diabetes mellitus
250   Diabetes mellitus
251   Other disorders of pancreatic internal secretion
252   Disorders of parathyroid gland
253   Disorders of the pituitary gland and its hypothalamic control
254   Diseases of thymus gland
255   Disorders of adrenal glands
256   Ovarian dysfunction
257   Testicular dysfunction
258   Polyglandular dysfunction and related disorders
259   Other endocrine disorders

ICD-9-CM, APPENDIX E

Nutritional deficiencies (260–269)

260	Kwashiorkor
261	Nutritional marasmus
262	Other severe protein-calorie malnutrition
263	Other and unspecified protein-calorie malnutrition
264	Vitamin A deficiency
265	Thiamine and niacin deficiency states
266	Deficiency of B-complex components
267	Ascorbic acid deficiency
268	Vitamin D deficiency
269	Other nutritional deficiencies

Other metabolic disorders and immunity disorders (270–279)

270	Disorders of amino-acid transport and metabolism
271	Disorders of carbohydrate transport and metabolism
272	Disorders of lipoid metabolism
273	Disorders of plasma protein metabolism
274	Gout
275	Disorders of mineral metabolism
276	Disorders of fluid, electrolyte, and acid-base balance
277	Other and unspecified disorders of metabolism
278	Obesity and other hyperalimentation
279	Disorders involving the immune mechanism

4. DISEASES OF BLOOD AND BLOOD-FORMING ORGANS

Diseases of the blood and blood-forming organs (280–289)

280	Iron deficiency anemias
281	Other deficiency anemias
282	Hereditary hemolytic anemias
283	Acquired hemolytic anemias
284	Aplastic anemia
285	Other and unspecified anemias
286	Coagulation defects
287	Purpura and other hemorrhagic conditions
288	Diseases of white blood cells
289	Other diseases of blood and blood-forming organs

5. MENTAL DISORDERS

Organic psychotic conditions (290–294)

290	Senile and presenile organic psychotic conditions
291	Alcoholic psychoses
292	Drug psychoses
293	Transient organic psychotic conditions
294	Other organic psychotic conditions (chronic)

Other psychoses (295–299)

295	Schizophrenic psychoses
296	Affective psychoses
297	Paranoid states
298	Other nonorganic psychoses
299	Psychoses with origin specific to childhood

Neurotic disorders, personality disorders, and other nonpsychotic mental disorders (300–316)

300	Neurotic disorders
301	Personality disorders
302	Sexual deviations and disorders
303	Alcohol dependence syndrome
304	Drug dependence
305	Nondependent abuse of drugs
306	Physiological malfunction arising from mental factors
307	Special symptoms or syndromes, not elsewhere classified
308	Acute reaction to stress
309	Adjustment reaction
310	Specific nonpsychotic mental disorders following organic brain damage
311	Depressive disorder, not elsewhere classified
312	Disturbance of conduct, not elsewhere classified
313	Disturbance of emotions specific to childhood and adolescence
314	Hyperkinetic syndrome of childhood
315	Specific delays in development
316	Psychic factors associated with diseases classified elsewhere

Mental retardation (317–319)

317	Mild mental retardation
318	Other specified mental retardation
319	Unspecified mental retardation

6. DISEASES OF THE NERVOUS SYSTEM AND SENSE ORGANS

Inflammatory diseases of the central nervous system (320–326)

320	Bacterial meningitis
321	Meningitis due to other organisms
322	Meningitis of unspecified cause
323	Encephalitis, myelitis, and encephalomyelitis
324	Intracranial and intraspinal abscess
325	Phlebitis and thrombophlebitis of intracranial venous sinuses
326	Late effects of intracranial abscess or pyogenic infection
327	Organic sleep disorders

Hereditary and degenerative diseases of the central nervous system (330–337)

330	Cerebral degenerations usually manifest in childhood
331	Other cerebral degenerations
332	Parkinson's disease
333	Other extrapyramidal disease and abnormal movement disorders
334	Spinocerebellar disease
335	Anterior horn cell disease
336	Other diseases of spinal cord
337	Disorders of the autonomic nervous system

Pain (338)

338	Pain, not elsewhere classified

Other headache syndromes (339)

339	Other headache syndromes

Other disorders of the central nervous system (340–349)

340	Multiple sclerosis
341	Other demyelinating diseases of central nervous system
342	Hemiplegia and hemiparesis
343	Infantile cerebral palsy
344	Other paralytic syndromes
345	Epilepsy
346	Migraine
347	Cataplexy and narcolepsy
348	Other conditions of brain
349	Other and unspecified disorders of the nervous system

Disorders of the peripheral nervous system (350–359)

350	Trigeminal nerve disorders
351	Facial nerve disorders
352	Disorders of other cranial nerves
353	Nerve root and plexus disorders
354	Mononeuritis of upper limb and mononeuritis multiplex
355	Mononeuritis of lower limb
356	Hereditary and idiopathic peripheral neuropathy
357	Inflammatory and toxic neuropathy
358	Myoneural disorders
359	Muscular dystrophies and other myopathies

Disorders of the eye and adnexa (360–379)

360	Disorders of the globe
361	Retinal detachments and defects
362	Other retinal disorders
363	Chorioretinal inflammations and scars and other disorders of choroid
364	Disorders of iris and ciliary body
365	Glaucoma
366	Cataract
367	Disorders of refraction and accommodation
368	Visual disturbances
369	Blindness and low vision
370	Keratitis
371	Corneal opacity and other disorders of cornea
372	Disorders of conjunctiva
373	Inflammation of eyelids
374	Other disorders of eyelids
375	Disorders of lacrimal system
376	Disorders of the orbit
377	Disorders of optic nerve and visual pathways
378	Strabismus and other disorders of binocular eye movements
379	Other disorders of eye

Diseases of the ear and mastoid process (380–389)

380	Disorders of external ear
381	Nonsuppurative otitis media and Eustachian tube disorders

382	Suppurative and unspecified otitis media
383	Mastoiditis and related conditions
384	Other disorders of tympanic membrane
385	Other disorders of middle ear and mastoid
386	Vertiginous syndromes and other disorders of vestibular system
387	Otosclerosis
388	Other disorders of ear
389	Hearing loss

7. DISEASES OF THE CIRCULATORY SYSTEM

Acute rheumatic fever (390–392)
390 Rheumatic fever without mention of heart involvement
391 Rheumatic fever with heart involvement
392 Rheumatic chorea

Chronic rheumatic heart disease (393–398)
393 Chronic rheumatic pericarditis
394 Diseases of mitral valve
395 Diseases of aortic valve
396 Diseases of mitral and aortic valves
397 Diseases of other endocardial structures
398 Other rheumatic heart disease

Hypertensive disease (401–405)
401 Essential hypertension
402 Hypertensive heart disease
403 Hypertensive renal disease
404 Hypertensive heart and renal disease
405 Secondary hypertension

Ischemic heart disease (410–414)
410 Acute myocardial infarction
411 Other acute and subacute form of ischemic heart disease
412 Old myocardial infarction
413 Angina pectoris
414 Other forms of chronic ischemic heart disease

Diseases of pulmonary circulation (415–417)
415 Acute pulmonary heart disease
416 Chronic pulmonary heart disease
417 Other diseases of pulmonary circulation

Other forms of heart disease (420–429)
420 Acute pericarditis
421 Acute and subacute endocarditis
422 Acute myocarditis
423 Other diseases of pericardium
424 Other diseases of endocardium
425 Cardiomyopathy
426 Conduction disorders
427 Cardiac dysrhythmias
428 Heart failure
429 Ill-defined descriptions and complications of heart disease

Cerebrovascular disease (430–438)
430 Subarachnoid hemorrhage
431 Intracerebral hemorrhage
432 Other and unspecified intracranial hemorrhage
433 Occlusion and stenosis of precerebral arteries
434 Occlusion of cerebral arteries
435 Transcient cerebral ischemia
436 Acute but ill-defined cerebrovascular disease
437 Other and ill-defined cerebrovascular disease
438 Late effects of cerebrovascular disease

Diseases of arteries, arterioles, and capillaries (440–448)
440 Atherosclerosis
441 Aortic aneurysm and dissection
442 Other aneurysm
443 Other peripheral vascular disease
444 Arterial embolism and thrombosis
445 Atheroembolism
446 Polyarteritis nodosa and allied conditions
447 Other disorders of arteries and arterioles
448 Diseases of capillaries

Diseases of veins and lymphatics, and other diseases of circulatory system (451–459)
451 Phlebitis and thrombophlebitis
452 Portal vein thrombosis
453 Other venous embolism and thrombosis
454 Varicose veins of lower extremities
455 Hemorrhoids
456 Varicose veins of other sites
457 Noninfective disorders of lymphatic channels
458 Hypotension
459 Other disorders of circulatory system

8. DISEASES OF THE RESPIRATORY SYSTEM

Acute respiratory infections (460–466)
460 Acute nasopharyngitis [common cold]
461 Acute sinusitis
462 Acute pharyngitis
463 Acute tonsillitis
464 Acute laryngitis and tracheitis
465 Acute upper respiratory infections of multiple or unspecified sites
466 Acute bronchitis and bronchiolitis

Other diseases of upper respiratory tract (470–478)
470 Deviated nasal septum
471 Nasal polyps
472 Chronic pharyngitis and nasopharyngitis
473 Chronic sinusitis
474 Chronic disease of tonsils and adenoids
475 Peritonsillar abscess
476 Chronic laryngitis and laryngotracheitis
477 Allergic rhinitis
478 Other diseases of upper respiratory tract

Pneumonia and influenza (480–488)
480 Viral pneumonia
481 Pneumococcal pneumonia [*Streptococcus pneumoniae* pneumonia]
482 Other bacterial pneumonia
483 Pneumonia due to other specified organism
484 Pneumonia in infectious diseases classified elsewhere
485 Bronchopneumonia, organism unspecified
486 Pneumonia, organism unspecified
487 Influenza
488 Influenza due to identified avian influenza virus

Chronic obstructive pulmonary disease and allied conditions (490–496)
490 Bronchitis, not specified as acute or chronic
491 Chronic bronchitis
492 Emphysema
493 Asthma
494 Bronchiectasis
495 Extrinsic allergic alveolitis
496 Chronic airways obstruction, not elsewhere classified

Pneumoconioses and other lung diseases due to external agents (500–508)
500 Coalworkers' pneumoconiosis
501 Asbestosis
502 Pneumoconiosis due to other silica or silicates
503 Pneumoconiosis due to other inorganic dust
504 Pneumopathy due to inhalation of other dust
505 Pneumoconiosis, unspecified
506 Respiratory conditions due to chemical fumes and vapors
507 Pneumonitis due to solids and liquids
508 Respiratory conditions due to other and unspecified external agents

Other diseases of respiratory system (510–519)
510 Empyema
511 Pleurisy
512 Pneumothorax
513 Abscess of lung and mediastinum
514 Pulmonary congestion and hypostasis
515 Postinflammatory pulmonary fibrosis
516 Other alveolar and parietoalveolar pneumopathy
517 Lung involvement in conditions classified elsewhere
518 Other diseases of lung
519 Other diseases of respiratory system

9. DISEASES OF THE DIGESTIVE SYSTEM

Diseases of oral cavity, salivary glands, and jaws (520–529)
520 Disorders of tooth development and eruption
521 Diseases of hard tissues of teeth
522 Diseases of pulp and periapical tissues
523 Gingival and periodontal diseases
524 Dentofacial anomalies, including malocclusion
525 Other diseases and conditions of the teeth and supporting structures
526 Diseases of the jaws
527 Diseases of the salivary glands
528 Diseases of the oral soft tissues, excluding lesions specific for gingiva and tongue
529 Diseases and other conditions of the tongue

Diseases of esophagus, stomach, and duodenum (530–538)
530 Diseases of esophagus
531 Gastric ulcer
532 Duodenal ulcer
533 Peptic ulcer, site unspecified
534 Gastrojejunal ulcer
535 Gastritis and duodenitis
536 Disorders of function of stomach
537 Other disorders of stomach and duodenum
538 Gastrointestinal mucositis (ulcerative)

Appendicitis (540–543)
540 Acute appendicitis
541 Appendicitis, unqualified
542 Other appendicitis
543 Other diseases of appendix

Hernia of abdominal cavity (550–553)
550 Inguinal hernia
551 Other hernia of abdominal cavity, with gangrene
552 Other hernia of abdominal cavity, with obstruction, but without mention of gangrene
553 Other hernia of abdominal cavity without mention of obstruction or gangrene

Noninfective enteritis and colitis (555–558)
555 Regional enteritis
556 Ulcerative colitis
557 Vascular insufficiency of intestine
558 Other noninfective gastroenteritis and colitis

Other diseases of intestines and peritoneum (560–569)
560 Intestinal obstruction without mention of hernia
562 Diverticula of intestine
564 Functional digestive disorders, not elsewhere classified
565 Anal fissure and fistula
566 Abscess of anal and rectal regions
567 Peritonitis
568 Other disorders of peritoneum
569 Other disorders of intestine

Other diseases of digestive system (570–579)
570 Acute and subacute necrosis of liver
571 Chronic liver disease and cirrhosis
572 Liver abscess and sequelae of chronic liver disease
573 Other disorders of liver
574 Cholelithiasis
575 Other disorders of gallbladder
576 Other disorders of biliary tract
577 Diseases of pancreas
578 Gastrointestinal hemorrhage
579 Intestinal malabsorption

10. DISEASES OF THE GENITOURINARY SYSTEM

Nephritis, nephrotic syndrome, and nephrosis (580–589)
580 Acute glomerulonephritis
581 Nephrotic syndrome
582 Chronic glomerulonephritis
583 Nephritis and nephropathy, not specified as acute or chronic
584 Acute renal failure
585 Chronic renal failure
586 Renal failure, unspecified
587 Renal sclerosis, unspecified
588 Disorders resulting from impaired renal function
589 Small kidney of unknown cause

Other diseases of urinary system (590–599)
590 Infections of kidney
591 Hydronephrosis
592 Calculus of kidney and ureter
593 Other disorders of kidney and ureter
594 Calculus of lower urinary tract
595 Cystitis
596 Other disorders of bladder
597 Urethritis, not sexually transmitted, and urethral syndrome
598 Urethral stricture
599 Other disorders of urethra and urinary tract

Diseases of male genital organs (600–608)
600 Hyperplasia of prostate
601 Inflammatory diseases of prostate
602 Other disorders of prostate
603 Hydrocele
604 Orchitis and epididymitis
605 Redundant prepuce and phimosis
606 Infertility, male
607 Disorders of penis
608 Other disorders of male genital organs

Disorders of breast (610–611)
610 Benign mammary dysplasias
611 Other disorders of breast
612 Deformity and disproportion of reconstructed breast

Inflammatory disease of female pelvic organs (614–616)
614 Inflammatory disease of ovary, fallopian tube, pelvic cellular tissue, and peritoneum
615 Inflammatory diseases of uterus, except cervix
616 Inflammatory disease of cervix, vagina, and vulva

Other disorders of female genital tract (617–629)
617 Endometriosis
618 Genital prolapse
619 Fistula involving female genital tract
620 Noninflammatory disorders of ovary, fallopian tube, and broad ligament
621 Disorders of uterus, not elsewhere classified
622 Noninflammatory disorders of cervix
623 Noninflammatory disorders of vagina
624 Noninflammatory disorders of vulva and perineum
625 Pain and other symptoms associated with female genital organs
626 Disorders of menstruation and other abnormal bleeding from female genital tract
627 Menopausal and postmenopausal disorders
628 Infertility, female
629 Other disorders of female genital organs

11. COMPLICATIONS OF PREGNANCY, CHILDBIRTH, AND THE PUERPERIUM

Ectopic and molar pregnancy and other pregnancy with abortive outcome (630–639)
630 Hydatidiform mole
631 Other abnormal product of conception
632 Missed abortion
633 Ectopic pregnancy
634 Spontaneous abortion
635 Legally induced abortion
636 Illegally induced abortion
637 Unspecified abortion
638 Failed attempted abortion
639 Complications following abortion and ectopic and molar pregnancies

Complications mainly related to pregnancy (640–649)
640 Hemorrhage in early pregnancy
641 Antepartum hemorrhage, abruptio placentae, and placenta previa
642 Hypertension complicating pregnancy, childbirth, and the puerperium
643 Excessive vomiting in pregnancy
644 Early or threatened labor
645 Prolonged pregnancy
646 Other complications of pregnancy, not elsewhere classified
647 Infective and parasitic conditions in the mother classifiable elsewhere but complicating pregnancy, childbirth, and the puerperium

648 Other current conditions in the mother classifiable elsewhere but complicating pregnancy, childbirth, and the puerperium
649 Other conditions or status of the mother complicating pregnancy, childbirth, or the puerperium

Normal delivery, and other indications for care in pregnancy, labor, and delivery (650–659)
650 Normal delivery
651 Multiple gestation
652 Malposition and malpresentation of fetus
653 Disproportion
654 Abnormality of organs and soft tissues of pelvis
655 Known or suspected fetal abnormality affecting management of mother
656 Other fetal and placental problems affecting management of mother
657 Polyhydramnios
658 Other problems associated with amniotic cavity and membranes
659 Other indications for care or intervention related to labor and delivery and not elsewhere classified

Complications occurring mainly in the course of labor and delivery (660–669)
660 Obstructed labor
661 Abnormality of forces of labor
662 Long labor
663 Umbilical cord complications
664 Trauma to perineum and vulva during delivery
665 Other obstetrical trauma
666 Postpartum hemorrhage
667 Retained placenta or membranes, without hemorrhage
668 Complications of the administration of anesthetic or other sedation in labor and delivery
669 Other complications of labor and delivery, not elsewhere classified

Complications of the puerperium (670–677)
670 Major puerperal infection
671 Venous complications in pregnancy and the puerperium
672 Pyrexia of unknown origin during the puerperium
673 Obstetrical pulmonary embolism
674 Other and unspecified complications of the puerperium, not elsewhere classified
675 Infections of the breast and nipple associated with childbirth
676 Other disorders of the breast associated with childbirth, and disorders of lactation
677 Late effect of complication of pregnancy, childbirth, and the puerperium

Other Maternal and Fetal Complications (678-679)
678 Other fetal conditions
679 Complications of in utero procedures

12. DISEASES OF THE SKIN AND SUBCUTANEOUS TISSUE

Infections of skin and subcutaneous tissue (680–686)
680 Carbuncle and furuncle
681 Cellulitis and abscess of finger and toe
682 Other cellulitis and abscess
683 Acute lymphadenitis
684 Impetigo
685 Pilonidal cyst
686 Other local infections of skin and subcutaneous tissue

Other inflammatory conditions of skin and subcutaneous tissue (690–698)
690 Erythematosquamous dermatosis
691 Atopic dermatitis and related conditions
692 Contact dermatitis and other eczema
693 Dermatitis due to substances taken internally
694 Bullous dermatoses
695 Erythematous conditions
696 Psoriasis and similar disorders
697 Lichen
698 Pruritus and related conditions

Other diseases of skin and subcutaneous tissue (700–709)
700 Corns and callosities
701 Other hypertrophic and atrophic conditions of skin
702 Other dermatoses
703 Diseases of nail
704 Diseases of hair and hair follicles
705 Disorders of sweat glands
706 Diseases of sebaceous glands
707 Chronic ulcer of skin
708 Urticaria
709 Other disorders of skin and subcutaneous tissue

13. DISEASES OF THE MUSCULOSKELETAL SYSTEM AND CONNECTIVE TISSUE

Arthropathies and related disorders (710–719)
710 Diffuse diseases of connective tissue
711 Arthropathy associated with infections
712 Crystal arthropathies
713 Arthropathy associated with other disorders classified elsewhere
714 Rheumatoid arthritis and other inflammatory polyarthropathies
715 Osteoarthrosis and allied disorders
716 Other and unspecified arthropathies
717 Internal derangement of knee
718 Other derangement of joint
719 Other and unspecified disorder of joint

Dorsopathies (720–724)
720 Ankylosing spondylitis and other inflammatory spondylopathies
721 Spondylosis and allied disorders
722 Intervertebral disc disorders
723 Other disorders of cervical region
724 Other and unspecified disorders of back

Rheumatism, excluding the back (725–729)
725 Polymyalgia rheumatica
726 Peripheral enthesopathies and allied syndromes
727 Other disorders of synovium, tendon, and bursa
728 Disorders of muscle, ligament, and fascia
729 Other disorders of soft tissues

Osteopathies, chondropathies, and acquired musculoskeletal deformities (730–739)
730 Osteomyelitis, periostitis, and other infections involving bone
731 Osteitis deformans and osteopathies associated with other disorders classified elsewhere
732 Osteochondropathies
733 Other disorders of bone and cartilage
734 Flat foot
735 Acquired deformities of toe
736 Other acquired deformities of limbs
737 Curvature of spine
738 Other acquired deformity
739 Nonallopathic lesions, not elsewhere classified

14. CONGENITAL ANOMALIES

Congenital anomalies (740–759)
740 Anencephalus and similar anomalies
741 Spina bifida
742 Other congenital anomalies of nervous system
743 Congenital anomalies of eye
744 Congenital anomalies of ear, face, and neck
745 Bulbus cordis anomalies and anomalies of cardiac septal closure
746 Other congenital anomalies of heart
747 Other congenital anomalies of circulatory system
748 Congenital anomalies of respiratory system
749 Cleft palate and cleft lip
750 Other congenital anomalies of upper alimentary tract
751 Other congenital anomalies of digestive system
752 Congenital anomalies of genital organs
753 Congenital anomalies of urinary system
754 Certain congenital musculoskeletal deformities
755 Other congenital anomalies of limbs
756 Other congenital musculoskeletal anomalies
757 Congenital anomalies of the integument
758 Chromosomal anomalies
759 Other and unspecified congenital anomalies

15. CERTAIN CONDITIONS ORIGINATING IN THE PERINATAL PERIOD

Maternal causes of perinatal morbidity and mortality (760–763)
760   Fetus or newborn affected by maternal conditions which may be unrelated to present pregnancy
761   Fetus or newborn affected by maternal complications of pregnancy
762   Fetus or newborn affected by complications of placenta, cord, and membranes
763   Fetus or newborn affected by other complications of labor and delivery

Other conditions originating in the perinatal period (764–779)
764   Slow fetal growth and fetal malnutrition
765   Disorders relating to short gestation and unspecified low birthweight
766   Disorders relating to long gestation and high birthweight
767   Birth trauma
768   Intrauterine hypoxia and birth asphyxia
769   Respiratory distress syndrome
770   Other respiratory conditions of fetus and newborn
771   Infections specific to the perinatal period
772   Fetal and neonatal hemorrhage
773   Hemolytic disease of fetus or newborn, due to isoimmunization
774   Other perinatal jaundice
775   Endocrine and metabolic disturbances specific to the fetus and newborn
776   Hematological disorders of fetus and newborn
777   Perinatal disorders of digestive system
778   Conditions involving the integument and temperature regulation of fetus and newborn
779   Other and ill-defined conditions originating in the perinatal period

16. SYMPTOMS, SIGNS, AND ILL-DEFINED CONDITIONS

Symptoms (780–789)
780   General symptoms
781   Symptoms involving nervous and musculoskeletal systems
782   Symptoms involving skin and other integumentary tissue
783   Symptoms concerning nutrition, metabolism, and development
784   Symptoms involving head and neck
785   Symptoms involving cardiovascular system
786   Symptoms involving respiratory system and other chest symptoms
787   Symptoms involving digestive system
788   Symptoms involving urinary system
789   Other symptoms involving abdomen and pelvis

Nonspecific abnormal findings (790–796)
790   Nonspecific findings on examination of blood
791   Nonspecific findings on examination of urine
792   Nonspecific abnormal findings in other body substances
793   Nonspecific abnormal findings on radiological and other examination of body structure
794   Nonspecific abnormal results of function studies
795   Nonspecific abnormal histological and immunological findings
796   Other nonspecific abnormal findings

Ill-defined and unknown causes of morbidity and mortality (797–799)
797   Senility without mention of psychosis
798   Sudden death, cause unknown
799   Other ill-defined and unknown causes of morbidity and mortality

17. INJURY AND POISONING

Fracture of skull (800–804)
800   Fracture of vault of skull
801   Fracture of base of skull
802   Fracture of face bones
803   Other and unqualified skull fractures
804   Multiple fractures involving skull or face with other bones

Fracture of spine and trunk (805–809)
805   Fracture of vertebral column without mention of spinal cord lesion
806   Fracture of vertebral column with spinal cord lesion
807   Fracture of rib(s), sternum, larynx, and trachea
808   Fracture of pelvis
809   Ill-defined fractures of bones of trunk

Fracture of upper limb (810–819)
810   Fracture of clavicle
811   Fracture of scapula
812   Fracture of humerus
813   Fracture of radius and ulna
814   Fracture of carpal bone(s)
815   Fracture of metacarpal bone(s)
816   Fracture of one or more phalanges of hand
817   Multiple fractures of hand bones
818   Ill-defined fractures of upper limb
819   Multiple fractures involving both upper limbs, and upper limb with rib(s) and sternum

Fracture of lower limb (820–829)
820   Fracture of neck of femur
821   Fracture of other and unspecified parts of femur
822   Fracture of patella
823   Fracture of tibia and fibula
824   Fracture of ankle
825   Fracture of one or more tarsal and metatarsal bones
826   Fracture of one or more phalanges of foot
827   Other, multiple, and ill-defined fractures of lower limb
828   Multiple fractures involving both lower limbs, lower with upper limb, and lower limb(s) with rib(s) and sternum
829   Fracture of unspecified bones

Dislocation (830–839)
830   Dislocation of jaw
831   Dislocation of shoulder
832   Dislocation of elbow
833   Dislocation of wrist
834   Dislocation of finger
835   Dislocation of hip
836   Dislocation of knee
837   Dislocation of ankle
838   Dislocation of foot
839   Other, multiple, and ill-defined dislocations

Sprains and strains of joints and adjacent muscles (840–848)
840   Sprains and strains of shoulder and upper arm
841   Sprains and strains of elbow and forearm
842   Sprains and strains of wrist and hand
843   Sprains and strains of hip and thigh
844   Sprains and strains of knee and leg
845   Sprains and strains of ankle and foot
846   Sprains and strains of sacroiliac region
847   Sprains and strains of other and unspecified parts of back
848   Other and ill-defined sprains and strains

Intracranial injury, excluding those with skull fracture (850–854)
850   Concussion
851   Cerebral laceration and contusion
852   Subarachnoid, subdural, and extradural hemorrhage, following injury
853   Other and unspecified intracranial hemorrhage following injury
854   Intracranial injury of other and unspecified nature

Internal injury of chest, abdomen, and pelvis (860–869)
860   Traumatic pneumothorax and hemothorax
861   Injury to heart and lung
862   Injury to other and unspecified intrathoracic organs
863   Injury to gastrointestinal tract
864   Injury to liver
865   Injury to spleen
866   Injury to kidney
867   Injury to pelvic organs
868   Injury to other intra-abdominal organs
869   Internal injury to unspecified or ill-defined organs

Open wound of head, neck, and trunk (870–879)
870   Open wound of ocular adnexa
871   Open wound of eyeball
872   Open wound of ear
873   Other open wound of head
874   Open wound of neck
875   Open wound of chest (wall)
876   Open wound of back
877   Open wound of buttock
878   Open wound of genital organs (external), including traumatic amputation
879   Open wound of other and unspecified sites, except limbs

Open wound of upper limb (880–887)
880 Open wound of shoulder and upper arm
881 Open wound of elbow, forearm, and wrist
882 Open wound of hand except finger(s) alone
883 Open wound of finger(s)
884 Multiple and unspecified open wound of upper limb
885 Traumatic amputation of thumb (complete) (partial)
886 Traumatic amputation of other finger(s) (complete) (partial)
887 Traumatic amputation of arm and hand (complete) (partial)

Open wound of lower limb (890–897)
890 Open wound of hip and thigh
891 Open wound of knee, leg [except thigh], and ankle
892 Open wound of foot except toe(s) alone
893 Open wound of toe(s)
894 Multiple and unspecified open wound of lower limb
895 Traumatic amputation of toe(s) (complete) (partial)
896 Traumatic amputation of foot (complete) (partial)
897 Traumatic amputation of leg(s) (complete) (partial)

Injury to blood vessels (900–904)
900 Injury to blood vessels of head and neck
901 Injury to blood vessels of thorax
902 Injury to blood vessels of abdomen and pelvis
903 Injury to blood vessels of upper extremity
904 Injury to blood vessels of lower extremity and unspecified sites

Late effects of injuries, poisonings, toxic effects, and other external causes (905–909)
905 Late effects of musculoskeletal and connective tissue injuries
906 Late effects of injuries to skin and subcutaneous tissues
907 Late effects of injuries to the nervous system
908 Late effects of other and unspecified injuries
909 Late effects of other and unspecified external causes

Superficial injury (910–919)
910 Superficial injury of face, neck, and scalp except eye
911 Superficial injury of trunk
912 Superficial injury of shoulder and upper arm
913 Superficial injury of elbow, forearm, and wrist
914 Superficial injury of hand(s) except finger(s) alone
915 Superficial injury of finger(s)
916 Superficial injury of hip, thigh, leg, and ankle
917 Superficial injury of foot and toe(s)
918 Superficial injury of eye and adnexa
919 Superficial injury of other, multiple, and unspecified sites

Contusion with intact skin surface (920–924)
920 Contusion of face, scalp, and neck except eye(s)
921 Contusion of eye and adnexa
922 Contusion of trunk
923 Contusion of upper limb
924 Contusion of lower limb and of other and unspecified sites

Crushing injury (925–929)
925 Crushing injury of face, scalp, and neck
926 Crushing injury of trunk
927 Crushing injury of upper limb
928 Crushing injury of lower limb
929 Crushing injury of multiple and unspecified sites

Effects of foreign body entering through orifice (930–939)
930 Foreign body on external eye
931 Foreign body in ear
932 Foreign body in nose
933 Foreign body in pharynx and larynx
934 Foreign body in trachea, bronchus, and lung
935 Foreign body in mouth, esophagus, and stomach
936 Foreign body in intestine and colon
937 Foreign body in anus and rectum
938 Foreign body in digestive system, unspecified
939 Foreign body in genitourinary tract

Burns (940–949)
940 Burn confined to eye and adnexa
941 Burn of face, head, and neck
942 Burn of trunk
943 Burn of upper limb, except wrist and hand
944 Burn of wrist(s) and hand(s)
945 Burn of lower limb(s)
946 Burns of multiple specified sites
947 Burn of internal organs
948 Burns classified according to extent of body surface involved
949 Burn, unspecified

Injury to nerves and spinal cord (950–957)
950 Injury to optic nerve and pathways
951 Injury to other cranial nerve(s)
952 Spinal cord injury without evidence of spinal bone injury
953 Injury to nerve roots and spinal plexus
954 Injury to other nerve(s) of trunk excluding shoulder and pelvic girdles
955 Injury to peripheral nerve(s) of shoulder girdle and upper limb
956 Injury to peripheral nerve(s) of pelvic girdle and lower limb
957 Injury to other and unspecified nerves

Certain traumatic complications and unspecified injuries (958–959)
958 Certain early complications of trauma
959 Injury, other and unspecified

Poisoning by drugs, medicinals and biological substances (960–979)
960 Poisoning by antibiotics
961 Poisoning by other anti-infectives
962 Poisoning by hormones and synthetic substitutes
963 Poisoning by primarily systemic agents
964 Poisoning by agents primarily affecting blood constituents
965 Poisoning by analgesics, antipyretics, and antirheumatics
966 Poisoning by anticonvulsants and anti-Parkinsonism drugs
967 Poisoning by sedatives and hypnotics
968 Poisoning by other central nervous system depressants and anesthetics
969 Poisoning by psychotropic agents
970 Poisoning by central nervous system stimulants
971 Poisoning by drugs primarily affecting the autonomic nervous system
972 Poisoning by agents primarily affecting the cardiovascular system
973 Poisoning by agents primarily affecting the gastrointestinal system
974 Poisoning by water, mineral, and uric acid metabolism drugs
975 Poisoning by agents primarily acting on the smooth and skeletal muscles and respiratory system
976 Poisoning by agents primarily affecting skin and mucous membrane, ophthalmological, otorhinolaryngological, and dental drugs
977 Poisoning by other and unspecified drugs and medicinals
978 Poisoning by bacterial vaccines
979 Poisoning by other vaccines and biological substances

Toxic effects of substances chiefly nonmedicinal as to source (980–989)
980 Toxic effect of alcohol
981 Toxic effect of petroleum products
982 Toxic effect of solvents other than petroleum-based
983 Toxic effect of corrosive aromatics, acids, and caustic alkalis
984 Toxic effect of lead and its compounds (including fumes)
985 Toxic effect of other metals
986 Toxic effect of carbon monoxide
987 Toxic effect of other gases, fumes, or vapors
988 Toxic effect of noxious substances eaten as food
989 Toxic effect of other substances, chiefly nonmedicinal as to source

Other and unspecified effects of external causes (990–995)
990 Effects of radiation, unspecified
991 Effects of reduced temperature
992 Effects of heat and light
993 Effects of air pressure
994 Effects of other external causes
995 Certain adverse effects, not elsewhere classified

Complications of surgical and medical care, not elsewhere classified (996–999)
996 Complications peculiar to certain specified procedures
997 Complications affecting specified body systems, not elsewhere classified
998 Other complications of procedures, not elsewhere classified
999 Complications of medical care, not elsewhere classified

ICD-9-CM, APPENDIX E

SUPPLEMENTARY CLASSIFICATION OF FACTORS INFLUENCING HEALTH STATUS AND CONTACT WITH HEALTH SERVICES (V01–V86)

Persons with potential health hazards related to communicable diseases (V01–V09)
V01   Contact with or exposure to communicable diseases
V02   Carrier or suspected carrier of infectious diseases
V03   Need for prophylactic vaccination and inoculation against bacterial diseases
V04   Need for prophylactic vaccination and inoculation against certain viral diseases
V05   Need for other prophylactic vaccination and inoculation against single diseases
V06   Need for prophylactic vaccination and inoculation against combinations of diseases
V07   Need for isolation and other prophylactic measures
V08   Asymptomatic human immunodeficiency virus [HIV] infection status
V09   Infection with drug-resistant microorganisms

Persons with potential health hazards related to personal and family history (V10–V19)
V10   Personal history of malignant neoplasm
V11   Personal history of mental disorder
V12   Personal history of certain other diseases
V13   Personal history of other diseases
V14   Personal history of allergy to medicinal agents
V15   Other personal history presenting hazards to health
V16   Family history of malignant neoplasm
V17   Family history of certain chronic disabling diseases
V18   Family history of certain other specific conditions
V19   Family history of other conditions

Persons encountering health services in circumstances related to reproduction and development (V20–V29)
V20   Health supervision of infant or child
V21   Constitutional states in development
V22   Normal pregnancy
V23   Supervision of high-risk pregnancy
V24   Postpartum care and examination
V25   Encounter for contraceptive management
V26   Procreative management
V27   Outcome of delivery
V28   Antenatal screening
V29   Observation and evaluation of newborns and infants for suspected condition not found

Liveborn infants according to type of birth (V30–V39)
V30   Single liveborn
V31   Twin, mate liveborn
V32   Twin, mate stillborn
V33   Twin, unspecified
V34   Other multiple, mates all liveborn
V35   Other multiple, mates all stillborn
V36   Other multiple, mates live- and stillborn
V37   Other multiple, unspecified
V39   Unspecified

Persons with a condition influencing their health status (V40–V49)
V40   Mental and behavioral problems
V41   Problems with special senses and other special functions
V42   Organ or tissue replaced by transplant
V43   Organ or tissue replaced by other means
V44   Artificial opening status
V45   Other postsurgical states
V46   Other dependence on machines
V47   Other problems with internal organs
V48   Problems with head, neck, and trunk
V49   Problems with limbs and other problems

Persons encountering health services for specific procedures and aftercare (V50–V59)
V50   Elective surgery for purposes other than remedying health states
V51   Aftercare involving the use of plastic surgery
V52   Fitting and adjustment of prosthetic device
V53   Fitting and adjustment of other device
V54   Other orthopedic aftercare
V55   Attention to artificial openings
V56   Encounter for dialysis and dialysis catheter care
V57   Care involving use of rehabilitation procedures
V58   Other and unspecified aftercare
V59   Donors

Persons encountering health services in other circumstances (V60–V69)
V60   Housing, household, and economic circumstances
V61   Other family circumstances
V62   Other psychosocial circumstances
V63   Unavailability of other medical facilities for care
V64   Persons encountering health services for specific procedures, not carried out
V65   Other persons seeking consultation without complaint or sickness
V66   Convalescence and palliative care
V67   Follow-up examination
V68   Encounters for administrative purposes
V69   Problems related to lifestyle

Persons without reported diagnosis encountered during examination and investigation of individuals and populations (V70–V82)
V70   General medical examination
V71   Observation and evaluation for suspected conditions
V72   Special investigations and examinations
V73   Special screening examination for viral and chlamydial diseases
V74   Special screening examination for bacterial and spirochetal diseases
V75   Special screening examination for other infectious diseases
V76   Special screening for malignant neoplasms
V77   Special screening for endocrine, nutritional, metabolic, and immunity disorders
V78   Special screening for disorders of blood and blood-forming organs
V79   Special screening for mental disorders and developmental handicaps
V80   Special screening for neurological, eye, and ear diseases
V81   Special screening for cardiovascular, respiratory, and genitourinary diseases
V82   Special screening for other conditions

Genetics (V83–V84)
V83   Genetic carrier status
V84   Genetic susceptibility to malignant neoplasm

Body Mass Index (V85)
V85   Body mass index

Estrogen Receptor Status (V86)
V86   Estrogen receptor status

Other specified personal exposures and history presenting hazards to health (V87)
V87   Other specified personal exposures and history presenting hazards to health

Acquired absence of other organs and tissue (V88)
V88   Acquired absence of other organs and tissue

Other suspected conditions not found (V89)
V89   Other suspected conditions not found

SUPPLEMENTARY CLASSIFICATION OF EXTERNAL CAUSES OF INJURY AND POISONING (E800–E899)

Railway accidents (E800–E807)
E800   Railway accident involving collision with rolling stock
E801   Railway accident involving collision with other object
E802   Railway accident involving derailment without antecedent collision
E803   Railway accident involving explosion, fire, or burning
E804   Fall in, on, or from railway train
E805   Hit by rolling stock
E806   Other specified railway accident
E807   Railway accident of unspecified nature

Motor vehicle traffic accidents (E810–E819)
E810   Motor vehicle traffic accident involving collision with train
E811   Motor vehicle traffic accident involving re-entrant collision with another motor vehicle
E812   Other motor vehicle traffic accident involving collision with another motor vehicle
E813   Motor vehicle traffic accident involving collision with other vehicle
E814   Motor vehicle traffic accident involving collision with pedestrian

E815 Other motor vehicle traffic accident involving collision on the highway
E816 Motor vehicle traffic accident due to loss of control, without collision on the highway
E817 Noncollision motor vehicle traffic accident while boarding or alighting
E818 Other noncollision motor vehicle traffic accident
E819 Motor vehicle traffic accident of unspecified nature

Motor vehicle nontraffic accidents (E820–E825)
E820 Nontraffic accident involving motor-driven snow vehicle
E821 Nontraffic accident involving other off-road motor vehicle
E822 Other motor vehicle nontraffic accident involving collision with moving object
E823 Other motor vehicle nontraffic accident involving collision with stationary object
E824 Other motor vehicle nontraffic accident while boarding and alighting
E825 Other motor vehicle nontraffic accident of other and unspecified nature

Other road vehicle accidents (E826–E829)
E826 Pedal cycle accident
E827 Animal-drawn vehicle accident
E828 Accident involving animal being ridden
E829 Other road vehicle accidents

Water transport accidents (E830–E838)
E830 Accident to watercraft causing submersion
E831 Accident to watercraft causing other injury
E832 Other accidental submersion or drowning in water transport accident
E833 Fall on stairs or ladders in water transport
E834 Other fall from one level to another in water transport
E835 Other and unspecified fall in water transport
E836 Machinery accident in water transport
E837 Explosion, fire, or burning in watercraft
E838 Other and unspecified water transport accident

Air and space transport accidents (E840–E845)
E840 Accident to powered aircraft at takeoff or landing
E841 Accident to powered aircraft, other and unspecified
E842 Accident to unpowered aircraft
E843 Fall in, on, or from aircraft
E844 Other specified air transport accidents
E845 Accident involving spacecraft

Vehicle accidents, not elsewhere classifiable (E846–E849)
E846 Accidents involving powered vehicles used solely within the buildings and premises of an industrial or commercial establishment
E847 Accidents involving cable cars not running on rails
E848 Accidents involving other vehicles, not elsewhere classifiable
E849 Place of occurrence

Accidental poisoning by drugs, medicinal substances, and biologicals (E850–E858)
E850 Accidental poisoning by analgesics, antipyretics, and antirheumatics
E851 Accidental poisoning by barbiturates
E852 Accidental poisoning by other sedatives and hypnotics
E853 Accidental poisoning by tranquilizers
E854 Accidental poisoning by other psychotropic agents
E855 Accidental poisoning by other drugs acting on central and autonomic nervous systems
E856 Accidental poisoning by antibiotics
E857 Accidental poisoning by anti-infectives
E858 Accidental poisoning by other drugs

Accidental poisoning by other solid and liquid substances, gases, and vapors (E860–E869)
E860 Accidental poisoning by alcohol, not elsewhere classified
E861 Accidental poisoning by cleansing and polishing agents, disinfectants, paints, and varnishes
E862 Accidental poisoning by petroleum products, other solvents and their vapors, not elsewhere classified
E863 Accidental poisoning by agricultural and horticultural chemical and pharmaceutical preparations other than plant foods and fertilizers
E864 Accidental poisoning by corrosives and caustics, not elsewhere classified

E865 Accidental poisoning from poisonous foodstuffs and poisonous plants
E866 Accidental poisoning by other and unspecified solid and liquid substances
E867 Accidental poisoning by gas distributed by pipeline
E868 Accidental poisoning by other utility gas and other carbon monoxide
E869 Accidental poisoning by other gases and vapors

Misadventures to patients during surgical and medical care (E870–E876)
E870 Accidental cut, puncture, perforation, or hemorrhage during medical care
E871 Foreign object left in body during procedure
E872 Failure of sterile precautions during procedure
E873 Failure in dosage
E874 Mechanical failure of instrument or apparatus during procedure
E875 Contaminated or infected blood, other fluid, drug, or biological substance
E876 Other and unspecified misadventures during medical care

Surgical and medical procedures as the cause of abnormal reaction of patient or later complication, without mention of misadventure at the time of procedure (E878–E879)
E878 Surgical operation and other surgical procedures as the cause of abnormal reaction of patient, or of later complication, without mention of misadventure at the time of operation
E879 Other procedures, without mention of misadventure at the time of procedure, as the cause of abnormal reaction of patient, or of later complication

Accidental falls (E880–E888)
E880 Fall on or from stairs or steps
E881 Fall on or from ladders or scaffolding
E882 Fall from or out of building or other structure
E883 Fall into hole or other opening in surface
E884 Other fall from one level to another
E885 Fall on same level from slipping, tripping, or stumbling
E886 Fall on same level from collision, pushing, or shoving, by or with other person
E887 Fracture, cause unspecified
E888 Other and unspecified fall

Accidents caused by fire and flames (E890–E899)
E890 Conflagration in private dwelling
E891 Conflagration in other and unspecified building or structure
E892 Conflagration not in building or structure
E893 Accident caused by ignition of clothing
E894 Ignition of highly inflammable material
E895 Accident caused by controlled fire in private dwelling
E896 Accident caused by controlled fire in other and unspecified building or structure
E897 Accident caused by controlled fire not in building or structure
E898 Accident caused by other specified fire and flames
E899 Accident caused by unspecified fire

Accidents due to natural and environmental factors (E900–E909)
E900 Excessive heat
E901 Excessive cold
E902 High and low air pressure and changes in air pressure
E903 Travel and motion
E904 Hunger, thirst, exposure, and neglect
E905 Venomous animals and plants as the cause of poisoning and toxic reactions
E906 Other injury caused by animals
E907 Lightning
E908 Cataclysmic storms, and floods resulting from storms
E909 Cataclysmic earth surface movements and eruptions

Accidents caused by submersion, suffocation, and foreign bodies (E910–E915)
E910 Accidental drowning and submersion
E911 Inhalation and ingestion of food causing obstruction of respiratory tract or suffocation
E912 Inhalation and ingestion of other object causing obstruction of respiratory tract or suffocation
E913 Accidental mechanical suffocation
E914 Foreign body accidentally entering eye and adnexa
E915 Foreign body accidentally entering other orifice

Other accidents (E916–E928)

E916 Struck accidentally by falling object
E917 Striking against or struck accidentally by objects or persons
E918 Caught accidentally in or between objects
E919 Accidents caused by machinery
E920 Accidents caused by cutting and piercing instruments or objects
E921 Accident caused by explosion of pressure vessel
E922 Accident caused by firearm missile
E923 Accident caused by explosive material
E924 Accident caused by hot substance or object, caustic or corrosive material, and steam
E925 Accident caused by electric current
E926 Exposure to radiation
E927 Overexertion and strenuous movements
E928 Other and unspecified environmental and accidental causes

Late effects of accidental injury (E929)

E929 Late effects of accidental injury

Drugs, medicinal and biological substances causing adverse effects in therapeutic use (E930–E949)

E930 Antibiotics
E931 Other anti-infectives
E932 Hormones and synthetic substitutes
E933 Primarily systemic agents
E934 Agents primarily affecting blood constituents
E935 Analgesics, antipyretics, and antirheumatics
E936 Anticonvulsants and anti-Parkinsonism drugs
E937 Sedatives and hypnotics
E938 Other central nervous system depressants and anesthetics
E939 Psychotropic agents
E940 Central nervous system stimulants
E941 Drugs primarily affecting the autonomic nervous system
E942 Agents primarily affecting the cardiovascular system
E943 Agents primarily affecting gastrointestinal system
E944 Water, mineral, and uric acid metabolism drugs
E945 Agents primarily acting on the smooth and skeletal muscles and respiratory system
E946 Agents primarily affecting skin and mucous membrane, ophthalmological, otorhinolaryngological, and dental drugs
E947 Other and unspecified drugs and medicinal substances
E948 Bacterial vaccines
E949 Other vaccines and biological substances

Suicide and self-inflicted injury (E950–E959)

E950 Suicide and self-inflicted poisoning by solid or liquid substances
E951 Suicide and self-inflicted poisoning by gases in domestic use
E952 Suicide and self-inflicted poisoning by other gases and vapors
E953 Suicide and self-inflicted injury by hanging, strangulation, and suffocation
E954 Suicide and self-inflicted injury by submersion [drowning]
E955 Suicide and self-inflicted injury by firearms and explosives
E956 Suicide and self-inflicted injury by cutting and piercing instruments
E957 Suicide and self-inflicted injuries by jumping from high place
E958 Suicide and self-inflicted injury by other and unspecified means
E959 Late effects of self-inflicted injury

Homicide and injury purposely inflicted by other persons (E960–E969)

E960 Fight, brawl, and rape
E961 Assault by corrosive or caustic substance, except poisoning

E962 Assault by poisoning
E963 Assault by hanging and strangulation
E964 Assault by submersion [drowning]
E965 Assault by firearms and explosives
E966 Assault by cutting and piercing instrument
E967 Child and adult battering and other maltreatment
E968 Assault by other and unspecified means
E969 Late effects of injury purposely inflicted by other person

Legal intervention (E970–E978)

E970 Injury due to legal intervention by firearms
E971 Injury due to legal intervention by explosives
E972 Injury due to legal intervention by gas
E973 Injury due to legal intervention by blunt object
E974 Injury due to legal intervention by cutting and piercing instruments
E975 Injury due to legal intervention by other specified means
E976 Injury due to legal intervention by unspecified means
E977 Late effects of injuries due to legal intervention
E978 Legal execution
E979 Terrorism

Injury undetermined whether accidentally or purposely inflicted (E980–E989)

E980 Poisoning by solid or liquid substances, undetermined whether accidentally or purposely inflicted
E981 Poisoning by gases in domestic use, undetermined whether accidentally or purposely inflicted
E982 Poisoning by other gases, undetermined whether accidentally or purposely inflicted
E983 Hanging, strangulation, or suffocation, undetermined whether accidentally or purposely inflicted
E984 Submersion [drowning], undetermined whether accidentally or purposely inflicted
E985 Injury by firearms and explosives, undetermined whether accidentally or purposely inflicted
E986 Injury by cutting and piercing instruments, undetermined whether accidentally or purposely inflicted
E987 Falling from high place, undetermined whether accidentally or purposely inflicted
E988 Injury by other and unspecified means, undetermined whether accidentally or purposely inflicted
E989 Late effects of injury, undetermined whether accidentally or purposely inflicted

Injury resulting from operations of war (E990–E999)

E990 Injury due to war operations by fires and conflagrations
E991 Injury due to war operations by bullets and fragments
E992 Injury due to war operations by explosion of marine weapons
E993 Injury due to war operations by other explosion
E994 Injury due to war operations by destruction of aircraft
E995 Injury due to war operations by other and unspecified forms of conventional warfare
E996 Injury due to war operations by nuclear weapons
E997 Injury due to war operations by other forms of unconventional warfare
E998 Injury due to war operations but occurring after cessation of hostilities
E999 Late effects of injury due to war operations

TABLE A

TABLE OF BACTERIAL FOOD POISONING

Bacteria Responsible	Description	Habitat	Types of Foods	Symptoms	Cause	Temperature Sensitivity
Staphylococcus aureus	Produces a heat-stable toxin.	Nose and throat of 30 to 50 percent of healthy population; also skin and superficial wounds.	Meat and seafood salads, sandwich spreads, and high salt foods.	Nausea, vomiting, and diarrhea within 4 to 6 hours. No fever.	Poor personal hygiene and subsequent temperature abuse.	No growth below 40° F. Bacteria are destroyed by normal cooking, but toxin is heat-stable.
Clostridium perfringens	Produces a spore and prefers low oxygen atmosphere. Live cells must be ingested.	Dust, soil, and gastrointestinal tracts of animals and man.	Meat and poultry dishes, sauces and gravies.	Cramps and diarrhea within 12 to 24 hours. No vomiting or fever.	Improper temperature control of hot foods and recontamination.	No growth below 40° F. Bacteria are killed by normal cooking, but a heat-stable spore can survive.
Clostridium botulinum	Produces a spore and requires a low oxygen atmosphere. Produces a heat-sensitive toxin.	Soils, plants, marine sediments, and fish.	Home-canned foods.	Blurred vision, respiratory distress, and possible DEATH.	Improper methods of home-processing foods.	Type E and Type B can grow at 38° F. Bacteria destroyed by cooking and the toxin is destroyed by boiling for 5 to 10 minutes. Heat-resistant spore can survive.
Vibrio parahaemolyticus	Requires salt for growth.	Fish and shellfish.	Raw and cooked seafood.	Diarrhea, cramps, vomiting, headache, and fever within 12 to 24 hours.	Recontamination of cooked foods or eating raw seafood.	No growth below 40° F. Bacteria killed by normal cooking.

Procedures
Volume 3

A

Abbe operation
 construction of vagina 70.61
  with graft or prosthesis 70.63
 intestinal anastomosis - *see* Anastomosis,
  intestine
Abciximab, infusion 99.20
Abdominocentesis 54.91
Abdominohysterectomy 68.49
 laparoscopic 68.41
Abdominoplasty 86.83
Abdominoscopy 54.21
Abdominouterotomy 68.0
 obstetrical 74.99
Abduction, arytenoid 31.69
AbioCor® total replacement heart 37.52
Ablation
 biliary tract (lesion) by ERCP 51.64
 endometrial (hysteroscopic) 68.23
 inner ear (cryosurgery) (ultrasound) 20.79
  by injection 20.72
 lesion
  esophagus 42.39
   endoscopic 42.33
  heart
   by peripherally inserted catheter
    37.34
   endovascular approach 37.34
   maze procedure (Cox-maze)
    endovascular approach 37.34
    open approach 37.33
    thoracoscopic approach 37.37
   thoracoscopic approach 37.37
  intestine
   large 45.49
    endoscopic 45.43
  large intestine 45.49
   endoscopic 45.43
  liver 50.26
   laparoscopic 50.25
   open 50.23
   percutaneous 50.24
  lung 32.26
   bronchoscopic thermoplasty 32.27
   open 32.23
   percutaneous 32.24
   thoracoscopic 32.25
  renal 55.35
   laparoscopic 55.34
   open 55.32
   percutaneous 55.33
 pituitary 07.69
  by
   Cobalt-60 92.32
   implantation (strontium-yttrium) (Y)
    NEC 07.68
    transfrontal approach 07.64
    transphenoidal approach 07.65
   proton beam (Bragg peak) 92.33
 prostate
  by
   cryoablation 60.62
   laser, transurethral 60.21
   radical cryosurgical ablation (RCSA)
    60.62
   radiofrequency thermotherapy 60.97
   transurethral needle ablation (TUNA)
    60.97
 tissue
  heart - *see* Ablation, lesion, heart
  liver - *see* Ablation, lesion, liver
  lung - *see* Ablation, lesion, lung
  renal - *see* Ablation, lesion, renal
Abortion, therapeutic 69.51
 by
  aspiration curettage 69.51
  dilation and curettage 69.01
  hysterectomy - *see* Hysterectomy
  hysterotomy 74.91

Abortion, therapeutic (*Continued*)
 by (*Continued*)
  insertion
   laminaria 69.93
   prostaglandin suppository 96.49
  intra-amniotic injection (saline) 75.0
Abrasion
 corneal epithelium 11.41
  for smear or culture 11.21
 epicardial surface 36.39
 pleural 34.6
 skin 86.25
Abscission, cornea 11.49
Absorptiometry
 photon (dual) (single) 88.98
Aburel operation (intra-amniotic injection for
  abortion) 75.0
Accouchement forcé 73.99
Acetabulectomy 77.85
Acetabuloplasty NEC 81.40
 with prosthetic implant 81.52
Achillorrhaphy 83.64
 delayed 83.62
Achillotenotomy 83.11
 plastic 83.85
Achillotomy 83.11
 plastic 83.85
Acid peel, skin 86.24
Acromionectomy 77.81
Acromioplasty 81.83
 for recurrent dislocation of shoulder 81.82
 partial replacement 81.81
 total replacement, NEC 81.80
  other 81.80
  reverse 81.88
Actinotherapy 99.82
Activities of daily living (ADL)
 therapy 93.83
 training for the blind 93.78
Acupuncture 99.92
 with smouldering moxa 93.35
 for anesthesia 99.91
Adams operation
 advancement of round ligament 69.22
 crushing of nasal septum 21.88
 excision of palmar fascia 82.35
Adenectomy - *see also* Excision, by site
 prostate NEC 60.69
 retropubic 60.4
Adenoidectomy (without tonsillectomy) 28.6
 with tonsillectomy 28.3
Adhesiolysis - *see also* Lysis, adhesions
 for collapse of lung 33.39
 middle ear 20.23
Adipectomy 86.83
Adjustment
 cardiac pacemaker program
  (reprogramming) - *omit code*
 cochlear prosthetic device (external
  components) 95.49
 dental 99.97
 gastric restrictive device (laparoscopic) 44.98
 occlusal 24.8
 orthopedic device (noninvasive)
  external fixator - *omit code*
 spectacles 95.31
Administration (of) - *see also* Injection
 Activase® 99.10
 adhesion barrier substance 99.77
 Alteplase (tPA, generic) 99.10
 Anistreplase (tPA, generic) 99.10
 antitoxins NEC 99.58
  botulism 99.57
  diphtheria 99.58
  gas gangrene 99.58
  scarlet fever 99.58
  tetanus 99.56
 Bender Visual-Motor Gestalt test 94.02
 Benton Visual Retention test 94.02
 DrotAA 00.11

Administration (*Continued*)
 Eminase® 99.10
 inhaled nitric oxide 00.12
 intelligence test or scale (Stanford-Binet)
  (Wechsler) (adult) (children) 94.01
  Minnesota Multiphasic Personality
   Inventory (MMPI) 94.02
  MMPI (Minnesota Multiphasic
   Personality Inventory) 94.02
 neuroprotective agent 99.75
 Proleukin® (low-dose) 99.28
  high-dose 00.15
 psychologic test 94.02
 Retavase® 99.10
 Reteplase (tPA, generic) 99.10
 Stanford-Binet test 94.01
 Streptase® 99.10
 Streptokinase (tPA, generic) 99.10
 Tenecteplase (tPA, generic) 99.10
 TNKase™ 99.10
 toxoid
  diphtheria 99.36
   with tetanus and pertussis, combined
    (DTP) 99.39
  tetanus 99.38
   with diphtheria and pertussis,
    combined (DTP) 99.39
 vaccine - *see also* Vaccination
  BCG 99.33
  measles-mumps-rubella (MMR) 99.48
  poliomyelitis 99.41
  TAB 99.32
 Wechsler
  Intelligence Scale (adult) (children) 94.01
  Memory Scale 94.02
 Xigris® 00.11
Adrenalectomy (unilateral) 07.22
 with partial removal of remaining gland
  07.29
 bilateral 07.3
  partial 07.29
  subtotal 07.29
 complete 07.3
 partial NEC 07.29
 remaining gland 07.3
 subtotal NEC 07.29
 total 07.3
Adrenalorrhaphy 07.44
Adrenalotomy (with drainage) 07.41
Advancement
 extraocular muscle 15.12
  multiple (with resection or recession) 15.3
 eyelid muscle 08.59
 eye muscle 15.12
  multiple (with resection or recession) 15.3
 graft - *see* Graft
 leaflet (heart) 35.10
 pedicle (flap) 86.72
 profundus tendon (Wagner) 82.51
 round ligament 69.22
 tendon 83.71
  hand 82.51
  profundus (Wagner) 82.51
 Wagner (profundus tendon) 82.51
AESOP® (Automated Endoscopic System for
  Optimal Positioning) - *see* category 17.4●
Albee operation
 bone peg, femoral neck 78.05
 graft for slipping patella 78.06
 sliding inlay graft, tibia 78.07
Albert operation (arthrodesis of knee) 81.22
Aldridge (-Studdiford) operation (urethral
  sling) 59.5
Alexander operation
 prostatectomy
  perineal 60.62
  suprapubic 60.3
 shortening of round ligaments 69.22
Alexander-Adams operation (shortening of
  round ligaments) 69.22

Alimentation, parenteral 99.29
Allograft - *see* Graft
Almoor operation (extrapetrosal drainage) 20.22
Altemeier operation (perineal rectal pull-through) 48.49
Alveolectomy (interradicular) (intraseptal) (radical) (simple) (with graft) (with implant) 24.5
Alveoloplasty (with graft or implant) 24.5
Alveolotomy (apical) 24.0
Ambulatory cardiac monitoring (ACM) 89.50
Ammon operation (dacryocystotomy) 09.53
Amniocentesis (transuterine) (diagnostic) 75.1
  with intra-amniotic injection of saline 75.0
Amniography 87.81
Amnioinfusion 75.37
Amnioscopy, internal 75.31
Amniotomy 73.09
  to induce labor 73.01
Amputation (cineplastic) (closed flap) (guillotine) (kineplastic) (open) 84.91
  abdominopelvic 84.19
  above-elbow 84.07
  above-knee (AK) 84.17
  ankle (disarticulation) 84.13
    through malleoli of tibia and fibula 84.14
  arm NEC 84.00
    through
      carpals 84.03
      elbow (disarticulation) 84.06
      forearm 84.05
      humerus 84.07
      shoulder (disarticulation) 84.08
      wrist (disarticulation) 84.04
    upper 84.07
  Batch-Spittler-McFaddin (knee disarticulation) 84.16
  below-knee (BK) NEC 84.15
    conversion into above-knee amputation 84.17
  Boyd (hip disarticulation) 84.18
  Callander's (knee disarticulation) 84.16
  carpals 84.03
  cervix 67.4
  Chopart's (midtarsal) 84.12
  clitoris 71.4
  Dieffenbach (hip disarticulation) 84.18
  Dupuytren's (shoulder disarticulation) 84.08
  ear, external 18.39
  elbow (disarticulation) 84.06
  finger, except thumb 84.01
    thumb 84.02
  foot (middle) 84.12
  forearm 84.05
  forefoot 84.12
  forequarter 84.09
  Gordon-Taylor (hindquarter) 84.19
  Gritti-Stokes (knee disarticulation) 84.16
  Guyon (ankle) 84.13
  hallux 84.11
  hand 84.03
  Hey's (foot) 84.12
  hindquarter 84.19
  hip (disarticulation) 84.18
  humerus 84.07
  interscapulothoracic 84.09
  interthoracoscapular 84.09
  King-Steelquist (hindquarter) 84.19
  Kirk (thigh) 84.17
  knee (disarticulation) 84.16
  Kutler (revision of current traumatic amputation of finger) 84.01
  Larry (shoulder disarticulation) 84.08
  leg NEC 84.10
    above knee (AK) 84.17
    below knee (BK) 84.15
    through
      ankle (disarticulation) 84.13
      femur (AK) 84.17
      foot 84.12

Amputation (Continued)
  leg NEC (Continued)
    through (Continued)
      hip (disarticulation) 84.18
      tibia and fibula (BK) 84.15
  Lisfranc
    foot 84.12
    shoulder (disarticulation) 84.08
  Littlewood (forequarter) 84.09
  lower limb NEC - *see also* Amputation, leg 84.10
  Mazet (knee disarticulation) 84.16
  metacarpal 84.03
  metatarsal 84.11
    head (bunionectomy) 77.59
  metatarsophalangeal (joint) 84.11
  midtarsal 84.12
  nose 21.4
  penis (circle) (complete) (flap) (partial) (radical) 64.3
  Pirogoff's (ankle amputation through malleoli of tibia and fibula) 84.14
  ray
    finger 84.01
    foot 84.11
    toe (metatarsal head) 84.11
  root (apex) (tooth) 23.73
    with root canal therapy 23.72
  shoulder (disarticulation) 84.08
  Sorondo-Ferre (hindquarter) 84.19
  S. P. Rogers (knee disarticulation) 84.16
  supracondylar, above-knee 84.17
  supramalleolar, foot 84.14
  Syme's (ankle amputation through malleoli of tibia and fibula) 84.14
  thigh 84.17
  thumb 84.02
  toe (through metatarsophalangeal joint) 84.11
  transcarpal 84.03
  transmetatarsal 84.12
  upper limb NEC - *see also* Amputation, arm 84.00
  wrist (disarticulation) 84.04
Amygdalohippocampectomy 01.59
Amygdalohippocampotomy 01.39
Amygdalotomy 01.39
Analysis
  cardiac rhythm device (AICD) (CRT-D) (CRT-P) (pacemaker) - *see* Interrogation
  character 94.03
  gastric 89.39
  psychologic 94.31
  transactional
    group 94.44
    individual 94.39
Anastomosis
  abdominal artery to coronary artery 37.17
  accessory-facial nerve 04.72
  accessory-hypoglossal nerve 04.73
  anus (with formation of endorectal ileal pouch) 45.95
  aorta (descending)-pulmonary (artery) 39.0
  aorta-renal artery 39.24
  aorta-subclavian artery 39.22
  aortoceliac 39.26
  aorto(ilio)femoral 39.25
  aortomesenteric 39.26
  appendix 47.99
  arteriovenous NEC 39.29
    for renal dialysis 39.27
  artery (suture of distal to proximal end) 39.31
    with
      bypass graft 39.29
        extracranial-intracranial [EC-IC] 39.28
      excision or resection of vessel - *see* Arteriectomy, with anastomosis, by site
    revision 39.49
  bile ducts 51.39

Anastomosis (Continued)
  bladder NEC 57.88
    with
      isolated segment of intestine 57.87 [45.50]
        colon (sigmoid) 57.87 [45.52]
        ileum 57.87 [45.51]
        open loop of ileum 57.87 [45.51]
      to intestine 57.88
        ileum 57.87 [45.51]
  bowel - *see also* Anastomosis, intestine 45.90
  bronchotracheal 33.48
  bronchus 33.48
  carotid-subclavian artery 39.22
  caval-mesenteric vein 39.1
  caval-pulmonary artery 39.21
  cervicoesophageal 42.59
  colohypopharyngeal (intrathoracic) 42.55
    antesternal or antethoracic 42.65
  common bile duct 51.39
  common pulmonary trunk and left atrium (posterior wall) 35.82
  cystic bile duct 51.39
  cystocolic 57.88
  epididymis to vas deferens 63.83
  esophagocolic (intrathoracic) NEC 42.56
    with interposition 42.55
    antesternal or antethoracic NEC 42.66
      with interposition 42.65
  esophagocologastric (intrathoracic) 42.55
    antesternal or antethoracic 42.65
  esophagoduodenal (intrathoracic) NEC 42.54
    with interposition 42.53
  esophagoenteric (intrathoracic) NEC - *see also* Anastomosis, esophagus, to intestinal segment 42.54
    antesternal or antethoracic NEC - *see also* Anastomosis, esophagus, antesternal, to intestinal segment 42.64
  esophagoesophageal (intrathoracic) 42.51
    antesternal or antethoracic 42.61
  esophagogastric (intrathoracic) 42.52
    antesternal or antethoracic 42.62
  esophagus (intrapleural) (intrathoracic) (retrosternal) NEC 42.59
    with
      gastrectomy (partial) 43.5
        complete or total 43.99
      interposition (of) NEC 42.58
        colon 42.55
        jejunum 42.53
        small bowel 42.53
    antesternal or antethoracic NEC 42.69
      with
        interposition (of) NEC 42.68
          colon 42.65
          jejunal loop 42.63
          small bowel 42.63
        rubber tube 42.68
      to intestinal segment NEC 42.64
        with interposition 42.68
        colon NEC 42.66
          with interposition 42.65
        small bowel NEC 42.64
          with interposition 42.63
    to intestinal segment (intrathoracic) NEC 42.54
      with interposition 42.58
      antesternal or antethoracic NEC 42.64
        with interposition 42.68
      colon (intrathoracic) NEC 42.56
        with interposition 42.55
        antesternal or antethoracic 42.66
          with interposition 42.65
      small bowel NEC 42.54
        with interposition 42.53
        antesternal or antethoracic 42.64
          with interposition 42.63
  facial-accessory nerve 04.72
  facial-hypoglossal nerve 04.71

Anastomosis *(Continued)*
    fallopian tube 66.73
        by reanastomosis 66.79
    gallbladder 51.35
        to
            hepatic ducts 51.31
            intestine 51.32
            pancreas 51.33
            stomach 51.34
    gastroepiploic artery to coronary artery 36.17
    hepatic duct 51.39
    hypoglossal-accessory nerve 04.73
    hypoglossal-facial nerve 04.71
    ileal loop to bladder 57.87 *[45.51]*
    ileoanal 45.95
    ileorectal 45.93
    inferior vena cava and portal vein 39.1
    internal mammary artery (to)
        coronary artery (single vessel) 36.15
            double vessel 36.16
        myocardium 36.2
    intestine 45.90
        large-to-anus 45.95
        large-to-large 45.94
        large-to-rectum 45.94
        large-to-small 45.93
        small-to-anus 45.95
        small-to-large 45.93
        small-to-rectal stump 45.92
        small-to-small 45.91
    intrahepatic 51.79
    intrathoracic vessel NEC 39.23
    kidney (pelvis) 55.86
    lacrimal sac to conjunctiva 09.82
    left-to-right (systemic-pulmonary artery) 39.0
    lymphatic (channel) (peripheral) 40.9
    mesenteric-caval 39.1
    mesocaval 39.1
    nasolacrimal 09.81
    nerve (cranial) (peripheral) NEC 04.74
        accessory-facial 04.72
        accessory-hypoglossal 04.73
        hypoglossal-facial 04.71
    pancreas (duct) (to) 52.96
        bile duct 51.39
        gall bladder 51.33
        intestine 52.96
        jejunum 52.96
        stomach 52.96
    pleurothecal (with valve) 03.79
    portacaval 39.1
    portal vein to inferior vena cava 39.1
    pulmonary-aortic (Pott's) 39.0
    pulmonary artery and superior vena cava 39.21
    pulmonary-innominate artery (Blalock) 39.0
    pulmonary-subclavian artery (Blalock-Taussig) 39.0
    pulmonary vein and azygos vein 39.23
    pyeloileocutaneous 56.51
    pyeloureterovesical 55.86
    radial artery 36.19
    rectum, rectal NEC 48.74
        stump to small intestine 45.92
    renal (pelvis) 55.86
        vein and splenic vein 39.1
    renoportal 39.1
    salpingothecal (with valve) 03.79
    splenic to renal veins 39.1
    splenorenal (venous) 39.1
        arterial 39.26
    subarachnoid-peritoneal (with valve) 03.71
    subarachnoid-ureteral (with valve) 03.72
    subclavian-aortic 39.22
    superior vena cava to pulmonary artery 39.21
    systemic-pulmonary artery 39.0
    thoracic artery (to)
        coronary artery (single) 36.15
            double 36.16
        myocardium 36.2

Anastomosis *(Continued)*
    ureter (to) NEC 56.79
        bladder 56.74
        colon 56.71
        ileal pouch (bladder) 56.51
        ileum 56.71
        intestine 56.71
        skin 56.61
    ureterocalyceal 55.86
    ureterocolic 56.71
    ureterovesical 56.74
    urethra (end-to-end) 58.44
    vas deferens 63.82
    veins (suture of proximal to distal end) (with bypass graft) 39.29
        with excision or resection of vessel - *see* Phlebectomy, with anastomosis, by site
        mesenteric to vena cava 39.1
        portal to inferior vena cava 39.1
        revision 39.49
        splenic and renal 39.1
    ventricle, ventricular (intracerebral) (with valve) - *see also* Shunt, ventricular 02.22
    ventriculoatrial (with valve) 02.32
    ventriculocaval (with valve) 02.32
    ventriculomastoid (with valve) 02.31
    ventriculopleural (with valve) 02.33
    vesicle - *see* Anastomosis, bladder
Anderson operation (tibial lengthening) 78.37
Anel operation (dilation of lacrimal duct) 09.42
Anesthesia
    acupuncture for 99.91
    cryoanalgesia nerve (cranial) (peripheral) 04.2
    spinal - *omit code*
Aneurysmectomy 38.60
    with
        anastomosis 38.30
            abdominal
                artery 38.36
                vein 38.37
            aorta (arch) (ascending) (descending) 38.34
            head and neck NEC 38.32
            intracranial NEC 38.31
            lower limb
                artery 38.38
                vein 38.39
            thoracic NEC 38.35
            upper limb (artery) (vein) 38.33
        graft replacement (interposition) 38.40
            abdominal
                aorta
                    endovascular approach 39.71
                        fenestrated (branching) graft 39.78
                    open approach 38.44
                        Zenith® Renu™ AAA graft 39.71
                artery 38.46
                vein 38.47
            aorta (arch) (ascending) (descending thoracic)
                abdominal 38.44
                thoracic 38.45
                thoracoabdominal 38.45 *[38.44]*
            head and neck NEC 38.42
            intracranial NEC 38.41
            lower limb
                artery 38.48
                vein 38.49
            thoracic NEC 38.45
            upper limb (artery) (vein) 38.43
    abdominal
        artery 38.66
        vein 38.67
    aorta (arch) (ascending) (descending) 38.64
    atrial, auricular 37.32
    head and neck NEC 38.62
    heart 37.32
    intracranial NEC 38.61

Aneurysmectomy *(Continued)*
    lower limb
        artery 38.68
        vein 38.69
    sinus of Valsalva 35.39
    thoracic NEC 38.65
    upper limb (artery) (vein) 38.63
    ventricle (myocardium) 37.32
Aneurysmoplasty - *see* Aneurysmorrhaphy
Aneurysmorrhaphy NEC 39.52
    by or with
        anastomosis - *see* Aneurysmectomy, with anastomosis, by site
        clipping 39.51
        coagulation 39.52
        electrocoagulation 39.52
        endovascular graft
            abdominal aorta 39.71
                fenestrated (branching) graft 39.78
            lower extremity artery(s) 39.79
            thoracic aorta 39.73
            upper extremity artery(s) 39.79
        excision or resection - *see also* Aneurysmectomy, by site
            with
                anastomosis - *see* Aneurysmectomy, with anastomosis, by site
                graft replacement - *see* Aneurysmectomy, with graft replacement, by site
        filipuncture 39.52
        graft replacement - *see* Aneurysmectomy, with graft replacement, by site
        methyl methacrylate 39.52
        suture 39.52
        wiring 39.52
        wrapping 39.52
    Matas' 39.52
Aneurysmotomy - *see* Aneurysmectomy
Angiectomy
    with
        anastomosis 38.30
            abdominal
                artery 38.36
                vein 38.37
            aorta (arch) (ascending) (descending) 38.34
            head and neck NEC 38.32
            intracranial NEC 38.31
            lower limb
                artery 38.38
                vein 38.39
            thoracic vessel NEC 38.35
            upper limb (artery) (vein) 38.33
        graft replacement (interposition) 38.40
            abdominal
                aorta 38.44
                artery 38.46
                vein 38.47
            aorta (arch) (ascending) (descending thoracic)
                abdominal 38.44
                thoracic 38.45
                thoracoabdominal 38.45 *[38.44]*
            head and neck NEC 38.42
            intracranial NEC 38.41
            lower limb
                artery 38.48
                vein 38.49
            thoracic vessel NEC 38.45
            upper limb (artery) (vein) 38.43
Angiocardiography (selective) 88.50
    carbon dioxide (negative contrast) 88.58
    combined right and left heart 88.54
    intra-operative coronary fluorescence vascular 88.59
    left heart (aortic valve) (atrium) (ventricle) (ventricular outflow tract) 88.53
        combined with right heart 88.54

Angiocardiography *(Continued)*
  right heart (atrium) (pulmonary valve)
      (ventricle) (ventricular outflow tract)
      88.52
    combined with left heart 88.54
  SPY, coronary 88.59
  vena cava (inferior) (superior) 88.51
Angiography (arterial) - *see also* Arteriography
    88.40
  by C.A.T. – *see* Scan, C.A.T., by site
  by computed tomography – *see* Scan, C.A.T.,
      by site
  by magnetic resonance – *see* Imaging,
      magnetic resonance, by site
  by radioisotope - *see* Scan, radioisotope, by
      site
  by ultrasound - *see* Ultrasonography,
      by site
  basilar 88.41
  brachial 88.49
  carotid (internal) 88.41
  celiac 88.47
  cerebral (posterior circulation) 88.41
  coronary NEC 88.57
    intra-operative fluorescence vascular
        88.59
  eye (fluorescein) 95.12
  femoral 88.48
  heart 88.50
  intra-abdominal NEC 88.47
  intracranial 88.41
  intrathoracic vessels NEC 88.44
  lower extremity NEC 88.48
  neck 88.41
  non-coronary, intra-operative fluorescence
      17.71
  placenta 88.46
  pulmonary 88.43
  renal 88.45
  specified artery NEC 88.49
  transfemoral 88.48
  upper extremity NEC 88.49
  veins - *see* Phlebography
  vertebral 88.41
Angioplasty (laser) - *see also* Repair, blood
    vessel

Note: Also use 00.40, 00.41, 00.42, or 00.43
to show the total number of vessels treated.
Use code 00.44 once to show procedure on a
bifurcated vessel.In addition, use 00.45,
00.46, 00.47, or 00.48 to show the number of
vascular stents inserted.
---

  balloon (percutaneous transluminal) NEC
      39.50
    coronary artery 00.66
  coronary 36.09
    open chest approach 36.03
    percutaneous transluminal (balloon)
        00.66
  percutaneous transluminal (balloon) (single
      vessel)
    basilar 00.62
    carotid 00.61
    cerebrovascular
      extracranial 00.62
      intracranial 00.61
    coronary (balloon) 00.66
    extracranial 00.61
    femoropopliteal 39.50
    iliac 39.50
    intracranial 00.62
    lower extremity NOS 39.50
    mesenteric 39.50
    peripheral NEC 39.50
    renal 39.50
    subclavian 39.50
    upper extremity NOS 39.50
    vertebral 00.61
      intracranial portion 00.62

Angioplasty *(Continued)*
    specified site NEC 39.50
      cerebrovascular
          extracranial 00.62
          intracranial 00.61
        peripheral 39.50
Angiorrhaphy 39.30
  artery 39.31
  vein 39.32
Angioscopy, percutaneous 38.22
  eye (fluorescein) 95.12
Angiotomy 38.00
  abdominal
      artery 38.06
      vein 38.07
  aorta (arch) (ascending) (descending) 38.04
  head and neck NEC 38.02
  intracranial NEC 38.01
  lower limb
      artery 38.08
      vein 38.09
  thoracic NEC 38.05
  upper limb (artery) (vein) 38.03
Angiotripsy 39.98
Ankylosis, production of - *see* Arthrodesis
Annuloplasty (heart) (posteromedial) 35.33
Anoplasty 49.79
  with hemorrhoidectomy 49.46
Anoscopy 49.21
Antebiogram - *see* Examination, microscopic
Antrectomy
  mastoid 20.49
  maxillary 22.39
    radical 22.31
  pyloric 43.6
Antrostomy - *see* Antrotomy
Antrotomy (exploratory) (nasal sinus) 22.2
  Caldwell-Luc (maxillary sinus) 22.39
    with removal of membrane lining 22.31
  intranasal 22.2
    with external approach (Caldwell-Luc)
        22.39
      radical 22.31
  maxillary (simple) 22.2
    with Caldwell-Luc approach 22.39
      with removal of membrane lining
          22.31
    external (Caldwell-Luc approach) 22.39
      with removal of membrane lining
          22.31
    radical (with removal of membrane
        lining) 22.31
Antrum window operation - *see* Antrotomy,
    maxillary
Aorticopulmonary window operation 39.59
Aortogram, aortography (abdominal)
    (retrograde) (selective) (translumbar)
    88.42
Aortoplasty (aortic valve) (gusset type) 35.11
Aortotomy 38.04
Apexcardiogram (with ECG lead) 89.57
Apheresis, therapeutic - *see* category 99.7●
Apicectomy
  lung 32.39
    thoracoscopic 32.30
  petrous pyramid 20.59
  tooth (root) 23.73
    with root canal therapy 23.72
Apicoectomy 23.73
  with root canal therapy 23.72
Apicolysis (lung) 33.39
Apicostomy, alveolar 24.0
Aponeurectomy 83.42
  hand 82.33
Aponeurorrhaphy - *see also* Suture, tendon
    83.64
  hand - *see also* Suture, tendon, hand 82.45
Aponeurotomy 83.13
  hand 82.11

Appendectomy (with drainage) 47.09
  incidental 47.19
    laparoscopic 47.11
  laparoscopic 47.01
Appendicectomy (with drainage) 47.09
  incidental 47.19
    laparoscopic 47.11
  laparoscopic 47.01
Appendicocecostomy 47.91
Appendicoenterostomy 47.91
Appendicolysis 54.59
  with appendectomy 47.09
    laparoscopic 47.01
    other 47.09
  laparoscopic 54.51
Appendicostomy 47.91
  closure 47.92
Appendicotomy 47.2
Application
  adhesion barrier substance 99.77
  anti-shock trousers 93.58
  arch bars (orthodontic) 24.7
    for immobilization (fracture) 93.55
  barrier substance, adhesion 99.77
  Barton's tongs (skull) (with synchronous
      skeletal traction) 02.94
  bone growth stimulator (surface)
      (transcutaneous) 99.86
  bone morphogenetic protein (Infuse™)
      (OP-1™) (recombinant) (rhBMP) 84.52
  Bryant's traction 93.44
    with reduction of fracture or dislocation -
        see Reduction, fracture *and*
        Reduction, dislocation
  Buck's traction 93.46
  caliper tongs (skull) (with synchronous
      skeletal traction) 02.94
  cast (fiberglass) (plaster) (plastic) NEC 93.53
    with reduction of fracture or dislocation -
        see Reduction, fracture *and*
        Reduction, dislocation
    spica 93.51
  cervical collar 93.52
    with reduction of fracture or dislocation -
        see Reduction, fracture *and*
        Reduction, dislocation
  clamp, cerebral aneurysm (Crutchfield)
      (Silverstone) 39.51
  croupette, croup tent 93.94
  crown (artificial) 23.41
  Crutchfield tongs (skull) (with synchronous
      skeletal traction) 02.94
  Dunlop's traction 93.44
    with reduction of fracture or dislocation -
        see Reduction, fracture *and*
        Reduction, dislocation
  elastic stockings 93.59
  electronic gaiter 93.59
  external fixator device (bone) 78.10
    carpal, metacarpal 78.14
    clavicle 78.11
    computer assisted (dependent) 84.73
    femur 78.15
    fibula 78.17
    humerus 78.12
    hybrid device or system 84.73
    Ilizarov type 84.72
    monoplanar system or device 84.71
    patella 78.16
    pelvic 78.19
    phalanges (foot) (hand) 78.19
    radius 78.13
    ring device or system 84.72
    scapula 78.11
    Sheffield type 84.72
    specified site NEC 78.19
    tarsal, metatarsal 78.18
    thorax (ribs) (sternum) 78.11
    tibia 78.17
    ulna 78.13
    vertebrae 78.19

A

Application *(Continued)*
  forceps, with delivery - *see* Delivery,
      forceps
  graft - *see* Graft
  gravity (G-) suit 93.59
  intermittent pressure device 93.59
  Jewett extension brace 93.59
  Jobst pumping unit (reduction of edema)
      93.59
  Lyman Smith traction 93.44
      with reduction of fracture or dislocation -
          see Reduction, fracture *and*
          Reduction, dislocation
  MAST (military anti-shock trousers)
      93.58
  Minerva jacket 93.52
  minifixator device (bone) - *see* category
      78.1 ●
  neck support (molded) 93.52
  obturator (orthodontic) 24.7
  orthodontic appliance (obturator) (wiring)
      24.7
  pelvic sling 93.44
      with reduction of fracture or dislocation - *see*
          Reduction, fracture *and* Reduction,
          dislocation
  peridontal splint (orthodontic) 24.7
  plaster jacket 93.51
      Minerva 93.52
  pressure
      dressing (bandage) (Gibney) (Robert
          Jones') (Shanz) 93.56
      trousers (anti-shock) (MAST) 93.58
  prosthesis for missing ear 18.71
  Russell's traction 93.44
      with reduction of fracture or dislocation -
          see Reduction, fracture *and*
          Reduction, dislocation
  splint, for immobilization (plaster)
      (pneumatic) (tray) 93.54
      with fracture reduction - *see* Reduction,
          fracture
  stereotactic head frame 93.59
  strapping (non-traction) 93.59
  substance, adhesion barrier 99.77
  Thomas collar 93.52
      with reduction of fracture or dislocation -
          see Reduction, fracture *and*
          Reduction, dislocation
  traction
      with reduction of fracture or dislocation -
          see Reduction, fracture *and*
          Reduction, dislocation
      adhesive tape (skin) 93.46
      boot 93.46
      Bryant's 93.44
      Buck's 93.46
      Cotrel's 93.42
      Dunlop's 93.44
      gallows 93.46
      Lyman Smith 93.44
      Russell's 93.44
      skeletal NEC 93.44
          intermittent 93.43
      skin, limbs NEC 93.46
      spinal NEC 93.42
          with skull device (caliper)
              (Crutchfield) (Gardner-Wells)
              (halo) (Vinke) (tongs) 93.41
              with synchronous insertion
                  02.94
      Thomas' splint 93.45
  Unna's paste boot 93.53
  vasopneumatic device 93.58
  Velpeau dressing 93.59
  Vinke tongs (skull) (with synchronous
      skeletal traction) 02.94
  wound dressing NEC 93.57
Aquapheresis 99.78
Arc lamp - *see* Photocoagulation
Arcuplasty 81.66

Arrest
  bone growth (epiphyseal) 78.20
      by stapling - *see* Stapling, epiphyseal plate
      femur 78.25
      fibula 78.27
      humerus 78.22
      radius 78.23
      tibia 78.27
      ulna 78.23
  cardiac, induced (anoxic) (circulatory) 39.63
  circulatory, induced (anoxic) 39.63
  hemorrhage - *see* Control, hemorrhage
Arslan operation (fenestration of inner ear)
    20.61
Arteriectomy 38.60
  with
      anastomosis 38.30
          abdominal 38.36
          aorta (arch) (ascending) (descending)
              38.34
          head and neck NEC 38.32
          intracranial NEC 38.31
          lower limb 38.38
          thoracic NEC 38.35
          upper limb 38.33
      graft replacement (interposition) 38.40
          abdominal
              aorta 38.44
          aorta (arch) (ascending) (descending
              thoracic) (thoracic)
              abdominal 38.44
              thoracic 38.45
              thoracoabdominal 38.45 *[38.44]*
          head and neck NEC 38.42
          intracranial NEC 38.41
          lower limb 38.48
          thoracic NEC 38.45
          upper limb 38.43
  abdominal 38.66
  aorta (arch) (ascending) (descending) 38.64
  head and neck NEC 38.62
  intracranial NEC 38.61
  lower-limb 38.68
  thoracic NEC 38.65
  upper limb 38.63
Arteriography (contrast) (fluoroscopic)
    (retrograde) 88.40
  by
      radioisotope - *see* Scan, radioisotope
      ultrasound (Doppler) - *see*
          Ultrasonography, by site
  aorta (arch) (ascending) (descending) 88.42
  basilar 88.41
  brachial 88.49
  carotid (internal) 88.41
  cerebral (posterior circulation) 88.41
  coronary (direct) (selective) NEC 88.57
      double catheter technique (Judkins)
          (Ricketts and Abrams) 88.56
      intra-operative fluorescence vascular
          88.59
      single catheter technique (Sones) 88.55
  Doppler (ultrasonic) - *see* Ultrasonography,
      by site
  femoral 88.48
  head and neck 88.41
  intra-abdominal NEC 88.47
  intrathoracic NEC 88.44
  lower extremity 88.48
  placenta 88.46
  pulmonary 88.43
  radioisotope - *see* Scan, radioisotope
  renal 88.45
  specified site NEC 88.49
  SPY, coronary 88.59
  superior mesenteric artery 88.47
  transfemoral 88.48
  ultrasound - *see* Ultrasonography, by site
  upper extremity 88.49
Arterioplasty - *see* Repair, artery
Arteriorrhaphy 39.31

Arteriotomy 38.00
  abdominal 38.06
  aorta (arch) (ascending) (descending)
      38.04
  head and neck NEC 38.02
  intracranial NEC 38.01
  lower limb 38.08
  thoracic NEC 38.05
  upper limb 38.03
Arteriovenostomy 39.29
  for renal dialysis 39.27
Arthrectomy 80.90
  ankle 80.97
  elbow 80.92
  foot and toe 80.98
  hand and finger 80.94
  hip 80.95
  intervertebral disc - *see* category 80.5 ●
  knee 80.96
  semilunar cartilage 80.6
  shoulder 80.91
  specified site NEC 80.99
  spine NEC 80.99
  wrist 80.93
Arthrocentesis 81.91
  for arthrography - *see* Arthrogram
Arthrodesis (compression) (extra-articular)
    (intra-articular) (with bone graft) (with
    fixation device) 81.20
  ankle 81.11
  carporadial 81.25
  cricoarytenoid 31.69
  elbow 81.24
  finger 81.28
  foot NEC 81.17
  hip 81.21
  interphalangeal
      finger 81.28
      toe NEC 77.58
          claw toe repair 77.57
          hammer toe repair 77.56
  ischiofemoral 81.21
  knee 81.22
  lumbosacral, lumbar NEC 81.08
      ALIF (anterior lumbar interbody fusion)
          81.06
      anterior column (interbody)
          anterolateral (anterior) technique 81.06
          posterior technique 81.08
      axial lumber interbody fusion [AxiaLIF®]
          81.08
      direct lateral interbody fusion [DLIF]
          81.06
      extreme lateral interbody fusion [XLIF®]
          81.06
      facet 81.07
      lateral transverse process technique 81.07
      PLIF (posterior lumbar interbody fusion)
          81.08
      TLIF (transforaminal lumbar interbody
          fusion) 81.08
  McKeever (metatarsophalangeal) 81.16
  metacarpocarpal 81.26
  metacarpophalangeal 81.27
  metatarsophalangeal 81.16
  midtarsal 81.14
  pantalar 81.11
  sacroiliac 81.08
  shoulder 81.23
  specified joint NEC 81.29
  spinal - *see also* Fusion, spinal 81.00
  subtalar 81.13
  tarsometatarsal 81.15
  tibiotalar 81.11
  toe NEC 77.58
      claw toe repair 77.57
      hammer toe repair 77.56
  triple 81.12
  wrist 81.26
Arthroendoscopy - *see* Arthroscopy
Arthroereisis, subtalar joint 81.18

◀ New   ◀▥ Revised   ~~deleted~~ Deleted   ● Use Additional Digit(s)   ▨ Omit code

Arthrogram, arthrography 88.32
  temporomandibular 87.13
Arthrolysis 93.26
Arthroplasty (with fixation device) (with
    traction) 81.96
  ankle 81.49
  carpals 81.75
    with prosthetic implant 81.74
  carpocarpal, carpometacarpal 81.75
    with prosthetic implant 81.74
  Carroll and Taber (proximal interphalangeal
    joint) 81.72
  cup (partial hip) 81.52
  Curtis (interphalangeal joint) 81.72
  elbow 81.85
    with prosthetic replacement (partial)
      (total) 81.84
  femoral head NEC 81.40
    with prosthetic implant 81.52
  finger(s) 81.72
    with prosthetic implant 81.71
  foot (metatarsal) with joint replacement 81.57
  Fowler (metacarpophalangeal joint) 81.72
  hand (metacarpophalangeal)
    (interphalangeal) 81.72
    with prosthetic implant 81.71
  hip (with bone graft) 81.40
    cup (partial hip) 81.52
    femoral head NEC 81.40
      with prosthetic implant 81.52
        with total replacement 81.51
      partial replacement 81.52
      total replacement 81.51
  interphalangeal joint 81.72
    with prosthetic implant 81.71
  Kessler (carpometacarpal joint) 81.74
  knee - see also Repair, knee 81.47
    prosthetic replacement (bicompartmental)
      (hemijoint) (partial) (total)
      (tricompartmental)
      (unicompartmental) 81.54
    revision 81.55
  metacarpophalangeal joint 81.72
    with prosthetic implant 81.71
  shoulder 81.83
    prosthetic replacement (partial) 81.81
      total, NEC 81.80
        other 81.80
        reverse 81.88
    for recurrent dislocation 81.82
  temporomandibular 76.5
  toe NEC 77.58
    with prosthetic replacement 81.57
    for hallux valgus repair 77.59
  wrist 81.75
    with prosthetic implant 81.74
      total replacement 81.73
Arthroscopy 80.20
  ankle 80.27
  elbow 80.22
  finger 80.24
  foot 80.28
  hand 80.24
  hip 80.25
  knee 80.26
  shoulder 80.21
  specified site NEC 80.29
  toe 80.28
  wrist 80.23
Arthrostomy - see also Arthrotomy 80.10
Arthrotomy 80.10
  as operative approach - omit code
  with
    arthrography - see Arthrogram
    arthroscopy - see Arthroscopy
    injection of drug 81.92
    removal of prosthesis without
        replacement - see Removal,
        prosthesis, joint structures
  ankle 80.17
  elbow 80.12

Arthrotomy (Continued)
  foot and toe 80.18
  hand and finger 80.14
  hip 80.15
  knee 80.16
  shoulder 80.11
  specified site NEC 80.19
  spine 80.19
  wrist 80.13
Artificial
  heart 37.52
    AbioCor® 37.52
    CardioWest™ (TAH-t) 37.52
  insemination 69.92
  kidney 39.95
  rupture of membranes 73.09
Arytenoidectomy 30.29
Arytenoidopexy 31.69
Asai operation (larynx) 31.75
Aspiration
  abscess - see Aspiration, by site
  anterior chamber, eye (therapeutic) 12.91
    diagnostic 12.21
  aqueous (eye) (humor) (therapeutic) 12.91
    diagnostic 12.21
  ascites 54.91
  Bartholin's gland (cyst) (percutaneous)
    71.21
  biopsy - see Biopsy, by site
  bladder (catheter) 57.0
    percutaneous (needle) 57.11
  bone marrow (for biopsy) 41.31
    from donor for transplant 41.91
    stem cell 99.79
  branchial cleft cyst 29.0
  breast 85.91
  bronchus 96.05
    with lavage 96.56
  bursa (percutaneous) 83.94
    hand 82.92
  calculus, bladder 57.0
  cataract 13.3
    with
      phacoemulsification 13.41
      phacofragmentation 13.43
        posterior route 13.42
  chest 34.91
  cisternal 01.01
  cranial (puncture) 01.09
  craniobuccal pouch 07.72
  craniopharyngioma 07.72
  cul-de-sac (abscess) 70.0
  curettage, uterus 69.59
    after abortion or delivery 69.52
    diagnostic 69.59
    to terminate pregnancy 69.51
  cyst - see Aspiration, by site
  diverticulum, pharynx 29.0
  endotracheal 96.04
    with lavage 96.56
  extradural 01.09
  eye (anterior chamber) (therapeutic)
    12.91
    diagnostic 12.21
  fallopian tube 66.91
  fascia 83.95
    hand 82.93
  gallbladder (percutaneous) 51.01
  hematoma - see also Aspiration, by site
    obstetrical 75.92
      incisional 75.91
  hydrocele, tunica vaginalis 61.91
  hygroma - see Aspiration, by site
  hyphema 12.91
  hypophysis 07.72
  intracranial space (epidural) (extradural)
    (subarachnoid) (subdural) (ventricular)
    01.09
  through previously implanted catheter
    or reservoir (Ommaya) (Rickham)
    01.02

Aspiration (Continued)
  joint 81.91
    for arthrography - see Arthrogram
  kidney (cyst) (pelvis) (percutaneous)
    (therapeutic) 55.92
    diagnostic 55.23
  liver (percutaneous) 50.91
  lung (percutaneous) (puncture) (needle)
    (trocar) 33.93
    thoracoscopic 33.20
  middle ear 20.09
    with intubation 20.01
  muscle 83.95
    hand 82.93
  nail 86.01
  nasal sinus 22.00
    by puncture 22.01
    through natural ostium 22.02
  nasotracheal 96.04
    with lavage 96.56
  orbit, diagnostic 16.22
  ovary 65.91
  percutaneous - see Aspiration, by site
  pericardium (wound) 37.0
  pituitary gland 07.72
  pleural cavity 34.91
  prostate (percutaneous) 60.91
  Rathke's pouch 07.72
  seminal vesicles 60.71
  seroma - see Aspiration, by site
  skin 86.01
  soft tissue NEC 83.95
    hand 82.93
  spermatocele 63.91
  spinal (puncture) 03.31
  spleen (cyst) 41.1
  stem cell 99.79
  subarachnoid space (cerebral) 01.09
  subcutaneous tissue 86.01
  subdural space (cerebral) 01.09
  tendon 83.95
    hand 82.93
  testis 62.91
  thymus 07.92
    thoracoscopic 07.95
  thyroid (field) (gland) 06.01
    postoperative 06.02
  trachea 96.04
    with lavage 96.56
    percutaneous 31.99
  tunica vaginalis (hydrocele) (percutaneous)
    61.91
  vitreous (and replacement) 14.72
    diagnostic 14.11
Assessment
  fitness to testify 94.11
  mental status 94.11
  nutritional status 89.39
  personality 94.03
  temperament 94.02
  vocational 93.85
Assistance
  cardiac - see also Resuscitation, cardiac
    extracorporeal circulation 39.61
  endotracheal respiratory - see category
    96.7●
  hepatic, extracorporeal 50.92
  respiratory (endotracheal) (mechanical) - see
    Ventilation, mechanical
Astragalectomy 77.98
Asymmetrogammagram - see Scan,
  radioisotope
Atherectomy
  cerebrovascular
    percutaneous
      extracranial vessel(s) 17.53
      intracranial vessel(s) 17.54
  coronary
    percutaneous transluminal
      17.55
  peripheral (noncoronary) 17.56

Atriocommissuropexy (mitral valve) 35.12
Atrioplasty NEC 37.99
  combined with repair of valvular and
      ventricular septal defects - see Repair,
      endocardial cushion defect
  septum (heart) NEC 35.71
Atrioseptopexy - see also Repair, atrial septal
      defect 35.71
Atrioseptoplasty - see also Repair, atrial septal
      defect 35.71
Atrioseptostomy (balloon) 35.41
Atriotomy 37.11
Atrioventriculostomy (cerebral-heart) 02.32
Attachment
  abutment (screw) for prosthetic ear device
      percutaneous 20.99
  eye muscle
      orbicularis oculi to eyebrow 08.36
      rectus to frontalis 15.9
  pedicle (flap) graft 86.74
      hand 86.73
      lip 27.57
      mouth 27.57
  pharyngeal flap (for cleft palate repair) 27.62
      secondary or subsequent 27.63

Attachment (Continued)
  prosthetic ear device, abutment 20.99
  retina - see Reattachment, retina
Atticoantrostomy (ear) 20.49
Atticoantrotomy (ear) 20.49
Atticotomy (ear) 20.23
Audiometry (Bekesy 5-tone) (impedance)
      (stapedial reflex response) (subjective)
      95.41
Augmentation
  bladder 57.87
  breast - see Mammoplasty, augmentation
  buttock ("fanny-lift") 86.89
  chin 76.68
  genioplasty 76.68
  mammoplasty - see Mammoplasty,
      augmentation
  outflow tract (pulmonary valve) (gusset
      type) 35.26
  in total repair of tetralogy of Fallot 35.81
  vocal cord(s) 31.0
Auriculectomy 18.39
Autograft - see Graft
Autologous - see Blood, transfusion
Autopsy 89.8

Autotransfusion (whole blood) 99.02 - see
      Blood, transfusion
Autotransplant, autotransplantation - see also
      Reimplantation
  adrenal tissue (heterotopic) (orthotopic)
      07.45
  kidney 55.61
  lung - see Transplant, transplantation, lung
      33.5●
  ovary 65.72
      laparoscopic 65.75
  pancreatic tissue 52.81
  parathyroid tissue (heterotopic) (orthotopic)
      06.95
  thyroid tissue (heterotopic) (orthotopic)
      06.94
  tooth 23.5
Avulsion, nerve (cranial) (peripheral) NEC
      04.07
  acoustic 04.01
  phrenic 33.31
  sympathetic 05.29
Azygography 88.63

B

Bacterial smear - see Examination, microscopic
Baffes operation (interatrial transposition of
      venous return) 35.91
Baffle, atrial or interatrial 35.91
Balanoplasty 64.69
Baldy-Webster operation (uterine suspension)
      69.22
Ballistocardiography 89.59
Balloon
  angioplasty - see Angioplasty, balloon
  pump, intra-aortic 37.61
  systostomy (atrial) 35.41
Ball operation
  herniorrhaphy - see Repair, hernia, inguinal
  undercutting 40.92
Bandage 93.37
  elastic 93.56
Banding
  gastric 44.68
      vertical 44.68
  pulmonary artery 38.85
Bankhart operation (capsular repair into
      glenoid, for shoulder dislocation) 81.82
Bardenheurer operation (ligation of innominate
      artery) 38.85
Barium swallow 87.61
Barkan operation (goniotomy) 12.52
  with goniopuncture 12.53
Barr operation (transfer of tibialis posterior
      tendon) 83.75
Barsky operation (closure of cleft hand)
      82.82
Basal metabolic rate 89.39
Basiotripsy 73.8
Bassett operation (vulvectomy with
      inguinal lymph node dissection)
      71.5 [40.3]
Bassini operation - see Repair, hernia,
      inguinal
Batch-Spittler-McFaddin operation (knee
      disarticulation) 84.16
Batista operation (partial ventriculectomy)
      (ventricular reduction) (ventricular
      remodeling) 37.35
Bearing surface, hip
  ceramic-on-ceramic 00.76
  ceramic-on-polyethylene 00.77
  metal-on-metal 00.75

Bearing surface, hip (Continued)
  metal-on-polyethylene 00.74
  oxidized zirconium -on-polyethylene 00.77
Beck operation
  aorta-coronary sinus shunt 36.39
  epicardial poudrage 36.39
Beck-Jianu operation (permanent gastrostomy)
      43.19
Behavior modification 94.33
Bell-Beuttner operation (subtotal abdominal
      hysterectomy) 68.39
  laparoscopic 68.31
Belsey operation (esophagogastric sphincter)
      44.65
Benenenti operation (rotation of bulbous
      urethra) 58.49
Berke operation (levator resection of eyelid)
      08.33
Bicuspidization of heart valve 35.10
  aortic 35.11
  mitral 35.12
Bicycle dynamometer 93.01
Biesenberger operation (size reduction of
      breast, bilateral) 85.32
  unilateral 85.31
Bifurcation, bone - see also Osteotomy 77.30
Bigelow operation (litholapaxy) 57.0
Bililite therapy (ultraviolet) 99.82
Billroth I operation (partial gastrectomy with
      gastroduodenostomy) 43.6
Billroth II operation (partial gastrectomy with
      gastrojejunostomy) 43.7
Binnie operation (hepatopexy) 50.69
Biofeedback, psychotherapy 94.39
Biopsy
  abdominal wall 54.22
  adenoid 28.11
  adrenal gland NEC 07.11
      closed 07.11
      open 07.12
      percutaneous (aspiration) (needle) 07.11
  alveolus 24.12
  anus 49.23
  appendix 45.26
  artery (any site) 38.21
  aspiration - see Biopsy, by site
  bile ducts 51.14
      closed (endoscopic) 51.14
      open 51.13
      percutaneous (needle) 51.12

Biopsy (Continued)
  bladder 57.33
      closed 57.33
      open 57.34
      transurethral 57.33
  blood vessel (any site) 38.21
  bone 77.40
      carpal, metacarpal 77.44
      clavicle 77.41
      facial 76.11
      femur 77.45
      fibula 77.47
      humerus 77.42
      marrow 41.31
      patella 77.46
      pelvic 77.49
      phalanges (foot) (hand) 77.49
      radius 77.43
      scapula 77.41
      specified site NEC 77.49
      tarsal, metatarsal 77.48
      thorax (ribs) (sternum) 77.41
      tibia 77.47
      ulna 77.43
      vertebrae 77.49
  bowel - see Biopsy, intestine
  brain NEC 01.13
      closed 01.13
      open 01.14
      percutaneous (needle) 01.13
  breast 85.11
      blind 85.11
      closed 85.11
      open 85.12
      percutaneous (needle) (Vimm-Silverman)
          85.11
  bronchus NEC 33.24
      brush 33.24
      closed (endoscopic) 33.24
      open 33.25
      transbronchoscopic needle aspiration
          (TBNA) 33.24
      Wang needle (transbronchoscopic)
          33.24
      washings 33.24
  bursa 83.21
  cardioesophageal (junction)
      44.14
      closed (endoscopic) 44.14
      open 44.15

◀ New   ◀▥ Revised   ~~deleted~~ Deleted   ● Use Additional Digit(s)   ▨ Omit code

A & B

Biopsy *(Continued)*
  cecum 45.25
    brush 45.25
    closed (endoscopic) 45.25
    open 45.26
  cerebral meninges NEC 01.11
    closed 01.11
    open 01.12
    percutaneous (needle) 01.11
  cervix (punch) 67.12
    conization (sharp) 67.2
  chest wall 34.23
  clitoris 71.11
  colon 45.25
    brush 45.25
    closed (endoscopic) 45.25
    open 45.26
  conjunctiva 10.21
  cornea 11.22
  cul-de-sac 70.23
  diaphragm 34.27
  duodenum 45.14
    brush 45.14
    closed (endoscopic) 45.14
    open 45.15
  ear (external) 18.12
    middle or inner 20.32
  endocervix 67.11
  endometrium NEC 68.16
    by
        aspiration curettage 69.59
        dilation and curettage
            69.09
    closed (endoscopic) 68.16
    open 68.13
  epididymis 63.01
  esophagus 42.24
    closed (endoscopic) 42.24
    open 42.25
  extraocular muscle or tendon 15.01
  eye 16.23
    muscle (oblique) (rectus) 15.01
  eyelid 08.11
  fallopian tube 66.11
  fascia 83.21
  fetus 75.33
  gallbladder 51.12
    closed (endoscopic) 51.14
    open 51.13
    percutaneous (needle) 51.12
  ganglion (cranial) (peripheral) NEC
    04.11
    closed 04.11
    open 04.12
    percutaneous (needle) 04.11
    sympathetic nerve 05.11
  gum 24.11
  heart 37.25
  hypophysis - *see also* Biopsy, pituitary
    gland 07.15
  ileum 45.14
    brush 45.14
    closed (endoscopic) 45.14
    open 45.15
  intestine NEC 45.27
    large 45.25
      brush 45.25
      closed (endoscopic) 45.25
      open 45.26
    small 45.14
      brush 45.14
      closed (endoscopic) 45.14
      open 45.15
  intra-abdominal mass 54.24
    closed 54.24
    percutaneous (needle) 54.24
  iris 12.22
  jejunum 45.14
    brush 45.14
    closed (endoscopic) 45.14
    open 45.15

Biopsy *(Continued)*
  joint structure (aspiration) 80.30
    ankle 80.37
    elbow 80.32
    foot and toe 80.38
    hand and finger 80.34
    hip 80.35
    knee 80.36
    shoulder 80.31
    specified site NEC 80.39
    spine 80.39
    wrist 80.33
  kidney 55.23
    closed 55.23
    open 55.24
    percutaneous (aspiration) (needle)
      55.23
  labia 71.11
  lacrimal
    gland 09.11
    sac 09.12
  larynx 31.43
    brush 31.43
    closed (endoscopic) 31.43
    open 31.45
  lip 27.23
  liver 50.11
    closed 50.11
    laparoscopic 50.14
    open 50.12
    percutaneous (aspiration) (needle) 50.11
    transjugular 50.13
    transvenous 50.13
  lung NEC 33.27
    brush 33.24
    closed (percutaneous) (needle) 33.26
      brush 33.24
      endoscopic 33.27
        brush 33.24
    endoscopic 33.27
      brush 33.24
    open 33.28
    thoracoscopic 33.20
    transbronchial 33.27
    transthoracic 33.26
  lymphatic structure (channel) (node) (vessel)
    40.11
  mediastinum NEC 34.25
    closed 34.25
    open 34.26
    percutaneous (needle) 34.25
  meninges (cerebral) NEC 01.11
    closed 01.11
    open 01.12
    percutaneous (needle) 01.11
    spinal 03.32
  mesentery 54.23
  mouth NEC 27.24
  muscle 83.21
    extraocular 15.01
    ocular 15.01
  nasopharynx 29.12
  nerve (cranial) (peripheral) NEC 04.11
    closed 04.11
    open 04.12
    percutaneous (needle) 04.11
    sympathetic 05.11
  nose, nasal 21.22
    sinus 22.11
      closed (endoscopic) (needle) 22.11
    open 22.12
  ocular muscle or tendon 15.01
  omentum
    closed 54.24
    open 54.23
    percutaneous (needle) 54.24
  orbit 16.23
    by aspiration 16.22
  ovary 65.12
    by aspiration 65.11
    laparoscopic 65.13

Biopsy *(Continued)*
  palate (bony) 27.21
    soft 27.22
  pancreas 52.11
    closed (endoscopic) 52.11
    open 52.12
    percutaneous (aspiration) (needle) 52.11
  pancreatic duct 52.14
    closed (endoscopic) 52.14
  parathyroid gland 06.13
  penis 64.11
  perianal tissue 49.22
  pericardium 37.24
  periprostatic 60.15
  perirectal tissue 48.26
  perirenal tissue 59.21
  peritoneal implant
    closed 54.24
    open 54.23
    percutaneous (needle) 54.24
  peritoneum
    closed 54.24
    open 54.23
    percutaneous (needle) 54.24
  periurethral tissue 58.24
  perivesical tissue 59.21
  pharynx, pharyngeal 29.12
  pineal gland 07.17
  pituitary gland 07.15
    transfrontal approach 07.13
    transsphenoidal approach 07.14
  pleura, pleural 34.24
    thoracoscopic 34.20
  prostate NEC 60.11
    closed (transurethral) 60.11
    open 60.12
    percutaneous (needle) 60.11
    transrectal 60.11
  rectum 48.24
    brush 48.24
    closed (endoscopic) 48.24
    open 48.25
  retroperitoneal tissue 54.24
  salivary gland or duct 26.11
    closed (needle) 26.11
    open 26.12
  scrotum 61.11
  seminal vesicle NEC 60.13
    closed 60.13
    open 60.14
    percutaneous (needle) 60.13
  sigmoid colon 45.25
    brush 45.25
    closed (endoscopic) 45.25
    open 45.26
  sinus, nasal 22.11
    closed (endoscopic) (needle) 22.11
    open 22.12
  skin (punch) 86.11
  skull 01.15
  soft palate 27.22
  soft tissue NEC 86.11
    closed (needle) (punch) 86.11
    open 83.21
  spermatic cord 63.01
  sphincter of Oddi 51.14
    closed (endoscopic) 51.14
    open 51.13
  spinal cord (meninges) 03.32
  spleen 41.32
    closed 41.32
    open 41.33
    percutaneous (aspiration) (needle)
      41.32
  stomach 44.14
    brush 44.14
    closed (endoscopic) 44.14
    open 44.15
  subcutaneous tissue (punch) 86.11
  supraglottic mass 29.12
  sympathetic nerve 05.11

Biopsy (Continued)
  tendon 83.21
    extraocular 15.01
    ocular 15.01
  testis NEC 62.11
    closed 62.11
    open 62.12
    percutaneous (needle) 62.11
  thymus 07.16
  thyroid gland NEC 06.11
    closed 06.11
    open 06.12
    percutaneous (aspiration) (needle) 06.11
      tongue 25.01
    closed (needle) 25.01
    open 25.02
  tonsil 28.11
  trachea 31.44
    brush 31.44
    closed (endoscopic) 31.44
    open 31.45
  tunica vaginalis 61.11
  umbilicus 54.22
  ureter 56.33
    closed (percutaneous) 56.32
      endoscopic 56.33
    open 56.34
    transurethral 56.33
  urethra 58.23
  uterus, uterine (endometrial) 68.16
    by
      aspiration curettage 69.59
      dilation and curettage 69.09
    closed (endoscopic) 68.16
    ligaments 68.15
      closed (endoscopic) 68.15
      open 68.14
    open 68.13
  uvula 27.22
  vagina 70.24
  vas deferens 63.01
  vein (any site) 38.21
  vulva 71.11
BiPAP 93.90
  delivered by
    endotracheal tube - *see* category 96.7●
    tracheostomy - *see* category 96.7●
BIS (bispectral index) monitoring 00.94 *[89.14]*
Bischoff operation (ureteroneocystostomy) 56.74
Bisection - *see also* Excision
  hysterectomy 68.39
    laparoscopic 68.31
  ovary 65.29
    laparoscopic 65.25
  stapes foot plate 19.79
    with incus replacement 19.11
Bischoff operation (spinal myelotomy) 03.29
Blalock operation (systemic-pulmonary anastomosis) 39.0
Blalock-Hanlon operation (creation of atrial septal defect) 35.42
Blalock-Taussig operation (subclavian-pulmonary anastomosis) 39.0
Blascovic operation (resection and advancement of levator palpebrae superioris) 08.33
Blepharectomy 08.20
Blepharoplasty - *see also* Reconstruction, eyelid 08.70
  extensive 08.44
Blepharorrhaphy 08.52
  division or severing 08.02
Blepharotomy 08.09
Blind rehabilitation therapy NEC 93.78
Block
  caudal - *see* Injection, spinal celiac ganglion or plexus 05.31
  dissection
    breast
      bilateral 85.46
      unilateral 85.45

Block (Continued)
  dissection (Continued)
    bronchus 32.6
    larynx 30.3
    lymph nodes 40.50
    neck 40.40
    vulva 71.5
  epidural, spinal - *see* Injection, spinal
  gasserian ganglion 04.81
  intercostal nerves 04.81
  intrathecal - *see* Injection, spinal
  nerve (cranial) (peripheral) NEC 04.81
  paravertebral stellate ganglion 05.31
  peripheral nerve 04.81
  spinal nerve root (intrathecal) - *see* Injection, spinal
  stellate (ganglion) 05.31
  subarachnoid, spinal - *see* Injection, spinal
  sympathetic nerve 05.31
  trigeminal nerve 04.81
Blood
  flow study, Doppler-type (ultrasound) - *see* Ultrasonography
  patch, spine (epidural) 03.95
  transfusion
    antihemophilic factor 99.06
    autologous
      collected prior to surgery 99.02
      intraoperative 99.00
      perioperative 99.00
      postoperative 99.00
      previously collected 99.02
      salvage 99.00
    blood expander 99.08
    blood surrogate 99.09
    coagulation factors 99.06
    exchange 99.01
    granulocytes 99.09
    hemodilution 99.03
    other substance 99.09
    packed cells 99.04
    plasma 99.07
    platelets 99.05
    serum, other 99.07
    thrombocytes 99.05
Blount operation
  femoral shortening (with blade plate) 78.25
    by epiphyseal stapling 78.25
Boari operation (bladder flap) 56.74
Bobb operation (cholelithotomy) 51.04
Bone
  age studies 88.33
  mineral density study 88.98
Bonney operation (abdominal hysterectomy) 68.49
  laparoscopic 68.41
Borthen operation (iridotasis) 12.63
Bost operation
  plantar dissection 80.48
  radiocarpal fusion 81.26
Bosworth operation
  arthroplasty for acromioclavicular separation 81.83
  fusion of posterior lumbar and lumbosacral spine 81.08
    for pseudarthrosis 81.38
  resection of radial head ligaments (for tennis elbow) 80.92
  shelf procedure, hip 81.40
Bottle repair of hydrocele, tunica-vaginalis 61.2
Boyd operation (hip disarticulation) 84.18
Brachytherapy
  intravascular 92.27
Brauer operation (cardiolysis) 37.10
Breech extraction - *see* Extraction, breech
Bricker operation (ileoureterostomy) 56.51
Brisement (forcé) 93.26
Bristow operation (repair of shoulder dislocation) 81.82
Brock operation (pulmonary valvotomy) 35.03

Brockman operation (soft tissue release for clubfoot) 83.84
Bronchogram, bronchography 87.32
  endotracheal 87.31
  transcricoid 87.32
Bronchoplasty 33.48
Bronchorrhaphy 33.41
Bronchoscopy NEC 33.23
  with biopsy 33.24
    lung 33.27
      brush 33.24
  fiberoptic 33.22
    with biopsy 33.24
      lung 33.27
        brush 33.24
  through tracheostomy 33.21
    with biopsy 33.24
      lung 33.27
        brush 33.24
Bronchospirometry 89.38
Bronchostomy 33.0
  closure 33.42
Bronchotomy 33.0
Browne (-Denis) **operation** (hypospadias repair) 58.45
Brunschwig operation (temporary gastrostomy) 43.19
Buckling, scleral 14.49
  with
    air tamponade 14.49
    implant (silicone) (vitreous) 14.41
    resection of sclera 14.49
    vitrectomy 14.49
    vitreous implant (silicone) 14.41
Bunionectomy (radical) 77.59
  with
    arthrodesis 77.52
    osteotomy of first metatarsal 77.51
    resection of joint with prosthetic implant 77.59
    soft tissue correction NEC 77.53
Bunnell operation (tendon transfer) 82.56
Burch procedure (retropubic urethral suspension for urinary stress incontinence) 59.5
Burgess operation (amputation of ankle) 84.14
Burn dressing 93.57
Burr holes 01.24
Bursectomy 83.5
  hand 82.31
Bursocentesis 83.94
  hand 82.92
Bursotomy 83.03
  hand 82.03
Burying of fimbriae in uterine wall 66.97
Bypass
  abdominal - coronary artery 36.17
  aortocoronary (catheter stent) (with prosthesis) (with saphenous vein graft) (with vein graft) 36.10
    one coronary vessel 36.11
    two coronary vessels 36.12
    three coronary vessels 36.13
    four coronary vessels 36.14
  arterial (graft) (mandril grown graft) (vein graft) NEC 39.29
    carotid-cerebral 39.28
    carotid-vertebral 39.28
    extracranial-intracranial [EC-IC] 39.28
    intra-abdominal NEC 39.26
    intrathoracic NEC 39.23
    peripheral NEC 39.29
  cardiopulmonary 39.61
    open 39.61
    percutaneous (closed) 39.66
  carotid-cerebral 39.28
  carotid-vertebral 39.28
  coronary - *see also* Bypass, aortocoronary 36.10
  extracranial-intracranial [EC-IC] 39.28

Bypass *(Continued)*
  gastric 44.39
    high 44.31
    laparoscopic 44.38
    Printen and Mason 44.31
  gastroduodenostomy (Jaboulay's) 44.39
    laparoscopic 44.38
    percutaneous [endoscopic] 44.32
  gastroenterostomy 44.39
    laparoscopic 44.38
  gastroepiploic - coronary artery 36.17
  gastrogastrostomy 44.39
    laparoscopic 44.38
  graft, pressurized treatment 00.16
  heart-lung (complete) (partial) 39.61
    open 39.61
    percutaneous (closed) 39.66
  high gastric 44.31
  ileo-jejunal 45.91
  internal mammary-coronary artery (single)
    36.15
    double vessel 36.16
  jejunal-ileum 45.91
  pulmonary 39.61
    open 39.61
    percutaneous (closed) 39.66
  shunt
    intestine
      large-to-large 45.94
      small-to-large 45.93
      small-to-small 45.91

Bypass *(Continued)*
  shunt *(Continued)*
    stomach 44.39
      high gastric 44.31
      laparoscopic 44.38
    terminal ileum 45.93
  vascular (arterial) (graft) (mandril grown
    graft) (vein graft) NEC 39.29
    aorta-carotid-brachial 39.22
    aorta-iliac-femoral 39.25
    aorta-renal 39.24
    aorta-subclavian-carotid 39.22
    aortic-superior mesenteric 39.26
    aortocarotid 39.22
    aortoceliac 39.26
    aortocoronary - *see also* Bypass,
      aortocoronary 36.10
    aortofemoral 39.25
    aortofemoral-popliteal 39.25
    aortoiliac 39.25
      to popliteal 39.25
    aortoiliofemoral 39.25
    aortomesenteric 39.26
    aortopopliteal 39.25
    aortorenal 39.24
    aortosubclavian 39.22
    axillary-brachial 39.29
    axillary-femoral (superficial) 39.29
    axillofemoral (superficial) 39.29
    carotid-cerebral 39.28
    carotid-vertebral 39.28

Bypass *(Continued)*
  vascular NEC *(Continued)*
    carotid to subclavian artery 39.22
    common hepatic-common iliac-renal
      39.26
    coronary - *see also* Bypass, aortocoronary
      36.10
    extracranial-intracranial [EC-IC] 39.28
    femoral-femoral 39.29
    femoroperoneal 39.29
    femoropopliteal (reversed saphenous
      vein) (saphenous) 39.29
    femorotibial (anterior) (posterior) 39.29
    iliofemoral 39.25
    ilioiliac 39.26
    internal mammary-coronary
      artery (single) 36.15
      double vessel 36.16
    intra-abdominal (arterial) NEC 39.26
      venous NEC 39.1
    intrathoracic NEC 39.23
    peripheral artery NEC 39.29
    popliteal-tibial 39.29
    renal artery 39.24
    splenorenal (venous) 39.1
    arterial 39.26
    subclavian-axillary 39.29
    subclavian-carotid 39.22
    subclavian-subclavian 39.22
    Y graft to renal arteries 39.24

C

Caldwell operation (sulcus extension) 24.91
Caldwell-Luc operation (maxillary sinusotomy)
  22.39
  with removal of membrane lining 22.31
Calibration, urethra 89.29
Calicectomy (renal) 55.4
Callander operation (knee disarticulation) 84.16
Caloric test, vestibular function 95.44
Calycectomy (renal) 55.4
Calyco-ileoneocystostomy 55.86
Calycotomy (renal) 55.11
Campbell operation
  bone block, ankle 81.11
  fasciotomy (iliac crest) 83.14
  reconstruction of anterior cruciate ligament
    81.45
Campimetry 95.05
Canaliculodacryocystorhinostomy 09.81
Canaliculoplasty 09.73
Canaliculorhinostomy 09.81
Canaloplasty, external auditory meatus 18.6
Cannulation - *see also* Insertion, catheter
  ampulla of Vater 51.99
  antrum 22.01
  arteriovenous 39.93
  artery 38.91
  caval-mesenteric vein 39.1
  cisterna chyli 40.61
  Eustachian tube 20.8
  lacrimal apparatus 09.42
  lymphatic duct, left (thoracic) 40.61
  nasal sinus (by puncture) 22.01
    through natural ostium 22.02
  pancreatic duct 52.92
    by retrograde endoscopy (ERP) 52.93
  renoportal 39.1
  sinus (nasal) (by puncture) 22.01
    through natural ostium 22.02
  splenorenal (venous) 39.1
    arterial 39.26
  thoracic duct (cervical approach) (thoracic
    approach) 40.61

Cannulization - *see* Cannulation
Canthocystostomy 09.82
Canthoplasty 08.59
Canthorrhaphy 08.52
  division or severing 08.02
Canthotomy 08.51
Capsulectomy
  joint - *see also* Arthrectomy 80.90
  kidney 55.91
  lens 13.65
    with extraction of lens 13.51
  ovary 65.29
    laparoscopic 65.25
Capsulo-iridectomy 13.65
Capsuloplasty - *see* Arthroplasty
Capsulorrhaphy 81.96
  with arthroplasty - *see* Arthroplasty
  ankle 81.94
  foot 81.94
  lower extremity NEC 81.95
  upper extremity 81.93
Capsulotomy
  joint - *see also* Division, joint capsule 80.40
    for claw toe repair 77.57
  lens 13.64
    with
      discission of lens 13.2
      removal of foreign body 13.02
        by magnet extraction 13.01
Cardiac
  mapping 37.27
  massage (external) (closed chest) 99.63
    open chest 37.91
  retraining 93.36
Cardiac support device (CSD) 37.41
Cardiectomy (stomach) 43.5
Cardiocentesis 37.0
Cardiography - *see also* Angiocardiography
  88.50
Cardiolysis 37.10
Cardiomyopexy 36.39
Cardiomyotomy 42.7
Cardio-omentopexy 36.39
Cardiopericardiopexy 36.39

Cardioplasty (stomach and esophagus)
  44.65
  stomach alone 44.66
    laparoscopic 44.67
Cardioplegia 39.63
Cardiopneumopexy 36.39
Cardiorrhaphy 37.49
Cardioschisis 37.12
Cardiosplenopexy 36.39
Cardiotomy (exploratory) 37.11
Cardiovalvulotomy - *see* Valvulotomy, heart
Cardioversion (external) 99.62
  atrial 99.61
CardioWest™ Total Temporary Artificial Heart
  (TAH-t) 37.52
Carotid pulse tracing with ECG lead 89.56
Carpectomy (partial) 77.84
  total 77.94
Carroll and Taber arthroplasty (proximal
  interphalangeal joint) 81.72
Casting (for immobilization) NEC 93.53
  with fracture-reduction - *see* Reduction,
    fracture
Castration
  female (oophorectomy, bilateral) 65.51
    laparoscopic 65.53
  male 62.41
C.A.T. (computerized axial tomography) -
  see also Scan, C.A.T. 88.38
Catheterization - *see also* Insertion,
  catheter
  arteriovenous 39.93
  artery 38.91
  bladder, indwelling 57.94
    percutaneous (cystostomy) 57.17
    suprapubic NEC 57.18
  bronchus 96.05
    with lavage 96.56
  cardiac (right) 37.21
    combined left and right 37.23
    left 37.22
      combined with right heart 37.23
    right 37.21
      combined with left heart 37.23

B & C

Catheterization (Continued)
central venous NEC 38.93
    peripherally inserted central catheter
        (PICC) 38.93
chest 34.04
    revision (with lysis of adhesions) 34.04
        thoracoscopic 34.06
    thoracoscopic 34.06
Eustachian tube 20.8
heart (right) 37.21
    combined left and right 37.23
    left 37.22
        combined with right heart 37.23
    right 37.21
        combined with left heart 37.23
hepatic vein 38.93
inferior vena cava 38.93
intercostal space (with water seal), for
        drainage 34.04
    revision (with lysis of adhesions) 34.04
        thoracoscopic 34.06
    thoracoscopic 34.06
lacrimonasal duct 09.44
laryngeal 96.05
nasolacrimal duct 09.44
pancreatic cyst 52.01
renal vein 38.93
Swan-Ganz (pulmonary) 89.64
transtracheal for oxygenation 31.99
umbilical vein 38.92
ureter (to kidney) 59.8
    for retrograde pyelogram 87.74
urethra, indwelling 57.94
vein NEC 38.93
    for renal dialysis 38.95
Cattell operation (herniorrhaphy) 53.51
Cauterization - see also Destruction, lesion, by
        site
anus NEC 49.39
    endoscopic 49.31
Bartholin's gland 71.24
broad ligament 69.19
bronchus 32.09
    endoscopic 32.01
canaliculi 09.73
cervix 67.32
chalazion 08.25
choroid plexus 02.14
conjunctiva 10.33
    lesion 10.32
cornea (fistula) (ulcer) 11.42
ear, external 18.29
endometrial implant - see Excision, lesion, by
        site
entropion 08.41
esophagus 42.39
    endoscopic 42.33
eyelid 08.25
    for entropion or ectropion 08.41
fallopian tube 66.61
    by endoscopy (hysteroscopy)
        (laparoscopy) 66.29
hemorrhoids 49.43
iris 12.41
lacrimal
    gland 09.21
    punctum 09.72
        for eversion 09.71
    sac 09.6
larynx 30.09
liver 50.29
lung 32.29
    endoscopic 32.28
    thoracoscopic 32.20
meibomian gland 08.25
nose, for epistaxis (with packing) 21.03
ovary 65.29
    laparoscopic 65.25
palate (bony) 27.31
pannus (superficial) 11.42
pharynx 29.39

Cauterization (Continued)
punctum, lacrimal 09.72
    for eversion 09.71
rectum 48.32
    radical 48.31
round ligament 69.19
sclera 12.84
    with iridectomy 12.62
skin 86.3
subcutaneous tissue 86.3
tonsillar fossa 28.7
urethra 58.39
    endoscopic 58.31
uterosacral ligament 69.19
uterotubal ostia 66.61
uterus 68.29
vagina 70.33
vocal cords 30.09
vulva 71.3
Cavernoscopy 34.21
Cavernostomy 33.1
Cavernotomy, kidney 55.39
Cavography (inferior vena cava) 88.51
CCM (implantation of cardiac contractility
        modulation)
    rechargeable pulse generator only 17.52
    total system 17.51
Cecectomy (with resection of terminal ileum)
    laparoscopic 17.32
    open and other 45.72
Cecil operation (urethral reconstruction) 58.46
Cecocoloplicopexy 46.63
Cecocolostomy 45.94
Cecofixation 46.64
Ceco-ileostomy 45.93
Cecopexy 46.64
Cecoplication 46.62
Cecorrhaphy 46.75
Cecosigmoidostomy 45.94
Cecostomy (tube) - see also Colostomy 46.10
Cecotomy 45.03
Celiocentesis 54.91
Celioscopy 54.21
Celiotomy, exploratory 54.11
Cell block and Papanicolaou smear - see
        Examination, microscopic
CentriMag® acute circulatory support device
        37.62
Cephalogram 87.17
    dental 87.12
    orthodontic 87.12
Cephalometry, cephalometrics 87.17
    echo 88.78
    orthodontic 87.12
    ultrasound (sonar) 88.78
    x-ray 87.81
Cephalotomy, fetus 73.8
Cerclage
    anus 49.72
    cervix 67.51
        transabdominal 67.51
        transvaginal 67.59
    isthmus uteri (cervix) 67.59
    retinal reattachment - see also Buckling,
        scleral 14.49
    sclera - see also Buckling, scleral 14.49
Cervicectomy (with synchronous colporrhaphy)
        67.4
Cervicoplasty 67.69
Cesarean section 74.99
    classical 74.0
    corporeal 74.0
    extraperitoneal 74.2
    fundal 74.0
    laparotrachelotomy 74.1
    Latzko 74.2
    low cervical 74.1
    lower uterine segment 74.1
    peritoneal exclusion 74.4
    specified type NEC 74.4
    supravesical 74.2

Cesarean section (Continued)
    transperitoneal 74.4
        classical 74.0
        low cervical 74.1
    upper uterine segment 74.0
    vaginal 74.4
    Waters 74.2
Chamberlain procedure - see Mediastinotomy
Chandler operation (hip fusion) 81.21
Change - see also Replacement
    cast NEC 97.13
        lower limb 97.12
        upper limb 97.11
    cystostomy catheter or tube 59.94
    gastrostomy tube 97.02
    length
        bone - see either category 78.2●
            Shortening, bone or category 78.3●
            Lengthening, bone
        muscle 83.85
            hand 82.55
        tendon 83.85
            hand 82.55
    nephrostomy catheter or tube 55.93
    pyelostomy catheter or tube 55.94
    splint 97.14
    tracheostomy tube 97.23
    ureterostomy catheter or tube 59.93
    urethral catheter, indwelling 57.95
Character analysis, psychologic 94.03
Charles operation (correction of lymphedema)
        40.9
Charnley operation (compression arthrodesis)
    ankle 81.11
    hip 81.21
    knee 81.22
Cheatle-Henry operation - see Repair, hernia,
        femoral
Check
    automatic implantable cardioverter/
        defibrillator (AICD) (interrogation
        only) 89.49
    CRT-D (cardiac resynchronization
        defibrillator) (interrogation only)
        89.49
    CRT-P (cardiac resynchronization
        pacemaker) (interrogation only)
        89.45
    pacemaker, artificial (cardiac) (function)
        (interrogation only) (rate) 89.45
        amperage threshold 89.48
        artifact wave form 89.46
        electrode impedance 89.47
        voltage threshold 89.48
    vision NEC 95.09
Cheiloplasty 27.59
Cheilorrhaphy 27.51
Cheilostomatoplasty 27.59
Cheilotomy 27.0
Chemical peel, skin 86.24
Chemocauterization - see also Destruction,
        lesion, by site
    corneal epithelium 11.41
    palate 27.31
Chemodectomy 39.89
Chemoembolization 99.25
Chemolysis
    nerve (peripheral) 04.2
    spinal canal structure 03.8
Chemoneurolysis 04.2
Chemonucleolysis (nucleus pulposus) 80.52
Chemopallidectomy 01.42
Chemopeel (skin) 86.24
Chemosurgery
    esophagus 42.39
        endoscopic 42.33
    Mohs' 86.24
    skin (superficial) 86.24
    stomach 43.49
        endoscopic 43.41
Chemothalamectomy 01.41

◄ New   ◄▏ Revised   ~~deleted~~ Deleted   ● Use Additional Digit(s)   ▨ Omit code

Chemotherapy - *see also* Immunotherapy
   Antabuse 94.25
   for cancer NEC 99.25
      brain wafer implantation 00.10
      CLO 17.70
      clofarabine 17.70
      CLOLAR® 17.70
      implantation of chemotherapeutic agent 00.10
      interstitial implantation 00.10
      intracavitary implantation 00.10
      wafer chemotherapy 00.10
   ithium 94.22
   methadone 94.25
   palate (bony) 27.31
Chevalier-Jackson operation (partial laryngectomy) 30.29
Child operation (radical subtotal pancreatectomy) 52.53
Cholangiocholangiostomy 51.39
Cholangiocholecystocholedochectomy 51.22
Cholangio-enterostomy 51.39
Cholangiogastrostomy 51.39
Cholangiogram 87.54
   endoscopic retrograde (ERC) 51.11
   intraoperative 87.53
   intravenous 87.52
   percutaneous hepatic 87.51
   transhepatic 87.53
Cholangiography - *see also* Cholangiogram 87.54
Cholangiojejunostomy (intrahepatic) 51.39
Cholangiopancreatography, endoscopic retrograde (ERCP) 51.10
Cholangiostomy 51.59
Cholangiotomy 51.59
Cholecystectomy (total) 51.22
   partial 51.21
      laparoscopic 51.24
   total 51.22
      laparoscopic 51.23
Cholecystenterorrhaphy 51.91
Cholecystocecostomy 51.32
Cholecystocholangiogram 87.59
Cholecystocolostomy 51.32
Cholecystoduodenostomy 51.32
Cholecystoenterostomy (Winiwater) 51.32
Cholecystogastrostomy 51.34
Cholecystogram 87.59
Cholecystoileostomy 51.32
Cholecystojejunostomy (Roux-en-Y) (with jejunojejunostomy) 51.32
Cholecystopancreatostomy 51.33
Cholecystopexy 51.99
Cholecystorrhaphy 51.91
Cholecystostomy NEC 51.03
   by trocar 51.02
Cholecystotomy 51.04
   percutaneous 51.01
Choledochectomy 51.63
Choledochoduodenostomy 51.36
Choledochoenterostomy 51.36
Choledochojejunostomy 51.36
Choledocholithotomy 51.41
   endoscopic 51.88
Choledocholithotripsy 51.41
   endoscopic 51.88
Choledochopancreatostomy 51.39
Choledochoplasty 51.72
Choledochorrhaphy 51.71
Choledochoscopy 51.11
Choledochostomy 51.51
Choledochotomy 51.51
Cholelithotomy 51.04
Chondrectomy 80.90
   ankle 80.97
   elbow 80.92
   foot and toe 80.98
   hand and finger 80.94
   hip 80.95
   intervertebral cartilage - *see* category 80.5●

Chondrectomy *(Continued)*
   knee (semilunar cartilage) 80.6
   nasal (submucous) 21.5
   semilunar cartilage (knee) 80.6
   shoulder 80.91
   specified site NEC 80.99
   spine - *see* category 80.5●
   wrist 80.93
Chondroplasty - *see* Arthroplasty
Chondrosternoplasty (for pectus excavatum repair) 34.74
Chondrotomy - *see also* Division, cartilage 80.40
   nasal 21.1
Chopart operation (midtarsal amputation) 84.12
Chordectomy, vocal 30.22
Chordotomy (spinothalamic) (anterior) (posterior) NEC 03.29
   percutaneous 03.21
   stereotactic 03.21
Ciliarotomy 12.55
Ciliectomy (ciliary body) 12.44
   eyelid margin 08.20
Cinch, cinching
   for scleral buckling - *see also* Buckling, scleral 14.49
   ocular muscle (oblique) (rectus) 15.22
      multiple (two or more muscles) 15.4
Cineangiocardiography - *see also* Angiocardiography 88.50
Cineplasty, cineplastic prosthesis
   amputation - *see* Amputation
   arm 84.44
   biceps 84.44
   extremity 84.40
      lower 84.48
      upper 84.44
   leg 84.48
Cineradiograph - *see* Radiography
Cingulumotomy (brain) (percutaneous radiofrequency) 01.32
Circumcision (male) 64.0
   female 71.4
CISH [classic infrafascial SEMM hysterectomy] 68.31
Clagett operation (closure of chest wall following open flap drainage) 34.72
Clamp and cautery, hemorrhoids 49.43
Clamping
   aneurysm (cerebral) 39.51
   blood vessel - *see* Ligation, blood vessel
   ventricular shunt 02.43
Clavicotomy 77.31
   fetal 73.8
Claviculectomy (partial) 77.81
   total 77.91
Clayton operation (resection of metatarsal heads and bases of phalanges) 77.88
Cleaning, wound 96.59
Clearance
   bladder (transurethral) 57.0
   pelvic
      female 68.8
      male 57.71
   prescalene fat pad 40.21
   renal pelvis (transurethral) 56.0
   ureter (transurethral) 56.0
Cleft lift 86.21
Cleidotomy 77.31
   fetal 73.8
Clipping
   aneurysm (basilar) (carotid) (cerebellar) (cerebellopontine) (communicating artery) (vertebral) 39.51
   arteriovenous fistula 39.53
   frenulum, frenum
      labia (lips) 27.91
      lingual (tongue) 25.91
   left atrial appendage 37.36
   tip of uvula 27.72
Clitoridectomy 71.4

Clitoridotomy 71.4
Clivogram 87.02
Closure - *see also* Repair
   abdominal wall 54.63
      delayed (granulating wound) 54.62
      secondary 54.61
      tertiary 54.62
   amputation stump, secondary 84.3
   anular disc 80.54
      with graft or prosthesis 80.53
   anulus fibrosus 80.54
      with graft or prosthesis 80.53
   aorticopulmonary fenestration (fistula) 39.59
   appendicostomy 47.92
   artificial opening
      bile duct 51.79
      bladder 57.82
      bronchus 33.42
      common duct 51.72
      esophagus 42.83
      gallbladder 51.92
      hepatic duct 51.79
      intestine 46.50
         large 46.52
         small 46.51
      kidney 55.82
      larynx 31.62
      rectum 48.72
      stomach 44.62
      thorax 34.72
      trachea 31.72
      ureter 56.83
      urethra 58.42
   atrial septal defect - *see also* Repair, atrial septal defect 35.71
      with umbrella device (King-Mills type) 35.52
      combined with repair of valvular and ventricular septal defects - *see* Repair, endocardial cushion defect
   bronchostomy 33.42
   cecostomy 46.52
   cholecystostomy 51.92
   cleft hand 82.82
   colostomy 46.52
   cystostomy 57.82
   diastema (alveolar) (dental) 24.8
   disrupted abdominal wall (postoperative) 54.61
   duodenostomy 46.51
   encephalocele 02.12
   endocardial cushion defect - *see also* Repair, endocardial cushion defect 35.73
   enterostomy 46.50
   esophagostomy 42.83
   fenestration
      aorticopulmonary 39.59
      septal, heart - *see also* Repair, heart, septum 35.70
   filtering bleb, corneoscleral (postglaucoma) 12.66
   fistula
      abdominothoracic 34.83
      anorectal 48.73
      anovaginal 70.73
      antrobuccal 22.71
      anus 49.73
      aorticopulmonary (fenestration) 39.59
      aortoduodenal 39.59
      appendix 47.92
      biliary tract 51.79
      bladder NEC 57.84
      branchial cleft 29.52
      bronchocutaneous 33.42
      bronchoesophageal 33.42
      bronchomediastinal 34.73
      bronchopleural 34.73
      bronchopleurocutaneous 34.73
      bronchopleuromediastinal 34.73

Closure *(Continued)*
  fistula *(Continued)*
    bronchovisceral 33.42
    bronchus 33.42
    cecosigmoidal 46.76
    cerebrospinal fluid 02.12
    cervicoaural 18.79
    cervicosigmoidal 67.62
    cervicovesical 57.84
    cervix 67.62
    cholecystocolic 51.93
    cholecystoduodenal 51.93
    cholecystoenteric 51.93
    cholecystogastric 51.93
    cholecystojejunal 51.93
    cisterna chyli 40.63
    colon 46.76
    colovaginal 70.72
    common duct 51.72
    cornea 11.49
        with lamellar graft (homograft) 11.62
            autograft 11.61
    diaphragm 34.83
    duodenum 46.72
    ear, middle 19.9
    ear drum 19.4
    enterocolic 46.74
    enterocutaneous 46.74
    enterouterine 69.42
    enterovaginal 70.74
    enterovesical 57.83
    esophagobronchial 33.42
    esophagocutaneous 42.84
    esophagopleurocutaneous 34.73
    esophagotracheal 31.73
    esophagus NEC 42.84
    fecal 46.79
    gallbladder 51.93
    gastric NEC 44.63
    gastrocolic 44.63
    gastroenterocolic 44.63
    gastroesophageal 42.84
    gastrojejunal 44.63
    gastrojejunocolic 44.63
    heart valve - *see* Repair, heart,
        valve
    hepatic duct 51.79
    hepatopleural 34.73
    hepatopulmonary 34.73
    ileorectal 46.74
    ileosigmoidal 46.74
    ileovesical 57.83
    ileum 46.74
    in ano 49.73
    intestine 46.79
        large 46.76
        small NEC 46.74
    intestinocolonic 46.74
    intestinoureteral 56.84
    intestinouterine 69.42
    intestinovaginal 70.74
    intestinovesical 57.83
    jejunum 46.74
    kidney 55.83
    lacrimal 09.99
    laryngotracheal 31.62
    larynx 31.62
    lymphatic duct, left (thoracic) 40.63
    mastoid (antrum) 19.9
    mediastinobronchial 34.73
    mediastinocutaneous 34.73
    mouth (external) 27.53
    nasal 21.82
        sinus 22.71
    nasolabial 21.82
    nasopharyngeal 21.82
    oroantral 22.71
    oronasal 21.82
    oval window (ear) 20.93
    pancreaticoduodenal 52.95
    perilymph 20.93

Closure *(Continued)*
  fistula *(Continued)*
    perineorectal 48.73
    perineosigmoidal 46.76
    perineourethroscrotal 58.43
    perineum 71.72
    perirectal 48.93
    pharyngoesophageal 29.53
    pharynx NEC 29.53
    pleura, pleural NEC 34.93
    pleurocutaneous 34.73
    pleuropericardial 37.49
    pleuroperitoneal 34.83
    pulmonoperitoneal 34.83
    rectolabial 48.73
    rectoureteral 56.84
    rectourethral 58.43
    rectovaginal 70.73
    rectovesical 57.83
    rectovesicovaginal 57.83
    rectovulvar 48.73
    rectum NEC 48.73
    renal 55.83
    reno-intestinal 55.83
    round window 20.93
    salivary (gland) (duct) 26.42
    scrotum 61.42
    sigmoidovaginal 70.74
    sigmoidovesical 57.83
    splenocolic 41.95
    stomach NEC 44.63
    thoracic duct 40.63
    thoracoabdominal 34.83
    thoracogastric 34.83
    thoracointestinal 34.83
    thorax NEC 34.73
    trachea NEC 31.73
    tracheoesophageal 31.73
    tympanic membrane - *see also*
        Tympanoplasty 19.4
    umbilicourinary 57.51
    ureter 56.84
    ureterocervical 56.84
    ureterorectal 56.84
    ureterosigmoidal 56.84
    ureterovaginal 56.84
    ureterovesical 56.84
    urethra 58.43
    urethroperineal 58.43
    urethroperineovesical 57.84
    urethrorectal 58.43
    urethroscrotal 58.43
    urethrovaginal 58.43
    uteroenteric 69.42
    uterointestinal 69.42
    uterorectal 69.42
    uteroureteric 56.84
    uterovaginal 69.42
    uterovesical 57.84
    vagina 70.75
    vaginocutaneous 70.75
    vaginoenteric 70.74
    vaginoperineal 70.75
    vaginovesical 57.84
    vesicocervicovaginal 57.84
    vesicocolic 57.83
    vesicocutaneous 57.84
    vesicoenteric 57.83
    vesicometrorectal 57.83
    vesicoperineal 57.84
    vesicorectal 57.83
    vesicosigmoidal 57.83
    vesicosigmoidovaginal 57.83
    vesicoureteral 56.84
    vesicoureterovaginal 56.84
    vesicourethral 57.84
    vesicourethrorectal 57.83
    vesicouterine 57.84
    vesicovaginal 57.84
    vulva 71.72
    vulvorectal 48.73

Closure *(Continued)*
  foramen ovale (patent) 35.71
    with
        prosthesis (open heart technique) 35.51
            closed heart technique 35.52
        tissue graft 35.61
  gastroduodenostomy 44.5
  gastrojejunostomy 44.5
  gastrostomy 44.62
  ileostomy 46.51
  jejunostomy 46.51
  laceration - *see also* Suture, by site
    liver 50.61
  laparotomy, delayed 54.62
  meningocele (spinal) 03.51
    cerebral 02.12
  myelomeningocele 03.52
  nephrostomy 55.82
  palmar cleft 82.82
  patent ductus arteriosus 38.85
  pelviostomy 55.82
  peptic ulcer (bleeding) (perforated) 44.40
  perforation
    ear drum - *see also* Tympanoplasty 19.4
    esophagus 42.82
    nasal septum 21.88
    tympanic membrane - *see also*
        Tympanoplasty 19.4
  proctostomy 48.72
  punctum, lacrimal (papilla) 09.91
  pyelostomy 55.82
  rectostomy 48.72
  septum defect (heart) - *see also* Repair, heart,
        septum 35.70
  sigmoidostomy 46.52
  skin (V-Y type) 86.59
  stoma
    bile duct 51.79
    bladder 57.82
    bronchus 33.42
    common duct 51.72
    esophagus 42.83
    gallbladder 51.92
    hepatic duct 51.79
    intestine 46.50
        large 46.52
        small 46.51
    kidney 55.82
    larynx 31.62
    rectum 48.72
    stomach 44.62
    thorax 34.72
    trachea 31.72
    ureter 56.83
    urethra 58.42
  thoracostomy 34.72
  tracheostomy 31.72
  ulcer (bleeding) (peptic) (perforated) 44.40
    duodenum 44.42
    gastric 44.41
    intestine (perforated) 46.79
    skin 86.59
    stomach 44.41
  ureterostomy 56.83
  urethrostomy 58.42
  vagina 70.8
  vascular
    percutaneous puncture - *omit code*
  vesicostomy 57.22
  wound - *see also* Suture, by site
    with graft - *see* Graft
    with tissue adhesive 86.59
Coagulation, electrocoagulation - *see also*
    Destruction, lesion, by site
  aneurysm (cerebral) (peripheral vessel)
      39.52
  arteriovenous fistula 39.53
  brain tissue (incremental) (radiofrequency)
      01.59
  broad ligament 69.19
  cervix 67.32

◀ New   ◀▦ Revised   ~~deleted~~ Deleted   ● Use Additional Digit(s)   ▦▦▦ Omit code

Coagulation, electrocoagulation *(Continued)*
 ear
  external 18.29
  inner 20.79
  middle 20.51
 fallopian tube 66.61
 gasserian ganglion 04.05
 nose, for epistaxis (with packing) 21.03
 ovary 65.29
  laparoscopic 65.25
 pharynx (by diathermy) 29.39
 prostatic bed 60.94
 rectum (polyp) 48.32
  radical 48.31
 retina (for)
  destruction of lesion 14.21
  reattachment 14.51
  repair for tear 14.31
 round ligament 69.19
 semicircular canals 20.79
 spinal cord (lesion) 03.4
 urethrovesical junction, transurethral 57.49
 uterosacral ligament 69.19
 uterus 68.29
 vagina 70.33
 vulva 71.3
Coating, aneurysm of brain 39.52
Cobalt-60 therapy (treatment) 92.23
Coccygectomy (partial) 77.89
 total 77.99
Coccygotomy 77.39
"Cocked hat" procedure (metacarpal
 lengthening and transfer of local flap)
 82.69
Cockett operation (varicose vein) lower limb
 38.59
 upper limb 38.53
Cody tack (perforation of footplate) 19.0
Coffey operation (uterine suspension) (Meig's
 modification) 69.22
Cole operation (anterior tarsal wedge
 osteotomy) 77.28
Colectomy (partial) (segmental) (subtotal)
 cecum (with terminal ileum)
  laparoscopic 17.32
  open and other 45.72
 laparoscopic 17.39
 left (Hartmann) (lower) (radical)
   laparoscopic 17.35
   open and other 45.75
 multiple segmental
  laparoscopic 17.31
  open and other 45.71
 open and other 45.79
 right (radical)
  laparoscopic 17.33
  open and other 45.73
 sigmoid
  laparoscopic 17.36
  open and other 45.76
 terminal ileum with cecum
  laparoscopic 17.32
  open and other 45.72
 total
  laparoscopic 45.81
  open 45.82
  other 45.83
  unspecified 45.83
 transverse
  laparoscopic 17.34
  open and other 45.74
Collapse, lung, surgical 33.39
 by
  destruction of phrenic nerve 33.31
  pneumoperitoneum 33.33
  pneumothorax, artificially-induced 33.32
  thoracoplasty 33.34
Collection, sperm for artificial insemination
 99.96
Collis-Nissen operation (hiatal hernia repair
 with esophagogastroplasty) 53.80

Colocentesis 45.03
Colocolostomy 45.94
 proximal to distal segment 45.79
Colocystoplasty 57.87 *[45.52]*
Colofixation 46.64
Coloileotomy 45.00
Colonna operation
 adductor tenotomy (first stage) 83.12
 hip arthroplasty (second stage) 81.40
 reconstruction of hip (second stage) 81.40
Colonoscopy 45.23
 with
  biopsy 45.25
   rectum 48.24
  stent - *see* Insertion, stent, colon
 fiberoptic (flexible) 45.23
 intraoperative 45.21
 through stoma (artificial) 45.22
 transabdominal 45.21
Colopexy 46.63
Coloplication 46.64
Coloproctostomy 45.94
Colorectosigmoidostomy 45.94
Colorectostomy 45.94
Colorrhaphy 46.75
Coloscopy - *see* Colonoscopy
Colosigmoidostomy 45.94
Colostomy (ileo-ascending) (ileotransverse)
 (perineal) (transverse) 46.10
 with anterior rectal resection 48.62
 delayed opening 46.14
 loop 46.03
 permanent (magnetic) 46.13
 temporary 46.11
Colotomy 45.03
Colpectomy 70.4
Colpoceliocentesis 70.0
Colpocentesis 70.0
Colpocleisis (complete) (partial) 70.8
Colpohysterectomy 68.59
 laparoscopically assisted (LAVH) 68.51
Colpoperineoplasty 70.79
 with repair of urethrocele 70.51
  with graft or prosthesis 70.53
Colpoperineorrhaphy 70.71
 following delivery 75.69
Colpopexy 70.77
 with graft or prosthesis 70.78
Colpoplasty 70.79
Colpopoiesis 70.61
 vaginal construction 70.61
  with graft or prosthesis 70.63
Colporrhaphy 70.71
 anterior (cystocele repair) 70.51
  with graft or prosthesis 70.54
 for repair of
  cystocele 70.51
   with rectocele 70.50
    with graft or prosthesis 70.53
  enterocele 70.92
   with graft or prosthesis 70.93
  rectocele 70.52
   with cystocele 70.50
    with graft or prosthesis 70.53
  urethrocele 70.51
   with graft or prosthesis 70.54
 posterior (rectocele repair) 70.52
  with graft or prosthesis 70.55
Colposcopy 70.21
Colpotomy 70.14
 for pelvic peritoneal drainage 70.12
Commando operation (radical glossectomy)
 25.4
Commissurotomy
 closed heart technique - *see* Valvulotomy,
  heart
 open heart technique - *see* Valvuloplasty,
  heart
Compression, trigeminal nerve 04.02
Conchectomy 21.69
Conchotomy 21.1

Conduction study, nerve 89.15
Conduitogram, ileum 87.78
Condylectomy - *see* category 77.8●
 mandible 76.5
Condylotomy NEC - *see also* Division, joint
 capsule 80.40
 mandible (open) 76.62
  closed 76.61
Conization
 cervix (knife) (sharp) (biopsy) 67.2
  by
   cryosurgery 67.33
   electroconization 67.32
Conjunctivocystorhinostomy 09.82
 with insertion of tube or stent 09.83
Conjunctivodacryocystorhinostomy (CDCR)
 09.82
 with insertion of tube or stent 09.83
Conjunctivodacryocystostomy 09.82
 with insertion of tube or stent 09.83
Conjunctivoplasty 10.49
Conjunctivorhinostomy 09.82
 with insertion of tube or stent 09.83
Constriction of globe, for scleral buckling - *see*
 also Buckling, scleral 14.49
Construction
 auricle, ear (with graft) (with implant) 18.71
 ear
  auricle (with graft) (with implant) 18.71
  meatus (osseous) (skin-lined) 18.6
 endorectal ileal pouch (H-pouch) (J-pouch)
  (S-pouch) (with anastomosis to anus)
  45.95
 esophagus, artificial - *see* Anastomosis,
  esophagus
 ileal bladder (open) 56.51
  closed 57.87 *[45.51]*
 ileal conduit 56.51
 larynx, artificial 31.75
 patent meatus (ear) 18.6
 penis (rib graft) (skin graft) (myocutaneous
  flap) 64.43
 pharyngeal valve, artificial 31.75
 urethra 58.46
 vagina, artificial 70.61
  with graft or prosthesis 70.63
 venous valves (peripheral) 39.59
Consultation 89.09
 comprehensive 89.07
 limited (single organ system) 89.06
 specified type NEC 89.08
Continuous positive airway pressure [CPAP]
 (non-invasive) 93.90
 delivered by
  endotracheal tube - *see* category 96.7●
  tracheostomy – *see* category 96.7●
Control
 atmospheric pressure and composition NEC
  93.98
  antigen-free air conditioning 93.98
  decompression chamber 93.97
  mountain sanatorium 93.98
 epistaxis 21.00
  by
   cauterization (and packing) 21.03
   coagulation (with packing) 21.03
   electrocoagulation (with packing) 21.03
   excision of nasal mucosa with grafting
    21.07
   ligation of artery 21.09
    ethmoidal 21.04
    external carotid 21.06
    maxillary (transantral) 21.05
   packing (nasal) (anterior) 21.01
    posterior (and anterior) 21.02
   specified means NEC 21.09
 hemorrhage 39.98
  abdominal cavity 54.19
  adenoids (postoperative) 28.7
  anus (postoperative) 49.95
  bladder (postoperative) 57.93

Control *(Continued)*
　hemorrhage *(Continued)*
　　chest 34.09
　　colon 45.49
　　　endoscopic 45.43
　　duodenum (ulcer) 44.49
　　　by
　　　　embolization (transcatheter)
　　　　　44.44
　　　　suture (ligation) 44.42
　　　endoscopic 44.43
　　esophagus 42.39
　　　endoscopic 42.33
　　gastric (ulcer) 44.49
　　　by
　　　　embolization (transcatheter)
　　　　　44.44
　　　　suture (ligation) 44.41
　　　endoscopic 44.43
　　intrapleural 34.09
　　　postoperative (recurrent) 34.03
　　laparotomy site 54.12
　　nose - *see also* Control, epistaxis 21.00
　　peptic (ulcer) 44.49
　　　by
　　　　embolization (transcatheter)
　　　　　44.44
　　　　suture (ligation) 44.40
　　　endoscopic 44.43
　　pleura, pleural cavity 34.09
　　　postoperative (recurrent) 34.03
　　postoperative NEC 39.98
　　postvascular surgery 39.41
　　prostate 60.94
　　specified site NEC 39.98
　　stomach - *see* Control, hemorrhage,
　　　gastric
　　thorax NEC 34.09
　　　postoperative (recurrent) 34.03
　　thyroid (postoperative) 06.02
　　tonsils (postoperative) 28.7
Conversion
　anastomosis - *see* Revision, anastomosis
　atrial rhythm (to sinus rhythm) 99.61
　cardiac rhythm NEC 99.69
　　to sinus rhythm 99.62
　gastrostomy to jejunostomy (endoscopic)
　　for feeding tube placement 46.32
　obstetrical position - *see* Version
Cooling, gastric 96.31
CorCap™ 37.41
Cordectomy, vocal 30.22
Cordopexy, vocal 31.69
Cordotomy
　spinal (bilateral) NEC 03.29
　　percutaneous 03.21
　vocal 31.3
Corectomy 12.12
Corelysis 12.35
Coreoplasty 12.35
Corneoconjunctivoplasty 11.53
Corpectomy, (vertebral) 80.99
　with diskectomy 80.99
Correction - *see also* Repair
　atresia
　　esophageal 42.85
　　　by magnetic forces 42.99
　　external meatus (ear) 18.6
　　nasopharynx, nasopharyngeal 29.4
　　rectum 48.0
　　tricuspid 35.94
　atrial septal defect - *see also* Repair, atrial
　　septal defect 35.71
　　combined with repair of valvular and
　　　ventricular septal defects - *see*
　　　　Repair, endocardial cushion defect
　blepharoptosis - *see also* Repair,
　　blepharoptosis 08.36
　bunionette (with osteotomy) 77.54

Correction *(Continued)*
　chordee 64.42
　claw toe 77.57
　cleft
　　lip 27.54
　　palate 27.62
　clubfoot NEC 83.84
　coarctation of aorta
　　with
　　　anastomosis 38.34
　　　graft replacement 38.44
　cornea NEC 11.59
　　refractive NEC 11.79
　　　epikeratophakia 11.76
　　　keratomileusis 11.71
　　　keratophakia 11.72
　　　radial keratotomy 11.75
　esophageal atresia 42.85
　　by magnetic forces 42.99
　everted lacrimal punctum 09.71
　eyelid
　　ptosis - *see also* Repair, blepharoptosis
　　　08.36
　　retraction 08.38
　fetal defect 75.36
　forcible, of musculoskeletal deformity NEC
　　93.29
　hammer toe 77.56
　hydraulic pressure, open surgery
　　　for penile inflatable prosthesis
　　　　64.99
　　urinary artificial sphincter 58.99
　intestinal malrotation 46.80
　　large 46.82
　　small 46.81
　inverted uterus - *see* Repair, inverted
　　　uterus
　lymphedema (of limb) 40.9
　　excision with graft 40.9
　　obliteration of lymphatics 40.9
　　transplantation of autogenous lymphatics
　　　40.9
　nasopharyngeal atresia 29.4
　overlapping toes 77.58
　palate (cleft) 27.62
　prognathism NEC 76.64
　prominent ear 18.5
　punctum (everted) 09.71
　spinal pseudarthrosis - *see* Refusion,
　　　spinal
　syndactyly 86.85
　tetralogy of Fallot
　　one-stage 35.81
　　partial - *see* specific procedure
　　total 35.81
　total anomalous pulmonary venous
　　　connection
　　one-stage 35.82
　　partial - *see* specific procedure
　　total 35.82
　transposition, great arteries, total 35.84
　tricuspid atresia 35.94
　truncus arteriosus
　　one-stage 35.83
　　partial - *see* specific procedure
　　total 35.83
　ureteropelvic junction 55.87
　ventricular septal defect - *see also* Repair,
　　　ventricular septal defect 35.72
　　combined with repair of valvular and
　　　atrial septal defects - *see* Repair,
　　　　endocardial cushion defect
Costectomy 77.91
　with lung excision - *see* Excision, lung
　associated with thoracic operation - *omit code*
Costochondrectomy 77.91
　associated with thoracic operation - *omit code*
Costosternoplasty (pectus excavatum repair)
　34.74

Costotomy 77.31
Costotransversectomy 77.91
　associated with thoracic operation -
　　omit code
Counseling (for) NEC 94.49
　alcoholism 94.46
　drug addiction 94.45
　employers 94.49
　family (medical) (social) 94.49
　marriage 94.49
　ophthalmologic (with instruction) 95.36
　pastoral 94.49
Countershock, cardiac NEC 99.62
Coventry operation (tibial wedge osteotomy)
　77.27
CPAP (continuous positive airway pressure)
　93.90
　delivered by
　　endotracheal tube - *see* category 96.7●
　　tracheostomy – *see* category 96.7●
Craniectomy 01.25
　linear (opening of cranial suture) 02.01
　reopening of site 01.23
　strip (opening of cranial suture) 02.01
Cranioclasis, fetal 73.8
Cranioplasty 02.06
　with synchronous repair of encephalocele
　　02.12
Craniotomy 01.24
　as operative approach - *omit code*
　fetal 73.8
　for decompression of fracture 02.02
　reopening of site 01.23
Craterization, bone - *see also* Excision, lesion,
　bone 77.60
Crawford operation (tarso-frontalis sling of
　eyelid) 08.32
Creation - *see also* Formation
　cardiac device (defibrillator) (pacemaker)
　　pocket
　　with initial insertion of cardiac
　　　device - *omit code*
　　new site (skin) (subcutaneous) 37.79
　conduit
　　apical-aortic (AAC) 35.93
　　ileal (urinary) 56.51
　　left ventricle and aorta 35.93
　　right atrium and pulmonary artery
　　　35.94
　　right ventricle and pulmonary (distal)
　　　artery 35.92
　　in repair of
　　　pulmonary artery atresia 35.92
　　　transposition of great vessels 35.92
　　　truncus arteriosus 35.83
　endorectal ileal pouch (H-pouch) (J-pouch)
　　(S-pouch) (with anastomosis to anus)
　　45.95
　esophagogastric sphincteric competence
　　NEC 44.66
　　laparoscopic 44.67
　Hartmann pouch - *see* Colectomy, by site
　interatrial fistula 35.42
　pericardial window 37.12
　pleural window, for drainage 34.09
　pocket
　　cardiac device (defibrillator) (pacemaker)
　　　with initial insertion of cardiac
　　　　device - *omit code*
　　　new site (skin) (subcutaneous) 37.79
　　loop recorder 37.79
　　thalamic stimulator pulse generator
　　　with initial insertion of battery
　　　　package - *omit code*
　　　new site (skin) (subcutaneous) 86.09
　shunt - *see also* Shunt
　　arteriovenous fistula, for dialysis 39.93
　　left-to-right (systemic to pulmonary
　　　circulation) 39.0

Creation (*Continued*)
  subcutaneous tunnel for esophageal
    anastomosis 42.86
    with anastomosis - *see* Anastomosis,
      esophagus, antesternal
  syndactyly (finger) (toe) 86.89
  thalamic stimulator pulse generator
    with initial insertion of battery
      package - *omit code*
    new site (skin) (subcutaneous) 86.09
  tracheoesophageal fistula 31.95
  window
    pericardial 37.12
    pleura, for drainage 34.09
Credé maneuver 73.59
Cricoidectomy 30.29
Cricothyreotomy (for assistance in breathing)
  31.1
Cricothyroidectomy 30.29
Cricothyrostomy 31.1
Cricothyrotomy (for assistance in breathing)
  31.1
Cricotomy (for assistance in breathing) 31.1
Cricotracheotomy (for assistance in breathing)
  31.1
Crisis intervention 94.35
Croupette, croup tent 93.94
Crown, dental (ceramic) (gold) 23.41
Crushing
  bone - *see* category 78.4●
  calculus
    bile (hepatic) passage 51.49
      endoscopic 51.88
    bladder (urinary) 57.0
    pancreatic duct 52.09
      endoscopic 52.94
  fallopian tube - *see also* Ligation, fallopian
    tube 66.39
  ganglion - *see* Crushing, nerve
  hemorrhoids 49.45
  nasal septum 21.88
  nerve (cranial) (peripheral) NEC 04.03
    acoustic 04.01
    auditory 04.01
    phrenic 04.03
      for collapse of lung 33.31
    sympathetic 05.0
    trigeminal 04.02
    vestibular 04.01
  vas deferens 63.71
Cryoablation - *see* Ablation
Cryoanalgesia nerve (cranial) (peripheral) 04.2
Cryoconization, cervix 67.33
Cryodestruction - *see* Destruction, lesion, by site
Cryoextraction, lens - *see also* Extraction,
  cataract, intracapsular 13.19
Cryohypophysectomy (complete) (total) - *see*
  also Hypophysectomy 07.69
Cryoleucotomy 01.32
Cryopexy, retinal - *see* Cryotherapy, retina
Cryoprostatectomy 60.62
Cryoretinopexy (for)
  reattachment 14.52
  repair of tear or defect 14.32
Cryosurgery - *see* Cryotherapy
Cryothalamectomy 01.41
Cryotherapy - *see also* Destruction, lesion, by
  site
  bladder 57.59
  brain 01.59
  cataract 13.19
  cervix 67.33
  choroid - *see* Cryotherapy, retina
  ciliary body 12.72
  corneal lesion (ulcer) 11.43
    to reshape cornea 11.79
  ear
    external 18.29
    inner 20.79

Cryotherapy (*Continued*)
  esophagus 42.39
    endoscopic 42.33
  eyelid 08.25
  hemorrhoids 49.44
  iris 12.41
  nasal turbinates 21.61
  palate (bony) 27.31
  prostate 60.62
  retina (for)
    destruction of lesion 14.22
    reattachment 14.52
    repair of tear 14.32
  skin 86.3
  stomach 43.49
    endoscopic 43.41
  subcutaneous tissue 86.3
  turbinates (nasal) 21.61
  warts 86.3
    genital 71.3
Cryptectomy (anus) 49.39
  endoscopic 49.31
Cryptorchidectomy (unilateral) 62.3
  bilateral 62.41
Cryptotomy (anus) 49.39
  endoscopic 49.31
Cuirass 93.99
Culdocentesis 70.0
Culdoplasty 70.92
  with graft or prosthesis 70.93
Culdoscopy (exploration) (removal of foreign
  body or lesion) 70.22
Culdotomy 70.12
Culp-Deweerd operation (spiral flap
  pyeloplasty) 55.87
Culp-Scardino operation (ureteral flap
  pyeloplasty) 55.87
Culture (and sensitivity) - *see* Examination,
  microscopic
Curettage (with packing) (with secondary
  closure) - *see also* Dilation and curettage
  adenoids 28.6
  anus 49.39
    endoscopic 49.31
  bladder 57.59
    transurethral 57.49
  bone - *see also* Excision, lesion, bone
    77.60
  brain 01.59
  bursa 83.39
    hand 82.29
  cartilage - *see also* Excision, lesion, joint
    80.80
  cerebral meninges 01.51
  chalazion 08.25
  conjunctiva (trachoma follicles) 10.33
  corneal epithelium 11.41
    for smear or culture 11.21
  ear, external 18.29
  eyelid 08.25
  joint - *see also* Excision, lesion, joint 80.80
  meninges (cerebral) 01.51
    spinal 03.4
  muscle 83.32
    hand 82.22
  nerve (peripheral) 04.07
    sympathetic 05.29
  sclera 12.84
  skin 86.3
  spinal cord (meninges) 03.4
  subgingival 24.31
  tendon 83.39
    sheath 83.31
      hand 82.21
  uterus (with dilation) 69.09
    aspiration (diagnostic) NEC 69.59
      after abortion or delivery 69.52
      to terminate pregnancy 69.51
    following delivery or abortion 69.02

Curette evacuation, lens 13.2
Curtis operation (interphalangeal joint
  arthroplasty) 81.72
Cutaneolipectomy 86.83
Cutdown, venous 38.94
Cutting
  nerve (cranial) (peripheral) NEC 04.03
    acoustic 04.01
    auditory 04.01
    root, spinal 03.1
    sympathetic 05.0
    trigeminal 04.02
    vestibular 04.01
  pedicle (flap) graft 86.71
  pylorus (with wedge resection) 43.3
  spinal nerve root 03.1
  ureterovesical orifice 56.1
  urethral sphincter 58.5
CVP (central venous pressure monitoring)
  89.62
Cyclectomy (ciliary body) 12.44
  eyelid margin 08.20
Cyclicotomy 12.55
Cycloanemization 12.74
Cyclocryotherapy 12.72
Cyclodialysis (initial) (subsequent) 12.55
Cyclodiathermy (penetrating) (surface) 12.71
Cycloelectrolysis 12.71
Cyclophotocoagulation 12.73
Cyclotomy 12.55
Cystectomy - *see also* Excision, lesion, by site
  gallbladder - *see* Cholecystectomy
  urinary (partial) (subtotal) 57.6
    complete (with urethrectomy) 57.79
    radical 57.71
      with pelvic exenteration (female)
        68.8
    total (with urethrectomy) 57.79
Cystocolostomy 57.88
Cystogram, cystography NEC 87.77
Cystolitholapaxy 57.0
Cystolithotomy 57.19
Cystometrogram 89.22
Cystopexy NEC 57.89
Cystoplasty NEC 57.89
Cystoproctostomy 57.88
Cystoprostatectomy, radical 57.71
Cystopyelography 87.74
Cystorrhaphy 57.81
Cystoscopy (transurethral) 57.32
  with biopsy 57.33
  for
    control of hemorrhage
      bladder 57.93
      prostate 60.94
    retrograde pyelography 87.74
  ileal conduit 56.35
  through stoma (artificial) 57.31
Cystostomy
  closed (suprapubic) (percutaneous) 57.17
  open (suprapubic) 57.18
  percutaneous (closed) (suprapubic) 57.17
  suprapubic
    closed 57.17
    open 57.18
Cystotomy (open) (for removal of calculi)
  57.19
Cystourethrogram (retrograde) (voiding)
  87.76
Cystourethropexy (by) 59.79
  levator muscle sling 59.71
  retropubic suspension 59.5
  suprapubic suspension 59.4
Cystourethroplasty 57.85
Cystourethroscopy 57.32
  with biopsy
    bladder 57.33
    ureter 56.33
Cytology - *see* Examination, microscopic

D

Dacryoadenectomy 09.20
  partial 09.22
  total 09.23
Dacryoadenotomy 09.0
Dacryocystectomy (complete) (partial) 09.6
Dacryocystogram 87.05
Dacryocystorhinostomy (DCR) (by intubation)
    (external) (intranasal) 09.81
Dacryocystostomy 09.53
Dacryocystosyringotomy 09.53
Dacryocystotomy 09.53
Dahlman operation (excision of esophageal
    diverticulum) 42.31
Dana operation (posterior rhizotomy) 03.1
Danforth operation (fetal) 73.8
Darrach operation (ulnar resection) 77.83
da Vinci® (S HD) Surgical System – see
    category 17.4●
Davis operation (intubated ureterotomy) 56.2
Deaf training 95.49
Debridement, NOS 86.28
  excisional, NOS 86.22
    abdominal wall 54.3
    bone - see also Excision, lesion, bone 77.60
      fracture - see Debridement, open
        fracture
    brain 01.59
    burn (skin) 86.22
    bursa 83.5
    cerebral meninges 01.51
    dental 96.54
    fascia 83.44
    flap graft 86.75
    graft (flap) (pedicle) 86.75
    heart valve (calcified) - see Valvuloplasty,
      heart
    infection (skin) 86.22
      nail bed or fold 86.27
    joint - see Excision, lesion, joint
    meninges (cerebral) 01.51
      spinal 03.4
    muscle 83.45
      hand 82.36
    nail 86.27
    nerve (peripheral) 04.07
    open fracture (compound) 79.60
      arm NEC 79.62
      carpal, metacarpal 79.63
      facial bone 76.2
      femur 79.65
      fibula 79.66
      foot NEC 79.67
      hand NEC 79.63
      humerus 79.61
      leg NEC 79.66
      phalanges
        foot 79.68
        hand 79.64
      radius 79.62
      specified site NEC 79.69
      tarsal, metatarsal 79.67
      tibia 79.66
      ulna 79.62
    patella 77.66
    pedicle graft 86.75
    skin or subcutaneous tissue (burn)
        (infection) (wound) 86.22
      cardioverter/defibrillator (automatic)
        pocket 37.79
      graft 86.75
      nail, nail bed, or nail fold 86.27
      pacemaker pocket 37.79
      pocket
        cardiac device NEC 37.79
        cardiac pacemaker 37.79
        cardioverter/defibrillator
          (automatic) 37.79
    skull 01.25
      compound fracture 02.02

Debridement, NOS (Continued)
  excisional, NOS (Continued)
    spinal cord (meninges) 03.4
    tendon 83.39
    VersaJet™ 86.28
    wound (skin) 86.22
  nonexcisional, NOS 86.28
    burn (skin) 86.28
    dental 96.54
    infection (skin) 86.28
    skin or subcutaneous tissue (burn)
        (infection) (wound) 86.28
    ultrasonic, ultrasound 86.28
    VersaJet™ 86.28
    wound (skin) 86.28
Decapitation, fetal 73.8
Decapsulation, kidney 55.91
Declotting - see also Removal, thrombus
  arteriovenous cannula or shunt
    39.49
Decompression
  anus (imperforate) 48.0
  biliary tract 51.49
    by intubation 51.43
      endoscopic 51.87
      percutaneous 51.98
  brain 01.24
  carpal tunnel 04.43
  cauda equina 03.09
  chamber 93.97
  colon 96.08
    by incision 45.03
    endoscopic (balloon) 46.85
  common bile duct 51.42
    by intubation 51.43
      endoscopic 51.87
      percutaneous 51.98
  cranial 01.24
    for skull fracture 02.02
  endolymphatic sac 20.79
  ganglion (peripheral) NEC 04.49
    cranial NEC 04.42
  gastric 96.07
  heart 37.0
  intestine 96.08
    by incision 45.00
    endoscopic (balloon) 46.85
  intracranial 01.24
  labyrinth 20.79
  laminectomy 03.09
  laminotomy 03.09
  median nerve 04.43
  muscle 83.02
    hand 82.02
  nerve (peripheral) NEC 04.49
    auditory 04.42
    cranial NEC 04.42
    median 04.43
    trigeminal (root) 04.41
  orbit - see also Orbitotomy 16.09
  pancreatic duct 52.92
    endoscopic 52.93
  pericardium 37.0
  rectum 48.0
  skull fracture 02.02
  spinal cord (canal) 03.09
  tarsal tunnel 04.44
  tendon (sheath) 83.01
    hand 82.01
  thoracic outlet
    by
      myotomy (division of scalenus
        anticus muscle) 83.19
      tenotomy 83.13
  trigeminal (nerve root) 04.41
Decortication
  arterial 05.25
  brain 01.51
  cerebral meninges 01.51
  heart 37.31
  kidney 55.91

Decortication (Continued)
  lung (partial) (total) 34.51
    thoracoscopic 34.52
  nasal turbinates - see Turbinectomy
  nose 21.89
  ovary 65.29
    laparoscopic 65.25
  periarterial 05.25
  pericardium 37.31
  ventricle, heart (complete) 37.31
Decoy, E2F 00.16
Deepening
  alveolar ridge 24.5
  buccolabial sulcus 24.91
  lingual sulcus 24.91
Defatting, flap or pedicle graft 86.75
Defibrillation, electric (external) (internal)
    99.62
  automatic cardioverter/defibrillator - see
    category 37.9●
de Grandmont operation (tarsectomy) 08.35
Delaying of pedicle graft 86.71
Delivery (with)
  assisted spontaneous 73.59
  breech extraction (assisted) 72.52
    partial 72.52
      with forceps to aftercoming head 72.51
    total 72.54
      with forceps to aftercoming head 72.53
    unassisted (spontaneous delivery) -
      omit code
  cesarean section - see Cesarean section
  Credé maneuver 73.59
  De Lee maneuver 72.4
  forceps 72.9
    application to aftercoming head (Piper)
      72.6
      with breech extraction
        partial 72.51
        total 72.53
    Barton's 72.4
    failed 73.3
    high 72.39
      with episiotomy 72.31
    low (outlet) 72.0
      with episiotomy 72.1
    mid 72.29
      with episiotomy 72.21
    outlet (low) 72.0
      with episiotomy 72.1
    rotation of fetal head 72.4
    trial 73.3
  instrumental NEC 72.9
    specified NEC 72.8
  key-in-lock rotation 72.4
  Kielland rotation 72.4
  Malstrom's extraction 72.79
    with episiotomy 72.71
  manually assisted (spontaneous) 73.59
  spontaneous (unassisted) 73.59
    assisted 73.59
  vacuum extraction 72.79
    with episiotomy 72.71
Delorme operation
  pericardiectomy 37.31
  proctopexy 48.76
  repair of prolapsed rectum 48.76
  thoracoplasty 33.34
Denervation
  aortic body 39.89
  carotid body 39.89
  facet, percutaneous (radiofrequency) 03.96
  ovarian 65.94
  paracervical uterine 69.3
  uterosacral 69.3
Denker operation (radical maxillary
    antrotomy) 22.31
Dennis-Barco operation - see Repair, hernia,
  femoral
Denonvillier operation (limited rhinoplasty)
    21.86

Densitometry, bone (serial) (radiographic)
  88.98
Depilation, skin 86.92
Derlacki operation (tympanoplasty) 19.4
Dermabond 86.59
Dermabrasion (laser) 86.25
  for wound debridement 86.28
Derotation - *see* Reduction, torsion
Desensitization
  allergy 99.12
  psychologic 94.33
Desmotomy - *see also* Division, ligament 80.40
Destruction
  breast 85.20
  chorioretinopathy - *see also* Destruction,
    lesion, choroid 14.29
  ciliary body 12.74
  epithelial downgrowth, anterior chamber
    12.93
  fallopian tube 66.39
    with
      crushing (and ligation) 66.31
        by endoscopy (laparoscopy) 66.21
      division (and ligation) 66.32
        by endoscopy (culdoscopy)
          (hysteroscopy) (laparoscopy)
          (peritoneoscopy) 66.22
      ligation 66.39
        with
          crushing 66.31
            by endoscopy (laparoscopy)
              66.21
          division 66.32
            by endoscopy (culdoscopy)
              (hysteroscopy)
              (laparoscopy)
              (peritoneoscopy) 66.22
  fetus 73.8
  hemorrhoids 49.49
    by
      cryotherapy 49.44
      sclerotherapy 49.42
  inner ear NEC 20.79
    by injection 20.72
  intervertebral disc (NOS) 80.50
    by injection 80.52
    by other specified method 80.59
    herniated (nucleus pulposus) 80.51
  LAA 37.36
  lacrimal sac 09.6
  left atrial appendage 37.36
  lesion (local)
    anus 49.39
      endoscopic 49.31
    Bartholin's gland 71.24
      by
        aspiration 71.21
        excision 71.24
        incision 71.22
        marsupialization 71.23
    biliary ducts 51.69
      endoscopic 51.64
    bladder 57.59
      transurethral 57.49
    bone - *see* Excision, lesion, bone
    bowel - *see* Destruction, lesion, intestine
    brain (transtemporal approach) NEC
      01.59
      by stereotactic radiosurgery 92.30
        cobalt 60 92.32
        linear accelerator (LINAC) 92.31
        multi-source 92.32
        particle beam 92.33
        particulate 92.33
        radiosurgery NEC 92.39
        single source photon 92.31
    breast NEC 85.20
    bronchus NEC 32.09
      endoscopic 32.01
    cerebral NEC 01.59
      meninges 01.51

Destruction (*Continued*)
  lesion (*Continued*)
    cervix 67.39
      by
        cauterization 67.32
        cryosurgery, cryoconization 67.33
        electroconization 67.32
    choroid 14.29
      by
        cryotherapy 14.22
        diathermy 14.21
        implantation of radiation source
          14.27
        photocoagulation 14.25
          laser 14.24
          xenon arc 14.23
        radiation therapy 14.26
    ciliary body (nonexcisional) 12.43
      by excision 12.44
    conjunctiva 10.32
      by excision 10.31
    cornea NEC 11.49
      by
        cryotherapy 11.43
        electrocauterization 11.42
        thermocauterization 11.42
    cul-de-sac 70.32
    duodenum NEC 45.32
      by excision 45.31
        endoscopic 45.30
      endoscopic 45.30
    esophagus (chemosurgery) (cryosurgery)
      (electroresection) (fulguration) NEC
      42.39
      by excision 42.32
        endoscopic 42.33
      endoscopic 42.33
    eye NEC 16.93
    eyebrow 08.25
    eyelid 08.25
      excisional - *see* Excision, lesion, eyelid
    heart
      by catheter ablation 37.34
      by endovascular approach 37.34
      by open approach 37.33
      by thoracoscopic approach 37.37
      left atrial appendage 37.36
    intestine (large) 45.49
      by excision 45.41
        endoscopic 45.43
          polypectomy 45.42
      endoscopic 45.43
        polypectomy 45.42
      small 45.34
        by excision 45.33
    intranasal 21.31
    iris (nonexcisional) NEC 12.41
      by excision 12.42
    kidney 55.39
      by marsupialization 55.31
    lacrimal sac 09.6
    larynx 30.09
    liver 50.29
    lung 32.29
      endoscopic 32.28
      thoracoscopic 32.20
    meninges (cerebral) 01.51
      spinal 03.4
    nerve (peripheral) 04.07
      sympathetic 05.29
    nose 21.30
      intranasal 21.31
      specified NEC 21.32
    ovary
      by
        aspiration 65.91
        excision 65.29
          laparoscopic 65.25
      cyst by rupture (manual) 65.93
    palate (bony) (local) 27.31
      wide 27.32

Destruction (*Continued*)
  lesion (*Continued*)
    pancreas 52.22
      by marsupialization 52.3
      endoscopic 52.21
    pancreatic duct 52.22
      endoscopic 52.21
    penis 64.2
    pharynx (excisional) 29.39
    pituitary gland
      by stereotactic radiosurgery 92.30
        cobalt 60 92.32
        linear accelerator (LINAC) 92.31
        multi-source 92.32
        particle beam 92.33
        particulate 92.33
        radiosurgery NEC 92.39
        single source photon 92.31
    rectum (local) 48.32
      by
        cryosurgery 48.34
        electrocoagulation 48.32
        excision 48.35
        fulguration 48.32
        laser (Argon) 48.33
        polyp 48.36
        radical 48.31
    retina 14.29
      by
        cryotherapy 14.22
        diathermy 14.21
        implantation of radiation source
          14.27
        photocoagulation 14.25
          laser 14.24
          xenon arc 14.23
        radiation therapy 14.26
    salivary gland NEC 26.29
      by marsupialization 26.21
    sclera 12.84
    scrotum 61.3
    skin NEC 86.3
    sphincter of Oddi 51.69
      endoscopic 51.64
    spinal cord (meninges) 03.4
    spleen 41.42
      by marsupialization 41.41
    stomach NEC 43.49
      by excision 43.42
        endoscopic 43.41
      endoscopic 43.41
    subcutaneous tissue NEC 86.3
    testis 62.2
    tissue of heart - *see* Excision, lesion,
      heart
    tongue 25.1
    urethra (excisional) 58.39
      endoscopic 58.31
    uterus 68.29
  nerve (cranial) (peripheral) (by
    cryoanalgesia) (by radiofrequency)
    04.2
  sympathetic, by injection of neurolytic
    agent 05.32
  neuroma
    acoustic 04.01
      by craniotomy 04.01
      by stereotactic radiosurgery
        92.30
        cobalt 60 92.32
        linear accelerator (LINAC)
          92.31
        multi-source 92.32
        particle beam 92.33
        particulate 92.33
        radiosurgery NEC 92.39
        single source photon 92.31
    cranial 04.07
    Morton's 04.07
    peripheral
      Morton's 04.07

Destruction *(Continued)*
  prostate (prostatic tissue)
    by
      cryotherapy 60.62
      microwave 60.96
      radiofrequency 60.97
      transurethral microwave thermotherapy
        (TUMT) 60.96
      transurethral needle ablation (TUNA)
        60.97
      TULIP (transurethral (ultrasound)
        guided laser induced
        prostatectomy) 60.21
      TUMT (transurethral microwave
        thermotherapy) 60.96
      TUNA (transurethral needle ablation)
        60.97
  semicircular canals, by injection 20.72
  vestibule, by injection 20.72
Detachment, uterosacral ligaments 69.3
Determination
  mental status (clinical) (medicolegal)
    (psychiatric) NEC 94.11
    psychologic NEC 94.09
  vital capacity (pulmonary) 89.37
Detorsion
  intestine (twisted) (volvulus) 46.80
    large 46.82
      endoscopic (balloon) 46.85
    small 46.81
  kidney 55.84
  ovary 65.95
  spermatic cord 63.52
    with orchiopexy 62.5
  testis 63.52
    with orchiopexy 62.5
  volvulus 46.80
    endoscopic (balloon) 46.85
Detoxification therapy 94.25
  alcohol 94.62
    with rehabilitation 94.63
    combined alcohol and drug 94.68
      with rehabilitation 94.69
  drug 94.65
    with rehabilitation 94.66
    combined alcohol and drug 94.68
      with rehabilitation 94.69
Devascularization, stomach 44.99
Device
  CorCap™ 37.41
  external fixator - *see* Fixator, external
Dewebbing
  esophagus 42.01
  syndactyly (fingers) (toes) 86.85
Dextrorotation - *see* Reduction, torsion
Dialysis
  hemodiafiltration, hemofiltration
    (extracorporeal) 39.95
  kidney (extracorporeal) 39.95
  liver 50.92
  peritoneal 54.98
  renal (extracorporeal) 39.95
Diaphanoscopy
  nasal sinuses 89.35
  skull (newborn) 89.16
Diaphysectomy - *see* category 77.8 ●
Diathermy 93.34
  choroid - *see* Diathermy, retina
  nasal turbinates 21.61
  retina
    for
      destruction of lesion 14.21
      reattachment 14.51
      repair of tear 14.31
  surgical - *see* Destruction, lesion, by site
  turbinates (nasal) 21.61
Dickson operation (fascial transplant)
  83.82
Dickson-Diveley operation (tendon
    transfer and arthrodesis to correct
    claw toe) 77.57

Dieffenbach operation (hip disarticulation)
  84.18
Dilation
  achalasia 42.92
  ampulla of Vater 51.81
    endoscopic 51.84
  anus, anal (sphincter) 96.23
  biliary duct
    endoscopic 51.84
    pancreatic duct 52.99
      endoscopic 52.98
    percutaneous (endoscopy) 51.98
    sphincter
      of Oddi 51.81
        endoscopic 51.84
      pancreatic 51.82
        endoscopic 51.85
  bladder 96.25
    neck 57.92
  bronchus 33.91
  cervix (canal) 67.0
    obstetrical 73.1
    to assist delivery 73.1
  choanae (nasopharynx) 29.91
  colon (endoscopic) (balloon) 46.85
    with insertion of colonic stent
      endoscopic 46.86
      other 46.87
  colostomy stoma 96.24
  duodenum (endoscopic) (balloon) 46.85
    with insertion of colonic stent
      endoscopic 46.86
      other 46.87
  endoscopic - *see* Dilation, by site
  enterostomy stoma 96.24
  esophagus (by bougie) (by sound) 42.92
  fallopian tube 66.96
  foreskin (newborn) 99.95
  frontonasal duct 96.21
  gastrojejunostomy site, endoscopic 44.22
  heart valve - *see* Valvulotomy, heart
  ileostomy stoma 96.24
  ileum (endoscopic) (balloon) 46.85
    with insertion of colonic stent
      endoscopic 46.86
      other 46.87
  intestinal stoma (artificial) 96.24
  intestine (endoscopic) (balloon) 46.85
    with insertion of colonic stent
      endoscopic 46.86
      other 46.87
  jejunum (endoscopic) (balloon) 46.85
    with insertion of colonic stent
      endoscopic 46.86
      other 46.87
  lacrimal
    duct 09.42
    punctum 09.41
  larynx 31.98
  lymphatic structure(s) (peripheral) 40.9
  nares 21.99
  nasolacrimal duct (retrograde) 09.43
    with insertion of tube or stent 09.44
  nasopharynx 29.91
  pancreatic duct 52.99
    endoscopic 52.98
  pharynx 29.91
  prostatic urethra (transurethral) (balloon)
    60.95
  punctum, lacrimal papilla 09.41
  pylorus
    by incision 44.21
    endoscopic 44.22
  rectum 96.22
  salivary duct 26.91
  sphenoid ostia 22.52
  sphincter
    anal 96.23
    cardiac 42.92
    of Oddi 51.81
      endoscopic 51.84

Dilation *(Continued)*
  sphincter *(Continued)*
    pancreatic 51.82
      endoscopic 51.85
    pylorus, endoscopic 44.22
      by incision 44.21
  Stenson's duct 26.91
  trachea 31.99
  ureter 59.8
    meatus 56.91
  ureterovesical orifice 59.8
  urethra 58.6
    prostatic (transurethral) (balloon) 60.95
  urethrovesical junction 58.6
  vagina (instrumental) (manual) NEC 96.16
  vesical neck 57.92
  Wharton's duct 26.91
  Wirsung's duct 52.99
    endoscopic 52.98
Dilation and curettage, uterus (diagnostic)
  69.09
  after
    abortion 69.02
    delivery 69.02
  to terminate pregnancy 69.01
Diminution, ciliary body 12.74
Disarticulation 84.91
  ankle 84.13
  elbow 84.06
  finger, except thumb 84.01
    thumb 84.02
  hip 84.18
  knee 84.16
  shoulder 84.08
  thumb 84.02
  toe 84.11
  wrist 84.04
Discectomy - *see* Diskectomy
Discission
  capsular membrane 13.64
  cataract (Wheeler knife) (Ziegler knife) 13.2
    congenital 13.69
    secondary membrane 13.64
  iris 12.12
  lens (capsule) (Wheeler knife) (Ziegler knife)
    (with capsulotomy) 13.2
  orbitomaxillary, radical 16.51
  pupillary 13.2
  secondary membrane (after cataract) 13.64
  vitreous strands (posterior approach) 14.74
    anterior approach 14.73
Discogram, diskogram 87.21
Discolysis (by injection) 80.52
Diskectomy (discectomy), intervertebral 80.51
  with corpectomy 80.99
  herniated (nucleus pulposus) 80.51
  percutaneous 80.59
Dispensing (with fitting)
  contact lens 95.32
  low vision aids NEC 95.33
  spectacles 95.31
Disruption
  blood brain barrier via infusion [BBBD] 00.19
Dissection - *see also* Excision
  aneurysm 38.60
  artery-vein-nerve bundle 39.91
  branchial cleft fistula or sinus 29.52
  bronchus 32.1
  femoral hernia 53.29
  groin, radical 40.54
  larynx block (en bloc) 30.3
  mediastinum with pneumonectomy 32.59
    thoracoscopic 32.50
  neck, radical 40.40
    with laryngectomy 30.4
    bilateral 40.42
    unilateral 40.41
  orbital fibrous bands 16.92
  pterygium (with reposition) 11.31
  radical neck - *see* Dissection, neck, radical
  retroperitoneal NEC 59.00

◀ New   ◀️ Revised   ~~deleted~~ Deleted   ● Use Additional Digit(s)   ▨ Omit code

Dissection *(Continued)*
  thoracic structures (block) (en bloc) (radical) (brachial plexus, bronchus, lobe of lung, ribs, and sympathetic nerves) 32.6
  vascular bundle 39.91
Distention, bladder (therapeutic) (intermittent) 96.25
Diversion
  biliopancreatic (BPD) 43.7 *[45.51] [45.91]*
    with duodenal switch 43.89 *[45.51] [45.91]*
    urinary
      cutaneous 56.61
      ileal conduit 56.51
      internal NEC 56.71
      ureter to
        intestine 56.71
        skin 56.61
      uretero-ileostomy 56.51
Diversional therapy 93.81
Diverticulectomy
  bladder (suprapubic) 57.59
    transurethral approach 57.49
  duodenum 45.31
    endoscopic 45.30
  esophagus 42.31
    endoscopic 42.33
  esophagomyotomy 42.7
  hypopharyngeal (by cricopharyngeal myotomy) 29.32
  intestine
    large 45.41
      endoscopic 45.43
    small 45.33
  kidney 55.39
  Meckel's 45.33
  pharyngeal (by cricopharyngeal myotomy) 29.32
  pharyngoesophageal (by cricopharyngeal myotomy) 29.32
  stomach 43.42
    endoscopic 43.41
  urethra 58.39
    endoscopic 58.31
Division
  Achilles tendon 83.11
  adductor tendon (hip) 83.12
  adhesions - *see* Lysis, adhesions
  angle of mandible (open) 76.62
    closed 76.61
  anterior synechiae 12.32
  aponeurosis 83.13
  arcuate ligament (spine) - *omit code*
  arteriovenous fistula (with ligation) 39.53
  artery (with ligation) 38.80
    abdominal 38.86
    aorta (arch) (ascending) (descending) 38.84
    head and neck NEC 38.82
    intracranial NEC 38.81
    lower limb 38.88
    thoracic NEC 38.85
    upper limb 38.83
  bladder neck 57.91
  blepharorrhaphy 08.02
  blood vessels, cornea 10.1
  bone - *see also* Osteotomy 77.30
  brain tissue 01.32
    cortical adhesions 02.91
  canaliculus 09.52
  canthorrhaphy 08.02
  cartilage 80.40
    ankle 80.47
    elbow 80.42
    foot and toe 80.48
    hand and finger 80.44
    hip 80.45
    knee 80.46
    shoulder 80.41
    specified site NEC 80.49
    spine 80.49
    wrist 80.43
  cerebral tracts 01.32

Division *(Continued)*
  chordae tendineae 35.32
  common wall between posterior left atrium and coronary sinus (with roofing of resultant defect with patch graft) 35.82
  congenital web
    larynx 31.98
    pharynx 29.54
  endometrial synechiae 68.21
  fallopian tube - *see* Ligation, fallopian tube
  fascia 83.14
    hand 82.12
  frenulum, frenum
    labial 27.91
    lingual 25.91
    tongue 25.91
  ganglion, sympathetic 05.0
  glossopharyngeal nerve 29.92
  goniosynechiae 12.31
  hypophyseal stalk - *see also* Hypophysectomy, partial 07.63
  iliotibial band 83.14
  isthmus
    horseshoe kidney 55.85
    thyroid 06.91
  joint capsule 80.40
    ankle 80.47
    elbow 80.42
    foot and toe 80.48
    hand and finger 80.44
    hip 80.45
    knee 80.46
    shoulder 80.41
    specified site NEC 80.49
    wrist 80.43
  labial frenum 27.91
  lacrimal ductules 09.0
  laryngeal nerve (external) (recurrent) (superior) 31.91
  ligament 80.40
    ankle 80.47
    arcuate (spine) - *omit code*
    canthal 08.36
    elbow 80.42
    foot and toe 80.48
    hand and finger 80.44
    hip 80.45
    knee 80.46
    palpebrae 08.36
    shoulder 80.41
    specified site NEC 80.49
    spine 80.49
      arcuate - *omit code*
      flavum - *omit code*
    uterosacral 69.3
    wrist 80.43
  ligamentum flavum (spine) - *omit code*
  meninges (cerebral) 01.31
  muscle 83.19
    hand 82.19
  nasolacrimal duct stricture (with drainage) 09.59
  nerve (cranial) (peripheral) NEC 04.03
    acoustic 04.01
    adrenal gland 07.42
    auditory 04.01
    glossopharyngeal 29.92
    lacrimal branch 05.0
    laryngeal (external) (recurrent) (superior) 31.91
    phrenic 04.03
      for collapse of lung 33.31
    root, spinal or intraspinal 03.1
    sympathetic 05.0
    tracts
      cerebral 01.32
      spinal cord 03.29
        percutaneous 03.21
    trigeminal 04.02
    vagus - *see also* Vagotomy 44.00
    vestibular 04.01

Division *(Continued)*
  otosclerotic process or material, middle ear 19.0
  papillary muscle (heart) 35.31
  patent ductus arteriosus 38.85
  penile adhesions 64.93
  posterior synechiae 12.33
  pylorus (with wedge resection) 43.3
  rectum (stricture) 48.91
  scalenus anticus muscle 83.19
  Skene's gland 71.3
  soft tissue NEC 83.19
    hand 82.19
  sphincter
    anal (external) (internal) 49.59
      left lateral 49.51
      posterior 49.52
    cardiac 42.7
    of Oddi 51.82
      endoscopic 51.85
    pancreatic 51.82
      endoscopic 51.85
  spinal
    cord tracts 03.29
      percutaneous 03.21
    nerve root 03.1
  symblepharon (with insertion of conformer) 10.5
  synechiae
    endometrial 68.21
    iris (posterior) 12.33
      anterior 12.32
  tarsorrhaphy 08.02
  tendon 83.13
    Achilles 83.11
    adductor (hip) 83.12
    hand 82.11
  trabeculae carneae cordis (heart) 35.35
  tympanum 20.23
  uterosacral ligaments 69.3
  vaginal septum 70.14
  vas deferens 63.71
  vein (with ligation) 38.80
    abdominal 38.87
    head and neck NEC 38.82
    intracranial NEC 38.81
    lower limb 38.89
      varicose 38.59
    thoracic NEC 38.85
    upper limb 38.83
    varicose 38.50
      abdominal 38.57
      head and neck NEC 38.52
      intracranial NEC 38.51
      lower limb 38.59
      thoracic NEC 38.55
      upper limb 38.53
  vitreous, cicatricial bands (posterior approach) 14.74
    anterior approach 14.73
Doleris operation (shortening of round ligaments) 69.22
D'Ombrain operation (excision of pterygium with corneal graft) 11.32
Domestic tasks therapy 93.83
Dopplergram, Doppler flow mapping - *see also* Ultrasonography
  aortic arch 88.73
  head and neck 88.71
  heart 88.72
  intraoperative transcranial 00.94
  thorax NEC 88.73
Dorrance operation (push-back operation for cleft palate) 27.62
Dotter operation (transluminal angioplasty) 39.59
Douche, vagina 96.44
Douglas' operation (suture of tongue to lip for micrognathia) 25.59
Downstream® System (AO therapy) (aqueous oxygen) 00.49

Doyle operation (paracervical uterine
    denervation) 69.3
Drainage
  by
      anastomosis - *see* Anastomosis
      aspiration - *see* Aspiration
      incision - *see* Incision
  abdomen 54.19
    percutaneous 54.91
  abscess - *see also* Drainage, by site and
      Incision, by site
    appendix 47.2
      with appendectomy 47.09
        laparoscopic 47.01
    parapharyngeal (oral) (transcervical) 28.0
    peritonsillar (oral) (transcervical) 28.0
    retropharyngeal (oral) (transcervical)
      28.0
    thyroid (field) (gland) 06.09
      percutaneous (needle) 06.01
      postoperative 06.02
    tonsil, tonsillar (oral) (transcervical) 28.0
  antecubital fossa 86.04
  appendix 47.91
    with appendectomy 47.09
      laparoscopic 47.01
    abscess 47.2
      with appendectomy 47.09
        laparoscopic 47.01
  axilla 86.04
  bladder (without incision) 57.0
    by indwelling catheter 57.94
      percutaneous suprapubic (closed)
        57.17
      suprapubic NEC 57.18
  buccal space 27.0
  bursa 83.03
    by aspiration 83.94
      hand 82.92
    hand 82.03
      by aspiration 82.92
    radial 82.03
    ulnar 82.03
  cerebrum, cerebral (meninges) (ventricle)
    (incision) (trephination) 01.39
    by
      anastomosis - *see* Shunt, ventricular
      aspiration 01.09
        through previously implanted
          catheter 01.02
  chest (closed) 34.04
    open (by incision) 34.09
    thoracoscopic 34.06
  cranial sinus (incision) (trephination) 01.21
    by aspiration 01.09
  cul-de-sac 70.12
    by aspiration 70.0
  cyst - *see also* Drainage, by site and
      Incision, by site
    pancreas (by catheter) 52.01
      by marsupialization 52.3
      internal (anastomosis) 52.4
    pilonidal 86.03
    spleen, splenic (by marsupialization)
      41.41
  duodenum (tube) 46.39
    by incision 45.01
  ear
    external 18.09
    inner 20.79
    middle (by myringotomy) 20.09
      with intubation 20.01
  epidural space, cerebral (incision)
    (trephination) 01.24
    by aspiration 01.09
  extradural space, cerebral (incision)
    (trephination) 01.24
    by aspiration 01.09
  extraperitoneal 54.0
  facial region 27.0
  fascial compartments, head and neck 27.0

Drainage (*Continued*)
  fetal hydrocephalic head (needling) (trocar)
    73.8
  fluid (blood) (cerebrospinal) (CSF)
    by
      external ventricular drain (EVD)
        placement 02.21
  gallbladder 51.04
    by
      anastomosis 51.35
      aspiration 51.01
      incision 51.04
  groin region (abdominal wall) (inguinal)
    54.0
    skin 86.04
    subcutaneous tissue 86.04
  hematoma - *see* Drainage, by site and
      Incision, by site
  hydrocephalic head (needling) (trocar) 73.8
  hypochondrium 54.0
    intra-abdominal 54.19
  iliac fossa 54.0
  infratemporal fossa 27.0
  intracranial space (epidural) (extradural)
    (incision) (trephination) 01.24
    by aspiration 01.09
    subarachnoid or subdural (incision)
      (trephination) 01.31
      by aspiration 01.09
  intraperitoneal 54.19
    percutaneous 54.91
  kidney (by incision) 55.01
    by
      anastomosis 55.86
      catheter 59.8
    pelvis (by incision) 55.11
  liver 50.0
    by aspiration 50.91
  Ludwig's angina 27.0
  lung (by incision) 33.1
    by punch (needle) (trocar) 33.93
  midpalmar space 82.04
  mouth floor 27.0
  mucocele, nasal sinus 22.00
    by puncture 22.01
    through natural ostium 22.02
  omentum 54.19
    percutaneous 54.91
  ovary (aspiration) 65.91
    by incision 65.09
    laparoscopic 65.01
  palmar space (middle) 82.04
  pancreas (by catheter) 52.01
    by anastomosis 52.96
  parapharyngeal 28.0
  paronychia 86.04
  parotid space 27.0
  pelvic peritoneum (female) 70.12
    male 54.19
  pericardium 37.0
  perigastric 54.19
    percutaneous 54.91
  perineum
    female 71.09
    male 86.04
  perisplenic tissue 54.19
    percutaneous 54.91
  peritoneum 54.19
    pelvic (female) 70.12
    percutaneous 54.91
  peritonsillar 28.0
  pharyngeal space, lateral 27.0
  pilonidal cyst or sinus 86.03
  pleura (closed) 34.04
    open (by incision) 34.09
    thoracoscopic 34.06
  popliteal space 86.04
  postural 93.99
  postzygomatic space 27.0
  pseudocyst, pancreas 52.3
    by anastomosis 52.4

Drainage (*Continued*)
  pterygopalatine fossa 27.0
  retropharyngeal 28.0
  scrotum 61.0
  skin 86.04
  spinal (canal) (cord) 03.09
    by anastomosis - *see* Shunt, spinal
    diagnostic 03.31
  spleen 41.2
    cyst (by marsupialization) 41.41
  subarachnoid space, cerebral (incision)
    (trephination) 01.31
    by aspiration 01.09
  subcutaneous tissue 86.04
  subdiaphragmatic 54.19
    percutaneous 54.91
  subdural space, cerebral (incision)
    (trephination) 01.31
    by aspiration 01.09
  subhepatic space 54.19
    percutaneous 54.91
  sublingual space 27.0
  submental space 27.0
  subphrenic space 54.19
    percutaneous 54.91
  supraclavicular fossa 86.04
  temporal pouches 27.0
  tendon (sheath) 83.01
    hand 82.01
  thenar space 82.04
  thorax (closed) 34.04
    open (by incision) 34.09
    thoracoscopic 34.06
  thyroglossal tract (by incision) 06.09
    by aspiration 06.01
  thyroid (field) (gland) (by incision)
    06.09
    by aspiration 06.01
    postoperative 06.02
  tonsil 28.0
  tunica vaginalis 61.0
  ureter (by catheter) 59.8
    by
      anastomosis NEC - *see also*
        Anastomosis, ureter 56.79
      incision 56.2
  ventricle (cerebral) (incision)
    by
      anastomosis - *see* Shunt, ventricular
      aspiration 01.09
        through previously implanted
          catheter 01.02
      extracranial ventricular shunt - *see*
        category 02.3
  vertebral column 03.09
Drawing test 94.08
Dressing
  burn 93.57
  ulcer 93.56
  wound 93.57
Drilling
  bone - *see also* Incision, bone 77.10
  ovary 65.99
Drotrecogin alfa (activated), infusion 00.11
Ductogram, mammary 87.35
Duhamel operation (abdominoperineal
  pull-through) 48.65
Duhrssen's
  incisions (cervix, to assist delivery)
    73.93
  operation (vaginofixation of uterus)
    69.22
Dunn operation (triple arthrodesis)
  81.12
Duodenectomy 45.62
  with
    gastrectomy - *see* Gastrectomy
    pancreatectomy - *see* Pancreatectomy
Duodenocholedochotomy 51.51
Duodenoduodenostomy 45.91
  proximal to distal segment 45.62

Duodenoileostomy 45.91
Duodenojejunostomy 45.91
Duodenoplasty 46.79
Duodenorrhaphy 46.71
Duodenoscopy 45.13
   through stoma (artificial) 45.12
   transabdominal (operative)
     45.11
Duodenostomy 46.39

Duodenotomy 45.01
Dupuytren operation
   fasciectomy 82.35
   fasciotomy 82.12
     with excision 82.35
   shoulder disarticulation
     84.08
Durabond 86.59
Duraplasty 02.12

Durham (-Caldwell) operation (transfer of
   biceps femoris tendon) 83.75
DuToit and Roux operation (staple
   capsulorrhaphy of shoulder) 81.82
DuVries operation (tenoplasty) 83.88
Dwyer operation
   fasciotomy 83.14
   soft tissue release NEC 83.84
   wedge osteotomy, calcaneus 77.28

E

E2F decoy 00.16
Eagleton operation (extrapetrosal drainage)
   20.22
ECG - see Electrocardiogram
Echocardiography 88.72
   intracardiac (heart chambers) (ICE) 37.28
   intravascular (coronary vessels) 00.24
   transesophageal 88.72
     monitoring (Doppler) (ultrasound)
      89.68
Echoencephalography 88.71
Echography - see Ultrasonography
Echogynography 88.79
Echoplacentogram 88.78
ECMO (extracorporeal membrane oxygenation)
   39.65
Eden-Hybinette operation (glenoid bone block)
   78.01
Educational therapy (bed-bound children)
   (handicapped) 93.82
EEG (electroencephalogram) 89.14
   monitoring (radiographic) (video) 89.19
Effler operation (heart) 36.2
Effleurage 93.39
EGD (esophagogastroduodenoscopy) 45.13
   with closed biopsy 45.16
Eggers operation
   tendon release (patellar retinacula) 83.13
   tendon transfer (biceps femoris tendon)
     (hamstring tendon) 83.75
EKG - see also Electrocardiogram 89.52
Elastic hosiery 93.59
Electrocardiogram (with 12 or more leads)
   89.52
   with vectorcardiogram 89.53
   fetal (scalp), intrauterine 75.32
   rhythm (with one to three leads) 89.51
Electrocautery - see also Cauterization
   cervix 67.32
   corneal lesion (ulcer) 11.42
   esophagus 42.39
     endoscopic 42.33
Electrocoagulation - see also Destruction, lesion,
   by site
   aneurysm (cerebral) (peripheral vessels)
     39.52
   cervix 67.32
   cystoscopic 57.49
   ear
     external 18.29
     inner 20.79
     middle 20.51
   fallopian tube (lesion) 66.61
     for tubal ligation - see Ligation, fallopian
      tube
   gasserian ganglion 04.02
   nasal turbinates 21.61
   nose, for epistaxis (with packing)
     21.03
   ovary 65.29
     laparoscopic 65.25
   prostatic bed 60.94
   rectum (polyp) 48.32
     radical 48.31

Electrocoagulation (Continued)
   retina (for)
     destruction of lesion 14.21
     reattachment 14.51
     repair of tear 14.31
   round ligament 69.19
   semicircular canals 20.79
   urethrovesical junction, transurethral 57.49
   uterine ligament 69.19
   uterosacral ligament 69.19
   uterus 68.29
   vagina 70.33
   vulva 71.3
Electrocochleography 20.31
Electroconization, cervix 67.32
Electroconvulsive therapy (ECT) 94.27
Electroencephalogram (EEG) 89.14
   monitoring (radiographic) (video) 89.19
     intraoperative 00.94
Electrogastrogram 44.19
Electrokeratotomy 11.49
Electrolysis
   ciliary body 12.71
   hair follicle 86.92
   retina (for)
     destruction of lesion 14.21
     reattachment 14.51
     repair of tear 14.31
   skin 86.92
   subcutaneous tissue 86.92
Electromyogram, electromyography (EMG)
   (muscle) 93.08
   eye 95.25
   urethral sphincter 89.23
Electronarcosis 94.29
Electronic gaiter 93.59
Electronystagmogram (ENG) 95.24
Electro-oculogram (EOG) 95.22
Electroresection - see also Destruction, lesion, by
   site
   bladder neck (transurethral) 57.49
   esophagus 42.39
     endoscopic 42.33
   prostate (transurethral) 60.29
   stomach 43.49
     endoscopic 43.41
Electroretinogram (ERG) 95.21
Electroshock therapy (EST) 94.27
   subconvulsive 94.26
Elevation
   bone fragments (fractured)
   orbit 76.79
   sinus (nasal)
     frontal 22.79
     maxillary 22.79
   skull (with debridement) 02.02
   spinal 03.53
   pedicle graft 86.71
Elliot operation (scleral trephination with
   iridectomy) 12.61
Ellis Jones operation (repair of peroneal
   tendon) 83.88
Ellison operation (reinforcement of collateral
   ligament) 81.44
Elmslie-Cholmeley operation (tarsal wedge
   osteotomy) 77.28

Eloesser operation
   thoracoplasty 33.34
   thoracostomy 34.09
Elongation - see Lengthening
Embolectomy 38.00
   with endarterectomy - see Endarterectomy
   abdominal
     artery 38.06
     vein 38.07
   aorta (arch) (ascending) (descending) 38.04
   arteriovenous shunt or cannula 39.49
   bovine graft 39.49
   head and neck NEC 38.02
   intracranial NEC 38.01
   lower limb
     artery 38.08
     vein 38.09
   mechanical
     endovascular
      head and neck 39.74
   pulmonary (artery) (vein) 38.05
   thoracic NEC 38.05
   upper limb (artery) (vein) 38.03
Embolization (transcatheter)
   adhesive (glue) 39.79
     head and neck 39.72
   arteriovenous fistula 39.53
     endovascular 39.72
   artery (selective) 38.80
     by
      endovascular approach 39.79
       head and neck vessels 39.72
        bare coils 39.75
        bioactive coils 39.76
       partial occlusion (balloon)
        (temporary) 39.77
      percutaneous transcatheter infusion
       99.29
     abdominal NEC 38.86
      duodenal (transcatheter) 44.44
      gastric (transcatheter) 44.44
      renal (transcatheter) 38.86
     aorta (arch) (ascending) (descending)
      38.84
      temporary therapeutic endovascular
       (balloon) (partial occlusion) 39.77
     duodenal (transcatheter) 44.44
     gastric (transcatheter) 44.44
     head and neck NEC 38.82
     intracranial NEC 38.81
     lower limb 38.88
     renal (transcatheter) 38.86
     thoracic NEC 38.85
     upper limb 38.83
     uterine (gelatin sponge) (gelfoam)
      (microspheres) (PVA) (spherical
      embolics) (without coil(s)) 68.25
   AVM, intracranial, endovascular approach
     39.72
   carotid cavernous fistula 39.53
   chemoembolization 99.25
   coil, endovascular 39.79
     head and neck 39.75
      bare coils 39.75
      bioactive coils 39.76
     uterine artery 68.24

Embolization *(Continued)*
vein (selective) 38.80
by
endovascular approach 39.79
head and neck 39.72
partial occlusion (balloon)
(temporary) 39.77
abdominal NEC 38.87
duodenal (transcatheter) 44.44
gastric (transcatheter) 44.44
duodenal (transcatheter) 44.44
gastric (transcatheter) 44.44
Embryotomy 73.8
EMG - *see* Electromyogram
Emmet operation (cervix) 67.61
Encephalocentesis - *see also* Puncture 01.09
fetal head, transabdominal 73.8
Encephalography (cisternal puncture)
(fractional) (lumbar)
(pneumoencephalogram) 87.01
Encephalopuncture 01.09
Encircling procedure - *see also* Cerclage
sclera, for buckling 14.49
with implant 14.41
Endarterectomy (gas) (with patch graft) 38.10
abdominal 38.16
aorta (arch) (ascending) (descending)
38.14
coronary artery - *see category* 36.0●
open chest approach 36.03
head and neck (open) NEC 38.12

> Note: Also use 00.40, 00.41, 00.42, or 00.43
> to show the total number of vessels treated.
> Use code 00.44 once to show procedure on a
> bifurcated vessel. In addition, use 00.45,
> 00.46, 00.47, or 00.48 to show the number of
> vascular stents inserted.

percutaneous approach, intracranial
vessel(s) 00.62
percutaneous approach, extracranial
vessel(s) 00.61
percutaneous approach, intracranial
vessel(s) 00.62
intracranial (open) NEC 38.11

> Note: Also use 00.40, 00.41, 00.42, or 00.43
> to show the total number of vessels treated.
> Use code 00.44 once to show procedure on a
> bifurcated vessel. In addition, use 00.45,
> 00.46, 00.47, or 00.48 to show the number of
> vascular stents inserted.

percutaneous approach, intracranial
vessel(s) 00.62
lower limb 38.18
thoracic NEC 38.15
upper limb 38.13
Endoaneurysmorrhaphy - *see also*
Aneurysmorrhaphy 39.52
by or with
endovascular graft
abdominal aorta 39.71
fenestrated (branching) graft 39.78
lower extremity artery(s) 39.79
thoracic aorta 39.73
upper extremity artery(s) 39.79
Endolymphatic (-subarachnoid) shunt 20.71
Endometrectomy (uterine) (internal) 68.29
bladder 57.59
cul-de-sac 70.32
Endoprosthesis
bile duct 51.87
femoral head (bipolar) 81.52
Endoscopy
with biopsy - *see* Biopsy, by site, closed
anus 49.21
biliary tract (operative) 51.11
by retrograde cholangiography (ERC)
51.11

Endoscopy *(Continued)*
biliary tract *(Continued)*
by retrograde cholangiopancreatography
(ERCP) 51.10
intraoperative 51.11
percutaneous (via T-tube or other tract)
51.98
with removal of common duct stones
51.96
bladder 57.32
through stoma (artificial) 57.31
bronchus NEC 33.23
with biopsy 33.24
fiberoptic 33.22
through stoma (artificial) 33.21
colon 45.23
through stoma (artificial) 45.22
transabdominal (operative) 45.21
cul-de-sac 70.22
ear 18.11
esophagus NEC 42.23
through stoma (artificial) 42.22
transabdominal (operative) 42.21
ileum 45.13
through stoma (artificial) 45.12
transabdominal (operative) 45.11
intestine NEC 45.24
large 45.24
fiberoptic (flexible) 45.23
through stoma (artificial) 45.22
transabdominal (intraoperative)
45.21
small 45.13
esophagogastroduodenoscopy (EGD)
45.13
with closed biopsy 45.16
through stoma (artificial) 45.12
transabdominal (operative) 45.11
jejunum 45.13
through stoma (artificial) 45.12
transabdominal (operative) 45.11
kidney 55.21
larynx 31.42
through stoma (artificial) 31.41
lung - *see* Bronchoscopy
mediastinum (transpleural) 34.22
nasal sinus 22.19
nose 21.21
pancreatic duct 52.13
pelvis 55.22
peritoneum 54.21
pharynx 29.11
rectum 48.23
through stoma (artificial) 48.22
transabdominal (operative) 48.21
sinus, nasal 22.19
stomach NEC 44.13
through stoma (artificial) 44.12
transabdominal (operative) 44.11
thorax (transpleural) 34.21
trachea NEC 31.42
through stoma (artificial) 31.41
transpleural
mediastinum 34.22
thorax 34.21
ureter 56.31
urethra 58.22
uterus 68.12
vagina 70.21
Enema (transanal) NEC 96.39
for removal of impacted feces 96.38
ENG (electronystagmogram) 95.24
Enlargement
aortic lumen, thoracic 38.14
atrial septal defect (pre-existing) 35.41
in repair of total anomalous pulmonary
venous connection 35.82
eye socket 16.64
foramen ovale (pre-existing) 35.41
in repair of total anomalous pulmonary
venous connection 35.82

Enlargement *(Continued)*
intestinal stoma 46.40
large intestine 46.43
small intestine 46.41
introitus 96.16
orbit (eye) 16.64
palpebral fissure 08.51
punctum 09.41
sinus tract (skin) 86.89
Enterectomy NEC 45.63
Enteroanastomosis
large-to-large intestine 45.94
small-to-large intestine 45.93
small-to-small intestine 45.91
Enterocelectomy 53.9
female 70.92
with graft or prosthesis 70.93
vaginal 70.92
with graft or prosthesis 70.93
Enterocentesis 45.00
duodenum 45.01
large intestine 45.03
small intestine NEC 45.02
Enterocholecystostomy 51.32
Enteroclysis (small bowel) 96.43
Enterocolectomy NEC 45.79
Enterocolostomy 45.93
Enteroentectropy 46.99
Enteroenterostomy 45.90
small-to-large intestine 45.93
small-to-small intestine 45.91
Enterogastrostomy 44.39
laparoscopic 44.38
Enterolithotomy 45.00
Enterolysis 54.59
laparoscopic 54.51
Enteropancreatostomy 52.96
Enterorrhaphy 46.79
large intestine 46.75
small intestine 46.73
Enterostomy NEC 46.39
cecum - *see also* Colostomy 46.10
colon (transverse) - *see also* Colostomy 46.10
loop 46.03
delayed opening 46.31
duodenum 46.39
loop 46.01
feeding NEC 46.39
percutaneous (endoscopic) 46.32
ileum (Brooke) (Dragstedt) 46.20
loop 46.01
jejunum (feeding) 46.39
loop 46.01
percutaneous (endoscopic) 46.32
sigmoid colon - *see also* Colostomy 46.10
loop 46.03
transverse colon - *see also* Colostomy 46.10
loop 46.03
Enterotomy 45.00
large intestine 45.03
small intestine 45.02
Enucleation - *see also* Excision, lesion, by site
cyst
broad ligament 69.19
dental 24.4
liver 50.29
ovarian 65.29
laparoscopic 65.25
parotid gland 26.29
salivary gland 26.29
skin 86.3
subcutaneous tissue 86.3
eyeball 16.49
with implant (into Tenon's capsule) 16.42
with attachment of muscles 16.41
EOG (electro-oculogram) 95.22
Epicardiectomy 36.39
Epididymectomy 63.4
with orchidectomy (unilateral) 62.3
bilateral 62.41
Epididymogram 87.93

◄ New   ◄▥ Revised   ~~deleted~~ Deleted   ● Use Additional Digit(s)   ▨ Omit code

Epididymoplasty 63.59
Epididymorrhaphy 63.81
Epididymotomy 63.92
Epididymovasostomy 63.83
Epiglottidectomy 30.21
Epikeratophakia 11.76
Epilation
  eyebrow (forceps) 08.93
    cryosurgical 08.92
    electrosurgical 08.91
  eyelid (forceps) NEC 08.93
    cryosurgical 08.92
    electrosurgical 08.91
  skin 86.92
Epiphysiodesis - *see also* Arrest, bone growth -
  see category 78.2●
Epiphysiolysis - *see also* Arrest, bone growth -
  see category 78.2●
Epiploectomy 54.4
Epiplopexy 54.74
Epiplorrhaphy 54.74
Episioperineoplasty 71.79
Episioperineorrhaphy 71.71
  obstetrical 75.69
Episioplasty 71.79
Episioproctotomy 73.6
Episiorrhaphy 71.71
  following episiotomy - *see* Episiotomy
  for obstetrical laceration 75.69
Episiotomy (with subsequent episiorrhaphy)
  73.6
  high forceps 72.31
  low forceps 72.1
  mid forceps 72.21
  nonobstetrical 71.09
  outlet forceps 72.1
EPS (electrophysiologic stimulation)
  as part of intraoperative testing - *omit code*
  catheter based invasive electrophysiologic
    testing 37.26
  device interrogation only without
    arrhythmia induction (bedside check)
    89.45-89.49
  noninvasive programmed electrical
    stimulation (NIPS) 37.20
Eptifibatide, infusion 99.20
Equalization, leg
  lengthening - *see* category 78.3●
  shortening - *see* category 78.2●
Equilibration (occlusal) 24.8
Equiloudness balance 95.43
ERC (endoscopic retrograde cholangiography)
  51.11
ERCP (endoscopic retrograde
  cholangiopancreatography) 51.10
  cannulation of pancreatic duct 52.93
ERG (electroretinogram) 95.21
ERP (endoscopic retrograde pancreatography)
  52.13
Eruption, tooth, surgical 24.6
Erythrocytapheresis, therapeutic 99.73
Escharectomy 86.22
Escharotomy 86.09
Esophageal voice training (postlaryngectomy)
  93.73
Esophagectomy 42.40
  abdominothoracocervical (combined)
    (synchronous) 42.42
  partial or subtotal 42.41
  total 42.42
Esophagocologastrostomy (intrathoracic) 42.55
  antesternal or antethoracic 42.65
Esophagocolostomy (intrathoracic) NEC 42.56
  with interposition of colon 42.55
  antesternal or antethoracic NEC 42.66
    with interposition of colon 42.65
Esophagoduodenostomy (intrathoracic) NEC
  42.54
  with
    complete gastrectomy 43.99
    interposition of small bowel 42.53

Esophagoenterostomy (intrathoracic) NEC - *see
  also* Anastomosis, esophagus, to intestinal
  segment 42.54
  antesternal or antethoracic - *see also*
    Anastomosis, esophagus, antesternal,
    to intestinal segment 42.64
Esophagoesophagostomy (intrathoracic) 42.51
  antesternal or antethoracic 42.61
Esophagogastrectomy 43.99
Esophagogastroduodenoscopy (EGD) 45.13
  with closed biopsy 45.16
  through stoma (artificial) 45.12
  transabdominal (operative) 45.11
Esophagogastromyotomy 42.7
Esophagogastropexy 44.65
Esophagogastroplasty 44.65
Esophagogastroscopy NEC 44.13
  through stoma (artificial) 44.12
  transabdominal (operative) 44.11
Esophagogastrostomy (intrathoracic) 42.52
  with partial gastrectomy 43.5
  antesternal or antethoracic 42.62
Esophagoileostomy (intrathoracic) NEC 42.54
  with interposition of small bowel 42.53
  antesternal or antethoracic NEC 42.64
    with interposition of small bowel 42.63
Esophagojejunostomy (intrathoracic) NEC
  42.54
  with
    complete gastrectomy 43.99
    interposition of small bowel 42.53
  antesternal or antethoracic NEC 42.64
    with interposition of small bowel
    42.63
Esophagomyotomy 42.7
Esophagoplasty NEC 42.89
Esophagorrhaphy 42.82
Esophagoscopy NEC 42.23
  by incision (operative) 42.21
  with closed biopsy 42.24
  through stoma (artificial) 42.22
  transabdominal (operative) 42.21
Esophagostomy 42.10
  cervical 42.11
  thoracic 42.19
Esophagotomy NEC 42.09
Estes operation (ovary) 65.72
  laparoscopic 65.75
Estlander operation (thoracoplasty) 33.34
ESWL (extracorporeal shockwave lithotripsy)
  NEC 98.59
  bile duct 98.52
  bladder 98.51
  gallbladder 98.52
  kidney 98.51
  Kock pouch (urinary diversion) 98.51
  renal pelvis 98.51
  specified site NEC 98.59
  ureter 98.51
Ethmoidectomy 22.63
Ethmoidotomy 22.51
Evacuation
  abscess - *see* Drainage, by site
  anterior chamber (eye) (aqueous) (hyphema)
    12.91
  cyst - *see also* Excision, lesion, by site
    breast 85.91
    kidney 55.01
    liver 50.29
  hematoma - *see also* Incision, hematoma
    obstetrical 75.92
    incisional 75.91
  hemorrhoids (thrombosed) 49.47
  pelvic blood clot (by incision) 54.19
  by
    culdocentesis 70.0
    culdoscopy 70.22
  retained placenta
    with curettage 69.02
    manual 75.4
  streptothrix from lacrimal duct 09.42

Evaluation (of)
  audiological 95.43
  cardiac rhythm device (CRT-D) (CRT-P)
    (AICD) (pacemaker) - *see* Interrogation
  criminal responsibility, psychiatric 94.11
  functional (physical therapy) 93.01
  hearing NEC 95.49
  orthotic (for brace fitting) 93.02
  prosthetic (for artificial limb fitting) 93.03
  psychiatric NEC 94.19
    commitment 94.13
  psychologic NEC 94.08
  testimentary capacity, psychiatric 94.11
Evans operation (release of clubfoot) 83.84
Evisceration
  eyeball 16.39
    with implant (into scleral shell) 16.31
  ocular contents 16.39
    with implant (into scleral shell) 16.31
  orbit - *see also* Exenteration, orbit 16.59
  pelvic (anterior) (posterior) (partial) (total)
    (female) 68.8
    male 57.71
Evulsion
  nail (bed) (fold) 86.23
  skin 86.3
  subcutaneous tissue 86.3
Examination (for)
  breast
    manual 89.36
    radiographic NEC 87.37
    thermographic 88.85
    ultrasonic 88.73
  cervical rib (by x-ray) 87.43
  colostomy stoma (digital) 89.33
  dental (oral mucosa) (peridontal) 89.31
    radiographic NEC 87.12
  enterostomy stoma (digital) 89.33
  eye 95.09
    color vision 95.06
    comprehensive 95.02
    dark adaptation 95.07
    limited (with prescription of spectacles)
    95.01
    under anesthesia 95.04
  fetus, intrauterine 75.35
  general physical 89.7
  glaucoma 95.03
  gynecological 89.26
  hearing 95.47
  microscopic (specimen) (of) 91.9●

> Note: Use the following fourth-digit
> subclassification with categories 90-91 to
> identify type of examination:
>
> 1   bacterial smear
> 2   culture
> 3   culture and sensitivity
> 4   parasitology
> 5   toxicology
> 6   cell block and Papanicolaou smear
> 9   other microscopic examination

    adenoid 90.3●
    adrenal gland 90.1●
    amnion 91.4●
    anus 90.9●
    appendix 90.9●
    bile ducts 91.0●
    bladder 91.3●
    blood 90.5●
    bone 91.5●
      marrow 90.6●
    brain 90.0●
    breast 91.6●
    bronchus 90.4●
    bursa 91.5●
    cartilage 91.5●
    cervix 91.4●
    chest wall 90.4●
    chorion 91.4●

Examination (*Continued*)
microscopic (*Continued*)
colon 90.9 ●
cul-de-sac 91.1 ●
dental 90.8 ●
diaphragm 90.4 ●
duodenum 90.8 ●
ear 90.3 ●
endocrine gland NEC 90.1 ●
esophagus 90.8 ●
eye 90.2 ●
fallopian tube 91.4 ●
fascia 91.5 ●
female genital tract 91.4 ●
fetus 91.4 ●
gallbladder 91.0 ●
hair 91.6 ●
ileum 90.9 ●
jejunum 90.9 ●
joint fluid 91.5 ●
kidney 91.2 ●
large intestine 90.9 ●
larynx 90.3 ●
ligament 91.5 ●
liver 91.0 ●
lung 90.4 ●
lymph (node) 90.7 ●
meninges 90.0 ●
mesentery 91.1 ●
mouth 90.8 ●
muscle 91.5 ●
musculoskeletal system 91.5 ●
nails 91.6 ●
nerve 90.0 ●
nervous system 90.0 ●
nose 90.3 ●
omentum 91.1 ●
operative wound 91.7 ●
ovary 91.4 ●
pancreas 91.0 ●
parathyroid gland 90.1 ●
penis 91.3 ●
perirenal tissue 91.2 ●
peritoneum (fluid) 91.1 ●
periureteral tissue 91.2 ●
perivesical (tissue) 91.3 ●
pharynx 90.3 ●
pineal gland 90.1 ●
pituitary gland 90.1 ●
placenta 91.4 ●
pleura (fluid) 90.4 ●
prostate 91.3 ●
rectum 90.9 ●
retroperitoneum 91.1 ●
semen 91.3 ●
seminal vesicle 91.3 ●
sigmoid 90.9 ●
skin 91.6 ●
small intestine 90.9 ●
specified site NEC 91.8 ●
spinal fluid 90.0 ●
spleen 90.6 ●
sputum 90.4 ●
stomach 90.8 ●
stool 90.9 ●
synovial membrane 91.5 ●
tendon 91.5 ●
thorax NEC 90.4 ●
throat 90.3 ●
thymus 90.1 ●
thyroid gland 90.1 ●
tonsil 90.3 ●
trachea 90.4 ●
ureter 91.2 ●
urethra 91.3 ●
urine 91.3 ●
uterus 91.4 ●
vagina 91.4 ●
vas deferens 91.3 ●
vomitus 90.8 ●
vulva 91.4 ●

Examination (*Continued*)
neurologic 89.13
neuro-ophthalmology 95.03
ophthalmoscopic 16.21
panorex, mandible 87.12
pelvic (manual) 89.26
instrumental (by pelvimeter) 88.25
pelvimetric 88.25
physical, general 89.7
postmortem 89.8
rectum (digital) 89.34
endoscopic 48.23
through stoma (artificial) 48.22
transabdominal 48.21
retinal disease 95.03
specified type (manual) NEC 89.39
thyroid field, postoperative 06.02
uterus (digital) 68.11
endoscopic 68.12
vagina 89.26
endoscopic 70.21
visual field 95.05
Exchange transfusion 99.01
intrauterine 75.2
Excision
aberrant tissue - *see* Excision, lesion, by site of tissue origin
abscess - *see* Excision, lesion, by site
accessory tissue - *see also* Excision, lesion, by site of tissue origin
lung 32.29
endoscopic 32.28
thoracoscopic 32.20
spleen 41.93
adenoids (tag) 28.6
with tonsillectomy 28.3
adenoma - *see* Excision, lesion, by site
adrenal gland - *see also* Adrenalectomy 07.22
ampulla of Vater (with reimplantation of common duct) 51.62
anal papilla 49.39
endoscopic 49.31
aneurysm (arteriovenous) - *see also* Aneurysmectomy 38.60
coronary artery 36.91
heart 37.32
myocardium 37.32
sinus of Valsalva 35.39
ventricle (heart) 37.32
anus (complete) (partial) 49.6
aortic subvalvular ring 35.35
apocrine gland 86.3
aponeurosis 83.42
hand 82.33
appendage, left atrial 37.36
appendiceal stump 47.09
laparoscopic 47.01
appendices epiploicae 54.4
appendix - *see also* Appendectomy
epididymis 63.3
testis 62.2
arcuate ligament (spine) - *omit code*
arteriovenous fistula - *see also* Aneurysmectomy 38.60
artery - *see also* Arteriectomy 38.60
Baker's cyst, knee 83.39
Bartholin's gland 71.24
basal ganglion 01.59
bile duct 51.69
endoscopic 51.64
bladder - *see also* Cystectomy
bleb (emphysematous), lung 32.29
endoscopic 32.28
thoracoscopic 32.20
blood vessel - *see also* Angiectomy 38.60
bone (ends) (partial), except facial - *see* category 77.8 ●
facial NEC 76.39
total 76.45
with reconstruction 76.44

Excision (*Continued*)
bone, except facial (*Continued*)
for graft (autograft) (homograft) - *see* category 77.7 ●
fragments (chips) - *see also* Incision, bone 77.10
joint - *see also* Arthrotomy 80.10
necrotic - *see also* Sequestrectomy, bone 77.00
heterotopic, from
muscle 83.32
hand 82.22
skin 86.3
tendon 83.31
hand 82.21
mandible 76.31
with arthrodesis - *see* Arthrodesis
total 76.42
with reconstruction 76.41
spur - *see* Excision, lesion, bone
total, except facial - *see* category 77.9 ●
facial NEC 76.45
with reconstruction 76.44
mandible 76.42
with reconstruction 76.41
brain 01.59
hemisphere 01.52
lobe 01.53
branchial cleft cyst or vestige 29.2
breast - *see also* Mastectomy 85.41
aberrant tissue 85.24
accessory 85.24
ectopic 85.24
nipple 85.25
accessory 85.24
segmental 85.23
supernumerary 85.24
wedge 85.21
broad ligament 69.19
bronchogenic cyst 32.09
endoscopic 32.01
bronchus (wide sleeve) NEC 32.1
buccal mucosa 27.49
bulbourethral gland 58.92
bulbous tuberosities (mandible) (maxilla) (fibrous) (osseous) 24.31
bunion - *see also* Bunionectomy 77.59
bunionette (with osteotomy) 77.54
bursa 83.5
hand 82.31
canal of Nuck 69.19
cardioma 37.33
carotid body (lesion) (partial) (total) 39.89
cartilage - *see also* Chondrectomy 80.90
intervertebral - *see* category 80.5 ●
knee (semilunar) 80.6
larynx 30.29
nasal (submucous) 21.5
caruncle, urethra 58.39
endoscopic 58.31
cataract - *see also* Extraction, cataract 13.19
secondary membrane (after cataract) 13.65
cervical
rib 77.91
stump 67.4
cervix (stump) NEC 67.4
cold (knife) 67.2
conization 67.2
cryoconization 67.33
electroconization 67.32
chalazion (multiple) (single) 08.21
cholesteatoma - *see* Excision, lesion, by site
choroid plexus 02.14
cicatrix (skin) 86.3
cilia base 08.20
ciliary body, prolapsed 12.98
clavicle (head) (partial) 77.81
total (complete) 77.91
clitoris 71.4

Excision *(Continued)*
  coarctation of aorta (end-to-end anastomosis) 38.64
    with
      graft replacement (interposition)
        abdominal 38.44
        thoracic 38.45
        thoracoabdominal 38.45 *[38.44]*
  common
    duct 51.63
    wall between posterior and coronary
        sinus (with roofing or resultant
        defect with patch graft) 35.82
  condyle - *see* category 77.8●
    mandible 76.5
  conjunctival ring 10.31
  cornea 11.49
    epithelium (with chemocauterization) 11.41
      for smear or culture 11.21
  costal cartilage 80.99
  cul-de-sac (Douglas') 70.92
    with graft or prosthesis 70.93
  cusp, heart valve 35.10
    aortic 35.11
    mitral 35.12
    tricuspid 35.14
  cyst - *see also* Excision, lesion, by site
    apical (tooth) 23.73
      with root canal therapy 23.72
    Baker's (popliteal) 83.39
    breast 85.21
    broad ligament 69.19
    bronchogenic 32.09
      endoscopic 32.01
    cervix 67.39
    dental 24.4
    dentigerous 24.4
    epididymis 63.2
    fallopian tube 66.61
    Gartner's duct 70.33
    hand 82.29
    labia 71.3
    lung 32.29
      endoscopic 32.28
      thoracoscopic 32.20
    mesonephric duct 69.19
    Morgagni
      female 66.61
      male 62.2
    mullerian duct 60.73
    nasolabial 27.49
    nasopalatine 27.31
      by wide excision 27.32
    ovary 65.29
      laparoscopic 65.25
    parovarian 69.19
    pericardium 37.31
    periodontal (apical) (lateral) 24.4
    popliteal (Baker's), knee 83.39
    radicular 24.4
    spleen 41.42
    synovial (membrane) 83.39
    thyroglossal (with resection of hyoid
        bone) 06.7
    urachal (bladder) 57.51
      abdominal wall 54.3
    vagina (Gartner's duct) 70.33
  cystic
    duct remnant 51.61
    hygroma 40.29
  dentinoma 24.4
  diaphragm 34.81
  disc, intervertebral NOS 80.50
    herniated (nucleus pulposus) 80.51
    other specified (diskectomy) 80.51
  diverticulum
    ampulla of Vater 51.62
    anus 49.39
      endoscopic 49.31
    bladder 57.59
      transurethral 57.49

Excision *(Continued)*
  diverticulum *(Continued)*
    duodenum 45.31
      endoscopic 45.30
    esophagus (local) 42.31
      endoscopic 42.33
    hypopharyngeal (by cricopharyngeal
        myotomy) 29.32
    intestine
      large 45.41
        endoscopic 45.43
      small NEC 45.33
    Meckel's 45.33
    pharyngeal (by cricopharyngeal
        myotomy) 29.32
    pharyngoesophageal (by cricopharyngeal
        myotomy) 29.32
    stomach 43.42
      endoscopic 43.41
    urethra 58.39
      endoscopic 58.31
    ventricle, heart 37.33
  duct
    mullerian 69.19
    paramesonephric 69.19
    thyroglossal (with resection of hyoid
        bone) 06.7
  ear, external (complete) NEC 18.39
    partial 18.29
      radical 18.31
  ectopic
    abdominal fetus 74.3
    tissue - *see also* Excision, lesion, by site of
        tissue origin
      bone, from muscle 83.32
      breast 85.24
      lung 32.29
        endoscopic 32.28
        thoracoscopic 32.20
      spleen 41.93
  empyema pocket, lung 34.09
  epididymis 63.4
  epiglottis 30.21
  epithelial downgrowth, anterior chamber
      (eye) 12.93
  epulis (gingiva) 24.31
  esophagus - *see also* Esophagectomy 42.40
  exostosis - *see also* Excision, lesion, bone
      77.60
    auditory canal, external 18.29
    facial bone 76.2
    first metatarsal (hallux valgus repair) - *see*
        Bunionectomy
  eye 16.49
    with implant (into Tenon's capsule) 16.42
      with attachment of muscles 16.41
  eyelid 08.20
    redundant skin 08.86
  falciform ligament 54.4
  fallopian tube - *see* Salpingectomy
  fascia 83.44
    for graft 83.43
      hand 82.34
    hand 82.35
      for graft 82.34
  fat pad NEC 86.3
    knee (infrapatellar) (prepatellar) 86.3
    scalene 40.21
  fibroadenoma, breast 85.21
  fissure, anus 49.39
    endoscopic 49.31
  fistula - *see also* Fistulectomy
    anal 49.12
    arteriovenous - *see also* Aneurysmectomy
        38.60
    ileorectal 46.74
    lacrimal
      gland 09.21
      sac 09.6
    rectal 48.73
    vesicovaginal 57.84

Excision *(Continued)*
  frenulum, frenum
    labial (lip) 27.41
    lingual (tongue) 25.92
  ganglion (hand) (tendon sheath) (wrist)
      82.21
    gasserian 04.05
    site other than hand or nerve 83.31
    sympathetic nerve 05.29
    trigeminal nerve 04.05
  gastrocolic ligament 54.4
  gingiva 24.31
  glomus jugulare tumor 20.51
  goiter - *see* Thyroidectomy
  gum 24.31
  hallux valgus - *see also* Bunionectomy
    with prosthetic implant 77.59
  hamartoma, mammary 85.21
  heart assist system - *see* Removal
  hematocele, tunica vaginalis 61.92
  hematoma - *see* Drainage, by site
  hemorrhoids (external) (internal) (tag)
      49.46
  heterotopic bone, from
    muscle 83.32
      hand 82.22
    skin 86.3
    tendon 83.31
      hand 82.21
  hydatid of Morgagni
    female 66.61
    male 62.2
  hydatid cyst, liver 50.29
  hydrocele
    canal of Nuck (female) 69.19
    male 63.1
    round ligament 69.19
    spermatic cord 63.1
    tunica vaginalis 61.2
  hygroma, cystic 40.29
  hymen (tag) 70.31
  hymeno-urethral fusion 70.31
  intervertebral disc - *see* Excision, disc,
      intervertebral (NOS) 80.50
  intestine - *see also* Resection, intestine
    for interposition 45.50
      large 45.52
      small 45.51
    large (total)
      for interposition 45.52
      laparoscopic 45.81
      local 45.41
        endoscopic 45.43
      open 45.82
      other 45.83
      segmental
        laparoscopic 17.39
        multiple
          laparoscopic 17.31
          open and other 45.71
        open and other 45.79
      unspecified 45.83
    small (total) 45.63
      for interposition 45.51
      local 45.33
      partial 45.62
      segmental 45.62
        multiple 45.61
  intraductal papilloma 85.21
  iris prolapse 12.13
  joint - *see also* Arthrectomy 80.90
  keloid (scar), skin 86.3
  LAA 37.36
  labia - *see* Vulvectomy
  lacrimal
    gland 09.20
      partial 09.22
      total 09.23
    passage 09.6
    sac 09.6
  left atrial appendage 37.36

Excision *(Continued)*
  lesion (local)
    abdominal wall 54.3
    accessory sinus - *see* Excision, lesion, nasal
      sinus
    adenoids 28.92
    adrenal gland(s) 07.21
    alveolus 24.4
    ampulla of Vater 51.62
    anterior chamber (eye) NEC 12.40
    anus 49.39
      endoscopic 49.31
    apocrine gland 86.3
    artery 38.60
      abdominal 38.66
      aorta (arch) (ascending) (descending
        thoracic) 38.64
        with end-to-end anastomosis 38.45
          abdominal 38.44
          thoracic 38.45
          thoracoabdominal 38.45 *[38.44]*
        with graft interposition graft
          replacement 38.45
          abdominal 38.44
          thoracic 38.45
          thoracoabdominal 38.45 *[38.44]*
      head and neck NEC 38.62
      intracranial NEC 38.61
      lower limb 38.68
      thoracic NEC 38.65
      upper limb 38.63
    atrium 37.33
    auditory canal or meatus, external 18.29
      radical 18.31
    auricle, ear 18.29
      radical 18.31
    biliary ducts 51.69
      endoscopic 51.64
    bladder (transurethral) 57.49
      open 57.59
      suprapubic 57.59
    blood vessel 38.60
      abdominal
        artery 38.66
        vein 38.67
      aorta (arch) (ascending) (descending)
        38.64
      head and neck NEC 38.62
      intracranial NEC 38.61
      lower limb
        artery 38.68
        vein 38.69
      thoracic NEC 38.65
      upper limb (artery) (vein) 38.63
    bone 77.60
      carpal, metacarpal 77.64
      clavicle 77.61
      facial 76.2
      femur 77.65
      fibula 77.67
      humerus 77.62
      jaw 76.2
        dental 24.4
      patella 77.66
      pelvic 77.69
      phalanges (foot) (hand) 77.69
      radius 77.63
      scapula 77.61
      skull 01.6
      specified site NEC 77.69
      tarsal, metatarsal 77.68
      thorax (ribs) (sternum) 77.61
      tibia 77.67
      ulna 77.63
      vertebrae 77.69
    brain (transtemporal approach) NEC
      01.59
      by stereotactic radiosurgery 92.30
        cobalt 60 92.32
        linear accelerator (LINAC) 92.31
        multi-source 92.32

Excision *(Continued)*
  lesion *(Continued)*
    brain NEC *(Continued)*
      by stereotactic radiosurgery
        (Continued)
        particle beam 92.33
        particulate 92.33
        radiosurgery NEC 92.39
        single source photon 92.31
    breast (segmental) (wedge) 85.21
    broad ligament 69.19
    bronchus NEC 32.09
      endoscopic 32.01
    cerebral (cortex) NEC 01.59
      meninges 01.51
    cervix (myoma) 67.39
    chest wall 34.4
    choroid plexus 02.14
    ciliary body 12.44
    colon 45.41
      endoscopic NEC 45.43
        polypectomy 45.42
    conjunctiva 10.31
    cornea 11.49
    cranium 01.6
    cul-de-sac (Douglas') 70.32
    dental (jaw) 24.4
    diaphragm 34.81
    duodenum (local) 45.31
      endoscopic 45.30
    ear, external 18.29
      radical 18.31
    endometrium 68.29
    epicardium 37.31
    epididymis 63.3
    epiglottis 30.09
    esophagus NEC 42.32
      endoscopic 42.33
    eye, eyeball 16.93
      anterior segment NEC 12.40
    eyebrow (skin) 08.20
    eyelid 08.20
      by
        halving procedure 08.24
        wedge resection 08.24
      major
        full-thickness 08.24
        partial-thickness 08.23
      minor 08.22
    fallopian tube 66.61
    fascia 83.39
      hand 82.29
    groin region (abdominal wall) (inguinal)
      54.3
      skin 86.3
      subcutaneous tissue 86.3
    gum 24.31
    heart 37.34
      Cox-maze, open 37.33
      maze, modified, endovascular 37.34
      maze, modified, open 37.33
      open 37.33
      other approach, closed 37.34
    hepatic duct 51.69
    inguinal canal 54.3
    intestine
      large 45.41
        endoscopic NEC 45.43
          polypectomy 45.42
      small NEC 45.33
    intracranial NEC 01.59
    intranasal 21.31
    intraspinal 03.4
    iris 12.42
    jaw 76.2
      dental 24.4
    joint 80.80
      ankle 80.87
      elbow 80.82
      foot and toe 80.88
      hand and finger 80.84

Excision *(Continued)*
  lesion *(Continued)*
    joint *(Continued)*
      hip 80.85
      knee 80.86
      shoulder 80.81
      specified site NEC 80.89
      spine 80.89
      wrist 80.83
    kidney 55.39
      with partial nephrectomy 55.4
    labia 71.3
    lacrimal
      gland (frontal approach) 09.21
      passage 09.6
      sac 09.6
    larynx 30.09
    ligament (joint) - *see also* Excision, lesion,
      joint 80.80
      broad 69.19
      round 69.19
      uterosacral 69.19
    lip 27.43
      by wide excision 27.42
    liver 50.29
    lung NEC 32.29
      by lung volume reduction surgery 32.22
      by wide excision 32.39
        thoracoscopic 32.30
      endoscopic 32.28
      thoracoscopic 32.20
    lymph structure(s) (channel) (vessel) NEC
      40.29
      node - *see* Excision, lymph, node
    mammary duct 85.21
    mastoid (bone) 20.49
    mediastinum 34.3
    meninges (cerebral) 01.51
      spinal 03.4
    mesentery 54.4
    middle ear 20.51
    mouth NEC 27.49
    muscle 83.32
      hand 82.22
      ocular 15.13
    myocardium 37.33
    nail 86.23
    nasal sinus 22.60
      antrum 22.62
        with Caldwell-Luc approach 22.61
        specified approach NEC 22.62
      ethmoid 22.63
      frontal 22.42
      maxillary 22.62
        with Caldwell-Luc approach 22.61
        specified approach NEC 22.62
      sphenoid 22.64
    nasopharynx 29.3●
    nerve (cranial) (peripheral) 04.07
      sympathetic 05.29
    nonodontogenic 24.31
    nose 21.30
      intranasal 21.31
      polyp 21.31
      skin 21.32
      specified site NEC 21.32
    odontogenic 24.4
    omentum 54.4
    orbit 16.92
    ovary 65.29
      by wedge resection 65.22
        laparoscopic 65.24
      that by laparoscope 65.25
    palate (bony) 27.31
      by wide excision 27.32
      soft 27.49
    pancreas (local) 52.22
      endoscopic 52.21
    parathyroid 06.89
    parotid gland or duct NEC 26.29
    pelvic wall 54.3

◄ New   ◄ Revised   ~~deleted~~ Deleted   ● Use Additional Digit(s)   Omit code

Excision *(Continued)*
  lesion *(Continued)*
    pelvirectal tissue 48.82
    penis 64.2
    pericardium 37.31
    perineum (female) 71.3
      male 86.3
    periprostatic tissue 60.82
    perirectal tissue 48.82
    perirenal tissue 59.91
    peritoneum 54.4
    perivesical tissue 59.91
    pharynx 29.39
      diverticulum 29.32
    pineal gland 07.53
    pinna 18.29
      radical 18.31
    pituitary (gland) - *see also*
        Hypophysectomy, partial 07.63
      by stereotactic radiosurgery 92.30
        cobalt 60 92.32
        linear accelerator (LINAC) 92.31
        multi-source 92.32
        particle beam 92.33
        particulate 92.33
        radiosurgery NEC 92.39
        single source photon 92.31
    pleura 34.59
    pouch of Douglas 70.32
    preauricular (ear) 18.21
    presacral 54.4
    prostate (transurethral) 60.61
    pulmonary (fibrosis) 32.29
      endoscopic 32.28
      thoracoscopic 32.20
    rectovaginal septum 48.82
    rectum 48.35
      polyp (endoscopic) 48.36
    retroperitoneum 54.4
    salivary gland or duct NEC 26.29
      en bloc 26.32
    sclera 12.84
    scrotum 61.3
    sinus (nasal) - *see* Excision, lesion, nasal
      sinus
    Skene's gland 71.3
    skin 86.3
      breast 85.21
      nose 21.32
      radical (wide) (involving underlying
        or adjacent structure) (with flap
        closure) 86.4
      scrotum 61.3
    skull 01.6
    soft tissue NEC 83.39
      hand 82.29
    spermatic cord 63.3
    sphincter of Oddi 51.62
      endoscopic 51.64
    spinal cord (meninges) 03.4
    spleen (cyst) 41.42
    stomach NEC 43.42
      endoscopic 43.41
        polyp 43.41
      polyp (endoscopic) 43.41
    subcutaneous tissue 86.3
      breast 85.21
    subgingival 24.31
    sweat gland 86.3
    tendon 83.39
      hand 82.29
      ocular 15.13
      sheath 83.31
        hand 82.21
    testis 62.2
    thorax 34.4
    thymus
      partial (open) (other) 07.81
        thoracoscopic 07.83
      total (open) (other) 07.82
        thoracoscopic 07.84

Excision *(Continued)*
  lesion *(Continued)*
    thyroid 06.31
      substernal or transsternal route 06.51
    tongue 25.1
    tonsil 28.92
    trachea 31.5
    tunica vaginalis 61.92
    ureter 56.41
    urethra 58.39
      endoscopic 58.31
    uterine ligament 69.19
    uterosacral ligament 69.19
    uterus 68.29
    vagina 70.33
    vein 38.60
      abdominal 38.67
      head and neck NEC 38.62
      intracranial NEC 38.61
      lower limb 38.69
      thoracic NEC 38.65
      upper limb 38.63
    ventricle (heart) 37.33
    vocal cords 30.09
    vulva 71.3
  ligament - *see also* Arthrectomy 80.90
    broad 69.19
    round 69.19
    uterine 69.19
    uterosacral 69.19
  ligamentum flavum (spine) - *omit code*
  lingual tonsil 28.5
  lip 27.43
  liver (partial) 50.22
  loose body
    bone - *see* Sequestrectomy, bone
    joint 80.10
  lung (with mediastinal dissection) 32.59
    accessory or ectopic tissue 32.29
      endoscopic 32.28
      thoracoscopic 32.20
    segmental 32.39
      thoracoscopic 32.30
    specified type NEC 32.29
      endoscopic 32.28
      thoracoscopic 32.20
    thoracoscopic 32.50
    volume reduction surgery 32.22
      biologic lung volume reduction
        (BLVR) - *see* category 33.7●
    wedge 32.29
      thoracoscopic 32.20
  lymph, lymphatic
    drainage area 40.29
      radical - *see* Excision, lymph, node,
        radical
      regional (with lymph node, skin,
        subcutaneous tissue, and fat)
        40.3
    node (simple) NEC 40.29
      with
        lymphatic drainage area (including
          skin, subcutaneous tissue,
          and fat) 40.3
        mastectomy - *see* Mastectomy,
          radical
        muscle and deep fascia - *see*
          Excision, lymph, node,
          radical
      axillary 40.23
        radical 40.51
        regional (extended) 40.3
      cervical (deep) (with excision of
        scalene fat pad) 40.21
        with laryngectomy 30.4
        radical (including muscle and deep
          fascia) 40.40
          bilateral 40.42
          unilateral 40.41
        regional (extended) 40.3
        superficial 40.29

Excision *(Continued)*
  lymph, lymphatic *(Continued)*
    node NEC *(Continued)*
      groin 40.24
        radical 40.54
        regional (extended) 40.3
      iliac 40.29
        radical 40.53
        regional (extended) 40.3
      inguinal (deep) (superficial) 40.24
        radical 40.54
        regional (extended) 40.3
      jugular - *see* Excision, lymph, node,
        cervical
      mammary (internal) 40.22
        external 40.29
          radical 40.59
          regional (extended) 40.3
        radical 40.59
          regional (extended) 40.3
      paratracheal - *see* Excision, lymph,
        node, cervical
      periaortic 40.29
        radical 40.52
        regional (extended) 40.3
      radical 40.50
        with mastectomy - *see* Mastectomy,
          radical
        specified site NEC 40.59
      regional (extended) 40.3
      sternal - *see* Excision, lymph, node,
        mammary
      structure(s) (simple) NEC 40.29
        radical 40.59
        regional (extended) 40.3
    lymphangioma (simple) - *see also* Excision,
      lymph, lymphatic, node, 40.29
    lymphocele 40.29
    mastoid - *see also* Mastoidectomy 20.49
    median bar, transurethral approach 60.29
    meibomian gland 08.20
    meniscus (knee) 80.6
      acromioclavicular 80.91
      jaw 76.5
      sternoclavicular 80.91
      temporomandibular (joint) 76.5
      wrist 80.93
    mullerian duct cyst 60.73
    muscle 83.45
      for graft 83.43
        hand 82.34
      hand 82.36
        for graft 82.34
    myositis ossificans 83.32
      hand 82.22
    nail (bed) (fold) 86.23
    nasolabial cyst 27.49
    nasopalatine cyst 27.31
      by wide excision 27.32
    neoplasm - *see* Excision, lesion, by site
    nerve (cranial) (peripheral) NEC 04.07
      sympathetic 05.29
    neuroma (Morton's) (peripheral nerve) 04.07
      acoustic
        by craniotomy 04.01
        by stereotactic radiosurgery 92.30
          cobalt 60 92.32
          linear accelerator (LINAC) 92.31
          multi-source 92.32
          particle beam 92.33
          particulate 92.33
          radiosurgery NEC 92.39
          single source photon 92.31
      sympathetic nerve 05.29
    nipple 85.25
      accessory 85.24
    odontoma 24.4
    orbital contents - *see also* Exenteration, orbit
      16.59
    osteochondritis dissecans - *see also* Excision,
      lesion, joint 80.80

Excision *(Continued)*
ovary - *see also* Oophorectomy
   partial 65.29
      by wedge resection 65.22
         laparoscopic 65.24
      that by laparoscope 65.25
Pancoast tumor (lung) 32.6
pancreas (total) (with synchronous
     duodenectomy) 52.6
   partial NEC 52.59
      distal (tail) (with part of body) 52.52
      proximal (head) (with part of body)
         (with synchronous
         duodenectomy) 52.51
      radical subtotal 52.53
      radical (one-stage) (two-stage) 52.7
      subtotal 52.53
paramesonephric duct 69.19
parathyroid gland (partial) (subtotal)
     NEC - *see also* Parathyroidectomy
     06.89
parotid gland - *see also* Excision, salivary
     gland 26.30
parovarian cyst 69.19
patella (complete) 77.96
   partial 77.86
pelvirectal tissue 48.82
perianal tissue 49.04
   skin tags 49.03
pericardial adhesions 37.31
periprostatic tissue 60.82
perirectal tissue 48.82
perirenal tissue 59.91
periurethral tissue 58.92
perivesical tissue 59.91
petrous apex cells 20.59
pharyngeal bands 29.54
pharynx (partial) 29.33
pilonidal cyst or sinus (open) (with partial
     closure) 86.21
pineal gland (complete) (total) 07.54
   partial 07.53
pituitary gland (complete) (total) - *see also*
     Hypophysectomy 07.69
pleura NEC 34.59
polyp - *see also* Excision, lesion, by site
   esophagus 42.32
      endoscopic 42.33
   large intestine 45.41
      endoscopic 45.42
   nose 21.31
   rectum (endoscopic) 48.36
   stomach (endoscopic) 43.41
preauricular
   appendage (remnant) 18.29
   cyst, fistula, or sinus (congenital)
     18.21
   remnant 18.29
prolapsed iris (in wound) 12.13
prostate - *see* Prostatectomy
pterygium (simple) 11.39
   with corneal graft 11.32
radius (head) (partial) 77.83
   total 77.93
ranula, salivary gland NEC 26.29
rectal mucosa 48.35
rectum - *see* Resection, rectum
redundant mucosa
   colostomy 45.41
      endoscopic 45.43
   duodenostomy 45.31
      endoscopic 45.30
   ileostomy 45.33
   jejunostomy 45.33
   perineum 71.3
   rectum 48.35
   vulva 71.3
renal vessel, aberrant 38.66
rib (cervical) 77.91
ring of conjunctiva around cornea
     10.31

Excision *(Continued)*
round ligament 69.19
salivary gland 26.30
   complete 26.32
   partial 26.31
   radical 26.32
scalene fat pad 40.21
scar - *see also* Excision, lesion, by site
   epicardium 37.31
   mastoid 20.92
   pericardium 37.31
   pleura 34.59
   skin 86.3
   thorax 34.4
secondary membrane, lens 13.65
seminal vesicle 60.73
   with radical prostatectomy 60.5
septum - *see also* Excision, by site
   uterus (congenital) 68.22
   vagina 70.33
sinus - *see also* Excision, lesion, by site
   nasal - *see* Sinusectomy
   pilonidal 86.21
   preauricular (ear) (radical) 18.21
   tarsi 80.88
   thyroglossal (with resection of hyoid
     bone) 06.7
   urachal (bladder) 57.51
     abdominal wall 54.3
Skene's gland 71.3
skin (local) 86.3
   for graft (with closure of donor site)
     86.91
   radical (wide) (involving underlying or
     adjacent structure) (with flap
     closure) 86.4
   tags
     perianal 49.03
     periauricular 18.29
soft tissue NEC 83.49
   hand 82.39
spermatocele 63.2
spinous process 77.89
spleen (total) 41.5
   accessory 41.93
   partial 41.43
stomach - *see* Gastrectomy
sublingual gland (salivary) - *see also* Excision,
     salivary gland 26.30
submaxillary gland - *see also* Excision,
     salivary gland 26.30
supernumerary
   breast 85.24
   digits 86.26
sweat gland 86.3
synechiae - *see also* Lysis, synechiae
   endometrial 68.21
tarsal plate (eyelid) 08.20
   by wedge resection 08.24
tattoo 86.3
   by dermabrasion 86.25
tendon (sheath) 83.42
   for graft 83.41
     hand 82.32
   hand 82.33
     for graft 82.32
thymus - *see also* Thymectomy 07.80
thyroglossal duct or tract (with resection of
     hyoid bone) 06.7
thyroid NEC - *see also* Thyroidectomy
     06.39
tongue (complete) (total) 25.3
   partial or subtotal 25.2
   radical 25.4
tonsil 28.2
   with adenoidectomy 28.3
   lingual 28.5
   tag 28.4
tooth NEC - *see also* Removal, tooth, surgical
     23.19
   from nasal sinus 22.60

Excision *(Continued)*
torus
   lingual 76.2
   mandible, mandibularis 76.2
   palate, palatinus 27.31
     by wide excision 27.32
trabeculae carneae cordis (heart) 35.35
trochanteric lipomatosis 86.83
tumor - *see* Excision, lesion, by site
ulcer - *see also* Excision, lesion, by site
   duodenum 45.31
     endoscopic 45.30
   stomach 43.42
     endoscopic 43.41
umbilicus 54.3
urachus, urachal (cyst) (bladder) 57.51
   abdominal wall 54.3
ureter, ureteral 56.40
   with nephrectomy - *see* Nephrectomy
   partial 56.41
   stricture 56.41
   total 56.42
ureterocele 56.41
urethra, urethral 58.39
   with complete cystectomy 57.79
   endoscopic 58.31
   septum 58.0
   stricture 58.39
     endoscopic 58.31
   valve (congenital) 58.39
     endoscopic (transurethral)
       (transvesical) 58.31
urethrovaginal septum 70.33
uterus (corpus) - *see also* Hysterectomy
     68.9
   cervix 67.4
     lesion 67.39
   lesion 68.29
   septum 68.22
uvula 27.72
vagina (total) 70.4
varicocele, spermatic cord 63.1
vein - *see also* Phlebectomy 38.60
   varicose 38.50
     abdominal 38.57
     head and neck NEC 38.52
     intracranial NEC 38.51
     lower limb 38.59
     ovarian 38.67
     thoracic NEC 38.55
     upper limb 38.53
verucca - *see also* Excision, lesion, by site
   eyelid 08.22
vesicovaginal septum 70.33
vitreous opacity 14.74
   anterior approach 14.73
vocal cord(s) (submucous) 30.22
vulva (bilateral) (simple) - *see also*
     Vulvectomy 71.62
wart - *see also* Excision, lesion, by site
   eyelid 08.22
wolffian duct 69.19
xanthoma (tendon sheath, hand) 82.21
   site other than hand 83.31
Excisional biopsy - *see* Biopsy
Exclusion
   LAA 37.36
   left atrial appendage 37.36
     percutaneous 37.36
     TigerPaw™ System 37.36
   pyloric
     laparoscopic 44.38
     open 44.39
Exenteration
   ethmoid air cells 22.63
   orbit 16.59
     with
       removal of adjacent structures
         16.51
       temporalis muscle transplant 16.59
       therapeutic removal of bone 16.52

Exenteration *(Continued)*
  pelvic (organs) (female) 68.8
    male 57.71
    petrous pyramid air cells 20.59
Exercise (physical therapy) NEC 93.19
  active musculoskeletal NEC 93.12
  assisting 93.11
    in pool 93.31
  breathing 93.18
  musculoskeletal
    active NEC 93.12
    passive NEC 93.17
  neurologic 89.13
  passive musculoskeletal NEC 93.17
  resistive 93.13
Exfoliation, skin, by chemical 86.24
Exostectomy - *see also* Excision, lesion, bone
    77.60
  first metatarsal (hallux valgus repair) - *see*
    Bunionectomy
  hallux valgus repair (with wedge
    osteotomy) - *see* Bunionectomy
Expiratory flow rate 89.38
Explant, explanation - *see* Removal
Exploration - *see also* Incision
  abdomen 54.11
  abdominal wall 54.0
  adrenal (gland) 07.41
    field 07.00
      bilateral 07.02
      unilateral 07.01
  artery 38.00
    abdominal 38.06
    aorta (arch) (ascending) (descending)
      38.04
    head and neck NEC 38.02
    intracranial NEC 38.01
    lower limb 38.08
    thoracic NEC 38.05
    upper limb 38.03
  auditory canal, external 18.02
  axilla 86.09
  bile duct(s) 51.59
    common duct 51.51
      endoscopic 51.11
      for
        relief of obstruction 51.42
          endoscopic 51.84
        removal of calculus 51.41
          endoscopic 51.88
      laparoscopic 51.11
    for relief of obstruction 51.49
      endoscopic 51.84
  bladder (by incision) 57.19
    endoscopic 57.32
      through stoma (artificial)
        57.31
  bone - *see also* Incision, bone 77.10
  brain (tissue) 01.39
  breast 85.0
  bronchus 33.0
    endoscopic - *see* Bronchoscopy
  bursa 83.03
    hand 82.03
  carotid body 39.89
  carpal tunnel 04.43
  choroid 14.9
  ciliary body 12.44
  colon 45.03
  common bile duct 51.51
    endoscopic 51.11
      for
        relief of obstruction 51.42
          endoscopic 51.84
        removal of calculus 51.41
          endoscopic 51.88
  coronary artery 36.99
  cranium 01.24
  cul-de-sac 70.12
    endoscopic 70.22
  disc space 03.09

Exploration *(Continued)*
  duodenum 45.01
    endoscopic - *see* Endoscopy, by site
  epididymis 63.92
  esophagus (by incision) NEC 42.09
    endoscopic - *see* Esophagoscopy
  ethmoid sinus 22.51
  eyelid 08.09
  fallopian tube 66.01
  fascia 83.09
    hand 82.09
  flank 54.0
  fossa (superficial) NEC 86.09
    pituitary 07.71
  frontal sinus 22.41
  frontonasal duct 96.21
  gallbladder 51.04
  groin (region) (abdominal wall) (inguinal) 54.0
    skin and subcutaneous tissue 86.09
  heart 37.11
  hepatic duct 51.59
  hypophysis 07.72
  ileum 45.02
  inguinal canal (groin) 54.0
  intestine (by incision) NEC 45.00
    large 45.03
    small 45.02
  intrathoracic 34.02
  jejunum 45.02
  joint structures - *see also* Arthrotomy 80.10
  kidney 55.01
    pelvis 55.11
  labia 71.09
  lacrimal
    gland 09.0
    sac 09.53
  laparotomy site 54.12
  larynx (by incision) 31.3
    endoscopic 31.42
  liver 50.0
  lung (by incision) 33.1
  lymphatic structure(s) (channel) (node)
    (vessel) 40.0
  mastoid 20.21
  maxillary antrum or sinus (Caldwell-Luc
    approach) 22.39
  mediastinum 34.1
    endoscopic 34.22
  middle ear (transtympanic) 20.23
  muscle 83.02
    hand 82.02
  neck - *see also* Exploration, thyroid 06.09
  nerve (cranial) (peripheral) NEC 04.04
    auditory 04.01
    root (spinal) 03.09
  nose 21.1
  orbit - *see also* Orbitotomy 16.09
  pancreas 52.09
    endoscopic 52.13
  pancreatic duct 52.09
    endoscopic 52.13
  pelvis (by laparotomy) 54.11
    by colpotomy 70.12
  penis 64.92
  perinephric area 59.09
  perineum (female) 71.09
    male 86.09
  peripheral vessels
    lower limb
      artery 38.08
      vein 38.09
    upper limb (artery) (vein) 38.03
  periprostatic tissue 60.81
  perirenal tissue 59.09
  perivesical tissue 59.19
  petrous pyramid air cells 20.22
  pilonidal sinus 86.03
  pineal (gland) 07.52
    field 07.51
  pituitary (gland) 07.72
    fossa 07.71

Exploration *(Continued)*
  pleura 34.09
  popliteal space 86.09
  prostate 60.0
  rectum - *see also* Proctoscopy 48.23
    by incision 48.0
  retroperitoneum 54.0
  retropubic 59.19
  salivary gland 26.0
  sclera (by incision) 12.89
  scrotum 61.0
  shunt
    ventriculoperitoneal at
      peritoneal site 54.95
      ventricular site 02.41
  sinus
    ethmoid 22.51
    frontal 22.41
    maxillary (Caldwell-Luc approach)
      22.39
    sphenoid 22.52
    tract, skin and subcutaneous tissue 86.09
  skin 86.09
  soft tissue NEC 83.09
    hand 82.09
  spermatic cord 63.93
  sphenoidal sinus 22.52
  spinal (canal) (nerve root) 03.09
  spleen 41.2
  stomach (by incision) 43.0
    endoscopic - *see* Gastroscopy
  subcutaneous tissue 86.09
  subdiaphragmatic space 54.11
  superficial fossa 86.09
  tarsal tunnel 04.44
  tendon (sheath) 83.01
    hand 82.01
  testes 62.0
  thymus (gland) 07.92
    field 07.91
    thoracoscopic 07.95
  thyroid (field) (gland) (by incision) 06.09
    postoperative 06.02
  trachea (by incision) 31.3
    endoscopic - *see* Tracheoscopy
  tunica vaginalis 61.0
  tympanum 20.09
    transtympanic route 20.23
  ureter (by incision) 56.2
    endoscopic 56.31
  urethra (by incision) 58.0
    endoscopic 58.22
  uterus (corpus) 68.0
    cervix 69.95
    digital 68.11
    postpartal, manual 75.7
  vagina (by incision) 70.14
    endoscopic 70.21
  vas deferens 63.6
  vein 38.00
    abdominal 38.07
    head and neck NEC 38.02
    intracranial NEC 38.01
    lower limb 38.09
    thoracic NEC 38.05
    upper limb 38.03
  vulva (by incision) 71.09
Exposure - *see also* Incision, by site
  tooth (for orthodontic treatment) 24.6
Expression, trachoma follicles 10.33
Exsanguination transfusion 99.01
Extension
  buccolabial sulcus 24.91
  limb, forced 93.25
  lingual sulcus 24.91
  mandibular ridge 76.43
Exteriorization
  esophageal pouch 42.12
  intestine 46.03
    large 46.03
    small 46.01

E & F

Exteriorization (*Continued*)
maxillary sinus 22.9
pilonidal cyst or sinus (open excision) (with partial closure) 86.21
Extirpation - *see also* Excision, by site
aneurysm - *see* Aneurysmectomy
arteriovenous fistula - *see* Aneurysmectomy
lacrimal sac 09.6
larynx 30.3
with radical neck dissection (with synchronous thyroidectomy) (with synchronous tracheostomy) 30.4
nerve, tooth - *see also* Therapy, root canal 23.70
varicose vein (peripheral) (lower limb) 38.59
upper limb 38.53
Extracorporeal
circulation (regional), except hepatic 39.61
hepatic 50.92
percutaneous 39.66
hemodialysis 39.95
membrane oxygenation (ECMO) 39.65
photopheresis, therapeutic 99.88
shockwave lithotripsy (ESWL) NEC 98.59
bile duct 98.52
bladder 98.51
gallbladder 98.52
kidney 98.51
renal pelvis 98.51
specified site NEC 98.59
ureter 98.51
Extracranial-intracranial bypass [EC-IC] 39.28
Extraction
breech (partial) 72.52
with forceps to aftercoming head 72.51
total 72.54
with forceps to aftercoming head 72.53
cataract 13.19
after cataract (by)
capsulectomy 13.65
capsulotomy 13.64
discission 13.64
excision 13.65
iridocapsulectomy 13.65
mechanical fragmentation 13.66

Extraction (*Continued*)
cataract (*Continued*)
after cataract (*Continued*)
needling 13.64
phacofragmentation (mechanical) 13.66
aspiration (simple) (with irrigation) 13.3
cryoextraction (intracapsular approach) 13.19
temporal inferior route (in presence of fistulization bleb) 13.11
curette evacuation (extracapsular approach) 13.2
emulsification (and aspiration) 13.41
erysiphake (intracapsular approach) 13.19
temporal inferior route (in presence of fistulization bleb) 13.11
extracapsular approach (with iridectomy) NEC 13.59
by temporal inferior route (in presence of fistulization bleb) 13.51
aspiration (simple) (with irrigation) 13.3
curette evacuation 13.2
emulsification (and aspiration) 13.41
linear extraction 13.2
mechanical fragmentation with aspiration by
posterior route 13.42
specified route NEC 13.43
phacoemulsification (ultrasonic) (with aspiration) 13.41
phacofragmentation (mechanical)
with aspiration by
posterior route 13.42
specified route NEC 13.43
ultrasonic (with aspiration) 13.41
rotoextraction (mechanical)
with aspiration by
posterior route 13.42
specified route NEC 13.43
intracapsular (combined) (simple) (with iridectomy) (with suction) (with zonulolysis) 13.19
by temporal inferior route (in presence of fistulization bleb) 13.11

Extraction (*Continued*)
cataract (*Continued*)
linear extraction (extracapsular approach) 13.2
phacoemulsification (and aspiration) 13.41
phacofragmentation (mechanical)
with aspiration by
posterior route 13.42
specified route NEC 13.43
ultrasonic 13.41
rotoextraction (mechanical)
with aspiration by
posterior route 13.42
specified route NEC 13.43
secondary membranous (after cataract) (by)
capsulectomy 13.65
capsulotomy 13.64
discission 13.64
excision 13.65
iridocapsulectomy 13.65
mechanical fragmentation 13.66
needling 13.64
phacofragmentation (mechanical) 13.66
common duct stones (percutaneous) (through sinus tract) (with basket) 51.96
fat for graft or banking 86.90
foreign body - *see* Removal, foreign body
kidney stone(s), percutaneous 55.03
with fragmentation procedure 55.04
lens (eye) - *see also* Extraction, cataract 13.19
Malstrom's 72.79
with episiotomy 72.71
menstrual, menses 69.6
milk from lactating breast (manual) (pump) 99.98
tooth (by forceps) (multiple) (single) NEC 23.09
with mucoperiosteal flap elevation 23.19
deciduous 23.01
surgical NEC - *see also* Removal, tooth, surgical 23.19
vacuum, fetus 72.79
with episiotomy 72.71
vitreous - *see also* Removal, vitreous 14.72

F

Face lift 86.82
Facetectomy 77.89
Facilitation, intraocular circulation NEC 12.59
Failed (trial) forceps 73.3
Family
counselling (medical) (social) 94.49
therapy 94.42
Farabeuf operation (ischiopubiotomy) 77.39
Fasanella-Servatt operation (blepharoptosis repair) 08.35
Fasciaplasty - *see* Fascioplasty
Fascia sling operation - *see* Operation, sling
Fasciectomy 83.44
for graft 83.43
hand 82.34
hand 82.35
for graft 82.34
palmar (release of Dupuytren's contracture) 82.35
Fasciodesis 83.89
hand 82.89
Fascioplasty - *see also* Repair, fascia 83.89
hand - *see also* Repair, fascia, hand 82.89
Fasciorrhaphy - *see* Suture, fascia
Fasciotomy 83.14
Dupuytren's 82.12
with excision 82.35

Fasciotomy (*Continued*)
Dwyer 83.14
hand 82.12
Ober-Yount 83.14
orbital - *see also* Orbitotomy 16.09
palmar (release of Dupuytren's contracture) 82.12
with excision 82.35
Fenestration
aneurysm (dissecting), thoracic aorta 39.54
aortic aneurysm 39.54
cardiac valve 35.10
chest wall 34.01
ear
inner (with graft) 20.61
revision 20.62
tympanic 19.55
labyrinth (with graft) 20.61
Lempert's (endaural) 19.9
operation (aorta) 39.54
oval window, ear canal 19.55
palate 27.1
pericardium 37.12
semicircular canals (with graft) 20.61
stapes foot plate (with vein graft) 19.19
with incus replacement 19.11
tympanic membrane 19.55
vestibule (with graft) 20.61
Ferguson operation (hernia repair) 53.00

Fetography 87.81
Fetoscopy 75.31
Fiberoscopy - *see* Endoscopy, by site
Fibroidectomy, uterine 68.29
Fick operation (perforation of foot plate) 19.0
Filipuncture (aneurysm) (cerebral) 39.52
Filleting
hammer toe 77.56
pancreas 52.3
Filling, tooth (amalgam) (plastic) (silicate) 23.2
root canal - *see also* Therapy, root canal 23.70
Fimbriectomy - *see also* Salpingectomy, partial 66.69
Uchida (with tubal ligation) 66.32
Finney operation (pyloroplasty) 44.29
Fissurectomy, anal 49.39
endoscopic 49.31
skin (subcutaneous tissue) 49.04
Fistulectomy - *see also* Closure, fistula, by site
abdominothoracic 34.83
abdominouterine 69.42
anus 49.12
appendix 47.92
bile duct 51.79
biliary tract NEC 51.79
bladder (transurethral approach) 57.84
bone - *see also* Excision, lesion, bone 77.60
branchial cleft 29.52
bronchocutaneous 33.42

◀ New   ◀ Revised   deleted Deleted   ● Use Additional Digit(s)   Omit code

Fistulectomy (Continued)
bronchoesophageal 33.42
bronchomediastinal 34.73
bronchopleural 34.73
bronchopleurocutaneous 34.73
bronchopleuromediastinal 34.73
bronchovisceral 33.42
cervicosigmoidal 67.62
cholecystogastroenteric 51.93
cornea 11.49
diaphragm 34.83
enterouterine 69.42
esophagopleurocutaneous 34.73
esophagus NEC 42.84
fallopian tube 66.73
gallbladder 51.93
gastric NEC 44.63
hepatic duct 51.79
hepatopleural 34.73
hepatopulmonary 34.73
intestine
large 46.76
small 46.74
intestinouterine 69.42
joint - see also Excision, lesion, joint 80.80
lacrimal
gland 09.21
sac 09.6
laryngotracheal 31.62
larynx 31.62
mediastinocutaneous 34.73
mouth NEC 27.53
nasal 21.82
sinus 22.71
nasolabial 21.82
nasopharyngeal 21.82
oroantral 22.71
oronasal 21.82
pancreas 52.95
perineorectal 71.72
perineosigmoidal 71.72
perirectal, not opening into rectum 48.93
pharyngoesophageal 29.53
pharynx NEC 29.53
pleura 34.73
rectolabial 71.72
rectourethral 58.43
rectouterine 69.42
rectovaginal 70.73
rectovesical 57.83
rectovulvar 71.72
rectum 48.73
salivary (duct) (gland) 26.42
scrotum 61.42
skin 86.3
stomach NEC 44.63
subcutaneous tissue 86.3
thoracoabdominal 34.83
thoracogastric 34.83
thoracointestinal 34.83
thorax NEC 34.73
trachea NEC 31.73
tracheoesophageal 31.73
ureter 56.84
urethra 58.43
uteroenteric 69.42
uterointestinal 69.42
uterorectal 69.42
uterovaginal 69.42
vagina 70.75
vesicosigmoidovaginal 57.83
vocal cords 31.62
vulvorectal 71.72
Fistulization
appendix 47.91
arteriovenous 39.27
cisterna chyli 40.62
endolymphatic sac (for decompression) 20.79
esophagus, external 42.10
cervical 42.11
specified technique NEC 42.19

Fistulization (Continued)
interatrial 35.41
labyrinth (for decompression) 20.79
lacrimal sac into nasal cavity 09.81
larynx 31.29
lymphatic duct, left (thoracic) 40.62
orbit 16.09
peritoneal 54.93
salivary gland 26.49
sclera 12.69
by trephination 12.61
with iridectomy 12.65
sinus, nasal NEC 22.9
subarachnoid space 02.22
thoracic duct 40.62
trachea 31.29
tracheoesophageal 31.95
urethrovaginal 58.0
ventricle, cerebral - see also Shunt, ventricular
02.22
Fistulogram
abdominal wall 88.03
chest wall 87.38
retroperitoneum 88.14
specified site NEC 88.49
Fistulotomy, anal 49.11
Fitting
arch bars (orthodontic) 24.7
for immobilization (fracture) 93.55
artificial limb 84.40
contact lens 95.32
denture (total) 99.97
bridge (fixed) 23.42
removable 23.43
partial (fixed) 23.42
removable 23.43
hearing aid 95.48
obturator (orthodontic) 24.7
ocular prosthetics 95.34
orthodontic
appliance 24.7
obturator 24.7
wiring 24.7
orthotic device 93.23
periodontal splint (orthodontic) 24.7
prosthesis, prosthetic device
above knee 84.45
arm 84.43
lower (and hand) 84.42
upper (and shoulder) 84.41
below knee 84.46
hand (and lower arm) 84.42
leg 84.47
above knee 84.45
below knee 84.46
limb NEC 84.40
ocular 95.34
penis (external) 64.94
shoulder (and upper arm) 84.41
spectacles 95.31
Five-in-one repair, knee 81.42
Fixation
bone
external, without reduction 93.59
with fracture reduction - see Reduction,
fracture
cast immobilization NEC 93.53
external fixator - see Fixator, external
splint 93.54
traction (skeletal) NEC 93.44
intermittent 93.43
internal (without fracture reduction) 78.50
with fracture reduction - see Reduction,
fracture
carpal, metacarpal 78.54
clavicle 78.51
femur 78.55
fibula 78.57
humerus 78.52
patella 78.56
pelvic 78.59

Fixation (Continued)
bone (Continued)
internal (Continued)
phalanges (foot) (hand) 78.59
radius 78.53
scapula 78.51
specified site NEC 78.59
tarsal, metatarsal 78.58
thorax (ribs) (sternum) 78.51
sternal fixation device with rigid
plates 84.94
tibia 78.57
ulna 78.53
vertebrae 78.59
breast (pendulous) 85.6
cardinal ligaments 69.22
cervical collar 93.52
duodenum 46.62
to abdominal wall 46.61
external (without manipulation for
reduction) 93.59
with fracture reduction - see Reduction,
fracture
cast immobilization NEC 93.53
pressure dressing 93.56
splint 93.54
strapping (non-traction) 93.59
traction (skeletal) NEC 93.44
intermittent 93.43
hip 81.40
ileum 46.62
to abdominal wall 46.61
internal
with fracture reduction - see Reduction,
fracture
without fracture reduction - see Fixation,
bone, internal
intestine 46.60
large 46.64
to abdominal wall 46.63
small 46.62
to abdominal wall 46.61
to abdominal wall 46.60
iris (bombé) 12.11
jejunum 46.62
to abdominal wall 46.61
joint - see Arthroplasty
kidney 55.7
ligament
cardinal 69.22
palpebrae 08.36
omentum 54.74
parametrial 69.22
plaster jacket 93.51
other cast 93.53
rectum (sling) 48.76
spine, with fusion - see also Fusion, spinal
81.00
spleen 41.95
splint 93.54
tendon 83.88
hand 82.85
testis in scrotum 62.5
tongue 25.59
urethrovaginal (to Cooper's ligament) 70.77
with graft or prosthesis 70.78
uterus (abdominal) (vaginal) (ventrofixation)
69.22
vagina 70.77
with graft or prosthesis 70.78
Fixator, external
computer assisted (dependent) 84.73
hybrid device or system 84.73
Ilizarov type 84.72
monoplanar system 84.71
ring device or system 84.72
Sheffield type 84.72
Flooding (psychologic desensitization) 94.33
Flowmetry, Doppler (ultrasonic) - see also
Ultrasonography
aortic arch 88.73

Flowmetry, Doppler *(Continued)*
  head and neck 88.71
  heart 88.72
  thorax NEC 88.73
Fluoroscopy - *see* Radiography
Fog therapy (respiratory) 93.94
Folding, eye muscle 15.22
  multiple (two or more muscles) 15.4
Foley operation (pyeloplasty) 55.87
Fontan operation (creation of conduit between right atrium and pulmonary artery) 35.94
Foraminotomy 03.09
Forced extension, limb 93.25
Forceps delivery - *see* Delivery, forceps
Formation
  adhesions
    pericardium 36.39
    pleura 34.6
  anus, artificial - *see* Colostomy
    duodenostomy 46.39
    ileostomy - *see* Ileostomy
    jejunostomy 46.39
      percutaneous (endoscopic) (PEJ) 46.32
  arteriovenous fistula (for kidney dialysis) (peripheral) (shunt) 39.27
    external cannula 39.93
  bone flap, cranial 02.03
  cardiac device (defibrillator) (pacemaker)
    pocket
      with initial insertion of cardiac device - *omit code*
      new site (skin) (subcutaneous) 37.79
  colostomy - *see* Colostomy
  conduit
    apical-aortic (AAC) 35.93
    ileal (urinary) 56.51
    left ventricle and aorta 35.93
    right atrium and pulmonary artery 35.94
    right ventricle and pulmonary (distal) artery 35.92
      in repair of
        pulmonary artery atresia 35.92
        transposition of great vessels 35.92
        truncus arteriosus 35.83
  endorectal ileal pouch (H-pouch) (J-pouch) (S-pouch) (with anastomosis to anus) 45.95
  fistula
    arteriovenous (for kidney dialysis) (peripheral shunt) 39.27
      external cannula 39.93
    bladder to skin NEC 57.18
      with bladder flap 57.21
      percutaneous 57.17
    cutaneoperitoneal 54.93
    gastric 43.19
      percutaneous (endoscopic) (transabdominal) 43.11
    mucous - *see* Colostomy
    rectovaginal 48.99
    tracheoesophageal 31.95
    tubulovalvular (Beck-Jianu) (Frank's) (Janeway) (Spivack's) (Ssabanejew-Frank) 43.19
    urethrovaginal 58.0
  ileal
    bladder
      closed 57.87 [45.51]
      open 56.51
    conduit 56.51
  interatrial fistula 35.42
  mucous fistula - *see* Colostomy
  pericardial
    baffle, interatrial 35.91
    window 37.12
  pleural window (for drainage) 34.09
  pocket
    cardiac device (defibrillator) (pacemaker)
      with initial insertion of cardiac device - *omit code*
      new site (skin) (subcutaneous) 37.79

Formation *(Continued)*
  pocket *(Continued)*
    loop recorder 37.79
    thalamic stimulator pulse generator
      with initial insertion of battery package - *omit code*
      new site (skin) (subcutaneous) 86.09
  pupil 12.39
    by iridectomy 12.14
  rectovaginal fistula 48.99
  reversed gastric tube (intrathoracic) (retrosternal) 42.58
    antesternal or antethoracic 42.68
  septal defect, interatrial 35.42
  shunt
    abdominovenous 54.94
    arteriovenous 39.93
    peritoneojugular 54.94
    peritoneo-vascular 54.94
    pleuroperitoneal 34.05
    transjugular intrahepatic portosystemic (TIPS) 39.1
  subcutaneous tunnel
    esophageal 42.86
      with anastomosis - *see* Anastomosis, esophagus, antesternal
    pulse generator lead wire 86.99
      with initial procedure - *omit code*
    thalamic stimulator pulse generator pocket
      with initial insertion of battery package - *omit code*
      new site (skin) (subcutaneous) 86.09
  syndactyly (finger) (toe) 86.89
  tracheoesophageal 31.95
  tubulovalvular fistula (Beck-Jianu) (Frank's) (Janeway) (Spivak's) (Ssabanejew-Frank) 43.19
  uretero-ileostomy, cutaneous 56.51
  ureterostomy, cutaneous 56.61
    ileal 56.51
  urethrovaginal fistula 58.0
  window
    pericardial 37.12
    pleural (for drainage) 34.09
      thoracoscopic 34.06
Fothergill (-Donald) operation (uterine suspension) 69.22
Fowler operation
  arthroplasty of metacarpophalangeal joint 81.72
  release (mallet finger repair) 82.84
  tenodesis (hand) 82.85
  thoracoplasty 33.34
Fox operation (entropion repair with wedge resection) 08.43
Fracture, surgical - *see also* Osteoclasis 78.70
  turbinates (nasal) 21.62
Fragmentation
  lithotriptor - *see* Lithotripsy
  mechanical
    cataract (with aspiration) 13.43
      posterior route 13.42
      secondary membrane 13.66
    secondary membrane (after cataract) 13.66
  ultrasonic
    cataract (with aspiration) 13.41
    stones, urinary (Kock pouch) 59.95
    urinary stones 59.95
      percutaneous nephrostomy 55.04
Franco operation (suprapubic cystotomy) 57.18
Frank operation (permanent gastrostomy) 43.19
Frazier (-Spiller) operation (subtemporal trigeminal rhizotomy) 04.02
Fredet-Ramstedt operation (pyloromyotomy) (with wedge resection) 43.3
Freeing
  adhesions - *see* Lysis, adhesions
  anterior synechiae (with injection of air or liquid) 12.32
  artery-vein-nerve bundle 39.91

Freeing *(Continued)*
  extraocular muscle, entrapped 15.7
  goniosynechiae (with injection of air or liquid) 12.31
  intestinal segment for interposition 45.50
    large 45.52
    small 45.51
  posterior synechiae 12.33
  synechiae (posterior) 12.33
    anterior (with injection of air or liquid) 12.32
  vascular bundle 39.91
  vessel 39.91
Freezing
  gastric 96.32
  prostate 60.62
Frenckner operation (intrapetrosal drainage) 20.22
Frenectomy
  labial 27.41
  lingual 25.92
  lip 27.41
  maxillary 27.41
  tongue 25.92
Frenotomy
  labial 27.91
  lingual 25.91
Frenulumectomy - *see* Frenectomy
Frickman operation (abdominal proctopexy) 48.75
Frommel operation (shortening of uterosacral ligaments) 69.22
Fulguration - *see also* Electrocoagulation and Destruction, lesion, by site
  adenoid fossa 28.7
  anus 49.39
    endoscopic 49.31
  bladder (transurethral) 57.49
    suprapubic 57.59
  choroid 14.21
  duodenum 45.32
    endoscopic 45.30
  esophagus 42.39
    endoscopic 42.33
  large intestine 45.49
    endoscopic 45.43
      polypectomy 45.42
  penis 64.2
  perineum, female 71.3
  prostate, transurethral 60.29
  rectum 48.32
    radical 48.31
  retina 14.21
  scrotum 61.3
  Skene's gland 71.3
  skin 86.3
  small intestine NEC 45.34
    duodenum 45.32
      endoscopic 45.30
  stomach 43.49
    endoscopic 43.41
  subcutaneous tissue 86.3
  tonsillar fossa 28.7
  urethra 58.39
    endoscopic 58.31
  vulva 71.3
Function
  study - *see also* Scan, radioisotope
    gastric 89.39
    muscle 93.08
      ocular 95.25
    nasal 89.12
    pulmonary - *see* categories 89.37
    renal 92.03
    thyroid 92.01
    urethral sphincter 89.23
Fundectomy, uterine 68.39
Fundoplication (esophageal) (Nissen's) 44.66
  laparoscopic 44.67
Fundusectomy, gastric 43.89

◀ New   ◀◀ Revised   ~~deleted~~ Deleted   ● Use Additional Digit(s)   ▨ Omit code

Fusion
- atlas-axis (spine) - *see* Fusion, spinal, atlas-axis
- bone - *see also* Osteoplasty 78.40
- cervical (spine) (C2 level or below) - *see* Fusion, spinal, cervical
- claw toe 77.57
- craniocervical - *see* Fusion, spinal, craniocervical
- dorsal, dorsolumbar - *see* Fusion, spinal, dorsal, dorsolumbar
- epiphyseal-diaphyseal - *see also* Arrest, bone growth 78.20
- epiphysiodesis - *see also* Arrest, bone growth 78.20
- hammer toe 77.56
- joint (with bone graft) - *see also* Arthrodesis 81.20
  - ankle 81.11
  - claw toe 77.57
  - foot NEC 81.17
  - hammer toe 77.56
  - hip 81.21
  - interphalangeal, finger 81.28
  - ischiofemoral 81.21
  - metatarsophalangeal 81.16
  - midtarsal 81.14
  - overlapping toe(s) 77.58
  - pantalar 81.11
  - spinal - *see also* Fusion, spinal 81.00
  - subtalar 81.13
  - tarsal joints NEC 81.17
  - tarsometatarsal 81.15
  - tibiotalar 81.11
  - toe NEC 77.58
    - claw toe 77.57
    - hammer toe 77.56
    - overlapping toe(s) 77.58

Fusion *(Continued)*
- lip to tongue 25.59
- lumbar, lumbosacral - *see* Fusion, spinal, lumbar, lumbosacral
- occiput-C2 (spinal) - *see* Fusion, spinal, occiput
- spinal, NOS (with graft) (with internal fixation) (with instrumentation) 81.00
  - anterior lumbar interbody fusion (ALIF) 81.06
  - atlas-axis (anterior transoral) (posterior) 81.01
    - for pseudarthrosis 81.31
  - axial lumber interbody fusion [AxiaLIF®] 81.08
  - cervical (C2 level or below) NEC 81.02
    - anterior column (interbody), anterolateral (anterior) technique 81.02
      - for pseudarthrosis 81.32
    - C1-C2 level (anterior) (posterior) 81.01
      - for pseudarthrosis 81.31
    - for pseudarthrosis 81.32
    - posterior column posterolateral (posterior) technique 81.03
      - for pseudarthrosis 81.33
  - craniocervical (anterior transoral) (posterior) 81.01
    - for pseudarthrosis 81.31
  - direct lateral interbody fusion [DLIF] 81.06
  - dorsal, dorsolumbar NEC 81.05
    - anterior column (interbody), anterolateral (anterior) (extracavitary) technique 81.04
      - for pseudarthrosis 81.34

Fusion *(Continued)*
- spinal, NOS *(Continued)*
  - dorsal, dorsolumbar NEC *(Continued)*
    - for pseudarthrosis 81.35
    - posterior column posterolateral (posterior) technique 81.05
      - for pseudarthrosis 81.35
  - extreme lateral interbody fusion [XLIF®] 81.06
  - facet 81.07
  - lumbar, lumbosacral NEC 81.08
    - anterior column (interbody) anterolateral (anterior) technique 81.06
      - for pseudarthrosis 81.36
    - posterior technique 81.08
      - for pseudarthrosis 81.38
    - lateral transverse process technique 81.07
      - for pseudarthrosis 81.37
    - posterior column, posterior (posterolateral) (transverse process) technique 81.07
  - number of vertebrae - *see* codes 81.62
  - occiput-C2 (anterior transoral) (posterior) 81.01
    - for pseudarthrosis 81.31
  - posterior lumbar interbody fusion (PLIF) 81.08
  - transforaminal lumbar interbody fusion (TLIF) 81.08

> Note: Also use either 81.62, as an additional code to show the total number of vertebrae fused.

- tongue (to lip) 25.59

G

Gait training 93.22
Galeaplasty 86.89
Galvanoionization 99.27
Games
- competitive 94.39
- organized 93.89

Gamma irradiation, stereotactic 92.32
Ganglionectomy
- gasserian 04.05
- lumbar sympathetic 05.23
- nerve (cranial) (peripheral) NEC 04.06
  - sympathetic 05.29
- sphenopalatine (Meckel's) 05.21
- tendon sheath (wrist) 82.21
  - site other than hand 83.31
- trigeminal 04.05

Ganglionotomy, trigeminal (radiofrequency) 04.02
Gant operation (wedge osteotomy of trochanter) 77.25
Garceau operation (tibial tendon transfer) 83.75
Gardner operation (spinal meningocele repair) 03.51
Gas endarterectomy 38.10
- abdominal 38.16
- aorta (arch) (ascending) (descending) 38.14
- coronary artery 36.09
- head and neck NEC 38.12
- intracranial NEC 38.11
- lower limb 38.18
- thoracic NEC 38.15
- upper limb 38.13

Gastrectomy (partial) (sleeve) (subtotal) NEC 43.89
- with
  - anastomosis (to) NEC 43.89
    - duodenum 43.6
    - esophagus 43.5
    - gastrogastric 43.89
    - jejunum 43.7
  - esophagogastrostomy 43.5
  - gastroduodenostomy (bypass) 43.6
  - gastroenterostomy (bypass) 43.7
  - gastrogastrostomy (bypass) 43.89
  - gastrojejunostomy (bypass) 43.7
  - jejunal transposition 43.81
- complete NEC 43.99
  - with intestinal interposition 43.91
- distal 43.6
- Hofmeister 43.7
- laparoscopic, vertical (sleeve) 43.82
- Polya 43.7
- proximal 43.5
- radical NEC 43.99
  - with intestinal interposition 43.91
- sleeve
  - laparoscopic 43.82
- total NEC 43.99
  - with intestinal interposition 43.91

Gastrocamera 44.19
Gastroduodenectomy - *see* Gastrectomy
Gastroduodenoscopy 45.13
- through stoma (artificial) 45.12
- transabdominal (operative) 45.11
Gastroduodenostomy (bypass) (Jaboulay's) 44.39
- with partial gastrectomy 43.6

Gastroenterostomy (bypass) NEC 44.39
- with partial gastrectomy 43.7
- laparoscopic 44.38
Gastrogastrostomy (bypass) 44.39
- with partial gastrectomy 43.89
- laparoscopic 44.38
Gastrojejunostomy (bypass) 44.39
- with partial gastrectomy 43.7
- laparoscopic 44.38
- percutaneous (endoscopic)
  - for bypass 44.32
  - for feeding tube placement 46.32
Gastrolysis 54.59
- laparoscopic 54.51
Gastropexy 44.64
Gastroplasty NEC 44.69
- laparoscopic 44.68
- vertical banded gastroplasty (VBG) 44.68
Gastroplication 44.69
- laparoscopic 44.68
Gastropylorectomy 43.6
Gastrorrhaphy 44.61
Gastroscopy NEC 44.13
- through stoma (artificial) 44.12
- transabdominal (operative) 44.11
Gastrostomy (Brunschwig's) (decompression) (fine caliber tube) (Kader) (permanent) (Stamm) (Stamm-Kader) (temporary) (tube) (Witzel) 43.19
- Beck-Jianu 43.19
- Frank's 43.19
- Janeway 43.19
- percutaneous (endoscopic) (PEG) 43.11
- Spivack's 43.19
- Ssabanejew-Frank 43.19
Gastrotomy 43.0
- for control of hemorrhage 44.49

Gavage, gastric 96.35
Gelman operation (release of clubfoot) 83.84
Genioplasty (augmentation) (with graft) (with
    implant) 76.68
    reduction 76.67
Ghormley operation (hip fusion) 81.21
Gifford operation
    destruction of lacrimal sac 09.6
    keratotomy (delimiting) 11.1
        radial (refractive) 11.75
Gill operation
    arthrodesis of shoulder 81.23
    laminectomy 03.09
Gill-Stein operation (carporadial arthrodesis)
    81.25
Gilliam operation (uterine suspension) 69.22
Gingivectomy 24.31
Gingivoplasty (with bone graft) (with soft
    tissue graft) 24.2
Girdlestone operation
    laminectomy with spinal fusion 81.00
    muscle transfer for claw toe repair 77.57
    resection of femoral head and neck (without
        insertion of joint prosthesis) 77.85
        with replacement prosthesis - see Implant,
            joint, hip
    resection of hip prosthesis 80.05
        with replacement prosthesis - see Implant,
            joint, hip
Girdlestone-Taylor operation (muscle transfer
    for claw toe repair) 77.57
Glenn operation (anastomosis of superior vena
    cava to right pulmonary artery) 39.21
Glenoplasty, shoulder 81.83
    with
        partial replacement 81.81
        total replacement, NEC 81.80
            other 81.80
            reverse 81.88
    for recurrent dislocation 81.82
Glomectomy
    carotid 39.89
    jugulare 20.51
Glossectomy (complete) (total) 25.3
    partial or subtotal 25.2
    radical 25.4
Glossopexy 25.59
Glossoplasty NEC 25.59
Glossorrhaphy 25.51
Glossotomy NEC 25.94
    for tongue tie 25.91
Glycoprotein IIB/IIIa inhibitor 99.20
Goebel-Frangenheim-Stoeckel operation
    (urethrovesical suspension) 59.4
Goldner operation (clubfoot release) 80.48
Goldthwaite operation
    ankle stabilization 81.11
    patellar stabilization 81.44
    tendon transfer for stabilization of patella
        81.44
Gonadectomy
    ovary
        bilateral 65.51
            laparoscopic 65.53
        unilateral 65.39
            laparoscopic 65.31
    testis
        bilateral 62.41
        unilateral 62.3
Goniopuncture 12.51
    with goniotomy 12.53
Gonioscopy 12.29
Goniospasis 12.59
Goniotomy (Barkan's) 12.52
    with goniopuncture 12.53
Goodal-Power operation (vagina) 70.8
Gordon-Taylor operation (hindquarter
    amputation) 84.19
GP IIB/IIIa inhibitor, infusion 99.20
Graber-Duvernay operation (drilling of
    femoral head) 77.15

Graft, grafting
    aneurysm 39.52
        endovascular
            abdominal aorta 39.71
                fenestrated (branching) graft 39.78
            lower extremity artery(s) 39.79
            thoracic aorta 39.73
            upper extremity artery(s) 39.79
    artery, arterial (patch) 39.58
        with
            excision or resection of vessel - see
                Arteriectomy, with graft
                replacement
            synthetic patch (Dacron) (Teflon) 39.57
            tissue patch (vein) (autogenous)
                (homograft) 39.56
    blood vessel (patch) 39.58
        with
            excision or resection of vessel - see
                Angiectomy, with graft
                replacement
            synthetic patch (Dacron) (Teflon) 39.57
            tissue patch (vein) (autogenous)
                (homograft) 39.56
    bone (autogenous) (bone bank) (dual onlay)
        (heterogeneous) (inlay) (massive
        onlay) (multiple) (osteoperiosteal)
        (peg) (subperiosteal) (with metallic
        fixation) 78.00
        with
            arthrodesis - see Arthrodesis
            arthroplasty - see Arthroplasty
            gingivoplasty 24.2
            lengthening - see Lengthening, bone
        carpals, metacarpals 78.04
        clavicle 78.01
        facial NEC 76.91
            with total ostectomy 76.44
        femur 78.05
        fibula 78.07
        humerus 78.02
        joint - see Arthroplasty
        mandible 76.91
            with total mandibulectomy 76.41
        marrow - see Transplant, bone, marrow
        nose - see Graft, nose
        patella 78.06
        pelvic 78.09
        pericranial 02.04
        phalanges (foot) (hand) 78.09
        radius 78.03
        scapula 78.01
        skull 02.04
        specified site NEC 78.09
        spine 78.09
            with fusion - see Fusion, spinal
        tarsal, metatarsal 78.08
        thorax (ribs) (sternum) 78.01
        thumb (with transfer of skin flap)
            82.69
        tibia 78.07
        ulna 78.03
        vertebrae 78.09
            with fusion - see Fusion, spinal
    breast (see also Mammoplasty) 85.89
        fat graft 85.55
    buccal sulcus 27.99
    cartilage (joint) - see also Arthroplasty
        nose - see Graft, nose
    chest wall (mesh) (silastic) 34.79
    conjunctiva (free) (mucosa) 10.44
        for symblepharon repair 10.41
    cornea - see also Keratoplasty 11.60
    dermal-fat 86.69
    dermal regenerative 86.67
    dura 02.12
    ear
        auricle 18.79
        external auditory meatus 18.6
        inner 20.61
        pedicle preparation 86.71

Graft, grafting (Continued)
    esophagus NEC 42.87
        with interposition (intrathoracic) NEC
            42.58
            antesternal or antethoracic NEC
                42.68
            colon (intrathoracic) 42.55
                antesternal or antethoracic 42.65
            small bowel (intrathoracic) 42.53
                antesternal or antethoracic 42.63
    eyebrow - see also Reconstruction, eyelid,
        with graft 08.69
    eyelid - see also Reconstruction, eyelid, with
        graft 08.69
        free mucous membrane 08.62
    eye socket (skin) (cartilage) (bone) 16.63
    fallopian tube 66.79
    fascia 83.82
        with hernia repair - see Repair, hernia
        eyelid 08.32
        hand 82.72
        tarsal cartilage 08.69
    fat pad NEC 86.89
        with skin graft - see Graft, skin, full-
            thickness
    flap (advanced) (rotating) (sliding) - see also
        Graft, skin, pedicle
        tarsoconjunctival 08.64
    hair-bearing skin 86.64
    hand
        fascia 82.72
        free skin 86.62
        muscle 82.72
        pedicle (flap) 86.73
        tendon 82.79
    heart, for revascularization - see category
        36.3 ●
    joint - see Arthroplasty
    larynx 31.69
    lip 27.56
        full-thickness 27.55
    lymphatic structure(s) (channel) (node)
        (vessel) 40.9
    mediastinal fat to myocardium 36.39
    meninges (cerebral) 02.12
    mouth, except palate 27.56
        full-thickness 27.55
    muscle 83.82
        hand 82.72
    myocardium, for revascularization 36.39
    nasolabial flaps 21.86
    nerve (cranial) (peripheral) 04.5
    nipple 85.86
    nose 21.89
        with
            augmentation 21.85
            rhinoplasty - see Rhinoplasty
            total reconstruction 21.83
        septum 21.88
        tip 21.86
    omentum 54.74
        to myocardium 36.39
    orbit (bone) (cartilage) (skin) 16.63
    outflow tract (patch) (pulmonary valve)
        35.26
        in total repair of tetralogy of Fallot 35.81
    ovary 65.92
    palate 27.69
        for cleft palate repair 27.62
    pedicle - see Graft, skin, pedicle
    penis (rib) (skin) 64.49
    pigskin 86.65
    pinch - see Graft, skin, free
    pocket - see Graft, skin, pedicle
    porcine 86.65
    postauricular (Wolff) 18.79
    razor - see Graft, skin, free
    rope - see Graft, skin, pedicle
    saphenous vein in aortocoronary bypass - see
        Bypass, aorto-coronary
    scrotum 61.49

Graft, grafting (*Continued*)
skin (partial-thickness) (split-thickness) 86.69
amnionic membrane 86.66
auditory meatus (ear) 18.6
dermal-fat 86.69
for breast augmentation 85.50
dermal regenerative 86.67
ear
auditory meatus 18.6
postauricular 18.79
eyelid 08.61
fat 86.87
flap - *see* Graft, skin, pedicle
free (autogenous) NEC 86.60
breast
deep inferior epigastric artery perforator (DIEP) flap, free 85.74
gluteal artery perforator [GAP] flap, free 85.76
superficial inferior epigastric artery (SIEA) flap, free 85.75
transverse rectus abdominis musculocutaneous (TRAM) flap, free 85.73
lip 27.56
thumb 86.62
for
pollicization 82.61
reconstruction 82.69
full-thickness 86.63
breast 85.83
hand 86.61
hair-bearing 86.64
eyelid or eyebrow 08.63
hand 86.62
full-thickness 86.61
heterograft 86.65
homograft 86.66
island flap 86.70
mucous membrane 86.69
eyelid 08.62
nose - *see* Graft, nose

Graft, grafting (*Continued*)
skin (*Continued*)
pedicle (flap) (tube) 86.70
advancement 86.72
attachment to site (advanced) (double) (rotating) (sliding) 86.74
hand (cross finger) (pocket) 86.73
lip 27.57
mouth 27.57
thumb 86.73
for
pollicization 82.61
reconstruction NEC 82.69
breast 85.84
deep inferior epigastric artery perforator (DIEP) flap, free 85.74
gluteal artery perforator (GAP) flap, free 85.76
latissimus dorsi myocutaneous flap 85.71
superficial inferior epigastric artery (SIEA) flap, free 85.75
transverse rectus abdominis musculocutaneous (TRAM) flap, free 85.73
transverse rectus abdominis myocutaneous (TRAM) flap, pedicled 85.72
defatting 86.75
delayed 86.71
design and raising 86.71
elevation 86.71
preparation of (cutting) 86.71
revision 86.75
sculpturing 86.71
transection 86.71
transfer 86.74
trimming 86.71
postauricular 18.79
rotation flap 86.70
specified site NEC 86.69
full-thickness 86.63

Graft, grafting (*Continued*)
tarsal cartilage 08.69
temporalis muscle to orbit 16.63
with exenteration of orbit 16.59
tendon 83.81
for joint repair - *see* Arthroplasty
hand 82.79
testicle 62.69
thumb (for reconstruction) NEC 82.69
tongue (mucosal) (skin) 25.59
trachea 31.79
tubular (tube) - *see* Graft, skin, pedicle
tunnel - *see* Graft, skin, pedicle
tympanum - *see also* Tympanoplasty 19.4
ureter 56.89
vagina
biological 70.94
synthetic 70.95
vein (patch) 39.58
with
excision or resection of vessel - *see* Phlebectomy, with graft replacement
synthetic patch (Dacron) (Teflon) 39.57
tissue patch (vein) (autogenous) (homograft) 39.56
vermilion border (lip) 27.56
Grattage, conjunctiva 10.31
Green operation (scapulopexy) 78.41
Grice operation (subtalar arthrodesis) 81.13
Grip, strength 93.04
Gritti-Stokes operation (knee disarticulation) 84.16
Gross operation (herniorrhaphy)
laparoscopic 53.43
with graft or prosthesis 53.42
other and open with graft or prosthesis 53.41
other open 53.49
Group therapy 94.44
Guttering, bone - *see also* Excision, lesion, bone 77.60
Guyon operation (amputation of ankle) 84.13

H

Hagner operation (epididymotomy) 63.92
Halsted operation - *see* Repair, hernia, inguinal
Hampton operation (anastomosis small intestine to rectal stump) 45.92
Hanging hip operation (muscle release) 83.19
Harelip operation 27.54
Harrison-Richardson operation (vaginal suspension) 70.77
with graft or prosthesis 70.78
Hartmann resection (of intestine) (with pouch) - *see* Colectomy, by site
Harvesting
bone marrow 41.91
fat for grafting or banking 86.90
stem cells 99.79
Hauser operation
achillotenotomy 83.11
bunionectomy with adductor tendon transfer 77.53
stabilization of patella 81.44
Heaney operation (vaginal hysterectomy) 68.59
laparoscopically assisted (LAVH) 68.51
Hearing aid (with battery replacement) 95.49
Hearing test 95.47
HeartMate® implantable heart assist system 37.66
HeartMate® II left ventricular assist system [LVAS] 37.66
Hegar operation (perineorrhaphy) 71.79
Heine operation (cyclodialysis) 12.55

Heineke-Mikulicz operation (pyloroplasty) 44.29
Heller operation (esophagomyotomy) 42.7
Hellström operation (transplantation of aberrant renal vessel) 39.55
Hemicolectomy
left
laparoscopic 17.35
open and other 45.75
right (extended)
laparoscopic 17.33
open and other 45.73
Hemicystectomy 57.6
Hemigastrectomy - *see* Gastrectomy
Hemiglossectomy 25.2
Hemilaminectomy (decompression) (exploration) 03.09
Hemilaryngectomy (anterior) (lateral) (vertical) 30.1
Hemimandibulectomy 76.31
Hemimastectomy (radical) 85.23
Hemimaxillectomy (with bone graft) (with prosthesis) 76.39
Heminephrectomy 55.4
Hemipelvectomy 84.19
Hemispherectomy (cerebral) 01.52
Hemithyroidectomy (with removal of isthmus) (with removal of portion of remaining lobe) 06.2
Hemodiafiltration (extracorporeal) 39.95
Hemodialysis (extracorporeal) 39.95
Hemodilution 99.03

Hemofiltration (extracorporeal) 39.95
Hemorrhage control - *see* Control, hemorrhage
Hemorrhoidectomy 49.46
by
cautery, cauterization 49.43
crushing 49.45
cryotherapy, cryosurgery 49.44
excision 49.46
injection 49.42
ligation 49.45
Hemostasis - *see* Control, hemorrhage
Henley operation (jejunal transposition) 43.81
Hepatectomy (complete) (total) 50.4
partial or subtotal 50.22
Hepatic assistance, extracorporeal 50.92
Hepaticocholangiojejunostomy 51.37
Hepaticocystoduodenostomy 51.37
Hepaticodochotomy 51.59
Hepaticoduodenostomy 51.37
Hepaticojejunostomy 51.37
Hepaticolithectomy 51.49
endoscopic 51.88
Hepaticolithotomy 51.49
endoscopic 51.88
Hepaticostomy 51.59
Hepaticotomy 51.59
Hepatocholangiocystoduodenostomy 51.37
Hepatocholedochostomy 51.43
endoscopic 51.87
Hepatoduodenostomy 50.69
Hepatogastrostomy 50.69
Hepatojejunostomy 50.69

G & H

Hepatolithotomy
  hepatic duct 51.49
  liver 50.0
Hepatopexy 50.69
Hepatorrhaphy 50.61
Hepatostomy (external) (internal) 50.69
Hepatotomy (with packing) 50.0
Hernioplasty - *see* Repair, hernia
Herniorrhaphy - *see* Repair, hernia
Herniotomy - *see* Repair, hernia
Heterograft - *see* Graft
Heterotransplant, heterotransplantation - *see*
  Transplant
Hey operation (amputation of foot) 84.12
Hey-Groves operation (reconstruction of
  anterior cruciate ligament) 81.45
Heyman operation (soft tissue release for
  clubfoot) 83.84
Heyman-Herndon (-Strong) operation
  (correction of metatarsus varus) 80.48
Hibbs operation (lumbar spinal fusion) - *see*
  Fusion, lumbar
Higgins operation - *see* Repair, hernia, femoral
High forceps delivery 72.39
  with episiotomy 72.31
Hill-Allison operation (hiatal hernia repair,
  transpleural approach) 53.80
Hinging, mitral valve 35.12
His bundle recording 37.29
Hitchcock operation (anchoring tendon of
  biceps) 83.88
Hofmeister operation (gastrectomy) 43.7
Hoke operation
  midtarsal fusion 81.14
  triple arthrodesis 81.12
Holth operation
  iridencleisis 12.63
  sclerectomy 12.65
Homans operation (correction of lymph-
  edema) 40.9
Homograft - *see* Graft
Homotransplant, homotransplantation - *see*
  Transplant
Hosiery, elastic 93.59
Hutch operation (ureteroneocystostomy) 56.74
Hybinette-Eden operation (glenoid bone block)
  78.01
Hydrocelectomy
  canal of Nuck (female) 69.19
  male 63.1

Hydrocelectomy (*Continued*)
  round ligament 69.19
  spermatic cord 63.1
  tunica vaginalis 61.2
Hydrotherapy 93.33
  assisted exercise in pool 93.31
  whirlpool 93.32
Hymenectomy 70.31
Hymenoplasty 70.76
Hymenorrhaphy 70.76
Hymenotomy 70.11
Hyperalimentation (parenteral) 99.15
Hyperbaric oxygenation 93.95
  wound 93.59
Hyperextension, joint 93.25
Hyperthermia NEC 93.35
  for cancer treatment (interstitial) (local)
    (radiofrequency) (regional)
    (ultrasound) (whole-body) 99.85
Hypnodrama, psychiatric 94.32
Hypnosis (psychotherapeutic) 94.32
  for anesthesia - *omit code*
Hypnotherapy 94.32
Hypophysectomy (complete) (total) 07.69
  partial or subtotal 07.63
    transfrontal approach 07.61
    transsphenoidal approach 07.62
  specified approach NEC 07.68
  transfrontal approach (complete) (total) 07.64
    partial 07.61
  transsphenoidal approach (complete) (total)
    07.65
    partial 07.62
Hypothermia (central) (local) 99.81
  gastric (cooling) 96.31
    freezing 96.32
  systemic (in open heart surgery) 39.62
Hypotympanotomy 20.23
Hysterectomy, NOS 68.9
  abdominal
    laparoscopic (total) (TLH) 68.41
    other (total) 68.49
    partial or subtotal (supracervical)
      (supravaginal) 68.39
    radical (modified) (Wertheim's) 68.69
      laparoscopic (total) [TLRH] 68.61
  supracervical 68.39
    classic infrafasical SEMM
      hysterectomy [CISH] 68.31
    laparoscopically assisted [LASH] 68.31

Hysterectomy, NOS (*Continued*)
  laparoscopic
    abdominal
      radical (total) (TLRH) 68.61
      total (TLH) 68.41
    supracervical (LASH) (LSH) 68.31
    total (TLH) 68.41
    vaginal, assisted (LAVH) 68.51
      radical (LRVH) 68.71
  radical
    abdominal
      laparoscopic 68.61
      other (modified) (Wertheim's) 68.69
    vaginal
      laparoscopic (LRVH) 68.71
      other 68.79
  vaginal (complete) (partial) (subtotal) (total)
    68.59
    laparoscopically assisted (LAVH) 68.51
    radical (Schauta) 68.79
      laparoscopic [LRVH] 68.71
Hysterocolpectomy (radical) (vaginal) 68.79
  abdominal 68.69
    laparoscopic 68.61
  laparoscopic 68.71
Hysterogram NEC 87.85
  percutaneous 87.84
Hysterolysis 54.59
  laparoscopic 54.51
Hysteromyomectomy 68.29
Hysteropexy 69.22
Hysteroplasty 69.49
Hysterorrhaphy 69.41
Hysterosalpingography gas (contrast) 87.82
  opaque dye (contrast) 87.83
Hysterosalpingostomy 66.74
Hysterostomatomy 68.12
Hysteroscopy 68.12
  with
    ablation
      endometrial 68.23
    biopsy 68.16
Hysterotomy (with removal of foreign body)
    (with removal of hydatidiform mole) 68.0
  for intrauterine transfusion 75.2
  obstetrical 74.99
    for termination of pregnancy 74.91
Hysterotrachelectomy 67.4
Hysterotracheloplasty 69.49
Hysterotrachelorrhaphy 69.41
Hysterotrachelotomy 69.95

I

IAEMT (intraoperative anesthetic effect
    monitoring and titration) 00.94 *[89.14]*
ICCE (intracapsular cataract extraction) 13.19
Ileal
  bladder
    closed 57.87 *[45.51]*
    open (ileoureterostomy) 56.51
  conduit (ileoureterostomy) 56.51
Ileocecostomy 45.93
Ileocolectomy
  laparoscopic 17.33
  open and other 45.73
Ileocolostomy 45.93
Ileocolotomy 45.00
Ileocystoplasty (isolated segment anastomosis)
    (open loop) 57.87 *[45.51]*
Ileoduodenotomy 45.01
Ileoectomy (partial) 45.62
  with cecectomy
    laparoscopic 17.32
    open and other 45.72
Ileoentectropy 46.99
Ileoesophagostomy 42.54

Ileoileostomy 45.91
  proximal to distal segment 45.62
Ileoloopogram 87.78
Ileopancreatostomy 52.96
Ileopexy 46.61
Ileoproctostomy 45.95
Ileorectostomy 45.93
Ileorrhaphy 46.73
Ileoscopy 45.13
  through stoma (artificial) 45.12
  transabdominal (operative) 45.11
Ileosigmoidostomy 45.93
Ileostomy 46.20
  continent (permanent) 46.22
    for urinary diversion 56.51
  delayed opening 46.24
  Hendon (temporary) 46.21
  loop 46.01
  Paul (temporary) 46.21
  permanent 46.23
    continent 46.22
  repair 46.41
  revision 46.41
  tangential (temporary) 46.21
  temporary 46.21

Ileostomy (*Continued*)
  transplantation to new site 46.23
  tube (temporary) 46.21
  ureteral
    external 56.51
    internal 56.71
Ileotomy 45.02
Ileotransversostomy 45.93
Ileoureterostomy (Bricker's) (ileal bladder)
    56.51
Imaging (diagnostic)
  by
    optical coherence tomography (OCT) - *see*
      OCT and Tomography, optical
      coherence
  diagnostic, not elsewhere classified 88.90
  endovascular ultrasound - *see* Imaging,
    intravascular ultrasound
  intraoperative
    iMRI - *see* Imaging, magnetic resonance
    intravascular - *see* Imaging, intravascular
      ultrasound
  intravascular ultrasound (IVUS) 00.29
    aorta 00.22
    aortic arch 00.22

◄ New   ◄═ Revised   ~~deleted~~ Deleted   ● Use Additional Digit(s)   ▨ Omit code

Imaging (Continued)
intravascular ultrasound (Continued)
carotid vessel 00.21
cerebral vessel, extracranial 00.21
coronary vessel 00.24
intrathoracic vessel 00.22
other specified vessel 00.28
peripheral vessel 00.23
renal vessel 00.25
vena cava (inferior) (superior) 00.22
magnetic resonance (nuclear) (proton) NEC
88.97
abdomen 88.97
bladder (urinary) 88.95
bone marrow blood supply 88.94
brain (brain stem) 88.91
intraoperative (iMRI) 88.96
real-time 88.96
chest (hilar) (mediastinal) 88.92
computer assisted surgery (CAS) with
MR/MRA 00.32
extremity (lower) (upper) 88.94
eye orbit 88.97
face 88.97
head NEC 88.97
musculoskeletal 88.94
myocardium 88.92
neck 88.97
orbit of eye 88.97
prostate 88.95
specified site NEC 88.97
spinal canal (cord) (spine) 88.93
VH™ - IVUS - see Imaging (diagnostic),
intravascular ultrasound (IVUS), by
site
virtual histology intravascular ultrasound -
see Imaging (diagnostic), intravascular
ultrasound (IVUS), by site
Immobilization (by)
with fracture-reduction - see Reduction,
fracture
bandage 93.59
bone 93.53
cast NEC 93.53
with reduction of fracture or dislocation -
see Reduction, fracture, and
Reduction, dislocation
device NEC 93.59
pressure dressing 93.56
splint (plaster) (tray) 93.54
with reduction of fracture or dislocation -
see Reduction, fracture, and
Reduction, dislocation
stereotactic head frame 93.59
strapping (non-traction) 93.59
Immunoadsorption
extracorporeal (ECI) 99.76
Immunization - see also Vaccination
allergy 99.12
autoimmune disease 99.13
BCG 99.33
brucellosis 99.55
cholera 99.31
diphtheria 99.36
DPT 99.39
epidemic parotitis 99.46
German measles 99.47
Hemophilus influenzae 99.52
influenza 99.52
measles 99.45
meningococcus 99.55
mumps 99.46
pertussis 99.37
plague 99.34
poliomyelitis 99.41
rabies 99.44
rubella 99.47
salmonella 99.55
smallpox 99.42
staphylococcus 99.55
TAB 99.32

Immunization (Continued)
tetanus 99.38
triple vaccine 99.48
tuberculosis 99.33
tularemia 99.35
typhoid-paratyphoid 99.32
typhus 99.55
viral NEC 99.55
whooping cough 99.37
yellow fever 99.43
Immunotherapy, antineoplastic 99.28
C-Parvum 99.28
Interferon 99.28
Interleukin-2 (low-dose) 99.28
high-dose 00.15
Levamisole 99.28
Proleukin (low-dose) 99.28
high-dose 00.15
Thymosin 99.28
Impella® percutaneous external heart assist
device 37.68
Implant, implantation
abdominal artery to coronary artery 36.17
artery
aortic branches to heart muscle 36.2
mammary to ventricular wall (Vineberg)
36.2
baffle, atrial or interatrial 35.91
biliary fistulous tract into stomach or
intestine 51.39
bipolar endoprosthesis (femoral head) 81.52
bladder sphincter, artificial (inflatable) 58.93
blood vessels to myocardium 36.2
bone growth stimulator (invasive)
(percutaneous) (semi-invasive) - see
category 78.9●
bone morphogenetic protein (Infuse™
(OP-1™) (recombinant) (rhBMP) 84.52
bone void filler 84.55
that with percutaneous vertebral
augmentation 81.66
that with percutaneous vertebroplasty
81.65
breast (for augmentation) (bilateral) 85.54
unilateral 85.53
cardiac contractility modulation (CCM)
rechargeable pulse generator only 17.52
total system 17.51
cardiac resynchronization device
defibrillator (biventricular) (BiV ICD)
(BiV pacemaker with defibrillator)
(BiV pacing with defibrillator)
(CRT-D) (device and one or more
leads) (total system) 00.51
left ventricular coronary venous lead
only 00.52
pulse generator only 00.54
pacemaker (BiV) (biventricular) (CRT-P)
(device and one or more leads)
(total system) 00.50
left ventricular coronary venous lead
only 00.52
pulse generator only 00.53
cardiac support device (CSD) 37.41
cardiomyostimulation system 37.67
cardioverter/defibrillator (automatic) 37.94
leads only (patch electrode) (pacing)
(sensing) 37.95
pulse generator only 37.96
total system 37.94
CCM (cardiac contractility modulation)
rechargeable pulse generator only 17.52
total system 17.51
chemotherapeutic agent 00.10
chest wall (mesh) (silastic) 34.79
chin (polyethylene) (silastic) 76.68
cochlear (electrode) 20.96
prosthetic device (electrode and receiver)
20.96
channel (single) 20.97
multiple 20.98

Implant, implantation (Continued)
cochlear (Continued)
prosthetic device (Continued)
electrode only 20.99
internal coil only 20.99
coil(s), endovascular 39.79
head or neck vessels
bare metal 39.75
bioactive 39.76
CorCap™ 37.41
cornea 11.73
CRT-D (biventricular defibrillator) (BiV ICD)
(BiV pacemaker with defibrillator)
(BiV pacing with defibrillator) (cardiac
resynchronization defibrillator) (device
and one or more leads) 00.51
left ventricular coronary venous lead only
00.52
pulse generator only 00.54
CRT-P (biventricular pacemaker) (BiV
pacemaker) (cardiac resynchronization
pacemaker) (device and one or more
leads) 00.50
left ventricular coronary venous lead only
00.52
pulse generator only 00.53
custodis eye 14.41
dental (endosseous) (prosthetic) 23.6
device
adjustable gastric band and port 44.95
bronchial device NOS 33.79
bronchial substance NOS 33.79
bronchial valve
multiple lobes 33.73
single lobe 33.71
cardiac support device (CSD) 37.41
CorCap™ 37.41
epicardial support device 37.41
Lap-Band™ 44.95
left atrial appendage 37.36
left atrial filter 37.36
left atrial occluder 37.36
MitraClip® percutaneous mitral valve
leaflet clip 35.97
prosthetic cardiac support device 37.41
sternal fixation device with rigid plates
84.94
subcutaneous for intracardiac or great
vessel hemodynamic monitoring
00.57
vascular access 86.07
ventricular support device 37.41
diaphragmatic pacemaker 34.85
Dynesys® 84.82
electrode(s)
brain 02.93
depth 02.93
foramen ovale 02.93
sphenoidal 02.96
cardiac (initial) (transvenous) 37.70
atrium (initial) 37.73
replacement 37.76
atrium and ventricle (initial) 37.72
replacement 37.76
epicardium (sternotomy or
thoracotomy approach) 37.74
left ventricular coronary venous
system 00.52
temporary transvenous pacemaker
system 37.78
during and immediately following
cardiac surgery 39.64
ventricle (initial) 37.71
replacement 37.76
carotid sinus 39.82
with synchronous pulse generator
implantation (total system)
39.81
depth 02.93
foramen ovale 02.93
gastric 04.92

Implant, implantation *(Continued)*
   electrode(s) *(Continued)*
      heart - *see also* Implant, electrode(s),
         cardiac 37.70
      intracranial 02.93
      osteogenic (invasive) for bone growth
         stimulation - *see* category 78.9●
      peripheral nerve 04.92
      sacral nerve 04.92
      sphenoidal 02.96
      spine 03.93
   electroencephalographic receiver
      brain 02.93
      intracranial 02.93
   electronic stimulator
      anus (subcutaneous) 49.92
      bladder 57.96
      bone growth (invasive) (percutaneous)
         (semi-invasive) 78.9●
      brain - *see* Implant, neurostimulator, brain
      carotid sinus 39.83
         with synchronous lead(s) implantation
            (total system) 39.81
      cochlear 20.96
         channel (single) 20.97
            multiple 20.98
      gastric 04.92
      intracranial - *see* Implant, neurostimulator,
         intracranial
      peripheral nerve - *see* Implant,
         neurostimulator, peripheral nerve
      phrenic nerve 34.85
      skeletal muscle 83.92
      spine - *see* Implant, neurostimulator,
         spine
      ureter 56.92
   electrostimulator - *see* Implant, electronic
      stimulator, by site
   endoprosthesis
      bile duct 51.87
      femoral head (bipolar) 81.52
      pancreatic duct 52.93
   endosseous (dental) 23.6
   epidural pegs 02.93
   epikeratoprosthesis 11.73
   epiretinal visual prosthesis 14.81
   estradiol (pellet) 99.23
   eye (Iowa type) 16.61
      integrated 16.41
   facial bone, synthetic (alloplastic) 76.92
   fallopian tube (Mulligan hood) (silastic tube)
      (stent) 66.93
      into uterus 66.74
   gastroepiploic artery to coronary artery 36.17
   hearing device, electromagnetic 20.95
   heart
      artificial 37.52
         total internal biventricular replacement
            system 37.52
            AbioCor® 37.52
            CardioWest™ (TAH-t) 37.52
      assist system
         CentriMag® – *see* Insertion, circulatory
            support device
         external heart assist device,
            percutaneous – *see* Insertion,
            circulatory support device
         external heart assist system, open
            approach 37.65
         extrinsic 37.68
         HeartMate® implantable heart assist
            system 37.66
         HeartMate® II left ventricular assist
            system [LVAS] 37.66
         Impella® percutaneous external
            circulatory assist device - *see*
            Insertion, circulatory support
            device
         implantable 37.66
         non-implantable – *see* Insertion,
            circulatory support device

Implant, implantation *(Continued)*
   heart *(Continued)*
      assist system *(Continued)*
         percutaneous external circulatory
            assist device – *see* Insertion,
            circulatory support device
         pulsation balloon 37.61
         pVAD (percutaneous VAD) – *see*
            Insertion, circulatory support
            device
         TandemHeart® - *see* Insertion,
            circulatory support device
         temporary non-implantable circulatory
            assist device - *see* Insertion,
            circulatory support device
         that for destination therapy (DT) 37.66
      auxiliary ventricle 37.62
      cardiac support device (CSD) 37.41
      circulatory assist system - *see* Implant,
         heart, assist system
      CorCap™ 37.41
      epicardial support device 37.41
      pacemaker - *see also* Implant, pacemaker,
         cardiac 37.80
      prosthetic cardiac support device 37.41
      total internal biventricular replacement
         system 37.52
      valve(s)
         prosthesis or synthetic device (partial)
            (synthetic) (total) 35.20
            aortic 35.22
            mitral 35.24
            pulmonary 35.26
            tricuspid 35.28
         tissue graft 35.20
            aortic 35.21
            mitral 35.23
            pulmonary 35.25
            tricuspid 35.27
      ventricular support device 37.41
   inert material
      breast (for augmentation) (bilateral) 85.54
         unilateral 85.53
      larynx 31.0
      nose 21.85
      orbit (eye socket) 16.69
         reinsertion 16.62
      scleral shell (cup) (with evisceration of
         eyeball) 16.31
         reinsertion 16.62
      Tenon's capsule (with enucleation of
         eyeball) 16.42
         with attachment of muscles 16.41
         reinsertion 16.62
      urethra 59.79
      vocal cord(s) 31.0
   infusion pump 86.06
   interbody spinal fusion device 84.51
   intracardiac or great vessel hemodynamic
      monitor, subcutaneous 00.57
   joint (prosthesis) (silastic) (Swanson type)
      NEC 81.96
      ankle (total) 81.56
         revision 81.59
      carpocarpal, carpometacarpal 81.74
      elbow (total) 81.84
         revision 81.97
      extremity (bioelectric) (cineplastic)
         (kineplastic) 84.40
         lower 84.48
            revision 81.59
         upper 84.44
            revision 81.97
      femoral (bipolar endoprosthesis) 81.52
         revision NOS 81.53
            acetabular and femoral components
               (total) 00.70
            acetabular component only 00.71
            acetabular liner and/or femoral
               head only 00.73
            femoral component only 00.72

Implant, implantation *(Continued)*
   joint NEC *(Continued)*
      femoral *(Continued)*
         revision NOS *(Continued)*
            femoral head only and/or
               acetabular liner 00.73
            total (acetabular and femoral
               components) 00.70
      finger 81.71
      hand (metacarpophalangeal)
         (interphalangeal) 81.71
         revision 81.97
      hip (partial) 81.52
         revision NOS 81.53
            acetabular and femoral components
              (total) 00.70
            acetabular component only 00.71
            acetabular liner and/or femoral
              head only 00.73
            femoral component only 00.72
            femoral head only and/or
              acetabular liner 00.73
            partial
               acetabular component only
                  00.71
               acetabular liner and/or femoral
                  head only 00.73
               femoral component only
                  00.72
               femoral head only and/or
                  acetabular liner 00.73
            total (acetabular and femoral
               components) 00.70
         total 81.51
            revision (acetabular and femoral
              components)
      interphalangeal 81.71
         revision 81.97
      knee (partial) (total) 81.54
         revision NOS 81.55
            femoral component 00.82
            partial
               femoral component 00.82
               patellar component 00.83
               tibial component 00.81
               tibial insert 00.84
            patellar component 00.83
            tibial component 00.81
            tibial insert 00.84
            total (all components) 00.80
      metacarpophalangeal 81.71
         revision 81.97
      shoulder (partial) 81.81
         revision 81.97
         total replacement, NEC 81.80
            other 81.80
            reverse 81.88
      toe 81.57
         for hallux valgus repair 77.59
         revision 81.59
      wrist (partial) 81.74
         revision 81.97
         total replacement 81.73
   kidney, mechanical 55.97
   Lap-Band™ 44.95
   larynx 31.0
   leads (cardiac) - *see* Implant, electrode(s),
      cardiac
   limb lengthening device, internal (NOS)
      84.54
      with kinetic distraction 84.53
   mammary artery
      in ventricle (Vineberg) 36.2
      to coronary artery (single vessel)
         36.15
         double vessel 36.16
   M-Brace™ 84.82
   Mulligan hood, fallopian tube 66.93
   nerve (peripheral) 04.79
   neuropacemaker - *see* Implant,
      neurostimulator, by site

◀ New   ◀▦ Revised   ~~deleted~~ Deleted   ● Use Additional Digit(s)   ▦ Omit code

Implant, implantation (Continued)
neurostimulator
electrodes
brain 02.93
gastric 04.92
intracranial 02.93
peripheral nerve 04.92
sacral nerve 04.92
spine 03.93
pulse generator (subcutaneous) 86.96
cranial 01.20
multiple array 86.95
rechargeable 86.98
single array 86.94
rechargeable 86.97
nose 21.85
Ommaya reservoir 02.22
orbit 16.69
reinsertion 16.62
outflow tract prosthesis (heart) (gusset type)
in
pulmonary valvuloplasty 35.26
total repair of tetralogy of Fallot 35.81
ovary into uterine cavity 65.72
laparoscopic 65.75
pacemaker
brain - see Implant, neurostimulator, brain
cardiac (device) (initial) (permanent) (replacement) 37.80
dual-chamber device (initial) 37.83
replacement 37.87
resynchronization device (biventricular pacemaker) (BiV pacemaker) (CRT-P)
device only (initial) (replacement) 00.53
total system (device and one or more leads) 00.50
transvenous lead into left ventricular coronary venous system 00.52
single-chamber device (initial) 37.81
rate responsive 37.82
replacement 37.85
rate responsive 37.86
temporary transvenous pacemaker system 37.78
during and immediately following cardiac surgery 39.64
carotid sinus 39.89
diaphragm 34.85
gastric 04.92
intracranial - see Implant, neurostimulator, intracranial
neural - see Implant, neurostimulator, by site
peripheral nerve - see Implant, neurostimulator, peripheral nerve
spine - see Implant, neurostimulator, spine
pancreas (duct) 52.96
penis, prosthesis (internal)
inflatable 64.97
non-inflatable 64.95
port, vascular access device 86.07
premaxilla 76.68
progesterone (subdermal) 99.23
prosthesis, prosthetic device
acetabulum (Aufranc-Turner) 81.52
ankle (total) 81.56
arm (bioelectric) (cineplastic) (kineplastic) 84.44
breast (bilateral) (Cronin) (Dow-Corning) (Perras-Pappillon) 85.54
unilateral 85.53
cardiac support device (CSD) (CorCap™) 37.41
cochlear 20.96
channel (single) 20.97
multiple 20.98

Implant, implantation (Continued)
prosthesis, prosthetic device (Continued)
epiretinal visual 14.81
extremity (bioelectric) (cineplastic) (kineplastic) 84.40
lower 84.48
upper 84.44
fallopian tube (Mulligan hood) (stent) 66.93
femoral head (Austin-Moore) (bipolar) (Eicher) (Thompson) 81.52
revision NOS 81.53
acetabular and femoral components (total) 00.70
acetabular component only 00.71
acetabular liner and/or femoral head only 00.73
femoral component only 00.72
femoral head only and/or acetabular liner 00.73
partial
acetabular component only 00.71
acetabular liner and/or femoral head only 00.73
femoral component only 00.72
femoral head only and/or acetabular liner 00.73
total (acetabular and femoral components) 00.70
joint (Swanson type) NEC 81.96
ankle (total) 81.56
carpocarpal, carpometacarpal 81.74
elbow (total) 81.84
finger 81.71
hand (metacarpophalangeal) (interphalangeal) 81.71
hip (partial) 81.52
revision NOS 81.53
acetabular and femoral components (total) 00.70
acetabular component only 00.71
acetabular liner and/or femoral head only 00.73
femoral component only 00.72
femoral head only and/or acetabular liner 00.73
partial
acetabular component only 00.71
acetabular liner and/or femoral head only 00.73
femoral component only 00.72
femoral head only and/or acetabular liner 00.73
total (acetabular and femoral components) 00.70
total 81.51
revision (acetabular and femoral components) 00.70
interphalangeal 81.71
knee (partial) (total) 81.54
revision NOS 81.55
femoral component 00.82
partial
femoral component 00.82
patellar component 00.83
tibial component 00.81
tibial insert 00.84
patellar component 00.83
tibial component 00.81
tibial insert 00.84
total (all components) 00.80
metacarpophalangeal 81.71
shoulder (partial) 81.81
total, NEC 81.80
other 81.80
reverse 81.88
toe 81.57
for hallux valgus repair 77.59
wrist (partial) 81.74
total 81.73

Implant, implantation (Continued)
prosthesis, prosthetic device (Continued)
leg (bioelectric) (cineplastic) (kineplastic) 84.48
lens 13.91
outflow tract (heart) (gusset type)
in
pulmonary valvuloplasty 35.26
total repair of tetralogy of Fallot 35.81
penis (internal) (non-inflatable) 64.95
inflatable (internal) 64.97
skin (dermal regenerative) (matrix) 86.67
testicular (bilateral) (unilateral) 62.7
pulsation balloon (phase-shift) 37.61
pump, infusion 86.06
radial artery 36.19
radioactive isotope 92.27
radium (radon) 92.27
retinal attachment 14.41
with buckling 14.41
Rheos™ carotid sinus baroreflex activation device 39.81
Rickham reservoir 02.22
silicone
breast (bilateral) 85.54
unilateral 85.53
skin (for filling of defect) 86.02
for augmentation NEC 86.89
spine NEC 84.59
facet replacement device(s) 84.84
interspinous process decompression device 84.80
pedicle-based dynamic stabilization device(s) 84.82
posterior motion preservation device(s) - see category 84.8●
stimoceiver - see Implant, neurostimulator, by site
stimulator
electrodes
carotid sinus (baroreflex activation device) 39.82
with synchronous pulse generator implantation (total system) 39.81
pulse generator
carotid sinus (baroreflex activation device) 39.83
with synchronous electrode(s) implantation (total system) 39.81
sudural
grids 02.93
strips 02.93
Swanson prosthesis (joint) (silastic) NEC 81.96
carpocarpal, carpometacarpal 81.74
finger 81.71
hand (interphalangeal) (metacarpophalangeal) 81.71
interphalangeal 81.71
knee (partial) (total) 81.54
revision 81.55
metacarpophalangeal 81.71
toe 81.57
for hallux valgus repair 77.59
wrist (partial) 81.74
total 81.73
systemic arteries into myocardium (Vineberg type operation) 36.2
Tandem™ heart 37.68
telescope (IMT) (miniature) 13.91
testicular prosthesis (bilateral) (unilateral) 62.7
tissue expander (skin) NEC 86.93
breast 85.95
tissue mandril (for vascular graft) 39.99
with
blood vessel repair 39.56
vascular bypass or shunt - see Bypass, vascular

Implant, implantation *(Continued)*
  tooth (bud) (germ) 23.5
    prosthetic 23.6
  umbrella, vena cava 38.7
  ureters into
    bladder 56.74
    intestine 56.71
      external diversion 56.51
    skin 56.61
  urethra
    for repair of urinary stress incontinence
      collagen 59.72
      fat 59.72
      polytef 59.72
  urethral sphincter, artificial (inflatable) 58.93
  urinary sphincter, artificial (inflatable) 58.93
  valve(s)
    endovascular – *see* Replacement, heart valve, by site
  vascular access device 86.07
  vitreous (silicone) 14.75
    for retinal reattachment 14.41
      with buckling 14.41
  vocal cord(s) (paraglottic) 31.98
  X Stop™ 84.80
Implosion (psychologic desensitization) 94.33
Incision (and drainage)
  with
    exploration - *see* Exploration
    removal of foreign body - *see* Removal, foreign body
  abdominal wall 54.0
    as operative approach - *omit code*
  abscess - *see also* Incision, by site
    antecubital fossa 86.04
    appendix 47.2
      with appendectomy 47.09
        laparoscopic 47.01
    axilla 86.04
    cheek 86.04
    extraperitoneal 54.0
    face 86.04
    gluteal 86.04
    groin region (abdominal wall) (inguinal) 54.0
      skin 86.04
      subcutaneous tissue 86.04
    hair follicle 86.04
    ischiorectal 49.01
    lip 27.0
    nailbed or nailfold 86.04
    neck 86.04
    omental 54.19
    paronychia 86.04
    perianal 49.01
    perigastric 54.19
    perineum (female) 71.09
      male 86.04
    perisplenic 54.19
    peritoneal NEC 54.19
      pelvic (female) 70.12
    popliteal space 86.04
    retroperitoneal 54.0
    sclera 12.89
    skin 86.04
    subcutaneous tissue 86.04
    subdiaphragmatic 54.19
    subhepatic 54.19
    submaxillary 86.04
    subphrenic 54.19
    supraclavicular fossa 86.04
    vas deferens 63.6
  adrenal gland 07.41
  alveolus, alveolar bone 24.0
  antecubital fossa 86.09
  anus NEC 49.93
    fistula 49.11
    septum 49.91
  appendix 47.2

Incision *(Continued)*
  artery 38.00
    abdominal 38.06
      aorta (arch) (ascending) (descending) 38.04
    head and neck NEC 38.02
    intracranial NEC 38.01
    lower limb 38.08
    thoracic NEC 38.05
    upper limb 38.03
  atrium (heart) 37.11
  auditory canal or meatus, external 18.02
  auricle 18.09
  axilla 86.09
  Bartholin's gland or cyst 71.22
  bile duct (with T or Y tube insertion) NEC 51.59
    common (exploratory) 51.51
      for
        relief of obstruction NEC 51.42
        removal of calculus 51.41
    for
      exploration 51.59
      relief of obstruction 51.49
  bladder 57.19
    neck (transurethral) 57.91
    percutaneous suprapubic (closed) 57.17
    suprapubic NEC 57.18
  blood vessel - *see also* Angiotomy 38.00
  bone 77.10
    alveolus, alveolar 24.0
    carpals, metacarpals 77.14
    clavicle 77.11
    facial 76.09
    femur 77.15
    fibula 77.17
    humerus 77.12
    patella 77.16
    pelvic 77.19
    phalanges (foot) (hand) 77.19
    radius 77.13
    scapula 77.11
    skull 01.24
    specified site NEC 77.19
    tarsals, metatarsals 77.18
    thorax (ribs) (sternum) 77.11
    tibia 77.17
    ulna 77.13
    vertebrae 77.19
  brain 01.39
    cortical adhesions 02.91
  breast (skin) 85.0
    with removal of tissue expander 85.96
  bronchus 33.0
  buccal space 27.0
  bulbourethral gland 58.91
  bursa 83.03
    hand 82.03
    pharynx 29.0
  carotid body 39.89
  cerebral (meninges) 01.39
    epidural or extradural space 01.24
    subarachnoid or subdural space 01.31
  cerebrum 01.39
  cervix 69.95
    to
      assist delivery 73.93
      replace inverted uterus 75.93
  chalazion 08.09
    with removal of capsule 08.21
  cheek 86.09
  chest wall (for extrapleural drainage) (for removal of foreign body) 34.01
    as operative approach - *omit code*
  common bile duct (for exploration) 51.51
    for
      relief of obstruction 51.42
      removal of calculus 51.41
  common wall between posterior left atrium and coronary sinus (with roofing of resultant defect with patch graft) 35.82

Incision *(Continued)*
  conjunctiva 10.1
  cornea 11.1
    radial (refractive) 11.75
  cranial sinus 01.21
  craniobuccal pouch 07.72
  cul-de-sac 70.12
  cyst
    dentigerous 24.0
    radicular (apical) (periapical) 24.0
  Duhrssen's (cervix, to assist delivery) 73.93
  duodenum 45.01
  ear
    external 18.09
    inner 20.79
    middle 20.23
  endocardium 37.11
  endolymphatic sac 20.79
  epididymis 63.92
  epidural space, cerebral 01.24
  epigastric region 54.0
    intra-abdominal 54.19
  esophagus, esophageal NEC 42.09
    web 42.01
  exploratory - *see* Exploration
  extradural space (cerebral) 01.24
  extrapleural 34.01
  eyebrow 08.09
  eyelid 08.09
    margin (trichiasis) 08.01
  face 86.09
  fallopian tube 66.01
  fascia 83.09
    with division 83.14
      hand 82.12
    hand 82.09
      with division 82.12
  fascial compartments, head and neck 27.0
  fistula, anal 49.11
  flank 54.0
  furuncle - *see* Incision, by site
  gallbladder 51.04
  gingiva 24.0
  gluteal 86.09
  groin region (abdominal wall) (inguinal) 54.0
    skin 86.09
    subcutaneous tissue 86.09
  gum 24.0
  hair follicles 86.09
  heart 37.10
    valve - *see* Valvulotomy
  hematoma - *see also* Incision, by site
    axilla 86.04
    broad ligament 69.98
    ear 18.09
    episiotomy site 75.91
    fossa (superficial) NEC 86.04
    groin region (abdominal wall) (inguinal) 54.0
      skin 86.04
      subcutaneous tissue 86.04
    laparotomy site 54.12
    mediastinum 34.1
    perineum (female) 71.09
      male 86.04
    popliteal space 86.04
    scrotum 61.0
    skin 86.04
    space of Retzius 59.19
    subcutaneous tissue 86.04
    vagina (cuff) 70.14
      episiotomy site 75.91
      obstetrical NEC 75.92
  hepatic ducts 51.59
  hordeolum 08.09
  hygroma - *see also* Incision, by site
    cystic 40.0
  hymen 70.11
  hypochondrium 54.0
    intra-abdominal 54.19
  hypophysis 07.72

Incision *(Continued)*
  iliac fossa 54.0
  infratemporal fossa 27.0
  ingrown nail 86.09
  intestine 45.00
    large 45.03
    small 45.02
  intracerebral 01.39
  intracranial (epidural space) (extradural
      space) 01.24
    subarachnoid or subdural space 01.31
  intraperitoneal 54.19
  ischiorectal tissue 49.02
    abscess 49.01
  joint structures - *see also* Arthrotomy 80.10
  kidney 55.01
    pelvis 55.11
  labia 71.09
  lacrimal
    canaliculus 09.52
    gland 09.0
    passage NEC 09.59
    punctum 09.51
    sac 09.53
  larynx NEC 31.3
  ligamentum flavum (spine) - *omit code*
  liver 50.0
  lung 33.1
  lymphangioma 40.0
  lymphatic structure (channel) (node) (vessel)
      40.0
  mastoid 20.21
  mediastinum 34.1
  meibomian gland 08.09
  meninges (cerebral) 01.31
    spinal 03.09
  midpalmar space 82.04
  mouth NEC 27.92
    floor 27.0
  muscle 83.02
    with division 83.19
      hand 82.19
    hand 82.02
      with division 82.19
  myocardium 37.11
  nailbed or nailfold 86.09
  nasolacrimal duct (stricture) 09.59
  neck 86.09
  nerve (cranial) (peripheral) NEC 04.04
    root (spinal) 03.1
  nose 21.1
  omentum 54.19
  orbit - *see also* Orbitotomy 16.09
  ovary 65.09
    laparoscopic 65.01
  palate 27.1
  palmar space (middle) 82.04
  pancreas 52.09
  pancreatic sphincter 51.82
    endoscopic 51.85
  parapharyngeal (oral) (transcervical) 28.0
  paronychia 86.09
  parotid
    gland or duct 26.0
    space 27.0
  pelvirectal tissue 48.81
  penis 64.92
  perianal (skin) (tissue) 49.02
    abscess 49.01
  perigastric 54.19
  perineum (female) 71.09
    male 86.09
  peripheral vessels
    lower limb
      artery 38.08
      vein 38.09
    upper limb (artery) (vein) 38.03
  periprostatic tissue 60.81
  perirectal tissue 48.81
  perirenal tissue 59.09
  perisplenic 54.19

Incision *(Continued)*
  peritoneum 54.95
    by laparotomy 54.19
    pelvic (female) 70.12
      male 54.19
  periureteral tissue 59.09
  periurethral tissue 58.91
  perivesical tissue 59.19
  petrous pyramid (air cells) (apex) (mastoid)
      20.22
  pharynx, pharyngeal (bursa) 29.0
    space, lateral 27.0
  pilonidal sinus (cyst) 86.03
  pineal gland 07.52
  pituitary (gland) 07.72
  pleura NEC 34.09
  popliteal space 86.09
  postzygomatic space 27.0
  pouch of Douglas 70.12
  prostate (perineal approach) (transurethral
      approach) 60.0
  pterygopalatine fossa 27.0
  pulp canal (tooth) 24.0
  Rathke's pouch 07.72
  rectovaginal septum 48.81
  rectum 48.0
    stricture 48.91
  renal pelvis 55.11
  retroperitoneum 54.0
  retropharyngeal (oral) (transcervical) 28.0
  salivary gland or duct 26.0
  sclera 12.89
  scrotum 61.0
  sebaceous cyst 86.04
  seminal vesicle 60.72
  sinus - *see* Sinusotomy
  Skene's duct or gland 71.09
  skin 86.09
    with drainage 86.04
    breast 85.0
    cardiac pacemaker pocket, new site 37.79
    ear 18.09
    nose 21.1
    subcutaneous tunnel for pulse generator
        lead wire 86.99
      with initial procedure - *omit code*
    thalamic stimulator pulse generator
        pocket, new site 86.09
      with initial insertion of battery
          package - *omit code*
    tunnel, subcutaneous for pulse generator
        lead wire 86.99
      with initial procedure - *omit code*
  skull (bone) 01.24
  soft tissue NEC 83.09
    with division 83.19
      hand 82.19
    hand 82.09
      with division 82.19
  space of Retzius 59.19
  spermatic cord 63.93
  sphincter of Oddi 51.82
    endoscopic 51.85
  spinal
    cord 03.09
    nerve root 03.1
  spleen 41.2
  stomach 43.0
  stye 08.09
  subarachnoid space, cerebral 01.31
  subcutaneous tissue 86.09
    with drainage 86.04
    tunnel
      esophageal 42.86
        with anastomosis - *see* Anastomosis,
            esophagus, antesternal
      pulse generator lead wire 86.99
        with initial procedure - *omit code*
  subdiaphragmatic space 54.19
  subdural space, cerebral 01.31
  sublingual space 27.0

Incision *(Continued)*
  submandibular space 27.0
  submaxillary 86.09
    with drainage 86.04
  submental space 27.0
  subphrenic space 54.19
  supraclavicular fossa 86.09
    with drainage 86.04
  sweat glands, skin 86.04
  temporal pouches 27.0
  tendon (sheath) 83.01
    with division 83.13
      hand 82.11
    hand 82.01
      with division 82.11
  testis 62.0
  thenar space 82.04
  thymus (open) (other) 07.92
    thoracoscopic 07.95
  thyroid (field) (gland) NEC 06.09
    postoperative 06.02
  tongue NEC 25.94
    for tongue tie 25.91
  tonsil 28.0
  trachea NEC 31.3
  tunica vaginalis 61.0
  umbilicus 54.0
  urachal cyst 54.0
  ureter 56.2
  urethra 58.0
  uterus (corpus) 68.0
    cervix 69.96
    for termination of pregnancy 74.91
    septum (congenital) 68.22
  uvula 27.71
  vagina (cuff) (septum) (stenosis) 70.14
    for
      incisional hematoma (episiotomy) 75.91
      obstetrical hematoma NEC 75.92
      pelvic abscess 70.12
  vas deferens 63.6
  vein 38.00
    abdominal 38.07
    head and neck NEC 38.02
    intracranial NEC 38.01
    lower limb 38.09
    thoracic NEC 38.05
    upper limb 38.03
  vertebral column 03.09
  vulva 71.09
    obstetrical 75.92
  web, esophageal 42.01
Incudectomy NEC 19.3
  with
    stapedectomy - *see also* Stapedectomy 19.19
    tympanoplasty - *see* Tympanoplasty
Incudopexy 19.19
Incudostapediopexy 19.19
  with incus replacement 19.11
Indentation, sclera, for buckling - *see also*
    Buckling, scleral 14.49
Indicator dilution flow measurement 89.68
Induction
  abortion
    by
      D and C 69.01
      insertion of prostaglandin suppository
          96.49
      intra-amniotic injection
          (prostaglandin) (saline) 75.0
    labor
      medical 73.4
      surgical 73.01
        intra- and extra-amniotic injection 73.1
        stripping of membranes 73.1
Inflation
  belt wrap 93.99
  Eustachian tube 20.8
  fallopian tube 66.8
    with injection of therapeutic agent 66.95
Infolding, sclera, for buckling - *see also*
    Buckling, scleral 14.49

Infraction, turbinates (nasal) 21.62
Infundibulectomy
  hypophyseal - *see also* Hypophysectomy,
      partial 07.63
  ventricle (heart) (right) 35.34
      in total repair of tetralogy of Fallot 35.81
Infusion (intra-arterial) (intravenous)
  4-Factor Prothrombin Complex Concentrate
      (00.96)
  with
      disruption of blood brain barrier [BBBD]
          00.19
  Abciximab 99.20
  antibiotic
      oxazolidinone class 00.14
  antineoplastic agent (chemotherapeutic) 99.25
      biological response modifier [BRM] 99.28
          cintredekin besudotox 99.28
          CLO 17.70
          clofarabine 17.70
          CLOLAR® 17.70
          high-dose interleukin-2 00.15
          low-dose interleukin-2 99.28
      biological response modifier [BRM],
          antineoplastic agent 99.28
      cintredekin besudotox 99.28
      high-dose interleukin-2 00.15
      low-dose interleukin-2 99.28
  cancer chemotherapy agent NEC 99.25
  cintredekin besudotox 99.28
  CLO 17.70
  clofarabine 17.70
  CLOLAR® 17.70
  drotrecogin alfa (activated) 00.11
  electrolytes 99.18
  enzymes, thrombolytic (streptokinase)
      (tissue plasminogen activator) (TPA)
      (urokinase)
      direct coronary artery 36.04
      intravenous 99.10
  Eptifibatide 99.20
  gamma globulin 99.14
  glucarpidase 00.95
  GP IIB/IIIa inhibitor 99.20
  hormone substance NEC 99.24
  human B-type natriuretic peptide (hBNP) 00.13
  IgG (immunoglobulin) 99.14
  immunoglobulin (IgG) (IVIG) (IVIg) 99.14
  immunosuppressive antibody therapy 00.18
  interleukin-2
      high-dose 00.15
      low-dose 99.28
  IVIG (immunoglobulin) (IVIg) 99.14
  Kcentra™ (00.96)
  lymphocyte 99.09
  nesiritide 00.13
  neuroprotective agent 99.75
  nimodipine 99.75
  nutritional substance - *see* Nutrition
  platelet inhibitor
      direct coronary artery 36.04
      intravenous 99.20
  Proleukin (low-dose) 99.28
      high-dose 00.15
  prophylactic substance NEC 99.29
  radioimmunoconjugate 92.28
  radioimmunotherapy 92.28
  radioisotope (liquid brachytherapy) (liquid
      I-125) 92.20
  recombinant protein 00.11
  reteplase 99.10
  therapeutic substance NEC 99.29
  thrombolytic agent (enzyme) (streptokinase)
      99.10
      with percutaneous transluminal
          angioplasty

Note: Also use 00.40, 00.41, 00.42, or 00.43
to show the total number of vessels treated.

          coronary 00.66
          non-coronary vessel(s) 39.50
          specified site NEC 39.50
          direct intracoronary artery 36.04

Infusion *(Continued)*
  tirofiban (HCL) 99.20
  vaccine
      tumor 99.28
  vasopressor 00.17
  Voraxaze® 00.95
Injection (into) (hypodermically)
      (intramuscularly) (intravenously) (acting
      locally or systemically)
  Actinomycin D, for cancer chemotherapy
      99.25
  adhesion barrier substance 99.77
  alcohol
      nerve - *see* Injection, nerve
      spinal 03.8
  anterior chamber, eye (air) (liquid)
      (medication) 12.92
  antibiotic 99.21
      oxazolidinone class 00.14
  anticoagulant 99.19
  anti-D (Rhesus) globulin 99.11
  antidote NEC 99.16
  anti-infective NEC 99.22
  antineoplastic agent (chemotherapeutic)
      NEC 99.25
      biological response modifier [BRM] 99.28
      cintredekin besudotox 99.28
      high-dose interleukin-2 00.15
      low-dose interleukin-2 99.28
  antivenin 99.16
  barrier substance, adhesion 99.77
  BCG
      for chemotherapy 99.25
      vaccine 99.33
  biological response modifier [BRM],
      antineoplastic agent 99.28
      cintredekin besudotox 99.28
      high-dose interleukin-2 00.15
      low-dose interleukin-2 99.28
  bone marrow 41.92
      transplant - *see* Transplant, bone, marrow
  breast (therapeutic agent) 85.92
      inert material (silicone) (bilateral) 85.52
      unilateral 85.51
  bursa (therapeutic agent) 83.96
      hand 82.94
  cancer chemotherapeutic agent 99.25
  caudal - *see* Injection, spinal
  cintredekin besudotox 99.28
  cortisone 99.23
  costochondral junction 81.92
  dinoprost-tromethine, intra-amniotic 75.0
  disc, intervertebral (herniated) 80.52
  ear, with alcohol 20.72
  electrolytes 99.18
  enzymes, thrombolytic (streptokinase)
      (tissue plasminogen activator) (TPA)
      (urokinase)
      direct coronary artery 36.04
      intravenous 99.10
  epidural, spinal - *see* Injection, spinal
  esophageal varices or blood vessel
      (endoscopic) (sclerosing agent) 42.33
  Eustachian tube (inert material) 20.8
  eye (orbit) (retrobulbar) 16.91
      anterior chamber 12.92
      subconjunctival 10.91
  fascia 83.98
      hand 82.96
  gamma globulin 99.14
  ganglion, sympathetic 05.39
      ciliary 12.79
      paravertebral stellate 05.39
  gel, adhesion barrier - *see* Injection, adhesion
      barrier substance
  globulin
      anti-D (Rhesus) 99.11
      gamma 99.14
      Rh immune 99.11
  glucarpidase 00.95
  heart 37.92

Injection *(Continued)*
  heavy metal antagonist 99.16
  hemorrhoids (sclerosing agent) 49.42
  hormone NEC 99.24
  human B-type natriuretic peptide (hBNP)
      00.13
  IgG (immunoglobulin) 99.14
  immune sera 99.14
  immunoglobulin (IgG) (IVIG) (IVIg) 99.14
  inert material - *see* Implant, inert material
  inner ear, for destruction 20.72
  insulin 99.17
  intervertebral space for herniated disc 80.52
  intra-amniotic
      for induction of
          abortion 75.0
          labor 73.1
  intrathecal - *see* Injection, spinal
  IVIG (immunoglobulin) (IVIg) 99.14
  joint (therapeutic agent) 81.92
      temporomandibular 76.96
  kidney (cyst) (therapeutic substance) NEC
      55.96
  larynx 31.0
  ligament (joint) (therapeutic substance) 81.92
  liver 50.94
  lung, for surgical collapse 33.32
  Methotrexate, for cancer chemotherapy 99.25
  nerve (cranial) (peripheral) 04.80
      agent NEC 04.89
          alcohol 04.2
          anesthetic for analgesia 04.81
              for operative anesthesia - *omit code*
          neurolytic 04.2
          phenol 04.2
      laryngeal (external) (recurrent) (superior)
          31.91
      optic 16.91
      sympathetic 05.39
          alcohol 05.32
          anesthetic for analgesia 05.31
          neurolytic agent 05.32
          phenol 05.32
  nesiritide 00.13
  neuroprotective agent 99.75
  nimodipine 99.75
  orbit 16.91
  pericardium 37.93
  peritoneal cavity
      air 54.96
      locally-acting therapeutic substance
          54.97
  platelet inhibitor
      direct coronary artery 36.04
      intravenous 99.20
  prophylactic substance NEC 99.29
  prostate 60.92
  radioimmunoconjugate 92.28
  radioimmunotherapy 92.28
  radioisotopes (intracavitary) (intravenous)
      92.28
  renal pelvis (cyst) 55.96
  retrobulbar (therapeutic substance) 16.91
      for anesthesia - *omit code*
  Rh immune globulin 99.11
  RhoGAM 99.11
  sclerosing agent NEC 99.29
      esophageal varices (endoscopic) 42.33
      hemorrhoids 49.42
      pleura 34.92
          treatment of malignancy (cytotoxic
              agent) 34.92 *[99.25]*
          with tetracycline 34.92 *[99.21]*
      varicose vein 39.92
      vein NEC 39.92
  semicircular canals, for destruction 20.72
  silicone - *see* Implant, inert material
  skin (sclerosing agent) (filling material)
      86.02
  soft tissue 83.98
      hand 82.96

Injection *(Continued)*
spinal (canal) NEC 03.92
alcohol 03.8
anesthetic agent for analgesia 03.91
for operative anesthesia - *omit code*
contrast material (for myelogram) 87.21
destructive agent NEC 03.8
neurolytic agent NEC 03.8
phenol 03.8
proteolytic enzyme (chymodiactin)
(chymopapain) 80.52
saline (hypothermic) 03.92
steroid NEC 03.92
spinal nerve root (intrathecal) - *see* Injection,
spinal
steroid NEC 99.23
subarachnoid, spinal - *see* Injection, spinal
subconjunctival 10.91
tendon 83.97
hand 82.95
testis 62.92
therapeutic agent NEC 99.29
thoracic cavity 34.92
thrombolytic agent (enzyme) (streptokinase)
99.10
with percutaneous transluminal
angioplasty

Note: Also use 00.40, 00.41, 00.42, or 00.43 to show the total number of vessels treated.

coronary 00.66
noncoronary vessels 39.50
specified site NEC 39.50
direct intracoronary artery 36.04
trachea 31.94
tranquilizer 99.26
tunica vaginalis (with aspiration) 61.91
tympanum 20.94
urethra (inert material)
for repair of urinary stress incontinence
collagen implant 59.72
endoscopic injection of implant 59.72
fat implant 59.72
polytef implant 59.72
vaccine
tumor 99.28
varices, esophagus (endoscopic) (sclerosing
agent) 42.33
varicose vein (sclerosing agent) 39.92
esophagus (endoscopic) 42.33
vestibule, for destruction 20.72
vitreous substitute (silicone) 14.75
for reattachment of retina 14.59
vocal cords 31.0
Voraxaze® 00.95
Inlay, tooth 23.3
Inoculation
antitoxins - *see* Administration, antitoxins
toxoids - *see* Administration, toxoids
vaccine - *see* Administration, vaccine
Insemination, artificial 69.92
Insertion
airway
esophageal obturator 96.03
nasopharynx 96.01
oropharynx 96.02
Allen-Brown cannula 39.93
antimicrobial envelope 17.81
aqueous drainage device (shunt) (stent)
12.67
arch bars (orthodontic) 24.7
for immobilization (fracture) 93.55
atrial septal umbrella 35.52
Austin-Moore prosthesis 81.52
baffle, heart (atrial) (interatrial) (intra-atrial)
35.91
bag, cervix (nonobstetrical) 67.0
after delivery or abortion 75.8
to assist delivery or induce labor 73.1
Baker's (tube) (for stenting) 46.85

Insertion *(Continued)*
balloon
gastric 44.93
heart (pulsation-type) (Kantrowitz) 37.61
intestine (for decompression) (for
dilation) 46.85
with insertion of colonic stent
endoscopic 46.86
other 46.87
band (adjustable)
gastric, laparoscopic 44.95
Lap-Band™ 44.95
Barton's tongs (skull) (with synchronous
skeletal traction) 02.94
bipolar endoprosthesis (femoral head) 81.52
Blakemore-Sengstaken tube 96.06
bone growth stimulator (invasive)
(percutaneous) (semi-invasive) - *see*
category 78.9●
bone morphogenetic protein (Infuse™)
(OP-1™) (recombinant) (rhBMP) 84.52
bone void filler 84.55
that with percutaneous vertebral
augmentation 81.66
that with percutaneous vertebroplasty
81.65
bougie, cervix, nonobstetrical 67.0
to assist delivery or induce labor 73.1
breast implant (for augmentation) (bilateral)
85.54
unilateral 85.53
bridge (dental) (fixed) 23.42
removable 23.43
bubble (balloon), stomach 44.93
caliper tongs (skull) (with synchronous
skeletal traction) 02.94
cannula
Allen-Brown 39.93
for extracorporeal membrane oxygenation
(ECMO) - *omit code*
nasal sinus (by puncture) 22.01
through natural ostium 22.02
pancreatic duct 52.92
endoscopic 52.93
vessel to vessel 39.93
cardiac resynchronization device
defibrillator (biventricular defibrillator)
(BiV ICD) (BiV pacemaker with
defibrillator) (BiV pacing with
defibrillator) (CRT- D) (device and
one or more leads) (total system)
00.51
left ventricular coronary venous lead
only 00.52
pulse generator only 00.54
pacemaker (biventricular pacemaker)
(BiV pacemaker) (CRT-P) (device
and one or more leads) (total
system) 00.50
left ventricular coronary venous lead
only 00.52
pulse generator only 00.53
cardiac support device (CSD) (CorCap™)
37.41
carotid artery stent(s) (stent graft) 00.63

Note: Also use 00.40, 00.41, 00.42, or 00.43 to show the total number of vessels treated. Use code 00.44 once to show procedure on a bifurcated vessel. In addition, use 00.45, 00.46, 00.47, or 00.48 to show the number of vascular stents inserted.

catheter
abdomen of fetus, for intrauterine
transfusion 75.2
anterior chamber (eye), for permanent
drainage
(glaucoma) 12.79
artery 38.91

Insertion *(Continued)*
catheter *(Continued)*
bile duct(s) 51.59
common 51.51
endoscopic 51.87
endoscopic 51.87
bladder, indwelling 57.94
suprapubic 57.18
percutaneous (closed) 57.17
bronchus 96.05
with lavage 96.56
central venous NEC 38.93
with guidance 38.97
for
hemodialysis 38.95
pressure monitoring 89.62
peripherally inserted central catheter
(PICC) 38.93
chest 34.04
revision (with lysis of adhesions)
34.04
thoracoscopic 34.06
thoracoscopic 34.06
cranial cavity 01.26
placement via burr hole(s) 01.28
esophagus (nonoperative) 96.06
permanent tube 42.81
intercostal (with water seal), for drainage
34.04
revision (with lysis of adhesions)
34.04
thoracoscopic 34.06
thoracoscopic 34.06
intracerebral 01.26
placement via burr hole(s) 01.28
NeuroFlo™ (partial abdominal aorta
occlusion) 39.77
spinal canal space (epidural)
(subarachnoid) (subdural) for
infusion of therapeutic or palliative
substances 03.90
Swan-Ganz (pulmonary) 89.64
temporary occlusion, abdominal aorta
39.77
transtracheal for oxygenation 31.99
vein NEC 38.93
for renal dialysis 38.95
chest tube 34.04
thoracoscopic 34.06
choledochohepatic tube (for decompression)
51.43
endoscopic 51.87
circulatory support device
CentriMag® 37.62
external heart assist device
biventricular 37.60
Impella® 37.68
percutaneous 37.68
temporary 37.62
non-implantable 37.62
pVAD (percutaneous VAD) 37.68
TandemHeart® 37.68
temporary non-implantable circulatory
assist device 37.62
cochlear prosthetic device - *see* Implant,
cochlear prosthetic device
contraceptive device (intrauterine) 69.7
CorCap™ 37.41
cordis cannula 54.98
coronary (artery)

Note: Also use 00.40, 00.41, 00.42, or 00.43 to show the total number of vessels treated. Use code 00.44 once to show procedure on a bifurcated vessel. In addition, use 00.45, 00.46, 00.47, or 00.48 to show the number of vascular stents inserted.

stent, drug-eluting 36.07
stent, non-drug-eluting 36.06
Crosby-Cooney button 54.98

Insertion *(Continued)*
CRT-D (biventricular defibrillator) (BiV ICD)
(BiV pacemaker with defibrillator)
(BiV pacing with defibrillator) (cardiac
resynchronization defibrillator) (device
and one or more leads) 00.51
left ventricular coronary venous lead only
00.52
pulse generator only 00.54
CRT-P (biventricular pacemaker) (BiV
pacemaker) (cardiac resynchronization
pacemaker) (device and one or more
leads) 00.50
left ventricular coronary venous lead only
00.52
pulse generator only 00.53
Crutchfield tongs (skull) (with synchronous
skeletal traction) 02.94
Davidson button 54.98
denture (total) 99.97
device
adjustable gastric band and port 44.95
bronchial device NOS 33.79
bronchial substance NOS 33.79
bronchial valve(s)
multiple lobes 33.73
single lobe 33.71
cardiac resynchronization - *see* Insertion,
cardiac resynchronization device
cardiac support device (CSD) 37.41
CorCap™ 37.41
epicardial support device 37.41
Lap-Band™ 44.95
left atrial appendage 37.90
left atrial filter 37.90
left atrial occluder 37.90
MitraClip® mitral leaflet clip 35.97
prosthetic cardiac support device 37.41
sternal fixation device with rigid plates
84.94
vascular access 86.07
ventricular support device 37.41
diaphragm, vagina 96.17
drainage tube
kidney 55.02
pelvis 55.12
renal pelvis 55.12
Dynesys® 84.82
elbow prosthesis (total) 81.84
revision 81.97
electrode(s)
bone growth stimulator (invasive)
(percutaneous) (semi-invasive) - *see*
category 78.9●
brain 02.93
depth 02.93
foramen ovale 02.93
sphenoidal 02.96
depth 02.93
foramen ovale 02.93
gastric 04.92
heart (initial) (transvenous) 37.70
atrium (initial) 37.73
replacement 37.76
atrium and ventricle (initial) 37.72
replacement 37.76
epicardium (sternotomy or
thoracotomy approach) 37.74
left ventricular coronary venous
system 00.52
temporary transvenous pacemaker
system 37.78
during and immediately following
cardiac surgery 39.64
ventricle (initial) 37.71
replacement 37.76
intracranial 02.93
osteogenic (for bone growth stimulation) -
see category 78.9●
peripheral nerve 04.92
sacral nerve 04.92

Insertion *(Continued)*
electrode(s) *(Continued)*
sphenoidal 02.96
spine 03.93
electroencephalographic receiver - *see*
Implant, electroencephalographic
receiver, by site
electronic stimulator - *see* Implant, electronic
stimulator, by site
electrostimulator - *see* Implant, electronic
stimulator, by site
endograft(s), endovascular graft(s)
endovascular, abdominal aorta 39.71
fenestrated (branching) 39.78
endovascular, head and neck vessels 39.72
endovascular, other vessels (for
aneurysm) 39.79
endovascular, thoracic aorta 39.73
endoprosthesis
bile duct 51.87
femoral head (bipolar) 81.52
pancreatic duct 52.93
envelope, antimicrobial 17.81
epidural pegs 02.93
external fixation device (bone) - *see* category
78.1●
eye valve implant 12.67
facial bone implant (alloplastic) (synthetic)
76.92
filling material, skin (filling of defect) 86.02
filter
vena cava (inferior) (superior)
(transvenous) 38.7
fixator, mini device (bone) - *see* category 78.1●
frame (stereotactic)
for radiosurgery 93.59
Gardner Wells tongs (skull) (with
synchronous skeletal traction) 02.94
gastric bubble (balloon) 44.93
globe, into eye socket 16.69
Greenfield filter 38.7
halo device (skull) (with synchronous
skeletal traction) 02.94
Harrington rod - *see also* Fusion, spinal, by
level
with dorsal, dorsolumbar fusion 81.05
Harris pin 79.15
heart
assist system - *see* Implant, heart assist
system
cardiac support device (CSD) 37.41
circulatory assist system - *see* Implant,
heart assist system
CorCap™ 37.41
epicardial support device 37.41
Impella® 37.68
pacemaker - *see* Insertion, pacemaker,
cardiac
prosthetic cardiac support device 37.41
pump (Kantrowitz) 37.62
valve - *see* Replacement, heart valve
ventricular support device 37.41
hip prosthesis (partial) 81.52
revision NOS 81.53
acetabular and femoral components
(total) 00.70
acetabular component only 00.71
acetabular liner and/or femoral head
only 00.73
femoral component only 00.72
femoral head only and/or acetabular
liner 00.73
partial
acetabular component only 00.71
acetabular liner and/or femoral
head only 00.73
femoral component only 00.72
femoral head only and/or
acetabular liner 00.73
total (acetabular and femoral
components) 00.70

Insertion *(Continued)*
hip prosthesis *(Continued)*
total 81.51
revision
acetabular and femoral components
(total) 00.70
total (acetabular and femoral
components) 00.70
Holter valve 02.22
Hufnagel valve - *see* Replacement, heart
valve
implant - *see* Insertion, prosthesis
infusion pump 86.06
interbody spinal fusion device 84.51
intercostal catheter (with water seal) for
drainage 34.04
revision (with lysis of adhesions) 34.04
thoracoscopic 34.06
intra-arterial blood gas monitoring system
89.60
intrauterine
contraceptive device 69.7
radium (intracavitary) 69.91
tamponade (nonobstetric) 69.91
Kantrowitz
heart pump 37.62
pulsation balloon (phase-shift) 37.61
keratoprosthesis 11.73
King-Mills umbrella device (heart) 35.52
Kirschner wire 93.44
with reduction of fracture or dislocation -
see Reduction, fracture *and*
Reduction, dislocation
knee prosthesis (partial (total) 81.54
revision NOS 81.55
femoral component 00.82
partial
femoral component 00.82
patellar component 00.83
tibial component 00.81
tibial insert 00.84
patellar component 00.83
tibial component 00.81
tibial insert 00.84
total (all components) 00.80
laminaria, cervix 69.93
Lap-Band™ 44.95
larynx, valved tube 31.75
leads - *see* Insertion, electrode(s)
lens, prosthetic (intraocular) 13.70
with cataract extraction, one-stage 13.71
secondary (subsequent to cataract
extraction) 13.72
limb lengthening device, internal, NOS
84.54
with kinetic distraction 84.53
loop recorder 37.79
metal staples into epiphyseal plate - *see also*
Stapling, epiphyseal plate 78.20
minifixator device (bone) - *see* category
78.1●
M-Brace™ 84.82
Mobitz-Uddin umbrella, vena cava 38.7
mold, vagina 96.15
Moore (cup) 81.52
myringotomy device (button) (tube) 20.01
with intubation 20.01
nasobiliary drainage tube (endoscopic)
51.86
nasogastric tube
for
decompression, intestinal 96.07
feeding 96.6
naso-intestinal tube 96.08
nasolacrimal tube or stent 09.44
nasopancreatic drainage tube (endoscopic)
52.97
neuropacemaker - *see* Implant,
neurostimulator, by site
neurostimulator - *see* Implant,
neurostimulator, by site

◀ New   ◀▥ Revised   ~~deleted~~ Deleted   ● Use Additional Digit(s)   Omit code

Insertion *(Continued)*
non-coronary vessel
stent(s) (stent graft)

Note: Also use 00.40, 00.41, 00.42, or 00.43 to show the total number of vessels treated. Use code 00.44 once to show procedure on a bifurcated vessel. In addition, use 00.45, 00.46, 00.47, or 00.48 to show the number of vascular stents inserted.

with
angioplasty 39.50
atherectomy 17.56
bypass - *omit code*
basilar 00.64
carotid 00.63
extracranial 00.64
intracranial 00.65
peripheral 39.90
bare, drug-coated 39.90
drug-eluting 00.55
vertebral 00.64
non-invasive (surface) (transcutaneous)
stimulator 99.86
obturator (orthodontic) 24.7
ocular implant
with synchronous
enucleation 16.42
with muscle attachment to implant 16.41
evisceration 16.31
following or secondary to
enucleation 16.61
evisceration 16.61
Ommaya reservoir 02.22
orbital implant (stent) (outside muscle cone) 16.69
with orbitotomy 16.02
orthodontic appliance (obturator) (wiring) 24.7
outflow tract prosthesis (gusset type) (heart)
in
pulmonary valvuloplasty 35.26
total repair of tetralogy of Fallot 35.81
pacemaker
brain - *see* Implant, neurostimulator, brain
cardiac (device) (initial) (permanent) (replacement) 37.80
dual-chamber device (initial) 37.83
replacement 37.87
during and immediately following cardiac surgery 39.64
resynchronization (biventricular pacemaker) (BiV pacemaker) (CRT-P) (device)
device only (initial) (replacement) 00.53
total system (device and one or more leads) 00.50
transvenous lead into left ventricular coronary venous system 00.52
single-chamber device (initial) 37.81
rate responsive 37.82
replacement 37.85
rate responsive 37.86
temporary transvenous pacemaker system 37.78
during and immediately following cardiac surgery 39.64
carotid 39.89
gastric 04.92
heart - *see* Insertion, pacemaker, cardiac
intracranial - *see* Implant, neurostimulator, intracranial
neural - *see* Implant, neurostimulator, by site
peripheral nerve - *see* Implant, neurostimulator, peripheral nerve
spine - *see* Implant, neurostimulator, spine

Insertion *(Continued)*
pacing catheter - *see* Insertion, pacemaker, cardiac
pack
auditory canal, external 96.11
cervix (nonobstetrical) 67.0
after delivery or abortion 75.8
to assist delivery or induce labor 73.1
rectum 96.19
sella turcica 07.79
vagina (nonobstetrical) 96.14
after delivery or abortion 75.8
palatal implant 27.64
penile prosthesis (internal) (non-inflatable) 64.95
inflatable (internal) 64.97
periodontal splint (orthodontic) 24.7
peripheral blood vessel - *see* non-coronary
pessary
cervix 96.18
to assist delivery or induce labor 73.1
vagina 96.18
pharyngeal valve, artificial 31.75
port, vascular access 86.07
prostaglandin suppository (for abortion) 96.49
prosthesis, prosthetic device
acetabulum (partial) 81.52
hip 81.52
revision NOS 81.53
acetabular and femoral components (total) 00.70
acetabular component only 00.71
acetabular liner and/or femoral head only 00.73
femoral component only 00.72
femoral head only and/or acetabular liner 00.73
partial
acetabular component only 00.71
acetabular liner and/or femoral head only 00.73
femoral component only 00.72
femoral head only and/or acetabular liner 00.73
total (acetabular and femoral components) 00.70
revision 81.53
ankle (total) 81.56
arm (bioelectric) (cineplastic) (kineplastic) 84.44
biliary tract 51.99
breast (bilateral) 85.54
unilateral 85.53
cardiac support device (CSD) (CorCap™) 37.41
chin (polyethylene) (silastic) 76.68
elbow (total) 81.84
revision 81.97
extremity (bioelectric) (cineplastic) (kineplastic) 84.40
lower 84.48
upper 84.44
fallopian tube 66.93
femoral head (Austin-Moore) (bipolar) (Eicher) (Thompson) 81.52
hip (partial) 81.52
revision NOS 81.53
acetabular and femoral components (total) 00.70
acetabular component only 00.71
acetabular liner and/or femoral head only 00.73
femoral component only 00.72
femoral head only and/or acetabular liner 00.73

Insertion *(Continued)*
prosthesis, prosthetic device *(Continued)*
hip *(Continued)*
revision NOS *(Continued)*
partial
acetabular component only 00.71
acetabular liner and/or femoral head only 00.73
femoral component only 00.72
femoral head only and/or acetabular liner 00.73
total (acetabular and femoral components) 00.70
total 81.51
revision
acetabular and femoral components (total) 00.70
total (acetabular and femoral components) 00.70
joint - *see* Arthroplasty
knee (partial) (total) 81.54
revision NOS 81.55
femoral component 00.82
partial
femoral component 00.82
patellar component 00.83
tibial component 00.81
tibial insert 00.84
patellar component 00.83
tibial component 00.81
tibial insert 00.84
total (all components) 00.80
leg (bioelectric) (cineplastic) (kineplastic) 84.48
lens 13.91
ocular (secondary) 16.61
with orbital exenteration 16.42
outflow tract (gusset type) (heart)
in
pulmonary valvuloplasty 35.26
total repair of tetralogy of Fallot 35.81
penis (internal) (noninflatable) 64.95
with
construction 64.43
reconstruction 64.44
inflatable (internal) 64.97
Rosen (for urinary incontinence) 59.79
shoulder
partial 81.81
revision 81.97
total, NEC 81.80
other 81.80
reverse 81.88
spine
artificial disc, NOS 84.60
cervical 84.62
nucleus 84.61
partial 84.61
total 84.62
lumbar, lumbosacral 84.65
nucleus 84.64
partial 84.64
total 84.65
thoracic (partial) (total) 84.63
other device 84.59
testicular (bilateral) (unilateral) 62.7
toe 81.57
hallux valgus repair 77.59
vagina
synthetic 70.95
pseudophakos - *see also* Insertion, lens 13.70
pump, infusion 86.06
radioactive isotope 92.27
radium 92.27
radon seeds 92.27,
Reuter bobbin (with intubation) 20.01
Rickham reservoir 02.22
Rosen prosthesis (for urinary incontinence) 59.79
Scribner shunt 39.93

Insertion *(Continued)*
  Sengstaken-Blakemore tube 96.06
  sensor (lead)
    intra-aneurysm sac pressure monitoring
        device 00.58
    intra-arterial, for continuous blood gas
        monitoring 89.60
    intracardiac or great vessel hemodynamic
        monitoring
      with lead 00.56
      without lead 38.26
  shunt - *see* Shunt
  sieve, vena cava 38.7
  skeletal muscle stimulator 83.92
  skull
    plate 02.05
    stereotactic frame 93.59
    tongs (Barton) (caliper) (Garder Wells)
        (Vinke) (with synchronous skeletal
        traction) 02.94
  spacer (cement) (joint) (methylmethacrylate)
      84.56
    spine 84.51
  sphenoidal electrodes 02.96
  spine
    bone void filler
      that with percutaneous vertebral
          augmentation 81.66
      that with percutaneous vertebroplasty
          81.65
    cage (BAK) 84.51
    facet replacement device(s) 84.84
    interbody spinal fusion device 84.51
    interspinous process decompression
        device 84.80
    non-fusion stabilization device - *see*
        category 84.8●
    pedicle-based dynamic stabilization
        device(s) 84.82
    posterior motion preservation device(s) -
        see category 84.8●
    spacer 84.51
  Spitz-Holter valve 02.2
  Steinmann pin 93.44
    with reduction of fracture or dislocation -
        see Reduction, fracture *and*
        Reduction, dislocation
  stent(s) (stent graft)
    aqueous drainage 12.67
    artery (bare) (bonded) (drug coated)
        (non-drug-eluting)

Note: Also use 00.40, 00.41, 00.42, or 00.43
to show the total number of vessels treated.
Use code 00.44 once to show procedure on a
bifurcated vessel. In addition, use 00.45,
00.46, 00.47, or 00.48 to show the number of
vascular stents inserted.

      basilar 00.64
      carotid 00.63
      cerebrovascular
        cerebral (intracranial) 00.65
        precerebral (extracranial) 00.64
          carotid 00.63
      coronary (bare) (bonded) (drug coated)
          (non-drug-eluting) 36.06
        drug-eluting 36.07
      extracranial 00.64
        carotid 00.63
      femoral artery, superficial 39.90
        drug-eluting 00.60
        non-drug-eluting 39.90
      intracranial 00.65
      non-coronary vessel
        basilar 00.64
        carotid 00.63
        extracranial 00.64
        femoral artery, superficial 39.90
          drug-eluting 00.60
          non-drug-eluting 39.90

Insertion *(Continued)*
  stent(s) *(Continued)*
    artery *(Continued)*
      non-coronary vessel *(Continued)*
        intracranial 00.65
        peripheral 39.90
          bare, drug-coated 39.90
          drug-eluting 00.55
        vertebral 00.64
      bile duct 51.43
        endoscopic 51.87
        percutaneous transhepatic 51.98
      colon
        endoscopic (fluoroscopic guidance)
            46.86
        other 46.87
      coronary (artery) (bare) (bonded) (drug
          coated) (non-drug-eluting) 36.06

Note: Also use 00.40, 00.41, 00.42, or 00.43
to show the total number of vessels treated.
Use code 00.44 once to show procedure on a
bifurcated vessel. In addition, use 00.45,
00.46, 00.47, or 00.48 to show the number of
vascular stents inserted.

      drug-eluting 36.07
      esophagus (endoscopic) (fluoroscopic)
          42.81
      mesenteric 39.90
        bare, drug-coated 39.90
        drug-eluting 00.55
      non-coronary vessel

Note: Also use 00.40, 00.41, 00.42, or 00.43
to show the total number of vessels treated.
Use code 00.44 once to show procedure on a
bifurcated vessel. In addition, use 00.45,
00.46, 00.47, or 00.48 to show the number of
vascular stents inserted.

      with angioplasty or atherectomy 39.50
      with bypass - *omit code*
      basilar 00.64
      carotid 00.63
      extracranial 00.64
      intracranial 00.65
      mesenteric 39.90
        bare, drug-coated 39.90
        drug-eluting 00.55
      peripheral 39.90
        bare, drug-coated 39.90
        drug-eluting 00.55
      renal 39.90
        bare, drug-coated 39.90
        drug-eluting 00.55
      vertebral 00.64
    pancreatic duct 52.92
      endoscopic 52.93
    peripheral 39.90

Note: Also use 00.40, 00.41, 00.42, or 00.43
to show the total number of vessels treated.
Use code 00.44 once to show procedure on a
bifurcated vessel. In addition, use 00.45,
00.46, 00.47, or 00.48 to show the number of
vascular stents inserted.

      bare, drug-coated 39.90
      drug-eluting 00.55
      femoral artery, superficial, drug-
          eluting 00.60
    precerebral 00.64

Note: Also use 00.40, 00.41, 00.42 or 00.43
to show the total number of vessels treated.
Use code 00.44 once to show procedure on a
bifurcated vessel. In addition, use 00.45,
00.46, 00.47, or 00.48 to show the number of
vascular stents inserted.

Insertion *(Continued)*
  stent(s) *(Continued)*
    renal 39.90
      bare, drug-coated 39.90
      drug-eluting 00.55
    subclavian 39.90

Note: Also use 00.40, 00.41, 00.42, or 00.43
to show the total number of vessels treated.
Use code 00.44 once to show procedure on a
bifurcated vessel. In addition, use 00.45,
00.46, 00.47, or 00.48 to show the number of
vascular stents inserted.

      bare, drug-coated 39.90
      drug-eluting 00.55
    tracheobronchial 96.05
    vertebral 00.64

Note: Also use 00.40, 00.41, 00.42, or 00.43
to show the total number of vessels treated.
Use code 00.44 once to show procedure on a
bifurcated vessel. In addition, use 00.45,
00.46, 00.47, or 00.48 to show the number of
vascular stents inserted.

  sternal fixation device with rigid plates
      84.94
  stimoceiver - *see* Implant, neurostimulator,
      by site
  stimulator for bone growth - *see* category
      78.9●
  subdural
    grids 02.93
    strips 02.93
  suppository
    prostaglandin (for abortion) 96.49
    vagina 96.49
  Swan-Ganz catheter (pulmonary) 89.64
  tampon
    esophagus 96.06
    uterus 69.91
    vagina 96.14
      after delivery or abortion 75.8
  Tandem™ heart 37.68
  telescope (IMT) (miniature) 13.91
  testicular prosthesis (bilateral) (unilateral)
      62.7
  tissue expander (skin) NEC 86.93
    breast 85.95
  tissue mandril (peripheral vessel) (Dacron)
      (Spark's type) 39.99
    with
      blood vessel repair 39.56
      vascular bypass or shunt - *see* Bypass,
          vascular
  tongs, skull (with synchronous skeletal
      traction) 02.94
  totally implanted device for bone growth
      (invasive) - *see* category 78.9●
  tube - *see also* Catheterization and Intubation
    bile duct 51.43
      endoscopic 51.87
    chest 34.04
      revision (with lysis of adhesions)
          34.04
        thoracoscopic 34.06
      thoracoscopic 34.06
    endotracheal 96.04
    esophagus (nonoperative) (Sengstaken)
        96.06
      permanent (silicone) (Souttar) 42.81
    feeding
      esophageal 42.81
      gastric 96.6
      nasogastric 96.6
    gastric
      by gastrostomy - *see* category 43.1●
      for
        decompression, intestinal 96.07
        feeding 96.6

Insertion (Continued)
  tube (Continued)
    intercostal (with water seal), for drainage
      34.04
      revision (with lysis of adhesions) 34.04
        thoracoscopic 34.06
    Miller-Abbott (for intestinal
      decompression) 96.08
    nasobiliary (drainage) 51.86
    nasogastric (for intestinal decompression)
      NEC 96.07
    naso-intestinal 96.08
    nasopancreatic drainage (endoscopic)
      52.97
    pancreatic duct 52.92
      endoscopic 52.93
    rectum 96.09
    stomach (nasogastric) (for intestinal
      decompression) NEC 96.07
      for feeding 96.6
    tracheobronchial 96.05
  umbrella device
    atrial septum (King-Mills) 35.52
    vena cava (Mobitz-Uddin) 38.7
  ureteral stent (transurethral) 59.8
    with ureterotomy 59.8 [56.2]
  urinary sphincter, artificial (AUS) (inflatable)
    58.93
  vaginal mold 96.15
  valve(s)
    bronchus
      multiple lobes 33.73
      single lobe 33.71
    Holter 02.22
    Hufnagel - see Replacement, heart valve
    pharyngeal (artificial) 31.75
    Spitz-Holter 02.22
    vas deferens 63.95
  vascular access device, totally implantable
    86.07
  vena cava sieve or umbrella 38.7
  Vinke tongs (skull) (with synchronous
    skeletal traction) 02.94
  X Stop™ 84.80
Instillation
  bladder 96.49
  digestive tract, except gastric gavage 96.43
  genitourinary NEC 96.49
  radioisotope (intracavitary) (intravenous)
    92.28
  thoracic cavity 34.92
Insufflation
  Eustachian tube 20.8
  fallopian tube (air) (dye) (gas) (saline) 66.8
    for radiography - see
      Hysterosalpingography
    therapeutic substance 66.95
  lumbar retroperitoneal, bilateral 88.15
Intercricothyroidotomy (for assistance in
  breathing) 31.1
Interleukin-2, infusion
  high-dose 00.15
  low-dose 99.28
Intermittent positive pressure breathing
  (IPPB) 93.91
Interposition operation
  esophageal reconstruction (intrathoracic)
    (retrosternal) NEC - see also
      Anastomosis, esophagus, with,
      interposition 42.58
  antesternal or antethoracic NEC - see also
    Anastomosis, esophagus, antesternal,
    with, interposition 42.68
  uterine suspension 69.21
Interrogation
  cardioverter-defibrillator, automatic (AICD)
    with catheter based invasive
      electrophysiologic testing 37.26
    with NIPS (arrhythmia induction) 37.20
    interrogation only (bedside device check)
      89.49

Interrogation (Continued)
  CRT-D (cardiac resynchronization
    defibrillator)
    with catheter based invasive
      electrophysiologic testing 37.26
    with NIPS (arrhythmia induction) 37.20
    interrogation only (bedside device check)
      89.49
  CRT-P (cardiac resynchronization
    pacemaker)
    with catheter based invasive
      electrophysiologic testing 37.26
    with NIPS (arrhythmia induction) 37.20
    interrogation only (bedside device check)
      89.45
  pacemaker
    with catheter based invasive
      electrophysiologic testing 37.26
    with NIPS (arrhythmia induction) 37.20
    interrogation only (bedside device check)
      89.45
Interruption
  vena cava (inferior) (superior) 38.7
Interview (evaluation) (diagnostic)
  medical, except psychiatric 89.05
    brief (abbreviated history) 89.01
    comprehensive (history and evaluation of
      new problem) 89.03
    limited (interval history) 89.02
    specified type NEC 89.04
  psychiatric NEC 94.19
    follow-up 94.19
    initial 94.19
    pre-commitment 94.13
Intimectomy 38.10
  abdominal 38.16
  aorta (arch) (ascending) (descending) 38.14
  head and neck NEC 38.12
  intracranial NEC 38.11
  lower limb 38.18
  thoracic NEC 38.15
  upper limb 38.13
Intraoperative anesthetic effect monitoring
  and titration (IAEMT) 00.94 [89.14]
Introduction
  orthodontic appliance 24.7
  therapeutic substance (acting locally or
    systemically) NEC 99.29
    bursa 83.96
      hand 82.94
    fascia 83.98
      hand 82.96
    heart 37.92
    joint 81.92
      temporomandibular 76.96
    ligament (joint) 81.92
    pericardium 37.93
    soft tissue NEC 83.98
      hand 82.96
    tendon 83.97
      hand 82.95
    vein 39.92
Intubation - see also Catheterization and
  Insertion
  bile duct(s) 51.59
    common 51.51
      endoscopic 51.87
    endoscopic 51.87
  esophagus (nonoperative) (Sengstaken) 96.06
    permanent tube (silicone) (Souttar) 42.81
  Eustachian tube 20.8
  intestine (for decompression) 96.08
  lacrimal for
    dilation 09.42
    tear drainage, intranasal 09.81
  larynx 96.05
  nasobiliary (drainage) 51.86
  nasogastric
    for
      decompression, intestinal 96.07
      feeding 96.6

Intubation (Continued)
  naso-intestinal 96.08
  nasolacrimal (duct) (with irrigation) 09.44
  nasopancreatic drainage (endoscopic) 52.97
  respiratory tract NEC 96.05
  small intestine (Miller-Abbott) 96.08
  stomach (nasogastric) (for intestinal
    decompression) NEC 96.07
    for feeding 96.6
  trachea 96.04
  ventriculocisternal 02.22
Invagination, diverticulum
  gastric 44.69
    laparoscopic 44.68
  pharynx 29.59
  stomach 44.69
    laparoscopic 44.68
Inversion
  appendix 47.99
  diverticulum
    gastric 44.69
      laparoscopic 44.68
    intestine
      large 45.49
        endoscopic 45.43
      small 45.34
    stomach 44.69
      laparoscopic 44.68
  tunica vaginalis 61.49
IOERT (intra-operative electron radiation
  therapy) 92.41
IOM (intra-operative neurophysiologic
  monitoring) 00.94
Ionization, medical 99.27
Iontherapy 99.27
Iontophoresis 99.27
Iridectomy (basal) (buttonhole) (optical)
  (peripheral) (total) 12.14
  with
    capsulectomy 13.65
    cataract extraction - see Extraction,
      cataract
    filtering operation (for glaucoma) NEC
      12.65
    scleral
      fistulization 12.65
      thermocauterization 12.62
      trephination 12.61
Iridencleisis 12.63
Iridesis 12.63
Irido-capsulectomy 13.65
Iridocyclectomy 12.44
Iridocystectomy 12.42
Iridodesis 12.63
Iridoplasty NEC 12.39
Iridosclerectomy 12.65
Iridosclerotomy 12.69
Iridotasis 12.63
Iridotomy 12.12
  by photocoagulation 12.12
  with transfixion 12.11
  for iris bombé 12.11
  specified type NEC 12.12
Iron lung 93.99
Irradiation
  gamma, stereotactic 92.32
Irrigation
  anterior chamber (eye) 12.91
  bronchus NEC 96.56
  canaliculus 09.42
  catheter
    ureter 96.46
    urinary, indwelling NEC 96.48
    vascular 96.57
    ventricular 02.41
    wound 96.58
  cholecystostomy 96.41
  cornea 96.51
    with removal of foreign body 98.21
  corpus cavernosum 64.98
  cystostomy 96.47

Irrigation *(Continued)*
 ear (removal of cerumen) 96.52
 enterostomy 96.36
 eye 96.51
  with removal of foreign body 98.21
 gastrostomy 96.36
 lacrimal
  canaliculi 09.42
  punctum 09.41
 muscle 83.02
  hand 82.02
 nasal
  passages 96.53
  sinus 22.00
 nasolacrimal duct 09.43
  with insertion of tube or stent
   09.44

Irrigation *(Continued)*
 nephrostomy 96.45
 peritoneal 54.25
 pyelostomy 96.45
 rectal 96.39
 stomach 96.33
 tendon (sheath) 83.01
  hand 82.01
 trachea NEC 96.56
 traumatic cataract 13.3
 tube
  biliary NEC 96.41
  nasogastric NEC 96.34
  pancreatic 96.42
 ureterostomy 96.46
 ventricular shunt 02.41
 wound (cleaning) NEC 96.59

Irving operation (tubal ligation) 66.32
Irwin operation - *see also* Osteotomy
 77.30
Ischiectomy (partial) 77.89
 total 77.99
Ischiopubiotomy 77.39
Isolation
 after contact with infectious disease
  99.84
 ileal loop 45.51
 intestinal segment or pedicle flap
  large 45.52
  small 45.51
Isthmectomy, thyroid - *see also* Thyroidectomy,
 partial 06.39
IVUS - *see* Ultrasound, intravascular, by site

J

Jaboulay operation (gastroduodenostomy)
 44.39
 laparoscopic 44.38
Janeway operation (permanent gastrostomy)
 43.19
Jatene operation (arterial switch) 35.84
Jejunectomy 45.62
Jejunocecostomy 45.93
Jejunocholecystostomy 51.32
Jejunocolostomy 45.93

Jejunoileostomy 45.91
Jejunojejunostomy 45.91
Jejunopexy 46.61
Jejunorrhaphy 46.73
Jejunostomy (feeding) 46.39
 delayed opening 46.31
 loop 46.01
 percutaneous (endoscopic) (PEJ) 46.32
 revision 46.41
Jejunotomy 45.02
Johanson operation (urethral reconstruction)
 58.46

Jones operation
 claw toe (transfer of extensor hallucis longus
  tendon) 77.57
  modified (with arthrodesis) 77.57
 dacryocystorhinostomy 09.81
 hammer toe (interphalangeal fusion) 77.56
  modified (tendon transfer with arthrodesis)
   77.57
 repair of peroneal tendon 83.88
Joplin operation (exostectomy with tendon
 transfer) 77.53

K

Kader operation (temporary gastrostomy) 43.19
Kasai portoenterostomy 51.37
Kaufman operation (for urinary stress
 incontinence) 59.79
Kazanjiian operation (buccal vestibular sulcus
 extension) 24.91
Kehr operation (hepatopexy) 50.69
Keller operation (bunionectomy) 77.59
Kelly (-Kennedy) operation (urethrovesical
 plication) 59.3
Kelly-Stoeckel operation (urethrovesical
 plication) 59.3
Kelotomy 53.9
Keratectomy (complete) (partial) (superficial)
 11.49
 for pterygium 11.39
  with corneal graft 11.32
Keratocentesis (for hyphema) 12.91
Keratomileusis 11.71
Keratophakia 11.72
Keratoplasty (tectonic) (with autograft) (with
 homograft) 11.60
 lamellar (nonpenetrating) (with homograft)
  11.62
  with autograft 11.61

Keratoplasty *(Continued)*
 penetrating (full-thickness) (with homograft)
  11.64
  with autograft 11.63
 perforating - *see* Keratoplasty, penetrating
 refractive 11.71
 specified type NEC 11.69
Keratoprosthesis 11.73
Keratotomy (delimiting) (posterior) 11.1
 radial (refractive) 11.75
Kerr operation (low cervical cesarean section)
 74.1
Kessler operation (arthroplasty,
 carpometacarpal joint) 81.74
Kidner operation (excision of accessory
 navicular bone) (with tendon transfer)
 77.98
Killian operation (frontal sinusotomy)
 22.41
Kineplasty - *see* Cineplasty
King-Steelquist operation (hind-quarter
 amputation) 84.19
Kirk operation (amputation through thigh)
 84.17
Kock pouch
 bowel anastomosis - *omit code*
 continent ileostomy 46.22

Kock pouch *(Continued)*
 cutaneous uretero-ileostomy 56.51
 ESWL (electrocorporeal shockwave
  lithotripsy) 98.51
 removal, calculus 57.19
 revision, cutaneous uretero-ileostomy
  56.52
 urinary diversion procedure 56.51
Kockogram (ileal conduitogram) 87.78
Kockoscopy 45.12
Kondoleon operation (correction of lymphedema) 40.9
Krause operation (sympathetic denervation)
 05.29
Kroener operation (partial salpingectomy)
 66.69
Kroenlein operation (lateral orbitotomy)
 16.01
Kronig operation (low cervical cesarean
 section) 74.1
Krunkenberg operation (reconstruction of
 below-elbow amputation) 82.89
Kuhnt-Szymanowski operation (ectropion
 repair with lid reconstruction)
 08.44
Kyphoplasty 81.66

L

Labbe operation (gastrotomy) 43.0
Labiectomy (bilateral) 71.62
 unilateral 71.61
Labyrinthectomy (transtympanic) 20.79
Labyrinthotomy (transtympanic) 20.79

Ladd operation (mobilization of intestine)
 54.95
Lagrange operation (iridosclerectomy) 12.65
Lambrinudi operation (triple arthrodesis) 81.12
Laminectomy (decompression) (for exploration)
 03.09
 as operative approach - *omit code*

Laminectomy *(Continued)*
 with
  excision of herniated intervertebral disc
   (nucleus pulposus) 80.51
  excision of other intraspinal lesion
   (tumor) 03.4
 reopening of site 03.02

Laminography - *see* Radiography
Laminoplasty, expansile 03.09
Laminotomy (decompression) (for exploration) 03.09
  as operative approach - *omit code*
  reopening of site 03.02
Langenbeck operation (cleft palate repair) 27.62
Laparoamnioscopy 75.31
Laparorrhaphy 54.63
Laparoscopy 54.21
  with
    biopsy (intra-abdominal) 54.24
      uterine ligaments 68.15
      uterus 68.16
    destruction of fallopian tubes - *see* Destruction, fallopian tube
Laparotomy NEC 54.19
  as operative approach - *omit code*
  exploratory (pelvic) 54.11
  reopening of recent operative site (for control of hemorrhage) (for exploration) (for incision of hematoma) 54.12
Laparotrachelotomy 74.1
Lapidus operation (bunionectomy with metatarsal osteotomy) 77.51
Larry operation (shoulder disarticulation) 84.08
Laryngectomy
  with radical neck dissection (with synchronous thyroidectomy) (with synchronous tracheostomy) 30.4
  complete (with partial laryngectomy) (with synchronous tracheostomy) 30.3
    with radical neck dissection (with synchronous thyroidectomy) (with synchronous tracheostomy) 30.4
  frontolateral partial (extended) 30.29
  glottosupraglottic partial 30.29
  lateral partial 30.29
  partial (frontolateral) (glottosupraglottic) (lateral) (submucous) (supraglottic) (vertical) 30.29
  radical (with synchronous thyroidectomy) (with synchronous tracheostomy) 30.4
  submucous (partial) 30.29
  supraglottic partial 30.29
  total (with partial pharyngectomy) (with synchronous tracheostomy) 30.3
    with radical neck dissection (with synchronous thyroidectomy) (with synchronous tracheostomy) 30.4
  vertical partial 30.29
  wide field 30.3
Laryngocentesis 31.3
Laryngoesophagectomy 30.4
Laryngofissure 30.29
Laryngogram 87.09
  contrast 87.07
Laryngopharyngectomy (with synchronous tracheostomy) 30.3
  radical (with synchronous thyroidectomy) 30.4
Laryngopharyngoesophagectomy (with synchronous tracheostomy) 30.3
  with radical neck dissection (with synchronous thyroidectomy) 30.4
Laryngoplasty 31.69
Laryngorrhaphy 31.61
Laryngoscopy (suspension) (through artificial stoma) 31.42
Laryngostomy (permanent) 31.29
  revision 31.63
  temporary (emergency) 31.1
Laryngotomy 31.3
Laryngotracheobronchoscopy 33.23
  with biopsy 33.24
Laryngotracheoscopy 31.42
Laryngotracheostomy (permanent) 31.29
  temporary (emergency) 31.1
Laryngotracheotomy (temporary) 31.1
  permanent 31.29

Laser - *see also* Coagulation, Destruction, *and* Photocoagulation by site
  angioplasty, percutaneous transluminal 39.59
    coronary - *see* Angioplasty, coronary
Laser interstitial thermal therapy (LITT) under guidance
  lesion
    brain 17.61
    breast 17.69
    head and neck 17.62
    liver 17.63
    lung 17.69
    prostate 17.69
    thyroid 17.62
Lash operation
  internal cervical os repair 67.59
  laparoscopic supracervical hysterectomy 68.31
LASIK (Laser-assisted in situ keratomileusis) 11.71
Latzko operation
  cesarean section 74.2
  colpocleisis 70.8
Lavage
  antral 22.00
  bronchus NEC 96.56
    diagnostic (endoscopic) bronchoalveolar lavage (BAL) (Mini-BAL) 33.24
  endotracheal 96.56
  gastric 96.33
  lung (total) (whole) 33.99
    diagnostic (endoscopic) bronchoalveolar lavage (BAL) 33.24
  nasal sinus(es) 22.00
    by puncture 22.01
    through natural ostium 22.02
  peritoneal (diagnostic) 54.25
  trachea NEC 96.56
Leadbetter operation (urethral reconstruction) 58.46
Leadbetter-Politano operation (ureteroneocystostomy) 56.74
LEEP (loop electrosurgical excision procedure) of cervix 67.32
Le Fort operation (colpocleisis) 70.8
LeMesurier operation (cleft lip repair) 27.54
Lengthening
  bone (with bone graft) 78.30
    femur 78.35
    for reconstruction of thumb 82.69
    specified site NEC 78.39 - *see also* category 78.3●
    tibia 78.37
    ulna 78.33
  extraocular muscle NEC 15.21
    multiple (two or more muscles) 15.4
  fascia 83.89
    hand 82.89
  hamstring NEC 83.85
  heel cord 83.85
  leg
    femur 78.35
    tibia 78.37
  levator palpebrae muscle 08.38
  muscle 83.85
    extraocular 15.21
      multiple (two or more muscles) 15.4
    hand 82.55
  palate 27.62
    secondary or subsequent 27.63
  tendon 83.85
    for claw toe repair 77.57
    hand 82.55
Leriche operation (periarterial sympathectomy) 05.25
Leucotomy, leukotomy 01.32
Leukopheresis, therapeutic 99.72
Lid suture operation (blepharoptosis) 08.31
Ligation
  adrenal vessel (artery) (vein) 07.43
  aneurysm 39.52

Ligation (Continued)
  appendages, dermal 86.26
  arteriovenous fistula 39.53
    coronary artery 36.99
  artery 38.80
    abdominal 38.86
    adrenal 07.43
    aorta (arch) (ascending) (descending) 38.84
    coronary (anomalous) 36.99
    ethmoidal 21.04
    external carotid 21.06
    for control of epistaxis - *see* Control, epistaxis
    head and neck NEC 38.82
    intracranial NEC 38.81
    lower limb 38.88
    maxillary (transantral) 21.05
    middle meningeal 02.13
    thoracic NEC 38.85
    thyroid 06.92
    upper limb 38.83
  atrium, heart 37.99
  auricle, heart 37.99
  bleeding vessel - *see* Control, hemorrhage
  blood vessel 38.80
    abdominal
      artery 38.86
      vein 38.87
    adrenal 07.43
    aorta (arch) (ascending) (descending) 38.84
    esophagus 42.91
      endoscopic 42.33
    head and neck 38.82
    intracranial NEC 38.81
    lower limb
      artery 38.88
      vein 38.89
    meningeal (artery) (longitudinal sinus) 02.13
    thoracic NEC 38.85
    thyroid 06.92
    upper limb (artery) (vein) 38.83
  bronchus 33.92
  cisterna chyli 40.64
  coronary
    artery (anomalous) 36.99
    sinus 36.39
  dermal appendage 86.26
  ductus arteriosus, patent 38.85
  esophageal vessel 42.91
    endoscopic 42.33
  ethmoidal artery 21.04
  external carotid artery 21.06
  fallopian tube (bilateral) (remaining) (solitary) 66.39
    by endoscopy (culdoscopy) (hysteroscopy) (laparoscopy) (peritoneoscopy) 66.29
    with
      crushing 66.31
        by endoscopy (laparoscopy) 66.21
      division 66.32
        by endoscopy (culdoscopy) (laparoscopy) (peritoneoscopy) 66.22
      Falope ring 66.39
        by endoscopy (laparoscopy) 66.29
    unilateral 66.92
  fistula, arteriovenous 39.53
    coronary artery 36.99
  gastric
    artery 38.86
    varices 44.91
      endoscopic 43.41
  hemorrhoids 49.45
  longitudinal sinus (superior) 02.13
  lymphatic (channel) (peripheral) 40.9
    thoracic duct 40.64
  maxillary artery 21.05

Ligation *(Continued)*
    meningeal vessel 02.13
    spermatic
        cord 63.72
            varicocele 63.1
        vein (high) 63.1
    splenic vessels 38.86
    subclavian artery 38.85
    superior longitudinal sinus 02.13
    supernumerary digit 86.26
    thoracic duct 40.64
    thyroid vessel (artery) (vein) 06.92
    toes (supernumerary) 86.26
    tooth 93.55
        impacted 24.6
    ulcer (peptic) (base) (bed) (bleeding vessel)
            44.40
        duodenal 44.42
        gastric 44.41
    ureter 56.95
    varices
        esophageal 42.91
            endoscopic 42.33
        gastric 44.91
            endoscopic 43.41
        peripheral vein (lower limb) 38.59
            upper limb 38.53
    varicocele 63.1
    vas deferens 63.71
    vein 38.80
        abdominal 38.87
        adrenal 07.43
        head and neck NEC 38.82
        intracranial NEC 38.81
        lower limb 38.89
        spermatic, high 63.1
        thoracic NEC 38.85
        thyroid 06.92
        upper limb 38.83
        varicose 38.50
            abdominal 38.57
            esophagus 42.91
                endoscopic 42.33
            gastric 44.91
                endoscopic 43.41
            head and neck 38.52
            intracranial NEC 38.51
            lower limb 38.59
            stomach 44.91
            thoracic NEC 38.55
            upper limb 38.53
    vena cava, inferior 38.7
    venous connection between anomalous
            vein to
        left innominate vein 35.82
        superior vena cava 35.82
    wart 86.26
Light coagulation - *see* Photocoagulation
Lindholm operation (repair of ruptured
        tendon) 83.88
Lingulectomy, lung 32.39
Linton operation (varicose vein)
        38.59
Lipectomy (subcutaneous tissue)
        (abdominal) (submental)
        86.83
Liposuction 86.83
Lip reading training 95.49
Lip shave 27.43
Lisfranc operation
    foot amputation 84.12
    shoulder disarticulation 84.08
Litholapaxy, bladder 57.0
    by incision 57.19
Lithotomy
    bile passage 51.49
    bladder (urinary) 57.19
    common duct 51.41
        percutaneous 51.96
    gallbladder 51.04
    hepatic duct 51.49

Lithotomy *(Continued)*
    kidney 55.01
        percutaneous 55.03
    ureter 56.2
Lithotripsy
    bile duct NEC 51.49
        extracorporeal shockwave (ESWL) 98.52
    bladder 57.0
        with ultrasonic fragmentation 57.0 *[59.95]*
        extracorporeal shockwave (ESWL) 98.51
    extracorporeal shockwave (ESWL) NEC
            98.59
        bile duct 98.52
        bladder (urinary) 98.51
        gallbladder 98.52
        kidney 98.51
        Kock pouch 98.51
        renal pelvis 98.51
        specified site NEC 98.59
        ureter 98.51
    gallbladder NEC 51.04
        endoscopic 51.88
        extracorporeal shockwave (ESWL) 98.52
    kidney 56.0
        extracorporeal shockwave (ESWL) 98.51
        percutaneous nephrostomy with
            fragmentation (laser) (ultrasound)
            55.04
    renal pelvis 56.0
        extracorporeal shockwave (ESWL) 98.51
        percutaneous nephrostomy with
            fragmentation (laser) (ultrasound)
            55.04
    ureter 56.0
        extracorporeal shock wave (ESWL) 98.51
LITT (laser interstitial thermal therapy) under
        guidance
    lesion
        brain 17.61
        breast 17.69
        head and neck 17.62
        liver 17.63
        lung 17.69
        prostate 17.69
        thyroid 17.62
Littlewood operation (forequarter amputation)
        84.09
LLETZ (large loop excision of the
        transformation zone) of cervix 67.32
Lloyd-Davies operation (abdominoperineal
        resection), NOS 48.50
    laparoscopic 48.51
    open 48.52
    other 48.59
Lobectomy
    brain 01.53
        partial 01.59
    liver (with partial excision of adjacent lobes)
        50.3
    lung (complete) 32.49
        partial 32.39
            thoracoscopic 32.30
        segmental (with resection of adjacent
            lobes) 32.49
            thoracoscopic 32.41
        thoracoscopic 32.41
    thyroid (total) (unilateral) (with removal of
        isthmus) (with removal of portion of
        remaining lobe) 06.2
        partial - *see also* Thyroidectomy, partial
            06.39
        substernal 06.51
        subtotal - *see also* Thyroidectomy, partial
            06.39
Lobotomy, brain 01.32
Localization, placenta 88.78
    by RISA injection 92.17
Longmire operation (bile duct anastomosis) 51.39
Loop ileal stoma (*see also* Ileostomy) 46.01
Loopogram 87.78
Looposcopy (ileal conduit) 56.35

Lord operation
    dilation of anal canal for hemorrhoids 49.49
    hemorrhoidectomy 49.49
    orchidopexy 62.5
Lower GI series (x-ray) 87.64
Lucas and Murray operation (knee arthrodesis
        with plate) 81.22
Lumpectomy
    breast 85.21
    specified site - *see* Excision, lesion, by site
Lymphadenectomy (simple) - *see also* Excision,
        lymph, node 40.29
Lymphadenotomy 40.0
Lymphangiectomy (radical) - *see also* Excision,
        lymph, node, by site, radical 40.50
Lymphangiogram
    abdominal 88.04
    cervical 87.08
    intrathoracic 87.34
    lower limb 88.36
    pelvic 88.04
    upper limb 88.34
Lymphangioplasty 40.9
Lymphangiorrhaphy 40.9
Lymphangiotomy 40.0
Lymphaticostomy 40.9
    thoracic duct 40.62
Lysis
    adhesions

> **Note:** blunt - *omit code*
>   digital - *omit code*
>   manual - *omit code*
>   mechanical - *omit code*
>   without instrumentation - *omit code*

        abdominal 54.59
            laparoscopic 54.51
        appendiceal 54.59
            laparoscopic 54.51
        artery-vein-nerve bundle 39.91
        biliary tract 54.59
            laparoscopic 54.51
        bladder (neck) (intraluminal) 57.12
            external 59.11
                laparoscopic 59.12
            transurethral 57.41
        blood vessels 39.91
        bone - *see* category 78.4●
        bursa 83.91
            by stretching or manipulation 93.28
            hand 82.91
        cartilage of joint 93.26
        chest wall 33.99
        choanae (nasopharynx) 29.54
        conjunctiva 10.5
        corneovitreal 12.34
        cortical (brain) 02.91
        ear, middle 20.23
        Eustachian tube 20.8
        extraocular muscle 15.7
        extrauterine 54.59
            laparoscopic 54.51
        eyelid 08.09
            and conjunctiva 10.5
        eye muscle 15.7
        fallopian tube 65.89
            laparoscopic 65.81
        fascia 83.91
            hand 82.91
                by stretching or manipulation
                93.26
        gallbladder 54.59
            laparoscopic 54.51
        ganglion (peripheral) NEC 04.49
            cranial NEC 04.42
        hand 82.91
            by stretching or manipulation 93.26
        heart 37.10
        intestines 54.59
            laparoscopic 54.51

Lysis (Continued)
  adhesions (Continued)
    iris (posterior) 12.33
      anterior 12.32
    joint (capsule) (structure) - see also
      Division, joint capsule 80.40
    kidney 59.02
      laparoscopic 59.03
    labia (vulva) 71.01
    larynx 31.92
    liver 54.59
      laparoscopic 54.51
    lung (for collapse of lung) 33.39
    mediastinum 34.99
    meninges (spinal) 03.6
      cortical 02.91
    middle ear 20.23
    muscle 83.91
      by stretching or manipulation 93.27
      extraocular 15.7
      hand 82.91
        by stretching or manipulation 93.26
    nasopharynx 29.54
    nerve (peripheral) NEC 04.49
      cranial NEC 04.42
      roots, spinal 03.6
      trigeminal 04.41
    nose, nasal 21.91
    ocular muscle 15.7

Lysis (Continued)
  adhesions (Continued)
    ovary 65.89
      laparoscopic 65.81
    pelvic 54.59
      laparoscopic 54.51
    penile 64.93
    pericardium 37.12
    perineal (female) 71.01
    peripheral vessels 39.91
    perirectal 48.81
    perirenal 59.02
      laparoscopic 59.03
    peritoneum (pelvic) 54.59
      laparoscopic 54.51
    periureteral 59.02
      laparoscopic 59.03
    perivesical 59.11
      laparoscopic 59.12
    pharynx 29.54
    pleura (for collapse of lung) 33.39
    spermatic cord 63.94
    spinal (cord) (meninges) (nerve roots) 03.6
    spleen 54.59
      laparoscopic 54.51
    tendon 83.91
      by stretching or manipulation 93.27
      hand 82.91
        by stretching or manipulation 93.26

Lysis (Continued)
  adhesions (Continued)
    thorax 34.99
    tongue 25.93
    trachea 31.92
    tubo-ovarian 65.89
      laparoscopic 65.81
    ureter 59.02
      with freeing or repositioning of ureter
        59.02
      intraluminal 56.81
      laparoscopic 59.03
    urethra (intraluminal) 58.5
    uterus 54.59
      intraluminal 68.21
      laparoscopic 54.51
      peritoneal 54.59
        laparoscopic 54.51
    vagina (intraluminal) 70.13
    vitreous (posterior approach) 14.74
      anterior approach 14.73
    vulva 71.01
  goniosynechiae (with injection of air or
    liquid) 12.31
  synechiae (posterior) 12.33
    anterior (with injection of air or liquid)
      12.32

M

Madlener operation (tubal ligation) 66.31
Magnet extraction
  foreign body
    anterior chamber, eye 12.01
    choroid 14.01
    ciliary body 12.01
    conjunctiva 98.22
    cornea 11.0
    eye, eyeball NEC 98.21
      anterior segment 12.01
      posterior segment 14.01
    intraocular (anterior segment) 12.01
    iris 12.01
    lens 13.01
    orbit 98.21
    retina 14.01
    sclera 12.01
    vitreous 14.01
Magnetic resonance imaging (nuclear) - see
  Imaging, magnetic resonance
Magnuson (-Stack) operation (arthroplasty for
  recurrent shoulder dislocation) 81.82
Mako Tactile Guidance System™ [TGS] - see
  category 17.4●
Malleostapediopexy 19.19
  with incus replacement 19.11
Malström's vacuum extraction 72.79
  with episiotomy 72.71
Mammaplasty - see Mammoplasty
Mammectomy - see also Mastectomy
  subcutaneous (unilateral) 85.34
    with synchronous implant 85.33
    bilateral 85.36
      with synchronous implant 85.35
Mammilliplasty 85.87
Mammography NEC 87.37
Mammoplasty 85.89
  with
    full-thickness graft 85.83
    muscle flap 85.85
    pedicle graft 85.84
    split-thickness graft 85.82
  amputative (reduction) (bilateral) 85.32
    unilateral 85.31

Mammoplasty (Continued)
  augmentation 85.50
    with
      breast implant (bilateral) 85.54
        unilateral 85.53
      injection into breast (bilateral) 85.52
        unilateral 85.51
  reduction (bilateral) 85.32
    unilateral 85.31
  revision 85.89
  size reduction (gynecomastia) (bilateral)
    85.32
    unilateral 85.31
Mammotomy 85.0
Manchester (-Donald) (-Fothergill) operation
  (uterine suspension) 69.22
Mandibulectomy (partial) 76.31
  total 76.42
    with reconstruction 76.41
Maneuver (method)
  Bracht 72.52
  Credé 73.59
  De Lee (key-in-lock) 72.4
  Kristeller 72.54
  Loveset's (extraction of arms in breech birth)
    72.52
  Mauriceau (-Smellie-Veit) 72.52
  Pinard (total breech extraction) 72.54
  Prague 72.52
  Ritgen 73.59
  Scanzoni (rotation) 72.4
  Van Hoorn 72.52
  Wigand-Martin 72.52
Manipulation
  with reduction of fracture or dislocation - see
    Reduction, fracture and Reduction,
    dislocation
  enterostomy stoma (with dilation) 96.24
  intestine (intra-abdominal) 46.80
    large 46.82
    small 46.81
  joint
    adhesions 93.26
      temporomandibular 76.95
    dislocation - see Reduction, dislocation
  lacrimal passage (tract) NEC 09.49

Manipulation (Continued)
  muscle structures 93.27
  musculoskeletal (physical therapy) NEC
    93.29
  nasal septum, displaced 21.88
  osteopathic NEC 93.67
    for general mobilization (general
      articulation) 93.61
    high-velocity, low-amplitude forces
      (thrusting) 93.62
    indirect forces 93.65
    isotonic, isometric forces 93.64
    low-velocity, high-amplitude forces
      (springing) 93.63
    to move tissue fluids 93.66
  rectum 96.22
  salivary duct 26.91
  stomach, intraoperative 44.92
  temporomandibular joint NEC 76.95
  ureteral calculus by catheter
    with removal 56.0
    without removal 59.8
  uterus NEC 69.98
    gravid 75.99
    inverted
      manual replacement (following
        delivery) 75.94
      surgical - see Repair, inverted uterus
Manometry
  esophageal 89.32
  spinal fluid 89.15
  urinary 89.21
Manual arts therapy 93.81
Mapping
  cardiac (electrophysiologic) 37.27
    doppler (flow) 88.72
    electrocardiogram only 89.52
Marckwald operation (cervical os repair) 67.59
Marshall-Marchetti (-Krantz) operation
  (retropubic urethral suspension) 59.5
Marsupialization - see also Destruction, lesion,
  by site
  cyst
    Bartholin's 71.23
    brain 01.59
    cervical (nabothian) 67.31

L & M

Marsupialization (Continued)
cyst (Continued)
dental 24.4
dentigerous 24.4
kidney 55.31
larynx 30.01
liver 50.21
ovary 65.21
laparoscopic 65.23
pancreas 52.3
pilonidal (open excision) (with partial closure) 86.21
salivary gland 26.21
spinal (intraspinal) (meninges) 03.4
spleen, splenic 41.41
lesion
brain 01.59
cerebral 01.59
liver 50.21
pilonidal cyst or sinus (open excision) (with partial closure) 86.21
pseudocyst, pancreas 52.3
ranula, salivary gland 26.21
Massage
cardiac (external) (manual) (closed) 99.63
open 37.91
prostatic 99.94
rectal (for levator spasm) 99.93
MAST (military anti-shock trousers) 93.58
Mastectomy (complete) (prophylactic) (simple) (unilateral) 85.41
with
excision of regional lymph nodes 85.43
bilateral 85.44
preservation of skin and nipple 85.34
with synchronous implant 85.33
bilateral 85.36
with synchronous implant 85.35
bilateral 85.42
extended
radical (Urban) (unilateral) 85.47
bilateral 85.48
simple (with regional lymphadenectomy) (unilateral) 85.43
bilateral 85.44
modified radical (unilateral) 85.43
bilateral 85.44
partial 85.23
radical (Halsted) (Meyer) (unilateral) 85.45
bilateral 85.46
extended (Urban) (unilateral) 85.47
bilateral 85.48
modified (unilateral) 85.43
bilateral 85.44
subcutaneous 85.34
with synchronous implant 85.33
bilateral 85.36
with synchronous implant 85.35
subtotal 85.23
Masters' stress test (two-step) 89.42
Mastoidectomy (cortical) (conservative) 20.49
complete (simple) 20.41
modified radical 20.49
radical 20.42
modified 20.49
simple (complete) 20.41
Mastoidotomy 20.21
Mastoidotympanectomy 20.42
Mastopexy 85.6
Mastoplasty - see Mammoplasty
Mastorrhaphy 85.81
Mastotomy 85.0
Matas operation (aneurysmorrhaphy) 39.52
Mayo operation
bunionectomy 77.59
herniorrhaphy
laparoscopic 53.43
with graft or prosthesis 53.42
other and open with graft or prosthesis 53.41
other open 53.49

Mayo operation (Continued)
vaginal hysterectomy 68.59
laparoscopically assisted (LAVH) 68.51
Maze procedure
Cox-maze, open 37.33
maze, modified, endovascular 37.34
maze, modified, open 37.33
Mazet operation (knee disarticulation) 84.16
McBride operation (bunionectomy with soft tissue correction) 77.53
McBurney operation - see Repair, hernia, inguinal
McCall operation (enterocele repair) 70.92
McCauley operation (release of clubfoot) 83.84
McDonald operation (encirclement suture, cervix) 67.59
McIndoe operation (vaginal construction) 70.61
with graft or prosthesis 70.63
McKeever operation (fusion of first metatarsophalangeal joint for hallux valgus repair) 77.52
McKissock operation (breast reduction) 85.33
McReynolds operation (transposition of pterygium) 11.31
McVay operation
femoral hernia - see Repair, hernia, femoral
inguinal hernia - see Repair, hernia, inguinal
Measurement
airway resistance 89.38
anatomic NEC 89.39
arterial blood gases 89.65
basal metabolic rate (BMR) 89.39
blood gases
arterial 89.65
continuous intra-arterial 89.60
venous 89.66
body 93.07
cardiac output (by)
Fick method 89.67
indicator dilution technique 89.68
oxygen consumption technique 89.67
thermodilution indicator 89.68
cardiovascular NEC 89.59
central venous pressure 89.62
coronary blood flow 89.69
fractional flow reserve (FFR) 00.59
intravascular pressure measurement 00.59
gastric function NEC 89.39
girth 93.07
intelligence 94.01
intracranial pressure 01.10
intraocular tension or pressure 89.11
as part of extended ophthalmologic work-up 95.03
intrauterine pressure 75.35
intravascular pressure 00.69
coronary 00.59
iliac 00.69
intra-abdominal 00.69
intrathoracic 00.67
aorta 00.67
aortic arch 00.67
carotid 00.67
mesenteric 00.69
peripheral 00.68
renal 00.69
limb length 93.06
lung volume 89.37
mixed venous blood gases 89.66
physiologic NEC 89.39
portovenous pressure 89.62
pulmonary airway flow, endoscopic 33.72
range of motion 93.05
renal clearance 89.29
respiratory NEC 89.38
skin fold thickness 93.07
skull circumference 93.07
sphincter of Oddi pressure 51.15

Measurement (Continued)
systemic arterial
blood gases 89.65
continuous intra-arterial 89.60
pressure 89.61
urine (bioassay) (chemistry) 89.29
vascular 89.59
venous blood gases 89.66
vital capacity (pulmonary) 89.37
Meatoplasty
ear 18.6
urethra 58.47
Meatotomy
ureter 56.1
urethra 58.1
internal 58.5
Mechanical ventilation - see Ventilation
Mediastinectomy 34.3
Mediastinoscopy 34.22
Mediastinotomy (Chamberlain procedure) 34.1
with pneumonectomy 32.59
thoracoscopic 32.50
Meloplasty, facial 86.82
Meningeorrhaphy (cerebral) 02.12
spinal NEC 03.59
for
meningocele 03.51
myelomeningocele 03.52
Meniscectomy (knee) NEC 80.6
acromioclavicular 80.91
sternoclavicular 80.91
temporomandibular (joint) 76.5
wrist 80.93
Menstrual extraction or regulation 69.6
Mentoplasty (augmentation) (with graft) (with implant) 76.68
reduction 76.67
Mesenterectomy 54.4
Mesenteriopexy 54.75
Mesenteriplication 54.75
Mesocoloplication 54.75
Mesopexy 54.75
Metatarsectomy 77.98
Metroplasty 69.49
Mid forceps delivery 72.29
Mikulicz operation (exteriorization of intestine) (first stage) 46.03
second stage 46.04
Miles operation (proctectomy), NOS 48.50
laparoscopic 48.51
open 48.52
other 48.59
Military anti-shock trousers (MAST) 93.58
Millard operation (cheiloplasty) 27.54
Miller operation
midtarsal arthrodesis 81.14
urethrovesical suspension 59.4
Millin-Read operation (urethrovesical suspension) 59.4
Mist therapy 93.94
Mitchell operation (hallux valgus repair) 77.51
MitraClip® mitral valve leaflet clip 35.97
Mobilization
joint NEC 93.16
mandible 76.95
neostrophingic (mitral valve) 35.12
spine 93.15
stapes (transcrural) 19.0
testis in scrotum 62.5
Mohs operation (chemosurgical excision of skin) 86.24
Molegraphy 87.81
Monitoring
BIS (bispectral index) monitoring 00.94 [89.14]
brain temperature 01.17
cardiac output (by)
ambulatory (ACM) 89.50
electrographic 89.54
during surgery - omit code
Fick method 89.67

Monitoring *(Continued)*
  cardiac output *(Continued)*
    Holter-type device 89.50
    indicator dilution technique 89.68
    intracardiac or great vessel hemodynamic
      sensor with lead 00.56
        sensor without lead 38.26
        subcutaneous device 00.57
    oxygen consumption technique 89.67
    specified technique NEC 89.68
    telemetry (cardiac) 89.54
    thermodilution indicator 89.68
    transesophageal (Doppler) (ultrasound) 89.68
  central venous pressure 89.62
  circulatory NEC 89.69
  continuous intra-arterial blood gas 89.60
  coronary blood flow (coincidence counting technique) 89.69
    fractional flow reserve (FFR) 00.59
    intravascular pressure measurement 00.59
  electroencephalographic 89.19
    intraoperative 00.94
    radio-telemetered 89.19
    video 89.19
  fetus (fetal heart)
    antepartum
      nonstress (fetal activity acceleration determinations) 75.34
      oxytocin challenge (contraction stress test) 75.35
      ultrasonography (early pregnancy) (Doppler) 88.78
    intrapartum (during labor) (extrauterine) (external) 75.34
      auscultatory (stethoscopy) - omit code
      internal (with contraction measurements) (ECG) 75.32
      intrauterine (direct) (ECG) 75.32
      phonocardiographic (extrauterine) 75.34
      pulsed ultrasound (Doppler) 88.78
      transcervical fetal oxygen saturation monitoring 75.38
      transcervical fetal SpO$_2$ monitoring 75.38
  Holter-type device (cardiac) 89.50
  IAEMT (intraoperative anesthetic effect monitoring and titration) 00.94 *[89.14]*
  intra-aneurysm sac pressure 00.58
  intracranial oxygen 01.16
  intracranial pressure 01.10
  intraoperative
    anesthetic effect monitoring and titration (IAEMT) 00.94 *[89.14]*
  intravascular pressure 00.69
    coronary 00.59
    iliac 00.69
    intra-abdominal 00.69

Monitoring *(Continued)*
  intravascular pressure *(Continued)*
    intrathoracic 00.67
      aorta 00.67
      aortic arch 00.67
      carotid 00.67
    mesenteric 00.69
    peripheral 00.68
    renal 00.69
  neurophysiologic
    intra-operative 00.94
  neurophysiologic (BAEP) (brainstem auditory evoked potentials) (EEG) (electroencephalogram) (electromyogram) (EMG) (MEP) (motor evoked potentials) (nerve conduction study) (somatosensory evoked potentials) (SSEP) (transcranial Doppler) 00.94
  partial pressure of brain oxygen (PbtO$_2$) 01.16
  pulmonary artery
    pressure 89.63
    wedge 89.64
  sleep (recording) - *see* categories 89.17
  systemic arterial pressure 89.61
    intra-aneursym sac pressure 00.58
  telemetry (cardiac) 89.54
  transesophageal cardiac output (Doppler) 89.68
  ventricular pressure (cardiac) 89.62
Moore operation (arthroplasty) 81.52
Moschowitz
  enterocele repair 70.92
    with graft or prosthesis 70.93
  herniorrhaphy - *see* Repair, hernia, femoral
  sigmoidopexy 46.63
Mountain resort sanitarium 93.98
Mouth-to-mouth resuscitation 93.93
Moxibustion 93.35
MRI - *see* Imaging, magnetic resonance
Muller operation (banding of pulmonary artery) 38.85
Multiple sleep latency test (MSLT) 89.18
Mumford operation (partial claviculectomy) 77.81
Musculoplasty - *see also* Repair, muscle 83.87
  hand - *see also* Repair, muscle, hand 82.89
Music therapy 93.84
Mustard operation (interatrial transposition of venous return) 35.91
Myectomy 83.45
  anorectal 48.92
  eye muscle 15.13
    multiple 15.3
  for graft 83.43
    hand 82.34
  hand 82.36
    for graft 82.34

Myectomy *(Continued)*
  levator palpebrae 08.33
  rectal 48.92
Myelogram, myelography (air) (gas) 87.21
  posterior fossa 87.02
Myelotomy
  spine, spinal (cord) (tract) (one-stage) (two-stage) 03.29
  percutaneous 03.21
Myocardiectomy (infarcted area) 37.33
Myocardiotomy 37.11
Myoclasis 83.99
  hand 82.99
Myomectomy (uterine) 68.29
  broad ligament 69.19
Myoplasty - *see also* Repair, muscle 83.87
  hand - *see also* Repair, muscle, hand 82.89
  mastoid 19.9
Myorrhaphy 83.65
  hand 82.46
Myosuture 83.65
  hand 82.46
Myotasis 93.27
Myotenontoplasty - *see also* Repair, tendon 83.88
  hand 82.86
Myotenoplasty - *see also* Repair, tendon 83.88
  hand 82.86
Myotenotomy 83.13
  hand 82.11
Myotomy 83.02
  with division 83.19
    hand 82.19
  colon NEC 46.92
    sigmoid 46.91
  cricopharyngeal 29.31
    that for pharyngeal (pharyngoesophageal) diverticulectomy 29.32
  esophagus 42.7
  eye (oblique) (rectus) 15.21
    multiple (two or more muscles) 15.4
  hand 82.02
    with division 82.19
  levator palpebrae 08.38
  sigmoid (colon) 46.91
Myringectomy 20.59
Myringodectomy 20.59
Myringomalleolabyrinthopexy 19.52
Myringoplasty (epitympanic, type I) (by cauterization) (by graft) 19.4
  revision 19.6
Myringostapediopexy 19.53
Myringostomy 20.01
Myringotomy (with aspiration) (with drainage) 20.09
  with insertion of tube or drainage device (button) (grommet) 20.01

N

Nailing, intramedullary
  with fracture reduction - *see* Reduction, fracture with internal fixation
  internal (without fracture reduction) 78.50
Narcoanalysis 94.21
Narcosynthesis 94.21
Narrowing, palpebral fissure 08.51
Nasopharyngogram 87.09
  contrast 87.06
Necropsy 89.8
Needleoscopy (fetus) 75.31
Needling
  Bartholin's gland (cyst) 71.21
  cataract (secondary) 13.64

Needling *(Continued)*
  fallopian tube 66.91
  hydrocephalic head 73.8
  lens (capsule) 13.2
  pupillary membrane (iris) 12.35
Nephrectomy (complete) (total) (unilateral) 55.51
  bilateral 55.54
  partial (wedge) 55.4
  remaining or solitary kidney 55.52
  removal transplanted kidney 55.53
Nephrocolopexy 55.7
Nephrocystanastomosis NEC 56.73
Nephrolithotomy 55.01
Nephrolysis 59.02
  laparoscopic 59.03

Nephropexy 55.7
Nephroplasty 55.89
Nephropyeloplasty 55.87
Nephropyeloureterostomy 55.86
Nephrorrhaphy 55.81
Nephroscopy 55.21
Nephrostolithotomy, percutaneous 55.03
Nephrostomy (with drainage tube) 55.02
  closure 55.82
  percutaneous 55.03
    with fragmentation (ultrasound) 55.04
Nephrotomogram, nephrotomography NEC 87.72
Nephrotomy 55.01
Nephroureterectomy (with bladder cuff) 55.51
Nephroureterocystectomy 55.51 *[57.79]*

Nerve block (cranial) (peripheral) NEC - *see also*
  Block, by site 04.81
Neurectasis (cranial) (peripheral) 04.91
Neurectomy (cranial) (infraorbital) (occipital)
  (peripheral) (spinal) NEC 04.07
  gastric (vagus) - *see also* Vagotomy
    44.00
  opticociliary 12.79
  paracervical 05.22
  presacral 05.24
  retrogasserian 04.07
  sympathetic - *see* Sympathectomy
  trigeminal 04.07
  tympanic 20.91
Neurexeresis NEC 04.07
Neuroablation
  radiofrequency 04.2
Neuroanastomosis (cranial) (peripheral) NEC
  04.74
  accessory-facial 04.72
  accessory-hypoglossal 04.73
  hypoglossal-facial 04.71

NeuroFlo™ catheter for partial (temporary)
  abdominal aorta occlusion 39.77
Neurolysis (peripheral nerve) NEC 04.49
  carpal tunnel 04.43
  cranial nerve NEC 04.42
  spinal (cord) (nerve roots) 03.6
  tarsal tunnel 04.44
  trigeminal nerve 04.41
Neuromonitoring
  intra-operative 00.94
Neuroplasty (cranial) (peripheral) NEC 04.79
  of old injury (delayed repair) 04.76
  revision 04.75
Neurorrhaphy (cranial) (peripheral) 04.3
Neurotomy (cranial) (peripheral) (spinal) NEC
  04.04
  acoustic 04.01
  glossopharyngeal 29.92
  lacrimal branch 05.0
  retrogasserian 04.02
  sympathetic 05.0
  vestibular 04.01

Neurotripsy (peripheral) NEC 04.03
  trigeminal 04.02
Nicola operation (tenodesis for recurrent
  dislocation of shoulder) 81.82
Nimodipine, infusion 99.75
NIPS (non-invasive programmed electrical
  stimulation) 37.20
Nissen operation (fundoplication of stomach)
  44.66
  laparoscopic 44.67
Noble operation (plication of small intestine)
  46.62
Norman Miller operation (vaginopexy) 70.77
  with graft or prosthesis 70.78
Norton operation (extraperitoneal cesarean
  section) 74.2
Nuclear magnetic resonance imaging - *see*
  Imaging, magnetic resonance
Nutrition, concentrated substances
  enteral infusion (of) 96.6
  parenteral, (total) 99.15
  peripheral parenteral 99.15

O

Ober (-Yount) operation (gluteal-iliotibial
  fasciotomy) 83.14
Obliteration
  bone cavity - *see also* Osteoplasty 78.40
  calyceal diverticulum 55.39
  canaliculi 09.6
  cerebrospinal fistula 02.12
  cul-de-sac 70.92
    with graft or prosthesis 70.93
  frontal sinus (with fat) 22.42
  lacrimal punctum 09.91
  lumbar pseudomeningocele 03.51
  lymphatic structure(s) (peripheral) 40.9
  maxillary sinus 22.31
  meningocele (sacral) 03.51
  pelvic 68.8
  pleural cavity 34.6
  sacral meningocele 03.51
  Skene's gland 71.3
  tympanomastoid cavity 19.9
  vagina, vaginal (partial) (total) 70.4
    vault 70.8
Occlusal molds (dental) 89.31
Occlusion
  artery
    by embolization - *see* Embolization, artery
    by endovascular approach - *see*
      Embolization, artery
    by ligation - *see* Ligation, artery
  fallopian tube - *see* Ligation, fallopian tube
  patent ductus arteriosus (PDA) 38.85
  vein
    by embolization - *see* Embolization, vein
    by endovascular approach - *see*
      Embolization, vein
    by ligation - *see* Ligation, vein
  vena cava (surgical) 38.7
Occupational therapy 93.83
OCT (optical coherence tomography)
  (intavascular imaging)
  coronary vessel(s) 38.24
  non-coronary vessel(s) 38.25
O'Donoghue operation (triad knee repair) 81.43
Odontectomy NEC - *see also* Removal, tooth,
  surgical 23.19
Oleothorax 33.39
Olshausen operation (uterine suspension) 69.22
Omentectomy 54.4
Omentofixation 54.74
Omentopexy 54.74
Omentoplasty 54.74

Omentorrhaphy 54.74
Omentotomy 54.19
Omphalectomy 54.3
Onychectomy 86.23
Onychoplasty 86.86
Onychotomy 86.09
  with drainage 86.04
Oophorectomy (unilateral) 65.39
  with salpingectomy 65.49
    laparoscopic 65.41
  bilateral (same operative episode) 65.51
    laparoscopic 65.53
    with salpingectomy 65.61
      laparoscopic 65.63
  laparoscopic 65.31
  partial 65.29
    laparoscopic 65.25
    wedge 65.22
      that by laparoscope 65.24
  remaining ovary 65.52
    laparoscopic 65.54
    with tube 65.62
      laparoscopic 65.64
Oophorocystectomy 65.29
  laparoscopic 65.25
Oophoropexy 65.79
Oophoroplasty 65.79
Oophororrhaphy 65.71
  laparoscopic 65.74
Oophorostomy 65.09
  laparoscopic 65.01
Oophorotomy 65.09
  laparoscopic 65.01
Opening
  bony labyrinth (ear) 20.79
  cranial suture 02.01
  heart valve
    closed heart technique - *see* Valvulotomy,
      by site
    open heart technique - *see* Valvuloplasty,
      by site
  spinal dura 03.09
Operation
  Abbe
    construction of vagina 70.61
      with graft or prosthesis 70.63
    intestinal anastomosis - *see* Anastomosis,
      intestine
  abdominal (region) NEC 54.99
  abdominoperineal, NOS 48.50
    laparoscopic 48.51
    open 48.52
    other 48.59

Operation (*Continued*)
  Aburel (intra-amniotic injection for abortion)
    75.0
  Adams
    advancement of round ligament 69.22
    crushing of nasal septum 21.88
    excision of palmar fascia 82.35
  adenoids NEC 28.99
  adrenal (gland) (nerve) (vessel) NEC 07.49
  Albee
    bone peg, femoral neck 78.05
    graft for slipping patella 78.06
    sliding inlay graft, tibia 78.07
  Albert (arthrodesis, knee) 81.22
  Aldridge (-Studdiford) (urethral sling) 59.5
  Alexander
    prostatectomy
      perineal 60.62
      suprapubic 60.3
    shortening of round ligaments of uterus
      69.22
  Alexander-Adams (shortening of round
    ligaments of uterus) 69.22
  Almoor (extrapetrosal drainage) 20.22
  Altemeier (perineal rectal pull-through)
    48.49
  Ammon (dacryocystotomy) 09.53
  Anderson (tibial lengthening) 78.37
  Anel (dilation of lacrimal duct) 09.42
  anterior chamber (eye) NEC 12.99
  anti-incontinence NEC 59.79
  antrum window (nasal sinus) 22.2
    with Caldwell-Luc approach 22.39
  anus NEC 49.99
  aortic body NEC 39.89
  aorticopulmonary window 39.59
  appendix NEC 47.99
  Arslan (fenestration of inner ear) 20.61
  artery NEC 39.99
  Asai (larynx) 31.75
  Baffes (interatrial transposition of venous
    return) 35.91
  Baldy-Webster (uterine suspension) 69.22
  Ball
    herniorrhaphy - *see* Repair, hernia,
      inguinal
    undercutting 49.02
  Bankhart (capsular repair into glenoid, for
    shoulder dislocation) 81.82
  Bardenheurer (ligation of innominate artery)
    38.85
  Barkan (goniotomy) 12.52
    with goniopuncture 12.53

Operation *(Continued)*
Barr (transfer of tibialis posterior tendon) 83.75
Barsky (closure of cleft hand) 82.82
Bassett (vulvectomy with inguinal lymph node dissection) 71.5 [40.3]
Bassini (herniorrhaphy) - *see* Repair, hernia, inguinal
Batch-Spittler-McFaddin (knee disarticulation) 84.16
Batista (partial ventriculectomy) (ventricular reduction) (ventricular remodeling) 37.35
Beck I (epicardial poudrage) 36.39
Beck II (aorta-coronary sinus shunt) 36.39
Beck-Jianu (permanent gastrostomy) 43.19
Bell-Beuttner (subtotal abdominal hysterectomy) 68.39
Belsey (esophagogastric sphincter) 44.65
Benenenti (rotation of bulbous urethra) 58.49
Berke (levator resection eyelid) 08.33
Biesenberger (size reduction of breast, bilateral) 85.32
unilateral 85.31
Bigelow (litholapaxy) 57.0
biliary (duct) (tract) NEC 51.99
Billroth I (partial gastrectomy with gastroduodenostomy) 43.6
Billroth II (partial gastrectomy with gastrojejunostomy) 43.7
Binnie (hepatopexy) 50.69
Bischoff (ureteroneocystostomy) 56.74
bisection hysterectomy 68.39
laparoscopic 68.31
Bishoff (spinal myelotomy) 03.29
bladder NEC 57.99
flap 56.74
Blalock (systemic-pulmonary anastomosis) 39.0
Blalock-Hanlon (creation of atrial septal defect) 35.42
Blalock-Taussig (subclavian-pulmonary anastomosis) 39.0
Blascovic (resection and advancement of levator palpebrae superioris) 08.33
blood vessel NEC 39.99
Blount
femoral shortening (with blade plate) 78.25
by epiphyseal stapling 78.25
Boari (bladder flap) 56.74
Bobb (cholelithotomy) 51.04
bone NEC - *see* category 78.4●
facial 76.99
injury NEC - *see* category 79.9●
marrow NEC 41.98
skull NEC 02.99
Bonney (abdominal hysterectomy) 68.49
laparoscopic 68.41
Borthen (iridotasis) 12.63
Bost
plantar dissection 80.48
radiocarpal fusion 81.26
Bosworth
arthroplasty for acromioclavicular separation 81.83
fusion of posterior lumbar spine 81.08
for pseudarthrosis 81.38
resection of radial head ligaments (for tennis elbow) 80.92
shelf procedure, hip 81.40
Bottle (repair of hydrocele of tunica vaginalis) 61.2
Boyd (hip disarticulation) 84.18
brain NEC 02.99
Brauer (cardiolysis) 37.10
breast NEC 85.99
Bricker (ileoureterostomy) 56.51
Bristow (repair of shoulder dislocation) 81.82
Brock (pulmonary valvulotomy) 35.03

Operation *(Continued)*
Brockman (soft tissue release for clubfoot) 83.84
bronchus NEC 33.98
Browne (-Denis) (hypospadias repair) 58.45
Brunschwig (temporary gastrostomy) 43.19
buccal cavity NEC 27.99
Bunnell (tendon transfer) 82.56
Burch procedure (retropubic urethral suspension for urinary stress incontinence) 59.5
Burgess (amputation of ankle) 84.14
bursa NEC 83.99
hand 82.99
bypass - *see* Bypass
Caldwell (sulcus extension) 24.91
Caldwell-Luc (maxillary sinusotomy) 22.39
with removal of membrane lining 22.31
Callander (knee disarticulation) 84.16
Campbell
bone block, ankle 81.11
fasciotomy (iliac crest) 83.14
reconstruction of anterior cruciate ligaments 81.45
canthus NEC 08.99
cardiac NEC 37.99
septum NEC 35.98
valve NEC 35.99
carotid body or gland NEC 39.89
Carroll and Taber (arthroplasty proximal interphalangeal joint) 81.72
Cattell (herniorrhaphy) 53.51
Cecil (urethral reconstruction) 58.46
cecum NEC 46.99
cerebral (meninges) NEC 02.99
cervix NEC 69.99
Chandler (hip fusion) 81.21
Charles (correction of lymphedema) 40.9
Charnley (compression arthrodesis)
ankle 81.11
hip 81.21
knee 81.22
Cheatle-Henry - *see* Repair, hernia, femoral
chest cavity NEC 34.99
Chevalier-Jackson (partial laryngectomy) 30.29
Child (radical subtotal pancreatectomy) 52.53
Chopart (midtarsal amputation) 84.12
chordae tendineae NEC 35.32
choroid NEC 14.9
ciliary body NEC 12.98
cisterna chyli NEC 40.69
Clagett (closure of chest wall following open flap drainage) 34.72
Clayton (resection of metatarsal heads and bases of phalanges) 77.88
clitoris NEC 71.4
cocked hat (metacarpal lengthening and transfer of local flap) 82.69
Cockett (varicose vein)
lower limb 38.59
upper limb 38.53
Cody tack (perforation of footplate) 19.0
Coffey (uterine suspension) (Meigs' modification) 69.22
Cole (anterior tarsal wedge osteotomy) 77.28
Collis-Nissen (hiatal hernia repair) 53.80
colon NEC 46.99
Colonna
adductor tenotomy (first stage) 83.12
hip arthroplasty (second stage) 81.40
reconstruction of hip (second stage) 81.40
commando (radical glossectomy) 25.4
conjunctiva NEC 10.99
destructive NEC 10.33
cornea NEC 11.99
Coventry (tibial wedge osteotomy) 77.27
Cox-maze procedure (ablation or destruction of heart tissue) - *see* maze procedure

Operation *(Continued)*
Crawford (tarso-frontalis sling of eyelid) 08.32
cul-de-sac NEC 70.92
Culp-Deweerd (spiral flap pyeloplasty) 55.87
Culp-Scardino (ureteral flap pyeloplasty) 55.87
Curtis (interphalangeal joint arthroplasty) 81.72
cystocele NEC 70.51
Dahlman (excision of esophageal diverticulum) 42.31
Dana (posterior rhizotomy) 03.1
Danforth (fetal) 73.8
Darrach (ulnar resection) 77.83
Davis (intubated ureterotomy) 56.2
de Grandmont (tarsectomy) 08.35
Delorme
pericardiectomy 37.31
proctopexy 48.76
repair of prolapsed rectum 48.76
thoracoplasty 33.34
Denker (radical maxillary antrotomy) 22.31
Dennis-Varco (herniorrhaphy) - *see* Repair, hernia, femoral
Denonvillier (limited rhinoplasty) 21.86
dental NEC 24.99
orthodontic NEC 24.8
Derlacki (tympanoplasty) 19.4
diaphragm NEC 34.89
Dickson (fascial transplant) 83.82
Dickson-Diveley (tendon transfer and arthrodesis to correct claw toe) 77.57
Dieffenbach (hip disarticulation) 84.18
digestive tract NEC 46.99
Doleris (shortening of round ligaments) 69.22
D'Ombrain (excision of pterygium with corneal graft) 11.32
Dorrance (push-back operation for cleft palate) 27.62
Dotter (transluminal angioplasty) 39.59
Douglas (suture of tongue to lip for micrognathia) 25.59
Doyle (paracervical uterine denervation) 69.3
Dühamel (abdominoperineal pull-through) 48.65
Duhrssen (vaginofixation of uterus) 69.22
Dunn (triple arthrodesis) 81.12
duodenum NEC 46.99
Dupuytren
fasciectomy 82.35
fasciotomy 82.12
with excision 82.35
shoulder disarticulation 84.08
Durham (-Caldwell) (transfer of biceps femoris tendon) 83.75
DuToit and Roux (staple capsulorrhaphy of shoulder) 81.82
DuVries (tenoplasty) 83.88
Dwyer
fasciotomy 83.14
soft tissue release NEC 83.84
wedge osteotomy, calcaneus 77.28
Eagleton (extrapetrosal drainage) 20.22
ear (external) NEC 18.9
middle or inner NEC 20.99
Eden-Hybinette (glenoid bone block) 78.01
Effler (heart) 36.2
Eggers
tendon release (patellar retinacula) 83.13
tendon transfer (biceps femoris tendon) (hamstring tendon) 83.75
Elliot (scleral trephination with iridectomy) 12.61
Ellis Jones (repair of peroneal tendon) 83.88
Ellison (reinforcement of collateral ligament) 81.44
Elmslie-Cholmeley (tarsal wedge osteotomy) 77.28

Operation *(Continued)*
  Eloesser
    thoracoplasty 33.34
    thoracostomy 34.09
  Emmet (cervix) 67.61
  endorectal pull-through 48.41
  epididymis NEC 63.99
  esophagus NEC 42.99
  Estes (ovary) 65.72
    laparoscopic 65.75
  Estlander (thoracoplasty) 33.34
  Evans (release of clubfoot) 83.84
  extraocular muscle NEC 15.9
    multiple (two or more muscles) 15.4
      with temporary detachment from
        globe 15.3
      revision 15.6
    single 15.29
      with temporary detachment from
        globe 15.19
  eyeball NEC 16.99
  eyelid(s) NEC 08.99
  face NEC 27.99
  facial bone or joint NEC 76.99
  fallopian tube NEC 66.99
  Farabeuf (ischiopubiotomy) 77.39
  Fasanella-Servatt (blepharoptosis repair)
    08.35
  fascia NEC 83.99
    hand 82.99
  female (genital organs) NEC 71.9
    hysterectomy NEC 68.9
  fenestration (aorta) 39.54
  Ferguson (hernia repair) 53.00
  Fick (perforation of footplate) 19.0
  filtering (for glaucoma) 12.79
    with iridectomy 12.65
  Finney (pyloroplasty) 44.29
  fistulizing, sclera NEC 12.69
  Foley (pyeloplasty) 55.87
  Fontan (creation of conduit between right
    atrium and pulmonary artery) 35.94
  Fothergill (-Donald) (uterine suspension)
    69.22
  Fowler
    arthroplasty of metacarpophalangeal joint
      81.72
    release (mallet finger repair) 82.84
    tenodesis (hand) 82.85
    thoracoplasty 33.34
  Fox (entropion repair with wedge resection)
    08.43
  Franco (suprapubic cystotomy) 57.19
  Frank (permanent gastrostomy) 43.19
  Frazier (-Spiller) (subtemporal trigeminal
    rhizotomy) 04.02
  Fredet-Ramstedt (pyloromyotomy) (with
    wedge resection) 43.3
  Frenckner (intrapetrosal drainage) 20.22
  Frickman (abdominal proctopexy) 48.75
  Frommel (shortening of uterosacral
    ligaments) 69.22
  Gabriel (abdominoperineal resection of
    rectum), NOS 48.50
    laparoscopic 48.51
    open 48.52
    other 48.59
  gallbladder NEC 51.99
  ganglia NEC 04.99
    sympathetic 05.89
  Gant (wedge osteotomy of trochanter)
    77.25
  Garceau (tibial tendon transfer) 83.75
  Gardner (spinal meningocele repair)
    03.51
  gastric NEC 44.99
  Gelman (release of clubfoot) 83.84
  genital organ NEC
    female 71.9
    male 64.99
  Ghormley (hip fusion) 81.21

Operation *(Continued)*
  Giffod
    destruction of lacrimal sac 09.6
    keratotomy (delimiting) 11.1
  Gill
    arthrodesis of shoulder 81.23
    laminectomy 03.09
  Gill-Stein (carporadial arthrodesis) 81.25
  Gilliam (uterine suspension) 69.22
  Girdlestone
    laminectomy with spinal fusion 81.00
    muscle transfer for claw toe 77.57
    resection of femoral head and neck
      (without insertion of joint
      prosthesis) 77.85
      with replacement prosthesis - *see*
        Implant, joint, hip
    resection of hip prosthesis 80.05
      with replacement prosthesis - *see*
        Implant, joint, hip
  Girdlestone-Taylor (muscle transfer for claw
    toe repair) 77.57
  glaucoma NEC 12.79
  Glenn (anastomosis of superior vena cava to
    right pulmonary artery) 39.21
  globus pallidus NEC 01.42
  Goebel-Frangenheim-Stoeckel
    (urethrovesical suspension) 59.4
  Goldner (clubfoot release) 80.48
  Goldthwaite
    ankle stabilization 81.11
    patella stabilization 81.44
    tendon transfer for patella dislocation
      81.44
  Goodall-Power (vagina) 70.4
  Gordon-Taylor (hindquarter amputation)
    84.19
  Graber-Duvernay (drilling femoral head)
    77.15
  Green (scapulopexy) 78.41
  Grice (subtalar arthrodesis) 81.13
  Gritti-Stokes (knee disarticulation) 84.16
  Gross (herniorrhaphy)
    laparoscopic 53.43
      with graft or prosthesis 53.42
    other and open with graft or prosthesis
      53.41
    other open 53.49
  gum NEC 24.39
  Guyon (amputation of ankle) 84.13
  Hagner (epididymotomy) 63.92
  Halsted - *see* Repair, hernia, inguinal
  Halsted mastectomy 85.45
  Hampton (anastomosis small intestine to
    rectal stump) 45.92
  hanging hip (muscle release) 83.19
  harelip 27.54
  Harrison-Richardson (vaginal suspension)
    70.77
    with graft or prosthesis 70.78
  Hartmann - *see* Colectomy, by site
  Hauser
    achillotenotomy 83.11
    bunionectomy with adductor tendon
      transfer 77.53
    stabilization of patella 81.44
  Heaney (vaginal hysterectomy) 68.59
    laparoscopically assisted (LAVH) 68.51
  heart NEC 37.99
    valve NEC 35.99
      adjacent structure NEC 35.39
  Hegar (perineorrhaphy) 71.79
  Heine (cyclodialysis) 12.55
  Heineke-Mikulicz (pyloroplasty) - *see*
    category 44.2●
  Heller (esophagomyotomy) 42.7
  Hellström (transplantation of aberrant renal
    vessel) 39.55
  hemorrhoids NEC 49.49
  Henley (jejunal transposition) 43.81
  hepatic NEC 50.99

Operation *(Continued)*
  hernia - *see* Repair, hernia
  Hey (amputation of foot) 84.12
  Hey-Groves (reconstruction of anterior
    cruciate ligament) 81.45
  Heyman (soft tissue release for clubfoot)
    83.84
  Heyman-Herndon (-Strong) (correction of
    metatarsus varus) 80.48
  Hibbs (lumbar spinal fusion) - *see* Fusion,
    lumbar
  Higgins - *see* Repair, hernia, femoral
  Hill-Allison (hiatal hernia repair,
    transpleural approach) 53.80
  Hitchcock (anchoring tendon of biceps)
    83.88
  Hofmeister (gastrectomy) 43.7
  Hoke
    midtarsal fusion 81.14
    triple arthrodesis 81.12
  Holth
    iridencleisis 12.63
    sclerectomy 12.65
  Homan (correction of lymphedema) 40.9
  Hutch (ureteroneocystostomy) 56.74
  Hybinette-Eden (glenoid bone block) 78.01
  hymen NEC 70.91
  hypopharynx NEC 29.99
  hypophysis NEC 07.79
  ileal loop 56.51
  ileum NEC 46.99
  intestine NEC 46.99
  iris NEC 12.97
    inclusion 12.63
  Irving (tubal ligation) 66.32
  Irwin - *see also* Osteotomy 77.30
  Jaboulay (gastroduodenostomy) 44.39
    laparoscopic 44.38
  Janeway (permanent gastrostomy) 43.19
  Jatene (arterial switch) 35.84
  jejunum NEC 46.99
  Johanson (urethral reconstruction) 58.46
  joint (capsule) (ligament) (structure) NEC
    81.99
    facial NEC 76.99
  Jones
    claw toe (transfer of extensor hallucis
      longus tendon) 77.57
      modified (with arthrodesis) 77.57
    dacryocystorhinostomy 09.81
    hammer toe (interphalangeal fusion)
      77.56
    modified (tendon transfer with
      arthrodesis) 77.57
    repair of peroneal tendon 83.88
  Joplin (exostectomy with tendon transfer)
    77.53
  Kader (temporary gastrostomy) 43.19
  Kaufman (for urinary stress incontinence)
    59.79
  Kazanjiian (buccal vestibular sulcus
    extension) 24.91
  Kehr (hepatopexy) 50.69
  Keller (bunionectomy) 77.59
  Kelly (-Kennedy) (urethrovesical plication)
    59.3
  Kelly-Stoeckel (urethrovesical plication) 59.3
  Kerr (cesarean section) 74.1
  Kessler (arthroplasty, carpometacarpal joint)
    81.74
  Kidner (excision of accessory navicular bone)
    (with tendon transfer) 77.98
  kidney NEC 55.99
  Killian (frontal sinusotomy) 22.41
  King-Steelquist (hindquarter amputation)
    84.19
  Kirk (amputation through thigh) 84.17
  Kock pouch
    bowel anastomosis - *omit code*
    continent ileostomy 46.22
    cutaneous uretero-ileostomy 56.51

Operation (Continued)

Kock pouch (Continued)

ESWL (electrocorporeal shock wave lithotripsy) 98.51

removal, calculus 57.19

revision, cutaneous uretero-ileostomy 56.52

urinary diversion procedure 56.51

Kondoleon (correction of lymphedema) 40.9

Krause (sympathetic denervation) 05.29

Kroener (partial salpingectomy) 66.69

Kroenlein (lateral orbitotomy) 16.01

Kronig (low cervical cesarean section) 74.1

Krukenberg (reconstruction of below-elbow amputation) 82.89

Kuhnt-Szymanowski (ectropion repair with lid reconstruction) 08.44

Labbe (gastrotomy) 43.0

labia NEC 71.8

lacrimal

gland 09.3

system NEC 09.99

Ladd (mobilization of intestine) 54.95

Lagrange (iridosclerectomy) 12.65

Lambrinudi (triple arthrodesis) 81.12

Langenbeck (cleft palate repair) 27.62

Lapidus (bunionectomy with metatarsal osteotomy) 77.51

Larry (shoulder disarticulation) 84.08

larynx NEC 31.98

Lash

internal cervical os repair 67.59

laparoscopic supracervical hysterectomy 68.31

Latzko

cesarean section, extraperitoneal 74.2

colpocleisis 70.8

Leadbetter (urethral reconstruction) 58.46

Leadbetter-Politano (ureteroneocystostomy) 56.74

Le Fort (colpocleisis) 70.8

LeMesurier (cleft lip repair) 27.54

lens NEC 13.90

Leriche (periarterial sympathectomy) 05.25

levator muscle sling

eyelid ptosis repair 08.33

urethrovesical suspension 59.71

urinary stress incontinence 59.71

lid suture (blepharoptosis) 08.31

ligament NEC 81.99

broad NEC 69.98

round NEC 69.98

uterine NEC 69.98

Lindholm (repair of ruptured tendon) 83.88

Linton (varicose vein) 38.59

lip NEC 27.99

Lisfranc

foot amputation 84.12

shoulder disarticulation 84.08

Littlewood (forequarter amputation) 84.09

liver NEC 50.99

Lloyd-Davies (abdominoperineal resection), NOS 48.50

laparoscopic 48.51

open 48.52

other 48.59

Longmire (bile duct anastomosis) 51.39

Lord

dilation of anal canal for hemorrhoids 49.49

hemorrhoidectomy 49.49

orchidopexy 62.5

Lucas and Murray (knee arthrodesis with plate) 81.22

lung NEC 33.99

lung volume reduction 32.22

biologic lung volume reduction (BLVR) - see category 33.7●

lymphatic structure(s) NEC 40.9

duct, left (thoracic) NEC 40.69

Madlener (tubal ligation) 66.31

Operation (Continued)

Magnuson (-Stack) (arthroplasty for recurrent shoulder dislocation) 81.82

male genital organs NEC 64.99

Manchester (-Donald) (-Fothergill) (uterine suspension) 69.22

mandible NEC 76.99

orthognathic 76.64

Marckwald (cervical os repair) 67.59

Marshall-Marchetti (-Krantz) (retropubic urethral suspension) 59.5

Matas (aneurysmorrhaphy) 39.52

Mayo

bunionectomy 77.59

herniorrhaphy

laparoscopic 53.43

with graft or prosthesis 53.42

other and open with graft or prosthesis 53.41

other open 53.49

vaginal hysterectomy 68.59

laparoscopically assisted (LAVH) 68.51

maze procedure (ablation or destruction of heart tissue)

by incision (open) 37.33

by median sternotomy 37.33

by peripherally inserted catheter 37.34

by thoracotomy without thoracoscope 37.33

endovascular approach 37.34

Mazet (knee disarticulation) 84.16

McBride (bunionectomy with soft tissue correction) 77.53

McBurney - see Repair, hernia, inguinal

McCall (enterocele repair) 70.92

with graft or prosthesis 70.93

McCauley (release of clubfoot) 83.84

McDonald (encirclement suture, cervix) 67.59

McIndoe (vaginal construction) 70.61

with graft or prosthesis 70.63

McKeever (fusion of first metatarsophalangeal joint for hallux valgus repair) 77.52

McKissock (breast reduction) 85.33

McReynolds (transposition of pterygium) 11.31

McVay

femoral hernia - see Repair, hernia, femoral

inguinal hernia - see Repair, hernia, inguinal

meninges (spinal) NEC 03.99

cerebral NEC 02.99

mesentery NEC 54.99

Mikulicz (exteriorization of intestine) (first stage) 46.03

second stage 46.04

Miles (complete proctectomy), NOS 48.50

laparoscopic 48.51

open 48.52

other 48.59

Millard (cheiloplasty) 27.54

Miller

midtarsal arthrodesis 81.14

urethrovesical suspension 59.4

Millin-Read (urethrovesical suspension) 59.4

Mitchell (hallux valgus repair) 77.51

Mohs (chemosurgical excision of skin) 86.24

Moore (arthroplasty) 81.52

Moschowitz

enterocele repair 70.92

with graft or prosthesis 70.93

herniorrhaphy - see Repair, hernia, femoral

sigmoidopexy 46.63

mouth NEC 27.99

Muller (banding of pulmonary artery) 38.85

Mumford (partial claviculectomy) 77.81

Operation (Continued)

muscle NEC 83.99

extraocular - see Operation, extraocular

hand NEC 82.99

papillary heart NEC 35.31

musculoskeletal system NEC 84.99

Mustard (interatrial transposition of venous return) 35.91

nail (finger) (toe) NEC 86.99

nasal sinus NEC 22.9

nasopharynx NEC 29.99

nerve (cranial) (peripheral) NEC 04.99

adrenal NEC 07.49

sympathetic NEC 05.89

nervous system NEC 05.9

Nicola (tenodesis for recurrent dislocation of shoulder) 81.82

nipple NEC 85.99

Nissen (fundoplication of stomach) 44.66

laparoscopic 44.67

Noble (plication of small intestine) 46.62

node (lymph) NEC 40.9

Norman Miller (vaginopexy) 70.77

with graft or prosthesis 70.78

Norton (extraperitoneal cesarean operation) 74.2

nose, nasal NEC 21.99

sinus NEC 22.9

Ober (-Yount) (gluteal-iliotibial fasciotomy) 83.14

obstetric NEC 75.99

ocular NEC 16.99

muscle - see Operation, extraocular muscle

O'Donoghue (triad knee repair) 81.43

Olshausen (uterine suspension) 69.22

omentum NEC 54.99

ophthalmologic NEC 16.99

oral cavity NEC 27.99

orbicularis muscle sling 08.36

orbit NEC 16.98

oropharynx NEC 29.99

orthodontic NEC 24.8

orthognathic NEC 76.69

Oscar Miller (midtarsal arthrodesis) 81.14

Osmond-Clark (soft tissue release with peroneus brevis tendon transfer) 83.75

ovary NEC 65.99

Oxford (for urinary incontinence) 59.4

palate NEC 27.99

palpebral ligament sling 08.36

Panas (linear proctotomy) 48.0

Pancoast (division of trigeminal nerve at foramen ovale) 04.02

pancreas NEC 52.99

pantaloon (revision of gastric anastomosis) 44.5

papillary muscle (heart) NEC 35.31

Paquin (ureteroneocystostomy) 56.74

parathyroid gland(s) NEC 06.99

parotid gland or duct NEC 26.99

Partsch (marsupialization of dental cyst) 24.4

Pattee (auditory canal) 18.6

Peet (splanchnic resection) 05.29

Pemberton

osteotomy of ilium 77.39

rectum (mobilization and fixation for prolapse repair) 48.76

penis NEC 64.98

Pereyra (paraurethral suspension) 59.6

pericardium NEC 37.99

perineum (female) NEC 71.8

male NEC 86.99

perirectal tissue NEC 48.99

perirenal tissue NEC 59.92

peritoneum NEC 54.99

periurethral tissue NEC 58.99

perivesical tissue NEC 59.92

pharyngeal flap (cleft palate repair) 27.62

secondary or subsequent 27.63

pharynx, pharyngeal (pouch) NEC 29.99

Operation *(Continued)*
  pineal gland NEC 07.59
  Pinsker (obliteration of nasoseptal telangiectasia) 21.07
  Piper (forceps) 72.6
  Pirogoff (ankle amputation through malleoli of tibia and fibula) 84.14
  pituitary gland NEC 07.79
  plastic - *see* Repair, by site
  pleural cavity NEC 34.99
  Politano-Leadbetter (ureteroneocystostomy) 56.74
  pollicization (with nerves and blood supply) 82.61
  Polya (gastrectomy) 43.7
  Pomeroy (ligation and division of fallopian tubes) 66.32
  Poncet
    lengthening of Achilles tendon 83.85
    urethrostomy, perineal 58.0
  Porro (cesarean section) 74.99
  posterior chamber (eye) NEC 14.9
  Potts-Smith (descending aorta-left pulmonary artery anastomosis) 39.0
  Printen and Mason (high gastric bypass) 44.31
  prostate NEC - *see also* Prostatectomy 60.69
    specified type 60.99
  pterygium 11.39
    with corneal graft 11.32
  Puestow (pancreaticojejunostomy) 52.96
  pull-through NEC 48.49
  pulmonary NEC 33.99
  push-back (cleft palate repair) 27.62
  Putti-Platt (capsulorrhaphy of shoulder for recurrent dislocation) 81.82
  pyloric exclusion 44.39
    laparoscopic 44.38
  pyriform sinus NEC 29.99
  "rabbit ear" (anterior urethropexy) (Tudor) 59.79
  Ramadier (intrapetrosal drainage) 20.22
  Ramstedt (pyloromyotomy) (with wedge resection) 43.3
  Rankin
    exteriorization of intestine 46.03
    proctectomy (complete), NOS 48.50
      laparoscopic 48.51
      open 48.52
      other 48.59
  Rashkind (balloon septostomy) 35.41
  Rastelli (creation of conduit between right ventricle and pulmonary artery) 35.92
    in repair of
      pulmonary artery atresia 35.92
      transposition of great vessels 35.92
      truncus arteriosus 35.83
  Raz-Pereyra procedure (bladder neck suspension) 59.79
  rectal NEC 48.99
  rectocele NEC 70.52
  re-entry (aorta) 39.54
  renal NEC 55.99
  respiratory (tract) NEC 33.99
  retina NEC 14.9
  Ripstein (repair of rectal prolapse) 48.75
  Rodney Smith (radical subtotal pancreatectomy) 52.53
  Roux-en-Y
    bile duct 51.36
    cholecystojejunostomy 51.32
    esophagus (intrathoracic) 42.54
    gastroenterostomy 44.39
      laparoscopic 44.38
    gastrojejunostomy 44.39
      laparoscopic 44.38
    pancreaticojejunostomy 52.96
  Roux-Goldthwait (repair of patellar dislocation) 81.44
  Roux-Herzen-Judine (jejunal loop interposition) 42.63

Operation *(Continued)*
  Ruiz-Mora (proximal phalangectomy for hammer toe) 77.99
  Russe (bone graft of scaphoid) 78.04
  Saemisch (corneal section) 11.1
  salivary gland or duct NEC 26.99
  Salter (innominate osteotomy) 77.39
  Sauer-Bacon (abdominoperineal resection), NOS 48.50
    laparoscopic 48.51
    open 48.52
    other 48.59
  Schanz (femoral osteotomy) 77.35
  Schauta (-Amreich) (radical vaginal hysterectomy) 68.79
    laparoscopic 68.71
  Schede (thoracoplasty) 33.34
  Scheie
    cautery of sclera 12.62
    sclerostomy 12.62
  Schlatter (total gastrectomy) 43.99
  Schroeder (endocervical excision) 67.39
  Schuchardt (nonobstetrical episiotomy) 71.09
  Schwartze (simple mastoidectomy) 20.41
  sclera NEC 12.89
  Scott
    intestinal bypass for obesity 45.93
    jejunocolostomy (bypass) 45.93
  scrotum NEC 61.99
  Seddon-Brooks (transfer of pectoralis major tendon) 83.75
  Semb (apicolysis of lung) 33.39
  seminal vesicle NEC 60.79
  Senning (correction of transposition of great vessels) 35.91
  Sever (division of soft tissue of arm) 83.19
  Sewell (heart) 36.2
  sex transformation NEC 64.5
  Sharrard (iliopsoas muscle transfer) 83.77
  shelf (hip arthroplasty) 81.40
  Shirodkar (encirclement suture, cervix) 67.59
  sigmoid NEC 46.99
  Silver (bunionectomy) 77.59
  Sistrunk (excision of thyroglossal cyst) 06.7
  Skene's gland NEC 71.8
  skin NEC 86.99
  skull NEC 02.99
  sling
    eyelid
      fascia lata, palpebral 08.36
      frontalis fascial 08.32
      levator muscle 08.33
      orbicularis muscle 08.36
      palpebrae ligament, fascia lata 08.36
      tarsus muscle 08.35
    fascial (fascia lata)
      eye 08.32
      for facial weakness (trigeminal nerve paralysis) 86.81
      palpebral ligament 08.36
      tongue 25.59
    tongue (fascial) 25.59
    urethra (suprapubic) 59.4
      retropubic 59.5
    urethrovesical 59.5
  Slocum (pes anserinus transfer) 81.47
  Sluder (tonsillectomy) 28.2
  Smith (open osteotomy of mandible) 76.62
  Smith-Peterson (radiocarpal arthrodesis) 81.25
  Smithwick (sympathectomy) 05.29
  Soave (endorectal pull-through) 48.41
  soft tissue NEC 83.99
    hand 82.99
  Sonneberg (inferior maxillary neurectomy) 04.07
  Sorondo-Ferré (hindquarter amputation) 84.19
  Soutter (iliac crest fasciotomy) 83.14
  Spalding-Richardson (uterine suspension) 69.22

Operation *(Continued)*
  spermatic cord NEC 63.99
  sphincter of Oddi NEC 51.89
  spinal (canal) (cord) (structures) NEC 03.99
  Spinelli (correction of inverted uterus) 75.93
  Spivack (permanent gastrostomy) 43.19
  spleen NEC 41.99
  S.P. Rogers (knee disarticulation) 84.16
  Ssabanejew-Frank (permanent gastrostomy) 43.19
  Stacke (simple mastoidectomy) 20.41
  Stallard (conjunctivocystorhinostomy) 09.82
    with insertion of tube or stent 09.83
  Stamm (-Kader) (temporary gastrostomy) 43.19
  Steinberg 44.5
  Steindler
    fascia stripping (for cavus deformity) 83.14
    flexorplasty (elbow) 83.77
    muscle transfer 83.77
  sterilization NEC
    female - *see also* specific operation 66.39
    male - *see also* Ligation, vas deferens 63.70
  Stewart (renal plication with pyeloplasty) 55.87
  stomach NEC 44.99
  Stone (anoplasty) 49.79
  Strassman (metroplasty) 69.49
    metroplasty (Jones modification) 69.49
    uterus 68.22
  Strayer (gastrocnemius recession) 83.72
  stress incontinence - *see* Repair, stress incontinence
  Stromeyer-Little (hepatotomy) 50.0
  Strong (unbridling of celiac artery axis) 39.91
  Sturmdorf (conization of cervix) 67.2
  subcutaneous tissue NEC 86.99
  sublingual gland or duct NEC 26.99
  submaxillary gland or duct NEC 26.99
  Summerskill (dacryocystorhinostomy by intubation) 09.81
  Surmay (jejunostomy) 46.39
  Swenson
    bladder reconstruction 57.87
    proctectomy 48.49
  Swinney (urethral reconstruction) 58.46
  Syme
    ankle amputation through malleoli of tibia and fibula 84.14
    urethrotomy, external 58.0
  sympathetic nerve NEC 05.89
  Taarnhoj (trigeminal nerve root decompression) 04.41
  Tack (sacculotomy) 20.79
  Talma-Morison (omentopexy) 54.74
  Tanner (devascularization of stomach) 44.99
  TAPVC NEC 35.82
  tarsus NEC 08.99
    muscle sling 08.35
  tendon NEC 83.99
    extraocular NEC 15.9
    hand NEC 82.99
  testis NEC 62.99
  tetralogy of Fallot
    partial repair - *see* specific procedure
    total (one-stage) 35.81
  Thal (repair of esophageal stricture) 42.85
  thalamus 01.41
    by stereotactic radiosurgery 92.32
      cobalt 60 92.32
      linear accelerator (LINAC) 92.31
      multi-source 92.32
      particle beam 92.33
      particulate 92.33
      radiosurgery NEC 92.39
      single source photon 92.31
  Thiersch
    anus 49.79
    skin graft 86.69
      hand 86.62

◄ New   ⇚ Revised   ~~deleted~~ Deleted   ● Use Additional Digit(s)   ▨ Omit code

Operation (Continued)

Thompson
cleft lip repair 27.54
correction of lymphedema 40.9
quadricepsplasty 83.86
thumb apposition with bone graft 82.69
thoracic duct NEC 40.69
thorax NEC 34.99
Thorek (partial cholecystectomy) 51.21
three-snip, punctum 09.51
thymus NEC 07.99
thoracoscopic, NEC 07.98
thyroid gland NEC 06.98
TKP (thermokeratoplasty) 11.74
Tomkins (metroplasty) 69.49
tongue NEC 25.99
flap, palate 27.62
tie 25.91
tonsil NEC 28.99
Torek (-Bevan) (orchidopexy) (first stage)
(second stage) 62.5
Torkildsen (ventriculocisternal shunt) 02.22
Torpin (cul-de-sac resection) 70.92
Toti (dacryocystorhinostomy) 09.81
Touchas 86.83
Touroff (ligation of subclavian artery) 38.85
trabeculae corneae cordis (heart) NEC 35.35
trachea NEC 31.99
Trauner (lingual sulcus extension) 24.91
truncus arteriosus NEC 35.83
Tsuge (macrodactyly repair) 82.83
Tudor "rabbit ear" (anterior urethropexy) 59.79
Tuffier
apicolysis of lung 33.39
vaginal hysterectomy 68.59
laparoscopically assisted (LAVH) 68.51
tunica vaginalis NEC 61.99
Turco (release of joint capsules in clubfoot) 80.48
Uchida (tubal ligation with or without fimbriectomy) 66.32
umbilicus NEC 54.99
urachus NEC 57.51
Urban (mastectomy) (unilateral) 85.47
bilateral 85.48
ureter NEC 56.99
urethra NEC 58.99
urinary system NEC 59.99
uterus NEC 69.99
supporting structures NEC 69.98
uvula NEC 27.79
vagina NEC 70.91
vascular NEC 39.99
vas deferens NEC 63.99
ligation NEC 63.71
vein NEC 39.99
vena cava sieve 38.7
vertebra NEC 78.49
vesical (bladder) NEC 57.99
vessel NEC 39.99
cardiac NEC 36.99
Vicq d'Azyr (larynx) 31.1
Vidal (varicocele ligation) 63.1
Vineberg (implantation of mammary artery into ventricle) 36.2
vitreous NEC 14.79
vocal cord NEC 31.98
von Kraske (proctectomy) 48.64
Voss (hanging hip operation) 83.19
Vulpius (-Compere) (lengthening of gastrocnemius muscle) 83.85
vulva NEC 71.8
Ward-Mayo (vaginal hysterectomy) 68.59
laparoscopically assisted (LAVH) 68.51
Wardill (cleft palate) 27.62
Waters (extraperitoneal cesarean section) 74.2
Waterston (aorta-right pulmonary artery anastomosis) 39.0

Operation (Continued)

Watkins (-Wertheim) (uterus interposition) 69.21
Watson-Jones
hip arthrodesis 81.21
reconstruction of lateral ligaments, ankle 81.49
shoulder arthrodesis (extra-articular) 81.23
tenoplasty 83.88
Weir
appendicostomy 47.91
correction of nostrils 21.86
Wertheim (radical hysterectomy) 68.69
laparoscopic 68.61
West (dacryocystorhinostomy) 09.81
Wheeler
entropion repair 08.44
halving procedure (eyelid) 08.24
Whipple (radical pancreaticoduodenectomy) 52.7
Child modification (radical subtotal pancreatectomy) 52.53
Rodney Smith modification (radical subtotal pancreatectomy) 52.53
White (lengthening of tendo calcaneus by incomplete tenotomy) 83.11
Whitehead
glossectomy, radical 25.4
hemorrhoidectomy 49.46
Whitman
foot stabilization (talectomy) 77.98
hip reconstruction 81.40
repair of serratus anterior muscle 83.87
talectomy 77.98
trochanter wedge osteotomy 77.25
Wier (entropion repair) 08.44
Williams-Richardson (vaginal construction) 70.61
with graft or prosthesis 70.63
Wilms (thoracoplasty) 33.34
Wilson (angulation osteotomy for hallux valgus) 77.51
window
antrum (nasal sinus) - see Antrotomy, maxillary
aorticopulmonary 39.59
bone cortex - see also Incision, bone 77.10
facial 76.09
nasoantral - see Antrotomy, maxillary
pericardium 37.12
pleural 34.09
Winiwarter (cholecystoenterostomy) 51.32
Witzel (temporary gastrostomy) 43.19
Woodward (release of high riding scapula) 81.83
Young
epispadias repair 58.45
tendon transfer (anterior tibialis) (repair of flat foot) 83.75
Yount (division of iliotibial band) 83.14
Zancolli
capsuloplasty 81.72
tendon transfer (biceps) 82.56
Ziegler (iridectomy) 12.14
Operculectomy 24.6
Ophthalmectomy 16.49
with implant (into Tenon's capsule) 16.42
with attachment of muscles 16.41
Ophthalmoscopy 16.21
Opponensplasty (hand) 82.56
Optical coherence tomography (OCT) (intravascular imaging)
coronary vessel(s) 38.24
non-coronary vessel(s) 38.25
Orbitomaxillectomy, radical 16.51
Orbitotomy (anterior) (frontal) (temporofrontal) (transfrontal) NEC 16.09
with
bone flap 16.01
insertion of implant 16.02

Orbitotomy (Continued)

Kroenlein (lateral) 16.01
lateral 16.01
Orchidectomy (with epididymectomy) (unilateral) 62.3
bilateral (radical) 62.41
remaining or solitary testis 62.42
Orchidopexy 62.5
Orchidoplasty 62.69
Orchidorrhaphy 62.61
Orchidotomy 62.0
Orchiectomy (with epididymectomy) (unilateral) 62.3
bilateral (radical) 62.41
remaining or solitary testis 62.42
Orchiopexy 62.5
Orchioplasty 62.69
Orthoroentgenography - see Radiography
Oscar Miller operation (midtarsal arthrodesis) 81.14
Osmond-Clark operation (soft tissue release with peroneus brevis tendon transfer) 83.75
Ossiculectomy NEC 19.3
with
stapedectomy - see also Stapedectomy 19.19
stapes mobilization 19.0
tympanoplasty 19.53
revision 19.6
Ossiculotomy NEC 19.3
Ostectomy (partial), except facial - see also category 77.8 ●
facial NEC 76.39
total 76.45
with reconstruction 76.44
first metatarsal head - see Bunionectomy
for graft (autograft) (homograft) - see also category 77.7 ●
mandible 76.31
total 76.42
with reconstruction 76.41
total, except facial - see also category 77.9 ●
facial NEC 76.45
with reconstruction 76.44
mandible 76.42
with reconstruction 76.41
Osteoarthrotomy - see also Osteotomy 77.30
Osteoclasis 78.70
carpal, metacarpal 78.74
clavicle 78.71
ear 20.79
femur 78.75
fibula 78.77
humerus 78.72
patella 78.76
pelvic 78.79
phalanges (foot) (hand) 78.79
radius 78.73
scapula 78.71
specified site NEC 78.79
tarsal, metatarsal 78.78
thorax (ribs) (sternum) 78.71
tibia 78.77
ulna 78.73
vertebrae 78.79
Osteolysis - see category 78.4 ●
Osteopathic manipulation - see also Manipulation, osteopathic 93.67
Osteoplasty NEC - see category 78.4 ●
with bone graft - see Graft, bone
for
bone lengthening - see Lengthening, bone
bone shortening - see Shortening, bone
repair of malunion or nonunion of fracture - see Repair, fracture, malunion or nonunion
carpal, metacarpal 78.44
clavicle 78.41

Osteoplasty NEC *(Continued)*
cranium NEC 02.06
with
flap (bone) 02.03
graft (bone) 02.04
facial bone NEC 76.69
femur 78.45
fibula 78.47
humerus 78.42
mandible, mandibular NEC 76.64
body 76.63
ramus (open) 76.62
closed 76.61
maxilla (segmental) 76.65
total 76.66
nasal bones 21.89
patella 78.46
pelvic 78.49
phalanges (foot) (hand) 78.49
radius 78.43
scapula 78.41
skull NEC 02.06
with
flap (bone) 02.03
graft (bone) 02.04
specified site NEC 78.49
tarsal, metatarsal 78.48
thorax (ribs) (sternum) 78.41
tibia 78.47
ulna 78.43
vertebrae 78.49
Osteorrhaphy - *see also* Osteoplasty 78.40
Osteosynthesis (fracture) - *see* Reduction, fracture
Osteotomy (adduction) (angulation) (block) (derotational) (displacement) (partial) (rotational) 77.30
carpals, metacarpals 77.34
wedge 77.24
clavicle 77.31
wedge 77.21
facial bone NEC 76.69
femur 77.35
wedge 77.25
fibula 77.37
wedge 77.27

Osteotomy *(Continued)*
humerus 77.32
wedge 77.22
mandible (segmental) (subapical) 76.64
angle (open) 76.62
closed 76.61
body 76.63
Gigli saw 76.61
ramus (open) 76.62
closed 76.61
maxilla (segmental) 76.65
total 76.66
metatarsal 77.38
wedge 77.28
for hallux valgus repair 77.51
patella 77.36
wedge 77.26
pelvic 77.39
wedge 77.29
phalanges (foot) (hand) 77.39
for repair of
bunion - *see* Bunionectomy
bunionette 77.54
hallux valgus - *see* Bunionectomy
wedge 77.29
for repair of
bunion - *see* Bunionectomy
bunionette 77.54
hallux valgus - *see* Bunionectomy
radius 77.33
wedge 77.23
scapula 77.31
wedge 77.21
specified site NEC 77.39
wedge 77.29
tarsal 77.38
wedge 77.28
thorax (ribs) (sternum) 77.31
wedge 77.21
tibia 77.37
wedge 77.27
toe 77.39
for repair of
bunion - *see* Bunionectomy
bunionette 77.54
hallux valgus - *see* Bunionectomy

Osteotomy *(Continued)*
toe *(Continued)*
wedge 77.29
for repair of
bunion - *see* Bunionectomy
bunionette 77.54
hallux valgus - *see* Bunionectomy
ulna 77.33
wedge 77.23
vertebrae 77.39
wedge 77.29
Otonecrectomy (inner ear) 20.79
Otoplasty (external) 18.79
auditory canal or meatus 18.6
auricle 18.79
cartilage 18.79
reconstruction 18.71
prominent or protruding 18.5
Otoscopy 18.11
Outfolding, sclera, for buckling - *see also* Buckling, scleral 14.49
Outfracture, turbinates (nasal) 21.62
Output and clearance, circulatory 92.05
Overdistension, bladder (therapeutic) 96.25
Overlapping, sclera, for buckling - *see also* Buckling, scleral 14.49
Oversewing
left atrial appendage (LAA) 37.36
pleural bleb 32.21
ulcer crater (peptic) 44.40
duodenum 44.42
stomach 44.41
Oxford operation (for urinary incontinence) 59.4
Oximetry
fetal pulse 75.38
Oxygenation 93.96
extracorporeal membrane (ECMO) 39.65
hyperbaric 93.95
wound 93.59
infusion therapy, Super 00.49
Oxygen therapy (catalytic) (pump) 93.96
hyperbaric 93.95
SuperSaturated 00.49

P

Pacemaker
cardiac - *see also* Insertion, pacemaker, cardiac
intraoperative (temporary) 39.64
temporary (during and immediately following cardiac surgery) 39.64
Packing - *see also* Insertion, pack
auditory canal 96.11
nose, for epistaxis (anterior) 21.01
posterior (and anterior) 21.02
rectal 96.19
sella turcica 07.79
vaginal 96.14
Palatoplasty 27.69
for cleft palate 27.62
secondary or subsequent 27.63
Palatorrhaphy 27.61
for cleft palate 27.62
Pallidectomy 01.42
Pallidoansotomy 01.42
Pallidotomy 01.42
by stereotactic radiosurgery 92.32
cobalt 60 92.32
linear accelerator (LINAC) 92.31
multi-source 92.32
particle beam 92.33
particulate 92.33

Pallidotomy *(Continued)*
by stereotactic radiosurgery *(Continued)*
radiosurgery NEC 92.39
single source photon 92.31
Panas operation (linear proctotomy) 48.0
Pancoast operation (division of trigeminal nerve at foramen ovale) 04.02
Pancreatectomy (total) (with synchronous duodenectomy) 52.6
partial NEC 52.59
distal (tail) (with part of body) 52.52
proximal (head) (with part of body) (with synchronous duodenectomy) 52.51
radical 52.53
subtotal 52.53
radical 52.7
subtotal 52.53
Pancreaticocystoduodenostomy 52.4
Pancreaticocystoenterostomy 52.4
Pancreaticocystogastrostomy 52.4
Pancreaticocystojejunostomy 52.4
Pancreaticoduodenectomy (total) 52.6
partial NEC 52.59
proximal 52.51
radical subtotal 52.53
radical (one-stage) (two-stage) 52.7
subtotal 52.53
Pancreaticoduodenostomy 52.96

Pancreaticoenterostomy 52.96
Pancreaticogastrostomy 52.96
Pancreaticoileostomy 52.96
Pancreaticojejunostomy 52.96
Pancreatoduodenectomy (total) 52.6
partial NEC 52.59
radical (one-stage) (two-stage) 52.7
subtotal 52.53
Pancreatogram 87.66
endoscopic retrograde (ERP) 52.13
Pancreatolithotomy 52.09
endoscopic 52.94
Pancreatotomy 52.09
Pancreolithotomy 52.09
endoscopic 52.94
Panendoscopy 57.32
specified site, other than bladder - *see* Endoscopy, by site
through artificial stoma 57.31
Panhysterectomy (abdominal) 68.49
laparoscopic 68.41
vaginal 68.59
laparoscopically assisted (LAVH) 68.51
Panniculectomy 86.83
Panniculotomy 86.83
Pantaloon operation (revision of gastric anastomosis) 44.5
Papillectomy, anal 49.39
endoscopic 49.31

◀ New ◀▥ Revised ~~deleted~~ Deleted ● Use Additional Digit(s) ▨ Omit code

Papillotomy (pancreas) 51.82
  endoscopic 51.85
Paquin operation (ureteroneocystostomy)
  56.74
Paracentesis
  abdominal (percutaneous) 54.91
  anterior chamber, eye 12.91
  bladder 57.11
  cornea 12.91
  eye (anterior chamber) 12.91
  thoracic, thoracis 34.91
  tympanum 20.09
    with intubation 20.01
Parasitology - *see* Examination, microscopic
Parathyroidectomy (partial) (subtotal) NEC
  06.89
  complete 06.81
  ectopic 06.89
  global removal 06.81
  mediastinal 06.89
  total 06.81
Parenteral nutrition, total 99.15
  peripheral 99.15
Parotidectomy 26.30
  complete 26.32
  partial 26.31
  radical 26.32
Partsch operation (marsupialization of dental
  cyst) 24.4
Passage - *see* Insertion and Intubation
Passage of sounds, urethra 58.6
Patch
  blood, spinal (epidural) 03.95
  graft - *see* Graft
  spinal, blood (epidural) 03.95
  subdural, brain 02.12
Patellapexy 78.46
Patellaplasty NEC 78.46
Patellectomy 77.96
  partial 77.86
Pattee operation (auditory canal) 18.6
Pectenotomy - *see also* Sphincterotomy, anal
  49.59
PDT (percutaneous dilatational tracheostomy) –
  see Tracheostomy
Pedicle flap - *see* Graft, skin, pedicle
Peet operation (splanchnic resection) 05.29
PEG (percutaneous endoscopic gastrostomy)
  43.11
PEGJJ (percutaneous [endoscopic]
  gastrojejunostomy) 44.32
PEJ (percutaneous endoscopic jejunostomy)
  46.32
Pelvectomy, kidney (partial) 55.4
Pelvimetry 88.25
  gynecological 89.26
Pelviolithotomy 55.11
Pelvioplasty, kidney 55.87
Pelviostomy 55.12
  closure 55.82
Pelviotomy 77.39
  to assist delivery 73.94
Pelvi-ureteroplasty 55.87
Pemberton operation
  osteotomy of ilium 77.39
  rectum (mobilization and fixation for
    prolapse repair) 48.76
Penectomy 64.3
Pereyra operation (paraurethral suspension)
  59.6
Perforation
  stapes footplate 19.0
Perfusion NEC 39.97
  carotid artery 39.97
  coronary artery 39.97
  for
    chemotherapy NEC 99.25
    hormone therapy NEC 99.24
  head 39.97
  hyperthermic (lymphatic), localized region
    or site 93.35

Perfusion NEC (*Continued*)
  intestine (large) (local) 46.96
    small 46.95
  kidney, local 55.95
  limb (lower) (upper) 39.97
  liver, localized 50.93
  neck 39.97
  subarachnoid (spinal cord) (refrigerated
    saline) 03.92
  total body 39.96
Pericardiectomy 37.31
Pericardiocentesis 37.0
Pericardiolysis 37.12
Pericardioplasty 37.49
Pericardiorrhaphy 37.49
Pericardiostomy (tube) 37.12
Pericardiotomy 37.12
Peridectomy 10.31
Perilimbal suction 89.11
Perimetry 95.05
Perineoplasty 71.79
Perineorrhaphy 71.71
  obstetrical laceration (current) 75.69
Perineotomy (nonobstetrical) 71.09
  to assist delivery - *see* Episiotomy
Periosteotomy - *see also* Incision, bone
  77.10
  facial bone 76.09
Perirectofistulectomy 48.93
Peritectomy 10.31
Peritomy 10.1
Peritoneocentesis 54.91
Peritoneoscopy 54.21
Peritoneotomy 54.19
Peritoneumectomy 54.4
Phacoemulsification (ultrasonic) (with
  aspiration) 13.41
Phacofragmentation (mechanical) (with
  aspiration) 13.43
  posterior route 13.42
  ultrasonic 13.41
Phalangectomy (partial) 77.89
  claw toe 77.57
  cockup toe 77.58
  hammer toe 77.56
  overlapping toe 77.58
  total 77.99
Phalangization (fifth metacarpal) 82.81
Pharyngeal flap operation (cleft palate repair)
  27.62
  secondary or subsequent 27.63
Pharyngectomy (partial) 29.33
  with laryngectomy 30.3
Pharyngogram 87.09
  contrast 87.06
Pharyngolaryngectomy 30.3
Pharyngoplasty (with silastic implant) 29.4
  for cleft palate 27.62
    secondary or subsequent 27.63
Pharyngorrhaphy 29.51
  for cleft palate 27.62
Pharyngoscopy 29.11
Pharyngotomy 29.0
Phenopeel (skin) 86.24
Phlebectomy 38.60
  with
    anastomosis 38.30
      abdominal 38.37
      head and neck NEC 38.32
      intracranial NEC 38.31
      lower limb 38.39
      thoracic NEC 38.35
      upper limb 38.33
    graft replacement 38.40
      abdominal 38.47
      head and neck NEC 38.42
      intracranial NEC 38.41
      lower limb 38.49
      thoracic NEC 38.45
      upper limb 38.43
  abdominal 38.67

Phlebectomy (*Continued*)
  head and neck NEC 38.62
  intracranial NEC 38.61
  lower limb 38.69
  thoracic NEC 38.65
  upper limb 38.63
  varicose 38.50
    abdominal 38.57
    head and neck NEC 38.52
    intracranial NEC 38.51
    lower limb 38.59
    thoracic NEC 38.55
    upper limb 38.53
Phlebogoniostomy 12.52
Phlebography (contrast) (retrograde)
  88.60
  by radioisotope - *see* Scan, radioisotope,
    by site
  adrenal 88.65
  femoral 88.66
  head 88.61
  hepatic 88.64
  impedance 88.68
  intra-abdominal NEC 88.65
  intrathoracic NEC 88.63
  lower extremity NEC 88.66
  neck 88.61
  portal system 88.64
  pulmonary 88.62
  specified site NEC 88.67
  vena cava (inferior) (superior) 88.51
Phleborrhaphy 39.32
Phlebotomy 38.99
Phonocardiogram, with ECG lead 89.55
Photochemotherapy NEC 99.83
  extracorporeal 99.88
Photocoagulation
  ciliary body 12.73
  eye, eyeball 16.99
  iris 12.41
  macular hole - *see* Photocoagulation,
    retina
  orbital lesion 16.92
  retina
    for
      destruction of lesion 14.25
      reattachment 14.55
      repair of tear or defect 14.35
    laser (beam)
      for
        destruction of lesion 14.24
        reattachment 14.54
        repair of tear or defect 14.34
    xenon arc
      for
        destruction of lesion 14.23
        reattachment 14.53
        repair of tear or defect 14.33
Photography 89.39
  fundus 95.11
Photopheresis, therapeutic 99.88
Phototherapy NEC 99.83
  newborn 99.83
  ultraviolet 99.82
Phrenemphraxis 04.03
  for collapse of lung 33.31
Phrenicectomy 04.03
  for collapse of lung 33.31
Phrenicoexeresis 04.03
  for collapse of lung 33.31
Phrenicotomy 04.03
  for collapse of lung 33.31
Phrenicotripsy 04.03
  for collapse of lung 33.31
Phrenoplasty 34.84
Physical medicine - *see* Therapy, physical
Physical therapy - *see* Therapy, physical
Physiotherapy, chest 93.99
PICC (peripherally inserted central catheter)
  38.93
Piercing ear, external (pinna) 18.01

Pigmenting, skin 86.02
Pilojection (aneurysm) (Gallagher) 39.52
Pinealectomy (complete) (total) 07.54
  partial 07.53
Pinealotomy (with drainage) 07.52
Pinning
  bone - *see* Fixation, bone, internal
  ear 18.5
Pinsker operation (obliteration of nasoseptal
    telangiectasia) 21.07
Piper operation (forceps) 72.6
Pirogoff operation (ankle amputation through
    malleoli of tibia and fibula) 84.14
Pituitectomy (complete) (total) - *see also*
    Hypophysectomy 07.69
Placentogram, placentography 88.46
  with radioisotope (RISA) 92.17
Planing, skin 86.25
Plantation, tooth (bud) (germ) 23.5
  prosthetic 23.6
Plasma exchange 99.07
Plasmapheresis, therapeutic 99.71
Plastic repair - *see* Repair, by site
Plasty - *see also* Repair, by site
  bladder neck (V-Y) 57.85
  skin (without graft) 86.89
  subcutaneous tissue 86.89
Platelet inhibitor (GP IIB/IIIa inhibitor only),
    infusion 99.20
Plateletpheresis, therapeutic 99.74
Play
  psychotherapy 94.36
  therapy 93.81
Pleating
  eye muscle 15.22
    multiple (two or more muscles) 15.4
  sclera, for buckling - *see also* Buckling, scleral
    14.49
Plethysmogram (carotid) 89.58
  air-filled (pneumatic) 89.58
  capacitance 89.58
  cerebral 89.58
  differential 89.58
  oculoplethysmogram 89.58
  penile 89.58
  photoelectric 89.58
  regional 89.58
  respiratory function measurement (body)
    89.38
  segmental 89.58
  strain-gauge 89.58
  thoracic impedance 89.38
  venous occlusion 89.58
  water-filled 89.58
Plethysmography
  CaverMap™ 89.58
  penile 89.58
Pleurectomy NEC 34.59
Pleurocentesis 34.91
Pleurodesis 34.6
  chemical 34.92
    with cancer chemotherapy substance
      34.92 [99.25]
      tetracycline 34.92 [99.21]
Pleurolysis (for collapse of lung) 33.39
Pleuropexy 34.99
Pleurosclerosis 34.6
  chemical 34.92
    with cancer chemotherapy substance
      34.92 [99.25]
      tetracycline 34.92 [99.21]
Pleurotomy 34.09
Plexectomy
  choroid 02.14
  hypogastric 05.24
Plication
  aneurysm
    heart 37.32
  annulus, heart valve 35.33
  bleb (emphysematous), lung 32.21
  broad ligament 69.22

Plication (*Continued*)
  diaphragm (for hernia repair) (thoracic
    approach) (thoracoabdominal
    approach) 53.81
  eye muscle (oblique) (rectus) 15.22
    multiple (two or more muscles) 15.4
  fascia 83.89
    hand 82.89
  inferior vena cava 38.7
  intestine (jejunum) (Noble) 46.62
  Kelly (-Stoeckel) (urethrovesical junction)
    59.3
  levator, for blepharoptosis 08.34
  ligament - *see also* Arthroplasty 81.96
    broad 69.22
    round 69.22
    uterosacral 69.22
  mesentery 54.75
  round ligament 69.22
  sphincter, urinary bladder 57.85
  stomach 44.69
    laparoscopic 44.68
  superior vena cava 38.7
  tendon 83.85
    hand 82.55
  tricuspid valve (with repositioning)
    35.14
  ureter 56.89
  urethra 58.49
  urethrovesical junction 59.3
  vein (peripheral) 39.59
  vena cava (inferior) (superior) 38.7
  ventricle (heart)
    aneurysm 37.32
Plicotomy, tympanum 20.23
Plombage, lung 33.39
Pneumocentesis 33.93
Pneumocisternogram 87.02
Pneumoencephalogram 87.01
Pneumogram, pneumography
  extraperitoneal 88.15
  mediastinal 87.33
  orbit 87.14
  pelvic 88.13
  peritoneum NEC 88.13
  presacral 88.15
  retroperitoneum 88.15
Pneumogynecography 87.82
Pneumomediastinography 87.33
Pneumonectomy (extended) (radical)
    (standard) (total) (with mediastinal
    dissection) 32.59
  partial
    complete excision, one lobe 32.49
    resection (wedge), one lobe 32.39
  thoracoscopic 32.50
Pneumonolysis (for collapse of lung) 33.39
Pneumonotomy (with exploration) 33.1
Pneumoperitoneum (surgically-induced)
    54.96
  for collapse of lung 33.33
  pelvic 88.12
Pneumothorax (artificial) (surgical) 33.32
  intrapleural 33.32
Pneumoventriculogram 87.02
Politano-Leadbetter operation
    (ureteroneocystostomy) 56.74
Politzerization, Eustachian tube 20.8
Pollicization (with carry over of nerves and
    blood supply) 82.61
Polya operation (gastrectomy) 43.7
Polypectomy - *see also* Excision, lesion, by site
  esophageal 42.32
    endoscopic 42.33
  gastric (endoscopic) 43.41
  large intestine (colon) 45.42
  nasal 21.31
  rectum (endoscopic) 48.36
Polysomnogram 89.17
Pomeroy operation (ligation and division of
    fallopian tubes) 66.32

Poncet operation
  lengthening of Achilles tendon 83.85
  urethrostomy, perineal 58.0
Porro operation (cesarean section) 74.99
Portoenterostomy (Kasai) 51.37
Positrocephalogram 92.11
Positron emission tomography (PET) - *see* Scan,
    radioisotope
Postmortem examination 89.8
Potts-Smith operation (descending aorta-left
    pulmonary artery anastomosis) 39.0
Poudrage
  intrapericardial 36.39
  pleural 34.6
PPN (peripheral parenteral nutrition)
    99.15
PPVI (percutaneous pulmonary valve
    implantation) 35.07
Preparation (cutting), pedicle (flap) graft
    86.71
Preputiotomy 64.91
Prescription for glasses 95.31
Pressurized
  graft treatment 00.16
Printen and Mason operation (high gastric
    bypass) 44.31
Probing
  canaliculus, lacrimal (with irrigation)
    09.42
  lacrimal
    canaliculi 09.42
    punctum (with irrigation) 09.41
  nasolacrimal duct (with irrigation) 09.43
    with insertion of tube or stent 09.44
  salivary duct (for dilation of duct) (for
    removal of calculus) 26.91
    with incision 26.0
Procedure - *see also* specific procedure
  diagnostic NEC
    abdomen (region) 54.29
    adenoid 28.19
    adrenal gland 07.19
    alveolus 24.19
    amnion 75.35
    anterior chamber, eye 12.29
    anus 49.29
    appendix 45.28
    biliary tract 51.19
    bladder 57.39
    blood vessel (any site) 38.29
    bone 78.80
      carpal, metacarpal 78.84
      clavicle 78.81
      facial 76.19
      femur 78.85
      fibula 78.87
      humerus 78.82
      marrow 41.38
      patella 78.86
      pelvic 78.89
      phalanges (foot) (hand) 78.89
      radius 78.83
      scapula 78.81
      specified site NEC 78.89
      tarsal, metatarsal 78.88
      thorax (ribs) (sternum) 78.81
      tibia 78.87
      ulna 78.83
      vertebrae 78.89
    brain 01.18
    breast 85.19
    bronchus 33.29
    buccal 27.24
    bursa 83.29
    canthus 08.19
    cecum 45.28
    cerebral meninges 01.18
    cervix 67.19
    chest wall 34.28
    choroid 14.19
    ciliary body 12.29

◄ New   ◄▥ Revised   ~~deleted~~ Deleted   ● Use Additional Digit(s)   ▨ Omit code

Procedure *(Continued)*
  diagnostic NEC *(Continued)*
    clitoris 71.19
    colon 45.28
    conjunctiva 10.29
    cornea 11.29
    cul-de-sac 70.29
    dental 24.19
    diaphragm 34.28
    duodenum 45.19
    ear
      external 18.19
      inner and middle 20.39
    epididymis 63.09
    esophagus 42.29
    Eustachian tube 20.39
    extraocular muscle or tendon 15.09
    eye 16.29
      anterior chamber 12.29
      posterior chamber 14.19
    eyeball 16.29
    eyelid 08.19
    fallopian tube 66.19
    fascia (any site) 83.29
    fetus 75.35
    gallbladder 51.19
    ganglion (cranial) (peripheral) 04.19
      sympathetic 05.19
    gastric 44.19
    globus pallidus 01.18
    gum 24.19
    heart 37.29
    hepatic 50.19
    hypophysis 07.19
    ileum 45.19
    intestine 45.29
      large 45.28
      small 45.19
    iris 12.29
    jejunum 45.19
    joint (capsule) (ligament) (structure) NEC
        81.98
      facial 76.19
    kidney 55.29
    labia 71.19
    lacrimal (system) 09.19
    large intestine 45.28
    larynx 31.48
    ligament 81.98
      uterine 68.19
    liver 50.19
    lung 33.29
    lymphatic structure (channel) (gland)
        (node) (vessel) 40.19
    mediastinum 34.29
    meninges (cerebral) 01.18
      spinal 03.39
    mouth 27.29
    muscle 83.29
      extraocular (oblique) (rectus) 15.09
      papillary (heart) 37.29
    nail 86.19
    nasopharynx 29.19
    nerve (cranial) (peripheral) NEC 04.19
      sympathetic 05.19
    nipple 85.19
    nose, nasal 21.29
      sinus 22.19
    ocular 16.29
      muscle 15.09
    omentum 54.29
    ophthalmologic 16.29
    oral (cavity) 27.29
    orbit 16.29
    orthodontic 24.19
    ovary 65.19
      laparoscopic 65.14
    palate 27.29
    pancreas 52.19
    papillary muscle (heart) 37.29
    parathyroid gland 06.19

Procedure *(Continued)*
  diagnostic NEC *(Continued)*
    penis 64.19
    perianal tissue 49.29
    pericardium 37.29
    periprostatic tissue 60.18
    perirectal tissue 48.29
    perirenal tissue 59.29
    peritoneum 54.29
    periurethral tissue 58.29
    perivesical tissue 59.29
    pharynx 29.19
    pineal gland 07.19
    pituitary gland 07.19
    pleura 34.28
    posterior chamber, eye 14.19
    prostate 60.18
    pulmonary 33.29
    rectosigmoid 48.29
    rectum 48.29
    renal 55.29
    respiratory 33.29
    retina 14.19
    retroperitoneum 59.29
    salivary gland or duct 26.19
    sclera 12.29
    scrotum 61.19
    seminal vesicle 60.19
    sigmoid 45.28
    sinus, nasal 22.19
    skin 86.19
    skull 01.19
    soft tissue 83.29
    spermatic cord 63.09
    sphincter of Oddi 51.19
    spine, spinal (canal) (cord) (meninges)
        (structure) 03.39
    spleen 41.39
    stomach 44.19
    subcutaneous tissue 86.19
    sympathetic nerve 05.19
    tarsus 09.19
    tendon NEC 83.29
      extraocular 15.09
    testicle 62.19
    thalamus 01.18
    thoracic duct 40.19
    thorax 34.28
    thymus 07.19
    thyroid gland 06.19
    tongue 25.09
    tonsils 28.19
    tooth 24.19
    trachea 31.49
    tunica vaginalis 61.19
    ureter 56.39
    urethra 58.29
    uterus and supporting structures
        68.19
    uvula 27.29
    vagina 70.29
    vas deferens 63.09
    vesical 57.39
    vessel (blood) (any site) 38.29
    vitreous 14.19
    vulva 71.19
  fistulizing, sclera NEC 12.69
  miscellaneous (nonoperative) NEC 99.99
  respiratory (nonoperative) NEC 93.99
  surgical - *see* Operation
Proctectasis 96.22
Proctectomy (partial) - *see also* Resection, rectum
    48.69
  abdominoperineal, NOS 48.50
    laparoscopic 48.51
    open 48.52
    other 48.59
  complete (Miles) (Rankin), NOS 48.50
    laparoscopic 48.51
    open 48.52
    other 48.59

Proctectomy *(Continued)*
  pull-through
    laparoscopic 48.42
    not otherwise specified 48.40
    open 48.43
    other 48.49
Proctoclysis 96.37
Proctolysis 48.99
Proctopexy (Delorme) 48.76
  abdominal (Ripstein) 48.75
Proctoplasty 48.79
Proctorrhaphy 48.71
Proctoscopy 48.23
  with biopsy 48.24
  through stoma (artificial) 48.22
  transabdominal approach 48.21
Proctosigmoidectomy - *see also* Resection,
    rectum 48.69
Proctosigmoidopexy 48.76
Proctosigmoidoscopy (rigid) 48.23
  with biopsy 48.24
  flexible 45.24
  through stoma (artificial) 48.22
  transabdominal approach 48.21
Proctostomy 48.1
Proctotomy (decompression) (linear) 48.0
Production - *see also* Formation *and* Creation
  atrial septal defect 35.42
  subcutaneous tunnel for esophageal
      anastomosis 42.86
    with anastomosis - *see* Anastomosis,
        esophagus, antesternal
Prognathic recession 76.64
Prophylaxis, dental (scaling) (polishing)
    96.54
Prostatectomy (complete) (partial) NEC 60.69
  loop 60.29
  perineal 60.62
  radical (any approach) 60.5
  retropubic (punch) (transcapsular) 60.4
  suprapubic (punch) (transvesical) 60.3
  transcapsular NEC 60.69
    retropubic 60.4
  transperineal 60.62
  transurethral 60.29
    ablation (contact) (noncontact) by laser
        60.21
    electrovaporization 60.29
    enucleative 60.29
    resection of prostate (TURP) 60.29
    ultrasound guided laser induced (TULIP)
        60.21
  transvesical punch (suprapubic) 60.3
Prostatocystotomy 60.0
Prostatolithotomy 60.0
Prostatotomy (perineal) 60.0
Prostatovesiculectomy 60.5
Protection (of)
  individual from his surroundings 99.84
  surroundings from individual 99.84
Psychoanalysis 94.31
Psychodrama 94.43
Psychotherapy NEC 94.39
  biofeedback 94.39
  exploratory verbal 94.37
  group 94.44
    for psychosexual dysfunctions 94.41
  play 94.36
  psychosexual dysfunctions 94.34
  supportive verbal 94.38
PTCA (percutaneous transluminal coronary
    angioplasty) - *see* Angioplasty, balloon,
    coronary
Ptyalectasis 26.91
Ptyalithotomy 26.0
Ptyalolithotomy 26.0
Pubiotomy 77.39
  assisting delivery 73.94
Pubococcygeoplasty 59.71
Puestow operation (pancreaticojejunostomy)
    52.96

P, Q, & R

Pull-through
abdomino-anal 48.49
abdominoperineal 48.49
Duhamel type 48.65
endorectal 48.41
Pulmowrap 93.99
Pulpectomy - *see also* Therapy, root canal 23.70
Pulpotomy - *see also* Therapy, root canal 23.70
Pump-oxygenator, for extracorporeal
circulation 39.61
percutaneous 39.66
Punch
operation
bladder neck, transurethral 57.49
prostate - *see* Prostatectomy
resection, vocal cords 30.22
Puncture
antrum (nasal) (bilateral) (unilateral)
22.01
artery NEC 38.98
for
arteriography - *see also* Arteriography
88.40
for
coronary arteriography - *see also*
Arteriography, coronary 88.57
percutaneous vascular closure -
omit code
bladder, suprapubic (for drainage) NEC
57.18
needle 57.11
percutaneous (suprapubic) 57.17
bursa 83.94
hand 82.92

Puncture *(Continued)*
cisternal 01.01
with contrast media 87.02
cranial 01.09
with contrast media 87.02
craniobuccal pouch 07.72
craniopharyngioma 07.72
fallopian tube 66.91
fontanel, anterior 01.09
heart 37.0
for intracardiac injection 37.92
hypophysis 07.72
iris 12.12
joint 81.91
kidney (percutaneous) 55.92
larynx 31.98
lumbar (diagnostic) (removal of dye) 03.31
lung (for aspiration) 33.93
nasal sinus 22.01
pericardium 37.0
pituitary gland 07.72
pleural cavity 34.91
Rathke's pouch 07.72
spinal 03.31
spleen 41.1
for biopsy 41.32
sternal (for bone marrow biopsy) 41.31
donor for bone marrow transplant 41.91
vein NEC 38.99
for
phlebography - *see also* Phlebography
88.60
transfusion - *see* Transfusion
ventricular shunt tubing 01.02

Pupillotomy 12.35
Push-back operation (cleft palate repair)
27.62
Putti-Platt operation (capsulorrhaphy of
shoulder for recurrent dislocation)
81.82
pVAD (percutaneous ventricular assist device)
37.68
Pyelogram (intravenous) 87.73
infusion (continuous) (diuretic) 87.73
percutaneous 87.75
retrograde 87.74
Pyeloileostomy 56.71
Pyelolithotomy 55.11
Pyeloplasty 55.87
Pyelorrhaphy 55.81
Pyeloscopy 55.22
Pyelostolithotomy, percutaneous 55.03
Pyelostomy 55.12
closure 55.82
Pyelotomy 55.11
Pyeloureteroplasty 55.87
Pylorectomy 43.6
Pyloroduodenotomy - *see* category 44.2●
Pyloromyotomy (Ramstedt) (with wedge
resection) 43.3
Pyloroplasty (Finney) (Heineke-Mikulicz)
44.29
dilation, endoscopic 44.22
by incision 44.21
not elsewhere classified 44.29
revision 44.29
Pylorostomy - *see* Gastrostomy

Q

Quadrant resection of breast 85.22
Quadricepsplasty (Thompson) 83.86
Quarantine 99.84
Quenuthoracoplasty 77.31
Quotient, respiratory 89.38

R

Rachicentesis 03.31
Rachitomy 03.09
Radiation therapy - *see also* Therapy, radiation
teleradiotherapy - *see* Teleradiotherapy
Radical neck dissection - *see* Dissection, neck
Radicotomy 03.1
Radiculectomy 03.1
Radiculotomy 03.1
Radiography (diagnostic) NEC 88.39
abdomen, abdominal (flat plate) NEC 88.19
wall (soft tissue) NEC 88.09
adenoid 87.09
ankle (skeletal) 88.28
soft tissue 88.37
bone survey 88.31
bronchus 87.49
chest (routine) 87.44
wall NEC 87.39
clavicle 87.43
computer assisted surgery (CAS) with
fluoroscopy 00.33
contrast (air) (gas) (radio-opaque substance)
NEC
abdominal wall 88.03
arteries (by fluoroscopy) - *see*
Arteriography

Radiography NEC *(Continued)*
contrast NEC *(Continued)*
bile ducts NEC 87.54
bladder NEC 87.77
brain 87.02
breast 87.35
bronchus NEC (transcricoid) 87.32
endotracheal 87.31
epididymis 87.93
esophagus 87.61
fallopian tubes
gas 87.82
opaque dye 87.83
fistula (sinus tract) - *see also* Radiography,
contrast, by site
abdominal wall 88.03
chest wall 87.38
gallbladder NEC 87.59
intervertebral disc(s) 87.21
joints 88.32
larynx 87.07
lymph - *see* Lymphangiogram
mammary ducts 87.35
mediastinum 87.33
nasal sinuses 87.15
nasolacrimal ducts 87.05
nasopharynx 87.06
orbit 87.14

Radiography NEC *(Continued)*
contrast NEC *(Continued)*
pancreas 87.66
pelvis
gas 88.12
opaque dye 88.11
peritoneum NEC 88.13
retroperitoneum NEC 88.15
seminal vesicles 87.91
sinus tract - *see also* Radiography, contrast,
by site
abdominal wall 88.03
chest wall 87.38
nose 87.15
skull 87.02
spinal disc(s) 87.21
trachea 87.32
uterus
gas 87.82
opaque dye 87.83
vas deferens 87.94
veins (by fluoroscopy) - *see* Phlebography
vena cava (inferior) (superior) 88.51
dental NEC 87.12
diaphragm 87.49
digestive tract NEC 87.69
barium swallow 87.61
lower GI series 87.64

◀ New ◀▥ Revised ~~deleted~~ Deleted ● Use Additional Digit(s) Omit code

Radiography NEC (*Continued*)
  digestive tract NEC (*Continued*)
    small bowel series 87.63
    upper GI series 87.62
  elbow (skeletal) 88.22
    soft tissue 88.35
  epididymis NEC 87.95
  esophagus 87.69
    barium-swallow 87.61
  eye 95.14
  face, head, and neck 87.09
  facial bones 87.16
  fallopian tubes 87.85
  foot 88.28
  forearm (skeletal) 88.22
    soft tissue 88.35
  frontal area, facial 87.16
  genital organs
    female NEC 87.89
    male NEC 87.99
  hand (skeletal) 88.23
    soft tissue 88.35
  head NEC 87.09
  heart 87.49
  hip (skeletal) 88.26
    soft tissue 88.37
  intestine NEC 87.65
  kidney-ureter-bladder (KUB) 87.79
  knee (skeletal) 88.27
    soft tissue 88.37
  KUB (kidney-ureter-bladder) 87.79
  larynx 87.09
  lower leg (skeletal) 88.27
    soft tissue 88.37
  lower limb (skeletal) NEC 88.29
    soft tissue NEC 88.37
  lung 87.49
  mandible 87.16
  maxilla 87.16
  mediastinum 87.49
  nasal sinuses 87.16
  nasolacrimal duct 87.09
  nasopharynx 87.09
  neck NEC 87.09
  nose 87.16
  orbit 87.16
  pelvis (skeletal) 88.26
    pelvimetry 88.25
    soft tissue 88.19
  prostate NEC 87.92
  retroperitoneum NEC 88.16
  ribs 87.43
  root canal 87.12
  salivary gland 87.09
  seminal vesicles NEC 87.92
  shoulder (skeletal) 88.21
    soft tissue 88.35
  skeletal NEC 88.33
    series (whole or complete) 88.31
  skull (lateral, sagittal or tangential
    projection) NEC 87.17
  spine NEC 87.29
    cervical 87.22
    lumbosacral 87.24
    sacrococcygeal 87.24
    thoracic 87.23
  sternum 87.43
  supraorbital area 87.16
  symphysis menti 87.16
  teeth NEC 87.12
    full-mouth 87.11
  thigh (skeletal) 88.27
    soft tissue 88.37
  thyroid region 87.09
  tonsils and adenoids 87.09
  trachea 87.49
  ultrasonic - *see* Ultrasonography
  upper arm (skeletal) 88.21
    soft tissue 88.35
  upper limb (skeletal) NEC 88.24
    soft tissue NEC 88.35

Radiography NEC (*Continued*)
  urinary system NEC 87.79
  uterus NEC 87.85
    gravid 87.81
  uvula 87.09
  vas deferens NEC 87.95
  wrist 88.23
  zygomaticomaxillary complex 87.16
Radioimmunotherapy 92.28
Radioisotope
  scanning - *see* Scan, radioisotope
  therapy - *see* Therapy, radioisotope
Radiology
  diagnostic - *see* Radiography
  therapeutic - *see* Therapy, radiation
Radiosurgery, stereotactic 92.30
  cobalt 60 92.32
  linear accelerator (LINAC) 92.31
  multi-source 92.32
  particle beam 92.33
  particulate 92.33
  radiosurgery NEC 92.39
  single source photon 92.31
Raising, pedicle graft 86.71
Ramadier operation (intrapetrosal drainage)
  20.22
Ramisection (sympathetic) 05.0
Ramstedt operation (pyloromyotomy) (with
  wedge resection) 43.3
Range of motion testing 93.05
Rankin operation
  exteriorization of intestine 46.03
  proctectomy (complete), NOS 48.50
    laparoscopic 48.51
    open 48.52
    other 48.59
Rashkind operation (balloon septostomy) 35.41
Rastelli operation (creation of conduit between
  right ventricle and pulmonary artery)
  35.92
  in repair of
    pulmonary artery atresia 35.92
    transposition of great vessels 35.92
    truncus arteriosus 35.83
Raz-Pereyra procedure (bladder neck
  suspension) 59.79
RCSA (radical cryosurgical ablation) of prostate
  60.62
Readjustment - *see* Adjustment
Reamputation, stump 84.3
Reanastomosis - *see* Anastomosis
Reattachment
  amputated ear 18.72
  ankle 84.27
  arm (upper) NEC 84.24
  choroid and retina NEC 14.59
    by
      cryotherapy 14.52
      diathermy 14.51
      electrocoagulation 14.51
      photocoagulation 14.55
        laser 14.54
        xenon arc 14.53
  ear (amputated) 18.72
  extremity 84.29
    ankle 84.27
    arm (upper) NEC 84.24
    fingers, except thumb 84.22
      thumb 84.21
    foot 84.26
    forearm 84.23
    hand 84.23
    leg (lower) NEC 84.27
    thigh 84.28
    thumb 84.21
    toe 84.25
    wrist 84.23
  finger 84.22
    thumb 84.21
  foot 84.26
  forearm 84.23

Reattachment (*Continued*)
  hand 84.23
  joint capsule - *see also* Arthroplasty 81.96
  leg (lower) NEC 84.27
  ligament - *see also* Arthroplasty
    uterosacral 69.22
  muscle 83.74
    hand 82.54
    papillary (heart) 35.31
  nerve (peripheral) 04.79
  nose (amputated) 21.89
  papillary muscle (heart) 35.31
  penis (amputated) 64.45
  retina (and choroid) NEC 14.59
    by
      cryotherapy 14.52
      diathermy 14.51
      electrocoagulation 14.51
      photocoagulation 14.55
        laser 14.54
        xenon arc 14.53
  tendon (to tendon) 83.73
    hand 82.53
    to skeletal attachment 83.88
      hand 82.85
  thigh 84.28
  thumb 84.21
  toe 84.25
  tooth 23.5
  uterosacral ligament(s) 69.22
  vessels (peripheral) 39.59
    renal, aberrant 39.55
  wrist 84.23
Recession
  extraocular muscle 15.11
    multiple (two or more muscles) (with
      advancement or resection) 15.3
  gastrocnemius tendon (Strayer operation)
    83.72
  levator palpebrae (superioris) muscle 08.38
  prognathic jaw 76.64
  tendon 83.72
    hand 82.52
Reclosure - *see also* Closure
  disrupted abdominal wall (postoperative)
    54.61
Reconstruction (plastic) - *see also* Construction
  and Repair, by site
  alveolus, alveolar (process) (ridge) (with
    graft or implant) 24.5
  artery (graft) - *see* Graft, artery
  artificial stoma, intestine 46.40
  auditory canal (external) 18.6
  auricle (ear) 18.71
  bladder 57.87
    with
      ileum 57.87 [*45.51*]
      sigmoid 57.87 [*45.52*]
  bone, except facial - *see also* Osteoplasty 78.40
    facial NEC 76.46
      with total ostectomy 76.44
    mandible 76.43
      with total mandibulectomy 76.41
  breast, total, NOS 85.70
    deep inferior epigastric artery perforator
      (DIEP) flap, free 85.74
    gluteal artery perforator (GAP) flap, free
      85.76
    latissimus dorsi myocutaneous flap 85.71
    other 85.79
    superficial inferior epigastric artery
      (SIEA) flap, free 85.75
    transverse rectus abdominis
      musculocutaneous (TRAM) flap,
      free 85.73
    transverse rectus abdominis
      myocutaneous (TRAM) flap,
      pedicled 85.72
  bronchus 33.48
  canthus (lateral) 08.59
  cardiac annulus 35.33

Reconstruction (Continued)
  chest wall (mesh) (silastic) 34.79
  cleft lip 27.54
  conjunctival cul-de-sac 10.43
    with graft (buccal mucous membrane)
        (free) 10.42
  cornea NEC 11.79
  diaphragm 34.84
  ear (external) (auricle) 18.71
    external auditory canal 18.6
    meatus (new) (osseous skin-lined) 18.6
    ossicles 19.3
    prominent or protruding 18.5
  eyebrow 08.70
  eyelid 08.70
    with graft or flap 08.69
      hair follicle 08.63
      mucous membrane 08.62
      skin 08.61
      tarsoconjunctival (one-stage)
          (two-stage) 08.64
    full-thickness 08.74
      involving lid margin 08.73
    partial-thickness 08.72
      involving lid margin 08.71
  eye socket 16.64
    with graft 16.63
  fallopian tube 66.79
  foot and toes (with fixation device) 81.57
    with prosthetic implant 81.57
  frontonasal duct 22.79
  hip (total) (with prosthesis) 81.51
  intraoral 27.59
  joint - see Arthroplasty
  lymphatic (by transplantation) 40.9
  mandible 76.43
    with total mandibulectomy 76.41
  mastoid cavity 19.9
  mouth 27.59
  nipple NEC 85.87
  nose (total) (with arm flap) (with forehead
      flap) 21.83
  ossicles (graft) (prosthesis) NEC 19.3
    with
        stapedectomy 19.19
        tympanoplasty 19.53
  pelvic floor 71.79
  penis (rib graft) (skin graft) (myocutaneous
      flap) 64.44
  pharynx 29.4
  scrotum (with pedicle flap) (with rotational
      flap) 61.49
  skin (plastic) (without graft) NEC 86.89
    with graft - see Graft, skin
  subcutaneous tissue (plastic) (without skin
      graft) NEC 86.89
    with graft - see Graft, skin
  tendon pulley (with graft) (with local tissue)
      83.83
    for opponensplasty 82.71
    hand 82.71
  thumb (osteoplastic) (with bone graft) (with
      skin graft) 82.69
  trachea (with graft) 31.75
  umbilicus
    laparoscopic 53.43
      with graft or prosthesis 53.42
    other and open with graft or prosthesis
        53.41
    other open 53.49
  ureteropelvic junction 55.87
  urethra 58.46
  vagina 70.62
    with graft or prosthesis 70.64
  vas deferens, surgically divided 63.82
Recontour, gingiva 24.2
Recreational therapy 93.81
Rectectomy - see also Resection, rectum 48.69
Rectopexy (Delorme) 48.76
  abdominal (Ripstein) 48.75
Rectoplasty 48.79

Rectorectostomy 48.74
Rectorrhaphy 48.71
Rectosigmoidectomy - see also Resection,
    rectum 48.69
  transsacral 48.61
Rectosigmoidostomy 45.94
Rectostomy 48.1
  closure 48.72
Red cell survival studies 92.05
Reduction - see also Excision, by site
  adipose tissue 86.83
  batwing arms 86.83
  breast (bilateral) 85.32
    unilateral 85.31
  bulbous tuberosities (mandible) (maxilla)
      (fibrous) (osseous) 24.31
  buttocks 86.83
  diastasis, ankle mortise (closed) 79.77
    open 79.87
  dislocation (of joint) (manipulation) (with
      cast) (with splint) (with traction
      device) (closed) 79.70
    with fracture - see Reduction, fracture, by
        site
    ankle (closed) 79.77
      open 79.87
    elbow (closed) 79.72
      open 79.82
    finger (closed) 79.74
      open 79.84
    foot (closed) 79.78
      open 79.88
    hand (closed) 79.74
      open 79.84
    hip (closed) 79.75
      open 79.85
    knee (closed) 79.76
      open 79.86
    open (with external fixation) (with
        internal fixation) 79.80
      specified site NEC 79.89
    shoulder (closed) 79.71
      open 79.81
    specified site (closed) NEC 79.79
      open 79.89
    temporomandibular (closed) 76.93
      open 76.94
    toe (closed) 79.78
      open 79.88
    wrist (closed) 79.73
      open 79.83
  elephantiasis, scrotum 61.3
  epistaxis - see also Control, epistaxis 21.00
  fracture (bone) (with cast) (with splint) (with
      traction device) (closed) 79.00
    with internal fixation 79.10
    alveolar process (with stabilization of
        teeth)
      mandible (closed) 76.75
        open 76.77
      maxilla (closed) 76.73
        open 76.77
      open 76.77
    ankle - see Reduction, fracture, leg
    arm (closed) NEC 79.02
      with internal fixation 79.12
      open 79.22
        with internal fixation 79.32
    blow-out - see Reduction, fracture, orbit
    carpal, metacarpal (closed) 79.03
      with internal fixation 79.13
      open 79.23
        with internal fixation 79.33
    epiphysis - see Reduction, separation
    facial (bone) NEC 76.70
      closed 76.78
      open 76.79
    femur (closed) 79.05
      with internal fixation 79.15
      open 79.25
        with internal fixation 79.35

Reduction (Continued)
  fracture (Continued)
    fibula (closed) 79.06
      with internal fixation 79.16
      open 79.26
        with internal fixation 79.36
    foot (closed) NEC 79.07
      with internal fixation 79.17
      open 79.27
        with internal fixation 79.37
    hand (closed) NEC 79.03
      with internal fixation 79.13
      open 79.23
        with internal fixation 79.33
    humerus (closed) 79.01
      with internal fixation 79.11
      open 79.21
        with internal fixation 79.31
    jaw (lower) - see also Reduction, fracture,
        mandible
      upper - see Reduction, fracture, maxilla
    larynx 31.64
    leg (closed) NEC 79.06
      with internal fixation 79.16
      open 79.26
        with internal fixation 79.36
    malar (closed) 76.71
      open 76.72
    mandible (with dental wiring) (closed)
        76.75
      open 76.76
    maxilla (with dental wiring) (closed)
        76.73
      open 76.74
    nasal (closed) 21.71
      open 21.72
    open 79.20
      with internal fixation 79.30
      specified site NEC 79.29
        with internal fixation 79.39
    orbit (rim) (wall) (closed) 76.78
      open 76.79
    patella (open) (with internal fixation)
        79.36
    phalanges
      foot (closed) 79.08
        with internal fixation 79.18
        open 79.28
          with internal fixation 79.38
      hand (closed) 79.04
        with internal fixation 79.14
        open 79.24
          with internal fixation 79.34
    radius (closed) 79.02
      with internal fixation 79.12
      open 79.22
        with internal fixation 79.32
    skull 02.02
    specified site (closed) NEC 79.09
      with internal fixation 79.19
      open 79.29
        with internal fixation 79.39
    spine 03.53
    tarsal, metatarsal (closed) 79.07
      with internal fixation 79.17
      open 79.27
        with internal fixation 79.37
    tibia (closed) 79.06
      with internal fixation 79.16
      open 79.26
        with internal fixation 79.36
    ulna (closed) 79.02
      with internal fixation 79.12
      open 79.22
        with internal fixation 79.32
    vertebra 03.53
    zygoma, zygomatic arch (closed) 76.71
      open 76.72
  fracture dislocation - see Reduction, fracture
  heart volume 37.35
  hemorrhoids (manual) 49.41

◀ New   ◀▥ Revised   ~~deleted~~ Deleted   ● Use Additional Digit(s)   ▦ Omit code

Reduction (*Continued*)
hernia - *see also* Repair, hernia
 manual 96.27
intussusception (open) 46.80
 with
  fluoroscopy 96.29
  ionizing radiation enema 96.29
  ultrasonography guidance 96.29
 hydrostatic 96.29
 large intestine 46.82
  endoscopic (balloon) 46.85
 pneumatic 96.29
 small intestine 46.81
lung volume 32.22
 biologic lung volume reduction (BLVR)
  - *see* category 33.7●
malrotation, intestine (manual) (surgical)
 46.80
 large 46.82
  endoscopic (balloon) 46.85
 small 46.81
mammoplasty (bilateral) 85.32
 unilateral 85.31
prolapse
 anus (operative) 49.94
 colostomy (manual) 96.28
 enterostomy (manual) 96.28
 ileostomy (manual) 96.28
 rectum (manual) 96.26
 uterus
  by pessary 96.18
  surgical 69.22
ptosis overcorrection 08.37
retroversion, uterus by pessary 96.18
separation, epiphysis (with internal fixation)
 (closed) 79.40
 femur (closed) 79.45
  open 79.55
 fibula (closed) 79.46
  open 79.56
 humerus (closed) 79.41
  open 79.51
 open 79.50
 specified site (closed) NEC - *see also*
  category 79.4●
  open - *see* category 79.5●
 tibia (closed) 79.46
  open 79.56
size
 abdominal wall (adipose) (pendulous)
  86.83
 arms (adipose) (batwing) 86.83
 breast (bilateral) 85.32
  unilateral 85.31
 buttocks (adipose) 86.83
 finger (macrodactyly repair) 82.83
 skin 86.83
 subcutaneous tissue 86.83
 thighs (adipose) 86.83
torsion
 intestine (manual) (surgical) 46.80
  large 46.82
   endoscopic (balloon) 46.85
  small 46.81
 kidney pedicle 55.84
 omentum 54.74
 spermatic cord 63.52
  with orchiopexy 62.5
 testis 63.52
  with orchiopexy 62.5
 uterus NEC 69.98
  gravid 75.99
ventricular 37.35
volvulus
 intestine 46.80
  large 46.82
   endoscopic (balloon) 46.85
  small 46.81
 stomach 44.92
Reefing, joint capsule - *see also* Arthroplasty
81.96

Re-entry operation (aorta) 39.54
Re-establishment, continuity - *see also*
 Anastomosis
bowel 46.50
fallopian tube 66.79
vas deferens 63.82
Referral (for)
psychiatric aftercare (halfway house)
 (outpatient clinic) 94.52
psychotherapy 94.51
rehabilitation
 alcoholism 94.53
 drug addiction 94.54
 psychologic NEC 94.59
 vocational 94.55
Reformation
cardiac pacemaker pocket, new site (skin)
 (subcutaneous) 37.79
cardioverter/defibrillator (automatic)
 pocket, new site (skin) (subcutaneous)
 37.79
chamber of eye 12.99
Refracture
bone (for faulty union) - *see also* Osteoclasis
 78.70
nasal bones 21.88
Refusion
spinal, NOS 81.30
 atlas-axis (anterior) (transoral) (posterior)
  81.31
 axial lumber interbody fusion [AxiaLIF®]
  81.38
 cervical (C2 level or below) NEC 81.32
  anterior column (interbody),
   anterolateral (anterior) technique
   81.32
  C1-C2 level (anterior) (posterior)
   81.31
  posterior column posterolateral
   (posterior) technique 81.33
 craniocervical (anterior) (transoral)
  (posterior) 81.31
 direct lateral interbody fusion [DLIF]
  81.36
 dorsal, dorsolumbar NEC 81.35
  anterior column (interbody),
   anterolateral (anterior)
   (extracavitary) technique
   81.34
  posterior column posterolateral
   (posterior) technique 81.35
 extreme lateral interbody fusion [XLIF®]
  81.36
 facet 81.37
 lumbar, lumbosacral NEC 81.38
  anterior column (interbody)
   anterolateral (anterior) technique
   81.36
   posterior technique 81.38
  anterior lumbar interbody fusion
   (ALIF) 81.36
  lateral transverse process technique
   81.37
  posterior column, posterior
   (posterolateral) (transverse
   process) technique 81.37
  posterior lumbar interbody fusion
   (PLIF) 81.38
  transforaminal lumbar interbody
   fusion (TLIF) 81.37
 number of vertebrae - *see* codes 81.62
 occiput– C2 (anterior) (transoral)
  (posterior) 81.31
 refusion NEC 81.39

Note: Also use either 81.62 as an additional
code to show the total number of vertebrae
fused.

Regional blood flow study 92.05
Regulation, menstrual 69.6

Rehabilitation programs NEC 93.89
alcohol 94.61
 with detoxification 94.63
 combined alcohol and drug 94.67
  with detoxification 94.69
drug 94.64
 with detoxification 94.66
 combined drug and alcohol 94.67
  with detoxification 94.69
sheltered employment 93.85
vocational 93.85
Reimplantation
adrenal tissue (heterotopic) (orthotopic)
 07.45
artery 39.59
 renal, aberrant 39.55
bile ducts following excision of ampulla of
 Vater 51.62
extremity - *see* Reattachment, extremity
fallopian tube into uterus 66.74
kidney 55.61
lung 33.5●
ovary 65.72
 laparoscopic 65.75
pancreatic tissue 52.81
parathyroid tissue (heterotopic) (orthotopic)
 06.95
pulmonary artery for hemitruncus repair
 35.83
renal vessel, aberrant 39.55
testis in scrotum 62.5
thyroid tissue (heterotopic) (orthotopic) 06.94
tooth 23.5
ureter into bladder 56.74
Reinforcement - *see also* Repair, by site
sclera NEC 12.88
 with graft 12.87
Reinsertion - *see also* Insertion or Revision
cystostomy tube 59.94
fixation device (internal) - *see also* Fixation,
 bone, internal 78.50
heart valve (prosthetic) 35.95
Holter (-Spitz) valve 02.42
implant (expelled) (extruded)
 eyeball (with conjunctival graft) 16.62
 orbital 16.62
nephrostomy tube 55.93
pyelostomy tube 55.94
ureteral stent (transurethral) 59.8
 with ureterotomy 59.8 [56.2]
ureterostomy tube 59.93
valve
 heart (prosthetic) 35.95
 ventricular (cerebral) 02.42
Relaxation - *see also* Release training 94.33
Release
carpal tunnel (for nerve decompression)
 04.43
celiac artery axis 39.91
central slip, extensor tendon hand (mallet
 finger repair) 82.84
chordee 64.42
clubfoot NEC 83.84
de Quervain's tenosynovitis 82.01
Dupuytren's contracture (by palmar
 fasciectomy) 82.35
 by fasciotomy (subcutaneous) 82.12
  with excision 82.35
Fowler (mallet finger repair) 82.84
joint (capsule) (adherent) (constrictive) - *see
 also* Division, joint capsule 80.40
laryngeal 31.92
ligament - *see also* Division, ligament 80.40
 median arcuate 39.91
median arcuate ligament 39.91
muscle (division) 83.19
 hand 82.19
nerve (peripheral) NEC 04.49
 cranial NEC 04.42
 trigeminal 04.41
pressure, intraocular 12.79

Release *(Continued)*
scar tissue
skin 86.84
stoma - *see* Revision, stoma
tarsal tunnel 04.44
tendon 83.13
hand 82.11
extensor, central slip (repair mallet finger) 82.84
sheath 83.01
hand 82.01
tenosynovitis 83.01
abductor pollicis longus 82.01
de Quervain's 82.01
external pollicis brevis 82.01
hand 82.01
torsion
intestine 46.80
large 46.82
endoscopic (balloon) 46.85
small 46.81
kidney pedicle 55.84
ovary 65.95
testes 63.52
transverse carpal ligament (for nerve decompression) 04.43
trigger finger or thumb 82.01
urethral stricture 58.5
Volkmann's contracture
excision of scar, muscle 83.32
fasciotomy 83.14
muscle transplantation 83.77
web contracture (skin) 86.84
Relief - *see* Release
Relocation - *see also* Revision
cardiac device (CRT-D) (CRT-P) (defibrillator) (pacemaker) pocket, new site (skin) (subcutaneous) 37.79
CRT-D pocket 37.79
CRT-P pocket 37.79
subcutaneous device pocket NEC 86.09
Remobilization
joint 93.16
stapes 19.0
Remodel
ventricle 37.35
Removal - *see also* Excision
Abrams bar (chest wall) 34.01
abscess - *see* Incision, by site
adenoid tag(s) 28.6
anal sphincter
with revision 49.75
without revision 49.76
arch bars (orthodontic) 24.8
immobilization device 97.33
arterial graft or prosthesis 39.49
arteriovenous shunt (device) 39.43
with creation of new shunt 39.42
artificial heart
internal biventricular replacement system 37.55
Barton's tongs (skull) 02.95
with synchronous replacement 02.94
bladder sphincter, artificial 58.99
with replacement 58.93
blood clot - *see also* Incision, by site
bladder (by incision) 57.19
without incision 57.0
kidney (without incision) 56.0
by incision 55.01
ureter
by incision 56.2
bone fragment (chip) - *see also* Incision, bone 77.10
joint - *see also* Arthrotomy 80.10
necrotic - *see also* Sequestrectomy, bone 77.00
joint - *see also* Arthrotomy 80.10
skull 01.25
with debridement of compound fracture 02.02

Removal *(Continued)*
bone growth stimulator - *see* category 78.6●
bony spicules, spinal canal 03.53
brace 97.88
breast implant 85.94
tissue expander 85.96
bronchial device or substance
endoscopic 33.78
calcareous deposit
bursa 83.03
hand 83.03
tendon, intratendinous 83.39
hand 82.29
calcification, heart valve leaflets - *see* Valvuloplasty, heart
calculus
bile duct (by incision) 51.49
endoscopic 51.88
laparoscopic 51.88
percutaneous 51.98
bladder (by incision) 57.19
without incision 57.0
common duct (by incision) 51.41
endoscopic 51.88
laparoscopic 51.88
percutaneous 51.96
gallbladder 51.04
endoscopic 51.88
laparoscopic 51.88
kidney (by incision) 55.01
without incision (transurethral) 56.0
percutaneous 55.03
with fragmentation (ultrasound) 55.04
renal pelvis (by incision) 55.11
percutaneous nephostomy 55.03
with fragmentation 55.04
transurethral 56.0
lacrimal
canaliculi 09.42
by incision 09.52
gland 09.3
by incision 09.0
passage(s) 09.49
by incision 09.59
punctum 09.41
by incision 09.51
sac 09.49
by incision 09.53
pancreatic duct (by incision) 52.09
endoscopic 52.94
perirenal tissue 59.09
pharynx 29.39
prostate 60.0
salivary gland (by incision) 26.0
by probe 26.91
ureter (by incision) 56.2
without incision 56.0
urethra (by incision) 58.0
without incision 58.6
caliper tongs (skull) 02.95
cannula
for extracorporeal membrane oxygenation (ECMO) - *omit code*
cardiac pacemaker (device) (initial) (permanent) (cardiac resynchronization device, CRT-P) 37.89
with replacement (by)
cardiac resynchronization pacemaker (CRT-P)
device only 00.53
total system 00.50
dual chamber device 37.87
single-chamber device 37.85
rate responsive 37.86
cardioverter/defibrillator pulse generator
without replacement (cardiac resynchronization defibrillator device (CRT-D)) 37.79

Removal *(Continued)*
cast 97.88
with reapplication 97.13
lower limb 97.12
upper limb 97.11
catheter (indwelling) - *see also* Removal, tube
bladder 97.64
cranial cavity 01.27
middle ear (tympanum) 20.1
ureter 97.62
urinary 97.64
CCM (cardiac contractility modulation)
without replacement (rechargeable pulse generator) (total system) 37.79
cerclage material, cervix 69.96
cerumen, ear 96.52
corneal epithelium 11.41
for smear or culture 11.21
coronary artery obstruction (thrombus) 36.09
direct intracoronary artery infusion 36.04
open chest approach 36.03
percutaneous transluminal (balloon)

> Note: Also use 00.40, 00.41, 00.42, or 00.43 to show the total number of vessels treated. Use code 00.44 once to show procedure on a bifurcated vessel. In addition, use 00.45, 00.46, 00.47, or 00.48 to show the number of vascular stents inserted.

Crutchfield tongs (skull) 02.95
with synchronous replacement 02.94
cyst - *see also* Excision, lesion, by site
dental 24.4
lung 32.29
endoscopic 32.28
thoracoscopic 32.20
cystic duct remnant 51.61
decidua (by)
aspiration curettage 69.52
curettage (D and C) 69.02
manual 75.4
dental wiring (immobilization device) 97.33
orthodontic 24.8
device (therapeutic) NEC 97.89
abdomen NEC 97.86
bronchus 33.78
valve 33.78
digestive system NEC 97.59
drainage - *see* Removal, tube
external fixation device 97.88
mandibular NEC 97.36
minifixator (bone) - *see* category 78.6●
for musculoskeletal immobilization NEC 97.88
genital tract NEC 97.79
head and neck NEC 97.39
intrauterine contraceptive 97.71
spine 80.09
thorax NEC 97.49
trunk NEC 97.87
urinary system NEC 97.69
diaphragm, vagina 97.73
drainage device - *see* Removal, tube
dye, spinal canal 03.31
ectopic fetus (from) 66.02
abdominal cavity 74.3
extraperitoneal (intraligamentous) 74.3
fallopian tube (by salpingostomy) 66.02
by salpingotomy 66.01
with salpingectomy 66.62
intraligamentous 74.3
ovarian 74.3
peritoneal (following uterine or tubal rupture) 74.3
site NEC 74.3
tubal (by salpingostomy) 66.02
by salpingotomy 66.01
with salpingectomy 66.62

Removal *(Continued)*
  electrodes
    bone growth stimulator - *see* category
      78.6⬤
    brain 01.22
      depth 01.22
        with synchronous replacement
          02.93
      foramen ovale 01.22
        with synchronous replacement
          02.93
      sphenoidal - *omit code*
      with synchronous replacement
        02.96
    cardiac pacemaker (atrial) (transvenous)
      (ventricular) 37.77
      with replacement 37.76
    carotid sinus 39.87
      with synchronous pulse generator
        removal (total system) 39.86
      with synchronous replacement
        39.82
    depth 01.22
      with synchronous replacement 02.93
    epicardial (myocardial) 37.77
      with replacement (by)
        atrial and/or ventricular lead(s)
          (electrode) 37.76
        epicardial lead 37.74
    epidural pegs 01.22
      with synchronous replacement 02.93
    foramen ovale 01.22
      with synchronous replacement 02.93
    gastric 04.93
      with synchronous replacement 04.92
    intracranial 01.22
      with synchronous replacement 02.93
    peripheral nerve 04.93
      with synchronous replacement 04.92
    sacral nerve 04.93
    sphenoidal - *omit code*
      with synchronous replacement 02.96
    spinal 03.94
      with synchronous replacement 03.93
    temporary transvenous pacemaker
      system - *omit code*
  electroencephalographic receiver (brain)
    (intracranial) 01.22
    with synchronous replacement 02.93
  electronic
    stimulator - *see* Removal, neurostimulator,
      by site
      bladder 57.98
      bone 78.6⬤
      skeletal muscle 83.93
        with synchronous replacement
          83.92
      ureter 56.94
  electrostimulator - *see* Removal, electronic,
    stimulator, by site
  embolus 38.00
    with endarterectomy - *see* Endarterectomy
    abdominal
      artery 38.06
      vein 38.07
    aorta (arch) (ascending) (descending)
      38.04
    arteriovenous shunt or cannula 39.49
    bovine graft 39.49
    head and neck vessel
      endovascular approach 39.74
      open approach, intracranial vessels
        38.01
      open approach, other vessels of head
        and neck 38.02
    intracranial vessel
      endovascular approach 39.74
      open approach, intracranial vessels
        38.01
      open approach, other vessels of head
        and neck 38.02

Removal *(Continued)*
  embolus *(Continued)*
    lower limb
      artery 38.08
      vein 38.09
    pulmonary (artery) (vein) 38.05
    thoracic vessel NEC 38.05
    upper limb (artery) (vein) 38.03
  embryo - *see* Removal, ectopic fetus
  encircling tube, eye (episcleral) 14.6
  epithelial downgrowth, anterior chamber
    12.93
  external fixation device 97.88
    mandibular NEC 97.36
    minifixator (bone) - *see* category 78.6⬤
  extrauterine embryo - *see* Removal, ectopic
    fetus
  eyeball 16.49
    with implant 16.42
      with attachment of muscles 16.41
  fallopian tube - *see* Salpingectomy
  feces (impacted) (by flushing) (manual) 96.38
  fetus, ectopic - *see* Removal, ectopic fetus
  fingers, supernumerary 86.26
  fixation device
    external 97.88
      mandibular NEC 97.36
      minifixator (bone) - *see* category 78.6⬤
    internal 78.60
      carpal, metacarpal 78.64
      clavicle 78.61
      facial (bone) 76.97
      femur 78.65
      fibula 78.67
      humerus 78.62
      patella 78.66
      pelvic 78.69
      phalanges (foot) (hand) 78.69
      radius 78.63
      scapula 78.61
      specified site NEC 78.69
      tarsal, metatarsal 78.68
      thorax (ribs) (sternum) 78.61
      tibia 78.67
      ulna 78.63
      vertebrae 78.69
  foreign body NEC - *see also* Incision, by site
    98.20
    abdominal (cavity) 54.92
      wall 54.0
    adenoid 98.13
      by incision 28.91
    alveolus, alveolar bone 98.22
      by incision 24.0
    antecubital fossa 98.27
      by incision 86.05
    anterior chamber 12.00
      by incision 12.02
        with use of magnet 12.01
    anus (intraluminal) 98.05
      by incision 49.93
    artificial stoma (intraluminal) 98.18
    auditory canal, external 18.02
    axilla 98.27
      by incision 86.05
    bladder (without incision) 57.0
      by incision 57.19
    bone, except fixation device - *see also*
      Incision, bone 77.10
      alveolus, alveolar 98.22
        by incision 24.0
    brain 01.39
      without incision into brain 01.24
    breast 85.0
    bronchus (intraluminal) 98.15
      by incision 33.0
    bursa 83.03
      hand 82.03
    canthus 98.22
      by incision 08.51
    cerebral meninges 01.31

Removal *(Continued)*
  foreign body NEC *(Continued)*
    cervix (intraluminal) NEC 98.16
      penetrating 69.97
    choroid (by incision) 14.00
      with use of magnet 14.01
      without use of magnet 14.02
    ciliary body (by incision) 12.00
      with use of magnet 12.01
      without use of magnet 12.02
    conjunctiva (by magnet) 98.22
      by incision 10.0
    cornea 98.21
      by
        incision 11.1
        magnet 11.0
    duodenum 98.03
      by incision 45.01
    ear (intraluminal) 98.11
      with incision 18.09
    epididymis 63.92
    esophagus (intraluminal) 98.02
      by incision 42.09
    extrapleural (by incision) 34.01
    eye, eyeball (by magnet) 98.21
      anterior segment (by incision) 12.00
        with use of magnet 12.01
        without use of magnet 12.02
      posterior segment (by incision) 14.00
        with use of magnet 14.01
        without use of magnet 14.02
      superficial 98.21
    eyelid 98.22
      by incision 08.09
    fallopian tube
      by salpingostomy 66.02
      by salpingotomy 66.01
    fascia 83.09
      hand 82.09
    foot 98.28
    gallbladder 51.04
    groin region (abdominal wall) (inguinal)
      54.0
    gum 98.22
      by incision 24.0
    hand 98.26
    head and neck NEC 98.22
    heart 37.11
    internal fixation device - *see* Removal,
      fixation device, internal
    intestine
      by incision 45.00
      large (intraluminal) 98.04
        by incision 45.03
      small (intraluminal) 98.03
        by incision 45.02
    intraocular (by incision) 12.00
      with use of magnet 12.01
      without use of magnet 12.02
    iris (by incision) 12.00
      with use of magnet 12.01
      without use of magnet 12.02
    joint structures - *see also* Arthrotomy 80.10
    kidney (transurethral) (by endoscopy)
      56.0
      by incision 55.01
      pelvis (transurethral) 56.0
        by incision 55.11
    labia 98.23
      by incision 71.09
    lacrimal
      canaliculi 09.42
        by incision 09.52
      gland 09.3
        by incision 09.0
      passage(s) 09.49
        by incision 09.59
      punctum 09.41
        by incision 09.51
      sac 09.49
        by incision 09.53

Removal *(Continued)*
  foreign body NEC *(Continued)*
    large intestine (intraluminal) 98.04
      by incision 45.03
    larynx (intraluminal) 98.14
      by incision 31.3
    lens 13.00
      by incision 13.02
        with use of magnet 13.01
    liver 50.0
    lower limb, except foot 98.29
      foot 98.28
    lung 33.1
    mediastinum 34.1
    meninges (cerebral) 01.31
      spinal 03.01
    mouth (intraluminal) 98.01
      by incision 27.92
    muscle 83.02
      hand 82.02
    nasal sinus 22.50
      antrum 22.2
        with Caldwell-Luc approach 22.39
      ethmoid 22.51
      frontal 22.41
      maxillary 22.2
        with Caldwell-Luc approach 22.39
      sphenoid 22.52
    nerve (cranial) (peripheral) NEC 04.04
      root 03.01
    nose (intraluminal) 98.12
      by incision 21.1
    oral cavity (intraluminal) 98.01
      by incision 27.92
    orbit (by magnet) 98.21
      by incision 16.1
    palate (penetrating) 98.22
      by incision 27.1
    pancreas 52.09
    penis 98.24
      by incision 64.92
    pericardium 37.12
    perineum (female) 98.23
      by incision 71.09
      male 98.25
        by incision 86.05
    perirenal tissue 59.09
    peritoneal cavity 54.92
    perivesical tissue 59.19
    pharynx (intraluminal) 98.13
      by pharyngotomy 29.0
    pleura (by incision) 34.09
    popliteal space 98.29
      by incision 86.05
    rectum (intraluminal) 98.05
      by incision 48.0
    renal pelvis (transurethral) 56.0
      by incision 56.1
    retina (by incision) 14.00
      with use of magnet 14.01
      without use of magnet 14.02
    retroperitoneum 54.92
    sclera (by incision) 12.00
      with use of magnet 12.01
      without use of magnet 12.02
    scrotum 98.24
      by incision 61.0
    sinus (nasal) 22.50
      antrum 22.2
        with Caldwell-Luc approach 22.39
      ethmoid 22.51
      frontal 22.41
      maxillary 22.2
        with Caldwell-Luc approach 22.39
      sphenoid 22.52
    skin NEC 98.20
      by incision 86.05
    skull 01.24
      with incision into brain 01.39
    small intestine (intraluminal) 98.03
      by incision 45.02

Removal *(Continued)*
  foreign body NEC *(Continued)*
    soft tissue NEC 83.09
      hand 82.09
    spermatic cord 63.93
    spinal (canal) (cord) (meninges) 03.01
    stomach (intraluminal) 98.03
      bubble (balloon) 44.94
      by incision 43.0
    subconjunctival (by magnet) 98.22
      by incision 10.0
    subcutaneous tissue NEC 98.20
      by incision 86.05
    supraclavicular fossa 98.27
      by incision 86.05
    tendon (sheath) 83.01
      hand 82.01
    testis 62.0
    thorax (by incision) 34.09
    thyroid (field) (gland) (by incision) 06.09
    tonsil 98.13
      by incision 28.91
    trachea (intraluminal) 98.15
      by incision 31.3
    trunk NEC 98.25
    tunica vaginalis 98.24
    upper limb, except hand 98.27
      hand 98.26
    ureter (transurethral) 56.0
      by incision 56.2
    urethra (intraluminal) 98.19
      by incision 58.0
    uterus (intraluminal) 98.16
    vagina (intraluminal) 98.17
      by incision 70.14
    vas deferens 63.6
    vitreous (by incision) 14.00
      with use of magnet 14.01
      without use of magnet 14.02
    vulva 98.23
      by incision 71.09
  gallstones
    bile duct (by incision) NEC 51.49
      endoscopic 51.88
    common duct (by incision) 51.41
      endoscopic 51.88
      percutaneous 51.96
    duodenum 45.01
    gallbladder 51.04
      endoscopic 51.88
      laparoscopic 51.88
    hepatic ducts 51.49
      endoscopic 51.88
    intestine 45.00
      large 45.03
      small NEC 45.02
    liver 50.0
  Gardner Wells tongs (skull) 02.95
    with synchronous replacement 02.94
  gastric band (adjustable), laparoscopic 44.97
  gastric bubble (balloon) 44.94
  granulation tissue - *see also* Excision, lesion, by site
    with repair - *see* Repair, by site
    cranial 01.6
    skull 01.6
  halo traction device (skull) 02.95
    with synchronous replacement 02.94
  heart assist system
    with replacement 37.63
    intra-aortic balloon pump (IABP) 97.44
    nonoperative 97.44
    open removal 37.64
    percutaneous external device 97.44
  heart replacement system
    internal biventricular 37.55
  hematoma - *see* Drainage, by site
  Hoffman minifixator device (bone) - *see* category 78.6●
  hydatidiform mole 68.0

Removal *(Continued)*
  impacted
    feces (rectum) (by flushing) (manual) 96.38
    tooth 23.19
    from nasal sinus (maxillary) 22.61
  implant
    breast 85.94
    cochlear prosthetic device 20.99
    cornea 11.92
    lens (prosthetic) 13.8
    middle ear NEC 20.99
    ocular 16.71
      posterior segment 14.6
    orbit 16.72
    retina 14.6
    tympanum 20.1
  implantable hemodynamic sensor (lead) and monitor device 37.79
  internal biventricular heart replacement system 37.55
  internal fixation device - *see* Removal, fixation device, internal
  intra-aortic balloon pump (IABP) 97.44
  intrauterine contraceptive device (IUD) 97.71
  joint (structure) NOS 80.90
    ankle 80.97
    elbow 80.92
    foot and toe 80.98
    hand and finger 80.94
    hip 80.95
    knee 80.96
    other specified sites 80.99
    shoulder 80.91
    spine 80.99
    toe 80.98
    wrist 80.93
  Kantrowitz heart pump 37.64
    nonoperative 97.44
  keel (tantalum plate), larynx 31.98
  kidney - *see also* Nephrectomy
    mechanical 55.98
    transplanted or rejected 55.53
  laminaria (tent), uterus 97.79
  leads (cardiac) - *see* Removal, electrodes, cardiac pacemaker
  lesion - *see* Excision, lesion, by site
  ligamentum flavum (spine) - *omit code*
  ligature
    fallopian tube 66.79
    ureter 56.86
    vas deferens 63.84
  limb lengthening device, internal - *see* category 78.6●
  loop recorder 86.05
  loose body
    bone - *see* Sequestrectomy, bone
    joint 80.10
  mesh (surgical) - *see* Removal, foreign body, by site
  lymph node - *see* Excision, lymph, node
  minifixator device (bone) - *see* category 78.6●
    external fixation device 97.88
  Mulligan hood, fallopian tube 66.94
    with synchronous replacement 66.93
  muscle stimulator (skeletal) 83.93
    with replacement 83.92
  myringotomy device or tube 20.1
  nail (bed) (fold) 86.23
    internal fixation device - *see* Removal, fixation device, internal
  necrosis
    skin 86.28
      excisional 86.22
  neuropacemaker - *see* Removal, neurostimulator, by site
  neurostimulator
    electrodes
      brain 01.22
        with synchronous replacement 02.93

◄ New   ◄▥ Revised   ~~deleted~~ Deleted   ● Use Additional Digit(s)   Omit code

Removal (*Continued*)
  neurostimulator (*Continued*)
    electrodes (*Continued*)
      gastric 04.93
      intracranial 01.22
        with synchronous replacement 02.93
      peripheral nerve 04.93
        with synchronous replacement 04.92
      sacral nerve 04.93
        with synchronous replacement 04.92
      spinal 03.94
        with synchronous replacement 03.93
    pulse generator (subcutaneous single array, multiple array) 86.05
      with synchronous replacement 86.96
        multiple array 86.95
          rechargeable 86.98
        single array 86.94
          rechargeable 86.97
    cranial 01.29
      with synchronous replacement 01.20
  nonabsorbable surgical material NEC - *see* Removal, foreign body, by site
  odontoma (tooth) 24.4
  orbital implant 16.72
  osteocartilagenous loose body, joint structures - *see also* Arthrotomy 80.10
  outer attic wall (middle ear) 20.59
  ovo-testis (unilateral) 62.3
    bilateral 62.41
  pacemaker
    brain (intracranial) - *see* Removal, neurostimulator
    cardiac (device) (initial) (permanent) 37.89
      with replacement
        dual-chamber device 37.87
        single-chamber device 37.85
          rate responsive 37.86
      electrodes (atrial) (transvenous) (ventricular) 37.77
        with replacement 37.76
      epicardium (myocardium) 37.77
        with replacement (by)
          atrial and/or ventricular lead(s) (electrode) 37.76
          epicardial lead 37.74
      temporary transvenous pacemaker system - *omit code*
    intracranial - *see* Removal, neurostimulator
    neural - *see* Removal, neurostimulator
    peripheral nerve - *see* Removal, neurostimulator
    spinal - *see* Removal, neurostimulator
  pack, packing
    dental 97.34
    intrauterine 97.72
    nasal 97.32
    rectum 97.59
    trunk NEC 97.85
    vagina 97.75
    vulva 97.75
  pantopaque dye, spinal canal 03.31
  patella (complete) 77.96
    partial 77.86
  pectus deformity implant device 34.01
  pelvic viscera, en masse (female) 68.8
    male 57.71
  pessary, vagina NEC 97.74
  pharynx (partial) 29.33
  phlebolith - *see* Removal, embolus
  placenta (by)
    aspiration curettage 69.52
    D and C 69.02
    manual 75.4
  plaque, dental 96.54

Removal (*Continued*)
  plate, skull 02.07
    with synchronous replacement 02.05
  polyp - *see also* Excision, lesion, by site
    esophageal 42.32
      endoscopic 42.33
    gastric (endoscopic) 43.41
    intestine 45.41
      endoscopic 45.42
    nasal 21.31
  prosthesis
    bile duct 51.95
      nonoperative 97.55
    cochlear prosthetic device 20.99
    dental 97.35
    epiretinal visual 14.82
    eye 97.31
    facial bone 76.99
    fallopian tube 66.94
      with synchronous replacement 66.93
    joint structures
      with replacement – *see* Revision, joint replacement by site
      without replacement
        ankle 80.07
        elbow 80.02
        foot and toe 80.08
        hand and finger 80.04
        hip 80.05
        knee 80.06
        shoulder 80.01
        specified site NEC 80.09
        spine 80.09
        unspecified site 80.00
        wrist 80.03
    lens 13.8
    penis (internal) without replacement 64.96
    Rheos™ carotid sinus baroreflex activation device 86.05
    Rosen (urethra) 59.99
    testicular, by incision 62.0
    urinary sphincter, artificial 58.99
      with replacement 58.93
  pseudophakos 13.8
  pterygium 11.39
    with corneal graft 11.32
  pulse generator
    cardiac pacemaker 37.86
    cardioverter/defibrillator 37.79
    carotid sinus 39.88
      with synchronous electrode removal (total system) 39.86
      with synchronous replacement 39.83
    neurostimulator - *see* Removal, neurostimulator, pulse generator
  pump assist device, heart 37.64
    with replacement 37.63
    nonoperative 97.44
  radioactive material - *see* Removal, foreign body, by site
  redundant skin, eyelid 08.86
  rejected organ
    kidney 55.53
    testis 62.42
  reservoir, ventricular (Ommaya) (Rickham) 02.43
    with synchronous replacement 02.42
  retained placenta (by)
    aspiration curettage 69.52
    D and C 69.02
    manual 75.4
  retinal implant 14.6
  Rheos™ carotid sinus baroreflex activation device 86.05
  rhinolith 21.31
  rice bodies, tendon sheaths 83.01
    hand 82.01
  Roger-Anderson minifixator device (bone) - *see* category 78.6 ●
  root, residual (tooth) (buried) (retained) 23.11
  Rosen prosthesis (urethra) 59.99

Removal (*Continued*)
  scleral buckle or implant 14.6
  Scribner shunt 39.43
  secondary membranous cataract (with iridectomy) 13.65
  secundines (by)
    aspiration curettage 69.52
    D and C 69.02
    manual 75.4
  sequestrum - *see* Sequestrectomy
  seton, anus 49.93
  Shepard's tube (ear) 20.1
  Shirodkar suture, cervix 69.96
  shunt
    arteriovenous 39.43
      with creation of new shunt 39.42
    lumbar-subarachnoid NEC 03.98
    pleurothecal 03.98
    salpingothecal 03.98
    spinal (thecal) NEC 03.98
    subarachnoid-peritoneal 03.98
    subarachnoid-ureteral 03.98
  silastic tubes
    ear 20.1
    fallopian tubes 66.94
      with synchronous replacement 66.93
  skin
    necrosis or slough 86.28
      excisional 86.22
      superficial layer (by dermabrasion) 86.25
  skull tongs 02.95
    with synchronous replacement 02.94
  spacer (cement) (joint) (methylmethacrylate) 84.57
  splint 97.88
  stent
    bile duct 97.55
    larynx 31.98
    ureteral 97.62
    urethral 97.65
  stimoceiver - *see* Removal, neurostimulator
  subdural
    grids 01.22
    strips 01.22
  supernumerary digit(s) 86.26
  suture(s) NEC 97.89
    abdominal wall 97.83
    by incision - *see* Incision, by site
    genital tract 97.79
    head and neck 97.38
    thorax 97.43
    trunk NEC 97.84
  symblepharon - *see* Repair, symblepharon
  temporary transvenous pacemaker system - *omit code*
  testis (unilateral) 62.3
    bilateral 62.41
    remaining or solitary 62.42
  thrombus 38.00
    with endarterectomy - *see* Endarterectomy
    abdominal
      artery 38.06
      vein 38.07
    aorta (arch) (ascending) (descending) 38.04
    arteriovenous shunt or cannula 39.49
    bovine graft 39.49
    coronary artery 36.09
    head and neck vessel NEC 38.02
    intracranial vessel NEC 38.01
    lower limb
      artery 38.08
      vein 38.09
    pulmonary (artery) (vein) 38.05
    thoracic vessel NEC 38.05
    upper limb (artery) (vein) 38.03
  tissue expander (skin) NEC 86.05
    breast 85.96
  toes, supernumerary 86.26
  tongs, skull 02.95
    with synchronous replacement 02.94

Removal *(Continued)*
tonsil tag 28.4
tooth (by forceps) (multiple) (single) NEC 23.09
  deciduous 23.01
  surgical NEC 23.19
    impacted 23.19
    residual root 23.11
    root apex 23.73
      with root canal therapy 23.72
trachoma follicles 10.33
T-tube (bile duct) 97.55
tube
  appendix 97.53
  bile duct (T-tube) NEC 97.55
  cholecystostomy 97.54
  cranial cavity 01.27
  cystostomy 97.63
  ear (button) 20.1
  gastrostomy 97.51
  large intestine 97.53
  liver 97.55
  mediastinum 97.42
  nephrostomy 97.61
  pancreas 97.56
  peritoneum 97.82
  pleural cavity 97.41
  pyelostomy 97.61
  retroperitoneum 97.81
  small intestine 97.52
  thoracotomy 97.41
  tracheostomy 97.37
  tympanostomy 20.1
  tympanum 20.1
  ureterostomy 97.62
ureteral splint (stent) 97.62
urethral sphincter, artificial 58.99
  with replacement 58.93
urinary sphincter, artificial 58.99
  with replacement 58.93
utricle 20.79
valve
  vas deferens 63.85
  ventricular (cerebral) 02.43
vascular graft or prosthesis 39.49
ventricular shunt or reservoir 02.43
  with synchronous replacement 02.42
Vinke tongs (skull) 02.95
  with synchronous replacement 02.94
vitreous (with replacement) 14.72
  anterior approach (partial) 14.71
  open sky technique 14.71
Wagner-Brooker minifixator device (bone) - *see* category 78.6 ●
wiring, dental (immobilization device) 97.33
  orthodontic 24.8
Renipuncture (percutaneous) 55.92
Renogram 92.03
Renotransplantation NEC 55.69

Note: To report donor source:
    cadaver 00.93
    live non-related donor 00.92
    live related donor 00.91
    live unrelated donor 00.92

Reopening - *see also* Incision, by site
blepharorrhaphy 08.02
canthorrhaphy 08.02
cilia base 08.71
craniotomy or craniectomy site 01.23
fallopian tube (divided) 66.79
iris in anterior chambers 12.97
laminectomy or laminotomy site 03.02
laparotomy site 54.12
osteotomy site - *see also* Incision, bone 77.10
  facial bone 76.09
tarsorrhaphy 08.02
thoracotomy site (for control of hemorrhage) (for examination) (for exploration) 34.03

Reopening *(Continued)*
thyroid field wound (for control of hemorrhage) (for examination) (for exploration) (for removal of hematoma) 06.02
Repacking - *see* Replacement, pack, by site
Repair
abdominal wall 54.72
adrenal gland 07.44
alveolus, alveolar (process) (ridge) (with graft) (with implant) 24.5
anal sphincter 49.79
  artificial sphincter
    implantation 49.75
    revision 49.75
  laceration (by suture) 49.71
    obstetric (current) 75.62
    old 49.79
aneurysm (false) (true) 39.52
  by or with
    clipping 39.51
    coagulation 39.52
    coil, NEC (endovascular approach) 39.79
      head and neck
        bare coils 39.75
        bioactive coils 39.76
    electrocoagulation 39.52
    excision or resection of vessel - *see also* Aneurysmectomy, by site
      with
        anastomosis - *see* Aneurysmectomy, with anastomosis, by site
        graft replacement - *see* Aneurysmectomy, with graft replacement, by site
    endovascular graft 39.79
      abdominal aorta 39.71
        fenestrated (branching) 39.78
      head and neck 39.72
      lower extremity artery(s) 39.79
      thoracic aorta 39.73
      upper extremity artery(s) 39.79
    filipuncture 39.52
    graft replacement - *see* Aneurysmectomy, with graft replacement, by site
    ligation 39.52
    liquid tissue adhesive (glue) 39.79
      endovascular approach 39.79
        head and neck 39.72
    methyl methacrylate 39.52
      endovascular approach 39.79
        head and neck 39.72
    occlusion 39.52
      endovascular approach 39.79
        head and neck 39.72
    suture 39.52
    trapping 39.52
    wiring 39.52
    wrapping (gauze) (methyl methacrylate) (plastic) 39.52
  coronary artery 36.91
  heart 37.32
  sinus of Valsalva 35.39
  thoracic aorta (dissecting), by fenestration 39.54
anomalous pulmonary venous connection (total)
  one-stage 35.82
  partial - *see* specific procedure
  total 35.82
anular disc 80.54
  with graft or prosthesis 80.53
anulus fibrosus 80.54
  with graft or prosthesis 80.53
anus 49.79
  laceration (by suture) 49.71
    obstetric (current) 75.62
    old 49.79

Repair *(Continued)*
aorta 39.31
aorticopulmonary window 39.59
arteriovenous fistula 39.53
  by or with
    clipping 39.53
    coagulation 39.53
    coil, NEC (endovascular approach) 39.79
      head and neck vessels
        bare coils 39.75
        bioactive coils 39.76
    division 39.53
    excision or resection - *see also* Aneurysmectomy, by site
      with
        anastomosis - *see* Aneurysmectomy, with anastomosis, by site
        graft replacement - *see* Aneurysmectomy, with graft replacement, by site
    ligation 39.53
      coronary artery 36.99
    occlusion 39.53
      endovascular approach 39.79
        head and neck 39.72
    suture 39.53
artery NEC 39.59
  by
    endovascular approach
      abdominal aorta 39.71
        fenestrated (branching) graft 39.78
      head and neck (total embolization or occlusion) 39.72
      other repair (of aneurysm) 39.79
      percutaneous repair of extracranial vessel(s) (for stent insertion) 00.61

Note: Also use 00.40, 00.41, 00.42, or 00.43 to show the total number of vessels treated. Use code 00.44 once to show procedure on a bifurcated vessel. In addition, use 00.45, 00.46, 00.47, or 00.48 to show the number of vascular stents inserted.

      percutaneous repair of intracranial vessel(s) (for stent insertion) 00.62

Note: Also use 00.40, 00.41, 00.42, or 00.43 to show the total number of vessels treated. Use code 00.44 once to show procedure on a bifurcated vessel. In addition, use 00.45, 00.46, 00.47, or 00.48 to show the number of vascular stents inserted.

      non-coronary percutaneous transluminal approach

Note: Also use 00.40, 00.41, 00.42, or 00.43 to show the total number of vessels treated. Use code 00.44 once to show procedure on a bifurcated vessel. In addition, use 00.45, 00.46, 00.47, or 00.48 to show the number of vascular stents inserted.

      angioplasty
        basilar 00.62
        carotid 00.61
        femoropopliteal 39.50
        iliac 39.50
        lower extremity NOS 39.50
        mesenteric 39.50
        renal 39.50
        upper extremity NOS 39.50
        vertebral 00.61
          intracranial portion 00.62
  atherectomy 17.56

Repair *(Continued)*
 artery NEC *(Continued)*
  with
   patch graft 39.58
    with excision or resection of
     vessel - *see* Arteriectomy, with
      graft replacement, by site
    synthetic (Dacron) (Teflon) 39.57
    tissue (vein) (autogenous)
     (homograft) 39.56
   suture 39.31
  coronary NEC 36.99
   by angioplasty - *see* Angioplasty,
    coronary
   by atherectomy
    percutaneous transluminal 17.55
 artificial opening - *see* Repair, stoma
 atrial septal defect 35.71
  with
   prosthesis (open heart technique) 35.51
    closed heart technique 35.52
   tissue graft 35.61
  combined with repair of valvular and
   ventricular septal defects - *see*
   Repair, endocardial cushion defect
  in total repair of total anomalous
   pulmonary venous connection
   35.82
 atrioventricular canal defect (any type)
  35.73
  with
   prosthesis 35.54
   tissue graft 35.63
 bifid digit (finger) 82.89
 bile duct NEC 51.79
  laceration (by suture) NEC 51.79
   common bile duct 51.71
 bladder NEC 57.89
  exstrophy 57.86
  for stress incontinence - *see* Repair, stress
   incontinence
  laceration (by suture) 57.81
   obstetric (current) 75.61
    old 57.89
  neck 57.85
 blepharophimosis 08.59
 blepharoptosis 08.36
  by
   frontalis muscle technique (with)
    fascial sling 08.32
    suture 08.31
   levator muscle technique 08.34
    with resection or advancement 08.33
   orbicularis oculi muscle sling 08.36
   tarsal technique 08.35
 blood vessel NEC 39.59
  with
   patch graft 39.58
    with excision or resection - *see*
     Angiectomy, with graft
     replacement
    synthetic (Dacron) (Teflon) 39.57
    tissue (vein) (autogenous)
     (homograft) 39.56
   resection - *see* Angiectomy
   suture 39.30
  coronary artery NEC 36.99
   by angioplasty - *see* Angioplasty,
    coronary
   by atherectomy
    percutaneous transluminal 17.55
  peripheral vessel NEC 39.59
   by angioplasty 39.50

Note: Also use 00.40, 00.41, 00.42, or 00.43 to show the total number of vessels treated. Use code 00.44 once to show procedure on a bifurcated vessel. In addition, use 00.45, 00.46, 00.47, or 00.48 to show the number of vascular stents inserted.

Repair *(Continued)*
 blood vessel NEC *(Continued)*
  peripheral vessel NEC *(Continued)*
   by atherectomy 17.56

Note: Also use 00.40, 00.41, 00.42, or 00.43 to show the total number of vessels treated. Use code 00.44 once to show procedure on a bifurcated vessel. In addition, use 00.45, 00.46, 00.47, or 00.48 to show the number of vascular stents inserted.

   by endovascular approach 39.79
  bone NEC - *see also* Osteoplasty - *see* category
   78.4●
   by synostosis technique - *see* Arthrodesis
  accessory sinus 22.79
  cranium NEC 02.06
   with
    flap (bone) 02.03
    graft (bone) 02.04
   for malunion, nonunion, or delayed
    union of fracture - *see* Repair,
    fracture, malunion or nonunion
  nasal 21.89
  skull NEC 02.06
   with
    flap (bone) 02.03
    graft (bone) 02.04
 bottle, hydrocele of tunica vaginalis
  61.2
 brain (trauma) NEC 02.92
 breast (plastic) - *see also* Mammoplasty
  85.89
 broad ligament 69.29
 bronchus NEC 33.48
  laceration (by suture) 33.41
 bunionette (with osteotomy) 77.54
 canaliculus, lacrimal 09.73
 canthus (lateral) 08.59
 cardiac pacemaker NEC 37.89
  electrode(s) (lead) NEC 37.75
 cardioverter/defibrillator (automatic)
  pocket, (skin) (subcutaneous)
  37.99
 cerebral meninges 02.12
 cervix 67.69
  internal os 67.59
   transabdominal 67.51
   transvaginal 67.59
  aceration (by suture) 67.61
   obstetric (current) 75.51
    old 67.69
 chest wall (mesh) (silastic) NEC 34.79
 chordae tendineae 35.32
 choroid NEC 14.9
  with retinal repair - *see* Repair, retina
 cisterna chyli 40.69
 claw toe 77.57
 cleft
  hand 82.82
  laryngotracheal 31.69
  lip 27.54
  palate 27.62
   secondary or subsequent 27.63
 coarctation of aorta - *see* Excision, coarctation
  of aorta
 cochlear prosthetic device 20.99
  external components only 95.49
 cockup toe 77.58
 colostomy 46.43
 conjunctiva NEC 10.49
  with scleral repair 12.81
  laceration 10.6
   with repair of sclera 12.81
  late effect of trachoma 10.49
 cornea NEC 11.59
  with
   conjunctival flap 11.53
   transplant - *see* Keratoplasty
  postoperative dehiscence 11.52

Repair *(Continued)*
 coronary artery NEC 36.99
  by angioplasty - *see* Angioplasty,
   coronary
  by atherectomy
   percutaneous transluminal 17.55
 cranium NEC 02.06
  with
   flap (bone) 02.03
   graft (bone) 02.04
 cusp, valve - *see* Repair, heart, valve
 cystocele 70.51
  with graft or prosthesis 70.54
  and rectocele 70.50
   with graft or prosthesis 70.53
 dental arch 24.8
 diaphragm NEC 34.84
 diastasis recti 83.65
 diastematomyelia 03.59
 ear (external) 18.79
  auditory canal or meatus 18.6
  auricle NEC 18.79
  cartilage NEC 18.79
  laceration (by suture) 18.4
  lop ear 18.79
  middle NEC 19.9
  prominent or protruding 18.5
 ectropion 08.49
  by or with
   lid reconstruction 08.44
   suture (technique) 08.42
   thermocauterization 08.41
   wedge resection 08.43
 encephalocele (cerebral) 02.12
 endocardial cushion defect 35.73
  with
   prosthesis (grafted to septa) 35.54
   tissue graft 35.63
 enterocele (female) 70.92
  with graft or prosthesis 70.93
  male 53.9
 enterostomy 46.40
 entropion 08.49
  by or with
   lid reconstruction 08.44
   suture (technique) 08.42
   thermocauterization 08.41
   wedge resection 08.43
 epicanthus (fold) 08.59
 epididymis (and spermatic cord) NEC
  63.59
  with vas deferens 63.89
 epiglottis 31.69
 episiotomy
  routine following delivery - *see*
   Episiotomy
  secondary 75.69
 epispadias 58.45
 esophagus, esophageal NEC 42.89
  fistula NEC 42.84
  stricture 42.85
 exstrophy of bladder 57.86
 eye, eyeball 16.89
  multiple structures 16.82
  rupture 16.82
  socket 16.64
   with graft 16.63
 eyebrow 08.89
  linear 08.81
 eyelid 08.89
  full-thickness 08.85
   involving lid margin 08.84
  laceration 08.81
   full-thickness 08.85
    involving lid margin 08.84
   partial-thickness 08.83
    involving lid margin 08.82
  linear 08.81
  partial-thickness 08.83
   involving lid margin 08.82
  retraction 08.38

Repair *(Continued)*
  fallopian tube (with prosthesis) 66.79
    by
      reanastomosis 66.79
      reimplantation into
        ovary 66.72
        uterus 66.74
      suture 66.71
  false aneurysm - *see* Repair, aneurysm
  fascia 83.89
    by or with
      arthroplasty - *see* Arthroplasty
      graft (fascial) (muscle) 83.82
        hand 82.72
        tendon 83.81
          hand 82.79
      suture (direct) 83.65
        hand 82.46
    hand 82.89
      by
        graft NEC 82.79
          fascial 82.72
          muscle 82.72
        suture (direct) 82.46
    joint - *see* Arthroplasty
  filtering bleb (corneal) (scleral) (by excision) 12.82
    by
      corneal graft - *see also* Keratoplasty 11.60
      scleroplasty 12.82
      suture 11.51
        with conjunctival flap 11.53
  fistula - *see also* Closure, fistula
    anovaginal 70.73
    arteriovenous 39.53
      clipping 39.53
      coagulation 39.53
        endovascular approach 39.79
          head and neck 39.72
      division 39.53
      excision or resection - *see also* Aneurysmectomy, by site
        with
          anastomosis - *see* Aneurysmectomy, with anastomosis, by site
          graft replacement - *see* Aneurysmectomy, with graft replacement, by site
      ligation 39.53
        coronary artery 36.99
      occlusion 39.53
        endovascular approach 39.79
          head and neck 39.72
      suture 39.53
    cervicovesical 57.84
    cervix 67.62
    choledochoduodenal 51.72
    colovaginal 70.72
    enterovaginal 70.74
    enterovesical 57.83
    esophagocutaneous 42.84
    ileovesical 57.83
    intestinovaginal 70.74
    intestinovesical 57.83
    oroantral 22.71
    perirectal 48.93
    pleuropericardial 37.49
    rectovaginal 70.73
    rectovesical 57.83
    rectovesicovaginal 57.83
    scrotum 61.42
    sigmoidovaginal 70.74
    sinus
      nasal 22.71
      of Valsalva 35.39
    splenocolic 41.95
    urethroperineovesical 57.84
    urethrovesical 57.84

Repair *(Continued)*
  fistula *(Continued)*
    urethrovesicovaginal 57.84
    uterovesical 57.84
    vagina NEC 70.75
    vaginocutaneous 70.75
    vaginoenteric NEC 70.74
    vaginoileal 70.74
    vaginoperineal 70.75
    vaginovesical 57.84
    vesicocervicovaginal 57.84
    vesicocolic 57.83
    vesicocutaneous 57.84
    vesicoenteric 57.83
    vesicointestinal 57.83
    vesicometrorectal 57.83
    vesicoperineal 57.84
    vesicorectal 57.83
    vesicosigmoidal 57.83
    vesicosigmoidovaginal 57.83
    vesicourethral 57.84
    vesicourethrorectal 57.83
    vesicouterine 57.84
    vesicovaginal 57.84
    vulva 71.72
    vulvorectal 48.73
  foramen ovale (patent) 35.71
    with
      prosthesis (open heart technique) 35.51
        closed heart technique 35.52
      tissue graft 35.61
  fracture - *see also* Reduction, fracture
    larynx 31.64
    malunion or nonunion (delayed)
      NEC - *see* category 78.4●
      with
        graft - *see* Graft, bone
        insertion (of)
          bone growth stimulator (invasive) - *see* category 78.9●
          internal fixation device 78.5●
        manipulation for realignment - *see* Reduction, fracture, by site, closed
        osteotomy
          with
            correction of alignment - *see* category 77.3●
            with internal fixation device - *see* categories 77.3● [78.5]●
            with intramedullary rod - *see* categories 77.3● [78.5]●
        replacement arthroplasty - *see* Arthroplasty
        sequestrectomy - *see* category 77.0●
        Sofield type procedure - *see* categories 77.3● [78.5]●
        synostosis technique - *see* Arthrodesis
    vertebra 03.53
  funnel chest (with implant) 34.74
  gallbladder 51.91
  gastroschisis 54.71
  great vessels NEC 39.59
    laceration (by suture) 39.30
      artery 39.31
      vein 39.32
  hallux valgus NEC 77.59
    resection of joint with prosthetic implant 77.59
  hammer toe 77.56
  hand 82.89
    with graft or implant 82.79
      fascia 82.72
      muscle 82.72
      tendon 82.79

Repair *(Continued)*
  heart 37.49
    assist system 37.63
    septum 35.70
      with
        prosthesis 35.50
        tissue graft 35.60
      atrial 35.71
        with
          prosthesis (open heart technique) 35.51
            closed heart technique 35.52
          tissue graft 35.61
        combined with repair of valvular and ventricular septal defects - *see* Repair, endocardial cushion defect
        in total repair of
          tetralogy of Fallot 35.81
          total anomalous pulmonary venous connection 35.82
          truncus arteriosus 35.83
      combined with repair of valvular defect - *see* Repair, endocardial cushion defect
      ventricular 35.72
        with
          prosthesis (open heart technique) 35.53
            closed heart technique 35.55
          tissue graft 35.62
        combined with repair of valvular and atrial septal defects - *see* Repair, endocardial cushion defect
        in total repair of
          tetralogy of Fallot 35.81
          total anomalous pulmonary venous connection 35.82
          truncus arteriosus 35.83
    total internal biventricular replacement system 37.52
    implantable battery 37.54
    implantable controller 37.54
    thoracic unit 37.53
    transcutaneous energy transfer [TET] device 37.54
    valve (cusps) (open heart technique) 35.10
      aortic (without replacement) 35.11
      combined with repair of atrial and ventricular septal defects - *see* Repair, endocardial cushion defect
      mitral (without replacement) 35.12
        with
          leaflet clip implant 35.97
          MitraClip® 35.97
        balloon, percutaneous 35.96
        endovascular repair with implant 35.97
        percutaneous with leaflet clip implant 35.97
      pulmonary (without replacement) 35.13
        in total repair of tetralogy of Fallot 35.81
      tricuspid (without replacement) 35.14
  hepatic duct 51.79
  hernia NEC 53.9
    anterior abdominal wall NEC (laparoscopic without graft or prosthesis) 53.59
      with prosthesis or graft
        laparoscopic 53.63
        other and open 53.69
    colostomy 46.42
    crural 53.29
    cul-de-sac (Douglas') 70.92

Repair *(Continued)*
  hernia NEC *(Continued)*
    diaphragmatic
      abdominal approach
        laparoscopic 53.71
        other and open 53.72
        unspecified 53.75
      thoracic, thoracoabdominal approach
          53.80
        laparoscopic 53.83
        other and open 53.84
    epigastric 53.59
      with prosthesis or graft 53.69
    esophageal hiatus
      abdominal approach
        laparoscopic 53.71
        other and open 53.72
        unspecified 53.75
      thoracic, thoracoabdominal approach
          53.80
    fascia 83.89
      hand 82.89
    femoral (unilateral) 53.29
      with prosthesis or graft 53.21
      bilateral 53.39
        with prosthesis or graft 53.31
    Ferguson 53.00
    Halsted 53.00
    Hill-Allison (hiatal hernia repair,
        transpleural approach) 53.80
    hypogastric 53.59
      with prosthesis or graft 53.69
    incisional 53.51
      laparoscopic with prosthesis or graft
          53.62
      other open with prosthesis or graft
          53.61
    inguinal (unilateral) 53.00
      with prosthesis or graft 53.05
      bilateral 53.10
        with prosthesis or graft 53.17
          laparoscopic 17.24
        direct
          laparoscopic with graft or
              prosthesis 17.21
          other and open (laparoscopic
              without graft or
              prosthesis) 53.11
            with prosthesis or graft 53.14
        direct and indirect
          laparoscopic with graft or
              prosthesis 17.23
          other and open (laparoscopic
              without graft or
              prosthesis) 53.13
            with prosthesis or graft
                53.16
        indirect
          laparoscopic with graft or
              prosthesis 17.22
          other and open (laparoscopic
              without graft or
              prosthesis) 53.12
            with prosthesis or graft
                53.15
      direct (unilateral)
        with prosthesis or graft 53.03
        and indirect (unilateral)
          laparoscopic with graft or
              prosthesis 17.11
          other and open (laparoscopic
              without graft or
              prosthesis) 53.01
            with prosthesis or graft
                53.03
        laparoscopic with graft or
            prosthesis 17.11
        other and open (laparoscopic
            without graft or prosthesis)
            53.01
          with prosthesis or graft 53.03

Repair *(Continued)*
  hernia NEC *(Continued)*
    inguinal *(Continued)*
      indirect (unilateral)
        laparoscopic with graft or
            prosthesis 17.12
        other and open (laparoscopic
            without graft or prosthesis)
            53.02
          with prosthesis or graft
              53.04
    internal 53.9
    ischiatic 53.9
    ischiorectal 53.9
    laparoscopic with graft or prosthesis,
        NOS 17.13
    lumbar 53.9
    manual 96.27
    obturator 53.9
    omental 53.9
    paraesophageal
      laparoscopic 53.71
      other and open 53.72
      unspecified 53.75
    parahiatal
      laparoscopic 53.71
      other and open 53.72
      unspecified 53.75
    paraileostomy 46.41
    parasternal 53.82
    paraumbilical
      laparoscopic 53.43
        with graft or prosthesis 53.42
      other and open with graft or prosthesis
          53.41
      other open 53.49
    pericolostomy 46.42
    perineal (enterocele) 53.9
    preperitoneal 53.29
    pudendal 53.9
    retroperitoneal 53.9
    sciatic 53.9
    scrotal - *see* Repair, hernia, inguinal
    spigelian 53.59
      with prosthesis or graft 53.69
    umbilical
      laparoscopic 53.43
        with graft or prosthesis 53.42
      other and open with graft or prosthesis
          53.41
      other open 53.49
    uveal 12.39
    ventral (laparoscopic without graft or
        prosthesis) 53.59
      with prosthesis or graft
        laparoscopic 53.63
        other and open 53.69
      incisional 53.51
        laparoscopic without graft or
            prosthesis 53.59
        other open with prosthesis or graft
            53.61
  hydrocele
    round ligament 69.19
    spermatic cord 63.1
    tunica vaginalis 61.2
  hymen 70.76
  hypospadias 58.45
  ileostomy 46.41
  ingrown toenail 86.23
  intestine, intestinal NEC 46.79
    fistula - *see* Closure, fistula,
        intestine
    laceration
      large intestine 46.75
      small intestine NEC 46.73
    stoma - *see* Repair, stoma
  inverted uterus NEC 69.29
    manual
      nonobstetric 69.94
      obstetric 75.94

Repair *(Continued)*
  inverted uterus NEC *(Continued)*
    obstetrical
      manual 75.94
      surgical 75.93
    vaginal approach 69.23
  iris (rupture) NEC 12.39
  jejunostomy 46.41
  joint (capsule) (cartilage) NEC - *see also*
      Arthroplasty 81.96
  kidney NEC 55.89
  knee (joint) NEC 81.47
    collateral ligaments 81.46
    cruciate ligaments 81.45
    five-in-one 81.42
    triad 81.43
  labia - *see* Repair, vulva
  laceration - *see* Suture, by site
  lacrimal system NEC 09.99
    canaliculus 09.73
    punctum 09.72
      for eversion 09.71
  laryngostomy 31.62
  laryngotracheal cleft 31.69
  larynx 31.69
    fracture 31.64
    laceration 31.61
  leads (cardiac) NEC 37.75
  ligament - *see also* Arthroplasty 81.96
    broad 69.29
    collateral, knee NEC 81.46
    cruciate, knee NEC 81.45
    round 69.29
    uterine 69.29
  lip NEC 27.59
    cleft 27.54
    laceration (by suture) 27.51
  liver NEC 50.69
    laceration 50.61
  lop ear 18.79
  lung NEC 33.49
  lymphatic (channel) (peripheral) NEC 40.9
    duct, left (thoracic) NEC 40.69
  macrodactyly 82.83
  mallet finger 82.84
  mandibular ridge 76.64
  mastoid (antrum) (cavity) 19.9
  meninges (cerebral) NEC 02.12
    spinal NEC 03.59
      meningocele 03.51
      myelomeningocele 03.52
  meningocele (spinal) 03.51
    cranial 02.12
  mesentery 54.75
  mouth NEC 27.59
    laceration NEC 27.52
  muscle NEC 83.87
    by
      graft or implant (fascia) (muscle) 83.82
        hand 82.72
      tendon 83.81
        hand 82.79
      suture (direct) 83.65
        hand 82.46
      transfer or transplantation (muscle)
          83.77
        hand 82.58
    hand 82.89
      by
        graft or implant NEC 82.79
          fascia 82.72
        suture (direct) 82.46
        transfer or transplantation (muscle)
            82.58
  musculotendinous cuff, shoulder 83.63
  myelomeningocele 03.52
  nasal
    septum (perforation) NEC 21.88
    sinus NEC 22.79
      fistula 22.71
  nasolabial flaps (plastic) 21.86

Repair *(Continued)*
  nasopharyngeal atresia 29.4
  nerve (cranial) (peripheral) NEC 04.79
    old injury 04.76
    revision 04.75
    sympathetic 05.81
  nipple NEC 85.87
  nose (external) (internal) (plastic) NEC - *see
    also* Rhinoplasty 21.89
    laceration (by suture) 21.81
  notched lip 27.59
  omentum 54.74
  omphalocele
    laparoscopic 53.43
      with graft or prosthesis 53.42
    other and open with graft or prosthesis
      53.41
    other open 53.49
  orbit 16.89
    wound 16.81
  ostium
    primum defect 35.73
      with
        prosthesis 35.54
        tissue graft 35.63
    secundum defect 35.71
      with
        prosthesis (open heart technique)
          35.51
          closed heart technique 35.52
        tissue graft 35.61
  ovary 65.79
    with tube 65.73
      laparoscopic 65.76
  overlapping toe 77.58
  pacemaker
    cardiac
      device (permanent) 37.89
      electrodes (leads) NEC 37.75
      pocket (skin) (subcutaneous) 37.79
  palate NEC 27.69
    cleft 27.62
      secondary or subsequent 27.63
    laceration (by suture) 27.61
  pancreas NEC 52.95
    Wirsung's duct 52.99
  papillary muscle (heart) 35.31
  patent ductus arteriosus 38.85
  pectus deformity (chest) (carinatum)
    (excavatum) 34.74
  pelvic floor NEC 70.79
    obstetric laceration (current) 75.69
    old 70.79
  penis NEC 64.49
    for epispadias or hypospadias 58.45
    inflatable prosthesis 64.99
    laceration 64.41
  pericardium 37.49
  perineum (female) 71.79
    laceration (by suture) 71.71
      obstetric (current) 75.69
      old 71.79
    male NEC 86.89
      laceration (by suture) 86.59
  peritoneum NEC 54.73
    by suture 54.64
  pharynx NEC 29.59
    laceration (by suture) 29.51
    plastic 29.4
  pleura NEC 34.93
  postcataract wound dehiscence 11.52
    with conjunctival flap 11.53
  pouch of Douglas 70.52
  primum ostium defect 35.73
    with
      prosthesis 35.54
      tissue graft 35.63
  prostate 60.93
  ptosis, eyelid - *see* Repair, blepharoptosis
  punctum, lacrimal NEC 09.72
    for correction of eversion 09.71

Repair *(Continued)*
  quadriceps (mechanism) 83.86
  rectocele (posterior colporrhaphy) 70.52
    with graft or prosthesis 70.55
    and cystocele 70.50
      with graft or prosthesis 70.53
  rectum NEC 48.79
    laceration (by suture) 48.71
    prolapse NEC 48.76
      abdominal approach 48.75
    STARR procedure 48.74
  retina, retinal
    detachment 14.59
      by
        cryotherapy 14.52
        diathermy 14.51
        photocoagulation 14.55
          laser 14.54
          xenon arc 14.53
        scleral buckling - *see also* Buckling,
          scleral 14.49
    tear or defect 14.39
      by
        cryotherapy 14.32
        diathermy 14.31
        photocoagulation 14.35
          laser 14.34
          xenon arc 14.33
  retroperitoneal tissue 54.73
  rotator cuff (graft) (suture) 83.63
  round ligament 69.29
  ruptured tendon NEC 83.88
    hand 82.86
  salivary gland or duct NEC 26.49
  sclera, scleral 12.89
    fistula 12.82
    staphyloma NEC 12.86
      with graft 12.85
  scrotum 61.49
  sinus
    nasal NEC 22.79
    of Valsalva (aneurysm) 35.39
  skin (plastic) (without graft) 86.89
    laceration (by suture) 86.59
  skull NEC 02.06
    with
      flap (bone) 02.03
      graft (bone) 02.04
  spermatic cord NEC 63.59
    laceration (by suture) 63.51
  sphincter ani 49.79
    laceration (by suture) 49.71
      obstetric (current) 75.62
      old 49.79
  spina bifida NEC 03.59
    meningocele 03.51
    myelomeningocele 03.52
  spinal (cord) (meninges) (structures) NEC
    03.59
    meningocele 03.51
    myelomeningocele 03.52
  spleen 41.95
  sternal defect 78.41
  stoma
    bile duct 51.79
    bladder 57.22
    bronchus 33.42
    common duct 51.72
    esophagus 42.89
    gallbladder 51.99
    hepatic duct 51.79
    intestine 46.40
      large 46.43
      small 46.41
    kidney 55.89
    larynx 31.63
    rectum 48.79
    stomach 44.69
      laparoscopic 44.68
    thorax 34.79
    trachea 31.74

Repair *(Continued)*
  stoma *(Continued)*
    ureter 56.62
    urethra 58.49
  stomach NEC 44.69
    laceration (by suture) 44.61
      laparoscopic 44.68
  stress incontinence (urinary) NEC
    59.79
    by
      anterior urethropexy 59.79
      Burch 59.5
      cystourethropexy (with levator muscle
        sling) 59.71
      injection of implant (fat) (collagen)
        (polytef) 59.72
      paraurethral suspension (Pereyra)
        59.6
      periurethral suspension 59.6
      plication of urethrovesical junction
        59.3
      pubococcygeal sling 59.71
      retropubic urethral suspension 59.5
      suprapubic sling 59.4
      tension free vaginal tape 59.79
      urethrovesical suspension 59.4
        gracilis muscle transplant 59.71
        levator muscle sling 59.71
    subcutaneous tissue (plastic) (without
      skin graft) 86.89
      laceration (by suture) 86.59
  supracristal defect (heart) 35.72
    with
      prosthesis (open heart technique)
        35.53
        closed heart technique 35.55
      tissue graft 35.62
  symblepharon NEC 10.49
    by division (with insertion of conformer)
      10.5
    with free graft 10.41
  syndactyly 86.85
  synovial membrane, joint - *see*
    Arthroplasty
  telecanthus 08.59
  tendon 83.88
    by or with
      arthroplasty - *see* Arthroplasty
      graft or implant (tendon) 83.81
        fascia 83.82
          hand 82.72
        hand 82.79
        muscle 83.82
          hand 82.72
      suture (direct) (immediate) (primary) -
        see also Suture, tendon 83.64
        hand 82.45
      transfer for transplantation (tendon)
        83.75
        hand 82.56
    hand 82.86
      by
        graft or implant (tendon) 82.79
        suture (direct) (immediate)
          (primary) - *see also* Suture,
          tendon, hand) 82.45
        transfer or transplantation (tendon)
          82.56
    rotator cuff (direct suture) 83.63
    ruptured NEC 83.88
      hand 82.86
    sheath (direct suture) 83.61
      hand 82.41
  testis NEC 62.69
  tetralogy of Fallot
    partial - *see* specific procedure
    total (one-stage) 35.81
  thoracic duct NEC 40.69
  thoracostomy 34.72
  thymus (gland) 07.93
  tongue NEC 25.59

◀ New   ◀▥ Revised   ~~deleted~~ Deleted   ● Use Additional Digit(s)   Omit code

Repair *(Continued)*
　tooth NEC 23.2
　　by
　　　crown (artificial) 23.41
　　　filling (amalgam) (plastic) (silicate) 23.2
　　　inlay 23.3
　total anomalous pulmonary venous connection
　　partial - *see* specific procedure
　　total (one-stage) 35.82
　trachea NEC 31.79
　　laceration (by suture) 31.71
　tricuspid atresia 35.94
　truncus arteriosus
　　partial - *see* specific procedure
　　total (one-stage) 35.83
　tunica vaginalis 61.49
　　laceration (by suture) 61.41
　tympanum - *see* Tympanoplasty
　ureter NEC 56.89
　　laceration (by suture) 56.82
　ureterocele 56.89
　urethra NEC 58.49
　　laceration (by suture) 58.41
　　　obstetric (current) 75.61
　　　　old 58.49
　　meatus 58.47
　urethrocele (anterior colporrhaphy) (female) 70.51
　　with graft or prosthesis 70.54
　　and rectocele 70.50
　　　with graft or prosthesis 70.53
　urinary sphincter, artificial (component) 58.99
　urinary stress incontinence - *see* Repair, stress incontinence
　uterus, uterine 69.49
　　inversion - *see* Repair, inverted uterus
　　laceration (by suture) 69.41
　　　obstetric (current) 75.50
　　　　old 69.49
　　ligaments 69.29
　　　by
　　　　interposition 69.21
　　　　plication 69.22
　uvula 27.73
　　with synchronous cleft palate repair 27.62
　vagina, vaginal (cuff) (wall) NEC 70.79
　　anterior 70.51
　　　with graft or prosthesis 70.54
　　　with posterior repair 70.50
　　　　with graft or prosthesis 70.53
　　cystocele 70.51
　　　with graft or prosthesis 70.54
　　　and rectocele 70.50
　　　　with graft or prosthesis 70.53
　　enterocele 70.92
　　　with graft or prosthesis 70.93
　　laceration (by suture) 70.71
　　　obstetric (current) 75.69
　　　　old 70.79
　　posterior 70.52
　　　with anterior repair 70.50
　　　　with graft or prosthesis 70.53
　　rectocele 70.52
　　　with graft or prosthesis 70.55
　　　and cystocele 70.50
　　　　with graft or prosthesis 70.53
　　urethrocele 70.51
　　　with graft or prosthesis 70.54
　　　and rectocele 70.50
　　　　with graft or prosthesis 70.53
　varicocele 63.1
　vas deferens 63.89
　　by
　　　anastomosis 63.82
　　　　to epididymis 63.83
　　　reconstruction 63.82
　　laceration (by suture) 63.81

Repair *(Continued)*
　vein NEC 39.59
　　by
　　　endovascular approach
　　　　head and neck (embolization or occlusion) 39.72
　　with
　　　patch graft 39.58
　　　　with excision or resection of vessel - *see* Phlebectomy, with graft replacement, by site
　　　　synthetic (Dacron) (Teflon) 39.57
　　　　tissue (vein) (autogenous) (homograft) 39.56
　　　suture 39.32
　ventricular septal defect 35.72
　　with
　　　prosthesis (open heart technique) 35.53
　　　　closed heart technique 35.55
　　　　in total repair of tetralogy of Fallot 35.81
　　　tissue graft 35.62
　　combined with repair of valvular and atrial septal defects - *see* Repair, endocardial cushion defect
　　in total repair of
　　　tetralogy of Fallot 35.81
　　　truncus arteriosus 35.83
　vertebral arch defect (spina bifida) 03.59
　vulva NEC 71.79
　　laceration (by suture) 71.71
　　　obstetric (current) 75.69
　　　　old 71.79
　Wirsung's duct 52.99
　wound (skin) (without graft) 86.59
　　abdominal wall 54.63
　　　dehiscence 54.61
　　postcataract dehiscence (corneal) 11.52

Replacement
　acetabulum (with prosthesis) 81.52
　ankle, total 81.56
　　revision 81.59
　aortic valve, NOS 35.22
　　with
　　　prosthesis 35.22
　　　tissue graft 35.21
　　　　endovascular 35.05
　　　endovascular (TAVI) (TAVR) (transarterial) (transcatheter) (transfemoral) (with tissue graft) 35.05
　　　transapical (intercostal) (transcatheter) (transthoracic) (transventricular) (with tissue graft) 35.06
　artery - *see* Graft, artery
　bag - *see* Replacement, pack or bag
　Barton's tongs (skull) 02.94
　bladder
　　with
　　　ileal loop 57.87 *[45.51]*
　　　sigmoid 57.87 *[45.52]*
　　sphincter, artificial 58.93
　bronchial device NOS 33.79
　bronchial substance NOS 33.79
　bronchial valve(s)
　　multiple lobes 33.73
　　single lobe 33.71
　caliper tongs (skull) 02.94
　cannula
　　arteriovenous shunt 39.94
　　pancreatic duct 97.05
　　vessel-to-vessel (arteriovenous) 39.94
　cardiac contractility modulation (CCM)
　　rechargeable pulse generator only 17.52
　　total system 17.51

Replacement *(Continued)*
　cardiac resynchronization device
　　defibrillator (biventricular defibrillator) (BiV ICD) (BiV pacemaker with defibrillator) (BiV pacing with defibrillator) (CRT-D) (device and one or more leads) (total system) 00.51
　　　left ventricular coronary venous lead only 00.52
　　　pulse generator only 00.54
　　pacemaker (biventricular pacemaker) (BiV pacemaker) (CRT-P) (device and one or more leads) (total system) 00.50
　　　left ventricular coronary venous lead only 00.52
　　　pulse generator only 00.53
　cardioverter/defibrillator (total system) 37.94
　　leads only (electrodes) (sensing) (pacing) 37.97
　　pulse generator only 37.98
　cast NEC 97.13
　　lower limb 97.12
　　upper limb 97.11
　catheter
　　bladder (indwelling) 57.95
　　cystostomy 59.94
　　external ventricular drain 02.21
　　ventricular shunt (cerebral) 02.42
　　wound 97.15
　CCM (cardiac contractility modulation)
　　rechargeable pulse generator only 17.52
　　total system 17.51
　CRT-D (biventricular defibrillator) (BiV ICD) (BiV pacemaker with defibrillator) (BiV pacing with defibrillator) (cardiac resynchronization defibrillator) (device and one or more leads) 00.51
　　left ventricular coronary venous lead only 00.52
　　pulse generator only 00.54
　CRT-P (biventricular pacemaker) (BiV pacemaker) (cardiac resynchronization pacemaker) (device and one or more leads) 00.50
　　left ventricular coronary venous lead only 00.52
　　pulse generator only 00.53
　Crutchfield tongs (skull) 02.94
　cystostomy tube (catheter) 59.94
　device
　　subcutaneous for intracardiac or great vessel hemodynamic monitoring 00.57
　diaphragm, vagina 97.24
　disc - *see* Replacement, intervertebral disc
　drain - *see also* Replacement, tube
　　vagina 97.26
　　vulva 97.26
　　wound, musculoskeletal or skin 97.16
　ear (prosthetic) 18.71
　elbow (joint), total 81.84
　electrode(s) - *see* Implant, electrode or lead by site or name of device
　　brain
　　　depth 02.93
　　　foramen ovale 02.93
　　　sphenoidal 02.96
　　carotid sinus 39.82
　　　with synchronous pulse generator replacement (total system) 39.81
　　depth 02.93
　　foramen ovale 02.93
　　gastric 04.92
　　intracranial 02.93
　　pacemaker - *see* Replacement, pacemaker, electrode(s)
　　peripheral nerve 04.92
　　sacral nerve 04.92

Replacement *(Continued)*
  electrode(s) *(Continued)*
    sphenoidal 02.96
    spine 03.93
  electroencephalographic receiver (brain)
    (intracranial) 02.93
  electronic
    cardioverter/defibrillator - *see*
      Replacement, cardioverter/
      defibrillator
    leads (electrode)(s) - *see* Replacement,
      electrode(s)
    stimulator - *see also* Implant, electronic
      stimulator, by site
      bladder 57.97
      muscle (skeletal) 83.92
      ureter 56.93
  electrostimulator - *see* Implant,
    electronic stimulator,
    by site
  enterostomy device (tube)
    large intestine 97.04
    small intestine 97.03
  epidural pegs 02.93
  femoral head, by prosthesis 81.52
    revision 81.53
  Gardner Wells tongs (skull) 02.94
  gastric band, laparoscopic 44.96
  gastric port device (subcutaneous) 44.96
  graft - *see* Graft
  halo traction device (skull) 02.94
  Harrington rod (with refusion of spine) - *see*
    Refusion, spinal
  heart
    artificial
      total internal biventricular replacement
        system 37.52
        implantable battery 37.54
        implantable controller 37.54
        thoracic unit 37.53
        transcutaneous energy transfer
          [TET] device 37.54
      total internal biventricular replacement
        system 37.52
        implantable battery 37.54
        implantable controller 37.54
        thoracic unit 37.53
        transcutaneous energy transfer [TET]
          device 37.54
    valve, NOS (with prosthesis) (with tissue
      graft) 35.20
      aortic, NOS 35.22
        with
          prosthesis 35.22
          tissue graft 35.21
            endovascular 35.05
        endovascular (TAVI) (TAVR)
          (transarterial) (transcatheter)
          (transfemoral) (with tissue
          graft) 35.05
        transapical (intercostal)
          (transcatheter) (transthoracic)
          (transventricular) (with tissue
          graft) 35.06
      endovascular, NOS 35.09
      mitral, NOS 35.24
        with
          prosthesis 35.24
          tissue graft 35.23
      poppet (prosthetic) 35.95
      pulmonary, NOS 35.26
        with
          prosthesis 35.26
          tissue graft 35.25
        endovascular (percutaneous) (PPVI)
          (TPVR) (transcatheter)
          (transfemoral) (transvenous)
          35.07
        transapical (intercostal)
          (transcatheter) (transthoracic)
          (transventricular) 35.08

Replacement *(Continued)*
  heart *(Continued)*
    valve, NOS *(Continued)*
      pulmonary, NOS *(Continued)*
        in total repair of tetralogy of Fallot
          35.81
      tricuspid, NOS 35.28
        with
          prosthesis 35.28
          tissue graft 35.27
  hip (partial) (with fixation device) (with
    prosthesis) (with traction) 81.52
    acetabulum 81.52
      revision 81.53
    femoral head 81.52
      revision 81.53
    total 81.51
      revision 81.53
  intervertebral disc
    artificial, NOS 84.60
      cervical 84.62
        nucleus 84.61
        partial 84.61
        total 84.62
      lumbar, lumbosacral 84.65
        nucleus 84.64
        partial 84.64
        total 84.65
      thoracic (partial) (total) 84.63
  inverted uterus - *see* Repair, inverted
    uterus
  iris NEC 12.39
  kidney, mechanical 55.97
  knee (bicompartmental) (hemijoint) (partial)
    (total) (tricompartmental)
    (unicompartmental) 81.54
    revision 81.55
  laryngeal stent 31.93
  leads (electrode)(s) - *see* Replacement,
    electrode(s)
  mechanical kidney 55.97
  mitral valve, NOS 35.24
    with
      prosthesis 35.24
      tissue graft 35.23
  Mulligan hood, fallopian tube 66.93
  muscle stimulator (skeletal) 83.92
  nephrostomy tube 55.93
  neuropacemaker - *see* Implant,
    neurostimulator, by site
  neurostimulator - *see also* Implant,
    neurostimulator, by site
    skeletal muscle 83.92
  pacemaker
    brain - *see* Implant, neurostimulator,
      brain
    cardiac device (initial) (permanent)
      dual-chamber device 37.87
      resynchronization - *see*
        Replacement, CRT-P
      single-chamber device 37.85
        rate responsive 37.86
    electrode(s), cardiac (atrial) (transvenous)
      (ventricular) 37.76
      epicardium (myocardium) 37.74
      left ventricular coronary venous
        system 00.52
    gastric - *see* Implant, neurostimulator,
      gastric
    intracranial - *see* Implant, neurostimulator,
      intracranial
    neural - *see* Implant, neurostimulator, by
      site
    peripheral nerve - *see* Implant,
      neurostimulator, peripheral nerve
    sacral nerve - *see* Implant,
      neurostimulator, sacral nerve
    spine - *see* Implant, neurostimulator,
      spine
    temporary transvenous pacemaker
      system 37.78

Replacement *(Continued)*
  pack or bag
    nose 97.21
    teeth, tooth 97.22
    vagina 97.26
    vulva 97.26
    wound 97.16
  pessary, vagina NEC 97.25
  prosthesis
    acetabulum 81.53
    arm (bioelectric) (cineplastic) (kineplastic)
      84.44
    biliary tract 51.99
    cochlear 20.96
    channel (single) 20.97
      multiple 20.98
    elbow 81.97
    epiretinal visual 14.83
    extremity (bioelectric) (cineplastic)
      (kineplastic) 84.40
      lower 84.48
      upper 84.44
    fallopian tube (Mulligan hood) (stent) 66.93
    femur 81.53
    leg (bioelectric) (cineplastic) (kineplastic)
      84.48
    penis (internal) (non-inflatable) 64.95
      inflatable (internal) 64.97
    pulmonary valve, NOS 35.26
      with
        prosthesis 35.26
        tissue graft 35.25
      endovascular (percutaneous) (PPVI)
        (TPVR) (transcatheter)
        (transfemoral) (transvenous) 35.07
      in total repair of tetralogy of Fallot 35.81
      transapical (intercostal) (transcatheter)
        (transthoracic) (transventricular)
        35.08
    pyelostomy tube 55.94
    rectal tube 96.09
    Rheos™ carotid sinus baroreflex activation
      device 39.81
    sensor (lead)
      intracardiac or great vessel hemodynamic
        monitoring 00.56
    shoulder NEC 81.83
      partial 81.81
      total, NEC 81.80
        other 81.80
        reverse 81.88
    skull
      plate 02.05
      tongs 02.94
    spacer (cement) (joint) (methylmethacrylate)
      84.56
    specified appliance or device NEC 97.29
    spinal motion preservation device
      facet replacement device(s) 84.84
      interspinous process device(s) 84.80
      pedicle-based dynamic stabilization
        device(s) 84.82
    splint 97.14
    stent
      bile duct 97.05
      fallopian tube 66.93
      larynx 31.93
      pancreatic duct 97.05
      trachea 31.93
    stimoceiver - *see* Implant, stimoceiver, by site
    stimulator
      electrode(s)
        carotid sinus 39.82
          with synchronous pulse generator
            replacement (total system)
            39.81
      pulse generator
        carotid sinus 39.83
          with synchronous electrode(s)
            replacement (total system)
            39.81

Replacement *(Continued)*
  subdural
    grids 02.93
    strips 02.93
  testis in scrotum 62.5
  tongs, skull 02.94
  tracheal stent 31.93
  tricuspid valve (with prosthesis) 35.28
    with tissue graft 35.27
  tube
    bile duct 97.05
    bladder 57.95
    cystostomy 59.94
    esophagostomy 97.01
    gastrostomy 97.02
    large intestine 97.04
    nasogastric 97.01
    nephrostomy 55.93
    pancreatic duct 97.05
    pyelostomy 55.94
    rectal 96.09
    small intestine 97.03
    tracheostomy 97.23
    ureterostomy 59.93
    ventricular (cerebral) 02.42
  umbilical cord, prolapsed 73.92
  ureter (with)
    bladder flap 56.74
    ileal segment implanted into bladder 56.89 [45.51]
  ureterostomy tube 59.93
  urethral sphincter, artificial 58.93
  urinary sphincter, artificial 58.93
  valve
    heart - *see also* Replacement, heart valve
      poppet (prosthetic) 35.95
    ventricular (cerebral) 02.42
  ventricular shunt (valve) 02.42
  Vinke tongs (skull) 02.94
  vitreous (silicone) 14.75
    for retinal reattachment 14.59

Replant, replantation - *see also* Reattachment
  extremity - *see* Reattachment, extremity
  penis 64.45
  scalp 86.51
  tooth 23.5

Reposition
  cardiac pacemaker
    electrode(s) (atrial) (transvenous) (ventricular) 37.75
    pocket 37.79
  cardiac resynchronization defibrillator (CRT-D) - *see* Revision, cardiac resynchronization defibrillator
  cardiac resynchronization pacemaker (CRT-P) - *see* Revision, cardiac resynchronization pacemaker
  cardioverter/defibrillator (automatic)
    lead(s) (epicardial patch) (pacing) (sensing) 37.75
    pocket 37.79
    pulse generator 37.79
  cilia base 08.71
  implantable hemodynamic sensor (lead) and monitor device 37.79
  iris 12.39
  neurostimulator
    leads
      subcutaneous, without device replacement 86.09
      within brain 02.93
      within or over gastric nerve 04.92
      within or over peripheral nerve 04.92
      within or over sacral nerve 04.92
      within spine 03.93
    pulse generator
      subcutaneous, without device replacement 86.09
  renal vessel, aberrant 39.55
  subcutaneous device pocket NEC 86.09

Reposition *(Continued)*
  thyroid tissue 06.94
  tricuspid valve (with plication) 35.14

Resection - *see also* Excision, by site
  abdominoendorectal (combined), NOS 48.50
    laparoscopic 48.51
    open 48.52
    other 48.59
  abdominoperineal (rectum), NOS 48.50
    pull-through (Altemeier) (Swenson) NEC 48.49
      Duhamel type 48.65
      laparoscopic 48.42
      not otherwise specified 48.40
      open 48.43
  alveolar process and palate (en bloc) 27.32
  aneurysm - *see* Aneurysmectomy
  aortic valve (for subvalvular stenosis) 35.11
  artery - *see* Arteriectomy
  bile duct NEC 51.69
    common duct NEC 51.63
  bladder (partial) (segmental) (transvesical) (wedge) 57.6
    complete or total 57.79
    lesion NEC 57.59
      transurethral approach 57.49
    neck 57.59
      transurethral approach 57.49
  blood vessel - *see* Angiectomy
  brain 01.59
    by
      stereotactic radiosurgery 92.30
        cobalt 60 92.32
        linear accelerator (LINAC) 92.31
        multi-source 92.32
        particle beam 92.33
        particulate 92.33
        radiosurgery NEC 92.39
        single source photon 92.31
    hemisphere 01.52
    lobe 01.53
  breast - *see also* Mastectomy
    quadrant 85.22
    segmental 85.23
  broad ligament 69.19
  bronchus (sleeve) (wide sleeve) 32.1
    block (en bloc) (with radical dissection of brachial plexus, bronchus, lobe of lung, ribs, and sympathetic nerves) 32.6
  bursa 83.5
    hand 82.31
  cecum (and terminal ileum)
    laparoscopic 17.32
    open and other 45.72
  cerebral meninges 01.51
  chest wall 34.4
  clavicle 77.81
  clitoris 71.4
  colon (partial) (segmental)
    ascending (cecum and terminal ileum)
      laparoscopic 17.32
      open and other 45.72
    cecum (and terminal ileum)
      laparoscopic 17.32
      open and other 45.72
    complete
      laparoscopic 45.81
      open 45.82
      other 45.83
      unspecified 45.83
    descending (sigmoid)
      laparoscopic 17.36
      open and other 45.76
    for interposition 45.52
    Hartmann
      laparoscopic 17.35
      open and other 45.75
    hepatic flexure
      laparoscopic 17.33
      open and other 45.73

Resection *(Continued)*
  colon *(Continued)*
    laparoscopic 17.39
    left radical (hemicolon)
      laparoscopic 17.35
      open and other 45.75
    multiple segmental
      laparoscopic 17.31
      open and other 45.71
    open and other 45.79
    right radical (hemicolon) (ileocolectomy)
      laparoscopic 17.33
      open and other 45.73
    segmental NEC
      laparoscopic 17.39
      multiple
        laparoscopic 17.31
        open and other 45.71
      open and other 45.79
    sigmoid
      laparoscopic 17.36
      open and other 45.76
    splenic flexure
      laparoscopic 17.35
      open and other 45.75
    total
      laparoscopic 45.81
      open 45.82
      other 45.83
      unspecified 45.83
    transverse
      laparoscopic 17.34
      open and other 45.74
  conjunctiva, for pterygium 11.39
    corneal graft 11.32
  cornual (fallopian tube) (unilateral) 66.69
    bilateral 66.63
  diaphragm 34.81
  endaural 20.79
  endorectal (pull-through) (Soave) 48.41
    combined abdominal, NOS 48.50
      laparoscopic 48.51
      open 48.52
      other 48.59
  esophagus (partial) (subtotal) - *see also* Esophagectomy 42.41
    total 42.42
  exteriorized intestine - *see* Resection, intestine, exteriorized
  fascia 83.44
    for graft 83.43
      hand 82.34
    hand 82.35
      for graft 82.34
  gallbladder (total) 51.22
  gastric (partial) (sleeve) (subtotal) NEC - *see also* Gastrectomy 43.89
    with anastomosis NEC 43.89
      esophagogastric 43.5
      gastroduodenal 43.6
      gastrogastric 43.89
      gastrojejunal 43.7
    complete or total NEC 43.99
      with intestinal interposition 43.91
    laparoscopic 43.82
    radical NEC 43.99
      with intestinal interposition 43.91
    wedge 43.42
      endoscopic 43.41
  hallux valgus (joint) - *see also* Bunionectomy
    with prosthetic implant 77.59
  hepatic
    duct 51.69
    flexure (colon)
      laparoscopic 17.33
      open and other 45.73
  infundibula, heart (right) 35.34
  intestine (partial) NEC
    cecum (with terminal ileum)
      laparoscopic 17.32
      open and other 45.72

Resection *(Continued)*
  intestine NEC *(Continued)*
    exteriorized (large intestine) 46.04
      small intestine 46.02
    for interposition 45.50
      large intestine 45.52
      small intestine 45.51
    hepatic flexure
      laparoscopic 17.33
      open and other 45.73
    ileum 45.62
      with cecum
        laparoscopic 17.32
        open and other 45.72
      laparoscopic 17.39
    large (partial) (segmental) NEC
      for interposition 45.52
      laparoscopic 17.39
      multiple segmental
        laparoscopic 17.31
        open and other 45.71
      other 45.79
      total
        laparoscopic 45.81
        open 45.82
        other 45.83
        unspecified 45.83
      unspecified 45.79
    left hemicolon
      laparoscopic 17.35
      open and other 45.75
    multiple segmental (large intestine)
      laparoscopic 17.31
      open and other 45.71
      small intestine 45.61
    open and other 45.79
    right hemicolon
      laparoscopic 17.33
      open and other 45.73
    segmental (large intestine)
      laparoscopic 17.39
      multiple
        laparoscopic 17.31
        open and other 45.71
      open and other 45.79
      small intestine 45.62
        multiple 45.61
    sigmoid
      laparoscopic 17.36
      open and other 45.76
    small (partial) (segmental) NEC
      45.62
      for interposition 45.51
      multiple segmental 45.61
      total 45.63
    total
      large intestine
        laparoscopic 45.81
        open 45.82
        other 45.83
        unspecified 45.83
      small intestine 45.63
  joint structure NEC - *see also* Arthrectomy
    80.90
  kidney (segmental) (wedge) 55.4
  larynx - *see also* Laryngectomy
    submucous 30.29
  lesion - *see* Excision, lesion, by site
  levator palpebrae muscle 08.33
  ligament - *see also* Arthrectomy 80.90
    broad 69.19
    round 69.19
    uterine 69.19
  lip (wedge) 27.43
  liver (partial) (wedge) 50.22
    lobe (total) 50.3
    total 50.4
  lung (wedge) NEC 32.29
    endoscopic 32.28
    segmental (any part) 32.39
      thoracoscopic 32.30

Resection *(Continued)*
  lung NEC *(Continued)*
    thoracoscopic 32.20
    volume reduction 32.22
      biologic lung volume reduction
        (BLVR) - *see* category 33.7●
  meninges (cerebral) 01.51
    spinal 03.4
  mesentery 54.4
  muscle 83.45
    extraocular 15.13
      with
        advancement or recession of other
          eye muscle 15.3
        suture of original insertion
          15.13
      levator palpebrae 08.33
      Muller's, for blepharoptosis 08.35
      orbicularis oculi 08.20
      tarsal, for blepharoptosis 08.35
    for graft 83.43
      hand 82.34
    hand 82.36
      for graft 82.34
    ocular - *see* Resection, muscle,
      extraocular
  myocardium 37.33
  nasal septum (submucous) 21.5
  nerve (cranial) (peripheral) NEC 04.07
    phrenic 04.03
      for collapse of lung 33.31
    sympathetic 05.29
    vagus - *see* Vagotomy
  nose (complete) (extended) (partial) (radical)
    21.4
  omentum 54.4
  orbitomaxillary, radical 16.51
  ovary - *see also* Oophorectomy
    wedge 65.22
      laparoscopic 65.24
  palate (bony) (local) 27.31
    by wide excision 27.32
    soft 27.49
  pancreas (total) (with synchronous
    duodenectomy) 52.6
    partial NEC 52.59
      distal (tail) (with part of body) 52.52
      proximal (head) (with part of body)
        (with synchronous
        duodenectomy) 52.51
      radical subtotal 52.53
    radical (one-stage) (two-stage) 52.7
      subtotal 52.53
  pancreaticoduodenal - *see also*
    Pancreatectomy 52.6
  pelvic viscera (en masse) (female) 68.8
    male 57.71
  penis 64.3
  pericardium (partial) (for)
    chronic constrictive pericarditis 37.31
    drainage 37.12
    removal of adhesions 37.31
  peritoneum 54.4
  pharynx (partial) 29.33
  phrenic nerve 04.03
    for collapse of lung 33.31
  prostate - *see also* Prostatectomy
    transurethral (punch) 60.29
  pterygium 11.39
  radial head 77.83
  rectosigmoid - *see also* Resection, rectum
    48.69
  rectum (partial) NEC 48.69
    with
      pelvic exenteration 68.8
      transsacral sigmoidectomy 48.61
    abdominoendorectal (combined), NOS
      48.50
      laparoscopic 48.51
      open 48.52
      other 48.59

Resection *(Continued)*
  rectum NEC *(Continued)*
    abdominoperineal, NOS 48.50
      laparoscopic 48.51
      open 48.52
      other 48.59
      pull-through NEC 48.49
        Duhamel type 48.65
        laparoscopic 48.42
        not otherwise specified 48.40
        open 48.43
    anterior 48.63
      with colostomy (synchronous) 48.62
    Duhamel 48.65
    endorectal 48.41
      combined abdominal, NOS 48.50
        laparoscopic 48.51
        open 48.52
        other 48.59
    posterior 48.64
    pull-through NEC 48.49
      endorectal 48.41
      laparoscopic 48.42
      not otherwise specified 48.40
      open 48.43
    STARR procedure 48.74
    submucosal (Soave) 48.41
      combined abdominal, NOS 48.50
        laparoscopic 48.51
        open 48.52
        other 48.59
  rib (transaxillary) 77.91
    as operative approach - *omit code*
    incidental to thoracic operation - *omit code*
  right ventricle (heart), for infundibular
    stenosis 35.34
  root (tooth) (apex) 23.73
    with root canal therapy 23.72
    residual or retained 23.11
  round ligament 69.19
  sclera 12.65
    with scleral buckling - *see also* Buckling,
      scleral 14.49
    lamellar (for retinal reattachment) 14.49
      with implant 14.41
  scrotum 61.3
  soft tissue NEC 83.49
    hand 82.39
  sphincter of Oddi 51.89
  spinal cord (meninges) 03.4
  splanchnic 05.29
  splenic flexure (colon) 45.75
  sternum 77.81
  stomach (partial) (sleeve) (subtotal)
    NEC - *see also* Gastrectomy 43.89
    with anastomosis NEC 43.89
      esophagogastric 43.5
      gastroduodenal 43.6
      gastrogastric 43.89
      gastrojejunal 43.7
    complete or total NEC 43.99
      with intestinal interposition 43.91
    fundus 43.89
    laparoscopic 43.82
    radical NEC 43.99
      with intestinal interposition 43.91
    wedge 43.42
      endoscopic 43.41
  submucous
    larynx 30.29
    nasal septum 21.5
    vocal cords 30.22
  synovial membrane (complete) (partial) - *see
    also* Synovectomy 80.70
  tarsolevator 08.33
  tendon 83.42
    hand 82.33
  thoracic structures (block) (en bloc) (radical)
    (brachial plexus, bronchus, lobes of
    lung, ribs, and sympathetic nerves)
    32.6

Resection *(Continued)*
thorax 34.4
tongue 25.2
wedge 25.1
tooth root 23.73
with root canal therapy 23.72
apex (abscess) 23.73
with root canal therapy 23.72
residual or retained 23.11
trachea 31.5
transurethral
bladder NEC 57.49
prostate 60.29
transverse colon
laparoscopic 17.34
open and other 45.74
turbinates - *see* Turbinectomy
ureter (partial) 56.41
total 56.42
uterus - *see* Hysterectomy
vein - *see* Phlebectomy
ventricle (heart) 37.35
infundibula 35.34
vesical neck 57.59
transurethral 57.49
vocal cords (punch) 30.22
Respirator, volume-controlled (Bennett)
(Byrd) - *see* Ventilation
Restoration
cardioesophageal angle 44.66
laparoscopic 44.67
dental NEC 23.49
by
application of crown (artificial) 23.41
insertion of bridge (fixed) 23.42
removable 23.43
extremity - *see* Reattachment, extremity
eyebrow 08.70
with graft 08.63
eye socket 16.64
with graft 16.63
tooth NEC 23.2
by
crown (artificial) 23.41
filling (amalgam) (plastic) (silicate)
23.2
inlay 23.3
Restrictive
gastric band, laparoscopic 44.95
Resurfacing, hip 00.86
acetabulum 00.87
with femoral head 00.85
femoral head 00.86
with acetabulum 00.85
partial NOS 00.85
acetabulum 00.87
femoral head 00.86
total (acetabulum and femoral head) 00.85
Resuscitation
artificial respiration 93.93
cardiac 99.60
cardioversion 99.62
atrial 99.61
defibrillation 99.62
external massage 99.63
open chest 37.91
intracardiac injection 37.92
cardiopulmonary 99.60
endotracheal intubation 96.04
manual 93.93
mouth-to-mouth 93.93
pulmonary 93.93
Resuture
abdominal wall 54.61
cardiac septum prosthesis 35.95
chest wall 34.71
heart valve prosthesis (poppet) 35.95
wound (skin and subcutaneous tissue)
(without graft) NEC 86.59
Retavase, infusion 99.10
Reteplase, infusion 99.10

Retightening (noninvasive)
external fixator device - *omit code*
Retinaculotomy NEC - *see also* Division,
ligament 80.40
carpal tunnel (flexor) 04.43
Retraining
cardiac 93.36
vocational 93.85
Retrogasserian neurotomy 04.02
Revascularization
cardiac (heart muscle) (myocardium) (direct)
36.10
with
bypass anastomosis
abdominal artery to coronary artery
36.17
aortocoronary (catheter stent)
(homograft) (prosthesis)
(saphenous vein graft) 36.10
one coronary vessel 36.11
two coronary vessels 36.12
three coronary vessels 36.13
four coronary vessels 36.14
gastroepiploic artery to coronary
artery 36.17
internal mammary-coronary artery
(single vessel) 36.15
double vessel 36.16
specified type NEC 36.19
thoracic artery-coronary artery
(single vessel) 36.15
double vessel 36.16
implantation of artery into heart
(muscle) (myocardium)
(ventricle) 36.2
indirect 36.2
specified type NEC 36.39
transmyocardial
endoscopic 36.33
endovascular 36.34
open chest 36.31
percutaneous 36.34
specified type NEC 36.32
thoracoscopic 36.33
Reversal, intestinal segment 45.50
large 45.52
small 45.51
Revision
amputation stump 84.3
current traumatic - *see* Amputation
anastomosis
biliary tract 51.94
blood vessel 39.49
gastric, gastrointestinal (with jejunal
interposition) 44.5
intestine (large) 46.94
small 46.93
pleurothecal 03.97
pyelointestinal 56.72
salpingothecal 03.97
subarachnoid-peritoneal 03.97
subarachnoid-ureteral 03.97
ureterointestinal 56.72
ankle replacement (prosthesis) 81.59
anterior segment (eye) wound (operative)
NEC 12.83
arteriovenous shunt (cannula) (for dialysis)
39.42
arthroplasty - *see* Arthroplasty
bone flap, skull 02.06
breast implant 85.93
bronchostomy 33.42
bypass graft (vascular) 39.49
abdominal - coronary artery 36.17
aortocoronary (catheter stent) (with
prosthesis) (with saphenous vein
graft) (with vein graft) 36.10
one coronary vessel 36.11
two coronary vessels 36.12
three coronary vessels 36.13
four coronary vessels 36.14

Revision *(Continued)*
bypass graft *(Continued)*
CABG - *see* Revision, aortocoronary
bypass graft
chest tube - *see* intercostal catheter
coronary artery bypass graft (CABG) - *see*
Revision, aortocoronary bypass
graft, abdominal - coronary artery
bypass, and internal mammary -
coronary artery bypass
intercostal catheter (with lysis of
adhesions) 34.04
thoracoscopic 34.06
internal mammary - coronary artery
(single) 36.15
double vessel 36.16
cannula, vessel-to-vessel (arteriovenous)
39.94
canthus, lateral 08.59
cardiac pacemaker
device (permanent) 37.89
electrode(s) (atrial) (transvenous)
(ventricular) 37.75
pocket 37.79
cardiac resynchronization defibrillator
(CRT-D)
device 37.79
electrode(s) 37.75
pocket 37.79
cardiac resynchronization pacemaker
(CRT-P)
device (permanent) 37.89
electrode(s) (atrial) (transvenous)
(ventricular) 37.75
pocket 37.79
cardioverter/defibrillator (automatic) pocket
37.79
cholecystostomy 51.99
cleft palate repair 27.63
colostomy 46.43
conduit, urinary 56.52
cystostomy (stoma) 57.22
disc - *see* Revision, intervertebral disc
elbow replacement (prosthesis) 81.97
enterostomy (stoma) 46.40
large intestine 46.43
small intestine 46.41
enucleation socket 16.64
with graft 16.63
esophagostomy 42.83
exenteration cavity 16.66
with secondary graft 16.65
extraocular muscle surgery 15.6
fenestration, inner ear 20.62
filtering bleb 12.66
fixation device (broken) (displaced) -
see also Fixation, bone, internal
78.50
flap or pedicle graft (skin) 86.75
foot replacement (prosthesis) 81.59
gastric anastomosis (with jejunal
interposition) 44.5
gastric band, laparoscopic 44.96
gastric port device
laparoscopic 44.96
gastroduodenostomy (with jejunal
interposition) 44.5
gastrointestinal anastomosis (with jejunal
interposition) 44.5
gastrojejunostomy 44.5
gastrostomy 44.69
laparoscopic 44.68
hand replacement (prosthesis) 81.97
heart procedure NEC 35.95
hip replacement NOS 81.53
acetabular and femoral components
(total) 00.70
acetabular component only 00.71
acetabular liner and/or femoral head
only 00.73
femoral component only 00.72

Revision *(Continued)*
  hip replacement NOS *(Continued)*
    femoral head only and/or acetabular
      liner 00.73
    partial
      acetabular component only 00.71
      acetabular liner and/or femoral head
        only 00.73
      femoral component only 00.72
      femoral head only and/or acetabular
        liner 00.73
      total (acetabular and femoral
        components) 00.70
  Holter (-Spitz) valve 02.42
  ileal conduit 56.52
  ileostomy 46.41
  intervertebral disc, artificial (partial) (total)
    NOS 84.69
    cervical 84.66
    lumbar, lumbosacral 84.68
    thoracic 84.67
  Jejunoileal bypass 46.93
  jejunostomy 46.41
  joint replacement
    acetabular and femoral components
      (total) 00.70
    acetabular component only 00.71
    acetabular liner and/or femoral head
      only 00.73
    ankle 81.59
    elbow 81.97
    femoral component only 00.72
    femoral head only and/or acetabular
      liner 00.73
    foot 81.59
    hand 81.97
    hip 81.53
      acetabular and femoral components
        (total) 00.70
      acetabular component only 00.71
      acetabular liner and/or femoral head
        only 00.73
      femoral component only 00.72
      femoral head only and/or acetabular
        liner 00.73
      partial
        acetabular component only 00.71
        acetabular liner and/or femoral
          head only 00.73
        femoral component only 00.72
        femoral head only and/or
          acetabular liner 00.73
        total (acetabular and femoral
          components) 00.70
    knee 81.55
    knee replacement NOS 81.55
      femoral component 00.82
      partial
        femoral component 00.82
        patellar component 00.83
        tibial component 00.81
        tibial insert 00.84
      patellar component 00.83
      tibial component 00.81
      tibial insert 00.84
      total (all components) 00.80
    lower extremity NEC 81.59
    toe 81.59
    upper extremity 81.97
    wrist 81.97
  knee replacement (prosthesis) NOS 81.55
    femoral component 00.82
    partial
      femoral component 00.82
      patellar component 00.83
      tibial component 00.81
      tibial insert 00.84
    patellar component 00.83
    tibial component 00.81
    tibial insert 00.84
    total (all components) 00.80

Revision *(Continued)*
  laryngostomy 31.63
  lateral canthus 08.59
  mallet finger 82.84
  mastoid antrum 19.9
  mastoidectomy 20.92
  nephrostomy 55.89
  neuroplasty 04.75
  ocular implant 16.62
  orbital implant 16.62
  pocket
    cardiac device (defibrillator) (pacemaker)
      with initial insertion of cardiac
        device - *omit code*
      new site (cardiac device pocket) (skin)
        (subcutaneous) 37.79
    carotid sinus stimulation pulse generator
      39.85
      with initial insertion of pulse generator
        - *omit code*
    intracardiac hemodynamic monitoring
      37.79
    subcutaneous device pocket NEC
      with initial insertion of generator or
        device - *omit code*
      new site 86.09
    thalamic stimulator pulse generator
      with initial insertion of battery
        package - *omit code*
      new site (skin) (subcutaneous) 86.09
  previous mastectomy site - *see* categories
    85.0
  proctostomy 48.79
  prosthesis
    acetabular and femoral components
      (total) 00.70
    acetabular component only 00.71
    acetabular liner and/or femoral head
      only 00.73
    ankle 81.59
    breast 85.93
    elbow 81.97
    epiretinal visual 14.83
    femoral component only 00.72
    femoral head only and/or acetabular
      liner 00.73
    foot 81.59
    hand 81.97
    heart valve (poppet) 35.95
    hip 81.53
      acetabular component only 00.71
      acetabular liner and/or femoral head
        only 00.73
      femoral component only 00.72
      femoral head only and/or acetabular
        liner 00.73
      partial
        acetabular component only
          00.71
        acetabular liner and/or femoral
          head only 00.73
        femoral component only 00.72
        femoral head only and/or
          acetabular liner 00.73
      acetabular and femoral components
        (total) 00.70
      total (acetabular and femoral
        components) 00.70
    knee NOS 81.55
      femoral component 00.82
      partial
        femoral component 00.82
        patellar component 00.83
        tibial component 00.81
        tibial insert 00.84
      patellar component 00.83
      tibial component 00.81
      tibial insert 00.84
      total (all components) 00.80
  lower extremity NEC 81.59
  shoulder 81.97

Revision *(Continued)*
  prosthesis *(Continued)*
    spine
      facet replacement device(s) 84.85
      interspinous process device(s) 84.81
      pedicle-based dynamic stabilization
        device(s) 84.83
    toe 81.59
    upper extremity 81.97
    wrist 81.97
  ptosis overcorrection 08.37
  pyelostomy 55.12
  pyloroplasty 44.29
  rhinoplasty 21.84
    scar
      skin 86.84
        with excision 86.3
  scleral fistulization 12.66
  shoulder replacement (prosthesis) 81.97
  shunt
    arteriovenous (cannula) (for dialysis)
      39.42
    lumbar-subarachnoid NEC 03.97
    peritoneojugular 54.99
    peritoneovascular 54.99
    pleurothecal 03.97
    salpingothecal 03.97
    spinal (thecal) NEC 03.97
    subarachnoid-peritoneal 03.97
    subarachnoid-ureteral 03.97
    ventricular (cerebral) 02.42
    ventriculoperitoneal
      at peritoneal site 54.95
      at ventricular site 02.42
  stapedectomy NEC 19.29
    with incus replacement (homograft)
      (prosthesis) 19.21
  stimulator
    electrode(s)
      carotid sinus 39.84
    pulse generator
      carotid sinus 39.85
  stoma
    bile duct 51.79
    bladder (vesicostomy) 57.22
    bronchus 33.42
    common duct 51.72
    esophagus 42.89
    gallbladder 51.99
    hepatic duct 51.79
    intestine 46.40
      large 46.43
      small 46.41
    kidney 55.89
    larynx 31.63
    rectum 48.79
    stomach 44.69
      laparoscopic 44.68
    thorax 34.79
    trachea 31.74
    ureter 56.62
    urethra 58.49
  tack operation 20.79
  toe replacement (prosthesis) 81.59
  tracheostomy 31.74
  tunnel
    pulse generator lead wire 86.99
      with initial procedure - *omit code*
  tympanoplasty 19.6
  uretero-ileostomy, cutaneous 56.52
  ureterostomy (cutaneous) (stoma) NEC 56.62
    ileal 56.52
  urethrostomy 58.49
  urinary conduit 56.52
  vascular procedure (previous) NEC 39.49
  ventricular shunt (cerebral) 02.42
  vesicostomy stoma 57.22
  wrist replacement (prosthesis) 81.97
Rhinectomy 21.4
Rhinocheiloplasty 27.59
  cleft lip 27.54

◀ New   ◀|| Revised   ~~deleted~~ Deleted   ● Use Additional Digit(s)   ▨ Omit code

Rhinomanometry 89.12
Rhinoplasty (external) (internal) NEC 21.87
  augmentation (with graft) (with synthetic
      implant) 21.85
  limited 21.86
  revision 21.84
  tip 21.86
  twisted nose 21.84
Rhinorrhaphy (external) (internal) 21.81
  for epistaxis 21.09
Rhinoscopy 21.21
Rhinoseptoplasty 21.84
Rhinotomy 21.1
Rhizotomy (radiofrequency) (spinal) 03.1
  acoustic 04.01
  trigeminal 04.02
Rhytidectomy (facial) 86.82
  eyelid
    lower 08.86
    upper 08.87
Rhytidoplasty (facial) 86.82
Ripstein operation (repair of prolapsed rectum)
    48.75
Robotic assisted surgery
  endoscopic 17.44
  laparoscopic 17.42

Robotic assisted surgery (Continued)
  open 17.41
  other and unspecified 17.49
  percutaneous 17.43
  thoracoscopic 17.45
Rodney Smith operation (radical subtotal
    pancreatectomy) 52.53
Roentgenography - see also Radiography
  cardiac, negative contrast 88.58
Rolling of conjunctiva 10.33
Root
  canal (tooth) (therapy) 23.70
    with
      apicoectomy 23.72
      irrigation 23.71
      resection (tooth) (apex) 23.73
        with root canal therapy 23.72
        residual or retained 23.11
Rotation of fetal head
  forceps (instrumental) (Kielland)
      (Scanzoni) (key-in-lock)
      72.4
  manual 73.51
Routine
  chest x-ray 87.44
  psychiatric visit 94.12

Roux-en-Y operation
  bile duct 51.36
  cholecystojejunostomy 51.32
  esophagus (intrathoracic) 42.54
  gastroenterostomy 44.39
    laparoscopic 44.38
  gastrojejunostomy 44.39
    laparoscopic 44.38
  pancreaticojejunostomy 52.96
Roux-Goldthwait operation (repair of
    recurrent patellar dislocation)
    81.44
Roux-Herzen-Judine operation (jejunal loop
    interposition) 42.63
Rubin test (insufflation of fallopian tube)
    66.8
Ruiz-Mora operation (proximal phalangectomy
    for hammer toe) 77.99
Rupture
  esophageal web 42.01
  joint adhesions, manual 93.26
  membranes, artificial 73.09
    for surgical induction of labor 73.01
  ovarian cyst, manual 65.93
Russe operation (bone graft of scaphoid) 78.04

S

Sacculotomy (tack) 20.79
Sacrectomy (partial) 77.89
  total 77.99
Saemisch operation (corneal section) 11.1
Salpingectomy (bilateral) (total) (transvaginal)
    66.51
  with oophorectomy 65.61
    laparoscopic 65.63
  partial (unilateral) 66.69
    with removal of tubal pregnancy 66.62
    bilateral 66.63
      for sterilization 66.39
        by endoscopy 66.29
  remaining or solitary tube 66.52
    with ovary 65.62
      laparoscopic 65.64
  unilateral (total) 66.4
    with
      oophorectomy 65.49
        laparoscopic 65.41
      removal of tubal pregnancy 66.62
      partial 66.69
Salpingography 87.85
Salpingohysterostomy 66.74
Salpingo-oophorectomy (unilateral) 65.49
  that by laparoscope 65.41
  bilateral (same operative episode) 65.61
    laparoscopic 65.63
  remaining or solitary tube and ovary 65.62
    laparoscopic 65.64
Salpingo-oophoroplasty 65.73
  laparoscopic 65.76
Salpingo-oophororrhaphy 65.79
Salpingo-oophorostomy 66.72
Salpingo-oophorotomy 65.09
  laparoscopic 65.01
Salpingoplasty 66.79
Salpingorrhaphy 66.71
Salpingosalpingostomy 66.73
Salpingostomy (for removal of non-ruptured
    ectopic pregnancy) 66.02
Salpingotomy 66.01
Salpingo-uterostomy 66.74
Salter operation (innominate osteotomy)
    77.39
Salvage (autologous blood) (intraoperative)
    (perioperative) (postoperative) 99.00

Sampling, blood for genetic determination of
    fetus 75.33
Sandpapering (skin) 86.25
Saucerization
  bone - see also Excision, lesion, bone 77.60
  rectum 48.99
Sauer-Bacon operation (abdominoperineal
    resection), NOS 48.50
  laparoscopic 48.51
  open 48.52
  other 48.59
Scalenectomy 83.45
Scalenotomy 83.19
Scaling and polishing, dental 96.54
Scan, scanning
  C.A.T. (computerized axial tomography)
      88.38
    with computer assisted surgery (CAS)
        00.31
    abdomen 88.01
    bone 88.38
      mineral density 88.98
    brain 87.03
    cardiac 87.41
    coronary 87.41
    head 87.03
    kidney 87.71
    skeletal 88.38
      mineral density 88.98
    thorax 87.41
  computerized axial tomography (C.A.T.) - see
      also Scan, C.A.T. 88.38
  C.T. - see Scan, C.A.T.
  gallium - see Scan, radioisotope
  liver 92.02
  MUGA (multiple gated acquisition) - see
      Scan, radioisotope
  positron emission tomography (PET) - see
      Scan, radioisotope
  radioisotope
    adrenal 92.09
    bone 92.14
      marrow 92.05
    bowel 92.04
    cardiac output 92.05
    cardiovascular 92.05
    cerebral 92.11
    circulation time 92.05
    eye 95.16

Scan, scanning (Continued)
  radioisotope (Continued)
    gastrointestinal 92.04
    head NEC 92.12
    hematopoietic 92.05
    intestine 92.04
    iodine-131 92.01
    kidney 92.03
    liver 92.02
    lung 92.15
    lymphatic system 92.16
    myocardial infarction 92.05
    pancreatic 92.04
    parathyroid 92.13
    pituitary 92.11
    placenta 92.17
    protein-bound iodine 92.01
    pulmonary 92.15
    radio-iodine uptake 92.01
    renal 92.03
    specified site NEC 92.19
    spleen 92.05
    thyroid 92.01
    total body 92.18
    uterus 92.19
  renal 92.03
  thermal - see Thermography
Scapulectomy (partial) 77.81
  total 77.91
Scapulopexy 78.41
Scarification
  conjunctiva 10.33
  nasal veins (with packing) 21.03
  pericardium 36.39
  pleura 34.6
    chemical 34.92
      with cancer chemotherapy substance
          34.92 [99.25]
      tetracycline 34.92 [99.21]
Schanz operation (femoral osteotomy) 77.35
Schauta (-Amreich) operation (radical vaginal
    hysterectomy) 68.79
  laparoscopic 68.71
Schede operation (thoracoplasty) 33.34
Scheie operation
  cautery of sclera 12.62
  sclerostomy 12.62
Schlatter operation (total gastrectomy)
    43.99

Schroeder operation (endocervical excision) 67.39
Schuchardt operation (nonobstetrical episiotomy) 71.09
Schwartze operation (simple mastoidectomy) 20.41
Scintiphotography - see Scan, radioisotope
Scintiscan - see Scan, radioisotope
Sclerectomy (punch) (scissors) 12.65
  for retinal reattachment 14.49
  Holth's 12.65
  trephine 12.61
    with implant 14.41
Scleroplasty 12.89
Sclerosis - see Sclerotherapy
Sclerostomy (Scheie's) 12.62
Sclerotherapy
  esophageal varices (endoscopic) 42.33
  hemorrhoids 49.42
  pleura 34.92
    treatment of malignancy (cytotoxic agent) 34.92 [99.25]
      with tetracycline 34.92 [99.21]
  varicose vein 39.92
  vein NEC 39.92
Sclerotomy (exploratory) 12.89
  anterior 12.89
    with
      iridectomy 12.65
      removal of vitreous 14.71
  posterior 12.89
    with
      iridectomy 12.65
      removal of vitreous 14.72
Scott operation
  intestinal bypass for obesity 45.93
  jejunocolostomy (bypass) 45.93
Scraping
  corneal epithelium 11.41
    for smear or culture 11.21
  trachoma follicles 10.33
Scrotectomy (partial) 61.3
Scrotoplasty 61.49
Scrotorrhaphy 61.41
Scrotomy 61.0
Scrub, posterior nasal (adhesions) 21.91
Sculpturing, heart valve - see Valvuloplasty, heart
Section - see also Division and Incision
  cesarean - see Cesarean section
  ganglion, sympathetic 05.0
  hypophyseal stalk - see also Hypophysectomy, partial 07.63
  ligamentum flavum (spine) - omit code
  nerve (cranial) (peripheral) NEC 04.03
    acoustic 04.01
    spinal root (posterior) 03.1
    sympathetic 05.0
    trigeminal tract 04.02
  Saemisch (corneal) 11.1
  spinal ligament 80.49
    arcuate - omit code
    flavum - omit code
  tooth (impacted) 23.19
Seddon-Brooks operation (transfer of pectoralis major tendon) 83.75
Semb operation (apicolysis of lung) 33.39
Senning operation (correction of transposition of great vessels) 35.91
Separation
  twins (attached) (conjoined) (Siamese) 84.93
    asymmetrical (unequal) 84.93
    symmetrical (equal) 84.92
Septectomy
  atrial (closed) 35.41
    open 35.42
    transvenous method (balloon) 35.41
  submucous (nasal) 21.5
Septoplasty NEC 21.88
  with submucous resection of septum 21.5
Septorhinoplasty 21.84

Septostomy (atrial) (balloon) 35.41
Septotomy, nasal 21.1
Sequestrectomy
  bone 77.00
    carpals, metacarpals 77.04
    clavicle 77.01
    facial 76.01
    femur 77.05
    fibula 77.07
    humerus 77.02
    nose 21.32
    patella 77.06
    pelvic 77.09
    phalanges (foot) (hand) 77.09
    radius 77.03
    scapula 77.01
    skull 01.25
    specified site NEC 77.09
    tarsals, metatarsals 77.08
    thorax (ribs) (sternum) 77.01
    tibia 77.07
    ulna 77.03
    vertebrae 77.09
  nose 21.32
  skull 01.25
Sesamoidectomy 77.98
Setback, ear 18.5
Sever operation (division of soft tissue of arm) 83.19
Severing of blepharorrhaphy 08.02
Sewell operation (heart) 36.2
Sharrard operation (iliopsoas muscle transfer) 83.77
Shaving
  bone - see also Excision, lesion, bone 77.60
  cornea (epithelium) 11.41
    for smear or culture 11.21
  patella 77.66
Shelf operation (hip arthroplasty) 81.40
Shirodkar operation (encirclement suture, cervix) 67.59
Shock therapy
  chemical 94.24
  electroconvulsive 94.27
  electrotonic 94.27
  insulin 94.24
  subconvulsive 94.26
Shortening
  bone (fusion) 78.20
    femur 78.25
    specified site NEC - see category 78.2●
    tibia 78.27
    ulna 78.23
  endopelvic fascia 69.22
  extraocular muscle NEC 15.22
    multiple (two or more muscles) 15.4
  eyelid margin 08.71
  eye muscle NEC 15.22
    multiple (two or more muscles) (with lengthening) 15.4
  finger (macrodactyly repair) 82.83
  heel cord 83.85
  levator palpebrae muscle 08.33
  ligament - see also Arthroplasty
    round 69.22
    uterosacral 69.22
  muscle 83.85
    extraocular 15.22
      multiple (two or more muscles) 15.4
    hand 82.55
  sclera (for repair of retinal detachment) 14.59
    by scleral buckling - see also Buckling, scleral 14.49
  tendon 83.85
    hand 82.55
  ureter (with reimplantation) 56.41
Shunt - see also Anastomosis and Bypass, vascular
  abdominovenous 54.94
  aorta-coronary sinus 36.39
  aorta (descending)-pulmonary (artery) 39.0

Shunt (Continued)
  aortocarotid 39.22
  aortoceliac 39.26
  aortofemoral 39.25
  aortoiliac 39.25
  aortoiliofemoral 39.25
  aortomesenteric 39.26
  aorto-myocardial (graft) 36.2
  aortorenal 39.24
  aortosubclavian 39.22
  apicoaortic 35.93
  aqueous drainage 12.67
  arteriovenous NEC 39.29
    for renal dialysis (by)
      anastomosis 39.27
      external cannula 39.93
  ascending aorta to pulmonary artery (Waterston) 39.0
  axillary-femoral 39.29
  carotid-carotid 39.22
  carotid-subclavian 39.22
  caval-mesenteric 39.1
  corpora cavernosa-corpus spongiosum 64.98
  corpora-saphenous 64.98
  descending aorta to pulmonary artery (Potts-Smith) 39.0
  endolymphatic (-subarachnoid) 20.71
  endolymph-perilymph 20.71
  extracranial-intracranial (EC-IC) 39.28
  femoroperoneal 39.29
  femoropopliteal 39.29
  iliofemoral 39.25
  ilioiliac 39.25
  intestinal
    large-to-large 45.94
    small-to-large 45.93
    small-to-small 45.91
  left subclavian to descending aorta (Blalock-Park) 39.0
  left-to-right (systemic-pulmonary artery) 39.0
  left ventricle (heart) (apex) and aorta 35.93
  lienorenal 39.1
  lumbar-subarachnoid (with valve) NEC 03.79
  mesocaval 39.1
  peritoneal-jugular 54.94
  peritoneo-vascular 54.94
  peritoneovenous 54.94
  pleuroperitoneal 34.05
  pleurothecal (with valve) 03.79
  portacaval (double) 39.1
  portal-systemic 39.1
  portal vein to vena cava 39.1
  pulmonary-innominate 39.0
  pulmonary vein to atrium 35.82
  renoportal 39.1
  right atrium and pulmonary artery 35.94
  right ventricle and pulmonary artery (distal) 35.92
    in repair of
      pulmonary artery atresia 35.92
      transposition of great vessels 35.92
      truncus arteriosus 35.83
  salpingothecal (with valve) 03.79
  semicircular subarachnoid 20.71
  spinal (thecal) (with valve) NEC 03.79
    subarachnoid-peritoneal 03.71
    subarachnoid-ureteral 03.72
  splenorenal (venous) 39.1
    arterial 39.26
  subarachnoid-peritoneal (with valve) 03.71
  subarachnoid-ureteral (with valve) 03.72
  subclavian-pulmonary 39.0
  subdural-peritoneal (with valve) 02.34
  superior mesenteric-caval 39.1
  systemic-pulmonary artery 39.0
  transjugular intrahepatic portosystemic [TIPS] 39.1
  vena cava to pulmonary artery (Green) 39.21

Shunt *(Continued)*
  ventricular (cerebral) (with valve) 02.22
    to
      abdominal cavity or organ 02.34
      bone marrow 02.39
      cervical subarachnoid space 02.22
      circulatory system 02.32
      cisterna magna 02.22
      extracranial site NEC 02.39
      gallbladder 02.34
      head or neck structure 02.31
      intracerebral site NEC 02.22
      lumbar site 02.39
      mastoid 02.31
      nasopharynx 02.31
      peritoneal 02.34
      thoracic cavity 02.33
      ureter 02.35
      urinary system 02.35
      venous system 02.32
  ventriculoatrial (with valve) 02.32
  ventriculocaval (with valve) 02.32
  ventriculocisternal (with valve) 02.22
  ventriculolumbar (with valve) 02.39
  ventriculomastoid (with valve) 02.31
  ventriculonasopharyngeal 02.31
  ventriculopleural (with valve) 02.33
Sialoadenectomy (parotid) (sublingual)
    (submaxillary) 26.30
  complete 26.32
  partial 26.31
  radical 26.32
Sialoadenolithotomy 26.0
Sialoadenotomy 26.0
Sialodochoplasty NEC 26.49
Sialogram 87.09
Sialolithotomy 26.0
Sieve, vena cava 38.7
Sigmoid bladder 57.87 [45.52]
Sigmoidectomy
  laparoscopic 17.36
  open and other 45.76
Sigmoidomyotomy 46.91
Sigmoidopexy (Moschowitz) 46.63
Sigmoidoproctectomy - *see also* Resection,
    rectum 48.69
Sigmoidoproctostomy 45.94
Sigmoidorectostomy 45.94
Sigmoidorrhaphy 46.75
Sigmoidoscopy (rigid) 48.23
  with biopsy 45.25
  flexible 45.24
  through stoma (artificial) 45.22
  transabdominal 45.21
Sigmoidosigmoidostomy 45.94
  proximal to distal segment
    laparoscopic 17.36
    open and other 45.76
Sigmoidostomy - *see also* Colostomy 46.10
Sigmoidotomy 45.03
Sign language 93.75
Silver operation (bunionectomy) 77.59
Sinogram
  abdominal wall 88.03
  chest wall 87.38
  retroperitoneum 88.14
Sinusectomy (nasal) (complete) (partial) (with
    turbinectomy) 22.60
  antrum 22.62
    with Caldwell-Luc approach 22.61
  ethmoid 22.63
  frontal 22.42
  maxillary 22.62
    with Caldwell-Luc approach 22.61
  sphenoid 22.64
Sinusotomy (nasal) 22.50
  antrum (intranasal) 22.2
    with external approach (Caldwell-Luc)
      22.39
      radical (with removal of membrane
        lining) 22.31

Sinusotomy *(Continued)*
  ethmoid 22.51
  frontal 22.41
  maxillary (intranasal) 22.2
    external approach (Caldwell-Luc) 22.39
      radical (with removal of membrane
        lining) 22.31
  multiple 22.53
  perinasal 22.50
  sphenoid 22.52
Sistrunk operation (excision of thyroglossal
    cyst) 06.7
Size reduction
  abdominal wall (adipose) (pendulous) 86.83
  arms (adipose) (batwing) 86.83
  breast (bilateral) 85.32
    unilateral 85.31
  buttocks (adipose) 86.83
  skin 86.83
  subcutaneous tissue 86.83
  thighs (adipose) 86.83
Skeletal series (x-ray) 88.31
SKyphoplasty 81.66
Sling - *see also* Operation, sling
  fascial (fascia lata)
    for facial weakness (trigeminal nerve
      paralysis) 86.81
      mouth 86.81
      orbicularis (mouth) 86.81
      tongue 25.59
  levator muscle (urethrocystopexy) 59.71
  pubococcygeal 59.71
  rectum (puborectalis) 48.76
  tongue (fascial) 25.59
Slitting
  canaliculus for
    passage of tube 09.42
    removal of streptothrix 09.42
  lens 13.2
  prepuce (dorsal) (lateral) 64.91
Slocum operation (pes anserinus transfer) 81.47
Sluder operation (tonsillectomy) 28.2
Small bowel series (x-ray) 87.63
Smith operation (open osteotomy of mandible)
    76.62
Smith-Peterson operation (radiocarpal
    arthrodesis) 81.25
Smithwick operation (sympathectomy) 05.29
Snaring, polyp, colon (endoscopic) 45.42
Snip, punctum (with dilation) 09.51
Soave operation (endorectal pull-through)
    48.41
Somatotherapy, psychiatric NEC 94.29
Sonneberg operation (inferior maxillary
    neurectomy) 04.07
Sorondo-Ferré operation (hindquarter
    amputation) 84.19
Soutter operation (iliac crest fasciotomy) 83.14
Spaulding-Richardson operation (uterine
    suspension) 69.22
Spectrophotometry NEC 89.39
  blood 89.39
  placenta 89.29
  urine 89.29
Spectroscopy
  intravascular 38.23
  near infrared (NIR) 38.23
Speech therapy NEC 93.75
Spermatocelectomy 63.2
Spermatocystectomy 60.73
Spermatocystotomy 60.72
Sphenoidectomy 22.64
Sphenoidotomy 22.52
Sphincterectomy, anal 49.6
Sphincteroplasty
  anal 49.79
    obstetrical laceration (current) 75.62
    old 49.79
  bladder neck 57.85
  pancreas 51.83
  sphincter of Oddi 51.83

Sphincterorrhaphy, anal 49.71
  obstetrical laceration (current) 75.62
  old 49.79
Sphincterotomy
  anal (external) (internal) 49.59
    left lateral 49.51
    posterior 49.52
  bladder (neck) (transurethral) 57.91
  choledochal 51.82
    endoscopic 51.85
  iris 12.12
  pancreatic 51.82
    endoscopic 51.85
  sphincter of Oddi 51.82
    endoscopic 51.85
  transduodenal ampullary 51.82
    endoscopic 51.85
Spinal anesthesia - *omit code*
Spinelli operation (correction of inverted
    uterus) 75.93
Spineoplasty 81.66
Spirometry (incentive) (respiratory) 89.37
Spivack operation (permanent gastrostomy)
    43.19
Splanchnicectomy 05.29
Splanchnicotomy 05.0
Splenectomy (complete) (total) 41.5
  partial 41.43
Splenogram 88.64
  radioisotope 92.05
Splenolysis 54.59
  laparoscopic 54.51
Splenopexy 41.95
Splenoplasty 41.95
Splenoportogram (by splenic arteriography)
    88.64
Splenorrhaphy 41.95
Splenotomy 41.2
Splinting
  dental (for immobilization) 93.55
    orthodontic 24.7
  musculoskeletal 93.54
  ureteral 56.2
Splitting - *see also* Division
  canaliculus 09.52
  lacrimal papilla 09.51
  spinal cord tracts 03.29
    percutaneous 03.21
  tendon sheath 83.01
    hand 82.01
Spondylosyndesis - *see also* Fusion, spinal 81.00
S.P. Rogers operation (knee disarticulation)
    84.16
Ssabanejew-Frank operation (permanent
    gastrostomy) 43.19
Stab, intercostal 34.09
Stabilization, joint - *see also* Arthrodesis
  patella (for recurrent dislocation) 81.44
Stacke operation (simple mastoidectomy) 20.41
Stallard operation
    (conjunctivocystorhinostomy) 09.82
  with insertion of tube or stent 09.83
Stamm (-Kader) operation (temporary
    gastrostomy) 43.19
Stapedectomy 19.19
  with incus replacement (homograft)
    (prosthesis) 19.11
  revision 19.29
    with incus replacement 19.21
Stapediolysis 19.0
Stapling
  artery 39.31
  blebs, lung (emphysematous) 32.21
  diaphysis - *see also* Stapling, epiphyseal plate
    78.20
  epiphyseal plate 78.20
    femur 78.25
    fibula 78.27
    humerus 78.22
    radius 78.23
    specified site NEC 78.29

Stapling *(Continued)*
  epiphyseal plate *(Continued)*
    tibia 78.27
    ulna 78.23
  gastric varices 44.91
  graft - *see* Graft
  left atrial appendage 37.36
  vein 39.32
STARR (stapled transanal rectal resection)
    48.74
StaXx® FX Structural Kyphoplasty System
    81.66
Steinberg operation 44.5
Steindler operation
  fascia stripping (for cavus deformity) 83.14
  flexorplasty (elbow) 83.77
  muscle transfer 83.77
Stereotactic radiosurgery 92.30
  cobalt 60 92.32
  linear accelerator (LINAC) 92.31
  multi-source 92.32
  particle beam 92.33
  particulate 92.33
  radiosurgery NEC 92.39
  single source photon 92.31
Stereotactic head frame application 93.59
Sterilization
  female - *see also* specific operation 66.39
  male NEC - *see also* Ligation, vas deferens
    63.70
Sternotomy 77.31
  as operative approach - *omit code*
  for bone marrow biopsy 41.31
Stewart operation (renal plication with
    pyeloplasty) 55.87
Stimulation (electronic) - *see also* Implant,
    electronic stimulator
  bone growth (percutaneous) - *see* category
    78.9 ●
    transcutaneous (surface) 99.86
  cardiac (external) 99.62
    internal 37.91
  carotid sinus 99.64
  CaverMap™ 89.58
  defibrillator
    as part of intraoperative testing - *omit code*
    catheter based invasive electrophysiologic
      testing 37.26
    device interrogation only without
      arrhythmia induction (bedside
      check) 89.45–89.49
    non-invasive programmed electrical
      stimulation (NIPS) 37.20
  electrophysiologic, cardiac
    as part of intraoperative testing - *omit code*
    catheter based invasive electrophysiologic
      testing 37.26
    device interrogation only without
      arrhythmia induction (bedside
      check) 89.45–89.49
    noninvasive programmed electrical
      stimulation (NIPS) 37.20
  nerve
    CaverMap™ 89.58
    penile 89.58
    peripheral or spinal cord, transcutaneous
      93.39
Stitch, Kelly-Stoeckel (urethra) 59.3
Stomatoplasty 27.59
Stomatorrhaphy 27.52
Stone operation (anoplasty) 49.79
Strapping (non-traction) 93.59
Strassman operation (metroplasty) 69.49
Strayer operation (gastrocnemius recession)
    83.72
Stretching
  eyelid (with elongation) 08.71
  fascia 93.28
  foreskin 99.95
  iris 12.63
  muscle 93.27

Stretching *(Continued)*
  nerve (cranial) (peripheral) 04.91
  tendon 93.27
Stripping
  bone - *see also* Incision, bone 77.10
  carotid sinus 39.89
  cranial suture 02.01
  fascia 83.14
    hand 82.12
  membranes for surgical induction of labor
    73.1
  meninges (cerebral) 01.51
    spinal 03.4
  saphenous vein, varicose 38.59
  subdural membrane (cerebral) 01.51
    spinal 03.4
  varicose veins (lower limb) 38.59
    upper limb 38.53
  vocal cords 30.09
Stromeyer-Little operation (hepatotomy) 50.0
Strong operation (unbridling of celiac artery
    axis) 39.91
Stryker frame 93.59
Study
  bone mineral density 88.98
  bundle of His 37.29
  color vision 95.06
  conduction, nerve (median) 89.15
  dark adaptation, eye 95.07
  electrophysiologic stimulation and
      recording, cardiac
    as part of intraoperative testing - *omit code*
    catheter based invasive electrophysiologic
      testing 37.26
    device interrogation only without
      arrhythmia induction (bedside
      check) 89.45–89.49
    noninvasive programmed electrical
      stimulation (NIPS) 37.20
  function - *see also* Function, study
    radioisotope - *see* Scan, radioisotope
  lacrimal flow (radiographic) 87.05
  ocular motility 95.15
  pulmonary
    airway flow measurement, endoscopic
      33.72
    function - *see* categories 89.37
  radiographic - *see* Radiography
  radio-iodinated triolein 92.04
  renal clearance 92.03
  spirometer 89.37
  tracer - *see also* Scan, radioisotope eye (P32)
    95.16
  ultrasonic - *see* Ultrasonography
  visual field 95.05
  xenon flow NEC 92.19
    cardiovascular 92.05
    pulmonary 92.15
Sturmdorf operation (conization of cervix) 67.2
Submucous resection
  larynx 30.29
  nasal septum 21.5
Summerskill operation
    (dacryocystorhinostomy by intubation)
    09.81
Surgery
  computer assisted (CAS) 00.39
    with robotics – *see* category 17.4 ●
    CAS with CT/CTA 00.31
    CAS with fluoroscopy 00.33
    CAS with MR/MRA 00.32
    CAS with multiple datasets 00.35
      imageless 00.34
      other CAS 00.39
    IGS - *see* Surgery, computer assisted
    image guided - *see* Surgery, computer
      assisted
    navigation (CT-free, IGN image guided,
      imageless) - *see* Surgery, computer
      assisted
  robotic assisted – *see* category 17.4 ●

Surmay operation (jejunostomy) 46.39
Suspension
  balanced, for traction 93.45
  bladder NEC 57.89
  diverticulum, pharynx 29.59
  kidney 55.7
  Olshausen (uterus) 69.22
  ovary 65.79
  paraurethral (Pereyra) 59.6
  periurethral 59.6
  urethra (retropubic) (sling) 59.5
  urethrovesical
    Goebel-Frangenheim-Stoeckel 59.4
    gracilis muscle transplant 59.71
    levator muscle sling 59.71
    Marshall-Marchetti (-Krantz) 59.5
    Millin-Read 59.4
    suprapubic 59.4
  uterus (abdominal or vaginal approach)
    69.22
  vagina 70.77
    with graft or prosthesis 70.78
Suture (laceration)
  abdominal wall 54.63
    secondary 54.61
  adenoid fossa 28.7
  adrenal (gland) 07.44
  aneurysm (cerebral) (peripheral) 39.52
  anus 49.71
    obstetric laceration (current) 75.62
    old 49.79
  aorta 39.31
  aponeurosis - *see also* Suture, tendon 83.64
  arteriovenous fistula 39.53
  artery 39.31
    percutaneous puncture closure - *omit code*
  bile duct 51.79
  bladder 57.81
    obstetric laceration (current) 75.61
  blood vessel NEC 39.30
    artery 39.31
      percutaneous puncture closure -
        omit code
    vein 39.32
  breast (skin) 85.81
  bronchus 33.41
  bursa 83.99
    hand 82.99
  canaliculus 09.73
  cecum 46.75
  cerebral meninges 02.11
  cervix (traumatic laceration) 67.61
    internal os, encirclement 67.59
    obstetric laceration (current) 75.51
      old 67.69
  chest wall 34.71
  cleft palate 27.62
  clitoris 71.4
  colon 46.75
  common duct 51.71
  conjunctiva 10.6
  cornea 11.51
    with conjunctival flap 11.53
  corneoscleral 11.51
    with conjunctival flap 11.53
  diaphragm 34.82
  duodenum 46.71
    ulcer (bleeding) (perforated) 44.42
      endoscopic 44.43
  dura mater (cerebral) 02.11
    spinal 03.59
  ear, external 18.4
  enterocele 70.92
    with graft or prosthesis 70.93
  entropion 08.42
  epididymis (and)
    spermatic cord 63.51
    vas deferens 63.81
  episiotomy - *see* Episiotomy
  esophagus 42.82
  eyeball 16.89

◀ New   ◀◀ Revised   ~~deleted~~ Deleted   ● Use Additional Digit(s)   �ढ Omit code

Suture *(Continued)*
  eyebrow 08.81
  eyelid 08.81
    with entropion or ectropion repair 08.42
  fallopian tube 66.71
  fascia 83.65
    hand 82.46
    to skeletal attachment 83.89
      hand 82.89
  gallbladder 51.91
  ganglion, sympathetic 05.81
  gingiva 24.32
  great vessel 39.30
    artery 39.31
    vein 39.32
  gum 24.32
  heart 37.49
  hepatic duct 51.79
  hymen 70.76
  ileum 46.73
  intestine 46.79
    large 46.75
    small 46.73
  jejunum 46.73
  joint capsule 81.96
    with arthroplasty - *see* Arthroplasty
      ankle 81.94
      foot 81.94
      lower extremity NEC 81.95
      upper extremity 81.93
  kidney 55.81
  labia 71.71
  laceration - *see* Suture, by site
  larynx 31.61
  ligament 81.96
    with arthroplasty - *see* Arthroplasty
    ankle 81.94
    broad 69.29
    Cooper's 54.64
    foot and toes 81.94
    gastrocolic 54.73
    knee 81.95
    lower extremity NEC 81.95
    sacrouterine 69.29
    upper extremity 81.93
    uterine 69.29
  ligation - *see* Ligation
  lip 27.51
  liver 50.61
  lung 33.43
  meninges (cerebral) 02.11
    spinal 03.59
  mesentery 54.75
  mouth 27.52
  muscle 83.65
    hand 82.46
    ocular (oblique) (rectus) 15.7
  nerve (cranial) (peripheral) 04.3
    sympathetic 05.81
  nose (external) (internal) 21.81
    for epistaxis 21.09
  obstetric laceration NEC 75.69
    bladder 75.61
    cervix 75.51
    corpus uteri 75.52
    pelvic floor 75.69
    perineum 75.69
    periurethral 75.69
    rectum 75.62
    sphincter ani 75.62
    urethra 75.61
    uterus 75.50
    vagina 75.69
    vulva 75.69
  omentum 54.64
  ovary 65.71
    laparoscopic 65.74
  palate 27.61
    cleft 27.62
  palpebral fissure 08.59
  pancreas 52.95

Suture *(Continued)*
  pelvic floor 71.71
    obstetric laceration (current) 75.69
  penis 64.41
  peptic ulcer (bleeding) (perforated) 44.40
  pericardium 37.49
  perineum (female) 71.71
    after delivery 75.69
      episiotomy repair - *see* Episiotomy
    male 86.59
  periosteum 78.20
    carpal, metacarpal 78.24
    femur 78.25
    fibula 78.27
    humerus 78.22
    pelvic 78.29
    phalanges (foot) (hand) 78.29
    radius 78.23
    specified site NEC 78.29
    tarsal, metatarsal 78.28
    tibia 78.27
    ulna 78.23
    vertebrae 78.29
  peritoneum 54.64
  periurethral tissue to symphysis pubis 59.5
  pharynx 29.51
  pleura 34.93
  rectum 48.71
    obstetric laceration (current) 75.62
  retina (for reattachment) 14.59
  sacrouterine ligament 69.29
  salivary gland 26.41
  scalp 86.59
    replantation 86.51
  sclera (with repair of conjunctiva) 12.81
  scrotum (skin) 61.41
  secondary
    abdominal wall 54.61
    episiotomy 75.69
    peritoneum 54.64
  sigmoid 46.75
  skin (mucous membrane) (without graft) 86.59
    with graft - *see* Graft, skin
    breast 85.81
    ear 18.4
    eyebrow 08.81
    eyelid 08.81
    nose 21.81
    penis 64.41
    scalp 86.59
      replantation 86.51
    scrotum 61.41
    vulva 71.71
  specified site NEC - *see* Repair, by site
  spermatic cord 63.51
  sphincter ani 49.71
    obstetric laceration (current) 75.62
    old 49.79
  spinal meninges 03.59
  spleen 41.95
  stomach 44.61
    ulcer (bleeding) (perforated) 44.41
      endoscopic 44.43
  subcutaneous tissue (without skin graft) 86.59
    with graft - *see* Graft, skin
  tendon (direct) (immediate) (primary) 83.64
    delayed (secondary) 83.62
      hand NEC 82.43
        flexors 82.42
    hand NEC 82.45
      delayed (secondary) 82.43
      flexors 82.44
        delayed (secondary) 82.42
    ocular 15.7
    rotator cuff 83.63
    sheath 83.61
      hand 82.41

Suture *(Continued)*
  tendon *(Continued)*
    supraspinatus (rotator cuff repair) 83.63
    to skeletal attachment 83.88
      hand 82.85
  Tenon's capsule 15.7
  testis 62.61
  thymus 07.93
  thyroid gland 06.93
  tongue 25.51
  tonsillar fossa 28.7
  trachea 31.71
  tunica vaginalis 61.41
  ulcer (bleeding) (perforated) (peptic) 44.40
    duodenum 44.42
      endoscopic 44.43
    gastric 44.41
      endoscopic 44.43
    intestine 46.79
    skin 86.59
    stomach 44.41
      endoscopic 44.43
  ureter 56.82
  urethra 58.41
    obstetric laceration (current) 75.61
  uterosacral ligament 69.29
  uterus 69.41
    obstetric laceration (current) 75.50
    old 69.49
  uvula 27.73
  vagina 70.71
    obstetric laceration (current) 75.69
    old 70.79
  vas deferens 63.81
  vein 39.32
  vulva 71.71
    obstetric laceration (current) 75.69
    old 71.79
Suture-ligation - *see also* Ligation
  blood vessel - *see* Ligation, blood vessel
Sweep, anterior iris 12.97
Swenson operation
  bladder reconstruction 57.87
  proctectomy 48.49
Swinney operation (urethral reconstruction) 58.46
Switch, switching
  coronary arteries 35.84
  great arteries, total 35.84
Syme operation
  ankle amputation through malleoli of tibia and fibula 84.14
  urethrotomy, external 58.0
Sympathectomy NEC 05.29
  cervical 05.22
  cervicothoracic 05.22
  lumbar 05.23
  periarterial 05.25
  presacral 05.24
  renal 05.29
  thoracolumbar 05.23
  tympanum 20.91
Sympatheticotripsy 05.0
Symphysiotomy 77.39
  assisting delivery (obstetrical) 73.94
  kidney (horseshoe) 55.85
Symphysis, pleural 34.6
Synchondrotomy - *see also* Division, cartilage 80.40
Syndactylization 86.89
Syndesmotomy - *see also* Division, ligament 80.40
Synechiotomy
  endometrium 68.21
  iris (posterior) 12.33
    anterior 12.32
Synovectomy (joint) (complete) (partial) 80.70
  ankle 80.77
  elbow 80.72

S

◀ New   ◀▌▌ Revised   ~~deleted~~ Deleted   ● Use Additional Digit(s)   ▨ Omit code

Synovectomy *(Continued)*
  foot and toe 80.78
  hand and finger 80.74
  hip 80.75
  knee 80.76
  shoulder 80.71

Synovectomy *(Continued)*
  specified site NEC 80.79
  spine 80.79
  tendon sheath 83.42
    hand 82.33
  wrist 80.73

Syringing
  lacrimal duct or sac 09.43
  nasolacrimal duct 09.43
    with
      dilation 09.43
      insertion of tube or stent 09.44

T

Taarnhoj operation (trigeminal nerve root decompression) 04.41
Tack operation (sacculotomy) 20.79
Tactile Guidance System™ [TGS] – *see* category 17.4●
Take-down
  anastomosis
    arterial 39.49
    blood vessel 39.49
    gastric, gastrointestinal 44.5
    intestine 46.93
    stomach 44.5
    vascular 39.49
    ventricular 02.43
  arterial bypass 39.49
  arteriovenous shunt 39.43
    with creation of new shunt 39.42
  cecostomy 46.52
  colostomy 46.52
  duodenostomy 46.51
  enterostomy 46.50
  esophagostomy 42.83
  gastroduodenostomy 44.5
  gastrojejunostomy 44.5
  ileostomy 46.51
  intestinal stoma 46.50
    large 46.52
    small 46.51
  jejunoileal bypass 46.93
  jejunostomy 46.51
  laryngostomy 31.62
  sigmoidostomy 46.52
  stoma
    bile duct 51.79
    bladder 57.82
    bronchus 33.42
    common duct 51.72
    esophagus 42.83
    gallbladder 51.92
    hepatic duct 51.79
    intestine 46.50
      large 46.52
      small 46.51
    kidney 55.82
    larynx 31.62
    rectum 48.72
    stomach 44.62
    thorax 34.72
    trachea 31.72
    ureter 56.83
    urethra 58.42
  systemic-pulmonary artery anastomosis 39.49
    in total repair of tetralogy of Fallot 35.81
  tracheostomy 31.72
  vascular anastomosis or bypass 39.49
  ventricular shunt (cerebral) 02.43
Talectomy 77.98
Talma-Morison operation (omentopexy) 54.74
Tamponade
  esophageal 96.06
  intrauterine (nonobstetric) 69.91
    after delivery or abortion 75.8
    antepartum 73.1
  vagina 96.14
    after delivery or abortion 75.8
    antepartum 73.1

Tanner operation (devascularization of stomach) 44.99
Tap
  abdomen 54.91
  chest 34.91
  cisternal 01.01
  cranial 01.09
  joint 81.91
  lumbar (diagnostic) (removal of dye) 03.31
  perilymphatic 20.79
  spinal (diagnostic) 03.31
  subdural (through fontanel) 01.09
  thorax 34.91
Tarsectomy 08.20
  de Grandmont 08.35
Tarsoplasty - *see also* Reconstruction, eyelid 08.70
Tarsorrhaphy (lateral) 08.52
  division or severing 08.02
Tattooing
  cornea 11.91
  skin 86.02
Tautening, eyelid for entropion 08.42
TAVI (transcatheter aortic valve implantation) 35.05
TAVR (transcatheter aortic valve replacement) 35.05
Telemetry (cardiac) 89.54
Teleradiotherapy
  beta particles 92.25
    intra-operative 92.41
  Betatron 92.24
  cobalt-60 92.23
  electrons 92.25
    intra-operative 92.41
  iodine-125 92.23
  linear accelerator 92.24
  neutrons 92.26
  particulate radiation NEC 92.26
  photons 92.24
  protons 92.26
  radioactive cesium 92.23
  radioisotopes NEC 92.23
Temperament assessment 94.02
Temperature gradient study - *see also* Thermography 88.89
Tendinoplasty - *see* Repair, tendon
Tendinosuture (immediate) (primary) - *see also* Suture, tendon 83.64
  hand - *see also* Suture, tendon, hand 82.45
Tendolysis 83.91
  hand 82.91
Tendoplasty - *see* Repair, tendon
Tenectomy 83.39
  eye 15.13
    levator palpebrae 08.33
    multiple (two or more tendons) 15.3
  hand 82.29
  levator palpebrae 08.33
  tendon sheath 83.31
    hand 82.21
Tenodesis (tendon fixation to skeletal attachment) 83.88
  Fowler 82.85
  hand 82.85
Tenolysis 83.91
  hand 82.91

Tenomyoplasty - *see also* Repair, tendon 83.88
  hand - *see also* Repair, tendon, hand 82.86
Tenomyotomy - *see* Tenonectomy
Tenonectomy 83.42
  for graft 83.41
    hand 82.32
  hand 82.33
    for graft 82.32
Tenontomyoplasty - *see* Repair, tendon
Tenontoplasty - *see* Repair, tendon
Tenoplasty - *see also* Repair, tendon 83.88
  hand - *see also* Repair, tendon, hand 82.86
Tenorrhaphy - *see also* Suture, tendon 83.64
  hand - *see also* Suture, tendon, hand 82.45
  to skeletal attachment 83.88
    hand 82.85
Tenosuspension 83.88
  hand 82.86
Tenosuture - *see also* Suture, tendon 83.64
  hand - *see also* Suture, tendon, hand 82.45
  to skeletal attachment 83.88
    hand 82.85
Tenosynovectomy 83.42
  hand 82.33
Tenotomy 83.13
  Achilles tendon 83.11
  adductor (hip) (subcutaneous) 83.12
  eye 15.12
    levator palpebrae 08.38
    multiple (two or more tendons) 15.4
  hand 82.11
  levator palpebrae 08.38
  pectoralis minor tendon (decompression thoracic outlet) 83.13
  stapedius 19.0
  tensor tympani 19.0
Tenovaginotomy - *see* Tenotomy
Tensing, orbicularis oculi 08.59
Termination of pregnancy
  by
    aspiration curettage 69.51
    dilation and curettage 69.01
    hysterectomy - *see* Hysterectomy
    hysterotomy 74.91
    intra-amniotic injection (saline) 75.0
Test, testing (for)
  14 C-Urea breath 89.39
  auditory function NEC 95.46
  Bender Visual-Motor Gestalt 94.02
  Benton Visual Retention 94.02
  cardiac (vascular)
    function NEC 89.59
    stress 89.44
      bicycle ergometer 89.43
      Masters' two-step 89.42
      treadmill 89.41
  Denver developmental (screening) 94.02
  fetus, fetal
    nonstress (fetal activity acceleration determinations) 75.34
    oxytocin challenge (contraction stress) 75.35
    sensitivity (to oxytocin) - *omit code*
  function
    cardiac NEC 89.59
    hearing NEC 95.46
    muscle (by)
      electromyography 93.08
      manual 93.04

◀ New   ◀▥ Revised   ~~deleted~~ Deleted   ● Use Additional Digit(s)   ▨ Omit code

Test, testing *(Continued)*
  function *(Continued)*
    neurologic NEC 89.15
    vestibular 95.46
      clinical 95.44
  glaucoma NEC 95.26
  hearing 95.47
    clinical NEC 95.42
  intelligence 94.01
  internal jugular-subclavian venous reflux
    89.62
  intracarotid amobarbital (Wada) 89.10
  Masters' two-step stress (cardiac) 89.42
  muscle function (by)
    electromyography 93.08
    manual 93.04
  neurologic function NEC 89.15
  neurophysiologic monitoring
    intra-operative 00.94
  nocturnal penile tumescence 89.29
  provocative, for glaucoma 95.26
  psychologic NEC 94.08
  psychometric 94.01
  radio-cobalt B12 Schilling 92.04
  range of motion 93.05
  rotation (Bárány chair) (hearing) 95.45
  sleep disorder function - *see* categories 89.17
  Stanford-Binet 94.01
  Thallium stress (transesophageal pacing)
    89.44
  tuning fork (hearing) 95.42
  Urea breath, (14 C) 89.39
  vestibular function NEC 95.46
    thermal 95.44
  Wada (hemispheric function) 89.10
  whispered speech (hearing) 95.42
TEVAP (transurethral electrovaporization of
  prostate) 60.29
Thalamectomy 01.41
Thalamotomy 01.41
  by stereotactic radiosurgery 92.32
    cobalt 60 92.32
    linear accelerator (LINAC) 92.31
    multi-source 92.32
    particle beam 92.33
    particulate 92.33
    radiosurgery NEC 92.39
    single source photon 92.31
Thal operation (repair of esophageal stricture)
  42.85
Theleplasty 85.87
Therapy
  Antabuse 94.25
  aqueous oxygen (AO) 00.49
  art 93.89
  aversion 94.33
  behavior 94.33
  Bennett respirator - *see* category 96.7●
  blind rehabilitation NEC 93.78
  Byrd respirator - *see* category 96.7●
  carbon dioxide 94.25
  cobalt-60 92.23
  conditioning, psychiatric 94.33
  continuous positive airway pressure (CPAP)
    93.90
    delivered by
      endotracheal tube - *see* category 96.7●
      tracheostomy – *see* category 96.7●
  croupette, croup tent 93.94
  daily living activities 93.83
    for the blind 93.78
  dance 93.89
  desensitization 94.33
  detoxification 94.25
  diversional 93.81
  domestic tasks 93.83
    for the blind 93.78
  Downstream® system 00.49
  educational (bed-bound children)
    (handicapped) 93.82
  electroconvulsive (ECT) 94.27

Therapy *(Continued)*
  electroshock (EST) 94.27
    subconvulsive 94.26
  electrotonic (ETT) 94.27
  encounter group 94.44
  extinction 94.33
  family 94.42
  fog (inhalation) 93.94
  gamma ray 92.23
  group NEC 94.44
    for psychosexual dysfunctions 94.41
  hearing NEC 95.49
  heat NEC 93.35
    for cancer treatment 99.85
  helium 93.98
  hot pack(s) 93.35
  hyperbaric oxygen 93.95
    wound 93.59
  hyperthermia NEC 93.35
    for cancer treatment 99.85
  individual, psychiatric NEC 94.39
    for psychosexual dysfunction 94.34
  industrial 93.89
  infrared irradiation 93.35
  inhalation NEC 93.96
    nitric oxide 00.12
  insulin shock 94.24
  intermittent positive pressure breathing
    (IPPB) 93.91
  IPPB (intermittent positive pressure
    breathing) 93.91
  leech 99.99
  lithium 94.22
  LITT (laser interstitial thermal therapy)
    under guidance
    lesion
      brain 17.61
      breast 17.69
      head and neck 17.62
      liver 17.63
      lung 17.69
      prostate 17.69
      thyroid 17.62
  maggot 86.28
  manipulative, osteopathic - *see also*
    Manipulation, osteopathic 93.67
  manual arts 93.81
  methadone 94.25
  mist (inhalation) 93.94
  music 93.84
  nebulizer 93.94
  neuroleptic 94.23
  nitric oxide 00.12
  occupational 93.83
  oxygen 93.96
    aqueous 00.49
    catalytic 93.96
    hyperbaric 93.95
      wound 93.59
    SuperSaturated 00.49
    wound (hyperbaric) 93.59
  paraffin bath 93.35
  physical NEC 93.39
    combined (without mention of
      components) 93.38
    diagnostic NEC 93.09
  play 93.81
    psychotherapeutic 94.36
  positive and expiratory pressure - *see*
    category 96.7●
  psychiatric NEC 94.39
    drug NEC 94.25
    lithium 94.22
  radiation 92.29
    contact (150 KVP or less) 92.21
    deep (200-300 KVP) 92.22
    electron, intra-operative 92.41
    high voltage (200-300 KVP) 92.22
    low voltage (150 KVP or less) 92.21
    megavoltage 92.24
    orthovoltage 92.22

Therapy *(Continued)*
  radiation *(Continued)*
    particle source NEC 92.26
    photon 92.24
    radioisotope (teleradiotherapy) 92.23
    retinal lesion 14.26
    superficial (150 KVP or less) 92.21
    supervoltage 92.24
  radioisotope, radioisotopic NEC 92.29
    implantation or insertion 92.27
    injection or instillation 92.28
    teleradiotherapy 92.23
  radium (radon) 92.23
  recreational 93.81
  rehabilitation NEC 93.89
  respiratory NEC 93.99
    bi-level positive airway pressure [BiPAP]
      93.90
      delivered by
        endotracheal tube - *see* category
          96.7●
        tracheostomy – *see* category 96.7●
    continuous positive airway pressure
      [CPAP] 93.90
      delivered by
        endotracheal tube - *see* category
          96.7●
        tracheostomy – *see* category 96.7●
    endotracheal respiratory assistance - *see*
      category 96.7●
    intermittent positive pressure breathing
      [IPPB] 93.91
    negative pressure (continuous) [CNP]
      93.99
    nitric oxide 00.12
    non-invasive positive pressure (NIPPV)
      93.90
    other continuous invasive (unspecified
      duration) 96.70
      for less than 96 consecutive hours
        96.71
      for 96 consecutive hours or more 96.72
    positive end expiratory pressure [PEEP]
      invasive - *see* category 96.7●
      non-invasive 93.90
  root canal 23.70
    with
      apicoectomy 23.72
      irrigation 23.71
  shock
    chemical 94.24
    electric 94.27
      subconvulsive 94.26
    insulin 94.24
  speech 93.75
    for correction of defect 93.74
  SuperOxygenation (SSO₂) 00.49
  SuperSaturated oxygen 00.49
  ultrasound
    heat therapy 93.35
    hyperthermia for cancer treatment 99.85
    physical therapy 93.35
    therapeutic - *see* Ultrasound
  ultraviolet light 99.82
Thermocautery - *see* Cauterization
Thermography 88.89
  blood vessel 88.86
  bone 88.83
  breast 88.85
  cerebral 88.81
  eye 88.82
  lymph gland 88.89
  muscle 88.84
  ocular 88.82
  osteoarticular 88.83
  specified site NEC 88.89
  vein, deep 88.86
Thermokeratoplasty 11.74
Thermoplasty
  bronchoscopic, bronchial (lung) 32.27
Thermosclerectomy 12.62

Thermotherapy (hot packs) (paraffin bath) NEC 93.35
  prostate
    by
      microwave 60.96
      radiofrequency 60.97
    transurethral microwave thermotherapy (TUMT) 60.96
    transurethral needle ablation (TUNA) 60.97
    TUMT (transurethral microwave thermotherapy) 60.96
    TUNA (transurethral needle ablation) 60.97
Thiersch operation
  anus 49.79
  skin graft 86.69
    hand 86.62
Thompson operation
  cleft lip repair 27.54
  correction of lymphedema 40.9
  quadricepsplasty 83.86
  thumb apposition with bone graft 82.69
Thoracectomy 34.09
  for lung collapse 33.34
Thoracentesis 34.91
Thoracocentesis 34.91
Thoracolysis (for collapse of lung) 33.39
Thoracoplasty (anterior) (extrapleural) (paravertebral) (posterolateral) (complete) (partial) 33.34
Thoracoscopy, transpleural (for exploration) 34.21
Thoracostomy 34.09
  for lung collapse 33.32
Thoracotomy (with drainage) 34.09
  as operative approach - omit code
  exploratory 34.02
Thoratec® implantable ventricular assist device (IVAD™) 37.66
Thoratec® ventricular assist device (VAD) system 37.66
Three-snip operation, punctum 09.51
Thrombectomy 38.00
  with endarterectomy - see Endarterectomy
  abdominal
    artery 38.06
    vein 38.07
  aorta (arch) (ascending) (descending) 38.04
  arteriovenous shunt or cannula 39.49
  bovine graft 39.49
  coronary artery 36.09
  head and neck vessel NEC 38.02
  intracranial vessel NEC 38.01
  lower limb
    artery 38.08
    vein 38.09
  mechanical
    endovascular
      head and neck 39.74
  pulmonary vessel 38.05
  thoracic vessel NEC 38.05
  upper limb (artery) (vein) 38.03
Thromboendarterectomy 38.10
  abdominal 38.16
  aorta (arch) (ascending) (descending) 38.14
  coronary artery 36.09
    open chest approach 36.03
  head and neck NEC 38.12
  intracranial NEC 38.11
  lower limb 38.18
  thoracic NEC 38.15
  upper limb 38.13
Thymectomy 07.80
  partial (open) (other) 07.81
    thoracoscopic 07.83
  total (open) (other) 07.82
    thoracoscopic 07.84
  transcervical 07.99
Thyrochondrotomy 31.3
Thyrocricoidectomy 30.29

Thyrocricotomy (for assistance in breathing) 31.1
Thyroidectomy NEC 06.39
  by mediastinotomy - see also Thyroidectomy, substernal 06.50
  with laryngectomy - see Laryngectomy
  complete or total 06.4
    substernal (by mediastinotomy) (transsternal route) 06.52
    transoral route (lingual) 06.6
  lingual (complete) (partial) (subtotal) (total) 06.6
  partial or subtotal NEC 06.39
    with complete removal of remaining lobe 06.2
    submental route (lingual) 06.6
    substernal (by mediastinotomy) (transsternal route) 06.51
  remaining tissue 06.4
  submental route (lingual) 06.6
  substernal (by mediastinotomy) (transsternal route) 06.50
    complete or total 06.52
    partial or subtotal 06.51
  transoral route (lingual) 06.6
  transsternal route - see also Thyroidectomy, substernal 06.50
  unilateral (with removal of isthmus) (with removal of portion of other lobe) 06.2
Thyroidorrhaphy 06.93
Thyroidotomy (field) (gland) NEC 06.09
  postoperative 06.02
Thyrotomy 31.3
  with tantalum plate 31.69
Tirofiban (HCL), infusion 99.20
Toilette
  skin - see Debridement, skin or subcutaneous tissue
  tracheostomy 96.55
Token economy (behavior therapy) 94.33
Tomkins operation (metroplasty) 69.49
Tomography - see also Radiography
  abdomen NEC 88.02
  cardiac 87.42
  computerized axial NEC 88.38
    abdomen 88.01
    bone 88.38
      quantitative 88.98
    brain 87.03
    cardiac 87.41
    coronary 87.41
    head 87.03
    kidney 87.71
    skeletal 88.38
      quantitative 88.98
    thorax 87.41
  head NEC 87.04
  kidney NEC 87.72
  lung 87.42
  optical coherence (intravascular imaging)
    coronary vessel(s) 38.24
    non-coronary vessel(s) 38.25
  thorax NEC 87.42
Tongue tie operation 25.91
Tonography 95.26
Tonometry 89.11
Tonsillectomy 28.2
  with adenoidectomy 28.3
Tonsillotomy 28.0
Topectomy 01.32
Torek (-Bevan) operation (orchidopexy) (first stage) (second stage) 62.5
Torkildsen operation (ventriculocisternal shunt) 02.2
Torpin operation (cul-de-sac resection) 70.92
Toti operation (dacryocystorhinostomy) 09.81
Touchas operation 86.83
Touroff operation (ligation of subclavian artery) 38.85
Toxicology - see Examination, microscopic
TPN (total parenteral nutrition) 99.15

Trabeculectomy ab externo 12.64
Trabeculodialysis 12.59
Trabeculotomy ab externo 12.54
Trachelectomy 67.4
Trachelopexy 69.22
Tracheloplasty 67.69
Trachelorrhaphy (Emmet) (suture) 67.61
  obstetrical 75.51
Trachelotomy 69.95
  obstetrical 73.93
Tracheocricotomy (for assistance in breathing) 31.1
Tracheofissure 31.1
Tracheography 87.32
Tracheolaryngotomy (emergency) 31.1
  permanent opening 31.29
Tracheoplasty 31.79
  with artificial larynx 31.75
Tracheorrhaphy 31.71
Tracheoscopy NEC 31.42
  through tracheotomy (stoma) 31.41
Tracheostomy (emergency) (temporary) (for assistance in breathing) 31.1
  mediastinal 31.21
  percutaneous dilatational
    other permanent 31.29
    temporary 31.1
  permanent NEC 31.29
  revision 31.74
Tracheotomy (emergency) (temporary) (for assistance in breathing) 31.1
  percutaneous dilatational
    other permanent 31.29
    temporary 31.1
  permanent 31.29
Tracing, carotid pulse with ECG lead 89.56
Traction
  with reduction of fracture or dislocation - see Reduction, fracture and Reduction, dislocation
  adhesive tape (skin) 93.46
  boot 93.46
  Bryant's (skeletal) 93.44
  Buck's 93.46
  caliper tongs 93.41
    with synchronous insertion of device 02.94
  Cortel's (spinal) 93.42
  Crutchfield tongs 93.41
    with synchronous insertion of device 02.94
  Dunlop's (skeletal) 93.44
  gallows 93.46
  Gardner Wells 93.41
    with synchronous insertion of device 02.94
  halo device, skull 93.41
    with synchronous insertion of device 02.94
  Lyman Smith (skeletal) 93.44
  manual, intermittent 93.21
  mechanical, intermittent 93.21
  Russell's (skeletal) 93.44
  skeletal NEC 93.44
    intermittent 93.43
  skin, limbs NEC 93.46
  spinal NEC 93.42
    with skull device (halo) (caliper) (Crutchfield) (Gardner Wells) (Vinke) (tongs) 93.41
      with synchronous insertion of device 02.94
  Thomas' splint 93.45
  Vinke tongs 93.41
    with synchronous insertion of device 02.94
Tractotomy
  brain 01.32
  medulla oblongata 01.32
  mesencephalon 01.32
  percutaneous 03.21

Tractotomy (Continued)
spinal cord (one-stage) (two-stage) 03.29
trigeminal (percutaneous) (radiofrequency) 04.02
Training (for) (in)
ADL (activities of daily living) 93.83
for the blind 93.78
ambulation 93.22
braille 93.77
crutch walking 93.24
dyslexia 93.71
dysphasia 93.72
esophageal speech (postlaryngectomy) 93.73
gait 93.22
joint movements 93.14
lip reading 93.75
Moon (blind reading) 93.77
orthoptic 95.35
prenatal (natural childbirth) 93.37
prosthetic or orthotic device usage 93.24
relaxation 94.33
speech NEC 93.75
esophageal type 93.73
for correction of defect 93.74
use of lead dog for the blind 93.76
vocational 93.85
TRAM (transverse rectus abdominis musculocutaneous) flap of breast
free 85.73
pedicled 85.72
Transactional analysis
group 94.44
individual 94.39
Transection - see also Division
artery (with ligation) - see also Division, artery 38.80
renal, aberrant (with reimplantation) 39.55
bone - see also Osteotomy 77.30
fallopian tube (bilateral) (remaining) (solitary) 66.39
by endoscopy 66.22
unilateral 66.92
isthmus, thyroid 06.91
muscle 83.19
eye 15.13
multiple (two or more muscles) 15.3
hand 82.19
nerve (cranial) (peripheral) NEC 04.03
acoustic 04.01
root (spinal) 03.1
sympathetic 05.0
tracts in spinal cord 03.29
trigeminal 04.02
vagus (transabdominal) - see also Vagotomy 44.00
pylorus (with wedge resection) 43.3
renal vessel, aberrant (with reimplantation) 39.55
spinal
cord tracts 03.29
nerve root 03.1
tendon 83.13
hand 82.11
uvula 27.71
vas deferens 63.71
vein (with ligation) - see also Division, vein 38.80
renal, aberrant (with reimplantation) 39.55
varicose (lower limb) 38.59
Transfer, transference
bone shaft, fibula into tibia 78.47
digital (to replace absent thumb) 82.69
finger (to thumb) (same hand) 82.61
to
finger, except thumb 82.81
opposite hand (with amputation) 82.69 [84.01]

Transfer, transference (Continued)
digital (Continued)
toe (to thumb) (with amputation) 82.69 [84.11]
to finger, except thumb 82.81 [84.11]
fat pad NEC 86.89
with skin graft - see Graft, skin, full-thickness
finger (to replace absent thumb) (same hand) 82.61
to
finger, except thumb 82.81
opposite hand (with amputation) 82.69 [84.01]
muscle origin 83.77
hand 82.58
nerve (cranial) (peripheral) (radial anterior) (ulnar) 04.6
pedicle graft 86.74
pes anserinus (tendon) (repair of knee) 81.47
tarsoconjunctival flap, from opposing lid 08.64
tendon 83.75
hand 82.56
pes anserinus (repair of knee) 81.47
toe-to-thumb (free) (pedicle) (with amputation) 82.69 [84.11]
Transfixion - see also Fixation
iris (bombé) 12.11
Transfusion (of) 99.03
antihemophilic factor 99.06
antivenin 99.16
autologous blood
collected prior to surgery 99.02
intraoperative 99.00
perioperative 99.00
postoperative 99.00
previously collected 99.02
salvage 99.00
blood (whole) NOS 99.03
expander 99.08
surrogate 99.09
bone marrow 41.00
allogeneic 41.03
with purging 41.02
allograft 41.03
with purging 41.02
autograft 41.01
with purging 41.09
autologous 41.01
with purging 41.09
coagulation factors 99.06
Dextran 99.08
exchange 99.01
intraperitoneal 75.2
in utero (with hysterotomy) 75.2
exsanguination 99.01
gamma globulin 99.14
granulocytes 99.09
hemodilution 99.03
intrauterine 75.2
packed cells 99.04
plasma 99.07
platelets 99.05
replacement, total 99.01
serum NEC 99.07
substitution 99.01
thrombocytes 99.05
Transillumination
nasal sinuses 89.35
skull (newborn) 89.16
Translumbar aortogram 88.42
Transplant, transplantation

Note: To report donor source:
cadaver 00.93
live non-related donor 00.92
live related donor 00.91
live unrelated donor 00.92

artery 39.59
renal, aberrant 39.55

Transplant, transplantation (Continued)
autotransplant - see Reimplantation
blood vessel 39.59
renal, aberrant 39.55
bone - see also Graft, bone 78.00
marrow 41.00
allogeneic 41.03
with purging 41.02
allograft 41.03
with purging 41.02
autograft 41.01
with purging 41.09
autologous 41.01
with purging 41.09
stem cell
allogeneic (hematopoietic) 41.05
with purging 41.08
autologous (hematopoietic) 41.04
with purging 41.07
cord blood 41.06
stem cell
allogeneic (hematopoietic) 41.05
with purging 41.08
autologous (hematopoietic) 41.04
with purging 41.07
cord blood 41.06
combined heart-lung 33.6
conjunctiva, for pterygium 11.39
corneal - see also Keratoplasty 11.60
dura 02.12
fascia 83.82
hand 82.72
finger (replacing absent thumb) (same hand) 82.61
to
finger, except thumb 82.81
opposite hand (with amputation) 82.69 [84.01]
gracilis muscle (for) 83.77
anal incontinence 49.74
urethrovesical suspension 59.71
hair follicles
eyebrow 08.63
eyelid 08.63
scalp 86.64
heart (orthotopic) 37.51
combined with lung 33.6
ileal stoma to new site 46.23
intestine 46.97
Islets of Langerhans (cells) 52.86
allotransplantation of cells 52.85
autotransplantation of cells 52.84
heterotransplantation 52.85
homotransplantation 52.84
kidney NEC 55.69
liver 50.59
auxiliary (permanent) (temporary) (recipient's liver in situ) 50.51
cells into spleen via percutaneous catheterization 38.91
lung 33.50
bilateral 33.50
combined with heart 33.6
double 33.52
single 33.51
unilateral 33.51
lymphatic structure(s) (peripheral) 40.9
mammary artery to myocardium or ventricular wall 36.2
muscle 83.77
gracilis (for) 83.77
anal incontinence 49.74
urethrovesical suspension 59.71
hand 82.58
temporalis 83.77
with orbital exenteration 16.59
nerve (cranial) (peripheral) 04.6
ovary 65.92
pancreas 52.80
heterotransplant 52.83
homotransplant 52.82

T

T & U

Transplant, transplantation *(Continued)*
  pancreas *(Continued)*
    Islets of Langerhans (cells) 52.86
      allotransplantation of cells 52.85
      autotransplantation of cells 52.84
      heterotransplantation 52.85
      homotransplantation 52.84
      reimplantation 52.81
  pes anserinus (tendon) (repair of knee)
    81.47
  renal NEC 55.69
    vessel, aberrant 39.55
  salivary duct opening 26.49
  skin - *see* Graft, skin
  spermatic cord 63.53
  spleen 41.94
  stem cells
    allogeneic (hematopoietic) 41.05
      with purging 41.08
    autologous (hematopoietic) 41.04
      with purging 41.07
    cord blood 41.06
  tendon 83.75
    hand 82.56
    pes anserinus (repair of knee) 81.47
    superior rectus (blepharoptosis) 08.36
  testis to scrotum 62.5
  thymus 07.94
  thyroid tissue 06.94
  toe (replacing absent thumb) (with
    amputation) 82.69 *[84.11]*
    to finger, except thumb 82.81 *[84.11]*
  tooth 23.5
  ureter to
    bladder 56.74
    ileum (external diversion) 56.51
      internal diversion only 56.71
    intestine 56.71
    skin 56.61
  vein (peripheral) 39.59
    renal, aberrant 39.55
  vitreous 14.72
    anterior approach 14.71
Transposition
  extraocular muscles 15.5
  eyelash flaps 08.63
  eye muscle (oblique) (rectus) 15.5

Transposition *(Continued)*
  finger (replacing absent thumb) (same hand)
    82.61
    to
      finger, except thumb 82.81
      opposite hand (with amputation) 82.69
        [84.01]
  interatrial venous return 35.91
  jejunal (Henley) 43.81
  joint capsule - *see also* Arthroplasty 81.96
  muscle NEC 83.79
    extraocular 15.5
    hand 82.59
  nerve (cranial) (peripheral) (radial anterior)
    (ulnar) 04.6
  nipple 85.86
  pterygium 11.31
  tendon NEC 83.76
    hand 82.57
  vocal cords 31.69
Transureteroureterostomy 56.75
Transversostomy - *see also* Colostomy 46.10
Trapping, aneurysm (cerebral) 39.52
Trauner operation (lingual sulcus extension)
  24.91
Trephination, trephining
  accessory sinus - *see* Sinusotomy
  corneoscleral 12.89
  cranium 01.24
  nasal sinus - *see* Sinusotomy
  sclera (with iridectomy) 12.61
Trial (failed) forceps 73.3
Trigonectomy 57.6
Trimming, amputation stump 84.3
Triple arthrodesis 81.12
Trochanterplasty 81.40
Tsuge operation (macrodactyly repair) 82.83
Tuck, tucking - *see also* Plication
  eye muscle 15.22
    multiple (two or more muscles) 15.4
  levator palpebrae, for blepharoptosis 08.34
Tudor "rabbit ear" operation (anterior
  urethropexy) 59.79
Tuffier operation
  apicolysis of lung 33.39
  vaginal hysterectomy 68.59
    laparoscopically assisted (LAVH) 68.51

TULIP (transurethral ultrasound guided laser
  induced prostectomy) 60.21
TUMT (transurethral microwave
  thermotherapy) of prostate 60.96
TUNA (transurethral needle ablation) of
  prostate 60.97
Tunnel, subcutaneous (antethoracic) 42.86
  esophageal 42.68
    with anastomosis - *see* Anastomosis,
      esophagus, antesternal 42.68
  pulse generator lead wire 86.99
    with initial procedure - *omit code*
Turbinectomy (complete) (partial) NEC
  21.69
  by
    cryosurgery 21.61
    diathermy 21.61
  with sinusectomy - *see* Sinusectomy
Turco operation (release of joint capsules in
  clubfoot) 80.48
TURP (transurethral resection of prostate)
  60.29
Tylectomy (breast) (partial) 85.21
Tympanectomy 20.59
  with tympanoplasty - *see* Tympanoplasty
Tympanogram 95.41
Tympanomastoidectomy 20.42
Tympanoplasty (type I) (with graft) 19.4
  with
    air pocket over round window 19.54
    fenestra in semicircular canal 19.55
    graft against
      incus or malleus 19.52
      mobile and intact stapes 19.53
    incudostapediopexy 19.52
  epitympanic, type I 19.4
  revision 19.6
  type
    II (graft against incus or malleus) 19.52
    III (graft against mobile and intact stapes)
      19.53
    IV (air pocket over round window)
      19.54
    V (fenestra in semicircular canal) 19.55
Tympanosympathectomy 20.91
Tympanotomy 20.09
  with intubation 20.01

U

UAE (uterine artery embolization), NOS
  68.25
  with
    coils 68.24
    particulate agent (gelatin sponge)
      (gelfoam) (microspheres)(polyvinyl
      alcohol) (PVA) (spherical embolics)
      68.25
Uchida operation (tubal ligation with or
  without fimbriectomy) 66.32
UFR (uroflowmetry) 89.24
Ultrafiltration 99.78
  hemodiafiltration 39.95
  hemodialysis (kidney) 39.95
  removal, plasma water 99.78
  therapeutic plasmapheresis 99.71
Ultrasonography
  abdomen 88.76
  aortic arch 88.73
  biliary tract 88.74
  breast 88.73
  deep vein thrombosis 88.77
  digestive system 88.74
  eye 95.13
  head and neck 88.71
  heart 88.72

Ultrasonography *(Continued)*
  intestine 88.74
  intravascular - *see* Ultrasound, intravascular
    (IVUS)
  lung 88.73
  midline shift, brain 88.71
  multiple sites 88.79
  peripheral vascular system 88.77
  retroperitoneum 88.76
  therapeutic - *see* Ultrasound
  thorax NEC 88.73
  total body 88.79
  urinary system 88.75
  uterus 88.79
    gravid 88.78
Ultrasound
  diagnostic - *see* Ultrasonography
  fragmentation (of)
    cataract (with aspiration) 13.41
    urinary calculus, stones (Kock pouch)
      59.95
  heart
    intracardiac (heart chambers) (ICE)
      37.28
    intravascular (coronary vessels) (IVUS)
      00.24
    non-invasive 88.72
  inner ear 20.79

Ultrasound *(Continued)*
  intravascular (IVUS) (VH™-IVUS) 00.29
    aorta 00.22
    aortic arch 00.22
    cerebral vessel, extracranial 00.21
    coronary vessel 00.24
    intrathoracic vessel 00.22
    other specified vessel 00.28
    peripheral vessel 00.23
    renal vessel 00.25
    vena cava (inferior) (superior) 00.22
    VH™-IVUS - *see* Ultrasound,
      intravascular, by site
    virtual histology intravascular
      ultrasound - *see* Ultrasound,
      intravascular, by site
  therapeutic
    head 00.01
    heart 00.02
    neck 00.01
    other therapeutic ultrasound 00.09
    peripheral vascular vessels 00.03
    vessels of head and neck 00.01
  therapy 93.35
Umbilectomy 54.3
Unbridling
  blood vessel, peripheral 39.91
  celiac artery axis 39.91

Uncovering - *see* Incision, by site
Undercutting
  hair follicle 86.09
  perianal tissue 49.02
Unroofing - *see also* Incision, by site
  external
      auditory canal 18.02
      ear NEC 18.09
  kidney cyst 55.39
UPP (urethral pressure profile) 89.25
Upper GI series (x-ray) 87.62
UPPP (uvulopalatopharyngoplasty) 27.69
  [29.4]
Uranoplasty (for cleft palate repair) 27.62
Uranorrhaphy (for cleft palate repair) 27.62
Uranostaphylorrhaphy 27.62
Urban operation (mastectomy) (unilateral)
  85.47
  bilateral 85.48
Ureterectomy 56.40
  with nephrectomy 55.51
  partial 56.41
  total 56.42
Ureterocecostomy 56.71
Ureterocelectomy 56.41
Ureterocolostomy 56.71
Ureterocystostomy 56.74
Ureteroenterostomy 56.71
Ureteroileostomy (internal diversion) 56.71
  external diversion 56.51
Ureterolithotomy 56.2
Ureterolysis 59.02
  with freeing or repositioning of ureter 59.02
  laparoscopic 59.03

Ureteroneocystostomy 56.74
Ureteropexy 56.85
Ureteroplasty 56.89
Ureteroplication 56.89
Ureteroproctostomy 56.71
Ureteropyelography (intravenous) (diuretic
      infusion) 87.73
  percutaneous 87.75
  retrograde 87.74
Ureteropyeloplasty 55.87
Ureteropyelostomy 55.86
Ureterorrhaphy 56.82
Ureteroscopy 56.31
  with biopsy 56.33
Ureterosigmoidostomy 56.71
Ureterostomy (cutaneous) (external) (tube)
  56.61
  closure 56.83
  ileal 56.51
Ureterotomy 56.2
Ureteroureterostomy (crossed) 56.75
  lumbar 56.41
  resection with end-to-end anastomosis 56.41
  spatulated 56.41
Urethral catheterization, indwelling 57.94
Urethral pressure profile (UPP) 89.25
Urethrectomy (complete) (partial) (radical)
  58.39
  with
      complete cystectomy 57.79
      pelvic exenteration 68.8
      radical cystectomy 57.71
Urethrocystography (retrograde) (voiding)
  87.76

Urethrocystopexy (by) 59.79
  levator muscle sling 59.71
  retropubic suspension 59.5
  suprapubic suspension 59.4
Urethrolithotomy 58.0
Urethrolysis 58.5
Urethropexy 58.49
  anterior 59.79
Urethroplasty 58.49
  augmentation 59.79
      collagen implant 59.72
      fat implant 59.72
      injection (endoscopic) of implant into
          urethra 59.72
      polytef implant 59.72
Urethrorrhaphy 58.41
Urethroscopy 58.22
  for control of hemorrhage of prostate 60.94
  perineal 58.21
Urethrostomy (perineal) 58.0
Urethrotomy (external) 58.0
  internal (endoscopic) 58.5
Uroflowmetry (UFR) 89.24
Urography (antegrade) (excretory)
      (intravenous) 87.73
  retrograde 87.74
Uteropexy (abdominal approach) (vaginal
      approach) 69.22
UVP (uvulopalatopharyngoplasty) 27.69 [29.4]
Uvulectomy 27.72
Uvulopalatopharyngoplasty (UPPP) 27.69
  [29.4]
Uvulotomy 27.71

V

Vaccination (prophylactic) (against) 99.59
  anthrax 99.55
  brucellosis 99.55
  cholera 99.31
  common cold 99.51
  disease NEC 99.55
      arthropod-borne viral NEC 99.54
  encephalitis, arthropod-borne viral 99.53
  German measles 99.47
  hydrophobia 99.44
  infectious parotitis 99.46
  influenza 99.52
  measles 99.45
  mumps 99.46
  paratyphoid fever 99.32
  pertussis 99.37
  plague 99.34
  poliomyelitis 99.41
  rabies 99.44
  Rocky Mountain spotted fever 99.55
  rubella 99.47
  rubeola 99.45
  smallpox 99.42
  Staphylococcus 99.55
  Streptococcus 99.55
  tuberculosis 99.33
  tularemia 99.35
  tumor 99.28
  typhoid 99.32
  typhus 99.55
  undulant fever 99.55
  yellow fever 99.43
Vacuum extraction, fetal head 72.79
  with episiotomy 72.71
VAD
  vascular access device - *see* Vascular access
      device, totally implantable
  ventricular assist device – *see* Implant, heart
      assist system

Vagectomy (subdiaphragmatic) - *see also*
      Vagotomy 44.00
Vaginal douche 96.44
Vaginectomy 70.4
Vaginofixation 70.77
  with graft or prosthesis 70.78
Vaginoperineotomy 70.14
Vaginoplasty 70.79
Vaginorrhaphy 70.71
  obstetrical 75.69
Vaginoscopy 70.21
Vaginotomy 70.14
  for
      culdocentesis 70.0
      pelvic abscess 70.12
Vagotomy (gastric) 44.00
  parietal cell 44.02
  selective NEC 44.03
      highly 44.02
      Holle's 44.02
      proximal 44.02
  truncal 44.01
Valvotomy - *see* Valvulotomy
Valvulectomy, heart - *see* Valvuloplasty,
  heart
Valvuloplasty
  heart, unspecified (without valve
      replacement) 35.10
  with prosthesis or tissue graft - *see*
      Replacement, heart, valve, by site
  aortic valve 35.11
      percutaneous (balloon) 35.96
  balloon, percutaneous 35.96
  combined with repair of atrial and
      ventricular septal defects - *see*
      Repair, endocardial cushion defect
  mitral valve
      balloon, percutaneous repair 35.96
      endovascular repair with implant
          35.97
      open, without replacement 35.12

Valvuloplasty (Continued)
  heart, unspecified (Continued)
      mitral valve (Continued)
          percutaneous repair
              with implant (leaflet clip) 35.97
              transcatheter repair with implant 35.97
      open heart technique 35.10
      percutaneous (balloon) 35.96
      pulmonary valve 35.13
          in total repair of tetralogy of Fallot
              35.81
          percutaneous (balloon) 35.96
      tricuspid valve 35.14
Valvulotomy
  heart (closed heart technique) (transatrial)
      (transventricular) 35.00
      aortic valve 35.01
      mitral valve 35.02
      open heart technique - *see* Valvuloplasty,
          heart
      pulmonary valve 35.03
          in total repair of tetralogy of Fallot
              35.81
      tricuspid valve 35.04
Varicocelectomy, spermatic cord 63.1
Varicotomy, peripheral vessels (lower limb)
  38.59
  upper limb 38.53
Vascular access device, totally implantable
  86.07
Vascular closure, percutaneous puncture -
  omit code
Vascularization - *see* Revascularization
Vasectomy (complete) (partial) 63.73
Vasogram 87.94
Vasoligation 63.71
  gastric 38.86
Vasorrhaphy 63.81
Vasostomy 63.6
Vasotomy 63.6
Vasotripsy 63.71

◀ New   ◀|||| Revised   ~~deleted~~ Deleted   ● Use Additional Digit(s)   ▨ Omit code   1193

Vasovasostomy 63.82
Vectorcardiogram (VCG) (with ECG) 89.53
Vectra® vascular access graft 86.07
Venectomy - *see* Phlebectomy
Venipuncture NEC 38.99
    for injection of contrast material - *see*
        Phlebography
Venography - *see* Phlebography
Venorrhaphy 39.32
Venotomy 38.00
    abdominal 38.07
    head and neck NEC 38.02
    intracranial NEC 38.01
    lower limb 38.09
    thoracic NEC 38.05
    upper limb 38.03
Venotripsy 39.98
Venovenostomy 39.29
Ventilation
    bi-level positive airway pressure [BiPAP]
      93.90
        delivered by
            endotracheal tube - *see* category 96.7●
            tracheostomy – *see* category 96.7●
    continuous positive airway pressure [CPAP]
      93.90
        delivered by
            endotracheal tube - *see* category 96.7●
            tracheostomy – *see* category 96.7●
    endotracheal respiratory assistance - *see*
        category 96.7●
    intermittent positive pressure breathing
      [IPPB] 93.91
    mechanical, NOS 93.90
        by endotracheal tube - *see* category 96.7●
        by tracheostomy - *see* category 96.7●
        endotracheal respiratory assistance - *see*
            category 96.7●
    invasive - *see* category 96.7●
    non-invasive [NIPPV] 93.90
    other continuous invasive (unspecified
      duration) 96.70
        for less than 96 consecutive hours
          96.71
        for 96 consecutive hours or more
          96.72
    negative pressure (continuous) [CNP] 93.99
    non-invasive positive pressure (NIPPV)
      93.90

Ventilation (*Continued*)
    positive end expiratory pressure [PEEP]
        invasive - *see* category 96.7●
        non-invasive 93.90
Ventriculectomy, heart
    partial 37.35
Ventriculocholecystostomy 02.34
Ventriculocisternostomy 02.22
Ventriculocordectomy 30.29
Ventriculogram, ventriculography (cerebral)
    87.02
    cardiac
        left ventricle (outflow tract) 88.53
            combined with right heart 88.54
        right ventricle (outflow tract) 88.52
            combined with left heart 88.54
        radionuclide cardiac 92.05
Ventriculomyocardiotomy 37.11
Ventriculoperitoneostomy 02.34
Ventriculopuncture 01.09
    through previously implanted catheter or
        reservoir (Ommaya) (Rickham) 01.02
Ventriculoseptopexy - *see also* Repair,
    ventricular septal defect 35.72
Ventriculoseptoplasty - *see also* Repair,
    ventricular septal defect 35.72
Ventriculostomy
    for
        external ventricular drainage (EVD) 02.21
        placement of ventricular catheter 02.21
        third (endoscopic) 02.22
Ventriculotomy
    cerebral 02.22
    heart 37.11
Ventriculoureterostomy 02.35
Ventriculovenostomy 02.32
Ventrofixation, uterus 69.22
Ventrohysteropexy 69.22
Ventrosuspension, uterus 69.22
VEP (visual evoked potential) 95.23
Version, obstetrical (bimanual) (cephalic)
    (combined) (internal) (podalic) 73.21
    with extraction 73.22
    Braxton Hicks 73.21
      with extraction 73.22
    external (bipolar) 73.91
    Potter's (podalic) 73.21
      with extraction 73.22
    Wigand's (external) 73.91

Version, obstetrical (*Continued*)
    Wright's (cephalic) 73.21
      with extraction 73.22
Vertebroplasty, percutaneous 81.65
Vesicolithotomy (suprapubic) 57.19
Vesicostomy 57.21
Vesicourethroplasty 57.85
Vesiculectomy 60.73
    with radical prostatectomy 60.5
Vesiculogram, seminal 87.92
    contrast 87.91
Vesiculotomy 60.72
Vestibuloplasty (buccolabial) (lingual) 24.91
Vestibulotomy 20.79
VH™-IVUS - *see* Ultrasound, intravascular, by
    site
Vicq D'azyr operation (larynx) 31.1
Vidal operation (varicocele ligation) 63.1
Vidianectomy 05.21
Villusectomy - *see also* Synovectomy 80.70
Vision check 95.09
Visual evoked potential (VEP) 95.23
Vitrectomy (mechanical) (posterior approach)
    14.74
    with scleral buckling 14.49
    anterior approach 14.73
Vocational
    assessment 93.85
    retraining 93.85
    schooling 93.82
Voice training (postlaryngectomy) 93.73
von Kraske operation (proctectomy) 48.64
Voss operation (hanging hip operation) 83.19
Vulpius (-Compere) operation (lengthening of
    gastrocnemius muscle) 83.85
Vulvectomy (bilateral) (simple) 71.62
    partial (unilateral) 71.61
    radical (complete) 71.5
    unilateral 71.61
V-Y operation (repair)
    bladder 57.89
      neck 57.85
    ectropion 08.44
    lip 27.59
    skin (without graft) 86.89
    subcutaneous tissue (without skin graft)
      86.89
    tongue 25.59

W

Wada test (hemispheric function) 89.10
Wang needle aspiration biopsy
    bronchus 33.24
    lung 33.27
Ward-Mayo operation (vaginal hysterectomy)
    68.59
    laparoscopically assisted (LAVH) 68.51
Washing - *see* Lavage and Irrigation
Waterston operation (aorta-right pulmonary
    artery anastomosis) 39.0
Watkins (-Wertheim) operation (uterus
    interposition) 69.21
Watson-Jones operation
    hip arthrodesis 81.21
    reconstruction of lateral ligaments, ankle
      81.49
    shoulder arthrodesis (extra-articular) 81.23
    tenoplasty 83.88
Webbing (syndactylization) 86.89
Weir operation
    appendicostomy 47.91
    correction of nostrils 21.86
Wertheim operation (radical hysterectomy)
    68.69
    laparoscopic 68.61

West operation (dacryocystorhinostomy)
    09.81
Wheeler operation
    entropion repair 08.44
    halving procedure (eyelid) 08.24
Whipple operation (radical
    pancreaticoduodenectomy) 52.7
    Child modification (radical subtotal
      pancreatectomy) 52.53
    Rodney Smith modification (radical subtotal
      pancreatectomy) 52.53
White operation (lengthening of tendo
    calcaneus by incomplete tenotomy) 83.11
Whitehead operation
    glossectomy, radical 25.4
    hemorrhoidectomy 49.46
Whitman operation
    foot stabilization (talectomy) 77.98
    hip reconstruction 81.40
    repair of serratus anterior muscle 83.87
    talectomy 77.98
    trochanter wedge osteotomy 77.25
Wier operation (entropion repair) 08.44
Williams-Richardson operation (vaginal
    construction) 70.61
    with graft or prosthesis 70.63
Wilms operation (thoracoplasty) 33.34

Wilson operation (angulation osteotomy for
    hallux valgus) 77.51
Window operation
    antrum (nasal sinus) - *see* Antrotomy,
      maxillary
    aorticopulmonary 39.59
    bone cortex - *see also* Incision, bone 77.10
    facial 76.09
    nasoantral - *see* Antrotomy, maxillary
    pericardium 37.12
    pleura 34.09
Winiwarter operation (cholecystoenterostomy)
    51.32
Wiring
    aneurysm 39.52
    dental (for immobilization) 93.55
      with fracture-reduction - *see* Reduction,
        fracture
    orthodontic 24.7
Wirsungojejunostomy 52.96
Witzel operation (temporary gastrostomy)
    43.19
Woodward operation (release of high riding
    scapula) 81.83
Wrapping, aneurysm (gauze) (methyl
    methacrylate) (plastic) 39.52

V & W

X

Xenograft 86.65
Xerography, breast 87.36
Xeromammography 87.36
Xiphoidectomy 77.81

X-ray
    chest (routine) 87.44
        wall NEC 87.39
    contrast - *see* Radiography, contrast
    diagnostic - *see* Radiography

X-ray *(Continued)*
    injection of radio-opaque substance - *see*
        Radiography, contrast
    skeletal series, whole or complete 88.31
    therapeutic - *see* Therapy, radiation

Y

Young operation
    epispadias repair 58.45
    tendon transfer (anterior tibialis) (repair of
        flat foot) 83.75
Yount operation (division of iliotibial band)
    83.14

Z

Zancolli operation
    capsuloplasty 81.72
    tendon transfer (biceps) 82.56

Zeus® Robotic Surgical System – *see* category
    17.4
Ziegler operation (iridectomy) 12.14
Zonulolysis (with lens extraction) - *see also*
    Extraction, cataract, intracapsular
    13.19

Z-plasty
    epicanthus 08.59
    eyelid - *see also* Reconstruction, eyelid 08.70
    hypopharynx 29.4
    skin (scar) (web contracture) 86.84
        with excision of lesion 86.3

X, Y & Z

Code also note: This instruction is used in the Tabular List for two purposes:

1) To code components of a procedure that are performed at the same time, and

2) To code the use of special adjunctive procedures or equipment.

Includes note: This note appears immediately under a two- or three-digit code title. The information further defines, or gives examples of, the contents of the category.

Excludes note: Terms following the word "Excludes" are to be coded elsewhere as indicated in each case.

◀ New   ◀▥ Revised   ~~deleted~~ Deleted   ● Use Additional Digit(s)   ▨ Omit code

CLASSIFICATION OF PROCEDURES

0. PROCEDURES AND INTERVENTIONS, NOT ELSEWHERE CLASSIFIED (00)

00 Procedures and interventions, Not Elsewhere Classified

● **00.0 Therapeutic ultrasound**

> **Excludes** *diagnostic ultrasound (non-invasive) (88.71–88.79)*
> *intracardiac echocardiography [ICE] (heart chamber(s)) (37.28)*
> *intravascular imaging (adjunctive) (00.21–00.29)*
>
> **Coding Clinic: 2002, Q4, P90-92**

00.01 Therapeutic ultrasound of vessels of head and neck
Anti-restenotic ultrasound
Intravascular non-ablative ultrasound

> **Excludes** *diagnostic ultrasound of:*
> *eye (95.13)*
> *head and neck (88.71)*
> *that of inner ear (20.79)*
> *ultrasonic:*
> *angioplasty of non-coronary vessel (39.50)*
> *embolectomy (38.01, 38.02)*
> *endarterectomy (38.11, 38.12)*
> *thrombectomy (38.01, 38.02)*

00.02 Therapeutic ultrasound of heart
Anti-restenotic ultrasound
Intravascular non-ablative ultrasound

> **Excludes** *diagnostic ultrasound of heart (88.72)*
> *ultrasonic ablation of heart lesion (37.34)*
> *ultrasonic angioplasty of coronary vessels (00.66, 36.09)*

00.03 Therapeutic ultrasound of peripheral vascular vessels
Anti-restenotic ultrasound
Intravascular non-ablative ultrasound

> **Excludes** *diagnostic ultrasound of peripheral vascular system (88.77)*
> *ultrasonic angioplasty of:*
> *non-coronary vessel (39.50)*

00.09 Other therapeutic ultrasound

> **Excludes** *ultrasonic:*
> *fragmentation of urinary stones (59.95)*
> *percutaneous nephrostomy with fragmentation (55.04)*
> *physical therapy (93.35)*
> *transurethral guided laser induced prostatectomy (TULIP) (60.21)*

● **00.1 Pharmaceuticals**

00.10 Implantation of chemotherapeutic agent
Brain wafer chemotherapy
Interstitial/intracavitary

> **Excludes** *injection or infusion of cancer chemotherapeutic substance (99.25)*
> ◆ Non-OR Procedure that affects MS-DRG assignment to MDC 01, MS-DRG 023
> **Coding Clinic: 2002, Q4, P93**

00.11 Infusion of drotrecogin alfa (activated)
Infusion of recombinant protein
Coding Clinic: 2002, Q4, P93-94

00.12 Administration of inhaled nitric oxide
Nitric oxide therapy
Coding Clinic: 2002, Q4, P94

00.13 Injection or infusion of nesiritide
Human B-type natriuretic peptide (hBNP)
Coding Clinic: 2002, Q4, P94

00.14 Injection or infusion of oxazolidinone class of antibiotics
Linezolid injection
Coding Clinic: 2002, Q4, P95

00.15 High-dose infusion interleukin-2 [IL-2]
Infusion (IV bolus, CIV) interleukin
Injection of aldesleukin

> **Excludes** *low-dose infusion interleukin-2 (99.28)*
> ◆ Non-OR Procedure that affects MS-DRG assignment to MDC 17, MS-DRG 837-838
> **Coding Clinic: 2003, Q4, P92**

00.16 Pressurized treatment of venous bypass graft [conduit] with pharmaceutical substance
Ex-vivo treatment of vessel
Hyperbaric pressurized graft [conduit]
Coding Clinic: 2004, Q4, P108

00.17 Infusion of vasopressor agent
Coding Clinic: 2004, Q4, P108-109

00.18 Infusion of immunosuppressive antibody therapy

> **Includes** during induction phase of solid organ transplantation
> monoclonal antibody therapy
> polyclonal antibody therapy
>
> **Coding Clinic: 2005, Q4, P101**

00.19 Disruption of blood brain barrier via infusion [BBBD]
Infusion of substance to disrupt blood brain barrier

> **Code also** chemotherapy (99.25)
>
> **Excludes** *other perfusion (39.97)*
>
> **Coding Clinic: 2007, Q4, P103-104**

● **00.2 Intravascular imaging of blood vessels**
Endovascular ultrasonography
Intravascular [ultrasound] imaging of blood vessels
Intravascular ultrasound (IVUS)
Virtual histology intravascular ultrasound (VH-IVUS)
Note: Real-time imaging of lumen of blood vessel(s) using sound waves

> **Code also** any synchronous diagnostic or therapeutic procedures
>
> **Excludes** *adjunct vascular system procedures, number of vessels treated (00.40–00.43)*
> *diagnostic procedures on blood vessels (38.21–38.29)*
> *diagnostic ultrasound of peripheral vascular system (88.77)*
> *intravascular imaging of vessel(s) by OCT (38.24–38.25)*
> *magnetic resonance imaging (MRI) (88.91–88.97)*
> *therapeutic ultrasound (00.01–00.09)*
>
> **Coding Clinic: 2004, Q4, P109-111**

00.21 Intravascular imaging of extracranial cerebral vessels
Common carotid vessels and branches
Intravascular ultrasound (IVUS), extracranial cerebral vessels

> **Excludes** *diagnostic ultrasound (non-invasive) of head and neck (88.71)*

00.22 Intravascular imaging of intrathoracic vessels
Aorta and aortic arch
Intravascular ultrasound (IVUS), intrathoracic vessels
Vena cava (superior) (inferior)

> **Excludes** *diagnostic ultrasound (non-invasive) of other sites of thorax (88.73)*

00.23 Intravascular imaging of peripheral vessels
Imaging of:
vessels of arm(s)
vessels of leg(s)
Intravascular ultrasound (IVUS), peripheral vessels

> **Excludes** *diagnostic ultrasound (non-invasive) of peripheral vascular system (88.77)*

◀ New   ◀▥ Revised   ~~deleted~~ Deleted   ● Use Additional Digit(s)   ✖ Valid O.R. Procedure
◆ Non-O.R. Procedure   ♀ Females Only   ♂ Males Only   OGCR Official Guidelines   **Coding Clinic**

1196

00.24 Intravascular imaging of coronary vessels
Intravascular ultrasound (IVUS), coronary vessels

> **Excludes** *diagnostic ultrasound (non-invasive) of heart (88.72)*
> *intracardiac echocardiography [ICE] (ultrasound of heart chamber(s)) (37.28)*

Coding Clinic: 2006, Q3, P8-9

00.25 Intravascular imaging of renal vessels
Intravascular ultrasound (IVUS), renal vessels
Renal artery

> **Excludes** *diagnostic ultrasound (non-invasive) of urinary system (88.75)*

00.28 Intravascular imaging, other specified vessel(s)

00.29 Intravascular imaging, unspecified vessel(s)

● **00.3 Computer assisted surgery [CAS]**
CT-free navigation
Image guided navigation (IGN)
Image guided surgery (IGS)
Imageless navigation
That without the use of robotic(s) technology

Code also diagnostic or therapeutic procedure

> **Excludes** *robotic assisted procedures (17.41–17.49)*
> *stereotactic frame application only (93.59)*

00.31 Computer assisted surgery with CT/CTA

00.32 Computer assisted surgery with MR/MRA
Coding Clinic: 2004, Q4, P111-113

00.33 Computer assisted surgery with fluoroscopy

00.34 Imageless computer assisted surgery

00.35 Computer assisted surgery with multiple datasets

00.39 Other computer assisted surgery
Computer assisted surgery NOS

● **00.4 Adjunct vascular system procedures**
Note: These codes can apply to both coronary and peripheral vessels. These codes are to be used in conjunction with other therapeutic procedure codes to provide additional information on the number of vessels upon which a procedure was performed and/or the number of stents inserted. As appropriate, code both the number of vessels operated on (00.40–00.43), and the number of stents inserted (00.45–00.48).

Code also any:
angioplasty (00.61–00.62, 00.66, 39.50)
atherectomy (17.53-17.56)
endarterectomy (38.10–38.18)
insertion of vascular stent(s) (00.55, 00.63–00.65, 36.06–36.07, 39.90)
other removal of coronary artery obstruction (36.09)

00.40 Procedure on single vessel
Number of vessels, unspecified

> **Excludes** *(aorto)coronary bypass (36.10–36.19)*
> *intravascular imaging of blood vessels (00.21–00.29)*

Coding Clinic: 2012, Q2, P15-16; 2011, Q4, P166-167; 2010, Q4, P113; Q2, P9; 2009, Q3, P13; Q2, P12; 2007, Q1, P17; 2006, Q3, P8-9; 2005, Q4, P69-72, 103-106

00.41 Procedure on two vessels

> **Excludes** *(aorto)coronary bypass (36.10–36.19)*
> *intravascular imaging of blood vessels (00.21–00.29)*

Coding Clinic: 2012, Q3, P6; 2006, Q4, P119; 2005, Q4, P101-106

00.42 Procedure on three vessels

> **Excludes** *(aorto)coronary bypass (36.10–36.19)*
> *intravascular imaging of blood vessels (00.21–00.29)*

00.43 Procedure on four or more vessels

> **Excludes** *(aorto)coronary bypass (36.10–36.19)*
> *intravascular imaging of blood vessels (00.21–00.29)*

◆Non-OR Procedure that affects MS-DRG assignment to MDC 05, MS-DRG 246, 248

00.44 Procedure on vessel bifurcation
Note: This code is to be used to identify the presence of a vessel bifurcation; it does not describe a specific bifurcation stent. Use this code only once per operative episode, irrespective of the number of bifurcations in vessels.

Coding Clinic: 2013, Q1, P6; 2006, Q4, P119

00.45 Insertion of one vascular stent
Number of stents, unspecified
Coding Clinic: 2011, Q4, P167; 2010, Q4, P113; 2009, Q3, P13; 2005, Q4, P69-72

00.46 Insertion of two vascular stents
Coding Clinic: 2012, Q3, P6; 2009, Q2, P12; 2005, Q4, P103-106

00.47 Insertion of three vascular stents
Coding Clinic: 2006, Q4, P119

00.48 Insertion of four or more vascular stents
◆Non-OR Procedure that affects MS-DRG assignment to MDC 05, MS-DRG 246, 248

00.49 SuperSaturated oxygen therapy
Aqueous oxygen (AO) therapy
SSO_2
SuperOxygenation infusion therapy

Code also any:
injection or infusion of thrombolytic agent (99.10)
insertion of coronary artery stent(s) (36.06-36.07)
intracoronary artery thrombolytic infusion (36.04)
number of vascular stents inserted (00.45-00.48)
number of vessels treated (00.40-00.43)
open chest coronary artery angioplasty (36.03)
other removal of coronary obstruction (36.09)
percutaneous transluminal coronary angioplasty [PTCA] (00.66)
procedure on vessel bifurcation (00.44)
transluminal coronary atherectomy (17.55)

> **Excludes** *other oxygen enrichment (93.96)*
> *other perfusion (39.97)*

Coding Clinic: 2008, Q4, P162-163

● **00.5 Other cardiovascular procedures**
Coding Clinic: 2008, Q3, P18; 2002, Q4, P95-101

✖ **00.50 Implantation of cardiac resynchronization pacemaker without mention of defibrillation, total system [CRT-P]**
BiV pacemaker
Biventricular pacemaker
Biventricular pacing without internal cardiac defibrillator
Implantation of cardiac resynchronization (biventricular) pulse generator pacing device, formation of pocket, transvenous leads including placement of lead into left ventricular coronary venous system, and intraoperative procedures for evaluation of lead signals.
That with CRT-P generator and one or more leads
Note: Device testing during procedure – *omit code*

> **Excludes** *implantation of cardiac resynchronization defibrillator, total system [CRT-D] (00.51)*
> *insertion or replacement of any type pacemaker device (37.80–37.87)*
> *replacement of cardiac resynchronization defibrillator pulse generator only [CRT-D] (00.54)*
> *replacement of cardiac resynchronization pacemaker pulse generator only [CRT-P] (00.53)*

Coding Clinic: 2008, Q3, P18; 2005, Q3, P3-9

Excludes   Includes   Use additional   Code also   Omit code

PROCEDURES AND INTERVENTIONS, NEC (00)

✷ 00.51 **Implantation of cardiac resynchronization defibrillator, total system [CRT-D]**
BiV defibrillator
BiV ICD
BiV pacemaker with defibrillator
BiV pacing with defibrillator
Biventricular defibrillator
Biventricular pacing with internal cardiac defibrillator
Implantation of a cardiac resynchronization (biventricular) pulse generator with defibrillator [AICD], formation of pocket, transvenous leads, including placement of lead into left ventricular coronary venous system, intraoperative procedures for evaluation of lead signals, and obtaining defibrillator threshold measurements.
That with CRT-D generator and one or more leads
Note: Device testing during procedure – *omit code*

Excludes *implantation of cardiac resynchronization pacemaker, total system [CRT-P] (00.50)*
implantation or replacement of automatic cardioverter/defibrillator, total system [AICD] (37.94)
replacement of cardiac resynchronization defibrillator pulse generator, only [CRT-D] (00.54)
Coding Clinic: 2012, Q2, P14-15; 2008, Q3, P18; 2007, Q1, P16-17x2; 2005, Q3, P3-9; 2002, Q4, P99-100

✷ 00.52 **Implantation or replacement of transvenous lead [electrode] into left ventricular coronary venous system**

Excludes *implantation of cardiac resynchronization defibrillator, total system [CRT-D] (00.51)*
implantation of cardiac resynchronization pacemaker, total system [CRT-P] (00.50)
initial insertion of transvenous lead [electrode] (37.70–37.72)
replacement of transvenous atrial and/or ventricular lead(s) [electrodes] (37.76)
MS-DRG: Refer to Part VI, Appendix E, Table 3, Cardioverter-Defibrillator Lead/Generator Reference Table
Coding Clinic: 2008, Q3, P18; 2005, Q3, P3-9

✷ 00.53 **Implantation or replacement of cardiac resynchronization pacemaker pulse generator only [CRT-P]**
Implantation of CRT-P device with removal of any existing CRT-P or other pacemaker device
Note: Device testing during procedure – *omit code*

Excludes *implantation of cardiac resynchronization pacemaker, total system [CRT-P] (00.50)*
implantation or replacement of cardiac resynchronization defibrillator pulse generator only [CRT-D] (00.54)
insertion or replacement of any type pacemaker device (37.80–37.87)
MS-DRG: Refer to Part VI, Appendix E, Table 3, Cardioverter-Defibrillator Lead/Generator Reference Table
Coding Clinic: 2005, Q3, P3-9

✷ 00.54 **Implantation or replacement of cardiac resynchronization defibrillator pulse generator device only [CRT-D]**
Implantation of CRT-D device with removal of any existing CRT-D, CRT-P, pacemaker, or defibrillator device
Note: Device testing during procedure – *omit code*

Excludes *implantation of automatic cardioverter/defibrillator pulse generator only (37.96)*
implantation of cardiac resynchronization defibrillator, total system [CRT-D] (00.51)
implantation or replacement of cardiac resynchronization pacemaker pulse generator only [CRT-P] (00.53)
MS-DRG: Refer to Part VI, Appendix E, Table 3, Cardioverter-Defibrillator Lead/Generator Reference Table
Coding Clinic: 2012, Q2, P13-15; 2005, Q3, P3-9; 2002, Q4, P100

00.55 **Insertion of drug-eluting stent(s) of other peripheral vessel(s)**
Endograft(s)   Stent grafts
Endovascular graft(s)
Code also any:
angioplasty of other non-coronary vessel(s) (39.50)
atherectomy of other non-coronary vessel(s) (17.56)
number of vascular stents inserted (00.45–00.48)
number of vessels treated (00.40–00.43)
procedure on vessel bifurcation (00.44)

Excludes *drug-coated peripheral stents, e.g., heparin coated (39.90)*
insertion of cerebrovascular stent(s) (00.63–00.65)
insertion of drug-eluting coronary artery stent (36.07)
insertion of drug-eluting stent(s) of superficial femoral artery (00.60)
insertion of non-drug-eluting stent(s):
coronary artery (36.06)
peripheral vessel (39.90)
that for other endovascular procedure (39.71-39.79)
Coding Clinic: 2012, Q4, P84-85; Q3, P13; 2002, Q4, P101-103

✷ 00.56 **Insertion or replacement of implantable pressure sensor with lead for intracardiac or great vessel hemodynamic monitoring**
Note: The sensor is physically connected by a lead to a separately implanted monitor.
Code also any associated implantation or replacement of subcutaneous monitor (00.57)

Excludes *circulatory monitoring (blood gas, arterial or venous pressure, cardiac output and coronary blood flow) (89.60–89.69)*
insertion of implantable pressure sensor without lead for intracardiac or great vessel hemodynamic monitoring (38.26)
MS-DRG: Refer to Part VI, Appendix E, Table 6, Lead/Device Reference Table
Coding Clinic: 2006, Q4, P119-120

◀ New   ◀≡ Revised   deleted Deleted   ● Use Additional Digit(s)   ✷ Valid O.R. Procedure
◆ Non-O.R. Procedure   ♀ Females Only   ♂ Males Only   OGCR Official Guidelines   **Coding Clinic**

1198

✖ **00.57 Implantation or replacement of subcutaneous device for intracardiac or great vessel hemodynamic monitoring**

Implantation of monitoring device with formation of subcutaneous pocket and connection to intracardiac pressure sensor via lead

Code also any associated insertion or replacement of implanted pressure sensor with lead (00.56)

MS-DRG: Refer to Part VI, Appendix E, Table 6, Lead/Device Reference Table

Coding Clinic: 2006, Q4, P119-120

00.58 Insertion of intra-aneurysm sac pressure monitoring device (intraoperative)

Insertion of pressure sensor during endovascular repair of abdominal or thoracic aortic aneurysm(s)

Coding Clinic: 2008, Q4, P163-165

00.59 Intravascular pressure measurement of coronary arteries

Includes   fractional flow reserve (FFR)

Code also any synchronous diagnostic or therapeutic procedures

Excludes   *intravascular pressure measurement of intrathoracic arteries (00.67)*

Coding Clinic: 2008, Q4, P163-165

● **00.6 Procedures on blood vessels**

Coding Clinic: 2004, Q4, P114-116

00.60 Insertion of drug-eluting stent(s) of superficial femoral artery

Code also any:
angioplasty of other non-coronary vessel(s) (39.50)
atherectomy of other non-coronary vessel(s) (17.56)
non-drug-eluting peripheral stents (39.90)
number of vascular stents inserted (00.45-00.48)
number of vessels treated (00.40-00.43)
procedure on vessel bifurcation (00.44)

Excludes   *insertion of drug-eluting stent(s) of other peripheral vessel (00.55)*
that for other endovascular procedure (39.71-39.79)

Coding Clinic: 2010, Q4, P113

✖ **00.61 Percutaneous angioplasty of extracranial vessel(s)**
Carotid
Vertebral

Code also any:
injection or infusion of thrombolytic agent (99.10)
number of vascular stents inserted (00.45–00.48)
number of vessels treated (00.40–00.43)
percutaneous atherectomy of extracranial vessel(s) (17.53)
percutaneous insertion of carotid artery stent(s) (00.63)
percutaneous insertion of other extracranial artery stent(s) (00.64)
procedure on vessel bifurcation (00.44)

Excludes   *angioplasty of other non-coronary vessel(s) (39.50)*
atherectomy of other non-coronary vessel(s) (17.56)
removal of cerebrovascular obstruction of vessel(s) by open approach (38.01–38.02, 38.11–38.12, 38.31–38.32, 38.41–38.42)

Coding Clinic: 2010, Q3, P17-18

✖ **00.62 Percutaneous angioplasty of intracranial vessel(s)**
Basilar artery
Intracranial portion of vertebral artery

Code also any:
injection or infusion of thrombolytic agent (99.10)
number of vascular stents inserted (00.45–00.48)
number of vessels treated (00.40–00.43)
percutaneous atherectomy of intracranial vessel(s) (17.54)
percutaneous insertion of intracranial stent(s) (00.65)
procedure on vessel bifurcation (00.44)

Excludes   *angioplasty of other non-coronary vessel(s) (39.50)*
atherectomy of other non-coronary vessel(s) (17.56)
removal of cerebrovascular obstruction of vessel(s) by open approach (38.01–38.02, 38.11–38.12, 38.31–38.32, 38.41–38.42)

MCE: Non-covered procedure except when combined with 00.65

Coding Clinic: 2011, Q4, P166; 2010, Q3, P18

00.63 Percutaneous insertion of carotid artery stent(s)

Includes the use of any embolic protection device, distal protection device, filter device, or stent delivery system

Non-drug-eluting stent

Code also any:
number of vascular stents inserted (00.45–00.48)
number of vessels treated (00.40–00.43)
percutaneous angioplasty of extracranial vessel(s) (00.61)
percutaneous atherectomy of extracranial vessel(s) (17.53)
procedure on vessel bifurcation (00.44)

Excludes   *angioplasty of other non-coronary vessel(s) (39.50)*
atherectomy of other non-coronary vessel(s) (17.56)
insertion of coil-retention or embolization stent (39.72)
insertion of drug-eluting peripheral vessel stent(s) (00.55)

◆ Non-OR Procedure that affects MS-DRG assignment to MDC 01, MS-DRG 034-036

Coding Clinic: 2010, Q3, P18

00.64 Percutaneous insertion of other extracranial artery stent(s)

Includes the use of any embolic protection device, distal protection device, filter device, or stent delivery system

Vertebral stent

Code also any:
number of vascular stents inserted (00.45–00.48)
number of vessels treated (00.40–00.43)
percutaneous angioplasty of extracranial vessel(s) (00.61)
percutaneous atherectomy of extracranial vessel(s) (17.53)
procedure on vessel bifurcation (00.44)

Excludes   *angioplasty of other non-coronary vessel(s) (39.50)*
atherectomy of other non-coronary vessel(s) (17.56)
insertion of coil-retention or embolization stent (39.72)
insertion of drug-eluting peripheral vessel stent(s) (00.55)

PROCEDURES AND INTERVENTIONS, NEC (00)

Excludes   Includes   Use additional   Code also   Omit code

PROCEDURES AND INTERVENTIONS, NEC (00)

00.65   **Percutaneous insertion of intracranial vascular stent(s)**

Basilar stent

Includes the use of any embolic protection device, distal protection device, filter device, or stent delivery system

Code also any:
number of vascular stents inserted (00.45–00.48)
number of vessels treated (00.40–00.43)
percutaneous angioplasty of intracranial vessel(s) (00.62)
percutaneous atherectomy of intracranial vessel(s) (17.54)
procedure on vessel bifurcation (00.44)

Excludes   *angioplasty of other non-coronary vessel(s) (39.50)*
atherectomy of other non-coronary vessel(s) (17.56)
insertion of coil-retention or embolization stent (39.72)
insertion of drug-eluting peripheral vessel stent(s) (00.55)

Coding Clinic: 2010, Q3, P18

✖ **00.66**   **Percutaneous transluminal coronary angioplasty [PTCA]**

Balloon angioplasty of coronary artery
Percutaneous coronary angioplasty NOS
PTCA NOS

Code also any:
injection or infusion of thrombolytic agent (99.10)
insertion of coronary artery stent(s) (36.06–36.07)
intracoronary artery thrombolytic infusion (36.04)
number of vascular stents inserted (00.45–00.48)
number of vessels treated (00.40–00.43)
procedure on vessel bifurcation (00.44)
SuperSaturated oxygen therapy (00.49)
transluminal coronary atherectomy (17.55)

Coding Clinic: 2012, Q3, P5; 2011, Q4, P167; 2010, Q2, P9; 2009, Q2, P12; 2007, Q1, P17; 2006, Q3, P8-9; 2005, Q4, 69-72, P101-103; 2004, Q1, P10; Q2, P3

00.67   **Intravascular pressure measurement of intrathoracic arteries**

Assessment of:
aorta and aortic arch
carotid

Code also any synchronous diagnostic or therapeutic procedures
Coding Clinic: 2008, Q4, P163-165

00.68   **Intravascular pressure measurement of peripheral arteries**

Other peripheral vessels
Vessels of arm(s)
Vessels of leg(s)

Code also any synchronous diagnostic or therapeutic procedures
Coding Clinic: 2008, Q4, P163-165

00.69   **Intravascular pressure measurement, other specified and unspecified vessels**

Iliac vessels
Intra-abdominal vessels
Mesenteric vessels
Renal vessels

Code also any synchronous diagnostic or therapeutic procedures

Excludes   *intravascular pressure measurement of:*
coronary arteries (00.59)
intrathoracic arteries (00.67)
peripheral arteries (00.68)

Coding Clinic: 2008, Q4, P163-165

● **00.7**   **Other hip procedures**
Coding Clinic: 2005, Q4, P106-113

✖ **00.70**   **Revision of hip replacement, both acetabular and femoral components**

Total hip revision

Code also any:
removal of (cement) (joint) spacer (84.57)
type of bearing surface, if known (00.74–00.77)

Excludes   *revision of hip replacement, acetabular component only (00.71)*
revision of hip replacement, femoral component only (00.72)
revision of hip replacement, Not Otherwise Specified (81.53)
revision with replacement of acetabular liner and/or femoral head only (00.73)

MCE: Bilateral procedure when 2+ different joint procedures are reported with principal diagnosis causes assigned to MDC 8

Coding Clinic: 2008, Q2, P3-4; 2008, Q1, P6; 2005, Q4, P110-112

✖ **00.71**   **Revision of hip replacement, acetabular component**

Partial, acetabular component only
That with:
exchange of acetabular cup and liner
exchange of femoral head

Code also any type of bearing surface, if known (00.74–00.77)

Excludes   *revision of hip replacement, both acetabular and femoral components (00.70)*
revision of hip replacement, femoral component (00.72)
revision of hip replacement, Not Otherwise Specified (81.53)
revision with replacement of acetabular liner and/or femoral head only (00.73)

Coding Clinic: 2005, Q4, P110-112

✖ **00.72**   **Revision of hip replacement, femoral component**

Partial, femoral component only
That with:
exchange of acetabular liner
exchange of femoral stem and head

Code also any type of bearing surface, if known (00.74–00.77)

Excludes   *revision of hip replacement, acetabular component (00.71)*
revision of hip replacement, both acetabular and femoral components (00.70)
revision of hip replacement, not otherwise specified (81.53)
revision with replacement of acetabular liner and/or femoral head only (00.73)

✖ **00.73**   **Revision of hip replacement, acetabular liner and/or femoral head only**

Code also any type of bearing surface, if known (00.74–00.77)

00.74   **Hip bearing surface, metal on polyethylene**

00.75   **Hip bearing surface, metal-on-metal**
Coding Clinic: 2006, Q4, P120-121

00.76   **Hip bearing surface, ceramic-on-ceramic**
Coding Clinic: 2005, Q4, P110-112

00.77   **Hip bearing surface, ceramic-on-polyethylene**

Hip bearing surface, oxidized zirconium-on-polyethylene

◀ New   ◀◀◀ Revised   ~~deleted~~ Deleted   ● Use Additional Digit(s)   ✖ Valid O.R. Procedure
◆ Non-O.R. Procedure   ♀ Females Only   ♂ Males Only   OGCR Official Guidelines   Coding Clinic

1200

● **00.8 Other knee and hip procedures**
    Note: Report up to two components using 00.81–00.83 to describe revision of knee replacements. If all three components are revised, report 00.80.
    Coding Clinic: 2005, Q4, P113-117

�ள **00.80 Revision of knee replacement, total (all components)**
        Replacement of femoral, tibial, and patellar components (all components)
        Code also any removal of (cement) (joint) spacer (84.57)
        Excludes *revision of only one or two components (tibial, femoral or patellar component) (00.81–00.84)*
        MCE: Bilateral procedure when 2+ different joint procedures are reported with principal diagnosis causes assigned to MDC 8
        Coding Clinic: 2008, Q1, P6

✧ **00.81 Revision of knee replacement, tibial component**
        Replacement of tibial baseplate and tibial insert (liner)
        Excludes *revision of knee replacement, total (all components) (00.80)*
        Coding Clinic: 2006, Q4, P103-104; 2005, Q4, P113-117

✧ **00.82 Revision of knee replacement, femoral component**
        That with replacement of tibial insert (liner)
        Excludes *revision of knee replacement, total (all components) (00.80)*
        Coding Clinic: 2006, Q3, P9-10; 2005, Q4, P113-117

✧ **00.83 Revision of knee replacement, patellar component**
        Excludes *revision of knee replacement, total (all components) (00.80)*

✧ **00.84 Revision of total knee replacement, tibial insert (liner)**
        Replacement of tibial insert (liner)
        Excludes *that with replacement of tibial component (tibial baseplate and liner) (00.81)*

✧ **00.85 Resurfacing hip, total, acetabulum and femoral head** 🕮
        Hip resurfacing arthroplasty, total
        MCE: Bilateral procedure when 2+ different joint procedures are reported with principal diagnosis causes assigned to MDC 8
        Coding Clinic: 2006, Q4, P121-122

✧ **00.86 Resurfacing hip, partial, femoral head** 🕮
        Hip resurfacing arthroplasty, NOS
        Hip resurfacing arthroplasty, partial, femoral head
        Excludes *that with resurfacing of acetabulum (00.85)*
        MCE: Bilateral procedure when 2+ different joint procedures are reported with principal diagnosis causes assigned to MDC 8

✧ **00.87 Resurfacing hip, partial, acetabulum** 🕮
        Hip resurfacing arthroplasty, partial, acetabulum
        Excludes *that with resurfacing of femoral head (00.85)*
        MCE: Bilateral procedure when 2+ different joint procedures are reported with principal diagnosis causes assigned to MDC 8

● **00.9 Other procedures and interventions**

    00.91 Transplant from live related donor
        Code also organ transplant procedure

    00.92 Transplant from live non-related donor
        Code also organ transplant procedure
        Coding Clinic: 2012, Q1, P13; 2008, Q2, P8-9; 2004, Q4, P116-117

    00.93 Transplant from cadaver
        Code also organ transplant procedure

    00.94 Intra-operative neurophysiologic monitoring
        Intra-operative neurophysiologic testing
        IOM
        Nerve monitoring
        Neuromonitoring
        That by:
            brainstem auditory evoked potentials [BAEP]
            electroencephalogram [EEG]
            electromyogram [EMG]
            motor evoked potentials [MEP]
            nerve conduction study
            somatosensory evoked potentials [SSEP]
            transcranial Doppler
        Includes cranial nerve, peripheral nerve and spinal cord testing performed intra-operatively
        Excludes *brain temperature monitoring (01.17)*
                  intracranial oxygen monitoring (01.16)
                  intracranial pressure monitoring (01.10)
                  plethysmogram (89.58)
        Coding Clinic: 2013, Q2, P9; 2011, Q1, P8; 2009, Q2, P3; 2007, Q4, P104-105

    00.95 Injection or infusion of glucarpidase
        Coding Clinic: 2012, Q4, P87

    00.96 Infusion of 4-Factor Prothrombin Complex Concentrate
        Infusion of 4F-PCC
        Excludes *transfusion of coagulation factors (99.06)*
                  transfusion of Factor IX complex (99.06)

Excludes   Includes   Use additional   Code also   Omit code

PROCEDURES AND INTERVENTIONS, NEC (00)

OPERATIONS ON THE NERVOUS SYSTEM (01–05)

(See Plates 86, 118, 472, 473, 500, 501, 502, 544, and 545 on pages 58–66.)

1. OPERATIONS ON THE NERVOUS SYSTEM (01–05)

● **01 Incision and excision of skull, brain, and cerebral meninges**

● **01.0 Cranial puncture**

01.01 Cisternal puncture
Cisternal tap
> **Excludes** *pneumocisternogram (87.02)*

01.02 Ventriculopuncture through previously implanted catheter
Puncture of ventricular shunt tubing

01.09 Other cranial puncture
Aspiration of:
    subarachnoid space
    subdural space
Cranial aspiration NOS
Puncture of anterior fontanel
Subdural tap (through fontanel)
Coding Clinic: 2009, Q3, P15-16; 2007, Q4, P105-107

● **01.1 Diagnostic procedures on skull, brain, and cerebral meninges**

01.10 Intracranial pressure monitoring
> **Includes** insertion of catheter or probe for monitoring
Coding Clinic: 2013, Q3, P11; 2009, Q3, P15-16; 2007, Q4, P105-107

01.11 Closed [percutaneous] [needle] biopsy of cerebral meninges
Burr hole approach

✖ **01.12 Open biopsy of cerebral meninges**

01.13 Closed [percutaneous] [needle] biopsy of brain
Burr hole approach
Stereotactic method
Coding Clinic: 1987, Mar-April, P9

✖ **01.14 Open biopsy of brain**
Coding Clinic: 2012, Q4, P81

✖ **01.15 Biopsy of skull**

01.16 Intracranial oxygen monitoring
Partial pressure of brain oxygen (PbtO$_2$)
> **Includes** insertion of catheter or probe for monitoring
Coding Clinic: 2013, Q3, P11; 2007, Q4, P105-107

01.17 Brain temperature monitoring
> **Includes** insertion of catheter or probe for monitoring
Coding Clinic: 2013, Q3, P11; 2007, Q4, P105-107

✖ **01.18 Other diagnostic procedures on brain and cerebral meninges**
> **Excludes** *brain temperature monitoring (01.17)*
>   *cerebral:*
>   *arteriography (88.41)*
>   *thermography (88.81)*
>   *contrast radiogram of brain (87.01–87.02)*
>   *echoencephalogram (88.71)*
>   *electroencephalogram (89.14)*
>   *intracranial oxygen monitoring (01.16)*
>   *intracranial pressure monitoring (01.10)*
>   *microscopic examination of specimen from nervous system and of spinal fluid (90.01–90.09)*
>   *neurologic examination (89.13)*
>   *phlebography of head and neck (88.61)*
>   *pneumoencephalogram (87.01)*
>   *radioisotope scan:*
>   *cerebral (92.11)*
>   *head NEC (92.12)*
>   *tomography of head:*
>   *C.A.T. scan (87.03)*
>   *other (87.04)*
Coding Clinic: 2013, Q3, P11; 1998, Q3, P12-13

✖ **01.19 Other diagnostic procedures on skull**
> **Excludes** *transillumination of skull (89.16)*
>   *x-ray of skull (87.17)*

● **01.2 Craniotomy and craniectomy**
> **Excludes** *decompression of skull fracture (02.02)*
>   *exploration of orbit (16.01–16.09)*
>   *that as operative approach –* omit code

✖ **01.20 Cranial implantation or replacement of neurostimulator pulse generator**
Code also any associated lead implantation (02.93)
> **Excludes** *implantation or replacement of subcutaneous neurostimulator pulse generator (86.94-86.98)*

✖ **01.21 Incision and drainage of cranial sinus**

✖ **01.22 Removal of intracranial neurostimulator lead(s)**
Code also any removal of neurostimulator pulse generator (86.05)
> **Excludes** *removal with synchronous replacement (02.93)*

✖ **01.23 Reopening of craniotomy site**

✖ **01.24 Other craniotomy**
Cranial:
    decompression
    exploration
    trephination
Craniotomy NOS
Craniotomy with removal of:
    epidural abscess
    extradural hematoma
    foreign body of skull
> **Excludes** *removal of foreign body with incision into brain (01.39)*
Coding Clinic: 2013, Q2, P18; 2010, Q4, P93; 1991, Q1, P14; 1984, July-Aug, P20

✖ **01.25 Other craniectomy**
Debridement of skull NOS
Sequestrectomy of skull
> **Excludes** *debridement of compound fracture of skull (02.02)*
>   *strip craniectomy (02.01)*
Coding Clinic: 2013, Q2, P18; 2006, Q1, P6

◀ New   ◀◫ Revised   ~~deleted~~ Deleted   ● Use Additional Digit(s)   ✖ Valid O.R. Procedure
◆ Non-O.R. Procedure   ♀ Females Only   ♂ Males Only   OGCR Official Guidelines   **Coding Clinic**

1202

01.26   **Insertion of catheter(s) into cranial cavity or tissue**
Code also any concomitant procedure (e.g. resection (01.59))
Excludes   *placement of intracerebral catheter(s) via burr hole(s) (01.28)*
Coding Clinic: 2009, Q3, P16x2; 2005, Q4, P117-119

01.27   **Removal of catheter(s) from cranial cavity or tissue**
Coding Clinic: 2005, Q4, P117-119

✖ **01.28**   **Placement of intracerebral catheter(s) via burr hole(s)**
Convection enhanced delivery
Stereotactic placement of intracerebral catheter(s)
Code also infusion of medication
Excludes   *insertion of catheter(s) into cranial cavity or tissue(s) (01.26)*
Coding Clinic: 2013, Q3, P11; 2009, Q3, P6; 2006, Q4, P122-123

✖ **01.29**   **Removal of cranial neurostimulator pulse generator**

● **01.3**   **Incision of brain and cerebral meninges**

✖ **01.31**   **Incision of cerebral meninges**
Drainage of:
    intracranial hygroma
    subarachnoid abscess (cerebral)
    subdural empyema

✖ **01.32**   **Lobotomy and tractotomy**
Division of:
    brain tissue
    cerebral tracts
Percutaneous (radiofrequency) cingulotomy

✖ **01.39**   **Other incision of brain**
Amygdalohippocampotomy
Drainage of intracerebral hematoma
Incision of brain NOS
Excludes   *division of cortical adhesions (02.91)*
Coding Clinic: 2009, Q4, P84

● **01.4**   **Operations on thalamus and globus pallidus**

✖ **01.41**   **Operations on thalamus**
Chemothalamectomy
Thalamotomy
Excludes   *that by stereotactic radiosurgery (92.30–92.39)*

✖ **01.42**   **Operations on globus pallidus**
Pallidoansectomy
Pallidotomy
Excludes   *that by stereotactic radiosurgery (92.30–92.39)*

● **01.5**   **Other excision or destruction of brain and meninges**

✖ **01.51**   **Excision of lesion or tissue of cerebral meninges**
Decortication of (cerebral) meninges
Resection of (cerebral) meninges
Stripping of subdural membrane of (cerebral) meninges
Excludes   *biopsy of cerebral meninges (01.11–01.12)*

✖ **01.52**   **Hemispherectomy**

✖ **01.53**   **Lobectomy of brain**

✖ **01.59**   **Other excision or destruction of lesion or tissue of brain**
Amygdalohippocampectomy
Curettage of brain
Debridement of brain
Marsupialization of brain cyst
Transtemporal (mastoid) excision of brain tumor
Excludes   *biopsy of brain (01.13–01.14)*
laser interstitial thermal therapy [LITT] of lesion or tissue of brain under guidance (17.61)
that by stereotactic radiosurgery (92.30–92.39)
Coding Clinic: 2005, Q4, P117-119; 1999, Q3, P7-8; Q1, P9-10; 1998, Q3, P12-13; Q1, P6-7; 1993, Q4, P33

✖ **01.6**   **Excision of lesion of skull**
Removal of granulation tissue of cranium
Excludes   *biopsy of skull (01.15)*
sequestrectomy (01.25)

● **02**   **Other operations on skull, brain, and cerebral meninges**

● **02.0**   **Cranioplasty**
Excludes   *that with synchronous repair of encephalocele (02.12)*

✖ **02.01**   **Opening of cranial suture**
Linear craniectomy
Strip craniectomy

✖ **02.02**   **Elevation of skull fracture fragments**
Debridement of compound fracture of skull
Decompression of skull fracture
Reduction of skull fracture
Code also any synchronous debridement of brain (01.59)
Excludes   *debridement of skull NOS (01.25)*
removal of granulation tissue of cranium (01.6)

✖ **02.03**   **Formation of cranial bone flap**
Repair of skull with flap

✖ **02.04**   **Bone graft to skull**
Pericranial graft (autogenous) (heterogenous)
Coding Clinic: 2013, Q2, P9; 2011, Q1, P8

✖ **02.05**   **Insertion of skull plate**
Replacement of skull plate
Coding Clinic: 2013, Q2, P9

✖ **02.06**   **Other cranial osteoplasty**
Repair of skull NOS
Revision of bone flap of skull
Coding Clinic: 2006, Q1, P6-7; 2005, Q1, P11; 1998, Q3, P9-10

✖ **02.07**   **Removal of skull plate**
Excludes   *removal with synchronous replacement (02.05)*

● **02.1**   **Repair of cerebral meninges**
Excludes   *marsupialization of cerebral lesion (01.59)*

✖ **02.11**   **Simple suture of dura mater of brain**

✖ **02.12**   **Other repair of cerebral meninges**
Closure of fistula of cerebrospinal fluid
Dural graft
Repair of encephalocele including synchronous cranioplasty
Repair of meninges NOS
Subdural patch
Coding Clinic: 2013, Q2, P9, P18

✖ **02.13**   **Ligation of meningeal vessel**
Ligation of:
    longitudinal sinus
    middle meningeal artery

✖ **02.14**   **Choroid plexectomy**
Cauterization of choroid plexus

● **02.2**   **Ventriculostomy**

✖ **02.21**   **Insertion or replacement of external ventricular drain [EVD]**
External ventricular drainage [EVD] setup
Replacement of external ventricular drain
Ventricular catheter placement for:
    drainage of cerebrospinal fluid [CSF]
    injection of medication or other substance
    sampling of cerebrospinal fluid [CSF]
Excludes   *extracranial ventricular shunt (02.31-02.35, 02.39)*
intracranial ventricular shunt (02.22)
other cranial puncture (01.09)
ventricular shunt replacement (02.41-02.43)
Coding Clinic: 2011, Q4, P161-162

✖ **02.22**   **Intracranial ventricular shunt or anastomosis**
Anastomosis of ventricle to:
    cervical subarachnoid space
    cistern magna
Insertion of Holter valve into intracranial system
Shunt between two intracranial ventricles
That by endoscopy
Third ventriculostomy
Ventriculocisternostomy

Excludes   Includes   Use additional   Code also   Omit code

OPERATIONS ON THE NERVOUS SYSTEM (01–05)

● **02.3 Extracranial ventricular shunt**

Includes that with insertion of valve

Coding Clinic: 1985, Sept-Oct, P12

✖ **02.31 Ventricular shunt to structure in head and neck**
Ventricle to nasopharynx shunt
Ventriculomastoid anastomosis
Coding Clinic: 2004, Q4, P111-113

✖ **02.32 Ventricular shunt to circulatory system**
Ventriculoatrial anastomosis
Ventriculocaval shunt

✖ **02.33 Ventricular shunt to thoracic cavity**
Ventriculopleural anastomosis

✖ **02.34 Ventricular shunt to abdominal cavity and organs**
Ventriculocholecystostomy
Ventriculoperitoneostomy

✖ **02.35 Ventricular shunt to urinary system**
Ventricle to ureter shunt

✖ **02.39 Ventricular shunt to extracranial site NEC**
Ventricle to bone marrow shunt

● **02.4 Revision, removal, and irrigation of ventricular shunt**

Excludes revision of distal catheter of ventricular shunt (54.95)

02.41 Irrigation and exploration of ventricular shunt
Exploration of ventriculoperitoneal shunt at ventricular site
Re-programming of ventriculoperitoneal shunt

✖ **02.42 Replacement of ventricular shunt**
Reinsertion of Holter valve
Revision of ventriculoperitoneal shunt at ventricular site

✖ **02.43 Removal of ventricular shunt**

● **02.9 Other operations on skull, brain, and cerebral meninges**

Excludes operations on:
pineal gland (07.17, 07.51–07.59)
pituitary gland [hypophysis] (07.13–07.15, 07.61–07.79)

✖ **02.91 Lysis of cortical adhesions**

✖ **02.92 Repair of brain**

✖ **02.93 Implantation or replacement of intracranial neurostimulator lead(s)**
Implantation, insertion, placement, or replacement of intracranial:
brain pacemaker [neuropacemaker]
depth electrodes
epidural pegs
electroencephalographic receiver
foramen ovale electrodes
intracranial electrostimulator
subdural grids
subdural strips
Code also any:
insertion of cranial implantation or replacement of neurostimulator pulse generator (01.20)
insertion of subcutaneous neurostimulator pulse generator (86.94-86.98)

✖ **02.94 Insertion or replacement of skull tongs or halo traction device**
Coding Clinic: 2001, Q3, P8; 1996, Q3, P14

02.95 Removal of skull tongs or halo traction device

02.96 Insertion of sphenoidal electrodes

✖ **02.99 Other**

Excludes chemical shock therapy (94.24)
electroshock therapy:
subconvulsive (94.26)
other (94.27)

● **03 Operations on spinal cord and spinal canal structures**
Code also any application or administration of an adhesion barrier substance (99.77)

● **03.0 Exploration and decompression of spinal canal structures**

✖ **03.01 Removal of foreign body from spinal canal**

✖ **03.02 Reopening of laminectomy site**

✖ **03.09 Other exploration and decompression of spinal canal**
Decompression:
laminectomy
laminotomy
Expansile laminoplasty
Exploration of spinal nerve root
Foraminotomy
Code also any synchronous insertion, replacement and revision of posterior spinal motion preservation device(s), if performed (84.80–84.85)

Excludes drainage of spinal fluid by anastomosis (03.71–03.79)
laminectomy with excision of intervertebral disc (80.51)
spinal tap (03.31)
that as operative approach – omit code

Coding Clinic: 2013, Q3, P13, Q2, P18, Q1, P7; 2008, Q4, P109-110; Q2, P12; 2007, Q4, P116-120; Q1, P10; 2004, Q3, P6-7; 2002, Q4, P109-110; 2002, Q2, P15; 1999, Q4, P13-14; 1995, Q2, P9-10; 1990, 1997, Q2, P6; Q2, P23

✖ **03.1 Division of intraspinal nerve root**
Rhizotomy

● **03.2 Chordotomy**

✖ **03.21 Percutaneous chordotomy**
Stereotactic chordotomy

✖ **03.29 Other chordotomy**
Chordotomy NOS
Tractotomy (one-stage) (two-stage) of spinal cord
Transection of spinal cord tracts

● **03.3 Diagnostic procedures on spinal cord and spinal canal structures**

03.31 Spinal tap
Lumbar puncture for removal of dye

Excludes lumbar puncture for injection of dye [myelogram] (87.21)

Coding Clinic: 2013, Q3, P13; 1990, Q2, P23

✖ **03.32 Biopsy of spinal cord or spinal meninges**

✖ **03.39 Other diagnostic procedures on spinal cord and spinal canal structures**

Excludes microscopic examination of specimen from nervous system or of spinal fluid (90.01–90.09)
x-ray of spine (87.21–87.29)

✖ **03.4 Excision or destruction of lesion of spinal cord or spinal meninges**
Curettage of spinal cord or spinal meninges
Debridement of spinal cord or spinal meninges
Marsupialization of cyst of spinal cord or spinal meninges
Resection of spinal cord or spinal meninges

Excludes biopsy of spinal cord or meninges (03.32)

Coding Clinic: 2013, Q3, P4; 2008, Q2, P10; 1995, Q3, P5-6

● **03.5 Plastic operations on spinal cord structures**

✖ **03.51 Repair of spinal meningocele**
Repair of meningocele NOS

✖ **03.52 Repair of spinal myelomeningocele**

✖ **03.53 Repair of vertebral fracture**
Elevation of spinal bone fragments
Reduction of fracture of vertebrae
Removal of bony spicules from spinal canal

Excludes percutaneous vertebral augmentation (81.66)
percutaneous vertebroplasty (81.65)

Coding Clinic: 2007, Q1, P20-21; 2004, Q4, P125-126; 2003, Q2, P22; 2002, Q2, P14; 1999, Q4, P12-13; 1996, Q3, P14

◀ New   ◀▥ Revised   ~~deleted~~ Deleted   ● Use Additional Digit(s)   ✖ Valid O.R. Procedure
◆ Non-O.R. Procedure   ♀ Females Only   ♂ Males Only   OGCR Official Guidelines   **Coding Clinic**

✳ **03.59 Other repair and plastic operations on spinal cord structures**
> Repair of:
>> diastematomyelia
>> spina bifida NOS
>> spinal cord NOS
>> spinal meninges NOS
>> vertebral arch defect
> Coding Clinic: 2008, Q4, P109-110

✳ **03.6 Lysis of adhesions of spinal cord and nerve roots**
> Coding Clinic: 1998, Q2, P18

● **03.7 Shunt of spinal theca**

> **Includes** that with valve

✳ **03.71 Spinal subarachnoid-peritoneal shunt**

✳ **03.72 Spinal subarachnoid-ureteral shunt**

✳ **03.79 Other shunt of spinal theca**
> Lumbar-subarachnoid shunt NOS
> Pleurothecal anastomosis
> Salpingothecal anastomosis
> Coding Clinic: 1997, Q1, P7

03.8 Injection of destructive agent into spinal canal
> Coding Clinic: 2003, Q2, P6

● **03.9 Other operations on spinal cord and spinal canal structures**

03.90 Insertion of catheter into spinal canal for infusion of therapeutic or palliative substances
> Insertion of catheter into epidural, subarachnoid, or subdural space of spine with intermittent or continuous infusion of drug (with creation of any reservoir)
>> Code also any implantation of infusion pump (86.06)

03.91 Injection of anesthetic into spinal canal for analgesia
> **Excludes** that for operative anesthesia — omit code
> Coding Clinic: 2010, Q3, P14; 2000, Q3, P15; 1999, Q1, P7-8; 1998, Q2, P18; 1985, Mar-April, P15; 1984, May-June, P14; 1984, July-Aug, P20

03.92 Injection of other agent into spinal canal
> Intrathecal injection of steroid
> Subarachnoid perfusion of refrigerated saline
> **Excludes** injection of:
>> contrast material for myelogram (87.21)
>> destructive agent into spinal canal (03.8)
> Coding Clinic: 2010, Q3, P14; 2003, Q2, P6; 2000, Q3, P15; 1998, Q2, P18

03.93 Implantation or replacement of spinal neurostimulator lead(s)
> Code also any insertion of neurostimulator pulse generator (86.94–86.98)
> Coding Clinic: 2000, Q1, P19-20

✳ **03.94 Removal of spinal neurostimulator lead(s)**
> Code also any removal of neurostimulator pulse generator (86.05)

03.95 Spinal blood patch

03.96 Percutaneous denervation of facet

✳ **03.97 Revision of spinal thecal shunt**
> Coding Clinic: 1999, Q2, P4

✳ **03.98 Removal of spinal thecal shunt**

✳ **03.99 Other**
> Coding Clinic: 1985, Mar-April, P15; 1984, May-June, P14; 1984, July-Aug, P20

● **04 Operations on cranial and peripheral nerves**

● **04.0 Incision, division, and excision of cranial and peripheral nerves**

> **Excludes** opticociliary neurectomy (12.79)
>> sympathetic ganglionectomy (05.21–05.29)

✳ **04.01 Excision of acoustic neuroma**
> That by craniotomy
> **Excludes** that by stereotactic radiosurgery (92.30–92.39)
> Coding Clinic: 1998, Q2, P20; 1995, Q2, P8

✳ **04.02 Division of trigeminal nerve**
> Retrogasserian neurotomy

✳ **04.03 Division or crushing of other cranial and peripheral nerves**
> **Excludes** that of:
>> glossopharyngeal nerve (29.92)
>> laryngeal nerve (31.91)
>> nerves to adrenal glands (07.42)
>> phrenic nerve for collapse of lung (33.31)
>> vagus nerve (44.00–44.03)
> Coding Clinic: 1998, Q2, P20

✳ **04.04 Other incision of cranial and peripheral nerves**

✳ **04.05 Gasserian ganglionectomy**

✳ **04.06 Other cranial or peripheral ganglionectomy**
> **Excludes** sympathetic ganglionectomy (05.21–05.29)

✳ **04.07 Other excision or avulsion of cranial and peripheral nerves**
> Curettage of peripheral nerve
> Debridement of peripheral nerve
> Resection of peripheral nerve
> Excision of peripheral neuroma [Morton's]
> **Excludes** biopsy of cranial or peripheral nerve (04.11–04.12)
> Coding Clinic: 1995, Q2, P8

● **04.1 Diagnostic procedures on peripheral nervous system**

04.11 Closed [percutaneous] [needle] biopsy of cranial or peripheral nerve or ganglion

✳ **04.12 Open biopsy of cranial or peripheral nerve or ganglion**

✳ **04.19 Other diagnostic procedures on cranial and peripheral nerves and ganglia**
> **Excludes** microscopic examination of specimen from nervous system (90.01–90.09)
>> neurologic examination (89.13)

04.2 Destruction of cranial and peripheral nerves
> Destruction of cranial or peripheral nerves by:
>> cryoanalgesia
>> injection of neurolytic agent
>> radiofrequency
> Radiofrequency ablation
> Coding Clinic: 2002, Q3, P10-11

✳ **04.3 Suture of cranial and peripheral nerves**

● **04.4 Lysis of adhesions and decompression of cranial and peripheral nerves**

✳ **04.41 Decompression of trigeminal nerve root**

✳ **04.42 Other cranial nerve decompression**
> Coding Clinic: 2002, Q3, P11-13; 1987, Mar-April, P8

✳ **04.43 Release of carpal tunnel**
> Coding Clinic: 1985, Nov-Dec, P11

✳ **04.44 Release of tarsal tunnel**

✳ **04.49 Other peripheral nerve or ganglion decompression or lysis of adhesions**
> Peripheral nerve neurolysis NOS
> Coding Clinic: 1993, Q2, P8

✳ **04.5 Cranial or peripheral nerve graft**

✳ **04.6 Transposition of cranial and peripheral nerves**
> Nerve transplantation

OPERATIONS ON THE NERVOUS SYSTEM (01–05)

● 04.7   **Other cranial or peripheral neuroplasty**
   ✖ 04.71   **Hypoglossal-facial anastomosis**
   ✖ 04.72   **Accessory-facial anastomosis**
   ✖ 04.73   **Accessory-hypoglossal anastomosis**
   ✖ 04.74   **Other anastomosis of cranial or peripheral nerve**
   ✖ 04.75   **Revision of previous repair of cranial and peripheral nerves**
   ✖ 04.76   **Repair of old traumatic injury of cranial and peripheral nerves**
   ✖ 04.79   **Other neuroplasty**
      Coding Clinic: 2006, Q1, P11

● 04.8   **Injection into peripheral nerve**
    Excludes   *destruction of nerve (by injection of neurolytic agent) (04.2)*
   04.80   **Peripheral nerve injection, not otherwise specified**
   04.81   **Injection of anesthetic into peripheral nerve for analgesia**
     Excludes   *that for operative anesthesia –* omit code
      Coding Clinic: 2000, Q1, P7-8
   04.89   **Injection of other agent, except neurolytic**
     Excludes   *injection of neurolytic agent (04.2)*

● 04.9   **Other operations on cranial and peripheral nerves**
   ✖ 04.91   **Neurectasis**
   ✖ 04.92   **Implantation or replacement of peripheral neurostimulator lead(s)**
     Code also any insertion of neurostimulator pulse generator (86.94–86.98)
     Excludes   *implantation or replacement of carotid sinus stimulation lead(s) (39.82)*
      Coding Clinic: 2007, Q2, P10-11; 2006, Q2, P5-6; 2004, Q2, P7; 2001, Q3, P16-17; 1996, Q3, P12
   ✖ 04.93   **Removal of peripheral neurostimulator lead(s)**
     Code also any removal of neurostimulator pulse generator (86.05)
      Coding Clinic: 2001, Q3, P16-17
   ✖ 04.99   **Other**

● 05   **Operations on sympathetic nerves or ganglia**
    Excludes   *paracervical uterine denervation (69.3)*
  ✖ 05.0   **Division of sympathetic nerve or ganglion**
    Excludes   *that of nerves to adrenal glands (07.42)*
● 05.1   **Diagnostic procedures on sympathetic nerves or ganglia**
    Coding Clinic: 2006, Q2, P7
   ✖ 05.11   **Biopsy of sympathetic nerve or ganglion**
   ✖ 05.19   **Other diagnostic procedures on sympathetic nerves or ganglia**
● 05.2   **Sympathectomy**
   ✖ 05.21   **Sphenopalatine ganglionectomy**
   ✖ 05.22   **Cervical sympathectomy**
   ✖ 05.23   **Lumbar sympathectomy**
   ✖ 05.24   **Presacral sympathectomy**
   ✖ 05.25   **Periarterial sympathectomy**
   ✖ 05.29   **Other sympathectomy and ganglionectomy**
     Excision or avulsion of sympathetic nerve NOS
     Sympathetic ganglionectomy NOS
     Excludes   *biopsy of sympathetic nerve or ganglion (05.11)*
       opticociliary neurectomy (12.79)
       periarterial sympathectomy (05.25)
       tympanosympathectomy (20.91)
● 05.3   **Injection into sympathetic nerve or ganglion**
    Excludes   *injection of ciliary sympathetic ganglion (12.79)*
   05.31   **Injection of anesthetic into sympathetic nerve for analgesia**
   05.32   **Injection of neurolytic agent into sympathetic nerve**
   05.39   **Other injection into sympathetic nerve or ganglion**
● 05.8   **Other operations on sympathetic nerves or ganglia**
   ✖ 05.81   **Repair of sympathetic nerve or ganglion**
   ✖ 05.89   **Other**
✖ 05.9   **Other operations on nervous system**

---

2.   OPERATIONS ON THE ENDOCRINE SYSTEM (06–07)

● 06   **Operations on thyroid and parathyroid glands**
    Includes   incidental resection of hyoid bone
  ● 06.0   **Incision of thyroid field**
    Excludes   *division of isthmus (06.91)*
   06.01   **Aspiration of thyroid field**
     Percutaneous or needle drainage of thyroid field
     Excludes   *aspiration biopsy of thyroid (06.11)*
       drainage by incision (06.09)
       postoperative aspiration of field (06.02)
   ✖ 06.02   **Reopening of wound of thyroid field**
     Reopening of wound of thyroid field for:
      control of (postoperative) hemorrhage
      examination
      exploration
      removal of hematoma
   ✖ 06.09   **Other incision of thyroid field**
     Drainage of hematoma by incision
     Drainage of thyroglossal tract by incision
     Exploration:
      neck by incision
      thyroid (field) by incision
     Removal of foreign body by incision
     Thyroidotomy NOS by incision
     Excludes   *postoperative exploration (06.02)*
       removal of hematoma by aspiration (06.01)

● 06.1   **Diagnostic procedures on thyroid and parathyroid glands**
   06.11   **Closed [percutaneous] [needle] biopsy of thyroid gland**
     Aspiration biopsy of thyroid
   ✖ 06.12   **Open biopsy of thyroid gland**
   ✖ 06.13   **Biopsy of parathyroid gland**
   ✖ 06.19   **Other diagnostic procedures on thyroid and parathyroid glands**
     Excludes   *radioisotope scan of:*
       parathyroid (92.13)
       thyroid (92.01)
       soft tissue x-ray of thyroid field (87.09)
✖ 06.2   **Unilateral thyroid lobectomy**
     Complete removal of one lobe of thyroid (with removal of isthmus or portion of other lobe)
     Hemithyroidectomy
     Excludes   *partial substernal thyroidectomy (06.51)*
● 06.3   **Other partial thyroidectomy**
   ✖ 06.31   **Excision of lesion of thyroid**
     Excludes   *biopsy of thyroid (06.11–06.12)*
       laser interstitial thermal therapy [LITT] of lesion or tissue of neck under guidance (17.62)
   ✖ 06.39   **Other**
     Isthmectomy
     Partial thyroidectomy NOS
     Excludes   *partial substernal thyroidectomy (06.51)*

◀ New   ◀▪▪ Revised   ~~deleted~~ Deleted   ● Use Additional Digit(s)   ✖ Valid O.R. Procedure
◆ Non-O.R. Procedure   ♀ Females Only   ♂ Males Only   OGCR Official Guidelines   **Coding Clinic**

1206

✖ **06.4   Complete thyroidectomy**
      Excludes *complete substernal thyroidectomy (06.52)*
                  that with laryngectomy (30.3–30.4)

● **06.5   Substernal thyroidectomy**
    ✖ **06.50   Substernal thyroidectomy, not otherwise specified**
    ✖ **06.51   Partial substernal thyroidectomy**
    ✖ **06.52   Complete substernal thyroidectomy**

✖ **06.6   Excision of lingual thyroid**
    Excision of thyroid by:
        submental route
        transoral route

✖ **06.7   Excision of thyroglossal duct or tract**

● **06.8   Parathyroidectomy**
    ✖ **06.81   Complete parathyroidectomy**
    ✖ **06.89   Other parathyroidectomy**
        Parathyroidectomy NOS
        Partial parathyroidectomy
        Excludes *biopsy of parathyroid (06.13)*

● **06.9   Other operations on thyroid (region) and parathyroid**
    ✖ **06.91   Division of thyroid isthmus**
        Transection of thyroid isthmus
    ✖ **06.92   Ligation of thyroid vessels**
    ✖ **06.93   Suture of thyroid gland**
    ✖ **06.94   Thyroid tissue reimplantation**
        Autotransplantation of thyroid tissue
    ✖ **06.95   Parathyroid tissue reimplantation**
        Autotransplantation of parathyroid tissue
        Coding Clinic: 1995, Q1, P9
    ✖ **06.98   Other operations on thyroid glands**
    ✖ **06.99   Other operations on parathyroid glands**

● **07   Operations on other endocrine glands**
    Includes operations on:
        adrenal glands
        pineal gland
        pituitary gland
        thymus
    Excludes *operations on:*
        aortic and carotid bodies (39.89)
        ovaries (65.0–65.99)
        pancreas (52.01–52.99)
        testes (62.0–62.99)

● **07.0   Exploration of adrenal field**
    Excludes *incision of adrenal (gland) (07.41)*
    ✖ **07.00   Exploration of adrenal field, not otherwise specified**
    ✖ **07.01   Unilateral exploration of adrenal field**
    ✖ **07.02   Bilateral exploration of adrenal field**

● **07.1   Diagnostic procedures on adrenal glands, pituitary gland, pineal gland, and thymus**
    07.11   Closed [percutaneous] [needle] biopsy of adrenal gland
    ✖ **07.12   Open biopsy of adrenal gland**
    ✖ **07.13   Biopsy of pituitary gland, transfrontal approach**
    ✖ **07.14   Biopsy of pituitary gland, transsphenoidal approach**
    ✖ **07.15   Biopsy of pituitary gland, unspecified approach**
    ✖ **07.16   Biopsy of thymus**
    ✖ **07.17   Biopsy of pineal gland**
    ✖ **07.19   Other diagnostic procedures on adrenal glands, pituitary gland, pineal gland, and thymus**
        Excludes *microscopic examination of specimen from endocrine gland (90.11–90.19)*
                  radioisotope scan of pituitary gland (92.11)

● **07.2   Partial adrenalectomy**
    ✖ **07.21   Excision of lesion of adrenal gland**
        Excludes *biopsy of adrenal gland (07.11–07.12)*
    ✖ **07.22   Unilateral adrenalectomy**
        Adrenalectomy NOS
        Excludes *excision of remaining adrenal gland (07.3)*
    ✖ **07.29   Other partial adrenalectomy**
        Partial adrenalectomy NOS
        Coding Clinic: 2005, Q2, P4-5

● **07.3   Bilateral adrenalectomy**
    Excision of remaining adrenal gland
    Excludes *bilateral partial adrenalectomy (07.29)*

● **07.4   Other operations on adrenal glands, nerves, and vessels**
    ✖ **07.41   Incision of adrenal gland**
        Adrenalotomy (with drainage)
    ✖ **07.42   Division of nerves to adrenal glands**
    ✖ **07.43   Ligation of adrenal vessels**
    ✖ **07.44   Repair of adrenal gland**
    ✖ **07.45   Reimplantation of adrenal tissue**
        Autotransplantation of adrenal tissue
    ✖ **07.49   Other**

● **07.5   Operations on pineal gland**
    ✖ **07.51   Exploration of pineal field**
        Excludes *that with incision of pineal gland (07.52)*
    ✖ **07.52   Incision of pineal gland**
    ✖ **07.53   Partial excision of pineal gland**
        Excludes *biopsy of pineal gland (07.17)*
    ✖ **07.54   Total excision of pineal gland**
        Pinealectomy (complete) (total)
    ✖ **07.59   Other operations on pineal gland**

● **07.6   Hypophysectomy**
    ✖ **07.61   Partial excision of pituitary gland, transfrontal approach**
        Cryohypophysectomy, partial transfrontal approach
        Division of hypophyseal stalk transfrontal approach
        Excision of lesion of pituitary [hypophysis] transfrontal approach
        Hypophysectomy, subtotal transfrontal approach
        Infundibulectomy, hypophyseal transfrontal approach
        Excludes *biopsy of pituitary gland, transfrontal approach (07.13)*
    ✖ **07.62   Partial excision of pituitary gland, transsphenoidal approach**
        Excludes *biopsy of pituitary gland, transsphenoidal approach (07.14)*
        Coding Clinic: 2013, Q1, P7; 1992, Q3, P13
    ✖ **07.63   Partial excision of pituitary gland, unspecified approach**
        Excludes *biopsy of pituitary gland NOS (07.15)*
    ✖ **07.64   Total excision of pituitary gland, transfrontal approach**
        Ablation of pituitary by implantation (strontium-yttrium) (Y) transfrontal approach
        Cryohypophysectomy, complete transfrontal approach
    ✖ **07.65   Total excision of pituitary gland, transsphenoidal approach**
    ✖ **07.68   Total excision of pituitary gland, other specified approach**
    ✖ **07.69   Total excision of pituitary gland, unspecified approach**
        Hypophysectomy NOS
        Pituitectomy NOS

OPERATIONS ON THE ENDOCRINE SYSTEM (06–07)

Excludes   Includes   Use additional   Code also   Omit code

● **07.7   Other operations on hypophysis**

�֍ **07.71   Exploration of pituitary fossa**

Excludes   *exploration with incision of pituitary gland (07.72)*

✖ **07.72   Incision of pituitary gland**
Aspiration of:
craniobuccal pouch
craniopharyngioma
hypophysis
pituitary gland
Rathke's pouch

✖ **07.79   Other**
Insertion of pack into sella turcica

● **07.8   Thymectomy**

✖ **07.80   Thymectomy, not otherwise specified**

✖ **07.81   Other partial excision of thymus**
Open partial excision of thymus

Excludes   *biopsy of thymus (07.16)*
thoracoscopic partial excision of thymus (07.83)

✖ **07.82   Other total excision of thymus**
Open total excision of thymus

Excludes   *thoracoscopic total excision of thymus (07.84)*

✖ **07.83   Thoracoscopic partial excision of thymus**

Excludes   *other partial excision of thymus (07.81)*
Coding Clinic: 2007, Q4, P108-109

✖ **07.84   Thoracoscopic total excision of thymus**

Excludes   *other total excision of thymus (07.82)*
Coding Clinic: 2007, Q4, P108-109

● **07.9   Other operations on thymus**

✖ **07.91   Exploration of thymus field**

Excludes   *exploration with incision of thymus (07.92)*

✖ **07.92   Other incision of thymus**
Open incision of thymus

Excludes   *thoracoscopic incision of thymus (07.95)*

✖ **07.93   Repair of thymus**

✖ **07.94   Transplantation of thymus**

✖ **07.95   Thoracoscopic incision of thymus**

Excludes   *other incision of thymus (07.92)*
Coding Clinic: 2007, Q4, P108-109

✖ **07.98   Other and unspecified thoracoscopic operations on thymus**

✖ **07.99   Other and unspecified operations on thymus**
Transcervical thymectomy

Excludes   *other thoracoscopic operations on thymus (07.98)*

(See Plates 81, 82, 87, and 90 on pages 67–71.)

03.   OPERATIONS ON THE EYE (08–16)

● **08   Operations on eyelids**

Includes   operations on the eyebrow

● **08.0   Incision of eyelid**

08.01   Incision of lid margin

08.02   Severing of blepharorrhaphy

08.09   Other incision of eyelid

● **08.1   Diagnostic procedures on eyelid**

✖ **08.11   Biopsy of eyelid**

08.19   Other diagnostic procedures on eyelid

● **08.2   Excision or destruction of lesion or tissue of eyelid**
Code also any synchronous reconstruction (08.61–08.74)

Excludes   *biopsy of eyelid (08.11)*

✖ **08.20   Removal of lesion of eyelid, not otherwise specified**
Removal of meibomian gland NOS

✖ **08.21   Excision of chalazion**

✖ **08.22   Excision of other minor lesion of eyelid**
Excision of:
verucca
wart

✖ **08.23   Excision of major lesion of eyelid, partial-thickness**
Excision involving one-fourth or more of lid margin, partial-thickness

✖ **08.24   Excision of major lesion of eyelid, full-thickness**
Excision involving one-fourth or more of lid margin, full-thickness
Wedge resection of eyelid
Coding Clinic: 2011, Q4, P135

✖ **08.25   Destruction of lesion of eyelid**

● **08.3   Repair of blepharoptosis and lid retraction**

✖ **08.31   Repair of blepharoptosis by frontalis muscle technique with suture**

✖ **08.32   Repair of blepharoptosis by frontalis muscle technique with fascial sling**

✖ **08.33   Repair of blepharoptosis by resection or advancement of levator muscle or aponeurosis**

✖ **08.34   Repair of blepharoptosis by other levator muscle techniques**

✖ **08.35   Repair of blepharoptosis by tarsal technique**

✖ **08.36   Repair of blepharoptosis by other techniques**
Correction of eyelid ptosis NOS
Orbicularis oculi muscle sling for correction of blepharoptosis

✖ **08.37   Reduction of overcorrection of ptosis**

✖ **08.38   Correction of lid retraction**

● **08.4   Repair of entropion or ectropion**

✖ **08.41   Repair of entropion or ectropion by thermocauterization**

✖ **08.42   Repair of entropion or ectropion by suture technique**

✖ **08.43   Repair of entropion or ectropion with wedge resection**

✖ **08.44   Repair of entropion or ectropion with lid reconstruction**

✖ **08.49   Other repair of entropion or ectropion**

● **08.5   Other adjustment of lid position**

✖ **08.51   Canthotomy**
Enlargement of palpebral fissure

✖ **08.52   Blepharorrhaphy**
Canthorrhaphy
Tarsorrhaphy

✖ **08.59   Other**
Canthoplasty NOS
Repair of epicanthal fold

● **08.6   Reconstruction of eyelid with flaps or grafts**

Excludes   *that associated with repair of entropion and ectropion (08.44)*

✖ **08.61   Reconstruction of eyelid with skin flap or graft**

✖ **08.62   Reconstruction of eyelid with mucous membrane flap or graft**

✖ **08.63   Reconstruction of eyelid with hair follicle graft**

✖ **08.64   Reconstruction of eyelid with tarsoconjunctival flap**
Transfer of tarsoconjunctival flap from opposing lid

✖ **08.69   Other reconstruction of eyelid with flaps or grafts**

◀ New   ◀◀◀ Revised   ~~deleted~~ Deleted   ● Use Additional Digit(s)   ✖ Valid O.R. Procedure
◆ Non-O.R. Procedure   ♀ Females Only   ♂ Males Only   OGCR Official Guidelines   **Coding Clinic**

1208

● 08.7 Other reconstruction of eyelid
> **Excludes** *that associated with repair of entropion and ectropion (08.44)*
> Coding Clinic: 1996, Q2, P11

✖ 08.70 Reconstruction of eyelid, not otherwise specified

✖ 08.71 Reconstruction of eyelid involving lid margin, partial-thickness

✖ 08.72 Other reconstruction of eyelid, partial-thickness

✖ 08.73 Reconstruction of eyelid involving lid margin, full-thickness

✖ 08.74 Other reconstruction of eyelid, full-thickness

● 08.8 Other repair of eyelid

08.81 Linear repair of laceration of eyelid or eyebrow

08.82 Repair of laceration involving lid margin, partial-thickness

08.83 Other repair of laceration of eyelid, partial-thickness

08.84 Repair of laceration involving lid margin, full-thickness

08.85 Other repair of laceration of eyelid, full-thickness

08.86 Lower eyelid rhytidectomy

08.87 Upper eyelid rhytidectomy
> Coding Clinic: 1996, Q2, P11

08.89 Other eyelid repair
> Coding Clinic: 2000, Q1, P22-23

● 08.9 Other operations on eyelids

✖ 08.91 Electrosurgical epilation of eyelid

✖ 08.92 Cryosurgical epilation of eyelid

✖ 08.93 Other epilation of eyelid

✖ 08.99 Other

● 09 Operations on lacrimal system

✖ 09.0 Incision of lacrimal gland
> Incision of lacrimal cyst (with drainage)

● 09.1 Diagnostic procedures on lacrimal system

✖ 09.11 Biopsy of lacrimal gland

✖ 09.12 Biopsy of lacrimal sac

✖ 09.19 Other diagnostic procedures on lacrimal system
> **Excludes** *contrast dacryocystogram (87.05)*
> *soft tissue x-ray of nasolacrimal duct (87.09)*

● 09.2 Excision of lesion or tissue of lacrimal gland

✖ 09.20 Excision of lacrimal gland, not otherwise specified

✖ 09.21 Excision of lesion of lacrimal gland
> **Excludes** *biopsy of lacrimal gland (09.11)*

✖ 09.22 Other partial dacryoadenectomy
> **Excludes** *biopsy of lacrimal gland (09.11)*

✖ 09.23 Total dacryoadenectomy

✖ 09.3 Other operations on lacrimal gland

● 09.4 Manipulation of lacrimal passage
> **Includes** *removal of calculus*
> *that with dilation*
> **Excludes** *contrast dacryocystogram (87.05)*

✖ 09.41 Probing of lacrimal punctum

✖ 09.42 Probing of lacrimal canaliculi

✖ 09.43 Probing of nasolacrimal duct
> **Excludes** *that with insertion of tube or stent (09.44)*

✖ 09.44 Intubation of nasolacrimal duct
> Insertion of stent into nasolacrimal duct
> Coding Clinic: 1994, Q2, P11

✖ 09.49 Other manipulation of lacrimal passage

● 09.5 Incision of lacrimal sac and passages

✖ 09.51 Incision of lacrimal punctum

✖ 09.52 Incision of lacrimal canaliculi

✖ 09.53 Incision of lacrimal sac

✖ 09.59 Other incision of lacrimal passages
> Incision (and drainage) of nasolacrimal duct NOS

● 09.6 Excision of lacrimal sac and passage
> **Excludes** *biopsy of lacrimal sac (09.12)*

● 09.7 Repair of canaliculus and punctum
> **Excludes** *repair of eyelid (08.81–08.89)*

✖ 09.71 Correction of everted punctum

✖ 09.72 Other repair of punctum

✖ 09.73 Repair of canaliculus

● 09.8 Fistulization of lacrimal tract to nasal cavity

✖ 09.81 Dacryocystorhinostomy [DCR]

✖ 09.82 Conjunctivocystorhinostomy
> Conjunctivodacryocystorhinostomy [CDCR]
> **Excludes** *that with insertion of tube or stent (09.83)*

✖ 09.83 Conjunctivorhinostomy with insertion of tube or stent

● 09.9 Other operations on lacrimal system

✖ 09.91 Obliteration of lacrimal punctum

✖ 09.99 Other
> Coding Clinic: 1994, Q2, P11

● 10 Operations on conjunctiva

✖ 10.0 Removal of embedded foreign body from conjunctiva by incision
> **Excludes** *removal of:*
> *embedded foreign body without incision (98.22)*
> *superficial foreign body (98.21)*

✖ 10.1 Other incision of conjunctiva

● 10.2 Diagnostic procedures on conjunctiva

✖ 10.21 Biopsy of conjunctiva

✖ 10.29 Other diagnostic procedures on conjunctiva

● 10.3 Excision or destruction of lesion or tissue of conjunctiva

✖ 10.31 Excision of lesion or tissue of conjunctiva
> Excision of ring of conjunctiva around cornea
> **Excludes** *biopsy of conjunctiva (10.21)*
> Coding Clinic: 2000, Q4, P41; 1996, Q3, P7

✖ 10.32 Destruction of lesion of conjunctiva
> **Excludes** *excision of lesion (10.31)*
> *thermocauterization for entropion (08.41)*

✖ 10.33 Other destructive procedures on conjunctiva
> Removal of trachoma follicles

● 10.4 Conjunctivoplasty

✖ 10.41 Repair of symblepharon with free graft
> Coding Clinic: 1996, Q3, P7

✖ 10.42 Reconstruction of conjunctival cul-de-sac with free graft
> **Excludes** *revision of enucleation socket with graft (16.63)*

✖ 10.43 Other reconstruction of conjunctival cul-de-sac
> **Excludes** *revision of enucleation socket (16.64)*

✖ 10.44 Other free graft to conjunctiva

✖ 10.49 Other conjunctivoplasty
> **Excludes** *repair of cornea with conjunctival flap (11.53)*

✖ 10.5 Lysis of adhesions of conjunctiva and eyelid
> Division of symblepharon (with insertion of conformer)

● 10.6 Repair of laceration of conjunctiva
> **Excludes** *that with repair of sclera (12.81)*

● 10.9 Other operations on conjunctiva

✖ 10.91 Subconjunctival injection
> Coding Clinic: 1996, Q3, P7

✖ 10.99 Other

OPERATIONS ON THE EYE (08–16)

Excludes Includes Use additional Code also Omit code

● 11 Operations on cornea
  ✖ **11.0 Magnetic removal of embedded foreign body from cornea**
       Excludes *that with incision (11.1)*
  ✖ **11.1 Incision of cornea**
       Incision of cornea for removal of foreign body
● ✖ **11.2 Diagnostic procedures on cornea**
    ✖ **11.21 Scraping of cornea for smear or culture**
    ✖ **11.22 Biopsy of cornea**
    ✖ **11.29 Other diagnostic procedures on cornea**
● ✖ **11.3 Excision of pterygium**
    ✖ **11.31 Transposition of pterygium**
    ✖ **11.32 Excision of pterygium with corneal graft**
    ✖ **11.39 Other excision of pterygium**
● ✖ **11.4 Excision or destruction of tissue or other lesion of cornea**
    ✖ **11.41 Mechanical removal of corneal epithelium**
         That by chemocauterization
         Excludes *that for smear or culture (11.21)*
         Coding Clinic: 2002, Q3, P20-21
    ✖ **11.42 Thermocauterization of corneal lesion**
    ✖ **11.43 Cryotherapy of corneal lesion**
    ✖ **11.49 Other removal or destruction of corneal lesion**
         Excision of cornea NOS
         Excludes *biopsy of cornea (11.22)*
● ✖ **11.5 Repair of cornea**
    ✖ **11.51 Suture of corneal laceration**
         Coding Clinic: 1996, Q3, P7
    ✖ **11.52 Repair of postoperative wound dehiscence of cornea**
    ✖ **11.53 Repair of corneal laceration or wound with conjunctival flap**
    ✖ **11.59 Other repair of cornea**
● ✖ **11.6 Corneal transplant**
       Excludes *excision of pterygium with corneal graft (11.32)*
    ✖ **11.60 Corneal transplant, not otherwise specified**
         Keratoplasty NOS
         Note: To report donor source - *see* codes 00.91–00.93
    ✖ **11.61 Lamellar keratoplasty with autograft**
    ✖ **11.62 Other lamellar keratoplasty**
    ✖ **11.63 Penetrating keratoplasty with autograft**
         Perforating keratoplasty with autograft
    ✖ **11.64 Other penetrating keratoplasty**
         Perforating keratoplasty (with homograft)
    ✖ **11.69 Other corneal transplant**
● ✖ **11.7 Other reconstructive and refractive surgery on cornea**
    ✖ **11.71 Keratomileusis**
         MCE: Non-covered procedure
    ✖ **11.72 Keratophakia**
         MCE: Non-covered procedure
    ✖ **11.73 Keratoprosthesis**
    ✖ **11.74 Thermokeratoplasty**
    ✖ **11.75 Radial keratotomy**
         MCE: Non-covered procedure
    ✖ **11.76 Epikeratophakia**
         MCE: Non-covered procedure
    ✖ **11.79 Other**
● ✖ **11.9 Other operations on cornea**
    ✖ **11.91 Tattooing of cornea**
    ✖ **11.92 Removal of artificial implant from cornea**
    ✖ **11.99 Other**
         Coding Clinic: 2002, Q3, P20-21

● 12 Operations on iris, ciliary body, sclera, and anterior chamber
       Excludes *operations on cornea (11.0–11.99)*
● ✖ **12.0 Removal of intraocular foreign body from anterior segment of eye**
    ✖ **12.00 Removal of intraocular foreign body from anterior segment of eye, not otherwise specified**
    ✖ **12.01 Removal of intraocular foreign body from anterior segment of eye with use of magnet**
    ✖ **12.02 Removal of intraocular foreign body from anterior segment of eye without use of magnet**
● ✖ **12.1 Iridotomy and simple iridectomy**
       Excludes *iridectomy associated with:*
         cataract extraction (13.11–13.69)
         removal of lesion (12.41–12.42)
         scleral fistulization (12.61–12.69)
    ✖ **12.11 Iridotomy with transfixion**
    ✖ **12.12 Other iridotomy**
         Corectomy   Iridotomy NOS
         Discission of iris
    ✖ **12.13 Excision of prolapsed iris**
    ✖ **12.14 Other iridectomy**
         Iridectomy (basal) (peripheral) (total)
● ✖ **12.2 Diagnostic procedures on iris, ciliary body, sclera, and anterior chamber**
    ✖ **12.21 Diagnostic aspiration of anterior chamber of eye**
    ✖ **12.22 Biopsy of iris**
    ✖ **12.29 Other diagnostic procedures on iris, ciliary body, sclera, and anterior chamber**
● ✖ **12.3 Iridoplasty and coreoplasty**
    ✖ **12.31 Lysis of goniosynechiae**
         Lysis of goniosynechiae by injection of air or liquid
    ✖ **12.32 Lysis of other anterior synechiae**
         Lysis of anterior synechiae:
            NOS
            by injection of air or liquid
    ✖ **12.33 Lysis of posterior synechiae**
         Lysis of iris adhesions NOS
    ✖ **12.34 Lysis of corneovitreal adhesions**
    ✖ **12.35 Coreoplasty**
         Needling of pupillary membrane
    ✖ **12.39 Other iridoplasty**
● ✖ **12.4 Excision or destruction of lesion of iris and ciliary body**
    ✖ **12.40 Removal of lesion of anterior segment of eye, not otherwise specified**
    ✖ **12.41 Destruction of lesion of iris, nonexcisional**
         Destruction of lesion of iris by:
            cauterization
            cryotherapy
            photocoagulation
    ✖ **12.42 Excision of lesion of iris**
         Excludes *biopsy of iris (12.22)*
    ✖ **12.43 Destruction of lesion of ciliary body, nonexcisional**
    ✖ **12.44 Excision of lesion of ciliary body**
● ✖ **12.5 Facilitation of intraocular circulation**
    ✖ **12.51 Goniopuncture without goniotomy**
    ✖ **12.52 Goniotomy without goniopuncture**
    ✖ **12.53 Goniotomy with goniopuncture**
    ✖ **12.54 Trabeculotomy ab externo**
    ✖ **12.55 Cyclodialysis**
    ✖ **12.59 Other facilitation of intraocular circulation**
         Coding Clinic: 1999, Q4, P13-14
● ✖ **12.6 Scleral fistulization**
       Excludes *exploratory sclerotomy (12.89)*
    ✖ **12.61 Trephination of sclera with iridectomy**
    ✖ **12.62 Thermocauterization of sclera with iridectomy**
    ✖ **12.63 Iridencleisis and iridotasis**
    ✖ **12.64 Trabeculectomy ab externo**

◀ New   ◀▥ Revised   ~~deleted~~ Deleted   ● Use Additional Digit(s)   ✖ Valid O.R. Procedure
◆ Non-O.R. Procedure   ♀ Females Only   ♂ Males Only   OGCR Official Guidelines   **Coding Clinic**

✼12.65 Other scleral fistulization with iridectomy

✼12.66 Postoperative revision of scleral fistulization procedure
　　　　Revision of filtering bleb
　　　　Excludes *repair of fistula (12.82)*
　　　　Coding Clinic: 2001, Q2, P16-17

✼12.67 Insertion of aqueous drainage device
　　　　Anterior chamber drainage device
　　　　Aqueous drainage shunt or stent
　　　　Eye valve implant
　　　　Filtration canal shunt or device

✼12.69 Other fistulizing procedure
　　　　Coding Clinic: 1996, Q3, P4

●12.7 Other procedures for relief of elevated intraocular pressure

✼12.71 Cyclodiathermy

✼12.72 Cyclocryotherapy

✼12.73 Cyclophotocoagulation

✼12.74 Diminution of ciliary body, not otherwise specified

✼12.79 Other glaucoma procedures
　　　　Coding Clinic: 1998, Q2, P16

●12.8 Operations on sclera
　　　　Excludes *those associated with:*
　　　　　　　retinal reattachment (14.41–14.59)
　　　　　　　scleral fistulization (12.61–12.69)

✼12.81 Suture of laceration of sclera
　　　　Suture of sclera with synchronous repair of conjunctiva

✼12.82 Repair of scleral fistula
　　　　Excludes *postoperative revision of scleral fistulization procedure (12.66)*

✼12.83 Revision of operative wound of anterior segment, not elsewhere classified
　　　　Excludes *postoperative revision of scleral fistulization procedure (12.66)*

✼12.84 Excision or destruction of lesion of sclera

✼12.85 Repair of scleral staphyloma with graft

✼12.86 Other repair of scleral staphyloma

✼12.87 Scleral reinforcement with graft

✼12.88 Other scleral reinforcement

✼12.89 Other operations on sclera
　　　　Exploratory sclerotomy

●12.9 Other operations on iris, ciliary body, and anterior chamber

✼12.91 Therapeutic evacuation of anterior chamber
　　　　Paracentesis of anterior chamber
　　　　Excludes *diagnostic aspiration (12.21)*

✼12.92 Injection into anterior chamber
　　　　Injection of:
　　　　　　air into anterior chamber
　　　　　　liquid into anterior chamber
　　　　　　medication into anterior chamber

✼12.93 Removal or destruction of epithelial downgrowth from anterior chamber
　　　　Excludes *that with iridectomy (12.41–12.42)*

✼12.97 Other operations on iris

✼12.98 Other operations on ciliary body

✼12.99 Other operations on anterior chamber

●13 Operations on lens

●13.0 Removal of foreign body from lens
　　　　Excludes *removal of pseudophakos (13.8)*

✼13.00 Removal of foreign body from lens, not otherwise specified

✼13.01 Removal of foreign body from lens with use of magnet

✼13.02 Removal of foreign body from lens without use of magnet

●13.1 Intracapsular extraction of lens
　　　　Code also any synchronous insertion of pseudophakos (13.71)

✼13.11 Intracapsular extraction of lens by temporal inferior route

✼13.19 Other intracapsular extraction of lens
　　　　Cataract extraction NOS
　　　　Cryoextraction of lens
　　　　Erysiphake extraction of cataract
　　　　Extraction of lens NOS

✼13.2 Extracapsular extraction of lens by linear extraction technique
　　　　Code also any synchronous insertion of pseudophakos (13.71)

✼13.3 Extracapsular extraction of lens by simple aspiration (and irrigation) technique
　　　　Irrigation of traumatic cataract
　　　　Code also any synchronous insertion of pseudophakos (13.71)

●13.4 Extracapsular extraction of lens by fragmentation and aspiration technique
　　　　Code also any synchronous insertion of pseudophakos (13.71)

✼13.41 Phacoemulsification and aspiration of cataract
　　　　Coding Clinic: 1996, Q3, P4; 1994, Q1, P16

✼13.42 Mechanical phacofragmentation and aspiration of cataract by posterior route
　　　　Code also any synchronous vitrectomy (14.74)

✼13.43 Mechanical phacofragmentation and other aspiration of cataract

●13.5 Other extracapsular extraction of lens
　　　　Code also any synchronous insertion of pseudophakos (13.71)

✼13.51 Extracapsular extraction of lens by temporal inferior route

✼13.59 Other extracapsular extraction of lens

●13.6 Other cataract extraction
　　　　Code also any synchronous insertion of pseudophakos (13.71)

✼13.64 Discission of secondary membrane [after cataract]

✼13.65 Excision of secondary membrane [after cataract]
　　　　Capsulectomy

✼13.66 Mechanical fragmentation of secondary membrane [after cataract]

✼13.69 Other cataract extraction

●13.7 Insertion of prosthetic lens [pseudophakos]
　　　　Excludes *implantation of intraocular telescope prosthesis (13.91)*

✼13.70 Insertion of pseudophakos, not otherwise specified

✼13.71 Insertion of intraocular lens prosthesis at time of cataract extraction, one-stage
　　　　Code also synchronous extraction of cataract (13.11–13.69)
　　　　Coding Clinic: 1996, Q3, P4

✼13.72 Secondary insertion of intraocular lens prosthesis

✼13.8 Removal of implanted lens
　　　　Removal of pseudophakos

●13.9 Other operations on lens
　　　　Coding Clinic: 2000, Q1, P9-10

✼13.90 Operation on lens, Not Elsewhere Classified

✼13.91 Implantation of intraocular telescope prosthesis
　　　　Implantable miniature telescope
　　　　Includes removal of lens, any method
　　　　Excludes *secondary insertion of ocular implant (16.61)*
　　　　Coding Clinic: 2006, Q4, P123-124

OPERATIONS ON THE EYE (08–16)

Excludes　　Includes　　Use additional　　Code also　　Omit code

● **14　Operations on retina, choroid, vitreous, and posterior chamber**
  ● **14.0　Removal of foreign body from posterior segment of eye**
      Excludes　*removal of surgically implanted material (14.6)*
      ✖ **14.00　Removal of foreign body from posterior segment of eye, not otherwise specified**
      ✖ **14.01　Removal of foreign body from posterior segment of eye with use of magnet**
      ✖ **14.02　Removal of foreign body from posterior segment of eye without use of magnet**
  ● **14.1　Diagnostic procedures on retina, choroid, vitreous, and posterior chamber**
      ✖ **14.11　Diagnostic aspiration of vitreous**
      ✖ **14.19　Other diagnostic procedures on retina, choroid, vitreous, and posterior chamber**
  ● **14.2　Destruction of lesion of retina and choroid**
      Includes　destruction of chorioretinopathy or isolated chorioretinal lesion
      Excludes　*that for repair of retina (14.31–14.59)*
      ✖ **14.21　Destruction of chorioretinal lesion by diathermy**
      ✖ **14.22　Destruction of chorioretinal lesion by cryotherapy**
      14.23　Destruction of chorioretinal lesion by xenon arc photocoagulation
      14.24　Destruction of chorioretinal lesion by laser photocoagulation
      14.25　Destruction of chorioretinal lesion by photocoagulation of unspecified type
      ✖ **14.26　Destruction of chorioretinal lesion by radiation therapy**
      ✖ **14.27　Destruction of chorioretinal lesion by implantation of radiation source**
      14.29　Other destruction of chorioretinal lesion
          Destruction of lesion of retina and choroid NOS
  ● **14.3　Repair of retinal tear**
      Includes　repair of retinal defect
      Excludes　*repair of retinal detachment (14.41–14.59)*
      ✖ **14.31　Repair of retinal tear by diathermy**
      ✖ **14.32　Repair of retinal tear by cryotherapy**
      14.33　Repair of retinal tear by xenon arc photocoagulation
      14.34　Repair of retinal tear by laser photocoagulation
          Coding Clinic: 1994, Q1, P17
      14.35　Repair of retinal tear by photocoagulation of unspecified type
      ✖ **14.39　Other repair of retinal tear**
  ● **14.4　Repair of retinal detachment with scleral buckling and implant**
      ✖ **14.41　Scleral buckling with implant**
          Coding Clinic: 1996, Q3, P6
      ✖ **14.49　Other scleral buckling**
          Scleral buckling with:
              air tamponade
              resection of sclera
              vitrectomy
          Coding Clinic: 1994, Q1, P16-17
  ● **14.5　Other repair of retinal detachment**
      Includes　that with drainage
      ✖ **14.51　Repair of retinal detachment with diathermy**
      ✖ **14.52　Repair of retinal detachment with cryotherapy**
      ✖ **14.53　Repair of retinal detachment with xenon arc photocoagulation**
      ✖ **14.54　Repair of retinal detachment with laser photocoagulation**
          Coding Clinic: 1987, Nov-Dec, P10
      ✖ **14.55　Repair of retinal detachment with photocoagulation of unspecified type**
      ✖ **14.59　Other**
  ✖ **14.6　Removal of surgically implanted material from posterior segment of eye**

  ● **14.7　Operations on vitreous**
      ✖ **14.71　Removal of vitreous, anterior approach**
          Open sky technique
          Removal of vitreous, anterior approach (with replacement)
      ✖ **14.72　Other removal of vitreous**
          Aspiration of vitreous by posterior sclerotomy
      ✖ **14.73　Mechanical vitrectomy by anterior approach**
          Coding Clinic: 1996, Q3, P4-5
      ✖ **14.74　Other mechanical vitrectomy**
          Posterior approach
          Coding Clinic: 2011, Q4, P106; 2010, Q2, P5; 1996, Q3, P5
      ✖ **14.75　Injection of vitreous substitute**
          Excludes　*that associated with removal (14.71–14.72)*
          Coding Clinic: 1998, Q1, P6; 1996, Q3, P5; 1994, Q1, P17
      ✖ **14.79　Other operations on vitreous**
          Coding Clinic: 1999, Q3, P12; 1999, Q1, P11; 1998, Q1, P6
  ● **14.8　Implantation of epiretinal visual prosthesis**
      14.81　Implantation of epiretinal visual prosthesis
          Note:　Includes lens removal if present, scleral buckling, vitrectomy, epiretinal membrane peeling and pericardial grafting
          Excludes　*implantation of intraocular telescope prosthesis (13.91)*
              other operations on retina, choroid, and posterior chamber (14.9)
              replacement of epiretinal visual prosthesis (14.83)
      14.82　Removal of epiretinal visual prosthesis
          Note:　Includes 360-degree limbal peritomy and vitrectomy if performed, and device extraction
          Excludes　*removal of eye prosthesis (97.31)*
      14.83　Revision or replacement of epiretinal visual prosthesis
          Note:　Includes tack replacement, device relocation, and replacement of pericardial grafting, if needed
          Excludes　*implantation of epiretinal visual prosthesis (14.81)*
  ✖ **14.9　Other operations on retina, choroid, and posterior chamber**
      Coding Clinic: 1996, Q3, P5; 1993, 5th Issue, P13-14

● **15　Operations on extraocular muscles**
  ● **15.0　Diagnostic procedures on extraocular muscles or tendons**
      ✖ **15.01　Biopsy of extraocular muscle or tendon**
      ✖ **15.09　Other diagnostic procedures on extraocular muscles and tendons**
  ● **15.1　Operations on one extraocular muscle involving temporary detachment from globe**
      ✖ **15.11　Recession of one extraocular muscle**
          Coding Clinic: 1996, Q3, P3-4
      ✖ **15.12　Advancement of one extraocular muscle**
      ✖ **15.13　Resection of one extraocular muscle**
          Coding Clinic: 1996, Q3, P4
      ✖ **15.19　Other operations on one extraocular muscle involving temporary detachment from globe**
          Excludes　*transposition of muscle (15.5)*
  ● **15.2　Other operations on one extraocular muscle**
      ✖ **15.21　Lengthening procedure on one extraocular muscle**
      ✖ **15.22　Shortening procedure on one extraocular muscle**
      ✖ **15.29　Other**
  ✖ **15.3　Operations on two or more extraocular muscles involving temporary detachment from globe, one or both eyes**
      Coding Clinic: 1996, Q3, P3-4x2
  ✖ **15.4　Other operations on two or more extraocular muscles, one or both eyes**
  ✖ **15.5　Transposition of extraocular muscles**
      Excludes　*that for correction of ptosis (08.31–08.36)*
  ✖ **15.6　Revision of extraocular muscle surgery**

◀ New　◀▥▥ Revised　~~deleted~~ Deleted　● Use Additional Digit(s)　✖ Valid O.R. Procedure
◆ Non-O.R. Procedure　♀ Females Only　♂ Males Only　OGCR Official Guidelines　**Coding Clinic**

✖ **15.7 Repair of injury of extraocular muscle**
  Freeing of entrapped extraocular muscle
  Lysis of adhesions of extraocular muscle
  Repair of laceration of extraocular muscle, tendon, or
    Tenon's capsule

✖ **15.9 Other operations on extraocular muscles and tendons**

● **16 Operations on orbit and eyeball**
  Excludes *reduction of fracture of orbit (76.78–76.79)*

● **16.0 Orbitotomy**

✖ **16.01 Orbitotomy with bone flap**
  Orbitotomy with lateral approach

✖ **16.02 Orbitotomy with insertion of orbital implant**
  Excludes *that with bone flap (16.01)*

✖ **16.09 Other orbitotomy**

✖ **16.1 Removal of penetrating foreign body from eye, not otherwise specified**
  Excludes *removal of nonpenetrating foreign body (98.21)*

● **16.2 Diagnostic procedures on orbit and eyeball**

✖ **16.21 Ophthalmoscopy**

✖ **16.22 Diagnostic aspiration of orbit**

✖ **16.23 Biopsy of eyeball and orbit**

✖ **16.29 Other diagnostic procedures on orbit and eyeball**
  Excludes *examination of form and structure of eye*
    (95.11–95.16)
    general and subjective eye examination
      (95.01–95.09)
    microscopic examination of specimen from
      eye (90.21–90.29)
    objective functional tests of eye
      (95.21–95.26)
    ocular thermography (88.82)
    tonometry (89.11)
    x-ray of orbit (87.14, 87.16)

● **16.3 Evisceration of eyeball**

✖ **16.31 Removal of ocular contents with synchronous implant into scleral shell**

✖ **16.39 Other evisceration of eyeball**

● **16.4 Enucleation of eyeball**

✖ **16.41 Enucleation of eyeball with synchronous implant into Tenon's capsule with attachment of muscles**
  Integrated implant of eyeball

✖ **16.42 Enucleation of eyeball with other synchronous implant**

✖ **16.49 Other enucleation of eyeball**
  Removal of eyeball NOS

● **16.5 Exenteration of orbital contents**

✖ **16.51 Exenteration of orbit with removal of adjacent structures**
  Radical orbitomaxillectomy

✖ **16.52 Exenteration of orbit with therapeutic removal of orbital bone**

✖ **16.59 Other exenteration of orbit**
  Evisceration of orbit NOS
  Exenteration of orbit with temporalis muscle transplant

● **16.6 Secondary procedures after removal of eyeball**
  Excludes *that with synchronous:*
    enucleation of eyeball (16.41–16.42)
    evisceration of eyeball (16.31)

✖ **16.61 Secondary insertion of ocular implant**

✖ **16.62 Revision and reinsertion of ocular implant**

✖ **16.63 Revision of enucleation socket with graft**

✖ **16.64 Other revision of enucleation socket**

✖ **16.65 Secondary graft to exenteration cavity**

✖ **16.66 Other revision of exenteration cavity**

✖ **16.69 Other secondary procedures after removal of eyeball**

● **16.7 Removal of ocular or orbital implant**

✖ **16.71 Removal of ocular implant**

✖ **16.72 Removal of orbital implant**

● **16.8 Repair of injury of eyeball and orbit**

✖ **16.81 Repair of wound of orbit**
  Excludes *reduction of orbital fracture (76.78–76.79)*
    repair of extraocular muscles (15.7)

✖ **16.82 Repair of rupture of eyeball**
  Repair of multiple structures of eye
  Excludes *repair of laceration of:*
    cornea (11.51–11.59)
    sclera (12.81)

✖ **16.89 Other repair of injury of eyeball or orbit**

● **16.9 Other operations on orbit and eyeball**
  Excludes *irrigation of eye (96.51)*
    prescription and fitting of low vision aids
      (95.31–95.33)
    removal of:
      eye prosthesis NEC (97.31)
      nonpenetrating foreign body from eye without
        incision (98.21)

  16.91 Retrobulbar injection of therapeutic agent
  Excludes *injection of radiographic contrast material*
    (87.14)
    opticociliary injection (12.79)

✖ **16.92 Excision of lesion of orbit**
  Excludes *biopsy of orbit (16.23)*

✖ **16.93 Excision of lesion of eye, unspecified structure**
  Excludes *biopsy of eye NOS (16.23)*

✖ **16.98 Other operations on orbit**

✖ **16.99 Other operations on eyeball**

OPERATIONS ON THE EYE (08–16)

3A. OTHER MISCELLANEOUS DIAGNOSTIC AND THERAPEUTIC PROCEDURES (17)

● **17 Other miscellaneous procedures**

● **17.1 Laparoscopic unilateral repair of inguinal hernia**
  Excludes *other and open unilateral repair of hernia (53.00 – 53.05)*
  Coding Clinic: 2008, Q4, P165-169

✖ **17.11 Laparoscopic repair of direct inguinal hernia with graft or prosthesis**
  Laparoscopic repair of direct and indirect inguinal hernia with graft or prosthesis

✖ **17.12 Laparoscopic repair of indirect inguinal hernia with graft or prosthesis**

✖ **17.13 Laparoscopic repair of inguinal hernia with graft or prosthesis, not otherwise specified**

● **17.2 Laparoscopic bilateral repair of inguinal hernia**
  Excludes *other and open bilateral repair of hernia (53.10 – 53.17)*
  Coding Clinic: 2008, Q4, P165-169

✖ **17.21 Laparoscopic bilateral repair of direct inguinal hernia with graft or prosthesis**

✖ **17.22 Laparoscopic bilateral repair of indirect inguinal hernia with graft or prosthesis**

✖ **17.23 Laparoscopic bilateral repair of inguinal hernia, one direct and one indirect, with graft or prosthesis**

✖ **17.24 Laparoscopic bilateral repair of inguinal hernia with graft or prosthesis, not otherwise specified**

Excludes   Includes   Use additional   Code also   Omit code

● **17.3   Laparoscopic partial excision of large intestine**

> **Excludes**   *other and open partial excision of large intestine (45.71- 45.79)*
>
> Coding Clinic: 2008, Q4, P169-172

✖ **17.31   Laparoscopic multiple segmental resection of large intestine**

✖ **17.32   Laparoscopic cecectomy**

✖ **17.33   Laparoscopic right hemicolectomy**

✖ **17.34   Laparoscopic resection of transverse colon**

✖ **17.35   Laparoscopic left hemicolectomy**

✖ **17.36   Laparoscopic sigmoidectomy**

✖ **17.39   Other laparoscopic partial excision of large intestine**

● **17.4   Robotic assisted procedures**

> Computer assisted robotic surgery
> Computer-enhanced robotic surgery
> Robotic procedure with computer assistance
> Surgeon-controlled robotic surgery
>
> Code first primary procedure
>
> **Excludes**   *computer assisted surgery (00.31-00.35, 00.39)*
>
> **Note:** This category includes use of a computer console with (3-D) imaging, software, camera(s), visualization and instrumentation *combined* with the use of robotic arms, device(s), or system(s) at the time of the procedure.
>
> Coding Clinic: 2008, Q4, P172-174

17.41   Open robotic assisted procedure
> Robotic assistance in open procedure

17.42   Laparoscopic robotic assisted procedure
> Robotic assistance in laparoscopic procedure
> Coding Clinic: 2009, Q3, P6

17.43   Percutaneous robotic assisted procedure
> Robotic assistance in percutaneous procedure

17.44   Endoscopic robotic assisted procedure
> Robotic assistance in endoscopic procedure

17.45   Thoracoscopic robotic assisted procedure
> Robotic assistance in thoracoscopic procedure

17.49   Other and unspecified robotic assisted procedure
> Robotic assistance in other and unspecified procedure
>
> **Excludes**   *endoscopic robotic assisted procedure (17.44)*
> *laparoscopic robotic assisted procedure (17.42)*
> *open robotic assisted procedure (17.41)*
> *percutaneous robotic assisted procedure (17.43)*
> *thoracoscopic robotic assisted procedure (17.45)*

● **17.5   Additional cardiovascular procedures**
> Coding Clinic: 2012, Q3, P13

✖ **17.51   Implantation of rechargeable cardiac contractility modulation [CCM], total system**

> **Note:** Device testing during procedure – *omit code*
> Implantation of CCM system includes formation of pocket, transvenous leads, including placement of leads, placement of catheter into left ventricle, intraoperative procedures for evaluation of lead signals, obtaining sensing threshold measurements, obtaining defibrillator threshold measurements.
>
> **Includes**   implantation of device with removal of existing device
>
> Code also any concomitant:
> coronary bypass (36.10 – 36.19)
> extracorporeal circulation (39.61)
> insertion or replacement of automatic cardioverter/defibrillator, total system [AICD] (37.94)
>
> **Excludes**   *implantation of CCM pulse generator only (17.52)*
>
> Coding Clinic: 2009, Q4, P141

✖ **17.52   Implantation or replacement of cardiac contractility modulation [CCM] rechargeable pulse generator only**

> Implantation of CCM device with removal of any existing CCM device
> **Note:** Device testing during procedure – *omit code*
> Code also any concomitant:
> revision of device pocket (37.79)
> revision of lead [electrode] (37.75)
> MS-DRG: Refer to Part VI, Appendix E, Table 3, Cardioverter-Defibrillator Lead/Generator Reference Table

✖ **17.53   Percutaneous atherectomy of extracranial vessel(s)**

> Directional atherectomy
> Excimer laser atherectomy
> Rotational atherectomy
> That by laser
> That by transluminal extraction
>
> Code also any:
> injection or infusion of thrombolytic agent (99.10)
> number of vascular stents inserted (00.45-00.48)
> number of vessels treated (00.40-00.43)
> percutaneous insertion of carotid artery stent(s) (00.63)
> percutaneous insertion of other extracranial artery stent(s) (00.64)
> procedure on vessel bifurcation (00.44)
>
> **Excludes**   *angioplasty of other non-coronary vessel(s) (39.50)*
> *atherectomy of intracranial vessel(s) (17.54)*
> *atherectomy of other non-coronary vessel(s) (17.56)*
> *removal of cerebrovascular obstruction of vessel(s) by open approach (38.01-38.02, 38.11-38.12, 38.31-38.32, 38.41-38.42)*

✖ **17.54   Percutaneous atherectomy of intracranial vessel(s)**

> Directional atherectomy
> Excimer laser atherectomy
> Rotational atherectomy
> That by laser
> That by transluminal extraction
>
> Code also any:
> injection or infusion of thrombolytic agent (99.10)
> number of vascular stents inserted (00.45-00.48)
> number of vessels treated (00.40-00.43)
> percutaneous insertion of intracranial vascular stent(s) (00.65)
> procedure on vessel bifurcation (00.44)
>
> **Excludes**   *angioplasty of other non-coronary vessel(s) (39.50)*
> *atherectomy of extracranial vessel(s) (17.53)*
> *atherectomy of other non-coronary vessel(s) (17.56)*
> *removal of cerebrovascular obstruction of vessel(s) by open approach (38.01-38.02, 38.11-38.12, 38.31-38.32, 38.41-38.42)*
>
> Coding Clinic: 2011, Q4, P167

✖ **17.55   Transluminal coronary atherectomy**

> Directional atherectomy
> Excimer laser atherectomy
> Rotational atherectomy
> That by laser
> That by percutaneous approach
> That by transluminal extraction
>
> Code also any:
> injection or infusion of thrombolytic agent (99.10)
> insertion of coronary artery stent (36.06-36.07)
> intracoronary artery thrombolytic infusion (36.04)
> number of vascular stents inserted (00.45-00.48)
> number of vessels treated (00.40-00.43)
> procedure on vessel bifurcation (00.44)
> SuperSaturated oxygen therapy (00.49)
> transluminal coronary angioplasty (00.66)
>
> Coding Clinic: 2011, Q4, P168

◀ New   ◀▥ Revised   ~~deleted~~ Deleted   ● Use Additional Digit(s)   ✖ Valid O.R. Procedure
◆ Non-O.R. Procedure   ♀ Females Only   ♂ Males Only   OGCR Official Guidelines   **Coding Clinic**

1214

✳ **17.56** **Atherectomy of other non-coronary vessel(s)**
Percutaneous transluminal atherectomy of:
  lower extremity vessels
  mesenteric artery
  renal artery
  upper extremity vessels

> **Includes**   directional atherectomy
>   excimer laser atherectomy
>   rotational atherectomy
>   that by laser
>   that by transluminal extraction

Code also any:
  injection or infusion of thrombolytic agent (99.10)
  insertion of drug-eluting peripheral vessel stent (00.55)
  insertion of non-drug-eluting peripheral vessel stent(s) or stent graft(s) (39.90)
  number of vascular stents inserted (00.45-00.48)
  number of vessels treated (00.40-00.43)
  procedure on vessel bifurcation (00.44)

> **Excludes**   *percutaneous angioplasty of extracranial or intracranial vessel(s) (00.61-00.62)*
> *percutaneous angioplasty of other non-coronary vessel(s) (39.50)*
> *percutaneous atherectomy of extracranial vessel(s) (17.53)*
> *percutaneous atherectomy of intracranial vessel(s) (17.54)*

● **17.6** **Laser interstitial thermal therapy [LITT] under guidance**
Focused laser interstitial thermal therapy [f-LITT] under MRI guidance
MRI-guided LITT

✳ **17.61** **Laser interstitial thermal therapy [LITT] of lesion or tissue of brain under guidance**
Focused laser interstitial thermal therapy [f-LITT] under MRI guidance
MRI-guided LITT of lesion or tissue of brain

> **Excludes**   *laser interstitial thermal therapy [LITT] of lesion or tissue of head under guidance (17.62)*

Coding Clinic: 2009, Q4, P144

✳ **17.62** **Laser interstitial thermal therapy [LITT] of lesion or tissue of head and neck under guidance**
Focused laser interstitial thermal therapy [f-LITT] under MRI guidance
MRI-guided LITT of lesion or tissue of head and neck

> **Excludes**   *laser interstitial thermal therapy [LITT] of lesion or tissue of brain under guidance (17.61)*

✳ **17.63** **Laser interstitial thermal therapy [LITT] of lesion or tissue of liver under guidance**
Focused laser interstitial thermal therapy [f-LITT] under MRI guidance
MRI-guided LITT of lesion or tissue of liver

✳ **17.69** **Laser interstitial thermal therapy [LITT] of lesion or tissue of other and unspecified site under guidance**
Focused laser interstitial thermal therapy [f-LITT] under MRI guidance
MRI-guided LITT of lesion or tissue of breast
MRI-guided LITT of lesion or tissue of lung
MRI-guided LITT of lesion or tissue of prostate

> **Excludes**   *laser interstitial thermal therapy [LITT] of lesion or tissue of brain under guidance (17.61)*
> *laser interstitial thermal therapy [LITT] of lesion or tissue of head and neck under guidance (17.62)*
> *laser interstitial thermal therapy [LITT] of lesion or tissue of liver under guidance (17.63)*

● **17.7** **Other diagnostic and therapeutic procedures**
17.70 **Intravenous infusion of clofarabine**

> **Excludes**   *injection or infusion of cancer chemotherapeutic substance (99.25)*

17.71 **Non-coronary intra-operative fluorescence vascular angiography [IFVA]**
Intraoperative laser arteriogram
SPY arteriogram
SPY arteriography

> **Excludes**   *intra-operative coronary fluorescence vascular angiography (88.59)*

Coding Clinic: 2010, Q4, P115

● **17.8** **Other adjunct procedures**
Note: These codes are to be used in conjunction with other therapeutic procedure codes to provide additional information on devices used as part of a procedure.

17.81 **Insertion of antimicrobial envelope**
Use of anti-microbial (mesh) (prophylactic antibiotics embedded) envelope with the insertion of cardiovascular implantable electronic devices (CIED)

Code first primary procedure:
insertion of cardiovascular implantable electronic device(s) [CIED] (00.51, 00.53, 00.54, 37.94, 37.96, 37.98)

Coding Clinic: 2011, Q4, P168

(See Plates 92 and 93 on pages 72–73.)
4. OPERATIONS ON THE EAR (18–20)

● **18** **Operations on external ear**

> **Includes**   operations on:
>   external auditory canal
>   skin and cartilage of:
>   auricle
>   meatus

● **18.0** **Incision of external ear**

> **Excludes**   *removal of intraluminal foreign body (98.11)*

18.01 **Piercing of ear lobe**
Piercing of pinna

18.02 **Incision of external auditory canal**

18.09 **Other incision of external ear**

● **18.1** **Diagnostic procedures on external ear**
18.11 **Otoscopy**
18.12 **Biopsy of external ear**
18.19 **Other diagnostic procedures on external ear**

> **Excludes**   *microscopic examination of specimen from ear (90.31–90.39)*

● **18.2** **Excision or destruction of lesion of external ear**
✳ **18.21** **Excision of preauricular sinus**
Radical excision of preauricular sinus or cyst

> **Excludes**   *excision of preauricular remnant [appendage] (18.29)*

18.29 **Excision or destruction of other lesion of external ear**
Cauterization of external ear
Coagulation of external ear
Cryosurgery of external ear
Curettage of external ear
Electrocoagulation of external ear
Enucleation of external ear
Excision of:
  exostosis of external auditory canal
  preauricular remnant [appendage]
Partial excision of ear

> **Excludes**   *biopsy of external ear (18.12)*
> *radical excision of lesion (18.31)*
> *removal of cerumen (96.52)*

Excludes   Includes   Use additional   Code also   Omit code

OTHER MISCELLANEOUS DIAGNOSTIC AND THERAPEUTIC PROCEDURES (17)

● **18.3 Other excision of external ear**
    Excludes *biopsy of external ear (18.12)*
  ✖ **18.31 Radical excision of lesion of external ear**
      Excludes *radical excision of preauricular sinus (18.21)*
  ✖ **18.39 Other**
      Amputation of external ear
      Excludes *excision of lesion (18.21–18.29, 18.31)*

  18.4 Suture of laceration of external ear

✖ **18.5 Surgical correction of prominent ear**
    Ear:
      pinning
      setback

✖ **18.6 Reconstruction of external auditory canal**
    Canaloplasty of external auditory meatus
    Construction [reconstruction] of external meatus of ear:
      osseous portion
      skin-lined portion (with skin graft)

● **18.7 Other plastic repair of external ear**
  ✖ **18.71 Construction of auricle of ear**
      Prosthetic appliance for absent ear
      Reconstruction:
        auricle
        ear
  ✖ **18.72 Reattachment of amputated ear**
  ✖ **18.79 Other plastic repair of external ear**
      Otoplasty NOS
      Postauricular skin graft
      Repair of lop ear
      Coding Clinic: 2003, Q3, P12-13

✖ **18.9 Other operations on external ear**
    Excludes *irrigation of ear (96.52)*
              packing of external auditory canal (96.11)
              removal of:
                cerumen (96.52)
                foreign body (without incision) (98.11)

● **19 Reconstructive operations on middle ear**
● **19.0 Stapes mobilization**
    Division, otosclerotic:
      material
      process
    Remobilization of stapes
    Stapediolysis
    Transcrural stapes mobilization
    Excludes *that with synchronous stapedectomy (19.11–19.19)*

● **19.1 Stapedectomy**
    Excludes *revision of previous stapedectomy (19.21–19.29)*
              stapes mobilization only (19.0)
  ✖ **19.11 Stapedectomy with incus replacement**
      Stapedectomy with incus:
        homograft
        prosthesis
  ✖ **19.19 Other stapedectomy**

● **19.2 Revision of stapedectomy**
  ✖ **19.21 Revision of stapedectomy with incus replacement**
  ✖ **19.29 Other revision of stapedectomy**

✖ **19.3 Other operations on ossicular chain**
    Incudectomy NOS
    Ossiculectomy NOS
    Reconstruction of ossicles, second stage

✖ **19.4 Myringoplasty**
    Epitympanic, type I
    Myringoplasty by:
      cauterization
      graft
    Tympanoplasty (type I)

● **19.5 Other tympanoplasty**
  ✖ **19.52 Type II tympanoplasty**
      Closure of perforation with graft against incus or malleus
  ✖ **19.53 Type III tympanoplasty**
      Graft placed in contact with mobile and intact stapes
      Coding Clinic: 1985, Mar-April, P15
  ✖ **19.54 Type IV tympanoplasty**
      Mobile footplate left exposed with air pocket between round window and graft
  ✖ **19.55 Type V tympanoplasty**
      Fenestra in horizontal semicircular canal covered by graft

✖ **19.6 Revision of tympanoplasty**

✖ **19.9 Other repair of middle ear**
    Closure of mastoid fistula
    Mastoid myoplasty
    Obliteration of tympanomastoid cavity

● **20 Other operations on middle and inner ear**
● **20.0 Myringotomy**
  ✖ **20.01 Myringotomy with insertion of tube**
      Myringostomy
  20.09 Other myringotomy
      Aspiration of middle ear NOS

  20.1 Removal of tympanostomy tube
    Coding Clinic: 1994, Q3, P7; 1987, Nov-Dec, P9

● **20.2 Incision of mastoid and middle ear**
  ✖ **20.21 Incision of mastoid**
  ✖ **20.22 Incision of petrous pyramid air cells**
  ✖ **20.23 Incision of middle ear**
      Atticotomy
      Division of tympanum
      Lysis of adhesions of middle ear
      Excludes *division of otosclerotic process (19.0)*
              stapediolysis (19.0)
              that with stapedectomy (19.11–19.19)

● **20.3 Diagnostic procedures on middle and inner ear**
  20.31 Electrocochleography
  ✖ **20.32 Biopsy of middle and inner ear**
  ✖ **20.39 Other diagnostic procedures on middle and inner ear**
      Excludes *auditory and vestibular function tests (89.13, 95.41–95.49)*
              microscopic examination of specimen from ear (90.31–90.39)

● **20.4 Mastoidectomy**
    Code also any:
      skin graft (18.79)
      tympanoplasty (19.4–19.55)
    Excludes *that with implantation of cochlear prosthetic device (20.96–20.98)*
  ✖ **20.41 Simple mastoidectomy**
  ✖ **20.42 Radical mastoidectomy**
  ✖ **20.49 Other mastoidectomy**
      Atticoantrostomy
      Mastoidectomy:
        NOS
        modified radical

● **20.5 Other excision of middle ear**
    Excludes *that with synchronous mastoidectomy (20.41–20.49)*
  ✖ **20.51 Excision of lesion of middle ear**
      Excludes *biopsy of middle ear (20.32)*
  ✖ **20.59 Other**
      Apicectomy of petrous pyramid
      Tympanectomy

◀ New   ◀▥ Revised   ~~deleted~~ Deleted   ● Use Additional Digit(s)   ✖ Valid O.R. Procedure
◆ Non-O.R. Procedure   ♀ Females Only   ♂ Males Only   OGCR Official Guidelines   **Coding Clinic**

● **20.6** **Fenestration of inner ear**
✖ **20.61** **Fenestration of inner ear (initial)**
Fenestration of:
labyrinth with graft (skin) (vein)
semicircular canals with graft (skin) (vein)
vestibule with graft (skin) (vein)
Excludes *that with tympanoplasty, type V (19.55)*
✖ **20.62** **Revision of fenestration of inner ear**
● **20.7** **Incision, excision, and destruction of inner ear**
✖ **20.71** **Endolymphatic shunt**
✖ **20.72** **Injection into inner ear**
Destruction by injection (alcohol):
inner ear
semicircular canals
vestibule
✖ **20.79** **Other incision, excision, and destruction of inner ear**
Decompression of labyrinth
Drainage of inner ear
Fistulization:
endolymphatic sac
labyrinth
Incision of endolymphatic sac
Labyrinthectomy (transtympanic)
Opening of bony labyrinth
Perilymphatic tap
Excludes *biopsy of inner ear (20.32)*
20.8 **Operations on Eustachian tube**
Catheterization of Eustachian tube
Inflation of Eustachian tube
Injection (Teflon paste) of Eustachian tube
Insufflation (boric acid-salicylic acid)
Intubation of Eustachian tube
Politzerization of Eustachian tube
● **20.9** **Other operations on inner and middle ear**
✖ **20.91** **Tympanosympathectomy**
✖ **20.92** **Revision of mastoidectomy**
Coding Clinic: 1998, Q2, P20

✖ **20.93** **Repair of oval and round windows**
Closure of fistula:
oval window
perilymph
round window
20.94 **Injection of tympanum**
✖ **20.95** **Implantation of electromagnetic hearing device**
Bone conduction hearing device
Excludes *cochlear prosthetic device (20.96–20.98)*
Coding Clinic: 2007, Q3, P5
✖ **20.96** **Implantation or replacement of cochlear prosthetic device, not otherwise specified**
Implantation of receiver (within skull) and insertion of electrode(s) in the cochlea
Includes mastoidectomy
Excludes *electromagnetic hearing device (20.95)*
✖ **20.97** **Implantation or replacement of cochlear prosthetic device, single channel**
Implantation of receiver (within skull) and insertion of electrode in the cochlea
Includes mastoidectomy
Excludes *electromagnetic hearing device (20.95)*
✖ **20.98** **Implantation or replacement of cochlear prosthetic device, multiple channel**
Implantation of receiver (within skull) and insertion of electrodes in the cochlea
Includes mastoidectomy
Excludes *electromagnetic hearing device (20.95)*
✖ **20.99** **Other operations on middle and inner ear**
Attachment of percutaneous abutment (screw) for prosthetic device
Repair or removal of cochlear prosthetic device (receiver) (electrode)
Excludes *adjustment (external components) of cochlear prosthetic device (95.49)*
fitting of hearing aid (95.48)
Coding Clinic: 2007, Q3, P5

(See Plates 49, 57, 58, and 61 on pages 74–77.)

5. **OPERATIONS ON THE NOSE, MOUTH, AND PHARYNX (21–29)**

● **21** **Operations on nose**
Includes operations on:
bone of nose
skin of nose
● **21.0** **Control of epistaxis**
21.00 **Control of epistaxis, not otherwise specified**
21.01 **Control of epistaxis by anterior nasal packing**
21.02 **Control of epistaxis by posterior (and anterior) packing**
Coding Clinic: 1995, Q1, P5
21.03 **Control of epistaxis by cauterization (and packing)**
✖ **21.04** **Control of epistaxis by ligation of ethmoidal arteries**
✖ **21.05** **Control of epistaxis by (transantral) ligation of the maxillary artery**
✖ **21.06** **Control of epistaxis by ligation of the external carotid artery**
✖ **21.07** **Control of epistaxis by excision of nasal mucosa and skin grafting of septum and lateral nasal wall**
✖ **21.09** **Control of epistaxis by other means**
Coding Clinic: 1995, Q1, P5
21.1 **Incision of nose**
Chondrotomy
Incision of skin of nose
Nasal septotomy

● **21.2** **Diagnostic procedures on nose**
21.21 **Rhinoscopy**
21.22 **Biopsy of nose**
21.29 **Other diagnostic procedures on nose**
Excludes *microscopic examination of specimen from nose (90.31–90.39)*
nasal:
function study (89.12)
x-ray (87.16)
rhinomanometry (89.12)
● **21.3** **Local excision or destruction of lesion of nose**
Excludes *biopsy of nose (21.22)*
nasal fistulectomy (21.82)
21.30 **Excision or destruction of lesion of nose, not otherwise specified**
21.31 **Local excision or destruction of intranasal lesion**
Nasal polypectomy
21.32 **Local excision or destruction of other lesion of nose**
Coding Clinic: 1989, Q2, P16
✖ **21.4** **Resection of nose**
Amputation of nose
✖ **21.5** **Submucous resection of nasal septum**
● **21.6** **Turbinectomy**
✖ **21.61** **Turbinectomy by diathermy or cryosurgery**
✖ **21.62** **Fracture of the turbinates**
✖ **21.69** **Other turbinectomy**
Excludes *turbinectomy associated with sinusectomy (22.31–22.39, 22.42, 22.60–22.64)*

Excludes   Includes   Use additional   Code also   Omit code

● **21.7　Reduction of nasal fracture**
　　　21.71　Closed reduction of nasal fracture
　　�876 **21.72　Open reduction of nasal fracture**
● **21.8　Repair and plastic operations on the nose**
　　　21.81　Suture of laceration of nose
　　�876 **21.82　Closure of nasal fistula**
　　　　　Nasolabial fistulectomy
　　　　　Nasopharyngeal fistulectomy
　　　　　Oronasal fistulectomy
　　�876 **21.83　Total nasal reconstruction**
　　　　　Reconstruction of nose with:
　　　　　　arm flap
　　　　　　forehead flap
　　�876 **21.84　Revision rhinoplasty**
　　　　　Rhinoseptoplasty
　　　　　Twisted nose rhinoplasty
　　�876 **21.85　Augmentation rhinoplasty**
　　　　　Augmentation rhinoplasty with:
　　　　　　graft
　　　　　　synthetic implant
　　�876 **21.86　Limited rhinoplasty**
　　　　　Plastic repair of nasolabial flaps
　　　　　Tip rhinoplasty
　　�876 **21.87　Other rhinoplasty**
　　　　　Rhinoplasty NOS
　　�876 **21.88　Other septoplasty**
　　　　　Crushing of nasal septum
　　　　　Repair of septal perforation
　　　　　Excludes　*septoplasty associated with submucous*
　　　　　　　　　　　resection of septum (21.5)
　　�876 **21.89　Other repair and plastic operations on nose**
　　　　　Reattachment of amputated nose
● **21.9　Other operations on nose**
　　　21.91　Lysis of adhesions of nose
　　　　　Posterior nasal scrub
　　�876 **21.99　Other**
　　　　　Excludes　*dilation of frontonasal duct (96.21)*
　　　　　　　　　　　irrigation of nasal passages (96.53)
　　　　　　　　　　　removal of:
　　　　　　　　　　　　intraluminal foreign body without
　　　　　　　　　　　　　incision (98.12)
　　　　　　　　　　　　nasal packing (97.32)
　　　　　　　　　　　replacement of nasal packing (97.21)

● **22　Operations on nasal sinuses**
　● **22.0　Aspiration and lavage of nasal sinus**
　　　22.00　Aspiration and lavage of nasal sinus, not otherwise specified
　　　22.01　Puncture of nasal sinus for aspiration or lavage
　　　22.02　Aspiration or lavage of nasal sinus through natural ostium
　● **22.1　Diagnostic procedures on nasal sinus**
　　　22.11　Closed [endoscopic] [needle] biopsy of nasal sinus
　　�876 **22.12　Open biopsy of nasal sinus**
　　　22.19　Other diagnostic procedures on nasal sinuses
　　　　　Endoscopy without biopsy
　　　　　Excludes　*transillumination of sinus (89.35)*
　　　　　　　　　　　x-ray of sinus (87.15–87.16)
　　　22.2　Intranasal antrotomy
　　　　　Excludes　*antrotomy with external approach (22.31–22.39)*
　● **22.3　External maxillary antrotomy**
　　�876 **22.31　Radical maxillary antrotomy**
　　　　　Removal of lining membrane of maxillary sinus
　　　　　　using Caldwell-Luc approach
　　�876 **22.39　Other external maxillary antrotomy**
　　　　　Exploration of maxillary antrum with Caldwell-Luc
　　　　　　approach

● **22.4　Frontal sinusotomy and sinusectomy**
　　�876 **22.41　Frontal sinusotomy**
　　�876 **22.42　Frontal sinusectomy**
　　　　　Excision of lesion of frontal sinus
　　　　　Obliteration of frontal sinus (with fat)
　　　　　Excludes　*biopsy of nasal sinus (22.11–22.12)*
● **22.5　Other nasal sinusotomy**
　　�876 **22.50　Sinusotomy, not otherwise specified**
　　�876 **22.51　Ethmoidotomy**
　　�876 **22.52　Sphenoidotomy**
　　�876 **22.53　Incision of multiple nasal sinuses**
● **22.6　Other nasal sinusectomy**
　　　　　Includes　that with incidental turbinectomy
　　　　　Excludes　*biopsy of nasal sinus (22.11–22.12)*
　　�876 **22.60　Sinusectomy, not otherwise specified**
　　�876 **22.61　Excision of lesion of maxillary sinus with Caldwell-Luc approach**
　　�876 **22.62　Excision of lesion of maxillary sinus with other approach**
　　�876 **22.63　Ethmoidectomy**
　　�876 **22.64　Sphenoidectomy**
● **22.7　Repair of nasal sinus**
　　�876 **22.71　Closure of nasal sinus fistula**
　　　　　Repair of oro-antral fistula
　　�876 **22.79　Other repair of nasal sinus**
　　　　　Reconstruction of frontonasal duct
　　　　　Repair of bone of accessory sinus
　　�876 **22.9　Other operations on nasal sinuses**
　　　　　Exteriorization of maxillary sinus
　　　　　Fistulization of sinus
　　　　　Excludes　*dilation of frontonasal duct (96.21)*

● **23　Removal and restoration of teeth**
　● **23.0　Forceps extraction of tooth**
　　　23.01　Extraction of deciduous tooth
　　　23.09　Extraction of other tooth
　　　　　Extraction of tooth NOS
　● **23.1　Surgical removal of tooth**
　　　23.11　Removal of residual root
　　　23.19　Other surgical extraction of tooth
　　　　　Odontectomy NOS
　　　　　Removal of impacted tooth
　　　　　Tooth extraction with elevation of mucoperiosteal
　　　　　　flap
　　　23.2　Restoration of tooth by filling
　　　23.3　Restoration of tooth by inlay
　● **23.4　Other dental restoration**
　　　23.41　Application of crown
　　　23.42　Insertion of fixed bridge
　　　23.43　Insertion of removable bridge
　　　23.49　Other
　　　23.5　Implantation of tooth
　　　23.6　Prosthetic dental implant
　　　　　Endosseous dental implant
　● **23.7　Apicoectomy and root canal therapy**
　　　23.70　Root canal, not otherwise specified
　　　23.71　Root canal therapy with irrigation
　　　23.72　Root canal therapy with apicoectomy
　　　23.73　Apicoectomy

◀ New　　◀▥ Revised　　~~deleted~~ Deleted　　● Use Additional Digit(s)　　�876 Valid O.R. Procedure
◆ Non-O.R. Procedure　　♀ Females Only　　♂ Males Only　　**OGCR** Official Guidelines　　**Coding Clinic**

● **24 Other operations on teeth, gums, and alveoli**

24.0 Incision of gum or alveolar bone
Apical alveolotomy

● **24.1 Diagnostic procedures on teeth, gums, and alveoli**

24.11 Biopsy of gum

24.12 Biopsy of alveolus

24.19 Other diagnostic procedures on teeth, gums, and alveoli

Excludes *dental:*
examination (89.31)
x-ray:
full-mouth (87.11)
other (87.12)
microscopic examination of dental specimen
(90.81–90.89)

✳ **24.2 Gingivoplasty**
Gingivoplasty with bone or soft tissue graft

● **24.3 Other operations on gum**

24.31 Excision of lesion or tissue of gum

Excludes *biopsy of gum (24.11)*
excision of odontogenic lesion (24.4)

24.32 Suture of laceration of gum

24.39 Other

✳ **24.4 Excision of dental lesion of jaw**
Excision of odontogenic lesion

✳ **24.5 Alveoloplasty**
Alveolectomy (interradicular) (intraseptal) (radical)
(simple) (with graft or implant)

Excludes *biopsy of alveolus (24.12)*
en bloc resection of alveolar process and palate
(27.32)

24.6 Exposure of tooth

24.7 Application of orthodontic appliance
Application, insertion, or fitting of:
arch bars
orthodontic obturator
orthodontic wiring
periodontal splint

Excludes *nonorthodontic dental wiring (93.55)*

24.8 Other orthodontic operation
Closure of diastema (alveolar) (dental)
Occlusal adjustment
Removal of arch bars
Repair of dental arch

Excludes *removal of nonorthodontic wiring (97.33)*

● **24.9 Other dental operations**

24.91 Extension or deepening of buccolabial or lingual sulcus

24.99 Other

Excludes *dental:*
debridement (96.54)
examination (89.31)
prophylaxis (96.54)
scaling and polishing (96.54)
wiring (93.55)
fitting of dental appliance [denture] (99.97)
microscopic examination of dental specimen
(90.81–90.89)
removal of dental:
packing (97.34)
prosthesis (97.35)
wiring (97.33)
replacement of dental packing (97.22)

● **25 Operations on tongue**

● **25.0 Diagnostic procedures on tongue**

25.01 Closed [needle] biopsy of tongue

✳ **25.02 Open biopsy of tongue**
Wedge biopsy

25.09 Other diagnostic procedures on tongue

✳ **25.1 Excision or destruction of lesion or tissue of tongue**

Excludes *biopsy of tongue (25.01–25.02)*
frenumectomy:
labial (27.41)
lingual (25.92)

Coding Clinic: 2002, Q2, P5-6

✳ **25.2 Partial glossectomy**

✳ **25.3 Complete glossectomy**
Glossectomy NOS
Code also any neck dissection (40.40–40.42)

✳ **25.4 Radical glossectomy**
Code also any:
neck dissection (40.40–40.42)
tracheostomy (31.1–31.29)

● **25.5 Repair of tongue and glossoplasty**

25.51 Suture of laceration of tongue

✳ **25.59 Other repair and plastic operations on tongue**
Fascial sling of tongue
Fusion of tongue (to lip)
Graft of mucosa or skin to tongue

Excludes *lysis of adhesions of tongue (25.93)*

Coding Clinic: 1997, Q1, P5

● **25.9 Other operations on tongue**

25.91 Lingual frenotomy

Excludes *labial frenotomy (27.91)*

25.92 Lingual frenectomy

Excludes *labial frenectomy (27.41)*

25.93 Lysis of adhesions of tongue

✳ **25.94 Other glossotomy**

✳ **25.99 Other**

● **26 Operations on salivary glands and ducts**

Includes operations on:
lesser salivary gland and duct
parotid gland and duct
sublingual gland and duct
submaxillary gland and duct

Code also any neck dissection (40.40–40.42)

26.0 Incision of salivary gland or duct

● **26.1 Diagnostic procedures on salivary glands and ducts**

26.11 Closed [needle] biopsy of salivary gland or duct

✳ **26.12 Open biopsy of salivary gland or duct**

26.19 Other diagnostic procedures on salivary glands and ducts

Excludes *x-ray of salivary gland (87.09)*

● **26.2 Excision of lesion of salivary gland**

✳ **26.21 Marsupialization of salivary gland cyst**

✳ **26.29 Other excision of salivary gland lesion**

Excludes *biopsy of salivary gland (26.11–26.12)*
salivary fistulectomy (26.42)

● **26.3 Sialoadenectomy**

✳ **26.30 Sialoadenectomy, not otherwise specified**

✳ **26.31 Partial sialoadenectomy**

✳ **26.32 Complete sialoadenectomy**
En bloc excision of salivary gland lesion
Radical sialoadenectomy

● **26.4 Repair of salivary gland or duct**

✳ **26.41 Suture of laceration of salivary gland**

✳ **26.42 Closure of salivary fistula**

✳ **26.49 Other repair and plastic operations on salivary gland or duct**
Fistulization of salivary gland
Plastic repair of salivary gland or duct NOS
Transplantation of salivary duct opening

● **26.9 Other operations on salivary gland or duct**

26.91 Probing of salivary duct

✳ **26.99 Other**

OPERATIONS ON THE NOSE, MOUTH, AND PHARYNX (21–29)

Excludes   Includes   Use additional   Code also   Omit code

OPERATIONS ON THE NOSE, MOUTH, AND PHARYNX (21–29)

● 27   Other operations on mouth and face
   Includes   operations on:
                 lips
                 palate
                 soft tissue of face and mouth, except tongue and
                      gingiva
   Excludes   operations on:
                 gingiva (24.0–24.99)
                 tongue (25.01–25.99)

✖ 27.0   **Drainage of face and floor of mouth**
         Drainage of:
              facial region (abscess)
              fascial compartment of face
              Ludwig's angina
         Excludes   drainage of thyroglossal tract (06.09)

✖ 27.1   **Incision of palate**

● 27.2   **Diagnostic procedures on oral cavity**
   ✖ 27.21   **Biopsy of bony palate**
   ✖ 27.22   **Biopsy of uvula and soft palate**
      27.23   **Biopsy of lip**
      27.24   **Biopsy of mouth, unspecified structure**
      27.29   **Other diagnostic procedures on oral cavity**
            Excludes   soft tissue x-ray (87.09)

● 27.3   **Excision of lesion or tissue of bony palate**
   ✖ 27.31   **Local excision or destruction of lesion or tissue of
             bony palate**
            Local excision or destruction of palate by:
                 cautery
                 chemotherapy
                 cryotherapy
            Excludes   biopsy of bony palate (27.21)
   ✖ 27.32   **Wide excision or destruction of lesion or tissue of
             bony palate**
            En bloc resection of alveolar process and palate

● 27.4   **Excision of other parts of mouth**
      27.41   **Labial frenectomy**
            Excludes   division of labial frenum (27.91)
   ✖ 27.42   **Wide excision of lesion of lip**
   ✖ 27.43   **Other excision of lesion or tissue of lip**
   ✖ 27.49   **Other excision of mouth**
            Excludes   biopsy of mouth NOS (27.24)
                         excision of lesion of:
                              palate (27.31–27.32)
                              tongue (25.1)
                              uvula (27.72)
                         fistulectomy of mouth (27.53)
                         frenectomy of:
                              lip (27.41)
                              tongue (25.92)
            Coding Clinic: 2005, Q2, P8-9

● 27.5   **Plastic repair of lip and mouth**
            Excludes   palatoplasty (27.61–27.69)
      27.51   **Suture of laceration of lip**
      27.52   **Suture of laceration of other part of mouth**
   ✖ 27.53   **Closure of fistula of mouth**
            Excludes   fistulectomy:
                              nasolabial (21.82)
                              oro-antral (22.71)
                              oronasal (21.82)
   ✖ 27.54   **Repair of cleft lip**
   ✖ 27.55   **Full-thickness skin graft to lip and mouth**
   ✖ 27.56   **Other skin graft to lip and mouth**
   ✖ 27.57   **Attachment of pedicle or flap graft to lip and mouth**
   ✖ 27.59   **Other plastic repair of mouth**

● 27.6   **Palatoplasty**
   ✖ 27.61   **Suture of laceration of palate**
   ✖ 27.62   **Correction of cleft palate**
            Correction of cleft palate by push-back operation
            Excludes   revision of cleft palate repair (27.63)
   ✖ 27.63   **Revision of cleft palate repair**
            Secondary:
                 attachment of pharyngeal flap
                 lengthening of palate
            Coding Clinic: 1996, Q1, P14
      27.64   **Insertion of palatal implant**
            Coding Clinic: 2004, Q4, P117-118
   ✖ 27.69   **Other plastic repair of palate**
            Code also any insertion of palatal implant (27.64)
            Excludes   fistulectomy of mouth (27.53)
            Coding Clinic: 1999, Q3, P22; 1997, Q1, P5; 1985, Mar-April, P12

● 27.7   **Operations on uvula**
   ✖ 27.71   **Incision of uvula**
   ✖ 27.72   **Excision of uvula**
            Excludes   biopsy of uvula (27.22)
   ✖ 27.73   **Repair of uvula**
            Excludes   that with synchronous cleft palate repair
                              (27.62)
                         uranostaphylorrhaphy (27.62)
   ✖ 27.79   **Other operations on uvula**
            Coding Clinic: 1992, Q3, P18; 1985, Mar-April, P12

● 27.9   **Other operations on mouth and face**
      27.91   **Labial frenotomy**
            Division of labial frenum
            Excludes   lingual frenotomy (25.91)
   ✖ 27.92   **Incision of mouth, unspecified structure**
            Excludes   incision of:
                              gum (24.0)
                              palate (27.1)
                              salivary gland or duct (26.0)
                              tongue (25.94)
                              uvula (27.71)
   ✖ 27.99   **Other operations on oral cavity**
            Graft of buccal sulcus
            Excludes   removal of:
                              intraluminal foreign body (98.01)
                              penetrating foreign body from mouth
                                   without incision (98.22)

● 28   **Operations on tonsils and adenoids**
   ✖ 28.0   **Incision and drainage of tonsil and peritonsillar structures**
            Drainage (oral) (transcervical) of:
                 parapharyngeal abscess
                 peritonsillar abscess
                 retropharyngeal abscess
                 tonsillar abscess
● 28.1   **Diagnostic procedures on tonsils and adenoids**
   ✖ 28.11   **Biopsy of tonsils and adenoids**
   ✖ 28.19   **Other diagnostic procedures on tonsils and adenoids**
            Excludes   soft tissue x-ray (87.09)
✖ 28.2   **Tonsillectomy without adenoidectomy**
            Coding Clinic: 1997, Q1, P5; 1990, Q2, P23
✖ 28.3   **Tonsillectomy with adenoidectomy**
            Coding Clinic: 2005, Q2, P16
✖ 28.4   **Excision of tonsil tag**
✖ 28.5   **Excision of lingual tonsil**
✖ 28.6   **Adenoidectomy without tonsillectomy**
            Excision of adenoid tag
✖ 28.7   **Control of hemorrhage after tonsillectomy and
         adenoidectomy**
            Coding Clinic: 2005, Q2, P16

◀ New   ◀▥ Revised   ~~deleted~~ Deleted   ● Use Additional Digit(s)   ✖ Valid O.R. Procedure
◆ Non-O.R. Procedure   ♀ Females Only   ♂ Males Only   OGCR Official Guidelines   **Coding Clinic**

● 28.9 Other operations on tonsils and adenoids
   ✖ 28.91 Removal of foreign body from tonsil and adenoid by incision
      Excludes *that without incision (98.13)*
   ✖ 28.92 Excision of lesion of tonsil and adenoid
      Excludes *biopsy of tonsil and adenoid (28.11)*
   ✖ 28.99 Other
      Coding Clinic: 1990, Q2, P23

● 29 Operations on pharynx
   Includes operations on:
      hypopharynx
      nasopharynx
      oropharynx
      pharyngeal pouch
      pyriform sinus
 ✖ 29.0 Pharyngotomy
   Drainage of pharyngeal bursa
   Excludes *incision and drainage of retropharyngeal abscess (28.0)*
      removal of foreign body (without incision) (98.13)
● 29.1 Diagnostic procedures on pharynx
   29.11 Pharyngoscopy
   29.12 Pharyngeal biopsy
      Biopsy of supraglottic mass
   29.19 Other diagnostic procedures on pharynx
      Excludes *x-ray of nasopharynx:*
        contrast (87.06)
        other (87.09)
 ✖ 29.2 Excision of branchial cleft cyst or vestige
   Excludes *branchial cleft fistulectomy (29.52)*

● 29.3 Excision or destruction of lesion or tissue of pharynx
   ✖ 29.31 Cricopharyngeal myotomy
      Excludes *that with pharyngeal diverticulectomy (29.32)*
   ✖ 29.32 Pharyngeal diverticulectomy
   ✖ 29.33 Pharyngectomy (partial)
      Excludes *laryngopharyngectomy (30.3)*
   ✖ 29.39 Other excision or destruction of lesion or tissue of pharynx
 ✖ 29.4 Plastic operation on pharynx
   Correction of nasopharyngeal atresia
   Excludes *pharyngoplasty associated with cleft palate repair (27.62–27.63)*
   Coding Clinic: 1999, Q3, P22; 1997, Q1, P5; 1992, Q3, P18; 1985, Mar-April, P12
● 29.5 Other repair of pharynx
   ✖ 29.51 Suture of laceration of pharynx
   ✖ 29.52 Closure of branchial cleft fistula
   ✖ 29.53 Closure of other fistula of pharynx
      Pharyngoesophageal fistulectomy
   ✖ 29.54 Lysis of pharyngeal adhesions
   ✖ 29.59 Other
● 29.9 Other operations on pharynx
   29.91 Dilation of pharynx
      Dilation of nasopharynx
   ✖ 29.92 Division of glossopharyngeal nerve
   ✖ 29.99 Other
      Excludes *insertion of radium into pharynx and nasopharynx (92.27)*
        removal of intraluminal foreign body (98.13)

6. OPERATIONS ON THE RESPIRATORY SYSTEM (30–34)

● 30 Excision of larynx
 ● 30.0 Excision or destruction of lesion or tissue of larynx
   ✖ 30.01 Marsupialization of laryngeal cyst
   ✖ 30.09 Other excision or destruction of lesion or tissue of larynx
      Stripping of vocal cords
      Excludes *biopsy of larynx (31.43)*
        laryngeal fistulectomy (31.62)
        laryngotracheal fistulectomy (31.62)
 ✖ 30.1 Hemilaryngectomy
 ● 30.2 Other partial laryngectomy
   ✖ 30.21 Epiglottidectomy
   ✖ 30.22 Vocal cordectomy
      Excision of vocal cords
   ✖ 30.29 Other partial laryngectomy
      Excision of laryngeal cartilage
 ✖ 30.3 Complete laryngectomy
   Block dissection of larynx (with thyroidectomy) (with synchronous tracheostomy)
   Laryngopharyngectomy
   Excludes *that with radical neck dissection (30.4)*
   Coding Clinic: 2012, Q1, P9-10
 ✖ 30.4 Radical laryngectomy
   Complete [total] laryngectomy with radical neck dissection (with thyroidectomy) (with synchronous tracheostomy)
   Coding Clinic: 2012, Q1, P9-10

● 31 Other operations on larynx and trachea
 31.0 Injection of larynx
   Injection of inert material into larynx or vocal cords
 31.1 Temporary tracheostomy
   Temporary percutaneous dilatational tracheostomy [PDT]
   Tracheotomy for assistance in breathing
   Code also any synchronous bronchoscopy, if performed (33.21–33.24, 33.27)
   ◆ Non-OR Procedure that affects MS-DRG assignment to MS-DRG 003-004, 011-013
   Coding Clinic: 2013, Q1, P19; 1997, Q1, P6
 ● 31.2 Permanent tracheostomy
   ✖ 31.21 Mediastinal tracheostomy
   ✖ 31.29 Other permanent tracheostomy
      Permanent percutaneous dilatational tracheostomy [PDT]
      Excludes *that with laryngectomy (30.3–30.4)*
      Code also any synchronous bronchoscopy, if performed (33.21–33.24, 33.27)
      Coding Clinic: 2013, Q1, P19; 2012, Q4, P84; 2005, Q2, P8-9; 2002, Q2, P6
 ✖ 31.3 Other incision of larynx or trachea
   Excludes *that for assistance in breathing (31.1–31.29)*
 ● 31.4 Diagnostic procedures on larynx and trachea
   31.41 Tracheoscopy through artificial stoma
      Excludes *that with biopsy (31.43–31.44)*
   31.42 Laryngoscopy and other tracheoscopy
      Excludes *that with biopsy (31.43–31.44)*
   31.43 Closed [endoscopic] biopsy of larynx
   31.44 Closed [endoscopic] biopsy of trachea
   ✖ 31.45 Open biopsy of larynx or trachea

OPERATIONS ON THE NOSE, MOUTH, AND PHARYNX (21–29)

Excludes   Includes   Use additional   Code also   Omit code

31.48　**Other diagnostic procedures on larynx**

> **Excludes** *contrast laryngogram (87.07)*
> *microscopic examination of specimen from larynx (90.31–90.39)*
> *soft tissue x-ray of larynx NEC (87.09)*

31.49　**Other diagnostic procedures on trachea**

> **Excludes** *microscopic examination of specimen from trachea (90.41–90.49)*
> *x-ray of trachea (87.49)*

✖ 31.5　**Local excision or destruction of lesion or tissue of trachea**

> **Excludes** *biopsy of trachea (31.44–31.45)*
> *laryngotracheal fistulectomy (31.62)*
> *tracheoesophageal fistulectomy (31.73)*

● 31.6　**Repair of larynx**

✖ 31.61　**Suture of laceration of larynx**

✖ 31.62　**Closure of fistula of larynx**
　　　　Laryngotracheal fistulectomy
　　　　Take-down of laryngostomy

✖ 31.63　**Revision of laryngostomy**

✖ 31.64　**Repair of laryngeal fracture**

✖ 31.69　**Other repair of larynx**
　　　　Arytenoidopexy
　　　　Graft of larynx
　　　　Transposition of vocal cords

> **Excludes** *construction of artificial larynx (31.75)*

● 31.7　**Repair and plastic operations on trachea**

✖ 31.71　**Suture of laceration of trachea**

✖ 31.72　**Closure of external fistula of trachea**
　　　　Closure of tracheotomy

✖ 31.73　**Closure of other fistula of trachea**
　　　　Tracheoesophageal fistulectomy

> **Excludes** *laryngotracheal fistulectomy (31.62)*

✖ 31.74　**Revision of tracheostomy**

✖ 31.75　**Reconstruction of trachea and construction of artificial larynx**
　　　　Tracheoplasty with artificial larynx

✖ 31.79　**Other repair and plastic operations on trachea**

● 31.9　**Other operations on larynx and trachea**

✖ 31.91　**Division of laryngeal nerve**

✖ 31.92　**Lysis of adhesions of trachea or larynx**

31.93　**Replacement of laryngeal or tracheal stent**

31.94　**Injection of locally-acting therapeutic substance into trachea**

31.95　**Tracheoesophageal fistulization**

✖ 31.98　**Other operations on larynx**
　　　　Dilation of larynx
　　　　Division of congenital web of larynx
　　　　Removal of keel or stent of larynx

> **Excludes** *removal of intraluminal foreign body from larynx without incision (98.14)*

✖ 31.99　**Other operations on trachea**

> **Excludes** *removal of:*
> *intraluminal foreign body from trachea without incision (98.15)*
> *tracheostomy tube (97.37)*
> *replacement of tracheostomy tube (97.23)*
> *tracheostomy toilette (96.55)*
> **Coding Clinic: 2010, Q3, P6**

● 32　**Excision of lung and bronchus**

> **Includes** rib resection as operative approach
> sternotomy as operative approach
> sternum-splitting incision as operative approach
> thoracotomy as operative approach

Code also any synchronous bronchoplasty (33.48)
Coding Clinic: 1988, Q4, P11

● 32.0　**Local excision or destruction of lesion or tissue of bronchus**

> **Excludes** *biopsy of bronchus (33.24–33.25)*
> *bronchial fistulectomy (33.42)*

32.01　**Endoscopic excision or destruction of lesion or tissue of bronchus**

✖ 32.09　**Other local excision or destruction of lesion or tissue of bronchus**

> **Excludes** *that by endoscopic approach (32.01)*

✖ 32.1　**Other excision of bronchus**
　　　Resection (wide sleeve) of bronchus

> **Excludes** *radical dissection [excision] of bronchus (32.6)*

● 32.2　**Local excision or destruction of lesion or tissue of lung**
Coding Clinic: 2006, Q4, P124-126

✖ 32.20　**Thoracoscopic excision of lesion or tissue of lung**
　　　　Thoracoscopic wedge resection
　　　　Coding Clinic: 2007, Q4, P109-113

✖ 32.21　**Plication of emphysematous bleb**

✖ 32.22　**Lung volume reduction surgery**
　　　　MCE: Limited coverage
　　　　Coding Clinic: 1997, Q1, P6; 1995, Q4, P64

✖ 32.23　**Open ablation of lung lesion or tissue**

✖ 32.24　**Percutaneous ablation of lung lesion or tissue**

✖ 32.25　**Thoracoscopic ablation of lung lesion or tissue**

> **Excludes** *thoracoscopic excision of lesion or tissue of lung (32.20)*

✖ 32.26　**Other and unspecified ablation of lung lesion or tissue**

> **Excludes** *bronchoscopic bronchial thermoplasty, ablation of smooth airway muscle (32.27)*

✖ 32.27　**Bronchoscopic bronchial thermoplasty, ablation of airway smooth muscle**

32.28　**Endoscopic excision or destruction of lesion or tissue of lung**

> **Excludes** *ablation of lung lesion or tissue:*
> *open (32.23)*
> *other (32.26)*
> *percutaneous (32.24)*
> *thoracoscopic (32.25)*
> *biopsy of lung (33.26–33.27)*

✖ 32.29　**Other local excision or destruction of lesion or tissue of lung**
　　　　Resection of lung:
　　　　　NOS
　　　　　wedge

> **Excludes** *ablation of lung lesion or tissue:*
> *open (32.23)*
> *other (32.26)*
> *percutaneous (32.24)*
> *thoracoscopic (32.25)*
> *biopsy of lung (33.26–33.27)*
> *laser interstitial thermal therapy [LITT] of lesion or tissue of lung under guidance (17.69)*
> *that by endoscopic approach (32.28)*
> *thoracoscopic excision of lesion or tissue of lung (32.20)*
> *wide excision of lesion of lung (32.3)*
> **Coding Clinic: 1999, Q3, P3-4**

◀ New　◀▥ Revised　~~deleted~~ Deleted　● Use Additional Digit(s)　✖ Valid O.R. Procedure
◆ Non-O.R. Procedure　♀ Females Only　♂ Males Only　OGCR Official Guidelines　Coding Clinic

1222

● **32.3 Segmental resection of lung**
  Partial lobectomy

  ✶ **32.30 Thoracoscopic segmental resection of lung**
    Coding Clinic: 2007, Q4, P109-113

  ✶ **32.39 Other and unspecified segmental resection of lung**
    Excludes *thoracoscopic segmental resection of lung (32.30)*

● **32.4 Lobectomy of lung**
  Lobectomy with segmental resection of adjacent lobes of lung

    Excludes *that with radical dissection [excision] of thoracic structures (32.6)*

  ✶ **32.41 Thoracoscopic lobectomy of lung**
    Coding Clinic: 2007, Q4, P109-113

  ✶ **32.49 Other lobectomy of lung**
    Excludes *thoracoscopic lobectomy of lung (32.41)*

● **32.5 Pneumonectomy**
  Excision of lung NOS
  Pneumonectomy (with mediastinal dissection)
  Coding Clinic: 1999, Q1, P6

  ✶ **32.50 Thoracoscopic pneumonectomy**
    Coding Clinic: 2007, Q4, P109-113

  ✶ **32.59 Other and unspecified pneumonectomy**
    Excludes *thoracoscopic pneumonectomy (32.50)*

✶ **32.6 Radical dissection of thoracic structures**
  Block [en bloc] dissection of bronchus, lobe of lung, brachial plexus, intercostal structure, ribs (transverse process), and sympathetic nerves

✶ **32.9 Other excision of lung**
    Excludes *biopsy of lung and bronchus (33.24–33.27)*
    pulmonary decortication (34.51)

● **33 Other operations on lung and bronchus**
    Includes rib resection as operative approach
    sternotomy as operative approach
    sternum-splitting incision as operative approach
    thoracotomy as operative approach

✶ **33.0 Incision of bronchus**

✶ **33.1 Incision of lung**
    Excludes *puncture of lung (33.93)*

● **33.2 Diagnostic procedures on lung and bronchus**

  ✶ **33.20 Thoracoscopic lung biopsy**
    Excludes *closed endoscopic biopsy of lung (33.27)*
    closed [percutaneous] [needle] biopsy of lung (33.26)
    open biopsy of lung (33.28)
    Coding Clinic: 2007, Q4, P109-113

  33.21 Bronchoscopy through artificial stoma
    Excludes *that with biopsy (33.24, 33.27)*

  33.22 Fiber-optic bronchoscopy
    Excludes *that with biopsy (33.24, 33.27)*
    Coding Clinic: 2004, Q1, P4-5; 1986, Sept-Oct, P11

  33.23 Other bronchoscopy
    Excludes *that for:*
    aspiration (96.05)
    biopsy (33.24, 33.27)
    Coding Clinic: 2002, Q3, P18; 1999, Q1, P6

  33.24 Closed [endoscopic] biopsy of bronchus
    Bronchoscopy (fiberoptic) (rigid) with:
      brush biopsy of "lung"
      brushing or washing for specimen collection
      excision (bite) biopsy
    Diagnostic bronchoalveolar lavage (BAL)
    Mini-bronchoalveolar lavage [mini-BAL]
    Transbronchoscopic needle aspiration [TBNA] of bronchus
    Excludes *closed biopsy of lung, other than brush biopsy of "lung" (33.26, 33.27)*
    whole lung lavage (33.99)
    Coding Clinic: 2011, Q3, P7-9; 2009, Q2, P8, 16; 2006, Q2, P20; 2004, Q3, P9; 2002, Q3, P16-17; 1991, Q3, P15; Q2, P15

✶ **33.25 Open biopsy of bronchus**
    Excludes *open biopsy of lung (33.28)*

  33.26 Closed [percutaneous] [needle] biopsy of lung
    Fine needle aspiration (FNA) of lung
    Transthoracic needle biopsy of lung (TTNB)
    Excludes *endoscopic biopsy of lung (33.27)*
    thoracoscopic lung biopsy (33.20)
    Coding Clinic: 1992, Q3, P12-13

  ✶ **33.27 Closed endoscopic biopsy of lung**
    Fiber-optic (flexible) bronchoscopy with fluoroscopic guidance with biopsy
    Transbronchial lung biopsy
    Transbronchoscopic needle aspiration [TBNA] of lung
    Excludes *brush biopsy of "lung" (33.24)*
    percutaneous biopsy of lung (33.26)
    thoracoscopic lung biopsy (33.20)
    Coding Clinic: 2011, Q3, P7-9; Q1, P18; 2009, Q2, P8, 16; 2004, Q3, P9; 2002, Q3, P16-17; 1991, Q3, P15; 1986, Sept-Oct, P11

  ✶ **33.28 Open biopsy of lung**
    Coding Clinic: 1999, Q3, P3-4; 1992, Q3, P12-13

  ✶ **33.29 Other diagnostic procedures on lung and bronchus**
    Excludes *bronchoalveolar lavage [BAL] (33.24)*
    contrast bronchogram:
      endotracheal (87.31)
      other (87.32)
    endoscopic pulmonary airway flow measurement (33.72)
    lung scan (92.15)
    magnetic resonance imaging (88.92)
    microscopic examination of specimen from bronchus or lung (90.41–90.49)
    routine chest x-ray (87.44)
    ultrasonography of lung (88.73)
    vital capacity determination (89.37)
    x-ray of bronchus or lung NOS (87.49)

● **33.3 Surgical collapse of lung**

  33.31 Destruction of phrenic nerve for collapse of lung

  33.32 Artificial pneumothorax for collapse of lung
    Thoracotomy for collapse of lung

  33.33 Pneumoperitoneum for collapse of lung

  ✶ **33.34 Thoracoplasty**

  ✶ **33.39 Other surgical collapse of lung**
    Collapse of lung NOS

● **33.4 Repair and plastic operation on lung and bronchus**

  ✶ **33.41 Suture of laceration of bronchus**

  ✶ **33.42 Closure of bronchial fistula**
    Closure of bronchostomy
    Fistulectomy:
      bronchocutaneous
      bronchoesophageal
      bronchovisceral
    Excludes *closure of fistula:*
      bronchomediastinal (34.73)
      bronchopleural (34.73)
      bronchopleuromediastinal (34.73)

  ✶ **33.43 Closure of laceration of lung**

  ✶ **33.48 Other repair and plastic operations on bronchus**

  ✶ **33.49 Other repair and plastic operations on lung**
    Excludes *closure of pleural fistula (34.73)*

OPERATIONS ON THE RESPIRATORY SYSTEM (30–34)

● **33.5 Lung transplant**
  Note: To report donor source - *see* codes 00.91–00.93
  Excludes *combined heart-lung transplantation (33.6)*

  Code also cardiopulmonary bypass [extracorporeal circulation] [heart-lung machine] (39.61)

✖ **33.50 Lung transplantation, not otherwise specified**
  MCE: Limited coverage

✖ **33.51 Unilateral lung transplantation**
  MCE: Limited coverage

✖ **33.52 Bilateral lung transplantation**
  Double-lung transplantation
  En bloc transplantation
    Code also cardiopulmonary bypass [extracorporeal circulation] [heart-lung machine] (39.61)
  MCE: Limited coverage

✖ **33.6 Combined heart-lung transplantation**
  Note: To report donor source - *see* codes 00.91–00.93
  Code also cardiopulmonary bypass [extracorporeal circulation] [heart-lung machine] (39.61)
  MCE: Limited coverage

● **33.7 Other endoscopic procedures in bronchus or lung**
  Excludes *insertion of tracheobronchial stent (96.05)*
  Coding Clinic: 2006, Q4, P126-127

  33.71 Endoscopic insertion or replacement of bronchial valve(s), single lobe
  Endobronchial airflow redirection valve
  Intrabronchial airflow redirection valve
    Excludes *endoscopic insertion or replacement of bronchial valve(s), multiple lobes (33.73)*
  Coding Clinic: 2008, Q4, P174-175

  33.72 Endoscopic pulmonary airway flow measurement
  Assessment of pulmonary airway flow
    Code also any diagnostic or therapeutic procedure if performed
  Coding Clinic: 2008, Q4, P174-175

  33.73 Endoscopic insertion or replacement of bronchial valve(s), multiple lobes
  Endobronchial airflow redirection valve
  Intrabronchial airflow redirection valve
    Excludes *endoscopic insertion or replacement of bronchial valve(s), single lobe (33.71)*

  33.78 Endoscopic removal of bronchial device(s) or substances

  33.79 Endoscopic insertion of other bronchial device or substances
  Biologic Lung Volume Reduction NOS (BLVR)

● **33.9 Other operations on lung and bronchus**
  33.91 Bronchial dilation
  Coding Clinic: 1997, Q1, P14

✖ **33.92 Ligation of bronchus**

✖ **33.93 Puncture of lung**
    Excludes *needle biopsy (33.26)*

✖ **33.98 Other operations on bronchus**
    Excludes *bronchial lavage (96.56)*
    removal of intraluminal foreign body from bronchus without incision (98.15)

✖ **33.99 Other operations on lung**
  Whole lung lavage
    Excludes *other continuous mechanical ventilation (96.70–96.72)*
    respiratory therapy (93.90–93.99)
  Coding Clinic: 2002, Q3, P17

● **34 Operations on chest wall, pleura, mediastinum, and diaphragm**
  Excludes *operations on breast (85.0–85.99)*
● **34.0 Incision of chest wall and pleura**
  Excludes *that as operative approach — omit code*

  34.01 Incision of chest wall
  Extrapleural drainage
    Excludes *incision of pleura (34.09)*
  Coding Clinic: 2000, Q3, P12; 1992, Q1, P13

✖ **34.02 Exploratory thoracotomy**

✖ **34.03 Reopening of recent thoracotomy site**

  34.04 Insertion of intercostal catheter for drainage
  Chest tube
  Closed chest drainage
  Revision of intercostal catheter (chest tube) (with lysis of adhesions)
    Excludes *thoracoscopic drainage of pleural cavity (34.06)*
  Coding Clinic: 2007, Q1, P14; 2003, Q2, P7-8; 1999, Q2, P12-13; Q1, P10; 1995, Q1, P5-6; 1992, Q1, P12

  34.05 Creation of pleuroperitoneal shunt

✖ **34.06 Thoracoscopic drainage of pleural cavity**
  Evacuation of empyema
  Coding Clinic: 2007, Q4, P109-113

  34.09 Other incision of pleura
  Creation of pleural window for drainage
  Intercostal stab
  Open chest drainage
    Excludes *thoracoscopy (34.21)*
    thoracotomy for collapse of lung (33.32)
  Coding Clinic: 2002, Q3, P22-23x2; 1994, Q1, P8

✖ **34.1 Incision of mediastinum**
  Excludes *mediastinoscopy (34.22)*
  mediastinotomy associated with pneumonectomy (32.5)

  Code also any biopsy, if performed

● **34.2 Diagnostic procedures on chest wall, pleura, mediastinum, and diaphragm**

✖ **34.20 Thoracoscopic pleural biopsy**
  Coding Clinic: 2007, Q4, P109-113

✖ **34.21 Transpleural thoracoscopy**
  Coding Clinic: 2002, Q3, P27

✖ **34.22 Mediastinoscopy**
  Code also any biopsy, if performed

  34.23 Biopsy of chest wall

  34.24 Other pleural biopsy
    Excludes *thoracoscopic pleural biopsy (34.20)*
  Coding Clinic: 2002, Q3, P22-23, 27

  34.25 Closed [percutaneous] [needle] biopsy of mediastinum

✖ **34.26 Open mediastinal biopsy**

✖ **34.27 Biopsy of diaphragm**

✖ **34.28 Other diagnostic procedures on chest wall, pleura, and diaphragm**
    Excludes *angiocardiography (88.50–88.58)*
    aortography (88.42)
    arteriography of:
      intrathoracic vessels NEC (88.44)
      pulmonary arteries (88.43)
    microscopic examination of specimen from chest wall, pleura, and diaphragm (90.41–90.49)
    phlebography of:
      intrathoracic vessels NEC (88.63)
      pulmonary veins (88.62)
    radiological examinations of thorax:
      C.A.T. scan (87.41)
      diaphragmatic x-ray (87.49)
      intrathoracic lymphangiogram (87.34)
      routine chest x-ray (87.44)
      sinogram of chest wall (87.38)
      soft tissue x-ray of chest wall NEC (87.39)
      tomogram of thorax NEC (87.42)
      ultrasonography of thorax 88.73)

◄ New ◄|||| Revised ~~deleted~~ Deleted ● Use Additional Digit(s) ✖ Valid O.R. Procedure
◆ Non-O.R. Procedure ♀ Females Only ♂ Males Only OGCR Official Guidelines Coding Clinic

� **34.29** **Other diagnostic procedures on mediastinum**

     Excludes *mediastinal:*
                pneumogram (87.33)
                x-ray NEC (87.49)

✻ **34.3** **Excision or destruction of lesion or tissue of mediastinum**

     Excludes *biopsy of mediastinum (34.25–34.26)*
                mediastinal fistulectomy (34.73)

✻ **34.4** **Excision or destruction of lesion of chest wall**

Excision of lesion of chest wall NOS (with excision of ribs)

     Excludes *biopsy of chest wall (34.23)*
                costectomy not incidental to thoracic procedure
                   (77.91)
                excision of lesion of:
                   breast (85.20–85.25)
                   cartilage (80.89)
                   skin (86.2–86.3)
                fistulectomy (34.73)

● **34.5** **Pleurectomy**

  ✻ **34.51** **Decortication of lung**

       Excludes *thoracoscopic decortication of lung (34.52)*

  ✻ **34.52** **Thoracoscopic decortication of lung**

       Coding Clinic: 2007, Q4, P109-113

  ✻ **34.59** **Other excision of pleura**

       Excision of pleural lesion

       Excludes *biopsy of pleura (34.24)*
                    pleural fistulectomy (34.73)

✻ **34.6** **Scarification of pleura**

Pleurosclerosis

     Excludes *injection of sclerosing agent (34.92)*

     Coding Clinic: 2012, Q3, P24; 1992, Q1, P12

● **34.7** **Repair of chest wall**

   34.71 **Suture of laceration of chest wall**

       Excludes *suture of skin and subcutaneous tissue alone*
                   (86.59)

   34.72 **Closure of thoracostomy**

  ✻ **34.73** **Closure of other fistula of thorax**

       Closure of:
          bronchopleural fistula
          bronchopleurocutaneous fistula
          bronchopleuromediastinal fistula

✻ **34.74** **Repair of pectus deformity**

     Repair of:
        pectus carinatum (with implant)
        pectus excavatum (with implant)
     Coding Clinic: 2004, Q2, P6-7

✻ **34.79** **Other repair of chest wall**

     Repair of chest wall NOS
     Coding Clinic: 2004, Q2, P6; 1987, Jan-Feb, P13

● **34.8** **Operations on diaphragm**

  ✻ **34.81** **Excision of lesion or tissue of diaphragm**

       Excludes *biopsy of diaphragm (34.27)*

  ✻ **34.82** **Suture of laceration of diaphragm**

  ✻ **34.83** **Closure of fistula of diaphragm**

       Thoracicoabdominal fistulectomy
       Thoracicogastric fistulectomy
       Thoracicointestinal fistulectomy

  ✻ **34.84** **Other repair of diaphragm**

       Excludes *repair of diaphragmatic hernia (53.7–53.82)*

  ✻ **34.85** **Implantation of diaphragmatic pacemaker**

  ✻ **34.89** **Other operations on diaphragm**

● **34.9** **Other operations on thorax**

   34.91 **Thoracentesis**

       Coding Clinic: 2012, Q4, P83

   34.92 **Injection into thoracic cavity**

       Chemical pleurodesis
       Injection of cytotoxic agent or tetracycline
       Instillation into thoracic cavity
       Requires additional code for any cancer
          chemotherapeutic substance (99.25)

       Excludes *that for collapse of lung (33.32)*

       Coding Clinic: 2012, Q3, P24; 2007, Q4, P109-113; Q1, P14; 1992,
                  Q1, P12; 1989, Q2, P17

  ✻ **34.93** **Repair of pleura**

  ✻ **34.99** **Other**

       Excludes *removal of:*
                   mediastinal drain (97.42)
                   sutures (97.43)
                   thoracotomy tube (97.41)

       Coding Clinic: 2000, Q1, P17; 1988, Q1, P9

(See Plates 141, 218, 219, 473, 500, 501, 502, 544, and 545 on pages 61–66 and 78–80.)

7.   OPERATIONS ON THE CARDIOVASCULAR SYSTEM (35–39)

● **35** **Operations on valves and septa of heart**

   Includes sternotomy (median) (transverse) as operative
                  approach
                thoracotomy as operative approach

   Code also any cardiopulmonary bypass [extracorporeal
       circulation] [heart-lung machine] (39.61)

● **35.0** **Closed heart valvotomy or transcatheter replacement of heart valve**

     Excludes *percutaneous (balloon) valvuloplasty (35.96)*

  ✻ **35.00** **Closed heart valvotomy, unspecified valve**

  ✻ **35.01** **Closed heart valvotomy, aortic valve**

  ✻ **35.02** **Closed heart valvotomy, mitral valve**

  ✻ **35.03** **Closed heart valvotomy, pulmonary valve**

  ✻ **35.04** **Closed heart valvotomy, tricuspid valve**

  ✻ **35.05** **Endovascular replacement of aortic valve**

       Note: Includes that with any balloon valvuloplasty;
          do not code separately
       Implantation of transcatheter aortic valve
       Replacement of aortic valve with tissue graft
          (autograft) (bioprosthetic) (heterograft)
          (homograft):
          transarterial approach
          transfemoral approach
       TAVI (transcatheter aortic valve implantation)
       TAVR (transcatheter aortic valve replacement)

       Excludes *open and other replacement of heart valve*
                   (35.20-35.28)

  ✻ **35.06** **Transapical replacement of aortic valve**

       Note: Includes that with any balloon valvuloplasty;
          do not code separately
       Implantation of transcatheter aortic valve
       Replacement of aortic valve with tissue graft
          (autograft) (bioprosthetic) (heterograft)
          (homograft):
          intercostal approach
          transventricular approach
       That via transthoracic exposure, i.e. thoracotomy,
          sternotomy, or subxiphoid approach

       Excludes *open and other replacement of heart valve*
                   (35.20-35.28)

Excludes   Includes   Use additional   Code also   Omit code

✖ **35.07** **Endovascular replacement of pulmonary valve**
Note: Includes that with any balloon valvuloplasty; do not code separately
Implantation of transcatheter pulmonary valve
PPVI (percutaneous pulmonary valve implantation)
Replacement of pulmonary valve:
transfemoral approach
transvenous approach
That within previously created right ventricle-to pulmonary artery conduit
TPVI (transcatheter pulmonary valve implantation)
Excludes   *open and other replacement of heart valve (35.20-35.28)*

✖ **35.08** **Transapical replacement of pulmonary valve**
Note: Includes that with any balloon valvuloplasty; do not code separately
Implantation of transcatheter pulmonary valve
Replacement of pulmonary valve:
intercostal approach
transventricular approach
That via transthoracic exposure, i.e. thoracotomy, sternotomy, or subxiphoid approach
Excludes   *open and other replacement of heart valve (35.20-35.28)*

✖ **35.09** **Endovascular replacement of unspecified heart valve**
Note: Includes that with any balloon valvuloplasty; do not code separately
Replacement of valve via:
intercostal approach
transventricular approach
Excludes   *open and other replacement of heart valve (35.20-35.28)*

● **35.1** **Open heart valvuloplasty without replacement**
Includes   open heart valvotomy
Excludes   *that associated with repair of:*
endocardial cushion defect (35.54, 35.63, 35.73)
percutaneous (balloon) valvuloplasty (35.96)
valvular defect associated with atrial and ventricular septal defects (35.54, 35.63, 35.73)
Code also cardiopulmonary bypass if performed [extracorporeal circulation] [heart-lung machine] (39.61)
Coding Clinic: 2008, Q2, P13

✖ **35.10** **Open heart valvuloplasty without replacement, unspecified valve**

✖ **35.11** **Open heart valvuloplasty of aortic valve without replacement**

✖ **35.12** **Open heart valvuloplasty of mitral valve without replacement**
Coding Clinic: 2010, Q3, P7; Q1, P7; 1997, Q1, P13; 1988, Q1, P10

✖ **35.13** **Open heart valvuloplasty of pulmonary valve without replacement**

✖ **35.14** **Open heart valvuloplasty of tricuspid valve without replacement**

● **35.2** **Open and other replacement of heart valve**
Includes   excision of heart valve with replacement
Code also cardiopulmonary bypass [extracorporeal circulation] [heart-lung machine] (39.61)
Excludes   *that associated with repair of:*
endocardial cushion defect (35.54, 35.63, 35.73)
valvular defect associated with atrial and ventricular septal defects (35.54, 35.63, 35.73)
transapical replacement of heart valve (35.06, 35.08)
transcatheter replacement of heart valve (35.05, 35.07)

✖ **35.20** **Open and other replacement of unspecified heart valve**
That with tissue graft or prosthetic implant
Excludes   *endovascular replacement of unspecified heart valve (35.09)*

✖ **35.21** **Open and other replacement of aortic valve with tissue graft**
Includes   that by:
autograft
heterograft
homograft
Excludes   *endovascular replacement of aortic valve (35.05)*
transapical replacement of aortic valve (35.06)
Coding Clinic: 1997, Q2, P8

✖ **35.22** **Open and other replacement of aortic valve**
Replacement of aortic valve, NOS
That with prosthetic (partial) (synthetic) (total)
Excludes   *endovascular replacement of aortic valve (35.05)*
transapical replacement of aortic valve (35.06)
Coding Clinic: 2011, Q4, P152; 2008, Q4, P177-180; 1996, Q1, P11

✖ **35.23** **Open and other replacement of mitral valve with tissue graft**
Includes   that by:
autograft
heterograft
homograft

✖ **35.24** **Open and other replacement of mitral valve**
Replacement of mitral valve, NOS
That with prosthetic (partial) (synthetic) (total)
Excludes   *percutaneous repair with implant or leaflet clip (35.97)*
Coding Clinic: 2009, Q3, P19; 1997, Q4, P54-55

✖ **35.25** **Open and other replacement of pulmonary valve with tissue graft**
Includes   that by:
autograft
heterograft
homograft
Excludes   *endovascular replacement of pulmonary valve (35.07)*
transapical replacement of pulmonary valve (35.08)
Coding Clinic: 2011, Q1, P24; 2007, Q1, P14-15; 2004, Q1, P16-17; 1997, Q2, P8

✖ **35.26** **Open and other replacement of pulmonary valve**
Replacement of pulmonary valve, NOS
That with prosthetic (partial) (synthetic) (total)
Excludes   *endovascular replacement of pulmonary valve (35.07)*
transapical replacement of pulmonary valve (35.08)

✖ **35.27** **Open and other replacement of tricuspid valve with tissue graft**
Includes   that by:
autograft
heterograft
homograft

✖ **35.28** **Open and other replacement of tricuspid valve**
Replacement of tricuspid valve, NOS
That with prosthetic (partial) (synthetic) (total)

● **35.3** **Operations on structures adjacent to heart valves**
Code also cardiopulmonary bypass [extracorporeal circulation] [heart-lung machine] (39.61)

✖ **35.31** **Operations on papillary muscle**
Division of papillary muscle
Reattachment of papillary muscle
Repair of papillary muscle

✖ **35.32** **Operations on chordae tendineae**
Division of chordae tendineae
Repair of chordae tendineae

✖ **35.33** **Annuloplasty**
Plication of annulus
Coding Clinic: 1997, Q1, P13; 1988, Q1, P10

✷ **35.34 Infundibulectomy**
    Right ventricular infundibulectomy

✷ **35.35 Operations on trabeculae carneae cordis**
    Division of trabeculae carneae cordis
    Excision of trabeculae carneae cordis
    Excision of aortic subvalvular ring

✷ **35.39 Operations on other structures adjacent to valves of heart**
    Repair of sinus of Valsalva (aneurysm)

● **35.4 Production of septal defect in heart**

  35.41 Enlargement of existing atrial septal defect
    Rashkind procedure
    Septostomy (atrial) (balloon)

✷ **35.42 Creation of septal defect in heart**
    Blalock-Hanlon operation

● **35.5 Repair of atrial and ventricular septa with prosthesis**

> **Includes** repair of septa with synthetic implant or patch

Code also cardiopulmonary bypass [extracorporeal circulation] [heart-lung machine] (39.61)

✷ **35.50 Repair of unspecified septal defect of heart with prosthesis**

> **Excludes** *that associated with repair of:*
> *endocardial cushion defect (35.54)*
> *septal defect associated with valvular defect (35.54)*

✷ **35.51 Repair of atrial septal defect with prosthesis, open technique**
    Atrioseptoplasty with prosthesis
    Correction of atrial septal defect with prosthesis
    Repair:
      foramen ovale (patent)
      with prosthesis ostium secundum defect with prosthesis

> **Excludes** *that associated with repair of:*
> *atrial septal defect associated with valvular and ventricular septal defects (35.54)*
> *endocardial cushion defect (35.54)*

✷ **35.52 Repair of atrial septal defect with prosthesis, closed technique**
    Insertion of atrial septal umbrella [King-Mills]
    Coding Clinic: 2005, Q2, 17-18; 1998, Q3, P11

✷ **35.53 Repair of ventricular septal defect with prosthesis, open technique**
    Correction of ventricular septal defect with prosthesis
    Repair of supracristal defect with prosthesis

> **Excludes** *that associated with repair of:*
> *endocardial cushion defect (35.54)*
> *ventricular defect associated with valvular and atrial septal defects (35.54)*

    Coding Clinic: 2007, Q1, P14-15

✷ **35.54 Repair of endocardial cushion defect with prosthesis**
    Repair:
      atrioventricular canal with prosthesis (grafted to septa)
      ostium primum defect with prosthesis (grafted to septa)
      valvular defect associated with atrial and ventricular septal defects with prosthesis (grafted to septa)

> **Excludes** *repair of isolated:*
> *atrial septal defect (35.51–35.52)*
> *valvular defect (35.20, 35.22, 35.24, 35.26, 35.28)*
> *ventricular septal defect (35.53)*

✷ **35.55 Repair of ventricular septal defect with prosthesis, closed technique**

● **35.6 Repair of atrial and ventricular septa with tissue graft**

Code also cardiopulmonary bypass [extracorporeal circulation] [heart-lung machine] (39.61)

✷ **35.60 Repair of unspecified septal defect of heart with tissue graft**

> **Excludes** *that associated with repair of:*
> *endocardial cushion defect (35.63)*
> *septal defect associated with valvular defect (35.63)*

✷ **35.61 Repair of atrial septal defect with tissue graft**
    Atrioseptoplasty with tissue graft
    Correction of atrial septal defect with tissue graft
    Repair:
      foramen ovale (patent) with tissue graft
      ostium secundum defect with tissue graft

> **Excludes** *that associated with repair of:*
> *atrial septal defect associated with valvular and ventricular septal defects (35.63)*
> *endocardial cushion defect (35.63)*

✷ **35.62 Repair of ventricular septal defect with tissue graft**
    Correction of ventricular septal defect with tissue graft
    Repair of supracristal defect with tissue graft

> **Excludes** *that associated with repair of:*
> *endocardial cushion defect (35.63)*
> *ventricular defect associate with valvular and atrial septal defects (35.63)*

✷ **35.63 Repair of endocardial cushion defect with tissue graft**
    Repair of:
      atrioventricular canal with tissue graft
      ostium primum defect with tissue graft
      valvular defect associated with atrial and ventricular septal defects with tissue graft

> **Excludes** *repair of isolated:*
> *atrial septal defect (35.61)*
> *valvular defect (35.20–35.21, 35.23, 35.25, 35.27)*
> *ventricular septal defect (35.62)*

● **35.7 Other and unspecified repair of atrial and ventricular septa**

Code also cardiopulmonary bypass [extracorporeal circulation] [heart-lung machine] (39.61)

✷ **35.70 Other and unspecified repair of unspecified septal defect of heart**
    Repair of septal defect NOS

> **Excludes** *that associated with repair of:*
> *endocardial cushion defect (35.73)*
> *septal defect associated with valvular defect (35.73)*

✷ **35.71 Other and unspecified repair of atrial septal defect**
    Repair NOS:
      atrial septum
      foramen ovale (patent)
      ostium secundum defect

> **Excludes** *that associated with repair of:*
> *atrial septal defect associated with valvular ventricular septal defects (35.73)*
> *endocardial cushion defect (35.73)*

✷ **35.72 Other and unspecified repair of ventricular septal defect**
    Repair NOS:
      supracristal defect
      ventricular septum

> **Excludes** *that associated with repair of:*
> *endocardial cushion defect (35.73)*
> *ventricular septal defect associated with valvular and atrial septal defects (35.73)*

OPERATIONS ON THE CARDIOVASCULAR SYSTEM (35-39)

Excludes   Includes   Use additional   Code also   Omit code

✖ **35.73** **Other and unspecified repair of endocardial cushion defect**
Repair NOS:
atrioventricular canal
ostium primum defect
valvular defect associated with atrial and ventricular septal defects

> **Excludes** *repair of isolated:*
> *atrial septal defect (35.71)*
> *valvular defect (35.20, 35.22, 35.24,*
> *35.26, 35.28)*
> *ventricular septal defect (35.72)*

● **35.8** **Total repair of certain congenital cardiac anomalies**
Note: For partial repair of defect [e.g. repair of atrial septal defect in tetralogy of Fallot] — *code to specific procedure*

✖ **35.81** **Total repair of tetralogy of Fallot**
One-stage total correction of tetralogy of Fallot with or without:
commissurotomy of pulmonary valve
infundibulectomy
outflow tract prosthesis
patch graft of outflow tract
prosthetic tube for pulmonary artery
repair of ventricular septal defect (with prosthesis)
take-down of previous systemic-pulmonary artery anastomosis

✖ **35.82** **Total repair of total anomalous pulmonary venous connection**
One-stage total correction of total anomalous pulmonary venous connection with or without:
anastomosis between (horizontal) common pulmonary trunk and posterior wall of left atrium (side-to-side)
enlargement of foramen ovale
incision [excision] of common wall between posterior left atrium and coronary sinus and roofing of resultant defect with patch graft (synthetic)
ligation of venous connection (descending anomalous vein) (to left innominate vein) (to superior vena cava)
repair of atrial septal defect (with prosthesis)

✖ **35.83** **Total repair of truncus arteriosus**
One-stage total correction of truncus arteriosus with or without:
construction (with aortic homograft) (with prosthesis) of a pulmonary artery placed from right ventricle to arteries supplying the lung
ligation of connections between aorta and pulmonary artery
repair of ventricular septal defect (with prosthesis)

✖ **35.84** **Total correction of transposition of great vessels, not elsewhere classified**
Arterial switch operation [Jatene]
Total correction of transposition of great arteries at the arterial level by switching the great arteries, including the left or both coronary arteries, implanted in the wall of the pulmonary artery

> **Excludes** *baffle operation [Mustard] [Senning] (35.91)*
> *creation of shunt between right ventricle and pulmonary artery [Rastelli] (35.92)*

● **35.9** **Other operations on valves and septa of heart**
Code also cardiopulmonary bypass, if performed [extracorporeal circulation] [heart-lung machine] (39.61)

✖ **35.91** **Interatrial transposition of venous return**
Baffle:
atrial
interatrial
Mustard's operation
Resection of atrial septum and insertion of patch to direct systemic venous return to tricuspid valve and pulmonary venous return to mitral valve

✖ **35.92** **Creation of conduit between right ventricle and pulmonary artery**
Creation of shunt between right ventricle and (distal) pulmonary artery

> **Excludes** *that associated with total repair of truncus arteriosus (35.83)*

Coding Clinic: 2007, Q1, P14-15

✖ **35.93** **Creation of conduit between left ventricle and aorta**
Creation of apicoaortic shunt
Shunt between apex of left ventricle and aorta
Coding Clinic: 2009, Q2, P8

✖ **35.94** **Creation of conduit between atrium and pulmonary artery**
Fontan procedure

✖ **35.95** **Revision of corrective procedure on heart**
Replacement of prosthetic heart valve poppet
Resuture of prosthesis of:
septum
valve

> **Excludes** *complete revision — code to specific procedure*
> *replacement of prosthesis or graft of:*
> *septum (35.50–35.63)*
> *valve (35.20–35.28)*

✖ **35.96** **Percutaneous balloon valvuloplasty**
Balloon dilation of valve

> **Excludes** *endovascular replacement of heart valve (35.05, 35.07)*
> *mitral valve repair with implant (35.97)*
> *transapical replacement of heart valve (35.06, 35.08)*

Coding Clinic: 2011, Q1, P24; 2010, Q3, P16; 2009, Q3, P19x3; 2004, Q3, P10

✖ **35.97** **Percutaneous mitral valve repair with implant**
Endovascular mitral valve repair
Implantation of mitral valve leaflet clip
Transcatheter mitral valve repair

> Code also any transesophageal echocardiography [TEE] (88.72)

> **Excludes** *percutaneous balloon valvuloplasty (35.96)*

Coding Clinic: 2010, Q4, P117

✖ **35.98** **Other operations on septa of heart**
Coding Clinic: 2007, Q1, P11-12

✖ **35.99** **Other operations on valves of heart**
Coding Clinic: 2009, Q3, P19

◀ New ◀▥ Revised ~~deleted~~ Deleted ● Use Additional Digit(s) ✖ Valid O.R. Procedure
◆ Non-O.R. Procedure ♀ Females Only ♂ Males Only OGCR Official Guidelines Coding Clinic

● **36 Operations on vessels of heart**

Includes sternotomy (median) (transverse) as operative approach
thoracotomy as operative approach

Code also any:
cardiopulmonary bypass, if performed [extracorporeal circulation] [heart-lung machine] (39.61)
injection or infusion of platelet inhibitor (99.20)
injection or infusion of thrombolytic agent (99.10)
Coding Clinic: 1990, Q2, P23-24; 1985, July-Aug, P8-9

● **36.0 Removal of coronary artery obstruction and insertion of stent(s)**
Coding Clinic: 1994, Q2, P14; 1993, 5th Issue, P3

✖ **36.03 Open chest coronary artery angioplasty**
Coronary (artery):
endarterectomy (with patch graft)
thromboendarterectomy (with patch graft)
Open surgery for direct relief of coronary artery obstruction

Excludes *that with coronary artery bypass graft (36.10–36.19)*

Code also any:
insertion of drug-eluting coronary stent(s) (36.07)
insertion of non-drug-eluting coronary stent(s) (36.06)
number of vascular stents inserted (00.45–00.48)
number of vessels treated (00.40–00.03)
procedure on vessel bifurcation (00.44)
Coding Clinic: 1994, Q1, P6; 1993, Q3, P7-8

36.04 Intracoronary artery thrombolytic infusion
That by direct coronary artery injection, infusion, or catheterization
Enzyme infusion
Platelet inhibitor

Excludes *infusion of platelet inhibitor (99.20)*
infusion of thrombolytic agent (99.10)
that associated with any procedure in 36.03
Coding Clinic: 2002, Q3, P20

36.06 Insertion of non-drug-eluting coronary artery stent(s)
Bare stent(s)
Bonded stent(s)
Drug-coated stent(s), i.e. heparin coated
Endograft(s)
Endovascular graft(s)
Stent grafts

Code also any:
number of vascular stents inserted (00.45– 00.48)
number of vessels treated (00.40–00.43)
open chest coronary artery angioplasty (36.03)
percutaneous transluminal coronary angioplasty [PTCA] (00.66)
procedure on vessel bifurcation (00.44)
transluminal coronary atherectomy (17.55)

Excludes *insertion of drug-eluting coronary artery stent(s) (36.07)*

◆Non-OR Procedure that affects MS-DRG assignment to MDC 05, MS-DRG 248-249
Coding Clinic: 2011, Q4, P167; 2009, Q2, P12; 2005, Q4, P69-72; 2001, Q2, P24; 2001, Q1, P9-10; 2000, Q1, P11-12; 1999, Q1, P17-18

36.07 Insertion of drug-eluting coronary artery stent(s)
Endograft(s)
Endovascular graft(s)
Stent graft(s)

Code also any:
number of vascular stents inserted (00.45– 00.48)
number of vessels treated (00.40–00.43)
open chest coronary artery angioplasty (36.03)
percutaneous transluminal coronary angioplasty [PTCA] (00.66)
procedure on vessel bifurcation (00.44)
transluminal coronary atherectomy (17.55)

Excludes *drug-coated stents, e.g., heparin coated (36.06)*
insertion of non-drug-eluting coronary artery stent(s) (36.06)

◆Non-OR Procedure that affects MS-DRG assignment to MDC 05, MS-DRG 246-247
Coding Clinic: 2012, Q3, P5; 2005, Q4, P103-106; 2002, Q4, P101-103

✖ **36.09 Other removal of coronary artery obstruction**
Coronary angioplasty NOS

Code also any:
number of vascular stents inserted (00.45–00.48)
number of vessels treated (00.40–00.43)
procedure on vessel bifurcation (00.44)

Excludes *that by open angioplasty (36.03)*
that by percutaneous transluminal coronary angioplasty [PTCA] (00.66)
transluminal coronary atherectomy (17.55)
Coding Clinic: 1990, Q2, P23

● **36.1 Bypass anastomosis for heart revascularization**
Note: Do not assign codes from series 00.40–00.43 with codes from series 36.10–36.19

Code also
cardiopulmonary bypass [extracorporeal circulation] [heart-lung machine] (39.61)
pressurized treatment of venous bypass graft [conduit] with pharmaceutical substance, if performed (00.16)
Coding Clinic: 2002, Q3, P3-91; 1993, Q3, P7-8; 1990, Q2, P24

✖ **36.10 Aortocoronary bypass for heart revascularization, not otherwise specified** 🔖
Direct revascularization:
cardiac with catheter stent, prosthesis, or vein graft
coronary with catheter stent, prosthesis, or vein graft
heart muscle with catheter stent, prosthesis, or vein graft
myocardial with catheter stent, prosthesis, or vein graft
Heart revascularization NOS

✖ **36.11 (Aorto)coronary bypass of one coronary artery** 🔖
Coding Clinic: 2002, Q3, P4-5,9; 1996, Q2, P7-8

✖ **36.12 (Aorto)coronary bypass of two coronary arteries** 🔖
Coding Clinic: 2007, Q4, P121-122; 2002, Q3, P8; 1999, Q4, P15-16; 1996, Q2, P7-8; 1993, 5th Issue, P17-24

✖ **36.13 (Aorto)coronary bypass of three coronary arteries** 🔖
Coding Clinic: 2002, Q3, P6-9; 1996, Q2, P7-8; 1993, 5th Issue, P17-24

✖ **36.14 (Aorto)coronary bypass of four or more coronary arteries** 🔖
Coding Clinic: 2002, Q3, P5; 1996, Q2, P7-8

✖ **36.15 Single internal mammary-coronary artery bypass** 🔖
Anastomosis (single):
mammary artery to coronary artery
thoracic artery to coronary artery
Coding Clinic: 2002, Q3, P4-9; 1999, Q4, P15-16; 1996, Q2, P7-8

OPERATIONS ON THE CARDIOVASCULAR SYSTEM (35–39)

OPERATIONS ON THE CARDIOVASCULAR SYSTEM (35–39)

✖ 36.16   **Double internal mammary-coronary artery bypass** 🔖
Anastomosis, double:
mammary artery to coronary artery
thoracic artery to coronary artery
Coding Clinic: 2002, Q3, P6,8-9; 1996, Q2, P7-8

✖ 36.17   **Abdominal - coronary artery bypass** 🔖
Anastomosis:
gastroepiploic - coronary artery

✖ 36.19   **Other bypass anastomosis for heart revascularization** 🔖
Coding Clinic: 1996, Q2, P7-8

✖ 36.2   **Heart revascularization by arterial implant**
Implantation of:
aortic branches [ascending aortic branches] into heart muscle
blood vessels into myocardium
internal mammary artery [internal thoracic artery] into:
heart muscle
myocardium
ventricle
ventricular wall
Indirect heart revascularization NOS

● 36.3   **Other heart revascularization**

✖ 36.31   **Open chest transmyocardial revascularization**

✖ 36.32   **Other transmyocardial revascularization**
Coding Clinic: 1998, Q4, P73-75

✖ 36.33   **Endoscopic transmyocardial revascularization**
Thoracoscopic transmyocardial revascularization
Coding Clinic: 2006, Q4, P127-128

✖ 36.34   **Percutaneous transmyocardial revascularization**
Endovascular transmyocardial revascularization
Coding Clinic: 2006, Q4, P127-128

✖ 36.39   **Other heart revascularization**
Abrasion of epicardium
Cardio-omentopexy
Intrapericardial poudrage
Myocardial graft:
mediastinal fat
omentum
pectoral muscles

● 36.9   **Other operations on vessels of heart**
Code also cardiopulmonary bypass [extracorporeal circulation] [heart-lung machine] (39.61)

✖ 36.91   **Repair of aneurysm of coronary vessel**
Coding Clinic: 2008, Q2, P13

✖ 36.99   **Other operations on vessels of heart**
Exploration of coronary artery
Incision of coronary artery
Ligation of coronary artery
Repair of arteriovenous fistula
Coding Clinic: 2003, Q3, P18; 1999, Q4, P15-16

● 37   **Other operations on heart and pericardium**
Code also any injection or infusion of platelet inhibitor (99.20)
Coding Clinic: 2007, Q1, P11-12

37.0   **Pericardiocentesis**

● 37.1   **Cardiotomy and pericardiotomy**
Code also cardiopulmonary bypass [extracorporeal circulation] [heart-lung machine] (39.61)

✖ 37.10   **Incision of heart, not otherwise specified**
Cardiolysis NOS

✖ 37.11   **Cardiotomy**
Incision of:
atrium
endocardium
myocardium
ventricle

✖ 37.12   **Pericardiotomy**
Pericardial window operation
Pericardiolysis
Pericardiotomy
Coding Clinic: 1995, Q3, P7

● 37.2   **Diagnostic procedures on heart and pericardium**

37.20   **Noninvasive programmed electrical stimulation (NIPS)**
Excludes *that as part of intraoperative testing – omit code*
catheter based invasive electrophysiologic testing (37.26)
device interrogation only without arrhythmia induction (bedside check) (89.45–89.49)
Coding Clinic: 2006, Q4, P128-129

37.21   **Right heart cardiac catheterization**
Cardiac catheterization NOS
Excludes *that with catheterization of left heart (37.23)*
◆ Non-OR Procedure that affects MS-DRG assignment to MDC 05, MS-DRG 216-218, 222-225, 233-234, 286-287
Coding Clinic: 2004, Q3, P10; 2003, Q3, P9-10; 1984, Nov-Dec, P12, 19; 1984, July-Aug, P19x2

37.22   **Left heart cardiac catheterization**
Excludes *that with catheterization of right heart (37.23)*
◆ Non-OR Procedure that affects MS-DRG assignment to MDC 05, MS-DRG 216-218, 222-225, 233-234, 286-287
Coding Clinic: 2013, Q2, P3; 2010, Q2, P9; 2006, Q1, P69-72; 2005, Q4, P69-72; Q2, P10-11, 17-18; Q3, P14; 2004, Q3, P10; Q2, P3; 2000, Q1, P21; 1993, 5th Issue, P17-24

37.23   **Combined right and left heart cardiac catheterization**
◆ Non-OR Procedure that affects MS-DRG assignment to MDC 05, MS-DRG 216-218, 222-225, 233-234, 286-287
Coding Clinic: 2007, Q1, P11-12; 2005, Q2, P17-18; 2004, Q3, P10; 2001, Q2, P8-9; 2000, Q1, P20-21; 1998, Q3, P11; 1996, Q1, P8; 1993, 5th Issue, P17-24; 1984, Nov-Dec, P19; 1984, July-Aug, P19

✖ 37.24   **Biopsy of pericardium**

37.25   **Biopsy of heart**
Coding Clinic: 2003, Q3, P16; 1994, Q3, P7-8

37.26   **Catheter based invasive electrophysiologic testing**
Electrophysiologic studies [EPS]
Code also any concomitant procedure
Excludes *that as part of intraoperative testing – omit code*
device interrogation only without arrhythmia induction (bedside check) (89.45–89.49)
His bundle recording (37.29)
noninvasive programmed electrical stimulation (NIPS) (37.20)
◆ Non-OR Procedure that affects MS-DRG assignment to MDC 05, MS-DRG 216-218, 246-251
Coding Clinic: 2003, Q3, P23; Q2, P19; 2002, Q1, P8-9; 1999, Q1, P3x21; 997, Q2, P10

37.27   **Cardiac mapping**
Code also any concomitant procedure
Excludes *electrocardiogram (89.52)*
His bundle recording (37.29)
◆ Non-OR Procedure that affects MS-DRG assignment to MDC 05, MS-DRG 246-251

37.28   **Intracardiac echocardiography**
Echocardiography of heart chambers
ICE
Code also any synchronous Doppler flow mapping (88.72)
Excludes *intravascular imaging of coronary vessels (intravascular ultrasound) (IVUS) (00.24)*

37.29   Other diagnostic procedures on heart and pericardium

Excludes *angiocardiography (88.50–88.58)*
cardiac function tests (89.41–89.69)
cardiovascular radioisotopic scan and
function study (92.05)
coronary arteriography (88.55–88.57)
diagnostic pericardiocentesis (37.0)
diagnostic ultrasound of heart (88.72)
x-ray of heart (87.49)

● **37.3   Pericardiectomy and excision of lesion of heart**

Code also cardiopulmonary bypass [extracorporeal
circulation] [heart-lung machine], if performed
(39.61)

✴ **37.31   Pericardiectomy**
Excision of:
adhesions of pericardium
constricting scar of:
epicardium
pericardium

✴ **37.32   Excision of aneurysm of heart**
Repair of aneurysm of heart

✴ **37.33   Excision or destruction of other lesion or tissue of
heart, open approach**
Ablation or incision of heart tissue (cryoablation)
(electrocautery) (laser) (microwave)
(radiofrequency) (resection) (ultrasound),
open chest approach
Cox-maze procedure
Maze procedure
That by median sternotomy
That by thoracotomy without use of thoracoscope

Excludes *ablation, excision, or destruction of lesion or*
tissue of heart:
endovascular approach (37.34)
thoracoscopic approach (37.37)
excision or destruction of left atrial
appendate (LAA) (37.36)
Coding Clinic: 2012, Q1, P14-15; 2010, Q3, P7; 2006, Q3, P13-14;
2003, Q4, P93-95; 1994, Q2, P12

✴ **37.34   Excision or destruction of other lesion or tissue of
heart, endovascular approach**
Ablation of heart tissue (cryoablation)
(electrocautery) (laser) (microwave)
(radiofrequency) (ultrasound), via peripherally
inserted catheter
Modified maze procedure, percutaneous approach

Excludes *ablation, excision or destruction of lesion of*
tissue of heart:
open approach (37.33)
thoracoscopic approach (37.37)
Coding Clinic: 2013, Q3, P10; 2012, Q1, P14-15; 2003, Q4,
P93-95; 2000, Q1, P20-21

✴ **37.35   Partial ventriculectomy**
Ventricular reduction surgery
Ventricular remodeling

Code also any synchronous:
mitral valve repair (35.02, 35.12)
mitral valve replacement (35.23–35.24)
MCE: Non-covered procedure
Coding Clinic: 2008, Q3, P9-10; 1997, Q4, P54-55

**37.36   Excision, destruction, or exclusion of left atrial
appendage (LAA)**

Includes clipping of left atrial appendage
oversewing of left atrial appendage
stapling of left atrial appendage
that by fastener or suture
thoracoscopic approach,
minithoracotomy approach,
percutaneous approach,
endovascular approach, or
subxiphoid approach

Code also any:
concomitant (open) procedure performed
fluoroscopy (87.49)
transesophageal echocardiography (TEE) (88.72)

Excludes *ablation, excision or destruction of lesion or*
tissue of heart, endovascular approach
(37.34)
excision or destruction of other lesion or
tissue of heart, thoracoscopic approach
(37.37)
insertion of left atrial appendage device
(37.90)
◆Non-OR Procedure that affects MS-DRG assignment to
MDC 05, MS-DRG 250-251
Coding Clinic: 2008, Q4, P176; 2006, Q3, P13-14

✴ **37.37   Excision or destruction of other lesion or tissue of
heart, thoracoscopic approach**
Ablation or incision of heart tissue (cryoablation)
(electrocautery) (laser) (microwave)
(radiofrequency) (resection) (ultrasound), via
thoracoscope
Modified maze procedure, thoracoscopic approach
That via thoracoscopically-assisted approach
(without thoracotomy) (with port access) (with
sub-xiphoid incision)

Excludes *ablation, excision or destruction of lesion or*
tissue of heart:
open approach (37.33)
endovascular approach (37.34)
thoracoscopic excision or destruction of left
atrial appendage [LAA] (37.36)
Coding Clinic: 2012, Q1, P14-15

● **37.4   Repair of heart and pericardium**
Coding Clinic: 1990, Q2, P24

✴ **37.41   Implantation of prosthetic cardiac support device
around the heart**
Cardiac support device (CSD)
Epicardial support device
Fabric (textile) (mesh) device
Ventricular support device on surface of heart

Code also any:
cardiopulmonary bypass [extracorporeal
circulation] [heart-lung machine] if
performed (39.61)
mitral valve repair (35.02, 35.12)
mitral valve replacement (35.23–35.24)
transesophageal echocardiography (88.72)

Excludes *circulatory assist systems (37.61–37.68)*
Coding Clinic: 2005, Q4, P119-120

✴ **37.49   Other repair of heart and pericardium**
Coding Clinic: 2008, Q3, P9-10

OPERATIONS ON THE CARDIOVASCULAR SYSTEM (35–39)

Excludes   Includes   Use additional   Code also   Omit code

OPERATIONS ON THE CARDIOVASCULAR SYSTEM (35–39)

●37.5 **Heart replacement procedures**
Coding Clinic: 2003, Q4, P96-98

✖37.51 **Heart transplantation**
Excludes *combined heart-lung transplantation (33.6)*
MCE: Limited coverage
Coding Clinic: 2008, Q4, P180-182; 2005, Q2, P14-15

✖37.52 **Implantation of total internal biventricular heart replacement system**
Artificial heart
Excludes *implantation of heart assist system [VAD] (37.62, 37.65, 37.66, 37.68)*
Note: This procedure includes substantial removal of part or all of the biological heart. Both ventricles are resected, and the native heart is no longer intact. Ventriculectomy is included in this procedure; do not code separately.
MCE: Non-covered procedure except when combined with V70.7. Limited coverage when combined with diagnosis V70.7

✖37.53 **Replacement or repair of thoracic unit of (total) replacement heart system**
Excludes *replacement and repair of heart assist system [VAD] (37.63)*
MCE: Non-covered procedure

✖37.54 **Replacement or repair of other implantable component of (total) replacement heart system**
Implantable battery
Implantable controller
Transcutaneous energy transfer [TET] device
Excludes *replacement and repair of heart assist system [VAD] (37.63)*
replacement or repair of thoracic unit of (total) replacement heart system (37.53)
MCE: Non-covered procedure

✖37.55 **Removal of internal biventricular heart replacement system**
Explantation of artificial heart
Code also any concomitant procedure, such as:
combined heart-lung transplantation (33.6)
heart transplantation (37.51)
implantation of internal biventricular heart replacement system (37.52)
Excludes *explantation [removal] of external heart assist system (37.64)*
explantation [removal] of percutaneous external heart assist device (97.44)
nonoperative removal of heart assist system (97.44)
that with replacement or repair of heart replacement system (37.53, 37.54)
Coding Clinic: 2008, Q4, P180-182

●37.6 **Implantation of heart and circulatory assist system(s)**
Excludes *implantation of prosthetic cardiac support system (37.41)*
Coding Clinic: 2008, Q4, P177-180; 2004, Q4, P118-120

✖37.60 **Implantation or insertion of biventricular external heart assist system**
Temporary cardiac support for both left and right ventricles, inserted in the same operative episode
Includes open chest (sternotomy) procedure for cannulae attachments
Note: Device (outside the body but connected to heart) with external circulation pump. Ventriculotomy is included; do not code separately.
Excludes *implantation of internal biventricular heart replacement system (artificial heart) (37.52)*
implant of pulsation balloon (37.61)
insertion of percutaneous external heart assist device (37.68)
insertion of temporary non-implantable extracorporeal circulatory assist device (37.62)

✖37.61 **Implant of pulsation balloon**
Coding Clinic: 2005, Q3, P14

✖37.62 **Insertion of temporary non-implantable extracorporeal circulatory assist device**
Insertion of heart assist system, NOS
Insertion of heart pump
Excludes *implantation of total internal biventricular heart replacement system [artificial heart] (37.52)*
implant of external heart assist system (37.65)
insertion of implantable extracorporeal heart assist system (37.66)
insertion of percutaneous external heart assist device (37.68)
removal of heart assist system (37.64)
Note: Includes explantation of this device; do not code separately.
Coding Clinic: 2003, Q4, P116-117; 1990, Q2, P23

✖37.63 **Repair of heart assist system**
Replacement of parts of an existing ventricular assist device (VAD)
Excludes *replacement or repair of other implantable component of (total) replacement heart system [artificial heart] (37.54)*
replacement or repair of thoracic unit of (total) replacement heart system [artificial heart] (37.53)

✖37.64 **Removal of external heart assist system(s) or device(s)**
Explantation of external device(s) providing left and right ventricular support
Explantation of single external device and cannulae
Excludes *explantation [removal] of percutaneous external heart assist device (97.44)*
nonoperative removal of heart assist system (97.44)
temporary non-implantable extracorporeal circulatory assist device (37.62)
that with replacement of implant (37.63)
Coding Clinic: 2008, Q4, P177-180

✱ **37.65 Implant of single ventricular (extracorporeal) external heart assist system**
Insertion of one device into one ventricle

Includes open chest (sternotomy) procedure for cannulae attachments

Excludes *implant of pulsation balloon (37.61)*
implantation of total internal biventricular heart replacement system (37.52)
insertion of implantable heart assist system (37.66)
insertion of implantation of two external VADs for simultaneous right and left heart support (37.60)
insertion of percutaneous external heart assist device (37.68)
that without sternotomy (37.62)

Note: Insertion or implantation of one external VAD for left or right heart support.
Note: Device (outside the body but connected to heart) with external circulation and pump.

✱ **37.66 Insertion of implantable heart assist system**
Axial flow heart assist system
Diagonal pump heart assist system
Left ventricular assist device (LVAD)
Pulsatile heart assist system
Right ventricular assist device (RVAD)
Rotary pump heart assist system
Transportable, implantable heart assist system
Ventricular assist device (VAD) not otherwise specified

Note: Device directly connected to the heart and implanted in the upper left quadrant of peritoneal cavity.
Note: This device can be used for either destination therapy (DT) or bridge-to-transplant (BTT).

Excludes *implant of pulsation balloon (37.61)*
implantation of total internal biventricular heart replacement system [artificial heart] (37.52)
insertion of percutaneous external heart assist device (37.68)

MCE: Limited coverage
Coding Clinic: 2003, Q4, P116-117; 1998, Q1, P8

✱ **37.67 Implantation of cardiomyostimulation system**
Note: Two-step open procedure consisting of transfer of one end of the latissimus dorsi muscle; wrapping it around the heart; rib resection; implantation of epicardial cardiac pacing leads into the right ventricle; tunneling and pocket creation for the cardiomyostimulator.
Coding Clinic: 1998, Q43, P75-76

✱ **37.68 Insertion of percutaneous external heart assist device**
Includes percutaneous [femoral] insertion of cannulae attachments
Circulatory assist device
Extrinsic heart assist device
pVAD
Percutaneous heart assist device
Coding Clinic: 2009, Q3, P12; 2008, Q2, P12

● **37.7 Insertion, revision, replacement, and removal of leads; insertion of temporary pacemaker system; or revision of cardiac device pocket**
Code also any insertion and replacement of pacemaker device (37.80–37.87)

Excludes *implantation or replacement of transvenous lead [electrode] into left ventricular cardiac venous system (00.52)*

37.70 Initial insertion of lead [electrode], not otherwise specified
Excludes *insertion of temporary transvenous pacemaker system (37.78)*
replacement of atrial and/or ventricular lead(s) (37.76)
◆Non-OR Procedure that affects MS-DRG assignment to MDC 01, 05, 21; refer to Part VI, Appendix E, Table 1, Pacemaker/Lead Device Reference Table and Table 3, Cardio-Defibrillator Lead/Generator Reference Table

37.71 Initial insertion of transvenous lead [electrode] into ventricle
Excludes *insertion of temporary transvenous pacemaker system (37.78)*
replacement of atrial and/or ventricular lead(s) (37.76)
◆Non-OR Procedure that affects MS-DRG assignment to MDC 01, 05, 21; refer to Part VI, Appendix E, Table 1, Pacemaker/Lead Device Reference Table and Table 3, Cardio-Defibrillator Lead/Generator Reference Table

37.72 Initial insertion of transvenous leads [electrodes] into atrium and ventricle
Excludes *insertion of temporary transvenous pacemaker system (37.78)*
replacement of atrial and/or ventricular lead(s) (37.76)
◆Non-OR Procedure that affects MS-DRG assignment to MDC 01, 05, 21; refer to Part VI, Appendix E, Table 1, Pacemaker/Lead Device Reference Table and Table 3, Cardio-Defibrillator Lead/Generator Reference Table
Coding Clinic: 2011, Q4, P168; 2008, Q4, P101-102; 1997, Q2, P4

37.73 Initial insertion of transvenous lead [electrode] into atrium
Excludes *insertion of temporary transvenous pacemaker system (37.78)*
replacement of atrial and/or ventricular lead(s) (37.76)
◆Non-OR Procedure that affects MS-DRG assignment to MDC 01, 05, 21; refer to Part VI, Appendix E, Table 1, Pacemaker/Lead Device Reference Table and Table 3, Cardio-Defibrillator Lead/Generator Reference Table

✱ **37.74 Insertion or replacement of epicardial lead [electrode] into epicardium**
Insertion or replacement of epicardial by:
sternotomy
thoracotomy

Excludes *replacement of atrial and/or ventricular lead(s) (37.76)*
MS-DRG: Refer to Part VI, Appendix E, Table 1, Pacemaker/Lead Device Reference Table and Table 3, Cardioverter-Defibrillator Lead/Generator Reference Table
Coding Clinic: 2007, Q1, P20; 2005, Q3, P3-9

OPERATIONS ON THE CARDIOVASCULAR SYSTEM (35–39)

Excludes   Includes   Use additional   Code also   Omit code

OPERATIONS ON THE CARDIOVASCULAR SYSTEM (35–39)

✖ **37.75 Revision of lead [electrode]**
Repair of electrode [removal with re-insertion]
Repositioning of lead(s) (AICD) (cardiac device)
(CRT-D) (CRT-P) (defibrillator) (pacemaker)
(pacing) (sensing) [electrode]
Revision of lead NOS
> **Excludes** *repositioning of temporary transvenous pacemaker system —* omit code
Coding Clinic: 2012, Q4, P82, 89; Q2, P14-15; 2005, Q3, P3-9; 1999, Q2, P11-12

✖ **37.76 Replacement of transvenous atrial and/or ventricular lead(s) [electrode]**
Removal or abandonment of existing transvenous or epicardial lead(s) with transvenous lead(s) replacement
> **Excludes** *replacement of epicardial lead [electrode] (37.74)*
MS-DRG: Refer to Part VI, Appendix E, Table 1, Pacemaker/Lead Device Reference Table and Table 3, Cardioverter-Defibrillator Lead/Generator Reference Table
Coding Clinic: 2005, Q3, P3-9

✖ **37.77 Removal of lead(s) [electrode] without replacement**
Removal:
epicardial lead (transthoracic approach)
transvenous lead(s)
> **Excludes** *removal of temporary transvenous pacemaker system —* omit code
> *that with replacement of:*
> *atrial and/or ventricular lead(s) [electrode] (37.76)*
> *epicardial lead [electrode] (37.74)*

37.78 Insertion of temporary transvenous pacemaker system
> **Excludes** *intraoperative cardiac pacemaker (39.64)*
Coding Clinic: 2005, Q3, P3-9; 1993, Q3, P12

✖ **37.79 Revision or relocation of cardiac device pocket**
Debridement and reforming pocket (skin and subcutaneous tissue)
Insertion of loop recorder
Relocation of pocket [creation of new pocket] pacemaker or CRT-P
Removal of cardiac device/pulse generator without replacement
Removal of the implantable hemodynamic pressure sensor (lead) and monitor device
Removal without replacement of cardiac resynchronization defibrillator device
Repositioning of implantable hemodynamic pressure sensor (lead) and monitor device
Repositioning of pulse generator
Revision of cardioverter/defibrillator (automatic) pocket
Revision of pocket for intracardiac hemodynamic monitoring
Revision or relocation of CRT-D pocket
Revision or relocation of pacemaker, defibrillator, or other implanted cardiac device pocket
> **Excludes** *removal of loop recorder (86.05)*
Coding Clinic: 2012, Q4, P89; 2005, Q3, P3-9; 1994, Q2, P10x2

● **37.8 Insertion, replacement, removal, and revision of pacemaker device**
> **Note:** Device testing during procedure – omit code
Code also any lead insertion, lead replacement, lead removal and/or lead revision (37.70–37.77)
> **Excludes** *implantation of cardiac resynchronization pacemaker [CRT-P] (00.50)*
> *implantation or replacement of cardiac resynchronization pacemaker pulse generator only [CRT-P] (00.53)*

✖ **37.80 Insertion of permanent pacemaker, initial or replacement, type of device not specified**
MS-DRG: Refer to Part VI, Appendix E, Table 1, Pacemaker/Lead Reference Table

37.81 Initial insertion of single-chamber device, not specified as rate responsive
> **Excludes** *replacement of existing pacemaker device (37.85–37.87)*
◆ Non-OR Procedure that affects MS-DRG assignment to MDC 01, 05, 21; refer to Part VI, Appendix E, Table 1, Pacemaker/Lead Device Reference Table

37.82 Initial insertion of single-chamber device, rate responsive
Rate responsive to physiologic stimuli other than atrial rate
> **Excludes** *replacement of existing pacemaker device (37.85–37.87)*
◆ Non-OR Procedure that affects MS-DRG assignment to MDC 01, 05, 21; refer to Part VI, Appendix E, Table 1, Pacemaker/Lead Device Reference Table

37.83 Initial insertion of dual-chamber device
Atrial ventricular sequential device
> **Excludes** *replacement of existing pacemaker device (37.85–37.87)*
◆ Non-OR Procedure that affects MS-DRG assignment to MDC 01, 05, 21; refer to Part VI, Appendix E, Table 1, Pacemaker/Lead Device Reference Table
Coding Clinic: 2011, Q4, P168; 2008, Q4, P101-102; 1997, Q2, P4; 1997, Q2, P4

✖ **37.85 Replacement of any type pacemaker device with single-chamber device, not specified as rate responsive**
MS-DRG: Refer to Part VI, Appendix E, Table 1, Pacemaker/Lead Reference Table

✖ **37.86 Replacement of any type of pacemaker device with single-chamber device, rate responsive**
Rate responsive to physiologic stimuli other than atrial rate
MS-DRG: Refer to Part VI, Appendix E, Table 1, Pacemaker/Lead Reference Table

✖ **37.87 Replacement of any type pacemaker device with dual-chamber device**
Atrial ventricular sequential device
MS-DRG: Refer to Part VI, Appendix E, Table 1, Pacemaker/Lead Reference Table

✖ **37.89 Revision or removal of pacemaker device**
Removal without replacement of cardiac resynchronization pacemaker device [CRT-P]
Repair of pacemaker device
> **Excludes** *removal of temporary transvenous pacemaker system —* omit code
> *replacement of existing pacemaker device (37.85–37.87)*
> *replacement of existing pacemaker device with CRT-P pacemaker device (00.53)*

● **37.9 Other operations on heart and pericardium**

37.90 Insertion of left atrial appendage device
Left atrial filter
Left atrial occluder
Transseptal catheter technique
◆ Non-OR Procedure that affects MS-DRG assignment to MDC 05, MS-DRG 250-251
Coding Clinic: 2004, Q4, P121-122

✖ **37.91 Open chest cardiac massage**
> **Excludes** *closed chest cardiac massage (99.63)*
Coding Clinic: 1988, Q4, P12

37.92 Injection of therapeutic substance into heart

37.93 Injection of therapeutic substance into pericardium

◀ New   ◀▥ Revised   ~~deleted~~ Deleted   ● Use Additional Digit(s)   ✖ Valid O.R. Procedure
◆ Non-O.R. Procedure   ♀ Females Only   ♂ Males Only   OGCR Official Guidelines   **Coding Clinic**

✳ **37.94** **Implantation or replacement of automatic cardioverter/defibrillator, total system [AICD]**
Implantation of defibrillator with leads (epicardial patches), formation of pocket (abdominal fascia) (subcutaneous), any transvenous leads, intraoperative procedures for evaluation of lead signals, and obtaining defibrillator threshold measurements
Techniques:
   lateral thoracotomy
   medial sternotomy
   subxiphoid procedure
Note: Device testing during procedure – *omit code*
Code also
   extracorporeal circulation, if performed (39.61)
   any concomitant procedure [e.g., coronary bypass (36.10–36.19) or CCM, total system (17.51)]
Excludes *implantation of cardiac resynchronization defibrillator, total system [CRT-D] (00.51)*
Coding Clinic: 2013, Q1, P11; 2012, Q4, P88; 2009, Q4, P141; 2003, Q2, P19; 2001, Q3, P5-7; 1999, Q3, P12-13; Q1, P3; 1994, Q2, P12

✳ **37.95** **Implantation of automatic cardioverter/defibrillator lead(s) only**
MS-DRG: Refer to Part VI, Appendix E, Table 3, Cardioverter-Defibrillator Lead/Generator Reference Table
Coding Clinic: 2012, Q4, P88

✳ **37.96** **Implantation of automatic cardioverter/defibrillator pulse generator only**
Note: Device testing during procedure – *omit code*
Excludes *implantation or replacement of cardiac resynchronization defibrillator, pulse generator device only [CRT-D] (00.54)*
MS-DRG: Refer to Part VI, Appendix E, Table 3, Cardioverter-Defibrillator Lead/Generator Reference Table
Coding Clinic: 2012, Q4, P88

✳ **37.97** **Replacement of automatic cardioverter/defibrillator lead(s) only**
Excludes *replacement of epicardial lead [electrode] into epicardium (37.74)*
replacement of transvenous lead [electrode] into left ventricular coronary venous system (00.52)
MS-DRG: Refer to Part VI, Appendix E, Table 3, Cardioverter-Defibrillator Lead/Generator Reference Table
Coding Clinic: 2012, Q4, P88; 2005, Q3, P3-9

✳ **37.98** **Replacement of automatic cardioverter/defibrillator pulse generator only**
Note: Device testing during procedure – *omit code*
Excludes *replacement of cardiac resynchronization defibrillator, pulse generator device only [CRT-D] (00.54)*
MS-DRG: Refer to Part VI, Appendix E, Table 3, Cardioverter-Defibrillator Lead/Generator Reference Table
Coding Clinic: 2012, Q4, P88; 1999, Q1, P3

✳ **37.99** **Other**
Excludes *cardiac retraining (93.36)*
conversion of cardiac rhythm (99.60–99.69)
implantation of prosthetic cardiac support device (37.41)
insertion of left atrial appendage device (37.90)
maze procedure (Cox-maze), open (37.33)
maze procedure, endovascular approach (37.34)
repositioning of pulse generator (37.79)
revision of lead(s) (37.75)
revision or relocation of pacemaker, defibrillator, or other implanted cardiac device pocket (37.79)
Coding Clinic: 2005, Q3, P3-9; Q2, P14-15; 1997, Q1, P12; 1994, Q1, P19; 1993, Q3, P12; 1989, Q1, P11

● **38** **Incision, excision, and occlusion of vessels**
Code also
   any application or administration of an adhesion barrier substance (99.77)
   cardiopulmonary bypass [extracorporeal circulation] [heart-lung machine] (39.61)
Excludes *that of coronary vessels (00.66, 36.03, 36.04, 36.09, 36.10–36.99)*
Coding Clinic: 1988, Q1, P11

The following fourth-digit subclassification is for use with appropriate categories in section 38.0, 38.1, 38.3, 38.5, 38.6, 38.8, and 38.9 according to site. Valid fourth-digits are in [brackets] at the end of each code/description.

0 **unspecified site**
1 **intracranial vessels**
   Cerebral (anterior) (middle)
   Circle of Willis
   Posterior communicating artery
2 **other vessels of head and neck**
   Carotid artery (common) (external) (internal)
   Jugular vein (external) (internal)
3 **upper limb vessels**
   Axillary
   Brachial
   Radial
   Ulnar
4 **aorta**
5 **other thoracic vessels**
   Innominate
   Pulmonary (artery) (vein)
   Subclavian
   Vena cava, superior
6 **abdominal arteries**
   Celiac
   Gastric
   Hepatic
   Iliac
   Mesenteric
   Renal
   Splenic
   Umbilical
   Excludes *abdominal aorta (4)*
7 **abdominal veins**
   Iliac
   Portal
   Renal
   Splenic
   Vena cava (inferior)
8 **lower limb arteries**
   Femoral (common) (superficial)
   Popliteal
   Tibial
9 **lower limb veins**
   Femoral
   Popliteal
   Saphenous
   Tibial

✳● **38.0** **Incision of vessel**
[0-9] Embolectomy
Thrombectomy
Excludes *endovascular removal of obstruction from head and neck vessel(s) (39.74)*
puncture or catheterization of any:
   artery (38.91, 38.98)
   vein (38.92–38.95, 38.99)
Coding Clinic: 2011, Q4, P109; 2003, Q1, P17-18; 1998, Q2, P23

Excludes   Includes   Use additional   Code also   Omit code

✖●**38.1** **Endarterectomy**
[0-6, 8]   Endarterectomy with:
    embolectomy
    patch graft
    temporary bypass during procedure
    thrombectomy
  Code also any:
    number of vascular stents inserted (00.45–00.48)
    number of vessels treated (00.40–00.43)
    procedure on vessel bifurcation (00.44)
    Coding Clinic: 2006, Q3, P20; 2002, Q1, P10-11; 2000, Q1, P16; 1999, Q2, P5; 1995, Q2, P16; 1985, Mar-April, P15

●**38.2** **Diagnostic procedures on blood vessels**
  Excludes *adjunct vascular system procedures (00.40–00.43)*

✖ **38.21** **Biopsy of blood vessel**
  38.22 **Percutaneous angioscopy**
    Excludes *angioscopy of eye (95.12)*

  38.23 **Intravascular spectroscopy**
    Intravascular chemography
    Near infrared (NIR) spectroscopy
    Includes spectroscopy of both coronary and peripheral vessels
    Excludes *intravascular imaging of:*
      coronary vessels (00.24, 38.24)
      peripheral vessels (00.23, 38.25)
    Coding Clinic: 2008, Q4, P182-183

  38.24 **Intravascular imaging of coronary vessel(s) by optical coherence tomography [OCT]**

  38.25 **Intravascular imaging of non-coronary vessel(s) by optical coherence tomograpy [OCT]**
    Excludes *intravascular imaging of coronary vessel(s) by OCT (38.24)*

✖ **38.26** **Insertion of implantable pressure sensor without lead for intracardiac or great vessel hemodynamic monitoring**
    Note: The sensor is a standalone device and is not physically connected to a separately implanted monitor.
    Leadless pressure sensor not physically connected to a separately implanted monitor
    Single device combination leadless pressure sensor with integral monitor for intracardiac or great vessel (or branch thereof) hemodynamic monitoring
    With or without internal batteries
    Without leads
    Excludes *circulatory monitoring (blood gas, arterial or venous pressure, cardiac output and coronary blood flow) (89.60-89.69)*
      hemodynamic monitoring system with sensor and separately implanted monitor (00.56 – 00.57)
      insertion or replacement of implantable pressure sensor with lead for intracardiac or great vessel hemodynamic monitoring (00.56)

✖ **38.29** **Other diagnostic procedures on blood vessels**
    Excludes *blood vessel thermography (88.86)*
      circulatory monitoring (89.61–89.69)
      contrast:
        angiocardiography (88.50–88.58)
        arteriography (88.40–88.49)
        phlebography (88.60–88.67)
      impedance phlebography (88.68)
      peripheral vascular ultrasonography (88.77)
      plethysmogram (89.58)
    Coding Clinic: 2000, Q3, P16; 1999, Q1, P7

✖●**38.3** **Resection of vessel with anastomosis**
[0-9]   Angiectomy
  Excision of:
    aneurysm (arteriovenous) with anastomosis
    blood vessel (lesion) with anastomosis
    Coding Clinic: 1985, Mar-April, P15; 1984, Nov-Dec, P10

✖●**38.4** **Resection of vessel with replacement**
[0-9]   Angiectomy
  Excision of:
    aneurysm (arteriovenous) or blood vessel (lesion) with replacement
  Partial resection with replacement
    Excludes *endovascular repair of aneurysm (39.71–39.79)*
    MS-DRG: Refer to Part VI, Appendix E, Table 2, Abdominal Aorta/Thoracic Vessel Resection Reference Table for 38.44 and 38.45
    Coding Clinic: 2008, Q2, P13; 2006, Q3, P15-16; 1999, Q2, P5-6; Q1, P15; 1992, Q3, P10-11; 1985, Mar-April, P15; 1984, Nov-Dec, P10

  Requires the use of one of the following fourth-digit subclassifications to identify site:

0	**unspecified site**
1	**intracranial vessels**
	Cerebral (anterior) (middle)
	Circle of Willis
	Posterior communicating artery
2	**other vessels of head and neck**
	Carotid artery (common) (external) (internal)
	Jugular vein (external) (internal)
3	**upper limb vessels**
	Axillary
	Brachial
	Radial
	Ulnar
4	**aorta, abdominal**
	Code also any thoracic vessel involvement (thoracoabdominal procedure) (38.45)
5	**thoracic vessels**
	Aorta (thoracic)
	Innominate
	Pulmonary (artery) (vein)
	Subclavian
	Vena cava, superior
	Code also any abdominal aorta involvement (thoracoabdominal procedure) (38.44)
6	**abdominal arteries**
	Celiac
	Gastric
	Hepatic
	Iliac
	Mesenteric
	Renal
	Splenic
	Umbilical
	Excludes *abdominal aorta (4)*
7	**abdominal veins**
	Iliac
	Portal
	Renal
	Splenic
	Vena cava (inferior)
8	**lower limb arteries**
	Femoral (common) (superficial)
	Popliteal
	Tibial
9	**lower limb veins**
	Femoral
	Popliteal
	Saphenous
	Tibial

✖●**38.5** **Ligation and stripping of varicose veins**
[0-3, 5, 7, 9] **Excludes** *ligation of varices:*
      esophageal (42.91)
      gastric (44.91)
    Coding Clinic: 1997, Q2, P7

◀ New   ◀█ Revised   ~~deleted~~ Deleted   ● Use Additional Digit(s)   ✖ Valid O.R. Procedure
◆ Non-O.R. Procedure   ♀ Females Only   ♂ Males Only   OGCR Official Guidelines   **Coding Clinic**

1236

✖ ● **38.6 Other excision of vessel**
[0-9]   Excision of blood vessel (lesion) NOS

> **Excludes** *excision of vessel for aortocoronary bypass*
> *(36.10–36.14)*
> *excision with:*
> *anastomosis (38.30–38.39)*
> *graft replacement (38.40–38.49)*
> *implant (38.40–38.49)*

Coding Clinic: 1995, Q3, P5-6; 1990, Q3, P17

✖ **38.7 Interruption of the vena cava**
Insertion of implant or sieve in vena cava
Ligation of vena cava (inferior) (superior)
Plication of vena cava
Coding Clinic: 2007, Q2, P5; 1994, Q2, P9

✖ ● **38.8 Other surgical occlusion of vessels**
[0-9]   Clamping of blood vessel
Division of blood vessel
Ligation of blood vessel
Occlusion of blood vessel

> **Excludes** *adrenal vessels (07.43)*
> *esophageal varices (42.91)*
> *gastric or duodenal vessel for ulcer (44.40–44.49)*
> *gastric varices (44.91)*
> *meningeal vessel (02.13)*
> *percutaneous transcatheter infusion embolization*
> *(99.29)*
> *spermatic vein for varicocele (63.1)*
> *surgical occlusion of vena cava (38.7)*
> *that for chemoembolization (99.25)*
> *that for control of (postoperative) hemorrhage:*
> *anus (49.95)*
> *bladder (57.93)*
> *following vascular procedure (39.41)*
> *nose (21.00–21.09)*
> *prostate (60.94)*
> *tonsil (28.7)*
> *thyroid vessel (06.92)*
> *transcatheter (infusion) (99.29)*

Coding Clinic: 2005, Q1, P14; 2003, Q1, P15-16; 2000, Q3, P16; 2005,
Q1, P14; 1999, Q1, P17-18; 1996, Q2, P7-8; 1996, Q1, P8; 1987,
Mar-April, P9

● **38.9 Puncture of vessel**

> **Excludes** *that for circulatory monitoring (89.60–89.69)*

38.91 Arterial catheterization
Coding Clinic: 2013, Q1, P5; 2005, Q1, P14; 1998, Q2, P24;
1995, Q1, P3; 1990, Q2, P23; 1988, Q1, P8; 1984,
May-June, P11

38.92 Umbilical vein catheterization

38.93 Venous catheterization, not elsewhere classified

> **Excludes** *that for cardiac catheterization*
> *(37.21–37.23)*
> *that for renal dialysis (38.95)*
> *that with guidance (electrocardiogram)*
> *(fluoroscopy) (ultrasound) (38.97)*

Coding Clinic: 2010, Q3, P14; 2000, Q3, P9; 1998, Q2, P24; 1996,
Q1, P5-6; 1992, Q2, P15-16; 1990, Q2, P24; 1985,
July-Aug, P11

38.94 Venous cutdown

38.95 Venous catheterization for renal dialysis

> **Excludes** *insertion of totally implantable vascular*
> *access device [VAD] (86.07)*

Coding Clinic: 2012, Q3, P6; 2008, Q4, P193; 1998, Q3, P13; 1994,
Q2, P11

38.97 Central venous catheter placement with guidance

> **Includes** guidance by:
> electrocardiogram
> fluoroscopy
> ultrasound

Coding Clinic: 2010, Q4, P121

38.98 Other puncture of artery

> **Excludes** *that for:*
> *arteriography (88.40–88.49)*
> *coronary arteriography (88.55–88.57)*

38.99 Other puncture of vein
Phlebotomy

> **Excludes** *that for:*
> *angiography of veins (88.60–88.68)*
> *extracorporeal circulation (39.61, 50.92)*
> *injection or infusion of:*
> *sclerosing solution (39.92)*
> *therapeutic or prophylactic*
> *substance (99.11–99.29)*
> *perfusion (39.96–39.97)*
> *phlebography (88.60–88.68)*
> *transfusion (99.01–99.09)*

Coding Clinic: 1988, Q1, P11

● **39 Other operations on vessels**

> **Excludes** *those on coronary vessels (36.03–36.99)*

✖ **39.0 Systemic to pulmonary artery shunt**
Descending aorta-pulmonary artery anastomosis (graft)
Left to right anastomosis (graft)
Subclavian-pulmonary anastomosis (graft)

> **Code also** cardiopulmonary bypass [extracorporeal
> circulation] [heart-lung machine] (39.61)

✖ **39.1 Intra-abdominal venous shunt**
Anastomosis:
mesocaval
portacaval
portal vein to inferior vena cava
splenic and renal veins
transjugular intrahepatic portosystemic shunt (TIPS)

> **Excludes** *peritoneovenous shunt (54.94)*

Coding Clinic: 2002, Q2, P4; 1993, Q4, P31; Q2, P8

● **39.2 Other shunt or vascular bypass**

> **Code also** pressurized treatment of venous bypass
> graft [conduit] with pharmaceutical substance, if
> performed (00.16)

✖ **39.21 Caval-pulmonary artery anastomosis**
> **Code also** cardiopulmonary bypass (39.61)

✖ **39.22 Aorta-subclavian-carotid bypass**
Bypass (arterial):
aorta to carotid and brachial
aorta to subclavian and carotid
carotid to subclavian

✖ **39.23 Other intrathoracic vascular shunt or bypass**
Intrathoracic (arterial) bypass graft NOS

> **Excludes** *coronary artery bypass (36.10–36.19)*

✖ **39.24 Aorta-renal bypass**

✖ **39.25 Aorta-iliac-femoral bypass**
Bypass:
aortofemoral
aortoiliac
aortoiliac to popliteal
aortopopliteal
iliofemoral [iliac-femoral]
Coding Clinic: 2003, Q1, P16-17; 1988, Q1, P10

✖ **39.26 Other intra-abdominal vascular shunt or bypass**
Bypass:
aortoceliac
aortic-superior mesenteric
common hepatic-common iliac-renal
Intra-abdominal arterial bypass graft NOS

> **Excludes** *peritoneovenous shunt (54.94)*

✖ **39.27 Arteriovenostomy for renal dialysis**
Anastomosis for renal dialysis
Formation of (peripheral) arteriovenous
fistula for renal [kidney] dialysis

> **Code also** any renal dialysis (39.95)

Coding Clinic: 2007, Q1, P18; 2006, Q1, P10-11; 1985, Sept-Oct,
P12

✖ **39.28 Extracranial-intracranial (EC-IC) vascular bypass**
MCE: Non-covered procedure
Coding Clinic: 1992, Q2, P7

OPERATIONS ON THE CARDIOVASCULAR SYSTEM (35–39)

Excludes   Includes   Use additional   Code also   Omit code

✖ **39.29　Other (peripheral) vascular shunt or bypass**
　　Bypass (graft):
　　　axillary-brachial
　　　axillary-femoral [axillofemoral] (superficial)
　　　brachial
　　　femoral-femoral
　　　femoroperoneal
　　　femoropopliteal (arteries)
　　　femorotibial (anterior) (posterior)
　　　popliteal
　　　vascular NOS

Excludes　*peritoneovenous shunt (54.94)*

Coding Clinic: 2003, Q1, P17-18; 2002, Q2, P8; Q1, P13; 1985, Sept-Oct, P13; 1984, July-Aug, P20

● **39.3　Suture of vessel**
　　Repair of laceration of blood vessel

Excludes　*any other vascular puncture closure device — omit code*
　　suture of aneurysm (39.52)
　　that for control of hemorrhage (postoperative):
　　　anus (49.95)
　　　bladder (57.93)
　　　following vascular procedure (39.41)
　　　nose (21.00–21.09)
　　　prostate (60.94)
　　　tonsil (28.7)

✖ **39.30　Suture of unspecified blood vessel**

✖ **39.31　Suture of artery**
　　Coding Clinic: 2012, Q4, P81-82; 2006, Q3, P9; 1998, Q2, P22

✖ **39.32　Suture of vein**

● **39.4　Revision of vascular procedure**

✖ **39.41　Control of hemorrhage following vascular surgery**

Excludes　*that for control of hemorrhage (post operative):*
　　anus (49.95)
　　bladder (57.93)
　　nose (21.00–21.09)
　　prostate (60.94)
　　tonsil (28.7)

✖ **39.42　Revision of arteriovenous shunt for renal dialysis**
　　Conversion of renal dialysis:
　　　end-to-end anastomosis to end-to-side
　　　end-to-side anastomosis to end-to-end
　　　vessel-to-vessel cannula to arteriovenous shunt
　　Removal of old arteriovenous shunt and creation of new shunt

Excludes　*replacement of vessel-to-vessel cannula (39.94)*

Coding Clinic: 1994, Q2, P15; 1993, Q4, P33

✖ **39.43　Removal of arteriovenous shunt for renal dialysis**

Excludes　*that with replacement [revision] of shunt (39.42)*

✖ **39.49　Other revision of vascular procedure**
　　Declotting (graft)
　　Revision of:
　　　anastomosis of blood vessel
　　　vascular procedure (previous)
　　Coding Clinic: 1999, Q2, P5; 1998, Q2, P17; 1994, Q2, P13, P15; 1993, Q4, P33

● **39.5　Other repair of vessels**
　　Coding Clinic: 2002, Q1, P13; 2000, Q4, P63-64; 1998, Q2, P17; 1996, Q4, P63

✖ **39.50　Angioplasty of other non-coronary vessel(s)**
　　Percutaneous transluminal angioplasty (PTA) of non-coronary vessels:
　　　Lower extremity vessels
　　　Mesenteric artery
　　　Renal artery
　　　Upper extremity vessels
　　Code also any:
　　　atherectomy of other non-coronary vessels(s) (17.56)
　　　injection or infusion of thrombolytic agent (99.10)
　　　insertion of drug-eluting peripheral vessel stent (00.55)
　　　insertion of non-drug-eluting peripheral vessel stent(s) or stent grafts(s) (39.90)
　　　number of vascular stents inserted (00.45–00.48)
　　　number of vessels treated (00.40–00.43)
　　　procedure on vessel bifurcation (00.44)

Excludes　*percutaneous angioplasty of extracranial or intracranial vessel(s) (00.61-00.62)*
　　percutaneous atherectomy of extracranial or intracranial vessel(s) (17.53-17.54)

Coding Clinic: 2012, Q3, P13; Q2, P15-16; 2010, Q4, P113; 2009, Q3, P13; 2006, Q4, P119; 2003, Q3, P10; 2001, Q2, P23x2, 24; 2000, Q2, P10-11; Q1, P12; 1993, 5th Issue, P11

✖ **39.51　Clipping of aneurysm**

Excludes　*clipping of arteriovenous fistula (39.53)*

✖ **39.52　Other repair of aneurysm**
　　Repair of aneurysm by:
　　　coagulation
　　　electrocoagulation
　　　filipuncture
　　　methyl methacrylate
　　　suture
　　　wiring
　　　wrapping

Excludes　*endovascular repair of aneurysm (39.71–39.79)*
　　re-entry operation (aorta) (39.54)
　　that with:
　　　graft replacement (38.40–38.49)
　　　resection (38.30–38.49, 38.60–38.69)

Coding Clinic: 2002, Q3, P25-27x2; 1999, Q1, P15-17 x2; 1988, Q1, P10

✖ **39.53　Repair of arteriovenous fistula**
　　Embolization of carotid cavernous fistula
　　Repair of arteriovenous fistula by:
　　　clipping
　　　coagulation
　　　ligation and division

Excludes　*repair of:*
　　　arteriovenous shunt for renal dialysis (39.42)
　　　head and neck vessels, endovascular approach (39.72)
　　that with:
　　　graft replacement (38.40–38.49)
　　　resection (38.30–38.49, 38.60–38.69)

Coding Clinic: 2006, Q3, P15-16; 2000, Q1, P8-9

✖ **39.54　Re-entry operation (aorta)**
　　Fenestration of dissecting aneurysm of thoracic aorta

　　Code also cardiopulmonary bypass [extracorporeal circulation] [heart-lung machine] (39.61)

✖ **39.55　Reimplantation of aberrant renal vessel**

◀ New　　◀▥ Revised　　~~deleted~~ Deleted　　● Use Additional Digit(s)　　✖ Valid O.R. Procedure
◆ Non-O.R. Procedure　　♀ Females Only　　♂ Males Only　　OGCR Official Guidelines　　**Coding Clinic**

✖ **39.56** **Repair of blood vessel with tissue patch graft**

Excludes *that with resection (38.40–38.49)*

Coding Clinic: 2004, Q1, P16-17

✖ **39.57** **Repair of blood vessel with synthetic patch graft**

Excludes *that with resection (38.40–38.49)*

✖ **39.58** **Repair of blood vessel with unspecified type of patch graft**

Excludes *that with resection (38.40–38.49)*

✖ **39.59** **Other repair of vessel**

Aorticopulmonary window operation
Arterioplasty NOS
Construction of venous valves (peripheral)
Plication of vein (peripheral)
Reimplantation of artery

Code also cardiopulmonary bypass [extracorporeal circulation] [heart-lung machine] (39.61)

Excludes *interruption of the vena cava (38.7)*
reimplantation of renal artery (39.55)
that with:
    graft (39.56–39.58)
    resection (38.30–38.49, 38.60–38.69)

Coding Clinic: 1993, Q4, P31-32; 5th Issue, P5; 1989, Q2, P17; 1985, July-Aug, P8-9; Mar-April, P15

● **39.6** **Extracorporeal circulation and procedures auxiliary to heart surgery**

39.61 **Extracorporeal circulation auxiliary to open heart surgery**

Artificial heart and lung
Cardiopulmonary bypass
Pump oxygenator

Excludes *extracorporeal hepatic assistance (50.92)*
extracorporeal membrane oxygenation [ECMO] (39.65)
hemodialysis (39.95)
percutaneous cardiopulmonary bypass (39.66)

Coding Clinic: 2010, Q3, P7; Q1, P14; 2009, Q2, P8; 2008, Q3, P9-10; 2006, Q2, P13; 2004, Q1, P16-17; 2002, Q3, P5; 1997, Q4, P54-55; 1997, Q2, P8; 1995, Q1, P5-6; 1993, 5th Issue, P17-24; 1990, Q2, P24; 1985, July-Aug, P8-9

39.62 **Hypothermia (systemic) incidental to open heart surgery**

Coding Clinic: 1995, Q1, P5-6

39.63 **Cardioplegia**

Arrest:
    anoxic
    circulatory

Coding Clinic: 1995, Q1, P5-6

39.64 **Intraoperative cardiac pacemaker**

Temporary pacemaker used during and immediately following cardiac surgery

Coding Clinic: 1995, Q1, P5-6

✖ **39.65** **Extracorporeal membrane oxygenation [ECMO]**

Excludes *extracorporeal circulation auxiliary to open heart surgery (39.61)*
percutaneous cardiopulmonary bypass (39.66)

Coding Clinic: 2011, Q4, P152; 1990, Q2, P23; 1989, Q2, P17

39.66 **Percutaneous cardiopulmonary bypass**

Closed chest

Excludes *extracorporeal circulation auxiliary to open heart surgery (39.61)*
extracorporeal hepatic assistance (50.92)
extracorporeal membrane oxygenation [ECMO] (39.65)
hemodialysis (39.95)

Coding Clinic: 1996, Q3, P11-12

● **39.7** **Endovascular procedures on vessel(s)**

Embolization
Endoluminal repair
Implantation
Occlusion
Removal
Repair

Excludes *angioplasty of other non-coronary vessel(s) (39.50)*
atherectomy of other non-coronary vessel(s) (17.56)
insertion of non-drug-eluting peripheral vessel stent(s) (39.90)
other repair of aneurysm (39.52)
percutaneous insertion of carotid artery stent(s) (00.63)
percutaneous insertion of intracranial stent(s) (00.65)
percutaneous insertion of other precerebral artery stent(s) (00.64)
resection of abdominal aorta with replacement (38.44)
resection of lower limb arteries with replacement (38.48)
resection of thoracic aorta with replacement (38.45)
resection of upper limb vessels with replacement (38.43)
temporary therapeutic partial occlusion of vessel (39.77)

Coding Clinic: 2000, Q4, P63-64

✖ **39.71** **Endovascular implantation of other graft in abdominal aorta**

Endovascular repair of abdominal aortic aneurysm with graft
Stent graft(s)

Code also intra-aneurysm sac pressure monitoring (intraoperative) (00.58)

Excludes *endovascular implantation of branching or fenestrated graft in aorta (39.78)*

Coding Clinic: 2013, Q1, P6; 2002, Q1, P13; 2000, Q4, P63-64

✖ **39.72** **Endovascular (total) embolization or occlusion of head and neck vessels**

Coil-retention stent
Embolization stent
Endograft(s)
Endovascular graft(s)
Liquid tissue adhesive (glue) embolization or occlusion
Other implant or substance for repair, embolization or occlusion
That for repair of aneurysm, arteriovenous malformation [AVM], or fistula

Excludes *embolization of head or neck vessels using bare coils (39.75)*
embolization of head or neck vessels using bioactive coils (39.76)
mechanical thrombectomy of pre-cerebral and cerebral vessels (39.74)

Coding Clinic: 2013, Q1, P8; 2002, Q4, P103-105

✖ **39.73** **Endovascular implantation of graft in thoracic aorta**

Endograft(s)
Endovascular graft(s)
Endovascular repair of defect of thoracic aorta with graft(s) or device(s)
Stent graft(s) or device(s)
That for repair of aneurysm, dissection, or injury

Excludes *fenestration of dissecting aneurysm of thoracic aorta (39.54)*

Code also intra-aneurysm sac pressure monitoring (intraoperative) (00.58)

Coding Clinic: 2005, Q4, P120-121

OPERATIONS ON THE CARDIOVASCULAR SYSTEM (35–39)

Excludes   Includes   Use additional   Code also   Omit code

✖ **39.74** **Endovascular removal of obstruction from head and neck vessel(s)**
Endovascular embolectomy
Endovascular thrombectomy of pre-cerebral and cerebral vessels
Mechanical embolectomy or thrombectomy

Code also:
any injection or infusion of thrombolytic agent (99.10)
number of vessels treated (00.40–00.43)
procedure on vessel bifurcation (00.44)

Excludes   *endarterectomy of intracranial vessels and other vessels of head and neck (38.11–38.12)*
occlusive endovascular embolization of head or neck vessel(s) using bare coils (39.75)
occlusive endovascular embolization of head or neck vessel(s) using bioactive coils (39.76)
open embolectomy or thrombectomy (38.01–38.02)
Coding Clinic: 2006, Q4, P129-130

✖ **39.75** **Endovascular embolization or occlusion of vessel(s) of head or neck using bare coils**
Bare metal coils
Bare platinum coils [BPC]
That for treatment of aneurysm, arteriovenous malformation [AVM] or fistula

✖ **39.76** **Endovascular embolization or occlusion of vessel(s) of head or neck using bioactive coils**
Biodegradable inner luminal polymer coils
Coil embolization or occlusion utilizing bioactive coils
Coils containing polyglycolic acid [PGA]
That for treatment of aneurysm, arteriovenous malformation [AVM] or fistula
Coding Clinic: 2009, Q4, P146

✖ **39.77** **Temporary (partial) therapeutic endovascular occlusion of vessel**
Includes   that of aorta
that by balloon catheter

Code also any:
diagnostic arteriogram (88.40-88.49)

Excludes   *any endovascular head or neck vessel procedure (39.72, 39.74-39.76)*
diagnostic procedures on blood vessels (38.21-38.29)
permanent endovascular procedure (39.79)

✖ **39.78** **Endovascular implantation of branching or fenestrated graft(s) in aorta**
Coding Clinic: 2013, Q1, P6

✖ **39.79** **Other endovascular procedures on other vessels**
Endograft(s)
Endovascular graft(s)
Liquid tissue adhesive (glue) embolization or occlusion
Other coil embolization or occlusion
Other implant or substance for repair, embolization or occlusion
Repair of aneurysm

Excludes   *abdominal aortic aneurysm resection [AAA] (38.44)*
endovascular implantation of graft in abdominal aorta (39.71)
endovascular implantation of graft in thoracic aorta (39.73)
endovascular embolization or occlusion of head and neck vessels, bare metal coils (39.75)
endovascular embolization or occlusion of head and neck vessels, bioactive coils (39.76)
insertion of drug-eluting peripheral vessel stent(s) (00.55)
insertion of non-drug-eluting peripheral vessel(s) (for other than aneurysm repair) (39.90)
non-endovascular repair of arteriovenous fistula (39.53)
other surgical occlusion of vessels - see category 38.8
percutaneous transcatheter infusion (99.29)
thoracic aortic aneurysm resection (38.45)
transcatheter embolization for gastric or duodenal bleeding (44.44)
uterine artery embolization with coils (68.24)
Coding Clinic: 2013, Q2, P7; 2012, Q2, P15-16; 2011, Q4, P138; 2010, Q2, P9; Q1, P21; 2009, Q2, P7; 2006, Q2, P22, 23x2; 2002, Q4, P103-105; 2001, Q3, P17-18

● **39.8** **Operations on carotid body, carotid sinus and other vascular bodies**
Excludes   *excision of glomus jugulare (20.51)*
Coding Clinic: 2007, Q2, P10-11

✖ **39.81** **Implantation or replacement of carotid sinus stimulation device, total system**
Carotid sinus baroreflex activation device
Implantation of carotid sinus stimulator and lead(s)
Includes   carotid explorations
Excludes   *implantation or replacement of carotid sinus stimulation lead(s) only (39.82)*
implantation or replacement of carotid sinus stimulation pulse generator only (39.83)

✖ **39.82** **Implantation or replacement of carotid sinus stimulation lead(s) only**
Excludes   *implantation or replacement of carotid sinus stimulation device, total system (39.81)*

✖ **39.83** **Implantation or replacement of carotid sinus stimulation pulse generator only**

> **Excludes** *implantation or replacement of carotid sinus stimulation device, total system (39.81)*
>
> Coding Clinic: 2010, Q4, P125

✖ **39.84** **Revision of carotid sinus stimulation lead(s) only**

Repair of electrode [removal with re-insertion]
Repositioning of lead(s) [electrode]
Coding Clinic: 2010, Q4, P124

✖ **39.85** **Revision of carotid sinus stimulation pulse generator**

Debridement and reforming pocket (skin and subcutaneous tissue)
Relocation of pocket [creation of new pocket]
Repositioning of pulse generator
Revision of carotid sinus stimulation pulse generator pocket

✖ **39.86** **Removal of carotid sinus stimulation device, total system**

✖ **39.87** **Removal of carotid sinus stimulation lead(s) only**

✖ **39.88** **Removal of carotid sinus stimulation pulse generator only**

✖ **39.89** **Other operations on carotid body, carotid sinus and other vascular bodies**

Chemodectomy
Denervation of:
    aortic body
    carotid body
Glomectomy, carotid

> **Excludes** *excision of glomus jugulare (20.51)*
>
> Coding Clinic: 2012, Q2, P10-11

● **39.9** **Other operations on vessels**

Coding Clinic: 1996, Q4, P63

39.90 **Insertion of non-drug-eluting, peripheral (non-coronary) vessel stent(s)**

Bare stent(s)
Bonded stent(s)
Drug-coated stent(s), i.e., heparin coated
Endograft(s)
Endovascular graft(s)
Endovascular recanalization techniques
Stent graft(s)

Code also any:
    non-coronary angioplasty or atherectomy (39.50)
    number of vascular stents inserted (00.45–00.48)
    number of vessels treated (00.40–00.43)
    procedure on vessel bifurcation (00.44)

> **Excludes** *insertion of drug-eluting peripheral vessel stent(s) (00.55)*
>   *percutaneous insertion of carotid artery stent(s) (00.63)*
>   *percutaneous insertion of intracranial stent(s) (00.65)*
>   *percutaneous insertion of other precerebral artery stent(s) (00.64)*
>   *that for aneurysm repair (39.71–39.79)*
>
> Coding Clinic: 2012, Q3, P13; 2009, Q3, P13; 2006, Q4, P119; 2001, Q2, P23-24; 2000, Q1, P12

✖ **39.91** **Freeing of vessel**

Dissection and freeing of adherent tissue:
    artery-vein-nerve bundle
    vascular bundle
Coding Clinic: 2002, Q3, P12-13

✖ **39.92** **Injection of sclerosing agent into vein**

> **Excludes** *injection:*
>   *esophageal varices (42.33)*
>   *hemorrhoids (49.42)*
>
> Coding Clinic: 1992, Q2, P17-18

✖ **39.93** **Insertion of vessel-to-vessel cannula**

Formation of:
    arteriovenous:
        fistula by external cannula
        shunt by external cannula

Code also any renal dialysis (39.95)
Coding Clinic: 1985, Sept-Oct, P12

✖ **39.94** **Replacement of vessel-to-vessel cannula**

Revision of vessel-to-vessel cannula

39.95 **Hemodialysis**

Artificial kidney   Hemofiltration
Hemodiafiltration   Renal dialysis

> **Excludes** *peritoneal dialysis (54.98)*
>
> Coding Clinic: 2008, Q4, P193; 2007, Q3, P11; 2004, Q1, P22; 2003, Q4, P111-112; 2001, Q2, P4-6, 13; 2000, Q4, P39-40; 1998, Q2, P20-21; 1986, Sept-Oct, P10-11

39.96 **Total body perfusion**

Code also substance perfused (99.21–99.29)

39.97 **Other perfusion**

Perfusion NOS
Perfusion, local [regional] of:
    carotid artery
    coronary artery
    head
    lower limb
    neck
    upper limb

Code also substance perfused (99.21–99.29)

> **Excludes** *perfusion of:*
>   *kidney (55.95)*
>   *large intestine (46.96)*
>   *liver (50.93)*
>   *small intestine (46.95)*
>   *SuperSaturated oxygen therapy (00.49)*
>
> Coding Clinic: 2013, Q3, P11; 2007, Q4, P103-104; 1996, Q3, P11-12

✖ **39.98** **Control of hemorrhage, not otherwise specified**

Angiotripsy
Control of postoperative hemorrhage NOS
Venotripsy

> **Excludes** *control of hemorrhage (postoperative):*
>   *anus (49.95)*
>   *bladder (57.93)*
>   *following vascular procedure (39.41)*
>   *nose (21.00–21.09)*
>   *prostate (60.94)*
>   *tonsil (28.7)*
>   *that by:*
>   *ligation (38.80–38.89)*
>   *suture (39.30–39.32)*

✖ **39.99** **Other operations on vessels**

> **Excludes** *injection or infusion of therapeutic or prophylactic substance (99.11–99.29)*
>   *transfusion of blood and blood components (99.01–99.09)*
>
> Coding Clinic: 1989, Q1, P11

OPERATIONS ON THE CARDIOVASCULAR SYSTEM (35–39)

Excludes   Includes   Use additional   Code also   Omit code

8. OPERATIONS ON THE HEMIC AND LYMPHATIC SYSTEM (40–41)

● **40 Operations on lymphatic system**
Coding Clinic: 1993, Q3, P12

✖ **40.0 Incision of lymphatic structures**

● **40.1 Diagnostic procedures on lymphatic structures**

✖ **40.11 Biopsy of lymphatic structure**
Transbronchoscopic needle aspiration [TBNA] of lymph node
Coding Clinic: 2010, Q3, P9; 2008, Q4, P90-91; 1984, Nov-Dec, P12

✖ **40.19 Other diagnostic procedures on lymphatic structures**
Excludes *lymphangiogram:*
abdominal (88.04)
cervical (87.08)
intrathoracic (87.34)
lower limb (88.36)
upper limb (88.34)
microscopic examination of specimen (90.71–90.79)
radioisotope scan (92.16)
thermography (88.89)

● **40.2 Simple excision of lymphatic structure**
Excludes *biopsy of lymphatic structure (40.11)*

✖ **40.21 Excision of deep cervical lymph node**

✖ **40.22 Excision of internal mammary lymph node**

✖ **40.23 Excision of axillary lymph node**
Coding Clinic: 2012, Q2, P4-5; 2002, Q2, P7

✖ **40.24 Excision of inguinal lymph node**

✖ **40.29 Simple excision of other lymphatic structure**
Excision of:
cystic hygroma
lymphangioma
Simple lymphadenectomy
Coding Clinic: 1999, Q1, P6

✖ **40.3 Regional lymph node excision**
Extended regional lymph node excision
Regional lymph node excision with excision of lymphatic drainage area including skin, subcutaneous tissue, and fat
Coding Clinic: 2012, Q1, P9-10; 1992, Q2, P7

● **40.4 Radical excision of cervical lymph nodes**
Resection of cervical lymph nodes down to muscle and deep fascia
Excludes *that associated with radical laryngectomy (30.4)*

✖ **40.40 Radical neck dissection, not otherwise specified**

✖ **40.41 Radical neck dissection, unilateral**
Coding Clinic: 2005, Q2, P8-9; 1999, Q2, P6-7

✖ **40.42 Radical neck dissection, bilateral**

● **40.5 Radical excision of other lymph nodes**
Excludes *that associated with radical mastectomy (85.45–85.48)*

✖ **40.50 Radical excision of lymph nodes, not otherwise specified**
Radical (lymph) node dissection NOS

✖ **40.51 Radical excision of axillary lymph nodes**

✖ **40.52 Radical excision of periaortic lymph nodes**

✖ **40.53 Radical excision of iliac lymph nodes**

✖ **40.54 Radical groin dissection**

✖ **40.59 Radical excision of other lymph nodes**
Excludes *radical neck dissection (40.40–40.42)*

● **40.6 Operations on thoracic duct**

✖ **40.61 Cannulation of thoracic duct**

✖ **40.62 Fistulization of thoracic duct**

✖ **40.63 Closure of fistula of thoracic duct**

✖ **40.64 Ligation of thoracic duct**

✖ **40.69 Other operations on thoracic duct**

✖ **40.9 Other operations on lymphatic structures**
Anastomosis of peripheral lymphatics
Dilation of peripheral lymphatics
Ligation of peripheral lymphatics
Obliteration of peripheral lymphatics
Reconstruction of peripheral lymphatics
Repair of peripheral lymphatics
Transplantation of peripheral lymphatics
Correction of lymphedema of limb, NOS
Excludes *reduction of elephantiasis of scrotum (61.3)*

● **41 Operations on bone marrow and spleen**
Coding Clinic: 1985, May-June, P18-19

● **41.0 Bone marrow or hematopoietic stem cell transplant**
Note: To report donor source - *see* codes 00.91–00.93
Excludes *aspiration of bone marrow from donor (41.91)*

✖ **41.00 Bone marrow transplant, not otherwise specified**

✖ **41.01 Autologous bone marrow transplant without purging**
Excludes *that with purging (41.09)*
MCE: Non-covered procedure only when principal or secondary diagnosis of 204.00, 205.00, 205.10, 205.11, 206.00, 207.00, 208.00

✖ **41.02 Allogeneic bone marrow transplant with purging**
Allograft of bone marrow with in vitro removal (purging) of T-cells
MCE: Non-covered procedure only when principal or secondary diagnosis of 203.00, 203.01

✖ **41.03 Allogeneic bone marrow transplant without purging**
Allograft of bone marrow NOS
MCE: Non-covered procedure only when principal or secondary diagnosis of 203.00, 203.01

✖ **41.04 Autologous hematopoietic stem cell transplant without purging**
Excludes *that with purging (41.07)*
MCE: Non-covered procedure only when principal or secondary diagnosis of 204.00, 205.00, 205.10, 205.11, 206.00, 207.00, 208.00

✖ **41.05 Allogeneic hematopoietic stem cell transplant without purging**
Excludes *that with purging (41.08)*
MCE: Non-covered procedure only when principal or secondary diagnosis of 203.00, 203.01
Coding Clinic: 2011, Q1, P24; 2009, Q1, P9

✖ **41.06 Cord blood stem cell transplant**

✖ **41.07 Autologous hematopoietic stem cell transplant with purging**
Cell depletion
MCE: Non-covered procedure only when principal or secondary diagnosis of 204.00, 205.00, 205.10, 205.11, 206.00, 207.00, 208.00
Coding Clinic: 2011, Q3, P6; 2006, Q2, P20-22

✖ **41.08 Allogeneic hematopoietic stem cell transplant**
Cell depletion
MCE: Non-covered procedure only when principal or secondary diagnosis of 203.00, 203.01

✖ **41.09 Autologous bone marrow transplant with purging**
With extracorporeal purging of malignant cells from marrow
Cell depletion
MCE: Non-covered procedure only when principal or secondary diagnosis of 204.00, 205.00, 205.10, 205.11, 206.00, 207.00, 208.00

41.1 Puncture of spleen
Excludes *aspiration biopsy of spleen (41.32)*

✖ **41.2 Splenotomy**

◀ New   ◀|||| Revised   ~~deleted~~ Deleted   ● Use Additional Digit(s)   ✖ Valid O.R. Procedure
◆ Non-O.R. Procedure   ♀ Females Only   ♂ Males Only   OGCR Official Guidelines   **Coding Clinic**

● 41.3   Diagnostic procedures on bone marrow and spleen

    41.31   Biopsy of bone marrow
        Coding Clinic: 1985, Jan-Feb, P15

    41.32   Closed [aspiration] [percutaneous] biopsy of spleen

    ✳ **41.33   Open biopsy of spleen**

    41.38   Other diagnostic procedures on bone marrow
        Excludes *microscopic examination of specimen from*
                bone marrow (90.61–90.69)
                radioisotope scan (92.05)

    41.39   Other diagnostic procedures on spleen
        Excludes *microscopic examination of specimen from*
                spleen (90.61–90.69)
                radioisotope scan (92.05)

● 41.4   Excision or destruction of lesion or tissue of spleen

    Code also any application or administration of an
    adhesion barrier substance (99.77)

    Excludes *excision of accessory spleen (41.93)*

    ✳ **41.41   Marsupialization of splenic cyst**

    ✳ **41.42   Excision of lesion or tissue of spleen**
        Excludes *biopsy of spleen (41.32–41.33)*

    ✳ **41.43   Partial splenectomy**

✳ 41.5   Total splenectomy
    Splenectomy NOS
    Code also any application or administration of an
    adhesion barrier substance (99.77)
        Coding Clinic: 2013, Q3, P12

● 41.9   Other operations on spleen and bone marrow
    Code also any application or administration of an
    adhesion barrier substance (99.77)

    41.91   Aspiration of bone marrow from donor for transplant
        Excludes *biopsy of bone marrow (41.31)*
        Coding Clinic: 1985, Jan-Feb, P15

    41.92   Injection into bone marrow
        Excludes *bone marrow transplant (41.00–41.03)*
        Coding Clinic: 1996, Q3, P17

    ✳ **41.93   Excision of accessory spleen**

    ✳ **41.94   Transplantation of spleen**

    ✳ **41.95   Repair and plastic operations on spleen**

    41.98   Other operations on bone marrow
        Coding Clinic: 2008, Q3, P19; 1994, Q3, P10

    ✳ **41.99   Other operations on spleen**

(See Plate 284 on page 81.)

9.   OPERATIONS ON THE DIGESTIVE SYSTEM (42–54)

● 42   Operations on esophagus

● 42.0   Esophagotomy

    ✳ **42.01   Incision of esophageal web**

    ✳ **42.09   Other incision of esophagus**
        Esophagotomy NOS
        Excludes *esophagomyotomy (42.7)*
                esophagostomy (42.10–42.19)

● 42.1   Esophagostomy

    ✳ **42.10   Esophagostomy, not otherwise specified**

    ✳ **42.11   Cervical esophagostomy**

    ✳ **42.12   Exteriorization of esophageal pouch**

    ✳ **42.19   Other external fistulization of esophagus**
        Thoracic esophagostomy
        Code also any resection (42.40–42.42)

● 42.2   Diagnostic procedures on esophagus

    ✳ **42.21   Operative esophagoscopy by incision**

    42.22   Esophagoscopy through artificial stoma
        Excludes *that with biopsy (42.24)*

    42.23   Other esophagoscopy
        Excludes *that with biopsy (42.24)*
        Coding Clinic: 2000, Q1, P20-21; 1998, Q3, P11

    42.24   Closed [endoscopic] biopsy of esophagus
        Brushing or washing for specimen collection
        Esophagoscopy with biopsy
        Suction biopsy of the esophagus
        Excludes *esophagogastroduodenoscopy [EGD] with*
                closed biopsy (45.16)

    ✳ **42.25   Open biopsy of esophagus**

    42.29   Other diagnostic procedures on esophagus
        Excludes *barium swallow (87.61)*
                esophageal manometry (89.32)
                microscopic examination of specimen from
                      esophagus (90.81–90.89)
        Coding Clinic: 1996, Q3, P12-13

● 42.3   Local excision or destruction of lesion or tissue of esophagus

    ✳ **42.31   Local excision of esophageal diverticulum**

    ✳ **42.32   Local excision of other lesion or tissue of esophagus**
        Excludes *biopsy of esophagus (42.24–42.25)*
                esophageal fistulectomy (42.84)

    42.33   Endoscopic excision or destruction of lesion or tissue of esophagus
        Ablation of esophageal neoplasm by endoscopic
            approach
        Control of esophageal bleeding by endoscopic
            approach
        Esophageal polypectomy by endoscopic approach
        Esophageal varices by endoscopic approach
        Injection of esophageal varices by endoscopic
            approach
        Excludes *biopsy of esophagus (42.24–42.25)*
                fistulectomy (42.84)
                open ligation of esophageal varices (42.91)
        Coding Clinic: 2012, Q4, P85

    ✳ **42.39   Other destruction of lesion or tissue of esophagus**
        Excludes *that by endoscopic approach (42.33)*

● 42.4   Excision of esophagus
    Excludes *esophagogastrectomy NOS (43.99)*

    ✳ **42.40   Esophagectomy, not otherwise specified**

    ✳ **42.41   Partial esophagectomy**
        Code also any synchronous:
            anastomosis other than end-to-end (42.51–42.69)
            esophagostomy (42.10–42.19)
            gastrostomy (43.11–43.19)

    ✳ **42.42   Total esophagectomy**
        Code also any synchronous:
            gastrostomy (43.11–43.19)
            interposition or anastomosis other than
                end-to-end (42.51–42.69)
        Excludes *esophagogastrectomy (43.99)*
        Coding Clinic: 1988, Q4, P11

Excludes   Includes   Use additional   Code also   Omit code

OPERATIONS ON THE DIGESTIVE SYSTEM (42–54)

● 42.5   **Intrathoracic anastomosis of esophagus**

> Code also any synchronous:
> esophagectomy (42.40–42.42)
> gastrostomy (43.1)

✖ 42.51   **Intrathoracic esophagoesophagostomy**

✖ 42.52   **Intrathoracic esophagogastrostomy**

✖ 42.53   **Intrathoracic esophageal anastomosis with interposition of small bowel**

✖ 42.54   **Other intrathoracic esophagoenterostomy**
> Anastomosis of esophagus to intestinal segment NOS

✖ 42.55   **Intrathoracic esophageal anastomosis with interposition of colon**

✖ 42.56   **Other intrathoracic esophagocolostomy**
> Esophagocolostomy NOS

✖ 42.58   **Intrathoracic esophageal anastomosis with other interposition**
> Construction of artificial esophagus
> Retrosternal formation of reversed gastric tube

✖ 42.59   **Other intrathoracic anastomosis of esophagus**
> Coding Clinic: 1988, Q4, P11

● 42.6   **Antesternal anastomosis of esophagus**

> Code also any synchronous:
> esophagectomy (42.40–42.42)
> gastrostomy (43.1)

✖ 42.61   **Antesternal esophagoesophagostomy**

✖ 42.62   **Antesternal esophagogastrostomy**

✖ 42.63   **Antesternal esophageal anastomosis with interposition of small bowel**

✖ 42.64   **Other antesternal esophagoenterostomy**
> Antethoracic:
> esophagoenterostomy
> esophagoileostomy
> esophagojejunostomy

✖ 42.65   **Antesternal esophageal anastomosis with interposition of colon**

✖ 42.66   **Other antesternal esophagocolostomy**
> Antethoracic esophagocolostomy

✖ 42.68   **Other antesternal esophageal anastomosis with interposition**

✖ 42.69   **Other antesternal anastomosis of esophagus**

✖ 42.7   **Esophagomyotomy**

● 42.8   **Other repair of esophagus**

42.81   **Insertion of permanent tube into esophagus**
> Coding Clinic: 1997, Q1, P15

✖ 42.82   **Suture of laceration of esophagus**

✖ 42.83   **Closure of esophagostomy**

✖ 42.84   **Repair of esophageal fistula, not elsewhere classified**
> **Excludes**   repair of fistula:
> bronchoesophageal (33.42)
> esophagopleurocutaneous (34.73)
> pharyngoesophageal (29.53)
> tracheoesophageal (31.73)

✖ 42.85   **Repair of esophageal stricture**

✖ 42.86   **Production of subcutaneous tunnel without esophageal anastomosis**

✖ 42.87   **Other graft of esophagus**
> **Excludes**   antesternal esophageal anastomosis with interposition of:
> colon (42.65)
> small bowel (42.63)
> antesternal esophageal anastomosis with other interposition (42.68)
> intrathoracic esophageal anastomosis with interposition of:
> colon (42.55)
> small bowel (42.53)
> intrathoracic esophageal anastomosis with other interposition (42.58)

✖ 42.89   **Other repair of esophagus**

● 42.9   **Other operations on esophagus**

✖ 42.91   **Ligation of esophageal varices**
> **Excludes**   that by endoscopic approach (42.33)

42.92   **Dilation of esophagus**
> Dilation of cardiac sphincter
> **Excludes**   intubation of esophagus (96.03, 96.06–96.08)

42.99   **Other**
> **Excludes**   insertion of Sengstaken tube (96.06)
> intubation of esophagus (96.03, 96.06–96.08)
> removal of intraluminal foreign body from esophagus without incision (98.02)
> tamponade of esophagus (96.06)

● 43   **Incision and excision of stomach**

> Code also any application or administration of an adhesion barrier substance (99.77)
> Coding Clinic: 1989, Q3, P14

✖ 43.0   **Gastrotomy**
> **Excludes**   gastrostomy (43.11–43.19)
> that for control of hemorrhage (44.49)

● 43.1   **Gastrostomy**

43.11   **Percutaneous [endoscopic] gastrostomy [PEG]**
> Percutaneous transabdominal gastrostomy
> Coding Clinic: 1994, Q2, P10-11

43.19   **Other gastrostomy**
> **Excludes**   percutaneous [endoscopic] gastrostomy [PEG] (43.11)
> Coding Clinic: 2012, Q2, P6; 1992, Q1, P13-14; 1989, Q3, P14

✖ 43.3   **Pyloromyotomy**

● 43.4   **Local excision or destruction of lesion or tissue of stomach**

43.41   **Endoscopic excision or destruction of lesion or tissue of stomach**
> Gastric polypectomy by endoscopic approach
> Gastric varices by endoscopic approach
> **Excludes**   biopsy of stomach (44.14–44.15)
> control of hemorrhage (44.43)
> open ligation of gastric varices (44.91)
> Coding Clinic: 1996, Q3, P10

✖ 43.42   **Local excision of other lesion or tissue of stomach**
> **Excludes**   biopsy of stomach (44.14–44.15)
> gastric fistulectomy (44.62–44.63)
> partial gastrectomy (43.5–43.89)

✖ 43.49   **Other destruction of lesion or tissue of stomach**
> **Excludes**   that by endoscopic approach (43.41)

✖ 43.5   **Partial gastrectomy with anastomosis to esophagus**
> Proximal gastrectomy

✖ 43.6   **Partial gastrectomy with anastomosis to duodenum**
> Billroth I operation
> Distal gastrectomy
> Gastropylorectomy

✖ 43.7   **Partial gastrectomy with anastomosis to jejunum**
> Billroth II operation
> Coding Clinic: 2003, Q3, P3-8

● 43.8   **Other partial gastrectomy**

✖ 43.81   **Partial gastrectomy with jejunal transposition**
> Henley jejunal transposition operation
> Code also any synchronous intestinal resection (45.51)

✖ 43.82   **Laparoscopic vertical (sleeve) gastrectomy**
> **Excludes**   laparoscopic banding (44.95)
> laparoscopic gastric restrictive procedure (44.95)
> MCE: Non-covered procedure

✖ 43.89   **Open and other partial gastrectomy**
> Partial gastrectomy with bypass gastrogastrostomy
> Sleeve resection of stomach
> **Excludes**   laparoscopic sleeve gastrectomy (43.82)
> Coding Clinic: 2003, Q3, P3-8

◀ New   ◀▥ Revised   ~~deleted~~ Deleted   ● Use Additional Digit(s)   ✖ Valid O.R. Procedure
◆ Non-O.R. Procedure   ♀ Females Only   ♂ Males Only   OGCR Official Guidelines   Coding Clinic

1244

● 43.9   **Total gastrectomy**
  ✖ 43.91   **Total gastrectomy with intestinal interposition**
  ✖ 43.99   **Other total gastrectomy**
        Complete gastroduodenectomy
        Esophagoduodenostomy with complete gastrectomy
        Esophagogastrectomy NOS
        Esophagojejunostomy with complete gastrectomy
        Radical gastrectomy

● 44   **Other operations on stomach**
      Code also any application or administration of an adhesion
        barrier substance (99.77)
● 44.0   **Vagotomy**
  ✖ 44.00   **Vagotomy, not otherwise specified**
        Division of vagus nerve NOS
  ✖ 44.01   **Truncal vagotomy**
  ✖ 44.02   **Highly selective vagotomy**
        Parietal cell vagotomy
        Selective proximal vagotomy
  ✖ 44.03   **Other selective vagotomy**
● 44.1   **Diagnostic procedures on stomach**
  ✖ 44.11   **Transabdominal gastroscopy**
        Intraoperative gastroscopy
        Excludes   *that with biopsy (44.14)*
    44.12   **Gastroscopy through artificial stoma**
        Excludes   *that with biopsy (44.14)*
    44.13   **Other gastroscopy**
        Excludes   *that with biopsy (44.14)*
    44.14   **Closed [endoscopic] biopsy of stomach**
        Brushing or washing for specimen collection
        Excludes   *esophagogastroduodenoscopy [EGD] with
                        closed biopsy (45.16)*
  ✖ 44.15   **Open biopsy of stomach**
    44.19   **Other diagnostic procedures on stomach**
        Excludes   *gastric lavage (96.33)
                        microscopic examination of specimen from
                          stomach (90.81–90.89)
                        upper GI series (87.62)*

● 44.2   **Pyloroplasty**
  ✖ 44.21   **Dilation of pylorus by incision**
    44.22   **Endoscopic dilation of pylorus**
        Dilation with balloon endoscope
        Endoscopic dilation of gastrojejunostomy site
        Coding Clinic: 2001, Q2, P17-18
  ✖ 44.29   **Other pyloroplasty**
        Pyloroplasty NOS
        Revision of pylorus
        Coding Clinic: 1999, Q3, P3
● 44.3   **Gastroenterostomy without gastrectomy**
  ✖ 44.31   **High gastric bypass**
        Printen and Mason gastric bypass
  ✖ 44.32   **Percutaneous [endoscopic] gastrojejunostomy**
        Bypass:
          gastroduodenostomy
        PEGJJ
        Excludes   *percutaneous (endoscopic) feeding
                        jejunostomy (46.32)*
  ✖ 44.38   **Laparoscopic gastroenterostomy** 🔗
        Bypass:
          gastroduodenostomy
          gastroenterostomy
          gastrogastrostomy
        Laparoscopic gastrojejunostomy without
          gastrectomy NEC
        Excludes   *gastroenterostomy, open approach (44.39)*
        Coding Clinic: 2004, Q4, P122

  ✖ 44.39   **Other gastroenterostomy** 🔗
        Bypass:
          gastroduodenostomy
          gastroenterostomy
          gastrogastrostomy
        Gastrojejunostomy without gastrectomy NOS
        Coding Clinic: 2003, Q3, P3-8; 2001, Q1, P16-17x2
● 44.4   **Control of hemorrhage and suture of ulcer of stomach or
      duodenum**
  ✖ 44.40   **Suture of peptic ulcer, not otherwise specified**
  ✖ 44.41   **Suture of gastric ulcer site**
        Excludes   *ligation of gastric varices (44.91)*
  ✖ 44.42   **Suture of duodenal ulcer site**
        Coding Clinic: 1987, Jan-Feb, P11
    44.43   **Endoscopic control of gastric or duodenal bleeding**
        Coding Clinic: 2004, Q2, P12-13; 1992, Q2, P17-18
    44.44   **Transcatheter embolization for gastric or duodenal
        bleeding**
        Excludes   *surgical occlusion of abdominal vessels
                        (38.86–38.87)*
    44.49   **Other control of hemorrhage of stomach or duodenum**
        That with gastrotomy
  ✖ 44.5   **Revision of gastric anastomosis**
        Closure of:
          gastric anastomosis
          gastroduodenostomy
          gastrojejunostomy
        Pantaloon operation
● 44.6   **Other repair of stomach**
  ✖ 44.61   **Suture of laceration of stomach**
        Excludes   *that of ulcer site (44.41)*
    44.62   **Closure of gastrostomy**
  ✖ 44.63   **Closure of other gastric fistula**
        Closure of:
          gastrocolic fistula
          gastrojejunocolic fistula
  ✖ 44.64   **Gastropexy**
  ✖ 44.65   **Esophagogastroplasty**
        Belsey operation
        Esophagus and stomach cardioplasty
  ✖ 44.66   **Other procedures for creation of esophagogastric
        sphincteric competence**
        Fundoplication
        Gastric cardioplasty
        Nissen's fundoplication
        Restoration of cardio-esophageal angle
        Excludes   *that by laparoscopy (44.67)*
        **Coding Clinic: 2012, Q3, P6; 2003, Q2, P12; 2001, Q2, P4, 5x2,
          6x3; 1998, Q3, P10**
  ✖ 44.67   **Laparoscopic procedures for creation of
        esophagogastric sphincteric competence**
        Fundoplication
        Gastric cardioplasty
        Nissen's fundoplication
        Restoration of cardio-esophageal angle
        Coding Clinic: 2004, Q4, P122
  ✖ 44.68   **Laparoscopic gastroplasty**
        Banding
        Silastic vertical banding
        Vertical banded gastroplasty (VBG)
        Code also any synchronous laparoscopic
          gastroenterostomy (44.38)
        Excludes   *insertion, laparoscopic adjustable gastric
                        band (restrictive procedure) (44.95)
                        other repair of stomach, open approach
                        (44.61–44.65, 44.69)*
        Coding Clinic: 2004, Q4, P123-124
  ✖ 44.69   **Other**
        Inversion of gastric diverticulum
        Repair of stomach NOS
        Coding Clinic: 2003, Q3, P3-8; 1999, Q3, P3; 1984, Nov-Dec, P13

Excludes   Includes   Use additional   Code also   Omit code

● **44.9   Other operations on stomach**
  ✖ **44.91   Ligation of gastric varices**
    Excludes   *that by endoscopic approach (43.41)*
  ✖ **44.92   Intraoperative manipulation of stomach**
    Reduction of gastric volvulus
  44.93   Insertion of gastric bubble (balloon)
    MCE: Non-covered procedure
  44.94   Removal of gastric bubble (balloon)
  ✖ **44.95   Laparoscopic gastric restrictive procedure** ✎
    Adjustable gastric band and port insertion
    Excludes   *laparoscopic gastroplasty (44.68)*
           other repair of stomach (44.69)
    Coding Clinic: 2004, Q4, P123-124
  ✖ **44.96   Laparoscopic revision of gastric restrictive procedure**
    Revision or replacement of:
      adjustable gastric band
      subcutaneous gastric port device
    Coding Clinic: 2004, Q4, P123-124
  ✖ **44.97   Laparoscopic removal of gastric restrictive device(s)**
    Removal of either or both:
      adjustable gastric band
      subcutaneous port device
    Excludes   *nonoperative removal of gastric restrictive*
           device(s) (97.86)
           open removal of gastric restrictive device(s)
           (44.99)
    Coding Clinic: 2004, Q4, P123-124
  ✖ **44.98   (Laparoscopic) adjustment of size of adjustable gastric restrictive device**
    Infusion of saline for device tightening
    Withdrawal of saline for device loosening
    Code also any:
      abdominal ultrasound (88.76)
      abdominal wall fluoroscopy (88.09)
      barium swallow (87.61)
    Coding Clinic: 2004, Q4, P123-124
  ✖ **44.99   Other**
    Excludes   *change of gastrostomy tube (97.02)*
           dilation of cardiac sphincter (42.92)
           gastric:
             cooling (96.31)
             freezing (96.32)
             gavage (96.35)
             hypothermia (96.31)
             lavage (96.33)
            insertion of nasogastric tube (96.07)
           irrigation of gastrostomy (96.36)
           irrigation of nasogastric tube (96.34)
           removal of:
             gastrostomy tube (97.51)
             intraluminal foreign body from stomach
               without incision (98.03)
            replacement of:
             gastrostomy tube (97.02)
             (naso-)gastric tube (97.01)
    Coding Clinic: 2004, Q3, P5; 1985, Jan-Feb, P14-15

● **45   Incision, excision, and anastomosis of intestine**
  Code also any application or administration of an adhesion
    barrier substance (99.77)
 ● **45.0   Enterotomy**
    Excludes   *duodenocholedochotomy (51.41–51.42, 51.51)*
           that for destruction of lesion (45.30–45.34)
           that of exteriorized intestine (46.14, 46.24, 46.31)
  ✖ **45.00   Incision of intestine, not otherwise specified**
  ✖ **45.01   Incision of duodenum**
  ✖ **45.02   Other incision of small intestine**
  ✖ **45.03   Incision of large intestine**
    Excludes   *proctotomy (48.0)*

● **45.1   Diagnostic procedures on small intestine**
  Code also any laparotomy (54.11–54.19)
  ✖ **45.11   Transabdominal endoscopy of small intestine**
    Intraoperative endoscopy of small intestine
    Excludes   *that with biopsy (45.14)*
  45.12   Endoscopy of small intestine through artificial stoma
    Excludes   *that with biopsy (45.14)*
  45.13   Other endoscopy of small intestine
    Esophagogastroduodenoscopy [EGD]
    Excludes   *that with biopsy (45.14, 45.16)*
    Coding Clinic: 2012, Q4, P84-85; 2004, Q3, P5
  45.14   Closed [endoscopic] biopsy of small intestine
    Brushing or washing for specimen collection
    Excludes   *esophagogastroduodenoscopy [EGD] with*
           closed biopsy (45.16)
  ✖ **45.15   Open biopsy of small intestine**
    Coding Clinic: 2005, Q2, P12; 2001, Q2, P9-11
  45.16   Esophagogastroduodenoscopy [EGD] with closed biopsy
    Biopsy of one or more sites involving esophagus,
      stomach, and/or duodenum
    Coding Clinic: 2005, Q3, P17-18
  45.19   Other diagnostic procedures on small intestine
    Excludes   *microscopic examination of specimen from*
           small intestine (90.91–90.99)
           radioisotope scan (92.04)
           ultrasonography (88.74)
           x-ray (87.61–87.69)

● **45.2   Diagnostic procedures on large intestine**
  Code also any laparotomy (54.11–54.19)
  ✖ **45.21   Transabdominal endoscopy of large intestine**
    Intraoperative endoscopy of large intestine
    Excludes   *that with biopsy (45.25)*
  45.22   Endoscopy of large intestine through artificial stoma
    Excludes   *that with biopsy (45.25)*
  45.23   Colonoscopy
    Flexible fiberoptic colonoscopy
    Excludes   *endoscopy of large intestine through*
           artificial stoma (45.22)
           flexible sigmoidoscopy (45.24)
           rigid proctosigmoidoscopy (48.23)
           transabdominal endoscopy of large intestine
             (45.21)
    Coding Clinic: 2005, Q3, P17-18; 1995, Q1, P3-4
  45.24   Flexible sigmoidoscopy
    Endoscopy of descending colon
    Excludes   *rigid proctosigmoidoscopy (48.23)*
  45.25   Closed [endoscopic] biopsy of large intestine
    Biopsy, closed, of unspecified intestinal site
    Brushing or washing for specimen collection
    Colonoscopy with biopsy
    Excludes   *proctosigmoidoscopy with biopsy (48.24)*
    Coding Clinic: 2003, Q1, P10-11
  ✖ **45.26   Open biopsy of large intestine**
  45.27   Intestinal biopsy, site unspecified
  45.28   Other diagnostic procedures on large intestine
  45.29   Other diagnostic procedures on intestine, site unspecified
    Excludes   *microscopic examination of specimen*
           (90.91–90.99)
           scan and radioisotope function study (92.04)
           ultrasonography (88.74)
           x-ray (87.61–87.69)

● **45.3**   **Local excision or destruction of lesion or tissue of small intestine**

    45.30   **Endoscopic excision or destruction of lesion of duodenum**

      Excludes   *biopsy of duodenum (45.14–45.15)*
          control of hemorrhage (44.43)
          fistulectomy (46.72)

    ✖ **45.31**   **Other local excision of lesion of duodenum**

      Excludes   *biopsy of duodenum (45.14–45.15)*
          fistulectomy (46.72)
          multiple segmental resection (45.61)
          that by endoscopic approach (45.30)

    ✖ **45.32**   **Other destruction of lesion of duodenum**

      Excludes   *that by endoscopic approach (45.30)*

    ✖ **45.33**   **Local excision of lesion or tissue of small intestine, except duodenum**
      Excision of redundant mucosa of ileostomy

      Excludes   *biopsy of small intestine (45.14–45.15)*
          fistulectomy (46.74)
          multiple segmental resection (45.61)

    ✖ **45.34**   **Other destruction of lesion of small intestine, except duodenum**
      Coding Clinic: 2012, Q3, P12

● **45.4**   **Local excision or destruction of lesion or tissue of large intestine**

    ✖ **45.41**   **Excision of lesion or tissue of large intestine**
      Excision of redundant mucosa of colostomy

      Excludes   *biopsy of large intestine (45.25–45.27)*
          endoscopic polypectomy of large intestine
          (45.42)
          fistulectomy (46.76)
          multiple segmental resection (17.31, 45.71)
          that by endoscopic approach (45.42–45.43)
      Coding Clinic: 1987, Nov-Dec, P11

    45.42   **Endoscopic polypectomy of large intestine**

      Excludes   *that by open approach (45.41)*
      Coding Clinic: 2011, Q3, P11; 2005, Q2, P16-17; 1990, Q2, P25

    45.43   **Endoscopic destruction of other lesion or tissue of large intestine**
      Endoscopic ablation of tumor of large intestine
      Endoscopic control of colonic bleeding

      Excludes   *endoscopic polypectomy of large intestine*
          (45.42)
      Coding Clinic: 2002, Q4, P61

    ✖ **45.49**   **Other destruction of lesion of large intestine**

      Excludes   *that by endoscopic approach (45.43)*
      Coding Clinic: 1987, Nov-Dec, P11

● **45.5**   **Isolation of intestinal segment**

      Code also any synchronous:
      anastomosis other than end-to-end (45.90–45.94)
      enterostomy (46.10–46.39)

    ✖ **45.50**   **Isolation of intestinal segment, not otherwise specified**
      Isolation of intestinal pedicle flap
      Reversal of intestinal segment

    ✖ **45.51**   **Isolation of segment of small intestine**
      Isolation of ileal loop
      Resection of small intestine for interposition
      Coding Clinic: 2005, Q2, P12-13x2; 2003, Q3, P3-8; Q2, P11-12; 2000, Q3, P7-8

    ✖ **45.52**   **Isolation of segment of large intestine**
      Resection of colon for interposition

● **45.6**   **Other excision of small intestine**

      Code also any synchronous:
      anastomosis other than end-to-end (45.90–45.93, 45.95)
      colostomy (46.10–46.13)
      enterostomy (46.10–46.39)

      Excludes   *cecectomy (17.32, 45.72)*
          enterocolectomy (17.39, 45.79)
          gastroduodenectomy (43.6–43.99)
          ileocolectomy (17.33, 45.73)
          pancreatoduodenectomy (52.51–52.7)

    ✖ **45.61**   **Multiple segmental resection of small intestine**
      Segmental resection for multiple traumatic lesions of small intestine

    ✖ **45.62**   **Other partial resection of small intestine**
      Duodenectomy
      Ileectomy
      Jejunectomy

      Excludes   *duodenectomy with synchronous*
          pancreatectomy (52.51–52.7)
          resection of cecum and terminal ileum
          (17.32, 45.72)
      Coding Clinic: 2010, Q1, P12; 2004, Q1, P10-11; 2003, Q1, P18

    ✖ **45.63**   **Total removal of small intestine**

● **45.7**   **Open and other partial excision of large intestine**

      Code also any synchronous:
      anastomosis other than end-to-end (45.92–45.94)
      enterostomy (46.10–46.39)

      Excludes   *laparoscopic partial excision of large intestine*
          (17.31–17.39)
      Coding Clinic: 2009, Q1, P10x2

    ✖ **45.71**   **Open and other multiple segmental resection of large intestine**
      Segmental resection for multiple traumatic lesions of large intestine

    ✖ **45.72**   **Open and other cecectomy**
      Resection of cecum and terminal ileum

    ✖ **45.73**   **Open and other right hemicolectomy**
      Ileocolectomy
      Right radical colectomy
      Coding Clinic: 2011, Q1, P15; 1999, Q3, P10-11

    ✖ **45.74**   **Open and other resection of transverse colon**

    ✖ **45.75**   **Open and other left hemicolectomy**

      Excludes   *proctosigmoidectomy (48.41–48.69)*
          second stage Mikulicz operation (46.04)
      Coding Clinic: 2002, Q4, P105-106

    ✖ **45.76**   **Open and other sigmoidectomy**
      Coding Clinic: 2010, Q3, P12; 1996, Q1, P9; 1989, Q3, P15; 2002, Q4, P105-106

    ✖ **45.79**   **Other and unspecified partial excision of large intestine**
      Enterocolectomy NEC
      Coding Clinic: 2009, Q1, P11; 2003, Q1, P18; 1997, Q3, P9-10; 1991, Q1, P11

● **45.8**   **Total intra-abdominal colectomy**
      Excision of cecum, colon, and sigmoid

      Excludes   *coloproctectomy (48.41–48.69)*
      Coding Clinic: 2013, Q2, P20-21; 2008, Q4, P169-172

    ✖ **45.81**   **Laparoscopic total intra-abdominal colectomy**

    ✖ **45.82**   **Open total intra-abdominal colectomy**

    ✖ **45.83**   **Other and unspecified total intra-abdominal colectomy**

OPERATIONS ON THE DIGESTIVE SYSTEM (42–54)

Excludes   Includes   Use additional   Code also   Omit code

OPERATIONS ON THE DIGESTIVE SYSTEM (42–54)

● **45.9 Intestinal anastomosis**

Code also any synchronous resection (45.31–45.8, 48.41–48.69)

> **Excludes**   *end-to-end anastomosis — omit code*

Coding Clinic: 1999, Q3, P10-11

�% **45.90 Intestinal anastomosis, not otherwise specified**

�% **45.91 Small-to-small intestinal anastomosis**
Coding Clinic: 2010, Q1, P12; 2003, Q3, P3-8

�% **45.92 Anastomosis of small intestine to rectal stump**
Hampton procedure
Coding Clinic: 2009, Q1, P5

�% **45.93 Other small-to-large intestinal anastomosis**
Coding Clinic: 2009, Q1, P5; 2003, Q1, P18; 1986, Nov-Dec, P11

�% **45.94 Large-to-large intestinal anastomosis**

> **Excludes**   *rectorectostomy (48.74)*

Coding Clinic: 2009, Q1, P5; 1989, Q3, P15

�% **45.95 Anastomosis to anus**
Formation of endorectal ileal pouch (H-pouch)
(J-pouch) (S-pouch) with anastomosis of small
intestine to anus
Coding Clinic: 2013, Q2, P20; 2005, Q2, P13-14

● **46 Other operations on intestine**

Code also any application or administration of an adhesion
barrier substance (99.77)

● **46.0 Exteriorization of intestine**

> **Includes**   loop enterostomy
> multiple stage resection of intestine

�% **46.01 Exteriorization of small intestine**
Loop ileostomy
Coding Clinic: 2013, Q2, P20-21

�% **46.02 Resection of exteriorized segment of small intestine**

�% **46.03 Exteriorization of large intestine**
Exteriorization of intestine NOS
First stage Mikulicz exteriorization of intestine
Loop colostomy

�% **46.04 Resection of exteriorized segment of large intestine**
Resection of exteriorized segment of intestine NOS
Second stage Mikulicz operation

● **46.1 Colostomy**

Code also any synchronous resection (45.49, 45.71–45.79, 45.8)

> **Excludes**   *loop colostomy (46.03)*
> *that with abdominoperineal resection of rectum (48.5)*
> *that with synchronous anterior rectal resection (48.62)*

�% **46.10 Colostomy, not otherwise specified**

�% **46.11 Temporary colostomy**

�% **46.13 Permanent colostomy**

   46.14 Delayed opening of colostomy

● **46.2 Ileostomy**

Code also any synchronous resection (45.34, 45.61–45.63)

> **Excludes**   *loop ileostomy (46.01)*

�% **46.20 Ileostomy, not otherwise specified**

�% **46.21 Temporary ileostomy**

�% **46.22 Continent ileostomy**

�% **46.23 Other permanent ileostomy**

   46.24 Delayed opening of ileostomy

● **46.3 Other enterostomy**

Code also any synchronous resection (45.61–45.8)

   46.31 Delayed opening of other enterostomy

   46.32 Percutaneous (endoscopic) jejunostomy [PEJ]
Endoscopic conversion of gastrostomy to
jejunostomy
Percutaneous (endoscopic) feeding enterostomy

> **Excludes**   *percutaneous [endoscopic]*
> *gastrojejunostomy (bypass) (44.32)*

Coding Clinic: 2010, Q3, P13

   46.39 Other
Duodenostomy
Feeding enterostomy
Coding Clinic: 1989, Q3, P15

● **46.4 Revision of intestinal stoma**

�% **46.40 Revision of intestinal stoma, not otherwise specified**
Plastic enlargement of intestinal stoma
Reconstruction of stoma of intestine
Release of scar tissue of intestinal stoma

> **Excludes**   *excision of redundant mucosa (45.41)*

�% **46.41 Revision of stoma of small intestine**

> **Excludes**   *excision of redundant mucosa (45.33)*

Coding Clinic: 2005, Q2, P11-12

�% **46.42 Repair of pericolostomy hernia**

�% **46.43 Other revision of stoma of large intestine**

> **Excludes**   *excision of redundant mucosa (45.41)*

Coding Clinic: 2002, Q2, P9-10

● **46.5 Closure of intestinal stoma**

Code also any synchronous resection (45.34, 45.49,
45.61–45.8)

�% **46.50 Closure of intestinal stoma, not otherwise specified**

�% **46.51 Closure of stoma of small intestine**

�% **46.52 Closure of stoma of large intestine**
Closure or take-down of:
cecostomy
colostomy
sigmoidostomy
Coding Clinic: 2009, Q1, P5; 2005, Q2, P4-5; 1997, Q3, P9-10;
1987, Nov-Dec, P8

● **46.6 Fixation of intestine**

�% **46.60 Fixation of intestine, not otherwise specified**
Fixation of intestine to abdominal wall

�% **46.61 Fixation of small intestine to abdominal wall**
Ileopexy

�% **46.62 Other fixation of small intestine**
Noble plication of small intestine
Plication of jejunum

�% **46.63 Fixation of large intestine to abdominal wall**
Cecocoloplicopexy
Sigmoidopexy (Moschowitz)

�% **46.64 Other fixation of large intestine**
Cecofixation
Colofixation

● **46.7 Other repair of intestine**

> **Excludes**   *closure of:*
> *ulcer of duodenum (44.42)*
> *vesicoenteric fistula (57.83)*

�% **46.71 Suture of laceration of duodenum**

�% **46.72 Closure of fistula of duodenum**

�% **46.73 Suture of laceration of small intestine, except
duodenum**
Coding Clinic: 2010, Q1, P12

�% **46.74 Closure of fistula of small intestine, except duodenum**

> **Excludes**   *closure of:*
> *artificial stoma (46.51)*
> *vaginal fistula (70.74)*
> *repair of gastrojejunocolic fistula (44.63)*

�% **46.75 Suture of laceration of large intestine**

�% **46.76 Closure of fistula of large intestine**

> **Excludes**   *closure of:*
> *gastrocolic fistula (44.63)*
> *rectal fistula (48.73)*
> *sigmoidovesical fistula (57.83)*
> *stoma (46.52)*
> *vaginal fistula (70.72–70.73)*
> *vesicocolic fistula (57.83)*
> *vesicosigmoidovaginal fistula (57.83)*

Coding Clinic: 1999, Q3, P8

�% **46.79 Other repair of intestine**
Duodenoplasty
Coding Clinic: 2011, Q3, P14

◀ New   ◀▥ Revised   ~~deleted~~ Deleted   ● Use Additional Digit(s)   ✕ Valid O.R. Procedure
◆ Non-O.R. Procedure   ♀ Females Only   ♂ Males Only   OGCR Official Guidelines   **Coding Clinic**

● **46.8 Dilation and manipulation of intestine**
Coding Clinic: 2003, Q1, P14-15; 1998, Q43, P82-83

✖ **46.80 Intra-abdominal manipulation of intestine, not otherwise specified**
Correction of intestinal malrotation
Reduction of:
intestinal torsion
intestinal volvulus
intussusception

Excludes *reduction of intussusception with:*
fluoroscopy (96.29)
ionizing radiation enema (96.29)
ultrasonography guidance (96.29)

✖ **46.81 Intra-abdominal manipulation of small intestine**
Coding Clinic: 2013, Q2, P4

✖ **46.82 Intra-abdominal manipulation of large intestine**
Coding Clinic: 2013, Q2, P4

46.85 Dilation of intestine
Dilation (balloon) of duodenum
Dilation (balloon) of jejunum
Endoscopic dilation (balloon) of large intestine
That through rectum or colostomy

Excludes *with insertion of colonic stent (46.86–46.87)*
Coding Clinic: 2007, Q3, P6-7; 1989, Q3, P15

46.86 Endoscopic insertion of colonic stent(s)
Colonoscopy (flexible) (through stoma) with
transendoscopic stent placement
Combined with fluoroscopic-guided insertion
Stent endoprosthesis of colon
Through the scope [TTS] technique

Excludes *other non-endoscopic insertion of colonic stent (46.87)*
Coding Clinic: 2009, Q4, P148

46.87 Other insertion of colonic stent(s)
Includes that by:
fluoroscopic guidance only
rectal guiding tube
non-endoscopic insertion

Code also any synchronous diagnostic procedure(s)

Excludes *endoscopic insertion of colonic stent (46.86)*

● **46.9 Other operations on intestines**

✖ **46.91 Myotomy of sigmoid colon**

✖ **46.92 Myotomy of other parts of colon**

✖ **46.93 Revision of anastomosis of small intestine**

✖ **46.94 Revision of anastomosis of large intestine**

46.95 Local perfusion of small intestine
Code also substance perfused (99.21–99.29)

46.96 Local perfusion of large intestine
Code also substance perfused (99.21–99.29)

✖ **46.97 Transplant of intestine**
Note: To report donor source - *see* codes
00.91–00.93
MCE: Limited coverage

✖ **46.99 Other**
Ileoentectomy

Excludes *diagnostic procedures on intestine*
(45.11–45.29)
dilation of enterostomy stoma (96.24)
intestinal intubation (96.08)
removal of:
intraluminal foreign body from large
intestine without incision (98.04)
intraluminal foreign body from small
intestine without incision (98.03)
tube from large intestine (97.53)
tube from small intestine (97.52)
replacement of:
large intestine tube or enterostomy device
(97.04)
small intestine tube or enterostomy
device (97.03)
Coding Clinic: 1999, Q3, P11; 1989, Q1, P11

● **47 Operations on appendix**
Includes appendiceal stump
Code also any application or administration of an adhesion
barrier substance (99.77)

● **47.0 Appendectomy**
Excludes *incidental appendectomy, so described*
laparoscopic (47.11)
other (47.19)
Coding Clinic: 1992, Q3, P12

✖ **47.01 Laparoscopic appendectomy**
Coding Clinic: 2001, Q1, P15-16; 1996, Q4, P64-65

✖ **47.09 Other appendectomy**
Coding Clinic: 1997, Q4, P52

● **47.1 Incidental appendectomy**
Coding Clinic: 1987, Jan-Feb, P11-12

✖ **47.11 Laparoscopic incidental appendectomy**

✖ **47.19 Other incidental appendectomy**
Coding Clinic: 2013, Q2, P4; 1996, Q4, P64-65;
1984, Nov-Dec, P12

✖ **47.2 Drainage of appendiceal abscess**
Excludes *that with appendectomy (47.0)*

● **47.9 Other operations on appendix**

✖ **47.91 Appendicostomy**

✖ **47.92 Closure of appendiceal fistula**

✖ **47.99 Other**
Anastomosis of appendix
Excludes *diagnostic procedures on appendix*
(45.21–45.29)
Coding Clinic: 2001, Q3, P16

● **48 Operations on rectum, rectosigmoid and perirectal tissue**
Code also any application or administration of an adhesion
barrier substance (99.77)
Coding Clinic: 1999, Q3, P8-9

✖ **48.0 Proctotomy**
Decompression of imperforate anus
Panas' operation [linear proctotomy]
Excludes *incision of perirectal tissue (48.81)*

✖ **48.1 Proctostomy**

● **48.2 Diagnostic procedures on rectum, rectosigmoid and
perirectal tissue**

✖ **48.21 Transabdominal proctosigmoidoscopy**
Intraoperative proctosigmoidoscopy
Excludes *that with biopsy (48.24)*

48.22 Proctosigmoidoscopy through artificial stoma
Excludes *that with biopsy (48.24)*

48.23 Rigid proctosigmoidoscopy
Excludes *flexible sigmoidoscopy (45.24)*
Coding Clinic: 2001, Q1, P8

48.24 Closed [endoscopic] biopsy of rectum
Brushing or washing for specimen collection
Proctosigmoidoscopy with biopsy
Coding Clinic: 2003, Q1, P12

✖ **48.25 Open biopsy of rectum**

48.26 Biopsy of perirectal tissue

**48.29 Other diagnostic procedures on rectum, rectosigmoid
and perirectal tissue**
Excludes *digital examination of rectum (89.34)*
lower GI series (87.64)
microscopic examination of specimen from
rectum (90.91–90.99)

● **48.3 Local excision or destruction of lesion or tissue of rectum**

48.31 Radical electrocoagulation of rectal lesion or tissue

48.32 Other electrocoagulation of rectal lesion or tissue
Coding Clinic: 1998, Q2, P18; 1987, Nov-Dec, P11

48.33 Destruction of rectal lesion or tissue by laser

48.34 Destruction of rectal lesion or tissue by cryosurgery

OPERATIONS ON THE DIGESTIVE SYSTEM (42–54)

| Excludes | Includes | Use additional | Code also | Omit code |

✖48.35 Local excision of rectal lesion or tissue
    Excludes *biopsy of rectum (48.24–48.25)*
      excision of perirectal tissue (48.82)
      hemorrhoidectomy (49.46)
      [endoscopic] polypectomy of rectum (48.36)
      rectal fistulectomy (48.73)

  48.36 [Endoscopic] polypectomy of rectum

●48.4 Pull-through resection of rectum
    Code also any synchronous anastomosis other than
    end-to-end (45.90, 45.92–45.95)
    Coding Clinic: 2008, Q4, P169-172

✖48.40 Pull-through resection of rectum, not otherwise
    specified
    Pull-through resection NOS
    Excludes *abdominoperineal pull-through NOS (48.50)*

✖48.41 Soave submucosal resection of rectum
    Endorectal pull-through operation

✖48.42 Laparoscopic pull-through resection of rectum

✖48.43 Open pull-through resection of rectum

✖48.49 Other pull-through resection of rectum
    Abdominoperineal pull-through
    Altemeier operation
    Swenson proctectomy
    Excludes *Duhamel abdominoperineal pull-through*
      (48.65)
      laparoscopic pull-through resection of
      rectum (48.42)
      open pull-through resection of rectum
      (48.43)
      pull-through resection of rectum, not
      otherwise specified (48.40)
    Coding Clinic: 2001, Q3, P8-9; 1999, Q2, P13

●48.5 Abdominoperineal resection of rectum
    Combined abdominoendorectal resection
    Complete proctectomy
    Includes with synchronous colostomy
    Code also any synchronous anastomosis other than
    end-to-end (45.90, 45.92–45.95)
    Excludes *Duhamel abdominoperineal pull-through (48.65)*
      that as part of pelvic exenteration (68.8)
    Coding Clinic: 2013, Q2, P20-21; 1997, Q2, P5

✖48.50 Abdominoperineal resection of the rectum, not
    otherwise specified

✖48.51 Laparoscopic abdominoperineal resection of the
    rectum

✖48.52 Open abdominoperineal resection of the rectum

✖48.59 Other abdominoperineal resection of the rectum
    Excludes *abdominoperineal resection of the rectum,*
      NOS (48.50)
      laparoscopic abdominoperineal resection of
      the rectum (48.51)
      open abdominoperineal resection of the
      rectum (48.52)

●48.6 Other resection of rectum
    Code also any synchronous anastomosis other than
    end-to-end (45.90, 45.92–45.95)

✖48.61 Transsacral rectosigmoidectomy

✖48.62 Anterior resection of rectum with synchronous
    colostomy
    Coding Clinic: 1997, Q2, P5

✖48.63 Other anterior resection of rectum
    Excludes *that with synchronous colostomy (48.62)*
    Coding Clinic: 1996, Q1, P9

✖48.64 Posterior resection of rectum

✖48.65 Duhamel resection of rectum
    Duhamel abdominoperineal pull-through

✖48.69 Other
    Partial proctectomy
    Rectal resection NOS
    Coding Clinic: 2005, Q2, P13-14; 1987, Jan-Feb, P11; 1986,
    Nov-Dec, P11

●48.7 Repair of rectum
    Excludes *repair of:*
      current obstetric laceration (75.62)
      vaginal rectocele (70.50, 70.52, 70.53, 70.55)

✖48.71 Suture of laceration of rectum

✖48.72 Closure of proctostomy

✖48.73 Closure of other rectal fistula
    Excludes *fistulectomy:*
      perirectal (48.93)
      rectourethral (58.43)
      rectovaginal (70.73)
      rectovesical (57.83)
      rectovesicovaginal (57.83)

✖48.74 Rectorectostomy
    Rectal anastomosis NOS
    Stapled transanal rectal resection (STARR)

✖48.75 Abdominal proctopexy
    Frickman procedure
    Ripstein repair of rectal prolapse

✖48.76 Other proctopexy
    Delorme repair of prolapsed rectum
    Proctosigmoidopexy
    Puborectalis sling operation
    Excludes *manual reduction of rectal prolapse (96.26)*

✖48.79 Other repair of rectum
    Repair of old obstetric laceration of rectum
    Excludes *anastomosis to:*
      large intestine (45.94)
      small intestine (45.92–45.93)
      repair of:
      current obstetrica laceration (75.62)
      vaginal rectocele (70.50, 70.52)

●48.8 Incision or excision of perirectal tissue or lesion
    Includes pelvirectal tissue
      rectovaginal septum

✖48.81 Incision of perirectal tissue
    Incision of rectovaginal septum

✖48.82 Excision of perirectal tissue
    Excludes *perirectal biopsy (48.26)*
      perirectofistulectomy (48.93)
      rectal fistulectomy (48.73)

●48.9 Other operations on rectum and perirectal tissue

✖48.91 Incision of rectal stricture

✖48.92 Anorectal myectomy

✖48.93 Repair of perirectal fistula
    Excludes *that opening into rectum (48.73)*
    Coding Clinic: 2007, Q1, P13

✖48.99 Other
    Excludes *digital examination of rectum (89.34)*
      dilation of rectum (96.22)
      insertion of rectal tube (96.09)
      irrigation of rectum (96.38–96.39)
      manual reduction of rectal prolapse (96.26)
      proctoclysis (96.37)
      rectal massage (99.93)
      rectal packing (96.19)
      removal of:
      impacted feces (96.38)
      intraluminal foreign body from rectum
      without incision (98.05)
      rectal packing (97.59)
      transanal enema (96.39)

OPERATIONS ON THE DIGESTIVE SYSTEM (42–54)

◀ New   ◀ Revised   deleted Deleted   ● Use Additional Digit(s)   ✖ Valid O.R. Procedure
◆ Non-O.R. Procedure   ♀ Females Only   ♂ Males Only   OGCR Official Guidelines   Coding Clinic

● **49 Operations on anus**

Code also any application or administration of an adhesion barrier substance (99.77)

● **49.0 Incision or excision of perianal tissue**

✖ **49.01 Incision of perianal abscess**
Coding Clinic: 2005, Q2, P10

✖ **49.02 Other incision of perianal tissue**
Undercutting of perianal tissue

Excludes *anal fistulotomy (49.11)*

49.03 Excision of perianal skin tags

✖ **49.04 Other excision of perianal tissue**

Excludes *anal fistulectomy (49.12)*
biopsy of perianal tissue (49.22)
Coding Clinic: 2001, Q1, P8

● **49.1 Incision or excision of anal fistula**

Excludes *closure of anal fistula (49.73)*

✖ **49.11 Anal fistulotomy**

✖ **49.12 Anal fistulectomy**

● **49.2 Diagnostic procedures on anus and perianal tissue**

49.21 Anoscopy

49.22 Biopsy of perianal tissue

49.23 Biopsy of anus

49.29 Other diagnostic procedures on anus and perianal tissue

Excludes *microscopic examination of specimen from anus (90.91–90.99)*

● **49.3 Local excision or destruction of other lesion or tissue of anus**
Anal cryptotomy
Cauterization of lesion of anus

Excludes *biopsy of anus (49.23)*
control of (postoperative) hemorrhage of anus (49.95)
hemorrhoidectomy (49.46)

49.31 Endoscopic excision or destruction of lesion or tissue of anus

✖ **49.39 Other local excision or destruction of lesion or tissue of anus**

Excludes *that by endoscopic approach (49.31)*
Coding Clinic: 2001, Q1, P8

● **49.4 Procedures on hemorrhoids**

49.41 Reduction of hemorrhoids

49.42 Injection of hemorrhoids

49.43 Cauterization of hemorrhoids
Clamp and cautery of hemorrhoids

✖ **49.44 Destruction of hemorrhoids by cryotherapy**

✖ **49.45 Ligation of hemorrhoids**
Coding Clinic: 2012, Q4, P81-82

✖ **49.46 Excision of hemorrhoids**
Hemorrhoidectomy NOS
Coding Clinic: 2007, Q1, P13

49.47 Evacuation of thrombosed hemorrhoids

✖ **49.49 Other procedures on hemorrhoids**
Lord procedure

● **49.5 Division of anal sphincter**

✖ **49.51 Left lateral anal sphincterotomy**

✖ **49.52 Posterior anal sphincterotomy**

✖ **49.59 Other anal sphincterotomy**
Division of sphincter NOS

✖ **49.6 Excision of anus**

● **49.7 Repair of anus**

Excludes *repair of current obstetric laceration (75.62)*

✖ **49.71 Suture of laceration of anus**

✖ **49.72 Anal cerclage**

✖ **49.73 Closure of anal fistula**

Excludes *excision of anal fistula (49.12)*

✖ **49.74 Gracilis muscle transplant for anal incontinence**

✖ **49.75 Implantation or revision of artificial anal sphincter**
Removal with subsequent replacement
Replacement during same or subsequent operative episode

✖ **49.76 Removal of artificial anal sphincter**
Explantation or removal without replacement

Excludes *revision with implantation during same operative episode (49.75)*

✖ **49.79 Other repair of anal sphincter**
Repair of old obstetric laceration of anus

Excludes *anoplasty with synchronous hemorrhoidectomy (49.46)*
repair of current obstetric laceration (75.62)
Coding Clinic: 1998, Q2, P16-17; 1997, Q1, P9-10

● **49.9 Other operations on anus**

Excludes *dilation of anus (sphincter) (96.23)*

✖ **49.91 Incision of anal septum**

✖ **49.92 Insertion of subcutaneous electrical anal stimulator**

✖ **49.93 Other incision of anus**
Removal of:
foreign body from anus with incision
seton from anus

Excludes *anal fistulotomy (49.11)*
removal of intraluminal foreign body without incision (98.05)

✖ **49.94 Reduction of anal prolapse**

Excludes *manual reduction of rectal prolapse (96.26)*

✖ **49.95 Control of (postoperative) hemorrhage of anus**

✖ **49.99 Other**

● **50 Operations on liver**

Code also any application or administration of an adhesion barrier substance (99.77)

✖ **50.0 Hepatotomy**
Incision of abscess of liver
Removal of gallstones from liver
Stromeyer-Little operation

● **50.1 Diagnostic procedures on liver**

50.11 Closed (percutaneous) [needle] biopsy of liver
Diagnostic aspiration of liver
Coding Clinic: 2005, Q3, P24; 1994, Q3, P11; 1988, Q4, P12

✖ **50.12 Open biopsy of liver**
Wedge biopsy
Coding Clinic: 2005, Q2, P13-14; 1984, Nov-Dec, P12

50.13 Transjugular liver biopsy
Transvenous liver biopsy

Excludes *closed (percutaneous) [needle] biopsy of liver (50.11)*
laparoscopic liver biopsy (50.14)
Coding Clinic: 2007, Q4, P113-114

✖ **50.14 Laparoscopic liver biopsy**

Excludes *closed (percutaneous) [needle] biopsy of liver (50.11)*
open biopsy of liver (50.12)
transjugular liver biopsy (50.13)
Coding Clinic: 2007, Q4, P113-114

✖ **50.19 Other diagnostic procedures on liver**

Excludes *laparoscopic liver biopsy (50.14)*
liver scan and radioisotope function study (92.02)
microscopic examination of specimen from liver (91.01–91.09)
transjugular liver biopsy (50.13)

Excludes   Includes   Use additional   Code also   Omit code

● **50.2　Local excision or destruction of liver tissue or lesion**
　　Coding Clinic: 2006, Q4, P124-126

✖ **50.21　Marsupialization of lesion of liver**

✖ **50.22　Partial hepatectomy**
　　Wedge resection of liver
　　Excludes　*biopsy of liver (50.11–50.12)*
　　　　　　　　hepatic lobectomy (50.3)

✖ **50.23　Open ablation of liver lesion or tissue**

✖ **50.24　Percutaneous ablation of liver lesion or tissue**

✖ **50.25　Laparoscopic ablation of liver lesion or tissue**

✖ **50.26　Other and unspecified ablation of liver lesion or tissue**

✖ **50.29　Other destruction of lesion of liver**
　　Cauterization of hepatic lesion
　　Enucleation of hepatic lesion
　　Evacuation of hepatic lesion
　　Excludes　*ablation of liver lesion or tissue:*
　　　　　　　　laparoscopic (50.25)
　　　　　　　　open (50.23)
　　　　　　　　other (50.26)
　　　　　　　　percutaneous (50.24)
　　　　　　　　laser interstitial thermal therapy [LITT]
　　　　　　　　　of lesion or tissue of liver under
　　　　　　　　　guidance (17.63)
　　　　　　　　percutaneous aspiration of lesion (50.91)
　　Coding Clinic: 2013, Q2, P13; 2003, Q2, P9

✖ **50.3　Lobectomy of liver**
　　Total hepatic lobectomy with partial excision of other lobe

✖ **50.4　Total hepatectomy**
　　Coding Clinic: 2008, Q2, P8-9

● **50.5　Liver transplant**
　　Note:　To report donor source - *see* codes 00.91–00.93

✖ **50.51　Auxiliary liver transplant**
　　Auxiliary hepatic transplantation leaving patient's
　　　own liver in situ
　　MCE: Non-Covered procedure

✖ **50.59　Other transplant of liver**
　　MCE: Limited coverage
　　Coding Clinic: 2013, Q2, P13; 2008, Q4, P120; Q2, P8-9

● **50.6　Repair of liver**

✖ **50.61　Closure of laceration of liver**

✖ **50.69　Other repair of liver**
　　Hepatopexy

● **50.9　Other operations on liver**
　　Excludes　*lysis of adhesions (54.5)*

50.91　Percutaneous aspiration of liver
　　Excludes　*percutaneous biopsy (50.11)*

50.92　Extracorporeal hepatic assistance
　　Liver dialysis
　　Coding Clinic: 2001, Q2, P21-22

50.93　Localized perfusion of liver

50.94　Other injection of therapeutic substance into liver

50.99　Other
　　Coding Clinic: 2013, Q2, P13

● **51　Operations on gallbladder and biliary tract**
　　Includes　operations on:
　　　　　　ampulla of Vater
　　　　　　common bile duct
　　　　　　cystic duct
　　　　　　hepatic duct
　　　　　　intrahepatic bile duct
　　　　　　sphincter of Oddi
　　Code also any application or administration of an adhesion
　　　barrier substance (99.77)

● **51.0　Cholecystotomy and cholecystostomy**

51.01　Percutaneous aspiration of gallbladder
　　Percutaneous cholecystotomy for drainage
　　That by: needle or catheter
　　Excludes　*needle biopsy (51.12)*

✖ **51.02　Trocar cholecystostomy**

✖ **51.03　Other cholecystostomy**

✖ **51.04　Other cholecystotomy**
　　Cholelithotomy NOS

● **51.1　Diagnostic procedures on biliary tract**
　　Excludes　*that for endoscopic procedures classifiable to 51.64,*
　　　　　　　　51.84–51.88, 52.14, 52.21, 52.93–52.94,
　　　　　　　　52.97–52.98
　　Coding Clinic: 1997, Q2, P7

51.10　Endoscopic retrograde cholangiopancreatography [ERCP]
　　Excludes　*endoscopic retrograde:*
　　　　　　　　cholangiography [ERC] (51.11)
　　　　　　　　pancreatography [ERP] (52.13)
　　Coding Clinic: 2003, Q3, P17-18; 2001, Q1, P8-9; 1999, Q2,
　　　P13-14; 1993, 5th Issue, P12

51.11　Endoscopic retrograde cholangiography [ERC]
　　Laparoscopic exploration of common bile duct
　　Excludes　*endoscopic retrograde:*
　　　　　　　　cholangiopancreatography [ERCP]
　　　　　　　　　(51.10)
　　　　　　　　pancreatography [ERP] (52.13)
　　Coding Clinic: 1996, Q1, P12-13; 1993, 5th Issue, P12; 1988, Q4,
　　　P7

51.12　Percutaneous biopsy of gallbladder or bile ducts
　　Needle biopsy of gallbladder

✖ **51.13　Open biopsy of gallbladder or bile ducts**

51.14　Other closed [endoscopic] biopsy of biliary duct or sphincter of Oddi
　　Brushing or washing for specimen collection
　　Closed biopsy of biliary duct or sphincter of Oddi by
　　　procedures classifiable to 51.10–51.11, 52.13

51.15　Pressure measurement of sphincter of Oddi
　　Pressure measurement of sphincter by procedures
　　　classifiable to 51.10–51.11, 52.13

✖ **51.19　Other diagnostic procedures on biliary tract**
　　Excludes　*biliary tract x-ray (87.51–87.59)*
　　　　　　　　microscopic examination of specimen from
　　　　　　　　biliary tract (91.01–91.09)

● **51.2　Cholecystectomy**

✖ **51.21　Other partial cholecystectomy**
　　Revision of prior cholecystectomy
　　Excludes　*that by laparoscope (51.24)*

✖ **51.22　Cholecystectomy**
　　Excludes　*laparoscopic cholecystectomy (51.23)*
　　Coding Clinic: 1997, Q4, P52; 1995, Q2, P11; 1993, 5th Issue, P11;
　　　1992, Q2, P16; 1988, Q4, P7

✖ **51.23　Laparoscopic cholecystectomy**
　　That by laser
　　Coding Clinic: 2008, Q4, P172-174; 1998, Q3, P10; 1997, Q4, P52;
　　　1996, Q1, P12-13; 1995, Q2, P11; 1994, Q3, P11

✖ **51.24　Laparoscopic partial cholecystectomy**
　　Coding Clinic: 1996, Q4, P69

● **51.3　Anastomosis of gallbladder or bile duct**
　　Excludes　*resection with end-to-end anastomosis*
　　　　　　　　(51.61–51.69)

✖ **51.31　Anastomosis of gallbladder to hepatic ducts**

✖ **51.32　Anastomosis of gallbladder to intestine**

✖ **51.33　Anastomosis of gallbladder to pancreas**

✖ **51.34　Anastomosis of gallbladder to stomach**

✖ **51.35　Other gallbladder anastomosis**
　　Gallbladder anastomosis NOS

✖ **51.36　Choledochoenterostomy**

✖ **51.37　Anastomosis of hepatic duct to gastrointestinal tract**
　　Kasai portoenterostomy
　　Coding Clinic: 2002, Q2, P12

✖ **51.39　Other bile duct anastomosis**
　　Anastomosis of bile duct NOS
　　Anastomosis of unspecified bile duct to:
　　　intestine　　　　pancreas
　　　liver　　　　　　stomach

◀ New　　◀ Revised　　deleted Deleted　　● Use Additional Digit(s)　　✖ Valid O.R. Procedure
◆ Non-O.R. Procedure　　♀ Females Only　　♂ Males Only　　OGCR Official Guidelines　　**Coding Clinic**

● **51.4   Incision of bile duct for relief of obstruction**

✖ **51.41   Common duct exploration for removal of calculus**

Excludes   *percutaneous extraction (51.96)*

Coding Clinic: 1996, Q1, P12-13; 1988, Q4, P7

✖ **51.42   Common duct exploration for relief of other obstruction**

✖ **51.43   Insertion of choledochohepatic tube for decompression**

Hepatocholedochostomy

Coding Clinic: 1988, Q4, P7

✖ **51.49   Incision of other bile ducts for relief of obstruction**

● **51.5   Other incision of bile duct**

Excludes   *that for relief of obstruction (51.41–51.49)*

✖ **51.51   Exploration of common duct**

Incision of common bile duct

Coding Clinic: 1996, Q1, P12

✖ **51.59   Incision of other bile duct**

● **51.6   Local excision or destruction of lesion or tissue of biliary ducts and sphincter of Oddi**

Code also anastomosis other than end-to-end (51.31, 51.36–51.39)

Excludes   *biopsy of bile duct (51.12–51.13)*

✖ **51.61   Excision of cystic duct remnant**

✖ **51.62   Excision of ampulla of Vater (with reimplantation of common duct)**

✖ **51.63   Other excision of common duct**

Choledochectomy

Excludes   *fistulectomy (51.72)*

51.64   Endoscopic excision or destruction of lesion of biliary ducts or sphincter of Oddi

Excision or destruction of lesion of biliary duct by procedures classifiable to 51.10–51.11, 52.13

Coding Clinic: 1993, 5th Issue, P14

✖ **51.69   Excision of other bile duct**

Excision of lesion of bile duct NOS

Excludes   *fistulectomy (51.79)*

● **51.7   Repair of bile ducts**

✖ **51.71   Simple suture of common bile duct**

✖ **51.72   Choledochoplasty**

Repair of fistula of common bile duct

✖ **51.79   Repair of other bile ducts**

Closure of artificial opening of bile duct NOS

Suture of bile duct NOS

Excludes   *operative removal of prosthetic device (51.95)*

● **51.8   Other operations on biliary ducts and sphincter of Oddi**

✖ **51.81   Dilation of sphincter of Oddi**

Dilation of ampulla of Vater

Excludes   *that by endoscopic approach (51.84)*

✖ **51.82   Pancreatic sphincterotomy**

Incision of pancreatic sphincter

Transduodenal ampullary sphincterotomy

Excludes   *that by endoscopic approach (51.85)*

✖ **51.83   Pancreatic sphincteroplasty**

51.84   Endoscopic dilation of ampulla and biliary duct

Dilation of ampulla and biliary duct by procedures classifiable to 51.10–51.11, 52.13

51.85   Endoscopic sphincterotomy and papillotomy

Sphincterotomy and papillotomy by procedures classifiable to 51.10–51.11, 52.13

Coding Clinic: 2003, Q3, P17.18; 1993, 5th Issue, P14

51.86   Endoscopic insertion of nasobiliary drainage tube

Insertion of nasobiliary tube by procedures classifiable to 51.10–51.11, 52.13

51.87   Endoscopic insertion of stent (tube) into bile duct

Endoprosthesis of bile duct

Insertion of stent into bile duct by procedures classifiable to 51.10–51.11, 52.13

Excludes   *nasobiliary drainage tube (51.86) replacement of stent (tube) (97.05)*

Coding Clinic: 2003, Q3, P17

51.88   Endoscopic removal of stone(s) from biliary tract

Laparoscopic removal of stone(s) from biliary tract

Removal of biliary tract stone(s) by procedures classifiable to 51.10–51.11, 52.13

Excludes   *percutaneous extraction of common duct stones (51.96)*

Coding Clinic: 2000, Q2, P11; 1997, Q2, P7; 1993, 5th Issue, P12

✖ **51.89   Other operations on sphincter of Oddi**

● **51.9   Other operations on biliary tract**

✖ **51.91   Repair of laceration of gallbladder**

✖ **51.92   Closure of cholecystostomy**

✖ **51.93   Closure of other biliary fistula**

Cholecystogastroenteric fistulectomy

✖ **51.94   Revision of anastomosis of biliary tract**

✖ **51.95   Removal of prosthetic device from bile duct**

Excludes   *nonoperative removal (97.55)*

51.96   Percutaneous extraction of common duct stones

Coding Clinic: 1988, Q4, P7

51.98   Other percutaneous procedures on biliary tract

Percutaneous biliary endoscopy via existing T-tube or other tract for:

dilation of biliary duct stricture

removal of stone(s) except common duct stone

exploration (postoperative)

Percutaneous transhepatic biliary drainage

Excludes   *percutaneous aspiration of gallbladder (51.01)*
percutaneous biopsy and/or collection of specimen by brushing or washing (51.12)
percutaneous removal of common duct stone(s) (51.96)

Coding Clinic: 1997, Q1, P14

✖ **51.99   Other**

Insertion or replacement of biliary tract prosthesis

Excludes   *biopsy of gallbladder (51.12–51.13)*
irrigation of cholecystostomy and other biliary tube (96.41)
lysis of peritoneal adhesions (54.5)
nonoperative removal of:
cholecystostomy tube (97.54)
tube from biliary tract or liver (97.55)

● **52   Operations on pancreas**

Includes   operations on pancreatic duct

Code also any application or administration of an adhesion barrier substance (99.77)

● **52.0   Pancreatotomy**

✖ **52.01   Drainage of pancreatic cyst by catheter**

Coding Clinic: 2011, Q3, P9

✖ **52.09   Other pancreatotomy**

Pancreatolithotomy

Excludes   *drainage by anastomosis (52.4, 52.96)*
incision of pancreatic sphincter (51.82)
marsupialization of cyst (52.3)

OPERATIONS ON THE DIGESTIVE SYSTEM (42–54)

Excludes   Includes   Use additional   Code also   Omit code

● 52.1   **Diagnostic procedures on pancreas**

  52.11   **Closed [aspiration] [needle] [percutaneous] biopsy of pancreas**

✖ 52.12   **Open biopsy of pancreas**

  52.13   **Endoscopic retrograde pancreatography [ERP]**

  Excludes   *endoscopic retrograde:*
  cholangiography [ERC] (51.11)
  cholangiopancreatography [ERCP]
  (51.10)
  that for procedures classifiable to
  51.14–51.15, 51.64, 51.84–51.88,
  52.14, 52.21, 52.92–52.94,
  52.97–52.98

  Coding Clinic: 1993, 5th Issue, P12

  52.14   **Closed [endoscopic] biopsy of pancreatic duct**
  Closed biopsy of pancreatic duct by procedures classifiable to 51.10–51.11, 52.13

✖ 52.19   **Other diagnostic procedures on pancreas**

  Excludes   *contrast pancreatogram (87.66)*
  endoscopic retrograde pancreatography
  [ERP] (52.13)
  microscopic examination of specimen from
  pancreas (91.01–91.09)

● 52.2   **Local excision or destruction of pancreas and pancreatic duct**

  Excludes   *biopsy of pancreas (52.11–52.12, 52.14)*
  pancreatic fistulectomy (52.95)

  52.21   **Endoscopic excision or destruction of lesion or tissue of pancreatic duct**
  Excision or destruction of lesion or tissue of pancreatic duct by procedures classifiable to 51.10–51.11, 52.13

✖ 52.22   **Other excision or destruction of lesion or tissue of pancreas or pancreatic duct**

✖ 52.3   **Marsupialization of pancreatic cyst**

  Excludes   *drainage of cyst by catheter (52.01)*

✖ 52.4   **Internal drainage of pancreatic cyst**
  Pancreaticocystoduodenostomy
  Pancreaticocystogastrostomy
  Pancreaticocystojejunostomy

● 52.5   **Partial pancreatectomy**

  Excludes   *pancreatic fistulectomy (52.95)*

✖ 52.51   **Proximal pancreatectomy**
  Excision of head of pancreas (with part of body)
  Proximal pancreatectomy with synchronous duodenectomy

✖ 52.52   **Distal pancreatectomy**
  Excision of tail of pancreas (with part of body)

✖ 52.53   **Radical subtotal pancreatectomy**
  Coding Clinic: 2001, Q1, P13

✖ 52.59   **Other partial pancreatectomy**

✖ 52.6   **Total pancreatectomy**
  Pancreatectomy with synchronous duodenectomy
  Coding Clinic: 2013, Q3, P12; 1996, Q4, P70-71

✖ 52.7   **Radical pancreaticoduodenectomy**
  One-stage pancreaticoduodenal resection with choledochojejunal anastomosis, pancreaticojejunal anastomosis, and gastrojejunostomy
  Two-stage pancreaticoduodenal resection (first stage) (second stage)
  Radical resection of the pancreas
  Whipple procedure

  Excludes   *radical subtotal pancreatectomy (52.53)*
  Coding Clinic: 2001, Q1, P13

● 52.8   **Transplant of pancreas**
  Note: To report donor source - *see* codes 00.91–00.93

✖ 52.80   **Pancreatic transplant, not otherwise specified**
  MS-DRG: Refer to Part VI, Appendix E, Table 5, Kidney/Pancreas Transplant Reference Table
  MCE: Non-covered procedure when reported alone (without 55.69); Limited coverage when combined with at least one principal or secondary diagnosis of 250.01, 250.03, 250.11, 250.13, 250.21, 250.23, 250.31, 250.33, 250.41, 250.43, 250.51, 250.53, 250.61, 250.63, 250.71, 250.73, 250.81, 250.83, 250.91, 250.93, 251.3
  MCE: Limited coverage

✖ 52.81   **Reimplantation of pancreatic tissue**

✖ 52.82   **Homotransplant of pancreas**
  MS-DRG: Refer to Part VI, Appendix E, Table 5, Kidney/Pancreas Transplant Reference Table
  MCE: Non-covered procedure when reported alone (without 55.69); Limited coverage when combined with at least one principal or secondary diagnosis of 250.01, 250.03, 250.11, 250.13, 250.21, 250.23, 250.31, 250.33, 250.41, 250.43, 250.51, 250.53, 250.61, 250.63, 250.71, 250.73, 250.81, 250.83, 250.91, 250.93
  MCE: Limited coverage

✖ 52.83   **Heterotransplant of pancreas**
  MCE: Non-covered procedure

  52.84   **Autotransplantation of cells of Islets of Langerhans**
  Homotransplantation of islet cells of pancreas
  ◆Non-OR Procedure that affects MS-DRG assignment to MDC 11, MS-DRG 673-675
  Coding Clinic: 1996, Q4, P70-71

  52.85   **Allotransplantation of cells of Islets of Langerhans**
  Heterotransplantation of islet cells of pancreas
  ◆Non-OR Procedure that affects MS-DRG assignment to MDC 11, MS-DRG 673-675
  Coding Clinic: 1996, Q4, P70-71

  52.86   **Transplantation of cells of Islets of Langerhans, not otherwise specified**

● 52.9   **Other operations on pancreas**

✖ 52.92   **Cannulation of pancreatic duct**

  Excludes   *that by endoscopic approach (52.93)*

  52.93   **Endoscopic insertion of stent (tube) into pancreatic duct**
  Insertion of cannula or stent into pancreatic duct by procedures classifiable to 51.10–51.11, 52.13

  Excludes   *endoscopic insertion of nasopancreatic*
  drainage tube (52.97)
  replacement of stent (tube) (97.05)
  Coding Clinic: 1997, Q2, P7

  52.94   **Endoscopic removal of stone(s) from pancreatic duct**
  Removal of stone(s) from pancreatic duct by procedures classifiable to 51.10–51.11, 52.13

✖ 52.95   **Other repair of pancreas**
  Fistulectomy of pancreas
  Simple suture of pancreas

✖ 52.96   **Anastomosis of pancreas**
  Anastomosis of pancreas (duct) to:
  intestine
  jejunum
  stomach

  Excludes   *anastomosis to:*
  bile duct (51.39)
  gallbladder (51.33)

52.97 Endoscopic insertion of nasopancreatic drainage tube
Insertion of nasopancreatic drainage tube by procedures classifiable to 51.10–51.11, 52.13
> **Excludes** *drainage of pancreatic cyst by catheter (52.01)*
> *replacement of stent (tube) (97.05)*

52.98 Endoscopic dilation of pancreatic duct
Dilation of Wirsung's duct by procedures classifiable to 51.10–51.11, 52.13

✖ **52.99 Other**
Dilation of pancreatic [Wirsung's] duct by open approach
Repair of pancreatic [Wirsung's] duct by open approach
> **Excludes** *irrigation of pancreatic tube (96.42)*
> *removal of pancreatic tube (97.56)*

● **53 Repair of hernia**
> **Includes** hernioplasty
> herniorrhaphy

Code also any application or administration of an adhesion barrier substance (99.77)
> **Excludes** *manual reduction of hernia (96.27)*

● **53.0 Other unilateral repair of inguinal hernia**
> **Excludes** *laparoscopic unilateral repair of inguinal hernia (17.11–17.13)*
> Coding Clinic: 1994, Q3, P8

✖ **53.00 Unilateral repair of inguinal hernia, not otherwise specified**
Inguinal herniorrhaphy NOS
Coding Clinic: 2008, Q4, P165-169; 2003, Q3, P10-11

✖ **53.01 Other and open repair of direct inguinal hernia**
Direct and indirect inguinal hernia
Coding Clinic: 1996, Q4, P65-66

✖ **53.02 Other and open repair of indirect inguinal hernia**

✖ **53.03 Other and open repair of direct inguinal hernia with graft or prosthesis**

✖ **53.04 Other and open repair of indirect inguinal hernia with graft or prosthesis**

✖ **53.05 Repair of inguinal hernia with graft or prosthesis, not otherwise specified**

● **53.1 Other bilateral repair of inguinal hernia**
> **Excludes** *laparoscopic bilateral repair of inguinal hernia (17.21–17.24)*

✖ **53.10 Bilateral repair of inguinal hernia, not otherwise specified**

✖ **53.11 Other and open bilateral repair of direct inguinal hernia**
Coding Clinic: 1988, Q1, P9

✖ **53.12 Other and open bilateral repair of indirect inguinal hernia**

✖ **53.13 Other and open bilateral repair of inguinal hernia, one direct and one indirect**

✖ **53.14 Other and open bilateral repair of direct inguinal hernia with graft or prosthesis**

✖ **53.15 Other and open bilateral repair of indirect inguinal hernia with graft or prosthesis**

✖ **53.16 Other and open bilateral repair of inguinal hernia, one direct and one indirect, with graft or prosthesis**

✖ **53.17 Bilateral inguinal hernia repair with graft or prosthesis, not otherwise specified**

● **53.2 Unilateral repair of femoral hernia**
✖ **53.21 Unilateral repair of femoral hernia with graft or prosthesis**
✖ **53.29 Other unilateral femoral herniorrhaphy**

● **53.3 Bilateral repair of femoral hernia**
✖ **53.31 Bilateral repair of femoral hernia with graft or prosthesis**
✖ **53.39 Other bilateral femoral herniorrhaphy**

● **53.4 Repair of umbilical hernia**
> **Excludes** *repair of gastroschisis (54.71)*

✖ **53.41 Other and open repair of umbilical hernia with graft or prosthesis**
✖ **53.42 Laparoscopic repair of umbilical hernia with graft or prosthesis**
✖ **53.43 Other laparoscopic umbilical herniorrhaphy**
✖ **53.49 Other open umbilical herniorrhaphy**
> **Excludes** *other laparoscopic umbilical herniorrhaphy (53.43)*
> *repair of umbilical hernia with graft or prosthesis (53.41, 53.42)*

● **53.5 Repair of other hernia of anterior abdominal wall (without graft or prosthesis)**
✖ **53.51 Incisional hernia repair**
Coding Clinic: 2003, Q3, P6
✖ **53.59 Repair of other hernia of anterior abdominal wall**
Repair of hernia:
epigastric
hypogastric
spigelian
ventral
That by laparoscopic approach
Coding Clinic: 1996, Q3, P15

● **53.6 Repair of other hernia of anterior abdominal wall with graft or prosthesis**
✖ **53.61 Other open incisional hernia repair with graft or prosthesis**
> **Excludes** *laparoscopic incisional hernia repair with graft or prosthesis (53.62)*
> Coding Clinic: 2006, Q2, P10-11
✖ **53.62 Laparoscopic incisional hernia repair with graft or prosthesis**
Coding Clinic: 2003, Q3, P11
✖ **53.63 Other laparoscopic repair of other hernia of anterior abdominal wall with graft or prosthesis**
✖ **53.69 Other and open repair of other hernia of anterior abdominal wall with graft or prosthesis**
> **Excludes** *other laparoscopic repair of other hernia of anterior abdominal wall with graft or prothesis (53.63)*

● **53.7 Repair of diaphragmatic hernia, abdominal approach**
✖ **53.71 Laparoscopic repair of diaphragmatic hernia, abdominal approach**
✖ **53.72 Other and open repair of diaphragmatic hernia, abdominal approach**
✖ **53.75 Repair of diaphragmatic hernia, abdominal approach, not otherwise specified**
> **Excludes** *laparoscopic repair of diaphragmatic hernia (53.71)*
> *other and open repair of diaphragmatic hernia (53.72)*

OPERATIONS ON THE DIGESTIVE SYSTEM (42–54)

Excludes   Includes   Use additional   Code also   Omit code

● 53.8   Repair of diaphragmatic hernia, thoracic approach

✖ 53.80   Repair of diaphragmatic hernia with thoracic approach, not otherwise specified
Thoracoabdominal repair of diaphragmatic hernia

✖ 53.81   Plication of the diaphragm

✖ 53.82   Repair of parasternal hernia

✖ 53.83   Laparoscopic repair of diaphragmatic hernia, with thoracic approach

✖ 53.84   Other and open repair of diaphragmatic hernia, with thoracic approach

Excludes   *repair of diaphragmatic hernia with thoracic approach, NOS (53.80)*

✖ 53.9   Other hernia repair
Repair of hernia: Repair of hernia:
ischiatic   omental
ischiorectal   retroperitoneal
lumbar   sciatic
obturator

Excludes   *relief of strangulated hernia with exteriorization of intestine (46.01, 46.03)*
repair of pericolostomy hernia (46.42)
repair of vaginal enterocele (70.92)

● 54   Other operations on abdominal region

Includes   operations on:
epigastric region
flank
groin region
hypochondrium
inguinal region
loin region
pelvic cavity
mesentery
omentum
peritoneum
retroperitoneal tissue space

Code also any application or administration of an adhesion barrier substance (99.77)

Excludes   *hernia repair (53.00–53.9)*
obliteration of cul-de-sac (70.92)
retroperitoneal tissue dissection (59.00–59.09)
skin and subcutaneous tissue of abdominal wall (86.01–86.99)
Coding Clinic: 1997, Q1, P11; 1987, Nov-Dec, P12

✖ 54.0   Incision of abdominal wall
Drainage of:
abdominal wall
extraperitoneal abscess
retroperitoneal abscess

Excludes   *incision of peritoneum (54.95)*
laparotomy (54.11–54.19)
Coding Clinic: 2006, Q2, P23-24; 2005, Q4, P74-77; 1993, 5th Issue, P9-10

● 54.1   Laparotomy

✖ 54.11   Exploratory laparotomy

Excludes   *exploration incidental to intra-abdominal surgery — omit code*
Coding Clinic: 1989, Q3, P14; 1988, Q4, P12; 1987, Jan-Feb, P11-12; 1984, Nov-Dec, P12

✖ 54.12   Reopening of recent laparotomy site
Reopening of recent laparotomy site for:
control of hemorrhage
exploration
incision of hematoma

✖ 54.19   Other laparotomy
Drainage of intraperitoneal abscess or hematoma

Excludes   *culdocentesis (70.0)*
drainage of appendiceal abscess (47.2)
exploration incidental to intra abdominal surgery — omit code
Ladd operation (54.95)
percutaneous drainage of abdomen (54.91)
removal of foreign body (54.92)
Coding Clinic: 2003, Q3, P16-17; 1992, Q1, P14

● 54.2   Diagnostic procedures of abdominal region

✖ 54.21   Laparoscopy
Peritoneoscopy

Excludes   *laparoscopic cholecystectomy (51.23)*
that incidental to destruction of fallopian tubes (66.21–66.29)
Coding Clinic: 1996, Q4, P64-66

✖ 54.22   Biopsy of abdominal wall or umbilicus

✖ 54.23   Biopsy of peritoneum
Biopsy of:
mesentery
omentum
peritoneal implant

Excludes   *closed biopsy of:*
omentum (54.24)
peritoneum (54.24)

54.24   Closed [percutaneous] [needle] biopsy of intra-abdominal mass
Closed biopsy of:
omentum
peritoneal implant
peritoneum

Excludes   *that of:*
fallopian tube (66.11)
ovary (65.11)
uterine ligaments (68.15)
uterus (68.16)
Coding Clinic: 1997, Q4, P57

54.25   Peritoneal lavage
Diagnostic peritoneal lavage

Excludes   *peritoneal dialysis (54.98)*
Coding Clinic: 1998, Q2, P19-20; 1993, Q4, P31

✖ 54.29   Other diagnostic procedures on abdominal region

Excludes   *abdominal lymphangiogram (88.04)*
abdominal x-ray NEC (88.19)
angiocardiography of venae cava (88.51)
C.A.T. scan of abdomen (88.01)
contrast x-ray of abdominal cavity (88.11–88.15)
intra-abdominal arteriography NEC (88.47)
microscopic examination of peritoneal and retroperitoneal specimen (91.11–91.19)
phlebography of:
intra-abdominal vessels NEC (88.65)
portal venous system (88.64)
sinogram of abdominal wall (88.03)
soft tissue x-ray of abdominal wall NEC (88.09)
tomography of abdomen NEC (88.02)
ultrasonography of abdomen and retroperitoneum (88.76)

✖ **54.3 Excision or destruction of lesion or tissue of abdominal wall or umbilicus**
Debridement of abdominal wall
Omphalectomy

> **Excludes** *biopsy of abdominal wall or umbilicus (54.22)*
> *size reduction operation (86.83)*
> *that of skin of abdominal wall (86.22, 86.26, 86.3)*

Coding Clinic: 1989, Q1, P11

✖ **54.4 Excision or destruction of peritoneal tissue**
Excision of:
appendices epiploicae
falciform ligament
gastrocolic ligament
lesion of:
mesentery
omentum
peritoneum
presacral lesion NOS
retroperitoneal lesion NOS

> **Excludes** *biopsy of peritoneum (54.23)*
> *endometrectomy of cul-de-sac (70.32)*

● **54.5 Lysis of peritoneal adhesions**
Freeing of adhesions of:
biliary tract
intestines
liver
pelvic peritoneum
peritoneum
spleen
uterus

> **Excludes** *lysis of adhesions of:*
> *bladder (59.11)*
> *fallopian tube and ovary*
> *laparoscopic (65.81)*
> *other (65.89)*
> *kidney (59.02)*
> *ureter (59.02)*

✖ **54.51 Laparoscopic lysis of peritoneal adhesions**
Coding Clinic: 2006, Q4, P130-134; 2003, Q3, P6-7; 1996, Q4, P65-66

✖ **54.59 Other lysis of peritoneal adhesions**
Coding Clinic: 2013, Q2, P4; 2010, Q1, P12; 2006, Q3, P15-16; 2003, Q3, P11; Q1, P14-15; 1996, Q4, P65-66; 1994, Q3, P8

● **54.6 Suture of abdominal wall and peritoneum**

✖ **54.61 Reclosure of postoperative disruption of abdominal wall**

✖ **54.62 Delayed closure of granulating abdominal wound**
Tertiary subcutaneous wound closure

✖ **54.63 Other suture of abdominal wall**
Suture of laceration of abdominal wall

> **Excludes** *closure of operative wound — omit code*

✖ **54.64 Suture of peritoneum**
Secondary suture of peritoneum

> **Excludes** *closure of operative wound — omit code*

● **54.7 Other repair of abdominal wall and peritoneum**

✖ **54.71 Repair of gastroschisis**
Coding Clinic: 2002, Q2, P9

✖ **54.72 Other repair of abdominal wall**

✖ **54.73 Other repair of peritoneum**
Suture of gastrocolic ligament

✖ **54.74 Other repair of omentum**
Epiplorrhaphy
Graft of omentum
Omentopexy
Reduction of torsion of omentum

> **Excludes** *cardio-omentopexy (36.39)*

Coding Clinic: 1987, Jan-Feb, P11

✖ **54.75 Other repair of mesentery**
Mesenteric plication
Mesenteropexy

● **54.9 Other operations of abdominal region**

> **Excludes** *removal of ectopic pregnancy (74.3)*

54.91 Percutaneous abdominal drainage
Paracentesis

> **Excludes** *creation of cutaneoperitoneal fistula (54.93)*

Coding Clinic: 2007, Q4, P95-96; 1999, Q3, P9; 1999, Q2, P14; 1998, Q3, P12; 1990, Q2, P25

✖ **54.92 Removal of foreign body from peritoneal cavity**
Coding Clinic: 1989, Q1, P11

✖ **54.93 Creation of cutaneoperitoneal fistula**
Coding Clinic: 1995, Q2, P10

✖ **54.94 Creation of peritoneovascular shunt**
Peritoneovenous shunt
Coding Clinic: 1988, Q1, P9

✖ **54.95 Incision of peritoneum**
Exploration of ventriculoperitoneal shunt at peritoneal site
Ladd operation
Revision of distal catheter of ventricular shunt
Revision of ventriculoperitoneal shunt at peritoneal site

> **Excludes** *that incidental to laparotomy (54.11–54.19)*

Coding Clinic: 2013, Q2, P4-5

54.96 Injection of air into peritoneal cavity
Pneumoperitoneum

> **Excludes** *that for:*
> *collapse of lung (33.33)*
> *radiography (88.12–88.13, 88.15)*

54.97 Injection of locally-acting therapeutic substance into peritoneal cavity

> **Excludes** *peritoneal dialysis (54.98)*

54.98 Peritoneal dialysis

> **Excludes** *peritoneal lavage (diagnostic) (54.25)*

Coding Clinic: 1993, Q4, P31

54.99 Other

> **Excludes** *removal of:*
> *abdominal wall suture (97.83)*
> *peritoneal drainage device (97.82)*
> *retroperitoneal drainage device (97.81)*

Coding Clinic: 1999, Q1, P4

OPERATIONS ON THE DIGESTIVE SYSTEM (42–54)

Excludes   Includes   Use additional   Code also   Omit code

10. OPERATIONS ON THE URINARY SYSTEM (55–59)

● **55 Operations on kidney**

> **Includes** operations on renal pelvis
>
> **Code also** any application or administration of an adhesion barrier substance (99.77)
>
> **Excludes** *perirenal tissue (59.00–59.09, 59.21–59.29, 59.91–59.92)*

● **55.0 Nephrotomy and nephrostomy**

> **Excludes** *drainage by:*
> *anastomosis (55.86)*
> *aspiration (55.92)*
> *incision of kidney pelvis (55.11–55.12)*

✖ **55.01 Nephrotomy**
> Evacuation of renal cyst
> Exploration of kidney
> Nephrolithotomy

✖ **55.02 Nephrostomy**
> Coding Clinic: 1997, Q2, P4; 1986, Sept-Oct, P11-12

✖ **55.03 Percutaneous nephrostomy without fragmentation**
> Nephrostolithotomy, percutaneous (nephroscopic)
> Percutaneous removal of kidney stone(s) by:
> basket extraction
> forceps extraction (nephroscopic)
> Pyelostolithotomy, percutaneous (nephroscopic)
> With placement of catheter down ureter
>
> **Excludes** *percutaneous removal by fragmentation (55.04)*
> *repeat nephroscopic removal during current episode (55.92)*
>
> Coding Clinic: 1996, Q2, P5

✖ **55.04 Percutaneous nephrostomy with fragmentation**
> Percutaneous nephrostomy with disruption of kidney stone by ultrasonic energy and extraction (suction) through endoscope
> With placement of catheter down ureter
> With fluoroscopic guidance
>
> **Excludes** *repeat fragmentation during current episode (59.95)*
>
> Coding Clinic: 1986, Sept-Oct, P11-12

● **55.1 Pyelotomy and pyelostomy**

> **Excludes** *drainage by anastomosis (55.86)*
> *percutaneous pyelostolithotomy (55.03)*
> *removal of calculus without incision (56.0)*

✖ **55.11 Pyelotomy**
> Exploration of renal pelvis
> Pyelolithotomy

✖ **55.12 Pyelostomy**
> Insertion of drainage tube into renal pelvis

● **55.2 Diagnostic procedures on kidney**

55.21 Nephroscopy

55.22 Pyeloscopy

55.23 Closed [percutaneous] [needle] biopsy of kidney
> Endoscopic biopsy via existing nephrostomy, nephrotomy, pyelostomy, or pyelotomy

✖ **55.24 Open biopsy of kidney**

✖ **55.29 Other diagnostic procedures on kidney**
> **Excludes** *microscopic examination of specimen from kidney (91.21–91.29)*
> *pyelogram:*
> *intravenous (87.73)*
> *percutaneous (87.75)*
> *retrograde (87.74)*
> *radioisotope scan (92.03)*
> *renal arteriography (88.45)*
> *tomography:*
> *C.A.T. scan (87.71)*
> *other (87.72)*

● **55.3 Local excision or destruction of lesion or tissue of kidney**
> Coding Clinic: 2006, Q4, P124-126

✖ **55.31 Marsupialization of kidney lesion**

✖ **55.32 Open ablation of renal lesion or tissue**

✖ **55.33 Percutaneous ablation of renal lesion or tissue**

✖ **55.34 Laparoscopic ablation of renal lesion or tissue**

✖ **55.35 Other and unspecified ablation of renal lesion or tissue**

✖ **55.39 Other local destruction or excision of renal lesion or tissue**
> Obliteration of calyceal diverticulum
>
> **Excludes** *ablation of renal lesion or tissue:*
> *laparoscopic (55.34)*
> *open (55.32)*
> *other (55.35)*
> *percutaneous (55.33)*
> *biopsy of kidney (55.23–55.24)*
> *partial nephrectomy (55.4)*
> *percutaneous aspiration of kidney (55.92)*
> *wedge resection of kidney (55.4)*
>
> Coding Clinic: 1996, Q1, P10-11

✖ **55.4 Partial nephrectomy**
> Calycectomy
> Wedge resection of kidney
>
> **Code also** any synchronous resection of ureter (56.40–56.42)

● **55.5 Complete nephrectomy**

> **Code also** any synchronous excision of:
> adrenal gland (07.21–07.3)
> bladder segment (57.6)
> lymph nodes (40.3, 40.52–40.59)

✖ **55.51 Nephroureterectomy**
> Nephroureterectomy with bladder cuff
> Total nephrectomy (unilateral)
>
> **Excludes** *removal of transplanted kidney (55.53)*
>
> Coding Clinic: 2005, Q2, P4-5

✖ **55.52 Nephrectomy of remaining kidney**
> Removal of solitary kidney
>
> **Excludes** *removal of transplanted kidney (55.53)*

✖ **55.53 Removal of transplanted or rejected kidney**
> Coding Clinic: 2008, Q4, P82-83

✖ **55.54 Bilateral nephrectomy**
> **Excludes** *complete nephrectomy NOS (55.51)*

● **55.6 Transplant of kidney**
> **Note:** To report donor source - *see* codes 00.91–00.93

✖ **55.61 Renal autotransplantation**

✖ **55.69 Other kidney transplantation**
> MS-DRG: Refer to Part VI, Appendix E, Table 5, Kidney/Pancreas Transplant Reference Table
> MCE: Limited coverage
> Coding Clinic: 2012, Q3, P17; 2004, Q4, P116-117; 1996, Q4, P70-71

✖ **55.7 Nephropexy**
> Fixation or suspension of movable [floating] kidney

● **55.8 Other repair of kidney**

✖ **55.81 Suture of laceration of kidney**

✖ **55.82 Closure of nephrostomy and pyelostomy**

✖ **55.83 Closure of other fistula of kidney**

✖ **55.84 Reduction of torsion of renal pedicle**

✖ **55.85 Symphysiotomy for horseshoe kidney**

✖ **55.86 Anastomosis of kidney**
> Nephropyeloureterostomy
> Pyeloureterovesical anastomosis
> Ureterocalyceal anastomosis
>
> **Excludes** *nephrocystanastomosis NOS (56.73)*

✖ **55.87 Correction of ureteropelvic junction**

✖ **55.89 Other**

◀ New   ◀▥ Revised   ~~deleted~~ Deleted   ● Use Additional Digit(s)   ✖ Valid O.R. Procedure
◆ Non-O.R. Procedure   ♀ Females Only   ♂ Males Only   **OGCR** Official Guidelines   **Coding Clinic**

● **55.9 Other operations on kidney**

    Excludes *lysis of perirenal adhesions (59.02)*

  ✖ **55.91 Decapsulation of kidney**
    Capsulectomy of kidney
    Decortication of kidney

  55.92 Percutaneous aspiration of kidney (pelvis)
    Aspiration of renal cyst
    Renipuncture

    Excludes *percutaneous biopsy of kidney (55.23)*

    Coding Clinic: 1984, Nov-Dec, P20

  55.93 Replacement of nephrostomy tube

  55.94 Replacement of pyelostomy tube

  55.95 Local perfusion of kidney

  55.96 Other injection of therapeutic substance into kidney
    Injection into renal cyst

  ✖ **55.97 Implantation or replacement of mechanical kidney**

  ✖ **55.98 Removal of mechanical kidney**

  ✖ **55.99 Other**

    Excludes *removal of pyelostomy or nephrostomy tube (97.61)*

● **56 Operations on ureter**

    Code also any application or administration of an adhesion barrier substance (99.77)

    Coding Clinic: 1986, Sept-Oct, P11-12

✖ **56.0 Transurethral removal of obstruction from ureter and renal pelvis**
    Removal of:
      blood clot from ureter or renal pelvis without incision
      calculus from ureter or renal pelvis without incision
      foreign body from ureter or renal pelvis without incision

    Excludes *manipulation without removal of obstruction (59.8)*
      that by incision (55.11, 56.2)
      transurethral insertion of ureteral stent for passage of calculus (59.8)

✖ **56.1 Ureteral meatotomy**

✖ **56.2 Ureterotomy**
    Incision of ureter for:
      drainage
      exploration
      removal of calculus

    Excludes *cutting of ureterovesical orifice (56.1)*
      removal of calculus without incision (56.0)
      transurethral insertion of ureteral stent for passage of calculus (59.8)
      urinary diversion (56.51–56.79)

    Coding Clinic: 1986, Sept-Oct, P10

● **56.3 Diagnostic procedures on ureter**

  56.31 Ureteroscopy

  56.32 Closed percutaneous biopsy of ureter

    Excludes *endoscopic biopsy of ureter (56.33)*

  56.33 Closed endoscopic biopsy of ureter
    Cystourethroscopy with ureteral biopsy
    Transurethral biopsy of ureter
    Ureteral endoscopy with biopsy through ureterotomy
    Ureteroscopy with biopsy

    Excludes *percutaneous biopsy of ureter (56.32)*

  ✖ **56.34 Open biopsy of ureter**

  56.35 Endoscopy (cystoscopy) (looposcopy) of ileal conduit

  ✖ **56.39 Other diagnostic procedures on ureter**

    Excludes *microscopic examination of specimen from ureter (91.21–91.29)*

● **56.4 Ureterectomy**

    Code also anastomosis other than end-to-end (56.51–56.79)

    Excludes *fistulectomy (56.84)*
      nephroureterectomy (55.51–55.54)

  ✖ **56.40 Ureterectomy, not otherwise specified**

  ✖ **56.41 Partial ureterectomy**
    Excision of lesion of ureter
    Shortening of ureter with reimplantation

    Excludes *biopsy of ureter (56.32–56.34)*

  ✖ **56.42 Total ureterectomy**

● **56.5 Cutaneous uretero-ileostomy**

  ✖ **56.51 Formation of cutaneous uretero-ileostomy**
    Construction of ileal conduit
    External ureteral ileostomy
    Formation of open ileal bladder
    Ileal loop operation
    Ileoureterostomy (Bricker's) (ileal bladder)
    Transplantation of ureter into ileum with external diversion

    Excludes *closed ileal bladder (57.87)*
      replacement of ureteral defect by ileal segment (56.89)

  ✖ **56.52 Revision of cutaneous uretero-ileostomy**
    Coding Clinic: 1996, Q3, P15; 1988, Q4, P7

● **56.6 Other external urinary diversion**

  ✖ **56.61 Formation of other cutaneous ureterostomy**
    Anastomosis of ureter to skin
    Ureterostomy NOS

  ✖ **56.62 Revision of other cutaneous ureterostomy**
    Revision of ureterostomy stoma

    Excludes *nonoperative removal of ureterostomy tube (97.62)*

● **56.7 Other anastomosis or bypass of ureter**

    Excludes *ureteropyelostomy (55.86)*

  ✖ **56.71 Urinary diversion to intestine**
    Anastomosis of ureter to intestine
    Internal urinary diversion NOS

    Code also any synchronous colostomy (46.10–46.13)

    Excludes *external ureteral ileostomy (56.51)*

  ✖ **56.72 Revision of ureterointestinal anastomosis**

    Excludes *revision of external ureteral ileostomy (56.52)*

  ✖ **56.73 Nephrocystanastomosis, not otherwise specified**

  ✖ **56.74 Ureteroneocystostomy**
    Replacement of ureter with bladder flap
    Ureterovesical anastomosis

  ✖ **56.75 Transureteroureterostomy**

    Excludes *ureteroureterostomy associated with partial resection (56.41)*

  ✖ **56.79 Other**

● **56.8 Repair of ureter**

  ✖ **56.81 Lysis of intraluminal adhesions of ureter**

    Excludes *lysis of periureteral adhesions (59.02–59.03)*
      ureterolysis (59.02–59.03)

  ✖ **56.82 Suture of laceration of ureter**

  ✖ **56.83 Closure of ureterostomy**

  ✖ **56.84 Closure of other fistula of ureter**

  ✖ **56.85 Ureteropexy**

  ✖ **56.86 Removal of ligature from ureter**

  ✖ **56.89 Other repair of ureter**
    Graft of ureter
    Replacement of ureter with ileal segment implanted into bladder
    Ureteroplication

OPERATIONS ON THE URINARY SYSTEM (55–59)

    Excludes   Includes   Use additional   Code also   Omit code

● 56.9   Other operations on ureter
    56.91   Dilation of ureteral meatus
    ✖ 56.92   Implantation of electronic ureteral stimulator
    ✖ 56.93   Replacement of electronic ureteral stimulator
    ✖ 56.94   Removal of electronic ureteral stimulator
       Excludes   *that with synchronous replacement (56.93)*
    ✖ 56.95   Ligation of ureter
    ✖ 56.99   Other
       Excludes   *removal of ureterostomy tube and ureteral catheter (97.62)*
            ureteral catheterization (59.8)

● 57   Operations on urinary bladder
    Code also any application or administration of an adhesion barrier substance (99.77)
    Excludes   *perivesical tissue (59.11–59.29, 59.91–59.92)*
            ureterovesical orifice (56.0–56.99)
    Coding Clinic: 1986, Sept-Oct, P11-12

    57.0   Transurethral clearance of bladder
       Drainage of bladder without incision
       Removal of:
          blood clots from bladder without incision
          calculus from bladder without incision
          foreign body from bladder without incision
       Excludes   *that by incision (57.19)*

● 57.1   Cystotomy and cystostomy
       Excludes   *cystotomy and cystostomy as operative approach — omit code*
    57.11   Percutaneous aspiration of bladder
    ✖ 57.12   Lysis of intraluminal adhesions with incision into bladder
       Excludes   *transurethral lysis of intraluminal adhesions (57.41)*
    57.17   Percutaneous cystostomy
       Closed cystostomy
       Percutaneous suprapubic cystostomy
       Excludes   *removal of cystostomy tube (97.63)*
            replacement of cystostomy tube (59.94)
    ✖ 57.18   Other suprapubic cystostomy
       Excludes   *percutaneous cystostomy (57.17)*
            removal of cystostomy tube (97.63)
            replacement of cystostomy tube (59.94)
    ✖ 57.19   Other cystotomy
       Cystolithotomy
       Excludes   *percutaneous cystostomy (57.17)*
            suprapubic cystostomy (57.18)
    Coding Clinic: 1986, Sept-Oct, P11-12

● 57.2   Vesicostomy
       Excludes   *percutaneous cystostomy (57.17)*
            suprapubic cystostomy (57.18)
    ✖ 57.21   Vesicostomy
       Creation of permanent opening from bladder to skin using a bladder flap
    ✖ 57.22   Revision or closure of vesicostomy
       Excludes   *closure of cystostomy (57.82)*

● 57.3   Diagnostic procedures on bladder
    57.31   Cystoscopy through artificial stoma
    57.32   Other cystoscopy
       Transurethral cystoscopy
       Excludes   *cystourethroscopy with ureteral biopsy (56.33)*
            retrograde pyelogram (87.74)
            that for control of hemorrhage (postoperative):
               bladder (57.93)
               prostate (60.94)
    Coding Clinic: 2011, Q1, P25; 2001, Q1, P14; 1984, May-June, P10

● 57.33   Closed [transurethral] biopsy of bladder
    ✖ 57.34   Open biopsy of bladder
       Coding Clinic: 2005, Q2, P12
    ✖ 57.39   Other diagnostic procedures on bladder
       Excludes   *cystogram NEC (87.77)*
            microscopic examination of specimen from bladder (91.31–91.39)
            retrograde cystourethrogram (87.76)
            therapeutic distention of bladder (96.25)

● 57.4   Transurethral excision or destruction of bladder tissue
    ✖ 57.41   Transurethral lysis of intraluminal adhesions
    ✖ 57.49   Other transurethral excision or destruction of lesion or tissue of bladder
       Endoscopic resection of bladder lesion
       Excludes   *transurethral biopsy of bladder (57.33)*
            transurethral fistulectomy (57.83–57.84)
    Coding Clinic: 1996, Q1, P10-11

● 57.5   Other excision or destruction of bladder tissue
       Excludes   *that with transurethral approach (57.41–57.49)*
    ✖ 57.51   Excision of urachus
       Excision of urachal sinus of bladder
       Excludes   *excision of urachal cyst of abdominal wall (54.3)*
    ✖ 57.59   Open excision or destruction of other lesion or tissue of bladder
       Endometrectomy of bladder
       Suprapubic excision of bladder lesion
       Excludes   *biopsy of bladder (57.33–57.34)*
            fistulectomy of bladder (57.83–57.84)

✖ 57.6   Partial cystectomy
    Excision of bladder dome
    Trigonectomy
    Wedge resection of bladder

● 57.7   Total cystectomy
    Includes   total cystectomy with urethrectomy
    ✖ 57.71   Radical cystectomy
       Pelvic exenteration in male
       Removal of bladder, prostate, seminal vesicles, and fat
       Removal of bladder, urethra, and fat in a female
       Code also any:
          lymph node dissection (40.3, 40.5)
          urinary diversion (56.51–56.79)
       Excludes   *that as part of pelvic exenteration in female (68.8)*
    ✖ 57.79   Other total cystectomy

● 57.8   Other repair of urinary bladder
       Excludes   *repair of:*
            current obstetric laceration (75.61)
            cystocele (70.50–70.51)
            that for stress incontinence (59.3–59.79)
    ✖ 57.81   Suture of laceration of bladder
    ✖ 57.82   Closure of cystostomy
    ✖ 57.83   Repair of fistula involving bladder and intestine
       Rectovesicovaginal fistulectomy
       Vesicosigmoidovaginal fistulectomy
    ✖ 57.84   Repair of other fistula of bladder
       Cervicovesical fistulectomy
       Urethroperineovesical fistulectomy
       Uterovesical fistulectomy
       Vaginovesical fistulectomy
       Excludes   *vesicoureterovaginal fistulectomy (56.84)*
    ✖ 57.85   Cystourethroplasty and plastic repair of bladder neck
       Plication of sphincter of urinary bladder
       V-Y plasty of bladder neck
    ✖ 57.86   Repair of bladder exstrophy

◀ New   ◀▥ Revised   ~~deleted~~ Deleted   ● Use Additional Digit(s)   ✖ Valid O.R. Procedure
◆ Non-O.R. Procedure   ♀ Females Only   ♂ Males Only   **OGCR** Official Guidelines   **Coding Clinic**

1260

✖ **57.87 Reconstruction of urinary bladder**
Anastomosis of bladder with isolated segment of ileum
Augmentation of bladder
Replacement of bladder with ileum or sigmoid [closed ileal bladder]
Code also resection of intestine (45.50–45.52)
Coding Clinic: 2005, Q2, P12-13x2; 2003, Q2, P11-12; 2000, Q3, P7-8

✖ **57.88 Other anastomosis of bladder**
Anastomosis of bladder to intestine NOS
Cystocolic anastomosis
Excludes *formation of closed ileal bladder (57.87)*

✖ **57.89 Other repair of bladder**
Bladder suspension, not elsewhere classified
Cystopexy NOS
Repair of old obstetric laceration of bladder
Excludes *repair of current obstetric laceration (75.61)*

● **57.9 Other operations on bladder**

✖ **57.91 Sphincterotomy of bladder**
Division of bladder neck
Coding Clinic: 1994, Q3, P12; 1990, Q2, P23

57.92 Dilation of bladder neck

✖ **57.93 Control of (postoperative) hemorrhage of bladder**

57.94 Insertion of indwelling urinary catheter

57.95 Replacement of indwelling urinary catheter

✖ **57.96 Implantation of electronic bladder stimulator**
MCE: Non-covered procedure

✖ **57.97 Replacement of electronic bladder stimulator**
MCE: Non-covered procedure

✖ **57.98 Removal of electronic bladder stimulator**
Excludes *that with synchronous replacement (57.97)*

✖ **57.99 Other**
Excludes *irrigation of:*
cystostomy (96.47)
other indwelling urinary catheter (96.48)
lysis of external adhesions (59.11)
removal of:
cystostomy tube (97.63)
other urinary drainage device (97.64)
therapeutic distention of bladder (96.25)

● **58 Operations on urethra**
Includes operations on:
bulbourethral gland [Cowper's gland]
periurethral tissue
Code also any application or administration of an adhesion barrier substance (99.77)

✖ **58.0 Urethrotomy**
Excision of urethral septum
Formation of urethrovaginal fistula
Perineal urethrostomy
Removal of calculus from urethra by incision
Excludes *drainage of bulbourethral gland or periurethral tissue (58.91)*
internal urethral meatotomy (58.5)
removal of urethral calculus without incision (58.6)

✖ **58.1 Urethral meatotomy**
Excludes *internal urethral meatotomy (58.5)*

● **58.2 Diagnostic procedures on urethra**
58.21 Perineal urethroscopy
58.22 Other urethroscopy
58.23 Biopsy of urethra
58.24 Biopsy of periurethral tissue
58.29 Other diagnostic procedures on urethra and periurethral tissue
Excludes *microscopic examination of specimen from urethra (91.31–91.39)*
retrograde cystourethrogram (87.76)
urethral pressure profile (89.25)
urethral sphincter electromyogram (89.23)

● **58.3 Excision or destruction of lesion or tissue of urethra**
Excludes *biopsy of urethra (58.23)*
excision of bulbourethral gland (58.92)
fistulectomy (58.43)
urethrectomy as part of:
complete cystectomy (57.79)
pelvic evisceration (68.8)
radical cystectomy (57.71)

58.31 Endoscopic excision or destruction of lesion or tissue of urethra
Fulguration of urethral lesion

58.39 Other local excision or destruction of lesion or tissue of urethra
Excision of:
congenital valve of urethra
lesion of urethra
stricture of urethra
Urethrectomy
Excludes *that by endoscopic approach (58.31)*

● **58.4 Repair of urethra**
Excludes *repair of current obstetric laceration (75.61)*

✖ **58.41 Suture of laceration of urethra**

✖ **58.42 Closure of urethrostomy**

✖ **58.43 Closure of other fistula of urethra**
Excludes *repair of urethroperineovesical fistula (57.84)*

✖ **58.44 Reanastomosis of urethra**
Anastomosis of urethra

✖ **58.45 Repair of hypospadias or epispadias**
Coding Clinic: 1997, Q3, P6; 1996, Q4, P34-35

✖ **58.46 Other reconstruction of urethra**
Urethral construction

✖ **58.47 Urethral meatoplasty**

✖ **58.49 Other repair of urethra**
Benenenti rotation of bulbous urethra
Repair of old obstetric laceration of urethra
Urethral plication
Excludes *repair of:*
current obstetric laceration (75.61)
urethrocele (70.50–70.51)
Coding Clinic: 2009, Q1, P5

✖ **58.5 Release of urethral stricture**
Cutting of urethral sphincter
Internal urethral meatotomy
Urethrolysis
Coding Clinic: 1997, Q1, P13-14

58.6 Dilation of urethra
Dilation of urethrovesical junction
Passage of sounds through urethra
Removal of calculus from urethra without incision
Excludes *urethral calibration (89.29)*
Coding Clinic: 2011, Q1, P25; 2001, Q1, P14; 1997, Q1, P13-14

OPERATIONS ON THE URINARY SYSTEM (55–59)

Excludes Includes Use additional Code also Omit code

● **58.9   Other operations on urethra and periurethral tissue**

✖ **58.91   Incision of periurethral tissue**
        Drainage of bulbourethral gland

✖ **58.92   Excision of periurethral tissue**
        Excludes   *biopsy of periurethral tissue (58.24)*
                    lysis of periurethral adhesions
                        laparoscopic (59.12)
                        other (59.11)

✖ **58.93   Implantation of artificial urinary sphincter [AUS]**
        Placement of inflatable:
            bladder sphincter
            urethral sphincter
        Removal with replacement of sphincter device
            [AUS]
        With pump and/or reservoir

✖ **58.99   Other**
        Removal of inflatable urinary sphincter without
            replacement
        Repair of inflatable sphincter pump and/or reservoir
        Surgical correction of hydraulic pressure of inflatable
            sphincter device
        Excludes   *removal of:*
                    intraluminal foreign body from urethra
                        without incision (98.19)
                    urethral stent (97.65)
        Coding Clinic: 2009, Q1, P5; 1995, Q4, P72-73

● **59   Other operations on urinary tract**
    Code also any application or administration of an adhesion
        barrier substance (99.77)

● **59.0   Dissection of retroperitoneal tissue**

✖ **59.00   Retroperitoneal dissection, not otherwise specified**

✖ **59.02   Other lysis of perirenal or periureteral adhesions**
        Excludes   *that by laparoscope (59.03)*

✖ **59.03   Laparoscopic lysis of perirenal or periureteral
        adhesions**
        Coding Clinic: 2006, Q4, P130-134

✖ **59.09   Other incision of perirenal or periureteral tissue**
        Exploration of perinephric area
        Incision of perirenal abscess

● **59.1   Incision of perivesical tissue**

✖ **59.11   Other lysis of perivesical adhesions**

✖ **59.12   Laparoscopic lysis of perivesical adhesions**

✖ **59.19   Other incision of perivesical tissue**
        Exploration of perivesical tissue
        Incision of hematoma of space of Retzius
        Retropubic exploration

● **59.2   Diagnostic procedures on perirenal and perivesical tissue**

✖ **59.21   Biopsy of perirenal or perivesical tissue**

✖ **59.29   Other diagnostic procedures on perirenal tissue,
        perivesical tissue, and retroperitoneum**
        Excludes   *microscopic examination of specimen from:*
                    perirenal tissue (91.21–91.29)
                    perivesical tissue (91.31–91.39)
                    retroperitoneum NEC (91.11–91.19)
                    retroperitoneal x-ray (88.14–88.16)

✖ **59.3   Plication of urethrovesical junction**
        Kelly-Kennedy operation on urethra
        Kelly-Stoeckel urethral plication

✖ **59.4   Suprapubic sling operation**
        Goebel-Frangenheim-Stoeckel urethrovesical suspension
        Millin-Read urethrovesical suspension
        Oxford operation for urinary incontinence
        Urethrocystopexy by suprapubic suspension

✖ **59.5   Retropubic urethral suspension**
        Burch procedure
        Marshall-Marchetti-Krantz operation
        Suture of periurethral tissue to symphysis pubis
        Urethral suspension NOS
        Coding Clinic: 1997, Q1, P11-12

✖ **59.6   Paraurethral suspension**
        Pereyra paraurethral suspension
        Periurethral suspension

● **59.7   Other repair of urinary stress incontinence**

✖ **59.71   Levator muscle operation for urethrovesical
        suspension**
        Cystourethropexy with levator muscle sling
        Gracilis muscle transplant for urethrovesical
            suspension
        Pubococcygeal sling

59.72   Injection of implant into urethra and/or bladder neck
        Collagen implant
        Endoscopic injection of implant
        Fat implant
        Polytef implant
        Coding Clinic: 1995, Q4, P72-73

✖ **59.79   Other**
        Anterior urethropexy
        Repair of stress incontinence NOS
        Tudor "rabbit ear" urethropexy
        Coding Clinic: 2001, Q2, P20; 2000, Q1, P14-15, 19-20; 1995, Q4,
                    P72-73

59.8   Ureteral catheterization
        Drainage of kidney by catheter
        Insertion of ureteral stent
        Ureterovesical orifice dilation
        Code also any ureterotomy (56.2)
        Excludes   *that for:*
                    retrograde pyelogram (87.74)
                    transurethral removal of calculus or clot from
                        ureter and renal pelvis (56.0)
        Coding Clinic: 2005, Q2, P12-13; 2003, Q2, P11-12; 2000, Q3, P7-8; 1994,
                    Q3, P8

● **59.9   Other operations on urinary system**
        Excludes   *nonoperative removal of therapeutic device*
                    (97.61–97.69)

✖ **59.91   Excision of perirenal or perivesical tissue**
        Excludes   *biopsy of perirenal or perivesical tissue*
                    (59.21)

✖ **59.92   Other operations on perirenal or perivesical tissue**

59.93   Replacement of ureterostomy tube
        Change of ureterostomy tube
        Reinsertion of ureterostomy tube
        Excludes   *nonoperative removal of ureterostomy tube*
                    (97.62)

59.94   Replacement of cystostomy tube
        Excludes   *nonoperative removal of cystostomy tube*
                    (97.63)

59.95   Ultrasonic fragmentation of urinary stones
        Shattered urinary stones
        Excludes   *percutaneous nephrostomy with*
                    fragmentation (55.04)
                    shock-wave disintegration (98.51)
        Coding Clinic: 1986, Sept-Oct, P11-12; 1984, Nov-Dec, P20

59.99   Other
        Excludes   *instillation of medication into urinary tract*
                    (96.49)
                    irrigation of urinary tract (96.45–96.48)
        Coding Clinic: 2008, Q2, P14

◀ New   ◀▥ Revised   ~~deleted~~ Deleted   ● Use Additional Digit(s)   ✖ Valid O.R. Procedure
◆ Non-O.R. Procedure   ♀ Females Only   ♂ Males Only   OGCR Official Guidelines   Coding Clinic

11. OPERATIONS ON THE MALE GENITAL ORGANS (60–64)

● **60 Operations on prostate and seminal vesicles**

    Includes operations on periprostatic tissue

    Code also any application or administration of an adhesion barrier substance (99.77)

    Excludes *that associated with radical cystectomy (57.71)*

✖ **60.0 Incision of prostate** ♂

    Drainage of prostatic abscess

    Prostatolithotomy

    Excludes *drainage of periprostatic tissue only (60.81)*

● **60.1 Diagnostic procedures on prostate and seminal vesicles**

    60.11 Closed [percutaneous] [needle] biopsy of prostate ♂

        Approach:

           transrectal

           transurethral

        Punch biopsy

    ✖ **60.12 Open biopsy of prostate** ♂

    60.13 Closed [percutaneous] biopsy of seminal vesicles ♂

        Needle biopsy of seminal vesicles

    ✖ **60.14 Open biopsy of seminal vesicles** ♂

    ✖ **60.15 Biopsy of periprostatic tissue** ♂

    ✖ **60.18 Other diagnostic procedures on prostate and periprostatic tissue** ♂

        Excludes *microscopic examination of specimen from prostate (91.31–91.39)*

               x-ray of prostate (87.92)

    ✖ **60.19 Other diagnostic procedures on seminal vesicles** ♂

        Excludes *microscopic examination of specimen from seminal vesicles (91.31–91.39)*

               x-ray:

                    contrast seminal vesiculogram (87.91)

                    other (87.92)

● **60.2 Transurethral prostatectomy**

    Excludes *local excision of lesion of prostate (60.61)*

    Coding Clinic: 1993, 5th Issue, P9; 1985, Sept-Oct, P10

    ✖ **60.21 Transurethral (ultrasound) guided laser induced prostatectomy (TULIP)** ♂

        Ablation (contact) (noncontact) by laser

        Coding Clinic: 1995, Q4, P71; 1994, Q2, P9; 1992, Q3, P13

    ✖ **60.29 Other transurethral prostatectomy** ♂

        Excision of median bar by transurethral approach

        Transurethral electrovaporization of prostate (TEVAP)

        Transurethral enucleative procedure

        Transurethral prostatectomy NOS

        Transurethral resection of prostate (TURP)

        Coding Clinic: 1997, Q3, P3; 1994, Q3, P12

✖ **60.3 Suprapubic prostatectomy** ♂

    Transvesical prostatectomy

    Excludes *local excision of lesion of prostate (60.61)*

             radical prostatectomy (60.5)

✖ **60.4 Retropubic prostatectomy** ♂

    Excludes *local excision of lesion of prostate (60.61)*

             radical prostatectomy (60.5)

✖ **60.5 Radical prostatectomy** ♂

    Prostatovesiculectomy

    Radical prostatectomy by any approach

    Excludes *cystoprostatectomy (57.71)*

    Coding Clinic: 1993, Q3, P12

● **60.6 Other prostatectomy**

    ✖ **60.61 Local excision of lesion of prostate** ♂

        Excludes *biopsy of prostate (60.11–60.12)*

               laser interstitial thermal therapy [LITT] of lesion or tissue of prostate under guidance (17.69)

    ✖ **60.62 Perineal prostatectomy** ♂

        Cryoablation of prostate

        Cryoprostatectomy

        Cryosurgery of prostate

        Radical cryosurgical ablation of prostate (RCSA)

        Excludes *local excision of lesion of prostate (60.61)*

    ✖ **60.69 Other** ♂

● **60.7 Operations on seminal vesicles**

    60.71 Percutaneous aspiration of seminal vesicle ♂

        Excludes *needle biopsy of seminal vesicle (60.13)*

    ✖ **60.72 Incision of seminal vesicle** ♂

    ✖ **60.73 Excision of seminal vesicle** ♂

        Excision of Müllerian duct cyst

        Spermatocystectomy

        Excludes *biopsy of seminal vesicle (60.13–60.14)*

               prostatovesiculectomy (60.5)

    ✖ **60.79 Other operations on seminal vesicles** ♂

● **60.8 Incision or excision of periprostatic tissue**

    ✖ **60.81 Incision of periprostatic tissue** ♂

        Drainage of periprostatic abscess

    ✖ **60.82 Excision of periprostatic tissue** ♂

        Excision of lesion of periprostatic tissue

        Excludes *biopsy of periprostatic tissue (60.15)*

● **60.9 Other operations on prostate**

    60.91 Percutaneous aspiration of prostate ♂

        Excludes *needle biopsy of prostate (60.11)*

    60.92 Injection into prostate test link ♂

    ✖ **60.93 Repair of prostate** ♂

    ✖ **60.94 Control of (postoperative) hemorrhage of prostate** ♂

        Coagulation of prostatic bed

        Cystoscopy for control of prostatic hemorrhage

    ✖ **60.95 Transurethral balloon dilation of the prostatic urethra** ♂

    ✖ **60.96 Transurethral destruction of prostate tissue by microwave thermotherapy** ♂

        Transurethral microwave thermotherapy (TUMT) of prostate

        Excludes *prostatectomy:*

               other (60.61–60.69)

               radical (60.5)

               retropubic (60.4)

               suprapubic (60.3)

               transurethral (60.21–60.29)

    ✖ **60.97 Other transurethral destruction of prostate tissue by other thermotherapy** ♂

        Radiofrequency thermotherapy

        Transurethral needle ablation (TUNA) of prostate

        Excludes *prostatectomy:*

               other (60.61–60.69)

               radical (60.5)

               retropubic (60.4)

               suprapubic (60.3)

               transurethral (60.21–60.29)

    ✖ **60.99 Other** ♂

        Excludes *prostatic massage (99.94)*

        Coding Clinic: 1990, Q3, P13

Excludes	Includes	Use additional	Code also	Omit code

● **61   Operations on scrotum and tunica vaginalis**
    61.0   Incision and drainage of scrotum and tunica vaginalis ♂
        Excludes   *percutaneous aspiration of hydrocele (61.91)*
● **61.1   Diagnostic procedures on scrotum and tunica vaginalis**
        61.11   Biopsy of scrotum or tunica vaginalis ♂
        61.19   Other diagnostic procedures on scrotum and tunica vaginalis ♂
✖ **61.2   Excision of hydrocele (of tunica vaginalis)** ♂
    Bottle repair of hydrocele of tunica vaginalis
        Excludes   *percutaneous aspiration of hydrocele (61.91)*
    61.3   Excision or destruction of lesion or tissue of scrotum ♂
    Fulguration of lesion of scrotum
    Reduction of elephantiasis of scrotum
    Partial scrotectomy of scrotum
        Excludes   *biopsy of scrotum (61.11)*
                  scrotal fistulectomy (61.42)
● **61.4   Repair of scrotum and tunica vaginalis**
        61.41   Suture of laceration of scrotum and tunica vaginalis ♂
      ✖ **61.42   Repair of scrotal fistula** ♂
      ✖ **61.49   Other repair of scrotum and tunica vaginalis** ♂
        Reconstruction with rotational or pedicle flaps
● **61.9   Other operations on scrotum and tunica vaginalis**
        61.91   Percutaneous aspiration of tunica vaginalis ♂
        Aspiration of hydrocele of tunica vaginalis
      ✖ **61.92   Excision of lesion of tunica vaginalis other than hydrocele** ♂
        Excision of hematocele of tunica vaginalis
      ✖ **61.99   Other** ♂
        Excludes   *removal of foreign body from scrotum without incision (98.24)*

● **62   Operations on testes**
  ✖ **62.0   Incision of testis** ♂
● **62.1   Diagnostic procedures on testes**
        62.11   Closed [percutaneous] [needle] biopsy of testis ♂
      ✖ **62.12   Open biopsy of testis** ♂
      ✖ **62.19   Other diagnostic procedures on testes** ♂
✖ **62.2   Excision or destruction of testicular lesion** ♂
    Excision of appendix testis
    Excision of cyst of Morgagni in the male
        Excludes   *biopsy of testis (62.11–62.12)*
✖ **62.3   Unilateral orchiectomy** ♂
    Orchidectomy (with epididymectomy) NOS
● **62.4   Bilateral orchiectomy**
    Male castration
    Radical bilateral orchiectomy (with epididymectomy)
    Code also any synchronous lymph node dissection (40.3, 40.5)
      ✖ **62.41   Removal of both testes at same operative episode** ♂
        Bilateral orchidectomy NOS
      ✖ **62.42   Removal of remaining testis** ♂
        Removal of solitary testis
✖ **62.5   Orchiopexy** ♂
    Mobilization and replacement of testis in scrotum
    Orchiopexy with detorsion of testis
    Torek (-Bevan) operation (orchidopexy) (first stage) (second stage)
    Transplantation to and fixation of testis in scrotum
● **62.6   Repair of testes**
        Excludes   *reduction of torsion (63.52)*
      ✖ **62.61   Suture of laceration of testis** ♂
      ✖ **62.69   Other repair of testis** ♂
        Testicular graft
✖ **62.7   Insertion of testicular prosthesis** ♂
● **62.9   Other operations on testes**
        62.91   Aspiration of testis ♂
        Excludes   *percutaneous biopsy of testis (62.11)*
        62.92   Injection of therapeutic substance into testis ♂
      ✖ **62.99   Other** ♂

● **63   Operations on spermatic cord, epididymis, and vas deferens**
  ● **63.0   Diagnostic procedures on spermatic cord, epididymis, and vas deferens**
        63.01   Biopsy of spermatic cord, epididymis, or vas deferens ♂
      ✖ **63.09   Other diagnostic procedures on spermatic cord, epididymis, and vas deferens** ♂
        Excludes   *contrast epididymogram (87.93)*
                contrast vasogram (87.94)
                other x-ray of epididymis and vas deferens (87.95)
✖ **63.1   Excision of varicocele and hydrocele of spermatic cord** ♂
    High ligation of spermatic vein
    Hydrocelectomy of canal of Nuck
✖ **63.2   Excision of cyst of epididymis** ♂
    Spermatocelectomy
✖ **63.3   Excision of other lesion or tissue of spermatic cord and epididymis** ♂
    Excision of appendix epididymis
        Excludes   *biopsy of spermatic cord or epididymis (63.01)*
✖ **63.4   Epididymectomy** ♂
        Excludes   *that synchronous with orchiectomy (62.3–62.42)*
● **63.5   Repair of spermatic cord and epididymis**
      ✖ **63.51   Suture of laceration of spermatic cord and epididymis** ♂
        63.52   Reduction of torsion of testis or spermatic cord ♂
        Excludes   *that associated with orchiopexy (62.5)*
      ✖ **63.53   Transplantation of spermatic cord** ♂
      ✖ **63.59   Other repair of spermatic cord and epididymis** ♂
    63.6   Vasotomy ♂
    Vasostomy
● **63.7   Vasectomy and ligation of vas deferens**
        63.70   Male sterilization procedure, not otherwise specified ♂
        MCE: Non-covered procedure
        63.71   Ligation of vas deferens ♂
        Crushing of vas deferens
        Division of vas deferens
        MCE: Non-covered procedure
        63.72   Ligation of spermatic cord ♂
        MCE: Non-covered procedure
        63.73   Vasectomy ♂
        MCE: Non-covered procedure
        Coding Clinic: 1998, Q2, P13
● **63.8   Repair of vas deferens and epididymis**
      ✖ **63.81   Suture of laceration of vas deferens and epididymis** ♂
      ✖ **63.82   Reconstruction of surgically divided vas deferens** ♂
      ✖ **63.83   Epididymovasostomy** ♂
      ✖ **63.84   Removal of ligature from vas deferens** ♂
      ✖ **63.85   Removal of valve from vas deferens** ♂
      ✖ **63.89   Other repair of vas deferens and epididymis** ♂
● **63.9   Other operations on spermatic cord, epididymis, and vas deferens**
        63.91   Aspiration of spermatocele ♂
      ✖ **63.92   Epididymotomy** ♂
      ✖ **63.93   Incision of spermatic cord** ♂
      ✖ **63.94   Lysis of adhesions of spermatic cord** ♂
      ✖ **63.95   Insertion of valve in vas deferens** ♂
      ✖ **63.99   Other** ♂

● **64   Operations on penis**
    Includes   operations on:
        corpora cavernosa
        glans penis
        prepuce
    64.0   Circumcision ♂
● **64.1   Diagnostic procedures on the penis**
      ✖ **64.11   Biopsy of penis** ♂
        64.19   Other diagnostic procedures on penis ♂

✖ **64.2** **Local excision or destruction of lesion of penis** ♂
    Excludes *biopsy of penis (64.11)*

✖ **64.3** **Amputation of penis** ♂

● **64.4** **Repair and plastic operation on penis**

✖ **64.41** **Suture of laceration of penis** ♂

✖ **64.42** **Release of chordee** ♂
    Coding Clinic: 1996, Q4, P34-35

✖ **64.43** **Construction of penis** ♂

✖ **64.44** **Reconstruction of penis** ♂

✖ **64.45** **Replantation of penis** ♂
    Reattachment of amputated penis

✖ **64.49** **Other repair of penis** ♂
    Excludes *repair of epispadias and hypospadias (58.45)*

✖ **64.5** **Operations for sex transformation, not elsewhere classified** ♂
    MCE: Non-covered procedure

● **64.9** **Other operations on male genital organs**

64.91 **Dorsal or lateral slit of prepuce** ♂

✖ **64.92** **Incision of penis** ♂

✖ **64.93** **Division of penile adhesions** ♂

64.94 **Fitting of external prosthesis of penis** ♂
    Penile prosthesis NOS

✖ **64.95** **Insertion or replacement of non-inflatable penile prosthesis** ♂
    Insertion of semi-rigid rod prosthesis into shaft of penis
    Excludes *external penile prosthesis (64.94)*
    inflatable penile prosthesis (64.97)
    plastic repair, penis (64.43–64.49)
    that associated with:
    construction (64.43)
    reconstruction (64.44)

✖ **64.96** **Removal of internal prosthesis of penis** ♂
    Removal without replacement of non-inflatable or inflatable penile prosthesis

✖ **64.97** **Insertion or replacement of inflatable penile prosthesis** ♂
    Insertion of cylinders into shaft of penis and placement of pump and reservoir
    Excludes *external penile prosthesis (64.94)*
    non-inflatable penile prosthesis (64.95)
    plastic repair, penis (64.43–64.49)
    Coding Clinic: 1990, Q2, P26

✖ **64.98** **Other operations on penis** ♂
    Corpora cavernosa-corpus spongiosum shunt
    Corpora-saphenous shunt
    Irrigation of corpus cavernosum
    Excludes *removal of foreign body:*
    intraluminal (98.19)
    without incision (98.24)
    stretching of foreskin (99.95)
    Coding Clinic: 1992, Q3, P9-10

✖ **64.99** **Other** ♂
    Excludes *collection of sperm for artificial insemination (99.96)*

---

12. OPERATIONS ON THE FEMALE GENITAL ORGANS (65–71)

● **65** **Operations on ovary**
    Code also any application or administration of an adhesion barrier substance (99.77)

● **65.0** **Oophorotomy**
    Salpingo-oophorotomy

✖ **65.01** **Laparoscopic oophorotomy** ♀

✖ **65.09** **Other oophorotomy** ♀

● **65.1** **Diagnostic procedures on ovaries**

✖ **65.11** **Aspiration biopsy of ovary** ♀

✖ **65.12** **Other biopsy of ovary** ♀

✖ **65.13** **Laparoscopic biopsy of ovary** ♀
    Coding Clinic: 1996, Q4, P66-67

✖ **65.14** **Other laparoscopic diagnostic procedures on ovaries** ♀

✖ **65.19** **Other diagnostic procedures on ovaries** ♀
    Excludes *microscopic examination of specimen from ovary (91.41–91.49)*

● **65.2** **Local excision or destruction of ovarian lesion or tissue**

✖ **65.21** **Marsupialization of ovarian cyst** ♀
    Excludes *that by laparoscope (65.23)*

✖ **65.22** **Wedge resection of ovary** ♀
    Excludes *that by laparoscope (65.24)*

✖ **65.23** **Laparoscopic marsupialization of ovarian cyst** ♀

✖ **65.24** **Laparoscopic wedge resection of ovary** ♀

✖ **65.25** **Other laparoscopic local excision or destruction of ovary** ♀

✖ **65.29** **Other local excision or destruction of ovary** ♀
    Bisection of ovary
    Cauterization of ovary
    Partial excision of ovary
    Excludes *biopsy of ovary (65.11–65.13)*
    that by laparoscope (65.25)

● **65.3** **Unilateral oophorectomy**
    Coding Clinic: 1995, Q3, P15

✖ **65.31** **Laparoscopic unilateral oophorectomy** ♀

✖ **65.39** **Other unilateral oophorectomy** ♀
    Excludes *that by laparoscope (65.31)*

● **65.4** **Unilateral salpingo-oophorectomy**

✖ **65.41** **Laparoscopic unilateral salpingo-oophorectomy** ♀
    Coding Clinic: 1996, Q4, P66-67

✖ **65.49** **Other unilateral salpingo-oophorectomy** ♀

● **65.5** **Bilateral oophorectomy**

✖ **65.51** **Other removal of both ovaries at same operative episode** ♀
    Female castration
    Excludes *that by laparoscope (65.53)*

✖ **65.52** **Other removal of remaining ovary** ♀
    Removal of solitary ovary
    Excludes *that by laparoscope (65.54)*

✖ **65.53** **Laparoscopic removal of both ovaries at same operative episode** ♀

✖ **65.54** **Laparoscopic removal of remaining ovary** ♀

● **65.6** **Bilateral salpingo-oophorectomy**

✖ **65.61** **Other removal of both ovaries and tubes at same operative episode** ♀
    Excludes *that by laparoscope (65.63)*
    Coding Clinic: 2012, Q4, P82; 1996, Q4, P64-65

✖ **65.62** **Other removal of remaining ovary and tube** ♀
    Removal of solitary ovary and tube
    Excludes *that by laparoscope (65.64)*

✖ **65.63** **Laparoscopic removal of both ovaries and tubes at same operative episode** ♀
    Coding Clinic: 2012, Q1, P3-5; 2009, Q3, P6; 2006, Q4, P130-134; 1996, Q4, P68

✖ **65.64** **Laparoscopic removal of remaining ovary and tube** ♀

Excludes   Includes   Use additional   Code also   Omit code

● 65.7 Repair of ovary
　　Excludes *salpingo-oophorostomy (66.72)*
　✖ 65.71 Other simple suture of ovary ♀
　　　Excludes *that by laparoscope (65.74)*
　✖ 65.72 Other reimplantation of ovary ♀
　　　Excludes *that by laparoscope (65.75)*
　✖ 65.73 Other salpingo-oophoroplasty ♀
　　　Excludes *that by laparoscope (65.76)*
　✖ 65.74 Laparoscopic simple suture of ovary ♀
　✖ 65.75 Laparoscopic reimplantation of ovary ♀
　✖ 65.76 Laparoscopic salpingo-oophoroplasty ♀
　✖ 65.79 Other repair of ovary ♀
　　　Oophoropexy
● 65.8 Lysis of adhesions of ovary and fallopian tube
　✖ 65.81 Laparoscopic lysis of adhesions of ovary and fallopian tube ♀
　　　Coding Clinic: 1996, Q4, P66-67
　✖ 65.89 Other lysis of adhesions of ovary and fallopian tube ♀
　　　Excludes *that by laparoscope (65.81)*
● 65.9 Other operations on ovary
　✖ 65.91 Aspiration of ovary ♀
　　　Excludes *aspiration biopsy of ovary (65.11)*
　✖ 65.92 Transplantation of ovary ♀
　　　Excludes *reimplantation of ovary*
　　　　　laparoscopic (65.75)
　　　　　other (65.72)
　✖ 65.93 Manual rupture of ovarian cyst ♀
　✖ 65.94 Ovarian denervation ♀
　✖ 65.95 Release of torsion of ovary ♀
　✖ 65.99 Other ♀
　　　Ovarian drilling
　　　Coding Clinic: 1986, Nov-Dec, P9
● 66 Operations on fallopian tubes
　　Code also any application or administration of an adhesion
　　　barrier substance (99.77)
● 66.0 Salpingotomy and salpingostomy
　✖ 66.01 Salpingotomy ♀
　✖ 66.02 Salpingostomy ♀
● 66.1 Diagnostic procedures on fallopian tubes
　✖ 66.11 Biopsy of fallopian tube ♀
　✖ 66.19 Other diagnostic procedures on fallopian tubes ♀
　　　Excludes *microscopic examination of specimen from*
　　　　　fallopian tubes (91.41–91.49)
　　　　　radiography of fallopian tubes (87.82–87.83,
　　　　　87.85)
　　　　　Rubin's test (66.8)
● 66.2 Bilateral endoscopic destruction or occlusion of fallopian tubes
　　Includes bilateral endoscopic destruction or occlusion of
　　　fallopian tubes by:
　　　　culdoscopy
　　　　endoscopy
　　　　hysteroscopy
　　　　laparoscopy
　　　　peritoneoscopy
　　　endoscopic destruction of solitary fallopian
　　　　tube
　✖ 66.21 Bilateral endoscopic ligation and crushing of fallopian tubes ♀
　　　MCE: Non-covered procedure
　✖ 66.22 Bilateral endoscopic ligation and division of fallopian tubes ♀
　　　MCE: Non-covered procedure
　✖ 66.29 Other bilateral endoscopic destruction or occlusion of fallopian tubes ♀
　　　MCE: Non-covered procedure

● 66.3 Other bilateral destruction or occlusion of fallopian tubes
　　Includes destruction of solitary fallopian tube
　　Excludes *endoscopic destruction or occlusion of fallopian*
　　　　tubes (66.21–66.29)
　✖ 66.31 Other bilateral ligation and crushing of fallopian tubes ♀
　　　MCE: Non-covered procedure
　✖ 66.32 Other bilateral ligation and division of fallopian tubes ♀
　　　Pomeroy operation
　　　MCE: Non-covered procedure
　✖ 66.39 Other bilateral destruction or occlusion of fallopian tubes ♀
　　　Female sterilization operation NOS
　　　MCE: Non-covered procedure
✖ 66.4 Total unilateral salpingectomy ♀
● 66.5 Total bilateral salpingectomy
　　Excludes *bilateral partial salpingectomy for sterilization*
　　　　(66.39)
　　　　that with oophorectomy (65.61–65.64)
　✖ 66.51 Removal of both fallopian tubes at same operative episode ♀
　✖ 66.52 Removal of remaining fallopian tube ♀
　　　Removal of solitary fallopian tube
● 66.6 Other salpingectomy
　　Includes salpingectomy by:
　　　　cauterization
　　　　coagulation
　　　　electrocoagulation
　　　　excision
　　Excludes *fistulectomy (66.73)*
　✖ 66.61 Excision or destruction of lesion of fallopian tube ♀
　　　Excludes *biopsy of fallopian tube (66.11)*
　✖ 66.62 Salpingectomy with removal of tubal pregnancy ♀
　　　Code also any synchronous oophorectomy (65.31,
　　　　65.39)
　　　Coding Clinic: 1995, Q3, P15; 1985, Sept-Oct, P14
　✖ 66.63 Bilateral partial salpingectomy, not otherwise specified ♀
　✖ 66.69 Other partial salpingectomy ♀
● 66.7 Repair of fallopian tube
　✖ 66.71 Simple suture of fallopian tube ♀
　✖ 66.72 Salpingo-oophorostomy ♀
　✖ 66.73 Salpingo-salpingostomy ♀
　✖ 66.74 Salpingo-uterostomy ♀
　✖ 66.79 Other repair of fallopian tube ♀
　　　Graft of fallopian tube
　　　Reopening of divided fallopian tube
　　　Salpingoplasty
　　　Coding Clinic: 1995, Q2, P10
　66.8 Insufflation of fallopian tube ♀
　　　Insufflation of fallopian tube with:
　　　　air
　　　　dye
　　　　gas
　　　　saline
　　　Rubin's test
　　Excludes *insufflation of therapeutic agent (66.95)*
　　　　that for hysterosalpingography (87.82–87.83)
　　　Coding Clinic: 1990, Q2, P26
● 66.9 Other operations on fallopian tubes
　66.91 Aspiration of fallopian tube ♀
　✖ 66.92 Unilateral destruction or occlusion of fallopian tube ♀
　　　Excludes *that of solitary tube (66.21–66.39)*
　✖ 66.93 Implantation or replacement of prosthesis of fallopian tube ♀
　✖ 66.94 Removal of prosthesis of fallopian tube ♀
　✖ 66.95 Insufflation of therapeutic agent into fallopian tubes ♀

◀ New　　◀‖‖ Revised　　deleted Deleted　　● Use Additional Digit(s)　　✖ Valid O.R. Procedure
◆ Non-O.R. Procedure　　♀ Females Only　　♂ Males Only　　OGCR Official Guidelines　　**Coding Clinic**

✖ **66.96** Dilation of fallopian tube ♀
✖ **66.97** Burying of fimbriae in uterine wall ♀
✖ **66.99** Other ♀
  Excludes *lysis of adhesions of ovary and tube*
    laparoscopic (65.81)
    other (65.89)
  Coding Clinic: 1994, Q2, P11

● **67** Operations on cervix
  Code also any application or administration of an adhesion barrier substance (99.77)
  67.0 Dilation of cervical canal ♀
    Excludes *dilation and curettage (69.01–69.09)*
      that for induction of labor (73.1)
  ● **67.1** Diagnostic procedures on cervix
    ✖ **67.11** Endocervical biopsy ♀
      Excludes *conization of cervix (67.2)*
    ✖ **67.12** Other cervical biopsy ♀
      Punch biopsy of cervix NOS
      Excludes *conization of cervix (67.2)*
    ✖ **67.19** Other diagnostic procedures on cervix ♀
      Excludes *microscopic examination of specimen from cervix (91.41–91.49)*
  ✖ **67.2** Conization of cervix ♀
    Excludes *that by:*
      cryosurgery (67.33)
      electrosurgery (67.32)
  ● **67.3** Other excision or destruction of lesion or tissue of cervix
    ✖ **67.31** Marsupialization of cervical cyst ♀
    ✖ **67.32** Destruction of lesion of cervix by cauterization ♀
      Electroconization of cervix
      LEEP (loop electrosurgical excision procedure)
      LLETZ (large loop excision of the transformation zone)
      Coding Clinic: 1998, Q1, P3
    ✖ **67.33** Destruction of lesion of cervix by cryosurgery ♀
      Cryoconization of cervix
    ✖ **67.39** Other excision or destruction of lesion or tissue of cervix ♀
      Excludes *biopsy of cervix (67.11–67.12)*
        cervical fistulectomy (67.62)
        conization of cervix (67.2)
  ✖ **67.4** Amputation of cervix ♀
    Cervicectomy with synchronous colporrhaphy
  ● **67.5** Repair of internal cervical os
    Coding Clinic: 2000, Q3, P11-12
    ✖ **67.51** Transabdominal cerclage of cervix ♀
    ✖ **67.59** Other repair of internal cervical os ♀
      Cerclage of isthmus uteri
      McDonald operation
      Shirodkar operation
      Transvaginal cerclage
      Excludes *laparoscopically assisted supracervical hysterectomy [LASH] (68.31)*
        transabdominal cerclage of cervix (67.51)
      Coding Clinic: 2008, Q4, P124-125
  ● **67.6** Other repair of cervix
    Excludes *repair of current obstetric laceration (75.51)*
    ✖ **67.61** Suture of laceration of cervix ♀
    ✖ **67.62** Repair of fistula of cervix ♀
      Cervicosigmoidal fistulectomy
      Excludes *fistulectomy:*
        cervicovesical (57.84)
        ureterocervical (56.84)
        vesicocervicovaginal (57.84)
    ✖ **67.69** Other repair of cervix ♀
      Repair of old obstetric laceration of cervix

● **68** Other incision and excision of uterus
  Code also any application or administration of an adhesion barrier substance (99.77)
  ✖ **68.0** Hysterotomy ♀
    Hysterotomy with removal of hydatidiform mole
    Excludes *hysterotomy for termination of pregnancy (74.91)*
  ● **68.1** Diagnostic procedures on uterus and supporting structures
    68.11 Digital examination of uterus ♀
      Excludes *pelvic examination, so described (89.26)*
        postpartal manual exploration of uterine cavity (75.7)
    68.12 Hysteroscopy ♀
      Excludes *that with biopsy (68.16)*
      Coding Clinic: 1990, Q2, P26
    ✖ **68.13** Open biopsy of uterus ♀
      Excludes *closed biopsy of uterus (68.16)*
    ✖ **68.14** Open biopsy of uterine ligaments ♀
      Excludes *closed biopsy of uterine ligaments (68.15)*
    ✖ **68.15** Closed biopsy of uterine ligaments ♀
      Endoscopic (laparoscopy) biopsy of uterine adnexa, except ovary and fallopian tube
    ✖ **68.16** Closed biopsy of uterus ♀
      Endoscopic (laparoscopy) (hysteroscopy) biopsy of uterus
      Excludes *open biopsy of uterus (68.13)*
      Coding Clinic: 2012, Q2, P18
    ✖ **68.19** Other diagnostic procedures on uterus and supporting structures ♀
      Excludes *diagnostic:*
        aspiration curettage (69.59)
        dilation and curettage (69.09)
        microscopic examination of specimen from uterus (91.41–91.49)
        pelvic examination (89.26)
        radioisotope scan of:
          placenta (92.17)
          uterus (92.19)
        ultrasonography of uterus (88.78–88.79)
        x-ray of uterus (87.81–87.89)
  ● **68.2** Excision or destruction of lesion or tissue of uterus
    ✖ **68.21** Division of endometrial synechiae ♀
      Lysis of intraluminal uterine adhesions
    ✖ **68.22** Incision or excision of congenital septum of uterus ♀
    ✖ **68.23** Endometrial ablation ♀
      Dilation and curettage
      Hysteroscopic endometrial ablation
    ✖ **68.24** Uterine artery embolization [UAE] with coils ♀
      Excludes *that without coils (68.25)*
    ✖ **68.25** Uterine artery embolization [UAE] without coils ♀
      Includes *that by:*
        gelatin sponge
        gelfoam
        microspheres
        particulate agent NOS
        polyvinyl alcohol [PVA]
        spherical embolics
      Excludes *that with coils (68.24)*
    ✖ **68.29** Other excision or destruction of lesion of uterus ♀
      Uterine myomectomy
      Excludes *biopsy of uterus (68.13, 68.16)*
        uterine fistulectomy (69.42)
      Coding Clinic: 2006, Q3, P18-19; 1996, Q1, P15

OPERATIONS ON THE FEMALE GENITAL ORGANS (65–71)

Excludes   Includes   Use additional   Code also   Omit code

1267

OPERATIONS ON THE FEMALE GENITAL ORGANS (65–71)

● **68.3**   **Subtotal abdominal hysterectomy**

  �48 **68.31**   **Laparoscopic supracervical hysterectomy [LSH]** ♀
       Classic infrafascial SEMM hysterectomy [CISH]
       Laparoscopically assisted supracervical
       hysterectomy [LASH]
       Coding Clinic: 2003, Q4, P98-99

  �48 **68.39**   **Other and unspecified subtotal abdominal
       hysterectomy** ♀
       Supracervical hysterectomy

       Excludes   *classic infrafascial SEMM hysterectomy
           [CISH] (68.31)
           laparoscopic supracervical hysterectomy
           [LSH] (68.31)*

● **68.4**   **Total abdominal hysterectomy**
     Code also any synchronous removal of tubes and ovaries
     (65.31–65.64)

     Excludes   *radical abdominal hysterectomy, any approach
        (68.61–68.69)*
     Coding Clinic: 1996, Q4, P64-65

  �48 **68.41**   **Laparoscopic total abdominal hysterectomy** ♀
       Total laparoscopic hysterectomy [TLH]
       Coding Clinic: 2012, Q1, P3-5; 2009, Q3, P6; 2006, Q4, P130-134

  �48 **68.49**   **Other and unspecified total abdominal
       hysterectomy** ♀
       Hysterectomy:
         extended

       Excludes   *laparoscopic total abdominal hysterectomy
           (68.41)*
       Coding Clinic: 2012, Q4, P82

● **68.5**   **Vaginal hysterectomy**
     Code also any synchronous:
       removal of tubes and ovaries (65.31–65.64)
       repair of cystocele or rectocele (70.50–70.52)
       repair of pelvic floor (70.79)

  �48 **68.51**   **Laparoscopically assisted vaginal hysterectomy
       (LAVH)** ♀
       Coding Clinic: 2012, Q1, P3-5; 1996, Q4, P68

  �48 **68.59**   **Other and unspecified vaginal hysterectomy** ♀

       Excludes   *laparoscopically assisted vaginal
           hysterectomy (LAVH) (68.51)
           radical vaginal hysterectomy (68.7)*

● **68.6**   **Radical abdominal hysterectomy**
     Code also any synchronous:
       lymph gland dissection (40.3, 40.5)
       removal of tubes and ovaries (65.31–65.64)

     Excludes   *pelvic evisceration (68.8)*

  �48 **68.61**   **Laparoscopic radical abdominal hysterectomy** ♀
       Laparoscopic modified radical hysterectomy
       Total laparoscopic radical hysterectomy [TLRH]
       Coding Clinic: 2006, Q4, P130-134

  �48 **68.69**   **Other and unspecified radical abdominal
       hysterectomy** ♀
       Modified radical hysterectomy
       Wertheim's operation

       Excludes   *laparoscopic total abdominal hysterectomy
           (68.41)
           laparoscopic radical abdominal hysterectomy
           (68.61)*

● **68.7**   **Radical vaginal hysterectomy**
     Code also any synchronous:
       lymph gland dissection (40.3, 40.5)
       removal of tubes and ovaries (65.31–65.64)

     Excludes   *abdominal hysterectomy, any approach
        (68.31–68.39, 68.41–68.49, 68.61–68.69,
        68.9)*

  �48 **68.71**   **Laparoscopic radical vaginal hysterectomy [LRVH]** ♀
       Coding Clinic: 2006, Q4, P130-134

  �48 **68.79**   **Other and unspecified radical vaginal hysterectomy** ♀
       Hysterocolpectomy
       Schauta operation

● **68.8**   **Pelvic evisceration** ♀
     Removal of ovaries, tubes, uterus, vagina, bladder, and
     urethra (with removal of sigmoid colon and rectum)
     Code also any synchronous:
       colostomy (46.12–46.13)
       lymph gland dissection (40.3, 40.5)
       urinary diversion (56.51–56.79)

● **68.9**   **Other and unspecified hysterectomy** ♀
     Hysterectomy, NOS

     Excludes   *abdominal hysterectomy, any approach
        (68.31–68.39, 68.41–68.49, 68.61–68.69)
        vaginal hysterectomy, any approach (68.51–68.59,
        68.71–68.79)*

● **69**   **Other operations on uterus and supporting structures**
     Code also any application or administration of an adhesion
     barrier substance (99.77)

● **69.0**   **Dilation and curettage of uterus**

     Excludes   *aspiration curettage of uterus (69.51–69.59)*

  �48 **69.01**   **Dilation and curettage for termination of pregnancy** ♀
       Coding Clinic: 1993, Q3, P6

  �48 **69.02**   **Dilation and curettage following delivery or
       abortion** ♀
       Coding Clinic: 1993, Q3, P6

  �48 **69.09**   **Other dilation and curettage** ♀
       Diagnostic D and C
       Coding Clinic: 1998, Q1, P4

● **69.1**   **Excision or destruction of lesion or tissue of uterus and
     supporting structures**

  �48 **69.19**   **Other excision or destruction of uterus and
       supporting structures** ♀

       Excludes   *biopsy of uterine ligament (68.14)*

● **69.2**   **Repair of uterine supporting structures**

  �48 **69.21**   **Interposition operation** ♀
       Watkins procedure

  �48 **69.22**   **Other uterine suspension** ♀
       Hysteropexy
       Manchester operation
       Plication of uterine ligament

  �48 **69.23**   **Vaginal repair of chronic inversion of uterus** ♀

  �48 **69.29**   **Other repair of uterus and supporting structures** ♀

● **69.3**   **Paracervical uterine denervation** ♀

● **69.4**   **Uterine repair**

     Excludes   *repair of current obstetric laceration (75.50–75.52)*

  ✈ **69.41**   **Suture of laceration of uterus** ♀

  ✈ **69.42**   **Closure of fistula of uterus** ♀

       Excludes   *uterovesical fistulectomy (57.84)*

  ✈ **69.49**   **Other repair of uterus** ♀
       Repair of old obstetric laceration of uterus

● **69.5**   **Aspiration curettage of uterus**

     Excludes   *menstrual extraction (69.6)*

  ✈ **69.51**   **Aspiration curettage of uterus for termination of
       pregnancy** ♀
       Therapeutic abortion NOS

  ✈ **69.52**   **Aspiration curettage following delivery or abortion** ♀

     69.59   **Other aspiration curettage of uterus** ♀
       Coding Clinic: 1998, Q1, P7

     69.6   **Menstrual extraction or regulation** ♀

     69.7   **Insertion of intrauterine contraceptive device** ♀

● **69.9**   **Other operations on uterus, cervix, and supporting structures**

     Excludes   *obstetric dilation or incision of cervix (73.1, 73.93)*

     69.91   **Insertion of therapeutic device into uterus** ♀

       Excludes   *insertion of:
           intrauterine contraceptive device (69.7)
           laminaria (69.93)
           obstetric insertion of bag, bougie, or pack
           (73.1)*

     69.92   **Artificial insemination** ♀

◀ New   ◀▬ Revised   ~~deleted~~ Deleted   ● Use Additional Digit(s)   ✖ Valid O.R. Procedure
◆ Non-O.R. Procedure   ♀ Females Only   ♂ Males Only   OGCR Official Guidelines   **Coding Clinic**

1268

69.93 Insertion of laminaria ♀
    Coding Clinic: 2010, Q2, P7

69.94 Manual replacement of inverted uterus ♀
    Excludes *that in immediate postpartal period (75.94)*

✖ **69.95** Incision of cervix ♀
    Excludes *that to assist delivery (73.93)*

69.96 Removal of cerclage material from cervix ♀

✖ **69.97** Removal of other penetrating foreign body from cervix ♀
    Excludes *removal of intraluminal foreign body from cervix (98.16)*

✖ **69.98** Other operations on supporting structures of uterus ♀
    Excludes *biopsy of uterine ligament (68.14)*

✖ **69.99** Other operations on cervix and uterus ♀
    Excludes *removal of:*
        foreign body (98.16)
        intrauterine contraceptive device (97.71)
        obstetric bag, bougie, or pack (97.72)
        packing (97.72)

● **70 Operations on vagina and cul-de-sac**
Code also any application or administration of an adhesion barrier substance (99.77)
Coding Clinic: 1990, Q2, P26

70.0 Culdocentesis ♀

● **70.1** Incision of vagina and cul-de-sac
    70.11 Hymenotomy ♀
    ✖ **70.12** Culdotomy ♀
    ✖ **70.13** Lysis of intraluminal adhesions of vagina ♀
    ✖ **70.14** Other vaginotomy ♀
        Division of vaginal septum
        Drainage of hematoma of vaginal cuff

● **70.2** Diagnostic procedures on vagina and cul-de-sac
    70.21 Vaginoscopy ♀
    70.22 Culdoscopy ♀
    ✖ **70.23** Biopsy of cul-de-sac ♀
    ✖ **70.24** Vaginal biopsy ♀
    ✖ **70.29** Other diagnostic procedures on vagina and cul-de-sac ♀

● **70.3** Local excision or destruction of vagina and cul-de-sac
    ✖ **70.31** Hymenectomy ♀
    ✖ **70.32** Excision or destruction of lesion of cul-de-sac ♀
        Endometrectomy of cul-de-sac
        Excludes *biopsy of cul-de-sac (70.23)*
    ✖ **70.33** Excision or destruction of lesion of vagina ♀
        Excludes *biopsy of vagina (70.24)*
                 vaginal fistulectomy (70.72–70.75)

✖ **70.4** Obliteration and total excision of vagina ♀
    Vaginectomy
    Excludes *obliteration of vaginal vault (70.8)*

● **70.5** Repair of cystocele and rectocele
    ✖ **70.50** Repair of cystocele and rectocele ♀
        Excludes *repair of cystocele and rectocele with graft or prosthesis (70.53)*
    ✖ **70.51** Repair of cystocele ♀
        Anterior colporrhaphy (with urethrocele repair)
        Excludes *repair of cystocele and rectocele with graft or prosthesis (70.53)*
                 repair of cystocele with graft or prosthesis (70.54)
        Coding Clinic: 1984, Nov-Dec, P20

✖ **70.52** Repair of rectocele ♀
    Posterior colporrhaphy
    Excludes *repair of cystocele and rectocele with graft or prosthesis (70.53)*
              repair of rectocele with graft or prosthesis (70.55)
              STARR procedure (48.74)
    Coding Clinic: 2006, Q1, P12

✖ **70.53** Repair of cystocele and rectocele with graft or prosthesis ♀
    Use additional code for biological substance (70.94) or synthetic substance (70.95), if known

✖ **70.54** Repair of cystocele with graft or prosthesis ♀
    Anterior colporrhaphy (with urethrocele repair)
    Use additional code for biological substance (70.94) or synthetic substance (70.95), if known

✖ **70.55** Repair of rectocele with graft or prosthesis ♀
    Posterior colporrhaphy
    Use additional code for biological substance (70.94) or synthetic substance (70.95), if known

● **70.6** Vaginal construction and reconstruction
    ✖ **70.61** Vaginal construction ♀
        Coding Clinic: 2006, Q3, P18-19
    ✖ **70.62** Vaginal reconstruction ♀
        Coding Clinic: 1984, Nov-Dec, P20
    ✖ **70.63** Vaginal construction with graft or prosthesis ♀
        Use additional code for biological substance (70.94) or synthetic substance (70.95), if known
        Excludes *vaginal construction (70.61)*
    ✖ **70.64** Vaginal reconstruction with graft or prosthesis ♀
        Use additional code for biological substance (70.94) or synthetic substance (70.95), if known
        Excludes *vaginal reconstruction (70.62)*

● **70.7** Other repair of vagina
    Excludes *lysis of intraluminal adhesions (70.13)*
              repair of current obstetric laceration (75.69)
              that associated with cervical amputation (67.4)
    ✖ **70.71** Suture of laceration of vagina ♀
        Coding Clinic: 1984, Nov-Dec, P20
    ✖ **70.72** Repair of colovaginal fistula ♀
    ✖ **70.73** Repair of rectovaginal fistula ♀
    ✖ **70.74** Repair of other vaginoenteric fistula ♀
    ✖ **70.75** Repair of other fistula of vagina ♀
        Excludes *repair of fistula:*
                 rectovesicovaginal (57.83)
                 ureterovaginal (56.84)
                 urethrovaginal (58.43)
                 uterovaginal (69.42)
                 vesicocervicovaginal (57.84)
                 vesicosigmoidovaginal (57.83)
                 vesicoureterovaginal (56.84)
                 vesicovaginal (57.84)
    ✖ **70.76** Hymenorrhaphy ♀
    ✖ **70.77** Vaginal suspension and fixation ♀
    ✖ **70.78** Vaginal suspension and fixation with graft or prosthesis ♀
        Use additional code for biological substance (70.94) or synthetic substance (70.95), if known
    ✖ **70.79** Other repair of vagina ♀
        Colpoperineoplasty
        Repair of old obstetric laceration of vagina

✖ **70.8** Obliteration of vaginal vault ♀
    LeFort operation

OPERATIONS ON THE FEMALE GENITAL ORGANS (65–71)

Excludes   Includes   Use additional   Code also   Omit code

● 70.9   Other operations on vagina and cul-de-sac
✖ 70.91   Other operations on vagina ♀
Excludes   *insertion of:*
diaphragm (96.17)
mold (96.15)
pack (96.14)
pessary (96.18)
suppository (96.49)
removal of:
diaphragm (97.73)
foreign body (98.17)
pack (97.75)
pessary (97.74)
replacement of:
diaphragm (97.24)
pack (97.26)
pessary (97.25)
vaginal dilation (96.16)
vaginal douche (96.44)

✖ 70.92   Other operations on cul-de-sac ♀
Obliteration of cul-de-sac
Repair of vaginal enterocele

✖ 70.93   Other operations on cul-de-sac with graft or prosthesis ♀
Repair of vaginal enterocele with graft or prosthesis
Use additional code for biological substance (70.94) or synthetic substance (70.95), if known

70.94   Insertion of biological graft ♀
Allogenic material or substance
Allograft
Autograft
Autologous material or substance
Heterograft
Xenogenic material or substance
Code first these procedures when done with graft or prosthesis:
Other operations on cul-de-sac (70.93)
Repair of cystocele (70.54)
Repair of cystocele and rectocele (70.53)
Repair of rectocele (70.55)
Vaginal construction (70.63)
Vaginal reconstruction (70.64)
Vaginal suspension and fixation (70.78)

70.95   Insertion of synthetic graft or prosthesis ♀
Artificial tissue
Code first these procedures when done with graft or prosthesis:
Other operations on cul-de-sac (70.93)
Repair of cystocele (70.54)
Repair of cystocele and rectocele (70.53)
Repair of rectocele (70.55)
Vaginal construction (70.63)
Vaginal reconstruction (70.64)
Vaginal suspension and fixation (70.78)

● 71   Operations on vulva and perineum
Code also any application or administration of an adhesion barrier substance (99.77)

● 71.0   Incision of vulva and perineum
✖ 71.01   Lysis of vulvar adhesions ♀
✖ 71.09   Other incision of vulva and perineum ♀
Enlargement of introitus NOS
Excludes   *removal of foreign body without incision (98.23)*

● 71.1   Diagnostic procedures on vulva
✖ 71.11   Biopsy of vulva ♀
✖ 71.19   Other diagnostic procedures on vulva ♀

● 71.2   Operations on Bartholin's gland
71.21   Percutaneous aspiration of Bartholin's gland (cyst) ♀
✖ 71.22   Incision of Bartholin's gland (cyst) ♀
✖ 71.23   Marsupialization of Bartholin's gland (cyst) ♀
✖ 71.24   Excision or other destruction of Bartholin's gland (cyst) ♀
✖ 71.29   Other operations on Bartholin's gland ♀

✖ 71.3   Other local excision or destruction of vulva and perineum ♀
Division of Skene's gland
Excludes   *biopsy of vulva (71.11)*
vulvar fistulectomy (71.72)
Coding Clinic: 2007, Q4, P90-91

✖ 71.4   Operations on clitoris ♀
Amputation of clitoris
Clitoridotomy
Female circumcision

✖ 71.5   Radical vulvectomy ♀
Code also any synchronous lymph gland dissection (40.3, 40.5)

● 71.6   Other vulvectomy
✖ 71.61   Unilateral vulvectomy ♀
Coding Clinic: 2006, Q2, P19
✖ 71.62   Bilateral vulvectomy ♀
Vulvectomy NOS

● 71.7   Repair of vulva and perineum
Excludes   *repair of current obstetric laceration (75.69)*
✖ 71.71   Suture of laceration of vulva or perineum ♀
✖ 71.72   Repair of fistula of vulva or perineum ♀
Excludes   *repair of fistula:*
urethroperineal (58.43)
urethroperineovesical (57.84)
vaginoperineal (70.75)
✖ 71.79   Other repair of vulva and perineum ♀
Repair of old obstetric laceration of vulva or perineum
Coding Clinic: 1997, Q1, P9-10

✖ 71.8   Other operations on vulva ♀
Excludes   *removal of:*
foreign body without incision (98.23)
packing (97.75)
replacement of packing (97.26)

✖ 71.9   Other operations on female genital organs ♀
Coding Clinic: 2004, Q4, P88-90; 2003, Q1, P13-14

◄ New   ◄|||| Revised   ~~deleted~~ Deleted   ● Use Additional Digit(s)   ✖ Valid O.R. Procedure
◆ Non-O.R. Procedure   ♀ Females Only   ♂ Males Only   OGCR Official Guidelines   Coding Clinic

1270

13. OBSTETRICAL PROCEDURES (72–75)

● **72 Forceps, vacuum, and breech delivery**

72.0 Low forceps operation ♀
Outlet forceps operation

72.1 Low forceps operation with episiotomy ♀
Outlet forceps operation with episiotomy

● **72.2 Mid forceps operation**

72.21 Mid forceps operation with episiotomy ♀

72.29 Other mid forceps operation ♀

● **72.3 High forceps operation**

72.31 High forceps operation with episiotomy ♀

72.39 Other high forceps operation ♀

72.4 Forceps rotation of fetal head ♀
DeLee maneuver
Key-in-lock rotation
Kielland rotation
Scanzoni's maneuver
    Code also any associated forceps extraction (72.0–72.39)

● **72.5 Breech extraction**

72.51 Partial breech extraction with forceps to aftercoming head ♀

72.52 Other partial breech extraction ♀

72.53 Total breech extraction with forceps to aftercoming head ♀

72.54 Other total breech extraction ♀

72.6 Forceps application to aftercoming head ♀
Piper forceps operation
    Excludes   partial breech extraction with forceps to aftercoming head (72.51)
    total breech extraction with forceps to aftercoming head (72.53)

● **72.7 Vacuum extraction**
    Includes   Malström's extraction

72.71 Vacuum extraction with episiotomy ♀

72.79 Other vacuum extraction ♀
    Coding Clinic: 2006, Q2, P5

72.8 Other specified instrumental delivery ♀

72.9 Unspecified instrumental delivery ♀

● **73 Other procedures inducing or assisting delivery**

● **73.0 Artificial rupture of membranes**

73.01 Induction of labor by artificial rupture of membranes ♀
Surgical induction NOS
    Excludes   artificial rupture of membranes after onset of labor (73.09)
    Coding Clinic: 2000, Q3, P5

73.09 Other artificial rupture of membranes ♀
Artificial rupture of membranes at time of delivery

73.1 Other surgical induction of labor ♀
Induction by cervical dilation
    Excludes   injection for abortion (75.0)
    insertion of suppository for abortion (96.49)

73.2 Internal and combined version and extraction

73.21 Internal and combined version without extraction ♀
Version NOS

73.22 Internal and combined version with extraction ♀

73.3 Failed forceps ♀
Application of forceps without delivery
Trial forceps

73.4 Medical induction of labor ♀
    Excludes   medication to augment active labor — omit code
    Coding Clinic: 2010, Q2, P7

● **73.5 Manually assisted delivery**

73.51 Manual rotation of fetal head ♀

73.59 Other manually assisted delivery ♀
Assisted spontaneous delivery
Crede maneuver
    Coding Clinic: 1998, Q4, P76-77

73.6 Episiotomy ♀
Episioproctotomy
Episiotomy with subsequent episiorrhaphy
    Excludes   that with:
    high forceps (72.31)
    low forceps (72.1)
    mid forceps (72.21)
    outlet forceps (72.1)
    vacuum extraction (72.71)
    Coding Clinic: 2008, Q4, P192; 2006, Q2, P5; 1992, Q1, P10-11

73.8 Operations on fetus to facilitate delivery ♀
Clavicotomy on fetus
Destruction of fetus
Needling of hydrocephalic head

● **73.9 Other operations assisting delivery**

73.91 External version ♀

73.92 Replacement of prolapsed umbilical cord ♀

73.93 Incision of cervix to assist delivery ♀
Dührssen's incisions

✖ **73.94 Pubiotomy to assist delivery** ♀
Obstetrical symphysiotomy

✖ **73.99 Other** ♀
    Excludes   dilation of cervix, obstetrical to induce labor (73.1)
    insertion of bag or bougie to induce labor (73.1)
    removal of cerclage material (69.96)

● **74 Cesarean section and removal of fetus**
Code also any synchronous:
hysterectomy (68.3–68.4, 68.6, 68.8)
myomectomy (68.29)
sterilization (66.31–66.39, 66.63)

✖ **74.0 Classical cesarean section** ♀
Transperitoneal classical cesarean section
    Coding Clinic: 2011, Q4, P133

✖ **74.1 Low cervical cesarean section** ♀
Lower uterine segment cesarean section
    Coding Clinic: 2001, Q1, P11-12

✖ **74.2 Extraperitoneal cesarean section** ♀
Supravesical cesarean section

✖ **74.3 Removal of extratubal ectopic pregnancy** ♀
Removal of:
ectopic abdominal pregnancy
fetus from peritoneal or extraperitoneal cavity following uterine or tubal rupture
    Excludes   that by salpingostomy (66.02)
    that by salpingotomy (66.01)
    that with synchronous salpingectomy (66.62)
    Coding Clinic: 1990, Q2, P25, 27; 1989, Q1, P11; 1985, Sept-Oct, P14

✖ **74.4 Cesarean section of other specified type** ♀
Peritoneal exclusion cesarean section
Transperitoneal cesarean section NOS
Vaginal cesarean section

● **74.9 Cesarean section of unspecified type**

✖ **74.91 Hysterotomy to terminate pregnancy** ♀
Therapeutic abortion by hysterotomy

✖ **74.99 Other cesarean section of unspecified type** ♀
Cesarean section NOS
Obstetrical abdominouterotomy
Obstetrical hysterotomy

OBSTETRICAL PROCEDURES (72–75)

● **75   Other obstetric operations**

75.0   Intra-amniotic injection for abortion ♀
Injection of:
   prostaglandin for induction of abortion
   saline for induction of abortion
Termination of pregnancy by intrauterine injection
> **Excludes**   *insertion of prostaglandin suppository for abortion*
> *(96.49)*

75.1   Diagnostic amniocentesis ♀

75.2   Intrauterine transfusion ♀
Exchange transfusion in utero
Insertion of catheter into abdomen of fetus for transfusion
Code also any hysterotomy approach (68.0)

● **75.3   Other intrauterine operations on fetus and amnion**
Code also any hysterotomy approach (68.0)

75.31   Amnioscopy ♀
Fetoscopy
Laparoamnioscopy
Coding Clinic: 2006, Q3, P16-18

75.32   Fetal EKG (scalp) ♀

75.33   Fetal blood sampling and biopsy ♀

75.34   Other fetal monitoring ♀
Antepartum fetal nonstress test
Fetal monitoring, not otherwise specified
> **Excludes**   *fetal pulse oximetry (75.38)*

75.35   Other diagnostic procedures on fetus and amnion ♀
Intrauterine pressure determination
> **Excludes**   *amniocentesis (75.1)*
> *diagnostic procedures on gravid uterus and*
> *placenta (87.81, 88.46, 88.78, 92.17)*

Coding Clinic: 2006, Q3, P16-18

� **75.36   Correction of fetal defect ♀**
OGCR Section I.C.10.a.2
> In cases when in utero surgery is performed on the
> fetus, a code from category 655 should be assigned
> identifying the fetal condition. Procedure code
> 75.36, Correction of fetal defect, should be assigned
> on the hospital inpatient record. No code from
> Chapter 15, the perinatal codes, should be used
> on the mother's record to identify fetal conditions.
> Surgery performed in utero on a fetus is still to be
> coded as an obstetric encounter.

75.37   Amnioinfusion ♀
Code also injection of antibiotic (99.21)
Coding Clinic: 1998, Q4, P76-77

75.38   Fetal pulse oximetry ♀
Transcervical fetal oxygen saturation monitoring
Transcervical fetal SpO_2 monitoring

75.4   Manual removal of retained placenta ♀
> **Excludes**   *aspiration curettage (69.52)*
> *dilation and curettage (69.02)*

Coding Clinic: 2006, Q3, P11

● **75.5   Repair of current obstetric laceration of uterus**

✻ **75.50   Repair of current obstetric laceration of uterus, not otherwise specified ♀**

✻ **75.51   Repair of current obstetric laceration of cervix ♀**

✻ **75.52   Repair of current obstetric laceration of corpus uteri ♀**
Coding Clinic: 2008, Q2, P7-8

● **75.6   Repair of other current obstetric laceration**
Code also episiotomy, if performed (73.6)
Coding Clinic: 2008, Q4, P192; 1992, Q1, P10-11

✻ **75.61   Repair of current obstetric laceration of bladder and urethra ♀**

75.62   Repair of current obstetric laceration of rectum and sphincter ani ♀

75.69   Repair of other current obstetric laceration ♀
Episioperineorrhaphy
Repair of:
   pelvic floor
   perineum
   vagina
   vulva
Secondary repair of episiotomy
Coding Clinic: 2008, Q4, P192; 2007, Q4, P125

75.7   Manual exploration of uterine cavity, postpartum ♀

75.8   Obstetric tamponade of uterus or vagina ♀
> **Excludes**   *antepartum tamponade (73.1)*

● **75.9   Other obstetric operations**

75.91   Evacuation of obstetrical incisional hematoma of perineum ♀
Evacuation of hematoma of:
   episiotomy
   perineorrhaphy

75.92   Evacuation of other hematoma of vulva or vagina ♀

✻ **75.93   Surgical correction of inverted uterus ♀**
Spintelli operation
> **Excludes**   *vaginal repair of chronic inversion of uterus*
> *(69.23)*

75.94   Manual replacement of inverted uterus ♀

✻ **75.99   Other ♀**
Coding Clinic: 2006, Q3, P16-18

(See Plates 244 and 509 on pages 82–83.)

14.   OPERATIONS ON THE MUSCULOSKELETAL SYSTEM (76–84)

● **76   Operations on facial bones and joints**
> **Excludes**   *accessory sinuses (22.00–22.9)*
> *nasal bones (21.00–21.99)*
> *skull (01.01–02.99)*

● **76.0   Incision of facial bone without division**

✻ **76.01   Sequestrectomy of facial bone**
Removal of necrotic bone chip from facial bone

✻ **76.09   Other incision of facial bone**
Reopening of osteotomy site of facial bone
> **Excludes**   *osteotomy associated with orthognathic*
> *surgery (76.61–76.69)*
> *removal of internal fixation device (76.97)*

● **76.1   Diagnostic procedures on facial bones and joints**

✻ **76.11   Biopsy of facial bone**

✻ **76.19   Other diagnostic procedures on facial bones and joints**
> **Excludes**   *contrast arthrogram of temporomandibular*
> *joint (87.13)*
> *other x-ray (87.11–87.12, 87.14–87.16)*

Coding Clinic: 1987, Nov-Dec, P12

✻ **76.2   Local excision or destruction of lesion of facial bone**
> **Excludes**   *biopsy of facial bone (76.11)*
> *excision of odontogenic lesion (24.4)*

◀ New   ◀ Revised   ~~deleted~~ Deleted   ● Use Additional Digit(s)   ✻ Valid O.R. Procedure
◆ Non-O.R. Procedure   ♀ Females Only   ♂ Males Only   OGCR Official Guidelines   **Coding Clinic**

● **76.3**   **Partial ostectomy of facial bone**
   �># **76.31**   **Partial mandibulectomy**
      Hemimandibulectomy
      Excludes   *that associated with temporomandibular*
           arthroplasty (76.5)
      Coding Clinic: 2005, Q2, P8-9
   ✷ **76.39**   **Partial ostectomy of other facial bone**
      Hemimaxillectomy (with bone graft or prosthesis)
      Coding Clinic: 1987, Jan-Feb, P14

● **76.4**   **Excision and reconstruction of facial bones**
   ✷ **76.41**   **Total mandibulectomy with synchronous reconstruction**
   ✷ **76.42**   **Other total mandibulectomy**
   ✷ **76.43**   **Other reconstruction of mandible**
      Excludes   *genioplasty (76.67–76.68)*
           that with synchronous total mandibulectomy
           (76.41)
      Coding Clinic: 2003, Q2, P13
   ✷ **76.44**   **Total ostectomy of other facial bone with synchronous reconstruction**
      Coding Clinic: 1993, Q3, P6
   ✷ **76.45**   **Other total ostectomy of other facial bone**
   ✷ **76.46**   **Other reconstruction of other facial bone**
      Excludes   *that with synchronous total ostectomy*
           (76.44)

✷ **76.5**   **Temporomandibular arthroplasty**
● **76.6**   **Other facial bone repair and orthognathic surgery**
      Code also any synchronous:
        bone graft (76.91)
        synthetic implant (76.92)
      Excludes   *reconstruction of facial bones (76.41–76.46)*
   ✷ **76.61**   **Closed osteoplasty [osteotomy] of mandibular ramus**
      Gigli saw osteotomy
   ✷ **76.62**   **Open osteoplasty [osteotomy] of mandibular ramus**
   ✷ **76.63**   **Osteoplasty [osteotomy] of body of mandible**
   ✷ **76.64**   **Other orthognathic surgery on mandible**
      Mandibular osteoplasty NOS
      Segmental or subapical osteotomy
      Coding Clinic: 2004, Q2, P9,10
   ✷ **76.65**   **Segmental osteoplasty [osteotomy] of maxilla**
      Maxillary osteoplasty NOS
   ✷ **76.66**   **Total osteoplasty [osteotomy] of maxilla**
   ✷ **76.67**   **Reduction genioplasty**
      Reduction mentoplasty
   ✷ **76.68**   **Augmentation genioplasty**
      Mentoplasty:
        NOS
        with graft or implant
   ✷ **76.69**   **Other facial bone repair**
      Osteoplasty of facial bone NOS

● **76.7**   **Reduction of facial fracture**
      Includes   internal fixation
      Code also any synchronous:
        bone graft (76.91)
        synthetic implant (76.92)
      Excludes   *that of nasal bones (21.71–21.72)*
   ✷ **76.70**   **Reduction of facial fracture, not otherwise specified**
   76.71   **Closed reduction of malar and zygomatic fracture**
   ✷ **76.72**   **Open reduction of malar and zygomatic fracture**
   76.73   **Closed reduction of maxillary fracture**
   76.74   **Open reduction of maxillary fracture**
   76.75   **Closed reduction of mandibular fracture**
   ✷ **76.76**   **Open reduction of mandibular fracture**
   ✷ **76.77**   **Open reduction of alveolar fracture**
      Reduction of alveolar fracture with stabilization of
      teeth

   76.78   **Other closed reduction of facial fracture**
      Closed reduction of orbital fracture
      Excludes   *nasal bone (21.71)*
   ✷ **76.79**   **Other open reduction of facial fracture**
      Open reduction of orbit rim or wall
      Excludes   *nasal bone (21.72)*

● **76.9**   **Other operations on facial bones and joints**
   ✷ **76.91**   **Bone graft to facial bone**
      Autogenous graft to facial bone
      Bone bank graft to facial bone
      Heterogenous graft to facial bone
   ✷ **76.92**   **Insertion of synthetic implant in facial bone**
      Alloplastic implant to facial bone
   76.93   **Closed reduction of temporomandibular dislocation**
   ✷ **76.94**   **Open reduction of temporomandibular dislocation**
   76.95   **Other manipulation of temporomandibular joint**
   76.96   **Injection of therapeutic substance into temporomandibular joint**
   ✷ **76.97**   **Removal of internal fixation device from facial bone**
      Excludes   *removal of:*
           dental wiring (97.33)
           external mandibular fixation device NEC
           (97.36)

   ✷ **76.99**   **Other**

● **77**   **Incision, excision, and division of other bones**
      Excludes   *laminectomy for decompression (03.09)*
           operations on:
             accessory sinuses (22.00–22.9)
             ear ossicles (19.0–19.55)
             facial bones (76.01–76.99)
             joint structures (80.00–81.99)
             mastoid (19.9–20.99)
             nasal bones (21.00–21.99)
             skull (01.01–02.99)

      The following fourth-digit subclassification is for use with
      appropriate categories in section 77 to identify the site. Valid
      fourth-digit categories are in brackets under each code.

0	**unspecified site**
1	**scapula, clavicle, and thorax [ribs and sternum]**
2	**humerus**
3	**radius and ulna**
4	**carpals and metacarpals**
5	**femur**
6	**patella**
7	**tibia and fibula**
8	**tarsals and metatarsals**
9	**other**
	Pelvic bones
	Phalanges (of foot) (of hand)
	Vertebrae

✷● **77.0**   **Sequestrectomy**
   [0-9]

✷● **77.1**   **Other incision of bone without division**
   [0-9]   Reopening of osteotomy site
      Excludes   *aspiration of bone marrow (41.31, 41.91)*
           removal of internal fixation device (78.60–78.69)
      Coding Clinic: 2002, Q1, P3-4

✷● **77.2**   **Wedge osteotomy**
   [0-9]   **Excludes**   *that for hallux valgus (77.51)*

✷● **77.3**   **Other division of bone**
   [0-9]   Osteoarthrotomy
      Excludes   *clavicotomy of fetus (73.8)*
           laminotomy or incision of vertebra (03.01–03.09)
           pubiotomy to assist delivery (73.94)
           sternotomy incidental to thoracic operation —
             omit code

OPERATIONS ON THE MUSCULOSKELETAL SYSTEM (76–84)

Excludes   Includes   Use additional   Code also   Omit code

OPERATIONS ON THE MUSCULOSKELETAL SYSTEM (76–84)

✳ ● **77.4 Biopsy of bone**
[0-9]   Coding Clinic: 2006, Q3, P13; 1998, Q2, P12

● **77.5 Excision and repair of bunion and other toe deformities**

✳ **77.51 Bunionectomy with soft tissue correction and osteotomy of the first metatarsal**

✳ **77.52 Bunionectomy with soft tissue correction and arthrodesis**

✳ **77.53 Other bunionectomy with soft tissue correction**

✳ **77.54 Excision or correction of bunionette**
        That with osteotomy

✳ **77.56 Repair of hammer toe**
        Filleting of hammer toe
        Fusion of hammer toe
        Phalangectomy (partial) of hammer toe

✳ **77.57 Repair of claw toe**
        Capsulotomy of claw toe
        Fusion of claw toe
        Phalangectomy (partial) of claw toe
        Tendon lengthening of claw toe

✳ **77.58 Other excision, fusion, and repair of toes**
        Cockup toe repair
        Overlapping toe repair
        That with use of prosthetic materials

✳ **77.59 Other bunionectomy**
        Resection of hallux valgus joint with insertion of prosthesis

✳ ● **77.6 Local excision of lesion or tissue of bone**
[0-9]   **Excludes** *biopsy of bone (77.40–77.49)*
        debridement of compound fracture (79.60–79.69)
Coding Clinic: 2013, Q3, P5; 2012, Q4, P83; 2010, Q4, P132; 2008, Q1, P3-4; 2004, Q4, P128-129; 2002, Q1, P3-49; 2001, Q3, P9; 2000, Q2, P18-19; 1999, Q1, P8-9

✳ ● **77.7 Excision of bone for graft**
[0-9]   Coding Clinic: 2013, Q2, P9; 2008, Q1, P5-6; 2007, Q2, P6; 2003, Q3, P19; 2003, Q2, P13; 2002, Q4, P107-110; 2002, Q2, P16; 2000, Q2, P12-13; 1999, Q4, P12-13; 1995, Q2, P9;1994, Q2, P7

✳ ● **77.8 Other partial ostectomy**
[0-9]   Condylectomy
        Excludes *amputation (84.00–84.19, 84.91)*
        arthrectomy (80.90–80.99)
        excision of bone ends associated with:
            arthrodesis (81.00–81.39, 81.62–81.66)
            arthroplasty (81.40–81.59, 81.71–81.85)
        excision of cartilage (80.5–80.6, 80.80–80.99)
        excision of head of femur with synchronous replacement (00.70–00.73, 81.51–81.53)
        hemilaminectomy (03.01–03.09)
        laminectomy (03.01–03.09)
        ostectomy for hallux valgus (77.51–77.59)
        partial amputation:
            finger (84.01)
            thumb (84.02)
            toe (84.11)
        resection of ribs incidental to thoracic operation — omit code
        that incidental to other operation — omit code
Coding Clinic: 2002, Q2, P8

✳ ● **77.9 Total ostectomy**
[0-9]   **Excludes** *amputation of limb (84.00–84.19, 84.91)*
        that incidental to other operation — omit code

● **78 Other operations on bones, except facial bones**

      Excludes *operations on:*
        accessory sinuses (22.00–22.9)
        facial bones (76.01–76.99)
        joint structures (80.00–81.99)
        nasal bones (21.00–21.99)
        skull (01.01–02.99)
Coding Clinic: 2002, Q2, P11
The following fourth-digit subclassification is for use with categories in section 78 to identify the site. Valid fourth-digit categories are in [brackets] under each code.

0	unspecified site
1	scapula, clavicle, and thorax [ribs and sternum]
2	humerus
3	radius and ulna
4	carpals and metacarpals
5	femur
6	patella
7	tibia and fibula
8	tarsals and metatarsals
9	other
	Pelvic bones
	Phalanges (of foot) (of hand)
	Vertebrae

✳ ● **78.0 Bone graft**
[0-9]   Bone:
        bank graft
        graft (autogenous) (heterogenous)
      That with debridement of bone graft site (removal of sclerosed, fibrous, or necrotic bone or tissue)
      Transplantation of bone
      Code also any excision of bone for graft (77.70–77.79)
      Excludes *that for bone lengthening (78.30–78.39)*
Coding Clinic: 2012, Q3, P11; 2006, Q4, P103-104; 1998, Q2, P12; 1994, Q3, P10; 1994, Q2, P7

✳ ● **78.1 Application of external fixator device**
[0-9]   Fixator with insertion of pins/wires/screws into bone
      Code also any type of fixator device, if known (84.71–84.73)
      Excludes *other immobilization, pressure, and attention to wound (93.51–93.59)*
Coding Clinic: 2005, Q4, P127-129; 1994, Q2, P5

✳ ● **78.2 Limb shortening procedures**
[0, 2-5, 7-9]   Epiphyseal stapling
      Open epiphysiodesis
      Percutaneous epiphysiodesis
      Resection/osteotomy

✳ ● **78.3 Limb lengthening procedures**
[0, 2-5, 7-9]   Bone graft with or without internal fixation devices or osteotomy
      Distraction technique with or without corticotomy/osteotomy
      Code also any application of an external fixation device (78.10–78.19)

78.4 ● Other repair or plastic operations on bone
[0-9]   Other operation on bone NEC
            Repair of malunion or nonunion fracture NEC
   Excludes   *application of external fixation device (78.10–78.19)*
                limb lengthening procedures (78.30–78.39)
                limb shortening procedures (78.20–78.29)
                osteotomy (77.3)
                reconstruction of thumb (82.61–82.69)
                repair of pectus deformity (34.74)
                repair with bone graft (78.00–78.09)
   Coding Clinic: 2013, Q1, P5; 2004, Q3, P9-10; 2002, Q3, P12; Q2, P14-16;
   1999, Q4, P22; 1997, Q1, P5; 1991, Q3, P20; Q2, P20

78.5 ● Internal fixation of bone without fracture reduction
[0-9]   Internal fixation of bone (prophylactic)
            Reinsertion of internal fixation device
            Revision of displaced or broken fixation device
   Excludes   *arthroplasty and arthrodesis (81.00–81.85)*
                bone graft (78.00–78.09)
                insertion of sternal fixation device with rigid plates
                   (84.94)
                limb shortening procedures (78.20–78.29)
                that for fracture reduction (79.10–79.19,
                   79.30–79.59)
   Coding Clinic: 2010, Q2, P6; 2004, Q3, P6-7; 2003, Q2, P15; 1999, Q4,
   P13-14; 1995, Q3, P12

78.6 ● Removal of implanted devices from bone
[0-9]   External fixator device (invasive)
            Internal fixation device
            Removal of bone growth stimulator (invasive)
            Removal of internal limb lengthening device
            Removal of pedicle screw(s) used in spinal fusion
   Excludes   *removal of cast, splint, and traction device*
                   (Kirschner wire) (Steinmann pin) (97.88)
                removal of posterior spinal motion preservation
                   (facet replacement, pedicle-based dynamic
                   stabilization, interspinous process) device(s)
                   (80.09)
                removal of skull tongs or halo traction device (02.95)
   Coding Clinic: 2003, Q2, P14; 2002, Q4, P110; 2000, Q2, P18-19; Q1,
   P15-16; 1995, Q1, P10

78.7 ● Osteoclasis
[0-9]

78.8 ● Diagnostic procedures on bone, not elsewhere
[0-9]   classified
   Excludes   *biopsy of bone (77.40–77.49)*
                magnetic resonance imaging (88.94)
                microscopic examination of specimen from bone
                   (91.51–91.59)
                radioisotope scan (92.14)
                skeletal x-ray (87.21–87.29, 87.43, 88.21–88.33)
                thermography (88.83)

78.9 ● Insertion of bone growth stimulator
[0-9]   Insertion of:
               bone stimulator (electrical) to aid bone healing
               osteogenic electrodes for bone growth stimulation
               totally implanted device (invasive)
   Excludes   *non-invasive (transcutaneous) (surface) stimulator*
                   (99.86)

79 ● Reduction of fracture and dislocation
   Includes   application of cast or splint reduction with insertion
                of traction device (Kirschner wire) (Steinmann
                pin)
   Code also any:
       application of external fixator device (78.10–78.19)
       type of fixator device, if known (84.71–84.73)
   Excludes   *external fixation alone for immobilization of fracture*
                   (93.51–93.56, 93.59)
                internal fixation without reduction of fracture
                   (78.50–78.59)
                operations on:
                   facial bones (76.70–76.79)
                   nasal bones (21.71–21.72)
                   orbit (76.78–76.79)
                   skull (02.02)
                   vertebrae (03.53)
                removal of cast or splint (97.88)
                replacement of cast or splint (97.11–97.14)
                traction alone for reduction of fracture (93.41–93.46)
   The following fourth-digit subclassification is for use with
   appropriate categories in section 79 to identify the site. Valid
   fourth-digit categories are in [brackets] under each code.

0	unspecified site	5	femur
1	humerus	6	tibia and fibula
2	radius and ulna		Leg NOS
	Arm NOS	7	tarsals and metatarsals
3	carpals and metacarpals		Foot NOS
	Hand NOS	8	phalanges of foot
4	phalanges of hand	9	other specified bone

79.0 ● Closed reduction of fracture without internal fixation
[0-9]   **Excludes**   *that for separation of epiphysis (79.40–79.49)*
            Coding Clinic: 2005, Q4, P127-129; 1989, Q3, P16; 1988, Q4, P11

79.1 ● Closed reduction of fracture with internal fixation
[0-9]   **Excludes**   *that for separation of epiphysis (79.40–79.49)*
            Coding Clinic: 1994, Q2, P6-7; 1993, Q4, P35; 1993, Q1, P27; 1984,
            May-June, P11

79.2 ● Open reduction of fracture without internal fixation
[0-9]   **Excludes**   *that for separation of epiphysis (79.50–79.59)*

79.3 ● Open reduction of fracture with internal fixation
[0-9]   **Excludes**   *that for separation of epiphysis (79.50–79.59)*
            Coding Clinic: 2012, Q2, P11-12; 2007, Q1, P3-8; 2004, Q1, P9; 1998, Q2,
            P12; 1994, Q3, P10; Q2, P5, 7

79.4 ● Closed reduction of separated epiphysis
[0-2, 5, 6, 9] Reduction with or without internal fixation

79.5 ● Open reduction of separated epiphysis
[0-2, 5, 6, 9] Reduction with or without internal fixation

79.6 ● Debridement of open fracture site
[0-9]   Debridement of compound fracture
            Coding Clinic: 1995, Q3, P12

79.7 ● Closed reduction of dislocation
   Includes   closed reduction (with external traction device)
   Excludes   *closed reduction of dislocation of*
                   temporomandibular joint (76.93)

   79.70 Closed reduction of dislocation of unspecified site
   79.71 Closed reduction of dislocation of shoulder
   79.72 Closed reduction of dislocation of elbow
   79.73 Closed reduction of dislocation of wrist
   79.74 Closed reduction of dislocation of hand and finger
   79.75 Closed reduction of dislocation of hip
   79.76 Closed reduction of dislocation of knee
   79.77 Closed reduction of dislocation of ankle
   79.78 Closed reduction of dislocation of foot and toe
   79.79 Closed reduction of dislocation of other specified sites

OPERATIONS ON THE MUSCULOSKELETAL SYSTEM (76–84)

Excludes	Includes	Use additional	Code also	Omit code

OPERATIONS ON THE MUSCULOSKELETAL SYSTEM (76–84)

● **79.8   Open reduction of dislocation**

   Includes open reduction (with internal and external
              fixation devices)

   Excludes *open reduction of dislocation of temporomandibular
             joint (76.94)*

✖ **79.80   Open reduction of dislocation of unspecified site**

✖ **79.81   Open reduction of dislocation of shoulder**

✖ **79.82   Open reduction of dislocation of elbow**

✖ **79.83   Open reduction of dislocation of wrist**

✖ **79.84   Open reduction of dislocation of hand and finger**

✖ **79.85   Open reduction of dislocation of hip**

✖ **79.86   Open reduction of dislocation of knee**

✖ **79.87   Open reduction of dislocation of ankle**
        Coding Clinic: 2004, Q1, P9

✖ **79.88   Open reduction of dislocation of foot and toe**

✖ **79.89   Open reduction of dislocation of other specified sites**

✖ ● **79.9   Unspecified operation on bone injury**
  [0-9]

● **80   Incision and excision of joint structures**

   Includes operations on:
             capsule of joint
             cartilage
             condyle
             ligament
             meniscus
             synovial membrane

   Excludes *cartilage of:*
             ear (18.01–18.9)
             nose (21.00–21.99)
             temporomandibular joint (76.01–76.99)

The following fourth-digit subclassification is for use with
appropriate categories in section 80 to identify the site:

0	unspecified site	6	knee
1	shoulder	7	ankle
2	elbow	8	foot and toe
3	wrist	9	other specified sites
4	hand and finger		Spine
5	hip		

✖ ● **80.0   Arthrotomy for removal of prosthesis without**
  [0-9] **replacement**

   Includes removal of posterior spinal motion
             preservation (dynamic stabilization,
             facet replacement, interspinous process)
             device(s)

Code also any:
   insertion of (cement) (joint) (methylmethacrylate) spacer
     (84.56)
   removal of (cement) (joint) (methylmethacrylate) spacer
     (84.57)

   Excludes *removal of pedicle screws used in spinal fusion
             (78.69)*
        Coding Clinic: 2012, Q3, P14-15; 2008, Q2, P3-5; 1997, Q2, P10; 1992, Q2,
        P18; 1990, Q2, P27

✖ ● **80.1   Other arthrotomy**
  [0-9] Arthrostomy

   Excludes *that for:*
             arthrography (88.32)
             arthroscopy (80.20–80.29)
             injection of drug (81.92)
             operative approach — omit code
        Coding Clinic: 2006, Q3, P22-23

✖ ● **80.2   Arthroscopy**
  [0-9]

● **80.3   Biopsy of joint structure**
  [0-9] Aspiration biopsy
        Coding Clinic: 2005, Q3, P13-14x2

✖ ● **80.4   Division of joint capsule, ligament, or cartilage**
  [0-9] Goldner clubfoot release
     Heyman-Herndon(-Strong) correction of metatarsus varus
     Release of:
       adherent or constrictive joint capsule
       joint
       ligament

   Excludes *symphysiotomy to assist delivery (73.94)*
             that for:
                carpal tunnel syndrome (04.43)
                tarsal tunnel syndrome (04.44)
        Coding Clinic: 2002, Q2, P16

● **80.5   Excision, destruction and other repair of intervertebral disc**
        Coding Clinic: 1986, Sept-Oct, P11-12

✖ **80.50   Excision or destruction of intervertebral disc,
        unspecified**
     Unspecified as to excision or destruction

✖ **80.51   Excision of intervertebral disc**
     Diskectomy
     Removal of herniated nucleus pulposus
     Level:
       cervical
       thoracic
       lumbar (lumbosacral)
     That by laminotomy or hemilaminectomy
     That with decompression of spinal nerve root at
       same level
     Requires additional code for any concomitant
       decompression of spinal nerve root at different
       level from excision site

   Code also any
     concurrent spinal fusion (81.00–81.09)
     repair of the anulus fibrosus (80.53–80.54)

   Excludes *intervertebral chemonucleolysis (80.52)*
             *laminectomy for exploration of intraspinal
               canal (03.09)*
             *laminotomy for decompression of spinal
               nerve root only (03.09)*
             *that for insertion of (non-fusion) spinal disc
               replacement device (84.60–84.69)*
             that with corpectomy, (vertebral) (80.99)
       Coding Clinic: 2009, Q2, P3; 2008, Q4, P183-184; Q4, P14-15;
       2008, Q1, P5-6; 2008, Q1, P3-5; 2007, Q1, P9; 2006, Q1,
       P12-13; 2004, Q4, P129-133; 2003, Q3, P12; 1996, Q1,
       P7 x2; 1995, Q2, P9

  80.52   Intervertebral chemonucleolysis
     With aspiration of disc fragments
     With diskography
     Injection of proteolytic enzyme into intervertebral
       space (chymopapain)

   Excludes *injection of anesthetic substance (03.91)*
             injection of other substances (03.92)

✖ **80.53   Repair of the anulus fibrosus with graft or prosthesis**
     Anular disc repair
     Closure (sealing) of the anulus fibrosus defect

   Includes microsurgical suture repair with fascial
             autograft
             soft tissue re-approximation repair with
             tension bands
             surgical mesh repair

   Code also any:
     application or administration of adhesion barrier
       substance, if performed (99.77)
     intervertebral discectomy, if performed (80.51)
     locally harvested fascia for graft (83.43)
     Coding Clinic: 2008, Q4, P183-184

◀ New   ◀▦ Revised   deleted Deleted   ● Use Additional Digit(s)   ✖ Valid O.R. Procedure
◆ Non-O.R. Procedure   ♀ Females Only   ♂ Males Only   OGCR Official Guidelines   Coding Clinic

1276

✖ **80.54** **Other and unspecified repair of the anulus fibrosus**
Anular disc repair
Closure (sealing) of the anulus fibrosus defect
Microsurgical suture repair without fascial autograft
Percutaneous repair of the anulus fibrosus

Code also any:
application or administration of adhesion barrier
substance, if performed (99.77)
intervertebral discectomy, if performed (80.51)
Coding Clinic: 2008, Q4, P183-184

✖ **80.59** **Other destruction of intervertebral disc**
Destruction NEC
That by laser
Coding Clinic: 2002, Q3, P10; 1989, Q1, P11; 1988, Q4, P11

✖ **80.6** **Excision of semilunar cartilage of knee**
Excision of meniscus of knee
Coding Clinic: 2003, Q2, P18; 2000, Q3, P4; 1996, Q2, P4; 1993, Q1, P23

✖ ● **80.7** **Synovectomy**
[0-9] Complete or partial resection of synovial membrane
Excludes *excision of Baker's cyst (83.39)*
Coding Clinic: 1984, Nov-Dec, P9

✖ ● **80.8** **Other local excision or destruction of lesion of joint**
[0-9] **Coding Clinic: 2008, Q1, P7**

✖ ● **80.9** **Other excision of joint**
[0-9] **Excludes** *cheilectomy of joint (77.80–77.89)*
excision of bone ends (77.80–77.89)
Coding Clinic: 2007, Q1, P20-21

● **81** **Repair and plastic operations on joint structures**
● **81.0** **Spinal fusion**
Includes arthrodesis of spine with:
bone graft
internal fixation

Code also:
any insertion of interbody spinal fusion device (84.51)
any insertion of recombinant bone morphogenetic
protein (84.52)
any synchronous excision of (locally) harvested bone for
graft (77.70–77.79)
the total number of vertebrae fused (81.62–81.64)

Note: Spinal fusion is classified by the anatomic portion
(column) fused and the technique (approach) used
to perform the fusion.

For the anterior column, the body (corpus) of
adjacent vertebrae are fused (interbody fusion).
The anterior column can be fused using an anterior,
lateral, or posterior technique.

For the posterior column, posterior structures of
adjacent vertebrae are fused (pedicle, lamina, facet,
transverse process, or "gutter" fusion). A posterior
column fusion can be performed using a posterior,
posterolateral, or lateral transverse technique.

Excludes *correction of pseudarthrosis of spine (81.30–81.39)*
refusion of spine (81.30–81.39)
Coding Clinic: 2009, Q2, P3

✖ **81.00** **Spinal fusion, not otherwise specified**
MS-DRG: Refer to Part VI, Appendix E, Table 4, Spinal
Fusion Reference Table

✖ **81.01** **Atlas-axis spinal fusion** 🔖
Craniocervical fusion by anterior, transoral, or
posterior technique
C1-C2 fusion by anterior, transoral, or posterior
technique
Occiput C2 fusion by anterior, transoral, or posterior
technique
MS-DRG: Refer to Part VI, Appendix E, Table 4, Spinal
Fusion Reference Table

✖ **81.02** **Other cervical fusion of the anterior column, anterior
technique** 🔖
Arthrodesis of C2 level or below:
anterior interbody fusion
anterolateral technique
MS-DRG: Refer to Part VI, Appendix E, Table 4, Spinal
Fusion Reference Table
**Coding Clinic: 2013, Q2, P26; 2003, Q4, P99-101; 2001, Q1, P6;
1996, Q1, P7x2**

✖ **81.03** **Other cervical fusion of the posterior column,
posterior technique** 🔖
Arthrodesis of C2 level or below, posterolateral
technique
MS-DRG: Refer to Part VI, Appendix E, Table 4, Spinal
Fusion Reference Table
Coding Clinic: 2013, Q2, P26

✖ **81.04** **Dorsal and dorsolumbar fusion of the anterior
column, anterior technique** 🔖
Arthrodesis of thoracic or thoracolumbar region:
anterior interbody fusion
anterolateral technique
Extracavitary technique
MS-DRG: Refer to Part VI, Appendix E, Table 4, Spinal
Fusion Reference Table
Coding Clinic: 2003, Q3, P19

✖ **81.05** **Dorsal and dorsolumbar fusion of the posterior
column, posterior technique** 🔖
Arthrodesis of thoracic or thoracolumbar region,
posterolateral technique
MS-DRG: Refer to Part VI, Appendix E, Table 4, Spinal
Fusion Reference Table

✖ **81.06** **Lumbar and lumbosacral fusion of the anterior
column, anterior technique** 🔖
Anterior lumbar interbody fusion (ALIF)
Arthrodesis of lumbar or lumbosacral region:
anterior interbody fusion
anterolateral technique
retroperitoneal
transperitoneal
Direct lateral interbody fusion [DLIF]
Extreme lateral interbody fusion [XLIF]
MS-DRG: Refer to Part VI, Appendix E, Table 4, Spinal
Fusion Reference Table
**Coding Clinic: 2008, Q2, P14-15; 2007, Q1, P9-10,20-21; 2002,
Q4, P107-108**

✖ **81.07** **Lumbar and lumbosacral fusion of the posterior
column, posterior technique** 🔖
Facet fusion
Posterolateral technique
Transverse process technique
MS-DRG: Refer to Part VI, Appendix E, Table 4, Spinal
Fusion Reference Table
Coding Clinic: 2009, Q2, P3; 2002, Q4, P108

✖ **81.08** **Lumbar and lumbosacral fusion of the anterior
column, posterior technique** 🔖
Arthrodesis of lumbar or lumbosacral region,
posterior interbody fusion
Axial lumbar interbody fusion [AxiaLIF]
Posterior lumbar interbody fusion (PLIF)
Transforaminal lumbar interbody fusion (TLIF)
MS-DRG: Refer to Part VI, Appendix E, Table 4, Spinal
Fusion Reference Table
**Coding Clinic: 2009, Q2, P3, 5; 2008, Q1, P5-6; 2006, Q1,
P12-14x2; 2005, Q4, P122-123; 2002, Q4, P107-110;
2000, Q2, P12-13; 1999, Q4, P12-13; 1995, Q2, P9**

OPERATIONS ON THE MUSCULOSKELETAL SYSTEM (76–84)

Excludes Includes Use additional Code also Omit code

● **81.1** **Arthrodesis and arthroereisis of foot and ankle**
  Includes arthrodesis of foot and ankle with:
    bone graft
    external fixation device

✖ **81.11** **Ankle fusion**
  Tibiotalar fusion

✖ **81.12** **Triple arthrodesis**
  Talus to calcaneus and calcaneus to cuboid and
  navicular

✖ **81.13** **Subtalar fusion**
  Excludes *arthroereisis (81.18)*

✖ **81.14** **Midtarsal fusion**

✖ **81.15** **Tarsometatarsal fusion**

✖ **81.16** **Metatarsophalangeal fusion**

✖ **81.17** **Other fusion of foot**

✖ **81.18** **Subtalar joint arthroereisis**
  Coding Clinic: 2005, Q4, P124

● **81.2** **Arthrodesis of other joint**
  Includes arthrodesis with:
    bone graft
    external fixation device
    excision of bone ends and compression

✖ **81.20** **Arthrodesis of unspecified joint**

✖ **81.21** **Arthrodesis of hip**

✖ **81.22** **Arthrodesis of knee**

✖ **81.23** **Arthrodesis of shoulder** 🖐

✖ **81.24** **Arthrodesis of elbow** 🖐

✖ **81.25** **Carporadial fusion**

✖ **81.26** **Metacarpocarpal fusion**

✖ **81.27** **Metacarpophalangeal fusion**

✖ **81.28** **Interphalangeal fusion**

✖ **81.29** **Arthrodesis of other specified joints**

● **81.3** **Refusion of spine**
  Includes arthrodesis of spine with:
    bone graft
    internal fixation
    correction of pseudarthrosis of spine

  Code also:
   any insertion of interbody spinal fusion device (84.51)
   any insertion of recombinant bone morphogenetic
    protein (84.52)
   any synchronous excision of (locally) harvested bone for
    graft (77.70–77.79)
   the total number of vertebrae fused (81.62–81.64)

  Note: Spine fusion is classified by the anatomic portion
    (column) fused and the technique (approach) used
    to perform the fusion.

    For the anterior column, the body (corpus) of
    adjacent vertebrae are fused (interbody fusion).
    The anterior column can be fused using an anterior,
    lateral, or posterior technique.

    For the posterior column, posterior structures of
    adjacent vertebrae are fused (pedicle, lamina, facet,
    transverse process, or "gutter" fusion). A posterior
    column fusion can be performed using a posterior,
    posterolateral, or lateral transverse technique.
  Coding Clinic: 2005, Q4, P122-123

✖ **81.30** **Refusion of spine, not otherwise specified**
  MS-DRG: Refer to Part VI, Appendix E, Table 4, Spinal
  Fusion Reference Table

✖ **81.31** **Refusion of atlas-axis spine** 🖐
  Craniocervical fusion by anterior, transoral, or
   posterior technique
  C1-C2 fusion by anterior, transoral, or posterior
   technique
  Occiput C2 fusion by anterior, transoral, or posterior
   technique
  MS-DRG: Refer to Part VI, Appendix E, Table 4, Spinal
  Fusion Reference Table

✖ **81.32** **Refusion of other cervical spine, anterior column,
anterior technique** 🖐
  Arthrodesis of C2 level or below:
   anterior interbody fusion
   anterolateral technique
  MS-DRG: Refer to Part VI, Appendix E, Table 4, Spinal
  Fusion Reference Table

✖ **81.33** **Refusion of other cervical spine, posterior column,
posterior technique** 🖐
  Arthrodesis of C2 level or below, posterolateral
   technique
  MS-DRG: Refer to Part VI, Appendix E, Table 4, Spinal
  Fusion Reference Table

✖ **81.34** **Refusion of dorsal and dorsolumbar spine, anterior
column, anterior technique** 🖐
  Arthrodesis of thoracic or thoracolumbar region:
   anterior interbody fusion
   anterolateral technique
  Extracavitary technique
  MS-DRG: Refer to Part VI, Appendix E, Table 4, Spinal
  Fusion Reference Table

✖ **81.35** **Refusion of dorsal and dorsolumbar spine, posterior
column, posterior technique** 🖐
  Arthrodesis of thoracic or thoracolumbar region,
   posterolateral technique
  MS-DRG: Refer to Part VI, Appendix E, Table 4, Spinal
  Fusion Reference Table

✖ **81.36** **Refusion of lumbar and lumbosacral spine, anterior
column, anterior technique** 🖐
  Anterior lumbar interbody fusion (ALIF)
  Arthrodesis of lumbar or lumbosacral region:
   anterior interbody fusion
   anterolateral technique
   retroperitoneal
   transperitoneal
  Direct lateral interbody fusion [DLIF]
  Extreme lateral interbody fusion [XLIF]
  MS-DRG: Refer to Part VI, Appendix E, Table 4, Spinal
  Fusion Reference Table

✖ **81.37** **Refusion of lumbar and lumbosacral spine, posterior
column, posterior technique** 🖐
  Facet fusion
  Posterolateral technique
  Transverse process technique
  MS-DRG: Refer to Part VI, Appendix E, Table 4, Spinal
  Fusion Reference Table

✖ **81.38** **Refusion of lumbar and lumbosacral spine, anterior
column, posterior technique** 🖐
  Arthrodesis of lumbar or lumbosacral region,
   posterior interbody fusion
  Axial lumbar interbody fusion [AxiaLIF]
  Posterior lumbar interbody fusion (PLIF)
  Transforaminal lumbar interbody fusion (TLIF)
  MS-DRG: Refer to Part VI, Appendix E, Table 4, Spinal
  Fusion Reference Table

✖ **81.39** **Refusion of spine, not elsewhere classified**
  MS-DRG: Refer to Part VI, Appendix E, Table 4, Spinal
  Fusion Reference Table

● **81.4** **Other repair of joint of lower extremity**
  Includes arthroplasty of lower extremity with:
    external traction or fixation
    graft of bone (chips) or cartilage
    internal fixation device

✖ **81.40** **Repair of hip, not elsewhere classified**

✖ **81.42** **Five-in-one repair of knee**
  Medial meniscectomy, medial collateral ligament
   repair, vastus medialis advancement,
   semitendinosus advancement, and pes
   anserinus transfer

✖ **81.43** **Triad knee repair**
  Medial meniscectomy with repair of the anterior
   cruciate ligament and the medial collateral
   ligament
  O'Donoghue procedure

✖ **81.44 Patellar stabilization**
Roux-Goldthwait operation for recurrent dislocation of patella

✖ **81.45 Other repair of the cruciate ligaments**

✖ **81.46 Other repair of the collateral ligaments**
Coding Clinic: 1995, Q1, P8

✖ **81.47 Other repair of knee**
Coding Clinic: 2013, Q2, P17; 2006, Q2, P13-14; 2003, Q2, P18; 2000, Q1, P12-13; 1996, Q2, P4; 1995, Q1, P8; 1993, Q3, P5

✖ **81.49 Other repair of ankle**
Coding Clinic: 2001, Q2, P14-15; 2000, Q3, P4

● **81.5 Joint replacement of lower extremity**
Note: Removal of prior prosthesis — *omit code*
Includes arthroplasty of lower extremity with:
external traction or fixation
graft of bone (chips) or cartilage
internal fixation device or prosthesis

✖ **81.51 Total hip replacement** 🏵
Replacement of both femoral head and acetabulum by prosthesis
Total reconstruction of hip
Code also any type of bearing surface, if known (00.74–00.77)
MCE: Bilateral procedure when 2+ different joint procedures are reported with principal diagnosis causes assigned to MDC 08
Coding Clinic: 2009, Q2, P3; 2004, Q4, P111-113; 1992, Q2, P18

✖ **81.52 Partial hip replacement** 🏵
Bipolar endoprosthesis
Code also any type of bearing surface, if known (00.74–00.77)
MCE: Bilateral procedure when 2+ different joint procedures are reported with principal diagnosis causes assigned to MDC 08
Coding Clinic: 1992, Q2, P18

✖ **81.53 Revision of hip replacement, not otherwise specified**
Revision of hip replacement, not specified as to components(s) replaced (acetabular, femoral, or both)
Code also any:
removal of (cement) (joint) spacer (84.57)
type of bearing surface, if known (00.74–00.77)
Excludes *revision of hip replacement, components specified (00.70–00.73)*
Coding Clinic: 2005, Q4, P106-113; 1997, Q3, P13

✖ **81.54 Total knee replacement** 🏵
Bicompartmental
Partial knee replacement
Tricompartmental
Unicompartmental (hemijoint)
MCE: Bilateral procedure when 2+ different joint procedures are reported with principal diagnosis causes assigned to MDC 08
Coding Clinic: 2013, Q3, P11, Q2, P17; 1985, Nov-Dec, P11

✖ **81.55 Revision of knee replacement, not otherwise specified**
Code also any removal of (cement) spacer (84.57)
Excludes *arthrodesis of knee (81.22)*
revision of knee replacement, components specified (00.80–00.84)
Coding Clinic: 2005, Q4, P113-117; 1997, Q2, P10

✖ **81.56 Total ankle replacement**
MCE: Bilateral procedure when 2+ different joint procedures are reported with principal diagnosis causes assigned to MDC 08

✖ **81.57 Replacement of joint of foot and toe**

✖ **81.59 Revision of joint replacement of lower extremity, not elsewhere classified**
Coding Clinic: 1988, Q1, P9

● **81.6 Other procedures on spine**
Note: Number of vertebrae
The vertebral spine consists of 25 vertebrae in the following order and number:
Cervical: C1 (atlas), C2 (axis), C3, C4, C5, C6, C7
Thoracic or Dorsal: T1, T2, T3, T4, T5, T6, T7, T8, T9, T10, T11, T12
Lumbar and Sacral: L1, L2, L3, L4, L5, S1
Coders should report only one code from the series 81.62 or 81.63 or 81.64 to show the total number of vertebrae fused on the patient.
Code also the level and approach of the fusion or refusion (81.00–81.08, 81.30–81.39)

81.62 Fusion or refusion of 2–3 vertebrae
Coding Clinic: 2009, Q2, P4; 2008, Q2, P14-15; 2008, Q1, P5-6; 2006, Q1, P12-14x2; 2005, Q4, P122-123

81.63 Fusion or refusion of 4–8 vertebrae
Coding Clinic: 2007, Q1, P20-21; 2003, Q4, P99-101

81.64 Fusion or refusion of 9 or more vertebrae
◆ Non-OR Procedure that affects MS-DRG assignment to MDC 08, MS-DRG 456-458

✖ **81.65 Percutaneous vertebroplasty**
Injection of bone void filler (cement) (polymethylmethacrylate) (PMMA) into the diseased or fractured vertebral body
Excludes *percutaneous vertebral augmentation (81.66)*
Coding Clinic: 2012, Q4, P84; 2008, Q2, P14-15; 2004, Q4, P125-126; 2002, Q2, P14-15

✖ **81.66 Percutaneous vertebral augmentation**
Insertion of inflatable balloon, bone tamp, or other device displacing (removing) (compacting) bone to create a space (cavity) (void) prior to the injection of bone void filler (cement) (polymethylmethacrylate) (PMMA) or other substance
Arcuplasty   Skyphoplasty
Kyphoplasty   Spineoplasty
Excludes *percutaneous vertebroplasty (81.65)*
Coding Clinic: 2008, Q2, P15; 2007, Q1, P3-8x2; 2006, Q3, P13; 2004, Q4, P125-126; 2002, Q2, P14

● **81.7 Arthroplasty and repair of hand, fingers and wrist**
Includes arthroplasty of hand and finger with:
external traction or fixation
graft of bone (chips) or cartilage
internal fixation device or prosthesis
Excludes *operations on muscle, tendon and fascia of hand (82.01–82.99)*

✖ **81.71 Arthroplasty of metacarpophalangeal and interphalangeal joint with implant**

✖ **81.72 Arthroplasty of metacarpophalangeal and interphalangeal joint without implant**
Coding Clinic: 1993, Q1, P28

✖ **81.73 Total wrist replacement**

✖ **81.74 Arthroplasty of carpocarpal or carpometacarpal joint with implant**

✖ **81.75 Arthroplasty of carpocarpal or carpometacarpal joint without implant**
Coding Clinic: 1993, Q3, P8

✖ **81.79 Other repair of hand, fingers and wrist**

● **81.8 Arthroplasty and repair of shoulder and elbow**
Includes arthroplasty of upper limb NEC with:
external traction or fixation
graft of bone (chips) or cartilage
internal fixation device or prosthesis

✖ **81.80 Other total shoulder replacement**
Excludes *reverse total shoulder replacement (81.88)*
Coding Clinic: 2008, Q2, P5-6

✖ **81.81 Partial shoulder replacement**

✖ **81.82 Repair of recurrent dislocation of shoulder**
Coding Clinic: 1995, Q3, P15

Excludes   Includes   Use additional   Code also   Omit code

� 81.83   **Other repair of shoulder** ⊗
   Coding Clinic: 2004, Q1, P12; 2002, Q4, P110; Q1, P9-10; 2001, Q4, P52; 2000, Q2, P14-15; 1993, Q3, P5

✶ 81.84   **Total elbow replacement**
   Partial elbow replacement

✶ 81.85   **Other repair of elbow** ⊗

✶ 81.88   **Reverse total shoulder replacement**
   Reverse ball-and-socket of the shoulder

   Excludes   *conversion of prior (failed) total shoulder replacement (arthroplasty) to reverse total shoulder replacement (81.97)*

● 81.9   **Other operations on joint structures**

   81.91   **Arthrocentesis**
      Joint aspiration

      Excludes   *that for:*
         arthrography (88.32)
         biopsy of joint structure (80.30–80.39)
         injection of drug (81.92)

   81.92   **Injection of therapeutic substance into joint or ligament**
      Coding Clinic: 2010, Q3, P14; 2000, Q2, P14-15; 1989, Q3, P16

✶ 81.93   **Suture of capsule or ligament of upper extremity**

      Excludes   *that associated with arthroplasty (81.71–81.75, 81.80–81.81, 81.84)*

✶ 81.94   **Suture of capsule or ligament of ankle and foot**

      Excludes   *that associated with arthroplasty (81.56–81.59)*

✶ 81.95   **Suture of capsule or ligament of other lower extremity**

      Excludes   *that associated with arthroplasty (81.51–81.55, 81.59)*

✶ 81.96   **Other repair of joint**

✶ 81.97   **Revision of joint replacement of upper extremity**
      Partial
      Removal of cement spacer
      Revision of arthroplasty of shoulder
      Total
      Coding Clinic: 2004, Q1, P12

✶ 81.98   **Other diagnostic procedures on joint structures**

      Excludes   *arthroscopy (80.20–80.29)*
         biopsy of joint structure (80.30–80.39)
         microscopic examination of specimen from joint (91.51–91.59)
         thermography (88.83)
         x-ray (87.21–87.29, 88.21–88.33)

✶ 81.99   **Other**

● 82   **Operations on muscle, tendon, and fascia of hand**

   Includes   operations on:
      aponeurosis
      synovial membrane (tendon sheath)
      tendon sheath

● 82.0   **Incision of muscle, tendon, fascia, and bursa of hand**

✶ 82.01   **Exploration of tendon sheath of hand**
      Incision of tendon sheath of hand
      Removal of rice bodies in tendon sheath of hand

      Excludes   *division of tendon (82.11)*

✶ 82.02   **Myotomy of hand**

      Excludes   *myotomy for division (82.19)*

✶ 82.03   **Bursotomy of hand**

   82.04   **Incision and drainage of palmar or thenar space**

✶ 82.09   **Other incision of soft tissue of hand**

      Excludes   *incision of skin and subcutaneous tissue alone (86.01–86.09)*

      Coding Clinic: 1987, Nov-Dec, P10

● 82.1   **Division of muscle, tendon, and fascia of hand**

✶ 82.11   **Tenotomy of hand**
      Division of tendon of hand

✶ 82.12   **Fasciotomy of hand**
      Division of fascia of hand

✶ 82.19   **Other division of soft tissue of hand**
      Division of muscle of hand

● 82.2   **Excision of lesion of muscle, tendon, and fascia of hand**

✶ 82.21   **Excision of lesion of tendon sheath of hand**
      Ganglionectomy of tendon sheath (wrist)

✶ 82.22   **Excision of lesion of muscle of hand**

✶ 82.29   **Excision of other lesion of soft tissue of hand**

      Excludes   *excision of lesion of skin and subcutaneous tissue (86.21–86.3)*

● 82.3   **Other excision of soft tissue of hand**
      Code also any skin graft (86.61–86.62, 86.73)

      Excludes   *excision of skin and subcutaneous tissue (86.21–86.3)*

✶ 82.31   **Bursectomy of hand**

✶ 82.32   **Excision of tendon of hand for graft**

✶ 82.33   **Other tenonectomy of hand**
      Tenosynovectomy of hand

      Excludes   *excision of lesion of:*
         tendon (82.29)
         sheath (82.21)

✶ 82.34   **Excision of muscle or fascia of hand for graft**

✶ 82.35   **Other fasciectomy of hand**
      Release of Dupuytren's contracture

      Excludes   *excision of lesion of fascia (82.29)*

✶ 82.36   **Other myectomy of hand**

      Excludes   *excision of lesion of muscle (82.22)*

✶ 82.39   **Other excision of soft tissue of hand**

      Excludes   *excision of skin (86.21–86.3)*
         excision of soft tissue lesion (82.29)

● 82.4   **Suture of muscle, tendon, and fascia of hand**

✶ 82.41   **Suture of tendon sheath of hand**

✶ 82.42   **Delayed suture of flexor tendon of hand**

✶ 82.43   **Delayed suture of other tendon of hand**

✶ 82.44   **Other suture of flexor tendon of hand**

      Excludes   *delayed suture of flexor tendon of hand (82.42)*

✶ 82.45   **Other suture of other tendon of hand**

      Excludes   *delayed suture of other tendon of hand (82.43)*

✶ 82.46   **Suture of muscle or fascia of hand**

● 82.5   **Transplantation of muscle and tendon of hand**

✶ 82.51   **Advancement of tendon of hand**

✶ 82.52   **Recession of tendon of hand**

✶ 82.53   **Reattachment of tendon of hand**

✶ 82.54   **Reattachment of muscle of hand**

✶ 82.55   **Other change in hand muscle or tendon length**

✶ 82.56   **Other hand tendon transfer or transplantation**

      Excludes   *pollicization of thumb (82.61)*
         transfer of finger, except thumb (82.81)

      Coding Clinic: 1999, Q2, P10; 1998, Q43, P39-40

✶ 82.57   **Other hand tendon transposition**
      Coding Clinic: 1993, Q3, P8; Q1, P28

✶ 82.58   **Other hand muscle transfer or transplantation**

✶ 82.59   **Other hand muscle transposition**

● 82.6   **Reconstruction of thumb**

      Includes   digital transfer to act as thumb
      Code also any amputation for digital transfer (84.01, 84.11)

✶ 82.61   **Pollicization operation carrying over nerves and blood supply**

✶ 82.69   **Other reconstruction of thumb**
      "Cocked-hat" procedure [skin flap and bone]
      Grafts:
         bone to thumb skin (pedicle) to thumb

● 82.7   **Plastic operation on hand with graft or implant**

✶ 82.71   **Tendon pulley reconstruction**
      Reconstruction for opponensplasty

✶ 82.72   **Plastic operation on hand with graft of muscle or fascia**

✶ 82.79   **Plastic operation on hand with other graft or implant**
      Tendon graft to hand

◀ New   ◀▥ Revised   ~~deleted~~ Deleted   ● Use Additional Digit(s)   ✶ Valid O.R. Procedure
◆ Non-O.R. Procedure   ♀ Females Only   ♂ Males Only   OGCR Official Guidelines   **Coding Clinic**

● **82.8 Other plastic operations on hand**
  ✳ **82.81 Transfer of finger, except thumb**
      Excludes *pollicization of thumb (82.61)*
      Coding Clinic: 2005, Q2, P7
  ✳ **82.82 Repair of cleft hand**
  ✳ **82.83 Repair of macrodactyly**
  ✳ **82.84 Repair of mallet finger**
  ✳ **82.85 Other tenodesis of hand**
      Tendon fixation of hand NOS
  ✳ **82.86 Other tenoplasty of hand**
      Myotenoplasty of hand
  ✳ **82.89 Other plastic operations on hand**
      Plication of fascia
      Repair of fascial hernia
      Excludes *that with graft or implant (82.71–82.79)*
● **82.9 Other operations on muscle, tendon, and fascia of hand**
    Excludes *diagnostic procedures on soft tissue of hand (83.21–83.29)*
  ✳ **82.91 Lysis of adhesions of hand**
      Freeing of adhesions of fascia, muscle, and tendon of hand
      Excludes *decompression of carpal tunnel (04.43)*
          that by stretching or manipulation only (93.26)
    82.92 Aspiration of bursa of hand
    82.93 Aspiration of other soft tissue of hand
      Excludes *skin and subcutaneous tissue (86.01)*
    82.94 Injection of therapeutic substance into bursa of hand
    82.95 Injection of therapeutic substance into tendon of hand
    82.96 Other injection of locally-acting therapeutic substance into soft tissue of hand
      Excludes *subcutaneous or intramuscular injection (99.11–99.29)*
  ✳ **82.99 Other operations on muscle, tendon, and fascia of hand**

● **83 Operations on muscle, tendon, fascia, and bursa, except hand**
    Includes operations on:
        aponeurosis
        synovial membrane of bursa and tendon sheaths
        tendon sheaths
    Excludes *diaphragm (34.81–34.89)*
        hand (82.01–82.99)
        muscles of eye (15.01–15.9)
● **83.0 Incision of muscle, tendon, fascia, and bursa**
  ✳ **83.01 Exploration of tendon sheath**
      Incision of tendon sheath
      Removal of rice bodies from tendon sheath
  ✳ **83.02 Myotomy**
      Excludes *cricopharyngeal myotomy (29.31)*
      Coding Clinic: 2008, Q4, P134-136
  ✳ **83.03 Bursotomy**
      Removal of calcareous deposit of bursa
      Excludes *aspiration of bursa (percutaneous) (83.94)*
  ✳ **83.09 Other incision of soft tissue**
      Incision of fascia
      Excludes *incision of skin and subcutaneous tissue alone (86.01–86.09)*
      Coding Clinic: 2009, Q1, P15
● **83.1 Division of muscle, tendon, and fascia**
  ✳ **83.11 Achillotenotomy**
  ✳ **83.12 Adductor tenotomy of hip**
  ✳ **83.13 Other tenotomy**
      Aponeurotomy
      Division of tendon
      Tendon release
      Tendon transection
      Tenotomy for thoracic outlet decompression

  ✳ **83.14 Fasciotomy**
      Division of fascia
      Division of iliotibial band
      Fascia stripping
      Release of Volkmann's contracture by fasciotomy
      Coding Clinic: 2006, Q4, P100-102
  ✳ **83.19 Other division of soft tissue**
      Division of muscle
      Muscle release
      Myotomy for thoracic outlet decompression
      Myotomy with division
      Scalenotomy
      Transection of muscle
● **83.2 Diagnostic procedures on muscle, tendon, fascia, and bursa, including that of hand**
  ✳ **83.21 Open biopsy of soft tissue**
      Excludes *biopsy of chest wall (34.23)*
          closed biopsy of skin and subcutaneous tissue (86.11)
  ✳ **83.29 Other diagnostic procedures on muscle, tendon, fascia, and bursa, including that of hand**
      Excludes *microscopic examination of specimen (91.51–91.59)*
          soft tissue x-ray (87.09, 87.38–87.39, 88.09, 88.35, 88.37)
          thermography of muscle (88.84)
● **83.3 Excision of lesion of muscle, tendon, fascia, and bursa**
    Excludes *biopsy of soft tissue (83.21)*
  ✳ **83.31 Excision of lesion of tendon sheath**
      Excision of ganglion of tendon sheath, except of hand
  ✳ **83.32 Excision of lesion of muscle**
      Excision of:
          heterotopic bone
          muscle scar for release of Volkmann's contracture
          myositis ossificans
  ✳ **83.39 Excision of lesion of other soft tissue**
      Excision of Baker's cyst
      Excludes *bursectomy (83.5)*
          excision of lesion of skin and subcutaneous tissue (86.3)
          synovectomy (80.70–80.79)
      Coding Clinic: 2010, Q3, P11; 2005, Q2, P3-4; 1997, Q2, P6
● **83.4 Other excision of muscle, tendon, and fascia**
  ✳ **83.41 Excision of tendon for graft**
  ✳ **83.42 Other tenonectomy**
      Excision of:
          aponeurosis
          tendon sheath
      Tenosynovectomy
  ✳ **83.43 Excision of muscle or fascia for graft**
      Coding Clinic: 2013, Q2, P9; 2011, Q1, P8
  ✳ **83.44 Other fasciectomy**
  ✳ **83.45 Other myectomy**
      Debridement of muscle NOS
      Scalenectomy
      Coding Clinic: 1999, Q1, P8-9
  ✳ **83.49 Other excision of soft tissue**
✳ **83.5 Bursectomy**
    Coding Clinic: 2006, Q2, P15x2; 1999, Q2, P10-11
● **83.6 Suture of muscle, tendon, and fascia**
  ✳ **83.61 Suture of tendon sheath**
  ✳ **83.62 Delayed suture of tendon**
  ✳ **83.63 Rotator cuff repair**
      Coding Clinic: 2011, Q4, P136; 2006, Q1, P6; 1993, Q2, P8
  ✳ **83.64 Other suture of tendon**
      Achillorrhaphy
      Aponeurorrhaphy
      Excludes *delayed suture of tendon (83.62)*
  ✳ **83.65 Other suture of muscle or fascia**
      Repair of diastasis recti

OPERATIONS ON THE MUSCULOSKELETAL SYSTEM (76–84)

● **83.7   Reconstruction of muscle and tendon**

> **Excludes**   *reconstruction of muscle and tendon associated with arthroplasty*

�֍ **83.71   Advancement of tendon**

�֍ **83.72   Recession of tendon**

✖ **83.73   Reattachment of tendon**

✖ **83.74   Reattachment of muscle**

✖ **83.75   Tendon transfer or transplantation**

✖ **83.76   Other tendon transposition**

✖ **83.77   Muscle transfer or transplantation**
> Release of Volkmann's contracture by muscle transplantation

✖ **83.79   Other muscle transposition**

● **83.8   Other plastic operations on muscle, tendon, and fascia**

> **Excludes**   *plastic operations on muscle, tendon, and fascia associated with arthroplasty*

✖ **83.81   Tendon graft**
> Coding Clinic: 2012, Q3, P11

✖ **83.82   Graft of muscle or fascia**
> Coding Clinic: 2013, Q2, P9; 2010, Q1, P14; 2001, Q3, P9

✖ **83.83   Tendon pulley reconstruction**

✖ **83.84   Release of clubfoot, not elsewhere classified**
> Evans operation on clubfoot

✖ **83.85   Other change in muscle or tendon length**
> Hamstring lengthening
> Heel cord shortening
> Plastic achillotenotomy
> Tendon plication

✖ **83.86   Quadricepsplasty**

✖ **83.87   Other plastic operations on muscle**
> Musculoplasty
> Myoplasty
> Coding Clinic: 1997, Q1, P9-10

✖ **83.88   Other plastic operations on tendon**
> Myotenoplasty
> Tendon fixation
> Tenodesis
> Tenoplasty
> Coding Clinic: 2013, Q2, P23

✖ **83.89   Other plastic operations on fascia**
> Fascia lengthening
> Fascioplasty
> Plication of fascia

● **83.9   Other operations on muscle, tendon, fascia, and bursa**

> **Excludes**   *nonoperative:*
> > *manipulation (93.25–93.29)*
> > *stretching (93.27–93.29)*

✖ **83.91   Lysis of adhesions of muscle, tendon, fascia, and bursa**
> **Excludes**   *that for tarsal tunnel syndrome (04.44)*

✖ **83.92   Insertion or replacement of skeletal muscle stimulator**
> Implantation, insertion, placement, or replacement of skeletal muscle:
> > electrodes
> > stimulator
> Coding Clinic: 1999, Q2, P10

✖ **83.93   Removal of skeletal muscle stimulator**

83.94   Aspiration of bursa

83.95   Aspiration of other soft tissue
> **Excludes**   *that of skin and subcutaneous tissue (86.01)*

83.96   Injection of therapeutic substance into bursa

83.97   Injection of therapeutic substance into tendon

83.98   Injection of locally-acting therapeutic substance into other soft tissue
> **Excludes**   *subcutaneous or intramuscular injection (99.11–99.29)*
> Coding Clinic: 2006, Q2, P11

✖ **83.99   Other operations on muscle, tendon, fascia, and bursa**
> Suture of bursa

● **84   Other procedures on musculoskeletal system**

● **84.0   Amputation of upper limb**

> **Excludes**   *revision of amputation stump (84.3)*

✖ **84.00   Upper limb amputation, not otherwise specified**
> Closed flap amputation of upper limb NOS
> Kineplastic amputation of upper limb NOS
> Open or guillotine amputation of upper limb NOS
> Revision of current traumatic amputation of upper limb NOS

✖ **84.01   Amputation and disarticulation of finger**
> **Excludes**   *ligation of supernumerary finger (86.26)*

✖ **84.02   Amputation and disarticulation of thumb**

✖ **84.03   Amputation through hand**
> Amputation through carpals

✖ **84.04   Disarticulation of wrist**

✖ **84.05   Amputation through forearm**
> Forearm amputation

✖ **84.06   Disarticulation of elbow**

✖ **84.07   Amputation through humerus**
> Upper arm amputation

✖ **84.08   Disarticulation of shoulder**

✖ **84.09   Interthoracoscapular amputation**
> Forequarter amputation

● **84.1   Amputation of lower limb**

> **Excludes**   *revision of amputation stump (84.3)*

✖ **84.10   Lower limb amputation, not otherwise specified**
> Closed flap amputation of lower limb NOS
> Kineplastic amputation of lower limb NOS
> Open or guillotine amputation of lower limb NOS
> Revision of current traumatic amputation of lower limb NOS

✖ **84.11   Amputation of toe**
> Amputation through metatarsophalangeal joint
> Disarticulation of toe
> Metatarsal head amputation
> Ray amputation of foot (disarticulation of the metatarsal head of the toe extending across the forefoot just proximal to the metatarsophalangeal crease)
> > **Excludes**   *ligation of supernumerary toe (86.26)*
> Coding Clinic: 2005, Q2, P7

✖ **84.12   Amputation through foot**
> Amputation of forefoot
> Amputation through middle of foot
> Chopart's amputation
> Midtarsal amputation
> Transmetatarsal amputation (amputation of the forefoot, including all the toes)
> > **Excludes**   *ray amputation of foot (84.11)*

✖ **84.13   Disarticulation of ankle**

✖ **84.14   Amputation of ankle through malleoli of tibia and fibula**

✖ **84.15   Other amputation below knee**
> Amputation of leg through tibia and fibula NOS

✖ **84.16   Disarticulation of knee**
> Batch, Spitler, and McFaddin amputation
> Mazet amputation
> S.P. Roger's amputation

✖ **84.17   Amputation above knee**
> Amputation of leg through femur
> Amputation of thigh
> Conversion of below-knee amputation into above-knee amputation
> Supracondylar above-knee amputation
> Coding Clinic: 2005, Q1, P16; 2003, Q3, P14-15; 1995, Q1, P10; 1988, Q4, P12

✖ **84.18   Disarticulation of hip**

✖ **84.19   Abdominopelvic amputation**
> Hemipelvectomy
> Hindquarter amputation

◀ New   ◀▥ Revised   d̶e̶l̶e̶t̶e̶d̶ Deleted   ● Use Additional Digit(s)   ✖ Valid O.R. Procedure
◆ Non-O.R. Procedure   ♀ Females Only   ♂ Males Only   OGCR Official Guidelines   **Coding Clinic**

1282

● **84.2** **Reattachment of extremity**
  ✖ **84.21** **Thumb reattachment**
  ✖ **84.22** **Finger reattachment**
  ✖ **84.23** **Forearm, wrist, or hand reattachment**
  ✖ **84.24** **Upper arm reattachment**
    Reattachment of arm NOS
  ✖ **84.25** **Toe reattachment**
  ✖ **84.26** **Foot reattachment**
  ✖ **84.27** **Lower leg or ankle reattachment**
    Reattachment of leg NOS
    Coding Clinic: 1995, Q1, P8
  ✖ **84.28** **Thigh reattachment**
  ✖ **84.29** **Other reattachment**
✖ **84.3** **Revision of amputation stump**
    Reamputation of stump
    Secondary closure of stump
    Trimming of stump

    Excludes *revision of current traumatic amputation [revision by further amputation of current injury] (84.00–84.19, 84.91)*
    Coding Clinic: 2005, Q1, P14,16; 1999, Q4, P15; 1998, Q4, P12; Q2, P15
● **84.4** **Implantation or fitting of prosthetic limb device**
  ✖ **84.40** **Implantation or fitting of prosthetic limb device, not otherwise specified**
  84.41 **Fitting of prosthesis of upper arm and shoulder**
  84.42 **Fitting of prosthesis of lower arm and hand**
  84.43 **Fitting of prosthesis of arm, not otherwise specified**
  ✖ **84.44** **Implantation of prosthetic device of arm**
  84.45 **Fitting of prosthesis above knee**
  84.46 **Fitting of prosthesis below knee**
  84.47 **Fitting of prosthesis of leg, not otherwise specified**
  ✖ **84.48** **Implantation of prosthetic device of leg**
● **84.5** **Implantation of other musculoskeletal devices and substances**
    Excludes *insertion of (non-fusion) spinal disc replacement device (84.60–84.69)*
  84.51 **Insertion of interbody spinal fusion device**
    Insertion of: cages (carbon, ceramic, metal, plastic or titanium)
      interbody fusion cage
      synthetic cages or spacers
      threaded bone dowels
    Code also refusion of spine (81.30–81.39)
    Code also spinal fusion (81.00–81.08)
    Coding Clinic: 2008, Q2, P14-15; 2007, Q1, P20-21; 2005, Q4, P122-123; 2004, Q1, P21-22; 2003, Q2, P20; 2002, Q4, P108-110
  84.52 **Insertion of recombinant bone morphogenetic protein rhBMP**
    That via collagen sponge, coral, ceramic and other carriers
    Code also primary procedure performed:
      fracture repair (79.00–79.99)
      spinal fusion (81.00–81.08)
      spinal refusion (81.30–81.39)
    Coding Clinic: 2009, Q2, P3; 2006, Q1, P13-14; 2002, Q4, P110-111
  84.53 **Implantation of internal limb lengthening device with kinetic distraction**
    Code also limb lengthening procedure (78.30–78.39)
    Coding Clinic: 2004, Q4, P127
  84.54 **Implantation of other internal limb lengthening device**
    Implantation of internal limb lengthening device, Not Otherwise Specified (NOS)
    Code also limb lengthening procedure (78.30–78.39)
    Coding Clinic: 2004, Q4, P127

84.55 **Insertion of bone void filler**
    Insertion of:
      acrylic cement (PMMA)
      bone void cement
      calcium based bone void filler
      polymethylmethacrylate (PMMA)
    Excludes *that with percutaneous vertebral augmentation (81.66)*
      that with percutaneous vertebroplasty (81.65)
    Coding Clinic: 2004, Q4, P128-129
84.56 **Insertion or replacement of (cement) spacer**
    Insertion or replacement of joint (methylmethacrylate) spacer
    Coding Clinic: 2013, Q3, P5; 2012, Q3, P14-15; 2008, Q2, P3-4; 2005, Q4, P124-125
84.57 **Removal of (cement) spacer**
    Removal of joint (methylmethacrylate) spacer
    Coding Clinic: 2008, Q2, P3-6; 2005, Q4, P124-125
✖ **84.59** **Insertion of other spinal devices**
    Excludes *initial insertion of pedicle screws with spinal fusion— omit code*
      insertion of facet replacement device(s) (84.84)
      insertion of interspinous process device(s) (84.80)
      insertion of pedicle-based dynamic stabilization device(s) (84.82)
    Coding Clinic: 2007, Q1, P9-10
● **84.6** **Replacement of spinal disc**
    Includes non-fusion arthroplasty of the spine with insertion of artificial disc prosthesis
  ✖ **84.60** **Insertion of spinal disc prosthesis, not otherwise specified**
    Replacement of spinal disc, NOS
    Includes diskectomy (discectomy)
  ✖ **84.61** **Insertion of partial spinal disc prosthesis, cervical**
    Nuclear replacement device, cervical
    Partial artificial disc prosthesis (flexible), cervical
    Replacement of nuclear disc (nucleus pulposus), cervical
    Includes diskectomy (discectomy)
  ✖ **84.62** **Insertion of total spinal disc prosthesis, cervical**
    Replacement of cervical spinal disc, NOS
    Replacement of total spinal disc, cervical
    Total artificial disc prosthesis (flexible), cervical
    Includes diskectomy (discectomy)
  ✖ **84.63** **Insertion of spinal disc prosthesis, thoracic**
    Artificial disc prosthesis (flexible), thoracic
    Replacement of thoracic spinal disc, partial or total
    Includes diskectomy (discectomy)
  ✖ **84.64** **Insertion of partial spinal disc prosthesis, lumbosacral**
    Nuclear replacement device, lumbar
    Partial artificial disc prosthesis (flexible), lumbar
    Replacement of nuclear disc (nucleus pulposus), lumbar
    Includes diskectomy (discectomy)
  ✖ **84.65** **Insertion of total spinal disc prosthesis, lumbosacral**
    Replacement of lumbar spinal disc, NOS
    Replacement of total spinal disc, lumbar
    Total artificial disc prosthesis (flexible), lumbar
    Includes diskectomy (discectomy)
    MCE: Non-covered procedure when beneficiary age >60
    Coding Clinic: 2004, Q4, P129-133
  ✖ **84.66** **Revision or replacement of artificial spinal disc prosthesis, cervical**
    Removal of (partial) (total) spinal disc prosthesis with synchronous insertion of new (partial) (total) spinal disc prosthesis, cervical
    Repair of previously inserted spinal disc prosthesis, cervical

OPERATIONS ON THE MUSCULOSKELETAL SYSTEM (76–84)

Excludes   Includes   Use additional   Code also   Omit code

✖ **84.67 Revision or replacement of artificial spinal disc prosthesis, thoracic**
    Removal of (partial) (total) spinal disc prosthesis with synchronous insertion of new (partial) (total) spinal disc prosthesis, thoracic
    Repair of previously inserted spinal disc prosthesis, thoracic

✖ **84.68 Revision or replacement of artificial spinal disc prosthesis, lumbosacral**
    Removal of (partial) (total) spinal disc prosthesis with synchronous insertion of new (partial) (total) spinal disc prosthesis, lumbosacral
    Repair of previously inserted spinal disc prosthesis, lumbosacral

✖ **84.69 Revision or replacement of artificial spinal disc prosthesis, not otherwise specified**
    Removal of (partial) (total) spinal disc prosthesis with synchronous insertion of new (partial) (total) spinal disc prosthesis
    Repair of previously inserted spinal disc prosthesis

● **84.7 Adjunct codes for external fixator devices**
    Code also any primary procedure performed:
        application of external fixator device (78.10, 78.12–78.13, 78.15, 78.17–78.19)
        reduction of fracture and dislocation (79.00–79.89)

  84.71 Application of external fixator device, monoplanar system
    Excludes   *other hybrid device or system (84.73)*
               ring device or system (84.72)
    Coding Clinic: 2005, Q4, P127-129

  84.72 Application of external fixator device, ring system
    Ilizarov type
    Sheffield type
    Excludes   *monoplanar device or system (84.71)*
               other hybrid device or system (84.73)

  84.73 Application of hybrid external fixator device
    Computer (assisted) (dependent) external fixator device
    Hybrid system using both ring and monoplanar devices
    Excludes   *monoplanar device or system, when used alone (84.71)*
               ring device or system, when used alone (84.72)

● **84.8 Insertion, replacement and revision of posterior spinal motion preservation device(s)**
    Dynamic spinal stabilization device(s)
    Includes   any synchronous facetectomy (partial, total) performed at the same level
    Code also any synchronous surgical decompression (foraminotomy, laminectomy, laminotomy), if performed (03.09)
    Excludes   *fusion of spine (81.00–81.08, 81.30–81.39)*
               insertion of artificial disc prosthesis (84.60– 84.69)
               insertion of interbody spinal fusion device (84.51)
    Coding Clinic: 2007, Q1, P9

✖ **84.80 Insertion or replacement of interspinous process device(s)**
    Interspinous process decompression device(s)
    Interspinous process distraction device(s)
    Excludes   *insertion or replacement of facet replacement device (84.84)*
               insertion or replacement of pedicle-based dynamic stabilization device (84.82)
    Coding Clinic: 2007, Q4, P116-120

✖ **84.81 Revision of interspinous process device(s)**
    Repair of previously inserted interspinous process device(s)
    Excludes   *revision of facet replacement device(s) (84.85)*
               revision of pedicle-based dynamic stabilization device (84.83)

✖ **84.82 Insertion or replacement of pedicle-based dynamic stabilization device(s)**
    Excludes   *initial insertion of pedicle screws with spinal fusion — omit code*
               insertion or replacement of facet replacement device(s) (84.84)
               insertion or replacement of interspinous process device(s) (84.80)
               replacement of pedicle screws used in spinal fusion (78.59)
    Coding Clinic: 2007, Q4, P116-120

✖ **84.83 Revision of pedicle-based dynamic stabilization device(s)**
    Repair of previously inserted pedicle-based dynamic stabilization device(s)
    Excludes   *removal of pedicle screws used in spinal fusion (78.69)*
               replacement of pedicle screws used in spinal fusion (78.59)
               revision of facet replacement device(s) (84.85)
               revision of interspinous process device(s) (84.81)

✖ **84.84 Insertion or replacement of facet replacement device(s)**
    Facet arthroplasty
    Excludes   *initial insertion of pedicle screws with spinal fusion — omit code*
               insertion or replacement of interspinous process device(s) (84.80)
               insertion or replacement of pedicle-based dynamic stabilization device(s) (84.82)
               replacement of pedicle screws used in spinal fusion (78.59)
    Coding Clinic: 2007, Q4, P116-120

✖ **84.85 Revision of facet replacement device(s)**
    Repair of previously inserted facet replacement device(s)
    Excludes   *removal of pedicle screws used in spinal fusion (78.69)*
               replacement of pedicle screws used in spinal fusion (78.59)
               revision of interspinous process device(s) (84.81)
               revision of pedicle-based dynamic stabilization device(s) (84.83)

● **84.9 Other operations on musculoskeletal system**
    Excludes   *nonoperative manipulation (93.25–93.29)*

✖ **84.91 Amputation, not otherwise specified**

✖ **84.92 Separation of equal conjoined twins**

✖ **84.93 Separation of unequal conjoined twins**
    Separation of conjoined twins NOS

✖ **84.94 Insertion of sternal fixation device with rigid plates**
    Excludes   *insertion of sternal fixation device for internal fixation of fracture (79.39)*
               internal fixation of bone without fracture reduction (78.59)
    Coding Clinic: 2010, Q4, P132

✖ **84.99 Other**

◀ New   ◀═ Revised   ~~deleted~~ Deleted   ● Use Additional Digit(s)   ✖ Valid O.R. Procedure
◆ Non-O.R. Procedure   ♀ Females Only   ♂ Males Only   OGCR Official Guidelines   **Coding Clinic**

1284

15. OPERATIONS ON THE INTEGUMENTARY SYSTEM (85–86)

● 85 Operations on the breast

> **Includes**   operations on the skin and subcutaneous tissue of:
> breast female or male
> previous mastectomy site female or male
> revision of previous mastectomy site

85.0 **Mastotomy**
Incision of breast (skin)
Mammotomy

> **Excludes**   *aspiration of breast (85.91)*
> *removal of implant (85.94)*

Coding Clinic: 2004, Q1, P3-4; 1990, Q2, P27

● 85.1 **Diagnostic procedures on breast**

85.11 **Closed [percutaneous] [needle] biopsy of breast**
Coding Clinic: 2000, Q2, P10; 1989, Q3, P17

✖ 85.12 **Open biopsy of breast**
Coding Clinic: 1989, Q3, P17; 1986, Mar-April, P11

85.19 **Other diagnostic procedures on breast**

> **Excludes**   *mammary ductogram (87.35)*
> *mammography NEC (87.37)*
> *manual examination (89.36)*
> *microscopic examination of specimen (91.61–91.69)*
> *thermography (88.85)*
> *ultrasonography (88.73)*
> *xerography (87.36)*

● 85.2 **Excision or destruction of breast tissue**

> **Excludes**   *mastectomy (85.41–85.48)*
> *reduction mammoplasty (85.31–85.32)*

✖ 85.20 **Excision or destruction of breast tissue, not otherwise specified**

> **Excludes**   *laser interstitial thermal therapy [LITT] of lesion or tissue of breast under guidance (17.69)*

✖ 85.21 **Local excision of lesion of breast**
Lumpectomy
Removal of area of fibrosis from breast

> **Excludes**   *biopsy of breast (85.11–85.12)*

Coding Clinic: 2012, Q3, P4; 1990, Q2, P27; 1989, Q3, P17; 1985, Sept-Oct, P12

✖ 85.22 **Resection of quadrant of breast**
Coding Clinic: 1985, Sept-Oct, P12

✖ 85.23 **Subtotal mastectomy**

> **Excludes**   *quadrant resection (85.22)*

Coding Clinic: 1992, Q2, P7; 1985, Sept-Oct, P12

✖ 85.24 **Excision of ectopic breast tissue**
Excision of accessory nipple

✖ 85.25 **Excision of nipple**

> **Excludes**   *excision of accessory nipple (85.24)*

● 85.3 **Reduction mammoplasty and subcutaneous mammectomy**
Coding Clinic: 1995, Q4, P79-80

✖ 85.31 **Unilateral reduction mammoplasty**
Unilateral:
amputative mammoplasty
size reduction mammoplasty

✖ 85.32 **Bilateral reduction mammoplasty**
Amputative mammoplasty
Reduction mammoplasty (for gynecomastia)

✖ 85.33 **Unilateral subcutaneous mammectomy with synchronous implant**

> **Excludes**   *that without synchronous implant (85.34)*

✖ 85.34 **Other unilateral subcutaneous mammectomy**
Removal of breast tissue with preservation of skin and nipple
Subcutaneous mammectomy NOS

✖ 85.35 **Bilateral subcutaneous mammectomy with synchronous implant**

> **Excludes**   *that without synchronous implant (85.36)*

✖ 85.36 **Other bilateral subcutaneous mammectomy**

● 85.4 **Mastectomy**

✖ 85.41 **Unilateral simple mastectomy**
Mastectomy:
NOS
complete

✖ 85.42 **Bilateral simple mastectomy**
Bilateral complete mastectomy

✖ 85.43 **Unilateral extended simple mastectomy**
Extended simple mastectomy NOS
Modified radical mastectomy
Simple mastectomy with excision of regional lymph nodes
Coding Clinic: 2012, Q2, P4-5; 1984, May-June, P11

✖ 85.44 **Bilateral extended simple mastectomy**

✖ 85.45 **Unilateral radical mastectomy**
Excision of breast, pectoral muscles, and regional lymph nodes [axillary, clavicular, supraclavicular]
Radical mastectomy NOS

✖ 85.46 **Bilateral radical mastectomy**

✖ 85.47 **Unilateral extended radical mastectomy**
Excision of breast, muscles, and lymph nodes [axillary, clavicular, supraclavicular, internal mammary, and mediastinal]
Extended radical mastectomy NOS

✖ 85.48 **Bilateral extended radical mastectomy**

● 85.5 **Augmentation mammoplasty**

> **Excludes**   *that associated with subcutaneous mammectomy (85.33, 85.35)*

Coding Clinic: 1995, Q4, P80

✖ 85.50 **Augmentation mammoplasty, not otherwise specified**

85.51 **Unilateral injection into breast for augmentation**

> **Excludes**   *injection of fat graft of breast (85.55)*

Coding Clinic: 1997, Q3, P13

85.52 **Bilateral injection into breast for augmentation**
Injection into breast for augmentation NOS

> **Excludes**   *injection of fat graft of breast (85.55)*

✖ 85.53 **Unilateral breast implant**
Coding Clinic: 2000, Q2, P18; 1998, Q2, P14

✖ 85.54 **Bilateral breast implant**
Breast implant NOS

✖ 85.55 **Fat graft to breast**
Autologous fat transplantation or transfer
Fat graft to breast NOS
Fat graft to breast with or without use of enriched graft
Micro-fat grafting

> **Includes**   extraction of fat for autologous graft

> **Excludes**   *that with reconstruction of breast (85.70–85.79)*

Coding Clinic: 2010, Q4, P115

✖ 85.6 **Mastopexy**

OPERATIONS ON THE INTEGUMENTARY SYSTEM (85–86)

● 85.7   **Total reconstruction of breast**
Coding Clinic: 2008, Q4, P185-187; 1993, Q1, P27-28

✖ 85.70   **Total reconstruction of breast, not otherwise specified**
Perforator flap, free

✖ 85.71   **Latissimus dorsi myocutaneous flap**

✖ 85.72   **Transverse rectus abdominis myocutaneous (TRAM) flap, pedicled**

Excludes   *transverse rectus abdominis myocutaneous (TRAM) flap, free (85.73)*

✖ 85.73   **Transverse rectus abdominis myocutaneous (TRAM) flap, free**

Excludes   *transverse rectus abdominis myocutaneous (TRAM) flap, pedicled (85.72)*
Coding Clinic: 2010, Q4, P115

✖ 85.74   **Deep inferior epigastric artery perforator (DIEP) flap, free**

✖ 85.75   **Superficial inferior epigastric artery (SIEA) flap, free**

✖ 85.76   **Gluteal artery perforator (GAP) flap, free**

✖ 85.79   **Other total reconstruction of breast**

Excludes   *deep inferior epigastric artery perforator (DIEP) flap, free (85.74)*
gluteal artery perforator (GAP) flap, free (85.76)
latissimus dorsi myocutaneous flap (85.71)
perforator flap, free (85.70)
superficial inferior epigastric artery (SIEA) flap, free (85.75)
total reconstruction of breast, not otherwise specified (85.70)
transverse rectus abdominis myocutaneous flap, free (85.73)
transverse rectus abdominis myocutaneous (TRAM) flap, pedicled (85.72)

● 85.8   **Other repair and plastic operations on breast**

Excludes   *that for:*
augmentation (85.50–85.54)
reconstruction (85.70–85.76, 85.79)
reduction (85.31–85.32)

85.81   **Suture of laceration of breast**

✖ 85.82   **Split-thickness graft to breast**

✖ 85.83   **Full-thickness graft to breast**

✖ 85.84   **Pedicle graft to breast**

✖ 85.85   **Muscle flap graft to breast**

✖ 85.86   **Transposition of nipple**
Coding Clinic: 1995, Q4, P79-80

✖ 85.87   **Other repair or reconstruction of nipple**

✖ 85.89   **Other mammoplasty**

● 85.9   **Other operations on the breast**

85.91   **Aspiration of breast**

Excludes   *percutaneous biopsy of breast (85.11)*

85.92   **Injection of therapeutic agent into breast**

Excludes   *that for augmentation of breast (85.51–85.52, 85.55)*

✖ 85.93   **Revision of implant of breast**
Coding Clinic: 1998, Q2, P14

✖ 85.94   **Removal of implant of breast**
Coding Clinic: 1998, Q2, P14; 1992, Q3, P4-5

✖ 85.95   **Insertion of breast tissue expander**
Insertion (soft tissue) of tissue expander (one or more) under muscle or platysma to develop skin flaps for donor use

✖ 85.96   **Removal of breast tissue expander**
Coding Clinic: 2000, Q2, P18

✖ 85.99   **Other**
Coding Clinic: 2012, Q2, P8; 1986, Nov-Dec, P9

● 86   **Operations on skin and subcutaneous tissue**

Includes   operations on:
hair follicles
male perineum
nails
sebaceous glands
subcutaneous fat pads
sudoriferous glands
superficial fossae

Excludes   *those on skin of:*
anus (49.01–49.99)
breast (mastectomy site) (85.0–85.99)
ear (18.01–18.9)
eyebrow (08.01–08.99)
eyelid (08.01–08.99)
female perineum (71.01–71.9)
lips (27.0–27.99)
nose (21.00–21.99)
penis (64.0–64.99)
scrotum (61.0–61.99)
vulva (71.01–71.9)

● 86.0   **Incision of skin and subcutaneous tissue**

86.01   **Aspiration of skin and subcutaneous tissue**
Aspiration of:
abscess of nail, skin, or subcutaneous tissue
hematoma of nail, skin, or subcutaneous tissue
seroma of nail, skin, or subcutaneous tissue
Coding Clinic: 1989, Q3, P16

86.02   **Injection or tattooing of skin lesion or defect**
Injection of filling material
Insertion of filling material
Pigmenting of skin of filling material

86.03   **Incision of pilonidal sinus or cyst**

Excludes   *marsupialization (86.21)*

86.04   **Other incision with drainage of skin and subcutaneous tissue**

Excludes   *drainage of:*
fascial compartments of face and mouth (27.0)
palmar or thenar space (82.04)
pilonidal sinus or cyst (86.03)
Coding Clinic: 2012, Q3, P4; 2009, Q1, P15; 2008, Q3, P8-9; 2004, Q4, P75-76

86.05   **Incision with removal of foreign body or device from skin and subcutaneous tissue**
Removal of carotid sinus baroreflex activation device
Removal of loop recorder
Removal of neurostimulator pulse generator (single array, dual array)
Removal of tissue expander(s) from skin or soft tissue other than breast tissue

Excludes   *removal of foreign body without incision (98.20–98.29)*
Coding Clinic: 1992, Q3, P9; 1986, Nov-Dec, P9

✖ 86.06   **Insertion of totally implantable infusion pump**

Code also any associated catheterization

Excludes   *insertion of totally implantable vascular access device (86.07)*
Coding Clinic: 1999, Q2, P4; 1993, 5th Issue, P11; 1988, Q1, P8

86.07   **Insertion of totally implantable vascular access device [VAD]**
Totally implanted port

Excludes   *insertion of totally implantable infusion pump (86.06)*

◆ Non-OR Procedure that affects MS-DRG assignment to MDC 09, MS-DRG 579-581; MDC 11, MS-DRG 673-675
Coding Clinic: 2011, Q3, P13; 2001, Q1, P13-14; 1996, Q1, P5-6x2; 1994, Q2, P11; 1993, 5th Issue, P11

◀ New   ◀ Revised   ~~deleted~~ Deleted   ● Use Additional Digit(s)   ✖ Valid O.R. Procedure
◆ Non-O.R. Procedure   ♀ Females Only   ♂ Males Only   OGCR Official Guidelines   **Coding Clinic**

1286

86.09   **Other incision of skin and subcutaneous tissue**
     Creation of thalamic stimulator pulse generator
       pocket, new site
     Escharotomy
     Exploration:
       sinus tract, skin
       superficial fossa
     Relocation of subcutaneous device pocket NEC
     Reopening subcutaneous pocket for device revision
       without replacement
     Undercutting of hair follicle

> **Excludes**   *creation of loop recorder pocket, new site,*
> *and insertion/relocation of device*
> *(37.79)*
> *creation of pocket for implantable,*
> *patient-activated cardiac event*
> *recorder and insertion/relocation of*
> *device (37.79)*
> *removal of catheter from cranial cavity*
> *(01.27)*
> *that for drainage (86.04)*
> *that of:*
>   *cardiac pacemaker pocket, new site*
>   *(37.79)*
>   *fascial compartments of face and mouth*
>   *(27.0)*

   ◆ Non-OR Procedure that affects MS-DRG assignment to
     MDC 09, MS-DRG 579-581
     Coding Clinic: 2005, Q1, P17; 2004, Q2, P3, 7-8x2; 1999, Q4,
     P21; 1995, Q3, P14; 1993, 5th Issue, P11; 1989, Q3,
     P17; 1985, July-Aug, P11; 1985, Mar-April, P15; 1984,
     May-June, P11, 14

● **86.1**   **Diagnostic procedures on skin and subcutaneous tissue**

   86.11   **Closed biopsy of skin and subcutaneous tissue**
       Coding Clinic: 2008, Q4, P97-100

   86.19   **Other diagnostic procedures on skin and**
      subcutaneous tissue

> **Excludes**   *microscopic examination of specimen*
> *from skin and subcutaneous tissue*
> *(91.61–91.79)*

● **86.2**   **Excision or destruction of lesion or tissue of skin and**
    subcutaneous tissue

   ✖ **86.21**   **Excision of pilonidal cyst or sinus**
       Marsupialization of cyst

> **Excludes**   *incision of pilonidal cyst or sinus (86.03)*

       Coding Clinic: 2011, Q3, P9

   ✖ **86.22**   **Excisional debridement of wound, infection, or burn**
       Removal by excision of:
         devitalized tissue
         necrosis
         slough

> **Excludes**   *debridement of:*
> *abdominal wall (wound) (54.3)*
> *bone (77.60–77.69)*
> *muscle (83.45)*
>   *of hand (82.36)*
> *nail (bed) (fold) (86.27)*
> *nonexcisional debridement of wound,*
>   *infection, or burn (86.28)*
> *open fracture site (79.60–79.69)*
> *pedicle or flap graft (86.75)*

     Coding Clinic: 2012, Q3, P4; 2008, Q3, P8-9; Q1, P3-4; 2006, Q3,
     P19-20; Q2, P11; 2005, Q2, P3-4; 2004, Q4, P138-139;
     Q2, P5; 2002, Q3, P23; Q1, P14-15; 2000, Q2, P9; 1999,
     Q1, P8-9; 1998, Q2, P15; 1995, Q3, P12; 1992, Q2, P17;
     1991, Q3, P18-19; Q2, P18-19; 1989, Q3, P16

86.23   **Removal of nail, nail bed, or nail fold**

86.24   **Chemosurgery of skin**
     Chemical peel of skin

✖ **86.25**   **Dermabrasion**
     That with laser

> **Excludes**   *dermabrasion of wound to remove embedded*
> *debris (86.28)*

86.26   **Ligation of dermal appendage**

> **Excludes**   *excision of preauricular appendage (18.29)*

86.27   **Debridement of nail, nail bed, or nail fold**
     Removal of:
       necrosis
       slough

> **Excludes**   *removal of nail, nail bed, or nail fold (86.23)*

86.28   **Nonexcisional debridement of wound, infection or**
    burn
     Debridement NOS
     Maggot therapy
     Removal of devitalized tissue, necrosis, and slough
       by such methods as:
         brushing
         irrigation (under pressure)
         scrubbing
         washing
     Ultrasonic debridement
     Water scalpel (jet)
     Coding Clinic: 2013, Q1, P15-16; 2011, Q4, P182; 2010, Q2, P11;
     2009, Q3, P13x3; 2007, Q1, P10-11; 2005, Q1, P14-15;
     2004, Q2, P5,6; 2003, Q2, P15; 2002, Q3, P23; 2001, Q2,
     P18; 1991, Q3, P18-19; Q2, P18-19

> **OGCR**   Section I.C.17.d
> Excisional debridement involves surgical removal
> or cutting away, as opposed to a mechanical
> (brushing, scrubbing, washing) debridement.
> For coding purposes, excisional debridement is
> assigned to code 86.22. Nonexcisional debridement
> is assigned to code 86.28.

● **86.3**   **Other local excision or destruction of lesion or tissue of skin**
    and subcutaneous tissue
     Destruction of skin by:
       cauterization cryosurgery
       fulguration
       laser beam
     That with Z-plasty

> **Excludes**   *adipectomy (86.83)*
> *biopsy of skin (86.11)*
> *wide or radical excision of skin (86.4)*
> *Z-plasty without excision (86.84)*

   ◆ Non-OR Procedure that affects MS-DRG assignment to MDC
     09, MS-DRG 579-581
     Coding Clinic: 1996, Q1, P9; 1995, Q3, P14; 1990, Q2, P27; 1989, Q1, P12

✖ **86.4**   **Radical excision of skin lesion**
     Wide excision of skin lesion involving underlying or
       adjacent structure

     Code also any lymph node dissection (40.3–40.5)

● **86.5**   **Suture or other closure of skin and subcutaneous tissue**

   86.51   **Replantation of scalp**

   86.59   **Closure of skin and subcutaneous tissue of other sites**
       Adhesives (surgical) (tissue)
       Staples
       Sutures

> **Excludes**   *application of adhesive strips (butterfly) —*
> *omit code*

       Coding Clinic: 2011, Q3, P13

OGCR   Section I.C.17.d
Excisional debridement involves surgical removal or cutting away, as
opposed to a mechanical (brushing, scrubbing, washing) debridement.
For coding purposes, excisional debridement is assigned to code
86.22. Nonexcisional debridement is assigned to code 86.28.

OPERATIONS ON THE INTEGUMENTARY SYSTEM (85–86)

Excludes   Includes   Use additional   Code also   Omit code

● **86.6   Free skin graft**

     Includes   excision of skin for autogenous graft

     Excludes   *construction or reconstruction of:*
          penis (64.43–64.44)
          trachea (31.75)
          vagina (70.61–70.64)

✖ **86.60   Free skin graft, not otherwise specified**

✖ **86.61   Full-thickness skin graft to hand**

     Excludes   *heterograft (86.65)*
          homograft (86.66)

✖ **86.62   Other skin graft to hand**

     Excludes   *heterograft (86.65)*
          homograft (86.66)

✖ **86.63   Full-thickness skin graft to other sites**

     Excludes   *heterograft (86.65)*
          homograft (86.66)

   86.64   Hair transplant

     Excludes   *hair follicle transplant to eyebrow or eyelash*
          (08.63)

✖ **86.65   Heterograft to skin**

     Pigskin graft   Porcine graft

     Excludes   *application of dressing only (93.57)*

     Coding Clinic: 2002, Q3, P23

✖ **86.66   Homograft to skin**

     Graft to skin of:
          amnionic membrane from donor skin from donor

✖ **86.67   Dermal regenerative graft**

     Artificial skin, NOS
     Creation of "neodermis"
     Decellularized allodermis
     Integumentary matrix implants
     Prosthetic implant of dermal layer of skin
     Regenerate dermal layer of skin

     Excludes   *heterograft to skin (86.65)*
          homograft to skin (86.66)

     Coding Clinic: 2010, Q3, P7-8; 2006, Q3, P19-20; 1998, Q43,
          P77-79

✖ **86.69   Other skin graft to other sites**

     Excludes   *heterograft (86.65)*
          homograft (86.66)

     Coding Clinic: 2010, Q1, P14; 1999, Q4, P15; 1998, Q43, P77-79

● **86.7   Pedicle grafts or flaps**

     Excludes   *construction or reconstruction of:*
          penis (64.43–64.44)
          trachea (31.75)
          vagina (70.61–70.64)

✖ **86.70   Pedicle or flap graft, not otherwise specified**

✖ **86.71   Cutting and preparation of pedicle grafts or flaps**

     Elevation of pedicle from its bed
     Flap design and raising
     Partial cutting of pedicle or tube
     Pedicle delay

     Excludes   *pollicization or digital transfer (82.61,*
          82.81)
          revision of pedicle (86.75)

     Coding Clinic: 2001, Q4, P66

✖ **86.72   Advancement of pedicle graft**
     Coding Clinic: 1999, Q3, P9-10

✖ **86.73   Attachment of pedicle or flap graft to hand**

     Excludes   *pollicization or digital transfer (82.61, 82.81)*

✖ **86.74   Attachment of pedicle or flap graft to other sites**

     Attachment by:
          advanced flap
          double pedicled flap
          pedicle graft
          rotating flap
          sliding flap
          tube graft

     Coding Clinic: 1999, Q3, P10; 1996, Q1, P15; 1993, Q2, P11

✖ **86.75   Revision of pedicle or flap graft**

     Debridement of pedicle or flap graft
     Defatting of pedicle or flap graft

● **86.8   Other repair and reconstruction of skin and subcutaneous tissue**

✖ **86.81   Repair for facial weakness**

✖ **86.82   Facial rhytidectomy**

     Face lift

     Excludes   *rhytidectomy of eyelid (08.86–08.87)*

✖ **86.83   Size reduction plastic operation**

     Liposuction
     Reduction of adipose tissue of:
          abdominal wall (pendulous)
          arms (batwing)
          buttock
          thighs (trochanteric lipomatosis)

     Excludes   *breast (85.31–85.32)*
          liposuction to harvest fat graft (86.90)

     Coding Clinic: 2006, Q2, P10-11

✖ **86.84   Relaxation of scar or web contracture of skin**

     Z-plasty of skin

     Excludes   *Z-plasty with excision of lesion (86.3)*

✖ **86.85   Correction of syndactyly**

✖ **86.86   Onychoplasty**

✖ **86.87   Fat graft of skin and subcutaneous tissue**

     Autologous fat transplantation or transfer
     Fat graft NOS
     Fat graft of skin and subcutaneous tissue with or
          without use of enriched graft
     Micro-fat grafting

     Includes   extraction of fat for autologous graft

     Excludes   *fat graft to breast (85.55)*

     Coding Clinic: 2013, Q1, P7

✖ **86.89   Other repair and reconstruction of skin and subcutaneous tissue**

     Excludes   *mentoplasty (76.67–76.68)*

     Coding Clinic: 2002, Q4, P107-108; 2000, Q1, P26; 1998, Q2, P20;
          1993, Q2, P11; 1992, Q2, P17

● **86.9   Other operations on skin and subcutaneous tissue**

✖ **86.90   Extraction of fat for graft or banking**

     Harvest of fat for extraction of cells for future use
     Liposuction to harvest fat graft

     Excludes   *that with graft at same operative episode*
          (85.55, 86.87)

✖ **86.91   Excision of skin for graft**

     Excision of skin with closure of donor site

     Excludes   *that with graft at same operative episode*
          (86.60- 86.69)

   86.92   Electrolysis and other epilation of skin

     Excludes   *epilation of eyelid (08.91–08.93)*

✖ **86.93   Insertion of tissue expander**

     Insertion (subcutaneous) (soft tissue) of expander
          (one or more) in scalp (subgaleal space), face,
          neck, trunk except breast, and upper and
          lower extremities for development of skin
          flaps for donor use

     Excludes   *flap graft preparation (86.71)*
          tissue expander, breast (85.95)

✖ **86.94   Insertion or replacement of single array neurostimulator pulse generator, not specified as rechargeable**

     Pulse generator (single array, single channel, single
          port) for intracranial, spinal, and peripheral
          neurostimulator

     Code also any associated lead implantation (02.93,
          03.93, 04.92)

     Excludes   *cranial implantation or replacement of*
          neurostimulator pulse generator
          (01.20)
          insertion or replacement of single array
          rechargeable neurostimulator pulse
          generator (86.97)

     Coding Clinic: 2004, Q4, P133-135

◀ New   ◀ᴵᴵᴵ Revised   ~~deleted~~ Deleted   ● Use Additional Digit(s)   ✖ Valid O.R. Procedure
◆ Non-O.R. Procedure   ♀ Females Only   ♂ Males Only   OGCR Official Guidelines   **Coding Clinic**

✖ **86.95** **Insertion or replacement of multiple array neurostimulator pulse generator, not specified as rechargeable**
> Pulse generator (multiple array, multiple channel, multiple port) for intracranial, spinal, and peripheral neurostimulator
>
> **Code also** any associated lead implantation (02.93, 03.93, 04.92)
>
> **Excludes** *cranial implantation or replacement of neurostimulator pulse generator (01.20)*
> *insertion or replacement of multiple array rechargeable neurostimulator pulse generator (86.98)*
> **Coding Clinic: 2004, Q4, P133-135**

✖ **86.96** **Insertion or replacement of other neurostimulator pulse generator**
> **Code also** any associated lead implantation (02.93, 03.93, 04.92)
>
> **Excludes** *cranial implantation or replacement of neurostimulator pulse generator (01.20)*
> *insertion of multiple array neurostimulator pulse generator (86.95, 86.98)*
> *insertion of single array neurostimulator pulse generator (86.94, 86.97)*
> **Coding Clinic: 2007, Q2, P10-11; 2006, Q2, P5-6; 2004, Q4, P133-135**

✖ **86.97** **Insertion or replacement of single array rechargeable neurostimulator pulse generator**
> Rechargeable pulse generator (single array, single channel, single port) for intracranial, spinal, and peripheral neurostimulator
>
> **Code also** any associated lead implantation (02.93, 03.93, 04.92)
>
> **Excludes** *cranial implantation or replacement of neurostimulator pulse generator (01.20)*
> **Coding Clinic: 2005, Q4, P130-131**

✖ **86.98** **Insertion or replacement of multiple array (two or more) rechargeable neurostimulator pulse generator**
> Rechargeable pulse generator (multiple array, multiple channel, multiple port) for intracranial, spinal, and peripheral neurostimulator
>
> **Code also** any associated lead implantation (02.93, 03.93, 04.92)
>
> **Excludes** *cranial implantation or replacement of neurostimulator pulse generator (01.20)*
> **Coding Clinic: 2005, Q4, P130-131**

86.99 **Other**
> **Excludes** *removal of sutures from:*
> *abdomen (97.83)*
> *head and neck (97.38)*
> *thorax (97.43)*
> *trunk NEC (97.84)*
> *wound catheter:*
> *irrigation (96.58)*
> *replacement (97.15)*

16. MISCELLANEOUS DIAGNOSTIC AND THERAPEUTIC PROCEDURES (87–99)

● **87** **Diagnostic Radiology**

  ● **87.0** **Soft tissue x-ray of face, head, and neck**
> **Excludes** *angiography (88.40–88.68)*

    87.01 **Pneumoencephalogram**

    87.02 **Other contrast radiogram of brain and skull**
> Pneumocisternogram
> Pneumoventriculogram
> Posterior fossa myelogram

    87.03 **Computerized axial tomography of head**
> C.A.T. scan of head
> **Coding Clinic: 2005, Q3, P12-13; 1999, Q3, P7-8**

    87.04 **Other tomography of head**

    87.05 **Contrast dacryocystogram**

    87.06 **Contrast radiogram of nasopharynx**

    87.07 **Contrast laryngogram**

    87.08 **Cervical lymphangiogram**

    87.09 **Other soft tissue x-ray of face, head, and neck**
> Noncontrast x-ray of:
> adenoid
> larynx
> nasolacrimal duct
> nasopharynx
> salivary gland
> thyroid region
> uvula
>
> **Excludes** *x-ray study of eye (95.14)*

  ● **87.1** **Other x-ray of face, head, and neck**
> **Excludes** *angiography (88.40–88.68)*

    87.11 **Full-mouth x-ray of teeth**

    87.12 **Other dental x-ray**
> Orthodontic cephalogram or cephalometrics
> Panorex examination of mandible
> Root canal x-ray

    87.13 **Temporomandibular contrast arthrogram**

    87.14 **Contrast radiogram of orbit**

    87.15 **Contrast radiogram of sinus**

    87.16 **Other x-ray of facial bones**
> X-ray of:
> frontal area
> mandible
> maxilla
> nasal sinuses
> nose
> orbit
> supraorbital area
> symphysis menti
> zygomaticomaxillary complex

    87.17 **Other x-ray of skull**
> Lateral projection of skull
> Sagittal projection
> Tangential projection

  ● **87.2** **X-ray of spine**

    87.21 **Contrast myelogram**

    87.22 **Other x-ray of cervical spine**

    87.23 **Other x-ray of thoracic spine**

    87.24 **Other x-ray of lumbosacral spine**
> Sacrococcygeal x-ray

    87.29 **Other x-ray of spine**
> Spinal x-ray NOS

  ● **87.3** **Soft tissue x-ray of thorax**
> **Excludes** *angiocardiography (88.50–88.58)*
> *angiography (88.40–88.68)*

    87.31 **Endotracheal bronchogram**

    87.32 **Other contrast bronchogram**
> Transcricoid bronchogram

    87.33 **Mediastinal pneumogram**

    87.34 **Intrathoracic lymphangiogram**

    87.35 **Contrast radiogram of mammary ducts**

    87.36 **Xerography of breast**

OPERATIONS ON THE INTEGUMENTARY SYSTEM (85–86)

Excludes   Includes   Use additional   Code also   Omit code

87.37   **Other mammography**
        Coding Clinic: 1989, Q3, P17

87.38   **Sinogram of chest wall**
        Fistulogram of chest wall

87.39   **Other soft tissue x-ray of chest wall**

● **87.4**   **Other x-ray of thorax**
      Excludes   *angiocardiography (88.50–88.58)*
                       angiography (88.40–88.68)

87.41   **Computerized axial tomography of thorax**
        C.A.T. scan of
           heart
           thorax
        Crystal linear scan of x-ray beam of thorax
        Electronic subtraction of thorax
        Photoelectric response of thorax
        Tomography with use of computer, x-rays, and
           camera of thorax

87.42   **Other tomography of thorax**
        Cardiac tomogram
        Excludes   *C.A.T. scan of heart (87.41)*

87.43   **X-ray of ribs, sternum, and clavicle**
        Examination for:
           cervical rib
           fracture

87.44   **Routine chest x-ray, so described**
        X-ray of chest NOS

87.49   **Other chest x-ray**
        X-ray of:
           bronchus NOS
           diaphragm NOS
           heart NOS
           lung NOS
           mediastinum NOS
           trachea NOS

● **87.5**   **Biliary tract x-ray**

87.51   **Percutaneous hepatic cholangiogram**
        Coding Clinic: 1990, Q2, P28

87.52   **Intravenous cholangiogram**

✖ **87.53**   **Intraoperative cholangiogram**
        Coding Clinic: 1996, Q1, P12-13; Q1, P12-13; 1990, Q2, P28

87.54   **Other cholangiogram**
        Coding Clinic: 1988, Q4, P7

87.59   **Other biliary tract x-ray**
        Cholecystogram

● **87.6**   **Other x-ray of digestive system**
87.61   **Barium swallow**
87.62   **Upper GI series**
87.63   **Small bowel series**
87.64   **Lower GI series**
87.65   **Other x-ray of intestine**
87.66   **Contrast pancreatogram**
87.69   **Other digestive tract x-ray**

● **87.7**   **X-ray of urinary system**
      Excludes   *angiography of renal vessels (88.45, 88.65)*

87.71   **Computerized axial tomography of kidney**
        C.A.T. scan of kidney

87.72   **Other nephrotomogram**

87.73   **Intravenous pyelogram**
        Diuretic infusion pyelogram

87.74   **Retrograde pyelogram**
87.75   **Percutaneous pyelogram**
87.76   **Retrograde cystourethrogram**
87.77   **Other cystogram**
87.78   **Ileal conduitogram**
87.79   **Other x-ray of the urinary system**
        KUB x-ray

● **87.8**   **X-ray of female genital organs**
87.81   **X-ray of gravid uterus** ♀
        Intrauterine cephalometry by x-ray
87.82   **Gas contrast hysterosalpingogram** ♀
87.83   **Opaque dye contrast hysterosalpingogram** ♀
87.84   **Percutaneous hysterogram** ♀
87.85   **Other x-ray of fallopian tubes and uterus** ♀
87.89   **Other x-ray of female genital organs** ♀

● **87.9**   **X-ray of male genital organs**
87.91   **Contrast seminal vesiculogram** ♂
87.92   **Other x-ray of prostate and seminal vesicles** ♂
87.93   **Contrast epididymogram** ♂
87.94   **Contrast vasogram** ♂
87.95   **Other x-ray of epididymis and vas deferens** ♂
87.99   **Other x-ray of male genital organs** ♂

● **88**   **Other diagnostic radiology and related techniques**
● **88.0**   **Soft tissue x-ray of abdomen**
      Excludes   *angiography (88.40–88.68)*

88.01   **Computerized axial tomography of abdomen**
        C.A.T. scan of abdomen
        Excludes   *C.A.T. scan of kidney (87.71)*
        Coding Clinic: 1998, Q2, P13

88.02   **Other abdomen tomography**
        Excludes   *nephrotomogram (87.72)*

88.03   **Sinogram of abdominal wall**
        Fistulogram of abdominal wall

88.04   **Abdominal lymphangiogram**

88.09   **Other soft tissue x-ray of abdominal wall**

● **88.1**   **Other x-ray of abdomen**
88.11   **Pelvic opaque dye contrast radiography**
88.12   **Pelvic gas contrast radiography**
        Pelvic pneumoperitoneum
88.13   **Other peritoneal pneumogram**
88.14   **Retroperitoneal fistulogram**
        Coding Clinic: 1998, Q3, P8-9
88.15   **Retroperitoneal pneumogram**
88.16   **Other retroperitoneal x-ray**
88.19   **Other x-ray of abdomen**
        Flat plate of abdomen
        Coding Clinic: 1999, Q3, P9

● **88.2**   **Skeletal x-ray of extremities and pelvis**
      Excludes   *contrast radiogram of joint (88.32)*

88.21   **Skeletal x-ray of shoulder and upper arm**
88.22   **Skeletal x-ray of elbow and forearm**
88.23   **Skeletal x-ray of wrist and hand**
88.24   **Skeletal x-ray of upper limb, not otherwise specified**
88.25   **Pelvimetry**
88.26   **Other skeletal x-ray of pelvis and hip**
88.27   **Skeletal x-ray of thigh, knee, and lower leg**
88.28   **Skeletal x-ray of ankle and foot**
        Coding Clinic: 2003, Q4, P110
88.29   **Skeletal x-ray of lower limb, not otherwise specified**

● **88.3**   **Other x-ray**
88.31   **Skeletal series**
        X-ray of whole skeleton
88.32   **Contrast arthrogram**
        Excludes   *that of temporomandibular joint (87.13)*
88.33   **Other skeletal x-ray**
        Excludes   *skeletal x-ray of:*
                extremities and pelvis (88.21–88.29)
                face, head, and neck (87.11–87.17)
                spine (87.21–87.29)
                thorax (87.43)

◀ New   ◀▥ Revised   ~~deleted~~ Deleted   ● Use Additional Digit(s)   ✖ Valid O.R. Procedure
◆ Non-O.R. Procedure   ♀ Females Only   ♂ Males Only   OGCR Official Guidelines   **Coding Clinic**

1290

88.34 Lymphangiogram of upper limb

88.35 Other soft tissue x-ray of upper limb

88.36 Lymphangiogram of lower limb

88.37 Other soft tissue x-ray of lower limb

Excludes *femoral angiography (88.48, 88.66)*

88.38 Other computerized axial tomography
C.A.T. scan NOS

Excludes *C.A.T. scan of:*
abdomen (88.01)
head (87.03)
heart (87.41)
kidney (87.71)
thorax (87.41)

Coding Clinic: 2005, Q3, P13-14

88.39 X-ray, other and unspecified

● 88.4 Arteriography using contrast material

Includes angiography of arteries
arterial puncture for injection of contrast
material
radiography of arteries (by fluoroscopy)
retrograde arteriography

Note: **The fourth-digit subclassification identifies the
site to be viewed, not the site of injection.**

Excludes *arteriography using:*
radioisotopes or radionuclides (92.01–92.19)
ultrasound (88.71–88.79)
fluorescein angiography of eye (95.12)

Coding Clinic: 1985, Nov-Dec, P14

88.40 Arteriography using contrast material, unspecified
site

88.41 Arteriography of cerebral arteries
Angiography of:
basilar artery
carotid (internal)
posterior cerebral circulation
vertebral artery

Coding Clinic: 2000, Q1, P16; 1999, Q1, P7; 1995, Q2, P12

88.42 Aortography
Arteriography of aorta and aortic arch

Coding Clinic: 2013, Q3, P3; 2010, Q2, P9; 1999, Q1, P17

88.43 Arteriography of pulmonary arteries

88.44 Arteriography of other intrathoracic vessels

Excludes *angiocardiography (88.50–88.58)*
*arteriography of coronary arteries
(88.55–88.57)*

88.45 Arteriography of renal arteries

88.46 Arteriography of placenta ♀
Placentogram using contrast material

88.47 Arteriography of other intra-abdominal arteries

Coding Clinic: 2009, Q2, P7; 2000, Q1, P18-19

88.48 Arteriography of femoral and other lower extremity
arteries

Coding Clinic: 2013, Q3, P3; 2006, Q2, P22-23; 2003, Q3, P10x2;
Q1, P17-18; 1996, Q2, P7-8; 1989, Q2, P17

88.49 Arteriography of other specified sites

Coding Clinic: 2010, Q2, P9

● 88.5 Angiocardiography using contrast material

Includes arterial puncture and insertion of arterial
catheter for injection of contrast material
cineangiocardiography
selective angiocardiography

Code also synchronous cardiac catheterization
(37.21–37.23)

Excludes *angiography of pulmonary vessels (88.43, 88.62)*

Coding Clinic: 2008, Q3, P18; 2002, Q3, P20

88.50 Angiocardiography, not otherwise specified

88.51 Angiocardiography of venae cavae
Inferior vena cavography
Phlebography of vena cava (inferior) (superior)

88.52 Angiocardiography of right heart structures
Angiocardiography of:
pulmonary valve
right atrium
right ventricle (outflow tract)

Excludes *intra-operative fluorescence vascular
angiography (88.59)*
*that combined with left heart
angiocardiography (88.54)*

◆Non-OR Procedure that affects MS-DRG assignment
to MDC 05, MS-DRG 216-218, 222-225,
233-234, 286-287

Coding Clinic: 2008, Q3, P18; 2007, Q1, P16-17

88.53 Angiocardiography of left heart structures
Angiocardiography of:
aortic valve
left atrium
left ventricle (outflow tract)

Excludes *intra-operative fluorescence vascular
angiography (88.59)*
*that combined with right heart
angiocardiography (88.54)*

◆Non-OR Procedure that affects MS-DRG assignment
to MDC 05, MS-DRG 216-218, 222-225,
233-234, 286-287

Coding Clinic: 2007, Q1, P11-12, 17; 2005, Q4, P69-72; Q3, P14;
2000, Q1, P20-21

88.54 Combined right and left heart angiocardiography

Excludes *intra-operative fluorescence vascular
angiography (88.59)*

◆Non-OR Procedure that affects MS-DRG assignment
to MDC 05, MS-DRG 216-218, 222-225,
233-234, 286-287

88.55 Coronary arteriography using a single catheter
Coronary arteriography by Sones technique
Direct selective coronary arteriography using a
single catheter

Excludes *intra-operative fluorescence vascular
angiography (88.59)*

◆Non-OR Procedure that affects MS-DRG assignment
to MDC 05, MS-DRG 216-218, 222-225,
233-234, 286-287

Coding Clinic: 2006, Q2, P25-26; 2002, Q3, P20; 1992, Q3, P10,
17-18

88.56 Coronary arteriography using two catheters
Coronary arteriography by:
Judkins technique
Ricketts and Abrams technique
Direct selective coronary arteriography using two
catheters

Excludes *intra-operative fluorescence vascular
angiography (88.59)*

◆Non-OR Procedure that affects MS-DRG assignment
to MDC 05, MS-DRG 216-218, 222-225,
233-234, 286-287

Coding Clinic: 2010, Q2, P13; 2006, Q3, P8-9; 2000, Q1, P20-21;
1992, Q3, P17-18; Q3, P10

88.57 Other and unspecified coronary arteriography
Coronary arteriography NOS

Excludes *intra-operative fluorescence vascular
angiography (88.59)*

◆Non-OR Procedure that affects MS-DRG assignment
to MDC 05, MS-DRG 216-218, 222-225,
233-234, 286-287

Coding Clinic: 2007, Q1, P15-16; 2006, Q2, P25-26; 2005, Q4,
P69-72; Q2, P10; Q3, P14; 2000, Q1, P21; 1992, Q3, P10,
17-18

88.58 Negative-contrast cardiac roentgenography
Cardiac roentgenography with injection of carbon
dioxide

◆Non-OR Procedure that affects MS-DRG assignment
to MDC 05, MS-DRG 216-218, 222-225,
233-234, 286-287

Excludes   Includes   Use additional   Code also   Omit code

88.59 Intra-operative coronary fluorescence vascular angiography
Intraoperative laser arteriogram (SPY)
SPY arteriogram
SPY arteriography
Coding Clinic: 2007, Q4, P121-122; 2006, Q2, P25-26

● **88.6 Phlebography**
Includes   angiography of veins
radiography of veins (by fluoroscopy)
retrograde phlebography
venipuncture for injection of contrast material
venography using contrast material

Note: **The fourth-digit subclassification (88.60–88.67) identifies the site to be viewed, not the site of injection.**

Excludes   *angiography using:*
radioisotopes or radionuclides (92.01–92.19)
ultrasound (88.71–88.79)
fluorescein angiography of eye (95.12)

88.60 Phlebography using contrast material, unspecified site

88.61 Phlebography of veins of head and neck using contrast material

88.62 Phlebography of pulmonary veins using contrast material

88.63 Phlebography of other intrathoracic veins using contrast material
Coding Clinic: 2008, Q3, P18

88.64 Phlebography of the portal venous system using contrast material
Splenoportogram (by splenic arteriography)

88.65 Phlebography of other intra-abdominal veins using contrast material
Coding Clinic: 2000, Q3, P9

88.66 Phlebography of femoral and other lower extremity veins using contrast material
Coding Clinic: 2006, Q2, P22-23

88.67 Phlebography of other specified sites using contrast material

88.68 Impedance phlebography

● **88.7 Diagnostic ultrasound**
Includes   echography
non-invasive ultrasound
ultrasonic angiography
ultrasonography

Excludes   *intravascular imaging (adjunctive) (IVUS) (00.21–00.29)*
that for intraoperative monitoring (00.94)
therapeutic ultrasound (00.01–00.09)
Coding Clinic: 2012, Q3, P6

88.71 Diagnostic ultrasound of head and neck
Determination of midline shift of brain
Echoencephalography

Excludes   *eye (95.13)*
Coding Clinic: 2002, Q1, P10-11; 1992, Q1, P11x2

88.72 Diagnostic ultrasound of heart
Echocardiography
Transesophageal echocardiography

Excludes   *echocardiography of heart chambers (37.28)*
intracardiac echocardiography (ICE) (37.28)
intravascular (IVUS) imaging of coronary vessels (00.24)
Coding Clinic: 2007, Q1, P11-12; 2005, Q2, P17-18; Q3, P14; 2004, Q4, P121-122; Q1, P16-17; 2000, Q1, P20-21; 1999, Q1, P6; 1998, Q3, P11

88.73 Diagnostic ultrasound of other sites of thorax
Aortic arch ultrasonography
Breast ultrasonography
Lung ultrasonography

88.74 Diagnostic ultrasound of digestive system

88.75 Diagnostic ultrasound of urinary system

88.76 Diagnostic ultrasound of abdomen and retroperitoneum
Coding Clinic: 1999, Q2, P14

88.77 Diagnostic ultrasound of peripheral vascular system
Deep vein thrombosis ultrasonic scanning

Excludes   *adjunct vascular system procedures (00.40–00.43)*
Coding Clinic: 1999, Q4, P17-18; Q1, P13; Q1, P12-13; 1993, 5th Issue, P5; 1992, Q1, P11

88.78 Diagnostic ultrasound of gravid uterus ♀
Intrauterine cephalometry:
echo
ultrasonic
Placental localization by ultrasound
Coding Clinic: 2010, Q2, P7; 2008, Q4, P124-125

88.79 Other diagnostic ultrasound
Ultrasonography of:
multiple sites
nongravid uterus
total body

● **88.8 Thermography**
88.81 Cerebral thermography

88.82 Ocular thermography

88.83 Bone thermography
Osteoarticular thermography

88.84 Muscle thermography

88.85 Breast thermography

88.86 Blood vessel thermography
Deep vein thermography

88.89 Thermography of other sites
Lymph gland thermography
Thermography NOS

● **88.9 Other diagnostic imaging**
Coding Clinic: 2006, Q2, P25-26

88.90 Diagnostic imaging, not elsewhere classified

88.91 Magnetic resonance imaging of brain and brain stem

Excludes   *intraoperative magnetic resonance imaging (88.96)*
laser interstitial thermal therapy [LITT] of lesion or tissue of brain under guidance (17.61)
real-time magnetic resonance imaging (88.96)
Coding Clinic: 2013, Q3, P11

88.92 Magnetic resonance imaging of chest and myocardium
For evaluation of hilar and mediastinal lymphadenopathy

Excludes   *laser interstitial thermal therapy [LITT] of lesion or tissue of breast under guidance (17.69)*
laser interstitial thermal therapy [LITT] of lesion or tissue of lung under guidance (17.69)
Coding Clinic: 2010, Q2, P13

88.93 Magnetic resonance imaging of spinal canal
Spinal cord levels:
cervical
thoracic
lumbar (lumbosacral)
Spinal cord
Spine

88.94 Magnetic resonance imaging of musculoskeletal
Bone marrow blood supply
Extremities (upper) (lower)

88.95 Magnetic resonance imaging of pelvis, prostate, and bladder

Excludes   *laser interstitial thermal therapy [LITT] of lesion or tissue of prostate under guidance (17.69)*

88.96   **Other intraoperative magnetic resonance imaging**
iMRI
Real-time magnetic resonance imaging
Coding Clinic: 2002, Q4, P111

88.97   **Magnetic resonance imaging of other and unspecified sites**
Abdomen
Eye orbit
Face
Neck

Excludes   *laser interstitial thermal therapy [LITT] of lesion or tissue of other and unspecified site under guidance (17.69)*

88.98   **Bone mineral density studies**
Dual photon absorptiometry
Quantitative computed tomography (CT) studies
Radiographic densitometry
Single photon absorptiometry

● **89**   **Interview, evaluation, consultation, and examination**

● **89.0**   **Diagnostic interview, consultation, and evaluation**

Excludes   *psychiatric diagnostic interview (94.11–94.19)*

89.01   **Interview and evaluation, described as brief**
Abbreviated history and evaluation

89.02   **Interview and evaluation, described as limited**
Interval history and evaluation

89.03   **Interview and evaluation, described as comprehensive**
History and evaluation of new problem

89.04   **Other interview and evaluation**

89.05   **Diagnostic interview and evaluation, not otherwise specified**

89.06   **Consultation, described as limited**
Consultation on a single organ system

89.07   **Consultation, described as comprehensive**

89.08   **Other consultation**

89.09   **Consultation, not otherwise specified**

● **89.1**   **Anatomic and physiologic measurements and manual examinations — nervous system and sense organs**

Excludes   *ear examination (95.41–95.49)*
eye examination (95.01–95.26)
the listed procedures when done as part of a general physical examination (89.7)

89.10   **Intracarotid amobarbital test**
Wada test

89.11   **Tonometry**

89.12   **Nasal function study**
Rhinomanometry

89.13   **Neurologic examination**

89.14   **Electroencephalogram**

Excludes   *that with polysomnogram (89.17)*
Coding Clinic: 2013, Q3, P11; 2005, Q3, P12-13

89.15   **Other nonoperative neurologic function tests**
Coding Clinic: 1995, Q3, P5-6; 1991, Q1, P14; 1987, Jan-Feb, P15-16

89.16   **Transillumination of newborn skull**

89.17   **Polysomnogram**
Sleep recording

89.18   **Other sleep disorder function tests**
Multiple sleep latency test [MSLT]

89.19   **Video and radio-telemetered electroencephalographic monitoring**
Radiographic EEG monitoring
Video EEG monitoring

Excludes   *intraoperative monitoring (00.94)*
Coding Clinic: 1992, Q1, P17; 1991, Q1, P14

● **89.2**   **Anatomic and physiologic measurements and manual examinations — genitourinary system**

Excludes   *the listed procedures when done as part of a general physical examination (89.7)*

89.21   **Urinary manometry**
Manometry through:
indwelling ureteral catheter
nephrostomy
pyelostomy
ureterostomy

89.22   **Cystometrogram**
Coding Clinic: 1990, Q2, P27

89.23   **Urethral sphincter electromyogram**
Coding Clinic: 1990, Q2, P27

89.24   **Uroflowmetry [UFR]**
Coding Clinic: 1990, Q2, P27

89.25   **Urethral pressure profile [UPP]**
Coding Clinic: 1990, Q2, P27

89.26   **Gynecological examination** ♀
Pelvic examination

89.29   **Other nonoperative genitourinary system measurements**
Bioassay of urine
Renal clearance
Urine chemistry

● **89.3**   **Other anatomic and physiologic measurements and manual examinations**

Excludes   *the listed procedures when done as part of a general physical examination (89.7)*

89.31   **Dental examination**
Oral mucosal survey
Periodontal survey

89.32   **Esophageal manometry**
Coding Clinic: 1996, Q3, P13

89.33   **Digital examination of enterostomy stoma**
Digital examination of colostomy stoma

89.34   **Digital examination of rectum**

89.35   **Transillumination of nasal sinuses**

89.36   **Manual examination of breast**

89.37   **Vital capacity determination**

Excludes   *endoscopic pulmonary airway flow measurement (33.72)*

89.38   **Other nonoperative respiratory measurements**
Plethysmography for measurement of respiratory function
Thoracic impedance plethysmography

Excludes   *endoscopic pulmonary airway flow measurement (33.72)*

89.39   **Other nonoperative measurements and examinations**
14 C-Urea breath test
Basal metabolic rate [BMR]
Gastric:
analysis
function NEC

Excludes   *body measurement (93.07)*
cardiac tests (89.41–89.69)
fundus photography (95.11)
limb length measurement (93.06)
Coding Clinic: 2001, Q2, P9-11; 2000, Q3, P9; 1996, Q3, P12-13; 1994, Q1, P18

● **89.4**   **Cardiac stress tests, pacemaker and defibrillator checks**

89.41   **Cardiovascular stress test using treadmill**
Coding Clinic: 1988, Q1, P11

89.42   **Masters' two-step stress test**
Coding Clinic: 1988, Q1, P11

89.43   **Cardiovascular stress test using bicycle ergometer**
Coding Clinic: 1988, Q1, P11

89.44   **Other cardiovascular stress test**
Thallium stress test with or without transesophageal pacing

MISCELLANEOUS DIAGNOSTIC AND THERAPEUTIC PROCEDURES (87—99)

Excludes   Includes   Use additional   Code also   Omit code

MISCELLANEOUS DIAGNOSTIC AND THERAPEUTIC PROCEDURES (87–99)

89.45 Artificial pacemaker rate check
Artificial pacemaker function check NOS
Bedside device check of pacemaker or cardiac
resynchronization pacemaker [CRT-P]
Interrogation only without arrhythmia induction

> **Excludes** *catheter based invasive electrophysiologic
> testing (37.26)*
> *noninvasive programmed electrical
> stimulation [NIPS] (arrhythmia
> induction) (37.20)*

Coding Clinic: 2010, Q3, P10; 2002, Q1, P3

89.46 Artificial pacemaker artifact wave form check

89.47 Artificial pacemaker electrode impedance check

**89.48 Artificial pacemaker voltage or amperage threshold
check**

**89.49 Automatic implantable cardioverter/defibrillator
(AICD) check**
Bedside check of an AICD or cardiac
resynchronization defibrillator [CRT-D]
Checking pacing thresholds of device
Interrogation only without arrhythmia induction

> **Excludes** *catheter based invasive electrophysiologic
> testing (37.26)*
> *noninvasive programmed electrical
> stimulation [NIPS] (arrhythmia
> induction) (37.20)*

Coding Clinic: 2004, Q4, P135-136; 2002, Q1, P9

● **89.5 Other nonoperative cardiac and vascular diagnostic procedures**

> **Excludes** *fetal EKG (75.32)*

Coding Clinic: 1984, July-Aug, P19

89.50 Ambulatory cardiac monitoring
Analog devices [Holter-type]
Coding Clinic: 1999, Q4, P21

89.51 Rhythm electrocardiogram
Rhythm EKG (with one to three leads)

89.52 Electrocardiogram
ECG NOS
EKG (with 12 or more leads)
Coding Clinic: 1988, Q1, P11

89.53 Vectorcardiogram (with ECG)

89.54 Electrographic monitoring
Telemetry

> **Excludes** *ambulatory cardiac monitoring (89.50)*
> *electrographic monitoring during surgery —
> omit code*

Coding Clinic: 1988, Q1, P11; 1984, Nov-Dec, P12

89.55 Phonocardiogram with ECG lead

89.56 Carotid pulse tracing with ECG lead

> **Excludes** *oculoplethysmography (89.58)*

89.57 Apexcardiogram (with ECG lead)
Coding Clinic: 1987, Jan-Feb, P15-16

89.58 Plethysmogram
Penile plethysmography with nerve stimulation

> **Excludes** *plethysmography (for):*
> *measurement of respiratory function
> (89.38)*
> *thoracic impedance (89.38)*

89.59 Other nonoperative cardiac and vascular measurements
Coding Clinic: 2010, Q2, P11; 2005, Q3, P21; 2004, Q4, P135-136;
2003, Q3, P23; 1992, Q2, P12

● **89.6 Circulatory monitoring**

> **Excludes** *electrocardiographic monitoring during surgery —
> omit code*
> *implantation or replacement of subcutaneous device for
> intracardiac hemodynamic monitoring (00.57)*
> *insertion or replacement of implantable pressure
> sensor (lead) for intracardiac hemodynamic
> monitoring (00.56)*

Coding Clinic: 1984, July-Aug, P19

89.60 Continuous intra-arterial blood gas monitoring
Insertion of blood gas monitoring system and
continuous monitoring of blood gases through
an intra-arterial sensor
Coding Clinic: 2002, Q4, P111-112

89.61 Systemic arterial pressure monitoring

> **Excludes** *intra-aneurysm sac pressure monitoring
> (intraoperative) (00.58)*
> *intravascular pressure measurement of
> intrathoracic arteries (00.67)*
> *intravascular pressure measurement of
> peripheral arteries (00.68)*

89.62 Central venous pressure monitoring

> **Excludes** *intravascular pressure measurement, other
> specified and unspecified vessels
> (00.69)*

89.63 Pulmonary artery pressure monitoring

> **Excludes** *pulmonary artery wedge monitoring (89.64)*

Coding Clinic: 1984, Nov-Dec, P19

89.64 Pulmonary artery wedge monitoring
Pulmonary capillary wedge [PCW] monitoring
Swan-Ganz catheterization
Coding Clinic: 1984, Nov-Dec, P19; July-Aug, P19

89.65 Measurement of systemic arterial blood gases

> **Excludes** *continuous intra-arterial blood gas
> monitoring (89.60)*

89.66 Measurement of mixed venous blood gases

**89.67 Monitoring of cardiac output by oxygen consumption
technique**
Fick method

89.68 Monitoring of cardiac output by other technique
Cardiac output monitor by thermodilution indicator

89.69 Monitoring of coronary blood flow
Coronary blood flow monitoring by coincidence
counting technique

> **Excludes** *intravascular pressure measurement of
> coronary arteries (00.59)*

89.7 General physical examination

89.8 Autopsy

● **90 Microscopic examination-I**
The following fourth-digit subclassification is for use with categories
in section 90 to identify type of examination:

> 1 bacterial smear
> 2 culture
> 3 culture and sensitivity
> 4 parasitology
> 5 toxicology
> 6 cell block and Papanicolaou smear
> 9 other microscopic examination

● **90.0 Microscopic examination of specimen from nervous system
and of spinal fluid**

● **90.1 Microscopic examination of specimen from endocrine gland,
not elsewhere classified**

● **90.2 Microscopic examination of specimen from eye**

● **90.3 Microscopic examination of specimen from ear, nose, throat,
and larynx**

● **90.4 Microscopic examination of specimen from trachea,
bronchus, pleura, lung, and other thoracic specimen, and of
sputum**

● **90.5 Microscopic examination of blood**

● **90.6 Microscopic examination of specimen from spleen and of
bone marrow**

● **90.7 Microscopic examination of specimen from lymph node and
of lymph**

● **90.8 Microscopic examination of specimen from upper
gastrointestinal tract and of vomitus**

● **90.9 Microscopic examination of specimen from lower
gastrointestinal tract and of stool**

◄ New   ◄ Revised   ~~deleted~~ Deleted   ● Use Additional Digit(s)   �ख़ Valid O.R. Procedure
◆ Non-O.R. Procedure   ♀ Females Only   ♂ Males Only   OGCR Official Guidelines   Coding Clinic

1294

● **91 Microscopic examination-II**

The following fourth-digit subclassification is for use with categories in section 91 to identify type of examination

> 1   bacterial smear
> 2   culture
> 3   culture and sensitivity
> 4   parasitology
> 5   toxicology
> 6   cell block and Papanicolaou smear
> 9   other microscopic examination

● **91.0 Microscopic examination of specimen from liver, biliary tract, and pancreas**

● **91.1 Microscopic examination of peritoneal and retroperitoneal specimen**

● **91.2 Microscopic examination of specimen from kidney, ureter, perirenal, and periureteral tissue**

● **91.3 Microscopic examination of specimen from bladder, urethra, prostate, seminal vesicle, perivesical tissue, and of urine and semen**

● **91.4 Microscopic examination of specimen from female genital tract ♀**
> Amnionic sac
> Fetus

● **91.5 Microscopic examination of specimen from musculoskeletal system and of joint fluid**
> Microscopic examination of:
> | | |
> |---|---|
> | bone | ligament |
> | bursa | muscle |
> | cartilage | synovial membrane |
> | fascia | tendon |

● **91.6 Microscopic examination of specimen from skin and other integument**
> Microscopic examination of:
> | | |
> |---|---|
> | hair | skin |
> | nails | |
>
> **Excludes**   *mucous membrane — code to organ site that of operative wound (91.71–91.79)*

● **91.7 Microscopic examination of specimen from operative wound**

● **91.8 Microscopic examination of specimen from other site**

● **91.9 Microscopic examination of specimen from unspecified site**

● **92 Nuclear medicine**

● **92.0 Radioisotope scan and function study**

92.01 Thyroid scan and radioisotope function studies
> Iodine-131 uptake
> Protein-bound iodine
> Radio-iodine uptake

92.02 Liver scan and radioisotope function study

92.03 Renal scan and radioisotope function study
> Renal clearance study

92.04 Gastrointestinal scan and radioisotope function study
> Radio-cobalt B12 Schilling test
> Radio-iodinated triolein study

92.05 Cardiovascular and hematopoietic scan and radioisotope function study
> Bone marrow scan or function study
> Cardiac output scan or function study
> Circulation time scan or function study
> Radionuclide cardiac ventriculogram scan or function study
> Spleen scan or function study
> **Coding Clinic: 1992, Q2, P7-8; 1988, Q1, P11**

92.09 Other radioisotope function studies

● **92.1 Other radioisotope scan**

92.11 Cerebral scan
> Pituitary

92.12 Scan of other sites of head
> **Excludes**   *eye (95.16)*

92.13 Parathyroid scan

92.14 Bone scan

92.15 Pulmonary scan

92.16 Scan of lymphatic system

92.17 Placental scan ♀

92.18 Total body scan

92.19 Scan of other sites

● **92.2 Therapeutic radiology and nuclear medicine**
> **Excludes**   *that for:*
> > *ablation of pituitary gland (07.64–07.69)*
> > *destruction of chorioretinal lesion (14.26–14.27)*

92.20 Infusion of liquid brachytherapy radioisotope
> I-125 radioisotope
> Intracavitary brachytherapy
> **Includes**   removal of radioisotope
> **Coding Clinic: 2005, Q4, P117-119; 2004, Q1, P3-5x2; 2000, Q1, P11-12; 1994, Q3, P11; 1994, Q2, P10**

92.21 Superficial radiation
> Contact radiation [up to 150 KVP]

92.22 Orthovoltage radiation
> Deep radiation [200–300 KVP]

92.23 Radioisotopic teleradiotherapy
> Teleradiotherapy using:
> > cobalt-60
> > iodine-125
> > radioactive cesium

92.24 Teleradiotherapy using photons
> Megavoltage NOS
> Supervoltage NOS
> Use of:
> > Betatron
> > linear accelerator

92.25 Teleradiotherapy using electrons
> Beta particles
> **Excludes**   *intra-operative electron radiation therapy (92.41)*

92.26 Teleradiotherapy of other particulate radiation
> Neutrons
> Protons NOS

✖ **92.27 Implantation or insertion of radioactive elements**
> Intravascular brachytherapy
> Code also incision of site
> **Excludes**   *infusion of liquid brachytherapy radioisotope (92.20)*
> **Coding Clinic: 2004, Q1, P3-5**

92.28 Injection or instillation of radioisotopes
> Injection or infusion of radioimmunoconjugate
> Intracavitary injection or instillation
> Intravenous injection or instillation
> Iodine-131 [I-131] tositumomab
> Radioimmunotherapy
> Ytrium-90 [Y-90] ibritumomab tiuxetan
> **Excludes**   *infusion of liquid brachytherapy radioisotope (92.20)*

92.29 Other radiotherapeutic procedure
> **Coding Clinic: 2013, Q1, P9; 2006, Q3, P14-15**

● **92.3 Stereotactic radiosurgery**
> Code also stereotactic head frame application (93.59)
> **Excludes**   *stereotactic biopsy*

92.30 Stereotactic radiosurgery, not otherwise specified
> ◆Non-OR Procedure that affects MS-DRG assignment to MDC 01, MS-DRG 040-042; MDC 10, MS-DRG 628-630; MDC 17, MS-DRG 823-825, 829-830

92.31 Single source photon radiosurgery
> High energy x-rays
> Linear accelerator (LINAC)
> ◆Non-OR Procedure that affects MS-DRG assignment to MDC 01, MS-DRG 040-042; MDC 10, MS-DRG 628-630; MDC 17, MS-DRG 823-825, 829-830

92.32 Multi-source photon radiosurgery
> Cobalt 60 radiation
> Gamma irradiation
> ◆Non-OR Procedure that affects MS-DRG assignment to MDC 01, MS-DRG 040-042; MDC 10, MS-DRG 628-630; MDC 17, MS-DRG 823-825, 829-830

MISCELLANEOUS DIAGNOSTIC AND THERAPEUTIC PROCEDURES (87–99)

Excludes	Includes	Use additional	Code also	Omit code

92.33 **Particulate radiosurgery**
Particle beam radiation (cyclotron)
Proton accelerator
◆ Non-OR Procedure that affects MS-DRG assignment to MDC 01, MS-DRG 040-042; MDC 10, MS-DRG 628-630; MDC 17, MS-DRG 823-825, 829-830

92.39 **Stereotactic radiosurgery, not elsewhere classified**
◆ Non-OR Procedure that affects MS-DRG assignment to MDC 01, MS-DRG 040-042; MDC 10, MS-DRG 628-630; MDC 17, MS-DRG 823-825, 829-830

● 92.4 **Intra-operative radiation procedures**

92.41 **Intra-operative electron radiation therapy**
IOERT
That using a mobile linear accelerator
Coding Clinic: 2007, Q4, P122

● 93 **Physical therapy, respiratory therapy, rehabilitation, and related procedures**

● 93.0 **Diagnostic physical therapy**

93.01 **Functional evaluation**

93.02 **Orthotic evaluation**

93.03 **Prosthetic evaluation**

93.04 **Manual testing of muscle function**
Coding Clinic: 1987, Jan-Feb, P15-16

93.05 **Range of motion testing**
Coding Clinic: 1987, Jan-Feb, P15-16

93.06 **Measurement of limb length**

93.07 **Body measurement**
Girth measurement
Measurement of skull circumference

93.08 **Electromyography**
Excludes *eye EMG (95.25)*
that for intraoperative monitoring (00.94)
that with polysomnogram (89.17)
urethral sphincter EMG (89.23)
Coding Clinic: 1987, Jan-Feb, P15-16

93.09 **Other diagnostic physical therapy procedure**

● 93.1 **Physical therapy exercises**
Coding Clinic: 1987, Jan-Feb, P15-16

93.11 **Assisting exercise**
Excludes *assisted exercise in pool (93.31)*

93.12 **Other active musculoskeletal exercise**

93.13 **Resistive exercise**

93.14 **Training in joint movements**

93.15 **Mobilization of spine**

93.16 **Mobilization of other joints**
Excludes *manipulation of temporomandibular joint (76.95)*

93.17 **Other passive musculoskeletal exercise**

93.18 **Breathing exercise**

93.19 **Exercise, not elsewhere classified**

● 93.2 **Other physical therapy musculoskeletal manipulation**

93.21 **Manual and mechanical traction**
Excludes *skeletal traction (93.43–93.44)*
skin traction (93.45–93.46)
spinal traction (93.41–93.42)

93.22 **Ambulation and gait training**

93.23 **Fitting of orthotic device**

93.24 **Training in use of prosthetic or orthotic device**
Training in crutch walking

93.25 **Forced extension of limb**

93.26 **Manual rupture of joint adhesions**

93.27 **Stretching of muscle or tendon**

93.28 **Stretching of fascia**

93.29 **Other forcible correction of deformity**
Coding Clinic: 1985, Nov-Dec, P11

● 93.3 **Other physical therapy therapeutic procedures**

93.31 **Assisted exercise in pool**

93.32 **Whirlpool treatment**

93.33 **Other hydrotherapy**

93.34 **Diathermy**

93.35 **Other heat therapy**
Acupuncture with smouldering moxa
Hot packs
Hyperthermia NEC
Infrared irradiation
Moxibustion
Paraffin bath
Excludes *hyperthermia for treatment of cancer (99.85)*

93.36 **Cardiac retraining**

93.37 **Prenatal training**
Training for natural childbirth

93.38 **Combined physical therapy without mention of the components**

93.39 **Other physical therapy**
Coding Clinic: 2005, Q2, P6-7; 2003, Q4, P105-106, 108-110; 1997, Q3, P12-13; 1991, Q3, P15; Q2, P15

● 93.4 **Skeletal traction and other traction**

93.41 **Spinal traction using skull device**
Traction using:
caliper tongs
Crutchfield tongs
halo device
Vinke tongs
Excludes *insertion of tongs or halo traction device (02.94)*
Coding Clinic: 2001, Q3, P8; 1996, Q3, P14

93.42 **Other spinal traction**
Cotrel's traction
Excludes *cervical collar (93.52)*

93.43 **Intermittent skeletal traction**

93.44 **Other skeletal traction**
Bryant's traction
Dunlop's traction
Lyman Smith traction
Russell's traction
Coding Clinic: 1989, Q3, P16

93.45 **Thomas' splint traction**

93.46 **Other skin traction of limbs**
Adhesive tape traction
Boot traction
Buck's traction
Gallows traction

● 93.5 **Other immobilization, pressure, and attention to wound**
Excludes *external fixator device (84.71–84.73)*
wound cleansing (96.58–96.59)

93.51 **Application of plaster jacket**
Excludes *Minerva jacket (93.52)*

93.52 **Application of neck support**
Application of:
cervical collar
Minerva jacket
molded neck support

93.53 **Application of other cast**

93.54 **Application of splint**
Plaster splint
Tray splint
Excludes *periodontal splint (24.7)*

93.55 **Dental wiring**
Excludes *that for orthodontia (24.7)*

93.56 **Application of pressure dressing**
Application of:
Gibney bandage
Robert Jones' bandage
Shanz dressing

93.57 **Application of other wound dressing**
Porcine wound dressing
Coding Clinic: 2012, Q3, P15; 2002, Q3, P23

◀ New   ◀▥ Revised   ~~deleted~~ Deleted   ● Use Additional Digit(s)   ✴ Valid O.R. Procedure
◆ Non-O.R. Procedure   ♀ Females Only   ♂ Males Only   OGCR Official Guidelines   **Coding Clinic**

1296

93.58   Application of pressure trousers
Application of:
anti-shock trousers
MAST trousers
vasopneumatic device
Coding Clinic: 1996, Q3, P13-14

93.59   Other immobilization, pressure, and attention to wound
Elastic stockings
Electronic gaiter
Intermittent pressure device
Oxygenation of wound (hyperbaric)
Stereotactic head frame application
Strapping (non-traction)
Velpeau dressing
Coding Clinic: 1999, Q3, P7-8; Q1, P12-13; 1991, Q1, P3-4; 1989, Q1, P12; 1988, Q4, P11

● **93.6   Osteopathic manipulative treatment**

93.61   Osteopathic manipulative treatment for general mobilization
General articulatory treatment

93.62   Osteopathic manipulative treatment using high-velocity, low-amplitude forces
Thrusting forces

93.63   Osteopathic manipulative treatment using low-velocity, high-amplitude forces
Springing forces

93.64   Osteopathic manipulative treatment using isotonic, isometric forces

93.65   Osteopathic manipulative treatment using indirect forces

93.66   Osteopathic manipulative treatment to move tissue fluids
Lymphatic pump

93.67   Other specified osteopathic manipulative treatment

● **93.7   Speech and reading rehabilitation and rehabilitation of the blind**

93.71   Dyslexia training

93.72   Dysphasia training

93.73   Esophageal speech training

93.74   Speech defect training

93.75   Other speech training and therapy
Coding Clinic: 2003, Q4, P105-106, 109-110; 1997, Q4, P35-37; Q3, P12-13

93.76   Training in use of lead dog for the blind

93.77   Training in braille or Moon

93.78   Other rehabilitation for the blind

● **93.8   Other rehabilitation therapy**

93.81   Recreation therapy
Diversional therapy
Play therapy
Excludes   play psychotherapy (94.36)

93.82   Educational therapy
Education of bed-bound children
Special schooling for the handicapped

93.83   Occupational therapy
Daily living activities therapy
Excludes   training in activities of daily living for the blind (93.78)
Coding Clinic: 2005, Q2, P6-7; 2003, Q4, P105-106, 108; 1997, Q3, P12-13

93.84   Music therapy

93.85   Vocational rehabilitation
Sheltered employment
Vocational:
assessment
retraining
training

93.89   Rehabilitation, not elsewhere classified
Coding Clinic: 2005, Q2, P6-7

● **93.9   Respiratory therapy**
Excludes   insertion of airway (96.01–96.05)
other continuous invasive (through endotracheal tube or tracheostomy) mechanical ventilation (96.70–96.72)
Coding Clinic: 2004, Q3, P3; 2002, Q1, P12.-13; 1998, Q3, P14

93.90   Non-invasive mechanical ventilation
Bi-level airway pressure
BiPAP without (delivery through) endotracheal tube or tracheostomy
CPAP without (delivery through) endotracheal tube or tracheostomy
Mechanical ventilation NOS
Non-invasive positive pressure (NIPPV)
Non-invasive PPV
NPPV
That delivered by non-invasive interface:
face mask
nasal mask
nasal pillow
oral mouthpiece
oronasal mask
Excludes   invasive (through endotracheal tube or tracheostomy) continuous mechanical ventilation (96.70–96.72)
Note: Patients admitted on non-invasive mechanical ventilation that subsequently require invasive mechanical ventilation; code both types of mechanical ventilation.
Coding Clinic: 2008, Q4, P187-190; Q1, P8-9; 2004, Q3, P3

93.91   Intermittent positive pressure breathing [IPPB]

93.93   Nonmechanical methods of resuscitation
Artificial respiration
Manual resuscitation
Mouth-to-mouth resuscitation
Coding Clinic: 2003, Q2, P17

93.94   Respiratory medication administered by nebulizer
Mist therapy

93.95   Hyperbaric oxygenation
Excludes   oxygenation of wound (93.59)

93.96   Other oxygen enrichment
Catalytic oxygen therapy
Cytoreductive effect
Oxygenators
Oxygen therapy
Excludes   oxygenation of wound (93.59)
SuperSaturated oxygen therapy (00.49)

93.97   Decompression chamber

93.98   Other control of atmospheric pressure and composition
Antigen-free air conditioning
Helium therapy
Excludes   inhaled nitric oxide therapy (INO) (00.12)
Coding Clinic: 2002, Q1, P14

93.99   Other respiratory procedures
Continuous negative pressure ventilation [CNP]
Postural drainage
Coding Clinic: 2003, Q4, P108-109; 1999, Q3, P11-12

● **94   Procedures related to the psyche**

● **94.0   Psychologic evaluation and testing**

94.01   Administration of intelligence test
Administration of:
Stanford-Binet
Wechsler Adult Intelligence Scale
Wechsler Intelligence Scale for Children

94.02   Administration of psychologic test
Administration of:
Bender Visual-Motor Gestalt Test
Benton Visual Retention Test
Minnesota Multiphasic Personality Inventory
Wechsler Memory Scale

94.03   Character analysis

94.08   Other psychologic evaluation and testing

94.09   Psychologic mental status determination, not otherwise specified

MISCELLANEOUS DIAGNOSTIC AND THERAPEUTIC PROCEDURES (87–99)

Excludes   Includes   Use additional   Code also   Omit code

● **94.1 Psychiatric interviews, consultations, and evaluations**
  94.11 Psychiatric mental status determination
    Clinical psychiatric mental status determination
    Evaluation for criminal responsibility
    Evaluation for testimentary capacity
    Medicolegal mental status determination
    Mental status determination NOS
  94.12 Routine psychiatric visit, not otherwise specified
  94.13 Psychiatric commitment evaluation
    Pre-commitment interview
  94.19 Other psychiatric interview and evaluation
    Follow-up psychiatric interview NOS

● **94.2 Psychiatric somatotherapy**
  94.21 Narcoanalysis
    Narcosynthesis
  94.22 Lithium therapy
  94.23 Neuroleptic therapy
  94.24 Chemical shock therapy
  94.25 Other psychiatric drug therapy
  94.26 Subconvulsive electroshock therapy
  94.27 Other electroshock therapy
    Electroconvulsive therapy (ECT)
    EST
  94.29 Other psychiatric somatotherapy

● **94.3 Individual psychotherapy**
  94.31 Psychoanalysis
  94.32 Hypnotherapy
    Hypnodrome
    Hypnosis
  94.33 Behavior therapy
    Aversion therapy
    Behavior modification
    Desensitization therapy
    Extinction therapy
    Relaxation training
    Token economy
  94.34 Individual therapy for psychosexual dysfunction
    Excludes *that performed in group setting (94.41)*
  94.35 Crisis intervention
  94.36 Play psychotherapy
  94.37 Exploratory verbal psychotherapy
  94.38 Supportive verbal psychotherapy
  94.39 Other individual psychotherapy
    Biofeedback

● **94.4 Other psychotherapy and counseling**
  94.41 Group therapy for psychosexual dysfunction
  94.42 Family therapy
  94.43 Psychodrama
  94.44 Other group therapy
  94.45 Drug addiction counseling
  94.46 Alcoholism counseling
  94.49 Other counseling

● **94.5 Referral for psychologic rehabilitation**
  94.51 Referral for psychotherapy
  94.52 Referral for psychiatric aftercare:
    That in:
      halfway house
      outpatient (clinic) facility
  94.53 Referral for alcoholism rehabilitation
  94.54 Referral for drug addiction rehabilitation
  94.55 Referral for vocational rehabilitation
  94.59 Referral for other psychologic rehabilitation

● **94.6 Alcohol and drug rehabilitation and detoxification**
  94.61 Alcohol rehabilitation
    ◆Non-OR Procedure that affects MS-DRG assignment to MDC 20, MS-DRG 895
  94.62 Alcohol detoxification
  94.63 Alcohol rehabilitation and detoxification
    ◆Non-OR Procedure that affects MS-DRG assignment to MDC 20, MS-DRG 895

  94.64 Drug rehabilitation
    ◆Non-OR Procedure that affects MS-DRG assignment to MDC 20, MS-DRG 895
  94.65 Drug detoxification
  94.66 Drug rehabilitation and detoxification
    ◆Non-OR Procedure that affects MS-DRG assignment to MDC 20, MS-DRG 895
  94.67 Combined alcohol and drug rehabilitation
    ◆Non-OR Procedure that affects MS-DRG assignment to MDC 20, MS-DRG 895
  94.68 Combined alcohol and drug detoxification
  94.69 Combined alcohol and drug rehabilitation and detoxification
    ◆Non-OR Procedure that affects MS-DRG assignment to MDC 20, MS-DRG 895

● **95 Ophthalmologic and otologic diagnosis and treatment**
● **95.0 General and subjective eye examination**
  95.01 Limited eye examination
    Eye examination with prescription of spectacles
  95.02 Comprehensive eye examination
    Eye examination covering all aspects of the visual system
  95.03 Extended ophthalmologic work-up
    Examination (for):
      glaucoma
      neuro-ophthalmology
      retinal disease
  ✖ **95.04 Eye examination under anesthesia**
    Code also type of examination
  95.05 Visual field study
  95.06 Color vision study
  95.07 Dark adaptation study
  95.09 Eye examination, not otherwise specified
    Vision check NOS

● **95.1 Examinations of form and structure of eye**
  95.11 Fundus photography
  95.12 Fluorescein angiography or angioscopy of eye
  95.13 Ultrasound study of eye
  95.14 X-ray study of eye
  95.15 Ocular motility study
  95.16 P32 and other tracer studies of eye

● **95.2 Objective functional tests of eye**
    Excludes *that with polysomnogram (89.17)*
  95.21 Electroretinogram [ERG]
  95.22 Electro-oculogram [EOG]
  95.23 Visual evoked potential [VEP]
  95.24 Electronystagmogram [ENG]
  95.25 Electromyogram of eye [EMG]
  95.26 Tonography, provocative tests, and other glaucoma testing

● **95.3 Special vision services**
  95.31 Fitting and dispensing of spectacles
  95.32 Prescription, fitting, and dispensing of contact lens
  95.33 Dispensing of other low vision aids
  95.34 Ocular prosthetics
  95.35 Orthoptic training
  95.36 Ophthalmologic counseling and instruction
    Counseling in:
      adaptation to visual loss
      use of low vision aids

● **95.4 Nonoperative procedures related to hearing**
  95.41 Audiometry
    Békésy 5-tone audiometry
    Impedance audiometry
    Stapedial reflex response
    Subjective audiometry
    Tympanogram
  95.42 Clinical test of hearing
    Tuning fork test
    Whispered speech test

◀ New   ◀▥ Revised   ~~deleted~~ Deleted   ● Use Additional Digit(s)   ✖ Valid O.R. Procedure
◆ Non-O.R. Procedure   ♀ Females Only   ♂ Males Only   OGCR Official Guidelines   **Coding Clinic**
1298

95.43   **Audiological evaluation**
  Audiological evaluation by:
    Bárány noise machine
    blindfold test
    delayed feedback
    masking
    Weber lateralization

95.44   **Clinical vestibular function tests**
  Thermal test of vestibular function

95.45   **Rotation tests**
  Bárány chair

95.46   **Other auditory and vestibular function tests**

95.47   **Hearing examination, not otherwise specified**

95.48   **Fitting of hearing aid**

> **Excludes**   *implantation of electromagnetic hearing device (20.95)*

95.49   **Other nonoperative procedures related to hearing**
  Adjustment (external components) of cochlear prosthetic device

● **96**   **Nonoperative intubation and irrigation**

  ● **96.0**   **Nonoperative intubation of gastrointestinal and respiratory tracts**

96.01   **Insertion of nasopharyngeal airway**

96.02   **Insertion of oropharyngeal airway**

96.03   **Insertion of esophageal obturator airway**

96.04   **Insertion of endotracheal tube**
  Coding Clinic: 2010, Q4, P80; 2009, Q2, P11; 2007, Q1, P11; 2006, Q2, P8-9; 2005, Q4, P83-89; Q3, P10-11; Q2, P19-20; 2003, Q2, P17; 1993, 5th Issue, P11

96.05   **Other intubation of respiratory tract**

> **Excludes**   *endoscopic insertion or replacement of bronchial device or substance (33.71, 33.79)*

  Coding Clinic: 1997, Q1, P14

96.06   **Insertion of Sengstaken tube**
  Esophageal tamponade

96.07   **Insertion of other (naso-)gastric tube**
  Intubation for decompression

> **Excludes**   *that for enteral infusion of nutritional substance (96.6)*

  Coding Clinic: 2008, Q4, P138-140

96.08   **Insertion of (naso-)intestinal tube**
  Miller-Abbott tube (for decompression)
  Coding Clinic: 2012, Q3, P23

96.09   **Insertion of rectal tube**
  Replacement of rectal tube

  ● **96.1**   **Other nonoperative insertion**

> **Excludes**   *nasolacrimal intubation (09.44)*

96.11   **Packing of external auditory canal**

96.14   **Vaginal packing ♀**

96.15   **Insertion of vaginal mold ♀**

96.16   **Other vaginal dilation ♀**

96.17   **Insertion of vaginal diaphragm ♀**

96.18   **Insertion of other vaginal pessary ♀**

96.19   **Rectal packing**

  ● **96.2**   **Nonoperative dilation and manipulation**

96.21   **Dilation of frontonasal duct**

96.22   **Dilation of rectum**

96.23   **Dilation of anal sphincter**

96.24   **Dilation and manipulation of enterostomy stoma**

96.25   **Therapeutic distention of bladder**
  Intermittent distention of bladder

96.26   **Manual reduction of rectal prolapse**

96.27   **Manual reduction of hernia**

96.28   **Manual reduction of enterostomy prolapse**
  Coding Clinic: 1987, Nov-Dec, P11

96.29   **Reduction of intussusception of alimentary tract**
  With:
    fluoroscopy
    ionizing radiation enema
    ultrasonography guidance
  Hydrostatic reduction
  Pneumatic reduction

> **Excludes**   *intra-abdominal manipulation of intestine, not otherwise specified (46.80)*

  Coding Clinic: 1998, Q43, P82-83

  ● **96.3**   **Nonoperative alimentary tract irrigation, cleaning, and local instillation**

96.31   **Gastric cooling**
  Gastric hypothermia

96.32   **Gastric freezing**

96.33   **Gastric lavage**

96.34   **Other irrigation of (naso-)gastric tube**

96.35   **Gastric gavage**

96.36   **Irrigation of gastrostomy or enterostomy**

96.37   **Proctoclysis**

96.38   **Removal of impacted feces**
  Removal of impaction:
    by flushing
    manually

96.39   **Other transanal enema**
  Rectal irrigation

> **Excludes**   *reduction of intussusception of alimentary tract by ionizing radiation enema (96.29)*

  Coding Clinic: 2012, Q3, P23

  ● **96.4**   **Nonoperative irrigation, cleaning, and local instillation of other digestive and genitourinary organs**

96.41   **Irrigation of cholecystostomy and other biliary tube**

96.42   **Irrigation of pancreatic tube**

96.43   **Digestive tract instillation, except gastric gavage**

96.44   **Vaginal douche ♀**

96.45   **Irrigation of nephrostomy and pyelostomy**

96.46   **Irrigation of ureterostomy and ureteral catheter**
  Coding Clinic: 1985, July-Aug, P15

96.47   **Irrigation of cystostomy**

96.48   **Irrigation of other indwelling urinary catheter**

96.49   **Other genitourinary instillation**
  Insertion of prostaglandin suppository
  Coding Clinic: 2001, Q1, P5

  ● **96.5**   **Other nonoperative irrigation and cleaning**

96.51   **Irrigation of eye**
  Irrigation of cornea

> **Excludes**   *irrigation with removal of foreign body (98.21)*

96.52   **Irrigation of ear**
  Irrigation with removal of cerumen

96.53   **Irrigation of nasal passages**

96.54   **Dental scaling, polishing, and debridement**
  Dental prophylaxis
  Plaque removal

96.55   **Tracheostomy toilette**

96.56   **Other lavage of bronchus and trachea**

> **Excludes**   *diagnostic bronchoalveolar lavage (BAL) (33.24)*
> *whole lung lavage (33.99)*

  Coding Clinic: 2002, Q3, P18

96.57   **Irrigation of vascular catheter**
  Coding Clinic: 1993, Q3, P5

96.58   **Irrigation of wound catheter**

96.59   **Other irrigation of wound**
  Wound cleaning NOS

> **Excludes**   *debridement (86.22, 86.27–86.28)*

  Coding Clinic: 2012, Q3, P4

96.6   **Enteral infusion of concentrated nutritional substances**

Excludes   Includes   Use additional   Code also   Omit code

● **96.7 Other continuous invasive mechanical ventilation**

Includes   BiPAP delivered through endotracheal tube or tracheostomy (invasive interface)
CPAP delivered through endotracheal tube or tracheostomy (invasive interface)
endotracheal respiratory assistance
invasive positive pressure ventilation [IPPV]
mechanical ventilation through invasive interface
that by tracheostomy
weaning of an intubated (endotracheal tube) patient

Excludes   *continuous negative pressure ventilation [CNP] (iron lung) (cuirass) (93.99)*
intermittent positive pressure breathing [IPPB] (93.91)
non-invasive bi-level positive airway pressure [BiPAP] (93.90)
non-invasive continuous positive airway pressure [CPAP] (93.90)
non-invasive positive pressure (NIPPV) (93.90)
that by face mask (93.90–93.99)
that by nasal cannula (93.90–93.99)
that by nasal catheter (93.90–93.99)

Code also any associated:
endotracheal tube insertion (96.04)
tracheostomy (31.1–31.29)

Note: Endotracheal Intubation

To calculate the number of hours (duration) of continuous mechanical ventilation during a hospitalization, begin the count from the start of the (endotracheal) intubation. The duration ends with (endotracheal) extubation.

If a patient is intubated prior to admission, begin counting the duration from the time of the admission. If a patient is transferred (discharged) while intubated, the duration would end at the time of transfer (discharge).

For patients who begin on (endotracheal) intubation and subsequently have a tracheostomy performed for mechanical ventilation, the duration begins with the (endotracheal) intubation and ends when the mechanical ventilation is turned off (after the weaning period).

Tracheostomy

To calculate the number of hours of continuous mechanical ventilation during a hospitalization, begin counting the duration when mechanical ventilation is started. The duration ends when the mechanical ventilator is turned off (after the weaning period).

If a patient has received a tracheostomy prior to admission and is on mechanical ventilation at the time of admission, begin counting the duration from the time of admission. If a patient is transferred (discharged) while still on mechanical ventilation via tracheostomy, the duration would end at the time of the transfer (discharge).

Coding Clinic: 2013, Q2, P25; 2008, Q4, P187-190; 2004, Q3, P3, 11; 2003, Q2, P17; 2002, Q2, P19; 1998, Q3, P14

96.70 Continuous invasive mechanical ventilation of unspecified duration
Invasive mechanical ventilation NOS
◆ Non-OR Procedure that affects MS-DRG assignment to MDC 04, MS-DRG 208
Coding Clinic: 1992, Q2, P13-14x3

96.71 Continuous invasive mechanical ventilation for less than 96 consecutive hours
◆ Non-OR Procedure that affects MS-DRG assignment to MDC 04, MS-DRG 208
Coding Clinic: 2013, Q1, P10; 2010, Q4, P80; 2009, Q2, P11; 2007, Q3, P7-8; 2006, Q2, P8-9x2; 2005, Q3, P10-11; 2004, Q3, P3, 11; 2003, Q2, P17; 2002, Q1, P12-13; 2001, Q1, P6-7; 1993, 5th Issue, P11; 1992, Q2, P13-14x3

96.72 Continuous invasive mechanical ventilation for 96 consecutive hours or more
◆ Non-OR Procedure that affects MS-DRG assignment to MS-DRG 003-004, MDC 04, MS-DRG 207, MDC 18, MS-DRG 870, MDC 22, MS-DRG 927, 933
Coding Clinic: 2013, Q1, P12; 2005, Q2, P19-20; 1992, Q2, P13-14x3

● **97 Replacement and removal of therapeutic appliances**

● **97.0 Nonoperative replacement of gastrointestinal appliance**

97.01 Replacement of (naso-)gastric or esophagostomy tube

97.02 Replacement of gastrostomy tube
Coding Clinic: 1997, Q1, P11

97.03 Replacement of tube or enterostomy device of small intestine
Coding Clinic: 2003, Q1, P10

97.04 Replacement of tube or enterostomy device of large intestine

97.05 Replacement of stent (tube) in biliary or pancreatic duct
Coding Clinic: 1999, Q2, P13-14

● **97.1 Nonoperative replacement of musculoskeletal and integumentary system appliance**

97.11 Replacement of cast on upper limb

97.12 Replacement of cast on lower limb

97.13 Replacement of other cast

97.14 Replacement of other device for musculoskeletal immobilization
Splinting
Strapping

97.15 Replacement of wound catheter

97.16 Replacement of wound packing or drain
Excludes   *repacking of:*
dental wound (97.22)
vulvar wound (97.26)

● **97.2 Other nonoperative replacement**

97.21 Replacement of nasal packing

97.22 Replacement of dental packing

97.23 Replacement of tracheostomy tube
Coding Clinic: 1987, Nov-Dec, P11

97.24 Replacement and refitting of vaginal diaphragm ♀

97.25 Replacement of other vaginal pessary ♀

97.26 Replacement of vaginal or vulvar packing or drain ♀

97.29 Other nonoperative replacements
Coding Clinic: 1999, Q3, P9; 1998, Q3, P12; 1985, Mar-April, P11

● **97.3 Nonoperative removal of therapeutic device from head and neck**

97.31 Removal of eye prosthesis
Excludes   *removal of ocular implant (16.71)*
removal of orbital implant (16.72)

97.32 Removal of nasal packing

97.33 Removal of dental wiring

97.34 Removal of dental packing

97.35 Removal of dental prosthesis

97.36 Removal of other external mandibular fixation device

97.37 Removal of tracheostomy tube

97.38 Removal of sutures from head and neck

97.39 Removal of other therapeutic device from head and neck
Excludes   *removal of skull tongs (02.94)*

● **97.4 Nonoperative removal of therapeutic device from thorax**

97.41 Removal of thoracotomy tube or pleural cavity drain
Coding Clinic: 1999, Q1, P10

97.42 Removal of mediastinal drain

97.43 Removal of sutures from thorax

◀ New   ◀▥ Revised   ~~deleted~~ Deleted   ● Use Additional Digit(s)   ✖ Valid O.R. Procedure
◆ Non-O.R. Procedure   ♀ Females Only   ♂ Males Only   OGCR Official Guidelines   **Coding Clinic**

97.44 **Nonoperative removal of heart assist system**
Explantation [removal] of circulatory assist device
Explantation [removal] of percutaneous external heart assist device
Intra-aortic balloon pump [IABP]
Removal of extrinsic heart assist device
Removal of pVAD
Removal of percutaneous heart assist device
Coding Clinic: 2001, Q4, P65

97.49 **Removal of other device from thorax**
> **Excludes** *endoscopic removal of bronchial device(s) or substances (33.78)*
Coding Clinic: 1986, Nov-Dec, P9

● 97.5 **Nonoperative removal of therapeutic device from digestive system**
97.51 **Removal of gastrostomy tube**
97.52 **Removal of tube from small intestine**
97.53 **Removal of tube from large intestine or appendix**
97.54 **Removal of cholecystostomy tube**
97.55 **Removal of T-tube, other bile duct tube, or liver tube**
Removal of bile duct stent
Coding Clinic: 2001, Q1, P8-9
97.56 **Removal of pancreatic tube or drain**
97.59 **Removal of other device from digestive system**
Removal of rectal packing

● 97.6 **Nonoperative removal of therapeutic device from urinary system**
97.61 **Removal of pyelostomy and nephrostomy tube**
97.62 **Removal of ureterostomy tube and ureteral catheter**
97.63 **Removal of cystostomy tube**
97.64 **Removal of other urinary drainage device**
Removal of indwelling urinary catheter
97.65 **Removal of urethral stent**
97.69 **Removal of other device from urinary system**

● 97.7 **Nonoperative removal of therapeutic device from genital system**
97.71 **Removal of intrauterine contraceptive device** ♀
97.72 **Removal of intrauterine pack** ♀
97.73 **Removal of vaginal diaphragm** ♀
97.74 **Removal of other vaginal pessary** ♀
97.75 **Removal of vaginal or vulvar packing** ♀
97.79 **Removal of other device from genital tract**
Removal of sutures

● 97.8 **Other nonoperative removal of therapeutic device**
97.81 **Removal of retroperitoneal drainage device**
97.82 **Removal of peritoneal drainage device**
Coding Clinic: 1993, 5th Issue, P8-9; 1990, Q2, P28; 1986, Sept-Oct, P12
97.83 **Removal of abdominal wall sutures**
97.84 **Removal of sutures from trunk, not elsewhere classified**
97.85 **Removal of packing from trunk, not elsewhere classified**
97.86 **Removal of other device from abdomen**
97.87 **Removal of other device from trunk**
97.88 **Removal of external immobilization device**
Removal of:
brace
cast
splint
97.89 **Removal of other therapeutic device**

● 98 **Nonoperative removal of foreign body or calculus**
● 98.0 **Removal of intraluminal foreign body from digestive system without incision**
> **Excludes** *removal of therapeutic device (97.51–97.59)*
98.01 **Removal of intraluminal foreign body from mouth without incision**
98.02 **Removal of intraluminal foreign body from esophagus without incision**

98.03 **Removal of intraluminal foreign body from stomach and small intestine without incision**
Coding Clinic: 1985, Jan-Feb, P14-15
98.04 **Removal of intraluminal foreign body from large intestine without incision**
98.05 **Removal of intraluminal foreign body from rectum and anus without incision**

● 98.1 **Removal of intraluminal foreign body from other sites without incision**
> **Excludes** *removal of therapeutic device (97.31–97.49, 97.61–97.89)*
98.11 **Removal of intraluminal foreign body from ear without incision**
98.12 **Removal of intraluminal foreign body from nose without incision**
98.13 **Removal of intraluminal foreign body from pharynx without incision**
98.14 **Removal of intraluminal foreign body from larynx without incision**
98.15 **Removal of intraluminal foreign body from trachea and bronchus without incision**
> **Excludes** *endoscopic removal of bronchial device(s) or substances (33.78)*
98.16 **Removal of intraluminal foreign body from uterus without incision** ♀
> **Excludes** *removal of intrauterine contraceptive device (97.71)*
98.17 **Removal of intraluminal foreign body from vagina without incision** ♀
98.18 **Removal of intraluminal foreign body from artificial stoma without incision**
98.19 **Removal of intraluminal foreign body from urethra without incision**

● 98.2 **Removal of other foreign body without incision**
> **Excludes** *removal of intraluminal foreign body (98.01–98.19)*
98.20 **Removal of foreign body, not otherwise specified**
98.21 **Removal of superficial foreign body from eye without incision**
98.22 **Removal of other foreign body without incision from head and neck**
Removal of embedded foreign body from eyelid or conjunctiva without incision
98.23 **Removal of foreign body from vulva without incision** ♀
98.24 **Removal of foreign body from scrotum or penis without incision** ♂
98.25 **Removal of other foreign body without incision from trunk except scrotum, penis, or vulva**
98.26 **Removal of foreign body from hand without incision**
Coding Clinic: 1987, Nov-Dec, P10
98.27 **Removal of foreign body without incision from upper limb, except hand**
98.28 **Removal of foreign body from foot without incision**
98.29 **Removal of foreign body without incision from lower limb, except foot**

● 98.5 **Extracorporeal shockwave lithotripsy [ESWL]**
Lithotriptor tank procedure
Disintegration of stones by extracorporeal induced shockwaves
That with insertion of stent
98.51 **Extracorporeal shockwave lithotripsy [ESWL] of the kidney, ureter, and/or bladder**
◆Non-OR Procedure that affects MS-DRG assignment to MDC 11, MS-DRG 691-692
98.52 **Extracorporeal shockwave lithotripsy [ESWL] of the gallbladder and/or bile duct**
MCE: Non-covered procedure
98.59 **Extracorporeal shockwave lithotripsy of other sites**
MCE: Non-covered procedure

Excludes   Includes   Use additional   Code also   Omit code

● **99　Other nonoperative procedures**

● **99.0　Transfusion of blood and blood components**

Code also for that done via catheter or cutdown (38.92-38.94)

99.00　Perioperative autologous transfusion of whole blood or blood components
Intraoperative blood collection
Postoperative blood collection
Salvage

99.01　Exchange transfusion
Transfusion:
exsanguination
replacement
Coding Clinic: 1989, Q2, P15

99.02　Transfusion of previously collected autologous blood
Blood component
Coding Clinic: 1990, Q1, P10; 1985, July-Aug, P16

99.03　Other transfusion of whole blood
Transfusion:
blood NOS
hemodilution
NOS

99.04　Transfusion of packed cells
Coding Clinic: 2011, Q4, P147; 2010, Q4, P80; 2006, Q4, P91-92

99.05　Transfusion of platelets
Transfusion of thrombocytes

99.06　Transfusion of coagulation factors
Transfusion of antihemophilic factor
Excludes infusion of 4-Factor Prothrombin Complex Concentrate (00.96)

99.07　Transfusion of other serum
Transfusion of plasma
Excludes injection [transfusion] of:
antivenin (99.16)
gamma globulin (99.14)
Coding Clinic: 1985, Nov-Dec, P14

99.08　Transfusion of blood expander
Transfusion of Dextran

99.09　Transfusion of other substance
Transfusion of:
blood surrogate
granulocytes
Excludes transplantation [transfusion] of bone marrow (41.00-41.09)
Coding Clinic: 2011, Q1, P24

● **99.1　Injection or infusion of therapeutic or prophylactic substance**
Includes injection or infusion given:
hypodermically acting locally or systemically
intramuscularly acting locally or systemically
intravenously acting locally or systemically
Coding Clinic: 2005, Q4, P101-103

99.10　Injection or infusion of thrombolytic agent
Alteplase
Anistreplase
Reteplase
Streptokinase
Tenecteplase
Tissue plasminogen activator (TPA)
Urokinase
Excludes aspirin — omit code
GP IIB/IIIa platelet inhibitors (99.20)
heparin (99.19)
SuperSaturated oxygen therapy (00.49)
warfarin — omit code
◆ Non-OR Procedure that affects MS-DRG assignment to MDC 01, MS-DRG 061-063
Coding Clinic: 2012, Q4, P85; Q2, P15-16; 2010, Q3, P5; 2006, Q2, P22; 2001, Q2, P8-9; Q2, P7-8, 23

99.11　Injection of Rh immune globulin
Injection of:
Anti-D (Rhesus) globulin
RhoGAM

99.12　Immunization for allergy
Desensitization

99.13　Immunization for autoimmune disease

99.14　Injection or infusion of immunoglobulin
Injection of immune sera
Injection or infusion of gamma globulin

99.15　Parenteral infusion of concentrated nutritional substances
Hyperalimentation
Total parenteral nutrition [TPN]
Peripheral parenteral nutrition [PPN]
Coding Clinic: 2003, Q4, P104-105

99.16　Injection of antidote
Injection of:
antivenin
heavy metal antagonist

99.17　Injection of insulin

99.18　Injection or infusion of electrolytes

99.19　Injection of anticoagulant
Excludes infusion of drotrecogin alfa (activated) (00.11)

● **99.2　Injection or infusion of other therapeutic or prophylactic substance**
Includes injection or infusion given:
hypodermically acting locally or systemically
intramuscularly acting locally or systemically
intravenously acting locally or systemically
Excludes SuperSaturated oxygen therapy (00.49)
Code also for:
injection (into):
breast (85.92)
bursa (82.94, 83.96)
intraperitoneal (cavity) (54.97)
intrathecal (03.92)
joint (76.96, 81.92)
kidney (55.96)
liver (50.94)
orbit (16.91)
other sites — see Alphabetic Index
perfusion:
NOS (39.97)
intestine (46.95, 46.96)
kidney (55.95)
liver (50.93)
total body (39.96)
Coding Clinic: 2004, Q4, P138; 2002, Q3, P20; 1998, Q43, P85-86

99.20　Injection or infusion of platelet inhibitor
Glycoprotein IIB/IIIa inhibitor
GP IIB/IIIa inhibitor
GP IIB-IIIa inhibitor
Excludes infusion of heparin (99.19)
injection or infusion of thrombolytic agent (99.10)
Coding Clinic: 2006, Q3, P8-9; 2004, Q2, P3

99.21　Injection of antibiotic
Excludes injection or infusion of oxazolidinone class of antibiotics (00.14)
Coding Clinic: 2010, Q3, P11; 1998, Q43, P76-77; 1990, Q2, P24; 1989, Q3, P16; 1987, Mar-April, P9

99.22　Injection of other anti-infective
Excludes injection or infusion of oxazolidinone class of antibiotics (00.14)

99.23　Injection of steroid
Injection of cortisone
Subdermal implantation of progesterone
Coding Clinic: 2000, Q3, P15; 1999, Q1, P7-8; 1996, Q3, P7; 1992, Q3, P9

99.24　Injection of other hormone
Coding Clinic: 2006, Q1, P9-10

◀ New　◀ Revised　deleted Deleted　● Use Additional Digit(s)　✖ Valid O.R. Procedure
◆ Non-O.R. Procedure　♀ Females Only　♂ Males Only　OGCR Official Guidelines　**Coding Clinic**

99.25 **Injection or infusion of cancer chemotherapeutic substance**
   Chemoembolization
   Injection or infusion of antineoplastic agent
   Use additional code for disruption of blood brain barrier, if performed [BBBD] (00.19)
   Excludes *immunotherapy, antineoplastic (00.15, 99.28)*
      implantation of chemotherapeutic agent (00.10)
      injection of radioisotope (92.28)
      injection or infusion of biological response modifier [BRM] as an antineoplastic agent (99.28)
      intravenous infusion of clofarabine (17.70)
   Coding Clinic: 2012, Q1, P13-14; 2009, Q4, P79; 2008, Q4, P82-83; 2007, Q4, P103-104; 2003, Q2, P6, 16-17; 2000, Q1, P23-24; 1999, Q1, P4; 1998, Q1, P6-7; 1996, Q3, P11-12; 1992, Q2, P6-7; Q1, P12; 1988, Q1, P8; 1986, Nov-Dec, P11; 1985, July-Aug, P11; 1984, May-June, P11

99.26 **Injection of tranquilizer**

99.27 **Iontophoresis**

99.28 **Injection or infusion of biological response modifier [BRM] as an antineoplastic agent**
   Immunotherapy, antineoplastic
   Infusion of cintredekin besudotox
   Interleukin therapy
   Low-dose interleukin-2 (IL-2) therapy
   Tumor vaccine
   Excludes *high-dose infusion interleukin-2 [IL-2] (00.15)*
   Coding Clinic: 2006, Q4, P122-123; 1999, Q2, P8; 1998, Q2, P10-11

99.29 **Injection or infusion of other therapeutic or prophylactic substance**
   Excludes *administration of neuroprotective agent (99.75)*
      immunization (99.31–99.59)
      infusion of blood brain barrier disruption substance (00.19)
      injection of sclerosing agent into:
         esophageal varices (42.33)
         hemorrhoids (49.42)
         veins (39.92)
      injection or infusion of human B-type natriuretic peptide (hBNP) (00.13)
      injection or infusion of nesiritide (00.13)
      injection or infusion of platelet inhibitor (99.20)
      injection or infusion of thrombolytic agent (99.10)
      uterine artery embolization without coils (68.25)
   Coding Clinic: 2012, Q4, P87; 2010, Q2, P5, 7, 14; Q1, P21-22; 2007, Q1, P11; 2004, Q4, P138; 2003, Q2, P10; 2002, Q3, P24-25; 2001, Q1, P15, 19-20; 2000, Q2, P14-15; Q1, P8-9, 18-19, 23-24; 1999, Q4, P17-18; 1998, Q2, P17-18, 23-24; Q1, P6; 1997, Q2, P11; 1996, Q3, P21; 1995, Q2, P12; 1990, Q2, P23-24; 1989, Q2, P17; 1988, Q1, P9; 1987, Sept-Oct, P11; 1984, Nov-Dec, P12

● **99.3** **Prophylactic vaccination and inoculation against certain bacterial diseases**

99.31 **Vaccination against cholera**

99.32 **Vaccination against typhoid and paratyphoid fever**
   Administration of TAB vaccine

99.33 **Vaccination against tuberculosis**
   Administration of BCG vaccine
   Coding Clinic: 1988, Q1, P8

99.34 **Vaccination against plague**

99.35 **Vaccination against tularemia**

99.36 **Administration of diphtheria toxoid**
   Excludes *administration of:*
      diphtheria antitoxin (99.58)
      diphtheria-tetanus-pertussis, combined (99.39)

99.37 **Vaccination against pertussis**
   Excludes *administration of diphtheria-tetanus-pertussis, combined (99.39)*

99.38 **Administration of tetanus toxoid**
   Excludes *administration of:*
      diphtheria-tetanus-pertussis, combined (99.39)
      tetanus antitoxin (99.56)

99.39 **Administration of diphtheria-tetanus-pertussis, combined**

● **99.4** **Prophylactic vaccination and inoculation against certain viral diseases**

99.41 **Administration of poliomyelitis vaccine**

99.42 **Vaccination against smallpox**

99.43 **Vaccination against yellow fever**

99.44 **Vaccination against rabies**

99.45 **Vaccination against measles**
   Excludes *administration of measles-mumps rubella vaccine (99.48)*

99.46 **Vaccination against mumps**
   Excludes *administration of measles-mumps rubella vaccine (99.48)*

99.47 **Vaccination against rubella**
   Excludes *administration of measles-mumps rubella vaccine (99.48)*

99.48 **Administration of measles-mumps-rubella vaccine**

● **99.5** **Other vaccination and inoculation**

99.51 **Prophylactic vaccination against the common cold**

99.52 **Prophylactic vaccination against influenza**

99.53 **Prophylactic vaccination against arthropod-borne viral encephalitis**

99.54 **Prophylactic vaccination against other arthropod-borne viral diseases**

99.55 **Prophylactic administration of vaccine against other diseases**
   Vaccination against:
      anthrax
      brucellosis
      Rocky Mountain spotted fever
      Staphylococcus
      Streptococcus
      typhus
   Coding Clinic: 1994, Q1, P19

99.56 **Administration of tetanus antitoxin**

99.57 **Administration of botulism antitoxin**

99.58 **Administration of other antitoxins**
   Administration of:
      diphtheria antitoxin
      gas gangrene antitoxin
      scarlet fever antitoxin

99.59 **Other vaccination and inoculation**
   Vaccination NOS
   Excludes *injection of:*
      gamma globulin (99.14)
      Rh immune globulin (99.11)
      immunization for:
      allergy (99.12)
      autoimmune disease (99.13)

MISCELLANEOUS DIAGNOSTIC AND THERAPEUTIC PROCEDURES (87–99)

Excludes   Includes   Use additional   Code also   Omit code

● **99.6 Conversion of cardiac rhythm**

> **Excludes** *open chest cardiac:*
> *electric stimulation (37.91)*
> *massage (37.91)*

99.60 Cardiopulmonary resuscitation, not otherwise specified
Coding Clinic: 1994, Q1, P16

99.61 Atrial cardioversion
Coding Clinic: 1993, Q3, P12

99.62 Other electric countershock of heart
Cardioversion:
NOS
external
Conversion to sinus rhythm
Defibrillation
External electrode stimulation
Coding Clinic: 2013, Q1, P10-11; 2007, Q1, P17-18

99.63 Closed chest cardiac massage
Cardiac massage NOS
Manual external cardiac massage

99.64 Carotid sinus stimulation

99.69 Other conversion of cardiac rhythm
Coding Clinic: 1988, Q4, P11

● **99.7 Therapeutic apheresis or other injection, administration, or infusion of other therapeutic or prophylactic substance**

99.71 Therapeutic plasmapheresis

> **Excludes** *extracorporeal immunoadsorption [ECI]*
> *(99.76)*

99.72 Therapeutic leukopheresis
Therapeutic leukocytapheresis

99.73 Therapeutic erythrocytapheresis
Therapeutic erythropheresis
Coding Clinic: 1994, Q1, P20-21

99.74 Therapeutic plateletpheresis

99.75 Administration of neuroprotective agent

99.76 Extracorporeal immunoadsorption
Removal of antibodies from plasma with protein A columns
Coding Clinic: 2002, Q4, P112-113

99.77 Application or administration of adhesion barrier substance
Coding Clinic: 2010, Q1, P21; 2002, Q4, P113

99.78 Aquapheresis
Plasma water removal
Ultrafiltration [for water removal]

> **Excludes** *hemodiafiltration (39.95)*
> *hemodialysis (39.95)*
> *therapeutic plasmapheresis (99.71)*

99.79 Other
Apheresis (harvest) of stem cells
Coding Clinic: 2008, Q3, P19; 2006, Q1, P12-14x2; 2005, Q1, P16-17; 1997, Q4, P55

● **99.8 Miscellaneous physical procedures**

99.81 Hypothermia (central) (local)

> **Excludes** *gastric cooling (96.31)*
> *gastric freezing (96.32)*
> *that incidental to open heart surgery (39.62)*
Coding Clinic: 2010, Q3, P14

99.82 Ultraviolet light therapy
Actinotherapy

99.83 Other phototherapy
Phototherapy of the newborn

> **Excludes** *extracorporeal photochemotherapy (99.88)*
> *photocoagulation of retinal lesion*
> *(14.23–14.25, 14.33–14.35,*
> *14.53–14.55)*
Coding Clinic: 1989, Q2, P15

99.84 Isolation
Isolation after contact with infectious disease
Protection of individual from his surroundings
Protection of surroundings from individual

99.85 Hyperthermia for treatment of cancer
Hyperthermia (adjunct therapy) induced by microwave, ultrasound, low energy radio frequency, probes (interstitial), or other means in the treatment of cancer

Code also any concurrent chemotherapy or radiation therapy
Coding Clinic: 1996, Q3, P11-12; 1989, Q3, P17

99.86 Non-invasive placement of bone growth stimulator
Transcutaneous (surface) placement of pads or patches for stimulation to aid bone healing

> **Excludes** *insertion of invasive or semi-invasive*
> *bone growth stimulators (device)*
> *(percutaneous electrodes)*
> *(78.90–78.99)*

99.88 Therapeutic photopheresis
Extracorporeal photochemotherapy
Extracorporeal photopheresis

> **Excludes** *other phototherapy (99.83)*
> *ultraviolet light therapy (99.82)*
Coding Clinic: 1999, Q2, P7-8

● **99.9 Other miscellaneous procedures**

99.91 Acupuncture for anesthesia

99.92 Other acupuncture

> **Excludes** *that with smouldering mox (93.35)*

99.93 Rectal massage (for levator spasm)

99.94 Prostatic massage ♂

99.95 Stretching of foreskin ♂

99.96 Collection of sperm for artificial insemination ♂

99.97 Fitting of denture

99.98 Extraction of milk from lactating breast ♀

99.99 Other
Leech therapy

◀ New ◀⃛ Revised ~~deleted~~ Deleted ● Use Additional Digit(s) ✖ Valid O.R. Procedure
◆ Non-O.R. Procedure ♀ Females Only ♂ Males Only OGCR Official Guidelines Coding Clinic

1304

Inpatient Procedures

2014 FINAL INPATIENT PROCEDURES

The following list is Addendum E of the Final Hospital Outpatient Prospective Payment System for Calendar Year 2014. These codes are only payable as inpatient procedures as displayed at http://www.cms.gov/apps/ama/license.asp?file=/Medicare/Medicare-Fee-for-Service-Payment/HospitalOutpatientPPS/Downloads/CMS-1601-FC-Addenda.zip

00176	01638	21180	22326	23920	27222	27580	32120	32815	33364
00192	01652	21182	22327	24900	27226	27590	32124	32820	33365
00211	01654	21183	22328	24920	27227	27591	32140	32850	33366
00214	01656	21184	22532	24930	27228	27592	32141	32851	33367
00215	01756	21188	22533	24931	27232	27596	32150	32852	33368
00452	01990	21194	22534	24940	27236	27598	32151	32853	33369
00474	11004	21196	22548	25900	27240	27645	32160	32854	33400
00524	11005	21247	22552	25905	27244	27646	32200	32855	33401
00540	11006	21255	22556	25915	27245	27702	32215	32856	33403
00542	11008	21268	22558	25920	27248	27703	32220	32900	33404
00546	15756	21343	22585	25924	27253	27712	32225	32905	33405
00560	15757	21344	22586	25927	27254	27715	32310	32906	33406
00561	15758	21346	22590	26551	27258	27724	32320	32940	33410
00562	16036	21347	22595	26553	27259	27725	32440	32997	33411
00567	19271	21348	22600	26554	27268	27727	32442	33015	33412
00580	19272	21366	22610	26556	27269	27880	32445	33020	33413
00604	19305	21422	22630	26992	27280	27881	32480	33025	33414
00622	19306	21423	22632	27005	27282	27882	32482	33030	33415
00632	19361	21431	22633	27025	27284	27886	32484	33031	33416
00670	19364	21432	22634	27030	27286	27888	32486	33050	33417
00792	19367	21433	22800	27036	27290	28800	32488	33120	33420
00794	19368	21435	22802	27054	27295	31225	32491	33130	33422
00796	19369	21436	22804	27070	27303	31230	32501	33140	33425
00802	20661	21510	22808	27071	27365	31290	32503	33141	33426
00844	20664	21615	22810	27075	27445	31291	32504	33202	33427
00846	20802	21616	22812	27076	27447	31360	32505	33203	33430
00848	20805	21620	22818	27077	27448	31365	32506	33236	33460
00864	20808	21627	22819	27078	27450	31367	32507	33237	33463
00865	20816	21630	22830	27090	27454	31368	32540	33238	33464
00866	20824	21632	22840	27091	27455	31370	32650	33243	33465
00868	20827	21705	22841	27120	27457	31375	32651	33250	33468
00882	20838	21740	22842	27122	27465	31380	32652	33251	33470
00904	20936	21750	22843	27125	27466	31382	32653	33254	33471
00908	20937	21810	22844	27130	27468	31390	32654	33255	33472
00932	20938	21825	22845	27132	27470	31395	32655	33256	33474
00934	20955	22010	22846	27134	27472	31584	32656	33257	33475
00936	20956	22015	22847	27137	27477	31587	32658	33258	33476
00944	20957	22110	22848	27138	27485	31725	32659	33259	33478
01140	20962	22112	22849	27140	27486	31760	32661	33261	33496
01150	20969	22114	22850	27146	27487	31766	32662	33265	33500
01212	20970	22116	22852	27147	27488	31770	32663	33266	33501
01214	21045	22206	22855	27151	27495	31775	32664	33300	33502
01232	21141	22207	22857	27156	27506	31780	32665	33305	33503
01234	21142	22208	22861	27158	27507	31781	32666	33310	33504
01272	21143	22210	22862	27161	27511	31786	32667	33315	33505
01274	21145	22212	22864	27165	27513	31800	32668	33320	33506
01402	21146	22214	22865	27170	27514	31805	32669	33321	33507
01404	21147	22216	23200	27175	27519	32035	32670	33322	33510
01442	21151	22220	23210	27176	27535	32036	32671	33330	33511
01444	21154	22224	23220	27177	27536	32096	32672	33332	33512
01486	21155	22226	23332	27178	27540	32097	32673	33335	33513
01502	21159	22318	23472	27181	27556	32098	32674	33361	33514
01634	21160	22319	23474	27185	27557	32100	32800	33362	33516
01636	21179	22325	23900	27187	27558	32110	32810	33363	33517

33518	33776	33977	35221	35571	37618	43135	43846	44310	46735
33519	33777	33978	35241	35583	37660	43279	43847	44314	46740
33521	33778	33979	35246	35585	37788	43282	43848	44316	46742
33522	33779	33980	35251	35587	38100	43300	43850	44320	46744
33523	33780	33981	35271	35600	38101	43305	43855	44322	46746
33530	33781	33982	35276	35601	38102	43310	43860	44345	46748
33533	33782	33983	35281	35606	38115	43312	43865	44346	46751
33534	33783	33990	35301	35612	38380	43313	43880	44602	47010
33535	33786	33991	35302	35616	38381	43314	43881	44603	47015
33536	33788	33992	35303	35621	38382	43320	43882	44604	47100
33542	33800	33993	35304	35623	38562	43324	44005	44605	47120
33545	33802	34001	35305	35626	38564	43325	44010	44615	47122
33548	33803	34051	35306	35631	38724	43326	44015	44620	47125
33572	33813	34151	35311	35632	38746	43330	44020	44625	47130
33600	33814	34401	35331	35633	38747	43331	44021	44626	47133
33602	33820	34451	35341	35634	38765	43340	44025	44640	47135
33606	33822	34502	35351	35636	38770	43341	44050	44650	47136
33608	33824	34800	35355	35637	38780	43350	44055	44660	47140
33610	33840	34802	35361	35638	39000	43351	44110	44661	47141
33611	33845	34803	35363	35642	39010	43352	44111	44680	47142
33612	33851	34804	35371	35645	39200	43360	44120	44700	47143
33615	33852	34805	35372	35646	39220	43361	44121	44715	47144
33617	33853	34806	35390	35647	39499	43400	44125	44720	47145
33619	33860	34808	35400	35650	39501	43401	44126	44721	47146
33641	33861	34812	35450	35654	39502	43405	44127	44800	47147
33645	33863	34813	35452	35656	39503	43410	44128	44820	47300
33647	33864	34820	35454	35661	39520	43415	44130	44850	47350
33660	33870	34825	35456	35663	39530	43425	44132	44899	47360
33665	33875	34826	35480	35665	39531	43460	44133	44900	47361
33670	33877	34830	35481	35666	39540	43496	44135	44960	47362
33675	33880	34831	35482	35671	39541	43500	44136	45110	47380
33676	33881	34832	35483	35681	39545	43501	44137	45111	47381
33677	33883	34833	35501	35682	39560	43502	44139	45112	47400
33681	33884	34834	35506	35683	39561	43520	44140	45113	47420
33684	33886	34900	35508	35691	39599	43605	44141	45114	47425
33688	33889	35001	35509	35693	41130	43610	44143	45116	47460
33690	33891	35002	35510	35694	41135	43611	44144	45119	47480
33692	33910	35005	35511	35695	41140	43620	44145	45120	47550
33694	33915	35013	35512	35697	41145	43621	44146	45121	47570
33697	33916	35021	35515	35700	41150	43622	44147	45123	47600
33702	33917	35022	35516	35701	41153	43631	44150	45126	47605
33710	33920	35045	35518	35721	41155	43632	44151	45130	47610
33720	33922	35081	35521	35741	42426	43633	44155	45135	47612
33722	33924	35082	35522	35800	42845	43634	44156	45136	47620
33724	33925	35091	35523	35820	42894	43635	44157	45395	47700
33726	33926	35092	35525	35840	42953	43640	44158	45397	47701
33730	33930	35102	35526	35870	42961	43641	44160	45400	47711
33732	33933	35103	35531	35901	42971	43644	44187	45402	47712
33735	33935	35111	35533	35905	43045	43645	44188	45540	47715
33736	33940	35112	35535	35907	43100	43771	44202	45550	47720
33737	33944	35121	35536	36660	43101	43772	44203	45562	47721
33750	33945	35122	35537	36822	43107	43773	44204	45563	47740
33755	33960	35131	35538	36823	43108	43774	44205	45800	47741
33762	33961	35132	35539	37140	43112	43775	44206	45805	47760
33764	33967	35141	35540	37145	43113	43800	44207	45820	47765
33766	33968	35142	35556	37160	43116	43810	44208	45825	47780
33767	33970	35151	35558	37180	43117	43820	44210	46705	47785
33768	33971	35152	35560	37181	43118	43825	44211	46710	47800
33770	33973	35182	35563	37182	43121	43832	44212	46712	47801
33771	33974	35189	35565	37215	43122	43840	44213	46715	47802
33774	33975	35211	35566	37616	43123	43843	44227	46716	47900
33775	33976	35216	35570	37617	43124	43845	44300	46730	48000

48001	50130	50825	56631	59120	61458	61591	62121	63265	92971
48020	50135	50830	56632	59121	61460	61592	62140	63266	92975
48100	50205	50840	56633	59130	61470	61595	62141	63267	92992
48105	50220	50845	56634	59135	61480	61596	62142	63268	92993
48120	50225	50860	56637	59136	61490	61597	62143	63270	99190
48140	50230	50900	56640	59140	61500	61598	62145	63271	99191
48145	50234	50920	57110	59325	61501	61600	62146	63272	99192
48146	50236	50930	57111	59350	61510	61601	62147	63273	99356
48148	50240	50940	57112	59514	61512	61605	62148	63275	99357
48150	50250	51525	57270	59525	61514	61606	62161	63276	99462
48152	50280	51530	57280	59620	61516	61607	62162	63277	99468
48153	50290	51550	57296	59830	61517	61608	62163	63278	99469
48154	50300	51555	57305	59850	61518	61609	62164	63280	99471
48155	50320	51565	57307	59851	61519	61610	62165	63281	99472
48400	50323	51570	57308	59852	61520	61611	62180	63282	99475
48500	50325	51575	57311	59855	61521	61612	62190	63283	99476
48510	50327	51580	57531	59856	61522	61613	62192	63285	99477
48520	50328	51585	57540	59857	61524	61615	62200	63286	99478
48540	50329	51590	57545	60254	61526	61616	62201	63287	99479
48545	50340	51595	58140	60270	61530	61618	62220	63290	99480
48547	50360	51596	58146	60505	61531	61619	62223	63295	0051T
48548	50365	51597	58150	60521	61533	61624	62256	63300	0052T
48551	50370	51800	58152	60522	61534	61630	62258	63301	0053T
48552	50380	51820	58180	60540	61535	61635	63043	63302	0075T
48554	50400	51840	58200	60545	61536	61680	63044	63303	0076T
48556	50405	51841	58210	60600	61537	61682	63050	63304	0078T
49000	50500	51865	58240	60605	61538	61684	63051	63305	0079T
49002	50520	51900	58267	60650	61539	61686	63077	63306	0080T
49010	50525	51920	58275	61105	61540	61690	63078	63307	0081T
49020	50526	51925	58280	61107	61541	61692	63081	63308	0092T
49040	50540	51940	58285	61108	61542	61697	63082	63700	0095T
49060	50545	51960	58293	61120	61543	61698	63085	63702	0098T
49062	50546	51980	58400	61140	61544	61700	63086	63704	0163T
49203	50547	53415	58410	61150	61545	61702	63087	63706	0164T
49204	50548	53448	58520	61151	61546	61703	63088	63707	0165T
49205	50600	54125	58540	61154	61548	61705	63090	63709	0169T
49215	50605	54130	58548	61156	61550	61708	63091	63710	0195T
49220	50610	54135	58605	61210	61552	61710	63101	63740	0196T
49255	50620	54390	58611	61250	61556	61711	63102	64752	0202T
49425	50630	54411	58700	61253	61557	61735	63103	64755	0219T
49428	50650	54417	58720	61304	61558	61750	63170	64760	0220T
49605	50660	54430	58740	61305	61559	61751	63172	64809	0235T
49606	50700	54650	58750	61312	61563	61760	63173	64818	0254T
49610	50715	55605	58752	61313	61564	61850	63180	64866	0255T
49611	50722	55650	58760	61314	61566	61860	63182	64868	0262T
49900	50725	55801	58822	61315	61567	61863	63185	65273	0266T
49904	50728	55810	58825	61316	61570	61864	63190	69155	0281T
49905	50740	55812	58940	61320	61571	61867	63191	69535	0293T
49906	50750	55815	58943	61321	61575	61868	63194	69554	0294T
50010	50760	55821	58950	61322	61576	61870	63195	69950	0309T
50040	50770	55831	58951	61323	61580	61875	63196	75952	0312T
50045	50780	55840	58952	61332	61581	62005	63197	75953	0318T
50060	50782	55842	58953	61333	61582	62010	63198	75954	G0341
50065	50783	55845	58954	61340	61583	62100	63199	75956	G0342
50070	50785	55862	58956	61343	61584	62115	63200	75957	G0343
50075	50800	55865	58957	61345	61585	62116	63250	75958	G0412
50100	50810	55866	58958	61440	61586	62117	63251	75959	G0414
50120	50815	56630	58960	61450	61590	62120	63252	92970	G0415
50125	50820								

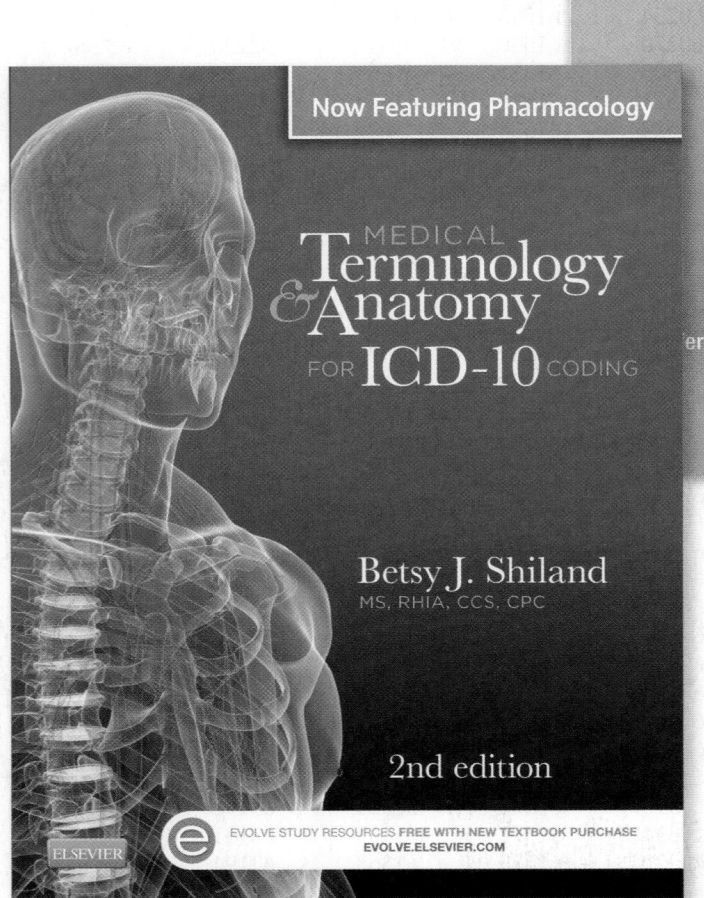